The GALE ENCYCLOPEDIA *of* MENTAL HEALTH

THIRD EDITION

The GALE ENCYCLOPEDIA of MENTAL HEALTH

THIRD EDITION

VOLUME

1

A–L

KRISTIN KEY, EDITOR

GALE
CENGAGE Learning

Detroit • New York • San Francisco • New Haven, Conn • Waterville, Maine • London

GALE
CENGAGE Learning®

Gale Encyclopedia of Mental Health, Third Edition

Project Editor: Kristin Key

Editorial: Tara Atterberry, Donna Batten, Jacqueline Longe, Kristin Mallegg, Brigham Narins, Joseph Palmisano, Bob Romaniuk, Alejandro Valtierra

Product Manager: Anne Marie Sumner

Editorial Support Services: Andrea Lopeman

Indexing Services: Laurie Andriot

Rights Acquisition and Management: Margaret Chamberlain-Gaston

Composition: Evi Abou-El-Seoud

Manufacturing: Wendy Blurton

Imaging: John Watkins

Product Design: Kristine Julien

LIBRARY OF CONGRESS CATALOGING-IN-PUBLICATION DATA

The Gale encyclopedia of mental health / Kristin Key, editor. -- 3rd ed.
p. cm.
Summary: "Alphabetically arranged encyclopedia (500 entries) that covers a wide variety of disorders, treatments, tests, and therapies, focused specifically on topics in mental health"– Provided by publisher.
Includes bibliographical references and index.
ISBN 978-1-4144-9012-0 (hardback) -- ISBN 978-1-4144-9013-7 (vol. 1) – ISBN 978-1-4144-9014-4 (vol. 2)
1. Psychiatry–Encyclopedias. 2. Mental illness–Encyclopedias.
I. Key, Kristin. II. Title: Encyclopedia of mental health.
RC437.G36 2012
616.89003–dc23
2011049279

Gale
27500 Drake Rd.
Farmington Hills, MI, 48331-3535

ISBN-13: 978-1-4144-9012-0 (set) ISBN-10: 1-4144-9012-7 (set)
ISBN-13: 978-1-4144-9013-7 (vol. 1) ISBN-10: 1-4144-9013-5 (vol. 1)
ISBN-13: 978-1-4144-9014-4 (vol. 2) ISBN-10: 1-4144-9014-3 (vol. 2)

This title is also available as an e-book.
ISBN-13: 978-1-4144-9015-1 ISBN-10: 1-4144-9015-1
Contact your Gale, a part of Cengage Learning sales representative for ordering information.

Printed in China
1 2 3 4 5 6 7 16 15 14 13 12

CONTENTS

ALPHABETICAL LIST OF ENTRIES

D

E

F

G

H

Q

R

S

PLEASE READ—IMPORTANT INFORMATION

The *Gale Encyclopedia of Mental Health, Third Edition* is a health reference product designed to inform and educate readers about mental health, mental disorders, and psychiatry. Gale, Cengage Learning believes the product to be comprehensive, but not necessarily definitive. It is intended to supplement, not replace, consultation with a physician or other healthcare practitioner. While Gale, Cengage Learning has made substantial efforts to provide information that is accurate, comprehensive, and up-to-date, Gale, Cengage Learning makes no representations or warranties of any kind, including without limitation, warranties of merchantability or fitness for a particular purpose, nor does it guarantee the accuracy, comprehensiveness, or timeliness of the information contained in this product. Readers should be aware that the universe of medical knowledge is constantly growing and changing, and that differences of opinion exist among authorities. Readers are also advised to seek professional diagnosis and treatment for any medical condition, and to discuss information obtained from this book with their healthcare provider.

INTRODUCTION

The *Gale Encyclopedia of Mental Health* is a valuable source of information on mental health. The *Encyclopedia* provides in-depth coverage of specific disorders recognized by the American Psychiatric Association in its *Diagnostic and Statistical Manual of Mental Disorders* (*DSM*), as well as other mental health conditions, diagnostic procedures and techniques, therapies, psychiatric medications, alternative treatments, legal concerns, and related topics.

SCOPE

The *Gale Encyclopedia of Mental Health* includes 500 entries on disorders, drugs, tests, and treatments. The *Encyclopedia* minimizes medical jargon and uses language that any reader can understand while still providing thorough coverage, making this text useful to consumers and students alike.

Entries follow a standardized format that provides information at a glance. Categories include:

Disorders and conditions

- Definition
- Demographics
- Description
- Causes and symptoms
- Diagnosis
- Treatment
- Prognosis
- Prevention

Drugs and herbs

- Definition
- Purpose
- Description
- Recommended dosage
- Precautions
- Side effects
- Interactions

Tests and procedures

- Definition
- Purpose
- Description
- Preparation
- Aftercare
- Risks
- Results

Treatments and therapies

- Definition
- Purpose
- Demographics
- Description
- Preparation
- Aftercare
- Risks

Other areas of discussion include Origins, Benefits, Research and general acceptance, and Training and certification, when applicable.

INCLUSION CRITERIA

A preliminary list of mental disorders and related topics was compiled from a wide variety of sources, including professional medical guides and textbooks as well as consumer guides and encyclopedias. An advisory board of professionals from a variety of healthcare fields, including psychology, psychiatry, pharmacy, and social work, evaluated the topics and made suggestions for updates and inclusion. The final selections were determined by Gale editors in conjunction with the advisory board.

ABOUT THE CONTRIBUTORS

The essays in this *Encyclopedia* were written by experienced medical writers, including physicians, pharmacists, and psychologists. All essays were reviewed by advisors to ensure that they are appropriate, up-to-date, and accurate.

HOW TO USE THIS BOOK

The *Gale Encyclopedia of Mental Health* has been designed with ready reference in mind.

- Straight **alphabetical arrangement** of topics allows users to locate information quickly.
- **Bold-faced terms** within entries direct the reader to related articles.
- **Cross-references** placed throughout the *Encyclopedia* direct readers to primary entries from alternate names, drug brand names, and related topics.
- Lists of **key terms** are provided where appropriate to define unfamiliar terms or concepts. A **glossary** of key terms is also included at the back of Volume 2.
- New to this edition, **Questions to Ask Your Doctor** sidebars provide sample questions that patients can ask their physicians.
- **Biographies** of key people recognized for their important work in the field of mental health are profiled in entry sidebars.
- **Resources** at the end of every entry direct readers to additional sources of information on a topic.
- Valuable **contact information** for organizations and support groups is included with each entry and compiled in the back of Volume 2.
- A comprehensive **general index** guides readers to all topics mentioned in the text.

GRAPHICS

The *Gale Encyclopedia of Mental Health* contains 240 color photographs, illustrations, charts, and tables.

ADVISORY BOARD

Several experts in mental health have provided invaluable assistance in the formulation of this encyclopedia, from defining the scope of coverage to reviewing individual entries for accuracy and accessibility. We would like to express our sincere thanks and appreciation for all of their contributions.

Thomas E. Backer
President
Human Interaction Research Institute
Associate Clinical Professor of Medical Psychology
School of Medicine
University of California, Los Angeles
Los Angeles, CA

Debra Franko
Professor, Author
Department of Counseling and Applied Educational Psychology, Bouvé College of Health Sciences
Northeastern University
Boston, MA

Irene S. Levine, PhD
Professor, Author
New York University School of Medicine
New York, NY

Susan Mockus, PhD
Medical Writer and Editor
Pawtucket, RI

Chitra Venkatasubramanian, MD
Clinical Assistant Professor, Neurology and Neurological Sciences
Stanford University School of Medicine
Palo Alto, CA

James E. Waun, MD, MA, RPh
Adjunct Assistant Professor of Clinical Pharmacy
Ferris State University
Associate Clinical Professor
Michigan State University
Registered Pharmacist
East Lansing, MI

Eric Zehr
Vice President
Addiction & Behavioral Services
Proctor Hospital
Peoria, IL

CONTRIBUTORS

Margaret Alic, PhD
Science Writer
Eastsound, WA

William Atkins
Medical Writer
Pekin, IL

Maria Eve Basile, PhD
Medical Writer
Roselle, NJ

Rosalyn Carson-DeWitt, MD
Medical Writer
Durham, NC

Laura Jean Cataldo, RN, EdD
Medical Writer
Myersville, MD

L. Lee Culvert
Medical Writer
Alna, ME

Tish Davidson, AM
Medical Writer
Fremont, CA

L. Fleming Fallon Jr., MD, DrPH
Professor of Public Health
Bowling Green University
Bowling Green, OH

Paula Ford-Martin
Medical Writer
Warwick, RI

Rebecca J. Frey, PhD
Research and Administrative Associate
East Rock Institute
New Haven, CT

Sandra L. Friedrich, MA
Science Writer
Clinical Psychology
Chicago, IL

Gary Gilles, MA
Medical Writer
Wauconda, IL

Clare Hanrahan
Medical Writer
Asheville, NC

Kelly Karpa, RPh, PhD
Assistant Professor
Department of Pharmacology
Pennsylvania State University College of Medicine
Hershey, PA

Monique Laberge, PhD
Research Associate
Department of Biochemistry and Biophysics
McGill University
Montreal, Quebec, Canada

Judy Leaver, MA
Behavioral Health Writer and Consultant
Washington, DC

Brenda Wilmoth Lerner, RN
Medical Editor and Writer
Montrose, AL

Mark A. Mitchell, MD
Medical Writer
Seattle, WA

Teresa G. Odle
Medical Writer
Albuquerque, NM

Jack Raber, PharmD
Principal
Clinipharm Services
Seal Beach, CA

Joan Schonbeck, RN
Medical Writer
Massachusetts Department of Mental Health
Marlborough, MA

Genevieve Slomski, PhD
Medical Writer
New Britain, CT

Heidi Splete
Freelance Writer
Washington, DC

Deanna M. Swartout-Corbeil, RN
Medical Writer
Thompsons Station, TN

Samuel Uretsky, PharmD
Medical Writer
Wantagh, NY

Ken R. Wells
Freelance Writer
Laguna Hills, CA

Emily Willingham, PhD
Freelance Writer
Austin, TX

A

AACAP *see* **American Academy of Child & Adolescent Psychiatry**

Abnormal Involuntary Movement Scale

Definition

The Abnormal Involuntary Movement Scale (AIMS) is a rating scale that was designed in the 1970s to measure involuntary movements known as **tardive dyskinesia** (TD). TD is a disorder that sometimes develops as a side effect of long-term treatment with neuroleptic (antipsychotic) medications.

Purpose

Tardive dyskinesia, a syndrome characterized by abnormal involuntary movements of the patient's face, mouth, trunk, or limbs, affects 20% to 30% of patients who have been treated for months or years with neuroleptic medications. Patients who are older, are heavy smokers, or have diabetes mellitus are at higher risk of developing TD. The movements of the patient's limbs and trunk are sometimes described as choreathetoid, a dance-like movement that repeats itself but does not have any type of rhythm.

The AIMS is used not only to detect tardive dyskinesia but also to follow the severity of a patient's TD over time. It is a valuable tool for clinicians who are monitoring the effects of long-term treatment with neuroleptic medications and for researchers studying the effects of these drugs. The AIMS is given every three to six months to monitor the patient for the development of TD. For most patients, TD develops three months after the initiation of neuroleptic therapy; in elderly patients, however, TD can develop after as little as one month.

Description

The AIMS was designed by W. Guy in 1976 and modified by M. R. Munetz and S. Benjamin in 1988. The test is performed by trained clinicians and can be completed in about 10 minutes. The AIMS has a total of twelve items rating involuntary movements of various areas of the patient's body. These items are rated on a five-point scale of severity from 0–4. The scale is rated from lowest to highest: 0 (none), 1 (minimal), 2 (mild), 3 (moderate), and 4 (severe).

The twelve items within the AIMS are generally grouped by function or body part affected:

- four items assess facial and oral movements (muscles of facial expression, such as movement of forehead, eyebrows, and cheeks; lips and peroral [relating to the mouth] area, expressions such as pouting or puckering; jaws, such as chewing, biting, or lateral movements; and tongue, such as ability to sustain movement)
- three items assess extremity and trunk movements (upper extremity, such as wrists, finger, hands, and arms; lower extremity, such as toes, ankles, knees, and legs; and trunk, such as neck, shoulders, and hips)
- three items assess global judgments, such as severity of distress from abnormal movements, incapacitation due to abnormal movements, and patient's awareness of abnormal movements
- two items assess problems of the gums and teeth (or dentures)

The majority of items refer to the body movements themselves. The clinician or rater will ask the patient about their body movements and will also observe the patient to note firsthand any unusual movements. If the patient has noticed any unusual movements of the mouth, face, hands, or feet, the clinician will want to know if the movements annoy the patient or interfere with daily activities. The patient is then observed for any movements while sitting in a chair with feet flat on

Abnormal Involuntary Movement Scale (AIMS)

Code: 0 = None, 1 = Minimal, 2 = Mild, 3 = Moderate, 4 = Severe

Movement ratings:

Rate highest severity observed in category I, II, III.
Rate movements that occur upon activation one point less than those observed spontaneously.
Circle movements as well as code number that applies.

I. Facial & oral movements	**1. Muscles of Facial Expression:** Movements of forehead, eyebrows, periorbital area, cheeks, including frowning, blinking, smiling, grimacing	0 1 2 3 4
	2. Lips and Perioral Area: Puckering, pouting, smacking	0 1 2 3 4
	3. Jaw: Biting, clenching, chewing, mouth opening, lateral movement	0 1 2 3 4
	4. Tongue: Rate only increases in movement both in and out of mouth. NOT inability to sustain movement. Darting in and out of mouth	0 1 2 3 4
II. Extremity movements	**5. Upper (arms, wrists, hands, fingers):** Include choreic movements (rapid objectively purposeless, irregular, spontaneous), atheoid movements. DO NOT INCLUDE TREMOR (repetitive, regular, rhythmic)	0 1 2 3 4
	6. Lower (legs, knees, ankles, toes): Lateral knee movement, foot tapping, heel dropping, foot squirming, inversion and eversion of foot	0 1 2 3 4
III. Trunk movements	**7. Neck, shoulders, and hips:** Rocking, twisting, squirming, pelvic gyrations	0 1 2 3 4
IV. Global judgment	**8. Severity of abnormal movements overall**	0 1 2 3 4
	9. Incapacitation due to abnormal movements	0 1 2 3 4
	10. Patient's awareness of abnormal movements. Rate only patient's report: No awareness = 0 Aware, no distress = 1 Aware, mild distress = 2 Aware, moderate distress = 3 Aware, severe distress = 4	0 1 2 3 4
V. Dental status	**11. Current problems with teeth and/or dentures?**	YES NO
	12. Are dentures usually worn?	YES NO
	13. Endentia?	YES NO
	14. Do movements disappear with sleep?	YES NO

Scale is available in the public domain; a self-evaluation tool is also provided online by the Center for Quality Assessment and Improvement in Mental Health (CQAIMH) at http://www.cqaimh.org/tool_sideeffect.html. *(Table by PreMediaGlobal. © 2012 Cengage Learning.)*

the floor, knees separated slightly with the hands on the knees. The clinician will instruct the patient to perform specific movements—first to open his or her mouth and stick out the tongue twice, and then to tap his or her thumb with each finger very rapidly for 10 to 15 seconds, the right hand first and then the left hand. While the patient performs these actions, the clinician will observe the patient's face and legs for any abnormal movements.

After the face and hands have been tested, the patient will be asked to flex (bend) and extend one arm at a time, and then stand up so that the clinician can observe the entire body for movements. When standing, the patient will need to extend both arms in front of the body with the palms facing downward while the trunk, legs, and mouth are again observed for signs of TD. The patient must then walk a few paces, and his or her gait and hands will be observed by the clinician twice.

To assess dental care, the patient must be calm and sitting in a firm chair that does not have arms, and the patient cannot have anything in his or her mouth. The clinician will ask the patient about the condition of his or her teeth and dentures, or if he or she is having any pain or discomfort from dentures.

Preparation

Preparation for the AIMS is neither necessary nor recommended by healthcare professionals.

Aftercare

There is no patient aftercare required for the AIMS, but follow-up exams are required every three to six months to monitor the effects of long-term treatment with neuroleptic medications and/or assess the severity of and treat any signs of TD.

KEY TERMS

Choreathetoid movements—Repetitive dance-like movements that do not have any type of rhythm.

Clozapine—A newer antipsychotic medication that is often given to patients who are developing signs of tardive dyskinesia.

Neuroleptic—Another name for the older antipsychotic medications, such as haloperidol (Haldol) and chlorpromazine (Thorazine).

Syndrome—A group of symptoms that together characterize a disease or disorder.

Tardive dyskinesia—Abbreviated as TD, a condition that involves involuntary movements of the tongue, jaw, mouth, face, or other groups of skeletal muscles that usually occurs either late in antipsychotic therapy or even after the therapy is discontinued; it may be irreversible.

Results

The total AIMS score is not reported to the patient. A rating of 2 or higher on the AIMS is considered evidence of TD. If the patient has mild TD in two areas or moderate movements in one area, then he or she should be given a **diagnosis** of TD. The AIMS is extremely reliable when it is administered by trained and experienced professionals.

If the patient's score on the AIMS suggests the diagnosis of TD, the clinician must consider whether the patient still needs to be on an antipsychotic medication, as sometimes the benefits of the drug may outweigh the risks. This question should be discussed with the patient and his or her family. If the patent requires ongoing treatment with antipsychotic drugs, a lower dose may be administered to see if it relieves the TD symptoms while still performing its intended function. Another option is to place the patient on a different medication, such as **clozapine** (Clozaril) or another atypical antipsychotic. Atypical antipsychotics are a newer class of medications that produce fewer side effects than older antipsychotic drugs.

See also Medication-induced movement disorders; Schizophrenia

Resources

BOOKS

American Psychiatric Association. *Diagnostic and Statistical Manual of Mental Disorders*. 4th ed., text rev. Washington, DC: American Psychiatric Association, 2000.

Loretz, Lorraine. *Primary Care Tools for Clinicians: A Compendium of Forms, Questionnaires, and Rating Scales for Everyday Practice*. St. Louis: Elsevier Mosby, 2005.

Pavuluri, Mani N., and Philip G. Janicak. *Handbook of Psychopharmacotherapy: A Life Span Approach*. Philadelphia: Lippincott Williams & Wilkins, 2004.

Sadock, Benjamin J., Virginia A. Sadock, and Pedro Ruiz, editors. *Kaplan & Sadock's Comprehensive Textbook of Psychiatry*. Philadelphia: Wolters Kluwer Health/Lippincott Williams & Wilkins, 2009.

Smith, David S. *Field Guide to Bedside Diagnosis*. Philadelphia: Lippincott Williams & Wilkins, 2007.

Stern, Theodore A., and John B. Herman, editors. *Massachusetts General Hospital Psychiatry Update and Board Preparation*. New York City: McGraw-Hill, 2004.

OTHER

Center for Quality Assessment and Improvement in Mental Health. "STABLE [STAndards for BipoLar Excellence Project] Resource Toolkit, Side-effects Monitoring: Abnormal Involuntary Movement Scale." http://www.cqaimh.org/pdf/tool_aims.pdf (accessed October 13, 2011).

ORGANIZATIONS

National Alliance for Research on Schizophrenia and Depression, 60 Cutter Mill Road, Suite 404, Great Neck, NY, 11021, (516) 829-0091, Fax: (516) 487-6930, info@narsad.org, http://www.narsad.org.

National Institute of Mental Health, 6001 Executive Boulevard, Room 8184, Bethesda, MD, 20892-9663, (301) 443-4513, (866) 615-6464, Fax: (301) 443-4279, nimhinfo@nih.gov, http://www.nimh.nih.gov.

Susan Hobbs, M.D.
William Atkins

Abuse

Definition

Abuse refers to harmful or injurious treatment of another human being that may include physical, sexual, verbal, psychological/emotional, intellectual, or spiritual maltreatment. Abuse may coexist with **neglect**, which is defined as failure to meet a dependent person's basic physical and medical needs, emotional deprivation, and/or desertion. Neglect is sometimes described as passive abuse.

Demographics

About 1.2 per 1,000 children suffer from **sexual abuse** yearly. Girls are more likely than boys to be abused sexually. According to a conservative estimate, 38% of

Percentage of stalking and harassment victimizations reported to the police, by victim gender

	Percentage of victims					
	All		Stalking		Harassment	
	Male	Female	Male	Female	Male	Female
Reported	20.6%	32.8%	36.8%	41.0%	6.8%	13.9%
Not reported	79.4%	67.2%	63.2%	59.0%	93.2%	86.1%
Number of victims	1,941,650	3,637,570	892,340	2,528,990	1,049,320	1,108,580

Note: Table excludes 4.5% of all male victims, 4.9% of all female victims, 0.1% of female stalking victims, 8% of male harassment victims, and 14.2% of female harassment victims due to missing data.

SOURCE: Baum, Katrina et al, *Stalking Victimization in the United States* (Washington, DC: Bureau of Justice Statistics, 2009).

(Table by PreMediaGlobal. © 2012 Cengage Learning.)

girls and 16% of boys are sexually abused before their eighteenth birthday. In 2009, there were an estimated 1,770 child deaths from abuse or neglect in the United States, indicating a rate of 2.34 children for every 100,000 in the population. Of the children who survive abuse, an estimated 20% have permanent physical injury. Younger children and children with birth defects, developmental delays, or chronic illnesses are at higher risk of being abused by parents or other caregivers.

Women are more likely than men to be the targets of abuse in adult life, and one in four women will experience domestic violence in her lifetime. It is estimated that four million women in the United States are involved in abusive marriages or relationships; moreover, about 33% of female murder victims are killed by their spouses or partners rather than by strangers.

About 3.4 million people suffer from a stalking incident yearly, and about 80% of stalking cases reported to police involve men stalking women. Half of all workplace bullies are women, and the majority of workplace bullies (81%) are bosses or supervisors. Research has demonstrated that female bullies tend to bully other women, while male bullies bully both men and women.

The costs of abuse to society run into billions of dollars annually in the United States alone. They include not only the direct costs of immediate medical and psychiatric treatment of abused people but also the indirect costs of learning difficulties, interrupted education, workplace absenteeism, and long-term health problems of abuse survivors.

Description

Abuse is a complex psychosocial problem that affects large numbers of people throughout the world. Although abuse was initially defined with regard to children when it first received sustained attention in the 1950s, clinicians and researchers now recognize that adults can suffer abuse under a number of different circumstances.

Physical abuse

Physical abuse refers to striking or beating another person with the hands or an object or assaulting a person with a knife, gun, or other weapon. Physical abuse also includes such behaviors as locking someone in a closet or other small space, gagging or tying someone up, or depriving someone of sleep. Physical abuse of infants or children may include shaking them, dropping them on the floor, or throwing them against the wall or other hard object.

Sexual abuse

Sexual abuse refers to inappropriate sexual contact between a child or adult and another person. Sexual abuse may include verbal remarks, fondling or kissing, or attempted or completed intercourse. Sexual contact between a child and a biological relative is known as incest, although some therapists extend the term to cover sexual contact between a child and any trusted caregiver, including relatives by marriage.

Verbal abuse

Verbal abuse refers to regular and consistent belittling, name-calling, labeling, or ridicule of a person. It may also include spoken threats. It is one of the most difficult forms of abuse to prove because it does not leave physical scars or other evidence, but it is nonetheless hurtful. Verbal abuse may occur in schools or workplaces as well as in homes among family members.

Emotional/psychological abuse

Emotional/psychological abuse covers a variety of behaviors that hurt or injure others even though no physical contact may be involved. In fact, emotional abuse is a stronger predictor than physical abuse of the likelihood of **suicide** attempts in later life. One form of emotional abuse is emotional blackmail, which involves making another person feel guilty until he or she does what is wanted. Other behaviors in this category include giving the silent treatment, shaming or humiliating someone, or committing an act intended to cause a person emotional pain, such as destroying a valued possession.

Intellectual/spiritual abuse

Intellectual/spiritual abuse refers to such behaviors as punishing people for having different intellectual interests or religious beliefs, preventing them from attending worship services, ridiculing their opinions, and the like.

Domestic violence

Domestic violence refers to the physical, emotional, and sexual abuse of a spouse or domestic partner. Early research into the problem of wife battering focused on middle-class couples, but it has since been recognized that spousal abuse can occur within couples of any socioeconomic status or sexual orientation.

Domestic violence illustrates the tendency of abusive people to attack anyone they perceive as vulnerable: Most men who batter women also abuse their children; some battered women abuse their children; and abusive humans are frequently cruel to animals.

Elder abuse

Elder abuse has become a subject of national concern in the last two decades. As older adults live longer, many become dependent for years on adult caregivers, who may be either their own adult children or nursing home personnel. Care of the elderly can be extremely stressful, especially if the older adult has **dementia**. Elder abuse may include physical hitting or slapping; withholding food or medications; tying individuals to a chair or bed; neglecting to bathe them or help them to the toilet; taking their personal possessions, including money or property; and restricting or cutting off their contacts with friends and relatives.

Stalking

Stalking, or the repeated pursuit or surveillance of another person by physical or electronic means, is defined as a crime in all 50 states. Many cases of stalking are extensions of domestic violence, in that the stalker attempts to track down a partner who left him or her. However, stalkers may also be casual acquaintances, workplace colleagues, or even total strangers. Stalking may include a number of abusive behaviors, including forced entry into a person's home; destruction of cars or other personal property; anonymous letters to a person's friends or employer; or repeated phone calls, letters, or e-mails.

Workplace bullying

Workplace **bullying** is, like stalking, increasingly recognized as interpersonal abuse. It should not be confused with sexual harassment or racial discrimination. Workplace bullying refers to verbal abuse of other workers; interfering with their work; withholding equipment or other resources needed to do their job; or invading their personal space, including touching them in a controlling manner.

Causes and symptoms

Causes

The causes of interpersonal abuse are complex and overlapping. Some of the most important factors are:

- Early learning experiences: This factor is sometimes described as the "life cycle" of abuse. Many abusive parents were themselves abused as children and have learned to see hurtful behavior as normal childrearing. At the other end of the life cycle, some adults who abuse their elderly parent are paying back the parent for abusing them in their early years.
- Ignorance of developmental timetables: Some parents have unrealistic expectations of children in terms of the appropriate age for toilet training, feeding themselves, and similar milestones; they may attack their children for not meeting these expectations.
- Economic stress: Many caregivers cannot afford part-time day care for children or dependent elderly parents, which would relieve some of their emotional strain. Even middle-class families can be financially stressed if they find themselves responsible for the costs of caring for elderly parents before their own children are financially independent.
- Lack of social support or social resources: Caregivers who have the support of an extended family, religious group, or close friends and neighbors are less likely to lose their self-control under stress.
- Substance abuse: Alcohol and mood-altering drugs do not cause abuse directly, but they weaken or remove a person's inhibitions against violence toward others. In addition, the cost of a drug habit often gives a person with a substance addiction another reason for resenting the needs of the dependent person. A majority of workplace bullies are substance addicts.
- Mental disorders: Depression, personality disorders, dissociative disorders, and anxiety disorders can all

affect parents' ability to care for their children appropriately. A small percentage of abusive parents or spouses are psychotic.

- Belief systems: Many men still think that they have a "right" to a relationship with a woman, and many people regard parents' rights over children as absolute.
- The role of bystanders: Research in the social sciences has shown that one factor that encourages abusers to continue their hurtful behavior is discovering that people who know about or suspect the abuse are reluctant to get involved. In most cases, bystanders are afraid of possible physical, social, or legal consequences for reporting abuse. The result, however, is that many abusers come to see themselves as invulnerable.

Symptoms

PHYSICAL AND NEUROBIOLOGICAL. In addition to such direct results of **trauma** as broken bones or ruptured internal organs, physically abused children often display retarded physical growth and poor coordination. Malnutrition may slow the development of the **brain** as well as produce such dietary deficiency diseases as rickets. In both children and adults, repeated trauma produces changes in the neurochemistry of the brain that affect memory formation. Instead of memories being formed in the normal way, which allows them to be modified by later experiences and integrated into a person's ongoing life, traumatic memories are stored as chaotic fragments of emotion and sensation that are sealed off from ordinary consciousness. These traumatic memories may then erupt from time to time in the form of flashbacks. Additionally, research has shown that adults who were abused during childhood have a greater likelihood of suffering from a number of health conditions throughout their lives, including allergies, asthma, bronchitis, arthritis, ulcers, and high blood pressure.

People who have suffered abuse also demonstrate a higher risk of developing psychiatric conditions, such as **depression**, anxiety, **substance abuse**, **personality disorders**, and suicidality.

COGNITIVE AND EMOTIONAL. Abused children develop distorted patterns of cognition (knowing) due to the emotional stress of abuse. As children, their language skills and academic performance lag behind those of other children, and they often display behavioral problems in the classroom setting. As adults, they may experience cognitive distortions that make it hard for them to distinguish between normal occurrences and abnormal ones or between important matters and relatively trivial ones. They often misinterpret other people's behavior and refuse to trust them. Both children and adults with abuse histories demonstrate low self-esteem and an inability to attach or bond with others. Emotional distortions include such patterns as being unable to handle strong feelings or being unusually tolerant of behavior from others that most people would protest.

SOCIAL AND EDUCATIONAL. The cognitive and emotional aftereffects of abuse have a powerful impact on adult educational, social, and occupational functioning. Children who are abused are often in physical and emotional pain at school; they cannot concentrate on schoolwork and consequently fall behind in their grades. They often find it hard to make or keep friends, and may be victimized by bullies or become bullies themselves. In adult life, abuse survivors are at risk of repeating childhood patterns through forming relationships with abusive spouses, employers, or professionals. Even though survivors may consciously want to avoid further abuse, they are often unconsciously attracted to people who remind them of their family of origin. Abused adults are also likely to fail to complete their educations, or they accept employment that is significantly below their actual level of ability. Adults who have previously suffered abuse also have a higher risk of displaying antisocial traits.

There are higher rates of teen pregnancy, juvenile delinquency, substance abuse, adult criminal behavior, and risk taking (with increased risks of sexually transmitted diseases) among people who have been abused. Ironically and tragically, abused children often grow up to be abusive parents, perpetuating the cycle of abuse.

Treatment

Treatment of the aftereffects of abuse must be tailored to the needs of the specific individual but usually involves a variety of long-term considerations that may include legal concerns, geographical relocation, and housing or employment as well as immediate medical or psychiatric care.

Medical and psychiatric

In addition to requiring immediate treatment for physical injuries, abused children and adults often need long-term **psychotherapy** in order to recover from specific mental disorders and to learn new ways of dealing with distorted thoughts and feelings. This approach to therapy is known as cognitive restructuring. Specific mental disorders that have been linked to childhood abuse include major depression, **bulimia nervosa**, **social phobia**, Munchausen syndrome by proxy, **generalized anxiety disorder**, **post-traumatic**

KEY TERMS

Cognitive restructuring—An approach to psychotherapy that focuses on helping patients examine distorted patterns of perceiving and thinking in order to change their emotional responses to people and situations.

Dementia—A group of symptoms (syndrome) associated with a progressive loss of memory and other intellectual functions that is serious enough to interfere with a person's ability to perform the tasks of daily life. Dementia impairs memory, alters personality, leads to deterioration in personal grooming, impairs reasoning ability, and causes disorientation.

Flashback—The reemergence of a traumatic memory as a vivid recollection of sounds, images, and sensations associated with the trauma. Those having the flashbacks typically feel as if they are reliving the event.

Incest—Unlawful sexual contact between people who are biologically related. Many therapists also use the term to refer to inappropriate sexual contact between members of a family, including stepparents and stepsiblings.

Stalking—The intentional pursuit or surveillance of another person, usually with the intent of forcing that person into a dating or marriage relationship. Stalking is punishable as a crime in all 50 states.

stress disorder, **borderline personality disorder**, **dissociative amnesia**, and **dissociative identity disorder**. Abused adults may develop post-traumatic **stress** disorder, major depression, or substance abuse disorders. Research is also focused on **genetic factors** as a partial explanation of the fact that some people appear to react more intensely than others to being abused.

In cases where abuse has reached levels that result in post-traumatic stress disorder (PTSD), medications may be useful for treating the accompanying anxiety, emotional outbursts, difficulty sleeping, and nightmares. Medications that have been used in this setting include antipsychotics, **antidepressants**, anxiolytics, and the blood pressure medication called prazosin, which has shown some utility in preventing **insomnia** and nightmares.

Legal considerations

Medical professionals and, increasingly, religious professionals are required by law to report **child abuse** to law enforcement officials, usually a child protection agency. Physicians are granted immunity from lawsuits for making such reports.

Adults in abusive situations may encounter a variety of responses from law enforcement or the criminal justice system. Many communities require police officers to arrest aggressors in domestic violence situations, and a growing number of small towns as well as cities have shelters for family members fleeing violent households. All major medical, educational, and legal professional societies, as well as mainstream religious bodies, have adopted strict codes of ethics and have procedures in place for reporting cases of abuse by their members.

Prevention

Prevention of abuse requires long-term social changes in attitudes toward violence, gender roles, and the relationship of the family to other institutions. Research in the structure and function of the brain may help to develop more effective treatments for the aftereffects of abuse and possibly new approaches to help break the intergenerational cycle of abuse. As of 2011, preventive measures included protective removal of children or elders from abusive households, legal penalties for abusive spouses and professionals, and education of the public about the nature and causes of abuse.

Resources

BOOKS

American Psychiatric Association. *Diagnostic and Statistical Manual of Mental Disorders.* 4th ed., Text rev. Washington, DC: American Psychiatric Association, 2000.

Bradley, W., et al. *Neurology in Clinical Practice.* 5th ed. Philadelphia: Butterworth-Heinemann, 2008.

Stern, Theodore A., et al. *Massachusetts General Hospital Comprehensive Clinical Psychiatry.* 1st ed. Philadelphia: Mosby Elsevier, 2008.

Weiner, William J., et al. *Neurology for the Non-Neurologist (Weiner, Neurology for the Non-Neurologist).* 6th ed. Baltimore: Lippincott Williams & Wilkins, 2010.

PERIODICALS

Asnes, A.G. "Managing Child Abuse: General Principles." *Pediatric Review* 31 (February 1, 2010): 47–55.

Falk, E. "Geriatricians and Psychologists: Essential Ingredients in the Evaluation of Elder Abuse and Neglect." *Journal of Elder Abuse and Neglect* 22 (July 10, 2010): 281–90.

Shipman, K. "Mental Health Treatment of Child Abuse and Neglect: The Promise of Evidence-based Practice." *Pediatric Clinics of North America* 56 (April 1, 2009): 417–28.

WEBSITES

Child Welfare Information Gateway. "Child Abuse and Neglect Fatalities: Statistics and Interventions." Last modified February 2011. http://www.childwelfare.gov/pubs/factsheets/fatality.pdf (accessed September 16, 2011).

"Domestic Violence." MedlinePlus. Last modified September 8, 2011. http://www.nlm.nih.gov/medlineplus/domestic-violence.html (accessed September 16, 2011).

U.S. Department of Health and Human Services, Administration on Children, Youth and Families. *Child Maltreatment 2004*. http://www.acf.hhs.gov/programs/cb/pubs/cm04/cm04.pdf (accessed September 16, 2011).

ORGANIZATIONS

American Academy of Child and Adolescent Psychiatry, 3615 Wisconsin Ave. NW, Washington, DC, 20016-3007, (202) 966-7300, Fax: (202) 966-2891, http://www.aacap.org.

Kempe Foundation, Gary Pavilion at Children's Hospital Colorado, Anschutz Medical Campus, 13123 E 16th Ave., B390, Denver, CO, 80045, (303) 864-5300, http://www.kempe.org.

National Coalition Against Domestic Violence, 1120 Lincoln St., Ste. 1603, Denver, CO, 80203, (303) 839-1852; TTY: (303) 839-1681, Fax: (303) 831-9251, http://www.ncadv.org.

National Institute of Mental Health, 6001 Executive Blvd., Rm. 8184, MSC 9663, Bethesda, MD, 20892-9663, (301) 433-4513; TTY: (301) 443-8431, Fax: (301) 443-4279, Toll-free: (866) 615-6464; TTY: (866) 415-8051, nimhinfo@nih.gov, http://www.nimh.nih.gov.

Rebecca Frey, PhD
Emily Jane Willingham, PhD
Rosalyn Carson-DeWitt

Acne excoriee *see* **Dermatillomania**

Acupressure

Definition

Acupressure is a form of touch therapy that uses the principles of **acupuncture** and traditional Chinese medicine (TCM). In acupressure, the same points on the body are used as in acupuncture, but they are stimulated with finger pressure instead of with the insertion of needles. Acupressure is used to relieve a variety of symptoms and pain.

Demographics

As of 2011, the cost of acupressure massage was, on average, \$60–\$70 per hour session. A visit to a Chinese medicine physician or acupuncturist can be more expensive, comparable to a visit to an allopathic physician if the practitioner is a certified medical doctor (MD). Insurance reimbursement varies widely, and consumers should inquire as to whether their policies cover alternative treatment, acupuncture, or massage therapy.

Purpose

In Chinese medicine, disease is viewed as an imbalance of the organs and chi in the body. The goal of acupressure, and also acupuncture, is to stimulate and unblock the circulation of chi by activating very specific points, called pressure points or *acupoints*.

Acupressure is used by Chinese medicine practitioners, acupuncturists, and massage therapists. Many massage schools in the United States include acupressure techniques as part of their bodywork programs. Shiatsu massage is very closely related to acupressure, involving the same points on the body and the same general principles, although it was developed over centuries in Japan rather than in China. Reflexology is a form of bodywork based on acupressure concepts. Jin Shin Do is a bodywork technique with an increasing number of practitioners in the United States that combines acupressure and shiatsu principles with qigong, Reichian theory, and **meditation**.

Description

Origins

Acupressure and related therapies (e.g., acupuncture, shiatsu massage) have their roots in Chinese medicine. One legend has it that acupuncture and acupressure evolved as early Chinese healers studied the puncture wounds of Chinese warriors, noting that certain points on the body created interesting results when stimulated. The oldest known text specifically on acupuncture points, the *Systematic Classic of Acupuncture*, dates to about 282 A.D.

Outside of Asian American communities, Chinese medicine remained virtually unknown in the United States until the 1970s, when Richard Nixon became the first U.S. president to visit China. On Nixon's trip, journalists were amazed to observe major operations being performed on patients without the use of anesthetics. Instead, fully conscious patients were being operated on with acupuncture needles inserted into them to control pain. At that time, a famous columnist for the *New York Times*, James Reston, had to undergo surgery and elected to use acupuncture for anesthesia. Later, he wrote some convincing stories on its effectiveness. Despite being neglected by mainstream medicine and the American Medical Association (AMA), acupuncture and Chinese medicine became an option for alternative medicine practitioners in the United States. In the early 2010s, millions of patients can attest to its effectiveness, and there are nearly 9,000 practitioners dispersed across all 50 states.

Acupressure and Chinese medicine

Chinese medicine views the body as a small part of the universe, subject to the laws and principles of

KEY TERMS

Acupoint—A pressure point stimulated in acupressure.

Chi—Basic life energy.

Meridian—A channel through which chi travels in the body.

Moxibustion—An acupuncture technique that involves burning of the herb moxa or mugwort.

Shiatsu—Japanese form of acupressure massage.

Yin/yang—Universal characteristics used to describe aspects of the natural world.

harmony and balance. Chinese medicine does not make as sharp a distinction as Western medicine does between mind and body. The Chinese system asserts that emotions and mental states are every bit as influential on disease as purely physical mechanisms, meaning that factors such as work, environment, and relationships affect a person's health. Chinese medicine also uses very different symbols and ideas to discuss the body and health. While Western medicine typically describes health as mainly physical and chemical processes, the Chinese use ideas of yin and yang, chi, and the organ system to describe health and the body.

YIN AND YANG. Everything in the universe has properties of yin and yang. Yin is associated with such attributes as cold, female, passive, downward, inward, dark, and wet. Yang is the opposite—hot, male, active, upward, outward, light, dry, and so on. Nothing is either completely yin or yang. These two principles always interact and affect each other. A healthy body possesses an equal balance of both yin and yang; disease occurs when there is too much or too little of either.

CHI. Chi (pronounced *chee*, also spelled *qi* or *ki* in Japanese shiatsu) is the fundamental life energy. It is found in food, air, water, and sunlight, and it travels through the body in channels called *meridians*. There are 12 major meridians in the body that transport chi, corresponding to the 12 main organs categorized by Chinese medicine.

ORGAN SYSTEM. Chinese medicine has developed intricate systems regarding how organs are related to physical and mental symptoms, and it has devised corresponding treatments using meridian and pressure point networks that are classified and numbered. Acupressure seeks to stimulate the points on the chi meridians that pass close to the skin, as these are the easiest to unblock and manipulate with finger pressure.

Physical examination

To get a complete **diagnosis** of which organs and meridian points are out of balance, a Chinese medicine practitioner will examine a patient very thoroughly, looking at physical, mental, and emotional activity; taking the pulse, usually at the wrists; examining the tongue and complexion; and observing the patient's demeanor and attitude. When the imbalance is located, the physician recommends specific pressure points for acupuncture or acupressure. If acupressure is recommended, the patient might opt for a series of treatments from a massage therapist.

Massage therapy

In massage therapy, acupressurists evaluate a patient's symptoms and overall health, but a massage therapist's diagnostic training is not as extensive as that of a TCM physician. In a massage therapy treatment, a person usually lies on a table or mat with thin clothing on. The acupressurist gently feels and palpates the abdomen and other parts of the body to determine energy imbalances. Then, the therapist works with different meridians throughout the body, depending on which organs are imbalanced in the abdomen. The therapist uses different types of finger movements and pressure on different acupoints, depending on whether the chi needs to be increased or dispersed at different points. The therapist observes and guides the energy flow through the patient's body throughout the session. Sometimes, special herbs (*Artemesia vulgaris* or moxa) may be placed on a point to warm it, a process called *moxibustion*. A session of acupressure is generally a very pleasant experience, and some people experience great benefit immediately. For more chronic conditions, several sessions may be necessary to relieve and improve conditions.

Self-treatment

Acupressure is easy to learn, and there are many good books that illustrate the position of acupoints and meridians on the body. The procedure can also be conducted anywhere, and it is a good form of treatment for spouses and partners to give to each other and for parents to perform on children for minor conditions. As effective as acupressure may be, it should not be used to the exclusion of allopathic methods that provide more reliable relief or cure for certain diseases and disorders.

While giving self-treatment or performing acupressure on another, a mental attitude of calmness and attention is important, as one person's energy can be used to help another's. Loose, thin clothing is recommended.

There are three general techniques for stimulating a pressure point:

- Tonifying is meant to strengthen weak chi and is done by pressing the thumb or finger into an acupoint with a firm, steady pressure, holding it for up to two minutes.
- Dispersing is meant to move stagnant or blocked chi, and the finger or thumb is moved in a circular motion or slightly in and out of the point for two minutes.
- Calming the chi in a pressure point utilizes the palm to cover the point and gently stroke the area for about two minutes.

There are many pressure points that are easily found and memorized to treat common ailments.

- For headaches and pain in the upper body, the "LI4" point is recommended. It is located in the web between the thumb and index finger, on the back of the hand. Using the thumb and index finger of the other hand, a person applies a pinching pressure until the point is felt and holds it for two minutes. Pregnant women should never press this point.
- To calm the nerves, a person finds the "CV12" point that is four thumb widths above the navel in the center of the abdomen. Calm the point with the palm, using gentle stroking for several minutes.
- For headaches and tension, a person locates the "GB20" points at the base of the skull in the back of the head, just behind the bones in back of the ears and then disperses these points for two minutes with the fingers or thumbs. The individual can also find the "yintang" point, which is in the middle of the forehead between the eyebrows and disperse it with gentle pressure for two minutes to clear the mind and to relieve headaches.

Benefits

Acupressure massage performed by a therapist can be very effective both as prevention and as a treatment for many health conditions. Unlike acupuncture, which requires a visit to a professional, acupressure can be performed by anyone. Acupressure techniques are fairly easy to learn and have been used to provide quick, cost-free, and effective relief from many symptoms. Acupressure points can also be stimulated to increase energy and feelings of well-being, reduce **stress**, stimulate the immune system, and alleviate sexual dysfunction.

Precautions

Acupressure is a safe technique, but it is not meant to replace professional health care. A physician should always be consulted when there are doubts about medical conditions. If a condition is chronic, a professional should be consulted; purely symptomatic treatment can exacerbate chronic conditions. Acupressure should not be applied to open wounds or to places that are swollen or inflamed. Areas of scar tissue, blisters, boils, rashes, or varicose veins should be avoided. Finally, certain acupressure points should not be stimulated on people with high or low blood pressure or on pregnant women.

QUESTIONS TO ASK YOUR DOCTOR

- What kind of results can I expect to feel with acupressure?
- What other type of treatment do you recommend for me?
- Will acupressure therapy interfere with my current medications?
- What symptoms or behaviors are important enough that I should seek immediate treatment?

Research and general acceptance

In general, Chinese medicine has been slow to gain acceptance in the West, mainly because it rests on ideas that differ from the Western scientific model. Western scientists have trouble with the idea of chi, the invisible energy of the body, and the idea that pressing on certain points can alleviate certain conditions seems incredible.

In trying to account for the action of acupressure, Western scientists have theorized that chi is actually part of the neuroendocrine system of the body. Celebrated orthopedic surgeon Robert O. Becker, who was twice nominated for the Nobel Prize, wrote a book on the subject called *Cross Currents: The Promise of Electromedicine; The Perils of Electropollution*. By using precise electrical measuring devices, Becker and his colleagues showed that the body has a complex web of electromagnetic energy and that traditional acupressure meridians and points contain amounts of energy that non-acupressure points do not.

The mechanisms of acupuncture and acupressure remain difficult to document in terms of the biochemical processes involved. Numerous testimonials are the primary evidence supporting the effectiveness of acupressure and acupuncture. Research and **clinical trials** continue to study the effectiveness of acupressure and acupuncture techniques in treating various health problems and in controlling pain.

Training and certification

There are two methods for becoming trained in the skill of acupressure. The first is training in traditional acupuncture and Chinese medicine, for which there are many schools and certifying bodies around the United States. The majority of acupressure practitioners are trained as certified massage therapists, either as acupressure or shiatsu specialists.

Resources

BOOKS

Kolster, Bernard C., and Astrid Waskowiak. *The Acupressure Atlas*. Rochester, VT: Healing Arts Press, 2007.

Vora, Devendra. *Health in Your Hands: Acupressure and Other Natural Therapies, Vol. 2*. Mumbai, India: Navneet, 2007.

Wright, Janet. *Reflexology and Acupressure*. London: Hamlyn Press, 2008.

PERIODICALS

Agarwal, A., et al. "Acupressure for Prevention of Pre-operative Anxiety: A Prospective, Randomised, Placebo Controlled Study." *Anaesthesia* (October 2005): 978–981.

Jamigorn, Mattawan, and Vorapong Phupong. "Acupressure and Vitamin B6 to Relieve Nausea and Vomiting in Pregnancy: A Randomized Study." *Archives of Gynecology and Obstetrics* (September 2007): 245–249.

"Non-Epidural Pain Relief." *The Informed Choice Initiative (Women's Edition)* (April 2007): 91–98.

OTHER

Wisconsin Department of Health Services. "Responding to Challenging Situations: Acupressure Points for Stress Relief." http://www.dhs.wisconsin.gov/caregiver/training/pdfcaregvtrng/respAcupressure.pdf (accessed November 14, 2011).

ORGANIZATIONS

Acupressure Institute, 1533 Shattuck Ave., Berkeley, CA, 94709, (800) 442-2232, http://www.acupressureinstitute.com.

American Massage Therapy Association, 500 Davis Street, Suite 900, Evanston, IL, 60201-4695, (847) 864-0123, (877) 905-0577, Fax: (847) 864-5196, info@amtamassage.org, http://www.amtamassage.org.

American Organization for Bodywork Therapies of Asia, 1010 Haddonfield-Berlin Rd., Suite 408, Voorhees, NJ, 08043-3514, (856) 782-1616, Fax: (856) 782-1653, office@aobta.org, http://www.aobta.org.

Jin Shin Do Foundation for Bodymind Acupressure, PO Box 416, Idyllwild, CA, 92549, (951) 659-5707, http://www.jinshindo.org.

Douglas Dupler
Laura Jean Cataldo, RN, Ed.D.

Acupuncture

Definition

Acupuncture, one of the main forms of treatment in traditional Chinese medicine (TCM), involves the use of sharp, thin needles that are inserted in the skin of the body at specific points where the flow of energy is thought to be blocked. This process is believed to adjust and alter the body's energy flow into healthier patterns and is used to treat a wide variety of illnesses and health conditions. As one of the many benefits thought to accrue from its use, acupuncture is believed by many people to help relieve symptoms of mental illness. The early development of acupuncture is also deep within the medical history of Japan, Korea, Vietnam, Taiwan, and other eastern Asian regions. Today, acupuncture remains a controversial subject regarding its therapeutic effectiveness in the field of Western medicine.

Purpose

In Chinese medicine, where acupuncture seems to have originated, disease is seen as imbalance in the organ system or chi meridians, and the goal of any remedy or treatment is to assist the body in re-establishing its innate harmony. Disease can be caused by internal factors such as emotions, external factors such as the environment and weather, and other factors such as injuries, **trauma**, diet, and germs. However, infection is seen not as primarily a problem with germs and viruses but as a weakness in the energy of the body that is allowing a sickness to occur. In Chinese medicine, no two illnesses are ever the same, as each body has its own characteristics of symptoms and balance. Acupuncture is used to open or adjust the flow of chi throughout the organ system, which will strengthen the body and prompt it to physically or mentally heal itself.

Mental illnesses, or mental health disorders, are psychiatric disorders that cause atypical behaviors that alter one's feelings, moods, or thinking. Types of mental illness include **bipolar disorder**, **depression**, **obsessive-compulsive disorder**, **panic disorder**, and **schizophrenia**. Acupuncturists claim that they can use the process of acupuncture to treat the causes of such mental problems by rebalancing the internal workings of the body. Acupuncture has been widely used in the world for many centuries—dating back to the first few centuries *B.C.*—but its effectiveness for anything other than the relief of pain and nausea has not yet been established within the medical community of the United States.

Demographics

Since mental disorders affect many people without regard to age, ethnic background, religion, or income,

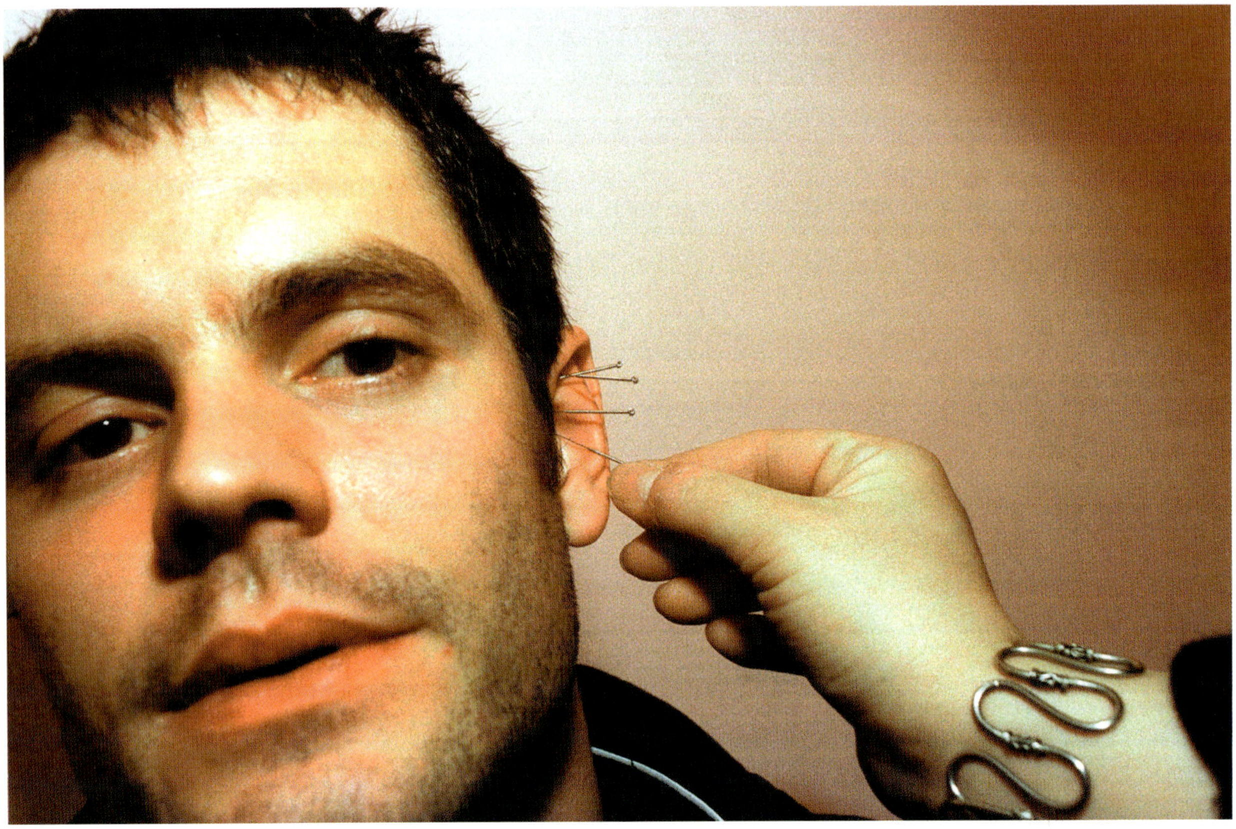

A recovering drug addict undergoes acupuncture treatment for withdrawal symptoms. *(© David Hoffman Photo Library/Alamy)*

they are a widespread problem in the United States and throughout the world. Consequently, acupuncture has become known as a method for treating such illnesses. The National Institutes of Health conducted a 2007 National Health Interview Survey that found about 3.1 million American adults and 150,000 children had used acupuncture in 2006. It also stated that over a six-year period, from 2002 through 2007, the frequency of acupuncture use among adults increased by about 0.3%, or approximately one million people.

As of 2011, more than 9,000 practitioners performed acupuncture within all 50 states of the United States and the District of Columbia. About 4,000 medical doctors (MDs) include it in their professional practices. Acupuncture has shown notable success in treating many conditions, and more than 15 million Americans have used it as a therapy. Acupuncture, however, remains largely unsupported by the medical establishment. The American Medical Association has been reluctant to encourage research, as the practice is based on concepts markedly unlike the Western scientific model.

Several forms of acupuncture are used in the United States. Japanese acupuncture uses extremely thin needles and does not incorporate herbal medicine in its practice. Auricular acupuncture, also called "auriculotherapy and ear acupuncture," uses acupuncture points only on the ear, which are believed to stimulate and balance internal organs. In France, where acupuncture is very popular and more widely accepted by the medical establishment, neurologist Paul Nogier (1908–1996) developed a system of acupuncture based on neuroendocrine theory rather than on traditional Chinese concepts, which has gained some use in the United States.

Description

Origins

The original text of Chinese medicine is the *Nei Ching, The Yellow Emperor's Classic of Internal Medicine*, which is estimated to be at least 2,500 years old. Thousands of books followed on the subject of Chinese healing, and its basic philosophies spread long ago to other Asian civilizations. Nearly all of the forms of Oriental medicine that are used in the West, including acupuncture, shiatsu, **acupressure** massage, and macrobiotics, are part of or have their roots in Chinese medicine. Legend has it that acupuncture developed when early Chinese physicians observed unpredicted effects of puncture wounds in Chinese warriors. The oldest known text on acupuncture, the *Systematic Classic of Acupuncture*, dates back to A.D. 282. Although acupuncture is its best-known technique, Chinese medicine traditionally uses herbal remedies, dietary therapy, lifestyle changes, and other means to treat patients.

In the early 1900s, only a few Western physicians who had visited China knew about and used acupuncture. Outside of Asian American communities, it remained virtually unknown until the 1970s, when Richard Nixon (1913–1994) became the first U.S. president to visit China. On Nixon's trip, journalists were amazed to observe major operations being performed on patients without the use of anesthetics. Instead, fully conscious patients were being operated on with only acupuncture needles inserted into them to control pain. During that time, a famous columnist for the *New York Times*, James Reston (1909–1995), had to undergo surgery in Beijing, China, and elected to use acupuncture for his post-operative pain instead of traditional pain medication. Reston later wrote some convincing stories on its effectiveness.

KEY TERMS

Acupressure—A form of massage using acupuncture points.

Auricular acupuncture—Acupuncture using only points found on the ears.

Chi—Basic life energy.

Mania—A condition of abnormally high irritability, arousal, or energy levels.

Meridian—A channel through which chi travels in the body.

Moxibustion—Acupuncture technique that involves burning the herb moxa or mugwort.

Tonification—Acupuncture technique for strengthening the body.

Yin/yang—Universal characteristics used to describe aspects of the natural world.

Basic ideas of Chinese medicine

Chinese medicine views the body as a small part of the universe, subject to universal laws and principles of harmony and balance. Chinese medicine does not draw a sharp line, as Western medicine does, between mind and body. The Chinese system believes that emotions and mental states are every bit as influential on disease as purely physical mechanisms and considers factors such as work, environment, lifestyle, and relationships as fundamental to the overall picture of a patient's health. Chinese medicine also uses very different symbols and ideas to discuss the body and health. While Western medicine typically describes health in terms of measurable physical processes made up of chemical reactions, the Chinese use the ideas of yin and yang, chi, the organ system, and the five elements to describe health and the body. To understand the ideas behind acupuncture, it is worthwhile to introduce some of these basic terms.

YIN AND YANG. According to Chinese philosophy, the universe and the body can be described by two separate but complementary principles, that of yin and yang. For example, in temperature, yin is cold and yang is hot. In gender, yin is female and yang is male. In activity, yin is passive and yang is active. In light, yin is dark and yang is bright. In direction, yin is inward and downward, and yang is outward and up. Nothing is ever completely yin or yang, but a combination of the two. These two principles are always interacting, opposing, and influencing each other. The goal of Chinese medicine is not to eliminate either yin or yang but to allow the two to balance each other and coexist harmoniously. For instance, if a person suffers from symptoms of high blood pressure, the Chinese system would say that the heart organ might have too much yang and would recommend methods either to reduce the yang or to increase the yin of the heart, depending on the other symptoms and organs in the body. Thus, acupuncture therapies seek to either increase or reduce yang or increase or reduce yin in particular regions of the body.

CHI. Another fundamental concept of Chinese medicine is that of chi (pronounced *chee*, also spelled *qi*). According to Chinese medicine, chi is the fundamental life energy of the universe. It is invisible and is found in the environment in air, water, food, and sunlight. In the body, it is the invisible vital force that creates and animates life. Humans are all born with inherited amounts of chi, and they also acquire chi from the food they eat and the air they breathe. The level and quality of a person's chi also depends on the state of physical, mental, and emotional balance. Chi travels through the body along channels called *meridians*.

THE ORGAN SYSTEM. In the Chinese system, there are twelve main organs: the lung, large intestine, stomach, spleen, heart, small intestine, urinary bladder, kidney, liver, gallbladder, pericardium, and "triple warmer," which represents the entire torso region. Each organ has chi energy associated with it, and each organ interacts with particular emotions on the mental level. As there are twelve organs, twelve types of chi can move through the body, and these move through twelve main channels or meridians. Chinese doctors connect symptoms to organs. That is, symptoms are caused by yin/yang imbalances in one or more organs or by an unhealthy flow of chi to or from one organ to another. Each organ has a different profile of symptoms it can manifest.

THE FIVE ELEMENTS. Another basis of Chinese medicine is the belief that the world and body are made up of five main elements: wood, fire, earth, metal, and water. These elements are all interconnected, and each element either generates or controls another element. For instance, water controls fire, and earth generates metal. Each organ is associated with one of the five elements. The Chinese system uses elements and organs to describe and treat conditions. For instance, the kidney is associated with water, and the heart is associated with fire. The two organs are related as water and fire are related. If the kidney is weak, then there might be a corresponding fire problem in the heart, so treatment might be made by acupuncture or herbs to cool the heart system and/or increase energy in the kidney system.

The Chinese have developed an intricate system that describes how organs and elements are related to physical and mental symptoms, and the above example is simple. Although this system sounds suspect to Western scientists, some interesting parallels have been observed. For instance, when mental illness occurs, Chinese medicine states that an imbalance has occurred within the body—either too much or too little yin and yang. It does not, however, treat mental illness as a particular disorder. Instead, acupuncturists treat the specific symptoms within each individual patient. Consequently, different patients, each with depression but with different symptoms, will receive a unique, customized treatment based on many different acupuncture points.

A visit to the acupuncturist

Typically, an acupuncturist first gets a thorough idea of a patient's medical history and symptoms, both physical and emotional, using a questionnaire and interview. Then the acupuncturist examines the patient to find further symptoms, looking closely at the tongue, the pulse at various points in the body, the complexion, general behavior, and other signs like coughs or pains. From this examination, the practitioner can determine patterns of symptoms that indicate which organs and areas are imbalanced. Depending on the problem, the acupuncturist inserts needles to manipulate chi on one or more of the twelve organ meridians. On these twelve meridians, there are nearly 2,000 points that can be used in acupuncture, with around 200 points being most frequently used by traditional acupuncturists. During an individual treatment, one to 20 needles may be used, depending on which meridian points are chosen.

Acupuncture needles are sterilized, and acupuncture is a very safe procedure. The depth of insertion of needles varies, depending on which chi channels are being treated. Some points barely go beyond superficial layers of skin, while some acupuncture points require a depth of 1–3 in. (3–8 cm) of needle. The needles generally do not cause pain. Patients sometimes report pinching sensations and often pleasant sensations, as the body experiences healing. Depending on the problem, the acupuncturist might spin or move the needles, or even pass a slight electrical current through some of them. *Moxibustion* may sometimes be used. Moxibustion is a process in which an herbal mixture (moxa or mugwort) is burned either like incense on the acupuncture point or on the end of the needle, a process believed to stimulate chi in a particular way. Acupuncturists also sometimes use *cupping*, during which small suction cups are placed on meridian points to stimulate them.

How long the needles are inserted also varies. Some patients require only a quick in-and-out insertion to clear problems and provide *tonification* (strengthening of health), while some other conditions might require needles to remain inserted up to an hour or more. The average visit to an acupuncturist takes about 30 minutes. The number of visits to the acupuncturist varies, with some conditions improving in one or two sessions, and others requiring a series of six or more visits over the course of weeks or months.

Costs for acupuncture vary, depending on whether the practitioner is a medical physician. Initial visits with non-MD acupuncturists can run from $50–$100, with follow-up visits usually costing less. Insurance reimbursement varies widely, depending on the company and state. Regulations tend to change frequently. Some states authorize Medicaid to cover acupuncture for certain conditions, and others have mandated that general coverage pay for acupuncture. Consumers should be aware of the provisions for acupuncture in their individual policies.

Preparation

Before you use an acupuncturist, make sure they are qualified. Health care providers, physicians and other traditional medical professionals can help to find reputable personnel within the acupuncture field. In addition, national acupuncture organizations can also be used as a referral. To be assured of the qualifications of an acupuncturist, check the person's credentials. A license is required to practice acupuncture in most states. Experience and education, especially in traditional medicine, should also be considered when selecting an acupuncturist.

Risks

Acupuncture is generally a safe procedure. If individuals are in doubt about a medical condition, more than one physician should be consulted. Individuals also should feel comfortable and confident that their acupuncturist is knowledgeable and properly trained.

The National Center for Complementary and Alternative Medicine (NCCAM), the American Medical Association (AMA), and other organizations from the United States have generally agreed that acupuncture is safe to be used when under the guidance of a trained practitioner who uses sterile needles. However, as of 2011, these U.S. organizations have declined to make statements as to the efficiency of acupuncture.

Results

The World Health Organization (WHO) recommends acupuncture as an effective treatment for over 40 medical problems, along with many mental illnesses such as nervous conditions. Acupuncture has been used in the treatment of alcoholism and **substance abuse**, which are often problems associated with mental illness.

Acupuncture, as related to the treatment of mental illness, has been researched by the medical community for many decades. For instance, as early as the 1970s, medical research has been conducted around the world concerning acupuncture and the treatment of depression. American **psychologist** John Allen, from the University of Arizona (Tucson), conducted one of these studies. Allen performed a double-blind randomized study of 34 women who were depressed as per the criteria of the ***Diagnostic and Statistical Manual of Mental Disorders*** *IV* (*DSM-IV*), which is a publication by the **American Psychiatric Association** that provides standards for the classification of mental disorders.

Dr. Allen divided the subjects into three treatment groups for eight weeks of study. The first group received acupuncture treatments specifically to treat their depression, while the second group received acupuncture for general treatment, and the third group did not receive acupuncture (control group). The group that received acupuncture specifically designed to treat depression showed marked improvement in their symptoms (43%) when compared to the other two groups (22% for the general acupuncture group and 14% for the no-treatment group). At the end of the study, only half of the participants were still classified as depressed by the *DSM-IV*.

Acupuncture has also been medically studied to help relieve symptoms due to **stress**. For instance, Drs. Shu-Ming Wang, Zeev N. Kain, and Paul F. White performed a study that was published during 2008 within the journal *Anesthesia & Analgesia*, a publication of the International Anesthesia Research Society. These American researchers from Yale University showed that auricular (ear) acupuncture helped to relive post-operative anxiety in children. An earlier study, also from Yale University researchers, showed that mothers of children about to have surgery had lower stress levels when acupuncture was performed.

Other studies have shown that acupuncture is effective at reducing symptoms associated with other mental illnesses and psychiatric disorders, such as depressive **neurosis**, **post-traumatic stress disorder**, schizophrenia, bipolar disorder, and mania, and symptoms often associated with such conditions as mood swings and **insomnia**. However, still other medical studies do not support these contentions, and further research into these applications is needed.

Research and general acceptance

Mainstream medicine has been slow to accept acupuncture. Research continues to produce conflicting results, and although more medical doctors are using the technique, the American Medical Association does not recognize it as a specialty. The reason for this position is that the mechanism of acupuncture is difficult to understand or measure scientifically, such as the invisible energy of chi in the body. Western medicine, admitting that acupuncture works in many cases, has theorized that the energy meridians are actually part of the nervous system and that acupuncture relieves pain by releasing endorphins, or natural painkillers, into the bloodstream. Despite the ambiguity in the biochemistry involved, acupuncture continues to show effectiveness in clinical tests, from reducing pain in chronic and acute illnesses to alleviating the symptoms of mental illnesses.

Medical research in acupuncture is growing. The National Center for Complementary and Alternative Medicine of the National Institutes of Health funds research in the use of acupuncture on a number of

QUESTIONS TO ASK YOUR DOCTOR

- What kind of results can I expect to feel with acupuncture?
- Can acupuncture hurt or injure me?
- What other type of treatment do you recommend for me?
- Will acupuncture interfere with my current medications?
- How long will it take to see results from my acupuncture treatment?

conditions, including pain and insomnia. When acupuncture is practiced by traditional medical professionals, its effectiveness to relieve pain is primarily believed to be due to acupuncture points being able to stimulate muscles, nerves, and connective tissue, which acts to increase the production of natural painkillers found within the body, and the increased flow of blood to these targeted locations.

Healthcare team roles

Medical acupuncture has evolved in the United States in an atmosphere that focuses on traditional Western methods, such as surgical techniques and pain management, and not as part of Chinese medicine overall. In the United States, medical practitioners sometimes incorporate acupuncture methods from China, Japan, Korea, and other countries as part of their complementary and alternative medicine (CAM) program. Generally, under such Western methods, a medical doctor (MD) or an osteopathic physician (DO) performs medical acupuncture.

Certain states permit only the practice of medical acupuncture. Practitioners complete their training as part of conventional medical school programs. Since any MD can legally perform acupuncture, the *American Academy of Medical Acupuncture* (AAMA) was chartered in 1987 to support the education and correct practice of physician-trained acupuncturists. Its members must be either MDs or DOs who have completed proper study of acupuncture techniques.

Resources

BOOKS

Filshie, Jacqueline. *Introduction to Medical Acupuncture.* Oxford, England: Churchill Livingstone, 2008.

Focks, Claudia. *Atlas of Acupuncture.* Oxford, England: Churchill Livingstone, 2008.

Landgren, Kajsa. *Ear Acupuncture: A Practical Guide.* Oxford, England: Churchill Livingstone, 2008.

Maciocia, Giovanni. *The Practice of Chinese Medicine: The Treatment of Diseases with Acupuncture and Chinese Herbs.* Oxford, England: Churchill Livingstone, 2008.

PERIODICALS

Hollifield M., et al. "Acupuncture for Post-traumatic Stress Disorder: A Randomized Controlled Pilot Trial." *Journal of Nervous and Mental Diseases* (June 2007): 504–513.

Mayhew, E., and E. Ernst. "Acupuncture for Fibromyalgia: A Systematic Review of Randomized Clinical Trials." *Rheumatology* (May 2007): 801–804.

Paterson, Charlotte. "Patients' Experiences of Western-style Acupuncture: The Influence of Acupuncture 'Dose', Self-care Strategies and Integration." *Journal of Health Services Research and Policy* (April 2007): 39–45.

Tillisch, Kirsten. "Complementary and Alternative Medicine for Gastrointestinal Disorders." *Clinical Medicine, Journal of the Royal College of Physicians* (June 2007): 224–227.

Wang, Shu-Ming, Zeev N. Kain, and Paul F. White. "Acupuncture Analgesia: II. Clinical Considerations." *Anesthesia & Analgesia* 106, no. 2 (2008): 611–621. http://www.anesthesia-analgesia.org/content/106/2/611.abstract?sid=ee00e4d9-924c-4a87-876b-e40570d7aa86 (accessed June 28, 2011).

WEBSITES

Acupuncture. Mayo Clinic. (December 11, 2009). http://www.mayoclinic.com/health/acupuncture/MY00946 (accessed June 28, 2011).

Acupuncture: An Introduction. National Center for Complimentary and Alternative Medicine. (March 22, 2011). http://nccam.nih.gov/health/acupuncture/introduction.htm#ususe (accessed June 28, 2011).

ORGANIZATIONS

American Academy of Medical Acupuncture, 1970 East Grand Avenue, El Segundo, CA, 90245, (310) 364-0193, administrator@medicalacupuncture.org, http://www.medicalacupuncture.org.

American Association of Acupuncture and Oriental Medicine, PO Box 162340, Sacramento, CA, 95816, Fax: (916) 443-4766, Toll-free: (866) 455-7999, http://www.aaaomonline.org.

National Certification Commission for Acupuncture and Oriental Medicine, 76 South Laura St., Suite 1290, Jacksonville, FL, 32202, (904) 598-1005, Fax: (904) 598-5001, http://www.nccaom.org.

Douglas Dupler
Teresa G. Odle
Laura Jean Cataldo, RN, Ed.D.
William A. Atkins, B.B., B.S., M.B.A.

Acute stress disorder

Definition

Acute **stress** disorder (ASD) is an anxiety disorder characterized by a cluster of dissociative and anxiety symptoms that occur within a month of a traumatic stressor. The diagnosis was added to the fourth edition of the ***Diagnostic and Statistical Manual of Mental Disorders*** *(DSM-IV)* in 1994 to distinguish time-limited reactions to **trauma** from the longer-lasting **post-traumatic stress disorder** (PTSD). Published by the **American Psychiatric Association**, the *DSM* contains diagnostic criteria, research findings, and treatment information for mental disorders and is the primary reference for mental health professionals in the United States. A fifth edition (*DSM-5*) is expected to publish in 2013.

Demographics

Acute responses to traumatic stressors are far more widespread in the general U.S. population than was first thought in 1980, when PTSD was introduced as a diagnostic category in the *DSM-III*. The National Comorbidity Survey, a major epidemiological study conducted between 1990 and 1992, estimated that the lifetime prevalence of trauma-related stress disorders among adult Americans was 7.8%, with women (10.4%) twice as likely as men (5%) to be diagnosed. These figures represented only a small proportion of adults who had experienced at least one traumatic event—60.7% of men and 51.2% of women. More than 10% of the men and 6% of the women reported experiencing four or more types of trauma in their lives.

As of 2011, the prevalence of ASD by itself in the general U.S. population was not known. A few studies of people exposed to traumatic events found rates of ASD between 14% and 33%. According to one study, some groups are at greater risk of developing ASD or PTSD, including people living in depressed urban areas or on Native American reservations (23%) and victims of violent crimes (58%).

The U.S. Department of Veterans Affairs has provided statistics on the rates of ASD in various traumatic situations. For instance, survivors of motor vehicle accidents experienced ASD in a range of 13% to 21%, whereas survivors of industrial accidents had a rate of about 5%, victims of violent assaults had an ASD rate of 13%, and survivors of mass shootings had a rate of approximately 33%.

Reported rates for ASD are likely still inaccurate, because the majority of victims recover within two weeks of the exposure to a traumatic event, so many of these incidences are not reported. However, the rate for ASD is most likely higher than PTSD, because if ASD takes longer than four weeks to resolve, its *DSM-IV* classification becomes PTSD.

Description

ASD, like PTSD, begins with exposure to a traumatic, horrifying, or terrifying event. Such events include combat (war), personal attack (e.g., mugging), natural disasters (e.g., earthquake, hurricane), and physical sexual assault (rape). Recent events associated with symptoms of ASD among survivors include the wars in Afghanistan and Iraq; Cyclone Nargis in Myanmar on May 1, 2008; and the Haiti earthquake on January 1, 2010. In March 2011, a strong earthquake and massive tsunami near Tohoku, Japan, caused a nuclear power plant disaster at the Fukushima Daiichi nuclear complex, about 150 miles (242 km) north of Tokyo. The sequence of disasters resulted in the death of more than 15,000 people, with 5,000 more injured. Thousands were missing, and even more were exposed to radioactivity. Hundreds of thousands of buildings and homes were destroyed or damaged in the disaster. The survivors experienced many physiological and psychological disorders, including ASD.

Unlike PTSD, ASD emerges sooner and abates more quickly; it is also marked by more dissociative symptoms, such as emotional detachment, **dissociative amnesia** (memory loss due to strong psychological stress), derealization (degraded, unreal perception of the external world), or **depersonalization** (deteriorated awareness of self). If left untreated, ASD is likely to progress to PTSD. Because ASD and PTSD share many symptoms, some researchers and clinicians question the validity of maintaining separate diagnostic categories. Others explain the conditions as two phases of an extended reaction to traumatic stress.

Causes and symptoms

Causes

The immediate cause of ASD is exposure to trauma—experiencing an extreme stressor involving a threat to life or the prospect of serious injury, witnessing an event that involves the death or serious injury of another person, or learning of the violent death or serious injury of a family member or close friend. The trauma's impact is determined by its cause, scope, and extent. Natural disasters (such as floods, earthquakes, or hurricanes) or accidents (airplane crashes, workplace explosions) are considered less traumatic than intentional human acts (such as **abuse** or murder) or terrorism. Terrorist-inflicted trauma appears to produce particularly high rates of ASD and PTSD in survivors and bystanders. The terrorist attacks on the United States on September 11, 2001, with the killing and injuring of thousands of people and the destruction of the Twin Towers of the World Trade Complex in New York City and the damage to the Pentagon outside of Washington, DC, is a prime example of terrorist-inflicted trauma that develops in people who survive and witness such events.

Although most people define trauma in terms of events such as war, terrorist attacks, and other events that result in vast loss of life, the leading cause of stress-related mental disorders in the United States is motor vehicle accidents. Most Americans are involved in a traffic accident at some point in their lives, and 25% of the population are involved in accidents resulting in serious injuries. Various studies in the 2000s and 2010s found that rates of ASD from traffic/motor vehicle accidents ranged from 13% to 21%, as provided by the Department of Veterans Affairs.

Several factors influence a person's risk of developing ASD after trauma:

- Age—Older adults are less likely to develop ASD, possibly because they have had more experience coping with painful or stressful events.
- Previous exposure—People who were abused or experienced trauma as children are more likely to develop ASD (or PTSD) as adults, because these may produce long-lasting biochemical changes in the central nervous system.
- Biological vulnerability—Twin studies indicate that certain abnormalities in brain hormone levels and brain structure are inherited, and that these increase a person's susceptibility to ASD following exposure to trauma.
- Support networks—People who have a network of close friends and relatives are less likely to develop ASD.
- Perception and interpretation—People who feel inappropriate responsibility for the trauma, regard the event as punishment for personal wrongdoing, or have generally negative or pessimistic worldviews are more likely to develop ASD than those who do not personalize the trauma or are able to maintain a balanced view of life.

Symptoms

Symptoms of ASD include:

- dissociative symptoms, including psychic numbing, feeling dazed or less aware of surroundings, derealization, depersonalization, and dissociative amnesia
- trauma reexperienced in the form of recurrent dreams, images, thoughts, illusions, or flashbacks
- avoidance of people, places, objects, conversations, and other stimuli reminiscent of the trauma (for example, refusal to drive after a traffic accident)
- hyperarousal or anxiety, including sleep problems, irritability, inability to concentrate, an intense startle response, hypervigilance, and physical restlessness (pacing the floor, fidgeting)
- significantly impaired social functions and/or the inability to do necessary tasks, including seeking help
- symptoms lasting at least two days and up to a maximum of four weeks and occurring within four weeks of the traumatic event

ASD symptoms are not caused by a substance, either by taking medication or abusing a drug, nor are they caused by a physiological condition. They do not meet the criteria of a **brief psychotic disorder** and do not represent the worsening of a mental disorder that the person had before the traumatic event.

People with ASD may show symptoms of **depression**, including difficulty enjoying activities that they previously found pleasurable, difficulty concentrating, and experiencing survivor's guilt for having survived an accident or escaped serious injury when others did not. The *DSM-IV-TR* notes that people diagnosed with ASD "often perceive themselves to have greater responsibility for the consequences of the trauma than is warranted" and may feel that they will not live out their normal life span. Many symptoms of ASD are also found in patients with PTSD.

Diagnosis

ASD symptoms typically develop within a month after the traumatic event; however, why some trauma survivors develop symptoms more rapidly than others remains unknown. Delayed symptoms are often triggered by a situation that resembles the original trauma.

ASD is usually diagnosed by matching the patient's symptoms to the *DSM* criteria. The symptoms must cause the patient great distress and must be severe enough to impair the patient's daily functioning. General questionnaires are in widespread use for diagnosing ASD, as well as clinical guidelines established in the United States, the United Kingdom, and, most recently, Australia. The Australian guidelines consist of a 19-point acute stress disorder scale, which appears to be effective in diagnosing ASD but frequently makes false-positive predictions of PTSD. The authors of the scale recommend that its use should be followed by a careful clinical evaluation.

Another measure to assess ASD is the acute stress disorder interview (ASDI), which has been validated against criteria provided by the *DSM-IV-TR*. It was validated by comparing its results with diagnoses made by clinicians experienced in differentiating ASM from PTSD. In addition, the acute stress disorder scale (ASDS) has been found to correlate with results from the ASDI, along with providing reliability, validity, and internal consistency.

Treatment

Therapy for ASM requires the use of several treatment modalities, as the disorder affects interpersonal relationships and occupational functioning as well as a patient's emotional and physical well-being. Usually, a therapist asks the patient to relate what happened during the incident and to describe the emotions felt at that time and experienced thereafter. Drugs may be prescribed but are usually limited to those necessary for treating specific symptoms.

KEY TERMS

Adjustment disorder—A disorder defined by the development of significant emotional or behavioral symptoms in response to a stressful event or series of events. Symptoms may include depressed mood, anxiety, and impairment of social and occupational functioning.

Depersonalization—A dissociative symptom in which individuals feel that their body is unreal, changing, or dissolving.

Derealization—A dissociative symptom in which the external environment is perceived as unreal or dreamlike.

Dissociation—A reaction to trauma in which the mind splits off certain aspects of the traumatic event from conscious awareness. It can affect the patient's memory, sense of reality, and sense of identity.

Dissociative amnesia—A dissociative disorder characterized by loss of memory for a period or periods of time, which may occur as a result of a traumatic event.

Exposure therapy—A form of cognitive-behavioral therapy in which patients suffering from phobias are exposed to their feared objects or situations while accompanied by the therapist. The length of exposure is gradually increased until the association between the feared situation and the patient's experienced panic symptoms is no longer present.

Flashback—The reemergence of a traumatic memory as a vivid recollection of sounds, images, and sensations associated with the trauma. The person having such a memory typically feels as if he or she is reliving the event.

Hyperarousal—A symptom of traumatic stress characterized by abnormally intense reactions to stimuli. A heightened startle response is one sign of hyperarousal.

Hypervigilance—A state of abnormally intense wariness or watchfulness that is found in survivors of trauma or long-term abuse. Hypervigilance is sometimes described as the feeling of being on red alert all the time.

Personalization—The tendency to refer large-scale events or general patterns of events to the self in inappropriate ways. For example, a person who regards the loss of a loved one in an accident as punishment for having quarreled with that person before the accident is said to be personalizing the event. This tendency increases a person's risk of developing ASD or PTSD after a traumatic event.

Psychic numbing—An inability to respond emotionally with normal intensity to people or situations; this numbing affects positive as well as negative emotions.

Supportive—An approach in psychotherapy that seeks to encourage or emotionally support the patient, as distinct from insight-oriented or educational approaches to treatment.

Survivor's guilt—A psychological reaction in trauma survivors that takes the form of guilt feelings for having survived or escaped a trauma without serious injury when others did not.

Therapeutic writing—A treatment technique in which patients are asked to write an account of the traumatic event and their emotional responses to it.

Medications

Specific drugs prescribed include **clonidine** (Catapres, Kapvay, Nexiclon), for hyperarousal; **propranolol** (Inderal), **clonazepam** (Ceberclon, Klonopin, Valpax), or **alprazolam** (Niravam, Xanax), for anxiety and panic reactions; **fluoxetine** (Prozac, Rapiflux, Sarafem, Selfemra), for avoidance symptoms; and **trazodone** (Desyrel, Oleptro, Trazon, Trialodine) or topiramate (Topamax, Topiragen), for **insomnia** and nightmares. **Antidepressants** may be prescribed if ASD progresses to PTSD. These medications may include **selective serotonin reuptake inhibitors (SSRIs)**, **monoamine oxidase inhibitors (MAOIs)**, or tricyclic antidepressants.

Psychotherapy

Cognitive-behavioral therapy, exposure therapy, therapeutic writing (**journal therapy**), and supportive therapy have been found effective in treating ASD. One variant of cognitive behavioral therapy, psychoeducational therapy, appears to be three to four times as effective as supportive therapy in preventing ASD from progressing to PTSD. This treatment combines cognitive restructuring of the traumatic event with exposure to disturbing images and techniques for anxiety management. In addition, it can help patients identify and reinforce positive aspects of their experience. For example, some people discover new strengths or talents in times of crisis or discover new spiritual resources.

Group and family therapies also help reinforce effective strategies for coping with the trauma and may reduce the risk of social isolation as a reaction to the trauma. They provide opportunities for patients to describe what happened and how they responded. As patients place their experience into a coherent narrative, they integrate the trauma into their lives as a whole, and, by telling their story, they receive support from their listeners.

Critical incident **stress management** (CISM) is a comprehensive crisis-intervention system in which a team of specially trained practitioners comes to the site of a traumatic event and provides several different forms of assistance. This assistance includes one-on-one crisis support; crisis management briefing, which is a 45–75-minute **intervention** for groups affected by the traumatic event; and critical incident stress debriefing, which is a structured group discussion of the event. CISM appears to be particularly helpful in preventing burnout and ASD among emergency service personnel, rescue personnel, police, and other caregivers who are involved in treating survivors of a traumatic event.

Alternative and complementary treatments

Many mainstream practitioners recommend holistic or naturopathic approaches to recovery from ASD, including good **nutrition** with appropriate dietary supplements and regular **exercise**. **Yoga** and some forms of body work or massage therapy are helpful in treating the muscle soreness and stiffness that is often a side effect of anxiety and insomnia related to ASD. Hydrotherapy is often helpful for post-traumatic muscular aches and cramps. A skilled naturopath may also recommend peppermint or other herbal preparations to calm the patient's digestive tract. In addition, prayer, **meditation**, or counseling with a spiritual advisor have been found to be helpful in treating patients with ASD whose belief systems have been affected by the traumatic event.

ASD in children

Very little is known about the prevalence of ASD or PTSD in children, and even less is known about the effectiveness of medications and **psychotherapy** in this age group. There were as of 2011 no standardized screens or diagnostic interviews in widespread use for assessing either ASD or PTSD in children, although a Child Post-traumatic Stress Reaction Index was published in 1992. One preliminary study recommended the cautious use of low doses of **imipramine** for treating children with ASD but noted that research in this area had barely begun.

Prognosis

Untreated ASD is highly likely to progress to PTSD. One team of Australian researchers found that 80% of persons diagnosed with ASD met criteria for PTSD six months later, and 75% met criteria for PTSD two years after the traumatic event.

QUESTIONS TO ASK YOUR DOCTOR

- Do I have acute stress disorder?
- What can I do to get better?
- Do I need medication?
- Do I need counseling?
- Do you think my ASD will progress into PTSD?

Clinicians in Norway compiled a list of four "early response" variables that appear to be effective predictors of ASD progressing to PTSD:

- the degree of the patient's sleep disturbance
- a strong startle reaction
- the degree of the patient's social withdrawal
- fear or phobia related to the site of the traumatic event

In addition to developing PTSD, people diagnosed with ASD are at increased risk of developing a **major depressive disorder**, particularly if their emotional responses to the trauma are marked by intense despair or hopelessness. Other possible developments are neglect of personal needs for health or safety and impulsive or needlessly risky behavior.

Prevention

Some forms of trauma, such as natural disasters and accidents, cannot be prevented. Traumas caused by human action require major social changes to reduce their frequency and severity, but given the increasing prevalence of trauma-related stress disorders around the world, these long-term changes are worth the effort. In the short run, educating people—particularly those in the helping professions—about the signs of critical incident stress may prevent some cases of exposure to trauma from developing into ASD and progressing to PTSD.

Resources

BOOKS

American Psychiatric Association. *Diagnostic and Statistical Manual of Mental Disorders,* 4th edition, text rev. Washington, DC: American Psychiatric Association, 2000.

Beers, Mark H., ed. *The Merck Manual of Diagnosis and Therapy*. Rahway, NJ: Merck, 2006.

Friedman, Matthew. *Post-traumatic and Acute Stress Disorders: The Latest Assessment and Treatment Strategies.* Kansas City, MO: Compact Clinicals, 2006.

Mendelsohn, Michaela, et al. *The Trauma Recovery Group: A Guide for Practitioners*. New York: Guilford Press, 2011.

Van der Kolk, Bessel A., Alexander C. McFarlane, and Lars Veisaeth, eds. *Traumatic Stress: The Effects of Overwhelming Experience on Mind, Body, and Society*. New York: Guilford Press, 2007.

WEBSITES

Australian Centre for Posttraumatic Mental Health. "Australian Guidelines for the Treatment of Adults with Acute Australian Stress Disorder and Posttraumatic Stress Disorder." September 10, 2007. http://www.nhmrc.gov.au/_files_nhmrc/file/publications/synopses/mh13.pdf (accessed September 7, 2011).

Gibson, Laura E. "Acute Stress Disorder." Department of Veteran Affairs. Last modified June 16, 2010. http://www.ptsd.va.gov/professional/pages/acute-stress-disorder.asp (accessed September 7, 2011).

Phillips, Katharine E. *Report of the DSM-V Anxiety, Obsessive-Compulsive Spectrum, Posttraumatic, and Dissociative Disorders Work Group*. American Psychiatric Association. April 2009. http://www.psych.org/MainMenu/Research/DSMIV/DSMV/DSMRevisionActivities/DSM-V-Work-Group-Reports/Anxiety-Obsessive-Compulsive-Spectrum-Posttraumatic-and-Dissociative-Disorders-Work-Group-Report.aspx (accessed September 7, 2011).

ORGANIZATIONS

American Academy of Experts in Traumatic Stress, 203 Deer Rd., Ronkonkoma, NY, 11779, (631) 543-2217, Fax: (631) 543-6977, info@aaets.org, http://www.aaets.org.

Anxiety Disorders Association of America, 8730 Georgia Ave., Silver Spring, MD, 20910, (240) 485-1001, http://www.adaa.org.

International Society for Traumatic Stress Studies, 111 Deer Lake Rd., Ste. 100, Deerfield, IL, 60015, (847) 480-9028, Fax: (847) 480-9282, http://www.istss.org.

National Institute of Mental Health, 6001 Executive Blvd., Rm. 8184, MSC 9663, Bethesda, MD, 20892-9663, (301) 433-4513; TTY: (301) 443-8431, (866) 615-6464; TTY: (866) 415-8051, Fax: (301) 443-4279, nimhinfo@nih.gov, http://www.nimh.nih.gov.

Rebecca J. Frey, PhD
William A. Atkins, BB, BS, MBA

Adapin *see* **Doxepin**

Addiction

Definition

Addiction is the compulsive need to use a habit-forming substance or the irresistible urge to engage in an activity or behavior, often despite harmful consequences. Persistent use leads to dependence and ultimately tolerance, or the need to increase the amount or duration of the substance or activity in order to achieve the same effect. Discontinuation of the addiction can lead to withdrawal, the unpleasant symptoms that arise when the addicted person is prevented from using the chosen substance or engaging in the behavior.

Demographics

Addiction to substances and activities is widespread in the United States, Canada, and internationally. **Substance abuse** and addiction cost Americans about $500 billion annually in healthcare costs, lost earnings, accidents, and crime. Every year, Americans experience more than 40 million debilitating illnesses or injuries as a result of tobacco, alcohol, and other addictive drug use. Likewise, about one in ten Canadians aged 15 or older are considered addicted to alcohol or drugs. Men are more than twice as likely as women to be addicted to a substance. Gender differences are much less pronounced among adolescents, however; teenage girls are almost as likely as boys to abuse a substance. Approximately 20% of people with addictions have other mental disorders, as well.

Nicotine dependence is the most common type of addiction. It is estimated that worldwide tobacco use results in at least five million deaths annually. Cigarette smoking is the leading preventable cause of death in the United States, accounting for about one out of every five deaths, with about 40,000 additional annual deaths caused by exposure to secondhand smoke. According to the Substance Abuse and Mental Health Services Administration's *National Survey on Drug Use and Health* (NSDUH), about 27.4% of Americans aged 12 or over were considered current users of tobacco products in 2010. About 8.3% of tobacco users were between the ages of 12 and 17, with the 18–25 demographic constituting the largest usage group (40.8% of users).

Alcoholism is the most common addiction to a psychoactive substance. Alcohol addiction affects both sexes and all races and nationalities. According to the 2010 *NSDUH*, 131.3 million Americans (51.8% of the population) reported having at least one alcoholic drink in the past 30 days. In addition, 58.6 million people (23.1%) reported having five or more drinks on the same occasion (**binge drinking**), and 16.9 million (6.7%) reported having five or more drinks on at least five occasions in the past 30 days (heavy **alcohol use**). Alcohol addiction rates are highest among young adults aged 18–29 and lowest among those 65 and older.

According to the 2010 *NSDUH*, 22.6 million Americans (8.9% of the population) age 12 and older reported using illicit drugs in the preceding month. The

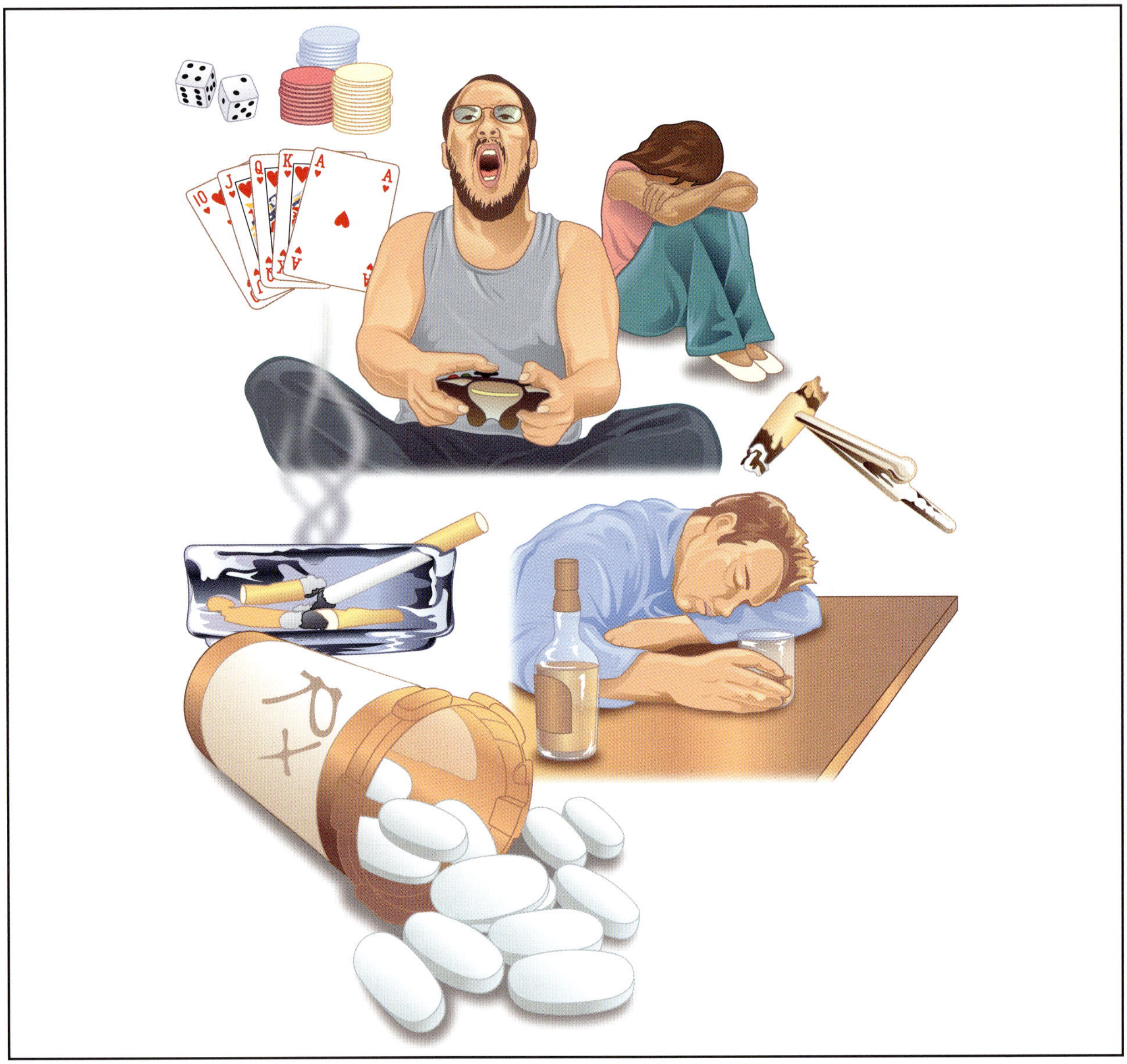

People can become addicted to a wide range of substances and activities. Represented in this illustration are gambling, video game, alcohol, and drug addictions. *(Illustration by Electronic Illustrators Group. © 2012 Cengage Learning.)*

most commonly abused drug was marijuana, followed by abuse of psychotherapeutic drugs (prescription pain relievers, **sedatives**, or stimulants used for nonmedical reasons).

Addictions most often first appear in adolescence. According to the survey, 10.1% of students ages 12–17 reported having used an illicit drug in the previous year. The use of illegal drugs among American teenagers declined between 2001 and 2008, thought it has risen slightly over the past few years. Cigarette smoking and alcohol use among American youth also declined significantly over the first decade of the twenty-first century.

Statistics on addictive activities (e.g., gambling, **sexual addiction**) are more difficult to obtain because these behaviors are less clearly defined than substance addiction. However, the National Council on Problem Gambling reported in 2010 that 85% of American adults have gambled at least once in their lifetimes, with 60% of the population gambling in any given year. Of these, about 1% are addicted to gambling, while another 2%–3% are considered problem gamblers. The rate of gambling addiction is related to access, with an estimated 6% of the population of Nevada being either problem or addicted gamblers. With an increase in legal gambling in the United States (only Utah and Hawaii do not have some form of legal gambling) and easy access to online gambling, the rate of gambling among teen and college-aged gamblers has increased by 600%.

Because there is no professional agreement on the definition of sexual addiction, the number of people considered to be addicted to sex is unknown. What is known is that sexual addiction is much more common in men than women. Persons addicted to sex are not necessarily sex offenders, nor are sex offenders necessarily sex addicts. Often, people addicted to sex have other mental health and impulse-control problems that contribute to their addictive behaviors.

Internet addiction is a new and growing phenomenon. The number of people addicted to the Internet is hard to pin down. One 2008 study estimated the rate at 8.2% of American Internet users. Other studies have estimated rates of 10% and 11% of Internet users in China and South Korea, respectively.

Description

Addiction most commonly refers to the compulsive use or abuse of or physical or psychological dependence on addictive substances, including:

- tobacco
- alcohol
- cocaine, including crack cocaine
- amphetamines, including methamphetamine or "crank," an extremely addictive substance
- heroin
- prescription medications

Prescription painkillers, such as the opiates Vicodin and OxyContin, have emerged as drugs of special concern because of their widespread use by high-school students.

Outside of substance use, the term "addiction" has been used to describe a wide and complex range of behaviors. These so-called process addictions are compulsive behaviors involving activities such as:

- gambling
- eating
- working
- exercising
- shopping or otherwise spending money
- sex
- Internet use

Most addictions are associated with mood modification. Initially, they make the addicted person feel better. Persons with addictions often describe a release of tension or feelings of euphoria when using the substance or engaging in the activity. Most addictions are progressive syndromes; without treatment, their severity increases over time. Furthermore, many addicts are addicted to more than one substance or activity. Addictions are characterized by frequent relapses—a return to using the abused substance or activity following a period of abstinence.

Substances can be both physically and psychologically addictive. Some substances are more addictive than others, either because they produce a rapid and intense change in mood or because they produce painful withdrawal symptoms when stopped suddenly. Drugs that are smoked or injected, giving an immediate but short-lived "high," tend to be more addictive than substances that are ingested.

The American Psychiatric Association's ***Diagnostic and Statistical Manual of Mental Disorders*** classifies substance abuse and dependence as psychological disorders that are considered major clinical syndromes (called "Axis I"). Over time, repeated drug use changes **brain** structure and function in fundamental

KEY TERMS

Addictive personality—The concept that addiction is the result of pre-existing character defects.

Dopamine—A neurotransmitter in the brain.

Methamphetamine (meth, methadrine, "speed")—A highly addictive medication that is used to treat attention deficit hyperactivity disorder and obesity but is widely abused as a stimulant.

Neurotransmitter—One of a group of chemicals secreted by a nerve cell (neuron) to carry a chemical message to another nerve cell, often as a way of transmitting a nerve impulse. Examples of neurotransmitters include acetylcholine, dopamine, serotonin, and norepinephrine.

Process addiction—Addiction to certain mood-altering behaviors, such as eating, gambling, sexual activity, overwork, and shopping.

Relapse—A recurrence of symptoms after a period of improvement or recovery.

Tolerance—The requirement for higher doses of a substance or more frequent engagement in an activity to achieve the same effect.

Withdrawal—The unpleasant, sometimes life-threatening physiological changes that occur due to the discontinuation of some drugs after prolonged regular use.

and long-lasting ways. Evidence suggests that these long-lasting brain changes are responsible for the distortions in cognitive and emotional functioning that characterize persons with addictions, particularly the **compulsion** to use drugs. This explains why many drug users cannot stop using by force of will alone.

Risk factors

Risk factors for addiction include:

- inherited factors
- adolescence
- addictive behavior in the home or among family members or peers
- early substance use
- early aggressive behavior
- academic failure
- lack of parental supervision
- poor social skills
- other mental disorders or illnesses
- substance abuse
- substance availability
- poverty

Causes and symptoms

For much of the twentieth century, addiction was viewed as a moral failing; today, addiction is widely viewed as a disease. The disease model of alcohol and drug addiction was first introduced in the late 1940s by E. M. Jellinek and was adopted by the American Medical Association in 1956. According to the disease model, the compulsion to use alcohol and/or drugs is genetically and physiologically based and, although the disease can be treated, it is progressive, chronic, and fatal if unchecked. However, some experts argue that addiction is better understood as a learned behavior, and that the negative behavior can be unlearned and replaced by learning new positive behaviors. The causes of addiction remain the subject of ongoing research and debate.

Causes

The initial positive consequences of substance use or a potentially addictive activity can "hook" a susceptible person and turn into an addiction. Addiction comes about through an array of changes in the brain and the strengthening of new memory connections. The anterior cingulate cortex in the frontal lobe of the brain is the area responsible for the long-term craving that triggers **relapse**.

Many experts believe that addictive substances and activities affect **neurotransmitters** in the brain. The primary pathway involved in the development and persistence of addiction is the brain reward or mesolimbic pathway, which operates via a neurotransmitter called **dopamine**. Dopamine pathways may interact with those of other neurotransmitters, including opioid pathways. These neuronal pathways have been identified as underlying both substance and process addictions.

Whatever the brain chemistry involved in addiction, it usually results from the interaction of several factors:

- Social learning. This may be the most important single factor in addiction and includes patterns of substance use and activities in the addict's family or subculture, peer pressure, and advertising or media influence.
- Availability. There are marked increases in addiction rates when tobacco, alcohol, or drugs are inexpensive or readily available.
- Individual development. Before the 1980s, addiction was blamed on an "addictive personality," which was described as escapist, impulsive, dependent, devious, manipulative, and self-centered. Although individual development may play a role in addiction, many doctors now believe that these character traits develop as a result of the addiction, rather causing the addiction.
- Genetic factors. It is estimated that genetic factors account for 40%–60% of an individual's vulnerability to addiction. Twin studies have shown that addiction has a strong inherited component. Some forms of addiction seem to run in families, and some people appear to be more vulnerable to addiction because of their body chemistry.

Symptoms

The continued use of an addictive substance or engagement in an addictive activity causes the body to adjust and develop tolerance. Increasing amounts of the substance or more frequent engagement in the activity are needed to produce the same effect. Some drug users can tolerate an amount of a substance that would be lethal in someone without a tolerance, though continued dosage increase will eventually reach fatal levels. If the drug is ceased, the person may experience a withdrawal syndrome. Symptoms of withdrawal vary but may include tremor, **insomnia**, agitation, aggression, vomiting, nightmares, and sweating. Long-term substance use may result in more serious symptoms; severe symptoms of withdrawal from alcohol and some drugs may include **seizures**, hallucinatory sensations, organ damage, and **dementia**. Even for addictions that do not involve substance use, persons may experience some symptoms of withdrawal when stopping the behavior or activity.

The inability to hold a steady job and disruptions of social and familial relationships are common behavioral symptoms of all types of addiction. Other behavioral symptoms include:

- participation in activity despite danger to self or others (e.g., driving under the influence)
- continuation of activity even though it has a negative effect on personal and social life and/or physical health
- significant time spent around the substance or activity, often in place of time spent previously on hobbies or events

Danger signs that may indicate the probable onset of addiction to alcohol or drugs include:

- a frequent desire to drink or use
- increasing consumption
- memory lapses (blackouts)
- morning drinking/drug use
- hiding use from family and coworkers
- using in secret

Alcoholic psychoses are symptoms of late-stage alcohol addiction and include:

- alcohol withdrawal delirium (delirium tremens)
- hallucinations
- Korsakoff's psychosis, an irreversible brain disorder involving severe memory loss

Diagnosis

Addictions usually are diagnosed by their symptoms and by lifestyle factors, such as when the addiction interferes with a person's life, personal relationships, work, and/or health. A physician, **psychologist**, or social worker usually makes a **diagnosis** of addiction based on the following criteria:

- a pattern of frequent and compulsive substance use or engagement in an activity
- preoccupation with acquiring and using an abused substance
- tolerance or escalation of the substance use or activity
- loss of willpower
- harmful consequences
- unmanageable lifestyle
- withdrawal symptoms

Examination

A physical examination may aid in diagnosis by probing for underlying conditions, such as **depression**, emotional upset, anxiety, or **stress**. A physician may also look for signs of malnutrition or other medical problems resulting from substance abuse.

Tests

Blood and urine tests may be ordered to check for substance use or for liver or other organ damage resulting from substance abuse.

Procedures

Imaging tests may be ordered to check for organ damage resulting from substance abuse.

Treatment

Addictions are notoriously difficult to treat. Treatment often requires a combination of medical, psychological, and social approaches.

Traditional

Although addiction treatment may be provided by practicing clinicians such as psychiatrists, psychologists, and **social workers**, it is more often provided by specialized addiction treatment programs and clinics. These programs usually rely upon confrontational tactics and re-education, often employing former or recovering addicts to treat newly admitted addicts. Residential settings can be effective in helping addicted individuals to stay away from the many cues, including people and places, that form the setting for their addiction. Substance addicts may need hospital treatment to manage withdrawal symptoms.

Individual or group **psychotherapy** is often helpful for treating addictions after the substance use or addictive activity has ceased. Many of the negative behaviors and personality problems associated with addictions disappear when the substance use or activity ceases. **Family therapy** can be helpful for addressing and changing "enabling behaviors" by family members who help maintain the addiction by providing money, food, shelter, and/or emotional support.

The effectiveness of addiction treatment based on behavioral and other psychotherapeutic methods is well-documented. Specific therapies to treat addiction include:

- cognitive-behavioral approaches, which aim to prevent relapse by helping addicts recognize, avoid, and cope with situations that encourage their addictions
- motivation-enhancing strategies, which utilize positive reinforcement and incentives
- motivational interviewing, which uses strategies that promote behavior changes
- solution-oriented and other brief therapy techniques
- harm-reduction approaches

Drugs

Research continues into pharmacological treatments for easing withdrawal and treating various addictions. Some promising drugs boost the levels of neurotransmitters in the brain. Medications that are used to treat addiction include:

- nicotine-replacement therapies, including gum, patches, and inhalers
- bupropion (Zyban), an antidepressant, for tobacco addiction
- varenicline, which blocks the pleasant effects of nicotine on the brain
- disulfiram (Antabuse) and acamprosate (Campral) for treating alcoholism
- naltrexone (Depade, ReVia) for preventing relapse in alcohol and opioid addicts
- methadone, which blocks the euphoric effect of opiates
- buprenorphine (Subutex) or buprenorphine and naloxone (Suboxone) to prevent withdrawal symptoms and to treat addiction to opioids, including heroin and narcotic painkillers
- sedatives for reducing anxiety and withdrawal symptoms
- antidepressants for treating underlying problems in addicts who have been "self-medicating"

Alternative

During the past several decades, alternatives to the complete abstinence model have arisen. Controlled-use programs allow addicted individuals to reduce their use without committing to complete abstinence. This alternative is highly controversial, and the prevailing belief is that recovery is only possible by committing to complete lifelong abstinence from all substance use.

Home remedies

Many people turn to **self-help groups** such as Alcoholics Anonymous (AA) and Narcotics Anonymous (NA) to treat their addictions. The approach of one addict helping another to stay "clean," with or without additional professional help, is widely accepted in the United States and around the world.

The most frequently recommended social outpatient treatment is the 12-step program. The number of visits to 12-step self-help groups exceeds the number of visits to all mental health professionals combined. There are 12-step groups for all major substance and process addictions.

The 12 steps consist of:

- admitting powerlessness over the addiction
- believing that a power greater than oneself can restore sanity
- making a decision to turn your will and your life over to the care of your higher power
- making a searching and fearless moral inventory of yourself
- admitting to your higher power, yourself, and another human being the exact nature of your wrongs
- becoming willing to have your higher power remove all of these defects from your character
- humbly asking your higher power to remove your shortcomings
- making a list of all persons harmed by your wrongs, and becoming willing to make amends to them all
- making direct amends to such people, whenever possible, except when to do so would injure them or others
- continuing to take personal inventory, and promptly admitting any future wrongdoings
- seeking to improve contact with the higher power of your understanding through meditation and prayer
- carrying the message of spiritual awakening to others, and practicing these principles in all of your affairs

Prognosis

The prognosis for recovery from any addiction depends on the substance or process, the individual's circumstances, and the underlying personality structure. Patterns of relapse tend to be very similar regardless of the specific addiction. Two-thirds of all relapses occur within the first 90 days following treatment. Substance abusers often make repeated attempts to quit before they are successful. Physical addictions alter a person's brain chemistry in ways that make it difficult to be exposed to the addictive substance again without relapsing, and cravings may persist for years. Between 40% and 60% of drug addicts relapse following treatment. Users of more than one drug have the worst prognosis for recovery.

Substance abuse can damage organs, including the brain and liver, and can lead to serious and even fatal illness, as well as mental disorders such as dementia. Drug addiction puts the addict at risk for:

- cardiovascular disease
- stroke
- cancer
- HIV/AIDS
- hepatitis B and C

QUESTIONS TO ASK YOUR DOCTOR

- Am I addicted to this substance/activity?
- What symptoms are associated with withdrawal?
- What are the risks of continued use and/or withdrawal?
- What are my treatment options?
- Am I likely to relapse?
- What role can my family play in my treatment?

- lung disease
- obesity
- other mental disorders

Prevention

Preventive approaches are most effective when targeted at young teenagers between the ages of 11 and 13. It is during these years that most young people are likely to first experiment with drugs and alcohol. Hence, reducing experimentation during this critical period holds promise for reducing the number of adults with addictions. Effective prevention programs focus on the concerns of young people with regard to the effects of tobacco, alcohol, and drugs. Training older adolescents to help younger adolescents resist peer pressure has shown considerable effectiveness in preventing experimentation.

Preventative measures against addiction include:

- fostering self-control and positive relationships
- promoting parental monitoring and support
- promoting anti-addiction policies
- educational programs for the public
- building strong communities

The most effective form of prevention appears to be a stable family that models responsible attitudes toward mood-altering substances and behaviors.

Resources

BOOKS

American Psychiatric Association. *Diagnostic and Statistical Manual of Mental Disorders (DSM-IV-TR)*, 4th ed., text rev. Washington, DC: American Psychiatric Association, 2000.

Califano, Joseph A., Jr. *High Society: How Substance Abuse Ravages America and What to Do About It*. New York: Public Affairs Press, 2007.

DiClemente, Carlo C. *Addiction and Change: How Addictions Develop and Addicted People Recover*. New York: Guilford Press, 2006.

Erickson, Carlton K. *The Science of Addiction: From Neurobiology to Treatment*. New York: W.W. Norton, 2007.

Hoffman, John, and Susan Froemke. *Addiction: Why Can't They Just Stop?* Emmaus, PA: Rodale Books, 2007.

PERIODICALS

Grant, Jon E., Judson A. Brewer, and Marc N. Potenza. "The Neurobiology of Substance and Behavioral Addictions." *CNS Spectrums* 11 (2006): 924–930.

Johnson, Brian, et al. "Reducing the Risk of Addiction to Prescribed Medications." *Psychiatric Times* (April 15, 2007): 35.

Kushlick, Danny. "Stopping the Conveyor Belt to Addiction: Addressing the Underlying Issues of Addiction Will Help Us to Tackle It." *New Statesman* (May 21, 2007): S4–S5.

Lobo, Daniela S. S., and James L. Kennedy. "The Genetics of Gambling and Behavioral Addictions." *CNS Spectrums* 11 (2006): 931–939.

WEBSITES

National Institute on Drug Abuse. "Drugs, Brains, and Behavior—The Science of Addiction." U.S. National Institutes of Health. http://www.nida.nih.gov/scienceofaddiction (accessed October 11, 2011).

ORGANIZATIONS

Al-Anon/Alateen, 1600 Corporate Landing Parkway, Virginia Beach, VA, 23454-5617, (757) 563-1600, Fax: (757) 563-1655, wso@al-anon.org, http://www.al-anon.alateen.org.

Alcoholics Anonymous, PO Box 459, New York, NY, 10163, (212) 870-3400, http://www.aa.org.

American Academy of Child and Adolescent Psychiatry, 3615 Wisconsin Avenue NW, Washington, DC, 20016-3007, (202) 966-7300, Fax: (202) 966-2891, http://www.aacap.org.

American Psychiatric Association, 1000 Wilson Boulevard, Suite 1825, Arlington, VA, 22209-3901, (703) 907-7300, (888) 35-PSYCH (357-7924), apa@psych.org, http://www.psych.org.

Centre for Addiction and Mental Health, 33 Russell St., Toronto, Ontario, Canada, M5S 2S1, (416) 535-8501, (800) 463-6273, http://www.camh.net.

National Council on Alcoholism and Drug Dependence, Inc., 244 East 58th Street, 4th Fl., New York, NY, 10022, (212) 269-7797, (800) NCA-CALL (622-2255), Fax: (212) 269-7510, national@mcadd.org, http://www.ncadd.org.

National Institute on Alcohol Abuse and Alcoholism (NIAAA), 5635 Fishers Lane, MSC 9304, Bethesda, MD, 20892-9304, (301) 443-3860, http://www.niaaa.nih.gov.

National Institute on Drug Abuse (NIDA), 6001 Executive Boulevard, Room 5213, Bethesda, MD, 20892-9561, (301) 443-1124, information@nida.nih.gov, http://www.drugabuse.gov/NIDAHome.html.

Barbara S. Sternberg, PhD
Emily Jane Willingham, PhD
Tish Davidson, AM

ADHD *see* **Attention deficit hyperactivity disorder**

Adjustment disorders

Definition

Adjustment disorders (ADs) are a group of disorders in which a person's psychological response to a stressor elicits symptoms that warrant clinical attention. This uniting feature of the adjustment disorders can manifest as emotional distress that exceeds what is an expected norm or as notable impairment of the person's functioning in the world, whether socially, academically, and/or occupationally.

Adjustment disorders are considered subthreshold mental disorders, which means that they are less well defined and share some of their features with other diagnostic categories. This relative vagueness of definition allows for the classification of psychiatric conditions that are clinically significant but do not meet the full criteria of major syndromes. Another way of explaining adjustment disorders is that they are located on a continuum between normal **stress** reactions and specific psychiatric disorders.

Demographics

Even though adjustment disorders are commonly diagnosed, there have been few large-scale epidemiological studies of adjustment disorders. Epidemiological studies seek to understand the source and development of disease. However, adjustment disorder appears to be common in the U.S. population; it has been estimated that about 22% of adults seeking outpatient psychological treatment have one of the subtypes of this disorder. As many as 70% of children in psychiatric inpatient settings may be diagnosed with an adjustment disorder. However, this statistic may be exaggerated; in a questionnaire sent to child psychiatrists in the early 1990s, 55% of the contacted psychiatrists admitted giving children the **diagnosis** of an adjustment disorder to avoid the **stigma** associated with other disorders.

In the early 2010s, there were no studies being conducted on the differences in the frequency of adjustment disorder in different racial or ethnic groups. However, some potential exists for bias in diagnosis, particularly when the diagnostic criteria concern abnormal responses to stressors. The ***Diagnostic and Statistical Manual of Mental Disorders***, fourth edition, text revision, also known as the *DSM-IV-TR*, specifies that clinicians must take a patient's cultural background into account when evaluating his or her responses to stressors. There is some evidence that patients with average to higher-than-average incomes are more often diagnosed with an AD than patients who lack socioeconomic stability or security.

Description

Typically, a person experiences a stressful event as one that changes his or her world in some fundamental way. An adjustment disorder indicates the person's significant difficulty in adjusting to the new reality. Subsets of this disorder make up the most frequent psychiatric diagnoses among mentally ill populations, with features that include diagnosis of adjustment disorder.

As a category of disorders, adjustment disorder first appeared in the revised third edition of the *Diagnostic and Statistical Manual of Mental Disorders* (*DSM-III-R*), and the term included nine subtypes. The *DSM-IV-TR* lists six subtypes of adjustment disorder, generally based on what feature best characterizes the person's symptoms. These six subtypes are: AD with depressed mood (thought to be the most common subtype), AD with anxiety, AD with mixed anxiety and depressed mood, AD with disturbance of conduct, AD with disturbance of emotions and conduct, and AD not otherwise specified (ADNOS). This last subtype is applied when one of the other five does not fit the specific symptoms of a given patient.

The criteria for these disorders also include time parameters. One of the criteria for diagnosing an adjustment disorder is that it is an acute response to stress lasting six or fewer months. In some special cases, the response can be chronic, lasting longer than six months, usually when the stressor has lasting consequences, such as divorce or death of a family member.

The stressful events that precipitate an adjustment disorder vary widely. Stressful events include the loss of a job, the end of a romantic relationship, a life transition such as a career change or retirement, the death of a pet, or a serious accident or sickness. Some are acute one-time stressors, such as relocating to a new area, while others are chronic, such as caring for a child with mental deficits or living in a crime-ridden neighborhood.

In spite of some disagreement among professionals about the validity of the diagnosis of adjustment disorder, many consider the category useful for three reasons: (1) an adjustment disorder may be an early sign of a major mental disorder and allow for early treatment and **intervention**; (2) adjustment disorders are situational or reactive and do not imply that the patient has an underlying **brain** disease; and (3) the category does not carry the social stigma associated with such diagnostic categories as major **depression** and is less likely to affect the individual's employment or educational opportunities.

Risk factors

Risk factors for adjustment disorders include:

- more than one stressful event within a relatively short time period
- history of abusive parenting, family disruption, fetal alcohol syndrome, or frequent moves in early childhood
- concurrent mental health problems
- exposure to war or criminal violence
- poverty, homelessness, or other difficult circumstances
- social isolation or absence of a family or friendship network
- presence of chronic physical illness

Causes and symptoms

Causes are various for adjustment disorders as are the symptoms.

Causes

As of 2011, the processes leading to disruption of an individual's ability to adapt to change were not well understood. In the initial edition of the *Diagnostic and Statistical Manual of Mental Disorders,* the identifiable stressor was described as "psychosocial," a category that excludes physical illnesses and natural disasters. In the *DSM-IV-TR*, the word "psychosocial" was deleted to make the point that any stressful event can lead to an adjustment disorder. It is important to recognize, however, that while adjustment disorders are triggered by external stressors, the symptoms result from the person's interpretation of and adaptation to the stressful event or circumstances. Beliefs, perceptions, fears, and expectations influence the development and symptoms of a given individual's adjustment disorder.

Symptoms

Unlike many other disorders categorized in the *DSM-IV-TR*, adjustment disorders do not have an accompanying clearly delineated symptom profile, which has led to their being perceived as a "transitional" diagnosis, awaiting the manifestation of symptoms more clearly related to some other better-defined disorder. This ambiguity arises from the difficulty in establishing what defines a reaction within the norms of a population. The *DSM-IV-TR* states that the symptoms of an adjustment disorder must appear within three months of a stressor and that they must meet at least one of the following criteria: (1) the distress is greater than what would be expected in response to that particular stressor; or (2) the individual experiences significant impairment in social relationships or in occupational or academic settings. Moreover, the symptoms cannot represent **bereavement** as normally experienced after the death of a loved one; cannot be an exacerbation of another, pre-existing disorder; and cannot meet the criteria for another disorder.

Each of the six subtypes of adjustment disorder is characterized by its own predominant symptoms.

- With depressed mood: The chief manifestations are feelings of sadness and depression, with a sense of accompanying hopelessness. The patient may be tearful and have uncontrollable bouts of crying.
- With anxiety: Patients are troubled by feelings of apprehension, nervousness, and worry. They may also feel jittery and unable to control their thoughts of doom. Children with this subtype may express fears of separation from parents or other significant people and may refuse to go to sleep alone or attend school.
- With mixed anxiety and depressed mood: Patients have a combination of symptoms from the previous two subtypes.
- With disturbance of conduct: Patients exhibit noticeable behavioral changes such as shoplifting, truancy, reckless driving, aggressive outbursts, or sexual promiscuity. Patients disregard the rights of others or previously followed rules of conduct with little concern, guilt, or remorse.
- With mixed disturbance of emotions and conduct: Patients exhibit sudden changes in behavior combined with feelings of depression or anxiety. They may feel or express guilt about the behavior but then repeat it shortly thereafter.
- With not otherwise specified: This subtype covers patients who are adjusting poorly to stress but who do not fit into the other categories. These patients may complain of physical illness and pull away from social contact.

Adjustment disorders may lead to **suicide** or suicidal thinking. Researchers also have found that the suicidal process moves faster and evolves more rapidly in patients with adjustment disorders than in those with major depression. Adjustment disorders may complicate the

KEY TERMS

Cognitive-behavioral therapy—An approach to psychotherapy that emphasizes the correction of distorted thinking patterns and changing one's behaviors accordingly.

Decision tree—A decision support model used in medical and psychiatric diagnosis that consists of a tree-like chart or diagram, including various symptoms, tentative diagnoses, diagnostic decisions, and their possible consequences.

Group therapy—Group interaction designed to provide support, correction through feedback, constructive criticism, and a forum for consultation and reference.

Interpersonal therapy—An approach that includes psychoeducation about the sick role and emphasis on the present and improving interpersonal dynamics and relationships. Interpersonal therapy is effective in treating adjustment disorders related to physical illness.

Psychosocial—An adjective that describes the emotional and social aspects of psychological disorders.

Solution-focused therapy—A type of therapy that involves concrete goals and an emphasis on future direction rather than past experiences.

Stressor—A stimulus or event that provokes a stress response in an organism. Stressors can be categorized as acute or chronic and as external or internal to the organism.

Subthreshold—A term used in psychiatry to describe a condition that has significant clinical features but does not meet the full criteria of major disorders. Adjustment disorders are considered subthreshold disorders.

Support group—A group whose primary purpose is the provision of empathy and emotional support for its members. Support groups are less formal and less goal-directed than those groups participating in group therapy.

treatment of other diseases when, for example, a sufferer loses interest in taking medication as prescribed or adhering to diet or **exercise** regimens.

An adjustment disorder can occur at any stage of life; however, the risk of an AD appears to increase during periods typically associated with major life changes, such as late adolescence, midlife, and retirement.

Diagnosis

Adjustment disorders are usually diagnosed as the result of an interview with a **psychiatrist**. The psychiatrist will take a history, including identification of the stressor that has triggered the adjustment disorder, and evaluate the patient's responses to the stressor. The patient's primary physician may give the person a thorough physical examination to rule out a previously undiagnosed medical illness.

The **American Psychiatric Association** considers adjustment disorder to be a residual category, meaning that the diagnosis is given only when an individual does not meet the criteria for a major mental disorder. For example, if a person fits the more stringent criteria for **major depressive disorder**, the diagnosis of adjustment disorder is not given. If the patient is diagnosed with an adjustment disorder but continues to have symptoms for more than six months after the stressor and its consequences have ceased, the diagnosis is changed to another mental disorder. The one exception to this time limit is situations in which the stressor itself is chronic or has enduring consequences. In that case, the adjustment disorder is considered chronic, and the diagnosis remains applicable beyond six months.

The lack of a diagnostic checklist or decision tree for adjustment disorders distinguishes these disorders from either **post-traumatic stress disorder** or **acute stress disorder**. All three require the presence of a stressor, but the latter two define the extreme stressor and specific patterns of symptoms. With adjustment disorder, the stressor may be any event that is significant to the patient, and the disorder may take different forms in different patients.

Adjustment disorders must also be distinguished from **personality disorders**, which are caused by enduring personality traits that are inflexible and cause social, interpersonal, and occupational impairment. A personality disorder that has not yet surfaced may be made worse by a stressor and may mimic an adjustment disorder. A clinician must separate relatively stable traits in a patient's personality from passing disturbances. In some cases, however, the patient may be given both diagnoses. Again, it is important for psychiatrists to be sensitive to the role of cultural factors in the presentation of the patient's symptoms.

If the stressor is a physical illness, diagnosis is further complicated. It is important to recognize the difference between an adjustment disorder and the direct physiological effects of a medical condition (e.g., the temporary functional impairment associated with chemotherapy). This distinction can be clarified through communication with the patient's physician or education about the medical condition and its treatment. For some individuals, however, both may occur and reinforce each other.

Examination

An office physical examination of a patient with an adjustment disorder usually will not lead to any significant findings unless the patient is suffering from a concurrent physical illness or injury.

Tests

There are no laboratory or imaging tests that can be used to diagnose adjustment disorder.

Treatment

Traditional, medicinal, and alternative treatments are used to help people with adjustment disorder.

Traditional

There have been few research studies of significant scope that compared the efficacy of different treatments for adjustment disorder. The relative lack of outcome studies is partially due to the lack of specificity in the diagnosis itself. Because there is such variability in the types of stressors involved in adjustment disorders, it has proven difficult to design effective studies. As a result, there is not yet a consensus regarding the most effective treatments for adjustment disorder.

There are, however, guidelines for effective approaches in treating people with adjustment disorders. Effective treatments include stress-reduction approaches, therapies that teach coping strategies for any stressors that cannot be reduced or removed, and groups that help patients build support networks of friends, family, and people in similar circumstances. **Psychodynamic psychotherapy** may be helpful in clarifying and interpreting the meaning of the stressor for a particular patient. For example, if the person has cancer, he or she may become more dependent on others, which may be threatening for people who place a high value on self-sufficiency. By exploring those feelings, the patient can then begin to recognize all that is not lost and regain a sense of self-worth.

Therapies that encourage the patient to express the fear, anxiety, rage, helplessness, and hopelessness of dealing with the stressful situation may be helpful. These approaches include **journal therapy**, certain types of **art therapy**, and movement or **dance therapy**. **Support groups** and **group therapy** allow patients to gain perspective on the adversity and establish relationships with others who share their problem. Psychoeducation

QUESTIONS TO ASK YOUR DOCTOR

- How can I tell the difference between a severe reaction to stress that is still within the normal range and an adjustment disorder?
- How many patients have you treated who were diagnosed with an adjustment disorder? What were their outcomes?
- What type of psychotherapy do you recommend for adjustment disorders?
- What is your opinion of spiritual or religious counseling?
- What is your opinion on the use of medications as part of the treatment plan?

and medical crisis counseling can assist individuals and families facing stress caused by a medical illness.

Short-term therapies such as **family therapy**, **cognitive-behavioral therapy**, solution-focused therapy, and **interpersonal therapy** have all been used with some success in treating adjustment disorder.

Drugs

Clinicians do not agree on the role of drugs in treating adjustment disorders. Some argue that medications are not necessary for adjustment disorders because of their brief duration. In addition, they maintain that drugs may be counterproductive by undercutting the patient's sense of responsibility and his or her motivation to find effective solutions. At the other end of the spectrum, other clinicians maintain that medication by itself is the best form of treatment, particularly for patients with medical conditions, those who are terminally ill, and those resistant to **psychotherapy**. Others advocate a middle ground of treatment that combines medication and psychotherapy.

Alternative

Spiritual and religious counseling can be helpful, particularly for people coping with existential issues related to physical illness or with moral conflicts related to difficult personal decisions (e.g., divorce, abortion, withdrawing life support from a dying family member).

Some herbal remedies appear to be helpful to some patients with adjustment disorders. For adjustment disorder with anxiety, a randomized controlled trial found that the 91 patients receiving euphytose (an herbal preparation containing a combination of plant extracts, including crataegus, ballota, passiflora, valeriana, cola, and paullinia) showed significant improvement over the 91 patients taking a placebo. There have been no reported follow-up studies confirming these findings.

Prognosis

Most adults who are diagnosed with adjustment disorder have a favorable prognosis. For most people, an adjustment disorder is temporary and will either resolve by itself or respond to treatment. For some, however, the stressor remains chronic and the symptoms may worsen. In addition, patients with adjustment disorders engage in deliberate self-harm at a rate that surpasses most other mental disorders. They may also be at an increased risk for future **substance abuse** disorders. Still other patients may develop a major depressive disorder even in the absence of an additional stressor.

Some studies have been conducted to follow up on patients five years after their initial diagnosis. At that time, 71% of adults were completely well with no residual symptoms, whereas 21% had developed a major depressive disorder or alcoholism. For children aged 8–13, adjustment disorder did not predict future psychiatric disturbances. For adolescents, however, the prognosis is grimmer. After five years, 43% had developed a major psychiatric disorder, often of far greater severity. These disorders included **schizophrenia**, **schizoaffective disorder**, major depression, substance use disorders, or personality disorders. In contrast to adults, the adolescents' behavioral symptoms and the type of adjustment disorder predicted future mental disorders.

Researchers have noted that once an adjustment disorder is diagnosed, psychotherapy, medication, or both can prevent the development of a more serious mental disorder. Effective treatment is critical, as adjustment disorders are associated with an increased risk of suicide attempts, completed suicide, substance abuse, and various unexplained physical complaints. Patients with chronic stressors may require ongoing treatment for continued symptom management. While patients may not become symptom-free, treatment can halt the progression toward a more serious mental disorder by enhancing the patient's ability to cope.

Prevention

In many cases, there is little possibility of preventing the stressors that trigger adjustment disorders. One preventive strategy that is helpful to many patients, however, is learning to be proactive in managing ordinary stress and maximizing problem-solving abilities when the patients are not in crisis. In addition, the general availability of counseling following a large-scale stressful event may ameliorate some stress responses.

Resources

BOOKS

American Psychiatric Association. *Diagnostic and Statistical Manual of Mental Disorders,* 4th ed., text rev. Washington, DC: APA, 2000.

Black, Donald W., and Nancy C. Andreasen. *Introductory Textbook of Psychiatry,* 5th ed. Arlington, VA: American Psychiatric Publishing, 2011.

Heidenreich, Pascal, and Isidor Pruter, eds. *Handbook of Stress: Causes, Effects, and Control.* Hauppauge, NY: Nova Science Publishers, 2009.

PERIODICALS

Baumeister, H., and K. Kufner. "Is It Time to Adjust the Adjustment Disorder Category?" *Current Opinion in Psychiatry* 22 (July 2009): 409–12.

Casey, P. "Adjustment Disorder: Epidemiology, Diagnosis, and Treatment." *CNS Drugs* 23 (November 1, 2009): 927–38.

Kar, N. "Psychological Impact of Disasters on Children: Review of Assessment and Interventions." *World Journal of Pediatrics* 5 (February 2009): 5–11.

WEBSITES

Mayo Clinic staff. "Adjustment Disorders." MayoClinic.com. March 17, 2011. http://www.mayoclinic.com/health/adjustment-disorders/DS00584 (accessed August 13, 2011).

Benton, Tami D., and Judith A. Ifeagwu. "Adjustment Disorders." Medscape Reference. January 12, 2009. http://emedicine.medscape.com/article/292759-overview (accessed August 13, 2011).

ORGANIZATIONS

American Psychiatric Association, 1000 Wilson Blvd., Ste. 1825, Arlington, VA, 22209-3901, (703) 907-7300, (888) 35-PSYCH (357-7924), apa@psych.org, http://www.psych.org.

Mental Health America, 2000 North Beauregard St., 6th Fl., Alexandria, VA, 22311, (703) 684-7722, (800) 969-6642; TTY: (800) 433-5959, Fax: (703) 684-5968, http://www.nmha.org.

National Alliance on Mental Illness (NAMI), 3803 N. Fairfax Drive, Ste. 100, Arlington, VA, 22203, (703) 524-7600, (800) 950-NAMI (6264), Fax: (703) 524-9094, http://www.nami.org.

National Institute of Mental Health, 6001 Executive Blvd., Rm. 8184, MSC 9663, Bethesda, MD, 20892-9663, (301) 443-4513; TTY: (301) 443-8431, (866) 615-6464; TTY: (866) 415-8051, Fax: (301) 443-4279, nimhinfo@nimh.gov, http://www.nimh.nih.gov.

Holly Scherstuhl, MEd
Emily Jane Willingham, PhD
Tish Davidson, AM

Adrenaline

Definition

Adrenaline (also known as epinephrine) is a hormone and neurotransmitter that the sympathetic nervous system releases as part of the body's "fight-or-flight" response. Adrenaline increases blood and oxygen flow to the muscles, releases stored energy from the liver and fat cells, and prepares the body for quick action.

Description

Synthesis

Epinephrine is an amine hormone. It is produced and released by a region in the central part of the adrenal gland called the adrenal medulla. In a multistep process, enzymes convert the amino acid tyrosine into the chemical L-dopa, which is converted to **dopamine** and then converted to norepinephrine. Epinephrine is synthesized from norepinephrine (noradrenaline) and released into the bloodstream.

Together, epinephrine and norepinephrine are known as the catecholamines. Epinephrine makes up about 80% of the catecholamines that are released as part of the body's **stress** response.

KEY TERMS

Adrenaline addiction—A drug-like response some people experience from participating in activities (such as skydiving or gambling) that trigger adrenaline release.

Beta blockers—Drugs that block beta-adrenergic receptors to reduce the actions of epinephrine, thereby lowering the heart rate and blood pressure.

Bronchioles—Tiny tubes in the lungs.

Catecholamines—A class of hormones that includes epinephrine and norepinephrine, which are involved in the fight-or-flight response.

Enzymes—Proteins that trigger chemical reactions in the body.

Glycogen—The form of glucose (sugar) that is stored in the liver and muscles.

Norepinephrine (noradrenaline)—A hormone produced by the adrenal gland, along with epinephrine, as part of the fight-or-flight response.

Tyrosine—The amino acid from which epinephrine is synthesized.

Mechanisms of action

When the body is confronted with a dangerous or stressful situation (such as a test for which someone has not studied or an encounter with a dangerous-looking individual), the fight-or-flight response is initiated. In order to act quickly, the body diverts energy away from areas where it is not needed to those where it is most required, such as the heart and muscles.

When the body senses a threat, the hypothalamus in the **brain** releases nerve signals to the adrenal medulla to release epinephrine and norepinephrine.

When released, the epinephrine circulates around the body through the bloodstream until it reaches its target organs—the heart, blood vessels, liver, and fat cells. The hormone binds to two different types of receptors: alpha-adrenergic and beta-adrenergic receptors. Each of these receptors triggers a different action within cells. Alpha receptors initiate smooth muscle contraction and blood vessel constriction, whereas beta receptors stimulate the heart muscle.

The release of epinephrine causes the following reactions in the body:

- The heart beats faster, pumping additional blood throughout the body and especially to the muscles, in preparation for action.
- Blood vessels constrict, raising the blood pressure.
- Small tubes in the lungs called bronchioles dilate to send more oxygen throughout the body.
- Glycogen (the stored form of glucose) is broken down into glucose in the liver and released.
- Fat stores are released from adipose tissue to be used for energy.
- Blood flow slows to the digestive tract, skin, and kidneys, where it is not needed as much.

History

The first people to identify the effects of epinephrine were British physician George Oliver (1841–1915) and endocrinologist Edward Albert Sharpey-Schafer (1850–1935). In 1894, they discovered that injecting an extract from the adrenal gland into the bloodstream of an animal raised its blood pressure. Then in 1901, Japanese chemist Jokichi Takamine (1854–1922) isolated and purified epinephrine from the adrenal medulla and patented it. British pharmacologist Henry Dale (1875–1968) began using the name adrenaline for the hormone.

Medication and adrenaline

Epinephrine can be isolated from the adrenal glands of animals and used for medical purposes. It can be injected into the heart to restart the heartbeats of people who are experiencing cardiac arrest. It can open the bronchioles of the lungs in people with asthma, or in those who have had severe allergic responses to food, medications, or other substances. Drugs called **beta blockers** are often given to patients to reduce anxiety. These drugs block beta-adrenergic receptors, slowing the heart rate and lowering blood pressure.

Adrenaline addiction

Some people may experience a drug-like high from participating in behaviors that trigger the body's fight-or-flight response. They are sometimes referred to as "adrenaline junkies" or "adrenaline addicts." For example, people who seek thrills, such as skydivers, mountain climbers, and extreme skiers, experience a rush of adrenaline from the knowledge that their actions could result in severe injury or even death. Compulsive gamblers often cite the reason for their **addiction** as less the desire to win than the physical rush they get from playing. Some people who steal feel that same type of adrenaline rush from the idea that they might be apprehended. The heightened sense of awareness, increased heartbeat, and rapid breathing that occur when the adrenal medulla releases adrenaline is similar to the high that people experience when taking drugs, and it can be similarly addictive.

Resources

BOOKS

Church, Matt. *Adrenaline Junkies and Serotonin Seekers: Balance Your Brain Chemistry to Maximize Energy, Stamina, Mental Sharpness, and Emotional Well-Being*. Berkeley, CA: Ulysses Press, 2004.

Goldstein, David S. *Adrenaline and the Inner World: An Introduction to Scientific Integrative Medicine*. Baltimore, MD: Johns Hopkins University Press, 2006.

Meyer, Jerrold S., and Linda F. Quenzer. *Psychopharmacology: Drugs, the Brain and Behavior*. Sunderland, MA: Sinauer Associates, Inc., 2005.

ORGANIZATIONS

American Psychiatric Association, 1000 Wilson Boulevard, Suite 1825, Arlington, VA, 22209-3901, (703) 907-7300, apa@psych.org, http://www.psych.org.

National Alliance on Mental Illness, 3803 N Fairfax Drive, Suite 100, Arlington, VA, 22203, (703) 524-7600, http://www.nami.org.

National Institute of Mental Health, 6001 Executive Blvd., Room 8184, MSC 9663, Bethesda, MD, 20892-9663, (301) 433-4513; TTY: (301) 443-8431, Fax: (301) 443-4279, Toll-free: (866) 615-6464; TTY: (866) 415-8051, nimhinfo@nih.gov, http://www.nimh.nih.gov.

Stephanie N. Watson

Adult ADHD

Definition

Adult **attention deficit hyperactivity disorder (ADHD)** is the form of ADHD present in persons over 18 years of age. The disorder is also known as adult ADD. ADHD (or ADD) is a disorder characterized by a persistent pattern of inattention and/or hyperactivity. It is estimated that about 60% of children diagnosed with ADHD will continue to have the disorder as adults.

There are three basic types of ADHD in adults as well as children: inattentiveness, impulsiveness, and a combination of the two.

Demographics

Estimates of the prevalence of adult ADHD in North America vary from 2% to 4.4%, or about 8.5 million adults in the United States and Canada. Relatively few of these people are diagnosed, however, so it is likely that the actual rate is higher. The worldwide prevalence of ADHD in adults is estimated to be about 5%; it appears to be higher in developed countries than in poorer ones.

While childhood ADHD affects more males than females (about 2:1), the gender ratio appears to become more even in adults. Some doctors think that the reason for this shift in the ratio is that girls are more likely to fit the inattentive childhood type of the disorder (ADHD-I) and are overlooked in classroom settings, while boys are more likely to exhibit the hyperactive form (ADHD-H) and come to the attention of their teachers and other adults. Adults with ADHD, however, are more likely to be inattentive than hyperactive; thus, women in this population are as likely as men to be diagnosed. Adult ADHD is thought to be equally common in all racial and ethnic groups.

Adult ADHD imposes economic costs on the persons who suffer from it as well as on society at large. A study done in 2004 reported that adults with ADHD who graduated from high school earned $11,000 less per year than their counterparts with the same level of education, while college graduates with adult ADHD earned $4,400 less per year than their counterparts without the disorder. The study estimated that adult ADHD costs the American economy $77 billion each year. For comparison, the annual cost of drug abuse is $58 billion; for alcohol abuse, $85 billion; and for **depression**, $43 billion.

Description

Although ADHD in children has been recognized as a mental disorder since the 1840s (when it was first described by a German physician in his own son), it was not considered

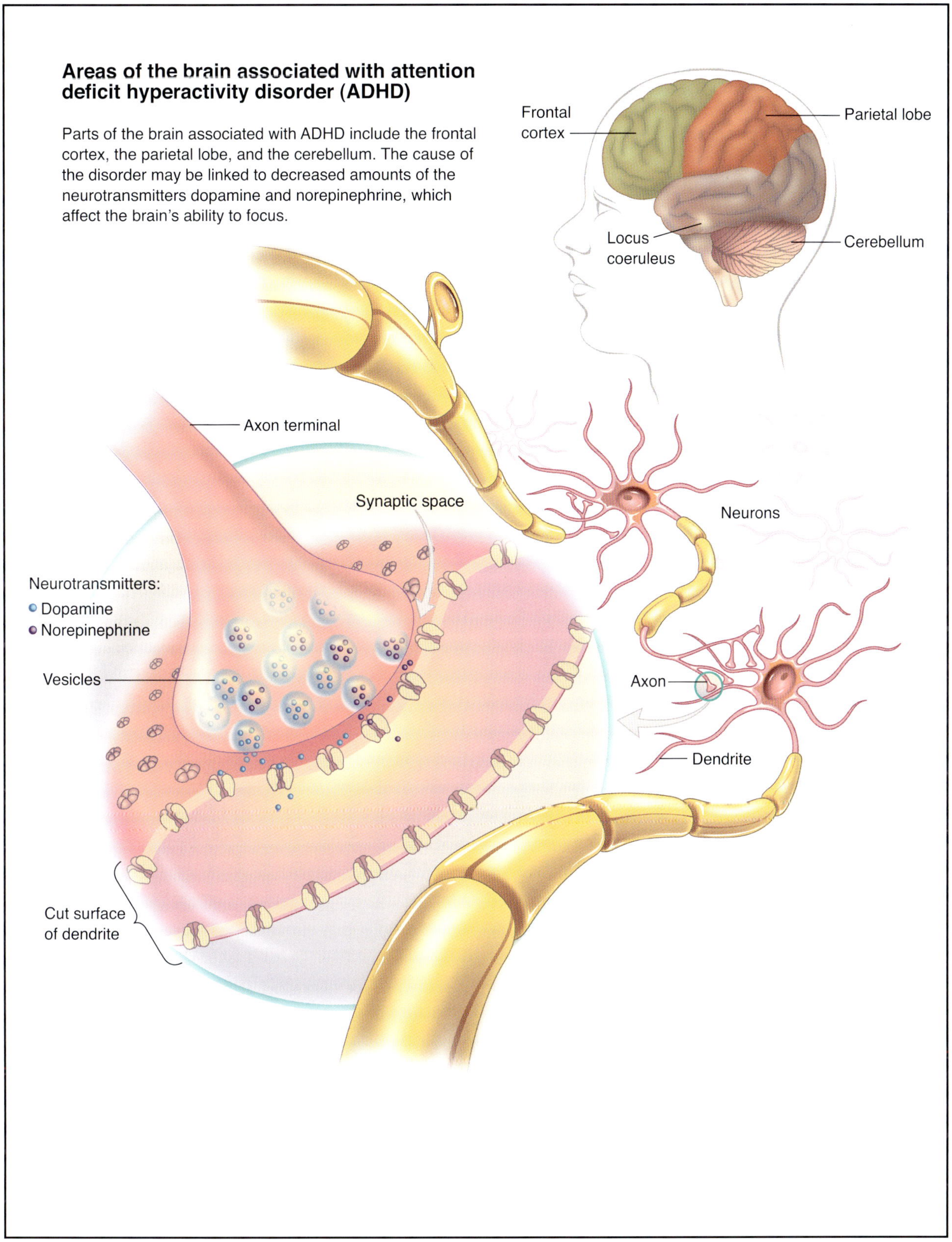

(Illustration by Electronic Illustrators Group. Reproduced by permission of Gale, a part of Cengage Learning.)

an appropriate **diagnosis** for adults until the 1970s, and formal diagnostic criteria for adult ADHD were not defined until 1987. One reason for the delay in recognizing the adult form of the disorder is that the symptoms of ADHD in adults are somewhat different from those in children; adults are less likely to display hyperactive behaviors. Adults with ADHD are more likely to say that they have trouble relaxing than feeling that they have to race around physically. Inattentiveness in an adult may take the form of forgetting meetings, work deadlines, or social get-togethers, and impulsiveness may take the form of moodiness, temper tantrums, or impatience in traffic jams. In addition, highly intelligent adults with ADHD are likely to have developed coping behaviors that mask their symptoms.

Adult ADHD can be summarized as a disorder affecting the person's executive functions, combined with difficulties in self-regulation and self-motivation. The executive functions are a set of mental abilities that control or manage other cognitive processes; they include the ability to plan ahead, to make decisions among several possible courses of action, to inhibit behaviors that are inappropriate in a specific setting, to choose appropriate behaviors, to think abstractly, and to use deductive reasoning. Adults with ADHD are likely to be seen by friends and coworkers as disorganized, unable to complete work assignments on time, easily distracted, overly emotional, or needing constant stimulation.

Risk factors

Risk factors for adult ADHD include:

- family history of the disorder
- having a mother who smoked, drank, or used drugs during pregnancy
- having a mother who was exposed to environmental toxins during pregnancy
- being born prematurely
- exposure to environmental toxins in childhood

Causes and symptoms

Causes

The causes of ADHD are not completely understood; however, studies of **brain** function using **positron emission tomography (PET)** scans indicate that the brains of children with ADHD may be structured differently from those of children without the disorder. More specifically, some researchers think that the parts of the brain that govern attentiveness do not have normal levels of **dopamine**, a chemical produced by the brain that allows nerve cells to transmit signals from one cell to another. Dopamine and another chemical called norepinephrine are **neurotransmitters** that play an important role in brain function. The uptake transporters for dopamine and norepinephrine are overly active in people with ADHD and clear these neurotransmitters from the connections between nerve cells much more rapidly than in normal individuals. The fact that medications that stimulate the release of dopamine are beneficial to patients with ADHD supports this theory.

There are also **genetic factors** involved in ADHD, though no specific causal gene has been identified as of 2011. It is known that the disorder runs in families; the parents and siblings of children with ADHD are two to eight times more likely to develop ADHD than the general population. The discovery through genome-wide association studies of a protein network implicated in adult ADHD may indicate that candidate genes for the disorder will be identified in the next few years.

Some researchers think that environmental toxins, particularly lead, and a mother's drinking or smoking during pregnancy are risk factors for ADHD. There is also some evidence that very low birth weight or premature birth may be risk factors for the disorder. It

KEY TERMS

Comorbidity—The presence of one or more disorders (or diseases) in a patient in addition to a primary disease or disorder.

Dopamine—A brain chemical that helps to regulate movement.

DSM—*Diagnostic and Statistical Manual of Mental Disorders*, a publication produced by the American Psychiatric Association and used by medical professionals in diagnosing mental disorders.

Executive functions—An umbrella term for the group of mental processes responsible for planning, abstract thinking, logical deduction, choosing appropriate behaviors and inhibiting inappropriate behaviors, and distinguishing between relevant and irrelevant sensory information.

Impairment—A physical or mental defect at the level of a major body system or organ.

Norepinephrine—Another brain chemical that affects a person's ability to pay attention.

Prevalence—The number of cases of a disease or disorder existing in a specific population at a given point in time.

Psychostimulant—A type of drug that increases the activity of the parts of the brain that produce dopamine.

is not known whether the emotional climate of a family contributes to the disorder, although some doctors think that mood or **anxiety disorders** in other family members may make a child's symptoms worse. Other theories proposing that ADHD is caused by head injuries, allergic reactions to food additives, or a diet high in sugary foods or energy drinks are considered unproven.

Symptoms

The symptoms of adult ADHD may appear in several areas of the person's life. Adults with ADHD are likely to have experienced trouble in the following areas:

- academic—underachievement in school, grade repetition, documented disciplinary infractions, incompletion of school, or frequently changed courses of study or educational institutions
- work—frequent changes of employment, history of frequent firing or poor performance reviews, difficulty moving up the employment ladder, or lower socioeconomic status
- social/legal—history of driving violations, including collisions, speeding, DUI citations, and other moving violations; use of illegal substances; heavy smoking; heavy alcohol consumption
- relationships—history of frequent breakups before marriage, repeated marriages, or frequent divorces; possible history of sexual promiscuity, unplanned pregnancy, and sexually transmitted diseases

Supervisors and coworkers may believe that the adult with ADHD does not listen to instructions, or they may resent having to finish the affected person's job assignments because he or she is easily distracted or cannot identify priorities. People related or married to an adult with ADHD often complain about having to cope with the consequences of the patient's impulsive behavior and poor decisions as well as his or her short temper, irritability, and irresponsibility.

Diagnosis

The diagnosis of adult ADHD is clinical, which means that it is based on the doctor's evaluation and judgment rather than the results of laboratory or imaging tests. Diagnosis is often complicated by the fact that between 50% and 80% of adults with ADHD have a concurrent mood or **substance abuse** disorder. In some cases, adults with ADHD consult a doctor because they are concerned about their work history, difficulties with schooling, or relationship problems; in other cases, they may seek help when they notice symptoms of ADHD in their child, or when the child is diagnosed with ADHD.

There are four major criteria for the diagnosis of adult ADHD:

- Specific symptoms. Adults with the inattentive form of ADHD may procrastinate, be indecisive, have difficulty recalling and organizing task-related materials, lose track of time, have difficulty managing time, avoid tasks or jobs that require sustained attention, have difficulty starting tasks or following through on them, and have trouble shifting attention from one task to another. Adults with the hyperactive/impulsive form of ADHD may choose only highly active, stimulating jobs; avoid uninteresting or sedentary work; moonlight at multiple jobs or work long hours; seek constant activity; become bored easily or act impatient; make impulsive decisions; frequently express irritation or lose their temper easily; and behave irresponsibly.
- Impairment in two or more areas of life (e.g., work, education, relationships, social situations). "Impairment" means that the adult's level of functioning is seriously affected by the behaviors.
- A persistent pattern of signs and symptoms beginning no later than age seven. Early recognition is essential for a later diagnosis of adult ADHD, as ADHD is not an adult-onset disorder. While it is not necessary for an adult to have been formally diagnosed with ADHD as a child, childhood symptoms of the disorder must be documented. Documentation may include school report cards; interviews with the adult's parents, if still living; or childhood symptoms self-reported by the adult.
- The symptoms cannot be better accounted for by another mental disorder. It is particularly important to evaluate the patient for mood disorders, because about 50% of adults diagnosed with ADHD have comorbid mood disorders.

Examination

A complete physical examination is important in order to rule out vision problems, hearing loss, seizure disorder, disorders of the thyroid gland, hypoglycemia (low blood sugar), or other possible physical causes of the patient's symptoms. It is also important for the doctor to be aware of any other medications that the patient may be taking for high blood pressure, diabetes, or other chronic physical disorders, as these may influence the choice of medications to treat the ADHD.

Tests

The physical examination is accompanied by a series of interviews with psychiatrists and psychologists. The patient may be given the Wechsler Adult Intelligence Scale (WAIS) or a similar test of intelligence and general knowledge in adults. The patient may also be given the **Structured Clinical Interview for DSM-IV** (SCID), which is an instrument used for the differential diagnosis of mental disorders according to *DSM-IV* categories. The SCID is useful in evaluating adult ADHD patients for comorbid mood, anxiety, or substance abuse disorders.

There are behavioral checklists and questionnaires for adult ADHD that doctors can use to narrow the diagnostic possibilities. A set of criteria called the Wender Utah Rating Scale (WURS) is commonly used to diagnose ADHD in adults:

- a history of ADHD in childhood
- hyperactivity and poor ability to focus or concentrate
- difficulty completing tasks
- mood swings
- difficulty controlling temper
- inability to handle stress
- impulsive behaviors

Another instrument that may be used in evaluating adults with ADHD is the Brown ADD Scale (BADDS) for adults. Based on Brown's model of ADHD as a disorder of executive functioning, the BADDS scale measures the patient's ability to function in six major areas:

- activation—organizing tasks and materials, estimating the time required, prioritizing tasks, and starting the work
- focus—focusing on a task and sustaining focus without being distracted
- effort—sustaining effort over long-term as well as short-term projects and remaining alert until the task is completed
- emotion—regulating and controlling emotions rather than allowing them to overwhelm thought processes and interfere with completing a task
- memory—accessing short-term memories and recalling as needed to complete a task
- action—thinking before acting impulsively, regulating the speed of work in order to complete tasks on time, and monitoring the context of interactions with other people

Procedures

In some cases, the doctor may recommend a CT scan or MRI to rule out head **trauma**, brain tumors, infections, seizure disorders, or other physical disorders that may affect the structure or functioning of the brain and produce symptoms resembling those of ADHD.

Treatment

Treatment for adults with ADHD is similar to that for children, namely, a combination of medications and **psychotherapy**. There are no surgical treatments recommended for ADHD.

Traditional

There are several different forms of psychotherapy that are reported to benefit adults diagnosed with ADHD. They include **cognitive-behavioral therapy** (CBT), which helps to correct poor self-image by encouraging the patient to look at and challenge the habits of negative thought and behavior. Relaxation training and **stress management** techniques to lower anxiety levels are also helpful. Patients who have particular difficulties with intimate relationships may be helped by **couples therapy** or **family therapy**.

Another approach to psychotherapy that is often recommended for adults with ADHD is behavioral coaching and job mentoring. The patient is taught such skills as time management; making reminder lists and keeping a calendar to organize and keep track of tasks; having one particular place in the home or office for such items as keys, bills, and other paperwork; and breaking down large or long-term tasks into smaller portions or time segments. In job mentoring, the patient is helped to gain a better understanding of workplace relationships—particularly what coworkers and supervisors reasonably should be able to expect of him or her—and ways to improve on-the-job functioning. However, coaching should not be considered a substitute for medication and formal psychotherapy.

Drugs

Medications are the mainstay of treatment for adult ADHD. The drugs most commonly prescribed are psychostimulants, which work by raising the level of dopamine and balancing the levels of other neurotransmitters in the patient's nervous system. These drugs are reported to benefit about 80% of patients. The psychostimulants most often prescribed for adults with ADHD are **methylphenidate** (Ritalin, Concerta, Daytrana, Metadate), **dextroamphetamine** (Dexedrine), **lisdexamfetamine** (Vyvanse), and dextroamphetamine-amphetamine (Adderall). Psychostimulants are available in both short-acting (about 4 hours) and long-acting (6 to 12 hours) forms; some adults with ADHD prefer the long-acting forms because they relieve concern about remembering to take another dose of medication during the day. Methylphenidate is also available in a long-acting patch form, sold under the trade name Daytrana. The patch is worn on the hip.

A newer drug that was approved by the U.S. Food and Drug Administration (FDA) in 2004 for the treatment of adult ADHD is **atomoxetine**, a

QUESTIONS TO ASK YOUR DOCTOR

- How can I tell whether I suffer from adult ADHD?
- My child has been recently diagnosed with ADHD. Does that mean that I also have the disorder?
- Have you ever treated an adult diagnosed with ADHD? Was their treatment successful?
- What is the difference between nonstimulant and psychostimulant medications?
- Can you recommend a coaching program for adults with ADHD?

nonstimulant. It was the only nonstimulant approved for this purpose as of 2011. Atomoxetine is a selective norepinephrine reuptake inhibitor sold under the trade name Strattera. Atomoxetine has a significant advantage over psychostimulants in that it is less likely to be abused, making it a good choice for patients with a history of substance abuse.

Patients with comorbid mood disorders may be prescribed antidepressant medications. The older tricyclic drugs have been found helpful in adults with ADHD, as has **venlafaxine** (Effexor), an antidepressant classified as a serotonin-norepinephrine reuptake inhibitor (SNRI). Another antidepressant found to benefit adult ADHD patients in **clinical trials** is **bupropion** (Wellbutrin), an atypical antidepressant that inhibits the reuptake of dopamine.

One important consideration for adult ADHD patients is to make sure that stimulants or other medications prescribed to treat the ADHD do not interact with other medications that the adult may be taking for chronic conditions such as high blood pressure, diabetes, anxiety disorders, and the like. In addition, adult athletes may need specialized medical therapy because many competitive sports bodies ban the use of psychostimulants.

As of mid 2011, there were 293 clinical trials of treatments for adult ADHD. Many of these are studies of the comparative effectiveness of medications already used to treat the disorder or studies of newer extended-release or long-acting formulations of these drugs. There were also several trials of investigational drugs, including **duloxetine** (Cymbalta), another norepinephrine reuptake inhibitor that was originally developed to treat major depression, and a drug identified only as PF-3654746. One study is investigating the effectiveness of massage therapy as a treatment for adult ADHD.

Alternative

Some forms of alternative medicine that have been suggested as treatments for adult ADHD include special **diets**, vitamin supplements, omega-3 fatty acids, and various herbal preparations (particularly **ginseng**, **ginkgo biloba** extract, or Chinese herbal medicines). There was no evidence as of 2011 that any of these alternative approaches was useful. There is some evidence, however, that **yoga** is a beneficial form of **exercise** for adults with ADHD, as it helps to teach focus, and the breathing exercises that are part of yoga are relaxing to many people.

Although some alternative practitioners have recommended medical marijuana as a short-term treatment for adult ADHD, most mainstream physicians disapprove its use because of the risk of substance abuse and a depressive disorder.

Prognosis

There was no cure for adult ADHD as of 2011, but the disorder usually can be managed, allowing the affected individual to improve functioning in daily life, including completing his or her education, forming stable relationships, and securing steady employment. Another benefit of treatment for ADHD is an improvement in the patient's self-esteem; perceived failures in various areas of life caused by the ADHD may cause low self-esteem and lead to mood or substance abuse disorders.

Prevention

There is no known way to prevent adult ADHD, because the causes of the disorder are still not completely understood.

Resources

BOOKS

American Psychiatric Association. *Diagnostic and Statistical Manual of Mental Disorders*. 4th ed., text rev. Washington, DC: American Psychiatric Association, 2000.

Barkley, Russell A. *Taking Charge of Adult ADHD*. New York: Guilford Press, 2010.

Brown, Thomas E. *Attention Deficit Disorder: The Unfocused Mind in Children and Adults*. New Haven, CT: Yale University Press, 2005.

Ramsay, J. Russell. *Nonmedication Treatments for Adult ADHD: Evaluating Impact on Daily Functioning and Well-Being*. Washington, DC: American Psychological Association, 2010.

Sarkis, Stephanie Moulton. *Adult ADD: A Guide for the Newly Diagnosed.* Oakland, CA: New Harbinger Publications, 2011.

Solanto, Mary V. *Cognitive-Behavioral Therapy for Adult ADHD: Targeting Executive Dysfunction*. New York: The Guilford Press, 2011.

PERIODICALS

Antshel, K.M., et al. "Advances in Understanding and Treating ADHD." *BMC Medicine* 9 (June 10, 2011): 72.

Bell, A.S. "A Critical Review of ADHD Diagnostic Criteria: What to Address in the DSM-V." *Journal of Attention Disorders* 15 (January 2011): 3–10.

Ermer, J.C., et al. "Pharmacokinetic Variability of Long-Acting Stimulants in the Treatment of Children and Adults with Attention-Deficit Hyperactivity Disorder." *CNS Drugs* 24 (December 1, 2010): 1009–25.

Haavik, J., et al. "Clinical Assessment and Diagnosis of Adults with Attention-Deficit/Hyperactivity Disorder." *Expert Review of Neurotherapeutics* 10 (October 2010): 1569–80.

Kutcher, J.S. "Treatment of Attention-Deficit Hyperactivity Disorder in Athletes." *Current Sports Medicine Reports* 10 (January–February 2011): 32–36.

Poelmans, G., et al. "Integrated Genome-wide Association Study Findings: Identification of a Neurodevelopmental Network for Attention Deficit Hyperactivity Disorder." *American Journal of Psychiatry* 168 (April 2011): 365–77.

Rösler, M., et al. "Attention Deficit Hyperactivity Disorder in Adults." *World Journal of Biological Psychiatry* 11 (August 2010): 684–98.

Rucklidge, J.J. "Gender Differences in Attention-deficit/ Hyperactivity Disorder." *Psychiatric Clinics of North America* 33 (June 2010): 357–73.

Wallis, D. "The Search for Biomarkers for Attention Deficit/ Hyperactivity Disorder." *Drug News and Perspectives* 23 (September 2010): 438–49.

WEBSITES

Adler, Lenard. "Adult ADHD" [3-1/2-minute video about ADHD in adults]. The Doctor's Channel. http://www.thedoctorschannel.com/video/2222.html?specialty=26 (accessed July 9, 2011).

"Adults Living with ADHD." National Alliance on Mental Illness (NAMI). http://www.nami.org/Template.cfm?Section=ADHD&Template=/ContentManagement/ContentDisplay.cfm&ContentID=106057 (accessed July 9, 2011).

"Attention-Deficit/Hyperactivity Disorder." U.S. Centers for Disease Control and Prevention (CDC). http://www.cdc.gov/ncbddd/adhd (accessed July 9, 2011).

Children and Adults with Attention-Deficit/Hyperactivity Disorder (CHADD). "What We Know: Diagnosis of ADHD in Adults." National Resource Center on ADHD. http://www.help4adhd.org/en/treatment/guides/WWK9 (accessed July 9, 2011).

Jaksa, Peter. "ADHD Fact Sheet." Attention Deficit Disorder Association (ADDA). http://www.add.org/?page=ADHD_Fact_Sheet (accessed July 10, 2011).

Mayo Clinic staff. "Adult ADHD (Attention-Deficit/Hyperactivity Disorder)." MayoClinic.com. http://www.mayoclinic.com/health/adult-adhd/DS01161 (accessed July 10, 2011).

National Institute of Mental Health. "Can Adults Have ADHD?" U.S. National Institutes of Health. http://www.nimh.nih.gov/health/publications/attention-deficit-hyperactivity-disorder/can-adults-have-adhd.shtml (accessed July 9, 2011).

ORGANIZATIONS

American Psychiatric Association, 1000 Wilson Boulevard, Suite 1825, Arlington, VA, 22209-3901, (703) 907-7300, apa@psych.org, http://www.psych.org.

Attention Deficit Disorder Association (ADDA), PO Box 7557, Wilmington, DE, 19803-9997, (800) 939-1019, info@add.org, http://www.add.org.

Centers for Disease Control and Prevention (CDC), 1600 Clifton Rd., Atlanta, GA, 30333, (800) 232-4636, cdcinfo@cdc.gov, http://www.cdc.gov.

Children and Adults with Attention-Deficit/Hyperactivity Disorder (CHADD), 8181 Professional Place, Suite 150, Landover, MD, 20785, (301) 306-7070, (800) 233-4050, Fax: (301) 306-7090, http://www.chadd.org.

National Alliance on Mental Illness (NAMI), 3803 N. Fairfax Dr., Suite 100, Arlington, VA, 22203, (703) 524-7600, (800) 950-NAMI, Fax: (703) 524-9094, http://www.nami.org.

National Institute of Mental Health (NIMH), 6001 Executive Boulevard, Room 8184, MSC 9663, Bethesda, MD, 20892-9663, (301) 443-4513, (866) 615-6464, Fax: (301) 443-4279, nimhinfo@nih.gov, http://www.nimh.nih.gov/index.shtml.

National Resource Center on ADHD, 8181 Professional Place, Suite 150, Landover, MD, 20785, (800) 233-4050, http://www.help4adhd.org.

Rebecca J. Frey, Ph.D.

Advance directives

Definition

An advance directive is a written document in which people clearly specify how medical decisions affecting them are to be made if they are unable to make them, or authorize a specific person to make such decisions for them. These documents are sometimes called living wills. Psychiatric advance directives serve the same purpose as general medical advance directives but are written by mental health consumers as a set of directions for others to follow prior to the onset of a period in which their decision making is impaired or an incapacitating crisis arises.

Description

Many states have passed laws related to medical advance directives and psychiatric advance directives. Advance directives usually fall into two categories: instruction directives and agent-driven directives. These two distinct documents may, in some cases, be combined into one form.

KEY TERMS

Conservator—Legal guardian.

Do Not Resuscitate order—A directive specifying that if an individual's heart stops, he or she should not receive cardiopulmonary resuscitation (CPR).

Proxy—An individual who makes decisions on behalf of another.

Instruction directives

An instruction directive is a written document that specifies the treatments individuals do and do not want, in the event that they become unable to make decisions about their care. These documents may indicate the affected individual's preferences about many aspects of treatment, including:

- people who should be contacted at a time of a medical or psychiatric crisis
- acceptable and unacceptable medications and dosages
- preferences for or against specific treatments such as tube feeding or breathing machines
- a Do Not Resuscitate order
- preferences about organ and tissue donation
- religious preferences

Agent-driven directives

An agent-driven directive may also be called a durable power of attorney. This directive is a signed, dated, and witnessed document that authorizes a designated person (usually a family member or close friend) to act as an agent or proxy. This empowers the proxy to make medical decisions for patients when they are deemed unable to make these decisions for themselves. The directive frequently includes the person's stated preferences in regard to treatment. Several states do not allow any of the following people to act as a person's proxy:

- the person's physician or other healthcare provider
- the staff of the healthcare facility(ies) providing the person's care
- guardians (often called conservators) of the person's financial affairs
- employees of federal agencies financially responsible for a person's care
- any person who serves as agent or proxy for 10 people or more

The person who is to act as the proxy should be familiar with the individual's expressed wishes about care and should understand how to work within the medical and mental health system.

Although most advance directives address situations arising from physical disability, according to Mental Health America, it has become increasingly accepted over the past 30 years for consumers of mental health services to know which treatments work best for them, and their opinions have become increasingly valued by those providing services. However, when mental health consumers become unable to make decisions or to give **informed consent** for treatments offered, others (including family, friends, judges, or care providers) make the decisions for them in crisis. In this situation, advance directives may be beneficial for people receiving care, as the legal document may protect them from unwanted treatment or **involuntary hospitalization**. In some states, the laws detail the content of psychiatric advance directives, which may include instructions about antipsychotic medication, **electroconvulsive therapy**, or hospital admission, and the naming of people who can act as surrogate decision makers if necessary.

Special concerns

In the United States, each state has specific laws about medical advance directives. How those laws apply to psychiatric advance directives can differ by state as well; a few states exclude psychiatric advance directives from their statutes altogether. The specific form the advance directive should take, the language it should use, and the number of witnesses required to make the document legal and binding vary from state to state; the document should be prepared by an attorney familiar with state advance directive requirements. In general, physicians and other healthcare professionals are expected to comply with the instructions of an advance directive, as long as those instructions are within the guidelines of accepted medical practice. It is recommended that people speak to their attorneys or physicians to ensure that their wishes are communicated in a form that is legally acceptable in their state.

In drafting an advance directive, the patient must be deemed lucid and able to communicate their wishes in order for the document to be valid. This assessment is generally done by a physician, although state laws vary, and some do not recognize this requirement.

Some other considerations associated with advance directives center on how they are implemented and whether or not a person who wants to complete one actually does so. Completing an advance directive can be difficult

QUESTIONS TO ASK YOUR DOCTOR

- Do you have an example of an advance directive from this state?
- What are some items you recommend putting into an advance directive?
- Could you explain some of the possible procedures I may wish to address in my advanced directive?
- Where should I file my advance directive?
- Can you put a copy in my file?
- Who else should I tell about my advance directive?

emotionally, and psychological, literacy, and informational barriers can exist. Various solutions have been suggested to address these problems, including a proposal for video-based advance directives in which individuals produce videotapes documenting their directives. In addition, even though as many as two-thirds of people with mental illness report that they would complete a psychiatric advance directive, only 4%–13% of outpatients receiving mental health treatment through public sector resources report having done so. A study published in the January 2011 issue of the American Psychiatric Association's journal *Psychiatric Services* found that, of more than 13,500 seniors living in nursing homes, patients with serious mental illnesses were 24% less likely to have prepared advance directives compared to residents with no mental illness. The study also noted that residents with mental illness were among the most likely groups to need advance directives, due to the high possibility of developing a disability and/or comorbid—co-occurring but unrelated—disorder. One proposal put forward to address this disconnect is the implementation of facilitated psychiatric advance directives involving a guided discussion and review of choices for completing an advance directive.

Resources

BOOKS

Kingsbury, Leigh Ann Creaney. *People Planning Ahead: A Guide to Communicating Healthcare and End of Life Wishes.* Washington, DC: American Association on Intellectual and Developmental Disabilities, 2009.

Swota, Alissa Hurwitz. *Culture, Ethics, and Advance Care Planning.* Lanham, MD: Lexington Books, 2009.

Thomas, Keri, and Ben Lobo, eds. *Advance Care Planning in End of Life Care.* Oxford: Oxford University Press, 2010.

PERIODICALS

Alfonso, Heather. "The Importance of Living Wills and Advance Directives." *Journal of Gerontological Nursing* 35, no. 10 (October 2009): 42–45.

Black, Kathy. "Promoting Advance Care Planning Through the National Healthcare Decisions Day Initiative." *Journal of Social Work in End-Of-Life and Palliative Care* 6, nos. 1–2 (January 2010): 11–26.

Pollack, Keshia M., Dan Morhaim, and Michael A. Williams. "The Public's Perspectives on Advance Directives: Implications for State Legislative and Regulatory Policy." *Health Policy* 96, no. 1 (June 2010): 57–63.

ORGANIZATIONS

American Bar Association, 321 N Clark St., Chicago, IL, 60654-7598, (800) 285-2221, http://www.americanbar.org.

American Hospital Association, 325 7th St. NW, Washington, DC, 20004-2802, (202) 638-1100, http://www.aha.org.

American Medical Association, 515 N State St., Chicago, IL, 60610, (800) 621-8335, http://www.ama-assn.org.

Joan Schonbeck, RN
Emily Jane Willingham, PhD
Tish Davidson, AM

Affect

Definition

Affect is a psychological term for an observable expression of emotion.

Description

A person's affect is the expression of emotion or feelings displayed to others through facial expressions, hand gestures, voice tone, and other emotional signs such as laughter or tears. Individual affect fluctuates according to emotional state. What is considered a normal range of affect, called the "broad affect," varies from culture to culture and even within a culture. Certain individuals may gesture prolifically while talking and display dramatic facial expressions in reaction to social situations or other stimuli. Others may show little outward response to social environments or interactions, expressing a narrow range of emotions.

There is some evidence that purposely changing affect can also bring about real changes in mood or feelings. Purposely making a face that is intended to display anger, for example, has been shown to actually increase the levels of anger and frustration. Although

KEY TERMS

Blunted affect—A lack of display of emotion or feelings, including monotone voice and expressionless face.

Labile affect—A display of frequently changing emotion or mood.

QUESTIONS TO ASK YOUR DOCTOR

- How do I know if I or my loved one is expressing a normal range of affect?
- What can I do if I feel my child is not displaying emotions normally?
- Can you recommend a psychologist or psychiatrist for an evaluation?

these changes are usually quite small, they suggest that affect is both a result of emotion and, in some cases, a cause of it.

People with psychological disorders may display variations in their affect. A "restricted" or "constricted" affect describes a mild restriction in the range or intensity of display of feelings. As the reduction in display of emotion becomes more severe, the term "blunted" affect may be applied. The absence of any exhibition of emotions is described as "flat" affect; the voice is monotone, the face expressionless, and the body immobile. "Labile" affect describes emotional instability or dramatic mood swings. When the outward display of emotion is out of context for the situation, such as laughter while describing pain or sadness, the affect is termed "inappropriate."

Resources

BOOKS

Balconi, Michela, ed. *Emotional Face Comprehension: Neuropsychological Perspectives.* New York: Nova Science, 2008.

Cole, Jonathan, and Henrietta Spalding. *The Invisible Smile: Living Without Facial Expression.* New York: Oxford University Press, 2009.

Mooney, Carla. *Mood Disorders.* San Diego, CA: Reference Point Press, 2010.

Reeve, Johnmarshall. *Understanding Motivation and Emotion,* 5th ed. Hoboken, NJ: John Wiley & Sons, 2009.

PERIODICALS

Bogaerts, Kathleen, et al. "Negative Affective Pictures Can Elicit Physical Symptoms in High Habitual Symptom Reporters." *Psychology and Health* 25, no. 6 (2010): 685–98.

Dowd, Haulie, Alex Zautra, and Michael Hogan. "Emotion, Stress, and Cardiovascular Response: An Experimental Test of Models of Positive and Negative Affect." *International Journal of Behavioral Medicine* 17, no. 3 (2010): 189–94.

ORGANIZATIONS

American Psychiatric Association, 1000 Wilson Blvd., Ste. 1825, Arlington, VA, 22209-3901, (703) 907-7300, apa@psych.org, http://www.psych.org.

American Psychological Association, 750 1st St. NE, Washington, DC, 20002-4242, (202) 336-5500; TDD/TTY: (202) 336-6123, (800) 374-2721, http://www.apa.org.

Tish Davidson, AM

Agoraphobia

Definition

Agoraphobia is an anxiety disorder characterized by intense fear related to being in situations from which escape might be difficult or embarrassing (e.g., being on a bus or train) or in which help might not be available in the event of a **panic attack** or panic symptoms. Panic is defined as extreme and unreasonable fear and anxiety.

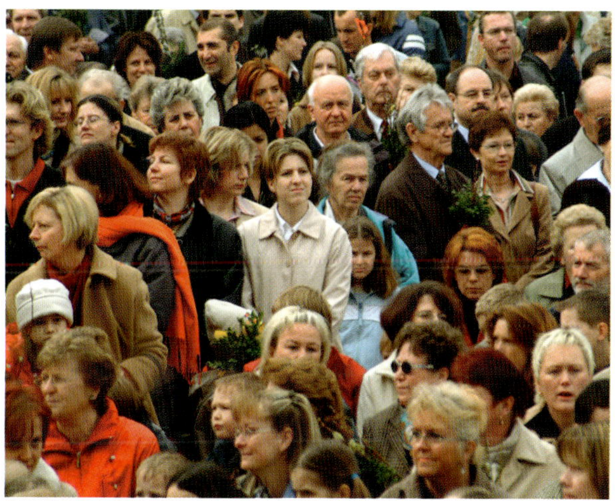

Agoraphobia is the fear of being trapped in a place where exiting may be difficult, such as in a crowd situation. *(© bildagentur-online.com/schneider/Alamy)*

Demographics

In general, phobias are the most common mental disorders in the U.S. population, affecting about 7% of adults, or 6.4 million Americans. Agoraphobia is one of the most common phobias, affecting between 2.7% and 5.8% of American adults. The onset of symptoms is most likely to occur between age 15 and age 35. The lifetime prevalence of agoraphobia is estimated at 5%–12%. Like most phobias, agoraphobia is two to four times more common in women than in men. The incidence of agoraphobia appears to be similar across racial and ethnic groups in the United States.

Description

The word "agoraphobia" comes from two Greek words that mean "marketplace" (agora) and "fear" (phobos). The anxiety associated with agoraphobia leads to avoidance of situations that involve being away from home alone, being in crowds, being on a bridge, or traveling by car or public transportation. Agoraphobia may intensify to the point that it interferes with a person's ability to take a job outside the home or to carry out such ordinary errands and activities as shopping for groceries or going out to a movie. According to the handbook used by mental health professionals to diagnose mental disorders, the ***Diagnostic and Statistical Manual of Mental Disorders***, fourth edition, text revision, also known as the *DSM-IV-TR,* individuals with agoraphobia typically are afraid of such symptoms as feeling dizzy, having an attack of diarrhea, fainting, or "going crazy."

The close association in agoraphobia between fear of being outside one's home and fear of having panic symptoms is reflected in the *DSM-IV-TR* classification of two separate disorders: **panic disorder** (PD) with agoraphobia and agoraphobia without PD. PD is characterized by sudden attacks of fear and panic. There may be no known reason for the occurrence of panic attacks; they are frequently triggered by fear-producing events or thoughts, such as driving or being in an elevator. PD is believed to be due to an abnormal activation of the body's hormonal system, causing a sudden fight-or-flight response.

People with agoraphobia appear to have two distinct types of anxiety: panic and the anticipatory anxiety related to fear of future panic attacks. The chief distinction between PD with agoraphobia and agoraphobia without PD is that individuals who are diagnosed with PD with agoraphobia meet all criteria for PD; in agoraphobia without PD, individuals are afraid of panic-like symptoms in public places, rather than full-blown panic attacks.

Proposed changes to the DSM for its fifth edition (*DSM-5*, 2013) include classifying agoraphobia as a separate and unique disorder, and removing it as a limiter for panic disorder. This revision recognizes that the two conditions may occur comorbidly, or at the same time, but considers them completely distinct.

Causes and symptoms

Causes

In the early 2010s, the causes of agoraphobia are viewed as complex and not completely understood. Research indicates several factors can contribute to the condition.

GENETIC. It has been known for some years that **anxiety disorders** tend to run in families. Recent research has confirmed earlier hypotheses that there is a genetic component to agoraphobia, and that it can be separated from susceptibility to PD. Researchers believe they have discovered a genetic locus on human chromosome 3 that governs a person's risk of developing agoraphobia. PD was found to be associated with two loci: one on human chromosome 1 and the other on chromosome 11q. Researchers concluded that agoraphobia and PD are both inheritable anxiety disorders that share some, but not all, of their genetic loci for susceptibility. If a person has a family member with agoraphobia, he or she is at higher risk of developing the disorder.

INNATE TEMPERAMENT. A number of researchers have pointed to inborn temperament as a broad vulnerability factor in the development of anxiety and mood disorders. In other words, a person's natural disposition or temperament may become a factor in developing a number of mood or anxiety disorders. Some people seem more sensitive throughout their lives to events, but upbringing and life history are also important factors in determining who will develop these disorders. Children who manifest what is known as behavioral inhibition (a group of behaviors that are displayed when the child is confronted with a new situation or unfamiliar people) in early infancy are at increased risk for developing more than one anxiety disorder in adult life, particularly if the inhibition remains over time. These behaviors include agitated movement (such as hyperextension), crying, and general irritability, followed by withdrawing, seeking comfort from a familiar person, and ceasing all action when noticing a new person or situation. Children of depressed or anxious parents are more likely to develop behavioral inhibition.

PHYSIOLOGICAL REACTIONS TO ILLNESS. Another factor in the development of PD and agoraphobia appears to be a history of respiratory disease. Some researchers have hypothesized that repeated episodes of respiratory disease can predispose a child to PD by making breathing difficult and lowering the threshold for feeling suffocated. It is also possible that respiratory diseases could generate fearful beliefs in the child's mind that would lead him or her to exaggerate the significance of respiratory symptoms.

LIFE EVENTS. About 42% of individuals diagnosed with agoraphobia report histories of real or feared separation from their parents or other caretakers in childhood. This statistic has been interpreted to mean that agoraphobia in adults is the aftermath of unresolved childhood separation anxiety. The fact that many individuals diagnosed with agoraphobia report that their first episode occurred after the death of a loved one, and the observation that other people with agoraphobia feel safe in going out as long as someone is with them, have been taken as supportive evidence of the separation anxiety hypothesis. However, there is little clinical research supporting this theory.

LEARNED BEHAVIOR. There are also theories about human learning that explain agoraphobia. It is thought that a person's initial experience of panic-like symptoms in a specific situation—for example, being alone in a subway station—may lead the person to associate physical symptoms of panic with all subway stations. Avoiding all subway stations would then reduce the level of the person's discomfort. Unfortunately, the avoidance strengthens the phobia because the person is unlikely to have the opportunity to test whether subway stations actually cause uncomfortable physical sensations. One of the most effective treatment modalities, exposure therapy, is based on the premise that phobias can be unlearned by reversing the pattern of avoidance.

SOCIAL FACTORS RELATED TO GENDER. Gender role socialization has been suggested as an explanation for the fact that the majority of individuals with agoraphobia are women. One form of this hypothesis maintains that some parents still teach girls to be fearful and timid about venturing out in public. Another version relates agoraphobia to the mother-daughter relationship, maintaining that mothers tend to give daughters mixed messages about becoming separate individuals. As a result, girls grow up with a more fragile sense of self and may stay within the physical boundaries of their home because they lack a firm sense of their internal psychological boundaries.

Symptoms

The symptoms of agoraphobia can be similar to those of specific phobia, and according to the *DSM-IV-TR*, **diagnosis** of agoraphobia "can be difficult because all of these conditions are characterized by avoidance of specific situations."

The symptoms of an episode of agoraphobia may include any or all of the following:

- trembling
- breaking out in sweat
- heart palpitations

KEY TERMS

Behavioral inhibition—A set of behaviors that appear in early infancy that are displayed when the child is confronted with a new situation or unfamiliar people. These behaviors include agitated movement, crying, and general irritability, followed by withdrawing, and seeking comfort from a familiar person. These behaviors are associated with an increased risk of social phobia and panic disorder in later life. Behavioral inhibition in children appears to be linked to anxiety and mood disorders in their parents.

Cognitive-behavioral therapy—A type of psychotherapy in which people learn to recognize and change negative and self-defeating patterns of thinking, feeling, and behavior.

Cognitive restructuring—An approach to psychotherapy that focuses on helping the individual examine distorted patterns of perceiving and thinking in order to change their emotional responses to people and situations.

Exposure therapy—A form of cognitive-behavioral therapy in which individuals with phobias are exposed to their feared objects or situations while accompanied by the therapist. The length of exposure is gradually increased until the association between the feared situation and the individual's experienced panic symptoms is no longer present.

Paresthesia—An abnormal sensation of tingling or "pins and needles." Paresthesia is a common panic-like symptom associated with agoraphobia.

Phobia—Irrational fear of places, things, or situations that lead to avoidance.

Specific phobia—A type of phobia in which the object or situation that arouses fear is clearly identifiable and limited. An older term for specific phobia is simple phobia.

- paresthesias (tingling or pins-and-needles sensations in the hands or feet)
- nausea
- fatigue
- rapid pulse or breathing rate
- a sense of impending doom

In most cases, the person with agoraphobia feels some relief from the symptoms after he or she has left the precipitating situation or returned home.

Diagnosis

The differential diagnosis of agoraphobia is described differently in *DSM-IV-TR* and in *International Classification of Diseases* (*ICD-10*), the European diagnostic manual. The *DSM-IV-TR* specifies that agoraphobia must be defined in relation to PD, and that the diagnoses of **specific phobias** and social phobias must be ruled out, a condition that will hold true for *DSM-5*. The *DSM-IV-TR* also specifies that the individual's symptoms must not be related to **substance abuse**; if they are related to a general medical condition, the individual must have excessive symptoms usually associated with that condition. For example, a person with Crohn's disease has realistic concerns about an attack of diarrhea in a public place and should not be diagnosed with agoraphobia unless the fear of losing bowel control is clearly exaggerated. The *DSM-IV-TR* description does not stipulate that a person must experience agoraphobia within a set number of circumstances in order to meet the diagnostic criteria.

In contrast, the European diagnostic manual primarily distinguishes between agoraphobia and delusional or obsessive disorders and depressive episodes. In addition, *ICD-10* specifies that the individual's anxiety must be restricted to or occur primarily within two out of four specific situations: in crowds, in public places, while traveling alone, or while traveling away from home. The primary area of agreement between the American and European diagnostic manuals is that both specify avoidance of the feared situation as a diagnostic criterion.

Diagnosis of agoraphobia is usually made by a physician or mental health professional after careful exclusion of other mental disorders and physical conditions or diseases that might be related to the individual's fears. Head injury, pneumonia, and withdrawal from certain medications can produce some of the symptoms of a panic attack. In addition, the physician may ask about caffeine intake as a possible dietary factor. Currently, there are no laboratory tests or diagnostic **imaging studies** that can be used to diagnose agoraphobia.

Furthermore, there are no widely used diagnostic interviews or screening instruments specifically for agoraphobia. Dutch researchers have developed a self-report questionnaire that promises to be helpful to doctors treating people with agoraphobia. The agoraphobic self-statements questionnaire (ASQ) is intended to evaluate thinking processes in individuals with agoraphobia, as distinct from their emotional responses.

Treatment

Treatment of agoraphobia usually consists of medication plus **cognitive-behavioral therapy** (CBT). Some individuals may be advised to cut down on or give up coffee or tea, as the caffeine in these beverages can contribute to their panic symptoms.

Drugs

Drugs that have been used with individuals diagnosed with agoraphobia include the benzodiazepine tranquilizers, the MAO inhibitors (**MAOIs**), tricyclic **antidepressants** (TCAs), and the **selective serotonin reuptake inhibitors** (**SSRIs**). In the past few years, the SSRIs have come to be regarded as the first-choice medication treatment because they have fewer side effects. The **benzodiazepines** have the disadvantage of increasing the symptoms of agoraphobia when they are withdrawn, as well as interfering with CBT. Benzodiazepines can decrease mental sharpness, making it difficult for individuals taking these drugs to focus in therapy sessions. The MAOIs require individuals to follow certain dietary guidelines; for example, patients must exclude aged cheeses, red wine, and certain types of beans. MAOIs are not widely prescribed. TCAs may produce such side effects as blurred vision, constipation, dry mouth, and drowsiness.

Psychotherapy

CBT is regarded as the most effective psychotherapeutic treatment for agoraphobia. The specific CBT approach that seems to work best with agoraphobia is exposure therapy. Exposure therapy is based on undoing the association that the individual originally formed between the panic symptoms and the feared situation. By being repeatedly exposed to the feared location or situation, the individual gradually learns that he or she is not in danger, and the anxiety symptoms fade away. The therapist typically explains the procedure of exposure therapy to the individual and reassures him or her that the exposure can be stopped at any time that his or her limits of toleration have been reached. The individual is then exposed in the course of a number of

QUESTIONS TO ASK YOUR DOCTOR

- Have possible physical causes of my panic symptoms been ruled out?
- Can you recommend a psychiatrist or psychologist?
- Should I reduce my caffeine consumption?
- Do you know of any support groups for individuals with agoraphobia in this area?
- How can I best provide support for my loved one with agoraphobia?

treatment sessions to the feared situation, usually for a slightly longer period each time. A typical course of exposure therapy takes about 12 weeks.

Another approach was used by German researchers who reported good results in treating individuals with agoraphobia with individual high-density exposure therapy. The individuals were exposed to their respective feared situations for an entire day for two to three weeks. One year later, the individuals had maintained their improvement.

Exposure treatment for agoraphobia may be combined with cognitive restructuring. This form of cognitive-behavioral therapy teaches individuals to observe the thoughts that they have in the feared situation, such as "I'll die if I have to go into that railroad station," and replace these thoughts with positive statements. In this example, the individual with agoraphobia might say to him- or herself, "I'll be just fine when I go in there to buy my ticket."

Although insight-oriented therapies have generally been considered relatively ineffective in treating agoraphobia, trials of brief **psychodynamic psychotherapy** in individuals with PD with agoraphobia indicate that this form of treatment may also be beneficial. One 2001 study of 21 individuals who participated in a 24-session course of treatment (twice weekly for 12 weeks) resulted in 16 experiencing remission of their agoraphobia, with no relapses at six-month follow-up. A larger 2007 study by the same group of researchers supported these initial findings.

Alternative and complementary treatments

Individuals diagnosed with agoraphobia have reported that alternative therapies, such as **hypnotherapy** and **music therapy**, were helpful in relieving symptoms of anxiety and panic. Ayurvedic medicine, **yoga**, religious practice, and guided imagery **meditation** have also been helpful.

Prognosis

The prognosis for untreated agoraphobia is considered poor by most European as well as most American physicians. The *DSM-IV-TR* remarks that little is known about the course of agoraphobia without PD but that anecdotal evidence indicates that it may persist for years with individuals becoming increasingly impaired. The *ICD-10* describes agoraphobia as "the most incapacitating of the phobic disorders," to the point that some individuals become completely housebound. With proper treatment, however, 90% of individuals diagnosed with agoraphobia can recover and resume a normal life.

Prevention

The **genetic factors** that appear to be implicated in the development of agoraphobia cannot be prevented. However, recent recognition of the link between anxiety and mood disorders in parents and vulnerability to phobic disorders in their children may help to identify children at risk and to develop appropriate preventive strategies for them.

Resources

BOOKS

Antony, Martin M., and Murray B. Stein. *Oxford Handbook of Anxiety and Related Disorders.* New York: Oxford University Press, 2009.

Leahy, Robert L. *Anxiety Free: Unravel Your Fears Before They Unravel You.* Carlsbad, CA: Hay House, 2009.

Starcevic, Vladan. *Anxiety Disorders in Adults: A Clinical Guide,* 2nd ed. New York: Oxford University Press, 2010.

PERIODICALS

Coelho, C. M., et al. "Specific Phobias in Older Adults: Characteristics and Differential Diagnosis." *International Psychogeriatrics* 22, no. 5 (August 2010): 702–11.

King, Anna, et al. "Nomophobia: The Mobile Phone in Panic Disorder with Agoraphobia: Reducing Phobias or Worsening of Dependence?" *Cognitive and Behavioral Neurology* 23, no. 1 (March 2010): 52–54.

Milrod, Barbara, et al. "A Pilot Open Trial of Brief Psychodynamic Psychotherapy for Panic Disorder." *Journal of Psychodynamic Therapy and Research* 10 (October 2001): 239–45.

———. "A Randomized Controlled Clinical Trial of Psychoanalytic Psychotherapy for Panic Disorder." *American Journal of Psychiatry* 164 (February 2007): 265–72.

Rosellini, Anthony, et al. "The Effects of Extraverted Temperament on Agoraphobia in Panic Disorder." *Journal of Abnormal Psychology* 119, no. 2 (May 2010): 420–26.

ORGANIZATIONS

American Academy of Child and Adolescent Psychiatry, 3615 Wisconsin Ave. NW, Washington, DC, 20016-3007, (202) 966-7300, Fax: (202) 966-2891, http://www.aacap.org.

American Psychiatric Association, 1000 Wilson Blvd., Ste. 1825, Arlington, VA, 22209-3901, (703) 907-7300, (888) 357-7924, apa@psych.org, http://www.psych.org.

American Psychological Association, 750 1st St. NE, Washington, DC, 20002-4242, (202) 336-5500, (800) 374-2721, apa@psych.org, http://www.apa.org.

Mental Health America, 2000 North Beauregard St., 6th Fl., Alexandria, VA, 22311, (703) 684-7722, (800) 969-6642, Fax: (703) 684-5968, http://www.nmha.org.

National Institute of Mental Health, 6001 Executive Blvd., Rm. 8184, MSC 9663, Bethesda, MD, 20892-9663, (301) 443-4513, (866) 615-6464, Fax: (301) 443-4279, nimhinfo@nimh.gov, http://www.nimh.nih.gov.

Rebecca Frey, Ph.D.
Ruth M. Wienclaw, Ph.D.
Tish Davidson, AM

AIMS *see* **Abnormal Involuntary Movement Scale**

Akineton *see* **Biperiden**

Alcoholics Anonymous *see* **Self-help groups**

Alcohol-induced persisting amnestic disorder *see* **Wernicke-Korsakoff syndrome**

Alcohol use and related disorders

Definition

The American Medical Association (AMA) defines alcoholism or alcohol (ethanol) dependence as "a primary, chronic disease with genetic, psychosocial, and environmental factors influencing its development and manifestations." Individuals with alcoholism develop emotional and physical dependence on alcoholic beverages, increased tolerance of the effects of alcohol, and withdrawal symptoms if alcohol consumption stops.

Demographics

The World Health Organization (WHO) estimates that about two billion people worldwide consume alcoholic beverages, and alcoholism is the most common **addiction** to a psychoactive substance. Alcohol addiction affects both sexes and all races and ethnicities. According to the 2009 National Survey on Drug Use and Health, 130.6 million Americans (51.9% of the population) reported having at least one alcoholic drink in the past 30 days. In addition, 59.6 million people (23.7%) reported having five or more drinks on the same occasion (**binge drinking**) and 17.1 million (6.8%) reported having five or more drinks on at least five occasions in the past 30 days (heavy alcohol use). According

Current, binge, and heavy alcohol use among persons aged 12 or older

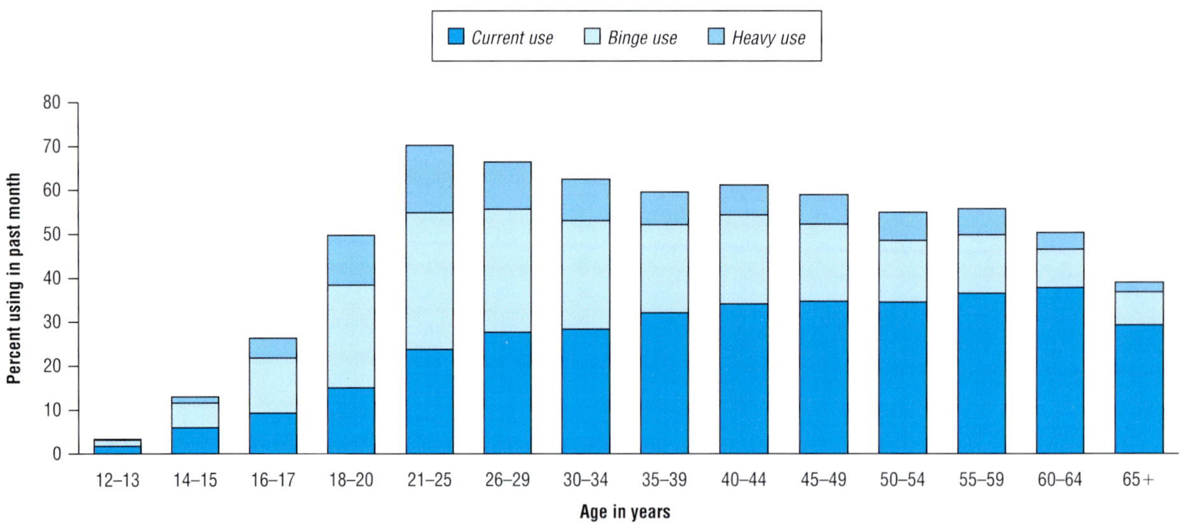

SOURCE: Substance Abuse and Mental Health Services Administration (SAMHSA), Office of Applied Studies, *Results from the 2009 National Survey on Drug Use and Health, Volume I: Summary of National Findings* (September 2010).

(Graph by PreMediaGlobal. © 2012 Cengage Learning.)

to a 2007 report from the Task Force on Community Preventive Services of the Centers for Disease Control and Prevention, excessive alcohol consumption in the United States is responsible for approximately 75,000 deaths per year, making it the third leading preventable cause of death. Alcohol addiction rates are highest among young adults aged 18–29 and lowest among those 65 and older.

Men are more than twice as likely to be alcohol dependent than women, but studies of female alcoholics indicate that women are at higher risk than men for serious health problems related to alcoholism. Because women tend to metabolize alcohol more slowly and have a lower percentage of body water and a higher percentage of body fat than men, they develop higher blood alcohol levels at a given amount of alcohol per pound of body weight. Thus, even though women typically begin to drink heavily at a later age than men, they often become dependent more rapidly. This relatively speedy progression of alcoholism in women is called telescoping. Smokers who are alcohol dependent are also much more likely to develop serious or fatal health problems associated with alcoholism.

Alcohol use by persons under age 21 is an important public health concern. In the United States, alcohol is the most commonly used and abused drug among youth. Although drinking under the age of 21 is against the law, people aged 12 to 20 years drink nearly 20% of all alcohol consumed in the United States. Much of this alcohol is consumed in the form of binge drinking.

At the other end of the age distribution, alcoholism among the elderly appears to be under-recognized. One-third of older persons with alcoholism develop the problem later in life, while the other two thirds grow older with the medical and psychosocial consequences of early onset alcoholism. Confusion and other signs of intoxication in an elderly person are also often misinterpreted as side effects of medications. In addition, the effects of alcohol may be increased in elderly patients because of physiological changes associated with aging. The elderly are at higher risk than younger people for becoming dependent on alcohol because their bodies do not absorb alcohol as efficiently; a 90-year-old who drinks the same amount of alcohol as a 20-year-old of the same sex will have a blood alcohol level 50% higher.

Description

Alcoholism is characterized by:

- a prolonged period of frequent, heavy alcohol use
- the inability to control drinking once it has begun
- physical dependence manifested by withdrawal symptoms when the individual stops using alcohol

Risk factors for alcoholism

- **Age:** Beginning drinking at a young age increases the risk of alcohol dependence.
- **Family history:** Children of alcohol-dependent parents are at greater risk of developing alcoholism.
- **Gender:** Males are more likely to become alcohol dependent than females, but women are at an increased risk of developing complications associated with alcoholism, such as liver disease.
- **Length of use:** Regular binge drinking over an extended period of time may result in alcohol dependence.
- **Mental health:** Persons afflicted by mental health disorders such as depression may be more likely to misuse alcohol or other substances.
- **Social and cultural factors:** Being surrounded by friends who routinely drink may increase a person's level of alcohol use. Alcohol consumption in the media may also influence personal drinking habits.

SOURCE: Mayo Clinic, "Alcoholism." Available online at: http://www.mayoclinic.com/health/alcoholism/DS00340 (accessed August 17, 2010).

(Table by PreMediaGlobal. Reproduced by permission of Gale, a part of Cengage Learning.)

- tolerance, or the need to use more and more alcohol to achieve the same effects
- a variety of social and/or legal problems arising from alcohol use

The effects of alcoholism are far reaching. Alcohol affects every body system, causing a wide range of health problems. Problems include poor **nutrition**; memory disorders; difficulty with balance and walking; liver disease (including cirrhosis and hepatitis); high blood pressure; muscle weakness (including the heart); heart rhythm disturbances; anemia; clotting disorders; decreased immunity to infections; gastrointestinal inflammation and irritation; acute and chronic problems with the pancreas; low blood sugar; high cholesterol; interference with fertility; increased risk of cancer of the liver, esophagus, and breast; weakened bones; sleep disturbances; anxiety; and **depression**. About 20% of adults admitted to the hospital (for any reason) are alcohol dependent.

On a personal level, alcohol abuse may lead to difficulties in marital and other relationships, domestic violence, **child abuse** or **neglect**, difficulty finding or keeping a job, impaired school or work performance, **homelessness**, or legal problems such as driving while intoxicated (DUI).

Risk factors

The risk of developing alcoholism has a definite genetic component. Studies have demonstrated that close relatives of people with alcoholism are more likely to become alcoholics themselves. This risk exists even for children adopted away from their biological families at birth and raised in a non-alcoholic adoptive family with no knowledge of their biological family's alcohol use. However, no specific gene for alcoholism has been found, and environmental factors (e.g., **stress**) and social factors (e.g., peer behavior, socializing patterns, and the availability of alcohol) are thought to play a role in whether a person becomes alcohol dependent. People who start drinking in their teens are at a much higher risk of developing alcohol dependency problems compared to people who start drinking at age 21 or older.

Causes and symptoms

Recently, some researchers have suggested that there are two distinct types of alcoholism. According to these researchers, type 1 alcoholism develops in adulthood, often in the early twenties. It is most often associated with the desire to relieve stress and anxiety and is not associated with any criminal or antisocial behavior. Type 2 alcoholism develops earlier, usually during the teenage years. Drinking is done primarily to get intoxicated. Type 2 alcoholism is associated with violence, destructiveness, and other criminal and antisocial behavior. Those who study alcoholism do not universally accept the distinction between these two types of alcoholism. Research continues in this area.

Causes

The cause of alcoholism is related to behavioral, biological, and **genetic factors**.

Behaviorally, alcohol consumption is related to internal or external feedback. Internal feedback is the internal state a person experiences during and after alcohol consumption. External feedback is made up of the cues that other people send the person when he or she drinks. Internal states pertaining to alcohol can include shame or hangover. Alcohol-related external cues can include reprimands, criticism, or encouragement. People may drink to the point of dependence because of peer pressure, for acceptance in a peer group, or because drinking is related to specific moods (e.g., easygoing, relaxed, calm, sociable) that are related to the formation of intimate relationships.

Biologically, repeated use of alcohol can impair the **brain** levels of a "pleasure" neurotransmitter called **dopamine**. **Neurotransmitters** are chemicals in the brain that pass impulses from one nerve cell to the next. When a person is dependent on alcohol, the areas of his or her brain that produce dopamine become depleted, and the individual can no longer enjoy the pleasures of everyday life—his or her brain chemistry is rearranged to depend on alcohol for transient euphoria (state of happiness).

Genetic studies have suggested that the GABA-A receptor alpha 2 subunit gene (GABRA2) and alcohol dehydrogenase (ADH) genes increase the risk for alcohol dependence. The GABRA genes are related to a receptor for gamma-amino butyric acid (GABA), a chemical in the central nervous system that is believed to mediate some of the physiological effects of alcohol. ADH is a chemical involved in the oxidation of alcohol in the body. These genes related to alcohol abuse can be passed from parents to their children.

The symptoms of alcoholism can be broken down into two major categories: symptoms of acute alcohol use, and symptoms of long-term alcohol use.

Immediate (acute) effects of alcohol use

Alcohol exerts a depressive effect on the brain. The blood-brain barrier does not prevent alcohol from entering the brain, so the brain alcohol level will quickly become equivalent to the blood alcohol level. In the brain, alcohol interacts with various neurotransmitters to alter nerve function. Alcohol's depressive effects result in difficulty walking, poor balance, slurring of speech, and generally poor coordination (accounting in part for the increased likelihood of injury). The affected person also may have impairment of peripheral vision. At higher alcohol levels, a person's breathing and heart rates may be slowed, and vomiting may occur (with a high risk of the vomit being breathed into the lungs, potentially resulting in aspiration pneumonia.) Still higher alcohol levels may result in coma and death.

Blood alcohol concentration (BAC) produces the following symptoms of central nervous system (CNS) depression at specific levels:

- 50 mg/dL: feelings of calm or mild drowsiness
- 50–150 mg/dL: loss of physical coordination. The legal BAC for drivers in most states is 80 mg/dL.
- 150–200 mg/dL: loss of mental faculties
- 300–400 mg/dL: unconsciousness
- Over 400 mg/dL: may be fatal

Effects of long-term (chronic) alcoholism

Long-term use of alcohol affects virtually every organ system of the body:

- Nervous system. An estimated 30%–40% of all men in their teens and twenties have experienced alcoholic blackout from drinking a large quantity of alcohol.

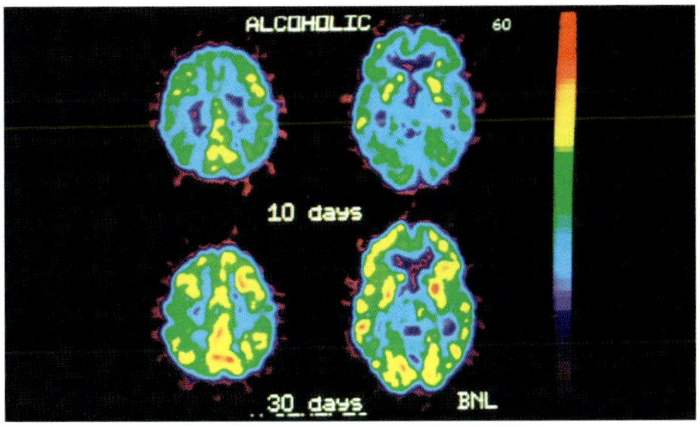

Colored positron emission tomography scans of a heavy drinker's brain during withdrawal from alcohol; the top shows brain activity after 10 days (yellow areas), and the bottom shows brain activity after 30 days without alcohol. *(© Pascal Goetgheluck/SPL/Photo Researchers, Inc.)*

This results in the loss of memory of the time surrounding the episode of drinking. Alcohol also causes sleep disturbances, so sleep quality is diminished. Numbness and tingling (paresthesia) may occur in the arms and legs. Wernicke's syndrome and Korsakoff's syndrome, which can occur together or separately, are due to the low thiamine (a B vitamin) levels found in many people with an alcohol dependence. Wernicke's syndrome results in disordered eye movements, very poor balance, and difficulty walking. Korsakoff's syndrome affects memory and prevents new learning from taking place.

- Gastrointestinal system. Alcohol-associated conditions include acid reflux, stomach ulcers, esophageal varices (enlarged blood vessels in the esophagus prone to bursting and hemorrhaging), diarrhea, pancreatitis, malnutrition, cirrhosis, and hepatitis.
- Blood. Alcohol may cause changes to all the types of blood cells. Red blood cells become abnormally large. White blood cells (important for fighting infections) decrease in number, resulting in a weakened immune system. This places alcohol-dependent individuals at increased risk for infections and may account in part for the increased risk of cancer faced by people with alcoholism. Platelets and blood clotting factors are affected, causing an increased risk of bleeding.
- Heart. Small amounts of alcohol cause a drop in blood pressure, but with increased consumption, alcohol raises blood pressure into a dangerous range (hypertension). High levels of fats circulating in the bloodstream increase the risk of heart disease. Heavy drinking results in an increase in heart size, weakening of the heart muscle, abnormal heart rhythms, a risk of blood clots forming within the chambers of the heart, and a greatly increased risk of stroke due to a blood clot entering the circulatory system and blocking a brain blood vessel.
- Reproductive system. Heavy drinking has a negative effect on fertility in both men and women. It decreases testicle and ovary size and interferes with both sperm and egg production.

People with chronic tolerance may appear to be sober (not intoxicated) even after consumption of alcohol quantities that could cause death in non-drinkers. People with alcohol dependence also develop alcohol withdrawal (a state of non-drinking) syndrome. The nervous system adapts to chronic ethanol exposure by increasing the activity of nerve-cell mechanisms that counteract alcohol's depressant effects. When drinking is abruptly reduced, the affected person develops disordered perceptions, **seizures**, and tremor (often accompanied by irritability, nausea, and vomiting). Tremor of the hands, known colloquially as "morning shakes," usually occurs in the morning due to overnight abstinence. The most serious manifestation of alcohol withdrawal syndrome is **delirium** tremens, which occurs in approximately 5% of people dependent on alcohol. Delirium tremens consists of agitation, disorientation, **insomnia**, hallucinations, **delusions**, intense sweating, fever, and increased heart rate (tachycardia). This state is a medical emergency because it can be fatal, and affected persons must be immediately hospitalized and treated with medications that control vital physiological functions.

In addition to physical symptoms, most persons with alcoholism have a history of psychiatric, occupational, financial, legal, or interpersonal problems. Alcohol misuse is the single most important predictor of violence between domestic partners as well as intergenerational violence within families. Since the early 1990s, most states have passed stricter laws against alcohol-impaired driving. These laws include such provisions as immediate license suspension for the first arrest for driving while impaired (DWI, also referred to as driving under the influence or DUI) and lowering the legal blood alcohol limit to 0.08 g/dL for adults and zero tolerance for drivers under age 21. Penalties for repeated DWI citations include prison sentences, house arrest with electronic monitoring, license plates that identify offending drivers, automobile confiscation, and putting a special ignition interlock on the offender's car. Deaths caused by a drunk driver may be punishable with prison time.

Alcoholism during pregnancy

A large body of evidence indicates that maternal alcohol consumption during pregnancy contributes adversely to a fetus's development. Abnormalities in infants and children associated with maternal alcohol consumption may include prenatal and postnatal physical retardation, neurological deficits (e.g., impaired attention control), intellectual disability, behavioral problems (e.g., impulsivity), skull or brain malformations, and facial malformations (e.g., a thin upper lip and elongated and flattened midface). These abnormalities, influenced by maternal alcohol consumption during pregnancy, are referred to as fetal alcohol effects (FAEs), or **fetal alcohol syndrome** (FAS) if a sufficient number of effects are apparent in the child.

FAS is the leading cause of intellectual disability in the United States. One to two of every 1,000 infants born in the United States are afflicted with FAS. Research studies that have followed infants with FAS and FAEs across time have found that many of these children continue to have cognitive difficulties (e.g., lower IQ scores, more learning problems, and poorer short-term memory functioning) and behavioral problems (e.g., high impulsivity and high activity level) into childhood and adolescence.

Diagnosis

The **diagnosis** of alcoholism is usually based on the patient's drinking history, a thorough physical examination, laboratory findings, and the results of psychodiagnostic assessment.

The ***Diagnostic and Statistical Manual of Mental Disorders***, 4th edition, text revision *(DSM-IV-TR)*, distinguishes between alcohol dependence and alcohol abuse largely on the basis of a compulsive element in alcohol dependence that is not present in alcohol abuse. Some psychiatrists differentiate between primary and secondary alcoholism. In primary alcoholism, the patient has no other major psychiatric diagnosis. In secondary alcoholism, the problem drinking is the patient's preferred way of medicating symptoms of another psychiatric disorder, such as depression, **schizophrenia**, **post-traumatic stress disorder**, or one of the **dissociative disorders**. Experts in other branches of medicine tend to emphasize patterns of, and attitudes toward, drinking in order to distinguish between nonproblematic use of alcohol and alcohol abuse or dependence.

The *DSM-IV-TR* requires three of the following traits to be present for a diagnosis of alcohol dependence:

- tolerance, meaning that a person becomes accustomed to consuming alcohol and must increase the amount in order to obtain the desired effect
- withdrawal, meaning that a person experiences unpleasant physical and psychological symptoms when he or she does not drink alcohol
- the tendency to drink more alcohol than one intends; being unable to avoid drinking or stop drinking once started
- devoting large blocks of time to acquiring and consuming alcohol
- unsuccessful attempts to reduce or stop alcohol use
- choosing to use alcohol at the expense of other important tasks or activities, such as work or family obligations
- drinking despite evidence of negative effects on one's physical and/or mental health

In order for a person to be diagnosed with alcohol abuse, one of the following four criteria must be met within a 12-month period. Because of drinking, a person repeatedly:

- fails to live up to his or her most important responsibilities at home, school, or work
- physically endangers himself or herself, or others (for example, by drinking and driving)
- gets into trouble with the law
- experiences difficulties in relationships or jobs

The proposed revisions for the *DSM-5* (5th edition) combine alcohol abuse and alcohol dependence and their respective diagnostic criteria into the single diagnosis of "alcohol use disorder."

Classification of alcohol use typically is based on the following five categories:

- Social drinkers. Individuals who use alcohol in minimal to moderate amounts to enhance meals or other social activities. They do not drink alone.
- Situational drinkers. These people rarely or never drink except during periods of stress. They are far more likely to drink alone than social drinkers.
- Problem drinkers. These individuals drink heavily, even when they are not under overwhelming stress. Their drinking causes some problems in their lives (e.g., DWI arrests), but they are capable of responding to warnings or advice from others.
- Binge drinkers. These drinkers uses alcohol in an out-of-control fashion at regular intervals. The binges may be planned. This pattern is a growing problem on many college campuses.
- Alcoholic drinkers. These are drinkers who have no control of any kind over their alcohol intake.

Other factors have complicated diagnosis of alcoholism in the United States, including: 1) the increasing

KEY TERMS

Acamprosate—Also called Campral, an anti-craving medication used since 1989 in Europe and since 2004 in the United States to reduce the craving for alcohol.

Alcohol Use Disorders Inventory Test (AUDIT)—A test for alcohol use developed by the World Health Organization (WHO). Its ten questions address three specific areas of drinking over a 12-month period: the amount and frequency of drinking, dependence upon alcohol, and problems that have been encountered due to drinking alcohol.

Behavioral therapy—Form of psychotherapy used to treat depression, anxiety disorders, phobias, and other forms of psychopathology.

Binge drinking—Consumption of five or more alcoholic drinks in a single, short period.

Blood-brain barrier—A network of blood vessels characterized by closely spaced cells that prevents many potentially toxic substances from penetrating the blood vessel walls to enter the brain. Alcohol is able to cross this barrier.

CAGE—A four-question assessment for the presence of alcoholism in both adults and children.

Detoxification—The phase of treatment during which a patient stops drinking and is monitored and cared for while he or she experiences withdrawal from alcohol.

Disulfiram—A medication that has been used since the late 1940s as part of a treatment plan for alcohol abuse. Disulfiram, which is sold under the trade name Antabuse, produces changes in the body's metabolism of alcohol that cause headaches, vomiting, and other unpleasant symptoms if the patient drinks even small amounts of alcohol.

Ethanol—The chemical name for beverage alcohol. It is also sometimes called ethyl alcohol or grain alcohol to distinguish it from isopropyl or rubbing alcohol.

Naltrexone—A medication originally developed to treat addiction to heroin or morphine that is also used to treat alcoholism. It works by reducing the craving for alcohol rather than by producing vomiting or other unpleasant reactions.

Neurotransmitter—One of a group of chemicals secreted by a nerve cell (neuron) to carry a chemical message to another nerve cell, often as a way of transmitting a nerve impulse. Examples of neurotransmitters include acetylcholine, dopamine, serotonin, and norepinephrine.

Relapse—A return to a disease state, after recovery appeared to be occurring. In alcoholism, relapse refers to a patient beginning to drink alcohol again after a period of avoiding alcohol.

Tolerance—A phenomenon during which a drinker becomes physically accustomed to a particular quantity of alcohol and requires ever-increasing quantities in order to obtain the same effects.

Withdrawal—Those signs and symptoms experienced by a person who has become physically dependent on a drug, experienced upon decreasing the drug's dosage or discontinuing its use.

tendency to combine alcohol with other drugs of abuse, sometimes called cross-addiction, and 2) the rising rates of alcohol abuse and dependence among children under 12 years of age.

Examination

A physician who suspects that a patient is abusing or dependent upon alcohol should perform a complete physical examination with appropriate laboratory tests, paying particular attention to liver function and the nervous system. Physical findings that suggest alcoholism include head injuries after age 18, broken bones after age 18, evidence of blackouts, frequent accidents or falls, puffy eyelids, flushed face, alcohol odor on the breath, shaky hands, slurred speech or tongue tremor, rapid involuntary eye movements (nystagmus), enlargement of the liver (hepatomegaly), hypertension, insomnia, and impotence (in males). Severe memory loss may point to advanced alcoholic damage to the central nervous system.

Tests

Several laboratory tests can be used to diagnose alcohol abuse and evaluate the presence of medical problems related to drinking. These tests include:

- Complete blood cell count (CBC). This test indicates the presence of anemia, which is common in alcoholics.
- Liver function tests. Tests for serum glutamine oxaloacetic transaminase (SGOT) and alkaline phosphatase can indicate alcohol-related injury to the liver. A high level (30 units) of gamma-glutamyltransferase (GGT) is a useful marker because it is found in 70% of heavy drinkers.

- Blood alcohol levels.
- Carbohydrate deficient transferrin (CDT) tests. This test should not be used as a screener, but it is useful in monitoring alcohol consumption in heavy drinkers (those who consume at least 60 grams of alcohol per day). When CDT is present, it indicates regular daily consumption of alcohol.

The results of these tests might not be accurate if the patient is abusing or is dependent on other substances.

Behavioral screening

Since some of the physical signs and symptoms of alcoholism can be produced by other drugs or disorders, screening tests can also help to determine the existence of a drinking problem. Several assessment instruments for alcoholism can either be self-administered or administered by a clinician. The CAGE test is a brief screening consisting of four questions:

- Have you ever felt the need to *cut down* on drinking?
- Have you ever felt *annoyed* by criticism of your drinking?
- Have you ever felt *guilty* about your drinking?
- Have you ever taken a morning *eye opener*?

One "yes" answer should raise a suspicion of alcohol abuse; two "yes" answers are considered a positive screen.

Other brief screens include the Alcohol Use Disorder Identification Test, or AUDIT, which also highlights some of the physical symptoms of alcohol abuse that doctors look for during a physical examination of the patient. The Michigan Alcoholism Screening Test, or MAST, is considered the diagnostic standard. It consists of 25 questions; a score of five or higher is considered to indicate alcohol dependency. The **Substance Abuse Subtle Screening Inventory** (SASSI), introduced in 1988, can be given in either group or individual settings in a paper-and-pencil or computerized format. The SASSI is available in an adolescent as well as an adult version from the SASSI Institute. Selection of an appropriate screen is important. Some brief screens may be inappropriate for widespread use in some subpopulations because of ethnic and gender bias.

Treatment

Traditional

Treatment of alcoholism often is a combination of inpatient and outpatient therapy, depending on the individual's alcohol history and physical condition. The person with alcoholism often resists the idea that he or she has an alcohol problem and needs to stop drinking. Treatment cannot be forced on adults unless imposed by a court of law. However, if the person is a danger to himself or herself or to others, immediate **hospitalization** may be possible without the individual's consent.

The first step in the treatment of alcoholism, called **detoxification**, involves helping the person stop drinking and ridding his or her body of the harmful (toxic) effects of alcohol. Because the person's brain and body have become accustomed to alcohol, he or she will most likely develop withdrawal symptoms and need to be supported through them. Withdrawal will be different for different individuals, depending on the severity of the alcoholism as measured by the quantity of alcohol ingested daily and the length of time the patient has been alcohol dependent.

Withdrawal symptoms can range from mild to life-threatening. Mild withdrawal symptoms include nausea, achiness, diarrhea, difficulty sleeping, sweatiness, anxiety, and trembling. This phase usually lasts no more than three to five days. More severe effects of withdrawal can include hallucinations in which a patient sees, hears, or feels something that is not actually present; seizures; an unbearable craving for more alcohol; confusion; fever; fast heart rate (tachycardia); high blood pressure (hypertension); and delirium (a fluctuating level of consciousness). Patients at the highest risk for the most severe symptoms of withdrawal are those with other medical problems, including malnutrition, liver disease, or Wernicke's syndrome. Severe withdrawal symptoms usually begin about three days after the individual's last drink and may last a variable number of days.

People going through mild withdrawal are monitored to make sure that more severe symptoms do not develop. Medications usually are unnecessary. Treatment of a patient suffering more severe effects of withdrawal may require sedative medications to relieve the discomfort of withdrawal and to avoid the potentially life-threatening complications of high blood pressure, fast heart rate, and seizures. Benzodiazepine drugs may be helpful in those patients experiencing hallucinations. If the patient vomits for an extended period, fluids may need to be given through a vein (intravenously, IV). Thiamine (a vitamin) is often included in the fluids, because thiamine levels are often very low in alcohol-dependent patients, and thiamine deficiency is responsible for the **Wernicke-Korsakoff syndrome**.

After the individual is no longer drinking and has passed through withdrawal, the next steps involve helping the individual avoid relapsing (the return to drinking). This phase of treatment is referred to as rehabilitation. It can continue for a lifetime. Many programs incorporate the family into rehabilitation therapy, because the family has likely been severely affected by the patient's drinking. Some therapists believe that family members, in an effort to deal with their loved one's drinking problem, develop patterns of behavior that unintentionally support or enable the patient's drinking. This situation is referred to as co-dependence. These patterns should be addressed in order to help successfully treat a person's alcoholism.

Sessions led by peers, in which recovering alcoholics meet regularly and provide support for each other's recoveries, are considered among the best methods of preventing a return to drinking. The best-known group following this model is Alcoholics Anonymous (AA), which uses a 12-step program and a buddy (sponsor) system to help people avoid drinking. The AA steps involve recognizing the destructive power that alcohol has held over the individual's life, looking to a higher power for help in overcoming the problem, reflecting on the ways in which the use of alcohol has hurt others and, if possible, making amends to those people. According to the **American Psychological Association** (APA), anyone, regardless of his or her religious beliefs or lack of religious beliefs, can benefit from participation in 12-step programs such as AA. The number of visits to 12-step **self-help groups** exceeds the number of visits to all mental health professionals combined.

Psychotherapy may also help affected persons to anticipate, understand, recognize, and prevent **relapse**. Along with **support groups**, behavioral therapy approaches typically include **cognitive-behavioral therapy** (CBT) and Motivated Enhancement Therapy (MET). CBT focuses on teaching alcoholics recognition and coping skills for craving states and high-risk situations that precipitate or trigger relapsing behaviors. MET can motivate patients to use their personal resources to initiate changes in behavior.

Drugs

Most drugs used to treat alcoholism fall into one of two groups: those that restrain the desire to drink by producing painful physical symptoms if the patient does drink, and those that appear to reduce the craving for alcohol directly. Several medications in the second category were originally developed to treat addiction to opioid substances (e.g., heroin and morphine). Drugs alone will not prevent relapse. They are most effective when used in conjunction with a self-help program and/or psychotherapy aimed at changing behavior.

ALCOHOL-SENSITIZING MEDICATIONS. The most commonly used alcohol-sensitizing agent is **disulfiram** (Antabuse), which has been used since the 1950s to deter alcoholics from drinking by the threat of a very unpleasant physical reaction if they do consume alcohol. The severity of the disulfiram/ethanol reaction (DER) depends on the amount of alcohol and disulfiram in the blood. A DER results when the drinker consumes alcohol because disulfiram inhibits the functioning of an enzyme called aldehyde dehydrogenase. This enzyme is needed to convert acetaldehyde, which is produced when the body begins to oxidize the alcohol. Without the aldehyde dehydrogenase, the patient's blood level of acetaldehyde rises, causing the symptoms associated with DER. The symptoms of the reaction include facial flushing, rapid heartbeat, palpitations, difficult breathing, lowered blood pressure, headaches, nausea, and vomiting. It was estimated that in 2008, 200,000 recovering alcoholics in the United States were taking disulfiram.

Another alcohol-sensitizing agent is calcium carbimide, which is marketed under the brand name Temposil. Calcium carbimide produces physiological reactions with alcohol, similar to those produced by disulfiram, but the onset of action is far more rapid, and the duration of action is much shorter.

ANTI-CRAVING MEDICATIONS. Another medication approved for the treatment of alcoholism is **naltrexone**, which appears to reduce the craving for alcohol. In addition, an injectable, long-acting form of naltrexone (**Vivitrol**) is available.

Acamprosate (Campral) is an anti-craving drug used in both the United States and Europe. It works by reducing the anxiety and insomnia that often occur when habitual drinkers become abstinent. Acamprosate has no psychotropic side effects nor any potential for abuse or dependence.

Other medications are available to treat the symptoms of alcohol withdrawal, such as shakiness, nausea, and sweating, that occur after someone with alcohol dependence stops drinking.

Clinical trial information is constantly updated by the National Institutes of Health, and the most recent information on alcoholism trials can be found at: http://clinicaltrials.gov/ct2/results?term=alcoholism

Alternative

Alternative treatments may be a helpful adjunct for the recovering alcoholic once the medical danger of withdrawal has passed. Stress is a drinking trigger for many people. Alternative therapies can help the recovering alcoholic eliminate or manage stress. These therapies include massage, **meditation**, **hypnotherapy**, **yoga**, and **acupuncture**.

Malnutrition caused by long-term alcohol use may be addressed by nutrition-oriented practitioners with careful attention to a healthy diet and the use of nutritional supplements such as vitamins A, B complex, and C, as well as certain fatty acids, amino acids, **zinc**, magnesium, and selenium.

Herbal treatments include milk thistle (*Silybum marianum*), which is thought to protect the liver against damage. Other herbs are thought to be helpful for the patient suffering through withdrawal. These include **lavender** (*Lavandula officinalis*), skullcap (*Scutellaria lateriflora*), **chamomile** (*Matricaria recutita*), peppermint (*Mentha piperita*), yarrow (*Achillea millefolium*), and **valerian** (*Valeriana officinalis*).

Prognosis

The prognosis for recovery from alcoholism varies widely. The usual course of the disorder is one of episodes of intoxication beginning in adolescence, with full-blown dependence by the mid-20s to mid-30s. The most common pattern is one of periodic attempts at abstinence alternating with relapses into uncontrolled drinking. On the other hand, it is thought that as many as 20% of persons diagnosed as alcohol dependent achieve long-term sobriety even without medical treatment.

It is difficult to compare the outcomes of the various treatment approaches to alcoholism, in part because their definitions of "success" vary. Some researchers count only total abstinence from alcohol as a successful outcome, while others regard curtailed drinking and better social adjustment as indicators of success. The role of genetic factors in the prognosis is still disputed. Available evidence suggests that such factors as the presence of a spouse, partner, or close friend in the alcoholic's life, or religious commitment can outweigh genetic vulnerability to the disorder.

Recovery from alcoholism is a lifelong process. The potential for relapse remains present and must be acknowledged and respected. Many individuals stop drinking and then relapse multiple times before attaining extended periods of sobriety. Statistics suggest that, among middle-class alcohol-dependent individuals in stable financial and family situations who have undergone treatment, 60% or more successfully stop drinking for at least one year.

Prevention

Prevention must begin at a young age, since the first instance of intoxication usually occurs during the teenage years. It is particularly important that teenagers who are at high risk for alcoholism—those with a family history of alcoholism, early or frequent use of alcohol, a tendency to drink to drunkenness, alcohol use that interferes with school work, a poor family environment, or a history of domestic violence—receive education about alcohol and its long-term effects. How this is best achieved, without alienating these young people and thus losing their attention, is the subject of continuing debate and study.

QUESTIONS TO ASK YOUR DOCTOR

- Can alcoholism be treated without medications?
- How can I best understand the factors that led to my alcoholism?
- Will I recover?
- Are lifestyle changes required?
- Are there associated conditions that also require treatment?

Resources

BOOKS

Benton, Sarah Allen. *Understanding the High-Functioning Alcoholic: Professional Views and Personal Insights.* Westport, CT: Praeger Publishers, 2009.

The Healing Project. *Voices of Alcoholism: The Healing Companion: Stories for Courage, Comfort and Strength.* Brooklyn, NY: LaChance Publishing, 2008.

Hedblom, Jack H. *Last Call: Alcoholism and Recovery.* Baltimore, MD: The Johns Hopkins University Press, 2007.

Jay, Jeff, and Debra Jay. *Love First: A Family's Guide to Intervention.* Center City, MN: Hazelden, 2008.

Maltzman, Irving. *Alcoholism: Its Treatments and Mistreatments.* Hackensack, NJ: World Scientific Publishing Co., 2008.

Tracy, Sarah W. *Alcoholism in America: From Reconstruction to Prohibition.* Baltimore, MD: The Johns Hopkins University Press, 2007.

OTHER

Substance Abuse and Mental Health Services Administration. "Faces of Change: Do I Have a Problem with Alcohol or Drugs?" U.S. Department of Health and Human Services. http://www.kap.samhsa.gov/products/brochures/pdfs/TIP35.pdf (accessed November 14, 2011).

WEBSITES

Centers for Disease Control and Prevention. "Fetal Alcohol Spectrum Disorders." http://www.cdc.gov/ncbddd/fasd/index.html (accessed November 14, 2011).

MedlinePlus. "Alcohol." U.S. National Library of Medicine, National Institutes of Health. http://www.nlm.nih.gov/medlineplus/alcohol.html (accessed November 14, 2011).

———. "Alcoholism." U.S. National Library of Medicine, National Institutes of Health. http://www.nlm.nih.gov/medlineplus/alcoholism.html (accessed November 14, 2011).

Thompson, Warren, R. Gregory Lande, and Raj K. Kalapatapu. "Alcoholism." Medscape Reference. June 9, 2011. http://emedicine.medscape.com/article/285913-overview (accessed November 14, 2011).

ORGANIZATIONS

Al-Anon/Alateen, 1600 Corporate Landing Parkway, Virginia Beach, VA, 23454-5617, (888) 4AL-ANON (425-2666), Fax: (757) 563-1655, wso@al-anon.org, http://www.al-anon.alateen.org.

Alcoholics Anonymous, http://www.aa.org, New York, NY, 10163, (212) 870-3400, http://www.aa.org.

National Council on Alcoholism and Drug Dependence, Inc., 244 East 58th Street 4th Floor, New York, NY, 10022, (212) 269-7797, 24-hour help line: (800) NCA-CALL Fax: (212) 269-7510, national@mcadd.org, http://www.ncadd.org.

National Institute on Alcohol Abuse and Alcoholism (NIAAA), 5635 Fishers Lane, MSC 9304, Bethesda, MD, 20892-9304, (301) 443-3860, http://www.niaaa.nih.gov.

Rebecca J. Frey, PhD
Joan Schonbeck, RN
Tish Davidson, AM

Alprazolam

Definition

Alprazolam is a tranquilizer. It belongs to a group of drugs called **benzodiazepines**. In the United States, alprazolam is sold under the brand name Xanax.

Purpose

The U.S. Food and Drug Administration (FDA) has approved alprazolam to treat anxiety, **panic disorder**, and anxiety associated with **depression**. Occasionally, alprazolam is used to treat alcohol withdrawal, but it is not FDA approved for this use and is not normally the first drug given when treating alcohol withdrawal symptoms.

Description

Alprazolam is classified as a benzodiazepine. Benzodiazepines are sedative-hypnotic drugs that help to relieve nervousness, tension, and other anxiety symptoms by slowing the central nervous system. To do this, they block the effects of a specific chemical involved in the transmission of nerve impulses in the **brain**, decreasing the excitement level of the nerve cells.

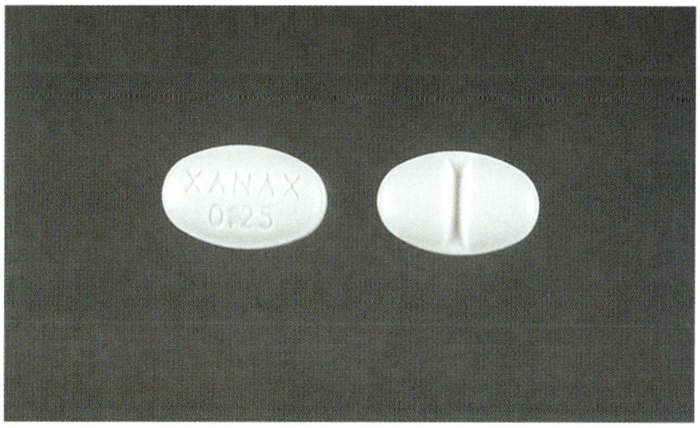

Xanax (alprazolam), 25 mg. *(U.S. Drug Enforcement Administration)*

All benzodiazepines cause sedation, including drowsiness and reduced mental alertness. However, one benefit of alprazolam is that it causes somewhat less drowsiness than many other benzodiazepine drugs.

Alprazolam comes in 0.25 mg, 0.5 mg, 1 mg and 2 mg tablets, and 1 mg/mL solution.

Recommended dosage

The recommended initial adult dose for anxiety is 0.25–0.5 mg taken three times daily. This dosage may be increased every three to four days to a maximum total of 4 mg daily. Dosage for alcohol withdrawal usually totals from 2–2.5 mg daily given in several small doses throughout the day.

The starting dose for treating panic disorder is 0.5 mg three times daily. This dosage may be increased every three to four days until the total daily dosage ranges from 2–10 mg. The total amount should be divided in at least three even daily doses. Average doses for anxiety associated with depression range from 2.5–3 mg daily, divided into even doses.

Precautions

Alprazolam should not be used by patients who are pregnant, have narrow angle glaucoma, take ketoconazole or itraconazole, or are allergic to this or any other benzodiazepine drug. The dose of alprazolam must be carefully regulated and individualized in the elderly (over age 60), people with liver or kidney disease, and those taking other medications used to treat mental disorders.

Because alprazolam is a nervous system and respiratory depressant, it should not be taken with other depressants, such as alcohol, other **sedatives**, sleeping pills, or tranquilizers. People taking this drug should not drive, operate dangerous machinery, or engage in hazardous activities that require mental alertness at least until they see how the drug affects them. Some patients taking alprazolam have engaged in "sleep driving," or operating a vehicle while sleeping, with no recollection of the event.

Alprazolam should be used under close physician supervision in patients with a history of **substance abuse**. Like other benzodiazepines, alprazolam can be habit forming. Risk and severity of dependence appears greater in patients taking doses larger than 4 mg daily. However, smaller doses may cause dependence if alprazolam is taken longer than 12 weeks. After four months, patients should be evaluated to see if they need to continue taking alprazolam.

Suddenly discontinuing alprazolam after several weeks may cause uncomfortable symptoms of withdrawal. Withdrawal symptoms in people who have taken alprazolam three months or longer may include **seizures**, anxiety, nervousness, and headache. Patients should discuss with their doctor how to gradually discontinue alprazolam use to avoid such symptoms.

Side effects

The most common side effects of alprazolam include sedation, dizziness, drowsiness, **insomnia**, and nervousness. The intensity of these side effects usually declines gradually and subsides in about eight weeks. A drop in blood pressure and an increase in heart rate may also occur in people who are taking alprazolam.

Decreased sex drive, menstrual disorders, and both weight gain and weight loss have been associated with use of alprazolam. People who experience the side effects of stomach upset, nausea, vomiting, and dry mouth should eat frequent, small meals and/or chew sugarless gum. Alprazolam has been associated with both diarrhea and constipation, as well as tremor, muscle cramps, vision disturbances, rash, and **amnesia** or memory loss.

Interactions

Alprazolam interacts with a long list of other medications. Anyone starting this drug should review the other medications they are taking with their physician and pharmacist for possible interactions. The most severe interactions occur with antifungal medications, such as ketoconazole, itraconazole, and fluconazole. These are associated with alprazolam toxicity (excessive sedation, **fatigue**, slurred speech, slowed reactions, and other types of psychomotor impairment).

Patients taking alprazolam should avoid eating grapefruit or drinking grapefruit juice due to potential adverse side effects.

Estrogens (female hormones), erythromycin (an antibiotic), **fluoxetine** (Prozac, Sarafem), cimetidine (Tagamet), isoniazid, and **disulfiram** (Antabuse) can increase the effects of alprazolam. Carbamazepine can make alprazolam less effective. When alprazolam is combined with other sedative drugs (tranquilizers, sleeping pills) or alcohol, its depressants effects are more intense. These combinations should be avoided.

KEY TERMS

Benzodiazepines—A group of central nervous system depressants used to relieve anxiety or to induce sleep.

Glaucoma—A group of eye diseases characterized by increased pressure within the eye significant enough to damage eye tissue and structures. If untreated, glaucoma results in blindness.

Resources

BOOKS

Kay, Jerald, Allan Tasman, and Jeffrey A. Lieberman. *Psychiatry: Behavioral Science and Clinical Essentials.* Philadelphia: W.B. Saunders Company, 2000.

Lacy, Charles F. *Drug Information Handbook with International Trade Names Index.* Hudson, OH: Lexi-Comp, Inc. 2011.

Pharmacia and Upjohn Company Staff. *Product Information: Xanax, Alprazolam.* Kalamazoo, MI: Pharmacia and Upjohn Company, 2011.

PERIODICALS

Yasui, N., et al. "Effects of Repeated Ingestion of Grapefruit Juice on the Single and Multiple Oral-Dose Pharmacokinetics and Pharmacodynamics of Alprazolam." *Psychopharmacology* 150, no. 2 (2000): 185–90.

WEBSITES

PubMed Health. "Alprazolam." U.S. National Library of Medicine. http://www.ncbi.nlm.nih.gov/pubmedhealth/PMH0000807 (accessed November 14, 2011).

Ajna Hamidovic, Pharm.D.

Alzheimer's disease

Definition

Alzheimer's disease (AD) is the most common form of **dementia** in those aged 65 and older. It is an irreversible and incurable progressive neurological disease caused by the degeneration and eventual death of a large number of neurons (nerve cells) in several areas of the **brain**, accompanied by diminished brain size. AD usually occurs in old age and begins with short-term memory loss. This is followed by the slow progressive loss of memory and cognitive and intellectual functions, leading to the deterioration of physical functioning and incapacitation.

Demographics

Alzheimer's disease is the most common degenerative brain disorder. It accounts for 50%–70% of all cases of dementia in the United States and for about 75% of all dementias in people over age 65. An estimated 5.1 million Americans have AD. The exact number is difficult to determine since AD is often misdiagnosed or not diagnosed until the disease is in its later stages. About 350,000 new cases of Alzheimer's disease are diagnosed each year in the United States, and approximately 65,800 people die from AD each year. It is the fourth-leading cause of death in American adults after heart disease, cancer, and **stroke**.

Alzheimer's rarely occurs before the age of 60. Early-onset AD, affecting people in their 30s, 40s, and 50s, accounts for only about 5% of total cases. About 3%–5% of men and women aged 65–74 have AD. About 20% of persons between 75 and 84 and nearly half of those over 85 have the disease. Slightly more women than men develop AD, which may be because women tend to live longer. About half of all nursing home patients in the United States have AD.

Alzheimer's disease appears to be more prevalent among African Americans, with estimates ranging from 14% to almost 100% higher than among Caucasian Americans. One study reported that the onset of AD in Hispanics occurs at an age that is, on average, five years younger than its onset in Caucasians.

The incidence of Alzheimer's in other developed countries is about the same as in the United States. In countries such as Japan that have a rapidly aging population with a higher percentage of people over 65, the incidence of AD is even higher than in the United States. In developing countries, the percentage of the

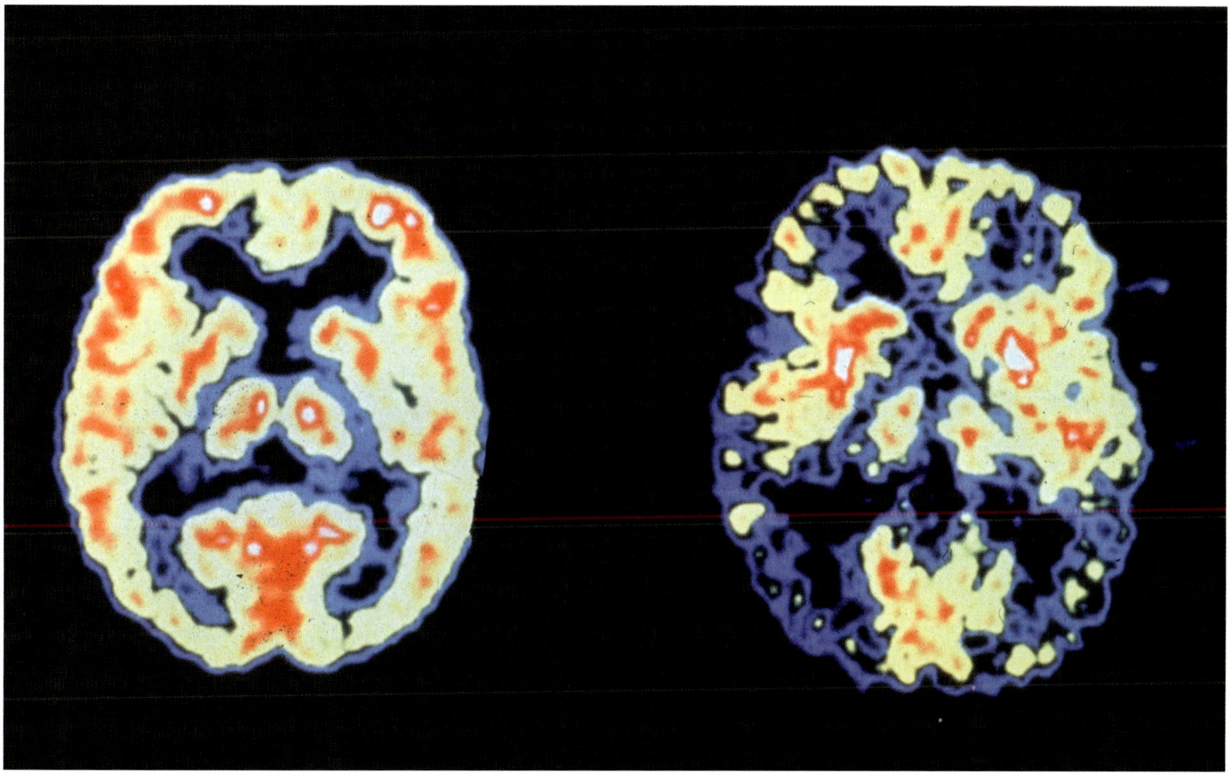

Colored positron emission tomography scans comparing a healthy brain (left) to a brain affected by Alzheimer's disease (yellow areas indicate brain activity). *(© Photo Researchers, Inc.)*

population with AD is lower because fewer people live to age 65. However, more than 50% of people with AD live in developing countries, and by 2025 this rate is expected to be above 70%.

The number of people afflicted with Alzheimer's is expected to more than triple by 2050, as the population ages and more people live longer. The number may be even higher than predicted, since recent research suggests that mild cognitive impairment observed in many elderly people may be early-stage Alzheimer's disease.

Description

In 1906 Alois Alzheimer (1864–1915), a German **psychiatrist** and neuroanatomist, was studying slides prepared from the brain of a 51-year-old woman, known as Frau D., who had died after suffering from dementia for several years. Her symptoms did not fit those of any brain disorder known at the time. Alzheimer found abnormal clumps of material—now called beta-amyloid plaques—and tangled bundles of fibers—neurofibrillary tangles—in Frau D.'s brain tissue. These plaques and tangles, found upon brain autopsy, constitute the diagnostic signature of Alzheimer's disease.

The plaques, sometimes called senile plaques, are sticky clumps or clusters of dead and dying neurons and other cellular debris surrounding insoluble deposits of beta-amyloid. The latter are fragments of a larger protein called amyloid precursor protein (APP) that was not processed properly. The plaques are located in between neurons and are believed to interfere with normal communication between neurons, eventually causing the nerve cells to die. The tangles are accumulations of twisted fragments of tau proteins inside neurons. Tau proteins normally bind and stabilize neurons. When tau proteins are damaged by the addition of phosphorus, a process called hyperphosphorylation, they form filaments that twist around each other to form neurofibrillary tangles that can no longer stabilize the neurons.

Increased beta-amyloid may cause the formation of neurofibrillary tangles. However, it is not known whether the plaques and tangles cause AD or are the result of it. Plaques and tangles occur as part of the normal aging process but are far less prevalent in normal brains than in the brains of AD patients. Because dementia had been associated with the elderly and Frau D. had been middle-aged, her disease was named presenile dementia and was thought to be a very rare disorder. It was not until the early 1950s that researchers at St. Elizabeth's Hospital in Washington, DC, came to realize that Alzheimer's disease is the single most common cause of dementia.

Scientists have since found other changes in the brains of AD patients. Connections between nerve cells are disrupted and nerve cells die in areas of the brain that are vital for memory and learning, including the hippocampus, which is a structure deep in the brain that controls short-term memory. Later, AD affects the cerebral cortex, particularly the areas responsible for language and reasoning. Eventually many areas of the brain become involved and atrophied (shrunken and dysfunctional).

The levels of the brain **neurotransmitters** norepinephrine, **serotonin**, and acetylcholine are also lower in AD. These chemicals transmit signals across the synapses, or gaps, between nerve cells. Many of the behavioral and psychiatric problems associated with AD are thought to result from low levels of these neurotransmitters. Acetylcholine and norepinephrine are important for many processes in the body, including digestion, blood vessel dilation and constriction, and regulation of heartbeat.

Public awareness of AD increased significantly when Ronald Reagan (1911–2004), the 40th president of the United States (1981–89), was diagnosed with the disease in 1994. He died from complications of AD in 2004 at the age of 93. Because of the growing numbers of people who are affected by AD, their increasing life expectancy, and the direct and indirect costs of their care, Alzheimer's disease is now considered to be a major public health concern.

Alzheimer's disease places severe emotional and financial burdens on patients and their families. In 2007, the annual cost of caring for a patient with AD was estimated at $18,400 for mild or early-stage conditions and at $36,100 for a patient with severe AD. The total annual cost of caring for AD patients in the United States was estimated to be at least $100 billion, including both direct patient costs and indirect costs, such as time lost from work by caregivers. On average, Medicare pays more than three times as much for the healthcare of a beneficiary with AD compared to a beneficiary without AD.

Risk factors

The most significant risk factor for AD is advancing age. The risk of developing AD begins to rise after age 65 and rises sharply after age 75. There are various other possible risk factors:

- About 25% of AD cases are considered to be familial Alzheimer's disease (FAD), defined as having symptoms of AD in at least three generations of a single family. About 2%–5% of all AD cases are familial early-onset FAD of one of three types (AD1, AD3, and

AD4), in which the disease develops before the age of 60—usually between the ages of 40 and 50, but sometimes as early as age 30. First-degree relatives of AD patients may have as much as a 20% lifetime risk of being affected by the disease. The risk to immediate relatives increases as more family members develop the disease. The remaining 75% of cases are sporadic Alzheimer's disease (SAD) with no clear family history.
- African American and Caribbean Hispanics who have mutations in a particular gene are at a higher than normal risk for AD, particularly if they have a family history of the disease.
- A family history of Parkinson's disease is a risk factor for AD.
- There is some evidence that neuronal damage from small strokes may be linked to AD.
- Studies have found a clear correlation between low educational and occupational attainment (employment in jobs that are not mentally challenging) and an increased risk for AD. Taking on less challenging rather than more challenging jobs as one grows older is also associated with a higher risk for AD.
- Studies on special breeds of genetically engineered (transgenic) mice have suggested high blood cholesterol levels may increase the rate of plaque deposition.
- Researchers suspect that a high-cholesterol, high-fat diet may increase the risk of AD. However, studies have not found cholesterol-lowering drugs to have any effect on AD onset.
- High systolic blood pressure combined with high blood cholesterol levels increases the risk of AD by three-to-four times.
- Obesity is a risk factor for AD.
- Mild cognitive impairment (MCI), which is characterized primarily by memory loss while other cognitive functions remain intact, increases the risk of AD. About 12% of people with MCI develop Alzheimer's disease each year. About 40% of people diagnosed with MCI have clear symptoms of AD after four years.
- High levels of an amino acid called homocysteine may be a risk factor for late-onset AD.
- Symptoms of AD may develop faster in people who have had a head trauma or hypothyroidism.
- Down syndrome patients over the age of 40 all develop the brain cell changes that are characteristic of Alzheimer's disease. Down syndrome–associated AD accounts for less than 1% of Alzheimer's cases.

Various environmental factors have been suspected of contributing to the development of AD. However, epidemiological studies have not borne out any links between AD and factors such as pollutants in drinking water, aluminum from commercial products, and metal dental fillings. Although higher-than-average levels of aluminum have been found in the brains of patients with AD, it now appears that this is a result rather than a cause of the disease.

Causes and symptoms

In most cases the cause of AD is unknown. It is most likely caused by a combination of genetic and environmental factors. Viral, immunological, and/or biochemical etiologies have also been proposed. Some studies link AD with an inability of the brain to metabolize sugar and use insulin effectively. Genetics almost certainly plays a role, even in sporadic AD. Brain inflammation and restriction of blood flow to the brain may play a role in the development of beta-amyloid plaques and neurofibrillary tangles. Highly reactive molecules called free radicals damage all types of cells through oxidative processes, especially brain cells, which have lower levels of protective antioxidants.

AD symptoms can be grouped into three categories: cognitive deficits or losses in brain function related to memory and learning, behavioral and psychiatric symptoms of dementia (BPSD), and difficulties with activities of daily life (ADL). For most of the twentieth century, studies of AD patients focused on cognitive symptoms. It was not until the 1980s and 1990s that researchers began to examine behavioral and psychiatric symptoms more closely.

There are four major cognitive deficits associated with AD:

- Amnesia (memory impairment). Patients may not be able to recall past events or form new memories, or both. A loss of the sense of time is also classified as amnesia.
- Aphasia (loss of language). Patients may not remember the names of objects and use words such as "thing" or "it" instead. They may echo what other people say or repeat a word or phrase over and over. Sometimes patients lose all language except curses.
- Apraxia (inability to perform voluntary movements). Patients with apraxia may have trouble putting on a hospital gown or brushing their teeth.
- Agnosia (inability to recognize familiar people and places). *Agnosia* comes from the Greek word meaning "to not know." Patients with agnosia may even fail to recognize their own face in a mirror.

Symptoms associated with BPSD include:

- Depression. Depression in AD is believed to result, at least in part, from lowered production of serotonin.

- Delusions (a false belief that is maintained even in the presence of evidence to the contrary). For example, AD patients may believe that someone is stealing from them when they cannot remember where they put something.
- Wandering. This behavior may result from becoming disoriented or lost, but sometimes AD patients wander for no apparent reason.
- Hallucinations (sensory experiences that seem real). Although hallucinations can affect any of the senses, most are visual or auditory. For example, AD patients may say that they see Martians in the corner of the room or hear the voices of their long-dead parents. Like delusions, hallucinations are believed to be related to the deterioration of brain tissue. However, sometimes they are caused by medications.
- Aggression (hitting, shoving, pushing, or threatening behavior)
- Agitation. Emotionally excited behavior (e.g., screaming, shouting, cursing, pacing, or fidgeting) that is disruptive or unsafe may result from brain tissue damage or be a symptom of depression. It is thought that the emotional overreactions of AD patients are related to destruction of neurons in the amygdala of the brain.

Personal-care symptoms (ADL) include difficulties with the following:

- eating, including simple cooking and washing dishes
- shopping for groceries and other necessities
- bathing, showering, or shaving
- grooming and dressing in clothing appropriate for the weather and activity
- toileting
- other aspects of personal hygiene such as teeth brushing, denture cleaning, or washing hair

Stages of AD

Although the rate of AD progression and specific symptoms vary with the individual, the general course of the progression is fairly consistent. Early-onset AD often progresses faster than the more common late-onset type. AD is generally considered to have seven stages:

- Stage 1: no decline in function yet noted. This includes individuals who may carry predictive gene mutations but have no symptoms and those who will develop AD by other mechanisms.
- Stage 2: generally normal functioning. The individual is aware of a subtle cognitive decline.
- Stage 3: early Alzheimer's disease. Patients have difficulty performing complex tasks that require cognitive skills.
- Stage 4: mild Alzheimer's disease. Patients require assistance with tasks such as paying bills or balancing a checkbook.
- Stage 5: moderate Alzheimer's disease. Patients require assistance in making everyday personal decisions such as choosing appropriate clothing or ordering from a restaurant menu.
- Stage 6: moderately severe Alzheimer's disease. Patients require assistance dressing, bathing, and using the toilet, and may have urinary and/or bowel incontinence.
- Stage 7: severe Alzheimer's disease. Vocabulary shrinks to a few words, followed by little or no verbal communication. The ability to walk is lost, followed by an inability to maintain a sitting posture in a chair. Eventually the patient experiences a profound lack of purposeful muscle control, is totally dependent for care, and cannot smile or hold up his or her head.

AD usually starts slowly with a very gradual decline that is termed "insidious." Some people are unaware of any impairment, blaming their forgetfulness on old age or "senior moments." Often the earliest symptoms are recognized only in hindsight by a friend or family member. Furthermore, since the present generation at risk for AD is the first in history to understand the implications of the disease, there are very powerful emotional reasons for attributing early signs of AD to normal aging, job **stress**, adjusting to retirement, and other less troubling factors. However, the insidious nature of AD onset is a characteristic that helps physicians to distinguish it from other causes of dementia, including **vascular dementia**.

Warning signs and symptoms

Key warning signs of early-stage AD include:

- repeatedly asking the same question
- repeatedly telling the same story, word for word
- memory loss that affects job performance
- loss of initiative
- inability to pay bills or balance a checkbook
- misplacing commonly used personal or household objects
- difficulty performing familiar tasks such as cooking, making repairs, or playing games such as cards or checkers
- poor or decreased judgment
- problems with abstract thinking
- getting lost in familiar surroundings
- relying on others to make decisions or answer questions
- disorientation of time and place

- problems with language
- mood or behavior changes
- personality changes
- neglecting personal hygiene—for example, not bathing or changing clothes regularly

The first symptoms of early-stage AD usually include forgetfulness, short-term memory loss, temporary episodes of spatial disorientation, groping for words, minor problems with arithmetic, and small errors in judgment, often accompanied by some anxiety, agitation, mild **depression**, and withdrawal. The patient may light the stove under a saucepan while forgetting to add the food or water, but most ADL are unaffected. Some patients can continue to operate a motor vehicle safely, although many people with early-stage AD voluntarily give up driving.

Everyone has occasional memory lapses that do not signify any change in cognitive function. Early-stage AD may begin with routine memory lapses—forgetting where one left the car keys—but progresses to more profound or disturbing lapses, such as forgetting that one has a car. Some AD patients are unaware that their memory is failing. Other patients are keenly aware of their memory loss and may become anxious and frustrated. Becoming lost or disoriented on a walk around the neighborhood becomes more likely as the disease progresses. Individuals with AD may forget the names of family members or forget what was said at the beginning of a sentence by the time they hear the end. Although the progression of memory loss varies, it eventually begins to interfere with daily activities.

Middle stage Alzheimer's typically begins two to three years after the initial onset. Patients begin to lose awareness of their cognitive deficits. Memory loss, especially of recent events, becomes more severe and is accompanied by moderate spatial and temporal disorientation, loss of ability to concentrate, aphasia, and increased anxiety. Severe language problems develop. Patients cannot understand or remember the names of objects. Their speech may not flow smoothly. Because of individual variation in disease progression, some patients may still be able to carry out routine behaviors and engage in generalized conversation. However, they can no longer drive a car, cook a meal, or read a newspaper. They are unable to work, plan and execute familiar tasks, and reason and exercise judgment. They may get lost easily and find simple activities confusing. The loss of cognitive functioning becomes impossible to ignore. Mood and personality are affected. Some people become angry or violent. Behavioral and psychiatric symptoms include agitation, wandering, temper tantrums, depression, and disorientation. Patients begin to lose their basic sense of personal identity. They may be at high risk for falls and other accidents. A small number of AD patients have vision problems. Although they frequently deny that they cannot see, autopsies confirm destruction in areas of the brain that process visual images.

Eventually, spatial and temporal disorientation becomes profound and may be accompanied by **delusions**, hallucinations, and **paranoia**. Patients may not recognize a family member or may accuse a spouse of infidelity. They may become uninhibited and confrontational. Some patients exhibit inappropriate sexual behaviors. AD patients may have trouble sleeping and suffer from nighttime confusion or agitation, called sunsetting or sundowner's syndrome. Some patients repeat words, thoughts, or movements, a behavior known as perseveration. Eventually they are unable to feed, bathe, dress, or groom themselves and cannot be left unattended.

In end-stage Alzheimer's disease, patients undergo general physical decline and lose control of many physical functions. **Seizures** and hypertonicity (increased muscle movements) are common. Bladder and bowel control is lost and stiffening muscles prevent walking. Patients who can walk often wander aimlessly and must be monitored for night wandering due to altered sleep patterns. Although some patients may use a wheelchair temporarily, eventually they become completely bedridden, unable even to sit up. Many patients are unable to talk. Abnormal jerking movements may occur for no reason or in response to touch or noises. Reflexes may be exaggerated and some patients experience whole body contractions known as generalized seizures.

Once the disease affects the brain stem, the basic processes of digestion, respiration, and excretion shut down. Patients may be unable to eat or swallow, and they sleep most of the time. Their hands and feet feel cold, breathing becomes shallow, and the patient is generally unresponsive. Death often results from infection, pneumonia, or malnutrition. Otherwise, breathing simply stops. From the onset of initial symptoms, disease progression can last up to 25 years, although the typical duration is 8 to 10 years.

Genetic profile

Familial early-onset Alzheimer's disease (FAD) accounts for fewer than 10% of AD cases. It can be caused by mutations in one of three genes. It is usually an autosomal dominant trait. Autosomal means that it affects males and females with equal frequency. Dominant means that it will affect individuals even if they inherited one copy of the mutated gene from one parent and a normal copy of the gene from the other parent. Individuals who have two copies of the mutant gene will pass on the gene to all of their children. If each parent has one copy of the mutant gene, there is a 75%

KEY TERMS

Acetylcholine—A neurotransmitter with effects that are generally opposite those of the neurotransmitters dopamine and norepinephrine. Acetylcholine dilates blood vessels, lowers blood pressure, and slows heartbeat.

Agitation—Excessive restlessness or emotional disturbance that is often associated with anxiety or psychosis; common in middle-stage AD.

Agnosia—Inability to recognize familiar people, places, and objects.

Amnesia—Partial or complete loss of memory or gaps in memory.

Amygdala—An almond-shaped brain structure of the limbic system that is activated in stressful situations and triggers fear.

Antioxidant—A substance that prevents the destructive effects of oxidative chemicals in the body.

Aphasia—Loss of language abilities.

Apolipoprotein E (APOE)—A protein that transports cholesterol throughout the body. One form of this protein, APOE e4, is associated with a 60% risk of late-onset AD.

Apraxia—An inability to perform purposeful movements that is not caused by paralysis or loss of feeling.

Autosomal dominant—A gene located on a chromosome other than the X or Y sex chromosomes, whose expression is dominant over that of a second copy of the same gene.

Beta-amyloid plaques—Senile plaques; structures in the brain, composed of dead or dying nerve cells and cell debris surrounding deposits of beta-amyloid protein, that are diagnostic of AD. Beta-amyloid forms when amyloid precursor protein (APP) is not broken down properly.

Brain stem—The part of the brain that connects to the spinal cord and controls most basic bodily functions. It is the last part of the brain to be destroyed by AD.

Cholinesterase inhibitors—Drugs that may slow the progression of AD by inhibiting the enzymes that break down acetylcholine.

Computed topography (CT) scan—A scan that uses x rays and a computer to form detailed images of a part of the body.

Delirium—A disturbance of consciousness marked by confusion, inattention, delusions, hallucinations, and agitation. It is distinguished from dementia by its relatively sudden onset and variation in the severity of symptoms.

Delusion—A persistent false belief held in the face of strong contradictory evidence.

Dementia—A group of symptoms (syndrome) associated with a chronic progressive impairment of memory, reasoning ability, and other intellectual functions; personality changes; deterioration in personal grooming; and disorientation.

Donepezil hydrochloride (Aricept)—A drug that increases the levels of acetylcholine in the brain.

Down syndrome—A genetic disorder characterized by an extra chromosome 21 (trisomy 21), intellectual disabilities, and susceptibility to early-onset AD.

Free radicals—Reactive atoms or molecules with unpaired electrons that damage cells, proteins, and DNA.

that any of their children will inherit the gene. If only one parent has one copy of the gene, each of their children has a 50% of inheriting the gene.

Identification of these three genes has led to the subdivision of familial early-onset AD into three categories:

- AD1 is a genetic defect in the amyloid precursor protein (APP) gene located on chromosome 21. Mutations in the APP gene are associated with AD onset between the ages of 55 and 60.
- AD3 is a genetic defect in the presenilin 1 (PSEN1) gene located on chromosome 14. Presenilin 1 may be one of the enzymes that clips APP into beta-amyloid. It also may be important for the functioning of synaptic connections between neurons.
- AD4 is an extremely rare genetic defect in the presenilin 2 (PSEN2) gene located on chromosome 1. Presenilin 2 is also involved in processing APP.

Mutations in PSEN1 and PSEN2 are associated with AD onset between the ages of 30 and 50. These three mutations result in the production of abnormal proteins and increased amounts of beta-amyloid. Together they account for approximately 50% of early-onset FAD.

Genetic disease—A disease caused by genes inherited from one or both parents.

Ginkgo—An herb from *Ginkgo biloba,* a shade tree native to China with fan-shaped leaves and fleshy seeds with edible kernels. Some alternative practitioners recommend ginkgo extract for preventing and treating AD.

Hallucination—False sensory perceptions, such as hearing sounds or seeing people or objects that are not there. Hallucinations can also affect the senses of smell, touch, and taste.

Hippocampus—A part of the brain's limbic system that is involved in memory formation and learning.

Insidious—Progressing gradually and inconspicuously, but with serious effects.

Magnetic resonance imaging (MRI)—An imaging technique that uses electromagnetic radiation and a computer to obtain detailed images of soft tissues such as the brain.

Mild cognitive impairment (MCI)—A transitional phase of memory loss in older people that precedes dementia or AD.

Neurofibrillary tangles—Accumulations of twisted protein fragments inside nerve cells in the brain that are diagnostic of AD.

Neurotransmitters—Chemicals that carry nerve impulses from one nerve cell to another. AD causes a drop in the production of several important neurotransmitters.

Norepinephrine—A neurotransmitter and adrenal hormone and the precursor of epinephrine.

Perseveration—Continuous involuntary repetition of speech or behavior.

Polygenic—A trait or disorder that is determined by several different genes. Most human characteristics, including height, weight, and general body build, are polygenic. Schizophrenia and late-onset AD are considered polygenic disorders.

Positron emission tomography (PET)—A medical imaging method capable of displaying the metabolic activity of organs and useful for investigating brain disorders.

Presenile dementia—The original name for Alzheimer's disease.

Presenilin (PSEN)—Proteins that are involved in processing amyloid precursor protein (APP). Mutations in the genes encoding these proteins can cause early-onset AD.

Pseudodementia—Depression with symptoms resembling those of dementia. The term "dementia of depression" is now preferred.

Serotonin—A neurotransmitter found in the brain and blood. Low levels of serotonin are associated with AD.

Sunsetting—Confusion or agitation in the evening.

Systolic—Referring to the rhythmic contraction of the heart (systole) as the blood in the chambers is forced out. Systolic blood pressure is blood pressure measured during the systolic phase.

Tau protein—A protein involved in maintaining the internal structure of nerve cells. Tau protein is damaged in AD and forms neurofibrillary tangles.

Tomography—A technique for producing a focused image of the structures at a specific depth within the body, while blurring details at other depths.

Sporadic AD (SAD) is considered a polygenic disorder because it is believed to result from the effects of multiple genes combined with environmental factors. This view is supported by research involving identical twins. Only one-third of identical twins of those with AD develop AD themselves. This suggests that factors other than genetic predisposition affect the development of SAD.

Down syndrome–associated Alzheimer's is another genetically determined form of AD. Normal individuals have two copies of each of the 22 human chromosomes, one copy from each parent. People with **Down syndrome**, also called trisomy 21, have three copies of chromosome 21, which results in brain changes that are similar to those that occur in both familial and sporadic AD. This is thought to be due to the overproduction of APP from the extra chromosome 21 APP gene.

Diagnosis

An early and accurate **diagnosis** of AD is important for developing strategies for managing symptoms and helping patients and their families plan for treatment, long-term care, and financial issues while the patient can still be involved in decision making. A diagnosis of AD also may help family members to avoid unnecessary anger and feelings of helplessness when dealing with the progression of the disease.

A diagnosis of AD is based upon the finding of slowly progressive dementia, exclusion of other possible causes for dementia, and brain-imaging studies that show changes in the structure of the brain, usually in the form of shrinkage. Possible AD is diagnosed when AD is considered to be the primary cause of the symptoms, but the diagnosis is complicated by the presence of another disorder. Probable AD is diagnosed when physicians and psychiatrists have ruled out all other disorders that could produce similar symptoms.

In 2011, new diagnostic criteria were proposed that identified three distinct stages of AD progression:

- preclinical Alzheimer's disease, revealed by tests such as brain scans before actual symptoms manifest
- mild cognitive impairment (MCI) due to Alzheimer's disease, identified as the beginning of cognitive difficulties before ADL is affected
- dementia due to Alzheimer's disease, the point at which the disease has progressed to impeding everyday life

The new criteria seek to more heavily incorporate physical testing, such as brain imaging, to better supplement observation and general cognitive and neurologic assessment.

Examination

Diagnosis of Alzheimer's disease can be quite complex and require consultations with various specialists. It requires a complete physical examination and medical and family history, including family members who have had AD and their ages of onset. The results of neurological exams are generally normal in early-stage AD. A complete evaluation of **alcohol use** and prescription and over-the-counter medication history, including alternative remedies, vitamins, herbal supplements, or illicit drugs, is necessary to rule out other causes of dementia, because more than 150 drugs can cause AD-like symptoms. Diagnosis is based upon clinical findings of otherwise unexplained slowly progressing dementia. FAD is diagnosed if there is a family history of the disease. Although AD almost always develops in Down syndrome patients over age 40, it may be difficult to determine whether further impairment is due to the Down syndrome or the progression of AD.

Other types of dementia, including some that are reversible, can cause symptoms similar to those of AD. Approximately 20% of patients originally suspected of having AD turn out to have some other disorder, about half of which are treatable:

- Multi-infarct vascular dementia is caused by strokes (blood clots in the brain) that lead to stepwise destruction of mental capacities.
- Diffuse white matter disease is a form of vascular dementia that can be diagnosed by magnetic resonance imaging (MRI) that reveals the generalized death of large parts of the brain.
- Parkinson's disease is a neurodegenerative condition that causes movement and functional abnormalities. Most Parkinson's patients have tremors and rigidity in their arms and legs.
- Alcohol-associated dementia is caused by nutritional deficiencies among people who abuse alcohol, especially malnutrition and deficiencies in vitamins B1 (thiamine) and B12 (cobalamin) and niacin (nicotinic acid). It is potentially reversible.
- Chronic use of certain drugs such as tranquilizers, sedatives, and pain relievers, as well as drug interactions, can cause potentially reversible dementia.
- Endocrine abnormalities (hormone imbalances), especially thyroid dysfunction, are less common causes of dementia. They can be diagnosed by blood tests.
- Chronic infections of the central nervous system, tertiary syphilis, trauma or injury to the brain, brain tumors, psychiatric conditions such as depression (pseudodementia or dementia of depression), and genetic and degenerative disorders other than AD can also cause dementia.

Evaluations for depression and **delirium** (reduced consciousness or awareness of one's environment) are particularly important components of the diagnostic process because, although they may be symptoms of AD, they can also be mistaken for AD. Depression and memory loss are both common among the elderly and a combination of the two can lead to a mistaken diagnosis of AD. Depression can be treated with drugs, although some **antidepressants** may worsen dementia, further complicating both diagnosis and treatment.

The clinical evaluation will assess cognitive impairment other than short-term memory loss. A family member or close friend of the patient often will be questioned about the onset and duration of symptoms. A neuropsychiatric examination may be performed to determine the pattern of cognitive impairment and probe the patient's level of functioning. Patients may be asked to write a sample check, describe how they answer the telephone, interpret sample traffic signs, or pick out items on a shopping list from a display.

Tests

Blood and urine tests are used to help rule out other causes of dementia. Genetic tests are available to detect genes known to cause AD, but they do not necessarily predict the development of AD.

Several types of oral and written tests are used to help diagnose AD and track its progression, including tests of mental status, functional abilities, memory, verbal fluency, and concentration. In early-stage AD, the results of these tests are usually within the normal range. The widely used mini-mental status examination (MMSE) is one such screening test. It is not particularly sensitive for detecting cognitive impairment in well-educated individuals who have previously functioned at a high level. It may also not yield accurate results for poorly educated individuals or cultural minorities. Another test, the clock test, asks patients to draw the face of a clock, possibly including a specific time such as 3:20. Patients with AD often put the numbers out of order, put them all in one part of the clock face instead of evenly spaced, or have difficulty drawing in the clock hands.

Occasionally, the patient's cerebrospinal fluid is tested for the levels of two proteins, Tau and a specific beta-amyloid protein fragment called A beta 42. Increased Tau protein and decreased A beta 42 in the cerebrospinal fluid are indicative of AD.

Procedures

Brain neuroimaging studies such as **positron emission tomography (PET)**, MRI, **single photon emission computed tomography** (SPECT) scans, or computed topography (CT) scans may be used to detect gross cerebral cortex atrophy due to brain cell death. **PET** scans can detect the earliest changes in brain structure. MRI scans are often performed on patients who are having problems with balance or gait. MRIs can detect diffuse atrophy that is often present in the cerebrum of the brain of AD patients. PET and SPECT scans can be used to evaluate patterns of glucose (sugar) metabolism in the brain to differentiate patterns characteristic of AD from those associated with vascular dementia and Pick's disease. PET scans are more precise than SPECT scans but are more expensive. However, imaging alone cannot diagnose AD. MRI and CT scans and electroencephalographs (EEGs), which measure the electrical activity in the brain, can be useful for excluding other causes of dementia such as stroke, subdural hematoma, and brain tumors.

Although a skilled physician can diagnose probable AD with 90% accuracy, a definitive diagnosis of Alzheimer's disease comes after the patient dies. A brain autopsy and examination of the brain tissue by a histopathologist can identify AD as the cause of death. The presence of a large number of beta-amyloid plaques and intraneuronal neurofibrillary tangles are considered diagnostic of AD. Antibodies that bind to the specific amyloid proteins are tagged with a fluorescent or colorimetric molecule and visualized in a microscope. In addition, the longer the disease has progressed, the smaller the brain is at death.

Treatment

There are several treatments for AD, including counseling, providing social and emotional support, and prescribing drugs to treat the symptoms.

Traditional

Although there is no cure for Alzheimer's disease, early diagnosis and prompt **intervention** can slow its progression and enable patients to function independently for a longer period. Healthcare professionals usually assess a patient's ADL to determine what type of care is needed. The mainstay of treatment is the establishment of daily routines, good nursing care and/or home-care strategies, and providing physical and emotional support. In the initial stages, counseling by a **psychologist** or an AD support group is recommended. The patient and caregiver should establish a relationship with a primary care provider so that illnesses, such as urinary or respiratory infections, can be properly diagnosed and treated rather than being simply attributed to the inevitable decline of AD. Neurological and behavioral aspects of AD, including anxiety, agitation, defiant behavior, **insomnia**, hallucinations, and seizures are treated as needed.

Treatment of AD is a very active area of research and the National Institutes of Health (NIH) and other agencies sponsor numerous **clinical trials** of new drugs and therapies. A list of current clinical trials enrolling volunteers can be found at: http://clinicaltrials.gov/ct2/results?term=Alzheimer.

Drugs

The most common drugs prescribed for AD are inhibitors of acetylcholinesterase and butylcholinesterase, enzymes that break down the neurotransmitters acetylcholine and butylcholine, respectively. The following medications increase levels of acetylcholine in the brain, thereby improving brain function in early-stage mild-to-moderate AD:

- galantamine (Razadyne, formerly known as Reminyl)
- rivastigmine (Exelon)
- donepezil hydrochloride (Aricept)

Aricept has been approved by the FDA to treat patients through all stages of AD. This drug may improve the individual's awareness of surroundings, as well as improve memory and cognitive function, though it is not a cure for

AD. It is offered as a tablet and should be taken whole, rather than crushed or chewed. It may be taken with or without food. Aricept must be taken regularly for the patient to receive the most beneficial effects of this medication.

Memantine (Namenda) is used to treat moderate-to-severe AD; it should not be used in patients with mild AD. It acts on glutamate, another brain neurotransmitter. This drug may also improve the individual's awareness of surroundings, as well as improve memory and cognitive function, though it is not a cure for AD. It is offered as a tablet or as an oral liquid and may initially be prescribed in gradually increasing dosages as directed by the physician. It may be taken with or without food. It is used alone or in combination with **donepezil**.

These drugs can modestly increase attention span, concentration, mental acuity, and information processing and improve the ability to perform normal ADL. They slow the progression of symptoms for about six months to one year in one-third to one-half of patients with AD. All have side effects, most often mild diarrhea, nausea, vomiting, muscle cramps, dizziness, headache, **fatigue**, and sleep disturbances. **Tacrine** (Cognex), the first such drug, is no longer prescribed because of the risk of liver toxicity.

The antioxidant vitamin E may delay AD onset by protecting neurons from free-radical damage. AD patients have lower blood levels of vitamin E than other adults of the same age. The Academy of Neurology has stated that vitamin E may indeed help with some symptoms of AD. One large two-year study of moderately affected AD patients found that taking 2000 IU (international units) of vitamin E daily significantly delayed disease progression as compared with patients taking a placebo. However, high levels of vitamin E can put patients at higher risk for bleeding disorders. Vitamin E therapy, in combination with cholinesterase inhibitors, has become the standard treatment for AD.

Drugs previously used to treat AD, including selegiline (a drug for Parkinson's disease), prednisone, estrogen, and nonsteroidal anti-inflammatory drugs (NSAIDs), have been found to be ineffective.

Medications can be prescribed to manage the behavioral and psychiatric symptoms of AD, which are often very stressful for caregivers. These medications are usually prescribed for the following specific symptoms:

- typical antipsychotics, usually haloperidol (Haldol), risperidone (Risperdal), olanzapine, or quetiapine, for anxiety, aggression, delusions, or hallucinations
- short-term antianxiety drugs, usually lorazepam (Ativan) or buspirone (BuSpar), for agitation
- a selective serotonin reuptake inhibitor (SSRI), such as citalopram or sertraline, at half the adult dosage, for depression, which is common in early-stage AD

Alzheimer's disease (AD) medications

Drug name (brand/generic)	Level of AD treated	Possible side effects
Aricept (donepezil)	All stages (mild, moderate, severe)	• Bruising • Confusion • Depression or anxiety • Dizziness • Extreme fatigue • Gastrointestinal upset, including vomiting • Pain, including joint pain and muscle cramps • Personality changes • Red, scaly, itchy skin • Strange dreams • Trouble sleeping
Exelon (rivastigmine)	Mild to moderate	• Confusion • Dizziness • Excessive perspiration • Gastrointestinal upset, including vomiting • Headache • Tremor • Trouble sleeping • Weakness and fatigue
Namenda (memantine)	Moderate to severe (should not be used to treat mild AD)	• Confusion • Constipation • Coughing • Dizziness • Fatigue • Headache • Pain • Vomiting
Razadyne (galantamine)	Mild to moderate	• Depression • Dizziness • Extreme fatigue • Gastrointestinal upset, including vomiting • Headache • Pale skin • Runny nose • Tremor • Trouble sleeping

(Table by PreMediaGlobal. © 2012 Cengage Learning.)

- acetaminophen or a very low dose of codeine for pain

Patients with AD are more susceptible to the side effects of medications, especially psychoactive drugs, and are usually given lower doses than younger adults. Physicians often recommend first trying to reduce behavioral symptoms with changes to the patient's environment.

Alternative

Antioxidants have shown some degree of effectiveness in treating AD, though further studies are needed. Antioxidants, in addition to vitamin E, include:

- vitamin C
- selenium

- green tea
- ginkgo biloba extract

Derived from the leaves of the *Ginkgo biloba* tree, ginkgo also increases blood and oxygen flow to the brain and has anti-inflammatory and neuroprotective effects. It has been used for many years in China, is widely prescribed in Europe for circulatory problems, and is the most common herbal treatment for AD. However, a large-scale, well-designed 2008 study found that ginkgo extract neither prevented nor delayed AD.

Other supplements for treating AD include huperzine A, thiamine (vitamin B1), cobalamin (vitamin B12), acetyl L-carnitine, **DHEA**, and folic acid, though none of these have yet been proven successful in clinical trials.

The incidence of AD is lower in countries with **diets** that are lower in calories and fats. There have been a few reports suggesting that diets rich in fish improve mental function in patients with AD or dementia, and AD patients treated with essential fatty acids have shown greater improvement in mood and mental function than patients on placebos. Because of its disease-preventing properties, red wine in moderation may also benefit AD patients. Patients with AD should avoid environmental toxins such as tobacco smoke.

A variety of other therapies may be beneficial in the treatment of psychological symptoms of AD:

- Music therapy has been found to calm agitated AD patients and improve mood; reduce chronic pain, depression, agitation, wandering, and feelings of isolation; and enhance long-term memory. Old familiar songs can be particularly effective in improving recall.
- Light therapy in the evening can help alleviate sleep-cycle disturbances.
- Supportive therapies include touch, compliments, and displays of affection.
- Sensory stimulation through massage and aromatherapy may be beneficial.
- Socio-environmental therapies include activities related to patient, previous interests and favorite foods, as well as pleasant surroundings.
- Insight-oriented psychotherapy addresses patients' awareness of their disease.
- Dance therapy, validation therapy, reminiscence therapy, and reality-oriented therapy have also been used with AD patients.

Home care

About 70% of AD patients are cared for at home, with the remainder residing in various types of institutions. Creative strategies are necessary to help the patient stay as independent as possible. Caregivers need their own support systems to minimize anger, despair, and burnout. Becoming familiar with likely future scenarios and considering financial and legal issues early on can ease the burden on both the patient and the family.

In the early stages of AD when memory loss is minimal, it is helpful for family and friends to interact with patients as much as possible, reminding them to eat, take their medication, keep their appointments, and help sustain daily living activities. Keeping records is helpful, particularly when there are several caregivers. The household should be organized so that important items can be found easily. The patient will need help in managing finances. Providing neighbors with a house key and setting up a schedule to check in on the patient are recommended. With the help of family, neighbors, and community resources, many people with early AD are able to maintain a successful lifestyle in their home environment for months or years.

Basic safety concerns for AD patients include:

- falls
- ingestion of dangerous substances
- wandering from home and becoming lost
- injury to one's self or others with sharp objects or fire
- the inability to respond rapidly to crisis situations

Often families have to modify their homes because of safety concerns. Possible modifications include:

- installing grab bars in bathrooms, bed rails, and clutter-free passageways
- unplugging and putting away electrical appliances when not in use
- storing matches, lighters, knives, or weapons out of reach
- lowering hot water heater temperature to avoid accidental scalding
- keeping a list of emergency numbers, including the poison control center and hospital emergency room, posted by the phone

Patients who have been diagnosed with AD should never be allowed to drive because of the risk of accidents or becoming disoriented. Some local chapters of the Alzheimer's Association offer help with transportation.

A calm, structured environment with simple orientation aids such as calendars and clocks can help reduce anxiety and increase safety. Labeling cabinets and drawers can help patients focus their attention. Signs can be posted reminding patients of important phone numbers and to turn off appliances and lock doors. Scheduling meals, bathing, and other activities at regular times and places provides routine and emotional security, since unfamiliar places and activities can be disorienting.

Caregivers should develop a daily routine and take advantage of periods during the day when the patient is less confused and more cooperative. The most severe symptoms often occur at night. Sleep disturbances may be minimized by keeping the patient engaged in activities during the day. Daily supervised walks are a good general exercise for people with AD.

A loss of grooming skills—mismatched clothing, unkempt hair, and decreased interest in personal hygiene—is often one of the early symptoms of AD. Caregivers, especially spouses, may find these changes embarrassing and difficult to handle. The caregiver will increasingly assume grooming responsibilities as the disease progresses.

Feeding may require using a colored plate to focus the patient's attention on the food. Finger foods may be preferable to the use of utensils. A nutritionist can give advice on well-balanced, easily prepared meals. Eventually the caregiver may need to feed the patient. As movement and swallowing become difficult, a feeding tube may be placed into the stomach through the abdominal wall.

Incontinence presents the most difficult problem for many caregivers and is a major reason for moving people with AD to nursing home care. In the early stages, limiting fluid intake and increasing the frequency of toileting can help. Careful attention to hygiene is important to prevent skin irritation and infection from soiled clothing.

Caregiver concerns

Family members or other caregivers have a difficult and stressful job, which becomes harder still as the disease progresses. Caring for dementia patients is significantly more demanding and time-consuming than caring for patients with other illnesses. Each day may bring new challenges as the patient's ability levels decrease and new patterns of behavior develop. Many caregivers find the constant but unpredictable demands extremely difficult. The personality changes of AD can be heartbreaking for family members as a loved one deteriorates, seeming to become a different person. As the disease progresses, the patient's behavior may become increasingly erratic. It may be impossible to leave a patient unattended for even a few minutes because the patient may wander off. Neighbors should always be informed of the person's condition. However, not all AD patients develop negative behaviors: some become gentle, spending increasing amounts of time in dreamlike states.

Caregivers often develop feelings of anger, resentment, guilt, and hopelessness. Depression is common and may need to be treated. Caregivers can become susceptible to illness, especially if they do not receive adequate support from family, friends, and community. **Support groups** can help caregivers deal with stress. The location and contact numbers for AD caregiver support groups are available from the Alzheimer's Association, local social service agencies, physicians, and pharmaceutical companies that manufacture the drugs used to treat AD.

Most families eventually need outside help to care for the AD patient. Personal care assistants, either volunteer or paid, may be available through local social service agencies. Adult daycare facilities are becoming increasingly common. Meal delivery, shopping assistance, or **respite** care may also be available. Special Alzheimer's disease facilities are available for both respite daycare and permanent long-term care.

The decision to move the patient to a nursing home is often one of the most difficult for the family, who may consider that they have failed in their obligations and are abandoning their loved one. Counsulting with a physician, clergy, or other trusted adviser can ease this transition. Selecting a nursing home may require a difficult balancing of costs, services, location, and availability. Keeping the entire family involved in the decision may help prevent further stress.

Social Security Disability, Medicare, Medicaid, or Supplemental Security Income may provide financial assistance but will not usually cover nursing home care indefinitely. Long-term care insurance, if purchased prior to diagnosis; reverse mortgages; or other financial devices may be appropriate.

Prognosis

There is no cure for Alzheimer's disease, and once the symptoms develop patients do not recover. The goal is to maintain cognitive and physical function for as long as possible. Although there is considerable variation in the rate of disease progression, symptoms continue to worsen, usually over a period of years. Eventually, loss of brain cells and brain damage result in the impairment of autonomic body functions, the failure of various organ systems, coma, and death. Most AD patients die within 8 to 10 years of diagnosis, although that interval can be as short as one year or as long as 20 years. The life expectancy of AD patients is increasing because the disease is generally being diagnosed at an earlier stage.

The most common cause of death among AD patients is infection. People with AD are often in poor health and may be malnourished, which puts them at increased risk of life-threatening infections such as pneumonia. They are also susceptible to other conditions and diseases of old age. The consequences of cancer, stroke, and heart disease can be more severe in patients with AD than in otherwise healthy people.

QUESTIONS TO ASK YOUR DOCTOR

- What are the indications that my loved one may have Alzheimer's disease?
- What diagnostic tests are needed for a thorough assessment?
- What treatment options do you recommend for my loved one?
- What kind of changes can I expect to see with the medications you have prescribed for my loved one?
- What are the side effects associated with the medications you have prescribed for my loved one?
- Should my loved one see a specialist? If so, what kind of specialist should I contact?
- What tests or evaluation techniques will you perform to see if treatment has been beneficial for my loved one?
- What physical or psychological limitations do you foresee?
- How does having Alzheimer's disease put my loved one at risk for other health conditions?
- What measures can be taken to prevent the progression of symptoms?
- Are there any new or experimental treatments available?
- Is my loved one eligible for any clinical trials?
- When should my loved one stop driving?
- What symptoms or adverse effects are important enough that I should seek immediate treatment?
- Can you recommend any support groups for me and my family?

Prevention

There is no known prevention for Alzheimer's disease. Several studies have suggested that high-fat and high-calorie diets may increase the risk of developing AD. Other possible risk factors include alcohol, salt, and refined carbohydrates. Some studies have found that fish consumption reduces the incidence of AD in Europe and North America, possibly due to the omega-3 fatty acids found in fish. It is also possible that staying physically and mentally active throughout life may lower the risk of AD.

Individuals with a history of Alzheimer's disease in their families may want to consider genetic counseling to clarify possible risk factors and determine the appropriateness of available genetic tests. Possessing a certain gene, the APOE e4 gene, is a risk factor for AD, but it is not considered useful for predicting whether a person will develop the disease. The National Institute on Aging has several reasons for not recommending using the test to screen people:

- It does not predict whether an individual will develop AD.
- There are ethical implications to testing for a disease that is currently incurable.
- It may have adverse psychological consequences for individuals and their families.
- It could lead to discrimination in employment or health insurance for carriers of the gene.

Research on the prevention of AD has focused on blocking the production of amyloid protein in the brain and on breaking down beta-amyloid after it is released from cells but before it has a chance to aggregate into insoluble plaques.

Healthcare team roles

Treatment of AD is a team effort, involving primary care physicians, nurses, imaging and laboratory technicians, gerontology specialists, psychiatrists, psychologists, and caregivers. Educating patients and caregivers about the nature of the disease and its progression usually falls on nursing staff. Nurses are also the first line of access for medical care and support groups. **Social workers**, counselors, and support group facilitators may provide emotional support, practical advice, and information about community resources. Specialized Alzheimer's disease facilities may be used for either respite daycare or permanent long-term care.

Resources

BOOKS

Calo-oy, Starr, and Bob Calo-oy. *Caregiving Tips A-Z, Alzheimer's & Other Dementias*. Fremont, CA: Orchard Publications, 2008.

Chan, A. P., ed. *Alzheimer's Disease Research Trends*. Hauppauge, NY: Nova Science, 2008.

Dawbarn, David, ed. *Neurobiology of Alzheimer's Disease*, 3rd ed. New York: Oxford University Press, 2007.

Doraiswamy, P. M., et al. *The Alzheimer's Action Plan: The Experts' Guide to the Best Diagnosis and Treatment for Memory Problems*. New York: St. Martin's Press, 2008.

Lerner, Adrienne. *Alzheimer's Disease*. Farmington Hills, MI: Greenhaven Press, 2008.

Mace, Nancy L., and Peter V. Rabins. *The 36-Hour Day: A Family Guide to Caring for Persons with Alzheimer*

Disease, Other Dementias, and Memory Loss in Later Life, 4th ed. Baltimore: Johns Hopkins University Press, 2006.

McCann-Beranger, Judith. *A Caregiver's Guide to Alzheimer's & Related Diseases*. New York: Bunim & Bannigan, 2008.

Sabbagh, Marwan. *The Alzheimer's Answer: Reduce Your Risk and Keep Your Brain Healthy*. Hoboken, NJ: Wiley, 2008.

Taylor, Richard. *Alzheimer's from the Inside Out*. Baltimore: Health Professions Press, 2006.

Whitehouse, Peter J., and Daniel George. *The Myth of Alzheimer's: What You Aren't Being Told About Today's Most Dreaded Diagnosis*. New York: St. Martin's Press, 2008.

PERIODICALS

Arnst, Catherine. "Is Alzheimer's a Form of Diabetes? If So, an Insulin-Centered Treatment Could Alter the Course of the Disease." *Bloomberg Business Week* (December 6, 2007). http://www.businessweek.com/magazine/content/07_51/b4063054323389.htm (accessed July 24, 2011).

Ault, Alicia. "Debate Continues Over Early Cognition Screening: Some Argue that Obtaining a Timely Baseline Could Offset Subsequent Delays in Diagnosing Alzheimer's." *Family Practice News* (December 15, 2007): 27.

Bain, L. J., Warren Barker, David A. Loewenstein, and Ranjan Duara. "Towards an Earlier Diagnosis of Alzheimer Disease." *Alzheimer Disease and Associated Disorders* 22, no. 2 (April-June 2008): 99–110.

Christensen, Daniel D., and Peter Lin. "Practical Treatment Strategies for Patients with Alzheimer's Disease." *Journal of Family Practice* (December 2007): 17–23.

Frisoni, Giovanni B., and Jennifer L. Whitwell. "How Fast Will It Go, Doc? New Tools for an Old Question from Patients with Alzheimer Disease." *Neurology* 70, no. 23 (June 2008): 2194–95.

Grady, Denise. "Finding Alzheimer's Before a Mind Fails." *New York Times* (December 26, 2007): A1+. http://www.nytimes.com/2007/12/26/health/26alzheimers.html?pagewanted=all (accessed July 24, 2011).

Guthrie, Catherine. "Is Alzheimer's a Form of Diabetes?" *Time Health* (October 18, 2007). http://www.time.com/time/health/article/0,8599,1673236,00.html (accessed July 24, 2011).

Ji, Hong-fang, and Hong-yu Zhang. "Multipotent Natural Agents to Combat Alzheimer's Disease: Functional Spectrum and Structural Features." *Acta Pharmacologica Sinica* (February 2008): 143–51.

Kontush, Anatol, and Svetlana Schekatolina. "An Update on Using Vitamin E in Alzheimer's Disease." *Expert Opinion on Drug Discovery* (February 2008): 261–71.

Palmer, Katie, et al. "Mild Cognitive Impairment in the General Population: Occurrence and Progression to Alzheimer Disease." *American Journal of Geriatric Psychiatry* 16, no. 7 (July 2008): 603–11.

Schwab, Claudia, and Patrick L. McGeer. "Inflammatory Aspects of Alzheimer Disease and Other Neurodegenerative Disorders." *American Journal of Alzheimer's Disease & Other Dementias* 13, no. 4 (May 2008): 359–69.

WEBSITES

"Alzheimer's Disease." *American Health Assistance Foundation*. Last modified June 6, 2011. http://www.ahaf.org/alzheimers (accessed July 29, 2011).

"Alzheimer's Disease." *MedlinePlus*. Last modified July 21, 2011. http://www.nlm.nih.gov/medlineplus/alzheimersdisease.html#cat25 (accessed July 29, 2011).

"Alzheimer's Disease." *NIH Senior Health*. Last modified March 30, 2010. http://nihseniorhealth.gov/alzheimersdisease/toc.html (accessed July 29, 2011).

Alzheimer's Disease Education and Referral Center. "Alzheimer's Disease: Unraveling the Mystery." *National Institute on Aging*. Last modified January 4, 2011. http://www.nia.nih.gov/Alzheimers/Publications/Unraveling (accessed July 29, 2011).

———. "New Research Illuminates Memory Loss and Early Dementia." *Connections* (Spring 2009). http://www.nia.nih.gov/Alzheimers/ResearchInformation/Newsletter/Spring2009/feature01.htm (accessed July 29, 2011).

Mayo Clinic Staff. "Alzheimer's Disease." MayoClinic.com. http://www.mayoclinic.com/print/alzheimers-disease/DS00161/DSECTION=all&METHOD=print (accessed July 29, 2011).

ORGANIZATIONS

Alzheimer's Association, 225 N Michigan Ave., 17th Fl., Chicago, IL, 60601-7633, (312) 335-8700, (800) 272-3900, Fax: (866) 699-1246, info@alz.org, http://www.alz.org.

Alzheimer's Disease Education and Referral Center, National Institute on Aging, PO Box 8250, Silver Spring, MD, 20907-8250, (800) 438-4380, adear@nia.nih.gov, http://www.nia.nih.gov/Alzheimers.

Alzheimer's Foundation of America, 322 8th Ave., 7th Fl., New York, NY, 10001, (866) 232-8484, Fax: (646) 638-1546, info@alzfdn.org, http://www.alzfdn.org.

American Academy of Neurology, 1080 Montreal Ave., St. Paul, MN, 55116, (800) 879-1960, http://www.aan.com.

American Health Assistance Foundation, 22512 Gateway Center Dr., Clarksburg, MD, 20871, (800) 437-2423, Fax: (301) 948-4403, info@ahaf.org, http://www.ahaf.org.

American Neurological Association, 5841 Cedar Lake Rd., Ste. 204, Minneapolis, MN, 55416, (952) 545-6284, http://www.aneuroa.org.

Family Caregiver Alliance, 180 Montgomery St., Ste. 900, San Francisco, CA, 94104, (415) 434-3388, (800) 445-8106, http://www.caregiver.org.

Fisher Center for Alzheimer's Research Foundation, One Intrepid Square, W 46th St. & 12th Ave., New York, NY, 10036, (800) 259-4636, http://foundationcenter.org.

Foundation for Health in Aging, 350 5th Ave., Ste. 801, New York, NY, 10118, (212) 755-6810, http://www.healthinaging.org.

National Institutes of Health, 9000 Rockville Pike, Bethesda, MD, 20892, (301) 496-4000, http://www.nih.gov.

National Institute of Neurological Disorders and Stroke, NIH Neurological Institute, PO Box 5801, Bethesda, MD, 20824, (301) 496-5751, (800) 352-9424, http://www.ninds.nih.gov.

National Library of Medicine, 8600 Rockville Pike, Bethesda, MD, 20894, http://www.nlm.nih.gov.

U.S. Administration on Aging, 1 Massachusetts Ave. NW, Washington, DC, 20001, (202) 401-4634, http://www.aoa.gov.

Bryan Richard Cobb, PhD
Ken R. Wells
Laura Jean Cataldo, RN, EdD

Amantadine

Definition

Amantadine is a synthetic antiviral agent that also has strong antiparkinsonian properties. It is sold in the United States under the brand name Symmetrel, and is also available under its generic name.

Purpose

Amantadine is used to treat a group of side effects (called parkinsonian side effects) that includes tremors, difficulty walking, and slack muscle tone. These side effects may occur in patients who are taking antipsychotic medications used to treat mental disorders such as **schizophrenia**. An unrelated use of amantadine is in the treatment of viral infections of some strains of influenza A.

Description

Some medicines, called antipsychotic drugs, that are used to treat schizophrenia and other mental disorders can cause side effects similar to the symptoms of Parkinson's disease. The patient does not have Parkinson's disease, but may experience shaking in muscles while at rest, difficulty with voluntary movements, and poor muscle tone.

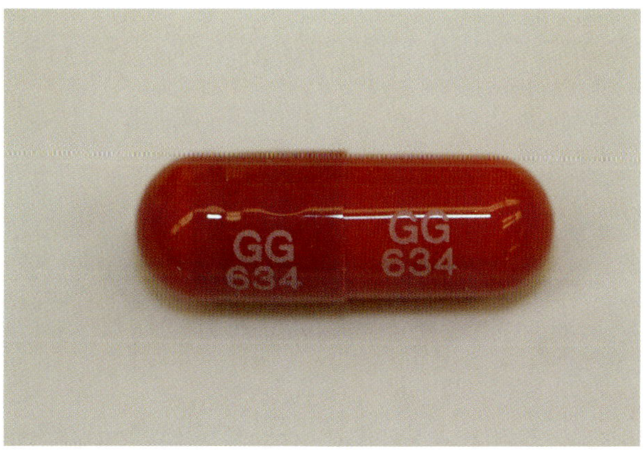

Amantadine hydrochloride, 100 mg. *(© Custom Medical Stock Photo, Inc. Reproduced by permission.)*

One way to eliminate these undesirable side effects is to stop taking the antipsychotic medicine. Unfortunately, the symptoms of the original mental disorder usually come back, so in most cases simply stopping the antipsychotic medication is not a reasonable option. Some drugs that control the symptoms of Parkinson's disease such as amantadine also control the parkinsonian side effects of antipsychotic medicines.

Amantadine works by restoring the chemical balance between **dopamine** and acetylcholine, two neurotransmitter chemicals in the **brain**. Taking amantadine along with the antipsychotic medicine helps to control symptoms of the mental disorder, while reducing parkinsonian side effects. Amantadine is in the same family of drugs (commonly known as anticholinergic drugs) as **biperiden** and **trihexyphenidyl**.

Recommended dosage

Amantadine is available in 100 mg tablets and capsules, as well as a syrup containing 50 mg of amantadine in each teaspoonful. For the treatment of drug-induced parkinsonian side effects, amantadine is usually given in a dose of 100 mg orally twice a day. Some patients may need a total daily dose as high as 300 mg. Patients who are taking other antiparkinsonian drugs at the same time may require lower daily doses of amantadine (e.g., 100 mg daily).

People with kidney disease or who are on hemodialysis must have their doses lowered. In these patients, doses may range from 100 mg daily to as little as 200 mg every seven days.

Precautions

Amantadine increases the amount of the neurotransmitter dopamine (a central nervous system stimulant) in the brain. Because of this, patients with a history of epilepsy or other seizure disorders should be carefully monitored while taking this drug. This is especially true in the elderly and in patients with kidney disease. Amantadine may cause visual disturbances and affect mental alertness and coordination. People should not operate dangerous machinery or motor vehicles while taking this drug.

Side effects

Five to ten percent of patients taking amantadine may experience the following nervous system side effects:

- dizziness or lightheadedness
- insomnia

KEY TERMS

Acetylcholine—A naturally occurring chemical in the body that transmits nerve impulses from cell to cell. It causes blood vessels to dilate, lowers blood pressure, and slows the heartbeat. Central nervous system well-being is dependent on a balance among the neurotransmitters acetylcholine, dopamine, serotonin, and norepinephrine.

Anticholinergic—Related to the ability of a drug to block the nervous system chemical acetylcholine. When acetylcholine is blocked, patients often experience dry mouth and skin, increased heart rate, blurred vision, and difficulty in urinating. In severe cases, blocking acetylcholine may cloud thinking and cause delirium.

Dopamine—A chemical in brain tissue that serves to transmit nerve impulses (is a neurotransmitter) and helps to regulate movement and emotions.

Neurotransmitter—A chemical in the brain that transmits messages between neurons, or nerve cells.

Parkinsonian—Related to symptoms associated with Parkinson's disease, a nervous system disorder characterized by abnormal muscle movement of the tongue, face, and neck; inability to walk or move quickly; walking in a shuffling manner; restlessness; and/or tremors.

- nervousness or anxiety
- impaired concentration

One to five percent of patients taking amantadine may experience the following nervous system side effects:

- irritability or agitation
- depression
- confusion
- lack of coordination
- sleepiness or nightmares
- fatigue
- headache

In addition, up to 1% of patients may experience hallucinations, euphoria (excitement), extreme forgetfulness, aggressive behavior, personality changes, or **seizures**. Seizures are the most serious of all the side effects associated with amantadine.

Gastrointestinal side effects may also occur in patients taking amantadine. Up to 10% of people taking this drug experience nausea and up to 5% have dry mouth, loss of appetite, constipation, and vomiting. In most situations, amantadine may be continued and these side effects treated symptomatically.

Between 1% and 5% of patients taking amantadine have also reported a bluish coloring of their skin (usually on the legs) that is associated with enlargement of the blood vessels (called livedo reticularis). This side effect usually appears within one month to one year of starting the drug and subsides within weeks to months after the drug is discontinued. People who think they may be experiencing this or other side effects from any medication should tell their physicians.

Interactions

Taking amantadine along with other drugs used to treat parkinsonian side effects may cause increased confusion or even hallucinations. The combination of amantadine and central nervous system stimulants (e.g., **amphetamines** or decongestants) may cause increased central nervous stimulation or increase the likelihood of seizures.

See also Medication-induced movement disorders

Resources

BOOKS

American Society of Health-System Pharmacists. *AHFS Drug Information 2008*. Bethesda, MD: American Society of Health-System Pharmacists, 2008.

PERIODICALS

Graham, Karen A., et al. "Double-Blind, Placebo-Controlled Investigation of Amantadine for Weight Loss in Subjects Who Gained Weight with Olanzapine." *American Journal of Psychiatry* 162, no. 9 (September 2005): 1744–46.

Silver, Henry, et al. "A Double-Blind, Cross-Over Comparison of the Effects of Amantadine or Placebo on Visuomotor and Cognitive Function Medicated Schizophrenia Patients." *International Clinical Psychopharmacology* 20, no. 6 (November 2005): 319–26.

Walsh, R. A., and A. E. Lang. "Multiple Impulse Control Disorders Developing in Parkinson's Disease after Initiation of Amantadine." *Movement Disorders* (September 27, 2011) [e-pub ahead of print]. http://dx.doi.org/10.1002/mds.23964 (accessed December 12, 2011).

OTHER

Enco Pharmaceuticals, Inc. "SYMMETREL (Amantadine Hydrochloride, USP) Tablets and Syrup." http://www.endo.com/PDF/symmetrel_pack_insert.pdf (accessed September 20, 2011).

Jack Raber, Pharm.D.
Ruth A. Wienclaw, PhD

Ambien *see* **Zolpidem**

American Academy of Child & Adolescent Psychiatry

Definition

The American Academy of Child and Adolescent Psychiatry (AACAP) is a 501 (c) (3) nonprofit medical organization that was founded in 1953 as an organization for practicing psychiatrists specializing in the care of youth. As of 2011, the AACAP represents over 7,500 physicians who treat the estimated 7–12 million American children and adolescents suffering from developmental or behavioral disorders. A major priority of the AACAP is expanding the workforce of specialists in adolescent and child psychiatry.

Purpose

The academy functions to establish and support ethical and professional standards in the practice of child and adolescent psychiatry; advocates for children, adolescents, and families with mental health needs; and promotes research and training to physicians and other healthcare providers. They strive to promote the healthy development of children, adolescents, and families, and to support psychiatrists working with child and adolescent populations.

Description

To qualify for membership in the academy, a person must be a doctor of medicine (MD) or a doctor of osteopathy (DO) who has completed four years of medical school; three years in an approved residency in medicine, neurology, and general psychiatry with adults; and two years of further training in psychiatric work with children, adolescents, and their families in an accredited residency in child and adolescent psychiatry. After completing these residency requirements, the candidate must then pass a certification examination in general psychiatry given by the American Board of Psychiatry and Neurology (ABPN). He or she is then eligible to take the additional certification examination in the subspecialty of child and adolescent psychiatry. Although the ABPN examinations are not required for practice, they are a further assurance of the physician's qualifications and competence.

The AACAP is governed by an elected council of 16 members; five of these members form the executive committee of the organization. Other members of the AACAP are able to join work groups, committees, and task forces (7 work groups and 60 committees were active as of 2011). Work groups and committees cover a wide variety of issues and special concerns ranging from continuing education, legal matters, religion and spirituality, and workforce issues to the special needs of adolescents (as distinct from younger children), Native American and minority youth, survivors of **trauma**, rural families, and military families. In addition to its internal committees, the academy works together with other medical professional organizations. It has a seat in the House of Delegates of the American Medical Association (AMA) and liaisons with the American Academy of Pediatrics (AAP), the **American Psychiatric Association** (APA), and the American Academy of Family Physicians (AAFP). The AACAP also sends representatives to such organizations as the National Alliance on Mental Illness (NAMI), Mental Health America, and the Federation of Families for Children's Mental Health.

Professional publications

The academy's strong commitment to furthering the understanding and treatment of children and adolescents is also reflected in the wide range of its publications, which include its official monthly, the *Journal of the American Academy of Child and Adolescent Psychiatry*, and a quarterly newsletter. The AACAP also provides information for the public in the form of *Facts for Families*, a collection of fact sheets providing frequently updated material discussing current psychiatric issues concerning children, adolescents, and their families. Topics include "Talking to Children about Terrorism and War," "Children and Video Games: Playing with Violence," "Children and Role Models," and "Psychotherapies for Children and Adolescents." The full collection is available in English and Spanish, with select translations also available in Malaysian, Polish, Icelandic, Arabic, Urdu, and Hebrew. In addition to *Facts for Families*, the academy has published two books for the general public, *Your Child* and *Your Adolescent*, and also provides online resource centers on a variety of mental health topics that affect children.

Resources

ORGANIZATIONS

American Academy of Child and Adolescent Psychiatry (AACAP), 3615 Wisconsin Avenue NW, Washington, DC, 20016-3007, (202) 966-7300, (800) 333-7636, Fax: (202) 966-2891, http://www.aacap.org.

American Academy of Family Physicians, 11400 Tomahawk Creek Pkwy., Leawood, KS, 66211-2672, (913) 906-6000, (800) 274-2237, Fax: (913) 906-6075, contactcenter@aafp.org, http://www.aafp.org.

American Academy of Pediatrics (AAP), 141 Northwest Point Boulevard, Elk Grove Village, IL, 60007, (847) 434-4000, Fax: (847) 434-8000, http://www.aap.org.

National Institute of Child Health and Human Development (NICHD), Bldg 31, Room 2A32, MSC 2425, 31 Center Drive, Bethesda, MD, 20847, (800) 370-2943; TTY: (888) 320-6942, Fax: (866) 760-5947, NICHDInformationResourceCenter@mail.nih.gov, http://www.nichd.nih.gov.

Laura Jean Cataldo, RN, Ed.D.

American Psychiatric Association

Definition

The American Psychiatric Association (APA) is a national medical society whose approximately 36,000 physician and medical student members specialize in the **diagnosis** and treatment of mental and emotional disorders. The oldest medical specialty society in the United States, the APA was begun in October 1844, when 13 physicians who specialized in the treatment of mental and emotional disorders met in Philadelphia and founded the Association of Medical Superintendents of American Institutions for the Insane. Their goals were to communicate professionally, cooperate in the collection of data, and improve the treatment of the mentally ill.

Purpose

More than one hundred and fifty years later, the APA's objectives are still designed to advance care for people with mental illnesses. Their mission is to improve treatment, rehabilitation, and care of the mentally ill and emotionally disturbed; to promote research, professional education in psychiatry and allied fields, and the prevention of psychiatric disabilities; to advance the standards of psychiatric services and facilities; to foster cooperation among those concerned with the medical, psychological, social, and legal aspects of mental health; to share psychiatric knowledge with other practitioners of medicine, scientists, and the public; and to promote the best interests of patients and others using mental health services.

Description

To be eligible to join the APA, a physician or resident must have graduated from a four-year program leading to an MD or DO degree, and have completed a residency program in psychiatry accredited by the Residency Review Committee for Psychiatry of the Accreditation Council for Graduate Medical Education (ACGME), the Royal College of Physicians and Surgeons of Canada (RCPS(C)), or the American Osteopathic Association (AOA). Applicants for membership must also provide a reference from a physician who is already a member of the APA.

The APA's annual meeting attracts more than 15,000 attendees and features hundreds of sessions and presenters. Additionally, the Association schedules more than 200 meetings each year among its councils, committees, and task forces to further advance the cause of mental health. The APA also offers a comprehensive continuing medical education program to its members.

Internal divisions of the APA include the Office of Minority and National Affairs, Early Career Psychiatrists, the Office of International Activities, women's programs, and minority and underrepresented group caucuses. The APA also operates several special interest groups and areas of study, including HIV psychiatry; disaster psychiatry; integrative medicine; and gay, lesbian, and bisexual health.

The APA has established the American Psychiatric Foundation (APF) as its philanthropic and educational arm. The Foundation seeks to educate the public about mental illness through workplacc programs and other initiatives. It also supports researchers, particularly in the fields of **schizophrenia** and minority mental health, and provides fellowships for qualified APA members, including an annual fellowship for a resident in psychiatry to work in a congressional office or committee.

Professional publications

The APA supports psychiatrists and their service to patients through such publications as the *American Journal of Psychiatry*, the oldest specialty journal in the United States, and *Psychiatric News*, the Association's official newsletter. The APA also publishes numerous books, specialty journals, and reports. American Psychiatric Publishing, Inc. (APP) is a fully owned subsidiary of the APA and offers hundreds of book titles as well as six specialty journals, including eBooks and eJournals. APP has two purposes—to serve as the distributor of publications of the APA and to publish books independent of APA policies and procedures. Since its founding in 1981, APP has evolved into a full-service publishing house, with editorial, production, marketing, and business staff.

The DSM

The ***Diagnostic and Statistical Manual of Mental Disorders*** is published by the APA and is the accepted guide by medical professionals for diagnosing mental health conditions and disorders. The *DSM* provides diagnostic criteria for approximately 300 mental health disorders. The fifth edition, or *DSM-5*, is being developed and is expected to publish in 2013.

Resources

WEBSITES

American Psychiatric Publishing. http://appi.org/Pages/default.aspx (accessed December 12, 2011).

ORGANIZATIONS

American Psychiatric Association, 1000 Wilson Blvd., Ste. 1825, Arlington, VA, 22209-3901, (703) 907-7300, apa@psych.org, http://www.psych.org.

American Psychological Association

Definition

The American Psychological Association (APA) was founded in July 1892 by three dozen members. As of 2011, it had more than 154,000 members and is both the world's largest association of psychologists and the major organization representing psychology in the Unites States. Presently chartered as a corporation in the District of Columbia, the APA considers itself a scientific as well as a professional organization. The APA restricts the use of the word "psychologist" to persons who hold doctorates in the field from accredited institutions, preferring to refer to persons with master's degrees in psychology as "clinicians," "counselors," or "specialists."

Purpose

The mission of the APA is to "advance the creation, communication, and application of psychological knowledge to benefit society and improve people's lives." The organization strives to support the growth of psychology as a science and advocates for the benefits of psychology in influencing public health and well-being.

Description

The APA is governed by a president, a board of directors, a council of representatives, and various boards and committees. It oversees several programs, including four directorates in science, practice, public interest, and education. The Science Directorate promotes the exchange of ideas and research findings through conventions, conferences, publications, and traveling museum exhibits. It also helps psychologists locate and obtain research funding, and its science advocacy program works for the enhancement of federal support for psychology, research, and teaching. The Practice Directorate promotes the practice of psychology and the availability of psychological care through legislative advocacy on such issues as health care reform, regulated state licensure, and pro bono services. The Public Interest Directorate supports the application of psychology to the advancement of human welfare through program and policy development; conference planning; and support of research, training, and advocacy in such areas as minority affairs, rural health, disability issues, women's issues, and lesbian and gay health. The Education Directorate serves to advance psychology in its work with educational institutions, including precollege as well as college and graduate programs; professional agencies; continuing education for APA members; and programs and initiatives in education.

The APA is subdivided into 54 divisions, which are specialized interest groups initiated by members. Topics include developmental psychology, clinical psychology, military psychology, child and family policy and practice, and **exercise** and sport psychology, as well as societies focused on specific age groups, genders, and ethnic groups. Each division has its own officers, publications, awards, and activities, and functions within the context of the APA.

In 1953, the APA started its foundation, the American Psychology Foundation (APF), with a donation of $500. The APF began its first public initiative in 1974, a study of gifted and talented youth. This program continues to add to the field of giftedness research through its publications and by attracting younger scholars to pursue research on gifted children. In the early 1990s, the APF underwent a major expansion program in order to support graduate and postdoctoral students in psychology. A fundraising campaign in 2000 increased the APF's grant-making capacity by more than 150% in just five years. The APF focuses on enhancing the field of psychology, whether through student development in the form of scholarships or research initiatives by way of grants. Funding programs include career development and education, child and family psychology, disaster relief, gay and lesbian psychology, international efforts, mental and physical health, **stigma** and prejudice, travel grants, violence prevention, and personal awards.

Professional publications

The APA's information dissemination efforts include the publication of books, including children's books; scientific and professional journals; magazines and newsletters, including *APA Monitor*, *gradPSYCH Magazine*, and *American Psychologist*; reports and brochures; and electronic databases, including *PsychINFO*, a worldwide computer database of psychological abstracts (not full-text articles) from the 1800s to the present that has provided references in psychology and related behavioral and social sciences since the 1970s.

The APA also hosts an annual convention, considered to be the world's largest meeting of psychologists.

Resources

BOOKS

Evans, Rand B., Virginia Staudt Sexton, and Thomas C. Cadwallader, eds. *The American Psychological Association: A Historical Perspective*. Washington, DC: American Psychological Association, 1992.

ORGANIZATIONS

American Psychological Association, 750 1st St. NE, Washington, DC, 20002-4242, (202) 336-5500; TDD/TTY: (202) 336-6123, (800) 374-2721, http://www.apa.org.

Amitriptyline

Definition

Amitriptyline is a medication used to treat various forms of **depression** and pain associated with the nerves (neuropathic pain), and to prevent migraine headaches. It is sold in the United States under the brand names Elavil and Endep.

Purpose

Amitriptyline helps relieve depression and pain. This medication, usually given at bedtime, also helps patients sleep better.

Description

Amitriptyline medication is one of several tricyclic **antidepressants**, so called because of the three-ring chemical structure common to these drugs. It acts to block reabsorption of **neurotransmitters** (chemicals that transmit nerve messages in the **brain**). Amitriptyline and the other tricyclic antidepressants are primarily used to treat mental depression but are increasingly being replaced by a newer and more effective group of antidepressant drugs called **selective serotonin reuptake inhibitors (SSRIs)**. Amitriptyline is sometimes prescribed to help treat pain associated with cancer. In addition, it is sometimes prescribed for various types of chronic pain. Tablets are available in 10, 25, 50, 70, and 150 mg doses.

Recommended dosage

The usual adult dose for pain management ranges from 10 mg to 150 mg at bedtime. Patients are generally

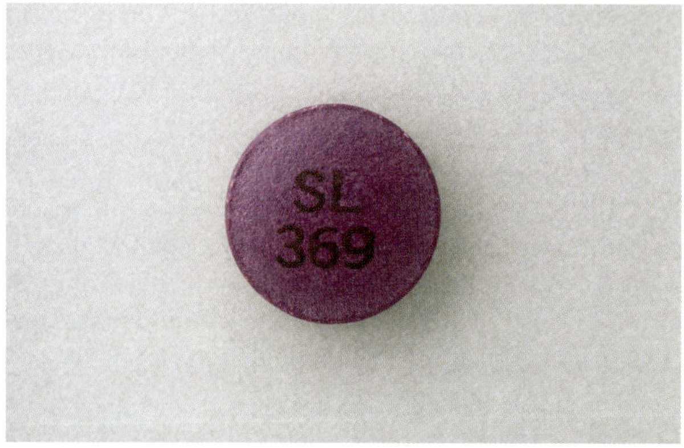

Amitriptyline, 75 mg. *(© Custom Medical Stock Photo, Inc. Reproduced by permission.)*

started on a low dose, and the amount may be increased as needed. Side effects, such as a dry mouth and drowsiness, may make it difficult to increase the dose in older adults. Bedtime dosing helps the patient sleep. Doctors generally prescribe 75–150 mg for depression. It is given at bedtime or in divided doses during the day. It may take 30 days for the patient to feel less depressed. Pain relief is usually noticed sooner than the mood change. Teens and older adults usually receive a lower dose. If the nightly dose is missed, it should not be taken the next morning. Taking amitriptyline during waking hours could result in noticeable side effects. Patients should check with their doctors if the daily dose is missed. Those on more than one dose per day should take a missed dose as soon as it is remembered but should not take two doses at the same time. While amitriptyline is usually administered orally, injectable amitriptyline is available. It should not be used in this form long term; patients should switch to tablets as soon as possible.

Precautions

Patients should not stop taking this medication suddenly. The dose should be decreased gradually, then discontinued. If the drug is stopped abruptly, the patient may experience headache, nausea, or discomfort throughout the body, and a worsening of original symptoms. The effects of the medication last for three to seven days after it has been stopped, and older patients usually are more prone to some side effects, such as drowsiness, dizziness, mental confusion, blurry vision, dry mouth, difficulty urinating, and constipation. Taking a lower dose may help resolve these problems. Patients may need to stop this medication before surgery.

Amitriptyline should not be given to anyone with allergies to the drug or to patients recovering from a heart attack. Patients taking the **monoamine oxidase inhibitors** (MAOIs) **tranylcypromine** (Parnate) or **phenelzine** (Nardil)– different types of antidepressants—should not use amitriptyline in combination. Amitriptyline should be administered with caution to patients with glaucoma, **seizures**, urinary retention, overactive thyroid, poor liver or kidney function, alcoholism, asthma, digestive disorders, enlarged prostate, seizures, or heart disease. Pregnant women should discuss the risks and benefits of this medication with their doctors, as fetal deformities have been associated with taking this drug during pregnancy. Women should not breastfeed while using amitriptyline.

This medication should not be given to children under 12 years of age. For adolescents and adults up to age 24, amitriptyline carries an increased risk of developing suicidal thoughts while taking the drug. Patients taking amitriptyline should be monitored for signs of worsening depression or other worrisome symptoms, such as increased agitation or aggression, panic attacks, extreme irritability, or frenzied behavior. If these symptoms are experienced by the patient or observed by a caregiver, the patient's physician should be contacted.

Side effects

Common side effects include dry mouth, drowsiness, constipation, and dizziness or lightheadedness when standing. Patients can suck on ice cubes or sugarless hard candy to combat the dry mouth. Increased fiber in the diet and additional fluids may help relieve constipation. Dizziness is usually caused by a drop in blood pressure when suddenly changing position. Patients should slowly rise from a sitting or lying position if dizziness is noticed. Amitriptyline may increase the risk of falls in older adults. Patients should not drive or operate machinery or appliances while under the influence of this drug. Alcohol and other central nervous system depressants can increase drowsiness. Amitriptyline may also produce blurry vision, irregular or fast heartbeat, high or low blood pressure, palpitations, and an increase or decrease in a diabetic patient's blood sugar levels. Patients' skin may become more sensitive to the sun, and thus direct sunlight should be avoided by wearing protective clothing and applying sunscreen with a protective factor of 15 or higher.

Amitriptyline may increase appetite, cause weight gain, or produce an unpleasant taste in the mouth. It may also cause diarrhea, vomiting, or heartburn. Taking this medication with food may decrease digestive side effects. Other less likely side effects include muscle tremors, nervousness, impaired sexual function, sweating, rash, itching, hair loss, ringing in the ears, and changes in the makeup of the patient's blood, including bone marrow suppression. Patients with **schizophrenia** may develop an increase in psychiatric symptoms.

KEY TERMS

Glaucoma—A group of eye diseases characterized by increased pressure within the eye, significant enough to damage eye tissue and structures. If untreated, glaucoma results in blindness.

Methylphenidate—A mild central nervous system stimulant that is used to treat hyperactivity.

Monoamine oxidase inhibitors (MAOIs)—A group of antidepressant drugs that decrease the activity of monoamine oxidase, a neurotransmitter found in the brain that affects mood.

Urinary retention—Excessive storage of urine in the body.

Interactions

Patients should always tell all doctors and dentists that they are taking this medication. It may decrease the effectiveness of some drugs used to treat high blood pressure and should not be taken with other antidepressants, epinephrine and other adrenaline-type drugs, or **methylphenidate**. Patients should not take over-the-counter medications without checking with their doctors. For instance, amitriptyline should not be taken with Tagamet (cimetidine) or Neosynephrine. Patients taking amitriptyline should avoid the dietary supplements **St. John's wort**, belladonna, henbane, and scopolia. Black tea may decrease the absorption of this drug. Patients should ingest the drug and tea at least two hours apart.

Resources

BOOKS

Consumer Reports and American Society of Health-System Pharmacists. *Consumer Reports Complete Drug Reference, 2009 ed.* Yonkers, NY: Consumers Reports, 2009.

Ellsworth, Allan J., et al. *Mosby's Medical Drug Reference*. St. Louis, MO: Mosby, 2007.

PERIODICALS

Frese, A., et al. "Pharmacologic Treatment of Central Post-Stroke Pain." *Clinical Journal of Pain* 22, no. 3 (March-April 2006): 252–60.

Mayers, Andrew G., and David S. Baldwin. "Antidepressants and Their Effect on Sleep." *Human Psychopharmacology: Clinical and Experimental* 20, no. 8 (December 2005): 533–59.

Miyasaki, J.M., et al. "Practice Parameter: Evaluation and Treatment of Depression, Psychosis, and Dementia in Parkinson Disease (an Evidence-Based Review): Report of the Quality Standards Subcommittee of the American Academy of Neurology." *Neurology* 66, no. 7 (April 2006): 996–1002.

Sterr, Andrea, et al. "Electroencephalographic Abnormalities Associated with Antidepressant Treatment: A Comparison of Mirtazapine, Venlafaxine, Citalopram, Reboxetine, and Amitriptyline." *Journal of Clinical Psychiatry* 67, no. 2 (February 2006): 325–26.

Veldhuijzen, D. S., et al. "Acute and Subchronic Effects of Amitriptyline on Processing Capacity in Neuropathic Pain Patients Using Visual Event-Related Potentials: Preliminary Findings." *Psychopharmacology* 183, no. 4 (2006): 462–70.

Vezmar, S., et al. "Pharmacokinetics and Efficacy of Fluvoxamine and Amitriptyline in Depression." *Journal of Pharmacological Sciences* 110, no. 1 (2009): 98–104.

WEBSITES

RevolutionHealth.com. "What is Elavil? (Amitriptyline)" July 2010. http://www.revolutionhealth.com/drugs-treatments/elavil (accessed September 20, 2011).

Mark Mitchell, MD
Ruth A. Wienclaw, PhD

Amnesia

Definition

Amnesia refers to the partial or total loss of memory. The loss may be temporary or permanent. Amnestic disorders are a group of disorders that involve loss of memories previously established, loss of the ability to create new memories, or loss of the ability to learn new information.

Demographics

The overall incidence of amnestic disorders is difficult to estimate. Amnestic disorders related to head injuries may affect people in any age group. Alcohol-induced amnestic disorder is most common in people over the age of 40 with histories of prolonged heavy **alcohol use**. Amnestic disorders resulting from the abuse of drugs other than alcohol are most common in people between the ages of 20 and 40. Transient global amnesia, in which people temporarily cannot recall recent events, usually appears in people over 50 with an estimated incidence of 23.5 cases per 100,000 people per year. Only 3% of people who experience transient global amnesia have symptoms that recur within a year. About 7% of all individuals over the age of 65 have some form of **dementia** that involves some degree of amnesia, as do about 50% of all individuals over the age of 85.

Description

Memory is the ability to retain and recall information. Memory can be subdivided into short-term memory, which involves holding information for one minute or less, and long-term memory, which involves holding onto information for more than one minute. Long-term memory can be further subdivided into recent memory, which involves new learning, and remote memory, which involves old information. In general, amnestic disorders more frequently involve deficits in new learning or recent memory.

There are a number of terms that are crucial to the understanding of amnestic disorders. In order to retain information, an individual must be able to pay close enough attention to the information that is presented; this is referred to as "registration." The process whereby memories are established is referred to as "encoding" or "storage." Retaining information in the long-term memory requires passage of time during which memory is consolidated. When an individual's memory is tested, retrieval is the process whereby the individual recalls the information from memory. Working memory is the ability to manipulate information from short-term memory in order to perform some function. Amnestic disorders may affect any or all of these necessary processes.

There are two types of amnesia: retrograde and anterograde. Retrograde amnesia refers to the loss of memories made prior to the onset of amnesia. Retrograde amnesia often occurs in conjunction with head injury and results in erasure of memory of events or information from some time period (ranging from seconds to months to the whole of a person's past) prior to the head injury. Over the course of recovery and rehabilitation from a head injury, memory may be restored or the period of amnesia may eventually shorten. Anterograde amnesia refers to the inability to recall events or facts introduced since the amnesia began (i.e., the inability to retain new memories). It is more common than retrograde amnesia. Although individuals with anterograde amnesia have difficulty with the establishment of memory from that time at which the amnesia started, they may clearly recall events that happened before the amnesia began. It is possible for a single individual to have both anterograde and retrograde amnesia depending on which part of the **brain** is damaged.

The diagnostic manual used by clinicians, ***Diagnostic and Statistical Manual of Mental Disorders***, fourth

KEY TERMS

Acetylcholine—A brain chemical or neurotransmitter that carries information throughout the nervous system.

Anterograde—Memory loss for information/ events occurring after the onset of the amnestic disorder.

Delirium—A condition characterized by waxing-and-waning episodes of confusion and agitation.

Dementia—A chronic condition in which thinking and memory are progressively impaired. Other symptoms may also occur, including personality changes and depression.

Electroconvulsive therapy—This type of therapy is used to treat major depression and severe mental illness that does not respond to medications. A measured dose of electricity is introduced into the brain in order to produce a convulsion. Electroconvulsive therapy is safe and effective.

Retrograde—Describes memory loss of information/events prior to the onset of the amnestic disorder.

Transient ischemic attack (TIA)—Temporary blockage of blood flow to the brain often resulting in slurred speech, vision disturbances, and loss of balance. The episode is brief and the damage is often short-term (not permanent); also called mini-stroke or warning stroke.

Wernicke-Korsakoff syndrome—A condition of the brain caused by alcohol abuse coupled with malnutrition; also called alcohol encephalopathy.

edition, text revision (*DSM-IV-TR*), lists three classifications of amnestic disorders: amnestic disorder due to a general medical condition, substance-induced persisting amnestic disorder, and amnestic disorder not otherwise specified.

Amnestic disorder due to a medical condition

The memory loss of amnestic disorder due to a general medical condition can be transient or chronic. This disorder can manifest as retrograde or anterograde loss. For **diagnosis**, individuals must experience impairment of social or occupational functioning that differs from their normal levels, and the memory loss cannot occur as part of dementia or **delirium**. The medical condition responsible must be confirmed by patient history or by physical exam or lab results.

Substance-induced persisting amnestic disorder

Substance-induced persisting amnestic disorder can occur with use of alcohol, **sedatives**, hypnotics, or anxiolytics. Methotrexate, a chemotherapy drug, can induce this condition, as can some toxins, including lead, mercury, carbon monoxide, insecticides, or industrial solvents. There are subtypes, including alcohol-induced persisting amnestic disorder. In the alcohol-induced form, the symptoms of **Wernicke-Korsakoff syndrome** may manifest as a result of the thiamine deficiency. Full recovery is not the norm with alcohol-induced amnestic disorder but is possible when caused by other drugs. The diagnostic criteria for the substance-induced form of amnestic disorder are similar to those for that induced by a general medical condition, except that the history should show exposure to the substance involved.

Amnestic disorder not otherwise specified

If the characteristics of the amnesia do not fit either of the above categories, the disorder is then classified as amnestic disorder not otherwise specified, generally because the causative agent/event is not known.

Dissociative amnesia

Dissociative amnesia is part of a different group of disorders, the **dissociative disorders**. It manifests as an inability to remember information that is personally important but possibly traumatic or stressful. It was previously called psychogenic amnesia. The memory impairment in this disorder is reversible, and memory loss can be of several types. It can be localized, in which the missing memory covers a defined period of time, or it can be selective, so that only bits and pieces of a situation are recalled. There are also three less common types: generalized (memories covering a lifetime are missing); continuous (memories are missing from a specific time period up to the present); and systematized (only memories from specific categories of information are missing, such as the names of family members). This disorder can arise in a person of any age.

Other types of amnesia

Transient global amnesia causes delirium (a period of waxing-and-waning confusion and agitation), anterograde amnesia, and retrograde amnesia for events and information from the several hours prior to the onset of the attack. It has no consistently identifiable cause, but researchers have suggested that migraine or transient ischemic attack (TIA) may be the trigger. The individual experiences sudden confusion and forgetfulness. Attacks can be as brief as 30 minutes or can last up to 24 hours. In severe attacks, an individual is completely disoriented and may also experience retrograde amnesia that extends back several years. While very frightening for the individual, transient global amnesia generally has an excellent prognosis for recovery, with no lasting memory deficit.

Childhood amnesia, a term coined by Anna Freud in the late 1940s, refers to the fact that most people cannot recall childhood experiences during the first three to five years of life. It has been suggested that this type of amnesia occurs because children and adults organize memories in different ways. The differences are based on the brain's physical development and communication among the different areas of the brain involved in developing memory. Others believe children begin remembering facts and events once they have accumulated enough experience to be able to relate experiences to each other.

Causes and symptoms

Amnesia has multiple causes. Most cases are traceable to brain injury related to physical **trauma**, disease, infection, and drug and alcohol abuse. In Wernicke-Korsakoff syndrome, for example, damage to the memory centers of the brain results from chronic use of alcohol coupled with malnutrition. Infections that damage brain tissue, such as encephalitis, also can cause amnesia, as can **stroke**. Other causes include various types of dementia (e.g., **Alzheimer's disease**), **traumatic brain injury** (e.g., concussion), accidents that involve oxygen deprivation to the brain or interruption of blood flow to the brain (e.g., ruptured aneurysms, near-drowning), tumors in the thalamus and/or hypothalamus, and **seizures**.

Sometimes procedures such as surgery or **electroconvulsive therapy** can produce amnesia. Dissociative amnesia is thought to be of psychological origin, caused by a psychological disorder or trauma.

Symptoms of amnestic disorders may include difficulty recalling remote events or information and/or difficulty learning and then recalling new information. In some cases, the individual is fully aware of the memory impairment and frustrated by it; in other cases, the individual may seem completely oblivious to the memory impairment or may even attempt to fill in the deficit in memory with confabulation. Depending on the underlying condition responsible for the amnesia, a number of other symptoms may be present as well.

Diagnosis

Diagnosis of amnestic disorders begins by establishing the level of orientation to person, place, and time. Do these individuals know who they are? Where they are? The day, date, and time? Can they recall common current events (e.g., identify the president)? Their responses may reveal information about the memory deficit. Family members or close friends may be an invaluable part of the examination, as they may provide some background information on the onset and progression of the memory loss as well as information regarding the individual's original level of functioning.

A variety of memory tests can be used to assess the ability to attend to information, utilize short-term memory, and store and retrieve information from long-term memory. Both verbal and visual memory should be tested. Verbal memory can be tested by working with an individual to memorize word lists and then testing recall after a certain amount of time has elapsed. Similarly, visual memory can be tested by asking an individual to locate several objects that were hidden in a room in the individual's presence.

Depending on what types of conditions are being considered, other tests may include blood tests, neuroimaging (CT, MRI, or **PET** scans of the brain), cerebrospinal fluid testing, and EEG testing.

Treatment

A neurologist and/or **psychiatrist** may be involved in diagnosing and treating amnestic disorders. Depending on the underlying condition responsible for the memory deficit, other specialists may be involved as well, such as occupational and speech and language therapists may be involved in rehabilitation programs for individuals who have amnestic disorders as part of their clinical picture.

Traditional

In some cases, treatment of the underlying disorder may help improve the accompanying amnesia. In mild cases of amnesia, rehabilitation may involve teaching memory techniques and encouraging the use of memory tools, such as association techniques, lists, notes, calendars, and timers. Memory exercises may be helpful. There are no specific drugs to treat amnesia. However, treatments for Alzheimer's disease and other dementias, such as **donepezil** (Aricept), are being studied to see if they may also be effective in treating amnestic disorders.

Prognosis

The prognosis is dependent on the underlying condition that has caused the memory deficit and on

QUESTIONS TO ASK YOUR DOCTOR

- What tests will you do to rule out medical conditions that might be causing or aggravating my loved one's amnestic disorder?
- How likely is it that this amnestic disorder is reversible or partially reversible?
- What kind of therapy might help my loved one regain some memories?
- Can you recommend a support group for caregivers of people with amnesia?

whether that condition has a tendency to progress or stabilize. Alzheimer's disease, for example, is relentlessly progressive, and the memory deficits that accompany this condition can be expected to worsen over time. Individuals who have memory deficits due to a brain tumor may have their symptoms improve after surgery to remove the tumor. Individuals with transient global amnesia can be expected to fully recover from their memory impairment within hours or days of its onset. In the case of some traumatic brain injuries, the amnesia may improve with time (as brain swelling decreases, for example), but some degree of amnesia for the events just prior to the moment of the injury may remain.

Prevention

Amnestic disorders are preventable in so far as brain injury can be prevented or minimized. Common sense approaches include wearing a helmet when bicycling, horseback riding, or participating in potentially dangerous sports; using automobile seat belts; and avoiding excessive alcohol or drug use. Brain infections should be treated swiftly and aggressively to minimize the damage due to swelling. Victims of strokes, brain aneurysms, and transient ischemic attacks should seek immediate medical treatment.

Resources

BOOKS

Bolzan, Scott, and Joan Bolzan. *My Life Deleted: A Memoir.* New York: HarperCollins, 2011.

Papanicolaou, Andrew C. *The Amnesias: A Clinical Textbook of Memory Disorders.* New York: Oxford University Press, 2006.

WEBSITES

"Amnesia." Mayo Clinic, October 10, 2009. http://www.mayoclinic.com/health/amnesia/DS01041 (accessed October 7, 2011).

"Memory." MedlinePlus. Last modified September 29, 2011. http://www.nlm.nih.gov/medlineplus/memory.html (accessed October 7, 2011).

Sucholeiki, Roy. "Transient Global Amnesia." Medscape Reference, June 16, 2010. http://emedicine.medscape.com/article/1160964-overview (accessed October 7, 2011).

ORGANIZATIONS

American Academy of Neurology, 1080 Montreal Ave., St. Paul, MN, 55116, (651) 695-2717, (800) 879-1960, Fax: (651) 879-2791, memberservices@aan.com, http://www.aan.com.

American Psychiatric Association, 1000 Wilson Blvd., Ste. 1825, Arlington, VA, 22209-3901, (703) 907-7300, apa@psych.org, http://www.psych.org.

National Institute of Neurological Disorders and Stroke, PO Box 5801, Bethesda, MD, 20824, (301) 496-5751; TTY: (301) 468-5981, (800) 352-9424, http://www.ninds.nih.gov.

Julia Barrett
Tish Davidson, AM

Amobarbitol *see* **Barbiturates**

Amoxapine

Definition

Amoxapine is an oral dibenzoxazepine-derivative tricyclic antidepressant. Formerly sold in the United States under the brand name Asendin, it is now manufactured and sold only under its generic name.

Purpose

Amoxapine is used primarily to treat **depression** and to treat the combination of symptoms of anxiety and depression. Like most **antidepressants** of this chemical and pharmacological class, amoxapine has also been used in limited numbers of patients to treat **panic disorder**, **obsessive-compulsive disorder**, **attention deficit hyperactivity disorder**, **enuresis** (bed-wetting), eating disorders such as **bulimia nervosa**, **cocaine addiction**, and the depressive phase of **bipolar disorder**. It has also been used to support **smoking cessation** programs.

Description

Tricyclic antidepressants act to change the balance of naturally occurring chemicals in the **brain** that regulate the transmission of nerve impulses between cells. Amoxapine acts primarily by increasing the concentration of norepinephrine and **serotonin** (chemicals that stimulate nerve cells) and, to a lesser extent, by blocking the action of another brain chemical, acetylcholine. Amoxapine shares most of the properties of other tricyclic antidepressants, such as **amitriptyline**, **clomipramine**, **desipramine**, **imipramine**, **nortriptyline**, **protriptyline**, and **trimipramine**. Studies comparing amoxapine with these other drugs have shown that amoxapine is no more or less effective than other antidepressants of its type. Its choice for treatment is as much a function of physician preference as any other factor.

The therapeutic effects of amoxapine, like other antidepressants, appear slowly. Maximum benefit is often not evident for at least two weeks after starting the drug. People taking amoxapine should be aware of this and continue taking the drug as directed, even if they do not see immediate improvement.

Recommended dosage

As with any antidepressant, amoxapine must be adjusted by the physician to produce the desired therapeutic effect. Amoxapine is available as 25 mg, 50 mg, 100 mg, and 150 mg oral tablets. Therapy is usually started at 100 to 150 mg per day and increased to 200 to 300 mg daily by the end of the first week. If no improvement is seen at this dose after two weeks, the physician may increase the dose up to 400 mg per day in outpatients, and up to 600 mg per day in hospitalized patients. Doses up to 300 mg may be given in single or divided doses. Doses of more than 300 mg per day should be divided in two or three doses daily.

Because of changes in drug metabolism of older patients, starting at about age 60, the initial dose of amoxapine should be adjusted downward to 50 to 75 mg per day and increased to 100 to 150 mg daily by the end of the first week. Some older patients may require up to 300 mg daily, but doses should never be increased beyond that.

Precautions

Like all tricyclic antidepressants, amoxapine should be used cautiously and with close physician supervision in people, especially the elderly, who have benign prostatic hypertrophy (prostate enlargement), urinary retention, and glaucoma, especially angle-closure glaucoma (the most severe form). Before starting treatment, people with these conditions should discuss the relative risks and benefits of treatment with their doctors to help determine whether amoxapine is the right antidepressant for them. Amoxapine also carries an increased risk of developing suicidal thoughts in children and adults up to age 24. All patients should be monitored for worsening depression or signs of self-harm, and physicians should be alerted to any changes in behavior.

One common problem with tricyclic antidepressants is sedation (drowsiness, lack of physical and mental alertness). This side effect is especially noticeable early in therapy. In most patients, sedation decreases or disappears entirely with time, but until then patients taking amoxapine should not perform hazardous activities requiring mental alertness or coordination. The sedative effect is increased when amoxapine is taken with other central nervous system depressants, such as alcoholic beverages, sleeping medications, other **sedatives**, or antihistamines. It may be dangerous to take amoxapine in combination with these substances. Amoxapine may increase the possibility of having **seizures**. Patients should tell their physician if they have a history of seizures, including seizures brought on by the abuse of drugs or alcohol. These people should use amoxapine only with caution and be closely monitored by their physician.

Amoxapine may increase heart rate and stress on the heart. It may be dangerous for people with cardiovascular disease, especially those who have recently had a heart attack, to take this drug or other tricyclic antidepressants. In rare cases where patients with cardiovascular disease must receive amoxapine, they should be monitored closely for cardiac rhythm disturbances and signs of cardiac stress or damage.

Side effects

Amoxapine shares side effects common to all tricyclic antidepressants. The most frequent of these are dry mouth, constipation, urinary retention, increased heart rate, sedation, irritability, dizziness, and decreased coordination. As with most side effects associated with tricyclic antidepressants, the intensity is highest at the beginning of therapy and tends to decrease with continued use.

Dry mouth, if severe to the point of causing difficulty speaking or swallowing, may be managed by dosage reduction or temporary discontinuation of the drug. Patients may also chew sugarless gum or suck on sugarless candy in order to increase the flow of saliva. Some artificial saliva products may give temporary relief.

Men with prostate enlargement who take amoxapine may be especially likely to have problems with urinary retention. Symptoms include having difficulty starting a urine flow and more difficulty than usual passing urine. In most cases, urinary retention is managed with dose reduction or by switching to another type of antidepressant. In extreme cases, patients may require treatment with bethanechol, a drug that reverses this particular side effect. People who think they may be experiencing any side effects from this or any other medication should tell their physicians.

KEY TERMS

Acetylcholine—A neurotransmitter with effects that are generally opposite those of the neurotransmitters dopamine and norepinephrine. Acetylcholine dilates blood vessels, lowers blood pressure, and slows heartbeat.

Anticholinergic—Related to the ability of a drug to block the nervous system chemical acetylcholine. When acetylcholine is blocked, patients often experience dry mouth and skin, increased heart rate, blurred vision, and difficulty urinating. In severe cases, blocking acetylcholine may cloud thinking and cause delirium.

Neurotransmitter—A naturally occurring chemical in the body that carries chemical messages to nerve cells, often by transmitting nerve impulses. Central nervous system well-being is dependent on a balance among the neurotransmitters acetylcholine, dopamine, serotonin, and norepinephrine.

Norepinephrine—A neurotransmitter in the brain that acts to constrict blood vessels and raise blood pressure. It works in combination with serotonin.

Serotonin—A widely distributed neurotransmitter that is found in blood platelets, the lining of the digestive tract, and the brain, and that works in combination with norepinephrine. It causes very powerful contractions of smooth muscle and is associated with mood, attention, emotions, and sleep. Low levels of serotonin are associated with depression.

Interactions

Dangerously high blood pressure has resulted from the combination of tricyclic antidepressants, such as amoxapine, and members of another class of antidepressants known as **monoamine oxidase inhibitors (MAOIs)**. Because of this, amoxapine should never be taken in combination with **MAOIs**. Patients taking any MAOIs, such as **phenelzine** sulfate (Nardil) or **tranylcypromine** sulfate (Parnate), should stop the MAOI and then wait at least 14 days before starting amoxapine or any other tricyclic antidepressant. The same holds true when discontinuing amoxapine and starting an MAOI.

Amoxapine may decrease the blood pressure–lowering effects of **clonidine**. Patients who take both drugs should be monitored for loss of blood pressure control, and the dose of clonidine should be increased as needed.

The sedative effects of amoxapine are increased by other central nervous system depressants, such as alcohol, sedatives, sleeping medications, or medications used for other mental disorders, such as **schizophrenia**. The anticholinergic effects of amoxapine are additive with other anticholinergic drugs, including **benztropine**, **biperiden**, **trihexyphenidyl**, and antihistamines.

Resources

BOOKS

American Society of Health-System Pharmacists. *AHFS Drug Information 2008*. Bethesda, MD: American Society of Health-System Pharmacists, 2008.

WEBSITES

PubMed Health. "Amoxapine." U.S. National Library of Medicine. http://www.ncbi.nlm.nih.gov/pubmedhealth/PMH0000609 (accessed December 12, 2011).

Jack Raber, Pharm.D.

Amphetamines

Definition

Amphetamines are a group of drugs that stimulate the central nervous system. Some of the brand names of amphetamines sold in the United States are Dexedrine, Biphetamine, Dexampex, Ferndex, Oxydess II, Spancap No. 1, Desoxyn, and Methampex. Some generic names of amphetamines include amphetamine, **dextroamphetamine**, and **methamphetamine**.

Purpose

Amphetamines stimulate the nervous system and are used in the treatment of **depression**, obesity, **attention deficit hyperactivity disorder** (ADHD), and **narcolepsy**, a disorder that causes individuals to fall asleep at inappropriate times during the day. Amphetamines are commonly abused as recreational drugs and are highly addictive.

Description

Amphetamines are usually given orally and their effects can last for hours. They produce their effects by altering chemicals that transmit nerve messages in the body. Use of amphetamines can cause considerable side effects and are especially toxic in large quantities.

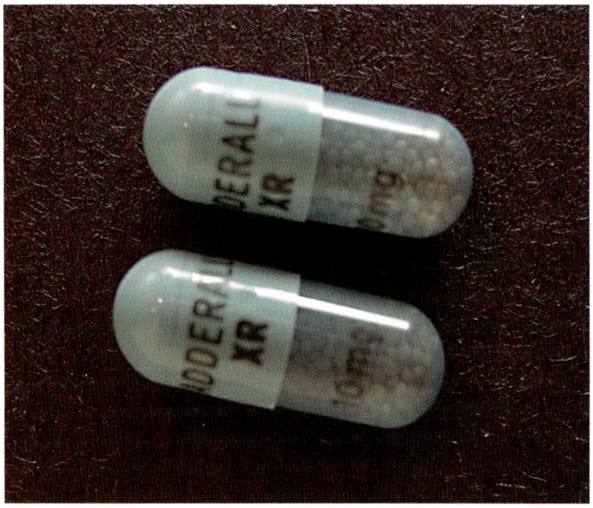

Adderall (dextroamphetamine and amphetamine), 10 mg.
(© Custom Medical Stock Photo, Inc. Reproduced by permission.)

Recommended dosage

Stimulants approved by the U.S. Food and Drug Administration (FDA) for treatment of ADHD are **methylphenidate** (sold under several trade names, including Ritalin), mixed amphetamine salts (trade name Adderall), and dextroamphetamine (trade name Dexedrine). These comparatively short-acting stimulants necessitate several doses through the day to maintain appropriate levels. Some long-acting forms are available, such as Ritalin LA and Adderall XR, and there is also a transdermal patch (trade name Daytrana) for delivery of methylphenidate through the skin.

The typical dose for amphetamines in the treatment of narcolepsy in adults ranges from 5 mg to 60 mg per day. These daily doses are usually divided into at least two small doses taken during the day. Doses usually start on the low end of the range and are increased until the desired effects occur. Children over the age of 12 years with narcolepsy receive 10 mg per day initially. Children between the ages of 6 and 12 years start with 5 mg per day. The typical dose for adults with obesity ranges from 5 mg to 30 mg per day given in divided doses. The medication is usually given about one-half hour to one hour before meals.

Precautions

Stimulant use in children with ADHD has been associated in some studies with sudden death in a small number of cases, leading to widespread concern; however, subsequent studies have found no difference in sudden death rates among children taking stimulants for ADHD and the general population using no medication. Use of these medications is not recommended for people who have known heart disease.

Another stimulant-related concern is the effects of these drugs on growth rate. Studies do indicate that while a child is taking stimulants, growth rate can slow. Some practitioners may recommend "drug holidays," in which the child stops taking the drug when circumstances require less focus or self-discipline, such as over a summer vacation. Studies indicate that the adverse effects on growth rate are eliminated by these drug holidays.

People who are taking amphetamines should not stop taking these drugs suddenly. The dose should be lowered gradually and then discontinued. Amphetamines should only be used while under the supervision of a physician. People should generally take the drug early in the day so that it does not interfere with sleep at night. Hazardous activities should be avoided until the person's condition has been stabilized with medication. The effects of amphetamines can last up to 20 hours after the medication has last been taken. Amphetamine therapy given to women for medical reasons does not present a significant risk of congenital disorders to the developing fetus. In such cases, a mild withdrawal in the newborn may occur. However, illicit use of amphetamines for nonmedical reasons presents a significant risk to the fetus and the newborn because of uncontrolled doses. Methamphetamine use during pregnancy, for example, has been associated with fetal growth retardation, premature birth, and heart and **brain** abnormalities.

Amphetamines are highly addictive and should be used only if alternative approaches have failed. They should be used with great caution in children under three years of age, anyone with a history of slightly elevated blood pressure, people with neurological tics, and individuals with Tourette syndrome. Individuals with a history of an overactive thyroid should not take amphetamines, nor should those with moderate-to-severe high blood pressure, the eye disease glaucoma, severe arteriosclerosis (hardening of the arteries), or psychotic symptoms (hallucinations and **delusions**). Individuals with a history of drug abuse, psychological agitation, or cardiovascular system disease also should not receive amphetamine therapy. In addition, patients who have taken a type of antidepressant called **monoamine oxidase inhibitors (MAOIs)** within the last 14 days should not receive amphetamines. **MAOIs** include **phenelzine** (Nardil) and **tranylcypromine** (Parnate).

Side effects

The most common side effects that are associated with amphetamines include the development of an irregular heartbeat, increased heart rate or blood pressure, dizziness, **insomnia**, restlessness, headache, shakiness, dry mouth, metallic taste, diarrhea, constipation, and weight loss. Other

KEY TERMS

Anticonvulsant drugs—Medications that relieve or prevent seizures.

Arteriosclerosis—A thickening, hardening, and loss of elasticity of the walls of the arteries.

Attention deficit hyperactivity disorder—A condition characterized by lack of concentration, impulsive or inappropriate behavior (relative to age level), and hyperactivity.

Congenital—Present at birth.

Glaucoma—A group of eye diseases characterized by increased pressure within the eye significant enough to damage eye tissue and structures. If untreated, glaucoma results in blindness.

Monoamine oxidase inhibitors (MAOIs)—A group of antidepressant drugs that decreases the activity of monoamine oxidase, a neurotransmitter in the brain that affects mood.

Tic—A sudden involuntary behavior that is difficult or impossible for the person to suppress. Tics may be either motor (related to movement) or vocal, and may become more pronounced under stress.

Tourette's syndrome—A neurological disorder characterized by multiple involuntary movements and uncontrollable vocalizations called tics that come and go over years, usually beginning in childhood and becoming chronic. Sometimes the tics include inappropriate language.

Tricyclic antidepressants—Antidepressant medications that have the common characteristic of a three-ring nucleus in their chemical structure. Imipramine and amitriptyline are examples of tricyclic antidepressants.

side effects can include changes in sexual drive, nausea, vomiting, allergic reactions, chills, depression, irritability, and other problems involving the digestive system. High doses, whether for medical purposes or illicit ones, can cause **addiction**, dependence, increased aggression, and, in some cases, psychotic episodes.

Interactions

Patients taking amphetamines should always tell their physicians and dentists that they are using this medication. Patients should consult their physicians before taking any over-the-counter medications while taking amphetamines. The interaction between over-the-counter cold medications with amphetamine is particularly dangerous, because this combination can significantly increase blood pressure. Such cold medications should be avoided when using amphetamines unless a physician has carefully analyzed the combination.

The combination of amphetamines and antacids slows down the ability of the body to eliminate the amphetamine. Furazolidone (Furoxone) combined with amphetamines can significantly increase blood pressure. Sodium bicarbonate can reduce the amount of amphetamine eliminated from the body, thereby dangerously increasing amphetamine levels in the body. Certain medications taken to control high blood pressure, including guanadrel (Hylorel) and guanethidine (Ismelin), MAOIs, and selegiline (Eldepryl) should not be used in conjunction with amphetamines. In addition, antihistamines, anticonvulsant drugs, and tricyclic **antidepressants** including **desipramine** (Norpramin) and **imipramine** (Tofranil) should not be combined with amphetamines.

Resources

BOOKS

Brunton, Laurence, Bruce Chabner, and Bjorn Knollman. *Goodman & Gilman's The Pharmacological Basis of Therapeutics*. 12th ed. New York: McGraw-Hill, 2010.

Consumer Reports and American Society of Health-System Pharmacists. *Consumer Reports Complete Drug Reference, 2009*. Yonkers, NY: Consumers Reports, 2009.

Ellsworth, Allan J., et al. *Mosby's Medical Drug Reference*. St. Louis, MO: Mosby, 2007.

Venes, Donald. *Taber's Cyclopedic Medical Dictionary*. 21st ed. Philadelphia: F.A. Davis Company, 2009.

PERIODICALS

Lopez, Frank A. "ADHD: New Pharmacological Treatments on the Horizon." *Journal of Developmental and Behavioral Pediatrics* 27, no. 5 (October 2006): 410–16.

Pliszka, Steven R. "Pharmacologic Treatment of Attention-Deficit/Hyperactivity Disorder: Efficacy, Safety, and Mechanisms of Action." *Neuropsychological Reviews* 17 (2007): 61–72. http://www.pathwayshrc.com.au/images/assets/pharmac%20adhd%20review.PDF (accessed November 9, 2011).

Sulzer, David, et al. "Mechanisms of Neurotransmitter Release by Amphetamines: A Review." *Progress in Neurobiology* 75 (2005): 406–33. http://www.sulzerlab.org/pdf_articles/Sulzer05AMPHreview.pdf (accessed November 9, 2011).

WEBSITES

Center for Substance Abuse Research. "Amphetamines." University of Maryland. http://www.cesar.umd.edu/cesar/drugs/amphetamines.asp (accessed September 29, 2011).

MedlinePlus. "Amphetamines." U.S. National Library of Medicine, National Institutes of Health. http://www.nlm.nih.gov/nlmhome.html (accessed September 29, 2011).

Mark Mitchell, MD
Emily Jane Willingham, PhD

Amphetamines and related disorders

Definition

Amphetamines are a group of powerful and highly addictive substances that dramatically affect the central nervous system. They induce a feeling of well-being and improve alertness, attention, and performance on various cognitive and motor tasks. Closely related are the so-called substitute amphetamines, which include MDMA (**ecstasy**) and **methamphetamine**. Finally, some over-the-counter drugs used as appetite suppressants also have amphetamine-like action. Amphetamine-related disorders refer to the effects of abuse, dependence, and acute intoxication stemming from inappropriate amphetamine and amphetamine-related drug usage.

Demographics

Amphetamine dependence and abuse occur at all levels of society, most commonly among 18- to 30-year-olds. Intravenous use is more common among individuals from lower socioeconomic groups and has a male-to-female ratio of three or four to one. Among people who do not use intravenously, males and females are relatively equally divided.

Of greatest recent concern has been the rise in the use of methamphetamine, although in some areas this increase has leveled off in recent years. The lifetime prevalence of methamphetamine abuse among U.S. students in grade 12 fell from 6.2% of respondents to 4.5% over two years in one recent government survey. However, in some metropolitan areas, including Atlanta, Denver, Honolulu, and Phoenix, use has increased, and there was a 15% increase in methamphetamine treatment admissions in St. Louis from 2004 to 2005. In some parts of Texas, this drug has replaced crack as a drug of choice. Another national survey found that 10.4 million Americans age 12 or older had tried methamphetamine at least once in their lives. The problem seems to be particularly severe in Western states, although it is spreading quickly in the South and Midwest, being reported as the fastest-growing problem in metropolitan Atlanta in 2006.

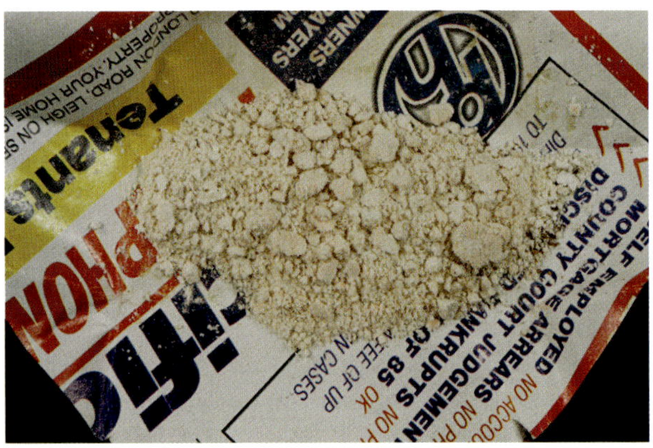

Amphetamine sulfate. *(© David Hoffman/Photo Library/Alamy)*

Nonmedical use of Adderall® in the past year among full-time college students aged 18 to 22, by selected demographic characteristics, 2006 and 2007

Race/ethnicity	
White	8.6%
Black or African American	1.0%
Asian	2.1%
Two or more races	2.7%
Hispanic	2.2%
Annual family income	
Less than $20,000	8.9%
$20,000 to $49,999	3.0%
$50,000 to $74,999	4.0%
$75,000 or more	6.0%

SOURCE: Substance Abuse and Mental Health Administration, Office of Applied Studies, *The NSDUH Report: Nonmedical Use of Adderall® among Full-Time College Students*, April 7, 2009.

(Table by PreMediaGlobal. © 2012 Cengage Learning.)

Description

Several amphetamines are currently available in the United States, including **dextroamphetamine** (Dexedrine) and **methylphenidate** (Ritalin). These Schedule II stimulants (those that the U.S. Drug Enforcement Administration considers to have medical usefulness and a high potential for abuse), known to be highly addictive, require a triplicate prescription that cannot be refilled. Amphetamines are also known as sympathomimetics, stimulants, and psychostimulants. Methamphetamine, the most common illegally produced amphetamine, goes by the street names of "speed," "meth," or "chalk." When it is smoked, it is called "ice," "crystal," "crank," or "glass." Methamphetamine is a white, odorless, bitter-tasting crystalline powder that dissolves in water or alcohol. Manufacture of methamphetamine in illegal laboratories has increased dramatically in recent years, leading to stricter laws governing the sale of products containing ephedrine or pseudoephedrine, the primary components of this drug.

The leaves of the East African bush *Catha edulis* can be chewed for their stimulant effects. This drug, cathinone, or "khat," has an effect on most of the central nervous system, in addition to providing the other properties of amphetamines. It is a stimulant drug similar in structure to amphetamines, with similar effects. The drug may be ingested by chewing the leaves, adding the leaves to food, or brewing the leaves and drinking as a tea. The stimulant effects are usually felt immediately and subside within three hours; however, they may last up to 24 hours. The potential for abuse and physical or psychological dependence is high, making this popular drug illegal in the United States.

Amphetamines intended for medical use were first used in nasal decongestants and bronchial inhalers. Early in the 1900s, they were also used to treat several medical and psychiatric conditions, including attention deficit disorders, obesity, **depression**, and **narcolepsy** (a rare condition in which individuals fall asleep at dangerous and inappropriate moments and cannot maintain normal alertness). They are still used to treat these disorders.

In the 1970s, governmental agencies initiated restrictions increasing the difficulty of obtaining amphetamines legally through prescription. During this same time period, a drug chemically related to the amphetamines began to be produced. This so-called designer drug, best known as "ecstasy" but also as MDMA, XTC, and Adam, has behavioral effects that combine amphetamine-like and hallucinogen-like properties.

The structure of amphetamines differs significantly from that of **cocaine**, even though both are stimulants with similar behavioral and physiological effects. Like cocaine, amphetamines result in an accumulation of the neurotransmitter **dopamine** in the prefrontal cortex. It is this excessive dopamine concentration that appears to produce the stimulation and feelings of euphoria experienced by the user. Cocaine is much more quickly metabolized and removed from the body, whereas amphetamines have a much longer duration of action. A large percentage of the drug remains unchanged in the body, leading to prolonged stimulant effects.

The handbook that mental health professionals use to diagnose mental disorders is the ***Diagnostic and Statistical Manual of Mental Disorders,*** also known as the *DSM.* The 2000 edition of this manual (the fourth edition, text revision, also known as *DSM-IV-TR*) describes four separate amphetamine-related disorders:

- Amphetamine dependence: Refers to chronic or episodic binges (known as "speed runs"), with brief drug-free periods of time in between use.
- Amphetamine abuse: Less severe than dependence. Individuals diagnosed with amphetamine abuse have milder, but nevertheless substantial, problems due to their drug usage.
- Amphetamine intoxication: Refers to serious maladaptive behavioral or psychological changes that develop during, or shortly after, use of an amphetamine or related substance.
- Amphetamine withdrawal: Refers to symptoms that develop within a few hours to several days after reducing or stopping heavy and prolonged amphetamine use. Withdrawal symptoms are, in general, opposite to those seen during intoxication and include fatigue, vivid and unpleasant dreams, insomnia or hypersomnia (too much sleep), increased appetite, and agitation or slowing down.

The fifth edition of the *Diagnostic and Statistical Manual of Mental Disorders,* also known as the *DSM-5* is due for publication in May 2013. Proposed changes to this edition include combining amphetamine abuse and amphetamine dependence into one condition, amphetamine use disorder.

Causes and symptoms

Causes

All amphetamines are rapidly absorbed when taken orally, and are even more rapidly absorbed when smoked, snorted, or injected. Tolerance develops with both standard and designer amphetamines, leading to the need for increasing doses.

Amphetamines produce their primary effects by causing the release of catecholamines, especially the nerve-signaling molecule or neurotransmitter dopamine, in the **brain**. These effects are particularly strong in areas of the brain associated with pleasure—specifically, the cerebral cortex and the limbic system, known as the "reward pathway." The effect on this pathway is probably responsible for the addictive quality of the amphetamines.

MDMA causes the release of the **neurotransmitters** dopamine and **serotonin** and the neurohormone norepinephrine. Serotonin is responsible for producing the hallucinogenic effects of the drug.

Symptoms

According to the *DSM-IV-TR,* symptoms of heavy, chronic, or episodic use of amphetamine, known as amphetamine dependence, can be very serious. Amphetamine dependence is characterized by compulsive drug seeking and drug use, leading to functional and molecular changes in the brain. Aggressive or violent behavior may occur, especially when high doses are ingested. Individuals may develop anxiety or paranoid ideas, or may experience terrifying psychotic episodes

KEY TERMS

Amphetamine abuse—An amphetamine problem in which the user experiences negative consequences from the use but has not reached the point of dependence.

Amphetamines—A group of powerful and highly addictive substances that stimulate the central nervous system. Amphetamines may be prescribed for various medical conditions but are often purchased illicitly and abused.

Catecholamine—A group of neurotransmitters synthesized from the amino acid tyrosine and released by the hypothalamic-pituitary-adrenal system in the brain in response to acute stress. The catecholamines include dopamine, serotonin, norepinephrine, and epinephrine.

Catha edulis—Leaves of an East African bush that can be chewed for their stimulant effect.

Dependence—A state in which a person requires a steady concentration of a particular substance to avoid experiencing withdrawal symptoms.

Designer amphetamines—Substances close in chemical structure to classic amphetamines that provide both stimulant and hallucinogenic effects.

Dopamine—A chemical in brain tissue that serves to transmit nerve impulses (i.e., a neurotransmitter) and helps to regulate movement and emotions. Large amounts of dopamine are released following ingestion of amphetamines.

Ecstasy—Best known of the so-called designer amphetamines, also known as "MDMA." It produces both stimulant and hallucinogenic effects.

Ephedrine—An amphetamine-like substance used as a nasal decongestant.

Formication—The sensation of bugs creeping on the skin.

Hyperthermia—Elevated body temperature resulting from ingestion of amphetamines.

Intoxication—The presence of significant behavioral or psychological changes following ingestion of a substance.

Methamphetamine—The most common illegally produced amphetamine.

Serotonin—A widely distributed neurotransmitter that is found in blood platelets, the lining of the digestive tract, and the brain, and that works in combination with norepinephrine. It causes very powerful contractions of smooth muscle and is associated with mood, attention, emotions, and sleep. Low levels of serotonin are associated with depression. Large amounts of serotonin are released after ingestion of MDMA.

"Speed run"—The episodic binging on amphetamines.

Withdrawal—Symptoms that occur when a drug is discontinued after prolonged regular use.

that resemble **schizophrenia**, with visual or auditory hallucinations, **delusions** such as the sensation of insects creeping on the skin (known as formication), hyperactivity, hypersexuality, confusion, and incoherence. Amphetamine-induced **psychosis** differs from true psychosis in that despite other symptoms, the disorganized thinking that is a hallmark of schizophrenia tends to be absent. Amphetamine dependence consistently affects relationships at home, school, and/or work.

Amphetamine abuse is less serious than dependence but can cause milder versions of the symptoms described above, as well as problems with family, school, and work. Legal problems may stem from aggressive behavior while using, or from obtaining drugs illegally. Individuals may continue to use despite the awareness that usage negatively impacts all areas of their lives.

Acute amphetamine intoxication begins with a "high" feeling that may be followed by feelings of euphoria. Users experience enhanced energy, becoming more outgoing and talkative, and more alert. Other symptoms include anxiety, tension, grandiosity, repetitive behavior, anger, fighting, and impaired judgment.

In both acute and chronic intoxication, individuals may experience dulled feelings, **fatigue**, sadness, and social withdrawal. These behavioral and psychological changes are accompanied by other signs and symptoms including increased or irregular heartbeat, dilation of the pupils, elevated or lowered blood pressure, heavy perspiring or chills, nausea and/or vomiting, motor agitation or retardation, muscle weakness, respiratory depression, and chest pain. Possible severe consequences include confusion, **seizures**, coma, and a variety of cardiovascular problems, including **stroke**. With amphetamine overdoses, death can result if treatment is not received immediately. Long-term abuse can lead to memory loss and contributes to increased transmission of hepatitis and HIV/AIDS, especially if users share needles. Impaired social and work functioning is another hallmark of both acute and chronic intoxication.

Following amphetamine intoxication, a "crash" occurs, characterized by symptoms of anxiety, shakiness, depressed mood, lethargy, fatigue, nightmares, headache, perspiring, muscle cramps, stomach cramps, and increased appetite. Withdrawal symptoms usually peak in two to four days and are gone within one week. The most serious withdrawal symptom is depression, which may be severe and lead to suicidal thoughts.

Use of so-called designer amphetamines, such as MDMA, leads to similar symptoms. Users also report a sense of feeling an unusual closeness with other people and enhanced personal comfort. They describe seeing an increased luminescence of objects in the environment, although these hallucinogenic effects are less than those caused by other **hallucinogens**, such as LSD. Some psychotherapists have suggested further research into the possible use of designer amphetamines in conjunction with **psychotherapy**. This idea is highly controversial.

As with other amphetamines, use of MDMA produces cardiovascular effects of increased blood pressure, heart rate, and heart oxygen consumption. People with pre-existing heart disease are at increased risk of cardiovascular catastrophe resulting from MDMA use. MDMA is not processed and removed from the body quickly and remains active for a long period of time. As a result, toxicity may rise dramatically when users take multiple doses over brief time periods, leading to harmful reactions such as dehydration, hyperthermia, and seizures.

MDMA tablets often contain other drugs, such as ephedrine, a stimulant, and dextromethorphan, a cough suppressant with PCP-like effects at high doses. These additives increase the harmful effects of MDMA. They also appear also to have toxic effects on the brain's serotonin system. In tests of learning and memory, people who use MDMA perform more poorly than people who do not use. Research with primates shows that MDMA can cause long-lasting brain damage. Exposure to MDMA during the period of pregnancy in which the fetal brain is developing is associated with learning deficits that last into adulthood.

Diagnosis

The *DSM* diagnostic criteria for amphetamine use disorder is as follows:

- use interferes with educational, occupational, or societal obligations (including home and family life)
- use causes dangerous situations (e.g., driving under the influence)
- use continues despite problems caused by the substance
- person experiences tolerance, withdrawal, and/or cravings
- substance is used in higher doses or for longer than originally intended
- use continues despite efforts to quit
- significant time is devoted to substance use
- use interferes with or replaces other activities
- use continues despite negative physical or psychological effects

At least two symptoms must occur within a 12-month period to be considered a disorder.

QUESTIONS TO ASK YOUR DOCTOR

- What risks are associated with amphetamine abuse?
- What symptoms are associated with amphetamine dependence?
- Does amphetamine dependence and abuse put me at risk for other health conditions?
- Can you recommend any treatment and support groups for me?

Treatment

According to the National Institute on Drug Abuse (NIDA), the most effective treatments for amphetamine **addiction** are cognitive-behavioral interventions. These are psychotherapeutic approaches that help individuals learn to identify and change their problematic patterns of thoughts and beliefs. As a result of changed thoughts and beliefs, feelings become more manageable and less painful. Interventions also help individuals increase their skills for coping with life's stressors. Amphetamine recovery groups and Narcotics Anonymous also appear to help.

No specific medications for amphetamine dependence are known to exist. On occasion, antidepressant medications can help combat the depressive symptoms frequently experienced by people who are newly abstinent from amphetamine use.

Overdoses of amphetamines are treated in established ways in emergency rooms. Because hyperthermia (elevated body temperature) and convulsions are common, emergency room treatment focuses on reducing body temperature and administering anticonvulsant medications.

Acute methamphetamine intoxication is often handled by observation in a safe, quiet environment. When extreme anxiety or panic is part of the reaction, treatment with antianxiety medications may be helpful. In cases of methamphetamine-induced psychoses, short-term use of antipsychotic medications is usually successful.

Prognosis

Classic amphetamines

According to the *DSM-IV-TR,* some individuals who develop abuse or dependence on amphetamines initiate use in an attempt to control their weight. Others become introduced through the illegal market. Dependence can occur very quickly when the substance is used intravenously or smoked. The few long-term data available show a tendency for people who have been dependent on amphetamines to decrease or stop using them after 8 to 10 years. This may result from the development of adverse mental and physical effects that emerge with long-term dependence. Few data are available on the long-term course of abuse.

Designer amphetamines

The NIDA reports that studies provide direct evidence that chronic use of MDMA causes brain damage in humans. Using advanced brain-imaging techniques, one study found that MDMA harms neurons that release serotonin. Serotonin plays an important role in regulating memory and other mental functions.

In a related study, researchers found that people who heavily use MDMA have memory problems that persist for at least two weeks after stopping use of the drug. Both studies strongly suggest that the extent of damage is directly related to the amount of MDMA used.

Prevention

In 1999, NIDA began a program known as the "Club Drug Initiative" in response to recent increases in abuse of MDMA and other drugs used in similar environments. This ongoing program seeks to increase awareness of the dangers of these drugs among teens, young adults, parents, and community members.

Research indicates a pervasive perception among users that MDMA is a "fun" drug with minimal risks. This myth might point to the main reason for the widespread increase in the drug's abuse. The Club Drug Initiative seeks to make the dangers of MDMA use far better known. Evidence of the program's initial success with this initiative might be seen in a growing perception by high school seniors that MDMA is a dangerous drug.

Resources

BOOKS

American Psychiatric Association. *Diagnostic and Statistical Manual of Mental Disorders.* 4th ed., text rev. Washington, DC: American Psychiatric Association, 2000.

American Psychological Association. *Publication Manual of the American Psychological Association.* 6th ed. Washington, DC: American Psychological Association, 2009.

Erickson, Carlton K, Ph.D. *Addiction Essentials: The Go-To Guide for Clinicians and Patients.* New York: W. W. Norton & Company, 2011.

PERIODICALS

Sulzer, David, et al. "Mechanisms of Neurotransmitter Release by Amphetamines: A Review." *Progress in Neurobiology* 75 (2005): 406–33.

WEBSITES

MedlinePlus. "Methamphetamine." U.S. National Library of Medicine, National Institutes of Health. http://www.nlm.nih.gov/medlineplus/methamphetamine.html (accessed November 14, 2011).

National Institute on Drug Abuse. "ClubDrugs.gov." http://www.clubdrugs.gov (accessed November 14, 2011).

———. "NIDA Infofacts: Methamphetamine." 2010. http://www.nida.nih.gov/Infofacts/methamphetamine.html (accessed November 14, 2011).

ORGANIZATIONS

American Psychological Association, 750 First Street NE, Washington, DC, 20003, (202) 336-5500, http://www.apa.org/index.aspx.

Narcotics Anonymous, PO Box 9999, Van Nuys, CA, 91409, (818) 773-9999, Fax: (818) 700-0700, http://www.na.org.

National Institute on Drug Abuse, 6001 Executive Blvd., Rm. 5213, Bethesda, MD, 20892, (301) 442-1124; Spanish: (240) 221-4007, information@nida.nih.gov, http://www.nida.nih.gov.

Substance Abuse and Mental Health Services Administration, 1 Choke Cherry Rd., Rockville, MD, 20857, (877) SAMHSA-7 (726-4727), (800) TTY: 487-4889, Fax: (240) 221-4292, SAMHSAInfo@samhsa.hhs.gov, http://www.samhsa.gov.

Barbara S. Sternberg, Ph.D.
Emily Jane Willingham, Ph.D.
Laura Jean Cataldo, RN, Ed.D.

Anafranil *see* **Clomipramine**

Anorexia nervosa

Definition

Anorexia nervosa (AN) is a psychiatric disorder characterized by an unrealistic fear of weight gain, conspicuous distortion of **body image**, and self-starvation. The individual is obsessed with becoming increasingly thinner and limits food intake to the point where health is compromised. The disorder can be fatal. The name comes from two Latin words that mean "nervous inability to eat."

The word *anorexia* alone literally means "loss of appetite" and is a symptom of several diseases. Anorexia nervosa is not a loss of appetite but the dangerous restriction of calories despite continuing hunger.

Demographics

Anorexia nervosa is a disorder of industrialized countries where food is abundant but the culture values a thin appearance. About 1% of Americans have AN, and diagnosed females outnumber males 10:1. In men, the disorder is more often diagnosed among homosexuals than heterosexuals. Some experts believe that the number of patients diagnosed represents only the most severe cases and that many more people have anorexic tendencies, but their symptoms do not rise to the level needed for a medical **diagnosis**.

Despite this belief, AN has the highest rate of death of all psychiatric disorders, based on data from a study published in the July 2011 issue of the *Archives of General Psychiatry*. In this study, which was a meta-analysis of 36 studies published between 1966 and 2010, people with AN were nearly six times more likely to die compared to healthy people. In addition, death rates among people with AN are twice as high as deaths in patients with **schizophrenia**, three times higher than patients with **bipolar disorder**, and four times higher than patients with major **depression**. When the data were broken out by age group, researchers found that individuals diagnosed with AN between ages 20 and 29 had an 18-fold risk of death compared to healthy people. By contrast, the risk of death was threefold when a diagnosis was made before the age of 15 years. The data suggest that one in five AN-related deaths is a **suicide**.

More than 95% of persons with AN are white, and about three-fourths come from households at the middle income level or above. Studies have found that the rate of AN in the United States is about double that in Europe.

Anorexia nervosa can occur in people as young as age 7 or may not develop until later in life. The most common ages of development are ages 14 and 18, which correspond with the ages of transitioning into and out of high school.

Description

Anorexia nervosa is often thought of as a modern problem, but the English physician Richard Morton first described it in 1689. AN is recognized as a psychiatric disorder in the ***Diagnostic and Statistical Manual of Mental Disorders*** (*DSM*), the handbook used by mental health professionals to diagnose mental disorders, published by the **American Psychiatric Association**.

Though most **diets** do not progress into AN, dieting is generally the starting point for future development of the disorder. As weight falls, the **obsession** with dieting increases. Affected persons may also increase physical exertion or **exercise** as weight decreases to lose even more weight. An affected person develops peculiar rules concerning exercise and eating. Patients with AN equate weight loss and avoidance of food with a sense of accomplishment and success. Weight gain is viewed as a sign of weakness ("succumbing to eating") and as failure. Eventually, the affected person becomes increasingly focused on losing weight and devotes most efforts to dieting and exercise.

Persons with AN may talk negatively about their bodies and appearance. Some are secretive about eating and will avoid eating in front of other people. They may develop abnormal eating habits such as chewing their food and then spitting it out, or they may have rigid ideas about "good" and "bad" foods (low- and high-calorie foods, respectively). AN is often concurrent with depression, **anxiety disorders**, and compulsive behavior.

There are two major subtypes of AN as classified by the *DSM*. The restrictive type involves weight loss solely through rigorously limiting the amount of calories eaten or by fasting. The person may exercise excessively or abuse drugs or herbal remedies claiming to increase the rate at which the body burns calories but does not engage in any purging behaviors. Individuals with the binge-eating/purging type eat and then purge themselves of the calories through self-induced vomiting, excessive laxative use, or abuse of diuretics or enemas. These behaviors are similar to those of **bulimia nervosa**, but patients with AN continue to restrict their diets severely when they are not binging and may fall to a very low weight, which is not common with bulimia.

Risk factors

Competitive athletes may be at risk of developing an eating disorder, especially in sports where weight is tied to performance. Jockeys, wrestlers, figure skaters, cross-country runners, and gymnasts (especially female gymnasts) have higher-than-average rates of AN. People such as actors, models, cheerleaders, and dancers (especially ballet dancers), whose performance is often tied to their appearance, are also at high risk of developing the disorder.

Other risk factors include:

- female gender
- perfectionism
- personality factors, including being eager to please other persons and having high expectations for oneself
- family history of eating disorders
- living in an industrialized society
- difficulty communicating negative emotions such as anger or fear
- difficulty resolving problems or conflict
- low self-esteem

Causes and symptoms

Causes

Anorexia nervosa is a complex disorder that does not have a single cause but appears to result from the interaction of cultural and biological factors. Research suggests that some people have a predisposition toward AN. The disorder develops after some event triggers the behavior, which then becomes self-reinforcing. The event might be a family member teasing about the person's weight, nagging about eating junk food, commenting on how clothes fit, or comparing the person unfavorably to someone else. Life events such as moving, starting a new school, breaking up with a partner, or even entering puberty can trigger anorexic behavior. Hereditary, psychological, and social factors also appear to play a role.

Research indicates that **genetic factors** play a role in more than half of AN cases. Twin studies show that if one twin has AN, the other has a greater likelihood of developing the disorder. Having a close relative, usually a mother or a sister, with AN also increases the likelihood of other (usually female) family members developing the disorder. Genetic factors can also predispose individuals to behaviors that make them susceptible to AN, such as perfectionism, **obsessive-compulsive disorder**, and anxiety.

Specialists in **family therapy** have demonstrated that dysfunctional family relationships and impaired family interaction can be associated with AN. Mothers of persons with AN tend to be intrusive, perfectionistic, overprotective, and have a fear of separation. Fathers of individuals with AN are often described as passive, withdrawn, moody, emotionally constricted, obsessive, and ineffective. Sociocultural factors include the messages given by society and the culture about women's roles and the thinness ideal for women's bodies. Developmental causes can include adolescent "acting out" or fear of adulthood transition.

Precipitating factors are often related to the developmental transitions common in adolescence. The onset of menstruation may be threatening in that it represents maturation or growing up. During this time in development, females gain weight as part of the developmental process, and this gain may cause a decrease in self-esteem. Development of AN could be a way that the adolescent retreats into childhood so as not to be burdened by maturity and physical concerns. Autonomy and independence struggles during adolescence may be acted out by developing AN. Some adolescents may develop AN because of their ambivalence about adulthood or because of feelings of loneliness, isolation, and abandonment.

There is some evidence that AN is linked to abnormal neurotransmitter activity in the part of the **brain** that controls pleasure and appetite. **Neurotransmitters** are also involved in other mental disorders such as depression.

KEY TERMS

Amenorrhea—Absence of the menses in a female who has begun to have menstrual periods.

Body dysmorphic disorder—A psychiatric disorder marked by preoccupation with an imagined physical defect.

Diuretic—A substance that removes water from the body by increasing urine production.

Electrolyte—Ions in the body that participate in metabolic reactions. The major human electrolytes are sodium (Na+), potassium (K+), calcium (Ca 2+), magnesium (Mg2+), chloride (Cl-), phosphate (HPO4 2-), bicarbonate (HCO3-), and sulfate (SO4 2-).

Hyperalimentation—A method of refeeding by infusing liquid nutrients and electrolytes directly into central veins through a catheter.

Lanugo—A soft, downy body hair that develops on the chest and arms of women with anorexia.

Neurotransmitter—One of a group of chemicals secreted by a nerve cell (neuron) to carry a chemical message to another nerve cell, often as a way of transmitting a nerve impulse. Examples of neurotransmitters are acetylcholine, dopamine, serotonin, and norepinephrine.

Purging—The use of vomiting, diuretics, or laxatives to clear the stomach and intestines after a binge.

Russell's sign—Scraped or raw areas on the patient's knuckles, caused by self-induced vomiting.

Superior mesenteric artery syndrome—A condition in which a person vomits after meals due to blockage of the blood supply to the intestine.

Research in this area is relatively new, and the findings are unclear. Also, people with AN tend to feel full sooner than other people. Some researchers believe that this is related to the fact that the stomach of people with AN tends to empty more slowly than normal; others think it may be related to the appetite control mechanism of the brain.

Although AN is still considered a disorder that largely affects women, its incidence in the male population is rising. Less is known about the causes of AN in males, but some risk factors are the same as for females. These include certain occupational goals (e.g., jockey) and increasing media emphasis on external appearance in men. Moreover, homosexual males are under pressure to conform to an ideal body weight that is less than the standard "attractive" weight for heterosexual males, which may increase the risk of dieting and weight concerns.

Symptoms

Symptoms of anorexic behavior include an overriding obsession with food and thinness that controls activities and eating patterns every hour of every day, and a refusal to admit that being severely underweight is dangerous to health.

Serious physical and psychological consequences of anorexic behavior include:

- excessive weight loss; loss of muscle
- stunted growth and delayed sexual maturation in preteens
- gastrointestinal complications, including liver damage, diarrhea, constipation, bloating, stomach pain
- cardiovascular complications, including irregular heartbeat, low pulse rate, cardiac arrest
- urinary system complications, including kidney damage, kidney failure, incontinence, urinary tract infections
- skeletal system complications, including loss of bone mass, increased risk of fractures, teeth eroded by stomach acid from repeat vomiting
- reproductive system complications in women, such as irregular menstrual periods, amenorrhea, infertility
- reproductive system complications in men, such as loss of sex drive, infertility
- fatigue, irritation, headaches, depression, anxiety, impaired judgment and thinking
- fainting, seizures, low blood sugar
- chronically cold hands and feet
- weakened immune system, swollen glands, increased susceptibility to infections
- development of fine hair called lanugo on the shoulders, back, arms, and face; head hair loss; blotchy, dry skin
- potentially life-threatening electrolyte imbalances
- coma
- increased risk of self-mutilation (cutting)
- increased risk of suicide
- death

Diagnosis

Diagnosis of AN is made when the individual meets the criteria for the disorder outlined in the *DSM*, fourth edition, text revision, also known as the *DSM-IV-TR*:

- extreme restriction of caloric intake resulting in significantly low weight (as determined after considering age, gender, level of development, and overall health)
- extreme fear of gaining weight or becoming fat, even when the individual is significantly underweight
- a distorted self-image that fuels a refusal to admit to being underweight, even when this is demonstrably true

The *DSM-IV-TR* includes in its diagnostic criteria the presence of amenorrhea, or three missed menstrual periods in a row after menstruation has been established, and a weight of less than 85% of the average weight for the patient's age and height group. These criteria have been proposed to be removed for the *DSM-5* (fifth edition, due to publish in 2013) as they are not consistent—some patients continue to have menstrual activity, and it is difficult to define low body weight with a specific numeric value.

Initial assessment usually includes a careful interview and patient history (clinical evaluation). A weight history, menstrual history, and description of daily food intake are important during initial evaluation. Risk factors and family history are also vital in suspected cases. Though patients may not admit to having AN, they may complain about related symptoms such as **fatigue**, headaches, dizziness, constipation, or frequent infections.

Tests

A physical examination begins with taking weight and blood pressure. Based on the physical exam, the physician may order laboratory tests, including a complete blood count (CBC), urinalysis, blood chemistries (to determine electrolyte levels), and liver function tests. Laboratory results can reveal anemia (low red blood cell count in the blood) and lowered white blood cells, pulse, blood pressure, and body temperature. The decreased temperature in extremities may cause a slight red-purple discoloration in limbs (acrocyanosis). The physician may also order an electrocardiogram to look for heart abnormalities. Other conditions, including metabolic disorders, brain tumors (especially hypothalamus and pituitary gland lesions), diseases of the digestive tract, and a condition called superior mesenteric artery syndrome, which can cause weight loss or vomiting after eating, may show symptoms similar to AN and need to be ruled out in medical evaluation.

The individual may be referred to a **psychiatrist** or **psychologist** for a mental status evaluation. The physician will evaluate factors such as whether the person is oriented in time and space, appearance, observable state of emotion (**affect**), attitude toward food and weight, delusional thinking, and thoughts of self-harm or suicide. This evaluation helps to distinguish between AN and other psychiatric disorders, including depression, schizophrenia, **social phobia**, obsessive-compulsive disorder, and **body dysmorphic disorder**. Three questionnaires that are often used are the Eating Attitudes Test (EAT), the Eating Disorder Examination, and the Eating Disorder Inventory (EDI). The disadvantage of these tests is that they may produce false-positive results, which means that a test result may indicate that test takers have AN when actually they do not.

Treatment

Persons affected with AN are often in **denial**, in that they do not see themselves as thin or in need of professional help. Education is important, as is engagement on the part of patients—a connection from the patients to the treatment, so that they agree to be actively involved. Engagement is a necessary but difficult task in the treatment of AN. If the affected persons' medical condition has deteriorated, **hospitalization** may be required. Initially, treatment objectives are focused on reversing behavioral abnormalities and nutritional deficiencies. Emotional support and reassurance that eating and caloric restoration will not make the person overweight are essential components during initial treatment sessions. Psychosocial (both psychological and social) issues and family dysfunction are also addressed, which may reduce the risk of relapsing behaviors or the recurrence of the disorder after a period of remission.

Traditional

Hospitalization is recommended for patients with any of the following characteristics:

- weight of 30% or more below normal, or weight loss over a three-month period of more than 30 pounds
- severely disturbed metabolism
- severe medical instability
- severe binging and purging
- signs of psychosis
- severe depression or risk of suicide
- family in crisis

Hospital inpatient care is first geared toward correcting problems that present as immediate medical crises, such as severe malnutrition, severe electrolyte imbalance, irregular heart beat, pulse below 45 beats per minute, or low body temperature. Patients are hospitalized if they are a high suicide risk, have severe clinical depression, or exhibit signs of an altered mental state. They may also need to be hospitalized to interrupt weight loss; stop the cycle of vomiting, exercising and/or laxative abuse; treat substance disorders; or for additional medical evaluation.

Day treatment or partial hospitalization, where the patient goes every day to an extensive treatment program, provides structured mealtimes, **nutrition** education, intensive therapy, medical monitoring, and supervision. If day treatment fails, the patient may need to be hospitalized or enter a full-time residential treatment facility.

Anorexia nervosa is a chronic disease and relapses are common and to be expected. Outpatient treatment provides medical supervision, **nutrition counseling**, self-help strategies, and **psychotherapy** after the patient has regained some weight and shows stability.

A nutrition consultant or dietitian is an essential part of the team needed to successfully treat AN. The first treatment concern is to get individuals medically stable by increasing calorie intake and balancing electrolytes. After that, nutritional therapy is needed to support the long process of recovery and stable weight gain. This is an intensive process involving nutrition education, meal planning, and nutrition monitoring, with the goal of developing a healthy relationship with food.

Psychotherapy

Medical **intervention** helps alleviate the immediate physical problems associated with AN, but if used alone it rarely changes behavior. Psychotherapy plays a major role in helping the patient understand and recover from AN. Several different types of psychotherapy may be used, depending on the individual's situation. Generally, the goal of psychotherapy is to help patients develop a healthy attitude toward their body and food. This may involve addressing the root causes of the anorexic behavior as well as the behavior itself.

Some types of psychotherapy have been successful in treating AN:

- Cognitive behavior therapy (CBT) is designed to change individuals' thoughts and feelings about their body and behaviors toward food, but it does not address why those thoughts or feelings exist. This therapy is relatively short-term.
- Psychodynamic therapy, also called psychoanalytic therapy, is a longer-term therapy that attempts to help individuals gain insight into the cause of the emotions that trigger anorexic behaviors.
- Interpersonal therapy is short-term therapy that helps individuals identify issues and problems in relationships. Individuals may be asked to look back at their family history to try to recognize problem areas and work toward resolving them.
- Family and couples therapy is helpful in dealing with other conflicts or disorders that may be perpetuating anorexic behavior. Family therapy is especially useful in helping parents with a child with AN or in helping parents become supportive of their child and facilitating such activities as designing a healthy eating plan for the child. Siblings of a young person with AN need support as well. Family therapy is the only therapy with strong empirical support for its effectiveness in treating AN.

A research study done at Stanford University Hospital and published in 2010 found that involving parents by putting them directly in charge of their child's

QUESTIONS TO ASK YOUR DOCTOR

- Does my loved one need to be hospitalized?
- How long do you think intensive treatment will take?
- Will my insurance pay for inpatient or outpatient treatment?
- What can we do to help?
- Can you refer us to a support group for families of persons with anorexia?

eating had a good rate of curing and preventing the redevelopment of anorexic behaviors. The program is very time intensive because the parent decides what the child must eat and then must sit at the table, sometimes for hours, until the child finishes the food. This is a departure from past practices in which parents were thought be a causative factor in the development of AN and were told not to monitor their child's eating habits.

Drugs

There is no medication that successfully treats the symptoms of AN, but a variety of medications may be prescribed to address secondary and comorbid conditions, such as physical problems caused by the eating disorder, depression, anxiety, and suicidal thoughts. The medications used vary depending on individual cases, but depression is common among persons with AN and is often treated with antidepressant drugs.

Prognosis

Anorexia nervosa is difficult to treat successfully. Medical stabilization, nutrition therapy, continued medical monitoring, and substantial psychiatric treatment give a person with AN the best chance of recovery. Estimates suggest that between 20% and 30% of people in treatment drop out too soon and have major relapses. Even those who stay in treatment **relapse** occasionally. Treating AN is often a long, slow, and expensive process. However, the longer the disorder remains untreated, the more difficult recovery is to achieve, with the consequences growing more severe. Many individuals with AN are willfully uncooperative and have difficulty being motivated to recover.

About half the people treated for AN recover completely and are able (though sometimes with difficulty) to maintain a normal weight. Of the remaining 50%, between 6% and 20% die. The most frequent causes of death associated with AN are starvation, electrolyte imbalance, heart failure, and suicide. About 20% remain dangerously underweight, and the rest remain thin. Long-term health complications are common.

Prevention

A nurturing and healthy family environment during developing years is particularly important. Recognition of the clinical signs with immediate treatment can possibly prevent disorder progression, and early diagnosis and treatment are correlated with a favorable outcome. Long-term goal setting should focus on three areas: learning new, healthy eating behaviors; learning to trust family members, friends, and health professionals who are trying to help; and learning emotional self-care so that healthy methods of coping with **stress** and pressure are exercised, rather than reverting to anorexic behavior.

Resources

BOOKS

Carleton, Pamela, and Deborah Ashin. *Take Charge of Your Child's Eating Disorder: A Physician's Step-By-Step Guide to Defeating Anorexia and Bulimia*. New York: Marlowe, 2007.

Heaton, Jeanne A., and Claudia J. Strauss. *Talking to Eating Disorders: Simple Ways to Support Someone Who Has Anorexia, Bulimia, Binge Eating or Body Image Issues*. New York, NY: New American Library, 2005.

Herzog, David B., Debra L. Franko, and Patricia Cable. *Unlocking the Mysteries of Eating Disorders*. New York: McGraw-Hill, 2007.

Liu, Aimee. *Gaining: The Truth About Life After Eating Disorders*. New York: Warner Books, 2007.

Messinger, Lisa, and Merle Goldberg. *My Thin Excuse: Understanding, Recognizing, and Overcoming Eating Disorders*. Garden City Park, NY: Square One, 2006.

Rubin, Jerome S., ed. *Eating Disorders and Weight Loss Research*. Hauppauge, NY: Nova Science, 2006.

Walsh, B. Timothy. *If Your Adolescent Has an Eating Disorder: An Essential Resource for Parents*. New York: Oxford University Press, 2005.

PERIODICALS

Arcelus, Jon, et al. "Mortality Rates in Patients With Anorexia Nervosa and Other Eating Disorders: A Meta-Analysis of 36 Studies." *Archives of General Psychiatry* 68, no. 7 (2011): 724–31. http://dx.doi.org/10.1001/archgenpsychiatry.2011.74 (accessed November 14, 2011).

Genders, R., and K. Tchanturia. "Cognitive Remediation Therapy (CRT) for Anorexia in Group Format: A Pilot Study." *Eating and Weight Disorders* 15, no. 4 (2010): e234–39.

Guillaume, S., et al. "Characteristics of Suicide Attempts in Anorexia and Bulimia Nervosa: A Case-control Study." *PLoS One* [Public Library of Science] 6, no. 8 (2011): e23578. http://dx.doi.org/10.1371/journal.pone.0023578 (accessed September 16, 2011).

Hudson, James, et al. "The Prevalence and Correlates of Eating Disorders in the National Comorbidity Survey Replication." *Biological Psychiatry* 61, no. 3 (2007): 348–58.

WEBSITES

American Psychological Association. "Eating Disorders." http://www.apa.org/helpcenter/eating.aspx (accessed September 16, 2011).

Bernstein, Bettina E. "Eating Disorder: Anorexia." Medscape Reference. October 14, 2010. http://emedicine.medscape.com/article/912187-overview (accessed September 16, 2011).

MedlinePlus. "Eating Disorders." U.S. National Library of Medicine, National Institutes of Health. March 17, 2011. http://www.nlm.nih.gov/medlineplus/eatingdisorders.html (accessed September 16, 2011).

ORGANIZATIONS

American Academy of Child and Adolescent Psychiatry, 3615 Wisconsin Ave., NW, Washington, DC, 20016-3007, (202) 966-7300, Fax: (202) 966-2891, http://aacap.org.

American Psychiatric Association, 1000 Wilson Blvd., Ste. 1825, Arlington, VA, 22209-3901, (703) 907-7300, apa@psych.org, http://www.psych.org.

American Psychological Association, 750 1st St., NE, Washington, DC, 20002-4242, (202) 336-5500; TDD/TTY: (202) 336-6123, (800) 374-2721, http://www.apa.org.

National Association of Anorexia Nervosa and Related Eating Disorders, PO Box 640, Naperville, IL, 60566, (630) 577-1330, anadhelp@anad.org, http://www.anad.org.

National Eating Disorders Association, 165 W 46th St., New York, NY, 10036, (212) 575-6200, (800) 931-2237, Fax: (212) 575-1650, info@NationalEatingDisorders.org, http://www.nationaleatingdisorders.org.

Tish Davidson, AM
Heidi Splete

Anosognosia

Definition

Anosognosia is a common but poorly understood neurological dysfunction in which a person who has suffered **brain** injury or damage is unable to recognize personal physical impairments or sensory, motor, perceptual, affective, or cognitive deficits.

Demographics

The majority of patients who suffer brain injury or damage may lack at least some degree of awareness of their physical or cognitive impairments. Reliable statistics are scarce, because often it is difficult to distinguish between anosognosia and a patients' desire to deny their illness or impairment. Nevertheless, it has been estimated that 10%–18% of **stroke** patients with partial or total paralysis on one side of their bodies (hemiparesis or hemiplegia) suffer from anosognosia. Other estimates put the incidence of anosognosia for hemiplegia (AHP) at 20%–30% of patients with one-sided paralysis following acute stroke. Furthermore, it has been estimated that about 50% of patients with **schizophrenia** and 40% of patients with **bipolar disorder** have an impaired awareness of their illness, and anosognosia is thought to be the single most important reason that such patients refuse medication. Some researchers estimate that up to 60% of individuals with mild cognitive impairment (MCI) and 81% of patients with **Alzheimer's disease** have some degree of anosognosia.

Description

Anosognosia has long been a source of fascination for cognitive scientists. In 1885, the Russian-Swiss neuropathologist Constantin von Monakow (1853–1930) described the case of a man with damage to the cerebral cortex of his brain who was unaware that he was blind. Gabriel Anton (1858–1933) wrote extensively of patients who were unaware of their severe neurological impairments. These included a man who, after damage to the right side of his brain, was unaware that he could not move his left limbs, had no feeling on his left side, and was blind in his left eye. The condition became known as Anton's syndrome. Although unawareness of blindness is sometimes referred to as Anton-Babinski syndrome, the term *anosognosia,* for the general lack of knowledge, awareness, or recognition of neurological deficits, was adopted in 1914 by the French neurologist Joseph Jules François Félix Babinski (1857–1932). The term is derived from the roots *a* (without), *noso* (illness), and *gnosia* (knowledge), meaning literally "to not know a disease." The terms *anosognosia, impaired awareness, unawareness of deficits,* and *lack of insight* are sometimes used interchangeably in the medical literature. Although **denial** of illness, in which a patient refuses to acknowledge their impairment or illness, is sometimes confused with anosognosia, the latter is caused by damage to the brain, whereas denial of illness is a psychological mechanism for managing disturbing emotions evoked by the illness or disability.

Anosognosia can be a lack of awareness of almost any type of neurological impairment or deficit that follows brain injury, including blindness, weakness or paralysis of the limbs, loss of speech or comprehension of words (aphasia), memory deficits, agnosia (the inability to recognize familiar objects or stimuli), or prosopagnosia (the inability to recognize faces). Anosognosia most often occurs in association with stroke, brain tumors, partial or total blindness or deafness arising from brain damage, Alzheimer's disease, Huntington's disease, schizophrenia, and bipolar disorder. However, anosognosia is not associated with mental confusion or other major cognitive disorders, nor is it directly related to sensory deficits.

The classic examples of anosognosia are patients who, after suffering a stroke in the right hemisphere of the brain, do not perceive that their left side is paralyzed. Such patients often insist that their left arm and leg are functioning normally, even after they fail at performing a simple task. For example, they will insist that they are raising both arms, even when they can see in a mirror that only their right arm is raised. Sometimes patients deny that a paralyzed limb belongs to them. The neurologist Oliver Sacks recounted the story of a patient who repeatedly fell out of bed from trying to throw his paralyzed leg to the floor—he thought that someone else's leg had been placed in his bed as a practical joke.

Anosognosia can be selective. A patient may be aware of one type of deficit, such as blindness in one visual field, but appear unaware of another deficit, such as paralysis of a limb. Anosognosia also can vary in degree. In its most extreme form, patients fail to recognize any impairment. In less extreme forms, patients may minimize the deficit or appear unconcerned about it, a condition referred to as anosodiaphoria.

Anosognosia is often associated with a behavioral syndrome called spatial neglect, which also can occur following brain injury. Spatial neglect refers to the inability to recognize, orient toward, or respond to stimuli, usually on the side of the body opposite the brain lesion.

Risk factors

Anosognosia is caused by injury to specific regions of the brain. Therefore, risk factors for the disorder are those associated with specific types of brain damage.

Causes and symptoms

Although the exact causes of anosognosia remain unclear, it is associated with brain damage, particularly to the right hemisphere. The frontal lobe and a part of the parietal lobe behind the frontal lobe appear to be most involved. The non-dominant parietal lobe (the right hemisphere in most people) is responsible for integrating the opposite side of the body with its environment. Thus, injury to the non-dominant lobe can lead to decreased awareness of the opposite side of the body and its environment. Some patients with anosognosia are also unable to recognize paralysis in others, suggesting that mirror neurons may be involved in such cases. Mirror neurons are brain cells that fire both when performing an action and when observing the action being performed by others.

KEY TERMS

Alzheimer's disease—A progressive, neurodegenerative disease characterized by loss of function and death of nerve cells in several areas of the brain, leading to loss of mental functions, such as memory and learning. Alzheimer's disease is the most common cause of dementia.

Aphasia—Loss of the ability to speak or understand language, due to brain injury or disease.

Bipolar disorder—A recurrent mood disorder, also known as manic-depressive disorder, in which patients have extreme mood swings from depression to mania or a mixture of both.

Cerebral cortex—The convoluted surface layer of the cerebrum or upper portion of the brain, which coordinates sensory and motor information.

Cognitive—Referring to conscious intellectual activity, including thinking, imagining, reasoning, remembering, and learning.

Confabulation—Using false or imagined details to explain physical phenomena or to fill in memory gaps.

Hemiplegia—Paralysis of one side of the body.

Lesion—An injured, diseased, or damaged area.

Mild cognitive impairment (MCI)—A transitional phase of memory loss in older people that precedes dementia or Alzheimer's disease.

Parietal lobe—The middle portion of each cerebral hemisphere of the brain; associated with bodily sensations.

Schizophrenia—A psychotic disorder characterized by loss of contact with one's environment, deterioration of everyday functioning, and personality disintegration.

Stroke—A sudden diminishing or loss of consciousness, sensation, or voluntary movement due to the rupture or obstruction of a blood vessel in the brain.

Vestibular system—The system that helps to maintain balance and orient the body.

Stroke and brain tumors affecting the right hemisphere are among the most common causes of anosognosia. Anosognosia accompanying Alzheimer's disease also may reflect impairment of the right prefrontal and/or frontal lobes and, in particular, the right inferior parietal area of the brain. Likewise, some evidence suggests that frontal lobe damage can cause anosognosia in patients with schizophrenia.

Symptoms of anosognosia not only vary among patients; they can even vary in the same patient at different times. Patients with anosognosia with hemiplegia can show varying degrees of awareness of their paralysis, ranging from anosodiaphoria—knowledge of, but indifference to, their paralysis—to complete unawareness, even in the face of confounding evidence. Patients sometimes fabricate explanations, called confabulations, for their paralyzed limbs. For example, they may claim that the paralyzed limb is far away from their body or belongs to someone else. They may even claim that someone else is lying in their bed, or may become violent toward the paralyzed limb.

Diagnosis

Examination

Anosognosia can usually be diagnosed by an interview and by the patient's behavior—for example, trying to walk despite paralysis. Patients may first be asked why they are in the hospital. If they do not acknowledge a deficit, such as paralysis, the physician may ask more specific questions about the affected body part. A patient with hemiplegia can be scored for anosognosia on a range from zero—readily acknowledging paralysis—to three, in which the patient firmly denies the problem, despite being unable to move a limb.

Anosognosia can be differentiated from denial of illness based on a patient's reaction to information about their deficit. Patients who are denying their impairment will indicate some awareness of the deficit. They will actively struggle to perform a requested task and usually become angry or resistant when confronted with information about their problem. In contrast, patients with anosognosia are unaware of their deficit, are puzzled when given information about it, and are usually indifferent or willing to try and perform a requested task. Sometimes patients with anosognosia admit to their deficit when initially confronted with information about it, but soon after they are again unaware of it. They may also confabulate. For example, patients with anosognosia with hemiplegia may explain that they are right-handed, so that their left arm is weaker, or they may claim that their paralyzed arm belongs to someone else.

QUESTIONS TO ASK YOUR DOCTOR

- Do you think that my loved one has anosognosia, or is there another cause for his/her symptoms?
- How is anosognosia diagnosed?
- What do you think caused the anosognosia?
- What is the prognosis?

Tests

Sometimes an anosognosia ratio (AR) is used to rate patients' awareness of their memory abilities. The AR compares patients' estimations of their memory abilities with objective memory scores and categorizes them as over-estimators, accurate estimators, or under-estimators. Anosognosia for memory loss is also diagnosed using the following scale:

- 1—readily admits memory loss
- 2—readily or inconsistently admits to a small degree of memory loss
- 3—is unaware of any impairment
- 4—angrily insists that there is no impairment of memory

Treatment

Traditional

Anosognosia often resolves over time. In long-term cases, cognitive therapy may be employed to train patients to cope with their impairment, although learning to cope may not relieve the anosognosia. Caloric reflex testing—stimulating the vestibular system by squirting cold water into the left ear canal—sometimes relieves anosognosia for a few hours. Although this effect is not understood, it may be that this intense stimulation of the vestibular system temporarily shifts the patient's awareness.

Drugs

Although there are no drug treatments for anosognosia, schizophrenic patients often become more aware of their illness when taking antipsychotic medications. Anosognosia in patients with bipolar disorder is even more likely to improve with medication.

Prognosis

Although anosognosia can continue indefinitely, in most cases it disappears over time. Some patients fluctuate, with increasing and decreasing periods of awareness of their deficit. However, in Alzheimer's patients, anosognosia often worsens as **dementia** progresses.

Anosognosia can have serious consequences. Patients with anosognosia usually make no attempt to compensate for their deficit, may be unwilling to participate in treatment or rehabilitation, and may suffer from increased post-stroke **depression**. Anosognosia appears to directly increase the incidence of violent behavior in patients with mental illnesses, in addition to effects attributable to medication non-adherence. Patients with severe mental illness and anosognosia may have to be coerced to take medication.

Prevention

There is no known method for preventing anosognosia. However, for patients with mental disorders, adherence to medication often relieves the condition.

Resources

BOOKS

Bayne, Tim, and Jordi Fernández. *Delusion and Self-Deception: Affective and Motivational Influences on Belief Formation.* New York: Psychological Press, 2009.

Berti, Anna, et al. "Motor Awareness and Motor Intention in Anosognosia for Hemiplegia." In *Sensorimotor Foundations of Higher Cognition,* edited by Patrick Haggard, Yves Rossetti, and Matsuo Kawato. New York: Oxford University Press, 2008.

Prigatano, George P. *The Study of Anosognosia.* New York: Oxford University Press, 2010.

Sacks, Oliver. *A Leg to Stand On.* New York: Quality Paperback Book Club, 1990.

PERIODICALS

Robbins, Matthew S., et al. "Anosognosia for Right Hemiplegia from Dominant Anterior Cerebral Artery Stroke." *Journal of the American Geriatrics Society* 57, no. 7 (July 2009): 1320–1322.

OTHER

Doty, Leilani. "Anosognosia (Unawareness of Decline or Difficulties)." AlzOnline.net. http://alzonline.phhp.ufl.edu/en/reading/Anosognosia.pdf (accessed November 19, 2010).

WEBSITES

"Anosognosia (Impaired Awareness of Illness)." Treatment Advocacy Center. http://www.treatmentadvocacycenter.org/index.php?option=com_content&task=view&id=469&Itemid=234 (accessed November 19, 2011).

ORGANIZATIONS

American Speech-Language-Hearing Association, 2200 Research Boulevard, Rockville, MD, 20850-3289, (301) 296-5700, (800) 638-8255, Fax: (301) 296-8580, actioncenter@asha.org, http://www.asha.org.

National Institute of Neurological Disorders and Stroke (NINDS), NIH Neurological Institute, PO Box 5801, Bethesda, MD, 20824, (301) 496-5751, (800) 352-9424, http://www.ninds.nih.gov/index.htm.

Treatment Advocacy Center, 200 N. Glebe Road, Suite 730, Arlington, VA, 22203, (703) 294-6001/6002, Fax: (703) 294-6010, info@treatmentadvocacycenter.org, http://www.treatmentadvocacycenter.org.

Ruvanee Pietersz Vilhauer, PhD
Margaret Alic, PhD

Antabuse *see* **Disulfiram**

Antianxiety drugs and abuse

Definition

Antianxiety drugs, or "anxiolytics," are powerful central nervous system (CNS) depressants that can slow normal **brain** function. They are often prescribed to reduce feelings of tension and anxiety and/or to bring about sleep. Antianxiety medications are among the most abused drugs in the United States, obtained both legally via prescription and illegally through the black market. These drugs are also known as **sedatives**.

Demographics

According to the Substance Abuse and Mental Health Services Administration's National Survey on Drug Use and Health, 7 million people (2.7%) aged 12 or older used prescription-type psychotherapeutic drugs in 2010. Of those, 2.4 million used psychotherapeutics nonmedically for the first time, averaging around 6,600 initiates per day. The average age for first nonmedical use of psychotherapeutics was 22, and females ages 12 to 17 were more likely than males of the same age group to be users of

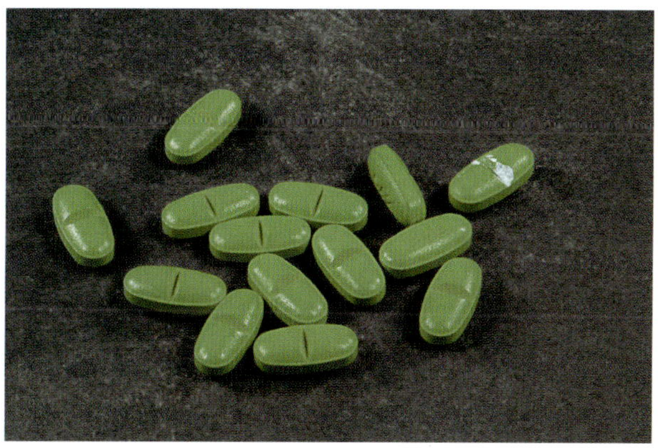

Rohypnol tablets. *(© David Hoffman Photo Library/Alamy)*

Percentage of U.S. adults (18+) reporting prescription antianxiety (anxiolytics, sedatives, and hypnotics) drug use in the past month, 1988–1994 and 2005–2008

	1988–1994	2005–2008
Total		
18 years and over, age-adjusted†	3.9	5.7
18 years and over, crude	3.6	5.8
Men		
18 years and over	2.6	4.3
18–44 years	*1.0	2.1
45–64 years	4.3	6.2
65 years and over	6.1	7.1
Women		
18 years and over	4.6	7.3
18–44 years	1.9	4.3
45–64 years	7.5	9.3
65 years and over	9.1	11.8

*Estimates are considered unreliable. Data preceded by an asterisk have a relative standard error of 20%–30%.
†Estimates are age-adjusted to the year 2000 standard population using three age groups: 18–44 years, 45–64 years, and 65 years and over.

SOURCE: Centers for Disease Control and Prevention, National Center for Health Statistics, *Health, United States, 2010*, February 2011.

(Table by PreMediaGlobal. © 2012 Cengage Learning.)

psychotherapeutics (3.7% versus 2.3%). When asked how they obtained the drugs, over one-half of the users admitted that the drugs came from a friend or relative for free. By race, American Indians or Alaska natives were the most likely to engage in this form of drug abuse, whereas African Americans were the least likely to do so.

Description

The drugs associated with this class of substance-related disorders are the **benzodiazepines** (e.g. **diazepam** [Valium], **chlordiazepoxide** [Librium], **alprazolam** [Xanax], **triazolam** [Halcion], and **estazolam** [ProSom]); the **barbiturates** (e.g., Seconal and pentobarbital [Nembutal]); and barbiturate-like substances, including Quaalude, Equanil, and Doriden. Any of these drugs is capable of producing either wakeful relief from tension or sleep, depending upon dosage. Some legal nonpsychiatric uses of antianxiety medications include medical treatment and prevention of **seizures** and use as muscle relaxants, anesthetics, and drugs to make other anesthetics work more effectively (known as adjuvants).

Although the types of central nervous system depressants work differently, they all produce a pleasant drowsy or calming effect. If used over a long period of time, tolerance develops, meaning larger doses are needed to achieve the initial effects. Continued use can lead to physical dependence and withdrawal symptoms when use is reduced or stopped. When combined with each other or other CNS depressants, such as alcohol, the effects are additive.

In addition to the drugs available in the United States by prescription, there are three other drugs that are predominantly central nervous system depressants with significant potential for abuse. These are:

- gamma hydroxybutyrate (GHB)
- flunitrazepam (Rohypnol)
- ketamine

GHB has been abused in the United States since about 1990 for its euphoric, sedative, and anabolic (bodybuilding) effects. It was widely available over the counter in health food stores until 1992. Bodybuilders used it to aid in reducing percentage of body fat and to build muscle. Street names for GHB include "Liquid ecstasy," "soap," "easy lay," and "Georgia home boy."

Rohypnol is of particular concern because of its use in date rape. When mixed with alcohol, Rohypnol can incapacitate its victims and prevent the person from resisting sexual assault. It can also lead to anterograde **amnesia**, in which individuals cannot remember what they experienced while under the influence. Rohypnol can be lethal when mixed with alcohol and/or other depressants. Rohypnol is not available by prescription in the United States, and it is illegal to import it. Even so, illegal use of Rohypnol started appearing in the United States in the early 1990s, when it became known as "rophies," "roofies," "roach," and "rope."

Ketamine is an anesthetic used predominately by veterinarians to treat animals. It can be injected or snorted. Ketamine goes by the street names of "Special K" or "Vitamin K." At certain doses, ketamine can cause dreamlike states and hallucinations. It has become particularly common in club and rave (large, all-night dance marathon) settings and has also been used as a date-rape drug. At high doses, it can cause **delirium**, amnesia, impaired motor functioning, high blood pressure, and **depression**. It can also cause potentially fatal respiratory problems.

Causes and symptoms

Causes

Antianxiety drugs can be taken orally to bring about a general calming or drowsy effect, usually experienced as pleasant. Abuse of antianxiety medication can develop with prolonged use, as tolerance grows relatively quickly. Increasing amounts of the drug are then needed to produce the initial effect. It is possible to become addicted to antianxiety drugs even when they are medically prescribed.

KEY TERMS

Abuse—A milder form of addiction than substance dependence. Generally, people who have been diagnosed with substance abuse do not experience the tolerance or withdrawal symptoms—the signs of physiological dependence—that people dependent on a substance experience.

Anxiolytic—A preparation or substance given to relieve anxiety; a tranquilizer.

Barbiturates—A class of medications (including Seconal and Nembutal) that causes sedation and drowsiness. They may be prescribed legally but may also be used as drugs of abuse.

Benzodiazepines—A group of central nervous system depressants used to relieve anxiety or to induce sleep.

Dependence—The adaptation of neurons and other physical processes to the use of a drug, followed by withdrawal symptoms when the drug is removed; physiological and/or psychological addiction.

Flunitrazepam (Rohypnol)—A central nervous system depressant that is not legal in the United States but is used as a date-rape drug.

Gamma hydroxybutyrate (GHB)—A central nervous system depressant that has been abused in the United States for euphoric, sedative, bodybuilding, and date-rape purposes.

Intoxication—The presence of significant problem behaviors or psychological changes following ingestion of a substance.

Ketamine—An anesthetic used predominately by veterinarians to treat animals that can be used as a date-rape drug.

Sedative—A medication that induces relaxation and sleep.

Tranquilizer—A medication that induces a feeling of calm and relaxation.

Withdrawal—Symptoms experienced by a person who is physically dependent on a drug when the drug use is discontinued.

A second cause of antianxiety drug abuse is their use when combined with other drugs, such as **cocaine**. It is not uncommon for a person abusing antianxiety drugs to pair the use of a stimulant, such as cocaine or **methamphetamine**, with a CNS depressant. The combination allows the user to feel alert for an extended period of time and then be able to come down from the high and even fall asleep.

Symptoms

Even when prescribed for medical reasons, an individual taking central nervous system depressants usually feels sleepy and uncoordinated during the first few days of treatment. As the body adjusts to the effects of the drug, these feelings begin to disappear. If the drug is used long term, the body develops tolerance, and increasing doses are needed to obtain the desired effect of general calming or drowsiness.

The use of antianxiety drugs can pose extreme danger when taken along with other medications that cause CNS depression, such as prescription pain medicines, some over-the-counter cold and allergy medications, and alcohol. Use of additional depressants can slow breathing and respiration and can lead to death.

Withdrawal from antianxiety medications can be dangerous if not done under medical supervision. The safest method of withdrawal involves a gradual reduction of dosage. Abrupt withdrawal from these medications can lead to seizures due to the sudden increase in brain activity.

Diagnosis

The manual used by mental health professionals to diagnose mental illnesses, the ***Diagnostic and Statistical Manual of Mental Disorders*** (*DSM*) includes specific diagnostic criteria for the four stages of substance abuse, which are:

- dependence
- abuse
- intoxication
- withdrawal

Substance dependence, the more severe form of **addiction**, is a group of cognitive, behavioral, and physiological symptoms associated with the continued use of the substance and includes both tolerance and withdrawal symptoms. Abuse is a less severe form of addiction that may also result in risky behavior, such as driving while under the influence. For example, individuals with an abuse disorder may miss work or school or get into arguments with parents or spouses about substance use. Such problems can easily escalate into full-blown dependence.

Intoxication refers to the presence of clinically significant problem behaviors or psychological changes, such as inappropriate sexual or aggressive behavior, mood swings, impaired judgment, or impaired social or work functioning, that develop during or shortly after use of an antianxiety medication. As with other CNS depressants such as alcohol, these behaviors may be accompanied by slurred speech, unsteady gait, memory or attention problems, poor coordination, and stupor or coma. Memory impairment is relatively common, especially a kind known as anterograde amnesia that resembles alcoholic blackouts.

Withdrawal is a characteristic syndrome that develops when use of the antianxiety medication is severely reduced or stopped abruptly. It is similar to abrupt cessation of heavy **alcohol use**. Symptoms may include increases in heart rate, respiratory rate, blood pressure or body temperature, sweating, hand tremor, **insomnia**, anxiety, nausea, and restlessness. Seizures may occur in perhaps as many as 20%–30% of individuals undergoing untreated withdrawal. In the more severe forms of withdrawal, hallucinations and delirium can occur. Withdrawal symptoms are generally the opposite of the acute effects experienced by first-time users of the drugs. Length of withdrawal varies depending upon the drug and may last as few as 10 hours or as long as three to four weeks. The longer the substance has been taken and the higher the dosages used, the more likely that withdrawal will be severe.

Treatment

According to the National Institute on Drug Abuse (NIDA), successful treatment for antianxiety medication addiction needs to incorporate several components. Counseling, particularly cognitive-behavioral counseling, focuses on helping addicted individuals identify and change the behaviors, attitudes, and beliefs that contributed to their drug usage. Combined with prescribed medications to make withdrawal safer and easier, counseling can help the addicted individual eventually make a full recovery. Often, it takes multiple courses of treatment before full recovery can be achieved. Various levels of care, from outpatient to residential care for up to 18 months, are available, depending upon need. Narcotics Anonymous also offers ongoing recovery support.

Prognosis

The most typical course of abuse according to the *DSM*, involves teens or young people in their early 20s who may escalate occasional use of antianxiety medications to the point at which they develop problems such as abuse or dependence. This is particularly likely for individuals who also abuse other substances. An initial pattern of use at parties can eventually lead to daily use and high degrees of tolerance.

A second course, observed somewhat less frequently, involves individuals who initially obtain medications by prescription, usually for treatment of anxiety or insomnia. Though the vast majority of people who use medications as prescribed do not go on to develop **substance abuse** problems, a small minority do. Again, tolerance develops and the need for higher dosages to reach the initial effects occurs. Individuals may justify their continued use on the basis of the original symptoms but engage in active substance seeking to ensure supply. Others at higher risk are those with alcohol dependence who might be given prescription antianxiety medications to reduce their anxiety or insomnia.

QUESTIONS TO ASK YOUR DOCTOR

- What risks are associated with antianxiety medications and antianxiety drug abuse?
- What symptoms are associated with antianxiety drug dependence?
- Does having antianxiety drug dependence and abuse put me at risk for other health conditions?
- Can you recommend any treatment and support groups for me?

Prevention

Healthcare professionals play a very important role in preventing and detecting abuse of prescription drugs. Primary care physicians, nurse practitioners, and pharmacists can all play a role.

It is estimated by the NIDA that approximately 70% of all Americans visit a healthcare provider at least once every two years. Thus, healthcare providers are in a unique position not only to prescribe medications as appropriate but also to identify **prescription drug abuse** when it exists and recommend appropriate treatment for recovery. Screening for substance abuse should be incorporated into routine history taking or when a patient currently exhibits symptoms associated with problem drug use.

Over time, providers should be alert to any increases in the amount of medication being used, which may be a sign of tolerance. They should also be aware that individuals addicted to prescription medications may engage in "doctor shopping"—that is, going from provider to provider in an effort to obtain multiple prescriptions of their abused drug.

Pharmacists can play a role in preventing prescription drug abuse as well. They should provide information and advice about the correct way to take prescribed medications and be alert to drug interactions. They can also play a role in detecting prescription fraud by noticing suspicious-looking prescription forms.

Resources

BOOKS

American Psychiatric Association. *Diagnostic and Statistical Manual of Mental Disorders.* 4th ed., Text rev. Washington, DC: American Psychiatric Association, 2000.

American Psychological Association. *Publication Manual of the American Psychological Association,* 6th ed. Washington, DC: American Psychological Association, 2009.

Erickson, Carlton K. *Addiction Essentials: The Go-To Guide for Clinicians and Patients.* New York: Norton, 2011.

PERIODICALS

Carter, Lawrence P., et al. "Relative Abuse Liability of GHB in Humans: A Comparison of Psychomotor, Subjective, and Cognitive Effects of Supratherapeutic Doses of Triazolam, Pentobarbital, and GHB." *Neuropsychopharmacology* 31, no. 11 (2006): 2537–51.

De Wit, Harriet, et al. "Evaluation of the Abuse Potential of Pagoclone, a Partial GABA-Sub(A) Agonist." *Journal of Clinical Psychopharmacology* 26, no. 3 (2006): 268–73.

McCabe, S. E., et al. "Medical Misuse of Controlled Medications Among Adolescents." *Archives of Pediatrics & Adolescent Medicine* 165, no. 8 (2011): 729–35.

Mintzer, Miriam Z., and R.R. Griffiths. "An Abuse Liability Comparison of Flunitrazepam and Triazolam in Sedative Drug Abusers." *Behavioural Pharmacology* 16, no. 7 (2005): 579–84.

WEBSITES

Smith, Melinda, Lawrence Robinson, and Jeanne Segal. "Antianxiety Medication." Helpguide.org. http://helpguide.org/mental/anxiety_medication_drugs_treatment.htm (accessed December 13, 2011).

ORGANIZATIONS

American Psychiatric Association, 1000 Wilson Blvd., Ste. 1825, Arlington, VA, 22209, (703) 907-7300, apa@psych.org, http://www.psych.org.

American Psychological Association, 750 1st St. NE, Washington, DC, 20003, (202) 336-5500, http://www.apa.org.

Anxiety Disorders Association of America, 8730 Georgia Ave., Ste. 600, Silver Spring, MD, 20910, (240) 485-1001, Fax: (240) 485-1035, http://www.adaa.org.

Mental Health America, 2000 N. Beauregard St., 6th Fl., Alexandria, VA, 22311, (703) 684-7722, (800) 969-6642, Fax: (703) 684-5968, http://www1.nmha.org.

National Alliance on Mental Illness, Colonial Place Three, 2107 Wilson Blvd., Ste. 300, Arlington, VA, 22201, (703) 524-7600, (800) 950-NAMI (6264), Fax: (703) 524-9094, http://www.nami.org.

National Institute on Drug Abuse, National Institutes of Health, 6001 Executive Blvd., Rm. 5213, Bethesda, MD, 20892, (301) 443-1124, information@nida.nih.gov, http://www.nida.nih.gov.

National Institute of Mental Health (NIMH), 6001 Executive Blvd., Rm. 8184, MSC 9663, Bethesda, MD, 20892, (301) 443-4513, (866) 615-6464, Fax: (301) 443-4279, nimhinfo@nih.gov, http://www.nimh.nih.gov.

Barbara S. Sternberg, PhD
Ruth A. Wienclaw, PhD
Laura Jean Cataldo, RN,EdD

Antidepressants

Definition

Antidepressants are medications that are used primarily to treat **depression** and depressive disorders.

Purpose

Antidepressant drugs are used to alleviate the symptoms of depression and are also sometimes used to treat other psychological disorders, including **anxiety disorders**, **seasonal affective disorder**, and some eating disorders. Because they are thought to increase the effectiveness of some pain medications, they are sometimes used in the treatment of migraine headaches. They may also be used as a component of **smoking cessation** programs and in the treatment of fibromyalgia and some types of **sleep disorders**.

Description

Depression is a serious condition that severely affects a person's quality of life. It is normal for a person to undergo brief periods of sadness or a general sense of feeling down. However, when these feelings do not subside, depression may be the cause. The three main depressive disorders include dysthymia, **major depressive disorder**, and **bipolar disorder**, which alternates between periods of "highs" (mania) and "lows" (depression). A person with major depressive disorder experiences five or more depressive symptoms for at least two weeks. These symptoms can include feelings of sadness, emptiness, guilt, or worthlessness; loss of interest in previously pleasurable activities; changes in eating and sleeping patterns; **fatigue**, lethargy, or agitation; difficulty concentrating; and suicidal thoughts. Antidepressant drugs are not the only treatment for depression; **psychotherapy** and other treatments are also independently effective in alleviating depression. Antidepressant drugs, if prescribed, are often used in combination with these other treatments.

The type of antidepressant medication prescribed depends on the particular array of symptoms a patient

Antidepressant medications (also used for anxiety disorders)

Generic name	Trade name	Drug class	FDA approved age
amitriptyline	Elavil	Tricyclic	18+
amoxapine	Asendin		18+
bupropion	Wellbutrin		18+
citalopram	Celexa	SSRI	18+
clomipramine	Anafranil	Tricyclic	10+ (for obsessive-compulsive disorder)
desipramine	Norpramin	Tricyclic	18+
desvenlafaxine	Pristiq	SNRI	18+
doxepin	Sinequan	Tricyclic	12+
duloxetine	Cymbalta	SNRI	18+
escitalopram	Lexapro	SSRI	18+; 12–17 for major depressive disorder
fluoxetine	Prozac	SSRI	8+
fluoxetine	Sarafem	SSRI	18+ (for premenstrual dysphoric disorder)
fluvoxamine	Luvox	SSRI	8+ (for obsessive-compulsive disorder)
imipramine	Tofranil	Tricyclic	6+ (for bedwetting in children)
imipramine pamoate	Tofranil-PM	Tricyclic	18+
isocarboxazid	Marplan	MAOI	18+
maprotiline	Ludiomil	Tricyclic	18+
mirtazapine	Remeron		18+
nortriptyline	Aventyl, Pamelor	Tricyclic	18+
paroxetine	Paxil	SSRI	18+
paroxetine mesylate	Pexeva	SSRI	18+
phenelzine	Nardil	MAOI	18+
protriptyline	Vivactil	Tricyclic	18+
selegiline transdermal	Emsam		18+
sertraline	Zoloft	SSRI	6+
tranylcypromine	Parnate	MAOI	18+
trazodone	Desyrel		18+
trimipramine	Surmontil	Tricyclic	18+
venlafaxine	Effexor	SNRI	18+

SOURCE: National Institute of Mental Health.

"Alphabetical List of Medications," available online at: http://www.nimh.nih.gov/health/publications/mental-health-medications/alphabetical-list-of-medications.shtml. *(Table by PreMediaGlobal. © 2012 Cengage Learning.)*

displays or reports. There are several different types of antidepressant drugs. All of them work by altering the level or activity of **neurotransmitters** in the **brain**. Neurotransmitters are chemicals that are released by neurons, or nerve cells. They attach to other neurons and activate them in various ways. Although antidepressant drugs affect communication between neurons within hours after these drugs are ingested, symptoms of depression usually improve only after a few weeks of taking the medication. Some people notice improvement in symptoms after two weeks, but most people notice a benefit only after six to eight weeks of using the medication. The reason for this delayed effect of antidepressants is not entirely clear. One theory is related to the finding that the changes in neurotransmitter activity caused by antidepressants increase the release of other chemicals, called neurotrophins, in the brain. In the normal brain, neurotrophins help neurons to grow and connect to other neurons. People with depression sometimes have shrinkage of neurons in parts of the brain. When more neurotrophins are present, neurons in these areas of the brain can grow.

The main classes of antidepressant drugs are tricyclic antidepressants, **monoamine oxidase inhibitors (MAOIs)**, **selective serotonin reuptake inhibitors (SSRIs)**, serotonin-norepinephrine reuptake inhibitors (SNRIs), and atypical antidepressants. A patient who does not improve with one type of antidepressant drug may sometimes be helped by another type of antidepressant, because different drugs work in different ways.

Tricyclic antidepressants

The first class of drugs used to treat depression was the tricyclic antidepressants. These drugs work by preventing neurons from reabsorbing the neurotransmitters **serotonin**, **dopamine**, and norepinephrine after they are released. This means that the neurotransmitters are able to remain in the gaps between neurons for a longer period of time, thus continuing to activate the neurons that receive them. Tricyclic antidepressants typically have more side effects than other types of antidepressants, because they can prevent nerve cells from functioning normally and additional neurotransmitters from working effectively. For example, they block the activity of histamine, a neurotransmitter that is involved in keeping people alert and awake. They also block the activity of acetylcholine, a neurotransmitter involved in many automatic body

Percentage of U.S. adults (18+) reporting prescription antidepressant drug use in the past month, 1988–1994 and 2005–2008

	1988–1994	2005–2008
Total		
18 years and over, age-adjusted†	2.4	11.1
18 years and over, crude	2.3	11.4
Men		
18 years and over	1.5	6.2
18–44 years	*1.0	3.6
45–64 years	*2.3	8.5
65 years and over	*2.3	10.0
Women		
18 years and over	3.1	16.2
18–44 years	2.3	11.9
45–64 years	4.6	21.9
65 years and over	3.5	17.3

*Estimates are considered unreliable. Data preceded by an asterisk have a relative standard error of 20%–30%.
†Estimates are age-adjusted to the year 2000 standard population using three age groups: 18–44 years, 45–64 years, and 65 years and over.

SOURCE: Centers for Disease Control and Prevention, National Center for Health Statistics, *Health, United States, 2010*, February 2011.

(Table by PreMediaGlobal. © 2012 Cengage Learning.)

functions. Specific tricyclic antidepressants include **imipramine** (Tofranil), **amitriptyline** (Elavil, Endep), **clomipramine** (Anafranil), **doxepin** (Sinequan, Adapin), **desipramine** (Norpramin), **nortriptyline** (Pamelor), **protriptyline** (Vivactil), and **trimipramine** (Surmontil).

MAOIs

The **monoamine oxidase inhibitors** are drugs that prevent neurotransmitters such as dopamine, serotonin, and norepinephrine from being broken down into inactive chemicals. This means that when **MAOIs** are used, more of these neurotransmitters are available to send messages in the brain. MAOIs can have potentially serious side effects, however, because they prevent the amino acid tyramine from being broken down. Tyramine is a chemical required by the body and is found in foods like aged cheese, smoked and pickled meats and fish, and raisins. If tyramine cannot be broken down, it can accumulate in the body, causing increased blood pressure and possibly **stroke**. Types of MAOIs include **isocarboxazid** (Marplan), **phenelzine** (Nardil), and **tranylcypromine** (Parnate).

SSRIs

The **selective serotonin reuptake inhibitors** work by preventing neurons from reabsorbing serotonin after it is released, so that the effect of serotonin on adjoining neurons is prolonged. The **SSRIs** include **citalopram** (Celexa), **escitalopram** (Lexapro), **fluoxetine** (Prozac), **fluvoxamine** (Luvox), **paroxetine** (Paxil), **sertraline** (Zoloft), and vilazodone (Viibryd). Vilazodone, a combination SSRI/5HT1A receptor agonist, was approved by the FDA in 2011 and may not cause some of the side effects common with other antidepressant medications, namely weight gain and sexual dysfunction.

SNRIs

Serotonin-norepinephrine reuptake inhibitors function similarly to SSRIs but block the absorption of both serotonin and norepinephrine, instead of just serotonin. Types of SNRIs include **desvenlafaxine** (Pristiq), **duloxetine** (Cymbalta), and **venlafaxine** (Effexor).

Atypical antidepressants

The atypical antidepressants are a miscellaneous collection of drugs with different chemical makeups than the other classes of antidepressants. Examples of atypical antidepressants include **bupropion** (Wellbutrin), **mirtazapine** (Remeron), and **trazodone** (Desyrel).

Recommended dosage

The dosage of antidepressants depends on the particular drug being prescribed, along with other factors such as the age of the patient, the patient's body chemistry, and the patient's body weight. Patients are usually started on a low dose to minimize side effects, and the dose is gradually increased over time to a level that is therapeutic. Newer antidepressants, however, may be started at the therapeutic dosage level.

Precautions

Use of antidepressant drugs may increase suicidal thoughts in children, adolescents, and adults through age 24. Healthcare practitioners and families of patients taking antidepressants should carefully monitor users for worsening depression, acts of self-harm, or other significant changes in behavior.

Antidepressants can precipitate mania in people who are susceptible to bipolar disorder. Healthcare practitioners typically take a detailed medical history before prescribing antidepressants. Various medical problems may affect the success or risks of antidepressants. These include—but are not limited to—angina, headaches, epilepsy, recent heart attacks or stroke, kidney disease, and diabetes. Some antidepressants may affect a fetus; pregnant women should inform their doctors about their condition before antidepressants are prescribed. Newborns of mothers who took SSRIs late in pregnancy displayed withdrawal symptoms, including tremor and respiratory problems. SSRIs may also put adults over the age of 65 at increased risk for fractures due to bone loss. Patients taking tricyclic antidepressants should carefully adhere to the dietary restrictions provided by their doctor in order to avoid potentially serious side effects. Patients who stop taking antidepressants may experience withdrawal symptoms if the drugs are abruptly discontinued.

Some medical professionals question the effectiveness of antidepressants. A 2008 review of antidepressant studies, published in *PLoS Medicine*, the journal of the Public Library of Science, concluded that for patients with mild-to-moderate depression, antidepressant drugs were not much more effective than placebos. Despite this, the number of people taking antidepressants has risen dramatically. A study published in the *Archives of General Psychiatry* revealed that use among persons aged 6 or older jumped from 5.8% of the U.S. population in 1996 to 10.1% in 2005 (27 million people). The U.S. Centers for Disease Control and Prevention estimates that 11% of adults (aged 18 or older) were prescribed antidepressants between 2005 and 2008. Because of the *PLoS* review and other studies, some feel that antidepressants may be overprescribed. Nevertheless, depression is not a condition that should be taken lightly, and patients should discuss all avenues with their physicians to find a treatment that works for them.

Side effects

People who take antidepressants may experience side effects. Though specific effects depend on the drug taken and the patient's characteristics, possible side effects include dry mouth, constipation, nausea, bladder problems, sexual problems, blurred vision, dizziness, daytime drowsiness, **insomnia**, increased heart rate, headache, nervousness, and agitation. Newer antidepressants, such as the SSRIs and SNRIs, are thought to have fewer and less troublesome side effects than the tricyclic antidepressants and the MAOIs.

Interactions

Antidepressants may result in dangerous side effects if taken in combination with other medications. There can also be dangerous side effects if different types of antidepressants are combined with each other; for instance, **serotonin syndrome** is a serious condition that can develop if there is too much serotonin in the body. Drugs that inhibit the absorption of serotonin should not be used in combination. Patients switching medications, such as from an SSRI to an MAOI (or vice versa), may need to wait a period of time before beginning the new medication. Patients should inform their doctor about all medications and herbal supplements they are taking before antidepressant drugs are prescribed and should follow dosing instructions exactly. Alcohol or other recreational drugs may decrease the effectiveness of antidepressants and should not be used in conjunction with the medication.

KEY TERMS

Acetylcholine—A neurotransmitter with effects that are generally opposite those of dopamine and norepinephrine. Acetylcholine dilates blood vessels, lowers blood pressure, and slows heartbeat.

Anxiety disorder—A type of psychological disorder characterized by unrealistic, irrational fear or intense anxiety.

Eating disorder—A type of psychological disorder characterized by disturbances in eating patterns, extreme concern about weight gain, and unhealthy efforts to control weight.

Fibromyalgia—A condition in which a person experiences chronic pain in the muscles and soft tissues around joints.

Mania—A state in which a person experiences intense excitement and euphoria.

Neurotransmitter—One of a group of chemicals secreted by a nerve cell (neuron) to carry a chemical message to another nerve cell, often as a way of transmitting a nerve impulse. Examples of neurotransmitters include acetylcholine, dopamine, serotonin, and norepinephrine.

Serotonin—5-Hydroxytryptamine; a substance that occurs throughout the body with numerous effects including neurotransmission in the brain. Inadequate amounts of serotonin are implicated in some forms of depression, obsessive-compulsive disorder, and anxiety disorders.

Stroke—A temporary loss of normal blood flow to an area of the brain, caused by blockage or rupture of a blood vessel.

See also Psychopharmacology; Star*D study

Resources

BOOKS

American Psychiatric Association. *Diagnostic and Statistical Manual of Mental Disorders*. 4th ed., text rev. Washington, DC: American Psychiatric Association, 2000.

Brenner, George M., and Craig W. Stevens. "Psychotherapeutic Drugs." Chap. 22 in *Pharmacology*. 3rd ed. Philadelphia: Saunders/Elsevier, 2010.

Diamond, Ronald, J. *Instant Psychopharmacology*. 3rd ed. New York: W.W. Norton and Company, 2009.

Dunbar, Katherine Read, ed. *Antidepressants*. Farmington Hills, MI: Greenhaven Press, 2006.

Kalat, James W. *Biological Psychology*. 10th ed. Belmont, CA: Wadsworth, 2009.

Kirsch, Irving. *The Emperor's New Drugs: Exploding the Antidepressant Myth*. New York: Basic Books, 2010.

PERIODICALS

Kirsch, Irving, et al. "Initial Severity and Antidepressant Benefits: A Meta-Analysis of Data Submitted to the Food and Drug Administration." *PLoS Medicine* 5, no. 2 (2008): e45. http://dx.doi.org/doi:10.1371/journal.pmed.0050045 (accessed September 20, 2011).

Kramer, Peter. "In Defense of Antidepressants." *New York Times*, July 9, 2011. http://www.nytimes.com/2011/07/10/opinion/sunday/10antidepressants.html?_r=1

Olfson, Mark, and Steven Marcus. "National Patterns in Antidepressant Medication Treatment." *Archives of General Psychiatry* 66, no. 8 (2009): 848–56. http://dx.doi.org/10.1001/archgenpsychiatry.2009.81 (accessed September 20, 2011).

Richards, J. Brent, et al. "Effect of Selective Serotonin Reuptake Inhibitors on the Risk of Fracture." *Archives of Internal Medicine* 167, no. 2 (2007): 188–94.

Szalavitz, Maia. "Antidepressants: Are They Effective or Just a Placebo?" *TIME*, June 3, 2010. http://www.time.com/time/health/article/0,8599,1991841,00.html (accessed September 20, 2011).

WEBSITES

MedlinePlus. "Antidepressants." U.S. National Library of Medicine, National Institutes of Health. http://www.nlm.nih.gov/medlineplus/antidepressants.html (accessed September 20, 2011).

National Institute of Mental Health. "Antidepressant Medications for Children and Adolescents: Information for Parents and Caregivers." National Institutes of Health. http://www.nimh.nih.gov/health/topics/child-and-adolescent-mental-health/antidepressant-medications-for-children-and-adolescents-information-for-parents-and-caregivers.shtml (accessed September 20, 2011).

———. "Mental Health Medications: What Medications Are Used to Treat Depression?" National Institutes of Health. http://www.nimh.nih.gov/health/publications/mental-health-medications/complete-index.shtml#pub5 (accessed September 20, 2011).

U.S. Food and Drug Administration. "Antidepressant Use in Children, Adolescents, and Adults." http://www.fda.gov/Drugs/DrugSafety/InformationbyDrugClass/UCM096273 (accessed September 20, 2011).

Ruvanee Pietersz Vilhauer, Ph.D.
James Waun

Antisocial personality disorder

Definition

Also known as psychopathy, sociopathy, dissocial personality disorder, or dyssocial personality disorder, antisocial personality disorder (APD) is a **diagnosis** applied to persons who routinely behave with little or no regard for the rights, safety, or feelings of others. This pattern of behavior is seen in children or young adolescents and can persist into adulthood.

The ***Diagnostic and Statistical Manual of Mental Disorders** (DSM)*, the handbook used by medical professionals in diagnosing mental disorders, classifies APD as one of six specific types of **personality disorders**, along with **avoidant personality disorder**, **borderline personality disorder**, **narcissistic personality disorder**, **obsessive-compulsive personality disorder**, and **schizotypal personality disorder**.

Demographics

Men are three times more likely to be diagnosed with antisocial personality disorder than women, according to the World Health Organization. Mental health professionals may diagnose 3%–30% of the population in clinical settings as having the disorder. The percentages may be even higher among prison inmates or persons in treatment for **substance abuse**. By some estimates, three-quarters of the prison population may meet the diagnostic criteria for APD.

Description

Men or women diagnosed with this personality disorder demonstrate few emotions beyond contempt for other people. Their lack of empathy is often combined with an inflated sense of self-worth and a superficial charm that tends to mask an inner indifference to the needs or feelings of others. Some studies indicate that people with APD can only mimic the emotions associated with committed love relationships and friendships that most people feel naturally.

People reared by parents with antisocial personality disorder or substance abuse disorders are more likely to develop APD than members of the general population. People with the disorder may be homeless, living in poverty, suffering from a concurrent substance abuse disorder, or piling up extensive criminal records, as antisocial personality disorder is associated with low socioeconomic status and urban backgrounds. Highly intelligent individuals with APD, however, may not come to the attention of the criminal justice or mental health care systems and may be underrepresented in diagnostic statistics.

Some legal experts and mental health professionals do not think that APD should be classified as a mental disorder on the grounds that the classification appears to excuse unethical, illegal, or immoral behavior. Despite these concerns, juries in the United States have consistently demonstrated that they do not regard a diagnosis of APD as exempting a person from prosecution or punishment for crimes committed.

Furthermore, some experts disagree with the categorization by the **American Psychiatric Association** (APA) of antisocial personality disorder. The APA considers the term "psychopathy" as synonymous with APD. However, some experts make a distinction between psychopathy and APD. Dr. Robert Hare, an authority on psychopathy and the originator of the **Hare Psychopathy Checklist**, claims that all persons with psychopathy have APD but not all individuals diagnosed with APD have psychopathy. Recent reports have made this distinction even clearer, suggesting that there is an emotional deficit component of psychopathy that is not necessarily present in people with APD. One expert review comments that only 25% of people diagnosed with APD or **conduct disorder**, a related condition seen in children, will show psychopathic tendencies.

Causes and symptoms

Causes

Studies of adopted children indicate that both genetic and environmental factors influence the development of APD, with heritability estimates ranging from 44% to 72%. Both biological and adopted children of people diagnosed with the disorder have an increased risk of developing it. Children born to parents diagnosed with APD but adopted into other families resemble their biological more than their adoptive parents in this regard. The environment of the adoptive home, however, may lower the child's risk of developing APD.

Researchers have linked antisocial personality disorder to childhood physical or **sexual abuse**, neurological disorders (which are often undiagnosed), and low IQ. Some experts have recently questioned the link between psychopathy, which these experts distinguish from APD, and early environmental **trauma**. As with other personality disorders, no one has identified any specific cause of antisocial personality disorder, and multiple factors are believed to affect the risk of APD developing. Persons diagnosed with APD also have an increased incidence of **somatization disorder** and substance-related disorders.

The fourth edition of the *DSM* (*DSM-IV-TR*) states that persons who show signs of conduct disorder with accompanying **attention deficit hyperactivity disorder** before the age of 10 have a greater chance of being diagnosed with APD as adults than do other children. The manual notes that abuse or **neglect** combined with erratic parenting or inconsistent discipline appears to increase the risk that a child diagnosed with conduct disorder will develop APD as an adult.

Brain imaging studies have identified some specific characteristics in the brains of people diagnosed with APD that suggest dysfunction of structures in the frontal and temporal lobes of the brain.

Symptoms

The central characteristic of antisocial personality disorder is an extreme disregard for the rights of other people. Individuals with APD lie and cheat to gain money or power. Their disregard for authority often leads to arrest and imprisonment. Because they have little regard for others and may act impulsively, they are frequently involved in fights. They show loyalty to few if any other people and are likely to seek power over others in order to satisfy sexual desires or economic needs.

People with APD often become effective "con artists." Those with well-developed verbal abilities can often charm and fool their victims, including unsuspecting or inexperienced therapists. People with APD have no respect for what others regard as societal norms or legal constraints. They may quit jobs on short notice, move to another city, or end relationships without warning and without what others would consider good reason. Criminal activities typically include theft, selling illegal drugs, and check fraud. Because persons with antisocial personality disorder make themselves their highest priority, they are quick to exploit others. They commonly rationalize these actions by dismissing their victims as weak, stupid, or unwary.

Some work has been done on the relationship between what are called "minor physical anomalies" and the presence of various disorders, including aggression disorders and psychopathy. The presence of these features—which include low-seated ears and adherent ear lobes—is associated with developmental derailments in the fetus at the end of the third trimester of pregnancy, and they have been linked with the development of conduct disorder and violence in adulthood. Studies directly examining their association, if any, with psychopathy or APD are lacking, but birth complications are known risk factors for violent and antisocial behaviors.

Diagnosis

The diagnosis of antisocial personality disorder is usually based on a combination of a careful medical as well as psychiatric history and an interview with the patient. The doctor will look for recurrent or repetitive patterns of antisocial behavior. He or she may use a diagnostic questionnaire for APD, such as the Hare Psychopathy Checklist-Revised or the self-reporting Psychopathic Personality Inventory, if the patient's history suggests the diagnosis. A person aged 18 years or older with a childhood history of disregard for the rights of others can be diagnosed as having APD if he or she gives evidence of three of the following seven behaviors associated with disregard for others:

- Fails to conform to social norms, as indicated by frequently performing illegal acts or pursuing illegal occupations.
- Deceives and manipulates others for selfish reasons, often in order to obtain money, sex, drugs, or power. This behavior may involve repeated lying, conning, or the use of false names.
- Fails to plan ahead or displays impulsive behavior, as indicated by a long succession of short-term jobs or frequent changes of address.
- Engages in repeated fights or assaults as a consequence of irritability and aggressiveness.
- Exhibits reckless disregard for safety of self or others.
- Shows a consistent pattern of irresponsible behavior, including failure to find and keep a job for a sustained length of time and refusal to pay bills or honor debts.
- Shows no evidence of sadness, regret or remorse for actions that have hurt others.

To meet *DSM-IV-TR* criteria for APD, a person must also have had some symptoms of conduct disorder before age 15, though this qualification may be removed in the fifth edition of the *DSM*. An adult 18 years or older who does not meet all the criteria for APD may be given a diagnosis of conduct disorder.

Antisocial behavior may appear in other mental disorders as well as in APD. These conditions must be distinguished from true APD. For instance, it is not uncommon for a person with a substance abuse disorder to lie to others in order to obtain money for drugs or alcohol. But unless indications of antisocial behavior were present during the person's childhood, he or she would not be diagnosed with antisocial personality disorder. People who meet the criteria for a substance abuse disorder as well as APD would be given a dual diagnosis.

Treatment

Antisocial personality disorder is highly unresponsive to any form of treatment, in part because persons with APD rarely seek treatment voluntarily. If they do seek help, it is usually in an attempt to find relief from **depression** or other forms of emotional distress. Although there are medications that are effective in treating some of the symptoms of the disorder, noncompliance with medication regimens or abuse of the drugs prevents the widespread use of these medications. The most successful treatment programs for APD are long-term structured residential settings in which the patient systematically earns privileges as he or she modifies behavior. In other words, if a person diagnosed with APD is placed in an environment in which they cannot victimize others, their behavior may improve. It is unlikely, however, that they would maintain good behavior if they left the disciplined environment.

If some form of individual **psychotherapy** is provided along with **behavior modification** techniques, the therapist's primary task is to establish a relationship with the patient, who has usually had very few healthy relationships in his or her life and is unable to trust others. The patient should be given the opportunity to establish positive relationships with as many people as possible and be encouraged to join **self-help groups** or prosocial organizations.

Unfortunately, these approaches are rarely if ever effective. Many persons with APD use therapy sessions to learn how to turn "the system" to their advantage. Their pervasive pattern of manipulation and deceit extends to all aspects of their life, including therapy. Generally, their behavior must be controlled in a setting where they know they have no chance of getting around the rules.

Prognosis

APD can follow a chronic and unremitting course from childhood or early adolescence into adult life. The impulsiveness that characterizes the disorder often leads to a jail sentence or an early death through accident, homicide, or **suicide**. There is some evidence that the worst behaviors that define APD diminish by midlife; the more overtly aggressive symptoms of the disorder occur less frequently in older patients. This improvement is especially true of criminal behavior but may apply to other antisocial acts as well.

Prevention

Measures intended to prevent antisocial personality disorder must begin with interventions in early childhood, before youths are at risk for developing conduct

KEY TERMS

Attention deficit hyperactivity disorder—A learning and behavioral disorder characterized by difficulty in sustaining attention, impulsive behavior, and excessive activity.

Conduct disorder—A behavioral and emotional disorder of childhood and adolescence in which children display physical aggression and infringe on or violate the rights of others. Youths diagnosed with conduct disorder may set fires, exhibit cruelty toward animals or other children, sexually assault others, or lie and steal for personal gain.

Psychopathy—A psychological syndrome that includes lack of a conscience or sense of guilt, lack of empathy, egocentricity, pathological lying, repeated violations of social norms, disregard of the law, shallow emotions, and a history of victimizing others.

Somatization disorder—A long-term condition in which a person has physical symptoms that involve more than one part of the body, but no physical cause can be found. The pain and symptoms are real and not faked.

Substance abuse disorder—Disorder that is characterized by an individual's need for more of a drug or alcohol than intended, an inability to stop using by choice, and an ongoing difficulty in recovering from the effects of the substance.

disorder. Preventive strategies include education for parenthood and other programs intended to lower the incidence of **child abuse**; Big Brother/Big Sister and similar mentoring programs to provide children at risk with adult role models of responsible and prosocial behavior; and further research into the **genetic factors** involved in APD.

Resources

BOOKS

American Psychiatric Association. *Diagnostic and Statistical Manual of Mental Disorders*. 4th ed., text rev. Washington, DC: American Psychiatric Publishing, 2000.

Black, Donald, W., and C. Lindon Larson. *Bad Boys, Bad Men: Confronting Antisocial Personality Disorder*. New York: Oxford University Press, 2000.

Cleckley, Hervey. *The Mask of Sanity*. 5th ed. Augusta, GA: Emily S. Cleckley, 1988.

Hare, Robert D. *Without Conscience: The Disturbing World of the Psychopaths Among Us*. New York: Guilford Press, 1999.

Lykken, David T. *The Antisocial Personalities*. Hillsdale, NJ: Lawrence Erlbaum Associates, 1995.

Simon, Robert I. *Bad Men Do What Good Men Dream: A Forensic Psychiatrist Illuminates the Darker Side of Human Behavior*. Washington, DC: American Psychiatric Association, 1996.

PERIODICALS

Abbott, Alison. "Into the Mind of a Killer." *Nature* 410 (2001): 296–98.

WEBSITES

Hare, Robert D. "'Without Conscience': Robert Hare's Web Site Devoted to the Study of Psychopathy." http://www.hare.org (accessed September 29, 2011).

MedlinePlus. "Antisocial Personality Disorder." U.S. National Library of Medicine, National Institutes of Health. http://www.nlm.nih.gov/medlineplus/ency/article/000921.htm (accessed September 29, 2011).

Dean A. Haycock, PhD
Emily Jane Willingham, PhD

Anxiety disorders

Definition

Anxiety disorders are a group of mental disturbances characterized by anxiety as a central or core symptom. Although anxiety is a commonplace experience, not everyone who experiences it has an anxiety disorder. Anxiety is associated with a wide range of physical illnesses, medication side effects, and other psychiatric disorders.

Prior to 1980, psychiatrists classified patients on the basis of a theory that defined anxiety as the outcome of the patient's unconscious conflicts. Subsequent revisions to the ***Diagnostic and Statistical Manual of Mental Disorders*** (*DSM*), the handbook used by medical professionals in diagnosing mental disorders, introduced and refined a new classification that considered recent discoveries about the biochemical and post-traumatic origins of some types of anxiety. The present definitions are based on the external and reported symptom patterns of the disorders rather than on theories about their origins.

Demographics

Anxiety disorders vary widely in their frequency of occurrence in the general population, age of onset, family patterns, and gender distribution. **Stress** and anxiety disorders caused by medical conditions or **substance**

abuse are less age- and gender-specific. Whereas **obsessive-compulsive disorder** (OCD) affects males and females equally, **generalized anxiety disorder** (GAD), **panic disorder**, and **specific phobias** all affect women more frequently than men. GAD and panic disorders are more likely to develop in young adults, whereas phobias and OCD often begin in childhood.

Description

Stimulated by real or imagined dangers, anxiety afflicts people of all ages and social backgrounds. When the anxiety results from irrational fears, it can disrupt or disable normal life. Some researchers believe anxiety is synonymous with fear, occurring in varying degrees and in situations in which people feel threatened by some danger. Others describe anxiety as an unpleasant emotion caused by unidentifiable dangers or dangers that, in reality, pose no threat. Unlike fear, which is caused by realistic, known dangers, anxiety can be more difficult to identify and to alleviate.

Rather than attempting to formulate a strict definition of anxiety, many psychologists simply make the distinction between normal anxiety and neurotic anxiety or anxiety disorders. Normal (sometimes called objective) anxiety occurs when people react appropriately to the situation causing the anxiety. For example, many people experience stage fright—the fear of speaking in front of large groups—or feel anxious on the first day at a new job. There is little, if any, real danger posed by either situation, yet each can stimulate intense anxiety that can affect or derail a person's desires or obligations. Despite these feelings, most people carry on and eventually adapt. In contrast, anxiety that is characteristic of anxiety disorders is disproportionately intense, and the anxious feelings interfere with a person's ability to carry out normal or desired activities.

Anxiety disorders are the most common form of mental disturbance in the United States. According to the Anxiety Disorders Association of America, as many as 40 million American adults are affected by anxiety disorders. These disorders can interfere with work, schooling, and family life. They also contribute to the high rates of alcohol and substance abuse among Americans. Anxiety disorders are an additional problem for health professionals because the physical symptoms of anxiety frequently bring people to primary care doctors or emergency rooms.

The fourth edition of the *DSM* (*DSM-IV-TR*) defines 12 types of anxiety disorders in the adult population. They can be grouped under the following headings:

- Panic disorders with or without **agoraphobia**. The chief characteristic of panic disorder is the occurrence of panic attacks coupled with fear of their recurrence. In clinical settings, agoraphobia is usually not a disorder by itself but is typically associated with some form of panic disorder. Patients with agoraphobia are afraid of places or situations in which they might have a panic attack and be unable to leave or to find help. Panic disorder affects approximately 2.7% of adults.
- Specific phobias. A phobia is an intense irrational fear of a specific object or situation that compels the individual to avoid it. Some phobias concern activities or objects that involve some risk (for example, flying or driving), but many are focused on harmless animals or other objects.
- Social phobia. Social phobia involves a fear of being humiliated, judged, or scrutinized. It manifests itself as a fear of performing certain functions in the presence of others, such as public speaking or using public lavatories.
- Obsessive-compulsive disorder (OCD). This disorder is marked by unwanted, intrusive, persistent thoughts or repetitive behaviors that reflect the patient's anxiety or attempts to control it. It affects about 1% of the population. About 6% of individuals who have OCD also have panic disorders.
- Stress disorders. These include **post-traumatic stress disorder** (PTSD) and **acute stress disorder**. Stress disorders are symptomatic reactions to traumatic events in the patient's life.
- Generalized anxiety disorder (GAD). GAD is the most commonly diagnosed anxiety disorder and occurs most frequently in young adults.
- Anxiety disorders due to known physiological causes. These include general medical conditions or substance abuse.
- Anxiety disorder not otherwise specified. This last category is not a separate type of disorder but is included to cover symptoms that do not meet the specific *DSM-IV* criteria for other anxiety disorders.

All *DSM* anxiety disorder diagnoses include a criterion of severity. The anxiety must be severe enough to interfere significantly with the patient's occupational or educational functioning, social activities or close relationships, and other customary activities.

Anxiety disorders in children and adolescents

DSM-IV defines one anxiety disorder as specific to children: **separation anxiety disorder**. This disorder is defined as anxiety regarding separation from home or family that is excessive or inappropriate for the child's age. In some children, separation anxiety takes the form of school avoidance.

Children and adolescents can also be diagnosed with panic disorder, phobias, generalized anxiety disorder, and the post-traumatic stress syndromes.

DSM-5

The members of the Anxiety, Obsessive-Compulsive Spectrum, Posttraumatic, and Dissociative Disorders Work Group, who are working on the latest revision to the *DSM* (*DSM-5*, 2013) have considered several changes to the diagnostic category of anxiety disorders. Potential changes include:

- making agoraphobia a separate and codable diagnosis rather than placing it within the context of panic disorder
- providing criteria for the assessment of panic attacks
- reclassifying OCD and the stress disorders (PTSD and acute stress disorder) as obsessive-compulsive and trauma- and stressor-related disorders, respectively

Causes and symptoms

The causes of anxiety include a variety of individual and general social factors and may produce physical, cognitive, emotional, or behavioral symptoms. The patients' ethnic or cultural backgrounds may influence their vulnerability to certain forms of anxiety. **Genetic factors** that lead to biochemical abnormalities may also play a role.

Anxiety in children may be caused by having experienced abuse, as well as by the factors that cause anxiety in adults.

Diagnosis

The diagnoses of anxiety disorders are complicated by the variety of causes of anxiety and the range of disorders that may include anxiety as a symptom. Before determining the specific course of treatment, the medical professional performs a complete evaluation of the patient. Symptoms are carefully analyzed as to their cause(s). Other conditions outside the realm of anxiety disorders may be secondary or primary factors in the **diagnosis**. Further, many patients with anxiety disorders have features or symptoms of more than one disorder. Patients whose anxiety is accounted for by another mental disorder, such as **schizophrenia** or major **depression**, are not diagnosed with an anxiety disorder.

Examination

A doctor examining an anxious patient usually begins by ruling out diseases that are known to cause anxiety and then proceeds to take the patient's medication history to exclude side effects of prescription drugs. Typically, doctors ask about caffeine consumption to see if the patient's dietary habits are a factor. The patient's work and family situations will also be discussed. Often, primary care physicians exhaust resources looking for medical causes for general patient complaints, which may indicate a physical illness. The Anxiety Disorders Association of American has published guidelines to aid physicians in diagnosing and managing generalized anxiety disorder.

Tests

There are no laboratory tests that can diagnose anxiety, although the doctor may order some specific tests to rule out other diseases and conditions, such as laboratory tests for blood sugar and thyroid function. Although there is no psychiatric test that can provide definite diagnoses of anxiety disorders, there are several short-answer interviews or symptom inventories that doctors can use to evaluate the intensity of a patient's anxiety and some of its associated features. These measures include the **Hamilton Anxiety Scale** and the Anxiety Disorders Interview Schedule (ADIS).

Treatment

Generally, anxiety disorders are treated with **psychotherapy**, medication, or both. The specific treatment process is determined based on the specific problem, along with the preference of the individual.

Traditional

Before treatment is begun, the patient should inform the medical professional of any medicines and other treatments being administered currently or in the past. For relatively mild anxiety disorders, psychotherapy alone may be sufficient. In general, doctors prefer to use a combination of medications and psychotherapy with more severely anxious patients. Most patients respond better to a combination of treatment methods than to either medications or psychotherapy alone.

Drugs

Medications are prescribed by medical professionals, usually psychiatrists, who sometimes provide psychotherapy services, both individually or as a member of a team (often consisting of counselors, **social workers**, and psychologists). The medications used for anxiety disorders generally include numerous types of **antidepressants**, **antianxiety drugs**, and beta blockers. Because of the variety of medications and treatment approaches available to treat anxiety disorders, the doctor cannot predict in advance which combination will be most helpful to a specific patient. In many cases, the doctor will need to try a new medication or treatment

Antianxiety medications[1]

Generic name	Trade name	FDA approved age
alprazolam	Xanax	18+
buspirone	BuSpar	18+
chlordiazepoxide	Librium	18+
clonazepam	Klonopin	18+
clorazepate	Tranxene	18+
diazepam	Valium	18+
lorazepam	Ativan	18+
oxazepam	(generic only)	18+

[1]All of these antianxiety medications are benzodiazepines, except buspirone.

SOURCE: National Institute of Mental Health.

"Alphabetical List of Medications," available online at: http://www.nimh.nih.gov/health/publications/mental-health-medications/alphabetical-list-of-medications.shtml. *(Table by PreMediaGlobal. © 2012 Cengage Learning.)*

over a six- to eight-week period in order to assess its effectiveness. Trying a few different treatment options does not necessarily mean that the patient cannot be helped or that the doctor is incompetent. In addition, medicines used during these periods help to control the problem while psychotherapy is being initiated.

ANTIDEPRESSANTS. Antidepressants are very effective for anxiety disorders. Under normal circumstances, antidepressants take from four to six weeks to become fully effective and symptoms begin to disappear. Some of the widely used antidepressants for anxiety disorders are:

- **Selective serotonin reuptake inhibitors** (SSRIs): These relatively new types of antidepressants work by changing the concentration of serotonin, a neurotransmitter, within the brain. SSRIs are commonly started at low doses, with higher doses coming at regular intervals until a proper plateau has been reached. These have fewer side effects than older antidepressants used for anxiety disorders. Side effects include nausea, nervousness, and sexual dysfunction, which usually fade with time. Types of frequently used SSRIs include citalopram (Celexa), escitalopram (Lexapro), fluoxetine (Prozac), paroxetine (Paxil), and sertraline (Zoloft).
- Tricyclics: These older antidepressants are as effective as SSRIs for anxiety disorders, except for obsessive-compulsive disorder (OCD). Dosages usually start small and gradually increase as needed. Symptoms include dizziness, dry mouth, drowsiness, and weight gain. Commonly used tricyclics are imipramine (Tofranil) and clomipramine (Anafranil).
- **Monoamine oxidase inhibitors** (MAOIs): The oldest type of antidepressants used for anxiety disorders, MAOIs have a number of side effects with a variety of foods and beverages that contain tyramine and numerous other types of medications (such as certain pain relievers, cold and allergy medications, and others). MAOIs can also interact with SSRIs and cause serious symptoms, including seizures and blood pressure and heart irregularities. Patients ought to seek further information from the attending physician with regards to these potential adverse interactions. The most frequently used MAOIs are isocarboxazid (Marplan), phenelzine (Nardil), and tranylcypromine (Parnate).

ANTIANXIETY DRUGS. **Benzodiazepines** are effective drugs that are used to counter anxiety. They may cause drowsiness in some patients. Benzodiazepines can be habit forming and are also needed in higher doses in order to be effective. For these two reasons, benzodiazepines are usually only used for short periods. Because of their habit-forming nature, they must be slowly reduced in amount before patients completely stop taking them. **Clonazepam** (Klonopin), **lorazepam** (Ativan), and **alprazolam** (Xanax) are types of benzodiazepines often prescribed for specific anxiety disorders. **Buspirone** (Buspar), within the drug group of azapirones, is a newer type of antianxiety drug that is used to treat generalized anxiety disorder (GAD).

BETA BLOCKERS. **Beta blockers**, which are also frequently used to treat physiological problems of the heart, are sometimes used to treat anxiety disorders. Physicians often use beta blockers when people have social phobias, such as fear of talking in front of an audience, in order to reduce anxiety in such situations. **Propranolol** (Inderal) is a commonly used beta blocker.

Psychotherapy

Psychotherapy can be effective at treating anxiety disorders when administered through a well-trained and experienced mental health professional. In addition, individuals with the problem must be actively engaged in their treatment; otherwise such therapy is unlikely to work.

Psychiatrists, **psychologists**, social workers, and counselors use cognitive-behavioral therapy (CBT) to help patients learn what is causing their specific problems and how to react to the symptoms when they occur. Each patient is considered a unique case and must be treated on an individualized basis for best results. For instance, a person with a **social phobia** is shown that heart attack–like symptoms are the result of the person's fear of speaking in front of people. The individual is provided with a proactive means to minimize fears when in social situations that provoke such problems. Likewise, people with other types of anxiety disorders are helped to

KEY TERMS

Agoraphobia—Abnormal anxiety regarding public places or situations from which the patient may wish to flee or in which he or she would be helpless in the event of a panic attack.

Compulsion—A repetitive or ritualistic behavior that a person performs to reduce anxiety. Compulsions often develop as a way of controlling or undoing obsessive thoughts.

Obsession—A repetitive or persistent thought, idea, or impulse that is perceived as inappropriate and distressing.

Panic attack—A time-limited period of intense fear accompanied by physical and cognitive symptoms. It may be unexpected or triggered by specific internal or external cues.

QUESTIONS TO ASK YOUR DOCTOR

- Do I have an anxiety disorder?
- What treatment plan is best for me?
- What medications should I use?
- Do I need counseling?

confront their fears and to desensitize themselves to anxiety-provoking situations.

Treatment in children and adolescents

A combination of CBT and medication has been found to be the most successful form of treatment for children aged 7–17. However, antidepressants should be used with caution in children and adolescents; some drugs are not recommended for children younger than 18, and children and adults up to age 24 are at increased risk of developing suicidal thoughts and behavior. **SSRIs** are prescribed more in children than other medications, including tricyclic antidepressants. Parents should discuss all treatment options with their child's physician and watch for signs of harmful behavior or worsening depression.

Alternative

Alternative treatments for anxiety cover a variety of approaches. **Meditation** and mindfulness training are thought to be beneficial to patients with phobias and panic disorder. Hydrotherapy is useful to some anxious patients because it promotes general relaxation of the nervous system. **Yoga**, aikido, tai chi, and **dance therapy** help patients work with the physical, as well as the emotional, tensions that either promote anxiety or are created by the anxiety.

Homeopathy and traditional Chinese medicine approach anxiety as a symptom of a systemic disorder. Homeopathic practitioners select a remedy based on other associated symptoms and the patient's general constitution. Chinese medicine regards anxiety as a blockage of *qi*, or vital force, inside the patient's body that is most likely to affect the lung and large intestine meridian flow. The practitioner of Chinese medicine chooses **acupuncture** point locations and/or herbal therapy to move the *qi* and rebalance the entire system in relation to the lung and large intestine.

Getting help

Although anxiety disorders are not always easy to diagnose, there are several reasons why it is important for patients with severe anxiety symptoms to get help. Anxiety does not always go away by itself and can progress to panic attacks, phobias, and episodes of depression. Untreated anxiety disorders may eventually lead to a diagnosis of major depression or interfere with the patient's education or ability to keep a job. In addition, many anxious patients develop addictions to drugs or alcohol when they try to "self-medicate" their symptoms. Moreover, since children learn ways of coping with anxiety from their parents, adults who get help for anxiety disorders are in a better position to help their families cope with factors that lead to anxiety than those who remain untreated. With appropriate treatment by medical professionals, most people with anxiety disorders can return to a normal daily life.

Prognosis

The prognosis for recovery depends on the specific disorder, the severity of the patient's symptoms, the specific causes of the anxiety, and the patient's degree of control over these causes.

Prevention

Anxiety is an unavoidable feature of human existence. However, humans have some power over their reactions to anxiety-provoking events and situations. Cognitive therapy and meditation or mindfulness training appear to be beneficial in helping people lower their long-term anxiety levels.

Resources

BOOKS

American Psychiatric Association. *Diagnostic and Statistical Manual of Mental Disorders.* 4th edition, text revised. Washington, DC: American Psychiatric Association, 2000.

Challem, Jack, and Melvyn Werbach. *The Food-Mood Solution: All-Natural Ways to Banish Anxiety, Depression, Anger, Stress, Overeating, and Alcohol and Drug Problems—and Feel Good Again.* Hoboken, NJ: Wiley, 2008.

Kase, Larina, and Deborah Roth Ledley. *Anxiety Disorders.* Hoboken, NJ: John Wiley and Sons, 2007.

Otto, Michael, and Stefan Hofmann, eds. *Avoiding Treatment Failures in the Anxiety Disorders (Series in Anxiety and Related Disorders).* New York: Springer, 2009.

National Institute of Mental Health. *Anxiety Disorders.* NIH Publication No. 06-3879. Bethesda, MD: NIMH, 2006.

Pelletier, Kenneth R. "Part II: CAM Therapies for Specific Conditions: Anxiety." In *The Best Alternative Medicine.* New York: Simon & Schuster, 2007.

PERIODICALS

Hofmann, Stefan, and Jasper A. J. Smits. "Cognitive-Behavioral Therapy for Adult Anxiety Disorders: A Meta-Analysis of Randomized Placebo-Controlled Trials." *Journal of Clinical Psychiatry* 69, no. 4 (April 2008): 621–32. http://www.ncbi.nlm.nih.gov/pmc/articles/PMC2409267 (accessed September 8, 2011).

WEBSITES

"Anxiety." MedlinePlus. http://www.nlm.nih.gov/medlineplus/anxiety.html (accessed September 8, 2011).

"Anxiety Disorders." American Psychiatric Association. http://www.dsm5.org/ProposedRevision/Pages/AnxietyDisorders.aspx (accessed September 8, 2011).

"PTSD. Stress and Resilience." National Institute of Mental Health. February 25, 2010. http://www.nimh.nih.gov/media/video/tuma-short-ptsd.shtml (accessed September 8, 2011).

"Treatment of Anxiety Disorders." National Institute of Mental Health. Last reviewed July 9, 2009. http://www.nimh.nih.gov/health/publications/anxiety-disorders/treatment-of-anxiety-disorders.shtml (accessed September 8, 2011).

Xiong, Glen L. "Hypochondriasis." Medscape Reference. Updated August 3, 2011. http://emedicine.medscape.com/article/290955-overview (accessed September 8, 2011).

Yates, William R. "Anxiety Disorders." Medscape Reference. Updated August 25, 2011. http://emedicine.medscape.com/article/286227-overview (accessed September 8, 2011).

ORGANIZATIONS

American Psychiatric Association, 1000 Wilson Blvd., Ste. 1825, Arlington, VA, 22209-3901, (703) 907-7300, apa@psych.org, http://www.psych.org.

American Psychological Association, 750 1st St., NE, Washington, DC, 20002-4242, (202) 336-5500; TDD/TTY: (202) 336-6123, (800) 374-2721, http://www.apa.org.

Anxiety Disorders Association of America, 8730 Georgia Ave., Silver Spring, MD, 20910, (240) 485-1001, Fax: (240) 485-1035, http://www.adaa.org.

Mental Health America, 2000 N. Beauregard St., 6th Fl., Alexandria, VA, 22311, (703) 684-7722, (800) 969-6642, Fax: (703) 684-5968, http://www1.nmha.org.

National Alliance on Mental Illness, 2107 Wilson Blvd., Ste. 300, Arlington, VA, 22201-3042, Fax: (703) 524-9094, (800) 950-6264, http://www.nami.org.

National Institute of Mental Health, 6001 Executive Blvd., Rm. 8184, MSC 9663, Bethesda, MD, 20892-9663, (301) 433-4513; TTY: (301) 443-8431, Fax: (301) 443-4279, (866) 615-6464; TTY: (866) 415-8051, nimhinfo@nih.gov, http://www.nimh.nih.gov.

Rebecca J. Frey, PhD
Teresa G. Odle
Laura Jean Cataldo, RN, EdD
William A. Atkins, BB, BS, MBA

Anxiety reduction techniques

Definition

Anxiety reduction techniques are learned skills that can be used by individuals to help overcome anxiety and its associated mental and physical symptoms, including tension, **stress**, worry, and nervousness. These techniques include relaxation, visualization and imagery, diaphragmatic breathing, stress inoculation, **meditation**, and **cognitive-behavioral therapy**.

Relaxation or progressive relaxation

This anxiety reduction technique is based on the premise that anxiety and stress are associated with muscle tension. When one achieves deep muscle relaxation, muscle tension is reduced, and this relaxed state is incompatible with anxiety.

Visualization and imagery

This anxiety reduction technique aids individuals in making a mental image of what they want to accomplish. For example, an individual might wish to release worries or concerns or create a relaxing image to escape momentarily from a stressful event.

Diaphragmatic breathing

This technique involves breathing sufficient amounts of air to help a person's blood fill with oxygen and be purified properly. In this technique, the individual breathes deeply from the diaphragm, which is located low in the chest near the abdomen. **Yoga** class instruction often includes teaching participants how to use breathing to reduce anxiety.

Stress inoculation

Stress inoculation training is a type of therapy that teaches clients to cope with anxiety and stressful situations by learning better functional patterns of self-talk. Self-talk, or what people tell themselves about stressful situations, can be habitual. For example, a person may take an ordinary event and automatically magnify its importance. Practices that counter self-talk help individuals to deal more effectively with anxiety and other stressful situations and to react to such problems in more positive ways.

Meditation

In this anxiety reduction technique, an individual is trained to focus his or her attention on one thing at a time. Meditation techniques focus on various physical sensations or mental images to neutralize troubling emotional and mental patterns and control them.

Cognitive-behavioral therapy

Cognitive-behavioral therapy (CBT) suggests various exercises that help individuals identify thoughts and beliefs that trigger anxiety. Once these thought patterns are identified, the individual learns techniques to help change negative thought patterns into healthier ones.

Purpose

The goal of learning and implementing anxiety reduction techniques is to reduce the intensity of anxiety. These techniques are also helpful in teaching people how to relax and manage stress. Many of the techniques are used in combination with each other. For example, a person may be taught diaphragmatic breathing while also engaging in relaxation techniques, a visualization and imagery exercise, or meditation.

Relaxation or progressive relaxation

Relaxation has been used to help women during childbirth and others dealing with chronic pain. Relaxation has also been used to treat muscle tension, muscle spasms, and neck and back pain and to decrease perspiration and respiratory rates. In addition, relaxation can help with **fatigue**, **depression**, **insomnia**, irritable bowel syndrome, high blood pressure, mild phobias, and **stuttering**.

Visualization and imagery

Visualization and imagery techniques have been helpful in treating general or specific anxiety, headaches, and muscle tension and spasms. They are also useful in reducing or eliminating pain and in the recovery from illnesses and injuries. Visualization and imagery techniques have also been used by athletes who want to achieve peak performance.

Diaphragmatic breathing

Diaphragmatic breathing has been found to help people reduce anxiety, depression, irritability, muscle tension, circulation, and fatigue.

Stress inoculation

Stress inoculation has been helpful in reducing interpersonal and general anxiety. For example, these techniques may be used when a person has an upcoming job interview, speech, or test. Stress inoculation has also been used to treat phobias, fear of heights, and chronic anger problems.

Meditation

Meditation has been used to treat and prevent high blood pressure, heart disease, **stroke**, migraine headaches, immunization diseases, obsessive thinking, attention problems, anxiety, depression, and anger control problems.

Cognitive-behavioral therapy

Cognitive-behavioral therapy (CBT) focuses on thought processes and belief systems. The overall goal of the approach is to identify problematic beliefs and thought patterns, which may be irrational or unrealistic, and replace them with more rational and realistic views.

Description

Anxiety reduction techniques are often practiced and demonstrated in therapy sessions with a trained professional. In addition, the person learning the techniques practices them regularly between therapy sessions.

Relaxation or progressive relaxation

In progressive relaxation, individuals are instructed to tighten and then relax various muscles. They either lie down or sit in a chair with their head supported. Each muscle group, such as face muscles, arm muscles, or leg muscles, is tensed for 5 to 7 seconds and then relaxed for 20 to 30 seconds. This action helps individuals recognize tense and relaxed muscles. This entire procedure is repeated one to five times and usually starts with the face muscles and moves to the foot muscles. When relaxation is used with chronic pain and childbirth, the techniques focus the person's attention on breathing and relaxing muscles as a distraction from the pain.

For mastery, relaxation techniques are typically practiced every day for one to two weeks. A person may engage in these techniques anywhere from 15 minutes to one hour per session. Sometimes, individuals record and replay instructions on tightening and relaxing various muscle groups until they become familiar with the muscle groups and establish a comfortable routine.

Visualization and imagery

The basic premise of visualization and imagery is that thoughts become reality. For example, if individuals think anxious thoughts, then they will become tense. The assumption of visualization and imagery is that people can use their imagination to assist them in feeling a certain way or performing a certain desired action. Programmed, receptive, and guided visualization are the basic types.

In programmed visualization, the person creates a vivid image, including sight, taste, sound, and smell. The individual then imagines a goal he or she wants to attain or some type of healing that is desired. In the visualization, the goal is achieved or the healing occurs.

An idea underlying both receptive visualization and guided visualization is that the person is seeking an answer to a life question or resolution to an issue, and the answer or resolution is within the person but is buried or inaccessible because of fear, doubt, or anxiety. These techniques are similar to dream interpretation and free association techniques used in **psychoanalysis** or psycho-dynamic therapy. For example, an individual may wonder whether he or she should remain in a current job. A proponent of these techniques would maintain that below the level of conscious thought, the person knows what he or she really wants to do but is not to listening to his or her desires or to act—the message is subconsciously being blocked. The goal of these techniques is to enable the person to relax and focus enough to receive that message, so that he or she can do what needs to be done.

In receptive visualization, the individual creates a peaceful mental scene. After the image is formed, the person asks a question and waits for the answer. To continue the job scenario, the person might imagine a beach and he ask the question, "Should I leave my job?" As the person continues to relax and remain in the scene, he or she may "hear" an answer blowing in the breeze or "see" a boat sailing away, which may be symbolic of the wish to leave a job.

In guided visualization, the person creates a vivid image, as in programmed visualization, but omits some important elements. The person then waits for the subconscious to supply the missing parts. For example, a computer programmer may wonder if he or she should stay in a present job or return to school for an advanced degree. When engaging in guided visualization, the person may visualize a cubicle at work, the pictures on the desk, the feel of the desk chair, and the sounds of people working beyond the cubicle, but he or she will omit an element from the scene. In this case, the element would be the computer. The person will then wait to see what the subconscious uses to replace the computer. Within the visualization, the computer may be replaced by books, which may represent a desire to return to school.

Visualization and imagery exercises work best when a person is relaxed. Exercises are typically practiced two to three times a day for 10 to 20 minutes at a time. How quickly an individual sees results can vary. Many people report immediate symptom relief. However, the personal goals a person sets, the power of his or her imagination, and the willingness to practice can all influence how rapidly benefits are obtained. Some people find it helpful to record and replay detailed descriptions of what they want to visualize or imagine.

Diaphragmatic breathing

Diaphragmatic breathing can be learned in minutes; however, the benefits may not be recognized until after

KEY TERMS

Depression—A psychiatric disorder that causes sleeplessness, lack of energy, poor concentration, hopelessness, and other negative feelings that may lead to thoughts of suicide.

Obsessive thinking—Thoughts that overcome a person's thought processes; a compulsive way of thinking in which the same thought repeats, preventing other thoughts.

Phobia—An irrational or illogical fear or hatred of something, such as fear of heights, confined spaces, or snakes.

Yoga—A physical, mental, and meditative discipline and practice that began in India.

Zen meditation—A discipline that teaches the mind to relax, which involves sitting in prescribed positions in order to calm the body and mind, with the goal to slow heart rate and breathing to reach a reflective meditative state.

ROLLO MAY (1909–1994)

Rollo May was the second of six children and the eldest son of Earl Tuttle, a field secretary at the Young Men's Christian Association, and Matie Boughton May, a homemaker. May grew up in Michigan in a family that had "more than its share of troubles." He later described his parents as "austere disciplinarians and anti-intellectuals" and portrayed their relationship as "discordant" and the precursor for his interest in psychology and counseling. His oldest sister was diagnosed as psychotic and spent time in mental hospitals.

His lectures on counseling and personality adjustment were published as his first book, *The Art of Counseling: How to Gain and Give Mental Health* (1939), which was well regarded. May studied psychology at Columbia University in New York City. While working on his dissertation in 1942 and still counseling, May was diagnosed with tuberculosis. This confrontation with his own mortality shaped his views on existentialism. While recuperating in upstate New York for almost two years, May wrote *The Meaning of Anxiety* (1950), which he considered the "watershed" event of his career. He stressed that anxiety can be a positive, motivating force for social and personal development and that people can use their inner resources for life choices. In 1953, May published *Man's Search for Himself*, a popular and critical success that established May as a leader of existentialist thinking in the United States.

By the early 1960s, May had become a leader in challenging behaviorism and psychoanalysis. He diverted from biological determinism and stressed by contrast the unique conscious elements in individual psychology. After moving to California in 1975, he resumed his private practice as a therapist. He also served in various capacities at the Saybrook Institute of the California School of Professional Psychology. More books and ideas followed: *Power and Innocence: A Search for the Sources of Violence* (1972), *The Courage to Create* (1975), *My Quest for Beauty* (1985), and *The Cry for Myth* (1991). May wrote more than fifteen books, many of which are directly related to his own experience and development. He was the recipient of the American Psychological Association's Gold Medal for his distinguished career in psychology, Phi Beta Kappa's Ralph Waldo Emerson Award, and the Whole Life Humanitarian Award.

several months of regular practice. When breathing from the diaphragm, clients are often told to lie down on a rug or blanket with their legs slightly apart, arms to the sides not touching the body, and eyes closed. Attention is brought to the breathing by placing one hand on the chest and the other hand on the abdomen area. The client is then instructed to breathe in through the nose and exhale out the mouth. Each time the client breathes in, he or she should try to breathe deeper. This should be practiced for a minimum of five minutes once or twice a day. Over a few weeks of practice, the time period should be increased to 20 minutes, and the activity can be performed while lying down, sitting, or standing.

Stress inoculation

As people go about their daily activities, they often talk to themselves. Stress inoculation uses this self-talk in helping clients decrease their anxiety and stress. Stress inoculation therapy works to turn the client's own thought patterns into a "vaccine" against stress-induced anxiety. The first step is to develop a list of stressful situations and arrange them from least to most stressful. Once anxiety-producing situations are identified, the client is taught to curb the anxiety-provoking thoughts and replace them with more positive coping thoughts. Once these new thoughts are learned, they can be tried out in real situations. The time it takes to replace habitual thoughts with new ones varies depending on the client's amount of practice and commitment to make this change.

Meditation

There are various forms of meditation. Depending on the type used, the individual focuses his or her attention in slightly different ways. For example, Zen meditation focuses on breathing, whereas in transcendental meditation, the person makes a sound or repeats a mantra selected to keep all other images and problems from intruding on his or her thoughts. With practice, a person can reach a meditative state and obtain its benefits within a few minutes.

Benefits

Anxiety reduction techniques are coping skills, designed to help people increase their calm and confidence. Used correctly, these skills help people maximize their

QUESTIONS TO ASK YOUR DOCTOR

- Where can I find more information on anxiety reduction techniques?
- What is the best type of anxiety reduction technique for my situation?
- What local organizations and individuals provide assistance on such techniques?
- Should I take medication along with using one or more of these techniques?

abilities to meet and move through the challenges of both everyday living and stress-provoking events. Reactive and self-defeating responses to everyday stressors or crises reduce or eliminate individuals' effective and positive responses. With these techniques, people can neutralize these negative responses in order to address constructively the situations that make them anxious.

Aftercare

After a person has learned and practiced anxiety reduction techniques, he or she may need additional instruction from a trained professional. Having a trained professional review these techniques can help reinforce what the person has already learned and been practicing. Furthermore, the person may identify aspects of the techniques that he or she is doing incorrectly, areas that need more attention or focus, and alternative methods of engaging in the techniques.

Risks

There are minimal risks associated with these techniques, but some physical problems may occur. For example, precautions should be taken when doing progressive relaxation and tensing the neck and back. In some cases, excessive tightening can cause muscle or spinal damage. Additionally, tightening various muscle groups, such as the toes or feet, can cause cramps. If physical problems occur, such as difficulty taking deep breaths, unusual muscle pain, or an increased level of anxiety, the individual should stop the activity and may want to consult a physician.

Results

In general, after engaging in anxiety reduction techniques, people report an increased sense of well-being and relaxation. People have a greater sense of self-control and greater confidence in being able to cope with stressful events. They are less fearful and are less likely to avoid stressful situations.

Progressive relaxation can reduce muscle tension. Engaging in relaxation may help to improve a person's energy level; it may reduce depression and anxiety as it increases the ability to retrieve information from memory.

With meditation, people often discover that they have some control over the thoughts that rise in their minds. Many begin to recognize dysfunctional patterns of thought and perceptions that have influenced their lives. Additionally, many people report a greater ability to manage their emotions and maintain stability. When a person meditates, he or she often suppresses the activity of the sympathetic nervous system, the part of the nervous system that activates the body for emergencies. Meditation also lowers a person's metabolism, heart, and breathing rates. Additionally, meditation decreases the chemicals in the body often associated with stress, such as **adrenaline**.

Abnormal results

Once a person begins to implement these anxiety reduction techniques effectively, he or she may discover old or hidden psychological pain. The individual may feel angry, frightened, or depressed, and it may be beneficial for him or her to talk to a friend, mental health professional, or meditation teacher.

Some people have difficulty with various aspects of the different techniques. For example, an individual may feel restless when first learning how to meditate or may feel as though a thousand thoughts are running through his or her mind. However, with practice and assistance from a trained professional, these difficulties will subside. People who feel frustrated or discouraged may simply need to find ways to make the practice of these techniques more comfortable. As is the case with many other skills, effectively reducing anxiety with these techniques requires patience and practice. If an individual does not practice these techniques regularly, the benefits will probably not be obtained.

Resources

BOOKS

Bourne, Edmund J. *The Anxiety and Phobia Workbook*, 5th ed. Oakland, CA: New Harbinger Publications, 2011.

Payne, Rosemary A., and Marie Donaghy. *Payne's Handbook of Relaxation Techniques: A Practical Handbook for the Health Care Professional.* Edinburgh: Churchill Livingstone/Elsevier, 2010.

Romas, John A., and Manoj Sharma. *Practical Stress Management: A Comprehensive Workbook for Managing Change and Promoting Health,* 5th ed. San Francisco: Pearson Benjamin Cummings, 2010.

Seaward, Brian Luke. *Essentials of Managing Stress.* Sudbury, MA: Jones and Bartlett, 2011.

PERIODICALS

Arch, Joanna J., and Michelle G. Craske. "Mechanisms of Mindfulness: Emotion Regulation Following a Focused Breathing Induction." *Behaviour Research and Therapy* 44, no. 12 (December 2006): 1849–58.

Bornas, Xavier, et al. "Changes in Heart Rate Variability of Flight Phobics During a Paced Breathing Task and Exposure to Fearful Stimuli." *International Journal of Clinical and Health Psychology* 6, no. 3 (September 2006): 549–63.

Hunt, Melissa, et al. "The Role of Imagery in the Maintenance and Treatment of Snake Fear." *Journal of Behavior Therapy and Experimental Psychiatry* 37, no. 4 (December 2006): 283–98.

Lundgren, Jesper, Sven G. Carlsson, and Ulf Berggren. "Relaxation Versus Cognitive Therapies for Dental Fear—A Psychophysiological Approach." *Health Psychology* 25, no. 3 (May 2006): 267–73.

Meuret, Alicia E., Thomas Ritz, Frank H. Wilhelm, and Walton T. Roth. "Voluntary Hyperventilation in the Treatment of Panic Disorder—Functions of Hyperventilation, Their Implications for Breathing Training, and Recommendations for Standardization." *Clinical Psychology Review* 25, no. 3 (May 2005): 285–306.

Rausch, Sarah M., Sandra E. Gramling, and Stephen M. Auerbach. "Effects of a Single Session of Large-Group Meditation and Progressive Muscle Relaxation Training on Stress Reduction, Reactivity, and Recovery." *International Journal of Stress Management* 13, no. 3 (August 2006): 273–90.

Roth, Walton T. "Physiological Markers for Anxiety: Panic Disorder and Phobias." *International Journal of Psychophysiology* 58, no. 2–3 (November–December 2005): 190–98.

WEBSITES

Ajmera, Ripa. "Different Anxiety Reduction Techniques." LiveStrong.com. February 26, 2010. http://www.livestrong.com/article/87730-different-anxiety-reduction-techniques (accessed August 13, 2011).

ORGANIZATIONS

American Psychiatric Association, 1000 Wilson Blvd., Ste. 1825, Arlington, VA, 22209-3901, (703) 907-7300, (888) 35-PSYCH (357-7924), apa@psych.org, http://www.psych.org.

American Psychological Association, 750 1st St. NE, Washington, DC, 20002, (202) 336-5500, (800) 374-2721; TDD/TTY: (202) 336-6123, http://www.apa.org.

Anxiety Disorders Association of America, 8730 Georgia Ave., Silver Spring, MD, 20910, (240) 485-1001, http://www.adaa.org.

National Institute of Mental Health, 6001 Executive Blvd., Rm. 8184, Bethesda, MD, 20892-9663, (301) 443-4513, (866) 615-6464, Fax: (301) 443-4279, nimhinfo@nih.gov, http://www.nimh.nih.gov.

Keith Beard, PsyD
Ruth A. Wienclaw, PhD
William Atkins

APA *see* **American Psychiatric Association; American Psychological Association**

Apathy

Definition

Apathy can be defined as an absence or suppression of emotion, feeling, concern or passion. Apathy is an indifference to things generally found to be exciting or moving.

Description

A strong connection exists between apathy and mental disorders. Apathy is one of the hallmark symptoms of **schizophrenia**. Many people with schizophrenia express little interest in the events surrounding them. Apathy can also occur in **depression** and depressive disorders. For example, people who are depressed and have **major depressive disorder** or **dysthymic disorder** often feel numb to events occurring around them, and do not derive pleasure from experiences that they once found enjoyable.

All people may experience periods of apathy. Disappointment and dejection are elements of life, and apathy is a normal way for humans to cope with such stresses—to be able to "shrug off" disappointments enables people to move forward and try other activities and achieve new goals. When the stresses pass, the apparent apathy also disappears. A period of apathy can also be viewed as a normal and transient phase through which many people pass. Long-term apathy and detachment, however, are not normal.

Apathy syndrome is being considered for inclusion in the fifth edition of the ***Diagnostic and Statistical Manual of Mental Disorders*** (*DSM*-5, 2013). Apathy syndrome is defined as a syndrome of primary motivational loss—that is, loss of motivation not attributable to emotional distress, intellectual impairment, or diminished level of consciousness.

Treatment

Transient apathy can be overcome. Friends and professionals may be able to assist individuals to develop an interest in their surroundings. Attitude is important. Persons who desire to overcome apathy have much higher odds of succeeding than do persons lacking a positive attitude.

Other than support, no specific treatment is needed for apathy, unless other more troubling disorders are also present.

The treatment of more persistent apathy (in a depressive disorder, for example), or the apathy that is characteristic of schizophrenia, may respond to treatment for the primary disorder. For depressive disorders, a number of **antidepressants** may be effective, including tricyclic antidepressants, **monoamine oxidase inhibitors (MAOIs)**, and **selective serotonin reuptake inhibitors (SSRIs)**. The tricyclic antidepressants include **amitriptyline** (Elavil), **imipramine** (Tofranil), and **nortriptyline** (Aventyl, Pamelor). **MAOIs** include **tranylcypromine** (Parnate) and **phenelzine** (Nardil). The most commonly prescribed **SSRIs** are **fluoxetine** (Prozac), **sertraline** (Zoloft), **paroxetine** (Paxil), **fluvoxamine** (Luvox), and **citalopram** (Celexa).

SCHIZOPHRENIA. For schizophrenia, the primary goal is to treat the more prominent symptoms (**positive symptoms**) of the disorder, such as the thought disorder and hallucinations that patients experience. Atypical antipsychotics are newer medications introduced in the 1990s that have been found to be effective for the treatment of schizophrenia. These medications include **clozapine** (Clozaril), **risperidone** (Risperdal), **quetiapine** (Seroquel), **ziprasidone** (Geodon), and **olanzapine** (Zyprexa). These newer drugs are more effective in treating the **negative symptoms** of schizophrenia (such as apathy) and have fewer side effects than the older antipsychotics. Most atypical antipsychotics, however, do have weight gain as a side effect, and patients taking clozapine must have their blood monitored periodically for signs of agranulocytosis, or a drop in the number of white blood cells.

Resources

BOOKS

Gelder, Michael, Paul Harrison, and Philip Cowen. *Shorter Oxford Textbook of Psychiatry*. 5th ed. New York: Oxford University Press, 2006.

PERIODICALS

Adams, K. B. "Depressive Symptoms, Depletion, or Developmental Change? Withdrawal, Apathy, and Lack of Vigor in the Geriatric Depression Scale." *Gerontologist* 41, no. 6 (2001): 768–777.

Clarke, Diana E., et al. "Apathy and Cognitive and Functional Decline in Community-Dwelling Older Adults: Results from the Baltimore ECA Longitudinal Study." *International Psychogeriatrics* 22, no. 5 (2010): 819–29.

Kalechstein, A. D., T. F. Newton, and A. H. Leavengood. "Apathy Syndrome in Cocaine Dependence." *Psychiatry Research* 109, no. 1 (2002): 97–100.

Landes, A. M., et al. "Apathy in Alzheimer's Disease." *Journal of the American Geriatric Society* 49, no. 12 (2001): 1700–1707.

Ramirez, S. M., et al. "Relationship of Numbing to Alexithymia, Apathy, and Depression." *Psychological Reports* 88, no. 1 (2001): 189–200.

Simon, Joe J., et al. "Neural Correlates of Reward Processing in Schizophrenia—Relationship to Apathy and Depression." *Schizophrenia Research* 118, nos. 1–3 (May 2010): 154–61.

ORGANIZATIONS

American Psychiatric Association, 1000 Wilson Blvd., Ste. 1825, Arlington, VA, 22209-3901, (703) 907-7300, apa@psych.org, http://www.psych.org.

American Psychological Association, 750 1st Street NE, Washington, DC, 20002-4242, (202) 336-5500; TDD/TTY: (202) 336-6123, (800) 374-2721, http://www.apa.org.

L. Fleming Fallon, Jr., M.D., Dr.P.H.

Aprepitant

Purpose

Aprepitant (brand name Emend) is a drug used to prevent stomachaches and vomiting in persons receiving cancer treatment (chemotherapy) or who have recently taken medicines to prevent pain during surgery (anesthesia). The drug also affects substances in the part of the **brain** associated with emotions, which has led scientists to question whether aprepitant could be used to treat certain mental disorders, particularly major **depression**.

Description

Aprepitant is classified as a substance P neurokin-1 (NK-1) receptor antagonist. This means that it blocks proteins called NK-1 receptors, which sit on cells in the brain region linked to gastrointestinal problems and the body's response to **stress**, anxiety, and depression. The receptors attach or bind to a naturally occurring chemical called substance P, which is found in higher amounts in persons with depression. Blocking the NK-1 receptors causes a decrease in the normal action of substance P that would otherwise be mediated by the NK-1 receptor.

Because aprepitant affects NK-1 receptors in the brain that are associated with emotions, and because it has shown activity in several animal models of depression, scientists had theorized that aprepitant might prove to be a powerful new antidepressant. In 1998, researchers reported that more than half of patients with depression who took aprepitant had an improvement in mood. The study involved 213 people who took the drug for six weeks. The scientists also discovered that the medicine worked as well as **paroxetine** (Paxil) in reducing anxiety.

In 2001, however, a larger trial involving 700 patients with mild-to-moderate depression failed to show that aprepitant worked any better than existing antidepressant medications. Additional studies also failed. In 2003, Merck & Company, the manufacturer of aprepitant, said it would no longer pursue the drug as a treatment for depression. The decision came just a few months after aprepitant received U.S. Food and Drug Administration (FDA) approval as a preventive for chemotherapy-related stomach upset.

Some researchers still investigate aprepitant as a possible treatment for depression, but **clinical trials** have failed to show that it is more effective in treating depression than existing **antidepressants** or even a placebo. A 2010 study found that although aprepitant antagonism, or blocking of NK-1 receptors, does affect emotional processing in humans, its effects are more limited and less consistent than the effects of other antidepressants. The use of aprepitant for other conditions that involve increased NK-1 receptor activity remains under investigation.

Resources

PERIODICALS

Alvaro, G., and R. Di Fabio. "Neurokinin 1 Receptor Antagonists—Current Prospects." *Current Opinion in Drug Discovery and Development* 10, no. 5 (2007): 613–21.

Herpfer, I., and K. Lieb. "Substance P Receptor Antagonists in Psychiatry: Rationale for Development and Therapeutic Potential." *CNS Drugs* 19, no. 4 (2005): 275–93.

Keller, M., et al. "Lack of Efficacy of the Substance P (Neurokinin 1 Receptor) Antagonist Aprepitant in the Treatment of Major Depressive Disorder." *Biological Psychiatry* 59, no. 3 (2006): 216–23.

Kelli Miller Stacy
Margaret Alic, PhD

Aricept *see* **Donepezil**

Aripiprazole

Definition

Aripiprazole (Abilify) is a newer generation antipsychotic medication. It was approved by the U.S. Food &

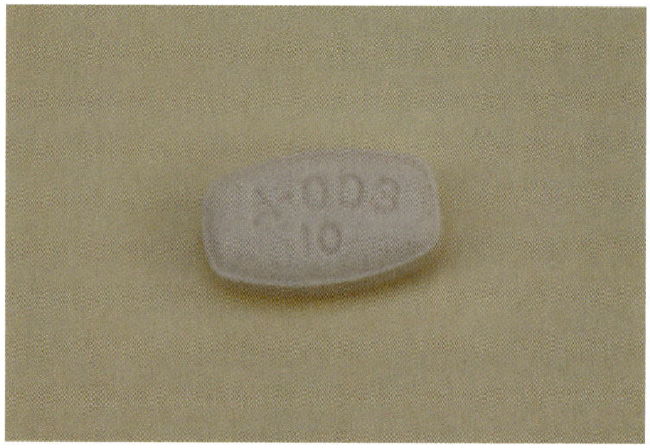

Abilify (aripiprazole), 10 mg. *(© Custom Medical Stock Photo, Inc. Reproduced by permission.)*

Drug Administration (FDA) in 2002 to treat **schizophrenia** symptoms. The symptoms of schizophrenia include hallucinations, **delusions**, **paranoia**, and social withdrawal. Aripiprazole is also FDA approved as a therapy for people with **bipolar disorder** who have had episodes of acute mania or mixed episodes of mania and **depression** but who have subsequently been stabilized for at least six weeks.

Purpose

Aripiprazole can be used short term to treat acute psychotic and manic states and agitation in **dementia**, as well as long term to treat chronic psychotic disorders such as schizophrenia. In the past, these conditions were typically treated with conventional antipsychotic drugs, such as phenothiazine, thioxanthene, and butyrophenone neuroleptics.

Although aripiprazole is primarily indicated for the treatment of adults, some studies suggest it also may be effective for children and adolescents with bipolar disorder. Researchers recommend a lower dose in younger patients. There is a risk of increased suicidal thoughts or actions, especially in children and adolescents taking aripiprazole and in patients with bipolar disorder.

Description

Aripiprazole is part of a class of drugs called atypical antipsychotics. Drugs in this class, which include **clozapine**, **olanzapine**, **quetiapine**, **risperidone**, and **ziprasidone**, are called "atypical" because of their relatively lower risk of certain types of adverse side effects compared to traditional antipsychotic drugs.

The exact mechanism by which aripiprazole and other atypical antipsychotic drugs work is unknown. Scientists believe that schizophrenia is caused by an imbalance of **dopamine** in the **brain**. Dopamine is a neurotransmitter that affects movement and balance. The theory is that aripiprazole acts as a partial agonist and antagonist, meaning that it binds to dopamine receptors in the brain and partially activates these receptors, while preventing dopamine from binding to and fully activating them. Conventional antipsychotic drugs, by contrast, act as full antagonists. These drugs completely block dopamine receptors and significantly interfere with dopamine transmission, which can cause severe movement side effects. Aripiprazole also affects another neurotransmitter, **serotonin**, which is involved in regulating mood and is also imbalanced in people with schizophrenia.

Although studies suggest that aripiprazole works well to treat psychotic conditions such as schizophrenia, less research has been conducted on how its effectiveness compares to that of conventional antipsychotic drugs.

Recommended dosage

Aripiprazole is only available by prescription. It is taken once a day by mouth as either a tablet or an oral solution. The oral solution is designed for older patients who have difficulty swallowing a tablet. Tablets range from 2 mg to 30 mg strengths. The oral solution is available in a 1 mg/mL solution. Aripiprazole can be taken with or without food. Some patients start on a low dose, and then their doctor increases the dose after approximately two weeks.

Precautions

Patients always need to read the accompanying medication guide before taking a prescribed drug. Aripiprazole may increase the risk for diabetes, and people who develop extreme thirst, frequent urination, or other diabetes symptoms while taking the drug should see a doctor for assessment. Because of potential interactions, people who are taking aripiprazole should tell their doctor if they have or are taking medications for any of the following conditions:

- Alzheimer's disease
- anxiety
- depression
- diabetes
- heart disease or heart failure
- high or low blood pressure
- human immunodeficiency virus (HIV)
- irritable bowel disease
- mental illness
- Parkinson's disease
- seizures
- stroke or mini-stroke
- surgery
- ulcers

Women who are pregnant, who intend to become pregnant, or who are nursing should ask their doctor before taking or discontinuing this drug. There is increased risk for extrapyramidal symptoms, a group of involuntary muscle **movement disorders**, and withdrawal symptoms in newborns whose mothers took aripiprazole during their third trimester of pregnancy. Symptoms include abnormal muscle tone, tremor, difficulty breathing and feeding, and agitation.

Because this medication may cause drowsiness and can impair judgment and motor skills, people who take it should take precautions when operating a motor vehicle or machinery. Alcohol can increase the sedative effects and is not advised for use in people who are taking aripiprazole. Also, people who take this drug should use caution when exercising, because aripiprazole can affect the body's ability to regulate temperature, potentially leading to overheating and dehydration.

This drug can increase the risk for a rare condition called **neuroleptic malignant syndrome** (NML). This condition, which is sometimes caused by drugs that interfere with the dopamine pathway, can raise body temperatures to potentially life-threatening levels.

Aripiprazole is not approved for the treatment of **psychosis** in elderly patients with dementia. The FDA in 2005 released a public health advisory warning patients and doctors against using aripiprazole and other atypical antipsychotics off-label. In studies, these drugs significantly increased the risk of death in older patients with dementia compared to placebo. Most of the deaths were associated with heart failure or infections such as pneumonia. In June 2008, the FDA required all manufacturers of antipsychotic drugs to create a warning label with information about this risk. Atypical antipsychotics also have been associated with an increased risk for **stroke** in elderly patients with dementia-related psychosis.

Aripiprazole can cause significant weight gain and the development of metabolic syndrome, the main characteristics of which are high cholesterol, increased blood pressure, insulin resistance or tolerance, or diabetes. Some practitioners use the diabetes drug metformin in patients who appear to be developing this syndrome, in an effort to avoid the development of diabetes and cardiovascular disease.

Side effects

Aripiprazole and other atypical antipsychotic drugs tend to cause fewer neurological side effects than the

KEY TERMS

Atypical antipsychotic—A class of newer-generation antipsychotic medications that are used to treat schizophrenia and other psychotic disorders.

Bipolar disorder—A brain disorder that causes extreme emotional shifts, from mania (elation or hyperactivity) to depression.

Delusions—A condition in which a person holds false beliefs despite evidence to the contrary.

Dementia—A loss of mental ability, often occurring with age, that can interfere with a person's ability to think clearly and function independently.

Dopamine—A chemical messenger in the brain that regulates movement and balance.

Extrapyramidal—Related to the motor system in the brain, the symptoms of which affect movement and coordination, including abnormal muscle movements and drooling.

Hallucinations—Seeing, hearing, feeling, smelling, or tasting things that do not exist.

Mania—A mood disorder in which a person may become impulsive or irritable and may exercise extremely poor judgment.

Neuroleptic malignant syndrome—A rare response to certain antipsychotic drugs, which can raise the body temperature to potentially life-threatening levels.

Off-label—The use of a prescription medication to treat conditions outside the indications approved by the U.S. Food and Drug Administration (FDA). It is legal for physicians to administer these drugs, but it is not legal for pharmaceutical companies to advertise drugs for off-label uses.

Paranoia—Condition in which a person has an irrational suspicion about another person or situation.

Partial agonist—A substance that partially activates a receptor in the brain while blocking the neurotransmitter for that receptor from binding to it.

Schizophrenia—A mental disorder in which a person experiences hallucinations and delusions and displays unusual behavior.

Serotonin—A chemical messenger in the brain that affects mood and emotion.

older antipsychotic drugs. In particular, they have a lower risk of extrapyramidal symptoms. However, the drug does have side effects. The most common side effects with aripiprazole are:

- anxiety
- constipation
- difficulty sleeping
- dizziness
- drowsiness
- headache
- nausea
- nervousness
- numbness
- tremor
- vomiting
- weight gain

Interactions

Aripiprazole can have potentially dangerous interactions with the following drugs:

- famotidine
- valproate
- lithium
- dextromethorphan
- warfarin
- omeprazole
- lorazepam

Patients should tell their physicians all of the drugs they are currently taking to avoid interactions.

Resources

BOOKS

Mondimore, Francis Mark. *Bipolar Disorder: A Guide for Patients and Families.* 2nd ed. Baltimore: Johns Hopkins University Press, 2006.

Stahl, Stephen M. *The Prescriber's Guide: Antipsychotics and Mood Stabilizers. Stahl's Essential Psychopharmacology.* Cambridge: Cambridge University Press, 2009.

Torrey, E. Fuller. *Surviving Schizophrenia: A Manual for Families, Patients, and Providers.* 5th ed. New York: Harper Collins, 2006.

ORGANIZATIONS

American Psychiatric Association, 1000 Wilson Blvd., Ste. 1825, Arlington, VA, 22209-3901, (703) 907-7300, apa@psych.org, http://www.psych.org.

National Alliance on Mental Illness, 2107 Wilson Blvd., Ste. 300, Arlington, VA, 22201-3042, Fax: (703) 524-9094, (800) 950-6264, http://www.nami.org.

National Institute of Mental Health, 6001 Executive Blvd., Rm. 8184, MSC 9663, Bethesda, MD, 20892-9663, (301) 433-4513; TTY: (301) 443-8431, Fax: (301) 443-4279, (866) 615-6464; TTY: (866) 415-8051, nimhinfo@nih.gov, http://www.nimh.nih.gov.

Stephanie N. Watson

Aromatherapy

Definition

Aromatherapy is the therapeutic use of plant-derived, aromatic essential oils to promote physical and psychological well-being. It is sometimes used in combination with massage and other therapeutic techniques as part of a holistic treatment approach.

Purpose

One of the basic concepts of mind/body medicine is that a positive frame of mind helps to keep people in good health. Aromatherapists maintain that essential oils derived from plants help people to slow down, relax from **stress**, and enjoy the sensory experiences of massage, warm water, and pleasant smells. Aromatherapy is thought to improve a person's mental outlook and sense of well-being by affecting the limbic system via the olfactory nerve, or the sense of smell. The limbic system is the area of the **brain** that regulates emotions. Relaxing and pleasant smells stimulate emotional responses of pleasure and relaxation. From a holistic perspective, aromatherapy is a form of preventive health care. Most aromatherapists believe that aromatherapy should be used as an adjunct to mainstream medical or psychiatric care, not as a substitute.

Aromatherapy is considered to be a useful complementary treatment for the relief of **depression**, anxiety, **insomnia**, **panic disorder**, stress-related physical disorders, menstrual cramps, and some gastrointestinal complaints. A recent Scottish study found that aromatherapy has a measurably calming effect on the symptoms of **dementia** in elderly people.

Aromatherapy can be used by itself or combined with Swedish massage, shiatsu, **acupressure**, reflexology, or **light therapy** to reinforce the positive results of these treatments.

Although there are professional aromatherapists as well as practitioners of holistic medicine who offer aromatherapy among their other services, people can also use aromatherapy at home as part of self-care. There are many guides to the various techniques of aromatherapy and the proper use of essential plant oils available in inexpensive paperback editions.

Description

Origins

Aromatic plants have been employed for their healing, preservative, and pleasurable qualities throughout recorded history in both the East and West. As early as 1500 B.C., the ancient Egyptians used waters, oils, incense, resins, and ointments scented with botanicals for their religious ceremonies.

There is evidence that the Chinese may have recognized the benefits of herbal and aromatic remedies much earlier. The oldest known herbal text, Shen Nung's *Pen Ts'ao* (c. 2700-3000 B.C.) catalogs over 200 botanicals. Ayurveda, a practice of traditional Indian medicine that dates back more than 2,500 years, also used aromatic herbs for treatment.

The Romans were well known for their use of fragrances. They bathed with botanicals and integrated them into their state and religious rituals. So did the Greeks, with a growing awareness of the medicinal properties of herbs. Greek physician and surgeon Pedanios Dioscorides, whose renown herbal text *De Materia Medica* (60 A.D.) was the standard textbook for Western medicine for 1,500 years, wrote extensively on the medicinal value of botanical aromatics. The *Medica* contained detailed information on some 500 plants and 4,740 separate medicinal uses for them, including an entire section on aromatics.

Written records of herbal distillation are found as early as the first century A.D., and around 1000 A.D., the noted Arab physician and naturalist Avicenna described the distillation of rose oil from rose petals and the medicinal properties of essential oils in his writings. However, it wasn't until 1937, when French chemist René-Maurice Gattefossé published *Aromatherapie: Les Huiles essentielles, hormones végé tales*, that aromatherapie, or aromatherapy, was introduced in Europe as a medical discipline. Gattefossé, who was employed by a French perfumeur, discovered the healing properties of **lavender** oil quite by accident when he suffered a severe burn while working and used the closest available liquid, lavender oil, to soak it.

In the late 20th century, French physician Jean Valnet used botanical aromatics as a front-line treatment for wounded soldiers in World War II. He wrote about his use of essential oils and their healing and antiseptic properties in his 1964 book *Aromatherapie, traitement des maladies par les essences des plantes*, which popularized the use of essential oils for medical and psychiatric treatment throughout France. Later, French biochemist Mauguerite Maury popularized the cosmetic benefits of essential oils, and in 1977 Robert Tisserand wrote the first English-language book on the subject, *The Art of Aromatherapy*, which introduced massage as an adjunct treatment to aromatherapy and sparked its popularity in the United Kingdom.

Types of essential oils

In aromatherapy, essential oils are carefully selected for their medicinal properties. As essential oils are absorbed into the bloodstream through application to the skin or inhalation, their active components trigger certain pharmalogical effects (e.g., pain relief).

In addition to physical benefits, aromatherapy has strong psychological benefits. The volatility of an oil, or the speed at which it evaporates in open air, is thought to be linked to its specific psychological effect. As a rule of thumb, oils that evaporate quickly are considered emotionally uplifting, while slowly-evaporating oils are thought to have a calming effect.

Some essential oils used in aromatherapy for mental health issues include:

- Roman chamomile (*Chamaemelum nobilis*). An anti-inflammatory and analgesic. Useful in treating otitis media (earache), skin conditions, menstrual pains, and depression.
- Clary sage (*Salvia sclarea*). This natural astringent is not only used to treat oily hair and skin, but is also said to be useful in regulating the menstrual cycle, improving mood, and controlling high blood pressure. Clary sage should not be used by pregnant women.
- Lavender (*Lavandula officinalis*). A popular aromatherapy oil that mixes well with most essential oils, lavender has a wide range of medicinal and cosmetic applications, including treatment of insect bites, burns, respiratory infections, intestinal discomfort, nausea, migraine, insomnia, depression, and stress.
- Neroli (bitter orange), (*Citrus aurantium*). Citrus oil extracted from bitter orange flower and peel and used to treat sore throat, insomnia, and stress- and anxiety-related conditions.
- Sweet orange (*Citrus sinensis*). An essential oil used to treat stomach complaints and known for its reported ability to lift the mood while relieving stress.

Essential oils contain active agents that can have potent physical effects. While some basic aromatherapy home treatments can be self-administered, medical aromatherapy should always be performed under the guidance of an aromatherapist, herbalist, massage therapist, nurse, or physician.

INHALATION. The most basic method of administering aromatherapy is direct or indirect inhalation of essential oils. Several drops of an essential oil can be applied to a tissue or handkerchief and gently inhaled. A small amount of essential oil can also be added to a bowl of hot water and used as a steam treatment. This technique is recommended when aromatherapy is used to treat respiratory and/or skin conditions. Aromatherapy steam devices are also available commercially. A warm bath containing essential oils can have the same effect as steam aromatherapy, with the added benefit of promoting relaxation. When used in a bath, water should be lukewarm rather than hot to slow the evaporation of the oil.

Essential oil diffusers, vaporizers, and light bulb rings can be used to disperse essential oils over a large area. These devices can be particularly effective in aromatherapy that uses essential oils to promote a healthier home environment. For example, eucalyptus and tea tree oil are known for their antiseptic qualities and are frequently used to disinfect sickrooms, and citronella and geranium can be useful in repelling insects.

DIRECT APPLICATION. Because of their potency, essential oils are diluted in a carrier oil or lotion before being applied to the skin to prevent an allergic skin reaction. The carrier oil can be a vegetable or olive based one, such as wheat germ or avocado. Light oils, such as safflower, sweet almond, grapeseed, hazelnut, apricot seed, or peach kernel, may be absorbed more easily by the skin. Standard dilutions of essential oils in carrier oils range from 2%–10%. However, some oils can be used at higher concentrations, while others should be diluted further for safe and effective use. The type of carrier oil used and the therapeutic use of the application may also influence how the essential oil is mixed. Individuals should seek guidance from a healthcare professional and/or aromatherapist when diluting essential oils.

Massage is a common therapeutic technique used in conjunction with aromatherapy to both relax the body and thoroughly administer the essential oil treatment. Essential oils can also be used in hot or cold compresses and soaks to treat muscle aches and pains (e.g., lavender and ginger). As a sore throat remedy, antiseptic and soothing essential oils (e.g., tea tree and **sage**) can be thoroughly mixed with water and used as a gargle or mouthwash.

INTERNAL USE. Some essential oils can be administered internally in tincture, infusion, or suppository form to treat certain symptoms or conditions; however, this treatment should never be self-administered. Essential oils should only be taken internally under the supervision of a qualified healthcare professional.

As nonprescription botanical preparations, the essential oils used in aromatherapy are typically not paid for by health insurance. The self-administered nature of the therapy controls costs to some degree. Aromatherapy treatment sessions from a professional aromatherapist are not covered by health insurance in most cases, although aromatherapy performed in conjunction with physical therapy, nursing, therapeutic massage, or other covered medical services may be covered. Individuals should check with their insurance provider to find out about their specific coverage.

Benefits

Aromatherapy offers diverse physical and psychological benefits, depending on the essential oil or oil combination and method of application used. Some common medicinal properties of essential oils used in aromatherapy include analgesic, antimicrobial, antiseptic, anti-inflammatory, astringent, sedative, antispasmodic, expectorant, diuretic, and sedative. Essential oils are used to treat a wide range of symptoms and conditions, including—but not limited to—gastrointestinal discomfort, skin conditions, menstrual pain and irregularities, stress-related conditions, mood disorders, circulatory problems, respiratory infections, and wounds.

Precautions

Individuals should only take essential oils internally under the guidance and close supervision of a health care professional. Some oils, such as eucalyptus, wormwood, and sage, should never be taken internally. Many essential oils are highly toxic and should not be used at all in aromatherapy. These include (but are not limited to) bitter almond, pennyroyal, mustard, sassafras, rue, and mugwort.

Citrus-based essential oils, including bitter and sweet orange, lime, lemon, grapefruit, and tangerine, are phototoxic, and exposure to direct sunlight should be avoided for at least four hours after their application.

Other essential oils, such as cinnamon leaf, black pepper, juniper, lemon, white camphor, eucalyptus blue gum, ginger, peppermint, pine needle, and thyme can be extremely irritating to the skin if applied in high enough concentration or without a carrier oil or lotion. Caution should always be exercised when applying essential oils topically. Individuals should never apply undiluted essential oils to the skin unless directed to do so by a trained healthcare professional and/or aromatherapist.

Individuals taking homeopathic remedies should avoid black pepper, camphor, eucalyptus, and peppermint essential oils. These oils may act as a remedy antidote to the homeopathic treatment.

KEY TERMS

Antiseptic—Inhibits the growth of microorganisms.

Bactericidal—An agent that destroys bacteria (e.g., *Staphylococci aureus, Streptococci pneumoniae, Escherichia coli, Salmonella enteritidis*).

Carrier oil—An oil used to dilute essential oils for use in massage and other skin care applications.

Contact dermatitis—Skin irritation as a result of contact with a foreign substance.

Enfleurage—A technique for extracting essential oils from flower petals by placing them on a layer of purified fat.

Essential oil—A volatile oil extracted from the leaves, fruit, flowers, roots, or other components of a plant and used in aromatherapy, perfumes, and foods and beverages.

Holistic—A practice of medicine that focuses on the whole patient, addressing the patient's social, emotional, and spiritual needs along with their physical treatment.

Limbic system—A group of structures in the brain that includes the amygdala, hippocampus, olfactory bulbs, and hypothalamus. The limbic system is associated with homeostasis and the regulation and arousal of emotions.

Maceration—A technique for extracting essential oils from plant leaves and stems by crushing the plant parts and soaking them in warm vegetable oil.

Olfactory nerve—The cranial nerve that regulates the sense of smell.

Phototoxic—Causes a harmful skin reaction when exposed to sunlight.

Remedy antidote—Certain foods, beverages, prescription medications, aromatic compounds, and other environmental elements that counteract the efficacy of homeopathic remedies.

Steam distillation—A process of extracting essential oils from plant products through a heating and evaporation process.

Volatile—Something that vaporizes or evaporates quickly when exposed to air.

Children should only receive aromatherapy treatment under the guidance of a trained aromatherapist or healthcare professional. Some essential oils may not be appropriate for treating children or may require additional dilution before use on children.

Certain essential oils should not be used by pregnant or nursing women or by people with specific illnesses or physical conditions. Individuals suffering from any chronic or acute health condition should inform their healthcare provider before starting treatment with any essential oil.

Asthmatic individuals should not use steam inhalation for aromatherapy, as it can aggravate their condition.

Essential oils are flammable, and should be kept away from heat sources.

Consumers should use caution when purchasing essential oils, as bargain oils are often adulterated, diluted, or synthetic. Pure essential oils can be expensive, and the cost of an oil will vary depending on its quality and availability.

QUESTIONS TO ASK YOUR DOCTOR

- In what way do you think aromatherapy will benefit me?
- What essential oils do you recommend?
- Will aromatherapy interact with my current medications?

Preparations

The method of extracting an essential oil varies by plant type. Common methods include water or steam distillation and cold pressing. Quality essential oils should be unadulterated and extracted from pure botanicals. Many aromatherapy oils on the market are synthetic and/or diluted, contain solvents, or are extracted from botanicals grown with pesticides or herbicides. To ensure best results, essential oils should be made from pure organic botanicals and labeled by their full botanical name. Oils should always be stored in dark bottles out of direct light.

Before using essential oils on the skin, individuals should perform a skin patch test by applying a small amount of the diluted oil behind the wrist and covering it with a bandage or cloth for up to 12 hours. If redness or irritation occurs, the oil should be diluted further and a second skin test performed, or it should be avoided altogether. Individuals should never apply undiluted essential oils to the skin unless advised to do so by a trained healthcare professional.

Risks

Side effects may occur and vary by the type of essential oil used. Citrus-based essential oils can cause heightened sensitivity to sunlight. Essential oils may also cause contact dermatitis, an allergic reaction characterized by redness and irritation. Anyone experiencing an allergic reaction to an essential oil should discontinue its use and contact their healthcare professional for further guidance. Individuals should do a small skin patch test with new essential oils before using them extensively.

Research & general acceptance

The antiseptic and bactericidal qualities of some essential oils (such as tea tree and peppermint) and their value in fighting infection has been detailed extensively in both ancient and modern medical literature.

Recent research in mainstream medical literature has also shown that aromatherapy has a positive psychological impact on patients. Several clinical studies involving both post-operative and chronically ill subjects showed that massage with essential oils can be helpful in improving emotional well-being and promoting the healing process.

Today, the use of holistic aromatherapy is widely accepted in Europe, particularly in Great Britain, where it is commonly used in conjunction with massage as both a psychological and physiological healing tool. In the United States, where aromatherapy is often misunderstood as solely a cosmetic treatment, the mainstream medical community has been slower to accept its use.

Training & certification

Certification or licensing is currently not required to become an aromatherapist in the United States; however, many states require that healthcare professionals who practice the "hands-on" therapies used in conjunction with aromatherapy (e.g., massage) to be licensed. There are state-licensed educational institutions that offer certificates and/or diplomas in aromatherapy training. Individuals interested in aromatherapy treatment from a professional aromatherapist may be able to obtain a referral from one of these institutions, or from their current healthcare provider.

Resources

BOOKS

Schiller, Carol, and David Schiller. *The Aromatherapy Encyclopedia: A Concise Guide to over 385 Plant Oils.* Laguna Beach, CA: Basic Health Publications, 2008.

PERIODICALS

van der Watt, G., and A. Janca. "Aromatherapy in Nursing and Mental Health Care." *Contemporary Nurse: A Journal for the Australian Nursing Profession* 30, no. 1 (2008): 69–75.

Yim, V. W., et al. "A Review on the Effects of Aromatherapy for Patients with Depressive Symptoms." *Journal of Alternative and Complementary Medicine* 15, no. 2 (2009): 187–95.

WEBSITES

National Institute of Complementary and Alternative Medicine. "Aromatherapy." National Institutes of Health. http://nccam.nih.gov/health/aromatherapy (accessed December 14, 2011).

ORGANIZATIONS

National Association of Holistic Aromatherapy, PO Box 1868, Banner Elk, NC, 28604, (828) 898-6161, Fax: (828) 898-1965, info@naha.org, http://www.naha.org.

Paula Ford-Martin
Laura Jean Cataldo, RN, Ed.D.

Artane *see* **Trihexyphenidyl**

Art therapy

Definition

Art therapy, sometimes called creative arts therapy or expressive arts therapy, encourages people to express and understand emotions through artistic outlets and the creative process.

Purpose

Art therapy provides participants with critical insight into their emotions, thoughts, and feelings. Key goals of the art therapy process include:

- Self-discovery—at its most successful, art therapy triggers an emotional catharsis, providing an outlet for otherwise internalized thoughts and feelings.
- Personal fulfillment—the creation of a tangible reward can build confidence and nurture feelings of self-worth. Personal fulfillment comes from both the creative and the analytical components of the artistic process.
- Empowerment—art therapy can help people visually express emotions and fears that they cannot express through conventional means, giving them some sense of control over these feelings.
- Relaxation and stress relief—chronic stress can be harmful to both mind and body. Stress can weaken and damage the immune system, cause insomnia and depression, and trigger circulatory problems (like high blood pressure and irregular heartbeat). When used alone or in combination with other relaxation techniques, such as guided imagery, art therapy can help relieve stress.
- Symptom relief and physical rehabilitation—art therapy can also help patients cope with pain. The therapy can promote physiological healing when patients identify and work through anger, resentment, and other emotional stressors. It is often prescribed to accompany pain control therapy for chronically and terminally ill patients.

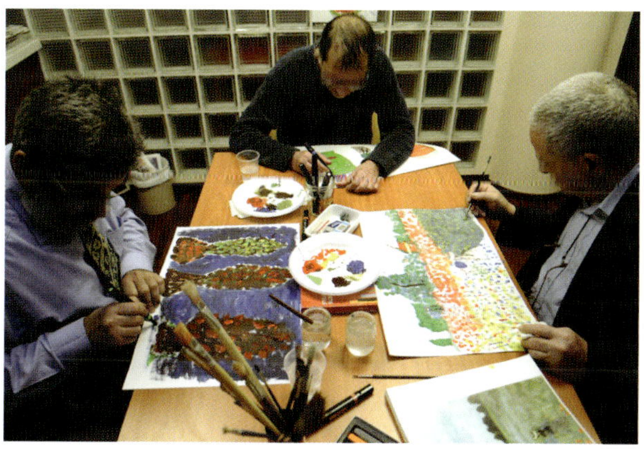

Three men participate in an art therapy session at a center for patients with Alzheimer's disease. *(© Durand Florence/ SIPA/newscom)*

Description

Art therapy, sometimes called expressive art or art psychology, encourages self-discovery and emotional growth. It is a two-part process, involving both the creation of art and the discovery of its meaning. Rooted in Sigmund Freud's and Carl Jung's theories of the subconscious and unconscious, art therapy is based on the assumption that visual symbols and images are the most accessible and natural form of communication to the human experience. Patients are encouraged to visualize and then create the thoughts and emotions that they cannot talk about. The resulting artwork is then reviewed and interpreted by the patient.

The "analysis" of the artwork produced in art therapy typically allows patients to gain some level of insight into their feelings and lets them work through these issues in a constructive manner. Art therapy is typically practiced with individual, group, or family **psychotherapy** (**talk therapy**). While a therapist may provide critical guidance for these activities, a key feature of effective art therapy is that the patient/artist, not the therapist, directs the interpretation of the artwork.

Origins

Humans have expressed themselves with symbols throughout history. Masks, ritual pottery, costumes, objects used in rituals, cave drawings, Egyptian hieroglyphics, and Celtic art and symbols are all visual records of self-expression and communication through art. Art has also been associated with spiritual power, and

KEY TERMS

Catharsis—Therapeutic discharge of emotional tension after recalling past events.

Mandala—A design, usually circular, that appears in religion and art. In Buddhism and Hinduism, the mandala has religious ritual purposes and serves as a yantra (a geometric emblem or instrument of contemplation).

Organic illness—A physically, biologically based illness.

artistic forms such as the Hindu and Buddhist mandala and Native American sand painting are considered powerful healing tools.

In the late nineteenth century, French psychiatrists Ambrose Tardieu and Paul-Max Simon both published studies on the similar characteristics of and symbolism in the artwork of the mentally ill. Tardieu and Simon viewed art therapy as an effective diagnostic tool to identify specific types of mental illness or traumatic events. Later, psychologists would use this diagnostic aspect to develop psychological drawing tests (e.g., the Draw-A-Man test, the Draw-A-Person Questionnaire [DAP.Q]) and projective personality tests involving visual symbol recognition (e.g., the **Rorschach inkblot test**, the **Thematic Apperception Test** [TAT], the Holtzman Inkblot Test [HIT]).

The growing popularity of milieu therapies at psychiatric institutions in the twentieth century was an important factor in the development of art therapy in the United States. Milieu therapies (or environmental therapies) focus on putting the patient in a controlled therapeutic social setting that provides the patient with opportunities to gain self-confidence and interact with peers in a positive way. Activities that encourage self-discovery and empowerment, such as art, music, dance, and writing, are important components of this approach.

Educator and therapist Margaret Naumburg was a follower of Freud and Jung and incorporated art into psychotherapy as a means for her patients to visualize and recognize the unconscious. She founded the Walden School in 1915, where she used students' artworks in psychological counseling. She published extensively on the subject and taught seminars on the technique at New York University in the 1950s. Today, she is considered the founder of art therapy in the United States.

In the 1930s, Karl, William, and Charles Menninger introduced an art therapy program at their Kansas-based psychiatric hospital, the Menninger Clinic. The Menninger Clinic employed a number of artists in residence in the following years, and the facility was also considered a leader in the art therapy movement through the 1950s and '60s. Other noted art therapy pioneers who emerged in the '50s and '60s included Edith Kramer, Hanna Yaxa Kwiatkowska (**National Institute of Mental Health**), and Janie Rhyne.

Art therapy has traditionally centered on visual mediums, like paintings, sculptures, and drawings. Some mental healthcare providers have now broadened the definition to include music, film, dance, writing, and other types of artistic expression.

Benefits

Art therapy can be a particularly useful treatment tool for children, who frequently have limited language skills. By drawing or using other visual means to express troublesome feelings, younger patients can begin to address these issues, even if they cannot identify or label these emotions with words. Art therapy is also valuable for adolescents and adults who are unable or unwilling to talk about thoughts and feelings.

Beyond its use in mental health treatment, art therapy is also used with traditional medicine to treat organic diseases and conditions. The connection between mental and physical health is well documented, and art therapy can promote healing by relieving **stress** and allowing the patient to develop coping skills.

Art therapy is often one part of a psychiatric inpatient or outpatient treatment program, and can take place in individual or **group therapy** sessions. Group art therapy sessions often take place in hospital, clinic, shelter, and community program settings. These group therapy sessions can have the added benefits of positive social interaction, empathy, and support from peers, which helps the artist learn that others share similar concerns and issues.

Precautions

Art materials and techniques should match the age and ability of the client. People with impairments, such as **traumatic brain injury** or a neurological condition, may have difficulties with the self-discovery portion of the art therapy process, depending on their level of functioning. However, they may still benefit from the sensory stimulation provided by art therapy and the pleasure they derive from artistic creation.

While art is accessible to all (with or without a therapist to guide the process), it may be difficult to tap the full potential of the interpretive component of art therapy without a therapist to guide the process. When art therapy is chosen as a therapeutic tool to cope with a physical condition, it should be treated as a supplemental therapy and not as a substitute for conventional medical treatments.

Preparation

Before starting art therapy, the therapist may have an introductory session with the client to discuss art therapy techniques and to give the client the opportunity to ask questions about the process. The client's comfort with the artistic process is critical to successful art therapy. The therapist will ensure that appropriate materials and space are available for the client, as well as an adequate amount of time for the session. If a person is exploring art as therapy without the guidance of a trained therapist, adequate materials, space, and time are still important factors in a successful creative experience.

The supplies used in art therapy are limited only by the artist's (and/or therapist's) imagination. Some of the materials often used include paper, canvas, poster board, assorted paints, inks, markers, pencils, charcoals, chalks, fabrics, string, adhesives, clay, wood, glazes, wire, bendable metals, and natural items (like shells, leaves, etc.). Providing artists with a variety of materials in assorted colors and textures can enhance their interest in the process and may result in a richer, more diverse exploration of their emotions in the resulting artwork. Appropriate tools such as scissors, brushes, erasers, easels, supply trays, glue guns, smocks or aprons, and cleaning materials are also essential.

An appropriate workspace should be available for the creation of art. Ideally, this should be a bright, quiet, comfortable place, with large tables, counters, or other suitable surfaces. The space can be as simple as a kitchen or office table, or as fancy as a specialized artist's studio.

The artist should have adequate time to become comfortable with and explore the creative process. This is especially true for people who do not consider themselves "artists" and who may be uncomfortable with the concept. If performed in a therapy group or one-on-one session, the art therapist should be available to answer general questions about materials and/or the creative process. However, the therapist should be careful not to influence the creation or interpretation of the work.

Research and general acceptance

A wide body of literature supports the use of art therapy in a mental health capacity. In mainstream medicine, as the mind-body connection between psychological well-being and physical health is further documented by studies in the field, art therapy continues to gain greater acceptance as a therapeutic technique for organic illness.

QUESTIONS TO ASK YOUR DOCTOR

- Do I have to be artistic to participate in art therapy?
- What are the benefits of art therapy over group therapy or counseling?
- How long will I need to participate in art therapy before I begin to see results?

Resources

BOOKS

Soneff, Sharon. *Art Journals and Creative Healing: Restoring the Spirit Through Self-Expression.* Minneapolis, MN: Quarry Books, 2008.

ORGANIZATIONS

American Art Therapy Association, 225 North Fairfax Street, Alexandria, VA, 22314, info@arttherapy.org, http://www.americanarttherapyassociation.org.

Paula Anne Ford-Martin

Asenapine

Definition

Asenapine, sold under the brand name Saphris, belongs to a class of drugs known as atypical antipsychotics, which are used to treat psychiatric disorders such as **schizophrenia**. Atypical antipsychotics work by altering the levels of the **neurotransmitters serotonin** and **dopamine**, which are involved in normal **brain** function and can affect the physiological states of **psychosis** and mania. Asenapine acts to inhibit the effects of serotonin and dopamine within the brain.

Purpose

Asenapine is an antipsychotic medication used in the treatment of schizophrenia and **bipolar disorder**. For schizophrenia, asenapine may be used to treat specific episodes or as maintenance therapy. In bipolar disorder, it may be used alone or in combination with mood stabilizer drugs, but it is not usually the first choice of medication.

Description

Asenapine works by antagonizing, or blocking, the signaling of neurotransmitters in the brain by binding their corresponding neurotransmitter receptors. Since the pathology of schizophrenia involves the overactivity of neurotransmitter signaling in some areas of the brain and underactivity in others, antipsychotics such as asenapine do not completely treat the disorder. The symptoms of schizophrenia known as **positive symptoms**, such as psychosis, are best treated with asenapine. The negative and cognitive symptoms such as withdrawal and difficulty reasoning are not as well addressed with asenapine. Similarly, the mania of bipolar disorder is better treated with asenapine than the **depression**.

Recommended dosage

Asenapine is taken as a tablet and is available in both flavored and unflavored preparations. The tablets are not crushed or chewed but are placed under the tongue to dissolve and enter the bloodstream. The available dosage forms are 5 mg and 10 mg. When used during an acute episode of schizophrenia, the 5 mg dose is taken twice a day. For maintenance in schizophrenia, the dose may be increased to 10 mg twice a day after at least a week on the 5 mg dose. When asenapine is used for bipolar disorder, the 10 mg dose is used twice a day as tolerated. If side effects develop or if other drugs are used in combination, the dose may be decreased to 5 mg twice a day. Side effects impacting the immune system may make a lower dose or discontinuation of the drug necessary. Persons with some types of severe liver disease may require dosage modifications.

Precautions

Atypical antipsychotics were developed for the purpose of avoiding some of the side effects often seen with older, conventional antipsychotic medications, such as **medication-induced movement disorders**. The atypical drugs do cause far fewer **movement disorders** than traditional medications but still have the potential to produce some disturbing movement-related effects. Patients taking asenapine must be monitored for the development of movement disorders as well as **neuroleptic malignant syndrome**, a dangerous reaction characterized by stiffness, mental status changes, and increased body temperature. However, asenapine is less likely to cause these disorders than many other types of antipsychotic medications.

Patients taking asenapine must have their immune system function monitored via periodic blood tests, as the drug can cause dangerous decreases in white blood cells. High blood sugar may also develop, especially in patients at risk for diabetes. Blood sugar is measured before initiating asenapine dosing and then monitored periodically. Asenapine carries a risk of low blood pressure and possible temporary loss of consciousness, especially in older or dehydrated patients rising quickly from a lying down position. Asenapine may also alter heart rhythm, potentially producing fatal arrhythmias.

Asenapine may not be appropriate for use or may require caution in patients with **dementia**, some heart abnormalities or disease, liver dysfunction, history of **stroke** or seizure, diabetes, immune dysfunction, patients who are dehydrated, and the elderly. Asenapine should not be used by women who are pregnant or trying to become pregnant, as some infants born to mothers who used asenapine during pregnancy exhibited withdrawal symptoms and muscle tremors. Because the safety of asenapine during breastfeeding is unknown, its use is not recommended.

In June 2008, the FDA announced a requirement for manufacturers of asenapine (and other antipsychotic drugs) to issue a warning label regarding the adverse effects of using antipsychotic drugs to treat behavioral problems in older individuals with dementia-related psychosis, including death. Studies showed that older adults with dementia taking antipsychotics such as asenapine were at increased risk of having a stroke or mini-stroke during treatment and, in some cases, of dying during treatment, though the reason for the finding was unclear. The use of asenapine in treating older adults with dementia-related psychosis is not approved by the FDA.

Side effects

Atypical antipsychotics such as asenapine are known for having fewer side effects than other types of older antipsychotic medications that act on neurotransmitter receptors in different parts of the brain. This is one reason why as a general class they tend to be the drug of choice in the treatment of schizophrenia. However, as with all medication, antipsychotics such as asenapine do have side effects. Sensitivity to asenapine varies among patients, and some patients may find that lower doses are more than their body system can tolerate. Common side effects of asenapine include dizziness, dry mouth, abdominal pain, increases

KEY TERMS

Bipolar disorder—A mood disorder marked by alternating episodes of extremely low mood (depression) and exuberant highs (mania).

Cognitive—Associated with thinking, learning, perception, awareness, and judgment.

Dopamine—A type of neurotransmitter involved in regulation of concentration, impulse control, judgment, mood, attention span, psychostimulation, disease states such as addiction, and depression.

Insomnia—Disorder involving disturbance of sleep.

Mania—Physiological state of hyperactivity experienced by patients with certain psychiatric illnesses involving inappropriate elevated mood, pressured speech, poor judgment, and sometimes psychotic episodes superimposed on the state of mania.

Negative symptoms—Symptoms of schizophrenia characterized by the absence or elimination of certain behaviors, such as initiative, speech, or affect.

Neuroleptic malignant syndrome—Dangerous reaction to antipsychotic medications that involves temperature instability, muscular rigidity, and altered mental status.

Neurotransmitter—One of a group of chemicals secreted by a nerve cell (neuron) to carry a chemical message to another nerve cell, often as a way of transmitting a nerve impulse. Examples of neurotransmitters include acetylcholine, dopamine, serotonin, and norepinephrine.

Neurotransmitter receptor—A physical recipient for chemicals called neurotransmitters. Receptors sit on the surface of cells that make up body tissues, and once bound to the neurotransmitter, they initiate the chemical signaling pathway associated with neurotransmitters.

Positive symptoms—Symptoms that are characterized by the production or presence of abnormal or excessive behaviors, including hallucinations and thought-process disorder.

Psychosis—A serious mental disorder characterized by defective or lost contact with reality, often with hallucinations or delusions.

Schizophrenia—A severe mental illness in which a person has difficulty distinguishing what is real from what is not real. It is often characterized by hallucinations, delusions, and withdrawal from people and social activities.

Serotonin—A type of neurotransmitter involved in regulation of the blood vessels, brain processes, and disease states such as depression.

in appetite, weight gain, **fatigue**, **insomnia**, irritability, anxiety, depression, joint pain, toothache, restless leg syndrome, reduced sense of touch, and alterations in liver enzymes. Antipsychotics such as asenapine that block dopamine receptors may cause an increase in prolactin, the hormone that causes lactation in women and impotence in men. Low blood pressure or a drop in blood pressure upon standing may result in loss of consciousness. Rare but serious potential side effects include severe movement disorders, high blood sugar or overt diabetes, stroke, severe difficulty swallowing, dangerous changes in heart rhythm, **seizures**, and changes in blood cells, including anemia and decreased immune function.

Interactions

Patients should make their doctor aware of all medications and supplements they are taking before using asenapine. Using alcohol while taking asenapine may create toxic reactions in the body and should be avoided. Drugs that affect the liver may alter the metabolism of asenapine, resulting in too much or too little of the drug in body. This could lead to increased side effects or even toxic doses. Likewise, asenapine may affect the metabolism of other drugs, leading to greater or lower doses than therapeutically desired.

Use of asenapine in combination with a number of other drugs may adversely affect heart rhythm; such drugs include the heart medications dronedarone and amiodarone, the chemotherapeutic toremifene, the antibiotics azithromycin and ciprofloxacin, the antifungal fluconazole, the antinausea drug ondansetron, and other antipsychotics such as **pimozide**. Using asenapine with certain blood pressure medications, such as enalapril and metoprolol, may cause dangerously low blood pressure. **Sedatives** such as codeine and herbal supplements such as calendula, capsicum, kava, and lemon balm may cause severe sedation in patients using asenapine. The herbal supplement chasteberry decreases the effectiveness of asenapine.

QUESTIONS TO ASK YOUR DOCTOR

- Should I eat before taking this medication?
- Will this medication interact with any of my other prescription medications?
- Are there any over-the-counter medications I should not take with this medicine?
- Will this medicine interact with any of my herbal supplements?
- What side effects should I watch for while taking this medication?
- Can I drink alcoholic beverages in the same time frame as taking this medication?
- Can I stop taking the medication right away or do I need to stop slowly?

Resources

BOOKS

Brunton, Laurence L., et al. *Goodman and Gilman's The Pharmacological Basis of Therapeutics*. 12th ed. New York: McGraw Hill Medical, 2011.

Stargrove, Mitchell Bebel, et al. *Herb, Nutrient, and Drug Interactions: Clinical Implications and Therapeutic Strategies*. St. Louis: Mosby, 2007.

PERIODICALS

Citrome, L. "A Systematic Review of Meta-Analyses of the Efficacy of Oral Atypical Antipsychotics for the Treatment of Adult Patients with Schizophrenia." *Expert Opinion of Pharmacotherapy* (October 17, 2011) [e-pub ahead of print]. http://dx.doi.org/10.1517/14656566.2011.626769 (accessed November 3, 2011).

Gonzalez, J. M., P. M. Thompson, and T. A. Moore. "Review of the Safety, Efficacy, and Side Effect Profile of Asenapine in the Treatment of Bipolar 1 Disorder." *Patient Preference and Adherence* 5 (2011): 333–41. http://dx.doi.org/10.2147/PPA.S10968 (accessed November 3, 2011).

ORGANIZATIONS

American College of Neuropsychopharmacology, 5034-A Thoroughbred Lane, Brentwood, TN, 37027, (615) 324-2360, Fax: (615) 523-1715, acnp@acnp.org, http://www.acnp.org/default.aspx.

American Society for Clinical Pharmacology and Therapeutics, 528 N Washington St., Alexandria, VA, 22314, (703) 836-6981, info@ascpt.org, http://www.ascpt.org.

National Institute of Mental Health, 6001 Executive Blvd., Rm. 8184, MSC 9663, Bethesda, MD, 20892-9663, (301) 443-4513; TTY: (301) 443-8431, Fax: (301) 443-4279, (866) 615-6464; TTY: (866) 415-8051, nimhinfo@nih.gov, http://www.nimh.nih.gov.

U.S. Food and Drug Administration, 10903 New Hampshire Ave., Silver Spring, MD, 20993-0002, (888) INFO-FDA (463-6332), http://www.fda.gov.

Maria Eve Basile, PhD

Asendin *see* **Amoxapine**

Asperger syndrome

Definition

Asperger syndrome (AS), which is also called Asperger disorder or autistic psychopathy, belongs to a group of childhood disorders known as **pervasive developmental disorders** (PDDs) or autistic spectrum disorders. AS was first described by Hans Asperger, an Austrian **psychiatrist**, in 1944. Asperger's work was unavailable in English before the mid-1970s; as a result, AS was often unrecognized in English-speaking countries until the late 1980s. Before the fourth edition of the American Psychiatric Association's ***Diagnostic and Statistical Manual of Mental Disorders*** (*DSM-IV*, 1994), there was no official definition of AS.

Demographics

According to the National Institute of Neurological Disorders and Stroke (NINDS), the rate of occurrence of AS is not well established. Estimates range from two out of every 10,000 children to one out of every 300, with boys affected up to four times more frequently than girls. Further research is required to obtain precise AS prevalence data. In addition, little research has been done on the populations of developing countries, and no information is available about the incidence of the disorder in different racial or ethnic groups.

Description

Children with AS learn to talk at the usual age and often have above-average verbal skills. They have normal or above-normal intelligence and the ability to take care of themselves. The distinguishing features of AS are problems with social interaction, particularly reciprocating and empathizing with the feelings of others; difficulties with nonverbal communication (e.g., facial expressions); peculiar speech habits that include repeated words or phrases and a flat, emotionless vocal tone; an apparent lack of "common sense"; a fascination with obscure or limited subjects (e.g., doorknobs, railroad schedules, astronomical data, etc.), often to the exclusion of other interests; clumsy and awkward physical movements; and

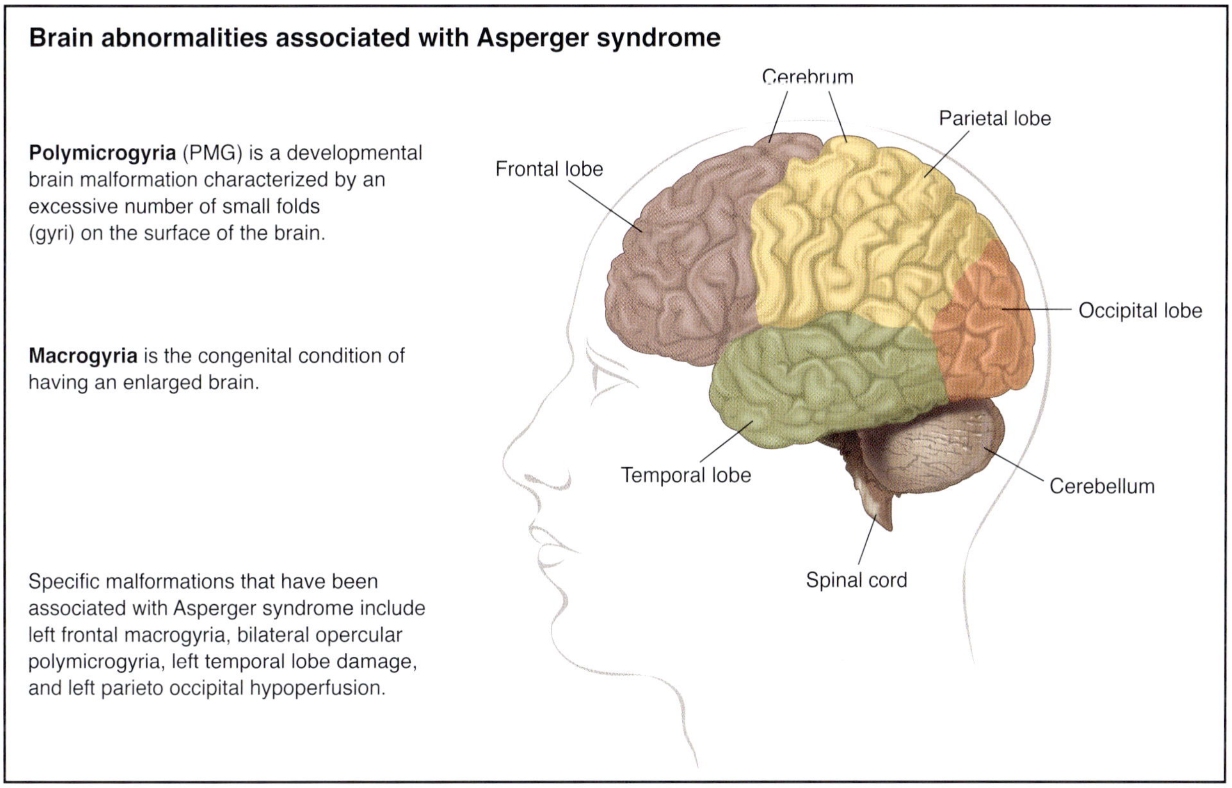

Possible brain malformations associated with Asperger syndrome. *(Illustration by Electronic Illustrators Group. Reproduced by permission of Gale, a part of Cengage Learning.)*

odd or eccentric behaviors, such as hand wringing or finger flapping, swaying or other repetitious whole-body movements, or watching spinning objects for long periods of time.

Risk factors

There is some indication that AS runs in families, particularly in families with histories of **depression** and **bipolar disorder**. Asperger noted that his initial group of patients had fathers with AS symptoms. Knowledge of the genetic profile as a risk factor continues to be limited.

Causes and symptoms

Asperger syndrome seems to run in families. **Imaging studies** have revealed differences in the structure and function of **brain** tissue. These changes appear to occur during embryonic brain development. As with **autism**, associations have been made between Asperger syndrome and a number of genes, many of which direct the formation of brain tissue and the communication between brain cells. A variety of environmental causes have also been postulated as causing Asperger syndrome, including advanced parental age, pesticides, and exposure to **valproic acid** (a seizure medication), though none of these have been proven. As with autism, although there has been popular uproar regarding a possible association between immunizations and the disorder, this association has been disproved. The research article that put forward this hypothesis has been publicly discredited, and a retraction has been printed.

In young children, the symptoms of AS typically include problems picking up social cues and understanding the basics of interacting with other children. These children may want friendships but find themselves unable to make friends. Most children with Asperger are diagnosed during the elementary school years, because the symptoms of the disorder become more apparent at this point. They include:

- poor pragmatic language skills, such as using incorrect tone or volume of voice for specific contexts or failing to understand the appropriate uses of humorous or slang expressions within social contexts
- problems with hand-eye coordination and other visual skills
- problems making eye contact with others
- learning difficulties, which may range from mild to severe
- tendency to become absorbed in a particular topic and not know when others are bored with the conversation

KEY TERMS

Autistic psychopathy—Hans Asperger's original name for Asperger syndrome. It is still used occasionally as a synonym for the disorder.

Gillberg's criteria—A six-item checklist for Asperger syndrome developed by Christopher Gillberg, a Swedish researcher. It is widely used as a diagnostic tool.

High-functioning autism (HFA)—A subcategory of autistic disorder consisting of children diagnosed with IQs of 70 or higher.

Nonverbal learning disability (NLD)—A learning disability syndrome identified in 1989 that may overlap with some of the symptoms of Asperger syndrome.

Pervasive developmental disorder (PDD)—Used by the American Psychiatric Association for individuals who meet some but not all of the criteria for autism.

- repetitive behaviors, such as counting a group of coins or marbles over and over, reciting the same song or poem several times, or buttoning and unbuttoning a jacket repeatedly

Adolescence is one of the most painful periods for young people with Asperger because social interactions are more complex in this age group and require more subtle social skills. Some boys with AS become frustrated while trying to relate to their peers and may become aggressive. Both boys and girls with the disorder are often quite naive for their age and easily manipulated by "street-wise" classmates. They are also more vulnerable than most youngsters to peer pressure.

Less research has been done regarding adults with AS. Some have serious difficulties with social and occupational functioning, but others are able to finish their schooling, join the workforce, and marry and have families.

Diagnosis

As of 2011, there were no blood tests or brain scans that could be used to diagnose AS. Until *DSM-IV* (1994), there was no "official" list of symptoms for the disorder, which made its **diagnosis** both difficult and inexact. Although most children with AS are diagnosed between five and nine years of age, many are not diagnosed until adulthood. Misdiagnoses are common; AS has been confused with such other neurological disorders as **Tourette syndrome** or with **attention deficit hyperactivity disorder (ADHD)**, **oppositional defiant disorder** (ODD), or **obsessive-compulsive disorder** (OCD). Some researchers think that AS overlaps some types of learning disability, such as the nonverbal learning disability (NLD) syndrome identified in 1989.

The inclusion of AS as a separate diagnostic category in *DSM-IV* was justified on the basis of a large international field trial of over one thousand children and adolescents. Nevertheless, the diagnosis of AS is also complicated by confusion with such other diagnostic categories as high-functioning (IQ 70) autism (HFA), and schizoid personality disorder of childhood. With regard to the latter, AS is not an unchanging set of personality traits but has a developmental dimension. AS is distinguished from HFA by the following characteristics:

- later onset of symptoms (usually around three years of age)
- early development of grammatical speech; the AS child's verbal IQ is usually higher than performance IQ (the reverse being the case in children with autism)
- less severe deficiencies in social and communication skills
- presence of intense interest in one or two topics
- physical clumsiness and lack of coordination
- family history of the disorder
- lower frequency of neurological disorders
- more positive outcome in later life

DSM-IV criteria for Asperger syndrome

DSM-IV specifies six diagnostic criteria for AS:

- The child's social interactions are impaired in at least two of the following ways: markedly limited use of nonverbal communication; lack of age-appropriate peer relationships; failure to share enjoyment, interests, or accomplishment with others; lack of reciprocity in social interactions.
- The child's behavior, interests, and activities are characterized by repetitive or rigid patterns, such as an abnormal preoccupation with one or two topics, or with parts of objects; repetitive physical movements; or rigid insistence on certain routines and rituals.
- The child's social, occupational, or educational functioning is significantly impaired.
- The child has normal age-appropriate language skills.
- The child has normal age-appropriate cognitive skills, self-help abilities, and curiosity about the environment.
- The child does not meet criteria for another specific PDD or schizophrenia.

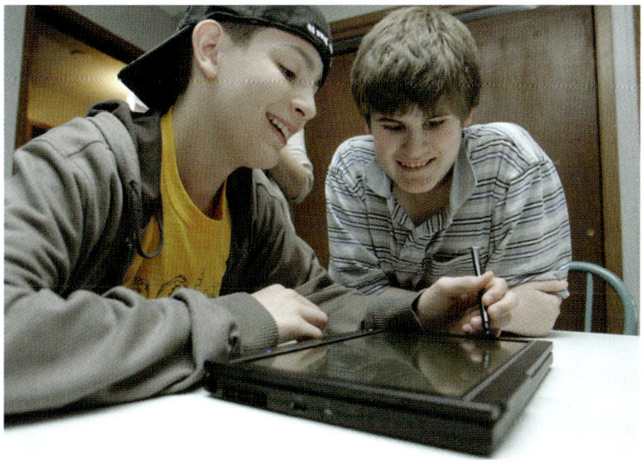

Two 14-year-old boys with Asperger syndrome attend an afterschool program for children with the disorder. *(© AP Images/Julie Koehn)*

Other diagnostic scales and checklists

Other instruments that have been used to identify children with AS include Gillberg's criteria, a six-item list compiled by a Swedish researcher that specifies problems in social interaction, a preoccupying narrow interest, forcing routines and interests on the self or others, speech and language problems, nonverbal communication problems, and physical clumsiness; and the Australian Scale for Asperger Syndrome, a detailed multi-item questionnaire developed in 1996.

Brain imaging findings

As of 2011, only a few structural abnormalities of the brain had been linked to AS. Findings include abnormally large folds in the brain tissue in the left frontal region, abnormally small folds in the operculum (a lid-like structure composed of portions of three adjoining brain lobes), and damage to the left temporal lobe. The first single photon emission tomography (SPECT) study of a patient with AS found a lower than normal blood supply in the left parietal area of the brain. Brain imaging studies on a larger sample of patients is the next stage of research.

Diagnostic coding changes in DSM-5

The diagnosis of Asperger syndrome has been complicated by its close relationship to the symptoms found in people with autistic disorders. As a result, researchers have had a great deal of difficulty determining prevalence and incidence statistics for Asperger syndrome, and clinicians have had difficulty accessing services for their patients. After re-evaluating the diagnostic criteria for AS, autism, and other related disorders, the panel charged with creating the fifth edition of the *DSM* (*DSM-5*), due out in May 2013, is expected to combine the diagnoses of Asperger syndrome, autism, **childhood disintegrative disorder**, and pervasive developmental disorder under the rubric of autism spectrum disorders. This change in the diagnostic coding has led to some controversy and will also lead to changes in the prevalence and incidence statistics for all of the affected disorders. The new categorization, however, may have the advantage of improved diagnostic consistency, with accompanying improvement in accessibility of services.

Treatment

There is no cure for AS and no single prescribed regimen for all affected patients. Specific treatments are based on the individual's symptom pattern.

Traditional

Individuals with Asperger syndrome often benefit from **psychotherapy**, particularly during adolescence, in order to help them cope with depression and other painful feelings related to their social difficulties. Treatment aims to help patients manage the major issues associated with the condition: lack of communication skills, obsessive routines, and physical clumsiness.

Therapists who are experienced in treating children with AS have found that the child should be allowed to proceed slowly in forming an emotional bond with the therapist. Too much emotional intensity at the beginning may be more than the child can handle. Behavioral approaches seem to work best with these children. **Play therapy** can be helpful in teaching the child to recognize social cues as well as lowering the level of emotional tension.

Communication and **social skills training** groups are also often used to help children with Asperger syndrome learn and then practice skills that may benefit them in the classroom, within their families, and in their efforts to connect to their peers.

Adults with AS are most likely to benefit from individual therapy using a cognitive behavioral approach, although many also attend **group therapy**. Some adults have been helped by working with speech therapists on their pragmatic language skills. A relatively new approach called behavioral coaching has been used to help adults with AS learn to organize and set priorities for their daily activities.

Drugs

The drugs that are recommended most often for children with AS are psychostimulants (**methylphenidate**,

pemoline), **clonidine**, or one of the tricyclic **antidepressants** (TCAs) for hyperactivity or inattention; **beta blockers**, neuroleptics, or lithium for anger, aggression, agitation, and irritability; **selective serotonin reuptake inhibitors (SSRIs)** or TCAs for rituals, repetitive behavior, depression, and preoccupations; and **SSRIs** or TCAs for anxiety and OCD-like symptoms. Low-dose **naltrexone** (a drug usually used to help alcoholics avoid drinking) has been shown to be useful in decreasing ritualistic, repetitive behaviors in people with Asperger syndrome. One alternative herbal remedy that has been tried with AS patients is **St. John's wort**.

Clinical trials

In 2011, 25 **clinical trials** for the treatment of Asperger syndrome were being sponsored by the National Institutes of Health (NIH) and other agencies.

One study (trial no. NCT00464477) was recruiting parents of children with a pervasive developmental disorder (including autism, autistic spectrum disorder, PDD-NOS, Asperger syndrome, childhood disintegrative disorder, and **Rett syndrome**) to participate in a study seeking to determine potential causes of these disorders. Other trials were evaluating drugs for treatment. For example, N-acetylcysteine was being tested for the improvement of the behavior problems often associated with autism spectrum disorders (NCT00453180). The potential beneficial effect of DMSA, an oral chelating agent that removes mercury and other metals from the body, was also being investigated (NCT00376194), as was the efficacy of **risperidone** in normalizing symptoms (NCT00352196). Other drugs being tested were **aripiprazole** (NCT00198055) and **citalopram** (NCT00086645). A **cognitive-behavioral therapy** (CBT) program was also being evaluated for treating anxiety symptoms, social problems, and adaptive behavior deficits in children with Asperger syndrome (NCT00280670).

Clinical trial information is constantly updated by NIH and the most recent information on AS trials can be found at: http://clinicaltrials.gov/ct2/results?term=Asperger+syndrome+

Prognosis

AS is a lifelong but stable condition. The prognosis for children with AS is generally good as far as intellectual development is concerned, though one challenge is equipping schools with the tools needed to meet special social needs. However, there is an increased risk of developing psychosis later in life.

QUESTIONS TO ASK YOUR DOCTOR

- Can Asperger syndrome be cured?
- What treatment options are available?
- How do they differ in terms of expected outcomes?
- Is drug therapy required?

Prevention

Effective prevention of Asperger syndrome awaits further genetic mapping together with ongoing research in the structures and functioning of the brain.

Resources

BOOKS

Attwood, T. *The Complete Guide to Asperger's Syndrome.* London: Jessica Kingsley, 2008.

Behrman R.E., et al. *Nelson Textbook of Pediatrics,* 18th ed. Philadelphia: Saunders, 2007.

Bradley, W., et al. *Neurology in Clinical Practice,* 5th ed. Philadelphia: Butterworth-Heinemann, 2008.

Carley, Michael John. *Asperger's from the Inside Out: A Supportive and Practical Guide for Anyone with Asperger's Syndrome.* New York: Perigee Trade, 2008.

Dubin, Nick, and Valerie Gaus. *Asperger Syndrome and Anxiety: A Guide to Successful Stress Management.* Philadelphia: Jessica Kingsley, 2009.

Gaus, Valerie L. *Cognitive-Behavioral Therapy for Adult Asperger Syndrome.* New York: Guilford Press, 2007.

Goetz, C.G. *Goetz's Textbook of Clinical Neurology,* 3rd ed. Philadelphia: Saunders, 2007.

Hagland, Carol. *Getting to Grips with Asperger Syndrome: Understanding Adults on the Autism Spectrum.* Philadelphia: Jessica Kingsley, 2009.

Marshack, Kathy J. *Life with a Partner or Spouse with Asperger Syndrome: Going over the Edge? Practical Steps to Saving You and Your Relationship.* Shawnee Mission, KS: Autism Asperger Publishing, 2009.

Patrick, Nancy J. *Social Skills for Teenagers and Adults with Asperger Syndrome: A Practical Guide to Day-to-day Life.* Philadelphia: Jessica Kingsley, 2008.

Robison, John Elder. *Look Me in the Eye: My Life with Asperger's.* New York: Three Rivers Press, 2008.

Silverman, Stephan M., and Rich Weinfeld. *School Success for Kids with Asperger's Syndrome: A Practical Guide for Parents and Teachers.* Waco, TX: Prufrock Press, 2007.

PERIODICALS

Bouxsein, K.J., et al. "A Comparison of General And Specific Instructions To Promote Task Engagement and Completion by a Young Man with Asperger Syndrome." *Journal of Applied Behavior Analysis* 41, no. 1 (2008): 113–16.

Fitzgerald, M. "Suicide and Asperger's Syndrome." *Crisis* 28, no. 1 (2007): 1–3.

Lopata, C., et al. "Motor and Visuomotor Skills of Children with Asperger's Disorder: Preliminary Findings." *Perceptual and Motor Skills* 104, no. 3, pt. 2 (2007): 1183–92.

Punshon, C., et al. "The Not Guilty Verdict: Psychological Reactions to a Diagnosis of Asperger Syndrome in Adulthood." *Autism* 13, no. 3 (2009): 265–83.

Rinehart, N.J., et al. "Brief Report: Inhibition of Return in Young People with Autism and Asperger's Disorder." *Autism* 12, no. 3 (2008): 249–60.

Ryburn, B., et al. "Asperger Syndrome: How Does It Relate to Non-verbal Learning Disability?" *Journal of Neuropsychology* 3, pt. 1 (2009): 107–23.

Sahlander, C., et al. "Motor Function in Adults with Asperger's Disorder: A Comparative Study." *Physiotherapy Theory and Practice* 24, no. 21 (2008): 73–81.

Senju, A., et al. "Mindblind Eyes: An Absence of Spontaneous Theory of Mind in Asperger Syndrome." *Science* 325, no. 5942 (2009): 883–85.

Tantam, D., and S. Girqis. "Recognition and Treatment of Asperger Syndrome in the Community." *British Medical Bulletin* 89 (2009): 41–62.

WEBSITES

"Asperger Syndrome." MedlinePlus. http://www.nlm.nih.gov/medlineplus/aspergerssyndrome.html (accessed October 10, 2010).

"Asperger Syndrome." National Institute of Child Health and Human Development. http://www.nichd.nih.gov/health/topics/asperger_syndrome.cfm (accessed October 10, 2010).

"Asperger Syndrome Information Page." National Institute of Neurological Disorders and Stroke. Last modified June 15, 2011. http://www.ninds.nih.gov/disorders/asperger/asperger.htm (accessed October 10, 2010).

ORGANIZATIONS

Autism Network International (ANI), PO Box 35448, Syracuse, NY, 13235-5448, http://autreat.com.

Autism Society of America, 4340 East-West Hwy., Ste. 350, Bethesda, MD, 20814, (301) 657-0881, (800) 328-8476, http://www.autism-society.org.

Global and Regional Asperger's Syndrome Partnership, 135 East 15th St., New York, NY, 10003, (646) 242-4003, info@grasp.org, http://www.grasp.org.

MAAP Services for Autism, Asperger Syndrome, and PDD, PO Box 524, Crown Point, IN, 46308, (219) 662-1311, Fax: (219) 662-0638, info@maapservices.org, http://www.maapservices.org.

National Institute of Mental Health, 6001 Executive Blvd., Rm. 8184, MSC 9663, Bethesda, MD, 20892-9663, (301) 433-4513; TTY: (301) 443-8431, Fax: (301) 443-4279, (866) 615-6464; TTY: (866) 415-8051, nimhinfo@nih.gov, http://www.nimh.nih.gov.

Rebecca J. Frey, PhD
Rosalyn Carson-DeWitt

Assertive community treatment

Definition

Assertive community treatment (ACT) is an integrative approach to treating severe mental illness, such as **schizophrenia**. Community-based, mobile teams provide patients with treatment and support services, including access to medication, counseling, education, and legal and financial support.

Purpose

ACT is aimed at older teenagers and adults with a mental illness that greatly impacts their ability to care for themselves and function at home or work. The intensive program traditionally helps patients with serious, long-term illnesses such as schizophrenia, **schizoaffective disorder**, or **bipolar disorder**, but ACT may also benefit those who have not had success with other outpatient treatment approaches or who have trouble accessing or adhering to other treatment regimens. ACT combines medication, counseling, rehabilitation, education, legal and financial support, and family assistance into one comprehensive program. Its goals aim to help people with mental illness recover in such areas as personal living (especially with regards to living independently), social interaction, relationships with friends and family members, and employment.

Description

Doctors Arnold J. Marx, Leonard I. Stein, Mary Ann Test, and additional colleagues pioneered the ACT program in the late 1960s in Madison, Wisconsin, as an alternative to admission to a psychiatric institution. While working at the Mendota State Hospital, now called the Mendota Mental Health Institute, the team noticed that patients who got better in the hospital often became sick again when reentering the community. They proposed that a round-the-clock program outside the hospital could provide the same ongoing support and therapy. In 1972, they put their theory to the test and formally launched ACT. The program is offered in many U.S. states and throughout Canada and the United Kingdom. The U.S. Department of Veterans Affairs also supports and has implemented ACT programs across the country.

Because ACT provides care outside of the doctor's office, usually in the comfort of the patient's home, the community-based program is sometimes referred to as a "hospital without walls." The cornerstone of each ACT program is a diverse team of nearly a dozen different healthcare specialists, including doctors, nurses, and counselors. Professionals involved with ACT include those with backgrounds and training in counseling, nursing, psychiatry, rehabilitation, social work, and other such relevant fields. The program provides support and care 24 hours a day, seven days a week, all year long.

Project leaders, called case managers, usually have fewer than 10 patients, which allows for highly individualized care. A patient is considered a "client" of the ACT team. ACT is different from other **community mental health** center (CMHC) services, which usually require the patient to visit a clinic for treatment. The ACT team comes to the client, and those who participate in ACT receive more personalized attention and may be in contact with the ACT team daily, as opposed to weekly or monthly. The ACT team provides all necessary care, including **substance abuse** treatment and rehabilitation. CMHC services often refer clients to an outside specialist for specific issues.

Key features

ACT has three key features: treatment, rehabilitation, and support services.

- The treatment of ACT may involve antipsychotic and antidepressant medicines, substance abuse therapy, counseling, and possible admission to a hospital for closer monitoring.
- The rehabilitation arm of the program helps the patient find volunteer work and paid employment and provides support for continuing education. Specialists teach patients new behaviors, such as how to structure schedules and perform daily activities.
- The support services advise patients on how to find legal and financial support, housing, transportation, and other services. Family members are taught how to cope with their loved one's illness and are provided with education materials. According to the Schizophrenia Patient Outcomes Research Team (PORT) study, funded by the National Institute of Mental Health and the Agency for Health Care Policy and Research, fewer than one in ten families of persons with schizophrenia receives such education and support.

Goals

ACT is targeted to persons with very severe mental illness that has led to repeated hospital and emergency room visits, **homelessness**, or jail time. According to the National Jail Association, about 700,000 persons with mental illness are incarcerated every year. ACT programs have helped such criminal offenders meet their legal obligations while providing medical support and rehabilitation services.

The ACT program aims to:

- relieve or cure symptoms of the disorder
- reduce or prevent repeated, severe episodes associated with the disorder
- enhance the client's quality of life
- improve functioning at work and in social settings
- encourage independence and teach necessary self-care skills
- reduce the burden of care on a patient's family by providing education and support

Benefits

Studies have shown that ACT and similar programs greatly reduce the number of hospital stays among those with severe mental illness. One study found that ACT not only reduced overall hospital admissions but also decreased the length of the hospital stays. ACT has been shown to improve patient functioning and encourage patients to stick to their treatment routines. The benefits

KEY TERMS

Antidepressant—A drug used to treat depression.

Antipsychotic—A drug used to treat serious mental disorders that cause hallucinations or delusions.

Bipolar disorder—A mental illness marked by alternating periods of excitement and depression; also called manic-depressive disorder.

Delusion—A false belief that persists despite evidence to the contrary.

Hallucination—A false or distorted sensory experience that appears to be real to the person experiencing it, such as seeing something that is not actually there.

Schizoaffective disorder—Schizophrenic symptoms occurring concurrently with a major depressive and/or manic episode.

Schizophrenia—A severe mental illness in which a person has difficulty distinguishing what is real from what is not real. It is often characterized by hallucinations, delusions, and withdrawal from people and social activities.

Substance abuse—Overuse of a drug or alcohol, which leads to addiction.

are reported to be particularly marked among those with a coexisting mental disorder and substance abuse problem, perhaps because such patients are at higher risk of **hospitalization** and complications.

Compared to those who are admitted to an institution, ACT clients have fewer symptoms, more positive social interactions, and spend less time unemployed. Experts say anywhere between 20% and 40% of people with the most severe and persistent mental illnesses would benefit from ACT.

Precautions

Because there are so many specialists on an ACT team, it can be costly. Some argue that the expense is justified, particularly when compared to the cost of an extended hospital stay. According to the National Alliance on Mental Illness (NAMI), ACT costs each participant between $9,000 and $14,000 a year, while hospital costs for an extended stay can exceed $100,000.

Preparation

Preparation involves locating an ACT program. There are a limited number of ACT teams in the United States. According to NAMI, only six states (Delaware, Idaho, Missouri, Rhode Island, Texas, and Wisconsin) offer statewide programs, though 19 other states offer test, or pilot, programs in specific communities. In different states, ACT may be known by different names; it is commonly referred to as the Program of Assertive Community Treatment (PACT), and many organizations use the terms interchangeably. Other names for ACT include community support programs (CSP) and mobile treatment teams (MTT). Regardless of the title, all ACT programs abide by standards set by NAMI.

Aftercare

ACT professionals work with patients without time limits in assertive community treatment programs. As such, patients are much better prepared when their treatment ends and aftercare begins.

Risks

The risk of relapse is always present for patients with mental illness. However, assertive community treatment has been proven to help reduce that risk and is considered an effective way, both from a medical and cost standpoint, to deal with severe and persistent mental illness. According to the Center for Behavioral Health Services and Criminal Justice Research, more than 25 randomized controlled trials have been conducted on ACT. The majority of these trials found ACT to be more effective than traditional care of patients with mental illness in the areas of decreased hospitalization, increased patient satisfaction, and improvement in housing stability and general quality of life. The biggest issue with ACT is that it is considered a largely underutilized form of treatment; NAMI estimates that up to 40% of adults with mental illness could be helped by ACT if it were available in their communities.

QUESTIONS TO ASK YOUR DOCTOR

- Does a local ACT program exist? If not, how far away is the nearest ACT program?
- Will my health insurance pay some or all of the expenses for ACT?
- Will I take medicine while going through ACT?
- What happens if ACT does not help me?

Resources

BOOKS

Johnson, Sandra J. *Assertive Community Treatment: Evidence-based Practice or Managed Recovery.* New Brunswick, NJ: Transaction Publishers, 2011.

PERIODICALS

Marshall, Max, and Austin Lockwood. "Assertive Community Treatment for People with Severe Mental Disorders." *Cochrane Database of Systematic Reviews* 2011, no. 4 (April): CD001089.

Rosen, Alan. "Assertive Community Treatment—Issues from Scientific and Clinical Literature with Implications for Practice." *Journal of Rehabilitation Research & Development* 44, no. 6 (2007): 813–26.

OTHER

Center for Behavioral Health Services and Criminal Justice Research. "Assertive Community Treatment: Intervention Fact Sheet." http://www.cbhs-cjr.rutgers.edu/pdfs/ACT_Fact_Sheet_2_09.pdf (accessed October 13, 2011).

WEBSITES

Assertive Community Treatment Association. "ACT History and Origins." http://www.actassociation.org/origins (accessed October 13, 2011).

Lehman, Anthony F., Donald M Steinwachs, et al. "The Schizophrenia Patient Outcomes Research Team (PORT) Treatment Recommendations—At Issue: Translating Research into Practice." Agency for Healthcare Research and Quality. http://www.ahrq.gov/clinic/schzrec.htm (accessed October 13, 2011).

National Alliance on Mental Illness. "Assertive Community Treatment (ACT)." http://www.nami.org/template.cfm?template=/contentManagement/contentDisplay.cfm&contentID=21056 (accessed October 13, 2011).

ORGANIZATIONS

Assertive Community Treatment Association, PO Box 2428, Brighton, MI, 48116, (810) 227-1859, Fax: (810) 227-5785, acta@actassociation.org, http://www.actassociation.org.

National Alliance on Mental Illness, 3803 North Fairfax Drive, Suite 100, Arlington, VA, 22203, (703) 524-7600, (800) 950-6264, Fax: (703) 524-9094, http://www.nami.org.

National Institute of Mental Health, 6001 Executive Boulevard, Room 8184, Bethesda, MD, 20892-9663, (301) 443-4513, (866) 615-6464, Fax: (301) 443-4279, nimhinfo@nih.gov, http://www.nimh.nih.gov.

Substance Abuse and Mental Health Services Administration, PO Box 2345, Bethesda, MD, 20847-2345, (877) 726-4727, Fax: (240) 221-4292, SAMHSAInfo@samhsa.hhs.gov, http://www.samhsa.org.

Kelli Miller Stacy
William Atkins

Assertiveness training

Definition

Assertiveness training is a form of behavior therapy designed to help people stand up for or empower themselves. The concept of assertiveness is a response that seeks to maintain an appropriate balance between passivity and aggression. Assertive responses promote fairness and equality in human interactions, based on a positive sense of respect for self and others. Assertiveness training may help individuals recover from daily pressures or aggravations experienced in social situations involving friends, parents, teachers, colleagues, or others.

Purpose

The purpose of assertiveness training is to teach people appropriate strategies for identifying and acting on their desires, needs, and opinions while remaining respectful of others. This form of training is tailored to the needs of specific participants and the situations they find particularly challenging. Assertiveness training is a broad approach that can be applied to many different personal, academic, healthcare, and work situations.

Description

Assertiveness training is often included within other programs, but "stand-alone" programs in self-assertion are offered in facilities like women's centers or college counseling centers. Corporate programs for new personnel sometimes offer assertiveness training as part of communication or teamwork groups, or as part of a program on sexual harassment.

Assertiveness training typically begins with an information-gathering exercise in which participants are asked to think about and list the areas in their life in which they have difficulty asserting themselves. Very often they will notice specific situations or patterns of behavior that they want to focus on during the course. The next stage in assertive training is usually "role-playing," which is designed to help participants practice clearer and more direct ways of communicating with others. The role-plays allow for practice and repetition of the new techniques, helping each person learn assertive responses by acting on them. Feedback is provided to improve the response, and the role-play is repeated. Eventually, each person is asked to practice assertive techniques in everyday life, outside the training setting. Role-plays usually incorporate specific problems for individual participants, such as difficulty speaking up to an overbearing boss, setting limits to intrusive friends, or stating a clear preference about dinner to a spouse. Role-plays often include examples of aggressive and passive responses, in addition to the assertive responses, to help participants distinguish between these extremes as they learn a new set of behaviors.

Assertiveness training promotes the use of "I" statements as a way to help individuals express their feelings and reactions to others. A commonly used model of an "I" statement is "when you _________, I feel ___________," to help the participant describe what they see the other person as doing, and how they feel about that action. "I" statements are often contrasted with "you" statements, which are usually not received well by others. For example, "When you are two hours late getting home from work, I feel both anxious and angry," is a less accusing communication than "You are a selfish and inconsiderate jerk for not telling me you would be two hours late." Prompts are often used to help participants learn new communication styles. This approach helps participants learn new ways of expressing themselves as well as how it feels to be assertive.

Learning specific techniques and perspectives such as self-observation skills, awareness of personal preferences, and assuming personal responsibility are important components of the assertiveness training process. Role-play and practice help with self-observation, while making lists can be a helpful technique for exploring personal preferences for those who may not have a good sense of their own needs and desires. Participants may be asked to list anything from their ten favorite movies or pieces of music to their favorite foods, places they would like to visit, subjects that interest them, and so on.

Origins

Assertiveness training has a decades-long history in mental health and personal growth groups, going back to the women's movement of the 1970s. The approach was introduced to encourage women to stand up for themselves appropriately in their interactions with others, particularly as they moved into graduate education and the workplace in greater numbers. The original association of assertiveness training with the women's movement in the United States grew out of the discovery of many women in the movement that they were hampered by their inability to be assertive. Today, assertiveness training is used in settings as diverse as schools, corporate boardrooms, and psychiatric hospitals, for purposes as varied as **substance abuse** treatment, **social skills training**, vocational programs, and responding to harassment. Psychological researchers at Southern Methodist University (Dallas, Texas) use a virtual-reality laboratory to teach women assertiveness skills to help prevent sexual victimization. U. S. psychologists Ernest Jouriles, Renee McDonald, and Lorelei Simpson found that women in a control group (without assertiveness training) were twice as likely to be victims of sexual victimization when compared to women who had participated in their assertiveness training.

Benefits

Learning to communicate in a clear and honest fashion helps strengthen interpersonal relationships. Specific areas of intervention and change in assertiveness training include conflict resolution, realistic goal setting, and stress management. In addition to emotional and psychological benefits, taking a more active approach to self-determination has been shown to have positive outcomes in many personal choices related to health, including being assertive in avoiding risky sexual situations, abstaining from using drugs or alcohol, and assuming responsibility for self-care if diagnosed with a chronic illness.

Precautions

There are a few precautions with assertiveness training. One potential caution would be to remain within assertive responses, rather than becoming aggressive. Some participants in assertiveness training programs who are just learning the techniques of appropriate assertiveness may "overdo" their new behaviors and come across as aggressive rather than assertive. Such overcompensation would most likely disappear with continued practice of the techniques.

One additional precaution about assertiveness training is that it should not be regarded as the equivalent of martial arts training or similar physical self-defense techniques. It is important to distinguish between contexts or situations in which verbal assertiveness is appropriate and useful, and those in which it is irrelevant. In some situations, a person's decision to leave the situation or seek help because they feel unsafe is preferable to a dangerous encounter.

Preparation

Preparation for assertiveness training varies from person to person. For some participants, prior preparation is not needed before practicing the techniques; for others, however, individual counseling or therapy may help prepare the individual for assertiveness training. For participants who may be more shy and feel uncomfortable saying "no" or speaking up for themselves, a brief course of individual therapy will help to prepare them psychologically and emotionally to use assertive techniques.

Aftercare

Aftercare can involve ongoing supportive therapy, again based on the individual's level of comfort in using the assertive techniques. For those who are comfortable using the techniques on their own, a supportive social network or occasional participation in a support group

KEY TERMS

Assertive—Confidently self-assured; able to express oneself constructively and directly.

Conflict resolution—Various methods used by psychologists and other such professionals to eliminate sources of conflict in patients.

Overcompensation—An attempt to overcome or correct a behavior by going too far in the opposite direction.

Role-playing—A technique used in assertiveness training and other forms of therapy in which participants act out roles relevant to real-life situations in order to change their attitudes and behaviors.

Stress management—A method used by medical professionals such as psychiatrists to reduce or eliminate stress (especially chronic stress) in patients' lives.

will be enough to help maintain the new behavioral patterns. The ultimate goal is for each participant to effectively self-monitor his or her use of assertive techniques on an ongoing basis.

Risks

There are minimal risks associated with assertiveness training. Personal relationships may be affected if those around the participant have difficulty accepting the changes in their friend or family member. This risk, however, is no greater than that associated with any other life change.

Another potential risk is that of overcompensating in the early stages of training by being too aggressive. With appropriate feedback, participants can usually learn to modify and improve their responses.

People who are very shy or self-conscious, or who were harshly treated as children, may experience anxiety during the training as they work toward speaking up and otherwise changing their behaviors. The anxiety may be uncomfortable but should decrease as the person becomes more comfortable with the techniques and receives encouragement from others in the program.

Results

An enhanced sense of well-being and more positive self-esteem are typical results from assertiveness training. Many participants report that they feel better about themselves and are more capable of handling the stresses of daily life. In addition, people who have participated in assertiveness training have a better sense of boundaries and are able to set appropriate and healthy limits with others. Being able to set appropriate limits (such as saying "no") helps people to avoid feeling victimized by others.

A healthy sense of self-determination and respect for others is the ultimate outcome of assertiveness training. Such a balance helps each person work better with others and make appropriate decisions for themselves.

See also Behavior modification

Resources

BOOKS

Bishop, Sue. *Develop Your Assertiveness*. London: Kogan Page, 2006.

Kemp, Jana. *NO!: How One Simple Word Can Transform Your Life*. New York: AMACOM, 2005.

Leman, Kevin. *Pleasers: Why Women Don't Have to Make Everyone Happy to be Happy*. Grand Rapids, MI: Revell, 2006.

McIntosh, Perry, and Richard A. Luecke. *Increase Your Influence at Work*. New York: American Management Association, 2011.

Newman, Susan. *The Book of No: 250 Ways to Say It—and Mean It—and Stop People-pleasing Forever*. New York: McGraw-Hill, 2006.

Townend, Anni. *Assertiveness and Diversity*. Basingstoke, UK: Palgrave Macmillan, 2007.

PERIODICALS

Hayakawa, M. "How Repeated 15-Minute Assertiveness Training Sessions Reduce Wrist Cutting in Patients with Borderline Personality Disorder." *American Journal of Psychotherapy* 63, no. 1 (2009): 41–51.

Lin, Y. R. "Evaluation of Assertiveness Training for Psychiatric Patients." *Journal of Clinical Nursing* 17, no. 21 (2008): 2875–83.

WEBSITES

Centre for Confidence and Well-Being. "Assertive Communication." http://www.centreforconfidence.co.uk/projects.php?pid=59 (accessed October 14, 2011).

Mayo Clinic staff. "Being Assertive: Reduce Stress, Communicate Better." MayoClinic.com. http://www.mayoclinic.com/health/assertive/SR00042 (accessed November 16, 2011).

Deanna Pledge, PhD
William Atkins

Assessment *see* **Psychological assessment and diagnosis**

Ativan *see* **Lorazepam**

Atomoxetine

Definition

Atomoxetine (Strattera) is a medication used to treat **attention deficit hyperactivity disorder (ADHD)**. Atomoxetine belongs to a class of drugs known as selective norepinephrine reuptake inhibitors (SNRIs), which specifically act on the neurological signaling chemical norepinephrine. Norepinephrine is a type of neurotransmitter involved in normal **brain** function and has an effect on mood and concentration.

Purpose

Atomoxetine is used to treat some of the symptoms of **ADHD** in both adults and children. It was the first nonstimulant drug approved by the U.S. Food and Drug

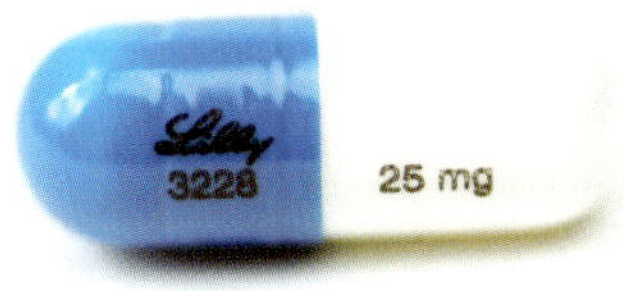

Strattera (atomoxetine), 25 mg. *(© Photo Researchers, Inc.)*

Administration for the treatment of ADHD, though the stimulants remain the mainstay of ADHD therapy. Atomoxetine is often used for patients with ADHD who develop too many side effects from stimulants or who cannot tolerate stimulants due to co-existing anxiety or **substance abuse**. Patients with Tourette syndrome may find that the stimulant medications used to treat ADHD worsen their tics; atomoxetine is useful in this scenario because it can treat the symptoms of ADHD without worsening co-existing tics. For patients with ADHD who also have co-existing **depression**, atomoxetine may have some antidepressant properties, though it has not officially been approved for use in treating depression. The decision to use atomoxetine alone or in combination with other drugs depends on the medical profile of the patient and individual health parameters.

Description

Atomoxetine has a therapeutic mechanism of action that is focused on the modulation of the natural body chemical norepinephrine. Norepinephrine is a type of neurotransmitter in the nervous system, a chemical that neurons use to signal one another in complex pathways for normal brain and body functioning. **Neurotransmitters** such as norepinephrine bind to chemical receptors on the surface of neurons (brain cells). Once bound to a receptor they affect physiological processes. The receptors activate a sequence of cellular events known as a chemical cascade or signaling pathway. Neurotransmitter signaling pathways are responsible for many regulatory processes, including neuronal signaling that affects mood and concentration.

During the signaling process, neurotransmitters such as norepinephrine travel from one neuron to the next. These chemicals need to cross a short space between the end of one neuron and the beginning of the next neuron, known as the synapse or synaptic space. Norepinephrine is released from the end of neuron one, crosses the synaptic space, and binds to a neurotransmitter-specific receptor on the surface of the next neuron (neuron two). Any extra norepinephrine that is left in the synaptic space is taken back up by neuron one in a process known as reuptake. The more neurotransmitters allowed to remain in the synaptic space, the more will eventually be allowed to bind to receptors on neuron two.

Selective norepinephrine reuptake inhibitors such as atomoxetine decrease the reuptake of the neurotransmitters by neuron one, allowing more norepinephrine to be present in the synapse. It is believed that a decrease in norepinephrine signaling contributes to disorders such as ADHD and depression. Atomoxetine mainly helps by increasing levels of norepinephrine, but it has some impact on the neurotransmitter **dopamine** in certain brain areas as well. Atomoxetine has little or no effect on the synaptic levels of other neurotransmitters such as **serotonin**.

The brain has discrete physiological areas that impact different functions of the mind and body. The area of the brain known as the prefrontal cortex affects attention span, judgment, response to external stimuli, memory, motor function, and impulse control. It is believed that increases in the available amounts of norepinephrine (and to a small degree dopamine) by drugs such as atomoxetine improve the symptoms of ADHD in the prefrontal cortex. Atomoxetine seems to function to improve the symptoms of ADHD without psychostimulation.

Recommended dosage

Atomoxetine is taken as an oral medication, usually in the morning, and often requires several weeks of therapy before ADHD symptoms improve. For adults, the dose is usually started at 40 mg for a few days, to allow the patient to adjust to the medication, and is then increased to 80 mg a day. Some patients will require the maximum dose of 100 mg a day for the best effect, but this dose should not be attempted until the patient does well on the 80 mg dose for three to four weeks. Children six years old and older and heavier than 154 lb. (70 kg) follow the same regimen but may have doses divided through the day to reduce the amount taken at any one time. Children who are older than six years and less than 70 kg are dosed based on weight. The usual starting dose is 0.5 mg per 2.2 lb. (1 kg) a day for several days, increased to 1.2 mg per kg

KEY TERMS

Bipolar disorder—Psychiatric mood disorder characterized by periods of manic behavior that may alternate with periods of depression; previously known as manic depressive disorder.

Cytochrome P450 (CYP450)—Enzymes present in the liver that metabolize drugs.

Dopamine—A type of neurotransmitter involved in regulation of concentration, impulse control, judgment, mood, attention span, psychostimulation, and disease states such as addiction, ADHD, and depression.

Glaucoma—Condition involving increased pressure within the eye that may cause damage and blindness.

Mania—Physiological state of hyperactivity experienced by patients with certain psychiatric illnesses involving inappropriate elevated mood, pressured speech, poor judgment, and sometimes psychotic episodes.

Monoamine oxidase inhibitors (MAOIs)—Type of antidepressant medication that affects various kinds of neurotransmitters, including serotonin.

Neurotransmitter—A chemical messenger that travels through the body and acts in the nervous system. Neurotransmitter signaling is responsible for a wide range of bodily processes and is often the target of medications involving the brain and cardiovascular system.

Neurotransmitter receptor—A physical recipient for chemicals called neurotransmitters. Receptors sit on the surface of cells that make up body tissues, and once bound to the neurotransmitter, they initiate the chemical signaling pathway associated with neurotransmitters.

Norepinephrine—A type of neurotransmitter involved in regulation of concentration, impulse control, judgment, mood, attention span, psychostimulation, and disease states such as ADHD and depression.

Nucleus accumbens—Area of the brain involved in psychostimulation and addiction.

Prefrontal cortex—Area of the brain involved in attention span, judgment, response to external stimuli, memory, motor function, and impulse control.

Serotonin—A type of neurotransmitter involved in regulation of the blood vessels, brain processes, and disease states such as depression.

Striatum—Area of the brain involved in psychostimulation and addiction.

Synapse—Physical space between neurons that allows the passage of neurotransmitters for chemical signaling pathways.

Tic—Involuntary movements (such as twitching or facial grimacing) or vocalizations (such as throat clearing or barking) associated with Tourette syndrome.

Tourette syndrome—An inherited neuropsychiatric disorder characterized by the development of both motor and vocal tics. The tics are preceded by a feeling of tension or urgency in the affected individual until the tic behavior is performed and relieves the perceived feeling of tension.

per day. The maximum dose in this population is 1.4 mg per kg per day.

Patients are frequently reassessed for the need for treatment, as drugs for ADHD are avoided unless absolutely necessary. The dose chosen depends on individual patient response to the medication regarding its effectiveness, and individual patient response to the medication regarding side effects. Patients are dosed at the lowest possible effective dose to avoid the development of adverse side effects. Slowly increasing the dose over time helps with minimizing side effects, and some side effects lessen with continued use. Some patients have altered metabolism of atomoxetine and require a slower pace for increasing the dose. Patients with liver impairment may not metabolize atomoxetine well and will require lower doses or may not be able to use the drug.

Precautions

Atomoxetine use is not without side effects or potential consequences. While many patients do well on atomoxetine, others are more sensitive to the medication and develop more side effects. Higher doses increase the risk of adverse effects, hence the lowest dose possible is used for treatment. Clinicians weigh the potential for benefit with atomoxetine treatment against the potential undesirable outcomes when making treatment decisions. Rare but serious reactions include very high blood pressure, glaucoma, loss of consciousness, heart arrhythmias, heart attack,

stroke, **seizures**, liver toxicity, and sudden death. Some patients develop increased aggressiveness, **psychosis**, mania, or suicidality in the first weeks of use before the intended therapeutic effects take place. Children are especially at risk for these behavioral side effects. Patients taking atomoxetine are monitored closely for behavioral changes, especially when starting treatment or after dose changes.

Atomoxetine may be contraindicated or may require caution in patients with uncontrolled hypertension, liver function impairment or liver disease, kidney function impairment, glaucoma, heart conditions or abnormalities, or seizure disorder. Kidney and liver function, as well as blood pressure, may be monitored while taking atomoxetine. Atomoxetine is discouraged from use in patients with **bipolar disorder**, as it is more likely to induce a state of mania in these individuals than in those without bipolar disorder. Atomoxetine is classified as category C for pregnancy, which means that either there are no adequate human or animal studies or that adverse fetal effects were found in animal studies, but there is no available human data. The decision whether to use category C drugs in pregnancy is generally based on weighing the critical needs of the mother against the risk to the fetus. Other lower category agents are used whenever possible. The safety of atomoxetine use during breastfeeding is unknown, so its use is not recommended.

Side effects

Atomoxetine has many negative side effects. It usually takes several weeks of medication for the treatment effect to occur, while the undesirable side effects may occur at the onset of treatment. Sensitivity to atomoxetine varies among patients, and some patients may find that even lower doses are more than their body system can tolerate. Common reactions include dry mouth, abdominal pain, nausea and vomiting, constipation, **insomnia**, **sleep disorders** and abnormal dreams, decreased appetite, changes in urination, **erectile dysfunction**, changes to the menstrual cycle, drowsiness, numbness and tingling in the extremities, dizziness, **fatigue**, hot flashes, increased blood pressure and heart rate, sweating, and palpitations.

Interactions

Patients should make their doctor aware of all medications and supplements they are taking before using atomoxetine. Using alcohol while taking atomoxetine may create toxic reactions in the body and should be avoided. Drugs that affect the liver may alter the metabolism of atomoxetine, resulting in too much or too little of the drug in the body. This could lead to increased side effects or even toxic doses. Likewise, atomoxetine may affect the metabolism of other drugs, leading to greater or lower doses than therapeutically desired.

Certain drugs may cause toxicity when used with atomoxetine, either through additive effects or through inhibition of metabolism, causing toxic levels of atomoxetine in the blood. Drugs that may cause toxicity with atomoxetine include **antidepressants** such as **bupropion** and **duloxetine**; the anti-ulcer drug cimetidine; cinacalcet, used to treat some endocrine disorders; some anticancer drugs, such as imatinib and nalotinib; caffeine; the heart drug amiodarone; certain antibiotics such as linezolid; and antipsychotics such as **haloperidol** and **thioridazine**. It is unknown which herbal supplements interact with atomoxetine.

Antidepressants called **monoamine oxidase inhibitors (MAOIs)** also increase the amounts of norepinephrine and dopamine left in the body and cannot be used concurrently with atomoxetine, as the combination may cause overstimulation of the central nervous system and toxicity. Switching drug treatment from an MAOI to atomoxetine may require a waiting period of up to two weeks between drugs. The antidepressant drug **maprotiline** may also have additive effects with atomoxetine that cause toxicity.

QUESTIONS TO ASK YOUR DOCTOR

- Can I take the full dose right away or do I need to slowly increase the dose up to the full amount?
- Can I stop taking the medication right away or do I need to slowly decrease the dose in order to go off the medication?
- When should I eat in reference to taking this medication?
- Will this medication interact with any of my other prescription medications?
- Are there any over-the-counter medications I should not take with this medicine?
- What side effects should I watch for?
- Can I drink alcoholic beverages in the same time frame as taking this medication?

Resources

BOOKS

Brunton, Laurence L., et al. *Goodman and Gilman's The Pharmacological Basis of Therapeutics.* 12th ed. New York: McGraw Hill Medical, 2011.

Stargrove, Mitchell Bebel, et al. *Herb, Nutrient, and Drug Interactions: Clinical Implications and Therapeutic Strategies.* St. Louis: Mosby, 2007.

ORGANIZATIONS

American College of Neuropsychopharmacology, 5034-A Thoroughbred Lane, Brentwood, TN, 37027, (615) 324-2360, Fax: (615) 523-1715, acnp@acnp.org, http://www.acnp.org/default.aspx

American Psychiatric Association, 1000 Wilson Blvd., Ste. 1825, Arlington, VA, 22209-3901, (703) 907-7300, apa@psych.org, http://www.psych.org

American Society for Clinical Pharmacology and Therapeutics, 528 N Washington St., Alexandria, VA, 22314, (703) 836-6981, info@ascpt.org, http://www.ascpt.org.

Mental Health America, 2000 N Beauregard St., 6th Fl., Alexandria, VA, 22311, (703) 684-7722, (800) 969-6642, Fax: (703) 684-5968, http://www.nmha.org.

Maria Eve Basile, PhD

Attachment disorder *see* **Reactive attachment disorder of infancy or early childhood**

Attention deficit hyperactivity disorder (ADHD)

Definition

Attention deficit hyperactivity disorder (ADHD) is a chronic developmental disorder characterized by attention problems, including distractibility, hyperactivity, impulsive behaviors, and the inability to remain focused on tasks or activities. Among its acronyms are AD/HD and ADD. Diagnosed in childhood, the disorder can continue into adulthood.

Demographics

ADHD is a psychiatric disorder that is generally diagnosed in children before the age of 7 years, although

Percentage of U.S. children aged 5–17 years diagnosed with attention deficit hyperactivity disorder (ADHD): 1998–2009

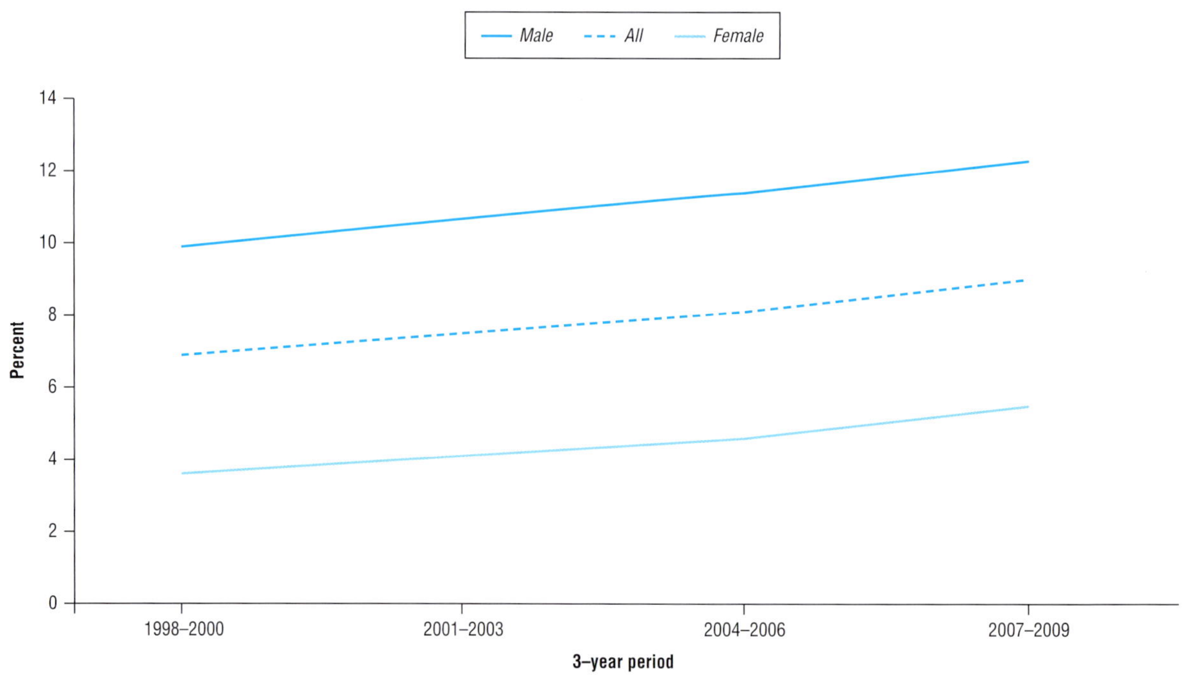

SOURCE: Akinbami, Lara J. et al, "Attention Deficit Hyperactivity Disorder among Children Aged 5–17 Years in the United States, 1998–2009," *NCHS Data Brief* [National Center for Health Statistics], no. 70 (August 2011).

(Graph by PreMediaGlobal. © 2012 Cengage Learning.)

its symptoms can continue into adulthood. The Centers for Disease Control and Prevention (CDC) states that about 9.5% of children from 4 to 17 years of age have been diagnosed in the United States with ADHD. The disorder is more common in boys (13.2%) than in girls (5.6%). In addition, approximately 4.7% of American adults have ADHD.

In the United States, from 2007 through 2008, the average rate of ADHD varied geographically from a low of 5.6% in Nevada, in the western part of the United States, to a high of 15.6% in the east-central state of North Carolina. The CDC also reported that the **diagnosis** rate of ADHD increased by an average of 3% per year from 1997 to 2006, and from 2003 to 2007, the annual rate was 5.6%.

Worldwide, 3%–5% of children are afflicted with ADHD, with rates ranging from less than 1% in the United Kingdom (which has strict standards for diagnosis) to 12% in some countries within South America. Up to 50% of those diagnosed in childhood continue to have symptoms into adulthood.

Description

ADHD, also called hyperkinetic disorder (HKD) outside of the United States, is the most commonly diagnosed neurological disorder in children. It is frequently diagnosed by the age of seven years; however, it can be diagnosed as early as two years. Although childhood ADHD has been studied extensively, less information is available on **adult ADHD**. Studies on adults have produced a wide range of conflicting results. One reason for the wide range of findings is that the hyperactive component of the disorder often becomes less noticeable as individuals mature and develop more self-control.

Three types of ADHD are recognized by the **American Psychiatric Association** and outlined in the ***Diagnostic and Statistical Manual of Mental Disorders***, fourth edition, text revised (*DSM-IV-TR*). These are:

- predominately hyperactive type, characterized by excessive physical activity (e.g., constant fidgeting, inability to stay seated, inability to engage in quiet play) and impulsive behaviors (e.g., interrupting, difficulty waiting in line)
- predominately inattentive type, characterized by inability to pay close attention to detail, stay on task, and organize tasks; sometimes referred to as attention deficit disorder (ADD)
- combined hyperactive and inattentive type, characterized by an inappropriately high activity level with a high level of distractibility

Causes and symptoms

Causes

Although the exact causes of ADHD are not known, it is clear that specific parts of the **brain** are involved, including the frontal cortex, parietal lobe, and possibly the cerebellum. Functional **magnetic resonance imaging** (fMRI) studies comparing the brains of children with ADHD and those without the disorder show that children with ADHD have weaker brain activation of the frontal area when responding to tasks that require inhibition. Researchers believe that this is related to an imbalance in certain **neurotransmitters** (the chemicals in the brain that carry messages between nerve cells), specifically deficits in the neurotransmitters **dopamine** and norepinephrine. Drugs used to treat ADHD make dopamine and/or norepinephrine more available in the brain.

ADHD also appears to have a hereditary component. Children with a parent or sibling with ADHD are two to eight times more likely to develop the disorder. Scientists have suggested at least 20 genes that may make a person more vulnerable to ADHD or contribute to the disorder in some way. As of 2011, these genes were being studied to learn more about whether they contribute to ADHD, and, if so, to what degree.

The condition is also more likely in children whose mothers smoke tobacco products, use drugs, or have been exposed to toxins. Pregnant women who smoke tobacco products are at increased risk to giving birth to a child with ADHD. Alcohol or drug use during pregnancy may also contribute to increased risk for ADHD. Children who are exposed to toxins are more likely to acquire developmental and behavioral problems associated with ADHD when compared to children who have never been exposed to toxins. One such toxin that has been scientifically shown to produce ADHD-like symptoms is the element lead (symbol Pb), which is sometimes found in paint from old homes and buildings.

A widely publicized study conducted by Benjamin F. Feingold (1899–1982) in the early 1970s suggested that allergies to certain foods and food additives caused the characteristic hyperactivity of children with ADHD. Although some children may have adverse reactions to certain foods that can affect their behavior (for example, a rash might temporarily cause a child to be distracted from other tasks), carefully controlled follow-up studies have uncovered no link between food allergies and ADHD. Some researchers believe that artificial coloring and food preservatives may contribute to hyperactive behavior as seen in ADHD, but no link has been proven. A popularly held misconception about food and ADHD is that the consumption of sugar causes hyperactive behavior. Studies have shown no link between sugar intake and ADHD. It is important to note, however, that a nutritionally balanced diet is important for normal development in all children.

Symptoms

Children with ADHD have short attention spans, becoming easily distracted or frustrated with tasks. Although they may be quite intelligent, their lack of focus frequently results in poor grades and difficulties in school. Children with ADHD act impulsively, taking action first and thinking later. They are constantly moving, running, climbing, squirming, and fidgeting, but they often have trouble with motor skills and, as a result, may be clumsy and awkward. Their clumsiness may extend to the social arena, where they are sometimes shunned due to their impulsive and intrusive behavior. Because of these symptoms, ADHD children are often troubled by low self-esteem and may have poor relationships.

Diagnosis

There is not a single test for ADHD. Psychiatrists and other mental health professionals use the criteria listed in the *DSM-IV-TR* as a guideline for determining the presence of the disorder. A diagnosis of ADHD requires the presence of at least six of the following symptoms of inattention or six or more symptoms of hyperactivity and impulsivity combined. These symptoms must occur before the age of seven years, be present in at least two different environments (e.g., home and school) for at least six months, and not be attributable to any other developmental or mental health disorder.

Signs of inattention include:

- fails to pay close attention to detail or makes careless mistakes in schoolwork or other activities
- has difficulty sustaining attention in tasks or activities
- does not appear to listen when spoken to
- does not follow through on instructions and does not finish tasks
- has difficulty organizing tasks and activities
- avoids or dislikes tasks that require sustained mental effort (e.g., homework)
- loses things necessary for tasks (e.g., books, tools)
- is easily distracted
- is forgetful in daily activities

Signs of hyperactivity and impulsivity include:

- fidgets with hands or feet or squirms in seat
- does not remain seated or is restless when expected to sit
- runs or climbs excessively when inappropriate (in adolescents and adults, feelings of restlessness)
- has difficulty playing quietly
- blurts out answers before the question has been completed
- has difficulty waiting (e.g., to take turns, to stand in line)
- interrupts and/or intrudes on others

Additional hyperactivity/impulsivity criteria proposed for the fifth edition of the *DSM* (*DSM-5*, 2013) include:

- acts without thinking, such as starting tasks without reading instructions or speaking without considering the consequences
- is impatient and acts restless when waiting for others
- is uncomfortable doing things slowly, often rushing to complete tasks
- finds it difficult to resist temptations or opportunities, even when they involve risk

Examination

The first step in determining if a child has ADHD is to consult with a pediatrician. The pediatrician can make an initial evaluation of the child's developmental maturity compared to other children in his or her age group. The physician also can perform a comprehensive physical examination to rule out any organic causes of ADHD symptoms, such as an overactive thyroid, vision problems, or hearing problems.

If an organic problem is not found, a **psychologist**, **psychiatrist**, neurologist, neuropsychologist, or learning specialist typically is consulted to perform a comprehensive ADHD assessment. A complete medical, family, social, psychiatric, and educational history is compiled from existing medical and school records and from interviews with parents and teachers. Interviews may also be conducted with the child, depending on his or her age. Along with these interviews, several clinical inventories may also be used, such as the Conners Rating Scales (Teacher's Questionnaire and Parent's Questionnaire), Child Behavior Checklist (CBCL), and the Barkley Home Situation Questionnaire. These inventories provide valuable information on the child's behavior in different settings and situations. In addition, the Wender Utah Rating Scale has been adapted for use in diagnosing ADHD in adults. Continuous Performance Tests, which involve tasks performed on a computer, may support a diagnosis of attention-deficit type ADHD but by themselves are not diagnostic.

As many as 50% to 60% of people diagnosed with ADHD also meet the diagnostic criteria for another major psychiatric disorder such as **anxiety disorders**, **depression**, **antisocial personality disorder**, **oppositional defiant disorder**, **bipolar disorder**, **substance**

abuse disorder, or **conduct disorder**. These individuals also have a high likelihood of having a learning disorder. Children with ADHD also sometimes have **Tourette syndrome**, which is a neurological disorder characterized by vocal tics or compulsive muscle spasms. A complete and comprehensive psychiatric assessment is critical to differentiate ADHD from other mood and behavioral disorders.

In the United States, public schools are required by federal law to offer free ADHD assessment upon request. A pediatrician also can provide a referral to a psychologist or pediatric psychiatrist for ADHD assessment. Parents should check with their insurance plans to see if these services are covered.

Treatment

The CDC reported that in 2007, 2.7 million children from the age of 4 to 17 years were on medication to treat ADHD. It also stated that of all the children diagnosed with ADHD, 66.3% were on medication. Concerning age, the CDC found that children from 11 to 17 years of age were more likely to take medication than children aged 4 to 10 years. In addition, boys were 2.8 times more likely to take medication than were girls. Treatment does not cure ADHD but has been found to help with its symptoms.

Therapy that addresses both psychological and social issues (called psychosocial therapy), usually combined with medications, is the treatment approach of choice to alleviate ADHD symptoms, and in younger children, therapy is preferred over medication. The combination of therapy and medication has proven to be the most effective treatment approach to ADHD. Most children who go through therapy for ADHD develop into normal functioning adults.

Drugs

Stimulant drugs, also known as psychostimulants, are considered the most effective medication for treating ADHD. These drugs generally increase the availability of neurotransmitters in the brain, which tends to reduce such symptoms as inattention, impulsivity, and hyperactivity. Drug therapy must be highly individualized with the benefits balanced against the risk of undesirable side effects. **Dextroamphetamine** (Dexedrine, Dextrostat), dextroamphetamine/amphetamine mixture (Adderall), **methylphenidate** (Concerta, Daytrana, Ritalin, Metadate), and **dexmethylphenidate** (Focalin) are common stimulant drug treatments. These drugs are available in both immediate release and extended release forms.

The use of the stimulant drug **pemoline** (Cylert) to treat ADHD was stopped in 2005 when the U.S. Food and Drug Administration (FDA) ruled that the risk of liver damage outweighed the benefits of this drug.

Attention deficit hyperactivity disorder (ADHD) medications[1]

Generic name	Trade name	FDA approved age
amphetamine	Adderall	3+
amphetamine (extended release)	Adderall XR	6+
atomoxetine	Strattera	6+
dexmethylphenidate	Focalin	6+
dexmethylphenidate (extended release)	Focalin XR	6+
dextroamphetamine	Dexedrine, Dextrostat	3+
guanfacine	Intuniv	6+
lisdexamfetamine dimesylate	Vyvanse	6+
methamphetamine	Desoxyn	6+
methylphenidate	Ritalin	6+
methylphenidate (extended release)	Metadate CD, Metadate ER, Ritalin SR	6+
methylphenidate (long-acting)	Ritalin LA, Concerta	6+
methylphenidate transdermal	Daytrana	6+
methylphenidate (oral solution and chewable tablets)	Methylin	6+

[1]All of these ADHD medications are stimulants, except atomoxetine and guanfacine.

SOURCE: National Institute of Mental Health.

"Alphabetical List of Medications," available online at: http://www.nimh.nih.gov/health/publications/mental-health-medications/alphabetical-list-of-medications.shtml. *(Table by PreMediaGlobal. © 2012 Cengage Learning.)*

Stimulant drugs may have adverse side effects in some children. These side effects include loss of appetite, **insomnia**, mood disturbance, headache, and gastrointestinal distress. Tics may also appear and should be monitored carefully. Psychotic reactions are among the more severe side effects. There is some evidence that long-term use of stimulant medication may interfere with physical growth and weight gain. Some experts feel that these effects are ameliorated by taking medication breaks (or "drug holidays") over school vacations or weekends. Increasingly, there is concern about long-term use of stimulant medications and their use of in very young children; their use is not recommended in children under age six unless absolutely necessary.

In the past, children who did not respond well to stimulant therapy were often given tricyclic **antidepressants** such as **desipramine** (Norpramin, Pertofane) and **imipramine** (Tofranil). These drugs are now rarely used, as they have a much higher risk of causing serious side effects, including cardiac arrhythmia (irregular heartbeat that can be life threatening).

Nonstimulant drugs are now the preferred choice for treating ADHD when stimulant drugs are found to be ineffective or when adverse side effects occur. Atomoxetine (Strattera) is a nonstimulant norepinephrine reuptake inhibitor. Its effect is to make norepinephrine remain in the brain longer, thus increasing the amount of norepinephrine available.

Other medications used to treat ADHD include some antidepressants (when stimulants or nonstimulants do not work or when a mood disorder is present in addition to ADHD). These include buproprion (Wellbutrin) and **venlafaxine** (Effexor), both atypical, nontricyclic antidepressants. **Clonidine** (Catapres) and **guanfacine** (Intuniv, Tenex), both systemic antihypertensive (blood pressure lowering) medications, also have been used to control aggression and hyperactivity in some ADHD children. They may also reduce symptoms such as tics or insomnia. However, these drugs can have serious side effects if taken with methylphenidate (Ritalin).

Generally, a child's response to medication will change with age and maturation, so ADHD symptoms should be monitored and prescriptions adjusted accordingly.

Therapies

It is important that drug treatment be carefully monitored and not be used exclusively in the management of ADHD. **Behavior modification** is often used in conjunction with drug therapy. Behavior modification uses a reward system to reinforce good behavior and task completion and can be implemented both in the classroom and at home. A tangible reward such as a sticker may be given to the child every time he or she completes a task or behaves in an acceptable manner. A chart system may be used to display the stickers and visually illustrate the child's progress. When a certain number of stickers are collected, the child may trade them in for a bigger reward such as a trip to the zoo or a day at the beach. The reward system stays in place until the good behavior becomes ingrained and is sustained without reward.

A variation of this technique, **cognitive-behavioral therapy**, works to decrease impulsive behavior by getting the child to recognize the connection between thoughts and behavior. Behavior is changed by altering negative thinking patterns.

Individual **psychotherapy** may help children with ADHD build self-esteem, give them a place to discuss their worries and anxieties, and help them gain insight into their behavior and feelings. **Family therapy** also may be beneficial in helping family members develop coping skills and in working through feelings of guilt or anger that the parents may be experiencing. Parenting skills training also helps parents to develop methods to better understand and deal with their children.

Social skills training can help children learn more appropriate behaviors while interacting with others. Many **support groups** are available around the country that help to provide a much needed network of information, education, and other types of support for children and their families.

Alternative treatment

A number of alternative treatments exist for ADHD. Although there is a lack of controlled studies to prove their efficacy, proponents report that they are successful in controlling symptoms in some ADHD patients. Nevertheless, none of these treatments meets the standards of safety and effectiveness required by conventional medicine. Some of the more popular alternative treatments are:

- EEG (electroencephalograph) biofeedback. By measuring brainwave activity and teaching the ADHD patient which type of brainwave is associated with attention, EEG biofeedback attempts to train patients to generate the desired brainwave activity.
- Dietary therapy. Based in part on the Feingold food allergy diet, dietary therapy focuses on a nutritional plan that is high in protein and complex carbohydrates and free of white sugar and salicylate-containing foods such as strawberries, tomatoes, and grapes. Zinc supplementation has shown positive results in alleviating symptoms of hyperactivity, impulsiveness, and social interaction problems, though additional research is needed.
- Herbal therapy. Herbal therapy uses a variety of natural remedies to address the symptoms of ADHD, such as ginkgo (*Ginkgo biloba*) for memory and mental sharpness and chamomile (*Matricaria recutita*) extract for calming. The safety of herbal remedies has not been demonstrated in controlled studies. For example, it is known that ginkgo may affect blood coagulation, but controlled studies have not yet evaluated the risk of the effect.
- Homeopathic medicine. The theory of homeopathic medicine is to treat the whole person at a core level. Constitutional homeopathic care requires consulting with a well-trained homeopath who has experience working with ADD and ADHD individuals.

Prognosis

Approximately 70% to 80% of ADHD patients treated with stimulant medication experience significant relief from symptoms, at least in the short term. Some children with ADHD seem to "outgrow" symptoms of the disorder in adolescence or early adulthood, whereas others retain some or all of their symptoms as adults. Some children diagnosed with ADHD also develop a conduct disorder. As many as 25% of adolescents with both ADHD and a conduct disorder go on to develop antisocial personality disorder and the criminal behavior, substance abuse, and high rate of **suicide** attempts that frequently accompany this psychiatric disorder.

Untreated, ADHD negatively affects a child's social and educational performance and can seriously damage his or her sense of self-esteem. Children with ADHD may have impaired relationships with their peers and be looked upon as social outcasts. They may be perceived as slow learners or troublemakers in the classroom. Siblings and even parents may develop resentful feelings toward the child.

Each child should have an individual educational plan (IEP) that outlines modifications to the regular mode of instruction that will facilitate the child's academic performance. Teachers must consider the needs of the child when giving instructions, making sure that they are well paced. They must also understand the origins of impulsive behavior—that the child is not deliberately trying to ruin a lesson or activity by acting unruly. Teachers should teach in a structured way, be comfortable with the remedial services the child may need, and be able to maintain good lines of communication with the parent.

Specialists should devise a series of compensatory strategies that will enable the child to cope with his or her attention deficit or hyperactivity. These strategies might include simple things like creating checklists of things to do before handing in assignments (name on top, check spelling, etc.), putting a clock on the child's desk to help structure time for activities, or covering the pictures on a page until the child has read the words so that he/she is not distracted.

Special assistance may not be limited to educational settings. Families frequently need help in coping with the demands and challenges of ADHD. The symptoms of inattention, shifting activities every five minutes, difficulty completing homework and household tasks, losing things, interrupting, not listening, rule breaking, constant talking, boredom, and irritability can take a toll on any family.

Parents may not understand how attention lapses or impulsivity affect daily functioning, and they might not be trained in the kind of techniques that help children with ADHD manage their behavior. Siblings may be resentful of what the child seems to "get away with" or the inordinate amount of attention he or she receives. The child with ADHD may be resentful of a younger sibling who is more accomplished at school or never seems to get in any trouble. Family interaction patterns may set up vicious cycles that become destructive and difficult to break.

Support groups for families are increasingly available through school districts and health care providers. Community colleges frequently offer courses in discipline and behavior management. Counseling services are available to complement any types of pharmacological treatment being used. There are a number of popular books available, which are informative and helpful.

KEY TERMS

Anxiety disorders—A group of psychological disorders that are all characterized by abnormal fear and/or excessive anxiety.

Bipolar disorder—A mood disorder marked by alternating episodes of extremely low mood (depression) and exuberant highs (mania).

Conduct disorder—A behavioral and emotional disorder of childhood and adolescence. Children with such a disorder act inappropriately, infringe on the rights of others, and violate societal norms.

Dopamine—A neurotransmitter that is involved in many brain activities, including movement and emotion.

Nervous tic—A repetitive, involuntary action, such as the twitching of a muscle or repeated blinking.

Neurotransmitter—One of a group of chemicals secreted by a nerve cell (neuron) to carry a chemical message to another nerve cell, often as a way of transmitting a nerve impulse. Examples of neurotransmitters are acetylcholine, dopamine, serotonin, and norepinephrine.

Norepinephrine—A type of neurotransmitter involved in regulation of concentration, impulse control, judgment, mood, attention span, and psychostimulation.

Oppositional defiant disorder—A disorder characterized by hostile, deliberately argumentative, and defiant behavior toward authority figures.

Tourette syndrome—A neurological disorder characterized by compulsive or vocal tics.

QUESTIONS TO ASK YOUR DOCTOR

- How do I know if my child has ADHD?
- What types of treatment do you recommend?
- What are the most serious side effects of medication?
- Can you refer my child to a therapist?
- Can you recommend any support groups for me and my family?

Prevention

There is no way to prevent attention deficit hyperactivity disorder. However, it is always wise for pregnant mothers to avoid the use of alcohol, drugs, and tobacco products to avoid medical problems with children later in life.

Resources

BOOKS

Alexander-Roberts, Colleen. *The AD/HD Parenting Handbook: Practical Advice for Parents From Parents*. 2nd ed. Lanham, MD: Taylor Trade, 2006.

American Psychiatric Association. *Diagnostic and Statistical Manual of Mental Disorders*. 4th ed., text rev. Washington, DC: American Psychiatric Association, 2000.

Brynie, Faith Hickman. *ADHD: Attention-Deficit Hyperactivity Disorder*. Minneapolis: Twenty-First Century Books, 2008.

Conners, Keith C. *Attention Deficit Hyperactivity Disorder in Children and Adolescents: The Latest Assessment and Treatment Strategies*. 4th ed. Kansas City, MO: Compact Clinicals, 2008.

Fitzgerald, Michael, Mark Bellgrove, and Michael Gill, eds. *Handbook of Attention-Deficit Hyperactivity Disorder*. Chichester, UK: John Wiley, 2007.

Gozal, David, and Dennis L. Molfese, eds. *Attention Deficit Hyperactivity Disorder: From Genes to Patients*. Totawa, NJ: Humana Press, 2005.

McBurnett, Keith, and Linda Pfiffner, eds. *Attention Deficit Hyperactivity Disorder: Concepts, Controversies, New Directions*. New York: Informa Healthcare, 2008.

PERIODICALS

Bálint, S., et al. "Neuropsychological Impairments in Adult Attention Deficit Hyperactivity Disorder: A Literature Review." *Psychiatric Hungary* 23, no. 5 (March 2008): 324–35.

Chen, Mandy, Carla M. Seipp, and Charlotte Johnston. "Mothers' and Fathers' Attributions and Beliefs in Families of Girls and Boys with Attention-Deficit/Hyperactivity Disorder." *Child Psychiatry and Human Development* 39, no. 1 (March 2008): 85–100.

Dennis, Tanya, et al. "Attention Deficit Hyperactivity Disorder: Parents' and Professionals' Perceptions." *Community Practitioner* 81, no. 3 (March 2008): 24–29.

Galéra, C., et al. "Early Risk Factors for Hyperactivity-Impulsivity and Inattention Trajectories from Age 17 Months to 8 Years." *Archives of General Psychiatry* 68, no. 12 (2011): 1267–75.

Sibley, Margaret H., et al. "Diagnosing ADHD in Adolescence." *Journal of Consulting and Clinical Psychology* (December 12, 2011) [e-pub ahead of print]. http://dx.doi.org/10.1037/a0026577 (accessed December 14, 2011).

WEBSITES

American Psychiatric Association. "A 10 Attention Deficit/Hyperactivity Disorder." DSM-5 Development. May 20, 2010. http://www.dsm5.org/ProposedRevisions/Pages/proposedrevision.aspx?rid=383 (accessed September 16, 2011).

Centers for Disease Control and Prevention. "Attention Deficit Hyperactivity Disorder (ADHD)." November 10, 2010. http://www.cdc.gov/ncbddd/adhd/data.html (accessed September 16, 2011).

Gordon, Selena. "New ADHD Guidelines Include Preschoolers, Older Children." HealthDay. October 16, 2011. http://www.healthfinder.gov/news/newsstory.aspx?Docid=657877 (accessed November 14, 2011).

Mayo Clinic staff. "Attention Deficit Hyperactivity Disorder (ADHD) in Children." MayoClinic.com. August 2, 2011. http://www.mayoclinic.com/health/adhd/DS00275 (accessed September 16, 2011).

MedlinePlus. "Attention Deficit Hyperactivity Disorder." U.S. National Library of Medicine, National Institutes of Health. June 23, 2011. http://www.nlm.nih.gov/medlineplus/attentiondeficithyperactivitydisorder.html (accessed September 16, 2011).

National Institute of Mental Health. "Attention Deficit Hyperactivity Disorder." July 5, 2011. http://www.nimh.nih.gov/health/publications/adhd/summary.shtml (accessed September 16, 2011).

ORGANIZATIONS

American Psychiatric Association, 1000 Wilson Blvd., Ste. 1825, Arlington, VA, 22209-3901, (703) 907-7300, apa@psych.org, http://www.psych.org.

American Psychological Association, 750 1st St. NE, Washington, DC, 20002-4242, (202) 336-5500; TDD/TTY: (202) 336-6123, (800) 374-2721, http://www.apa.org.

Attention Deficit Disorder Association, PO Box 7557, Wilmington, DE, 19803-9997, (800) 939-1019, info@add.org, http://www.add.org.

Children and Adults with Attention Deficit/Hyperactivity Disorder, 8181 Professional Place, Ste. 150, Landover, MD, 20785, (301) 306-7070, Fax: (301) 306-7090, (800) 233-4050, http://www.chadd.org.

Tish Davidson, AM
Laura Jean Cataldo, RN, EdD
William A. Atkins, BB, BS, MBA

Autism

Definition

Autism is a complex developmental disorder distinguished by difficulties with social interaction, verbal and nonverbal communication, and behavioral problems, including repetitive behaviors and narrow focus of interest.

Demographics

Estimates suggest that about 1 of every 110 children in the United States is affected by autism. Autism is almost four times more likely to be diagnosed in males. Autism is a disorder that is found worldwide, and it is not specific to any one socio-economic, ethnic, or racial group. In identical twins, if one twin has autism, there is a 60%–90% chance that the other twin will have it as well. In fraternal twins, this chance drops to 0%–24%. Previous estimates stated that parents who had one child with autism had a 5% chance of having a second child with the condition, but research published in 2011 by the journal *Pediatrics* suggested that this figure could actually be as high as 19%.

Description

Classic autism is one of several disorders categorized as autism spectrum disorders (ASD). Other ASDs include **Asperger syndrome**, **Rett syndrome**, **childhood disintegrative disorder**, and pervasive developmental disorder. As of 2011, the classification of autism and autism spectrum disorders was being re-evaluated by the **American Psychiatric Association** for revision in the fifth edition of the ***Diagnostic and Statistical Manual of Mental Disorders*** (*DSM-5*, 2013). It has been proposed that Asperger syndrome be eliminated as a separate **diagnosis**. Instead, Asperger syndrome, autism, childhood disintegrative disorder, and pervasive developmental disorder not otherwise specified (PPD-NOS) would be grouped under a single classification, termed "autism spectrum disorder." This proposal was controversial and as of 2011 remained unresolved. *DSM-5* is expected to publish in 2013.

Autism usually manifests before children are three years old, and it continues throughout their lifetime. The severity of the condition varies among individuals, ranging from the most severe (extremely unusual, repetitive, self-injurious, and aggressive behavior) to very mild. No autistic children are alike in the manifestation of their symptoms, so treatment options must be devised to treat each child individually. Autism cannot be cured but is treatable. With early diagnosis and intensive therapy, children with autism may be able to lead healthy, full lives.

Risk factors

Being a boy increases one's risk for autism; boys are 3–4 times as likely as girls to have the condition. There may be some **genetic factors** involved, as autism runs in some families. Certain **brain** conditions also increase the risk of having autism, including tuberous sclerosis, **Tourette syndrome**, epilepsy, and fragile X syndrome. Being born to a father who is older than 40 seems to increase the risk of autism. Research on mothers' ages was expected as of 2011. Despite popular concern, vaccines have not been proven to increase the risk of autism. The original research article that proposed the correlation has been discredited, and a retraction has been printed in the journal.

Causes and symptoms

Researchers know that autism is a complex brain disorder that affects the way brain tissue grows and the way brain cells communicate with each other. More than 20 genes have been identified as associated with autism. Studies have implicated several causes for the disorder, including genetic errors and possible environmental triggers (such as pesticide exposure), but more

Number of U.S. students with autism, 2000–2009

	Ages 3 to 5	Ages 6 to 11	Ages 12 to 17	Ages 18 to 21	Ages 6 to 21	Total (3–21)
2000	14,065	52,460	22,502	4,633	79,595	93,660
2002	19,039	74,707	37,260	6,702	118,669	137,708
2004	25,929	97,374	59,474	9,576	166,424	192,353
2006	35,111	125,944	85,666	12,984	224,594	259,705
2008	44,977	161,236	112,972	18,610	292,818	337,795
2009	47,204	182,446	128,345	22,443	333,234	380,438

SOURCE: Data Accountability Center, Individuals with Disabilities Education Act (IDEA).

Number of U.S. students with autism, ages 3–21, as reported to the Individuals with Disabilities Education Act (IDEA). Data captured by the Data Accountability Center and available online at http://www.ideadata.org/PartBChildCount.asp. *(Table by PreMediaGlobal.*

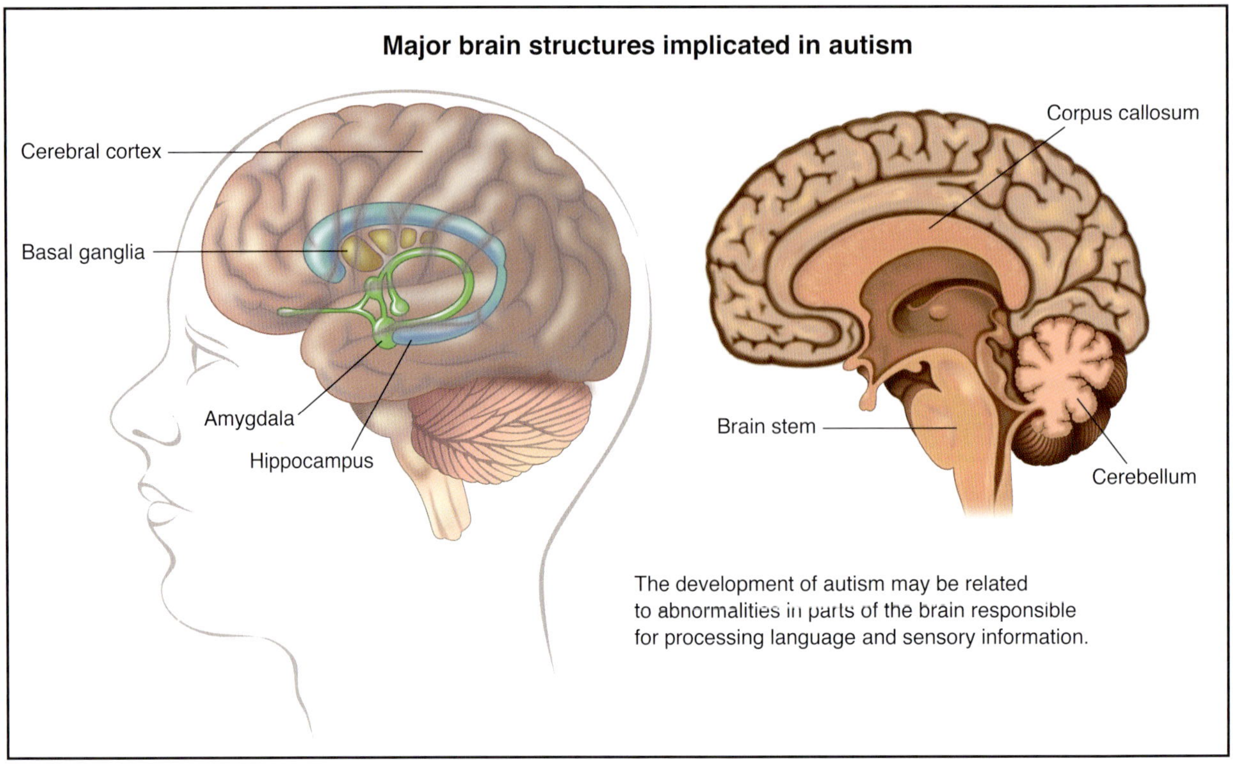

(Illustration by Electronic Illustrators Group. Reproduced by permission of Gale, a part of Cengage Learning.)

investigation is needed. Studies have found abnormalities in several parts of the brain that are believed to have occurred during fetal development. The problem may be centered in the parts of the brain responsible for processing language and information from the senses.

Profound problems with social interaction are the most common symptoms of autism and the most visible. Children with autism have different ways of learning and experiencing their environment. They often have more acute reactions to sensory stimulation such as sound and touch. This results in avoidance of eye contact, physical contact, and oftentimes an aversion to music and other sounds. It is perhaps the way children with autism experience their world that causes difficulties with social interaction, language, and nonverbal communication.

Human beings are social creatures, and social interaction is present from birth onward. Children with autism have difficulty making social connections. When infants can follow an object or person with their gaze, it is considered a developmental milestone. Children with autism tend to avoid eye contact altogether. They do not actively cuddle or hug, but rather they passively accept physical contact or they shy away from it. They may become rigid or flaccid when they are held, cry when picked up, and show little interest in human contact. Such children do not lift their arms in anticipation of being picked up. These children may appear to have formed no attachment to their parents and do not learn typical childhood games, such as peek-a-boo.

Children with autism do not readily learn social cues. They do not know when or how to react to specific social situations or exchanges. Because of this, they tend to look at and respond to different situations similarly. They do not understand that others have different perspectives and, as a result, seem to lack empathy.

Because of their problems socially and the inability to translate social interactions appropriately, children with autism seem to have uncontrolled emotional outbursts, expressing themselves in a manner that does not suit the specific social situation of the moment.

Language problems

Verbal communication problems vary greatly for autistic children. Some children do not speak at all. Some will only use one or two words at a time. Some autistic children may develop vocabulary only to lose it. Others may develop an extensive vocabulary but will have difficulty sustaining a natural, back-and-forth conversation. Children with autism tend to talk in a sing-song voice or more robotically, without emotional inflections. They do not take body language into consideration and take what is being said quite literally.

KEY TERMS

Antidepressants—A type of medication that is used to treat depression; it is also sometimes used to treat autism.

Asperger syndrome—A condition in which individuals have autistic behavior but no problems with language and no clinically significant cognitive delay.

Fragile X syndrome—A genetic condition related to the X chromosome that affects mental, physical, and sensory development.

Major tranquilizers—A group of drugs that includes the psychotropic or neuroleptic drugs, sometimes used to help people with autism. They carry significant risk of side effects, including parkinsonism and movement disorders and should be prescribed with caution.

Opiate blockers—A type of drug that blocks the effects of natural opiates in the system. This type of drug makes some people, including some people with autism, appear more responsive to their environment.

Phenylketonuria (PKU)—An enzyme deficiency present at birth that disrupts metabolism and causes brain damage. This rare inherited defect may be linked to the development of autism.

Rubella—Also known as German measles. When a woman contracts rubella during pregnancy, her developing infant may be damaged. One of the problems that may result is autism.

Stimulants—A class of drugs, including Ritalin, used to treat people with autism. They may make children calmer and better able to concentrate, but they also may limit growth or have other side effects.

Tuberous sclerosis—A genetic disease that causes skin problems, seizures, and intellectual disabilities. Autism occurs more often in individuals with tuberous sclerosis.

Because of their impinged language skills and the inability to express their needs, autistic children seem to act inappropriately to get what they need. They may grab something without asking or blurt out statements.

Restricted interests and activity

Language and social problems inhibit social play for children with autism. They do not engage in imaginative play and role playing and instead focus on repetition, some focusing on a subject of interest intensely.

Children with autism often stick to a rigid daily routine. Any variance to the routine may be upsetting to them and result in an extreme emotional response. Repetitive physical behaviors such as rocking, spinning, and arm flapping are also characteristic of autism. The repetitive behaviors are often self-soothing responses to sensory stimulation from the outside world.

Sensory problems

The sensory world poses a real problem to many autistic children, who seem overwhelmed by their own senses. Children with autism may ignore objects or become obsessed with them, continually watching the object or the movement of their fingers over it. Some children with autism may react to sounds by banging their head or flapping their fingers. Some high-functioning autistic adults who have written books about their childhood experiences report that sounds were often excruciating to them, forcing them to withdraw from their environment.

Diagnosis

There is no medical test for diagnosing autism. Diagnosis is made after careful observation and screening by parents, caregivers, and physicians. Early diagnosis is beneficial in treating the symptoms of autism. Some early warning signs are:

- avoiding eye contact
- avoiding physical contact such as hugs
- inability to play make-believe
- not pointing out interesting objects
- not responding to conversation directed at them
- practicing excessively repetitive behaviors
- repeating words or phrases
- losing skills and/or language after learning them

Once parents feel there is a problem or their pediatrician has identified developmental problems during well-baby checkups, they can seek out a developmental pediatrician for further diagnosis. There are several screening tests used. They are:

- Childhood Autism Rating Scale (CARS)—a test based on a 15-point scale where specific behaviors are observed by the physician
- Checklist for Autism in Toddlers (CHAT)—a test to detect autism in 18-month-olds that utilizes

questionnaires filled out by both the parents and the pediatrician

- Autism Screening Questionnaire—a 40-item questionnaire for diagnosing children four and older
- Screening Test for Autism in Two-Year-Olds—a direct observation of three skill areas, including play, motor imitation, and joint attention

Some children have a few of the symptoms of autism but not enough to be diagnosed with the "classical" form of the condition. Children who have autistic behavior but no problems with language may be diagnosed with Asperger syndrome by using the Autism Spectrum Screening Questionnaire, the Australian Scale for Asperger syndrome, or the Childhood Asperger Syndrome Test. Children who have no initial symptoms but who begin to show autistic behavior as they get older might be diagnosed with childhood disintegrative disorder (CDD), another autistic spectrum disorder. It is also important to rule out other problems that seem similar to autism.

Treatment

Because the symptoms of autism can vary greatly from one person to the next, there is not a single treatment that works for all individuals. A spectrum of interventions, including behavioral and educational training, diet and **nutrition**, alternative medicine and therapies, and medication, should be utilized and adjusted to treat each individual. The most strongly recommended treatment option is behavioral and educational training. Early **intervention** and treatment is key to helping autistic children grow into productive adults.

Educational and behavioral treatment

Several educational and behavioral treatments are:

- Applied Behavior Analysis (ABA)
- speech therapy
- occupational therapy, including sensory integration therapy
- social skills therapy, including play therapy

Typically, behavioral techniques are used to help the child respond and decrease symptoms. This might include positive **reinforcement** to boost language and social skills. This training includes structured, skill-oriented instruction designed to improve social and language abilities. Training needs to begin as early as possible, since early intervention appears to positively influence brain development.

Most autistic children respond to intervention at home as well as at school. Schools focus on areas in which the child may be delayed, such as in speech or socialization. As children with autism grow and move to different phases of childhood and adolescence, parents in collaboration with educators and physicians need to adapt the treatment to suit the needs of their child.

Medication

No single medication treats symptoms of autism; however, some medications have been used to combat specific needs in autistic children. Drugs can control epilepsy, which affects up to 20% of people with autism. Medication can also treat anxiety, **depression**, and hyperactivity. Medication must be individualized and adjusted as individuals develop.

Five types of drugs are sometimes prescribed to help the behavior problems of people with autism:

- stimulants, such as methylphenidate (Ritalin), can help with symptoms of hyperactivity and inattention
- antidepressants, such as fluvoxamine (Luvox), can help with symptoms of depression, anxiety, repetitive/ritualistic behaviors, and obsessive/compulsive-type symptoms
- opiate blockers, such as naltrexone (ReVia), may also improve ritualistic behaviors
- antipsychotics may be used to improve irritability and dampen aggression
- tranquilizers may be used to calm irritability and aggression and to quell anxiety

In 2010, reports were published regarding use of the drug **memantine**, traditionally used to treat Alzheimer's patients, in a study conducted by Michael Amen at Ohio State University. The study's hypothesis rested in similarities between autism and **Alzheimer's disease**, both of which involve a malfunction in the brain involving the chemical glutamate, which affects the patient's speech and interaction. While most drugs for autism only focus on lessening symptoms such as hyperactivity or repetitive actions, this study was designed to help improve communication, one of the core issues of autism. As of 2011, additional studies were ongoing.

Alternative treatment

Some parents report success with megavitamin therapy. Some studies have shown that vitamin B_6 with magnesium improves eye contact and speech and lessens tantrum behavior. Vitamin B_6 causes fewer side effects than other medications and is considered

QUESTIONS TO ASK YOUR DOCTOR

- How severe is my child's autism?
- Does my child have any associated medical problems that will need treatment along with autism?
- What sort of behaviors can I expect from my child?
- Is my child eligible for any early intervention programs available locally?
- What can I do at home to best help my child?
- What should I tell my other children/relatives/friends about this disorder?

safe when used in appropriate doses. However, not many health practitioners advocate its use in the treatment of autism, citing that the studies showing its benefit are flawed.

DMG (DIMETHYLGLYCINE). DMG (dimethylglycine), which is available in many health food stores, is legally classified as a food, not as a vitamin or drug. Some researchers claim that it improves speech in children with autism. Those who respond to this treatment will usually do so within a week. Again, many doctors do not feel that the studies are adequate to promote this treatment.

DIET. Many parents have seen beneficial effects from a gluten-free and casein-free diet. Gluten is found in the seeds of cereal plants such as wheat, barley, oats, and rye. Casein is a protein found in milk. Often people have sensitivities to these substances without realizing it. Many foods contain these substances as an ingredient; however, there are growing numbers of gluten-free and casein-free foods available for people that would like to eliminate them from their **diets**. Parents interested in using diet as a treatment should discuss with their child's doctor how to initiate an elimination diet.

EXERCISE. One researcher found that vigorous **exercise** (20 minutes or longer, three or four days a week) seems to decrease hyperactivity, aggression, self-injury, and other autistic symptoms.

Prognosis

Autism is treatable but not curable. With appropriate treatments adjusted as the patient ages, the symptoms of autism seem to improve. For the best prognosis, parents and caregivers should focus on providing the best therapies possible in order for children to develop to their highest potential. Because the incidence of autism seems to be increasing worldwide, enough so that the Centers for Disease Control and Prevention has voiced concern about its prevalence, there is more awareness of autism and more ongoing research efforts. People with autism have a normal life expectancy, and with proper intervention they can lead full lives.

Prevention

Until the cause of autism is discovered, prevention is not possible.

Resources

BOOKS

Behrman R.E., et al. *Nelson Textbook of Pediatrics.* 18th ed. Philadelphia: Saunders, 2007.

Bradley, W., et al. *Neurology in Clinical Practice.* 5th ed. Philadelphia: Butterworth-Heinemann, 2008.

Coplan, James. *Making Sense of Autistic Spectrum Disorders: Create the Brightest Future for Your Child with the Best Treatment Options.* New York: Bantam Books, 2010.

Glasberg, Beth. *Stop That Seemingly Senseless Behavior: FBA-Based Interventions for People with Autism.* Bethesda, MD: Woodbine House, 2008.

Offit, Paul A. *Autism's False Prophets: Bad Science, Risky Medicine, and the Search for a Cure.* New York: Columbia University Press, 2008.

PERIODICALS

Inglese, M. "Caring for Children with Autism Spectrum Disorder. Part I: Prevalence, Etiology, and Core Features." *Journal of Pediatric Nursing* 24 (2009): 41–48.

Ozonoff S., et al. "Recurrence Risk for Autism Spectrum Disorders: A Baby Siblings Research Consortium Study." *Pediatrics* 128, no. 3 (2011): e488–e495. http://dx.doi.org/10.1542/peds.2010-2825 (accessed October 11, 2011).

Pina-Camacho, L., et al. "Autism Spectrum Disorder: Does Neuroimaging Support the DSM-5 Proposal for a Symptom Dyad? A Systematic Review of Functional Magnetic Resonance Imaging and Diffusion Tensor Imaging Studies." *Journal of Autism and Developmental Disorders* (September 20, 2011) [e-pub ahead of print]. http://dx.doi.org/10.1007/s10803-011-1360-4 (accessed November 14, 2011).

Rice, C. "The Changing Prevalence of the Autism Spectrum Disorders." *American Family Physician* 29 (2011): 486–89.

WEBSITES

American Academy of Child and Adolescent Psychiatry. "Autism Resource Center." http://www.aacap.org/cs/Autism.ResourceCenter (accessed October 11, 2011).

Mayo Clinic staff. "Autism." MayoClinic.com. May 27, 2010. http://www.mayoclinic.com/print/autism/DS00348 (accessed October 11, 2011).

MedlinePlus. "Autism." U.S. National Library of Medicine, National Institutes of Health. April 7, 2011. http://www.nlm.nih.gov/medlineplus/autism.html (accessed October 11, 2011).

National Institute of Neurological Disorders and Stroke. "Autism Fact Sheet." U.S. National Institutes of Health. http://www.ninds.nih.gov/disorders/autism/detail_autism.htm (accessed November 14, 2011).

ORGANIZATIONS

American Academy of Child and Adolescent Psychiatry, 3615 Wisconsin Ave. NW, Washington, DC, 20016-3007, (202) 966-7300, Fax: (202) 966-2891, http://aacap.org.

American Psychiatric Association, 1000 Wilson Blvd., Ste. 1825, Arlington, VA, 22209-3901, (703) 907-7300, apa@psych.org, http://www.psych.org.

Autism Network International, PO Box 35448, Syracuse, NY, 13235-5448, http://autreat.com.

Autism Society of America, 4340 East-West Hwy., Ste. 350, Bethesda, MD, 20814, (301) 657-0881, (800) 328-8476, http://www.autism-society.org.

Autism Speaks, 1 East 33rd Street, 4th Fl., New York, NY, 10016, (212) 252-8584, Fax: (212) 252-8676, (888) AUTISM2 (288-4762), contactus@autismspeaks.org, http://www.autismspeaks.org.

Carol A. Turkington
Tish Davidson, AM
Rosalyn Carson-DeWitt

Autism spectrum disorders *see* **Asperger syndrome; Autism; Childhood disintegrative disorder; Pervasive developmental disorders**

Aventyl *see* **Nortriptyline**

Aversion therapy

Definition

Aversion therapy is a type of **cognitive-behavioral therapy** (CBT) in which an undesirable or harmful behavior is paired with an aversive or noxious stimulus in an attempt to reduce or eliminate the undesirable behavior. A form of classical conditioning, aversion therapy is based on the theory that the patient will eventually avoid the behavior because it has come to be associated with pain, unpleasantness, or unhappiness.

Purpose

The purpose of aversion therapy is to decrease or eliminate undesirable behaviors. Aversion therapy has been used since 1932 to treat alcohol and drug abuse, and this is remains its most common application. In addition to alcohol, aversion therapy is used to treat addictions to marijuana, **amphetamines** such as crystal meth, and opiates, including oxycodone and other prescription painkillers. It also is sometimes used to treat smoking, gambling **addiction**, **kleptomania** (the **compulsion** to steal), **paraphilias** (socially unacceptable sexual practices), and violent behaviors. Mild aversion therapy, followed by positive **reinforcement**, has been successfully used to treat **pica**—the compulsion to eat non-foods, such as paper or dirt, which affects 10%–32% of children between the ages of one and six, as well as some women during pregnancy. Aversion therapy is also sometimes used in conjunction with dermatologic and psychiatric treatments for dermatitis artefacta—the deliberate and conscious self-infliction of skin lesions. Aversion therapy is a common self-help treatment for such benign habits as nail biting or even writer's block.

Description

Like other behavioral therapies, aversion therapy is based on learning theory—the concept that all behaviors are learned and that, under the right circumstances, undesirable behaviors can be unlearned. Aversion therapy is an application of the branch of learning theory called classical conditioning. The best-known example of classical conditioning is Pavlov's dogs, who were conditioned to salivate in response to a bell by repeatedly pairing bell-ringing with feeding.

Unlike insight-oriented therapies, which focus on revealing unconscious motives in order to produce change, aversion therapy focuses on changing a specific behavior by matching it with an unpleasant or aversive stimulus. The unpleasant feelings or sensations eventually come to be associated with the undesirable behavior, causing the behavior to decrease in frequency or stop altogether. Aversion therapy differs from aversive procedures, which are behavioral therapies based on operant conditioning and in which the aversive stimulus, usually called a punishment, is presented after the behavior rather than together with it.

The particulars of aversion therapy depend on the behavior to be changed and the aversive stimulus. The therapy may be administered on either an inpatient or outpatient basis and either alone as a single **intervention** or as part of a multifaceted treatment program. In addition to pairing the undesirable behavior with aversive stimuli, aversion therapy sometimes pairs avoidance of the behavior with positive images, such as employment, education, or other socially appropriate activities.

Aversion therapy for alcohol or drug addiction attempts to change positive emotional associations with the substance to negative associations with the sight, smell, or taste of the abused substance. The most commonly administered aversion therapy is the use of an emetic or vomiting-producing medication to discourage alcohol consumption. **Disulfiram** (DSF) (Antabuse) is approved by the U.S. Food and Drug Administration (FDA) and has been used for alcohol-aversion therapy for more than half a century. DSF inhibits the enzyme aldehyde dehydrogenase (ALDH), which breaks down alcohol in the body. Inhibition of ALDH results in the buildup of acetaldehyde, which causes a violent noxious reaction—such as flushing, nausea, vomiting, and palpitations—when alcohol is consumed.

Various aversion therapies to help smokers to quit have been attempted with little success. The only method that has met with any success at all is rapid smoking, in which patients rapidly chain smoke cigarettes until they become sick. This method is not recommended because it is unhealthy and only occasionally successful.

Classical aversion therapy involves the administration of electric shocks. In the past, shocks were inflicted by the therapist. In the early 2010s, if electroshock aversion therapy is used, patients shock themselves using a portable battery-operated device, usually attached to their arm or leg. The shock level is uncomfortable and perhaps even painful, but not intensely painful, dangerous, or damaging. Patients shock themselves while thinking about the undesirable behavior. Sometimes pictures or other props associated with the behavior are used to reinforce the imagined behavior. Eventually the patient may become uncomfortable thinking about the behavior and the desire to engage in it may lessen or disappear.

Other aversion therapies are also self-administered. An example of a self-help aversion therapy is putting red pepper or a bitter substance on one's fingernails to discourage nail biting. Another type involves practicing a mildly painful technique, such as holding one's breath until it becomes uncomfortable, when faced with temptation or an urge for the undesirable behavior. This method has been used to treat kleptomania. Other self-help methods for minor undesirable behaviors include snapping an elastic band on the wrist when an undesirable thought or temptation is present.

A technique called **covert sensitization** or covert conditioning, developed by the American **psychologist** Joseph Cautela, is a less intrusive form of aversion therapy. Rather than using chemical aversions (such as Antabuse) or electroshock, covert sensitization utilizes imagined aversions. For example, images of an undesirable behavior, such as smoking, might be systematically paired with images of aversive stimuli, such as nausea and vomiting.

Benefits

Aversion therapy can be moderately successful for reducing or eliminating certain undesirable behaviors, especially at the outset of drug or alcohol rehabilitation. Drug and alcohol users link various environmental stimuli, such as taste, smell, sight, or surroundings, with pleasure associated with substance use. Aversive stimuli under medically supervised conditions can substitute these positive emotional associations with negative associations such as nausea and vomiting. Studies have found that aversion therapy can result in significantly improved rates of drug or alcohol abstinence. Aversion therapy has been found to be less effective for **smoking cessation**.

Covert sensitization has been used successfully to treat alcoholism, cigarette smoking, compulsive gambling, and juvenile delinquency. One study of six different cases found covert sensitization to be a fast and cost-effective treatment for a fingernail biter, a marijuana smoker, a cigarette smoker, an alcoholic, an obese patient, and a chocolate addict. All six patients eliminated their undesirable behavior and maintained abstinence throughout the follow-up period.

Precautions

Some aversion therapies, especially electroshock therapy, are potentially dangerous and should only be practiced in specialized clinics under the supervision of an experienced medical professional. Electroshock equipment should be of the highest quality, and the patient should be in control of the intensity at all times. Most importantly, aversion therapy should never be used coercively.

During the twentieth century, aversion therapy frequently involved pairing undesirable thoughts or behaviors with electric shocks of mild (faradic) but varying intensities or with potent emetics. Sometimes the consequences were disastrous, including fatalities, mental illness, and **suicide**. In some of the most egregious examples, electroshock aversion therapy was used to attempt to "cure" homosexuality. Patients were shown erotic same-sex images and if they became aroused, they received electric shocks, sometimes to the genitalia.

KEY TERMS

Antabuse—Trade name for disulfiram (DSF), a chemical used to treat alcoholism by causing a severe physiological reaction to any amount of alcohol.

Aversant—A chemical or medication with unpleasant effects that is used in aversion therapy.

Aversion—A strong feeling of unpleasantness, dislike, or disgust; stimulated in aversion therapy to reduce or eliminate an undesirable behavior.

Classical conditioning—A psychological process in which a neutral stimulus is repeatedly paired with a stimulus that produces a specific response, until the previously neutral stimulus also produces the response.

Cognitive-behavioral therapy (CBT)—A type of psychotherapy in which people learn to recognize and change negative and self-defeating patterns of thinking and behavior.

Compliance—Adherence to a treatment plan or medication regimen.

Covert sensitization or conditioning—A form of aversion therapy in which the patient imagines or views images of an undesirable behavior, followed by imagining or viewing images of an aversive consequence.

Dermatitis artefacta—A disorder characterized by the deliberate and conscious self-infliction of skin lesions.

Emetic—A medication that causes vomiting; usually used to treat poisoning but also used in aversion therapy.

Faradic—A type of discontinuous alternating electric current sometimes used in aversion therapy; named for the nineteenth-century British physicist Michael Faraday.

Operant conditioning—A psychological process in which a desired behavior or increasingly close approximations of the desired behavior are followed with positive or rewarding stimuli.

Paraphilia—Unusual or socially unacceptable sexual thoughts or behaviors.

Pica—Abnormal cravings for or eating of non-food substances, such as ashes or chalk, caused by mental illness or a nutritional deficiency.

Stimulus—An agent that directly elicits a response, such as a thought, emotion, or action, including images, smells, sounds, words, or ideas. In aversion therapy, the stimulus is typically a mild electric shock or a medication that produces unpleasant effects.

Sometimes patients could stop the shock and the image was replaced with an opposite-sex image. With another type of aversion therapy, patients were injected with a nausea-inducing drug while looking at images of homosexual activity and with a euphoria-inducing drug while viewing images of heterosexual activity. These types of aversion therapy were not only ineffectual but were later considered abusive. Both the **American Psychological Association** and the **American Psychiatric Association** declare aversion therapy for homosexuality to be a violation of professional guidelines and codes of conduct. The practice is illegal in some countries.

Although the use of electroshock is now rare, aversion therapy remains controversial. Although the foul odors, nasty tastes, and loud noises that are sometimes employed as aversive stimuli may be merely unpleasant, chemicals and medications can be physically painful and in some cases can cause severe illness. Antabuse may cause severe reactions if even a very small amount alcohol is inadvertently consumed in a sauce or vinegar within a few weeks of taking the drug. Alcohol-containing medications applied to the skin or fumes containing alcohol can also cause reactions.

There are also ethical concerns about aversion therapy. Social critics and the general public alike often consider this type of treatment to be punitive and morally objectionable. In the past, aversion therapy was sometimes used to treat mental illnesses, such as **schizophrenia**, as well as intellectual and developmental disabilities, with negative consequences. Advocates for special patient populations have called for an end to the use of all aversive stimuli, arguing that all aversive procedures are coercive and use an unnecessary degree of control or manipulation to modify behavior. These concerns have frequently been portrayed in the media. Anthony Burgess's 1962 novel *A Clockwork Orange* (and the subsequent Stanley Kubrick film) depicted a particularly brutal, and ultimately unsuccessful, form of aversion therapy for violent criminal behavior. Aversion conditioning was also explored in Aldous Huxley's 1932 novel

QUESTIONS TO ASK YOUR DOCTOR

- Would you recommend that I undergo aversion therapy? Why or why not?
- What would be involved in my aversion therapy?
- Are there unpleasant side effects to aversion therapy?
- Is aversion therapy likely to be successful?

Brave New World, in Ken Kesey's 1962 novel and the subsequent film *One Flew Over the Cuckoo's Nest*, and in the film *A Beautiful Mind*, about John Forbes Nash Jr., the Nobel Laureate in economics whose schizophrenia was treated with aversion therapy.

In addition to ethical considerations, the unpleasant effects of aversion therapy often lead to poor **compliance**, high treatment dropout rates, and potentially hostile and aggressive patients. Studies have generally shown that aversion therapy, even for **substance abuse**, is significantly less effective than positive behavioral change therapies that focus on rewards.

Preparation

In general, no particular preparation is required for aversion therapy. However, Antabuse should never be given to a patient who has consumed alcohol within at least the past 12 hours.

Aftercare

Most aversion therapies do not require aftercare. However, reactions to Antabuse can occur up to two weeks after treatment, so it is very important that patients treated with this drug avoid all contact with alcohol, including alcohol-containing fumes.

Risks

Aversion therapy with chemicals or medications has the potential to worsen heart, lung, or gastrointestinal problems. Some patients undergoing aversion therapy, especially treatment with powerful chemical or pharmacological aversive stimuli, have become negative, hostile, or aggressive. Electroshock aversion therapy may increase anxiety and anxiety-related symptoms that can interfere with the conditioning process, leading to decreased acceptance of the treatment. Finally, aversion therapy has great potential for patient abuse.

Research and general acceptance

Although aversion therapy has some adherents, especially for treating substance abuse, there is widespread opposition to the practice, both among clinicians and the general public. In addition to ethical objections, there are very few studies indicating its effectiveness. In general, operant conditioning with positive rewards is considered more effective and less intrusive than aversion therapy. However, covert sensitization may be moderately effective, is nonintrusive, and does not carry the same risks as other types of aversion therapy.

Resources

BOOKS

Spiegler, Michael D., and David C. Guevremont. *Contemporary Behavior Therapy*. Belmont, CA: Wadsworth, Cengage Learning, 2010. See esp. chap. 7, "Deceleration Behavior Therapy: Differential Reinforcement, Punishment, and Aversion Therapy."

PERIODICALS

"Smoking Cessation Interventions and Strategies." *Australian Nursing Journal* 16, no. 6 (December 2008/January 2009): 29–32.

Witkiewitz, Katie, and G. Alan Marlatt. "Behavioral Therapy Across the Spectrum." *Alcohol Research & Health* 33, no. 4 (2011): 313–19. http://pubs.niaaa.nih.gov/publications/arh334/313-319.htm (accessed December 15, 2011).

WEBSITES

"Aversion Therapy Treatment." Schick Shadel Hospital. http://schickshadel.com/programs/aversion_therapy_treatment.php (accessed September 8, 2011).

ORGANIZATIONS

American Psychological Association, 750 1st St., NE, Washington, DC, 20002-4242, (202) 336-5500; TDD/TTY: (202) 336-6123, (800) 374-2721, http://www.apa.org.

Mental Health America, 2000 N Beauregard St., 6th Fl., Alexandria, VA, 22311, (703) 684-7722, (800) 969-6642, Fax: (703) 684-5968, http://www.nmha.org.

John Garrison, PhD
Emily Jane Willingham, PhD
Margaret Alic, PhD

Avoidant personality disorder

Definition

Avoidant personality disorder (AvPD), also referred to as anxious personality disorder or anxious (avoidant) personality disorder, is characterized by hypersensitivity to rejection and criticism, desire for uncritical acceptance by others, social withdrawal despite a desire for affection and acceptance, and low self-esteem. The behavior patterns associated with avoidant personality disorder are persistent and severe, impairing a person's ability to work with others or maintain social relationships.

Demographics

Avoidant personality disorder appears to be as frequent in males as in females. It affects between 0.5% and 1.0% of adults in the general North American population, but it has been diagnosed in approximately 10% of clinical outpatients.

Description

People who are diagnosed with avoidant personality disorder desire to be in relationships with others but lack the skills and confidence needed to engage in social interactions. In order to protect themselves from anticipated criticism or ridicule, they withdraw from other people. This avoidance of interaction tends to isolate them from meaningful relationships and serves to reinforce their feelings of nervousness and awkwardness in social situations.

The behavior of people with avoidant personality disorder is characterized by social withdrawal, **shyness**, distrustfulness, and emotional distance. People with AvPD tend to be very cautious when they speak, and they convey a general impression of awkwardness in their manner. Most are highly self-conscious and self-critical about their problems relating to others.

There are varying levels of avoidant personality disorder. Some persons may be shy or social phobic and avoid forming relationships entirely. Others may be able to form relationships but have difficulty sustaining them in the long term. If a person with AvPD can manage long-term relationships, he or she may be unable to sever them when needed (e.g., moving out of his or her parent's house).

Causes and symptoms

Causes

The cause of avoidant personality disorder is not clearly defined and may be influenced by a combination of social, genetic, and biological factors. Avoidant personality traits typically appear in childhood, with signs of excessive shyness and fear when the child confronts new people and situations. These characteristics are developmentally appropriate emotions for children, however, and do not necessarily mean that a pattern of avoidant personality disorder will continue into adulthood. When shyness, unfounded fear of rejection, hypersensitivity to criticism, and a pattern of social avoidance persist and intensify through adolescence and young adulthood, a **diagnosis** of avoidant personality disorder is often indicated.

Many persons diagnosed with avoidant personality disorder have had painful early experiences of chronic parental criticism and rejection. The need to bond with the rejecting parent makes the avoidant person hungry for relationships but their longing gradually develops into a defensive shell of self-protection against repeated parental criticisms. Ridicule or rejection by peers further reinforces the young person's pattern of social withdrawal and contributes to their fear of social contact.

Symptoms

The ***Diagnostic and Statistical Manual of Mental Disorders,*** (fourth edition, text revision or *DSM-IV-TR*) specifies seven diagnostic criteria for avoidant personality disorder:

- The person avoids occupational activities that require significant interpersonal contact. Job interviews or promotions may be turned down because the person's own perceptions of his or her abilities do not match the job description.
- The person is reluctant to participate in social involvement without clear assurance that he or she will be accepted. People with this disorder assume other people are not safe to trust until proven otherwise. Others must offer repeated support and encouragement in order to persuade them to participate in a social event.
- The person fears being shamed or ridiculed in close relationships. As a result, people with this disorder become overly alert to behavioral cues that may indicate disapproval or rejection. They will flee a situation in which they believe that others might turn against them.
- The person is preoccupied with being criticized or rejected. Much mental and physical energy is spent brooding about and avoiding situations perceived as "dangerous."
- The person is inhibited in unfamiliar social situations due to feelings of inadequacy. Low self-esteem undermines his or her confidence in meeting and conversing with new acquaintances.
- The person regards him- or herself as socially inept. This self-disparagement is especially apparent when the person must make social contacts with strangers. People with avoidant personality disorder perceive themselves as unappealing or inferior to others.

- The person is reluctant to take social risks, in order to avoid possible humiliation. Persons with AvPD seek interactions that promise the greatest amount of acceptance while minimizing the likelihood of embarrassment or rejection. They might go to a school dance, for example, but remain in one corner chatting with close friends rather than going out on the dance floor with someone they do not know well.

Diagnosis

Many individuals exhibit some avoidant behaviors at one point or another in their lives. Occasional feelings of self-doubt and fear in new and unfamiliar social or personal relationships are not unusual, nor are they unhealthy, as these situations may trigger feelings of inadequacy and the wish to hide from social contact in even the most self-confident individuals. An example would be the anxious hesitancy of a new immigrant in a country with a different language and customs. Avoidant characteristics are regarded as meeting the diagnostic criteria for a personality disorder only when they begin to have a long-term negative impact on the affected person; they lead to functional impairment by significantly altering occupational choice or lifestyle, or otherwise impinging on quality of life; and they cause significant emotional distress.

Avoidant personality disorder can occur in conjunction with other social phobias, mood and **anxiety disorders**, and **personality disorders**. The diagnosis may be complicated by the fact that avoidant personality disorder may be either the cause or result of other mood and anxiety disorders. For example, individuals who have **major depressive disorder** may begin to withdraw from social situations and experience feelings of worthlessness, symptoms that are also prominent features of avoidant personality disorder. On the other hand, the insecurity and isolation that are symptoms of avoidant personality disorder can trigger feelings of **depression**.

The characteristics of avoidant personality disorder may resemble those found in both schizoid and schizotypal personality disorders. Persons with these disorders are prone to social isolation. Those diagnosed with avoidant personality disorder, however, differ from those with schizoid or schizotypal disorder, because they want to have relationships with others but are prevented by their social insecurities. Persons diagnosed with schizoid and schizotypal personality disorders, on the other hand, usually prefer social isolation.

Personality disorders are usually diagnosed following a complete medical history and an interview with the patient. Although there are no laboratory tests for personality disorders, the doctor may give the patient a physical examination to rule out the possibility that a general medical condition is affecting the patient's behavior. For example, people with disorders of the digestive tract may avoid social occasions for fear of a sudden attack of diarrhea or the need to vomit. If the interview with the patient suggests a diagnosis of avoidant personality disorder, the doctor may administer a diagnostic questionnaire or another type of assessment tool.

Assessment tools helpful in diagnosing avoidant personality disorder include:

- **Minnesota Multiphasic Personality Inventory** (MMPI)
- Millon Clinical Multiaxial Inventory (MCMI)
- Rorschach Psychodiagnostic Test
- **Thematic Apperception Test** (TAT)

In diagnosis, it is important to distinguish between the fear of rejection that characterizes avoidant personality disorder from the inability to form relationships that characterizes schizoid patients. Similarly, it is important to distinguish between the fear of relationships characteristic of AvPD and a healthy, natural desire to be alone.

Proposed changes for the fifth edition of the *DSM* (*DSM-5*, 2013) include reorganizing the category of personality disorders (other disorders include **antisocial personality disorder**, **borderline personality disorder**, **narcissistic personality disorder**, **obsessive-compulsive personality disorder**, and **schizotypal personality disorder**). The specific diagnostic criteria for avoidant personality disorder will change but will still center on the same core symptoms—impairments in identity, self-direction, empathy, and intimacy, along with the traits of withdrawal, avoidance, absence of enjoyment in life, and anxiety.

Treatment

The general goal of treatment in avoidant personality disorder is improvement of self-esteem and confidence. As the patient's self-confidence and social skills improve, he or she will become more resilient to potential or real criticism by others.

Psychodynamically oriented therapies

These approaches are usually supportive; the therapist empathizes with the patient's strong sense of shame and inadequacy in order to create a relationship of trust. Therapy usually moves slowly at first, because persons with avoidant personality disorder are mistrustful of others. Treatment that probes into their emotional state too quickly may result in more protective withdrawal by the patient. As trust is established and the patient feels safer discussing details of his or her situation, the patient may be able to draw important connections between his or her deeply felt sense of shame and the resultant behavior in social situations.

Cognitive-behavioral therapy

Cognitive-behavioral therapy (CBT) may be helpful in treating individuals with avoidant personality disorder. This approach assumes that faulty thinking patterns underlie the personality disorder, and therefore focuses on changing distorted cognitive patterns by examining the validity of the assumptions behind them. If a patient feels inferior to his or her peers, a cognitive therapist would test the reality of these assumptions by asking the patient to name friends and family who enjoy his or her company, or to describe past social encounters that were fulfilling. By showing the patient that others value his or her company and that social situations can be enjoyable, the irrationality of the patient's social fears and insecurities are exposed. This process is known as cognitive restructuring.

Group therapy

Group therapy helps provide patients with social experiences that expose them to feedback from others in a safe, controlled environment. Persons with avoidant personality disorder may, however, be reluctant to enter group therapy due to their fear of social rejection. The empathetic environment of the group setting can help each member overcome his or her social anxieties. **Social skills training** can also be incorporated into group therapy to enhance social awareness and feedback.

Family and marital therapy

Family or couple therapy can be helpful for a patient who wants to break out of a family pattern that reinforces the avoidant behavior. The focus of marital therapy would include attempting to break the cycle of rejection, criticism or ridicule that typically characterizes most avoidant marriages. Other strategies include helping the couple to develop constructive ways of relating to one another without shame.

Medications

The use of **monoamine oxidase inhibitors (MAOIs)** has proven useful in helping patients with avoidant personality disorder to control symptoms of social unease and experience initial success. The major drawback of these medications is limitations on the patient's diet. People taking **MAOIs** must avoid foods containing a substance known as tyramine, which is found in most cheeses, liver, red wines, sherry, vermouth, beans with broad pods, soy sauce, sauerkraut, and meat extracts.

KEY TERMS

Cognitive restructuring—An approach to psychotherapy that focuses on helping patients examine distorted patterns of perception and thought in order to change their emotional responses to people and situations.

Monoamine oxidase inhibitors (MAOIs)—A group of antidepressant drugs that decreases the activity of monoamine oxidase, a neurotransmitter found in the brain that affects mood. MAOIs are also used in the treatment of avoidant personality disorder.

Supportive—An approach to psychotherapy that seeks to encourage the patient or offer emotional support to him or her, as distinct from insight-oriented or educational approaches to treatment.

Prognosis

Higher-functioning persons with avoidant personality disorder can generally be expected to improve their social awareness and improve their social skills to some degree. Because of the significant social fear and deep-seated feelings of inferiority, these patterns usually do not change dramatically. Lower-functioning persons are likely to drop out of treatment if they become too anxious.

Prevention

Since avoidant personality disorder usually originates in the patient's family of origin, the only known preventive measure is a nurturing, emotionally stimulating, and expressive family environment.

Resources

BOOKS

American Psychiatric Association. *Diagnostic and Statistical Manual of Mental Disorders*. 4th ed., text rev. Washington, DC: American Psychiatric Publishing, 2000.

Kantor, Martin. *Distancing: Avoidant Personality Disorder*, Revised and expanded. Westport, CT: Praeger, 2003.

Newman, Cory F., and Randy Fingerhut. "Psychotherapy for Avoidant Personality Disorder." In *Oxford Textbook of Psychotherapy*, edited by Glen O. Gabbard, Judith S. Beck, and Jeremy Holmes. Oxford, UK: Oxford University Press, 2005.

Pretzer, James , Barbara Fleming, and Karen M. Simon. *Clinical Applications of Cognitive Therapy*. 2nd ed. New York: Springer, 2004.

Rasmussen, Paul R. *The Personality-Guided Cognitive-Behavioral Therapy*. Washington, DC: American Psychological Association, 2005.

Silverstein, Marshall L. *Disorders of the Self: A Personality-Guided Approach*. Washington, DC: American Psychological Association, 2007.

PERIODICALS

Carter, S. A., and K. D. Wu. "Relations among Symptoms of Social Phobia Subtypes, Avoidant Personality Disorder, Panic, and Depression." *Behavior Therapy* 41, no. 1 (2010): 2–13.

Emmelkamp, Paul M., et al. "Comparison of Brief Dynamic and Cognitive-Behavioural Therapies in Avoidant Personality Disorder." *British Journal of Psychiatry* 189, no. 1 (July 2006): 60–64.

Hopwood, C. J., et al. "Hierarchical Relationships Between Borderline, Schizotypal, Avoidant and Obsessive-Compulsive Personality Disorders." *Acta Psychiatrica Scandinavica* 113, no. 5 (May 2006): 430–39.

Huprich, Steven K. "Differentiating Avoidant and Depressive Personality Disorders." *Journal of Personality Disorders* 19, no. 6 (December 2005): 659–73.

Huprich, Steven K., Mark Zimmerman, and Iwona Chelminski. "Disentangling Depressive Personality Disorder from Avoidant, Borderline, and Obsessive-Compulsive Personality Disorders." *Comprehensive Psychiatry* 47, no. 4 (July–August 2006): 298–306.

Olssøn, Ingrid, and Alv A. Dahl. "Avoidant Personality Problems—Their Association with Somatic and Mental Health, Lifestyle, and Social Network. A Community-Based Study." *Comprehensive Psychiatry* (December 5, 2011) [e-pub ahead of print]. http://dx.doi.org/10.1016/j.comppsych.2011.10.007 (accessed December 15, 2011).

Ralevski, E., et al. "Avoidant Personality Disorder and Social Phobia: Distinct Enough to Be Separate Disorders?" *Acta Psychiatrica Scandinavica* 112, no. 3 (September 2005): 208–14.

Reich, James. "Avoidant Personality Disorder and its Relationship to Social Phobia." *Current Psychiatry Reports* 11, no. 1 (2009): 89–93. http://dx.doi.org/10.1007/s11920-009-0014-0 (accessed December 14, 2011).

Ripoll, L. H., J. Triebwasser, and L.J. Siever. "Evidence-Based Pharmacotherapy for Personality Disorders." *International Journal of Neuropsychopharmacology* 14, no. 9 (2011): 1257–88.

ORGANIZATIONS

American Psychiatric Association, 1000 Wilson Blvd., Ste. 1825, Arlington, VA, 22209-3901, (703) 907-7300, apa@psych.org, http://www.psych.org.

Gary Gilles, MA
Paula Ford-Martin, MA
Ruth A. Wienclaw, PhD

B

Barbiturates

Definition

Barbiturates are a large class of drugs used primarily for sedation, general anesthesia, and as a treatment for some types of epilepsy. In the past, barbiturates were used to sedate people with anxiety and similar disorders, but they have been largely replaced by **benzodiazepines**. The most drugs within the barbiturate family are the generics of amobarbital, aprobarbital, butabarbital, butalbital, mephobarbital, methohexital, pentobarbital, phenobarbital, and secobarbital.

Purpose

Barbiturates have been used to sedate patients prior to surgery as well as to produce general anesthesia, to induce sleep in patients with **insomnia**, to sedate patients with **anxiety disorders**, and to treat some forms of epilepsy. These drugs are highly addictive and are often abused as recreational drugs. Although still commercially available, barbiturates such as amobarbital, pentobarbital, and secobarbital are no longer routinely recommended for insomnia because of their ability to cause dependence, tolerance, and withdrawal. In general, barbiturates lose their efficacy when they are used to treat insomnia on a daily basis for more than two weeks. These drugs also have significant side effects when taken in large doses and can cause respiratory failure and death. Because of the high potential for abuse and adverse side effects, newer medicines, primarily benzodiazepines, have largely replaced barbiturates. Barbiturates still in use include butabarbital and secobarbital to treat insomnia and phenobarbital to treat **seizures**.

Description

The therapeutic effects of barbiturates as a class of drugs are all related to their ability to depress the central nervous system, producing sedation. At high enough doses and with certain preparations, they can induce sleep. Barbiturates were commonly prescribed in the 1960s and 1970s for treating anxiety and insomnia but were largely abused. Because the prescription of barbiturates has declined with the advent of safer drugs, rates of abuse have declined as well; however, a study presented at the American Association for Geriatric Psychiatry annual meeting in 2010 revealed that barbiturates are the primary drug used in geriatric suicides.

Some generic barbiturates (and their brand names) are:

- amobarbital (Amytal Sodium)
- amobarbital/secobarbital combination (Tuinal)
- aprobarbital (Alurate)
- butabarbital (Busodium, Butisol Sodium)
- butalbital (Fiorinal), hexobarbital (Sombulex)
- mephobarbital (Mebaral)
- methohexital (Brevital)
- pentobarbital (Nembutal)
- phenobarbital (Luminal)
- secobarbital (Seconal)
- talbutal (Lotusate)
- thiobarbital (Ibition)

Recommended dosage

Butabarbital is taken before bed if used to treat insomnia or may be taken up to four times a day to treat anxiety. Secobarbital is also taken for insomnia. For both conditions, usage should be evaluated after 7–10 days; if symptoms have not improved within two weeks, it is not likely that the condition will improve by continued use of the drug. Phenobarbital may be taken up to three times a day to treat uncontrolled seizures. Patients should never take more than the prescribed dose, nor should they take the drugs for longer than the intended time.

Precautions

Barbiturate abuse can occur when taking these drugs for a long period of time, in higher than prescribed doses, or without a prescription. Long-term barbiturate use should be avoided unless there is a strong medical need, such as uncontrolled seizures. Abuse of barbiturates can lead to **addiction**, along with serious impairment and distress to both mind and body. Women addicted to barbiturates while pregnant can give birth to addicted babies who may suffer withdrawal symptoms after birth. Symptoms of withdrawal in babies and adults include tremor, insomnia, and general agitation. Severe withdrawal in adults may progress to hallucinations and **psychosis**. Because of the severe risks associated with barbiturate use, it is against U.S. law to use these drugs without a prescription from a medical professional, and when a condition requires long-term drug use, alternative medications should be prescribed whenever possible.

Children who are hyperactive should not receive phenobarbital or other barbiturates. Paradoxically, some children become stimulated and hyperactive after receiving barbiturates.

The use of barbiturates in the elderly (over age 65 years) should be watched closely. Elderly patients must be carefully monitored for confusion, agitation, **delirium**, and excitement if they take barbiturates. Barbiturates should be avoided in elderly patients who are receiving drugs for other mental disorders such as **schizophrenia** or **depression**.

Women should be aware that barbiturate use can make hormonal birth control pills containing estrogen less effective. Women should not use barbiturates during pregnancy unless absolutely necessary. In these cases, they should take the minimum amount required to control the problem. Barbiturate use by pregnant women has been associated with increased risk of fetal damage, newborn bleeding problems, bleeding during childbirth, and, if occurring in the final three months of gestation, dependency in the newborn with attendant withdrawal effects after birth. One study has found a potential link between barbiturate use during pregnancy and **brain** tumors in the infant. Women who are breastfeeding should not take barbiturates because these drugs enter the breast milk and may cause serious side effects in the nursing baby.

People should not drive, operate heavy equipment, or perform other activities requiring mental alertness while taking barbiturates. Some patients taking butabarbital or secobarbital for insomnia have engaged in sleep-related behaviors, including eating, talking, and even driving while asleep, with no recollection of the events. If barbiturates are being used to treat insomnia, they should only be taken when the patient is able to have a full night's sleep (seven to eight hours).

KEY TERMS

Benzene—A colorless toxic liquid with a chemical formula of C_6H_6, where C stands for carbon and H for hydrogen.

Benzodiazepines—A group of drugs used to induce sleep, relieve anxiety, produce sedation, and prevent seizures; generally, such drugs are used as hypnotics in high doses, anxiolytics in medium does, and sedatives in low doses.

Diazepine—A seven-membered unsaturated heterocyclic compound with two nitrogen atoms and three double bonds.

Dependence—A state in which a person requires a steady concentration of a particular substance to avoid experiencing withdrawal symptoms.

Epilepsy—A medical condition involving episodes of irregular electrical discharge within the brain that causes impairment or loss of consciousness, followed by convulsions.

Recreational drugs—The use of a drug with the intention of creating a psychoactive (heightened) mental experience; for the most part, such use is illegal.

Tolerance—The requirement for higher doses of a substance or more frequent engagement in an activity to achieve the same effect.

Side effects

The most common side effect of barbiturate use is drowsiness. Less common side effects include agitation, confusion, breathing difficulties, abnormally low blood pressure, nausea, vomiting, constipation, lowered body temperature, decreased heart rate, movement difficulty, nightmares, anxiety, nervousness, mental depression, and dizziness. Rare but reported side effects include fever, headache, anemia, allergic reactions, and liver damage.

Interactions

Patients should always tell their doctor and dentist when they are taking barbiturates. Barbiturates should generally not be taken with other drugs used to treat mental disorders. In addition, patients should inform their healthcare providers about any health or medical problems, especially a history of alcohol or drug abuse or problems with anemia, asthma, diabetes, hyperthyroid, or kidney or liver disease, among others.

QUESTIONS TO ASK YOUR DOCTOR

- Why are you prescribing this medication?
- What alternative medications are available?
- What are the possible side effects?
- How long will I need to take the medication?

There are a number of drugs that barbiturates should not be combined with, because the barbiturates may increase the rate of breakdown of these drugs, thus reducing their availability to the body. These drugs include oral corticosteroids such as predisolone, methylprednisolone, prednisone, or dexamethasone; estrogen and oral contraceptives; blood-thinning medications such as warfarin (Coumadin); the antibiotic doxycycline (Vibramycin); and anticonvulsants such as phenytoin (Dilantin). Barbiturates may also lower the amount of absorption of vitamins D and K.

Because barbiturates work on the central nervous system, they may add to the effects of alcohol and other drugs that slow the central nervous system, such as antihistamines, cold medicine, allergy medicine, sleep aids, medicine for seizures, tranquilizers, some pain relievers, and muscle relaxants. They may also add to the effects of anesthetics, including those used for dental procedures. The combined effects of barbiturates and alcohol or other CNS depressants (drugs that slow the central nervous system) can be very dangerous, leading to unconsciousness and even death. Individuals who are taking barbiturates should not drink alcohol and should check with their physician before taking any medicines classified as CNS depressants.

Taking an overdose of barbiturates or combining barbiturates with alcohol or other central nervous system depressants can cause unconsciousness and even death. Anyone who shows signs of an overdose or a reaction to combining barbiturates with alcohol or other drugs should get emergency medical help immediately. Signs include:

- severe drowsiness
- breathing problems
- slurred speech
- staggering
- slow heartbeat
- excessive confusion
- severe weakness

Resources

BOOKS

Goodman, Louis S., et al. *Goodman & Gilman's The Pharmacological Basis of Therapeutics,* 12th ed. New York: McGraw-Hill Medical, 2011.

Henn, Debra, and Deborah de Eugenio, eds. *Barbiturates.* New York: Chelsea House, 2007.

Karch, A. M. *Lippincott's Nursing Drug Guide.* Springhouse, PA: Lippincott Williams & Wilkins, 2007.

Liska, Ken. *Drugs and the Human Body: With Implications for Society.* Upper Saddle River, NJ: Pearson Prentice Hall, 2009.

Preston, J., et al. *Handbook of Clinical Psychopharmacology for Therapists.* Oakland, CA: New Harbinger, 2008.

WEBSITES

"Barbiturate Abuse." Drugs.com. http://www.drugs.com/cg/barbiturate-abuse.html (accessed October 7, 2011).

"Barbiturate Intoxication and Overdose, Systemic." MedlinePlus. http://www.nlm.nih.gov/medlineplus/ency/article/000951.htm (accessed October 7, 2011).

Cooper, Jeffrey S. "Toxicity, Sedative-Hypnotics." Medscape Reference. http://www.emedicine.com/emerg/topic525.htm (accessed October 7, 2011).

Harrison, Pam. "Barbiturates Still Drugs of Choice in Geriatric Suicide." Medscape News, March 11, 2010. http://www.medscape.com/viewarticle/718354 (accessed October 7, 2011).

ORGANIZATIONS

American Psychiatric Association, 1000 Wilson Blvd., Ste. 1825, Arlington, VA, 22209-3901, (703) 907-7300, apa@psych.org, http://www.psych.org.

Anxiety Disorders Association of America, 8730 Georgia Ave., Silver Spring, MD, 20910, (240) 485-1001, Fax: (240) 485-1035, http://www.adaa.org.

Mental Health America, 2000 N. Beauregard St., 6th Fl., Alexandria, VA, 22311, (703) 684-7722, (800) 969-6642, Fax: (703) 684-5968, http://www1.nmha.org.

National Alliance on Mental Illness, 3803 N Fairfax Dr., Ste. 100, Arlington, VA, 22203, (703) 524-7600, http://www.nami.org.

National Institute of Mental Health, 6001 Executive Blvd., Rm. 8184, MSC 9663, Bethesda, MD, 20892-9663, (301) 443-4513; TTY: (301) 443-8431, Fax: (301) 443-4279, (866) 615-6464; TTY: (866) 415-8051, nimhinfo@nih.gov, http://www.nimh.nih.gov.

Mark Mitchell, MD
Emily Jane Willingham, PhD
William A. Atkins, BB, BS, MBA

BDI, BDI-II *see* **Beck Depression Inventory**

Beck Depression Inventory

Definition

The Beck Depression Inventory (BDI) is a series of 21 multiple-choice questions developed to measure the intensity, severity, and depth of depressive symptoms in patients aged 13 to 80 years. The questionnaire can be filled out by the patient as a self-reported test or administered verbally by a trained professional. The BDI also helps measure symptoms related to depression such as **fatigue**, irritability, guilt, weight loss, and **apathy**. A shorter form is also available; it is composed of seven questions and is designed for administration by primary care providers.

KEY TERMS

Cognitive therapy—A psychiatric treatment that focuses on changing cognitive beliefs and thinking patterns to produce behavioral change.

Depression—A mental condition in which a person feels extremely sad and loses interest in life; symptoms may include sleep problems, loss of appetite, loss of concentration, and, in severe cases, attempts at self-harm or suicide.

Dysthymia—A less severe but chronic (ongoing) form of depression.

Purpose

The BDI was first developed by American **psychiatrist** Aaron T. Beck—from the Beck Institute for Cognitive Therapy and Research and the Department of Psychiatry at the University of Pennsylvania (Philadelphia)—who is considered a pioneer in cognitive therapy. The purpose of the BDI is to detect, assess, and monitor changes in depressive symptoms among people in a mental health care setting. Its primary goal is to determine the primary cause of **depression** in patients.

Description

The BDI was first developed and published in 1961. It was adapted in the 1970s and copyrighted in 1978 (BDI-1A). A second (and latest) version of the inventory (BDI-II) was developed and published in 1996 to reflect changes in the fourth (IV) edition, text revised (TR) version of the ***Diagnostic and Statistical Manual of Mental Disorders*** (*DSM-IV-TR*), a handbook that mental health professionals use to diagnose mental disorders. (The fifth edition [*DSM-5*] is being developed for publication in May 2013.) Beck, along with Doctors Robert A. Steer and Gregory K. Brown, authored the BDI-II.

The long form of the BDI is composed of 21 questions or items, each with four possible responses. Each response is assigned a score ranging from zero to three, indicating the severity of the symptom that the patient has experienced over the past two weeks. A version designed for use by primary care providers (BDI-PC) is composed of seven self-reported items.

The BDI is divided into two subscales. The affective subscale consists of eight items that measure psychological, or mood, symptoms. The eight characteristics contained within this subscale address negative thoughts involving:

- failure
- pessimism
- guilt
- self-punishment
- self-dislike (self-dissatisfaction)
- self-criticism
- suicide
- worthlessness

The remaining 13 characteristics focus on somatic, or physical, symptoms. They consist of negative feelings representing:

- agitation
- irritability
- sadness
- crying/tearfulness
- loss of pleasure
- loss of interest (social withdrawal)
- loss of interest in sex (loss of libido)
- tiredness/fatigue
- loss of energy
- trouble concentrating
- indecisiveness
- change in appetite (especially weight loss)
- change in sleep patterns (especially insomnia)

The BDI is also used to detect depressive symptoms in a primary care setting. The BDI usually takes between five and ten minutes to complete as part of a psychological or medical examination.

Preparation

Preparation for the Beck Depression Inventory test is not necessary nor recommended by the medical community.

Aftercare

Depending on the results of the BDI, aftercare will involve treating the depression or depressive disorder.

Precautions

The BDI is designed for use by trained professionals. In order to achieve accurate results, it should be administered by a knowledgeable mental health professional who is trained in its use and interpretation. Like other tests that measure depression using inputs from patients, there is a risk of patients understating or exaggerating their symptoms.

Results

The sum of all BDI item scores indicates the severity of depression. The test is scored differently for the general population and for individuals who have been clinically diagnosed with depression. For the general population, a score of 21 or over represents depression. For people who have been clinically diagnosed, BDI-II scores from 0 to 13 represent minimal depressive symptoms, scores of 14 to 19 indicate mild depression, scores of 20 to 28 indicate moderate depression, and scores of 29 to 63 indicate severe depression. (BDI-II scores differ from those of the original BDI.) The BDI can distinguish between different subtypes of depressive disorders, such as major depression and dysthymia (a less severe form of depression).

The BDI has been extensively tested for content validity, concurrent validity, and construct validity. The BDI has content validity—the extent to which items of a test are representative of that which is to be measured—because it was constructed from a consensus among clinicians about depressive symptoms displayed by psychiatric patients. Concurrent validity is a measure of the extent to which a test concurs with already existing standards; at least 35 studies have shown concurrent validity between the BDI and such measures of depression as the **Hamilton Depression Scale** and the **Minnesota Multiphasic Personality Inventory**-D. Tests for construct validity—the degree to which a test measures an internal construct or variable—have shown the BDI to be related to medical symptoms, anxiety, **stress**, loneliness, sleep patterns, alcoholism, suicidal behaviors, and adjustment among youth.

QUESTIONS TO ASK YOUR DOCTOR

- How will the Beck Depression Inventory help me solve my depression?
- How does the BDI work?
- Is the BDI able to diagnose severe or minor cases of depression?

Factor analysis, a statistical method used to determine underlying relationships between variables, has also supported the validity of the BDI. The BDI can be interpreted as one syndrome (depression) composed of three factors: negative attitudes toward self, performance impairment, and somatic (bodily) disturbance.

The BDI has also been extensively tested for reliability, following established standards for psychological tests first published in 1985. Internal consistency has been estimated successfully by over 25 studies in many populations. The BDI has been shown to be valid and reliable, with results corresponding to clinician ratings of depression in more than 90% of all cases.

Higher BDI scores have been shown in a few studies to be inversely related to educational attainment; the BDI, however, does not consistently correlate with gender, race, or age.

The BDI is one of the most widely used assessment tests by medical professionals and researchers for measuring depressive symptoms.

See also Cognitive-behavioral therapy

Resources

BOOKS

American Psychiatric Association. *Diagnostic and Statistical Manual of Mental Disorders*. 4th ed., text rev. Washington, DC: American Psychiatric Association, 2000.

Beck, Aaron T., and Brad A. Alford. *Depression: Causes and Treatments*. Philadelphia: University of Pennsylvania Press, 2009.

Clark, David A., and Aaron T. Beck. *Cognitive Therapy of Anxiety Disorders: Science and Practice*. New York: Guilford Press, 2010.

Clark, David A., Aaron T. Beck, and Brad A. Alford. *Scientific Foundations of Cognitive Theory and Therapy of Depression*. New York City: John Wiley & Sons, 2003.

Nezu, Arthur, George F. Ronan, and Elizabeth A. Meadows, editors. *Practitioner's Guide to Empirically Based*

Measures of Depression. New York City: Springer Publishing Company, 2006.

PERIODICALS

Konstantinidis, A., et al. "A Comparison of the Major Depression Inventory (MDI) and the Beck Depression Inventory (BDI) in Severely Depressed Patients." *International Journal of Psychiatry in Clinical Practice* 15, no. 1 (2011): 56–61.

Mehl, Matthias R. "The Lay Assessment of Subclinical Depression in Daily Life." *Psychological Assessment* 18, no. 3 (September 2006): 340–45.

Quilty, L. C., K. A. Zhang, and R. M. Bagby. "The Latent Symptom Structure of the Beck Depression Inventory-II in Outpatients with Major Depression." *Psychological Assessment* 22, no. 3 (2010): 603–8.

Snijders, A. H., M. M. Robertson, and M. Orth. "Beck Depression Inventory is a Useful Screening Tool for Major Depressive Disorder in Gilles de la Tourette Syndrome." *Journal of Neurology, Neurosurgery & Psychiatry* 77, no. 6 (June 2006): 787–89.

Stulz, N, and P. Crits-Christoph. "Distinguishing Anxiety and Depression in Self-Report: Purification of the Beck Anxiety Inventory and Beck Depression Inventory-II." *Journal of Clinical Psychiatry* 66, no. 9 (2010): 927–40.

WEBSITES

Pearson Assessments. "Beck Depression Inventory®—II (BDI®—II)." http://www.pearsonassessments.com/HAIWEB/Cultures/en-us/Productdetail.htm?Pid=015-8018-370 (accessed November 16, 2010).

University of Pennsylvania, Perelman School of Medicine, Department of Psychiatry. "Aaron T. Beck, M.D." http://www.med.upenn.edu/suicide/beck/index.html (accessed October 14, 2011).

ORGANIZATIONS

American Psychiatric Association, 1000 Wilson Boulevard, Suite 1825, Arlington, VA, 22209-3901, (703) 907-7300, apa@psych.org, http://www.psych.org.

American Psychological Association, 750 First Street NE, Washington, DC, 20002, (202) 336-5500, (800) 374-2721, http://www.apa.org.

Depression and Bipolar Support Alliance, 730 North Franklin Street, Suite 501, Chicago, IL, 60654-7225, (800) 826-3632, Fax: (312) 642-7243, http://www.dbsalliance.org.

National Alliance on Mental Illness, 3803 North Fairfax Drive, Suite 100, Arlington, VA, 22203, (703) 524-7600, (800) 950-6264, Fax: (703) 524-9094, http://www.nami.org.

National Institute of Mental Health, 6001 Executive Boulevard, Room 8184, MSC 9663, Bethesda, MD, 20892-9663, (301) 443-4513, (866) 615-6464, Fax: (301) 443-4279, nimhinfo@nih.gov, http://www.nimh.nih.gov.

Michael Polgar, PhD
Ruth A. Wienclaw, PhD
William Atkins

Bed-wetting *see* **Enuresis**

Behavioral addiction *see* **Process addiction**

Behavioral neurology *see* **Neuropsychiatry**

Behavioral self-control training *see* **Self-control strategies**

Behavior modification

Definition

Behavior modification is an empirically based psychological treatment approach founded on the principles of operant conditioning. The goal is to replace undesirable behaviors with more desirable ones through positive or negative **reinforcement** of adaptive behavior. During behavior modification, various methods may be used to produce positive change. Such methods include **aversion therapy**, desensitization, and **biofeedback**, which may include such features as physical and mental persuasion (coercion), positive reinforcement (rewards), negative reinforcement (punishment), medication use, **psychotherapy**, and others.

Purpose

Behavior modification is used to treat a variety of problems in both adults and children. It was developed so that educational and treatment techniques could be used on an individualized basis while still conforming to a standard format. The process of behavior modification includes five key steps:

- Decision: Decide what the patient should do to eliminate the problem.
- Program: Devise a program to weaken or eliminate undesirable behavior and strengthen desirable behavior.
- Treatment: Carry out a treatment program according to established principles and guidelines.
- Record: Keep detailed and objective records.
- Alteration: Alter any part of the program if further progress can be made.

Behavior modification has been successfully used to treat **obsessive-compulsive disorder** (OCD), **attention deficit hyperactivity disorder (ADHD)**, phobias, **enuresis** (bed-wetting), anxiety disorder, and **separation anxiety disorder**, among others.

Description

Behavior modification is based on the principles of operant conditioning, which were developed by American behaviorist B. F. Skinner (1904–90). Skinner formulated the concept of operant conditioning, through which behavior could be shaped by reinforcement (or the lack of it). Skinner considered his concept applicable to a wide range of both human and animal behaviors and introduced operant conditioning to the general public in his 1938 book, *The Behavior of Organisms*. Behavior modification is distinguished by a focus on behavior and its consequences. Other related forms of therapy, such as **cognitive-behavioral therapy**, may take into account internal motivation and feelings as well.

Key concepts of behavior modification are:

- attribution
- biases
- self-perception
- cognitive dissonance
- learned helpfulness
- motivation
- stress reduction or tolerance

Techniques

Techniques used in behavior modification include:

- Systematic desensitization, which treats disturbances that have identifiable sources, such as a paralyzing fear of closed spaces; usually involves training the individual to relax in the presence of fear-producing stimuli.
- Aversion therapy, which treats bad habits by breaking (stopping) them with various techniques—such as applying electric shock when the bad habit appears—so as to change the habit from being perceived as positive to negative.
- Biofeedback, which treats disturbed behavior that has physical symptoms—for instance, monitoring blood pressure or heartbeat rate and rewarding the individual when positive change occurs, such as decrease in heartbeat rate.

One widely used behavior modification technique is positive reinforcement, which encourages certain behaviors through a system of rewards. In behavior therapy, it is common for the therapist to draw up a contract with the client establishing the terms of the reward system. The system can consist of goals, rewards, and consequences. In addition to being practiced either consciously or unconsciously by educators and parents, this system also has come in to widespread use as a way to address behaviors in children with attention deficit hyperactivity disorder (ADHD).

KEY TERMS

Anxiety—Worry or tension in response to real or imagined stress, danger, or dreaded situations. Physical reactions such as fast pulse, sweating, trembling, fatigue, and weakness may accompany anxiety.

Attention deficit hyperactivity disorder (ADHD)—A learning and behavioral disorder characterized by difficulty in sustaining attention, impulsive behavior, and excessive activity.

Cognitive dissonance—A conflict of anxiety resulting from the difference in one's beliefs and one's actions.

Conduct disorder—A behavioral and emotional disorder of childhood and adolescence in which children display physical aggression and infringe on or violate the rights of others. Youths diagnosed with conduct disorder may set fires, exhibit cruelty toward animals or other children, sexually assault others, or lie and steal for personal gain.

Enuresis—Involuntary urination.

Obsessive-compulsive disorder (OCD)—An anxiety disorder in which individuals cannot prevent themselves from dwelling on unwanted thoughts, acting on urges, or performing repetitious rituals, such as washing their hands or checking to make sure they turned off the lights.

Behavior modification also can discourage unwanted behavior through either negative reinforcement or punishment. Negative reinforcement refers to an undesirable response that stops only when the desired behavior is performed. Punishment is the application of an aversive or unpleasant stimulus in reaction to a particular behavior. For example, for children, this could be the removal of television privileges when they disobey a parent or teacher.

The removal of reinforcement altogether is called extinction. Extinction eliminates the incentive for unwanted behavior by withholding the expected response. A widespread parenting technique based on extinction is the time-out, in which children are separated from the group when they misbehave. This technique removes the expected reward of adult attention.

Attention deficit hyperactivity disorder

Behavior modification is important when treating children and adolescents with attention deficit hyperactivity disorder (ADHD), which is a developmental

B. F. SKINNER (1904–90)

American behavioral psychologist Burrhus Frederic (B. F.) Skinner was born in Susquehanna, Pennsylvania. Skinner became interested in behaviorist psychology after reading the works of John Watson and Ivan Pavlov. He entered Harvard University (Cambridge, Massachusetts) as a graduate student in psychology in 1928 and received his degree three years later. While at Harvard, he laid the foundation for a new system of behavioral analysis through his research in the field of animal learning, using unique experimental equipment of his own design.

Skinner's most successful and well-known apparatus, the Skinner Box, was a cage in which a laboratory rat could, by pressing on a bar, activate a mechanism that would drop a food pellet into the cage. Another device recorded each press of the bar, producing a permanent record of experimental results without the presence of a tester. Skinner analyzed the rats' bar-pressing behavior by varying his patterns of reinforcement (feeding) to learn their responses to different schedules, including random ones.

Using this box to study how rats "operated on" their environment led Skinner to formulate the principle of operant conditioning through which an experimenter can gradually shape the behavior of a subject by manipulating its responses through reinforcement or lack of it. In contrast to Pavlovian, or response, conditioning, which depends on an outside stimulus, Skinner's operant conditioning depends on the subject's responses themselves. Skinner introduced the concept of operant conditioning in his first book, *The Behavior of Organisms* (1938). His ideas eventually became so influential that the American Psychological Association created a separate division of studies related to them (Division 25: The Experimental Analysis of Behavior), and four journals of behaviorist research were established.

Skinner's work also was influential in the clinical treatment of mental and emotional disorders. In the late 1940s, he began to develop the behavior modification method in which subjects receive a series of small rewards for desired behavior. Considered a useful technique for psychologists and psychiatrists with deeply disturbed patients, behavior modification has also been widely used by the general population in overcoming obesity, shyness, speech problems, addiction to smoking, and other problems.

Extending his ideas to the realm of philosophy, Skinner concluded that all behavior was the result of either positive or negative reinforcement, meaning that the existence of free will was merely an illusion. To explore the social ramifications of his behaviorist principles, he wrote the novel *Walden Two* (1948), which depicted a utopian society in which all reinforcement was positive. While detractors of this controversial work regarded its vision of social control through strict positive reinforcement as totalitarian, the 1967 founding of the Twin Oaks Community in Virginia was inspired by Skinner's ideas. Skinner elaborated further on his ideas about positive social control in his book *Beyond Freedom and Dignity* (1971), which critiques the notion of human autonomy, arguing that many actions ascribed to free will are performed due to necessity.

disorder that is characterized by attention problems and hyperactivity often occurring before the age of seven years. Medical professionals often combine medication with behavior modification techniques to manage ADHD. Such techniques may involve child-behavior training by parents, behavior modification by academics within the classroom, and placement in special education classes and situations. Positive reinforcement may be used to encourage good behavior, while negative reinforcement is often used to discourage bad behavior.

Anxiety

Anxiety disorders can be effectively controlled by a variety of behavior modification techniques. Such disorders include **generalized anxiety disorder** (GAD), **panic disorder** (and panic disorder with **agoraphobia**), phobias (such as social anxiety disorder), obsessive-compulsive disorder (OCD), **post-traumatic stress disorder** (PTSD), separation anxiety disorder, and childhood anxiety disorder.

Eating disorders

Eating disorders such as **anorexia nervosa**, **binge eating disorder**, and **bulimia nervosa** have been successfully treated with behavior modification. Obesity has also been shown to respond well to behavior modification, and structured behavioral programs have been established for the treatment of both obesity and eating disorders. Medical research is ongoing to study behavior modification techniques with respect to the systematic manipulation of all factors relating to eating and exercise. Many studies have shown that undergoing behavior modification treatment for an average of 18 weeks is as effective as losing a modest amount of weight safely through diet and exercise, and most of the time the weight is kept off without **relapse**.

Conduct disorders

Treatment of **conduct disorder** (CD) among children has been shown to be effective when behavioral parent training programs are implemented. Children with CD do not understand the difference between right and wrong, and behavioral modification programs help them to develop and understand that distinction. Such programs are frequently performed at home under the guidance of medical professionals. The problem areas of the child, such as aggression, deceitfulness, and inappropriate behavior, are targeted.

Benefits

Behavior modification works to address and correct negative behaviors, thus helping to improve the quality of individuals' lives and their success in society, at work, and in school.

Precautions

It is important to use a credentialed and licensed therapist. A therapist who has not had the proper training can force the client to move through the process too quickly or not provide adequate treatment. Clients should have a comfortable and trusting relationship with their therapist.

Preparation

Searching for a therapist may take time and effort, just as it does when looking for any healthcare professional. Both the National Association of Cognitive-Behavioral Therapists and the Association for Behavioral and Cognitive Therapies have information on their websites on how to find a behavior modification therapist.

Aftercare

Behavior modification techniques are often continued by parents or other caregivers after therapy has ended. Such at-home care is necessary in order to reinforce the lessons learned.

QUESTIONS TO ASK YOUR DOCTOR

- Can you refer me to a good behavior modification therapist?
- Do you believe that behavior modification therapy will help my type of problem?
- How long can I expect to be in therapy?

Risks

Behavior modification has been proven effective. However, some criticize its methods for its (sometimes) overuse of punishment. Rather than changing behavior, behavior modification is sometimes thought to instill in children the sense of avoiding being punished rather than actually modifying behavior. Consequently, behavior modification is sometimes thought to be a form of control; that is, a person is punished if behaviors are not improved. Many psychologists, therapists, and **social workers** who administer behavior modification attempt to use positive reinforcement five times more frequently than negative reinforcement, what is called a 5:1 ratio of positive to negative responses. A harsher criticism of behavior modification comes from some people who believe it is not ethical to deliberately change behavior in others. Whether such criticism is valid or not, it does exist in some realms of psychology.

Controversy also surrounds the use of electroshock treatment as negative reinforcement. Electroshock therapy was used in the 1980s as a treatment for **autism** and other developmental disorders but was soon replaced by less invasive treatments. Though it is not common, the practice still exists and may be used when other treatments prove unsuccessful. Proponents of the treatment claim that the therapy is given when the patients pose a danger to themselves or others and that it is chosen to avoid serious self-harm. Such patients may suffer from **intellectual disability** disorders and may not know the extent or consequences of their actions. Opponents of the treatment raise the ethical question of whether such practice is a form of torture. Electroshock therapy is not a preferred form of behavior modification.

Resources

BOOKS

Gaus, Valerie L. *Cognitive-Behavioral Therapy for Adult Asperger Syndrome.* New York: Guilford Press, 2007.

Kaiser, Barbara, and Judy Sklar Rasminsky. *Challenging Behavior in Young Children: Understanding, Preventing, and Responding Effectively*. Upper Saddle River, NJ: Pearson, 2012.

Martin, G., and J. Pear. *Behavior Modification: What It Is and How to Do It,* 8th ed. Upper Saddle River, NJ: Pearson Prentice Hall, 2007.

Miltenberger, Raymond G. *Behavior Modification: Principles and Procedures,* 4th ed. Belmont, CA: Thomson Wadsworth, 2008.

PERIODICALS

Leaf, Justin B., et al. "A Program Description of a Community-Based Intensive Behavioral Intervention Program for Individuals with Autism Spectrum Disorders." *Education & Treatment of Children* 34, no. 2 (2011): 259–85.

Pilkington, Ed. "Shock Tactics: Treatment or Torture?" *The Guardian*, March 12, 2011. http://www.guardian.co.uk/society/2011/mar/12/electric-shock-school-matthew-israel (accessed September 8, 2011).

OTHER

Ahern, Laurie, and Eric Rosenthal. *Torture not Treatment: Electric Shock and Long-Term Restraint in the United States on Children and Adults with Disabilities at the Judge Rotenberg Center.* Washington, DC: Mental Disability Rights International, 2010. http://www.mdri.org/PDFs/USReportandUrgentAppeal.pdf (accessed September 8 2011).

WEBSITES

"Cognitive-Behavioral Therapy." National Alliance on Mental Health, June 2003. http://www.nami.org/Template.cfm?Section=About_Treatments_and_Supports&template=/ContentManagement/ContentDisplay.cfm&ContentID=7952 (accessed September 8, 2011).

"Strategies for Teaching Students with Behavioral Disorders." West Virginia University. Last updated April 20, 2007. http://www.as.wvu.edu/~scidis/behavior.html (accessed September 8, 2011).

ORGANIZATIONS

American Psychiatric Association, 1000 Wilson Blvd., Ste. 1825, Arlington, VA, 22209-3901, (703) 907-7300, apa@psych.org, http://www.psych.org.

Association for Behavioral and Cognitive Therapies, 305 7th Ave., 16th Fl., New York, NY, 10001, (212) 647-1890, Fax: (212) 647-1865, (866) 615-6464, http://www.abct.org.

National Association of Cognitive-Behavioral Therapists, PO Box 2195, Weirton, WV, 26062, (304) 723-3982, (800) 853-1135, nacbt@nacbt.org, http://www.nacbt.org.

National Institute of Mental Health, 6001 Executive Blvd., Rm. 8184, MSC 9663, Bethesda, MD, 20892-9663, (301) 433-4513; TTY: (301) 443-8431, Fax: (301) 443-4279, (866) 615-6464; TTY: (866) 415-8051, nimhinfo@nih.gov, http://www.nimh.nih.gov.

Emily Jane Willingham, PhD
Tish Davidson, AM
Brenda Lerner
William Atkins, BB, BS, MBA

Behavior therapy *see* **Cognitive-behavioral therapy**

Benadryl *see* **Diphenhydramine**

Bender Gestalt Test

Definition

The Bender Gestalt Test (BGT), or the Bender Visual Motor Gestalt Test, is a **psychological assessment** instrument used to evaluate visual-motor functioning and visual perception skills in both children and adults. The format of the test consists of the reproduction (copying) by the participant of simple line drawings (geometric designs). Scores on the test are used to identify possible organic **brain** damage and the degree of maturation of the nervous system. The Bender Gestalt was developed by American **psychiatrist** and child neuropsychiatrist Lauretta Bender (1897–1987) in the late nineteenth century.

Bender published the monograph "A Visual Motor Gestalt and Its Clinical Use" in 1935. Concentrating within the psychological and psychiatric field of child neurology, she included the psychological test within the publication. At that time, it consisted of figures drawn on three-inch by five-inch cards, which were derived from the work of Czech-born American **psychologist** Max Wertheimer (1880–1943). Test takers were asked to copy each figure onto a blank piece of paper and to reproduce each figure as well as they could. The results of the test, which normally took from seven to ten minutes, were based on accuracy of the resultant figures and other such relevant factors. The American Orthopsychiatric Association originally published the BGT. In the 1990s, the Riverside Publishing Company acquired the test.

The revised Bender Gestalt Test—the Bender Visual-Motor Gestalt Test, Second Edition (Bender-Gestalt II)—was first published in 2003. Drs. Scott L. Decker and Gary G. Brannigan authored the latest revision based on a sample of over 4,000 individuals, from 4 years of age to over 85 years of age, representing the population of the United States as it stood in the 2000 U.S. census. The revised psychological test battery features an expanded age range and a more comprehensive assessment of visual-motor skills.

Purpose

The Bender Gestalt Test is a widely used assessment tool, both in the United States and internationally, for measuring cognitive abilities and to assess brain dysfunction.

It remains a popular psychological test because it is simple to use, is brief to administer, and has proven effective for a wide range of ages (from three to over 85 years). It is also frequently used within inpatient psychiatric locations because of its ability to differentiate between serious mental disorders and brain impairment. The Bender-Gestalt II is also beneficial for recognizing cognitive decline in older adults.

The Bender Gestalt Test is used to evaluate visual-motor maturity and integration skills, style of responding, reaction to frustration, ability to correct mistakes, planning and organizational skills, and motivation. Copying figures requires fine motor skills, the ability to discriminate between varying elements of visual stimuli, the capacity to integrate visual skills with motor skills, and the ability to shift attention from the original design to what is being drawn.

The Bender-Gestalt II is used to assess the maturation of visuomotor perceptions of children and adults. It is used to offer perspective into many psychological conditions such as **Alzheimer's disease** (AD), **attention deficit hyperactivity disorder (ADHD)**, **autism**, giftedness, learning disabilities, and intellectual disabilities. Its primary purposes are to:

- furnish information to help clarify the development and neuropsychological functioning of the test taker
- disclose level of competence of visual-motor perceptions, which is related to language and intelligence functions
- provide information on the participant including the ability to take the test, attitude while completing it, physical ability and aptitude during the test, and drawing ability and technique
- impart early (screening) recognition as to psychological and neuropsychological impairment

Description

The Bender Gestalt Test is an individually administered pencil-and-paper test used to make a **diagnosis** of brain injury. The original Bender Gestalt Test contains nine geometric figures drawn in black. These figures, sometimes called stimulus cards, are presented to the examinee one at a time; then, the examinee is asked to copy the unique figure onto a blank sheet of paper with the card still in sight. Examinees are allowed to erase but may not use any mechanical aids (such as rulers). The popularity of this test among clinicians is most likely due to the short amount of time it takes to administer and score. The average amount of time to complete the test is five to ten minutes.

The Bender Gestalt Test lends itself to several variations in administration. One method requires the examinee to view each card for five seconds, after which the card is removed. Then, the examinee draws the figure from memory. Another variation involves having the examinee draw the figures by following the standard procedure. The examinee is then given a clean sheet of paper and asked to draw as many figures as he or she can recall. In a third variation, the test is given to a group, rather than to an individual. Note that these variations were not part of the original test. In addition, one of the most popular scoring systems used with the BGT is the Bender-Gestalt Test for Young Children, which was developed by American clinical child psychologist and school psychologist Elizabeth Munsterberg Koppitz (1919–1983).

The Bender-Gestalt Test II contains 16 figures and is designed to be given to people from 3 years of age to over 85 years, a small extension of the age range from the previous edition. In addition, it has a new recall procedure for visual-motor (visuomotor) memory that assures a more comprehensive assessment of such skills. It also includes new supplemental tests of simple motor and perceptual ability to help identify motor-visual deficits. An optional timed component of the test allows the administrator to time each drawing. In addition, the revised test contains new norms for copy and recall procedures. Overall, it is considered a quick way to adequately measure both visual-motor development and psychological functioning. The main test takes between five and ten minutes to administer. A period of five minutes is usually needed to complete each of the supplemental visual and motor tests. The revised scoring system for the BGT-II was developed based on research conducted on several other scoring systems, including the Global Scoring System.

The Koppitz Developmental Scoring System (Koppitz-II), authored by Dr. Cecil Reynolds, is also available to be used with the Bender-Gestalt II. The Koppitz-II has been expanded in the scope of its scoring, along with a better reliability in its scoring system for all age levels. The scoring system has been normed based on a nationally stratified representative sample (as based on the U.S. census) of children and adults (a total of 3,600 people) from all parts of the United States, determined by community size, ethnicity, geographic region, socioeconomic condition, and other important factors.

Precautions

The Bender Gestalt Test and the revised test should not be administered to an individual with severe visual impairment unless his or her vision has been adequately corrected with eyeglasses or contact lenses. Additionally, the test should not be given to an examinee with a severe motor impairment, as the impairment would affect his or her ability to draw the geometric figures correctly. The test scores might thereby be distorted.

KEY TERMS

Alzheimer's disease—A degenerative medical disorder that adversely affects the brain and causes dementia within the later years of life.

Attention deficit hyperactivity disorder—A condition involving hyperactivity in children, characterized by an inability to concentrate and inappropriate or impulsive behaviors.

Autism—A neuropsychological problem that usually begins before the age of three years and develops with respect to disorders involving speech and language, interpretation of the world, social interactions and the formation of relationships, and reaction to stimuli. Repetitive behaviors are often seen within the condition.

Visuomotor—Pertaining to visual and motor processes.

The Bender Gestalt Test has been criticized for being used to assess problems with organic factors in the brain. This criticism stems from the lack of specific signs on the Bender Gestalt Test that are definitively associated with brain injury or the diagnosis of brain injury. As such, the Bender Gestalt Test should never be used in isolation. When making a diagnosis, results from the Bender Gestalt Test should be used in conjunction with other medical, developmental, educational, psychological, and neuropsychological information.

Finally, psychometric testing requires administration and evaluation by a clinically trained examiner. If a scoring system is used, the examiner should carefully evaluate its reliability and validity, as well as the normative sample being used. A normative sample is a group within a population who take a test and represent the larger population. This group's scores on a test are then used to create "norms" with which the scores of test takers are compared.

Results

A scoring system does not have to be used to interpret performance on either form of the Bender Gestalt Test, though there are several reliable and valid scoring systems available. Many of the available scoring systems focus on specific-type difficulties experienced by the test taker. The following difficulties may indicate poor visual-motor abilities in the test taker:

- angular difficulty—increasing, decreasing, distorting, or omitting an angle in a figure
- bizarre doodling—adding peculiar components to the drawing that have no relationship to the original Bender Gestalt figure
- closure difficulty—difficulty closing open spaces on a figure, or connecting various parts of the figure, resulting in a gap in the copied figure
- cohesion—drawing a part of a figure larger or smaller than shown on the original figure and out of proportion with the rest of the figure; may also include drawing a figure or part of a figure significantly out of proportion with other figures
- collision—crowding the designs or allowing the end of one design to overlap or touch a part of another design
- contamination—occurs when a previous figure, or part of a figure, influences the examinee's completion of the current figure; for example, combining two different Bender Gestalt figures
- fragmentation—destroying part of the figure by not completing it, or breaking up the figures in ways that entirely lose the original design
- impotence—occurs when the examinee draws a figure inaccurately but seems to recognize the error, then makes several unsuccessful attempts to improve the drawing
- irregular line quality or lack of motor coordination—drawing rough lines, particularly when the examinee shows a tremor motion
- line extension—adding or extending a part of the copied figure that was not on the original figure
- omission—failing to connect the parts of a figure adequately or reproducing only parts of a figure
- overlapping difficulty—problems in drawing portions of figures that overlap, simplifying the drawing at the point that it overlaps, sketching or redrawing the overlapping portions, or otherwise distorting the figure at the point where it overlaps
- perseveration—increasing, prolonging, or continuing the number of units in a figure; for example, drawing significantly more dots or circles than shown on the original figure
- retrogression—substituting more primitive figures for the original design; for example, substituting solid lines or loops for circles, dashes for dots, dots for circles, or circles for dots, or filling in circles
- rotation—rotating a figure or part of a figure by 45° or more; also includes when the examinee rotates the stimulus card that is being copied.
- scribbling—drawing primitive lines that have no relationship to the original Bender Gestalt figure
- simplification—replacing a part of the figure with a more simplified figure, not due to maturation (Drawings that are primitive in terms of maturation would be categorized under "retrogression.")

QUESTIONS TO ASK YOUR DOCTOR

- Is the Bender Gestalt Test an appropriate assessment test for me? My children?
- Should other psychological tests be used in combination with the Bender Gestalt Test?
- What is the next step after taking the test?
- Is the test reliable?
- Does the Bender Gestalt Test help to evaluate mental decline in older adults?

- superimposition of design—drawing one or more of the figures on top of each other
- workover—reinforcing, increasing pressure, or overworking a line or lines in a whole or partial figure

Additionally, observing the examinee's behavior while drawing the figures can provide the examiner with an informal evaluation and data that can supplement the formal evaluation of the examinee's visual and perceptual functioning. For example, if an examinee takes a large amount of time to complete the geometric figures, it may suggest a slow, methodical approach to tasks, compulsive tendencies, or depressive symptoms. If an examinee rapidly completes the test, this could indicate an impulsive style.

Resources

BOOKS

Brannigan, Gary G., and Scott L. Decker. *Bender Visual-Motor Gestalt Test*. Itasca, IL: Riverside Publishing, 2003.

Hutt, M. L. *The Hutt Adaptation of the Bender Gestalt Test*. New York: Grune and Stratton, 1985.

Kaufman, Alan, S., and Elizabeth O. Lichtenberger. *Assessing Adolescent and Adult Intelligence*. Hoboken, NJ: John Wiley, 2006.

Koppitz, E. M. *The Bender Gestalt Test for Young Children*. Vol. 2. New York: Grune and Stratton, 1975.

Pascal, G. R., and B. J. Suttell. *The Bender Gestalt Test: Quantification and Validation for Adults*. New York: Grune and Stratton, 1951.

Sattler, Jerome M. "Assessment of Visual-Motor Perception and Motor Proficiency." In *Assessment of Children: Behavioral and Clinical Applications*. 4th ed. San Diego: Jerome M. Sattler, Publisher, Inc., 2002.

Watkins, E. O. *The Watkins Bender Gestalt Scoring System*. Novato, CA: Academic Therapy, 1976.

WEBSITES

"Bender Visual-Motor Gestalt Test, Second Edition (Bender-Gestalt II." Pearson. http://www.pearsonassessments.com/HAIWEB/Cultures/en-us/Productdetail.htm?Pid=015-8064-127&Mode=summary (May 19, 2011).

"Bender Visual-Motor Gestalt Test, Second Edition (Bender Gestalt II)." Western Psychological Services. http://portal.wpspublish.com/portal/page?_pageid=53,126639&_dad=portal&_schema=PORTAL (May 19, 2011).

"KOPPITZ-2: Koppitz Developmental Scoring System for the Bender Gestalt Test—Second Ed." Pro-Ed Inc. http://www.proedinc.com/customer/productView.aspx?ID=3724 (May 20, 2011).

"Koppitz Developmental Scoring System for the Bender Gestalt Test, Second Edition (KOPPITZ-2)." Riverside Publishing. http://www.riversidepublishing.com/koppitz2 (May 20, 2011).

ORGANIZATIONS

American Geriatrics Society, 40 Fulton St., 18th Fl., New York, NY, 10038, (212) 308-1414, Fax: (212) 832-8646, info@americangeriatrics.org, http://www.americangeriatrics.org.

American Psychiatric Association, 1000 Wilson Boulevard, Suite 1825, Arlington, VA, 22209, (888) 357-7924, apa@psych.org, http://www.psych.org.

National Institute on Aging, Building 31, Room 5C27, 31 Center Drive, MSC 2292, Bethesda, MD, 20892, (301) 496-1752, (800) 222-4225 (TTY), Fax: (301) 496-1072, http://www.nia.nih.gov.

National Institute of Mental Health, 6001 Executive Boulevard, Room 8184, MSC 9663, Bethesda, MD, 20892-9663, (301) 443-4513, (866) 615-6464, Fax: (301) 443-4279, nimhinfo@nih.gov, http://www.nimh.nih.gov.

National Institute of Neurological Disorders and Stroke, PO Box 5801, Bethesda, MD, 20824, (301) 496-5751. TTY: (301) 468-5981, (800) 352-9424, http://www.ninds.nih.gov.

Keith Beard, Psy.D.
William Atkins

Benzodiazepines

Definition

Benzodiazepines are medicines that help relieve nervousness, tension, and other symptoms by slowing the central nervous system.

Purpose

Benzodiazepines are a class of **antianxiety drugs**. While anxiety is a normal response to stressful situations, some people have unusually high levels of anxiety that can interfere with everyday life. Benzodiazepines help bring anxious feelings under control and also relieve other troubling symptoms of anxiety, such as pounding heartbeat, breathing problems, irritability, nausea, and faintness.

Physicians may sometimes prescribe benzodiazepines for other conditions, such as muscle spasms, epilepsy and other seizure disorders, phobias, **panic disorder**, withdrawal from alcohol, and sleeping problems. However, this medicine should not be used every day for sleep problems that last more than a few days. If used this way, the drug loses its effectiveness within a few weeks.

Description

The family of antianxiety drugs known as benzodiazepines includes **alprazolam** (Xanax), **chlordiazepoxide** (Librium), **diazepam** (Valium), and **lorazepam** (Ativan). These medicines take effect fairly quickly, starting to work within an hour after they are taken. Benzodiazepines are available only with a physician's prescription and are available in tablet, capsule, liquid, or injectable forms.

Recommended dosage

The recommended dosage depends on the type of benzodiazepine, its strength, and the condition for which it is being taken. Doses may be different for different people. Check with the physician who prescribed the drug or the pharmacist who filled the prescription for the correct dosage.

Always take benzodiazepines exactly as directed. Never take larger or more frequent doses, and do not take the drug for longer than directed. If the medicine does not seem to be working, check with the physician who prescribed it. Do not increase the dose or stop taking the medicine unless the physician says to do so. Stopping the drug suddenly may cause withdrawal symptoms, especially if it has been taken in large doses or over a long period. People who are taking the medicine for seizure disorders may have **seizures** if they stop taking it suddenly. If it is necessary to stop taking the medicine, check with a physician for directions on how to stop. The physician may recommend tapering down gradually to reduce the chance of withdrawal symptoms or other problems.

KEY TERMS

Anxiety—Worry or tension in response to real or imagined stress, danger, or dreaded situations. Physical reactions, such as fast pulse, sweating, trembling, fatigue, and weakness may accompany anxiety.

Central nervous system—The brain and spinal cord.

Dependence—A state in which a person requires a steady concentration of a particular substance to avoid experiencing withdrawal symptoms.

Epilepsy—A brain disorder with symptoms that include seizures.

Glaucoma—A condition in which pressure in the eye is abnormally high. If not treated, glaucoma may lead to blindness.

Myasthenia gravis—A chronic disease with symptoms that include muscle weakness and sometimes paralysis.

Panic disorder—A disorder in which people have sudden and intense attacks of anxiety in certain situations. Symptoms such as shortness of breath, sweating, dizziness, chest pain, and extreme fear often accompany the attacks.

Phobia—An intense, abnormal, or illogical fear of something specific, such as heights or open spaces.

Seizure—A sudden attack, spasm, or convulsion.

Sleep apnea—A condition in which a person temporarily stops breathing during sleep.

Tolerance—The requirement for higher doses of a substance or more frequent engagement in an activity to achieve the same effect.

Withdrawal symptoms—A group of physical or mental symptoms that may occur when a person suddenly stops using a drug to which he or she has become dependent.

Precautions

Seeing a physician regularly while taking benzodiazepines is important, especially during the first few months of treatment. The physician will check to make sure the medicine is working as it should and will note any unwanted side effects. People who take benzodiazepines to relieve nervousness, tension, or symptoms of panic disorder should check with their physicians every two to three months to make sure they still need to keep taking the medicine. Benzodiazepines do have some addictive potential, and long-term use of benzodiazepines may result in dependence and tolerance, so it is important that therapy is monitored.

Patients who are taking benzodiazepines for sleep problems should check with their physicians if their symptoms do not improve after seven to ten days. Sleep problems that last longer than this may be a sign of another medical problem. If the medication works successfully and is stopped, patients may have trouble sleeping for the first few nights, but this effect should only be temporary.

Some people feel drowsy, dizzy, light-headed, or less alert when using benzodiazepines. The drugs may also cause clumsiness or unsteadiness. When the medicine is taken at bedtime, these effects may even occur the next morning, producing a "hangover" effect. Persons should not drive, use machines, or participate in any other hazardous activity after taking benzodiazepines until they know how the drugs affect them. In general, older people and children are more sensitive to the effects of benzodiazepines, which may increase the chance of side effects.

Benzodiazepines may cause behavior changes in some people, similar to those seen in people who act differently when they drink alcohol. More extreme changes, such as confusion, agitation, and hallucinations, also are possible. If a person starts having strange or unusual thoughts or exhibiting strange behavior while taking this medicine, he or she should contact the prescribing physician.

Some benzodiazepines increase the likelihood of birth defects. Using these medicines during pregnancy may also cause the baby to become dependent on them, resulting in withdrawal symptoms after birth. When taken late in pregnancy or around the time of labor and delivery, these drugs can cause other problems in the newborn baby, such as weakness, breathing problems, slow heartbeat, and body temperature problems. Women who are breast-feeding their babies should also not use this medicine without checking with their physicians, as benzodiazepines may pass into breast milk.

Because benzodiazepines work on the central nervous system, they may add to the effects of alcohol and other drugs that slow down the central nervous system (CNS depressants). Such drugs include antihistamines, cold medicine, allergy medicine, sleep aids, medicine for seizures, tranquilizers, some pain relievers, and muscle relaxants. They may also add to the effects of anesthetics, including those used for dental procedures. These effects may last several days after the treatment with benzodiazepines ends. The combined effects of benzodiazepines and alcohol or other CNS depressants can be very dangerous, leading to unconsciousness or even death. Anyone taking benzodiazepines should not drink alcohol and should check with his or her physician before using any CNS depressants. Anyone who shows signs of an overdose or of the effects of combining benzodiazepines with alcohol or other drugs should get immediate emergency help. Warning signs include slurred speech or confusion, severe drowsiness, staggering, and profound weakness.

People with certain medical conditions or who are taking certain other medicines can have problems if they take benzodiazepines. Patients should let their doctors know if they have any of these conditions:

- current or past drug or alcohol abuse
- depression
- severe mental illness
- epilepsy or other seizure disorders
- swallowing problems
- chronic lung disease such as emphysema, asthma, or chronic bronchitis
- kidney disease
- liver disease
- brain disease
- glaucoma
- hyperactivity
- myasthenia gravis
- porphyria
- sleep apnea
- allergies

Side effects

The most common side effects are dizziness, lightheadedness, drowsiness, clumsiness, unsteadiness, and slurred speech. These problems usually go away as the body adjusts to the drug and do not require medical treatment unless they persist or they interfere with normal activities.

More serious side effects are not common but may occur. If any of the following side effects occur, patients should check with the physician who prescribed the medicine as soon as possible:

- behavior changes
- memory problems
- difficulty concentrating
- confusion
- depression
- seizures (convulsions)
- hallucinations
- sleep problems
- increased nervousness, excitability, or irritability
- involuntary movements of the body, including the eyes
- low blood pressure
- unusual weakness or tiredness
- skin rash or itching
- unusual bleeding or bruising
- yellow skin or eyes
- sore throat
- sores in the mouth or throat

- fever and chills

Patients who take benzodiazepines for a long time or at high doses may notice side effects for several weeks after they stop taking the drug. They should check with their physicians if these or other troublesome symptoms occur:

- irritability
- nervousness
- sleep problems

Other rare side effects may occur. Patients who experience unusual symptoms during or after treatment with benzodiazepines should contact their physician.

Interactions

Benzodiazepines may interact with a variety of other medicines. When this happens, the effects of one or both of the drugs may change or the risk of side effects may be greater. Persons taking benzodiazepines should let their physician know all other medicines they are currently taking. Among the drugs that may interact with benzodiazepines are:

- CNS depressants, such as medicine for allergies, colds, hay fever, and asthma
- sedatives
- tranquilizers
- prescription pain medicines
- muscle relaxants
- seizure medications
- sleep aids
- barbiturates
- anesthetics

Other medications may interact with benzodiazepines. Patients should check with their physician or pharmacist before combining benzodiazepines with any other prescription or nonprescription (over-the-counter) medicines.

Resources

BOOKS

American Psychiatric Association. *Diagnostic and Statistical Manual of Mental Disorders*. 4th ed., text rev. Washington, DC: American Psychiatric Publishing, 2000.

Brunton, Laurence, Bruce Chabner, and Bjorn Knollman. *Goodman & Gilman's The Pharmacological Basis of Therapeutics* 12th ed. New York: McGraw-Hill, 2010.

Doble, Adam, Ian Martin, and David J. Nutt. *Calming the Brain: Benzodiazepines and Related Drugs from Laboratory to Clinic*. London: Informa Healthcare, 2003.

PERIODICALS

Lader, Malcolm. "Benzodiazepines Revisited—Will We Ever Learn?" *Addiction* 106, no. 12 (2011): 2086–109. http://dx.doi.org/10.1111/j.1360-0443.2011.03563.x (accessed December 15, 2011).

Mugunthan, K., T. McGuire, and P. Glasziou. "Minimal Interventions to Decrease Long-Term use of Benzodiazepines in Primary Care: A Systematic Review and Meta-Analysis." *British Journal of General Practice* 61, no. 590 (2011): 573–80.

ORGANIZATIONS

U.S. Food and Drug Administration, 10903 New Hampshire Ave., Silver Spring, MD, 20993-0002, (888) INFO-FDA (463-6332), http://www.fda.gov.

Nancy Ross-Flanigan

Benztropine

Definition

Benztropine is classified as an antiparkinsonian agent. It is sold in the United States under the brand name Cogentin and is also available under its generic name.

Purpose

Benztropine is used to treat a group of side effects (called parkinsonian side effects) that includes tremors, difficulty walking, and slack muscle tone. These side effects may occur in patients who are taking antipsychotic medications used to treat mental disorders such as **schizophrenia**.

Description

Some medicines used to treat schizophrenia and other mental disorders, called antipsychotic drugs, can cause side effects that are similar to the symptoms of Parkinson's disease. Patients do not have Parkinson's disease but experience similar symptoms, such as shaking in muscles while at rest, difficulty with voluntary movements, and poor muscle tone.

One way to eliminate these undesirable side effects is to stop taking the antipsychotic medicine. Unfortunately, the symptoms of the original mental disorder usually come back, so simply stopping the antipsychotic medication is not a reasonable option in most cases. Some drugs that control the symptoms of Parkinson's disease, such as benztropine, also control the parkinsonian side effects of antipsychotic medicines.

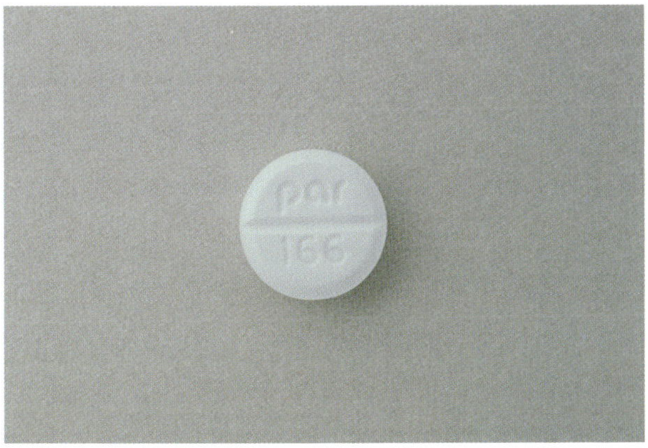

Cogentin (benztropine), 2 mg. *(© Custom Medical Stock Photo, Inc. Reproduced by permission.)*

Benztropine works by restoring the chemical balance between **dopamine** and acetylcholine, two neurotransmitter chemicals in the **brain**. Taking benztropine along with the antipsychotic medicine helps to control symptoms of the mental disorder, while reducing parkinsonian side effects. Benztropine is in the same family of drugs (commonly known as anticholinergic drugs) as **biperiden** and **trihexyphenidyl**.

Recommended dosage

Benztropine is available in 0.5, 1.0, and 2.0 mg tablets and in an injectable form containing 2 mg in each 2 mL glass container. For the treatment of tremors, poor muscle tone, and similar side effects, benztropine should be started at a dose of 1 to 2 mg orally. In cases of severe side effects, benztropine can be given as an intramuscular injection two to three times daily or as needed. Parkinson-like side effects caused by antipsychotic drugs may come and go, so benztropine may not be needed on a regular basis. Benztropine may also be prescribed to prevent these side effects before they actually occur. This is called a prophylactic (preventative) therapy.

Precautions

Benztropine should never be used in children under age three. It should be used cautiously and with close physician supervision in older children and in the elderly. Like all anticholinergic drugs, benztropine decreases the body's ability to sweat and cool itself. People who are unaccustomed to being outside in hot weather should take care to stay as cool as possible and drink extra fluids. People who are chronically ill, have a central nervous system disease, or who work outside during hot weather may need to avoid taking benztropine.

People who have the following medical problems may experience increased negative side effects when taking benztropine. Those who have these problems should discuss their conditions with their physician before starting the drug:

- glaucoma, especially closed-angle glaucoma
- intestinal obstruction
- prostate enlargement
- urinary bladder obstruction

Although rare, some patients experience euphoria while taking benztropine and may abuse it for this reason. Euphoria can occur at doses only two to four times the normal daily dose. Patients with a history of drug abuse should be observed carefully for benztropine abuse.

Side effects

Although benztropine helps to control the side effects of antipsychotic drugs, it can produce side effects of its own. A person taking benztropine may have some of the following reactions, which may vary in intensity:

- dry mouth
- dry skin
- blurred vision
- nausea or vomiting
- constipation
- disorientation
- drowsiness
- irritability
- increased heart rate
- urinary retention

Dry mouth, if severe to the point of causing difficulty speaking or swallowing, may be managed by reducing or temporarily discontinuing benztropine. Chewing sugarless gum or sucking on sugarless candy may also help to increase the flow of saliva. Some artificial saliva products may give temporary relief.

Men with prostate enlargement may be especially prone to urinary retention. Symptoms of this problem include having difficulty starting a urine flow and more difficulty passing urine than usual. This side effect may be severe and require discontinuation of the drug. Urinary retention may require catheterization. People who think they may be experiencing any side effects from this or any other medication should tell their physicians.

Patients who take an overdose of benztropine are treated with forced vomiting, removal of stomach contents and stomach washing, activated charcoal, and respiratory support if needed. They are also given physostigmine, an antidote for anticholinergic drug poisoning.

KEY TERMS

Acetylcholine—A naturally occurring chemical in the body that transmits nerve impulses from cell to cell. It causes blood vessels to dilate, lowers blood pressure, and slows the heartbeat. Central nervous system well-being is dependent on a balance among the neurotransmitters acetylcholine, dopamine, serotonin, and norepinephrine.

Anticholinergic—Related to the ability of a drug to block the nervous system chemical acetylcholine. When acetylcholine is blocked, patients often experience dry mouth and skin, increased heart rate, blurred vision, and difficulty urinating. In severe cases, blocking acetylcholine may cloud thinking and cause delirium.

Catheterization—Placing a tube in the bladder so that it can be emptied of urine.

Dopamine—A chemical in brain tissue that serves to transmit nerve impulses (is a neurotransmitter) and helps to regulate movement and emotions.

Neurotransmitter—A chemical in the brain that transmits messages between neurons, or nerve cells.

Parkinsonian—Related to symptoms associated with Parkinson's disease, a nervous system disorder characterized by abnormal muscle movement of the tongue, face, and neck; inability to walk or move quickly; walking in a shuffling manner; restlessness; and/or tremors.

Interactions

When drugs such as benztropine are taken with **antidepressants** such as **amitriptyline**, **imipramine**, **trimipramine**, **desipramine**, **nortriptyline**, **protriptyline**, **amoxapine**, and **doxepin**, or with many antihistamines that also have anticholinergic properties, the effects and side effects of benztropine are usually intensified.

Drugs such as benztropine decrease the speed with which food moves through the stomach and intestines. Because of this, the absorption of other drugs being taken may be enhanced by benztropine. Patients receiving benztropine should be alerted to unusual responses to other drugs they might be taking and report any changes to their physicians.

Resources

BOOKS

American Society of Health-System Pharmacists. *AHFS Drug Information 2008*. Bethesda, MD: American Society of Health-System Pharmacists, 2008.

Preston, John D., John H. O'Neal, and Mary C. Talaga. *Handbook of Clinical Psychopharmacology for Therapists*. 5th ed. Oakland, CA: New Harbinger Publications, 2008.

PERIODICALS

de Leon, Jose. "Letter to the Editor: Benztropine Equivalents for Antimuscarinic Medication." *American Journal of Psychiatry*. 162, no. 3 (March 2005): 627.

WEBSITES

MedlinePlus. "Benztropine Mesylate Oral." U.S. National Library of Medicine, National Institutes of Health. http://www.nlm.nih.gov/medlineplus/druginfo/meds/a682155.html (accessed December 15, 2011).

Jack Raber, Pharm.D.
Ruth A. Wienclaw, PhD

Bereavement

Definition

Bereavement is the emotional state caused by any major loss, such as the death of a loved one.

Demographics

Almost everyone experiences bereavement at some point in their lives. Many people undergo multiple bereavements. Although it is a normal part of life, some people suffer major complications of bereavement. Between 17% and 27% of people experience depressive illness during their first year of bereavement. One study found that 10% of bereaved people met the criteria for complicated **grief** disorder. Another study found that 9% of bereaved people met the criteria for **major depressive disorder** four months after their loss and 5.7% met the criteria for **post-traumatic stress disorder** (PTSD).

Description

The English word *bereavement* comes from an ancient Germanic root meaning "to rob" or "to seize by violence." *Mourning* refers to the public rituals or symbols of bereavement, including funeral services and the wearing of black. *Grief* refers to the personal experience of loss, including physical and emotional symptoms. Whereas public expressions of mourning are usually short-lived, grief caused by bereavement is a process that can last months or even years.

Bereavement is a complex experience and no two people respond in exactly the same way. Reactions to death are influenced by many factors, including ethnic and religious traditions, relationships with the deceased, personal beliefs about an afterlife, the cause of death and whether it was sudden or expected, and the deceased's age. Furthermore, the death of a loved one inevitably confronts adults and older adolescents with their own mortality. Because of this emotional complexity and variety of responses, most physicians and counselors advise bereaved people to trust their own feelings and grieve in ways that seem most helpful to them.

Grief counselors recognize that bereavement has two dimensions—the actual loss and symbolic losses. For example, parents who lose a child suffer a series of symbolic losses in addition to the child's death, such as the knowledge that their child will never graduate from high school, marry, or have children.

There are several generally recognized stages or phases of uncomplicated bereavement and grief, although for most people, bereavement feels like an emotional roller coaster rather than a sequence of stages. People may experience none, some, or all of the phases in any order, or they may vacillate between them.

- Avoidance, shocked disbelief, or denial usually lasts for about two weeks after the initial bereavement. Symptoms may include emotional numbness, deep sighing, breathlessness, choking, and loss of appetite and strength.
- As awareness of the loss develops, the bereaved may enter a confrontational phase, which typically lasts several months and includes pain and suffering, deep sadness, weeping, guilt, panic, confusion, anger, despair, blaming others, a sense of helplessness, and physical symptoms of stress.
- The bargaining phase is an attempt to somehow reverse the loss.
- Depression often sets in at about six months after the initial bereavement. Survivors may lose interest in life and become socially isolated.
- In the resolution, accommodation, or acceptance phase, which usually occurs within one to two years, people adjust to their loss and to life without the loved one, learn to cope with new roles and responsibilities, and possibly even redefine their identity.

Not all feelings and experiences associated with bereavement are negative. If the deceased was suffering from illness, some bereaved people may feel relief that the deceased's suffering has ended. Some people find that bereavement, though difficult, is a time of personal growth. They may develop a new appreciation of life and increased self-esteem as they master new tasks and adjust to the experience of carrying on independently.

Although bereavement is a normal part of life and not a psychiatric disorder, it is one of life's most stressful experiences. Bereavement is associated with a high risk for psychological distress, social isolation, physical illness, and death. The fourth edition of the ***Diagnostic and Statistical Manual of Mental Disorders*** (*DSM-IV*) classifies bereavement as a condition that may require clinical attention, since it can lead to major depressive disorder or PTSD. Since the early 1990s, thanatologists—specialists in issues related to death and dying—have identified two types of bereavement grief that do not resolve normally with the passage of time: complicated and traumatic grief. Complicated grief disorder is also referred to as atypical or abnormal grief, pathologic grief, or pathologic mourning. Outside sources have proposed that complicated grief disorder be included in the *DSM-5*, and the **American Psychiatric Association** has adapted the suggestion under the name bereavement related disorder in the proposed additions to the appendix for further study. Traumatic grief is a type of complicated grief that occurs following a loved one's death from an accident, **suicide**, homicide, disaster, or war.

Risk factors

Reactions to bereavement are influenced by many factors, including the personality of the bereaved, their relationship to the deceased, the manner of death, and cultural background. There are considerable differences among cultural groups in the ways that bereavement is expressed and in the duration of normal bereavement.

Risk factors for complicated or traumatic grief include:

- being unprepared for an untimely loss
- physical or mental suffering of the victim
- excessive dependence on the deceased
- difficulties with personal attachments or lack of emotional support
- media intrusiveness or frustration with the justice system in cases of traumatic bereavement
- lack of closure when a person is missing and/or presumed dead
- guilt, shame, and/or anger after a suicide
- disenfranchised grief over a loss that cannot be openly acknowledged, such as a secret relationship
- guilt or shame over grief for an animal

Causes and symptoms

Although the loss of a spouse or beloved friend or relative is the most common cause of bereavement, other losses—such as permanent injury, divorce, or the death of a pet—can also cause bereavement. Bereavements such as miscarriage or abortion or a loved one's **diagnosis** of **Alzheimer's disease** are referred to as "silent losses."

Mental symptoms of bereavement may include:

- sadness, anxiety, irritability, apathy, anger, fear, and mood swings
- feelings of helplessness and low self-esteem
- flashbacks and hallucinations of the deceased
- confusion and preoccupation with the deceased, resulting in poor judgment or lack of insight
- suicidal thoughts, which occur in as many as 54% of survivors up to six months after their loss
- homicidal thoughts

Physical symptoms of bereavement may include:

- poor personal hygiene and grooming
- changes in appetite and weight
- dehydration
- low energy
- fatigue
- loss of interest in sex
- sleep disturbances
- chest or throat pain
- palpitations
- headache
- hair loss
- nausea and vomiting
- gastrointestinal distress
- aches and pains
- lowered immunity

Bereavement in children

Children experience bereavement differently than adolescents and adults. Preschool children do not usually understand the finality and irreversibility of death. They may talk or act as if the deceased family member or pet will wake up or return. Children between the ages of five and nine are better able to understand the finality of death, but they tend to assume it will not affect them and are shocked by a death in their immediate family. In addition to physical symptoms of bereavement, children may regress to an earlier stage—for example, acting like an infant, with baby talk or wanting to drink from a baby bottle.

Complicated or traumatic grief

Complicated grief is an abnormally intense and prolonged response to bereavement. Whereas most people move through a period of bereavement, those with complicated grief remain in chronic mourning and are unable to function normally, accept their loss, or make the necessary adjustments for living effectively without their loved one. They cannot stop longing for the deceased and may feel that a part of them died along with the loved one. They experience persistent distressing thoughts about the deceased and may feel bitter and agitated. Although these reactions are normal during the initial months of bereavement, persistence of such symptoms beyond six months may be indicative of a pathological condition. People with complicated grief may start to behave like the deceased, mimic symptoms of their illness, act recklessly, or talk about joining their loved one in death. Although complicated grief can coexist with clinical **depression**, it is a distinct disorder.

Traumatic grief results from a sudden event involving violence, suffering, mutilation, or multiple deaths that appears to be random or preventable. Symptoms of traumatic grief are similar to those of PTSD and can include muscle tension, an exaggerated startle response, hallucinations, flashbacks, avoidance of certain situations, marked irritability, and interference with sleep and concentration.

Bereavement related disorder

Bereavement related disorder is another name for complicated grief disorder, but the *DSM-5* diagnostic criteria require that symptoms extend beyond 12 months after the death. Persons experiencing bereavement related disorder struggle with social interaction and have yet to establish or maintain a self-identity without the deceased present. They may find it difficult to make any type of plans, avoid places or people that remind them of the deceased, and continue to experience extreme and persistent longing. Traumatic grief is classified as traumatic bereavement.

Diagnosis

Abnormal bereavement can be identified through examination and tests.

Examination

Bereavement is a normal response to a death or other loss. Although in the initial months people often have symptoms that are characteristic of clinical depression or major depressive disorder, medical diagnosis is usually not necessary unless the symptoms last for more than two

KEY TERMS

Bibliotherapy—The use of books (usually self-help or problem-solving) to improve one's understanding of personal problems and/or to heal painful feelings.

Biofield healing—A general term for alternative therapies that are based on the belief that the human body is surrounded by an energy field (aura) that reflects the condition of the body and spirit. Rebalancing or repairing the energy field is thought to bring about healing in mind and body. Reiki, therapeutic touch, polarity balancing, SHEN therapy, and certain forms of color therapy are considered types of biofield healing.

Complicated grief—An abnormal response to bereavement that includes unrelieved yearning for the deceased, the total loss of positive beliefs or worldview, and general dysfunction.

Disenfranchised grief—Grief that is not openly expressed because the bereavement cannot be publicly acknowledged.

Mourning—The public expression of bereavement, including funerals and other rituals, special clothing, and symbolic gestures.

Post-traumatic stress disorder (PTSD)—A psychological reaction that continues long after a highly stressful event and is characterized by depression, anxiety, flashbacks, and nightmares.

Thanatologist—A specialist in the study of death and psychological mechanisms for coping with death.

Traumatic grief—Grief resulting from bereavement under traumatic circumstances, such as natural or transportation disasters, acts of terrorism, and murder.

months and the person experiences persistent feelings of guilt, thoughts of death, or feelings of unworthiness, or is unable to perform normal activities.

Tests

Various psychological inventories and questionnaires can be used to diagnose PTSD, major depression, or **acute stress disorder**. There are also specific questionnaires for diagnosing complicated grief.

Treatment

Abnormal bereavement can be treated with psychological therapy and with prescribed medications.

Traditional

Normal bereavement does not usually require formal treatment. However, many people choose to participate in bereavement or grief **support groups**. These are particularly helpful for guiding people through common but painful problems, such as disposing of the deceased's possessions, celebrating holidays, and coping with anniversaries. Individual and group **psychotherapy**, as well as support groups, are used to treat patients with complicated or traumatic grief or PTSD.

Drugs

Recent research suggests that antidepressant medication can help with bereavement. Complicated or traumatic grief and PTSD are also treated with antianxiety and sleep-inducing medications.

Alternative

Various alternative therapies are used to treat sleep disturbances and other symptoms of bereavement:

- meditation
- movement therapies, such as yoga and tai chi
- therapeutic touch, Reiki, and other forms of biofield healing
- bibliotherapy and journaling
- music and art therapy
- hydrotherapy
- massage therapy

Home remedies

The single most important factor in healing from bereavement is the support of others. Bereaved people are advised to face and express their feelings. Focusing on positive aspects of life and trying to find meaning in the loss are helpful coping strategies. Bereaved people often continue some form of relationship with the deceased, such as attachment to physical reminders, prayer, sensing the presence of the deceased in one's life, or commemorative festivals and rituals, such as the Day of the Dead celebration in Mexico.

Bereaved children should be reassured of their safety and the safety of their loved ones. They should be encouraged to express their feelings. Adults should ensure that bereaved children do not have any

QUESTIONS TO ASK YOUR DOCTOR

- Are my feelings and physical symptoms a normal response to bereavement?
- How long should I expect these symptoms to continue?
- Are there medications that might help me?
- Is there a bereavement support group that you can recommend?

misconceptions concerning their loss, but children should not be overloaded with facts or exposed to disturbing television images. Their daily routines should remain as normal as possible.

Prognosis

Most people progress through the stages of grieving within a few months to two years, without clinical **intervention**. Painful emotions diminish in intensity over time, eventually becoming episodic. Feelings of bereavement may reemerge with anniversaries and holidays or poignant memories. Nevertheless, bereavement can induce permanent personal changes, both positive and negative. Complicated or traumatic grief may take three or more years to resolve, even with appropriate treatment.

Prevention

Bereavement is a normal response to loss, and loss is a universal human experience. Normal grieving following bereavement should be allowed to run its course. Most bereavement counselors maintain that attempting to stifle or shorten the grief process is more likely to cause emotional difficulties in the long run. However, it is important to maintain one's physical health during bereavement.

Resources

BOOKS

American Psychiatric Association. *Diagnostic and Statistical Manual of Mental Disorders,* 4th ed., text rev. Washington, DC: American Psychiatric Association, 2000.

Bonanno, George A. *The Other Side of Sadness: What the New Science of Bereavement Tells Us About Life After Loss.* New York: Basic Books, 2009.

Hood, Ann. *Comfort: A Journey Through Grief.* New York: Norton, 2008.

Okun, Barbara, and Joseph Nowkinski. *Saying Goodbye: How Families Can Find Renewal Through Loss.* New York: Berkley, 2011.

Schechter, Harold. *The Whole Death Catalog: A Lively Guide to the Bitter End.* New York: Ballantine, 2009.

Stroebe, Margaret S., ed. *Handbook of Bereavement Research and Practice: Advances in Theory and Intervention.* Washington, DC: American Psychological Association, 2008.

PERIODICALS

Brent, David, et al. "The Incidence and Course of Depression in Bereaved Youth 21 Months After the Loss of a Parent to Suicide, Accident, or Sudden Natural Death." *American Journal of Psychiatry* 166, no. 7 (July 2009): 786–94.

Mahon, Margaret M. "Taking It to the Street . . . and the Hospital, the School, and the Workplace: Bereavement Research in the 21st Century." *Gerontologist* 29, no. 2 (April 2009): 285–91.

Shear, M. K., et al. "Complicated Grief and Related Bereavement Issues for DSM-5." *Depression and Anxiety* 28 (February 2011): 103–117.

Van der Houwen, Karolijne, et al. "Risk Factors for Bereavement Outcome: A Multivariate Approach." *Death Studies* 34, no. 3 (March 2010): 195–220.

OTHER

Harper, Linda R. "Healing After the Loss of Your Pet." Best Friends Animal Society. http://www.bestfriends.org/theanimals/pdfs/allpets/PetLossHarper.pdf (accessed September 8, 2011).

WEBSITES

American Academy of Child and Adolescent Psychiatry. "Children and Grief." *Facts for Families.* Last updated March 2011. http://www.aacap.org/cs/root/facts_for_families/children_and_grief (accessed September 8, 2011).

American Academy of Child and Adolescent Psychiatry. "When a Pet Dies." *Facts for Families.* Last updated March 2011. http://www.aacap.org/cs/root/facts_for_families/when_a_pet_dies (accessed September 8, 2011).

Burnett, Lynn Barkley. "Grief and Bereavement." eMedicine Health.com. http://www.emedicinehealth.com/grief_and bereavement/article_em.htm (accessed September 8, 2011).

Lubit, Roy, H. "Acute Treatment of Disaster Survivors." Medscape Reference. Last updated April 25, 2011. http://emedicine.medscape.com/article/295003-overview (accessed September 8, 2011).

National Organization for Victim Assistance. "Survivors of Homicide Victims." National Organization of Parents of Murdered Children. http://www.pomc.com/survivor.cfm (accessed September 8, 2011).

Smith, Melinda, Ellen Jaffe-Gill, and Jeanne Segal. "Coping with Grief and Loss: Support for Grieving and Bereavement." Helpguide.org. Last updated March 2011. http://

www.helpguide.org/mental/grief_loss.htm (accessed September 8, 2011).

ORGANIZATIONS

American Academy of Child and Adolescent Psychiatry, 3615 Wisconsin Ave., NW, Washington, DC, 20016-3007, (202) 966-7300, Fax: (202) 966-2891, http://www.aacap.org.

American Hospice Foundation, 2120 L St., NW, Ste. 200, Washington, DC, 20037, (202) 223-0204, (800) 347-1413, Fax: (202) 223-0208, http://www.americanhospice.org.

American Psychiatric Association, 1000 Wilson Blvd., Ste. 1825, Arlington, VA, 22209-3901, (703) 907-7300, apa@psych.org, http://www.psych.org.

Compassionate Friends, PO Box 3696, Oak Brook, IL, 60522, (630) 990-0010, (877) 969-0010, Fax: (630) 990-0246, http://www.compassionatefriends.org.

Dougy Center, PO Box 86852, Portland, OR, 97286, (503) 775-5683, (866) 775-5683, help@dougy.org, http://www.grievingchild.org.

Mental Health America, 2000 N. Beauregard St., 6th Fl., Alexandria, VA, 22311, (703) 684-7722, (800) 969-6642, Fax: (703) 684-5968, info@mentalhealthamerica.net, http://www.mentalhealthamerica.net.

National Institute of Mental Health, 6001 Executive Blvd., Rm. 8184, MSC 9663, Bethesda, MD, 20892-9663, (301) 443-4513; TTY: (301) 443-8431, Fax: (301) 443-4279, (866) 615-6464; TTY: (866) 415-8051, nimhinfo@nih.gov, http://www.nimh.nih.gov.

Tragedy Assistance Program for Survivors, 1777 F St., NW, Ste. 600, Washington, DC, 20006, (202) 588-TAPS (8277), (800) 959-TAPS (8277), Fax: (202) 509-8282, info@taps.org, http://www.taps.org.

Rebecca Frey, PhD
Ruvanee Pietersz Vilhauer, PhD
Margaret Alic, PhD

Beta blockers

Definition

Beta blockers, also known as beta antagonists, are a class of drugs that were first developed for the treatment of certain heart conditions and hypertension. Beta blockers were later found to be useful in treating glaucoma, migraine headaches, and some psychiatric disorders such as performance anxiety, tremors secondary to lithium, and **medication-induced movement disorders** that are caused by some antipsychotic drugs. There are a number of beta blockers approved for use in the United States, including acebutolol, bisoprolol, nadolol, **propranolol**, and metoprolol, which have various trade names. Propranolol is the most commonly used in psychiatric practice.

Purpose

Beta blockers are proven effective in the treatment of performance anxiety, lithium-induced tremors, and neuroleptic-induced akathisia (a physical condition caused by certain antipsychotic drugs). Beta blockers have sometimes been used with **benzodiazepines** in treating alcohol withdrawal.

Description

Beta blockers act on that part of the central nervous system that controls mental alertness, lung function, heart rate, and blood vessels. Although there is more than one mechanism by which beta blockers work in anxiety states, the most beneficial result probably arises from the fact that beta blockers slow the heart to a normal rate and rhythm. Persons with performance anxiety, for example, would not experience the usual chest tightness and rapid heart rate that is associated with such acts as public speaking or acting.

Certain antipsychotic medications known as neuroleptics can cause an unwanted effect called akathisia, which is the inability to sit, stand still, or remain inactive. Patients are restless, and in severe cases may pace constantly and forcefully and repeatedly stomp their feet. Beta blockers can sometimes treat this condition with a lower incidence of side effects than other drugs.

Recommended dosage

Propranolol is available in several different forms. Tablets are available, as are an oral solution and an injectable form. Dosage varies considerably depending on the reason for taking the drug and the age of the person. A physician will determine the appropriate dosage, although some examples include:

- For one-time usage to treat performance anxiety, a single dose ranging from 10–40 mg taken a half hour before the performance (e.g., public speaking) is typical.
- For lithium-induced tremors that cannot be controlled by reducing caffeine intake or administering the dosage of lithium at bedtime, propranolol at a dose of 20–160 mg daily may be given in two or three evenly divided doses.
- For akathisia caused by antipsychotic medications, propranolol can be administered at doses of 10–30 mg three times daily.

Precautions

Because of their ability to narrow airways, beta blockers, especially propranolol, should not be taken by

KEY TERMS

Akathisia—Agitated or restless movement, usually affecting the legs. Movement is accompanied by a sense of discomfort and an inability to sit, stand still, or remain inactive for periods of time. Akathisia is a common side effect of some neuroleptic (antipsychotic) medications.

Benzodiazepines—A group of central nervous system depressants used to relieve anxiety or to induce sleep.

Tremor—Involuntary shaking of the hands and arms.

people with asthma and chronic obstructive pulmonary disease (COPD). If there is an urgent need to use beta blockers in persons with respiratory problems, atenolol or metoprolol are the beta blockers of choice, as they are less likely to have this side effect. However, even these drugs should be used with caution. Patients with congestive heart failure, or certain cardiac conduction abnormalities such as a heart block, should also use beta blockers with caution.

Beta blockers should be used with close physician monitoring in people with diabetes, since the symptoms of low blood sugar (increased heart rate, light-headedness, and abnormal perspiration) may be not be recognized by patients.

Side effects

Beta blockers can cause undesired decreases in blood pressure and are typically not given if blood pressure is 90/60 mm Hg or less. Beta blockers can also cause an undesired drop in heart rate. People whose resting heart rate is less than 55 beats per minute should not take beta blockers.

Occasionally, beta blockers can cause rash, weakness, nausea, vomiting, and stomach discomfort.

Interactions

Each medication in the class of beta blockers has the potential to interact with a multitude of other medications. Anyone starting beta-blocker therapy should review the other medications they are taking with their physician and pharmacist for possible interactions. Patients should always inform all of their healthcare providers, including dentists, that they are taking beta blockers.

Resources

PERIODICALS

Huh, J., D. Goebert, J. Takeshita, B. Y. Lu, and M. Kang. "Treatment of Generalized Anxiety Disorder: A Comprehensive Review of the Literature for Psychopharmacologic Alternatives to Newer Antidepressants and Benzodiazepines." *The Primary Care Companion to CNS Disorders* 13, no. 2 (2011).

WEBSITES

National Institute of Mental Health. "What Medications are Used to Treat Anxiety Disorders?" U.S. National Institutes of Health. http://www.nimh.nih.gov/health/publications/mental-health-medications/what-medications-are-used-to-treat-anxiety-disorders.shtml (accessed October 31, 2011).

Ajna Hamidovic, Pharm.D.
Emily Jane Willingham, PhD

Bibliotherapy

Definition

Bibliotherapy is a form of therapy in which structured readings are used as an adjunct to **psychotherapy**. Such readings can be used to reinforce learning or insights gained in the therapeutic session or to give individuals additional professional resources to help in personal growth and development.

Purpose

The goal of bibliotherapy is to broaden and deepen the patient's understanding of the particular problem that requires treatment. The written materials may educate the patient about the disorder itself or be used to increase the patient's acceptance of a proposed treatment. Many people find that the opportunity to read about their problem outside the therapist's office facilitates active participation in their treatment and promotes a stronger sense of personal responsibility for recovery. In addition, many are relieved to find that others have had the same disorder or problem and have coped successfully with or recovered from it. From the therapist's standpoint, providing patients with specific information or assignments to be completed outside regular in-office sessions speeds the progress of therapy.

The goals of bibliotherapy include the following:

- provide information or insight
- stimulate discussion about problems
- communicate new values or attitudes
- create awareness of the existence of the problem in the wider population
- provide potential solutions to problems

Bibliotherapy has been applied in a variety of settings to many kinds of people with psychological problems. Practitioners have reported successful use of bibliotherapy in treating people with eating disorders, anxiety and mood disorders, **agoraphobia**, alcohol and **substance abuse**, and stress-related physical disorders.

Description

In most settings, bibliotherapy is used as an adjunct to more traditional forms of psychotherapy. Practitioners of cognitive-behavioral therapies are among the most enthusiastic supporters of bibliotherapy, particularly in the development of individualized treatment protocols, including workbooks, for specific disorders. For example, patients with eating disorders, especially **bulimia nervosa**, often benefit from receiving educational information appropriate to their stage of recovery, such as books or articles about cultural biases regarding weight, attractiveness, and dieting. This information helps patients better understand the rationale for their treatment and to work on new skills or behavioral changes more effectively.

Benefits

For many people, additional information or workbooks can be used in private to reinforce their commitment to getting better. People who lack the time or finances to attend regular psychotherapy sessions at a practitioner's office often find that bibliotherapy can bridge the gap between infrequent appointments. Further, the nature of the disorder itself may sometimes preclude in-office treatment, such as for people suffering from agoraphobia. Current research indicates that a bibliotherapeutic approach can be highly effective in helping people with agoraphobia better understand and cope with their symptoms.

Precautions

Bibliotherapy is an adjunct to psychotherapy. It is not intended as a replacement for psychotherapy or as a self-help treatment. In addition, bibliotherapy is not likely to be useful with patients who have thought disorders, psychoses, limited intellectual ability, dyslexia, or active resistance to treatment. As with any form of treatment, bibliotherapy is effective only if it actively engages the patient's desire for and belief in recovery.

KEY TERMS

Adjunct—A form of treatment that is not strictly necessary but is helpful to a therapy regimen.

Cognitive-behavioral therapy—An approach to psychotherapy that emphasizes the correction of distorted thinking patterns and changing one's behaviors accordingly.

Dyslexia—A type of reading disorder.

Regimen—A regulated course of treatment for a medical or mental disorder.

Aftercare

Unlike many standard forms of psychotherapy, bibliotherapeutic approaches often include specific examples of ways to deal with relapses or setbacks. As long as the patients keep these materials, they have easy access to resources for getting back on track.

Risks

People who use self-help manuals without professional guidance run the risk of misapplying techniques or misdiagnosing their problems.

Results

As with any form of treatment, bibliotherapy is effective only if it actively engages the client's desire for and belief in recovery. For many people, additional information or workbooks can be used in private to reinforce their commitment to getting better. People who lack the time or finances to attend regular psychotherapy sessions at a practitioner's office often find that bibliotherapy can bridge the gap between infrequent appointments. Further, the nature of the disorder itself may sometimes preclude in-office treatment, such as for people suffering from agoraphobia. Current research indicates that a bibliotherapeutic approach can be highly effective in helping people with agoraphobia better understand and cope with their symptoms.

Resources

BOOKS

Hipsky, Shellie Jacobs. *The Drama Discovery Curriculum: Bibliotherapy and Theater Games for Students with Emotional and Behavioral Challenges*. Lancaster, PA: Proactive Publications, 2006.

VandenBos, Gary R. ed. *APA Dictionary of Psychology*. Washington, DC: American Psychological Association, 2006.

White, John R., and Arthur S. Freeman, eds. "Introduction." In *Cognitive-Behavioral Group Therapy for Specific Problems and Populations*, edited by John R. White and Arthur S. Freeman. Washington, DC: American Psychological Association, 2000.

PERIODICALS

Carlbring, Per, et al. "An Open Study of Internet-Based Bibliotherapy with Minimal Therapist Contact via Email for Social Phobia." *Clinical Psychologist* 10, no. 1 (March 2006): 30–38.

Febbraro, Greg A. R. "An Investigation Into the Effectiveness of Bibliotherapy and Minimal Contact Interventions in the Treatment of Panic Attacks." *Journal of Clinical Psychology* 61, no. 6 (June 2005): 763–79.

Floyd, Mark, et al. "Two-Year Follow-Up of Bibliotherapy and Individual Cognitive Therapy for Depressed Older Adults." *Behavior Modification* 30, no. 3 (May 2006): 281–94.

Foster, Tom. "Read All About It: Guided Bibliotherapy for Depression in Adults." *Irish Journal of Psychological Medicine* 23, no. 3 (September 2006): 111–13.

Heath, Melissa Allen, et al. "Bibliotherapy: A Resource to Facilitate Emotional Healing and Growth." *School Psychology International* 26 no. 5 (December 2005): 563–80.

Norcross, John C. "Integrating Self-Help Into Psychotherapy: 16 Practical Suggestions." *Professional Psychology: Research and Practice* 37, no. 6 (December 2006): 683–93.

Pehrsson, Dale E., and P. A. McMillen. "Bibliotherapy Evaluation Tool: Grounding Counselors in the Therapeutic Use of Literature." *Arts in Psychotherapy* 32, no. 1 (2005): 47–59.

Rapee, Ronald M., Maree J. Abbott, and Heidi J. Lyneham. "Bibliotherapy for Children With Anxiety Disorders Using Written Materials for Parents: A Randomized Controlled Trial." *Journal of Consulting and Clinical Psychology* 74, no. 3 (June 2006): 436–44.

Reeves, T., and J. M. Stace. "Improving Patient Access and Choice: Assisted Bibliotherapy for Mild to Moderate Stress/Anxiety in Primary Care." *Journal of Psychiatric and Mental Health Nursing* 12, no. 3 (June 2005): 341–46.

Thomas, S. P. "Bibliotherapy: New Evidence of Effectiveness." *Issues in Mental Health Nursing* 32, no. 4 (2011): 191.

Jane A. Fitzgerald, PhD
Ruth A. Wienclaw, PhD

Binge drinking

Definition

Binge drinking is the rapid consumption of alcohol with the goal of intoxication. In the past, binge drinking was usually considered to be heavy, out-of-control drinking, usually alone, for periods of up to several days. Binge drinking is now more often defined by the quantity of alcohol consumed on a single occasion. The National Advisory Council of the National Institute on Alcohol Abuse and Alcoholism (NIAAA) defines binge drinking as reaching a blood alcohol concentration (BAC) of at least 0.08 grams per deciliter, which generally corresponds to five drinks within about two hours for adult males and four drinks for adult females.

Demographics

Binge drinking is common in most parts of the world, and alcohol consumption, including binge drinking, is a major cause of death. Every year, more than

Alcohol use among college-age students, 2009

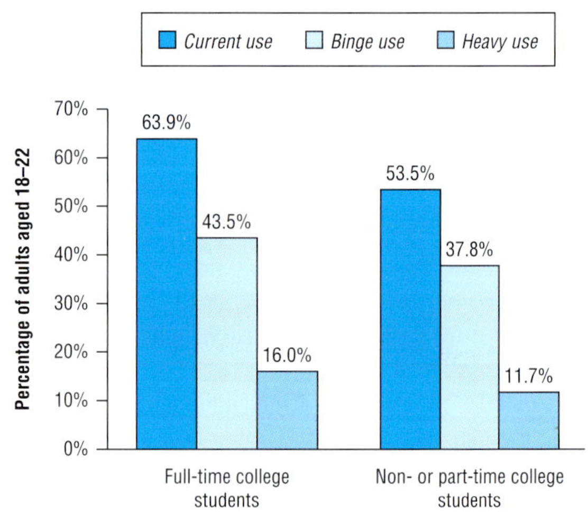

Current use: At least one drink during the past 30 days.
Binge use: Five or more drinks within the same period, at least once during the past 30 days.
Heavy use: Five or more drinks within the same period, during five or more of the past 30 days.

SOURCE: Substance Abuse and Mental Health Services Administration (SAMHSA), Office of Applied Studies, *Results from the 2009 National Survey on Drug Use and Health, Volume I: Summary of National Findings* (September 2010).

(Graph by PreMediaGlobal. © 2012 Cengage Learning.)

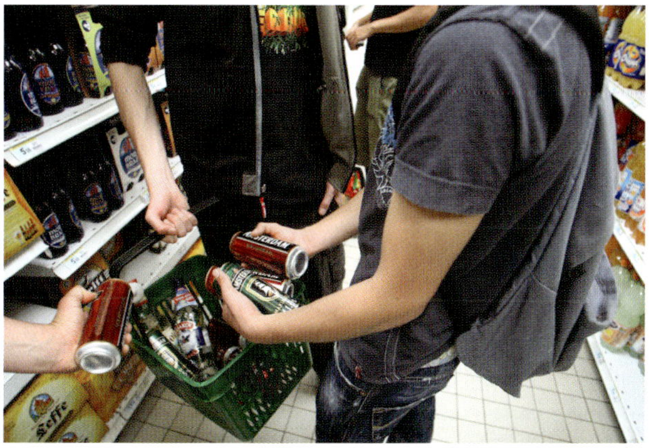

A group of young adults buys alcohol. Consuming five or more drinks (or four for women) within a short time period is considered binge drinking. *(© Photopqr/Ouest France/ Marc Ollivier/newscom)*

33 million adult Americans binge drink. According to national surveys released in 2010 and reported by the U.S. Centers for Disease Control and Prevention, 75% of the alcohol consumed by U.S. adults is consumed by binge drinking. Among Americans who drink, almost one in three adults and two out of three high school students binge drink. Among American adults who drink to excess, approximately 92% report binge drinking at least once in a 30-day period. Binge drinking is more prevalent in males (21% vs. 10% of females). Among non-Hispanic whites, 16% binge drink, compared with 10% of non-Hispanic blacks. Binge drinking varies greatly from state to state, with estimates of binge drinking by adults ranging from 6.8% in Tennessee to 23.9% in Wisconsin. Binge drinkers are 14 times more likely than other drinkers to drive while alcohol impaired.

Although 70% of binge-drinking episodes in the United States involve adults aged 26 and older, binge drinking by high school and college students is of particular concern. Binge drinking accounts for approximately 90% of all alcohol consumed by Americans under the age of 21, and 51% of 18–20-year-olds who drink alcohol binge drink, the highest proportion for any age group.

Although binge drinking among young people appears to be increasing in many countries, binge drinking by U.S. college students has remained stable over time. Rates vary with the individual school, from 1% to more than 70% of students. Overall, more than 40% of U.S. college students of all ages report binge drinking at least once during an average two-week period. Every year, an estimated 30,000 American college students require medical treatment for alcohol overdose. Among students who drive at least once a week, 13% report driving after having at least five drinks, and within all age groups, persons who binge drink are 14 times more likely to drive while under the influence.

Description

Binge drinking is generally recognized as a harmful—and potentially life-threatening—practice, but there is no universally accepted definition of what constitutes binge drinking. Some U.S. researchers prefer the phrase "episodic heavy drinking," referring to at least five consecutive drinks for men and at least four for women on at least one occasion in a two-week period. Three or more such episodes within two weeks constitute heavy binge drinking. In many European countries, however, binge drinking is defined by significantly more than four or five drinks. There is also considerable variation in the definition of a standard drink. Furthermore, alcohol is metabolized at different rates. A person's BAC is affected by body weight, the duration of time in which alcohol is consumed, and concurrent food intake. To account for these factors, the NIAAA has redefined binge drinking as a pattern of consumption that brings the BAC to 0.08 gram percent or above. However, all definitions of binge drinking include drinking to the point of intoxication.

One standard drink is generally defined as:

- 12 fluid ounces (fl oz) of regular beer
- 8–9 fl oz of malt liquor
- 5 fl oz of table wine
- 3–4 fl oz of fortified wine, such as sherry or port
- 2–3 fl oz of cordial, liqueur, or aperitif
- 1.5 fl oz (one jigger or shot) of brandy or 80-proof spirits (hard liquor)

The acceptability of binge drinking varies in different cultures. In some societies, binge drinking and intoxication are considered normal. In most cultures that tolerate drinking, binge drinking is more acceptable for males than for females and may even be considered a male rite of passage. Binge drinking may also be acceptable on certain occasions, such as wedding celebrations, wakes, or sports tournaments.

Binge drinking is associated with numerous social problems. It increases the likelihood of high-risk behaviors, such as driving under the influence; engaging in unplanned, unsafe, unprotected, or nonconsensual sex; accidents or injuries due to loss of physical coordination; and aggression or violence. People that binge drink are more likely to miss school or work and to perform less productively because of hangovers. They may engage in inappropriate interpersonal behaviors that negatively affect their relationships. Schools with high rates of binge drinking have higher rates of property damage and verbal, physical, and sexual violence.

Binge drinking is associated with a variety of adverse health effects, including cardiovascular problems such as atrial fibrillation. Binge drinking by pregnant women can directly harm their unborn babies and cause **fetal alcohol syndrome** or another fetal alcohol spectrum disorder. Binge drinking is also associated with liver disease, neurological damage, sexual dysfunction, and poor control of diabetes. Finally, binge drinking can cause potentially fatal alcohol poisoning.

Risk factors

Risk factors for binge drinking include **stress**, **sexual abuse**, and mental illness. Additional risk factors for college students include having engaged in binge drinking in high school and residing in a sorority or fraternity. Low-priced, easily available alcohol is strongly correlated with binge drinking by college students. Binge drinking rates among college students correlate with those of adults living in the same state—36% in the ten states with the lowest rates of adult binge drinking compared with 53% in the ten highest adult–binge drinking states.

Causes and symptoms

The causes of binge drinking can be psychological or social. Many people binge drink to escape stress or personal problems. Other binge drinkers, especially young people, report that they engage in the practice because of peer pressure, for social status, or to fit in with a drinking culture. Bars, liquor stores, and advertising promote drinking as an attractive activity.

The rise in popularity of inexpensive alcoholic energy drinks, which contain caffeine and other stimulants in addition to high alcohol levels, led to a frightening increase in binge drinking in the late 2000s, especially among college students. These products appear to be designed to support binge drinking, as the stimulants enable drinkers to stay awake and consume more alcohol, rather than passing out. Numerous hospitalizations and several deaths led some colleges and states to ban the drinks, and because the safety of such supplements in combination with alcohol had not been approved by the U.S. Food and Drug Administration (FDA), manufacturers were required by the FDA to remove caffeine from the beverages.

Although binge drinkers are not necessarily alcohol dependent, three out of five frequent binge drinkers may meet the criteria for alcohol abuse and one in five may be alcohol dependent. Some studies indicate that people who have three or more binge-drinking episodes within a two-week period display some symptoms of alcoholism.

Alcohol poisoning can be a potentially life-threatening consequence of binge drinking. Alcohol poisoning affects involuntary reflexes, including breathing and the gag reflex. An impaired gag reflex can cause drinkers to choke on their own vomit. Other signs of alcohol poisoning include:

- extreme confusion
- seizures
- unconsciousness
- slow or irregular breathing
- lowered body temperature
- pale or bluish skin

KEY TERMS

Alcoholic energy drink—Caffeinated alcoholic beverages; malt liquors which, in addition to high alcohol content, have added caffeine and sometimes other stimulants.

Alcohol poisoning—A potentially life-threatening condition caused by consuming large amounts of alcohol over a short period, negatively affecting heart rate, breathing, and the gag reflex.

Atrial fibrillation—A condition in which the upper chamber of the heart quivers instead of pumping in an organized way.

Blood alcohol concentration or content (BAC)—A measure of the amount of alcohol in the body; in most states, legal alcohol intoxication is defined as a BAC of at least 0.08 grams per deciliter of blood.

Cognitive-behavioral therapy (CBT)—A type of psychotherapy in which people learn to recognize and change negative and self-defeating patterns of thinking and behavior.

Fetal alcohol spectrum disorders—A range of birth defects, including intellectual disability, poor growth, nervous system dysfunctions, and malformations, that result from heavy maternal alcohol consumption during pregnancy.

Tolerance—The body's adjustment to a drug such as alcohol, requiring increasingly higher quantities to produce the same effects.

Withdrawal—The unpleasant, sometimes life-threatening, physiological changes that can occur due to the discontinuation of alcohol or drugs after prolonged regular use.

Diagnosis

Examination

Although people usually recover from binge drinking by "sleeping it off," alcohol poisoning is a medical emergency that requires immediate attention. The physician will check for signs and symptoms of alcohol poisoning. It is important that medical personnel be informed as to the amount and type of alcohol consumed over a specific period of time.

Tests

Blood tests are used to determine blood alcohol levels and other signs of alcohol toxicity, such as low blood sugar. A urine test may help to confirm a **diagnosis** of alcohol poisoning.

Treatment

The most important treatment for binge drinking is to stop drinking. Binge drinkers should never be allowed to drive. If alcohol poisoning is suspected, it is important to stay with the person and try to keep them conscious until medical help arrives. If they are vomiting, they should be kept in a sitting position if possible, or, if lying down, have their head turned to one side to prevent choking. Patients with alcohol poisoning must be carefully monitored to prevent breathing and gagging problems. Oxygen therapy may be required, as well as intravenous fluids to prevent dehydration.

Traditional

Patients who are physically dependent on alcohol may require medical treatment for managing symptoms of alcohol withdrawal. Counseling may be required to address the underlying reasons for alcohol abuse. Groups such as Alcoholics Anonymous (AA) have a proven track record of helping people with drinking problems. Alcoholism is also treated with **cognitive-behavioral therapy** (CBT) or interactional group **psychotherapy** based on a 12-step program. Severe cases may require **hospitalization** or treatment in a substance-abuse rehabilitation facility.

Drugs

Anxiolytic drugs are sometimes prescribed to control anxiety symptoms that accompany alcohol withdrawal. The FDA has approved three medications for the treatment of alcoholism:

- disulfiram (Antabuse) causes illness if alcohol is consumed
- naltrexone (Depade, ReVia) acts on the brain to reduce the craving for alcohol
- acamprosate (Canpral) reduces withdrawal symptoms

Prognosis

Binge drinking is particularly dangerous for young people whose brains are still developing. Young people are more likely than adults to engage in risky behaviors when binge drinking, leading to automobile accidents, violence, sexually transmitted diseases, and unplanned pregnancies. Binge drinking disrupts sleep patterns, making it harder to concentrate in school, and binge drinkers are more likely to drop out of school. Studies have shown that teens who binge drink throughout high school are more likely to be overweight and have high blood pressure by the age of 24. Binge drinking can cause people to become angry or moody and socially isolated. Frequent binge drinking can induce tolerance, so that more alcohol is required to achieve a particular level of intoxication. Over time, binge drinking can cause liver disease, heart disease, and other chronic conditions, as well as **stroke** and certain cancers. Binge drinking by pregnant women can cause fetal alcohol spectrum disorders and other harm to their babies. Severe alcohol poisoning can lead to irreversible **brain** damage or death. Finally, binge drinking may be a precursor to alcohol dependence.

Prevention

Evidence demonstrates that parental influence and family values are very powerful determinants of drinking behavior. School- and community-based educational programs, starting in middle school if not before, teach alcohol awareness and stress the dangers of binge drinking. Many colleges and universities have alcohol awareness and prevention programs, beginning with freshman orientation. Peer-to-peer counseling and interactive programs can be particularly effective. Alcohol awareness programs can also be directed toward workplaces and promoted in the mainstream media. Healthcare providers and social service workers should educate their patients and clients.

Social norms approaches teach that activities such as binge drinking are not socially acceptable. Social norming has been shown to be especially effective in reducing binge drinking among young people. For example, many young people believe that binge drinking is much more prevalent than it actually is, and correcting this misconception can discourage the practice.

One study found that in seven states that had at least four laws targeting high-volume alcohol sales, campus binge-drinking rates were lower—33% compared to 48% in states without such laws. States with other alcohol-control policies also had lower rates of college binge drinking. Other interventions that have been shown to help prevent binge drinking in college students include:

- increasing the cost of alcoholic beverages through taxation

QUESTIONS TO ASK YOUR DOCTOR

- Does my pattern of alcohol consumption qualify as binge drinking?
- What is a safe level of alcohol consumption?
- Is there a program or group that could help me control my binge drinking?

- limiting the number of retail alcohol outlets within a given area
- consistently enforcing laws against underage drinking and drunk driving
- screening and counseling students for alcohol abuse

Bars and restaurants can also play a role in reducing binge drinking. Atmosphere, such as lighting and music, can affect how much and how fast patrons drink. Serving alcohol at a slower rate, offering food and nonalcoholic drinks, and especially refusing to serve intoxicated customers and preventing them from driving are business practices that help discourage binge drinking.

Resources

BOOKS

Bakewell, Lisa. *Alcohol Information for Teens*. 2nd ed. Detroit: Omnigraphics, 2009.

Dowdall, George W. *College Drinking: Reframing a Social Problem*. Westport, CT: Praeger, 2009.

Marczinski, Cecile A., Estee C. Grant, and Vincent J. Grant. *Binge Drinking in Adolescents and College Students*. Hauppauge, NY: Nova Science, 2009.

Roloff, Tamara L. *Alcoholism*. Detroit: Greenhaven, 2010.

Young, Amy M., et al. "Drinking Like a Guy: Frequent Binge Drinking among Undergraduate Women." In: *The American Drug Scene: An Anthology*, edited by James A. Inciardi and Karen McElrath. 5th ed. New York: Oxford University Press, 2008.

PERIODICALS

Howland, Jonathan, et al. "The Effects of Binge Drinking on College Students' Next-Day Academic Test-Taking Performance and Mood State." *Addiction* 105, no. 4 (April 2010): 655–665.

Reinberg, Steven. "Binge Drinking, Hypertension a Deadly Combo." *U.S. News & World Report*, August 19, 2010. http://health.usnews.com/health-news/family-health/heart/articles/2010/08/19/binge-drinking-hypertension-a-deadly-combo (accessed October 14, 2011).

Roy-Bornstein, Carolyn. "Underage Drinking." *Pediatrics for Parents* 26 (March/April 2010): 11–12.

WEBSITES

Center for Science in the Public Interest. "Binge Drinking on College Campuses." http://www.cspinet.org/booze/collfact1.htm (accessed December 11, 2010).

Nemours Foundation. "Binge Drinking." TeensHealth.org. http://kidshealth.org/teen/drug_alcohol/alcohol/binge_drink.html (accessed December 1, 2011).

U.S. Centers for Disease Control and Prevention. "Alcohol and Public Health Fact Sheets: Binge Drinking." http://www.cdc.gov/alcohol/fact-sheets/binge-drinking.htm (accessed December 1, 2011).

———. "CDC Vital Signs: Binge Drinking." http://www.cdc.gov/vitalsigns/BingeDrinking/index.html (accessed October 14, 2011).

———. "1 in 4 High School Students and Young Adults Report Binge Drinking." http://www.cdc.gov/media/pressrel/2010/r101005.html (accessed December 1, 2011).

U.S. Food and Drug Administration. "Caffeinated Alcoholic Beverages." U.S. Department of Health and Human Services. http://www.fda.gov/Food/FoodIngredientsPackaging/ucm190366.htm (accessed December 2, 2011).

ORGANIZATIONS

International Center for Alcohol Policies, 1519 New Hampshire Avenue NW, Washington, DC, 20036, (202) 986-1159, Fax: (202) 986-2080, info@icap.org, http://www.icap.org.

National Institute on Alcohol Abuse and Alcoholism (NIAAA), 5635 Fishers Lane, MSC 9304, Bethesda, MD, 20892-9304, (301) 443-3860, http://www.niaaa.nih.gov.

Substance Abuse and Mental Health Services Administration, 1 Choke Cherry Road, Rockville, MD, 20857, (877) SAMHSA-7 (726-4727), Fax: (240) 221-4292, SAMHSAInfo@samhsa.hhs.gov, http://www.samhsa.gov.

U.S. Centers for Disease Control and Prevention, 1600 Clifton Road, Atlanta, GA, 30333, (800) CDC-INFO (232-4636), cdcinfo@cdc.gov, http://www.cdc.gov.

Jill U. Adams
Margaret Alic, PhD

Binge eating disorder

Definition

Binge eating disorder (BED) is a serious eating disorder characterized by frequent consumption of a large amount of food over a limited period of time, such as one or two hours. BED is also known as compulsive overeating.

Demographics

Binge eating disorder is the most commonly diagnosed eating disorder, affecting 3.5% of women and 2% of men at some point in their adult lives.

Although it often begins in late adolescence or early twenties, BED is also common during middle age. As many as one-half of people attending weight-loss clinics are binge eaters. Although BED affects blacks and whites equally, there has been little research on binge eating by other racial or ethnic groups.

Data from a 2011 study conducted by the National Institutes of Mental Health showed that the lifetime prevalence of binge eating disorder in teens is 1.6% (approximately 300,000 teens). The study was based on interviews with more than 10,000 adolescents aged 13 to 18 years. The study data also showed that rates of binge eating disorder, as well as bulimia, have approximately doubled since 1990, while the rates of anorexia have remained fairly stable. More girls were affected by binge eating disorder than boys, and approximately 15% of any teens with binge eating disorder had attempted **suicide**.

Description

Although most people overeat on occasion, BED is a pattern of frequently recurring abnormal overeating, which is different from continuous snacking and often occurs in the absence of hunger. Although the duration of each binge may vary significantly, binge eating is characterized by the inability to stop eating during each episode and a feeling of being out of control. A binge typically ends only when all of the desirable binge foods have been consumed or when the person feels too full to continue. Binge eaters generally eat very fast and alone—usually out of embarrassment—and suffer strong negative feelings such as guilt, shame, or **depression** following the binge.

Many eating disorder specialists define BED as overeating that occurs at least twice a week for at least three months and that has a negative effect on an individual's health, relationships, and/or daily activities. However, BED is a relatively new area of research, and many aspects of the disorder remain unclear.

In the revised fourth edition of the ***Diagnostic and Statistical Manual of Mental Disorders*** (*DSM-IV-TR*), the **American Psychiatric Association** (APA) defines the better known—but less common—eating disorders, **anorexia nervosa** and **bulimia nervosa**, as psychiatric disorders with formal diagnostic criteria. BED is classified as an eating disorder not otherwise specified (EDNOS) and has no diagnostic criteria. It has been proposed that BED be included as a specific disorder in the fifth edition of the *DSM*, *DSM-5* (2013). This is important because the classification can affect both recommended therapies and health insurance coverage for treatment. However, the proposal has proved controversial.

The proposed diagnostic criteria state that individuals must experience binge eating episodes at least once a week for three months to be diagnosed with binge eating disorder.

Some experts believe that binge eating should be classified as an obesity-related behavior. However, not all binge eaters are obese and not all obese people are binge eaters. Furthermore, binge eaters are far more likely to report significant mood problems, especially depression, and greater dissatisfaction with their weight and shape, as compared to persons with obesity.

Other experts believe that binge eating is a subtype of bulimia. Bulimia is characterized by episodes of binge eating followed by self-induced purging through vomiting; abuse of laxatives, diuretics, or enemas; fasting; or **compulsive exercise**. Although persons with BED often attempt to diet between binges, they do not purge extra calories. They also do not exhibit anorexic or self-starving behaviors, which may occur in persons with bulimia.

Risk factors

Risk factors for binge eating are similar to risk factors for other eating disorders. These include:

- a family history of eating disorders
- frequent dieting, especially rigorous diets or frequently gaining and losing large amounts of weight (weight cycling)
- preoccupation with weight and body image
- impulsiveness or poor impulse control
- low self-esteem and negative self-talk
- difficulty expressing feelings appropriately and managing anger
- a history of sexual abuse
- depression, which can be both a risk factor for binge eating and a result of binge eating

Causes and symptoms

Like other eating disorders, BED has multiple causes. Some people appear to be genetically predisposed to binge eating. Researchers believe that this may be related to abnormalities in **brain neurotransmitters** that help regulate appetite. Binge-eating episodes may occur in response to strong negative emotions, such as depression or anxiety, or to less defined feelings of distress or tension. People who binge eat are far more likely than others to describe themselves as experiencing personal and work problems and as being hypersensitive to the opinions of others. Like with bulimia, persons with BED are more likely than others to be diagnosed with major depression, substance-related disorders, and **personality disorders**. Binge eating is often triggered by stress—sometimes the **stress** is caused by very restrictive **diets**, but often the stress is caused by social and cultural factors, such as family conflicts or dysfunctional relationships. Pressure felt by cultural and media messages that promote being thin as desirable can also result in binge eating, which is used as a coping mechanism. Some patients report that their binges are related to the ingestion of certain "trigger foods," usually carbohydrates.

Whatever the cause, bingeing appears to temporarily alleviate uncomfortable or painful feelings. While bingeing, patients typically describe themselves as "numb" or "spaced out." Their relief is short-lived, leading to repeated bingeing. The out-of-control eating is a frightening experience for most people, and they usually feel embarrassed and ashamed about their bingeing. In the aftermath of a binge, many people experience overwhelming feelings of guilt, self-disgust, anxiety, and depression. They vow never to binge again but are unable to prevent it.

Symptoms of binge eating can be difficult to detect. The eating often occurs in private, and the eater tends to be secretive about food. Specific symptoms of binge eating include:

- feeling out of control and unable to stop eating
- continuing to eat despite feeling full or even painfully uncomfortable
- eating abnormally large amounts of food at one sitting, sometimes as many as 3,000–10,000 calories in a short period
- eating abnormally fast
- eating alone or in secret
- hoarding food and hiding empty food containers
- constant dieting without weight loss
- obsessive concern with weight
- depression
- anxiety
- substance abuse

KEY TERMS

Anorexia nervosa—A serious eating disorder that primarily affects young women in their teens and early twenties and is characterized by a pathological fear of gaining weight. Anorexia causes disturbed eating behavior and can lead to severe weight loss and malnutrition.

Bulimia nervosa—A serious eating disorder that primarily affects young women and is characterized by compulsive overeating followed by purging, usually self-induced vomiting or the use of laxatives or diuretics.

Cognitive-behavioral therapy (CBT)—A type of psychotherapy in which people learn to recognize and change negative and self-defeating patterns of thinking and behavior.

Electrolytes—Ions—such as sodium, potassium, calcium, magnesium, chloride, phosphate, bicarbonate, and sulfate—that are dissolved in bodily fluids such as blood and regulate or affect most metabolic processes.

Neurotransmitters—Chemicals that carry impulses between nerve cells (neurons), including acetylcholine, dopamine, serotonin, and norepinephrine.

Selective serotonin reuptake inhibitors (SSRIs)—A class of antidepressants that works by blocking the reabsorption of serotonin by brain cells, raising the level of the chemical in the brain.

Serotonin—5-Hydroxytryptamine; a neurotransmitter present throughout the body, especially in the brain. Inadequate amounts of serotonin have been implicated in numerous disorders, including depression and obsessive-compulsive disorder.

Triglycerides—A type of fat in the blood. High levels of triglycerides can increase the risk of coronary artery disease.

Weight cycling—Repeatedly gaining and losing weight.

Diagnosis

Diagnosis requires examination, tests, and compiling relevant personal information.

Examination

Diagnosis should include a physical examination and medical history, although binge eating disorder is often diagnosed and treated by a **psychiatrist** or **psychologist**. Diagnosis can be difficult. Binge eaters often go to extremes to hide how much they eat. They may, for example, buy snack food at the grocery store and eat it in the car before they get home or buy food in secret and hoard it. Although diagnosis usually begins with a personal and family history, including eating habits and **exercise**, binge eaters may lie about their eating.

Tests

Physicians usually order standard laboratory tests, including a complete blood count (CBC), urinalysis, and blood tests to check levels of cholesterol, triglycerides, and electrolytes. Additional tests, such as thyroid function, may be ordered to rule out other disorders. If the patient is obese, tests may be performed for obesity-related conditions, such as diabetes, cardiovascular disease, and sleep apnea.

Procedures

The assessment process may include a questionnaire, such as the Eating Disorder Examination Questionnaire. There are several clinical inventories or scales that are used to assess depressive symptoms, including the **Hamilton Depression Scale** (HAM-D) and the **Beck Depression Inventory** (BDI). These tests are usually administered in an office setting.

Treatment

There are various approaches in treating BED; however, for the best results, patients must want to stop binge eating.

Traditional

BED is usually treated most effectively by a combination of **psychotherapy** and **group therapy**. However, physicians are more likely to concentrate on weight-control issues, using drugs, diet, and **nutrition counseling** to reduce the health risks of obesity-related diseases. Although **nutrition** counseling and meal planning may help control weight, they do not address the impulse to binge eat. Psychologists are more likely to treat behavior and thought patterns that cause abnormal eating, since obesity may be easier to treat once bingeing behavior is controlled.

Several types of psychotherapy may be effective for treating BED. **Cognitive-behavioral therapy** (CBT) is a relatively short-term therapy designed to confront and change thoughts and feelings about one's body and behaviors toward food. It does not address the origins of those thoughts and feelings, but rather explores **self-control strategies** and the development of skills for coping with emotional distress. **Interpersonal therapy** is short-term therapy to help identify and resolve specific relationship issues and problems and has been shown to be successful in the treatment of BED. Dialectical behavior therapy (DBT) utilizes structured private and group sessions for reducing behaviors that interfere with quality of life, finding alternate solutions to current problem situations, and learning to regulate emotions. **Family therapy** is helpful for treating children who binge eat. It teaches strategies for reducing conflict, disorder, and stress that can trigger binge eating.

Drugs

There are no drugs specifically approved by the U.S. Food and Drug Administration (FDA) for treating binge eating. However, the FDA has approved **antidepressants** called **selective serotonin reuptake inhibitors (SSRIs)**, such as **fluoxetine** (Prozac) and **sertraline** (Zoloft), for the treatment of bulimia, which involves binge-eating behavior. These medications increase **serotonin** levels in the brain and are thought to affect the body's sense of fullness. **SSRIs** are often prescribed for BED, regardless of whether there are signs of depression. Tricyclic antidepressants (TCAs) and appetitive suppressants may be prescribed for BED, but their use is rare. The anticonvulsant topiramate (Topamax), which is normally used to control **seizures**, has been found to reduce binge-eating episodes, but this drug can have serious side effects.

Alternative

Alternative treatments for binge eating often focus on curbing concurrent depression. Herbal remedies that may ease symptoms of depression include **5-HTP**, **DHEA**, **saffron**, and **St. John's wort**; kava-kava root may reduce symptoms of anxiety. Relaxation exercises and techniques that may help reduce binge-eating episodes triggered by stress or depression include **music therapy**, **yoga**, and other forms of relaxation.

Home remedies

Although weight-loss programs are helpful for some people with BED, they generally are not recommended until after BED treatment, since low-calorie diets can trigger binge eating. Weight-loss programs generally do not address binge-eating triggers to the same extent as psychotherapy. Weight loss should be medically supervised.

Self help programs, including books and manuals, videos, and **support groups**, can be helpful for treating BED. A 2010 study of patients with at least one binge-eating episode per week found that 64% of patients who attended eight therapy sessions utilizing a six-step self-help program were binge free after one year. This compared with 45% of patients who were given only basic healthy eating information and informed of available services.

Self-help programs are cost-effective as well. In another 2010 study of 123 patients with binge eating disorder, a guided self-help program was significantly more cost effective than simply providing patients with options for treatment. The cost to society in terms of binge-free days and workplace productivity was significantly reduced in the **intervention** group, with a savings of more than $26,000 per quality of life year.

Home remedies for binge eating include eating breakfast, avoiding diets, getting appropriate essential nutrients, and keeping less food in the home. Binge eaters are also advised to exercise and seek support from friends and family members.

QUESTIONS TO ASK YOUR DOCTOR

- Should I be concerned about binge eating if I am not overweight?
- What are the health consequences of binge eating?
- Will I need both medication and psychotherapy?
- Can you recommend a therapist?
- Is there anything my friends and family can do to help me overcome my binge eating?
- Can you refer me to a support group for binge eating?
- Will my insurance cover my medical and psychological treatment?

Prognosis

Overall rates of recovery are higher for BED than for bulimia. Some people find that simply the act of seeking help or taking a placebo improves their control over binge eating. This is one reason why some medical professionals do not accept binge eating as a genuine disorder. In any case, binge-eating relapses are common in response to stressful life events.

Prevention

Binge eating is difficult to prevent, since its causes are unclear, and it can be difficult to detect. Prevention strategies include:

- eating small meals every three or four hours to avoid hunger
- tracking food intake
- avoiding eating alone
- avoiding using food for comfort in times of stress
- monitoring negative self-talk and practicing positive self-talk
- spending time doing something enjoyable every day
- staying busy without becoming frantic or stressed
- being aware of situations that invite bingeing and looking for ways to avoid or defuse such situations
- avoiding extreme diets
- teaching children to have healthy attitudes toward their weight, appearance, and diet
- avoiding comparisons or teasing about body size and shape
- loving and accepting family members for who they are
- being alert for signs of low self-esteem, anxiety, depression, and drug or alcohol abuse, and seeking help if signs appear

Resources

BOOKS

Agras, W. Stewart. *Overcoming Eating Disorders: A Cognitive-Behavioral Therapy Approach for Bulimia Nervosa and Binge-Eating Disorder,* 2nd ed. New York: Oxford University Press, 2008.

American Psychiatric Association. *Diagnostic and Statistical Manual of Mental Disorders (DSM-IV-TR),* 4th ed., text rev. Washington, DC: American Psychiatric Association, 2000.

Bulik, Cynthia M. *Crave: Why You Binge Eat and How to Stop.* New York: Walker, 2009.

Favor, Lesli J. *Food as Foe: Nutrition and Eating Disorders.* New York: Marshall Cavendish Benchmark, 2008.

Herzog, David B., Debra L. Franko, and Patricia Cable. *Unlocking the Mysteries of Eating Disorders.* New York: McGraw-Hill, 2007.

Lawton, Sandra Augustyne. *Eating Disorders Information for Teens,* 2nd ed. Detroit: Omnigraphics, 2009.

Mitchell, James E. *Binge-Eating Disorder: Clinical Foundations and Treatment.* New York: Guilford, 2008.

Schulherr, Susan. *Eating Disorders for Dummies.* Hoboken, NJ: Wiley, 2008.

Seles, Monica. *Getting a Grip: On My Body, My Mind, My Self.* New York: Avery, 2009.

Silverstein, Alvin, Virginia B. Silverstein, and Laura Silverstein Nunn. *The Eating Disorders Update: Understanding Anorexia, Bulimia, and Binge Eating.* Berkeley Heights, NJ: Enslow, 2009.

PERIODICALS

Ellin, Abby. "Redefining an Eating Disorder." *New York Times* (January 19, 2010): D5.

Hellmich, Nanci. "Treatment for Binge Eating Need Not Be Extensive or Expensive Study: 64% Stopped with Six-Step Plan." *USA Today* (April 6, 2010): D4.

Lynch, Frances, et al. "Cost-effectiveness of Guided Self-help Treatment for Recurrent Binge Eating." *Journal of Consulting and Clinical Psychology* 78, no. 3 (June 2010): 322–33.

Mond, Jonathan M., Carol B. Peterson, and Phillipa J. Hay. "Prior Use of Extreme Weight-Control Behaviors in a Community Sample of Women with Binge Eating Disorder or Subthreshold Binge Eating Disorder: A Descriptive Study." *International Journal of Eating Disorders* 43, no. 5 (July 2010): 440–46.

Moon, Kenneth T. "Comparison of Psychological Treatments for Binge Eating Disorder." *American Family Physician* 82, no. 5 (September 1, 2010): 534.

Roberto, Christina A., et al. "Binge Eating, Purging, or Both: Eating Disorder Psychopathology Findings from an Internet Community Survey." *International Journal of Eating Disorders* 43, no. 8 (December 2010): 724–31.

Treasure, Janet, Angélica M. Claudino, and Nancy Zucker. "Eating Disorders." *Lancet* 375, no. 9714 (February 13–19, 2010): 583–93.

WEBSITES

"Binge-Eating Disorder." MayoClinic.com. October 9, 2010. http://www.mayoclinic.com/health/binge-eating-disorder/DS00608 (accessed September 16, 2011).

Doheny, Kathleen. "Study: Eating Disorders in Teens Are Common." WebMD. March 7, 2011. http://www.webmd.com/mental-health/anorexia-nervosa/news/20110307/study-eating-disorders-in-teens-are-common (accessed September 16, 2011).

"Eating Disorders." MedlinePlus. November 30, 2010. http://www.nlm.nih.gov/medlineplus/eatingdisorders.html (accessed September 16, 2011).

ORGANIZATIONS

American Psychological Association, 750 1st St. NE, Washington, DC, 20002-4242, (202) 336-5500, (800) 374-2721, http://www.apa.org.

National Association of Anorexia Nervosa and Associated Disorders, PO Box 640, Naperville, IL, 60566, (630) 577-1330, anadhelp@anad.org, http://www.anad.org.

National Eating Disorders Association, 165 W 46th St., New York, NY, 10036, (212) 575-6200, (800) 931-2237, Fax: (212) 575-1650, info@NationalEatingDisorders.org, http://www.nationaleatingdisorders.org.

Overeaters Anonymous, PO Box 44020, Rio Rancho, NM, 87174-4020, (505) 891-2664, Fax: (505) 891-4320, http://www.oa.org.

Weight-control Information Network, 1 WIN Way, Bethesda, MD, 20892-3665, (202) 828-1025, (877) 946-4627, Fax: (202) 828-1028, win@info.niddk.nih.gov, http://win.niddk.nih.gov/index.htm.

Tish Davidson, AM
Margaret Alic, PhD
Heidi Splete

Biofeedback

Definition

Biofeedback, or applied psychophysiological feedback, is a patient-guided treatment that teaches an individual to control muscle tension, pain, body temperature, **brain** waves, and other bodily functions and processes through relaxation, visualization, and other cognitive control techniques. Biological signals such as heart rate, skin temperature, or brain activity are measured and "fed back," or returned, to the patient in order for the patient to develop techniques for manipulating them.

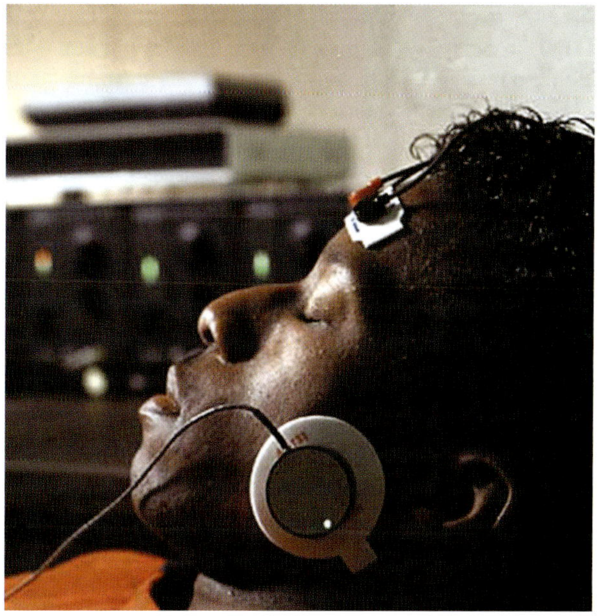

A patient undergoes biofeedback. *(© Will & Deni McIntyre/Photo Researchers, Inc.)*

Purpose

The purpose of biofeedback is to enhance an individual's awareness of physical reactions to physical, emotional, or psychological **stress**, and their ability to influence their own physiological responses. The overall purpose is to develop self-regulation skills that play a role in improving health and well-being.

Description

Biofeedback is an important part of understanding the relationship between physical state and thoughts, feelings, and behaviors. Prior to beginning any biofeedback training, individuals may need a comprehensive psychological, educational, and/or medical assessment. Biofeedback can be used in conjunction with nonmedical treatments, such as **psychotherapy**, **cognitive-behavioral therapy**, and behavioral treatment strategies.

Biofeedback has been used as a part of a comprehensive treatment approach with a number of conditions, including chronic pain, irritable bowel syndrome (IBS), temporomandibular joint disorder (TMJ), Raynaud's syndrome, epilepsy, **attention deficit hyperactivity disorder** (ADHD), anxiety, migraine headaches, **depression**, **traumatic brain injury**, and **sleep disorders**.

Conditions related to stress are also treated using biofeedback, such as certain types of headaches, high blood pressure, bruxism (teeth grinding), **post-traumatic stress disorder** (PTSD), eating disorders, **substance abuse**, and some **anxiety disorders**. In treatment of stress-related conditions, biofeedback is often used in combination with relaxation training. Sometimes, biofeedback is used to help individuals learn how to experience deeper relaxation, such as in childbirth education or general **stress management** programs. Such training is referred to as biofeedback-assisted relaxation training. Even for individuals who can achieve relaxation through other strategies such as **meditation** or relaxation, biofeedback can be a valuable added technique. Biofeedback offers special advantages, such as allowing the clinician to track closely the places where an individual tenses up and helping the individual learn what thoughts and feelings are associated with the tension.

Origins

In 1961, Neal Miller, an experimental **psychologist**, suggested that autonomic nervous system responses (for instance, heart rate, blood pressure, gastrointestinal activity, regional blood flow) could be under voluntary control. The results of his experiments showed that such autonomic processes were controllable. This work led to the creation of biofeedback therapy. Miller's work was expanded by other researchers. In the 1970s, UCLA researcher Barry Sterman established that both cats and monkeys could be trained to control their brain wave patterns. Sterman used his techniques on human patients with epilepsy and was able to reduce **seizures** by 60% with the use of biofeedback. Other researchers published reports of their use of biofeedback in the treatment of cardiac arrhythmias, headaches, Raynaud's syndrome, and excess stomach acid, and as a tool for teaching deep relaxation. Since the early work of Miller and Sterman, biofeedback has developed into a front-line behavioral treatment for an even wider range of disorders and symptoms.

How biofeedback works

Biofeedback utilizes electronic sensors, or electrodes, attached to various parts of the body to detect changes in physical responses. Visual or auditory signals, such as a light display or a series of beeps, then inform the individual of these changes. While the individual views or listens to feedback, he or she begins to recognize thoughts, feelings, and mental images that influence his or her physical reactions. By monitoring this mind-body connection, the individual can use the same thoughts, feelings, and mental images as cues or reminders to become more relaxed or to change heartbeat, brain wave patterns, body temperature, and other body functions. The individual uses trial-and-error to change the signals in the desired direction. For example, individuals trying to control their blood pressure levels may see a light flash whenever the pressure drops below a certain level. They may then try to remember what their thoughts and feelings were at the moment and deliberately maintain them to keep the blood pressure level low.

Three stages of biofeedback training

- Awareness of the problematic physical response: Individuals may complete a psychophysiological stress profile (PSP) to identify how their bodies respond to a variety of stressors and determine their ability to overcome undesired physical reactions. Doing so involves a period of rest, stress, and recovery. For example, various sensors are attached to various parts of the body, and a baseline measurement lasting from two to four minutes records physical responses. The individual then goes through a standard set of stressors (such as rapid math calculations or running in place), each lasting from two to four minutes. This activity is followed by another relaxation period to determine the length of the recovery period.
- Using signals from the biofeedback equipment to control physical responses: The individual is assisted in reaching certain goals related to managing a specific physical response.
- Transferring control from biofeedback equipment or the healthcare professional: Individuals learn to identify triggers that alert them to implement their new-found self-regulation skills.

Types of biofeedback equipment

- Electromyograph (EMG): Sensors (or electrodes) placed on the skin on pertinent parts of the body monitor electrical activity in muscles, specifically tension. This is the most frequently used biofeedback method in the treatment of various neurologic disorders such as stroke, cerebral palsy, traumatic brain injury, and multiple sclerosis. In children and adolescents, EMG may be used to treat tension headaches, enuresis, and encopresis. In treating TMJ or bruxism, EMG sensors are placed on jaw muscles. Chronic stress is treated by monitoring muscle tension in various places on the body.
- Galvanic skin response (GSR): Sensors on the fingers monitor perspiration. This is also referred to as obtaining a skin conductance level (SCL). GSR may be used in the treatment of anxiety, phobias, stress, and sleep problems.
- Temperature or thermal sensors: Sensors monitor body temperature and changes in blood flow. Changes in hand temperature, for example, can indicate relaxation when there is increased blood flow to the skin. Temperature biofeedback may be useful for treating

migraine headache, Raynaud's disorder, and anxiety disorders.

- Heart rate sensors: A pulse monitor placed on the fingertip monitors pulse rate. Increases in heart rate are associated with emotional arousal, such as being angry or fearful. Decreases in heart rate are associated with relaxation.
- Capnometry (CAP): Respiratory sensors monitor oxygen intake and carbon dioxide output. This differentiates correct breathing from problematic breathing practices. Breath control training may be used to treat panic attacks, asthma, and a variety of stress-related conditions.
- Electroencephalographs (EEG) or neurofeedback: Sensors attached to the scalp monitor brain wave activity in different parts of the brain. It may be used to treat conditions with proven or suspected impact on brain wave patterns such as seizure disorders or epilepsy, ADHD, learning disabilities, migraine headaches, traumatic brain injury, and sleep disorders.

Biofeedback is geared toward whatever a person finds most appealing and understandable and is provided in several formats such as auditory, visual, or multimedia. Audio feedback, which may take the form of changes in tone and pitch, is useful because visual attention is not necessary. Visual feedback can be provided in various forms such as bar or line graphs on a computer screen. Initially, it was thought that over time computer signals could become boring or visually unappealing. In response to this suspicion, Barry Bittman developed Mindscope in 1992, which displays video scenes with realistic sounds on a high definition television set connected to a computer. Physical responses detected by the biofeedback equipment control an engaging audiovisual environment of beautiful and realistic scenes. Clarity, perspective, motion, and sounds improve as individuals deepen their relaxation. For children and adolescents, this may be described as a video game for the body. Visual displays for EMG biofeedback may include sports such as basketball, baseball, and golf, where the individual plays against the computer.

The setting in which biofeedback training takes place can vary. Sometimes the clinician, client, and equipment are in the same room. Sometimes the client sits in a comfortable chair in a semi-dark, quiet room while the clinician is in another room with the equipment. In this arrangement, the clinician and client may communicate using an intercom.

In some cases, children and adolescents may reach the desired level of control in three to five sessions. Depending on the condition, biofeedback training may require a series of sessions for several days or weeks. In general, it takes 10–15 sessions at the lower end and 40–50 sessions at the higher end.

KEY TERMS

Anxiety—Experienced as a troubled feeling, a sense of dread, fear of the future, or distress over a possible threat to a person's physical or mental well-being.

Attention deficit hyperactivity disorder (ADHD)—A developmental disorder characterized by distractibility, hyperactivity, impulsive behaviors, and the inability to remain focused on tasks or activities.

Cognitive-behavioral therapy—Psychotherapy technique designed to help people change their attitudes, perceptions, and patterns of thinking.

Benefits

Through biofeedback training, individuals learn to control targeted physical responses (such as increased heart rate) and, over time, are able to recognize what is required to reduce problematic symptoms. Eventually, the external biofeedback becomes unnecessary as the individual learns to perceive internal physical responses and make the desired changes. The individual then has a powerful, portable, and self-administered treatment tool to deal with problematic symptoms that arise in response to anxiety, depression, stress, or other conditions.

Sometimes, biofeedback is used to help individuals learn how to experience deeper relaxation, such as in childbirth education or general stress management programs. Such training is referred to as biofeedback-assisted relaxation training. Even for individuals who can achieve relaxation through other strategies such as meditation or relaxation, biofeedback offers special advantages, such as allowing the clinician to track closely the places where an individual tenses up and helping the individual learn what thoughts and feelings are associated with the tension.

Precautions

Biofeedback depends on the motivation and active participation of participants. Thus, it may not be suitable for individuals with low motivation who are not willing to take a highly active role in treatment, such as those who have depression. Also, since biofeedback focuses on initiating behavioral changes, individuals inclined to examine their past to alleviate problems and symptoms may benefit more from other treatment types, such as psychotherapy. Individuals with cognitive impairment may be unable to remain engaged in the treatment, depending on their level of functioning. Also, individuals with a pacemaker or other implanted electrical devices should inform their health-care professional before entering biofeedback training, as certain types of biofeedback sensors may interfere with the devices. Patients with specific pain symptoms in which the cause is unknown should have a thorough medical examination to rule out underlying diseases or conditions before starting biofeedback training. Biofeedback can be used in combination with conventional therapies; however, while it can be used in combination with conventional medical treatment for illnesses such as cancer and diabetes, it should not replace those treatments.

The use of biofeedback techniques to treat an array of disorders has been extensively described in the medical literature. Controlled studies for some applications are limited, such as for the treatment of menopausal symptoms and premenstrual disorder (PMS). There is also some debate over the effectiveness of biofeedback in ADHD treatment. While many therapists, counselors, and mental health professionals have reported great success in treating patients with ADHD by using neurofeedback techniques, some critics attribute this positive therapeutic impact to a placebo effect.

There is also some debate among mental health professionals as to whether biofeedback should be considered a first-line treatment for some mental illnesses and to what degree other treatments, such as medication, should be employed as an adjunct therapy.

Research on the success of biofeedback in treating certain conditions is inconclusive or needs to be validated. Some research studies use a small number of participants, which makes it difficult to generalize the results for a larger population. Also, many conditions have different subtypes with a variety of psychological, social, and physical causes. This fact, combined with research design concerns, makes it difficult to compare research studies. For example, while most studies have reported positive outcomes in the treatment of alcohol abuse and dependence, problems with methods and statistical analyses have called study results into question. Also, its effectiveness in treating opiate abuse or dependence has not been consistently shown, as with its use in treating menopausal hot flashes, and there are limitations in studies relating to its use in cancer treatment. Continued research is needed to further evaluate and improve different biofeedback techniques for various conditions.

QUESTIONS TO ASK YOUR DOCTOR

- What are the indications that biofeedback would be a useful treatment approach for my condition?
- What kind of results can be determined with biofeedback treatment?
- How long will biofeedback treatment take?
- Will insurance cover biofeedback treatment?

Preparation

Biofeedback is most successful when individuals are motivated to learn. It is useful for people who have difficulty relaxing, even when they make efforts to do so. A receptive and open attitude, or "passive volition," is important for attaining desired responses rather than actively focusing on attaining them. It is important that individuals are willing to practice regularly at home to apply the skill to everyday life. Establishing a foundation of trust and confidence in the health care professional is an important component of biofeedback training.

Before beginning biofeedback training, an initial consultation is conducted to record medical history, treatment background, and biofeedback goals. The procedure is explained to provide a clear understanding of how and why the training can be helpful. The individual may be shown the equipment and told where the electrodes will be placed and how they work.

Before electrodes are placed on the body, the skin surface must be adequately prepared by using alcohol preparation pads to remove oils, makeup, and dead skin cells that may interfere with the biofeedback signal. An electrode paste is then applied to the sensor, or a small adhesive pad may be used to attach the sensor to the skin. Heart rate, temperature, and GSR monitors may be placed on the fingertip with a Velcro or elastic band. With CAP, the tip of a small, flexible, plastic tube is positioned in the nostril using tape. An individual may be taught several forms of biofeedback initially, and then the training may be tailored to the individual's preference.

The biofeedback trainer must have technical skill, an understanding of basic anatomy and physiology, knowledge of various conditions, and familiarity with computer hardware and software. The **American Psychological Association** views biofeedback as a proficiency area—master's and doctoral level training programs are available through a variety of sources, and certification is available through the Biofeedback Certification Institute of America.

Aftercare

There is no aftercare for biofeedback. Individuals apply what they learn during the sessions, and in this way, they help control their responses to stressors.

Risks

There are no known side effects with properly administered biofeedback.

Resources

BOOKS

Cade, Maxwell C., and Nona Coxhead. *The Awakened Mind: Biofeedback and the Development of Higher States of Awareness.* New York: Element Books, 2011.

Coben, Robert, and James R. Evans, eds. *Neurofeedback and Neuromodulation Techniques and Applications.* San Diego, CA: Academic Press, 2010.

Kotsirilos, Vicki, et al. *A Guide to Evidence-based Integrative and Complementary Medicine.* New York: Churchill Livingstone, 2011.

Miller, Eric B. *Bio-Guided Music Therapy: A Practitioner's Guide to the Clinical Integration of Music and Biofeedback.* Philadelphia: Jessica Kingsley, 2011.

Robbins, Jim. *A Symphony in the Brain: The Evolution of the New Brain Wave Biofeedback.* New York: Grove Press, 2008.

Swingle, Paul G. *Biofeedback for the Brain: How Neurotherapy Effectively Treats Depression, ADHD, Autism, and More.* Piscataway, NJ: Rutgers University Press, 2008.

ORGANIZATIONS

Association for Applied Psychotherapy and Biofeedback, 10200 W 44th Ave., Ste. 304, Wheat Ridge, CO, 80033, (303) 422-8436, (800) 477-8892, aapb@resourcecenter.com, http://www.aapb.org.

Biofeedback Certification International Alliance, 10200 W 44th Ave., Ste. 310, Wheat Ridge, CO, 80033, (303) 420-2902, (866) 908-8713, Fax: (303) 422-8894, info@bcia.org, http://www.bcia.org.

Joneis Thomas, PhD
Laura Jean Cataldo, RN, EdD

Biperiden

Definition

Biperiden is classified as an antiparkinsonian agent. It is sold in the United States under the brand name of Akineton.

Purpose

Biperiden is used to treat a group of side effects (called parkinsonian side effects) that includes tremors, difficulty walking, and slack muscle tone. These side effects may occur in patients who are taking antipsychotic medications used to treat mental disorders such as **schizophrenia**.

Description

Some medicines used to treat schizophrenia and other mental disorders, called antipsychotic drugs, can cause side effects that are similar to the symptoms of Parkinson's disease. The patient does not have Parkinson's disease may experience similar symptoms, including shaking in muscles while at rest, difficulty with voluntary movements, and poor muscle tone.

One way to eliminate these undesirable side effects is to stop taking the antipsychotic medicine. Unfortunately, the symptoms of the original mental disorder usually come back, so in most cases simply stopping the antipsychotic medication is not a reasonable option. Some drugs such as biperiden that control the symptoms of Parkinson's disease also control the parkinsonian side effects of antipsychotic medicines.

Biperiden works by restoring the chemical balance between **dopamine** and acetylcholine, two neurotransmitter chemicals in the **brain**. Taking biperiden along with the antipsychotic medicine helps to control symptoms of the mental disorder, while reducing parkinsonian side effects. Biperiden is in the same family of drugs (commonly known as anticholinergic drugs) as **benztropine**, **amantadine**, and **trihexyphenidyl**.

Recommended dosage

Biperiden is available in 2 mg tablets. For the treatment of tremor, poor muscle tone, and other parkinsonian side effects, the dose of biperiden is 2 mg orally taken one to three times daily. The side effects caused by antipsychotic drugs may come and go, so biperiden may not be needed on a regular basis. Biperiden may also be prescribed to prevent these side effects before they actually occur. This is called as prophylactic (preventative) therapy.

Precautions

Biperiden should never be used in children under age three. It should be used cautiously and with close physician supervision in older children and in the elderly. Biperiden, like all anticholinergic drugs, decreases sweating and the body's ability to cool itself. People who are unaccustomed to being outside in hot weather should take care to stay as cool as possible and drink extra fluids. People who are chronically ill, have a central nervous system disease, or who work outside during hot weather may need to avoid taking biperiden.

People who have the following medical problems may experience increased negative side effects when taking biperiden. Anyone with these problems should discuss their condition with their physician before starting the drug:

- glaucoma, especially closed-angle glaucoma
- intestinal obstruction
- prostate enlargement
- urinary bladder obstruction

Although rare, some patients experience euphoria while taking biperiden and may abuse it for this reason. Euphoria can occur at doses only two to four times the normal daily dose. Patients with a history of drug abuse should be observed carefully for biperiden abuse.

Side effects

Although biperiden helps control the side effects of antipsychotic drugs, it can produce side effects of its own. A person taking biperiden may have some of the following side effects, which may vary in intensity:

- dry mouth
- dry skin
- blurred vision
- nausea or vomiting
- constipation
- disorientation
- drowsiness
- irritability
- increased heart rate
- urinary retention

Dry mouth, if severe to the point of causing difficulty in speaking or swallowing, may be managed by dosage reduction or temporary discontinuation of the drug. Chewing sugarless gum or sucking on sugarless candy may also help to increase the flow of saliva. Some artificial saliva products may give temporary relief.

Men with prostate enlargement may be especially prone to urinary retention. Symptoms of this problem include having difficulty starting a urine flow and more difficulty passing urine than usual. This side effect may be severe and require discontinuation of the drug. Urinary retention may require catheterization. People who think they may be experiencing any side effects from this or any other medication should tell their physicians.

KEY TERMS

Acetylcholine—A naturally occurring chemical in the body that transmits nerve impulses from cell to cell. It causes blood vessels to dilate, lowers blood pressure, and slows the heartbeat. Central nervous system well-being is dependent on a balance among the neurotransmitters acetylcholine, dopamine, serotonin, and norepinephrine.

Anticholinergic—Related to the ability of a drug to block the nervous system chemical acetylcholine. When acetylcholine is blocked, patients often experience dry mouth and skin, increased heart rate, blurred vision, and difficulty urinating. In severe cases, blocking acetylcholine may cloud thinking and cause delirium.

Catheterization—Placing a tube in the bladder so that it can be emptied of urine.

Dopamine—A chemical in brain tissue that serves to transmit nerve impulses (a neurotransmitter) and helps to regulate movement and emotions.

Neurotransmitter—A chemical in the brain that transmits messages between neurons, or nerve cells.

Parkinsonian—Related to symptoms associated with Parkinson's disease, a nervous system disorder characterized by abnormal muscle movement of the tongue, face, and neck; inability to walk or move quickly; walking in a shuffling manner; restlessness; and/or tremors.

Patients who take an overdose of biperiden are treated with forced vomiting, removal of stomach contents and stomach washing, activated charcoal, and respiratory support if needed. They are also given physostigmine, an antidote for anticholinergic drug poisoning.

Interactions

When drugs such as biperiden are taken with **antidepressants** such as **amitriptyline**, **imipramine**, **trimipramine**, **desipramine**, **nortriptyline**, **protriptyline**, **amoxapine**, and **doxepin**, as well as with many antihistamines that also have anticholinergic properties, the effects of biperiden are usually intensified.

Drugs such as biperiden decrease the speed with which food moves through the stomach and intestines. Because of this, it is possible that the absorption of some drugs may be enhanced by biperiden. Patients receiving biperiden should be observed for unusual responses to other drugs they might be taking.

Resources

BOOKS

American Society of Health-System Pharmacists. *AHFS Drug Information 2008*. Bethesda, MD: American Society of Health-System Pharmacists, 2008.

DeVane, C. Lindsay, Pharm.D. "Drug Therapy for Mood Disorders." In *Fundamentals of Monitoring Psychoactive Drug Therapy*. Baltimore: Williams and Wilkins, 1990.

Jack Raber, Pharm.D.

Biphetamine *see* **Amphetamines**

Bipolar disorder

Definition

Bipolar disorder, formerly known as manic **depression**, is a psychiatric disorder characterized by severe and unusual changes in energy level, mood, and interactions with others. The mood swings associated with bipolar disorder are unpredictable and range from mania (elevated or irritable mood) to depression (a mood characterized by loss of interest and sadness). Bipolar disorder causes significant impairment in social, occupational, and general functioning.

Demographics

According to the National Institutes of Mental Health (NIMH), in 2008 the lifetime prevalence rate of bipolar disorder in the United States was 1%–1.6%. Other statistics suggest that 1.0% of the population has bipolar disorder type I, and 1.1% of the population has bipolar disorder type II. About another 2.4%–4.7% of the population has subthreshold bipolar disorder, meaning that these individuals show characteristics of the disorder but do not rise to the level of formal **diagnosis**. Internationally, the lifetime prevalence of reported bipolar disorder ranges from 0.3%–1.5%.

No racial differences in distribution exist. While bipolar type I occurs equally in both sexes, bipolar II and rapid-cycling bipolar disorder are more common in females than in males. The average age of onset of bipolar disorder is 25; however, about 1% of adolescents and 0.2%–0.4% of children have been diagnosed with the bipolar disorder. Controversy exists about diagnosing the disorder in these groups. Because of the complexity of the disorder, a correct diagnosis can be delayed, and between 20%–30% of adults with bipolar disorder report having had undiagnosed symptoms in childhood or adolescence.

Description

Bipolar disorder is characterized by alternating manic episodes, in which the individual feels abnormally euphoric, optimistic, and energetic, and depressive periods, in which the individual feels sad, hopeless, guilty, and sometimes suicidal. Manic or depressive periods may last for days, weeks, or months and run the spectrum from mild to severe. These episodes may be separated by periods of emotional stability during which the individual functions normally.

Bipolar I disorder is characterized by at least one **manic episode** without a major depressive episode. Manic episodes are the "high" of the manic-depressive cycle. A person experiencing a manic episode often has feelings of self-importance, elation, talkativeness, increased sociability, and a desire to embark on goal-oriented activities, coupled with the characteristics of irritability, impatience, impulsiveness, hyperactivity, and a decreased need for sleep. Usually this manic period is followed by a period of severe depression, although a few individuals may not experience a major depressive episode. Mixed states, where both manic or hypomanic symptoms and depressive symptoms occur at the same time, also may occur (e.g., the racing thoughts of mania with the listlessness of depression). Dysphoric mania, characterized by anger and irritability, is common, particularly in adolescents.

Bipolar II disorder is characterized by major depressive episodes alternating with episodes of **hypomania**, a milder form of mania. A bipolar depressive episode may be difficult to distinguish from a unipolar major depressive episode. Patients with bipolar depression tend to have extremely low energy, slowed mental and physical processes, and more profound **fatigue** (for example, **hypersomnia**, a sleep disorder marked by a need for excessive sleep or sleepiness when awake) than people with unipolar depression.

Cyclothymia refers to the cycling of hypomanic episodes with less severe depression that does not reach major depressive proportions. Some people with cyclothymia develop bipolar I or II disorder later in life.

A phenomenon known as rapid cycling occurs in up to 20% of bipolar individuals. In rapid cycling, at least four manic and depressive moods swings must occur within 12 months. In some cases of ultra-rapid cycling, the individual may bounce between manic and depressive states several times within a 24-hour period. This condition is very hard to distinguish from mixed states.

Risk factors

According to the Mayo Clinic, 60% of bipolar cases have a family history of the disease. The Child and

Adolescent Bipolar Foundation (CABF) reports that the risk for a child of one bipolar parent to develop the disorder is 15%–30%. If both parents have bipolar disorder, the risk for each child increases to 50%–75%. The risk in siblings and fraternal twins is 15%–25%. The risk in identical twins, who share the same genes, is approximately 70%. Research in identical twins indicates that both genes and other factors play a role in developing bipolar disorder.

Women who have given birth may also be at increased risk of developing subsequent episodes in the immediate period after giving birth.

Causes and symptoms

Causes

Although the source of bipolar disorder has not been clearly identified, a number of genetic and environmental factors appear to be involved in triggering episodes. Bipolar disorder has an inherited component, as children who have at least one parent with bipolar disorder are more likely to develop the disorder. Several studies have uncovered possible genetic connections to the predisposition for bipolar disorder. A large study done in Sweden reported in 2009 that **schizophrenia** and bipolar disorder appeared to share similar genetic causes.

No specific gene mutations have been identified that consistently show up in bipolar patients. However, there appears to be a potential genetic correlation between bipolar disorder and mutations in specific regions of chromosomes 13, 18, and 21. The building blocks of genes, called nucleotides, are normally arranged in a specific order and quantity. If these nucleotides are repeated in a redundant fashion, a genetic abnormality often results. Some evidence exists for an abnormal type of nucleotide sequence (CAG/CTG repeats) on chromosome 18 in patients with bipolar II disorder. However, not all bipolar patients have this mutation, and the presence of this sequence does not worsen the disorder or change the age of onset.

People with bipolar disorder tend to have other psychiatric disorders. **Oppositional defiant disorder** (ODD) and **attention deficit hyperactivity disorder** (ADHD) are among the most common. Over half of patients diagnosed with bipolar disorder have a history of **substance abuse**. A high rate of association exists between **cocaine** abuse and bipolar disorder. The emotional and physical highs and lows of cocaine use correspond to the manic depression cycle of the bipolar patient, making the disorder difficult to diagnose.

For some bipolar patients, manic and depressive episodes coincide with seasonal changes. Depressive episodes are typical during winter and fall, and manic episodes are more probable in the spring and summer months.

Brain imaging studies suggest that there are physical changes in the brains of people with bipolar disorder. It is hypothesized that **dopamine** and other **neurotransmitters** involved in mood may be involved. The possible role of hormonal imbalances in bipolar disorder is another area of investigation. Further research is needed to determine which genes are involved in bipolar disorder. It is likely that both genetic and environmental factors contribute to the disease.

Symptoms

Bipolar disorder causes recurrent dramatic mood swings that range from manic highs to depressive lows. There are often periods of normal mood in between episodes of mania and depression. Severe changes in energy and behavior accompany the swings in mood.

Manic episode symptoms include:

- increased energy, activity, and restlessness
- excessively high, euphoric mood
- extreme irritability and reactivity
- racing thoughts and fast speech that jump from one topic to another, known as a flight of ideas
- distractibility due to unimportant events and the inability to concentrate
- low perceived need for sleep
- unrealistic beliefs in personal abilities, powers, or importance
- poor judgment and impulsive behaviors
- increased sexual drive
- provocative, intrusive, or aggressive behavior
- denial that anything is wrong

Depressive episode symptoms include:

- persistent sad, anxious, or empty mood
- feelings of irritability, hopelessness, or negative mood
- feelings of guilt, worthlessness, or helplessness
- inability to take pleasure in activities
- fatigue
- inability to concentrate
- poor judgment
- extreme sleep patterns
- extreme appetite changes that result in weight change
- chronic pain or physical discomfort in the absence of physical illness or injury
- thoughts or attempts of suicide

Some people with bipolar II disorder have depressive episodes concurrent with mood reactivity and can switch from depression to hypomania. Hypomania is characterized by a mild or moderate level of mania. Because hypomania is less severe, it may be associated with increased functioning and enhanced productivity. However, hypomania is not a normal state of mind. Without proper treatment, hypomania may eventually progress into severe mania or switch into depression. Severe episodes of mania or depression may also include symptoms of **psychosis**. Psychotic symptoms include visual or auditory hallucinations and **delusions** (illogical and false but strongly held beliefs). Psychotic symptoms in bipolar disorder tend to reflect the current extreme mood episode. During mania, psychotic delusions may include grandiosity, such as believing one has special powers of flight or extreme financial wealth or power. During depressive episodes, delusions may include paranoid fears of being poisoned or the belief that one has committed a terrible crime. Because of these psychotic symptoms, bipolar disorder is sometimes mistaken for schizophrenia.

Some people with bipolar disorder display a mixed state of symptoms. A mixed bipolar state is characterized by symptoms of agitation, sleeplessness, appetite changes, psychosis, and suicidal tendencies. A depressed and hopeless mood may occur in conjunction with extreme energy. Signs of bipolar disorder may also be demonstrated outside of mental illness symptoms in behaviors such as alcohol or drug abuse, poor work performance, strained interpersonal relationships, or excessive promiscuity. Symptoms of bipolar disorder with postpartum onset usually occur within four weeks following childbirth. Bipolar disorder with a seasonal pattern displays symptoms related to seasonal change and latitude. The prevalence of the season-specific bipolar symptoms increases with higher latitudes and winter months.

Bipolar symptoms often present differently in children and adolescents. Manic episodes in these age groups are typically characterized by more psychotic features than in adults, which may lead to a misdiagnosis of schizophrenia. Children and adolescents also tend toward irritability and aggressiveness instead of elation. Further, symptoms tend to be chronic (ongoing) rather than acute (episodic). Bipolar children are easily distracted, impulsive, and hyperactive, which can lead to a misdiagnosis of ADHD. Furthermore, their aggression often leads to violence, which may be misdiagnosed as a **conduct disorder**. Complicating the picture is the fact that ADHD and conduct disorders are often present concurrently in children with bipolar disorder.

School problems are frequently encountered in children and adolescents with bipolar disorder. Teachers, **social workers**, and counselors who are knowledgeable about bipolar disorder and familiar with its symptoms can be helpful in describing behaviors seen in the classroom to parents and clinicians so that appropriate evaluation, diagnosis, and **intervention** may be determined. Modifications in portions of the daily schedule and some academic accommodations for this population may be helpful in the school environment.

KEY TERMS

Cyclothymia—A milder form of bipolar disorder characterized by alternating hypomania and less severe depressive episodes.

Dopamine—A neurotransmitter and the precursor of norepinephrine.

Neuroprotective—Conveying some form of protection to the nervous system from injury.

Neurotransmitter—One of a group of chemicals secreted by a nerve cell (neuron) to carry a chemical message to another nerve cell, often as a way of transmitting a nerve impulse. Examples of neurotransmitters include acetylcholine, dopamine, serotonin, and norepinephrine.

Nucleotides—Building blocks of genes, which are arranged in specific order and quantity.

Off-label use—The use of a prescription medication to treat conditions outside the indications approved by the U.S. Food and Drug Administration (FDA). It is legal for physicians to administer these drugs, but it is not legal for pharmaceutical companies to advertise drugs for off-label uses.

Rapid cycling—Four or more manic, hypomanic, mixed, or depressive episodes within a 12-month period.

Schizophrenia—A severe mental disorder in which a person loses touch with reality and has illogical thoughts, delusions, hallucinations, behavioral problems, and other disturbances.

Selective serotonin reuptake inhibitors (SSRIs)—A class of antidepressants that works by blocking the reabsorption of serotonin in brain cells, raising the level of the chemical in the brain. SSRIs include fluoxetine (Prozac) and sertraline hydrochloride (Zoloft).

Diagnosis

Bipolar disorder usually is diagnosed and treated by a **psychiatrist** and/or a **psychologist** with medical assistance. In addition to an interview, several clinical inventories or scales may be used to assess the patient's mental status and determine the presence of bipolar symptoms. These include the Millon Clinical Multiaxial Inventory III (MCMI-III), **Minnesota Multiphasic Personality Inventory** II (MMPI-2), the Internal State Scale (ISS), the Self-Report Manic Inventory (SRMI), and the Young Mania Rating Scale (YMRS). The tests are verbal and/or written and are administered in both hospital and outpatient settings. Taking a detailed family history is also important in making the diagnosis of bipolar disorder because it often runs in families. Laboratory tests for drug and **alcohol use** may be done to rule out other causes of the behavior.

Psychologists and psychiatrists typically use the criteria listed in the ***Diagnostic and Statistical Manual of Mental Disorders*** (*DSM*) published by the **American Psychiatric Association** to definitively diagnose bipolar disorder. The *DSM* describes a manic episode as an abnormally elevated (or elevated and irritable mood) lasting a period of at least one week that is distinguished by at least three of the mania symptoms. If the mood of the patient is irritable and not elevated, four of the symptoms are required.

Although some clinicians find the criteria too rigid, a hypomanic diagnosis requires a duration of at least four days with at least three of the symptoms indicated for manic episodes (four if mood is irritable and not elevated). The *DSM* notes that unlike manic episodes, hypomanic episodes do not cause a marked impairment in social or occupational functioning, do not require **hospitalization**, and do not have psychotic features. In addition, because hypomanic episodes are characterized by high energy and goal-directed activities, often resulting in a positive outcome and perceived in a positive manner by the patient (e.g., as a time of heightened creativity or work output), bipolar II disorder can go undiagnosed.

Substance abuse, thyroid disease, and use of prescription or over-the-counter medication can mask or mimic the presence of bipolar disorder. In cases of substance abuse, the patient must undergo a period of **detoxification** and abstinence before a mood disorder is diagnosed and treatment begins.

Treatment

Treatment for bipolar disorder relies primarily on prescribed drugs, though psychotherapy and other treatments may be administered in conjunction with medication.

Drugs

Medication is the most effective treatment for bipolar disorder. A combination of mood-stabilizing agents, **antidepressants**, antipsychotics, and anticonvulsants may be used for long-term regulation of manic and depressive episodes. In the acute phase, the choice of medication for bipolar disorder is dependent on the stage or type of current episode. Many drugs are used to treat an acute manic episode, primarily the antipsychotics and **benzodiazepines** (e.g., **lorazepam**, **clonazepam**). In the presence of psychotic symptoms, atypical antipsychotics may be used to treat psychotic symptoms and acute mania and contribute to mood stabilization. For depressive episodes, antidepressants may be used. Medications may be added temporarily to treat episodes of mania or depression that break through despite mood-stabilizer treatment.

Mood-stabilizing drugs dampen the extremes of manic and depressive episodes. Lithium (Cibalith-S, Eskalith, Lithane, Lithobid, Lithonate, Lithotabs) was the first mood stabilizer approved by the U.S. Food and Drug Administration (FDA) for the treatment of mania and the prevention of both manic and depressive episodes. Lithium is a first-line medication used in the long-term preventative treatment of extreme mood episodes in bipolar disorder. It has been demonstrated to play a neuroprotective role in brain function. Because lithium takes up to ten days to reach a therapeutic level in the bloodstream, it sometimes is prescribed in conjunction with neuroleptics and/or benzodiazepines to provide more immediate relief of a manic episode. Lithium also has been shown to be effective in regulating bipolar depression, but it is not recommended for mixed mania. Lithium may not be an effective long-term treatment option for rapid cyclers, who typically develop a tolerance for it or may not respond to it. Possible side effects of the drug include weight gain, thirst, nausea, and hand tremors. Prolonged lithium use also may cause hyperthyroidism (a disorder in which the thyroid is overactive, which may cause heart palpitations, nervousness, the presence of goiter, sweating, and a wide array of other symptoms) and abnormalities in liver function.

In addition to lithium, the following drugs are commonly used to treat bipolar disorders:

- Carbamazepine (Tegretol, Atretol) is an anticonvulsant drug often prescribed in conjunction with other mood-stabilizing agents. The drug may be used to treat bipolar patients who have not responded well to lithium therapy. Blurred vision and abnormal eye movement are two possible side effects of carbamazepine therapy.
- Divalproex sodium (Depakote) is one of the few drugs available that has been proven effective in treating

rapid cycling bipolar and mixed states patients. Valproate, an anticonvulsant, is prescribed alone or in combination with carbamazepine and/or lithium. Stomach cramps, indigestion, diarrhea, hair loss, appetite loss, nausea, and unusual weight loss or gain are some of the common side effects of valproate.

- Risperidone (Risperdal) may be used for short-term (usually no more than three weeks) treatment of acute mania associated with bipolar disorder. It may be given in conjunction with lithium or valproate. Side effects include weight gain, sedation, and abnormally low blood pressure upon rising from lying down (orthostatic hypotension).
- Quetiapine (Seroquel) is a newer antipsychotic that acts on neurotransmitters in the brain. It appears to have fewer side effects than some of the older antipsychotics.
- Olanzapine (Zyprexa, Zydis) may be used to treat acute manic episodes in individuals with bipolar I. Its mechanism of action is not clear. Side effects include orthostatic hypotension (low blood pressure when rising to a standing position).
- Symbyax, a combination of olanzapine and fluoxetine, was the first drug approved by the FDA specifically to treat bipolar disorder.

Because antidepressants may stimulate manic episodes in some bipolar patients, their use in bipolar disorder is controversial. Typically used as short-term treatment, antidepressants are not specifically approved for treating depression associated with bipolar disorder but may be prescribed off-label. **Selective serotonin reuptake inhibitors (SSRIs)** or, less often, **monoamine oxidase inhibitors** (MAO inhibitors) may be prescribed for episodes of bipolar depression. Tricyclic antidepressants used to treat unipolar depression may trigger rapid cycling in bipolar patients and are, therefore, not a preferred treatment option for bipolar depression.

Antidepressants commonly prescribed for bipolar disorder include:

- SSRIs such as fluoxetine (Prozac), sertraline (Zoloft), and paroxetine (Paxil). SSRIs treat depression by regulating levels of serotonin, a neurotransmitter. Anxiety, diarrhea, drowsiness, headache, sweating, nausea, sexual problems, and insomnia are all possible side effects of SSRIs.
- MAOIs such as tranylcypromine (Parnate) and phenelzine (Nardil). MAOIs block the action of monoamine oxidase (MAO), an enzyme in the central nervous system. Patients taking MAOIs must eliminate foods high in tyramine (found in aged cheeses and meats) from their diet to avoid hypotensive side effects.
- Bupropion (Wellbutrin), a heterocyclic antidepressant. The exact neurochemical mechanism of the drug is not known, but it has been effective in regulating bipolar depression in some patients. Side effects of bupropion include agitation, anxiety, confusion, tremor, dry mouth, fast or irregular heartbeat, headache, and insomnia.

Other drugs may be used in conjunction with a long-term pharmaceutical treatment plan:

- Long-acting benzodiazepines such as clonazepam (Klonopin) and alprazolam (Xanax) may be used for rapid treatment of manic symptoms to calm and sedate patients until mania or hypomania have waned and mood-stabilizing agents can take effect. Sedation is a common effect, and clumsiness, lightheadedness, and slurred speech are other possible side effects of benzodiazepines.
- Neuroleptics such as chlorpromazine (Thorazine) and haloperidol (Haldol) also may be used to control mania while a mood stabilizer such as lithium or valproate takes effect. Because neuroleptic side effects can be severe (difficulty in speaking or swallowing, paralysis of the eyes, loss of balance control, muscle spasms, severe restlessness, stiffness of arms and legs, tremors in fingers and hands, twisting movements of body, and weakness of arms and legs), benzodiazepines are generally preferred over neuroleptics.

Clozapine (Clozaril) is an atypical antipsychotic medication used to control manic episodes in patients who have not responded to typical mood stabilizing agents. The drug has also been a useful prophylactic, or preventative treatment, in some bipolar patients. Common side effects of clozapine are tachycardia (rapid heart rate), hypotension, constipation, and weight gain. Agranulocytosis, a potentially serious but reversible condition in which the white blood cells that typically fight infection in the body are destroyed, is a possible side effect of clozapine. Patients treated with the drug should undergo weekly blood tests to monitor white blood cell counts.

Many individuals suffer from **sleep deprivation** during the manic portion of bipolar disorder. When this occurs, chemical activity in the brain is altered, lowering the production of melatonin (a naturally occurring hormone important for stimulating sleep). Research is ongoing to look at the effects of melatonin in regulating the sleep-wake cycle for persons with bipolar disorder.

Treatment for children with bipolar disorder generally includes **psychotherapy** (including behavioral therapy and family-inclusive therapy) as well as medication therapy. Children may respond to psychiatric medication differently than adults do, so clinicians may choose to limit the dosage and duration of medication during which the child is monitored closely for medication benefits and side effects. Parents are often encouraged to note changes in behavior, mood, and sleep patterns of their child to aid in evaluation of medications and psychotherapy. In addition, psychologists and psychiatrists generally work closely with parents and the child to educate them about the illness.

Electroconvulsive therapy

Electroconvulsive therapy (ECT) has been successful in treating both unipolar and bipolar depression and mania. However, ECT usually is employed after all pharmaceutical treatment options have been explored in patients with severe depression and suicidal thoughts. ECT is given under anesthesia, and patients are given a muscle relaxant medication to prevent convulsions. The treatment consists of a series of electrical pulses that move into the brain through electrodes on the patient's head. Although the exact mechanisms behind the success of ECT therapy are not known, it is believed that this electrical current alters the electrochemical processes of the brain, consequently relieving depression. Headaches, muscle soreness, nausea, and confusion are possible side effects immediately following an ECT procedure. Temporary memory loss has also been reported in ECT patients. In bipolar patients, ECT is often used in conjunction with drug therapy.

Psychosocial interventions

Psychosocial interventions include both patient education and psychotherapy. It is important for patients to receive social support and illness management skills. Family and friends must be aware of the high rates of social dysfunction and marital discord. Involvement in national **support groups** is advisable (e.g., Depression and Bipolar Support Alliance, National Alliance on Mental Illness).

Psychoeducation usually focuses on all of the following:

- assessment of parameters that will have an impact on the outcome of patient's disease
- implementation of boundaries and requirements of treatment
- implementation of a personal cost-benefit analysis concerning specific treatment directions
- implementation of a follow-up program
- implementation of future directions, which may include adjustment or change interventions

Genetic counseling should be included in **family education** programs since the predisposition for this disorder has been genetically proven to increase among first-degree relatives.

Alternative and complementary treatment

Alternative treatments for bipolar disorder generally are used as complementary treatments to conventional therapies. General recommendations for controlling bipolar symptoms include maintaining a calm environment, avoiding over stimulation, getting plenty of rest and regular **exercise**, and eating a healthy diet.

Chinese herbs may help to soften mood swings. Traditional Chinese medicine (TCM) remedies are prescribed based on the patient's overall constitution and the presentation of symptoms. These remedies can help to stabilize moods, not just treat swings in mood. A TCM practitioner might recommend a mixture called the Iron Filings Combination, which includes the Chinese herbs asparagus, ophiopogon, fritillaria, arisaema, orange peel, polygala, acorus, forsythia, hoelen, fu-shen, scrophularia, uncaria stem, salvia, and iron filings to treat certain types of mania in the bipolar patient. There are other formulas for depression. A trained practitioner should guide all of these remedies.

Acupuncture can be used to help maintain a more even temperament.

Biofeedback is effective in helping some patients control such symptoms as irritability, poor self control, racing thoughts, and sleep problems.

A diet low in vanadium, a mineral found in meats and other foods, and high in vitamin C may be helpful in reducing depression.

Individuals using herbal remedies in addition to traditional pharmaceuticals should tell their physician, as some herbal remedies interact with conventional drugs, either heightening or depressing their effect. Recommended herbal remedies to ease depressive episodes may include damania (*Turnera diffusa*), **ginseng** (*Panax ginseng*), kola (*Cola nitida*), lady's slipper (*Cypripedium calceolus*), **lavender** (*Lavandula angustifolia*), lime blossom (*Tilia x vulgaris*), oats (*Avena sativa*), rosemary (*Rosmarinus officinalis*), skullcap (*Scutellaria laterifolia*), **St. John's wort** (*Hypericum perforatum*), **valerian** (*Valeriana officinalis*), and vervain (*Verbena officinalis*).

Prognosis

While most patients show some positive response to treatment, response varies widely, from full recovery to a complete lack of response to all drug and/or ECT therapy. Drug therapies frequently need adjustment to achieve the maximum benefit for the patient. Bipolar disorder is a chronic, recurrent illness in over 90% of

QUESTIONS TO ASK YOUR DOCTOR

- How will the prescribed medications help me?
- When should I take the medications? Should I take them with food?
- What if I miss a dose?
- What are the possible side effects of these medications and what can be done about them?
- How long before the medications take effect and what types of improvement should I expect?
- Are there specific risks to these medications?
- Can I choose to discontinue the medications?
- Are there foods, other medications, supplements, or activities that I should avoid?
- How will my other medical conditions affect the treatment?
- Are there dietary, physical activity, or lifestyle changes that might help with my bipolar episodes?
- Are there alternative treatments for bipolar disorder?
- What type of psychotherapy might useful?
- Are there support groups available for bipolar disorder?

people with the disorder. The disorder requires lifelong observation and treatment after diagnosis. According to the World Health Organization, bipolar disorder is the sixth-leading cause of disability worldwide.

Suicide is the major complication of bipolar disorder and is related to the duration of the depressive episode. Some 25%–50% of individuals with bipolar disorder attempt suicide, and 11% complete the suicide attempt. The longer the depressive episode lasts, the higher the risk of suicidal tendencies. Alcoholics and patients with other chronic medical diseases are particularly prone to planning and implementing a suicide attempt.

The groups of individuals most likely to carry out a suicide attempt are:

- individuals overwhelmed by life problems (attempts in this group tend to be related to aggression and impulsive behaviors, not depressive episodes)
- individuals attempting to control others
- individuals with a chronic medical illness
- individuals with other severe types of psychotic illness, delusions, or paranoia
- individuals with a concurrent substance abuse problem

Prevention

The ongoing medical management of bipolar disorder is critical to preventing **relapse**, or recurrence, of manic episodes. Even in carefully controlled treatment programs, bipolar patients may experience recurring episodes of the disorder. Patient education in the form of psychotherapy or **self-help groups** is crucial for training bipolar patients to recognize signs of mania and depression and to take an active part in their treatment program.

Resources

BOOKS

American Psychiatric Association. *Diagnostic and Statistical Manual of Mental Disorders.* 4th ed., text rev. Washington, DC: American Psychiatric Association, 2000.

American Psychological Association. *Publication Manual of the American Psychological Association,* 6th ed. Washington, DC: American Psychological Association, 2009.

Fast, Julie A. *Loving Someone with Bipolar Disorder: Understanding and Helping Your Partner,* 2nd ed. Oakland, CA: New Harbinger, 2012.

Haycock, Dean. *The Everything Health Guide to Adult Bipolar Disorder,* 2nd ed. Avon, MA: Adams Media, 2010.

Mondimore, Francis M. *Bipolar Disorder: A Guide for Patients and Families,* 2nd ed. Baltimore: Johns Hopkins University Press, 2006.

Otto, Michael, et al. *Living with Bipolar Disorder.* New York: Oxford University Press, 2011.

WEBSITES

"Bipolar Disorder." *MedlinePlus.* Last updated September 23, 2011. http://www.nlm.nih.gov/medlineplus/bipolardisorder.html (accessed October 3, 2011).

"Bipolar Disorder." *National Institute of Mental Health.* http://www.nimh.nih.gov/health/topics/bipolar-disorder/index.shtml (accessed October 3, 2011).

ORGANIZATIONS

American Academy of Child and Adolescent Psychiatry, 3615 Wisconsin Ave. NW, Washington, DC, 20016-3007, (202) 966-7300, Fax: (202) 966-2891, http://aacap.org.

American Psychiatric Association, 1000 Wilson Blvd., Ste. 1825, Arlington, VA, 22209-3901, (703) 907-7300, apa@psych.org, http://www.psych.org.

American Psychological Association, 750 1st St., NE, Washington, DC, 20002-4242, (202) 336-5500; TDD/TTY: (202) 336-6123, (800) 374-2721, http://www.apa.org.

Child & Adolescent Bipolar Foundation, 820 Davis St., Suite 520, Evanston, IL, 60201, info@thebalancedmind.org, http://www.thebalancedmind.org.

Depression and Bipolar Support Alliance, 730 N Franklin St., Ste. 501, Chicago, IL, 60654-7225, (800) 826-3632, Fax: (312) 642-7243, http://www.dbsalliance.org.

Mental Health America, 2000 N Beauregard St., 6th Fl., Alexandria, VA, 22311, (703) 684-7722, (800) 969-6642, Fax: (703) 684-5968, http://www.nmha.org.

National Alliance on Mental Illness, 3803 N Fairfax Dr., Ste. 100, Arlington, VA, 22203, (703) 524-7600, http://www.nami.org.

National Institute of Mental Health, 6001 Executive Blvd., Rm. 8184, MSC 9663, Bethesda, MD, 20892-9663, (301) 433-4513; TTY: (301) 443-8431, Fax: (301) 443-4279, (866) 615-6464; TTY: (866) 415-8051, nimhinfo@nih.gov, http://www.nimh.nih.gov.

National Institutes of Health, 9000 Rockville Pike, Bethesda, MD, 20892, (301) 496-4000; TTY: (301) 402-9612, http://www.nih.gov.

Maria Basile, PhD
Laura Jean Cataldo, RN, EdD

Body dysmorphic disorder

Definition

Body dysmorphic disorder (BDD) is defined by the **American Psychiatric Association** in its ***Diagnostic and Statistical Manual of Mental Disorders*** *(DSM)* as a condition marked by excessive preoccupation with an imaginary or minor defect in a facial feature or localized part of the body. The diagnostic criteria specify that the condition must be sufficiently severe to cause a decline in the patient's social, occupational, or educational functioning. The most common cause of this decline is the time lost to obsessing about the "defect." Proposed changes for the fifth edition of the *DSM* (*DSM-5*, 2013) include moving BDD to the category of obsessive-compulsive and related disorders. Previously, BDD was classified as a somatoform disorder—disorders characterized by physical complaints that appear to be medical in origin but that cannot be explained in terms of a physical disease, the results of **substance abuse**, or by another mental disorder.

Although cases of BDD have been reported in the psychiatric literature from a number of different countries for over a century, the disorder was first defined as a formal diagnostic category by the *DSM-III-R* in 1987. The word "dysmorphic" comes from two Greek words: *dys*, which means "bad" or "ugly," and *morphos*, which means "shape" or "form." BDD was previously known as dysmorphophobia.

Demographics

BDD is thought to affect 1%–2% of the population in the United States and Canada, although some doctors think that it is underdiagnosed because it coexists so often with **depression** and other disorders. In addition, individuals are often ashamed of grooming rituals and other behaviors associated with BDD and may avoid telling their doctor about them.

The usual age of onset of BDD is late childhood or early adolescence; the average age of individuals diagnosed with the disorder is 17, although the disorder may develop in older individuals who become preoccupied with the physical effects of aging. The disorder affects men and women equally, but there are no reliable data regarding racial or ethnic differences in the incidence of the disorder. BDD has a high rate of comorbidity, which means that people diagnosed with the disorder are likely to be diagnosed with another psychiatric disorder, most commonly major depression, **social phobia**, or **obsessive-compulsive disorder** (OCD). About half of all men (but not women) diagnosed with BDD also have a substance abuse disorder. About 29% of individuals with BDD eventually try to commit **suicide**.

Description

BDD is characterized by an unusually exaggerated degree of worry or concern about a specific part of the face or body (such as the nose or breasts), rather than the general size or shape of the body. It is distinguished from **anorexia nervosa** and **bulimia nervosa**, where patients are preoccupied with their overall weight and body shape. Studies have found that between 40% and 76% of people with BDD seek nonpsychiatric treatments such as cosmetic surgery or dermatological treatments, and the rates of people with BDD among all cosmetic surgery patients range from 7% to 15%; rates are similar in dermatology practices.

Since the first publication of *DSM-IV* in 1994, some psychiatrists have suggested that a subtype of BDD exists, which they termed muscle dysmorphia. Muscle dysmorphia is marked by excessive concern with one's muscularity and/or fitness. Persons with muscle dysmorphia spend unusual amounts of time working out in gyms or exercising rather than obsessing about a feature such as the skin or nose. Muscle dysmorphia is more prevalent among males. To accommodate muscle dysmorphia as a classification, the *DSM-IV-TR* has added references regarding body build and excessive weightlifting to DSM-IV's description of BDD, and the proposed changes for *DSM-5* include muscle dysmorphia as a specifier in the diagnostic criteria for BDD. The muscle dysmorphia version of BDD is associated with higher suicide rates and higher rates of substance abuse.

BDD and muscle dysmorphia can both be described as disorders resulting from the patient's distorted **body image**. Body image refers to the mental picture individuals have of their outward appearance, including size, shape, and form. It has two major components: how people perceive their physical appearance and how they feel about their body. Significant distortions in self-perception can lead to intense body dissatisfaction and dysfunctional behaviors aimed at improving appearance. Some patients with BDD are aware that their concerns are excessive; others do not have this degree of insight. About 50% of patients diagnosed with BDD also meet the criteria for a **delusional disorder**, which is characterized by beliefs that are not based in reality. The *DSM-5* revised description of body dysmorphic disorder emphasizes that the individual performs repetitive behaviors such as mirror checking, skin picking, or comparing themselves to others. Learning to control these repetitive behaviors can be crucial to a BDD treatment plan.

Causes and symptoms

Causes

The causes of BDD fall into two major categories, neurobiological and psychosocial.

NEUROBIOLOGICAL CAUSES. Research indicates that patients diagnosed with BDD have **serotonin** levels that are lower than normal. Serotonin is a neurotransmitter—a chemical produced by the **brain** that helps to transmit nerve impulses across the junctions between nerve cells. Low serotonin levels are associated with depression and other mood disorders. However, because these studies are conducted after the person has been diagnosed with BDD, it is not possible to know whether the low serotonin levels cause the BDD or are an effect of the disorder.

PSYCHOSOCIAL CAUSES. A young person's family of origin has a powerful influence on his or her vulnerability to BDD. Children whose parents are themselves obsessed with appearance, dieting, and/or bodybuilding, or who are highly critical of their children's looks, are at greater risk of developing BDD.

An additional factor in some young people is a history of childhood **trauma** or abuse. Buried feelings about the abuse or traumatic incident emerge in the form of **obsession** about a part of the face or body. This "reassignment" of emotions from the unacknowledged true cause to another issue is called displacement. For example, an adolescent who frequently felt overwhelmed in childhood by physically abusive parents may develop a preoccupation with muscular strength and power.

Another important factor in the development of BDD is the influence of the mass media in developed countries, particularly the role of advertising in spreading images of supposedly physically perfect men and women. Impressionable children and adolescents absorb the message that anything short of physical perfection is unacceptable. They may then develop distorted perceptions of their own faces and bodies.

Symptoms

The central symptom of BDD is excessive concern with a specific facial feature or body part. The parts of the body most frequently involved are the skin, hair, nose, teeth, breasts, eyes, and even eyebrows, but any feature can be a focus of the obsession.

Other symptoms of body dysmorphic disorder include:

- Ritualistic behavior. Ritualistic behavior refers to actions that the patient performs to manage anxiety and that take up excessive amounts of his or her time. Patients are typically upset if someone or something interferes with or interrupts their ritual. In the context of BDD, ritualistic behaviors may include exercise or makeup routines, assuming specific poses or postures in front of a mirror, or skin picking (dermatillomania).
- Camouflaging the "problem" feature or body part with makeup, hats, or clothing. Camouflaging appears to be the single most common symptom among persons with BDD, occurring in 94% of patients.
- Abnormal behavior around mirrors, car bumpers, large windows, or other reflective surfaces. A majority of patients diagnosed with BDD frequently check their appearance in mirrors or spend long periods of time doing so. A minority, however, react in the opposite fashion and avoid mirrors whenever possible.
- Frequently requesting reassurance from others (related to appearance).
- Frequently comparing one's appearance to others.
- Avoiding activities outside the home, including school and social events.

BDD patients have high rates of self-destructive behavior, including performing surgery on themselves at home (liposuction followed by skin stapling, sawing down teeth, and removing facial scars with sandpaper) and attempted or completed suicide. Many are unable to remain in school, form healthy relationships, or keep steady jobs. In one group of 100 patients diagnosed with BDD, 48% had been hospitalized for psychiatric reasons, and 30% had made at least one suicide attempt.

The loss of functioning resulting from BDD can have serious consequences for the patient's future. Adolescents with BDD often cut school and may be reluctant to participate in sports, join church- or civic-sponsored youth groups, or hold part-time or summer jobs. One study found that 32% of participants had missed work for at least a week in the previous month because of their BDD, while 32% of those still in school had missed classes for a week. Adults with muscle dysmorphia have been known to turn down job promotions to have more time to work out in their gym or fitness center. The economic consequences of BDD also include overspending on cosmetics, clothing, or plastic surgery.

Diagnosis

The **diagnosis** of BDD in children and adolescents is often made by physicians in family practice, as they are more likely to have developed long-term relationships of trust with the patient. With adults, it is often specialists in dermatology, cosmetic dentistry, or plastic surgery who may suspect that the patient has BDD because of frequent requests for repeated or unnecessary procedures. The diagnosis is made on the basis of the patient's history together with the physician's observations of the patient's overall mood and conversation patterns. People with BDD often come across to others as generally anxious and worried. In addition, the patient's dress or clothing styles, if attempting to hide the "problem" feature, may suggest a diagnosis of BDD.

Several questionnaires are used for assessing the presence of BDD. Researchers sometimes use a semi-structured interview called the BDD Data Form to collect information about the disorder from patients. This form includes demographic information, information about body areas of concern and the history and course of the illness, and the patient's history of **hospitalization** or suicide attempts, if any. Another diagnostic questionnaire frequently used to identify BDD patients is the Structured Clinical Interview for DSM-III-R Disorders, or SCID-II. Other questionnaires used in assessments include the Yale-Brown Obsessive Compulsive Scale Modified for Body Dysmorphic Disorder and the Body Dysmorphic Disorder Examination.

There are no brain **imaging studies** or laboratory tests used to diagnose BDD. Some studies using brain imaging have identified some characteristics similar to those seen in obsessive-compulsive disorder, although studies are not in complete agreement on whether these findings are diagnostic of BDD.

Treatment

The standard treatment regimen for body dysmorphic disorder is a combination of medications and **psychotherapy**. Surgical, dental, or dermatologic treatments have been found ineffective and in some cases may exacerbate symptoms. In one study, cosmetic surgeons reported that 40% of their patients with BDD had made legal or physical threats against them.

Medications

The medications most frequently prescribed for patients with BDD are the **selective serotonin reuptake inhibitors (SSRIs)**, most commonly **fluoxetine** (Prozac) or **sertraline** (Zoloft). Other **SSRIs** that have been used with this group of patients include **fluvoxamine** (Luvox) and **paroxetine** (Paxil). Only fluoxetine is approved by the FDA for use in children; another SSRI, **escitalopram** (Lexapro), is approved for use in adolescents aged 12 and up.

The relatively high rate of positive responses to SSRIs among BDD patients led to the hypothesis that the disorder has a neurobiological component related to serotonin levels in the body. An associated finding is that patients with BDD require higher dosages of SSRI medications to be effective than patients who are being treated for depression with these drugs.

According to experts at the Mayo Clinic in Rochester, Minnesota, it is important for BDD patients to continue to take their medications even when they are feeling better, because symptoms may suddenly recur. It is also important to attend psychotherapy sessions consistently.

Psychotherapy

The most effective approach to psychotherapy with BDD patients is **cognitive-behavioral therapy**, of which cognitive restructuring is one component. Because the disorder is related to **delusions** about one's appearance, cognitive-oriented therapy that challenges inaccurate self-perceptions is more effective than purely supportive approaches. Relaxation techniques also work well with BDD patients when they are combined with cognitive restructuring.

Prognosis

The *DSM-IV-TR* notes that the disorder "has a fairly continuous course, with few symptom-free intervals, although the intensity of symptoms may wax and wane over time."

Prevention

Given the pervasive influence of the mass media in contemporary Western societies, the best preventive strategy involves challenging those afflicted with the disorder and who consequently have unrealistic images of attractive people. Parents, teachers, primary healthcare professionals, and other adults who work with young people can point out and discuss the pitfalls of trying to look "perfect." In addition, parents or other adults can educate themselves about BDD and its symptoms, and should pay attention to any warning signs in their children's dress or behavior. They also can modulate their own behaviors of pointing out or highlighting physical "imperfections" in themselves or in their children, because there is a link between parents with such concerns and children with BDD.

Resources

BOOKS

American Psychiatric Association. *Diagnostic and Statistical Manual of Mental Disorders.* 4th ed., Text rev. Washington, DC: American Psychiatric Association, 2000.

PERIODICALS

Carey, Paul, et al. "SPECT Imaging of Body Dysmorphic Disorder." *Journal of Neuropsychiatry Clinical Neuroscience* 16 (2004): 357–59.

Crerand, Canice E., et al. "Nonpsychiatric Medical Treatment of Body Dysmorphic Disorder." *Psychosomatics* 46 (2005): 549–55.

Hunt, T. J., O. Thienhaus, and A. Ellwood. "The Mirror Lies: Body Dysmorphic Disorder." *American Family Physician* 78, no. 2 (2008: 217–22.

Leone, James E., Edward J. Sedory, and Kimberly A. Gray. "Recognition and Treatment of Muscle Dysmorphia and Related Body Image Disorders." *Journal of Athletic Training* 40 (2005): 352–59.

Phillips, Katharine A., et al. "Demographic Characteristics, Phenomenology, Comorbidity, and Family History in 200 Individuals with Body Dysmorphic Disorder." *Psychosomatics* 46 (2005): 317–26.

Phillips, Katharine A., and S.L. McElroy. "Personality Disorders and Traits in Patients with Body Dysmorphic Disorder." *Comparative Psychiatry* 41 (2000): 229–36.

Pope, Courtney G., et al. "Clinical Features of Muscle Dysmorphia Among Males with Body Dysmorphic Disorder." *Body Image* 2 (2005): 395–400.

WEBSITES

Mayo Clinic staff. "Body Dysmorphic Disorder." MayoClinic.com. http://www.mayoclinic.com/health/body-dysmorphic-disorder/DS00559 (accessed December 16, 2011).

ORGANIZATIONS

American Academy of Child and Adolescent Psychiatry, 3615 Wisconsin Ave., NW, Washington, DC, 20016-3007, (202) 966-7300, Fax: (202) 966-2891, http://aacap.org.

American Psychological Association, 750 1st St., NE, Washington, DC, 20002-4242, (202) 336-5500; TDD/TTY: (202) 336-6123, (800) 374-2721, http://www.apa.org.

Rebecca Frey, PhD
Emily Jane Willingham, PhD
Heidi Splete

Body image

Definition

Body image is a mental opinion or description that individuals have of their own physical appearance. It is a subjective concept, based on comparisons to socially constructed standards or ideals. Perception of body image among people can range from very negative to very positive. Depending on age and other factors, the degree of concern with body image can also vary widely among individuals.

Individuals who have a poor body image perceive their body as unattractive to others, whereas those with a good body image view their body as attractive to others. Their views may or may not accurately reflect the person's actual appearance or parallel how others judge a person's body—for instance, people may consider an individual attractive, when at the same time that individual views him- or herself as unattractive.

Description

Scientists have found that body image is first formed as an infant during contact or lack of contact with people such as parents and family members. Physical contact in the form of hugs, kisses, and other forms of affection can help develop an early positive body image. Lack of loving contact can have the opposite effect, forming an early negative body image.

Negative body image

Body image, especially among individuals as they go through puberty (a stage of physical and mental development that allows for sexual reproduction and causes transformation in the physical body shape), can become a problem under certain circumstances. For example, parents who are overly concerned with their children's weight and appearance may cause their children to develop negative concepts of their body. Other parents who are preoccupied with their own weight and appearance can indirectly lead their children toward being critical of their bodies. A child's peers can exert pressure, urging each other to attain a certain ideal figure or criticizing individuals who somehow do not measure up to their expectations. Media depictions of models and actors and popular discussion of celebrities in terms of their physical appearance also shape young people's perceptions about ideal body type. Body image is also closely associated with self-esteem, which is defined as the amount of value or personal worth individuals subjectively feel they have.

As puberty nears, children become increasingly focused on their physical appearance. An adolescent may mature more quickly or slowly than his or her peers. Any deviation from the perceived "ideal" can result in a negative body image, and adolescents may diet, **exercise**, or use **steroids**, stimulants, or laxatives to counter their own negative self-concept and achieve the body image they desire. Some teenage girls are even having plastic surgery (with parental permission) to "correct" what they perceive as flaws in their appearance.

Distorted body images in adolescence can lead to a number of disorders, such as **anorexia nervosa**, **bulimia nervosa**, or **body dysmorphic disorder**, a severe, clinically recognized condition characterized by an obsession with illusory body image. The behaviors that accompany these psychological disorders can be life threatening if taken to the extreme. Body image disorders are often accompanied by additional psychological problems such as **depression** or anxiety and thoughts of **suicide**. For some individuals, body image eventually becomes an all-consuming preoccupation.

Teens are especially concerned about how other people view them, and they can be more sensitive to aspects of body image and vulnerable to external pressures as they experience physiological changes. Males may be overly concerned with height when they see females of their same age who are growing taller, and females may feel sensitive about their height and weight as their bodies develop.

According to the National Eating Disorders Association, 91% of young college women report having been on at least one diet. Seventy percent of young college men report being unhappy with their body image, with 32% of all college men stating that they have dieted once or more than once. Other studies show similar percentages among young adults, which help to support the contention that young people are concerned with body image and that they generally aspire to be slim.

Differences among men and women

Concern with body image is generally more important to women than it is to men. Women usually are more critical of their overall body and individual parts of their body than are men. However, the gap between the two genders has been narrowing over recent years as men become more concerned with their body image.

Poor body image is often affected by feelings of being overweight, especially with women. Men, by contrast, often desire more muscle mass when considering their body image. Their desire to be more masculine is connected to a desire to add muscle mass and improve muscle definition. Poor body image can lead to fad dieting, obesity, and eating disorders, along with low self-esteem, depression, anxiety, and general emotional distress. However, for the most part, people with good exercise habits, positive personal and sexual lives, and excellent emotional and mental states have better and more accurate perceptions of their body image than people without those characteristics and experiences.

Causes and symptoms

Causes of negative body image

Body image can be affected by outside influences. Media sources, such as television, the Internet, and magazines, often portray people closer to the commonly accepted ideal body type than the average body type in order to sell their products and services. Consequently, people—especially older children and young adults—are overly influenced and swayed by such depictions of body image. According to the Association of Body Image and Disordered Eating (ABIDE), the average U.S. citizen is exposed to about 5,000 advertising messages every day. Studies of network television commercials have shown that attractiveness is a desirable trait that advertisers regularly use to convince viewers to purchase their products.

Family life can also affect a person's perception of body image. Parents who criticize their children about the way they look, talk, or act may have a negative effect on the development of self-esteem in their offspring.

Young people may also be affected by the comments of peers when it comes to their body image. Teasing conveys negative values about a person. Racial, sexual, and other types of teasing can have a negative impact on body image and self-esteem. Children may urge their peers to conform to trends in clothing, language, and other cultural aspects, all of which can potentially hurt a person's body image.

Symptoms of negative body image

Exaggerated and distorted concerns with body image have been linked in medical studies with decreases in self-esteem and increases in dieting and eating disorders, including anorexia nervosa, **binge eating disorder**, and bulimia. Bulimia is an eating disorder marked by episodes of binge eating followed by one or more behaviors to control weight, most commonly self-induced vomiting, laxative abuse, fasting, or excessive exercise. The disorder is rare in children under age 14. It is estimated to occur in between 1%–3% of high school– and college-aged women in the United States.

People with extreme body image problems may have body dysmorphic disorder (BDD), which involves a distorted body image without any eating disorders. Body dysmorphic disorder was recognized as a psychiatric disorder in 1997, although its symptoms have been exhibited in patients for more than 100 years. The disorder involves **obsession** and complete preoccupation with an imagined or mild physical flaw. It is known to occur in 1%–2% of Americans, but it is thought to be underdiagnosed because it often occurs in conjunction with other psychiatric disorders such as major depression and **obsessive-compulsive disorder**. Excessive preoccupation with body image and an obsession with positive body image has also been associated with the personality disorder narcissism (self-admiration or an overestimation about one's appearance).

Diagnosis

Within the field of **psychoanalysis**, a person's body image is often measured by asking individuals to rate parts of their body (such as face, stomach, and buttocks) with respect to a series of pictures representing an ideal body image. The difference in the rating between an individual's current body image and a perceived ideal body image is generally considered the amount that individuals are dissatisfied with their body.

Prevention

Without a healthy regard for one's self, people can often become very self-conscious of their body image. Feelings of depression, anxiety, and isolation may occur. With low self-esteem and body image problems, some people use alcohol or drugs to offset those negative feelings. Others turn away from their regular activities and their usual friends, becoming withdrawn and showing lack of interest in themselves and the world around them.

A person may recover from negative body image by attempting to accept things that cannot be changed and working on things that realistically could be improved. In some cases, outside help is needed in the form of a guidance counselor, parent, coach, religious leader, or someone else that is trusted and accepting of personal feelings. Crisis hotlines are also available to help with such problems.

Resources

BOOKS

Knoblich, Gunther, et al., eds. *Human Body Perception from the Inside Out.* Oxford, UK: Oxford University Press, 2005.

Messinger, Lisa, and Merle Goldberg. *My Thin Excuse: Understanding, Recognizing, and Overcoming Eating Disorders.* Garden City Park, NY: Square One Publishers, 2006.

Preester, Helena, and Veroniek Knockaert, eds. *Body Image and Body Schema: Interdisciplinary Perspectives.* Philadelphia: John Benjamins Publishing Co., 2005.

Wilhelm, Sabine. *Feeling Good About the Way You Look: A Program for Overcoming Body Image Problems.* New York: Guilford Publications, Inc., 2006.

Wykes, Maggie, and Barrie Gunter. *The Media and Body Image: If Looks Could Kill.* Thousand Oaks, CA: Sage Publications Ltd., 2005.

WEBSITES

Ahmed, Iqbal, et al. "Psychiatric Manifestations of Body Dysmorphic Disorder." Medscape Reference. http://www.emedicine.com/med/topic3124.htm (accessed September 30, 2011).

MedlinePlus. "Anorexia Nervosa." U.S. National Library of Medicine, National Institutes of Health. http://www.nlm.nih.gov/medlineplus/ency/article/000362.htm (accessed September 30, 2011).

———. "Bulimia." U.S. National Library of Medicine, National Institutes of Health. http://www.nlm.nih.gov/medlineplus/ency/article/000341.htm (accessed September 30, 2011).

ORGANIZATIONS

Academy for Eating Disorders, 111 Deer Lake Rd., Suite 100, Deerfield, IL, 60015, (847) 498-4274, Fax: (847) 480-9282, info@aedweb.org, http://www.aedweb.org.

National Association of Anorexia Nervosa and Associated Disorders, Inc, PO Box 640, Naperville, IL, 60566, (630) 577-1333, anadhelp@anad.org, http://www.anad.org.

National Eating Disorders Association, 165 West 46th Street, New York, NY, 10036, (1-800) 931-2237, info@NationalEating-Disorders.org, http://www.nationaleatingdisorders.org.

National Institute of Mental Health, 6001 Executive Blvd., Room 8184, MSC 9663, Bethesda, MD, 20892-9663, (301) 443-4513, (866) 615-6464, Fax: (301)443-4279, nimhinfo@nih.gov, http://www.nimh.nih.gov.

Tish Davidson, AM
Laura Jean Cataldo, RN, EdD

Body integrity identity disorder

Definition

Body integrity identity disorder (BIID) is a condition in which a person who is not psychotic seeks the elective amputation of one or more limbs (or body parts). In most cases the limb or body part is healthy, not malformed, and

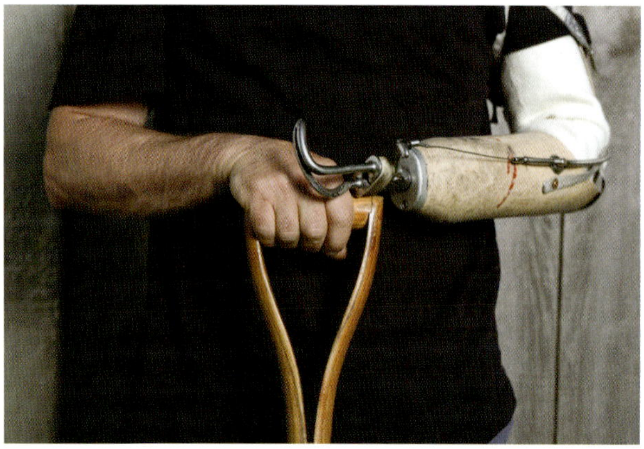

Persons with body integrity identity disorder experience an intense desire to have one (or more) limbs amputated. *(© iStockPhoto.com/Michael Courtney)*

functioning normally. People with BIID have an idealized image of themselves as amputees and wish to have their actual body altered to conform to this image.

Demographics

Most psychiatrists consider BIID a very rare disorder; a book published in 2000 by **psychologist** Gregg Furth (1945–) identified about 200 people with BIID, and a case study published in 2005 by **psychiatrist** Michael First (1956–) estimated a few thousand people worldwide. Internet sources claim that there are at least several thousand persons in Canada and the United States alone who have the disorder, but these estimates are not substantiated. Exact statistics and demographics are difficult to obtain. The majority of persons with BIID in early medical studies appear to be middle-aged Caucasian males with above-average levels of education; women accounted for only 4 of the 52 subjects profiled in First's case study. The mean age in the study was 48 years, with the youngest person 23 years old and the oldest 77.

Although no one has compiled an exhaustive survey of the body parts most likely to be chosen for amputation by persons with BIID, First's preliminary work indicates that the left leg above the knee is the most common choice, followed by fingers or toes. In his work, First maintains that people with BIID are very specific about the disability they desire or the number of limbs they want to have amputated, and the point at which they want the limb(s) removed.

Description

BIID was originally called *apotemnophilia*, a term coined by psychologist John Money (1921–2006) in 1977. The word comes from three Greek terms meaning "away from," "to cut," and "love of." Money maintained that persons with apotemnophilia had a sexual motivation for desiring amputation and considered the disorder a paraphilia, or sexual desire for unusual or extreme (and in some cases illegal) objects or situations. Since most persons with BIID do not report sexual feelings associated with their desire for amputation, apotemnophilia is now used only to refer to a condition in which a person cannot be aroused or sexually satisfied unless they obtain the desired procedure. Furth, who co-authored the 1977 article with Money, suggested supplementing apotemnophilia with *amputee identity disorder* in order to distinguish between persons who do report a sexual interest in amputation and those who do not. Furth considers himself to have amputee identity disorder and made headlines in 1999 when he went to Scotland to consult a surgeon who had already performed two amputations on healthy persons.

The term *body integrity identity disorder* was introduced by First, who served as the editor of the ***Diagnostic and Statistical Manual of Mental Disorders***, fourth edition, text revised (*DSM-IV-TR*) and who has been involved in the development of the fifth edition (*DSM-5*, 2013). BIID is not yet recognized by the *DSM*, but First supports the addition. He maintains that BIID is a more accurate name for the disorder because the condition (in his opinion) includes people who feel a need for blindness, deafness, or other disability, or paralysis or other impairment of a limb rather than amputation.

It is important to distinguish BIID from **body dysmorphic disorder** (BDD), a condition with which it is often confused because of the similarity of the names. Another reason for the confusion is that some psychiatrists initially favored adding BIID to *DSM-5* as a subtype of body dysmorphic disorder. Other researchers, however, have noted a core distinction between the two conditions. People diagnosed with BDD are excessively concerned about supposed defects in their body shape, facial features, or other aspects of their physical appearance and want to improve the features they find distressing, whereas people with BIID do not perceive the body part that they want amputated as defective or embarrassing. BIID is more nearly like **gender identity disorder** in that the person with BIID perceives their limb as incongruent with their sense of self, similar to the way in which a person with gender identity disorder perceives their biological sex as alien to their sense of self.

BIID is difficult to describe because most people—including those who have had to have a limb amputated because of traumatic injury or complications of diabetes—think of amputation as a frightening and upsetting experience. The notion that someone would consider the removal of a limb as a necessary expression of their sense of self seems absurd to the general majority. It also sounds paradoxical when a person with BIID claims that they need to have a limb (or sensory ability) removed in order to feel "complete." Moreover, many amputees report feelings of anger toward people with BIID because they feel that those with BIID are minimizing the suffering of someone who had no choice about amputation.

Another source of difficulty in describing and understanding BIID is that it has developed its own vocabulary for people who have the disorder or are attracted to someone who does. "Devotees" are people who are sexually attracted to amputees or disabled people, although some people in this group prefer to call themselves "admirers." "Wannabes" are people who have an obsessional need for amputation or impairment but have not yet had a procedure to bring it about, whereas "realized wannabes" are those who finally achieved the amputation or impairment they desired. "Pretenders" are people with BIID who use crutches, eye patches, wheel chairs, or similar devices or props in public in order to feel disabled. There is reportedly a considerable overlap among these groups, with many devotees also being pretenders or wannabes.

People with BIID frequently report having the desire for amputation from an early age. One of First's subjects reported having a desire to amputate his leg at age three or four; another man stated that his desire for amputation began in kindergarten, when he had a schoolmate who was missing his left hand and became curious about what it might be like to lose his own hand. Others with BIID maintain that they first became aware of their interest in amputation in early adolescence. There are relatively few who maintain that they were adults when they first experienced an interest in amputation or disability.

Risk factors

There were three suggested risk factors for BIID as of 2011: exposure to an amputee at an early age (three to four years), male sex, and abnormality or malfunction of the parietal lobe of the cerebral cortex.

Causes and symptoms

Causes

There is little agreement among medical professionals about the cause(s) of BIID. Some of the theories that have been proposed include:

- Imprinting. This term refers to the theory that some susceptible children who encounter an amputee at an early age are imprinted with amputation as part of their own mental picture of an ideal body.
- An unloving or dysfunctional home life. This theory holds that people with BIID feel unloved or ignored as children and come to think that amputation or disability will secure them the love they need.
- A defect in the parietal lobe of the cerebral cortex. Some preliminary studies carried out in the early 2000s at the Center for Brain and Cognition of the University of California, San Diego, suggest that people with BIID may have a neurological disorder involving proprioception, which is the body's internal sense of its position in space and of the location of various parts of the body in relation to one another. The parietal lobe of the cerebral cortex is thought to govern the brain's inner body mapping function. If the neurological theory is correct, an abnormality in the parietal lobe would mean that the person with BIID's brain fails to include the limb that he or she wants amputated in its mapping of the person's physical form.
- Conditions in the general culture at a specific point in time. This viewpoint is associated with the work of Ian Hacking, a historian of science who coined the phrase "looping effect" to explain how the classification of a mental disorder affects the behavior of people who decide that they fit that category. In other words, the definition of a new diagnostic category allows some people to reinterpret their past or present experiences in the light of that category, and then to think about actions they would not have considered earlier—such as requesting amputation.
- An extension of extreme body modification. Body modification comprises such practices as body piercing, tattoos, breast implants, and other surgical alterations of the body for aesthetic purposes. Some psychiatrists think that BIID may simply represent extreme body modification carried one step further; however, most persons who identify themselves as having BIID reject this explanation.

There was no evidence as of 2011 that BIID runs in families or that it has a genetic basis.

Symptoms

There is no universally accepted list of BIID symptoms, and not all persons who maintain that they have BIID will experience every symptom. However, some of the signs and symptoms most frequently identified as characteristic of BIID include:

- a feeling of incompleteness as an able-bodied individual, coupled with a feeling of certainty that one will feel "whole" or "complete" after obtaining the needed amputation or other impairment

KEY TERMS

Anecdotal—Based on personal experience or reported individual observations unverified by controlled experiments.

Apotemnophilia—A word coined by John Money in 1977 to describe the condition now known as body integrity identity disorder. Money originally thought that BIID had a sexual component, hence the Greek root *philia* at the end of the word.

Body dysmorphic disorder (BDD)—A psychiatric disorder in which the affected person is excessively preoccupied with a perceived defect in his or her physical appearance.

Cerebral cortex—The outer layer of the cerebrum (forebrain), composed of gray matter and containing sensory, motor, and association areas.

Devotee—Someone who is sexually attracted to amputees or disabled persons.

Ethics—The branch of philosophy that deals with questions of morality (good and evil, right and wrong).

Paraphilia—The medical term for a condition in which a person is sexually aroused by nonhuman objects, animals, corpses, children and other nonconsenting partners, or specific individuals or situations that are not part of normative stimulation.

Pretender—A person with BIID who uses assistive devices or other props in public in order to appear disabled.

Proprioception—A person's normal sense of posture, balance, direction of movement, and location in space.

Transabled—A word coined by people with BIID to express their need to be disabled.

Wannabe—A person with BIID who feels a need for an amputation or impairment.

- a very specific notion of the amputation or disability required
- feelings of intense envy when encountering another person with the needed disability or amputation
- feelings of intense shame regarding the need for the amputation or disability, due to the belief that no one else could possibly understand the condition
- repeated episodes of depression and possibly suicidal thoughts
- rehearsal for the needed amputation or disability by pretending (imitating the desired disability)
- failure of psychotherapy or medications to alleviate the feelings
- in some cases, plotting to injure oneself in order to achieve the needed amputation or other impairment

Diagnosis

There were no formal diagnostic criteria for BIID as of 2011, though the disorder is recognized by the medical community. There are also no psychological tests or inventories to screen for the disorder. Given the fact that many people with BIID are afraid to discuss their feelings, most cases seem to come to the attention of therapists only when the patient brings up the subject.

Treatment

Treatment of BIID is highly controversial. Most patients with the disorder maintain that **psychotherapy** and medications do not help, although some observe that psychotherapy has been beneficial in helping them deal more effectively with other problems in their lives. A few wannabes report that pretending helps them cope to some extent with their BIID.

Surgery

Most persons with BIID maintain that surgery is the only effective treatment for their condition. In fact, BIID first came to the attention of the general public in 2000 with media reports of Robert Smith, a surgeon in Scotland who agreed to amputate the healthy legs of two patients with BIID. Smith maintained that he performed the operations to head off the possibility that the patients would otherwise resort to self-amputation or other dangerous measures. There had been several highly publicized cases of such behavior in the late 1990s, including a man who lost his life from a botched amputation performed by a surgeon who had lost his license twenty years previously, and a man in Wisconsin who had constructed a homemade guillotine in 1999 to amputate his left arm. Other persons with BIID have packed their limbs in dry ice in order to require a surgeon to amputate them, or have blown off the unwanted limb with shotguns. Smith was forced to give up performing amputations for BIID because of the public fury that resulted from his operations.

Surgery as therapy for BIID raises a number of ethical questions. One is whether people have an absolute right to do anything they wish to their own bodies, and whether surgeons should be obligated to carry out their wishes. Moreover, unlike plastic surgery to improve a person's appearance, surgical removal of a limb or other body part may decrease the amputee's ability to work or otherwise function in society. Should taxpayers be expected to support those who intentionally seek amputation because of a psychological disorder? In addition, given the increasing scarcity of healthcare resources, should surgeons be asked to divert time and attention from patients with life-threatening emergencies in order to perform elective amputations? Last, amputation is irreversible, which concerns many surgeons who are afraid of lawsuits if the BIID patient regrets the procedure afterward. Although Smith's two patients and others who succeeded in achieving the amputation or disability they sought maintain that they are finally at peace with themselves, therapists who have studied BIID still recommend medications and psychotherapy as the first line of treatment.

There were no **clinical trials** of psychotherapy, medications, or other treatments for BIID as of 2011.

Prognosis

As no large-scale research studies of BIID had been conducted as of 2011, information about its prognosis is purely anecdotal (individual reports unverified by formal controlled experiments). One website for people with BIID maintains that the disorder becomes worse as people grow older and their need for amputation intensifies.

Prevention

There is no known way to prevent BIID, because the condition is still not understood.

Resources

BOOKS

Furth, Gregg M., and Robert Smith. *Amputee Identity Disorder: Information, Questions, Answers, and Recomendations about Self-Demand Amputation*. Bloomington, IN: AuthorHouse, 2000.

Hacking, Ian. *Mad Travelers: Reflections on the Reality of Transient Mental Illnesses*. Charlottesville, VA: University Press of Virginia, 1998.

Smith, Stephen W., and Ronan Deazley, eds. *The Legal, Medical and Cultural Regulation of the Body: Transformation and Transgression*. Burlington, VT: Ashgate, 2009.

PERIODICALS

Elliott, Carl. "A New Way to Be Mad." *The Atlantic*, December 2000. http://www.theatlantic.com/magazine/archive/2000/12/a-new-way-to-be-mad/4671 (accessed August 4, 2011).

Ellison, Jesse. "Cutting Desire." *Newsweek*, May 28, 2008. http://www.newsweek.com/2008/05/28/cutting-desire.html (accessed August 4, 2011).

First, M.B. "Desire for Amputation of a Limb: Paraphilia, Psychosis, or a New Type of Identity Disorder?" *Psychological Medicine* 35 (June 2005): 919–928.

Henig, Robin M. "At War with Their Bodies, They Seek to Sever Limbs." *New York Times*, March 22, 2005. http://query.nytimes.com/gst/fullpage.html?res=9C0CE4-D61E3CF931A15750C0A9639C8B63&pagewanted=all (accessed August 4, 2011).

Müller, S. "Body Integrity Identity Disorder (BIID)—Is the Amputation of Healthy Limbs Ethically Justified?" *American Journal of Bioethics* 9 (January 2009): 36–43.

Patrone, D. "Disfigured Anatomies and Imperfect Analogies: Body Integrity Identity Disorder and the Supposed Right to Self-demanded Amputation of Healthy Body Parts." *Journal of Medical Ethics* 35 (September 2009): 541–545.

Phillips, K.A., et al. "Body Dysmorphic Disorder: Some Key Issues for DSM-V." *Depression and Anxiety* 27 (June 2010): 573–591.

WEBSITES

Dotinga, Randy. "Out on a Limb" [account of Gregg Furth's search for a surgeon to amputate his right leg]. Salon.com. August 29, 2000. http://www.salon.com/health/feature/2000/08/29/amputation (accessed July 14, 2011).

Mulvihill, Karen, and Karlie Pouliot. "Determined to Amputate: One Man's Struggle with Body Integrity Identity Disorder." FOXNews.com. May 20, 2009. http://www.foxnews.com/story/0,2933,520811,00.html (accessed July 14, 2011).

O'Connor, Sean. *Transabled.org* (blog). http://transabled.org (accessed August 2, 2011).

"Whole: A Documentary" [2003 documentary film about BIID]. http://www.whole-documentary.com (accessed July 15, 2011).

ORGANIZATIONS

American Psychiatric Association, 1000 Wilson Boulevard, Suite 1825, Arlington, VA, 22209-3901, (703) 907-7300, apa@psych.org, http://www.psych.org.

Center for Brain and Cognition, University of California, San Diego, 109 Mandler Hall, 9500 Gilman Drive, La Jolla, CA, 92093-0109, (858) 534-6240, Fax: (858) 534-7190, ramalab@ucsd.edu, http://cbc.ucsd.edu/index.html.

Rebecca J. Frey, Ph.D.

Bodywork therapies

Definition

Bodywork therapies comprise body-based approaches to treatment that emphasize manipulation and realignment of the body's structure in order to improve its function as well as the client's mental outlook. These therapies typically combine a relatively passive phase, in which the client receives deep-tissue bodywork or postural correction from an experienced instructor or practitioner, and a more active period of movement education, in which the client practices sitting, standing, and moving about with better alignment of the body and greater ease of motion.

Bodywork should not be equated only with massage. Massage therapy is one form of bodywork, but in massage therapy, practitioners use oil or lotion to reduce the friction between their hands and the client's skin. In most forms of bodywork, little if any lubrication is used, as the goal of this type of hands-on treatment is to warm, relax, and stretch the fascia (a band or sheath of connective tissue that covers, supports, or connects the muscles and the internal organs) and underlying layers of tissue.

Purpose

The purpose of bodywork therapy is the correction of problems in the client's overall posture, connective tissue, and/or musculature in order to bring about greater ease of movement, less discomfort, and a higher level of energy in daily activity. Some forms of bodywork have as a secondary purpose the healing or prevention of repetitive stress injuries, particularly for people whose occupations require intensive use of specific parts of the body (e.g., dancers, musicians, professional athletes, and opera singers). Bodywork may also heal or prevent specific musculoskeletal problems, such as lower back pain or neck pain.

Bodywork therapies are holistic in that they stress increased self-awareness and intelligent use of one's body as one of the goals of treatment. Some of these therapies use verbal discussion, visualization, or **guided imagery** along with movement education to help clients break old patterns of moving and feeling. Although most bodywork therapists do not address mental disorders directly in their work with clients, they are often knowledgeable about the applications of bodywork to such specific emotions as **depression**, anger, or fear.

Although some bodywork therapies, such as Rolfing or Hellerwork, offer programs structured around a specific number or sequence of lessons, all therapies emphasize individualized treatment and respect for the uniqueness of each individual's body. Bodywork instructors or practitioners typically work with clients on a one-to-one basis, as distinct from a group or classroom approach.

Demographics

Massage therapy, under which many forms of bodywork are often counted, was estimated be a $16–20 billion industry in 2008. Bodywork therapies have become increasingly mainstream since the 1980s, and the industry is estimated to still be growing at a rapid pace.

Description

The following are brief descriptions of some popular bodywork therapies.

Alexander technique

The Alexander technique was developed by the Australian actor F. Matthias Alexander (1869–1955), who had voice problems that were not helped by available medical treatments. Alexander decided to set up a number of mirrors so that he could watch himself during a performance from different angles. He found that he was holding his head and neck too far forward and that these unconscious patterns were the source of the tension in his body that was harming his voice. He then developed a method for teaching others to observe the patterns of tension and stress in their posture and movement and to correct these patterns with a combination of hands-on guidance and visualization exercises. The Alexander technique is included in the curricula of the Juilliard School of Music and many other drama and music schools around the world, because performing artists are particularly vulnerable to repetitive stress injuries if they hold or move their bodies incorrectly.

In an Alexander technique session, the client works one-on-one with an instructor who uses verbal explanations as well as guided movement. Often referred to as "explorations," the sessions last about 30 minutes. Although most clients see positive changes after only two or three sessions, teachers of the technique recommend a course of 20–30 sessions so that new movement skills can be learned and changes maintained.

Rolfing

Rolfing, which is also called Rolf therapy or structural integration, is a holistic system of bodywork that uses deep manipulation of the body's soft tissue to realign and balance the body's myofascial (muscular and connective tissue) structure. It was developed by Ida Rolf (1896–1979), a biochemist who became interested in the structure of the human body after an accident damaged her health. Rolf studied with an osteopath as well as with practitioners of other forms of alternative medicine and developed her own technique of body movement, which she called structural integration. Rolfing is an approach that seeks to counteract the effects of gravity, which tends to pull the body out of alignment over time and cause the connective tissues to stiffen and contract.

Rolfing treatment begins with the "Basic Ten," a series of ten sessions each lasting 60–90 minutes, spaced a week or more apart. After a period of integration, the client may undertake advanced treatment sessions. "Tune-up" sessions are recommended every six months. In Rolfing sessions, practitioners use their fingers, hands, knuckles, or elbows to rework the connective tissue over the client's entire body. The deep tissues are worked until they become pliable, which allows the muscles to lengthen and return to their proper alignment. Rolfing treatments are done on a massage table, with the client wearing only undergarments.

Hellerwork

Hellerwork is a bodywork therapy developed by Joseph Heller, a former NASA engineer who became a certified Rolfer in 1972 and started his own version of structural integration, called Hellerwork, in 1979. Heller describes his program as "a powerful system of somatic education and structural bodywork" delivered in a series of eleven sessions. Hellerwork is similar to Rolfing in that it begins with manipulation of the deep tissues of the body. Heller, however, decided that physical realignment of the body by itself is insufficient, so he extended his system to include movement education and guided dialogue to promote self-awareness.

The bodywork aspect of Hellerwork is intended to release the tension that exists in the fascia, which is the sheath or layer of connective tissue that covers, supports, or connects the muscles and internal organs of the body. Fascia is flexible and moist in its normal state, but the effects of gravity and ongoing physical stresses lead to misalignments that cause the fascia to become rigid. The first hour of a Hellerwork session is devoted to deep connective tissue bodywork in which the Hellerwork practitioner uses his or her hands to release tension in the client's fascia. The bodywork is followed by movement education, which includes the use of video feedback to help clients learn movement patterns that will help to keep their bodies in proper alignment. The third component of Hellerwork is dialogue, which is intended to help clients become more aware of the relationships between their emotions and attitudes and their body.

Tragerwork

Trager psychophysical integration, which is often called simply Tragerwork, was developed by Milton Trager (1908–1977), who was born with a spinal deformity and earned a medical degree in his middle age after working out an approach to healing chronic pain. Tragerwork is based on the theory that many illnesses are caused by tension patterns that are held in the unconscious mind as much as in the tissues of the body; clients are advised to think of Tragerwork sessions as "learning experiences" rather than "treatments." Tragerwork sessions are divided into bodywork, which is referred to as tablework, and an **exercise** period. Trager practitioners use their hands during tablework to perform a variety of gentle motions—rocking, shaking, vibrating, and gentle stretching—intended to help the client release patterns of tension by experiencing how it feels to move freely and effortlessly on one's own. Following the tablework, clients are taught how to perform simple dance-like exercises called "Mentastics," for practice at home. Tragerwork sessions take between 60–90 minutes, and clients are advised to spend 10–15 minutes three times a day doing the Mentastics exercises.

Feldenkrais method

The Feldenkrais method, like Hellerwork, refers to its approach as "somatic education." Developed by Moshe Feldenkrais (1904–1984), a scientist and engineer who was also a judo instructor, the Feldenkrais method consists of two major applications: awareness through movement (ATM) lessons, a set of verbally directed exercise lessons intended to engage the client's intelligence as well as physical perception, and functional integration (FI), in which a Feldenkrais practitioner works with the client one-on-one, guiding the client through a series of movements that alter habitual patterns and convey new learning directly to the neuromuscular system. Functional integration is done with the client fully clothed, lying or sitting on a low padded table.

Perhaps the most distinctive feature of the Feldenkrais method is its emphasis on new patterns of thinking, attention, cognition, and imagination as byproducts of new patterns of physical movement. It is the most intellectually oriented of the various bodywork therapies and has been described as a combination of motor development, biomechanics, psychology, and martial arts. The Feldenkrais method is the form of bodywork that has been most extensively studied by mainstream medical researchers.

Trigger point therapy

Trigger point therapy, which is sometimes called myotherapy, is a treatment for pain relief in the musculoskeletal system based on the application of pressure to trigger points in the client's body. Trigger points are defined as hypersensitive spots or areas in the muscles that cause pain when subjected to stress, whether the cause is an occupational injury, a disease, or emotional stress. Trigger points are not necessarily in the same location where the client feels pain.

Myotherapy is a two-step process. In the first step, the therapist locates the client's trigger points and applies pressure to them. This step relieves pain and also relaxes the muscles associated with it. In the second part of the therapy session, the client learns a series of exercises that progressively stretch the muscles that have been relaxed by the therapist's pressure. Most clients need fewer than 10 sessions to benefit from myotherapy. One distinctive feature of trigger point therapy is that clients are asked to bring a relative or trusted friend to learn the pressure technique and the client's personal trigger points. This so-called buddy system helps the client to maintain the benefits of the therapy in the event of a **relapse**.

Shiatsu

Shiatsu is the oldest form of bodywork therapy, having been practiced for centuries in Japan as part of traditional medical treatment. It is also the type of bodywork most commonly requested by clients in Western countries as well as in East Asia. The word *shiatsu* itself is a combination of two Japanese words that mean "pressure" and "finger." Shiatsu resembles **acupuncture** in its use of the basic concepts of *ki,* the vital energy that flows throughout the body, and the meridians, or 12 major pathways that channel ki to the various organs of the body. In Asian terms, shiatsu works by unblocking and rebalancing the distribution of ki in the body. In the categories of Western medicine, shiatsu may stimulate the release of endorphins, which are chemical compounds that block the receptors in the **brain** that perceive pain.

A shiatsu treatment begins with the practitioner's assessment of the client's basic state of health, including posture, vocal tone, complexion color, and condition of hair. This evaluation is used together with ongoing information about the client's energy level gained through the actual bodywork. The shiatsu practitioner works with the client lying fully clothed on a futon. The practitioner seeks out the meridians in the client's body through finger pressure and stimulates points along the meridians known as *tsubos.* The tsubos are centers of high energy where the ki tends to collect. Pressure on the tsubos results in a release of energy that rebalances the energy level throughout the body.

Craniosacral therapy

Craniosacral therapy, or CST, is a form of treatment that originated with William Sutherland, an American osteopath of the 1930s who theorized that the manipulative techniques that osteopaths were taught could be applied to the skull. Sutherland knew from his medical training that the skull is not a single piece of bone but consists of several bones that meet at seams and that the cerebrospinal fluid that bathes the brain and spinal cord has a natural rise-and-fall rhythm. Sutherland experimented with gentle manipulation of the skull in order to correct imbalances in the distribution of the cerebrospinal fluid. Contemporary craniosacral therapists practice manipulation not only of the skull but also of the meningeal membranes that cover the brain and spinal cord and sometimes of the facial bones. Many practitioners of CST are also osteopaths.

In CST, the patient lies on a massage table while the therapist gently palpates, or presses, the skull and spine. If the practitioner is also an osteopath, he or she will take a complete medical history as well. The therapist also "listens" to the cranial rhythmic impulse or rhythmic pulsation of the cerebrospinal fluid with his or her hands. Interruptions of the normal flow by abnormalities caused by tension or injury are diagnostic clues to the practitioner. Once he or she has identified the cause of the abnormal rhythm, the skull and spinal column are gently manipulated to restore the natural rhythm of the cranial impulse. Craniosacral therapy appears to be particularly useful in treating physical disorders of the head, including migraine headaches, ringing in the ears, sinus problems, and injuries of the head, neck, and spine. In addition, patients rarely require extended periods of CST treatments.

Benefits

Benefits from bodywork include deep relaxation, improved posture, greater ease and spontaneity of movement, greater range of motion for certain joints, greater understanding of the structures and functions of the body and their relationship to emotions, and release of negative emotions.

Many persons also report healing or improvement of specific conditions, including migraine headaches, repetitive stress injuries, osteoarthritis, **insomnia**, sprains and bruises, sports injuries, stress-related illnesses, sciatica, post-pregnancy problems, menstrual cramps, temporomandibular joint disorders, lower back pain, whiplash injuries, disorders of the immune system, asthma, depression, digestive problems, chronic **fatigue**, and painful scar tissue. The Alexander technique has been reported to ease the process of childbirth by improving the mother's postural alignment prior to delivery.

Some studies of the Feldenkrais method have found that its positive effects on subjects' self-esteem, mood, and anxiety symptoms are more significant than its effects on body function.

Precautions

Persons who are seriously ill, acutely feverish, or suffering from a contagious infection should wait until

KEY TERMS

Bodywork—Any technique involving hands-on massage or manipulation of the body.

Endorphins—A group of peptide compounds released by the body in response to stress or traumatic injury. Endorphins react with opiate receptors in the brain to reduce or relieve pain sensations. Shiatsu is thought to work by stimulating the release of endorphins.

Fascia (plural, fasciae)—A band or sheath of connective tissue that covers, supports, or connects the muscles and the internal organs.

Ki—The Japanese spelling of *qi,* the traditional Chinese term for vital energy or the life force.

Meridians—In traditional Chinese medicine, a network of pathways or channels that convey *ki* through the body.

Movement education—The active phase of bodywork, in which clients learn to move with greater freedom and to maintain the proper alignment of their bodies.

Osteopathy—A system of medical practice that believes that the human body can make its own remedies to heal infection. It originally used manipulative techniques but also added surgical, hygienic, and medicinal methods when needed. Doctors of osteopathy are referred to as osteopaths or DOs.

Repetitive stress injury (RSI)—A type of injury to the musculoskeletal and nervous systems associated with occupational strain or overuse of a specific part of the body. Bodywork therapies are often recommended to people suffering from RSIs.

Somatic education—Used in both Hellerwork and the Feldenkrais method to describe the integration of bodywork with self-awareness, intelligence, and imagination.

Structural integration—The term used to describe the method and philosophy of life associated with Rolfing. Its fundamental concept is the vertical line.

Tsubo—In shiatsu, a center of high energy located along one of the body's meridians. Stimulation of the *tsubos* during a shiatsu treatment is thought to rebalance the flow of vital energy in the body.

they have recovered before beginning a course of bodywork. As a rule, types of bodywork that involve intensive manipulation or stretching of the deeper layers of body tissue are not suitable for persons who have undergone recent surgery or have recently suffered severe injury. In the case of Tragerwork, shiatsu, and trigger point therapy, clients should inform the therapist of any open wounds, bruises, or fractures so that the affected part of the body can be avoided during treatment. Craniosacral therapy, the Feldenkrais method, and the Alexander technique involve gentle touch and do not require any special precautions.

Individuals recovering from **abuse** or receiving treatment for any post-traumatic syndrome or dissociative disorder should consult their therapist before undertaking bodywork. Although bodywork is frequently recommended as an adjunctive treatment for these disorders, it can also trigger flashbacks if the bodywork therapist touches a part of the patient's body associated with the abuse or **trauma**. Many bodywork therapists, however, are well informed about post-traumatic symptoms and disorders and are able to adjust their treatments accordingly.

Preparation

Bodywork usually requires little preparation on the client's or patient's part, except for partial undressing for Rolfing, trigger point therapy, and Hellerwork.

Aftercare

Aftercare for shiatsu, trigger point therapy, and craniosacral therapy consists of a brief period of rest after the treatment.

Some bodywork approaches involve various types of long-term aftercare. Rolfing clients return for advanced treatments or tune-ups after a period of integrating the changes in their bodies resulting from the Basic Ten sessions. Tragerwork clients are taught Mentastics exercises to be done at home. The Alexander technique and the Feldenkrais approach assume that clients will continue to practice their movement and postural changes for the rest of their lives. Trigger point therapy clients are asked to involve friends or relatives who can help them maintain the benefits of the therapy after the treatment sessions are over.

Risks

The deep tissue massage and manipulation in Rolfing and Hellerwork are uncomfortable for many people, particularly during the first few sessions. There are, however, no serious risks of physical injury from any form of bodywork that is administered by a trained practitioner of the specific treatment. As mentioned,

QUESTIONS TO ASK YOUR DOCTOR

- Is bodywork therapy right for me?
- What type of bodywork therapy would you recommend?
- Do I have any injuries that would preclude bodywork therapy?
- Are there any local practitioners whom you recommend?
- Have any of your other patients tried this type of bodywork therapy? What were their experiences?
- Is bodywork therapy covered by my insurance?

however, bodywork therapies that involve intensive manipulation or stretching of the deeper layers of body tissue are not suitable for persons who have undergone recent surgery or have recently suffered severe injury.

Research and general acceptance

There is very little peer-reviewed scientific research on the effectiveness of bodywork therapies. Some studies have suggested that massage may be effective in alleviating a variety of symptoms when used in conjunction with more traditional treatments. Additional rigorous scientific study is needed to determine if bodywork therapies are more or less effective than traditional massage therapy and to discover what mechanisms underlie this effectiveness.

Training and certification

The training and certification requirements for bodywork therapy differ substantially depending on the type of therapy. Many therapies have professional associations that provide training and certification to their members. Individuals looking for a practitioner of bodywork therapy should find out if there is a professional organization for that type of therapy and what kinds of certifications are available. Responsible therapists should always be willing to provide and explain their professional credentials.

Resources

BOOKS

Benjamin, Patricia J. *Pearson's Massage Therapy: Blending Art with Science.* Upper Saddle River, NJ: Pearson, 2011.

King, Hollis H., Michael M. Patterson, and Wilfrid Janig, eds. *The Science and Clinical Application of Manual Therapy.* Edinburgh: Churchill Livingstone/Elsevier, 2010.

Stager, Leslie. *Nurturing Massage for Pregnancy: A Practical Guide to Bodywork for the Perinatal Cycle.* Baltimore: Lippincott Williams & Wilkins, 2010.

PERIODICALS

Chaitow, Leon. "Has Osteopathy a Role to Play in the Treatment of Flu?" *Journal of Bodywork & Movement Therapies* 14, no. 1 (January 2010): 1–2.

Field, Tiffany, et al. "Benefits of Combining Massage Therapy with Group Interpersonal Psychotherapy in Prenatally Depressed Women." *Journal of Bodywork & Movement Therapies* 13, no. 4 (October 2009): 297–303.

Fries, Christopher J. "Classification of Complementary and Alternative Medical Practices: Family Physicans' Ratings of Effectiveness." *Canadian Family Physician* 54, no. 11 (November 2008): 1570–71.

ORGANIZATIONS

American Massage Therapy Association, 500 Davis St., Evanston, IL, 60201, (877) 905-2700, http://www.amtamassage.org.

Associated Bodywork & Massage Professionals, 25188 Genesee Trail Rd., Golden, CO, 80401, (800) 458-2267, Fax: (800) 667-8260, http://www.abmp.com.

Rebecca Frey
Rosalyn Carson-DeWitt, MD
Tish Davidson, AM

Borderline personality disorder

Definition

Borderline personality disorder (BPD) is a serious mental illness characterized by an inability to regulate emotional responses and moods, impacting self-image and interpersonal relationships. BPD can result in impulsive, self-harming, and suicidal behaviors; **substance abuse**; eating disorders; and the disruption of family life.

Demographics

BPD accounts for 30%–60% of all diagnosed **personality disorders**. According to the National Institutes of Mental Health, approximately 2% of Americans suffer from BPD. About 20% of all psychiatric hospitalizations are due to BPD. The disorder usually becomes evident in early adulthood, with a typical age of onset of 18 years. BPD is rarely initially diagnosed in people over age 40. Though as many as 80% of patients treated for

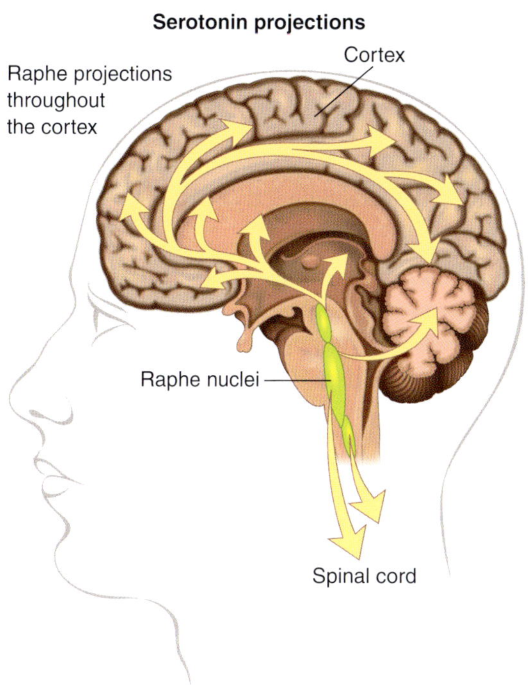

Borderline personality disorder

Diagnostic criteria for borderline personality disorder

Affective (mood-related) symptoms

1. Unstable mood caused by brief but intense episodes of depression, irritability, or anxiety
2. Chronic feelings of emptiness
3. Inappropriate and intense anger or difficulty controlling anger

Impulsive symptoms

4. Impulsive behavior in at least two areas (e.g., spending money, substance abuse, binge eating)
5. Recurrent suicidal behavior, gestures, or threats, or recurring acts of self-mutilation
6. Pattern of unstable and intense interpersonal relationships

Interpersonal symptoms

7. Extreme, persistently unstable perception of self
8. Frantic efforts to avoid abandonment

Cognitive symptoms

9. Stress-related paranoia and/or feeling disconnected from oneself

The Diagnostic and Statistical Manual of Mental Disorders states that the presence of five or more symptoms is necessary to diagnose BPD.

Diagnostic criteria for borderline personality disorder according to the *Diagnostic and Statistical Manual of Mental Disorders* (*DSM-IV-TR*). *(Illustration by Electronic Illustrators Group. Reproduced by permission of Gale, a part of Cengage Learning.)*

BPD are female, this gender bias is less obvious in samples from community populations, suggesting that women may be more likely than men to seek treatment. BPD appears to be equally common among all races and ethnicities. Although the suicidal thinking and **suicide** attempts that are characteristic of BPD are less common in traditional societies, they are becoming increasingly common both in modern societies and in traditional societies that are undergoing rapid change.

Description

The term "borderline" in BPD is now considered a misnomer. It was originally used by the **psychologist** Adolf Stern in the 1930s to describe patients with neuroses that bordered on **psychosis**. Today the term more often refers to borderline states of consciousness that BPD patients may feel when they are experiencing dissociative symptoms—feelings of disconnection from oneself. People with BPD and other personality disorders often utilize coping strategies or defense mechanisms to deny responsibility for their emotions and behaviors.

BPD is a complex disorder with many manifestations. One major feature of BPD is a defense mechanism called "splitting," in which patients alternate between idealizing the significant people in their lives as flawless and devaluing them as unfair and uncaring. Their unrealistic expectations of others inevitably lead to disappointment and unstable interpersonal relationships. Another defense mechanism is referred to as "projective identification," in which patients attribute their own feelings to others and behave in ways that reinforce those attributes. When BPD patients' hostilities are reciprocated, they do not realize that it is due to their own hostility.

BPD results in a high degree of interpersonal conflict, estrangement of family and friends, and divorce. It is also linked to substance abuse, eating disorders, and a history of physical, sexual, or emotional abuse. Self-injury and suicide attempts are common among BPD patients.

Risk factors

Abuse or other childhood **trauma**, such as separation, **neglect**, or abandonment, is a major risk factor for BPD. According to the **National Institute of Mental Health**, studies have found that between 40% and 71% of patients diagnosed with BPD report having been sexually abused as children, most often by someone who was not their primary caregiver. However, most abused children do not develop BPD, and many BPD patients

KEY TERMS

Attention deficit hyperactivity disorder (ADHD)—Conditions characterized by age-inappropriate attention span, hyperactivity, and impulsive behavior.

Bipolar disorder—A recurrent mood disorder, also known as manic-depressive disorder, in which patients have extreme mood swings from depression to mania or a mixture of both.

Cognitive—Conscious intellectual activity, including thinking, imagining, reasoning, remembering, and learning.

Cognitive-behavioral therapy (CBT)—A type of psychotherapy in which people learn to recognize and change negative and self-defeating patterns of thinking and behavior.

Depression—A mental condition in which a person feels extremely sad and loses interest in life. A depressed person may have problems with appetite, sleep, concentration, and daily functioning. Severe depression can lead to suicide attempts.

Dialectical behavior therapy (DBT)—A type of cognitive-behavioral therapy designed specifically to treat borderline personality disorder.

Dissociative—Disconnection from oneself.

Eating disorder—A condition characterized by an abnormal attitude towards food, altered appetite control, and unhealthy eating habits.

Neurotransmitters—Chemicals that transmits nerve impulses from one nerve cell to another.

Opioids—A group of endogenous polypeptides in the brain that bind to opiate receptors.

Post-traumatic stress disorder (PTSD)—A psychological response to a highly stressful event; typically characterized by depression, anxiety, flashbacks, nightmares, and avoidance of reminders of the traumatic experience.

Psychodynamic—Mental, emotional, or motivational forces or processes that affect mental state and behavior, especially unconscious processes that develop in early childhood.

Psychosis—A serious mental disorder, such as schizophrenia, characterized by loss of contact with reality.

Schizophrenia—A psychotic disorder characterized by loss of contact with one's environment, deterioration of everyday functioning, and personality disintegration.

Serotonin—A neurotransmitter located primarily in the brain, blood serum, and stomach membrane.

were not abused as children. Rather, abuse appears to act as a trigger in people who are genetically predisposed to BPD. Studies of twins suggest that at least some features of BPD, especially mood instability and impulsivity, are highly heritable.

Causes and symptoms

The biological basis of BPD is an area of active research. Recent studies suggest that BPD may involve differences in the functioning of the brain's endogenous opioid system, which helps regulate emotions. BPD may also involve disruptions in signaling pathways in the **brain**, involving the **neurotransmitters serotonin**, norepinephrine, and acetylcholine, which help regulate emotions such as anxiety, sadness, irritability, and anger. Feelings of inadequacy and self-loathing arising from childhood abuse or neglect appear to contribute to the development of BPD. It has been theorized that the idealized demands that adults with BPD make on themselves and others are attempts to compensate for care and nurturing denied in childhood.

BPD was first defined as a disorder in the third edition of the American Psychiatric Association's ***Diagnostic and Statistical Manual of Mental Disorders*** (*DSM-III*), published in 1980 and revised in subsequent editions. The revised fourth edition, *DSM-IV-TR,* requires that at least five symptoms be present for a **diagnosis** of BPD. However some clinicians suggest that a diagnosis should require symptoms from each of the three following dimensions or groupings:

- The affective dimension includes mood-related symptoms, such as brief—but intense—episodes of depression, irritability, anxiety, and, especially, inappropriate outbursts of sarcasm, anger, and/or physical violence. The level of mood instability can be a strong predictor of suicide attempts. Other affective symptoms include chronic feelings of emptiness.
- The impulsive dimension includes impulsive behaviors in at least two areas, such as spending money, sex, substance abuse, reckless driving, or binge eating. Impulsive symptoms also include recurrent suicidal threats, gestures, or behaviors, as well as recurring acts of self-mutilation, such as cutting or burning, which

result from a combination of impulsivity and rapid and intense mood swings. These latter self-harming behaviors are not generally considered suicidal, but rather serve a personal purpose, such as providing relief from an extreme emotional state.

- The interpersonal dimension includes a pattern of intense but unstable interpersonal relationships, characterized by alternating idealization and devaluation or "love-hate." It also includes a persistently unstable self-image or sense of self and frantic efforts to avoid real or perceived abandonment.

There are also cognitive criteria for diagnosis of BPD that include stress-related, short-lived **paranoia** and/or severe dissociative symptoms—feeling disconnected from oneself, as if observing one's actions from the outside. Symptoms tend to be exacerbated by feelings of isolation and lack of social support. Patients may frantically try to avoid being alone. These symptoms can lead to frequent changes in relationships, jobs, long-term goals, or gender identity. Studies have found that as many as 40% of patients with BPD report having semi-psychotic thoughts and short delusional periods, and that the presence of psychotic symptoms can be a predictor of self-harming behaviors.

Although BPD symptoms can be similar to symptoms of the better known—but less common—schizophrenic and bipolar disorders, the intense episodes of anxiety, **depression**, or anger with BPD usually last only hours, rather than days or weeks. However, these episodes may be associated with impulsive aggression, substance abuse, or self-injury. Although patients with BPD may experience auditory hallucinations, they are aware that they are hallucinating, unlike patients with **schizophrenia**.

BPD is sometimes difficult to diagnose in adolescence, since symptoms such as impulsive and experimental behaviors, insecurity, and mood swings are common in teenagers. Some researchers have further suggested that BPD is not a defined pathological condition but rather overlapping symptoms of other personality disorders.

Diagnosis

Clinicians diagnose BPD on the basis of interviews with the patient and a complete personality assessment. With the patient's permission, family members and friends also may be interviewed. The clinician may require that symptoms that have been consistently present over time match at least five of the nine criteria in the *DSM-IV-TR*. The clinician should rule out chronic substance abuse and/or medical conditions, especially central nervous system disorders, which can cause similar symptoms. The clinician will attempt to identify problems that often occur in conjunction with BPD, including mood disorders such as depression or anxiety, **post-traumatic stress disorder** (PTSD), eating disorders, or **attention deficit hyperactivity disorder** (ADHD).

Treatment

Traditional

Individuals with BPD seek psychiatric help and **hospitalization** at a much higher rate than people with other personality disorders, perhaps because of their fear of abandonment and their search for idealized interpersonal relationships. **Psychotherapy** is the treatment of choice for BPD, and patients often require long-term services. Dialectical behavior therapy (DBT), a type of **cognitive-behavioral therapy** (CBT), has emerged as an effective therapy for individuals with suicidal tendencies. This treatment focuses on decreasing self-harming behaviors and building self-confidence and coping skills through a combination of **social skills training**, mood awareness, meditative exercises, and education about the disorder. **Group therapy** is a component of DBT and is an option for some BPD patients, although patients may feel threatened by the idea of "sharing" their therapist with others.

The nature of BPD makes it a challenging disorder to treat effectively. The therapist-patient relationship is subject to the same inappropriate and unrealistic demands that individuals with BPD place on all of their significant personal relationships. Individuals with BPD are often chronic treatment seekers, who become easily frustrated when they feel that the therapist is not providing adequate attention or empathy. Symptomatic anger, impulsivity, and self-destructive behaviors can further impede the therapist-patient relationship. In addition, some BPD patients may resent any progress in therapy because of their fear of abandonment or of ending the therapist relationship. Addressing the high incidence of suicidal thoughts and tendencies in BPD patients is also a major therapeutic challenge.

Drugs

Medications are often used in conjunction with psychotherapy to treat symptoms of BPD. **Antidepressants**, especially those that enhance the activity of the neurotransmitter serotonin, can improve emotional symptoms. Mood-stabilizing drugs that enhance the activity of gamma-aminobutyric acid (GABA), the primary inhibitory neurotransmitter in the brain, may help with BPD mood swings. In severe cases, antipsychotic drugs may be prescribed. Some patients take several different medications, each designed to address a different manifestation of BPD. However, drugs are rarely effective without individual and group or **family therapy**.

QUESTIONS TO ASK YOUR DOCTOR

- What type of psychotherapy might be appropriate for my condition?
- Are there community resources that might be of help to me?
- What medications might help manage my symptoms?
- Are there resources available for my family and friends?
- Is there a hotline or other number I can call if I am having suicidal thoughts?
- Do you know a therapist who is trained in DBT?

Alternative

Several new psychotherapies have been developed for treating BPD; however, little research on their efficacy has been conducted. Schema therapy combines CBT with techniques from psychodynamic therapies to examine repetitive life patterns or schemas. Mentalization therapy is geared toward helping patients perceive the minds of others as distinct from their own, thereby enabling them to reassess their perceptions of reality. Transference-focused psychotherapy (TFP) is a psychodynamic treatment that attempts to correct patients' perceptions of their therapist and other important people in their lives.

Home remedies

BPD is a serious disorder that requires extensive mental health services and possibly medications. However, because symptoms of the illness are usually focused on interpersonal relationships, family members may need support and therapy as well.

Prognosis

Treatments for BPD have improved in recent years, and many patients are eventually able to lead productive lives. Symptoms of the disorder usually peak in young adulthood and frequently stabilize after age 30, with symptoms improving in later adulthood, especially by about age 40. However, individuals with BPD are at very high risk for suicide attempts. Although estimates vary widely, some studies have found that as many as 80% of those with BPD attempt suicide at least once, and as many as 10% complete suicide. Although suicidal behavior usually peaks when patients are in their mid-20s, most completed suicides occur among patients over 30 and most often involve those who have experienced no improvement after numerous attempts at treatment. BPD patients with a diagnosed depressive disorder have a much higher risk of suicide and require swift diagnosis and appropriate **intervention**. Adults with BPD also are at higher risk for becoming victims of violence, including rape. This may be due to poor judgment and impulsive behaviors that result in patients choosing inappropriate partners and dangerous lifestyles and environments.

Prevention

BPD is thought to result from a complex of causes, and there is no known prevention, other than ensuring a safe and nurturing childhood environment for those at risk for the disorder. Prompt, appropriate treatment for BPD is crucial for preventing the worsening of symptoms and suicidal behaviors.

Resources

BOOKS

American Psychiatric Association. *Diagnostic and Statistical Manual of Mental Disorders (DSM-IV-TR)*, 4th ed., text rev. Washington, DC: American Psychiatric Association, 2000.

Elliot, Charles H., and Laura L. Smith. *Borderline Personality Disorder for Dummies.* Hoboken, NJ: Wiley, 2009.

Krawitz, Roy, and Wendy Jackson. *Borderline Personality Disorder.* New York: Oxford University Press, 2008.

Mason, Paul T., and Randi Kreger. *Stop Walking on Eggshells: Taking Your Life Back When Someone You Care About Has Borderline Personality Disorder,* 2nd ed. Oakland, CA: New Harbinger, 2010.

Porr, Valerie. *Overcoming Borderline Personality Disorder: A Family Guide for Healing and Change.* New York: Oxford University Press, 2010.

PERIODICALS

Bandelow, Borwin, et al. "Borderline Personality Disorder: A Dysregulation of the Endogenous Opioid System?" *Psychological Review* 117, no. 2 (April 2010): 623–636.

Buckner, Randy A., et al. "Early Family Environment, Borderline Personality Symptoms, and Somatic Preoccupation Among Internal Medicine Outpatients." *Comprehensive Psychiatry* (May–June 2009), 221–225.

Eichelman, Burr. "Borderline Personality Disorder, PTSD, and Suicide." *American Journal of Psychiatry* 167, no. 10 (October 2010): 1152–1154.

Neacsiu, Andrada D., Shireen L. Rizvi, and Marsha M. Linehan. "Dialectical Behavior Therapy Skills Use as a Mediator and Outcome of Treatment for Borderline Personality Disorder." *Behaviour Research and Therapy* 48, no. 9 (September 2010): 832–839.

Prossin, Alan R., et al. "Dysregulation of Regional Endogenous Opioid Function in Borderline Personality Disorder." *American Journal of Psychiatry* 167, no. 8 (August 2010): 925–934.

Raven, Christopher. "Borderline Personality Disorder: Still a Diagnosis of Exclusion?" *Mental Health Today* (June 2009): 26–31.

Samuel, D. B., et al. "Conceptual Changes to the Definition of Borderline Personality Disorder Proposed for DSM-5." *Journal of Abnormal Psychology* (August 29, 2011) [e-pub ahead of print].

WEBSITES

"Borderline Personality Disorder." Mental Health America. http://www.mentalhealthamerica.net/go/information/get-info/borderline-personality-disporder (accessed November 29, 2010).

"Borderline Personality Disorder." National Institute of Mental Health. August 24, 2010. http://www.nimh.nih.gov/health/publications/borderline-personality-disorder-fact-sheet/index.shtml (accessed November 29, 2010).

"Frequently Asked Questions." BPDCentral. http://www.bpdcentral.com/faqs.shtml (accessed November 29, 2010).

"Treatment of Borderline Personality Disorder." Facing the Facts/BPDFamily.com. August 3, 2010. http://www.bpdfamily.com/bpdresources/nk_a107.htm (accessed November 30, 2010).

ORGANIZATIONS

American Psychiatric Association, 1000 Wilson Blvd., Ste. 1825, Arlington, VA, 22209-3901, (703) 907-7300, apa@psych.org, http://www.psych.org.

Mental Health America, 2000 N. Beauregard St., 6th Fl., Alexandria, VA, 22311, (703) 684-7722, (800) 969-6642, Fax: (703) 684-5968, http://www.nmha.org.

National Education Alliance for Borderline Personality Disorder, PO Box 974, Rye, NY, 10580.info@neabpd.com, http://www.borderlinepersonalitydisorder.com.

National Institute of Mental Health, 6001 Executive Blvd., Room 8184, MSC 9663, Bethesda, MD, 20892-9663, (301) 443-4513, (866) 615-6464, Fax: (301) 443-4279, nimhinfo@nih.gov, http://www.nimh.nih.gov.

Personality Disorders Awareness Network, 490 Sun Valley Dr., Ste. 205, Roswell, GA, 30076, (770) 642-4236 x61, Fax: (770) 642-4239, info@pdan.org, http://www.pdan.org.

Treatment and Research Advancements National Association for Personality Disorder, 23 Greene St., New York, NY, 10013, (212) 966-6514, (888) 4-TARA-APD, http://www.tara4bpd.org.

Laith Farid Guilli, MD
Margaret Alic, PhD

Brain

Definition

The brain is the part of the central nervous system (CNS) located inside the skull. It is made up of nerve cells (neurons) and supporting glial cells. Along with the spinal cord and network of nerves, the brain controls information flow throughout the body; voluntary actions such as walking, reading, and talking; involuntary (autonomic) reactions such as breathing and digestion; and cognitive functions such as thinking, learning, and memory.

Description

The human brain is a soft, shiny, grayish-white, mushroom-shaped structure. The gray matter of the brain consists primarily of nerve cell bodies, and the white matter consists primarily of long nerve cell processes called axons that are covered with myelin sheaths. Neurons carry information in the brain and throughout the nervous system in the form of brief electrical impulses. When an impulse reaches the end of an axon, **neurotransmitters** are released at junctions called synapses. These chemicals bind to receptors on the receiving neurons, triggering the continuation of the impulse.

During embryonic development, the gray matter grows faster than the white and folds in on itself, giving rise to convoluted ridges, called gyri, and grooves or valleys, called sulci, thereby creating a large surface area. At birth, the average infant's brain weighs 13.7 oz (390 g); by age 15, it has nearly reached its full adult size of about 3 lb (1.4 kg).

The brain is protected by the skull and three layers of membrane called the meninges, which also cover and protect the spinal cord. The major divisions of the brain are the brain stem, cerebellum, diencephalon, and cerebrum. The latter consists of two large, paired cerebral hemispheres.

Brain stem

The brain stem sits at the base of the brain and connects the brain with the spinal cord. The spinal cord conducts sensory and motor nerve impulses between the brain and the peripheral nervous system. Ascending nerve pathways carry the information through the brain stem to the rest of the brain, and descending nerve pathways carry information from higher brain regions to peripheral nerves to coordinate motor function. In addition, twelve pairs of cranial nerves originate in the underside of the brain, primarily in the brain stem, and exit the skull through openings. These nerves carry information to and from the sensory organs and muscles of the head and neck and the organs of the chest and upper gastrointestinal tract. The brain stem consists of the medulla oblongata, pons, and midbrain.

MEDULLA OBLONGATA. The medulla oblongata is closest to the spinal cord. It is vaguely scoop-shaped, with longitudinal grooves corresponding to numerous nerve tracts. Every nerve transmission between the brain and spinal cord passes through the medulla. The fibers on

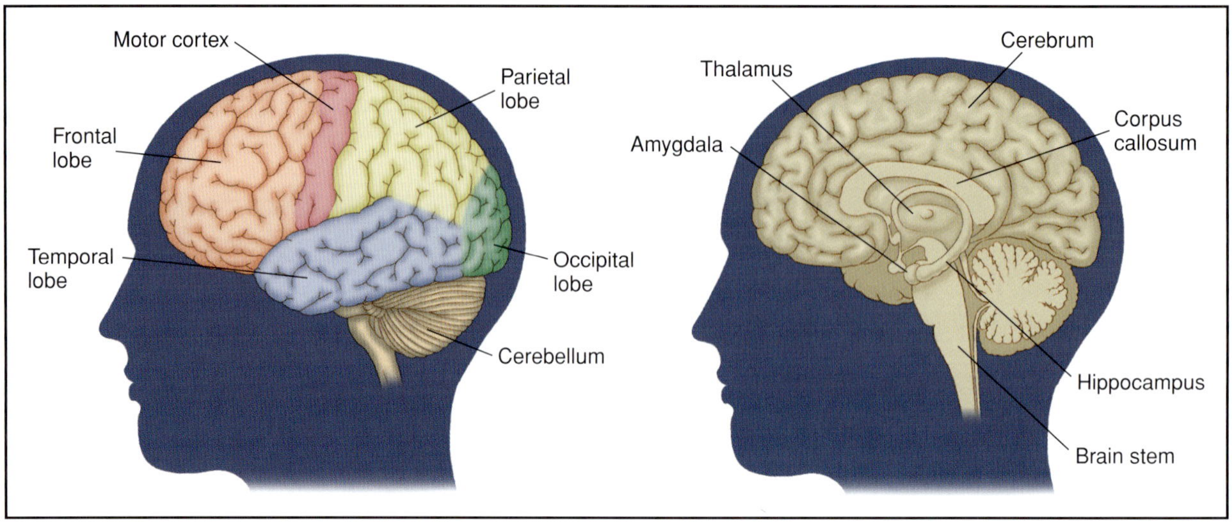

Diagram showing the exterior (left) and interior (right) anatomy of the human brain. *(Illustration by Frank Forney. Reproduced by permission of Cengage Learning.)*

the right side of the medulla cross to the left and those on the left cross to the right. Thus, each side of the brain controls the opposite side of the body. The medulla regulates vital body functions, such as heartbeat, breathing rate, and dilation of blood vessels, and helps coordinate swallowing, vomiting, hiccupping, coughing, and sneezing.

PONS. The pons, Latin for "bridge," conducts messages between the spinal cord and the rest of the brain and between different parts of the brain. It is involved in motor control, sensory analysis, and consciousness levels and sleep. Some structures within the pons are linked to the cerebellum and are involved in movement and posture.

MIDBRAIN. The midbrain or mesencephalon is the smallest and most anterior portion of the brain stem. It conveys impulses between the cerebral cortex, pons, and spinal cord, and has visual and audio reflex centers that are involved in eye and head movements. The anterior portion of the midbrain includes the cerebral peduncle, a large bundle of axons extending from the cerebral cortex through the brain stem that are important for voluntary motor function.

Diencephalon

The diencephalon, or "between brain," lies between the midbrain and the cerebral hemispheres and connects the cerebral hemispheres to the limbic system. It consists of the thalamus and hypothalamus.

The thalamus is a large body of gray matter at the top of the diencephalon, positioned deep within the forebrain. Axons from every sensory system except olfaction (smell) enter the thalamus and relay sensory information to the cerebral cortex. The thalamus also has some motor functions and regulates some emotions and memory.

The hypothalamus controls a number of body functions and helps regulate the endocrine or hormonal system through control of the pituitary gland. The hypothalamus controls the autonomic nervous system, including body temperature, heartbeat, and digestion; emotional responses including anger and aggression; thirst and hunger; and circadian rhythms including sleep.

Cerebrum

Constituting nearly 90% of the brain's weight, the cerebrum is formed by the cerebral hemispheres, which are connected by a bundle of white matter called the corpus callosum.

Each cerebral hemisphere has a somewhat different function. The left hemisphere works mainly in speech and language comprehension, logic, writing, and arithmetic. The right hemisphere is more involved with spatial relations, symbolism, art, and imagination. Because damage to the left hemisphere is more likely to cause language deficits, it is commonly referred to as the dominant hemisphere. Nearly all right-handed people and most left-handed people have a left-dominant brain, though some people have a right-dominant brain or language function that is more equally distributed between the hemispheres.

The basal ganglia are four masses of gray matter located deep within each of the cerebral hemispheres. They modulate the output of the frontal cortex involving motor function, as well as cognition and motivation. The corpus striatum is the major point of entry into the basal ganglia circuitry, receiving input from almost all cortical areas. The corpus striatum is subdivided into the caudate nucleus, putamen, and globus pallidus.

The hemispheres are covered by the gray matter of the cerebral cortex. The cortex accounts for about 40% of the brain's total mass, with a surface area of over 1 sq yd. (about 1 sq m). It is the site of the highest level of neural functioning, including higher motor functions, perception, language, cognition, emotion, and memory.

The cerebral cortex is divided into four major lobes. The frontal lobe contains the primary motor cortex and premotor area, involved in voluntary movement; Broca's area, involved in writing and speech; and the prefrontal cortex, involved in personality, insight, and foresight. The parietal lobe contains the primary somatosensory cortex, which is involved in tactile and positioning information, as well as areas affecting spatial orientation and language comprehension. The temporal lobe contains the primary auditory cortex; Wernicke's area, involved in language comprehension and meaning; and areas involved in the higher processing of visual input, along with the aspects of learning and memory associated with the limbic system. The occipital lobe contains the primary visual cortex and the visual association cortex.

Cerebellum

The cerebellum is located below the cerebrum and behind the brain stem. It is butterfly shaped, with the "wings" forming the two cerebellar hemispheres; the two halves are connected by the vermis. The cerebellum coordinates many neuromuscular functions, such as balance, movement, and posture. Disorders of or damage to the cerebellum often result in ataxia (problems with coordination), dysarthria (unclear speech due to lack of muscle control), and nystagmus (uncontrollable jerking of the eyeballs).

Limbic system

The limbic system is sometimes referred to as the "emotional brain." It is involved in drive-related behavior, memory, and emotional responses, including feeding, defense, and sexuality. The limbic system includes the limbic lobe, which is buried within the cerebrum and includes portions of the frontal, parietal, and temporal lobes. It also includes the amygdalae—one of the four basal ganglia of each hemisphere—which are involved in memory, emotion, and fear. The amygdalae lie beneath the surface of the temporal lobes where they cause a bulge called the uncus. The other structures of the limbic system are the hippocampi of the cerebral hemispheres and the thalamus and hypothalamus of the diencephalon.

The hippocampus, referred to as the "gateway to memory," is involved in learning and memory functions. It converts short-term memory into more permanent memory and is involved in the storage and retrieval of long-term memory and recall of learned spatial associations. The hippocampus is a curved sheet of cortex folded into the basal medial portion of the temporal lobe. It is divided into three multilayered sections, the dentate gyrus, hippocampus proper, and subiculum, with the latter situated as a transitional zone between the other two. The dentate gyrus receives input from the cortex and sends output to the hippocampus proper, which then sends output to the subiculum.

Nervous tracts

Tracts are groups or bundles of nerve fibers that constitute an anatomical and functional unit. Commissural tracts, such as the corpus callosum, connect the cerebral hemispheres. Association tracts make connections within the same hemisphere. Projection tracts connect the brain with the spinal cord. Sensory tracts project upward from the spinal cord into regions of the brain. Motor tracts project down from the brain into the spinal cord, bringing motor output information to the periphery. The internal capsule is the major structure carrying ascending and descending nerve projection fibers to and from the cerebral cortex.

Meninges and ventricular systems

The meninges are membranes that cover and protect the central nervous system (CNS), enclosing the cerebrospinal fluid (CSF) that buoys up the brain. The three membranes of the meninges are the thick external dura mater, which supplies mechanical strength; the middle web-like, delicate arachnoid mater, which forms a protective barrier and space for CSF circulation, and the internal pia mater, which is continuous with all the contours of the brain and forms CSF. The dura mater contains six major venous sinuses that drain the cerebral veins and several smaller sinuses.

Dural venous sinuses are formed in spaces where the two layers of the dura mater separate. The superior sagittal sinus, straight sinus, and right and left transverse sinuses meet in a structure called the confluence of the sinuses. Venous blood circulation follows a pathway through the superior sagittal and straight sinuses into the confluence and then through the transverse sinuses. Each transverse sinus carries venous blood along an S-shaped course until it empties into the internal jugular vein. The major dural sinuses also connect with several smaller sinuses.

The arachnoid mater follows the general shape of the brain. The space between the arachnoid mater and pia

KEY TERMS

Amygdala—One of the four basal ganglia in each cerebral hemisphere, consisting of a mass of gray matter in the roof of the lateral ventricle; part of the limbic system.

Anterior—Situated toward the head or front.

Axon—The long process that conducts impulses away from the nerve cell body.

Brain stem—The part of the brain that connects the forebrain and cerebrum to the spinal cord; consisting of the midbrain, pons, and medulla oblongata.

Central nervous system (CNS)—The brain and spinal cord.

Cerebellum—The part of the brain between the brain stem and back of the cerebrum, consisting of two lateral lobes and a median lobe, and involved especially in muscle coordination and maintenance of bodily equilibrium.

Cerebral cortex—The convoluted surface gray matter of the cerebrum that coordinates motor and sensory information and cognitive function.

Cerebrospinal fluid (CSF)—The fluid that circulates through the central nervous system to maintain uniform pressure on the brain and spinal cord.

Cerebrum—The enlarged, forward portion overlying the rest of the brain, consisting of the two cerebral hemispheres and connecting structures, and responsible for conscious mental processes.

Cognition—Conscious intellectual activity, including thinking, imagining, reasoning, remembering, and learning.

Corpus callosum—(plural, corpora callosa) A thick bundle of nerve fibers lying deep in the brain that connects the two cerebral hemispheres and coordinates their functions.

Diencephalon—The "between brain" or "interbrain" beneath the cerebral hemispheres and consisting of the thalamus and hypothalamus.

Glial cells—The support cells of nervous tissue, especially in the brain, spinal cord, and ganglia, interspersed between signal-transmitting neurons. There are three main types of neuroglia: astrocytes, oligodendrocytes, and microglia.

Gyri—Convoluted ridges between the sulci or grooves on the surface of the brain.

Hippocampus—A part of the limbic system that extends over the floor of the descending horn of each lateral ventricle and is important for forming, storing, and processing memory.

Hypothalamus—Part of the diencephalon beneath the thalamus that controls the autonomic nervous system and regulates hormone production by the adjacent pituitary gland.

Limbic system—Brain structures, including the hypothalamus, hippocampi, and amygdalae, that are involved in emotion and motivation.

Meninges—The three membranes that enclose the brain and spinal cord, consisting of the dura mater, arachnoid mater, and pia mater.

Myelin—A white, fatty substance that covers and protects nerves.

Neuron—Cells that transmit and receive nerve impulses; consisting of a cell body and multiple projections called dendrites or solitary axons that conduct impulses to and from the cell body.

Neurotransmitter—A chemical, such as dopamine, norepinephrine, or serotonin, that transmits nerve impulses across synapses.

Peripheral nerve—A nerve in a distant location from the brain that receives information in the form of an impulse from the brain and spinal cord.

Pituitary gland—A small endocrine organ in the brain that is associated with various hormones that control and regulate other endocrine organs. The pituitary affects most basic bodily functions, including growth and development.

Sulci—The furrows or grooves on the surface of the brain between convolutions.

Synapse—The space at which a nerve impulse passes from one neuron to the next.

Thalamus—The largest portion of the diencephalon, which relays impulses, especially sensory impulses, to and from the cerebral cortex.

Ventricular system—The system of small cavities in the brain that forms, circulates, and drains the cerebrospinal fluid.

mater is called the subarachnoid space and contains CSF. CSF enters venous circulation through small protrusions into the venous sinus called arachnoid villi. The pia mater forms part of the choroid plexus, a highly convoluted and vascular membranous material that lies within the ventricular system of the brain and is responsible for most CSF production.

The brain contains four ventricles. Each cerebral hemisphere contains a long, C-shaped lateral ventricle that communicates with the narrow, slit-shaped third ventricle of the diencephalon. The third ventricle communicates with the tent-shaped fourth ventricle of the pons and medulla, which protrudes into the cerebellum. CSF flows in a specific pattern that allows newly formed CSF to replace the old several times daily. The CSF is formed in the lateral ventricles, flows into the third and then the fourth ventricle, into basal cisterns, up and over the cerebral hemispheres, and into the arachnoid villi, where it is drained into a venous sinus for return to the venous system. Some CSF is diverted from the basal cisterns into the subarachnoid space of the spinal cord.

Studying the brain

Neurons carry information through the nervous system in the form of brief electrical impulses called action potentials. When an impulse reaches the end of an axon, neurotransmitters are released at junctions called synapses. The neurotransmitters are chemicals that bind to receptors on the receiving neurons, triggering the continuation of the impulse. Fifty different neurotransmitters have been discovered since the first was identified in 1920. By studying the chemical effects of neurotransmitters in the brain, scientists have developed treatments for mental disorders and are learning more about how drugs affect the brain.

Electroencephalogram

Technology provides useful tools for researching the brain and helping patients with brain disorders. An electroencephalogram (EEG) records brain waves, which are produced by electrical activity in the brain. It is obtained by positioning electrodes on the head and amplifying the waves with an electroencephalograph. EEGs are valuable in diagnosing brain diseases such as epilepsy and tumors.

Magnetic resonance imaging (MRI)

Using a magnetic field to display the living brain at various depths, **magnetic resonance imaging** can produce very clear and detailed pictures of brain structures. These images, which often appear as cross-sectional slices, are obtained by altering the main magnetic field of a specific brain area. MRI is particularly valuable in diagnosing damage to soft tissues, such as areas affected by head **trauma**. MRI also reveals tumors and other types of brain lesions.

Positron emission tomography (PET)

During a **positron emission tomography** scan, a technician injects the patient with a small amount of a substance, such as glucose, that is marked with a radioactive tag. By tracking the radioactive substance as it travels to the brain, physicians can see almost immediately where glucose is consumed in the brain. This indicates brain activity, an important factor in diagnosing epilepsy, **Alzheimer's disease**, or Parkinson's disease. **PET** is also valuable in locating tumors and brain areas that have been affected by a **stroke** or blood clot.

Researchers have developed a molecule, abbreviated FDDNP, that binds to the plaques and protein tangles that characterize Alzheimer's disease in the brain. This molecule also is fluorescent, and after injection of a solution of FDDNP into a patient, clinicians can use PET to capture an image of the brain showing where it has bound and is fluorescing. In this way, they can distinguish a brain even with mild cognitive impairment when compared to a brain with no cognitive impairment and also can distinguish mild impairment from Alzheimer's disease.

Magnetoencephalography (MEG)

Magnetoencephalography measures the electromagnetic fields created between neurons as electrochemical information is passed along. Of all brain scanning methods, MEG provides the most accurate indicator of nerve cell activity, which can be measured in milliseconds. By combining an MRI with MEG, clinicians can get a noninvasive look at the brain that is especially useful in diagnosing epilepsy or migraines. MEG also helps identify specific brain areas involved with different tasks. Any movement by the patient—wiggling the toes, for example—appears on the computer screen immediately as concentric colored rings. This pinpoints brain signals even before the toes are actually wiggled. Researchers foresee that these techniques could someday help paralysis victims move by supplying information on how to stimulate their muscles or indicating the signals needed to control an artificial limb.

Computed axial tomography scan (CT or CAT)

Computed tomography scans use x rays to produce a picture of the targeted area of the body in cross sections. Clinicians may use a dye that creates a contrast between tissues to highlight a specific area of interest for the scan. In the brain, this type of scan can be used to identify an area of stroke or hemorrhage, causes of headache, and causes of lost sensory or motor function. This test may also be used in the **diagnosis** of other disorders involving the brain, including **delirium**, **dementia**, and **schizophrenia**.

Resources

BOOKS

Ashwell, Ken W. S. *Anatomica: The Complete Home Medical Reference*. Richmond Hill, Ontario: Firefly, 2010.

Carter, Rita, et al. *The Human Brain Book*. New York: DK Pub., 2009.

PERIODICALS

Brenninkmeijer, Jonna. "Taking Care of One's Brain: How Manipulating the Brain Changes People's Selves." *History of the Human Sciences* 23, no. 1 (February 2010): 107–26.

Dekosky, Steven T., Milos D. Ikonomovic, and Sam Gandy. "Traumatic Brain Injury—Football, Warfare, and Long-Term Effects." *New England Journal of Medicine* 363, no. 14 (September 30, 2010): 1293–96.

Ogilvie, Megan. "Genesis: The Life of the Brain." *Toronto Star*, (July 10, 2010): IN.1.

Raichle, Marcus E. "The Brain's (Dark Energy)." *Scientific American* 201, no. 3 (March 2010): 44.

Small, Gary W., et al. "PET of Brain Amyloid and Tau in Mild Cognitive Impairment." *The New England Journal of Medicine* 355 (2006): 2652–63.

WEBSITES

Chudler, Eric H. "Brain Facts and Figures." Neuroscience for Kids. http://faculty.washington.edu/chudler/facts.html (accessed September 30, 2011).

MedlinePlus. "Brain Diseases." U.S. National Library of Medicine, National Institutes of Health. http://www.nlm.nih.gov/medlineplus/braindiseases.html (accessed September 30, 2011).

U.S. National Institute of Mental Health. "Neuroimaging and Mental Illness: A Window Into the Brain." http://www.nimh.nih.gov/health/publications/neuroimaging-and-mental-illness-a-window-into-the-brain/neuroimaging-and-mental-illness-a-window-into-the-brain.shtml (accessed September 30, 2011).

U.S. National Institute of Neurological Disorders and Stroke. "Brain Basics: Know Your Brain." http://www.ninds.nih.gov/disorders/brain_basics/know_your_brain.htm (accessed September 30, 2011).

ZERO TO THREE: National Center for Infants, Toddlers and Families. "Early Experiences Matter." http://main.zerotothree.org/site/PageServer?pagename=ter_key_brainFAQ (accessed September 30, 2011).

ORGANIZATIONS

National Institute of Mental Health, 6001 Executive Blvd., Room 8184, MSC 9663, Bethesda, MD, 20892-9663, (301) 433-4513; TTY: (301) 443-8431, (866) 615-6464; TTY: (866) 415-8051, Fax: (301) 443-4279, nimhinfo@nih.gov, http://www.nimh.nih.gov.

National Institute of Neurological Disorders and Stroke, PO Box 5801, Bethesda, MD, 20824, (301) 496-5751; TTY: (301) 468-5981, (800) 352-9424, http://www.ninds.nih.gov.

Breathing-related sleep disorder

Definition

Breathing-related sleep disorder is marked by sleep disruption from abnormal breathing during sleep. The most common complaint of individuals with breathing-related sleep disorder is excessive daytime sleepiness, brought on by frequent interruptions of nocturnal, or nighttime, sleep. A less frequent complaint is **insomnia** or inability to sleep. About two-thirds of people with this disorder experience daytime sleepiness, and one-third experience an inability to sleep.

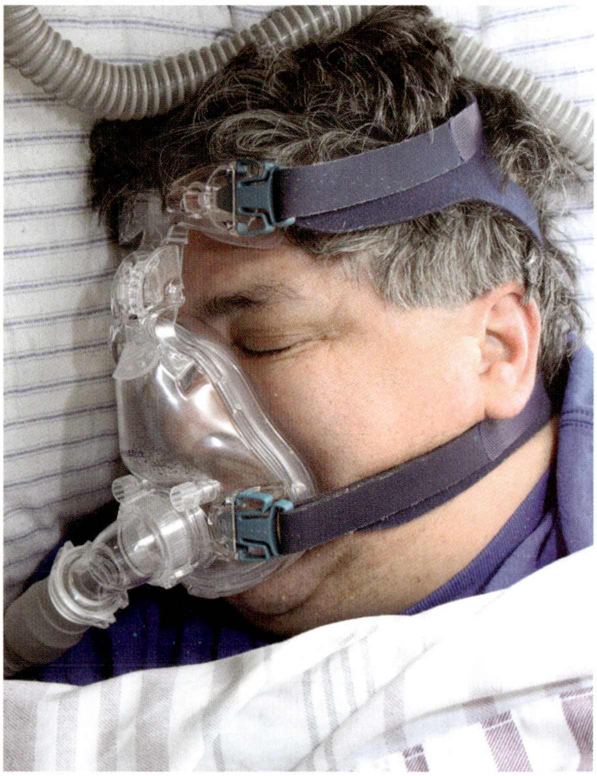

An individual undergoes the continuous positive airway pressure (CPAP) test for sleep apnea. *(© Custom Medical Stock Photo, Inc. Reproduced by permission.)*

Mental health professionals use the ***Diagnostic and Statistical Manual of Mental Disorders***, also known as the *DSM* to diagnose mental disorders. In the fourth edition, text revision *(DSM-IV-TR)*, breathing-related sleep disorder is listed as one of several different primary **sleep disorders**. Within the category of primary sleep disorders, it is classified as one of the dyssomnias, which are characterized by irregularities in the quality, timing, and amount of sleep.

The *DSM-IV-TR* lists three types of breathing-related sleep disorder: obstructive sleep apnea syndrome (the most common type), central sleep apnea syndrome, and central alveolar hypoventilation syndrome.

The fifth edition of the *DSM* (*DSM-5*, 2013) proposes placing breathing-related sleep disorder under wake-sleep disorders and dividing it into obstructive sleep apnea hypopnea syndrome, primary central sleep apnea, and primary alveolar hypoventilation.

Demographics

The National Center on Sleep Disorder Research estimates that between 40 and 70 million Americans experience chronic or intermittent sleep-related disorders. The majority of patients with the obstructive sleep apnea type of breathing-related sleep disorder are overweight, middle-aged males. Four percent of middle-aged men and 2% of middle-aged women meet the criteria for obstructive sleep apnea. Among children, the male-to-female ratio is 1:1. Prevalence of breathing-related sleep disorder among children peaks between two and eight years of age.

Description

The most common feature of any breathing-related sleep disorder is interruption of the person's sleep, leading to excessive daytime sleepiness. When the regular nighttime sleep of individuals is frequently interrupted, sleepiness at other times of the day is the usual result. People with breathing-related sleep disorder often find that they feel sleepy during relaxing activities such as reading or watching a movie. With extreme cases, those with this condition may feel so sleepy that they fall asleep during activities that require alertness, such as talking, walking, or driving.

Other people with breathing-related sleep disorder report having insomnia, or the inability to sleep. Patients also find that their sleep does not refresh them; they may awaken frequently during sleep, or have difficulty breathing while sleeping or lying down.

The two sleep apnea syndromes that are listed as subtypes of breathing-related sleep disorder are characterized by episodes of airway blockage or breathing cessation during sleep. Sleep apnea is potentially deadly. Central alveolar hypoventilation syndrome is distinguished from the other two subtypes of breathing-related sleep disorder by the fact that shallow breathing causes reduced oxygen content of the blood. The alveoli, which are the tiny air sacs in the lung tissue, cannot oxygenate the blood efficiently because those with this disorder are not breathing deeply enough. Shallow breathing often occurs when people are awake and is common in severely overweight individuals.

Causes and symptoms

Causes

Many people with the obstructive sleep apnea syndrome subtype of breathing-related sleep disorder are overweight. The symptoms often grow worse as their weight increases. People who have obstructive sleep apnea and are not overweight often have breathing passages that are narrowed by swollen tonsils, abnormally large adenoids, or other abnormalities of the various structures of the mouth and throat. The fundamental underlying cause appears to be a narrow or collapsible airway with a loss of muscle tone in the airway during sleep.

Central sleep apnea syndrome is often associated with cardiac or neurological conditions affecting airflow regulation. It is a disorder that occurs most frequently in elderly patients.

Patients diagnosed with central alveolar hypoventilation syndrome experience a breathing impairment related to abnormally low arterial oxygen levels.

Symptoms

Obstructive sleep apnea syndrome, which is the most common type of breathing-related sleep disorder, is marked by frequent episodes of upper airway obstruction during sleep. Patients with this syndrome alternate between loud snores or gasps and silent periods that usually last for 20–30 seconds. The snoring is caused by the partial blockage of the airway. The silent periods are caused by complete obstruction of the airway, which makes the patient's breathing stop. These periods of breathing cessation can last between 10 seconds and one minute.

Obstructive sleep apnea syndrome is also common in children with enlarged tonsils. The symptoms of any breathing-related sleep disorder in children are often subtle and more difficult to diagnose. Children under five years are more likely to demonstrate nighttime symptoms such as apnea and breathing difficulties. Children over five years are more likely to demonstrate daytime symptoms such as sleepiness and attention difficulties.

People with central sleep apnea syndrome experience periods when the oxygenation of blood in the lungs temporarily stops during sleep, but they do not suffer airway obstruction. Although these patients may snore, their snoring is usually mild and not a major complaint.

Central alveolar hypoventilation syndrome is characterized by excessive sleepiness and insomnia.

Diagnosis

A **diagnosis** of breathing-related sleep disorder usually requires a thorough physical examination of the patient. The patient may be referred to an otorhinolaryngologist (a doctor who specializes in disorders of the ear, nose, and throat) for a detailed evaluation of the upper respiratory tract. The physical examination is followed by observation of the patient in a sleep clinic or laboratory. Breathing patterns, including episodes of snoring and apnea, are evaluated when the patient is connected to a device called a polysomnogram. The polysomnogram uses a set of electrodes to measure several different body functions associated with sleep, including heart rate, eye movements, **brain** waves, muscle activity, breathing, changes in blood oxygen concentration, and body position. Interviews are also conducted with the patients and their partners.

To meet criteria for the diagnosis of breathing-related sleep disorder, patients must experience interruptions of sleep leading to insomnia or excessive sleepiness that have been determined to result from one of the following sleep-related breathing conditions: obstructive sleep apnea syndrome, central sleep apnea syndrome, or central alveolar hypoventilation syndrome.

The disturbance in sleep must also not be attributed to another mental disorder, to a general medical condition not related to breathing, or to the direct effects on the body of a prescription medication or drug of abuse.

Treatment

Weight loss is key to effective treatment of overweight people with breathing-related sleep disorder. It is often considered the first step in treating any disorder involving sleep apnea. Increased **exercise** and reduced-calorie **diets** are the most important components of an effective weight loss regimen.

Another approach to addressing sleep apnea is a postural change during sleep, called "positional therapy." The U.S. Food and Drug Administration (FDA) has approved a pillow that is supposed to aid in preventing the sleeper from assuming a supine (on the back) position, which may worsen sleep apnea. Postural alarms are being marketed to warn the sleeper, but many people try home-based approaches to ensure that they do not flip onto their backs during sleep. One study found that sleeping on the back with the torso elevated may result in reduced apneas but recommended that patients trying this option use foam pillows rather than soft pillows, which can push the chin onto the chest and worsen apnea.

Oral appliances may be effective for people who have mild apnea. The most common of these is the mandibular advancement device (also called MAD), which pushes the lower jaw forward, keeping the airway open.

Continuous positive airway pressure therapy, also known as CPAP therapy, is a popular form of treatment for the obstructive sleep apnea subtype of breathing-related sleep disorder. CPAP therapy, which has been in use since 1981, involves the use of a high-pressure blower that delivers continuous air flow to a mask worn by the patient during sleep. The airflow from the CPAP blower is often very effective in reducing or eliminating sleep apnea episodes. CPAP treatment is, however, inconvenient and somewhat noisy for anyone who must share a bedroom with the patient. Patients do not always comply with this form of treatment because they may find it to be too constrictive and cumbersome. In addition, they may experience mask discomfort, nasal congestion, and nose and throat dryness. Proper mask fitting and a humidifier can help to alleviate some side effects. A couple of alternative forms of CPAP may improve **compliance** by improving comfort, including bi-level positive airway pressure, which has two sets of air pressures that it delivers, one for exhalation and one for inhalation, to make using the device more comfortable. Another product is the C-Flex, which provides flexible positive airway pressure, alternating pressures for inhalation and exhalation on a breath-by-breath basis. The company that produces the C-Flex received FDA permission to market its product in 2004. CPAPs, as medical devices, must be obtained through a doctor's prescription.

There are no medications that directly target sleep apnea.

Surgery to relieve airway obstruction may be performed in some cases. If the airway obstruction is related to anatomical structures that narrow the airway, surgical reshaping of the soft palate and uvula (a small, conical-shaped piece of tissue attached to the middle of the soft palate) may be performed. Another surgical procedure that is sometimes conducted on very obese patients with obstructive sleep apnea is a tracheostomy, or an artificial opening made in the windpipe. This operation has a number of unpleasant side effects, however, and so is usually reserved for patients whose breathing-related disorder is life threatening.

KEY TERMS

Alveolar—Pertaining to alveoli, which are tiny air sacs at the ends of the small air passages in the lungs.

Apnea—A brief suspension or interruption of breathing.

Dyssomnia—A type of sleep disorder characterized by a problem with the amount, quality, or timing of the patient's sleep.

Hypoventilation—An abnormally low level of blood oxygenation in the lungs.

Polysomnogram—A machine that is used to diagnose sleep disorders by measuring and recording a variety of body functions related to sleep, including heart rate, eye movements, brain waves, muscle activity, breathing, changes in blood oxygen concentration, and body position.

Syndrome—A group of symptoms that together characterize a disease or disorder.

Tracheostomy—A surgical procedure in which an artificial opening is made in the patient's windpipe to relieve airway obstruction.

Patients with sleep apnea are advised to abstain from alcohol and sedative medications, which are often given to patients who display any type of sleeping irregularities. Alcohol and **sedatives** often increase the likelihood of upper airway problems during sleep.

Prognosis

Breathing-related sleep disorder often has a gradual long-term progression and a chronic course. For this reason, many people have the disorder for years before seeking treatment. For many, symptoms worsen during middle age, causing people to seek treatment at that point.

Successful treatment of other conditions, such as obesity, common cardiovascular and cerebrovascular comorbidities, or enlarged tonsils in children, often aids in the treatment of breathing-related sleep disorder. Weight loss often leads to spontaneous resolution of the disorder. Because **depression** has been found at high rates among people with sleep apnea (as high as 64% in some studies), any assessments should evaluate for the presence of depression to aid in improving the prognosis.

Prevention

Because overweight people are more likely to develop the more common obstructive sleep apnea type of breathing-related sleep disorder, a good preventive measure is effective weight management. Good general health and treatment of related physiological conditions are also effective in preventing the disorder.

Resources

BOOKS

American Psychiatric Association. *Diagnostic and Statistical Manual of Mental Disorders*. 4th ed., text rev. Washington, DC: American Psychiatric Publishing, 2000.

Buysse, Daniel J., Charles M. Morin, and Charles F. Reynolds III. "Sleep Disorders." In *Treatments of Psychiatric Disorders*, edited by Glen O. Gabbard. Washington, DC: American Psychiatric Publishing, 2010.

Buysse, Daniel J. *Sleep Disorders and Psychiatry*. Washington, DC: American Psychiatric Publishing, 2010.

Pollak, Charles P., Michael Thorpy, and Jan Yager. *The Encyclopedia of Sleep and Sleep Disorders*. New York: Facts on File, 2009.

PERIODICALS

Aloia, Mark S., et al. "Treatment Adherence and Outcomes in Flexible vs. Standard Continuous Positive Airway Pressure Therapy." *Chest* 127 (2005): 2085–93.

Dauvilliers, Yves, and A. Buguet. "Hypersomnia." *Dialogues in Clinical Neuroscience* 7, no. 4 (2005): 347–56.

Haba-Rubio, José. "Psychiatric Aspects of Organic Sleep Disorders." *Dialogues in Clinical Neuroscience* 7, no. 4 (2005): 335–46.

Lloberes, Patricia, et al. "Predictive Factors of Quality-of-life Improvement and Continuous Positive Airway Pressure Use in Patients with Sleep Apnea-Hypopnea Syndrome: Study at 1 Year." *Chest* 126, no. 4 (October 2004): 1241–47.

WEBSITES

Cataletto, Mary E., et al. "Breathing-Related Sleep Disorder." Medscape Reference. http://emedicine.medscape.com/article/291807-overview (accessed September 30, 2011).

U.S. National Heart Lung and Blood Institute. "What is Sleep Apnea?" http://www.nhlbi.nih.gov/health/dci/Diseases/SleepApnea/SleepApnea_WhatIs.html (accessed September 30, 2011).

ORGANIZATIONS

American Sleep Apnea Association, 6856 Eastern Ave. NW, Ste. 203, Washington, DC, (202) 293-3650, Fax: (202) 293-3656, http://www.sleepapnea.org.

American Sleep Disorders Association, 6301 Bandel Rd. NW, Ste. 101, Rochester, MN, 55901, http://www.asda.org.

National Center on Sleep Disorders Research, 6701 Rockledge Drive, Bethesda, MD, (301) 435-0199, Fax: (301) 480-3451, http://www.nhlbi.nih.gov.

National Sleep Foundation, 1010 N Glebe Rd., Ste. 310, Arlington, VA, 22201, (703) 243-1697, nsf@sleepfoundation.org, http://www.sleepfoundation.org.

Ali Fahmy, PhD
Emily Jane Willingham, PhD

Brief psychotic disorder

Definition

Brief psychotic disorder is a short-term **psychosis** lasting between one day and one month, with complete recovery following the episode. It is characterized by at least one symptom of psychosis, such as **delusions**, hallucinations, incoherence, severely disorganized thinking or behavior, or catatonic behavior.

Demographics

Although the incidence of brief psychotic disorder is not known, it is relatively rare in the United States and other developed countries. One study of 221 patients admitted to U.S. hospitals for a first-time psychotic episode found that only 9% were experiencing brief psychoses. Although mental disorders with psychotic symptoms lasting longer than one month, such as **schizophrenia**, are more prevalent in developed nations, the incidence of brief psychotic reactions and disorders appears to be up to ten-fold higher in the developing world. Some clinicians believe that brief psychotic disorder is more common among those of lower socioeconomic status, as well as among immigrants. An international epidemiological study found that brief psychotic disorder was twice as common in women as in men. In the United States, the incidence in women is more than two-fold higher than in men. Brief psychotic disorder is more common in adolescents and young adults in their twenties and thirties than in older adults. Stress-induced brief psychotic disorder most often affects adults in their twenties through their forties.

Description

Brief psychotic disorder is a **diagnosis** that is more common and better studied in Scandinavia and other parts of Western Europe than in the United States. It is defined as one or more temporary symptoms of psychosis that are not attributable to a physical disease, a clinical diagnosis of mental illness, a reaction to medication, or intoxication with drugs or alcohol. In contrast to **schizophreniform disorder**, which lasts at least one month but less than six months, and schizophrenia, which lasts longer than six months, brief psychotic disorder lasts from one day to one month. Patients may or may not be aware of their psychoses. As with all psychotic disorders, brief psychotic disorder can be severely disruptive and can potentially lead to violence or **suicide**.

There are several types of brief psychotic disorder:

- Stress-induced psychosis, also called brief psychotic disorder with obvious stressor or brief reactive psychosis, is by far the most common type. It occurs under circumstances of severe stress or trauma, such as divorce, bereavement, combat, natural disaster, an accident, or violent assault. Normal functioning generally returns once the stress is relieved, support becomes available, or the patient develops coping skills.
- Defense mechanism in personality disorder is a brief psychotic disorder that sometimes develops when individuals with personality disorders face severe stress.
- Brief psychotic disorder without obvious stressor occurs in the absence of an apparent stress or trauma.
- Postpartum psychosis occurs in women, usually within four weeks of giving birth, and is thought to be associated with dramatic hormonal changes that occur with childbirth and in the immediate postpartum period. Postpartum psychosis is often misdiagnosed and treated inappropriately. In severe cases, it can result in infanticide or suicide.
- Early-stage schizophrenia is often misdiagnosed as brief psychotic disorder.

Culture not only influences the form of a psychotic reaction, but it also determines what is considered to be psychotic. Behaviors that are viewed as psychotic or bizarre in one culture may be acceptable in another. A diagnosis of brief psychotic disorder requires that the symptoms or behaviors are not an acceptable manifestation of culture or religion and are not part of a religious practice or **meditation**. Individuals within a community or culture may exhibit behavior that is attributable to a particular cause or stimulus, such as cabin fever, witchcraft, or spiritual possession, or that may be the result of a culturally specific phobia, such as fear of sinning in a religious community or fear of being cold in tropical climates. These are known as culture-bound syndromes or culturally defined disorders. Another example is *koro,* which occurs in some parts of Asia and is a delusional **obsession** with the possibility that the genitals will retract or shrink into the body. Unrecognizable speech patterns or "speaking in tongues," which sometimes occurs as part of a religious experience, is also an example of a culture-bound syndrome.

Risk factors

A preexisting personality disorder—antisocial, paranoid, narcissistic, borderline, or schizotypal—appears to be a major risk factor for brief psychotic disorder in response to stressful situations. There is some evidence that brief psychotic disorder is more common in families with a history of mood disorders, such as **depression** or **bipolar disorder**.

Causes and symptoms

The precise causes of brief psychotic disorder are unclear. The majority of cases are triggered by an extremely stressful or traumatic event, and there is some evidence that susceptibility has a genetic basis. It also has been suggested that people with **personality disorders** may be physiologically or psychologically vulnerable to the development of psychotic symptoms. Psychodynamic theories suggest that the disorder may be caused by poor coping skills, particularly in individuals with personality disorders. Coping skills are defense mechanisms that can protect a person from dangerous fantasies and can act as an escape in overwhelmingly stressful situations. These circumstances can include family- or work-associated conflicts, accidents, severe illness, loss of a loved one, immigration difficulties, or traumatic events. Postpartum psychosis is thought to be caused by rapid hormonal changes immediately following childbirth, coupled with **stress**.

The ***Diagnostic and Statistical Manual of Mental Disorders*** (DSM) provides three major criteria for brief psychotic disorder:

- At least one positive symptom of psychosis, from the following symptoms: delusions; hallucinations; disorganized speech that is strange, peculiar, or difficult to comprehend; disorganized (bizarre or childlike) behavior; or catatonic behavior.
- Limited duration, with psychotic symptoms occurring for at least one day but less than one month and with eventual return to normal level of functioning.
- Symptoms that are not biologically influenced or attributable to another disorder—that is, symptoms not occurring as part of a mood disorder, schizoaffective disorder, or schizophrenia; not due to intoxication with drugs or alcohol; not due to an adverse reaction to a medication; and not due to a physical injury or medical illness.

Delusions are a classic feature of psychosis. Delusions are strongly held irrational or unrealistic beliefs that are extremely difficult to change, even in the face of contradictory evidence. Delusions can be paranoid or persecutory, wherein the delusional person is excessively suspicious or believes that he or she is the victim of a conspiracy. Delusions can also be unjustified grandiose beliefs that exaggerate one's importance, such as believing oneself to be a famous person or hold an enviable position. Grandiose delusions often have religious overtones, such as believing one's self to be the Virgin Mary. Delusions also can involve elaborate love fantasies (called erotomanic delusions) or extreme and irrational jealousy. Somatic delusions, from *soma,* the Greek word for body, are erroneous but strongly held beliefs about the characteristics or functioning of one's body; for example, refusing to eat because of the conviction that one's throat muscles are completely paralyzed and that only liquids can be swallowed.

Hallucinations are false perceptions. They can occur in various forms that parallel the human senses. Auditory hallucinations—usually hearing voices—are the most common hallucinations. Auditory-visual hallucinations involve both hearing and seeing what is not present. Visual hallucinations can also occur alone. Somatic hallucinations are bodily sensations, such as smelling nonexistent odors or feeling something on or under one's skin.

Incoherence or disorganized speech is distorted speech that is peculiar or difficult to comprehend. It may involve mixing words together in no coherent order, responses that are irrelevant or strange in the context of a conversation, or echolalia (repeating another person's exact words either immediately or after a delay of minutes or hours).

Disorganized or bizarre thought patterns and behaviors can range from childlike behaviors, such as skipping, singing, or hopping in inappropriate circumstances, to unusual practices, such as **hoarding** food or wrapping one's head and clothing with aluminum foil. Catatonic behaviors can be either strange bodily movements or lack of movement. Catalepsy is motionless **catatonia**, in which the patient may remain in the same position for hours. Rapid or persistently repeated movements, frequent grimacing and strange facial expressions, and unusual gestures are the opposite symptom.

Brief psychotic disorder is often accompanied by severe agitation, fear, or anger, and agitated patients are more likely to harm themselves or others. Other symptoms that may be associated with brief psychotic behavior include:

- changes in weight, energy level, or eating or sleeping habits
- indecision
- rapid mood changes and emotional volatility
- uncooperativeness
- disorientation or confusion
- impaired concentration and attention
- poor insight or judgment
- bizarre dress
- screaming or muteness

KEY TERMS

Bipolar disorder—A recurrent mood disorder, in which patients have extreme mood swings from depression to mania or a mixture of both.

Catatonia—Psychomotor disturbances that can include stupor, rigidity, muteness, or purposeless and bizarre movements.

Delusion—A persistent false belief held in the face of strong contradictory evidence.

Echolalia—A pathological repetition of what others say.

Hallucination—False sensory perceptions; hearing sounds or seeing people or objects that are not present. Hallucinations can also affect the senses of smell, touch, and taste.

Koro—A culture-specific syndrome involving a belief that one's external genitalia are shrinking or retracting and may disappear, occurring primarily in Southeast Asia.

Personality disorder—A psychopathological condition in which a person's patterns and behaviors are considered deviant or nonadaptive, but without neurosis or psychosis.

Psychodynamic—Mental, emotional, or motivational forces or processes that affect mental state and behavior, especially unconscious processes that develop in early childhood.

Psychosis—A serious mental disorder, such as schizophrenia, characterized by loss of contact with reality.

Schizophrenia—A psychotic disorder characterized by loss of contact with one's environment, deterioration of everyday functioning, and personality disintegration.

Schizophreniform disorder—A psychosis resembling schizophrenia, but lasting only between one and six months.

- memory impairment
- physical or verbal aggression
- suicidal or homicidal thoughts or behaviors

Diagnosis

The cause of the symptoms helps to determine whether the person is described as having brief psychotic disorder. If the psychotic symptoms appear as a result of a physical disease, a reaction to medication, or intoxication with drugs or alcohol, then the unusual behaviors are not classified as brief psychotic disorder.

Examination

If a physical examination reveals no biological basis for the symptoms, the patient may be referred to a **psychiatrist**. Brief psychotic disorder is usually diagnosed by interviewing the patient and possibly family members. The diagnostician usually performs a semi-structured interview called a **mental status examination**, which evaluates the patient's ability to concentrate, remember, realistically understand the situation, and think logically. Past history and/or the identification of a specific stressful event, particularly in patients with personality disorders, further suggests a diagnosis of brief psychotic disorder. Psychotic symptoms that persist for longer than one month require a different diagnosis.

Tests

Laboratory tests may be used to distinguish brief psychotic disorder from various other medical conditions. Blood alcohol levels and urine drug screening may be used to rule out substance-induced causes.

Procedures

In some cases, **imaging studies** such as x rays, **computed tomography** (CT) scans, or **magnetic resonance imaging** (MRI) may be necessary to rule out physical causes for the symptoms. An electroencephalogram (EEG) to measure **brain** waves may be performed.

Treatment

Various treatments are used for brief psychotic disorder.

Traditional

Although brief psychotic disorder is usually treated with drugs, supportive therapy or **psychotherapy** may be helpful in reducing anxiety and educating the patient about psychiatric illness. **Talk therapy** may also help the patient cope with the stress that precipitated the psychosis. Patients with acute psychosis may require **hospitalization**, both for evaluation and safety concerns. Aggressive patients may require brief seclusion or restraint. Once the psychosis has passed, individual, family, or **group therapy** may help the patient cope with stress and conflict and improve self-confidence and self-esteem.

Drugs

Antipsychotic medications are very effective at decreasing or ending brief psychotic episodes.

Haloperidol (Haldol) is commonly used for psychotic symptoms that are accompanied by agitation. It is often administered by injection. However, injected **ziprasidone** (Geodon) may be more effective and better tolerated than haloperidol. Other conventional antipsychotics that may be prescribed are **thiothixene** (Navane), thorazine, **fluphenazine** (Prolixin), **trifluoperazine** (Stelazine), **perphenazine** (Trilafon), and **thioridazine** (Mellaril). Newer-generation atypical antipsychotics are generally taken daily as tablets, capsules, or liquid by patients who are not agitated. These antipsychotics include **olanzapine** (Zyprexa), **quetiapine** (Seroquel), **paliperidone** (Invega), **risperidone** (Risperdal), and **clozapine** (Clozaril). Although these drugs can be taken for a longer period than haloperidol, they should not be used for more than one month. In addition to antipsychotics, drugs to decrease anxiety, such as **lorazepam** (Ativan) or **diazepam** (Valium), or to slow activity, such as **diphenhydramine** (Benadryl), may be prescribed. Hormones may be prescribed for postpartum psychosis.

Alternative

Symptoms of brief psychotic disorder that may be part of a culture-bound syndrome are usually most effectively treated by societal norms. For example, bathing in a sacred river might be the usual method of curing a psychotic-like state in a particular culture.

Home remedies

In cases in which the symptoms of brief psychotic disorder only minimally interfere with a patient's functioning and the specific trigger is known, elimination of the stressor may be sufficient treatment.

Prognosis

By definition, brief psychotic disorder resolves within a month. If the disorder was triggered by major stress or a traumatic experience and the patient had no previous psychiatric problems, the prognosis is good, and the disorder is unlikely to recur. European studies have found that 50%–80% of patients with brief psychotic disorder do not suffer major psychiatric problems in the future. However, the prognosis is poor in cases in which a triggering event cannot be identified, if the patient suffers from a personality disorder, or if the episode proves to be a prelude to schizophrenia or bipolar disorder. Patients with personality disorders may suffer from intermittent brief psychotic disorder throughout their lives.

Prevention

Early diagnosis and treatment of brief psychotic disorder can minimize disruptions to the patient's life. In the case of severe stressors, such as natural disasters or terrorist attacks, strong social support and immediate post-crisis counseling may prevent the development of brief psychotic disorder in susceptible people. Women who experience postpartum psychosis may choose to not have additional children or may be prescribed preventative antipsychotic medication during future postpartum periods.

QUESTIONS TO ASK YOUR DOCTOR

- Why do you believe that my symptoms constitute brief psychotic disorder?
- What medication will you prescribe?
- How long before the medication takes effect?
- Do you recommend therapy as well as medication?
- Is the psychotic disorder likely to recur?

Resources

BOOKS

American Psychiatric Association. *Diagnostic and Statistical Manual of Mental Disorders (DSM-IV-TR)*, 4th ed., text rev. Washington, DC: American Psychiatric Association, 2000.

Dziegielewski, Sophia F. *DSM-IV-TR in Action,* 2nd ed. Hoboken, NJ: John Wiley & Sons, 2010.

PERIODICALS

Correll, C. U., et al. "Predictors of Remission, Schizophrenia, and Bipolar Disorder in Adolescents with Brief Psychotic Disorder or Psychotic Disorder not Otherwise Specified Considered at Very High Risk for Schizophrenia." *Journal of Child and Adolescent Psychopharmacology* 18, no. 5 (2008): 475–90.

WEBSITES

MedlinePlus. "Brief Reactive Psychosis." U.S. Library of Medicine, National Institutes of Health. February 7, 2010. http://www.nlm.nih.gov/medlineplus/ency/article/001529.htm (accessed July 24, 2011).

———. "Haloperidol." U.S. Library of Medicine, National Institutes of Health. May 16, 2011. http://www.nlm.nih.gov/medlineplus/druginfo/meds/a682180.html (accessed July 24, 2011).

Memon, Mohammed A., and Michael Larson. "Brief Psychotic Disorder." Medscape Reference. May 15, 2009. http://emedicine.medscape.com/article/294416-overview (accessed July 24, 2011).

ORGANIZATIONS

AGS Foundation for Health in Aging, Empire State Bldg., 350 5th Ave., Ste. 801, New York, NY, 10018, (212) 755-

6810, (800) 563-4916, Fax: (212) 832-8646, http://www.healthinaging.org.

American Psychological Association, 750 1st St. NE, Washington, DC, 20002-4242, (202) 336-5500, (800) 374-2721, http://www.apa.org.

Mental Health America, 2000 N Beauregard St., 6th Fl., Alexandria, VA, 22311, (703) 684-7722, (800) 969-6642, Fax: (703) 684-5968, http://www.nmha.org.

National Alliance on Mental Illness, 3803 N Fairfax Dr., Ste. 100, Arlington, VA, 22203, (703) 524-7600, (800) 950-6264, Fax: (703) 524-9094, http://www.nami.org.

Deborah Rosch Eifert, PhD
Ruth A. Wienclaw, PhD
Margaret Alic, PhD

Bulimia nervosa

Definition

Bulimia nervosa is an eating disorder characterized by binge eating and engaging in inappropriate ways of counteracting the bingeing (using laxatives, for example) to prevent weight gain. The word "bulimia" is the Latin form of the Greek word *boulimia*, which means "extreme hunger." A binge is consuming a larger amount of food within a limited period of time than most people would eat in similar circumstances. Most people with bulimia report feelings of loss of control associated with bingeing, and some have mildly dissociative experiences in the course of a binge, which means that they feel disconnected from themselves and from reality when they binge.

The handbook mental health professionals use to aid in **diagnosis** is the ***Diagnostic and Statistical Manual of Mental Disorders***. The fourth edition, text revision, also known as the *DSM-IV-TR,* categorizes bulimia nervosa as an eating disorder, along with **anorexia nervosa**.

Demographics

Bulimia nervosa affects between 1% and 3% of women in developed countries; its prevalence is thought to have increased markedly since 1970. The rates are similar across cultures in the United States, Japan, the United Kingdom, Australia, South Africa, Canada, France, Germany, and Israel. About 80% to 90% of patients with bulimia are female. The average age at onset among women with bulimia is 14 and among men, 18. Homosexual men appear to be as vulnerable to developing bulimia as heterosexual women, while lesbians are less vulnerable.

Bulimia was previously thought to primarily affect Caucasian women in the United States, but recent studies indicate that this is no longer the case; the rates among African American and Hispanic women have risen faster than the rate of bulimia for the female population as a whole. One report indicates that the chief difference between African American and Caucasian women with bulimia is that African American patients are less likely to eat restricted **diets** between episodes of binge eating.

Description

Bulimia nervosa is classified into two subtypes according to the methods used to prevent weight gain after a binge. The purging subtype of bulimia is characterized by the use of self-induced vomiting, laxatives, enemas, or diuretics (pills that induce urination); in the nonpurging subtype, fasting or overexercising is used to compensate for binge eating.

The onset of bulimia nervosa is most common in late adolescence or early adult life. Dieting efforts and body dissatisfaction, however, often occur in the teenage years. For these reasons, bulimia is often described as a developmental disorder. Genetic researchers have identified specific genes linked to susceptibility to eating disorders, and the environmental primary factor in the development of bulimia nervosa is **stress** related to the onset of puberty. Girls who have strongly negative feelings about their bodies in response to puberty are at high risk for developing bulimia.

The binge eating associated with bulimia begins most often after a period of strict dieting. Most people with bulimia develop purging behaviors in response to the bingeing. Vomiting is used by 80%–90% of patients diagnosed with bulimia. The personal accounts of recovered bulimics suggest that most "discover" vomiting independently as a way of ridding themselves of the food rather than learning about it from other adolescents. Vomiting is often done to relieve an uncomfortable sensation of fullness in the stomach following a binge as well as to prevent absorption of the calories in the food. Vomiting is frequently induced by stimulating the gag reflex at the back of the throat by touching the area with the fingers or a toothbrush, but a minority of patients use syrup of ipecac to induce vomiting. Regular use of syrup of ipecac has severe medical consequences, including dehydration, muscle weakness, diarrhea, and serious heart problems that can lead to death. About one-third of bulimics use laxatives after binge eating to empty the digestive tract, and a minority use diuretics or enemas. Purging behaviors lead to a series of digestive and metabolic disturbances that then reinforce the behaviors.

A small proportion of bulimics **exercise** excessively (**compulsive exercise**) or fast after a binge instead of purging.

Patients with bulimia may come to the attention of a **psychiatrist** or **psychologist** because they develop medical or dental complications due to the eating disorder. In some cases, the patient's dentist is the "case finder," because the sulfuric acid that comes up from the stomach during vomiting wears away at tooth enamel. Many times, however, the person with bulimia seeks help, although often not until years after the disorder develops.

Causes and symptoms

Causes

The primary etiological model for bulimia, proposed by psychologist Eric Stice, cites the following factors as the main predictors of bulimia:

- pressure to be thin, whether from society and the media at large or from peers
- an internalization of the belief that thin is the ideal body type
- body dissatisfaction based on this belief
- dieting or other restrictive actions in an attempt to lose weight
- negative affect, based on the initial body dissatisfaction

Because the motivation for weight loss is tied to a desire to meet a fictional ideal and not an actual medical need to lose weight, results are unsatisfactory, as they are not addressing the actual problem. Both dieting and negative affect increase the risk for eating disorder behaviors, particularly bulimic symptoms such as binge eating and compensatory behaviors. Along with sociocultural pressures, familial and **genetic factors** may contribute to the desire to be thin and the development of an eating disorder.

SOCIOCULTURAL CAUSES. Emphasis in the mass media on slenderness in women as the primary criterion of beauty and desirability is commonly noted in studies of bulimia. Historians of fashion have remarked that the standard of female attractiveness has changed over the past half century in the direction of increased thinness; some have commented that actress Marilyn Monroe would have been considered "fat" by contemporary standards. The ideal female figure is not only unattainable by the vast majority of women but is lighter than the standards associated with good health by insurance companies. In 1965, the average model weighed 8% less than the average American woman; by 2001, she weighed 25% less. Recent news reports have focused on this **obsession** with thinness in the fashion industry because of the deaths of several models from eating disorders. One major fashion group in Spain went so far as to set a minimum body mass index for models on its catwalks in 2006 after a model died during a show in South America of causes apparently related to an eating disorder.

Nutrition experts have pointed to the easy availability of foods high in processed carbohydrates in developed countries as a social factor that contributes to the incidence of bulimia. One study found that subjects who were given two slices of standard mass-produced white bread with some jelly had their levels of **serotonin** increased temporarily by 450%. This finding suggests that bulimics who binge on ice cream, bread, cookies, pizza, and fast food items that are high in processed carbohydrates are simply manipulating their neurochemistry in a highly efficient manner. The incidence of bulimia may be lower in developing countries because diets that are high in vegetables and whole-grain products but low in processed carbohydrates do not affect serotonin levels in the **brain** as rapidly or as effectively.

Some overweight or obese individuals who are starting a new diet may develop bulimia as a coping strategy. In addition, individuals who are perfectionists and struggle with the cultural focus on thinness are at greater risk, as are persons involved in sports or occupations that require strict weight control, such as gymnastics, figure skating, horse jockeying, wrestling, ballet, or modeling.

FAMILIAL FACTORS. A number of recent studies point to the interpersonal relationships in the family of origin (the patient's family while growing up) as a factor in the later development of bulimia. People with bulimia are more likely than people with anorexia to have been sexually abused in childhood; studies have found that abnormalities in blood levels of serotonin (a neurotransmitter associated with mood disorders) and cortisol (the primary stress hormone in humans) in bulimic patients with a history of childhood **sexual abuse** resemble those in patients with **post-traumatic stress disorder** (PTSD). Post-traumatic stress disorder is a mental disorder that can develop after someone has experienced a traumatic event (sexual assault, for example) and is unable to process and move beyond that event. The disorder is characterized by disturbingly realistic flashbacks of the traumatic event.

A history of eating conflicts and struggles over food in the family of origin is also a risk factor for the development of bulimia nervosa, whether the parents or siblings were overweight or obese or had an eating disorder. Personal accounts by recovered bulimics frequently describe parents who were preoccupied with food or dieting. Fathers appear to be as influential as mothers in this regard. A recent study focusing on girls suggests that the influence of the father may be related to the father's own concerns and body preoccupations and that this influence may be stronger as a child gets older. Other risk factors identified in a 2007 study, which followed the children from birth, were a low activity level in early childhood and rapid eating in later childhood. In addition, and not surprisingly, peer and parental teasing about body weight or shape also increase risk, as does having a familial history of **substance abuse**.

GENETICS. Several studies have obtained results pointing to a genetic understructure for eating disorders, including bulimia. Studies investigating the relationship between characteristics of bulimia in families and their correlation with patterns of gene expression have linked bulimia to genes on human chromosome 10.

Symptoms

The *DSM-IV-TR* specifies that bingeing and the inappropriate attempts to compensate for it must occur twice a week for three months on average to meet the diagnostic criteria for bulimia nervosa. However, recent studies have shown that individuals who reported these behaviors once a week were clinically similar to those who reported such behaviors twice a week. A revision for the upcoming *DSM-5* (fifth edition, 2013) proposes changing the minimum frequency of these activities to once a week to meet the criteria for bulimia nervosa.

A second criterion of bulimia nervosa is exaggerated concern with body shape and weight. Bulimia can be distinguished from **body dysmorphic disorder** (BDD) by the fact that people with BDD usually focus on a specific physical feature—most commonly a facial feature—rather than overall shape and weight. Bulimics do, however, resemble patients with BDD in that they have distorted body images.

Bulimia is associated with a number of physical symptoms. Binge eating by itself rarely causes serious medical complications, but it is associated with nausea, abdominal distension and cramping, slowed digestion, and weight gain.

Self-induced vomiting, by contrast, may have serious medical consequences, including the following:

- Erosion of tooth enamel, particularly on the molars and maxillary incisors. Loss of tooth enamel is irreversible.
- Enlargement of the salivary glands.
- Scars and calloused areas on the knuckles from contact with the teeth.
- Irritation of the throat and esophagus from contact with stomach acid.
- Tearing of mucous membranes in the upper gastrointestinal tract or perforation of the esophagus and stomach wall. Perforation of part of the digestive tract is a rare complication of bulimia and is potentially fatal.
- Electrolyte imbalances. The loss of fluids from repeated vomiting and laxative abuse can deplete the body's stores of hydrogen chloride, potassium, sodium, and magnesium. Hypokalemia (abnormally low levels of potassium in the blood) is a potential medical emergency that can lead to muscle cramps, seizures, and heart arrhythmias.

Other physical symptoms associated with bulimia include irregular menstrual periods or amenorrhea; petechiae (pinhead-sized bruises from capillaries ruptured by increased pressure due to vomiting) in the skin around the eyes, and rectal prolapse (the lowering of the rectum from its usual position).

Diagnosis

The diagnosis of bulimia nervosa is made on the basis of a physical examination, a psychiatric assessment, the patient's eating history, and the findings of laboratory tests. Patients who do not meet the full criteria for bulimia nervosa may be given the diagnosis of subsyndromal bulimia or of an eating disorder not otherwise specified (EDNOS).

Physical examination

Patients suspected of having bulimia nervosa should be given a complete physical examination because the disorder has so many potential medical complications. In addition, most bulimics are close to normal weight or only slightly overweight, and so the presence of the disorder is not outwardly apparent. The examination should include not only vital signs and an assessment of the patient's height and weight relative to age, but also a check for such signs of bulimia as general hair loss, abdominal soreness, swelling of the parotid glands, telltale scars on the back of the hand, petechiae, edema, and teeth that look ragged or "moth-eaten."

Psychiatric assessment

Psychiatric assessment of patients with bulimia usually includes four components:

- a thorough history of body weight, eating patterns, diets, typical daily food intake, methods of purging (if used), and concept of ideal weight
- a history of the patient's significant relationships with parents, siblings, and peers, including any present or past physical, emotional, or sexual abuse

- a history of previous psychiatric treatment (if any) and assessment of any comorbid (occurring at the same time as the bulimia) mood, anxiety, substance abuse, or personality disorders
- administration of standardized instruments that measure attitudes toward eating, body size, and weight (e.g., the Eating Disorder Examination, the Eating Disorder Inventory, the Eating Attitude Test [EAT], the Kids' Eating Disorder Survey [KEDS])

Laboratory findings

Laboratory tests ordered for patients suspected of having bulimia usually include a complete blood cell count, blood serum chemistry, thyroid tests, and urinalysis. If necessary, the doctor may also order a chest x ray and an electrocardiogram (EKG). Typical findings in patients with bulimia include low levels of chloride and potassium in the blood and higher than normal levels of amylase, a digestive enzyme found in saliva.

Treatment

Treatment for bulimia nervosa typically involves several therapy approaches. However, bulimia treatment is complicated by several factors.

First, patients diagnosed with bulimia nervosa frequently have coexisting psychiatric disorders, such as major **depression**, **dysthymic disorder**, **anxiety disorders**, substance abuse disorders, or **personality disorders**. In the case of depression, the mood disorder may either precede or follow the onset of bulimia; with bulimia, the prevalence of depression is 40%–70%. With regard to substance abuse, about 30% of patients diagnosed with bulimia nervosa abuse either alcohol or stimulants over the course of the eating disorder. The personality disorders most often diagnosed in patients with bulimia are borderline, narcissistic, histrionic, and antisocial. **Borderline personality disorder** is a disorder characterized by stormy interpersonal relationships, unstable self-image, and impulsive behavior. People with **narcissistic personality disorder** believe that they are extremely important and are unable to have empathy for others. Individuals with **histrionic personality disorder** seek attention almost constantly and are very emotional. **Antisocial personality disorder** is characterized by a disregard for others' rights—people with this disorder often deceive and manipulate others. Although patients may have both bulimia nervosa and anorexia nervosa, a number of clinicians have noted that patients with predominate bulimia tend to develop impulsive and unstable personality disturbances, whereas patients with predominate anorexia tend to be more obsessional and perfectionistic. Estimates of the prevalence of personality disorders among patients with bulimia range between 2% and 50%. The clinician must then decide whether to treat the eating disorder and the comorbid conditions concurrently or sequentially. It is generally agreed, however, that a substance abuse disorder, if present, must be treated before the bulimia can be effectively managed. It is also generally agreed that mood disorders and bulimia can be treated concurrently, often using antidepressant medication along with therapy.

Second, the limitations on treatment imposed by **managed care** complicate the treatment of bulimia nervosa. When the disorder first received attention in the 1970s, patients with bulimia were often hospitalized until the most significant physical symptoms of the disorder could be treated. Few patients with bulimia are hospitalized today, with the exception of medical emergencies related to electrolyte imbalances and gastrointestinal injuries associated with the eating disorder. Most treatment protocols for bulimia nervosa now reflect cost-containment measures.

Medications

The most common medications given to patients are **antidepressants**, because bulimia is so closely associated with depression. Short-term medication trials of tricyclic antidepressants (particularly **desipramine**, **imipramine**, and **amitriptyline**) have shown promise in reducing episodes of binge eating and vomiting, but these medications are rarely used. The **monoamine oxidase inhibitors** are not recommended as initial medications for patients diagnosed with bulimia because of their side effects. The most promising results have been obtained with the **selective serotonin reuptake inhibitors**, or **SSRIs**. **Fluoxetine** (Prozac) was approved in 1998 by the U.S. Food and Drug Administration (FDA) for the treatment of bulimia nervosa. Effective dosages of fluoxetine are higher for the treatment of bulimia than they are for the treatment of depression. Although a combination of medication and **cognitive-behavioral therapy** is more effective in treating most patients with bulimia than medication alone, one team of researchers reported success with fluoxetine by itself in treating some patients who had not responded to **psychotherapy**.

Ondansetron (Zofran), a drug that was originally developed to control nausea from chemotherapy and radiation therapy for cancer, blocks serotonin reuptake and also works to inhibit vomiting. It has shown some patients in ameliorating symptoms of bulimia nervosa.

In addition to antidepressant or antinausea medications, such acid-reducing medications as cimetidine and ranitidine may be given to patients with bulimia to relieve discomfort in the digestive tract associated with irritation caused by stomach acid.

Psychotherapy

Cognitive-behavioral therapy (CBT) is regarded as the most successful psychotherapeutic approach to bulimia nervosa. CBT is intended to interrupt the faulty thinking processes associated with bulimia, such as preoccupations with food and weight, black-and-white thinking ("all or nothing" thinking, or thinking thoughts only at extreme ends of a spectrum), and low self-esteem, as well as such behaviors as the binge-purge cycle. Patients are first helped to regain control over their food intake by keeping food diaries and receiving feedback about their meal plans, symptom triggers, and nutritional balance, as well as learning the associations between thoughts, feelings, and behaviors. They are then taught to challenge rigid thought patterns through cognitive restructuring techniques and by receiving **assertiveness training** and practice in identifying and expressing their feelings in words rather than through distorted eating patterns. About 50% of patients treated with CBT are able to stop bingeing and purging. Of the remaining half, some show partial improvement and a small minority do not respond at all. Part of CBT involves setting goals to focus on at home. These goals for patients include taking things one day at a time, not blaming themselves, and spending time with supportive friends and family members.

Family therapy is sometimes recommended as an additional mode of treatment for patients with bulimia who come from severely troubled or food-obsessed families, which can increase their risk of relapsing. Family therapy can also be helpful for adolescents with bulimia nervosa as a first-line approach to addressing the disorder.

Other mainstream therapies

Medical nutrition therapy (MNT) is a recognized component of the treatment of eating disorders. Effective MNT for patients with bulimia involves an understanding of cognitive-behavioral therapy as well as the registered dietitian's usual role of assisting the physician with monitoring the patient's physical symptoms, laboratory values, and vital signs. In the treatment of bulimia, the dietitian's specialized knowledge of nutrition may be quite helpful in dealing with the myths about food and fad diets that many bulimic patients believe. The dietitian's most important task, however, is helping patients to normalize their eating patterns to break the deprivation/bingeing cycle that is characteristic of bulimia nervosa. Calorie intake is usually based on retaining the patients' weight to prevent hunger, because hunger increases susceptibility to bingeing.

Alternative and complementary treatments

Alternative therapies that have been shown to be helpful for some patients in relieving the anxiety and muscular soreness associated with bulimia nervosa are **acupuncture**, massage therapy, hydrotherapy, and shiatsu. However, it should be noted that there is no empirical evidence for the effectiveness of these treatments.

Herbal remedies that have been used to calm digestive upsets in patients with bulimia include teas made from **chamomile** or peppermint. Peppermint helps to soothe the intestines by slowing down the rate of smooth muscle contractions (peristalsis). Chamomile has been used to help expel gas from the digestive tract, a common complaint of persons with bulimia. Both herbs have a wide margin of safety.

Some patients with bulimia have responded well to **yoga** because its emphasis on focused breathing and **meditation** calls attention to and challenges the distorted thought patterns that characterize bulimia. In addition, the stretching and bending movements that are part of a yoga practice help to displace negative thoughts focused on the body's outward appearance with positive appreciation of its strength and agility. Last, because yoga is noncompetitive, it allows participants to explore the uniqueness of their bodies rather than constantly comparing themselves to other people.

Prognosis

The prognosis of bulimia depends on several factors, including age at onset, types of purging behaviors used (if any), and the presence of other psychiatric conditions or disorders. As with any eating disorder, bulimia can be treated most effectively if it is identified as soon as possible. In many cases, the disorder becomes a chronic (long-term) condition; 20%–50% of patients have symptoms for at least five years in spite of treatment. The usual pattern is an alternation between periods of remission and new episodes of bingeing. Patients whose periods of remission last for a year or longer have a better prognosis; patients diagnosed with major depression or personality disorders have a less favorable prognosis. Overall, however, the prognosis for full recovery from bulimia nervosa is considered relatively poor compared to other eating disorders.

Bulimia nervosa appears to produce changes in the functioning of the serotonin system in the brain. Researchers at the University of Pittsburgh who compared brain images taken by **positron emission**

tomography (PET) from women with bulimia who had been in remission for a year or longer with brain images from healthy women found that the women with bulimia did not have a normal age-related decline in serotonin binding. Because serotonin helps to regulate mood, appetite, and impulse control, the study may help to explain why some women may be more susceptible to developing bulimia than others.

In addition, data from one study suggest that bulimia and other eating disorders can have a negative impact on infertility. In a review of surveys from more than 11,000 pregnant women, those with past or current eating disorders were more than twice as likely to have undergone some type of infertility treatment to help them become pregnant. The study was published in August 2011 in the *British Journal of Obstetrics and Gynecology.*

Prevention

Although a genetic link to bulimia has been identified, there are currently no gene-based preventive measures. With regard to family influences, the overwhelming majority of studies have found that the most important preventive measure that can be taken is the establishment of healthful eating patterns and attitudes toward food in the family of origin.

Resources

BOOKS

American Psychiatric Association. *Diagnostic and Statistical Manual of Mental Disorders.* 4th ed., Text rev. Washington, DC: American Psychiatric Association, 2000.

Herzog, David B., et al. *Unlocking the Mysteries of Eating Disorders.* New York: McGraw-Hill, 2007.

PERIODICALS

Agras, Stewart W., et al. "Childhood Risk Factors for Thin Body Preoccupation and Social Pressure to Be Thin." *Journal of the American Academy of Child and Adolescent Psychiatry* 46 (2007): 171–78.

Bulik, Cynthia M. "Exploring the Gene: Environment Nexus in Eating Disorders." *Journal of Psychiatry and Neuroscience* 30 (2005): 335–39.

Crow, S. J., et al. "Increased Mortality in Bulimia Nervosa and Other Eating Disorders." *American Journal of Psychiatry* 166 (December 2009): 1342–46.

Engler, P.A. "Predicting Eating Disorder Group Membership: An Examination and Extension of the Sociocultural Model." *Behavior Therapy* 37, no. 1 (2006): 69–79.

Hudson, James I., Eva Hiripi Jr., Harrison G. Pope, and Ronald C. Kessler. "The Prevalence and Correlates of Eating Disorders in the National Comorbidity Survey Replication." *Biological Psychiatry* 61, no. 3 (2007): 348–358.

Little, J.W. "Eating Disorders: Dental Implications." *Oral Surgery, Oral Medicine, Oral Pathology, Oral Radiology, and Endodontics* 93 (February 2002): 138–43.

Schmidt, U., et al. "A Randomized Controlled Trial of Family Therapy and Cognitive Behavior Therapy Guided Self-Care for Adolescents with Bulimia Nervosa and Related Disorders." *American Journal of Psychiatry* 164, no. 4 (2007): 591–98.

Steinhausen, Hans-Christoph, and Sandy Weber. "The Outcome of Bulimia Nervosa: Findings From One-Quarter Century of Research." *American Journal of Psychiatry* 166, no. 12 (2009): 1331–41. http://dx.doi.org/10.1176/appi.ajp.2009.09040582 (accessed September 16, 2011).

Van den Eyndea, Frederique, and Ulrike Schmidta. "Treatment of Bulimia Nervosa and Binge Eating Disorder." *Psychiatry* 7, no. 4 (2008): 161–66.

WEBSITES

Mayo Clinic staff. "Bulimia Nervosa." MayoClinic.com. February 23, 2010. http://www.mayoclinic.com/health/bulimia/DS00607 (accessed November 14, 2011).

National Alliance on Mental Illness. "Bulimia Nervosa." http://www.nami.org/Template.cfm?Section=by_illness&template=/ContentManagement/ContentDisplay.cfm&ContentID=102972 (accessed November 14, 2011).

WomensHealth.gov. "Bulimia Nervosa Fact Sheet." U.S. Department of Health and Human Services. http://www.womenshealth.gov/publications/our-publications/fact-sheet/bulimia-nervosa.cfm (accessed November 14, 2011).

ORGANIZATIONS

American Academy of Child and Adolescent Psychiatry, 3615 Wisconsin Ave., NW, Washington, DC, 20016-3007, (202) 966-7300, Fax: (202) 966-2891, http://aacap.org.

Center for the Study of Anorexia and Bulimia, 1841 Broadway, 4th Fl., New York, NY, 10023, (212) 333-3444, Fax: (212) 333-5444, casb@icpnyc.org, http://www.csabnyc.org.

National Association of Anorexia Nervosa and Related Eating Disorders, PO Box 640, Naperville, IL, 60566, (630) 577-1330, anadhelp@anad.org, http://www.anad.org.

National Eating Disorders Association, 165 W 46th St., New York, NY, 10036, (212) 575-6200, (800) 931-2237, Fax: (212) 575-1650, info@NationalEatingDisorders.org, http://www.nationaleatingdisorders.org.

Rebecca Frey, PhD
Emily Jane Willingham, PhD
Heidi Splete

Bullying

Definition

Bullying is a persistent pattern of threatening, harassing, or aggressive behavior directed toward another person or persons who are perceived as smaller, weaker, or less powerful. Although often thought of as a childhood phenomenon, bullying can occur wherever people interact,

Child victims of bullying, during the past 12 months and in their lifetime, by gender, age, and type of bullying, 2008*

	Past 12 months	Lifetime
Physical bullying	**13.2**	**21.6**
Females	12.8	22.4
Males	16.7	25.9
2–5 yrs.	19.1	20.4
6–9 yrs.	21.5	28.0
10–13 yrs.	10.7	19.9
14–17 yrs.	8.0	28.5
Psychological bullying (e.g., teasing)	**19.7**	**29.5**
Females	23.5	35.5
Males	20.6	30.6
2–5 yrs.	13.5	14.6
6–9 yrs.	30.4	38.4
10–13 yrs.	27.8	39.6
14–17 yrs.	15.8	38.4
Internet bullying	**1.8**	**2.5**
Females	3.4	4.5
Males	1.6	2.3
2–5 yrs.	0.0	0.0
6–9 yrs.	0.0	0.0
10–13 yrs.	2.6	3.2
14–17 yrs.	5.6	7.9

*Data given as percentage of children surveyed; 4,549 total (2,276 female and 2,273 male).

SOURCE: Finkelhor, D., H. Turner, S. Ormrod, and S.L. Hamby. "Violence, Abuse, and Crime Exposure in a National Sample of Children and Youth." *Pediatrics* 124, no. 5 (2009): 1411–23.

(Table by PreMediaGlobal. © 2012 Cengage Learning.)

most often observable in the workplace and in the home in adults. Bullying is also called harassment.

Demographics

Bullying in children

Bullying among children is a persistent and substantial problem that requires serious attention. According to a study published in 2001 by the Kaiser Family Foundation and Nickelodeon Television, 55% of 8–11-year-olds and 68% of 12–15-year-olds said that bullying is a "big problem" for people their age. Seventy-four percent of the 8–11-year-olds and 86% of the 12–15-year-olds also reported that children were bullied or teased at their school. These statistics were essentially unchanged in 2011. Children at greatest risk of being bullied are those who are perceived as social isolates or outcasts by their peers, have a history of changing schools, have poor social skills or a desire to fit in "at any cost," are defenseless, or are viewed by their peers as being different.

A study of more than 16,000 children in the sixth through tenth grades conducted for the National Institute of Child Health and Human Development found that nearly 60% of the children responding had been victims of rumors. More than 50% of the children reported that they had been the victims of sexual harassment. A Canadian study reported in 2010 that cyberbullying is also a common problem, with 49% of children in a sample of 2,200 students reporting being bullied on the Internet and 34% admitting to bullying others online.

The National Center for Education Statistics (NCES) of the U.S. Department of Education found that white, non-Hispanic children were more likely to report being the victims of bullying than black or other non-Hispanic children. Younger children were more likely to report being bullied than older children, and children attending schools with gangs were more likely to report being bullied than children in schools without a major gang presence. No differences were found in these patterns between public and private schools. Fewer children reported bullying in schools that were supervised by police officers, security officers, or staff hallway monitors. Victims of bullying were more likely to be criminally victimized at school than were other children. Victims of bullying were more afraid of being attacked both at school and elsewhere and more likely to avoid certain areas of school (for example, the cafeteria, hallways or stairs, or restrooms) or activities where bullying was more likely to take place. Significantly, victims of bullies were more likely to report that they carried weapons to school for protection.

Children who are identified as bullies by the time they are eight years of age are six times more likely than other children to have a criminal conviction by the time they are 24 years old. Bullying behavior may also be accompanied by other inappropriate behavior, including criminal, delinquent, or gang behavior.

Bullying in the workplace

Although research has been conducted on workplace bullying in Europe for some time, the topic has only recently become of interest in the United States. The nonprofit Workplace Bullying Institute conducted two surveys in 2010 with over 6,000 respondents. It defined workplace bullying as "repeated mistreatment: sabotage by others that prevented work from getting done, verbal **abuse**, threatening conduct, intimidation and humiliation" and compared statistics to its 2007 survey. The 2010 survey found that 35% of workers have experienced bullying first hand (37% in 2007); 62% of bullies are men and 58% of targets are women; women bullies target women in 80% of cases; and the majority (68%) of bullying is same-gender harassment.

Prevalence and characteristics of U.S. workplace bullying, 2007 and 2010

	Prevalence (%)		18–29 yrs.		30–49 yrs.		50–54 yrs.		Hispanic		African American		Caucasian		Asian American	
Bullying characteristics	**2007**	**2010**	**2007**	**2010**	**2007**	**2010**	**2007**	**2010**	**2007**	**2010**	**2007**	**2010**	**2007**	**2010**	**2007**	**2010**
Currently bullied or bullied in the past year	12.6	8.8	18.5	27.0	16.8	50.0	9.9	23.0		12.7		11.0		7.9		8.8
Not currently bullied but bullied in the past (more than one year ago)	24.2	25.7		22.0		47.0		30.0		23.5		27.6		25.7		9.7
Witnessed only	12.3	15.5		29.0		49.0		22.0	14.0	12.3	21.1	7.9	10.8	16.8	8.5	37.6
Male targets of bullying	43.3	42.0														
Female targets of bullying	56.7	58.0														
Male bullies	60.0	62.0														
Female bullies	40.0	38.0														
Female bullies targeting women	71.0	80.0														
Female bullies targeting men	28.7	20.0														
Male bullies targeting women	46.5	45.5														
Male bullies targeting men	53.5	55.5														

SOURCE: Workplace Bullying Institute, *The WBI U.S. Workplace Bullying Survey*, 2010.

(Table by PreMediaGlobal. © 2012 Cengage Learning.)

Description

There are many forms of bullying in both children and adults. Bullies may intimidate or harass their victims physically through hitting, pushing, or other physical violence; verbally through such actions as threats or name calling; or psychologically through spreading rumors (both live and online), making sexual comments or gestures, or excluding the victim from desired activities.

There are many reasons to stop bullying. Bullying interferes with school performance, and children who are afraid of being bullied are more likely to miss school or drop out. Bullied children frequently experience developmental harm and fail to reach their full physiological, social, and academic potentials. Children who are bullied grow increasingly insecure and anxious and have persistently decreased self-esteem and greater **depression** than their peers, often even as adults. Children and adolescents have even been known to commit **suicide** as a result of being bullied; this tragic outcome has been referred to by some writers as "bullycide."

People who are bullies as children often become bullies as adults. Bullying behavior in the home is called "child abuse" or "spousal abuse." Bullying also occurs in prisons, churches, summer camps, college or boarding school dormitories, and other social groups or group living situations.

Recently, attention has been turned to the topic of bullying in the workplace, defined as occurring when bosses and organizational peers bully those whom they perceive as weaker or inferior. Those bullied at work often become perceived as ineffective, thus abrogating their career success and influencing their earning potential. Victims of workplace bullying often change jobs in search of a less hostile environment because organizations are frequently not sensitive to the issue of workplace bullying or are not equipped to deal with it adequately or justly.

Cyberbullying

Bullying does not need to occur in person: cyberbullying is a persistent pattern of threatening, harassing, or aggressive behavior carried out online. The widespread popularity of cell phones and other mobile devices means that cyberbullying can be carried out anonymously without the need for a computer. Cyberbullying can take a number of different forms:

- sending hurtful or threatening messages directly to the victim via e-mail or phone texting
- spreading rumors about the victim to others via e-mail or other forms of messaging
- setting up websites, posting videos, or creating pages on social media to hurt or humiliate the victim

Cyberbullying is increasingly considered a particularly damaging form of bullying because it can be carried on 24/7, can be shared with a wide number of people (an example would be a video that "goes viral" on YouTube), and is hard to undo due to a number of online services that archive Internet sites.

Some researchers maintain that cyberbullies fall into several different categories and do not necessarily resemble the classic schoolyard bully. While some cyberbullies are power-hungry or vengeful, others may just be bored and looking for something to do for online entertainment. Another common type of cyberbully is the inadvertent bully, typically an adolescent who doesn't think before sending a message or who is so invested in online role-playing that he or she fails to understand that the recipient of such a message may take it seriously.

Another reason for concern about cyberbullying is that electronic communication itself has the potential to intensify situations that are already touchy, because the absence of face-to-face contact makes it harder for the cyberbully to "see" the humanity of the victim. E-mail messages and texting lack vocal tone, making it easier to increase the hostility and aggressiveness of text messages. There have been several notable cases of electronic messaging escalating into real-world violence, such as the "Facebook murder" that occurred in Florida in April 2011, in which a 15-year-old boy was lured into an ambush by his former girlfriend via text messages.

Risk factors

Warning signs and factors that may indicate risk for being or becoming a bully include:

- lack of impulse control (frequent loss of temper, extreme impulsiveness, easily becoming frustrated, extreme mood swings)
- family factors (physical abuse or violence within the family, substance or alcohol abuse within the family, overly permissive parenting, lack of clear limits, inadequate parental supervision, harsh/corporal punishment, child abuse, inconsistent parenting)
- behavioral symptoms (gang affiliation, name calling or abusive language, carrying a weapon, hurting animals, abusing alcohol or drugs, making serious threats, vandalizing or damaging property, frequent physical fighting)

Causes and symptoms

There is no evidence to support the theory that there is a genetic component to bullying behavior. Particularly in children, bullying appears to result from the bully's copying the actions of role models who bully others. According to the Centers for Disease Control and Prevention (CDC), this pattern frequently occurs when bullies come from a home in which one parent bullies another or one or both parents bully the children. When such behavior is modeled for children with such personality traits as lack of impulse control or aggression, they are particularly prone to bullying behavior, which often continues into adulthood.

Bullying in children

According to the U.S. Department of Health and Human Services, children with dominant personalities and who are more impulsive and active are more prone to becoming bullies than children without these traits. Bullies also often have a history of emotional or behavioral problems. Victims of bullying, on the other hand, tend to be more anxious, insecure, and socially isolated than their peers and often lack age-appropriate social skills. The probability of victimization can be compounded when the victim has low self-esteem due to physical characteristics (for example, the victim believes her/himself to be unattractive, is disfigured in some way, or is outside the normal range for height or weight) or personal problems (for example, health problems or physical or mental disability).

Symptoms or indications that a child may be being bullied include:

- social withdrawal or isolation (few or no friends; feeling isolated, sad, and alone; feeling picked on or persecuted; feeling rejected or not liked; having poor social skills)
- somatic complaints (frequent complaints about illness; displaying victim body language, including hanging head, hunching shoulders, and avoiding eye contact)
- avoidant behavior (not wanting to go to school, skipping classes or school)
- affective reactions (crying easily; having mood swings; talking about hopelessness, running away, or suicide)
- physical clues (bringing home damaged possessions or reporting that belongings were "lost")
- behavior changes (changes in eating or sleeping patterns)
- aggressive behavior (threatening violence to self or others, taking or attempting to take a weapon to school)

Each child will react to bullying in a different manner, and some children will react with only a few of these symptoms. These differences, however, do not mean that bullying is not severe or that **intervention** is not needed.

Bullying in the workplace

Bullying in the workplace is usually motivated by political rather than personal reasons. Workers may compete for promotions, raises, and other honors. In an attempt to climb the ladder of success, some individuals do what they can to not only present themselves in a good light to their superiors, but also to make one or more coworkers seem unworthy or inept. Bullying bosses demonstrate poor leadership styles and poor motivational skills, frequently attempting to further either their own or the company's agenda through harassment, belittling, or other negative behaviors.

Common tactics used by workplace bullies include:

- discounting/belittling the victim in public (making statements such as "that's silly" in response to the victim's ideas, disregarding evidence of satisfactory or superlative work done by victim, taking credit for victim's work)
- making false accusations (rumors about victim, lies about victim's performance)
- harassing the victim (verbal putdowns based on gender, race, disability)
- isolating the victim (encouraging others to turn against victim, socially or physically isolating the victim from others)
- nonverbal aggression (staring, glaring, silent treatment)
- sabotaging the victim's work
- unequal treatment (retaliating against victim who files a complaint, making up arbitrary rules for victim to follow, assigning undesirable work as a punishment, making unreasonable/unreachable goals or deadlines for victim, performing a constructive discharge of duties)

Diagnosis

Bullying, in itself, is not a mental disorder, although aggressive or harassing behavior may be symptomatic of a number of disorders, particularly **antisocial personality disorder**. There are, however, a number of criteria to help determine whether someone is a bully. First, to qualify as bullying, the bully's behavior must be intended to cause physical or psychological harm to the other person. Second, bullying behavior is not an isolated incident but results in a consistent pattern of such behavior over time. Third, bullying occurs where there is an imbalance of power whereby the bully has more physical or psychological power than the victim. Harassing behavior is not considered to be bullying if it occurs between individuals of equal strength and status or if it is a one-time event.

Bullying behavior in children can include any of the following behaviors:

- dominance (enjoying feeling powerful and in control, seeking to dominate or manipulate others, being a poor winner or loser)
- lack of empathy (deriving satisfaction from the fears, pain, or discomfort of others; enjoying conflict between others; displaying intolerance of or prejudice toward others)

KEY TERMS

Bullycide—Suicide attributed to the victim's having been bullied.

Cyberbullying—The use of electronic devices, including computers, cell phones, and other mobile devices, to bully by means of hurtful messages, spreading rumors, or misusing social media.

- negative emotions or violence (displaying uncontrolled anger or a pattern of impulsive and chronic hitting, intimidating, or aggressive behavior)
- lack of responsibility (blaming others for his/her problems)
- other behaviors (using drugs or alcohol, hiding bullying behavior from adults, having a history of discipline problems)

Victims of bullying, whether children or adults, may need to be assessed and treated if they need help responding to, or recovering from, bullying.

Treatment

If bullying behavior is symptomatic of an underlying mental disorder such as **conduct disorder** or antisocial personality disorder, treatment should first address the underlying disorder. For situations in which bullying behavior is not part of a pattern associated with an underlying mental disorder, treatment and establishing organizational or familial processes for dealing with it are required.

Bullying in children

If parent(s) suspect that their child is a bully, help can be sought from mental health professionals and school counselors. Taking the child to a child **psychologist** and participating in **family therapy** as appropriate can help teach a bully better interpersonal skills. Contacting the school counselor or a child psychologist is also an appropriate step in helping the victims of bullies.

If parents suspect that their child may be being bullied, they should make sure that he or she understands that the problem is not his or her fault and that he or she does not have to face the situation alone. Parents can discuss ways to deal with bullies, including walking away, being assertive, and getting help. Parents should also encourage the child to report bullying behavior to a

QUESTIONS TO ASK YOUR DOCTOR

- I didn't grow up with cell phones and social media. What should I tell my children to help them protect themselves against cyberbullying?
- Have you ever treated a child or teenager who developed a physical or mental disorder because of bullying? What was the outcome?
- Have you ever treated or referred an adult who was suffering from workplace bullying?

teacher, counselor, or other trusted adult. However, parents should not try to resolve the situation themselves but should contact the school to report the behavior and to seek recommendations for further assistance.

Dealing with cyberbullying

Cyberbullying requires some different approaches than face-to-face bullying because of the nature of electronic messages and also because cyberbullying can involve legal penalties for the bully. Some practical tips for dealing with cyberbullying include:

- Save evidence of harassing e-mails and other forms of cyberbullying. These can be forwarded to a parent or trusted friend, or saved on a flash drive.
- Report cyberbullying to the service provider. Many social networking sites as well as phone companies and e-mail providers take reports of cyberbullying seriously and will block the bully's account.
- Use the block setting on cell phones or other mobile devices to stop the cyberbully from sending messages.
- Use passwords to protect online e-mail accounts and cell phones, and change the passwords frequently.

Bullying in the workplace

Bullying in the workplace can be minimized if the organization develops and enforces antiharassment policies and procedures. These should include a stated definition on what constitutes harassment, creating and implementing a disciplinary system to punish the bully rather than the victim, and instituting a formal grievance system to report workplace bullying. Other measures that can be taken include inclusiveness and harassment training, awareness training to educate employees on how to spot bullying behavior, and offering courses in conflict resolution, anger management, or **assertiveness training**.

Bullies are not the only ones needing help. The intention of a bully is to harm the other person; victims, therefore, may experience a number of negative consequences from being the victim of a bully. If the behavior associated with being a victim persists after the bullying situation has been resolved, or if the situation continues without just resolution, victims should be assessed for depression and/or an anxiety disorder (if their symptoms warrant) and should receive the appropriate treatment.

Prevention

To help keep a child from becoming a bully, it is important to be a role model for nonviolent behavior. Parents should also clearly communicate to the child that bullying behavior is not acceptable—clear limits should be established for acceptable behavior, and consequences for ignoring the limits should be defined. Teaching good social skills, including efficacious conflict-resolution skills and anger management skills, can also help potential bullies learn alternative socially acceptable behaviors.

Recent attention in the media to student suicides related to bullying as well as school shootings and similar acts of violence has prompted a search for new approaches to the problem. One approach involves making it easier for students to break the "code of silence" that makes them reluctant to inform on their peers. Safe2Tell is an anonymous 24/7 hotline that some communities have set up that allows students to report bullying, plans to attack the school, and other forms of violent behavior.

A more comprehensive approach is the Olweus (pronounced ohl-VAY-us) Bullying Prevention Program (OBBP), a systems-change approach designed by a Norwegian educator named Dan Olweus in 1983 and tested in both Norway and the United States for over 25 years. The program is designed to improve peer relations and make schools safer, more positive places for students to learn and develop. Goals of the program include reducing existing bullying problems among students, preventing new bullying problems, and achieving better peer relations at school. As of 2011, the OBBP approach had been used with over 40,000 students in both countries and was reported to reduce bullying rates by up to 50%. Designed for long-term use in elementary, middle, and junior high schools, the program includes a questionnaire about bullying for students to answer as well as training for teachers, school administrators, parents, and community leaders.

The program does not utilize conflict-resolution or peer-mediation techniques, because it believes that these approaches assume that the parties involved are equal in power or status, whereas bullying is based on power imbalances. According to proponents of the Olweus program, it reduces vandalism as well as bullying and other forms of antisocial behavior in the schools where it has been tried. It has also been successfully used in summer camps, sports teams, and other organizations for children and adolescents.

Resources

BOOKS

Hamilton, Jill, ed. *Bullying and Hazing*. Detroit, MI: Greenhaven Press, 2008.

Monks, Claire P., and Iain Coyne, eds. *Bullying in Different Contexts*. New York: Cambridge University Press, 2011.

Olweus, Dan, et al. *Olweus Bullying Prevention Program: Schoolwide Guide*. Center City, MN: Hazelden, 2007.

Pennsylvania Bar Institute. *Surviving the Schoolyard Battlefield*. Mechanicsburg, PA: PBI, 2008.

Spivet, Bonnie. *Stopping Cyberbullying*. New York: PowerKids Press, 2012.

PERIODICALS

Blosnich, J., and R. Bossarte. "Low-level Violence in Schools: Is There an Association between School Safety Measures and Peer Victimization?" *Journal of School Health* 81 (February 2011): 107–113.

Centers for Disease Control and Prevention (CDC). "Bullying among Middle School and High School Students—Massachusetts, 2009." *Morbidity and Mortality Weekly Report* 60 (April 22, 2011): 465–471.

Johnson, S.L. "An Ecological Model of Workplace Bullying: A Guide for Intervention and Research." *Nursing Forum* 46 (April 2011): 55–63.

Meloni, M., and M. Austin. "Implementation and Outcomes of a Zero Tolerance of Bullying and Harassment Program." *Australian Health Review* 35 (February 2011): 92–94.

Mishna, F., et al. "Cyber Bullying Behaviors among Middle and High School Students." *American Journal of Orthopsychiatry* 80 (July 2010): 362–374.

Olweus, D., and S.P. Limber. "Bullying in School: Evaluation and Dissemination of the Olweus Bullying Prevention Program." *American Journal of Orthopsychiatry* 80 (January 2010): 124–134.

Payne, S.R., and D.S. Elliott. "Safe2Tell(®) : An Anonymous, 24/7 Reporting System for Preventing School Violence." *New Directions for Youth Development* 129 (March 2011): 103–111.

Stagg, S.J., and D. Sheridan. "Effectiveness of Bullying and Violence Prevention Programs." *Journal of the American Association of Occupational Health Nurses* 58 (October 2010): 419–424.

Waasdorp, T.E., et al. "A Multilevel Perspective on the Climate of Bullying: Discrepancies Among Students, School Staff, and Parents." *Journal of School Violence* 10 (January 1, 2011): 115–132.

Wang, J., et al. "Cyber and Traditional Bullying: Differential Association with Depression." *Journal of Adolescent Health* 48 (April 2011): 415–417.

WEBSITES

ABC News. "Teen Triangle and Facebook Feud Lead to Murder of 15-Year-Old Florida Boy." http://abcnews.go.com/US/teen-triangle-leads-vicious-murder-15-year-florida/story?id=13422887 (accessed May 24, 2011).

American Academy of Child and Adolescent Psychiatry (AACAP) Facts for Families. "Bullying." http://www.aacap.org/cs/root/facts_for_families/bullying (accessed May 23, 2011).

Hazelden Foundation. "An Overview of the Olweus Bullying Prevention Program" (10-minute video). http://www.youtube.com/watch?v=P9C5wJ6uAk0 (accessed May 23, 2011).

Olweus Bullying Prevention Program. "What Is Bullying?" http://www.olweus.org/public/bullying.page (accessed May 22, 2011).

StopBullying.gov Home Page. http://www.stopbullying.gov (accessed May 21, 2011).

STOP Cyberbullying. "What Methods Work with the Different Kinds of Cyberbullies?" http://www.stopcyberbullying.org/parents/howdoyouhandleacyberbully.html (accessed May 22, 2011).

TeensHealth. "Cyberbullying." http://kidshealth.org/teen/school_jobs/bullying/cyberbullying.html (accessed May 22, 2011).

TeensHealth. "Dealing with Bullying." http://kidshealth.org/teen/your_mind/problems/bullies.html (accessed May 22, 2011).

Workplace Bullying Institute Home Page. http://www.workplacebullying.org (accessed May 22, 2011).

ORGANIZATIONS

Act Against Bullying, PO Box 57962, London, United Kingdom W4 2TG, (44) 208 995 9500, info@actagainstbullying.org, http://www.actagainstbullying.org/index.htm.

American Academy of Child and Adolescent Psychiatry (AACAP), 3615 Wisconsin Avenue, NW, Washington, DC, United States, 20016-3007, (202) 966-7300, Fax: (202) 966-2891, http://www.aacap.org.

Hazelden Foundation, PO Box 11, Center City, MN, United States, 55012-0011, (651) 213-4200, (800) 257-7810, info@hazelden.org, http://www.hazelden.org.

Olweus Bullying Prevention Program, (800) 328-9000, olweusinfo@hazelden.org, http://www.olweus.org/public/index.page.

STOP Cyberbullying, (201) 463-8663, parry@aftab.com, http://www.stopcyberbullying.org/index2.html.

Workplace Bullying Institute (WBI), PO Box 29915, Bellingham, WA, United States, 98228 http://www.workplacebullying.org.

Ruth A. Wienclaw, Ph.D.
Rebecca J. Frey, Ph.D.

Bupropion

Definition

Bupropion is an antidepressant drug used to elevate mood and promote recovery of a normal range of emotions in patients with depressive disorders. In addition, bupropion is used to as an aid in **smoking cessation** treatment. In the United States, bupropion is sold as an antidepressant under the brand name Wellbutrin. As a smoking cessation treatment, the drug is marketed under the brand name Zyban.

Purpose

Bupropion is approved by the U.S. Food and Drug Administration (FDA) to treat **depression** and **seasonal affective disorder** and to aid in smoking cessation. It may have therapeutic uses in **panic disorder** and **attention deficit hyperactivity disorder (ADHD)** but as of 2011 was not FDA approved for those indications.

Description

Bupropion is a nontricyclic antidepressant drug. Until the 1980s, tricyclic **antidepressants** were the mainstay of the pharmacological treatment of depression, but they had unwanted side effects, including sedation, dizziness, fainting, and weight gain. Bupropion was one of the first antidepressants to be developed by pharmaceutical researchers seeking drugs effective in treating depression but without the unwanted actions of the tricyclic antidepressants.

The exact way that bupropion works in the **brain** is not understood. Its mechanism of action appears to be different from that of most other antidepressant drugs, although bupropion does act on some of the same **neurotransmitters** and neurotransmission pathways. Neurotransmitters are naturally occurring chemicals that regulate the transmission of nerve impulses from one cell to another. Mental well-being is partially dependent on maintaining the proper balance among the various neurotransmitters in the brain. Bupropion may restore normal emotional feelings by counteracting abnormalities of neurotransmission that occur in depressive disorders.

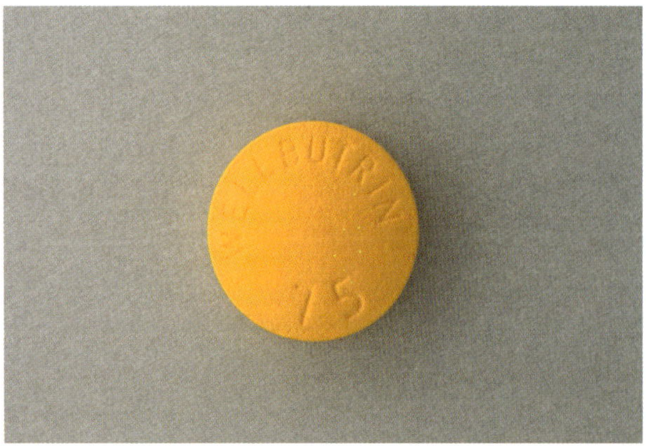

Wellbutrin (bupropion), 75 mg. *(© Custom Medical Stock Photo, Inc. Reproduced by permission.)*

Bupropion is less likely to cause weight gain and adverse effects on blood pressure and the heart, compared to other antidepressants. However, it is more likely to trigger epileptic **seizures**.

Recommended dosage

The usual adult dose of bupropion (Wellbutrin) is 100 mg, taken three times per day, with at least six hours between doses. The sustained-release form of the drug (Wellbutrin SR) is taken as 150 mg twice a day with at least eight hours between doses. An extended-release, once-daily dose (Wellbutrin XL) is also available and is usually taken in the morning. For smoking cessation, bupropion (Zyban) is taken as 150 mg sustained-release tablets twice a day, with at least eight hours between doses. Bupropion treatment should be started at a lower dose, then gradually increased to a therapeutic dosage as directed by the physician. Generally, the total dosage should not exceed 300 mg per day, except as directed by the physician.

The therapeutic effects of bupropion, like other antidepressants, appear slowly. Maximum benefit is often not evident for several weeks after starting the drug. People taking bupropion should be aware of this and continue taking the drug as directed even if they do not see immediate improvement in mood.

Since higher doses of bupropion increase the risk of seizures, no more than 150 mg should be given at any one time, and the total daily dosage should not be increased by more than 100 mg every three days. Increasing the dosage gradually also minimizes any agitation, restlessness, and **insomnia** that may occur.

Healthy elderly patients do not appear to be more sensitive to side effects of bupropion than younger adults and do not require reduced doses. Certain medical conditions, especially liver and kidney disease, may necessitate dose reduction. Although bupropion has been taken by children and adolescents under age 18, it has not yet been systematically studied in these age groups.

Precautions

Bupropion is more likely to trigger epileptic seizures than other antidepressants. The drug should not be given

KEY TERMS

Anxiety—An emotion that can be experienced as a troubled feeling, sense of dread, fear of the future, or distress over a perceived threat to a person's physical or mental well-being.

Attention deficit hyperactivity disorder (ADHD)—A developmental disorder characterized by distractibility, hyperactivity, impulsive behaviors, and the inability to remain focused on tasks or activities.

Depression—A mental state characterized by feelings of sadness, despair, discouragement, and low energy, sometimes accompanied by oversleeping and/or overeating.

Insomnia—Having difficulty falling asleep and/or staying asleep.

Seizure—A convulsion or uncontrolled discharge of nerve cells that may spread to other cells throughout the brain.

to patients who have a history of epilepsy, take other medication to help control seizures, or have some other condition associated with seizures, such as head **trauma** or alcoholism. Nevertheless, less than 1% of healthy people taking bupropion at the recommended dose have seizures. The possibility of seizures is increased at higher doses and following a sudden increase in dose. Patients should minimize alcohol intake while taking bupropion, since alcohol consumption increases the chance of seizures.

Because of the possibility of overdose, potentially suicidal patients should be given only small quantities of the drug at one time. Increases in blood pressure have occurred in patients taking bupropion along with **nicotine** treatment for smoking cessation. Monitoring blood pressure is recommended in such cases. Excessive stimulation, agitation, insomnia, and anxiety have been troublesome side effects for some patients, especially when treatment is first begun or when the dose is increased. Such adverse effects may be less intense and less frequent when the dose is increased gradually.

When taken for smoking cessation, some patients have developed severe neuropsychiatric symptoms, including aggression, depression, mania, panic attacks, and suicidal thoughts and actions. As with other antidepressants, children and adults up to 24 years of age are at increased risk for developing suicidal thoughts and actions. It is generally not advised for children under the age of 18 to take bupropion, but in some cases it may be the best treatment available. Patients should consult with their doctor and read the medication guide before starting treatment with bupropion.

It has not been determined whether bupropion is safe to take during pregnancy. Pregnant women should take bupropion only if necessary. The drug is secreted in breast milk. Women taking bupropion should consult their physicians about risks associated with breast-feeding.

Side effects

Bupropion is a very mild stimulant and may cause insomnia, agitation, confusion, restlessness, and anxiety. These effects may be more pronounced at the beginning of therapy and after dose increases. Headache, dizziness, and tremor may occur. Despite its stimulating effects, bupropion may also cause sedation.

Weight loss is more common with bupropion than weight gain, but both have been reported. Other negative side effects include:

- excessive sweating
- dry mouth
- sore throat
- nausea
- vomiting
- decreased appetite
- constipation
- blurred vision
- rapid heart rate

Interactions

Bupropion should not be administered along with other medications that lower the seizure threshold, such as **steroids** and the asthma medication theophylline. Many psychiatric medications also lower the seizure threshold. **Monoamine oxidase inhibitors (MAOIs)**, another type of antidepressant medication, should not be taken with bupropion or two weeks before starting the drug. Adverse effects may increase in patients taking levodopa and other medications for Parkinson's disease along with bupropion. Patients should inform their doctors about all other medications they are taking before starting this drug.

Nicotine patch therapy may be administered concurrently with bupropion in smoking cessation treatment. If this is done, blood pressure must be monitored, since increased blood pressure has been reported with this combination of medications.

Certain drugs, especially those eliminated by the liver, may interfere with the elimination of bupropion from the

QUESTIONS TO ASK YOUR DOCTOR

- What kind of changes can I expect to see or feel with this medication?
- Does it matter what time of day I take this medication? If so, what is the recommendation?
- Should I take this medication with or without food?
- What are the side effects associated with this medication?
- Will this medication interact or interfere with other medications I am currently taking?
- What symptoms or adverse effects are important enough that I should seek immediate treatment?

body, causing higher blood levels and increased side effects. Conversely, bupropion may delay the elimination of other medicines, including many antidepressants, antipsychotic drugs, and heart medications, resulting in higher blood levels and potentially increased side effects.

Resources

BOOKS

Albers, Lawrence J., Rhoda K. Hahn, and Christopher Reist. *Handbook of Psychiatric Drugs, 2011 Edition.* Laguna Hills, CA: Current Clinical Strategies, 2010.

American Society of Health-System Pharmacists. *AHFS Drug Information 2011.* Bethesda, MD: ASHP, 2011.

Baldwin, Robert C. *Depression in Later Life.* New York: Oxford University Press, 2010.

Graham, George. *The Disordered Mind: An Introduction to Philosophy of Mind and Mental Illness.* New York: Routledge, 2010.

Holland, Leland Norman, and Michael Patrick Adams. *Core Concepts in Pharmacology.* 3rd ed. New York: Prentice Hall, 2011.

North, Carol, and Sean Yutzy. *Goodwin and Guze's Psychiatric Diagnosis.* New York: Oxford University Press, 2010.

O'Connor, Richard. *Undoing Depression: What Therapy Doesn't Teach You and Medication Can't Give You.* 2nd ed. New York: Little, Brown, 2010.

Preston, John D., John H. O'Neal, and Mary C. Talaga. *Handbook of Clinical Psychopharmacology for Therapists.* 6th ed. Oakland, CA: New Harbinger, 2010.

PERIODICALS

Lader, M. "Foreword. A Comprehensive Review of Bupropion." *Clinical Drug Investigation* 19, no. 31, supplement 1 (2011): 1–3.

Little, John T., et al. "Bupropion and Venlafaxine Responders Differ in Pretreatment Regional Cerebral Metabolism in Unipolar Depression." *Biological Psychiatry* 57, no. 3 (February 2005): 220–28.

Thase, Michael E., et al. "Remission Rates Following Antidepressant Therapy with Bupropion or Selective Serotonin Reuptake Inhibitors: A Meta-Analysis of Original Data From 7 Randomized Controlled Trials." *Journal of Clinical Psychiatry* 66, no. 8 (August 2005): 974–81.

ORGANIZATIONS

American Academy of Clinical Toxicology, 6728 Old McLean Village Dr., McLean, VA, 22101, (703) 556-9222, Fax: (703) 556-8729, admin@clintox.org, http://www.clintox.org.

American Psychiatric Association, 1000 Wilson Blvd., Ste. 1825, Arlington, VA, 22209-3901, (703) 907-7300, apa@psych.org, http://www.psych.org.

American Society for Clinical Pharmacology and Therapeutics, 528 N Washington St., Alexandria, VA, 22314, (703) 836-6981, info@ascpt.org, http://www.ascpt.org.

American Society for Pharmacology and Experimental Therapeutics, 9650 Rockville Pike, Bethesda, MD, 20814-3995, (301) 634-7060, http://www.aspet.org.

Depression and Bipolar Support Alliance, 730 N Franklin St., Ste. 501, Chicago, IL, 60654, (800) 826-3632, Fax: (312) 642-7243, http://www.dbsalliance.org.

National Alliance on Mental Illness, 2107 Wilson Blvd., Ste. 300, Arlington, VA, 22201-3042, Fax: (703) 524-9094, (800) 950-6264, http://www.nami.org.

National Institute of Mental Health, 6001 Executive Blvd., Rm. 8184, MSC 9663, Bethesda, MD, 20892-9663, (301) 433-4513; TTY: (301) 443-8431, Fax: (301) 443-4279, (866) 615-6464; TTY: (866) 415-8051, nimhinfo@nih.gov

Richard Kapit, MD
Ruth A. Wienclaw, PhD
Laura Jean Cataldo, RN, EdD

BuSpar *see* **Buspirone**

Buspirone

Definition

Buspirone is an antianxiety (anxiolytic) drug sold in the United States under the brand name BuSpar. It is also available under its generic name.

Purpose

Buspirone is used for the treatment of generalized **anxiety disorders** and for short-term relief of symptoms of anxiety.

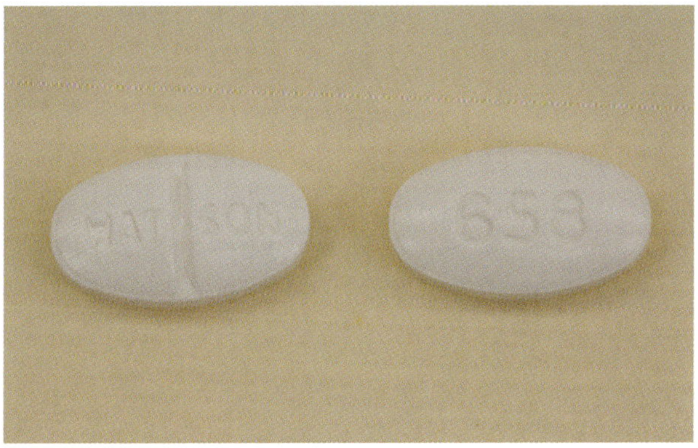

Buspirone, 10 mg. *(© Custom Medical Stock Photo, Inc. Reproduced by permission.)*

Description

Buspirone's mechanism of action is unclear but probably involves actions on such central nervous system chemicals as **dopamine**, **serotonin**, acetylcholine, and norepinephrine. These chemicals are called **neurotransmitters** and are involved in the transmission of nervous impulses from cell to cell. Mental well-being is partially dependent on maintaining a balance among different neurotransmitters.

Buspirone's actions are different from the common class of **sedatives** called **benzodiazepines**. The primary actions of benzodiazepines are to reduce anxiety, relax skeletal muscles, and induce sleep. The earliest drugs in this class were **chlordiazepoxide** (Librium) and **diazepam** (Valium). The mechanism of buspirone's action is also different from **barbiturates** such as phenobarbital. Unlike benzodiazepines, buspirone has no anticonvulsant or muscle-relaxant properties, and unlike benzodiazepines or barbiturates it does not have strong sedative properties. If **insomnia** is a component of the patient's anxiety disorder, a sedative/hypnotic drug may be taken along with buspirone at bedtime. Buspirone also diminishes anger and hostility for most people. Unlike benzodiazepines, which may aggravate anger and hostility in some patients (especially older patients), buspirone may help patients with anxiety who also have a history of aggression

The benefits of buspirone take a long time to become evident. Unlike benzodiazepines, with which the onset of action and time to maximum benefit are short, patients must take buspirone for three to four weeks before feeling the maximum benefit of the drug. In some cases, four to six weeks of treatment may be required. Patients should be aware of this and continue to take the drug as prescribed even if they think they are not seeing any improvement.

Buspirone is available in 5, 10, 15, and 30 mg tablets.

KEY TERMS

Anxiety—An emotion that can be experienced as a troubled feeling, sense of dread, fear of the future, or distress over a possible threat to a person's physical or mental well-being.

Depression—A mental state characterized by feelings of sadness, despair, and discouragement.

Insomnia—Having difficulty falling asleep or remaining asleep.

Neurotransmitter—A chemical that aids or alters the transmission of impulses between the points that connect nerves.

Serotonin—A chemical messenger in the brain thought to play a role in mood regulation.

Recommended dosage

The usual starting dose of this drug is 10 to 15 mg per day. This total amount is divided into two or three doses. For example, a dose of 5 mg may be given two or three times per day to make a total dose of 10 to 15 mg per day. The dose may be increased in increments of 5 mg daily every two to four days. Most patients respond to a dose of 15 to 30 mg daily. Patients should not take a total dose of more than 60 mg daily. When patients are receiving certain other drugs in addition to buspirone, starting doses of buspirone may need to be lowered (e.g., 2.5 mg twice daily), and any dosage increase should be done with caution and under close physician supervision. Dosages may need to be reduced in patients with kidney or liver problems.

Precautions

Buspirone is less sedating (it causes less drowsiness and mental sluggishness) than other **antianxiety drugs**. However, some patients may still experience drowsiness and mental impairment. Because it is impossible to predict which patients may experience sedation with buspirone, those starting this drug should not drive or operate machinery until they know how the drug will affect them.

Patients who have been taking benzodiazepines for a long time should be gradually withdrawn from them while they are being switched over to buspirone. They should also be observed for symptoms of benzodiazepine withdrawal.

Patients with kidney damage should take buspirone with caution in close consultation with their physician. They may require a lower dosage of buspirone to prevent buildup of the drug in the body. Patients with severe

QUESTIONS TO ASK YOUR DOCTOR

- What kind of changes can I expect to see or feel with this medication?
- Does it matter what time of day I take this medication? If so, what is the recommendation?
- Should I take this medication with or without food?
- What are the side effects associated with this medication?
- Will this medication interact or interfere with other medications I am currently taking?
- What symptoms or adverse effects are important enough that I should seek immediate treatment?

kidney disease should not take buspirone. Patients with liver damage should likewise be monitored for a buildup of buspirone and have their doses lowered if necessary.

Side effects

The most common side effects associated with buspirone involve the nervous system. Ten percent of patients may experience dizziness, drowsiness, and headache, and another 5% may experience **fatigue**, nervousness, insomnia, and light-headedness. Patients may also experience:

- excitement
- depression
- anger
- hostility
- confusion
- nightmares or other sleep disorders
- lack of coordination
- tremor
- numbness of the extremities

Although buspirone is considered nonsedating, some patients experience drowsiness and lack of mental alertness at higher doses, especially early in therapy. In most patients, these side effects decrease with time.

The following side effects have also been associated with buspirone:

- nausea (up to 8% of patients)
- dry mouth, abdominal distress, gastric distress, diarrhea, and constipation (up to 5% of patients)
- rapid heart rate and palpitations (up to 2% of patients)
- blurred vision (up to 2% of patients)
- increased or decreased appetite
- flatulence
- nonspecific chest pain
- rash
- irregular menstrual periods and/or breakthrough bleeding

Interactions

Patients should avoid drinking grapefruit juice while on buspirone, as it inhibits the metabolism of the drug, resulting in potentially toxic amounts of the substance in the bloodstream.

Dangerously high blood pressure has resulted from the combination of buspirone and members of another class of **antidepressants** known as **monoamine oxidase inhibitors (MAOIs)**. Because of this, buspirone should never be taken in combination with MAOIs. Patients taking any MAOIs, such as **phenelzine** sulfate (Nardil) or **tranylcypromine** sulfate (Parnate), should stop the MAOIs and wait at least 14 days before starting buspirone. The same holds true when discontinuing buspirone and starting any MAOIs.

Certain drugs that affect the liver may alter the metabolism of buspirone. Examples of such drugs are erythromycin, a broad-spectrum antibiotic; itraconazole, an oral antifungal agent; and **nefazodone**, an antidepressant. When these drugs are combined with buspirone, buspirone concentrations may increase to the point of toxicity (poisoning). These combinations should either be avoided or doses of buspirone decreased to compensate for this interaction.

Resources

BOOKS

Albers, Lawrence J., Rhoda K. Hahn, and Christopher Reist. *Handbook of Psychiatric Drugs.* Laguna Hills, CA: Current Clinical Strategies, 2010.

American Society of Health-System Pharmacists. *AHFS Drug Information 2011.* Bethesda, MD: ASHP, 2011.

Graham, George. *The Disordered Mind: An Introduction to Philosophy of Mind and Mental Illness.* New York: Routledge, 2010.

Holland, Leland Norman, and Michael Patrick Adams. *Core Concepts in Pharmacology.* 3rd ed. New York: Prentice Hall, 2011.

North, Carol, and Sean Yutzy. *Goodwin and Guze's Psychiatric Diagnosis.* New York: Oxford University Press, 2010.

Preston, John D., John H. O'Neal, and Mary C. Talaga. *Handbook of Clinical Psychopharmacology for Therapists.* 6th ed. Oakland, CA: New Harbinger, 2010.

PERIODICALS

Baldwin, David S., and Claire Polkinghorn. "Evidence-based Pharmacotherapy of Generalized Anxiety Disorder." *International Journal of Neuropsychopharmacology* 8, no. 2 (June 2005): 293–302.

Buydens-Branchey, Laure, Marc Branchey, and Christine Reel-Brander. "Efficacy of Buspirone in the Treatment of Opioid Withdrawal." *Journal of Clinical Psychopharmacology* 25, no. 3 (June 2005): 230–36.

Helvink, Badalin, and Suzanne Holroyd. "Buspirone for Stereotypic Movements in Elderly with Cognitive Impairment." *Journal of Neuropsychiatry and Clinical Neurosciences* 18, no. 2 (Spring 2006): 242–44.

McRae, Aimee L., Kathleen T. Brady, and Rickey E. Carter. "Buspirone for Treatment of Marijuana Dependence: A Pilot Study." *American Journal on Addictions* 15, no. 5 (September/October 2006): 404.

Quitkin, Frederick, et al. "Medication Augmentation after the Failure of SSRIs for Depression." *New England Journal of Medicine* 354, no. 12 (March 2006): 1243–52.

Verster, Joris C., Dieuwke S. Veldhuijzen, and Edmund R Volkerts. "Is It Safe to Drive a Car When Treated with Anxiolytics? Evidence from On-the-Road Driving Studies During Normal Traffic." *Current Psychiatry Reviews* 1, no. 2 (June 2005): 215–25.

WEBSITES

PubMed Health. "Buspirone." U.S. National Library of Medicine. http://www.ncbi.nlm.nih.gov/pubmedhealth/PMH0000876 (accessed December 17, 2011).

ORGANIZATIONS

American Academy of Clinical Toxicology, 6728 Old McLean Village Dr., McLean, VA, 22101, (703) 556-9222 Fax: (703) 556-8729, admin@clintox.org, http://www.clintox.org.

American Academy of Family Physicians, 11400 Tomahawk Creek Pkwy., Leawood, KS, 66211-2672, (913) 906-6000, (800) 274-2237, Fax: (913) 906-6075, contactcenter@aafp.org, http://www.aafp.org.

American Psychiatric Association, 1000 Wilson Blvd., Ste. 1825, Arlington, VA, 22209-3901, (703) 907-7300, apa@psych.org, http://www.psych.org.

American Society for Clinical Pharmacology and Therapeutics, 528 N Washington St., Alexandria, VA, 22314, (703) 836-6981, info@ascpt.org, http://www.ascpt.org.

Anxiety Disorders Association of America, 8730 Georgia Ave., Silver Spring, MD, 20910, (240) 485-1001, Fax: (240) 485-1035, http://www.adaa.org.

National Alliance on Mental Illness, 2107 Wilson Blvd., Ste. 300, Arlington, VA, 22201-3042, Fax: (703) 524-9094, (800) 950-6264, http://www.nami.org.

National Institute of Mental Health, 6001 Executive Blvd., Rm. 8184, MSC 9663, Bethesda, MD, 20892-9663, (301) 433-4513; TTY: (301) 443-8431, Fax: (301) 443-4279, (866) 615-6464; TTY: (866) 415-8051, nimhinfo@nih.gov, http://www.nimh.nih.gov.

Jack Raber, PharmD
Ruth A. Wienclaw, PhD
Laura Jean Cataldo, RN, EdD

C

Caffeine-related disorders

Definition

Caffeine is a white, bitter crystalline alkaloid derived from coffee or tea. It belongs to a class of compounds called xanthines, its chemical formula being 1,3,7-trimethylxanthine. Caffeine is classified together with **cocaine** and **amphetamines** as an analeptic, or central nervous system stimulant. Coffee is the most abundant source of caffeine, although caffeine is also found in tea, cocoa, and cola beverages as well as in over-the-counter and prescription medications for pain relief.

In the clinician's handbook for diagnosing mental disorders (the ***Diagnostic and Statistical Manual of Mental Disorders***, known as the *DSM-IV-TR*), caffeine-related disorders are classified under the rubric of substance-related disorders. *DSM-IV-TR* specifies four caffeine-related disorders: caffeine intoxication, caffeine-induced anxiety disorder, caffeine-induced sleep disorder, and caffeine-related disorder not otherwise specified. A fifth disorder, caffeine withdrawal, was listed as being considered for further study in the *DSM-IV* and is proposed to be included as a **diagnosis** in the fifth edition (*DSM-5*, 2013).

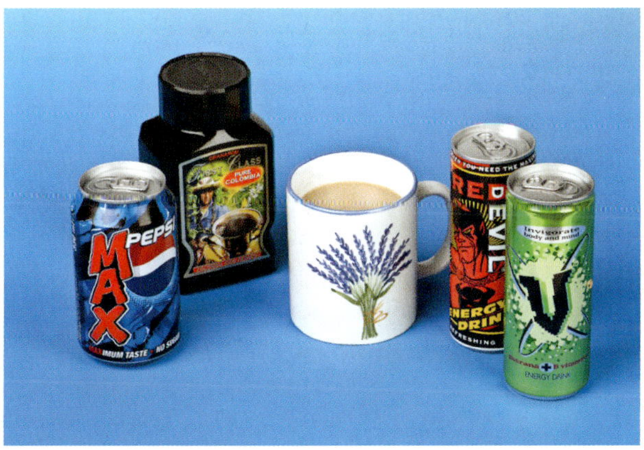

Many different products contain caffeine, including coffee, tea, colas, and energy drinks. *(© Martyn F. Chillmaid/Photo Researchers, Inc.)*

Demographics

The general population of the United States has a high level of caffeine consumption, with an average intake of 200 mg per day. About 85% of the population uses caffeine in any given year. Among adults in the United States, about 30% consume 500 mg or more of caffeine each day. These figures are lower, however, than the figures for Sweden, the United Kingdom, and other parts of Europe, where the average daily consumption of caffeine among all adults is 400 mg or higher. In developing countries, the average consumption of caffeine is much lower, about 50 mg per day.

In the United States, levels of caffeine consumption among all races and ethnic groups are related to age, with usage beginning in the late teens and rising until the early 30s. Caffeine consumption tapers off in adults over 40 and decreases in adults over 65. Caffeine intake is higher among males than among females in North America.

Description

Caffeine-related disorders are often unrecognized for a number of reasons, including caffeine's "low profile" as a drug of abuse. Consumption of drinks containing caffeine is unregulated by law and is nearly universal in the United States; one well-known textbook of pharmacology refers to caffeine as "the most widely used psychoactive drug in the world." In many countries, coffee is a social lubricant as well as a stimulant; the "coffee break" is a common office ritual, and many people find it difficult to imagine eating a meal in a fine restaurant without having coffee at some point during the meal. It is estimated that 10–12 billion lb. (4–5 billion kg) of coffee are consumed worldwide each year.

People often underestimate the amount of caffeine they consume on a daily basis because they think of caffeine only in connection with coffee; however, tea, cocoa, and

Approximate amounts of caffeine in popular products

	Size	Amount of caffeine
Sprite, Fanta, 7 UP	12 oz (355 mL)	0 mg
Tea, decaffeinated	8 oz (240 mL)	1–4 mg
Coffee, decaffeinated, brewed	8 oz (240 mL)	2–12 mg
Hershey's Milk Chocolate	1.55 oz (43 g)	9 mg
Tea, green, brewed	8 oz (240 mL)	15 mg
Barq's Root Beer	12 oz (355 mL)	23 mg
Hershey's Special Dark Chocolate	1.45 oz (41 g)	31 mg
Coca-Cola Classic	12 oz (355 mL)	35 mg
Pepsi	12 oz (355 mL)	36–38 mg
Tea, black, brewed	8 oz (240 mL)	40–120 mg
Sunkist Orange, regular or diet	12 oz (355 mL)	41 mg
Dr Pepper	12 oz (355 mL)	42–44 mg
Diet Coke	12 oz (355 mL)	47 mg
Mountain Dew	12 oz (355 mL)	54 mg
Coffee, espresso	1 oz (30 mL)	58–75 mg
Excedrin® extra-strength headache	1 tablet	65 mg
Red Bull energy drink	8.3 oz (245 mL)	76 mg
SoBe No Fear energy drink	8 oz (240 mL)	83 mg
Coffee, brewed	8 oz (240 mL)	95–200 mg
5-hour ENERGY® drink	2 oz (59 mL)	138 mg
Monster Energy drink	16 oz (473 mL)	160 mg
NO-DOZ® maximum-strength caffeine	1 tablet	200 mg

(Table by PreMediaGlobal. © 2012 Cengage Learning.)

some types of soft drinks (such as colas) also contain significant amounts of caffeine. In one British case study, a teenager who was hospitalized with muscle weakness, nausea, vomiting, diarrhea, and weight loss was found to have caffeine intoxication caused by drinking about 2 gal. (8 L) of cola on a daily basis for the two years. She had been consuming over a gram of caffeine per day. Chocolate bars and coffee-flavored yogurt or ice cream are additional sources of measurable amounts of caffeine.

Caffeine has some legitimate medical uses in athletic training and in the relief of tension-type headaches. It is available in over-the-counter (OTC) preparations containing aspirin or acetaminophen for pain relief as well as in such OTC stimulants as NoDoz and Vivarin. It is also available in energy drinks and supplements and more recently in alcoholic beverages, though the latter is considered unsafe by the U.S. Food and Drug Administration (FDA), who in 2010 ordered several manufacturers of caffeinated alcoholic beverages to cease production. Some beverages are still available, but the effects of caffeine and alcohol have not been sufficiently tested, and the full extent of possible adverse effects is not yet known.

In comparison to other drugs of abuse, caffeine is less likely to produce the same degree of physical or psychological dependence. Few coffee or tea drinkers report loss of control over caffeine intake, or significant difficulty in reducing or stopping consumption of beverages and food items containing caffeine. Still, a research team at Johns Hopkins regards caffeine as a model drug for understanding **substance abuse** and dependence. The team maintains that 9%–30% of caffeine consumers in the United States may be caffeine-dependent, according to *DSM* criteria for substance dependency.

Pharmacological aspects of caffeine

An outline of the effects of caffeine on the central nervous system (CNS) and other organ systems of the body may be helpful in understanding its potential for physical dependence. When a person drinks a beverage (or eats food) containing caffeine, the caffeine is absorbed from the digestive tract without being broken down. It is rapidly distributed throughout the tissues of the body by means of the bloodstream. If a pregnant woman drinks a cup of coffee or tea, the caffeine in the drink will cross the placental barrier and enter the baby's bloodstream.

When the caffeine reaches the **brain**, it increases the secretion of norepinephrine, a neurotransmitter that is associated with the so-called "fight or flight" **stress** response. The rise in norepinephrine levels and the increased activity of the neurons, or nerve cells, in many other areas of the brain helps to explain why the symptoms of caffeine intoxication resemble the symptoms of a **panic attack**.

The effects of caffeine are thought to occur as a result of competitive antagonism at adenosine receptors. Adenosine is a water-soluble compound of adenine and ribose; it functions to modulate the activities of nerve cells and produces a mild sedative effect when it activates certain types of adenosine receptors. Caffeine competes with adenosine to bind at these receptors and counteracts the sedative effects of the adenosine. If the person stops drinking coffee, the adenosine has no competition for activating its usual receptors and may produce a sedative effect that is experienced as **fatigue** or drowsiness.

Caffeine can produce a range of physical symptoms following ingestion of as little as 100 mg, although amounts of 250 mg or higher are usually needed to produce symptoms that meet the criteria of caffeine intoxication.

Causes and symptoms

Causes

The immediate cause of caffeine intoxication and other caffeine-related disorders is consumption of an amount of caffeine sufficient to produce the symptoms specified by the *DSM* as criteria for the disorder. The precise amount of caffeine necessary to produce symptoms varies from person to person depending on body size and degree of tolerance to caffeine. Tolerance of the stimulating effects of caffeine builds up rapidly in humans; mild withdrawal symptoms have been reported in persons who were drinking as little as one to two cups of coffee per day.

Some people may find it easier than others to consume large doses of caffeine because they are insensitive to its taste. Caffeine tastes bitter to most adults, which may serve to limit their consumption of coffee and other caffeinated beverages. Slightly more than 30% of the American population, however, has an inherited inability to taste caffeine.

Symptoms

CAFFEINE INTOXICATION. The symptoms of caffeine intoxication are similar to those of an anxiety disorder and include:

- restlessness
- nervousness
- excitement
- insomnia
- flushed face
- diuresis (increased urinary output)
- gastrointestinal disturbance
- muscle twitching
- talking or thinking in a rambling manner
- tachycardia (rapid heartbeat) or disturbances of heart rhythm (arrhythmias)
- periods of inexhaustibility
- psychomotor agitation

Some people have experienced ringing in the ears or seeing flashes of light at doses of caffeine above 250 mg. Profuse sweating and diarrhea are also possible symptoms. High short-term consumption of caffeine can produce or worsen gastrointestinal problems, occasionally leading to peptic ulcers or hematemesis (vomiting blood). Doses of caffeine higher than 10 g may produce respiratory failure, **seizures**, and eventually death.

In addition to the symptoms produced by high short-term doses, long-term consumption of caffeine has been associated with fertility problems and with bone loss in women leading to osteoporosis in old age. Some studies have found that pregnant women who consume more than 150 mg per day of caffeine have an increased risk of miscarriage and low birth weight babies, but the findings are complicated by the fact that most women who drink large amounts of coffee during pregnancy are also heavy smokers. Some researchers believe that long-term consumption of caffeine is implicated in cardiovascular diseases but acknowledge that further research is required.

On the other hand, moderate doses of caffeine improve athletic performance as well as alertness. Caffeine in small doses can relieve tension headaches, and one study found that a combination of ibuprofen and caffeine was more effective in relieving tension headaches than either ibuprofen alone or a placebo. Coffee consumption also appears to lower the risk of alcoholic and nonalcoholic cirrhosis of the liver.

CAFFEINE WITHDRAWAL. Symptoms of caffeine withdrawal include:

- headache
- fatigue
- depression or irritable mood
- lack of concentration
- nausea or vomiting, or general aches and pains

DRUG INTERACTIONS. Caffeine is often combined with aspirin or acetaminophen in over-the-counter and prescription analgesics (pain relievers). It can also be combined with ibuprofen. On the other hand, certain groups of drugs should not be combined with caffeine or taken with beverages containing caffeine. Oral contraceptives, cimetidine (Tagamet), mexiletine (Mexitil), and **disulfiram** (Antabuse) interfere with the breakdown of caffeine in the body. Caffeine interferes with the body's absorption of iron, and with drugs that regulate heart rhythm, including quinidine and **propranolol** (Inderal). Caffeine may produce serious side effects when taken together with **monoamine oxidase inhibitors (MAOIs)** or with certain decongestant medications.

Combinations of ephedra and caffeine have been used in weight-loss programs because they produce greater weight loss than can be achieved by caloric restriction alone. However, side effects of supplements containing ephedra and caffeine include **insomnia**, high blood pressure (hypertension), anxiety, irritability, and, if used in the long-term, chronic fatigue. The combination may be linked to more serious side effects, including death due to altered heart rhythm, but further research is needed to determine whether the combination alone is actually causal in such adverse events.

Practitioners of homeopathy have traditionally advised patients not to drink beverages containing caffeine in the belief that caffeine "antidotes" homeopathic remedies. Contemporary homeopaths disagree on the antidoting effects of caffeine, observing that homeopathy is used widely and effectively in Europe and that Europeans tend to drink strong espresso coffee more frequently than Americans.

Diagnosis

Diagnosis of a caffeine-related disorder is usually based on the patient's recent history, a physical examination, or laboratory analysis of body fluids. In addition to medical evidence, the examiner will rule out other mental disorders, particularly manic episodes, **generalized anxiety disorder**, **panic disorder**, amphetamine intoxication, or withdrawal from **sedatives**, tranquilizers, sleep medications, or **nicotine**. All of these disorders or syndromes may produce symptoms resembling those of caffeine intoxication. In most cases, the temporal relationship of the symptoms to high levels of caffeine intake establishes the diagnosis. The examiner may consider the possibility of **depression** during the differential diagnosis, as many people with depression and eating disorders self-medicate with caffeine.

Caffeine intoxication

To meet the *DSM* criteria for caffeine intoxication, a person must develop five or more of the twelve symptoms identified; the symptoms must cause significant distress or impair the person's social or occupational functioning; and the symptoms must not be caused by a medical disorder, an anxiety disorder, or another mental disorder. Because people develop tolerance to caffeine fairly quickly with habitual use, caffeine intoxication is most likely to occur in those who consume caffeine infrequently or who have recently increased their intake significantly.

Caffeine-induced anxiety and sleep disorders

DSM criteria for caffeine-induced anxiety and **sleep disorders** specify that the symptoms of anxiety and insomnia respectively must be more severe than the symptoms associated with caffeine intoxication. In addition, the anxiety or insomnia must be severe enough to require separate clinical attention.

Caffeine withdrawal

The *DSM-5* diagnostic criteria for caffeine withdrawal is met if a person drinks caffeine daily over an extended period of time and experiences at least three of the symptoms of caffeine withdrawal once consumption is ceased (within 24 hours). As with caffeine intoxication, the symptoms must cause significant distress or impair the person's social or occupational function and must not be caused by another disorder, including physical or mental disorders.

Treatment

Treatment of caffeine-related disorders involves lowering consumption levels or abstaining from beverages containing caffeine. If withdrawal symptoms are experienced, they usually resolve quickly as the body adjusts to the absence of caffeine.

Caffeine consumption has the advantage of having relatively weak (compared to alcohol or cigarettes) social **reinforcement**, in the sense that one can easily choose a noncaffeinated or decaffeinated beverage in a restaurant or at a party without attracting comment. Thus, physical dependence on caffeine is less complicated by the social factors that reinforce nicotine and other drug habits.

Prognosis

With the exception of acute episodes of caffeinism, most people recover from caffeine intoxication without great difficulty.

Prevention

Prevention of caffeine-related disorders requires awareness of the caffeine content of caffeinated beverages, OTC drugs, and other sources of caffeine; monitoring daily intake; and substituting caffeinated coffee, tea, or soft drinks for the decaffeinated versions of these beverages.

Resources

BOOKS

American Psychiatric Association. *Diagnostic and Statistical Manual of Mental Disorders*. 4th ed., text rev. Washington, DC: American Psychiatric Publishing, 2000.

"Anxiety Due to a Physical Disorder or a Substance." In *The Merck Manual of Diagnosis and Therapy*, edited by Robert S. Porter and Justin L. Kaplan. Whitehouse Station, NJ: Merck Sharp & Dohme, 2011.

Murray, Michael, and Joseph Pizzorno. *Encyclopedia of Natural Medicine*. New York: Three Rivers Press, 1997.

O'Brien, Charles P. "Drug Addiction and Drug Abuse." In *Goodman & Gilman's The Pharmacological Basis of Therapeutics*, edited by Laurence Brunton, Bruce Chabner, and Bjornn Knollman, 12th ed. New York: McGraw-Hill, 2010.

Pelletier, Kenneth R. "Naturopathic Medicine: 'Do No Harm'." In *The Best Alternative Medicine*. New York: Touchstone, 2002.

PERIODICALS

Corrao, G., et al. "Coffee, Caffeine, and the Risk of Liver Cirrhosis." *Annals of Epidemiology* 11 (October 2001): 458–465.

De Valck, E., and R. Cluydts. "Slow-Release Caffeine as a Countermeasure to Driver Sleepiness Induced by Partial Sleep Deprivation." *Journal of Sleep Research* 10, no. 3 (September 2001): 203–209.

Diamond, S., T.K. Balm, and F.G. Freitag. "Ibuprofen Plus Caffeine in the Treatment of Tension-Type Headache." *Clinical Pharmacology and Therapeutics* 68, no. 3 (2000): 312–319.

Griffiths, R.R., and A.L. Chausmer. "Caffeine as a Model Drug of Dependence: Recent Developments in Understanding Caffeine Withdrawal, the Caffeine Dependence Syndrome, and Caffeine Negative Reinforcement." *Japanese Journal of Psychopharmacology* 20, no. 5 (November 2000): 223–231.

MacFadyen, L., D. Eadie, and T. McGowan. "Community Pharmacists' Experience of Over-the-Counter Medicine Misuse in Scotland." *Perspectives in Public Health* 121, no. 3 (September 2001): 185–192.

Preboth, Monica. "Effect of Caffeine on Exercise Performance." *American Family Physician* 61 (May 1, 2000): 628.

Rapurl, P.B., et al. "Caffeine Intake Increases the Rate of Bone Loss in Elderly Women and Interacts with Vitamin D Receptor Genotypes." *American Journal of Clinical Nutrition* 74, no. 5 (November 2001): 694–700.

Rumpler, William, et al. "Oolong Tea Increases Metabolic Rate and Fat Oxidation in Men." *Journal of Nutrition* 131, no. 11 (November 1, 2001): 2848–2852.

Sardao, V. A., P. J. Oliveira, and A. J. Moreno. "Caffeine Enhances the Calcium-Dependent Cardiac Mitochondrial Permeability Transition: Relevance for Caffeine Toxicity." *Toxicology and Applied Pharmacology* 179, no. 1 (February 2002): 50–56.

ORGANIZATIONS

American College of Sports Medicine, PO Box 1440, Indianapolis, IN, 46206-1440, (317) 637-9200, Fax: (317) 634-7817, http://www.acsm.org.

American Dietetic Association, 120 South Riverside Plz., Ste. 2000, Chicago, IL, 60606, (312) 899-0040, (800) 877-1600, http://www.eatright.org.

Center for Science in the Public Interest, 1220 L St. NW, Ste. 300, Washington, DC, 20005, (202) 332-9110, Fax: (202) 265-4954, http://www.cspinet.org.

U.S. Food and Drug Administration, 10903 New Hampshire Ave., Silver Spring, MD, 20993-0002, (888) INFO-FDA (463-6332), http://www.fda.gov.

Rebecca J. Frey, PhD

Cannabis and related disorders

Definition

Cannabis, more commonly called marijuana, refers to the several varieties of *Cannabis sativa*, or Indian hemp plant, that contain the psychoactive drug delta-9-tetrahydrocannabinol (THC). Cannabis-related disorders refer to problems associated with the use of substances derived from this plant.

Demographics

Marijuana is the most commonly used illicit drug in the United States. As with most other illicit drugs, cannabis use disorders appear more often in males and are most common among people between the ages of 18 and 30 years.

Statistics from 2010, published in the *National Survey on Drug Use and Health*, revealed that 17.4 million Americans over the age of 12 had used marijuana a minimum of one time in the previous month. The percentage of persons using marijuana has increased consistently since 2007, and approximately 60% of illicit drug users only smoke marijuana.

Experts are particularly concerned by the increase in daily or near daily use (defined as using marijuana at least 20 times in the previous 30 day period) among students in eighth, tenth, and twelfth grade. The National Institute of Drug Abuse conducts an annual nationwide study of eighth-, tenth-, and twelfth-grade students and young adults, known as the *Monitoring the Future Study*. The results track back to the 1970s, when marijuana use was at an all-time high. After a drastic dip, use started to climb again from 1992 to 1998. In 2010, roughly 15% of eighth graders, 27% of tenth graders, and 35% of twelfth graders had used marijuana in the past 12 months, with all three usage rates on a pattern of gradual incline (at rates of 1%, 3%, and 6%, respectively).

The Drug Abuse Warning Network, operated by the **Substance Abuse and Mental Health Services Administration** (SAMHSA), tracks data on emergency room admissions related to substance use, including cannabis. An estimated 376,467 people were admitted to U.S. emergency departments in 2009 as a result of marijuana use, with almost a third of patients under the age of 21

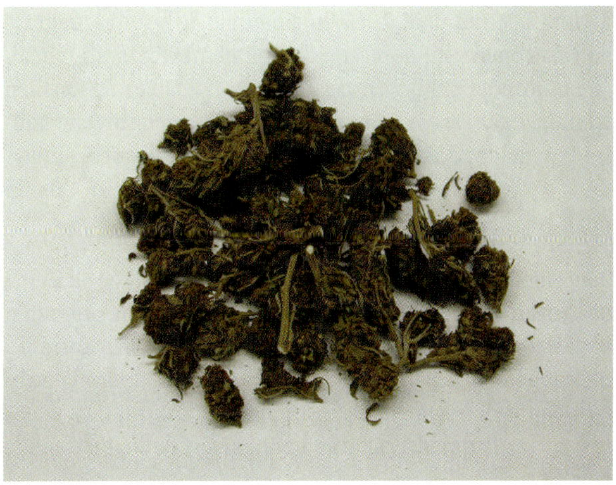

Cannabis (marijuana). *(U.S. Drug Enforcement Administration)*

Consequences of marijuana abuse

Acute (present during intoxication)

- Impairs short-term memory
- Impairs attention, judgment, and other cognitive functions
- Impairs coordination and balance
- Increases heart rate
- Psychotic episodes

Persistent (lasting longer than intoxication, but may not be permanent)

- Impairs memory and learning skills
- Sleep impairment

Long-term (cumulative effects of chronic abuse)

- Can lead to addiction
- Increases risk of chronic cough, bronchitis
- Increases risk of schizophrenia in vulnerable individuals
- May increase risk of anxiety, depression, and amotivational syndrome*

*These are often reported co-occurring symptoms/disorders with chronic marijuana use. However, research has not yet determined whether marijuana is causal or just associated with these mental problems.

SOURCE: U.S. Department of Health and Human Services, National Institute on Drug Abuse, "Marijuana Abuse," *Research Report Series*, September 2010.

(Table by PreMediaGlobal. Reproduced by permission of Gale, a part of Cengage Learning.)

(109,967). (However, it should be noted that amounts may include the use of marijuana with another drug.)

Description

Cannabis—in the form of marijuana, hashish (a dried resinous material that seeps from cannabis leaves and is more potent than marijuana), or other cannabinoids—is considered the most commonly used illegal substance in the world. Its effects have been known for thousands of years and were described as early as the fifth century B.C., when the Greek historian Herodotus told of a tribe of nomads who, after inhaling the smoke of roasted hemp seeds, emerged from their tent excited and shouting for joy.

Cannabis is a short form of the Latin name for the hemp plant, *Cannabis sativa*. All parts of the plant contain psychoactive substances, with THC making up the highest percentage. The most potent parts are the flowering tops and the dried, blackish-brown residue that comes from the leaves known as "hashish" or "hash."

There are more than 200 slang terms for marijuana, including "pot," "herb," "weed," "Mary Jane," "grass," "tea," and "ganja." It is usually chopped and/or shredded and rolled into a cigarette or "joint," or is placed in a pipe or a water pipe and smoked. One alternative method of using marijuana involves adding it to foods and eating it, such as baking it into brownies. It can also be brewed as a tea. Marijuana is also used in "blunts"—cigarettes emptied of their tobacco content and filled with a combination of marijuana and another drug such as crack **cocaine**.

Between 1840 and 1900, European and American medical journals published numerous articles on the therapeutic uses of marijuana. It was recommended as an appetite stimulant, muscle relaxant, painkiller, sedative, and anticonvulsant. As late as 1913, Sir William Osler recommended it highly for treatment of migraine. Public opinion changed, however, as alternative medications such as aspirin, opiates, and **barbiturates** became available. In 1937, the United States passed the Marijuana Tax Act, which made the drug essentially impossible to obtain for medical purposes.

The debate over the use of marijuana as a medicine continues today. THC is known to successfully treat nausea caused by cancer treatment drugs, stimulate the appetites of persons diagnosed with acquired immune deficiency syndrome (AIDS), and possibly assist in the treatment of glaucoma. Its use as a medicinal agent is still, however, highly controversial. As of 2011, medical marijuana was legally available in sixteen states: Alaska, Arizona, California, Colorado, District of Columbia, Delaware, Hawaii, Maine, Michigan, Montana, Nevada, New Jersey, New Mexico, Oregon, Rhode Island, Vermont, and Washington. Possession limits and ability to cultivate at home vary by state.

Cannabis use is generally perceived as benign, but a number of concerning research studies suggest that it has some potentially serious side effects. In addition to the known side effect of amotivational syndrome, some studies have shown an increased risk of psychotic disorders among cannabis users. While these associations have been demonstrated, causality is still unclear. The question remains as to whether individuals with these disorders are more likely to use cannabis, or whether individuals who use cannabis have a potentially higher risk of developing these disorders.

Cannabis-related disorders reflect the problematic use of cannabis products to varying degrees. These disorders include:

- Cannabis dependence—the compulsive need to use the drug, coupled with problems associated with chronic drug use.
- Cannabis abuse—periodic use that may cause legal problems; problems at work, home, or school; or danger when driving.
- Cannabis intoxication—the direct effects of acute cannabis use and reactions that accompany it, such as feeling "high," euphoria, sleepiness, lethargy, impairment in

short-term memory, stimulated appetite, impaired judgment, distorted sensory perceptions, impaired motor performance, and other symptoms.

Causes and symptoms

Causes

Cannabis-related disorders share many of the same root causes with disorders related to other addictive substances. The initial desire for a "high," combined with the widely held perception that cannabis use is not dangerous, often leads to experimentation in the teen years. It is believed that the greater availability, higher potency, and lower price of cannabis in recent years have all contributed to the increase in cannabis-related disorders.

Symptoms

CANNABIS DEPENDENCE AND ABUSE. The handbook used by mental health professionals to diagnose mental disorders is the ***Diagnostic and Statistical Manual of Mental Disorders***, also known as the *DSM-IV-TR*. This manual states that the central features of cannabis dependence are compulsive use, tolerance of its effects, and withdrawal symptoms. Use may interfere with family, school, and work, and may cause legal problems.

Regular cannabis smokers may show many of the same respiratory symptoms as tobacco smokers. These include daily cough and phlegm, chronic bronchitis, and more frequent chest colds. Marijuana smoke is known to contain 50%–70% more carcinogens than tobacco smoke. Continued use can lead to abnormal functioning of the lung tissue, which may be injured or destroyed by the cannabis smoke.

Recent research indicates that smoking marijuana has the potential to cause severe increases in heart rate and blood pressure, particularly if combined with cocaine use. Even with marijuana use alone, however, during one study the heart rate of subjects increased an average of 29 beats per minute when smoking marijuana. Additionally, heart attack risk is increased fourfold within the first hour of smoking marijuana.

A study of heavy marijuana users has shown that critical skills related to attention, memory, and learning can be impaired, even after use is discontinued for at least 24 hours. Compared to light users, heavy users made more errors on tasks and had more difficulty sustaining attention and shifting attention when required. They also had more difficulty registering, processing, and using information. These findings suggest that the greater impairment in mental functioning among heavy users is most likely due to an alteration of **brain** activity directly produced by the marijuana use.

Recent studies have found that babies born to mothers who used marijuana during pregnancy were smaller than those born to non-using mothers. Smaller babies are more likely to develop health problems. Additionally, nursing mothers who use marijuana pass some of the THC to the babies in their breast milk. Research shows that use of marijuana during the first month of breast-feeding can impair an infant's motor development.

Cannabis abuse is characterized by less frequent use and less severe problems. However, as with cannabis dependence, abuse can interfere with performance at school or work, cause legal problems, and interfere with motor activities such as driving or operating machinery; fatal traffic accidents are more common among individuals testing positive for cannabis use.

CANNABIS INTOXICATION. Cannabis intoxication refers to the occurrence of problematic behaviors or psychological changes that develop during, or shortly after, cannabis use. Intoxication usually starts with a "high" feeling followed by euphoria, inappropriate laughter, and feelings of grandiosity. Other symptoms include sedation, lethargy, impaired short-term memory, difficulty with motor tasks, impaired judgment, distorted sensory perceptions, and the feeling that time is passing unusually slowly. Sometimes severe anxiety, feelings of **depression**, or social withdrawal may occur. Along with these symptoms, common signs of cannabis intoxication include red eyes, increased appetite, dry mouth, and increased heart rate. Sometimes continued use is associated with weight gain as a result of increased appetite.

CANNABIS WITHDRAWAL. Recent research challenges the notion that cannabis use is not physically addictive. In fact, "cannabis withdrawal disorder" is a proposed addition for the fifth edition of the *DSM* (*DSM-5*, 2013). According to the NIDA, daily cannabis users experience withdrawal symptoms including irritability, stomach pain, aggression, and anxiety. Many frequent cannabis users are believed to continue using in order to avoid these unpleasant symptoms. Long-term use may lead to changes in the brain similar to those seen with long-term use of other addictive substances.

Diagnosis

Diagnosis of cannabis-related disorders is made in a number of ways. Intoxication is easiest to diagnose because of clinically observable signs, including reddened eye membranes, increased appetite, dry mouth, and increased heart rate. It is also diagnosed by the presence of problematic behavioral or psychological changes, such as impaired motor coordination, judgment, anxiety, euphoria, and social withdrawal. Occasionally, panic attacks may occur, and there may be impairment of short-term memory. Lowered immune system resistance, lowered testosterone levels in males, and chromosomal damage may also occur. Psychologically, chronic use of marijuana has been associated with a loss of ambition known as "amotivational syndrome."

Cannabis use is often paired with the use of other addictive substances, especially **nicotine**, alcohol, and cocaine. Marijuana may be mixed and smoked with opiates, phencyclidine (PCP or angel dust), or hallucinogenic drugs. Individuals who regularly use cannabis often report physical and mental lethargy and an inability to experience pleasure when not intoxicated (known as anhedonia). If taken in sufficiently high dosages, cannabinoids have psychoactive effects similar to **hallucinogens** such as lysergic acid diethylamide (LSD), and individuals using high doses may experience adverse effects that resemble hallucinogen-induced "bad trips." Paranoid ideation is another possible effect of heavy use, and, occasionally, hallucinations and **delusions** occur. Highly intoxicated individuals may feel as if they are outside their body (**depersonalization**) or as if what they are experiencing isn't real (derealization).

Urine tests can usually identify metabolites of cannabinoids. Because cannabinoids are fat soluble, they remain in the body for extended periods. Individuals who have used cannabis may show positive urine tests for as long as two to four weeks after using. Tests that analyze strands of hair can detect past marijuana use over an even longer period, up to three months. Examination of the nasopharynx and bronchial lining may also show clinical changes due to cannabis use.

Treatment

Treatment options for individuals with cannabis-related disorders are identical to those available for people with alcohol and other **substance abuse** disorders. The goal of treatment is abstinence. Treatment approaches range from inpatient **hospitalization**, drug and alcohol rehabilitation facilities, and various outpatient programs. Twelve-step programs such as Narcotics Anonymous are also treatment options. For heavy users experiencing withdrawal symptoms, treatment with antianxiety and/or antidepressant medications may assist in the treatment process.

Prognosis

According to the *DSM-IV-TR*, cannabis dependence and abuse tend to develop over a period of time. They may, however, develop more rapidly among young people with other emotional problems. Most people who become dependent begin using regularly. Over time, both frequency and amount increase. With chronic use, there can be a decrease in, or loss of, the pleasurable effects of the substance, along with increased feelings of anxiety and/or depression. As with alcohol and nicotine, cannabis use tends to begin early in the course of substance abuse, and many people later go on to develop dependence on other illicit substances. Because of this, cannabis has been referred to as a "gateway" drug, although this view is highly controversial, as not all cannabis users advance to other drugs. There is much that remains unknown about the social, psychological, and neurochemical basis of drug-use progression, and it is unclear whether marijuana use actually causes individuals to go on to use other illicit substances.

One of the long-term effects of chronic use has been termed "amotivational syndrome." This refers to the observation that many heavy, chronic users seem unambitious in relation to school and/or career. More serious consequences of cannabis use involve the acute or chronic development of psychotic or mood disorders. Some studies have suggested an association between cannabis use and sudden-onset **psychosis**, **schizophrenia**, or **bipolar disorder**, or an increased chance of **relapse** of an already-established psychiatric disorder. While a causative link has not been proven, there is some concern that cannabis use could either unmask a genetic predisposition for these psychiatric disorders or precipitate a relapse in vulnerable individuals.

Prevention

Many drug-education programs focus strongly on discouraging marijuana experimentation among young teenagers. A study reported by the NIDA indicated that high-sensation seekers—individuals who seek out new, emotionally intense experiences and are willing to take risks to obtain these experiences—are at greater risk for using marijuana and other drugs, and for using them at an earlier age. To counter this risk, the NIDA developed a series of dramatic public service announcements (PSAs) for national television that aired during programs that would appeal to high-sensation seekers, such as action-oriented television shows. The PSAs were aired in a limited television area, and the results were monitored. Marijuana use declined substantially among teens in these areas during the PSA campaigns, and long-term effects were shown for several months afterwards. In one county, marijuana use decreased by 38%, and in another, by 26.7%.

Other initiatives in prevention include drug-education programs like the D.A.R.E. (Drug Awareness and

Resistance Education) program, which targets fifth graders. D.A.R.E. and other antidrug programs focus on peer pressure resistance and the use of older teens who oppose drug use as models of a drug-free lifestyle. These programs show mixed results.

Resources

BOOKS

American Psychiatric Association. *Diagnostic and Statistical Manual of Mental Disorders*. 4th ed., text rev. Washington, DC: American Psychiatric Association, 2000.

Emmett, David, and Graeme Nice. *What You Need to Know about Cannabis: Understanding the Facts*. London; Philadelphia: Jessica Kingsley Publishers, 2009.

Maisto, Stephen A., Mark Galizio, and Gerard J. Connors. *Drug Use and Abuse*. 6th ed. Belmont, CA: Wadsworth, Cengage Learning, 2011. See esp. chap. 11, "Marijuana."

Schuckit, Marc A. *Drug and Alcohol Abuse: A Clinical Guide to Diagnosis and Treatment*. 6th ed. New York: Springer, 2010.

PERIODICALS

"Adverse Effects of Cannabis." *Prescrire International* 20, no. 112 (January 2011): 18–23.

Allsop, D.J., et al. "The Cannabis Withdrawal Scale Development: Patterns and Predictors of Cannabis Withdrawal and Distress." *Drug and Alcohol Dependence* (July 2, 2011) [e-pub ahead of print].

Copeland, J., and W. Swift. "Cannabis Use Disorder: Epidemiology and Management." *International Review of Psychiatry* 21 (April 1, 2009): 96–103.

Fernández-Artamendi S., et al. "Cannabis and Mental Health." *Actas Españolas de Psiquiatría* 39, no. 3 (2011): 180–90.

McLaren, J., et al. "Assessing Evidence for a Causal Link between Cannabis and Psychosis: A Review of Cohort Studies." *International Journal of Drug Policy* 21, no. 1 (2010): 10–19.

WEBSITES

National Cannabis Prevention and Information Centre. "Cannabis Research" [monthly bibliography of resesarch articles related to cannabis]. http://ncpic.org.au/ncpic/publications/cannabis-research (accessed September 7, 2011).

Substance Abuse and Mental Health Services Administration (SAMHSA). "Drug Abuse Warning Network (DAWN)." http://dawninfo.samhsa.gov (accessed September 7, 2011).

University of Michigan. "Monitoring the Future: A Continuing Study of American Youth." http://monitoringthefuture.org (accessed September 7, 2011).

ORGANIZATIONS

American Council for Drug Education, 50 Jay St., Brooklyn, NY, 11201, (646) 505-2061, acde@phoenixhouse.org, http://www.acde.org.

Narcotics Anonymous, PO Box 9999, Van Nuys, CA, 91409, (818) 773-9999, Fax: (818) 700-0700, http://www.na.org.

National Cannabis Prevention and Information Centre (NCPIC), PO Box 684, Randwick NSW 2031, Australia +61 2 9385 0208, info@ncpic.org.au, http://ncpic.org.au.

National Institute on Drug Abuse, 6001 Executive Blvd., Rm. 5213, Bethesda, MD, 20892, (301) 442-1124; Spanish: (240) 221-4007, information@nida.nih.gov, http://www.nida.nih.gov.

National Organization for the Reform of Marijuana Laws (NORML), 1600 K St. NW, Washington, DC, 20006, (202) 483-5500, Fax: (202) 483-0057, norml@norml.org, http://norml.org.

Substance Abuse and Mental Health Services Administration, 1 Choke Cherry Rd., Rockville, MD, 20857, (877) SAMHSA-7 (726-4727), (800) 487-4889 (TTY), Fax: (240) 221-4292, SAMHSAInfo@samhsa.hhs.gov, http://www.samhsa.gov.

Barbara S. Sternberg, PhD
Rosalyn Carson-DeWitt, MD

Capgras syndrome

Definition

Capgras syndrome (CS) is a relatively rare delusion of negative identification in which the patient believes that an individual or individuals well-known to him or her is an almost identical physiological double. CS is also known as the "illusion of doubles" and the "illusion of false recognition."

Demographics

Reported cases of CS have focused on adults, although a few cases have been reported with younger adults. It was once thought that CS is a disorder occurring only in women. However, cases have also been reported in men.

CS is related to numerous underlying causes including central nervous system disorders, **dementia**, and **psychosis**. The demographics of CS vary with the underlying cause.

Description

Capgras syndrome was named for the French **psychiatrist** Jean Capgras in 1923. In CS, the object of the delusion is typically a person with whom the patient is either particularly familiar or has an emotional tie, however, cases have been reported of the delusion being extended to pets and even inanimate objects, such as letters or a teacup. The term "syndrome"—a group of symptoms characterizing a disorder—as applied to CS is misleading; CS is more accurately described as a symptom associated with multiple physiological and psychological disorders.

Causes and symptoms

The literature is divided as to whether CS is psychological or physiological in nature. Historically, CS was thought to be a purely psychological condition. More recently, however, the focus has shifted, and CS is now considered by many clinicians to be a disorder of the central nervous system. It is estimated that between 21% and 40% of CS cases stem from physiological disorders including dementia, head **trauma**, epilepsy, and cerebrovascular disease. Neuroimaging data suggest a link between CS and abnormalities of the right hemisphere of the **brain**. In fact, the literature supports the conclusion that CS can be a symptom of virtually any central nervous system disorder.

CS has been observed in association with various systemic illnesses including vitamin B12 deficiency, chicken encephalitis, and diseases of the thyroid, parathyroid, and liver. CS has also been found associated with the use of various drugs, including morphine and **diazepam** (Valium). CS has been observed following transient physiological disturbances such as pneumocystis pneumonia in an HIV-positive patient, migraine headache, overdose of a bronchial dilator containing **adrenaline** and adropinemethonitrate, and interictal psychosis of epilepsy.

Diagnosis

Most clinicians regard CS as a symptom associated with numerous underlying causes rather than a syndrome in the classical sense of the term. **Diagnosis** should be based on psychological and personality testing as well as neuroradiological testing to determine the underlying cause rather than relying purely on behavioral descriptions.

CS can occur at any time during a psychosis and is not currently considered to be an essential element of any psychological disorder. It is impossible to predict the occurrence of CS based on the course of the overall psychopathology.

Treatment

CS is typically treated with a combination of antipsychotic medication and supportive psychological therapy in which stronger areas of mental and behavioral processes are used to overcome weaker areas of functioning. Patients presenting with CS stemming from psychosis have been found to improve on **pimozide** even when nonresponsive to **haloperidol**. CS stemming from physiological causes is best treated by treating the underlying disorder.

KEY TERMS

Central nervous system—The brain and spinal cord.

Delusion—A false idea held despite all evidence to the contrary.

Dementia—Deterioration of intellect, reasoning ability, memory, and will resulting from organic brain disease.

Interictal—Occurring between seizures.

Psychosis—A mental illness that markedly interferes with the patient's ability to deal with the demands of everyday life. Psychosis is characterized by loss of contact with reality, often accompanied by delusions and hallucinations.

Prognosis

The symptoms of CS have been found in most, but not all, cases to clear shortly after the remission of the psychosis. In the case of **depression**, however, the symptoms of CS persist longer than those of other syndromes of doubles (syndrome of Frégoli, syndrome of intermetamorphosis, syndrome of subjective doubles). The symptoms of CS invariably recur when there is a **relapse** of the basic psychotic condition with which they were associated.

Prevention

CS is an uncommon occurrence associated with a range of disorders both psychological and physiological in nature. Prevention of CS is actually a question of preventing the underlying disorder resulting in CS. There are no investigations under way concerning the prevention of CS.

Resources

BOOKS

Fewtrell, David, and Kieron O'Connor. "Capgras Syndrome and Delusions of Misidentification." in *Clinical Phenomenology and Cognitive Psychology*. New York: Routledge, 1995.

PERIODICALS

Devavrat, Joshi, et al. "Capgras Syndrome in Postictal Delirium." *Psychiatry* 7, no. 3 (March 2010) 37–39.

Ruth A. Wienclaw, PhD

Carbamazepine

Definition

Carbamazepine is an anticonvulsant that is structurally related to tricyclic **antidepressants** such as **amitriptyline** and **imipramine**. In the United States, carbamazepine is sold under the trade names Tegretol and Carbatrol.

Purpose

Carbamazepine is effective in the treatment of psychomotor and grand mal **seizures** and a type of facial pain called trigeminal neuralgia and, in combination with other drugs, for psychiatric disorders such as mania and extreme aggression. Carbamazepine is also occasionally used to control pain in persons with cancer.

Description

Carbamazepine was first marketed as an antiseizure medication and as a first-line treatment for trigeminal neuralgia. Because it was later noted to be effective in patients with certain psychiatric disorders, psychiatrists began combining it with other drugs such as lithium and major tranquilizers in severe cases of bipolar disease and aggressive behavior that could not be managed with single-drug therapy.

Carbamazepine is available in 100 mg chewable tablets, 200 mg capsules, and a suspension at 100 mg per 5 mL of liquid.

Recommended dosage

When used to treat seizure disorders or psychiatric disease, the recommended initial dosage of carbamazepine is 200 mg two times each day. The effectiveness of carbamazepine may decline with time, so if needed, the daily dosage may be increased by 200 mg once each week. Total daily dosages should not exceed 1,000 mg in children between the ages of 12 and 15 years. Total daily dosages for adults should not exceed 1,200 mg. Carbamazepine doses should be taken with meals.

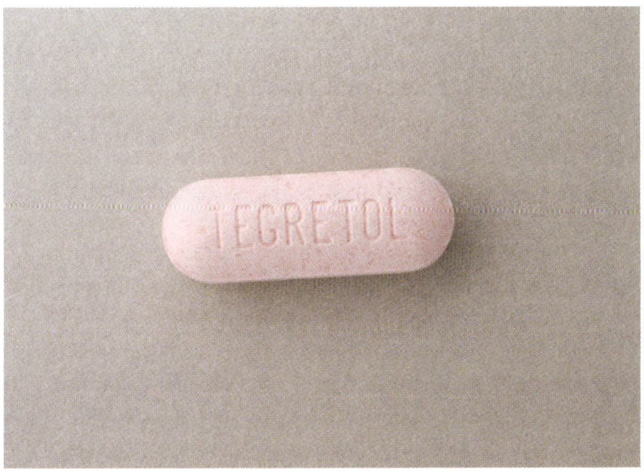

Carbamazepine, 200 mg. *(© Custom Medical Stock Photo, Inc. Reproduced by permission.)*

Precautions

Because carbamazepine may affect mental alertness, especially early in therapy, patients receiving this drug should be cautioned about operating dangerous machinery or driving a car until the drug's effects can be fully evaluated.

Carbamazepine should be used with caution in persons who also experience other types of seizure disorders such as atypical absence seizures. Among such individuals, carbamazepine usage has been associated with an increased risk of initiating, rather than controlling, generalized convulsions.

Carbamazepine should never be discontinued abruptly unless another treatment for seizures is initiated at the same time. If this does not happen, acute withdrawal of carbamazepine may result in seizures.

Carbamazepine has been reported to cause aplastic anemia, which generally does not respond to treatment. The bone marrow of persons with aplastic anemia does not produce adequate amounts of red blood cells, white blood cells, and platelets. Blood counts should be monitored in individuals using this drug. Some people with previously diagnosed **depression** of the bone marrow should not take carbamazepine. Patients should also be alert for signs and symptoms of bone marrow toxicity such as fever, sore throat, infection, mouth sores, easy bruising, or bleeding which occurs just under the skin.

Carbamazepine may cause birth defects and should be avoided by women who are pregnant. An effective contraceptive method should be used by sexually active women who are taking carbamazepine. It is important to note that this medication may decrease the effectiveness of oral contraceptives. The drug can cross into breast milk and should be avoided by women who are breast-feeding.

Side effects

The most commonly reported adverse reactions to carbamazepine are dizziness, drowsiness, unsteadiness, nausea, and vomiting. These are more common when therapy is just beginning. Carbamazepine may also cause a skin rash or sensitivity to the sun as well as blurred vision.

Interactions

Blood levels of carbamazepine may be reduced when it is used in combination with other drugs such as phenobarbital, phenytoin, or primidone. This means that inadequate amounts of carbamazepine are available to the body, limiting the ability of the drug to control seizure activity or treat psychiatric disease. Carbamazepine also causes reductions in the blood levels of the following drugs when they are used simultaneously: phenytoin, warfarin, doxycycline, **haloperidol**, **valproic acid**, and theophylline.

The simultaneous administration of carbamazepine with erythromycin, cimetidine, propoxyohene, isoniacid, **fluoxetine** and calcium channel blockers such as nifedipine and verapamil may increase the blood level of carbamazepine to a toxic range.

The simultaneous use of carbamazepine and oral contraceptives may increase the possibility that the oral contraceptive will not be effective in preventing pregnancy. Some physicians recommend that a different method of contraception be used while carbamazepine is being taken.

People taking carbamazepine should not drink grapefruit juice. Grapefruit juice slows the breakdown of carbamazepine, increasing the concentration of carbamazepine in the bloodstream.

Due to the potential of many interactions with other drugs, individuals should consult with a physician or pharmacist prior to starting any new medications either bought over the counter or initiated by another physician.

Resources

BOOKS

El-Mallakh, Rif S. "Lithium and Antiepileptic Drugs in Bipolar Depression." In *Bipolar Depression: A Comprehensive Guide*. Washington, DC: American Psychiatric Publishing, 2006.

Foreman, John C., and Torben Johansen. *Textbook of Receptor Pharmacology*. 2nd ed. Boca Raton, FL: CRC Press, 2002.

Page, Clive P., et al. *Integrated Pharmacology*. 3rd ed. St. Louis, MO: Elsevier, 2006.

Preston, John D., John H. O'Neal, and Mary C. Talaga. *Handbook of Clinical Psychopharmacology for Therapists*. 5th ed. Oakland, CA: New Harbinger Publications, 2008.

PERIODICALS

Bowden, Charles L., and Nancy U. Karren. "Anticonvulsants in Bipolar Disorder." *Australian and New Zealand Journal of Psychiatry* 40, no. 5 (May 2006): 386–93.

Cepeda, M. Soledad, and John T. Farrar. "Economic Evaluation of Oral Treatments for Neuropathic Pain." *Journal of Pain* 7, no. 2 (February 2006): 119–28.

DeBattista, Charles, and Alan F. Schatzberg. "Psychotropic Dosing and Monitoring Guidelines." *Primary Psychiatry* 13, no. 6 (June 2006): 61–81.

El-Mallakh, Rif, et al. "Bipolar II Disorder: Current and Future Treatment Options." *Annals of Clinical Psychiatry* 18, no. 4 (October–December. 2006): 259–66.

Gamble, C., et al. "A Meta-Analysis of Individual Patient Responses to Lamotrigine or Carbamazepine Monotherapy." *Neurology* 66, no. 9 (May 9, 2006): 1310–17.

Gayatri, N. A., and J. H. Livingston. "Aggravation of Epilepsy by Anti-Epileptic Drugs." *Developmental Medicine and Child Neurology* 48, no. 5 (May 2006): 394–98.

Ginsberg, Lawrence D. "Carbamazepine Extended-Release Capsules Use in Bipolar Disorder: Efficacy and Safety in Adult Patients." *Annals of Clinical Psychiatry* 18 (Suppl. 1) (May 2006): 9–14.

———. "Outcomes and Length of Treatment with Carbamazepine Extended-Release Capsules in Bipolar Disorder." *Annals of Clinical Psychiatry* 18 (Suppl. 1) (May 2006): 15–18.

———. "Predictors of Response to Carbamazepine Extended-Release Capsules Treatment in Bipolar Disorder." *Annals of Clinical Psychiatry* 18 (Suppl. 1) (May 2006): 23–26.

———. "Safety of Carbamazepine Extended-Release Capsules in Bipolar Disorder Polypharmacy." *Annals of Clinical Psychiatry* 18 (Suppl. 1) (May 2006): 19–22.

Nasrallah, Henry A., Terence A. Ketter, and Amir H. Kalali. "Carbamazepine and Valproate for The treatment of Bipolar Disorder: A Review of the Literature." *Journal of Affective Disorders* 95, no. 1 (October 2006): 69–78.

Zhang, Zhang-Jin, et al. "Adjunctive Herbal Medicine with Carbamazepine for Bipolar Disorders: A Double-Blind, Randomized, Placebo-Controlled Study." *Journal of Psychiatric Research* 41, no. 3–4 (April–June 2007): 360–69.

ORGANIZATIONS

American Academy of Clinical Toxicology, 6728 Old McLean Village Dr., McLean, VA, 22101, (703) 556-9222, Fax: (703) 556-8729, admin@clintox.org, http://www.clintox.org.

American Psychiatric Association, 1000 Wilson Blvd., Ste. 1825, Arlington, VA, 22209-3901, (703) 907-7300, apa@psych.org, http://www.psych.org.

American Society for Clinical Pharmacology and Therapeutics, 528 N Washington St., Alexandria, VA, 22314, (703) 836-6981, info@ascpt.org, http://www.ascpt.org.

U.S. Food and Drug Administration, 10903 New Hampshire Ave., Silver Spring, MD, 20993-0002, (888) INFO-FDA (463-6332), http://www.fda.gov.

L. Fleming Fallon, Jr., MD, DrPH
Ruth A. Wienclaw, PhD

Carbatrol *see* **Carbamazepine**

CASE *see* **Clinical Assessment Scales for the Elderly**

Case management

Definition

Case management is a system for managing and delivering health care with the goal of improving the quality and continuity of care and decreasing cost. Case management includes coordinating all necessary medical and mental health care as well as any associated support services.

Purpose

Case management tries to enhance access to care and improve the continuity and efficiency of services. Depending on the specific setting and locale, case managers are responsible for a variety of tasks, ranging from linking clients to services to actually providing intensive clinical or rehabilitative programs. Case management consists of four specific functions, including assessment of need, care planning, implementation, and regular review, after which the cycle begins again. Other core functions include outreach to engage clients in services, assessing individual needs, arranging requisite support services (such as housing, benefit programs, job training, etc.), monitoring medication and use of services, and advocating for client rights and entitlements.

Case management is not a time-limited service, but is intended to be ongoing. Wrap-around case management refers to efforts that are made prior to hospital admission, throughout **hospitalization**, and continuing after discharge, providing support within all dimensions of the patient's life.

In particular, case management in mental health is intended to decrease the need for hospitalization or readmission after hospitalization; to help people reintegrate into the community after hospitalization; to improve **compliance** to complicated medical regimens, particularly among psychiatric patients; and to help with socialization and daily functioning. Providing these types of case management services to the chronically mentally ill is believed to be less taxing on the economy than repeated or lengthy hospitalizations, and ongoing research is exploring this premise.

Description

Over the past 50 years, there have been fundamental changes in the system of mental health care in the United States. In the 1950s, mental health care for people with severe and persistent mental illnesses (like **schizophrenia**, **bipolar disorder**, severe **depression**, and **schizoaffective disorder**) was provided almost exclusively by large public mental hospitals. Created as part of a reform movement, these state hospitals provided a wide range of basic life supports in addition to mental health treatment, including housing, meals, clothing, and laundry services, and varying degrees of social and **vocational rehabilitation**.

During the latter half of the same decade, the introduction of neuroleptic medication provided symptomatic management of seriously disabling psychoses. This breakthrough, along with other subsequent reforms in mental health policy (including the introduction of Medicare and Medicaid in 1965 and the Supplemental Security Income [SSI] program in 1974), provided incentives for policy makers to discharge patients to the community and transfer state mental health expenditures to the federal government.

These advances—coupled with new procedural safeguards for involuntary patients, court decisions establishing the right to treatment in the least restrictive setting, and changed philosophies of care—led to widespread **deinstitutionalization**.

As a result of deinstitutionalization policies, the number of patients discharged from hospitals has risen, and the average length of stay for newly admitted patients has decreased. An increasing number of patients are never admitted at all, but are diverted to a more complex and decentralized system of community-based care. Case management was designed to remedy the confusion created by multiple care providers in different settings, and to assure accessibility, continuity of care, and accountability for individuals with long-term disabling mental illnesses. In addition, legislation has mandated that patients be managed in the "least restrictive environment" (that is, within a community setting). This is believed to be both therapeutically and economically preferable.

Models of case management

The two models of case management mentioned most often in mental health literature are **assertive community treatment** (ACT) and intensive case management. A third model, clinical case management, refers to a program where the case manager assigned to a client also functions as their primary therapist.

ASSERTIVE COMMUNITY TREATMENT. The ACT model (referred to in other locations as PACT, or Program of Assertive Community Treatment) originated in an inpatient research unit at Mendota State Hospital in Madison, Wisconsin, in the late 1960s. The program's architects, Arnold Marx, MD, Leonard Stein, MD, and Mary Ann Test, PhD, sought to create a "hospital without walls." In this model, teams of 10–12 professionals—including case managers, a **psychiatrist**, nurses, **social workers**, and vocational specialists—are assigned ongoing responsibility 24 hours a day, 7 days a week, 365 days a year, for a caseload of approximately 10 clients with severe and persistent mental illnesses.

ACT uses multidisciplinary teams with low client-to-staff ratios, practices assertive outreach, provides in-vivo services (in the client's own setting) and **crisis intervention** (as necessary), emphasizes assisting clients in managing their illness, assists with activities of daily living (ADL) skills, and promotes relationship building, emotional support, and an orientation, whenever possible, toward providing clients with services rather than linking them to other providers.

Compared to other psychosocial interventions, the ACT program has a remarkably strong evidence base. Twenty-five randomized controlled **clinical trials** have demonstrated that these programs reduce hospitalization, **homelessness**, and inappropriate hospitalization; increase housing stability; control psychiatric symptoms; and improve quality of life, especially among individuals who are high users of mental health services. However, despite ACT's widespread acceptance and proven success, statewide programs had only been implemented in six states as of 2011.

INTENSIVE CASE MANAGEMENT. Intensive case management practices are typically targeted to individuals with the greatest service needs, including individuals with a history of multiple hospitalizations, people dually diagnosed with **substance abuse** problems, individuals with mental illness who have been involved with the criminal justice system, and individuals who are both homeless and severely mentally ill.

In 2000, Richard Schaedle and Irwin Epstein conducted a survey of 22 experts and found that although intensive case management shares many critical ingredients with ACT programs, its elements are not as clearly articulated. Another distinction between intensive case management and ACT appears to be that the latter relies more heavily on a team versus individual approach. In addition, intensive case managers are more likely to "broker" treatment and rehabilitation services rather than provide them directly. Finally, intensive case management programs are more likely to focus on client strengths, empowering clients to fully participate in all treatment decisions.

CLINICAL CASE MANAGEMENT. A meta-analytic study comparing ACT and clinical case management found that although the generic approach resulted in increased hospital admissions, it significantly decreased the length of stay. This suggests that the overall impact of clinical case management is positive. Consistent with prior research, the study concluded that both ACT and high-quality clinical case management should be essential features of any mental health service system. One of the greatest tragedies of deinstitutionalization has been that most families often become de facto case managers for their family members, without any training or support. In recent years, many case management programs have expanded their teams to successfully utilize consumers as peer counselors and family members as outreach workers. The programs have also been adapted to serve older individuals with severe and persistent mental illnesses. While the ACT model offers the strongest evidential base for its effectiveness, research into the clinical and service system outcomes of this and other models of case management is ongoing.

Case management for children and adolescents

Case management is also used to coordinate care for children with serious emotional disturbances—diagnosed mental health problems that substantially disrupt a child's ability to function socially, academically, and emotionally. Although not a formal **diagnosis** in the ***Diagnostic and Statistical Manual of Mental Disorders*** (*DSM*), the handbook published by the **American Psychiatric Association** and used by mental health professionals to diagnose mental disorders, the term "serious emotional disturbance" is commonly used by states and the federal government to identify children with the greatest service needs. Although the limited research on case management for children and youth with serious emotional disturbances has been primarily focused on service use rather than clinical outcomes, there is growing evidence that case management is an effective **intervention** for this population.

Case management models used for children vary considerably. One model, called "wraparound," helps families develop a plan to address the child's individual needs across multiple life domains (home and school, for example). Research on the effectiveness of this model is still in an early stage. Another model, known as the children and youth intensive case management or expanded broker model, had been evaluated in two controlled studies. Findings suggest that this broker/advocacy model results in behavioral improvements and fewer days in hospital settings.

Funding

The effectiveness of any case management program depends upon the availability of high-quality treatment and support services in a given community, the structure

KEY TERMS

Bipolar disorder—A mood disorder marked by alternating episodes of extremely low mood (depression) and exuberant highs (mania). Also known as manic–depression disorder.

De facto—Acting as; fulfilling a role, even though the occupation of the role is not legally recognized.

Schizophrenia—A severe mental illness in which a person has difficulty distinguishing what is real from what is not real. It is often characterized by hallucinations, delusions, and withdrawal from people and social activities.

and coordination of the service system, and on the ability of an individual or family to pay for care either through private insurance or (more often) through public benefit and entitlement programs. Though the Centers for Medicaid and Medicare Services previously permitted the use of Medicaid funds for ACT, the program has since changed its policies regarding all of the types of services that have fallen under the title of "case management." Medicaid has limited its definition of reimbursable services to exclude direct service provision. Reimbursable services are restricted to assessment, planning, referrals, and monitoring of service delivery. This backlash has extended to the types of case management referred to as "community support." These types of services are also excluded for payment under Medicaid, due to an inability to exercise sufficient cost containment or verification. As a result, some community programs continue to operate under various time-limited grants, but their funding is constantly threatened. Ongoing research is attempting to prove both therapeutic efficacy and financial economy of these types of programs, in an effort to secure more stable support for the expansion and support. Possible financial benefits include the savings realized from keeping patients out of jails, hospitals, and emergency rooms. Compared to traditional outpatient programs, case management also offers a level of care that is far more comprehensive and humane for treating persons with mental illness.

Resources

BOOKS

Lloyd, Chris, Robert King, Frank Deane, and Kevin Gournay, eds. *Clinical Management in Mental Health Services*. Oxford, UK: Wiley-Blackwell, 2009.

Longhofer, Jeffrey, Paul M. Kubek, and Jerry Floersch. *On Being and Having a Case Manager*. New York: Columbia University Press, 2010.

Rapp, Charles A., and Richard J. Goscha. *The Strength Model: Case Management and People with Psychiatric Disabilities* New York: Oxford University Press, 2006.

PERIODICALS

Angell, Beth, and Colleen Mahoney. "Reconceptualizing the Case Management Relationship in Intensive Treatment: A Study of Staff Perceptions and Experiences." *Adminstration and Policy in Mental Health and Mental Health Services Research* 34, no. 2 (2007): 172–88.

Rosenthal, David A., et al. "A Survey of Current Disability Management Practice: Emerging Trends and Implications for Certification." *Rehabilitation Counseling Bulletin* 50, no. 2 (2007): 76–86.

Shattell M. "Assertive Community Treatment and the Physical Health Needs of Persons with Severe Mental Illness: Issues around Integration of Mental Health and Physical Health." *Journal of American Psychiatric Nurses Association* 34, no. 2 (2011): 57–63.

Wright-Berryman, J. "A Review of Consumer-provided Services on Assertive Community Treatment and Intensive Case Management Teams: Implications for Future Research and Practice." *Journal of American Psychiatric Nurses Association* 17 (2011): 37–44.

WEBSITES

National Alliance on Mental Illness. "Assertive Community Treatment (ACT)." http://www.nami.org/about/pact.htm (accessed September 7, 2011).

ORGANIZATIONS

Assertive Community Treatment Association, PO Box 2428, Brighton, MI, 48116, (810) 227-1859, Fax: (810) 227-5785, acta@actassociation.org, http://www.actassociation.org.

Irene S. Levine, PhD
Ruth A. Wienclaw, PhD
Rosalyn Carson-DeWitt

CAT *see* **Children's Apperception Test**

Catapres *see* **Clonidine**

Catatonia

Definition

Associated with a large number of serious mental and physical illnesses, catatonia is a condition marked by changes in muscle tone or activity. Two distinct sets of symptoms are characteristic of this condition. In catatonic stupor, the individual experiences a deficit of motor (movement) activity that can render him/her motionless.

KEY TERMS

Barbiturates—A group of medicines that slow breathing and lower the body temperature and blood pressure. They can be habit forming and are now used chiefly for anesthesia.

Benzodiazepines—A group of medicines that help reduce anxiety (especially before surgery) and to help people sleep.

Electroconvulsive therapy—A therapy used to treat major depression and severe mental illness that does not respond to medications. A measured dose of electricity is introduced into the brain in order to produce a convulsion. Electroconvulsive therapy is safe and effective.

Mutism—The inability or refusal to speak.

Negativism—Behavior characterized by resistance, opposition, and refusal to cooperate with requests, even the most reasonable ones.

Neuroleptic drugs—Antipsychotic drugs, including major tranquilizers, used in the treatment of psychoses such as schizophrenia.

Catatonic excitement, or excessive movement, is associated with violent behavior directed toward oneself or others.

Demographics

According to the ***Diagnostic and Statistical Manual of Mental Disorders***, fourth edition, text revision (*DSM-IV-TR*) between 5% and 9% of all psychiatric inpatients show some catatonic symptoms. Of these, 25–50% are associated with mood disorders, 10–15% are associated with **schizophrenia**, and the remainder are associated with other mental disorders.

Description

Catatonia is described in the *DSM-IV-TR,* as having what may seem like contradictory symptoms. In catatonic stupor, motor activity may be reduced to zero. Patients diagnosed with a catatonic disorder may maintain their body position for hours, days, weeks, or even months at a time. Individuals avoid bathing and grooming, make little or no eye contact with others, may be mute and rigid, and initiate no social behaviors. In catatonic excitement, the individual is extremely hyperactive, although the activity seems to have no purpose. Violence toward him/herself or others may be seen.

Catatonia can be categorized as intrinsic or extrinsic. If the condition has an identifiable cause, it is designated as extrinsic. If no cause can be determined following physical examination, laboratory testing, and history taking, the illness is considered to be intrinsic.

Features of catatonia may also be seen in **neuroleptic malignant syndrome** (NMS), which is an uncommon (but potentially lethal) reaction to some medications used to treat major mental illnesses, specifically antipsychotic drugs such as **haloperidol** (Haldol). NMS is considered a medical emergency since 25% of untreated cases result in death. Catatonia can also be present in individuals who may have a number of other physical and emotional conditions such as drug intoxication, **depression**, and schizophrenia. It is most commonly associated with mood disorders.

Depression with catatonic features

Individuals who are severely depressed may show disturbances of motor behavior; they may be essentially immobile or exhibit excessive but seemingly random motor activity. Extreme negativism, elective mutism (choosing not to speak), peculiar movements, mimicking words or phrases, or mimicking movements may also be part of the picture. In their most extreme forms, catatonic stupor and catatonic excitement may necessitate supervision so that the individual does not hurt him- or herself or others. Catatonic behaviors may also be seen in persons with other mood disorders, such as manic or mixed-mood states; these are also known as bipolar I and bipolar II disorders.

Catatonic schizophrenia

The catatonic type of schizophrenia is characterized by severe psychomotor disturbance. Individuals with this disorder show extreme immobility. They may stay in the same position for hours, days, weeks, or longer. The position they assume may be unusual and appear uncomfortable to the observer. If another person moves part of the catatonic individual's body, such as a limb, he or she may maintain the position into which they are placed, a condition known as "waxy flexibility." Sometimes catatonia presents itself as excessive motor activity, but the activity seems purposeless and does not appear to fit with what is happening in the environment. In its most severe forms, whether stupor or excitement, the individual may need close supervision to keep from injuring him- or herself or others.

Catatonic disorder due to general medical condition

Individuals with catatonia due to a medical condition may show symptoms similar to persons with catatonic schizophrenia and catatonic depression. However, the cause is believed to be physiological. Certain infectious, metabolic, or neurological diseases, such as encephalitis, may cause catatonic symptoms that can be either temporary or permanent. They may also appear as side effects of various medications, including several drugs of abuse.

Causes and symptoms

The causes of catatonia are largely unknown, although research indicates that **brain** structure and function are altered in this condition. While this and other information point to a physical cause, none had been proven as of 2011. A variety of medical conditions also may lead to catatonia, including head **trauma**, cerebrovascular disease, encephalitis, and certain metabolic disorders. NMS is an adverse side effect of certain antipsychotic drugs.

A variety of symptoms are associated with catatonia. Among the more common are echopraxia (imitation of the gestures of others) and echolalia (parrot-like repetition of words spoken by others). Other signs and symptoms include violence directed toward one's self, the assumption of inappropriate posture, **selective mutism**, negativism, facial grimaces, and animal-like noises.

Catatonic stupor is marked by immobility and a behavior known as *cerea flexibilitas* (waxy flexibility), in which the individual can be made to assume bizarre (and sometimes painful) postures that they will maintain for extended periods. The individual may become dehydrated and malnourished because food and liquids are refused. In extreme situations such individuals must be fed through a tube. Catatonic excitement is characterized by hyperactivity and violence; the individual may harm him- or herself or others. On rare occasions, isolation or restraint may be needed to ensure the individual's safety and the safety of others.

Diagnosis

Recognition of catatonia is made on the basis of specific movement symptoms. These include odd ways of walking such as walking on tiptoes or ritualistic pacing and, rarely, hopping and skipping. Repetitive odd movements of the fingers or hands, as well as imitating the speech or movements of others also may indicate that catatonia is present. There are no laboratory or other tests that can be used to positively diagnose this condition, but medical and neurological tests are necessary to rule out underlying lesions or disorders that may be causing the observed symptoms.

Treatment

Treatment of catatonia includes medications such as **benzodiazepines** (which are the preferred treatment) and rarely **barbiturates**. Antipsychotic drugs may be appropriate in some cases but often cause catatonia to worsen. **Electroconvulsive therapy** may prove beneficial for clients who do not respond to medication. If these approaches are unsuccessful, treatment may be redirected to attempts to control the signs and symptoms of the illness.

QUESTIONS TO ASK YOUR DOCTOR

- What kinds of tests will you do to rule out an underlying medical reason for my loved one's catatonia?
- What precautions can I take to make sure my loved one does not injure himself or herself?
- Does my loved one need inpatient treatment?
- What are the side effects of the drugs you are prescribing for my loved one?
- How soon can I expect to see improvement?

Prognosis

Catatonia usually responds quickly to medication interventions.

Prevention

There is no known way to prevent catatonia, because the cause has not yet been identified. Research efforts continue to explore possible origins. Avoiding excessive use of neuroleptic drugs can help minimize the risk of developing catatonic-like symptoms.

Resources

BOOKS

American Psychiatric Association. *Diagnostic and Statistical Manual of Mental Disorders,* 4th ed., text rev. Washington, DC: American Psychiatric Association, 2000.

Black, Donald W., and Nancy C. Andreasen. *Introductory Textbook of Psychiatry,* 5th ed. Arlington, VA: American Psychiatric Publishing, 2011.

Fink, Max, and Michael Alan Taylor. *A Clinician's Guide to Diagnosis and Treatment.* New York: Cambridge University Press, 2003.

Frisch, Noreen Cavan, and Lawrence E. Frisch. *Psychiatric Mental Health Nursing,* 4th ed. Clifton Park, NY: Delmar Publishers, 2011.

WEBSITES

Brasic, James R. "Catatonia." Medscape Reference. October 8, 2010. http://emedicine.medscape.com/article/1154851-overview (accessed July 29, 2011).

ORGANIZATIONS

American Psychiatric Association, 1000 Wilson Blvd., Ste. 1825, Arlington, VA, 22209-3901, (703)907-7300, (888) 357-7924, apa@psych.org, http://www.psych.org.

Mental Health America, 2000 N Beauregard St., 6th Fl., Alexandria, VA, 22311, (703) 684-7722, (800) 969-6642, Fax: (703) 684-5968, http://www.nmha.org.

National Alliance on Mental Illness, 3803 N Fairfax Dr., Ste. 100, Arlington, VA, 22203, (703) 524-7600, (800) 950-6264, Fax: (703) 524-9094, http://www.nami.org.

National Institute of Mental Health, 6001 Executive Blvd., Rm. 8184, MSC 9663, Bethesda, MD, 20892-9663, (301) 443-4513, (866) 615-6464, Fax: (301) 443-4279, nimhinfo@nimh.gov, http://www.nimh.nih.gov.

Donald G. Barstow, RN
Tish Davidson, AM

Catatonic disorders

Definition

Catatonic disorders are a group of symptoms characterized by disturbances in motor (muscular movement) behavior that may have either a psychological or a physiological basis. The condition itself is called **catatonia**.

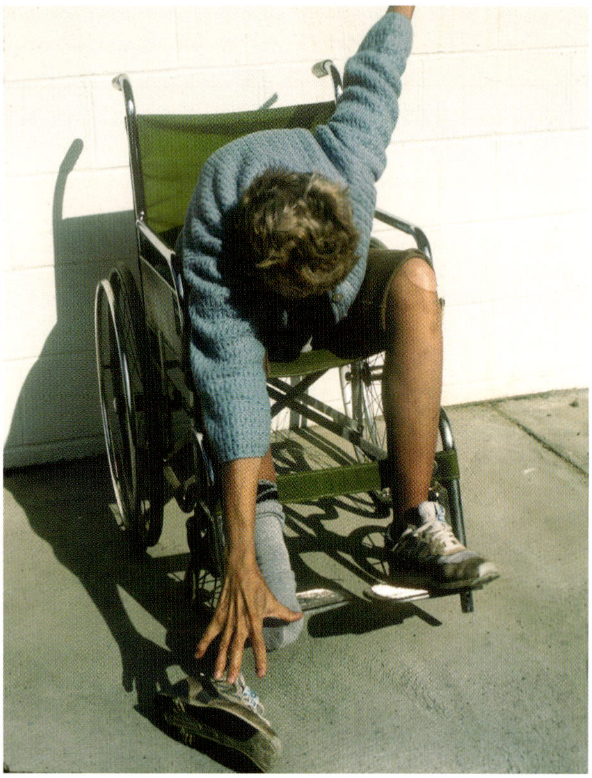

A patient with catatonic schizophrenia. *(© Photo Researchers, Inc.)*

Demographics

According to the ***Diagnostic and Statistical Manual of Mental Disorders***, fourth edition, text revision (*DSM-IV-TR*), between 5% and 9% of all psychiatric inpatients show some catatonic symptoms. Of these, 25%–50% are associated with mood disorders, 10%–15% are associated with **schizophrenia**, and the remainder are associated with other mental disorders. Catatonic symptoms also can occur in a wide variety of general medical conditions, including infectious, metabolic, and neurological disorders. They may also appear as side effects of various medications, including several drugs of abuse.

Description

The **psychiatrist** Karl Ludwig Kahlbaum first described catatonic symptoms in 1874. Kahlbaum described catatonia as a disorder characterized by unusual motor symptoms. His description of individuals with catatonic behaviors remains accurate to this day. Kahlbaum carefully documented the symptoms and the course of the illness, providing a natural history of this unusual disorder.

The *DSM-IV-TR* describes catatonia as having what may seem like contradictory symptoms. Catatonic stupor is characterized by slowed motor activity, often to the point of being motionless and appearing unaware of surroundings. Persons affected may hold their body in a single rigid position for hours, days, weeks, or even months at a time. People in semi-immobile catatonic states may allow a postural change and then "freeze" in the new posture, or may resist attempts at change. Patients may exhibit negativism, which means that they resist all attempts to be moved, or all instructions or requests to move, without any apparent motivation. In less severe situations, individuals may avoid bathing and grooming, make little or no eye contact with others, may be mute and rigid, and initiate no social behaviors. They may display a complete lack of verbalization, or echolalia (repeating or echoing heard phrases or sentences). In catatonic excitement, the condition can manifest as excessive movement and hyperactivity, such as frantic running up and down a flight of stairs or repetitive pacing. Individuals in the excited state may even try to harm themselves or others.

This range in symptoms may have its root in the fact that catatonia has a variety of causes. Because of this, catatonia is considered a condition, not a **diagnosis**. Some experts argue that, rather than being a discrete and describable classification, catatonia may instead be a collection of various illnesses without common specificities. Catatonia has been associated with a laundry list of disorders, including psychotic disorders, depressive disorders, dementias, and reactive disorders. In the *DSM*, catatonia is recognized as a symptom of schizophrenia, **schizophreniform disorder**, **schizoaffective disorder**, **psychosis**, **bipolar disorder**, depressive disorders, and general medical conditions.

DSM-IV types of catatonic disorder

CATATONIC SCHIZOPHRENIA. A characteristic of the disorders associated with schizophrenia is severe disturbance in motor behavior. Individuals with catatonic schizophrenia often show extreme immobility. They may stay in the same position for hours, days, weeks, or longer. The position they assume may be unusual and appear uncomfortable to the observer; for example, a person with catatonic schizophrenia may stand on one leg like a stork or hold one arm outstretched for a long time. If an observer moves a hand or limb of the catatonic person's body, he or she may maintain the new position. This condition is known as *cerea flexibilitas*, or waxy flexibility. In other situations, a person with catatonic schizophrenia may be extremely active, but the activity appears bizarre, purposeless, and unconnected to the situation or surroundings.

DEPRESSION WITH CATATONIC FEATURES. People who are severely depressed may show disturbances of motor behavior resembling those of patients diagnosed with catatonic schizophrenia. These people with **depression** may remain virtually motionless or move around in an extremely vigorous, but apparently random, fashion. Other parts of the symptomatic picture may include extreme negativism, elective mutism (choosing not to speak), peculiar movements, and echolalia or echopraxia (imitating another person's movements). These behaviors may require caregivers to supervise patients to ensure they do not harm themselves or others.

MOOD DISORDERS AND CATATONIA. Catatonic behaviors also may occur in people with other mood disorders. People experiencing manic or mixed mood states (a simultaneous combination of manic and depressive symptoms) may at times exhibit either the immobility or agitated random activity seen in catatonia.

CATATONIC DISORDER DUE TO A GENERAL MEDICAL CONDITION. People with catatonic disorder due to a medical condition show symptoms similar to those of catatonic schizophrenia and catatonic depression, except that the cause is believed to be related to an underlying medical condition. Neurological diseases such as encephalitis may cause catatonic symptoms that can be temporary or lasting. Overall, at least 35 distinct medical and neurological illnesses have been associated with catatonia. In addition to encephalitis, other common causative agents include structural damage to the central nervous system, metabolic disturbances, **seizures**, and exposure to some drugs.

DSM-5

Proposed changes for the fifth edition of the DSM (DSM-5, 2013) classify catatonia as a specifier for other conditions, including schizophrenia and mood disorders, rather than as its own diagnosis. The catatonia may also be of unknown origin or be related to **substance abuse** (such as in **substance-induced psychotic disorder**).

Causes and symptoms

Causes

The causes of catatonia are largely unknown, although research indicates that the brain's structure and function are altered in this condition. While this and other information point to a physical cause, none has yet been proven. Although the initiating factors of catatonia can vary greatly, research has hypothesized some common underlying mechanisms. There may be imbalances or problems in regulating signaling among nerves in the central nervous system, involving **neurotransmitters** (nerve signaling molecules) such as **dopamine** and **serotonin**. In addition, some **brain imaging studies** have found an enlarged cerebral cortex and reduced cerebellum in some people with catatonia, although this is not a consistent finding. People who have emerged from catatonic states report having had intense emotions, including uncontrollable anxiety and paralyzing fear. Others also report having experienced depression, euphoria, or aggression while in the catatonic state.

Symptoms

CATATONIC SCHIZOPHRENIA. Catatonic schizophrenia manifests with prominent motor symptoms and abnormalities. These symptoms, as given in the *DSM-IV-TR*, include:

- catalepsy, or motionlessness maintained over a long period of time
- catatonic excitement, marked by agitation and seemingly pointless movement
- catatonic stupor, with markedly slowed motor activity, often to the point of immobility and seeming unawareness of the environment
- catatonic rigidity, in which a rigid position is assumed and held against all outside efforts to change it
- catatonic posturing, in which a bizarre or inappropriate posture is assumed and maintained over a long period of time

KEY TERMS

Dopamine—A neurochemical made in the brain that is involved in many brain activities, including movement and emotion.

Neurotransmitter—One of a group of chemicals secreted by a nerve cell (neuron) to carry a chemical message to another nerve cell, often as a way of transmitting a nerve impulse. Examples of neurotransmitters include acetylcholine, dopamine, serotonin, and norepinephrine.

Serotonin—5-Hydroxytryptamine; a substance that occurs throughout the body with numerous effects including neurotransmission. Low serotonin levels are associated with mood disorders, particularly depression and obsessive-compulsive disorder.

- waxy flexibility, in which a limb or other body part of a catatonic person can be moved into another position that is then maintained (the body part is said to feel as if it were made of wax)
- akinesia, or absence of physical movement

DEPRESSION WITH CATATONIC FEATURES. Within the category of mood disorders, catatonic symptoms are most commonly associated with bipolar I disorder. Bipolar I disorder is a mood disorder involving periods of mania interspersed with depressive episodes. Symptoms of catatonic excitement, such as random activity unrelated to the environment or the repetition of words, phrases, and movements may occur during manic phases. Catatonic immobility may appear during the most severe phase of the depressive cycle. The actual catatonic symptoms are indistinguishable from those seen in catatonic schizophrenia. It is also possible for catatonic symptoms to occur in conjunction with other mood disorders, including bipolar II disorder (involving a milder form of mania called **hypomania**), mixed disorders (involving simultaneous mania and depression), and major depressive disorders.

CATATONIC DISORDER DUE TO GENERAL MEDICAL CONDITION. Symptoms of catatonic disorder caused by medical conditions are indistinguishable from those that occur in schizophrenia and mood disorders. Unlike individuals with schizophrenia, however, those with catatonic symptoms due to a medical condition demonstrate greater insight and awareness into their illness and symptoms. They have periods of clear thinking, and their **affect** (emotional response) is generally appropriate to the circumstances. Neither of these conditions is true of patients with schizophrenia or severe depression.

Diagnosis

Recognition of catatonia is made on the basis of specific movement symptoms. These include odd ways of walking, such as walking on tiptoes or ritualistic pacing, or, rarely, hopping and skipping. Repetitive odd movements of the fingers or hands or imitating the speech or movements of others also may indicate that catatonia is present. There are no laboratory or other tests that can be used to positively diagnose this condition, but medical and neurological tests are necessary to rule out underlying lesions or disorders that may be causing the observed symptoms.

Catatonic schizophrenia may be diagnosed when the patient's other symptoms include thought disorder, inappropriate affect, and a history of peculiar behavior and dysfunctional relationships. Catatonic symptoms associated with a mood disorder may be diagnosed when patients have a prior history of mood disorder or after careful psychiatric evaluation.

Treatment

Drugs

Treatment for catatonic symptoms can rely on drug-based approaches or on **electroconvulsive therapy** (ECT). **Benzodiazepines** (e.g., **lorazepam**) have often been the first-line treatment approach, although response to this therapy varies a great deal. One study has found that use of lorazepam was not effective in treating chronic catatonia, and there are other concerns about using benzodiazepines, including the fact that withdrawal from these drugs has itself been associated with inducing catatonia.

Other drugs that have been applied in cases of catatonia include antipsychotics. As with benzodiazepines, there are some concerns that the attempted cure could also be causative; these drugs have also been associated with precipitating catatonic episodes. However, the perceived reduction in rates of catatonic schizophrenia has accompanied the introduction and increasing use of these drugs.

Electroconvulsive therapy

ECT, or electroconvulsive therapy, elicits negative reactions from many people, as it involves the administration of an electric shock to the brain to precipitate a seizure. However, some psychiatrists maintain that it is a safe and effective approach and is an appropriate treatment for catatonia, especially if patients fail to respond adequately to drug therapy.

Prognosis

The prognosis for a person with catatonia varies with the cause underlying the disorder. With disorders such as

QUESTIONS TO ASK YOUR DOCTOR

- What kinds of tests will you do to rule out an underlying medical reason for my loved one's catatonia?
- What precautions can I take to make sure my loved one does not injure him/herself?
- Does my loved one need inpatient treatment?
- What are the side effects of the drugs you are prescribing?
- How soon can I expect to see improvement?

alcohol abuse disorder or affective disorder, the prognosis for resolution is relatively good; however, when catatonia accompanies schizophrenia, there is an association with earlier and higher levels of mortality. In one systematic review, the authors ranked associated catatonic disorders with their relative prognoses from best to worst, as follows: depression with catatonia, periodic catatonia, cycloid psychoses with catatonia, bipolar disorder with catatonia, catatonic schizophrenia, and non-catatonic schizophrenia. The choice of treatment also can influence prognosis.

Prevention

There are no specific preventive measures for most causes of catatonia. Infectious disease can sometimes be prevented. Catatonic symptoms caused by medications or drugs of abuse usually can be reversed by suspending use of the drug.

Resources

BOOKS

American Psychiatric Association. *Diagnostic and Statistical Manual of Mental Disorders*. 4th ed., text rev. Washington, DC: American Psychiatric Publishing, 2000.

Black, Donald W., and Nancy C. Andreasen. *Introductory Textbook of Psychiatry*. 5th ed. Arlington, VA: American Psychiatric Publishing, 2011.

Fink, Max, and Michael Alan Taylor. *A Clinician's Guide to Diagnosis and Treatment*. New York: Cambridge University Press, 2006.

Frisch, Noreen Cavan, and Lawrence E. Frisch. *Psychiatric Mental Health Nursing*. 4th ed. Farmington Hills, MI: Cengage Learning, 2011.

WEBSITES

Brasic, James R. "Catatonia." Medscape Reference. http://emedicine.medscape.com/article/1154851-overview (accessed October 1, 2011).

ORGANIZATIONS

American Psychiatric Association, 1000 Wilson Blvd., Ste. 1825, Arlington, VA, 22209-3901, (703) 907-7300, (888) 35-PSYCH (357-7924), apa@psych.org, http://www.psych.org.

Mental Health America, 2000 N Beauregard St., 6th Fl., Alexandria, VA, 22311, (703) 684-7722, (800) 969-6642, Fax: (703) 684-5968, http://www.nmha.org.

National Alliance on Mental Illness, 3803 N Fairfax Dr., Ste. 100, Arlington, VA, 22203, (703) 524-7600, (800) 950-NAMI (6264), Fax: (703) 524-9094, http://www.nami.org.

National Institute of Mental Health, 6001 Executive Blvd., Rm. 8184, MSC 9663, Bethesda, MD, 20892-9663, (301) 433-4513; TTY: (301) 443-8431, (866) 615-6464; TTY: (866) 415-8051, Fax: (301) 443-4279, nimhinfo@nih.gov, http://www.nimh.nih.gov.

Barbara Sternberg, PhD
Emily Jane Willingham, PhD
Tish Davidson, AM

CATIE

Definition

The Clinical Antipsychotic Trials of Intervention Effectiveness (CATIE) **Schizophrenia** Study was a set of **clinical trials** funded by the **National Institute of Mental Health** (NIMH) and coordinated by the University of North Carolina at Chapel Hill. The main CATIE trials were conducted between December 2000 and December 2004. According to the description of the study posted at ClinicalTrials.gov, the study was to consist of three phases: Phase I, subdivided into a Phase IA and Phase IB, to last up to 18 months; Phase II, to last 6 months; and Phase III, for patients who discontinue Phase II, no time limit specified.

Several ancillary studies, most notably the CATIE-Alzheimer's Disease (CATIE-AD) clinical trials, were conducted during the later phases of the main CATIE trials. The other studies include: a comparison of different antipsychotics for patients with schizophrenia at increased risk of cardiovascular disease; a study of the optimal medications for patients with schizophrenia; and a pilot study of metformin (a drug developed to treat type 2 diabetes) as a treatment for patients with schizophrenia who had gained weight while taking antipsychotic drugs. These studies were conducted between 2007 and 2010.

Purpose

The purpose of the early CATIE studies was to evaluate the effectiveness and side effects of newer antipsychotic drugs (sometimes called "atypical antipsychotics"), which have fewer side effects, but are more expensive, in comparison to conventional antipsychotic drugs in the treatment of schizophrenia. One of the purposes of the study was to help doctors maximize the benefits of antipsychotic drugs while minimizing their negative side effects.

Demographics

The CATIE study was open to participants from 18 to 65 years of age who had been diagnosed with schizophrenia using the ***Diagnostic and Statistical Manual of Mental Disorders***, Fourth Edition, Text Revision (*DSM-IV-TR*), and who were able to use oral medications. The initial estimated enrollment was 1,600 patients. Of the 1,460 patients who were actually enrolled in the CATIE study, 74% were male, 40% were nonwhite, and 12% were Hispanic. The mean (average) age of CATIE participants was 40.6 years. The average length of time participants had had schizophrenic episodes was 14.4 years. Participants in the study were treated at 54 different clinical sites across the country and reflected the range of people in the United States suffering from schizophrenia.

People who were intolerant of the drugs used in the trials, pregnant or breastfeeding, having their first schizophrenic episode, or diagnosed with **dementia** or intellectual disability rather than schizophrenia were excluded from the study.

Description

The primary CATIE study was designed for people with schizophrenia who might benefit from a change in their antipsychotic medication. Atypical antipsychotic medications frequently have fewer serious adverse side effects than conventional antipsychotics but are considerably more expensive. The CATIE study was an attempt to investigate scientifically the effectiveness of the newer drugs in comparison with the conventional antipsychotic drug **perphenazine** (Trilafon). All drugs used in the CATIE study had been previously approved by the U.S. Food and Drug Administration (FDA). The atypical antipsychotic drugs under investigation in the study were:

- clozapine (Clozaril)
- olanzapine (Zyprexa)
- quetiapine (Seroquel)
- risperidone (Risperdal)
- ziprasidone (Geodon)

Aripiprazole (Abilify), another atypical antipsychotic drug, was not approved by the FDA in time to be included in the study. No placebos were used in the study.

All drugs evaluated in the CATIE study had already undergone clinical trials by the representative pharmaceutical companies in order to get FDA approval to market each drug. Although these studies were appropriately rigorous to earn FDA approval, they typically had a limited number of participants, tested only two or three drugs per study, and lasted only four to eight weeks.

As compared to the clinical trials previously conducted by the pharmaceutical companies, the CATIE study lasted for 18 months and enrolled over 1,400 participants. This longer in-depth study allowed researchers to study drug actions and side effects in more detail and to examine longer-term effects of their use. Although the pharmaceutical companies donated the medications for the study and advised the researchers of optimal dosages, they had no other input into the design, implementation, analysis, or interpretation of the study results.

Study participants were randomly assigned to the experimental treatments in a double-blind study. "Double-blind" means that the doctors administering the drugs were not able to choose which medication their patients received, and that none of the researchers, administering physicians, or patients knew which treatment the patients were receiving. This study design helped ensure that preconceived expectations about the effectiveness of any of the drugs did not affect the outcome of the study. Patients were randomly assigned to either of the atypical antipsychotics or the control conventional antipsychotic. Patients continued on the assigned drug for 18 months or until the drug failed to continue to control their symptoms or produced intolerable side effects, or the patients decided to stop the medication or withdraw from the study.

Previous research has shown that patients taking antipsychotic medication are better off than those not doing so, and that staying on antipsychotic medication is critical to controlling the symptoms of schizophrenia and preventing a **relapse**. Therefore, one of the primary measures of success in the CATIE study was how long patients benefited from the medication to which they were assigned and how long before they decided it needed to be changed. When patients decided that the medication was not effective, researchers recorded the reasons the medication was stopped (for example, because the medication no longer controlled the symptoms, or the side effects were intolerable). Other data collected included the effects of the medications on the symptoms of schizophrenia and level of the patient's functioning on the medication.

Results

The study found that the conventional antipsychotic generally was equally effective and tolerated as well as the newer and more expensive atypical antipsychotic medications. Of the atypical antipsychotics, **olanzapine** performed somewhat better than the other drugs in the study. Patients on this drug were less likely to be hospitalized for psychotic relapse and tended to stay on their medication longer than patients taking other antipsychotic drugs in the study. However, patients on olanzapine also tended to gain significant amounts of weight and experienced other metabolic changes associated with diabetes, compared to patients taking the other drugs in the study.

Nearly 75% of the patients in the CATIE study switched to a different medication during the course of the study. Participants who stopped taking the medication for any reason were given the opportunity to continue in the study in one of two ways. In the so-called efficacy pathway, patients who discontinued an atypical antipsychotic because it was not sufficiently effective were randomly assigned to receive another atypical antipsychotic to help determine what treatment should be chosen for such patients. In the tolerability pathway, patients who discontinued their medication because of side effects were allowed to receive another medication in order to help determine the next best choice for patients who experience adverse side effects with an atypical antipsychotic. The conventional antipsychotic (perphenazine) was not included in this second phase of the study, because researchers had not expected the conventional medication to work as well as the newer drugs when they designed the study.

Most of the participants in the Phase II efficacy pathway study had not benefited from their first antipsychotic medication and had worse symptoms than they did at the beginning of the study. These participants also tended to have worse symptoms than those participants in the tolerability pathway study. **Clozapine** was very effective for this group and worked significantly better than the other atypical antipsychotics. Forty-four percent of participants in this part of the study were able to stay on their medication for the remainder of the study. Participants on the efficacy pathway stayed on their medication for an average of 10 months as compared to three months for those taking the other atypical antipsychotics. In addition, most of these participants had greater symptom relief than participants taking the other medications.

As in Phase I of the study, in the tolerability pathway of the Phase II study, a high rate (74%) of patients stopped taking their medication. However, 35% of the Phase II participants in the tolerability study who took olanzapine or **risperidone** continued taking their medication until the end of the study. Only 23% of participants taking **ziprasidone** and 16% of participants taking **quetiapine** in the Phase I study were able to continue throughout the entire 18 months.

The results of the Phase II study show that the choice of a different medication for patients who stop taking an antipsychotic medication depends on their reason for stopping the first medication. Participants who stopped taking their antipsychotic medication in Phase I because it was not adequately controlling their symptoms were more likely to stay on their medication if they were switched to olanzapine or risperidone rather than quetiapine or ziprasidone. There was no difference among the four medications tested in Phase II, however, for participants who had stopped taking their Phase I medication because they experienced adverse side effects.

The CATIE study has several major implications. First, the results of Phase I of the study show that it is worthwhile to start patients on less-expensive conventional antipsychotic medications before trying the atypicals. Specifically, physicians and patients should consider perphenazine as an alterative to atypical antipsychotics because of its similar effectiveness and its lower price.

The CATIE study results can also be used to help select a different antipsychotic medication for those patients who were not successfully treated on another antipsychotic. The results of the Phase II study show that the reason for stopping the first medication should be considered when choosing another medication.

The study results also show that clozapine is often a good choice of medication for patients who do not respond well to other antipsychotic medications. In Phase II of the study, clozapine was more effective in controlling symptoms than the other atypical antipsychotics under evaluation. For patients whose symptoms are not well controlled on clozapine, olanzapine and risperidone tend to be more effective than ziprasidone or quetiapine. However, the side effects of these drugs must be taken into account.

The CATIE study did not reveal a clear path of next treatment for those patients who had discontinued use of an antipsychotic due to adverse side effects. In such cases, it is important to balance the degree of symptom control from the drug with the nature of its side effects. For example, olanzapine tended to result in considerable weight gain and metabolic problems, whereas ziprasidone consistently resulted in weight loss and improvement of metabolic disorders. Of the drugs tested, risperidone had the fewest adverse side effects.

KEY TERMS

Ancillary—Subordinate or secondary.

C-reactive protein (CRP)—A protein whose levels in blood rise rapidly in response to inflammation. It can be measured to test for the presence of inflammation and response to treatment; it is also used as a rough indication of a patient's risk of heart disease.

Double-blind study—A study in which neither the individual subjects nor the researchers know who is in the control group and the experimental group.

Herpes simplex virus type 1 (HSV-1)—A virus that causes cold sores. Infection with HSV-1 appears to be correlated with an increased risk of cognitive deficits in schizophrenia patients.

Insulin resistance—A condition in which a person's natural insulin becomes less effective in lowering the blood sugar level.

Metformin—A drug developed to treat type 2 diabetes that has been used experimentally to treat weight gain in patients with schizophrenia.

Off-label—Referring to the use of a prescription medication for an unapproved reason to use it, an unapproved age group, or an unapproved dosage level.

Placebo—An inert substance or sham treatment given to a control group in a clinical trial to test the effectiveness of the real medication or treatment.

Tardive dyskinesia—A disorder characterized by involuntary and repetitive body movements that sometimes develops after long-term use of antipsychotic medications.

CATIE phase III results

CATIE subjects who had discontinued taking antipsychotics in phases I and II of the CATIE study were eligible to participate in phase III. They were offered a choice of nine antipsychotic regimens with assistance from their study doctor. The options included eight single-medication regimens (oral aripiprazole, clozapine, olanzapine, perphenazine, quetiapine, risperidone, ziprasidone, or long-acting injectable **fluphenazine** decanoate) or a combination of any two drugs on the list.

The phase III study enrolled 270 subjects out of 410 who were eligible. Only a small number selected either fluphenazine or perphenazine. The remaining seven options were chosen by 30 to 40 patients each. The researchers reported that the patients who chose clozapine or combination antipsychotic treatment were the most symptomatic, while those who selected aripiprazole and ziprasidone had the highest body mass index. The researchers concluded that combination antipsychotic therapy warrants further study. The phase III study was also the first CATIE report regarding aripiprazole, which was not available when the study began and was not included in previous phases of the study.

NIMH reconsiderations (2006)

In December 2006, the *American Journal of Psychiatry* published an article written by the CATIE researchers on the cost-effectiveness of the older antipsychotic drugs in comparison to the more expensive atypical antipsychotics. According to the NIMH, the article raised a number of questions regarding reimbursement policies for antipsychotic medications. At the time the article was published, antipsychotics were the fourth largest group of medications prescribed in the United States, with an annual cost of $10 billion. The atypical antipsychotics represented 90% of that sum, costing 10 times as much as the older drugs. About 80% of the cost for these drugs was borne by the public sector. The NIMH wished to clarify some of the implications of the cost-effectiveness data:

- People's responses to antipsychotic drugs are highly individual; therefore, the most effective drug for a given patient is the best choice whether it is the least expensive or not. The CATIE study showed that a "one-size-fits-all" approach to the treatment of schizophrenia is unworkable.
- One of the purposes of the CATIE study was to expand the range of medication choices available to patients by examining whether the older antipsychotics are still useful, rather than restricting access to any antipsychotic drug.
- The CATIE study lasted only 18 months, which is not long enough to determine whether patients are at increased risk of tardive dyskinesia, diabetes, or other long-term effects of some of the older antipsychotic drugs.

The CATIE-Alzheimer's Disease (CATIE-AD) Study

The CATIE-Alzheimer's Disease (CATIE-AD) study, funded by the NIMH, was a placebo-controlled clinical trial of three atypical antipsychotics. The study evaluated the effectiveness of antipsychotic medications in treating patients diagnosed with **Alzheimer's disease** (AD), as these drugs had been used off-label in managing the symptoms of AD and other dementias. Their safety as well their efficacy in treating AD was not clear, however. The CATIE-AD study was carried out at 42 sites around the United States. The 421 patients who participated were recruited between 2000 and December 2003 and had to manifest one or more of four symptoms of AD: hallucinations, agitation, aggressive behavior, or **delusions**. The three drugs that were tested in the CATIE-AD study were three atypical antipsychotics: risperidone (Risperdal), olanzapine (Zyprexa), and quetiapine (Seroquel). Patients who chose to discontinue the antipsychotic they were given in phase I of the AD trial could choose a different antipsychotic or **citalopram** (an antidepressant) in phase II.

The study was completed in 2005 and released its first reports in 2006. While some Alzheimer's patients appeared to benefit from the antipsychotic medications, others discontinued them because of their side effects. On the whole, the researchers concluded that the atypical antipsychotics were no more effective than a placebo in treating AD when side effects were taken into consideration. In addition, a follow-up study published in 2009 reported that the patients gained weight, particularly those who had taken olanzapine or quetiapine, and showed an increase in blood cholesterol levels. The researchers stated that patients with AD given any atypical antipsychotic to manage behavioral problems should be closely monitored for metabolic changes.

Later ancillary studies conducted by CATIE investigators

There were three ancillary studies conducted between 2007 and 2010 by researchers who had participated in the primary CATIE study:

- The METS study. This was a 16-week clinical trial of metformin, a drug prescribed for patients with diabetes to increase insulin sensitivity, as a possible treatment for weight gain related to taking antipsychotic medications.
- The Comparison of Antipsychotics for Metabolic Problems (CAMP) study. This study sought to find whether individuals with schizophrenia taking atypical antipsychotics at increased risk of heart disease (measured by body mass index and blood cholesterol levels) would benefit by switching to antidepressant therapy.
- Comparison of optimal treatments for schizophrenia. This was a clinical trial of three different antipsychotics (olanzapine, perphenazine, and aripiprazole) in combination with other drugs to reduce the side effects of the antipsychotic medications.

QUESTIONS TO ASK YOUR DOCTOR

- What is your opinion of participation in clinical trials?
- What is your opinion of the CATIE study?
- Have you ever treated a patient diagnosed with schizophrenia? If so, what medications did they take, and did they stay on them?
- Do you think antipsychotic medications are effective as a treatment for Alzheimer's?

Research and general acceptance

The CATIE study continues to stimulate questions regarding the long-term side effects of antipsychotic drugs as well as their comparative effectiveness. Researchers studying the effects of antipsychotic medications on certain biomarkers associated with an increased risk of cardiovascular disorders reported in 2009 that C-reactive protein (CRP) emerged as a useful marker of increased risk in schizophrenia patients, and that olanzapine had the most noticeable effect in raising the patients' CRP levels. A report published in 2010 noted the contribution of the CATIE study to the issue of metabolic disorders in schizophrenia patients taking antipsychotics, particularly the high rate of insulin resistance in these patients.

A 2011 report noted that some of the drugs tested in the CATIE study were superior to others in relieving symptoms of **depression** in patients with schizophrenia who suffered a major depressive episode. A study of **tardive dyskinesia** in schizophrenia patients that was also published in 2011 made use of CATIE data to show that the presence or course of tardive dyskinesia in patients diagnosed with it was not correlated with any specific antipsychotic drug nor with the length of time between the patient's beginning to take the drug and discontinuing its use. Last, a third 2011 study reported a correlation between evidence of herpes simplex virus type 1 (HSV-1) infection and neurocognitive deficits in the patients in the original CATIE study. The patient sample included all 1,308 patients for whom baseline blood samples were still available.

Resources

BOOKS

American Psychiatric Association. *Diagnostic and Statistical Manual of Mental Disorders.* 4th ed., Text rev. Washington, DC: American Psychiatric Association, 2000.

Meyer, Jonathan M., and Henry A. Nasrallah, eds. *Medical Illness and Schizophrenia*, 2nd ed. Washington, DC : American Psychiatric Pub., 2009.

Stroup, T. Scott, and Jeffrey A. Lieberman, eds. *Antipsychotic Trials in Schizophrenia: The CATIE Project*. New York: Cambridge University Press, 2010.

VandenBos, Gary R., ed. *APA Dictionary of Psychology*. Washington, DC: American Psychological Association, 2007.

PERIODICALS

Addington, D.E., et al. "Impact of Second-generation Antipsychotics and Perphenazine on Depressive Symptoms in a Randomized Trial of Treatment for Chronic Schizophrenia." *Journal of Clinical Psychiatry* 72 (January 2011): 75–80.

Caroff, S.N., et al. "Treatment Outcomes of Patients with Tardive Dyskinesia and Chronic Schizophrenia." *Journal of Clinical Psychiatry* 72 (March 2011): 295–303.

Hermes, E., et al. "The Association between Weight Change and Symptom Reduction in the CATIE Schizophrenia Trial." *Schizophrenia Research* 128 (May 2011): 166–170.

Khan, A.Y., et al. "The Adjunctive Use of Metformin to Treat or Prevent Atypical Antipsychotic-induced Weight Gain: A Review." *Psychiatric Practice* 16 (September 2010): 289–296.

Meyer, J.M. "Antipsychotics and Metabolics in the Post-CATIE Era." *Current Topics in Behavioral Neurosciences* 4 (2010): 23–42.

Meyer, J.M., et al. "Inflammatory Markers in Schizophrenia: Comparing Antipsychotic Effects in Phase 1 of the Clinical Antipsychotic Trials of Intervention Effectiveness Study." *Biological Psychiatry* 66 (December 1, 2009): 1013–1022.

Miller, E.A., et al. "Assessing the Relationship between Health Utilities, Quality of life, and Health Care Costs in Alzheimer's Disease: The CATIE-AD Study." *Current Alzheimer Research* 7 (June 2010): 348–357.

Rosenheck, R. A., et al. "Cost-Effectiveness of Second-Generation Antipsychotics and Perphenazine in a Randomized Trial of Treatment for Chronic Schizophrenia." *American Journal of Psychiatry* 163 (December 2006): 2080–2089.

Stroup, T.S., et al. "Results of Phase 3 of the CATIE Schizophrenia Trial." *Schizophrenia Research* 107 (January 2009): 1–12.

Swanson, J.W., et al. "Alternative Pathways to Violence in Persons with Schizophrenia: The Role of Childhood Antisocial Behavior Problems." *Law and Human Behavior* 32 (June 2008): 228–240.

Yolken, R.H., et al. "Serological Evidence of Exposure to Herpes Simplex Virus type 1 Is Associated with Cognitive Deficits in the CATIE Schizophrenia Sample." *Schizophrenia Research* 128 (May 2011): 61–65.

Zheng, L., et al. "Metabolic Changes Associated with Second-generation Antipsychotic Use in Alzheimer's Disease Patients: The CATIE-AD Study." *American Journal of Psychiatry* 166 (May 2009): 583–590.

WEBSITES

CATIE Home Page, University of North Carolina School of Medicine. http://www.catie.unc.edu/index.html (accessed May 15, 2011).

ClinicalTrials.gov. "CATIE–Schizophrenia Trial." July 2, 2007. http://www.clinicaltrials.gov/ct/show/NCT00014001?order=1 (accessed May 12, 2011).

ClinicalTrials.gov. "Comparison of Antipsychotics for Metabolic Problems in the Treatment of People With Schizophrenia or Schizoaffective Disorder (CAMP)." November 12, 2010. http://www.clinicaltrials.gov/show/NCT00423878 (accessed May 16, 2011).

ClinicalTrials.gov. "Comparison of Optimal Antipsychotic Treatments for Schizophrenia." July 2, 2007. http://www.clinicaltrials. gov/ct2/show/NCT00802100 (accessed May 16, 2011).

ClinicalTrials.gov. "The Use of Metformin in the Treatment of Antipsychotic-Induced Weight Gain in Schizophrenia (The METS Study)." November 12, 2010. http://www.clinicaltrials.gov/show/NCT00816907 (accessed May 16, 2011).

National Institute of Mental Health (NIMH). "Clinical Antipsychotic Trials of Intervention Effectiveness (CATIE)." December 7, 2011. http://www.nimh.nih.gov/trials/practical/catie/index.shtml (accessed May 12, 2011).

National Institute of Mental Health (NIMH) Health Topics. "Schizophrenia." http://www.nimh.nih.gov/health/topics/schizophrenia/index.shtml (accessed May 12, 2011).

ORGANIZATIONS

Alzheimer's Disease Education and Referral Center of the National Institute on Aging (ADEAR), PO Box 8250, Silver Spring, MD, 20907, Fax: (301) 495-3334, (800) 438-4380, http://www.nia.nih.gov/Alzheimers/ContactUs.htm, http://www.nia.nih.gov/Alzheimers.

National Institute of Mental Health (NIMH), 6001 Executive Boulevard, Room 8184, MSC 9663, Bethesda, MD, 20892-9663, (301) 443-4513, Fax: (301) 443-4279, (866) 615-6464, nimhinfo@nih.gov, http://www.nimh.nih.gov/index.shtml.

University of North Carolina School of Medicine, Department of Psychiatry, 110 Conner Drive, Suite 4, Chapel Hill, NC, 27514, (919) 929-7449, http://www.psychiatry.unc.edu.

Ruth A. Wienclaw, PhD
Rebecca J. Frey, PhD

CAT scan *see* **Computed tomography**

Causes of mental illness *see* **Origin of mental illnesses**

Celexa *see* **Citalopram**

Chamomile

Definition

Since about 3000 BCE in Ancient Egypt, chamomile has been grown and used in various healing applications, including as a medicine to ease **depression** and anxiety.

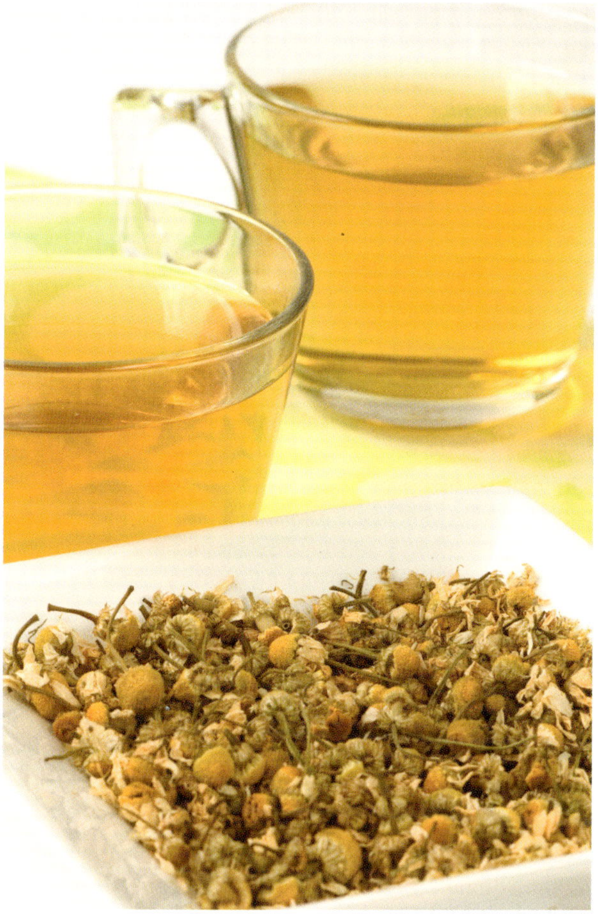

Dried chamomile flowers. *(© iStockPhoto.com/Magdalena Kucova)*

The plant is related to the daisy family; it has strongly scented foliage and flowers with white petals and yellow centers. The name *chamomile* is derived from two Greek words that mean "ground" and "apple," because chamomile leaves smell somewhat like apples and because the plant grows close to the ground. Chamomile is used as a homeopathic remedy for certain mental health conditions.

Purpose

The traditional German description of chamomile is *alles zutraut*, which means that the plant "is good for everything." Chamomile has been used internally for a wide variety of complaints, such as a treatment for parasitic worms (anthelmintic), to prevent or expel gas (carminative), to reduce inflammation (anti-inflammatory), and to control infection (antiseptic). Chamomile has also been used internally as an antispasmodic, to relieve intestinal cramping, digestive disorders, menstrual cramps, **premenstrual syndrome** (PMS), headache, and other stress-related disorders; and as a sedative, often in the form of tea, to treat anxiety and insomnia.

External uses (as **aromatherapy**) of chamomile for mental health conditions include blending its essential oil with **lavender** or rose for scenting perfumes, candles, creams, or other aromatherapy products intended to calm or relax the user's mind and body and reduce anxiety.

Description

There are two varieties of chamomile commonly used in herbal preparations for internal use and for aromatherapy (external use). One is called Roman chamomile (*Anthemis nobilis*), with contemporary sources in Belgium and southern England. Roman chamomile grows to a height of 9 in. (23 cm) or less and is frequently used as a ground cover along garden paths because of its pleasant apple scent. It is also called English chamomile, ground apple, whig plant, and common chamomile.

German chamomile (*Matricaria recutita*) is grown extensively in Germany, Hungary, and parts of the former Soviet Union. It is also sometimes medically called *Matricaria chamomilla,* along with common names such as Hungarian chamomile, wild chamomile, sweet false chamomile, and others. German chamomile grows to a height of about 3 ft. (1 m) and is the variety most commonly cultivated in the United States, where it is used medicinally.

Even though they are very different species of plant, the Roman and German versions of chamomile seem to have similar calming properties, which may help alleviate anxiety and **stress**, produce mild sedation, and reduce restlessness and irritability.

The chamomile flowers are harvested for both internal and external use. Chamomile flowers can be dried and used directly in teas and homemade topical preparations, but they are also available commercially in prepackaged tea bags and in capsule form. The essential oil of chamomile is pressed from the leaves as well as the flowers; it costs about $22–$35 for 5 mL. Chamomile is also available as a liquid extract.

The chemically active components of chamomile are alpha bisabobol, chamozulene, polyines, tannin, coumarin, flavonoids, and apigenin. However, no single component has been credited with all the major healing properties of whole chamomile; it is assumed that the various components work together to produce the plant's beneficial effects.

Chamomile seems to have a calming effect on people with such problems as anxiety, depression, and stress. Anxiety such as is found in generalized anxiety syndrome is a common mental health disorder that, according to the **National Institute of Mental Health**, affects about 40 million adults in the United States each year. These people often become fearful or stressed in situations that most people find normal.

Research

A study published in the *Journal of Clinical Psychopharmacology* (August 2009) showed that chamomile capsules may help to reduce symptoms of anxiety, particularly those caused by **generalized anxiety disorder** (GAD). Researchers from the University of Pennsylvania conducted a randomized, double-blind, placebo-controlled study to see if chamomile extract helped reduce symptoms in 57 participants with mild to moderate GAD. The eight-week study divided the patients into two groups: one receiving chamomile capsules containing 220 mg of pharmaceutical-grade extract from German chamomile, and the other receiving placebo capsules that were scented to smell like chamomile. Doses of the chamomile capsules were adjusted upward during the study for some participants, based on their scores on the Hamilton Anxiety Rating (HAMA) and similar tests. The researchers found that the HAMA scores for the people taking the chamomile capsules were lower than for those in the control group, meaning their anxiety had been reduced. The study concluded that the difference between the two groups was "clinically meaningful and statistically significant." The study was the first controlled clinical trial of chamomile extract for GAD, so additional studies are needed to support its findings.

Recommended dosage

No standard dosage has been made for chamomile within the medical or homeopathic community. The following are approximate guidelines. Children may be given 1–2 mL of a glycerin preparation of German chamomile three times a day; or 2–4 oz. (57–100 g) of tea, one to three times a day, depending on the child's weight. It is often used to calm a baby unwilling to fall asleep. Chamomile may also be applied to bath water or as massage oil for a baby. In addition, it may be sprayed into the air of a baby's room by diluting 12 drops of it per ounce of distilled water. In all cases, the smell of chamomile helps to calm the baby. Most importantly, though, parents should not give chamomile or any other herbal or health supplement to a child without first consulting with the child's doctor or other medical professional.

Adults may take a tea made from 0.7–1 oz. (2–3 g) of dried chamomile steeped in a cup of boiling water for five to ten minutes, three to four times daily. Alternately, adults may take 5 mL of 1:5 dilution of chamomile tincture three times daily.

Precautions

Despite its multitude of uses, chamomile has not been proven clinically effective in treating any conditions, such as those involving mental illness. Studies are ongoing; however, few studies have been conducted on the relationship between chamomile and its calming effect on people with such problems as anxiety and stress.

Because chamomile is related botanically to the ragweed plant, persons who are highly allergic to ragweed should use chamomile with caution. People who are allergic to such flowers as aster, chrysanthemum, marigold, daisy, or sunflower should avoid chamomile. Some plants such as celery also can produce adverse reactions when taken with chamomile. In addition, people with asthma should avoid chamomile because it can increase asthmatic symptoms. People who want to use chamomile need to discuss doing so with a doctor.

Chamomile is generally safe to drink when prepared using the recommended quantity of dried flowers. Highly concentrated tea made from Roman chamomile has been reported to cause nausea; this reaction is caused by a compound found in Roman chamomile called anthemic acid.

Women who are pregnant or could become pregnant should not use chamomile, according to medical persons at the University of Maryland Medical Center, because its use may increase the risk of miscarriage. In addition, mothers who are breastfeeding their newborn infant should not use chamomile because it could harm the baby.

Chamomile contains a small amount of warfarin so it produces mild blood thinning effects. Therefore, persons taking warfarin (Coumadin) or similar blood-thinning medications such as ardeparin (Normiflo), dalteparin (Fragmin), danaparoid (Orgaran), or enoxaparin (Lovenox) should use chamomile only after consulting their physician, as it may intensify the effects of anticoagulant drugs. Persons on blood-thinning medications may not be able to take chamomile or may require monitoring by a physician. These individuals need to talk with a doctor before using chamomile.

The U.S. Food and Drug Administration (FDA) does not evaluate chamomile with regards to its effectiveness, purity, or safety. In addition, regulation of the manufacturing process for chamomile products is not conducted in the United States. Users need to purchase chamomile from only reliable sources to minimize dangers within such products.

Side effects

Generally, chamomile is considered safe. However, it can cause side effects such as allergic reactions in people who are sensitive to ragweed and other substances. A doctor should be contacted immediately if an allergic reaction to chamomile occurs such as tightness in the chest, hives, rash, itching, skin irritation, vomiting, and wheezing. The side effects of chamomile over the

KEY TERMS

Allergic reaction—A physiological reaction to certain substances, such as ragweed or grass, that occurs when a susceptible person comes into close proximity with the substance.

Antispasmodic—A preparation given to relieve intestinal cramping and relax the smooth muscles of the internal organs; to relieve digestive disorders, menstrual cramps, premenstrual syndrome (PMS), headache, and other stress-related disorders.

Warfarin—A blood-thinning drug. People taking blood thinners should not take chamomile.

long term has not been determined by the medical community.

Interactions

Chamomile can increase the effects of anticoagulant medications. In addition, its tannin content may interfere with iron absorption. Chamomile may also add to the effects of **benzodiazepines**, including **diazepam** (Valium), **lorazepam** (Ativan, Temesta), and midazolam (Dormicum, Hypnovel, Versed). It could also adversely interact with **sedatives**, antiplatelet drugs, aspirin, nonsteroidal anti-inflammatory drugs (NSAIDs, such as ibuprofen and naproxen), and other drugs. Chamomile could also interact with supplements such as **ginkgo biloba**, garlic, saw palmetto, **St. John's wort**, and **valerian**.

Further, chamomile should not be taken two weeks before or after surgery. When considering whether to use chamomile, it is always advisable to seek the help of a primary healthcare professional such as the family doctor. In addition, advice from an expert in herbal/health supplements can also be useful.

Resources

BOOKS

Arrowsmith, Nancy. *Essential Herbal Wisdom: A Complete Exploration of 50 Remarkable Herbs.* Woodbury, MN: Llewellyn, 2009.

Mayo Clinic Book of Alternative Medicine. New York: Time Home Entertainment, 2007.

McGilvery, Carole, and Jimi Reed. *The Illustrated Practical Handbook of Aromatherapy: The Power of Essential Aromatic Oils to Relax Your Body and Mind and Relieve Common Ailments.* London: Lorenz, 2007.

PDR for Herbal Medicines. 4th ed. Montvale, NJ: Thomson, 2007.

PERIODICALS

Amsterdam, J.D., et al. "A Randomized, Double-blind, Placebo-controlled Trial of Oral Matricaria Recutita (Chamomile) Extract Therapy for Generalized Anxiety Disorder." *Journal of Clinical Psychopharmacology* 29, no. 4 (August 2009): 378–82.

WEBSITES

"Chamomile." *Network of Care for Behavioral Health.* October 26, 2010. http://cuyahoga.oh.networkofcare.org/mh/library/hwdetail.cfm?hwid=ug1993spec (accessed August 24, 2011).

Griffin, R. Morgan. "Chamomile." *WebMD.* http://www.webmd.com/vitamins-and-supplements/lifestyle-guide-11/supplement-guide-chamomile (accessed August 24, 2011).

Keville, Kathy. "Aromatherapy: Chamomile." *Discovery.* http://health.howstuffworks.com/wellness/natural-medicine/aromatherapy/aromatherapy-chamomile.htm (accessed August 24, 2011).

Miller, Alicia. "Anxiety & Chamomile." *LiveStrong.com.* http://www.livestrong.com/article/240729-anxiety-chamomile (accessed August 24, 2011).

"Study Shows Chamomile Capsules Ease Anxiety Symptoms." *National Institutes of Health.* http://nccam.nih.gov/news/newsletter/2010_may/chamomileanxiety.htm (accessed August 24, 2011).

ORGANIZATIONS

American Botanical Council, 6200 Manor Rd., Austin, TX, 78723, (512) 926-4900, Fax: (512) 926-2345, abc@herbalgram.org, http://www.herbalgram.org.

American Psychiatric Association, 1000 Wilson Blvd., Ste. 1825, Arlington, VA, 22209-3901, (703) 907-7300, apa@psych.org, http://www.psych.org.

American Psychological Association, 750 1st St., NE, Washington, DC, 20002-4242, (202) 336-5500; TDD/TTY: (202) 336-6123, (800) 374-2721, http://www.apa.org.

National Association for Holistic Aromatherapy, PO Box 1868, Banner Elk, NC, 28604, (828) 898-6161, Fax: (828) 898-1965, info@naha.org, http://www.naha.org.

Rebecca J. Frey, PhD
William A. Atkins, BB, BS, MBA

Child abuse

Definition

Child abuse, sometimes called child maltreatment, describes four types of actions toward children: physical abuse, **sexual abuse**, psychological abuse, and **neglect**. In many cases, the same child experiences more than one type of **abuse**. The abusers can be parents or other family members, caregivers such as

Child abuse victims with a reported disability or mental health problem, 2009

Type of disability	Number of children abused	Percentage of total child abuse victims	Number of states reporting
Behavior problem	14,202	2.9	36
Emotional disturbance	9,928	2.1	43
Learning disability	5,011	1.0	38
Intellectual disability	2,100	0.4	41
Physical disability	3,273	0.7	27
Visual or hearing impairment	1,938	0.4	37
Other medical conditions	17,062	3.5	41
Total number of child abuse victims with a disabilty	**53,514**	**11.1**	**42**
Total number of child abuse victims	**484,076**		**42**

SOURCE: U.S. Department of Health and Human Services, Administration for Children and Families, Administration on Children, Youth and Families, Children's Bureau, *Child Maltreatment* 2009 (2010).

Report available online at http://www.acf.hhs.gov/programs/cb/pubs/cm09/cm09.pdf. *(Table by PreMediaGlobal. © 2012 Cengage Learning.)*

teachers or babysitters, acquaintances (including other children), and, in very rare instances, strangers.

Demographics

Child abuse was once viewed as a minor social problem in the United States. However, in the late twentieth century, issues of child welfare came under scrutiny by the media, law enforcement, and healthcare professionals. This increase in awareness led to a sharp rise in the number of reported cases of child abuse. Today, child abuse is recognized as a problem that occurs among households of all racial, ethnic, and income levels, although the incidence of reported cases is higher in low-income households where adult caregivers experience greater **financial stress** and social difficulties, have less education and less understanding of child development, and may have less access to social services. In addition, children of parents who are substance abusers are more likely to experience abuse than children living in households where there is no **substance abuse**. Many child abusers were themselves abused as children.

Statistically, it is difficult to find reliable national figures for cases of child abuse because each state keeps its own records and has its own definitions of what constitutes abuse. Child abuse almost always occurs in private, and because abuse often is hidden from view and its victims may be too young or too frightened to speak out, experts suggest that its true prevalence is probably greater than official data indicates. The majority of children are abused by their parents, so the child may feel that they have no advocate for their well being. However, based on information reported by states to the U.S. Department of Health and Human Services Administration for Children and Families, in 2009, approximately 702,000 children were victims of child abuse. Of those, 78% were victims of neglect, 18% were physically abused, 10% suffered sexual abuse, 8% were psychologically or emotionally maltreated, 2% experienced medical neglect, and 10% suffered other types of abuse, including congenital drug **addiction** (existing at birth). An estimated 1,770 children died as a result of abuse or neglect.

Description

There are four types of child abuse: physical (intentional infliction of injury or pain), sexual (any sexual activity, even if there is no physical contact), psychological (verbal or emotional abuse), and neglect (failure to provide for the child's basic needs).

Physical abuse

Physical abuse is the nonaccidental infliction of physical injury to a child. Legal definitions of physical child abuse vary from state to state, but injuries requiring medical attention typically are regarded as abusive. Physical abuse takes many forms, including cuts, bruises, burns, broken bones, poisoning, and internal injuries. Nonetheless, difficulties associated with defining the line between discipline and abuse are well known. Many states explicitly note that spanking "when administered in a reasonable manner" does not constitute abuse. Thus, how severely parents can inflict physical punishment upon their children without it being considered abusive remains subject to interpretation.

The physical abuser is usually a family member or other caregiver and is likely to be male. The injuries can be inflicted by such actions as punching, kicking, biting, burning, or beating, or by use of a weapon such as a baseball bat or knife. A rare form of physical abuse is Munchausen syndrome by proxy, in which a caregiver (most often the mother) seeks attention by intentionally making the child sick or appear to be sick.

Sexual abuse

Children are sexually abused when they experience contact that is for the sexual gratification of an adult or a significantly older or dominant child when they are younger than the legal age of consent or at a stage of development at which they do not possess sufficient maturity to understand the nature of the acts and therefore to provide **informed consent**. Abusers may use coercion or deceptive manipulation, but often physical force is not necessary since the perpetrator is likely to be someone with whom the child has a trusting relationship and who is in a position of authority over the child. In many states, sexual activity is automatically assumed to be abuse when a defined age difference exists between the older abuser and the younger (minor) victim independent of any consent the victim may have given.

Sexual behaviors can include touching the breasts, genitals, and buttocks while the victim is either dressed or undressed. Sexually abusive behavior also includes cunnilingus, fellatio, or penetration of the vagina or anus with sexual organs or objects. However, sexual abuse does not have to involve any actual touching. Children can be coerced into disrobing and exposing themselves or watching adults disrobe or engage in sexual activity. Pornographic photography or videography also are forms of sexual abuse of children.

Sexual abuse victims can be either boys or girls, though most, but not all, perpetrators are male. Despite publicity surrounding cases where a child is sexually assaulted by a stranger, almost all sexual abuse against children is perpetrated by a family member (e.g. father, stepfather, aunt, uncle, sibling, cousin) or family intimate (e.g., live-in partner or friend of the parent). Perpetrators go to great lengths to conceal sexual abuse. Children who have been sexually abused may not report the behavior due to threats, shame, or to a lack of understanding of what has happened.

Rape is the most violent form of sexual abuse. An act of sexual intercourse is considered rape when

- will is overcome by force or fear, whether from threats, use of weapons, violence, or use of drugs;
- mental impairment renders the victim incapable of rational judgment; or
- the victim is below the legal age established for consent.

Psychological abuse

Abuse of children is not limited to the physical body. Psychological abuse encompasses rejecting, ignoring, criticizing, belittling, humiliating, threatening with violence, or otherwise terrorizing the child, all of which have the effect of eroding the child's self-esteem and sense of security. This type of abuse can also include isolating the child from friends or other family members or destroying the child's property.

Psychological abuse may be the result of actions not directed specifically at the child. The prevalence of domestic violence exposes children to intimidating and frightening scenes every day. Many children live in homes where domestic violence is an ongoing problem that they witness regularly, often as a result of being "caught in the middle" of a parental altercation. Children who observe violence react with many of the same psychological symptoms as children who have experienced it directly.

Psychological abuse often accompanies other types of abuse. It is difficult to prove and rarely is reported.

Neglect

Neglect is the failure to satisfy a child's basic needs and can assume many forms. Physical neglect is the failure (beyond the constraints imposed by poverty) to provide adequate food, clothing, shelter, or supervision. Children may live in filthy conditions or situations where food is not provided, or where they develop infections or other medical conditions that go untreated. Failure to send children to school or otherwise provide for their education may also be considered neglect. Psychological neglect is the failure to satisfy a child's normal psychological needs and/or behavior that damages a child's normal psychological development (e.g., permitting drug abuse in the home, having the child witness domestic violence).

Risk factors

The greatest risk factor for abuse is being young; the most child fatalities due to abuse or neglect are in children younger than age four. Children who are disabled and those who are nonrhythmic (have unpredictable eating and sleeping patterns) are also more likely to be abused. Similarly, children who are distractible, impulsive, or who have high activity levels are more likely to experience physical abuse.

Causes and symptoms

Causes

SOCIOCULTURAL FACTORS. Poverty is the sociocultural factor most strongly linked to abuse. Although

Child abuse victims by age, 2009

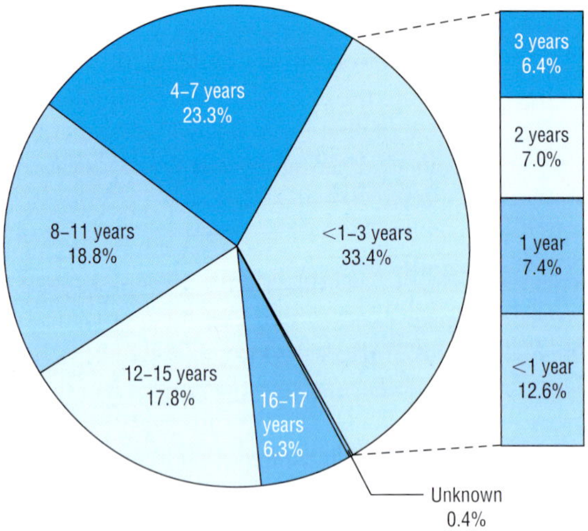

SOURCE: U.S. Department of Health and Human Services, Administration for Children and Families, Administration on Children, Youth and Families, Children's Bureau, *Child Maltreatment 2009* (2010).

Report available online at http://www.acf.hhs.gov/programs/cb/pubs/cm09/cm09.pdf. *(Chart by PreMediaGlobal. © 2012 Cengage Learning.)*

physical abuse occurs at all income levels, it happens more often in very poor families. It is possible that abuse in middle- and upper-class families is less likely to be reported or recognized by an outside source, such as a family physician, than abuse in poorer families, where the abuse may be realized when the victim is treated in an emergency room or public clinic setting. Even with such reporting bias, however, poverty seems strongly linked to abuse, possibly due to the frustrating effects of poverty on the parents. Physical crowding is also associated with abuse, a condition more likely to occur in poverty. If too many people share a small living space, severe punishment of children as a means of maintaining control is more likely.

Job loss and dissatisfaction are other factors often associated with child abuse. Higher rates of abuse exist in military compared to non-military families. It is generally felt that the link between these environmental stressors and abuse is strengthened by the absence of social support networks that might otherwise buffer the family against adversity. Having no one to assist with child care or no one to question the use of severe discipline increases the chance that a parent may injure a child.

Perpetrators of sexual abuse in children, or pedophiles, exist in all economic and cultural groups. Psychologically, however, they share certain traits. Pedophiles often have a history of being abused themselves, and abusing other children seems to be triggered by increased life stressors such as marital problems, job layoffs, or abuse of drugs.

CAREGIVER FACTORS. Parents who abuse their children are likely to be younger than the average parent and are more likely to be single parents. Having a mental illness, such as **depression**, or abusing drugs or alcohol also makes a parent more likely to abuse his or her child. Parents who were themselves abused as children are more likely to abuse their own children, though not every parent who was abused becomes an abuser; some parents go to great lengths to ensure that they never harm their children.

Abusive parents socialize differently from nonabusive parents. Nonabusive parents tend to use ignoring or time-out procedures, whereas abusive parents tend to shout, threaten, and spank. Some forms of child abuse escalate over time, with the parent spanking harder and more frequently to get the same effect or resorting to abuse to get results. Female caregivers inflict more soft tissue injuries, broken bones, and internal injuries than male caregivers. Severe injuries from a single, explosive incident in which the child is shaken, thrown, or struck are more likely to involve male caregivers.

Abusive parents often expect their children to perform behaviors that they are not yet capable of performing. Parents who abuse young children expect them to be able to control their impulses, recall and obey complex parental rules, and perform mature chains of behavior such as getting up, washing, and getting dressed by themselves. Nonabusive parents recognize that toddlers and preschool children are incapable of such behaviors. Understanding the limitations of a young child's memory, ability to follow instructions, impulse control, and attention span is essential to developing reasonable expectations for the child. Parents who expect behavior a child cannot deliver are apt to progressively increase their control techniques in order to get the child to comply.

Abusive discipline is often the result of the belief that the young child is deliberately misbehaving to cause the parent difficulty. Parents who adopt this belief make claims such as that their 18-month-old could stay clean if she wanted to but dirties her clothing just to make more work for the mother. Abusive parents who believe a child has chosen to misbehave inflict more punishment on their children than parents who accurately recognize when a child's behavior is not intentional. Such abusive parents believe that effective parenting involves maintaining tight control over the child, which is often linked to the application of force.

Another belief abusive parents often hold is that their children should engage in reciprocal parenting. They believe that if they sometimes comfort, wait on, and take care of the child, the child should do the same for them. Such beliefs stem from the abusive parents' lack of awareness of children's developmental capabilities and possibly the parents' own immaturity or lack of support from other adults. Regardless of the source, when such expectations are not met by the child, the parent often responds with anger and hostility.

EMOTIONAL FACTORS. Anger is the most frequent trigger for parental abuse. Abusive parents appear to have a lower threshold for childish behaviors than average parents. Thus, child behaviors that are merely irritating to average parents are infuriating to abusive parents. Finally, abusive parents may have less control over their anger than nonabusive parents, either because they are unaware of their level of anger, because they are chronically angry, or because they lack anger management skills.

When considering how emotion influences child abuse, it seems important to consider positive emotions as well. Abusive parents consider their children less rewarding than nonabusive parents. In observation, abusive parents touch their children less, cuddle them less, less frequently call the affectionate names ("honey," "sweetheart"), and smile less at their children. Nonabusive parents respond flexibly to their children, letting the child lead the play interaction. Even in play, abusive parents have expectations that their children seem unable or unwilling to fulfill, making play a disagreeable chore rather than a rewarding endeavor. Abusive parents seem trapped by their own lack of skills, limited developmental understanding, inappropriate expectations, high negative emotion, and low enjoyment of the child.

Symptoms

Although these signs do not necessarily indicate that a child has been abused, they may help adults recognize that something is wrong. The possibility of abuse should be investigated if a child shows a number of these symptoms, or any of them to a marked degree.

Physical abuse:

- unexplained recurrent injuries or burns
- improbable excuses or refusal to explain injuries
- wearing clothes to cover injuries, even in hot weather
- refusal to undress for gym
- bald patches
- chronic running away
- fear of medical help or examination
- self-destructive tendencies
- aggression toward others
- fear of physical contact; shrinking back if touched
- admitting excessive punishment (such as a child being beaten every night to make him/her study)
- fear of suspected abuser being contacted

Sexual abuse:

- overly affectionate or knowledgeable in a sexual way inappropriate to the child's age
- medical problems such as chronic itching, pain in the genitals, venereal diseases
- development of depression, self-mutilation, suicide attempts, overdoses, anorexia, or other severe actions
- attempts at running away
- personality changes such as becoming insecure or clingy
- regressing to younger behavior patterns such as thumb-sucking or bringing out discarded cuddly toys
- sudden loss of appetite or engaging in compulsive eating
- social isolation or withdrawal
- inability to concentrate
- lack of trust or fear for someone they know well, such as not wanting to be alone with a babysitter or specific family member
- anxiety about clothing being removed
- wetting the bed or having nightmares
- drawing sexually explicit pictures
- trying to be "ultra-good" or perfect; overreacting to criticism

Psychological abuse:

- physical, mental, and psychological developmental lags
- sudden speech disorders
- continual self-depreciation (e.g.,"I'm stupid, ugly, worthless," etc.)
- overreaction to mistakes
- extreme fear of any new situation
- inappropriate response to pain (e.g., "I deserve this")
- neurotic behavior (e.g., rocking, hair twisting, self-mutilation)
- extremes of passivity or aggression

Neglect:

- constant hunger
- poor personal hygiene

- no social relationships
- constant tiredness
- poor state of clothing
- compulsive scavenging
- emaciation
- untreated medical problems
- destructive tendencies

A child may be subjected to a combination of different kinds of abuse. It is also possible that a child may show no outward signs and hide what is happening from everyone.

Diagnosis

Doctors and many other professionals who work with children are required by law to report suspected abuse to their state's Child Protective Services (CPS) agency. Abuse investigations often are a group effort involving medical personnel, **social workers**, police officers, and others. Some hospitals and communities maintain child protection teams that respond to cases of possible abuse. Careful questioning of the parents is crucial, as is interviewing the child (if he or she is capable of being interviewed). Trained investigators must ensure, however, that their questioning does not further traumatize the child and also that their style of questioning does not prompt the child to give the answers the child thinks the questioner wants rather than accurate answers. A physical examination for signs of physical or sexual abuse or of neglect is necessary and may include x rays, blood tests, and other procedures.

Treatment

Notification of the appropriate authorities, treatment of the child's injuries, and protecting the child from further harm are the immediate priorities in abuse cases. If the child does not require hospital treatment, protection often involves placing him or her with relatives, in a group home, or in foster care. Once the immediate concerns are dealt with, it becomes essential to determine how the child's long-term medical, psychological, educational, and other needs can best be met. This process involves evaluating not only the child's needs but also the needs of the family (e.g., drug abuse counseling, parental skills training, anger management training). The authorities also must determine whether other children living in the same household have been abused. On investigation, signs of physical abuse are discovered in about 20% of other children living in the abused child's household.

Prognosis

Child abuse often has lifelong consequences. Research shows that abused children and adolescents are more likely to do poorly in school and experience depression, extreme anger, antisocial personality traits, and other psychiatric problems. They also are more likely to become promiscuous, abuse drugs and alcohol, run away, and attempt **suicide**. As adults, they often have trouble establishing intimate relationships.

Most children who have been abused experience some symptoms of **post-traumatic stress disorder** (PTSD). PTSD in children and adolescents may be acute or delayed, meaning that the child may experience symptoms immediately or not until after a period of time has passed, perhaps when the child feels safe. Symptoms may include re-experiencing the abusive episodes at some level, feeling emotionally numb, or feeling the physiological effects of fear (elevated heart rate, abnormal breathing patterns, and so forth). Children may experience disassociation and appear to "space out" when reminded of the abuse or perpetrator. They may become enraged or feel guilt at having provoked the episodes or survived them. They may have invasive memories, repeated behaviors, or fears related to the abusive situations. They may act out some of their issues in play—punishing the bad guy or victimizing another character when playing with dolls or action figures. In severe cases of chronic **trauma**, the child may develop serious or prolonged disassociation or depression. Severe and chronic abuse has also been implicated in cases of multiple personality disorder.

Once the abuse has stopped, some of these symptoms can be treated with some form of counseling or therapy, but full recovery may be a lifelong task. Adults who have been abused as children may have to face issues long after the abuse has stopped, such as when they enter into sexual relationships or when they raise their own children. Long-term therapy by a professional trained in working with abused children and adults offers the best chance of overcoming childhood abuse.

Prevention

There are many barriers to changing abusive parental behavior. Most abusive parents' own histories suggest that strong physical discipline is the preferred model of parenting, and most abusive parents live in families and neighborhoods in which violence is not only condoned but viewed as a necessary vehicle for interpersonal influence. The stressors that are omnipresent in abusive parents' lives contribute to high levels of anger and depression, which prevent the parent from experiencing enjoyment of the child. Further, when a parent responds with strong physical discipline, the child's misbehavior typically stops, at least for that moment, reinforcing the parent's behavior.

It may be preferable to prevent the development of abusive parenting by instituting early interventions to provide parental skills, alter developmental knowledge, change unreasonable parenting expectations, and block the steady build-up of anger and extinguishing of affection for the child. Prevention programs now target teenagers before pregnancy as well as young mothers to try to break the cycle of abuse.

Government efforts to prevent abuse include home-visitor programs aimed at high-risk families and school-based efforts to teach children how to respond to attempted sexual abuse. Psychological abuse prevention has been promoted through the media.

When children reach age three, parents should begin teaching them about "bad touches" and about confiding in a suitable adult if they are touched or treated in a way that makes them uneasy. Parents also need to exercise caution in hiring babysitters and other caregivers. Anyone who suspects abuse should report those suspicions to the police or his or her local CPS agency. Prevent Child Abuse America (listed in references) is an excellent source of information on the many **support groups** and other organizations that help abused and at-risk children and their families. One of these organizations, Parents Anonymous, sponsors local **self-help groups** throughout the United States, Canada, and Europe.

Resources

WEBSITES

MedlinePlus. "Child Abuse." U.S. National Library of Medicine, National Institutes of Health. May 19, 2011. http://www.nlm.nih.gov/medlineplus/childabuse.html (accessed October 1, 2011).

U.S. Department of Health and Human Services. "Child Welfare Information Gateway." http://www.childwelfare.gov (accessed October 1, 2011).

ORGANIZATIONS

Childhelp National Child Abuse Hotline, (800) 4-A-CHILD (422-4453), TDD: (800) 2-A-CHILD (222-4453).

Parents Anonymous, Inc, 675 West Foothill Blvd., Suite 220, Claremont, CA, 91711-3475, (909) 621-6184, Fax: (909) 625-6304, Parentsanonymous@parentsanonymous.org, http://www.parentsanonymous.org.

Prevent Child Abuse America, 228 South Wabash Ave., 10th Floor, Chicago, IL, 60604, (312) 663-3520, Fax: (312) 939-8962, mailbox@preventchildabuse.org, http://www.preventchildabuse.org.

Rape, Abuse and Incest National Network (RAINN), (800) 656-HOPE (4673), http://www.rainn.org/get-help/national-sexual-assault-online-hotline.

Tish Davidson, AM

Childhood bipolar disorder *see* **Juvenile bipolar disorder**

Childhood depression *see* **Juvenile depression**

Childhood disintegrative disorder

Definition

Childhood disintegrative disorder (CDD) is a developmental disorder that resembles severe **autism**. Children with CDD undergo normal development for at least two years, followed by permanent loss of their previously acquired language, motor, adaptive, and social skills. CDD is also known as Heller (or Heller's) syndrome, **dementia** infantilis, and disintegrative **psychosis**.

Demographics

CDD is very rare, affecting only 1–2 out of every 100,000 children. In contrast, autism affects about 20 children per 10,000, and pervasive developmental disorder not otherwise specified (PDD-NOS) affects 30 per 10,000. However, CDD may be underdiagnosed because of its similarities to other developmental disorders. Although CDD is about four times more common in boys than in girls, it was long thought be equally common in both genders, because girls with **Rett syndrome** were often misdiagnosed with CDD. The average age of CDD **diagnosis** is 3.9 years.

Description

Childhood disintegrative disorder was first described by Thomas Heller, an Austrian educator, in 1908. It is a complex and poorly understood condition that affects many different areas of development. Children with CDD develop normally in all areas—language comprehension and speech, nonverbal communication, gross- and fine-motor skills, social relationships, play, and self-care—for at least their first two years. At some point before the age of ten, but usually between three and four years, they begin to lose their previously acquired skills. The losses may be gradual, occurring over a period of six to nine months or longer. Losses can also occur very rapidly, over days or weeks.

CDD is classified as a pervasive developmental disorder (PDD), along with autism, **Asperger syndrome**, Rett syndrome, and PDD-NOS. These conditions may also be collectively referred to as autism spectrum

KEY TERMS

Adaptive behavior—A person's ability to accomplish tasks and adapt to and function in an environment.

Amyloid—A waxy material, made up primarily of protein, that accumulates in organs and tissues with conditions such as Alzheimer's disease.

Asperger syndrome—A developmental disorder that is similar to mild autism. It is characterized by impaired social interaction, repetitive patterns of behavior, and restricted interests, but with normal language and cognitive development and often above-average abilities in a narrow field.

Autism—A variable developmental disorder that includes an impaired ability to communicate and form normal social relationships.

Autism spectrum disorder (ASD)—A range of disorders that includes classic autism, with Asperger syndrome at the mild end of the spectrum and childhood disintegrative disorder at the severe end.

Autoimmune disease—Disorders caused when the immune system's antibodies or T cells attack the body's own molecules, cells, or tissues.

Catatonia—Psychomotor disturbances that can include stupor, rigidity, muteness, or purposeless and bizarre movements.

Epilepsy—A chronic nervous system disorder that typically causes temporary behavior changes, uncontrolled shaking, loss of attention, or unconsciousness.

Fine motor skills—Control of the smaller muscles of the body, especially in the hands, feet, and head, for activities such as writing and crafts.

Gross motor skills—Control of the large muscles of the body, including the arms, legs, back, abdomen, and torso, for activities such as sitting, crawling, walking, and running.

Pervasive developmental disorder (PDD)—A group of five disorders—including Asperger syndrome, autism, Rett disorder, childhood disintegrative disorder (CDD), and pervasive developmental disorder not otherwise specified (PDD-NOS)—that are characterized by developmental delays or impairments.

Rett syndrome—An inherited progressive neurodevelopmental disorder that affects females, usually beginning in infancy, and is characterized by cognitive and motor deterioration, slow brain growth, and intellectual disability.

Schizophrenia—A psychotic disorder characterized by loss of contact with one's environment, deterioration of everyday functioning, and personality disintegration.

disorders (ASD), and CDD is sometimes classified as the severest form of ASD. However, the onset of CDD is usually somewhat later than the onset of autism (classical ASD), and autism does not usually involve the dramatic developmental regression that is characteristic of CDD.

CDD was listed as a separate diagnosis in the fourth edition of the ***Diagnostic and Statistical Manual of Mental Disorders***, text revised (*DSM-IV-TR*), the handbook used by medical professionals in diagnosing mental disorders. Proposed changes for the fifth edition (*DSM-5, 2013*) subsume CDD into the criteria for autism spectrum disorder. The decision came after a review of existing cases of CDD, which failed to provide enough evidence to support CDD as a distinct diagnosis from regressive autism. Still, the proposal to subsume CDD and the other **pervasive developmental disorders** into one category has been met with controversy.

Risk factors

Risk factors for CDD appear to be both genetic and environmental. Genetic risk factors may include a family history of autism, Asperger syndrome, or rolandic epilepsy. Environmental risk factors may include exposure to viruses, especially prenatal exposure to rubella, cytomegalovirus, or herpes simplex, or other infections such as toxoplasmosis. Exposure to toxins, premature birth, and birth **trauma** may also be potential risk factors.

Causes and symptoms

The cause of CDD is unknown. It may result from a combination of genetic susceptibility, possibly involving autoimmunity, and prenatal or postnatal **stress**, including infection, exposure to toxins, or birth trauma. Autoimmune responses occur when the immune system attacks the body's own components. CDD appears to involve deposition of amyloid in the **brain** and disruption of nerve transmission in the brain. It also may involve the immune system chemical interleukin-1 or the brain chemical beta-endorphin.

CDD often occurs in conjunction with other conditions, such as tuberous sclerosis, which causes noncancerous brain tumors; lipid storage diseases, in which excess fats build up in the brain and nervous system; and subacute sclerosing panencephalitis, a chronic brain infection. Other conditions commonly associated with CDD include autoimmune disorders, allergies, asthma, food sensitivities, and gastrointestinal disorders. CDD is sometimes associated with **seizures** and occasionally with brain disorders such as leukodystrophy or Schilder's disease.

CDD may begin with unexplained changes in behavior, such as anxiety, agitation, or unprovoked anger. Behavioral changes are followed by loss of communication, social, and motor skills. Children may stop speaking and communicating nonverbally or revert to single or repeated words. Some 90% of children with CDD lose the ability to feed and wash themselves, lose bowel and/or bladder control, and develop nonspecific overactivity. Essentially all children with CDD lose social skills. They may reject all social interaction and withdraw into themselves. Aggressiveness and tantrums are common. Children may withdraw from physical contact and lose the ability to be consoled. They may perform strange repetitive behaviors known as motor stereotypes or mannerisms, such as head bobbing, rocking, or spinning. They may fixate on certain objects or activities and have trouble with any changes in routine and in transitioning from one activity to another. They also may have difficulty transitioning from wakefulness to sleep and develop **insomnia**. Many children with CDD develop catatonia—a fixed posture or body position. Although the regression eventually stops, children do not usually regain their lost skills.

Diagnosis

A diagnosis of CDD requires that a child regresses dramatically in at least two of the following areas, although most children regress in multiple areas:

- receptive language skills (nonverbal and verbal comprehension)
- expressive language skills (spoken language)
- social or self-help skills, known as adaptive behavior
- imaginary play and playing with peers
- motor skills, including a decline in the ability to walk or grasp objects
- bowel or bladder control, if previously established

Examination

The first signs of CDD may be detected by a pediatrician performing a developmental screening during a routine well-child visit. Developmental screenings utilize parent reports, as well as the physician's observations of the child's language, motor, social, play, and self-help skills. More often, however, parents consult their pediatrician because of suspected developmental delay or the child's loss of previously acquired skills.

The physician will conduct a physical examination to check for conditions such as epilepsy. If a developmental disorder is suspected, the child is usually referred to a team of childhood development specialists for in-depth testing to differentiate CDD from other PDDs, as well as from **schizophrenia**. The team may include a child **psychologist** or **psychiatrist**, a neurologist, a pediatrician specializing in behavior and development, a hearing specialist or audiologist, a speech therapist, a physical therapist, and an occupational therapist.

Because CDD follows at least two years of normal development, medical records, parents' reports, baby books, photo albums, and home videos are important for documenting previous developmental milestones. A family medical history may also be relevant.

Tests

Blood tests will include a complete blood cell count (CBC), genetic tests for chromosome abnormalities and inherited diseases or conditions, and screens for heavy metal poisoning, such as mercury, arsenic, and especially lead, which can cause nervous system damage, developmental delays, behavior problems, and hearing loss. Blood tests will also measure thyroid, kidney, and liver function. Glucose tolerance and HIV testing will be performed. Urine testing may also be involved.

The child will undergo vision and hearing tests. Detailed communication and language tests will evaluate the child's verbal and nonverbal communications skills, including speech rhythms and tone, comprehension, facial expressions, body language, gestures, and social clues. A behavior inventory may utilize any of various rating scales and checklists to evaluate social interactions; play skills; responses to visual, auditory, and touch stimuli in the environment; and diagnostic behaviors such as repetitive movements.

Developmental tests determine a child's developmental age by measuring:

- gross motor skills, including walking, running, jumping, climbing, and throwing
- fine motor skills, including use of hands and fingers to manipulate objects such as pencils, scissors, and buttons
- sensory skills, including responses to sights, sounds, taste, touch, and smell
- play skills, including playing with other children and adults, as well as toys and other objects, and whether play is imaginative, goal-oriented, or purposeful

- self-care skills, including feeding, dressing, toileting, and toothbrushing
- cognitive skills, including attention, concentration, following directions, thinking, and problem solving

Specific tests may include:

- Children's Autism Rating Scale (CARS)
- Kaufman Assessment Battery for Children (KABC), an intelligence and mental processing evaluation
- other intelligence tests
- Vineland Adaptive Behavior Scale
- PDD Behavior Inventory to assess responses to intervention
- occupational therapy evaluation to determine tactile sensitivity, such as responses to touching and hugging, and to assess motor delays
- educational and achievement testing, including verbal and nonverbal communication

Procedures

Imaging procedures, such as x rays, **magnetic resonance imaging** (MRI), **positron emission tomography (PET)**, or **computed tomography** (CT) scans, will rule out brain tumors, head trauma, or anatomical abnormalities. Electrical activity in the brain is measured with an electroencephalogram (EEG), including a sleep EEG. About 50% of children with CDD have abnormal EEGs. EEGs can also help rule out seizure disorders.

Treatment

Traditional

Treatment for CDD is very similar to treatment for autism, with early and intense educational interventions that are highly structured and behavior-based. Behavior therapies require a consistent approach by psychologists; speech, physical, and occupational therapists; teachers; parents; and caregivers to help the child learn or relearn sensory integration and language, social, and self-care skills. Behavior therapy uses rewards to reinforce desirable behaviors and discourage problem behaviors. Family supportive therapy is also usually required.

Drugs

Various medications may be used to treat CDD. Atypical antipsychotics and drugs for anxiety or **depression**, such as selective **serotonin** or norepinephrine reuptake inhibitors (**SSRIs**, SNRIs), have been widely used to treat behavior and mood problems in children with CDD and can sometimes control severe problems, such as repetitive movements or aggression. Anticonvulsants may help control seizures. Sometimes very low-dose and carefully monitored treatment with stimulants or non-stimulants, such as **methylphenidate** or **atomoxetine**, can improve severely impaired attention. **Haloperidol** and **risperidone** are approved by the U.S. Food and Drug Administration (FDA) for treating irritability in childhood autism and may also help with aggression and hyperactivity. Many children and especially adolescents with CDD have impaired sleep-wake cycles and chronic **sleep deprivation** can aggravate aggressive behaviors. Sleep cycles can sometimes be improved by a melatonin agonist such as agomelatine. However, many of these drugs can have potentially serious side effects in children with CDD. Preliminary studies have suggested that corticosteroids may improve language and slow the progression of CDD. Other recent studies have indicated that **memantine**, a drug for treating **Alzheimer's disease** symptoms, may be useful for CDD.

Alternative

Various complementary therapies used for ASD may be applicable to CDD. These include art and **music therapy** and sensory integration—a technique used by occupational therapists to help normalize sensory experiences. Special **diets** and vitamin and mineral supplements are also commonly used with autistic children. However, there is no evidence that alternative treatments such as cranial manipulation or dietary therapies are useful for CDD or any other ASD. Parents who decide to try a special diet for their child should consult with a nutritionist before and after, to prevent or reverse diet-induced vitamin, mineral, or caloric changes. It is particularly important that children with CDD receive adequate **nutrition** to prevent growth retardation.

Home remedies

CDD is a devastating disorder that places tremendous burden and stress on families and caregivers. Parents must be educated in supporting their child's treatments. They must learn and practice set routines that help prevent emotional outbursts and temper tantrums. Families require regular **respite** care to provide time away from the child and the stress of CDD. However, finding appropriate service providers for children with CDD can be difficult, especially outside of large cities. **Support groups** for families can help reduce isolation and frustration, and autism support groups and organizations include CDD families in their services.

Prognosis

Children with CDD have a very poor prognosis. By the age of ten, most children have impairments similar to

QUESTIONS TO ASK YOUR DOCTOR

- What are the possible causes of my child's symptoms?
- What tests will be performed?
- Should we see a specialist?
- What treatments do you recommend?
- What is my child's prognosis?

severe autism, and lost skills are not usually regained. Only about 20% of children with CDD regain their ability to speak in sentences. The risk of seizures increases with age, peaking during adolescence. Most adults with CDD remain dependent on full-time caregivers or are institutionalized.

Prevention

There is no known prevention for CDD. Some experts believe that enriching experiences during critical stages of brain development might potentially overcome genetic predispositions. Disruption of psychosocial development at earlier stages may result in even more severe impairment.

Resources

BOOKS

Hegde, M. N. *Hegde's PocketGuide to Communication Disorders*. Clifton Park, NY: Thomson Delmar Learning, 2008.

Pierangelo, Roger, and George A. Giuliani. *Teaching Students with Autism Spectrum Disorders*.Thousand Oaks, CA: Corwin Press, 2008.

Woliver, Robbie. *Alphabet Kids from ADD to Zellweger Syndrome: A Guide to Developmental, Neurobiological and Psychological Disorders for Parents and Professionals*. Philadelphia: Jessica Kingsley, 2009.

PERIODICALS

Homan, K.J., M. W. Mellon, D. Houlihan, and M. Z. Katusic. "Brief Report: Childhood Disintegrative Disorder: A Brief Examination of Eight Case Studies." *Journal of Autism and Developmental Disorders* 41, no. 4 (2011): 497–504.

Mordekar, S. R., et al. "Corticosteroid Treatment of Behaviour, Language and Motor Regression in Childhood Disintegrative Disorder." *European Journal of Paediatric Neurology* 13, no. 4 (July 2009): 367–69.

Palomo, R., et al. "A Case Study of Childhood Disintegrative Disorder using Systematic Analysis of Family Home Movies." *Journal of Autism and Developmental Disorders* 38, no. 10 (November 2008): 1853–1858.

WEBSITES

Bernstein, Bettina E. "Childhood Disintegrative Disorder." Medscape Reference. http://emedicine.medscape.com/article/916515-overview (accessed December 9, 2011).

Mayo Clinic Staff. "Childhood Disintegrative Disorder." MayoClinic.com. September 16, 2010. http://www.mayoclinic.com/print/childhood-disintegrative-disorder/DS00801 (accessed December 9, 2011).

MedlinePlus. "Childhood Disintegrative Disorder." U.S. National Library of Medicine, National Institutes of Health. http://www.nlm.nih.gov/medlineplus/ency/article/001535.htm (accessed December 9, 2011).

ORGANIZATIONS

Autism Society, 4340 East-West Hwy., Ste. 350, Bethesda, MD, 20814, (301) 657-0881, (800) 3-AUTISM (328-8476), http://www.autism-society.org.

National Institute of Child Health and Human Development Information Resource Center, PO Box 3006, Rockville, MD, 20847, (800) 370-2943, Fax: (866) 760-5947, NICHDInformationResourceCenter@mail.nih.gov, http://www.nichd.nih.gov.

National Institute of Neurological Disorders and Stroke, NIH Neurological Institute, PO Box 5801, Bethesda, MD, 20824, (301) 496-5751, (800) 352-9424, http://www.ninds.nih.gov/index.htm.

Tish Davidson, AM
Margaret Alic, PhD

Childhood onset fluency disorder
see **Stuttering**

Children's Apperception Test (CAT)

Definition

The Children's Apperception Test (CAT) is a widely used projective thematic personality test for children aged three through ten, which analyzes the stories that children tell about pictures.

Purpose

The primary purpose of the CAT is to assess a child's personality, self-image, and view of the world, by analyzing responses to standardized pictorial stimuli. The CAT is most often used to identify and diagnose personality and emotional disorders in children. It is rarely used as the sole basis of a clinical **psychological assessment**. Rather, it is usually one of a battery of tests, including other projective tests, that supplement information obtained from interviews with the child and parents. The CAT is designed to reveal information about children's perceptions and imaginations, to help psychologists and psychiatrists understand their conscious and unconscious needs, motives, attitudes, emotions, and conflicts.

The CAT was originally developed to examine so-called psychosexual conflicts that arise at different stages of child development, including relationship issues, sibling rivalry, and aggression. However, in recent years, the CAT has come into widespread use as a general method for describing personality and assessing maturity, as well as measuring psychological health. The CAT is used in clinical, educational, and research settings. Because pictures form the content of the CAT, it is used throughout the world.

The CAT is used to reveal and assess:

- personality traits
- maturity
- life stresses
- perceptions of reality
- defenses
- aggressive tendencies
- self-control
- judgment
- degree of autonomy or independence
- psychodynamic processes

Description

The CAT is a type of personality assessment called a projective test, similar to Rorschach inkblots and the popular **Thematic Apperception Test** (TAT). Projection, a concept that originated with Sigmund Freud, is a psychological mechanism by which humans' unconscious needs, motives, and emotions are projected onto the external world and control behavior. People come to believe that these feelings are actually being expressed by the external environment and are directed back at them. Whereas cognitive tests utilize intellectual measures of a person's knowledge of the world, projective storytelling techniques, like the CAT, are open ended and encourage the free expression of thoughts and feelings that reveal personality traits.

The CAT is always administered to individual children by a trained professional, usually a **psychiatrist**, **psychologist**, social worker, or specially trained pediatrician or teacher. It may be administered as a component of therapy or as a play technique. It is not timed, but usually takes 20–45 minutes. The test must be administered in a quiet room, free of distractions.

First, the examiner establishes a rapport with the child. The child is then shown ten black-and-white picture cards, one at a time in a particular sequence, and asked to describe each situation and make up a story about the picture, with a beginning, middle, and end. For example, the child may be asked to describe what preceded the scene in the picture, how the characters in the picture are feeling, and what might happen next. The pictures have been chosen to encourage storytelling related to situations such as family life, school, illness, injury, competition, and **body image**. The examiner may choose to use only selected pictures. The child's stories are expected to reveal information about relationships with family and peers, feelings about school, and self-confidence and self-esteem. The stories may also reveal a child's anxieties and fears and psychological defenses in a variety of contexts, including school, play, and body image.

The original CAT, now referred to as the CAT-A for animals or simply the CAT, was designed specifically for younger children, who, it was thought, would more readily identify with drawings of animals. The CAT-A pictures are designed to appeal to a child's imagination and encourage storytelling. The animals are pictured within human social settings. Most involve animals interacting with their environment and are meant to represent needs that a child can identify. Pictures include:

- baby chicks seated around a table with an adult chicken in the background
- a baby bear and a large bear playing tug-of-war
- a mouse peering through a peephole at a lion seated on a throne
- a mother kangaroo with one baby kangaroo in her pouch and an older baby kangaroo beside her
- two baby bears sleeping in a small bed in front of a larger bed with two bulges in it
- a baby bear lying next to two large bears in a cave
- a ferocious tiger leaping at a monkey climbing a tree
- two adult monkeys sitting on a sofa and another adult monkey talking to a baby monkey
- a rabbit sitting on a child's bed, as seen through a doorway
- a puppy being spanked by an adult dog in front of a bathroom

Using the example of the ferocious tiger and the monkey, one child might tell a story about them playing a game. However, another child might talk about the heroic monkey escaping from the evil tiger. This could represent the child's fear of aggression or need to escape punishment.

A supplement, the CAT-S, was first published in 1952 and was designed to elicit more specific responses from children. It includes pictures of children in family situations, such as birth, death, prolonged illness, or separation from parents.

KEY TERMS

Apperception—The process of understanding something in terms of previous experience.

Cognitive—Conscious intellectual activity, including thinking, imagining, reasoning, remembering, and learning.

Defense—An unconscious mental process that protects the conscious mind from unacceptable or painful thoughts, impulses, or desires. Examples of defenses include denial, rationalization, projection, and repression. Some defenses are considered to represent lower levels of maturation than others; thus identifying a child's defenses may be helpful in evaluating his or her level of psychological maturity.

Ego—In Freudian psychology, the conscious, rational part of the mind that experiences and reacts to the outside world.

Personality test—Various standardized tasks that are used to determine aspects of personality or emotional status.

Projective test—A psychological test for assessing thinking patterns, observational abilities, attitudes, and feelings, based on open-ended responses to ambiguous stimuli; often used to evaluate personality disorders.

Psychodynamic—Mental, emotional, or motivational forces or processes that affect mental state and behavior, especially unconscious processes that develop in early childhood.

Psychosexual conflicts—In Freudian categories, internal conflicts related to problems at a particular stage of childhood development. Freud associated each developmental stage with a particular part of the human body, such as the mouth or the phallus.

Reliability—The ability of a test to yield consistent, repeatable results.

Rorschach test—A popular projective psychological test, in which a subject's interpretation of a series of ten standard inkblots are used to assess personality and emotional traits and diagnose disorders.

Sibling rivalry—Competition among brothers and sisters in a nuclear family. It is considered to be an important influence in shaping the personalities of children who grow up in middle-class Western societies but less relevant in traditional African and Asian cultures.

Superego—According to Freud, the part of the mind that represents traditional parental and societal values. The superego is the source of guilt feelings.

Thematic Apperception Test (TAT)—A clinical psychology projective test for diagnostic, psychodynamic, and personality assessments, based on responses to black and white pictures.

Validity—The ability of a test to measure accurately what it claims to measure.

The CAT-H was first published in 1965. It consists of ten pictures of human children and adults in the same common social situations that are depicted with animals in the original CAT. It is used with children who identify more readily with people than with animals, especially seven-to-ten-year-olds who view the animal pictures as childish. The CAT-H is also commonly used for research purposes. An important difference between the CAT-A and the CAT H is that gender identity is more ambiguous in the animal pictures, enabling children to relate to all of the young animals rather than just those of their own gender, as in the CAT-H.

The complete CAT kit includes the CAT-A, CAT-H, and CAT-S picture cards and manuals, recording and analysis banks, and the "Haworth Schedule of Adaptive Mechanisms in CAT Responses." The latter is a checklist developed by Mary Haworth to aid in the qualitative analysis of CAT stories and to help formulate rough quantitative measures.

Origins

The CAT was originally developed in 1949 by the psychiatrist, psychoanalyst, and psychologist Leopold Bellak and his then-wife, Sonya Baychok Sorel Bellak. It was designed as a downward extension of the TAT for children aged three through ten. The TAT had been developed in the 1930s by the psychologists Henry A. Murray and Christiana D. Morgan. Murray believed that people's needs affect the ways in which they interact with their environment. Like the CAT, the TAT utilizes a picture interpretation technique to reveal aspects of personality and interpersonal relationships. In particular, the TAT was designed to reveal the strengths of people's needs and drives—especially their need for achievement and recognition—as well as emotions, conflicts, complexes, and unconscious fantasies. The TAT is used with adults and children aged ten and older. It consists of a series of 31 pictures portraying people in common—but ambiguous—situations, in order to elicit oral or written stories about relationships and social situations.

Preparation

The CAT should be administered, scored, and interpreted only by a trained and experienced mental health professional who is knowledgeable in the psychological theories behind the test. It is recommended that the examiner obtain a child's personal, psychological, educational, and medical histories before administering the CAT. This ensures that the examiner has a context for interpreting the child's responses. For example, stories of loss or **grief** might be considered abnormal responses or a cause for concern unless the examiner knows that the child's pet has just died.

Risks

Although many decades of experience with the CAT have indicated that it can provide accurate and useful information about personality traits, emotions, and needs, many experts remain critical of it and other projective tests, questioning their reliability, validity, and usefulness as diagnostic tools. The CAT, in particular, has been criticized for its lack of objective scoring, its reliance on the examiner's methods and bias, and results that may be inconsistent. Critics have also questioned its validity or effectiveness at measuring the traits it purports to assess, such as needs, conflicts, and motivations.

Interpretations of CAT responses are very subjective. A child's stories or the examiner's interpretations of the stories can lead to an improper **diagnosis**. Some critics also maintain that cultural and language differences between the examiner and the child can affect CAT results. Studies have found that the gender, race, and socioeconomic class of the examiner and of the child affect both the child's stories and the examiner's interpretations. For these reasons, the CAT is often referred to as an assessment tool rather than a test, and is normally used only in conjunction with other psychological assessments designed for children. It is very important that parents seek a second opinion or have their child assessed by other methods before reaching decisions based on the CAT. In addition to all of these concerns, many parents have reported that the CAT did not provide any new information about their child.

Results

The CAT is not quantitatively scored, because, as with other projective tests, there are a wide range of responses. The basic stories that a child tells are recorded, and the occurrence or lack of various thematic elements is noted on a form. Each story is analyzed in depth to reveal the child's needs, attitudes, emotions, conflicts, and response patterns. The examiner summarizes personality traits and attitudes and conflicts that are revealed by each story.

The important story components that are analyzed include the:

- main theme and conflicts
- main character or protagonist
- protagonist's primary needs or motivations
- protagonist's anxieties, fears, and conflicts
- relationship of the protagonist to his or her immediate environment
- child's perceptions of the external world, as revealed by the characters in the stories
- child's ego integration, or perception of and adaptation to reality
- functioning of the child's superego, or semi-conscious system of morality or conscience

Like other projective tests, the CAT does not have a standardized method of administration or norms for interpretation. Although the CAT is designed to be interpreted according to psychoanalytical theories, the examiner has a great deal of flexibility, and interpretation is often influenced by the examiner's preferred theories or biases.

QUESTIONS TO ASK YOUR DOCTOR

- Should my child be given the CAT or other projective psychological tests?
- Who will administer the CAT?
- Will I be informed of my child's responses on the CAT?
- How will my child's CAT responses be interpreted?
- What other psychological and diagnostic tests should my child have?

Resources

BOOKS

Bellak, Leopold, and David M. Abrams. *The Thematic Apperception Test, the Children's Apperception Test, and the Senior Apperception Technique in Clinical Use.* 6th ed. Boston: Allyn and Bacon, 1997.

Bellak, Leopold, and Sonya Sorel Bellak. *Children's Apperception Test (C.A.T.).* Oxford, England: C.P.S., 1949.

Bellak, Leopold. *The Thematic Apperception Test and the Children's Apperception Test in Clinical Use*. Oxford, England: Grune & Stratton, 1954.

Chandler, Louis A. "The Need-Threat Analysis: A Scoring System for the Children's Apperception Test." In *A Handbook of Clinical Scoring Systems for Thematic Apperceptive Techniques,* edited by Sharon Rae Jenkins. New York: Routledge, 2007.

Teglasi, Hedwig. *Essentials of TAT and Other Storytelling Assessments*. 2nd ed. Hoboken, NJ: John Wiley & Sons, 2010.

PERIODICALS

Berant, Ety, Mario Mikulincer, and Phillip R. Shaver. "Mothers' Attachment Style, Their Mental Health, and Their Children's Emotional Vulnerabilities: A 7-Year Study of Children With Congenital Heart Disease." *Journal of Personality* 76, no. 1 (February 2008): 31–66.

Lis, A. "The Children's Apperception Test Evaluation Form: Initial Data." *Psychological Reports* 96, no. 3, Pt. 1 (June 2005): 755–68.

WEBSITES

Center for Psychological Studies, Nova Southeastern University. "Children's Apperception Test." http://www.cps.nova.edu/~cpphelp/CAT.html (accessed October 1, 2011).

ORGANIZATIONS

American Psychological Association, 750 1st St. NE, Washington, DC, 20002-4242, (202) 336-5500; TDD/TTY: (202) 336-6123, (800) 374-2721, http://www.apa.org.

Center for Psychological Studies, Nova Southeastern University, 3301 College Ave., Fort Lauderdale-Davie, FL, 33314-7796, (800) 541-6682, ext. 25700, http://www.cps.nova.edu.

Margaret Alic, PhD

Children's Depression Inventory

Definition

The Children's Depression Inventory (CDI) is a symptom-oriented instrument for assessing cognitive (thoughts), affective (emotions), and behavioral (psychological) signs of depression in children between the ages of seven and 17 years. The CDI differentiates between **major depressive disorder** (a severe case of depression) and **dysthymic disorder** (a less severe form of depression) in children. The basic CDI consists of 27 items, but a 10-item short form (CDI-S) is also available for use as a screener (a test for screening patients). The 27-item test analyzes depressive symptoms such as depressed mood, lack of hedonic (pleasure) capacity, and interpersonal behaviors. The reading level for the CDI is first grade.

The updated version of the CDI, the Children's Depression Inventory 2 (CDI-2), is based on the original CDI—retaining many of its best features—but adds several important improvements to its predecessor that were based on reports taken from parents, children and adolescents, and teachers. For instance, the CDI-2 includes new items that concentrate on the fundamental aspects of childhood depression. It also includes measurement scales that are considered more reliable and valid. The norms established by the CDI-2 are also updated, taken from a more recent sample of the U.S. population. This sample is said to be more representative of the U.S. population than the previous version. In addition, the revised CDI contains normative samples of the Parent and Teacher forms.

Purpose

First developed in 1992 by Maria Kovacs, professor of psychiatry at the University of Pittsburgh School of Medicine, the CDI was intended to assist in the difficult **diagnosis** of depression in young children. One complication was that depression was regarded as an adult disorder until the 1970s. It was thought that children's nervous systems were not sufficiently mature to manifest the neurochemical changes in **brain** function associated with depression.

The **National Institute of Mental Health** (NIMH) estimated that as many as 2.5% of children and 8.3% of adolescents under the age of 18 years in the United States have depression. A study sponsored by the NIMH of 9- to 17-year-olds found that 6.0% developed depression in a six-month period, with 4.9% diagnosed as having major depression. Research also indicates that children and adolescents experience the onset of depression at earlier ages than previous generations, are more likely to experience recurrences, and are more likely to experience severe depression as adults.

The CDI is intended to be used by clinicians and counselors in order to detect and evaluate the symptoms of a major depressive disorder or dysthymic disorder in children or adolescents and to distinguish between children with those disorders and children with other psychiatric conditions. Such professionals also use it to support diagnoses and treatment planning. The CDI can be administered repeatedly in order to measure changes in the depression over time and to evaluate the results of treatment for depressive disorders. It is regarded as adequate for assessing the severity of the depressive symptoms.

The CDI has also been used in research studies of the epidemiology of depression in children as well as studies of dissociative symptoms and post-traumatic syndromes in children. It has been rated as having adequate to excellent psychometric properties by research psychologists.

Kovacs authored the CDI-2 as well. The CDI-2 measures affective, cognitive, and behavioral symptoms of depression in school-aged children and adolescents.

Description

CDI

The CDI is self-rated, which means that the children or adolescents being evaluated record their answers to the questions on the test sheet, as distinct from giving verbal answers to questions that are then analyzed and recorded by the examiner. The basic CDI takes approximately 15 minutes to complete, while the CDI-S (the short form) takes about five minutes. Other self-rated instruments for assessing depression in children are the **Beck Depression Inventory** (BDI) and the Weinberg Screening Affective Scale (WSAS).

The CDI was standardized with the help of 1,266 children from various U.S. public schools in Florida. In all, 592 males (from the ages of seven to 15 years) and 674 females (from the ages of seven to 16 years) participated in the standardization process from grade levels of two through eight. Approximately 77% of the participants were Caucasian-Americans, and about 23% were African Americans, American Indians, and Hispanics. In addition, most of the children were from middle-class socioeconomic backgrounds, and about 20% of them came from single-parent homes. The children were divided into two age groups (7–11 years, and 12–17 years) and separated by gender (sex).

The original CDI is divided into five subscales that measure different symptom groups of depression. These subscales are:

- negative mood (anger and/or irritability)
- interpersonal difficulties (problems making and keeping social relationships)
- negative self-esteem (feelings of inadequacy in performing normal daily activities)
- ineffectiveness (lack of or reduced motivation in completing tasks)
- anhedonia (absence or decreased presence of pleasure and joy)

Each question on the CDI consists of three possible responses; the children or adolescents being evaluated select the response that most closely describes themselves over the preceding two weeks. The CDI is designed to make quantitative measurements of the following symptoms of depression: mood disturbances; capacity for enjoyment; depressed self-evaluation; disturbances in behavior toward other people; and vegetative symptoms, which include **fatigue**, oversleeping, having difficulty with activities requiring effort, and other symptoms of passivity or inactivity. The CDI is designed to assess children at numerous locations such as schools, guidance clinics, physician offices, and psychiatric offices.

CDI-2

The age range for the revised test, CDI-2, is also seven to 17 years, with an administration time of 5–15 minutes. The CDI-2 is teacher-completed, parent-completed, or youth-completed. In addition, online, software, and paper-and-pencil versions are available, with the first two versions computer-scored and the last one hand-scored. All versions are scored using the Multi-Health Systems (MHS) QuikScore™ format. Within the paper-and-pencil version, the administrator writes an evaluation on external layers of the form, which is later transferred to a hidden grid within internal layers. The internal layers are used to tabulate the results. With the other two versions, Response/E-Paper forms are available.

The CDI-2 can be completed on the Web and can be scored there, too. Administrators are linked via the Internet to an organization sponsoring the test taker, and correspondence can be sent to a website requested by each recipient. Once the test is completed, the organization can download the score through an E-Paper form.

A software program can be acquired for use with the CDI-2. The test-taker first completes a paper-and-pencil version of the test, and then the responses are transferred onto the software program, which performs the scoring procedure.

The scales for the CDI-2 include: emotional problems and functional problems. Subscales include: negative mood, negative self-esteem, ineffectiveness, and interpersonal problems. Three reports are also available: the Assessment Report, the Progress Report, and the Comparative Report. The Assessment Report provides results from one administrator, whereas the Progress Report gives an overview of changes that have occurred over time from the administration of up to four administrators. The Comparative Report provides an overview of symptoms from the test-taker taken from the responses of up to five administrators.

The various inventory forms for reporting of the results from the CDI-2 include: the Self Report (which is a full-length version of the CDI-2), the Self Report (Short), the Teacher Report, and the Parent Report. Each assesses the presence and severity of depression and its symptoms. The full-length Self Report version is used when a more descriptive assessment is needed to determine depressive symptoms. It contains 28 items, and includes both scales and all four subscales. It normally takes less than 15 minutes to complete.

The short form Self Report contains only 12 items, takes about half the time to complete when compared to the full form, and takes 5–10 minutes to administer. It is used when less of an assessment is needed. Both forms of the Self Report require only a first-grade reading level. In addition, both have test-takers make a mark for each specific statement that best describes their feelings or behavior over the past two weeks.

The Teacher and Parents forms are comparable with the short form, but its instructions are altered for its specific administrator (teacher or parent). The strength of the results for both forms is that they maximize the administrator's ability to observe depressive symptoms. For the Parent form, the mother, father, or caregiver is asked to rate the child on factors relating to the environment around the home and with the family itself over the past two weeks. For the Teacher form, the child's teacher concentrates on the academic, emotional behavior, and social characteristics of the child while in the classroom over the previous two weeks. Both forms provide a Total Score and two scale scores: Emotional Problems and Functional Problems.

The CDI-2 was normalized from a sample of 1,100 children ranging from ages of seven to 17 years, who lived in 26 states in the United States (with a similar number of states in each of the four major geographical regions of the country). The sample size was evenly distributed according to age and gender. Fifty males and 50 females filled each of the 11 age categories. In addition, the U.S. census for 2000 was used to find a representative sample of people based on race and ethnicity. Data from 319 children diagnosed with **attention deficit hyperactivity disorder (ADHD)**, **conduct disorder** (CD), **generalized anxiety disorder** (GAD), major depressive disorder (MDD), or **oppositional defiant disorder** (ODD) were also included.

Preparation

Preparation for the CDI is neither necessary nor recommended by the medical community.

KEY TERMS

Attention deficit hyperactivity disorder—A condition involving hyperactivity in children, often causing the inability to concentrate and inappropriate or impulsive behaviors.

Conduct disorder—A psychiatric disorder characterized by a distinct pattern of repetitious behavior, which is considered abnormal in everyday society and often derogatory to others.

Depression—A psychiatric disorder involving feelings of hopelessness and symptoms of fatigue, sleeplessness, suicidal tendencies, and poor concentration.

Dysthymia—A form of depression with persistent symptoms such as fatigue, insomnia, loss of appetite, and problems with self-esteem, but considered not severe enough to be classified as a psychosis (psychiatric disorder involving loss of contact with reality).

Generalized anxiety disorder—An anxiety disorder characterized by daily irrational worry that is often also excessive and uncontrolled.

Oppositional defiant disorder—A psychiatric disorder characterized by an ongoing pattern of excessively hostile, angry, and disobedient behavior that is directed toward authority figures.

Aftercare

The Child Depression Inventory, both its original form and the revised form, is one way that the medical community can accurately identify depression in children and adolescents. Once depression is identified it is much easier to treat such patients.

Risks

The CDI and CDI-2 share certain drawbacks with other self-report measures used in children, namely that children do not have the same level of ability as adults to understand and report strong internal emotions. However, children have the same ability as adults to modify their answers on the CDI/CDI-2 and similar tests to reflect what they think are the desired answers rather than what they actually feel. This phenomenon is variously known as "faking good" or "faking bad," depending on the bias of the modified answers. Some researchers have also observed that children who do not have age-appropriate reading skills may receive an inaccurate diagnosis on the basis of their CDI/CDI-2 score.

QUESTIONS TO ASK YOUR DOCTOR

- How will the Children's Depression Inventory 2 help me solve my child's depression?
- How does the CDI-2 work?
- Is the CDI-2 able to diagnose severe or minor cases of depression?
- Will the results the CDI-2 help inform what treatment to use?
- What other tests are well suited to supplement this test?

Precautions

Because depressive symptoms fluctuate somewhat in children as well as in adults, the author of the test recommends retesting children who score positive on the CDI/CDI-2, with a two- to four-week interval between the test and the retest. A child who screens positive on the CDI/CDI-2 should receive a comprehensive diagnostic evaluation by a licensed mental health professional. The evaluation should include interviews with the child or adolescent; the parents or other caregivers; and, when possible, such other observers as teachers, social service personnel, or the child's primary care physician.

Results

For each item within the CDI, the administrator scores according to the following: 0 equals an absence of symptoms; 1 equals mild symptoms; and 2 equals definite symptoms. Scoring consists of a total score and five sub-scores, which are determined by age and gender. The total score has a minimum possible score of 0 and a maximum possible value of 54. The sub-scores are named: negative mood, interpersonal difficulties, negative self-esteem, ineffectiveness, and anhedonia. The test administrator totals the responses and plots them onto a profile form. A score that falls below a cutoff point, or is 1.0–2.0 standard deviations above the mean, is considered to be positive for depression. The administrator can use a QuickScore™ Form as a help in scoring.

The results of the CDI should be evaluated only by a trained professional **psychologist** or **psychiatrist**, and not by a parent, teacher, school nurse, or other such untrained persons.

Parental Concerns

The CDI and the CDI 2 are both short and easy assessment tests to administer. They can be administered to one child or many children. The CDI/CDI-2 test is considered to possess excellent psychometric properties; that is, it is able to accurately and reliably measure depression when administered by a trained professional. Many research studies have supported these conclusions in the assessment of depression in children and adolescents.

Resources

BOOKS

American Psychiatric Association. *Diagnostic and Statistical Manual of Mental Disorders.* 4th ed., Text rev. Washington, DC: American Psychiatric Association, 2000.

Beers, Mark H., et al. *The Merck Manual of Diagnosis and Therapy.* Whitehouse Station, NJ: Merck Research Laboratories, 2006.

Clark, David A., and Aaron T. Beck. *Cognitive Therapy of Anxiety Disorders: Science and Practice.* New York: Guilford Press, 2010.

Clark, David A., Aaron T. Beck, and Brad A. Alford. *Scientific Foundations of Cognitive Theory and Therapy of Depression.* New York: John Wiley & Sons, 2003.

Nezu, Arthur, George F. Ronan, and Elizabeth A. Meadows, eds. *Practitioner's Guide to Empirically Based Measures of Depression.* New York: Springer, 2006.

VandenBos, Gary R., ed. *APA Dictionary of Psychology.* Washington, DC: American Psychological Association, 2007.

WEBSITES

"Children's Depression Inventory (CDI)." Nova Southeastern University. http://www.cps.nova.edu/~cpphelp/CDI.html (accessed October 7, 2011).

"Children's Depression Inventory (CDI)." Pearson Assessments. http://psychcorp.pearsonassessments.com/haiweb/cultures/en-us/productdetail.htm?pid=015-8044-762&Community =CA_Psych_Settings_Military (accessed October 7, 2011).

"Children's Depression Inventory 2." Mental Health Systems (MHS). http://www.mhs.com/product.aspx?gr=edu&prod=cdi2&id=overview#top (accessed May 20, 2011).

"Children's Depression Inventory 2 (CDI-2)." Pearson. http://www.pearsonpsychcorp.com.au/productdetails/448 (accessed October 7, 2011).

"Children's Depression Inventory 2 (CDI-2)." Western Psychological Services. http://portal.wpspublish.com/portal/page?_ pageid=53,272957&_dad=portal&_schema=PORTAL (accessed October 7, 2011).

"Depression." National Institute of Mental Health. http://www.nimh.nih.gov/health/publications/depression/complete-index.shtml (accessed October 7, 2011).

"Newsmaker: Maria Kovacs." *Pittsburgh Tribune-Review,* July 16, 2010. http://www.pittsburghlive.com/x/pittsburghtrib/news/cityregion/s_690591.html (accessed May 20, 2011).

ORGANIZATIONS

American Academy of Child and Adolescent Psychiatry, 3615 Wisconsin Ave. NW, Washington, DC, 20016-3007, (202) 966-7300, Fax: (202) 966-2891, http://aacap.org.

American Psychiatric Association, 1000 Wilson Blvd., Ste. 1825, Arlington, VA, 22209-3901, (703) 907-7300, apa@psych.org, http://www.psych.org.

American Psychological Association, 750 1st St. NE, Washington, DC, 20002-4242, (202) 336-5500; TDD/TTY: (202) 336-6123, (800) 374-2721, http://www.apa.org.

Depression and Bipolar Support Alliance, 730 N Franklin St., Ste. 501, Chicago, IL, 60654, (800) 826-3632, Fax: (312) 642-7243, http://www.dbsalliance.org.

National Institute of Mental Health, 6001 Executive Blvd., Rm. 8184, MSC 9663, Bethesda, MD, 20892-9663, (301) 433-4513; TTY: (301) 443-8431, Fax: (301) 443-4279, (866) 615-6464; TTY: (866) 415-8051, nimhinfo@nih.gov, http://www.nimh.nih.gov.

Rebecca J. Frey, PhD
William A. Atkins

Chloral hydrate

Definition

Chloral hydrate is a drug used to help sedate persons before and after surgery, to help relieve anxiety or tension, and to promote sleep in individuals with **insomnia**. It is sold in the United States under the brand names Aquachloral, Aquachloral Supprettes, and Noctec, as well as its generic name. In the United States, chloral hydrate has largely been replaced by other medications.

Purpose

Chloral hydrate is considered a controlled substance in the United States and is only available with a prescription. Because of a potential for **addiction** with long-term use, chloral hydrate is given only occasionally to help sedate persons before and after surgery, primarily children. Historically, it has been used to treat insomnia and anxiety but has since been replaced by other drugs.

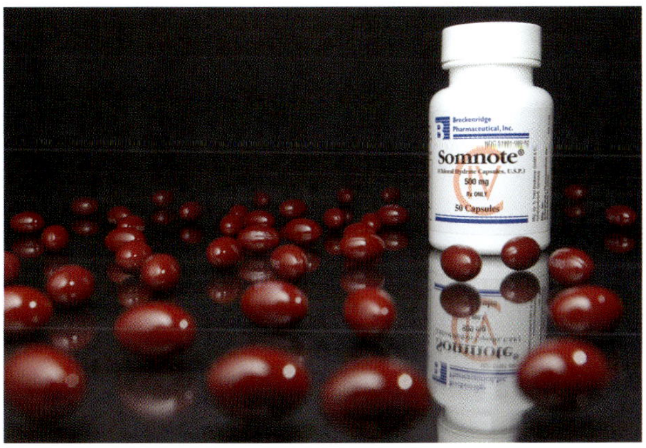

Somnote (chloral hydrate). *(© Bloomberg/Getty Images)*

Description

Chloral hydrate is classified as a sedative-hypnotic drug. The mechanism by which this drug works is not completely understood. It is believed that a chemical produced by chloral hydrate, called trichloroethanol, causes a mild depressive effect on the **brain**.

Recommended dosage

Chloral hydrate is available in oral and suppository forms. The oral form includes both capsules and syrup. Adults usually receive 500–1,000 mg taken 15–30 minutes before bedtime or surgery. These dosages are for hypnotic effects. For sedative effects, 250 mg is usually taken three times daily after meals. Total daily dosage should not be more than 2 g (2,000 mg). The hypnotic dose for children is usually 50 mg for every kilogram of body weight. The maximum amount per single dose is 1 g. Daily dosage is usually divided into several smaller doses and taken throughout the day. The sedative dose is typically one-half of the hypnotic dose. The syrup form should be combined with a half glass of fruit juice or water. The capsules should be taken with a full glass of water or juice to help prevent stomach upset.

The typical dose using suppositories is 500 to 1,000 mg at bedtime for adults to address trouble sleeping, and 325 mg three times a day for daytime sedation in adults. When given to children in preparation for a medical procedure, the dose is calculated based on body weight, usually at 50 mg per kilogram. If used to calm children before a nonsurgical procedure, such as **electroencephalography**, the dose is usually reduced to 25 mg per kilogram of body weight.

Precautions

Patients taking this drug for more than a few days should be monitored by a physician to ensure that significant side effects are not developing. Patients should not stop taking chloral hydrate suddenly. Instead, the dosage should be gradually decreased over time. Chloral hydrate should not be combined with other central nervous depressants, such as alcohol, antihistamines, and tranquilizers, as the effects will be increased.

Chloral hydrate should be used with great caution only where necessary in persons with a history of heart disease, severe kidney disease, or severe liver disease; people with gastrointestinal problems or porphyria; persons with a history of drug abuse; and in the elderly.

It should be used with caution in pregnant women and in women who are nursing. Chloral hydrate, like most drugs, can be taken in excess to the point of overdose. Signs of overdose include difficulty in swallowing, extreme weakness, confusion, **seizures**, extreme drowsiness, low body temperature, staggering, changes in heart rate, and breathing problems.

Side effects

Uncommon but serious side effects of chloral hydrate use include skin rash or hives, confusion, **hallucination**, and excessive excitement. The development of any of these side effects should be promptly reported to a doctor.

Less serious but more common side effects of chloral hydrate use include nausea, stomach pain, and vomiting. Other less common side effects include diarrhea, light-headedness, dizziness, drowsiness, and clumsiness.

Interactions

Because of additive depressant effects on the central nervous system, this drug should not be combined with alcohol. Likewise, chloral hydrate should not be combined with tricyclic **antidepressants** or with the blood-thinning drug warfarin (Coumadin). The prescribing physician should be made aware of any other drugs or medications the patient is taking to avoid complications.

Resources

BOOKS

Brunton, Laurence, Bruce Chabner, and Bjorn Knollman. *Goodman & Gilman's The Pharmacological Basis of Therapeutics*. 12th ed. New York: McGraw-Hill, 2010.

Consumer Reports and American Society of Health-System Pharmacists. *Consumer Reports Complete Drug Reference*. Yonkers, NY: Consumers Reports, 2009.

Ellsworth, Allan J., et al. *Mosby's Medical Drug Reference*. St. Louis, MO: Mosby, 2007.

Venes, Donald. *Taber's Cyclopedic Medical Dictionary*. 21st ed. Philadelphia: F.A. Davis Company, 2009.

WEBSITES

3-RX.com. "Chloral Hydrate." http://www.3-rx.com/drugs/detailed/chloral-hydrate/default.php (accessed October 1, 2011).

MedlinePlus. "Chloral Hydrate (Systemic)." U.S. National Library of Medicine. National Institutes of Health. http://www.nlm.nih.gov/medlineplus/druginfo/medmaster/a682201.html (accessed October 1, 2011).

Mark Mitchell, MD
Emily Jane Willingham, PhD

Chlordiazepoxide

Definition

Chlordiazepoxide is used to treat anxiety and also to control agitation brought on by alcohol withdrawal. It is a member of the benzodiazepine family of compounds, which slow the central nervous system to ease tension or nervousness. In the United States, it is sold under the trade names of Librium and Librax, and as Limbitrol when in combination with another drug, **amitriptyline**.

Purpose

Chlordiazepoxide is used for the short-term relief of symptoms of anxiety and the management of **anxiety disorders**. It is also used for treating symptoms of withdrawal from acute alcoholism and alcoholic intoxication. When combined with amitriptyline, it is used to treat **depression** that accompanies anxiety or tension.

Description

Chlordiazepoxide is useful when treating anxiety for short periods of time. It has sedative properties that are effective for these brief periods of use. In addition, it is occasionally used to stimulate appetites and is a weak analgesic. Its precise mechanism of action is unknown, and several hours are needed for peak levels of the drug to be achieved. Chlordiazepoxide is available in 5, 10, and 25 mg capsules.

Recommended dosage

The recommended dosage varies with **diagnosis**. The lowest possible dosage that provides relief from symptoms should be used as the drug has a high potential for causing physiological and psychological dependence. When used in adults for the treatment of moderate anxiety, the usual oral dosage is 5–10 mg three or four

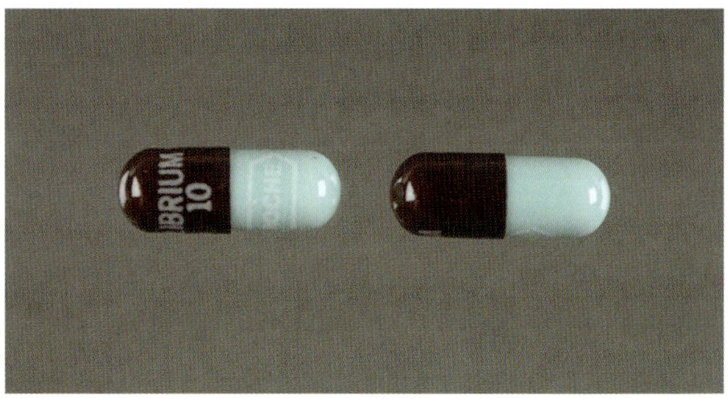

Librium (chlordiazepoxide), 10 mg. *(U.S. Drug Enforcement Administration)*

KEY TERMS

Anterograde amnesia—The inability to form new memories.

Anxiety—An emotion that can be experienced as a troubled feeling, sense of dread, fear of the future, or distress over a possible threat to a person's physical or mental well-being.

Depression—A mental state characterized by feelings of sadness, despair, discouragement, and low energy, sometimes accompanied by oversleeping and/or overeating.

times per day. When used for the treatment of more severe anxiety and anxiety disorders, the usual oral dosage is 20–25 mg three or four times per day. When used by older persons, or to relieve symptoms of preoperative apprehension or anxiety, the usual oral dosage is 5 mg two to four times per day. If used as a preoperative medication, the usual dosage is 50–100 mg via intramuscular (IM) injection. When used to treat symptoms of acute alcoholism, the usual initial oral dosage is 50–100 mg, repeated as needed until agitation is adequately controlled. The recommended maximum dosage is 300 mg per day. The usual dosage for children is 5 mg two to four times per day.

Precautions

Persons with suicidal tendencies should be closely monitored, as chlordiazepoxide may lower the threshold for action in attempting **suicide**. Children and adolescents up to 24 years of age are especially at risk when taking the chlordiazepoxide/amitriptyline combination, as are individuals with a history or family history of **bipolar disorder**. The drug has a high potential for causing physiological or psychological dependence.

Benzodiazepines, including chlordiazepoxide, carry the risk of inducing anterograde **amnesia** (the loss of the ability to make new memories). Chlordiazepoxide is slow to metabolize and is not generally advised for use in the elderly, as the slow elimination rate can lead to accumulation in the body, producing prolonged effects. This is especially dangerous to elderly patients, who are at risk for falls.

In the early 2000s, there were cases in which pills originating overseas but sold over the counter in the United States contained chlordiazepoxide. A case from 2001 involved ingredients shipped from Asia for pill manufacture in California, and another case from 2006 involved pills from Brazil. Both resulted in warnings to consumers by the U.S. Food and Drug Administration (FDA). In the case involving Brazil, the products—marketed as dietary/weight loss supplements under the names Emagrece Sim and Herbathin—were available for sale over the Internet and imported and distributed by a Florida company. Because of the serious possibility of interactions with medication and vitamins and the lack of quality control, taking these pills was considered dangerous. The FDA advised consumers who had these products to return them to the distributor.

Side effects

Other than physiological and psychological dependence, few adverse effects have been reported. The most commonly reported include drowsiness, confusion, and movement difficulties. These are most common among older persons. Occasionally, transient loss of consciousness has been reported.

Other adverse effects include:

- edema (abnormal accumulation of fluid in bodily tissues)
- minor menstrual irregularities
- nausea
- constipation
- changes in libido (sex drive)

Also, chlordiazepoxide may impair mental or physical skills needed to perform complex motor tasks. For this reason, persons using this drug are advised not to drive automobiles or operate machinery.

This drug is known to increase the risk of birth defects in the fetus when taken by a woman during the first three months of pregnancy, and it also can cause dependency in the developing baby that can result in withdrawal symptoms following birth. Chlordiazepoxide passes into the breast milk and can cause breathing trouble and slow heartbeat in babies.

Interactions

Chlordiazepoxide may increase the effect of alcohol or other substances that depress central nervous system functions. For this reason, they should not be used at the same time. A small number of reports of interaction with oral anticoagulants have been received, and it may exacerbate porphyria, which is a group of inherited disorders in which there is abnormally increased production of substances called porphyrins. Any medications, prescribed or over the counter, should be brought to the attention of a doctor or pharmacist by individuals considering taking chlordiazepoxide.

QUESTIONS TO ASK YOUR DOCTOR

- What kind of changes can I expect to see or feel with this medication?
- Does it matter what time of day I take this medication? If so, what is the recommendation?
- Should I take this medication with or without food?
- What are the side effects associated with this medication?
- Will this medication interact or interfere with other medications I am currently taking?
- What symptoms or adverse effects are important enough that I should seek immediate treatment?

Resources

BOOKS

Albers, Lawrence J., Rhoda K. Hahn, and Christopher Reist. *Handbook of Psychiatric Drugs.* Laguna Hills, CA: Current Clinical Strategies, 2010.

American Society of Health-System Pharmacists. *AHFS Drug Information 2011.* Bethesda, MD: ASHP, 2011.

Graham, George. *The Disordered Mind: An Introduction to Philosophy of Mind and Mental Illness.* New York: Routledge, 2010.

Holland, Leland Norman, and Michael Patrick Adams. *Core Concepts in Pharmacology.* 3rd ed. New York: Prentice Hall, 2011.

North, Carol, and Sean Yutzy. *Goodwin and Guze's Psychiatric Diagnosis.* New York: Oxford University Press, 2010.

Preston, John D., John H. O'Neal, and Mary C. Talaga. *Handbook of Clinical Psychopharmacology for Therapists.* 6th ed. Oakland, CA: New Harbinger, 2010.

PERIODICALS

Alexopoulou A., A. Michael, and S.P. Dourakis. "Acute Thrombocytopenic Purpura in a Patient Treated with Chlordiazepoxide and Clidinium." *Archives of Internal Medicine* 161, no. 14 (2001): 1778–79.

ORGANIZATIONS

American Academy of Clinical Toxicology, 6728 Old McLean Village Dr., McLean, VA, 22101, (703) 556-9222, Fax: (703) 556-8729, admin@clintox.org, http://www.clintox.org.

American Academy of Family Physicians, 11400 Tomahawk Creek Pkwy., Leawood, KS, 66211-2672, (913) 906-6000, (800) 274-2237, Fax: (913) 906-6075, contactcenter@aafp.org, http://www.aafp.org.

American Medical Association, 515 N State St., Chicago, IL, 60610, (312) 464-5000, (800) 621-8335, http://www.ama-assn.org.

American Psychiatric Association, 1000 Wilson Blvd., Ste. 1825, Arlington, VA, 22209-3901, (703) 907-7300, apa@psych.org, http://www.psych.org.

American Society for Clinical Pharmacology and Therapeutics, 528 N Washington St., Alexandria, VA, 22314, (703) 836-6981, info@ascpt.org, http://www.ascpt.org.

Anxiety Disorders Association of America, 8730 Georgia Ave., Silver Spring, MD, 20910, (240) 485-1001, Fax: (240) 485-1035, http://www.adaa.org.

Mental Health America, 2000 N. Beauregard St., 6th Fl., Alexandria, VA, 22311, (703) 684-7722, (800) 969-6642, Fax: (703) 684-5968, http://www1.nmha.org.

National Alliance on Mental Illness, 2107 Wilson Blvd., Ste. 300, Arlington, VA, 22201-3042, Fax: (703) 524-9094, (800) 950-6264, http://www.nami.org.

National Institute of Mental Health, 6001 Executive Blvd., Rm. 8184, MSC 9663, Bethesda, MD, 20892-9663, (301) 433-4513; TTY: (301) 443-8431, Fax: (301) 443-4279, (866) 615-6464; TTY: (866) 415-8051, nimhinfo@nih.gov, http://www.nimh.nih.gov.

L. Fleming Fallon, Jr., MD, DrPH
Emily Jane Willingham, PhD
Laura Jean Cataldo, RN, EdD

Chlorpromazine

Definition

Chlorpromazine is an antipsychotic drug. It is a member of the phenothiazine family of compounds and is used to alleviate the symptoms and signs of **psychosis**. Psychosis is a form of severe mental illness characterized by hallucinations, **delusions**, agitation, unusual behavior, and loss of contact with reality. In the United States,

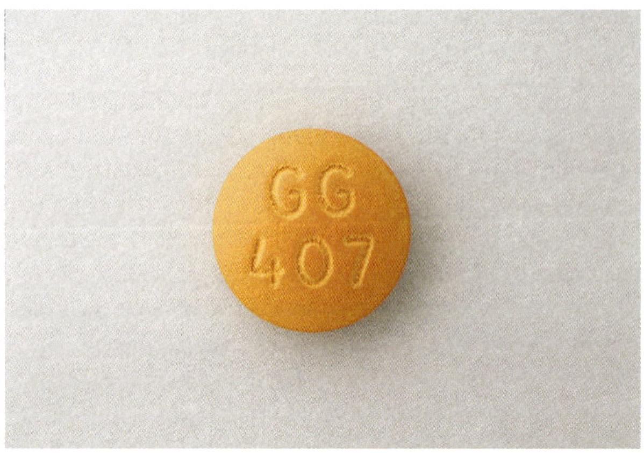

Chlorpromazine, 50 mg. *(© Custom Medical Stock Photo, Inc. Reproduced by permission.)*

HEINZ EDGAR LEHMANN (1911–1999)

Heinz Edgar Lehmann was a German-born Canadian psychiatrist best known for his use of chlorpromazine for the treatment of schizophrenia in the 1950s. Born in Berlin, Germany, he was educated at the University of Freiburg, the University of Marburg, the University of Vienna, and the University of Berlin. He emigrated to Canada in 1937. In 1947, he was appointed clinical director of Montreal's Douglas Hospital. From 1971 to 1975, he was the chairman of the McGill University Department of Psychiatry. In 1976, he was made an Officer of the Order of Canada. In 1970, he was made a fellow of the Royal Society of Canada. He was inducted into the Canadian Medical Hall of Fame in 1998. In 1999, the Canadian College of Neuropsychopharmacology established the Heinz Lehmann award in his honor, given in recognition of outstanding contributions to research in neuropsychopharmacology in Canada.

chlorpromazine is also sold under the brand name Thorazine.

Purpose

Chlorpromazine is principally used to reduce the signs and symptoms of psychosis. For this purpose, the drug is used in **schizophrenia** and the manic phase of bipolar (formerly manic-depressive) disorder. The drug is also used in the management of severe behavioral disorders with aggression, combativeness, or excessive excitability. Chlorpromazine may sometimes be used as a sedative in nonpsychotic patients with excessive anxiety and agitation. In addition, the drug has been used to relieve nausea, vomiting, and persistent hiccups.

Description

Chlorpromazine was the first antipsychotic drug. It is not an exaggeration to say that the development of this medication began a revolution in the treatment of severe mental illness, which continues in the twenty-first century. Patients with schizophrenia and other psychoses, who once would have been considered hopelessly untreatable and relegated to the back wards of state institutions, are often able, as a result of treatment with chlorpromazine or similar medications, to live in the community and lead fuller lives.

The discovery of chlorpromazine resulted from efforts of pharmaceutical researchers in the first half of the twentieth century to develop sedative medications. Several drugs of a chemical class known as phenothiazines were investigated and shown to be effective **sedatives**, but they had little effect on agitated patients with psychosis. A new phenothiazine drug, chlorpromazine, was synthesized in France in 1950 and was tested on such patients. In 1952, two French psychiatrists, Jean Delay and Pierre Deniker, announced that the drug exerted a specific effect in diminishing the symptoms and signs of psychosis in patients with severe mental illnesses.

The mechanism of action of chlorpromazine occurs primarily through its interactions with proteins on the cells that take messages from **dopamine**, a nerve signaling molecule, and send them to other cells.

Chlorpromazine, when sold under the name Thorazine, is available in many forms: tablets of 10, 25, 50, 100, and 200 mg; spansules (sustained release capsules) of 30, 75, and 150 mg; ampules for injection of 25 and 50 mg; a multidose vial of 10 mL of 25 mg/mL; syrup 10mg/5mL, 4 fl oz.; and suppositories of 25 and 100 mg. Generic chlorpromazine manufacturers may supply a somewhat different set of dosages and products.

Recommended dosage

For acutely disturbed adult patients diagnosed with a psychosis, such as schizophrenia or mania, the usual daily dosage ranges from 100 mg to 1,000 mg per day. Some patients may require a higher dosage. There is great variation in individual dosage requirements for chlorpromazine and for other antipsychotic medications. It is usually advisable to begin with a lower dosage and increase the dosage until sufficient reduction of symptoms is achieved. Maximum reduction of symptoms may take many weeks of continued treatment. Because of the possibility of side effects, which may be severe, lower dosages should be used in outpatients, children, the elderly, and patients with serious health problems. For nonpsychotic patients with excessive anxiety or agitation, amounts used are generally less than 200 mg per day, divided into two or three doses.

Precautions

Elderly patients (those over age 65), especially women, and patients receiving long-term antipsychotic treatment are prone to develop **tardive dyskinesia**. This syndrome consists of involuntary, uncoordinated movements that may not disappear or may only partially improve after the drug is stopped. Tardive dyskinesia involves involuntary movements of the tongue, jaw,

KEY TERMS

Anxiety—An emotion that can be experienced as a troubled feeling, sense of dread, fear of the future, or distress over a possible threat to a person's physical or mental well-being.

Bipolar disorder—A mood disorder marked by alternating episodes of extremely low mood (depression) and exuberant highs (mania), also known as manic-depressive disorder.

Delusions—Irrational beliefs that defy normal reasoning and remain firm even when overwhelming proof is presented to dispute them. Delusions are distinct from culturally or religiously based beliefs that may be seen as untrue by outsiders.

Epilepsy—A disorder associated with disturbed electrical discharges in the central nervous system that cause seizures.

Extrapyramidal symptoms—A group of side effects associated with antipsychotic medications and characterized by involuntary muscle movements, including contraction and tremor.

Schizophrenia—A major mental illness marked by psychotic symptoms, including hallucinations, delusions, and severe disruptions in thinking.

Seizure—A convulsion, or uncontrolled discharge of nerve cells that may spread to other cells throughout the brain.

mouth, or face or other groups of skeletal muscles and may also appear after chlorpromazine use has stopped. There is no known effective treatment for tardive dyskinesia, although gradual (but rarely complete) improvement may occur over a long period. The need for long-term antipsychotic medication should be weighed against the risk of developing tardive dyskinesia, which increases with duration of treatment.

Neuroleptic malignant syndrome (NMS), a dangerous condition with high fever, muscular rigidity, rapid pulse, sweating, and altered mental state, may occur with antipsychotic medication. NMS requires immediate medical treatment.

Phenothiazine drugs, such as chlorpromazine, may cause sedation and may interfere with driving and other tasks requiring alertness. They may increase the effects of alcohol and sedatives. The adverse effects of chlorpromazine may be increased in people with diseases of the heart, liver, or kidney, or other debilitating illnesses. Phenothiazines may lower the seizure threshold, making it more likely that a seizure will occur in people who have a history of **seizures**. People with epilepsy may require adjustment of their antiseizure medications. Chlorpromazine may cause acute muscle spasms, particularly of the head and neck, and sudden decreases of blood pressure. Patients may need to be hospitalized during the initial phase of treatment, particularly when receiving high doses or treatment by injection.

Chlorpromazine reduces the body's ability to sweat, thus interfering with the regulation of body temperature. This may be a problem for some people in very hot weather. The problem most commonly occurs in elderly people in hot buildings without air conditioning. Body temperature may reach fatal levels. People taking chlorpromazine should be aware of the possibility of developing hyperthermia (high body temperature) in very hot weather. They should seek cool places in hot weather.

Children may be especially susceptible to neurologic reactions to phenothiazines, such as muscle spasms. Elderly patients may be particularly sensitive to sedation, low blood pressure, and other side effects. These patients should start with lower doses and increase their dosage gradually under physician supervision. Chlorpromazine may decrease salivation in older patients, predisposing them to tooth decay, gum disease, and mouth infections. Candy and other sugary foods should be limited, and oral hygiene should be maintained.

Chlorpromazine, like all phenothiazines, should not be taken by pregnant women because these drugs harm the developing fetus. Babies born to mothers who took chlorpromazine during pregnancy may develop extrapyramidal symptoms (EPS) and withdrawal symptoms, including agitation, trouble breathing, and difficulty feeding. Breastfeeding is not recommended while a woman is taking the drug. Phenothiazines are secreted in breast milk and may cause harm to nursing infants.

Chlorpromazine is associated with an increased risk of death when used in elderly patients with **dementia**. In June 2008, the U.S. Food and Drug Administration (FDA) announced a requirement for manufacturers of chlorpromazine (and other antipsychotic drugs) to add a warning label to their packaging stating this risk. The reason for the increase was unclear in studies, but most deaths were found to be related either to cardiovascular complications or complications associated with infection. Chlorpromazine is not approved by the FDA for the treatment of behavior problems in older adults with dementia, and patients in this category (or caregivers of patients in this category) should discuss the risks of taking chlorpromazine with their physician.

Chlorpromazine also carries the risk of potentially fatal heart arrhythmias.

QUESTIONS TO ASK YOUR DOCTOR

- What kind of changes can I expect to see or feel with this medication?
- Does it matter what time of day I take this medication? If so, what is the recommendation?
- Should I take this medication with or without food?
- What are the side effects associated with this medication?
- Will this medication interact or interfere with other medications I am currently taking?
- What symptoms or adverse effects are important enough that I should seek immediate treatment?

Side effects

Chlorpromazine and other phenothiazines may cause many side effects. The following more common side effects are grouped by the body system affected:

- cardiovascular: decreases of blood pressure, especially on arising, which may cause dizziness or fainting; rapid heart rate and changes in heart rhythm and electrocardiogram
- nervous system: sedation, muscle spasms of the head and neck, muscle rigidity, restlessness, tremors, slowed movement, shuffling gait, increased seizure tendency
- digestive system: dry mouth, nausea, constipation, abnormal liver tests
- autonomic: blurred vision, nasal congestion, reduced sweating, difficulty urinating, problems with ejaculation, impotence
- hormonal: lactation, breast enlargement
- skin: rashes, sensitivity to sunlight
- body as a whole: weight gain

Interactions

Chlorpromazine interacts with a long list of other medications. Individuals who are starting this drug should review the other medications they are taking with their physician and pharmacist for possible interactions. Chlorpromazine and other phenothiazines may intensify the effects of drugs causing sedation, including alcohol, **barbiturates**, narcotic pain medications, minor tranquilizers, and antihistamines. Similarly, chlorpromazine may cause excessive reductions of blood pressure in patients taking other medicines that lower blood pressure. Chlorpromazine may also intensify side effects of drugs that cause blurred vision, dry mouth, diminished sweating in hot weather, and constipation. Many other antipsychotics and **antidepressants** cause such effects.

Chlorpromazine may enhance the effects of medications that lower the seizure threshold, such as steroid drugs, the asthma medication theophylline, and many other psychiatric drugs. Patients with epilepsy may require dosage adjustments of their antiseizure medications. The effectiveness of medications for Parkinson's disease may be reduced by chlorpromazine and other antipsychotics. The likelihood of changes in heart rhythm may be increased when the drug is taken with other medications that have the same effect, including other antipsychotic drugs, antidepressants, certain heart medicines, and erythromycin.

Certain drugs that are eliminated by the liver may interfere with the elimination of chlorpromazine from the body, causing higher blood levels and increased side effects. Chlorpromazine may delay the elimination of other medicines, including many antidepressants, antipsychotic drugs, and heart medications, resulting in higher levels of these other medications and possibly increased side effects.

Resources

BOOKS

Albers, Lawrence J., Rhoda K. Hahn, and Christopher Reist. *Handbook of Psychiatric Drugs.* Laguna Hills, CA: Current Clinical Strategies, 2010.

American Society of Health-System Pharmacists. *AHFS Drug Information 2011.* Bethesda, MD: ASHP, 2011.

Graham, George. *The Disordered Mind: An Introduction to Philosophy of Mind and Mental Illness.* New York: Routledge, 2010.

Holland, Leland Norman, and Michael Patrick Adams. *Core Concepts in Pharmacology.* 3rd ed. New York: Prentice Hall, 2011.

Miklowitz, David J. *Bipolar Disorder: A Family-Focused Treatment Approach.* 2nd ed. New York: Guilford Press, 2010.

North, Carol, and Sean Yutzy. *Goodwin and Guze's Psychiatric Diagnosis.* New York: Oxford University Press, 2010.

Preston, John D., John H. O'Neal, and Mary C. Talaga. *Handbook of Clinical Psychopharmacology for Therapists.* 6th ed. Oakland, CA: New Harbinger, 2010.

PERIODICALS

Rosenbloom, Michael. "Chlorpromazine and the Psychopharmacologic Revolution." *Journal of the American Medical Association* 287 (2002): 1860–61. Available online at http://jama.ama-assn.org/cgi/content/full/287/14/1860 (accessed August 25, 2011).

ORGANIZATIONS

American Academy of Clinical Toxicology, 6728 Old McLean Village Dr., McLean, VA, 22101, (703) 556-9222, Fax: (703) 556-8729, admin@clintox.org, http://www.clintox.org.

American Academy of Family Physicians, 11400 Tomahawk Creek Pkwy., Leawood, KS, 66211-2672, (913) 906-6000, (800) 274-2237, Fax: (913) 906-6075, contactcenter@aafp.org, http://www.aafp.org.

American Medical Association, 515 N State St., Chicago, IL, 60610, (312) 464-5000, (800) 621-8335, http://www.ama-assn.org.

American Psychiatric Association, 1000 Wilson Blvd., Ste. 1825, Arlington, VA, 22209-3901, (703) 907-7300, apa@psych.org, http://www.psych.org.

American Psychological Association, 750 1st St., NE, Washington, DC, 20002-4242, (202) 336-5500; TDD/TTY: (202) 336-6123, (800) 374-2721, http://www.apa.org.

American Society for Clinical Pharmacology and Therapeutics, 528 N Washington St., Alexandria, VA, 22314, (703) 836-6981, info@ascpt.org, http://www.ascpt.org.

Anxiety Disorders Association of America, 8730 Georgia Ave., Silver Spring, MD, 20910, (240) 485-1001, Fax: (240) 485-1035, http://www.adaa.org.

Depression and Bipolar Support Alliance, 730 N Franklin St., Ste. 501, Chicago, IL, 60654, (800) 826-3632, Fax: (312) 642-7243, http://www.dbsalliance.org.

Mental Health America, 2000 N Beauregard St., 6th Fl., Alexandria, VA, 22311, (703) 684-7722, (800) 969-6642, Fax: (703) 684-5968, http://www1.nmha.org.

National Alliance on Mental Illness, 2107 Wilson Blvd., Ste. 300, Arlington, VA, 22201-3042, Fax: (703) 524-9094, (800) 950-6264, http://www.nami.org.

National Institute of Mental Health, 6001 Executive Blvd., Rm. 8184, MSC 9663, Bethesda, MD, 20892-9663, (301) 443-4513; TTY: (301) 443-8431, Fax: (301) 443-4279, (866) 615-6464; TTY: (866) 415-8051, nimhinfo@nih.gov, http://www.nimh.nih.gov.

U.S. National Library of Medicine, 8600 Rockville Pike, Bethesda, MD, 20894, (301) 594-5983, (888) 346-3656; TDD: (800) 735-2258, Fax: (301) 402-1384, http://www.nlm.nih.gov.

Richard Kapit, MD
Ruth A. Wienclaw, PhD
Laura Jean Cataldo, RN, EdD

Chronic motor or vocal tic disorder *see* **Tic disorders**

Chronic pain *see* **Pain disorder**

Cigarettes *see* **Nicotine and related disorders**

Circadian rhythm sleep disorder

Definition

Circadian rhythm sleep disorder (CRSD) is any of several persistent or recurring patterns of sleep disruption that result from an altered circadian rhythm or sleep-wake cycle. CRSD leads to **insomnia** or excessive sleepiness during waking hours, resulting in impaired functioning.

Demographics

More than 70 million Americans are estimated to have some form of sleep disorder. Among CRSDs, delayed sleep phase usually begins during adolescence, affecting up to 7% of teens. Without treatment, delayed sleep phase may continue and is believed to affect up to 4% of adults. Jet-lag and shift-work CRSDs usually cause the most severe symptoms in late-middle-aged and elderly people. An estimated 14% of Americans perform shift work and up to 60% of night-shift workers have CRSD. Non-24-hour sleep-wake syndrome is probably the rarest CRSD, most often affecting people who are totally blind.

Description

There are more than 80 recognized **sleep disorders**, usually classified into seven primary groups, including CRSD, insomnia, sleep-related breathing problems, and **hypersomnia**. CRSD is a dyssomnia (having irregularities in the quality, timing, and amount of sleep) caused by alterations in circadian rhythms or a mismatch between natural circadian rhythms and external signals or demands.

Circadian rhythms are physiological, mental, and behavioral changes that occur over a period of approximately 24 hours. "Circadian" is Latin for "around a day." Most circadian rhythms are controlled by the body's master biological clock, the suprachiasmatic nucleus (SCN), located in the hypothalamus of the **brain**. Light hitting the retina of the eye sends signals through the optic nerve to the SCN. In response to light, the SCN signals the pineal gland to stop producing the hormone melatonin. After dark, melatonin levels rise and cause drowsiness. The SCN synchronizes other bodily functions, such as temperature, hormone secretion, urine production, and blood pressure, with the sleep-wake cycle. Although most people actually have a 25-hour biological clock, sunlight or other bright light normally resets the SCN to follow the sun's 24-hour cycle. To some extent, circadian rhythms can also be affected by external time cues, such as an alarm clock or meals.

Although classifications of CRSDs vary, the major types are:

- delayed sleep phase
- jet lag
- shift-work-induced
- non-24-hour sleep-wake syndrome
- medical-condition-induced
- drug- or substance-induced
- other unspecified

CRSDs cause insomnia and/or excessive drowsiness and interfere with occupational, social, and other functioning. Shift-work CRSD is of particular concern because workplace accidents tend to increase in number and severity during the night shift. Mistakes by fatigued night-shift workers can contribute to medical errors and to major industrial accidents.

The ***Diagnostic and Statistical Manual of Mental Disorders***, a handbook used by mental health professionals to diagnose mental disorders, defines circadian rhythm sleep disorder as one of several primary sleep-wake disorders.

Risk factors

Stress is a risk factor for various types of CRSD. CRSD also is common in people with **dementia**, who often sleep erratically and in snatches. Delayed sleep phase sometimes runs in families. Risk factors for jet lag include frequent flying, crossing multiple time zones, and flying east, thereby "losing" time. Night-shift workers, especially those who switch to a normal sleep schedule on days off and those who work rotating shifts, are especially at risk for CSRD. Having a more erratic biological clock may be a risk factor for substance-induced CRSD.

Causes and symptoms

Sometimes the cause of a CRSD is apparent, as with jet lag, shift work, and non-24-hour sleep-wake syndrome in the blind. In other cases the cause of CRSD is less obvious. Delayed sleep phase is often caused by stress. Various medical conditions can cause CRSD. Dementia can weaken circadian rhythms. Liver disease can also cause delayed sleep phase due to toxin buildup in the blood.

Many drugs and other substances, including alcohol, can cause CRSD. Some drugs cause early sleep, resulting in earlier awakening and an advanced sleep rhythm. The same medication may cause sleepiness in one person and insomnia in another. Herbs; vitamins and minerals; supplements such as tryptophan; antihistamines; allergy, cold, and flu remedies; sleeping pills; muscle relaxants; pain medications; some **antidepressants**; antianxiety and antipsychotic medications; drugs for Parkinson's disease: seizure medications; blood pressure, cholesterol, and heart medications; and chemotherapy can all cause drug-induced CRSD. Caffeine can cause delayed sleep phase or an irregular sleep-wake rhythm. Other stimulants, weight-control medications, **steroids**, and some asthma medications also can cause delayed sleep phase.

Symptoms of CRSD take different forms:

- Delayed sleep phase disorder causes falling asleep late, such as in the early morning, and awakening late, a cycle that is very difficult to change.
- Advanced sleep phase disorder causes falling asleep early and awakening early each day.
- Irregular sleep-wake rhythm is characterized by sleeping off and on over a 24-hour period.
- Jet lag can involve insomnia, daytime fatigue or sleepiness, early waking, general malaise, and various other symptoms. It occurs within one or two days of crossing at least two time zones, especially when traveling in an easterly direction.

KEY TERMS

Chronotherapy—A sleep disorder treatment that involves adjusting sleep and wake times to reset one's biological clock.

Circadian rhythm—An approximately 24-hour cycle of physiological and behavioral activity.

Dementia—A group of symptoms (syndrome) associated with chronic progressive impairment of memory, reasoning ability, and other intellectual functions; personality changes; deterioration in personal grooming; and disorientation.

Dyssomnia—Irregularities in the timing, length, and quality of sleep.

Insomnia—Prolonged or abnormal inability to obtain adequate sleep.

Melatonin—A hormone involved in regulation of the sleep-wake cycle and other circadian rhythms.

Pineal gland—A small endocrine gland in the brain that produces melatonin.

Sleep hygiene—Beneficial behavior and environmental choices that precede sleep and tend to help produce a good night's sleep.

Suprachiasmatic nucleus (SCN)—A pair of nerve clusters in the hypothalamus in the brain that receives light input from the retina via the optic nerve and regulates circadian rhythms.

- Shift workers are more likely to experience both insomnia and daytime sleepiness. They may have impaired performance, relationship problems, irritability, and depression, and are at increased risk for heart, digestive, mental, and emotional problems. They have almost twice the risk of falling asleep while driving.
- Free-running (non-entrained) CRSD is a non-24-hour sleep-wake syndrome, in which sleep occurs somewhat later each day. Blind people whose retinas cannot detect light often have lifelong CRSD, since their circadian rhythms follow their innate 25-hour clock, pushing sleep and wake times further back each day.
- Unspecified CRSD can cause daytime and evening sleepiness or insomnia. People with irregular sleep patterns have difficulty knowing when they will fall asleep and wake up.

Diagnosis

A **diagnosis** of CRSD requires that the sleep disturbance not be related to normal adjustments in response to a schedule change. It also must be persistent or recurring and result in family, social, or occupational problems.

Examination

The physician will perform a physical exam, including a neurological exam, and take a medical history, including past and present drug, alcohol, and medication use. Patients usually keep a sleep diary of their sleep and wake-up times for a period of several weeks, as well as the timing of any medications or other substances they take. They may use the Epworth Sleepiness Scale to rate their sleep. Patients with constant jet lag or other serious CRSDs may choose to consult a sleep specialist.

Tests

Blood tests may be performed if the physician suspects a neurological condition or other medical problem. Drug tests may be performed if substance-induced CRSD is suspected. Body temperature and melatonin levels may be measured.

Procedures

Computed tomography (CT) scans or **magnetic resonance imaging** (MRI) may be performed to detect medical conditions underlying CRSD. Some patients wear an actigraph on their wrists for one to two weeks. This device records active and inactive periods throughout the 24-hour day. In severe cases, patients may undergo direct observation in a sleep lab. However, overnight sleep studies are not usually required to diagnose CRSD unless the patient is at risk for another sleep disorder. A polysomnogram charts brain waves, heart beat, muscle activity, breathing, and arm and leg movements during sleep in the laboratory.

Treatment

Various treatments are used for DRSD, chosen in light of the specific causes of the problem.

Traditional

Treatment of CRSD depends on the type and cause. Education about good sleep hygiene and behavior counseling can be helpful. Mild cases of delayed sleep phase often resolve simply by following strict sleep and wake times. More severe cases may require incremental changes, for example, going to sleep 15–30 minutes earlier each day until an appropriate pattern is achieved. Sometimes a night of **sleep deprivation** is prescribed to reset the biological clock. Chronotherapy may include delaying sleep for three hours each night until the sleep-wake cycle has rotated around the clock. Drug-induced CRSD may involve changing or stopping a medication. Detailed sleep logs are often used to monitor progress during treatment.

Drugs

Melatonin is often used to treat jet lag and other CRSDs. Timing of the medication depends on symptoms, but generally melatonin is taken 20–60 minutes before the desired sleep time. Although some studies have found higher doses to be better at promoting sleep, doses as small as 0.5 mg may be as effective as doses of 5 mg or more. Tasimelteon, which acts like melatonin, is also used to treat CRSD. Other drugs for preventing or treating jet lag and other CRSDs include nonbenzodiazepines—such as **zolpidem** (Ambien), eszopiclone (Lunesta), and **zaleplon** (Sonata)—and **benzodiazepines**, such as **triazolam** (Halcion).

Alternative

Melatonin is available as a nutritional supplement for jet lag, shift work, and delayed sleep phase, and to improve night-time sleep in the blind. However, most melatonin supplements are high-dosage, and melatonin can build up in the body with unknown effects. Therefore, most experts discourage non-medically supervised use of melatonin supplements.

There are various other alternative treatments for jet lag. Although some frequent fliers use **aromatherapy** or homeopathy, **light therapy**, which involves exposing the eyes to light for a specific amount of time, is especially useful for jet-lagged travelers who are indoors out of the sunlight in a different time zone. There are various types of light therapy, including an artificial bright light, a light box or desk lamp, a full-spectrum lamp that simulates sunlight, or a light visor worn on the head. A dawn simulator that gradually brightens to simulate sunrise can help with waking up. Exposure to a special, very bright light close to the desired wake-up time can help reset the biological clock to a new time zone.

Home remedies

Sunlight is the best way to reset one's biological clock and maintain a regular sleep-wake cycle. Online jet-lag calculators can help determine the best time for light exposure. For example, after flying from New York to Paris, travelers are advised to obtain light exposure between 11:20 A.M. and 2 P.M. on the first day and between 8:20 A.M. and 11 A.M. on the second day. Light should be avoided between 9 A.M. and 11:20 A.M. on the first day and between 6 A.M. and 8:20 A.M. on the second day. A sleep mask or sleeping with the blinds or drapes closed can help. Dark glasses can block out light during the day. By the third or fourth day, one's biological clock should be reset to local time, especially if combined with **exercise** such as walking or jogging. Caffeine can help counter daytime sleepiness but can also make it more difficult to sleep if consumed within six hours of bedtime. If staying for a week or more in the new time zone, travelers should sleep during appropriate times for that zone.

Jet-lag **diets** are effective for some people. These often involve alternating days of feasting and fasting and high-protein and low-protein meals. Eating more high-protein foods during waking hours and more carbohydrates before sleep may also be effective.

Shift workers benefit the most from a regular work schedule. If schedule rotations cannot be avoided, it is preferable to rotate forward, with shifts becoming progressively later. Sleeping environments should be free of daytime light and noise.

Prognosis

Patients with delayed sleep phase often have great difficulty changing their sleep patterns or maintaining a preferred pattern. Jet-lag and shift-work symptoms disappear with a return to one's usual schedule and environment or adjustment to the new schedule. It is estimated that it takes about one day per time zone to recover from jet lag. Some research suggests that the human body never completely adapts to shift work, especially when there is a reversion to a normal sleep schedule on days off.

Prevention

Good sleep behavior (called sleep hygiene) is important for maintaining sleep-wake cycles.

QUESTIONS TO ASK YOUR DOCTOR

- Do you think I have a circadian rhythm sleep disorder or some other type?
- What do you think is causing my sleep disorder?
- Do you recommend melatonin supplements?
- What measures can I take to reset my biological clock?
- What is my prognosis?

Maintaining a regular sleep-wake cycle can help prevent problems even in people who are susceptible to altered circadian rhythms. Stresses such as long-distance travel, shift work, and sleep-disrupting lifestyles should be avoided if possible.

Methods for preventing or reducing jet lag include:

- getting plenty of rest before traveling
- gradually adjusting sleeping and eating schedules before leaving home—to earlier if traveling east and to later if traveling west
- arriving at one's destination a few days early to adjust to the change
- adjusting light exposure appropriately
- following the local sleeping schedule
- drinking plenty of water to prevent dehydration and avoiding caffeine and alcohol
- sleeping on airplanes if arriving at night and staying awake if arriving in the daytime

Methods for reducing CRSD in shift workers include:

- nap-friendly workplace policies
- brightly lit workplaces
- avoiding shift changes and rotations
- wearing dark glasses to block sunlight after work
- keeping the same sleep-wake schedule on days off
- using an eye mask and ear plugs to eliminate light and noise when sleeping
- avoiding caffeine near bedtime
- avoiding alcohol

Resources

BOOKS

Foldvary-Schaefer, Nancy. *The Cleveland Clinic Guide to Sleep Disorders.* New York: Kaplan, 2009.

Lee-Chiong, Teofilo L., ed. *Sleep Medicine Essentials.* Hoboken, NJ: Wiley-Blackwell, 2009.

Wright, Kenneth P., ed. *Circadian Rhythm Sleep Disorders.* Philadelphia: Saunders, 2009.

PERIODICALS

Chang, Anne-Marie, et al. "Sleep Timing and Circadian Phase in Delayed Sleep Phase Syndrome." *Journal of Biological Rhythms* 24, no. 4 (August 2009): 313–21.

Rajaratnam, Shantha M. W., et al. "Melatonin Agonist Tasimelteon (VEC-162) for Transient Insomnia after Sleep-Time Shift: Two Randomised Controlled Multi-centre Trials." *Lancet* 373, no. 9662 (February 7–13, 2009): 482–91.

Sack, Robert L. "Jet Lag." *New England Journal of Medicine* 362 (February 4, 2010): 440–47.

WEBSITES

Mayo Clinic Staff. "Jet Lag Disorder." MayoClinic.com. July 10, 2010. http://www.mayoclinic.com/health/jet-lag/DS01085 (accessed July 25, 2011).

National Institute of General Medical Sciences. "Circadian Rhythms Fact Sheet." April 23, 2011. http://www.nigms.nih.gov/Publications/Factsheet_CircadianRhythms.htm (accessed July 25, 2011).

National Institute of Neurological Disorders and Stroke. "Brain Basics: Understanding Sleep." May 21, 2007. http://www.ninds.nih.gov/disorders/brain_basics/understanding_ sleep.htm#circadian_rhythms (accessed July 25, 2011).

"Shift Work and Sleep." National Sleep Foundation. http://www.sleepfoundation.org/article/sleep-topics/shift-work-and-sleep (accessed July 25, 2011).

ORGANIZATIONS

American Academy of Sleep Medicine, 2510 N Frontage Rd., Darien, IL, 60561, (630) 737-9700, Fax: (630) 737-9790, inquiries@aasmnet.org, http://www.aasmnet.org.

National Heart, Lung, and Blood Institute, NHLBI Health Information Center, PO Box 30105, Bethesda, MD, 20824-0105, (301) 592-8573, Fax: (240) 629-3246, nhlbiinfo@nhlbi.nih.gov, http://www.nhlbi.nih.gov.

National Sleep Foundation, 1010 N. Glebe Road, Ste. 310, Arlington, VA, 22201, (703) 243-1697, nsf@sleepfoundation.org, http://www.sleepfoundation.org.

Ali Fahmy, PhD
Margaret Alic, PhD

Citalopram

Definition

Citalopram is a selective **serotonin** reuptake inhibitor (SSRI) antidepressant drug that is sold in the United States under brand name Celexa.

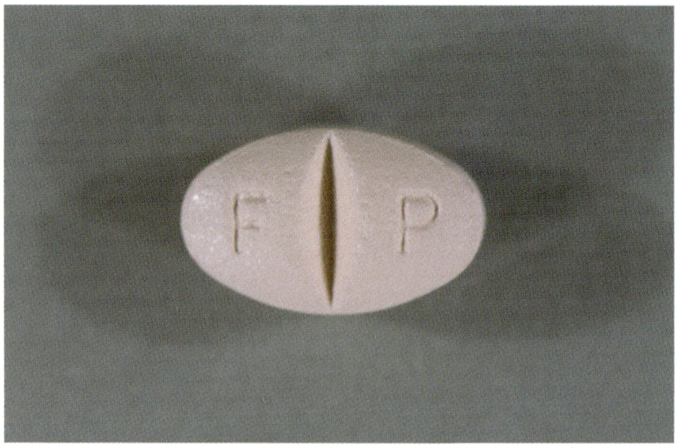

Citalopram, 20 mg. *(© Custom Medical Stock Photo, Inc. Reproduced by permission.)*

Purpose

Citalopram is approved by the U.S. Food and Drug Administration (FDA) for the treatment of **depression**. Possible off-label uses include the treatment of **panic disorder**, **obsessive-compulsive disorder**, alcoholism, **social phobia**, **post-traumatic stress disorder**, eating disorders, and **premenstrual dysphoric disorder**; however, these uses are not approved by the FDA.

Description

Serotonin is a **brain** chemical that carries nerve impulses from one nerve cell to another. Researchers think that depression and certain other mental disorders may be caused, in part, because there is not enough serotonin being released and transmitted in the brain. Like the other SSRI **antidepressants**, **fluoxetine** (Prozac), **sertraline** (Zoloft), and **paroxetine** (Paxil), citalopram increases the level of brain serotonin (also known as 5-HT). Increased serotonin levels in the brain may be beneficial in patients with obsessive-compulsive disorder, alcoholism, certain types of headaches, post-traumatic stress disorder (PTSD), premenstrual tension and mood swings, and panic disorder.

Citalopram is available in 20 mg, 40 mg, and 60 mg tablets.

Recommended dosage

The daily dosage of citalopram for depression is 20–60 mg. The initial dosage is usually 20 mg per day. This dosage may then be increased to 40 mg per day at an interval of no less than one week. Most patients experience relief from depression at this dosage and do not require more than 40 mg per day. The dosage is taken once daily, either in the morning or in the evening.

Patients who are being treated for panic disorder receive doses ranging from 20–60 mg daily. A dosage of

KEY TERMS

Anxiety—An emotion that can be experienced as a troubled feeling, sense of dread, fear of the future, or distress over a possible threat to a person's physical or mental well-being.

Depression—A mental state characterized by feelings of sadness, despair, discouragement, and low energy, sometimes with oversleeping and/or overeating.

Insomnia—The inability to fall asleep or remain asleep.

Off-label use—Drugs approved by the Food and Drug Administration (FDA) for specific uses, legally prescribed by physicians for other "off-label" uses. It is not legal for pharmaceutical companies to advertise drugs for off-label uses.

20–30 mg daily appears to be optimal for the treatment of many patients with panic disorders.

Precautions

Patients who are allergic to citalopram, any other SSRI drug, or any component of the preparation should not take citalopram.

Patients with liver problems and elderly patients (over age 65) need to take smaller amounts of the drug. Dosage for these patients should start at 20 mg but can be increased to 40 mg daily if needed. Patients with kidney problems do not need dosage adjustments. Patients with history of mania, **suicide** attempts, or seizure disorders should start citalopram with caution and only under close physician supervision. Children and young people up to age 24 are at higher risk of developing suicidal thoughts and actions, and, in general, children under 18 are not advised to take citalopram.

Side effects

More than 15% of patients develop **insomnia** while taking citalopram. Nausea and dry mouth occur in about 20% patients being treated with citalopram. Patients also experience tremor, anxiety, agitation, yawning, headaches, dizziness, restlessness, and sedation with citalopram therapy. These side effects usually diminish or disappear with continued use of the drug, although it may take up to four weeks for this to occur.

A drop in blood pressure and increased heart rate have been associated with citalopram use. In general, patients do not experience weight gain or loss after starting citalopram.

Sexual dysfunction, which includes decreased sex drive in women and difficulty ejaculating in men, is associated with the use of citalopram. In some patients, it may take up to 12 weeks for these side effects to disappear. In some patients these sexual side effects never resolve. If sexual side effects continue, the dose of citalopram may be reduced. Patients can also have drug holidays when the weekend dose is either decreased or skipped, or they can discuss with their physician the risks and benefits of switching to another antidepressant.

Interactions

Citalopram interacts with many other medications. Individuals who are starting this drug should review the other medications they are taking with their physician and pharmacist for possible interactions. Patients should always inform all their healthcare providers, including dentists, that they are taking citalopram.

Certain antifungal medications such as itraconazole, fluconazole, ketoconazole, as well as the antibiotic erythromycin, can increase the levels of citalopram in the body. This can cause increased side effects. Levomethadyl, a medication used to treat opioid dependence, may cause toxicity to the heart if used together with citalopram.

Serious side effects called **serotonin syndrome** have resulted from the combination of antidepressants such as citalopram and members of another class of antidepressants known as **monoamine oxidase inhibitors (MAOIs)**. Serotonin syndrome usually consists of at least three of the following symptoms: diarrhea, fever, sweatiness, mood or behavior changes, overactive reflexes, fast heart rate, restlessness, and shivering or shaking. Because of this syndrome, citalopram should never be taken in combination with **MAOIs**. MAOIs include **isocarboxazid**, nialamide, pargyline, selegiline, **phenelzine**, procarbazine, iproniazid, and clorgyline. Patients taking any MAOIs, should stop the MAOI then wait at least 14 days before starting citalopram or any other antidepressant. The same holds true when discontinuing citalopram and starting an MAOI.

Buspirone, an antianxiety medication, should not be used together with citalopram. Ginkgo and **St. John's wort**, herbal supplements that are common in the United States, should not be taken together with citalopram.

Use of citalopram, as with other **SSRIs**, may increase the risk of gastrointestinal bleeding. Patients should inform their doctors if they are taking anticoagulants (blood thinners).

QUESTIONS TO ASK YOUR DOCTOR

- What kind of changes can I expect to see or feel with this medication?
- Does it matter what time of day I take this medication? If so, what is the recommendation?
- Should I take this medication with or without food?
- What are the side effects associated with this medication?
- Will this medication interact or interfere with other medications I am currently taking?
- What symptoms or adverse effects are important enough that I should seek immediate treatment?

Resources

BOOKS

Albers, Lawrence J., Rhoda K. Hahn, and Christopher Reist. *Handbook of Psychiatric Drugs.* Laguna Hills, CA: Current Clinical Strategies, 2010.

American Society of Health-System Pharmacists. *AHFS Drug Information 2011.* Bethesda, MD: ASHP, 2011.

Baldwin, Robert C. *Depression in Later Life.* New York: Oxford University Press, 2010.

Graham, George. *The Disordered Mind: An Introduction to Philosophy of Mind and Mental Illness.* New York: Routledge, 2010.

Holland, Leland Norman, and Michael Patrick Adams. *Core Concepts in Pharmacology.* 3rd ed. New York: Prentice Hall, 2011.

North, Carol, and Sean Yutzy. *Goodwin and Guze's Psychiatric Diagnosis.* New York: Oxford University Press, 2010.

O'Connor, Richard. *Undoing Depression: What Therapy Doesn't Teach You and Medication Can't Give You.* 2nd ed. New York: Little, Brown, 2010.

Preston, John D., John H. O'Neal, and Mary C. Talaga. *Handbook of Clinical Psychopharmacology for Therapists.* 6th ed. Oakland, CA: New Harbinger, 2010.

ORGANIZATIONS

American Academy of Clinical Toxicology, 6728 Old McLean Village Dr., McLean, VA, 22101, (703) 556-9222, Fax: (703) 556-8729, admin@clintox.org, http://www.clintox.org.

American Academy of Family Physicians, 11400 Tomahawk Creek Pkwy., Leawood, KS, 66211-2672, (913) 906-6000, (800) 274-2237, Fax: (913) 906-6075, contactcenter@aafp.org, http://www.aafp.org.

American Medical Association, 515 N State St., Chicago, IL, 60610, (312) 464-5000, (800) 621-8335, http://www.ama-assn.org.

American Psychiatric Association, 1000 Wilson Blvd., Ste. 1825, Arlington, VA, 22209-3901, (703) 907-7300, apa@psych.org, http://www.psych.org.

American Psychological Association, 750 1st St., NE, Washington, DC, 20002-4242, (202) 336-5500; TDD/TTY: (202) 336-6123, (800) 374-2721, http://www.apa.org.

American Society for Clinical Pharmacology and Therapeutics, 528 N Washington St., Alexandria, VA, 22314, (703) 836-6981, info@ascpt.org, http://www.ascpt.org.

Anxiety Disorders Association of America, 8730 Georgia Ave., Silver Spring, MD, 20910, (240) 485-1001, Fax: (240) 485-1035, http://www.adaa.org.

Depression and Bipolar Support Alliance, 730 N Franklin St., Ste. 501, Chicago, IL, 60654, (800) 826-3632, Fax: (312) 642-7243, http://www.dbsalliance.org.

Mental Health America, 2000 N Beauregard St., 6th Fl., Alexandria, VA, 22311, (703) 684-7722, (800) 969-6642, Fax: (703) 684-5968, http://www1.nmha.org.

National Alliance on Mental Illness, 2107 Wilson Blvd., Ste. 300, Arlington, VA, 22201-3042, Fax: (703) 524-9094, (800) 950-6264, http://www.nami.org.

National Institute of Mental Health, 6001 Executive Blvd., Rm. 8184, MSC 9663, Bethesda, MD, 20892-9663, (301) 443-4513; TTY: (301) 443-8431, Fax: (301) 443-4279, (866) 615-6464; TTY: (866) 415-8051, nimhinfo@nih.gov, http://www.nimh.nih.gov.

U.S. National Library of Medicine, 8600 Rockville Pike, Bethesda, MD, 20894, (301) 594-5983, (888) 346-3656; TDD: (800) 735-2258, Fax: (301) 402-1384, http://www.nlm.nih.gov.

Ajna Hamidovic, PharmD
Laura Jean Cataldo, RN, EdD

Client-centered therapy *see* **Person-centered therapy**

Clinical Antipsychotic Trials of Intervention Effectiveness *see* **CATIE**

Clinical Assessment Scales for the Elderly

Definition

The Clinical Assessment Scales for the Elderly, often abbreviated as CASE, is a comprehensive diagnostic tool used to determine and measure the presence of acute mental disorders and other psychopathologic conditions in elderly adults. It is published by PAR, Inc. (Lutz, Florida, United States).

Purpose

The CASE is used to determine the presence of mental disorders in an elderly person as defined by the ***Diagnostic and Statistical Manual of Mental Disorders***. (*DSM*) The *DSM* is the basic reference work consulted by mental health professionals when making a **diagnosis**. The CASE, which is used with adults between the ages of 55 and 90, consists of a self-report form (labeled Form S) in which the person answers questions about himself or herself related to various scales. The test can be administered to an individual or to a group. If the elderly adult is unable to complete the form because of cognitive or physical deficiencies, an other-rating form (labeled Form R) is provided for use by a knowledgeable caregiver, such as a spouse, child, sibling, or healthcare worker. The person elected to take the test should be able to complete it within 40 minutes.

The CASE is not always used specifically for diagnosing mental disorders. It may be administered simply as a general assessment tool to gain insight about an elderly person. It may serve as a neurological screening tool to rule out other problems. The test makers also claim that it can be used as an early screening tool for **dementia**, opening the door for elderly adults to receive medications to slow the progress of **Alzheimer's disease**.

Description

The Clinical Assessment Scales for the Elderly were developed and written by American psychologists Cecil R. Reynolds (1952–) and Erin D. Bigler. The most recent version of the test was published in 2001. It is designed based on the fourth (IV) edition, text revision (TR) of the *DSM* (*DSM-IV-TR*). (The fifth edition [*DSM-5*] will be published in May 2013.) The CASE was normalized using a sample of approximately 2,000 adults in the United States from the ages of 55 to 90 (taken from the U.S. census). One thousand participants were used for each of the two test forms.

The CASE consists of 10 clinical scales that assess the following: Anxiety (ANX); Cognitive Competence (COG); **Depression** (DEP); Fear of Aging (FOA); Obsessive-Compulsiveness (OCD); **Paranoia** (PAR); Psychoticism (PSY); Somatization (SOM); Mania (MAN); and **Substance Abuse** (SUB). These scales were developed to eliminate (or, at least, minimize) any biases associated with gender and ethnicity. The degree to which an elderly person exhibits symptoms in these areas can help a mental health professional with the process of differential diagnosis for a mental disorder.

The CASE also includes three validity scales: L scale (measures positive/negative dissimulation and distortion); F scale (measures infrequently endorsed items); and V scale (measures random responses, failure to comprehend items, and lack of cooperation by patients). Generally, these scales are helpful in evaluating the consistency/inconsistency of a person's responses and whether the person is faking his or her answers.

KEY TERMS

Depression—A psychiatric disorder involving feelings of hopelessness and symptoms of fatigue, sleeplessness, suicidal tendencies, and poor concentration.

Diagnostic and Statistical Manual of Mental Disorders—A handbook that mental health professionals use to diagnose mental disorders. The current edition is the fourth edition, text revision (*DSM-IV-TR*); the fifth edition (*DSM-5*) is being developed and is expected to be published in May 2013.

Psychopathology—The study of the causes and development of psychiatric disorders in humans.

The person who is completing the CASE, whether using the self-rating form or the other-rating form, responds to the test's written items. The test usually takes 20 to 40 minutes to finish, but it is not timed. People are generally given as much time as they need to complete it. The scoring of the CASE takes approximately 10 minutes.

A shorter version of the test, called the Clinical Assessment Scales for the Elderly-Short Form (CASE-SF), is also available when a faster assessment is needed. In addition, the Short Form is sometimes used as a preliminary assessment to determine whether a more comprehensive or other type of evaluation is needed. The CASE-SF, administered either individually or within a group, takes 10 to 20 minutes to complete and includes all ten of the clinical scales. It also includes two of the CASE validity scales: F and V scales.

Preparation

Preparation for the Clinical Assessment Scales for the Elderly is neither necessary nor recommended by the medical community.

Aftercare

The Clinical Assessment Scales for the Elderly is one way that the medical community can accurately identify the presence of mental disorders within elderly patients. Once

QUESTIONS TO ASK YOUR DOCTOR

- How will the Clinical Assessment Scales for the Elderly help?
- How does the CASE work?
- How will the CASE help if we find out that mental illness is not present?
- Will the CASE be able to provide any further insight into the problem?
- Will it be able to rule out other problems?

the CASE is completed, it is much easier to treat such patients.

Benefits

The CASE has been shown to be nearly free of any ethnic and gender biases. In fact, studies of gender and ethnic biases have shown that the test is basically free of such biases for the following three ethnic groups: Caucasians, African Americans, and Hispanics. The test also contains three validity scales to identify feigning (the act of test-takers trying to hide their disorder) and for use in forensic assessments (the analysis of results for the purposes relating to crime or litigation). The test has been shown to have good reliability and validity. Construct validity for the Form S of the CASE was performed using correlations from the **Minnesota Multiphasic Personality Inventory** 2 (MMPI-2), the Back Depression Inventory (BDI), the Beck Hopelessness Scale (BHS), and both the State and Trait scales of the State-Trait Anxiety Inventory (STAI).

Results

Scoring for the CASE is relatively simple. Scores are calculated for each scale and it is then compared to age-appropriate scores to determine the presence or severity of symptoms. For example, if a person scores high on the Depression scale, this information could be used as part of an overall diagnosis for a *DSM-IV-TR* depressive disorder. A person scoring high on the Psychoticism scale may have a psychotic disorder. For any specific *DSM-IV-TR* diagnosis to be made, however, all of the required criteria for that disorder must be met. The results from the CASE may satisfy only some of the requirements.

The Fear of Aging scale assesses the person's degree of apprehension or concern about the aging process. It is not necessarily related to a particular *DSM-IV-TR* disorder. Information about a person's fear of aging, however, may be helpful during the diagnostic process. It may also be useful information for a psychotherapist or other counselor, to understand the patient's concerns or to measure progress in therapy.

See also Figure drawings; House-Tree-Person Test

Resources

BOOKS

American Psychiatric Association. *Diagnostic and Statistical Manual of Mental Disorders.* 4th edition, Text revision. Washington, DC: American Psychiatric Association, 2000.

Reynolds, Cecil R., and Erin D. Bigler. *Clinical Assessment Scales for the Elderly.* San Antonio, TX: The Psychological Corporation, 2001.

WEBSITES

"Cecil Reynolds." Texas A & M University. http://directory.cehd.tamu.edu/view.epl?nid=c-reynolds (accessed November 19, 2010).

"Clinical Assessment Scales for the Elderly™ (CASE™)." PAR, Inc. http://www4.parinc.com/Products/Product.aspx?ProductID=CASE (accessed November 19, 2010).

"Clinical Assessment Scales for the Elderly™ Short Form (CASE-SF™)." PAR, Inc. http://www4.parinc.com/Products/Product.aspx?ProductID=CASE-SF (accessed November 19, 2010).

"Erin David Bigler." Brigham Young University. http://psychology.byu.edu/Faculty/EBigler/Home.dhtml (accessed November 19, 2010).

ORGANIZATIONS

American Psychiatric Association, 1000 Wilson Blvd., Ste. 1825, Arlington, VA, 22209-3901, (703) 907-7300, apa@psych.org, http://www.psych.org.

American Psychological Association, 750 1st St., NE, Washington, DC, 20002, (202) 336-5500, (800) 374-2721, http://www.apa.org.

Depression and Bipolar Support Alliance, 730 N Franklin St., Ste. 501, Chicago, IL, 60654-7225, (800) 826-3632, Fax: (312) 642-7243, http://www.dbsalliance.org.

National Institute of Mental Health, 6001 Executive Boulevard, Room 8184, MSC 9663, Bethesda, MD, 20892-9663, (301) 443-4513, (866) 615-6464, Fax: (301) 443-4279, nimhinfo@nih.gov, http://www.nimh.nih.gov.

Ali Fahmy, PhD
Emily Jane Willingham, PhD
William Atkins

Clinical trials

Definition

A clinical trial is a controlled scientific experiment designed to determine the effectiveness of a treatment in curing or lessening the symptoms of a disease or disorder.

Description

Clinical trials typically are used to assess the effectiveness of a new treatment in comparison with the current standard of care or an existing treatment for a disease or disorder. For example, before a new drug is approved by the U.S. Food and Drug Administration (FDA) for release and use in the United States, the drug must first undergo rigorous testing to determine (a) whether or not it is effective in treating the disorder, and (b) what side effects may result from the drug use that make it inadvisable or dangerous to some or all potential patients.

Clinical trials are research studies designed according to professional standards using scientific methods. In clinical trials, as many variables as possible are controlled to determine the effects of the drug or treatment option. For example, a simple experiment to test the effectiveness of a new drug for epilepsy might include the following steps. First, researchers typically randomly divide the research subjects into two groups: one group that receives the new drug, and the other group that receives the conventional drug or treatment. The group receiving the new drug is called the experimental group, and the group receiving no treatment or conventional treatment is called the control group. Researchers then collect baseline data on the symptoms of the subjects prior to treatment, such as number and frequency of **seizures**. This phase of the experiment is called the pretest. After the pretest data are collected, the researchers give the new drug (the independent variable) to the experimental group while not changing the treatment of the control group. After an appropriate amount of time for the drug to take effect, the subjects are tested again using the same criteria as were used for the pretest to determine any difference between the two groups as a result of the drug (dependent variable). When all the data are collected, they are statistically analyzed to determine whether there is a reasonable basis to say that the effects of the new drug are significantly different from the effects of the old treatment (or no treatment) and not due to chance variations. This basic research design can be made more complicated to simultaneously answer multiple research questions, such as what dose of the new medication is most effective, whether increasing dosage levels of the medication results in more side effects, whether the drug is effective for some demographic groups but not others (e.g., only works well on adult females but not on adult males), or to compare several treatments at once.

There are several general types of clinical trials:

- treatment trials that test the relative effectiveness of new drugs or treatments or combinations of drugs and/or treatments
- prevention trials that investigate ways to prevent a disease in individuals who have not previously had it or to prevent its return in individuals who have
- diagnostic trials that seek to find better ways to diagnose a disorder or illness
- screening trials to determine the best way to detect a disease or disorder
- quality-of-life trials that investigate how to make life easier or more normal for those with a chronic illness

Clinical trials typically have four phases. In Phase I, the experimental drug or treatment is tested on a small group of people to investigate its safety, determine a recommended dosage or range, and identify potential side effects. In Phase II, the experimental drug or treatment is tested on a larger group of people to further determine its effectiveness and safety. Phase III clinical trials examine the drug or treatment from an even wider perspective. The experimental drug or treatment is given to large groups of people to confirm the findings of the previous studies on a larger population. Phase III clinical trials are also often used to compare the relative effectiveness of treatments and gather safety information. Finally, Phase IV clinical trials are run after a drug has been marketed. At that time, a drug may undergo further studies to examine its risks, benefits, and optimal use.

KEY TERMS

Bias—When a point of view prevents impartial judgment on issues relating to the subject of that point of view.

Clinical—Pertaining to or founded on observation and treatment of participants, as distinguished from theoretical or basic science.

Food and Drug Administration (FDA)—The U.S. Department of Health and Human Services agency responsible for ensuring the safety and effectiveness of all drugs, biologics, vaccines, and medical devices. The FDA also works with the blood banking industry to safeguard the nation's blood supply.

Placebo—An inactive pill, liquid, or powder that has no treatment value.

Randomization—A method based on chance by which study participants are assigned to a treatment group.

Recruiting—Period during which a trial is attempting to identify and enroll participants.

Considerations before entering a clinical trial as a subject

Clinical trials are necessary to help ensure the safety and effectiveness of a drug or treatment before it is put into general use. In addition, joining a clinical trial as a research subject may be of potential benefit to patients who have exhausted available treatment options without success. Clinical trials give patients the opportunity to try a new drug or treatment that may help their condition when conventional methods have failed. However, certain things must be considered before joining a clinical trial as a subject.

First, there is no guarantee that subjects in clinical trials will receive the new drug or treatment. They may be randomly placed in the control group where they receive a placebo or conventional treatment rather than the new drug or treatment. There is no way to tell whether one will be in the experimental group or the control group. Frequently, even researchers or people administrating the treatment do not know which group the subject is in (this is called a double-blind study) so that their expectations will not unintentionally bias the results. Therefore, all other available treatment options should typically be tried before joining a clinical trial as a subject.

In addition, there is always the possibility of encountering unknown negative side effects from the new drug or treatment. For this reason, subjects in clinical trials are required to read, understand, and sign **informed consent** documents. The decision to join a clinical trial as a subject should always be made in conjunction with one's health care provider in order to reduce the risk of negative side effects from the treatment.

Individuals should be well informed and have a good understanding of the following prior to making a decision about participating:

- the purpose of the study
- their role in the study
- any risks, discomforts, or potential inconveniences involved
- potential conflicts of interest
- the time involved, the number of visits required, and the length of the study
- any ethical issues relating to personal information, privacy, photography, tape recording, use of information, and confidentiality

Availability of participation with NIH.gov

The research hospital of the National Institutes of Health (NIH) is located at the NIH Clinical Center in Bethesda, Maryland. New or improved medical treatments, medications, and therapies, are actualized through ongoing clinical research performed at this center. One key component in attaining information and scientific discovery is participation in the many clinical trials by volunteers. Recruitment is ongoing for sick or healthy participants. To find out more about medical research studies, various clinical trials, and availability in participating in a clinical trial with NIH, contact the Patient Recruitment and Public Liaison Office at 1-800-411-1222 or visit their website: http://www.cc.nih.gov/participate.shtml.

Resources

BOOKS

American Society of Health-System Pharmacists. *AHFS Drug Information 2011.* Bethesda, MD: American Society of Health-System Pharmacists, 2011.

Holland, Leland Norman, and Michael Patrick Adams. *Core Concepts in Pharmacology,* 3rd ed. New York: Prentice Hall, 2011.

WEBSITES

ClinicalTrials.gov. http://www.clinicaltrials.gov/ct/action/GetStudy.

ORGANIZATIONS

National Institutes of Health (NIH), 9000 Rockville Pike, Bethesda, MD, 20892, (301) 496-4000, http://www.nih.gov/index.html.

U.S. National Library of Medicine, 8600 Rockville Pike, Bethesda, MD, 20894, http://www.nlm.nih.gov/medlineplus/medlineplus.html.

Ruth A. Wienclaw, PhD
Laura Jean Cataldo, RN, EdD

Clomipramine

Definition

Clomipramine is an antidepressant drug used primarily to alleviate obsessions and compulsions in patients with **obsessive-compulsive disorder**. Clomipramine is also used in the treatment of depressive disorders and in a number of other psychiatric and medical conditions. In the United States, the drug has also been known by the brand name Anafranil.

Purpose

Clomipramine is principally used in the treatment of the obsessions and compulsions of obsessive-compulsive disorder (OCD), when these symptoms greatly disrupt patients' daily activities. Obsessions are repetitive

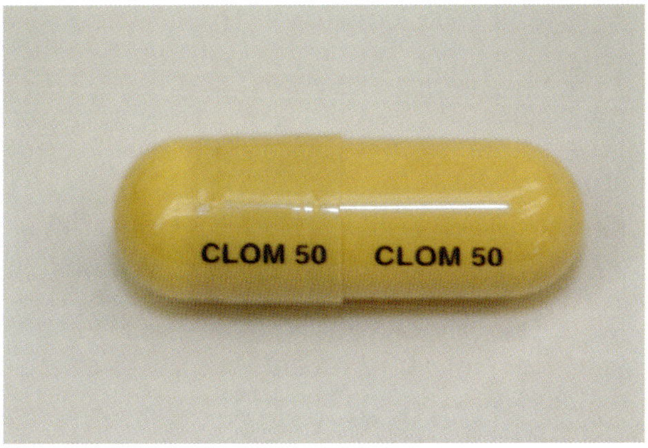

Clomipramine, 50 mg. *(© Custom Medical Stock Photo, Inc. Reproduced by permission.)*

thoughts and impulses, and compulsions are repetitive behaviors. Patients with OCD find these experiences inappropriate, distressing, and time-consuming.

Clomipramine may also be used in the treatment of depressive disorders, especially when associated with obsessions and compulsions, and in **panic disorder**, pain management, sleep attacks (**narcolepsy** and cataplexy), and **anorexia nervosa**. The drug may help to reduce compulsive behaviors in a variety of disorders with such symptoms, including **trichotillomania** (hair pulling), onychophagia (nail biting), **Tourette syndrome** (tics and vocalizations), and childhood **autism**.

Description

Clomipramine is one of the tricyclic **antidepressants**, so-called because of the three-ring chemical structure common to these drugs. In the 1940s and 1950s, pharmaceutical researchers synthesized a number of new compounds for possible medical use as antihistamines and **sedatives**. After testing in animal experiments, a few of these substances were selected for human study. One potential drug, the tricyclic compound **imipramine**, was not useful in calming agitation, but it had a striking effect in improving the mood of certain patients with **depression**.

Since the discovery of imipramine, many other tricyclic antidepressants have been developed with somewhat different pharmacological activities and side effect profiles. Within this group of drugs, clomipramine is exceptionally potent in affecting levels of **serotonin** in the **brain**. In this action, it is similar to serotonin-selective antidepressant drugs, such as **fluoxetine** (Prozac), which act specifically on serotonin levels and are effective in OCD. Serotonin is a messenger chemical (neurotransmitter) involved in transmitting signals between nerve cells. Clomipramine reduces the effects on serotonin transmission in depression and OCD symptoms.

Recommended dosage

For adults, clomipramine is administered in dosages up to a maximum of 250 mg per day. Starting with a dose of 25 mg, the dosage is increased during the first two weeks to 100 mg per day. If needed, it is further increased gradually over the next several weeks. The initial dose is low to avoid side effects, and it is increased slowly to permit the patient to develop tolerance or adapt to side effects that may occur.

Older patients (over age 65), children, and adolescents are more sensitive to the side effects and toxicities of tricyclic antidepressants such as clomipramine. The maximum daily dose is usually lower for elderly patients than for younger adults. For children and adolescents, the maximum recommended daily dose is the lesser of 100 mg or 3 mg per kg of body weight.

Precautions

Seizures are the most important risk associated with clomipramine. Among patients taking the drug for six months or more, more than 1% may experience seizures. The risk of seizure increases with larger doses, and seizures have been reported to occur following abrupt discontinuation of the medication. Caution and physician supervision are required if the patient has a history of epilepsy or some other condition associated with seizures, such as brain damage or alcoholism.

Clomipramine and other tricyclic antidepressants often cause drowsiness. Activities requiring alertness, such as driving, should be avoided until patients understand how the drug affects them. Dizziness or lightheadedness may occur on arising from a seated position, due to sudden decreases in blood pressure. Fainting may also occur. Patients with glaucoma may find their condition worsened. Persons with heart disease should use tricyclic antidepressants with caution due to a possibility of adverse effects on heart rhythm.

Studies have found that some antidepressant drugs, including clomipramine, may increase the chances of suicidal thoughts in children and adults up to age 24. Patients taking clomipramine should be monitored, regardless of age, for worsening depression or other adverse changes in behavior.

It has not been determined whether clomipramine is safe to take during pregnancy, and the patient's need for this medicine should be balanced against the possibility of harm to the fetus. Tricyclic antidepressants may be secreted in breast milk and may cause sedation and depress the breathing of a nursing infant.

Side effects

Clomipramine may cause many side effects. Initially, the side effects of tricyclic drugs may be more pronounced, but sensitivity often decreases with continued treatment. Some of the more common side effects are:

- headache
- confusion
- nervousness
- restlessness
- sleep difficulties
- numbness
- tingling sensations
- tremors
- twitches
- nausea
- loss of appetite
- indigestion
- constipation
- blurred vision
- increased sweating
- difficulty urinating (especially in men with prostate enlargement)
- menstrual pain
- ejaculatory difficulty
- impotence
- decreased sex drive
- fatigue
- weight gain

Sensitivity to ultraviolet light may increase, and sunburns may occur more easily. Patients may also develop dry mouth due to decreased saliva, possibly contributing to the development of tooth decay, gum disease, and mouth infections. Patients should avoid sweets, sugary beverages, and chewing gum containing sugar.

Less commonly, tricyclic drugs may cause adverse effects on almost any organ or system of the body, particularly the blood, hormones, kidney, and liver. Patients should consult their physicians if symptoms develop or bodily changes appear.

Interactions

Tricyclic antidepressants such as clomipramine may interact with many other drugs. Patients should inform their physicians about all other drugs they are taking before starting treatment.

Clomipramine may intensify the effects of other drugs that act on serotonin levels, possibly producing **serotonin syndrome**, a rare but dangerous condition with fever, sweating, tremors, and changes in mental state. Drugs that may interact this way include other antidepressants, especially **selective serotonin reuptake inhibitors (SSRIs)** and **monoamine oxidase inhibitors (MAOIs)**. These drugs should not be taken within two weeks of taking clomipramine. Other drugs to avoid are lithium, **alprazolam** (Xanax), fenfluramine (Pondimin), amphetamine, dextromethorphan (used in cough suppressants), meperidine (Demerol), and tramadol (Ultram).

KEY TERMS

Autonomic—The part of the nervous system that governs the heart, involuntary muscles, and glands.

Cataplexy—A symptom of narcolepsy marked by a sudden episode of muscle weakness triggered by strong emotions. The muscle weakness may cause the person's knees to buckle, or the head to drop. In severe cases, the patient may become paralyzed for a few seconds or minutes.

Epilepsy—A neurological disorder characterized by the onset of seizures. Seizures are caused by a disturbance in the electrical activity in the brain and can cause loss of consciousness, muscle spasms, rhythmic movements, abnormal sensory experiences, or altered mental states.

Kilogram—A metric unit of weight. It equals 2.2 lb.

Monoamine oxidase inhibitors (MAOIs)—A group of antidepressant drugs that decreases the activity of monoamine oxidase, a neurotransmitter found in the brain that affects mood.

Neurotransmitter—A chemical in the brain that transmits messages between neurons, or nerve cells.

Serotonin—A widely distributed neurotransmitter that is found in blood platelets, the lining of the digestive tract, and the brain, and that works in combination with norepinephrine. It causes very powerful contractions of smooth muscle, and is associated with mood, attention, emotions, and sleep. Low levels of serotonin are associated with depression.

Tricyclic drugs may intensify the effects of other drugs causing sedation, including alcohol, **barbiturates**, narcotic pain medications, minor tranquilizers, and antihistamines. Tricyclics may cause excessive reductions of blood pressure in patients taking blood pressure medicine, especially upon standing from a sitting or reclined position. Conversely, these drugs may interfere with the pressure-reducing effects of certain other blood pressure medicines and may necessitate an adjustment in dosage. Tricyclics may interact with thyroid medications to produce abnormalities of heart rhythm. Concurrent use of tricyclic antidepressants with other psychiatric medicines may result in intensification of certain side effects.

Certain drugs may interfere with the elimination of tricyclic antidepressants from the body, causing higher blood levels and increased side effects. This effect may occur with cimetidine (Tagamet), other antidepressants, **methylphenidate** (Ritalin, Concerta), and some antipsychotic medications.

Resources

BOOKS

Maina, Giuseppe, Umberto Albert, and Filippo Bogetto. "Obsessive-Compulsive Disorder Resistant to Pharmacological Treatment." In *Obsessive-Compulsive Disorder Research,* edited by B.E. Ling. Hauppauge, NY: Nova Science Publishers, 2005, 171–99.

Preston, John D., John H. O'Neal, and Mary C. Talaga. *Handbook of Clinical Psychopharmacology for Therapists*. 5th ed. Oakland, CA: New Harbinger Publications, 2008.

Simpson, H. Blair, and Michael R. Liebowitz. "Combining Pharmacotherapy and Cognitive-Behavioral Therapy in the Treatment of OCD." In *Concepts and Controversies in Obsessive-Compulsive Disorder,* by Jonathan Abramowitz and Arthur C. Houts. New York: Springer Science, 2005, 359–76.

PERIODICALS

Anderson, Shawanda W., and Marvin B. Booker. "Cognitive Behavioral Therapy Versus Psychosurgery for Refractory Obsessive-Compulsive Disorder." Letter in *Journal of Neuropsychiatry and Clinical Neurosciences* 18, no. 1 (February 2006): 129.

Fineberg, Naomi A., and Tim M. Gale. "Evidence-Based Pharmacotherapy of Obsessive-Compulsive Disorder." *International Journal of Neuropsychopharmacology* 8, no. 1 (March 2005): 107–29.

Foa, Edna B., et al. "Randomized, Placebo-Controlled Trial of Exposure and Ritual Prevention, Clomipramine, and Their Combination in the Treatment of Obsessive-Compulsive Disorder." *American Journal of Psychiatry* 162, no. 1 (January 2005): 151–61.

Shavitt, Roseli G., et al. "Clinical Features Associated with Treatment Response in Obsessive-Compulsive Disorder." *Comprehensive Psychiatry* 474 (2006): 276–81.

Simpson, Helen Blair, et al. "Response Versus Remission in Obsessive-Compulsive Disorder." *Journal of Clinical Psychiatry* 67, no. 2 (February 2006): 269–76.

ORGANIZATIONS

American Academy of Child and Adolescent Psychiatry, 3615 Wisconsin Ave. NW, Washington, DC, 20016-3007, (202) 966-7300, Fax: (202) 966-2891, http://aacap.org.

American Academy of Clinical Toxicology, 6728 Old McLean Village Dr., McLean, VA, 22101, (703) 556-9222, Fax: (703) 556-8729, admin@clintox.org, http://www.clintox.org.

American College of Neuropsychopharmacology, 5034-A Thoroughbred Ln., Brentwood, TN, 37027, (615) 324-2360, Fax: (615) 523-1715, acnp@acnp.org, http://www.acnp.org/default.aspx.

American Psychiatric Association, 1000 Wilson Blvd., Ste. 1825, Arlington, VA, 22209-3901, (703) 907-7300, apa@psych.org, http://www.psych.org.

Richard Kapit, MD
Ruth A. Wienclaw, PhD

Clonazepam

Definition

Clonazepam belongs to a group of drugs called benzodiazepines. **Benzodiazepines** are medications that help relieve nervousness, tension, symptoms of anxiety, and some types of **seizures** by slowing the central nervous system. In the United States, clonazepam is sold under brand name Klonopin.

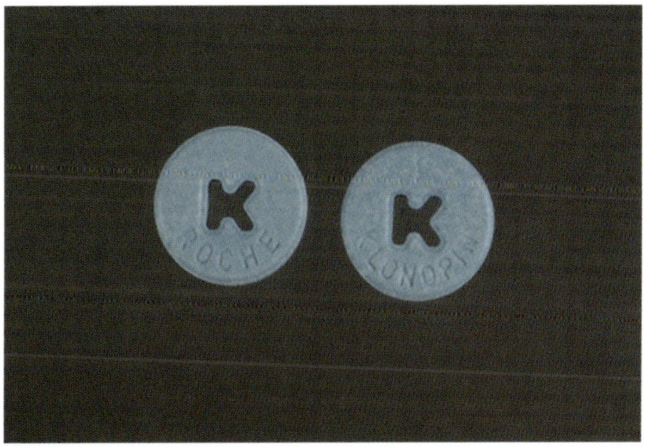

Klonopin (clonazepam), 1 mg. *(U.S. Drug Enforcement Administration)*

Purpose

Clonazepam is approved by the U.S. Food and Drug Administration (FDA) for the treatment of **panic disorder** and some types of epilepsy. It may also be used off-label to treat **social phobia**, mania, **post-traumatic stress disorder** (PTSD), and **medication-induced movement disorders**, a side effect of some antipsychotic drugs. It is legal for physicians to administer drugs for off-label uses, but these uses are not approved by the FDA.

Description

Clonazepam belongs to a group of drugs called benzodiazepines. Benzodiazepines are sedative-hypnotic drugs that help to relieve nervousness, tension, anxiety symptoms, and seizures by slowing the central nervous system. To do this, they block the effects of a specific chemical involved in the transmission of nerve impulses in the **brain**, decreasing the excitement level of the nerve cells.

When clonazepam is used to treat panic disorder, it is more sedating than **alprazolam**, another benzodiazepine drug used to treat panic disorder. However, unlike alprazolam, clonazepam may trigger depressive episodes in patients with a previous history of **depression**. In people who experience social phobia, treatment with clonazepam reduces the rate of depression. The use of clonazepam for social phobia is considered an off-label use—a use that is legal when prescribed by a physician but that is not approved by the FDA.

Clonazepam comes in 0.5 mg, 1.0 mg, and 2.0 mg tablets.

Recommended dosage

For panic disorder, the initial recommended dose is 0.25 mg twice daily. This dose can be increased every three days in increments of 0.125–0.25 mg twice daily. The target dose for panic disorder is 1.0 mg per day, although some people benefit from doses up to a maximum of 4.0 mg per day. When a person stops taking clonazepam, the drug should be gradually discontinued by decreasing the dose by 0.125 mg twice daily every three days.

Although clonazepam is not FDA approved for the treatment of PTSD, doses in the range of 0.25–3.0 mg daily appear to help treat symptoms of this disorder. Daily dosages for the treatment of social phobia range from 1.0–2.5 mg, while the dosage to control mania may be as high as 10.0 mg daily.

Precautions

Women who are pregnant should not use clonazepam, because it may harm the developing fetus. Clonazepam should never be taken by people who have had an allergic reaction to it or another benzodiazepine drug such as **diazepam** (Valium). People with narrow-angle glaucoma or severe liver disease should not take clonazepam. People who have kidney disease may need to take a reduced dosage of the drug. Saliva production may increase while taking clonazepam. Because of this, people with respiratory disease or an impaired gag reflex should use clonazepam with close physician supervision.

Because clonazepam is a nervous system depressant, it should not be taken with other such depressants, such as alcohol, other **sedatives**, sleeping pills, or tranquilizers. People taking clonazepam may feel unusually drowsy and mentally sluggish when they first start taking the drug. They should not drive, operate machinery, or engage in activities that require mental alertness until they see how clonazepam affects them. Because of a loss of coordination, elderly patients are at risk for falls. This excessive sedation usually goes away after a short time on the drug.

People who have underlying depression should be closely monitored while taking clonazepam, especially if they are at risk for attempting **suicide**. Clonazepam treatment should not be stopped abruptly, as patients may experience withdrawal symptoms including tremor, **insomnia**, anxiety, and seizures. Clonazepam can be habit-forming.

Side effects

The main side effects of clonazepam are sedation, dizziness, impaired coordination, depression, and **fatigue**. Some people experience decreased sex drive while taking clonazepam. The drug may also cause short-term memory loss or **amnesia**.

A small number of people develop sinus problems and upper respiratory tract infections while taking clonazepam. One of the side effects of clonazepam may be increased salivation. This may cause some people to start coughing while taking clonazepam. Clonazepam may also cause anorexia and dry mouth. It may cause either constipation or diarrhea. There are a few reports of clonazepam causing menstrual irregularities or blurred vision.

Interactions

Clonazepam may increase the sedative effects of other drugs that depress the central nervous system such as certain strong pain medicines (opiates such as codeine, oxycodone, hydromorphone) and antihistamines (found in many cold and allergy medications).

KEY TERMS

Anorexia—Loss of appetite or unwillingness to eat. Can be caused by medications, depression, and/or many other factors.

Benzodiazepines—A group of central nervous system depressants used to relieve anxiety or to induce sleep.

Glaucoma—A group of eye diseases characterized by increased pressure within the eye, significant enough to damage eye tissue and structures. If untreated, glaucoma results in blindness.

The sedative effect is also increased if clonazepam is taken with alcohol.

Disulfiram (Antabuse), a medication used to treat alcohol dependence, increases the effect of clonazepam. Medications that make clonazepam ineffective include phenobarbital, phenytoin, **carbamazepine**, theophylline, rifampin, and rifabutin.

Resources

BOOKS

Lacy, Charles F., Leonard L. Lance, and Laura L. Armstrong. *Lexi-Comp's Drug Information Handbook*. Hudson, OH: Lexi-Comp, 2010.

Preston, John D., John H. O'Neal, and Mary C. Talaga. *Handbook of Clinical Psychopharmacology for Therapists*. 5th ed. Oakland, CA: New Harbinger Publications, 2008.

PERIODICALS

Nardi, Antonio E., and Giampaolo Perna. "Clonazepam in the Treatment of Psychiatric Disorders: An Update." *International Clinical Psychopharmacology* 21, no. 3 (May 2006): 131–42.

Paparrigopoulos, Thomas J. "REM Sleep Behaviour Disorder: Clinical Profiles and Pathophysiology." *International Review of Psychiatry* 17, no. 4 (August 2005): 293–300.

ORGANIZATIONS

American Academy of Child and Adolescent Psychiatry, 3615 Wisconsin Ave. NW, Washington, DC, 20016-3007, (202) 966-7300, Fax: (202) 966-2891, http://aacap.org.

American Academy of Clinical Toxicology, 6728 Old McLean Village Dr., McLean, VA, 22101, (703) 556-9222, Fax: (703) 556-8729, admin@clintox.org, http://www.clintox.org.

American College of Neuropsychopharmacology, 5034-A Thoroughbred Ln., Brentwood, TN, 37027, (615) 324-2360, Fax: (615) 523-1715, acnp@acnp.org, http://www.acnp.org/default.aspx.

American Psychiatric Association, 1000 Wilson Blvd., Ste. 1825, Arlington, VA, 22209-3901, (703) 907-7300, apa@psych.org, http://www.psych.org.

Ajna Hamidovic, PharmD
Ruth A. Wienclaw, PhD

Clonidine

Definition

Clonidine belongs to a class of drugs called central alpha-adrenergic agonists. In the United States, clonidine tablets are sold under the brand name Catapres and clonidine skin patches are sold under the brand name Catapres-TTS. The tablets are also available generically. There is an injectable form that is administered directly into the spinal cord for the treatment of postoperative pain.

Purpose

Clonidine tablets and patches are approved by the U.S. Food and Drug Administration (FDA) for the treatment of high blood pressure. In addition, clonidine has been found to be useful in the treatment of alcohol, opiate, and **nicotine** withdrawal syndromes, **attention deficit hyperactivity disorder (ADHD)**, and **Tourette syndrome**, which is one of the **tic disorders**.

Clonidine is also useful in treating neuropathic pain, which is usually characterized as a sensation of tingling, burning, or shooting pain in the limbs that may come and go quickly and erratically. Clonidine gel used topically (on the skin) provides analgesia to the affected painful

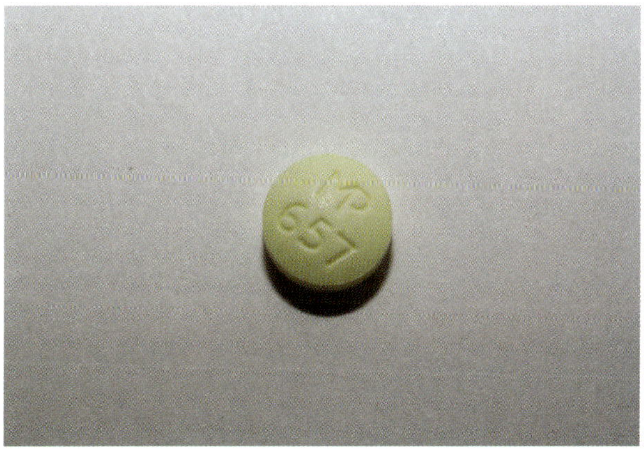

Clonidine, 0.1 mg. *(© Custom Medical Stock Photo, Inc. Reproduced by permission.)*

nerves, and though the mechanism of action is not well known, it is thought that the drug may decrease a local release of norepinephrine at the site of the nerve fibers, which stops the sensitized nerve fibers from causing pain.

Other indications

Other uses of clonidine are:

- treatment of dysmenorrhea (painful cramps during menstrual period)
- hypertensive crisis
- hot flashes associated with menopause
- as a diagnostic tool in the diagnosis of pheochromocytoma (a tumor of the adrenal glands that may be accompanied by high blood pressure, a fast heart rate, and changes in the endocrine system)

Other indications and benefits in the use of clonidine may be identified by further research. **Clinical trials** in the use of this drug for pain, anxiety, hypertension, and other conditions are ongoing.

Description

Clonidine was synthesized in the 1960s and was initially tested as a nasal decongestant. In the United States, clonidine was first used to treat hypertension, although it has also been investigated for treatment of different neuropsychiatric disorders. Clonidine works on specific nerve cells in the **brain** that are responsible for lowering blood pressure, slowing heart rate, and decreasing the body's reaction to the withdrawal of chemicals such as alcohol, opiates, and nicotine. Because of this, clonidine is often used to treat the symptoms of drug, alcohol, and nicotine withdrawal.

Clonidine is beneficial in opiate withdrawal because it treats symptoms commonly associated with that condition (watery eyes and nose, diarrhea, irritability). For this condition, clonidine is often used alone. For the treatment of alcohol withdrawal, clonidine is usually combined with benzodiazepine tranquilizers such as Librium, Valium, Xanax, or Ativan.

Several studies of treatment for **smoking cessation** showed patients treated with clonidine had decreased nicotine craving. Clonidine skin patches appear to be more effective than tablets for this condition. Both dermal patches and tablets are effective in the treatment of Tourette syndrome and **ADHD**.

Clonidine tablets are available in 0.1 mg, 0.2 mg, and 0.3 mg strengths. Clonidine skin patches are available in 0.1 mg, 0.2 mg, and 0.3 mg per day patches. Each patch lasts seven days.

KEY TERMS

Attention deficit hyperactivity disorder (ADHD)—A developmental disorder characterized by distractibility, hyperactivity, impulsive behaviors, and the inability to remain focused on tasks or activities.

Tourette syndrome—An abnormal condition that causes uncontrollable facial grimaces and tics and arm and shoulder movements. Tourette syndrome is perhaps best known for uncontrollable vocal tics that include grunts, shouts, and use of obscene language (coprolalia).

Recommended dosage

Dosages of 0.4–0.6 mg have been used for the treatment of alcohol withdrawal. Total daily dosage for the treatment of opiate withdrawal range between 0.5 and 1.4 mg, depending on the stage as well as the severity of withdrawal symptoms. If the clonidine patch is used to treat nicotine withdrawal symptoms, dosages that deliver 0.1–0.2 mg daily are used. For oral therapy (tablets), a total dosage of 0.2–0.4 mg daily is taken in divided doses.

Pediatric doses of clonidine are calculated based on the child's body weight. Clonidine dosage for ADHD in children is 5 micrograms per kilogram of body weight per day orally in four divided doses. Children who require a daily dosage of 0.2 mg usually can use the 0.3 mg dermal patch. If ADHD is associated with sleep disturbances, low to moderate doses of clonidine can be taken at bedtime. Oral doses in children with Tourette syndrome range from 3–6 micrograms per kilogram of body weight per day divided into two-to-four even doses.

Precautions

Clonidine should not be used by people who have a known allergy to this drug. If a person has underlying **depression**, clonidine should be used with caution and under close physician supervision.

Clonidine should not be abruptly withdrawn, but rather slowly decreased over several days to avoid withdrawal symptoms. Withdrawal symptoms include an increase in blood pressure, irritability, nervousness, **insomnia**, and headache. Because of the possibility of withdrawal, clonidine should not be used in patients who are unwilling or unable to follow the prescribing information.

Clonidine should be used only with caution and close physician supervision in patients with chronic renal

QUESTIONS TO ASK YOUR DOCTOR

- What kind of changes can I expect to see or feel with this medication?
- Does it matter what time of day I take this medication? If so, what is the recommendation?
- Should I take this medication with or without food?
- What are the side effects associated with this medication?
- Will this medication interact or interfere with other medications I am currently taking?
- What symptoms or adverse effects are important enough that I should seek immediate treatment?

failure, coronary artery disease, and in patients with preexisting eye problems. People with kidney disease may need to take a reduced dosage. Clonidine should not be used by pregnant women, except in the rare case where the benefits of taking clonidine outweigh the risks to the developing fetus.

Side effects

The most common side effect associated with clonidine is dizziness accompanying sudden changes in position such as standing up rapidly. In order to avoid this, patients should stand up slowly. People using the dermal patch may develop rash, hair loss, a burning sensation on the skin, or other skin irritations where the patch is applied. Switching to tablets may not completely eliminate these skin problems.

Clonidine can cause dry mouth, constipation, nausea, daytime sleepiness, weakness, and lethargy. These side effects may take several weeks to disappear. In some cases, these side effects can be eliminated with dosage readjustment. In addition, clonidine may cause eye dryness, loss of sex drive, and decreased sexual activity.

If patients experience weight gain in the beginning of therapy, they can expect this side effect to decline over a period of several days to weeks.

Interactions

Clonidine's blood pressure–lowering effects may be enhanced by other drugs that also lower blood pressure. Conversely, the blood pressure–lowering effects of clonidine may be negated by many **antidepressants**.

Resources

BOOKS

American Society of Health-System Pharmacists. *AHFS Drug Information 2011.* Bethesda, MD: ASHP, 2011.

Holland, Leland Norman, and Michael Patrick Adams. *Core Concepts in Pharmacology.* 3rd ed. New York: Prentice Hall, 2011.

Preston, John D., John H. O'Neal, and Mary C. Talaga. *Handbook of Clinical Psychopharmacology for Therapists.* 6th ed. Oakland, CA: New Harbinger, 2010.

PERIODICALS

Favrat, B., et al. "Opioid Antagonist Detoxification under Anaesthesia Versus Traditional Clonidine Detoxification Combined with an Additional Week of Psychosocial Support: A Randomized Clinical Trial." *Drug and Alcohol Dependence* 81, no. 2 (February 2006): 109–16.

Friemoth, Jerry. "What Is the Most Effective Treatment for ADHD in Children?" *Journal of Family Practice* 54, no. 2 (February 2005): 166–68.

Marsch, Lisa A., et al. "Comparison of Pharmacological Treatments for Opioid-Dependent Adolescents: A Randomized Controlled Trial." *Archives of General Psychiatry* 62, no. 10 (October 2005): 1157–64.

Ponizovsky, Alexander M., et al. "Well-Being, Psychosocial Factors, and Side-Effects Among Heroin-Dependent Inpatients after Detoxification Using Buprenorphine Versus Clonidine." *Addictive Behaviors* 31, no. 11 (November 2006): 2002–13.

Schnoes, Connie J., et al. "Pediatric Prescribing Practices for Clonidine and Other Pharmacologic Agents for Children with Sleep Disturbance." *Clinical Pediatrics* 45, no. 3 (April 2006): 229–38.

ORGANIZATIONS

American Academy of Clinical Toxicology, 6728 Old McLean Village Dr., McLean, VA, 22101, (703) 556-9222, Fax: (703) 556-8729, admin@clintox.org, http://www.clintox.org.

American Academy of Family Physicians, 11400 Tomahawk Creek Pkwy., Leawood, KS, 66211-2672, (913) 906-6000, (800) 274-2237, Fax: (913) 906-6075, contactcenter@aafp.org, http://www.aafp.org.

American Psychiatric Association, 1000 Wilson Blvd., Ste. 1825, Arlington, VA, 22209-3901, (703) 907-7300, apa@psych.org, http://www.psych.org.

National Institutes of Health, 9000 Rockville Pike, Bethesda, MD, 20892, (301) 496-4000; TTY: (301) 402-9612, http://www.nih.gov.

U.S. National Library of Medicine, 8600 Rockville Pike, Bethesda, MD, 20894, (301) 594-5983, (888) 346-3656; TDD: (800) 735-2258, Fax: (301) 402-1384, http://www.nlm.nih.gov.

Ajna Hamidovic, PharmD
Ruth A. Wienclaw, PhD
Laura Jean Cataldo, RN, EdD

Clorazepate

Definition

Clorazepate is a medication that belongs to a family of drugs called benzodiazepines—a group of pharmacologically active compounds used to produce a calming effect by relieving anxiety and tension. In the United States, clorazepate is sold under brand names Tranxene and Gen-XENE.

Purpose

Clorazepate is used for the treatment of anxiety and alcohol withdrawal. Clorazepate is also an adjunct in the management of partial **seizures**.

Description

Clorazepate binds to different sites in the **brain**, causing them to shift into a state that is less excitable. The drug is very effective in treating anxiety and **anxiety disorders**. Moreover, anxiety associated with undergoing surgical procedures is controlled with clorazepate. Clorazepate alone is not effective in treating seizures; however, if used along with other standard seizure medications, such as phenobarbital, primidone, phenytoin, **carbamazepine**, and **valproic acid**, better seizure control may be achieved. Convulsions and anxiety associated with alcohol withdrawal are controlled with clorazepate.

Clorazepate is available in two formulations. Clorazepate tablets come in 3.75 mg, 7.5 mg, and 15.0 mg doses, while slow-release tablets, administered once daily, are available in 11.25 mg and 22.5 mg strengths. Capsules are available in 3.75 mg, 7.5 mg, and 15.0 mg strengths.

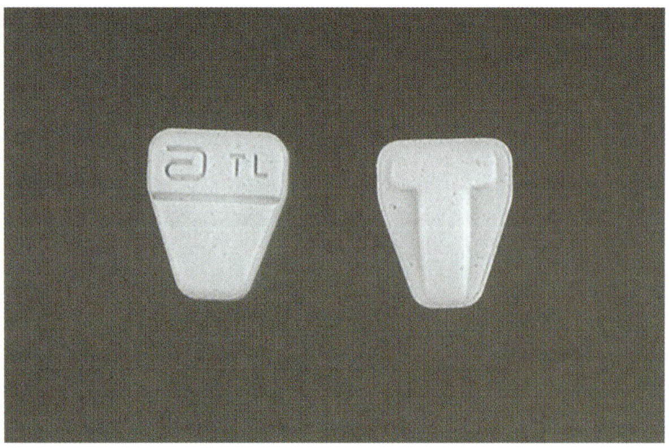

Tranxene (clorazepate), 75 mg. *(U.S. Drug Enforcement Administration)*

Recommended dosage

If used for anxiety, the dose of clorazepate usually is 15–60 mg daily in divided dose intervals. Usually, however, the average dose is 30 mg daily given in two to four doses. If slow-release formulation is used, the dose of either 11.25 mg or 22.5 mg is usually administered at bedtime. Slow-release products should not be used to initiate therapy. Doses may be lower in elderly patients and patients with liver or kidney problems.

Doses of clorazepate for the management of seizures differ in adult and pediatric populations. Patients 9–12 years of age should be started on 3.75–7.5 mg twice daily. This dose should be increased by no more than 3.75 mg weekly. The maximum dose per day is 60 mg administered in two to three divided doses. Children older than 12 and adults should receive 7.5 mg two to three times daily. This can be increased to a higher dose by adding 7.5 mg at weekly intervals. The total daily dose should not exceed 90 mg daily administered in 2–3 doses. In patients undergoing alcohol withdrawal, the first dose is 30 mg. Treatment is continued with 15 mg two to four times daily for the maximum dose of 90 mg in one day. Once maximum dose is achieved, the dose is gradually decreased over subsequent days.

Precautions

Pregnant women should not take clorazepate. Patients who have narrow-angle glaucoma should not take clorazepate, as this may worsen their condition. Clorazepate should not be used in patients younger than nine years of age.

If **depression** coexists with anxiety, clorazepate should be used with caution as it can worsen existing depression and increase the risk of **suicide**. Patients should be cautioned against engaging in activities requiring mental alertness, such as driving or operating machinery, since clorazepate causes drowsiness and dizziness. Clorazepate is a long-acting drug and it may take time for its effects to diminish. Some cases of "sleep driving," or operating a vehicle while asleep, have been reported. Elderly patients are also at increased risk for falls, due to loss of coordination.

Abrupt discontinuation of clorazepate has been associated with withdrawal symptoms and seizures. Hence, doses of clorazepate should be slowly decreased in patients who have been taking clorazepate continuously over several weeks. Other withdrawal symptoms may include nervousness, **insomnia**, irritability, diarrhea, and muscle aches.

Side effects

The most common side effects include drowsiness, dizziness, and confusion. There are a few reports about behavioral changes associated with the use of clorazepate and they include rage, depression, irritability, and aggression.

Other side effects include vision disturbances—such as blurred and double vision—decreased libido, nausea, vomiting, either decreased or increased appetite, and diarrhea or constipation. Clorazepate may also cause short-term memory loss or **amnesia**. In a few cases, clorazepate has been associated with liver toxicity where patients developed jaundice or fever. It is also known to cause a rash.

Interactions

Simultaneous use of clorazepate and dong quai, a Chinese herb, has been associated with excessive muscle relaxation and central nervous system depression. Other herbs that should not be used with clorazepate are **ginkgo biloba** and **kava kava**.

Omeprazole, a medication used to treat heartburn, should not be used together with clorazepate. **Valerian**, an herb used as a sleep aid, binds to the same receptors in the brain as clorazepate; thus, the desired effects of clorazepate may not be seen in patients taking it and valerian at the same time.

Clorazepate may increase the effects of other drugs that cause drowsiness. These drugs include antihistamines (such as Benadryl), **sedatives** (usually used to treat insomnia), pain relievers, anxiety and seizure medicines, and muscle relaxants. Alcohol combined with clorazepate also causes excessive drowsiness and should not be used. Grapefruit and grapefruit juice should also be avoided, as it may slow the metabolism of the drug in the body, prolonging the effects and potentially causing overdose if the drug is continually taken.

Resources

BOOKS

Preston, John D., John H. O'Neal, and Mary C. Talaga. *Handbook of Clinical Psychopharmacology for Therapists*. 5th ed. Oakland, CA: New Harbinger Publications, 2008.

PERIODICALS

Lelong-Boulouard, Véronique, et al. "Interactions of Buprenorphine and Dipotassium Clorazepate on Anxiety and Memory Functions in the Mouse." *Drug and Alcohol Dependence* 85, no. 2 (November 8, 2006): 103–13.

Millan, Mark J., et al. "Anxiolytic Properties of Agomelatine, an Antidepressant with Melatoninergic and Serotonergic Properties: Role of 5-HT2C Receptor Blockade." *Psychopharmacology* 177, no. 4 (February 2005): 448–58.

Quentin, Thomas, et al. "Clorazepate Affects Cell Surface Regulation of Delta and Kappa Opioid Receptors, Thereby Altering Buprenorphine-Induced Adaptation in the Rat Brain." *Brain Research* 1063, no. 1 (November 2005): 84–95.

Rowlett, James K., et al. "Anti-Conflict Effects of Benzodiazepines in Rhesus Monkeys: Relationship with Therapeutic Doses in Humans and Role of GABA-Sub(A) Receptors." *Psychopharmacology* 184, no. 2 (January 2006): 201–11.

ORGANIZATIONS

American Academy of Child and Adolescent Psychiatry, 3615 Wisconsin Ave. NW, Washington, DC, 20016-3007, (202) 966-7300, Fax: (202) 966-2891, http://aacap.org.

American Academy of Clinical Toxicology, 6728 Old McLean Village Dr., McLean, VA, 22101, (703) 556-9222, Fax: (703) 556-8729, admin@clintox.org, http://www.clintox.org.

American College of Neuropsychopharmacology, 5034-A Thoroughbred Ln., Brentwood, TN, 37027, (615) 324-2360, Fax: (615) 523-1715, acnp@acnp.org, http://www.acnp.org/default.aspx.

American Psychiatric Association, 1000 Wilson Blvd., Ste. 1825, Arlington, VA, 22209-3901, (703) 907-7300, apa@psych.org, http://www.psych.org.

Ajna Hamidovic, PharmD
Ruth A. Wienclaw, PhD

Clozapine

Definition

Clozapine is an antipsychotic drug used to alleviate the symptoms and signs of schizophrenia—a form of severe mental illness—that is characterized by hallucinations, **delusions**, unusual behavior, and loss of contact

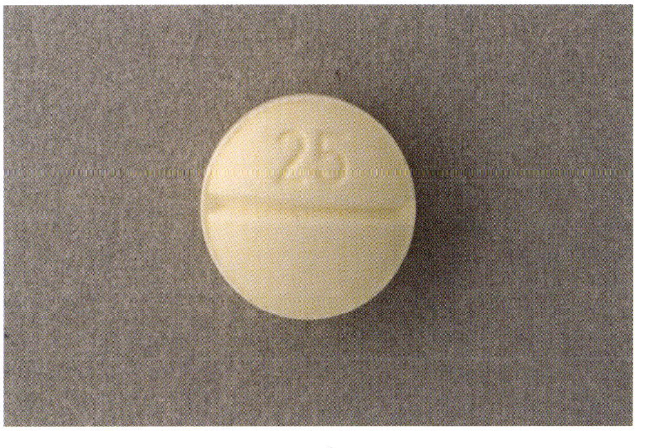

Clozaril (clozapine), 25 mg. *(© Custom Medical Stock Photo, Inc. Reproduced by permission.)*

with reality. In the United States, the drug is also known by the brand name Clozaril.

Purpose

Clozapine is principally used to reduce the signs and symptoms of severe schizophrenic illness. The drug is intended for use in patients with severe **schizophrenia** who have not responded to any other antipsychotic drug. Clozapine is also used in patients with severe schizophrenia when other antipsychotic medications have caused intolerable side effects.

Description

Clozapine is considered an atypical antipsychotic drug. Atypical antipsychotics differ from typical antipsychotics in their effectiveness in schizophrenia and their profile of side effects. Clozapine may reduce the signs and symptoms of schizophrenia in a large proportion of patients with treatment-resistant schizophrenia who do not respond to typical antipsychotics. Moreover, the drug is less likely than typical antipsychotics to cause **tardive dyskinesia** and other extrapyramidal (pertaining to a neural network in the **brain**) side effects. Tardive dyskinesia is a syndrome of involuntary, uncoordinated movements that may not disappear or may only partially improve after the drug is stopped. Tardive dyskinesia involves involuntary movements of the tongue, jaw, mouth or face, or other groups of skeletal muscles. The incidence of tardive dyskinesia increases with increasing age and with increasing dosage. It may also appear after the use of the antipsychotic has stopped. Women are at greater risk than men for developing tardive dyskinesia. There is no known effective treatment for this syndrome, although gradual (but rarely complete) improvement may occur over a long period.

Clozapine was the first atypical antipsychotic drug to be developed. In the late 1980s, clozapine was tested in severely ill patients with schizophrenia who had been treated with a typical antipsychotic drug but had not shown much improvement. A significant proportion of these patients improved as a result of treatment with clozapine.

The superiority of clozapine in patients resistant to treatment is considered an important advance, but the drug is not without problems. Clozapine is generally considered the most toxic of the antipsychotic drugs. It causes agranulocytosis, a life-threatening depletion of white blood cells, in 1%–2% of patients. It also causes epileptic **seizures** and adverse effects on the heart and blood pressure more frequently than other antipsychotic medicines. Clozapine is usually reserved for the most severely ill patients with schizophrenia who have not responded to other treatments. Other atypical antipsychotic drugs were developed subsequently and are considered safer to use than clozapine.

The mechanisms of action of antipsychotic drugs are not completely understood. The effect of clozapine is believed to be related to its actions in blocking neurotransmission due to the **neurotransmitters dopamine** and **serotonin** in a region of the brain called the limbic system, which is involved with emotions and motivation. The actions of clozapine may target the limbic system more specifically than those of typical antipsychotic drugs.

In 2005, the effectiveness of clozapine was evaluated in the Clinical Antipsychotic Trials of Intervention Effectiveness (**CATIE**) Schizophrenia Study. This study evaluated the effectiveness and side effects of atypical antipsychotics, including clozapine, in comparison to a conventional antipsychotic drug in the treatment of schizophrenia. Phase I of the study found that the newer antipsychotics were not significantly more effective than the less expensive, conventional antipsychotic medications. In Phase II of the study, it was found that participants who had not benefited from their first antipsychotic medication tended to be effectively treated by clozapine. For those patients, clozapine worked significantly better than other atypical antipsychotics; the conventional antipsychotic, however, was not included in this phase of the study.

The study results also showed that clozapine is often a good choice of medication for patients who do not respond well to other antipsychotic medications. Clozapine was more effective in controlling symptoms than the other atypical antipsychotics under evaluation. For patients whose symptoms were not well-controlled on clozapine, **olanzapine** and **risperidone** tended to be more effective than **ziprasidone** or **quetiapine**.

As many as 20%–60% of patients have schizophrenia that is treatment resistant, making the management of schizophrenia a challenge for clinicians. Whereas inadequate response to clozapine treatment is frequently encountered in practice, augmentation strategies are sometimes employed. Drug augmentation studies have been ongoing to study and evaluate the effect of adding additional antipsychotic drugs to a patient's regimen of treatment with clozapine. In the early 2000s, the results of drug augmentation studies showed only marginal therapeutic benefit.

Augmenting clozapine with other drugs such as risperidone may minimize some symptoms associated with schizophrenia; however, the effectiveness of augmentation therapy overall remains inconclusive. Continued studies were considered needed to research

KEY TERMS

Delusions—Irrational beliefs that defy normal reasoning and remain firm even when overwhelming proof is presented to dispute them. Delusions are distinct from culturally or religiously based beliefs that may be seen as untrue by outsiders.

Epilepsy—A disorder associated with disturbed electrical discharges in the central nervous system that cause seizures.

Extrapyramidal symptoms—A group of side effects associated with antipsychotic medications and characterized by involuntary muscle movements, including contraction and tremor.

Off-label use—Drugs in the United States, approved by the Food and Drug Administration (FDA) for specific uses based on the results of clinical trials, and then legally prescribed by physicians for other "off-label" uses. It is not legal for pharmaceutical companies to advertise drugs for off-label uses.

Schizophrenia—A major mental illness marked by psychotic symptoms, including hallucinations, delusions, and severe disruptions in thinking.

Seizure—A convulsion or uncontrolled discharge of nerve cells that may spread to other cells throughout the brain.

and demonstrate the effects of augmenting clozapine with other drugs aimed at diminishing the symptoms of schizophrenia.

Recommended dosage

Clozapine is available as 25 mg and 100 mg tablets. The usual dosage of clozapine is 300–600 mg per day; however, some patients may require daily dosages of up to 900 mg. To minimize side effects, the initial dose of clozapine is 12.5 mg (one-half tablet) twice a day, and the dose is increased by 25–50 mg each day, until the dose reaches 300–450 mg per day. The daily dosage of the drug is then determined based on the individual patient's response, but increases should not exceed 100 mg once or twice a week.

Precautions

Clozapine may cause agranulocytosis, a life-threatening depletion of white blood cells. The blood cells affected by clozapine defend the body against infections by bacteria and other microorganisms, and patients with agranulocytosis are subject to severe infections. Clozapine treatment is reserved for the most severely ill patients with schizophrenia who have not responded to other treatments. Clozapine is available only through a distribution system that assures close monitoring of white blood cells. Patients must have white blood cell counts determined before starting treatment, then once every week for the first six months, once every other week after that, and once a week for the first month after clozapine treatment is stopped.

Clozapine may cause epileptic seizures in about 5% of patients. The frequency of seizures goes up as the dose of the drug is increased. Usually, patients who experience seizures on clozapine discontinue the drug or reduce the dose. **Neuroleptic malignant syndrome** (NMS), a dangerous condition with high fever, muscular rigidity, rapid pulse, sweating, and altered mental state, may occur with all antipsychotic medications, including clozapine. NMS requires immediate medical treatment.

Clozapine frequently causes sedation and may interfere with driving and other tasks requiring alertness. The drug may increase the effects of alcohol and **sedatives**. Clozapine may cause low blood pressure and sudden drops in blood pressure on standing up, which may cause dizziness or fainting. Elevated heart rate may occur in 25% of patients; this effect may be a serious risk for patients with heart disease. Clozapine-induced fever, unrelated to any illness, may occur. The fever usually subsides within a few days, but it may require discontinuing the drug.

Clozapine may cause myocarditis (heart inflammation). Symptoms may be similar to the flu and include chest pain, **fatigue**, fever, joint pain, and leg swelling. If any of these or other unusual side effects develop, patients should contact their physician immediately.

Clozapine and other antipsychotic drugs are associated with an increased risk of death when used in elderly patients with **dementia**. In June 2008, the U.S. Food and Drug Administration (FDA) announced a requirement for manufacturers of clozapine (and other antipsychotic drugs) to add a warning label to their packaging stating this risk. The reason for the increase was unclear in studies, but most deaths were found to be related to either cardiovascular complications or complications associated with infection. Clozapine is not approved by the FDA for the treatment of behavior problems in older adults with dementia, and patients in this category (or caregivers of patients in this category) should discuss the risks of taking clozapine with their physician. Elderly patients may also be particularly sensitive to sedation, low blood pressure, and other side effects.

Clozapine should be used in pregnant women only when strictly necessary. Babies born to mothers who took clozapine during their pregnancy may be at risk for extrapyramidal symptoms (EPS) and symptoms of withdrawal, including agitation, trouble breathing, and difficulty feeding. Clozapine may be secreted in breast milk, and breastfeeding may not be advisable. Clozapine has a higher risk of adverse side effects in children and adolescents but may be necessary if other treatments are not effective.

Side effects

Clozapine may cause many side effects. The following side effects are grouped by the body system affected:

- cardiovascular: decreases of blood pressure, especially on arising from a seated or lying position, which may cause dizziness or fainting; rapid heart rate; changes in heart rhythm; and electrocardiogram
- nervous system: sedation, increased seizure tendency
- digestive system: increased appetite, excessive salivation, nausea, constipation, abnormal liver tests, elevated blood sugar
- autonomic: blurred vision, exacerbation of glaucoma, dry mouth, nasal congestion, decreased sweating, difficulty urinating, particularly in men with enlarged prostate
- skin: rashes
- body as a whole: weight gain, fever

Interactions

Clozapine may interact with many other drugs. Patients (or their caregivers) should inform the physician in charge about all other drugs the patient is taking before the patient starts treatment. Because of the risk of agranulocytosis, clozapine should not be given along with medications that suppress production of blood cells.

Clozapine may intensify the effects of drugs causing sedation, including alcohol, **barbiturates**, narcotic pain medications, minor tranquilizers, and antihistamines. Similarly, clozapine may cause excessive reductions of blood pressure in patients taking other medicines that lower blood pressure. Clozapine may also intensify side effects of drugs that cause blurred vision, dry mouth, diminished sweating in hot weather, and constipation. Many other antipsychotics and **antidepressants** cause such side effects.

Clozapine may increase the effects of other medications that also lower seizure threshold (make it more likely to have seizures), such as steroid drugs, the asthma medication theophylline, and many other psychiatric drugs. Patients with epilepsy may require adjustment in their dosage of antiseizure medications. Lithium may increase the risk of seizures and other nervous system adverse effects when given with clozapine.

Certain drugs that are eliminated by the liver may interfere with the elimination of clozapine from the body, causing higher blood levels and increased side effects. Conversely, clozapine may interfere with the elimination of other drugs that are eliminated by the liver. Antidepressants that affect brain serotonin levels may increase blood levels of clozapine, possibly causing increased side effects.

QUESTIONS TO ASK YOUR DOCTOR

- What kind of changes can I expect to see or feel with this medication?
- Does it matter what time of day I take this medication? If so, what is the recommendation?
- Should I take this medication with or without food?
- What are the side effects associated with this medication?
- Will this medication interact or interfere with other medications I am currently taking?
- What symptoms or adverse effects are important enough that I should seek immediate treatment?

Resources

BOOKS

Albers, Lawrence J., Rhoda K. Hahn, and Christopher Reist. *Handbook of Psychiatric Drugs.* Laguna Hills, CA: Current Clinical Strategies, 2010.

American Society of Health-System Pharmacists. *AHFS Drug Information 2011.* Bethesda, MD: ASHP, 2011.

Graham, George. *The Disordered Mind: An Introduction to Philosophy of Mind and Mental Illness.* New York: Routledge, 2010.

Holland, Leland Norman, and Michael Patrick Adams. *Core Concepts in Pharmacology.* 3rd ed. New York: Prentice Hall, 2011.

Preston, John D., John H. O'Neal, and Mary C. Talaga. *Handbook of Clinical Psychopharmacology for Therapists.* 6th ed. Oakland, CA: New Harbinger, 2010.

PERIODICALS

Brunette, Mary F., et al. "Clozapine Use and Relapses of Substance Use Disorder Among Patients with Co-occurring Schizophrenia and Substance Use Disorders." *Schizophrenia Bulletin* 32, no. 4 (October 2006): 637–43.

Essock, S.M., et al. "Effectiveness of Switching Antipsychotic Medications." *American Journal of Psychiatry* 163, no. 12 (December 2006): 2090–95.

Gogtay, N., and J. Rapoport. "Clozapine Use in Children and Adolescents." *Expert Opinion on Pharmacotherapy* 9, no. 3 (February 2008): 459–65.

Lamberti, J. Steven, et al. "Prevalence of the Metabolic Syndrome Among Patients Receiving Clozapine." *American Journal of Psychiatry* 163, no. 7 (July 2006): 1273–76.

Lieberman, J.A., et al. "Effectiveness of Antipsychotic Drugs in Patients with Chronic Schizophrenia." *New England Journal of Medicine* 353, no. 12 (September 22, 2005): 1209–23.

Luchins, Daniel J. "In the Aftermath of CATIE: How Should Administrators Value Atypical Antipsychotic Medications?" *Administration and Policy in Mental Health and Mental Health Services Research* 33, no. 5 (September 2006): 541–43.

McEvoy, J.P., et al. "Effectiveness of Clozapine versus Olanzapine, Quetiapine, and Risperidone in Patients with Chronic Schizophrenia Who Did Not Respond to Prior Atypical Antipsychotic Treatment." *American Journal of Psychiatry* 163, no. 4 (April 2006): 600–610.

Miodownik, Chanoch, et al. "The Effect of Sudden Clozapine Discontinuation on Management of Schizophrenic Patients: A Retrospective Controlled Study." *Journal of Clinical Psychiatry* 67, no. 8 (August 2006): 1204–1208.

Rocha, Fábio Lopes, and Cláudia Hara. "Benefits of Combining Aripiprazole to Clozapine: Three Case Reports." *Progress in Neuropsychopharmacology and Biological Psychiatry* 30, no. 6 (July 2006): 1167–69.

Shaw, Philip, and Judith L. Rapoport. "Decision Making about Children with Psychotic Symptoms: Using the Best Evidence in Choosing a Treatment." *Journal of the American Academy of Child and Adolescent Psychiatry* 45, no. 11 (November 2006): 1381–86.

Shaw, Philip, et al. "Childhood-Onset Schizophrenia: A Double-Blind, Randomized Clozapine-Olanzapine Comparison." *Archives of General Psychiatry* 63, no. 7 (July 2006): 721–30.

ORGANIZATIONS

American Academy of Clinical Toxicology, 6728 Old McLean Village Dr., McLean, VA, 22101, (703) 556-9222, Fax: (703) 556-8729, admin@clintox.org, http://www.clintox.org.

American Academy of Family Physicians, 11400 Tomahawk Creek Pkwy., Leawood, KS, 66211-2672, (913) 906-6000, (800) 274-2237, Fax: (913) 906-6075, contactcenter@aafp.org, http://www.aafp.org.

American Medical Association, 515 N State St., Chicago, IL, 60610, (312) 464-5000, (800) 621-8335, http://www.ama-assn.org.

American Psychiatric Association, 1000 Wilson Blvd., Ste. 1825, Arlington, VA, 22209-3901, (703) 907-7300, apa@psych.org, http://www.psych.org.

American Psychological Association, 750 1st St., NE, Washington, DC, 20002-4242, (202) 336-5500; TDD/TTY: (202) 336-6123, (800) 374-2721, http://www.apa.org.

American Society for Clinical Pharmacology and Therapeutics, 528 N Washington St., Alexandria, VA, 22314, (703) 836-6981, info@ascpt.org, http://www.ascpt.org.

Anxiety Disorders Association of America, 8730 Georgia Ave., Silver Spring, MD, 20910, (240) 485-1001, Fax: (240) 485-1035, http://www.adaa.org.

Depression and Bipolar Support Alliance, 730 N Franklin St., Ste. 501, Chicago, IL, 60654, (800) 826-3632, Fax: (312) 642-7243, http://www.dbsalliance.org.

Mental Health America, 2000 N. Beauregard St., 6th Fl., Alexandria, VA, 22311, (703) 684-7722, (800) 969-6642, Fax: (703) 684-5968, http://www1.nmha.org.

National Alliance on Mental Illness, 2107 Wilson Blvd., Ste. 300, Arlington, VA, 22201-3042, Fax: (703) 524-9094, (800) 950-6264, http://www.nami.org.

National Institute of Mental Health, 6001 Executive Blvd., Rm. 8184, MSC 9663, Bethesda, MD, 20892-9663, (301) 433-4513; TTY: (301) 443-8431, Fax: (301) 443-4279, (866) 615-6464; TTY: (866) 415-8051, nimhinfo@nih.gov, http://www.nimh.nih.gov.

National Institutes of Health, 9000 Rockville Pike, Bethesda, MD, 20892, (301) 496-4000; TTY: (301) 402-9612, http://www.nih.gov.

U.S. National Library of Medicine, 8600 Rockville Pike, Bethesda, MD, 20894, (301) 594-5983, (888) 346-3656; TDD: (800) 735-2258, Fax: (301) 402-1384, http://www.nlm.nih.gov.

Richard Kapit, MD
Ruth A. Wienclaw, PhD
Laura Jean Cataldo, RN, EdD

Clozaril *see* **Clozapine**

Cocaine and related disorders

Definition

Cocaine is extracted from the coca plant, which grows in Central and South America. The substance is processed into many forms for use as an illegal drug of abuse. Cocaine is dangerously addictive, and users of the drug experience a "high"—a feeling of euphoria or intense happiness, along with hypervigilance, increased sensitivity, irritability or anger, impaired judgment, and anxiety.

Forms of the drug

In its most common form, cocaine is a whitish crystalline powder that produces feelings of euphoria when ingested. In powder form, cocaine is known by such street names as "coke," "blow," "C," "flake," "snow" and "toot." It is most commonly inhaled or snorted. It may also be dissolved in water and injected.

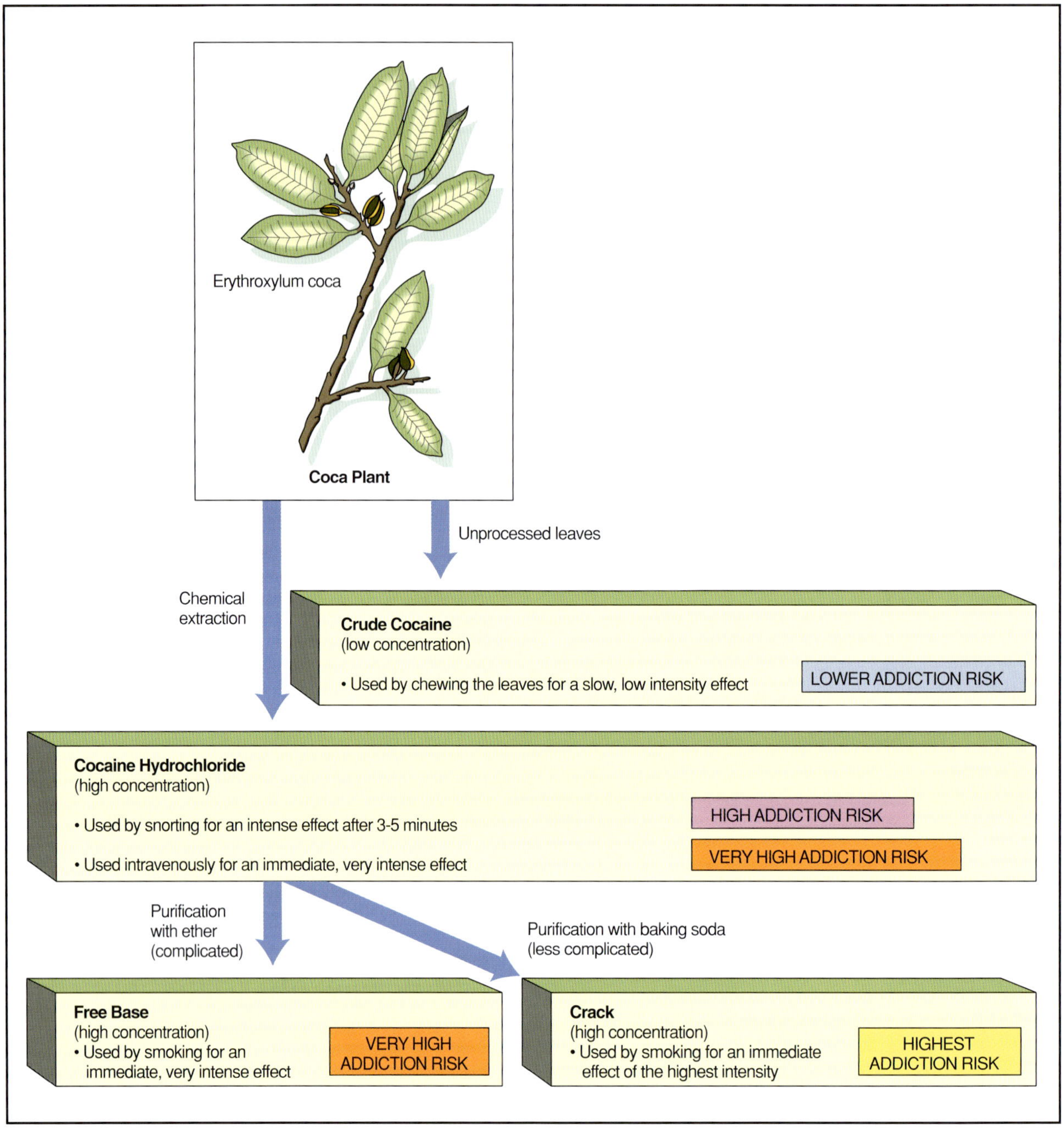

Various forms of cocaine (including the coca plant) and the addiction risks associated with them. *(Illustration by Hans & Cassady.)*

Crack is a form of cocaine that can be smoked and that produces an immediate, more intense, and more short-lived high. It comes in off-white chunks or chips called "rocks."

In addition to their stand-alone use, both cocaine and crack are often mixed with other substances. Cocaine may be mixed with methcathinone to create a "wildcat." Cigars may be hollowed out and filled with a mixture of crack and marijuana. Either cocaine or crack used in conjunction with heroin is called a "speedball." Cocaine used together with alcohol represents the most common fatal two-drug combination.

Demographics

The patterns of cocaine abuse in the United States have changed much over the past thirty years. They have been changing in other parts of the world as well, including South America and Western

Europe. In the United States, several studies have attempted to track drug abuse in many different populations. The studies include: the Monitoring the Future Study (MTF); the National Household Survey on Drug Abuse (NHSDA); the Drug Abuse Warning Network (DAWN), which gets reports from emergency rooms and medical examiners' offices on drug-related cases and deaths; and Arrestee Drug Abuse Monitoring (ADAM), which gets information on urine samples obtained from people who have been arrested.

In the annual MTF study, cocaine use among high-school seniors had declined from 13.1% in 1985 to 3.1% in 1992—the lowest it had been since 1975, when the survey was first implemented. The rate of cocaine use began to rise again and peaked at 5.5% in 1997. The NHSDA found that the levels of cocaine use declined over the same time period. The decline in the rates has been thought to be due in part to education about the risks of cocaine abuse.

The incidence of new crack cocaine users has also decreased. There was a minimal decline in the numbers of excessive cocaine users between the years 1985 and 1997. The Epidemiologic Catchment Area (ECA) studies done in the early 1980s combined cocaine dependence with cocaine abuse and found that one-month to six-month prevalence rates for cocaine abuse and dependence were low or could not be measured. The lifetime rate of cocaine abuse was 0.2%.

A 1997 study from The National Institute on Drug Abuse indicates that among outpatients who abuse substances, 55% abuse cocaine.

Cocaine abuse affects both genders and many different populations across the United States. Males are one-and-a-half to two times more likely to abuse cocaine than females. Cocaine began as a drug of the upper classes in the 1970s; now the socioeconomic status of cocaine users has shifted. Cocaine is more likely to be abused by the economically disadvantaged because it is easy for them to get, and it is inexpensive ($10 for a small bag of crack cocaine). These factors have led to increased violence (people who are cocaine dependent may become involved in illegal activity, such as drug dealing, in order to acquire funds for their habit) and higher rates of acquired immune deficiency (AIDS) among disadvantaged populations.

A National Survey on Drug Use and Health (NSDUH) survey reports that in 2009, 4.8 million Americans age 12 and older had abused cocaine in any form. Adults 18 to 25 years of age have a higher rate of cocaine use than any other age group.

Description

Cocaine-related disorders form a very broad topic. According to the mental health clinician's handbook, ***Diagnostic and Statistical Manual of Mental Disorders***, fourth edition, text revised (also known as the *DSM-IV-TR*), the broad category of cocaine-related disorders can be subdivided into two categories: cocaine use disorders and cocaine-induced disorders. Cocaine use disorders include cocaine dependence and cocaine abuse. Cocaine-induced disorders include:

- cocaine intoxication
- cocaine withdrawal
- cocaine intoxication delirium
- cocaine-induced psychotic disorder, with delusions
- cocaine-induced psychotic disorder, with hallucinations
- cocaine-induced mood disorder
- cocaine-induced anxiety disorder
- cocaine-induced sexual dysfunction
- cocaine-induced sleep disorder
- cocaine-related disorder not otherwise specified

The fifth edition of the *DSM*, also known as the *DSM-5* is due for publication in 2013. This edition may include proposed changes and revisions to some current diagnostic criteria for psychiatric diagnoses, including combining "Substance Abuse," and "Dependence," into a single disorder, thus modifying "Cocaine Abuse," and "Cocaine Dependence," to a title of "Cocaine Use Disorder."

Cocaine use disorders

COCAINE ABUSE. For the cocaine abuser, the use of the substance leads to maladaptive behavior over a 12-month period. The person may fail to meet responsibilities at school, work, or home. The cocaine abuse impairs the affected person's judgment, and he or she puts himself or herself in physical danger to use the substance. For example, the individual may use cocaine in an unsafe environment. The person who abuses cocaine may be arrested or charged with possession of the substance, yet continue to use cocaine despite all of the personal and legal problems that may result.

COCAINE DEPENDENCE. Cocaine dependence is even more serious than cocaine abuse. Dependence is a maladaptive behavior that, over a three-month period, has caused the affected individual to experience tolerance for, and withdrawal symptoms from, cocaine. Tolerance is the need to increase the amount of cocaine intake to achieve the same desired effect. In other words, someone who is dependent on cocaine needs more cocaine to produce the same "high" that a lesser amount produced in the past. The dependent person also experiences cocaine withdrawal. Withdrawal symptoms develop within hours or days after cocaine use that has been heavy and prolonged and then abruptly stopped. The symptoms include irritable mood and two or more of the following symptoms: **fatigue**, nightmares, difficulty sleeping or too much sleep, elevated appetite, agitation (restlessness), or slowed physical movements. The onset of withdrawal symptoms can cause a person to use more cocaine to avoid these painful and uncomfortable symptoms. The dependent person uses larger amounts of cocaine for longer periods of time than intended. He or she cannot cut back on the use of the substance, often has a difficult time resisting cocaine when it is available, and may abandon work or school to spend more time acquiring and planning to acquire more cocaine. The individual continues to use cocaine despite the negative effects it has on family life, work, and school.

Cocaine-induced disorders

COCAINE INTOXICATION. Cocaine intoxication occurs after recent cocaine use. The person experiences a feeling of intense happiness, hypervigilance, increased sensitivity, irritability or anger, with impaired judgement, and anxiety. The intoxication impairs the person's ability to function at work or school or in social situations. Two or more of the following symptoms are present immediately after the use of cocaine:

- enlarged pupils
- elevated heart rate
- elevated or lowered blood pressure
- chills and increased sweating
- nausea or vomiting
- weight loss
- agitation or slowed movements
- weak muscles
- chest pain
- coma
- confusion
- irregular heartbeat
- depressed respiration
- seizures
- odd postures
- odd movements

COCAINE WITHDRAWAL. Withdrawal symptoms develop within hours or days after cocaine use that has been heavy and prolonged and then abruptly stopped. The symptoms include irritable mood and two or more of the following symptoms: fatigue, nightmares, difficulty sleeping or too much sleep, elevated appetite, agitation (restlessness), or slowed physical movements.

COCAINE-INDUCED DELIRIUM. According to the *DSM-IV-TR*, several criteria must be met in order for a health care professional to establish the **diagnosis** of cocaine-induced **delirium**. Patients have a disturbance of their level of consciousness or awareness, evidenced by drowsiness or an inability to concentrate or pay attention. Patients also experience a change in their cognition (ability to think) evidenced by a deficit in their language or their memory. For example, these patients may forget where they have placed an item, or their speech may be confusing. These symptoms have rapid onset within hours or days of using cocaine, and the symptoms fluctuate throughout the course of the day. These findings cannot be explained by **dementia** (state of impaired thought processes and memory that can be caused by various diseases and conditions), and the doctor must not be able to recognize a physical reason that can account for the symptoms other than cocaine intoxication.

COCAINE-INDUCED PSYCHOTIC DISORDER, WITH DELUSIONS. The person with this disorder has experienced intoxication or withdrawal from cocaine within a month from the time he or she begins to experience **delusions** (beliefs that the person continues to maintain, despite evidence to the contrary). In order for this state to be considered cocaine-induced psychotic disorder, these symptoms cannot be due to another condition or substance.

COCAINE-INDUCED PSYCHOTIC DISORDER, WITH HALLUCINATIONS. This condition is the same as cocaine-induced psychotic disorder with delusions, except that this affected individual experiences hallucinations instead of delusions. Hallucinations can be described as hearing and seeing things that are not real.

COCAINE-INDUCED MOOD DISORDER. The person with this disorder has experienced intoxication or withdrawal from cocaine within a month from the time he or she begins to experience depressed, elevated, or irritable mood with **apathy** (lack of empathy for others, and lack of showing a broad range of appropriate emotions).

COCAINE-INDUCED ANXIETY DISORDER. The person with this disorder has experienced intoxication or withdrawal from cocaine within a month from the time he or she begins to experience anxiety, panic attacks, obsessions, or compulsions. Panic attacks are discrete episodes of intense anxiety. Persons affected with panic attacks may experience accelerated heart rate, shaking or trembling, sweating, shortness of breath, or fear of going crazy or losing control, as well as other symptoms. An

obsession is an unwelcome, uncontrollable, persistent idea, thought, image, or emotion that a person cannot help thinking even though it creates significant distress or anxiety. A **compulsion** is a repetitive, excessive, meaningless activity or mental exercise which a person performs in an attempt to avoid distress or worry.

COCAINE-INDUCED SEXUAL DYSFUNCTION. The person with this disorder has experienced intoxication or withdrawal from cocaine within a month from the time he or she begins to experience sexual difficulties, and these difficulties are deemed by the clinician to be due directly to the cocaine use. Substance-induced sexual difficulties can range from impaired desire, impaired arousal, impaired orgasm, or sexual pain.

COCAINE-INDUCED SLEEP DISORDER. This disorder is characterized by difficulty sleeping (**insomnia**) during intoxication or increased sleep duration when patients are in withdrawal.

COCAINE-RELATED DISORDER NOT OTHERWISE SPECIFIED. This classification is reserved for clinicians to use when a cocaine disorder that the clinician sees does not fit into any of the above categories.

KEY TERMS

Anxiety—Can be experienced as a troubled feeling, a sense of dread, fear of the future, or distress over a possible threat to a person's physical or mental well-being.

Depression—A mental state characterized by feelings of sadness, despair, and discouragement.

Dopamine—A chemical in brain tissue that serves to transmit nerve impulses and helps to regulate movement and emotions.

Hallucinations—To hear, see, or otherwise sense things that are not real. Hallucinations can result from nervous system abnormalities, mental disorders, or the use of certain drugs.

Panic attack—A period of intense fear or discomfort with a feeling of doom and a desire to escape. The person may shake, sweat, be short of breath, and experience chest pain.

Causes and symptoms

Causes

BIOCHEMICAL/PHYSIOLOGICAL CAUSES. Twin studies have demonstrated that there is a higher rate of cocaine abuse in identical twins as compared to fraternal twins. This indicates that **genetic factors** contribute to the development of cocaine abuse. This finding also indicates, however, that unique environmental factors contribute to the development of cocaine abuse as well. (If genes alone determined who would develop cocaine dependence, 100% of the identical twins with the predisposing genes would develop the disorder. However, because the results show only a relationship, or a correlation, between genetics and cocaine use among twins, these results indicate that other factors must be at work as well.) Studies have also shown that disorders like **attention deficit hyperactivity disorder** (ADHD), **conduct disorder**, and **antisocial personality disorder** all have genetic components, and since patients who abuse cocaine have a high incidence of these diagnoses, they may also be genetically predisposed to abusing cocaine.

REINFORCEMENT. Learning and conditioning also play a unique role in the perpetuation of cocaine abuse. Each inhalation and injection of cocaine causes pleasurable feelings that reinforce the drug-taking procedure. In addition, the patient's environment plays a role in cueing and reinforcing the experience in the patient's mind. The association between cocaine and environment is so strong that many people recovering from cocaine **addiction** report that being in an area where they used drugs brings back memories of the experience and makes them crave drugs. Specific areas of the **brain** are thought to be involved in cocaine craving, including the amygdala (a part of the brain that controls aggression and emotional reactivity) and the prefrontal cortex (a part of the brain that regulates anger, aggression, and the brain's assessment of fear, threats, and danger).

Symptoms

The following list is a summary of the acute (short-term) physical and psychological effects of cocaine on the body:

- blood vessels constrict
- elevated heart rate
- elevated blood pressure
- a feeling of intense happiness
- elevated energy level
- a state of increased alertness and sensory sensitivity
- elevated anxiety
- panic attacks
- elevated self-esteem
- diminished appetite
- spontaneous ejaculation and heightened sexual arousal
- psychosis (loss of contact with reality)

The following list is a summary of the chronic (long-term) physical and psychological effects of cocaine on the body:

- depressed mood
- irritability
- physical agitation
- decreased motivation
- difficulty sleeping
- hypervigilance
- elevated anxiety
- panic attacks
- hallucinations
- psychosis

Diagnosis

If a mental health clinician suspects cocaine use, he or she may ask the patient specifically about swallowing, injecting, or smoking the substance. Urine and blood testing will also be conducted to determine the presence of the substance. Doctors may talk to friends or relatives concerning the patient's drug use, especially for cases in which the physician suspects that the patient is not being entirely honest about substance use. The clinician may also investigate a patient's legal history for drug arrests that may give clues to periods of **substance abuse** to which the patient will not admit.

Differential diagnosis

Differential diagnosis is the process of distinguishing one condition from other, similar conditions. The cocaine abuse disorder is easily confused with other substance abuse disorders and various forms of mental illness.

The symptoms of cocaine intoxication, such as increased talkativeness, poor sleep, and the intense feelings of happiness, are similar to the symptoms for **bipolar disorder**, so the urine toxification screening test may play a key role in the diagnosis. Patients with cocaine intoxication with hallucinations and delusions can be mistaken for schizophrenic patients instead, further emphasizing the importance of the urine and blood screens. As part of establishing the diagnosis, the physician must also rule out PCP (phencyclidine) intoxication and Cushing's disease (an endocrine disorder of excessive cortisol production). Withdrawal symptoms are similar to those of the patient with major **depression**. For this reason, the clinician may ask the patient about his or her mood during times of abstinence from drug use to discern whether any true mood disorders are present. If cocaine use is causing depression, the depression should resolve within a couple of weeks of stopping drug use.

Laboratory testing

The breakdown products of cocaine remain in the urine. The length of time that they remain depends on the dose of cocaine, but most doses would not remain in the urine longer than a few days. Cocaine can also be found in other bodily fluids such as blood, saliva, sweat, and hair, and these provide better estimates as to recent cocaine use. The hair can hold evidence that a patient has been using drugs for weeks to months. **Positron emission tomography (PET)** and single-photon emission **computed tomography** (SPECT) are different kinds of **imaging studies**. Both kinds of scans look at the amount of blood that is flowing to the brain. When these images are taken of the brains of people who abuse cocaine, the resulting scans can reveal abnormalities in certain sections of the brain. The brains of people addicted to cocaine shrink, or atrophy.

Neuropsychological assessment

Neuropsychological testing is also an important tool for examining the effects of toxic substances on brain functioning. Some physicians may use neuropsychological assessments to reveal patients' cognitive and physical impairment after cocaine use. Neuropsychological testing assesses brain functioning through structured and systematic behavioral observation. Neuropsychological tests are designed to examine a variety of cognitive abilities, including speed of information processing, attention, memory, and language. An example of a task that a physician might ask the patient to complete as part of a neuropsychological examination is to name as many words beginning with a particular letter as the patient can in one minute. Patients who abuse cocaine often have difficulty completing tasks, such as the one described, that require concentration and memory.

Treatment

Psychological and social interventions

TREATMENT SETTINGS. Not all patients who abuse cocaine need to resort to long-term treatment. Treatment length varies with the degree that a person is dependent on the substance. If the patient has other psychiatric conditions, such as major depression or **schizophrenia**, or has significant medical complications of cocaine abuse, then he or she is more likely to require higher-intensity treatment. Residential programs or therapeutic communities may be helpful, particularly in more severe cases. Patients typically spend six to 12 months in such programs, which may also include vocational training and other features. The availability of such treatment, as well as medical insurance's ability to cover treatment, are all issues that affect the patient's access to treatment.

PSYCHOTHERAPY. A wide range of behavioral interventions have been successfully used to treat cocaine addiction. The approach used must be tailored to the specific needs of each individual patient, however.

Contingency management rewards drug abstinence (confirmed by urine testing) with points or vouchers that patients can exchange for such things as an evening out or membership in a gym. **Cognitive-behavioral therapy** helps users learn to recognize and avoid situations most likely to lead to cocaine use and to develop healthier ways to cope with stressful situations.

Supportive therapy helps patients to modify their behavior by preventing **relapse** by taking actions such as staying away from drug-using friends and from neighborhoods or situations where cocaine is abundant.

Self-help groups like Narcotics Anonymous (NA) or Cocaine Anonymous (CA) are helpful for many recovering substance abusers. CA is a twelve-step program for cocaine abusers, modeled after Alcoholics Anonymous (AA). **Support groups** and **group therapy** led by a therapist can be helpful because other addicts can share coping and relapse-prevention strategies. The group's support can help patients face devastating changes and life issues. Some experts recommend that patients be cocaine-free for at least two weeks before participating in a group, but other experts argue that a two-week waiting period is unnecessary and counterproductive. Group counseling sessions led by drug counselors who are in recovery themselves are also useful for some people overcoming their addictions. These group counseling sessions differ from group therapy in that the people in a counseling group are constantly changing.

The National Institute of Drug Abuse conducted a study comparing different forms of **psychotherapy**: patients who had both group drug counseling and individual drug counseling had improved outcomes. Patients who had cognitive-behavioral therapy stayed in treatment longer.

Medications

Many medications—greater than twenty—have been tested, but none has been found to reduce the intensity of withdrawal. **Dopamine** agonists like **amantadine** and bromocriptine and tricyclic **antidepressants** such as **desipramine** have failed in studies to help treat symptoms of cocaine withdrawal or intoxication.

QUESTIONS TO ASK YOUR DOCTOR

- What risks are associated with cocaine abuse?
- What symptoms are associated with cocaine dependence?
- Does having cocaine dependence and abuse put me at risk for other health conditions?
- Can you recommend any treatment and support groups for me?

Alternative therapy

Alternative techniques, such as **acupuncture**, EEG **biofeedback**, and visualization, may be useful in treating addiction when combined with conventional treatment approaches.

Prognosis

Not all cocaine abusers become dependent on the drug. However, even someone who only uses occasionally can experience the harmful effects (interpersonal relationship conflicts, work or school difficulties) of using cocaine, and even occasional use is enough to addict. In the course of a person's battle with cocaine abuse, he or she may vary the forms of the drug that he or she uses. A person may use the inhaled form at one time and the injected form at another, for example.

Many studies of short-term outpatient treatment over a six month to two-year period indicate that people addicted to cocaine have a better chance of recovering than people who are addicted to heroin. A study of veterans who participated in an inpatient or day hospital treatment program that lasted 28 days revealed that about 60% of people who were abstinent at four months were able to maintain their abstinence at seven months.

Having a good social support network greatly improves the prognosis for recovery from cocaine abuse and dependence.

Prevention

Efforts to prevent cocaine abuse, as well as any substance abuse, begin with prevention programs that are based in schools or in the workplace, heath care clinics, criminal justice systems, and public housing. Programs such as Students Taught Awareness (STAR) are cost-effective and have reduced the rates of substance abuse in the schools. These school-based programs also foster parental involvement and education about substance abuse issues. The juvenile justice system also implements drug-prevention programs. Even many workplaces provide drug screening and treatment and counseling for those who test positive. Employers may also provide workshops on substance abuse prevention. The United States Department of Housing and Urban Development (HUD) also sponsors drug-prevention programs.

Resources

BOOKS

American Psychiatric Association. *Diagnostic and Statistical Manual of Mental Disorders.* 4th ed., Text rev. Washington, DC: American Psychiatric Association, 2000.

American Psychological Association. *Publication Manual of the American Psychological Association,* 6th ed. Washington, DC: American Psychological Association, 2009.

Erickson, Carlton K. *Addiction Essentials: The Go-To Guide for Clinicians and Patients.* New York: W. W. Norton & Company, 2011.

Sadock, Benjamin J., Virginia Alcott Sadock, and Pedro Ruiz, eds. *Kaplan and Sadock's Comprehensive Textbook of Psychiatry,* 2nd ed. New York: Lippincott Williams & Wilkins, 2009.

PERIODICALS

Adinoff, Byron, et al. "Limbic Response to Procaine in Cocaine Addicted Subjects." *American Journal of Psychiatry* (March 2001): 390-398.

Held, Gale A. "Linkages Between Substance Abuse Prevention and Other Human Services Literature Review." National Institute on Drug Abuse (NIDA) (June 1998).

Jacobsen, Leslie K., et al. "Quantitative Morphology of the Caudate and Putamen in Patients With Cocaine Dependence." *American Journal of Psychiatry* (March 2000): 486-489.

Kampman, Kyle M., et al. "Amantadine in the Treatment of Cocaine-Dependent Patients With Severe Withdrawal Symptoms." *American Journal of Psychiatry* (December 2000): 2052-2054.

WEBSITES

Leshner, Alan. "Cocaine Abuse and Addiction." *National Institute on Drug Abuse Research Report Series.* NIH Publication Number 99-4342. Washington, D.C: U.S. Government Printing Offices, 1999, revised September 2010. http://www.drugabuse.gov/ResearchReports/Cocaine/Cocaine.html (accessed December 19, 2011).

ORGANIZATIONS

American Academy of Addiction Psychiatry (AAAP), 400 Massasoiti Ave., Ste. 307, 2nd Fl., East Providence, RI, 02914, (401) 524-3076, Fax: (401) 272-0922, http://www.aaap.org.

American Psychiatric Association, 1000 Wilson Blvd., Ste. 1825, Arlington, VA, 22209, (703) 907-7300, apa@psych.org, http://www.psych.org.

American Psychological Association, 750 First Street NE, Washington, DC, 20003, (202) 336-5500, http://www.apa.org/index.aspx.

Cocaine Anonymous World Services (CAWS), 21720 S Wilmington Ave., Ste. 304, Long Beach, CA, 90810, (301) 559-5833, http://www.ca.org.

National Institute on Drug Abuse, 6001 Executive Blvd., Rm. 5213, Bethesda, MD, 20892, (301) 442-1124; Spanish: (240) 221-4007, information@nida.nih.gov, http://www.nida.nih.gov.

Substance Abuse and Mental Health Services Administration, 1 Choke Cherry Rd., Rockville, MD, 20857, (877) SAMHSA-7 (726-4727), (800) TTY: 487-4889, Fax: (240) 221-4292, SAMHSAInfo@samhsa.hhs.gov, http://www.samhsa.gov.

Susan Hobbs, MD
Peter Gregutt
Laura Jean Cataldo, RN, EdD

Cogentin *see* **Benztropine**

Cognex *see* **Tacrine**

Cognistat

Definition

The Cognistat is a standardized neurobehavioral screening test. It is a test that examines neurological (**brain** and central nervous system) health in relation to a person's behavior.

Purpose

As a screening test, the Cognistat may be administered to identify basic strengths and weaknesses so that further tests (if necessary) can be selected, and the data provided by the Cognistat can then be used as preliminary data against which scores from other tests given may be compared. Cognistat results have been used in a number of arenas, most notably in behavioral medicine. For example, Cognistat results may be useful to track cognitive decline (decreased thinking and reasoning abilities) in patients with organic brain disorders, to develop helpful strategies for cognitive problems associated with **schizophrenia**, and to help distinguish among terminally ill cancer patients those with **depression** and anxiety versus those with cognitive impairment.

Description

The Cognistat usually takes less than 45 minutes to complete, and the test explores, quantifies, and describes performance in central areas of brain-behavior relations: level of consciousness, orientation, attention, language, constructional ability, memory, calculations and reasoning. The subareas of language are spontaneous speech, comprehension, repetition, and naming. The subareas of reasoning are similarities and judgment. Exploration occurs through interactive behavioral tasks that rely on perception, cognitive processing, and motor skills. The test is more quickly administered to higher than lower functioning individuals by providing a difficult screening item at the beginning of each section. Only when a screening item is missed are the metric, or more remedial, items applied, usually from easiest to most difficult within that section.

The test begins with the examiner asking general questions of the test taker (name, address, age, etc.), and while these questions are being answered, the examiner is subjectively assessing the test taker's level of consciousness. The examiner then asks general questions to confirm the test taker's level of orientation, meaning that the test taker is correctly oriented to place and time—he or she knows what day it is and where he or she is. To test the examinee's attention and memory, the test taker will be asked to repeat a series of digits and the first part of a verbal memory task will be given. (This task will be asked about again later in the test.)

The language section begins with a sample of spontaneous speech derived by asking for a description of a detailed line drawing. The language comprehension section requires responses to simple commands that involve manipulation of common objects placed before the examinee. In the language repetition subtest, the test taker is asked to repeat short phrases and simple sentences. In naming, the last of the language subtests, the screening item differs in form from the metric (easier) items. In the screening item, the examiner holds up an object and asks the test taker to name its four major parts, as the examiner points to them one after another. If the test taker fails, he or she is asked to name eight separate objects, one after another represented by line drawings.

In the next section, constructional ability, the screening item is a visual memory task wherein a stimulus sheet is presented for ten seconds, and the examinee is asked to draw the stimuli from memory. The test taker is then asked to assemble plastic tiles into designs, one after another, as each is shown on a card. Faster completion yields greater points. After the constructional items, the test taker is asked to recall the verbal memory items presented earlier. For items he or she cannot recall, the examiner provides prompts, or clues.

The calculations section is composed of simple verbal mathematics, and is followed by the reasoning section, which includes two subtests. The first consists of associative thinking items known as similarities. In similarities items, the examinee is asked to explain how

KEY TERMS

Screening test—A test given as a preliminary tool, that helps to later target a more thorough analysis.

Standardized test—A test that follows a regimented structure, and each individual's scores may be compared with those of groups of people. In the case of the Cognistat, test taker's scores can be compared to groups of young adults, middle-aged adults, the geriatric, and people who have undergone neurosurgery.

two concepts are alike. Greater points are awarded if their concept is abstract rather than concrete. The final subtest on the Cognistat is the judgment subtest of the reasoning section. In the judgment subtest, the examinee is asked to answer questions that demonstrate practical judgment in solving basic problem scenarios. Scores for this subtest are weighted based on their appropriateness. There is only one fully appropriate response to each item.

The test booklet provides space for listing medications, and for noting comments about any physical deficits and the examinee's impression of his or her own performance.

Risks

The Cognistat is more sensitive than many similar tests, but considers a limited sample of behavior at a brief point in time. Thus, its results are not generalizable and should not be viewed as conclusive indicators of the areas being assessed. It is important that the examiner be properly trained in the use of the test. Test takers may be affected by test-related discomfort or performance anxiety. This may be particularly true when prior to testing, the examinee was not fully aware of his or her deficits, especially deficits that become more apparent as testing progresses. The test's reliability has not been fully documented. Further research and standardization data is needed.

Results

When test administration is complete, the examiner tallies the points earned in each section, and plots them on the cognitive status profile located on the front of the test booklet. On the profile, numerical scores are described to fall within the normal or impaired range. The impaired range is broken down into mild, moderate and severe. An individual's scores can also be compared to standardization group data, and his or her profile may be compared to five case study profiles presented in the test guide. The few items that do not allow for quantitative analysis—the sample of spontaneous speech, for example—are factored into the interpretation of results by the examiner. There is no mechanism for transforming raw scores into percentiles or standard scores, and the test is not designed to generate one main score.

Resources

BOOKS

Northern California Neurobehavioral Group, Inc. *2011 Cognistat and Cognistat Assessment System Manual*. Fairfax, CA: 2011.

PERIODICALS

Nazem, Sarra, et al. "Montreal Cognitive Assessment Performance in Patients with Parkinson's Disease with 'Normal' Global Cognition According to Mini-Mental State Examination Score." *Journal of the American Geriatric Society* 57, no. 2 (February 2009) 304–308.

WEBSITES

Cognistat.com. http://www.cognistat.com (accessed October 30, 2011).

Geoffrey G. Grimm, PhD, LPC

Cognitive-behavioral therapy

Definition

Cognitive-behavioral therapy (CBT) is an action-oriented form of psychosocial therapy that assumes that maladaptive, or faulty, thinking patterns cause maladaptive behavior and negative emotions. (Maladaptive behavior is behavior that is counter-productive or interferes with everyday living.) The treatment focuses on changing individuals' thoughts (cognitive patterns) in order to change their behavior and emotional state. CBT can be employed with both adults and children.

Purpose

Theoretically, cognitive-behavioral therapy can be employed in any situation in which there is a pattern of unwanted behavior accompanied by distress and impairment. CBT differs from other traditional forms of supportive **psychotherapy** in that it is time-limited and does not attempt to understand the etiology of the disorder. Instead, it works to change dysfunctional, ingrained thought patterns that lead to dysfunctional behaviors. The entire process is often accomplished in 6–20 one-hour sessions.

CBT is a recommended treatment option for a number of mental disorders, including affective (mood) disorders, **personality disorders**, **social phobia**, **obsessive-compulsive disorder** (OCD), eating disorders, **substance abuse**, anxiety or **panic disorder**, **agoraphobia**, **post-traumatic stress disorder** (PTSD), and **attention deficit hyperactivity disorder (ADHD)**. Newer applications include treating **stuttering**. It is also frequently used as a tool for dealing with chronic pain for patients with illnesses such as rheumatoid arthritis, back problems, and cancer. Patients with **sleep disorders** may also find cognitive-behavioral therapy a useful treatment for **insomnia**. Some research has shown CBT alone to have better efficacy than medication alone in the treatment of these disorders; other research shows that a combination of CBT and medication offers the greatest benefit. Research supports the use of CBT (without medication) as a first-line treatment for a number of disorders, including binge eating, insomnia, and some **anxiety disorders**.

Precautions

CBT may not be suitable for some patients. Those who do not have a specific behavioral issue they wish to address and whose goals for therapy are to gain insight into the past may be better served by psychodynamic therapy. Patients must also be willing to take an active role in the treatment process.

Cognitive-behavioral **intervention** may be inappropriate for some severely psychotic patients and for cognitively impaired patients (for example, patients with organic **brain** disease or a **traumatic brain injury**), depending on their level of functioning. Some research has refuted the use of CBT in **schizophrenia** and **bipolar disorder**, although there has also been research that suggests that CBT can be useful in improving the negative and **positive symptoms** of schizophrenia, decreasing hospitalizations, and improving **compliance** with the medical regimens of both schizophrenia and bipolar disorder.

Description

CBT combines the individual goals of cognitive therapy and behavioral therapy.

Pioneered by psychologists Aaron Beck and Albert Ellis in the 1960s, cognitive therapy assumes that maladaptive behaviors and disturbed mood or emotions are the result of inappropriate or irrational thinking patterns, called automatic thoughts. Instead of reacting to the reality of a situation, individuals react to their own distorted viewpoint of the situation. For example, a person may conclude that he is "worthless" simply because he failed an exam or did not get a date. Cognitive therapists attempt to make their patients aware of these distorted thinking patterns, or cognitive distortions, and change them (a process termed cognitive restructuring).

Behavioral therapy, or **behavior modification**, trains individuals to replace undesirable behaviors with healthier behavioral patterns. Unlike psychodynamic therapies, it does not focus on uncovering or understanding the unconscious motivations that may be behind the maladaptive behavior. In other words, strictly behavioral therapists do not try to find out why their patients behave the way they do, they just teach them to change the behavior.

CBT integrates the cognitive restructuring approach of cognitive therapy with the behavioral modification techniques of behavioral therapy. The therapist works with the patient to identify both the thoughts and the behaviors that are causing distress and to change those thoughts in order to readjust the behavior. In some cases, the patient may have certain fundamental core beliefs, called schemas, which are flawed and require modification. For example, a patient with **depression** may be avoiding social contact with others and experiencing considerable emotional distress because of his or her isolation. When questioned why, the patient may reveal that he or she is afraid of rejection or of what others may do or say. Upon further exploration, the patient and therapist may discover that the patient's real fear is not rejection, but the belief that he or she is uninteresting and unlovable. The therapist might test the reality of that assertion by having the patient name friends and family who love him or her and enjoy the patient's company. By showing the patient that others value him or her, the therapist both exposes the irrationality of the patient's beliefs and provides him or her with a new model of thought to change old behavior patterns. In this case, the person learns to think, "I am an interesting and lovable person; therefore, I should not have difficulty making new friends in social situations." If enough "irrational cognitions" are changed, the patient may experience considerable relief from his depression.

A number of different techniques may be employed in CBT to help patients uncover and examine their thoughts and change their behaviors. They include:

- Behavioral homework assignments. Cognitive-behavioral therapists frequently request that their patients complete homework assignments between therapy sessions. These may consist of real-life "behavioral experiments" where patients are encouraged to try out new responses to situations discussed in therapy sessions.
- Cognitive rehearsal. The patient imagines a difficult situation and the therapist guides him through the step-by-step process of facing and successfully dealing with it. The patient then works on practicing, or rehearsing, these steps mentally. Ideally, when the situation arises in real life, the patient will draw on the rehearsed behavior to address it.
- Journal. Patients are asked to keep a detailed diary recounting their thoughts, feelings, and actions when specific situations arise. The journal helps to make patients aware of their maladaptive thoughts and to show their consequences on behavior. In later stages of therapy, it may serve to demonstrate and reinforce positive behaviors.
- Modeling. The therapist and patient engage in role-playing exercises in which the therapist acts out appropriate behaviors or responses to situations.
- Conditioning. The therapist uses reinforcement to encourage a particular behavior. For example, a child with ADHD gets a gold star every time he stays focused on tasks and accomplishes certain daily chores. The gold star reinforces and increases the desired behavior by identifying it with something positive. Reinforcement can also be used to extinguish unwanted behaviors by imposing negative consequences.
- Systematic desensitization. Patients imagine a situation they fear, while the therapist employs techniques to help them relax, helping them cope with their fear reaction and eventually eliminate the anxiety altogether. For example, patients in treatment for agoraphobia, or fear of open or public places, will relax and then picture themselves on the sidewalk outside of their house. In their next session, they may relax and then imagine a visit to a crowded shopping mall. The imagery of the anxiety-producing situations gets progressively more intense until, eventually, the therapist and patient approach the anxiety-causing situation in real-life (a "graded exposure"), perhaps by visiting a mall. Exposure may be increased to the point of "flooding," providing maximum exposure to the real situation. By repeatedly pairing a desired response (relaxation) with a fear-producing situation (open, public spaces), patients gradually become desensitized to the old response of fear and learns to react with feelings of relaxation.
- Validity testing. Patients are asked to test the validity of the automatic thoughts and schemas they encounter. The therapist may ask patients to defend or produce evidence that a schema is true. If the patients are unable to meet the challenge, the faulty nature of the schema is exposed.

- Aversive conditioning. This technique employs the principles of classical conditioning to lessen the appeal of a behavior that is difficult to change because it is either habitual or temporarily rewarding. Patients are exposed to an unpleasant stimulus while engaged in or thinking about the behavior in question. Eventually the behavior itself becomes associated with unpleasant rather than pleasant feelings. One treatment method used with alcoholics is the administration of a nausea-inducing drug together with an alcoholic beverage to produce an aversion to the taste and smell of alcohol by having it become associated with nausea. Studies investigating use of these aversive conditioning approaches have not identified a high level of therapeutic effectiveness. According to the American Psychiatric Association, aversion therapy should be practiced only in specialized centers. In counterconditioning, a maladaptive response is weakened by the strengthening of a response that is incompatible with it. A well-known type of counterconditioning is systematic desensitization, which counteracts the anxiety connected with a particular behavior or situation by inducing a relaxed response to it instead. This method is often used in the treatment of people who are afraid of flying.

Initial treatment sessions are typically spent explaining the basic tenets of CBT to patients and establishing a positive working relationship between therapist and patient. CBT is a collaborative, action-oriented therapy effort. As such, it empowers patients by giving them an active role in the therapy process and discourages any overdependence on the therapist that may occur in other therapeutic relationships. Therapy is typically administered in an outpatient setting in either an individual or group session. Therapists include psychologists, clinical **social workers**, counselors, or psychiatrists. Treatment is relatively short in comparison to some other forms of psychotherapy, usually lasting no longer than 16 weeks. Many insurance plans provide reimbursement for cognitive-behavioral therapy services. Because coverage is dependent on the disorder or illness the therapy is treating, patients should check with their individual plans.

Rational-emotive behavior therapy

Rational-emotive behavior therapy (REBT) is a popular variation of cognitive-behavioral therapy developed in 1955 by **psychologist** Albert Ellis. REBT is based on the belief that individuals' past experiences shape their belief system and thinking patterns. People form illogical, irrational thinking patterns that become the cause of both their negative emotions and of further irrational ideas. REBT focuses on helping patients discover these irrational beliefs that guide their behavior and replace them with rational beliefs and thoughts in order to relieve their emotional distress.

There are ten basic irrational assumptions that trigger maladaptive emotions and behaviors:

- It is a necessity for an adult to be loved and approved of by almost everyone for virtually everything.
- A person must be thoroughly competent, adequate, and successful in all respects.
- Certain people are bad, wicked, or villainous and should be punished for their sins.
- It is catastrophic when things are not going the way one would like.
- Human unhappiness is externally caused. People have little or no ability to control their sorrows or to rid themselves of negative feelings.
- It is right to be terribly preoccupied with and upset about something that may be dangerous or fearsome.

KEY TERMS

Automatic thoughts—Thoughts that automatically come to mind when a particular situation occurs. Cognitive-behavioral therapy seeks to challenge automatic thoughts.

Cognitive restructuring—The process of replacing maladaptive thought patterns with constructive thoughts and beliefs.

Maladaptive—Unsuitable or counterproductive; for example, maladaptive behavior is inappropriate to a given situation.

Psychodynamic therapy—A therapeutic approach that assumes dysfunctional or unwanted behavior is caused by unconscious, internal conflicts and focuses on gaining insight into these motivations.

Relaxation technique—A technique used to relieve stress. Exercise, biofeedback, hypnosis, and meditation are all effective relaxation tools. Relaxation techniques are used in cognitive-behavioral therapy to teach patients new ways of coping with stressful situations.

Schemas—Fundamental core beliefs or assumptions that are part of the perceptual filter people use to view the world. Cognitive-behavioral therapy seeks to change maladaptive schemas.

- It is easier to avoid facing many of life's difficulties and responsibilities than it is to undertake more rewarding forms of self-discipline.
- The past is all-important. Because something once strongly affected someone's life, it should continue to do so indefinitely.
- People and things should be different from the way they are. It is catastrophic if perfect solutions to the grim realities of life are not immediately found.
- Maximal human happiness can be achieved by inertia and inaction or by living passively and without commitment.

Meichenbaum's self-instructional approach

Psychologist Donald Meichenbaum pioneered the self-instructional, or "self-talk," approach to CBT in the 1970s. This approach focuses on changing what people say to themselves, both internally and out loud. It is based on the belief that an individual's actions follow directly from this self-talk. This type of therapy emphasizes teaching patients coping skills that they can use in a variety of situations to help themselves. The technique used to accomplish this is self-instructional inner dialogue, a method of talking through a problem or situation as it occurs.

Preparation

Patients may seek therapy independently or be referred for treatment by a primary physician, psychologist, or **psychiatrist**. Because the patient and therapist work closely together to achieve specific therapeutic objectives, it is important that their working relationship is comfortable and their goals are compatible. Prior to beginning treatment, the patient and therapist should meet for a consultation session, or mutual interview. The consultation gives the therapist the opportunity to make an initial assessment of the patient and recommend a course of treatment and goals for therapy. It also gives the patient an opportunity to find out important details about the therapist's approach to treatment, professional credentials, and any other issues of interest.

In some managed-care clinical settings, an intake interview or evaluation is required before a patient begins therapy. The intake interview is used to evaluate the patient and assign the person to a therapist. It may be conducted by a psychiatric nurse, counselor, or social worker.

Results

Many patients who undergo CBT successfully learn how to replace their maladaptive thoughts and behaviors with positive ones that facilitate individual growth and happiness. CBT may be used in conjunction with pharmaceutical and other treatment interventions, so overall success rates are difficult to gauge. However, success rates of 65% or more have been reported with CBT alone as a treatment for panic attacks and agoraphobia. Although many of the conditions that are responsive to CBT may **relapse**, follow-up sessions can be effective, even on an as-needed basis, and often require fewer sessions than the initial round of treatment.

QUESTIONS TO ASK YOUR DOCTOR

- What kind of therapy is right for me?
- Does insurance usually cover this kind of treatment?
- How often should I attend therapy?
- How long will my treatment last before I see results?

Resources

BOOKS

Beck, Judith S. *Cognitive Behavior Therapy: Basics and Beyond*. 2nd ed. New York: Guilford Press, 2011.

Craske, Michelle G. *Cognitive-Behavioral Therapy*. Washington, DC: American Psychological Association, 2010.

PERIODICALS

Freedman S. "Cognitive Behavior Therapy for Panic Disorder." *Israeli Journal Psychiatry and Related Sciences* 46 (2009): 251–56.

Manicavasgar V. "Mindfulness-based Cognitive Therapy vs. Cognitive Behaviour Therapy as a Treatment for Non-melancholic Depression." *Journal of Affective Disorders* 130 (2011): 138–44.

McManus F. "A Demonstration of the Efficacy of Two of the Components of Cognitive Therapy for Social Phobia." *Journal of Anxiety Disorders* 23 (2009): 496–503.

WEBSITES

"Psychotherapies." National Institutes of Health. August 16, 2010. http://www.nimh.nih.gov/health/topics/psychotherapies/index.shtml (accessed October 11, 2011).

ORGANIZATIONS

Albert Ellis Institute, 45 East 65th St., New York, NY, 10021, (212) 535-0822, (800) 323-4738, Fax: (212) 249-3582, info@albertellis.org, http://www.rebt.org.

Association for Behavioral and Cognitive Therapies, 305 7th Ave., 16th Fl., New York, NY, 10001, (212) 647-1890, Fax: (212) 647-1865, (866) 615-6464, http://www.abct.org.

Beck Institute for Cognitive Behavior Therapy, 1 Belmont Ave., Ste. 700, Bala Cynwyd, PA, 19004, (610) 664-3020, Fax: (610) 709-5336, info@beckinstitute.org, http://www.beckinstitute.org.

Paula Anne Ford-Martin
Brenda W. Lerner

Cognitive problem-solving skills training

Definition

Cognitive problem-solving skills training (CPSST) is a behavioral treatment that attempts to decrease or eliminate inappropriate or disruptive behaviors in children. The training emphasizes teaching children coping mechanisms so that they can react to situations in calm and rational ways. Using both cognitive and behavioral techniques and focusing on the child more than on the parents or the family unit, CPSST helps the child gain the ability to self-manage thoughts and feelings and interact appropriately with others by developing new perspectives and solutions. The basis of the treatment is the underlying principle that children lacking constructive ways to address the environment have problematic behaviors; teaching children positive problem solving and challenging dysfunctional thoughts improves functioning.

Purpose

The goal of CPSST is to reduce or terminate inappropriate, dysfunctional behaviors in children by expanding their "behavioral repertoire," including ways of cognitive processing. The behavioral repertoire is the range of ways of behaving that an individual possesses. With certain disorders, such as **conduct disorder**, **intermittent explosive disorder**, **oppositional defiant disorder**, antisocial behaviors, aggressive acting out, or **attention deficit hyperactivity disorder** with disruptive behavior, the number of ways of interpreting reality and responding to the world are limited and involve primarily negative responses. Although CPSST originally focused on children with problem behaviors or poor relationships with others, it has generalized its focus to a variety of different disorders in children and adults (though most of the treatment research is focused on children).

Description

The therapist conducts individual CPSST sessions with the child, usually once a week for 45 minutes to an hour, typically for several months to a year. The cognitive portion of the treatment involves changing false views of daily situations, confronting irrational interpretations of others' actions, challenging the unhelpful assumptions that typically underlie the individual's problem behaviors, and generating alternative solutions to problems. For example, if meeting with a child who has received a school suspension for becoming physically enraged at a teacher, the therapist will start by exploring the situation with the child, asking what thoughts and feelings were experienced. The child might state, "My teacher hates me. I'm always getting sent to the principal and she yells at me all the time." The therapist will try to help the child explore the supporting evidence for the "my teacher hates me" notion based on things seen or heard in the classroom. The ultimate goal is to help the child shift his or her perceptions so that, instead of seeing the student-teacher negative interactions as something external to the self, the child comes to see his or her part in the problem. This discussion also helps the child to see that he or she can help influence the outcome of the student/teacher interactions. When the child makes a global, stable, and negative attribution about why the interactions with the teacher are negative—where the attitude of the teacher is the cause of the problems—the child loses the sense of having any efficacy and is liable to show poorer behavior. By changing the child's perceptions and examining different options for the child's responses, the child recognizes that changing his or her own behavior can produce positive outcomes.

The behavioral aspect of CPSST involves **modeling** positive behaviors, role-playing challenging situations, and rewarding improvement in behavior, as well as providing corrective feedback on alternative and more appropriate ways of handling situations. In each session, the child is coached on problem-solving techniques, including brainstorming a number of possible solutions to difficulties, evaluating solutions, and planning the steps involved in gaining a desired goal (also called "means-end thinking"). For instance, when discussing a conflict, the therapist might help the child come up with some techniques for handling future situations, such as visualizing a calming scene, using a mediator to work out the issue, or avoiding problematic behaviors. The options generated would be discussed and evaluated as to how practical they are and how to implement them.

After a session, the child is given therapy homework, which might include implementing these newer ways of thinking and behaving in specific types of problematic situations, such as in school, with peers, or at home. The child might be asked to keep track of negative, externalizing thoughts by maintaining a written record of them for several days. The therapist may ask the child to try one of the new options and compare the results against past experiences. Typically, the between-sessions work begins with the conditions that appear the easiest in which to implement new behaviors, gradually progressing to more complex or challenging circumstances.

Although the bulk of the sessions involve the individual child and the therapist, the parents are brought into the therapy for a portion of the work. The parents observe the therapist and the child as they practice the new skills and are educated on how to assist the child outside of the sessions. Parents learn how to correctly remind the child to use the CPSST techniques for problem solving in daily living and assist the child with the steps involved in applying these skills. Parents are also coached on how to promote the positive behaviors by rewarding their occurrence with praise, extra attention, points toward obtaining a reward desired by the child, stickers or other small indicators of positive behavior, additional privileges, or hugs and other affectionate gestures. The scientific term for the rewarding of desired behavior is "positive reinforcement," referring to consequences that cause the desired target behavior to increase.

In research studies of outcomes, CPSST has been found to be effective in changing children's behavior. Changes in behavior have been shown to persist long term (one year) after completion of treatment. Success in altering undesirable behaviors is enhanced when CPSST is combined with **parent management training**. Parent management training is the in-depth education of parents or other primary caretakers in applying behavioral techniques such as positive **reinforcement** in their parenting.

Preparation

Parents and older children can prepare for cognitive problem-solving skills training by researching the topic before attending sessions. In addition, parents can practice positive behavior as a supplement to CPSST. Such behaviors will often help children learn how to deal with situations in more appropriate ways.

KEY TERMS

Attention deficit hyperactivity disorder (ADHD)—A persistent pattern of inattention, hyperactivity and/or impulsiveness, typically found in children.

Conduct disorder—A behavioral and emotional disorder of childhood and adolescence, characterized by socially inappropriate behaviors.

Dysfunctional—Degraded ability or inability to function emotionally.

Intermittent explosive disorder—A disorder characterized by uncontrolled anger and rage, especially when the situation is not seen as appropriate for such behaviors by normally acting persons.

Modeling—A behavioral therapy technique in which a patient first observes and then imitates a desired behavior.

Oppositional defiant disorder—A consistent public pattern of actions that display defiance and hostility toward authorities.

Precautions

The CPSST is considered to be a good way to minimize or eliminate inappropriate or disruptive behaviors in children when administered by a trained professional. Parents should seek therapists with solid credentials and experience. CPSST may not work the first time and may need to be repeated, along with additional counseling. If parent management training was not included initially, it may likely be included in repeat sessions of CPSST.

Results

While individual results vary, problematic behaviors are reduced or eliminated in many children.

See also Behavior modification; Token economy system

Resources

BOOKS

Beauchaine, Theodore P., and Stephen P. Hinshaw, eds. *Child and Adolescent Psychopathology*. Hoboken, NJ: John Wiley and Sons, 2008.

D'Zurilla, Thomas J., and Arthur M. Nezu. *Problem-Solving Therapy: A Positive Approach to Clinical Intervention*. New York: Springer, 2007.

Macdonald, Alasdair J. *Solution-Focused Therapy: Theory, Research and Practice*. Los Angeles: SAGE, 2007.

Murphy, John J. *Solution-Focused Counseling in Schools.* Alexandria, VA: American Counseling Association, 2008.

Nelson, Thorana S., and Frank N. Thomas, eds. *Handbook of Solution-Focused Brief Therapy: Clinical Applications.* New York: Haworth Press, 2007.

Weisz, John R., and Alan E. Kazdin, eds. *Evidence-Based Psychotherapies for Children and Adolescents.* New York: The Guilford Press, 2010.

PERIODICALS

Thomas, Christopher R. "Evidence-Based Practice for Conduct Disorder Symptoms." *Journal of the American Academy of Child and Adolescent Psychiatry* 45 (2006): 109–14.

ORGANIZATIONS

Association for Behavioral and Cognitive Therapies, 305 7th Avenue, 16th Floor, New York, NY, 10001, (212) 647-1890, Fax: (212) 647-1865, http://www.abct.org.

Deborah RoschEifert, PhD
Emily Jane Willingham, PhD

Cognitive remediation

Definition

Cognitive remediation is a teaching process that targets areas of neuropsychological functioning involved in learning and basic day-to-day functioning. This terminology can be confusing because some researchers use the phrase "cognitive remediation" to refer to environmental adjustments meant to ease cognitive requirements.

Cognitive remediation as a behavioral treatment is an approach designed to address cognitive deficits through neural rehabilitation. This approach relies on the idea, demonstrated in many recent studies of humans and primates, that the **brain** can circumvent damage or loss through repetition of the same activity. Through repetition, neurocognitive abilities, such as working memory, attention, problem solving, and cognitive flexibility and functioning, can be improved. Cognitive remediation usually uses computers to provide exercises to improve patients' neuropsychological skills.

Cognitive remediation (CR) is also different from the similarly sounding cognitive remediation therapy (CRT). Cognitive remediation focuses on improving the underlying neuropsychological functions that provide for memory, attention, abstract thinking, and other such concepts. In cognitive remediation therapy, the focus is on applying more effective patterns of thinking to behaviors or emotional problems.

Purpose

The primary purpose of cognitive remediation is to minimize cognitive deficits. The main goals of cognitive remediation are to bolster specific cognitive capacities that are weak. It is distinguished from a compensatory approach that seeks to get around a cognitive deficit by use of compensating strategies, such as using a notebook as a memory support in memory loss. Cognitive remediation has been applied in those who have had a **traumatic brain injury** (a **stroke**, tumor, or head injury); in those who have learning disabilities; and in people who have **schizophrenia**, **depression**, and **bipolar disorder**. For example, people with schizophrenia and other psychotic disorders often have trouble maintaining an attentive state, along with memory and problem-solving problems. Cognitive remediation can help to solve such problems. It has also been successful in treating people with **anorexia nervosa**, an eating disorder. Cognitive remediation can also be used for the treatment of alcohol and **substance abuse** disorders.

For people with brain injury, remediation typically targets the following neuropsychological functions: attention and concentration, memory, planning, monitoring one's work or behavior, and making adjustments based on feedback. For instance, individuals with a brain injury may repeat a series of letters, showing that with practice they are able to repeat longer lists. Remediation is also used to help children and adults cope with learning disabilities. Learning disabilities can interfere with progress in reading; in understanding and communicating through spoken language; in writing; in arithmetic; in understanding such nonverbal information as telling time or understanding visual information; and in comprehending social interactions and cues. Difficulties with concentration, problem solving, organization, identifying errors, and using feedback effectively are also areas that can be treated with cognitive remediation. People with schizophrenia sometimes exhibit cognitive impairment, and cognitive remediation therapy has shown promise in addressing these losses.

Description

People with cognitive problems (or deficits) have difficulties with such routine activities as remembering the appointments for the day or where they have placed their wallet or purse. They may also have problems organizing their personal life and professional lives, along with their living space. Because of such disorganization, they often misplace belongings.

Cognitive deficits occur in many forms and situations. Individuals who have had a traumatic brain injury may work with a remediator using computer programs that target one area at a time, such as attention. The individual is then helped to generalize what is learned from the program to real life. This **intervention** is usually done at a hospital, although it is not limited to clinical settings. Remediation for this group of people is considered helpful but not curative. It is typically practiced by a neuropsychologist.

Remediation for individuals with learning disabilities aims to bolster a particular area of learning or adaptation, such as in academics or socialization. Although the intervention varies according to the disability and the individual's profile of strengths and weaknesses, the remediator will make use of the person's stronger capacities to bolster the weaker ones. For example, individuals might need help with written language because they frequently omit words from their sentences. Once it has been determined that their oral language (both receptive and expressive) is adequate and that the motor aspect of writing is intact, the remediator has an idea of the individuals' strengths and weaknesses in the area of writing. In this case, the remediator makes use of their stronger auditory (hearing-related) skills to build up the capacity to translate spoken language into written (visual) language. Specifically, the remediator might read aloud a sentence written by the person (with omissions) and ask the person to identify the mistakes the person hears. The omission is identified by hearing it and then the individual is shown on paper the place where the word is missing. In this way, individuals with these deficits can learn to identify errors visually that they can already identify through the auditory modality of listening. This particular exercise fosters visual awareness of errors, which is a symptom or outcome of the deeper problem of translating language from oral to visual form.

This process can also be achieved with computer-assisted tasks. These methods focus on gradually increasing the difficulty level and complexity of the cognitive functions being applied.

The process continues with diminishing degrees of assistance. Specifically, after individuals become more skillful in matching visual omissions with the auditory ones read by the remediator, they begin to read the sentences aloud and identify the words that are missing from the sentences on the page. In the next step, they begin to read their work silently with the same kind of scrutiny as in the previous exercise. In this manner, remediation fosters both learning and internalizing a cognitive capacity.

Cognitive remediation sessions for learning disabilities usually take place twice a week. This type of intervention is practiced by psychologists, neuropsychologists, special educators, and learning specialists.

KEY TERMS

Anorexia nervosa—An eating disorder characterized by denial of a healthy body weight, a distorted image of appearance, and steadfast refusal to eat much food for a fear of gaining weight.

Bipolar disorder—A mood disorder characterized by abnormally high energy levels and moodiness, usually without depression.

Depression—A psychiatric disorder involving feelings of hopelessness and symptoms of fatigue, sleeplessness, suicidal tendencies, and poor concentration.

Schizophrenia—A serious mental disorder involving degraded thinking and emotions, often associated with hallucinations or sensory awareness of stimuli that are not present, as in hearing voices that are not there.

Stimulant abuse disorders—Also called stimulant use disorders, any disorder that involves the abuse of stimulants that affect the central nervous system.

The depth and breadth of the intervention varies according to the remediator's professional training and particular area of expertise. Some professionals specialize in working with certain types of learning disabilities; some, like psychologists, may incorporate their understanding of emotional difficulties within their work as a cognitive remediator.

Cognitive remediation can also take a strategy-oriented approach, in which the patient practices tasks that require strategizing (to plan or decide on a plan of action).

Cognitive deficits can be pinpointed by various assessment tests administered by psychological professionals. One such assessment is the Brief Assessment of Cognition in Schizophrenia (BACS). Another one is the MATRICS Consensus Cognitive Battery (MCCB). Both can identify an individual's cognitive problems and also can pinpoint what areas (conditions) need to be improved.

Schizophrenia

A study ("A Meta-Analysis of Cognitive Remediation in Schizophrenia") published in the *American Journal of Psychiatry* in December 2007, evaluated whether cognitive remediation was beneficial for improving the symptoms, cognitive abilities, and psychosocial functioning of 1,151 patients with schizophrenia. The meta-analytical study of 26 randomized, controlled trials concluded that cognitive remediation did produce "significant improvement" for all three factors. In addition, when adjunctive psychiatric rehabilitation with used with cognitive remediation with respect to psychosocial functioning, the researchers saw that the effects were much stronger than when cognitive remediation was used alone.

They concluded that, "Cognitive remediation produces moderate improvements in cognitive performance and, when combined with psychiatric rehabilitation, also improves functional outcomes."

Anorexia nervosa

Studies done by British **psychologist** Kate Tchanturia and others have focused on the use of cognitive remediation therapy in treating anorexia nervosa. In studies, patients generally received ten 45-minute sessions, with assessments before and after therapy. Tchanturia reported that preliminary results suggested that cognitive remediation may be especially successful in patients who have not had results with other forms of therapies, largely because CRT focuses on cognitive tasks and not food or related emotions. The patients found the tasks enjoyable and thus were more likely to participate, and they had a sense of achievement in applying their new thinking strategies to their behaviors, such as eating patterns.

Benefits

When remediation is targeting the problem area accurately and individuals are actively engaging in the process, then progress should be evident in the skill area targeted, in the participants' awareness of their area of difficulty, and in their awareness of some techniques and strategies that are helpful.

Cognitive remediation programs can help to improve impaired cognitive skills that interfere with daily activities. Cognitive deficits may not be eliminated, but they can be controlled and minimized with effective strategies. These are best accomplished with the help of trained professionals.

Precautions

Cognitive remediation is not suitable as a substitute for medical treatments or for the various types of **psychotherapy**. Instead, it is to be used as a complement treatment for mental disorders such as **attention deficit hyperactivity disorder** (ADHD) in children, brain injuries, early-stage **dementia** in older people, schizophrenia, and depression.

QUESTIONS TO ASK YOUR DOCTOR

- How effective is cognitive remediation in cases like mine?
- Are there any underlying medical or psychological concerns that need to be corrected before we proceed with CR?
- Should I take any assessment tests?
- Will I need CR for a short or long time? What will happen if I stop CR?

When cognitive remediation is used, the medical professional administering it must make sure the patient is clinically stable. During the process, the patient must be actively involved in the treatment process. A clinically unstable person may not be able to concentrate for twenty minutes or more, which is essential for successfully conducting cognitive remediation.

Preparation

Before remediation can begin, individuals being treated must receive a neuropsychological or in-depth psychological evaluation in order to identify the underlying neuropsychological capacities (i.e., language, memory, attention, visual perception, visual spatial abilities, motor abilities) that are interfering with their acquiring the needed skills. The evaluation is also intended to rule out emotional difficulties as the primary cause of learning problems. Children with learning disabilities frequently experience feelings of inadequacy and low self-esteem that need to be addressed. If psychological difficulties, however, are the main reason for their academic struggles, individuals should be treated with psychotherapy rather than cognitive remediation.

Aftercare

A plan of aftercare is sometimes necessary in order to return individuals to a community living style. Aftercare is normally monitored by a healthcare professional so that progress can be observed and modifications to the aftercare plan can be easily implemented, if needed. Aftercare may continue until skills are satisfactorily improved and maintained in real life situations.

Risks

Cognitive remediation may not succeed in all cases. The amount of success depends in part on the severity of the problem, along with the **diagnosis**, the specific illness, and various socio-environmental concerns. Medical studies have confirmed that improvements delivered by cognitive remediation may be temporary.

Resources

BOOKS

Evers, Rebecca B. *Planning Effective Instruction for Students with Learning and Behavior Problems.* Upper Saddle River, NJ: Pearson, 2011.

Tchanturia, Kate, and James Lock. "Cognitive Remediation Therapy for Eating Disorders: Development, Refinement and Future Directions." In *Current Topics in Behavioral Neurosciences.* Vol. 6 of *Behavioral Neurobiology of Eating Disorders.* New York: Springer, 2011.

Wilson, Mike, ed. *Disabilities Affecting Learning.* Farmington Hills, MI: Greenhaven Press, 2010.

PERIODICALS

Hylton, Hilary. "A Drug to End Drug Addiction." *Time Magazine* (January 9, 2008). http://www.time.com/time/health/article/0,8599,1701864,00.html (accessed September 16, 2011).

Keefe, R.S., et al. "The Relationship of the Brief Assessment of Cognition in Schizophrenia (BACS) to Functional Capacity and Real-world Functional Outcome." *Journal of Clinical and Experimental Neuropsychology* 2 (February 28, 2006): 260–69. http://www.ncbi.nlm.nih.gov/pubmed/16484097 (accessed September 16, 2011).

Lindenmayer, Jean-Pierre. "A Randomized Controlled Trial of Cognitive Remediation Among Inpatients With Persistent Mental Illness." *Psychiatric Services* 59 (March 2008): 241–47. http://dx.doi.org/10.1176/appi.ps.59.3.241 (accessed September 9, 2011).

McGurk, Susan R., et al. "A Meta-Analysis of Cognitive Remediation in Schizophrenia." *American Journal of Psychiatry* 164, no. 12 (December 2009): 1791–1802. http://dx.doi.org/10.1176/appi.ajp.2007.07060906 (accessed September 9, 2011).

Medalia, Alice. "Cognitive Remediation for Psychiatric Patients." *Psychiatric Times, UBM Medica* (March 9, 2009). http://www.psychiatrictimes.com/display/article/10168/1386195 (accessed September 16, 2011).

Tchanturia, Kate, Helen Davies, and Iain C. Campbell. "Cognitive Remediation Therapy for Patients with Anorexia Nervosa: Preliminary Findings." *Annals of General Psychiatry* 6, no. 14 (2007). http://dx.doi.org/10.1186/1744-859X-6-14 (accessed September 9, 2011).

WEBSITES

"Learning Disabilities Online." LDonline.com. http://www.ldonline.org (accessed September 16, 2011).

Medalia, Alice. "Question: What Is Cognitive Remediation and for Whom Is It Helpful?" Columbia Psychiatry. http://asp.cumc.columbia.edu/psych/asktheexperts/ask_the_experts_inquiry.asp?SI=300 (accessed September 16, 2011).

Vocci, Frank. *Cognitive Remediation in the Treatment of Stimulant Abuse Disorders: A Research Agenda.* APA PsycNET Direct. (December 2008). http://psycnet.apa.org/?fa=main.doiLanding&doi=10.1037/a0014101 (accessed September 16, 2011).

ORGANIZATIONS

American Psychiatric Association, 1000 Wilson Blvd., Ste. 1825, Arlington, VA, 22209-3901, (703) 907-7300, apa@psych.org, http://www.psych.org.

American Psychological Association, 750 1st St., NE, Washington, DC, 20002-4242, (202) 336-5500; TDD/TTY: (202) 336-6123, (800) 374-2721, http://www.apa.org.

Susan Fine, PsyD
Emily Jane Willingham, PhD
William Atkins, BB, BS, MBA

Cognitive retraining

Definition

Cognitive retraining is a therapeutic strategy that seeks to improve or restore a person's cognitive skills. These skills include paying attention, remembering, organizing, reasoning and understanding, problem solving, decision making, and higher level cognitive (thinking) abilities. These skills are all interrelated. Cognitive retraining is one aspect of cognitive rehabilitation, a comprehensive approach to restoring such skills after a **traumatic brain injury** or other disability.

Purpose

The purpose of cognitive retraining is the reduction of cognitive problems associated with **brain** injury, other disabilities or disorders, and aging. Cognitive retraining aims to decrease the everyday problems faced by individuals with cognitive difficulties, thereby improving the quality of their lives.

Description

The techniques of cognitive retraining are best known for their use with persons who have suffered a brain injury. However, cognitive retraining has also been used in patients with **dementia** (including **Alzheimer's disease**), **schizophrenia**, **attention deficit hyperactivity disorder (ADHD)**, **learning disorders**, **obsessive-compulsive disorder** (OCD), and cognitive changes associated with aging. Professionals from a variety of fields, such as psychology, psychiatry, occupational therapy, and **speech-language pathology**, may be involved in cognitive retraining.

There are generally two parts in the process of cognitive retraining: restoring the cognitive skill that was lost or degraded, and learning to use alternative strategies to compensate for the degraded skill. In the first part, repetitive exercises are used to strengthen skills that have been degraded or lost, such as concentration, memory, judgment, or problem solving. In the second part, strategies are taught to the patient in order to cope (or compensate) with weakened cognitive skills. In some cases, the degraded skills are restored to their normal level.

Cognitive retraining includes a considerable amount of repetitive practice that targets the skills of interest. In fact, repetition is essential for the newly retrained skills to become automatic. Regular feedback is another important element of cognitive retraining, as is the use of rewards. Retraining usually begins with simpler skills and proceeds to more complicated ones. The therapist may address cognitive skills while the person is practicing real-life tasks, in an effort to improve their performance of these tasks. In fact, practicing skills in the ways and settings they will be used in real life is critical to the success of retraining efforts. The length of time for cognitive training varies according to the type and extent of the injury and the type of retraining skills used. For example, retraining memory may take months or years. In contrast, it may take only a few days or weeks to retrain someone to organize his or her home or workplace.

The use of computerization for cognitive retraining has become an increasingly common practice. In particular, researchers have focused on developing a "mixed-reality" system, producing a virtual reality environment for the person undergoing rehabilitation. This system, called in one study a "Human Experience Modeler," places the patient in a context similar to reality—such as home or work—except that the stimuli can be controlled and the patient's experiences captured with automated feedback provided. These approaches have shown some promising success in pilot studies.

Types of cognitive retraining

Types of cognitive retraining include:

- Attention and concentration retraining. This type of cognitive retraining aims to improve several abilities, including focusing attention, dividing attention, maintaining attention while reducing the effects of boredom and fatigue, and resisting distraction. Attention has been considered the foundation of other more complicated cognitive skills and is an important skill for cognitive retraining. This area of cognitive retraining has been widely researched and has been shown to improve patients' abilities in various tasks related to attention.
- Memory retraining. Memory retraining involves teaching the patient several strategies that can be used to recall certain types of information. For example, rhymes may be used as a memory aid. A series of numbers, such as a phone number with an area code, may be broken down into smaller groups. A person may be taught to go through each letter of the alphabet until he or she remembers someone's name. Both memory and organization problems are common and often disabling after head injury.
- Organizational skills retraining. This approach is used when the person has difficulty keeping track of or finding items, doing tasks in a set order, and/or doing something in a timely manner. Strategies may include having one identified place for an item. In addition, the person can be taught to keep the items that are used most frequently closer to him or her (the front or the lower shelves of a cabinet, drawer, closet, or desk, for example). Items that are often used together (such as comb and brush, toothbrush and toothpaste) are placed beside each other. Items may be put into categories (allocating decorations to a specific holiday, such as the Fourth of July or Thanksgiving). These strategies help individuals function better in their home or work environment.
- Reasoning. Reasoning refers to the ability to connect and organize information in a logical, rational way. Reasoning retraining techniques include listing the facts or reality of a situation; excluding irrelevant facts or details; putting the steps to solve a problem in a logical order; and avoiding irrational thinking, such as jumping to conclusions based on incomplete information, or focusing on the negative aspects of the situation and ignoring the positive. When the person can connect relevant information in a logical way, they are better able to understand or comprehend it.

KEY TERMS

Attention deficit hyperactivity disorder (ADHD)—A condition found mostly in children with primary symptoms of an inability to concentrate, inappropriate behaviors, and impulsiveness.

Cognitive—Related to the acquisition of knowledge (learning).

Depression—A psychiatric disorder involving feelings of hopelessness and symptoms of fatigue, sleeplessness, suicidal tendencies, and poor concentration.

Obsessive-compulsive disorder (OCD)—A disorder that involves excess anxiety; emotions of fear, worry, and apprehension; and repetitious behaviors and obsessions.

Schizophrenia—A mental disorder involving degraded thinking and emotions.

- Problem solving. Problem-solving retraining aims to help people define a problem, come up with possible solutions to it, discuss the solution(s) with others and listen to their advice, review the various possible solutions from many perspectives, and evaluate whether the problem was solved after going through these steps. This sequence may be repeated several times until the problem is solved. This process is referred to as "SOLVE," from the first letter of the name of each step: Specify, Options, Listen, Vary, and Evaluate. The "SOLVE" technique is more appropriate for use with individuals at a higher level of functioning.
- Decision making. Decision-making retraining is used when a person must choose from a number of options. The goal of this retraining is to help him or her consider the decision thoroughly before taking any action. The considerations may range from such practical matters as money, people, and rules and policies to personality issues.
- Executive skills. Executive skills retraining refers to teaching individuals how to monitor themselves, control their thinking and actions, think in advance, set goals, manage time, act in socially acceptable ways, and transfer skills to new situations. These are higher-level cognitive skills. Charts and videotapes may be used to monitor behavior, and a variety of questions, tasks, and games may be used in retraining these skills.

Preparation

Cognitive retraining usually takes place in a quiet room without distractions. It is important for the person to feel relaxed and calm while they are being retrained in cognitive skills. Engaging in cognitive retraining is not recommended when someone is emotional distressed—e.g., after the recent loss of a loved one. The therapist usually evaluates the patient's level of cognitive skills and the extent of their cognitive problems before retraining begins. This evaluation provides a way to monitor improvement by comparing the patient's skill levels during and after retraining to his or her skill levels before retraining. Cognitive retraining requires patience and persistence on the part of everyone involved.

Aftercare

The therapist will try to promote the transfer of skills learned using cognitive retraining techniques to the settings of the patient's everyday life. Training may be continued until the patient's skills are improved, transferred to, and maintained in real world activities.

QUESTIONS TO ASK YOUR DOCTOR

- Will cognitive retraining help me (or my loved one) to recover fully?
- If I don't recover completely, how can I cope with my condition?
- How long will it take to go through cognitive retraining?
- Can you advise me on the best type of cognitive retraining in my particular case?
- Will my health insurance pay for cognitive retraining?

Precautions

The extent to which a person with a brain injury can recover from or compensate for cognitive problems varies with the person and their injury. Therapy must be tailored to each individual's needs and abilities. Some cognitive retraining techniques require higher levels of skill and, therefore, they would be more suitable for persons who have made some progress in their recovery. In addition, a person's moods and emotions have an effect on their cognitive skills. Someone who is depressed, for example, may need **psychotherapy** and/or medication before he or she can engage in and benefit from cognitive retraining. Some persons with brain injuries may find it difficult to transfer a skill learned in one setting, such as a clinic, to another setting, such as their home. Although a specific individual may show some improvement on training tasks, his or her cognitive skills may not be considered improved or restored unless there is some evidence that the skills have been transferred to everyday settings and can be maintained over time. It is important for the therapist, patient, and the patient's friends or family members not to assume that improvement on training exercises and tests automatically leads to transfer of the skills to real-life settings.

Results

Cognitive retraining may be considered successful if performance on a behavior related to a particular cognitive skill has improved. It is ultimately successful if it helps the injured person improve his or her functioning and meet his or her needs in real-life situations and settings.

Positive results are more likely obtained when caregivers are trained and educated as part of the patient's therapy. The strategies used for cognitive retraining should be familiar to caregivers, and they should encourage such strategies for the overall improvement of the patient. Improvement may take time, and it helps when the patient has an understanding support system in place.

Resources

BOOKS

Parenté, Rick, and Douglas Herrmann. *Retraining Cognition: Techniques and Applications*. Austin, TX: PRO-ED, 2010.

Schutz, Larry E. *Head Injury Recovery in Real Life*. San Diego, CA: Plural, 2010.

Silver, Jonathan M., Thomas W. McAllister, and Stuart C. Yudofsky, eds. *Textbook of Traumatic Brain Injury*. Washington, DC: American Psychiatric Association, 2011.

PERIODICALS

Buhlmann, Ulrike, et al. "Cognitive Retraining for Organizational Impairment in Obsessive-Compulsive Disorder." *Psychiatry Research* 144 (2006): 109–16.

Fidopiastis, C. M., et al. "Human Experience Modeler: Context-Driven Cognitive Retraining to Facilitate Transfer of Learning." *CyberPsychology and Behavior* 9 (2006): 183–87.

WEBSITES

American Brain Tumor Association. "Cognitive Retraining." http://www.abta.org/Becoming_Well_Again_Through../Cognitive_Retraining/199 (accessed November 21, 2011).

Joneis Thomas, PhD
Emily Jane Willingham, PhD

Cognitive self-regulation *see* **Self-control strategies**

Cognitive therapy *see* **Cognitive-behavioral therapy**

Communication disorders *see* **Expressive language disorder; Mixed receptive-expressive language disorder; Phonological disorder; Social communication disorder; Stuttering**

Community mental health

Definition

Community mental health is an approach to providing access to professional mental health care in local communities. It includes services offered through public mental health programs, public health departments, community mental health centers, private programs, medical clinics, hospitals, religious organizations, colleges and other educational institutions, and neighborhood centers. Community mental health assessment has evolved into a field of research called "psychiatric epidemiology," which determines the prevalence of various mental disorders in specific communities, with the goal of developing appropriate community mental health programs and evaluating their effectiveness.

Purpose

The primary purpose of community mental health is to decrease the need for inpatient and hospital-based mental health services as well as to supplement those services, and to help patients become successfully reintegrated into society. Community mental health services are generally dispersed among a variety of local facilities and programs, rather than isolating patients from their communities by segregating them in centralized hospitals. The goal of community mental health programs is to be more responsive to local needs and more accessible to more people. They also help alleviate "psychiatric boarding," in which patients with mental illnesses are confined in overcrowded hospital emergency departments. Community mental health centers (CMHCs) provide valuable services to people who may otherwise not have access to mental health care, especially low-income youth and families in urban and rural areas throughout the United States.

Community mental health can address a wide range of problems. Many programs, including residential, day, and outpatient treatment, are involved in transitioning patients from institutions or from parents' homes to independent or semi-independent living situations. Some programs provide diagnostic and treatment services for a wide variety of mental disorders. Others refer clients to psychologists or psychiatrists. Community mental health may provide emergency care for suicidal patients, for patients with acute **panic disorder**, or for victims and witnesses of natural disasters and other violent or traumatic events. Some community mental health programs provide **substance abuse** treatment. However, the high demand for community mental health services and the lack of adequate funding have meant that patients might not have timely access to the community-based care that they require.

Demographics

There is a tremendous need for community mental health services throughout the United States. This need skyrockets in times of **economic stress** and recession. In most states, the primary clients of community mental health services are Medicaid recipients. However, it has been estimated that as many as two-thirds of American children and teens—more than six million children—do not receive the mental health services that they need. A survey of juvenile detention facilities found that two-thirds were holding children who were awaiting community mental health services. Some of these children were as young as seven. Over a six-month period, almost 15,000 young people were being held in detention until community mental health services became available, at a very high cost to American taxpayers. These detention facilities are generally not equipped to provide care for mentally ill youth, some of whom may pose a danger to themselves or others.

Community mental health, particularly when it is integrated into other community-based organizations, can be particularly relevant for racial and ethnic minorities in the United States. African Americans are much more likely to turn to family or to their religious or social communities for emotional support than to seek professional help. African Americans also generally have less access to mental health care, even though they are disproportionately more likely to experience circumstances that increase the risk of developing a mental illness. These circumstances include **homelessness**, exposure to violence, and children in foster care or otherwise in the child welfare system.

Asian Americans and Pacific Islanders have higher rates of depressive symptoms than white Americans but have the lowest rates of utilization of mental health services. Southeast Asians, especially refugees, have particularly high rates of **depression** and **post-traumatic stress disorder** (PTSD). Their need for outpatient mental health services is twice that of the general Asian American population.

Latinos are also at higher risk for depression, anxiety, and substance abuse. American-born Latinos and long-term residents have significantly higher rates of psychiatric disorders, especially substance abuse, compared with recent immigrants. Like African Americans, Latinos are far less likely than others to seek mental health services, especially from specialized mental health facilities. In part, this appears to be related to the severe shortage of Latino and Spanish speaking mental health care providers.

Description

The services included in community mental health programs depend on the state and local area. The focus of community mental health is on preventing psychiatric **hospitalization** and in assisting in the transition out of inpatient care. Some states offer only very limited community mental health services. Others offer a wide range of services for children, adults, and families. These may include mental health screening and assessment, psychological testing, psychiatric evaluations, individual **psychotherapy**, group psychotherapy, psychiatric medications, family and **couples therapy**, family psychological and educational counseling, peer support programs, **respite** care, **case management**, jail diversion, integrated treatment for co-existing disorders, and crisis interventions. Some community mental health programs provide supportive housing, supported employment, and even longer-term and inpatient care. A 24-hour crisis hotline or emergency psychiatric services are important components of community mental health. These may be provided in conjunction with a local hospital.

Community mental health services may be available for severely emotionally disturbed youth or for those who have been traumatized by **sexual abuse** or violence and require specialized interventions. Juveniles suspected of mental illness may be referred to community mental health programs by the courts. Community mental health also may include multidisciplinary assessments of parents with mental illness who are suspected of, or have been accused of, child maltreatment. Some programs include victims' services for child and adult crime victims and their families.

Some community mental health programs include intensive case management services for ending chronic homelessness and substance abuse. These services may include job and life-skills training, employment referrals, housing options, meals, substance abuse treatment, and other rehabilitation services. Special services may also be available for older adults, including adult day respite, home-meal delivery, housekeeping, and emergency home response, as well as screenings for nursing home placement or veterans' services, and assistance in transitions from nursing homes to independent- or assisted-living arrangements.

Programs may include the training of community mental health professionals. In addition to these specialists, community mental health may involve psychiatrists, including child and geriatric psychiatrists, clinical psychologists, clinical **social workers**, nurse practitioners, psychiatric nurses, counselors, clergy, recreational and occupational therapists, and **assertive community treatment** (ACT) teams. ACT is a community-based treatment approach for assisting in the recovery and rehabilitation of patients with severe and persistent mental illnesses.

Although some community mental health programs are based in stand-alone CMHCs, programs located within community groups or churches can reach populations that might not otherwise seek mental health services. They also can increase awareness of mental health issues and resources and reduce stigmas associated with mental disorders. Some community mental health programs are school-based, linking mental health providers with teachers and family advocates for treating children with disruptive behavior disorders. Community mental health can also be associated with:

- outpatient psychiatric clinics
- community rehabilitation programs
- community support programs
- adult daycare centers
- day treatment centers
- home health agencies
- club programs
- foster care programs
- sheltered workshops
- group and private homes

Eligibility for community mental health services varies by state and local area. In general, people in crises and children and adults with severe mental illnesses are given first priority. During times of budgetary restraint, the first to be cut from community mental health services are often those who are not enrolled in Medicaid, so as to preserve federal Medicaid matching funds. Approximately 2% of public mental health funding comes from Medicare, which, in addition to senior citizens, serves younger people with disabilities. Unlike Medicaid, Medicare does not cover many community-based services and requires co-payments for outpatient mental health treatment. In addition to Medicaid and Medicare, community mental health services may accept private insurance or offer a sliding fee scale based on ability to pay. The State Children's Health Insurance Program (SCHIP) may or may not provide the same range of mental health services as Medicaid, depending on the state. Some county and municipal local governments administer and partially fund community mental health for their residents.

Origins

During the 1960s, in response to the increased availability of psychiatric medications and an outcry over involuntary commitments, public psychiatric hospitals began reducing their populations or closing completely. Mentally ill patients were released into the community to live independently. The Community Mental Health Centers Act of 1963 aimed to create a comprehensive community mental health system to serve this population, providing prevention, early treatment, and continuity of care within larger communities and promoting the social integration of people with mental health needs. However, the programs were never adequately funded, and many planned community mental health services never materialized.

KEY TERMS

Assertive community treatment (ACT)—A service-delivery model for providing comprehensive, highly individualized, locally based treatment directly to patients with serious, persistent mental illnesses.

Community Mental Health Clinic (CMHC)—A community-based provider of limited or comprehensive mental health services; usually at least partially publicly funded.

Epidemiology—A field of medical science dealing with the incidence, distribution, and control of disease in a population.

Medicaid—A joint state and federal program for providing medical care for low-income children and families.

Medicare—The U.S. government healthcare system for those aged 65 and over.

Post-traumatic stress disorder (PTSD)—A psychological response to a highly stressful event; typically characterized by depression, anxiety, flashbacks, nightmares, and avoidance of reminders of the traumatic experience.

Psychiatric boarding—The practice of holding mentally ill patients in emergency department corridors and waiting areas, because of the lack of hospital beds or other facilities.

Respite care—Temporary care of a patient to provide caregivers with a period of physical, mental, and emotional rest.

State Children's Health Insurance Program; SCHIP; CHIP—A state-administered health insurance program for lower- and middle-income children who are without private health insurance and whose family incomes are above the Medicaid eligibility limits.

Initially, CMHCs provided outpatient care to people with less severe, episodic, or acute mental health problems. Soon they were also caring for the deinstitutionalized chronically mentally ill. With the repeal of the Mental Health Systems Act and with federal funding for CMHCs replaced by block grants to the states in the early 1980s, the system deteriorated further. Subsequent programs to provide for community mental health were relatively short-lived and impacted only a few urban centers. As a result, vast numbers of persons with mental illness have become homeless or are incarcerated in prisons.

QUESTIONS TO ASK YOUR DOCTOR

- Would community mental health services be helpful for me?
- What type of community mental health services should I pursue?
- What community mental health services are available in my area?
- Am I eligible for community mental health?
- What type of community mental health provider will I be able to see?

As of the early twenty-first century, the U.S. **Substance Abuse and Mental Health Services Administration** was continuing to fund the Comprehensive Community Mental Health Services for Children and Their Families Program. This community mental health program provides youth (from birth through age 21) and their families with cultural- and language-appropriate evidence-based mental health services and support. The National Council for Community Behavioral Healthcare advocates for improved public policies in mental and behavioral health, and offers state-of-the-science education and practice improvement resources for the personnel of community mental health programs. It has also pioneered the implantation of Mental Health First Aid USA to educate the public about the signs and symptoms of mental disorders.

Common problems

In the early 2010s, states and the federal government were attempting to deal with economic problems and massive budget deficits in part by further slashing community mental health funding and restricting eligibility for services. At the same time, the demand for mental health services was rising dramatically. Increasingly, law enforcement agencies were forced to provide emergency services for the mentally ill—services that had previously been provided by community mental health programs. In addition, managed behavioral health care and the strict use of medical management techniques decreased access to community care, resulting in more patients in crisis and increased utilization of hospital emergency departments. Low reimbursement rates under Medicaid and Medicare further reduced community mental health services. Coverage for antipsychotic drugs was reduced or eliminated. Some experts warned that the entire mental health system in the United States was on the verge of collapse.

Resources

BOOKS

Altman, Neil. *The Analyst in the Inner City: Race, Class, and Culture Through a Psychoanalytic Lens,* 2nd ed. New York: Routledge, 2010.

Fernando, Suman, and Frank Keating. *Mental Health in a Multi-Ethnic Society: A Multidisciplinary Handbook,* 2nd ed. New York: Routledge, 2009.

Kay, Jerald, and Victor Schwartz. *Mental Health Care in the College Community.* Hoboken, NJ: Wiley-Blackwell, 2010.

Moritsugu, John, Frank Y. Wong, and Karen Grover Duffy. *Community Psychology,* 4th ed. Boston: Allyn & Bacon, 2010.

Nelson, Geoffrey B., and Isaac Prilleltensky. *Community Psychology: In Pursuit of Liberation and Well-Being,* 2nd ed. New York: Palgrave Macmillan, 2010.

Roberts, Albert R., and Kenneth Yeager. *Pocket Guide to Crisis Intervention.* New York: Oxford University Press, 2009.

Schinke, Steven Paul. *Behavioral Methods in Social Welfare: Helping Children, Adults, and Families in Community Settings.* New Brunswick: Aldine Transaction, 2009.

PERIODICALS

Alakeson, Vidhya, Nalini Pande, and Michael Ludwig. "A Plan to Reduce Emergency Room 'Boarding' of Psychiatric Patients." *Health Affairs* 29, no. 9 (September 2010): 1637–1642.

Bloom, Joseph D. "'The Incarceration Revolution': The Abandonment of the Seriously Mentally Ill to Our Jails and Prisons." *Journal of Law, Medicine & Ethics* 38, no. 4 (Winter 2010): 727–734.

Duncan, Tracey M., Maureen Davey, and Adam Davey. "Transporting Functional Family Therapy to Community-Based Programs." *Family Journal* 19, no. 1 (January 2011): 41–46.

Saylers, Michelle P., et al. "Integrating Assertive Community Treatment and Illness Management and Recovery for Consumers with Severe Mental Illness." *Community Mental Health Journal* 46, no. 4 (August 2010): 319–329.

Zezima, Katie. "State Cuts Put Officers on Front Lines of Mental Care." *New York Times* (December 5, 2010): A32.

OTHER

NAMI State Advocacy. "Public Mental Health Service Funding: An Overview." National Alliance on Mental Illness. January 2010. http://www.nami.org/Content/NavigationMenu/State_Advocacy/About_the_Issue/Funding.pdf (accessed January 11, 2011).

WEBSITES

"African American Community Mental Health Fact Sheet." National Alliance on Mental Illness. http://www.nami.org/Template.cfm?Section=Fact_Sheets1&Template=/

ContentManagement/ContentDisplay.cfm&ContentID=53812 (accessed January 11, 2011).

Kortrijk, H. E., et al. “Treatment Outcome in Patients Receiving Assertive Community Treatment.” *Community Mental Health Journal* 46, no. 4 (August 2010). http://www.springerlink.com/content/510q277x50364725/full text.html (accessed January 12, 2011).

National Alliance on Mental Illness. “Assertive Community Treatment (ACT).” About Treatments & Supports. http://www.nami.org/Template.cfm?Section=About_Treatments_and_Supports&template=/ContentManagement/ContentDisplay.cfm&ContentID=8075 (accessed January 12, 2011).

ORGANIZATIONS

American Psychiatric Association, 1000 Wilson Blvd., Ste. 1825, Arlington, VA, 22209-3901, (703) 907-7300, apa@psych.org, http://www.psych.org.

National Alliance on Mental Illness, 3803 N. Fairfax Dr., Ste. 100, Arlington, VA, 22203, (703) 524-7600, (800) 950-NAMI (6264), Fax: (703) 524-9094, http://www.nami.org.

National Council for Community Behavioral Healthcare, 1701 K St. NW, Ste. 400, Washington, DC, 20006, (202) 684-7457, Fax: (202) 386-9391, communications@thenationalcouncil.org, http://www.TheNationalCouncil.org.

National Institute of Mental Health, 6001 Executive Blvd., Room 8184, MSC 9663, Bethesda, MD, 20892-9663, (301) 443-4513, (866) 615-6464, Fax: (301)443-4279, nimhinfo@nih.gov, http://www.nimh.nih.gov.

Substance Abuse and Mental Health Services Administration, 1 Choke Cherry Rd., Rockville, MD, 20857, (877) SAMHSA-7 (726-4727), Fax: (240) 221-4292, SAMHSAInfo@samhsa.hhs.gov, http://www.samhsa.gov.

Michael Polgar, PhD
Emily Jane Willingham, PhD
Margaret Alic, PhD

Compliance

Definition

Compliance with appropriate, recommended, and prescribed mental health treatments simply means that a person is following a doctor’s orders. Compliance is more likely when there is agreement and confidence regarding the medical **diagnosis** and prognosis. Compliance is complicated by uncertainty about the nature of an illness and/or the effects of certain treatments, particularly medications. Some practitioners argue that the concept of “compliance” is paternalistic and does not include the patient enough in the decision-making process. Many recent studies have focused more on the concept of shared decision making with a strong relationship between the patient and practitioner. Either way, the nature of this relationship can be a strong determinant of how well a patient adheres to an agreed-upon course.

In everyday usage, the term compliance means deference and obedience, elevating the authority of medical expertise. Alternatively, adherence to medical advice refers to a somewhat more informed and equitable decision by a patient to stick with appropriate medical treatment. In any case, a mental health treatment cannot be effective or even evaluated if a patient does not follow a doctor’s orders. A mental health treatment that is effective for one disorder may not be beneficial for other disorders, and diagnoses may evolve over time, complicating the issue of compliance.

Description

From a health provider’s viewpoint, for medical treatments to have their desired effects, complying or conforming to treatments is absolutely necessary. The concept of medication management reflects this idea that the provider is responsible and in control, while the patient is a docile body who is incapacitated by disease or condition. From the perspective of health patients, adherence to medical treatment is enhanced when there is a good healthcare relationship and when patients openly share their health beliefs and experience of illness with their provider.

Problems with compliance

In mental health care, uncertainty about compliance is a challenging source of variation in the effectiveness of treatments. Noncompliance can represent a significant risk and cost to the medical system. For providers, partial compliance or discontinuation of medications represents the difficulty of maintaining treatment successes over time. Problems with compliance are often attributed to the patient, but may also reflect the appropriateness of a medication or treatment.

Compliance rates

Rates of compliance with mental health appointments are the greatest challenge (estimated in one hospital at 91%), while medication noncompliance is the second most challenging problem in the treatment of persons with mental illness. Mental health medication compliance can be determined by questioning patients, counting pills or prescriptions, and through drug monitoring with urine, blood, or other test measures. Overall, recent research estimates compliance to be 58%. Patients who report lower rates are often considered unreliable indicators of compliance, while physicians report higher rates. Compliance with antidepressant medications is higher, on average (65%). Mental health medication compliance rates are only somewhat lower than medication compliance in other types of health care, which have been estimated at 76%.

Explaining variation in compliance

Research in psychiatry, psychology, and sociology provides many explanations for variations in compliance. In psychiatry, clinical problems such as drug or alcohol abuse are sometimes used to explain noncompliance. Patients may also discontinue taking medications because of unwanted side effects. Health beliefs and patient-provider relationships are also recognized. In psychology and sociology, health beliefs and behaviors (in context of family, work, etc.) may enhance or limit compliance. If an individual's family member supports medication compliance, and the individual believes in the medicine's benefits, compliance may be enhanced (similar to a placebo effect). If an individual feels that a medicine makes him or her drowsy and affects work, compliance may be reduced. People who have limited access to or trust in doctors or medical science, and people whose faith precludes them from certain types of medical care, are less likely to comply with treatment recommendations.

To a large extent, patient compliance is a direct reflection of the quality of the doctor-patient relationship. When health-care provider and patient achieve a successful treatment alliance, as is advocated as part of the shared decision-making approach, and when the treatment is practical and beneficial for both the provider and the patient, cooperation reduces concerns about treatment for both parties. When patients are empowered and motivated to improve their health with the help of a doctor, compliance or adherence to treatment is higher. When there is distrust, disagreement, or misunderstanding involved, as when mental health status is uncertain or treatment side effects are unwelcome, compliance is lower. One British study found that patients with mental disorders were likely to prefer the form of treatment recommended by psychiatrists with whom they had good relationships, even if the treatment itself was painful. Some patients preferred **electroconvulsive therapy** (ECT) to tranquilizers for **depression** because they had built up trusting relationships with the doctors who used ECT, and perceived the doctors who recommended medications as bullying and condescending. Because noncompliant patients are less likely to continue in care, they are also less likely to find helpful providers or successful treatments. Thus, noncompliance with treatment may become a self-fulfilling cycle.

Compliance is higher when treatments, including medications, help patients feel better, when a family supports the treatment, and when taking medication prevents **relapse** of symptoms. However, people may be distressed by potential side effects of any medication, including those psychiatric medications that limit functioning. Limited functioning through drowsiness, also a problem of the older generation of antihistamines, is the best example. It is an effect of many medicines, particularly those for mental disorders. Other unwelcome side effects of various psychiatric medications include weight gain, involuntary movements such as muscle twitching, and impaired coordination. Patients may feel embarrassed about taking medication, especially medications for illnesses that have a strong social **stigma** associated with them; may have difficulty getting a prescription for medication; and may have financial problems paying for treatment or medication. In some cases, when a patient is noncompliant or perceived to be at odds with treatment recommendations, they may risk losing autonomy over medical decisions. When at risk to self or others, people who are medication noncompliant may be pressured or forced to take medication at the risk of being involuntarily hospitalized.

Multiple challenges in mental health care

Compliance rates reflect the proportion of individuals in treatment who have the highest possibility of successful treatment. Noncompliance rates reflect those individuals who have either discontinued or avoided treatment, and thus have lower probabilities of treatment success. Sometimes patients do not want to get rid of their symptoms (mania, for example), or patients may not consider their experiences (symptoms) to be indicative of a disorder. In addition, successful mental health care is hampered by the fact that many people with mental health problems either do not use or lack access to mental health care.

The **Substance Abuse** and Mental Health Services Administration's National Survey on Drug Use and Health found in 2008 that just over half (58.7%) of adults in the United States with a serious mental illness received treatment for a mental health problem. Therefore, compliance with treatment is part of a larger national challenge to provide quality mental health care and to use it well.

Resources

BOOKS

Horwitz, Allan. *Creating Mental Illness*. Chicago: University of Chicago Press, 2002.

Pescosolido, Bernice, and Carol Boyer. "How Do People Come to Use Mental Health Services?" In *A Handbook of the Sociology of Mental Health: Social Contexts, Theories, and Systems,* by Allan Horwitz. Cambridge: Cambridge University Press, 1999.

Pescosolido, Bernice, Carol Boyer, and Keri Lubell. "The Social Dynamics of Responding to Mental Health Problems." In *The Sociology of Mental Illness*. by Jane D. McLeod and Eric R. Wright. New York: Oxford University Press. 2009.

PERIODICALS

Adams, Jared R., and Robert E. Drake. "Shared Decision-Making and Evidence-Based Practice." *Community Mental Health Journal* 42, no. 1 (February 2006): 87–105.

Bebbington, P. E. "The Content and Context of Compliance." *International Clinical Psychopharmacology* 9, no. 5 (Suppl. 1995): 41–50.

Centorrino, Franca, et al. "Factors Associated with Noncompliance with Psychiatric Outpatient Visits." *Psychiatric Services* 52 (March 2001): 378–80.

Day, J.C., et al. "Attitudes Toward Antipsychotic Medication." *Archives of General Psychiatry* 62, no. 7 (July 2005) 717–24.

Helbling, Josef, et al. "Attitudes to Antipsychotic Drugs and their Side Effects: A Comparison Between General Practitioners and the General Population." *BioMed Central Psychiatry* 6 (2006): 42.

Wang, Philip, Olga Demler, and Ronald Kessler. "Adequacy of Treatment for Serious Mental Illness in the United States." *American Journal of Public Health* 92, no. 1 (2002): 92–98.

ORGANIZATIONS

American Psychiatric Association, 1000 Wilson Blvd., Ste. 1825, Arlington, VA, 22209-3901, (703) 907-7300, apa@psych.org, http://www.psych.org.

American Sociological Association, 1430 K Street, NW, Ste. 600, Washington, DC, 20005, http://www.asanet.org.

National Institute of Mental Health, 6001 Executive Blvd., Room 8184, MSC 9663, Bethesda, MD, 20892-9663, (301) 433-4513; TTY: (301) 443-8431, Fax: (301) 443-4279, (866) 615-6464; TTY: (866) 415-8051, nimhinfo@nih.gov, http://www.nimh.nih.gov.

Substance Abuse and Mental Health Services Administration Referral Resource, 1 Choke Cherry Rd., Rockville, MD, 20857, (877) SAMHSA-7 (726-4727), (800) TTY: 487-4889, Fax: (240) 221-4292, SAMHSAInfo@samhsa.hhs.gov, http://www.samhsa.gov.

Michael Polgar, PhD
Emily Jane Willingham, PhD

Compulsion

Definition

A compulsion is a behavior or mental act performed to help reduce anxiety or distress.

Description

Compulsions are not voluntary activities and are not performed for pleasure. Instead, a person with a compulsion feels the need to engage in a particular behavior to relieve the **stress** and discomfort which would become overwhelming if the activity were not performed in a specific, repeated manner. Examples of compulsive motor activities are washing hands until raw, repeatedly checking the security of a locked door, and arranging and rearranging items in a set order. Some examples of compulsory mental acts are counting or silently repeating specific words. If a person troubled by compulsions is unable to perform such activities, stress and discomfort increase. The performance of the acts relieves distress, but only temporarily.

Often, compulsions are not acts that could logically be expected to relieve or prevent the fears that inspire them. For example, a person might feel compelled to count numbers in a certain order to "undo" the perceived damage or threat that follows a thought or behavior, or might check to make sure a door is locked every few minutes. Compulsions, in some cases, are attempts to undo obsessions and are usually not successful.

Resources

BOOKS

VandenBos, Gary R. ed. *APA Dictionary of Psychology.* Washington, DC: American Psychological Association, 2006.

Dean A. Haycock, PhD
Ruth A. Wienclaw, PhD

Compulsive exercise

Definition

Compulsive exercise is a disorder marked by excessively long and frequent athletic workouts as a form of weight control or excellence in sports. It is frequently associated with such eating disorders as **anorexia nervosa** and **bulimia nervosa**. Compulsive exercise is also known as hypergymnasia and anorexia athletica, and some researchers refer to it as exercise abuse, exercise bulimia, or exercise addiction. It is not recognized as a disorder in the ***Diagnostic and Statistical Manual of Mental Disorders*** *(DSM)* but is included as a symptom of bulimia nervosa.

Demographics

Compulsive exercising is most common in adolescents and young adults in North America, and more common in young women than in young men. It is more common among competitive athletes at the high-school and college levels than other youth. Among adult males, it is estimated that about 10% of competitive runners and 10% of bodybuilders are exercise addicts. Exact statistics for any age group are difficult to obtain, however, because of disagreements among doctors as to whether compulsive exercising is always associated with other disorders or whether it should be identified as a primary disorder.

Description

Compulsive exercise or exercise **addiction** is characterized by a need to work out physically longer than is needed to maintain fitness or is recommended by a coach or trainer. Although there is no exact length of time specified as a criterion for exercise addiction, some experts consider two hours or longer to be a starting point for evaluating student athletes. In addition to excessive time spent working out, often to the detriment of relationships and school or work obligations, the person who is exercising compulsively feels depressed or anxious when he or she cannot exercise, and exercises in spite of injury, illness, extreme weather, or medical advice in order to relieve the negative feelings.

Compulsive exercise has been associated with eating disorders, particularly bulimia nervosa and anorexia nervosa in women, and with **body dysmorphic disorder** in men. It has also been associated with distortions of **body image** and **obsessive-compulsive disorder** (OCD). More recently, however, researchers have identified persons in whom the compulsive exercising is primary—that is, the **compulsion** exists by itself rather than being secondary to poor body image, disordered eating, or another mental disorder. There are documented cases of persons who exercise excessively for the sake of feeling a temporary euphoria that is sometimes called "runner's high." The "high" results from the release of endorphins, which are chemicals produced by the pituitary gland and hypothalamus that function as natural analgesics (pain relievers) and produce a general sense of well-being.

Risk factors

Risk factors for compulsive exercise include:

- pre-existing anorexia or bulimia nervosa
- pressure from parents or coaches to excel in a sport
- participation in a sport or dance program that requires or encourages weight control or classifies athletes by weight (e.g., classical ballet, gymnastics, figure skating, wrestling, horse racing, rowing, or running)
- female sex among adolescents or male sex among adults
- existing compulsive behavior problems (e.g., shopping, gambling, Internet addiction)
- general attitude of perfectionism or a need to be the best in all aspects of life
- a strong need to feel in control
- having parents who are obsessed with their own appearance or figure flaws
- having parents who frequently criticize the weight or body shape of other family members

Causes and symptoms

Causes

Compulsive exercising is thought to be a multifactorial disorder; that is, it is the end result of a number of different factors in most people who have the disorder rather than having a single cause. The causes that have been identified include:

- the influence of mass media images of "perfect" bodies and advanced athletic performances; the omnipresence of television, social media, Internet videos, and sports- or fitness-related magazines makes these images hard to avoid
- pressures within the child's family or school athletic program to do well in competitive athletic activities
- in some families, obsession with physical fitness coupled with fear of obesity
- history of anxiety or depression in the family
- personal history of low self-esteem

There was no indication as of 2011 that compulsive exercise is inherited or has genetic causes.

Symptoms

The symptoms of compulsive exercise include the following:

- The person does not enjoy the exercise but feels a sense of obligation instead; he or she feels driven to exercise in spite of illness, injury, or bad weather conditions (including extreme heat), or in spite of the impact of long periods of exercise on school, work, or relationships.
- The exercise has a compulsive or ritualistic quality—the person's workout becomes a way to deal with feelings of stress or anxiety. If the person misses a workout one day, he or she might perform two workouts the following day.
- The exercise functions as a purging behavior—as compensation or punishment for eating "too much."

- The person develops symptoms of withdrawal—insomnia, changes in appetite, moodiness, or difficulty concentrating on schoolwork or other work—if the exercise is reduced or stopped.
- The person has recently lost a significant amount of weight or is underweight for his or her height; in females, amenorrhea (cessation of normal menstrual periods) may occur.
- The person bases his or her self-esteem on the length and number of workouts completed and is frequently dissatisfied with his or her athletic accomplishments.
- The person exercises alone in order to hide the length of the workout or to avoid having their routine disturbed.

Compulsive exercise may also produce physical symptoms, particularly if the person is combining it with a weight-reduction diet or the use of laxatives and self-induced vomiting. One common physical disorder is overtraining, which develops when an athlete does not allow enough time for rest and recovery between hard training sessions. Under normal circumstances, improvements in strength, endurance, and overall fitness take place after the rest period. This process of improvement may take days to complete. If the athlete returns to hard training with inadequate rest, his or her performance will hit a plateau and eventually decline. This decline will occur much more rapidly if the athlete is also suffering from jet lag, an infectious illness, menstruation, or poor **nutrition**.

The symptoms of overtraining have been variously ascribed to microtrauma to muscle tissue, protein deficiency, breakdown of muscle tissue due to reduced calorie intake, stress on the nervous system, and elevated levels of cortisol (a hormone associated with stress) in the body for long periods of time. Some specific symptoms of overtraining include:

- persistent muscle soreness
- unusual and long-lasting fatigue
- an elevated resting heart rate
- increased incidence of injuries
- increased susceptibility to illness
- increased irritability and moodiness

Female dancers and athletes are at risk for a gender-specific disorder known as "female athlete triad." The triad is a group of three disorders often found together in female athletes, consisting of disordered eating leading to low energy availability, amenorrhea, and low bone density leading to osteoporosis. Girls and women with the triad are at increased risk of stress fractures and overuse injuries as well as **depression**, anxiety, and a weakened immune system.

KEY TERMS

Amenorrhea—Absence of menstrual periods in a woman of reproductive age. Excessive exercise can lead to amenorrhea in females.

Body dysmorphic disorder—A mental disorder marked by obsession with real (but minor) or imagined flaws in the shape or appearance of one's body. It is sometimes referred to as "imagined ugliness."

Body image—In medicine, the sum of a person's perceptions of, beliefs about, and emotional attitudes toward his or her body.

Cortisol—A steroid hormone produced by the adrenal gland that is released in response to stress. Cortisol suppresses the immune system and slows down bone formation.

Endorphins—Neurotransmitters produced by the pituitary gland that can relieve pain and produce a feeling of well-being.

Female athlete triad—A group of three disorders often found together in female athletes, consisting of disordered eating, amenorrhea, and osteoporosis.

Runner's high—A feeling of exhilaration that occurs when a period of strenuous exercise activates the release of endorphins. While typically associated with long-distance runners, the experience of such a high has been reported by dancers and athletes in other sports.

Diagnosis

There are no formal diagnostic criteria for compulsive exercise. **Diagnosis** depends on the person's level of awareness of the problem; observations by parents, coaches, teachers, or other family members; and the primary physician's knowledge of the warning signs of compulsive exercise. In many cases, the patient's history will provide clues, particularly amenorrhea in women or a history of sudden weight loss, frequent infections, and sports-related injuries in both sexes.

Examination

The doctor will check the patient's weight, heart rate, and blood pressure as part of a standard office examination. He or she may also check for soft-tissue or joint injuries if compulsive exercise is suspected. If the examination and patient history suggest compulsive exercising, the doctor may ask the patient directly about the frequency and length of workouts and average daily calorie intake.

Tests

The doctor may order imaging tests to check for stress fractures or blood and urine tests to rule out other causes of **fatigue** and weight loss.

Although there are no criteria for compulsive exercise in the *DSM*, there are a few questionnaires that have been devised since the 1990s to screen people for exercise addiction. One tool is the Exercise Addiction Inventory (EAI), short form (1996), which consists of six questions:

1. Exercise is the most important thing in my life.
2. There have been conflicts between me and my partner (or other family members) over my exercise.
3. I use exercise to change my moods.
4. Over time, I have increased the amount of exercise I do each day.
5. I feel moody and irritable if I miss an exercise session.
6. If I cut down on the amount of exercise and then start again, I always end up exercising as often as I did before.

The person is instructed to rate each item on a five-point scale, with 1 representing "Disagree Strongly," and 5 representing "Agree Strongly." A score of 24 or higher indicates that the person is at high risk for exercise addiction.

Another self-administered questionnaire is the Exercise Dependence Scale (EDS), a 21-item questionnaire designed in 2001 for persons 18 and older. It takes about five minutes to complete. The subject is instructed to rate each item on a six-point scale, with 1 indicating "Never," and 6 indicating "Always." The EDS was modeled on the criteria for substance dependency as set forth in *DSM-IV*. The lower the person's score, the greater the likelihood of exercise dependency.

Treatment

Treatment of compulsive exercise is usually carried out by a team that includes a physical therapist, nutritionist, the person's coach or trainer, and a psychotherapist, as well as the person's primary care doctor. Psychotherapy—particularly cognitive-behavioral therapy—has been found helpful in providing patients with a more balanced perspective on physical exercise. The nutritionist can help the person plan a balanced diet, while the physical therapist and trainer can assist the person in designing a workout schedule that will keep him or her fit without feeding the compulsion.

Patients who are diagnosed with an eating disorder as well as compulsive exercise may also be treated with **antidepressants**, most commonly the class of drugs known as **selective serotonin reuptake inhibitors (SSRIs)**.

QUESTIONS TO ASK YOUR DOCTOR

- How can I tell whether I am at risk for compulsive exercising?
- How much exercising is too much? When does it become a disorder?
- How can I tell whether my child is beginning to work out compulsively?
- Have you ever treated a patient for compulsive exercising? If so, was the treatment effective?
- What is your opinion of inventories and questionnaires for compulsive exercise?
- Do you think that compulsive exercise should be considered a distinctive disorder?

Prognosis

The prognosis for compulsive exercise depends on the person's age and whether the condition is primary or secondary. In most cases, recovery from compulsive exercise is a process that takes several months to several years. In general, compulsive exercise that is a primary disorder has a better prognosis than compulsive exercise associated with an eating disorder.

Prevention

Parents are the first line of preventing compulsive exercise in children. Specific suggestions include:

- Setting a good example of self-acceptance; don't obsess over appearance and perceived flaws.
- Avoid criticizing the weight or body shape of other family members. Even teasing remarks can hurt a teenager who may be struggling with other issues.
- Don't pressure children to excel in sports; accept that different children have different levels of athletic ability, and reassure them that it is perfectly acceptable to participate in a sport without being a star.
- Choose forms of exercise that the whole family can enjoy together (e.g., hiking, swimming, cycling, beach

volleyball), to reduce the temptation for one member to exercise alone.

- When appropriate, remind children that the images of "perfect" bodies on television or the Internet are often altered by various photographic techniques and are unrealistic ideals for most people.

Resources

BOOKS

Currie-McGhee, Leanne. *Exercise Addiction*. Detroit, MI: Lucent Books, 2011.

Morgan, John F. *The Invisible Man: A Self-Help Guide for Men with Eating Disorders, Compulsive Exercise and Bigorexia*. New York: Routledge, 2008.

Szabo, Attila. *Addiction to Exercise: A Symptom or a Disorder?* New York: Nova Science, 2010.

PERIODICALS

Bewell-Weiss, C.V., and J.C. Carter. "Predictors of Excessive Exercise in Anorexia Nervosa." *Comprehensive Psychiatry* 51 (November–December 2010): 566–571.

Boecker, H., et al. "The Runner's High: Opioidergic Mechanisms in the Human Brain." *Cerebral Cortex* 18 (November 2008): 2523–2531.

Dalle Grave, R. "Features and Management of Compulsive Exercising in Eating Disorders." *The Physician and Sports Medicine* 37 (October 2009): 20–28.

Goodwin, H., et al. "Psychometric Evaluation of the Compulsive Exercise Test (CET) in an Adolescent Population: Links with Eating Psychopathology." *European Eating Disorders Review* 19 (May–June 2011): 269–279.

Homan, K. "Athletic-ideal and Thin-Ideal Internalization as Prospective Predictors of Body Dissatisfaction, Dieting, and Compulsive Exercise." *Body Image* 7 (June 2010): 240–245.

Meyer, C., et al. "Compulsive Exercise and Eating Disorders." *European Eating Disorders Review* 19 (May–June 2011): 174–189.

Smith, A.M., and A.A. Link. "Sport Psychology and the Adolescent Athlete." *Pediatric Annals* 39 (May 2010): 310–316.

Villella, C., et al. "Behavioural Addictions in Adolescents and Young Adults: Results from a Prevalence Study." *Journal of Gambling Studies* 27 (June 2011): 203–214.

White, J., and E. Hallowell. "Examination of a Sociocultural Model of Excessive Exercise among Male and Female Adolescents." *Body Image* 7 (June 2010): 227–233.

WEBSITES

American Running Association (ARA). "Know the Signs of Unhealthy Exercise Addiction." Active.com. http://www.active.com/running/Articles/Know_the_signs_of_unhealthy_exercise_addiction.htm (accessed July 24, 2011).

Female Athlete Triad Coalition. http://www.femaleathletetriad.org (accessed July 23, 2011).

Nemours. "Compulsive Exercise." KidsHealth.org. http://kidshealth.org/parent/emotions/behavior/compulsive_exercise.html (accessed July 22, 2011).

ORGANIZATIONS

American College of Sports Medicine (ACSM), PO Box 1440, Indianapolis, IN, 46206-1440, (317) 637-9200, Fax: (317) 634-7817, http://www.acsm.org/AM/Template.cfm?Section=Home.

American Council on Exercise (ACE), 4851 Paramount Dr., San Diego, CA, 92123, (858) 576-6500, Fax: (858) 576-6564, (888) 825-3636, http://www.acefitness.org/default.aspx.

American Psychiatric Association, 1000 Wilson Blvd., Ste. 1825, Arlington, VA, 22209-3901, (703) 907-7300, apa@psych.org, http://www.psych.org.

American Running Association (ARA), 4405 East-West Hwy., Ste. 405, Bethesda, MD, 20814, Fax: (301) 913-9520, (800) 776-2732 x 13, http://www.americanrunning.org/m/contact/, http://www.americanrun ning.org.

National Eating Disorders Association (NEDA), 165 W 46th St., New York, NY, 10036, (212) 575-6200, Fax: (212) 575-1650, (800) 931-2237, info@NationalEatingDisorders.org, http://www.nationaleatingdisorders.org.

National Institute of Mental Health (NIMH), 6001 Executive Blvd., Rm. 8184, MSC 9663, Bethesda, MD, 20892-9663, (301) 443-4513, Fax: (301) 443-4279, (866) 615-6464, nimhinfo@nih.gov, http://www.nimh.nih.gov/index.shtml.

Rebecca J. Frey, PhD

Compulsive gambling *see* **Gambling disorder**

Computed tomography

Definition

Computed tomography (CT) scanning, also called x-ray computed tomography scanning and computerized axial tomography (CAT) scanning, is a diagnostic tool that provides views (images) of internal body structures using x rays. In 1980, about three million CT scans were performed in the United States. That number increased to over 70 million in 2007. In the field of mental health, a CT scan may be used when a patient seeks help for symptoms that could possibly be attributed to a medical (physiologic, as opposed to psychologic) cause.

Purpose

CT scans are used to image bone, soft tissues, fluids, and air. Since the 1990s, CT equipment has become more affordable and available. CT scans have become the imaging examination of choice for the diagnoses of most

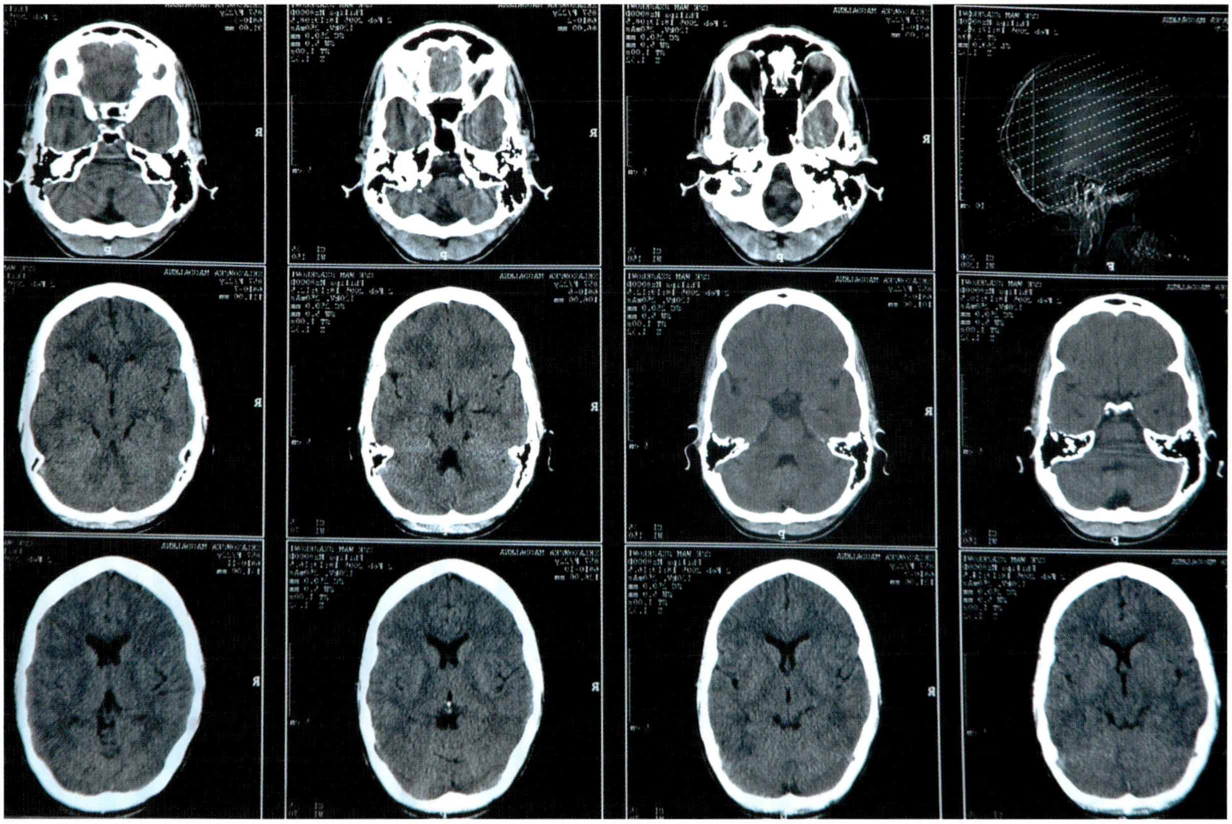

Computed tomography (CT) scan of a human brain. *(© Konrad Zelazowski/Alamy)*

solid tumors. Because the computerized image is sharp, focused, and three-dimensional, many structures can be better differentiated (visualized) when compared with standard x rays. About one-half of all diagnostic CT scans performed on adults are on the body (including the chest, abdomen, spine, and extremities), with another one-third on the head. Approximately three out of four scans are performed in the hospital, with one out of four within a single-specialty practice environment.

Common indications for CT scans include:

- Sinus. The CT scan can show details of sinusitis, bone fractures, and the presence of bony tumor involvement. Physicians may order a CT scan of the sinuses to provide an accurate map for surgery.
- Brain. Brain CT scans can detect hematomas (blood clotted mass), tumors, strokes, aneurysms (a blood vessel that ruptures), and degenerative or infected brain tissue. The introduction of CT scanning, especially spiral CT, has helped reduce the need for more invasive procedures such as cerebral angiography (inserting a wire through an artery to where it will reach brain vessels for visualization in real time).
- Body. CT scans of the chest, abdomen, spine, and extremities can detect the presence of tumors, enlarged lymph nodes, abnormal collection of fluid, and vertebral disc disease. These scans can also be helpful in evaluating the extent of bone breakdown in osteoporosis.
- Heart and aorta. CT scans can focus on the thoracic (chest) or abdominal aorta to locate aneurysms and other possible aortic diseases.
- Chest. CT scans of the chest are useful in distinguishing tumors and in detailing accumulation of fluid in chest infections.

It is important to note that CT scans alone are not used to diagnose mental disorders. Their primary function in this role is ensuring that psychological symptoms cannot be attributed to physical causes (such as a **brain** tumor) or as a supplement to a psychiatric exam. Mental health diagnoses are largely symptom based, despite physical changes in the brain.

Description

Computed tomography is the combination of focused x-ray beams and the computerized production of an image. CT applies the more general process of tomography, which is any type of imaging procedure that uses any type of electromagnetic radiation to generate sections of an object. Thus, by generating a series of two-dimensional x-ray images taken around a single-axis of rotation, a three-dimensional image of an object, such as a portion of the human body, is produced. Introduced in the early 1970s, CT has advanced rapidly and is now widely used, sometimes in the place of standard x rays.

CT procedure

A CT scan may be performed in a hospital or outpatient imaging center. Although the equipment looks large and intimidating, it is very sophisticated and fairly comfortable. The patient is asked to lie on a gantry, or narrow table, that slides into the center of the scanner. The scanner looks like a doughnut and is round in the middle, which allows the x-ray beam to rotate around the patient. The scanner section may also be tilted slightly to allow for certain cross-sectional angles.

The gantry moves very slightly as the precise adjustments for each sectional image are made. A technologist watches the procedure from a window and views the images on a computer screen. Generally, patients are alone during the procedure, though exceptions are sometimes made for pediatric patients. Communication is possible via an intercom system.

It is essential that the patient lie very still during the procedure to prevent motion blurring. In some studies, such as chest CTs, the patient will be asked to hold his or her breath during image capture.

Following the procedure, films of the images are usually printed for the radiologist and referring physician to review. A radiologist can also interpret CT examinations on the computer screen. The procedure time will vary in length depending on the area being imaged. Average study times are from 30 to 60 minutes. Some patients may be concerned about claustrophobia (a feeling of being "closed in"), but the width of the "doughnut" portion of the scanner is wide enough to ease many patients' fears. Doctors may consider giving **sedatives** to patients who have severe claustrophobia or difficulty lying still (such as small children).

The CT image

While traditional x-ray machines image organs in two dimensions, often resulting in organs in the front of the body being superimposed over those in the back, CT scans allow for a more three-dimensional effect. CT images can be likened to slices in a loaf of bread. Precise sections of the body can be located and imaged as cross-sectional views. The screen before the technologist shows a computer's analysis of each section detected by the x-ray beam, so various densities of tissue can be easily distinguished.

Contrast agents

Contrast agents are often used in CT exams and in other radiology procedures to illuminate certain details of anatomy more clearly. Some contrasts are natural, such as air or water. A water-based contrast agent is sometimes administered for specific diagnostic purposes. Barium sulfate is commonly used in gastroenterology procedures. The patient may drink this contrast or receive it in an enema. Oral or rectal contrast is usually given when examining the abdomen or cells, but not when scanning the brain or chest. Iodine is the most widely used intravenous contrast agent and is given through an intravenous needle.

If contrast agents are used in the CT exam, these will be administered several minutes before the study begins. Patients undergoing abdominal CT may be asked to drink a contrast medium. Some patients may experience a salty taste, flushing of the face, warmth or slight nausea, or hives from an intravenous contrast injection. Technologists and radiologists have the equipment and training to help patients through these minor reactions and to handle more severe reactions. Severe reactions to contrast are rare but do occur.

Types of CT scans

SPIRAL CT SCANS. The spiral CT scan is advantageous over traditional CT because it allows for the continuous re-creation of images. While traditional CT allows the technologist to take slices at very small and precise intervals one after the other, spiral CT stays in motion and allows for a continuous flow of images, without stopping the scanner to move to the next image slice. A major advantage of spiral CT is the ability to reconstruct images anywhere along the length of the study area. Because the procedure is faster, patients are required to lie still for shorter periods of time. The ability to image contrast more rapidly after it is injected, when it is at its highest level, is another advantage of spiral CT's high speed.

ELECTRON BEAM TOMOGRAPHY. Electron beam CT scans are another type of CT technology that can be used to detect calcium buildup in arteries. These calcium deposits are potential risk factors for coronary artery disease. Electron beam CT scans take pictures more quickly than conventional CTs, and are therefore better able to produce clear images of the heart as it pumps blood.

Some facilities have spiral, electron, and conventional CT available. Although spiral is more advantageous for many applications, conventional CT is still a precise method for imaging many tissues and structures. The physician will evaluate which type of CT works best for the specific exam purpose.

SINGLE PHOTON EMISSION CT SCANS. Single photon emission computerized tomography (SPECT) scans are used in research and may assist in diagnosing brain disorders such as **Alzheimer's disease** and Parkinson's disease. SPECT scans use gamma-ray emitting radioisotopes (radioactive isotopes) as the method for producing images of active regions of the brain. The process begins by injecting the brain with a radioactive tracer. Because the tracer remains concentrated—it does not spread out in the brain—it lasts up to one minute. This advantage means that such a scan can be performed quickly. It is especially useful for scanning the brains of epileptic patients, because the scan can be produced after an epileptic seizure has passed.

New technologies

A new generation of CT scanning equipment was developed in the late 2000s and is expected to dramatically increase the quality and safety of CT scans. One example, the Siemens CT machine or "Somatom Definition Flash" dual-source computed tomography scanner, is able to scan a patient more than twice as fast as conventional equipment. A single scan can be completed within 43 cm/s with a temporal resolution of 75 ms. A complete scan can be performed in about 250 ms. This new technology does not require the patient to hold their breath during the scan and is especially useful in **trauma** cases when quick analysis is needed.

The first system to be installed in a medical center within the United Sates occurred at the Mayo Clinic in Rochester, Minnesota, in 2009. In addition, the dose of radiation impinging on a patient's heart is much lower than current systems. Traditional systems output from 8 to 40 mSv (units of radiation), while the new Siemens instrument produces only 1 mSv.

Precautions

Pregnant women or those who could possibly be pregnant should not have a CT scan, particularly a full body or abdominal scan, unless the diagnostic benefits outweigh the risks. If the exam is necessary for obstetric purposes, technologists are instructed not to repeat films if there are errors. Pregnant patients receiving a CT scan or any x-ray exam away from the abdominal area may be protected by a lead apron; most radiation, known as scatter, travels through the body, however, and is not totally blocked by the apron.

KEY TERMS

Electromagnetic radiation—Radiation including gamma rays, x rays, ultraviolet light, visible light, infrared radiation, microwaves, and radio waves.

Tomography—A scanning technique that uses electromagnetic radiation (such as gamma rays or x rays) or ultrasound to produce a three-dimensional image of the structure.

Tumor—An abnormal growth of body cells, which may be malignant (harmful) or benign (harmless).

X ray—A type of electromagnetic radiation, between gamma rays and ultraviolet, with a wavelength of between 0.01 and 10 nm.

Contrast agents are often used in CT exams, though some types of tumors are better seen without it. Patients should discuss the use of contrast agents with their doctor, and should be asked to sign a consent form prior to the administration of contrast. One of the common contrast agents, iodine, can cause allergic reactions. Patients who are known to be allergic to iodine or shellfish should inform the physician prior to the CT scan; a combination of medications can be given to such patients before the scan to prevent or minimize the reaction. Contrast agents may also put patients with diabetes at risk of kidney failure, particularly those taking the medication metformin (Fortamet, Glucophage, Glumetza, Riomet), an oral antidiabetic drug.

Radiation exposure from a CT scan is similar to, though higher than, that of a conventional x ray. Although there is risk to pregnant women, the risk to other adults is minimal and it should produce no effects. Severe contrast reactions are rare, but they are still a risk of CT procedures.

Though some hospitals offer full-body CT scans as a preventative measure in screening disease, it is not recommended in healthy individuals. The U.S. Food and Drug Administration (FDA) advises individuals to consider both the risks and benefits of full-body screening and to discuss the procedure thoroughly with their physician.

Preparation

If a contrast medium is administered, the patient may be asked to fast for about four to six hours prior to the procedure. Patients will usually be given a gown (like a typical hospital gown) to be worn during the procedure.

QUESTIONS TO ASK YOUR DOCTOR

- Will I need to have someone with me during the imaging scan? Will this person need to drive me home?
- What special precautions should be taken with a child?
- Should I especially be concerned with scans to my brain? How about other organs of my body?
- Should I expect any side effects?
- How many CT scans is it safe to undergo in any one year? How far apart should they be spaced?
- How will this scan help in the diagnosis of my disorder?

All metal and jewelry should be removed to avoid artifacts on the film. Depending on the type of study, patients may also be required to remove dentures.

Aftercare

Generally, no aftercare is required following a CT scan. Immediately following the exam, the technologist will continue to watch the patient for possible adverse contrast reactions. Patients are instructed to advise the technologist of any symptoms, particularly respiratory difficulty. The site of contrast injection will be bandaged and may feel tender following the exam.

Results

Normal findings on a CT exam show bone, the most dense tissue, as white areas. Tissues and fat will show as various shades of gray, and fluids will be gray or black. Air will also look black. Intravenous, oral, and rectal contrasts appear as white areas. The radiologist can determine if tissues and organs appear normal by the sensitivity of the gray shadows. Abnormal results may show different characteristics of tissues within organs. Accumulations of blood or other fluids where they do not belong may be detected. Radiologists can differentiate among types of tumors throughout the body by viewing details of their makeup.

Brain studies

The precise differences in density allowed by CT scan can clearly show tumors, strokes, or lesions in the brain area as altered densities. These lighter or darker areas on the image may indicate a tumor or hematoma within the brain and skull area. Different types of tumors can be identified by the presence of edema (fluid), by the tissue's density, or by studying blood vessel location and activity. The speed and convenience of CT often allows for detection of hemorrhage (bleeding) before symptoms even occur.

Resources

BOOKS

Armstrong, Peter, Martin L. Wastie, and Andrea G. Rockall. *Diagnostic Imaging*. Chichester, UK: Wiley-Blackwell, 2009.

Birkfellner, Wolfgang. *Applied Medical Image Processing: A Basic Course*. Boca Raton, FL: Taylor & Francis, 2011.

Frank, Eugene D. *Merrill's Atlas of Radiographic Positioning & Procedures*. St. Louis: Elsevier/Mosby, 2012.

Romans, Lois E. *Computed Tomography for Technologists: A Comprehensive Text*. Baltimore: Wolters Kluwer Health/ Lippincott Williams & Wilkins, 2011.

Seeram, Euclid. *Computed Tomography: Physical Principles, Clinical Applications and Quality Control*. St. Louis: Saunders/Elsevier, 2009.

PERIODICALS

Brenner, David J., and Eric J. Hall. "Computed Tomography—An Increasing Source of Radiation Exposure." *The New England Journal of Medicine* 357 (November 29, 2007): 2277–84. http://www.nejm.org/doi/full/10.1056/NEJMra072149 (accessed October 31, 2011).

WEBSITES

Mayo Clinic staff. "CT Scan." MayoClinic.com. January 12, 2011. http://www.mayoclinic.com/health/ct-scan/MY00309 (accessed October 31, 2011).

MedlinePlus. "Cranial CT Scan." U.S. National Library of Medicine. November 22, 2010. http://www.nlm.nih.gov/medlineplus/ency/article/003786.htm (accessed October 31, 2011).

U.S. Food and Drug Administration. "Computed Tomography." U.S. Department of Health and Human Services. http://www.fda.gov/Radiation-EmittingProducts/RadiationEmittingProductsandProcedures/MedicalImaging/MedicalX-Rays/ucm115317.htm (accessed October 31, 2011).

———. "Full-Body CT Scans: What you Need to Know." April 6, 2010. http://www.fda.gov/Radiation-EmittingProducts/RadiationEmittingProductsandProcedures/MedicalImaging/MedicalX-Rays/ucm115340.htm (accessed October 31, 2011).

ORGANIZATIONS

American College of Radiology, 1891 Preston White Drive, Reston, VA, 22091, (703) 648-8900, http://www.acr.org.

Laith Farid Gulli, MD
Teresa G. Norris, RN
William A. Atkins, BB, BS, MBA

Conduct disorder

Definition

Conduct disorder (CD), also sometimes called disruptive behavior disorder, is a childhood and adolescent behavior disorder characterized by aggressive and destructive activities (for example, fighting, **bullying**, lying, and stealing) that cause serious disruptions in the child's natural environments such as home, school, church, or neighborhood. The overriding feature of conduct disorder is the repetitive and persistent pattern of defiant or impulsive behaviors that violate societal norms and the rights of other people. Such long-term behavior and personality problems often lead to problems later in life, such as illegal drug use, further antisocial behaviors, criminal activities and legal problems.

Demographics

Studies of conduct disorder worldwide have found that overall rates are 4.6% of boys and 4.5% of girls. In the United States, it is one of the most prevalent categories of mental health problems of children, with rates estimated at 5% of children, with about 9% for males and 2% for females. According to the U.S. **Substance Abuse and Mental Health Services Administration**, in 2009, 1%–4% of 9- to 17-year-old children were affected by CD. Because of a discrepancy among mental health experts as to the exact definition of conduct disorder, estimates from other sources vary from as low as 2% to as high as 16% of children in the United States, with most of the cases developing in children in their late childhood or early teenage years. Statistics suggest the disorder is more likely to affect boys than girls. In addition, children are at more risk of CD when **child abuse** is part of their past, drug or alcohol **addiction** is found among their parents and caregivers, family conflicts are frequent, genetic defects are present within the family, and poverty is part of their experience.

Description

The specific behaviors used to produce a **diagnosis** of conduct disorder are often categorized into four groups: aggressive conduct that causes or threatens physical harm to other people or animals, nonaggressive behavior that causes property damage or loss, deceitfulness or theft, and serious violations of rules. In addition, two subtypes of conduct disorder can be delineated based on the age at which symptoms first appear. Childhood-onset type is appropriate for children showing at least one of the behaviors in question before the age of ten years. Adolescent onset type is defined by the absence of any conduct disorder criteria before the age of ten years. Severity may be described as mild, moderate, or severe, depending on the number of problems exhibited and their impact on other people.

Youngsters who show symptoms (most often aggression) before the age of ten years may also exhibit oppositional behavior and peer relationship problems. When they also show persistent conduct disorder and then develop adult **antisocial personality disorder**, they should be distinguished from individuals who had no symptoms of conduct disorder before age ten. The childhood type is more highly associated with heightened aggression, male gender, **oppositional defiant disorder**, and a family history of antisocial behavior.

The individual behaviors that can be observed when conduct disorder is diagnosed may be problematic and chronic. They tend to occur frequently and are distressingly consistent across time, settings, and families. Not surprisingly, these children function poorly in a variety of places. In fact, the behaviors clustered within the term "conduct disorder" account for a majority of clinical referrals, classroom detentions or other sanctions, being asked to stop participating in numerous activities, and can be extremely difficult (even impossible) for parents to manage.

The negative consequences of conduct disorder, particularly childhood onset, may include illicit drug use, dropping out of school, violent behavior, severe family conflict, and frequent delinquent acts. Such behaviors often result in the child's eventual placement out of the home, in special education, and/or the juvenile justice system. There is evidence that the rates of disruptive behavior disorders may be as high as 50% in youth in public sectors of care such as juvenile justice, alcohol and drug services, schools for youths with serious emotional disturbances, child welfare, and mental health.

Other mental problems are also frequently associated with conduct disorder, such as **attention deficit hyperactivity disorder** (ADHD), antisocial personality disorder (APD), **major depressive disorder** (MDD), **learning disorders**, thought disorders, **substance abuse**, mood disorders, **post-traumatic stress disorder** (PTSD), and **bipolar disorder** (BD).

The financial costs of crime and correction for repeated juvenile offenses by youth with conduct disorder are extensive. The social costs include citizens' fear of such behaviors, loss of a sense of safety, and disruptions in classrooms that interfere with other children's opportunity to learn. The costs to the child and the child's family are enormous in terms of the emotional and other resources needed to address the consequences of the constellation of symptoms that define conduct disorder.

Causes and symptoms

Various determinants tend to be present in children with conduct disorder, and it is possible there may be a genetic predisposition to this disorder. Symptoms recur among children exhibiting this disorder.

Causes

There is no known direct cause for conduct disorder. However, many determinants are proposed to explain how conduct disorder becomes present within children. These determinants include various types of factors:

- biological: such as problems during pregnancy, injuries to the brain early in life, or other mental illnesses such as anxiety disorders that contribute to CD
- environmental: factors such as a dysfunctional family life, lack of discipline in school or home, physical or mental abuse, or traumatic experiences
- genetics: often times other family members have mental illnesses or are substance or alcohol abusers
- social: poor parenting of a child can lead to conduct disorder, along with poverty or low socioeconomic status and being seen as an outcast by other students or peers

The frustrating behavior of youngsters with conduct disorder frequently leads to blaming, labeling, and other unproductive activities. Children who are "acting out" do not inspire sympathy or the benefit of the doubt. Further, other children often ostracize them. Parents of such children are often blamed as poor disciplinarians or bad parents. As a result, parents of children with conduct disorder may be reluctant to engage with schools or other authorities. At the same time, there is a strong correlation between children diagnosed with conduct disorder and a significant level of family dysfunction, poor parenting practices, an overemphasis on coercion and hostile communication patterns, verbal and physical aggression, and a history of maltreatment.

A possible genetic component may exist as a factor in conduct disorder, which has been traditionally viewed as a behavioral disorder. One study with adopted children in the mid-1990s looked at the relationship between birth parents with antisocial personality disorder and adverse adoptive home environments. When both of these adverse conditions occurred, there was significantly increased aggressiveness and conduct disorder in the adopted children. That was not the case if there was no indication of antisocial personality disorder in the birth parents. This finding, which has been supported in studies in the 2000s and 2010s, has important implications for prevention and **intervention** of conduct disorders and its associated conditions of substance abuse and aggressiveness.

Symptoms

Conduct disorder has many varied symptoms among children who have this mental disorder. Symptoms are commonly divided into four general groups: destructive behavior, aggressive behavior, violation of rules, and deceitful behavior. Some of the more common activities (which may fall into more than one of these groups) that are seen within people with CD are:

- destroying or vandalizing property such as intentionally setting a building on fire (arson)
- doing physical harm to others, such as fighting, bullying
- using dangerous weapons such as guns and knives
- being cruel to people or animals
- forcing others to have sex or having sex at an early age
- stealing, shoplifting, or breaking into cars or homes
- having wide mood swings
- running away
- getting into trouble repeatedly
- skipping school, truancy
- playing pranks on people
- lying to get something desired or to avoid doing something
- abusing alcohol or illegal drugs
- having few friends
- having little remorse (without guilt feelings) for bad behaviors

Diagnosis

Testing does not help diagnose conduct disorder. Such a diagnosis is solely based on the child's history. A comprehensive evaluation should be undertaken to find out if co-existing conditions exist, such as anxiety, mood disorders, learning problems, PTSD, ADHD, and others. Further, behavior that represents conduct disorder is more serious than simple adolescent exuberance, rebellion, or immaturity. The fourth edition, text revised, of the ***Diagnostic and Statistical Manual of Mental Disorders*** (*DSM-IV-TR*) indicates that for conduct disorder to be diagnosed, the patient must be shown to have repeatedly violated rules, age-appropriate social norms, and the rights of others for a period of at least twelve months. This is shown by three or more of the following behaviors, with at least one having taken place in the previous six months: aggression to people or animals, property destruction, lying or theft, and serious rule violations.

Aggression to people or animals includes:

- engaging in frequent bullying or threatening behavior
- often starting fights
- using a weapon that could cause serious injury (gun, knife, club, broken glass)
- showing physical cruelty to people
- showing physical cruelty to animals
- engaging in theft with confrontation (armed robbery, extortion, mugging, purse snatching)
- forcing sex upon someone

Property destruction includes deliberately setting fires to cause serious damage and/or deliberately destroying the property of others by means other than fire setting.

Lying or theft includes:

- breaking into a building, car, or house belonging to someone else
- frequently lying or breaking promises for gain or to avoid obligations (called "conning")
- stealing valuables without confrontation (burglary, forgery, shop lifting)

Serious rule violations include:

- beginning before the age of 13 years, frequently staying out at night against parents' wishes
- running away from parents overnight twice or more or once for an extended period
- engaging in frequent truancy beginning before the age of 13 years

Mild severity means there are few problems with conduct beyond those needed to make a diagnosis and all of the problems cause little harm to other people. Moderate severity means the number and effect of the conduct problems is between the extremes of mild and severe. Severe is indicated if there are many more conduct symptoms than are needed to make the diagnosis (more than three in the previous twelve months or more than one in the previous six months), or the behaviors cause other people considerable harm.

It is generally diagnosed when somebody, often a child in school, comes to the attention of authorities (school, law enforcement, and others) most often because of behavior. The person might then be referred to a **psychiatrist** or **psychologist** for assessment and diagnosis. It is unlikely that any sort of specific test is given; rather, the individual would have to meet the criteria as defined by the *DSM-IV-TR*. Usually there is a history of acting out in school, neighborhood, home, and other social settings. Court-ordered treatment would likely occur if the person comes to the attention of the police and if a crime is committed. A judge might order treatment as an alternative to jail or before a sentence is served.

Treatment

Treatment is much more successful when the child's parents or caregivers are actively involved in the process. When such members are participating, parents or caregivers at home can carry out CD techniques started by the medical professional. However, when the family is part of the problem, the child is often taken away from the disruptive environment and placed in a more stable and healthy one. Many places are available that provide such stable environments while at the same time providing behavioral modification treatment. Two of these are wilderness programs and boot camps. Medication may also be a part of the treatment.

Earlier treatments of youth with conduct disorder relied on legal processes to declare a child in need of supervision or treatment and thus able to be placed in residential settings established for this purpose. While residential placements may still be used, recent treatment models have relied less on such restrictive procedures. The increased visibility and sophistication of the consumer movement, comprising families of children and youth with mental health disorders, has brought pressure to bear on treatment providers. Such action helps to stop blaming families, to stop removing children from their families for services, to focus instead on strengths and assets in both the child and the child's family, and to use community-based interventions in several domains in which the child and family live.

Community-based interventions, sometimes called wrap-around services, attempt to handle the child within the child's natural environment in a comprehensive and flexible way. The idea is to target a range of child, parent, family, and social system factors associated with a child's behavioral problems. This approach has been successful in modifying antisocial behavior, reducing rates of restrictive placement, and lowering the cost of services.

For the most part, conduct disorder is treated based on the age of the child, the disorder's severity, and the ability of the child to deal with it on a daily basis. Treatment is usually complicated for both the patient and the administrator, especially if the patient is unwilling to cooperate due to mistrust or fear of authority figures.

The treatment process usually includes **psychotherapy**, which is used to help the child express problems and control feelings in socially acceptable ways. Specific types of psychotherapy used to treat CD are **cognitive-behavioral therapy**, which helps to improve the thinking processes and problem-solving abilities within the patient, along with anger management and impulse control, and **family therapy**, which helps to improve interactions among family members. Treatment may also include special education classes for those children having learning problems. The attending medical professional may instruct the parents or caretakers as to special educational and management programs that need to be used at home and in school. Medication is sometimes used and may be effective in controlling aggression. Most drugs used for it are also used to treat the symptoms of other mental illnesses such as **depression** and ADHD.

One treatment program that has been used with some success is child cognitive behavioral treatment and skills training, which trains children with conduct disorder in anger-coping, peer coping, and problem-solving skills.

Parent management training and family therapy are also used to treat conduct disorder. Parents learn to apply behavioral principles effectively, how to play with their children, and how to teach them new skills.

Generally, a variety of treatment modes are used to address such a complex disorder. Severe antisocial behavior on the part of the child and adverse parenting practices on the part of parents and caregivers may cause the family to stop treatment before it can be effective or before meaningful change can be achieved. Treatment takes quite long because new attitudes and behaviors must be ingrained in the child. The earlier treatment begins and the longer it is applied, the more successful the results tend to be for the child.

Prognosis

Early identification and appropriate, innovative, and comprehensive treatment will improve the course of conduct disorder and possibly prevent a host of negative outcomes that are associated with it. Unfortunately, the **stigma** of treatment and the undiagnosed problems of many parents prevent many families from seeking treatment. Instead their children come into contact with the juvenile and criminal justice system.

In addition, children with more severe symptoms or other mental problems or other illnesses (such as drug abuse) have the lowest chance of improving from conduct disorder. They may be unable to adapt to the complexities of being an adult and may have persistent problems in various aspects of their life.

Prevention

Prognosis may best be improved by prevention of conduct disorder before it becomes so resistant to treatment. Research indicates that early intervention holds the greatest promise. It incorporates several components such as child tutoring, classroom intervention, peer training, social-cognitive skills training, parent training, and family problem solving.

Other studies have included early parent or family interventions, school based interventions, and community interventions. Again, these include a variety of elements, including parent training that includes education about normal child development, child problem solving, and family communication skills training. Research is still needed to determine where and when to target specific preventive interventions.

For the most part, improving the condition of the child helps to prevent the occurrence of CD, such as making sure the child is in a positive environment that emphasizes good behaviors and minimizes bad behaviors.

KEY TERMS

Antisocial personality disorder—A condition characterized by pervasive disregard for the rights of others that begins in childhood and often continues into adulthood.

Attention deficit hyperactivity disorder—A condition characterized by lack of concentration, impulsive or inappropriate age-related behavior, and hyperactivity.

Bipolar disorder—A condition characterized by extreme mood swings, from euphoria to depression.

Learning disorder—A condition characterized by difficulty in learning that has an unknown cause.

Major depressive disorder—A condition characterized by low mood, low self-esteem, and loss of pleasure or interest in everyday activities.

Mood disorders—A group of conditions characterized by pronounced disturbances in the state of mind.

Post-traumatic stress disorder—A condition resulting from severe emotional trauma (such as from war or natural disaster) and characterized by flashbacks, low energy, anxiety, depression, and sleep disturbances.

Substance abuse—The excessive consumption of an illegal drug or other substance that has a pronounced effect on the mind or body but without any therapeutic application.

Thought disorder—A condition characterized by incomprehensible language, either written or spoken.

QUESTIONS TO ASK YOUR DOCTOR

- Does my child have conduct disorder?
- What treatment plan is best?
- What medications should be used?
- Does my child need counseling?
- Will you be able to help my child?
- Is there support available for parents?

Resources

BOOKS

American Psychiatric Association. *Diagnostic and Statistical Manual of Mental Disorders*, 4th ed., text rev. Washington, DC: American Psychiatric Association, 2000.

Leeming, David A., Kathryn Madden, and Stanton Marlan, eds. *Encyclopedia of Psychology and Religion*. New York: Springer, 2010.

Morrison, James. *DSM-IV Made Easy: The Clinician's Guide to Diagnosis*. New York: Guilford Press, 2006.

WEBSITES

"Conduct Disorder." American Academy of Child and Adolescent Psychology. Last updated July 2004. http://aacap.org/page.ww?name=Conduct+Disorder& section= Facts+for+Families (accessed September 8, 2011).

"Conduct Disorder." MedlinePlus. Last updated February 28, 2011. http://www.nlm.nih.gov/medlineplus/ency/article/000919.htm (accessed September 8, 2011).

"Helping Children and Youth with Conduct Disorder and Oppositional Defiant Disorder: Systems of Care." U.S. Substance Abuse and Mental Health Services Administration, January 2006. http://store.samhsa.gov/product/Helping-Children-and-Youth-With-Conduct-Disorder-and-Oppositional-Defiant-Disorder-Systems-of-Care/SMA06-4200 (accessed September 8, 2011).

"Mental Health and Conduct Disorder." WebMD. http://www.webmd.com/mental-health/mental-health-conduct-disorder (accessed September 8, 2011).

ORGANIZATIONS

American Academy of Child and Adolescent Psychiatry, 3615 Wisconsin Ave., NW, Washington, DC, 20016-3007, (202) 966-7300, Fax: (202) 966-2891, http://aacap.org.

American Psychiatric Association, 1000 Wilson Blvd., Ste. 1825, Arlington, VA, 22209-3901, (703) 907-7300, apa@psych.org, http://www.psych.org.

Federation of Families for Children's Mental Health, 9605 Medical Center Dr., Rockville, MD, 20850, (240) 403-1901, Fax: (240) 403-1909, ffcmh@ffcmh.org, http://ffcmh.org.

Mental Health America, 2000 N. Beauregard St., 6th Fl., Alexandria, VA, 22311, (703) 684-7722, (800) 969-6642, Fax: (703) 684-5968, http://www1.nmha.org.

National Alliance on Mental Illness, 2107 Wilson Blvd., Ste. 300, Arlington, VA, 22201-3042, Fax: (703) 524-9094, (800) 950-6264, http://www.nami.org.

National Institute of Mental Health, 6001 Executive Blvd., Rm. 8184, MSC 9663, Bethesda, MD, 20892-9663, (301) 433-4513; TTY: (301) 443-8431, Fax: (301) 443-4279, (866) 615-6464; TTY: (866) 415-8051, nimhinfo@nih.gov, http://www.nimh.nih.gov.

Judy Leaver, MA
William Atkins, BB, BS, MBA

Conners' Rating Scales

Definition

Developed by Dr. C. Keith Conners, PhD, the latest version of the Conners' Rating Scales (CRS) is the Conners' Rating Scales–Third Edition, or Conners 3. The Conners 3 is a set of paper and pencil screening questionnaires designed to be completed by parents, teachers, and students to assist in evaluating children and teenagers for **attention deficit hyperactivity disorder (ADHD)** and related behavioral, emotional, and learning problems.

Purpose

The Conners 3 is used as part of a comprehensive examination and is designed to be easily administered and scored. Both the long and short versions serve as tools to assist in determining whether children or teenagers between the ages of 6 and 18 years might have **ADHD** or another disorder, such as **oppositional defiant disorder** or **conduct disorder**. In addition, a self-report form is used to assess children or teenagers between the ages of 8 and 18 years.

Description

The Conners 3 is available in long and short versions for parents (or caregivers) and teachers, along with a self-report version that is completed by the student. The long version takes approximately 20 minutes to complete, while the short version usually takes about 10 minutes. The ADHD Index is completed in less than five minutes. The Conners 3 is normalized based on gender-specific, age-stratified norms from a large, nationally representative sample of the U.S. population. Specifically, it was normalized using ratings from approximately 1,200 parents, 1,200 teachers, and 1,000 children and adolescent reports. The normative data was taken over a one-year period based on the age of the children and adolescents and was separated by gender. The standardization sample of the U.S. population was based on ethnicity, gender, parent education, and race.

The Conners 3 has been improved over the previous edition, the CRS-Revised (CRS-R), with respect to the following:

- updated normative data
- unlimited use when computer scoring is selected
- better focus on ADHD
- modified age range (6–18 years, as opposed to 6–17 years for previous versions)
- expanded number of scales, including two additional *DSM-IV-TR* symptom scales (*Diagnostic and Statistical Manual of Mental Disorders*, fourth edition, text revision)
- new screener items to identify any possible anxiety or depression
- availability of impairment items, which measure the problem's impact
- use of critical items that identify children who need immediate attention
- guidance in planning and monitoring interventions

Conners 3 includes six empirical scales concerning hyperactivity/impulsivity, executive functioning, learning difficulties, aggression, peer relations, and family relations. The *DSM-IV-TR* symptom scales assess the possibility of various disorders, including three types of ADHD (hyperactive/impulsive, inattentive, or combined), oppositional defiant disorder, and conduct disorder, the later two of which are new to the third edition. The Conners 3 also comprises three validity scales, also new to the third edition, and a rational scale, which assesses inattention.

The short form includes the strongest items from the long form, which are hyperactivity/impulsivity, inattention, executive functioning, learning problems, aggression, peer relations, and positive and negative impressions.

The Conners 3 also includes two indexes, the global index and the ADHD index. Each is composed of ten items. The global index measures general psychopathology, whereas the ADHD index aims to help distinguish children with ADHD from those without the condition. It is also a recommended test for the screening of large numbers of children or teenagers and is a good way to measure the effectiveness of treatment or the response to **intervention** in such children and teens.

KEY TERMS

Attention deficit hyperactivity disorder (ADHD)—A persistent pattern of inattention, hyperactivity and/or impulsiveness; the pattern is more frequent and severe than is typically observed in people at a similar level of development.

Diagnostic and Statistical Manual of Mental Disorders—The handbook that mental health professionals use to diagnose mental disorders.

Executive function—The cognitive processes that facilitate mental control, such as planning, problem solving, ability to change, prioritization, and self control.

The long version for parents contains 110 items, while the long version for teachers contains 115 items. The parents' short version contains 43 items, and the teachers' short version has 39. The self-report scale contains 59 items in the long form and 39 items in the short form. The forms span multiple pages, and numbers circled on the front or back page are automatically transferred to a middle section for use by a clinician. The clinician transfers the circled scores into appropriate scales on the middle form and totals each scale at the bottom of the page. The parent and teacher scales are written at the equivalent of a fourth-to-fifth grade reading level. The self-report scale for children is written at the third-grade reading level.

Preparation

The long form is recommended for an initial evaluation, because it more thoroughly assesses the *DSM* diagnostic criteria and may better identify specific needs of a child as compared to the short form. However, the short form is beneficial when an evaluation needs to be done on a timely basis or when many tests will be performed over a specific period (such as when the professional administrator wishes to monitor progress).

Precautions

As with all psychological evaluation instruments, the Conners 3 is not perfect. There is a risk of obtaining false positives (incorrectly diagnosing the disorder) or false negatives (failing to identify the disorder). Therefore, the information obtained from completed forms should not be used in isolation, but should be one piece of a complex evaluation that includes a clinical interview with the

> **QUESTIONS TO ASK YOUR DOCTOR**
>
> - What should I do next if the CRS finds that my child has ADHD?
> - What qualifications should I look for in a professional administering the CRS?
> - What other tests are available for diagnosing ADHD?

child, other diagnostic measures such as a computerized continuous performance test, and patient self-reports—for those old enough and with sufficient reading ability to do so. Although the Conners 3 can be readily administered and scored by a nonprofessional, a professional, such as a **psychologist** or counselor, who is familiar with the scales should facilitate the test to ensure accurate results.

Previous versions of the Conners' scales (earlier than CRS-R, which preceded Conners 3) were criticized by those claiming disparity between results obtained in different ethnic groups. This version, along with CRS-R, should dispel this concern, since it was "normed" using data from thousands of subjects crossing all cultural and ethnic boundaries. The technical manual for CRS-R even contains separate normative information for specific ethnic groups. However, there are generally no or statistically insignificant differences between age and gender groups.

Results

After transferring the raw scores to the various scales and totaling them, the total of each scale is transferred to another form designed to graphically portray the results. The clinician must be careful to transpose the raw scores to the correct age group column within each major scale. Each of these column scores can then be converted to a T-score. T-scores are standardized scores with a mean of 50 and a standard deviation of 10. These can be further converted to percentile scores as needed.

As a rule, T-scores above 60 are cause for concern and have interpretive value. Interpretable scores range from a low T-score of 61 (mildly atypical) to above 70 (markedly atypical). However, again, this information should not be used in isolation to make a **diagnosis**.

The Conners 3 can be hand scored or computer scored. A Hand-Scored Kit and a Software Kit are both available. The Software Kit provides for unlimited computer scoring with Web links to the *DSM-IV-TR* diagnostic criteria, along with an Assessment Report (total score and symptom count score), Feedback Report (assessment summary), and Progress Report (result comparison when administered more than once).

Resources

BOOKS

Austin, Vance L., and Daniel T. Sciarra. *Children and Adolescents with Emotional and Behavior Disorders.* Boston: Merrill, 2010.

Hammerness, Paul Graves. *ADHD.* Westport, CT: Greenwood Press, 2008.

McLeod, Jane D, and Eric R. Wright, editors. *The Sociology of Mental Illness: A Comprehensive Reader.* New York: Oxford University Press, 2010.

Shepherd, Terry L. *Working with Students with Emotional and Behavior Disorders: Characteristics and Teaching Strategies.* Upper Saddle River, NJ: Merrill, 2010.

WEBSITES

Pearson. "C. Keith Conners [biography]." PsychCorp.co.uk. http://www.psychcorp.co.uk/Psychology/ChildMental-Health/ChildADDADHDBehaviour/ConnersEarlyChild-hood(ConnersEC)/Authors/CKeithConners.aspx (accessed November 23, 2011).

Pearson Assessments. "Conners Third Edition (Conners 3) [product page]." http://www.pearsonassessments.com/HAIWEB/Cultures/en-us/Productdetail.htm?Pid=Conners_3 (accessed November 23, 2011).

ORGANIZATIONS

Children and Adults with Attention Deficit/Hyperactivity Disorder, 8181 Professional Place, Ste. 150, Landover, MD, 20785, (301) 306-7070, Fax: (301) 306-7090, http://www.chadd.org

Substance Abuse and Mental Health Services Administration Referral Resource, 1 Choke Cherry Rd., Rockville, MD, 20857, (877) SAMHSA-7 (726-4727), (800) TTY: 487-4889, Fax: (240) 221-4292, SAMHSAInfo@samhsa.hhs.gov, http://www.samhsa.gov.

Jack H. Booth, PsyD
William A. Atkins

Conversion disorder

Definition

Conversion disorder is defined by the ***Diagnostic and Statistical Manual of Mental Disorders***, fourth edition, text revision, also known as the *DSM-IV-TR*, as a mental disorder whose central feature is the appearance of symptoms affecting the patient's senses or voluntary movements that suggest a neurological or general medical disease or condition. Other terms that have sometimes been used for conversion disorder include pseudoneurologic syndrome, hysterical **neurosis**, and psychogenic disorder. The *Diagnostic and Statistical Manual of Mental Disorders (DSM-5*, 2013) proposes changing the name of conversion disorder to functional neurological symptoms.

Demographics

The lifetime prevalence rates of conversion disorder in the general population are estimated to fall between 2.5 and 500 per 100,000 people. Differences among estimates reflect differences in the method of **diagnosis** as well as regional population differences. In terms of clinical populations, conversion disorder is diagnosed in 5–14% of general hospital patients; 1–3% of outpatient referrals to psychiatrists; and 5–25% of psychiatric outpatients. The frequency among clinical populations overall is reported between 20 and 120 per 100,000 patients.

Among adults, women diagnosed with conversion disorder outnumber men by a 2:1 to 10:1 ratio; among children, however, the gender ratio is closer to 1:1. Less-educated people and those of lower socioeconomic status are more likely to develop conversion disorder; race by itself does not appear to be a factor. There is, however, a major difference between the populations of developing and developed countries. In developing countries, the prevalence of conversion disorder may run as high as 31%.

Conversion disorder is a major reason for visits to primary care practitioners. One study of health care utilization estimated that 25–72% of office visits to primary care doctors involved psychological distress that takes the form of somatic (physical) symptoms. Another study estimated that at least 10% of all medical treatments and diagnostic services were ordered for patients with no evidence of organic disease. Conversion disorder carries a high economic price tag. Patients who convert their emotional problems into physical symptoms spend nine times as much for health care as people who do not somatosize; and 82% of adults with conversion disorder stop working because of their symptoms. The annual bill for conversion disorder in the United States comes to $20 billion, not counting absenteeism from work and disability payments.

Description

The *DSM-IV-TR* classifies conversion disorder as one of the **somatoform disorders**, first classified as a group of mental disorders by the *DSM III* in 1980. Somatoform disorders are marked by persistent physical symptoms that cannot be fully explained by a medical condition, **substance abuse**, or other mental disorder, but rather seem to stem from psychological issues or conflicts.

Conversion disorder has a complicated history that helps to explain the number of different names for it. Two eminent neurologists of the nineteenth century, Jean-Martin Charcot in Paris, France, and Josef Breuer in Vienna, Austria, were investigating what was then called hysteria, a disorder primarily affecting women (the term "hysteria" comes from the Greek word for uterus or womb). Women diagnosed with hysteria had frequent emotional outbursts and a variety of neurologic symptoms, including paralysis, fainting spells, convulsions, and temporary loss of sight or hearing. Pierre Janet (one of Charcot's students), and Breuer independently came to the same conclusion about the cause of hysteria—that it resulted from psychological **trauma**. Janet, in fact, coined the term "dissociation" to describe the altered state of consciousness experienced by many patients who were diagnosed with hysteria.

The next stage in the study of conversion disorder was research into the causes of "combat neurosis" in World War I (1914–1918) and World War II (1939–1945). Many of the symptoms observed in "shell-shocked" soldiers were identical to those of "hysterical" women. Two of the techniques still used in the treatment of conversion disorder, hypnosis and narcotherapy, were introduced as therapies for combat veterans. The various terms used by successive editions of the *DSM* and the *ICD* (the European equivalent of *DSM*) for conversion disorder reflect its association with hysteria and dissociation. The first edition of the *DSM* (1952) used the term "conversion reaction." The *DSM-II* (1968) called the disorder "hysterical neurosis (conversion type)," and the *DSM-III* (1980), *DSM-III-R* (1987), and *DSM-IV* (1994) have all used the term "conversion disorder." *ICD-10* refers to it as "dissociative (conversion) disorder."

DSM-IV-TR (2000) specifies six criteria for the diagnosis of conversion disorder. They are:

- The patient has one or more symptoms or deficits affecting the senses or voluntary movement that suggest a neurological or general medical disorder.
- The onset or worsening of the symptoms was preceded by conflicts or stressors in the patient's life.
- The symptom is not faked or produced intentionally.
- The symptom cannot be fully explained as the result of a general medical disorder, substance intake, or a behavior related to the patient's culture.

- The symptom is severe enough to interfere with the patient's schooling, employment, or social relationships, or is serious enough to require a medical evaluation.
- The symptom is not limited to pain or sexual dysfunction, does not occur only in the context of somatization disorder, and is not better accounted for by another mental disorder.

The *DSM-IV-TR* lists four subtypes of conversion disorder: conversion disorder with motor symptom or deficit; with sensory symptom or deficit; with **seizures** or convulsions; and with mixed presentation.

Although conversion disorder is most commonly found in individuals, it sometimes occurs in groups. One such instance occurred in 1997 in a group of three young men and six adolescent women of the Embera, an indigenous tribe in Colombia. The young people believed that they had been put under a spell or curse and developed dissociative symptoms that were not helped by antipsychotic medications or traditional herbal remedies. They were cured when shamans from their ethnic group came to visit them. The episode was attributed to psychological **stress** resulting from rapid cultural change.

Another example of group conversion disorder occurred in Iran in 1992. Ten girls out of a classroom of 26 became unable to walk or move normally following tetanus inoculations. Although the local physicians were able to treat the girls successfully, public health programs to immunize people against tetanus suffered an immediate negative impact. One explanation of group conversion disorder is that an individual who is susceptible to the disorder is typically more affected by suggestion and easier to hypnotize than the average person.

Causes and symptoms

Causes

The immediate cause of conversion disorder is a stressful event or situation that leads the patient to develop bodily symptoms as symbolic expressions of a long-standing psychological conflict or problem.

Two terms that are used in connection with the causes of conversion disorder are primary gain and secondary gain. Primary gain refers to the lessening of the anxiety and communication of the unconscious wish that the patient derives from the symptom(s). Secondary gain refers to the interference with daily tasks, removal from the uncomfortable situation, or increased attention from significant others that the patient obtains as a result of the symptom(s).

Physical, emotional, or **sexual abuse** can be a contributing cause of conversion disorder in both adults and children. In a study of 34 children who developed pseudoseizures, 32% had a history of **depression** or sexual abuse, and 44% had recently experienced a parental divorce, death, or violent quarrel. At least one study, however, has found no consistent association between dissociation and sexual or physical abuse. In the adult population, conversion disorder may be associated with mobbing, a term that originated among European psychiatrists and industrial psychologists to describe psychological abuse in the workplace. One American woman who quit her job because of mobbing was unable to walk for several months. Adult males sometimes develop conversion disorder during military basic training. Conversion disorder may also develop in adults as a long-delayed after effect of childhood abuse. A team of surgeons reported on the case of a patient who went into a psychogenic coma following a throat operation. The surgeons found that she had been repeatedly raped as a child by her father, who stifled her cries by smothering her with a pillow.

Symptoms

In general, symptoms of conversion disorder are not under the patient's conscious control, and are frequently mysterious and frightening to the patient. The symptoms usually have an acute onset, but sometimes worsen gradually.

The most frequent forms of conversion disorder in Western countries include:

- Pseudoparalysis. In pseudoparalysis, the patient loses the use of half of his/her body or of a single limb. The weakness does not follow anatomical patterns and is often inconsistent upon repeat examination.
- Pseudosensory syndromes. Patients with these syndromes often complain of numbness or lack of sensation in various parts of their bodies. The loss of sensation typically follows the patient's notion of their anatomy, rather than known characteristics of the human nervous system.
- Pseudoseizures. These are the most difficult symptoms of conversion disorder to distinguish from their organic equivalents. Between 5% and 35% of patients with pseudoseizures also have epilepsy. Electroencephalograms (EEGs) and the measurement of serum prolactin levels are useful in distinguishing pseudoseizures from epileptic seizures.
- Pseudocoma. Pseudocoma is also difficult to diagnose. Because true coma may indicate a life-threatening

condition, patients must be given standard treatments for coma until the diagnosis can be established.

- Psychogenic movement disorders. These can mimic myoclonus, parkinsonism, dystonia, dyskinesia, and tremor. Doctors sometimes give patients with suspected psychogenic movement disorders a placebo medication to determine whether the movements are psychogenic or the result of an organic disorder.
- Pseudoblindness. Pseudoblindness is one of the most common forms of conversion disorder related to vision. Placing a mirror in front of the patient and tilting it from side to side can often be used to determine pseudoblindness, because humans tend to follow the reflection of their eyes.
- Pseudodiplopia. Pseudodiplopia, or seeing double, can usually be diagnosed by examining the patient's eyes.
- Pseudoptosis. Ptosis, or drooping of the upper eyelid, is a common symptom of myasthenia gravis and a few other disorders. Some people can cause their eyelids to droop voluntarily with practice. The diagnosis can be made on the basis of the eyebrow; in true ptosis, the eyebrows are lifted, whereas in pseudoptosis they are lowered.
- Hysterical aphonia. Aphonia refers to loss of the ability to produce sounds. In hysterical aphonia, the patient's cough and whisper are normal, and examination of the throat reveals normal movement of the vocal cords.

Psychiatrists working in various parts of the Middle East and Asia report that the symptoms of conversion disorder as listed by the *DSM-IV* and the *ICD-10* do not fit well with the symptoms of the disorder most frequently encountered in their patient populations.

Diagnosis

Conversion disorder is one of the few mental disorders that appears to be overdiagnosed, particularly in emergency departments. There are numerous instances of serious neurologic illness that were initially misdiagnosed as conversion disorder. Newer techniques of diagnostic imaging have helped to lower the rate of medical errors. In addition, functional **magnetic resonance imaging** (MRI) has identified specific areas of the **brain** that show differential activation in cases of conversion disorder, and imaging findings may eventually be useful in distinguishing conversion disorder.

Diagnostic issues

Diagnosis of conversion disorder is complicated by its coexistence with physical illness in as many as 60% of patients. Alternatively explained, a diagnosis of conversion disorder does not exclude the possibility of a concurrent organic disease. The examining doctor will usually order a mental health evaluation when conversion disorder is suspected, as well as x rays, other **imaging studies** that may be useful, and appropriate laboratory tests. The doctor will also take a thorough patient history that will include the presence of recent stressors in the patient's life, as well as a history of abuse. Children and adolescents are usually asked about their school experiences, one question they are asked is whether a recent change of school or an experience related to school may have intensified academic pressure.

In addition, there are a number of bedside tests that doctors can use to distinguish between symptoms of conversion disorder and symptoms caused by physical diseases. These may include the drop test, in which a "paralyzed" arm is dropped over the patient's face. In conversion disorder, the arm will not strike the face. Other tests include applying a mildly painful stimulus to a "weak" or "numb" part of the body. The patient's pulse rate will typically rise in cases of conversion disorder, and he or she will usually pull back the limb that is being touched.

Factors suggesting a diagnosis of conversion disorder

The doctor can use a list of factors known to be associated with conversion disorder to assess the likelihood that a specific patient may have the disorder:

- Age. Conversion disorder is rarely seen in children younger than six years or adults over 35 years.
- Sex. The female:male ratio for the disorder ranges between 2:1 and 10:1. It is thought that higher rates of conversion disorder in women may reflect the greater vulnerability of females to abuse.
- Residence. People who live in rural areas are more likely to develop conversion disorder than those who live in cities.
- Level of education. Conversion disorder occurs less often among sophisticated or highly educated people.
- Family history. Children sometimes develop conversion disorder from observing their parents' reactions to stressors. This process is known as social modeling.
- A recent stressful change or event in the patient's life.

An additional feature suggesting conversion disorder is the presence of *la belle indifférence*. The French phrase refers to an attitude of relative unconcern on the patient's part about the symptoms or their implications. La belle indifférence is, however, much more common in adults

KEY TERMS

Aphonia—Inability to speak caused by a functional disturbance of the voice box or vocal cords.

(la) Belle indifférence—A psychiatric symptom sometimes found in patients with conversion disorder, in which the patient shows a surprising lack of concern about the nature or implications of his/her physical symptom(s).

Conversion—In psychiatry, a process in which a repressed feeling, impulse, thought, or memory emerges in the form of a bodily symptom.

Diplopia—A disorder of vision in which a single object appears double. Diplopia is sometimes called double vision.

Dyskinesia—Difficulty in performing voluntary muscular movements.

Dystonia—A neurological disorder characterized by involuntary muscle spasms. The spasms can cause a painful twisting of the body and difficulty walking or moving.

Electroencephalogram (EEG)—A test that measures the electrical activity of the brain by means of electrodes placed on the scalp or in the brain itself.

Factitious disorder—A type of mental disturbance in which patients intentionally act physically or mentally ill without obvious benefits. It is distinguished from malingering by the absence of an obvious motive, and from conversion disorder by intentional production of symptoms.

Hysteria—In nineteenth-century psychiatric use, a neurotic disorder characterized by violent emotional outbursts and disturbances of the sensory and motor (movement-related) functions. The term "hysterical neurosis" is still used by some psychiatrists as a synonym for conversion disorder.

Malingering—Knowingly pretending to be physically or mentally ill to avoid some unpleasant duty or responsibility, or for economic benefit.

Myoclonus—An abrupt spasm or twitching in a muscle or group of muscles.

Narcotherapy—A form of psychotherapy that involves the administration of a drug that makes the patient drowsy.

Primary gain—In psychiatry, the principal psychological reason for the development of a patient's symptoms. In conversion disorder, the primary gain from the symptom is the reduction of anxiety and the exclusion of an inner conflict from conscious awareness.

Pseudoseizure—A fit that resembles an epileptic seizure but is not associated with abnormal electrical discharges in the patient's brain.

Psychogenic—Originating in the mind, or in a mental process or condition. The term "psychogenic" is sometimes used as a synonym for "conversion."

Ptosis—Drooping of the upper eyelid.

Secondary gain—A term that refers to other benefits that a patient obtains from a conversion symptom. For example, a patient's loss of function in an arm might require other family members to do the patient's share of household chores; or they might give the patient more attention and sympathy than he or she usually receives.

Shaman—In certain indigenous tribes or groups, a person who acts as an intermediary between the natural and supernatural worlds. Shamans are regarded as having the power or ability to cure illnesses.

Social modeling—A process of learning behavioral and emotional-response patterns from observing one's parents or other adults. Some researchers think that social modeling plays a part in the development of conversion disorder in children.

Somatoform disorders—A group of psychiatric disorders in the *DSM-IV-TR* classification that are characterized by external physical symptoms or complaints that are related to psychological problems rather than organic illness. Conversion disorder is classified as a somatoform disorder.

Stressor—A stimulus or event that provokes a stress response in an organism. Stressors can be categorized as acute or chronic, and as external or internal to the organism.

with conversion disorder than in children or adolescents. Patients in these younger age groups are much more likely to react to their symptoms with fear or hopelessness. A recent review of the published reports of la belle indifférence found that this feature was not useful in discriminating conversion disorder from physically based disease because of muddy definitions and application of it in diagnosis.

Medical conditions that mimic conversion symptoms

It is important for the doctor to rule out serious medical disorders in patients who appear to have conversion symptoms. At least one study has found an approximately 4% rate of misdiagnosis of an actual physical problem as a conversion disorder. The following disorders must be considered in the differential diagnosis:

- multiple sclerosis (blindness resulting from optic neuritis)
- myasthenia gravis (muscle weakness)
- periodic paralysis (muscle weakness)
- myopathies (muscle weakness)
- polymyositis (muscle weakness)
- Guillain-Barré syndrome (motor and sensory symptoms)

Treatment

Patients diagnosed with conversion disorder frequently benefit from a team approach to treatment and from a combination of treatment modalities. A team approach is particularly beneficial if the patient has a history of abuse, or if he or she is being treated for a concurrent physical condition or illness.

Medications

While there are no drugs for the direct treatment of conversion disorder, medications are sometimes given to patients to treat the anxiety or depression that may be associated with conversion disorder.

Psychotherapy

Psychodynamic psychotherapy is sometimes used with children and adolescents to help them gain insight into their symptoms. Cognitive-behavioral approaches have also been tried, with good results. **Family therapy** is often recommended for younger patients whose symptoms may be related to family dysfunction. **Group therapy** appears to be particularly useful in helping adolescents to learn social skills and coping strategies, and to decrease their dependency on their families.

Inpatient treatment

Hospitalization is sometimes recommended for children with conversion disorders who are not helped by outpatient treatment. Inpatient treatment also allows for a more complete assessment of possible coexisting organic disorders, and for the child to improve his or her level of functioning outside of an abusive or otherwise dysfunctional home environment.

Alternative and complementary therapies

Alternative and complementary therapies that have been shown to be helpful in the treatment of conversion disorder include hypnosis, relaxation techniques, visualization, and **biofeedback**.

Prognosis

The prognosis for recovery from conversion disorder is highly favorable. Patients who have clearly identifiable stressors in their lives, acute onset of symptoms, and a short interval between symptom onset and treatment have the best prognosis. Of patients hospitalized for the disorder, over half recover within two weeks. Between 20% and 25% will **relapse** within a year. The individual symptoms of conversion disorder are usually self-limited and do not lead to lasting disabilities; however, patients with hysterical aphonia, paralysis, or visual disturbances, have better prognoses for full recovery than those with tremor or pseudoseizures.

Prevention

The incidence of conversion disorder in adults is likely to continue to decline with rising levels of formal education and the spread of basic information about human psychology. Prevention of conversion disorder in children and adolescents depends on better strategies for preventing abuse.

Resources

BOOKS

American Psychiatric Association. *Diagnostic and Statistical Manual of Mental Disorders*. 4th ed., text rev. Washington, DC: American Psychiatric Publishing, 2000.

"Conversion Disorder." In *The Merck Manual of Diagnosis and Therapy*, edited by Robert S. Porter and Justin L. Kaplan. Whitehouse Station, NJ: Merck Sharp & Dohme Corp., 2011.

Davenport, Noa, Ruth D. Schwartz, and Gail P. Elliott. *Mobbing: Emotional Abuse in the American Workplace*. Ames, IA: Civil Society Publishing, 1999.

Dorland's Pocket Medical Dictionary. Philadelphia: Elsevier Health Sciences, 2012.

Herman, Judith. *Trauma and Recovery: The Aftermath of Violence—from Domestic Abuse to Political Terror*. 14th printing. New York: Basic Books, 1997.

Pelletier, Kenneth R. "Sound Mind, Sound Body: MindBody Medicine Comes of Age." In *The Best Alternative Medicine*. New York: Touchstone, 2002.

World Health Organization (WHO). *The ICD-10 Classification of Mental and Behavioural Disorders*. Geneva: WHO, 1993.

PERIODICALS

Al-Sharbati, Marwan M., et al. "A Case of Bilateral Ptosis with Unsteady Gait: Suggestibility and Culture in Conversion Disorder." *International Journal of Psychiatry in Medicine* 31, no. 2 (2001): 225–32.

Campo, John V. "Case Study: Negative Reinforcement and Behavioral Management of Conversion Disorder." *Journal of the American Academy of Child and Adolescent Psychiatry* 39, no. 6 (June 2000): 787–90.

Glick, T.H., T.P. Workman, and S. V. Gaufberg. "Suspected Conversion Disorder: Foreseeable Risks and Avoidable Errors." *Academy of Emergency Medicine* 7, no. 11 (November 2000): 1272–77.

Haghighi, S.S., and S. Meyer. "Psychogenic Paraplegia in a Patient with Normal Electrophysiologic Findings." *Spinal Cord* 39, no. 12 (December 2001): 664–67.

Isaac, Mohan, and Prabhat K. Chand. "Dissociative and Conversion Disorders: Defining Boundaries." *Current Opinion in Psychiatry* 19, no. 1 (January 2006): 61–66.

Meyers, Timothy J., Bruce W. Jafek, and Arlen D. Meyers. "Recurrent Psychogenic Coma Following Tracheal Stenosis Repair." *Archives of Otolaryngology—Head & Neck Surgery* 125, no. 11 (November 1999): 1267–69.

Moene, F. C., et al. "Organic Syndromes Diagnosed as Conversion Disorder: Identification and Frequency in a Study of 85 Patients." *Journal of Psychosomatic Research* 49, no. 1 (July 2000): 7–12.

Mori, S., et al. "Psychogenic Hearing Loss with Panic Anxiety Attack After the Onset of Acute Inner Ear Disorder." *ORL Journal of Otorhinolaryngology and Related Specialties* 64, no. 1 (January–February 2002): 41–44.

Pineros, Marion, Diego Rosselli, Claudia Calderon. "An Epidemic of Collective Conversion and Dissociation Disorder in an Indigenous Group of Colombia: Its Relation to Cultural Change." *Social Science & Medicine* 46, no. 11 (January 1998): 1425–28.

Shaibani, Aziz, and Marwan N. Sabbagh. "Pseudoneurologic Syndromes: Recognition and Diagnoses." *American Family Physician* 57, no. 10 (May 15, 1998): 2485–94.

Stone, Jon, et al. "Systematic Review of Misdiagnosis of Conversion Symptom and 'Hysteria'" *British Medical Journal* 331 (2005): 989.

Stone, Jon, Roger Smyth, Alan Carson, Charles Warlow, and Michael Sharpe. "La Belle Indifference in Conversion Symptoms and Hysteria." *British Journal of Psychiatry* 188 (2006): 204–209.

Syed, E.U., et al. "Conversion Disorder: Difficulties in Diagnosis Using DSM-IV/ICD-10." *Journal of the Pakistan Medical Association* 51, no. 4 (April 2001): 143–45.

Wyllie, Elaine, et al. "Psychiatric Features of Children and Adults with Pseudoseizures." *Archives of Pediatrics & Adolescent Medicine* 153 (March 1999): 244–48.

Yasamy, M.T., A. Bahramnezhad, H. Ziaaddini. "Post-Vaccination Mass Psychogenic Illness in an Iranian Rural School." *Eastern Mediterranean Health Journal* 5 (July 1999): 710–16.

ORGANIZATIONS

American Academy of Child and Adolescent Psychiatry, 3615 Wisconsin Ave. NW, Washington, DC, 20016-3007, (202) 966-7300, Fax: (202) 966-2891, http://aacap.org.

National Institute of Mental Health, 6001 Executive Blvd., Room 8184, MSC 9663, Bethesda, MD, 20892-9663, (301) 433-4513; TTY: (301) 443-8431, Fax: (301) 443-4279, (866) 615-6464; TTY: (866) 415-8051, nimhinfo@nih.gov, http://www.nimh.nih.gov.

Rebecca J. Frey, PhD
Emily Jane Willingham, PhD

Co-occurring disorders

Definition

Co-occurring disorders are sets of mental illnesses that appear together in a single individual. They include a **substance abuse** disorder with at least one other Axis I or Axis II mental illness. The five Axes are standard diagnostic categories established by the **American Psychiatric Association** (APA). In co-occurring disorders, an Axis I substance abuse disorder is always present simultaneously with at least one other mental health disorder from Axis I or II. Another name for co-occurring disorders is dual **diagnosis**, although this may include more than two diagnoses. Dual diagnosis, in this case, means "more than one." Yet another name given this condition is co-morbidity, with morbidity meaning "illness."

Demographics

Children of alcoholics and of drug-addicted individuals are more likely to have co-occurring disorders than America's general population. In addition, patients with **depression** are more at risk for substance abuse and alcohol abuse disorders than people having no mental illness. In addition, the U.S. Department of Health and Human Services has found that people who have received public assistance under welfare-reform programs experienced an average of three or four severe mental disorders (SMDs) in addition to substance abuse, without receiving adequate treatment. The affected homeless population suffers similar circumstances, while youth and the aged are also affected by co-occurring disorders.

Among youth, disruptive behavior disorders occur more frequently with than without substance abuse disorders. Older adults with depression or anxiety are at higher risk for substance and alcohol abuse than middle-aged adults. Seniors may be grieving losses of family, friends, and employment. They may drink or misuse drugs to rid themselves of pain and the complications of poverty. Co-occurring disorders complicate the management of any memory problems they may have, slowing metabolism, arthritis, hypertension, diabetes, **Alzheimer's disease** and other dementias, and various additional health problems. Further, because women generally outlive men, co-occurring disorders and related physical problems are more prevalently becoming the maladies of older women. However, they also affect veterans and people with eating disorders.

Description

The term substance abuse includes substance-use disorders on a continuum from experimentation, to regular use, to drug dependence and **addiction**. Substances include prescription drugs, over-the-counter medications, marijuana, **cocaine**, heroin, mescaline (peyote), glues (sniffing), spray-can aerosols (huffing), and other categories. Substance abuse is the usual co-occurring disorder among adults with SMDs such as **bipolar disorder**, other psychoses, and depression.

Causes and symptoms

Depression itself is the most common mental illness coexisting with physical disorders. Further, depression often occurs among patients with substance abuse, whereas substance abuse can coexist with anxiety, **post-traumatic stress disorder** (PTSD), **personality disorders**, and eating disorders. Co-occurring disorders result in serious problems, such as higher rates of illness **relapse** than in cases of only one mental illness; increased numbers of hospitalizations; and higher risks for violence, incarceration, **homelessness**, **suicide**, and exposure to major infections such as HIV and hepatitis.

Substance or alcohol abuse may co-occur with eating disorders, because such patients self-medicate feelings of shame, anxiety, extreme hunger, and self-hate commonly experienced in eating disorders. This further complicates their recovery. Finally, many military veterans experience anxiety, depression, and/or post-traumatic **stress** disorder (PTSD) at the same time they have a history of substance abuse or alcoholism. Unfortunately, assessment, treatment, and prevention services for veterans have been inadequate.

According to statistics compiled by the U.S. **Substance Abuse and Mental Health Services Administration** (SAMHSA), 10 million Americans or more will develop at least one mental illness together with a substance abuse disorder in any one-year period. The APA has learned that 7% of the American population, or 21 million people, have a full-blown **psychosis** at any given time. Co-occurring disorders affect a full 50% of all individuals who have severe mental disorders such as psychoses. Kessler et al. recently found in a controlled study that 55% of the general population may experience one mental illness, 22% from two, and 23% from three co-occurring disorders. This translates to 69 million Americans having three co-occurring disorders.

SAMSHA has found that the prevalence of co-occurring disorders has increased during the last three decades. Named in the early 1980s, dual diagnoses considered most likely to occur among either youth and young adults with **schizophrenia** or people with bipolar disorder, all of whom showed a history of drug abuse and/or alcohol abuse. The medical opinion was that a person's entrance into the drug culture was the cause of another mental illness. Currently, it is thought that one or more mental disorders occur first, followed by drugs or alcohol used in self-medicating behavior used to cover unwanted mental symptoms.

Diagnosis

Careful assessment by a licensed professional and therapeutic team is necessary to plan effective treatment

KEY TERMS

Axis—One of five diagnostic categories of the American Psychiatric Association that are used for mental health diagnoses. Axis I describes the clinical syndrome or major diagnosis; Axis II lists developmental disorders or intellectual disability and personality disorders; Axis III lists physical disorders; Axis IV includes the severity of psychosocial stressors for the individual; and Axis V describes an individual's highest level of functioning currently and in the past 12 months.

Intervention—A confrontation of a substance abuser by a group of interested people who propose immediate medical treatment. An intervention is also a method of treatment used in therapy.

Substance abuse—Illicit, inaccurate, or recreational use of either prescription or illegal drugs. Alcohol can also be abused as a substance but has its own category, alcohol abuse.

Welfare-to-Work—Several American public reforms of the late 1990s and early 2000s, designed to move individuals from public assistance to paying jobs.

strategies. This begins with a detailed medical history and clinical interviews of the patient and family members to establish related health and behavioral patterns and substance or alcohol abuse history. Because **denial** is an inherent aspect of the problem, a battery of psychiatric tests can uncover mental illnesses. These tests include the **Minnesota Multiphasic Personality Inventory** (MMPI), Rorschach and other inkblot tests, other personality and projective tests, and the **Wechsler intelligence scales**. A number of substance abuse checklists can help determine substance- and alcohol-related disorders.

Treatment

Despite evidence of the high prevalence of dual diagnoses, the U.S. mental health and substance abuse systems have run separate programs, causing confusion. Failure to combine services for coordinated treatment means prolonged suffering and expense for patients, families, insurance companies, the U.S. health care system, and public assistance and disability programs. In light of welfare reform and health care improvements, the 1990s provided many programs for these patients, often more holistic and supported by federal funding for targeting ex-offenders and welfare-to-work populations.

The key factors in an integrated treatment program are (1) treatment must be approached in stages; (2) assertive outreach leads to higher client-retention rates; (3) motivational interventions accompanied by education, counseling, and social support; (4) viewing recovery as a long-term, community-based process; (5) effecting a comprehensive strategy; and (6) cultural sensitivity and cultural competence.

For many dual diagnosis patients, the criminal justice system is their last stop. Many jailed youth fail to be diagnosed. Their behavior mandated their incarceration, and mental health assessment was not considered. The juvenile and adult justice systems have become the treatment providers, but treatment is not always an option. Two-thirds (67%) of incarcerated youth with substance abuse disorders have one or more additional mental illnesses. The coexistence of a **conduct disorder** and/or attention deficit–type disorders with substance abuse results in a serious disability. However, a dual-diagnosis patient in the criminal justice system may never receive psychiatric evaluation or treatment.

One specific problem with treatments for dual diagnoses is that most mental health treatments are designed, tested, and validated through controlled studies of individuals who have only one mental diagnosis. These treatments might not be as effective when there are two or more mental disorders. However, individually prescribed treatment plans have been successful in using these specific components:

- Planned therapeutic interventions: The client is engaged and persuaded to participate in rehabilitation. In planned group and individual therapies, the patients are given coping skills and support toward managing their illnesses.
- Psychological counseling: This includes both cognitive (thinking) and behavioral skills to change negative thinking patterns and unwanted behaviors. It can include role-playing and homework.
- Social counseling: This includes support groups, group therapy, and family therapy facilitated by professionals. It includes diversity and sensitivity training and cultural competency instruction.
- Health-related education: This helps clients commit to managing their illnesses. It requires an acceptance of, and commitment to, a long-term supervised recovery process.
- Aggressive follow-up: A treatment team provides intensive, frequent patient follow-up with meetings in the patient's workplace and home as well as in the case manager's office.
- Comprehensive treatment: This holistic treatment targets education, health, employment, personal behavior patterns, stress management, peer networks, family, housing, financial skills, spiritual life, and other aspects.

Additional considerations

Alcoholics Anonymous, Al-Anon, Narcotics Anonymous, and similar 12-step programs frequently supplement treatment for substance abuse and co-occurring disorders. However, their success cannot be quantitatively validated, because they are anonymous. Further, the direct confrontation of an engagement **intervention** and that of ongoing 12-step programs can be too threatening for mental health patients. The primary care physician or therapist must decide the most appropriate strategies for each patient.

The use of psychiatric drugs to alter mood or behavior is understandably controversial in substance abuse recovery, so treatments such as **support groups** for co-occurring disorders can be more effective than drug therapies.

Prognosis

The prognosis for co-occurring disorders depends on the prognosis of the separate disorders occurring in a specific patient, along with the combined effects of those

QUESTIONS TO ASK YOUR DOCTOR

- What risks are associated with co-occurring disorders?
- What symptoms are associated with co-occurring disorders?
- Does having co-occurring disorders put me at risk for other health conditions?
- Can you recommend any treatments or support groups?

disorders. Dual diagnoses usually present a worse overall health outlook than a single mental illness.

New studies and additional research are ongoing to learn more about co-occurring disorders. **Clinical trials** surrounding the use of various pharmacological and non-pharmacological treatment therapies are ongoing. Individuals who wish to participate can find a list of clinical trials currently enrolling volunteers at http://clinicaltrials.gov. There is no cost to the patient to participate in a clinical trial.

Prevention

Early preventative education, screening, assessment, diagnosis, and treatment are vital to the health of a person experiencing or at risk for co-occurring disorders. Appropriate health-promotion education is useful and necessary in alerting the general populations to the risks and signs of co-occurring disorders and in helping themselves maintain good mental hygiene.

Resources

BOOKS

American Psychiatric Association. *Diagnostic and Statistical Manual of Mental Disorders,* 4th ed., Text rev. Washington, DC: American Psychiatric Association, 2000.

American Psychological Association. *Publication Manual of the American Psychological Association,* 6th ed. Washington, DC: American Psychological Association, 2009.

Erickson, Carlton K, Ph.D. *Addiction Essentials: The Go-To Guide for Clinicians and Patients.* New York: W. W. Norton & Company, 2011.

PERIODICALS

Kessler, Ronald C., et al. "Prevalence, Severity, and Comorbidity of 12-month DSM-IV Disorders in the National Comorbidity Survey Replication." *Archive of General Psychiatry* 62 (2005): 617–627.

Roszak, Dennis J. "Mental Illness Starts Early in Life, but Treatment Often Begins Decades Later." *Hospitals & Health Networks* 79, no. 7 (2005): 130.

Saxena, Shekhar, and Jose Manoel Bertolote. "Co-occurring Depression & Physical Disorders: Need for an Adequate Response from the Health Care System." *Indian Journal of Medical Research.* 122, no. 4 (2005): 273–276.

Watkins, Katherine E., et al. "Prevalence and Characteristics of Clients with Co-occurring Disorders in Outpatient Substance Abuse Treatment." *American Journal of Drug and Alcohol Abuse* 30, no. 4 (2004): 749–764.

WEBSITES

ClinicalTrials.gov. http://www.clinicaltrials.gov/ct/action/GetStudy.

ORGANIZATIONS

American Psychiatric Association, 1000 Wilson Boulevard, Suite 1825, Arlington, VA, 22209, (703) 907-7300, apa@psych.org, http://www.psych.org.

Dual Recovery Anonymous, PO Box 8107, Prairie Village, KS, 66208, (913) 991-2703, http://www.draonline.org/index.html.

Mental Health America, 2000 N. Beauregard Street, 6th Floor, Alexandria, VA, 22311, (703) 684-7722, (800) 969-6642, Fax: (703) 684-5968, http://www1.nmha.org.

National Alliance on Mental Illness (NAMI), Colonial Place Three, 2107 Wilson Blvd., Suite 300, Arlington, VA, 22201, (703) 524-7600, (800) 950-NAMI (6264) Fax: (703) 524-9094, http://www.nami.org.

National Institute of Mental Health (NIMH), 6001 Executive Boulevard, Room 8184, MSC 9663, Bethesda, MD, 20892, (301) 443-4513, (866) 615-6464, Fax: (301) 443-4279, nimhinfo@nih.gov, http://www.nimh.nih.gov/index.shtml.

Patty Inglish, MS
Laura Jean Cataldo, RN, EdD

Couples therapy

Definition

Couples therapy is psychological treatment for couples dealing with relationship problems and issues.

Purpose

The purpose of couples therapy is to improve a relationship and overcome problems and distress within the relationship. Couples therapy can address a wide range of problems between partners, including incompatibility, poor communication, lack of intimacy, and sexual difficulties. It may also address psychological disorders affecting one or both partners, such as **depression**, anxiety, **schizophrenia**, alcoholism, or domestic violence. Couples therapy identifies the causes of dissatisfaction and distress in a relationship and devises and implements a treatment plan for improving or alleviating symptoms and establishing a healthier level of functioning within the relationship.

Description

Couples therapy works to resolve issues affecting a couple's relationship. Couples therapy is available from psychologists, psychiatrists, and psychotherapists, many of whom specialize in treating intimate relationships. There are also proprietary commercial couples therapy programs and organized groups, as well as do-it-yourself couples therapy programs available on the Internet or as smartphone applications.

Types of couples therapy include:

- traditional behavioral
- integrative behavioral
- cognitive-behavioral
- emotionally or emotion focused
- psychoanalytic or psychodynamic
- object relations
- ego analytical
- structural strategic
- systemic
- Gottman method
- educational and preventative

Behavioral therapy models are based on rewarding and reinforcing desired behaviors. Traditional behavioral couples therapy (TBCT or BCT) assumes a link between relationship distress and aversive behaviors or lack of positive **reinforcement** and attempts to decrease negative or punishing interactions and increase positive exchanges. Behavioral therapy models focus on environmental influences, the influences of individual and couple histories, and relationship behaviors. A cornerstone of BCT is helping partners identify, address, and attempt to change problematic patterns of interaction. BCT also emphasizes listening to one's partner, expressing needs without accusation, asking for behavior changes, and developing problem-solving skills.

Integrative behavioral couples therapy (IBCT) was developed in the 1990s by psychologists Andrew Christensen and Neil Jacobson, based on their observations that some couples are unable or unwilling to change or make changes that are short-lived or emotionally unsatisfying for one partner. IBCT aims to increase emotional acceptance and understanding by each partner and to change those patterns that are bothersome to both partners, while building on BCT models of improving behavior, communication, and problem solving. IBCT tends to be more flexible and individualized for specific problems than BCT. In particular, IBCT focuses on repetitious interactions and problems that are causing relationship distress, such as the "demand-withdraw" pattern of interaction identified by Christensen. In this pattern, one partner (more often the woman) identifies a problem and nags the other about it, while the other partner (more often the man) withdraws or avoids the issue. This pattern of behavior has become a major focus of couples therapy, since it correlates directly with relationship dissatisfaction. IBCT also examines larger relationship patterns and how past issues, including those stemming from childhood, affect those patterns.

KEY TERMS

Behavioral couples therapy (BCT)—Traditional behavioral couples therapy (TBCT); relationship therapy based on behavioral psychology models.

Cognition—Conscious intellectual activity, including thinking, imagining, reasoning, remembering, and learning.

Cognitive-behavioral therapy (CBT)—A type of psychotherapy in which people learn to recognize and change negative and self-defeating patterns of thinking and behavior.

Emotionally focused therapy for couples (EFT-C)—A widely used, evidence-based system of therapy, developed in the 1980s by Leslie Greenberg and Susan Johnson, that emphasizes the individual emotions of each partner.

Integrative behavioral couples therapy (IBCT)—A widely used and more flexible and individualized form of behavioral couples therapy, developed by Andrew Christensen and Neil Jacobson in the 1990s.

Introjection—The unconscious incorporation of ideas or attitudes into one's personality or the turning toward oneself of the love or hostility felt for another.

Psychoanalytic—Understanding human motivations, emotions, and mental processes according to theories and concepts originally developed by Sigmund Freud.

Psychodynamic—Mental, emotional, or motivational forces or processes that affect mental state and behavior, especially unconscious processes that develop in early childhood.

Cognitive-behavioral couples therapy, also based on the BCT model, assumes that emotional and behavioral dysfunction in relationships is related to inappropriate information processing, such as "jumping to conclusions" and negative cognitive appraisals. Therefore, it focuses on increasing awareness of perceptions, assumptions, attributions, and/or standards in relationship interactions and on uncovering negative thought forms that drive negative behaviors.

Emotionally or emotion focused therapy for couples (EFT-C) was developed by Leslie Greenberg and Susan Johnson in the 1980s. It has been widely adopted by family therapists as well as couples therapists. EFT-C views emotion and cognition (thinking) as interdependent, with emotion as a primary driver of interpersonal expression. In the EFT-C model, distress stems from the unexpressed and unacknowledged emotional needs of each partner, leading to negative interactions and dysfunction. EFT-C helps couples acknowledge, assess, and express emotions related to their distress. It emphasizes each partner's anger, sadness, shame, and fear, as well as positive emotions, including love and compassion, rather than focusing on interactional processes. EFT-C emphasizes responsiveness to the emotional needs of each partner when discussing and resolving conflicts and recognizing and appreciating interdependence and the need for attachment between partners. Greenberg further argues that conflict results from breakdowns in both the ability to soothe one's self and to soothe one's partner and that the abilities to self-soothe and to regulate one's emotional responses are essential for disrupting negative relationship patterns and beginning to experience the relationship in new ways. Partners who can regulate their own distress are less likely to attack or withdraw.

Psychoanalytic or psychodynamic couples therapy is based on the model that early childhood experiences determine, in part, relationship behaviors. Thus, it attempts to reveal unresolved childhood conflicts with parental figures and connect these with relationship interactions. At the core of this model are the processes of introjection and childhood separation and individuation from maternal interaction. One of the goals of psychoanalytic couples therapy is to separate present feelings from those of one's childhood.

Object relations couples therapy creates a neutral, impartial environment for understanding the distortions and internalized conflicts that each partner brings to the relationship in the form of dysfunctional behaviors. This model proposes that an unconscious desire for a "mothering figure" is the central motivation for selection and attachment to a mate and that this induces further repression of poorly developed aspects of personality or "lost parts."

Ego analytic couples therapy proposes that dysfunction originates in an inability to recognize intolerance, invalidation of sensitivities, and relationship problems themselves. It further proposes that relationship problems fall into two major categories—dysfunctions brought to the relationship from early childhood experiences and **trauma** and feelings of disentitlement on the part of one partner, often due to shame or guilt. Ego analytic therapy uses methods that foster the communication of important feelings.

Structural strategic couples therapy views relationships as progressing through developmental stages. Problems reflect difficulty coping with life changes, either external or personal, and resisting change in the relationship despite dissatisfaction, preferring instead to attempt to maintain status quo baseline functioning. This therapy challenges negative perceptions, encourages positive perceptions through role playing, and presents alternative possibilities and behaviors.

Systemic couples therapy examines the rules and roles adopted by the couple, especially those that have become dysfunctional. The goal is to understand how those patterns shape the relationship and how they can be changed.

The Gottman method, developed by psychologists John and Julie Gottman, is based on the observation that happy couples behave like good friends and handle conflicts in positive ways. The goal of Gottman therapy is to learn more positive means of expression when confronting the inevitable conflicts in a relationship.

Educational and preventative couples therapy attempts to establish good communication early in a relationship. There are several evidence-based programs that focus on open communication, listening skills, and relationship training. The Prevention and Relationship Enhancement Program (PREP) program has been in use since 1989 and is practiced by mental health professionals, lay people, and clergy in 28 countries. The Couples Communication Program involves an "awareness wheel" and a "listening wheel" to help couples trace their issues and learn to listen to one another. The Practical Application of Intimate Relationship Skills (PAIRS) program explores couples' past emotional issues and how these shape their current interactions, with a focus on listening and tackling problems.

Benefits

Couples therapy can help relieve symptomatic behaviors that are causing problems and distress. Therapy can lead to healthier and more appropriate interactions and behaviors. Couples may increase their awareness and develop new relationship skills, particularly when both partners have a reasonable and sincere willingness to confront problems in a positive manner and change patterns of behavior.

Precautions

Couples should seek out a mental health professional who specializes in couples therapy and with whom both partners feel comfortable and able to develop a trusting relationship. A sincere desire to improve relationship patterns, change behaviors, and work with the process is essential for successful couples therapy. Both partners must be honest and cooperative, forthcoming with all necessary information, and willing to keep all appointments.

Preparation

In preparing for couples therapy, both partners must understand that cooperation, honesty, and emotional openness are essential, and both partners should have the desire to modify or change dysfunctional behaviors. Partners should also understand that positive results cannot be guaranteed. During the initial session, the therapist typically performs an extensive assessment that includes in-depth information gathering about the primary problem or problems. The assessment also includes information about occupations, schooling, employment, childhood development, parental history, **substance abuse**, and religion, and the medical, legal, and psychological histories of both partners. Further psychological tests and measurements may be indicated for either or both partners. Following the assessment, the therapist typically suggests a course of treatment.

Aftercare

Couples therapy usually lasts several months or longer, until the relationship is functioning at a level that is satisfactory to both partners and adequate skills have been developed for dealing with conflict. The couple should be alert for a return of old behavior patterns. Relapse-prevention techniques can be employed, and couples are advised to return to therapy if symptoms of **relapse** appear. Sometimes follow-up visits or long-term therapy are required.

Risks

Couples therapy rarely makes a relationship worse. The major risk is that the relationship fails to improve or that dysfunctional patterns return. These circumstances tend to develop when there is a breakdown in the new skills developed during therapy or if one of the partners is resistant to long-term change or cannot overcome self-defeating behaviors.

QUESTIONS TO ASK YOUR DOCTOR

- What type of couples therapy do you recommend?
- What are the advantages of this type of couples therapy?
- What is typically involved in couples therapy?
- How long do you anticipate our couples therapy will last?
- What outcomes have you experienced with couples therapy?

Research and general acceptance

There has been a great deal of research on different types of couples therapy. A 2010 study conducted by Christensen and colleagues, which compared TBCT and IBCT with chronically and severely distressed couples, found that both types yielded a high rate of satisfaction immediately after treatment. Two years after treatment, about 70% of the IBCT-treated couples reported relationship satisfaction, a very high success rate compared with other types of couples therapy. After five years, about one-half of the couples had maintained significantly improved relationships, about one-fourth of the relationships were as distressed as before treatment, and about one-fourth of the couples had separated or divorced. The study did not include follow-up sessions that would normally occur during a crisis or relapse. The U.S. Department of Veterans Affairs has chosen IBCT as its evidence-based **psychotherapy** for couples **intervention**. Christensen intends to make IBCT strategies available to couples as a free online program.

Resources

BOOKS

Abraham, Laurie. *The Husbands and Wives Club: A Year in the Life of a Couples Therapy Group.* New York: Simon & Schuster, 2010.

Baucom, Donald H., Kurt Hahlweg, and Mariann Grawe-Gerber, eds. *Enhancing Couples: The Shape of Couple Therapy to Come.* Cambridge, MA: Hogrefe, 2010.

Greenberg, Leslie S., and Rhonda N. Goldman. *Emotion-Focused Couples Therapy: The Dynamics of Emotion, Love, and Power.* Washington, DC: American Psychological Association, 2008.

Hoistad, Jan. *Romance Rehab: 10 Steps to Rescue Your Relationship.* New York: Sterling, 2010.

Knudson-Martin, Carmen, and Anne Rankin Mahoney. *Couples, Gender, and Power: Creating Change in Intimate Relationships.* New York: Springer, 2009.

O'Leary, K. Daniel, and Erica M. Woodin. *Psychological and Physical Aggression in Couples: Causes and Interventions.* Washington, DC: American Psychological Association, 2009.

Rastogi, Mudita, and Volker K. Thomas. *Multicultural Couple Therapy.* Los Angeles: Sage, 2009.

Schulz, Marc S., ed. *Strengthening Couple Relationships for Optimal Child Development: Lessons from Research and Intervention.* Washington, DC: American Psychological Association, 2010.

PERIODICALS

Christensen, Andrew, et al. "Marital Status and Satisfaction Five Years Following a Randomized Clinical Trial Comparing Traditional Versus Integrative Behavioral Couple Therapy." *Journal of Consulting and Clinical Psychology* 78, no. 2 (April 2010): 225–35.

DeAngelis, Tori. "The Couples Doctor." *Monitor on Psychology* 42, no. 1 (January 2011): 46. http://www.apa.org/monitor/2011/01/christensen.aspx (accessed July 25, 2011).

Garfield, Robert. "Male Emotional Intimacy: How Therapeutic Men's Groups Can Enhance Couples Therapy." *Family Process* 49, no. 1 (March 2010): 109–22.

Greenberg, Leslie, Serine Warwar, and Wanda Malcolm. "Emotion-Focused Couples Therapy and the Facilitation of Forgiveness." *Journal of Marital and Family Therapy* 36, no. 1 (January 2010): 28–42.

Johnson, Susan, and Dino Zuccarini. "Integrating Sex and Attachment in Emotionally Focused Couple Therapy." *Journal of Marital and Family Therapy* 36, no. 4 (October 2010): 431–45.

Luscombe, Belinda. "Honey, Can You Hear Me Now?" *Time* 176, no. 21 (November 22, 2010). http://www.time.com/time/magazine/article/0,9171,2030914,00.html (accessed July 25, 2011).

Tambling, Rachel B., and Lee N. Johnson. "Client Expectations About Couple Therapy." *American Journal of Family Therapy* 38, no. 4 (July 2010): 322–33.

ORGANIZATIONS

American Association for Marriage and Family Therapy, 112 S Alfred St., Alexandria, VA, 22314, (703) 838-9808, Fax: (703) 838-9805, http://www.aamft.org.

American Psychological Association, 750 1st St. NE, Washington, DC, 20002-4242, (202) 336-5500, (800) 374-2721, http://www.apa.org.

Interpersonal Communication Programs, 30772 Southview Dr., no. 200, Evergreen, CO, 80439, (303) 674-2051, (800) 328-5099, Fax: (303) 674-4283, icp@comskills.com, http://www.couplecommunication.com.

PAIRS Foundation, 1675 Market St., Ste. 207, Weston, FL, 33326, (877) PAIRS-4U, info@pairs.com, http://www.pairs.com.

Laith Farid Gulli, MD
Kathleen Berrisford, MSCSW, CAC
Emily Jane Willingham, PhD
Margaret Alic, PhD

Covert sensitization

Definition

Covert sensitization is a form of behavior therapy in which an undesirable behavior is paired with an unpleasant image in order to eliminate that behavior.

Purpose

As with other **behavior modification** therapies, covert sensitization is a treatment grounded in learning theory—one of the basic tenets being that all behavior is learned and that undesirable behaviors can be unlearned under the right circumstances. Covert sensitization is one of a group of behavior therapy procedures classified as covert conditioning, in which an aversive stimulus in the form of a nausea- or anxiety-producing image is paired with an undesirable behavior to change that behavior. It is best understood as a mixture of both the classical and the operant conditioning categories of learning. Based on research begun in the 1960s, psychologists Joseph Cautela and Albert Kearney published the 1986 classic *The Covert Conditioning Handbook*, which remains a definitive treatise on the subject.

The goal of covert sensitization is to directly eliminate the undesirable behavior itself, unlike insight-oriented psychotherapies that focus on uncovering unconscious motives in order to produce change. The behaviors targeted for modification are often referred to as "maladaptive approach behaviors," which includes behaviors such as alcohol abuse, drug abuse, and smoking; pathological gambling; overeating; sexual deviations, and sexually based nuisance behaviors such as obscene phone calling. The type of behavior to be changed and the characteristics of the aversive imagery to be used influence the treatment, which is usually administered in an outpatient setting either by itself or as a component of a multimodal program. Self-administered homework assignments are almost always part of the treatment package. Some therapists incorporate covert sensitization with hypnosis in the belief that outcome is enhanced.

Description

The patient being treated with covert sensitization can expect a fairly standard set of procedures. The therapist begins by assessing the problem behavior, and will most likely measure frequency, severity, and the environment in which it occurs. Depending upon the type of behavior to be changed, some therapists may also take treatment measures before, during, and after physiological arousal (such as heart rate) to better

KEY TERMS

Covert—Concealed, hidden, or disguised.

Operant—Conditioning in which the desired response is reinforced by an introduced stimulus.

Sensitization—To make sensitive or susceptible.

assess treatment impact. Although the therapeutic relationship is not the focus of treatment, the behavior therapist believes that good rapport will facilitate a more successful outcome and strives to establish positive but realistic expectations. Also, a positive relationship is necessary to establish patient confidence in the rationale for exposure to the discomfort of unpleasant images.

The therapist will explain the treatment rationale and protocol. Patient understanding and consent are important, since, by intention, he or she will be asked to experience images that arouse unpleasant and uncomfortable physical and psychological associations. The therapist and patient collaborate in creating a list of aversive images uniquely meaningful to the patient that will be applied in the treatment. Standard aversive images include vomiting, snakes, spiders, vermin, and embarrassing social consequences. An aversive image is then selected appropriate to the target problem behavior. Usually, the image with the most powerful aversive response is chosen. The patient is instructed on how to relax—an important precursor to generating intense imagery. The patient is then asked to relax and imagine approaching the situation where the undesirable behavior occurs (for example, purchasing donuts prior to overeating).

If the patient has a difficult time imagining the scene, the image may be presented verbally by the therapist. As the patient imagines getting closer to the situation (donut store), he or she is asked to clearly imagine an unpleasant consequence (such as vomiting) just before indulging in the undesirable behavior (purchasing donuts and overeating). The scene must be imagined with sufficient vividness that a sense of physiological discomfort or high anxiety is actually experienced. Then the patient imagines leaving the situation and experiencing considerable relief. The patient learns to associate unpleasant sensations (nausea and vomiting) with the undesirable behavior, leading to decreased desire and avoidance of the situation in the future. An alternative behavior incompatible with the problem behavior may be recommended (eat fruit when hungry for a donut).

The patient is given the behavioral homework assignment to practice self-administering the treatment. The patient is told to alternate the aversive scenes with scenes of self-controlled restraint in which he or she rejects the undesirable behavior before indulging in it, thus avoiding the aversive stimulus. The procedure is practiced several times with the therapist in the office, and the patient practices the procedure 10 to 20 times during each home session between office sessions. The patient is then asked to practice in the actual situation, imagining the aversive consequences and avoiding the situation. With much variation, and depending upon the nature of the behavior targeted for change, the patient may see the therapist anywhere from 5 to 20 sessions over a period of a few weeks to several months. The treatment goal is to eliminate the undesirable behavior altogether.

Aftercare

Patients completing covert sensitization treatment are likely to be asked by the therapist to return periodically over the following six to twelve months or longer, for booster sessions to prevent **relapse**.

Risks

Covert sensitization is comparatively risk-free. This is in contrast to the medical and ethical concerns raised by some other aversive procedures such as **aversion therapy**, in which potent chemical and pharmacological stimulants may be used as aversants.

Results

Depending upon the objectives established at the beginning of treatment, patients successfully completing covert sensitization might expect to stop the undesirable behavior. If they practice **relapse prevention** techniques, they can expect to maintain the improvement. Although this treatment may appear to be relatively simple, it has been found to be quite effective for treating many circumscribed problem behaviors.

Resources

BOOKS

Cautela, Joseph, and Albert Kearney. *The Covert Conditioning Handbook*. New York: Brooks/Cole Publishing Co., 1993.

Kaplan, Harold, and Benjamin Sadock, eds. *Synopsis of Psychiatry*. 10th ed. Baltimore: Lippincott Williams & Wilkins, 2007.

Plaud, Joseph, and Georg Eifert, eds. *From Behavior Theory to Behavior Therapy*. Boston: Allyn and Bacon, 1998.

ORGANIZATIONS

Association for Behavioral and Cognitive Therapies, 305 Seventh Ave., 16th Floor, New York, NY, 10001-6008, (212) 647-1890, Fax: (212) 647-1865, http://www.abct.org.

John Garrison, PhD

Creative therapies *see* **Art therapy; Dance therapy; Journal therapy; Music therapy**

Creutzfeldt-Jakob disease *see* **Dementia**

KEY TERMS

Bipolar disorder—A mood disorder characterized by abnormally high energy levels and moodiness, usually without depression.

Depression—A psychiatric disorder involving feelings of hopelessness and symptoms of fatigue, sleeplessness, suicidal tendencies, and poor concentration.

Schizophrenia—A mental disorder involving degraded thinking and emotions.

Crisis housing

Definition

Crisis housing (or sometimes also called crisis residential services) consists of supervised short-term residential alternatives to **hospitalization** for adults with serious mental illnesses or children with serious emotional or behavioral disturbances. Treatment for such crisis services consists of unlocked, non-hospital facilities in a round-the-clock setting.

Purpose

The purpose of crisis housing is to avoid hospitalization and to stabilize the patient. During this time, a determination is made as to the next steps to take for the recovery of the patient. The course of most serious mental illness (such as **schizophrenia**, **bipolar disorder**, severe **depression**, and **borderline personality disorder**) is cyclical, typically characterized by periods of relative well-being, interrupted by periods of deterioration or **relapse**. When relapse occurs, the individual generally exhibits florid symptoms that require immediate psychiatric attention and treatment. More often than not, relapse is caused by the individual's failure to comply with a prescribed medication regimen (not taking medication regularly, not taking the amount or dose prescribed, or not taking it all). Relapse can also be triggered during periods of great **stress** or can even occur spontaneously, without any marked changes in lifestyle or medication regimen. When these crises recur, the goal of treatment is to stabilize the individual as soon as possible, since research suggests that relapsing patients are also more likely to attempt **suicide**.

Description

Over the past 40 years, crisis housing programs have evolved as short-term, less costly, and less restrictive residential alternatives to hospitalization. Intended to divert individuals from emergency rooms, jails, and hospitals into community-based treatment settings, they offer intensive crisis support to individuals and their families. Services include **diagnosis**, assessment, and treatment (including medication stabilization); rehabilitation; and links to community-based services. These programs are intended to stabilize the individual as rapidly as possible—usually between 8 and 60 days—so they can return to their home or residence in the community.

Some of the earliest crisis housing programs include Soteria House and La Posada, which began in northern California in the 1970s, and the START (short-term acute residential treatment) program, which began in San Diego, California, in 1980. While programs vary from location to location, most offer acute services 24 hours a day, seven days a week, in a small noninstitutional residential setting. Adequate structure and supervision is provided by an interdisciplinary team of professionals and other trained workers.

Beginning the day they arrive, residents help develop their own plans for recovery and continued care in the community. Patients receive state-of-the art psychopharmacological treatment and other cognitive-behavioral interventions. Residents are encouraged to play an active role in the operation of the household, including meal preparation. The home-like environment is helpful in lessening the **stigma** and sense of failure that often occurs when someone needs to return to an inpatient psychiatric unit.

Similarly, in the case of seriously emotionally disturbed children and adolescents, the goal of crisis housing is to avert visits to the emergency room or hospitalization by stabilizing the individual in as normal a setting as possible. Compared to these services for adults, there is typically greater emphasis placed on involving families and schools in planning for community-based care after discharge.

Evaluations of several of these programs suggest that they may provide high-quality treatment and care at a lower cost than hospitals. In 2008, a study published by the *American Journal of Community Psychology* found that people with serious psychiatric conditions got better faster and paid less money when at a facility using a "consumer-managed residential program" (CRP), as opposed to staying at a traditional psychiatric hospital. Crisis housing is not currently available in all communities, although it is becoming more widely available.

Preparation

A wide variety of crisis housing programs exist in the United States. Some patients go into crisis housing after being directly released from psychiatric emergency rooms at hospitals or other such medical facilities. Other patients use crisis housing after being briefly admitted into a hospital, in what is considered a "step down" program that slowly treats such patients with a number of steps designed to return their lives to normalcy. Still others admit themselves directly, or do so with the help of a trusted medical professional, while bypassing such medical facilities all together. Physicians and other medical professionals, such as psychologists, help to monitor these patients. In addition, in some of the more difficult cases, treatment is over a longer period of time (around 30 to 60 days), while in other simpler cases the period is much shorter (less than 12 days).

Aftercare

Once the short-term crisis housing care has been completed, the patient has become more stable and is now ready for further help based on their stay at such crisis housing facilities.

Risks

There are always risks when interacting with people with serious mental illnesses or chronic emotional or behavioral disturbances. However, the crisis housing setting has been shown to be an effective way to treat such people in the short-term.

Results

Medical studies have shown over the past forty years that crisis housing produces outcomes that are equal to or better than inpatient services (such as psychiatric hospitals). In addition, these studies have found that the costs of such crisis housing programs are also less expensive than with inpatient facilities; in fact, such research has shown that costs can be 25%–75% less. Recent publications involving such comparisons show that even the most difficult cases can be successfully treated at crisis housing facilities.

QUESTIONS TO ASK YOUR DOCTOR

- How long will I need to stay at crisis housing?
- Could you explain further what is meant by crisis housing?
- Will my health insurance pay for such services?
- Will I be able to leave crisis housing if I wish?
- Will you be able to see me while I'm in crisis housing?

See also Bipolar disorder; Borderline personality disorder; Crisis intervention; Schizophrenia

Resources

BOOKS

Beck, Aaron T., and Brad A. Alford. *Depression: Causes and Treatments.* Philadelphia: University of Pennsylvania Press, 2009.

Clark, David A., and Aaron T. Beck. *Cognitive Therapy of Anxiety Disorders: Science and Practice.* New York: Guilford Press, 2010.

Clark, David A., Aaron T. Beck, and Brad A. Alford. *Scientific Foundations of Cognitive Theory and Therapy of Depression.* New York: John Wiley & Sons, 2003.

Johnson, Sandra J. *Assertive Community Treatment: Evidence-based Practice or Managed Recovery.* New Brunswick, NJ: Transaction, 2011.

Nezu, Arthur, George F. Ronan, and Elizabeth A. Meadows, editors. *Practitioner's Guide to Empirically Based Measures of Depression.* New York: Springer Publishing Company, 2006.

Tolman, Anton O. *Depression In Adults: The Latest Assessment And Treatment Strategies.* Kansas City, MO: Compact Clinicals, 2005.

Torrey, E. Fuller. *Surviving Schizophrenia: A Manual for Families, Consumers and Providers,* 5th ed. New York: Collins, 2006.

VandenBos, Gary R., editor. *APA Dictionary of Psychology.* Washington, DC: American Psychological Association, 2007.

PERIODICALS

Hawthorne, W.B., et al. "A Randomized Trial of Short-Term Acute Residential Treatment for Veterans." *Psychiatric Services* 56 (2005): 1379–86.

OTHERS

"Crisis Residential Facilities Healthier Than Psychiatric Hospitals?—Study Finds More Mental Health Improvements At Consumer-Managed Program." Medical News Today. August 19, 2008. http://www.medicalnewstoday.com/articles/118619.php (accessed November 23, 2010).

Crisis Residential Programs. California Institute for Mental Health. http://www.cimh.org/downloads/handouts/November%2016%202005%20Crisis%20Residential%20Services1.doc (accessed November 24, 2010).

ORGANIZATIONS

American Psychiatric Association, 1000 Wilson Blvd., Ste. 1825, Arlington, VA, 22209-3901, (703) 907-7300, apa@psych.org, http://www.psych.org.

American Psychological Association, 750 lst St., NE, Washington, DC, 20002, (202) 336-5500, (800) 374-2721, http://www.apa.org.

Depression and Bipolar Support Alliance, 730 North Franklin St., Ste. 501, Chicago, IL, 60654-7225, (800) 826-3632, Fax: (312) 642-7243, http://www.dbsalliance.org.

National Alliance on Mental Illness, 3803 North Fairfax Dr., Ste. 100, Arlington, VA, 22203, (703) 524-7600, (800) 950-6264, Fax: (703) 524-9094, http://www.nami.org.

National Institute of Mental Health, 6001 Executive Blvd., Rm 8184, MSC 9663, Bethesda, MD, 20892-9663, (301) 443-4513, (866) 615-6464, Fax: (301) 443-4279, nimhinfo@nih.gov, http://www.nimh.nih.gov.

Irene S. Levine, PhD
Emily Jane Willingham, PhD

Crisis intervention

Definition

Crisis **intervention** refers to methods used to offer immediate, short-term help to individuals who experience an event that produces emotional, mental, physical, and behavioral distress or problems. A crisis can be any situation in which an individual perceives a sudden loss of ability to use effective problem-solving and coping skills. Any number of events or circumstances can be considered crises, including life-threatening situations such as natural disasters (e.g., earthquakes, tornadoes, hurricanes), sexual assault or other criminal victimization, medical illness, mental illness, thoughts of **suicide** or homicide, or loss of or drastic changes in relationships (e.g., death of a loved one or divorce).

Purpose

Crisis intervention has several purposes. It aims to reduce the intensity of an individual's emotional, mental, physical, and behavioral reactions to a crisis. Another purpose is to help individuals return to their level of functioning before the crisis. Functioning may be improved above and beyond this by developing new coping skills and eliminating ineffective ways of coping, such as withdrawal, isolation, and **substance abuse**. In this way, individuals are better equipped to cope with future difficulties. Through talking about what happened, and the feelings about what happened, while developing ways to cope and solve problems, crisis intervention aims to assist individuals in recovering from crises and to prevent serious long-term problems from developing. Research documents positive outcomes for crisis intervention, such as decreased distress and improved problem solving.

Description

Individuals are more open to receiving help during crises. A person may have experienced the crisis within the last 24 hours or within a few weeks before seeking help. Crisis intervention is conducted in a supportive manner. The length of time for crisis intervention may range from one session to several weeks, with the average being four weeks. Crisis intervention is not sufficient for individuals with long-standing problems. Session length may range from 20 minutes to two or more hours. Crisis intervention is appropriate for children, adolescents, and younger and older adults. It can take place in a range of settings, such as hospital emergency rooms, crisis centers, counseling centers, mental health clinics, schools, correctional facilities, and other social service agencies. Local and national telephone hotlines are available to address crises related to suicide, domestic violence, sexual assault, and other concerns. They are usually available 24 hours a day, seven days a week.

Responses to crisis

A typical crisis intervention progresses through several phases. It begins with an assessment of what happened during the crisis and the individual's responses to it. There are certain common patterns of response to most crises. An individual's reaction to a crisis can include emotional reactions (e.g., fear, anger, guilt, **grief**), mental reactions (e.g., difficulty concentrating, confusion, nightmares), physical reactions (e.g., headaches, dizziness, **fatigue**, stomach problems), and behavioral reactions (e.g., sleep and appetite problems, isolation, restlessness). Assessment of the individual's potential for suicide and/or homicide is also conducted. Information about the individual's strengths, coping skills, and social support networks is obtained as well.

Education

There is an educational component to crisis intervention. It is critical for individuals to be informed about various responses to crises and informed that they are having normal reactions to an abnormal situation.

Individuals will also be told that the responses are temporary. Although there is not a specific time that people can expect to recover from crises, individuals can help recovery by engaging in coping and problem-solving skills.

Coping and problem solving

Other elements of crisis intervention include helping individuals understand the crisis and their response to it as well as becoming aware of and expressing feelings, such as anger and guilt. Exploring coping strategies is a major focus of crisis intervention. Strategies that the individuals previously used, but that have not been used to deal with the current crisis, may be enhanced or bolstered. Also, new coping skills may be developed. Coping skills may include relaxation techniques and **exercise** to reduce body tension and **stress** as well as putting thoughts and feelings on paper through journal writing instead of keeping them inside. In addition, options for social support or spending time with people who provide a feeling of comfort and caring are addressed. Another central focus of crisis intervention is problem solving. This process involves thoroughly understanding the problem and the desired changes, considering alternatives for solving the problem, discussing the pros and cons of alternative solutions, selecting a solution and developing a plan to try it out, and evaluating the outcome. Cognitive therapy, which is based on the notion that thoughts can influence feelings and behavior, can be used in crisis intervention.

In the final phase of crisis intervention, the professional will review changes the individual made in order to point out that it is possible to cope with difficult life events. Continued use of the effective coping strategies that reduced distress will be encouraged. Assistance will be provided in making realistic plans for the future, particularly in terms of dealing with potential future crises. Signs that the individual's condition is worsening or "red flags" will be discussed. Information will be provided about resources for additional help should the need arise. A telephone follow-up may be arranged for some agreed-upon time.

Preparation

There are many ways to prepare and intervene in a crisis, with results that can vary widely, depending on the severity of the crisis and other such related factors. Some of these ways to deal with the crisis include (1) suicide intervention, (2) critical incident stress debriefing and management, and (3) medical crisis counseling.

Suicide intervention

PURPOSE. Suicidal behavior is the most frequent mental health emergency. The goal of crisis intervention in that case is to keep the individual alive so that a stable state can be reached, and alternatives to suicide can be explored. In other words, the goal is to help the individual reduce distress and survive the crisis.

ASSESSMENT. Suicide intervention begins with an assessment of how likely it is that the individual will attempt suicide in the immediate future. This assessment has various components. The professional will evaluate whether or not the individual has a plan for how the act would be attempted, how deadly the method is (e.g., shooting, overdosing), whether means are available (e.g., access to weapons), and whether the plan is detailed and specific versus vague. The professional will also assess the individual's emotions, such as **depression**, hopelessness, hostility, and anxiety. Past suicide attempts as well as completed suicides among family and friends will be assessed. The nature of any current crisis event or circumstance will be evaluated, such as loss of physical abilities because of illness or accident, unemployment, and loss of an important relationship.

TREATMENT PLAN. A written safekeeping contract may be obtained. This is a statement indicating that individuals will not commit suicide and that they agree to various actions, such as notifying their clinician, family, friends, or emergency personnel, should thoughts of committing suicide again arise. The contract may also include coping strategies that the individuals agree to engage in to reduce distress. If the individuals state that they are not able to do this, then it may be determined that medical assistance is required and voluntary, or involuntary psychiatric **hospitalization** may be implemented. Most individuals with thoughts of suicide do not require hospitalization and respond well to outpatient treatment. Educating family and friends and seeking their support are important aspects of suicide intervention. Individual therapy, **family therapy**, substance abuse treatment, and/or psychiatric medication may be recommended.

KEY TERMS

Coping—In psychology, a term that refers to a person's patterns of response to stress.

Critical incident—Also known as a "crisis event." An event that is stressful enough to overwhelm the coping skills of a person or group.

Stress—A physical and psychological response that results from being exposed to a demand or pressure.

Stressor—A stimulus or event that provokes a stress response in an organism. Stressors can be categorized as acute or chronic, and as external or internal to the organism.

Critical incident stress debriefing and management

DEFINITION. Critical incident stress debriefing (CISD) uses a structured, small-group format to discuss a distressing crisis event. It is the best-known and most widely used debriefing model. Critical incident **stress management** (CISM) refers to a system of interventions that includes CISD as well as other interventions, such as one-on-one crisis intervention, **support groups** for family and significant others, stress-management education programs, and follow-up programs. Originally designed to be used with high-risk professional groups, such as emergency services, public safety, disaster response, and military personnel, it can be used with any population, including children. A trained personnel team conducts this intervention. The team usually includes professional support personnel, such as mental health professionals and clergy. In some settings, peer support personnel, such as emergency services workers, will be part of the debriefing team. It is recommended that a debriefing occur after the first 24 hours following a crisis event, but before 72 hours have passed since the incident.

PURPOSE. This process aims to prevent excessive emotional, mental, physical, and behavioral reactions and **post-traumatic stress disorder** (PTSD) from developing in response to a crisis. Its goal is to help individuals recover as quickly as possible from the stress associated with a crisis.

PHASES OF CISD. There are seven phases to a formal CISD:

1. Introductory remarks: The team sets the tone and rules for the discussion, and encourages participant cooperation.
2. Fact phase: Participants describe what happened during the incident.
3. Thought phase: Participants state the first or main thoughts while going through the incident.
4. Reaction phase: Participants discuss the elements of the situation that were worst.
5. Symptom phase: Participants describe the symptoms of distress experienced during or after the incident.
6. Teaching phase: The team provides information and suggestions that can be used to reduce the impact of stress.
7. Re-entry phase: The team answers participants' questions and makes summary comments.

PRECAUTIONS. Some concern has been expressed in the research literature about the effectiveness of CISD. It has been thought that as long as the provider(s) of CISD have been properly trained, the process should be helpful to individuals in distress. If untrained personnel conduct CISD, then it may result in harm to the participants. CISD is neither **psychotherapy** nor a substitute for it. It is not designed to solve all problems presented during the meeting. In some cases, a referral for follow-up assessment and/or treatment is recommended to individuals after a debriefing.

Medical crisis counseling

Medical crisis counseling is a brief intervention used to address psychological (anxiety, fear, and depression) and social (family conflicts) problems related to chronic illness in the health care setting. It uses coping techniques and builds social support to help patients manage the stress of being newly diagnosed with a chronic illness or suffering a worsening of a medical condition. It aims to help patients understand their reactions as normal responses to a stressful circumstance and to help them function better. Preliminary studies of medical crisis counseling indicate that one to four sessions may be needed. Research is also promising in terms of its effectiveness at decreasing patients' levels of distress and improving their functioning.

QUESTIONS TO ASK YOUR DOCTOR

- What is crisis intervention?
- How will it help me? Why do I need it?
- How long will I need crisis intervention?
- Will my health insurance pay for such services?
- Will I be able to stop crisis intervention at any time if I wish?
- How will I know when I am no longer in need of crisis intervention?

Aftercare

After the short-term crisis has subsided, and crisis intervention is completed, the patient has become more stable and is now ready for further professional assistance based on help provided during this critical time in their lives.

Risks

There are always risks when interacting with people with serious mental illnesses or chronic emotional or behavioral disturbances. However, crisis intervention has been shown to be an effective way to help such people in the short term.

Results

As with any type of interaction with individuals going through an emotional, mental, physical, or behavioral crisis, risks can and do occur. However, with the proper professional help, along with use of established and proven procedures, success is likely achieved during crisis intervention.

Resources

BOOKS

Echterling, Lennis G., Jack Presbury, and J. Edson McKee. *Crisis Intervention: Promoting Resilience and Resolution in Troubled Times.* Upper Saddle River, NJ: Prentice Hall, 2004.

Hendricks, James E., Jerome B. McKean, and Cindy Gillespie Hendricks. *Crisis Intervention: Contemporary Issues for On-Site Interveners.* 3rd ed. Springfield, IL: Charles C. Thomas Publisher, 2003.

Jackson-Cherry, Lisa R, and Bradley T. Erford. *Crisis Intervention and Prevention.* Upper Saddle River, NJ: Pearson, 2010.

James, Richard K. *Crisis Intervention Strategies.* Belmont, CA: Thomson Brooks/Cole, 2008.

Roberts, Albert R. *Crisis Intervention Handbook: Assessment, Treatment, and Research.* New York: Oxford University Press, 2005.

Stone, Howard W. *Crisis Counseling.* Minneapolis: Fortress Press, 2009.

Thyer, Bruce A. "'Tis a Consummation Devoutly to Be Wished." *Foundations of Evidence-Based Social Work Practice,* Albert R. Roberts, and Kenneth R. Yeager, eds. New York: Oxford University Press, 2006.

Wiger, Donald E., and Kathy J. Harowski. *Essentials of Crisis Counseling and Intervention.* New York: John Wiley & Sons, 2003.

PERIODICALS

Allen, Andrea, and others. "An Empirically Informed Intervention for Children Following Exposure to Severe Hurricanes." *The Behavior Therapist* 29, no. 6 (Sept. 2006): 118–24.

Basoglu, Metin, Ebru Salcioglu, and Maria Livanou. "A Randomized Controlled Study of Single-Session Behavioural Treatment of Earthquake-Related Post-Traumatic Stress Disorder Using an Earthquake Simulator." *Psychological Medicine* 37, no. 2 (Feb. 2007): 203–13.

Bruffaerts, Ronny, Marc Sabbe, and Koen Demyttenaere. "Who Visits the Psychiatric Emergency Room for the First Time?" *Social Psychiatry and Psychiatric Epidemiology* 41, no. 7 (July 2006): 580–86.

Everly, George S., Jr., and others. "Introduction to and Overview of Group Psychological First Aid." *Brief Treatment and Crisis Intervention* 6, no. 2 (May 2006): 130–36.

Gard, Betsy A., and Josef I. Ruzek. "Community Mental Health Response to Crisis." *Journal of Clinical Psychology* 62, no. 8 (Aug. 2006): 1029–41.

Roberts, Albert R. "Applying Roberts' Triple ABCD Model in the Aftermath of Crisis-Inducing and Trauma-Inducing Community Disasters." *International Journal of Emergency Mental Health* 8, no. 3 (Summer 2006): 175–82.

Roberts, Albert R. "Juvenile Offender Suicide: Prevalence, Risk Factors, Assessment, and Crisis Intervention Protocols." *International Journal of Emergency Mental Health* 8, no. 4 (Fall 2006): 255–66.

Singer, Jonathan B. "Making Stone Soup: Evidence-Based Practice for a Suicidal Youth With Comorbid Attention Deficit/Hyperactivity Disorder and Major Depressive Disorder." *Brief Treatment and Crisis Intervention* 6, no. 3 (Aug. 2006): 234–47.

Stapleton, Amy B., et al. "Effects of Medical Crisis Intervention on Anxiety, Depression, and Posttraumatic Stress Symptoms: A Meta-Analysis." *Psychiatric Quarterly* 77, no. 3 (Sept. 2006): 231–38.

Vingilis, Evelyn, et al. "Process and Outcome Evaluation of an Emergency Department Intervention for Persons with Mental Health Concerns Using a Population Health Approach." *Administration and Policy in Mental Health and Mental Health Services Research* 34, no. 2 (Mar. 2007): 160–71.

WEBSITES

American Psychiatric Association. "Disaster Psychiatry Tools." http://www.psych.org/Resources/DisasterPsychiatry.aspx (accessed November 14, 2011).

Mentor Research Institute. "What Is Crisis Counseling?" CrisisCounseling.org. October 10, 2006. http://www.crisiscounseling.org/Handouts/Whatiscrisiscounseling.htm (accessed November 24, 2011).

ORGANIZATIONS

Disaster Psychiatry Outreach, PO Box 1228, One Gustave L. Levy Place, New York, NY, 10029-6574, (646) 233-1215, info@disasterpsych.org, http://www.disasterpsych.org.

Substance Abuse and Mental Health Services Administration, 1 Choke Cherry Rd., Rockville, MD, 20857, (877) 726-4727, http://www.samhsa.gov.

Joneis Thomas, PhD
Ruth A. Wienclaw, PhD

Cyclothymic disorder

Definition

Cyclothymic disorder, also known as cyclothymia, is a relatively mild form of bipolar II disorder characterized by mood swings that may appear to be almost within the normal range of emotions. These mood swings range from mild **depression** (dysthymia) to mania of low intensity (**hypomania**).

Demographics

Patients with cyclothymic disorder are estimated to constitute 3%–10% of all psychiatric outpatients. They may be particularly well represented among those with complaints about marital and interpersonal difficulties. In the general population, the lifetime chance of developing cyclothymic disorder is about 1%. The actual percentage of the general population with cyclothymia is probably somewhat higher, however, as many patients may not be aware that they have a treatable disease or seek treatment if they do.

Cyclothymic disorder frequently coexists with **diagnosis** of cyclothymic disorder. The female-to-male ratio in cyclothymic disorder is approximately 3:2. It is estimated that 50%–75% of all patients develop the disorder between the ages of 15 and 25.

Description

Cyclothymic disorder, a symptomatically mild form of bipolar II disorder, involves mood swings ranging from mild depression to mild mania. It is possible for cyclothymia to go undiagnosed, and for individuals with the disorder to be unaware that they have a treatable disease. Individuals with cyclothymia may experience episodes of low-level depression, known as dysthymia; or periods of intense energy, creativity, and/or irritability, known as hypomania; or they may alternate between both mood states. Like other bipolar disorders, cyclothymia is a chronic illness characterized by mood swings that can occur as often as every day and last for several days, weeks, or months. Individuals with this disorder are never free of symptoms of either hypomania or mild depression for more than two months at a time.

Persons with cyclothymic disorder differ in the relative proportion of depressive versus hypomanic episodes that they experience. Some individuals have more frequent depressive episodes, whereas others are more likely to feel hypomanic. Most individuals who seek help for the disorder alternate between feelings of mild depression and intense irritability. Those who feel energized and creative when they are hypomanic and find their emotionally low periods tolerable may never seek treatment.

Causes and symptoms

Causes

Controversy exists over whether cyclothymic disorder is truly a mood disorder in either biological or psychological terms, or whether it belongs in the class of disorders known as **personality disorders**. Despite this controversy, most of the evidence from biological and genetic research supports the placement of cyclothymia within the mood disorder category.

Genetic data provide strong support that cyclothymia is indeed a mood disorder. About 30% of all patients with cyclothymia have family histories of bipolar I disorder, which involves full-blown manic episodes alternating with periods of relative emotional stability. Full-blown depressive episodes are frequently, but not always, part of the picture in bipolar I disorder. Reviews of the family histories of bipolar I patients show a tendency toward illnesses that alternate across generations: bipolar I in one generation, followed by cyclothymia in the next, followed again by bipolar I in the third generation. The general prevalence of cyclothymia in families with bipolar I diagnoses is much higher than in families with other mental disorders or in the general population. It has been reported that about one-third of patients with cyclothymic disorder subsequently develop a major mood disorder.

Most psychodynamic theorists believe that the psychosocial origins of cyclothymia lie in early traumas and unmet needs dating back to the earliest stages of childhood development. Hypomania has been described as a deficiency of self-criticism and an absence of inhibitions. The patient is believed to use **denial** to avoid external problems and internal feelings of depression. Hypomania is also believed to be frequently triggered by profound interpersonal loss. The false feeling of euphoria (giddy or intense happiness) that arises in such instances serves as a protection against painful feelings of sadness, and even possibly anger against the lost loved one.

Symptoms

The symptoms of cyclothymic disorder are identical to those of bipolar I disorder except that they are usually less severe. It is possible, however, for the symptoms of cyclothymia to be as intense as those of bipolar I, but of shorter duration. About one-half of all patients with cyclothymic disorder have depression as their major symptom. These persons are most likely to seek help for their symptoms, especially during their depressed episodes. Other patients with cyclothymic disorder experience primarily hypomanic symptoms. They are less likely to seek help than those who suffer primarily from depression. Almost all patients with cyclothymic disorder have periods of mixed symptoms (both depression and hypomania together) during which time they are highly irritable.

Cyclothymic disorder usually causes disruption in all areas of the person's life. Most individuals with this disorder are unable to succeed in their professional or personal lives as a result of their symptoms. However, a few who primarily display hypomanic episodes are high achievers who work long hours and require little sleep. A person's ability to manage the symptoms of the disorder depends upon a number of personal, social, and cultural factors.

The lives of most people diagnosed with cyclothymic disorder are difficult. The cycles of the disorder tend to be much shorter than in bipolar I. In cyclothymic disorder, mood changes are irregular and abrupt, and can occur within hours. While there are occasional periods of normal mood, the unpredictability of the patient's feelings and behavior creates great **stress** not only for the patient but for those who must live or work with him/her. Patients often feel that their moods are out of control. During mixed periods, when they are highly irritable, they may become involved in unprovoked arguments with family, friends, and coworkers, causing stress to all around them.

It is common for cyclothymic disorder patients to abuse alcohol and/or other drugs as a means of self-medicating. It is estimated that about 5%–10% of all patients with cyclothymic disorder also have substance dependence.

Diagnosis

Since the symptoms tend to be mild, a diagnosis of cyclothymic disorder is usually not made until a person with the disorder is sufficiently disturbed by the symptoms or their consequences to seek help. While there currently are no laboratory tests or **imaging studies** that can detect the disorder, the patient will usually undergo a general physical examination to rule out general medical conditions that are often associated with depressed mood. The patient will also be given a **psychological assessment** to evaluate his/her symptoms, mental state, behaviors, and other relevant data. If the patient's history or other aspects of his or her behavior during the assessment suggest the diagnosis of cyclothymic disorder, friends or family members of the patient may be interviewed to gather additional data.

The manual used by mental health professionals to diagnose mental illnesses is called the ***Diagnostic and Statistical Manual of Mental Disorders***, also known as the *DSM*. The *DSM* specifies six criteria that must be met for a diagnosis of cyclothymic disorder. They are:

- Numerous episodes of hypomania and depression that are not severe enough to be considered major depression. These episodes must have occurred for at least two years in adults or one year in children and adolescents.
- During this period, the individual has not been free from either hypomania or mild depression for more than two months at a time.
- Neither major depression nor mania has been present during the first two years of the disorder. (After the two years, manic or depressive episodes may surface.)
- The individual does not have another disorder such as schizophrenia, schizoaffective disorder, or delusional disorder.
- The symptoms are not due to the direct effects of substance use (such as a drug of abuse or a prescribed medication) or to a medical condition.
- The symptoms cause significant impairment in the patient's social, occupational, family, or other important areas of life functioning.

The *DSM-5* (2013) proposed criteria has added specifiers to account for cyclothymic disorder with mixed features (formerly mixed episodes, or symptoms of mania and major depression concurrently), rapid cycling, anxiety, **suicide** risk, seasonal pattern, and postpartum onset.

Treatment

Traditional

Psychotherapy with individuals diagnosed with cyclothymic disorder is best directed toward increasing the patients' awareness of their condition and helping them develop effective coping strategies for mood swings. Often, considerable work is needed to improve the patient's relationships with family members and workplace colleagues because of damage done to these relationships during hypomanic episodes. Because cyclothymic disorder is a lifelong condition, psychotherapy is also a long-term commitment. Working with families of cyclothymic patients, whether individually or in **family therapy** sessions, can help them adjust more effectively to the patients' mood swings as well. Other forms of therapy include **cognitive-behavioral therapy**, which focuses on identifying triggers and changing behaviors, and **group therapy**, where patients with cyclothymic disorder can relate their experiences.

Drugs

Medication is an important component of treatment for cyclothymic disorder. A class of drugs known as antimanic medications, or mood stabilizers, is usually the first line of treatment for these patients. Lithium (Eskalith, Lithobid) is considered a first-line treatment for hypomanic episodes; other drugs include **carbamazepine** (Tegretol) and sodium valproate (Depakene). **Valproic acid** (Depakene), **divalproex sodium** (Depakote), and **lamotrigine** (Lamictal), all anticonvulsant or antiseizure medications, may be given to help prevent mood swings. Antidepressant medications are generally not recommended for treating cyclothymic disorder and

KEY TERMS

Bipolar I disorder—A major mood disorder characterized by full-blown manic episodes, often interspersed with episodes of major depression.

Bipolar II disorder—Disorder with major depressive episodes and mild manic episodes known as hypomania.

Borderline personality disorder—A severe and usually life-long mental disorder characterized by violent mood swings and severe difficulties in sustaining interpersonal relationships.

Cyclothymia—An alternate name for cyclothymic disorder.

Denial—A psychological defense mechanism that reduces anxiety by excluding recognition of an addiction or similar problem from the conscious mind.

Dysthymia—Depression of low intensity.

Hypomania—A milder form of mania that is characteristic of bipolar II disorder.

Psychodynamic theorists—Therapists who believe that the origins of mental problems lie in a person's internal conflicts and complexes.

Psychosocial—A term that refers to the emotional and social aspects of psychological disorders.

should be used with caution, as the use of **antidepressants** may induce hypomanic or full-blown manic episodes. An estimated 40%–50% of all patients with cyclothymic disorder treated with antidepressants experience such episodes.

Quetiapine (Seroquel), a member of a class of drugs known as atypical antipsychotics, was approved by the U.S. Food and Drug Administration (FDA) in 2008 to treat the depressive and manic episodes of **bipolar disorder** and may have some application for treating cyclothymic disorder.

Prognosis

While some patients later diagnosed with cyclothymic disorder were considered sensitive, hyperactive, or moody as children, the onset of cyclothymic disorder usually occurs gradually during the patient's late teens or early twenties. Often school performance becomes a problem along with difficulty establishing peer relationships. Approximately one-third of all patients with cyclothymic disorder develop a major mood disorder during their lifetime, usually bipolar II disorder.

Prevention

Cyclothymic disorder appears to have a strong genetic component. It is far more common among the first-degree biological relatives of persons with bipolar I disorder than among the general population. At this time, there are no known effective preventive measures that can reduce the risk of developing cyclothymic disorder. Genetic counseling, which assists a couple in understanding their risk of producing a child with the disorder, may be of some help.

Resources

BOOKS

American Psychiatric Association. *Diagnostic and Statistical Manual of Mental Disorders*. 4th ed., text rev. Washington, DC: American Psychiatric Publishing, 2000.

Drevets, Wayne C., and Richard D. Todd. "Depression, Mania, and Related Disorders." In *Adult Psychiatry*, edited by Eugene H. Rubin and Charles F. Zorumski. 2nd ed. Malden, MA: Blackwell Publishing, 2005.

PERIODICALS

Andlin-Sobocki, Patrik, and Hans-Ulrich Wittchen. "Cost of Affective Disorders in Europe." *European Journal of Neurology* 12, Supplement (June 2005): 34–38.

Bisol, Luísa W., and Diogo R. Lara. "Low-dose Quetiapine for Patients with Dysregulation of Hyperthymic and Cyclothymic Temperaments." *Journal of Psychopharmacology* 24, no. 3 (March 2010): 421–24. http://dx.doi.org/10.1177/0269881108097715 (accessed September 1, 2011).

ORGANIZATIONS

American Psychiatric Association, 1000 Wilson Blvd., Ste. 1825, Arlington, VA, 22209-3901, (703) 907-7300, apa@psych.org, http://www.psych.org.

Mental Health Foundation, PO Box 322, Albany, NY, 12201. info@mentalhealthfoundation.net, http://www.mentalhealthfoundation.net.

Barbara S. Sternberg, PhD
Ruth A. Wienclaw, PhD

Cylert *see* **Pemoline**

Cymbalta *see* **Duloxetine**

D

Dalmane *see* **Flurazepam**

Dance therapy

Definition

Dance therapy is a type of **psychotherapy** that uses movement to further the social, cognitive, emotional, and physical development of the individual. Dance therapists work with people who have many kinds of emotional problems, intellectual deficits, and life-threatening illnesses. They are employed in psychiatric hospitals, daycare centers, mental health centers, prisons, special schools, and private practice. They work with people of all ages in both group and individual therapy. Some dance therapists also engage in research.

Dance therapists try to help people develop communication skills, a positive self-image, and emotional stability.

Origins

Dance therapy began as a profession in the 1940s with the work of Marian Chace (1896–1970). A modern dancer, Chace began teaching dance after ending her career with the Denishawn Dance Company in 1930. In her classes, she noticed that some of her students were more interested in the emotions they expressed while dancing (loneliness, **shyness**, fear) than the mechanics of the moves. She encouraged them by emphasizing freedom of movement more than technique.

In time, doctors in the community started sending her patients. They included antisocial children, people with movement problems, and those with psychiatric illnesses. Eventually, Chace became part of the staff of St. Elizabeth's Hospital in Washington, DC. She was the first dance therapist employed in a formal position by the federal government. Chace worked with the emotionally troubled patients at St. Elizabeth's and tried to get them to reach out to others through dance. Some of them had **schizophrenia**, and others were former servicemen suffering from **post-traumatic stress disorder**. Success for these patients meant being able to participate with their class in moving to rhythmic music. Chace is quoted as having said, "This rhythmic action in unison with others results in a feeling of well-being, relaxation, and good fellowship."

Marian Chace eventually studied at the Washington School of Psychiatry and began making treatment decisions about her patients along with other members of the St. Elizabeth's medical team. Her work attracted many followers and the first dance therapy interns began learning and teaching dance therapy at St. Elizabeth's in the 1950s.

Other dancers, such as Trudi Schoop and Mary Whitehouse, began using dance therapy in the 1940s to help people feel more comfortable with themselves and their bodies. Whitehouse later became a Jungian analyst and an influential member of the dance therapy community. She developed a process called "movement in-depth," an extension of her understanding of dance, movement, and depth psychology. She helped found the contemporary movement practice called authentic movement. In this type of movement, founded on the principles of Jungian analysis, patients dance out their feelings about an internal image, often one that can help them understand their past or their current struggles. Whitehead's student, Janet Alder furthered Whitehead's work in authentic movement by establishing the Mary Starks Whitehouse Institute in 1981.

In 1966, dance therapy was formally recognized when the American Dance Therapy Association (ADTA) was formed.

Description

There are more than 1,200 dance therapists in the United Sates and in many foreign countries. Like other mental health professionals, they use a wide range of techniques to help their patients. Some of the major schools

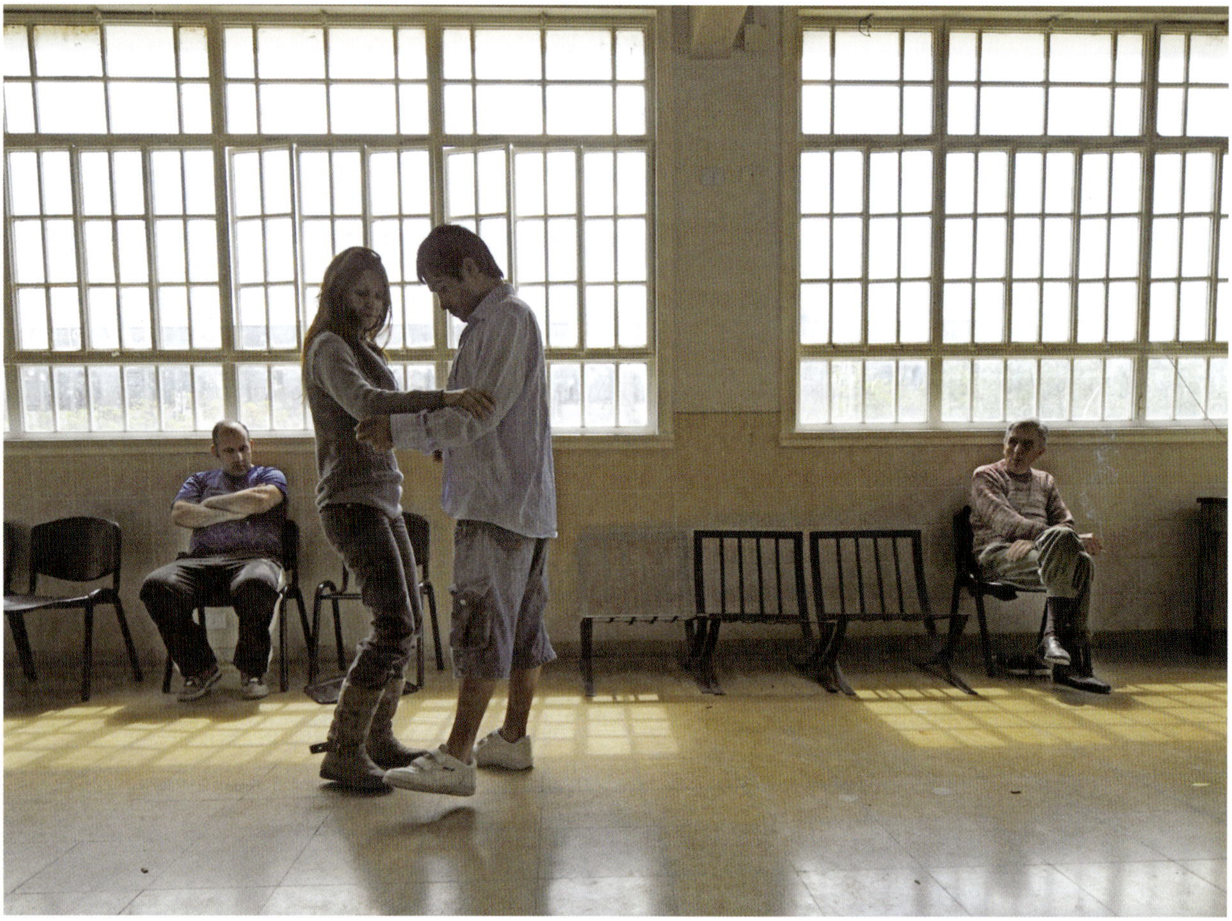

A patient and a nurse dance during a tango therapy session at a neuropsychiatric hospital in Argentina. *(© Daniel Garcia/AFP/Getty Images)*

of thought in dance therapy are the Freudian approach, Jungian technique, and object relations orientation. Many therapists, however, do not adhere to just one school but use techniques from various types of dance therapy.

The authentic movement technique is derived from the Jungian method of analysis, in which people work with recurring images in their thoughts or dreams to derive meaning from their life. Instead of asking the patient to dance out certain emotions, the therapist instructs the patient to move when he or she feels the inner impulse. The moves are directed by the patient, and the therapist is a noncritical witness to the movement. The moves are supposed to emerge from the patient's subconscious. Similarly, in Freudian technique, dance therapists work with patients to uncover feelings hidden deep in the subconscious by expressing those feelings through dance.

In object relations technique, the therapist often helps the patient examine personal problems by considering the primary initial relationship with the patient's parents. Emotions are expressed in a physical way. For instance, a patient might work out his fears of abandonment by repeatedly coming close to and dancing at a distance from the therapist.

Dance therapists sometimes use other types of therapy along with dance, such as visual art or drama. Therapists also discuss what happens during a dancing session by spending time in **talk therapy**. Dance therapists use visualizations during sessions, too. For example, the therapist might instruct patients to imagine they are on a beautiful, peaceful beach as they dance.

In one frequently used technique, the therapist mirrors the movements of the patient as he or she expresses important emotions. This is especially powerful in one-on-one therapy. It is thought that this device provides a sense of safety and validates the patient's emotions.

The underlying premise of dance therapy is that when people dance, they are expressing highly significant emotions. A fist thrust out in anger into the air or a head bent in shame has deep significance to a dance therapist. Through dance therapy, the theory is, patients are able to more easily express painful, frightening emotions and can move past them. After experiencing dance therapy, they can talk about their feelings more freely and remove barriers they have erected between themselves and other people. The hope is that eventually they can go on to live psychologically healthy lives.

Benefits

Dance therapy can be helpful to a wide range of patients—from psychiatric patients to those with cancer to lonely elderly people. Dance therapy is often an easy way for individuals to express emotions, even when their experience is so traumatic they cannot talk about it. It is frequently used with rape victims and survivors of other forms of **sexual abuse** and incest. It can also help people with physical deficits improve their self-esteem and learn balance and coordination.

Dance therapists also work with people who have chronic health problems and life-threatening diseases to help them deal with pain, fear of death, and changes in their body. Many people with such illnesses find dance therapy classes to be a way to relax, get away from their pain and emotional difficulties for a while, and express feelings about taboo subjects (such as impending death).

Dance therapy is suitable for people who are not accomplished dancers and may even be good for those who are clumsy on the dance floor. The emphasis in dance therapy is on free movement, not restrictive steps, and expressing one's true emotions. Children who cannot master difficult dances or cannot sit still for traditional psychotherapy often benefit from free-flowing dance therapy. Even older people who cannot move well or are confined to wheelchairs can participate in dance therapy. All they need to do is move in some way to the rhythm of the music.

Dance therapy can be useful in a one-on-one situation, in which the therapist works with only one patient to provide a safe place to express emotions. Classes can help provide emotional support, enhanced communication skills, and appropriate physical boundaries (a skill that is vital for sexual abuse victims).

Preparations

People who want to use dance therapy should find a qualified therapist. The ADTA provides lists of qualified therapists. Individuals who try dance therapy benefit especially if they have an open mind and a willingness to participate.

KEY TERMS

Authentic movement—A type of movement that is influenced heavily by Jungian analysis and works by analyzing the internal images of the patient. Patients are also urged to dance only when they feel the impulse to move.

Freudian analysis—A psychological treatment based on the theories developed by Sigmund Freud, in which the therapist seeks to help the patient resolve conflicts and traumas buried in the subconscious.

Jungian analysis—A psychological treatment based on the theories of Carl Jung, in which the patient strives to understand the internal, often mythic images in thoughts and dreams.

Psychotherapy—A psychological treatment that seeks to resolve traumas and emotional conflicts, often by discussing them and emotionally reliving difficult past events.

Test anxiety—A name for the stress and intensity of emotional upset that students experience before they take exams.

Precautions

Qualified dance therapists should have completed a graduate program in dance therapy approved by the ADTA and should be registered with the ADTA. They should be able to dance, and they should have extensive training in psychology.

Side effects

There are no known side effects from dance therapy.

Research & general acceptance

Dance therapy was once dismissed as an ineffective, feel good treatment, but it is now more respected. Many research studies have proven that dance therapy can be an effective tool to help people overcome psychological problems.

In one study, older people with cognitive deficits showed that dance therapy could significantly increase their functional abilities. Patients improved their balance, rhythmic discrimination, mood, and social interaction.

In 1999, a pilot study of 21 university students showed that those who took a series of four or five group dance therapy sessions in a period of two weeks

> **QUESTIONS TO ASK YOUR DOCTOR**
>
> - Do I have any physical limitations that would prohibit my undertaking dance therapy?
> - What kind of changes can I expect to see or feel with dance therapy?
> - Will dance therapy interfere with my current medications?
> - Can you recommend any support groups for me and my family?

significantly reduced their test anxiety as measured by the Test Anxiety Inventory. Afterwards, the subjects reported that their dance movement experience was positive and provided them with psychological insight. The researchers concluded that dance therapy could be a viable method of treatment for students who suffer from overwhelming test anxiety and should be researched further.

In another study presented at the ADTA national conference, dance therapist Donna Newman-Bluestein reported success in using techniques of dance therapy with cardiac patients. In a **stress reduction** class, health professionals used dance therapy methods to teach body awareness, relaxation, self-expression, creativity, and empathy. According to Newman-Bluestein, the dance therapy techniques helped the patients deal with such stressful emotions as anger, increased their self-awareness, made them more relaxed, and helped them adjust emotionally to having heart disease.

Training & certification

Dance therapists should have dance experience and a liberal arts background with coursework in psychology in their undergraduate degree. Professional dance therapy training takes place on the graduate level. A qualified dance therapist has received a graduate degree from a school approved by the ADTA or has a master's degree in dance or psychology and has taken additional dance therapy credits.

After graduation, dance therapists can become registered with the ADTA, meaning that they are qualified to practice. After two years they may receive an additional recognition when they become a registered Academy of Dance therapist. They can then teach dance therapy and can supervise interns.

Dance therapists can also obtain psychological credentials by taking a test and becoming registered by the National Board for Certified Counselors.

Resources

BOOKS

Brooke, Stephanie L., ed. *The Use of the Creative Therapies With Autism Spectrum Disorders*. Springfield, IL: Charles C. Thomas Publisher, 2009.

Chaiklin, Sharon, and Hilda Wengrower, eds. *The Art and Science of Dance/Movement Therapy: Life is Dance*. New York: Routledge, 2009.

Rennie, Jeanette, ed. *Learning Disability: Physical Therapy Treatment and Management, A Collaborative Approach*. West Sussex, England: John Wiley & Sons, 2009.

PERIODICALS

Brody, Jane. "Dancing Shoes Replace the Therapist's Couch." *The New York Times* (18 October 1995): C13.

Erwin-Grabner, Tracy, et al. "Effectiveness of Dance/Movement Therapy on Reducing Test Anxiety." *American Journal of Dance Therapy* 21, no. 1 (Spring/Summer 1999) 19–34.

Gold, D.T., et al. "Factors Associated with Persistence with Teriparatide Therapy: Results from the DANCE Observational Study." *Journal of Osteoporosis* 2011: 314970.

ORGANIZATIONS

American Dance Therapy Association, 10632 Little Patuxent Parkway, Ste. 108, Columbia, MD, 21044, (410) 997-4040, Fax: (410) 997-4048, http://www.adta.org.

Barbara Boughton
Laura Jean Cataldo, RN, EdD

Deinstitutionalization

Definition

Deinstitutionalization is a long-term trend wherein fewer people reside as patients in mental hospitals and fewer mental health treatments are delivered in public hospitals. This trend is directly due to the process of closing public hospitals and the ensuing transfers of patients to community-based mental health services in the late twentieth century. It represents the dissipation of patients over a wider variety of healthcare settings and geographic areas. Deinstitutionalization also illustrates evolution in the structure, practice, experiences, and purposes of mental health care in the United States.

Demographics

The trend called deinstitutionalization forces some individuals who have previously been housed within mental institutions, for such problems as **bipolar disorder**, **depression**, and **schizophrenia**, to take care of themselves without professional help or to rely on other means than such institutions. In most cases, these individuals receive comparable help within local community settings, such as shelters or nursing homes. However, in a few circumstances, these individuals become homeless. Sometimes, without proper preparation for life in society, they break the law and end up in jail or prison. In other cases, they become victims of criminals. The more fortunate ones seek refuge with family and friends who provide them support.

Description

History

In the United States in the nineteenth century, hospitals were built to house and care for people with chronic illness, and mental health care was a local responsibility. As with most chronic illness, **hospitalization** did not always provide a cure. Individual states assumed primary responsibilities for mental hospitals beginning in 1890. In the first part of the twentieth century, while mental health treatments had very limited efficacy, many patients received custodial care in state hospitals. Custodial care refers to care in which the patient is watched and protected, but a cure is not sought.

After the founding of the National Institutes of Mental Health (NIMH), new psychiatric medications were developed and introduced into state mental hospitals beginning in 1955. These new medicines brought new hope, and helped address some of the symptoms of mental disorders.

President John F. Kennedy's 1963 **Community Mental Health** Centers Act accelerated the trend toward deinstitutionalization with the establishment of a network of community mental health centers. In the 1960s, with the introduction of Medicare and Medicaid, the federal government assumed an increasing share of responsibility for the costs of mental health care. That trend continued into the 1970s with the implementation of the Supplemental Security Income program in 1974. State governments helped accelerate deinstitutionalization, especially of elderly people. In the 1960s and 1970s, state and national policies championed the need for comprehensive community mental health care, though this ideal was slowly and only partially realized.

Beginning in the 1980s, **managed care** systems began to review systematically the use of inpatient hospital care for mental health. Both public concerns and private health insurance policies generated financial incentives to admit fewer people to hospitals and discharge inpatients more rapidly, limit the length of patient stays, or to transfer responsibility to less costly forms of care.

Indicators and trends

Many statistical indicators show the amount of inpatient hospital care for persons with mental illness decreased during the latter half of the twentieth century, while the total volume of mental health care increased.

A patient care episode is a specific measure of the volume of care provided by an organization or system. It begins when a person visits a healthcare facility for treatment and ends when the person leaves the facility. In 1955 77% of all patient care episodes in mental health organizations took place in 24-hour hospitals. By 1994, although the numbers of patient care episodes increased by more than 500%, only 26% of mental health treatment episodes were in these hospitals. The timing of this trend varied across different states and regions, but it was consistent across a variety of indicators.

The number of inpatient beds available to each group of 100,000 civilians decreased from over 200 beds in 1970 to less than 50 in 1992. The average number of patients in psychiatric hospitals decreased from over 2,000 in 1958 to about 500 in 1978. While adjusted per-capita spending on mental health rose from $16.53 in 1969 to $19.33 in 1994, the portion of funds spent on state and county mental hospitals fell from $9.11 to $4.56.

In 2009, according to the U.S. Centers for Disease Control and Prevention (CDC), 3.2% of adults in the United States, who were not living within mental institutions, had serious psychological distress. The CDC also stated that 67% of residents in nursing homes had mental disorders, approximately 996,000 people within the country.

Transinstitutionalization

Trends toward deinstitutionalization also reflect shifting demographics and boundaries of care. For example, decreases in inpatient mental health care can be complemented by increases in outpatient mental health care. Decreases in inpatient mental health care can also be paired with increases in other forms of care, such as social welfare, criminal justice, or nursing home care. Thus, deinstitutionalization is part of a process sometimes called transinstitutionalization, the transfer of institutional populations from hospitals to jails, nursing homes, and shelters.

Causes and consequences

Causes

Deinstitutionalization, originally and idealistically portrayed by advocates and consumers as a liberating, humane policy alternative to restrictive care, may also be

KEY TERMS

Bipolar disorder—A mood disorder characterized by abnormally high energy levels and moodiness, usually without depression.

Depression—A psychiatric disorder involving feelings of hopelessness and symptoms of fatigue, sleeplessness, suicidal tendencies, and poor concentration.

Mental disorder—A psychiatric disorder of mental faculties.

Schizophrenia—A mental disorder involving degraded thinking and emotions.

interpreted as a series of health policy reforms that are associated with the gradual demise of mental health care dependent on large, state-supported hospitals. Deinstitutionalization is often attributed to decreased need for hospital care and to the advent of new psychiatric medicines.

Consequences

Ideally, deinstitutionalization represents more humane and liberal treatment of mental illness in community-based settings. Pragmatically, it represents a change in the scope of mental health care from longer, custodial inpatient care to shorter outpatient care.

The process of deinstitutionalization, combined with the scarcity of community-based care, is also associated with the visible problems of **homelessness**. Between 30% and 50% of homeless people in the United States are people with mental illness, and people with mental illness are disproportionate among the homeless.

Diagnosis

Deinstitutionalization also describes the adjustment process whereby people with illness are removed from the effects of life within institutions. Since people may become socialized to highly structured institutional environments, they often adapt their social behavior to institutional conditions. Therefore, adjusting to life outside of an institution may be difficult.

Treatment

Defined experientially, deinstitutionalization allows individuals to regain freedom and empower themselves through responsible choices and actions. With the assistance of **social workers** and through psychiatric rehabilitation, former inpatients can adjust to everyday life outside of institutional rules and expectations. This aspect of deinstitutionalization promotes hope and recovery, ongoing debates over the best structure and process of mental health service delivery notwithstanding.

Prognosis

Differing views exist among mental health professionals, advocacy groups, citizens, public officials, family members, and others as to what is best for individuals with intellectual disabilities. Discussions continue as to the most efficient and beneficial ways to deal with these individuals.

In 2007, Dr. Benedetto Saraceno, as the director of Mental Health and **Substance Abuse** within the World Health Organization (WHO), commented on the effectiveness of community based health services. Dr. Saraceno stated, "Not only are community mental health services more accessible to people living with severe mental disabilities, these are also more effective in taking care of their needs compared to mental hospitals. Community mental health services are also likely to have less possibilities for **neglect** and violations of human rights, which are too often encountered in mental hospitals."

However, in too many cases an effective network of these community mental health services are not available to help people with severe mental disabilities. Dr. Saraceno urged all countries to provide such networks for the nearly 54 million people with severe mental disorders around the world.

In whatever manner the United States and other countries proceed with regards to handling mental illness—through deinstitutionalization or other such means—mental illness has been proven to be a significant negative component on the health and productivity of people throughout the world. For instance, a comprehensive 2004 study (updated in 2008) called the Global Burden of Disease (GBD), conducted by WHO, the World Bank, and Harvard University, found that mental illness contributes about 15% to all diseases within economies of developed countries.

Prevention

The problem of mental health, especially homelessness, is partially addressed through prevention programs, which are generally considered less costly and more effective than previous programs. Although deinstitutionalization programs have helped with regards to mental illness, there is still much to do and much still wrong with the system. Barriers, such as lack of knowledge and prejudices, still exist concerning mentally ill people. Community based services such as those provided from day-care centers, schools, and community centers continue to improve on the mental health issue in the United States and around the world. These institutions help to enhance the ongoing process of deinstitutionalization.

Resources

BOOKS

Johnson, Sandra J. *Assertive Community Treatment: Evidence-based Practice or Managed Recovery.* New Brunswick, NJ: Transaction, 2011.

McLeod, Jane D., and Eric R. Wright, editors. *The Sociology of Mental Illness: A Comprehensive Reader.* New York City: Oxford University Press, 2010.

Moritsugu, John, Frank Y. Wong, and Karen Grover Duffy. *Community Psychology.* Boston: Allyn & Bacon, 2010.

Scheid, Teresa L., and Tony N. Brown, eds. *A Handbook for the Study of Mental Health: Social Contexts, Theories, and Systems.* Cambridge: Cambridge University Press, 2010.

Torrey, E. Fuller. *The Insanity Offense: How America's Failure to Treat the Seriously Mentally Ill Endangers its Citizens.* New York City, W.W. Norton, 2008.

VandenBos, Gary R., editor. *APA Dictionary of Psychology.* Washington, DC: American Psychological Association, 2007.

WEBSITES

Centers for Disease Control and Prevention. "Mental Health." http://www.cdc.gov/nchs/fastats/mental.htm (accessed December 2, 2011).

National Institutes of Mental Health. "Mental Health Topics: Statistics." August 6, 2009. http://www.nimh.nih.gov/health/topics/statistics/index.shtml (accessed December 2, 2011).

World Health Organization. "Community Mental Health Services will Lessen Social Exclusion, says WHO." June 1, 2007. http://www.who.int/mediacentre/news/notes/2007/np25/en/index.html (accessed December 2, 2011).

——— "Global Burden of Disease." October 27, 2010. http://www.who.int/topics/global_burden_of_disease/en (accessed December 2, 2011).

ORGANIZATIONS

American Psychiatric Association, 1000 Wilson Blvd., Ste. 1825, Arlington, VA, 22209-3901, (703) 907-7300, apa@psych.org, http://www.psych.org.

American Psychological Association, 750 1st St. NE, Washington, DC, 20002-4242, (202) 336-5500; TDD/TTY: (202) 336-6123, (800) 374-2721, http://www.apa.org.

American Sociological Association, 1430 K St. NW, Ste. 600, Washington, DC, 20005, (202) 383-9005, Fax: (202) 638-0882, http://www.asanet.org.

National Institute of Mental Health, 6001 Executive Blvd., Rm. 8184, MSC 9663, Bethesda, MD, 20892-9663, (301) 433-4513; TTY: (301) 443-8431, Fax: (301) 443-4279, (866) 615-6464; TTY: (866) 415-8051, nimhinfo@nih.gov, http://www.nimh.nih.gov.

Substance Abuse and Mental Health Services Administration Referral Resource, 1 Choke Cherry Rd., Rockville, MD, 20857, (877) SAMHSA-7 (726-4727), (800) TTY: 487-4889, Fax: (240) 221-4292, SAMHSAInfo@samhsa.hhs.gov, http://www.samhsa.gov.

Michael Polgar, PhD

Delirium

Definition

Delirium is a medical condition characterized by a general disorientation accompanied by cognitive impairment, mood shift, self-awareness, and inability to focus and maintain attention. The change occurs over a short period of time—hours to days—and the disturbance in consciousness fluctuates throughout the day.

Demographics

Children, possibly because of their immature **brain** development and physiological differences from adults, can be particularly susceptible to delirium. This susceptibility is most common in association with fevers or some kinds of medications (such as anticholinergics, medications used for motor control problems). A child in a state of delirium may exhibit behavior that can be mistaken for willful lack of cooperation.

The elderly are also particularly sensitivity to delirium, also probably because of differences in physiology as the body ages. Being male and elderly enhances this risk.

Description

The word delirium comes from the Latin *delirare*. In its Latin form, the word means to become crazy or to rave. A phrase often used to describe delirium is "clouding of consciousness," meaning the person has a diminished awareness of their surroundings. In the ***Diagnostic and Statistical Manual of Mental Disorders***, fourth edition, text revision (*DSM-IV-TR*), delirium is categorized based on its assumed causes; for example, "Substance-Induced Delirium." Disorders involving delirium are listed in the same section as those involving **dementia**, but the two conditions differ in several characteristics. Dementia, for example, may exhibit a longer developmental process and is typically accompanied by multiple cognitive deficits.

While the delirium is active, the person tends to fade in and out of lucidity, meaning that he or she will sometimes appear to know what's going on, but at other times may show disorientation to time, place, person, or situation. The longer the delirium goes untreated, the more progressive the disorientation becomes. It usually begins with disorientation to time, during which a patient will declare it to be morning, even though it may be late at night. Later, the person may state that he or she is in a different place rather than at home or in a hospital bed. Still later, the patient may not recognize loved ones, close friends, or relatives, or may insist that a visitor is someone else altogether. Finally, the patient may not recognize the reason for his or her **hospitalization**. This waxing and waning of consciousness is often worse at the end of a day, a phenomenon known as "sundowning."

A delirious patient has a difficult time with most mental operations, including understanding, judgement, and inference. Because the patient cannot maintain awareness of his or her environment, disorientation can result. Nevertheless, disorientation and memory loss are not essential to the **diagnosis** of delirium; the inability to focus and maintain attention, however, is essential to rendering a correct diagnosis. Left unchecked, delirium tends to transition from inattention to increased levels of lethargy, leading to torpor, stupor, and coma. In its other form, delirious patients become agitated and almost hypervigilant, with a dramatically altered sleep-wake cycle that fluctuates between great guardedness and **hypersomnia** (excessive drowsiness) during the day and wakefulness during the night. Delirious patients may also experience hallucinations of the visual, auditory, or tactile type. In such cases, the patient will see things others cannot see, hear things others cannot hear, and/or feel things that others cannot feel, such as feeling as though his or her skin is crawling. In short, the extremes of delirium range from the appearance of simple confusion and **apathy** to anxiety, agitation, and hyperactivity, with some patients experiencing both ends of the spectrum during a single episode. If delirium is suspected, it is imperative that an evaluation occurs quickly, because if left untreated, the condition can progress to death.

Causes and symptoms

Causes

While the symptoms of delirium are numerous and varied, the causes of delirium fall into four basic categories: medical, chemical, surgical, or neurological. The *DSM* attributes the causes of delirium to either a general (or multiple) medical condition or to substance use or withdrawal, which includes delirium as a side effect of medication. Delirium is often associated with factors that result in a disturbance of the normal sleep-wake cycle.

METABOLIC CAUSES. Many metabolic disorders, such as hypothyroidism, hyperthyroidism, hypokalemia, and anoxia, can cause delirium. For example, hypothyroidism (the thyroid gland emits reduced levels of thyroid hormones) brings about a change in emotional responsiveness, which can appear similar to depressive symptoms and cause a state of delirium. Other metabolic sources of delirium involve the dysfunction of the pituitary gland, pancreas, adrenal glands, and parathyroid glands. It should be noted that when a metabolic imbalance goes unattended, the brain may suffer irreparable damage.

DELIRIUM AND MEDICATION. One of the most frequent causes of delirium in the elderly is overmedication. The use of medications such as tricyclic **antidepressants** and antiparkinsonian medications can bring about an anticholinergic toxicity and subsequent delirium. In addition to the anticholinergic drugs, other drugs that can be the source of a delirium are:

- anticonvulsants, used to treat epilepsy
- antihypertensives, used to treat high blood pressure
- cardiac glycosides, such as Digoxin, used to treat heart failure
- cimetidine, used to reduce the production of stomach acid
- disulfiram, used in the treatment of alcoholism
- insulin, used to treat diabetes
- opiates, used to treat pain
- phencyclidine (PCP), used originally as an anesthetic but later removed from the market; now only produced and used illicitly
- salicylates, found in aspirin
- steroids, sometimes used to prevent muscle wasting in bedridden or other immobile patients

Additionally, systemic poisoning by chemicals or compounds such as carbon monoxide, lead, mercury, or other industrial chemicals can cause delirium.

DELIRIUM AND OTHER SUBSTANCES. Alcohol is the most widely used and most well known of the drugs whose withdrawal symptoms include delirium. Delirium onset from the abstinence of alcohol in a chronic user can begin within three days of cessation of drinking. The term *delirium tremens* is used to describe this form of delirium. The resulting symptoms of this delirium are similar in nature to other delirious states but may be preceded by clear-headed auditory hallucinations. In other words, the delirium has not begun, but the patient may experience auditory hallucinations. Delirium tremens may develop soon after and can have ominous consequences, with as many as 15% of those affected dying.

OTHER CAUSES OF DELIRIUM. Some of the structural causes of delirium include vascular blockage, subdural hematoma, and brain tumors. Any of these can damage the brain and cause delirium, whether as a direct result of the condition or by way of a secondary complication, such as oxygen deprivation. Some patients become delirious following surgery. This can be due to any of several factors, such as effects of anesthesia, infections, or a metabolic imbalance.

Infectious diseases can also cause delirium. Commonly diagnosed diseases such as urinary tract infections, pneumonia, or fever from a viral infection can induce delirium. Additionally, diseases of the liver, kidney, lungs, and cardiovascular system can cause delirium, as can infections specific to the brain. Even a deficiency of thiamine (vitamin B_1) can be a trigger for delirium.

Symptoms

Symptoms of delirium are often those associated with the disturbed sleep-wake cycle and include a confused state of mind accompanied by poor attention, impaired recent memory, irritability, inappropriate behavior (e.g., use of vulgar language with lack of a history of such behavior), and anxiety and fearfulness. In some cases, the person can appear to be psychotic, fostering illusions, **delusions**, hallucinations, and/or **paranoia**. In other cases, the patient may simply appear to be withdrawn and apathetic. In still other cases, the patient may become agitated and restless, be unable to remain in bed, and feel a strong need to pace the floor. This restlessness and hyperactivity can alternate with periods of apparent stupor.

Diagnosis

The diagnosis of delirium relies on a distinction of its occurrence from dementia. It should be determined not to arise from previously existing dementia. Other features include identifying it as a loss of clarity about the environment (inattention), sudden changes in cognition (e.g., disorientation), and a relatively sudden onset (compared to dementia).

Diagnosis of some cases of delirium may not occur at all; whether or not delirium is diagnosed in a patient depends on how it is manifested. If the person is an elderly, postoperative patient who appears quiet and apathetic, the condition may go undiagnosed. However, if the patient presents with the agitated, uncooperative type of delirium, it will certainly be noticed. In any case, where there is sudden onset of a confused state accompanied by a behavioral change, delirium should be considered, though this is not intended to imply that such a diagnosis will be made easily.

The psychotic features of delirium may be mistaken for another primary mental illness such as **schizophrenia** or a **manic episode**, such as that associated with **bipolar disorder**. However, there are major differences between these diagnoses and delirium. In people who have schizophrenia, their odd behavior, stereotyped motor activity, or abnormal speech persists in the absence of disorientation like that seen with delirium. The schizophrenic appears alert, and although delusions and/or hallucinations persist, he or she could be formally tested. In contrast, the delirious patient appears hapless and disoriented between episodes of lucidity. The delirious patient may not be testable. A manic episode could be misconstrued for agitated delirium, but consistency of elevated mood would contrast sharply to the less consistent mood of the delirious patient. Delirium should always be considered when there is a rapid onset and especially when the patient fluctuates between an aware state and a confused state.

Because delirium can be superimposed into a pre-existing dementia, the most often posed question when diagnosing delirium is whether the person might have dementia instead. Both cause disturbances of memory, but a person with dementia does not reflect the disturbance of consciousness present in someone with delirium. Expert history taking is a must in differentiating dementia from delirium. Dementia is insidious in nature and progresses slowly, while delirium begins with a sudden onset and acute symptoms. A person with dementia may appear clear-headed but can harbor delusions not elicited during an interview. There is not the typical fluctuation of consciousness in dementia that manifests itself in delirium. It has been stated that, as a general rule, delirium comes and goes, but dementia comes and stays. Delirium rarely lasts more than a month. The clinician must be prepared to rule out **factitious disorder** and **malingering** as possible causes for the delirium, as well.

Frequent mental status examinations conducted at various times throughout the day may be required to render a diagnosis of delirium. This assessment is generally done using the **Mini-Mental State Examination** (MMSE). This abbreviated form of **mental status examination** assesses the patient's orientation, registration, attention and concentration, recall, language, and spatial perception. Another tool for use in diagnosing delirium is the Delirium Rating Scale-Revised-98, although studies regarding its ability to differentiate different types of delirium have not been undertaken. Yet another diagnostic tool is the Memorial Delirium Assessment Scale, or MDAS. One tool that does not require patient participation is the Confusion Assessment Method, or CAM.

When a state of delirium is confirmed, the clinician is faced with the task of making the diagnosis in appropriate context to its cause. If the delirium is caused by a general medical condition, the clinician must identify the source of the delirium within the diagnosis. For example, if the delirium is caused by liver dysfunction, in which the liver cannot rid the system of toxins and allows them to enter the system and thus the brain, the diagnosis would be delirium due to hepatic encephalopathy. Delirium may also be caused by a substance such as alcohol. To render a diagnosis of alcohol intoxication delirium, the cognitive symptoms would be more exaggerated than those found in intoxication syndrome. If the delirium is caused by withdrawal from alcohol, the diagnosis would be alcohol withdrawal delirium (delirium tremens could be a feature of this diagnosis).

There may be instances in which delirium has multiple causes, such as when a patient has a head **trauma** and liver failure, or viral encephalitis and alcohol withdrawal. When delirium comes from multiple sources, a diagnosis of delirium precedes each medical condition that contributes.

Treatment

Treating delirium means treating the underlying illness that is its basis. This could include correcting any chemical disparities within the body, such as electrolyte imbalances; treating an infection; reducing a fever; or removing or discontinuing a medication or toxin. A review of anticholinergic effects of medications administered to the patient should take place. It is suggested that **sedatives** and hypnotic-type medications not be used; however, despite the fact that they can sometimes contribute to delirium, in cases of agitated delirium, the benefits may outweigh the risks. Medications that are often used to treat agitated delirium include **haloperidol**, **thioridazine**, and **risperidone**. These can reduce the psychotic features and curb some of the volatility of the patient, but they only treat the symptoms of the delirium, not the source. **Benzodiazepines** (medications that slow the central nervous system to relax the patient) can assist in controlling agitated patients, but, since they can contribute to delirium, should be used in the lowest therapeutic doses possible. The reduction and discontinuance of all psychotropic drugs should be the goal of treatment and occur as soon as possible to permit recovery and viable assessment of the patient.

Prognosis

If a quick diagnosis and treatment of delirium occur, the condition is frequently reversible. However, if the condition goes unchecked or is treated too late, there is a high incidence of mortality or permanent brain damage. The underlying illness may respond quickly to a treatment regimen, but improvement in mental functioning may lag behind, especially in the elderly. Moreover, one study disclosed that one group of elderly survivors of

KEY TERMS

Anoxia—Lack of oxygen.

Anticholinergic toxicity—A poisonous effect brought about by ingestion of medications or other toxins that block acetylcholine receptors. When these receptors are blocked, the person taking the medication may find that he or she gets overheated, has dry mouth, has blurry vision, and retains urine.

Coma—Unconsciousness.

Factitious disorder—A false or exaggerated disorder in which the physical or psychological symptoms are controlled or produced by the patient.

Hyperthyroidism—Condition resulting from the thyroid glands secreting excessive thyroid hormone, causing an increased basal metabolic rate and an increased need for food to meet the demand of the metabolic activity; generally, however, weight loss results.

Hypervigilant—Extreme attention and focus to both internal and external stimuli.

Hypokalemia—Abnormally low levels of potassium in the blood. Hypokalemia is a potential medical emergency, as it can lead to disturbances in of the heart rhythm.

Stupor—A trance-like state that causes a person to appear numb to their environment.

Subdural hematoma—Active bleeding or a blood clot inside the dura (leathery covering of the brain). This bleeding or clot causes swelling of the brain and if left untreated can cause death.

Torpor—Sluggishness or inactivity.

Tricyclic antidepressants—Antidepressant medications that have the common characteristic of a three-ring nucleus in their chemical structure. Imipramine and amitriptyline are examples of tricyclic antidepressants.

Vascular—Pertaining to the bloodstream (arteries, veins, and blood vessels).

delirium, at three years following hospital discharge, had a 33% higher rate of death than other patients. Delirium is a medical emergency that requires prompt attention to avoid the potential for permanent brain damage and death.

Resources

BOOKS

American Psychiatric Association. *Diagnostic and Statistical Manual of Mental Disorders*. 4th ed., text rev. Washington, DC: American Psychiatric Publishing, 2000.

First, Michael B., and Allan Tasman. *Clinical Guide to the Diagnosis and Treatment of Mental Disorders*. 2nd ed. Hoboken, NJ: Wiley, 2010.

Kaplan, Harold, and Benjamin Sadock, eds. *Synopsis of Psychiatry*. 10th ed. Baltimore: Lippincott Williams & Wilkins, 2007.

Miller, Bruce L., and Bradley F. Boeve, eds. *The Behavioral Neurology of Dementia*. New York: Cambridge University Press, 2009.

Porter, Robert S., and Justin L. Kaplan, eds. *The Merck Manual of Diagnosis and Therapy*. 19th ed. Whitehouse Station, NJ: Merck Research Laboratories, 2011.

PERIODICALS

de Rooij, S.E., et al. "Clinical Subtypes of Delirium and Their Relevance for Daily Clinical Practice." *International Journal of Geriatric Psychiatry* 20, no. 7 (July 2005): 609–615.

Han, J.H., et al. "Delirium in Older Emergency Department Patients: Recognition, Risk Factors, and Psychomotor Subtypes." *Academic Emergency Medicine* 16, no. 3 (March 2009) 193–200.

Katz, Ira R., et al. "Validating the Diagnosis of Delirium and Evaluating its Association With Deterioration Over a One-Year Period." *American Journal of Geriatric Psychiatry* 9 (Spring 2001): 148–159.

Mayo-Smith, Michael F., et al. "Management of Alcohol Withdrawal Delirium." *Archives of Internal Medicine* 164, no. 13 (July 12, 2004). http://archinte.ama-assn.org/cgi/content/full/164/13/1405 (accessed October 3, 2011).

Trzepacz, Paula T., et al. "Validation of The Delirium Rating Scale-Revised-98: Comparison with the Delirium Rating Scale and the Cognitive Test for Delirium." *Journal of Neuropsychiatry and Clinical Neuroscience* 13 (May 2001): 229–242.

Webster, Robert, and Suzanne Holroyd. "Prevalence of Psychotic Symptoms in Delirium." *Psychosomatics* 41 (December 2000): 519–522.

WEBSITES

U.S. National Cancer Institute. "Cognitive Disorders and Delirium (PDQ)." http://www.cancer.gov/cancertopics/pdq/supportivecare/delirium/healthprofessional/allpages (accessed October 3, 2011).

Jack H. Booth, PsyD

Delusional disorder

Definition

Delusional disorder is a psychotic condition characterized by recurrent or persistent non-bizarre **delusions**, without other obvious symptoms of mental illness. Delusions are false beliefs, based on a mistaken interpretation of reality. The beliefs are held with strong conviction, even in the face of contradictory proof. Non-bizarre delusions are plausible, in that there is a small possibility that they could be true under other circumstances.

Demographics

Delusional disorder is rare, with a lifetime risk of less than one in 1,000. The estimated prevalence in adults is 0.03%. In contrast, the prevalence of **schizophrenia** is estimated at 1%. However, delusional disorder may account for 1%–2% of psychiatric hospital admissions. The age at onset ranges from 18–90 years, with a mean age of 40 years. Delusional disorder, especially late-onset, is more prevalent in females than in males.

Description

Individuals with delusional disorder typically do not appear abnormal, unless they are discussing aspects of their lives that are affected by delusions. They may realize that their beliefs are unusual and, therefore, often choose not to discuss them with others. However, they may make unusual day-to-day choices based on their delusions. For example, people who are under the delusion that the government is spying on them might refuse to use a telephone or credit card. Although they may find their delusional reality distressing, they are not necessarily aware that there is anything abnormal about their thought processes or functioning. They usually attribute any problems or obstacles, such as having trouble getting a job or maintaining a romantic relationship, to their delusional reality. Using the government example, people may believe that there is nothing wrong except for government interference in their lives and that, if that ceased, their other problems would disappear.

People with delusional disorder do not usually have major mood or emotional problems. They rarely, if ever, hallucinate. When hallucinations do occur, they are components of the delusional belief. For example, people who believe that their internal organs are rotting may hallucinate smells or sensations related to that delusion.

There are various forms of delusional disorder:

- Paranoid or persecutory delusional disorder is the most common type. People believe that others are plotting against them and want to harm them or their loved ones. Persecutory delusions go far beyond symptoms of a paranoid personality. They often involve elaborate plots for spying, poisoning, or murder. People with paranoid delusions may even seek legal redress against their imagined enemies.
- Jealous delusions usually involve imagined infidelity on the part of a spouse or romantic partner, based on minimal or even contrary evidence. A person with delusional jealousy may try to restrict a partner's activities. This type of delusional disorder is most likely to be associated with violent behavior.
- Erotomanic delusions involve the belief that someone, usually a celebrity or person of higher status, is secretly in love with the deluded person. Erotomanic delusions are more common in women than in men. They can lead to stalking or even violence against the other person or against a perceived romantic rival.
- Grandiose delusions are an unjustified conviction in one's own importance or uniqueness. Grandiose delusions can take many forms, such as believing that one holds an exalted position, has connections to a famous person or deity, is very wealthy or knowledgeable, or has extraordinary powers or abilities.
- Somatic delusions involve excessive, irrational concerns about bodily functioning, such as an imagined physical deformity or illness, infestation with parasites or insects, or the conviction that one is emitting a foul stench. People with somatic delusions often avoid others and seek medical treatment for their imagined afflictions.
- Mixed-type delusions involve more than one of the above types.
- Unspecified delusions do not fit any of the above categories.

Unless their delusions result in illegal behavior or affect work or daily activities, people may adapt well enough to navigate life effectively without coming to clinical attention. The decision to seek medical help may result from a desire to reduce feelings of **depression**, anxiety, fear, or rage caused by the delusions, rather than from recognition that the beliefs are delusional. Persons with delusional disorder may be perceived as being angry and threatening. Rarely, they may become violent, usually toward someone who plays a part in the delusion, most often a spouse or sexual partner.

Although delusions can be a component of various psychotic disorders, in conditions such as schizophrenia, the delusions are usually bizarre or impossible, such as believing oneself to be controlled by an external force or having strange thoughts inserted into one's **brain**. Therefore, some researchers contend that delusional disorder is not a psychotic disorder, but rather a type of depression that may respond better to **antidepressants** or therapies for treating depression. Accepted cultural or religious beliefs are not delusions, regardless of how bizarre or delusional they may appear to nonbelievers. Because so many different disorders can cause delusions and because a **diagnosis** of delusional disorder is relatively subjective, some clinicians believe that the focus should be on treating the delusional thinking rather than on diagnosis.

Risk factors

Having close family members with delusional disorder or paranoid personality traits appears to be a risk factor for delusional disorder. Family members with other types of mental illness, such as schizophrenia or schizoaffective or mood disorders, do not seem to increase the risk of delusional disorder.

Causes and symptoms

The cause of delusional disorder is unknown. Its increased incidence among closely related individuals suggests that there is an inherited or genetic component to the disorder. A number of studies have found differences in the functioning of certain brain regions in individuals with delusional disorder. Patients with delusional disorder tend to have neurological activity consistent with continually threatening conditions, whereas non-delusional people exhibit such patterns only under conditions that could truly be interpreted as threatening.

It has been suggested that delusional disorder results from dysfunctional cognitive processing or thought patterns. Delusions may arise from distorted perceptions or understandings of one's environment, particularly with regard to other people and to the causes of unusual or negative events. Studies have found that delusional individuals make inferences and formulate theories about reality based on less information than would normally be required. This "jumping to conclusions" can lead to delusional interpretations of ordinary events and a tendency to view life as a series of threatening events. For example, developing flu-like symptoms during a week when new people move into the neighborhood might lead a delusional person to the conclusion that the new neighbors are the source of the infection. The patient might not consider alternative explanations, such as a family member with the flu or co-workers recently out with the flu. Other research has found that those who are

KEY TERMS

Agitation—Excessive restlessness or emotional disturbance that is often associated with anxiety or psychosis.

Cognition—Conscious intellectual activity, including thinking, imagining, reasoning, remembering, and learning.

Delusion—A persistent false belief held in the face of strong contradictory evidence.

Dementia—A group of symptoms (syndrome) associated with chronic progressive impairment of memory, reasoning ability, and other intellectual functions; personality changes; deterioration in personal grooming; disorientation; and sometimes delusions.

Erotomania—The false belief that one is the object of another's love or sexual desire.

Hallucination—False sensory perceptions; hearing sounds or seeing people or objects that are not there. Hallucinations can also affect the senses of smell, touch, and taste.

Psychotic—Pertaining to a serious mental disorder, such as schizophrenia, characterized by loss of contact with reality.

Schizoaffective disorder—Having symptoms of both schizophrenia and bipolar disorder.

Schizophrenia—A psychotic disorder characterized by loss of contact with one's environment, deterioration of everyday functioning, and personality disintegration.

prone to delusions interpret other people differently. Their interpretations of how others view them tend to be distorted.

There may also be motivations or defense mechanisms underlying delusions. Delusional disorder in susceptible people occasionally appears to be precipitated by difficulties in coping with life or maintaining high self-esteem. In order to maintain a positive self-image, people sometimes regard others as the cause of their personal difficulties. Over time, this can become an established pattern of thought, leading to delusional disorder.

The primary symptom of delusional disorder is persistent delusions or fixed beliefs about other people, situations, or conditions, which are plausible but false. The American Psychiatric Association's ***Diagnostic and Statistical Manual of Mental Disorders***, fourth edition, text revision (*DSM-IV-TR*), specifies the criteria for delusional disorder as non-bizarre delusions that:

- persist for at least one month and are resistant to change
- are not part of a cultural or religious belief
- occur in the absence of obvious peculiar or bizarre behavior
- occur without hallucinations or with rare hallucinations that relate directly to the delusion
- occur without concurrent mood episodes or episodes that are brief relative to the duration of the delusion
- occur in the absence of memory loss; medical illness; or drug-, alcohol-, or medication-related effects that are associated with the delusions

Diagnosis

Delusions are common symptoms of many other psychiatric illnesses, such as schizophrenia and **schizoaffective disorder**. **Dementia** caused by the deterioration of brain tissue, such as **Alzheimer's disease**, can result in delusions. Delusions can also occur as a result of brain tumors or injury or drug or alcohol reactions. Therefore, diagnosis of delusional disorder involves, in part, the elimination of other causes for the delusions. For example, the absence of persistent hallucinations may rule out schizophrenia or schizoaffective disorder and the absence of memory loss can rule out dementia.

Because delusions occur in many different disorders, some clinician-researchers have argued that there is little usefulness in focusing on what diagnosis the person has been given. Those who ascribe to this view believe it is more important to focus on the symptom of delusional thinking and find ways to have an effect on delusions, whether they occur in delusional disorder or schizophrenia or schizoaffective disorder. Many **psychotherapy** techniques used in delusional disorder come from symptom-focused (as opposed to diagnosis-focused) researcher-practitioners.

Examination

The clinician will perform a physical examination and obtain a medical history. The patient interview focuses on current situations and past history. With the patient's permission, family members or friends may be interviewed. A semi-structured interview, called a **mental status examination**, may be used to assess the patient's concentration, memory, understanding, and logical thinking. The mental status examination is intended to reveal peculiar thought processes. However, delusional people often conceal their thoughts because they know they are unusual. They may resist diagnosis and treatment because they are convinced of the reality of their delusions.

Tests

Various tests may be performed to rule out other physical or mental disorders. The Peters Delusion Inventory (PDI) is a psychological test for identifying and understanding delusional thinking, although it is more commonly used in research than in clinical practice.

Procedures

An electroencephalogram (EEG) may be taken to record brain activity. **Imaging studies** such as **magnetic resonance imaging** (MRI) or **computed tomography** (CT) scans may be performed if an underlying medical or neurological problem is suspected.

Treatment

Treatment of delusional disorder can be difficult, especially if the delusions are long-lasting. Patients may not believe that they have a mental disorder and may be resistant to treatment. **Hospitalization** is usually counterproductive, since it will reinforce paranoid delusions, but sometimes partial hospitalization or day-treatment programs are required.

Traditional

Psychotherapy, especially cognitive therapy, is usually the most effective treatment for delusional disorder, especially when it focuses on symptoms. **Family therapy** may also be beneficial. The therapist usually begins by concentrating on concrete life problems and goals and reinforcing positive outcomes to improve the patient's self-confidence and self-esteem. Therapies that stress social skills and behavior- and solution-oriented goals are usually more effective than therapies that focus on self-knowledge and insight or that directly challenge the delusions. Once a supportive and trusting relationship is established, the therapist takes gentle advantage of any doubts the patient has about the delusions, beginning with the least-significant aspects. Only then can the therapist begin to draw attention to differences between the delusions and reality. Using empathy and hypothetical questions, the therapist helps the patient generate alternative, evidence-based explanations and reach logical conclusions. If the patient is unwilling to relinquish even the smallest delusional belief, the therapy will probably be very long-term. In any case, therapy is likely to last at least six to 12 months.

Drugs

Antipsychotic medications, particularly in conjunction with psychotherapy, can be helpful for delusional disorder, though patients who do not acknowledge having a disorder may be unwilling to begin or maintain treatment with antipsychotics. Atypical, also called novel or newer-generation, antipsychotic medications, such as **risperidone** (Risperdal), **quetiapine** (Seroquel), and **olanzapine** (Zyprexa), can be effective with some patients. These are generally taken orally on a daily basis for a relatively long term. Response to antipsychotics for delusional disorder appears to follow the "rule of thirds"—about one-third of patients respond somewhat positively, one-third show little change, and one-third worsen or are unable to comply with the drug regimen.

Antipsychotics can be particularly useful for ending episodes of acute agitation. Agitation is a state of frantic activity, accompanied by anger or exaggerated fearfulness, which increases the risk that patients will harm themselves or others. Agitation is a typical response to severe or harsh confrontation about delusions. Agitation can also result from preventing patients from performing inappropriate acts that they view as urgent in light of their delusional realities. In emergency situations, patients may be given an injection of **haloperidol** (Haldol), usually in combination with other medications to decrease anxiety and slow activity, such as **lorazepam** (Ativan).

Alternative

Self-help or **support groups** or nonprofessional interventions are not generally appropriate for patients with delusional disorder. Delusional people are usually suspicious and mistrustful of others and their motivations. This attitude makes group dynamics difficult and possibly counterproductive.

Prognosis

The prognosis for delusional disorder varies. Sometimes the delusions disappear in a short time. In other cases, delusions persist for months or years, perhaps varying in intensity and significance. In general, about 33%–50% of cases resolve completely; about 10% show some improvement of symptoms, although irrational beliefs continue; and about 30%–40% of cases persist with no improvement. The prognosis depends largely on the level of conviction with regard to the delusions and openness to information that contradicts the delusions. Reluctance to accept treatment worsens the prognosis. However, some people with ongoing delusional disorder continue to function reasonably well over the long term.

QUESTIONS TO ASK YOUR DOCTOR

- Do you think I have delusional disorder? Why?
- What type of psychotherapy do you recommend?
- Do I need to take antipsychotic medications?
- What are the possible side effects of these medications?
- What is my prognosis?

Prevention

There are no known preventions for delusional disorder.

Resources

BOOKS

American Psychiatric Association. *Diagnostic and Statistical Manual of Mental Disorders (DSM-IV-TR)*, 4th ed., text rev. Washington, DC: American Psychiatric Association, 2000.

Freeman, Daniel, Richard P. Bentall, and Philippa A. Garety. *Persecutory Delusions: Assessment, Theory, and Treatment.* New York: Oxford University Press, 2008.

Kantor, Martin. *Understanding Paranoia: A Guide for Professionals, Families, and Sufferers.* Westport, CT: Praeger, 2008.

PERIODICALS

Dimopoulos, N. P., C. I. Mitsonis, and V. V. Psarra. "Delusional Disorder, Somatic Type Treated with Aripiprazole-Mirtazapine Combination." *Journal of Psychopharmacology* 22, no. 7 (September 2008): 812–14.

Easton, Judith A., Todd K. Shackelford, and Lucas D. Schipper. "Delusional Disorder—Jealous Type: How Inclusive are the *DSM-IV* Diagnostic Criteria?" *Journal of Clinical Psychology* 64, no. 3 (March 2008): 264–75.

WEBSITES

"Delusional Disorder." October 27, 2009. Aetna InteliHealth. http://www.intelihealth.com/IH/ihtPrint/WSIHW000/24479/31787.html?hide=t&k=basePrint (accessed July 25, 2011).

"Delusional Disorder." PsychCentral. June 1, 2010. http://psychcentral.com/disorders/sx11.htm (accessed July 25, 2011).

National Institute of Mental Health. "Delusional (Paranoid) Disorder." Associates in Counseling and Child Guidance. http://accg.net/delusional_paranoid_disorder.htm (accessed July 25, 2011).

ORGANIZATIONS

American Psychiatric Association, 1000 Wilson Blvd., Ste. 1825, Arlington, VA, 22209-3901, (703) 907-7300, apa@psych.org, http://www.psych.org.

American Psychological Association, 750 1st St. NE, Washington, DC, 20002-4242, (202) 336-5500, (800) 374-2721, http://www.apa.org.

Mental Health America, 2000 N. Beauregard St., 6th Fl., Alexandria, VA, 22311, (703) 684-7722, (800) 969-6642, Fax: (703) 684-5968, http://www.nmha.org.

National Alliance on Mental Illness, 3803 N Fairfax Dr., Ste. 100, Arlington, VA, 22203, (703) 524-7600, (800) 950-6264, Fax: (703) 524-9094, http://www.nami.org.

National Institute of Mental Health, 6001 Executive Blvd., Rm. 8184, MSC 9663, Bethesda, MD, 20892-9663, (301) 443-4513, (866) 615-6464, Fax: (301)443-4279, nimhinfo@nih.gov, http://www.nimh.nih.gov.

Deborah Rosch Eifert, PhD
Margaret Alic, PhD

Delusions

Definition

Delusions are unshakeable false beliefs. They are irrational, defy normal reasoning, and remain firm even in the face of overwhelming proof to the contrary. Delusions are psychotic symptoms that are often accompanied by hallucinations and/or feelings of **paranoia**, which act to strengthen the delusions.

Demographics

Delusions can be symptoms of many physical and mental disorders, as well as reactions to some medications. The prevalence of **schizophrenia**, which usually includes delusions, is estimated at 1% of the population, with delusions and hallucinations in males usually beginning between the ages of 16 and 30. Women tend to develop schizophrenia later, with 25% of cases appearing after age 45. Schizophrenia affects men and women equally and the incidence is similar in various racial and ethnic groups around the world.

Other common disorders that may involve delusions include **bipolar disorder**, **depression**, **dementia**, and some types of alcohol and drug abuse. Most people with **Alzheimer's disease** eventually develop delusions.

Other disorders that cause delusions are quite rare. The estimated prevalence of delusional disorder—in which delusions are the only or the primary symptom—is 0.025%–0.03% in adults. **Shared psychotic disorder** usually occurs only in long-term relationships in which a dominant partner with a psychotic disorder induces delusions in the more submissive partner. It also can occur among groups of people closely involved with a psychotic person. Postpartum **psychosis** occurs following approximately 0.01% of births, usually within the first four weeks.

Description

Delusions are most often symptoms of psychotic disorders, in which the patient has a diminished or distorted sense of reality. Neurological and physical illnesses and some medications can also cause delusions. Delusions are distinct from acceptable cultural- or religious-based beliefs, regardless of how irrational these may seem to outsiders. Delusions are unrelated to individual intelligence levels.

Delusions sometimes are difficult to distinguish from overvalued or unreasonable ideas. Overvalued ideas may be present in **anorexia nervosa**, **obsessive-compulsive disorder**, **body dysmorphic disorder**, and **hypochondriasis**. However, with overvalued or unreasonable ideas, people usually have at least some level of doubt as to the validity of their ideas. People with delusions are absolutely convinced that their delusions are real.

Most people with schizophrenia have delusions and delusions are the primary symptom of **delusional disorder**. Delusions also may occur with:

- schizoaffective disorder
- schizophreniform disorder
- brief psychotic disorder
- substance-induced psychotic disorder
- shared psychotic disorder
- postpartum psychosis
- bipolar disorder or mania
- major depressive disorder with psychotic features or delusional depression
- personality disorders, including schizotypal, paranoid, and sometimes borderline
- delirium
- Alzheimer's disease and other dementias
- Parkinson's disease, Huntington's disease, and certain chromosomal disorders
- HIV and other brain infections
- some types of epilepsy
- stroke
- brain tumors or cysts
- traumatic brain injury

Delusions are categorized as either bizarre or non-bizarre and mood-congruent or mood-incongruent. Bizarre delusions are completely implausible, with no association with reality, such as the belief that aliens have removed one's **brain**. Non-bizarre delusions are false beliefs that would be possible under some circumstances, such as the mistaken belief that one is under constant police surveillance. Delusional disorder always involves non-bizarre delusions. A mood-congruent delusion is consistent with either a depressive or manic state. For example, a depressed person may believe that the world is coming to an end. Someone in a manic state might believe that he is a famous person or has special talents or abilities. A mood-incongruent delusion is inconsistent with both depression or mania or is mood-neutral, such as a depressed person who believes that thoughts are being inserted into her mind by some outside force, person, or group ("thought insertion").

Delusions can fall into various categories:

- Paranoid or persecutory delusions—the belief that others are plotting against the individual or are out to cause harm—are the most common type of delusion. Sometimes persecutory delusions are isolated and fragmented. Often they are well-organized belief systems, called systematized delusions, that involve elaborate plots for ruining one's reputation or spying on, poisoning, drugging, or murdering the victim. Systematized delusions can be so broad and complex as to explain every aspect of one's life.
- Jealous delusions usually involve imagined infidelity on the part of a spouse or romantic partner. A person with delusional jealousy may try to restrict a partner's activities. This type of delusion is most likely to be associated with violent behavior.
- Erotomanic delusions involve the belief that someone, usually a celebrity, famous person, or person perceived as having a higher status, is secretly in love with the deluded person. These delusions can lead to stalking or even violence against the other person or a perceived romantic rival.
- Grandiose delusions are an unjustified conviction in one's own importance and uniqueness. These can take many forms, such as believing that one holds an exalted position, has connections to a famous person or deity, is very wealthy or knowledgeable, has extraordinary powers or abilities, or has a special mission in life. People may believe that they are rock stars or Jesus Christ. More often, people believe that they have great but under-recognized accomplishments.
- Somatic delusions involve excessive and irrational concerns about bodily functioning, such as an imagined illness, physical deformity, infestation with parasites or insects, or a conviction that one is emitting a foul stench.

- Mixed type delusions have characteristics of more than one type.
- Unspecified delusions do not fit any of the above categories.

Delusions are also categorized by theme. A monothematic delusion is a single delusional belief or a few false beliefs that all relate to one theme. People with polythematic delusions have a variety of unrelated delusional beliefs. Delusions can have any theme, but there are certain common themes:

- A delusion of control is the belief that another person, group, or external force controls one's thoughts, feelings, impulses, or behavior. People may believe that aliens are controlling their bodily movements. Thought broadcasting (the belief that one's thoughts are being heard aloud), thought insertion, and thought withdrawal (the belief that an outside force, person, or group is removing or extracting a one's thoughts) are other examples of control delusions.
- A mind-reading delusion is the belief that other people are aware of one's thoughts.
- Nihilistic delusions involve the absence or nonexistence of self, parts of oneself, others, or the world. Nihilistic delusions sometimes involve the end of the world.
- A delusion of guilt, sin, or self-accusation is intense false remorse. People may believe that they have committed a horrible crime and should be punished severely or are convinced that they are responsible for a natural disaster, such as fire, flood, or earthquake.
- A delusion of reference is the false belief that insignificant remarks, events, or objects have personal meaning or significance. For example, people may believe that they are receiving special messages from their television. Although the messages are usually negative, they also can be grandiose.
- Religious delusions have a religious or spiritual content. They may be combined with other delusions, such as grandiose delusions (for example, the belief that one has been chosen by God), delusions of control, or delusions of guilt. Beliefs that are acceptable within a person's religious or cultural background are not delusions.
- The Capgras delusion is the belief that an imposter has been substituted for a close relation, such as a spouse, sibling, parent, or child.

Risk factors

Risk factors for delusions depend on the underlying cause. A family history is an important risk factor for many psychotic disorders. **Stress** and low self-esteem also are risk factors for delusions. Shared psychotic disorder most often occurs in couples who are reclusive or socially isolated.

Causes and symptoms

Although delusions are usually caused by an underlying disorder, illness, or drug reaction, the precise causes are unknown. Genetics, neurological or brain chemistry abnormalities, and psychological mechanisms may all play a role.

Delusions suggest an abnormality in thought content, patterns, or processes. They may result from distorted perceptions and understanding of one's environment, particularly with regard to other people and the causes of unusual or negative events. Studies have found that individuals with delusions make inferences and formulate theories about reality based on less information than would normally be required. This "jumping to conclusions" can lead to delusional interpretations of ordinary events. In some cases, delusions may be caused by poor coping skills. **Brief psychotic disorder** in susceptible individuals is usually triggered by an extremely stressful or traumatic event. It is sometimes argued that psychiatric delusions develop through normal cognitive processes for understanding unusual or difficult experiences.

There may be motivations or defense mechanisms underlying some delusions. It is often assumed that paranoid delusions are caused by low self-esteem. In order to maintain a positive self-image, people sometimes regard others as the cause of their personal difficulties. Over time, this can become an established pattern of thought.

Some studies have indicated that delusions may be generated by abnormalities in the limbic system, the portion of the brain on the inner edge of the cerebral cortex that helps regulate emotions. People with schizophrenia have imbalances in **serotonin** and dopamine—neurotransmitters in the brain—that affect reactions to stimuli, which can lead to delusions. Patients with delusional disorder tend to have neurological activity consistent with continually threatening conditions.

Delusions can be caused by drugs such as **amphetamines**, **cocaine**, and phencyclidine (PCP). Delusions can occur both during use and withdrawal from drugs or alcohol. Some prescription drugs, including stimulants, **steroids**, and medications for Parkinson's disease, can cause delusions.

Symptoms depend on the type of delusion. Paranoid delusions are very common in older adults with schizophrenia or dementia. People who believe that they are being poisoned may develop strange eating habits or try to avoid food completely, which can lead to malnutrition. People who believe that their possessions are being stolen may hide things. People who are overly suspicious or believe they are being persecuted may isolate themselves from others. Patients with delusional depression may have somatic delusions or delusions of

KEY TERMS

Alzheimer's disease—A progressive, neurodegenerative disease characterized by loss of function and death of nerve cells in several areas of the brain, leading to loss of mental functions, such as memory and learning. Alzheimer's disease is the most common cause of dementia.

Bipolar disorder—A recurrent mood disorder, also known as manic-depressive disorder, in which patients have extreme mood swings from depression to mania or a mixture of both.

Cognitive—Conscious intellectual activity, including thinking, imagining, reasoning, remembering, and learning.

Dementia—A group of symptoms (syndrome) associated with chronic progressive impairment of memory, reasoning ability, and other intellectual functions; personality changes; deterioration in personal grooming; disorientation; and sometimes delusions.

Hallucinations—False sensory perceptions; hearing sounds or seeing people or objects that are not there. Hallucinations can also affect the senses of smell, touch, and taste.

Limbic system—The brain structures involved in memory, emotion, and motivation, including the hippocampus and hypothalamus.

Mania—Psychotic excitement, hyperactivity, disorganized behavior, and/or elevated mood; the manic phase of bipolar disorder.

Neurotransmitters—Chemicals that carry impulses between nerve cells (neurons), including acetylcholine, dopamine, serotonin, and norepinephrine.

Paranoia—An unfounded or exaggerated distrust of others.

Personality disorder—A psychopathological condition in which a person's patterns and behaviors are considered deviant or non-adaptive, but without neurosis or psychosis.

Psychosis—A serious mental disorder, such as schizophrenia, characterized by loss of contact with reality.

Schizoaffective disorder—Having symptoms of both schizophrenia and bipolar disorder.

Schizophrenia—A psychotic disorder characterized by loss of contact with one's environment, deterioration of everyday functioning, and personality disintegration.

Schizophreniform disorder—A psychosis resembling schizophrenia, but lasting only between one and six months.

Shared psychotic disorder—Also known as folie à deux, shared psychotic disorder is a rare condition in which an otherwise healthy person, or secondary case, shares delusions with a primary case—a person with schizophrenia or another psychotic disorder who has well-established delusions.

guilt. Patients with psychotic depression may pose a danger to themselves or others.

People with delusions often resist **diagnosis** and treatment. Because of their firm convictions in their delusions, they do not believe that there is anything abnormal about their thoughts or behaviors. In many cases of shared psychotic disorder, only one partner will seek treatment.

Diagnosis

Examination

Diagnosis usually involves identifying the underlying cause of the delusions. This includes a complete physical examination and medical history. A mental health professional, usually a **psychiatrist** or **psychologist**, uses specially designed interviews and assessments to evaluate mental status and diagnose psychotic disorders. Family members or friends also may be interviewed.

Tests

Clinical inventories and other tests are used to evaluate mental status. Specific tests for underlying physical illnesses or drug reactions may be conducted.

Procedures

Imaging procedures may be used to detect brain tumors or abnormalities. An electroencephalogram (EEG) may be used to measure brain activity.

Treatment

Traditional

Treatment depends on the underlying cause of the delusions. **Psychotherapy**, cognitive therapy, and **family therapy** may be options. Treatment for shared psychotic disorder includes separating the secondary case from the primary partner. **Hospitalization** may be necessary for severe delusions. The healthcare provider may need to hear the person express delusional thoughts before ordering **involuntary hospitalization**. Sometimes **electroconvulsive therapy** (ECT) is used to treat delusions, especially conditions that fail to respond to drug treatment or psychotherapy. ECT can be especially effective for psychotic depression.

Drugs

Both conventional and new-generation or atypical antipsychotics can effectively treat delusions, although side effects are common. Antipsychotics include **thioridazine** (Mellaril), **haloperidol** (Haldol), **chlorpromazine** (Thorazine), **clozapine** (Clozaril), **risperidone** (Risperdal), **olanzapine** (Zyprexa), **quetiapine** (Seroquel), and **fluphenazine** (Prolixin Decanoate). Some of these drugs block both serotonin and **dopamine**. Antipsychotics are usually started at low dosages and are gradually increased every few days. Sometimes patients need to try several different drugs to maximize effectiveness and minimize side effects. Older adults who **relapse** after initial treatment may have to continue on antipsychotics indefinitely. Tranquilizers or **sedatives**, such as **lorazepam** (Ativan) or **diazepam** (Valium), may be used to treat anxiety, agitation, or **insomnia** accompanying delusions.

Home care

People with delusions must be treated with finesse. Trust is very important. Rather than directly confronting or arguing about the impossibility of a delusion, family members and friends should acknowledge distresses caused by the delusion, reassure the patient, respond to his or her feelings, and attempt to distract the patient with other topics or activities.

Prognosis

The prognosis for delusions depends on the underlying cause. Delusions caused by schizophrenia usually disappear within a few weeks of treatment with antipsychotics, and the shorter the duration of delusions and hallucinations, the better the long-term prognosis. Although psychotic depression is a very serious and potentially dangerous condition, depressive symptoms other than delusions are more likely to continue or return following treatment. With appropriate treatment, delusional disorder can be relieved in up to 50% of patients. However, because of their strong belief in the reality of their delusions and a lack of insight into their condition, individuals with this disorder may never seek treatment. With shared psychotic disorder, the induced delusions in the secondary partner usually disappear when the individuals are separated.

QUESTIONS TO ASK YOUR DOCTOR

- What do you think is causing my delusions?
- What types of physical and psychiatric diagnostic tests do I need?
- What are my treatment options?
- What are the expected effects of my prescribed medications?
- What are the side effects associated with these medications?

Prevention

There are no known means for preventing delusions. However, early diagnosis and treatment can help minimize disruptions and long-term effects.

Resources

BOOKS

DeLisi, Lynn E. *100 Questions & Answers About Schizophrenia: Painful Minds,* 2nd ed. Sudbury, MA: Jones & Bartlett, 2009.

Graham, George. *The Disordered Mind: An Introduction to Philosophy of Mind and Mental Illness.* New York: Routledge, 2010.

Wootton, Tom, et al. *Bipolar In Order: Looking At Depression, Mania, Hallucination, and Delusion from the Other Side.* Tiburon, CA: Bipolar Advantage, 2010.

PERIODICALS

Coltheart, Max, Robyn Langdon, and Ryan McKay. "Delusional Belief." *Annual Review of Psychology* 62 (2011): 271–298.

Lincoln, Tania M., et al. "Is Fear of Others Linked to an Uncertain Sense of Self? The Relevance of Self-Worth, Interpersonal Self-Concepts, and Dysfunctional Beliefs to Paranoia." *Behavior Therapy* 41, no. 2 (June 2010): 187–197.

Rhodes, John, and Simon Jakes. "Perspectives on the Onset of Delusions." *Clinical Psychology and Psychotherapy* 17, no. 2 (March/April 2010): 136–146.

OTHER

Duckworth, Ken. "Understanding Schizophrenia and Recovery." National Alliance on Mental Illness. http://www.nami.org/Content/Microsites316/NAMI_PA,_Cumberland_and_Perry_Cos_/Discussion_Groups559/No_Active_Discussion_Groups_for_this_Site/NAMI_Schizophrenia_Aug08.pdf (accessed December 18, 2010).

WEBSITES

Cleveland Clinic. "Shared Psychotic Disorder." June 8, 2009. http://my.clevelandclinic.org/disorders/psychotic_disorder/hic_shared_psychotic_disorder.aspx (accessed December 19, 2010).

"Delusional Disorder." October 27, 2009. Aetna InteliHealth. http://www.intelihealth.com/IH/ihtPrint/WSIHW000/24479/31787.html?hide=t&k=basePrint (accessed December 16, 2010).

Mental Health America. "Paranoia and Paranoid Disorders." http://www.nmha.org/go/paranoia (accessed December 18, 2010).

———. "Schizophrenia: What You Need to Know." http://www.mentalhealthamerica.net/go/information/get-info/schizophrenia/schizophrenia-what-you-need-to-know (accessed December 18, 2010).

National Institute of Mental Health. "Schizophrenia." http://www.nimh.nih.gov/health/publications/schizophrenia/complete-index.shtml (accessed December 19, 2010).

ORGANIZATIONS

American Psychiatric Association, 1000 Wilson Blvd., Ste. 1825, Arlington, VA, 22209, (703) 907-7300, apa@psych.org, http://www.psych.org.

Mental Health America, 2000 N. Beauregard St., 6th Fl., Alexandria, VA, 22311, (703) 684-7722, (800) 969-6642, Fax: (703) 684-5968, http://www.nmha.org.

National Alliance on Mental Illness, 3803 N. Fairfax Dr., Ste. 100, Arlington, VA, 22203, (703) 524-7600, (800) 950-NAMI (6264), Fax: (703) 524-9094, http://www.nami.org.

National Institute of Mental Health, 6001 Executive Blvd., Rm. 8184, MSC 9663, Bethesda, MD, 20892, (301) 443-4513, (866) 615-6464, Fax: (301) 443-4279, nimhinfo@nih.gov, http://www.nimh.nih.gov.

Paula Anne Ford-Martin
Laura Jean Cataldo, RN, EdD
Jennifer Hahn, PhD
Margaret Brantley
Margaret Alic, PhD

Dementia

Definition

Dementia is a condition characterized by a progressive, irreversible decline in mental ability, accompanied by changes in behavior, personality, and, in the late stage, motor functions. There is commonly a loss of memory and the skills required to carry out activities of daily living. The changes are severe enough to seriously impair the person's ability to function or to interact socially and include changes due to diseases (e.g., Alzheimer's and Creutzfeldt-Jakob diseases), changes due to **stroke** (**vascular dementia**) or repeated blows to the head (dementia pugilistica, as experienced by boxers), and damage due to long-term alcohol abuse. There are over 70 different types of dementia, but **Alzheimer's disease** (AD) is considered the form that causes the most complications.

Demographics

The demographic distribution of dementia varies somewhat according to its cause. Recent research indicates that dementia in many individuals has overlapping causes, so it is not always easy to assess the true rates of occurrence of the different types. For example, Alzheimer's disease and multi-infarct dementia are found together in about 15%–20% of cases.

Alzheimer's disease

According to the Alzheimer's Association (AA), AD is the sixth-leading cause of death in the United States and the fifth-leading cause of death for persons 65 years of age or older. Data collected between 2000 and 2008 showed a decline in the death rates of most major diseases; however, the death rate for AD increased by 66% over this same time frame.

The prevalence of dementia increases rapidly with age. It affects about 1% of people from the age of 60 to 64 years and approximately doubles every five years after age 60, affecting 30% to 50% of adults by age 85. In total, AD afflicts approximately 5.4 million individuals in the United States, two-thirds of whom are women. Researchers do not know yet whether the sex ratio simply reflects the fact that women tend to live longer than men or whether female gender is itself a risk factor for AD. Some studies suggest that the risk for dementia is higher among African Americans and Hispanic Americans than it is for Caucasians. More than half of all nursing home admissions occur because of dementia. Surveys have found that dementia is the condition most feared by older adults in the United States.

Multi-infarct dementia

Multi-infarct dementia (MID), also called vascular dementia, is responsible for 15%–20% of cases of dementia (not counting cases in which it coexists with AD). Unlike AD, MID is more common in men than in women. Diabetes, high blood pressure, a history of smoking, and heart disease are all risk factors for MID. Researchers in Sweden have suggested that MID is underdiagnosed and may coexist with other dementias more frequently than is presently recognized.

Dementia with Lewy bodies

Dementia with Lewy bodies (DLB), also called by various other names such as Lewy body dementia, is now thought to be the second most common form of dementia after Alzheimer's disease. However, because researchers do not completely understand the relationship between Lewy bodies, AD, and Parkinson's disease, the demographic distribution is unclear.

Other dementias

Frontal lobe dementia (FLD), Pick's disease (also called Pick's dementia), Huntington disease, Parkinson's disease, human immunodeficiency virus (HIV) infection, alcoholism, head **trauma**, and other causes of dementia account for about 10% of all cases. In FLD and Pick's disease, women appear to be affected slightly more often than men. Dementia pugilistic, a dementia typically occurring in boxers that develops due to repeated head injury, is thought to affect at least 15% of boxers and has been increasingly found in other contact sports, such as football.

Description

The definition of dementia has become more inclusive over the past several decades. Whereas earlier descriptions of dementia emphasized memory loss, the current ***Diagnostic and Statistical Manual of Mental Disorders*** (*DSM-IV-TR*, fourth edition, text revised) of the **American Psychiatric Association** (APA) defines dementia as an overall decline in intellectual function, including difficulties with language, simple calculations, planning and judgment, and abstract reasoning, as well as loss of memory. Dementia is not caused simply by aging, although it is quite common in older people. Many researchers regard it as resulting from injuries, infections, **brain** diseases, tumors, biochemical changes within the brain, or other disorders. Most recently, researchers have found a possible connection between dementia and **attention deficit hyperactivity disorder (ADHD)**. Argentine researchers reported in 2010 that adults with symptoms of **ADHD** are more than three times more likely than other adults to develop Lewy body dementia later in life, though further research is needed.

Risk factors

Genetic factors play a role in several types of dementia, but the importance of these factors in the development of the dementia varies considerably. AD is known, for example, to have an autosomal (non–sex related) dominant pattern in most early-onset cases as well as in some late-onset cases, and to show different degrees of penetrance (frequency of expression) in late-life cases. Researchers have not yet discovered how the genes associated with dementia interact with other risk factors to produce or trigger the dementia. One nongenetic risk factor under investigation in 2011 was exposure to toxic substances in the environment.

Causes and symptoms

Causes

Dementia can be caused by as many as 80 different diseases and conditions, ranging from dietary deficiencies and metabolic disorders to head injuries and inherited diseases. Types of dementia and their causes include:

- Primary dementia. These dementias are characterized by damage to or wasting away of the brain tissue itself. They include AD, Pick's disease, and frontal lobe dementia.
- Multi-infarct dementia. Also called vascular dementia, this type is caused by blood clots in the small blood vessels of the brain. When the clots cut off the blood supply to the brain tissue, the brain cells are damaged and may die.
- Lewy body dementia. Lewy bodies are areas of injury found on damaged nerve cells in certain parts of the brain. They are associated with AD and Parkinson's disease, but researchers do not yet know whether dementia with Lewy bodies is a distinct type of dementia or a variation of AD or Parkinson's disease.
- Dementia related to alcoholism or exposure to heavy metals (e.g., arsenic, antimony, bismuth, mercury).
- Dementia related to infectious diseases. These infections may be caused by viruses (e.g., HIV, viral encephalitis), spirochetes (e.g., Lyme disease, syphilis), or prions (e.g., Creutzfeldt-Jakob disease).
- Dementia related to abnormalities in the structure of the brain. These may include a buildup of spinal fluid in the brain (hydrocephalus), tumors, or blood collecting beneath the membrane that covers the brain (subdural hematoma).
- Dementia caused by injury. These include dementia pugilistica, also called chronic traumatic encephalopathy, which results from repeated head injury, or post-traumatic dementia, which results from one severe traumatic brain injury. Symptoms may not appear until years after the injury.

Dementia may also be associated with **depression**, low levels of thyroid hormone, niacin, or vitamin (B_{12}) deficiency. Dementia related to these conditions is often reversible.

EARLY-ONSET ALZHEIMER'S DISEASE. In early-onset AD, which accounts for 2%–7% of cases of AD, the symptoms develop before age 60 years. Early-onset AD usually is caused by an inherited genetic mutation and is prevalent in persons with **Down syndrome**.

LATE-ONSET ALZHEIMER'S DISEASE. Research indicates that late-onset AD, also called sporadic AD, is a polygenic disorder; that is, its development is influenced by more than one gene. As of 2011, at least seven genes were associated with the development of AD. Finding genetic risk factors like these helps scientists better understand how AD develops and identify possible treatments to study. Specifically, the National Institute on Aging supports several major genetics research programs, including the Alzheimer's Disease Genetics Study, the Alzheimer's Disease Genetics Consortium, the Dominantly Inherited Alzheimer Network (DIAN), and the National Cell Repository for Alzheimer' Disease (NCRAD). The Alzheimer's Disease Genetics Constortium helps to collect and conduct GWAS for tens of thousands of samples from people who have late-onset AD.

MULTI-INFARCT DEMENTIA. While the chief risk factors for MID are high blood pressure (hypertension), advanced age, smoking, diabetes mellitus (diabetes), hypercholesterolemia (high cholesterol), and cardiovascular and cerebrovascular disease, there is an inherited form of MID called CADASIL, which stands for cerebral autosomal dominant arteriopathy with subcortical infarcts and leukoencephalopathy. CADASIL can cause psychiatric disturbances and severe headaches as well as dementia.

Several studies have documented a link between elevated levels of an amino acid called homocysteine in the blood and the risk of developing dementia, primarily vascular dementia. As homocysteine concentration can be modified by diet, the finding proposes the theory that at least one risk factor for dementia may be controllable.

FRONTAL LOBE DEMENTIAS. Researchers think that between 25% and 50% of cases of FLD involve genetic factors. Pick's disease appears to have a much smaller genetic component than FLD. It is not yet known what other risk factors combine with inherited traits to influence the development of frontal lobe dementias.

FAMILIAL BRITISH DEMENTIA. Familial British dementia (FBD) is a rare autosomal dominant disorder that was first reported in the 1940s in a large British family extending over nine generations. FBD resembles AD in that the individual develops a progressive dementia related to amyloid deposits in the brain. In 1999, a mutated gene that produces the amyloid responsible for FBD was discovered on human chromosome. It was reported in 2009 that this mutation results in the production of an amyloidogenic fragment called amyloid-Bri (ABri). Studies of this mutation are yielding further clues as to the development of both FBD and AD.

CREUTZFELDT-JAKOB DISEASE. Although Creutzfeldt-Jakob disease (CJD) is caused by the random mutations in prion proteins, researchers think that 5%–15% of cases may have a genetic component, where the mutations are inherited. The genetic (hereditary) component of its cause is called familial CJD, or fCJD.

Symptoms

Dementia is marked by a gradual impoverishment of thought and other mental activities, regardless of its cause. Losses eventually affect virtually every aspect of mental functioning. Specific symptoms may vary depending on the type of dementia.

ALZHEIMER'S DISEASE. Dementia related to AD often progresses slowly; it may be accompanied by irritability, wide mood swings, and personality changes in the early stage. In second-stage AD, the individual typically gets lost easily, is completely disoriented with regard to time and space, and may become angry, uncooperative, or aggressive. In final-stage AD, the individual is completely bedridden, has lost control over bowel and bladder functions, and may be unable to swallow or eat. The risk of **seizures** increases as the individual progresses from early to end-stage AD. Death usually results from an infection or malnutrition.

MULTI-INFARCT DEMENTIA. In MID, symptoms are more likely to occur after age 70. In the early stages, the individual retains his or her personality more fully than an individual with AD. Another distinctive feature of this type of dementia is that it often progresses in a stepwise fashion; that is, the individual shows rapid changes in functioning but then remains at a plateau for a while rather than showing a continuous decline. The symptoms of MID may also have a "patchy" quality; that is, some of the individual's mental functions may be severely affected while others remain relatively undamaged. Specific symptoms of MID include exaggerated reflexes, an abnormal gait (manner of walking), loss of bladder or bowel control, and inappropriate laughing or crying.

DEMENTIA WITH LEWY BODIES. This type of dementia may combine some features of AD, such as severe memory loss and confusion, with certain symptoms associated with Parkinson's disease, such as stiff muscles, a shuffling gait, and trembling or shaking of the hands. Visual hallucinations may be one of the first symptoms of dementia with Lewy bodies.

FRONTAL LOBE DEMENTIAS. The frontal lobe dementias are gradual in onset. Pick's disease is most likely to develop in persons between the ages of 40 and

60, while FLD typically begins before age 65. The first symptoms of FLD often include socially inappropriate behavior (e.g., rude remarks, sexual gestures, lack of personal hygiene). Individuals often are obsessed with eating and may put non-food items in their mouths, as well as make frequent sucking or smacking noises. In the later stages of FLD or Pick's disease, the individual may develop muscle weakness, twitching, and **delusions** or hallucinations.

CREUTZFELDT-JAKOB DISEASE. The dementia associated with CJD occurs most often in persons between ages 40 and 60. It is typically preceded by a period of several weeks in which the individual complains of unusual tiredness, anxiety, loss of appetite, or difficulty concentrating. The first sign that a person may have CJD is rapidly advancing dementia, which leads to memory loss, hallucinations, and personality changes. These symptoms are followed with irregular movements of the body, seizures, rigid posture, speech problems, and balance/coordination dysfunction. This type of dementia usually progresses much more rapidly than other dementias, usually over a span of a few months.

Diagnosis

In some cases, a patient's primary physician may be able to diagnose dementia; in many instances, however, the patient will be referred to a neurologist or a specialist in geriatric medicine. The differential **diagnosis** of dementia is complicated because of the number of possible causes, because more than one cause may be present, and because dementia can coexist with other conditions such as depression and **delirium**. Delirium is a temporary disturbance of consciousness marked by confusion, restlessness, inability to focus attention, hallucinations, or delusions. In elderly people, delirium is frequently a side effect of surgery, medications, infectious illnesses, or dehydration. Delirium can be distinguished from dementia by the fact that delirium usually comes on suddenly (in a few hours or days) and may vary in severity—it is often worse at night. Dementia develops much more slowly, over a period of months or years, and the patient's symptoms are relatively stable. It is possible for a person to have delirium and dementia at the same time.

Another significant diagnostic distinction in elderly patients is the distinction between dementia and age-associated memory impairment (AAMI). Older people with AAMI have a mild degree of memory loss; they do not learn new information as quickly as younger people, and they may take longer to recall a certain fact or to balance their checkbook, but they do not have the degree of memory impairment that characterizes dementia and do not get progressively worse. Other problems that may be mistakenly labeled as dementia include delirium, **psychosis**, depression, and the side effects of various medications.

The *DSM-IV-TR* specifies that certain criteria must be met for an individual to be diagnosed with dementia. One criterion is significant weakening of the individual's memory with regard to learning new information as well as recalling previously learned information. In addition, the individual must be found to have one or more of the following disturbances:

- Loss of language function (aphasia). People with dementia may use vague words like "it" or "thing," often because they cannot recall the exact name of an object. They also may echo what other people say, or repeat a word or phrase over and over. People in the later stages of dementia may stop speaking completely.
- Loss of the ability to perform intentional movements even though the person is not paralyzed, has not lost their sense of touch, and knows what they are trying to do (apraxia). For example, an individual with apraxia may stop brushing their teeth or have trouble tying their shoelaces.
- Loss of the ability to recognize objects even though the person's sight and sense of touch are normal (agnosia). People with severe agnosia may fail to recognize family members or their own face reflected in a mirror.
- Problems with abstract thinking and complex behavior. This criterion refers to the loss of the ability to make plans, carry out the steps of a task in the proper order, make appropriate decisions, evaluate situations, show good judgment, etc. For example, a person with dementia might light a stove burner under a saucepan before putting food or water in the pan or be unable to record checks and balance his or her checkbook.

The *DSM-IV-TR* also specifies that these disturbances must be severe enough to cause problems in the person's daily life, and these disturbances they must represent a decline from a previously higher level of functioning.

A new edition of the *DSM* (*DSM-5*) is expected to publish in May 2013. Proposed changes for the fifth edition include replacing the diagnosis of dementia (and all related forms) with the diagnosis of major neurocognitive disorder, which will be further broken down by various causes (e.g., major neurocognitive disorder associated with Alzheimer's disease, vascular disease, etc.). A condition is considered to be a major cognitive disorder if a person exhibits great cognitive deficits in at least one (but typically in two or more) of the following areas:

- complex attention
- executive ability
- learning and memory
- language
- visual construction and perception
- social cognition

Examination

PATIENT HISTORY. The doctor will begin by taking a full history, including the patient's occupation and educational level as well as medical history. The occupational and educational history allows the examiner to make a more accurate assessment of the extent of the patient's memory loss and other evidence of intellectual decline. In some cases, the occupational history may indicate exposure to heavy metals or other toxins. A complete medical history allows the doctor to assess possibilities such as delirium, depression, alcohol-related dementia, dementia related to head injury, or dementia caused by infection. It is particularly important for the doctor to have a list of all the patient's medications, including over-the-counter preparations, because of the possibility that the patient's symptoms are related to side effects.

MENTAL STATUS EXAMINATION. A **mental status examination** (MSE) evaluates the patient's ability to communicate, follow instructions, recall information, and perform simple tasks involving movement and coordination, as well as his or her emotional state and general sense of space and time. The MSE includes the doctor's informal evaluation of the patient's appearance, vocal tone, facial expressions, posture, and gait, as well as formal questions or instructions. A common form that has been used since 1975 is the Folstein Mini-Mental Status Examination, or MMSE. Questions that are relevant to diagnosing dementia include asking the patient to count backward from 100 by 7s, to make change, to name the current president, to repeat a short phrase after the examiner, to draw a clock face or geometric figure, and to follow a set of instructions involving movement (e.g., throwing a ball or folding paper). The examiner may test the patient's abstract reasoning ability by asking him or her to explain a familiar proverb or may test the patient's judgment by asking about a problem with a common-sense solution, such as what a person should do when a prescription runs out.

NEUROLOGICAL EXAMINATION. A neurological examination includes an evaluation of the patient's cranial nerves and reflexes. The cranial nerves govern the ability to speak as well as to see, hear, taste, and smell. The patient may be asked to stick out the tongue, follow the examiner's finger with the eyes, raise the eyebrows, etc. The patient is also asked to perform certain actions that test coordination and spatial orientation, such as touching the nose with the eyes closed. The doctor will usually touch or tap certain areas of the body, such as the knee or the sole of the foot, to test the patient's reflexes. Failure to respond to the touch or tap may indicate damage to certain parts of the brain.

Tests

LABORATORY TESTS. Blood and urine samples are collected in order to rule out such conditions as thyroid deficiency, niacin (vitamin B_{12}) deficiency, heavy metal poisoning, liver disease, HIV infection, syphilis, anemia, medication reactions, or kidney failure. A lumbar puncture (spinal tap) may be done to rule out neurosyphilis.

DIAGNOSTIC IMAGING. The patient may be given a CT (**computed tomography**) scan or MRI (**magnetic resonance imaging**) scan to detect evidence of strokes, disintegration of the brain tissue in certain areas, blood clots or tumors, a buildup of spinal fluid, or bleeding into the brain tissue. **PET** (**positron emission tomography**) or SPECT (**single photon emission computed tomography**) imaging is not used routinely to diagnose dementia, but may be used to rule out AD or frontal lobe degeneration if a patient's CT or MRI scan is inconclusive.

Treatment

Traditional

Traditional methods for treating dementia are proven to be effective at slowing some of the symptoms associated with dementia. In some cases, cognitive function can be improved but not corrected. Some types of dementia respond better to treatment than others. In all cases, proper care and support for the individual afflicted with dementia is helpful, whether it is provided at home or in an institution.

REVERSIBLE AND RESPONSIVE DEMENTIAS. Some types of dementia are reversible, and a few types respond to specific treatments related to their causes. Dementia related to dietary deficiencies or metabolic disorders is treated with the appropriate vitamins or thyroid medication. Dementia related to HIV infection often responds well to zidovudine (Retrovir), a drug given to prevent the AIDS (acquired immune deficiency syndrome) virus from replicating. MID is usually treated by controlling the patient's blood pressure and/or diabetes; while treatments for these disorders cannot undo damage already caused to brain tissue, they can slow the progress of the dementia. Patients with alcohol-related dementia often improve over the long term if they are able to stop drinking. Dementias related to head injuries, hydrocephalus, and tumors are treated by surgery.

It is important to evaluate and treat elderly patients for depression, because the symptoms of depression in older people often mimic dementia. This condition is sometimes called pseudodementia. In addition, patients with both depression and dementia often show some improvement in intellectual functioning when the depression is treated.

IRREVERSIBLE DEMENTIAS. There are no medications or surgical techniques that can cure AD, the frontal lobe dementias, multi-infarct dementia, or dementia with Lewy bodies. There are also no treatments that reverse or stop the progression of these dementias.

Early **intervention** may help to minimize complications and allow the patient to compensate for the alterations in functioning, resulting in an improved quality of life. It may also allow the patient and family to plan for the future and to identify resources.

BEHAVIORAL TREATMENT. Behavioral approaches may be used to reduce the frequency or severity of problem behaviors such as aggression or socially inappropriate conduct. Problem behavior may be a reaction to frustration or over-stimulation. Understanding and modifying the situations that trigger problem behaviors can be effective; strategies may include breaking down complex tasks such as dressing or feeding into simpler steps, or reducing the amount of activity in the environment to avoid confusion and agitation. Pleasurable activities such as crafts, games, and music can provide therapeutic stimulation and improve mood.

HOME MODIFICATION. Modifying the environment can increase safety and comfort while decreasing agitation. Home modifications for safety include removal or lock-up of hazards such as sharp knives, dangerous chemicals, and tools. Childproof latches may be used to limit access as well. Bed rails and bathroom safety rails can be important safety measures. Confusion may be reduced with the use of simpler decorative schemes and the presence of familiar objects. Covering or disguising doors may reduce the tendency to wander. Positioning the bed in view of the bathroom can decrease incontinence.

LONG-TERM CARE. Long-term institutional care may be required for persons with dementia, as profound cognitive losses often precede death by a number of years. Early planning for the financial burden of nursing home care is critical. Useful information about financial planning for long-term care is available through the Alzheimer's Association.

Family members or others caring for a person with dementia are often subject to extreme **stress** and may develop feelings of anger, resentment, guilt, and hopelessness, in addition to the sorrow they feel for their loved one and for themselves. Depression is an extremely common consequence of being a full-time caregiver for a person with dementia. **Support groups** can be an important way to deal with the stress of caregiving. Contact numbers are available from the Alzheimer's Association; they may also be available through a local social service agency.

The primary goals of treatment for progressive dementias are to preserve as much functioning and independence as possible and to maintain quality of life as long as possible. Caring for a person with dementia can be difficult and complex. The patient must cope with functional and cognitive limitations, while family members or other caregivers must assume increasing responsibility for the person's physical needs. The patient and family should be educated early on in the disease progression to help them anticipate and plan for inevitable changes.

Drugs

Periodically, new drugs are studied for the treatment of dementia. The only drugs approved by the U.S. Food and Drug Administration (FDA) as of 2011 for the symptomatic treatment of AD were **tacrine** (Cognex), **donepezil** (Aricept), **rivastigmine** (Exelon), **galantamine** (Lycoremine, Nivalin, Razadyne, Razadyne ER, Reminyl), and **memantine** (Namenda). The first four are called cholinesterase inhibitors (which prevents the breakdown of acetylcholine, a chemical in the brain that is thought to help with memory and thinking), while the last one is classified as an uncompetitive low-to-moderate affinity N-methyl-D-aspartate (NMDA) receptor antagonist. The cholinesterase inhibitor drugs may provide temporary improvement in cognitive functioning for a fairly large percentage of patients with mild-to-moderate AD. Memantine is prescribed for moderate-to-severe AD only. Doctors sometimes prescribe both types of drugs for their patients. However, drug therapy can be complicated by forgetfulness, especially if the drug must be taken several times a day. New treatments for AD continue to be researched through **clinical trials**; as of August 2011, there were more than 100 active clinical trials for AD and other dementias.

Psychotic symptoms, including **paranoia**, delusions, and hallucinations, may be treated with antipsychotic drugs such as **haloperidol**, **chlorpromazine**, **risperidone**, and **clozapine**. Side effects of these drugs can be

KEY TERMS

Agnosia—Loss of the ability to recognize objects by use of the physical senses.

Amyloid—A waxy translucent substance, composed mostly of protein, that forms plaques (abnormal deposits) in the brain.

Aphasia—Loss of previously acquired ability to speak, or to understand written or spoken language.

Apraxia—Impairment of the ability to make purposeful movements, but not paralysis or loss of sensation.

Creutzfeldt-Jakob disease—A degenerative disease of the central nervous system caused by a prion, or "slow virus."

Delirium—A disturbance of consciousness marked by confusion, difficulty paying attention, delusions, hallucinations, or restlessness. It can be distinguished from dementia by its relatively sudden onset and variation in the severity of the symptoms.

Dementia pugilistica—A delayed-onset form of dementia caused by repeated head injury; often occurs in boxers.

Hematoma—An accumulation of blood, often clotted, in a body tissue or organ, usually caused by a break or tear in a blood vessel.

Huntington disease—A midlife-onset inherited disorder characterized by progressive dementia and loss of control over voluntary movements. It is sometimes called Huntington's chorea.

Hydrocephalus—The excess accumulation of cerebrospinal fluid around the brain, often causing enlargement of the head.

Lewy bodies—Areas of injury found on damaged nerve cells in certain parts of the brain associated with dementia.

Multi-infarct dementia—Dementia caused by damage to brain tissue resulting from a series of blood clots or clogs in the blood vessels. It is also called vascular dementia.

Parkinson's disease—A disease of the nervous system most common in people over 60, characterized by a shuffling gait, trembling of the fingers and hands, and muscle stiffness. It may be related in some way to Lewy body dementia.

Pick's disease—A rare type of primary dementia that affects the frontal lobes of the brain. It is characterized by a progressive loss of social skills, language, and memory, leading to personality changes and sometimes loss of moral judgment.

Pseudodementia—A term for a depression with symptoms resembling those of dementia. The term dementia of depression is now preferred.

significant. **Antianxiety drugs** such as **diazepam** (Valium) may improve behavioral symptoms, especially agitation and anxiety, although **buspirone** (BuSpar) has fewer side effects. The anticonvulsant **carbamazepine** (Tegretol) is sometimes prescribed for agitation. Depression is treated with **antidepressants**, usually beginning with **selective serotonin reuptake inhibitors (SSRIs)** such as **fluoxetine** (Prozac) or **paroxetine** (Paxil). In general, medications are administered cautiously in the lowest possible effective doses to individuals with dementia in order to minimize side effects. Supervision of taking medications is generally required.

Research is ongoing on how the brain and AD are intertwined and how studies of the brain are leading to advances in the diagnosis and treatment of AD and other dementias. Swiss researchers reported in 2011 in the *Journal of Neuroscience* that new technologies, such as digital holographic microscopy (DHM), allow researchers to more thoroughly observe neuron activity in the brain, allowing for better testing of the effects of AD drugs.

Alternative therapies

No alternative therapies have been found to conclusively prevent, reverse, or slow dementias except for those caused by nutrient deficiencies. However, some alternative therapies may help treat the specific symptoms associated with dementia. **Aromatherapy** and **music therapy** have shown promise for relieving symptoms of agitation and promoting calm in patients with dementia. **Sage** and **ginkgo biloba** have also shown some effectiveness in clinical trials with treating symptoms of AD and dementia, respectively. Though past studies touted the success of ginkgo biloba, new research released in 2009 found the herb to make little difference in the cognitive health of participants of a large-scale study. Further research is needed to test the efficacy of herbal and nutritional supplements in treating symptoms of dementia.

Prognosis

The prognosis for reversible dementia related to nutritional or thyroid problems is usually good once the

QUESTIONS TO ASK YOUR DOCTOR

- What type of dementia does my loved one have?
- How far advanced is the dementia?
- What, if anything, can be done to slow the dementia or treat accompanying symptoms?
- How long can I expect my loved one to be able to remain at home?
- What can I do to make my home safe for my loved one?
- Can you refer me to a support group for caregivers of people with dementia?
- Do you know of any adult daycare programs available for people with dementia?

cause has been identified and treated. The prognoses for dementias related to alcoholism or HIV infection depend on the patient's age and the severity of the underlying disorder.

For those with irreversible progressive dementia, the outlook often includes slow deterioration in mental and physical capacities ending in death. Eventually, help is often required when swallowing, walking, and even sitting become difficult. Aid can consist of preparing special **diets** that can be more easily consumed and making surroundings safe in case of falls. Lift assists in areas such as the bathroom can also be useful. On average, people with AD live eight years past their diagnosis, with a range from 1–20 years. Patients with frontal lobe dementia or Pick's disease live on average between five and ten years after diagnosis. The course of Creutzfeldt-Jakob disease is much more rapid, with patients living between 5 and 12 months after diagnosis. Vascular dementia is usually progressive, with death resulting from stroke, infection, or heart disease.

Prevention

Dementia caused by repeated blows to the head can be prevented by avoiding sports where head trauma is common. Alcohol abuse–related dementia can be prevented by avoiding excessive alcohol consumption or minimized by receiving early treatment for alcoholism. Good **nutrition** can prevent nutrient-deficiency dementia. Unfortunately, most forms of dementia cannot be prevented.

Resources

BOOKS

American Psychiatric Association. *Diagnostic and Statistical Manual of Mental Disorders*. 4th ed., text rev. Washington, DC: American Psychiatric Association, 2000.

Dziegielewski, Sophia F. *DSM-IV-TR in Action*. Hoboken, NJ: John Wiley & Sons, 2010.

Hardman, Lizabeth. *Dementia*. Detroit: Lucent, 2009.

Mendelson, Scott D. *Beyond Alzheimer's: How to Avoid the Modern Epidemic of Dementia*. Lanham, MD: M. Evans, 2009.

Miller, Bruce, and Bradley F. Boeve, editors. *The Behavioral Neurology of Dementia*. Cambridge, UK: Cambridge University Press, 2009.

Schulte-Markwort, Michael, Kathrin Marutt, and Peter Riedesser, eds. *Cross-walks ICD-10-DSM IV-TR: A Synopsis of Classifications of Mental Disorders*. Cambridge, MA: Hogrefe & Huber, 2003.

Steele, Cynthia. *Dementia Care*. New York: McGraw-Hill Medical, 2010.

Stoppe, Gabriela, ed. *Competence Assessment in Dementia*. Germany: Springer, 2008.

PERIODICALS

Jourdain, Pascal, et al. "Determination of Transmembrane Water Fluxes in Neurons Elicited by Glutamate Ionotropic Receptors and by the Cotransporters KCC2 and NKCC1: A Digital Holographic Microscopy Study." *The Journal of Neuroscience* 31, no. 33 (2011): 11846–54.

Snitz, Beth E., et al. "Ginkgo Biloba for Preventing Cognitive Decline in Older Adults: A Randomized Trial." *Journal of the American Medical Association* 302, no. 24 (2009): 2663–70. http://dx.doi.org/10.1001/jama.2009.1913 (accessed November 1, 2011).

WEBSITES

Alzheimer's Association. "Alzheimer's Facts and Figures." 2011. http://www.alz.org/alzheimers_disease_facts_and_figures.asp (accessed August 24, 2011).

———. "Medications for Memory Loss." November 16, 2011. http://www.alz.org/alzheimers_disease_standard_prescriptions.asp (accessed December 12, 2011).

Delacourte, André. "Familial British dementia." Alzheimer Europe. October 9, 2009. http://www.alzheimer-europe.org/Dementia/Other-forms-of-dementia/Neuro-Degenerative-Diseases/Familial-British-dementia (accessed August 23, 2011).

Mayo Clinic staff. "Dementia." MayoClinic.com. April 16, 2011. http://www.mayoclinic.com/health/dementia/DS01131 (accessed August 26, 2011).

MedlinePlus. "Dementia." U.S. National Library of Medicine, National Institutes of Health. http://www.nlm.nih.gov/medlineplus/dementia.html (accessed August 26, 2011).

U.S. National Institute of Aging. "Alzheimer's Disease Genetics Fact Sheet." U.S. National Institutes of Health. June 2011. http://www.nia.nih.gov/Alzheimers/Publications/geneticsfs.htm (accessed August 23, 2011).

ORGANIZATIONS

Alzheimer Europe, 145, route de Thionville, LuxembourgL-2611, 35229 79 70, Fax: 35229 79 72, info@alzheimer-europe.org, http://www.alzheimer-europe.org.

Alzheimer's Association, 225 North Michigan Avenue, Floor 17, Chicago, IL, 10118, (313) 335-8700, Fax: (313) 699-1246, info@alz.org, http://www.alz.org.

American Geriatrics Society, 40 Fulton St., 18th Fl., New York, NY, 10038, (212) 308-1414, Fax: (212) 832-8646, info@americangeriatrics.org, http://www.americangeriatrics.org.

Center for the Study of Traumatic Encephalopathy, (617) 638-6143, cbaugh@bu.edu, http://www.bu.edu/cste.

National Institute on Aging, Building 31, Room 5C27, 31 Center Drive, MSC 2292, Bethesda, MD, 20892, (301) 496-1752, Fax: (301) 496-1072, (800) 222-4225, http://www.nia.nih.gov.

National Institute of Mental Health, 6001 Executive Boulevard, Room 8184, MSC 9663, Bethesda, MD, 20892-9663, (301) 443-4513, Fax: (301) 443-4279, (866) 615-6464, nimhinfo@nih.gov, http://www.nimh.nih.gov.

National Institute of Neurological Disorders and Stroke, PO Box 5801, Bethesda, MD, 20824, (301) 496-5751, (800) 352-9424, http://www.ninds.nih.gov.

Deanna M. Swartout-Corbeil, RN
Tish Davidson, AM
William Atkins, BB, BS, MBA

Dementia of the Alzheimer's type *see* **Alzheimer's disease**

Denial

Definition

Denial is refusal to acknowledge the existence or severity of unpleasant external realities or internal thoughts and feelings.

Description

Theory of denial

In psychology, denial is a concept originating with the psychodynamic theories of Sigmund Freud (1856-1939), founder of the discipline of **psychoanalysis**. According to Freud, three mental dynamics, or motivating forces, influence human behavior: the id, ego, and superego. The id consists of basic survival instincts and what Freud believed to be the two dominant human drives: sex and aggression. If the id were the only influence on behavior, humans would exclusively seek to increase pleasure, decrease pain, and achieve immediate gratification of desires. The ego consists of logical and rational thinking. It enables humans to analyze the realistic risks and benefits of a situation, to tolerate some pain for future profit, and to consider alternatives to the impulse-driven behavior of the id. The superego consists of moralistic standards and forms the basis of the conscience. Although the superego is essential to a sense of right and wrong, it can also include extreme, unrealistic ideas about what one should and should not do.

These three forces all have different goals (id, pleasure; ego, reality; superego, morality) and continually strive for dominance, resulting in internal conflict. This conflict produces anxiety. The ego, which functions as a mediator between the two extremes of the id and the superego, attempts to reduce this anxiety by using defense mechanisms. Defense mechanisms are indirect ways of dealing or coping with anxiety, such as explaining problems away or blaming others for problems. Denial is one of many defense mechanisms. It entails ignoring or refusing to believe an unpleasant reality. Defense mechanisms protect one's psychological well-being in traumatic situations, or in any situation that produces anxiety or conflict. However, they do not resolve the anxiety-producing situation and, if overused, can lead to psychological disorders. Although Freud's model of the id, ego, and superego is not emphasized by most psychologists today, defense mechanisms are still regarded as potentially maladaptive behavioral patterns that may lead to psychological disorders.

Examples of denial

Death is a common occasion for denial. When someone learns of the sudden, unexpected death of a loved one, at first he or she may not be able to accept the reality of this loss. The initial denial protects that person from the emotional shock and intense **grief** that often accompanies news of death. Chronic or terminal illnesses also encourage denial. People with such illnesses may think, "It's not so bad; I'll get over it," and refuse to make any lifestyle changes.

Denial can also apply to internal thoughts and feelings. For instance, some children are taught that anger is wrong in any situation. As adults, if these individuals experience feelings of anger, they are likely to deny their feelings to others. Cultural standards and expectations can encourage denial of subjective experience. Men who belong to cultures with extreme notions of masculinity may view fear as a sign of weakness and deny internal feelings of fear. Some cultures are thought to discourage the acknowledgment of mental illness, resulting in individuals denying their psychological symptoms and often developing physical symptoms instead.

Certain **personality disorders** tend to be characterized by denial more than others. For example, those with **narcissistic personality disorder** deny information that suggests they are not perfect. Antisocial behavior is characterized by denial of the harm done to others (such as with sexual offenders or substance abusers).

Denial can also be exhibited on a large scale—among groups, cultures, or even nations. Lucy Bregman gives an example of national denial of imminent mortality in the 1950s: school children participated in drills where they hid under desks in preparation for atomic attacks. Another example of large-scale denial is the recent assertion by some that the World War II Holocaust never occurred.

TREATMENT OF DENIAL. Denial is treated differently in different types of therapy. In psychoanalytic therapy, denial is regarded as an obstacle to progress that must eventually be confronted and interpreted. Timing is important, however. Psychoanalytic therapists wait until clients appear emotionally ready or have some degree of insight into their problems before confronting them. In the humanistic and existential therapies, denial is considered the framework by which clients understand their world. Not directly confronting denial, therapists assist clients in exploring their world view and considering alternative ways of being. In cognitive-behavioral therapies, denial is not regarded as an important phenomenon. Rather, denial would suggest that an individual has not learned the appropriate behaviors to cope with a stressful situation. Therapists assist individuals in examining their current thoughts and behaviors and devising strategic ways to make changes.

Traditional treatment programs for **substance abuse** and other addictions view denial as a central theme. Such programs teach that in order to overcome addiction, one must admit to being an alcoholic or addict. Those who are unable to accept such labels are informed they are in denial. Even when the labels are accepted, individuals are still considered to be in denial if they do not acknowledge the severity of their addictions. From this perspective, progress cannot be made until individuals recognize the extent of their denial and work toward acceptance. There is much controversy in the field of addictions regarding the role of denial and how it should be addressed. Traditional programs such as these stress direct confrontation. Other professionals do not insist on the acceptance of labels. They believe that denial should be worked through more subtly, empathically focusing on the personal reasons surrounding denial and seeking to strengthen the desire to change. This subtle form of addressing denial is known as motivational enhancement therapy, and can be used with other types of disorders as well.

KEY TERMS

Antisocial behavior—Behavior characterized by high levels of anger, aggression, manipulation, or violence.

Cognitive-behavioral therapies—An approach to psychotherapy that emphasizes the correction of distorted thinking patterns and changing one's behaviors accordingly.

Defense mechanisms—Indirect strategies used to reduce anxiety rather than directly facing the issues causing the anxiety.

Dependent personality disorder—Personality disorder characterized by a constant, unhealthy need to be liked and appreciated by others at all costs.

Ego—In Freudian psychology, the conscious, rational part of the mind that experiences and reacts to the outside world.

Humanistic and existential therapies—Therapies that focus on achieving one's full potential, guided by subjective experience.

Id—A construct in Freudian psychodynamic theory that represents the irrational, self-centered aspects of human thought.

Motivational enhancement therapy—Therapy that focuses on increasing motivation for change by empathically comparing and contrasting the consequences and benefits of changing or not changing.

Narcissistic personality disorder—Personality characterized by continually exaggerating one's own positive qualities and refusing to recognize personal defects or flaws.

Psychoanalytic therapy—Therapy based on the psychodynamic theory of Sigmund Freud.

Psychodynamic—Referring to the motivational forces, unconscious as well as conscious, that form human attitudes and behavior.

Superego—According to Freud, the part of the mind that represents traditional parental and societal values. The superego is the source of guilt feelings.

Resources

BOOKS

Bregman, Lucy. *Beyond Silence and Denial: Death and Dying Reconsidered.* Louisville, Kentucky: Westminster John Knox Press, 1999.

Millon, Theodore, et al. *Personality Disorders in Modern Life.* 2nd ed. New York: John Wiley and Sons, 2004.

PERIODICALS

Cramer, Phebe, and Melissa A. Brilliant. "Defense Use and Defense Understanding in Children." *Journal of Personality* 69, no. 2 (2001): 291–321.

Parker, Gordon, Gemma Gladstone, and Kuan Tsee Chee. "Depression in the Planet's Largest Ethnic Group: The Chinese." *American Journal Of Psychiatry* 158, no. 6 (June 2001): 857–864.

Schneider, Sandra L., and Robert C. Wright. "The FoSOD: A Measurement Tool for Reconceptualizing the Role of Denial in Child Molesters." *Journal of Interpersonal Violence* 16, no. 6 (2001): 545–564.

ORGANIZATIONS

American Psychoanalytic Association, 309 East 49th Street, New York, NY, 10017-1601, (212) 752-0450, Fax: (212) 593-0571, info@apsa.org, http://www.apsa.org.

Sandra L. Friedrich, MA

Depacon *see* **Divalproex sodium**

Depakene *see* **Divalproex sodium; Valproic acid**

Depakote *see* **Divalproex sodium**

Dependent personality disorder

Definition

Dependent personality disorder (DPD) is characterized by an excessive need to be taken care of or to depend upon others. Persons with this disorder are typically submissive and display clinging behavior toward those from whom they fear separation.

Dependent personality disorder is one of several **personality disorders** listed in the standard reference guide for mental disorders, the ***Diagnostic and Statistical Manual of Mental Disorders,*** the fourth edition, text revision (*DSM-IV-TR*). Changes for the fifth edition of the *DSM* (*DSM-5*, 2013) propose that DPD be represented and diagnosed by a combination of core impairment in personality functioning and specific pathological personality traits, rather than as a specific type.

Demographics

DPD is rarely, if ever, diagnosed in children or adolescents because of their inherent dependence on others resulting from their age and developmental limitations.

DPD is one of the most frequently diagnosed personality disorders. It occurs equally in men and women, and usually appears in early- to middle-age adulthood.

Description

Persons with DPD are docile, passive, and nonassertive. They exert a great deal of energy to please others, are self-sacrificing, and constantly attempt to elicit the approval of others. They are reluctant to express disagreement with others and are often willing to go to abnormal lengths to win the approval of those on whom they rely. They are readily influenced and can be taken advantage of easily. This **compliance** and reliance upon others leads to a subtle message that someone should assume responsibility for significant areas of the patient's life. This is often displayed as helplessness, even for completion of seemingly simple tasks.

Patients with DPD have a low level of confidence in their own intelligence and abilities. They often have difficulty making decisions and undertaking projects on their own. They are prone to be pessimistic and self-doubting, and to belittle their own accomplishments. They shy away from responsibility in occupational settings.

Affected individuals are uneasy being alone and are preoccupied with the fear of being abandoned or rejected by others. Their moods are characterized by frequent bouts of anxiety or fearfulness; generally, their demeanor is sad. Their style of thinking is naïve and uncritical, and lacks discretion.

Causes and symptoms

Causes

It is commonly thought that the development of dependency in people with dependent personality disorder is a result of over-involvement and intrusive behavior by their primary caretakers. Caretakers may foster dependence in the child to meet their own dependency needs and may reward extreme loyalty but reject attempts the child makes towards independence. Families of those with DPD often do not express their emotions, are controlling, and demonstrate poorly defined relational roles within the family unit.

Individuals with DPD often have been socially humiliated by others in their developmental years. They may carry significant doubts about their abilities to perform tasks, to take on new responsibilities, and generally to function independently of others. This reinforces their suspicions that they are incapable of living autonomously. In response to these feelings, they portray helplessness in order to elicit caregiving behavior from some people in their lives.

Symptoms

The *DSM-IV-TR* specifies eight diagnostic criteria for DPD. Individuals with this disorder:

- Have difficulty making common decisions. They typically need an excessive amount of advice and reassurance before they can make even simple decisions, such as the clothing to wear on a given day.
- Need others to assume responsibility for them. Because they view themselves as incapable of being autonomous, they withdraw from adult responsibilities by acting passive and helpless. They allow others to take the initiative for many areas of their life. Adults with this disorder typically depend on a parent or spouse to make major decisions for them, such as where to work or live, or with whom to be friends.
- Have difficulty expressing disagreement with others. Disagreeing with others is often viewed as too risky. It might sever the support or approval of those they upon whom they depend. They are often overly agreeable because they fear alienating other people.
- Have difficulty initiating or doing things on their own. They lack self-confidence and believe they need help to begin or sustain tasks. They often present themselves as inept and unable to understand or accomplish the task at hand.
- Go to excessive lengths to obtain support or nurturing from others. They may even volunteer to do unpleasant tasks if they believe that doing so will evoke a positive response from others. They may subject themselves to great personal sacrifice or tolerate physical, verbal, or sexual abuse in their quest to get what they believe they need from others.
- Feel helpless when alone. Because they feel incapable of caring for themselves, they experience significant anxiety when alone. To avoid being alone, they may spend time with people with whom they have little interest.
- Quickly seek a new relationship when a previous one ends. When a marriage, dating, or other close relationship ends, there is typically an urgency to find a new relationship that will provide the support of the former relationship.
- Are preoccupied with fears of being left to take care of themselves. Their greatest fear is to be left alone and to be responsible for themselves. Even as adults, their dependence upon others may appear childlike.

Diagnosis

Age and cultural factors should be considered in diagnosing DPD. Certain cultural norms suggest a submissive, polite, or dependent posture in relating to the opposite sex or authority figures. DPD should only be diagnosed when it meets the specific criteria and is clearly outside one's cultural norms.

The **diagnosis** of DPD is based on a clinical interview to assess symptomatic behavior. Other assessment tools helpful in confirming the diagnosis include:

- The Dependent Personality Questionnaire
- Minnesota Multiphasic Personality Inventory (MMPI-2)
- Millon Clinical Multi-axial Inventory (MCMI-II)
- Rorschach Psychodiagnostic Test
- Thematic Apperception Test (TAT)

For a person to be diagnosed with DPD, at least five of the eight symptoms described must be the present, and these symptoms must begin by early adulthood and be evident in a variety of contexts.

The diagnosis of dependent personality disorder must be distinguished from **borderline personality disorder**, since there are common characteristics. Borderline personality disorder is characterized by fear of abandonment, as well, but with feelings of emptiness and rage. In contrast, the dependent personality responds to this fear of abandonment with submissiveness and searches for a replacement relationship to maintain dependency.

Likewise, persons with **histrionic personality disorder** have a strong need for reassurance and approval and may appear childlike in their clinging behavior. Histrionics are characterized by a gregarious demeanor and make active demands for attention, while dependents respond with docile and self-deprecating behavior.

Avoidant personality disorder can also be confused with DPD. Both are characterized by feelings of inadequacy, oversensitivity to criticism, and a frequent need for assurance. However, these patients typically have such an intense fear of rejection that they instinctively withdraw until they are certain of acceptance. Dependents, in contrast, actually seek out contact with others because they need the approval of others.

Treatment

The general goal of treatment is to increase the individual's sense of autonomy and ability to function independently.

Psychodynamically oriented therapies

A long-term approach to psychodynamic treatment can be successful, but may lead to heightened dependencies and difficult separation in the therapeutic relationship over time. The preferred approach is a time-limited treatment plan consisting of a predetermined number of sessions. This has been proved to facilitate the exploration process of dependency issues more effectively than long-term therapy in most patients.

Cognitive-behavioral therapy

Cognitive-behavioral approaches attempt to increase the affected person's ability to act independently of others, improve their self-esteem, and enhance the quality of their interpersonal relationships. Often, patients play an active role in setting goals. Methods often used in **cognitive-behavioral therapy** (CBT) include assertiveness and **social skills training** to help reduce reliance on others, including the therapist.

Interpersonal therapy

Treatment using an interpersonal approach can be useful because the individual is usually receptive to treatment and seeks help with interpersonal relationships. The therapist can help the patient explore their long-standing patterns of interacting with others, and understand how these have contributed to dependency issues. The goal is to show the patient the high price they pay for this dependency, and to help them develop healthier alternatives. **Assertiveness training** and learning to identify feelings is often used to heighten improve interpersonal behavior.

Group therapy

When a person is highly motivated to see growth, a more interactive therapeutic group can be successful in helping to explore passive-dependent behavior. If the individual is socially reluctant or impaired in assertiveness, decision making, or negotiation, a supportive decision-making group is more appropriate. Time-limited assertiveness-training groups with clearly defined goals have been proven to be effective.

Family and marital therapy

Individuals with DPD are usually brought to therapy by their parents. They are often young adults who are struggling with neurotic or psychotic symptoms. The goal of **family therapy** is often to untangle the enmeshed family relationships, which usually elicits considerable resistance by most family members unless all are in therapy.

Marital therapy can be productive in helping couples reduce the anxiety of both partners, who have dependency needs that arise in the relationship.

Medications

Individuals with DPD can experience anxiety and depressive disorders as well. In these cases, it may prove useful to use **antidepressants** or **antianxiety drugs**. Unless the anxiety or **depression** is severe enough to warrant a primary diagnosis, medications are generally not recommended for treatment. Persons with DPD may become overly dependent on any medication used.

KEY TERMS

Millon Clinical Multiaxial Inventory (MCMI-II)—A self-report instrument designed to help the clinician assess *DSM-IV*-related personality disorders and clinical syndromes. It provides insight into 14 personality disorders and 10 clinical syndromes.

Minnesota Multiphasic Personality Inventory (MMPI-2)—A comprehensive assessment tool widely used to diagnosed personality disorders.

Rorschach Psychodiagnostic Test—This series of 10 "ink blot" images allows the patient to project their interpretations, which can be used to diagnose particular disorders.

Thematic Apperception Test (TAT)—A projective test using stories and descriptions of pictures to reveal some of the dominant drives, emotions, sentiments, conflicts, and complexes of a personality.

Prognosis

The general prognosis for individuals with DPD is good. Persons who enter treatment can learn to become more autonomous, and improved functioning can be expected.

Prevention

Although prevention of the disorder might not be possible, treatment of DPD can sometimes allow a person who is prone to this disorder to learn more productive ways of dealing with situations.

Resources

BOOKS

American Psychiatric Association. *Diagnostic and Statistical Manual of Mental Disorders*. 4th ed., text rev. Washington, DC: American Psychiatric Publishing, 2000.

Millon, Theodore, and Roger Davis. *Disorders of Personality: DSM IV and Beyond*. New York: John Wiley and Sons, 1996.

Porter, Robert S., and Justin L. Kaplan, eds. *The Merck Manual of Diagnosis and Therapy*. 19th ed. Whitehouse Station, NJ: Merck Research Laboratories, 2011.

Sperry, Len. *Handbook of Diagnosis and Treatment of DSM-IV Personality Disorders*. 2nd ed. New York: Routledge, 2003.

PERIODICALS

Tyrer, P., J. Morgan, and D. Cicchetti. "The Dependent Personalilty Questionnaire (DPQ): A Screening Instrument for Dependent Personality." *International Journal of Social Psychiatry* 50, no. 1 (March 2004): 10–17.

WEBSITES

MedlinePlus. "Dependent Personality Disorder." U.S. National Library of Medicine, National Institutes of Health. http://medlineplus.nlm.nih.gov/medlineplus/ency/article/000941.htm (accessed October 3, 2011).

ORGANIZATIONS

American Psychiatric Association, 1000 Wilson Blvd., Suite 1825, Arlington, VA, 22209-3901, (703) 907-7300, apa@psych.org, http://www.psych.org.

International Society for the Study of Personality Disorders, University of Michigan Health System, Psychiatry MCHC-6, Box 5295, 1500 East Medical Center Drive, Ann Arbor, MI, 48109-5295, (734) 936-8316, Fax: (734) 936-9761, http://www.isspd.com.

National Institute of Mental Health, 6001 Executive Blvd., Room 8184, MSC 9663, Bethesda, MD, 20892-9663, (301) 433-4513; TTY: (301) 443-8431, (866) 615-6464; TTY: (866) 415-8051, Fax: (301) 443-4279, nimhinfo@nih.gov, http://www.nimh.nih.gov.

Gary Gilles, MA
Emily Jane Willingham, PhD

Depersonalization and depersonalization disorder

Definition

Depersonalization disorder (sometimes called "depersonalization neurosis") is a dissociative disorder marked by persistent or repeated feelings of disconnect or detachment from one' body. Depersonalization is a state in which the individual ceases to perceive the reality of the self or the environment. The patient feels that his or her body is unreal, is changing, or is dissolving; or that he or she is outside of the body.

Demographics

The lifetime prevalence of depersonalization disorder in the general population is unknown, possibly because many people are made anxious by episodes of depersonalization and are afraid to discuss them with a primary care physician. One survey done by the National Institutes of Mental Health (NIMH) indicates that about half of the adults in the United States have had one or two brief episodes of depersonalization in their lifetimes, usually resulting from severe **stress**. About a third of people exposed to life-threatening dangers develop brief periods of depersonalization, as do 40% of psychiatric inpatients. Estimates of the prevalence of depersonalization disorder in the general population range from 2.4% to 20%.

Depersonalization disorder is diagnosed about twice as often in women as in men. It is not known whether this sex ratio indicates that women are at greater risk for the disorder or if they are more likely to seek help for its symptoms, or both. Little information is available about the incidence of the disorder in different racial or ethnic groups.

Description

Depersonalization disorder is classified by the ***Diagnostic and Statistical Manual of Mental Disorders***, fourth edition, text revision, also known as the *DSM-IV-TR*, as one of the **dissociative disorders**. These are mental disorders in which the normally well-integrated functions of memory, identity, perception, and consciousness are separated (dissociated). The dissociative disorders are usually connected to recent or past **trauma**, or with an intense internal conflict that forces the mind to separate incompatible or unacceptable knowledge, information, or feelings. In depersonalization disorder, the patient's self-perception is disrupted. Patients feel as if they are external observers of their own lives, or that they are detached from their own bodies.

Depersonalization as a symptom may occur in the **diagnosis** of depersonalization disorder if the episodes of depersonalization occur only during panic attacks or following a traumatic stressor.

A person with depersonalization disorder experiences subjective symptoms of unreality that make him or her uneasy and anxious. "Subjective" is a word that refers to the thoughts and perceptions inside an individual's mind, as distinct from the objects of those thoughts and perceptions outside the mind. Because depersonalization is a subjective experience, many people who have chronic or recurrent episodes of depersonalization are afraid others will not understand if they try to describe what they are feeling, or will think they are "crazy." As a result, depersonalization disorder may be underdiagnosed because the symptom of depersonalization is underreported.

The symptom of depersonalization can also occur in normal individuals under circumstances such as **sleep deprivation**, the use of certain anesthetics, experimental conditions in a laboratory (experiments involving weightlessness, for example), and emotionally stressful situations (such as taking an important academic examination or being in a traffic accident). One such example involves some of the rescue personnel from the September 11, 2001, terrorist attacks on the World Trade Center and the Pentagon. These individuals experienced episodes of depersonalization after a day and a half without sleep. A more commonplace example is the use of nitrous oxide, or "laughing gas," as an anesthetic during oral surgery. Many dental patients report a sense of unreality or feeling of being outside their bodies during nitrous oxide administration.

To further complicate the matter, depersonalization may be experienced in different ways by different individuals. Common descriptions include a feeling of being outside one's body; "floating on the ceiling looking down at myself;" feeling as if one's body is dissolving or changing; feeling as if one is a machine or robot; an "unreal" feeling that one is in a dream or that one "is on automatic pilot." Most patients report a sense of emotional detachment or uninvolvement, or a sense of emotional numbing. Depersonalization is distinct from a dissociative symptom called derealization, in which people perceive the external world as unreal, dreamlike, or changing. The various ways that people experience depersonalization are related to their bodies or their sense of self.

Depersonalization is a common experience in the general adult population. However, when a patient's symptoms of depersonalization are severe enough to cause significant emotional distress, or interfere with normal functioning, the criteria of the *DSM-IV-TR* for depersonalization disorder are met.

Causes and symptoms

Causes

Depersonalization disorder, like dissociative disorders in general, has been regarded as the result of severe **abuse** in childhood. This can be of a physical, emotional, and/or sexual nature.

Trauma and emotional abuse in particular are strong predictors of depersonalization disorder in adult life, as well as of depersonalization as a symptom in other mental disorders. Analysis of one study of 49 patients diagnosed with depersonalization disorder indicated much higher scores than the control subjects for the total amount of emotional abuse endured and for the maximum severity of this type of abuse. The researchers concluded that emotional abuse has been relatively neglected by psychiatrists compared to other forms of childhood trauma.

It is thought that abuse in childhood or trauma in adult life may account for the distinctive cognitive (knowledge-related) profile of patients with depersonalization disorder. These patients have significant difficulties in focusing their attention, with spatial reasoning, and with short-term visual and verbal memory. However, they have intact reality testing. (Reality testing refers to a person's ability to distinguish between their internal experiences and the objective reality of persons and objects in the outside world.) Otherwise stated, a patient with depersonalization disorder may experience his/her body as unreal, but knows that "feelings aren't facts." The *DSM-IV-TR* specifies intact reality testing as a diagnostic criterion for depersonalization disorder.

The causes of depersonalization disorder are not completely understood. Recent advances in **brain** imaging and other forms of neurological testing, however, have confirmed that depersonalization disorder is a distinct diagnostic entity and should not be considered a subtype of **post-traumatic stress disorder** (PTSD). A recent study using brain-imaging techniques found that patients with depersonalization disorder do not process emotional information in the same way as healthy controls, and their differences on brain imaging reflect their reported reduced or absent emotional response to verbal material that normally would elicit strong emotion, such as "There is a bomb inside the parcel."

NEUROBIOLOGICAL. In the past few years, several features of depersonalization disorder have been traced to differences in brain functioning. A group of British researchers found that the emotional detachment that characterizes depersonalization is associated with a lower level of nerve-cell responses in regions of the brain that are responsible for emotional feeling; and an increased level of nerve-cell responses was found in regions of the brain related to emotional regulation.

A group of American researchers concluded that patients with depersonalization disorder had different patterns of response to tests of the hypothalamic-pituitary-adrenal axis (HPA; the part of the brain involved in the "fight-or-flight" reaction to stress) than did patients with PTSD. Other tests by the same research team showed that patients with depersonalization disorder can be clearly distinguished from patients with major **depression** by tests of the functioning of the HPA axis.

Other neurobiological studies involving **positron emission tomography (PET)** measurements of glucose (sugar) metabolism in different areas of the brain found that patients with depersonalization disorder appear to have abnormal functioning of the sensory cortex. The sensory cortex is the part of the brain that governs the senses of sight, hearing, and perceptions of the location of one's body in space. These studies indicate that depersonalization is a symptom that involves differences in sensory perception and subjective experiences. In the study of patients and their processing of emotional information, it was found that patients showed a similar response in the visual cortex to emotional and neutral verbal information. They did not appear to distinguish these two classes of material, which could either be because they have an overall reduced emotional response or because their response to neutral material is enhanced.

HISTORICAL. Depersonalization disorder may be a reflection of changes in people's sense of self or personal identity within Western cultures since the eighteenth century. Historians of psychiatry have noted that whereas some mental disorders, such as depression, have been reported since the beginnings of Western medicine, no instances of the dissociative disorders were recorded before the 1780s. It seems that changes in social institutions and the structure of the family since the mid-eighteenth century may have produced a psychological structure in Westerners that makes individuals increasingly vulnerable to self disorders—as they are now called. Experiences of the unreality of one's body or one's self, such as those that characterize depersonalization disorder, presuppose a certain notion of how the self is presumed to feel. The emphasis on individualism and detachment from one's family is a mark of adult maturity in contemporary Western societies that appears to be a contributing factor to the frequency of dissociative symptoms and disorders.

Symptoms

Although the *DSM-IV-TR* does not specify a list of primary symptoms of depersonalization, clinicians generally consider the triad of emotional numbing, changes in visual perception, and altered experience of one's body to be important core symptoms of depersonalization disorder.

The *DSM-IV-TR* notes that patients with depersonalization disorder frequently score high on measurements of hypnotizability.

Diagnosis

The diagnosis of depersonalization disorder is usually a diagnosis of exclusion. The doctor will take a detailed medical history, give the patient a physical examination, and order blood and urine tests in order to rule out depersonalization resulting from epilepsy, **substance abuse**, medication side effects, or recent periods of sleep deprivation.

There are several standard diagnostic questionnaires that may be given to evaluate the presence of a dissociative disorder. The Dissociative Experiences Scale (DES) is a frequently administered self-report screener for dissociation. The **Structured Clinical Interview for DSM-IV** Dissociative Disorders, or SCID-D, can be used to make the diagnosis of depersonalization disorder distinct from the other dissociative disorders defined by *DSM-IV*. The SCID-D is a semistructured interview, which means that the examiner's questions are open-ended and allow the patient to describe experiences of depersonalization in some detail—distinct from simple yes-or-no answers.

In addition to these instruments, a six-item Depersonalization Severity Scale, or DSS, has been developed to discriminate between depersonalization disorder and other dissociative or post-traumatic disorders, and to measure the effects of treatment in patients.

Treatment

Depersonalization disorder sometimes resolves on its own without treatment. Specialized treatment is recommended only if the symptoms are persistent, recurrent, or upsetting to the patient. Insight-oriented **psychodynamic psychotherapy**, cognitive behavior therapy, and hypnosis have been demonstrated to be effective with some patients. There is, however, no single form of **psychotherapy** that is effective in treating all patients diagnosed with depersonalization disorder.

Medications that have been helpful to patients with depersonalization disorder include the benzodiazepine tranquilizers, such as **lorazepam** (Ativan), **clorazepate** (Tranxene), and **alprazolam** (Xanax), and the tricyclic **antidepressants**, such as **amitriptyline** (Elavil), **doxepin** (Sinequan), and **desipramine** (Norpramin).

KEY TERMS

Abuse—Physical, emotional, or sexual harm.

Depersonalization neurosis—Another name for depersonalization disorder.

Derealization—A dissociative symptom in which the external environment is perceived as unreal or dreamlike.

Dissociation—A reaction to trauma in which the mind splits off certain aspects of the traumatic event from conscious awareness. Dissociation can affect the patient's memory, sense of reality, and sense of identity.

Dissociative disorders—A group of disorders marked by the separation (dissociation) of perception, memory, personal identity, and consciousness. Depersonalization disorder is one of five dissociative disorders defined by *DSM-IV-TR*.

Hypothalamic-pituitary-adrenal (HPA) system—A part of the brain involved in the human stress response. The HPA system releases cortisol, the primary human stress hormone, and neurotransmitters that activate other brain structures associated with the fight-or-flight reaction. The HPA system appears to function in abnormal ways in patients diagnosed with depersonalization disorder. It is sometimes called the HPA axis.

Reality testing—A phrase that refers to a person's ability to distinguish between subjective feelings and objective reality. A person who knows that their body is real even though they may be experiencing it as unreal, for example, is said to have intact reality testing. Intact reality testing is a *DSM-IV-TR* criterion for depersonalization disorder.

Selective serotonin reuptake inhibitors (SSRIs)—Commonly prescribed drugs for treating depression. SSRIs affect the chemicals that nerves in the brain use to send messages to one another.

Serotonin—A widely distributed neurotransmitter that is found in blood platelets, the lining of the digestive tract, and in the brain where it works in combination with norepinephrine. It causes very powerful contractions of smooth muscle, and is associated with mood, attention, emotions, and sleep. Low levels of serotonin are associated with depression.

Stress—A physical and psychological response that results from being exposed to a demand or pressure.

Stressor—A stimulus or event that provokes a stress response in an organism. Stressors can be categorized as acute or chronic, and as external or internal to the organism.

Subjective—Referring to a person's unique internal thoughts and feelings, as distinct from the objects of those thoughts and feelings in the external world.

Tricyclic antidepressants (TCAs)—Antidepressant medications that have the common characteristic of a three-ring nucleus in their chemical structure. Imipramine and amitriptyline are examples of tricyclic antidepressants.

Selective serotonin reuptake inhibitors (SSRIs), which include **fluoxetine** (Prozac), **sertraline** (Zoloft), and **paroxetine** (Paxil), may also be effective. **SSRIs** affect levels of the brain chemicals that nerve cells use to send messages to each another. These chemical messengers, called (**neurotransmitters**), are released by one nerve cell and taken up by others. If the receiving cell does not take up the chemical, the sending cell will take it up, a process called "reuptake." SSRIs work by preventing the reuptake of **serotonin**, leaving more serotonin for nerve signaling. Serotonin signaling is associated with feelings of well-being.

Unfortunately, there have been very few well-designed studies comparing different medications for depersonalization disorder. Because depersonalization disorder is frequently associated with trauma, effective treatment must include other stress-related symptoms, as well.

Relaxation techniques have been reported to be a beneficial adjunctive treatment for persons diagnosed with depersonalization disorder, particularly for those who are worried about their sanity.

Prognosis

The prognosis for recovery from depersonalization disorder is good. Most patients recover completely, particularly those who developed the disorder in connection with traumas that can be explored and resolved in treatment. A few patients develop a chronic form of the disorder; this is characterized by periodic episodes of depersonalization in connection with stressful events in their lives.

Prevention

Some clinicians think that depersonalization disorder has an undetected onset in childhood, even though most patients first appear for treatment as adolescents or young adults. Preventive strategies could include the development of screening techniques for identifying children at risk, as well as further research into the effects of emotional abuse on children.

Further neurobiological research may lead to the development of medications or other treatment modalities for preventing, as well as treating, depersonalization.

Resources

BOOKS

American Psychiatric Association. *Diagnostic and Statistical Manual of Mental Disorders*. 4th ed., text rev. Washington, DC: American Psychiatric Publishing, 2000.

"Depersonalization Disorder." In *The Merck Manual of Diagnosis and Therapy*, edited by Robert S. Porter. Whitehouse Station, NJ: Merck Sharp & Dohme, 2011.

Ellenberger, Henri. *The Discovery of the Unconscious: The History and Evolution of Dynamic Psychiatry*. New York: Basic Books, 1981.

Herman, Judith. *Trauma and Recovery*. 14th printing. New York: Basic Books, 1997.

Physicians' Desk Reference 2011. 66th ed. Montvale, NJ: PDR Network, 2011.

Stout, Martha. *The Myth of Sanity: Tales of Multiple Personality in Everyday Life*. New York: Penguin Books, 2002.

PERIODICALS

Berrios, G. E., and M. Sierra. "Depersonalization: A Conceptual History." *Historical Psychiatry* 8, no. 30 Pt 2 (June 1997): 213–29.

Guralnik, O., J. Schmeidler, and D. Simeon. "Feeling Unreal: Cognitive Processes in Depersonalization." *American Journal of Psychiatry* 157 (January 2000): 103–109.

Lambert, M. V., et al. "Visual Imagery and Depersonalisation." *Psychopathology* 34, no. 5 (Sept.–Oct. 2001): 259–64.

Medford, Nicholas, et al. "Emotional Memory in Depersonalization Disorder: A Functional MRI Study." *Psychiatry Research* 148 (December 1, 2006): 93–102.

Phillips, M.L., et al. "Depersonalization Disorder: Thinking Without Feeling." *Psychiatry Research* 108, no. 3 (December 30, 2001): 145–60.

Sierra, M., and G.E. Berrios. "The Phenomenological Stability of Depersonalization: Comparing the Old with the New." *Journal of Nervous and Mental Disease* 189, no. 9 (September 2001): 629–36.

Sierra, M., et al. "Lamotrigine in the Treatment of Depersonalization Disorder." Letter to the editor in *Journal of Clinical Psychiatry* 62 (October 2001): 826–27.

Simeon, D., D.J. Stein, and E. Hollander. "Treatment of Depersonalization Disorder with Clomipramine." *Biological Psychiatry* 44, no. 4 (August 15, 1998): 302–303.

Simeon, D., et al. "Feeling Unreal: A PET Study of Depersonalization Disorder." *American Journal of Psychiatry* 157 (November 2000): 1782–88.

Simeon, D., et al. "Hypothalamic-Pituitary-Adrenal Axis Dysregulation in Depersonalization Disorder." *Neuropsychopharmacology* 25, no. 5 (November 2001): 793–95.

Simeon, D., et al. "Personality Factors Associated with Dissociation: Temperament, Defenses, and Cognitive Schemata." *American Journal of Psychiatry* 159 (March 2002): 489–91.

Simeon, D., et al. "The Role of Childhood Interpersonal Trauma in Depersonalization Disorder." *American Journal of Psychiatry* 158 (July 2001): 1027–33.

Simeon, D., O. Guralnik, and J. Schmeidler. "Development of a Depersonalization Severity Scale." *Journal of Traumatic Stress* 14, no. 2 (April 2001): 341–49.

Spitzer, Carsten, et al. "Recent Developments in the Theory of Dissociation." *World Psychiatry* 5, no. 2 (June 2006): 82–86.

Stanton, B.R., et al. "Basal Activity of the Hypothalamic-Pituitary-Adrenal Axis in Patients with Depersonalization Disorder." *Psychiatry Research* 104, no. 1 (October 10, 2001): 85–89.

Zanarini, M.C., et al. "The Dissociative Experiences of Borderline Patients." *Comprehensive Psychiatry* 41, no. 3 (May–June 2000): 223–27.

WEBSITES

Mayo Clinic staff. "Dissociative Disorders." MayoClinic.com. March 3, 2011. http://www.mayoclinic.com/health/dissociative-disorders/DS00574/DSECTION=5 (accessed October 3, 2011).

ORGANIZATIONS

International Society for the Study of Trauma and Dissociation, 8400 Westpark Dr., 2nd Fl., McLean, VA, 22102, (703) 610-9037, Fax: (703) 610-0234, http://www.isst-d.org.

International Society for Traumatic Stress Studies, 111 Deer Lake Rd., Ste. 100, Deerfield, IL, 60015, (847) 480-9028, Fax: (847) 480-9282, http://www.istss.org.

National Institute of Mental Health, 6001 Executive Blvd., Room 8184, MSC 9663, Bethesda, MD, 20892-9663, (301) 433-4513; TTY: (301) 443-8431, Fax: (301) 443-4279, (866) 615-6464; TTY: (866) 415-8051, nimhinfo@nih.gov, http://www.nimh.nih.gov.

National Organization for Rare Disorders, 55 Kenosia Ave., PO Box 1968, Danbury, CT, 06813-1968, (203) 744-0100, Fax: (203) 798-2291, (800) 999-6673, http://www.rarediseases.org.

Rebecca J. Frey, PhD
Emily Jane Willingham, PhD

Depression

Definition

Depression is the general name for a family of illnesses known as depressive disorders. As an illness, depression can affect not only the personal mood and internal thoughts of a person, but also the outwardly physical functions of affected individuals. In a depressive state, an individual may have diminished feelings, behaviors, or thoughts, along with a general lack of mental and physical health. Depression can include one or all of the following feelings: anxiety, emptiness, hopelessness, guilt, irritability, restlessness, or sadness. In addition, depressive disorders usually result from a combination of genetic, environmental, and psychological factors.

The American Psychiatric Association's *Diagnostic and Statistical Manual of Mental Disorders (DSM)* provides descriptions and standards for mental disorders. The *DSM* defines a major depressive episode (MDE) as a period of two weeks or longer during which there is either depressed mood or loss of interest or pleasure and at least four other symptoms that reflect a change in functioning, such as problems with sleep, eating, energy, concentration, and self-image.

Demographics

Depression is one of the leading causes of disability in the United States. According to the U.S. **National Institute of Mental Health** (NIMH), approximately 9.5% of adult Americans (those aged 18 years or older, about 18.8 million adults as of 2010) have some type of depressive disorder. In all, the National Institutes of Health (NIH) declares that about 20 million people in the United States are depressed. For young people in college, one out of every four students in the country has some type of diagnosable mental illness. Even small children in elementary schools have been diagnosed with depressive symptoms.

Depressive disorders

Diagnosis	Symptoms	Treatment
Sadness	Transient, normal depressive response or mood change due to stress.	Emotional support
Bereavement	Sadness related to a major loss that persists for less than two months after the loss. Thoughts of death and morbid preoccupation with worthlessness are also present.	Emotional support, counseling
Sadness problem	Sadness or irritability that begins to resemble major depressive disorder, but lower in severity and more transient.	Support, counseling, medication possible
Adjustment disorder with depressed mood	Symptoms include depressed mood, tearfulness, and hopelessness, and occur within three months of an identifiable stressor. Symptoms resolve in six months.	Psychotherapy, medication
Major depressive disorder	A depressed or irritable mood or diminished pleasure as well as three to seven of the following criteria almost daily for two weeks. The criteria include: recurrent thoughts of death and suicidal ideation, weight loss or gain, fatigue or energy loss, feelings of worthlessness, diminished ability to concentrate, insomnia or hypersomnia, and feeling hyper and jittery or abnormally slow.	Psychotherapy, medication
Dysthymic disorder	Depressed mood for most of the day, for more days than not, for one year, including the presence of two of the following symptoms: poor appetite or overeating, insomnia/hypersomnia, low energy/fatigue, poor concentration, and feelings of hopelessness. Symptoms are less severe than those of a major depressive episode but are more persistent.	Psychotherapy, medication
Bipolar I disorder, most recent episode depressed	Current major depressive episode with a history of one manic or mixed episode. (Manic episode is longer than four days and causes significant impairment in normal functioning.) Moods are not accounted for by another psychiatric disorder.	Psychotherapy, medication
Bipolar II disorder, recurrent major depressive episodes with hypomanic episodes	Presence or history of one major depressive episode and one hypomanic episode (similar to manic episode but shorter and less severe). Symptoms are not accounted for by another psychiatric disorder and cause clinically significant impairment in functioning.	Psychotherapy, medication

SOURCE: Academy of American Family Physicians, http://www.aafp.org.

Types of depressive disorders. *(Table by PreMediaGlobal. Reproduced by permission of Gale, a part of Cengage Learning.)*

The U.S. Centers for Disease Control and Prevention (CDC) states that at the end of 2010, 4.1% of American adults met the criteria for major depression. Geographically, depression is more prevalent in the southeastern states than in any other region of the United States. The CDC also states that depression is more likely to occur in people 45 to 64 years of age, women, African Americans, Hispanics, and non-Hispanic persons of other races or multiple races. People with less than a high-school education are also at greater risk of being depressed, as are persons who have undergone a divorce. In addition, individuals who are unable to work or unemployed are more likely to be depressed, along with those without health insurance.

Depression within the United States is increasing on an annual basis. Internationally, depression is estimated to become the second most common health problem in the world by 2020. According to the NIMH, many people have more than one mental disorder at any given time. Nearly half of those with any mental disorder meet criteria for two or more disorders.

That women experience depression at a rate of almost twice that of men may be partially explained by the greater willingness of women to seek psychological treatment, but this does not explain the entire discrepancy. Many physical events specific to women, such as menstruation, pregnancy, miscarriage, the postpartum period, and menopause are recognized as factors contributing to depression in women. Women in the United States may face environmental stresses with a higher frequency than do men. For instance, most single-parent households are headed by women; women still provide the majority of child and elder care, even in two-income families; and women are generally paid less than men, so financial concerns may be greater.

Particular demographic problems associated with depression include depression in the elderly (**late-life depression**) and depression in children and adolescents (**juvenile depression**). One common belief is that depression is normal in elderly people. This is not the case, although increasing age and the absence of interpersonal relationships are associated with depression. Because of this misconception, depressive disorders in the elderly population often go undiagnosed and untreated. Similarly, many parents often ignore the symptoms of a depressive disorder in their children, assuming that these symptoms are merely a phase that the child will later outgrow.

Description

Everyone feels sadness, **grief**, or despair at some point in their lives. However, unlike these normal, transient emotional states, a depressive disorder is not a temporary bout of "feeling down," but rather a serious disease that should be recognized and treated as a medical condition. Without treatment, a depressive disorder can persist, and its symptoms can go on for weeks, months, or even years.

Depression is quite widespread and one of the leading causes of disability in the world. Commonly recognized symptoms of all types of depressive disorders are recurring feelings of sadness and guilt; changes in sleeping patterns, such as **insomnia** or oversleeping; changes in appetite; decreased mental and physical energy; unusual irritability; the inability to enjoy once-favored activities; difficulty working; and thoughts of death or **suicide**. If only these "down" symptoms are experienced, the individual may have a unipolar depressive disorder such as dysthymia or major depression. If the depressed periods alternate with extreme "up" periods, the individual may have a **bipolar disorder**.

Dysthymia

Dysthymia is a relatively mild depressive disorder that is characterized by the presence of two or more of the symptoms listed above. The symptoms are not severe enough to disable the affected individual but are long-term (chronic) and may last for several years. *Dysthymia* is a compound word originating in Greek that means ill or bad (*dys-*) soul, mind, or spirit (*thymia*). Individuals affected with dysthymia often also experience episodes of major depression at some point in their lives.

Major depression

In major depression, the affected individual has five or more symptoms and experiences one or more prolonged episodes of depression that last longer than two weeks. These episodes disrupt the ability of the affected individual to the point that the person is unable to function. Individuals experiencing an episode of major depression often entertain suicidal thoughts, the presence of which contributes to this disorder being quite serious. Major depression should not be confused with a grief reaction such as that associated with the death of a loved one. Some individuals affected by major depression may experience only a single bout of disabling depression in their lifetimes. More commonly, affected individuals experience recurrent disabling episodes throughout their lives.

Other depressive disorders

The fifth edition of the *DSM* (*DSM-5*, 2013) proposes to include the following depressive disorders:

- disruptive mood dysregulation disorder
- major depressive disorder, single episode
- major depressive disorder, recurrent

- chronic depressive disorder (dysthymia)
- premenstrual dysphoric disorder
- mixed anxiety/depression
- substance-induced depressive disorder
- depressive disorder associated with a known general medical condition
- other specified depressive disorder
- unspecified depressive disorder

Previously, depressive disorders and bipolar disorder, a condition that alternates between periods of extreme excitement (mania) and periods of depression, were both classified as mood disorders. The proposed *DSM-5* changes divide the two into new categories, depressive disorders and bipolar and related disorders.

Causes and symptoms

Causes

Depressive disorders are believed to be related to genetic imbalances in **brain** chemistry, particularly in relation to the chemicals that carry signals between brain cells (**neurotransmitters**), as well as the hormones released by parts of the brain. **Serotonin** and norepinephrine are two important neurotransmitters. Disruption of the brain's circuits in areas involved with emotions, appetite, sexual drive, and sleep is a likely cause of the dysfunctions associated with depressive disorders. Thus, some of the newest treatments for depression are drugs that are known to affect brain chemistry.

There are also many non-genetic factors that cause depression, including stressful environments or situations, certain illnesses, and precipitating conditions, such as the loss of a close relationship. Alcohol abuse and the use of **sedatives**, **barbiturates**, narcotics, or other drugs can cause depression due to their effect on brain chemistry.

Symptoms

Individuals affected with depressive disorders display a wide range of symptoms. These symptoms vary in severity from person to person and vary over time in a single affected individual.

Symptoms that characterize a depressive state include:

- feelings of hopelessness
- feelings of guilt
- feelings of worthlessness
- a persistently sad or anxious mood
- restlessness or irritability
- a loss of interest in activities that were once considered pleasurable
- difficulty concentrating, remembering, or making decisions
- sleep disorders, including insomnia, early-morning awakening, and/or oversleeping

KEY TERMS

Bipolar disorder—Formerly called "manic depression," this psychological disorder is characterized by periods of mania followed by periods of depression.

Cognitive/behavioral therapies—Psychological counseling that focuses on changing the behavior of the patient.

Dysthymia—A psychological condition of chronic depression that is not disabling but prevents the individual from functioning at his or her full capacity.

Electroconvulsive therapy—A psychological treatment in which a series of controlled electrical impulses are delivered to the brain in order to induce a seizure.

Grief reaction—The normal depression felt after a traumatic major life occurrence, such as the loss of a loved one.

Interpersonal therapies—Also called "talking therapy," this type of psychological counseling is focused on determining how dysfunctional interpersonal relationships of the affected individual may be causing or influencing symptoms of depression.

Major depression—A psychological condition in which the patient experiences one or more disabling attacks of depression lasting two or more weeks.

Polygenic—A trait, characteristic, or condition that depends on the activity of more than one gene for its emergence or expression.

Psychodynamic therapies—A form of psychological counseling that seeks to determine and resolve the internal conflicts that may be causing an individual to experience the symptoms of depression.

Psychotherapy—Psychological counseling that seeks to determine the underlying causes of a patient's depression. The form of this counseling may be cognitive/behavioral, interpersonal, or psychodynamic.

- constant fatigue
- eating disorders, including weight loss or overeating
- suicidal thoughts and/or tendencies
- recurrent physical symptoms that do not respond to the normal treatments of these symptoms, such as headaches, digestive problems, and chronic pain

Diagnosis

Depression is notoriously difficult to diagnose because its symptoms are not readily apparent to the medical professional unless the patient first recognizes and admits to them. Once the individual seeks help for his or her symptoms, the first step in the **diagnosis** of a depressive disorder is a complete physical examination to rule out any medical conditions, viral infections, or currently used medications that may produce effects similar to those seen in depression. Alcohol or other drug abuse as a possible cause of the observed symptoms should also be investigated. Once a physical basis for these symptoms is eliminated, a complete psychological exam should be undertaken. This examination consists of a **mental status examination**, a complete history of both current and previously experienced symptoms, and a family history.

The mental status examination is used to determine whether a more severe psychotic condition is evident. This mental status examination will also determine whether the depressive disorder has caused changes in speech, thought patterns, or memory, which may indicate the presence of a depressive disorder. The complete psychological exam also includes a complete history of the symptoms being experienced by the affected individual. This history includes the onset of the symptoms, their duration, and whether the affected individual has had similar symptoms in the past. In the case of past symptoms, a treatment history should be completed to assess whether these symptoms previously responded to treatment, and if so, which treatments were effective. The final component of the complete psychological exam is the family history. In cases where the affected individual has similarly affected family members, a treatment history should also be completed, as thoroughly as possible, for these family members.

The diagnostic criteria for a major depressive episode (MDE) according to the DSM are:

- At least five of the following symptoms present during the same two-week period, nearly every day, and representing a change from previous functioning. At least one of the symptoms is either depressed mood or loss of interest or pleasure; the remaining four include
  1. depressed mood (alternatively, irritable mood in children and adolescents)
  2. markedly diminished interest or pleasure in all, or almost all, activities
  3. significant weight loss when not dieting, or weight gain or decrease or increase in appetite
  4. insomnia or hypersomnia
  5. psychomotor agitation or retardation
  6. fatigue or loss of energy
  7. feelings of worthlessness or excessive or inappropriate guilt
  8. diminished ability to think or concentrate, or indecisiveness
  9. recurrent thoughts of death (not just fear of dying), recurrent suicidal thoughts without a specific plan, or a suicide attempt or a specific plan for committing suicide
- The symptoms significantly disturb functions of daily life, such as social and occupational activities, and are not attributed to another medical condition (mental or physical).
- The symptoms are not a side effect of a substance (drug or prescribed medication) nor caused by an antidepressant treatment (e.g., electroshock therapy).

The *DSM-IV-TR* (fourth edition, text revised) accounts for periods of **bereavement** in what is referred to as the "grief exclusion." Feelings of grief after the loss of a loved one are similar to symptoms of depression, but a normal period of bereavement is not considered an acceptable basis for a diagnosis of depression. The *DSM-5* proposed changes eliminate the grief exclusion, the rationale being that there is not enough evidence to support the loss of a loved one as unique from other serious stressors experienced in life, such as rape, divorce, or cancer; all of these situations are likely to produce depressive symptoms, at least temporarily. This proposal is controversial, as supporters of the grief exclusion believe that its removal stigmatizes bereavement by allowing it to be diagnosed as an MDE.

Dysthymia

A diagnosis of dysthymia, or chronic depressive disorder, requires that the depression occur consistently for at least two years, or at least one year of irritability in children. Depression must be accompanied by two or more symptoms:

- loss of appetite or overeating
- insomnia or hypersomnia
- fatigue
- low self-esteem
- loss of concentration or reduced ability to make decisions
- sense of hopelessness

The symptoms cannot have more than a two-month lapse during the two-year period, cannot be caused by another psychotic or medical disorder, cannot be the result of a substance (drug or medication), and must significantly impair daily functioning.

Mixed anxiety/depression

Mixed anxiety/depression requires that the patient experience three or four symptoms of an MDE (including depressed mood), accompanied by distressing anxiety. Anxious distress requires two or more of the following: irrational worries, constant unpleasant worries, inability to relax, motor tension, and the consistent fear that something terrible will happen.

Treatment

Treatment of depression is on a case-by-case basis that is largely dependent on the outcome of the psychological examination. Some mildly affected individuals respond fully to **psychotherapy** and do not require medication. Some individuals affected with moderate or severe depression benefit from antidepressant medication. Most affected individuals respond best to a combination of antidepressant medication and psychotherapy—the medication to provide relatively rapid relief from the symptoms of depression and the psychotherapy to learn effective ways to manage and cope with problems and issues that may cause the continuation of symptoms or the onset of new symptoms of depression.

Various types of antidepressant medications are available for the treatment of depressive disorders. Many individuals affected by depression will go through a variety of **antidepressants**, or antidepressant combinations, before the best medication and dosage for them is identified. Almost all antidepressant medications must be taken regularly for at least two months before the full therapeutic effects are realized. A full course of medication is generally no shorter than six to nine months to prevent recurrence of the symptoms. In individuals affected with bipolar disorder or chronic major depression, medication may have to be continued throughout the remainder of their lives. These time-related conditions often pose problems in the management of individuals affected with depressive disorder. Many individuals who have a depressive disorder discontinue their medications before the fully prescribed course, for a variety of reasons. Some affected individuals feel side effects of the medications prior to feeling any benefits; others do not feel that the medication is helping, because of the delay between the initiation of the treatment and the feelings of symptom relief; and, many feel better prior to the full course and so cease taking the medication.

The three most commonly prescribed antidepressant drug classes consist of the older tricyclics (TCAs) and the two relatively new drug classes: the **selective serotonin reuptake inhibitors (SSRIs)** and the **monoamine oxidase inhibitors (MAOIs)**. The most common TCAs are: **amitriptyline** (Elavil), **clomipramine** (Anafranil), **desipramine** (Norpramin, Pertofrane), **doxepin** (Sinequan, Adapin), **imipramine** (Tofranil, Janimine), **nortriptyline** (Pamelor, Aventyl), **protriptyline** (Vivactil), and **trimipramine** (Surmontil). The most common **SSRIs** are: **citalopram** (Celexa), **fluoxetine** (Prozac), **fluvoxamine** (Luvox), **paroxetine** (Paxil), and **sertraline** (Zoloft). The most common **MAOIs** are: **phenelzine** (Nardil) and **tranylcypromine** (Parnate).

Many antidepressant medications cause side effects, such as agitation, bladder problems, blurred vision, constipation, drowsiness, dry mouth, headache, insomnia, nausea, nervousness, or sexual problems. Most of these side effects wear off as the treatment course progresses. The tricyclics cause more severe side effects than the newer SSRIs or MAOIs.

In the most severely affected individuals, or where antidepressant medications either have not worked or cannot be taken, **electroconvulsive therapy** (ECT) may be considered. In the ECT procedure, electrodes are placed on specific locations on the head to deliver electrical stimulation to the brain. Electrical stimulation is designed to trigger a brief seizure. These **seizures** generally last approximately 30 seconds. The patient does not consciously feel the stimulations. ECT has been much improved in recent years; specifically, it is no longer the electroshock treatment of nightmares, and its deleterious effects on long-term memory have been reduced. ECT treatments are generally administered several times a week as necessary to control the symptoms being experienced.

Several short-term (10- to 20-week) psychotherapies have also been demonstrated to be effective in the treatment of depressive disorders. These include interpersonal and **cognitive-behavioral therapy**. Interpersonal therapies focus on the interpersonal relationships of the affected individual that may both cause and heighten the depression. Cognitive-behavioral therapy focuses on how the affected individual may be able to change his or her patterns of thinking or behaving that may lead to episodes of depression. Psychodynamic therapies, which generally are not short-term psychotherapies, seek to treat the individual with a depressive disorder through a resolution of internal conflicts. Psychodynamic therapies are generally not initiated during major depressive episodes or until the symptoms of depression are significantly improved by medication or one of the short-term psychotherapies.

Alternative

St. John's wort (Hypericum perforatum) is used throughout Europe to treat depressive symptoms. Unlike traditional prescription antidepressants, this herbal anti-depressant has few reported side effects. Results on the success of St. John's wort are conflicting: a review of 37 **clinical trials** comparing St. John's wort to antidepressants discovered that St. John's wort is most beneficial to persons with mild depression. The herb provided minimal effects similar to a placebo in those with major depression. However, later studies have found more positive results in using St. John' wort to treat major depression. Because supplements are not regulated by the FDA in the same way as conventional medications, care should be taken when selecting herbal treatments.

5-hydroxytryptophan (5-HT, **5-HTP**) is a precursor to serotonin and is available as a supplement. Most of the commercially available 5-HTP is extracted from the plant Griffonia simplicifolia. In several small studies, treatment with 5-HTP significantly improved depression in more than half of the patients. However, some users of 5-HTP have developed eosinophilia-myalgia syndrome (EMS), a serious medical condition characterized by myalgia and blood abnormalities. It is unclear whether the EMS was caused by the use of 5-HTP, a contaminant discovered in some 5-HTP products, or an external factor. Until more research is done, the U.S. National Library of Medicine's and National Institutes of Health's MedlinePlus service advises against using 5-HTP

Clinical trials

In May 2011, the NIH ClinicalTrials.gov website showed 2,260 clinical trials for depression—classified as ongoing (recruiting volunteers or active but not recruiting), completed, or unknown status—along with 2,243 trials for depressive disorders and 912 clinical trials for major depressive disorders. NIH constantly updates clinical trial information. The most recent information on depression trials can be found at: http://clinicaltrials.gov/search/open/condition=%22Depression%22.

Prognosis

Over 80% of individuals affected with a depressive disorder have demonstrated improvement after receiving the appropriate combination of treatments. One significant tragedy associated with depression is the failure of many affected individuals to realize that they have a treatable medical condition. Some affected individuals who do not receive treatment may recover completely on their own (without professional medical assistance), but most will suffer needlessly. A small number of individuals with depressive disorder do not respond to treatment.

QUESTIONS TO ASK YOUR DOCTOR

- What is causing my depression?
- How severe is my depression?
- Could my depression be caused by another condition or underlying disease?
- How safe are antidepressants? Are there side effects from them? What about long-term side effects?
- How long will it take before the antidepressants begin to work?
- Are antidepressant medicines addictive?
- Can I be treated for depression without medicines?
- Is depression hereditary? Should I be concerned that I will pass depression to my children?

Prevention

Depression is not always preventable. However, persons can minimize depression's impact on their lives by recognizing the symptoms of depression and seeking help right away from a medical professional. **Stress** is an early warning sign that depression may occur. It is important to control stresses encountered in life. A social support network in the form of friends and family can help to control stress. Maintain interactions with people, whether professionally or personally. Isolation from the outside world adds to the risk of depression.

Depression is treatable, but the key to alleviating the worse forms of depression is to discuss symptoms openly with a family doctor or other trusted medical practitioner. Treating physical or mental issues is also likely to help reduce the occurrence of depression. Maintaining a high level of self-esteem will help to reduce the risk of depression or help to counter bouts of depression.

Besides seeking professional help, depression can be lessened in risk by enjoying life, eating a well-balanced and healthy diet, getting plenty of **exercise**, sleeping a sufficient number of hours each night, balancing work and personal life, and adhering to a healthy lifestyle. If feeling generally overwhelmed or stressed, seek help from self-help books, relaxation techniques (such as **yoga**, **meditation**, or tai chi), or **support groups**. A medical professional, such as a **psychologist**, can help in locating such resources. Stress can often be alleviated by eliminating unnecessary to-dos and by adding structure to daily activities (such as maintaining a list of activities and tasks to be accomplished).

Resources

BOOKS

Aguirre, Blaise A. *Depression.* Westport, CT: Greenwood Press, 2008.

Bjornlund, Lydia. *Depression.* Detroit: Lucent Books, 2010.

Gordon, James S. *Unstuck: Your Guide to the Seven-Stage Journey Out of Depression.* New York: Penguin Press, 2008.

Karp, David A. *Is It Me or My Meds?: Living with Antidepressants.* Cambridge: Harvard University Press, 2007.

Katon, Wayne, et al. *The Depression Helpbook.* Boulder, CO: Bull, 2008.

Knaus, William J. *The Cognitive Behavioral Workbook for Depression: A Step-by-step Program.* Oakland, CA: New Harbinger Publications, 2006.

Luciani, Joseph J. *Self-Coaching: The Powerful Program to Beat Anxiety and Depression,* 2nd edition, New York: Wiley, 2006.

Williams, Mark, et al. *The Mindful Way through Depression: Freeing Yourself from Chronic Unhappiness.* New York: The Guilford Press, 2007.

PERIODICALS

Adamek, M. E., and G. Y. Slater. "Depression and Anxiety." *Journal of Gerontological Social Work* 50, suppl. 1 (2008): 153–189.

American College of Physicians. "Summaries for patients. Use of drugs to treat depression: guidelines from the American College of Physicians." *Annals of Internal Medicine* 149, no. 10 (November 2008): I56.

"Check your vitamin D intake to avoid multiple health consequences. Three 2008 studies link low vitamin D levels to depression, hip fractures, and increased risk of death." *Health News* 14, no. 11 (November 2008): 9–10.

Gartlehner, G., et al., "Comparative benefits and harms of second-generation antidepressants: background paper for the American College of Physicians." *Annals of Internal Medicine* 149, no. 10 (November 2008): 734–750.

Kozasa, E. H., et al. "Evaluation of Siddha Samadhi Yoga for anxiety and depression symptoms: a preliminary study." *Psychological Reports* 103, no. 1 (August 2008): 271–274.

Krishnan, V., and E. J. Nestler. "The molecular neurobiology of depression." *Nature* 455, no. 7215 (October 2008): 894–902.

Luijendijk, H. J., et al. "Incidence and recurrence of late-life depression." *Archives of General Psychiatry* 65, no. 12 (December 2008): 1394–1401.

Mouchet-Mages, S., and F. J. Bayle. "Sadness as an integral part of depression." *Dialogues in Clinical Neuroscience* 10, no. 3 (2008): 321–327.

Paykel, E. S. "Basic concepts of depression." *Dialogues in Clinical Neuroscience* 10, no. 3 (2008): 279–289.

OTHER

Kendler, Kenneth S. [No title listed; article explains rationale behind removal of the grief exclusion criterion.] http://www.dsm5.org/about/Documents/grief%20exclusion_Kendler.pdf (accessed July 28, 2011).

WEBSITES

Centers for Disease Control and Prevention. "An Estimated 1 in 10 U.S. Adults Report Depression." March 31, 2011. http://www.cdc.gov/Features/dsDepression (accessed May 11, 2011).

First, Michael B., Ronald W. Pies, and Sidney Zisook. "Depression or Bereavement? Defining the Distinction." Medscape News. http://www.medscape.com/viewarticle/740333 (accessed July 28, 2011).

MedlinePlus. "Depression." U.S. Library of Medicine, National Institutes of Health. May 8, 2011. http://www.nlm.nih.gov/medlineplus/depression.html (accessed May 12, 2011).

National Institute of Mental Health. "Depression." http://www.nimh.nih.gov/health/publications/depression/complete-index.shtml (accessed May 11, 2011).

———. "Women and Depression: Discovering Hope." August 31, 2010. http://www.nimh.nih.gov/health/publications/depression-what-every-woman-should-know/summary.shtml (accessed May 12, 2011).

WomensHealth.gov. "Depression." March 17, 2010. http://womenshealth.gov/faq/depression.cfm (accessed May 12, 2011).

ORGANIZATIONS

American Psychiatric Association (APA), 1000 Wilson Boulevard, Suite 1825, Arlington, VA, 22209, (888) 357-7924, apa@psych.org, http://www.psych.org.

Depression and Bipolar Support Alliance, 730 N. Franklin Street, Suite 501, Chicago, IL, 60654-7225, (800) 826-3632, Fax: (312) 642-7243, info@dbsalliance.org, http://www.dbsalliance.org.

Mental Health America, 2000 N. Beauregard Street, 6th Floor, Alexandria, VA, 22311, (703) 684-7722, (800) 969-6642, Fax: (703) 684-5968, http://www.nmha.org.

National Institute of Mental Health (NIMH), 6001 Executive Boulevard, Bethesda, MD, 20892-9663, (301) 443-4513, (866) 615-6464, Fax: (301) 443-4279, nimhinfor@nih.gov, http://www.nimh.nih.gov.

Substance Abuse and Mental Health Services Administration, 1 Choke Cherry Road, Rockville, MD, 20857, (877) 726-4727, http://www.samhsa.gov.

Paul A. Johnson
Monique Laberge, PhD
William Atkins

Dermatillomania

Definition

Dermatillomania, also called psychogenic excoriation (skin removal), neurotic excoriation, acne excoriée, pathological skin picking (PSP), and compulsive skin picking, is characterized by excessive picking, scratching, or squeezing of skin. Dermatillomania is hypothesized to be an impulse control disorder related to **obsessive-compulsive disorder** (OCD), **body dysmorphic disorder** (BDD), and/or **depression**. Dermatillomania can, therefore, be distinguished from other dermatological diseases that are influenced by psychological factors (e.g., psoriasis or alopecia) because it is a dermatological manifestation of a psychiatric syndrome.

Demographics

Dermatillomania is probably underdiagnosed in the general population, partly because persons with the disorder can often hide its visible evidence under clothing or makeup, and partly because most are embarrassed to report the disorder to their doctors. In addition, children with the disorder may not think of their skin picking as abnormal. Estimates range from 1% to 5.4% of the general population in Canada and the United States, with women more likely to develop the disorder than men. The female/male ratio is variously given as 1.2:1 to 9:1. About 2% of patients seen in U.S. dermatology clinics are diagnosed with compulsive skin picking.

Estimates differ about the age range of patients with dermatillomania. Some researchers report that older children and adolescents are the most susceptible age group, whereas other observers report that the mean age at onset of the disorder is 30 to 45 years of age.

Humans are not the only species in which skin picking behavior has been reported. It has also been observed in horses, birds, cats, and dogs, and in laboratory rats given **amphetamines**.

Description

Behaviors associated with dermatillomania include excessive excoriation of skin at multiple sites that are easily reachable. Excoriation may be triggered by and occur at sites of skin lesions (e.g., acne, scabs, insect bites) or in response to such skin sensations as dryness, tingling, or pain. In some cases the skin picking is associated with **cocaine** or **methamphetamine addiction**, in that the abuse of these drugs sometimes results in a sensation known as formication, or the feeling that insects are crawling on or under the skin. Prescription drugs known to cause formication include **methylphenidate** (Ritalin) and eszopiclone (Lunesta).

The face is the most common site of excoriation that is usually performed with the fingers or fingernails but may involve the teeth or such other instruments as tweezers, pins, or blades. Other parts of the body that are commonly affected include the gums, lips, upper back, shoulders, scalp, abdomen, chest, and the fingernails, cuticles, and toenails. Excoriation may occur in brief bouts (less than 5 minutes) or for extended periods of time as long as 12 hours and is usually worse in the evening.

Impulse control disorders in general are characterized by irresistible impulses to commit acts that may be harmful to the self or others. Feelings of tension or anxiety may precede these acts that may then be followed by pleasure or gratification following the performance of the act. Guilt or regret may or may not be felt subsequent to the act. A person experiencing dermatillomania is likely to be under substantial distress and may feel embarrassed about the excoriating behavior. Social functioning may be severely affected, especially sports participation and other functions in which skin lesions will be exposed. Excoriation may result in varied medical complications, including bleeding, ulcers, infections, and temporary or permanent disfigurement.

Risk factors

Risk factors for dermatillomania include:

- female sex
- age between 8 and 40
- history of childhood abuse
- present abuse of cocaine, methamphetamine, or other stimulant drugs
- high stress level in the family, school, or workplace
- being diagnosed with a mood or anxiety disorder; between 48% and 79% of patients who pick their skin meet the criteria for a mood disorder, and 65% meet the criteria for an anxiety disorder
- being diagnosed with BDD; one study reported that 27% of patients with BDD pick at their skin
- having certain internal disorders that affect the skin, such as diabetes, lymphoma, hyperthyroidism, liver disease, anemia, or uremia

As far as is known, race or ethnicity is not a risk factor for dermatillomania.

Causes and symptoms

Causes

The causes of dermatillomania are still debated and discussed by dermatologists as well as psychiatrists, as is the disorder's relationship to mood, anxiety, impulse control, and **substance abuse** disorders. In some cases

KEY TERMS

Dermatologist—A physician who specializes in the diagnosis and treatment of disorders of the skin, scalp, hair, and nails.

Excoriation—The medical term for abrasion of the upper layer of skin caused by mechanical means, most often scratching or picking.

Formication—The medical term for the sensation of insects crawling on or under the skin. The English word is taken from *formica*, the Latin word for "ant."

Lesion—Any abnormality in or injury to a body tissue. It is derived from the Latin word for "injury."

Scabies—A contagious skin infection in humans and other animals caused by a tiny parasite that burrows under the skin and causes intense itching.

Unna sleeve—A dressing made of gauze impregnated with glycerin, zinc oxide, and calamine that can be used to protect skin injured by compulsive picking from further injury. It is named for the German dermatologist who invented it.

the onset of the disorder is triggered by an insect bite, itchy rash, acne, or other skin disorder, but in other cases there is no underlying skin disease or blemish when the patient first begins to pick at the skin. In some cases the skin picking is associated with emotional **stress**, but in others it is an unconscious process. Some patients report that their skin picking has a ritualistic quality, whereas others report being in a dissociated state during their skin picking episodes.

There was no evidence as of 2011 that **brain** abnormalities or **genetic factors** were involved in the disorder.

Symptoms

The most noticeable external symptom of dermatillomania is the appearance of scratches, scabs, open sores, and/or bruises on areas of the skin that are pulled, squeezed, or picked at. Some of the lesions may appear to be partially healed and reopened. There may or may not be visible bleeding.

Diagnosis

The **diagnosis** is made on the basis of a combination of patient history, office examination of the skin lesions, and direct questioning about skin picking. The patient may or may not volunteer information about the self-injurious behavior. There are a few online self-tests about skin picking, and the patient may seek help after taking the test. The doctor will ask about stress levels, drug use, a history of skin disorders (if any), and a history of mood, anxiety, or impulse control disorders as part of the history-taking.

Dermatillomania was not formally included in ***Diagnostic and Statistical Manual of Mental Disorders***, fourth edition, text revision (*DSM-IV-TR*), although it is proposed for inclusion under the name "Skin picking disorder" in *DSM-5*, due for publication in 2013. The editors of *DSM-5* have proposed the following diagnostic criteria for skin picking disorder:

- There is recurrent skin picking resulting in the appearance of skin lesions.
- The skin picking or pulling "causes clinically significant distress or impairment in social, occupational, or other important areas of functioning."
- The skin picking is not due directly to the physiological effects of a substance or a general medical condition that affects the skin.
- The skin picking is not restricted to the symptoms of another psychiatric disorder, such as BDD or delusional disorder.

As of 2011, the *DSM-5* development group was debating adding a fifth criterion to address the actual urges to engage in skin picking or failed attempts at resisting skin picking.

Examination

The patient's primary care physician may be able to identify lesions created by skin picking but may also refer the patient to a dermatologist for an office examination, particularly if the patient also has acne, eczema, or another skin disorder. The dermatologist can usually distinguish skin excoriations caused by compulsive skin picking from other skin disorders because the lesions are typically clean and linear with irregular borders. They are similar in size and shape to one another and occur on parts of the body that the patient can easily scratch. They are generally distributed on both sides of the body in a symmetrical pattern.

Tests

In some cases the dermatologist may take a small sample of skin to rule out scabies, a fungal infection, or other organic skin disorder. The doctor may also order a complete blood cell count, fasting blood glucose level, or urine test to rule out diabetes, anemia, or other systemic disorders. Imaging tests are not useful in diagnosing dermatillomania.

Treatment

Treatment for compulsive skin picking is usually multimodal, involving a combination of medications and **psychotherapy**.

Drugs

Case reports and small trials have examined the efficacy of various types of drugs for dermatillomania: **antidepressants**, including the **selective serotonin reuptake inhibitors** (**SSRIs**, such as **fluvoxamine**) and the tricyclics (**doxepin** and **clomipramine**), opiate antagonists (**naltrexone**), typical antipsychotics (**pimozide**), and atypical antipsychotics (**olanzapine**, **aripiprazole**). Some patients are reportedly helped by **gabapentin**, a drug originally developed to treat epilepsy that is also used to relieve neuropathic pain.

Another approach that works well for some patients is the use of an Unna sleeve or Unna boot to protect the affected part of the body while the patient is receiving psychotherapy and medications for the compulsive skin picking. Named for the German dermatologist Paul Unna (1850–1929), the Unna sleeve (or boot) is a gauze wrapping impregnated with a mixture of glycerin, **zinc** oxide, and calamine to promote healing. It has been used in the treatment of burns and venous ulcers as well as neurotic excoriation.

Psychotherapy

Behavioral treatments, including psychotherapy and hypnosis, have been examined for effectiveness in dermatillomania. Small-scale studies or case reports have suggested that habit reversal therapy (HRT), a form of **cognitive-behavioral therapy** in which a program of self-monitoring is paired with practicing a competing response, is effective. In HRT, the patient is taught first to be mindful of the situations or events that trigger the skin-picking episodes and then to practice alternative behaviors when the triggers are present. Other forms of psychotherapy, in which behavioral and emotional as well as topical therapies are practiced, can also be effective, as is **group therapy** for the disorder.

Alternative

Some patients with compulsive skin picking are helped by mindfulness **meditation** as an adjunct to HRT. Others report that the relaxation response, breathing exercises, and other **stress reduction** techniques are helpful.

QUESTIONS TO ASK YOUR DOCTOR

- Have you ever treated a patient with dermatillomania?
- What is your opinion of habit reversal training as a treatment for the disorder?
- What do you think causes the disorder?
- Why do you think women are at increased risk of dermatillomania?

Prognosis

Dermatillomania is often a long-term psychiatric problem—the mean duration of symptoms is between 5 and 21 years—but is not known to be fatal. It is, however, not well researched. One team of researchers in Minnesota reported in late 2010 that patients with dermatillomania are on average more severely impaired than patients with **trichotillomania**. There were only eight **clinical trials** of treatments for dermatillomania as of 2011; five were trials of various drugs (**escitalopram**, dronabinol, **lamotrigine**, and n-acetyl cysteine), and three trials were testing the effectiveness of cognitive behavioral interventions.

Large-scale outcome studies of dermatillomania are lacking, although some researchers suggest that visiting a dermatologist prior to experiencing symptoms for one year results in a better prognosis. Permanent scarring and complications from infection of the tissues injured by skin picking are possible. In addition, the chronic rebuilding of the injured tissues has been suggested to be a potential causative factor for skin cancer.

Prevention

There is no known way to prevent dermatillomania because its underlying causes or triggers are not well understood.

Resources

BOOKS

Aboujaoude, Elias, and Lorrin M. Koran. *Impulse Control Disorders*. New York: Cambridge University Press, 2010.

Grant, Jon E., ed. *Trichotillomania, Skin Picking, and Other Body-focused Repetitive Behaviors*. Washington, DC: American Psychiatric Publishing, 2012.

PERIODICALS

Grant, J.E., et al. "A Double-blind, Placebo-controlled Trial of Lamotrigine for Pathological Skin Picking: Treatment Efficacy and Neurocognitive Predictors of Response."

Journal of Clinical Psychopharmacology 30 (2010): 396–403.

Harris, S.S., et al. "Pathologic Grooming Behavior: Facial Dermatillomania." *Cutis* 87 (2011): 14–18.

Odlaug, Bryan L., and Jon E. Grant. "Pathologic Skin Picking." *American Journal of Drug and Alcohol Abuse* 36 (2010): 296–303.

Odlaug, Bryan L., and Jon E. Grant. "Quality of Life and Clinical Severity in Pathological Skin Picking and Trichotillomania." *Journal of Anxiety Disorders* 24, no. 8 (2010): 823–29.

Paley, K., et al. "Unna Sleeve for Neurotic Excoriations." *Cutis* 85 (2010): 149–52.

Schuck, K., et al. "The Effects of Brief Cognitive-behaviour Therapy for Pathological Skin Picking: A Randomized Comparison to Wait-list Control." *Behaviour Research and Therapy* 49 (2011): 11–17.

Snorrason, I., et al. "Motor Inhibition, Reflection Impulsivity, and Trait Impulsivity in Pathological Skin Picking." *Behavior Therapy* 42 (2011): 521–32.

Turner, B.T., et al. "The Skin Picking Impact Project: Phenomenology, Interference, and Treatment Utilization of Pathological Skin Picking in a Population-based Sample." *Journal of Anxiety Disorders* 25 (2011): 88–95.

OTHER

Hayden, Lisa. "Scars of Shame" [three-minute trailer for a documentary about dermatillomania produced by the National Film Board of Canada]. http://www.youtube.com/watch?v=UGjhx7OGcGU (accessed October 14, 2011).

WEBSITES

"Body Dysmorphic Disorder." Mayo Clinic. November 5, 2010. http://www.mayoclinic.com/health/body-dysmorphic-disorder/DS00559 (accessed October 14, 2011).

"Compulsive Skin Picking." DermNetNZ. Last updated June 28, 2011. http://dermnetnz.org/systemic/skin-picking.html (accessed October 14, 2011).

"Compulsive Skin Picking." OCD Center of Los Angeles. http://www.ocdla.com/compulsiveskinpicking.html (accessed October 14, 2011).

"Dermatillomania/Compulsive Skin Picking Test." OCD Center of Los Angeles. http://www.ocdla.com/dermatillomania-compulsive-skin-picking-test.html (accessed October 14, 2011).

"F 04 Skin Picking Disorder." American Psychiatric Association. DSM-5 Development. May 19, 2010. http://www.dsm5.org/ProposedRevision/Pages/proposedrevision.aspx?rid=401 (accessed October 14, 2011).

Scheinfeld, Noah S. "Neurotic Excoriations." Medscape. August 3, 2011. http://emedicine.medscape.com/article/1122042-overview (accessed October 14, 2011).

ORGANIZATIONS

American Academy of Dermatology, PO Box 4014, Schaumburg, IL, 60168, (847) 240-1280, Fax: (847) 240-1859, (866) 503-SKIN, http://www.aad.org.

American Psychiatric Association, 1000 Wilson Blvd., Ste. 1825, Arlington, VA, 22209-3901, (703) 907-7300, apa@psych.org, http://www.psych.org.

American Psychological Association, 750 1st St. NE, Washington, DC, 20002-4242, (202) 336-5500; TDD/TTY: (202) 336-6123, (800) 374-2721, http://www.apa.org.

National Institute of Mental Health, 6001 Executive Blvd., Rm. 8184, MSC 9663, Bethesda, MD, 20892-9663, (301) 433-4513; TTY: (301) 443-8431, Fax: (301) 443-4279, (866) 615-6464; TTY: (866) 415-8051, nimhinfo@nih.gov, http://www.nimh.nih.gov.

OCD Center of Los Angeles, 11620 Wilshire Blvd., Ste. 890, Los Angeles, CA, 90025, (310) 824-5200, http://www.ocdla.com/contactus.html, http://www.ocdla.com/index.html.

Andrew J. Bean, PhD
Rebecca J. Frey, PhD

Desensitization *see* **Systematic desensitization**

Desipramine

Definition

Desipramine is an antidepressant drug used to elevate mood and promote recovery of a normal range of emotions in patients with depressive disorders. In addition, desipramine has uses in a number of other psychiatric and medical conditions. In the United States, the drug is also known by its brand name, Norpramin.

Purpose

Desipramine is known principally as an antidepressant drug used to promote recovery of depressed patients. It also

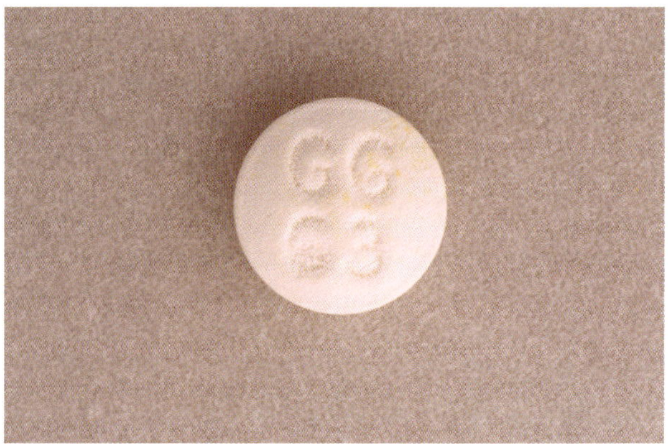

Desipramine. *(© Custom Medical Stock Photo, Inc. Reproduced by permission.)*

has therapeutic uses in **panic disorder**, pain management, **attention deficit hyperactivity disorder (ADHD)**, sleep attacks (**narcolepsy** and cataplexy), binge eating, and for **cocaine** craving in the treatment of **addiction**.

Description

Desipramine is one of the tricyclic **antidepressants**, so-called because of the three-ring chemical structure common to these drugs. Until the late 1980s, desipramine and other tricyclic antidepressants, such as **imipramine**, formed the mainstay of the pharmacological treatment of depressive disorders.

The therapeutic action of antidepressants is not completely understood. It is known that these drugs boost the levels of certain messenger chemicals, called **neurotransmitters**, which are involved in transmitting signals between nerve cells in the **brain**. This action may help to restore normal emotional feelings by counteracting abnormalities of nerve signal transmission that occur in depressive disorders.

Desipramine is one of a large number of tricyclic antidepressant compounds. Each was developed for somewhat differing pharmacological effects and side-effect profiles. The effects of desipramine are similar to those of other tricyclics, although some patients may find one drug of this group more effective or more tolerable than another. It is available as Norpramin in 10, 25, 50, 75, 100, and 150 mg tablets, although generic manufacturers may supply a somewhat different set of dosages.

Recommended dosage

For adults, desipramine is usually administered in dosages of 100–200 mg per day. Doses ranging from 75 mg to 300 mg per day are sometimes prescribed. The initial daily dose is usually low to avoid side effects, and it is usually increased, as necessary, until a therapeutic effect is achieved. Desipramine may be administered in divided doses or a single daily dose.

Geriatric patients, children, and adolescents are more sensitive to the side effects and toxicities of tricyclic antidepressants than other people. For geriatric patients, the dose may range from 25 mg to 100 mg per day. For children 6–12 years old, the recommended dose ranges from 10 mg to 30 mg per day in divided doses. For adolescents, daily dosages range from 25 mg to 50 mg but may be increased up to 100 mg, if needed.

Precautions

Because desipramine and other tricyclic antidepressants may cause drowsiness, activities requiring alertness, such as driving, may be impaired. Patients should avoid such activities until they understand how the drug affects them. Dizziness or lightheadedness may occur when standing due to sudden decreases in blood pressure. Fainting may also occur. Patients with glaucoma may find their condition aggravated. Among patients with epilepsy, **seizures** may become more frequent. Persons with heart disease should use tricyclic antidepressants with caution due to a possibility of adverse effects on heart rhythm.

Studies have found that some antidepressant drugs, including desipramine, may increase the chances of suicidal thoughts in children and adults up to age 24. Patients taking desipramine should be monitored, regardless of age, for worsening **depression** or other adverse changes in behavior.

It has not been determined whether desipramine is safe to take during pregnancy, and the patient's need for this medicine should be balanced against the possibility of harm to the fetus. Tricyclic antidepressants may be secreted in breast milk and may cause sedation and depressed breathing in a nursing infant.

Side effects

Desipramine may cause many side effects. Initially, the side effects of tricyclic drugs may be more pronounced, but sensitivity may decrease with continued treatment. Some of the more common side effects include **fatigue**, confusion, nervousness, restlessness, sleep difficulties, numbness, tingling sensations, tremors, blurred vision, difficulty urinating (especially in men with prostate enlargement), constipation, rashes, and weight gain. Sensitivity to ultraviolet light may be increased, and sunburns may occur more easily. Sweating may be reduced, causing sensitivity to heat and hot weather. Patients may also develop dry mouth due to decreased saliva, possibly contributing to the development of tooth decay, gum disease, and mouth infections. Patients should avoid sweets, sugary beverages, and chewing gum containing sugar.

Less commonly, tricyclic drugs may cause adverse effects on almost any organ or system of the body, particularly the blood, hormones, kidney, and liver. Patients should consult their physicians if symptoms develop or bodily changes occur.

Interactions

Tricyclic antidepressants such as desipramine may interact with many other drugs. Patients should inform their physicians about all other drugs they are taking. Tricyclic drugs may intensify the effects of drugs causing

KEY TERMS

Autonomic—The part of the nervous system that governs the heart, involuntary muscles, and glands.

Cataplexy—A symptom of narcolepsy marked by a sudden episode of muscle weakness triggered by strong emotions. The muscle weakness may cause the person's knees to buckle, or the head to drop. In severe cases, the patient may become paralyzed for a few seconds or minutes.

Epilepsy—A neurological disorder characterized by the onset of seizures. Seizures are caused by a disturbance in the electrical activity in the brain and can cause loss of consciousness, muscle spasms, rhythmic movements, abnormal sensory experiences, or altered mental states.

Glaucoma—A group of eye diseases characterized by increased pressure within the eye significant enough to damage eye tissue and structures. If untreated, glaucoma results in blindness.

Neurotransmitter—A chemical in the brain that transmits messages between neurons, or nerve cells.

sedation, including alcohol, **barbiturates**, narcotic pain medications, minor tranquilizers, and antihistamines. Tricyclics may cause excessive drops in blood pressure in patients taking blood-pressure medicine, especially upon sitting up or standing. Conversely, these drugs may interfere with the pressure-reducing effects of certain other blood pressure medicines. Tricyclics may interact with thyroid medications to produce heart rhythm abnormalities. Also, they may increase seizure tendency in patients with epilepsy, requiring adjustment of anti-epileptic medication. Concurrent use of tricyclic antidepressants with other antidepressants or other psychiatric medicines may result in intensification of certain side effects.

Certain drugs may interfere with the elimination of tricyclic antidepressants from the body causing higher blood levels and increased side effects. This effect may occur with cimetidine (Tagamet), other antidepressants, **methylphenidate** (Ritalin, Concerta), and some antipsychotic medications. Patients taking **monoamine oxidase inhibitors (MAOIs)** should tell their physicians before starting desipramine (or vice-versa). They will likely need to wait a period of at least 14 days after their last MAOI dosage before beginning treatment with desipramine.

Resources

BOOKS

Preston, John D., John H. O'Neal, and Mary C. Talaga. *Handbook of Clinical Psychopharmacology for Therapists*. 5th ed. Oakland, CA: New Harbinger Publications, 2008.

PERIODICALS

Amitai, Yona, and Henri Frischer. "Excess Fatality from Desipramine in Children and Adolescents." *Journal of the American Academy of Child and Adolescent Psychiatry* 45, no. 1 (January 2006): 54–60.

DeRubeis, Robert J., et al. "Cognitive Therapy vs Medications in the Treatment of Moderate to Severe Depression." *Archives of General Psychiatry* 62, no. 4 (April 2005): 409–16.

Mayers, Andrew G., and David S. Baldwin. "Antidepressants and Their Effect on Sleep." *Human Psychopharmacology: Clinical and Experimental* 20, no. 8 (December 2005): 533–59.

McDowell, David, et al. "Desipramine Treatment of Cocaine-Dependent Patients with Depression: A Placebo-Controlled Trial." *Drug and Alcohol Dependence* 80, no. 2 (November 2005): 209–21.

Musselman, Dominique L., et al. "Double-Blind, Multicenter, Parallel-Group Study of Paroxetine, Desipramine, or Placebo in Breast Cancer Patients (stages I, II, III, and IV) with Major Depression." *Journal of Clinical Psychiatry* 67, no. 2 (February 2006): 288–96.

Rains, Adrienne, L. Scahill, and V. Hamrin. "Nonstimulant Medications for the Treatment of ADHD." *Journal of Child and Adolescent Psychiatric Nursing* 19, no. 1 (February 2006): 44–47.

Walsh, B. Timothy, Robyn Sysko, and Michael K. Parides. "Early Response to Desipramine Among Women with Bulimia Nervosa." *International Journal of Eating Disorders* 39, no. 1 (January 2006): 72–75.

Wilens, Timothy E., et al. "Blood Pressure Changes Associated with Medication Treatment of Adults with Attention-Deficit/Hyperactivity Disorder." *Journal of Clinical Psychiatry* 66, no. 2 (February 2005): 253–59.

ORGANIZATIONS

American Academy of Child and Adolescent Psychiatry, 3615 Wisconsin Ave. NW, Washington, DC, 20016-3007, (202) 966-7300, Fax: (202) 966-2891, http://aacap.org.

American Academy of Clinical Toxicology, 6728 Old McLean Village Dr., McLean, VA, 22101, (703) 556-9222, Fax: (703) 556-8729, admin@clintox.org, http://www.clintox.org.

American College of Neuropsychopharmacology, 5034-A Thoroughbred Lane, Brentwood, TN, 37027, (615) 324-2360, Fax: (615) 523-1715, acnp@acnp.org, http://www.acnp.org.

American Psychiatric Association, 1000 Wilson Blvd., Ste. 1825, Arlington, VA, 22209-3901, (703) 907-7300, apa@psych.org, http://www.psych.org.

Richard Kapit, MD
Ruth A. Wienclaw, PhD

Desoxyn *see* **Amphetamines**

Desvenlafaxine

Definition

Desvenlafaxine, sold under the brand name Pristiq, is a medication used to treat **depression**. This medication belongs to a class of drugs known as selective **serotonin** norepinephrine reuptake inhibitors (SNRIs), which affect the **neurotransmitters** serotonin and norepinephrine. These chemicals are involved in normal **brain** function and are associated with clinical depression.

Purpose

Desvenlafaxine is approved for the treatment of clinical depression, though other potential uses were being explored as of 2011. Desvenlafaxine is the synthetic form of a metabolite of the antidepressant **venlafaxine**. It was developed based on the theory that a significant portion of the therapeutical benefits of venlafaxine may have come from this metabolite. Desvenlafaxine is expected to have fewer interactions with other medications than venlafaxine due to differences in how it is metabolized. Whether there is an advantage in taking desvenlafaxine instead of venlafaxine is debated.

Description

Desvenlafaxine works by acting on the neurotransmitters serotonin and norepinephrine, chemicals in the body that help regulate normal brain and body functioning. Neurotransmitters such as serotonin and norepinephrine bind to chemical receptors on the surface of the brain. Once bound to their designated receptor, they begin to affect physiological processes. It is believed that a decrease in serotonin and norepinephrine contributes to illnesses such as depression and **anxiety disorders**; SNRIs help counteract this by increasing the actions of the neurotransmitters, though desvenlafaxine has a larger impact on serotonin than norepinephrine.

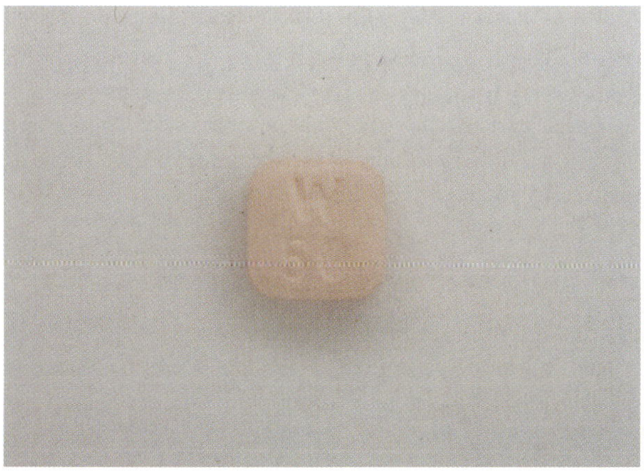

Desvenlafaxine (Pristiq), 50 mg. *(© Custom Medical Stock Photo, Inc. Reproduced by permission.)*

Whether a patient is going to benefit from taking an SNRI medication may have a genetic component. Individual response to each SNRI varies greatly. The initial trial of an SNRI can be difficult, because adverse side effects may occur before the patient begins to see the benefits of the medication, which may be frustrating to the patient. A drug that works best for one patient may not work for another patient, and having no success with one SNRI does not mean that a patient will have the same results with another SNRI. Finding which SNRI is going to work for a patient may require a trial of multiple drugs until an effective agent is identified. Generally, a drug is used for 4–6 weeks before a decision is made regarding its effectiveness. If the drug has shown some benefit but the healthcare provider thinks that it could be improved, the dose may be increased if the patient is able to tolerate it.

Recommended dosage

Desvenlafaxine is taken as an oral medication. The dosage used may vary depending on how an individual patient responds. If side effects develop that are not tolerable, the patient may require a lower dose. Desvenlafaxine is usually dosed at 50 mg daily. Higher doses rarely result in better therapeutic effects and increase the risk of adverse side effects. Elderly patients tend to develop side effects more easily and may be more sensitive to the effects of the medication; these populations may require dosing every other day. Patients with impaired liver or kidney function impacting metabolism require lower doses or less frequent dosing to avoid toxicity. Slowly increasing the dose may help minimize side effects, and some side effects may abate with continued use. Patients are periodically reassessed to determine whether there is need for continued treatment with desvenlafaxine. SNRIs, including desvenlafaxine, need to be slowly tapered off if discontinued to avoid withdrawal symptoms.

Precautions

Antidepressant drugs, including desvenlafaxine, have been associated with an increased risk of suicidal thoughts and behaviors in children and adults up to age 24. Any

KEY TERMS

Bipolar disorder—A mood disorder marked by alternating episodes of extremely low mood (depression) and exuberant highs (mania).

Glaucoma—Condition involving increased pressure within the eye that may cause damage and blindness.

Mania—Physiological state of hyperactivity experienced by patients with certain psychiatric illnesses involving inappropriate elevated mood, pressured speech, poor judgment, and sometimes psychotic episodes superimposed on the state of mania.

Metabolite—Chemical compound that occurs as a result of a parent drug being broken down and metabolized in the body. A metabolite may be a medically active or inactive compound, depending on the drug in question.

Monoamine oxidase inhibitors (MAOIs)—Type of antidepressant medication that affects various kinds of neurotransmitters including serotonin.

Neurotransmitter—One of a group of chemicals secreted by a nerve cell (neuron) to carry a chemical message to another nerve cell, often as a way of transmitting a nerve impulse. Examples of neurotransmitters include acetylcholine, dopamine, serotonin, and norepinephrine.

Neurotransmitter receptor—A physical recipient for chemicals called neurotransmitters. Receptors sit on the surface of cells that make up body tissues, and once bound to the neurotransmitter, they initiate the chemical signaling pathway associated with neurotransmitters.

Selective serotonin norepinephrine reuptake inhibitors (SNRIs)—Drug class that acts to specifically inhibit the reuptake of serotonin and norepinephrine in the neuronal synapse with little effect on other types of neurotransmitters, thereby decreasing side effects associated with broader acting drugs.

Selective serotonin reuptake inhibitors (SSRIs)—Drug class that acts to specifically inhibit the reuptake of serotonin only in the neuronal synapse with little effect on other types of neurotransmitters, thereby decreasing side effects associated with broader acting drugs.

Serotonin—A type of neurotransmitter involved in regulation of the blood vessels, brain processes, and disease states such as depression.

Serotonin syndrome—A potentially life threatening drug reaction involving an excess of the neurotransmitter serotonin, usually occurring when too many medications that increase serotonin are taken together, such as antimigraine triptans and certain antidepressants.

Synapse—Physical space between neurons that allows the passage of neurotransmitters for chemical signaling pathways.

patient taking an antidepressant drug should be monitored for changes in behavior and worsening depression. If treatment with desvenlafaxine is ceased, it should be slowly discontinued to avoid the development of SNRI discontinuation syndrome. Such withdrawal symptoms include flu-like symptoms, anxiety, agitation, vivid or bizarre dreams, **insomnia**, nausea, vomiting, diarrhea, sense of imbalance, chills, **fatigue**, dizziness, headache, numbness and tingling of the extremities, and other sensory disturbances. Discontinuation syndrome may be avoided if the dose is properly reduced over time.

SNRI overdose may result in a condition known as **serotonin syndrome**. Serotonin overdose may be caused by taking multiple drugs that increase the amount of serotonin signaling in the body. Symptoms of serotonin overdose range from mild to life-threatening, depending on the individual situation. Symptoms may include high blood pressure, high fever, nausea, diarrhea, headache, sweating, increased heart rate, tremor, muscle twitching, **delirium**, shock, coma, and death.

Desvenlafaxine may be contraindicated or may require caution in use in patients with uncontrolled hypertension, liver function impairment or liver disease, kidney function impairment, seizure disorder, bleeding disorders, glaucoma, dehydration, history of alcohol abuse, and in patients younger than 25 years of age or the elderly. Kidney and liver function, as well as blood pressure and behavioral changes, may be monitored while patients are taking desvenlafaxine. SNRIs such as desvenlafaxine are discouraged for use in patients with **bipolar disorder**, as the drugs can induce a state of mania in these individuals. There are selective conditions under which a doctor may prescribe an SNRI such as desvenlafaxine to a bipolar patient, but only for a short period and under careful monitoring. Desvenlafaxine is classified as category C for pregnancy, which means that either there are no adequate human or animal studies or that adverse fetal effects were found in animal studies, but there is no available human data. The decision whether or not to use category C drugs in pregnancy is generally based on weighing the critical needs of the mother against the risk to the fetus. Other lower category agents are used whenever possible. The safety of desvenlafaxine use during breast-feeding is unknown and, therefore, its use is not recommended.

Side effects

SNRIs tend to have fewer side effects than other types of older antidepressant medications, but side effects may still occur. Common side effects of desvenlafaxine include nausea and vomiting, headache, dizziness, fatigue, constipation or diarrhea, sexual dysfunction, sweating, dry mouth, shakiness, tremor, palpitations, loss of appetite, weight changes, hot flashes, chills, elevated blood pressure, vision changes, ringing in the ears, anxiety, abnormal dreams, and insomnia. Rare but serious potential side effects include mania, worsened depression and suicidality, **seizures**, serotonin syndrome, discontinuation syndrome, electrolyte imbalances, lung damage or disease, urinary retention, skin reactions, abnormal bleeding, liver damage, and glaucoma.

Interactions

Patients should make their doctor aware of all medications and supplements they are taking before using desvenlafaxine. Using alcohol while taking desvenlafaxine may create toxic reactions and should be avoided. Drugs that affect the liver may alter the metabolism of desvenlafaxine and may result in too much or to little of the drug in the body, though this possibility is less of a concern than with other drugs.

SNRIs should not be used with other drugs that inhibit the absorption of serotonin, such as **selective serotonin reuptake inhibitors (SSRIs)**. **Antidepressants** called **monoamine oxidase inhibitors (MAOIs)** also increase the amount of serotonin should not be used concurrently with desvenlafaxine. Patients taking **MAOIs** should stop and wait at least 14 days before starting treatment with desvenlafaxine; switching from desvenlafaxine to an MAOI may require a waiting period of up to five weeks.

Other drugs that increase serotonin in the body include sumatriptan (Imitrex), used to treat migraine headaches; the antipsychotics **chlorpromazine** and **fluphenazine**; and the herbal supplements yohimbe and **St. John's wort**. Diuretics (water pills) such as hydrochlorothiazide, diet pills such as sibutramine (Meridia), caffeine, certain diabetes drugs such as sulfonylureas, mood stabilizers such as **valproic acid**, and antipsychotics such as **haloperidol** and **clozapine** should not be used with desvenlafaxine to avoid potentially toxic effects. There is increased risk of internal bleeding when desvenlafaxine is used with anticoagulant drugs such as aspirin, warfarin, or large doses of the herbal supplements red clover, dong quai, **ginkgo biloba**, feverfew, or concentrated green tea.

QUESTIONS TO ASK YOUR DOCTOR

- Can I take the full dose right away or do I need to slowly increase the dose up to the full amount?
- Can I stop taking the medication right away or do I need to stop slowly?
- Should I eat before taking this medication?
- Will this medication interact with any of my other prescription medications? Over-the-counter medications? Herbal supplements?
- What side effects should I watch for while taking this medication?
- Can I drink alcoholic beverages in the same time frame as taking this medication?

Resources

BOOKS

Brunton, Laurence L., et al. *Goodman and Gilman's The Pharmacological Basis of Therapeutics*. 12th ed. New York: McGraw Hill Medical, 2011.

Stargrove, Mitchell Bebel, et al. *Herb, Nutrient, and Drug Interactions: Clinical Implications and Therapeutic Strategies*. St. Louis: Mosby, 2007.

PERIODICALS

Tourian, K. A., et al. "A 10-Month, Open-Label Evaluation of Desvenlafaxine in Outpatients with Major Depressive Disorder." *Primary Care Companion to CNS Disorders* 13, no. 2 (2011): e1–e10.

WEBSITES

PubMed Health. "Desvenlafaxine." U.S. National Library of Medicine. http://www.ncbi.nlm.nih.gov/pubmedhealth/PMH0000449 (accessed November 3, 2011).

ORGANIZATIONS

American College of Neuropsychopharmacology, 5034-A Thoroughbred Lane, Brentwood, TN, 37027, (615) 324-2360, Fax: (615) 523-1715, acnp@acnp.org, http://www.acnp.org/default.aspx.

American Society for Clinical Pharmacology and Therapeutics, 528 N Washington St., Alexandria, VA, 22314, (703) 836-6981, info@ascpt.org, http://www.ascpt.org.

Mental Health America, 2000 N Beauregard St., 6th Fl., Alexandria, VA, 22311, (703) 684-7722, (800) 969-6642, Fax: (703) 684-5968, http://www.nmha.org.

U.S. Food and Drug Administration, 10903 New Hampshire Ave., Silver Spring, MD, 20993-0002, (888) INFO-FDA (463-6332), http://www.fda.gov.

Maria Eve Basile, PhD

Desyrel *see* **Trazodone**

Detoxification

Definition

Detoxification is a process in which the body is allowed to free itself of a drug. During this period, the symptoms of withdrawal are also treated. Detoxification is the primary step in any drug treatment program and is used as the initial phase in treating alcohol, heroin, inhalant, sedative, and hypnotic addictions.

Purpose

Detoxification is only the first step in the long-term recovery of alcoholics and drug addicts. The immediate purposes of detoxification are to clear the toxins out of the body and help the patient achieve a substance-free condition. Detoxification treatment also aims to relieve the physical symptoms of withdrawal and treat any comorbid medical or psychiatric disorders. For the recovering person to stay abstinent on a long-term basis, detoxification needs to lead into long-term community residential program treatment or outpatient drug treatment lasting three to six months.

Demographics

Alcohol and **substance abuse** are common disorders in the general adult population in North America. The lifetime prevalence of alcoholism in American adults is estimated to be between 13.7% and 23.5%. At any one time, approximately 15.2 million Americans aged 12 and older are alcohol-dependent. There are 1.2 million hospital admissions for problems related to alcohol abuse each year in the United States. Estimates of drug dependence are more difficult to compile because the abuse of specific drugs fluctuates over time and is affected by social trends. It was thought that 3.9 million Americans were dependent on illicit drugs as of early 2010.

There is a considerable gap between the number of people who need treatment for alcohol and substance abuse and the number who actually receive it. The NIH estimates that in 2007, 23.2 million Americans aged 12 or older needed treatment for an illicit drug or **alcohol use** problem, but only 3.9 million received treatment at a specialized substance abuse facility.

The number of people undergoing detoxification is also difficult to estimate because the process has a "revolving-door" quality; that is, many persons with alcohol or drug addictions do not go on to the second phase of recovery from substance abuse. They do not maintain sobriety or freedom from drugs for more than a few days or weeks, and may require detoxification several times within a calendar year. Risk factors for repeated episodes of detoxification include:

- homelessness
- underlying mental illness
- personality disorder
- lack of support from family, friends, or other support community
- unemployment
- low level of education
- involvement with the criminal justice system
- multiple addictions
- male sex

Description

The body, when allowed to be free from drugs, detoxifies itself through its normal metabolic processes. Withdrawal symptoms are treated during this process so that the patient will be comfortable while the body detoxifies itself.

The process of substance addiction

Before discussing detoxification, it may be useful to understand how the body becomes addicted and why withdrawal symptoms are experienced. In physical **addiction** or dependence, as a person uses a substance or chemical over a long period of time, his or her body chemistry changes. Once a substance enters the body through drinking, smoking, injecting, or inhaling, it travels through the bloodstream to the **brain**. The brain has a complex reward system built in; when people engage in activities that are important for survival (such as eating), special nerve cells in the brain release chemicals (**neurotransmitters**, including **dopamine**) that induce feelings of pleasure. Because of this reward system in the brain, humans are programmed to want to repeat actions that elicit those pleasant sensations. In other words, feelings of pleasure reinforce certain activities or behaviors. Addictive substances interfere with this reward system. Some drugs mimic the effects of a natural chemical, some block the communication between nerve cells, and some substances trigger a larger-than-normal release of neurotransmitters like dopamine. The result of this interference is that dependent drug users physically need the drug to feel pleasure. As they become more dependent, their bodies become less responsive to the substance and need more of it to get the desired response—a phenomenon called tolerance. Also as a result of the interference with the brain's system, when the dependent user does not have the drug in his or her system, feelings of **depression** or unpleasant withdrawal symptoms may be experienced. These consequences also reinforce the substance use. People dependent on substances resort to using more drugs to avoid the depression or the withdrawal symptoms.

Withdrawal symptoms

The symptoms and severity of these symptoms vary from one substance to another.

ALCOHOL. After a person who has used alcohol heavily for a long time stops drinking, he or she may experience increased heart rate, shaking, difficulty sleeping, nausea, restlessness, anxiety, and even **seizures**. The affected person may also experience hallucinations (seeing, hearing, or feeling something that is not actually present). In some cases, **delirium** tremens (DTs) may occur as part of the withdrawal. Delirium tremens is a violent delirium (fading in and out of consciousness) with tremors, increased motor activity, visual hallucinations, disorientation, confusion, and fever that happens 48–96 hours after the alcohol-dependent person has had his or her last drink. These symptoms can last anywhere from three to 10 days. This state is a medical emergency because it could be fatal.

HEROIN AND OTHER OPIATES. Heroin is part of a family of drugs called opiates or **opioids**, which are made up of drugs that come from the seeds of the Asian poppy (e.g., heroin, opium, and morphine) and also manufactured drugs that act like the natural drugs (meperidine or Demerol). Symptoms of opiate withdrawal include restlessness, **insomnia**, anxiety, irritability, loss of appetite, diarrhea, abdominal cramps, nausea, sweating, chills, and runny eyes and nose.

SEDATIVES AND HYPNOTICS. **Sedatives** and hypnotics are drug families that are often considered in one group called the sedative-hypnotics. These drugs depress or slow down the body's functions, and can be used to calm anxiety or to induce sleep. When taken in high doses or when abused, these drugs can cause unconsciousness or death. These drugs include **barbiturates** and **benzodiazepines**. Some barbiturates are amobarbital (Amytal), pentobarbital (Nembutal), and secobarbital (Seconal). Some benzodiazepines include **diazepam** (Valium), **chlordiazepoxide** (Librium), and **lorazepam** (Ativan). When a person dependent on these drugs stops taking them suddenly, he or she might experience restlessness, muscle cramps, anxiety, insomnia, irritability, paranoid behavior, and even seizures or death.

Alcohol detoxification

Patients being detoxified from alcohol can safely be treated with rest, **nutrition**, vitamins, and thiamin (a B vitamin whose absorption is affected by alcohol abuse). Detoxification can be completed in an inpatient setting, or patients may participate in intensive outpatient (day hospital) treatment. People with mild or moderate withdrawal symptoms undergo detoxification over a five-day period and receive a benzodiazepine or phenobarbital to help ease the withdrawal symptoms. Delirium tremens can be treated with very high-dose benzodiazepines (such as chlordiazepoxide or diazepam) or with antipsychotic medications such as Haldol (**haloperidol**). The patient usually receives medication at doses high enough to give 60 mg or more of the medication over a 24- to 36-hour period, and the doses of these medications are gradually decreased by 20% each day. Patients who have liver disease, **dementia**, or patients who are over the age of 65 or with significant medical problems may receive lorazepam for the withdrawal symptoms.

Heroin detoxification

Patients with heroin dependence may receive help with their detoxification in one of two forms. Opioid agonists are drugs that act like heroin in the patient's body but do not provide the same "high," and are given in gradually decreasing doses. Because these medications "act" like heroin, the person does not experience withdrawal symptoms. Some examples of this kind of medication are **methadone** and levo-alpha-acetylmethadol (LAAM); buprenorphine is a partial opioid agonist, which means that it acts like heroin or methadone, but it limits the effects of opioids so that higher doses produce no greater effects. It is available as a monotherapy (meaning it is the only drug taken) or in combination with another drug, naloxone, as therapy for heroin detoxification. Some studies have found that bupreno-porphine shows promise in treating pregnant women for opiate addiction; however, the current standard of care remains methadone replacement for pregnant women. The second form of help for patients undergoing heroin detoxification is the use of a drug, such as **clonidine** (Catapres), that blocks some of the withdrawal symptoms. There is also a controversial method of heroin detoxification called ultra-rapid opioid detoxification under anesthesia/sedation, and there is an experimental method using a medication called lofexidine.

METHADONE SUBSTITUTION. Methadone substitution can occur in outpatient or inpatient settings, and is a method of detoxification that involves helping patients off substances such as heroin by substituting these substances with methadone to ease the withdrawal symptoms, and gradually decreasing the dose until no methadone is needed for the symptoms. Patients may begin with a dose of methadone that is between 20 mg and 40 mg per day. The initial dose may be adjusted so that the most beneficial dose can be discovered, based on the patient's withdrawal symptoms. The dose is then gradually decreased over the next several days. The decrease in methadone dosage is called tapering. If the detoxification is being completed in an inpatient setting, the methadone dose can be tapered more quickly, because medical staff can closely monitor patients for withdrawal, and detoxification can be achieved in about five to 10 days. However, in the case of outpatient detoxification, the taper has to be done much more slowly to assure that the patient does not have an adverse reaction or **relapse** (use the drug of abuse again) to treat their withdrawal symptoms. The dose may be decreased about 10% per week initially until a dose of 20 mg is reached. Then the dose can be decreased by 3% per week for the rest of the time that the patient needs to be detoxified. Patients are usually comfortable with the slow decrease of the medication until the dose gets below 20 mg/day. At that point, patients tend to become fearful of being off opioids and having symptoms of withdrawal.

Clonidine is used much more frequently than methadone in detoxification. Methadone is used frequently as long-term maintenance treatment for heroin addiction.

BUPRENORPHINE. Buprenorphine is another medication that is used during opioid detoxification. Because it also acts like heroin in the body, the patient does not experience the withdrawal symptoms as the heroin is being eliminated from the body. It is given as an intramuscular injection or intravenously. It begins to work within 15 minutes and its effects last six hours. It is given as part of three phases of detoxification: induction, stabilization, and maintenance. Induction is the initiation of buprenoporphine therapy, which is administered once the patient has not used opiates for 12 to 24 hours. During stabilization, the dose may be adjusted as the patient stops having cravings or experiences fewer side effects. The length of the maintenance phase varies depending on the needs of the individual, and ends with medically supervised withdrawal. This drug has shown greater effectiveness than other replacement therapies in treating opiate withdrawal.

CLONIDINE. Clonidine is a medication that decreases many of the symptoms of opioid withdrawal. Patients may require nonsteroidal anti-inflammatory drugs (NSAIDS, such as ibuprofen) for the treatment of muscle aches. Clonidine's major side effects include sedation and hypotension (low blood pressure) because it is used to treat high blood pressure. Patients undergoing detoxification using clonidine will have their blood pressure and pulse checked regularly. The starting dose of clonidine is 0.1–0.3 mg every four to six hours—the maximum amount that can be given in one day is 1 mg. During days two through four of the detoxification, the dose of clonidine is adjusted to control the withdrawal symptoms. Again, however, the dose cannot exceed the maximum dose. On the fifth day of detoxification, the dose may be slowly tapered.

The clonidine patch is a transdermal patch, allowing the drug to be delivered through the skin and exposing the patient to a constant amount of the drug over a seven-day period. It also allows the person to experience a more comfortable heroin detoxification. It comes in three doses: 0.1 mg, 0.2 mg, and 0.3 mg. Patients who use the clonidine patch need to have both the patch on and take oral clonidine during the first two days of the detoxification, because it takes the patch two days to reach a steady state and be effective. The patient takes oral clonidine 0.2 mg three times a day, and the weight of the patient determines the dose of the patch. On day two, the amount of clonidine that the patient takes by mouth is reduced by half and then it is completely stopped after day three. After seven days, the patch is removed and replaced with a patch that is half the amount of the original dose. The patch is continued for as long as the patient continues to have symptoms of withdrawal. Blood pressure is monitored for the patient using the patch, as well. The detoxification process in general takes about seven days using clonidine.

CLONIDINE-NALTREXONE ULTRA-RAPID DETOXIFICATION. Clonidine-naltrexone ultra-rapid detoxification has been attempted as a faster means of detoxification than using clonidine alone, and a similar "ultra-fast" method in combination with anesthesia has also been tested. These approaches remain quite controversial, and published clinical data supporting their efficacy are lacking, as are controlled trials. Anesthesia-assisted detoxification may even have adverse effects, especially in patients with co-occurring disorders.

LOFEXIDINE. Lofexidine is used experimentally in the United Kingdom for opioid detoxification. It appears to cause less sedation and fewer cases of low blood pressure than clonidine. In the United States, the National Institute of Drug Abuse (NIDA) is conducting studies on treatments using this drug in combination with **naltrexone**.

Mixed substance abuse

Mixed substance abuse (also called polysubstance abuse) occurs when individuals abuse more than one substance. Many doctors prefer to use phenobarbital to detoxify patients with polysubstance abuse problems. Patients receiving phenobarbital may receive a test dose, and then based on his or her tolerance and symptoms, the dose will be adjusted. Patients cannot receive more than 600 mg of phenobarbital a day. After two to three days, once the patient is doing well, the dose can be reduced by 30–60 mg. Whether detoxification for polysubstance abusers will be completed on an inpatient or outpatient status depends on the drugs the patient abuses.

Benzodiazepines

These medications are often used to help patients during detoxification, but these substances themselves can be abused and addictive. Patients who have taken a prescribed benzodiazepine for two weeks, even in a therapeutic dose, need to be safely detoxified with a slow taper. The amount of drug the person takes is dropped by 10%–25% every week if the patient has minimal withdrawal symptoms. If the patient has taken very high doses for long periods of time, he or she is at increased risk for addiction. If the person has been taking a benzodiazepine medication for years, it can take months before he or she can get off the drug. Anticonvulsant medications like **carbamazepine** (Tegretol) and **divalproex sodium** (Depakote) can be used to make the detoxification process faster and more comfortable for the patient.

Benefits

All approaches to detoxification benefit patients by treating the physical symptoms of withdrawal from alcohol or drugs and by preparing patients for the later phases of recovery from substance abuse.

Specific benefits of inpatient detoxification programs include:

- Ongoing medical supervision of withdrawal symptoms.
- Separation from substance-abusing companions and environments.
- Prevention of easy access to alcohol or drugs.

Specific benefits of outpatient detoxification programs include:

- Lower expense.
- Less time-consuming.
- Patient can maintain normal employment and family routines.
- Patient can often enter second-phase rehabilitation in the same facility as first-phase detoxification.

Precautions

When individuals are physically dependent on a substance, they experience withdrawal symptoms when they abstain from the drug. Withdrawal symptoms vary with each drug of abuse, but can be severe, and even dangerous. Patients who want to overcome their dependence need help managing the withdrawal symptoms. The patient's medical team strives to get the patient off a substance on which he or she is physically dependent, while treating the withdrawal symptoms.

Pregnant women cannot be detoxified from opiates (also called narcotics, including morphine, heroin, and similar drugs) because strict detoxification can increase the risk of spontaneous abortion or premature birth. These women can be treated with methadone as an alternative. Methadone acts as a replacement for the heroin in the woman's body, but the methadone does not provide the "high" that the heroin provides. In addition, methadone is safer for the fetus than heroin.

To be an effective first step of treatment, detoxification must be an individualized process because patients have varying needs. Aspects used in determining treatment options include the type of substance(s) the person is abusing, whether more than one substance is involved, the severity of the withdrawal syndrome; and whether inpatient or outpatient detoxification is preferable for the particular patient. Outpatient detoxification is not safe for patients who:

- have delirium tremens or other potentially life-threatening complications of withdrawal
- have such serious associated medical conditions as cirrhosis, inflammation of the pancreas, or gastrointestinal bleeding
- are judged to be suicidal or homicidal
- are in difficult family or employment situations
- cannot travel to the treatment facility on a daily basis

Preparation

The first step in any detoxification, regardless of the substance, is a physical exam and history taken by a physician. This information gathering and examination will help the treatment team assess the patient's overall health. In general, the healthier the patient is, the better the chances are that the patient will experience a detoxification without serious or life-threatening complications. Patients also need to give urine and blood samples to test for drugs and alcohol.

Aftercare

After the patient has completed detoxification, he or she needs further treatment either at an outpatient, inpatient, residential, or day hospital program in order to remain drug-free for the long term. Patients are treated by trained health care professionals, and some patients are also counseled by people who are recovering from addiction themselves. Many patients benefit from 12-step programs or **self-help groups**, such as Alcoholics Anonymous (AA) or Narcotics Anonymous (NA).

Most opioid users are treated with ambulatory or outpatient detoxification or residential treatment followed by outpatient counseling. Some people who have abused opioids and have undergone detoxification and counseling are able to remain drug-free. Many, however, relapse, even after receiving **psychotherapy**. People recovering from opioid addiction can receive methadone or LAAM as maintenance therapy to prevent relapse. Similar to the aid these medications can give patients during detoxification, when taken daily as a therapy they continue to "act" as heroin, keeping the withdrawal symptoms from appearing. Methadone maintenance therapy can be provided through either residential or therapeutic communities and outpatient drug-free programs. Methadone maintenance treatment therapy is controversial, however, because it does not cure the person's addiction—it replaces it with another substance. Proponents of methadone maintenance therapy argue that people receiving methadone are able to function much better in society than people addicted to heroin. Because their drug-seeking behavior is reduced, these patients can become productive at work and their interpersonal relations improve.

People recovering from alcoholism can also benefit from counseling and support after detoxification, and a maintenance therapy is available to them, as well. **Disulfiram** (Antabuse) is a medication that interferes with the body's breakdown and processing of alcohol. When alcohol is consumed while a patient is taking disulfiram, the medication makes the effects of the alcohol much worse than the patient would normally experience; facial flushing, headache, nausea, and vomiting occurs, even if alcohol is consumed in a small amount. In order for disulfiram to be effective, the patient must want this kind of **reinforcement** to maintain abstinence and must be committed to it. Patients also must note that any form of alcohol can trigger the undesired effects, including cooking wine or mouthwash with alcohol. This drug, when used in combination with buprenorphine, also appears to be effective in treating **cocaine** addiction in people who also are addicted to heroin.

Risks

When benzodiazepines are the drug of addiction, they must be discontinued and cannot be given on an outpatient basis because of their potential for abuse. For all patients undergoing detoxification, benzodiazepine use must be monitored carefully because of the potential for new addiction. Elderly patients undergoing detoxification and receiving benzodiazepines must be monitored closely because they are more sensitive to the sedating effects of these drugs and are also more prone to falls while receiving these drugs. If benzodiazepines are not discontinued gradually, patients can have withdrawal symptoms such as irritability, poor sleep, agitation and seizures. Ultrarapid opioid detoxification under anesthesia/sedation is a serious procedure. Patients have died undergoing this procedure, and it remains controversial.

It should also be noted that many substances used in detoxification can themselves cause addiction. An example of this risk has already been given with benzodiazepines—these medications ease withdrawal symptoms during detoxification, but patients can become addicted to these medications, as well.

Results

Normal results for a well-managed detoxification would include freedom from the drug of addiction and ability to enter long-term treatment.

Success rates vary among people recovering from substance abuse. As might be expected, patients who successfully complete a full treatment program after detoxification (that includes counseling, psychotherapy, **family therapy**, and/or **group therapy** or some combination of those therapy types) achieve higher rates of success at remaining drug-free. Patients who were addicted for shorter periods of time and patients who spend longer periods in treatment are generally more successful at remaining abstinent from drugs over the long term.

Studies indicate that people who abuse alcohol and who want to stop have a higher chance of success if they undergo inpatient detoxification versus outpatient detoxification.

One abnormal result that may occur is that patients who received nasogastric or tracheal tubes for opioid detoxification under anesthesia may experience adverse effects or complications. These patients are at risk for: **trauma** to their lips, vocal cords, larynx, and teeth; nosebleeds; high blood pressure; elevated heart rate; irregular heartbeat; and vomiting, which can lead to aspiration pneumonia.

KEY TERMS

Agonist—A chemical that reproduces the mechanism of action of a neurotransmitter.

Antagonist—A substance whose actions counteract the effects of or work in the opposite way from another chemical or drug.

Buprenorphine—A medication that blocks some of the withdrawal effects during heroin detoxification.

Detoxification—A process in which the body is allowed to free itself of a drug while the symptoms of withdrawal are treated. It is the primary step in any treatment program for drug or alcohol abuse.

Disulfiram—A medication that helps reinforce abstinence in people who are recovering from alcohol abuse. If a person taking disulfiram drinks even a small amount of alcohol, he or she experiences facial flushing, headache, nausea, and vomiting.

Lofexidine—A medication approved for use in Great Britain to aid the opioid detoxification process.

Methadone—A drug often prescribed legally as a replacement for heroin. It induces a slight high but blocks heroin from producing a more powerful euphoric effect. It may be used in heroin detoxification to ease the process, or it may be used daily after detoxification as maintenance therapy. Methadone maintenance therapy is controversial.

Withdrawal—Symptoms experienced by a person who has become physically dependent on a drug, experienced when the drug use is discontinued.

An additional abnormal result would be a new addiction as a consequence of the detoxification.

After the detoxification is completed, a patient may relapse. Support is critical for the patient to continue long-term therapy and successfully overcome addiction.

See also Addiction; Disease concept of chemical dependency

Resources

BOOKS

Fisher, Gary L., and Nancy A. Roget, eds. *Encyclopedia of Substance Abuse Prevention, Treatment, and Recovery*. Los Angeles: Sage, 2008.

Galanter, Marc, and Herbert D. Kleber, eds. *The American Psychiatric Publishing Textbook of Substance Abuse Treatment*. 4th ed. Washington, DC: American Psychiatric Publishing, 2008.

Jaffe, Jerome H., et al. "Substance-Related Disorders." In *Comprehensive Textbook of Psychiatry*, edited by Benjamin J. Sadock and Virginia A. Sadock. 7th ed. Philadelphia: Lippincott Williams and Wilkins, 2000.

Matthews, John. "Substance-Related Disorders: Cocaine and Narcotics." In *Psychiatry Update and Board Preparation* edited by Thomas A. Stern and John B. Herman. New York: McGraw Hill, 2000.

Porter, Robert S., and Justin L. Kaplan, eds. *The Merck Manual of Diagnosis and Therapy*. 19th ed. Whitehouse Station, NJ: Merck Research Laboratories, 2011.

PERIODICALS

Frydrych, L.M., et al. "Self-help Program Components and Linkage to Aftercare Following Inpatient Detoxification." *Journal of Addictive Diseases* 28, no. 1 (January 2009): 21–27.

Fuller, Richard K., and Susanne Hiller-Sturmhofel. "Alcoholism Treatment in the United States: An Overview." *Alcohol Research and Health* 23 (Spring 1999): 69–77.

Khantzian, Edward J. "Methadone Treatment for Opioid Dependence." *American Journal of Psychiatry* 157 (November 2000): 1895–96.

Preuss, U.W., et al. "Personality Disorders in Alcohol-dependent Individuals: Relationship with Alcohol Dependence Severity." *European Addiction Research* 15, no. 4 (April 2009): 188–95.

Shreeram, S.S., Timothy McDonald, and Sylvia Dennison. "Psychosis After Ultrarapid Opiate Detoxification." *American Journal of Psychiatry* 158 (June 2001): 970.

WEBSITES

Buprenorphine Information Center, Center for Substance Abuse Treatment. "Buprenorphine." U.S. Substance Abuse and Mental Health Services Administration. http://buprenorphine.samhsa.gov/about.html (accessed October 3, 2011.)

Center for Substance Abuse Treatment. "Detoxification and Substance Abuse Treatment." U.S. Substance Abuse and Mental Health Services Administration. Treatment Improvement Protocol (TIP) Series 45. DHHS Publication No. (SMA) 06-4131, 2006. http://store.samhsa.gov/product/Detoxification-and-Substance-Abuse-Treatment/SMA06-4226 (accessed October 3, 2011).

Mathias, Robert. "Alcohol-Treatment Medication May Reduce Cocaine Abuse Among Heroin Treatment Patients." U.S. National Institute on Drug Abuse. NIDA Notes (16). 2005. http://archives.drugabuse.gov/NIDA_Notes/NNVol16N1/Alcohol.html (accessed October 3, 2011).

MedlinePlus. "Opiate Withdrawal." U.S. National Library of Medicine. National Institutes of Health. September 28, 2011. http://www.nlm.nih.gov/medlineplus/ency/article/000949.htm (accessed October 3, 2011).

Trachtenberg, Alan I., and Michael F. Fleming. "Diagnosis and Treatment of Drug Abuse in Family Practice." U.S. National Institute on Drug Abuse. NIDA Research Monograph. 2005. http://archives.drugabuse.gov/diagnosis-treatment/diagnosis.html (accessed October 3, 2011).

U.S. National Institute of Drug Abuse. "Effectiveness of Lofexidine to Prevent Stress-Related Opiate Relapse

During Naltrexone Treatment." http://clinicaltrials.gov/ct/gui/show/NCT00142909;jsessionid=0B14CF2553B3CC2A2D16FE2652613D76?order=48 (accessed October 3, 2011).

ORGANIZATIONS

Alcoholics Anonymous (AA) World Services, Inc, PO Box 459, New York, NY, 10163, (212) 870-3400, http://www.aa.org.

American Council on Alcoholism, http://www.aca-usa.org.

American Society of Addiction Medicine, 4601 N. Park Ave., Upper Arcade #101, Chevy Chase, MD, 20815, (301) 656-3920, Fax: (301) 656-3815, email@asam.org, http://www.asam.org.

Hazelden Foundation, PO Box 11, Center City, MN, 55012-0011, info@hazelden.org, http://www.hazelden.org.

National Institute on Alcohol Abuse and Alcoholism, 5635 Fishers Lane, MSC 9304, Bethesda, MD, 20892-9304, http://www.niaaa.nih.gov.

National Institute on Drug Abuse, 6001 Executive Blvd., Room 5213, Bethesda, MD, 20892-9561, http://www.nida.nih.gov.

Susan Hobbs, MD
Emily Jane Willingham, PhD

Developmental coordination disorder

Definition

Developmental coordination disorder is diagnosed when children do not develop normal motor coordination (coordination of movements involving the voluntary muscles).

Demographics

It is estimated that as many as 6% of children between the ages of five and 11 have developmental coordination disorder. Males and females are thought to be equally likely to have this disorder, although males may be more likely to be diagnosed. Developmental coordination disorder and speech-language disorders seem to be closely linked, although it is not clear why this is the case. Children with one disorder are more likely to have the other as well.

Description

Developmental coordination disorder has been known by many other names, some of which are still used today. It has been called clumsy child syndrome, clumsiness, developmental disorder of motor function, and congenital maladroitness. Developmental coordination disorder is usually first recognized when a child fails to reach such normal developmental milestones as walking or beginning to dress him- or herself.

Children with developmental coordination disorder often have difficulty performing tasks that involve both large and small muscles, including forming letters when they write, throwing or catching balls, and buttoning buttons. Children who have developmental coordination disorder generally have developed normally in all other ways. The disorder can, however, lead to social or academic problems for children. Because of their underdeveloped coordination, they may choose not to participate in activities on the playground. This avoidance can lead to conflicts with or rejection by their peers. Also, children who have problems forming letters when they write by hand, or drawing pictures, may become discouraged and give up academic or artistic pursuits even though they have normal intelligence.

Causes and symptoms

The symptoms of developmental coordination disorder vary greatly from child to child. The general characteristic is that the child has abnormal development of one or more types of motor skills when the child's age and intelligence quotient (IQ) are taken into account. In some children these coordination deficiencies manifest as an inability to tie shoes or catch a ball, while in other children they appear as an inability to draw objects or properly form printed letters.

Some investigators believe that there are different subtypes of developmental coordination disorder. While there is disagreement over how to define these different subtypes, they can provide a useful framework for the categorization of symptoms. There are six general groups of symptoms. These include:

- general unsteadiness and slight shaking
- an at-rest muscle tone that is below normal
- muscle tone that is consistently above normal
- inability to move smoothly because of problems putting together the subunits of the whole movement
- inability to produce written symbols
- visual perception problems related to development of the eye muscles

Children can have one or more of these types of motor difficulties.

Developmental coordination disorder usually becomes apparent when children fail to meet normal developmental milestones. Some children with developmental coordination disorder do not learn large motor skills such as walking, running, and climbing until a much later point in time than their peers. Others have problems with such small muscle skills as learning to fasten buttons, close or open zippers, or tie shoes. Some children have problems learning how to handle silverware properly. In others the disorder does not appear until they are expected to learn how to write in school. Some children just look clumsy and often walk into objects or drop things.

There are no known causes of developmental coordination disorder. There are, however, various theories about its possible causes. Some theories attribute the disorder to biological causes. Some of the possible biological causes include such prenatal complications as fetal malnutrition. Low birth weight or prematurity are thought to be possible causes, but there is no hard evidence supporting these claims.

Diagnosis

The **diagnosis** of developmental coordination disorder is most commonly made when a child's parents or teachers notice that he or she is lagging behind peers in learning motor skills, is having learning problems in school, or has frequent injuries from falls and other accidents resulting from clumsiness. In most cases, the child's pediatrician will perform a physical examination in order to rule out problems with eyesight or hearing that interfere with muscular coordination, and to rule out disorders of the nervous system. In addition to a medical examination, a learning specialist or child **psychiatrist** may be consulted to rule out other types of learning disabilities.

The types of motor impairment that lead to a diagnosis of developmental coordination disorder are somewhat vague, as the disorder has different symptoms in different children. There are many ways in which this kind of motor coordination problem can manifest itself, all of which may serve as criteria for a diagnosis of developmental coordination disorder. The core of the diagnosis rests on the child's being abnormally clumsy. To make this determination, the child's motor coordination must be compared to that of other children of a similar age and intelligence level.

The difference between a child who has developmental coordination disorder and one who is simply clumsy and awkward can be hard to determine. For a child to be diagnosed with developmental coordination disorder there must be significant negative consequences for the child's clumsiness. The negative effects may be seen in the child's performance in school, activities at play, or other activities that are necessary on a day-to-day basis. Also, for developmental coordination disorder to be diagnosed, the child's problems with motor coordination cannot result from such general medical conditions as muscular dystrophy, and cannot result directly from an intellectual disability. Some criteria require that the child have an IQ of at least 70 to be diagnosed with developmental coordination disorder.

Treatment

No treatments are known to work for all cases of developmental coordination disorder. Experts recommend that a specialized course of treatment, possibly involving work with an occupational therapist, be drawn up to address the needs of each child. Many children can be effectively helped in special education settings to work more intensively on such academic problems as letter formation. For other children, physical education classes designed to improve general motor coordination, with emphasis on skills the child can use in playing with peers, can be very successful. Any kind of physical training that allows the child to safely practice motor skills and motor control may be helpful.

It is important for children who have developmental coordination disorder to receive individualized therapy, because for many children the secondary problems that result from extreme clumsiness can be very distressing. Children who have developmental coordination disorder often have problems playing with their peers because of an inability to perform the physical movements involved in many games and sports. Unpopularity with peers or exclusion from their activities can lead to low self-esteem and poor self-image. Children may go to great lengths to avoid physical education classes and similar situations in which their motor coordination deficiencies might be noticeable. Treatments that focus on skills that are useful on the playground or in the gymnasium can help to alleviate or prevent these problems.

Children with developmental coordination disorder also frequently have problems writing letters and doing sums, or performing other motor activities required in the classroom—including coloring pictures, tracing designs, or making figures from modeling clay. These children may become frustrated by their inability to master tasks that their classmates find easy and may stop trying or become disruptive. Individualized programs designed to help children master writing or skills related to arts and crafts may help them regain confidence and interest in classroom activities.

Prognosis

For many people, developmental coordination disorder lasts into adulthood. Through specialized attention and teaching techniques it is possible over time for many children to develop the motor skills that they lack. Some

KEY TERMS

Maladroitness—Another word for awkwardness or clumsiness.

Motor skills—Skills pertaining to or involving muscular movement.

children, however, never fully develop the skills they need. Although many children improve their motor skills significantly, in most cases their motor skills will never match those of their peers at any given age.

Prevention

There is no known way to prevent developmental coordination disorder, although a healthy diet throughout pregnancy and regular prenatal care may help, as they help to prevent many childhood problems.

Resources

BOOKS

American Psychiatric Association. *Diagnostic and Statistical Manual of Mental Disorders*. 4th ed., text rev. Washington, DC: American Psychiatric Publishing, 2000.

Sadock, Benjamin J., and Virginia A. Sadock, eds. *Comprehensive Textbook of Psychiatry*. Vol. 2. 7th ed. Philadelphia: Lippincott Williams and Wilkins, 2000.

PERIODICALS

Rasmussen, Peder, and Christopher Gillberg. "Natural Outcome of ADHD with Developmental Coordination Disorder at Age 22 Years: A Controlled, Longitudinal, Community-Based Study." *Journal of the American Academy of Child and Adolescent Psychiatry* 39, no. 11 (November 2000): 1424–31.

Smyth, Mary M., Heather I. Anderson, and A. Churchill. "Visual Information and the Control of Reaching in Children: A Comparison Between Children With and Without Developmental Coordination Disorder." *Journal of Motor Behavior* 33, no. 3 (September 2001): 306–320.

WEBSITES

MedlinePlus. "Developmental Coordination Disorder." U.S. National Library of Medicine, National Institutes of Health. http://www.nlm.nih.gov/medlineplus/ency/article/001533.htm (accessed October 4, 2011).

ORGANIZATIONS

American Academy of Pediatrics, 141 Northwest Point Blvd., Elk Grove Village, IL, 60007-1098, (847) 434-4000, Fax: (847) 434-4000, http://www.aap.org.

Tish Davidson, AM
Emily Jane Willingham, PhD

Developmental disorders *see* **Pervasive developmental disorders**

Developmental reading disorder *see* **Reading disorder**

Deviance *see* **Paraphilias**

Dexedrine *see* **Amphetamines; Dextroamphetamine**

Dexmethylphenidate

Definition

Dexmethylphenidate (Focalin) is a medication used to treat **attention deficit hyperactivity disorder (ADHD)**. It belongs to the class of drugs known as central nervous system (CNS) stimulants and acts on the neurological signaling chemicals norepinephrine and **dopamine**. Norepinephrine and dopamine are types of neurotransmitter involved in normal **brain** function and have an effect on mood, concentration, and impulse control.

Purpose

Dexmethylphenidate is used to treat some of the symptoms of **ADHD** in both adults and children six years old and older. It is a CNS stimulant that improves memory, concentration, and impulse control and belongs to the category of drug that remains the mainstay of ADHD therapy. The first drug chosen for ADHD is often **methylphenidate** (Ritalin), but patients that do not do well on methylphenidate are usually given

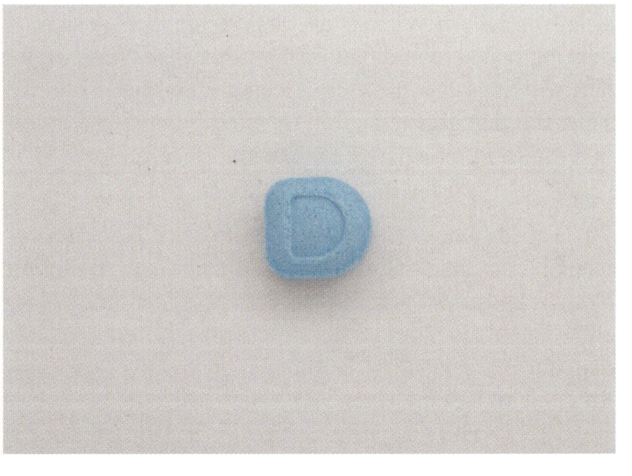

Focalin (dexmethylphenidate), 2.5 mg. *(© Custom Medical Stock Photo, Inc. Reproduced by permission.)*

dexmethylphenidate as a second-line drug. Dexmethylphenidate is available as an extended release medication, which reduces the need for re-dosing through the school or work day. It is used for patients in whom this is a priority. Because the capsules can be opened and the drug sprinkled on meals, it can be used in patients who have trouble swallowing pills. For patients with ADHD who also have co-existing **depression**, dexmethylphenidate may have some antidepressant properties and may be useful for patients who have both ADHD and depression at the same time. However, dexmethylphenidate has not officially been approved for use in treating depression.

Description

Dexmethylphenidate has a therapeutic mechanism of action that is focused on the modulation of the natural body chemicals norepinephrine and dopamine. Norepinephrine and dopamine are types of **neurotransmitters** in the nervous system, chemicals that neurons use to signal one another in complex pathways for normal brain and body functioning. Neurotransmitters bind to chemical receptors on the surface of neurons (brain cells). Once bound to a receptor they affect physiological processes. The receptors activate a sequence of cellular events known as a chemical cascade or signaling pathway.

Neurotransmitter signaling pathways are responsible for many regulatory processes, including neuronal signaling that affects mood, concentration, and impulse control. During the signaling process, neurotransmitters such as norepinephrine and dopamine travel from one neuron to the next. These chemicals need to cross a short space between the end of one neuron and the beginning of the next neuron known as the synapse or synaptic space. For example, norepinephrine is released from the end of neuron one, crosses the synaptic space, and binds to a neurotransmitter-specific receptor on the surface of the next neuron (neuron two). Any extra norepinephrine that is left in the synaptic space is taken back up by neuron one in a process known as reuptake. The more neurotransmitter allowed to remain in the synaptic space, the more will eventually be allowed to bind to receptors on neuron two and participate in the signaling process.

Neurotransmitter reuptake inhibitors such as dexmethylphenidate decrease the reuptake of norepinephrine and dopamine by neuron one, allowing more neurotransmitter to be present in the synapse and, therefore, more neurotransmitter signaling to occur. It is believed that a decrease in norepinephrine signaling contributes to disorders such as ADHD and depression. It is thought that dexmethylphenidate increases signaling of norepinephrine and dopamine by both inhibiting reuptake from the synapse and by increasing the amount released into the synapse. This has an impact on areas of the brain that involve attention span, judgment, response to external stimuli, memory, motor function, mental focus, and impulse control.

Recommended dosage

Dexmethylphenidate is given as an oral medication in pill form, but it may be sprinkled on food as well. Doses are taken early in the day with a full glass of water; doses are not taken in the evening. Patients are frequently reassessed for the need for treatment, as drugs for ADHD are avoided unless absolutely necessary. The dose chosen depends on individual patient response to the medication regarding its effectiveness, and individual patient response to the medication regarding side effects. Patients are dosed at the lowest possible effective dose to avoid the development of adverse side effects. Slowly increasing the dose over time helps with minimizing side effects.

The dose of dexmethylphenidate in both adults and children six years old and greater is started at 2.5 mg taken twice a day. The dose is increased by 5 mg or 10 mg increments every week for a maximum of 20 mg a day. The extended release formulation of dexmethylphenidate is given orally once a day at a dose of 10–30 mg. The dose is started low at 5 mg once a day taken in the morning and increased in increments of 5 mg a day over seven days to the desired dose. The maximum dose for the extended release form is 30 mg per day. Dosing of both the regular and extended release form is altered if the patient was previously taking methylphenidate and is switching to dexmethylphenidate. In this scenario the patient starts taking dexmethylphenidate at 50% of the current methylphenidate daily dose and is increased as needed from there. Doses are given at least four hours apart. Doses are lowered if side effects become intolerable.

Precautions

Dexmethylphenidate is a potentially habit-forming medication and should not be used for longer periods or at higher doses than prescribed. Patients are often given "drug holidays"—for example, when school is over for the summer—during which they forgo medication to avoid the development of adverse effects. Caution is used in patients with a history of **substance abuse**.

There is an association between ADHD and **Tourette syndrome**. Patients with Tourette syndrome often have involuntary movements or vocalizations known as tics. Patients who have Tourette syndrome and ADHD may find that the stimulant medications used to treat ADHD worsen their tics. Caution must be used in treating patients with motor tics, Tourette syndrome, or a family history of the disorder. Dexmethylphenidate may not be appropriate for use in these patients.

KEY TERMS

Bipolar disorder—Psychiatric mood disorder characterized by periods of manic behavior that may alternate with periods of depression, also known as manic depressive disorder.

Cytochrome P450 (CYP450)—Enzymes present in the liver that metabolize drugs.

Dopamine—A type of neurotransmitter involved in regulation of concentration, impulse control, judgment, mood, attention span, psychostimulation, and disease states such as addiction, ADHD, and depression.

Glaucoma—Condition involving increased pressure within the eye that may cause damage and blindness.

Mania—Physiological state of hyperactivity experienced by patients with certain psychiatric illnesses involving inappropriate elevated mood, pressured speech, poor judgment, and sometimes psychotic episodes superimposed on the state of mania.

Monoamine oxidase inhibitors (MAOIs)—Type of antidepressant medication that affects various kinds of neurotransmitters including serotonin.

Neurotransmitter—A chemical messenger that travels through the body and acts in the nervous system. Neurotransmitter signaling is responsible for a wide range of bodily processes and is often the target of medications involving the brain and cardiovascular system.

Neurotransmitter receptor—A physical recipient for chemicals called neurotransmitters. Receptors sit on the surface of cells that make up body tissues, and once bound to the neurotransmitter, they initiate the chemical signaling pathway associated with neurotransmitters.

Norepinephrine—A type of neurotransmitter involved in regulation of concentration, impulse control, judgment, mood, attention span, psychostimulation, and disease states such as ADHD and depression.

Synapse—Physical space between neurons that allows the passage of neurotransmitters for chemical signaling pathways.

Tic—Involuntary movements (such as twitching or facial grimacing) or vocalizations (such as throat clearing or barking) associated with Tourette syndrome.

Tourette syndrome—An inherited neuropsychiatric disorder characterized by the development of both motor and vocal tics. The tics are preceded by a feeling of tension or urgency in the affected individual until the tic behavior is performed and relieves the perceived feeling of tension.

Some patients taking dexmethylphenidate develop increased aggressiveness, **psychosis**, mania, or suicidal behavior in the first weeks of use. Children are especially at risk for these behavioral side effects. Patients taking dexmethylphenidate should be monitored closely for behavioral changes, especially when starting treatment or after dose changes. Dexmethylphenidate is discouraged from use in patients with **bipolar disorder**, as it is more likely to induce a state of mania in these individuals than in those without bipolar disorder.

Dexmethylphenidate may lower seizure threshold in some patients and may not be appropriate for use in patients with seizure disorder. Dexmethylphenidate may be contraindicated or may require caution in use in patients with hyperthyroidism, high blood pressure, liver function impairment or liver disease, kidney function impairment, heart conditions or abnormalities, and glaucoma. Cardiac function, heart rate, and blood pressure may be monitored while taking dexmethylphenidate. Blood cell parameters and growth progression (in pediatric patients) may need to be monitored with prolonged use, as growth retardation may occur with prolonged use.

Dexmethylphenidate is classified as category C for pregnancy, which means that either there are no adequate human or animal studies or that adverse fetal effects were found in animal studies, but there is no available human data. The decision whether to use category C drugs in pregnancy is generally based on weighing the critical needs of the mother against the risk to the fetus. Other lower category agents are used whenever possible. The safety of dexmethylphenidate use during breastfeeding is listed as probably safe, but data are limited and caution is advised.

Side effects

Dexmethylphenidate has many negative side effects. Sensitivity to dexmethylphenidate varies among patients, and some patients may find even lower doses are more than their body system can tolerate. Common reactions include abdominal discomfort or pain, dizziness,

insomnia, anxiety, headache, decreased appetite, changes in blood pressure and heart rate, weight loss, and visual disturbances. Dry mouth and throat pain are especially likely with the extended release formulation.

Rare but serious reactions include toxic skin reactions, blood disorders, heart arrhythmias, heart attack, **stroke**, **seizures**, and sudden death.

Interactions

Patients should make their doctor aware of all medications and supplements they are taking before using dexmethylphenidate. Using alcohol while taking dexmethylphenidate may create toxic reactions in the body and should be avoided. Dexmethylphenidate is metabolized by a set of liver enzymes known as cytochrome P450 (CYP450). There are many subtypes of CYP450 enzymes and dexmethylphenidate interacts with multiple subtypes. Drugs that induce or activate these enzymes may increase the metabolism of dexmethylphenidate. This results in lower levels of therapeutic medication, thereby negatively affecting treatment. Drugs that act to inhibit the action of CYP450 may cause undesired increased levels of dexmethylphenidate in the body. This could lead to increased side effects or even toxic doses. Likewise dexmethylphenidate may affect the metabolism of other drugs, leading to greater or lower doses than therapeutically desired. For example, dexmethylphenidate may inhibit the metabolism of the anticonvulsant medication phenytoin and the anticoagulant medication warfarin, causing increased levels of these drugs in the blood and toxicity. The anticonvulsant medication **carbamazepine** may lower levels of dexmethylphenidate present in the blood by inducing its metabolism, causing lower levels of dexmethylphenidate than therapeutically desired.

Certain drugs may cause toxicity when used with dexmethylphenidate, either through additive effects that cause serious side effects or through inhibition of dexmethylphenidate metabolism that cause toxic levels of dexmethylphenidate in the blood. Caffeine may cause toxicity with dexmethylphenidate by increasing the risk of heart rhythm abnormalities and excess nervous system stimulation. There have been rare reports of sudden cardiac death when dexmethylphenidate was used with the blood pressure drug **clonidine**. Use of the antipsychotic **pimozide** with dexmethylphenidate increases the risk of motor tics as a side effect of medication. Many **antidepressants** interact with dexmethylphenidate. The antidepressant **bupropion** increases risk of seizures when used with dexmethylphenidate. The antidepressant **venlafaxine** may cause greater than expected weight loss when used with dexmethylphenidate. Antidepressants called **monoamine oxidase inhibitors (MAOIs)** also increase the amount of norepinephrine and dopamine released into the synapse and cannot be used with dexmethylphenidate as it may cause overstimulation of the central nervous system and toxicity. Switching drug treatment for an individual patient from an MAOI to dexmethylphenidate may require a waiting period of up to two weeks between drugs. The antibiotic linezolid also impacts **MAOIs** and requires the same caution. Many diet drugs such as sibutramine may have additive effects with dexmethylphenidate that cause toxicity. It is unknown which herbal supplements interact with dexmethylphenidate.

QUESTIONS TO ASK YOUR DOCTOR

- Can I take the full dose right away or do I need to slowly increase the dose?
- Can I stop taking the medication right away or do I need to slowly decrease the dose?
- When should I eat in reference to taking this medication?
- What time of day should I take this medication?
- How long should I take this medication before I am reassessed?
- Will this medication interact with any of my other prescription medications?
- Are there any over-the-counter medications I should not take with this medicine?
- What are the side effects I should watch for?
- Can I drink alcoholic beverages in the same time frame as taking this medication?

Resources

BOOKS

Brunton, Laurence L., et al. *Goodman and Gilman's The Pharmacological Basis of Therapeutics.* 12th ed. New York: McGraw Hill Medical, 2011.

Stargrove, Mitchell Bebel, et al. *Herb, Nutrient, and Drug Interactions: Clinical Implications and Therapeutic Strategies.* St. Louis: Mosby, 2007.

ORGANIZATIONS

American College of Neuropsychopharmacology, 5034-A Thoroughbred Lane, Brentwood, TN, 37027, (615) 324-2360, Fax: (615) 523-1715, acnp@acnp.org, http://www.acnp.org/default.aspx.

American Psychiatric Association, 1000 Wilson Blvd., Ste. 1825, Arlington, VA, 22209-3901, (703) 907-7300, apa@psych.org, http://www.psych.org.

American Society for Clinical Pharmacology and Therapeutics, 528 N Washington St., Alexandria, VA, 22314, (703) 836-6981, info@ascpt.org, http://www.ascpt.org.

Mental Health America, 2000 N Beauregard St., 6th Fl., Alexandria, VA, 22311, (703) 684-7722, (800) 969-6642, Fax: (703) 684-5968, http://www.nmha.org.

Maria Eve Basile, PhD

Dextroamphetamine

Definition

Dextroamphetamine, sold under the brand name Dexedrine, is a medication used to treat **attention deficit hyperactivity disorder (ADHD)** and the sleep disorder **narcolepsy**. It belongs to the class of drugs known as central nervous system (CNS) stimulants and works by altering levels of the **neurotransmitters** norepinephrine and **dopamine**. Norepinephrine and dopamine are types of neurotransmitters involved in normal **brain** function and have an effect on mood, energy level, concentration, appetite, and impulse control.

Purpose

Dextroamphetamine is used to treat some of the symptoms of **ADHD** in both adults and children. This CNS stimulant improves memory, concentration, and impulse control, and belongs to the category of drug that remains the mainstay of ADHD therapy. For patients with ADHD who also have co-existing **depression**, dextroamphetamine may have some antidepressant properties, though it has not been approved by the U.S. Food and Drug Administration for this purpose. Dextroamphetamine has been approved for use in treating narcolepsy, a condition where patients experience uncontrollable sleep attacks during the day, and is one of the main treatments for this disorder. Dextroamphetamine is available as an extended release medication, which reduces the need for re-dosing throughout the school or work day. It is also available combined with the drug amphetamine in a combination pill (Adderall). The choice of using dextroamphetamine alone or in combination with other drugs depends on the medical profile of the patient.

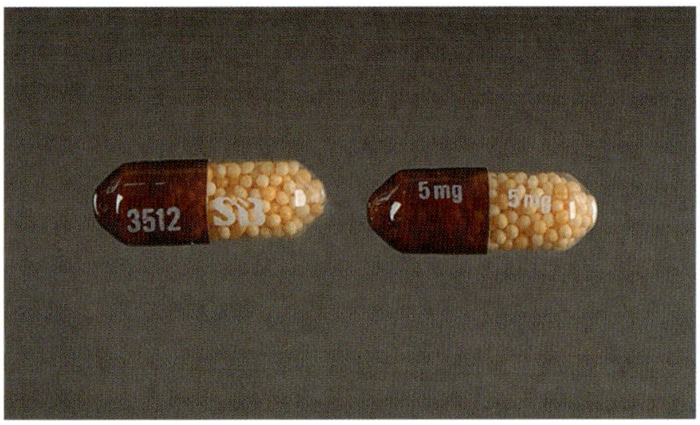

Dexedrine (dextroamphetamine), 5 mg. *(U.S. Drug Enforcement Administration)*

Description

Dextroamphetamine works by affecting the neurotransmitters norepinephrine and dopamine. Neurotransmitters are chemicals that neurons (brain cells) use to communicate with one another. It is believed that lower levels of norepinephrine and dopamine contribute to disorders such as ADHD and depression, so dextroamphetamine helps prevent the absorption of these neurotransmitters. The increase in norepinephrine and dopamine has an impact on areas of the brain that involve attention span, judgment, response to external stimuli, memory, motor function, mental focus, and impulse control.

Recommended dosage

Dextroamphetamine is given as an oral medication in pill form. Doses are taken early in the day with a full glass of water; doses are not taken in the evening. Patients are frequently reassessed for the need for treatment, as stimulant medications like dextroamphetamine are generally avoided unless absolutely necessary. The dose chosen depends on individual patient response to the medication regarding its effectiveness, and individual patient response to the medication regarding side effects. Patients are dosed at the lowest possible effective dose to avoid adverse side effects, and slowly increasing the dose may help with minimizing side effects.

The dose of dextroamphetamine for treating ADHD in both adults and children six years old and older is started at 5 mg taken once or twice a day. The dose is increased slowly after the first week as needed up to 40 mg per day, divided throughout the day. The maximum allowable dose is 60 mg per day. Similar doses are used to treat narcolepsy in adults and children greater than six years of age. Children three to five years of age being treated for ADHD are given lower doses of dextroamphetamine, beginning from 2.5 mg and slowly working up to 40 mg per day as needed. If multiple doses are used during a day, they should be taken at least four hours apart. If adverse side effects occur, doses may be lowered.

Precautions

Dextroamphetamine is a potentially habit forming medication and should never be used for longer periods or at higher doses than prescribed. Patients are often given drug “holidays”—for example, when school is over for the summer—during which they forgo medication to help avoid developing a dependence on the drug. Because of its addictive potential, caution is used in patients with a history of **substance abuse**. Dextroamphetamine causes a withdrawal syndrome when stopped abruptly; when discontinuing use, the medication should be tapered off gradually.

There is an association between ADHD and **Tourette syndrome**. Patients with Tourette syndrome often have involuntary movements or vocalizations known as tics. Patients who have Tourette syndrome with ADHD may find that the stimulant medications used to treat ADHD worsen their tics. Caution must be used in treating patients with motor tics, Tourette syndrome, or a family history of the disorder. Dextroamphetamine may not be appropriate for use in these patients.

Rare but serious reactions include severe elevations in blood pressure, heart arrhythmias, heart attack, **stroke**, **seizures**, and sudden death. Some patients develop increased aggressiveness, **psychosis**, mania, or suicidality in the first weeks of use. Children are especially at risk for these behavioral side effects. Patients taking dextroamphetamine are monitored closely for behavioral changes, especially when starting treatment or after dose changes. Growth retardation may occur with prolonged use.

Dextroamphetamine may be contraindicated or may require caution in use in patients with high blood pressure, blood vessel disease, heart rhythm abnormalities, heart conditions or structural abnormalities, certain thyroid disorders, liver function impairment or liver disease, kidney function impairment, or glaucoma. Dextroamphetamine may lower seizure threshold in some patients and may not be appropriate for use in patients with seizure disorder. Cardiac function, heart rate, and blood pressure may be monitored while taking dextroamphetamine. Dextroamphetamine is discouraged from use in patients with **bipolar disorder**, as it is more likely to induce a state of mania in these individuals than in those without bipolar disorder.

Dextroamphetamine is classified as a category C drug for pregnancy, which means either that there are no adequate human or animal studies or that adverse fetal effects were found in animal studies, but there is no available human data. The decision of whether to use category C drugs in pregnancy is generally based on weighing the critical needs of the mother against the risk to the fetus. Other lower category agents are used whenever possible. Some data suggest that dextroamphetamine may be unsafe for use during breast-feeding, and its use is not recommended.

Side effects

Sensitivity to dextroamphetamine varies between patients, and some patients may find that even lower doses are more than their body system can tolerate. Common reactions include dizziness, **insomnia**, anxiety, restlessness, euphoria, headache, decreased appetite, weight loss, changes in blood pressure and heart rate, palpitations, tremor, dry mouth, unpleasant taste, diarrhea or constipation, tic exacerbation, impotence, sexual dysfunction, and visual disturbances.

KEY TERMS

Dopamine—A type of neurotransmitter involved in regulation of concentration, impulse control, judgment, mood, attention span, psychostimulation, and disease states such as addiction, ADHD, and depression.

Glaucoma—Condition involving increased pressure within the eye that may cause damage and blindness.

Mania—Physiological state of hyperactivity experienced by patients with certain psychiatric illnesses involving inappropriate elevated mood, pressured speech, poor judgment, and sometimes psychotic episodes superimposed on the state of mania.

Monoamine oxidase inhibitors (MAOIs)—Type of antidepressant medication that affects various kinds of neurotransmitters including serotonin.

Narcolepsy—Condition involving increased daytime sleepiness in the form of uncontrollable sleep attacks that interfere with normal functioning.

Neurotransmitter—One of a group of chemicals secreted by a nerve cell (neuron) to carry a chemical message to another nerve cell, often as a way of transmitting a nerve impulse. Examples of neurotransmitters include acetylcholine, dopamine, serotonin, and norepinephrine.

Norepinephrine—A type of neurotransmitter involved in regulation of concentration, impulse control, judgment, mood, attention span, psychostimulation, and disease states such as ADHD and depression.

Tic—Involuntary movements (such as twitching or facial grimacing) or vocalizations (such as throat clearing or barking) associated with Tourette syndrome.

Tourette syndrome—An inherited neuropsychiatric disorder characterized by the development of both motor and vocal tics. The tics are preceded by a feeling of tension or urgency in the affected individual until the tic behavior is performed and relieves the perceived feeling of tension.

QUESTIONS TO ASK YOUR DOCTOR

- Can I take the full dose right away or do I need to slowly increase the dose?
- Can I stop taking the medication right away or do I need to slowly decrease the dose?
- Should I eat before taking this medication?
- What time of day should I take this medication?
- How long should I take this medication before I am reassessed?
- Will this medication interact with any of my other prescription medications?
- Are there any over-the-counter medications I should not take with this medicine?
- What side effects should I watch for?
- Can I drink alcoholic beverages in the same time frame as taking this medication?

Interactions

Patients should make their doctor aware of all medications and supplements they are taking before using dextroamphetamine. Using alcohol while taking dextroamphetamine may create toxic reactions in the body and should be avoided. Drugs that affect the liver may alter the metabolism of dextroamphetamine, resulting in too much or too little of dextroamphetamine in the body. This could lead to increased side effects or even toxic doses. Likewise, dextroamphetamine may affect the metabolism of other drugs, leading to greater or lower doses than therapeutically desired.

Certain drugs used in combination with dextroamphetamine may cause serious heart rhythm abnormalities, excess nervous system stimulation, or blood pressure changes. Such substances include caffeine, marijuana derivatives, the obesity drug sibutramine, some migraine medications such as ergotamines, and decongestants such as phenylephrine. Use of the antipsychotic **pimozide** with dextroamphetamine increases the risk of motor tics as a side effect of medication. Use of certain other antipsychotics such as **fluphenazine** increases risk of psychosis. Antacids and the glaucoma and diuretic drug acetazolamide decrease the excretion of dextroamphetamine from the body and may cause toxic levels to accumulate.

Many **antidepressants** interact with dextroamphetamine. The antidepressant **bupropion** increases risk of seizures when used with dextroamphetamine. **Venlafaxine** may cause greater than expected weight loss when used with dextroamphetamine. Antidepressants called **monoamine oxidase inhibitors (MAOIs)** also increase the levels of norepinephrine and dopamine in the brain and should not be used with dextroamphetamine, as the combination may cause overstimulation of the central nervous system and toxicity. Patients taking **MAOIs** will need to stop taking the MAOI for at least 14 days before starting treatment with dextroamphetamine (or vice versa). Many herbal supplements may also interact with dextroamphetamine and cause toxicity, including green tea and **ginseng**.

Resources

BOOKS

Brunton, Laurence L., et al. *Goodman and Gilman's The Pharmacological Basis of Therapeutics.* 12th ed. New York: McGraw Hill Medical, 2011.

Stargrove, Mitchell Bebel, et al. *Herb, Nutrient, and Drug Interactions: Clinical Implications and Therapeutic Strategies.* St. Louis: Mosby, 2007.

ORGANIZATIONS

American Society for Clinical Pharmacology and Therapeutics, 528 N Washington St., Alexandria, VA, 22314, (703) 836-6981, info@ascpt.org, http://www.ascpt.org.

Mental Health America, 2000 N Beauregard St., 6th Fl., Alexandria, VA, 22311, (703) 684-7722, (800) 969-6642, Fax: (703) 684-5968, http://www.nmha.org.

National Institute of Mental Health, 6001 Executive Blvd., Rm. 8184, MSC 9663, Bethesda, MD, 20892-9663, (301) 433-4513; TTY: (301) 443-8431, Fax: (301) 443-4279, (866) 615-6464; TTY: (866) 415-8051, nimhinfo@nih.gov, http://www.nimh.nih.gov.

U.S. Food and Drug Administration, 10903 New Hampshire Ave., Silver Spring, MD, 20993-0002, (888) INFO-FDA (463-6332), http://www.fda.gov.

Maria Eve Basile, PhD

DextroStat *see* **Dextroamphetamine**

DHEA

Definition

Dehydroepiandrosterone (DHEA) is a precursor (prohormone) of the sex hormones estrogen and testosterone. It is a steroid produced naturally by the adrenal glands and is also sold as a dietary supplement.

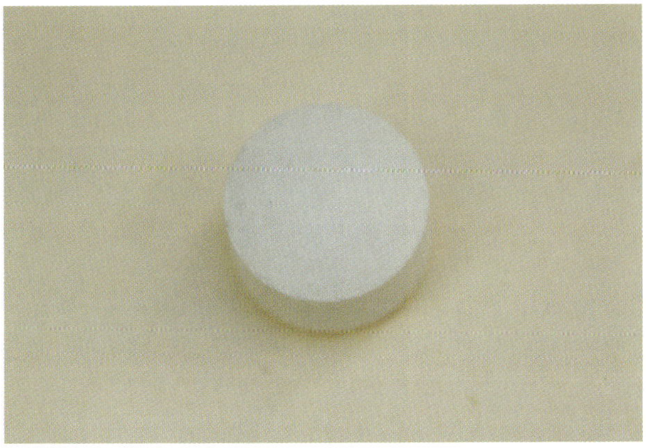

DHEA supplement. *(© Custom Medical Stock Photo, Inc. Reproduced by permission.)*

Purpose

Many claims have been made for DHEA, including that it fights aging, burns fat, increases muscle mass, boosts the immune system, eliminates symptoms of menopause, prevents **Alzheimer's disease**, and can treat everything from inflammatory bowel syndrome to **cocaine** withdrawal. There is little or highly questionable evidence to support most of these claims. DHEA does have medical uses in treating adrenal insufficiency (Addison's disease) and systemic lupus erythematosus (SLE).

Description

DHEA is a supplement with a long history of controversy. In the 1980s, it was promoted by supplement makers as a so-called miracle product that could improve athletic performance, build muscle, burn fat, restore sexual potency, and prevent aging. Many of these claims are still made by supplement makers today. In 1985, the U.S. Food and Drug Administration (FDA) banned DHEA for sale in the United States because of its potential for abuse and the high risk of serious side effects. DHEA was also banned by several sports organizations, including the International Olympic Committee and the National Football League. In 1994, the U.S. Congress passed the Dietary Supplement Health and Education Act (DSHEA). Under this law, DHEA met the definition of a dietary supplement and could once again be sold without a prescription in the United States.

DSHEA regulates supplements such as DHEA in the same way that food is regulated. Like food manufacturers, manufacturers of dietary supplements do not have to prove that their product is either safe or effective before it can be sold to the public. Manufacturers of conventional pharmaceutical drugs, must prove both safety and effectiveness in humans before a new drug is approved for use. With dietary supplements, the burden of proof falls on the FDA to show that the supplement is either unsafe or ineffective before it can be restricted or banned. Information about a supplement's safety and effectiveness is normally gathered only after people using the product develop health problems or complain that the product does not work. In the mid-2000s, there was pressure to reclassify DHEA as a hormone and ban its over-the-counter sale, but dietary supplement manufacturers have fought this move. Federal law requires that all manufacturers of dietary supplements and over-the-counter drugs report consumer complaints of adverse events (negative side effects) to the FDA. This requirement makes accumulating information on the safety of DHEA faster and easier.

DHEA is produced mainly in the adrenal glands. These are small, compact hormone-producing tissues located just above each kidney. The adrenal glands convert cholesterol into DHEA and release it into the bloodstream. DHEA is also produced in smaller amounts by the testes, liver, and possibly the **brain**.

DHEA is a prohormone, meaning that the body can convert it into several different hormones, including the female hormone estrogen and the male hormone testosterone. During development, the fetal adrenal glands produce large amounts of DHEA. After birth, production drops and remains low during childhood. As adulthood approaches, the rate of DHEA production increases, reaching a peak between ages 25 and 30. From age 30 on, the level of DHEA declines steadily until age 80; elderly men have only about 10% as much DHEA in their blood as they did at age 25.

Some researchers, observing the relationship between aging and decreased levels of DHEA, hypothesized the decrease in DHEA caused age-related problems such as cardiovascular disease, decreased sexual function, and **dementia**. They theorized that aging could be delayed by using dietary supplements to restore DHEA levels to those of a younger person. This hypothesis has not been tested, yet DHEA has been promoted as a supplement that can increase longevity and ward off a number of age-related changes.

Researchers tend to be much more cautious. For one thing, humans and other primates (apes, monkeys) produce substantial amounts of DHEA, but common laboratory animals such as rats and mice produce almost none. Therefore, it is unclear whether results of testing DHEA in lab animals can be applied to humans. Some researchers have spoken out against supplement makers, complaining that their research has been taken out of context, misrepresented, or just plain altered to support the claims of manufacturers selling DHEA, especially those selling over the Internet.

DHEA remains of great interest to researchers. **Clinical trials** are underway to determine safety and effectiveness of DHEA in a variety of situations.

DHEA's role in health care

DHEA has two uses accepted by practitioners of conventional medicine. Under supervision of a physician, DHEA has been used to successfully treat Addison's disease. Addison's disease is the result of adrenal insufficiency. The adrenal glands do not produce enough hormones. DHEA supplements simply replace what the body should be making.

DHEA has also been used by physicians to treat symptoms of systemic lupus erythematosus (SLE). SLE is a complicated autoimmune disease in which the body attacks and damages its own tissues. It is not clear why DHEA improves SLE symptoms such as joint pain and inflammation of the tissue surrounding the heart, but the majority of clinical trials in humans support this use.

There is mixed evidence to support two other claims for DHEA—that it helps with weight loss and that it relieves **depression** symptoms. A rigorous study led by researchers at the Mayo Clinic and published in 2006, found no anti-aging effects in elderly participants who took DHEA for two years. There were no measurable improvements in muscle strength, body fat, physical performance, insulin sensitivity, or quality of life.

Dietary supplement manufacturers continue to use unsubstantiated claims about DHEA that appeal to individuals searching for the fountain of youth. These include claims that DHEA improves memory, eliminates or improves symptoms of Alzheimer's disease, prevents cardiovascular disease, increases bone density, treats chronic **fatigue** syndrome, treats cocaine withdrawal, improves symptoms of Crohn's disease and inflammatory bowel syndrome, slows the development of AIDS, restores fertility, cures **erectile dysfunction**, treats symptoms of menopause such as hot flashes, helps manage **schizophrenia**, increases muscle strength and athletic performance, stimulates the immune system, prevents skin aging, and treats the symptoms of fibromyalgia. There are no independent, controlled, rigorous studies to support any of these uses. The National Center for Complementary and Alternative Medicine (NCCAM) does not recommend the use of DHEA supplements as a means to improve any health problems. The National Institute for Aging (NIA) advises against the use of DHEA supplements due to the lack of evidence proving any form of anti-aging benefit.

KEY TERMS

Depression—A mental state characterized by feelings of sadness, despair, and discouragement.

Insomnia—Waking in the middle of the night and having difficulty returning to sleep or waking too early in the morning.

Schizophrenia—A major mental illness marked by psychotic symptoms, including hallucinations, delusions, and severe disruptions in thinking.

Use of DHEA in mental health

DHEA has been determined as "possibly effective" for treatment in schizophrenia by the *Natural Medicines Comprehensive Database,* which rates effectiveness based on scientific evidence, noting that DHEA may be more effective in women than men who have schizophrenia. Additionally, the organization has given DHEA a rating of "insufficient evidence to rate effectiveness" for treatment in depression, noting that there is some (insufficient) evidence that DHEA may improve mood and help lessen symptoms associated with depression. More evidence is needed to rate DHEA for these uses.

Clinical trials regarding the effect of DHEA on depression and for anxiety symptoms of schizophrenia suggest that DHEA may be of some benefit for use in these conditions; however, further study is needed before a firm conclusion can be drawn. The long-term effects of taking DHEA are not known.

Certain drugs used in mental health, including **chlorpromazine** (Thorazine), **quetiapine** (Seroquel), and **alprazolam** (Xanax), may increase or decrease DHEA levels in the body. Further research is needed to determine the effects of DHEA administration if used by individuals taking psychiatric medication.

Clinical trials have looked at levels of naturally occurring DHEA in the body in individuals with anxiety disorder, schizophrenia, or **schizoaffective disorder**. Current information regarding participation in a clinical trial is available at the website of the NIH Clinical center (http://www.cc.nih.gov/participate).

Recommended dosage

DHEA is sold as a dietary supplement in the form of tablets, capsules, and a liquid injection. Dosage range is 25–250 mg per day. An independent study of DHEA supplements found that many supplements contained amounts of DHEA ranging from none to one and a half times the amount described on the label.

Administration and dosage of DHEA for Addison's disease or SLE is determined by a physician, who will also obtain ongoing blood tests to monitor levels of hormones in the body. The typical dosage of DHEA for Addison's disease is 25–50 mg daily and for SLE, 200 mg daily.

Precautions

People under age 40 should not take DHEA supplements.

DHEA should never be given to children. Parents should keep this and all drugs and supplements stored safely out of reach of children to prevent accidental poisoning.

Pregnant women should not take DHEA. There is some evidence that it can induce early labor. The effect on the developing fetus is unknown.

Breastfeeding women should avoid DHEA supplementation because DHEA passes into breast milk and may affect development of the infant.

People who have a high risk of developing estrogen- or testosterone-sensitive cancers, such as breast cancer or prostate cancer, should not take DHEA supplements. DHEA is converted into estrogen or testosterone. These hormones appear to stimulate the growth of certain cancers.

Athletes should be aware that some athletic governing bodies ban DHEA supplement use and test for abnormally high levels of DHEA as part of routine drug testing.

Side effects

DHEA supplementation in healthy people can cause major side effects. Many of these come about because of the conversion of DHEA into high levels of testosterone and estrogen. These include:

- masculinization of women, including deepening voice and increased body hair
- menstrual irregularities in women
- feminization of men, including, enlarged breasts and shrunken testicles
- decreased HDL ("good") cholesterol
- high blood pressure (hypertension)
- liver damage

Less serious side effects include acne, increased sweating, breast tenderness, **insomnia**, nausea, and abdominal pain.

QUESTIONS TO ASK YOUR DOCTOR

- What kind of changes can I expect to see or feel when taking DHEA?
- Does it matter what time of day I take DHEA? If so, what is the recommendation?
- Should I take DHEA with or without food?
- What are the side effects associated with DHEA?
- Will DHEA interact or interfere with other medications I am currently taking?
- What symptoms or adverse effects are important enough that I should seek immediate treatment?

Interactions

High levels of DHEA may interfere with the way the liver processes certain drugs. As a result, these drugs may accumulate in the body in high levels and cause adverse effects or be more rapidly deactivated and not produce a therapeutic response. Drugs that may be affected by high levels of DHEA are anticonvulsants, antipsychotics, corticosteroids, oral contraceptives, hormone replacement therapy drugs, insulin, and drugs to treat insomnia.

Resources

BOOKS

Ahmed, Nessar. *Clinical Biochemistry*. New York: Oxford University Press, 2011.

Ritsner, Michael S, ed. *Handbook of Schizophrenia Spectrum Disorders*. New York: Springer, 2011.

Sharon, Michael. *Nutrient A-Z: A User's Guide to Foods, Herbs, Vitamins, Minerals & Supplements*, 4th ed. New York: Carlton, 2009.

Watson, Ronald Ross, ed. *DHEA in Human Health and Aging*. Boca Raton, FL: CRC Press, 2011.

PERIODICALS

Arlt, Wiebke. "Androgen Therapy in Women." *European Journal of Endocrinology* 154, no. 1 (2006): 1–11. Available at http://eje-online.org/cgi/content/full/154/1/1 (accessed October 3, 2011).

Arnold, Julia T., and Marc R. Blackman. "Does DHEA Exert Direct Effects on Androgen and Estrogen Receptors, and Does It Promote or Prevent Prostate Cancer?" *Endocrinology* 146, no. 11 (2005): 4565–67. Available at http://endo.endojournals.org/cgi/content/full/146/11/4565 (accessed October 3, 2011).

WEBSITES

Boyles, Salynn. "Anti-Aging Hormone a Bust, Study Shows." WebMd.com. October 18, 2006. http://www.webmd.com/healthy-aging/news/20061018/antiaging-hormone-bust-study-shows (accessed October 3, 2011).

"DHEA." *MayoClinic.com*. Mayo Clinic. Last modified August 1, 2011. http://www.mayoclinic.com/health/dhea/NS_patient-dhea (accessed October 3, 2011).

"DHEA." Medline Plus. Last updated July 8, 2011. http://www.nlm.nih.gov/medlineplus/druginfo/natural/patient-dhea.html (accessed October 3, 2011).

"Dehydroepiandrosterone: Overview." University of Maryland Medical Center, April 4, 2002. http://www.umm.edu/altmed/articles/dehydroepiandrosterone-000299.htm (accessed October 3, 2011).

"Menopausal Symptoms and CAM." National Center for Complementary and Alternative Medicine, January 2008. http://nccam.nih.gov/health/menopause/menopausesymptoms.htm (accessed October 3, 2011).

ORGANIZATIONS

National Center for Complementary and Alternative Medicine, 9000 Rockville Pike, Bethesda, MD, 20892, (888) 644-6226, http://nccam.nih.gov.

National Institute on Aging, Bldg. 31, Rm. 5C27, 31 Center Drive, MSC 2292, Bethesda, MD, 20892, (301) 496-1752, (888) TTY: (800) 222-4225, Fax: (301) 496-1072, http://www.nia.nih.gov.

Office of Dietary Supplements, National Institutes of Health, 6100 Executive Blvd., Rm. 3B01, MSC 7517, Bethesda, MD, 20892-7517, (301) 435-2920, Fax: (301) 480-1845, ods@nih.gov, http://dietary-supplements.info.nih.gov.

Tish Davidson, AM
Laura Jean Cataldo, RN, EdD

Diagnosis

Definition

Diagnosis can be defined as the identification and labeling of a disease based on its signs and symptoms. Mental health clinicians (psychiatrists, psychologists, and psychiatric nurse practitioners) diagnose mental disorders using the criteria listed in the ***Diagnostic and Statistical Manual of Mental Disorders***, also known as the *DSM*, published by the **American Psychiatric Association** (APA). The *DSM* is a reference work consulted by psychiatrists, psychologists, physicians in clinical practice, **social workers**, medical and nursing students, pastoral counselors, and other professionals in health care and social services. The version of the *DSM* used as of 2012 is the fourth edition, text revision (*DSM-IV-TR*); a fifth edition of the *DSM* (*DSM-5*) is scheduled for publication in 2013.

According to the *DSM*, the term "mental disorder" is unfortunate because it implies that a mental disorder is separate from a physical illness, when actually, according to the APA, researchers and scientists now know that the distinction is not clear. The APA argues that "there is much 'physical' in 'mental disorders' and much 'mental' in 'physical disorders,'" but continues to use the term "mental disorders" because a better term has not yet been found. The APA defines a mental disorder as "a clinically significant behavioral or psychological syndrome or pattern that occurs in an individual and that is associated with present distress or disability or with a significantly increased risk of suffering death, pain, disability, or an important loss of freedom" (though this definition is being revised for the *DSM-5*).

Purpose

One of the main purposes of psychiatric diagnosis is to guide treatment planning. If doctors know that a particular disorder has been treated effectively with a specific drug or therapy, then the best practice can be applied to future diagnoses. Diagnosis also helps to establish a prognosis for the patient and his or her family, and it helps enable communication among healthcare professionals (including insurers) involved in the patient's care. Additionally, a formal diagnosis, as recognized by the *DSM*, may be necessary in order for insurers to pay for medical services. (The APA maintains, however, that the *DSM* diagnostic categories should not be used in courtroom proceedings for the purpose of establishing a defendant's legal guilt or innocence.)

Description

The process of psychiatric diagnosis varies according to the patient's overall health condition, behavioral problems (if any), and the setting of the examination. For example, a patient being examined in an emergency room with obvious signs of drug or alcohol intoxication and related injuries will require a physical work-up first, whereas a patient voluntarily consulting a **psychiatrist** about recent changes in mood or problems with memory can usually be evaluated in a series of clinical interviews. The APA's published *Practice Guideline for the Psychiatric Evaluation of Adults*, second edition (2010), outlines the basic parts of a psychiatric interview:

- reason for the evaluation (given by the patient and/or concerned others)
- history of the present illness (symptoms, severity, length of time involved)
- past psychiatric history
- history of alcohol or substance abuse

- general medical history
- developmental, psychosocial, and educational history (includes sexual orientation, marital status, children, religious or spiritual beliefs, educational level, family and social support network)
- military and occupational history
- legal history
- family history
- review of systems (ROS) (a checklist of physical symptoms related to the various organ systems in the body—ear, nose, and throat; respiratory; cardiovascular; gastrointestinal; genitourinary; musculoskeletal; skin and hair; neurological; serves to identify problems that may have a physical rather than psychiatric origin)
- physical examination

The second part of the psychiatric examination consists of a **mental status examination** (MSE), an assessment of the patient's general level of functioning, and any psychiatric tests that the examiner thinks may be necessary to establish or rule out a specific diagnosis. These tests may include a structured interview like the SCID (Structured Clinical Interview for Diagnoses) or one or more inventories for the patient to complete in the office.

In some cases the interviewer will need to consult others (bystanders, first responders, family members) to obtain necessary information about the patient's present condition and past history.

Precautions

The act of labeling a mental disorder may have unintended effects for the person with the disorder. Although the *DSM* states that its diagnoses do not label people, in reality, many people who have received diagnoses of mental disorders may feel affected by the label their disorder has been given. People diagnosed with mental disorders may feel stigmatized, and that others' perceptions of them, as well as their self-perceptions, have changed as a result of their diagnosis.

Patients who are considered a threat to their own safety and that of others may require medication (usually benzodiazepine tranquilizers or antipsychotic drugs) or (as a last resort) physical restraints before a psychiatric evaluation can be completed. Patients who are judged to be dangerous to themselves or others can be hospitalized against their will, and law enforcement notified.

Risks

The primary risk of psychiatric diagnosis is the possibility of misdiagnosis by an inexperienced interviewer or by the lack of time needed for a thorough evaluation.

KEY TERMS

Mental status examination (MSE)—A clinical evaluation in which the doctor assesses the patient's external appearance, attitude, behavior, mood and affect, speech, thought processes, thought content, perception, cognition, insight (or lack thereof), and judgment.

Review of systems (ROS)—A systematic checklist of the various organ systems in the human body—ear, nose, and throat; respiratory; cardiovascular; gastrointestinal; genitourinary; musculoskeletal; skin and hair; neurological—used to ensure that all relevant physical signs and symptoms have been taken into account during a medical or psychiatric evaluation.

Stigma—Any personal attribute that causes a person to be socially shamed, avoided, or discredited. Mental disorders are a common cause of stigma.

Resources

BOOKS

American Psychiatric Association. *Diagnostic and Statistical Manual of Mental Disorders*. 4th ed., text rev. Washington, DC: American Psychiatric Publishing, 2000.

———. *Practice Guideline for the Psychiatric Evaluation of Adults*. 2nd ed. Washington, DC: American Psychiatric Association, 2010.

Freeman, Hugh, ed. *A Century of Psychiatry*. London: Mosby, 1999.

North, Carol, and Sean Yutzy. *Goodwin and Guze's Psychiatric Diagnosis*. New York: Oxford University Press, 2010.

Regier, Darrel A., et al., eds. *The Conceptual Evolution of DSM-5*. Washington, DC: American Psychiatric Publishing, 2010.

PERIODICALS

Broome, M., and L. Bortolotti. "What's Wrong with 'Mental' Disorders? A Commentary on 'What Is a Mental/Psychiatric Disorder? From DSM-IV to DSM-V' by Stein et al. (2010)." *Psychological Medicine* 40, no. 11 (November 2010): 1783–1785.

Ronningstam, E. "Narcissistic Personality Disorder in DSM-V—In Support of Retaining a Significant Diagnosis." *Journal of Personality Disorders* 25, no. 2 (April 2011): 248–259.

Shear, M.K., et al. "Complicated Grief and Related Bereavement Issues for DSM-5." *Depression and Anxiety* 28, no. 2 (February 2011): 103–117.

Stein, D.J., et al. "What Is a Mental/Psychiatric Disorder? From DSM-IV to DSM-V." *Psychological Medicine* 40, no. 11 (November 2010): 1759–1765.

van Emmerich, Arnold A.P., and J.H. Kamphuis. "Testing a DSM-5 Reformulation of Posttraumatic Stress Disorder: Impact on Prevalence and Comorbidity Among Treatment-seeking Civilian Trauma Survivors." *Journal of Traumatic Stress* 24, no. 2 (April 2011): 213–217.

Verhoeff, B., and G. Glas. "The Search for Dysfunctions. A Commentary on 'What Is a Mental/Psychiatric Disorder? From DSM-IV to DSM-V' by Stein et al (2010)." *Psychological Medicine* 40, no. 11 (November 2010): 1787–1788.

Woods, S.W., et al. "DSM-5 and the 'Psychosis Risk Syndrome': The DSM-5 Proposal Is Better Than DSM-IV." *Psychosis* 2, no. 3 (October 2010): 187–190.

WEBSITES

American Psychiatric Association. "Definition of a Mental Disorder." DSM-5 Development. http://www.dsm5.org/ProposedRevisions/Pages/proposedrevision.aspx?rid=465 (accessed October 4, 2011).

Merck Manual for Healthcare Professionals. "Behavioral Emergencies." The Merck Manuals Online Medical Library. June 2008. http://www.merckmanuals.com/professional/sec15/ch195/ch195d.html (accessed October 4, 2011).

———. "Routine Psychiatric Assessment." http://www.merckmanuals.com/professional/sec15/ch195/ch195b.html (accessed October 4, 2011).

ORGANIZATIONS

American Psychiatric Association (APA), 1000 Wilson Boulevard, Suite 1825, Arlington, VA, 22209-3901, (703) 907-7300, apa@psych.org, http://www.psych.org.

National Institute of Mental Health (NIMH), 6001 Executive Boulevard, Room 8184, MSC 9663, Bethesda, MD, 20892-9663, (301) 443-4513, Fax: (301) 443-4279, (866) 615-6464, nimhinfo@nih.gov, http://www.nimh.nih.gov/index.shtml.

Rebecca J. Frey, PhD

Diagnostic and Statistical Manual of Mental Disorders

Definition

The *Diagnostic and Statistical Manual of Mental Disorders* (*DSM*), published by the **American Psychiatric Association**, is a reference work used by psychiatrists, psychologists, physicians, clinical researchers, regulatory agencies, health insurance companies, and other professionals to diagnose and access standard classification codes for a comprehensive list of mental disorders. Its use is varied, from promoting effective **diagnosis**, treatment, and quality of care to facilitating medical recordkeeping. The *DSM* is divided into three major parts: diagnostic classification, diagnostic criteria sets, and descriptive text.

Purpose

The stated purpose of the *DSM* is threefold: to provide "a helpful guide to clinical practice," to "facilitate research and improve communication among clinicians and researchers," and to serve as "an educational tool for teaching psychopathology."

Description

As of 2012, the version of the *DSM* most commonly in use was the fourth edition, text revised (*DSM-IV-TR*). A fifth edition was planned for release in 2013 (*DSM-5*). The changes of the *DSM*, over its five editions, can be summarized as follows:

- a move away from defining mental disorders by their causes toward defining them as clusters of symptoms
- coordination with the World Health Organization (WHO)'s *International Classification of Diseases* (ICD)
- increased use of field trials and statistical analysis in evaluating the adequacy of diagnostic terms and criteria

Origins of the DSM

The concept of the *DSM* dates back to the 1840s, when the U.S. Census Bureau attempted for the first time to count the numbers of patients confined in mental hospitals. American **psychologist** Isaac Ray (1807–81), superintendent of the Butler Hospital in Rhode Island, presented a paper at the 1849 meeting of the Association of Medical Superintendents of American Institutions for the Insane (the forerunner of the present American Psychiatric Association), in which he called for a uniform system of naming, classifying, and recording cases of mental illness. The same plea was made in 1913 by Dr. James May to the same organization, which by then had renamed itself the American Medico-Psychological Association. In 1933, the New York Academy of Medicine and the Medico-Psychological Association compiled the first edition of the *Statistical Manual for Mental Diseases*, which was also adopted by the American Neurological Association. The *Statistical Manual* went through several editions between 1933 and 1952, when the first edition of the *Diagnostic and Statistical Manual of Mental Disorders* appeared. The task of compiling mental hospital statistics was turned over to the then-newly formed **National Institute of Mental Health** (NIMH) in 1949.

DSM-I and *DSM-II*

The *DSM-I*, which appeared in 1952, maintained the coding system of earlier American manuals. Many of the disorders in this edition were termed "reactions," a term borrowed from Swiss **psychiatrist** Adolf Meyer (1866–1950). Meyer viewed mental disorders as reactions of an individual's personality to a combination of psychological, social, and biological factors. *DSM-I* also incorporated the nomenclature for disorders developed by the U.S. Army and modified by the Veterans Administration (VA) to treat the postwar mental health problems of service personnel and veterans. The VA classification system grouped mental problems into three large categories: psychophysiological, personality, and acute disorders.

DSM-II, which was published in 1968, represented the first attempt to coordinate the *DSM* with the *ICD*. *DSM-II* appeared before the ninth edition of the *ICD*, or *ICD-9*, which was published in 1975. *DSM-II* continued the *DSM-I*'s psychoanalytical approach to the etiology of the nonorganic mental disorders and **personality disorders**.

DSM-III, DSM-III-R and *DSM-IV*

DSM-III, which was published in 1980 after six years of preparatory work, represented a major break with the first two editions of the *DSM*. *DSM-III* introduced the present descriptive symptom-based approach to mental disorders, added lists of explicit diagnostic criteria, removed references to the etiology of disorders, did away with the term "neurosis," and established the present multi-axial system of symptom evaluation. This sweeping change originated in an effort begun in the early 1970s by a group of psychiatrists at the medical school of Washington University in St. Louis, Missouri, to improve the state of research in American psychiatry. The St. Louis group began by drawing up a list of "research diagnostic criteria" for **schizophrenia**, a disorder that can manifest itself in a variety of ways. The group was concerned primarily with the identification of markers for schizophrenia that would allow the disease to be studied at other research sites without introducing errors by using different types of patients in different centers.

What happened with *DSM-III*, *DSM-III-R*, and *DSM-IV* was that a tool for scholarly investigation of a few mental disorders was transformed into a diagnostic method applied to all mental disorders without further distinction. The leaders of this transformation were biological psychiatrists who wanted to empty the diagnostic manual of terms and theories associated with hypothetical or explanatory concepts. The transition from an explanatory approach to mental disorders to a descriptive or phenomenological one in the period between *DSM-II* and *DSM-III* is sometimes called the "neo-Kraepelinian revolution"; another term that has been applied to the orientation represented in *DSM-III* and its successors is *empirical*, which denotes reliance on experience or experiment alone, without recourse to theories or hypotheses. The word occurs repeatedly in the description of "The DSM-IV Revision Process" in the Introduction to *DSM-IV-TR*.

DSM-IV built upon the research generated by the empirical orientation of *DSM-III*. By the early 1990s, most psychiatric diagnoses had an accumulated body of published studies or data sets. Publications up through 1992 were reviewed for *DSM-IV*, which was published in 1994. Conflicting reports or lack of evidence were handled by data re-analyses and field trials. The NIMH sponsored 12 *DSM-IV* field trials together with the National Institute on Drug Abuse (NIDA) and the National Institute on Alcohol Abuse and Alcoholism (NIAAA). The field trials compared the diagnostic criteria sets of *DSM-III*, *DSM-III-R*, *ICD-10* (which had been published in 1992), and the proposed criteria sets for *DSM-IV*. The field trials recruited subjects from a variety of ethnic and cultural backgrounds, in keeping with a new concern for cross-cultural applicability of diagnostic standards. In addition to its inclusion of culture-specific syndromes and disorders, *DSM-IV* represented much closer cooperation and coordination with the World Health Organization experts who had worked on *ICD-10*. A modification of *ICD-10* for clinical practitioners, the *ICD-10-CM*, was introduced in the United States in 2004.

Multi-axial and biopsychosocial approach

The *DSM-III* introduced a system of five axes or dimensions for assessing all aspects of a patient's mental and emotional health. The multi-axial system was designed to provide a more comprehensive picture of complex or concurrent mental disorders. According to the *DSM-IV-TR*, the system was also intended to "promote the application of the biopsychosocial model in clinical, educational, and research settings." The reference to the biopsychosocial model is significant, because it indicates that the *DSM-IV-TR* does not reflect the view of any specific "school" or tradition within psychiatry regarding the cause or origin (etiology) of mental disorders. In other words, the *DSM-IV-TR* is theoretical in its approach to diagnosis and classification—the axes and categories do not represent any overarching theory about the sources or fundamental nature of mental disorders.

The biopsychosocial approach was originally proposed by American psychiatrist George L. Engel (1913–1999) in 1977 as a way around the disputes between psychoanalytically and biologically oriented psychiatrists who were splitting the field in the 1970s. The introduction to *DSM-IV-TR* is explicit about the manual's intentions to be "applicable in a wide variety of contexts" and "used by clinicians and researchers of many different orientations (e.g., biological, psychodynamic, cognitive, behavioral, interpersonal, family/systems)."

The atheoretical stance of the *DSM-IV-TR* is also significant in that it underlies the manual's approach to the legal implications of mental illness. *DSM* notes the existence of an "imperfect fit between questions of ultimate concern to the law and the information contained in a clinical diagnosis." What is meant here is that the *DSM-IV-TR* diagnostic categories do not meet forensic standards for defining a "mental defect," "mental disability," or similar terms. Because *DSM-IV-TR* states that "inclusion of a disorder in the classification . . . does not require that there be knowledge about its etiology," it advises legal professionals against basing decisions about a person's criminal responsibility, competence, or degree of behavioral control on *DSM* diagnostic categories.

The five diagnostic axes specified by *DSM-IV-TR* are:

- Axis I: clinical disorders, including anxiety disorders, mood disorders, schizophrenia, and other psychotic disorders
- Axis II: personality disorders and intellectual disability, including notations about problematic aspects of the patient's personality that fall short of the criteria for a personality disorder
- Axis III: general medical conditions, including diseases or disorders that may be related physiologically to the mental disorder; that are sufficiently severe to affect the patient's mood or functioning; or that influence the choice of medications for treating the mental disorder
- Axis IV: psychosocial and environmental problems, including conditions or situations that influence the diagnosis, treatment, or prognosis of the patient's mental disorder, such as family or relationship problems, social problems, educational or occupational problems, housing problems, financial problems, problems with access to health care, legal problems, and other problems (war, disasters, etc.)
- Axis V: global assessment of functioning

Rating the patient's general level of functioning is intended to help the doctor draw up a treatment plan and evaluate treatment progress. The primary scale for Axis V is the global assessment of functioning (GAF) scale, which measures a patient's level of functioning on a scale of 1–100. *DSM-IV-TR* includes three specialized global scales in its appendices: the social and occupational functioning assessment scale (SOFAS), the defensive functioning scale (DFS), and the global assessment of relational functioning (GARF) scale. For instance, the GARF is a measurement of the maturity and stability of the relationships within a family or between a couple.

Diagnostic categories

DSM-IV-TR. The Axis I clinical disorders of the *DSM-IV-TR* are divided among 15 categories: disorders usually first diagnosed in infancy, childhood, or adolescence; **delirium**, **dementia**, amnestic, and other cognitive disorders; medical disorders due to a general medical condition; substance-related disorders; schizophrenia and other psychotic disorders; mood disorders; **anxiety disorders**; **somatoform disorders**; factitious disorders; **dissociative disorders**; sexual and gender identity disorders; eating disorders; **sleep disorders**; **impulse control disorders** not elsewhere classified; and **adjustment disorders**.

The diagnostic categories of *DSM-IV-TR* are essentially symptom-based, or, as the manual puts it, based "on criteria sets with defining features." Another term that is sometimes used to describe this method of classification is phenomenological. A phenomenological approach to classification is one that emphasizes externally observable phenomena rather than their underlying nature or origin.

DSM-5. Proposed changes for the *DSM-5* include revised diagnostic categories, increasing the total to 20: neurodevelopmental disorders; schizophrenia spectrum and other psychotic disorders; bipolar and related disorders; depressive disorders; anxiety disorders; obsessive-compulsive and related disorders; trauma- and stressor-related disorders; dissociative disorders; somatic symptom disorders; feeding and eating disorders; elimination disorders; sleep-wake disorders; **sexual dysfunctions**; gender dysphoria; disruptive, impulse control, and conduct disorders; substance use and addictive disorders; neurocognitive disorders; personality disorders; **paraphilias**; and other disorders.

Medical model of mental disorders

Another important characteristic of the *DSM-IV-TR* classification system is its dependence on the medical model of mental disorders. Such terms as "psychopathology," "mental illness," "differential diagnosis," and "prognosis" are all borrowed from medical practice. The medical model as it came to dominate psychiatry can be traced back to the work of Emil Kraepelin (1856–1926), a German psychiatrist whose *Handbuch der Psychiatrie* ("Handbook of Psychiatry") was the first basic textbook in the field and introduced the first nosology, or systematic classification, of mental disorders. Prior to its adoption, mental illness was attributed to supernatural or moral causes (desire to engage in bad behavior). By the early 1890s, Kraepelin's handbook was being used in medical schools across Europe. He updated and revised it periodically to accommodate new findings, including a disease (**Alzheimer's disease**) that he named after one of his clinical assistants, Aloysius (Alois) Alzheimer (1864–1915). The 1907 edition of Kraepelin's handbook included 15 categories, most of which were still used over a century later. Kraepelin's work was also significant because it represented a biologically based view of mental disorders, as opposed to the psychoanalytical approach of Sigmund Freud. Kraepelin thought that mental disorders could ultimately be traced to organic diseases of the **brain** rather than disordered emotions or psychological processes. The controversy between these two perspectives dominated psychiatric research and practice until well after World War II (1939–45).

Textual revisions in DSM-IV-TR

The text-revised edition of the *DSM-IV*, published in 2000, does not represent either a fundamental change in the basic classification structure of *DSM-IV* or the addition of new diagnostic entities. The textual revisions that were made to the 1994 edition of *DSM-IV* included:

- correction of factual errors
- review of currency of information
- changes to reflect research published after 1992, which was the last year included in the literature review prior to the publication of *DSM-IV*
- improvements to enhance the educational value of *DSM-IV*
- updated *ICD* diagnostic codes, some of which were changed in 1996

Criticisms of DSM-IV *and* DSM-IV-TR

One reason for a new edition of the *DSM* (*DSM-5*) is the number of criticisms of the fourth edition of the manual, such as:

- The medical model underlying the empirical orientation of *DSM-IV* reduces human beings to "one-dimensional" sources of data; it does not encourage practitioners to treat the whole person.
- The medical model perpetuates the social stigma attached to mental disorders.
- The symptom-based criteria sets have led to an endless multiplication of mental conditions and disorders. The unwieldy size of *DSM-IV* is a common complaint of doctors in clinical practice—a volume that was only 119 pages long in its second (1968) edition has swollen to 886 pages in less than thirty years.
- The symptom-based approach has also made it easier to politicize the process of defining new disorders for inclusion in *DSM* or dropping older ones. The inclusion of post-traumatic stress disorder (PTSD) and the deletion of homosexuality as a disorder are often cited as examples of this concern for political correctness.
- The criteria sets of *DSM-IV* incorporate implicit (implied but not expressly stated) notions of human psychological well-being that do not allow for ordinary diversity among people. Some of the diagnostic categories of *DSM-IV* come close to defining various temperamental and personality differences as mental disorders.
- The *DSM-IV* criteria do not distinguish adequately between poor adaptation to ordinary problems of living and true psychopathology. One by-product of this inadequacy is the suspiciously high rates of prevalence reported for some mental disorders. One observer remarked that "it is doubtful that 28% or 29% of the population would be judged [by managed care plans] to need mental health treatment in a year."
- The diagnostic classes defined by *DSM-IV* hinder efforts to recognize disorders that run across classes. For example, PTSD has more in common with respect to etiology and treatment with the dissociative disorders than it does with the anxiety disorders with which it is grouped. Another example is body dysmorphic disorder, which resembles the obsessive-compulsive disorders more than it does the somatoform disorders.
- The current classification is deficient in acknowledging disorders of uncontrolled anger, hostility, and aggression. Even though inappropriate expressions of anger and aggression lie at the roots of major social problems, only one *DSM-IV* disorder (intermittent explosive disorder) is explicitly concerned with them. In contrast, entire classes of disorders are devoted to depression and anxiety.
- The emphasis of *DSM-IV* on biological psychiatry has contributed to the widespread popular notion that most problems of human life can be solved by taking pills.
- The current approach to diagnosing mental disorders takes a categorical, rather than dimensional (continuum), perspective on symptoms of mental illness.

Alternative nosologies

A number of different nosologies or schemes of classification have been proposed to replace the current descriptive model of mental disorders.

THE DIMENSIONAL MODEL. Dimensional alternatives to *DSM-IV* would replace the categorical classification now in use with a recognition that mental disorders lie on a continuum with both mildly disturbed and normal behavior, rather than being qualitatively distinct. For example, the personality disorders of Axis II are increasingly regarded as extreme variants of common personality characteristics. In the dimensional model, patients would be identified in terms of their position on a specific dimension of cognitive or affective capacity rather than placed in a categorical "box."

THE HOLISTIC MODEL. The holistic approach to mental disorders places equal emphasis on social and spiritual as well as pharmacological treatments. A biochemist that was diagnosed with schizophrenia and eventually recovered compared the reductionism of the biological model of his disorder with the empowering qualities of holistic approaches. He stressed the healing potential in treating patients as whole persons rather than as isolated collections of nervous tissue with chemical imbalances, stating that "the major task in recovering from mental illness is to regain social roles and identities. This entails focusing on the individual and building a sense of responsibility and self-determination."

THE ESSENTIAL OR PERSPECTIVAL MODEL. The third and most complex alternative model is associated with the medical school of Johns Hopkins University (Baltimore, Maryland), where it is taught as part of the medical curriculum. This model identifies four broad perspectives that can be used to identify the distinctive characteristics of mental disorders, which are often obscured by the present categorical classifications.

The four perspectives are:

- Disease. This perspective works with categories and accounts for physical diseases or damage to the brain that produces psychiatric symptoms. It accounts for such disorders as Alzheimer's disease or schizophrenia.
- Dimensions. This perspective addresses disorders that arise from the combination of a cognitive or emotional weakness in the patient's constitution and a life experience that challenges the individual's vulnerability.
- Behaviors. This perspective is concerned with disorders associated with something that the patient is doing (alcoholism, drug addiction, eating disorders, etc.) that has become a dysfunctional way of life.
- Life story. This perspective focuses on disorders related to what the patient has encountered in life, such as events that have injured the person's hopes and aspirations.

In the Johns Hopkins model, each perspective has its own approach to treatment: the disease perspective seeks to cure or prevent disorders rooted in biological disease processes; the dimensional perspective attempts to strengthen constitutional weaknesses; the behavioral perspective seeks to interrupt the problematic behaviors and assist patients in overcoming their appeal; and the life story perspective offers help in "rescripting" a person's life narrative, usually through cognitive behavioral treatment.

DSM-5

The fifth edition of the *DSM* is slated for publication in May 2013. Aside from changes to specific sets of diagnostic criteria, the *DSM-5* is set to undergo a major organizational revision. Other changes are being made to correct perceived errors within criteria sets identified in the *DSM-IV*, and several diagnostic codes are being updated to coincide with updates to the *ICD-9-CM* coding system.

One of the most recognizable changes involves the title—the use of Roman numerals in previous editions is being abandoned, so the fifth edition will be the first to use Arabic numerals. Other considerations include whether to abandon the previous axis framework and consolidate the first three axes into a single axis that covers all psychiatric and medical diagnoses. This would be done in order to parallel the way the *ICD-10* is organized. Simultaneously, Axis IV (psychosocial issues such as housing or economic issues) is being reviewed in order to bring it into line with the *ICD*.

Other notable changes include collapsing a number of currently separate disorders (**Asperger syndrome**, **childhood disintegrative disorder**, and pervasive developmental disorder) under the rubric of **autism** spectrum disorder; creating a single "addiction and related disorders" category to replace **substance abuse** and dependence; including a behavioral addictions category to describe gambling; the inclusion of new **suicide** scales; the creation of risk syndromes that will help improve early recognition of evolving disorders; finer distinctions between childhood **bipolar disorder**, childhood **oppositional defiant disorder**, and newer diagnoses, such as **disruptive mood dysregulation disorder**; and honing of the criteria for eating disorders, as well as including **binge eating disorder**. The exclusion of diagnoses present in prior editions and the addition of several new disorders is already prompting controversy.

While feedback has been solicited in response to the proposed changes, controversy continues to cloud the new edition's development. Concerns about transparency of the task force has plagued the *DSM-5*'s development, and various interest groups are vocal in their support or opposition to changes to the diagnostic criteria. Interested users can follow the development of the *DSM-5* on its website: http://www.dsm5.org.

KEY TERMS

Amnestic—Having to do with, or related to, amnesia.

Biological psychiatry—An approach to psychiatry that emphasizes the biological and biochemical factors in mental illness; it tends to favor drug treatments for mental disorders rather than psychotherapy.

Biopsychosocial model—An approach to human health that holds that a combination of biological, psychological, and social factors should be taken into account when evaluating a patient rather than physical factors alone.

Delirium—A temporary mental problem characterized by confusion, restlessness, and (sometimes) hallucinations, which can be caused by a brain injury, fever, or other such accidents or maladies.

Dementia—A deterioration of cognitive/intellectual abilities, including memory, while other brain activities, such as bodily movements and senses, appear to be normal; sometimes also called senility.

Depression—A psychiatric disorder involving feelings of hopelessness and symptoms of fatigue, sleeplessness, suicidal tendencies, and poor concentration.

Empirical—Based on information gathered by scientific observation or experiments, as distinct from pure theory.

Forensic—Pertaining to legal matters or courtroom proceedings.

Medical model of mental illness—An approach to psychiatric diagnosis and treatment patterned on the process of diagnosis and treatment of physical disease.

Mental disorder—A psychiatric disorder of mental faculties.

Schizophrenia—A severe mental illness in which a person has difficulty distinguishing what is real from what is not real. It is often characterized by hallucinations, delusions, language and communication disturbances, and withdrawal from people and social activities.

Resources

BOOKS

American Psychiatric Association. *Diagnostic and Statistical Manual of Mental Disorders*. 4th ed., text rev. Washington, DC: American Psychiatric Association, 2000.

Borch-Jacobsen, Mikkel. *Making Minds and Madness: From Hysteria to Depression*. Cambridge, UK: Cambridge University Press, 2009.

Peterson, David B. *Psychological Aspects of Functioning, Disability, and Health*. New York: Springer, 2011.

Regier, Darrel A., et al., eds. *The Conceptual Evolution of DSM-5*. Washington, DC: American Psychiatric Publishing, 2011.

PERIODICALS

First, Michael B. "DSM-5 Proposals for Mood Disorders: A Cost-Benefit Analysis." *Current Opinions in Psychiatry* 29 (December 12, 2010): 1–9.

Happ, F. "Criteria, Categories, and Continua: Autism and Related Disorders in DSM-5." *Journal of the American Academy of Child and Adolescent Psychiatry* 50 (June 2011): 540–42.

Woods, Scott W. "The Case for Including Attenuated Psychotic Symptoms Syndrome in DSM-5 as a Psychosis Risk Syndrome." *Schizophrenia Research* 123, no. 2–3 (November 2010): 199–207.

WEBSITES

American Psychiatric Association. "DSM-5 Development: Frequently Asked Questions." http://www.dsm5.org/about/Pages/faq.aspx (accessed September 16, 2011).

World Health Organization. "International Classification of Diseases (ICD)." http://www.who.int/classifications/icd/en (accessed September 16, 2011).

ORGANIZATIONS

American Psychiatric Association, 1000 Wilson Blvd., Ste. 1825, Arlington, VA, 22209-3901, (703) 907-7300, apa@psych.org, http://www.psych.org.

Rebecca J. Frey, PhD
William A. Atkins, PhD

Diastat AcuDial *see* **Diazepam**

Diazepam

Definition

Diazepam is a mild tranquilizer in the class of drugs known as **benzodiazepines**. It is most commonly sold in the United States under the brand name Valium. The generic form of this drug is also available.

Purpose

Diazepam is used on a short-term basis to treat patients with mild to moderate anxiety. It is also used to treat some types of **seizures** (epilepsy), muscle spasms, nervous tension, and symptoms relating to alcohol withdrawal.

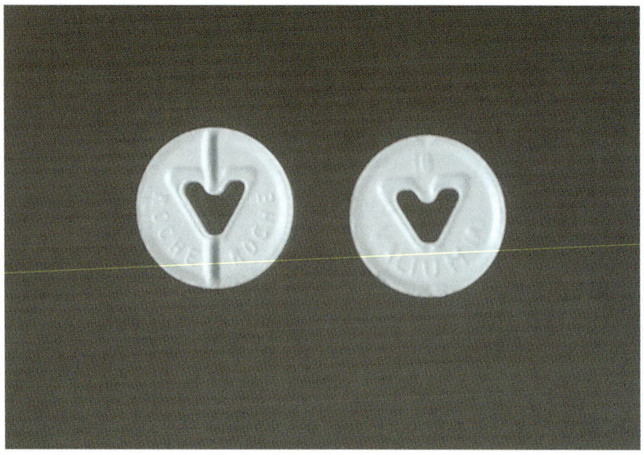

Valium (diazepam), 10 mg. *(U.S. Drug Enforcement Administration)*

Description

Diazepam is one of many chemically related tranquilizers in the class of drugs called benzodiazepines. Benzodiazepines are sedative-hypnotic drugs that help to relieve nervousness, tension, and other anxiety symptoms by slowing the central nervous system. To do this, they block the effects of a specific chemical involved in the transmission of nerve impulses in the **brain**, decreasing the excitement level of the nerve cells. All benzodiazepines, including diazepam, cause sedation, drowsiness, and reduced mental and physical alertness.

Recommended dosage

The typical dose of diazepam used to treat anxiety or seizures in healthy adults ranges from a total of 6 mg to 40 mg per day given in three or four doses. People over age 60 are usually given lower doses in the range of 4–10 mg per day to treat anxiety or nervous tension. For acute treatment of seizures, a higher dose of diazepam is given intravenously (directly into the vein) only in a controlled medical setting such as a hospital or emergency room. For alcohol withdrawal, the typical dose is a total of 30–40 mg per day given in three or four doses.

The typical dose for a child over age six months with anxiety or seizures is a total of 3–10 mg per day divided into several doses. In general, children receive lower doses of diazepam even when they have a body weight equivalent to a small adult. Diazepam is usually taken as a pill, but an injectable form is sometimes used when a serious seizure is in progress or when muscle spasms are severe. There is a liquid oral form of the drug available, and diazepam is also available as a rectal gel, marketed as Diastat AcuDial.

KEY TERMS

Anterograde amnesia—The inability to form new memories.

Anxiety—An emotion that can be experienced as a troubled feeling, sense of dread, fear of the future, or distress over a possible threat to a person's physical or mental well-being.

Epilepsy—A disorder associated with disturbed electrical discharges in the central nervous system that cause seizures.

Seizure—A convulsion or uncontrolled discharge of nerve cells that may spread to other cells throughout the brain.

Precautions

The elderly, children, and those with significant health problems need to be carefully evaluated before receiving diazepam. Children under the age of six months should not take diazepam. In addition, people with a history of liver disease, kidney disease, or those with low levels of a protein in the blood called albumin need to be carefully assessed before starting this drug.

The sedative effects of diazepam are cumulative and long lasting. People taking diazepam should not drive, operate dangerous machinery, or engage in hazardous activities that require mental alertness, because diazepam can cause drowsiness. Alcohol and any drugs that treat mental illness should not be used when taking this medication. People who have previously had an allergic reaction to any dosage level of diazepam or any other benzodiazepine drug should not take diazepam. People with acute narrow-angle glaucoma should not take diazepam.

The prescribing physician should be consulted regularly if diazepam is taken consistently for more than two weeks. Diazepam and other drugs in this class can be habit-forming. Diazepam can become a drug of abuse and should be used with caution in patients with a history of **substance abuse**. People taking diazepam should not stop taking the drug abruptly. Doing so can lead to withdrawal effects such as shaking, stomach cramps, nervousness, and irritability.

Diazepam may carry the risk of anterograde **amnesia**.

Individuals using diazepam in the form of rectal gel (Diastat AcuDial), should check the prefilled syringe applicator tip (without removing the cap) for cracks. The U.S. Food and Drug Administration (FDA) issued an alert in 2006 addressing this concern; cracks in the

QUESTIONS TO ASK YOUR DOCTOR

- What kind of changes can I expect to see or feel with this medication?
- Does it matter what time of day I take this medication? If so, what is the recommendation?
- Should I take this medication with or without food?
- What are the side effects associated with this medication?
- Will this medication interact or interfere with other medications I am currently taking?
- What symptoms or adverse effects are important enough that I should seek immediate treatment?

applicator tip have been known to occur, allowing medication to leak out and compromising the amount of medication in the syringe. This situation could result in the syringe not containing enough medication to treat a seizure. Cracks can occur over time so it is important to check syringes on a regular basis to ensure they are acceptable for use.

Side effects

Anxiety, irregular heartbeat, forgetfulness, mental **depression**, and confusion are side effects that could require prompt medical attention. However, these side effects are not common when taking diazepam. Even more unusual but serious events are behavior changes, low blood pressure, muscle weakness, and jaundice (yellowing of the eyes or skin). More common but less serious side effects include drowsiness, clumsiness, slurred speech, and dizziness. Rare among these less serious side effects are stomach cramps, headache, muscle spasm, nausea, vomiting, and dry mouth.

Once a person stops taking diazepam, the following side effects could occur from withdrawal: sleeping difficulties, nervousness, and irritability. Less common side effects from withdrawal include:

- confusion
- abdominal cramps
- mental depression
- sensitivity to light
- nausea
- shaking
- increased sweating

Rarely seen side effects include seizures, hallucinations, and feelings of distrust in the patient.

Interactions

Diazepam interacts with a long list of other medications. Individuals who are starting this drug should review the other medications they are taking with their physician and pharmacist for possible interactions. Patients should always inform all their healthcare providers, including dentists, that they are taking diazepam. Diazepam can add to the depressive effects of other central nervous system depressant drugs (for example, alcohol, other tranquilizers, or sleeping pills) when taken together. In severe cases, this effect can result in death.

Several drugs reduce the ability of diazepam to be broken down and cleared from the body, which results in higher levels of the drug in the blood and increases the probability that side effects will occur. These drugs include several antibiotics, such as erythromycin; anti-stomach acid drugs, such as cimetidine (Tagamet); and antifungal drugs, such as fluconazole. Alcohol should not be used when taking diazepam and other benzodiazepine drugs. There may also be an interaction between this drug and grapefruit juice. Other drugs that are used to treat mental disorders should not be combined with diazepam unless the patient is under the careful supervision and monitoring of a doctor.

Those who rely on urine tests to monitor blood sugar should know that this drug can produce false results with tests using Clinistix and Diastix and that they should instead use TesTape for urine testing of sugar.

Resources

BOOKS

Albers, Lawrence J., Rhoda K. Hahn, and Christopher Reist. *Handbook of Psychiatric Drugs.* Laguna Hills, CA: Current Clinical Strategies, 2010.

American Society of Health-System Pharmacists. *AHFS Drug Information 2011.* Bethesda, MD: ASHP, 2011.

Aminoff, Michael J., ed. *Neurology and General Medicine.* 4th ed. New York: Churchill Livingstone, 2007.

Devinsky, Orrin. *Epilepsy: Patient and Family Guide.* 3rd ed. New York: Demos Medical, 2007.

Holland, Leland Norman, and Michael Patrick Adams. *Core Concepts in Pharmacology.* 3rd ed. New York: Prentice Hall, 2011.

Kuzniecky, Ruben, ed. *Epilepsy 101: The Ultimate Guide for Patients and Families.* Leona, NJ: Medicus Press, 2009.

Panayiotopoulos, C.P. *Antiepileptic Drugs, Pharmacopoeia.* New York: Springer, 2010.

Patsalos, Philip N., and Blaise F.D. Bourgeois. *The Epilepsy Prescriber's Guide to Antiepileptic Drugs.* New York: Cambridge University Press, 2010.

Preston, John D., John H. O'Neal, and Mary C. Talaga. *Handbook of Clinical Psychopharmacology for Therapists.* 6th ed. Oakland, CA: New Harbinger, 2010.

Shorvon, Simon. *Handbook of Epilepsy Treatment.* 3rd ed. New York: Wiley-Blackwell, 2010.

Tatum, William O., Peter W. Kaplan, and Pierre Jallon. *Epilepsy A to Z: A Concise Encyclopedia.* 2nd ed. New York: Demos Medical, 2009.

ORGANIZATIONS

American Academy of Clinical Toxicology, 6728 Old McLean Village Dr., McLean, VA, 22101, (703) 556-9222, Fax: (703) 556-8729, admin@clintox.org, http://www.clintox.org.

American Academy of Family Physicians, 11400 Tomahawk Creek Pkwy., Leawood, KS, 66211-2672, (913) 906-6000, (800) 274-2237, Fax: (913) 906-6075, contactcenter@aafp.org, http://www.aafp.org.

American Medical Association, 515 N State St., Chicago, IL, 60610, (312) 464-5000, (800) 621-8335, http://www.ama-assn.org.

American Psychiatric Association, 1000 Wilson Blvd., Ste. 1825, Arlington, VA, 22209-3901, (703) 907-7300, apa@psych.org, http://www.psych.org.

American Psychological Association, 750 1st St., NE, Washington, DC, 20002-4242, (202) 336-5500; TDD/TTY: (202) 336-6123, (800) 374-2721, http://www.apa.org.

American Society for Clinical Pharmacology and Therapeutics, 528 N Washington St., Alexandria, VA, 22314, (703) 836-6981, info@ascpt.org, http://www.ascpt.org.

Anxiety Disorders Association of America, 8730 Georgia Ave., Silver Spring, MD, 20910, (240) 485-1001, Fax: (240) 485-1035, http://www.adaa.org.

Depression and Bipolar Support Alliance, 730 N Franklin St., Ste. 501, Chicago, IL, 60654, (800) 826-3632, Fax: (312) 642-7243, http://www.dbsalliance.org.

Mental Health America, 2000 N. Beauregard St., 6th Fl., Alexandria, VA, 22311, (703) 684-7722, (800) 969-6642, Fax: (703) 684-5968, http://www1.nmha.org.

National Alliance on Mental Illness, 2107 Wilson Blvd., Ste. 300, Arlington, VA, 22201-3042, Fax: (703) 524-9094, (800) 950-6264, http://www.nami.org.

National Institute of Mental Health, 6001 Executive Blvd., Rm. 8184, MSC 9663, Bethesda, MD, 20892-9663, (301) 433-4513; TTY: (301) 443-8431, Fax: (301) 443-4279, (866) 615-6464; TTY: (866) 415-8051, nimhinfo@nih.gov, http://www.nimh.nih.gov.

National Institutes of Health, 9000 Rockville Pike, Bethesda, MD, 20892, (301) 496-4000; TTY: (301) 402-9612, http://www.nih.gov.

U.S. National Library of Medicine, 8600 Rockville Pike, Bethesda, MD, 20894, (301) 594-5983, (888) 346-3656; TDD: (800) 735-2258, Fax: (301) 402-1384, http://www.nlm.nih.gov.

Mark Mitchell, MD
Emily Jane Willingham, PhD
Laura Jean Cataldo, RN, EdD

Diets

Definition

Special diets are designed to help individuals make changes in their usual eating habits or food selection. Some special diets involve changes in the overall diet, such as diets for people needing to gain or lose weight or eat more healthfully. Other special diets are designed to help individuals limit or avoid certain foods or dietary components that could interfere with the activity of a medication. Still other special diets are designed to counter nutritional effects of certain medications.

Purpose

Special diets are used in the treatment of people with certain mental disorders for the following reasons:

- identify and correct disordered eating patterns
- prevent or correct nutritional deficiencies or excesses
- prevent interactions between foods or nutrients and medications

Description

Special types of diets or changes in eating habits have been suggested for people with certain mental disorders. In some disorders, such as eating disorders or **substance abuse**, dietary changes are an integral part of therapy. In other disorders, such as attention deficit hyperactivity disorder, various proposed diets have questionable therapeutic value.

Many medications for mental disorders can affect appetite or nutrition-related functions such as saliva production, ability to swallow, bowel function, and activity level. Changes in diet or food choices may be required to help prevent negative effects of medications.

Finally, interactions can occur between some medications used to treat people with mental disorders and certain foods or nutritional components of the diet. For example, grapefruit and apple juice can interact with some specific psychotropic drugs (medications taken for psychiatric conditions) and should be avoided by individuals taking those medicines. Tyramine, a natural substance found in aged or fermented foods, can interfere with the functioning of **monoamine oxidase inhibitors (MAOIs)** and must be restricted in individuals using these types of medications. A person's preexisting medical condition and nutritional needs should be taken into account when designing any special diet.

KEY TERMS

Attention deficit hyperactivity disorder (ADHD)—A developmental disorder characterized by distractibility, hyperactivity, impulsive behaviors, and the inability to remain focused on tasks or activities.

Depression—A mental state characterized by feelings of sadness, despair, and discouragement.

Food allergy—An abnormal reaction to a food eaten or touched. A food allergy is related to the immune system.

Special diets for specific disorders

Eating disorders

The two main types of eating disorders are **anorexia nervosa** and **bulimia nervosa**. Individuals with anorexia nervosa starve themselves, whereas individuals with bulimia nervosa usually have normal or slightly above normal body weight but engage in binge eating followed by purging with laxatives, vomiting, or **exercise**.

Special diets for individuals with eating disorders focus on restoration of normal body weight and control of bingeing and purging. These diets are usually carried out under the supervision of a multidisciplinary team, including a physician, **psychologist**, and dietitian.

The overall dietary goal for individuals with anorexia nervosa is to restore a healthy body weight. An initial goal might be to stop weight loss and improve food choices. Energy intake is then increased gradually until normal weight is restored. Because individuals with anorexia nervosa have an intense fear of gaining weight and becoming fat, quantities of foods eaten are increased very slowly so that the patient will continue treatments and therapy.

The overall dietary goal for individuals with bulimia nervosa is to gain control over eating behavior and to achieve a healthy body weight. An initial goal is to stabilize weight and eating patterns to help individuals gain control over the binge-purge cycle. Meals and snacks are eaten at regular intervals to lessen the possibility that hunger and fasting will trigger a binge. Once eating behaviors have been stabilized, energy intake can be gradually adjusted to allow individuals to reach a normal body weight healthfully.

For individuals with either anorexia nervosa or bulimia, continued follow-up and support are required after normal weight and eating behaviors are restored, particularly since the rate of **relapse** is high. In addition to dietary changes, **psychotherapy** is an essential part of the treatment of eating disorders and helps individuals deal with fears and misconceptions about body weight and eating behavior.

Attention deficit hyperactivity disorder

Attention deficit hyperactivity disorder (ADHD) accounts for a substantial portion of referrals to child mental health services. Children with **ADHD** are inappropriately active, easily frustrated or distracted, impulsive, and have difficulty sustaining concentration. Usual treatment of ADHD involves medication, behavioral management, and education.

Many dietary factors have been proposed as causes of ADHD, including sugar, food additives, and food allergies. In the 1970s the Feingold diet became popular for treatment of ADHD. The Feingold diet excludes artificial colorings and flavorings, natural sources of chemicals called salicylates (found in fruits), and preservatives called BHT and BHA. Although scientific evidence does not support the effectiveness of the Feingold diet, a modified Feingold diet, including fruits, has been shown to be nutritionally balanced and should not be harmful as long as the child continues to receive conventional ADHD treatment also.

A high intake of sugar and sugary foods has also been implicated as a cause of ADHD. Although carefully controlled studies have shown no association between sugar and ADHD, diets high in sugar should be discouraged because they are often low in other nutrients and can contribute to dental problems.

Food allergies have also been implicated as a cause of ADHD, and some groups have suggested using elimination diets to treat ADHD. Elimination diets omit foods that most commonly cause allergies in children, such as eggs, milk, peanuts, or shellfish. Although research does not support the value of elimination diets for all children with ADHD, children with specific food allergies can become irritable and restless. Children with a suspected food allergy should be evaluated by an allergist.

Stimulant medications used to treat ADHD, such as **methylphenidate** (Ritalin), can cause appetite loss (anorexia) and retard growth, although some research suggests that a child's ultimate height appears not to be affected by stimulant medications. As a precaution, children on such medicines should receive close monitoring of growth patterns, and parents should carefully observe their child's appetite and interest in meals and snacks. Providing regular meals and snacks, even when the child is not hungry, can help to assure adequate growth.

Mood disorders

Mood disorders include both **depression** (unipolar disorder) and episodes of mania followed by depression (**bipolar disorder**). Both types of disorders can affect appetite and eating behavior.

Although some individuals with depression eat more than usual and gain weight, depression more often causes loss of appetite and weight loss. As individuals with depression lose interest in eating and social relationships, they often skip meals and ignore feelings of hunger. Unintentional weight losses of up to 15% of body mass can occur.

Treatment with antidepressant medications often reverses weight loss and restores appetite and interest in eating. If individuals have lost a significant amount of weight, they may need to follow a high-calorie diet to restore weight to normal levels and replaced nutritional deficiencies. High-calorie diets usually include three balanced meals from all the food groups and several smaller snacks throughout the day. A protein/calorie supplement may also be necessary for some individuals.

Depression is sometimes treated with **MAOIs**. Individuals on these medications need to follow a tyramine-restricted diet.

Individuals with mania are often treated with lithium. Sodium and caffeine intake can affect lithium levels in the blood, and intake of these should not suddenly be increased or decreased. Weight gain can occur in response to some antidepressant medications and lithium.

Schizophrenia

Individuals with **schizophrenia** can have hallucinations, delusional thinking, and bizarre behavior. These distorted behaviors and thought processes can also be extended to **delusions** and hallucinations about food and diet, making people with schizophrenia at risk for poor **nutrition**.

Individuals with schizophrenia may believe that certain foods are poisonous or have special properties. They may think they hear voices telling them not to eat. Some may eat huge quantities of food thinking that it gives them special powers. Individuals with untreated schizophrenia may lose a significant amount of weight. Delusional beliefs and thinking about food and eating usually improve once individuals are started on medication to treat schizophrenia.

Substance abuse

Substance abuse can include abuse of alcohol, cigarettes, marijuana, **cocaine**, or other drugs. Individuals abusing any of these substances are at risk for nutritional problems. Many of these substances can reduce appetite, decrease absorption of nutrients into the body, and cause individuals to make poor food choices.

Special diets used for withdrawal from substance abuse are designed to correct any nutritional deficiencies that have developed, aid in the withdrawal of the substance, and prevent the individual from making unhealthy food substitutions as the addictive substance is withdrawn. For example, some individuals may compulsively overeat when they stop smoking, leading to weight gain. Others may substitute caffeine-containing beverages such as soda or coffee for an addictive drug. Such harmful substitutions should be discouraged, emphasizing well-balanced eating combined with adequate rest, **stress management**, and regular exercise. Small, frequent meals and snacks that are rich in vitamins and minerals from healthful foods should be provided. Fluid intake should be generous, but caffeine-containing beverages should be limited.

Individuals withdrawing from alcohol may need extra thiamin supplementation, either intravenously or through a multivitamin supplement because alcohol metabolism in the body requires extra thiamin. Individuals taking drugs to help them avoid alcohol will need to avoid foods with even small amounts of alcohol.

Common withdrawal symptoms and dietary suggestions for coping with these symptoms include:

- Appetite loss: Eat small, frequent meals and snacks; limit caffeine; and use nutritional supplements if necessary.
- Appetite increase: Eat regular meals; eat a variety of foods; and limit sweets and caffeine.
- Diarrhea: Eat moderate amounts of fresh fruits, vegetables, concentrated sugars, juices, and milk and increase intake of cereal fiber.
- Constipation: Drink plenty of fluids; increase fiber in the diet; and increase physical activity.
- Fatigue: Eat regular meals; limit sweets and caffeine; and drink plenty of fluid.

Dietary considerations and medications

Medications that affect body weight

Many medications used to treat mental disorders promote weight gain. These include:

- anticonvulsants (divalproex)

- certain types of antidepressants (amitriptyline)
- antipsychotic medications (clozapine, olanzapine, quetiapine, and risperidone)

Dietary treatments for individuals taking these medications should focus on a balanced, low-fat diet coupled with an increase in physical activity to counter the side effects of these medications. Nutrient-rich foods such as fruits, vegetables, and whole grain products should be emphasized in the diet, whereas sweets, fats, and other foods high in energy but low in nutrients should be limited. Regular physical activity can help limit weight gain caused by these medications.

Some medications can cause loss of appetite, restlessness, and weight loss. Individuals on such medications should eat three balanced meals and several smaller snacks of protein and calorie-rich foods throughout the day. Eating on a regular schedule rather than depending on appetite can help prevent weight loss associated with loss of appetite.

Medications that affect gastrointestinal function

Many psychiatric medications can affect gastrointestinal functioning. Some drugs can cause dry mouth, difficulty swallowing, constipation, altered taste, heartburn, diarrhea, or nausea. Consuming frequent smaller meals, drinking adequate fluids, modifying texture of foods if necessary, and increasing fiber content of foods can help counter gastrointestinal effects of medications.

Monoamine oxidase inhibitors

Individuals being treated with MAOIs such as **tranylcypromine**, **phenelzine**, and **isocarboxazid**, must carefully follow a tyramine-restricted diet. Tyramine, a nitrogen-containing substance normally present in certain foods, is usually broken down in the body by oxidase. However, in individuals taking MAOIs, tyramine is not adequately broken down and builds up in the blood, causing the blood vessels to constrict and increasing blood pressure.

Tyramine is normally found in many foods, especially protein-rich foods that have been aged or fermented, pickled, or bacterially contaminated. Cheese is especially high in tyramine. A tyramine intake of less than 5 mg daily is recommended. A diet that includes even just 6 mg of tyramine can increase blood pressure; a diet that provides 25 mg of tyramine can cause life-threatening increases in blood pressure.

TYRAMINE-RESTRICTED DIET. Tyramine is found in aged, fermented, and spoiled food products. The tyramine content of a specific food can vary greatly depending on storage conditions, ripeness, or contamination. Reaction to tyramine-containing foods in individuals taking MAOIs can also vary greatly depending on what other foods are eaten with the tyramine-containing food, the length of time between MAOI dose and eating the food, and individual characteristics such as weight or age.

Foods to avoid on a tyramine-controlled diet include:

- all aged and mature cheeses or cheese spreads, including foods made with these cheeses, such as salad dressings, casseroles, or certain breads
- any outdated or nonpasteurized dairy products
- dry fermented sausages such as summer sausage, pepperoni, salami, or pastrami
- smoked or pickled fish
- nonfresh meat or poultry
- leftover foods containing meat or poultry
- tofu and soy products
- overripe, spoiled, or fermented fruits or vegetables
- sauerkraut
- fava or broad beans
- soups containing meat extracts or cheese
- gravies containing meat extracts or nonfresh meats
- tap beer
- nonalcoholic beer
- yeast extracts
- soy sauce
- liquid powdered protein supplements

Perishable refrigerated items such as milk, meat, or fruit should be eaten within 48 hours of purchase. Any spoiled food and food stored in questionable conditions should not be eaten.

Lithium

Lithium is often used to treat individuals with mania. Lithium can cause nausea, vomiting, anorexia, diarrhea, and weight gain. Almost one-half of individuals taking lithium gain weight.

Individuals taking lithium should maintain a fairly constant intake of sodium (found in table salt and other food additives) and caffeine in their diet. If an individual restricts sodium intake, less lithium is excreted in the urine and blood lithium levels rise. If an individual increases caffeine intake, more lithium is excreted in the urine and blood levels of lithium fall.

Anticonvulsant medications

Sodium caseinate and calcium caseinate can interfere with the action and effectiveness of some anticonvulsants. Individuals taking these drugs should read labels carefully to avoid foods containing these additives.

Psychotropic medications

Some psychotropic medications, such as **amitriptyline**, can decrease absorption of the vitamin riboflavin from food. Good food sources of riboflavin include milk and milk products, liver, red meat, poultry, fish, whole grain, and enriched breads and cereals. Riboflavin supplements may also be needed.

Other psychotropic drugs, such as **fluvoxamine**, **sertraline**, **nefazodone**, **alprazolam**, **triazolam**, midazolam, **carbamazepine**, and **clonazepam**, interact with grapefruit juice, so individuals taking these drugs must take care to avoid grapefruit juice. In some cases, apple juice must be avoided as well. Patients should discuss potential drug interactions with their doctors or pharmacists.

Caffeine-restricted diet

Caffeine is a stimulant and can interfere with the actions of certain medications. People taking lithium and people recovering from addictions may be asked by their treatment team to monitor (and, in the case of addictions, restrict) their caffeine intake. Foods and beverages high in caffeine include:

- chocolate
- cocoa mix and powder
- chocolate ice cream, milk, and pudding
- coffee
- cola beverages
- tea

Alcohol-restricted diet

Alcohol interacts with some medications used to treat mental disorders. In the case of alcoholism recovery, the negative interaction resulting from the combination of one medication (**disulfiram** or Antabuse) and alcohol consumption is actually part of treatment for some people. (The medication causes an extremely unpleasant reaction when any alcohol is consumed, reinforcing or rewarding the avoidance of alcohol.)

When individuals are taking medication that requires that they avoid alcohol, foods containing alcohol must be avoided as well as beverage alcohol. The following foods contain small amounts of alcohol:

- flavor extracts, such as vanilla, almond, or rum
- cooking wines
- candies or cakes prepared or filled with liqueur
- apple cider
- cider and wine vinegar
- commercial eggnog
- béarnaise or bordelaise sauces
- desserts such as crepes suzette or cherries jubilee
- teriyaki sauce
- fondues

QUESTIONS TO ASK YOUR DOCTOR

- How can I tell if I am getting the right nutrients?
- What types of diagnostic tests do I need?
- What dietary changes, if any, would you recommend for me?
- What changes in my eating regimen would you recommend?
- What kind of changes can I expect to see with the medications you have prescribed for me?
- What tests or evaluation techniques can you perform to see if my nutritional choices promote a healthy condition?
- What symptoms are important enough that I should seek immediate treatment?

Resources

BOOKS

Bean, Dianne. *Nutrition Ambition: Reaching Your Wellness Goals, Ages 8–12,* 2nd ed. Winter Park, FL: Baux, 2009.

Bender, David A. *A Dictionary of Food and Nutrition.* New York: Oxford University Press, 2009.

Cousens, Gabriel. *Conscious Eating,* 2nd ed. Berkley, CA: North Atlantic Books, 2009.

Plant, Jane, and Gill Tidey. *Eating for Better Health.* New York: Virgin Books, 2010.

Robertson, Cathie. *Safety, Nutrition and Health in Early Education,* 4th ed. Florence, KY: Wadsworth, 2009.

Shils, Maurice E. *Modern Nutrition in Health and Disease,* 11th ed. New York: Lippincott Williams & Wilkins, 2012.

Virani, Adil S., et al., eds. *Clinical Handbook of Psychotropic Drugs,* 19th ed. Cambridge, MA: Hogrefe, 2011.

PERIODICALS

Daubenmier, Jennifer J., et al. "The Contribution of Changes in Diet, Exercise, and Stress Management to Changes in Coronary Risk in Women and Men in the Multisite Cardiac Lifestyle Intervention Program." *Annals of Behavioral Medicine* 33, no. 1 (2007): 57–68.

Groesz, Lisa M., and Eric Stice. "An Experimental Test of the Effects of Dieting on Bulimic Symptoms: The Impact of Eating Episode Frequency." *Behaviour Research and Therapy* 45, no. 1 (2007): 49–62.

Hagler, Athena S., et al. "Psychosocial Correlates of Dietary Intake Among Overweight and Obese Men." *American Journal of Health Behavior* 31, no. 1 (2007): 3–12.

Jabs, Jennifer, and Carol M. Devine. "Time Scarcity and Food Choices: An Overview." *Appetite* 47, no. 2 (2006): 196–204.

Leung, Newman, and Emma Price. "Core Beliefs in Dieters and Eating Disordered Women." *Eating Behaviors* 8, no. 1 (2007): 65–72.

Mobbs, Charles V., et al. "Low-Carbohydrate Diets Cause Obesity, Low-Carbohydrate Diets Reverse Obesity: A Metabolic Mechanism Resolving the Paradox." *Appetite* 48, no. 2 (2007): 135–38.

Payne, Martha E., et al. "Vascular Nutritional Correlates of Late-Life Depression." *American Journal of Geriatric Psychiatry* 14, no. 9 (2006): 787–95.

ORGANIZATIONS

American Academy of Family Physicians, 11400 Tomahawk Creek Pkwy., Leawood, KS, 66211-2672, (913) 906-6000, (800) 274-2237, Fax: (913) 906-6075, contactcenter@aafp.org, http://www.aafp.org.

American Dietetic Association, 120 South Riverside Plaza, Ste. 2000, Chicago, IL, 60606, (312) 899-0040, (800) 877-1600, http://www.eatright.org.

American Psychiatric Association, 1000 Wilson Blvd., Ste. 1825, Arlington, VA, 22209-3901, (703) 907-7300, apa@psych.org, http://www.psych.org.

American Psychological Association, 750 1st St. NE, Washington, DC, 20002-4242, (202) 336-5500; TDD/TTY: (202) 336-6123, (800) 374-2721, http://www.apa.org.

National Eating Disorders Association, 165 W 46th St., New York, NY, 10036, (212) 575-6200, Fax: (212) 575-1650, (800) 931-2237, http://www.nationaleatingdisorders.org.

Nancy Gustafson, MS, RD, FADA, ELS
Ruth A. Wienclaw, PhD
Laura Jean Cataldo, RN, EdD

Diphenhydramine

Definition

Diphenhydramine is an antihistamine used in psychiatric medicine to treat **medication-induced movement disorders**, such as may be caused by antipsychotic drugs. When used for this purpose, diphenhydramine is prescribed in the generic form. It is used in general medicine to treat allergies and allergic reactions (sold over-the-counter as Benadryl), motion sickness, **insomnia**, cough, and nausea.

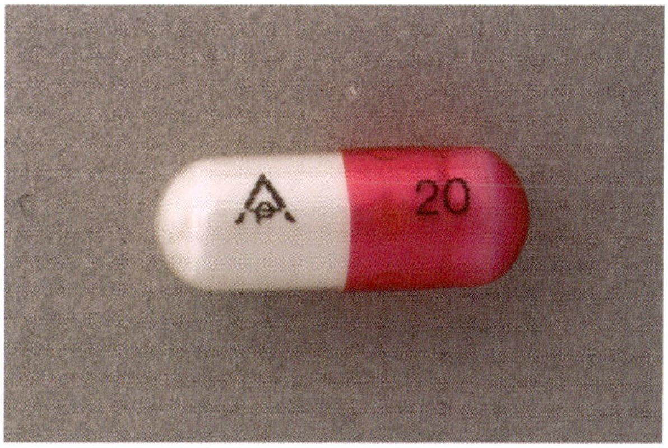

Benadryl (diphenhydramine). *(© Custom Medical Stock Photo, Inc. Reproduced by permission.)*

Purpose

Phenothiazines are sometimes used to treat psychotic disorders such as **schizophrenia**. As a side effect, these drugs may cause tremors and abnormal involuntary movements of the muscles, referred to as extrapyramidal neurologic **movement disorders**. Diphenhydramine is used to control these symptoms. It is may be used to treat the stiffness and tremor of Parkinson's disease and may induce sleep.

Description

Diphenhydramine is easily absorbed when taken by mouth and is readily distributed throughout the body. Maximal effect occurs approximately one hour after swallowing the drug and continues for four to six hours. Diphenhydramine seems to compete with the chemical histamine for specific receptor sites on cells in the **brain** and central nervous system. This means that it achieves its therapeutic effect by taking the place of the neurotransmitter histamine on these cells.

Recommended dosage

The dosage of diphenhydramine must be adjusted according to the needs of individuals and their responses. Adults are generally given 25–50 mg orally, three to four times daily. Diphenhydramine may be administered through a vein or injected deep within a muscle. The usual dosage is 10–50 mg per injection, although some people may require 100 mg. The total daily dosage should not exceed 400 mg. People who forget to take a dose of this drug should skip the dose and take the next one at the regularly scheduled time. They should not double up subsequent doses if one is missed.

People should not take diphenhydramine if they are taking other preparations that contain antihistamines unless specifically directed to do so by a physician.

Precautions

People with peptic ulcer disease, bowel obstructions, an enlarged prostate, angle closure glaucoma, or difficulty urinating due to a blockage in the bladder should not use diphenhydramine without close physician supervision and monitoring. People with asthma, heart disease, high blood pressure, or an overactive thyroid should use this drug with caution. Before taking diphenhydramine, people with these conditions should discuss the risks and benefits of this drug with their doctor. Individuals should not take diphenhydramine for several days before an allergy test, as it will interfere with the results.

Elderly people are more sensitive to the sedating effects of diphenhydramine. The drug may also lower blood pressure, which can cause dizziness and lightheadedness when switching from a seated to a standing position. Older patients should move slowly when rising to a standing position to prevent fainting.

Drowsiness commonly occurs after taking diphenhydramine. This effect may be more pronounced if alcohol or any other central nervous system depressant, such as a tranquilizer or pain medication, is also taken. People taking the drug should not drive, operate machinery, or perform tasks requiring mental alertness until the effects of the medication have worn off.

Side effects

Diphenhydramine may cause dizziness, difficulties with coordination, confusion, restlessness, nervousness, difficulty sleeping, blurry or double vision, ringing in the ears, headache, or convulsions. Stomach distress is a relatively common side effect of diphenhydramine. Some people may develop poor appetites, nausea, vomiting, diarrhea, or constipation. Individuals also may experience low blood pressure, heart palpitations, rapid or irregular heartbeats, frequent urination, or difficulty urinating. Urine may be retained in the bladder. Thickened lung secretions are common among older persons. Other side effects include hives, a rash, sensitivity to the sun, and a dry mouth and nose.

Interactions

Alcohol, pain medications, sleeping pills, tranquilizers, and **antidepressants** may make the drowsiness associated with diphenhydramine more severe. Diphenhydramine should not be used by persons taking hay-fever medicines, **sedatives**, narcotics, anesthetics, **barbiturates**, or muscle relaxants.

KEY TERMS

Anticholinergic—Related to the ability of a drug to block the nervous system chemical acetylcholine. When acetylcholine is blocked, patients often experience dry mouth and skin, increased heart rate, blurred vision, and difficulty in urinating. In severe cases, blocking acetylcholine may cloud thinking and cause delirium.

Antihistamine—A medication used to alleviate allergy or cold symptoms such as runny nose, itching, hives, watering eyes, or sneezing.

Extrapyramidal movement disorders—Involuntary movements that occur as a side effect of some psychiatric medications.

Histamine—Substance released during allergic reactions.

Hypokinesia—A condition of abnormally diminished motor activity.

Parkinson's disease—A disease of the nervous system most common in people over 60, characterized by a shuffling gait, trembling of the fingers and hands, and muscle stiffness.

Parkinsonism—A condition caused by the destruction of the brain cells that produce dopamine (a neurotransmitter); characterized by tremors of the fingers and hands, a shuffling gait, and muscular rigidity.

Phenothiazine—A class of drugs widely used in the treatment of psychosis.

Resources

BOOKS

Foreman, John C., and Torben Johansen. *Textbook of Receptor Pharmacology*. 2nd ed. Boca Raton, FL: CRC Press, 2002.

Page, Clive P., et al. *Integrated Pharmacology*. 3rd ed. St. Louis, MO: Elsevier, 2006.

Preston, John D., John H. O'Neal, and Mary C. Talaga. *Handbook of Clinical Psychopharmacology for Therapists*. 5th ed. Oakland, CA: New Harbinger Publications, 2008.

PERIODICALS

Grillon, Christian, et al. "The Benzodiazepine Alprazolam Dissociates Contextual Fear from Cued Fear in Humans as Assessed by Fear-Potentiated Startle." *Biological Psychiatry* 60, no. 7 (October 1, 2006): 760–66.

Khoromi, Suzan, et al. "Topiramate in Chronic Lumbar Radicular Pain." *Journal of Pain* 6, no. 12 (December 2005): 829–36.

Scaife, J.C., et al. "Sensitivity of Late-Latency Auditory and Somatosensory Evoked Potentials to Threat of Electric Shock and the Sedative Drugs Diazepam and Diphenhydramine in Human Volunteers." *Journal of Psychopharmacology* 20, no. 4 (November 1, 2008): 828–35.

Turner, Claire, Alison D. F. Handford, and Anthony N. Nicholson. "Sedation and Memory: Studies with a Histamine H-1 Receptor Antagonist." *Journal of Psychopharmacology* 20, no. 4 (July 2006): 506–17.

ORGANIZATIONS

American Academy of Family Physicians, 11400 Tomahawk Creek Pky., Leawood, KS, 66211-2672, (913) 906-6000, (800) 274-2237, Fax: (913) 906-6075, contactcenter@-aafp.org, http://www.aafp.org.

American Parkinson Disease Association, Inc, 135 Parkinson Ave., Staten Island, NY, 10305, (718) 981-8001, Fax: (718) 981-4399, apda@apdaparkinson.org, http://www.apdaparkinson.com.

American Psychiatric Association, 1000 Wilson Blvd., Ste. 1825, Arlington, VA, 22209-3901, (703) 907-7300, apa@psych.org, http://www.psych.org.

American Society for Clinical Pharmacology and Therapeutics, 528 North Washington St., Alexandria, VA, 22314, (703) 836-6981, http://www.ascpt.org.

American Society for Pharmacology and Experimental Therapeutics, 9650 Rockville Pike, Bethesda, MD, 20814-3995, (301) 634-7060, Fax: (301) 634-7061, http://www.aspet.org.

Parkinson's Disease Foundation, 1359 Broadway, Ste. 1509, New York, NY, 10018, (212) 923-4700, Fax: (212) 923-4778, info@pdf.org, http://www.pdf.org.

U.S. Food and Drug Administration, 10903 New Hampshire Ave., Silver Spring, MD, 20993-0002, (888) INFO-FDA (463-6332), http://www.fda.gov.

L. Fleming Fallon, Jr, MD, DrPH
Ruth A. Wienclaw, PhD

Disease concept of chemical dependency

Definition

Disease concept of chemical dependency is the concept that a disorder (such as chemical dependency) is like a disease and has a characteristic set of signs, symptoms, and natural history (clinical course, or outcome).

Description

The disease concept has long been accepted by the medical community. The concept proposes that a disease is characterized by a specific set of signs and symptoms and that the disease, if left untreated, will progress to some endpoint or outcome (clinical course). However, controversy arises when the medical community is faced with new abnormal conditions, owing mostly to the new technologies in genetic engineering. This controversy becomes especially apparent when examining psychological disorders.

In the past, psychological disorders were thought in general to be due to both psychological and social abnormalities. Although these psychosocial problems are still of utmost importance, researchers have since discovered that many psychological disorders, such as alcoholism, also have genetic causes. Recent studies have identified a genetic area (locus) where a gene is located that can transmit alcoholism from affected father to son. Mental health professionals also know from clinical experience that alcoholics demonstrate a characteristic set of specific signs and symptoms. Additionally, it is well established that the ultimate clinical course for untreated alcoholism is death. Therefore alcoholism, once thought to be a disorder of those with a weak will, or "party people" can now be characterized as a disease.

There is compelling evidence that other chemical dependencies may also have biological causes. All psychoactive mood-altering drugs (alcohol, **cocaine**, marijuana, heroin, etc.) act in specific sites in the **brain** and on a specific neurotransmitter (a chemical that delivers impulses from one nerve cell to another) called **dopamine**. These mood-altering substances cause dopamine depletion, inducing an abnormality in nerve cells that "hijacks" the cells into chemical dependence. In other words, the substance introduced in the body affects the dopamine in a way that makes the affected individual unable to experience everyday pleasures—the individual instead needs that substance to experience pleasure. Thus the individual's driving force is any drug that can provide some kind of transient happiness (euphoria). In fact, the gene for alcoholism is located in the dopamine molecule. This can further suggest that chemical dependencies may have a medical (biological) cause.

The disease concept of chemical dependency is gaining worldwide acceptance, but does have some critics who argue instead that **addiction** must be understood as a general pattern of behavior, not as a medical problem. Advocates of the disease concept of chemical dependency model maintain that the identification of biological causes or correlations is crucially important for treatment. They argue that if clinicians can understand the intricate details concerning the mechanisms associated with drug effects, then measures to interrupt the effects can be devised. These interventions can be both medical (developing new drugs to chemically block effects of illicit drugs) and psychological.

According to the disease concept model, psychological **intervention** includes a vital educational component that teaches people with chemical dependency the concept of understanding addiction as disease. As a result of this understanding, affected people then view their dependency as a disease, similar to other diseases with a biological cause (heart disease, cancer, high blood pressure), and with a specific set of signs and symptoms and an outcome in the future (clinical course). Proponents of this approach believe that this understanding can help affected people to follow treatment recommendations, and can reduce shame and guilt commonly associated with chemical dependence. Alcoholics Anonymous is a prominent example of an organization that embodies the disease concept of chemical dependency.

Resources

PERIODICALS

Kampman, Kyle M. "New Medications for the Treatment of Cocaine Dependence." *Psychiatry* 2, no. 12, (December 2005) 44–48.

Stanger, Catherine. "Behavioral and Emotional Problems Among Children of Drug Abusers." *Psychiatric Times* 20, no. 2 (February 1, 2003).

WEBSITES

U.S. National Institute on Drug Abuse. "Addition Is a Chronic Disease." http://archives.drugabuse.gov/about/welcome/aboutdrugabuse/chronicdisease (accessed November 14, 2011).

U.S. National Institute on Drug Abuse. "Drugs, Brains, and Behavior—The Science of Addiction." http://www.nida.nih.gov/scienceofaddiction (accessed November 14, 2011).

Laith Farid Gulli, MD

Disorder of written expression

Definition

Disorder of written expression, formerly called developmental expressive writing disorder, is a learning disability in which a person's ability to communicate in writing is substantially below the level normally expected based on the individual's age, intelligence, life experiences, educational background, or physical impairments. This disability affects both the physical reproduction of letters and words and the organization of thoughts and ideas in written compositions.

Demographics

Several studies have estimated that between 3% and 5% of students have disorder of written expression. However, it is difficult to separate this disorder from other **learning disorders**. Deficits in written work may be attributed to reading, language, or attention disorders, limited educational background, or lack of fluency in the language of instruction. Disorder of written expression unassociated with any other learning disability is rare. It commonly occurs in conjunction with **reading disorder** or **mathematics disorder**.

Description

Disorder of written expression is one of the more poorly understood learning disabilities. Learning disabilities that manifest themselves only in written work were first described in the late 1960s. These early studies described three main types of written disorders:

- inability to form letters and numbers correctly, also called dysgraphia
- inability to write words spontaneously or from dictation
- inability to organize words into meaningful thoughts

There are several difficulties in studying disorder of written expression and in implementing a remedial program. Disorder of written expression usually appears in conjunction with other reading or language disabilities, making it hard to separate manifestations of the disability related only to written expression. Delays in attention, visual-motor integration, visual processing, and expressive language may also contribute to writing disorders. Also, there are no standard tests specifically designed to evaluate disorder of written expression.

Causes and symptoms

Causes

The causes of disorder of written expression are unknown. Different manifestations of the disorder may have different causes. For example, people who cannot form letters correctly on the page (dysgraphia) may have delays in hand-eye coordination and difficulties concentrating. People who are unable to write words from memory or dictation appear to have deficits in their visual memory. They cannot remember what the words look like. People who produce legible script but cannot organize their thoughts on paper may have cognitive processing problems. Because disorder of written expression is a little-studied disorder, specific causes have not yet been determined.

Symptoms

Symptoms that suggest disorder of written expression include:

- poor or illegible handwriting
- poorly formed letters or numbers
- excessive spelling errors
- excessive punctuation errors
- excessive grammar errors
- sentences that lack logical cohesion
- paragraphs and stories that are missing elements and that do not make sense or lack logical transitions
- deficient writing skills that significantly impact academic achievement or daily life

These symptoms must be evaluated in light of the person's age, intelligence, educational experience, and cultural or life experience. Written expression must be substantially below the level of samples produced by others of the same age, intelligence, and background. Normally, several of the symptoms are present simultaneously.

Diagnosis

There are no specific tests to diagnose disorder of written expression. This disorder is not normally diagnosed before age eight because of the variability with which children acquire writing skills. It is most commonly diagnosed in the fourth or fifth grade, although it can be noted and diagnosed as soon as the first grade. Requests for testing usually originate with a teacher or parent who notes multiple symptoms of the disorder in a child's writing.

Several standardized tests accurately reflect spelling abilities, but do not assess other writing skills with the same reliability. Tests that might be helpful in diagnosing disorder of written expression include the Diagnostic Evaluation of Writing Skills (DEWS), the Test of Early Written Language (TEWL), and the Test of Adolescent Language.

However, assessment using standardized tests is not enough to make a **diagnosis** of disorder of written expression. In addition, a qualified evaluator should compare multiple samples of the student's written work with the written work normally expected from students of comparable backgrounds. The person being evaluated may also be asked to perform tasks such as writing from dictation or copying written material as part of diagnostic testing.

Treatment

Little is known about how to treat disorder of written expression. Intense writing remediation may help, but no specific method or approach to remediation has proved particularly successful. Since disorder of written expression usually occurs in conjunction with other learning disabilities, treatment is often directed at those better-understood learning problems.

Prognosis

Little is known about the long-term outcome for people with disorder of written expression. However, it appears that those who have this disorder may develop low self-esteem and social problems related to their lack of academic achievement. Later in life they may be more likely to drop out of school and may find employment opportunities that require writing skills to be closed to them.

Prevention

There are no known ways to prevent disorder of written expression.

Resources

BOOKS

American Psychiatric Association. *Diagnostic and Statistical Manual of Mental Disorders*. 4th ed., text rev. Washington, DC: American Psychiatric Publishing, 2000.

Sadock, Benjamin J., and Virginia A. Sadock, eds. *Comprehensive Textbook of Psychiatry*. Vol. 2. 7th ed. Philadelphia: Lippincott Williams and Wilkins, 2000.

OTHER

International Dyslexia Association. "Just the Facts: Dysgraphia." Fact Sheet #82. http://ldanh.org/docs/fact sheets4.27.04/dysgraphia.pdf (accessed October 5, 2011).

WEBSITES

MedlinePlus. "Disorders of Written Expression." U.S. National Library of Medicine. National Institutes of Health. November 14, 2010. http://www.nlm.nih.gov/medlineplus/ ency/article/001543.htm (accessed October 5, 2011).

U.S. National Institute for Neurological Disorders and Stroke. "NINDS Dysgraphia Information Page." http://www. ninds.nih.gov/disorders/dysgraphia/dysgraphia.htm (accessed October 5, 2011).

ORGANIZATIONS

American Academy of Child and Adolescent Psychiatry , 3615 Wisconsin Ave. NW, Washington, DC, 20016-3007, (202) 966-7300, Fax: (202) 966-2891, http://aacap.org.

Learning Disabilities Association of America, 4156 Library Rd., Pittsburgh, PA, 15234-1349, (412) 341-1515, http:// www.ldanatl.org.

National Center for Learning Disabilities, 381 Park Ave. S, Ste. 1401, New York, NY, 10016, (212) 545-7510, Fax: (212) 545-9665, (888) 575-7373, http://www.ncld.org.

Tish Davidson, AM
Emily Jane Willingham, PhD

Disruptive behavior disorder *see* **Conduct disorder**

Disruptive mood dysregulation disorder

Definition

Disruptive mood dysregulation disorder (DMDD) is a new category of childhood mood disorder proposed for the fifth edition of the ***Diagnostic and Statistical Manual of Mental Disorders*** (*DSM-5*, 2013). The disorder is defined by the *DSM* as a chronically unhappy mood in children over the age of six accompanied by frequent outbursts of rage that are more intense than the temper tantrums seen in toddlers.

Demographics

The demographics of the disorder are unknown, as it is a fairly new **diagnosis** and has not yet undergone field testing. It is possible, however, that some children diagnosed with **juvenile bipolar disorder** actually have DMDD. Prior to the 1990s, **bipolar disorder** (BD) in children was considered an extremely rare condition. Beginning in the late 1990s, a team of researchers at Harvard began to think that a diagnosis of bipolar disorder better accounted for chronic irritability and moodiness in children—many of whom had already been diagnosed with **attention deficit hyperactivity disorder (ADHD)**. The number of children diagnosed with bipolar disorder increased 4,000% between 1994 and 2003, according to a 2007 study published in the *Archives of General Psychiatry*.

As of 2011, approximately one million children in the United States had been diagnosed with bipolar disorder; about two-thirds of these children were boys. This finding was puzzling to some psychiatrists for two reasons: first, the gender ratio of bipolar disorder in adults is closer to 50/50, and second, many people diagnosed with BD as children do not meet the criteria for the diagnosis as adults. The latter was an especially unusual finding, as BD is considered a lifelong disorder. Conversely, most people diagnosed with BD as adults did not experience uncontrolled anger issues as children, prompting questions as to whether or not another disorder might account for the childhood symptoms.

Description

Disruptive mood dysregulation disorder is a new disorder proposed for inclusion in the *DSM-5*, although symptoms of the condition have been recognized since the *DSM-III* was published in 1980. Prior to the 1990s, most children with anger management problems were diagnosed as having **conduct disorder**. The problem was that most treatments, including behavioral therapy, had a low record of success in treating conduct disorder. The Harvard psychiatrists evaluated a group of children diagnosed with **ADHD** with severe anger problems and realized that the symptoms might be better accounted for in a mood disorder rather than an impulse control disorder; this realization led them to label the condition as childhood bipolar disorder. Because bipolar disorder can be treated with medications, specifically atypical antipsychotics, some hypothesized that the diagnosis would be more agreeable to insurance companies, who were more willing to reimburse the cost of medications than of psychotherapies, and to parents, who found some relief in believing that their troubled child had a biologically based disorder. The annual sales of atypical antipsychotics for children rose sharply in the United States, from $402,000 in 2000 to $6.8 million by 2006.

In order to diagnose children with bipolar disorder, the Harvard group had to change one of the criteria for BD in adults to accommodate a different symptom profile in children with anger issues. To meet the diagnosis of BD, an adult must be identified as having episodes of mania (a state of abnormal irritability, elevated mood, or high energy lasting for a week or longer) as well as episodes of **depression** and periods of normal mood. The children who were studied in the early 1990s did not have manic episodes lasting for several days or a month, so the researchers redefined manic episodes in children as very brief and very frequent outbursts of temper or aggressive behavior. This redefinition meant that children who were simply overly excitable while they were going through a difficult period of adjustment (geographical relocation, a new school, or death or divorce in the family) were at risk of being labeled as having bipolar disorder. The diagnosis of childhood BD did not account for situational stressors or developmental differences among children.

Children diagnosed with juvenile bipolar disorder may also face issues later in life due to the **stigma** attached to the diagnosis, especially since it is understood to be a lifelong condition. Labeling a child as bipolar risks causing difficulties for the child later in life, such as when he or she seeks admission to college or applies for a job. Further, the atypical antipsychotics have potentially severe side effects that include rapid weight gain, an increased risk of type 2 diabetes, and a shortened lifespan. In addition, there is some evidence that they have an effect on the development of the nervous system in growing children.

KEY TERMS

Mania—A state in which a person has an abnormally elevated ("high") or irritable mood or energy level that is not caused by a medical illness or drugs of abuse.

Stigma—Any personal attribute that causes a person to be socially shamed, avoided, or discredited. Mental disorders are a common cause of stigma.

DMDD is considered a preliminary disorder, as its acceptance is not yet widespread within the psychiatric community. If the incidence of juvenile bipolar disorder is truly overestimated, the diagnosis of DMDD will be helpful in finding effective treatments, especially if children are unnecessarily taking medication for bipolar disorder. However, DMDD has prompted debate within the psychiatric field.

Causes and symptoms

The causes of DMDD were not known as of 2011. There is evidence, however, that the condition can be differentiated from bipolar disorder in that it does not seem to run in families or have a genetic basis.

The core symptoms of DMDD are temper outbursts consisting of verbal or physical aggression that are out of proportion to the triggering situation or event and inappropriate to the child's developmental level. The child also displays irritable, angry, grumpy, or sad moods in between the angry outbursts.

Diagnosis

There are no laboratory, genetic, or imaging tests that can be used to diagnose DMDD. The diagnosis is made on the basis of the child psychiatrist's clinical judgment. Children with a previous diagnosis of bipolar disorder may be rediagnosed with DMDD; the co-director of the Children's Hospital Boston's mood disorder program cites diagnosing 65% and 80% of children previously diagnosed with bipolar disorder who were brought to them for a second opinion with DMDD.

The proposed *DSM* diagnostic criteria for DMDD are as follows:

- Criterion A: The child displays severe and recurrent temper outbursts in response to stress. Outbursts may take the form of verbal or physical attacks on people, pets, or objects. The outbursts must be considered inappropriate for the situation and for the child's level of development.
- Criterion B: Outbursts occur at least three times a week (on average).
- Criterion C: Between outbursts, the child's mood is persistently grumpy, irritable, or sad, to the extent that it is noticed by others.
- Criterion D: The child exhibits the symptoms of criteria A through C for at least 12 months, and any symptom-free periods must last no longer than 3 months.
- Criterion E: The symptoms occur in at least two environments (e.g., home or school) and are considered extreme in at least one of the environments.
- Criterion F: The child is at least six years old.
- Criterion G: The onset of the symptoms occurs before age 10.
- Criterion H: The child does not meet the criteria for a manic episode.
- Criterion I: The behaviors do not occur in the context of a psychotic disorder, do not better meet the criteria for another diagnosis, and are not due to a general medical or neurological condition. The diagnosis of DMDD may, however, coexist with another disorder, including ADHD, conduct disorder, or oppositional defiant disorder.

The present definition of DMDD has been criticized by some child psychiatrists on the grounds that in essence it turns a single symptom—temper outbursts—into a complete syndrome. As a result, the new disorder overlaps with the definitions of several other childhood disorders and is not clearly differentiated from them. Also, the current diagnostic criteria do not take into consideration the great variability in what are considered appropriate expressions of temper across children, developmental phases, families, and subcultures—what is considered a severe outburst in some families or cultures might be less extreme in others.

Treatment

There was no standard approach to treatment for DMDD as of 2011, because the disorder had only been recently identified. Some psychiatrists have suggested a multidimensional approach to therapy, using medications only sparingly, prescribing **antidepressants** rather than antipsychotics, and focusing on helping the child deal with life's challenges without giving in to explosive temper outbursts.

There was one clinical research study of mood dysregulation in children under way as of mid-2011.

QUESTIONS TO ASK YOUR DOCTOR

- Have you ever treated a child with disruptive mood dysregulation disorder?
- What treatment options are available?
- Should my child see a specialist?

The trial was studying the effectiveness of **risperidone** (Risperdal), an atypical antipsychotic, as a treatment for the disorder.

Prognosis

The prognosis of DMDD was not known as of 2011. While many child psychiatrists expect that children with this disorder will have some problems lasting into adulthood, they will not have bipolar disorder (if DMDD is the true cause of their symptoms). It should be noted, however, that bipolar disorder is a serious condition, and if a child exhibits symptoms of juvenile bipolar disorder, they should not be ignored.

Prevention

Because the causes of DMDD are not yet identified, it is not yet known how to prevent DMDD.

Resources

BOOKS

American Psychiatric Association. *Diagnostic and Statistical Manual*. 4th ed., text rev. Washington, DC: American Psychiatric Association, 2000.

Kaplan, Stuart L. *Your Child Does Not Have Bipolar Disorder: How Bad Science and Good Public Relations Created the Diagnosis*. Santa Barbara, CA: Praeger, 2011.

McDonnell, Mary Ann, and Janet Wozniak. *Is Your Child Bipolar?: The Definitive Resource on How to Identify, Treat, and Thrive with a Bipolar Child*. New York: Bantam, 2008.

Papolos, Demitri, and Janice Papolos. *The Bipolar Child: The Definitive and Reassuring Guide to Childhood's Most Misunderstood Disorder*, 3rd ed. New York: Broadway Books, 2006.

PERIODICALS

Carlson, Gabrielle A. "Who Are the Children With Severe Mood Dysregulation, a.k.a. 'Rages?'" *American Journal of Psychiatry* 164 (August 1, 2007): 1140–42.

Moreno, C., et al. "National Trends in the Outpatient Diagnosis and Treatment of Bipolar Disorder in Youth." *Archives of General Psychiatry* 64 (September 2007): 1032–1039.

Olson, Jeremy. "Bipolar Label Soars Among Kids." *Minneapolis Star-Tribune*, June 23, 2011. http://www.startribune.com/lifestyle/wellness/124136764.html?page=all&prepage=1&c=y#continue (accessed August 11, 2011).

Parens, E., and J. Johnston. "Controversies Concerning the Diagnosis and Treatment of Bipolar Disorder in Children." *Child and Adolescent Psychiatry and Mental Health* 4 (March 10, 2010). http://www.ncbi.nlm.nih.gov/pmc/articles/PMC2846895/?tool=pubmed (accessed August 11, 2011).

Stringaris, A. "Irritability in Children and Adolescents: A Challenge for DSM-5." *European Child and Adolescent Psychiatry* 20 (February 2011): 61–66.

OTHER

American Psychiatric Association, Childhood and Adolescent Disorders Work Group. "Justification for Temper Dysregulation Disorder with Dysphoria." DSM-5 Development. http://www.dsm5.org/Proposed%20Revision%20Attachments/Justification%20for%20Temper%20Dysregulation%20Disorder%20with%20Dysphoria.pdf (accessed July 16, 2011).

WEBSITES

American Psychiatric Association. "D 00 Disruptive Mood Dysregulation Disorder." DSM-5 Development. http://www.dsm5.org/proposedrevisions/pages/proposedrevision.aspx?rid=397 (accessed July 16, 2011).

Child and Adolescent Psychiatry Consulting. "Bipolar Disorder versus Temper Dysregulation Disorder." http://www.drjenna.net/disorders-and-treatments/bipolar-disorder/bipolar-disorder-versus-temper-dysregulation-disorder (accessed July 16, 2011).

Children's Hospital Boston. "Q & A: Bipolar Disorder vs. Temper Dysregulation Disorder with Dysphoria." *Pediatric Views*. http://www.childrenshospital.org/views/aug10/bipolar_disorder_vs_temper_dysregulation_disorder_with_dysphoria.html (accessed July 16, 2011).

Frances, Allen. "DSM5 Temper Dysregulation—Good Intentions, Bad Solution." Psychology Today. http://www.psychologytoday.com/blog/dsm5-in-distress/201004/dsm5-temper-dysregulation-good-intentions-bad-solution (accessed July 15, 2011).

Spiegel, Alix. "Children Labeled 'Bipolar' May Get A New Diagnosis." National Public Radio (NPR). http://www.npr.org/templates/story/story.php?storyId=123544191 (accessed July 16, 2011).

ORGANIZATIONS

American Academy of Child and Adolescent Psychiatry (AACAP), 3615 Wisconsin Avenue, NW, Washington, DC, 20016-3007, (202) 966-7300, Fax: (202) 966-2891, http://www.aacap.org.

American Psychiatric Association, 1000 Wilson Boulevard, Suite 1825, Arlington, VA, 22209-3901, (703) 907-7300, apa@psych.org, http://www.psych.org.

Rebecca J. Frey, PhD

Dissociation and dissociative disorders

Definition

The dissociative disorders are a group of mental disorders that affect consciousness and cause significant interference with a patient's general functioning, including in social relationships and employment.

Demographics

The dissociative disorders vary in their severity and the suddenness of onset. It is difficult to give statistics for their frequency in the United States because they are a relatively new category and are often misdiagnosed. Studies suggest a frequency of pathological dissociation in the general North American population of between 2% and 3.3%. In Europe, reported rates are lower, at 0.3% in the nonclinical population and between 1.8% and 2.9% in student populations. Among psychiatric patients, the frequency is much higher, between 5.4% and 12.7%, and it also is higher in groups with specific psychiatric diagnoses; for example, frequency among women with eating disorders can be as high as 48.6%.

Description

In order to have a clear picture of these disorders, dissociation should first be understood. Dissociation is a mechanism that allows the mind to separate or compartmentalize certain memories or thoughts from normal consciousness. These split-off mental contents are not erased, however, and may resurface spontaneously or be triggered by objects or events in the person's environment.

Dissociation occurs along a spectrum of severity, and experiencing dissociation does not necessarily mean that a person has a dissociative disorder or other mental illness. A mild degree of dissociation occurs with some physical stressors; people who have gone without sleep for a long period of time, have had "laughing gas" for dental surgery, or have been in a minor accident often have brief dissociative experiences. Other examples of mild dissociation include becoming involved in a book or movie so completely that surroundings or the passage of time are not noticed, or driving on the highway and passing several exits without recollection. Dissociation is related to hypnosis in that hypnotic trance also involves a temporarily altered state of consciousness. Most patients with dissociative disorders are highly hypnotizable.

People in other cultures sometimes have dissociative experiences in the course of religious or other group activities (in certain trance states). These occurrences should not be judged against what is considered "normal" in the United States.

The pathological forms of dissociation have been dichotomized into the categories of detachment and compartmentalization. Specific characteristics distinguish each of these, although there can be overlap. Patients who have the compartmentalized type of dissociation do not engage in conscious integration of mental systems and do not or cannot consciously access certain areas of memory or information that would normally be available. This type of dissociation can occur in **conversion disorder** or **dissociative amnesia**.

A person exhibiting the detachment form of a dissociation disorder experiences the altered state of consciousness that is more commonly associated with the concept of dissociation. In such cases, the feelings of **depersonalization** are not merely transient, brief manifestations brought on by causes such as a lack of sleep. People with dissociation disorder may exhibit a flat affect (lack of or reduced presentation of mood or emotion) and may experience the sensation of being out of their own bodies. This type of dissociation is present in **depersonalization disorder**.

Dissociative amnesia

Dissociative **amnesia** is a disorder in which the distinctive feature is the patient's inability to remember important personal information to a degree that cannot be explained by normal forgetfulness. In many cases, it is a reaction to a traumatic accident or witnessing a violent crime. Patients with dissociative amnesia may develop depersonalization or trance states as part of the disorder, but they do not experience a change in identity.

Dissociative fugue

Dissociative fugue is a disorder in which a person temporarily loses his or her sense of personal identity and travels to another location where he or she may assume a new identity. Again, this condition usually follows a major stressor or **trauma**. Apart from an inability to recall their past or personal information, patients with dissociative fugue do not behave strangely or appear disturbed to others. Cases of dissociative fugue are more common in wartime or in communities disrupted by a natural disaster.

Depersonalization disorder

Depersonalization disorder is a disturbance in which the patient's primary symptom is a sense of detachment from the self. Depersonalization as a symptom (not as a disorder) is quite common in college-age populations.

It is often associated with **sleep deprivation** or recreational drug use. It may be accompanied by derealization (where objects in an environment appear altered). Patients sometimes describe depersonalization as feeling "like a robot" or as watching themselves from the outside. Depersonalization disorder may also involve feelings of numbness or loss of emotional affect.

Dissociative identity disorder (DID)

Dissociative identity disorder (DID) (formerly multiple personality disorder) is considered the most severe dissociative disorder and involves all of the major dissociative symptoms. People with this disorder have more than one personality state, and the personality state controlling the person's behavior changes from time to time. Often, a stressor will cause the change in personality state. The various personality states have separate names, temperaments, gestures, and vocabularies. This disorder is often associated with severe physical or **sexual abuse**, especially abuse during childhood. Women are diagnosed with this disorder more often than men.

Dissociative disorder not otherwise specified (DDNOS)

DDNOS is a diagnostic category ascribed to patients with dissociative symptoms that do not meet the full criteria for a specific dissociative disorder.

Risk factors

Risk factors for developing a dissociative disorder include possessing an innate ability to dissociate easily, experiencing repeated episodes of severe physical or sexual abuse in childhood, lacking the support to counteract abusive relative(s), and being influenced by relatives with dissociative symptoms or disorders.

The relationship of dissociative disorders to childhood abuse has led to intense controversy and lawsuits concerning the accuracy of childhood memories. The brain's storage, retrieval, and interpretation of memories are still not fully understood. Controversy also exists regarding how much individuals presenting dissociative disorders have been influenced by books and movies to describe a certain set of symptoms (scripting).

Causes and symptoms

Causes

Moderate or severe forms of dissociation can be caused by such traumatic experiences as childhood abuse, combat, criminal attacks, or involvement in a natural or transportation disaster. Patients with **acute stress disorder**, **post-traumatic stress disorder**, conversion disorder, or **somatization disorder** may develop dissociative symptoms. Recent studies of trauma indicate that the human **brain** stores traumatic memories in a different way than normal memories. Traumatic memories are not processed or integrated into a person's ongoing life in the same fashion as normal memories. Instead, they are dissociated, or split off, and may erupt into consciousness from time to time without warning. The affected person cannot control or "edit" these memories. Over a period of time, these two sets of memories, the normal and the traumatic, may coexist as parallel sets without ever being combined or blended. In extreme cases, different sets of dissociated memories may cause people to develop separate personalities for these memories (dissociative identity disorder).

Symptoms

AMNESIA. Amnesia in a dissociative disorder is marked by gaps in a patient's memory for long periods of time or for traumatic events. Doctors can distinguish this type of amnesia from loss of memory caused by head injuries or drug intoxication, because the amnesia is "spotty" and related to highly charged events and feelings.

DEPERSONALIZATION. Depersonalization is a dissociative symptom in which the patient feels that his or her body is unreal, is changing, or is dissolving. Some patients experience depersonalization as being outside their bodies or watching a movie of themselves.

DEREALIZATION. Derealization is a dissociative symptom in which the external environment is perceived as unreal. The patient may see walls, buildings, or other objects as changing in shape, size, or color. In some cases, the patient may feel that other persons are machines or robots, though the patient is able to acknowledge the unreality of this feeling.

IDENTITY DISTURBANCES. Patients with dissociative fugue, DDNOS, or DID often experience confusion about their identities or even assume new identities. Identity disturbances result from the patient having compartmentalized entire personality traits or characteristics as well as memories. When a stressful or traumatic experience triggers the reemergence of these dissociated parts, the patient may act differently, answer to a different name, or appear confused by his or her surroundings.

Diagnosis

Examination

When a doctor is evaluating a patient with dissociative symptoms, he or she will first rule out any physical conditions that might produce those symptoms. These conditions include epilepsy, head injuries, brain disease, side effects of medications, **substance abuse**, intoxication, AIDS, **dementia** complex, or recent periods of extreme physical stress and sleeplessness. In some cases, the doctor may give the patient an electroencephalogram (EEG) to eliminate epilepsy or other seizure disorders.

Tests

If the patient appears to have no physical conditions, the doctor will then test to rule out psychotic disturbances, including **schizophrenia**. Psychological tests such as the Dissociative Experiences Scale (DES) may also help narrow the **diagnosis**. If the patient has a high score on this test, he or she can be evaluated further with the Dissociative Disorders Interview Schedule (DDIS) or the Structured Clinical Interview for *DSM-IV* Dissociative Disorders (SCID-D). It is also possible for doctors to measure a patient's hypnotizability as part of a diagnostic evaluation.

Treatment

Studies now suggest that treatment of a specific dissociative disorder should be based on whether or not the manifestations are considered the compartmentalized type or the detachment type. Treatment recommendations for the compartmentalized types of disorders include focusing on reactivating and integrating the isolated mental compartments, possibly through hypnosis. To address detachment-based dissociation, therapies may include identifying triggers for the detached state and determining how to stop the triggers and/or stop the detached condition when it is triggered. Standard approaches for these tactics may include **cognitive-behavioral therapy**.

Drugs

Some doctors prescribe tranquilizers or **antidepressants** for the anxiety and/or **depression** that often accompanies dissociative disorders. However, patients with dissociative disorders are at risk for abusing or becoming dependent on medications.

Alternative

Patients with dissociative disorders often require treatment by a therapist with some specialized understanding of dissociation. This background is particularly important if the patient's symptoms include identity problems. Many patients with dissociative disorders are helped by both group and individual treatment.

Hypnosis is frequently recommended as a method of treatment for dissociative disorders, partly because hypnosis is related to the process of dissociation. Hypnosis may help patients recover repressed ideas and memories. Therapists treating patients with DID sometimes use hypnosis in the process of "fusing" the patient's alternate personalities.

Prognosis

Prognoses for dissociative disorders vary. Recovery from dissociative fugue is usually rapid. Dissociative amnesia may resolve quickly, but can become a chronic disorder in some patients. Depersonalization disorder, DDNOS, and DID are usually chronic conditions. DID often requires five or more years of treatment for recovery.

Prevention

Since the primary cause of dissociative disorders is thought to involve extended periods of humanly inflicted trauma, prevention depends on the elimination of physical and psychological abuse.

KEY TERMS

Amnesia—A general medical term for loss of memory that is not due to ordinary forgetfulness. Amnesia can be caused by head injuries, brain disease, or epilepsy, as well as by dissociation.

Depersonalization—A dissociative symptom in which patients feel that their bodies are unreal, are changing, or are dissolving.

Derealization—A dissociative symptom in which the external environment is perceived as unreal.

Dissociation—A reaction to trauma in which the mind splits off certain aspects of the traumatic event from conscious awareness. Dissociation can affect the patient's memory, sense of reality, and sense of identity.

Fugue—A dissociative experience during which those affected travel away from home, have amnesia regarding their past, and may be confused about their identity but otherwise appear normal.

Hypnosis—The means by which a state of extreme relaxation and suggestibility is induced. Hypnosis is used to treat amnesia and identity disturbances that occur in dissociative disorders.

Multiple personality disorder (MPD)—An older term for dissociative identity disorder (DID).

Trauma—A disastrous or life-threatening event that can cause severe emotional distress, including dissociative symptoms and disorders.

Resources

BOOKS

Courtois, Christine A., and Julian D. Ford, eds. *Treating Complex Traumatic Stress Disorders: An Evidence-Based Guide*. New York: The Guilford Press, 2009.

Graham, George. *The Disordered Mind: An Introduction to Philosophy of Mind and Mental Illness*. New York: Routledge, 2010.

North, Carol, and Sean Yutzy. *Goodwin and Guze's Psychiatric Diagnosis*. New York: Oxford University Press, 2010.

Shams, M.D.K. *Human Relation and Personified Relational Disorders*. Raleigh, NC: lulu.com, 2009.

ORGANIZATIONS

American Psychiatric Association, 1000 Wilson Blvd., Ste. 1825, Arlington, VA, 22209-3901, (703) 907-7300, apa@psych.org, http://www.psych.org.

American Psychological Association, 750 1st Street NE, Washington, DC, 20002-4242, (202) 336-5500; TDD/TTY: (202) 336-6123, (800) 374-2721, http://www.apa.org.

Mental Health America, 2000 N Beauregard St., 6th Fl., Alexandria, VA, 22311, (703) 684-7722, (800) 969-6642, Fax: (703) 684-5968, http://www1.nmha.org.

National Alliance on Mental Illness, 3803 N Fairfax Dr., Ste. 100, Arlington, VA, 22203, (703) 524-7600, Fax: (703) 524-9094, http://www.nami.org.

National Institute of Mental Health, 6001 Executive Blvd., Rm. 8184, MSC 9663, Bethesda, MD, 20892-9663, (301) 433-4513; TTY: (301) 443-8431, (866) 615-6464; TTY: (866) 415-8051, Fax: (301) 443-4279, nimhinfo@ nih.gov, http://www.nimh.nih.gov.

Rebecca J. Frey, PhD
Emily Jane Willingham, PhD
Laura Jean Cataldo, RN, EdD

Dissociative amnesia

Definition

Dissociative **amnesia** is classified by the ***Diagnostic and Statistical Manual of Mental Disorders***, fourth edition, text revision (*DSM-IV-TR*), as one of the **dissociative disorders**, which are mental disorders in which the normally well-integrated functions of memory, identity, perception, or consciousness are separated (dissociated). The dissociative disorders are usually associated with **trauma** in the recent or distant past, or with an intense internal conflict that forces the mind to separate incompatible or unacceptable knowledge, information, or feelings. In dissociative amnesia, the continuity of the patient's memory is disrupted. Patients with dissociative amnesia have recurrent episodes in which they forget important personal information or events, usually connected with trauma or severe **stress**. The information that is lost to the patient's memory is usually too extensive to be attributed to ordinary absentmindedness or forgetfulness related to aging. Dissociative amnesia was formerly called psychogenic amnesia.

Amnesia is a symptom of other medical and mental disorders; however, the patterns of amnesia differ depending on the cause of the disorder. Amnesia associated with head trauma is typically both retrograde (the patient has no memory of events shortly before the head injury) and anterograde (the patient has no memory of events after the injury). The amnesia that is associated with seizure disorders is sudden onset. Amnesia in patients with **delirium** or **dementia** occurs in the context of extensive disturbances of the patient's cognition (knowing), speech, perceptions, emotions, and behaviors. Amnesia associated with **substance abuse**, which is sometimes called a blackout, typically affects only short-term memory and is irreversible. In dissociative amnesia, in contrast to these other conditions, the patient's memory loss is almost always anterograde, which means that it is limited to the period following the traumatic event(s). In addition, patients with dissociative amnesia do not have problems learning new information.

Demographics

Dissociative amnesia can appear in patients of any age past infancy. Its true prevalence is unknown. In recent years, there has been an intense controversy among therapists regarding the increase in case reports of dissociative amnesia and the accuracy of the memories recovered. Some maintain that the greater awareness of dissociative symptoms and disorders among psychiatrists has led to the identification of cases that were previously misdiagnosed. Other therapists maintain that dissociative disorders are overdiagnosed in people who are extremely vulnerable to suggestion.

It should be noted that psychiatrists in the United States and Canada have significantly different opinions of dissociative disorder diagnoses. On the whole, Canadian psychiatrists, both French- and English-speaking, have serious reservations about the scientific validity and diagnostic status of dissociative amnesia and dissociative identity disorder. Only 30% of Canadian psychiatrists think that these two dissociative disorders should be included in the *DSM-IV-TR* without reservation; and only 13% think that here is strong scientific support for the validity of these diagnoses.

Description

Patients with dissociative amnesia usually report a gap or series of gaps in their recollection of their life history. The gaps are usually related to episodes of **abuse** or equally severe trauma, although some persons with dissociative amnesia also lose recall of their own **suicide** attempts, episodes of **self-mutilation**, or violent behavior.

Five different patterns of memory loss have been reported in patients with dissociative amnesia:

- Localized. The patient cannot recall events that took place within a limited period of time (usually several hours or one to two days) following a traumatic event. For example, some survivors of the World Trade Center attacks do not remember how they got out of the damaged buildings or what streets they took to get away from the area.
- Selective. The patient can remember some, but not all, of the events that took place during a limited period of time. For example, a veteran of D-Day (June 6, 1944) may recall some details, such as eating a meal on the run or taking prisoners, but not others (seeing a close friend hit or losing a commanding officer).
- Generalized. The person cannot recall anything in his/her entire life. Persons with generalized amnesia are usually found by the police or taken by others to a hospital emergency room.
- Continuous. The amnesia covers the entire period without interruption from a traumatic event in the past to the present.
- Systematized. The amnesia covers only certain categories of information, such as all memories related to a certain location or to a particular person.

Most patients diagnosed with dissociative amnesia have either localized or selective amnesia. Generalized amnesia is extremely rare. Patients with generalized, continuous, or systematized amnesia are usually eventually diagnosed as having a more complex dissociative disorder, such as **dissociative identity disorder**.

Causes and symptoms

Causes

The primary cause of dissociative amnesia is stress associated with traumatic experiences that the patient has either survived or witnessed. These may include such major life stressors as serious financial problems, the death of a parent or spouse, extreme internal conflict, and guilt related to serious crimes or turmoil caused by difficulties with another person.

Susceptibility to hypnosis appears to be a predisposing factor in dissociative amnesia. Thus far, no specific genes have been associated with vulnerability to dissociative amnesia.

Some personality types and character traits seem to be risk factors for dissociative disorders. A group of researchers in the United States has found that persons diagnosed with dissociative disorders have much higher scores for immature psychological defenses than normal subjects.

Symptoms

The central symptom of dissociative amnesia is loss of memory for a period or periods of time in the patient's life. The memory loss may take a variety of different patterns.

Other symptoms that have been reported in patients diagnosed with dissociative amnesia include the following:

- confusion
- emotional distress related to the amnesia, usually in direct proportion to the importance of what has been forgotten or the consequences of forgetting
- mild depression

Some patients diagnosed with dissociative amnesia have problems or behaviors that include disturbed interpersonal relationships, sexual dysfunction, employment problems, aggressive behaviors, self-mutilation, or suicide attempts.

Diagnosis

The diagnosis of dissociative amnesia is usually a diagnosis of exclusion. The doctor will take a detailed medical history, give the patient a physical examination, and order blood and urine tests, as well as an electroencephalogram (EEG) or head x ray to rule out memory loss resulting from seizure disorders, substance abuse (including abuse of **inhalants**), head injuries, or medical conditions, such as **Alzheimer's disease** or delirium associated with fever.

Some conditions, such as age-related memory impairment (AAMI), may be ruled out on the basis of the patient's age. **Malingering** can usually be detected in patients who are faking amnesia because they typically exaggerate and dramatize their symptoms; they have obvious financial, legal, or personal reasons (for example, draft evasion) for pretending loss of memory. In addition, patients with genuine dissociative amnesia usually score high on tests of hypnotizability. The examiner may administer the Hypnotic Induction Profile (HIP) or a similar measure that evaluates whether the patient is easily hypnotized. This enables the examiner to rule out malingering or **factitious disorder**.

There are several standard diagnostic questionnaires that may be given to evaluate the presence of a dissociative disorder. The Dissociative Experiences Scale (DES) is a frequently administered self-report screener for all forms of dissociation. The Structured Clinical Interview for the *DSM-IV-TR* Dissociative Disorders (SCID-D) can be used to make the diagnosis of dissociative amnesia distinct from the other dissociative disorders defined by the *DSM-IV-TR*. The SCID-D is a semi-structured interview, which means that the examiner's questions are open-ended and allow the patient to describe experiences of amnesia in some detail, as distinct from simple "yes" or "no" answers.

Diagnosis of dissociative amnesia in children before the age of puberty is complicated by the fact that inability to recall the first four to five years of one's life is a normal feature of human development. As part of the differential diagnosis, a physician who is evaluating a child in this age group will rule out inattention, **learning disorders**, oppositional behavior, **psychosis**, and seizure disorders or head trauma. To make an accurate diagnosis, several different people (such as teachers, therapists, **social workers**, or the child's primary care physician) may be asked to observe or evaluate the child.

Treatment

Treatment of dissociative amnesia usually requires two distinct periods or phases of **psychotherapy**.

Psychotherapy

Psychotherapy for dissociative amnesia is supportive in its initial phase. It begins with creating an atmosphere of safety in the treatment room. Very often, patients gradually regain their memories when they feel safe with and supported by the therapist. This rapport does not mean that they necessarily recover their memories during therapy sessions; one study of 90 patients with dissociative amnesia found that most of them had their memories return while they were at home alone or with family or close friends. The patients denied that their memories were derived from a therapist's suggestions, and a majority of them were able to find independent evidence or corroboration of their childhood abuse.

If the memories do not return spontaneously, hypnosis or sodium amytal (a drug that induces a semi-hypnotic state) may be used to help recover them.

After the patient has recalled enough of the missing past to acquire a stronger sense of self and continuity in their life history, the second phase of psychotherapy commences. During this phase, the patient deals more directly with the traumatic episode(s), and recovery from its aftereffects. Studies of the treatments for dissociative amnesia in combat veterans of World War I (1914–1918) found that recovery and cognitive integration of dissociated traumatic memories within the patient's overall personality were more effective than treatment methods that focused solely on releasing feelings.

Medications

At present, there are no therapeutic agents that prevent amnestic episodes or that cure dissociative amnesia itself. Patients may, however, be given **anti-depressants** or other appropriate medications for treatment of the **depression**, anxiety, **insomnia**, or other symptoms that may accompany dissociative amnesia.

Legal implications

Dissociative amnesia poses a number of complex issues for the legal profession. The disorder has been cited by plaintiffs in cases of recovered memories of abuse leading to lawsuits against the perpetrators of the abuse. Dissociative amnesia has also been cited as a defense in cases of murder of adults as well as in cases of neonatricide (murder of an infant shortly after birth). Part of the problem is the adversarial nature of courtroom procedure in the United States, but it is generally agreed that judges and attorneys need better guidelines regarding dissociative amnesia in defendants and plaintiffs.

Prognosis

The prognosis for recovery from dissociative amnesia is generally good. The majority of patients eventually recover the missing parts of their past, either by spontaneous re-emergence of the memories or through hypnosis and similar techniques. A minority of patients are never able to reconstruct their past; they develop a chronic form of dissociative amnesia. The prognosis for a specific patient depends on a combination of his or her present life circumstances; the presence of other mental disorders; and the severity of stresses or conflicts associated with the amnesia.

Prevention

Strategies for the prevention of **child abuse** might lower the incidence of dissociative amnesia in the general population. There are no effective preventive strategies for dissociative amnesia caused by traumatic experiences in adult life in patients without a history of childhood abuse.

KEY TERMS

Age-associated memory impairment (AAMI)—A condition in which an older person has some memory loss and takes longer to learn new information. AAMI is distinguished from dementia because it is not progressive and does not represent a serious decline from the person's previous level of functioning. Benign senescent forgetfulness is another term for AAMI.

Anterograde amnesia—Amnesia for events that occurred after a physical injury or emotional trauma but before the present moment. Anterograde amnesia typically occurs in dissociative amnesia.

Defense—An unconscious mental process that protects the conscious mind from unacceptable or painful thoughts, impulses, or desires. Examples of defenses include denial, rationalization, projection, and repression.

Delirium—A disturbance of consciousness marked by confusion, difficulty paying attention, delusions, hallucinations, or restlessness. It can be distinguished from dissociative amnesia by its relatively sudden onset and variation in the severity of the symptoms.

Dementia—A group of symptoms (syndrome) associated with a progressive loss of memory and other intellectual functions that is serious enough to interfere with a person's ability to perform the tasks of daily life. Dementia impairs memory, alters personality, leads to deterioration in personal grooming, impairs reasoning ability, and causes disorientation.

Depersonalization—A dissociative symptom in which the patient feels that his or her body is unreal, is changing, or is dissolving.

Derealization—A dissociative symptom in which the external environment is perceived as unreal or dreamlike.

Dissociation—A reaction to trauma in which the mind splits off certain aspects of the traumatic event from conscious awareness. Dissociation can affect the patient's memory, sense of reality, and sense of identity.

Factitious disorder—A type of mental disturbance in which patients intentionally act physically or mentally ill without obvious benefits. It is distinguished from malingering by the absence of an obvious motive, and from conversion disorder by intentional production of symptoms.

Malingering—Knowingly pretending to be physically or mentally ill to avoid some unpleasant duty or responsibility, or for economic benefit.

Retrograde amnesia—Amnesia for events that occurred before a traumatic injury. Retrograde amnesia is not usually found in patients with dissociative amnesia.

Supportive—An approach to psychotherapy that seeks to encourage the patient or offer emotional support to him or her, as distinct from insight-oriented or educational approaches to treatment.

Resources

BOOKS

American Psychiatric Association. *Diagnostic and Statistical Manual of Mental Disorders*. 4th ed., text rev. Washington, DC: American Psychiatric Publishing, 2000.

"Dissociative Amnesia." In *The Merck Manual of Diagnosis and Therapy*, edited by Robert S. Porter and Justin L. Kaplan. 19th ed. Whitehouse Station, NJ: Merck Research Laboratories, 2011.

Ellenberger, Henri. *The Discovery of the Unconscious: The History and Evolution of Dynamic Psychiatry*. New York: Basic Books, 1981.

Herman, Judith. *Trauma and Recovery*. 14th printing. New York: Basic Books, 1997.

Stout, Martha. *The Myth of Sanity: Tales of Multiple Personality in Everyday Life*. New York: Penguin Books, 2002.

PERIODICALS

Brandt, J., and W.G. Van Gorp. "Functional ('psychogenic') Amnesia." *Seminars in Neurology* 26, no. 3 (July 2006): 331–40.

Brown, P., O. Van der Hart, and M. Graafland. "Trauma-Induced Dissociative Amnesia in World War I Combat Soldiers. II. Treatment Dimensions." *Australia and New Zealand Journal of Psychiatry* 33 (1999): 392–98. Available online at http://www.onnovdhart.nl/articles/amnesiaWW1_2.pdf (accessed November 9, 2011).

Carrion, V. G., and H. Steiner. "Trauma and Dissociation in Delinquent Adolescents." *Journal of the American Academy of Child and Adolescent Psychiatry* 39, no. 3 (2000): 353–59.

Chu, J.A., et al. "Memories of Childhood Abuse: Dissociation, Amnesia, and Corroboration." *American Journal of Psychiatry* 156 (1999): 749–55.

Durst, R., A. Teitelbaum, and R. Aronzon. "Amnestic State in a Holocaust Survivor Patient: Psychogenic Versus Neurological Basis." *Israel Journal of Psychiatry and Related Sciences* 36, no. 1 (1999): 47–54.

Lalonde, J. K., et al. "Canadian and American Psychiatrists' Attitudes Toward Dissociative Disorders Diagnoses." *Canadian Journal of Psychiatry* 46, no. 5 (June 2001): 407–12. Available online at http://ww1.cpa-apc.org:8080/Publications/Archives/CJP/2001/June/original.asp (accessed November 9, 2011).

Miller, P.W., et al. "An Unusual Presentation of Inhalant Abuse with Dissociative Amnesia." *Veterinary and Human Toxicology* 44, no. 1 (February 2002): 17–19.

Pope, Harrison G., Jr. "Recovered Memories of Childhood Abuse: The Royal College of Psychiatrists Issues Important Precautions." *British Medical Journal* 316 (February 14, 1998): 713. Available online at http://www.bmj.com/content/316/7130/488.full?sid=5c9caa33-0a45-4fb0-9980-a057abd9e57e (accessed November 9, 2011).

Porter, S., et al. "Memory for Murder. A Psychological Perspective on Dissociative Amnesia in Legal Contexts." *International Journal of Law and Psychiatry* 24 (January–February 2001): 23–42.

Simeon, D., et al. "Personality Factors Associated with Dissociation: Temperament, Defenses, and Cognitive Schemata." *American Journal of Psychiatry* 159 (March 2002): 489–91.

Spinelli, M. G. "A Systematic Investigation of 16 Cases of Neonaticide." *American Journal of Psychiatry* 158 (May 2001): 811–13.

"Symposium: Science and Politics of Recovered Memories." Special issue of *Ethics and Behavior* 8, no. 2 (1998).

Zanarini, M.C., et al. "The Dissociative Experiences of Borderline Patients." *Comprehensive Psychiatry* 41, no. 3 (May–June 2000): 223–27.

WEBSITES

National Alliance on Mental Illness. "Dissociative Disorders." June 2000. http://www.nami.org/Content/ContentGroups/Helpline1/Dissociative_Disorders.htm (accessed October 5, 2011).

ORGANIZATIONS

International Society for the Study of Trauma and Dissociation, 8400 Westpark Dr., 2nd Fl., McLean, VA, 22102, (703) 610-9037, Fax: (703) 610-0234, http://www.isst-d.org.

International Society for Traumatic Stress Studies, 111 Deer Lake Rd., Ste. 100, Deerfield, IL, 60015, (847) 480-9028, Fax: (847) 480-9282, http://www.istss.org.

National Institute of Mental Health, 6001 Executive Blvd., Room 8184, MSC 9663, Bethesda, MD, 20892-9663, (301) 433-4513; TTY: (301) 443-8431, Fax: (301) 443-4279, (866) 615-6464; TTY: (866) 415-8051, nimhinfo@nih.gov, http://www.nimh.nih.gov.

National Organization for Rare Disorders, 55 Kenosia Ave., PO Box 1968, Danbury, CT, 06813-1968, (203) 744-0100, Fax: (203) 798-2291, (800) 999-6673, http://www.rarediseases.org.

Rebecca Frey, PhD
Emily Jane Willingham, PhD

Dissociative fugue

Definition

Dissociative fugue is a rare condition in which a person suddenly, without planning or warning, travels far from home or work and leaves behind a past life. Patients show signs of **amnesia** and have no conscious understanding or knowledge of the reason for the flight. The condition is usually associated with severe **stress** or **trauma**. Because people cannot remember all or part of their past, at some point they become confused about their identity and the situations in which they find themselves. In rare cases, they may take on new identities. The **American Psychiatric Association** (APA) classifies dissociative fugue as one of four **dissociative disorders**, along with **dissociative amnesia**, **dissociative identity disorder**, and **depersonalization disorder**.

Demographics

Dissociative fugue is a rare disorder estimated to affect just 0.2% of the population, nearly all of them adults. More people may experience dissociative fugue during or in the aftermath of serious accidents, wars, natural disasters, or other highly traumatic or stressful events.

Description

The key feature of dissociative fugue is "sudden, unexpected travel away from home or one's customary place of daily activities, with inability to recall some or all of one's past," according to the APA. The travels associated with the condition can last for a few hours or as long as several months. Some individuals have traveled thousands of miles from home while in a state of dissociative fugue. (The word *fugue* stems from the Latin word for flight—*fugere*.) At first, people experiencing the condition may appear completely normal. With time, however, confusion appears. This confusion may result from the realization that they cannot remember the past. Those affected may suddenly realize that they do not belong where they find themselves.

During an episode of dissociative fugue, those affected may take on new identities, complete with a new name. They may even establish new homes and ties to their communities. More often those affected realize something is wrong not long after fleeing—in a matter of hours or days. In such cases, they may phone home for help, or come to the attention of police after becoming distressed at finding themselves unexplainably in unfamiliar surroundings.

Dissociative fugue is distinct from dissociative identity disorder (DID). In cases of DID, which previously was called multiple personality disorder, those affected lose memory of events that take place when one of several distinct identities takes control of them. If the person with dissociative fugue assumes a new identity, it does not coexist with other identities, as is typical of DID. Repeated instances of apparent dissociative fugue are more likely a symptom of DID, not true dissociative fugue.

Causes and symptoms

Causes

Episodes of dissociative fugue are often associated with very stressful events. Traumatic experiences, such as war or natural disasters, seem to increase the incidence of the disorder. Other, more personal types of stress might also lead to the unplanned travel and amnesia characteristic of dissociative fugue. The shocking death of a loved one or seemingly unbearable pressures at work or home, for example, might cause some people to run away for brief periods and blank out their pasts.

Symptoms

People in the midst of dissociative fugue episodes may appear to have no psychiatric symptoms at all or to be only slightly confused. Therefore, for a time, it may be very difficult to spot someone experiencing a fugue. After a while, however, patients show significant signs of confusion or distress because they cannot remember recent events, or they realize a complete sense of identity is missing. This amnesia is a characteristic symptom of the disorder.

Diagnosis

The ***Diagnostic and Statistical Manual of Mental Disorders***, 4th edition, text revision, also known as the *DSM-IV-TR*, lists four criteria for diagnosing dissociative fugue:

- unexplained and unexpected travel from a person's usual place of living and working along with partial or complete amnesia
- uncertainty and confusion about one's identity, or in rare instances, the adoption of a new identity
- the flight and amnesia that characterize the fugue are not related exclusively to DID, nor is it the result of substance abuse or a physical illness
- an episode must result in distress or impairment severe enough to interfere with the ability of the patient to function in social, work, or home settings

Accurate **diagnosis** typically must wait until the fugue is over and the person has sought help or has been brought to the attention of mental health care providers. The diagnosis can then be made using the patient's history and reconstruction of events that occurred before, during, and after the patient's excursion.

KEY TERMS

Amnesia—A general medical term for loss of memory that is not due to ordinary forgetfulness. Amnesia can be caused by head injuries, brain disease, or epilepsy, as well as by dissociation.

Dissociation—A reaction to trauma in which the mind splits off certain aspects of the traumatic event from conscious awareness. Dissociation can affect the patient's memory, sense of reality, and sense of identity.

Treatment

Psychotherapy, sometimes involving hypnosis, is often effective in the treatment of dissociative fugue. With support from therapists, patients are encouraged to remember past events by learning to face and cope with the stressful experiences that precipitated the fugue. Because the cause of the fugue is usually a traumatic event, it is often necessary to treat disturbing feelings and emotions that emerge when the patient finally faces the trauma. The troubling events that drove them to run and forget about their past may, when remembered, result in **grief**, **depression**, fear, anger, remorse, and other psychological states that require therapy.

Prognosis

The prognosis for dissociative fugue is often good. Not many cases last longer than a few months and many people make quick recoveries. In more serious cases, patients may take longer to recover memories of the past.

Resources

BOOKS

Allen, Thomas E., et al. *A Primer on Mental Disorders: A Guide for Educators, Families, and Students.* Lanham, MD: Scarecrow Press, 2001.

American Psychiatric Association. *Diagnostic and Statistical Manual of Mental Disorders.* 4th ed., text rev. Washington, DC: American Psychiatric Publishing, 2000.

"Dissociative Fugue." In *The Merck Manual of Diagnosis and Therapy*, edited by Robert S. Porter and Justin L. Kaplan. 19th ed. Whitehouse Station, NJ: Merck Research Laboratories, 2011.

ORGANIZATIONS

American Psychiatric Association, 1000 Wilson Blvd., Ste. 1825, Arlington, VA, 22209-3901, (703) 907-7300, apa@psych.org, http://www.psych.org.

International Society for the Study of Trauma and Dissociation, 8400 Westpark Drive, Second Floor, McLean, VA, 22102, (703) 610-9037, Fax: (703) 610-0234, http://www.isst-d.org.

National Alliance on Mental Illness, 3803 N Fairfax Drive, Ste. 100, Arlington, VA, 22203, (703) 524-7600, http://www.nami.org.

New York Online Access to Health, http://www.noah-health.org/en/mental/disorders/dissociative.html.

Dean A. Haycock, PhD
Emily Jane Willingham, PhD

Dissociative identity disorder

Definition

Previously known as multiple personality disorder, dissociative identity disorder (DID) is a condition in which those affected have more than one distinct identity or personality state. At least two of these personalities repeatedly assert themselves to control the behavior of the affected person. Each personality state has a distinct name, past, identity, and self-image.

Psychiatrists and psychologists use a handbook called the ***Diagnostic and Statistical Manual of Mental Disorders***, fourth edition, text revision (*DSM-IV-TR*) to diagnose mental disorders. In this handbook, DID is classified as a dissociative disorder. Other mental disorders in this category include **depersonalization disorder**, **dissociative fugue**, and **dissociative amnesia**. The nature of DID and even its existence is debated by psychiatrists and psychologists.

Demographics

Studies in North America and Europe indicate that as many as 5% of patients in psychiatric wards have undiagnosed DID. Partially hospitalized patients and outpatients may have an even higher incidence. For every man diagnosed with DID, eight or nine women are diagnosed. Among children, boys and girls diagnosed with DID are pretty closely matched 1:1. No one is sure why this discrepancy between diagnosed adults and children exists.

Description

"Dissociation" describes a state in which the integrated functioning of a person's identity, including consciousness, memory, and awareness of surroundings, is disrupted or eliminated. Dissociation is a mechanism that allows the mind to separate or compartmentalize certain memories or thoughts from normal consciousness. These memories are not erased, but are buried and may resurface at a later time. Dissociation is related to hypnosis in that hypnotic trance also involves a temporarily altered state of consciousness. In severe, impairing dissociation, individuals experience a lack of awareness of important aspects of their identities.

The phrase "dissociative identity disorder" replaced "multiple personality disorder" because the new name emphasizes the disruption of a person's identity that characterizes the disorder. People with the illness are consciously aware of one aspect of their personality or self while being totally unaware of, or dissociated from, other aspects of it. This is a key feature of the disorder. It requires only two distinct identities or personality states to qualify as DID, but there have been cases in which 100 distinct alternate personalities, or alters, were reported. Fifty percent of patients with DID harbor fewer than 11 identities.

Because the alters alternate in controlling the consciousness and behavior of the individual, patients experience long gaps in memory—gaps that far exceed typical episodes of forgetting that occur in those unaffected by DID.

Despite the presence of distinct personalities, one primary identity exists in many cases. The primary identity uses the name the patient was born with and tends to be quiet, dependent, depressed, and guilt-ridden. The alters have their own names and unique traits. They are distinguished by different temperaments, likes, dislikes, manners of expression, and even physical characteristics such as posture and body language. It is not unusual for patients with DID to have alters of different genders, sexual orientations, ages, or nationalities. It typically takes just seconds for one personality to replace another but the shift can be gradual in rarer instances. In either case, the emergence of one personality, and the retreat of another, is often triggered by a stressful event.

People with DID tend to have other severe disorders as well, such as **depression**, **substance abuse**, **borderline personality disorder**, and eating disorders, among others. The degree of impairment ranges from mild to severe, and complications may include **suicide** attempts, **self-mutilation**, violence, or drug abuse.

Left untreated, DID can last a lifetime. Treatment for the disorder consists primarily of individual **psychotherapy**.

Causes and symptoms

Causes

The severe dissociation that characterizes patients with DID is currently understood to result from a set of causes:

- an innate ability to dissociate easily
- repeated episodes of severe physical or sexual abuse in childhood
- lack of supportive or comforting people to counteract abusive relative(s)
- influence of other relatives with dissociative symptoms or disorders

The primary cause of DID appears to be severe and prolonged **trauma** experienced during childhood. This trauma can be associated with emotional, physical, or **sexual abuse**, or some combination. One theory is that young children, faced with a routine of torture, sexual abuse, or **neglect**, dissociate themselves from their trauma by creating separate identities or personality states. Manufactured alters may suffer while primary identities "escape" the unbearable experiences. Dissociation, which is easy for young children to achieve, becomes a useful defense. This strategy displaces the suffering onto another identity. Over time, children, who on average are around six years old at the time of the appearance of the first alter, may create many more.

There is considerable controversy about the nature, and even the existence, of DID. The causes are disputed, with some experts identifying extensive trauma in childhood as causative, while others maintain that the cause of the disorder is iatrogenic, or introduced by the news media or therapist. In this latter form, mass media or therapists plant the seeds that patients suppressed memories and dissociation severe enough to have created separate personalities. One cause for the skepticism is the alarming increase in reports of the disorder since the 1980s; more cases of DID were reported between 1981 and 1986 than in the previous 200 years combined. In some cases, people reporting DID and recovered memory became involved in lawsuits related to the recovered memories, only to find that the memories were not, in fact, real. Another disorder, false memory syndrome, then becomes the explanation. Thus, an area of contention is the notion of suppressed memories, a crucial component in DID. Many experts in memory research say that it is almost impossible for anyone to remember things that happened before the age of three, the age when some patients with DID supposedly experience abuse, but the brain's storage, retrieval, and interpretation of childhood memories are still not fully understood. The relationship of **dissociative disorders** to childhood abuse has led to intense controversy and lawsuits concerning the accuracy of childhood memories. Because childhood trauma is a factor in the development of DID, some doctors think it may be a variation of **post-traumatic stress disorder** (PTSD). In both DID and PTSD, dissociation is a prominent mechanism.

Symptoms

The major dissociative symptoms experienced by patients with DID are **amnesia**, **depersonalization**, derealization, and identity disturbances.

AMNESIA. Amnesia in patients with DID is marked by gaps in their memory for long periods of their past, and, in some cases, their entire childhood. Most patients with DID have amnesia, or "lose time," for periods when another personality is "out." They may report finding items in their house that they cannot remember having purchased, finding notes written in different handwriting, or other evidence of unexplained activity.

DEPERSONALIZATION. Depersonalization is a dissociative symptom in which patients feel that their bodies are unreal, are changing, or are dissolving. Some patients with DID experience depersonalization as feeling outside of their bodies, or as watching a movie of themselves.

DEREALIZATION. Derealization is a dissociative symptom in which patients perceive the external environment as unreal. Patients may see walls, buildings, or other objects as changing in shape, size, or color. Patients with DID may fail to recognize relatives or close friends.

IDENTITY DISTURBANCES. People with DID usually have a main personality that psychiatrists refer to as the "host." This is generally not the person's original personality but is rather one developed in response to childhood trauma. It is usually this personality that seeks psychiatric help. Patients with DID are often frightened by their dissociative experiences, which can include losing awareness of hours or even days, meeting people who claim to know them by another name, or feeling "out of body."

Psychiatrists refer to the phase of transition between alters as the "switch." After a switch, people with DID assume whole new physical postures, voices, and vocabularies. Specific circumstances or stressful situations may bring out particular identities. Some patients have histories of erratic performance in school or in their jobs caused by the emergence of alternate personalities during examinations or other stressful situations. Each alternate identity takes control one at a time, denying control to the others. Patients vary with regard to their alters' awareness of one another. One alter may not acknowledge the existence of others or it may criticize other alters. At times during therapy, one alter may allow another to take control.

Diagnosis

The *DSM-IV-TR* lists four diagnostic criteria for identifying DID and differentiating it from similar disorders:

- Traumatic stressor: Patients have been exposed to catastrophic events involving actual or threatened death or injury, or a serious physical threat to themselves or others. During exposure to the trauma, their emotional response was marked by intense fear, feelings of helplessness, or horror. In general, stressors caused intentionally by human beings (genocide, rape, torture, abuse, etc.) are experienced as more traumatic than accidents, natural disasters, or "acts of God."
- The demonstration of two or more distinct identities or personality states in an individual. Each separate identity must have its own way of thinking about, perceiving, relating to, and interacting with the environment and self.
- Two of the identities assume control of the patient's behavior, one at a time and repeatedly.
- Extended periods of forgetfulness lasting too long to be considered ordinary forgetfulness.
- Determination that the above symptoms are not due to drugs, alcohol, or other substances and that they cannot be attributed to any other general medical condition. It is also necessary to rule out fantasy play or imaginary friends when considering a diagnosis of DID in children.

Proper **diagnosis** of DID is complicated because some of the symptoms of DID overlap with symptoms of other mental disorders. Misdiagnoses are common and include depression, **schizophrenia**, borderline personality disorder, **somatization disorder**, and **panic disorder**.

Because the extreme dissociative experiences related to this disorder can be frightening, people with the disorder may go to emergency rooms or clinics because they fear they are going insane.

When a doctor is evaluating a patient for DID, the first step is to rule out physical conditions that sometimes produce amnesia, depersonalization, or derealization. These conditions include head injuries, **brain** disease (especially seizure disorders), side effects from medications, substance abuse or intoxication, AIDS **dementia** complex, or recent periods of extreme physical stress and sleeplessness. In some cases, the doctor may give the patient an electroencephalograph (EEG) to exclude epilepsy or other seizure disorders. The physician also must consider whether the patient is **malingering** and/or offering fictitious complaints.

If the patient appears to be physically healthy, the doctor will next rule out psychotic disturbances, including schizophrenia. Many patients with DID are misdiagnosed as having schizophrenia because they may "hear" their alters "talking" inside their heads. Doctors who suspect DID can use a screening test called the Dissociative Experiences Scale (DES). Patients with high scores on this test can be evaluated further with the Dissociative Disorders Interview Schedule (DDIS) or the Structured Clinical Interview for Dissociative Disorders (SCID-D).

Treatment

Treatment of DID may last for five to seven years in adults and usually requires several different treatment methods.

Psychotherapy

Ideally, patients with DID should be treated by a therapist with specialized training in dissociation. This specialized training is important because the patient's personality switches can be confusing or startling. In addition, many patients with DID have hostile or suicidal alter personalities. Most therapists who treat patients with DID have rules or contracts for treatment that include such issues as responsibility for the patient's safety. Psychotherapy for patients with DID typically has several stages: an initial phase for uncovering and "mapping" the patient's alters; a phase of treating the traumatic memories and "fusing" the alters; and a phase of consolidating the patient's newly integrated personality.

Most therapists who treat multiples, or patients with DID, recommend further treatment after personality integration, on the grounds that the patients have not learned the social skills that most people acquire in adolescence and early adult life. In addition, **family therapy** is often recommended to help families understand DID and the changes that occur during personality reintegration.

Many patients with DID are helped by **group therapy** as well as individual treatment, provided that the group is limited to people with dissociative disorders. Patients with DID sometimes have setbacks in mixed therapy groups because other patients are bothered or frightened by their personality switches.

Medications

Some doctors prescribe tranquilizers or **antidepressants** for patients with DID because their alter personalities may have anxiety or mood disorders. However, other therapists who treat patients with DID prefer to keep medications to a minimum because these patients

KEY TERMS

Alter—An alternate or secondary personality in a person with dissociative identity disorder. Each alter has a unique way of looking at and interacting with the world.

Amnesia—A general medical term for loss of memory that is not due to ordinary forgetfulness. Amnesia can be caused by head injuries, brain disease, or epilepsy, as well as by dissociation.

Borderline personality disorder—A severe and usually lifelong mental disorder characterized by violent mood swings and severe difficulties in sustaining interpersonal relationships.

Depersonalization—A dissociative symptom in which patients feel that their bodies are unreal, are changing, or are dissolving.

Derealization—A dissociative symptom in which the external environment is perceived as unreal.

Dissociation—A reaction to trauma in which the mind splits off certain aspects of the traumatic event from conscious awareness. Dissociation can affect a patient's memory, sense of reality, and sense of identity.

Host—The dominant or main alter in a person with DID.

Hypnosis—The means by which a state of extreme relaxation and suggestibility is induced. Hypnosis is used to treat amnesia and identity disturbances that occur in people with dissociative disorders.

Malingering—Knowingly pretending to be physically or mentally ill to avoid some unpleasant duty or responsibility, or for economic benefit.

Multiple personality disorder (MPD)—An older term for dissociative identity disorder (DID).

Panic disorder—An anxiety disorder in which an individual experiences sudden, debilitating attacks of intense fear.

Post-traumatic stress disorder (PTSD)—A disorder caused by an extremely stressful or traumatic event (such as rape, act of war, or natural disaster), in which the trauma victim is haunted by flashbacks. In the flashbacks, the event is reexperienced in the present. Other symptoms include nightmares and feelings of anxiety.

Primary personality—The core personality of a patient with DID.

Schizophrenia—A severe mental illness in which a person has difficulty distinguishing what is real from what is not real. It is often characterized by hallucinations, delusions, language and communication disturbances, and withdrawal from people and social activities.

Shift—The transition of control from one alter to another in a person with DID. Usually shifts occur rapidly, within seconds, but in some cases a more gradual changeover is observed. Also referred to as a switch.

Somatization disorder—A type of mental disorder in which the patient has physical complaints that serve as coping strategies for emotional distress.

Trauma—A disastrous or life-threatening event that can cause severe emotional distress.

can easily become psychologically dependent on drugs. In addition, many patients with DID have at least one alter who abuses drugs or alcohol, substances that are dangerous in combination with most tranquilizers.

Hypnosis

Although not always necessary, hypnosis (or **hypnotherapy**) is a standard method of treatment for patients with DID. Hypnosis may help patients recover repressed ideas and memories. Further, hypnosis can also be used to control problematic behaviors that many patients with DID exhibit, such as self-mutilation, or eating disorders like **bulimia nervosa**. In the later stages of treatment, the therapist may use hypnosis to "fuse" the alters as part of the patient's personality integration process.

Prognosis

Unfortunately, no systematic studies of the long-term outcome of DID currently exist. Some therapists believe that the prognosis for recovery is excellent for children and good for most adults. Although treatment takes several years, it is often ultimately effective. As a general rule, the earlier the patient is diagnosed and properly treated, the better the prognosis. Patients may find they are bothered less by symptoms as they advance into middle age, with some relief beginning to appear in the late 40s. Stress or substance abuse, however, can cause a **relapse** of symptoms at any time.

Prevention

Prevention of DID requires **intervention** in abusive families and treating children with dissociative symptoms as early as possible.

Resources

BOOKS

Acocella, Joan. *Creating Hysteria: Women and Multiple Personality Disorder*. San Francisco, CA: Jossey-Bass Publishers, 1999.

Alderman, Tracy, and Karen Marshall. *Amongst Ourselves, A Self-Help Guide to Living with Dissociative Identity Disorder*. Oakland, CA: New Harbinger Publications, 1998.

American Psychiatric Association. *Diagnostic and Statistical Manual of Mental Disorders*. 4th ed., text rev. Washington, DC: American Psychiatric Publishing, 2000.

Saks, Elyn R., and Stephen H. Behnke. *Jekyll on Trial: Multipersonality Disorder and Criminal Law*. New York: New York University Press, 1997.

PERIODICALS

Gleaves, D. H., M. C. May, and E. Cardena. "An Examination of the Diagnostic Validity of Dissociative Identity Disorder." *Clinical Psychology Review* 21, no. 4 (June 2001): 577–608.

Lalonde, J. K., et al. "Canadian and American Psychiatrists' Attitudes Toward Dissociative Disorders Diagnoses." *Canadian Journal of Psychiatry* 46, no. 5 (June 2001): 407–12.

Spitzer, Carsten, et al. "Recent Developments in the Theory of Dissociation." *World Psychiatry* 5, no. 2 (June 2006): 82–86.

Stickley, T., and R. Nickeas. "Becoming One Person: Living with Dissociative Identity Disorder." *Journal of Psychiatric and Mental Health Nursing* 13, no. 2 (April 2006): 180–87.

WEBSITES

Mayo Clinic. "Dissociative Disorders." http://www.mayoclinic.com/health/dissociative-disorders/DS00574/DSECTION=5 (accessed October 3, 2011).

Merck Manual for Healthcare Professionals. "Dissociative Identity Disorder." The Merck Manuals Online Medical Library. June 2008. http://www.merckmanuals.com/professional/psychiatric_disorders/dissociative_disorders/dissociative_identity_disorder.html#v1026117 (accessed October 5, 2011).

ORGANIZATIONS

American Psychiatric Association, 1000 Wilson Blvd., Ste. 1825, Arlington, VA, 22209-3901, (703) 907-7300, apa@psych.org, http://www.psych.org.

International Society for the Study of Trauma and Dissociation, 8400 Westpark Dr., 2nd Fl., McLean, VA, 22102, (703) 610-9037, Fax: (703) 610-0234, http://www.isst-d.org.

National Alliance on Mental Illness, 3803 N Fairfax Drive, Ste. 100, Arlington, VA, 22203, (703) 524-7600, http://www.nami.org.

Rebecca J. Frey, PhD
Dean A. Haycock, PhD
Emily Jane Willingham, PhD

Disulfiram

Definition

Disulfiram is an aldehyde dehydrogenase inhibitor. It prohibits the activity of aldehyde dehydrogenase, an enzyme found in the liver. In the United States, disulfiram is sold under brand name Antabuse.

Purpose

Disulfiram is used as a conditioning treatment for alcohol dependence. When taken with alcohol, disulfiram causes many unwanted and unpleasant effects, and the fear of these is meant to condition the patient to avoid alcohol.

Description

Two Danish physicians who were investigating disulfiram for its potential benefits to destroy parasitic worms took disulfiram and became sick at a cocktail party. After a series of pharmacological and clinical studies, it was determined that disulfiram interacts with alcohol.

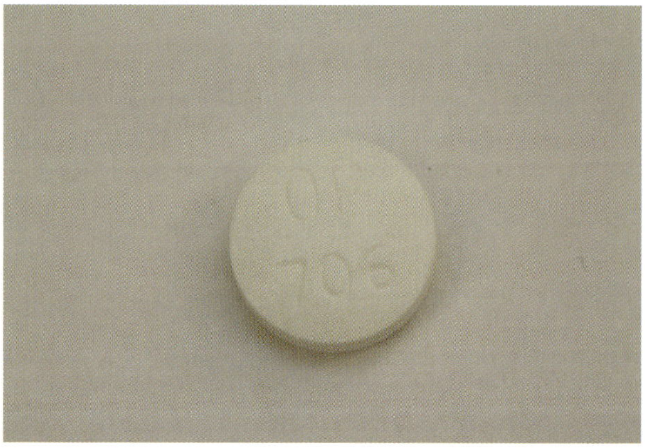

Antabuse (disulfiram), 250 mg. *(© Custom Medical Stock Photo, Inc. Reproduced by permission.)*

Disulfiram by itself is not toxic. If taken with alcohol, however, it alters certain steps in the breakdown of alcohol. When alcohol is ingested, it is converted first to a chemical called acetaldehyde. Acetaldehyde is further broken down into acetate. In order for acetaldehyde to be broken down into acetate, aldehyde dehydrogenase needs to be active. Disulfiram is an aldehyde dehydrogenase inhibitor. Since disulfiram blocks the activity of aldehyde dehydrogenase, acetaldehyde cannot be broken down and the levels of acetaldehyde become five to ten times higher than the normal levels. This causes uncomfortable effects that encourage the person to avoid alcohol.

Disulfiram comes in a 250 mg and 500 mg tablet.

Recommended dosage

Disulfiram therapy should be started only after the patient has abstained from alcohol for at least 12 hours. The initial dose may be as high as 500 mg taken once daily. If the medication is sedating, the dose can be administered in the evening. Ideally, the daily dose should be taken in the morning—the time the resolve not to drink may be strongest. The initial dosing period can last for one to two weeks.

A maintenance dose can range anywhere from 125–500 mg daily with the average dose being 250 mg daily. Disulfiram therapy should continue until full recovery. This may take months to years, depending upon the patient's response and motivation to stop using alcohol. The duration of disulfiram's activity is 14 days after discontinuation, and patients need to avoid alcohol for this period of time.

Precautions

Before beginning therapy, patients should be carefully evaluated for their intellectual capacity to understand the goal of therapy, which can be described as behavioral modification with negative **reinforcement**. Patients with history of **psychosis**, severe myocardial disease, and coronary occlusion should not take disulfiram. People with diabetes taking disulfiram are at an increased risk for complications. Severe liver failure has been associated with the use of disulfiram in patients with or without a prior history of liver problems. People with advanced or severe liver disease should not take disulfiram. Disulfiram should never be given to patients who are in a state of alcohol intoxication or without the patient's knowledge. Those patients with history of **seizures**, hypothyroidism, or nephritis need to use disulfiram with caution and close monitoring.

KEY TERMS

Coronary occlusion—Blockage of the arteries supplying blood to the heart.

Hypothyroidism—Thyroid gland that is abnormally low-functioning. A lowered metabolic rate results.

Jaundice—A yellowing of the skin caused by excess bilirubin in the blood; a liver disorder.

MAO inhibitors—A group of antidepressant drugs that decrease the activity of monoamine oxidase, a neurotransmitter found in the brain that affects mood.

Myocardial disease—Disease of the muscular layer of the heart wall.

Nephritis—Inflammation of the kidney.

Psychosis—Severe state characterized by loss of contact with reality and deterioration in normal social functioning; examples are schizophrenia and paranoia. Psychosis is usually one feature of an overarching disorder, not a disorder in itself. (Plural: psychoses)

Besides avoiding alcohol, patients should also avoid any products containing alcohol. This includes many cold syrups, tonics, and mouthwashes. Patients should not even use topical preparations that contain alcohol such as perfume and aftershave lotion.

Side effects

The most common side effect of disulfiram includes drowsiness and **fatigue**. Many patients experience metallic or garlic-like aftertaste, but most patients develop tolerance to this effect.

In addition, disulfiram is associated with impotence. This is most common in doses of 500 mg daily. Disulfiram can cause blurred vision, skin discoloration, inflammation of the skin, increased heart rate, and mental changes.

During the first three months of therapy, patients should have their liver function evaluated. Patients need to be monitored for the signs of jaundice, nausea, vomiting, abdominal pain, light stools, and dark urine as these may be the signs of liver damage due to disulfiram. The signs of alcohol ingestion include flushing, headache, nausea, vomiting and abdominal pain.

Interactions

Disulfiram can make cisapride, **benzodiazepines**, astemizole, cyclosporine, erythromycin, and cholesterol-lowering drugs called statins more toxic. Disulfiram in combination with isoniazid, **monoamine oxidase inhibitors (MAOIs)** (such as phenelzine and **tranylcypromine**), metronidazole, omeprazole and tricyclic **antidepressants** may cause adverse central nervous system effects.

In addition, disulfiram may raise the concentrations of the medications theophylline and phenytoin in the body. Patients taking warfarin (a blood-thinning drug) are at an increased risk of bleeding. Disulfiram should never be used with tranylcypromine and amprenavir oral solution.

Disulfiram may react even with small amounts of alcohol found in over-the-counter cough and cold preparations and any medication that comes in an elixir form.

Resources

BOOKS

Lacy, Charles F. *Drug Information Handbook with International Trade Names Index*. Hudson, OH: Lexi-Comp, Inc. 2011.

Taylor, David, Carol Paton, and Shitij Kapur. *The Maudsley Prescribing Guidelines Tenth Edition*. London: Informa Healthcare, 2009.

PERIODICALS

Berglund, Mats. "A Better Widget? Three Lessons for Improving Addiction Treatment from a Meta-Analytical Study." *Addiction* 100, no. 6 (June 2005): 742–50.

Boothby, Lisa, A., and Paul L. Doering. "Acamprosate for the Treatment of Alcohol Dependence." *Clinical Therapeutics* 27, no. 6 (June 2005): 695–714.

Buonopane, Alessandra, and Ismene L. Petrakis. "Pharmacotherapy of Alcohol Use Disorders." *Substance Use and Misuse* 40, no. 13–14 (2005): 2001–20, 2043–-48.

Krampe, Henning, et al. "Follow-Up of 180 Alcoholic Patients for Up to 7 Years After Outpatient Treatment: Impact of Alcohol Deterrents on Outcome." *Alcoholism: Clinical and Experimental Research* 30, no. 1 (January 2006): 86–95.

Kulig, Clark C., and Thomas P. Beresford. "Hepatitis C in Alcohol Dependence: Drinking Versus Disulfiram." *Journal of Addictive Diseases* 24, no. 2 (2005): 77–89.

Nava, Felice, et al. "Comparing Treatments of Alcoholism on Craving and Biochemical Measures of Alcohol Consumptions." *Journal of Psychoactive Drugs* 38, no. 3 (September 2006): 211–17.

Petrakis, Ismene L., et al. "Naltrexone and Disulfiram in Patients with Alcohol Dependence and Comorbid Psychiatric Disorders." *Biological Psychiatry* 57, no. 10 (May 15, 2005): 1128–37.

Sofuoglu, Mehmet, and Thomas R. Kosten. "Novel Approaches to the Treatment of Cocaine Addiction." *CNS Drugs* 19, no. 1 (2005): 13–25.

Suh, Jesse J., et al. "The Status of Disulfiram: A Half of a Century Later." *Journal of Clinical Psychopharmacology* 26, no. 3 (June 2006): 290–302.

Ajna Hamidovic, PharmD
Ruth A. Wienclaw, PhD

Divalproex sodium

Definition

Divalproex sodium is an anticonvulsant (anti-seizure) drug. It is also used to treat mania and to help prevent migraine headaches. It is sold under multiple brand names in the United States, including Depacon, Depakene, Depakote, and Depakote Sprinkle.

Purpose

Divalproex sodium is effective in the treatment of epilepsy, particularly for preventing simple, complex (petit mal), absence, mixed, and tonic-clonic (grand mal) **seizures**. Divalproex sodium is also used to treat the manic phase of **bipolar disorder** (also called manic-depressive disorder) in adults, and to prevent migraine headache in adults.

Description

Divalproex sodium is chemically compounded from sodium valproate and **valproic acid** in a 1:1 ratio.

Divalproex sodium is thought to work by increasing the levels of a **brain** neurotransmitter called gamma-aminobutyric acid (GABA). GABA is an inhibitory

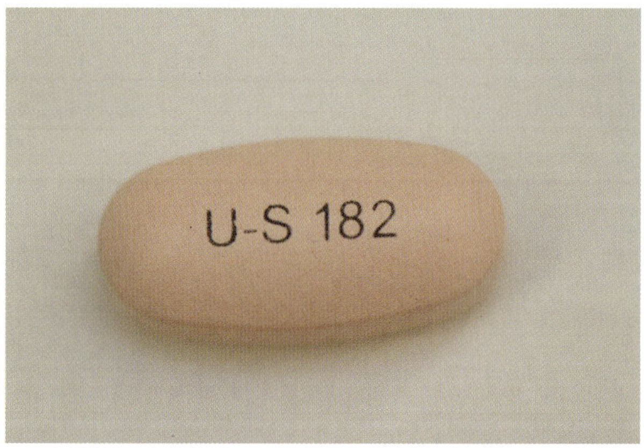

Divalproex sodium, 500 mg. *(© Custom Medical Stock Photo, Inc. Reproduced by permission.)*

KEY TERMS

Absence seizures—Also called a petit mal seizure; characterized by abrupt, short-term lack of conscious activity or other abnormal change in behavior.

Epilepsy—A disorder associated with disturbed electrical discharges in the central nervous system that cause seizures.

Seizure—A convulsion, or uncontrolled discharge of nerve cells that may spread to other cells throughout the brain.

Tonic-clonic seizure—A seizure involving the entire body, characterized by unconsciousness, muscle contraction, and rigidity, also called grand mal or generalized seizures.

Trigeminal neuralgia—A disorder of the trigeminal nerve that causes severe facial pain.

neurotransmitter, which means that its presence makes it harder for nerve cells (neurons) in the brain to become activated (fire). It is believed that increasing GABA's inhibitory action on brain neurons accounts for the ability of divalproex sodium to decrease seizures, curb manic behaviors, and decrease the frequency of migraine headaches.

Divalproex sodium was discovered to decrease the likelihood of seizure in 1963. In 1978 the U.S. Food and Drug Administration (FDA) approved it for this use. Other uses for divalproex sodium were researched and approved subsequently, including use against mania (1995) and use to decrease migraine headache frequency. Divalproex sodium's 1995 approval as an anti-mania medication was considered an exciting advance, since it represented the first new drug introduced for this use in 25 years.

Recommended dosage

Divalproex sodium is available in tablets of 125 mg, 250 mg, and 500 mg. Divalproex sodium is also available in 125 mg capsules, in a 500 mg extended release tablet, and in a syrup containing 250 mg active drug per 5 mL.

Divalproex sodium therapy is usually started at 10–15 mg per 2.2 lb. (1 kg) of body weight per day. Dosages are then increased until seizures seem to be well controlled. This effect is usually achieved at averages under 60 mg per kg per day.

To treat mania, divalproex sodium is usually started at a daily dose of about 750 mg.

For migraine prevention, divalproex sodium is started at 250 mg, twice per day. In some patients, this dose will be raised to a total of 1,000 mg per day.

Precautions

Before taking divalproex sodium, patients should read the medication guide. A greater risk of liver damage exists in patients with kidney disease, known liver disease, Addison's disease, blood diseases, children under the age of two, patients with organic brain diseases (such as Alzheimer's, Parkinson's, slow virus infections, Huntington's chorea, or multiple sclerosis), patients with metabolic disorders present at birth, patients with severe seizure disorders and accompanying intellectual disability, and patients who are taking several other anticonvulsant drugs.

Because divalproex sodium can affect a patient's blood by dropping the platelet (a type of blood cell that affects clotting) count and interfering with coagulation (clotting) capability, both platelet count and coagulation parameters should be verified before a patient starts the medication and at intervals throughout its use.

Divalproex sodium is known to cause an increased risk of birth defects when taken during pregnancy. Children born to mothers who took divalproex sodium during their pregnancy tend to score lower on cognitive exams, including IQ tests, than children whose mothers took other anticonvulsants and not divalproex sodium (or related medications) when pregnant. Individuals and their healthcare provider must weigh the potential risks and benefits of using this medication during pregnancy. Women who take this medicine should not breast-feed, since a small amount will pass into the breast milk.

Divalproex sodium causes drowsiness and impairs alertness in some individuals. Patients just beginning to use the medication should avoid driving and using dangerous machinery until they determine how the drug affects them. The sedative effects are increased in the presence of alcohol, so patients should avoid drinking while taking medicines containing divalproex sodium.

Side effects

Some of the more common side effects of divalproex sodium are:

- mild stomach cramps
- change in menstrual cycle
- diarrhea
- loss of hair

- indigestion
- change in appetite
- nausea and vomiting
- trembling in the hands and arms

These side effects usually go away as the patient's body becomes accustomed to the medication.

Another common side effect of this medication is weight gain. Individuals taking divalproex sodium should focus on a balanced, low-fat diet coupled with an increase in physical activity to counter this side effect. Nutrient-rich foods such as fruits, vegetables, and whole grain products should be emphasized in the diet, whereas sweets, fats, and other foods high in carbohydrates but low in nutrients should be limited. Regular physical activity can help limit weight gain caused by this medication.

Less common side effects include:

- severe stomach cramps or continued nausea and vomiting
- changes in mood, behavior, or thinking
- double vision or seeing spots
- severe fatigue
- easy bruising or unusual bleeding
- yellow cast to the skin or the whites of the eyes (jaundice)
- odd eye movements
- increased seizures

Patients who notice these symptoms should check with their doctor to see if their dosage or medication needs to be adjusted.

Rare side effects that should be checked out by a doctor include:

- clumsiness
- difficulty with balance
- constipation
- dizziness
- drowsiness
- headache
- skin rash
- agitation
- restlessness
- irritability

QUESTIONS TO ASK YOUR DOCTOR

- What kind of changes can I expect to see or feel with this medication?
- Does it matter what time of day I take this medication? If so, what is the recommendation?
- Should I take this medication with or without food?
- What are the side effects associated with this medication?
- Will this medication interact or interfere with other medications I am currently taking?
- What symptoms or adverse effects are important enough that I should seek immediate treatment?

Interactions

Divalproex sodium is metabolized (broken down) in the liver. Other drugs that are metabolized in the liver can have too low or too high concentrations in the body when taken with divalproex sodium. Levels of divalproex sodium may be increased when taken with felbamate, isoniazid, salicylates (aspirin-containing medications), clarithromycin, erythromycin, and troleandomycin. Divalproex sodium may increase levels of **carbamazepine**, phenytoin, **lamotrigine**, nimodipine, phenobarbital, and zidovudine. Use with **clonazepam** may cause absence seizures. Cholestyramine and colestipol may reduce the absorption and the blood levels of divalproex sodium.

Resources

BOOKS

Aminoff, Michael J., ed. *Neurology and General Medicine.* 4th ed. New York: Churchill Livingstone, 2007.

Brunton, Laurence, Bruce A. Chabner, and Bjorn Knollman. *Goodman & Gilman's The Pharmacological Basis of Therapeutics.* 12th ed. New York: McGraw-Hill, 2010.

Devinsky, Orrin. *Epilepsy: Patient and Family Guide.* 3rd ed. New York: Demos Medical, 2007.

Diamond, Seymour, and Merle Lea Diamond. *A Patient's Guide to Headache and Migraine.* 2nd ed. Newtown, PA: Handbooks in Health Care, 2009.

Kuzniecky, Ruben, ed. *Epilepsy 101: The Ultimate Guide for Patients and Families.* Leona, NJ: Medicus Press, 2009.

Miklowitz, David Jay. *Bipolar Disorder: A Family-focused Treatment Approach.* 2nd ed. New York: Guilford Press, 2010.

Panayiotopoulos, C.P. *Antiepileptic Drugs, Pharmacopoeia.* New York: Springer, 2010.

Patsalos, Philip N., and Blaise F.D. Bourgeois. *The Epilepsy Prescriber's Guide to Antiepileptic Drugs.* New York: Cambridge University Press, 2010.

Shorvon, Simon. *Handbook of Epilepsy Treatment.* 3rd ed. New York: Wiley-Blackwell, 2010.

Tatum, William O., Peter W. Kaplan, and Pierre Jallon. *Epilepsy A to Z: A Concise Encyclopedia.* 2nd ed. New York: Demos Medical, 2009.

ORGANIZATIONS

American Academy of Neurology, 1080 Montreal Ave., St. Paul, MN, 55116, (651) 695-2717, (800) 879-1960, Fax: (651) 879-2791, memberservices@aan.com, http://www.aan.com.

American Epilepsy Society, 342 N Main St., West Hartford, CT, 06117-2507, (860) 586-7505, Fax: (860) 586-7550, http://www.aesnet.org.

American Neurological Association, 5841 Cedar Lake Rd., Ste. 204, Minneapolis, MN, 55416, (952) 545-6284, ana@llmsi.com, http://www.aneuroa.org.

American Psychiatric Association, 1000 Wilson Blvd., Ste. 1825, Arlington, VA, 22209-3901, (703) 907-7300, apa@psych.org, http://www.psych.org.

American Psychological Association, 750 1st St., NE, Washington, DC, 20002-4242, (202) 336-5500; TDD/TTY: (202) 336-6123, (800) 374-2721, http://www.apa.org.

Epilepsy Foundation, 8301 Professional Pl., Landover, MD, 20785-7223, (800) 332-1000, Fax: (301) 577-2684, http://epilepsyfoundation.org.

National Headache Foundation, 820 N Orleans St., Ste. 217, Chicago, IL, 60610, (312) 274-2650, (888) 643-5552, info@headaches.org, http://www.headaches.org.

National Institutes of Health, 9000 Rockville Pike, Bethesda, MD, 20892, (301) 496-4000; TTY: (301) 402-9612, http://www.nih.gov.

U.S. National Library of Medicine, 8600 Rockville Pike, Bethesda, MD, 20894, (301) 594-5983, (888) 346-3656; TDD: (800) 735-2258, Fax: (301) 402-1384, http://www.nlm.nih.gov.

Rosalyn Carson-Dewitt, MD
Laura Jean Cataldo, RN, EdD

DMDD *see* **Disruptive mood dysregulation disorder**

Dolophine *see* **Methadone**

Domestic abuse *see* **Abuse**

Domestic violence *see* **Abuse**

Donepezil

Definition

Donepezil is a drug approved by the U.S. Food and Drug Administration (FDA) to treat symptoms of **dementia** associated with **Alzheimer's disease**. In the United States, donepezil is sold under the trade name Aricept.

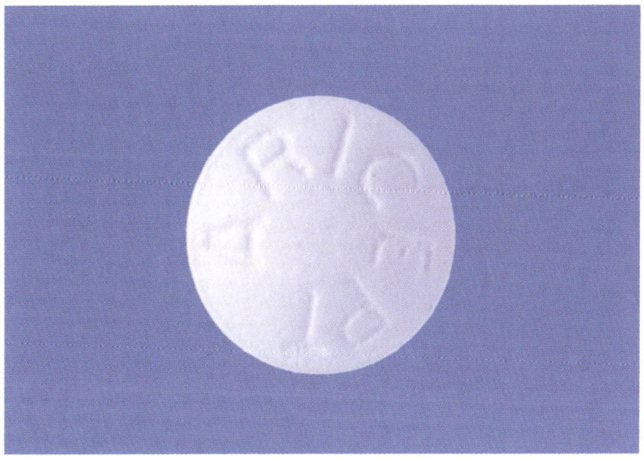

Aricept (donepezil). *(© Custom Medical Stock Photo, Inc. Reproduced by permission.)*

Purpose

Donepezil is used to help treat symptoms in individuals with Alzheimer's disease. The drug may cause small improvements in dementia for a short period of time, but donepezil does not stop the progression of Alzheimer's disease.

Description

Donepezil is in a class of drugs known as cholinesterase inhibitors. Drugs in this class prevent the breakdown of acetylcholine, a neurotransmitter that helps facilitate nerve impulses within the **brain**. In Alzheimer's disease, cells in specific regions of the brain die, meaning they are no longer able to transmit nerve impulses. By sustaining the concentration of acetylcholine in the brain, donepezil and other cholinesterase inhibitors help maintain the transmission of nerve impulses.

Donepezil is available as tablets in two different strengths. It is the only cholinesterase inhibitor approved by the FDA to treat all stages of Alzheimer's disease, from mild to severe.

Recommended dosage

The initial dosage of donepezil is 5 mg taken at bedtime. This dose should be continued for four to six weeks. The dosage may then be increased to 10 mg at bedtime, but there is no clear evidence that the higher dosage is more beneficial. The higher dosage is also likely to cause more side effects.

Precautions

People with certain heart conditions, stomach ulcers, bladder obstruction, asthma, chronic obstructive pulmonary disease, or a history of **seizures** should use

KEY TERMS

Acetylcholine—A naturally occurring chemical in the body that transmits nerve impulses from cell to cell. It causes blood vessels to dilate, lowers blood pressure, and slows the heartbeat. Central nervous system well-being is dependent on a balance among acetylcholine, dopamine, serotonin, and norepinephrine.

Dementia—A group of symptoms (syndrome) associated with a progressive loss of memory and other intellectual functions that is serious enough to interfere with a person's ability to perform the tasks of daily life. Dementia impairs memory, alters personality, leads to deterioration in personal grooming, impairs reasoning ability, and causes disorientation.

Neurotransmitter—A chemical in the brain that transmits messages between neurons, or nerve cells.

donepezil with caution under close physician supervision, as the drug may worsen or aggravate these conditions. Patients taking donepezil should be reassessed periodically to determine whether the drug is providing any benefits. When caregivers feel the drug is no longer beneficial, it may be stopped.

Side effects

More than 5% of people taking donepezil experience difficulty sleeping, dizziness, nausea, diarrhea, muscle cramps, headache, or other pains. Diarrhea, nausea, and vomiting occur more often with the 10 mg dose than the 5 mg dosage. These adverse effects are usually mild, short-lived, and typically subside when the drug is stopped. Other less common side effects include abnormal dreams, **depression**, drowsiness, fainting, loss of appetite, weight loss, frequent urination, arthritis, and easy bruising. Donepezil may slow heart rate, increase acid in the stomach, make urination difficult, cause breathing difficulties, and may increase the risk of seizures in persons with a history of seizure disorder.

Interactions

Research has found that the effects of donepezil on Alzheimer's disease may be enhanced through combination therapy with **memantine** (Namenda). Studies have shown that the use of memantine in combination therapy with donepezil is frequently more effective than the use of donepezil alone in the treatment of moderate to severe Alzheimer's disease. Using memantine and donepezil in combination therapy does not affect the pharmacokinetics of either drug. **Clinical trials** have shown such combination therapy to be both safe and effective, although the safety precautions for both drugs must be considered before combination therapy is undertaken.

Many drugs may alter the effects of donepezil; likewise, donepezil may alter the action of other drugs. Drugs such as dicyclomine, phenytoin, **carbamazepine**, dexamethasone, rifampin, or phenobarbital may lessen the effects of donepezil. Other drugs such as bethanechol, ketoconazole, or quinidine may increase some of the side effects associated with donepezil. When donepezil and nonsteroidal anti-inflammatory drugs such as ibuprofen (Advil) or naproxen (Aleve) are used together, there may be an increased tendency to develop stomach ulcers. Donepezil may increase the side effects associated with use of **fluvoxamine**, an antidepressant. If succinylcholine, a drug commonly used during anesthesia, is used with donepezil, prolonged muscle paralysis may result.

Resources

BOOKS

Ellsworth, Allan J., et al. *Mosby's Medical Drug Reference*. St. Louis, MO: Mosby, 2007.

VandenBos, Gary R. ed. *APA Dictionary of Psychology*. Washington, DC: American Psychological Association, 2006.

Wolters Kluwer Health. *Drug Facts and Comparisons 2012*. 66th ed. St. Louis: Lippincott, Williams & Wilkins, 2011.

PERIODICALS

Asp, Elissa, et al. "Verbal Repetition in Patients with Alzheimer's Disease Who Receive Donepezil." *International Journal of Geriatric Psychiatry* 21, no. 5 (May 2006): 426–31.

Chen, Xiying, et al. "Donepezil Effects on Cerebral Blood Flow in Older Adults with Mild Cognitive Deficits." *Journal of Neuropsychiatry & Clinical Neurosciences* 18, no. 2 (May 2006): 178–85.

Cholongitas, Evangelos, Chrysoula Pipili, and Maria Dasenaki. "Recurrence of Upper Gastrointestinal Bleeding After Donepezil Administration." *Alzheimer Disease and Associated Disorders* 20, no. 4 (October–December 2006): 326.

Cummings, Jeffrey L., Thomas McRae, and Richard Zhang. "Effects of Donepezil on Neuropsychiatric Symptoms in Patients with Dementia and Severe Behavioral Disorders." *American Journal of Geriatric Psychiatry* 14, no. 7 (July 2006): 605–12.

Feldman, Howard H., Frederick A. Schmitt, and Jason T. Olin. "Activities of Daily Living in Moderate-to-Severe Alzheimer Disease: An Analysis of the Treatment Effects of

Memantine in Patients Receiving Stable Donepezil Treatment." *Alzheimer Disease and Associated Disorders* 20, no. 4 (October–December 2006): 263–68.

Hogan, David B. "Donepezil for Severe Alzheimer's Disease." *The Lancet* 367, no. 9516 (April 1, 2006): 1031–32.

Kitabayashi, Yurinosuke, et al. "Donepezil-Induced Nightmares in Mild Cognitive Impairment." *Psychiatry and Clinical Neurosciences* 60, no. 1 (February 2006): 123–24.

Maruyama, Masahiro, et al. "Benefits of Combining Donepezil Plus Traditional Japanese Herbal Medicine on Cognition and Brain Perfusion in Alzheimer's Disease: A 12-Week Observer-Blind, Donepezil Monotherapy Controlled Trial." *Journal of the American Geriatrics Society* Letter to the editor, 54, no. 5 (May 2006): 869–71.

Mazeh, D., et al. "Donepezil for Negative Signs in Elderly Patients with Schizophrenia: An Add-On, Double-Blind, Crossover, Placebo-Controlled Study." *International Psychogeriatrics* 18, no. 3 (September 2006): 429–36.

Ringman, John M., and Jeffrey L. Cummings. "Current and Emerging Pharmacological Treatment Options for Dementia." *Behavioural Neurology* 17, no. 1 (2006): 5–16.

Schredl, M., et al. "The Effect of Donepezil on Sleep in Elderly, Healthy Persons: A Double-Blind Placebo-Controlled Study." *Pharmacopsychiatry* 39, no. 6 (November 2006): 205–208.

Stiles, Melissa M., and Sandra Martin. "Does Treatment with Donepezil Improve Memory for Patients With Mild Cognitive Impairment?" *Journal of Family Practice* 55, no. 5 (May 2006): 435–36. Available online at http://www.jfponline.com/Pages.asp?AID=4104&UID= (accessed November 11, 2011).

Tariot, Pierre N., et al. "Memantine Treatment in Patients with Moderate to Severe Alzheimer Disease Already Receiving Donepezil: A Randomized Controlled Trial." *Journal of the American Medical Association* 291, no. 3 (January 21, 2004): 317–24. Available online at http://jama.ama-assn.org/content/291/3/317.full (accessed November 9, 2011).

Winblad, Bengt, et al. "Donepezil in Patients with Severe Alzheimer's Disease: Double-Blind, Parallel-Group, Placebo-Controlled Study." *The Lancet* 367, no. 9516 (April 1, 2006): 1057–65.

Wong, Shelley. "The Safety of Donepezil in Treating Vascular Dementia." *CNS Spectrums* 11, no. 9 (September 2006): 658–61.

OTHER

Eisai Co., Ltd. "Aricept Prescribing and Patient Information." http://www.aricept.com/assets/pdf/AriceptComboFullPI-November2010.pdf (accessed October 5, 2011).

WEBSITES

Alzheimer's Association. "Medications for Memory Loss." http://www.alz.org/alzheimers_disease_standard_prescriptions.asp (accessed November 14, 2011).

Kelly Karpa, RPh, PhD
Ruth A. Wienclaw, PhD

Dopamine

Definition

Dopamine, identified as a central nervous system agent in 1959, is a neurotransmitter (nerve-signaling molecule) the body makes from the amino acid tyrosine. Dopamine in turn serves as the molecule the body uses to make **adrenaline** and noradrenaline. In addition to operating in nervous system signaling, it also acts as a hormone in an area of the **brain** called the hypothalamus, regulating release of the hormone prolactin, which is involved in parenting behavior and milk production. The body regulates dopamine' activity in the brain in part by using proteins called dopamine transporters, which can take up dopamine and dump it back into a cell, preventing the signaling molecule from exerting its activity. The body also has five types of proteins, called dopamine receptors, responsible for recognizing the dopamine molecule, binding to it, and transmitting its signal to the cell. Dopamine is at the center of the development of a number of psychiatric disorders, including **addiction** and **schizophrenia**, and it also plays a prominent role in the manifestations of Parkinson's disease.

Description

The brain produces dopamine in three primary areas: the substantia nigra, the ventral tegmental area, and the arcuate nucleus. The first two are of particular interest in terms of psychiatric disorders; the arcuate nucleus is associated with dopamine's role as a neurohormone in prolactin regulation.

Disorders associated with dopamine signaling have a biological basis in the brain that appears to be site-specific. The brain has four major dopamine signaling pathways.

- The mesocortical pathway connects the ventral tegmental area to the cortex, the part of the brain involved in cognition and that may play a role in motivation. This pathway features in hypotheses of dopamine's association with schizophrenia.
- The mesolimbic pathway also begins in the ventral tegmental area, which is linked to the nucleus accumbens, the largest component of the ventral striatum. Much research has associated the nucleus accumbens and the mesolimbic pathway with brain reward processes and addiction and also with different aspects of schizophrenia.
- The nigrostriatal pathway connects the dopamine-producing nigrostriatal area with the striatum and plays a high-profile role in the development of Parkinson's symptoms.

- The tuberoinfundibular pathway involves the hypothalamus and dopamine as a neurohormone.

In terms of neuropsychiatric disorders, dopamine is probably best known as the neurotransmitter underlying the development and persistence of addiction as part of the mesolimbic reward pathway. Experiences people find rewarding, such as food or sex, can become associated with increased dopamine, as can some pathological behaviors, such as compulsive gambling. Some drugs also directly elicit an increase in dopamine, setting off the reward pathway and leading to more use of the drug. Ultimately, some people become addicted to substances or behaviors because of the dopamine release they trigger and the feelings of euphoria or tension relief that can follow the release.

Anatomically, these distinct dopamine-signaling pathways, variously involved in specific pathologies, may overlap with one another. For example, there is some comorbidity among schizophrenia, **depression**, and drug dependence and some anatomical overlap in the dopamine-signaling areas of the brain underlies this.

Dopamine receptors

The dopamine receptors, the five proteins responsible for receiving the dopamine signal for a cell, are divided into two general classes: those that are D1-like, and those that are D2-like. Of the five, the D1A through D1D and D5 receptors are all D1-like, and the D2, D3, and D4 receptors fall into the D2-like category. The distribution of these receptors differs in different dopamine-related areas of the brain. For example, the ventral striatum and limbic cortex of the mesolimbic pathway have more D2-like receptors, and D2 and D4 receptors are more closely associated with people with **substance abuse** problems. The dorsal striatum, involved in dopamine-related disorders such as Parkinson's, has more D2- than D1-like receptors. But in the prefrontal cortex, where dopamine-signaling dysfunction is associated with schizophrenia, the ratio of D1-like receptors to D2-like receptors is higher. The two general classes of receptors have opposite effects at the molecular level, but they act together in complex ways.

Dopamine and schizophrenia

A proposed explanation for the manifestations of schizophrenia is the "dopamine hypothesis of schizophrenia." This hypothesis implicates dopamine-signaling dysfunction along different dopamine pathways in the symptoms associated with schizophrenia. The hypothesis finds its origins in the fact that antipsychotic medications (also called "neuroleptics") exert their effects by blocking or inhibiting D2 receptors. The mesolimbic pathway may be involved, a conclusion based on studies showing a link between dysfunction of this system and the **delusions** and hallucinations of schizophrenia, with an increase in striatal dopamine in association with these occurrences. On the other hand, the mesocortical pathway is also probably involved because of its role in working memory, memorization, and manipulation of spatial information, all of which are affected in schizophrenia. A decrease in dopamine in the prefrontal area, which is linked to the ventral tegmental area in the mesocortical pathway, appears to lead to the cognitive deficits of schizophrenia. In addition, the nigrostriatal pathway may be involved: there is an increase in dopamine transmission from the substantia nigra to the striatum in people with schizophrenia.

Dopamine, the brain reward system, and addiction

The nucleus accumbens (in the ventral striatum and part of the mesolimbic pathway) is the focal point of dopamine's involvement in the brain's reward pathway and addiction. There is an increase in dopamine release in the nucleus accumbens in addiction, and activity in this area is a target of models exploring the mechanisms of behavioral or substance addictions. Human **imaging studies**, which have become quite revelatory in terms of the biological underpinnings of psychiatric disorders, show that endogenous release of dopamine in the striatum is correlated with drug-induced feelings of pleasure. For example, a dose of amphetamine or of alcohol will promote dopamine release in the ventral striatum. Dopamine also is associated with the cravings of addiction and may play a role in the significance an addicted person may assign to cues that others perceive as neutral (known as salience). This system has also been implicated in process or behavioral addiction.

Dopamine and movement and repetitive disorders

Dopamine's role in the extrapyramidal (movement and coordination) symptoms of Parkinson's is seated in a shortage of the neurotransmitter in the nigrostriatal pathway, specifically involving the putamen and caudate nucleus. Tourette syndrome, a condition characterized by onset in childhood, involuntary tics, stereotypic behaviors, and repetitive thoughts and rituals, is also seated in the dorsal striatum. This syndrome can occur as a comorbidity with **obsessive-compulsive disorder** and/or **attention deficit hyperactivity disorder** (ADHD), which some studies also have associated with dopamine-signaling dysfunction.

Dopamine and mood disorders

Changes in dopamine signaling may contribute to symptoms of depression, such as an inability to experience pleasure or loss of motivation. Although low levels of dopamine binding to the D2 receptor are associated with social anxiety, an increase in dopamine can be associated

KEY TERMS

D1, D2, etc.—Dopamine receptor proteins.

Mesolimbic pathway—The "reward pathways" of the brain.

Nucleus accumbens—A part of the brain involved in the mesolimbic reward pathway, which receives dopamine signaling from the ventral tegmental area.

Ventral tegmental area—Produces dopamine and signals to the nucleus accumbens and the rest of the striatum.

with the hypersocial behavior of someone experiencing the manic aspects of **bipolar disorder**.

Drugs related to dopamine/dopamine receptor regulation

Drugs may act at any point along a dopamine-signaling pathway. L-dopa, used in treating Parkinson's, is a dopamine precursor that is synthesized into dopamine in the brain and ameliorates the effects of low dopamine levels in the dorsal striatum. **Monoamine oxidase inhibitors (MAOIs)** block the activity of the enzyme that breaks down dopamine; these may be used as **antidepressants** and can affect dopamine-related pathways. Antipsychotics are divided into two classes, the typical and atypical antipsychotics, and can target different types of dopamine receptors. Atypical antipsychotics, including **clozapine**, may target the D4 receptor more strongly than the D2. Bromocriptine targets D2 and is a partial inhibitor of D1. The recently approved aripiprazole is a partial dopamine agonist (mimic), and **amantadine** is also a dopamine agonist.

Resources

BOOKS

American Psychiatric Association. *Diagnostic and Statistical Manual of Mental Disorders*. 4th ed., text rev. Washington, DC: American Psychiatric Publishing, 2000.

PERIODICALS

Franken, Ingmar H.A., Jan Booij, and Wim van den Brink. "The Role of Dopamine in Human Addiction: From Reward to Motivated Attention." *European Journal of Pharmacology* 526 (2005): 199–206.

Grant, Jon E., Judson A. Brewer, and Marc N. Potenza. "The Neurobiology of Substance and Behavioral Addictions." *CNS Spectrum* 11, no. 12 (December 2006): 924–930.

Greene, James G. "Gene Expression Profiles of Brain Dopamine Neurons and Relevance to Neuropsychiatric Disease." *Journal of Physiology* 575, Pt. 2 (September 1, 2006): 411–416.

Kienast, T., and A. Heinz. "Dopamine and the Diseased Brain." *CNS and Neurological Disorders—Drug Targets* 5, no. 1 (February 2006): 109–131.

Totterdell, Susan. "The Anatomy of Comorbid Neuropsychiatric Disorders Based on Cortico-limbic Synaptic Interactions." *Neurotoxicity Research* 10, no. 2 (October 2006): 65–85.

WEBSITES

MedlinePlus. "Schizophrenia." U.S. National Library of Medicine. National Institutes of Health http://www.nlm.nih.gov/medlineplus/schizophrenia.html (accessed October 5, 2011).

U.S. National Institute of Mental Health. "Schizophrenia." http://www.nimh.nih.gov/healthinformation/schizophreniamenu.cfm (accessed October 5, 2011).

Emily Jane Willingham, PhD

Doral *see* **Quazepam**

Down syndrome

Definition

Down syndrome, or trisomy 21, is a genetic disorder caused by the presence of an extra copy of chromosome 21 or by a portion of chromosome 21 translocated (attached) to another chromosome in one of the affected

Incidence of medical conditions associated with Down syndrome

Disorder	Incidence
Infertility	>99% in men; absence of ovulation in 30% of women
Mental retardation	>95%
Growth retardation	>95%
Alzheimer's disease	Affects up to 75% by age 60
Ophthalmic (eye) disorders	60%
Hearing loss	40%–75%
Congenital heart defects	40%

Rarer complications include epilepsy (5%–10%), gastrointestinal malformations (5%), hypothyroidism (5%), and leukemia (1%).

SOURCE: American Academy of Family Physicians, "Down Syndrome: Prenatal Risk Assessment and Diagnosis."

Report available online at http://www.aafp.org/afp/20000815/825.html. *(Table by PreMediaGlobal. © 2012 Cengage Learning.)*

child's parents. It is not inherited in most cases but is caused by a random genetic abnormality. The disorder is named for John Langdon Haydon Down (1828–1896) a British doctor who pioneered the care and education of children with the syndrome that now bears his name, as well as publishing the first scientific description of it in 1866. The cause of Down syndrome was finally identified in 1959 by Jérôme Lejeune (1926–1994), a French pediatrician and geneticist.

Down syndrome was sometimes referred to in the past as Mongolian idiocy or mongolism because the facial features of some children with the syndrome were thought to resemble those of people from Mongolia. In 1965 the World Health Organization (WHO) stated that *mongolism* should no longer be used as a synonym for Down syndrome, following a request from the organization's Mongolian delegate. Mongolism is presently considered a disrespectful term and should not be used in discussions of the condition, although the word still occasionally appears in print.

Demographics

Down syndrome is the most common human chromosomal abnormality. It occurs in about one in every 733 to 800 live births in the United States, or about 5,400 children per year. The rate is higher among children born to older parents, fathers as well as mothers. The mother's age is a risk factor for Down syndrome, rising from one chance in 1,562 in mothers 24 or younger to one in 19 in mothers over 45. Recent studies indicate that the father's age is also a factor; men 42 years and older are at increased risk of fathering a child with trisomy 21. These babies, however, represent only about a quarter of those conceived with trisomy 21. The condition is linked to so many heart defects and other problems that affect survival before birth that about 75% of fetuses conceived with Down syndrome are miscarried.

Down syndrome occurs with equal frequency in all races and ethnic groups worldwide. Boys are slightly more likely to be affected than girls; the gender ratio is 1.2:1. As of 2011, there were about 400,000 people with Down syndrome living in the United States.

Humans are not the only species affected by the syndrome; comparable conditions have been identified in mice and chimpanzees.

Description

The additional genetic material in Down syndrome results in characteristic physical features and intellectual disability. The average IQ scores of children with the syndrome are between 35 and 70. Characteristic facial features include a head that is smaller than average, upward-slanting eyes with a skin fold in the upper eyelid called an epicanthic fold, and a flattened nose. The hands are short and broad with short fingers, and they often have a single crease across the palm. Another characteristic feature of Down syndrome is hypotonia, which is the medical term for poor muscle tone. Children with Down syndrome often need extensive physical therapy in order to learn to walk and move normally, and are at increased risk of obesity as they grow older. In addition, normal growth is slowed; most of these children never reach full adult height. The average height for adult men with Down syndrome is 5 ft. 1 in. (1.5 m); for women, 4 ft. 9 in. (1.4 m).

Between 40% and 60% of infants with Down syndrome are born with severe heart defects; others have blockages of the esophagus and small intestine. These defects may require surgery shortly after birth. These children are also at increased risk of childhood leukemia.

Adolescents and adults with Down syndrome are more likely than other people to develop health problems that include frequent sinus and ear infections, cataracts, gastrointestinal reflux disease (GERD), hearing problems, sleep apnea, dislocated hips, and hypothyroidism.

Risk factors

There are three known risk factors for having a child with Down syndrome:

- Mother older than 35 years of age and/or father older than 42.
- Having a previous child with Down syndrome. A woman who has borne one child with the syndrome has about a 1% chance of having a second child with the condition.
- Either parent being a carrier of the genetic translocation for Down syndrome.

There are no lifestyle or environmental factors known to cause Down syndrome.

Causes and symptoms

Causes

Down syndrome results from genetic errors during the formation of germ cells (eggs and sperm) or during cell division shortly after the egg is fertilized by the sperm. The most common form of Down syndrome, responsible for about 95% of cases, occurs when an egg or sperm carrying two copies of chromosome 21 is involved in conception. The reason for the extra copy in

KEY TERMS

Chorionic villus sampling (CVS)—A prenatal test that involves taking a small sample of the placenta, the organ that forms inside the uterus during pregnancy and supplies the baby with oxygen and nutrients carried by the blood.

Chromosome—A microscopic thread-like structure found within each cell of the body and consists of a complex of proteins and DNA. Humans have 46 chromosomes arranged into 23 pairs. Changes in either the total number of chromosomes or their shape and size (structure) may lead to physical or mental abnormalities.

Congenital—Present at birth.

Epicanthic fold—A fold in the inner corner of the skin of the upper eyelid, found in about half of children with Down syndrome. The epicanthic fold is found in many people of Mongolian origin and is one of the features that led to earlier writers referring to Down syndrome as mongolism.

Germ cell—A cell involved in reproduction. In humans the germ cells are the sperm (male) and egg (female). Unlike other cells in the body, germ cells contain only half the standard number of chromosomes.

Hypotonia—The medical term for poor muscle tone.

Intellectual disability—Significant impairment in intellectual function and adaptation in society. Usually associated with an intelligence quotient (IQ) below 70.

Karyotype—A standard arrangement of photographic or computer-generated images of chromosome pairs from a cell in ascending numerical order, from largest to smallest.

Mosaic—A term referring to a genetic situation in which a person's cells do not have the exact same composition of chromosomes. In Down syndrome, this may mean that some cells have a normal number (46) of chromosomes while other cells have an abnormal 47 chromosomes.

Nondisjunction—Nonseparation of a chromosome pair during either meiosis or mitosis.

Translocation—The transfer of one part of a chromosome to another chromosome during cell division. A balanced translocation occurs when pieces from two different chromosomes exchange places without loss or gain of any chromosome material. An unbalanced translocation involves the unequal loss or gain of genetic information between two chromosomes.

Trisomy—The condition of having three identical chromosomes, instead of the normal two, in a cell.

Tubal ligation—A surgical procedure in which a woman's fallopian tubes are cut or blocked to prevent an egg from reaching the uterus for fertilization.

the abnormal germ cell is a genetic error called nondisjunction. During the normal process of germ cell formation, the paired chromosomes in the cell divide so that each daughter cell has only one member of the pair. In nondisjunction, one daughter cell gets both members of the chromosome pair and the other cell has none. If a germ cell carrying two copies of chromosome 21 is fertilized by a normal germ cell from the other parent, the child will have three copies of chromosome 21. This genetic error is called a full trisomy 21.

Some children with Down syndrome have some body cells with the extra copy of chromosome 21 and some body cells without the extra copy. This condition is called mosaic trisomy 21. It is thought to result from random errors in cell division during the early stages of fetal development. Mosaic trisomy 21 accounts for about 2% of children with Down syndrome.

About 3% of cases of Down syndrome occur in families with carriers. A part of chromosome 21 may become attached to chromosome 14 either before or at the moment of conception. This type of genetic error is called a balanced translocation because there is no extra material from chromosome 21. A person with this type of translocation looks normal and develops normally; however, he or she has an increased risk of having a child with full trisomy 21.

Symptoms

The extra chromosome 21 affects almost every organ system in the body. Some physical indications of Down syndrome in an infant include:

- an additional skin fold at the inner corner of upper eyelid (epicanthic fold)
- a short neck
- white spots on the iris of the eye known as Brushfield spots
- a round face

- ears that are smaller than normal
- a flattened area at the back of the head
- missing teeth or delayed development of teeth
- protruding tongue and a tendency to breathe through the mouth
- an extra-wide space between the big toe and second toe

Diagnosis

Most babies with Down syndrome are diagnosed at birth on the basis of their physical features. The **diagnosis** can be confirmed by a blood test and karyotype.

Tests

Down syndrome can be screened for and diagnosed before birth. Screening tests are used to estimate the chance that an individual woman will have a baby with Down syndrome. A test called the maternal serum alpha-fetoprotein test (MSAFP) is offered to all pregnant women under the age of 35. If the mother decides to have this test, it is performed between 15 and 22 weeks of pregnancy. The MSAFP screen measures a protein and two hormones that are normally found in maternal blood during pregnancy. A specific pattern of these hormones and protein can indicate an increased risk for having a baby born with Down syndrome. However, this is only a risk-assessment test; MSAFP cannot diagnose Down syndrome directly. Women found to have an increased risk of their babies being affected with Down syndrome are offered amniocentesis. The MSAFP test can detect up to 60% of all babies who will be born with Down syndrome.

Ultrasound screening for Down syndrome is also available. This is generally performed in the mid-trimester of pregnancy. Abnormal growth patterns characteristic of Down syndrome such as growth retardation, heart defects, duodenal atresia, T-E fistula, shorter than normal long-bone lengths, and extra folds of skin along the back of the neck of the developing fetus may all be observed via ultrasonic imaging.

The only way to definitively establish (with about 99% accuracy) the presence or absence of Down syndrome in a developing baby is to test a tissue sample during the pregnancy itself. Testing is usually done either by amniocentesis or chorionic villus sampling (CVS). All women under the age of 35 at high risk for having a baby affected with Down syndrome via an MSAFP screen and all mothers over the age of 35 are offered either CVS or amniocentesis. In CVS, a tiny tube is inserted into the opening of the uterus to retrieve a small sample of the placenta (the organ that attaches the growing baby to the mother via the umbilical cord, and provides oxygen and **nutrition**). In amniocentesis, a small amount of the fluid in which the baby is floating is withdrawn with a long thin needle. CVS may be performed as early as 10 to 12 weeks into a pregnancy. Amniocentesis is generally not performed until at least the fifteenth week. Both CVS and amniocentesis carry small risks of miscarriage. Approximately 1% of women miscarry after undergoing CVS testing, while approximately 0.5% miscarry after undergoing amniocentesis. Both amniocentesis and CVS allow the baby's own karyotype to be determined.

Treatment

Physical issues

There is no cure for Down syndrome. Medical and surgical treatment of children with trisomy 21 is highly individualized. Infants with heart defects or obstructions in the esophagus and digestive tract usually need immediate surgery. Older children require periodic checkups for cataracts, hearing loss, and thyroid problems. Some children need special medications and diuretics for heart problems, and most need to be monitored for frequent infections, particularly ear infections and pneumonia.

ALTERNATIVE. The National Down Syndrome Society (NDSS) notes that various alternative therapies, including pituitary extract, glutamic acid, thyroid hormone, 5-hydroxytryptophan, dimethyl sulfoxide (DMSO), dihydroepiandosterone, sicca cell therapy, vitamin and mineral supplements, and growth hormone have been recommended at various times as treatments for Down syndrome. Sicca cell therapy, also known as dry cell therapy, consists of injections of dried cells taken from fetal or newborn animals under the skin or into the muscle. This treatment has been shown to be dangerous.

The NDSS discourages parents from trying alternative therapies that claim to "normalize" their child's appearance or boost his or her intelligence. There is no harm, however, in using such complementary and alternative approaches as **art therapy**, **music therapy**, pet therapy, or certain types of movement therapy, provided the child enjoys the activity and the therapist is qualified to work with children who have Down syndrome.

Developmental issues

It is not possible to tell at birth whether a baby with Down syndrome will be severely disabled or will have low-normal intelligence. Individualized assessment of the child is critical to providing opportunities for full development. In general, children with mosaic Down syndrome have higher IQ scores than children with full trisomy 21. There are many adults with the syndrome who are able to hold jobs and live independently; some have become successful artists, actors, and singers. In addition, community and family support allows people with Down syndrome to have rich, meaningful relationships.

In general, children with Down syndrome develop on a slower timetable than other children. Some typical developmental milestones for children with Down syndrome are as follows, with the normal milestone in parentheses for purposes of comparison:

- Baby sits up without assistance: 6–30 months (5–9 months).
- Crawls: 8–22 months (6–12 months).
- Stands up: 1–3.25 years (8–17 months).
- Walks without assistance: 1–4 years (9–18 months).
- Says first word: 1–4 years (1–3 years).
- Uses first two-word phrase: 2–7.5 years (15–32 months).
- Smiles at people: 1.5–5 months (1–3 months).
- Eats with fingers: 10–24 months (7–14 months).
- Eats with a spoon: 13–39 months (12–20 months).
- Toilet trained: 2–7 years (16–42 months).
- Dresses self without assistance: 3.5–8.5 years (3.25–5 years).

It is important to keep this distinctive developmental timetable in mind because it affects psychiatric evaluation of mental health issues in children with Down syndrome.

At one time children with Down syndrome were either institutionalized or put in special education programs apart from other children. In the early 2010s, however, the emphasis in treatment is to give these children as many opportunities as possible to go to school with other children in their age group and participate in sports, group activities, and other aspects of social life during the growing years. Some community groups help families deal with the emotional effects of raising a child with Down syndrome. Schools are required to provide services to children with Down syndrome, sometimes in separate special education classrooms, and sometimes in regular classrooms (their presence in regular classrooms is called mainstreaming or inclusion).

Child development specialists recommend that children diagnosed with Down syndrome receive early **intervention**, which is a systematic program of therapy, exercises, and activities mandated by the Individuals with Disabilities Education Act (IDEA) of 2004. Early intervention can begin any time after birth up to age three; the 2004 amendments to IDEA allow states to continue early intervention programs until the child is eligible to enter kindergarten. Each state has its own set of regulations for early intervention. The most common types of early intervention treatments for infants with Down syndrome are physical therapy, speech and language therapy, and occupational therapy.

Mental health issues

In general, children with Down syndrome are at greater risk of developing a mental disorder than other children. Childhood behavioral problems in affected children are similar to those in other children; however, they typically appear at a later age and last longer. For example, the temper tantrums associated with the "terrible twos" in most children may not appear in a child with Down syndrome until age four. To make sure that a child with Down syndrome receives an accurate diagnostic evaluation for behavioral problems or other mental health issues, parents should:

- Make sure that the problem is not caused by or associated with a physical condition or disorder. Because children with Down syndrome can have disorders ranging from visual deficits and hearing loss to digestive disorders and anemia, their mood and behavior are often affected by physical complaints.
- Check to see whether there are stressors at home or in the school that are affecting the child and whether the stress level can be lowered.
- Work with a child psychologist or behavioral pediatrician on a behavior treatment plan based on the ABCs of behavior (Antecedent, Behavior, and Consequence of the behavior).

There were 33 trials of treatments for mental health issues in children with Down syndrome under way as of 2011. Most are trials of social skills therapy, **donepezil**, or vitamin therapy. There are also several trials of new screening and diagnostic measures for mothers at risk of having a child with Down syndrome.

The most common behavioral problems in children with Down syndrome are wandering away from home and oppositional or stubborn behavior. Oppositional behavior is often related to frustration with language and communication difficulties; in many cases this issue can be resolved by finding ways to help the child communicate more effectively, such as by using assistive communication devices.

DEMENTIA. As people with Down syndrome age, they face an increased chance of developing **Alzheimer's disease** (sometimes referred to as **dementia** or senility). Most people have a 12% chance of developing Alzheimer's, but almost all people with Down syndrome will have either Alzheimer's or a similar type of dementia by the age of 50. Alzheimer disease causes the brain to shrink and to break down. The number of brain cells decreases, and abnormal deposits and structural arrangements occur. This process results in a loss of brain functioning and eventual death. A study published by a group of Japanese researchers in 2011 reported that donepezil, a drug given to treat Alzheimer's, is also beneficial to patients with low IQs.

ATTENTION DEFICIT HYPERACTIVITY DISORDER. **Attention deficit hyperactivity disorder (ADHD)** is more common in children with Down syndrome than in the general population, although it usually appears at a later age. One study reported in 2011 that the prevalence of **ADHD** in the sample of children with Down syndrome was 49%. It is important to rule out an anxiety disorder or difficulties with processing language as possible reasons for the child's difficulties with attention. The treatment for ADHD in children with Down syndrome is the same as that for other children.

AUTISM SPECTRUM DISORDERS. As with ADHD, **autism** spectrum disorders manifest in children with Down syndrome at a later age, usually around six to eight years of age. It is estimated that 5% to 7% of children with Down syndrome also have autism spectrum disorders. Treatment is the same as for other children with autism; but it is important for the child to be identified as early as possible so that he or she can receive appropriate services in a timely fashion.

OBSESSIVE-COMPULSIVE DISORDER. Children with Down syndrome are more likely to develop OCD than other children. Symptoms usually develop at a later age than in other children but are often more intense. The obsessive behaviors typically take such forms as rearranging beads, insisting on sitting in the same chair all the time, or playing with belts, shoelaces, or other items of clothing.

DEPRESSION. **Depression** is reported to be more common in children as well as adults with Down syndrome, although it is often underdiagnosed and undertreated. Reasons for the increased risk of depression include the effects of physical disorders, differences in brain structure and function, language difficulties, and greater vulnerability in adult life to the loss of friends and family members. Antidepressant medications, **psychotherapy**, and **electroconvulsive therapy** (ECT) have all been reported to be effective in treating depression in patients with Down syndrome.

SEXUALITY AND FERTILITY. Girls with Down syndrome begin to menstruate on average at age 12-1/2, which is close to the same age as their peers in the general population, although some begin as early as 10 or as late as 14. About 50% of women with Down syndrome are fully capable of having children, although menopause typically begins around age 40. Between 35% and 50% of children born to mothers with Down syndrome are likely to have trisomy 21 or other developmental disabilities.

Boys with Down syndrome reach puberty at about the same age as their peers in the general population. There is limited information about fertility in males with Down syndrome, although there were at least two proven cases of paternity as of 2011. Most researchers believe that adult males with Down syndrome have lower sperm counts than other men. It is not known whether males with Down syndrome are more likely to father children who have the syndrome. Adult males with Down syndrome should always use contraception unless they have decided to start a family.

Given the increased life expectancy of people with Down syndrome and the ability of many to find employment and live in the community, education about human intimacy and sexuality is an important part of their transition to adult life. This education should include information about **sexual abuse**: how to recognize it, how to prevent it, and how to report it.

People with Down syndrome are as susceptible to sexually transmitted diseases as other adolescents and young adults, and need to be taught about the use of condoms and other contraceptives. Young women with Down syndrome can use any method of contraception of their choice without medical risk; however, the chosen method must be appropriate to the individual's ability to use it effectively. With regard to tubal ligation, many states have laws restricting access to this procedure for women with intellectual or developmental disabilities. If tubal ligation is considered, the woman with Down syndrome should be involved in the decision as much as possible.

Prognosis

People with Down syndrome have a shortened life expectancy in addition to a high risk of early Alzheimer's disease; they often show a noticeable loss of mental function by age 30. About 85% of babies born with trisomy 21 survive the first year of life, but only 50% will live to reach age 60. This is a great improvement, however, as the life expectancy of a person with Down syndrome was only 25 years as recently as 1980.

Congenital heart disorders are one reason for the present high mortality rate, as are vulnerability to infections, a high rate of disorders of the digestive tract, and premature aging. Children with Down syndrome are also more likely to develop leukemia than other children. In spite of these risks, the prognosis for a baby born with Down syndrome is better than ever before. Because of

> **QUESTIONS TO ASK YOUR DOCTOR**
>
> - Have you ever treated a child with Down syndrome? An adult?
> - What is your opinion of early intervention for children with the syndrome?
> - Do you think researchers will ever discover a cure for the syndrome?
> - Have you ever referred a couple for genetic counseling regarding their risk of having a baby with the syndrome?

modern medical treatments, including antibiotics to treat infections, and surgery to treat heart defects and duodenal atresia, the life expectancy of people with Down syndrome has greatly increased.

Prevention

There is no known way to prevent Down syndrome, because most cases of the syndrome are caused by a spontaneous mutation. Women can take steps before and during pregnancy to have a healthy pregnancy. Steps include taking a daily multivitamin with folic acid (400 micrograms), not smoking, and not drinking alcohol during pregnancy. Once a couple has had one baby with Down syndrome, they are often concerned about the likelihood of future offspring also being born with the disorder.

When a baby with Down syndrome has the type that results from a translocation, it is possible that one of the two parents is a carrier of a balanced translocation. A carrier has rearranged chromosomal information and can pass it on, but he or she does not have an extra chromosome and is not affected with the disorder. When one parent is a carrier of a translocation, the chance of future offspring having Down syndrome is greatly increased. The specific risk can be assessed by a genetic counselor. Adults who are concerned that they may have a balanced translocation of chromosome 21 can choose to have a karyotype to see whether their chromosomes are in fact abnormal. Pregnant women over 35 should have tests during the first trimester (three-month period) of pregnancy to screen for the syndrome.

Resources

BOOKS

Burack, Jacob A., et al., eds. *Oxford Handbook of Intellectual Disability and Development*, 2nd ed. New York: Oxford University Press, 2011.

Chicoine, Brian, and Dennis McGuire. *Guide to Good Health for Teens and Adults with Down Syndrome*. Bethesda, MD: Woodbine House, 2010.

Goldstein, Sam, and Cecil R. Reynolds, eds. *Handbook of Neurodevelopmental and Genetic Disorders in Children*, 2nd ed. New York: Guilford Press, 2011.

Royston, Angela. *Explaining Down Syndrome*. Mankato, MN: Smart Apple Press, 2010.

Simons, Jo Ann. *The Down Syndrome Transition Handbook: Charting Your Child's Course to Adulthood*. Bethesda, MD: Woodbine House, 2010.

Skallerup, Susan J., ed. *Babies with Down Syndrome: A New Parents' Guide*, 3rd ed. Bethesda, MD: Woodbine House, 2008.

PERIODICALS

Calles, J.L., Jr. "Cognitive-adaptive Disabilities." *Pediatric Clinics of North America* 58 (February 2011): 189–203.

Couzens, D., et al. "Cognitive Development and Down Syndrome: Age-related Change on the Stanford-Binet Test (Fourth Edition)." *American Journal on Intellectual and Developmental Disabilities* 116 (May 2011): 181–204.

Ekstein, S., et al. "Down Syndrome and Attention-Deficit/Hyperactivity Disorder (ADHD)." *Journal of Child Neurology* (May 31, 2011) [e-pub. ahead of print].

Gray, L., et al. "The Continuing Challenge of Diagnosing Autism Spectrum Disorder in Children with Down Syndrome." *Child Care, Health and Development* 37 (July 2011): 459–461.

Kondoh, T., et al. "Donepezil Significantly Improves Abilities in Daily Lives of Female Down Syndrome Patients with Severe Cognitive Impairment: A 24-week Randomized, Double-blind, Placebo-controlled Trial." *International Journal of Psychiatry in Medicine* 41 (January 2011): 71–89.

Landt, J., et al. "Age-related Changes in Plasma Dehydroepiandrosterone Levels in Adults with Down's Syndrome and the Risk of Dementia." *Journal of Neuroendocrinology* 23 (May 2011): 450–455.

Rissman, R.A., and W.C. Mobley. "Implications for Treatment: GABAA Receptors in Aging, Down Syndrome and Alzheimer's Disease." *Journal of Neurochemistry* 117 (May 2011): 613–622.

Urv, T.K., et al. "Psychiatric Symptoms in Adults with Down Syndrome and Alzheimer's Disease." *American Journal on Intellectual and Developmental Disabilities* 115 (July 2010): 265–276.

Walker, J.C., et al. "Depression in Down Syndrome: A Review of the Literature." *Research in Developmental Disabilities* 32 (September-October 2011): 1432–1440.

WEBSITES

Chen, Harold. "Genetics of Down Syndrome." Medscape. November 29, 2011. http://emedicine.medscape.com/article/943216-overview (accessed December 12, 2011).

Mayo Clinic. "Down Syndrome." Medscape. November 29, 2011. http://www.mayoclinic.com/health/down-syndrome/DS00182 (accessed December 12, 2011).

National Human Genome Research Institute (NHGRI). "Learning about Down Syndrome." http://www.genome.gov/19517824 (accessed August 23, 2011).

National Institute of Child Health and Human Development (NICHD). "Down Syndrome." http://www.nichd.nih.gov/health/topics/Down_Syndrome.cfm (accessed August 23, 2011).

Patterson, Bonnie. "Managing Behavior." National Down Syndrome Society (NDSS). http://www.ndss.org/index.php?option=com_ content&view=article&id=69&Itemid=90 (accessed December 15, 2011).

Virginia Commonwealth University Life Sciences. "On Down Syndrome." [9-1/2 minute video about the condition.] http://www.youtube.com/watch?v=bEV kbuooXo4 (accessed August 23, 2011).

ORGANIZATIONS

American Academy of Child and Adolescent Psychiatry (AACAP), 3615 Wisconsin Avenue, N.W., Washington, DC, United States, 20016-3007, (202) 966-7300, Fax: (202) 966-2891, http://www.aacap.org.

American Psychiatric Association (APA), 1000 Wilson Boulevard, Suite 1825, Arlington, VA, United States, 22209-3901, (703) 907-7300, apa@psych.org, http://www.psych.org.

National Down Syndrome Society (NDSS), 666 Broadway, 8th Floor, New York, NY, United States, 10012, Fax: (212) 979-2873, (800) 221-4602, info@ndss.org, http://www.ndss.org/index.php.

National Human Genome Research Institute (NHGRI), Building 31, Room 4B09, 31 Center Drive, MSC 2152, 9000 Rockville Pike, Bethesda, MD, United States, 20892-2152, (301) 402-0911, Fax: (301) 402-2218, http://www.genome.gov.

National Institute of Child Health and Human Development Information Resource Center, PO Box 3006, Rockville, MD, United States, 20847, Fax: (866) 760-5947, (800) 370-2943, NICHDInformationResourceCenter@mail.nih.gov, http://www.nichd.nih.gov.

Rebecca J. Frey, PhD

Doxepin

Definition

Doxepin is a tricyclic antidepressant. It is sold in the United States under the brand name Sinequan and is also available under its generic name.

Purpose

Doxepin is used primarily to treat **depression** and to treat the combination of symptoms of anxiety and depression. Like most **antidepressants**, doxepin has also been used to treat **panic disorder**, **obsessive-compulsive disorder**,**attention deficit hyperactivity disorder** (ADHD), **enuresis** (bed-wetting), eating disorders such as **bulimia nervosa**, **cocaine** dependency, and the depressive phase of bipolar (manic-depressive) disorder. It has also been used to support **smoking cessation** programs.

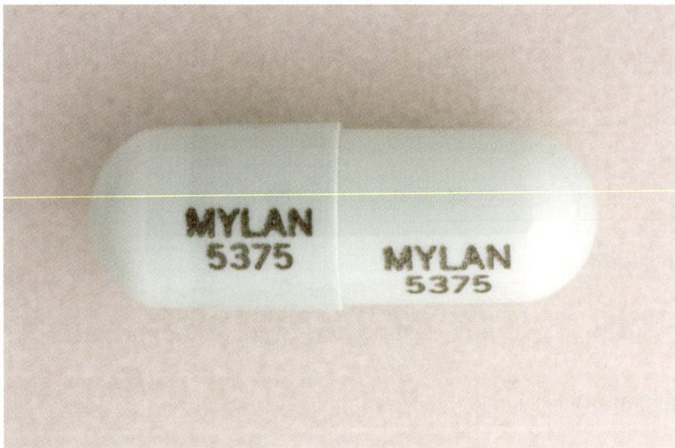

Doxepin. *(© Custom Medical Stock Photo, Inc. Reproduced by permission.)*

Description

Doxepin acts to change the balance of naturally occurring chemicals in the **brain** that regulate the transmission of nerve impulses between cells. Its action primarily increases the concentration of norepinephrine and **serotonin** (both chemicals that stimulate nerve cells) and, to a lesser extent, blocks the action of another brain chemical, acetylcholine. Although not technically a tricyclic antidepressant, doxepin shares most of the properties of these drugs, which include **amitriptyline**, **clomipramine**, **desipramine**, **imipramine**, **nortriptyline**, **protriptyline**, and **trimipramine**. Studies comparing doxepin with these other drugs have shown that doxepin is no more or less effective than other antidepressants of its type. Its choice for treatment is as much a function of physician preference as any other factor.

The therapeutic effects of doxepin, like other antidepressants, appear slowly. Maximum benefit is often not evident for at least two weeks after starting the drug. People taking doxepin should be aware of this and continue taking the drug as directed even if they do not see immediate improvement.

Recommended dosage

As with any antidepressant, doxepin must be carefully adjusted by the physician to produce the desired therapeutic effect. Doxepin is available as 10 mg, 25 mg, 50 mg, 75 mg, 100 mg, and 150 mg oral capsules as well as an oral concentrate solution containing 10 mg of drug in each milliliter of solution.

Therapy is usually started at 30–150 mg per day and gradually increased to 300 mg daily if needed. There is little evidence that doses above 300 mg daily provide any additional benefits. Amounts up to 150 mg may be taken as a single dose at bedtime to decrease daytime sleepiness. Doses of more than 150 mg per day should be divided into two or three doses and taken throughout the day.

In patients over age 60, therapy should be maintained at the low end of the dosing range and increased cautiously and with physician supervision. Patients with organic brain syndrome (psychiatric symptoms of **dementia** often seen in elderly patients) generally require daily doses of only 25–50 mg.

If the oral concentrate of doxepin is used, each dose should be diluted in at least 4 oz (120 mL) of milk, orange, prune, tomato, pineapple, or grapefruit juice just before administration. Doxepin is not compatible with many carbonated beverages and should not be diluted in them.

Precautions

As with other tricyclic antidepressants, doxepin should be used cautiously and with close physician supervision in people, especially the elderly, who have benign prostatic hypertrophy, urinary retention, and glaucoma, especially angle-closure glaucoma (the most severe form). Before starting treatment, people with these conditions should discuss the relative risks and benefits of treatment with their doctors to help determine if doxepin is the right antidepressant for them.

Several antidepressants, including doxepin, have been found to potentially increase the risk of suicidal thoughts and actions in patients younger than 25. All persons taking doxepin, regardless of age, should be monitored for signs of worsening depression or self-harm.

Doxepin may increase heart rate and stress on the heart. It may be dangerous for people with cardiovascular disease, especially those who have recently had a heart attack, to take this drug or other antidepressants in the same pharmacological class. In rare cases where patients with cardiovascular disease must receive doxepin, they should be monitored closely for cardiac rhythm disturbances and signs of cardiac stress or damage. Doxepin may also increase the possibility of having **seizures**. Patients should tell their physician if they have a history of seizures, including seizures brought on by the abuse of drugs or alcohol. These people should use doxepin only with caution and be closely monitored by their physician.

A common problem with antidepressants is sedation (drowsiness, lack of physical and mental alertness). This side effect is especially noticeable early in therapy. In most patients, sedation decreases or disappears entirely with time, but until then patients taking doxepin should not perform activities requiring mental alertness, such as driving or operating machinery.

Doxepin should not be taken by nursing mothers because it is secreted into breast milk and may cause side effects in the nursing infant.

Side effects

Doxepin shares the side effects of tricyclic antidepressants. The most frequent of these are dry mouth, constipation, urinary retention, increased heart rate, sedation, irritability, dizziness, and decreased coordination. As with most side effects associated with tricyclic antidepressants, the intensity is highest at the beginning of therapy and tends to decrease with continued use.

Dry mouth, if severe to the point of causing difficulty speaking or swallowing, may be managed by dosage reduction or temporary discontinuation of the drug. Patients may also chew sugarless gum or suck on sugarless candy in order to increase the flow of saliva. Some artificial saliva products may give temporary relief.

Men with prostate enlargement who take doxepin may be especially likely to have problems with urinary retention. Symptoms include having difficulty starting a urine flow and more difficulty than usual passing urine. In most cases, urinary retention is managed with dose reduction or by switching to another type of antidepressant. In extreme cases, patients may require treatment with bethanechol, a drug that reverses this particular side effect. People who think they may be experiencing any side effects from this or any other medication should tell their physicians.

Interactions

Dangerously high blood pressure has resulted from the combination of antidepressants such as doxepin and members of another class of antidepressants known as **monoamine oxidase inhibitors (MAOIs)**. Because of this, doxepin should never be taken in combination with **MAOIs**. Patient's taking any MAOIs, for example Nardil (**phenelzine** sulfate) or Parnate (**tranylcypromine** sulfate), should stop the MAOI then wait at least 14 days before starting doxepin or any tricyclic antidepressant. The same holds true when discontinuing doxepin and starting an MAOI.

Doxepin may decrease the blood pressure–lowering effects of **clonidine**. Patients who take both drugs should be monitored for loss of blood-pressure control and the dose of clonidine increased as needed.

KEY TERMS

Acetylcholine—A naturally occurring chemical in the body that transmits nerve impulses from cell to cell. Generally, it has opposite effects from dopamine and norepinephrine; it causes blood vessels to dilate, lowers blood pressure, and slows the heartbeat. Central nervous system well-being is dependent on a balance among acetylcholine, dopamine, serotonin, and norepinephrine.

Anticholinergic—Related to the ability of a drug to block the nervous system chemical acetylcholine. When acetylcholine is blocked, patients often experience dry mouth and skin, increased heart rate, blurred vision, and difficulty urinating. In severe cases, blocking acetylcholine may cloud thinking and cause delirium.

Benign prostate hypertrophy—Enlargement of the prostate gland.

Norepinephrine—A neurotransmitter in the brain that acts to constrict blood vessels and raise blood pressure. It works in combination with serotonin.

Organic brain syndrome—A class of disorders characterized by progressive deterioration of mental processes caused by temporary brain dysfunction or permanent brain damage. Symptoms include delusions, dementia, amnesia, and delirium that are not caused by drugs, alcohol, or as a side effect of medication.

Serotonin—A widely distributed neurotransmitter that is found in blood platelets, the lining of the digestive tract, and the brain, and that works in combination with norepinephrine. It causes very powerful contractions of smooth muscle, and is associated with mood, attention, emotions, and sleep. Low levels of serotonin are associated with depression.

The sedative effects of doxepin are increased by other central nervous system depressants such as alcohol, **sedatives**, sleeping medications, antihistamines, or medications used for other mental disorders such as **schizophrenia**. The anticholinergic effects of doxepin are additive with other anticholinergic drugs such as **benztropine**, **biperiden**, **trihexyphenidyl**, and antihistamines.

Resources

BOOKS

American Society of Health-System Pharmacists. *AHFS Drug Information 2008*. Bethesda, MD: American Society of Health-System Pharmacists, 2008.

DeVane, C. Lindsay, Pharm.D. "Drug Therapy for Mood Disorders." In *Fundamentals of Monitoring Psychoactive Drug Therapy*. Baltimore: Williams and Wilkins, 1990.

Jack Raber, PharmD

Draw-a-person test *see* **Figure drawings**

DSM *see* **Diagnostic and Statistical Manual of Mental Disorders**

Dual diagnosis *see* **Co-occurring disorders**

Duloxetine

Definition

Duloxetine is a medication used to treat a variety of nervous system oriented illnesses, including **depression** and neuropathic pain. Neuropathic pain is pain generated by the nervous system, also known as neurogenic pain. Duloxetine belongs to a class of drugs known as selective **serotonin** norepinephrine reuptake inhibitors (SSNRI), which specifically acts on two chemicals called serotonin and norepinephrine. These chemicals are types of neurotransmitter involved in normal **brain** function. These **neurotransmitters** can affect the physiological state of clinical depression as well as neuropathic pain.

Purpose

Duloxetine can be used to treat a broad range of mood and stress-related psychiatric illnesses as well as illnesses involving neuropathic pain. It is mainly used to treat clinical depression, **generalized anxiety disorder** (GAD), and pain associated with diabetic peripheral neuropathy or fibromyalgia. Choice of using duloxetine

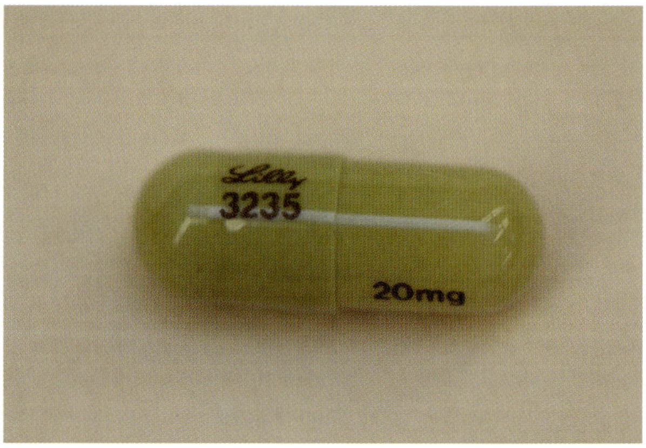

Cymbalta (duloxetine), 20 mg. *(© Custom Medical Stock Photo, Inc. Reproduced by permission.)*

alone or in combination with other drugs depends on the medical disorder and individual health parameters.

Description

Duloxetine has a therapeutic mechanism of action that is focused on the modulation of the natural body chemicals serotonin and norepinephrine. Serotonin and norepinephrine are types of neurotransmitters in the nervous system, chemicals that neurons use to signal one another in complex pathways for normal brain and body functioning. Neurotransmitters like serotonin and norepinephrine bind to chemical receptors on the surface of neurons (brain cells). Once bound to a receptor they affect physiological processes.

The receptors activate a sequence of cellular events known as a chemical cascade or signaling pathway. Neurotransmitter signaling pathways are responsible for many regulatory processes including neuronal signaling that affects mood and pain. During the signaling process, neurotransmitters such as serotonin travel from one neuron to the next. These chemicals need to cross a short space between the end of one neuron and the beginning of the next neuron known as the synapse or synaptic space. Serotonin or norepinephrine is released from the end of neuron one, crosses the synaptic space, and binds to a neurotransmitter-specific receptor on the surface of the next neuron (neuron two). Any extra serotonin or norepinephrine that is left in the synaptic space is taken back up by neuron one in a process known as reuptake. The more neurotransmitter allowed to remain in the synaptic space, the more will eventually be allowed to bind to receptors on neuron two and participate in the signaling process.

Selective serotonin and norepinephrine reuptake inhibitors like duloxetine decrease the reuptake of these neurotransmitters by neuron one, allowing more serotonin or norepinephrine to be present in the synapse and, therefore, more neurotransmitter signaling to occur. It is believed that a decrease in serotonin and norepinephrine signaling contributes to illness such as depression and **anxiety disorders**. Selective serotonin and norepinephrine reuptake inhibitors help by increasing signaling, with little effect on the synaptic levels of other neurotransmitters. An increase in serotonin and norepinephrine in the spinal cord is believed to inhibit the signaling of neurogenic pain pathways, hence their use in controlling pain associated with diabetic neuropathy or fibromyalgia.

Whether a patient is going to benefit from any SSNRI medication may have a genetic component. Individual response to each SSNRI varies greatly, and these drugs tend to require several weeks to take effect. The initial trial of an SSNRI can be difficult because the side effects begin right away while the beneficial effects take up to two weeks to develop. The particular SSNRI that works best for one patient may have no effect on another patient. Also, having no response to one SSNRI does not mean that a patient will not have a good therapeutic response to another SSNRI. Finding which SSNRI is going to work for a patient may require a trial of multiple drugs until an effective agent is found. Generally, an agent is attempted for four to six weeks before concluding it will not have an effect and switching to another agent. If there is an effect but the healthcare provider judges it could be improved, the dose is often increased as the patient is able to tolerate. Duloxetine is often the SSNRI of initial choice, because it is effective and generally well tolerated by many patients.

Recommended dosage

Duloxetine is taken as an oral medication. The dosage used varies depending on the medical condition being treated, individual patient response to the medication regarding its effectiveness, and individual patient response to the medication regarding side effects. Some people naturally require a higher dose of duloxetine in order to achieve the desired effect. Other patients require a lower dose either for effect or because they quickly develop side effects that are not tolerable.

Duloxetine used for **major depressive disorder** and generalized anxiety disorder is usually dosed at 60 mg daily. Duloxetine used for neuropathic pain in diabetic neuropathy or fibromyalgia is dosed similarly. This dose can be taken in one pill or in increments of 30 mg twice daily if a patient tolerates smaller doses better than large ones. Patients may start at a lower 30 mg daily dose for the first week of treatment and gradually work their way up to the dose needed for effect in 10 mg weekly implements or may go directly to a 60 mg daily dose after a week at 30 mg per day. The elderly are usually started at a lower dose, due to their increased sensitivity to these medications and their side effects. The maximum dose that may be used is 120 mg per day, but doses higher than 60 mg per day have rarely been shown to improve symptoms further and may not be tolerable to the patient. Patients are dosed at the lowest possible effective dose to avoid the development of adverse side effects. Slowly increasing the dose over time helps with minimizing side effects, and some side effects become lessened with continued use. Patients are periodically reassessed to determine whether there is need for continued treatment with duloxetine. All SSNRIs, including duloxetine, need to be slowly tapered off if discontinued, to avoid a discontinuation withdrawal syndrome.

Precautions

SSNRIs have many side effects. It usually takes several weeks of medication for the treatment effect to occur, while the undesirable side effects may occur at the onset of treatment. When an SSNRI is prescribed to a patient with a disease like major depression or severe pain, this time lapse in beneficial versus adverse effects may be difficult for patient **compliance** with treatment. The classic description is patients who are already feeling depressed or in pain take an SSNRI, experience side effects and so feel worse, all while being told that they will eventually get better. This situation can be frustrating for patients with depression or severe pain. Fortunately, SSNRIs do help many people and have fewer overall side effects than some older medications used for the same purpose. Great benefit may be gained if a patient is able to get past the first couple weeks of treatment.

It takes some time to determine whether a particular SSNRI such as duloxetine will work for an individual patient. Each SSNRI is tried for four to six weeks to determine whether it is the appropriate agent for a patient. Having one SSNRI fail in treatment for an individual patient does not mean that another SSNRI will not work for that person. Sometimes multiple drugs need to be attempted under physician care before the proper treatment is found for a patient. Duloxetine has a high success rate and is often chosen as the first SSNRI to try for a patient.

When a patient discontinues the use of duloxetine, the dose needs to be tapered down slowly. SSNRIs have little to no abuse potential. However, if an SSNRI is abruptly discontinued without tapering, there may be symptoms of withdrawal known as SSNRI discontinuation syndrome. Withdrawal symptoms of this syndrome may include flu-like symptoms, anxiety, agitation, vivid or bizarre dreams, **insomnia**, nausea, vomiting, diarrhea, sense of imbalance, chills, **fatigue**, dizziness, headache, numbness and tingling of the extremities, and other sensory disturbances. Discontinuation syndrome may be avoided completely if the dose of duloxetine is properly tapered down over time.

SSNRI overdose may result in a condition known as **serotonin syndrome**, also called serotonin toxicity, serotonin poisoning, and serotonin storm. Serotonin overdose may be caused by taking multiple drugs that increase the amount of serotonin signaling in the body. While chemical signaling pathways are a part of normal brain function, over-activation can be dangerous. Drugs that increase serotonin signaling may do so by increasing the amount of serotonin available to bind to and activate receptors or by directly activating serotonin receptors. These drugs can cause serotonin overdose if used at the same time or in time periods too close together. Symptoms of serotonin overdose may range from mild to life-threatening, depending on the individual situation. Symptoms may include high blood pressure, high fever, nausea, diarrhea, headache, sweating, increased heart rate, tremor, muscle twitching, **delirium**, shock, coma, and death.

Duloxetine may be contraindicated or may require caution in use in patients with uncontrolled hypertension, liver function impairment or liver disease, kidney function impairment, seizure disorder, bleeding disorders, glaucoma, dehydration, history of alcohol abuse, and in patients under 25 years of age or the elderly. Kidney and liver function, as well as blood pressure and behavioral changes, may be monitored while taking duloxetine. SSNRIs such as duloxetine are discouraged from use in patients with **bipolar disorder**, as they can induce a state of mania in these individuals. There are selective conditions under which a doctor may prescribe an SSNRI such as duloxetine to a bipolar patient for a short period of time under careful monitoring. Duloxetine is classified as category C for pregnancy, which means either there are no adequate human or animal studies; or that adverse fetal effects were found in animal studies, but there is no available human data. The decision whether or not to use category C drugs in pregnancy is generally based on weighing the critical needs of the mother against the risk to the fetus. Other lower category agents are used whenever possible. The safety of duloxetine use during breast-feeding is unknown and its use is not recommended.

Side effects

SSNRIs are known for having fewer side effects than other types of older antidepressant medications that act on many types of neurotransmitter, which is one reason why they tend to be the drug of choice in treatment of depression. However, as with all medication, SSNRIs such as duloxetine do have side effects. Sensitivity to duloxetine varies among patients, and some patients may find lower doses are more than their body system can tolerate. Common side effects of duloxetine include nausea, headache, dizziness, constipation, sexual dysfunction, diarrhea, sweating, dry mouth, shakiness, tremor, loss of appetite, weight changes, hot flashes, elevated blood pressure, yawning, anxiety, and insomnia. Rare but serious potential side effects include mania, worsened depression and suicidality, **seizures**, serotonin syndrome, discontinuation syndrome, electrolyte imbalances, urinary retention, skin reactions, abnormal bleeding, liver damage, and glaucoma.

Interactions

Patients should make their doctor aware of all medications and supplements they are taking before using duloxetine. Using alcohol while taking duloxetine may create toxic reactions in the body and should be

KEY TERMS

Bipolar disorder—Psychiatric mood disorder characterized by periods of manic behavior that may alternate with periods of depression, also known as manic depressive disorder.

Cytochrome P450 (CYP450)—Enzymes present in the liver that metabolize drugs.

Diabetic peripheral neuropathy—Complication of long–term diabetes involving damage to nerves in the periphery (outside of the brain and spinal cord) that may include symptoms such as numbness and burning pain.

Fibromyalgia—Chronic condition in which patients experience widespread musculoskeletal pain and fatigue; an amplified neuropathic pain pathway may be involved.

Glaucoma—Condition involving increased pressure within the eye that may cause damage and blindness.

Mania—Physiological state of hyperactivity experienced by patients with certain psychiatric illnesses involving inappropriate elevated mood, pressured speech, poor judgment, and sometimes psychotic episodes superimposed on the state of mania.

Monoamine oxidase inhibitors (MAOIs)—Type of antidepressant medication that affects various kinds of neurotransmitters including serotonin.

Neuropathic pain—State of pain also known as neurogenic pain that is caused by neurotransmitter signaling in nervous system pain pathways between either the peripheral nervous system or the spinal cord and the brain.

Neurotransmitter—A chemical messenger that travels through the body and acts in the nervous system. Neurotransmitter signaling is responsible for a wide range of bodily processes and is often the target of medications involving the brain and cardiovascular system.

Neurotransmitter receptor—A physical recipient for chemicals called neurotransmitters. Receptors sit on the surface of cells that make up body tissues, and once bound to the neurotransmitter, they initiate the chemical signaling pathway associated with neurotransmitters.

Selective serotonin norepinephrine reuptake inhibitors (SSNRI)—Drug class that acts to specifically inhibit the reuptake of serotonin and norepinephrine in the neuronal synapse with little effect on other types of neurotransmitters, thereby decreasing side effects associated with broader acting drugs.

Selective serotonin reuptake inhibitors (SSRI)—Drug class that acts to specifically inhibit the reuptake of serotonin only in the neuronal synapse with little effect on other types of neurotransmitters, thereby decreasing side effects associated with broader acting drugs.

Serotonin—A type of neurotransmitter involved in regulation of the blood vessels, brain processes, and disease states such as depression.

Serotonin syndrome—A potentially life threatening drug reaction involving an excess of the neurotransmitter serotonin, usually occurring when too many medications that increase serotonin are taken together such as antimigraine triptans and certain antidepressants.

Synapse—Physical space between neurons that allows the passage of neurotransmitters for chemical signaling pathways.

avoided. Duloxetine is metabolized by a set of liver enzymes known as cytochrome P450 (CYP450). There are many subtypes of CYP450 enzymes and duloxetine interacts with multiple subtypes. Drugs that induce or activate these enzymes may increase the metabolism of duloxetine. This results in lower levels of therapeutic medication, thereby negatively affecting treatment. Drugs that act to inhibit the action of CYP450 may cause undesired increased levels of duloxetine in the body. This could lead to increased side effects or even toxic doses. Likewise duloxetine may affect the metabolism of other drugs, leading to greater or lower doses than therapeutically desired.

SSNRIs such as duloxetine should not be used at the same time as other medications that increase levels of serotonin in the neuronal synapse. Too much serotonin signaling may lead to the medical condition serotonin syndrome, which can be severe and life threatening. **Antidepressants** called **selective serotonin reuptake inhibitors (SSRIs)** are similar to duloxetine, except for lacking effects on the neurotransmitter norepinephrine, and should not be used concurrently due to additive effects. Antidepressants called **monoamine oxidase inhibitors (MAOIs)** increase the amount of serotonin released into the synapse and cannot be used concurrently with duloxetine. Switching drug treatment for an

QUESTIONS TO ASK YOUR DOCTOR

- Can I take the full dose right away or do I need to slowly increase the dose?
- Can I stop taking the medication right away or do I need to slowly decrease the dose?
- When should I eat in reference to taking this medication?
- What time of day should I take this medication?
- How long should I take this medication before I am reassessed?
- Will this medication interact with any of my other prescription medications?
- Are there any over-the-counter medications I should not take with this medicine?
- What are the side effects I should watch for?
- Can I drink alcoholic beverages in the same time frame as taking this medication?

individual patient from an MAOI to duloxetine may require a waiting period of up to two weeks between drugs. Switching from duloxetine to an MAOI may require a waiting period of up to five weeks duration. Another example of a medication that has additive serotonin effects with duloxetine is sumatriptan (Imitrex). Sumatriptan is used to treat migraine headaches and acts directly on serotonin receptors in the brain to activate their serotonin signaling pathway. The combination of an SSNRI increasing the amount of serotonin available to activate serotonin receptor signaling pathways, and sumatriptan directly activating serotonin receptor signaling pathways, may produce undesirable additive effects or overdose. Other drugs that cannot be combined with duloxetine due to risk of serotonin syndrome are the antipsychotics **chlorpromazine** and **fluphenazine**, as well as the herbal supplements yohimbe and **St. John's wort**.

By inhibiting specific subtypes of CYP450, SSNRIs such as duloxetine may dangerously increase the levels of other drugs in the body that would have otherwise been metabolized by the CYP450. Duloxetine may inhibit the metabolism of heart drugs such as **propranolol**, known as **beta blockers**, causing increased toxic levels of propranolol in the blood. Other drugs may cause toxicity when used with duloxetine, either through additive effects or through inhibition of duloxetine metabolism causing toxic levels of duloxetine in the blood. Drugs that may cause toxicity with duloxetine include diuretics (water pills) such as hydrochlorothiazide, diet pills such as sibutramine (Meridia), caffeine, the heart drug amiodarone, certain antibiotics such as ciprofloxacin and linezolid, mood stabilizers such as lithium, antipsychotics such as **haloperidol** and **clozapine**, and certain anti-seizure drugs such as phenytoin. There is increased risk of internal bleeding when duloxetine is used with anticoagulant drugs such as aspirin, warfarin, or large doses of the herbal supplements red clover, **ginkgo biloba**, feverfew, or concentrated green tea. Duloxetine cannot be combined with the antipsychotic medications **pimozide** (Orap) or **thioridazine** (Mellaril) due to dangerous cardiac complications.

Resources

BOOKS

Brunton, Laurence L., et al. *Goodman and Gilman's The Pharmacological Basis of Therapeutics.* 12th ed. New York: McGraw Hill Medical, 2011.

Stargrove, Mitchell Bebel, et al. *Herb, Nutrient, and Drug Interactions: Clinical Implications and Therapeutic Strategies.* St. Louis: Mosby, 2007.

ORGANIZATIONS

American College of Neuropsychopharmacology, 5034-A Thoroughbred Lane, Brentwood, TN, 37027, (615) 324-2360, Fax: (615) 523-1715, acnp@acnp.org, http://www.acnp.org.

American Psychiatric Association, 1000 Wilson Blvd., Ste. 1825, Arlington, VA, 22209-3901, (703) 907-7300, apa@psych.org, http://www.psych.org.

American Society for Clinical Pharmacology and Therapeutics, 528 N Washington St., Alexandria, VA, 22314, (703) 836-6981, info@ascpt.org, http://www.ascpt.org.

Mental Health America, 2000 N Beauregard St., 6th Fl., Alexandria, VA, 22311, (703) 684-7722, (800) 969-6642, Fax: (703) 684-5968, http://www.nmha.org.

Maria Eve Basile, PhD

Dyslexia *see* **Reading disorder**

Dyspareunia

Definition

Dyspareunia is painful sexual intercourse. The same term is used whether the pain results from a medical or a psychosocial problem. Dyspareunia may be diagnosed in men and women, although the **diagnosis** is rare in men;

when it does occur in men, it is almost always caused by a physical problem.

Because of the prevalence of this problem among women in the context of psychosocial associations, only women's experiences are emphasized.

Demographics

About 15% of women may have pain with intercourse at some point in their lives. About 1–2% have true dyspareunia. The incidence is much higher in women who have been raped or otherwise sexually abused. Dyspareunia in men is rare.

Description

Dyspareunia is any pain experienced any time before, during, or following sexual intercourse. The pain may be located in the genitals or within the pelvis. It is not unusual for women to occasionally have pain during intercourse. This is not true dyspareunia.

A woman who has dyspareunia often also has **vaginismus**. Vaginismus is an involuntary tightening of the vaginal muscles in response to penetration. It can make intercourse painful or impossible.

The professional's handbook, the ***Diagnostic and Statistical Manual of Mental Disorders***, fourth edition, text revised (*DSM-IV-TR*), classifies this condition as a sexual dysfunction. There is considerably controversy about whether or not dyspareunia should continue to be classified as it has been in the *DSM-IV*, with some practitioners arguing for its reclassification in the *DSM-5* as a **pain disorder**. The *DSM-5* (to be published in 2013) proposes subsuming dyspareunia into a new disorder: Genito-Pelvic Pain/Penetration Disorder. It also proposes listing dyspareunia in males as a diagnosis not elsewhere specified because of the infrequent use of this diagnosis in males.

Causes and symptoms

Causes

Psychosocial causes of dyspareunia include:

- Prior sexual trauma. Many women who have been raped or sexually abused as children may have dyspareunia. Even when a woman wishes to have sex with someone later, the act of intercourse may trigger memories of the trauma and interfere with her enjoyment of the act. Vaginismus often occurs in such situations.
- Guilt, anxiety, or tension about sex. Any of these can cause tense vaginal muscles and also prevent arousal from occurring. People who were raised with the idea that sex is bad may be more prone to have this problem. Fear of pregnancy may make arousal difficult.
- Prior physical trauma to the vaginal area. Women who have had an accidental injury or surgery in the vaginal area may become sensitive to penetration. Vaginismus is common in these cases.
- Depression or anxiety in general. Either of these can lead to loss of interest in sex. This can be experienced by either sex.
- Problems in a relationship. Dyspareunia may occur when a woman feels her sexual partner is abusive or emotionally distant, she is no longer attracted to her partner, or she fears her partner is no longer attracted to her. Men, too, can lose interest in sex because of prior emotional trauma in a relationship; however, the result is usually impotence, rather than dyspareunia.
- Vasocongestion, which can occur when either partner frequently becomes aroused but does not reach orgasm. Vasocongestion is a pooling of blood in dilated blood vessels. Normally, the pelvic area becomes congested with blood when a person becomes sexually aroused. This congestion goes away quickly after orgasm. If there is no orgasm, the congestion takes much longer to resolve.

Any of these factors may cause painful sex. The affected person may then associate pain with sex and find it even harder to relax and become aroused in the future.

Symptoms

The *DSM-IV* diagnostic criteria for dyspareunia are as follows:

- Recurrent or persistent genital pain associated with sexual intercourse in either a male or a female.
- The disturbance causes marked distress or interpersonal difficulty.
- The disturbance is not caused exclusively by vaginismus or lack of lubrication, is not better accounted for by another Axis I disorder (except another sexual dysfunction), and is not due exclusively to the direct physiological effects of a substance (such as a drug of abuse or a medication) or a general medical condition.

The most common symptom of dyspareunia from psychosocial causes is pain at the vaginal opening as the penis enters the vagina. Entry may be difficult, and the pain may be burning or sharp. The woman may have a sense of being "dry." Pain may continue or ease as thrusting continues.

Vasocongestion can cause an aching pain in the pelvic area that persists for hours after intercourse. Pain with orgasm, or pain deep in the pelvis with thrusting, is more likely to be a sign of a medical problem but can result from lack of arousal and tension.

A person who experiences pain during sex may feel embarrassed or ashamed. Dyspareunia can cause problems in relationships or lead to the affected person's avoiding relationships altogether.

Diagnosis

About 30% to 40% of all women who seek help from a sexual counselor for dyspareunia have a clear physical cause identified as the reason for their pain. Examples of possible physical causes are infections, sexually transmitted diseases (STDs), estrogen deficiencies, and vulvar vestibulitis (severe pain during vaginal penetration).

A full family and sexual history can help pinpoint possible psychosocial causes. A psychological evaluation can determine the cause of the problem. Women who have been raped or abused may also have **post-traumatic stress disorder** (PTSD) or **generalized anxiety disorder**.

There are two types of dyspareunia. Lifelong or primary dyspareunia means that the condition has been present for the entire sexual life of the affected person. This type is usually associated with **sexual abuse**, being raised to believe that sex is bad, fear of sex, or a painful first sexual experience. Acquired or secondary dyspareunia begins after a period of normal sexual function. It often has a medical cause, but it may be a result of some sort of **trauma**, such as rape.

Treatment

Some studies have found that treatments that approach dyspareunia resulting from vulvar vestibulitis syndrome as a pain disorder, rather than as a sexual dysfunction, are quite effective in reducing the symptoms of pain.

Counseling is often helpful to identify and reframe negative feelings about sex. **Couples therapy** can help improve communication between partners and resolve problems that may be a factor in the sexual relationship. Women who have been abused or raped may benefit from counseling techniques designed to help overcome fears and issues caused by traumatic experiences.

Sex therapy may be offered to provide information about the physical aspects of arousal and orgasm. A sex therapist will also offer suggestions for how to improve sexual technique. For example, increasing time for foreplay and allowing the woman to control when and how penetration occurs can help her to relax and become aroused more easily.

Women who also have vaginismus may be given a set of devices they can use at home to dilate the opening of the vagina. Affected women start with a very small device and gradually work up to a penis-sized device, proceeding to a larger size only when they can use the smaller one without pain or fear. This retrains the vaginal muscles and helps the involuntary muscle tightening of vaginismus.

Use of a vaginal lubricant, at least temporarily, may be helpful in some women to reduce anxiety about possible pain.

There are no specific medications that treat dyspareunia. Medications that increase blood flow or relax muscles may be helpful in some cases.

KEY TERMS

Vaginismus—An involuntary tightening of the vaginal muscles that makes sexual intercourse painful, difficult, or impossible.

Vasocongestion—A pooling of blood in dilated blood vessels.

Vulvar vestibulitis syndrome (VVS)—Thought to be the most frequent cause of dyspareunia in premenopausal women. A chronic, persistent clinical syndrome, it is characterized by severe pain on vestibular touch or attempted vaginal entry.

Prognosis

With treatment, the chance of overcoming dyspareunia and having an enjoyable sexual life is good. Treatment can take several months, particularly in the case of survivors of a violent trauma such as rape.

Resources

BOOKS

Hales Robert E., Stuart C. Yudofsky, and John A. Talbott, eds. *The American Psychiatric Press Textbook of Psychiatry*. 3rd ed. Washington, DC: American Psychiatric Press, 1999.

Sadock, Benjamin J., and Virginia A. Sadock, eds. *Comprehensive Textbook of Psychiatry*. Vol. 2. 7th ed. Philadelphia: Lippincott Williams and Wilkins, 2000.

PERIODICALS

Binik, Yitzchak M. "Should Dyspareunia be Retained as a Sexual Dysfunction in DSM-V. A Painful Classification Decision." *Archives of Sexual Behavior* 34, no. 1 (February 2005): 11–21.

Heim, Lori J. "Evaluation and Differential Diagnosis of Dyspareunia." *American Family Physician* 63:8 (April 15, 2001): 1535–44. Available online at http://www.aafp.org/afp/20010415/1535.html (accessed November 9, 2011).

WEBSITES

American Academy of Family Physicians. "Dyspareunia: Painful Sex for Women." *Familydoctor.org*. August 2004. http://familydoctor.org/669.xml (accessed October 5, 2011).

Martirosyan, Armen E. "Dyspareunia (Painful Sexual Intercourse)." Armenian Medical Network. http://www.health.am/diseases/more/dyspareunia_painful_sexual_intercourse (accessed October 5, 2011).

MedlinePlus. "Female Sexual Dysfunction." U.S. National Library of Medicine, National Institutes of Health. March 5, 2007. http://www.nlm.nih.gov/medlineplus/ency/article/003151.htm (accessed October 5, 2011).

Jody Bower, MSW
Emily Jane Willingham, PhD

Dysthymic disorder

Definition

Dysthymic disorder is defined as a mood disorder with chronic (long-term) depressive symptoms that are present most of the day, more days than not, for a period of at least two years.

Demographics

The lifetime prevalence has been estimated to be 4.1% for women and 2.2% for men, with an overall rate of 1.5% of people over age 18 in the U.S. population affected in a given year. This percentage, in actual numbers, is about 3.3 million adults. In adults, dysthymic disorder is more common in women than in men and research suggests that the prevalence in the age group 25 to 64 years is 6% for women. In children, dysthymic disorder can occur equally among both genders. The median age of onset is 31 years.

Description

Everyone experiences feelings of unhappiness and sadness occasionally. When these depressed feelings start to dominate everyday life and cause physical and mental deterioration, the feelings become known as depressive disorders. Depressive disorders can be categorized as **major depressive disorder** or dysthymic disorder. Individuals who have dysthymic disorder have had their depressive symptoms for years—they often cannot pinpoint exactly when they started to feel depressed. People with dysthymic disorder may describe to their doctor feelings of hopelessness, lowered self-esteem, poor concentration, indecisiveness, decreased motivation, sleeping too much or too little, or eating too much or too little. Symptoms are present often and for the whole day and are typically present for at least two years.

Causes and symptoms

Causes

The causes of **depression** are complex and not yet completely understood. Sleep abnormalities, hormones, **neurotransmitters** (chemicals that communicate impulses from one nerve cell to another), upbringing, heredity, and stressors (significant life changes or events that cause **stress**) all have been implicated as causes of depression.

Dysthymic disorder occurs in approximately 25% to 50% of persons who have sleep abnormalities that include reduced rapid eye movement (REM) sleep and impaired sleep continuity. REM sleep is an essential component of the sleep cycle and quality of sleep.

There is some evidence that suggests a correlation with hormonal imbalances of cortisol or thyroid hormones. In many adults, levels of cortisol (a stress hormone) are elevated during acute depressive periods and return to normal when the person is no longer depressed. In children and adolescents, experimental results have been quite inconsistent, although there is some evidence that hypersecretion of cortisol is associated with more severe depressive symptoms and with a higher likelihood of recurrence of depression. A lack of thyroid hormone mimics depression quite well, and thyroid hormone levels are routinely checked in patients with recent-onset depression.

In depression, there appears to be abnormal excess or inhibition of signals that control mood, thoughts, pain, and other sensations. Some studies suggest an imbalance of the neurotransmitter called **serotonin**. It is assumed that the reason **antidepressants** are effective is that they correct these chemical imbalances. For example, the **selective serotonin reuptake inhibitors (SSRIs)**, one class of antidepressant medications that includes **fluoxetine** (Prozac), appears to establish a normal level of serotonin. As the name implies, the drug inhibits the reuptake of the serotonin neurotransmitter from the gaps between nerve cells, thus increasing neurotransmitter action, alleviating depressive symptoms.

A child's upbringing may also be key in the development of dysthymic disorder. For example, it is speculated that if a person is abused and neglected throughout childhood and adolescence, a pattern of low self-esteem and negative thinking may emerge, and, from that, a lifelong pattern of depression may follow.

Heredity seems to play a role in the development of depressive disorders. People with major depression in their immediate family are up to three times more likely to have the disorder themselves. It would seem that biological and **genetic factors** may make certain individuals more prone to depressive disorders, but that environmental circumstances, or stressors, may then trigger the disorder.

Symptoms

The mental health professional's handbook to aid in patient **diagnosis** is the ***Diagnostic and Statistical Manual of Mental Disorders***, fourth edition, text revision (*DSM-IV-TR*). The *DSM-IV-TR* has established a list of criteria that can indicate a diagnosis. These criteria include:

- Depressed mood for most of the day, more days than not.
- When depressed, two (or more) of the following are also present: decreased appetite or overeating, too much or too little sleep, low energy level, low self-esteem, decreased ability to concentrate, difficulty making decisions, and/or feelings of hopelessness.
- During the two years of the disorder, the patient has never been without symptoms listed for more than two months at a time.
- No major depressive episode (a more severe form of depression) has been present during the first two years of the disorder.
- There has never been a manic disorder, and criteria for a less severe depression called cyclothymic disorder has never been established.
- The disorder does not exclusively occur with psychosis, schizophrenia, or delusional illnesses.
- The symptoms of depression cause clinically significant impairment and distress in occupational, social, and general functioning.

Dysthymic disorder can be described as "early onset" (onset before age 21 years), "late onset" (onset is age 21 years or older), and "with atypical features" (features that are not commonly observed).

The *DSM-5* (2013) proposes changing the name of the disorder to chronic depressive disorder and eliminating the exclusion of a major depressive episode from its list of criteria for diagnoses.

Diagnosis

To diagnose a patient with this disorder, the *DSM-IV-TR* criteria must be met, and evaluation of this is accomplished through an extensive psychological interview and evaluation. The affected person seeking the clinician's help usually exhibits symptoms of irritability, feelings of worthlessness and hopelessness, crying spells, decreased sex drive, agitation, and thoughts of death. The clinician must rule out any possible medical conditions that can cause depressed affect. (Affect can be defined as the expression of emotion displayed to others through facial expressions, hand gestures, tone of voice, etc.) The diagnosis cannot be made if depression occurs during an active course of **psychosis**, **delusions**, **schizophrenia**, or **schizoaffective disorder**. If **substance abuse** is determined as the cause of depression, then a diagnosis of substance-induced mood disorder can be established.

Further psychological tests that can be administered to help in the diagnostic process include the **Beck Depression Inventory** and the **Hamilton Depression Scale**.

Treatment

The goals of treatment include remission of symptoms and psychological and social recovery.

Medications

Studies suggest some treatment success with medications such as tricyclic antidepressants (TCAs) or monoaminoxidase inhibitors (**MAOIs**). Medications can be effective in patients who have depression due to sleep abnormalities. Some tricyclic antidepressants include **amitriptyline** (Elavil), **imipramine** (Tofranil), and **nortriptyline** (Aventyl, Pamelor), and some MAOIs include **tranylcypromine** (Parnate) and **phenelzine** (Nardil), although these are not considered first-line use antidepressants. **Selective serotonin reuptake inhibitors** (**SSRIs**) are recommended during initial treatment planning after a definitive diagnosis is well established. The most commonly prescribed SSRIs are fluoxetine (Prozac), **sertraline** (Zoloft), **paroxetine** (Paxil), **fluvoxamine** (Luvox), and **citalopram** (Celexa). Trials are currently ongoing to assess the effects of several other drugs on the symptoms of dysthymic disorder.

Psychological therapies

Clinical reports suggest that **cognitive-behavioral therapy**, interpersonal **psychotherapy**, or **family therapy** can be effective with concurrent antidepressant medication to treat the symptoms of depression. In these therapies, the goal is to help the patient develop healthy problem-solving and coping skills.

Prognosis

Dysthymic disorder often begins in late childhood or adolescence. The disorder follows a chronic (long-term) course. The development of a more major form of clinical depression called major depressive disorder among children with dysthymic disorder is significant. Childhood onset of dysthymic disorder is considered an early indicator for recurrent mood disorder that may even have more severe clinical symptoms in the patient's future. Patients with this disorder usually have impaired emotional, social, and physical functioning.

In general, the clinical course of dysthymic disorder is not promising. Causes of a poorer outcome include not completing treatment, noncompliance with medication intake, and lack of willingness to change behaviors that promote a depressed state. However, patients can do very well with a short course of medications if they have a desire to follow psychotherapy treatment recommendations.

If left untreated, dysthymic disorder can result in significant financial and occupational losses. People with this disorder tend to isolate themselves by restricting daily activities and spending days in bed. Patients often complain of poor health and incur more disability days when compared to the general population. Higher rates of successful outcome occur in people who undergo psychotherapy and treatment with appropriate medications.

Prevention

There is no known prevention for dysthymic disorder. Early **intervention** for children with depression may be effective in arresting the development of more severe problems.

Resources

BOOKS

Goldman, Lee, and Andrew I. Schafer, eds. *Goldman's Cecil Medicine*, 24th ed. Philadelphia: Elsevier, 2011.

Tasman, Allan, et al., eds. *Psychiatry*. 3rd ed. New York: Wiley and Sons, 2008.

PERIODICALS

Brown, C. S. "Depression and Anxiety Disorders." *Obstetrics and Gynecology Clinics of North America* 28, no. 2 (June 2001): 241–68.

Youdim, Moussa B.H., Dale Edmondson, and Keith F. Tipton. "The Therapeutic Potential of Monoamine Oxidase Inhibitors." *Nature Reviews Neuroscience* 7, no. 4 (2006): 295–309.

WEBSITES

U.S. National Institute of Mental Health. "The Invisible Disease: Depression." NIH Publication 01-4591. Updated 2002. http://www.intelihealth.com/IH/ihtIH?t=29391&c=192252&p=~br,IHC|~st,8596|~r,EMIHC277|~b,*|&d=dmtContent (accessed October 5, 2011).

U.S. National Institute of Mental Health. "Dysthymic Disorder Among Adults." http://www.nimh.nih.gov/statistics/1DD_ADULT.shtml (accessed October 5, 2011).

Laith Farid Gulli, MD
Linda Hesson, MA, LLP, CAC
Emily Jane Willingham, PhD

E

Eating disorders *see* **Anorexia nervosa; Binge eating disorder; Bulimia nervosa**

Economic and financial stress

Definition

Economic and financial **stress** is stress caused by a person's money or financial situation and is generally a reaction to the threat or worry of not having enough money to meet basic living needs. This perceived threat, known as a stressor, may result from an unanticipated situation or event that threatens a person's financial stability, or it may be experienced by those who have not yet been able to obtain financial stability.

Demographics

According to the American Psychological Association's *Stress in America* report, in 2010, 76% of Americans cited money as a source of stress. Additional stressors included the general economy (65%), work (70%), and job stability (49%). Women were more likely to stress over money and the economy than men (79% compared to 74% and 68% compared to 61%, respectively). Among different age groups, adults aged 19–64 were more likely to name money as their top source of stress than seniors (65+), who cited the economy.

Description

Economic and financial stress may be arise from a number of circumstances, such as losing a job, moving, going to college, applying for a loan, incurring credit debt, having a child, or buying a house, to name a few. One of the potential factors in developing financial stress is a perceived sense of loss of control, especially when the circumstances surrounding financial stress are unpreventable or unforeseen. A person with a financial "safety net," who can maintain control of his or her life in the event of a layoff or loss of investments, for example, will experience relatively less stress and anxiety from the adverse event. Also, persons who consider their socioeconomic status to be based not only on financial resources but on other factors such as social connections and educational level may feel more optimistic when facing the threat of a financial disruption.

Most approaches to understanding stress emphasize that the cognitive evaluation of an event—that is, how a person thinks about the event—is what leads to the reaction of stress or no stress. After an adverse event, such as the loss of a job, the person evaluates the effects of the event and the amount of resources he or she has to deal with the adversity. If the strength of the resources—financial, social, and psychological—is greater than the strength of the adversity—reduced income—there is less stress. However, if the strength of the adversity is greater than the strength of the resources, there is greater stress. The amount of money a person needs is relative—as a person becomes accustomed to having less, the change in the standard of living starts to feel normal, and what is perceived as normal does not generally cause stress.

Relative deprivation

People tend to compare their circumstances with their peers. If a person perceives him- or herself to have less than friends or neighbors, the person may feel that his or her finances are inadequate. This is known as relative deprivation. Relative deprivation suggests that our evaluation of what is "normal" does not only rest on our own experience but is affected by the experience of others.

Learned helplessness

Another psychological effect of stress is learned helplessness. If rats in a cage receive an electric shock, they will move from the place of the shock to another part of the cage. However, if they receive a shock no matter where in the cage they go, they will lie down and accept the shock. When faced with a stressor, humans look for ways to deal

Percentage of American adults (age 18+) experiencing debt stress, 2009–2011

HOW OFTEN DO YOU WORRY ABOUT THE TOTAL AMOUNT YOU (AND YOUR SPOUSE/PARTNER) OWE IN OVERALL DEBT?

	May/June 2009	November 2009	May 2010	November 2010	June 2011
All/most of the time	19%	23%	21%	20%	20%
All of the time	9%	11%	10%	9%	9%
Most of the time	10%	12%	11%	11%	11%
Some of the time	29%	27%	28%	25%	29%
Hardly ever/not at all	47%	45%	49%	52%	46%
Hardly ever	26%	20%	23%	23%	20%
Not at all	22%	25%	25%	29%	26%
No debt	5%	4%	2%	3%	5%
Don't know	*	*	*	*	*
Refused	*	*	*	*	1%
Total number of persons interviewed	**1,000**	**1,006**	**1,002**	**1,000**	**1,001**

HOW MUCH STRESS DOES THE TOTAL DEBT YOU CARRY CAUSE YOU (AND YOUR SPOUSE/PARTNER)?

	May/June 2009	November 2009	May 2010	November 2010	June 2011
Great deal/quite a bit of stress	17%	22%	20%	18%	16%
Great deal of stress	8%	12%	10%	7%	8%
Quite a bit of stress	9%	11%	10%	11%	8%
Some stress	29%	28%	26%	23%	31%
Not very much/no stress at all	54%	49%	53%	59%	53%
Not very much stress	28%	23%	25%	26%	23%
No stress at all	27%	26%	28%	33%	30%
Don't know	*	*	*	*	*
Refused	-	1%	*	*	1%
Total number of persons interviewed	**941**	**964**	**976**	**973**	**956**

SOURCE: GfK Roper Public Affairs & Corporate Communications, "A Telephone Survey of the American General Population (Ages 18+)," *The AP-GfK Poll*, June 2011.

Report available online at http://surveys.ap.org/data%5CGfK%5CAP-GfK%20Poll_About%20DSI%20072011.pdf. *(Table by PreMediaGlobal. © 2012 Cengage Learning.)*

with the threat, but if attempts all fail, learned helplessness—often in the form of depression—can develop. Anyone demonstrating the symptoms of agitation, lethargy, and **depression** in response to an aversive financial event may be experiencing economic and financial stress.

Finances and satisfaction with life

Money and financial stability do not necessarily equate with happiness. Satisfaction with life is considered a good resource against stress, although it may not prevent stress completely. A measure of satisfaction with life, as developed by **psychologist** Ed Diener, considers conditions such as having few regrets and achieving major goals. In the United States, for example, income has increased over the years while measures of happiness have remained stable. Since the 1930s, the U.S. government has reported the average per-person income, and since the late 1950s, the National Opinion Research Center has asked participants in a survey study how happy they considered themselves. Although the buying power of individual Americans has steadily increased by nearly three times since 1957, the number of persons describing themselves as "very happy" has remained at close to 30%. If more money led to more happiness, the percentage of people rating themselves as "very happy" should have increased in relation to the increase in disposable income. Happiness is not connected directly with the amount of money one has, and among those who are meeting at least their basic needs (food, shelter), there is no correlation between the amount of income and satisfaction with life.

Risk factors

In general, anyone who misjudges his or her financial security is at risk for economic and financial stress. Those who either do not make financial goals or who strive for unrealistic financial goals are also at risk for economic and financial stress. Further, people who continuously live beyond their means will eventually face the consequences that lead to economic and financial stress.

Causes and symptoms

It is a common perception that an aversive financial event is the cause of the economic and financial stress.

KEY TERMS

"Fight-or-flight" response—A function of the autonomic nervous system that prepares the brain to make an immediate decision to deal with a sudden threat.

Learned helplessness—The tendency to give up on solving a problem when efforts appear to bring no results.

Meditation—Technique of concentration for relaxing the mind and body.

Relative deprivation—The tendency to base one's criteria for normalcy on comparisons with neighbors and relatives.

"Satisfaction with Life"—Term coined by psychologist Ed Diener as a level of satisfaction determined by acceptance of the past, contentment with the present, and optimism for the future.

Socioeconomic status—Perceived status of an individual, family or community based on average income, education level, and social status.

However, the unpleasant event itself is not a stressor—it is the subjective evaluation of the event as a threat that makes it a stressor. As the stock market dips, a multimillionaire might lose more money in one day than most people make in a lifetime. Although unpleasant, this event is not a threat to the multimillionaire, who does not have to change his/her lifestyle or daily pattern.

The physiological effects of stress are the release of hormones usually reserved for reactions to physical danger. When faced with life-threatening situations, the body responds with a "fight-or-flight" reaction—the decision to fight the threat or run away. Natural selection developed "fight or flight" to increase survivability in the face of environmental threats to life. However, modern humans have been shown to react similarly to psychological and social threats. These physiological reactions over time can reduce the efficiency of the immune system. Symptoms of the "fight-or-flight" response include involuntary muscle contractions, increased heart rate, and trouble breathing.

Treatment

Economic and financial stress may be alleviated by finding a solution to the perceived problem. For instance, if the stressor is loss of a job, then searching for a new job may help reduce the stress. If the stressor is credit card debt, cutting up the credit cards to avoid accumulating further debt may help ease anxiety. If the stress persists and begins to interfere with activities of daily life, such as fulfilling familial responsibilities or social zing with friends, the person may wish to see a doctor or therapist to learn about other treatment options.

General treatments for stress

TRADITIONAL. Traditional **psychotherapy** focuses on the patient understanding his or her financial situation clearly. The humanistic approach to counseling encourages individuals to recognize their personal value, which may help counteract any feelings of diminished worth based on financial difficulties. Humanistic counseling often leads participants to more social interactions, which can shift their focus from a financial perspective to deriving pleasure from relationships.

DRUGS. Doctors do not usually prescribe drugs for treatment of commonplace stress brought on by financial difficulties. Some patients may use over-the-counter analgesics but should still discuss this option with their physician. If the stress becomes unmanageable, the doctor might prescribe an antianxiety medication.

ALTERNATIVE. Alternative **stress management** techniques are widely used and are easy for people to do at home. A person might keep a daily record of the onset of stress-related reactions, noting the exact time of the onset, whatever thoughts he or she might had at the onset, and any events that prompted the onset. A therapist can then help the patient evaluate the record and identify any unknown stressors. If the patient recognizes that he or she is putting too much value into these stressors, including financial worries, then the stress reactions may be reduced.

Other alternative therapies include **meditation**, relaxation techniques, massage, **yoga**, **exercise**, **aromatherapy**, and more.

Home remedies

The best thing a person can do to treat financial stress is to organize his or her financial situation. Balancing the household budget is a great first step in regaining control of finances. The person should analyze his or her monthly spending and identify costs that are necessities (e.g., rent, food, bills) and those that are luxuries (dinners out, entertainment). By allotting a portion of income each month to cover all of the necessities, the person is able to see how much is left for luxuries, helping avoid unnecessary spending.

Prevention

Though some circumstances surrounding economic and financial stress are not preventable, such as the state of the national economy or job layoffs, creating and following a budget can help to prevent some financial stress. Saving money, even a little bit at a time, can also help to prevent stress and may help to relieve stress when an unforeseen financial event does arise.

Resources

BOOKS

Durand, V. Mark, and David H. Barlow. *Essentials Of Abnormal Psychology*. Belmont, CA: Wadsworth, Cengage Learning, 2010.

PERIODICALS

Belluck, Pam. "Coping with Financial Stress." *New York Times* (April 8, 2009). http://www.nytimes.com/2009/04/09/health/09stressbox.html (accessed November 3, 2011).

Bruzzese, Anita. "Job, Retirement, Financial Stress Takes Toll on Baby Boomers." *USA Today* (September 9, 2011). http://www.usatoday.com/money/jobcenter/workplace/bruzzese/2011-09-07-tips-to-cope-with-baby-boomers-financial-personal-stresses_n.htm (accessed November 3, 2011).

Wrosch, Carsten, Jutta Heckhausen, and Margie E. Lachman. "Primary and Secondary Control Strategies for Managing Health and Financial Stress Across Adulthood." *Psychology and Aging* 15, no. 3 (2000): 387–99.

OTHER

American Psychological Association. *Stress in America 2010*. Washington, DC: American Psychological Association, 2010. http://www.apa.org/news/press/releases/stress/national-report.pdf (accessed November 3, 2010).

Turner, Jo. "Coping with Financial Stress." University of Florida Extension, Institute of Food and Agricultural Sciences. http://miami-dade.ifas.ufl.edu/old/programs/efnep/publications/Coping-with-Financial-Stress.PDF (accessed November 3, 2011).

WEBSITES

American Psychological Association. "Psychology Topics: Money." http://www.apa.org/topics/money/index.aspx (accessed November 3, 2011).

Cox, Lauren. "Financial Stress: How Bad Can it Get?" ABC News (September 24, 2008). http://abcnews.go.com/Health/story?id=5867963&page=1#.TrMxY3LMqQw (accessed November 3, 2011).

ORGANIZATIONS

American Institute of Stress, 124 Park Avenue, Yonkers, NY, 10703, (914) 963-1200, stress125@optonline.net, http://www.stress.org.

American Psychological Association, 750 1st St. NE, Washington, DC, 20002-4242, (202) 336-5500; TDD/TTY: (202) 336-6123, (800) 374-2721, http://www.apa.org.

National Institute of Mental Health, 6001 Executive Blvd., Rm. 8184, MSC 9663, Bethesda, MD, 20892-9663, (301) 443-4513, (866) 615-6464, nimhinfo@nih.gov, http:// www.nimh.nih.gov.

Ray F. Brogan, PhD

Ecstasy

Definition

Ecstasy is the popular name for the synthetic, psychoactive drug 3,4-methylenedioxymethamphetamine, or MDMA. It is chemically similar to **methamphetamine** and the hallucinogen mescaline. MDMA acts both as a stimulant and psychedelic, producing an energizing effect as well as distortions in time and perception and enhanced enjoyment from tactile experiences. MDMA exerts its primary effects in the **brain** on neurons that use the chemical **serotonin** to communicate with other neurons. The serotonin system plays an important role in regulating mood, aggression, sexual activity, sleep, and sensitivity to pain. Ecstasy has a large number of other street names. These include Adam, B-bombs, bean, Blue Nile, clarity, crystal, decadence, disco biscuit, E, essence, Eve, go, hug drug, Iboga, love drug, morning shot, pollutants, Rolls Royce, Snackies, speed for lovers, sweeties, wheels, X, and XTC.

Demographics

Ecstasy is one of a group of drugs known as club drugs, because the drug is used primarily in dance clubs, at raves, and at dances on college and high school campuses. Use is more common in urban areas. Most users of ecstasy are white teenagers and young adults from middle- and upper-class households. The U.S. Office of National Drug Control Policy reports that, according to the National Survey on Drug Use and Health (NSDUH), in 2010, an estimated 695,000 Americans had used MDMA in the past

Emergency department visits involving ecstasy, 2008

Drugs taken	Number of visits
Ecstasy only	3,968
Ecstasy in combination with other drugs	13,897
One other drug	5,584
Two other drugs	2,682
Three other drugs	2,502
Four or more other drugs	3,129
Total ecstasy-related visits	**17,865**

The drugs most commonly used with ecstasy were marijuana (38.2% of cases), alcohol (38.1%), and cocaine (31.8%).

SOURCE: Substance Abuse and Mental Health Services Administration, Center for Behavioral Health Statistics and Quality, "Emergency Department Visits Involving Ecstasy," *The DAWN Report* (March 24, 2011).

Available online at http://oas.samhsa.gov/2k11/DAWN027/Ecstasy.htm. *(Table by PreMediaGlobal. © 2012 Cengage Learning.)*

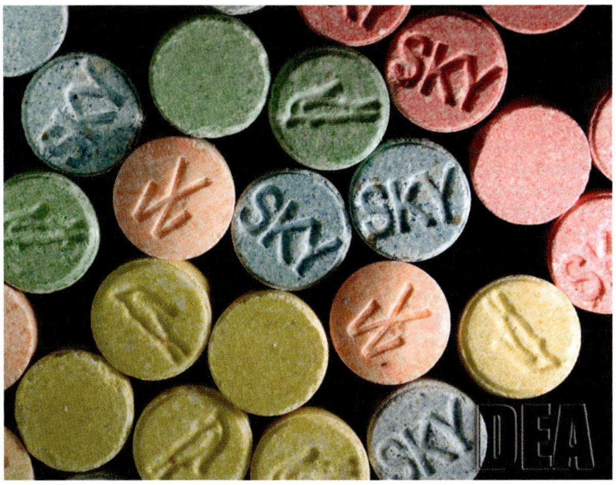

Ecstasy tablets. *(U.S. Drug Enforcement Administration)*

month (considered to be current users of ecstasy), with almost one million Americans using ecstasy for the first time in 2010.

Although the use of ecstasy by teenagers and young adults rose between 1996 and 2002, use appeared to decrease over subsequent years. *Monitoring the Future*, a study conducted every year by the University of Michigan and funded by the National Institute on Drug Abuse (NIDA), surveys middle- and high-school students on their drug use. In 2010, the survey found that 2.4% of eighth graders, 4.7% of tenth graders, and 4.5% of twelfth graders surveyed reported that they had used ecstasy at least once in the past year. In contrast, in 2002, 4.3% of eighth graders, 6.6% of tenth graders, and 10.5% of twelfth graders reported having used ecstasy.

Description

MDMA was first synthesized in 1912 by the German pharmaceutical company Merck. Merck patented the drug in 1914. The U.S. military conducted some studies of MDMA in the 1950s, but the public knew virtually nothing about the drug until the 1970s. In the early 1970s, a few psychotherapists and psychiatrists began to explore the therapeutic uses of MDMA. They believed that they could help people benefit more from treatment if they combined doses of MDMA with **psychotherapy**. The number of clinicians who used MDMA as an adjunct to psychotherapy grew in the next few years.

The name "ecstasy" was coined in the early 1980s, when distributors began to envision a larger market for the drug. Ecstasy became popular as a club drug and was often sold in nightclubs and bars. Because of reports of increases in the recreational use of ecstasy and scientific reports suggesting that the related drug MDA could cause brain damage, the U.S. Drug Enforcement Administration (DEA) banned both ecstasy and 3,4-methylenedioxyamphetamine (MDA) in the mid-1980s. Following the ban on ecstasy, a lawsuit was filed against the DEA by a group of physicians who believed that ecstasy has therapeutic value. Despite the lawsuit, the DEA ban on ecstasy became permanent. As of 2011, ecstasy was classified as a Schedule I drug. Schedule I drugs are considered to have high potential for abuse and no currently accepted medical value. They are not considered safe for use even under medical supervision. It is illegal to use, sell, or manufacture ecstasy in the United States. Ecstasy that is seized by the DEA is manufactured mainly in the Netherlands, Belgium, and Canada, although some is also illegally made in laboratories in the United States.

The recreational use of ecstasy continued to increase despite the DEA ban. Through the late 1980s and 1990s, ecstasy began to be used widely at raves, which are all-night dance parties often held in warehouses and attended by large numbers of young people.

Ecstasy is sometimes described as an "entactogen," because it gives users feelings of peacefulness, acceptance, empathy, euphoria, and closeness to others. Ecstasy is typically synthesized from precursor chemicals such as piperonyl methylketone, piperonal, isosafrole, or safrole. Safrole is an essential oil that is found in the tree *Sassafras albidum*, which grows in the eastern United States, and in the tree *Ocotea pretiosa*, which grows in South America. Safrole is also found in nutmeg, dill, parsley seed, crocus, **saffron**, vanilla beans, and calamus.

Some people use a product called herbal ecstasy. The main constituents of herbal ecstasy are legal herbs that are stimulants such as ephedra, guarana, and caffeine. Other herbs and vitamins may also be included. Herbal ecstasy is sold in tablet form as Cloud 9, Herbal Bliss, Ritual Spirit, Herbal X, GWM, Rave Energy, Ultimate Xphoria, and X. The quantities of ephedrine and caffeine in the tablets can vary widely. Although people who take herbal ecstasy believe it to be a legal, safe alternative to ecstasy, there are reports of numerous adverse effects, including severe reactions such as high blood pressure, **seizures**, heart attacks, strokes, and death.

Method of administration

Most users take ecstasy orally. Users also sometimes inhale or inject it. Although ecstasy is available as a capsule or a powder, it usually is sold in tablet form. The tablets are available in different colors, shapes, and sizes, and are often imprinted with logos such as smiley faces, clover leaves, cartoon characters, or the logos of popular commercial brands, such as those for clothing or automobiles. On average, an ecstasy tablet has about 100 mg of MDMA. However, the MDMA content in tablets can vary a great deal. Pure MDMA salt, which is a white, bitter-tasting substance, is usually not the only ingredient in ecstasy tablets. The MDMA in ecstasy tablets is often blended with other drugs such as caffeine, aspirin, dextromethorphan, ephedrine, methamphetamine, and MDA.

Psychotherapeutic use of ecstasy

Some psychiatrists and psychotherapists still advocate for the therapeutic use of ecstasy. While most of these professionals believe that recreational use of ecstasy is likely to be unsafe, they argue that small doses of unadulterated MDMA can be used effectively as an adjunct to psychotherapy, when used once or twice in a controlled therapeutic setting. They believe that MDMA is beneficial because it can help patients put aside their anxiety and fear and explore psychological issues that would normally be too painful to confront. Although ecstasy-assisted psychotherapy may also be indicated in other situations, it is thought to be particularly helpful in the treatment of **post-traumatic stress disorder** (PTSD) and to help people with terminal illness deal with the fear of dying.

Long-term damage resulting from MDMA use

MDMA causes the release of the **neurotransmitters dopamine** and serotonin and the neurohormone norepinephrine. Research on the long-term effects of MDMA has mainly focused on cognition and behavioral changes related to serotonin levels.

The NIDA reports that studies provide direct evidence that chronic use of MDMA causes brain damage in humans. Using advanced brain imaging techniques, one study found that MDMA harms neurons that release serotonin (serotonin plays an important role in regulating memory and other mental functions). In a related study, researchers found that people who use MDMA heavily have memory problems that persist for at least two weeks after stopping use of the drug. Both studies strongly suggest that the extent of damage is directly related to the amount of MDMA used.

Another study, reported by the *Journal of Neurology Neurosurgery and Psychiatry* on April 6, 2011, supported the hypothesis that long-term users of ecstasy are at risk for brain damage. The study included a total of 17 men; 10 who were in their 20s and were long-term users of ecstasy, and 7 in their 20s who had never used the drug. In a study performed by a group of Dutch researchers, magnetic resonance imaging (MRI) brain scans of the ecstasy users showed an approximate 10% shrinkage in the volume of the hippocampus (a portion of the brain responsible for the functions of learning and memory). The brain scans revealed that the ecstasy users (having taken ecstasy tablets over a six-and-a-half year period) had about 10.5% less hippocampal volume than non-users of ecstasy, as well as a lower (about 4.6% on average) proportion of grey matter in the brain, suggesting that long-term effects of ecstasy may not be limited to the hippocampus. Researchers noted as well that shrinkage of the hippocampus is already known as one finding in older patients who have diseases associated with cognitive impairment, such as **Alzheimer's disease**.

Animal studies indicate that repeated doses of MDMA show long-term decreases in concentrations of serotonin and that ecstasy may cause long-term brain damage from severe damage to brain cells. Brain scans and **psychological assessment** of humans using ecstasy suggest that damage to brain cells may cause memory loss or psychological problems due to destruction of serotonin-producing neurons in the brain. In addition, damage to neurons that regulate dopamine may cause motor disturbances in humans (such as in Parkinson's disease), resulting in tremors, unsteady gait, and paralysis.

Use of MDMA produces cardiovascular effects of increased blood pressure, heart rate, and heart oxygen consumption. People with pre-existing heart disease are at increased risk for cardiovascular catastrophe resulting from MDMA use. Toxicity may rise dramatically when users take multiple doses over brief periods, leading to harmful reactions such as dehydration, hyperthermia, and seizures. Long-term abuse can lead to memory loss.

MDMA tablets often contain other drugs, such as ephedrine, a stimulant, and dextromethorphan, a cough suppressant with PCP-like effects at high doses. These additives increase the harmful effects of MDMA. They also appear to have toxic effects on the brain's serotonin system. In tests of learning and memory, people who use MDMA perform more poorly than people who do not use it. Research with primates shows that MDMA can cause long-lasting brain damage. Exposure to MDMA during the period of pregnancy in which the fetal brain is developing is associated with learning deficits that last into adulthood.

Causes and symptoms

Like other drug use, the decision to use ecstasy results from complex combinations of factors such as genetic predisposition to risk taking, family history, **stress**, and peer pressure.

Ecstasy is absorbed quickly after it is taken orally, and it can be detected in the blood within about 30 minutes. It typically has its effect within 20–60 minutes after it is ingested. The average time for onset of effects is 30 minutes. It has its peak effects about 60–90 minutes after it is ingested. The main effects of ecstasy last about 3–5 hours. Women are more sensitive to ecstasy than men and are more likely to experience an optimal effect of the drug at a lower dose, in proportion to body weight, than men.

Ecstasy mimics the effects of the neurotransmitter serotonin, activating cell receptors in the brain that normally respond to serotonin. Serotonin is involved in many processes in the body, including the regulation of mood, aggression, sexual activity, sleep, sensitivity to pain, and eating. MDMA also causes the release of serotonin, as well as the neurotransmitters norepinephrine and dopamine. The levels of hormones such as cortisol, prolactin, and testosterone increase when ecstasy is used. The level of vasopressin, a hormone that is involved in elevating blood pressure and retaining water in the body, also increases.

Ecstasy users report intensely pleasurable experiences after taking ecstasy. They feel euphoric and are more aware of sensory stimuli. Users often wear fluorescent jewelry or accessories and use mentholated ointments or sprays to enhance the sensory effects they experience. Users of ecstasy usually feel socially uninhibited and close to other people. They find that they have an increased sense of empathy. They also claim to become emotionally open and have exceptionally clear insight into themselves. Time perception may become distorted. Because ecstasy has a stimulant effect, users often feel energetic and can remain awake for long periods. Ecstasy increases sensuality, but it does not directly increase sexual drive or appetite. However, because it decreases inhibitions and makes users more open to others, users sometime engage in sexual activity after taking ecstasy. Men sometimes experience delayed orgasms, although orgasms may be more intense than usual.

Ecstasy users sometimes have undesirable experiences. In one research study, about 25% of users reported having gone through at least one occasion when ecstasy use resulted in unpleasant experiences and body sensations. Short-term adverse reactions that have been reported include dilated pupils, unusual sensitivity to bright light, headache, sweating, increased heart rate, tooth grinding (bruxism), spasms of the jaw muscle (trismus), loss of appetite, nausea, muscle aches, **fatigue**, dizziness, vertigo, thirst, numbness, tingling skin, retention of urine, staggering gait (ataxia), unsteadiness, tics, tremors, restlessness, agitation, **paranoia**, and nystagmus. Research has shown that driving a car under the influence of ecstasy is unsafe.

The scientific literature on the effects of ecstasy is somewhat inconsistent. This is partly because well-controlled studies cannot be carried out on ecstasy use. However, many in the scientific community agree that brain levels of serotonin increase when ecstasy is ingested and that they decrease after an episode of ecstasy use. The depletion of serotonin is thought to cause "midweek blues." This term refers to the lethargy, concentration and memory problems, and depressed mood that many ecstasy users experience for a few days after taking the drug. Other changes that occur for a few days after ecstasy use are increased feelings of aggressiveness, unsociability, irritability, decreased appetite, and poor sleep. Some researchers have reported that chronic, heavy ecstasy use is associated with **sleep disorders**, **depression**, high levels of anxiety, impulsiveness and hostility, and problems with memory and attention. Memory and attention deficits may continue for up to 6 months after drug use is stopped, but symptoms are reported to remit after 6 to 12 months. The extent of cognitive deficits may depend on the number of tablets taken per occasion of use.

Ecstasy causes body temperature to increase. Abnormal increases in body temperature are more likely when the user is in a hot environment, such as on a crowded dance floor. A number of ecstasy-related deaths have been reported that are attributable to drug-induced increases in body temperature. Several users who later died were admitted to hospitals with abnormally high temperatures, ranging from 104°F (40°C) to 109°F (43°C). The immediate cause of death in these users was damage to organs such as the liver and heart. Other deaths have occurred because of water intoxication, which can develop when ecstasy users drink too much water to combat hyperthermia. The increase in vasopressin that accompanies the use of ecstasy makes excessive water intake particularly dangerous. Water intoxication results in decreased levels of sodium in the blood, which can be fatal.

Ecstasy users appear to develop tolerance to the drug with repeated use, needing more of it to achieve the effect they desire. Novice users tend to take one or two tablets per session, whereas highly experienced users may take more than three tablets per session. The use of increased doses may exacerbate the amphetamine-like effects of the drug. Heavy users sometimes binge use, either by taking several tablets simultaneously or by repeatedly taking tablets during a single session that may last up to 48 hours. In such binging sessions, users may go without sleep or food and sometimes consume up to 20 tablets. In some cases, binge users snort powdered ecstasy or inject it. Binging on ecstasy can result in consequences such as

KEY TERMS

Catecholamines—Family of neurotransmitters containing dopamine, norepinephrine and epinephrine, produced and secreted by cells of the adrenal medulla and the brain. Catecholamines have excitatory effects on smooth muscle cells of the vessels that supply blood to the skin and mucous membranes and have inhibitory effects on smooth muscle cells located in the wall of the gut, the bronchial tree of the lungs, and the vessels that supply blood to skeletal muscle. There are two different main types of receptors for these neurotransmitters, called alpha and beta adrenergic receptors. Catecholamines are also known as adrenergic neurotransmitters.

Dopamine—A neurochemical made in the brain that is involved in many brain activities, including movement and emotion.

Neurotransmitter—One of a group of chemicals secreted by a nerve cell (neuron) to carry a chemical message to another nerve cell, often as a way of transmitting a nerve impulse. Examples of neurotransmitters are acetylcholine, dopamine, serotonin, and norepinephrine.

Norepinephrine—A hormone released by nerve cells and the adrenal medulla that causes constriction of blood vessels. Norepinephrine also functions as a neurotransmitter.

Serotonin—5-Hydroxytryptamine; a substance that occurs throughout the body with numerous effects, including neurotransmission. Low serotonin levels are associated with mood disorders, particularly depression and obsessive-compulsive disorder.

loss of appetite, weight loss, days off from work, and depression.

Diagnosis

Diagnosis of ecstasy use is difficult, because the effects tend to wear off after a few hours and because individuals who use ecstasy often use other drugs as well, making the effects difficult to separate.

Treatment

There are no drug treatments for ecstasy use. Behavioral interventions have proved most successful. In **cognitive-behavioral therapy**, users learn to recognize, manage, and avoid situations most likely to lead to illicit drug use, and develop healthy ways to cope with stressful situations. Ecstasy is psychologically addictive in as many as 43% of users, so issues of dependency must be addressed, as must the use of other drugs in conjunction with ecstasy use.

Prognosis

There are scientific and political debates about whether ecstasy causes long-term damage to the human brain. Some researchers and drug enforcement agencies claim that ecstasy is a dangerous drug capable of causing irreversible brain damage, and other researchers suggest that claims of irreversible neurotoxicity in humans are exaggerated and unproven. Because of ethical considerations, ecstasy cannot be given to people who do not use it to study its effects on the brain. However, studies of brain function are sometimes carried out in people who already take ecstasy, using brain-imaging technology. These types of studies are methodologically complex, and results are interpretable in various ways. Therefore, controversy continues about the potential long-term effects of ecstasy on the human brain.

Studies conducted on rats and monkeys have shown that high doses of ecstasy can have long-term negative effects on neurons that contain serotonin. Serotonin levels become depleted in these animals, and serotonin-containing nerves become damaged. The degeneration of neurons is exacerbated when the animals are placed in high-temperature environments. In these types of studies, animals are usually given very high doses of ecstasy, and the drug is usually injected. Some researchers have argued that the results of these animal studies cannot be extrapolated to human users, who use much lower doses and typically ingest the drug orally.

Methodological and ethical problems in ecstasy research

Scientific research on ecstasy use has some limitations. Because ecstasy is classified as a Schedule I drug, researchers cannot easily conduct controlled experimental studies by administering MDMA to people in laboratories. Additionally, people who use ecstasy often use other drugs, such as heroin, **cocaine**, and ketamine, either deliberately or as a result of using contaminated ecstasy. Therefore, it is difficult to determine whether effects observed in users are due to the current or previous use of these other drugs, the use of ecstasy, or the combination of ecstasy with other drugs. Scientists also cannot easily determine whether effects noted in ecstasy users are due to drug use or the personal characteristics of people who choose to use ecstasy recreationally.

Although psychiatrists and psychotherapists used ecstasy in the 1970s as an adjunct to psychotherapy, no controlled **clinical trials** were conducted at the time that could provide evidence for its therapeutic efficacy. After ecstasy became classified as a Schedule I drug, it became difficult for researchers to study its psychotherapeutic uses, because institutional review boards typically do not approve research studies that have the potential for causing harm to humans who participate in them.

Prevention

Social networks and peer pressure play major roles in starting ecstasy use. Peer-led education about the risks of ecstasy is thought to be more effective than adult-led education programs.

Resources

BOOKS

Erickson, Carlton K. *Addiction Essentials: The Go-To Guide for Clinicians and Patients.* New York: Norton, 2011.

Galanter, Marc, and Herbert D. Kleber, eds. *Textbook of Substance Abuse Treatment,* 2nd ed. Washington, DC: American Psychiatric Press, 2008.

Holland, Julie, ed. *Ecstasy: The Complete Guide.* Kindle edition. Rochester, VT: Park Street Press, 2010.

Iversen, Leslie. *Speed, Ecstasy, Ritalin: The Science of Amphetamines.* Oxford: Oxford University Press, 2006.

PERIODICALS

Den Hollander, Bjørnar, et al. "Preliminary Evidence of Hippocampal Damage in Chronic Users of Ecstasy." *Journal of Neurology Neurosurgery and Psychiatry* 28, no. 3 (2011): 1136.

Dumont, G.J.H., and R.J. Verkes. "A Review of Acute Effects of 3,4-Methylenedioxymethamphetamine in Healthy Volunteers." *Journal of Psychopharmacology* 20, no. 2 (2006): 176.

Gahlinger, Paul M. "Club Drugs: MDMA, Gamma-hydroxybutyrate (GHB), Rohypnol, and Ketamine." *American Family Physician* 69, no. 11 (2004): 2619.

Watkins, Katherine E., et al. "An Update on Adolescent Drug Use: What School Counselors Need to Know." *Professional School Counseling* 10, no. 2 (2006): 131–39.

WEBSITES

"Club Drugs." MedlinePlus. Last updated September 2, 2011. http://www.nlm.nih.gov/medlineplus/clubdrugs.html (accessed October 3, 2011).

"Ecstasy: What We Know and Don't Know About MDMA: A Scientific Review." National Institute on Drug Abuse, July 2001. http://www.drugabuse.gov/Meetings/MDMA/MDMAExSummary.html (accessed October 3, 2011).

Finefrock, Douglas C., Mai Kim Lai, and Karen Tonya Mason. "Club Drugs." eMedicinehealth, October 17, 2005. http://www.emedicinehealth.com/club_drugs/article_em.htm (accessed October 3, 2011).

Hahn, In-Hei. "MDMA Toxicity." Medscape Reference, January 26, 2009. http://emedicine.medscape.com/article/821572-overview (accessed October 3, 2011).

ORGANIZATIONS

American Psychological Association, 750 1st St. NE, Washington, DC, 20002-4242, (202) 336-5500; TDD/TTY: (202) 336-6123, (800) 374-2721, http://www.apa.org.

National Clearinghouse on Alcohol and Drug Information, PO Box 2345, Rockville, MD, 20847, (877) SAMHSA-7; Spanish: (877) 767-8432; TDD: (800) 487-4889, Fax: (240) 221-4292, http://ncadi.samhsa.gov.

National Council on Alcoholism and Drug Dependence, Inc., 244 E 58th St., 4th Fl., New York, NY, 10022, (212) 269-7797, (800) NCA-CALL, Fax: (212) 269-7510, national@mcadd.org, http://www.ncadd.org.

National Institutes of Health, 9000 Rockville Pike, Bethesda, MD, 20892, (301) 496-4000; TTY: (301) 402-9612, http://www.nih.gov.

U.S. National Library of Medicine, 8600 Rockville Pike, Bethesda, MD, 20894, (301) 594-5983, (800) 735-2258, Fax: (301) 402-1384, http://www.nlm.nih.gov.

Barbara S. Sternberg, PhD
Emily Jane Willingham, PhD
Laura Jean Cataldo, RN, EdD

EEG *see* **Electroencephalography**

Effexor *see* **Venlafaxine**

Elavil *see* **Amitriptyline**

Elder abuse

Definition

Elder **abuse** is a general term used to describe harmful acts toward an elderly adult, such as physical abuse, **sexual abuse**, emotional or psychological abuse, financial exploitation, and **neglect**, including self-neglect.

Demographics

Results from the National Elder Abuse Incidence Study, funded in part by the Administration on Aging, suggest that over 500,000 people 60 years of age and older are abused or neglected each year in the United States. It was also found that four times as many incidents of abuse, neglect, or self-neglect are never reported, causing researchers to estimate that as many as two million elderly persons in the United States are abused each year. In 90% of the cases, the abusers were

Types of elder abuse

Type†	Description	Examples
Financial exploitation	Illegal or improper use of an older adult's funds, property, or assets	Cashing checks without authorization, forging signatures, misusing or stealing money or possessions
Neglect	Refusal or failure to fulfill any part of a person's obligation or duties to an older adult	Refusing or failing to provide an older adult with such necessities as food, water, clothing, shelter, personal hygiene, medicine, comfort, personal safety, and other essentials
Physical abuse	Use of physical force that may result in bodily injury, physical pain, or impairment	Striking with an object, hitting, pushing, shoving
Psychological abuse±	Infliction of anguish, pain, or distress through verbal or nonverbal acts	Verbal assaults, insults, threats, intimidation, humiliation, and harassment
Sexual abuse	Nonconsensual sexual contact of any kind	Unwanted touching, rape, sodomy, coerced nudity

†Federal and state law may define these terms differently.
±Psychological abuse can also be referred to as verbal or emotional abuse.

SOURCE: U.S. Government Accountability Office, *Elder Justice: Stronger Federal Leadership Could Enhance National Response to Elder Abuse*, a report to the chairman, Senate Special Committee on Aging, U.S. Senate, March 2011.

Report available online at http://www.gao.gov/new.items/d11208.pdf. *(Table by PreMediaGlobal. © 2012 Cengage Learning.)*

found to be family members, and most often were the adult children or spouses of those abused. In addition, equal numbers of men and women have been identified as the abusers. However, women, especially those over 80 years of age, tend to be victimized more than men.

Description

Elder abuse can take place anywhere, but the two main settings addressed by law are domestic settings, such as the elder's home or the caregiver's home, and institutional settings, such as a nursing home or group home. In general, there are five basic types of elderly abuse: physical, sexual, emotional or psychological, financial, and neglect. Data from the National Center on Elder Abuse (NCEA) indicate that more than one-half of the cases reported involve some kind of neglect, whereas 1 in 7 cases involve physical abuse. It is considered neglect when a caretaker deprives an elderly person of the necessary care needed in order to avoid physical or mental harm. Sometimes the behavior of an elderly person threatens his or her own health; in those cases, the abuse is called self-neglect. Physical abuse refers to physical force that causes bodily harm to an elderly person, such as slapping, pushing, kicking, pinching, or burning.

Adult Protective Services estimates of elder abuse reports received, investigations, and substantiations (proven cases) in state fiscal year 2009

	Number in state fiscal year 2009	Number of states responding
Reports received†	357,000	31
Investigations	292,000	33
Substantiations	95,000	27

†States provided data on reports received prior to any screening for eligibility.

SOURCE: U.S. Government Accountability Office, *Elder Justice: Stronger Federal Leadership Could Enhance National Response to Elder Abuse*, a report to the chairman, Senate Special Committee on Aging, U.S. Senate, March 2011.

Report available online at http://www.gao.gov/new.items/d11208.pdf. *(Table by PreMediaGlobal. © 2012 Cengage Learning.)*

About 1 in 8 cases of elderly abuse involve some form of financial exploitation, which is defined as the use of an elderly person's resources without his or her consent. The NCEA defines emotional and psychological abuse of a senior as causing anguish, pain, or distress through verbal or nonverbal acts, such as verbal assaults, insults, intimidation, and humiliation, for example. Isolating elderly persons from their friends and family as well as giving them the silent treatment are two other forms of emotional and psychological abuse. Any kind of non-consensual sexual contact with an elderly person that takes place without his or her consent is considered sexual abuse.

Causes and symptoms

Elder abuse is a complex problem that can be caused by many factors. According to the NCEA, social isolation and mental impairment are two factors of elder abuse. Studies show that people advanced in years, such as in their eighties, with a high level of frailty and dependency, are more likely to be victims of elder abuse than people who are younger and better equipped to stand up for themselves. Because spouses make up a large percentage of elder abusers, at least 40% statistically, some research has been done in the area, which shows that a pattern of domestic violence is associated with many of the cases. The risk of elder abuse appears to be especially high when adult children live with their elderly parents for financial reasons or because they have personal problems, such as drug dependency or mental illness. Some experts have speculated that elderly people living in rural areas with their caretakers may have a higher risk of being abused than city dwellers. The idea behind this theory is that the opportunity exists for the abuse to occur, but there is less likelihood that the abuser will be caught. More research in this very important area is needed in order to illuminate the relationship between these factors.

The NCEA identifies the following as signs of elder abuse:

- Bruises, pressure marks, broken bones, abrasions, and burns may indicate physical abuse or neglect.
- Unexplained withdrawal from normal activities and unusual depression may be indicators of emotional abuse.
- Bruises around the breasts or genital area, as well as unexplained bleeding around the genital area, may be signs of sexual abuse.
- Large withdrawals of money from an elder's bank account, sudden changes in a will, and the sudden disappearance of valuable items may be indications of financial exploitation.
- Bedsores, poor hygiene, unsanitary living conditions, and unattended medical needs may be signs of neglect.
- Failure to take necessary medicines, leaving a burning stove unattended, poor hygiene, confusion, unexplained weight loss, and dehydration may all be signs of self-neglect.

Effects on the abused can be devastating. Victims of elder abuse have the potential to experience extensive and debilitating loss, including financial loss associated with the loss of a home or loss of life savings. In addition, they may suffer loss of health and preventative care, resulting in deleterious mental and physical well-being. Many of these victims suffer loss that is difficult to quantify such as loss of independence, security, and dignity, while feeling **grief**, **depression**, and helplessness.

Victims of nursing home abuse or neglect are especially vulnerable. Nursing homes are regulated by state agencies and are mandated to have staff who are licensed, trained, supervised, and responsible for safe and compassionate treatment of individuals in their care. In the event of any kind of abuse (known or just in question), families may choose to retain an attorney with a background in nursing home and elder abuse issues to assist in determining the possibility of abuse and to help in negotiating appropriate action.

KEY TERMS

Mortality rate—A measure of the number of deaths in a specific population, usually expressed per 1,000 per year.

National Center on Elder Abuse (NCEA)—Association directed by the U.S. Administration on Aging dedicated to the prevention of elder mistreatment; a resource center, assisting at national, state and local levels.

National Committee for the Prevention of Elder Abuse (NCPEA)—Association established in 1988 and dedicated to assuring the safety, security, and dignity of elderly citizens; also serves to provide information and education relating to the prevention of elder abuse.

Diagnosis

The National Committee for the Prevention of Elder Abuse notes that Adult Protective Services (APS) caseworkers are often on the front lines when it comes to elderly abuse. People being abused or those who believe abuse is taking place can turn to their local APS office for help. The APS routinely screens calls, keeps all information confidential, and, if necessary, sends a caseworker out to conduct an investigation. In the event that a **crisis intervention** is needed, the APS caseworker can arrange for any necessary emergency treatment. If it is unclear whether elder abuse has taken place, the APS caseworker can serve as a liaison between the elderly person and other community agencies.

According to the National Committee for the Prevention of Elder Abuse, "professionals in the field of aging are often the first to discover signs of elder abuse." Providing encouragement and advice, they play a critical role in educating others with regard to the needs of the elderly. They provide valuable support to the victims of abuse and also monitor high-risk situations and gather important information that can help confirm that abuse has taken place.

Some people might think that a person who has cognitive impairment might be unable to describe mistreatment; however, that is not the case. In fact, guidelines set by the American Medical Association call for "routine questions about abuse and neglect even among patients with cognitive impairment in order to improve the identification of cases and implement appropriate treatment and referral." Rather than an inability to describe mistreatment, what might stop an elderly person from reporting abuse is a sense of embarrassment or fear of retaliation. To complicate matters, differences exist among cultural groups regarding what defines abuse.

Most states have established laws that define elder abuse and require healthcare providers to report any cases they encounter with penalties attached for failing to do so. Indeed, statistics show that healthcare providers, for example, report almost 25% of the known cases of elder abuse. Therefore, physicians play a very important role in identifying and treating elders who have been abused. Yet only 1 of every 13 cases of elder abuse are estimated to be reported by physicians. There may be several reasons for this pattern. In some cases, the problem may simply go unnoticed, especially if the physician has no obvious reason to suspect any wrongdoing. In other cases, the patient may hide or deny the problem.

In recent years, much media attention has been focused on elderly abuse that takes place in institutional settings. Anyone who believes that a loved one is being abused while in a nursing home or other institutional setting should contact the authorities for assistance immediately.

Treatment

Treatment of elderly persons who have been abused may involve medical care, for treating any injuries; psychotherapy, for treating the emotional trauma; and legal action.

Prognosis

The mortality rate of elderly persons who have been mistreated is higher than the mortality rate of an elderly person who has not experienced abuse. Nonetheless, numerous success stories exist regarding interventions. **Social workers** and healthcare professionals, as well as concerned citizens from a variety of backgrounds, have played a key role in identifying and obtaining treatment for abused elders.

The NCEA and other groups associated with preventing elder abuse work to carry out public awareness activities to increase national awareness and prevention of elder abuse and maintain efforts to secure safe care for elder individuals. Engaging in public awareness campaigns with state, regional, and national organizations is ongoing, including ad campaigns, dissemination of resource materials, and public education on this topic. The NCEA urges individuals, families, organizations, and businesses to join them in preventing elder mistreatment.

Prevention

Planning for the future is one of the best ways to avoid elder abuse. Older persons should consider a variety of retirement options, ones that will encourage safety as well as independence. It is important to stay active in the community. Avoiding isolation minimizes the likelihood that abuse will occur. Individuals ought to seek professional counsel when necessary; it is important for everyone to know their rights and to be advocates on their own behalf.

QUESTIONS TO ASK YOUR DOCTOR

- What are the indications that my loved one may be a victim of elder abuse?
- What examinations are needed for a thorough assessment?
- What measures can be taken to prevent elder abuse?
- How can the quality of life of my loved one be improved?
- Can you recommend an organization that will provide me with additional information about elder abuse?

Resources

BOOKS

Brogden, Mike, and Preeti Nijhar. *Crime, Abuse and the Elderly.* Portland OR: Willan, 2011.

Buchanan, Paul D. *Protecting the Shadow: A Year Inside an Adult Protective Services.* Wellesley, MA: Branden Books, 2011.

Payne, Brian K. *Crime and Elder Abuse,* 3rd ed. Springfield, IL: Charles C. Thomas, 2011.

Pyrek, Kelly M. *Healthcare Crime: Investigating Abuse, Fraud, and Homicide by Caregivers.* Boca Raton, FL: CRC Press, 2011.

WEBSITES

The National Elder Abuse Incidence Study, September 1998. http://www.aoa.gov/AoARoot/AoA_Programs/Elder_Rights/Elder_Abuse/docs/ABuseReport_Full.pdf (accessed October 3, 2011).

"Signs of Nursing Home Abuse." Nursing Home Abuse Center. http://www.nursinghomeabusecenter.org/signs-of-abuse.html (accessed October 3, 2011).

ORGANIZATIONS

American Academy of Family Physicians, 11400 Tomahawk Creek Pkwy., Leawood, KS, 66211-2672, (913) 906-6000, (800) 274-2237, Fax: (913) 906-6075, contactcenter@aafp.org, http://www.aafp.org.

American Medical Association, 515 N State St., Chicago, IL, 60610, (312) 464-5000, (800) 621-8335, http://www.ama-assn.org.

National Alliance on Mental Illness, 3803 N Fairfax Dr., Ste. 100, Arlington, VA, 22203, (703) 524-7600, http://www.nami.org.

National Center on Elder Abuse. Administration on Aging, 1 Massachusetts Ave. NW, Washington, DC, 20001, (202) 619-0724, Fax: (202) 357-3555, asainfo@asa.hhs.gov, http://www.aoa.gov.

National Committee for the Prevention of Elder Abuse, 151 1st Ave., No. 93, New York, NY, 10003, (800) 677-1116, Fax: (212) 420-6026, http://www.preventelderabuse.org.

U.S. National Library of Medicine, 8600 Rockville Pike, Bethesda, MD, 20894, http://www.nlm.nih.gov.

LeeAnn Paradise
Laura Jean Cataldo, RN, EdD

Electroconvulsive therapy

Definition

Electroconvulsive therapy (ECT) is a procedure in which a patient is treated by using controlled low-dose electric currents to induce a seizure. Also known as electroshock therapy, ECT is classified along with **vagus nerve stimulation**, repetitive **transcranial magnetic stimulation**, **magnetic seizure therapy**, and deep **brain** stimulation as a form of brain stimulation therapy.

Purpose

The purpose of ECT is to produce a convulsion that may relieve symptoms associated with such mental illnesses as **major depressive disorder**, treatment-resistant **depression**, **bipolar disorder**, severe mania, acute **psychosis**, and **catatonia**.

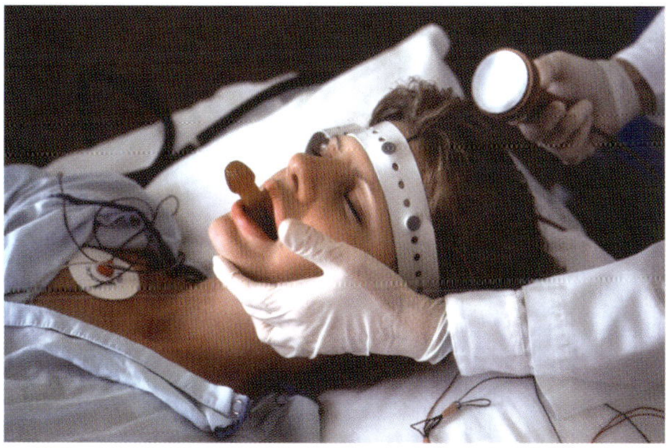

A woman prepares to receive electroconvulsive therapy (ECT), a treatment for depression. ECT works by inducing seizures in the brain; the rubber mouthpiece will keep the patient from biting down on her teeth or her tongue during the procedure. *(© Photo Researchers, Inc.)*

ECT is also used as a treatment of last resort for patients with Parkinson's disease, **Tourette syndrome**, and treatment-resistant **obsessive-compulsive disorder**.

Demographics

The demographics of ECT vary widely around the world: Some countries consider it a safe and effective treatment for severe depression and other mental disorders and have strict guidelines regarding its administration (United States, United Kingdom), whereas other countries either do not permit its use (Slovenia) or severely restrict it (Italy, the Netherlands). One problem has to do with the shortage of anesthesiologists in some countries, resulting in ECT being administered without anesthesia (Japan, India). Other countries permit the administration of ECT without the patient's **informed consent**.

Statistics about the use of ECT in the United States are difficult to obtain because some states require hospitals to report its use and others do not. The **American Psychiatric Association** estimated in the late 1990s that about 100,000 people received ECT each year, with wide variations in different parts of the country. ECT is used more often in private than in public hospitals, and minority patients are underrepresented among those receiving ECT. About 70% of patients receiving ECT in the United States are women, but this figure is usually explained as a result of the fact that more women than men are diagnosed with severe or treatment-resistant depression. The most recent figures from the United Kingdom indicate that 12,000 persons receive ECT each year.

Description

ECT uses low-dose electric currents together with anesthesia, muscle relaxants, and oxygen to produce a mild generalized seizure or convulsion. With repeated administration, usually over a period of weeks, ECT may be effective in relieving symptoms of several mental illnesses.

The American Psychiatric Association's *Practice Guidelines for the Treatment of Psychiatric Disorders* discusses the use of ECT in the treatment of major depressive disorder, bipolar disorder, and **schizophrenia**. It is most closely associated with the treatment of severe depression. Historically, ECT was the treatment of choice for depression when a patient with severe depression or psychotic symptoms was at increased risk of committing **suicide** and had not responded to other treatments. The third edition of the APA practice guide to the treatment of depression, published in November 2010, notes that "Electroconvulsive therapy has the highest rates of response and remission of any form of antidepressant treatment, with 70%–90% of those treated showing improvement.... The proportion of patients with major depressive disorder who respond to ECT is still greater than the proportion who respond to antidepressant medication. In addition, ECT has been associated with significant improvements in health-related quality of life." The guide also notes that patients with catatonia, **neuroleptic malignant syndrome**, and parkinsonism may benefit from the procedure.

According to the APA, the normal course of treatment for patients receiving ECT is 2–3 treatments per week for a total of 6–12 treatments in most cases. The total rarely exceeds 20 treatments. Premature termination of ECT is associated with a worse prognosis.

Although antidepressant medications are effective in many cases, they may take 2–6 weeks to begin to work. In addition, some patients with mania and schizophrenia may not be able to tolerate the side effects of the antipsychotic medications used to treat these disorders. For these individuals, ECT is an option. ECT is also indicated when patients need a treatment that brings about rapid improvement because they are refusing to eat or drink or presenting some other danger to themselves.

ECT is also recommended for certain subgroups of patients diagnosed with depression. Many elderly patients, for example, respond better to ECT than to antidepressant medications. Pregnant women are another subgroup that may benefit from ECT. Because ECT does not harm a fetus as some medications might, pregnant women with severe depression can choose ECT for relief of their depressive symptoms.

As of 2011, other treatments, such as transcranial magnetic stimulation (TMS), were becoming available and replacing ECT in some cases. According to experts at the Mayo Clinic, ECT and TMS have both benefits and drawbacks, and some patients are more likely to benefit from ECT than from TMS.

Origins

ECT was introduced in 1938 by two Italian psychiatrists, Ugo Cerletti (1877–1963) and Lucio Bini (1908–1964). According to Cerletti, the idea of using electroshocks to treat schizophrenia by inducing a convulsion came to him while observing slaughterhouse workers in Rome use electric shocks to anesthetize cattle before cutting their throats. The shocks caused the animals to have epileptic convulsions, which rendered them unable to resist the butchers. Cerletti thought that electroshocks might help schizophrenics, because it was noted in the 1930s that patients with epilepsy rarely developed schizophrenia. After experimenting on animals, Cerletti and his colleague Bini used ECT for the first time on a human patient, a homeless man with schizophrenia, in April 1938. The treatment was successful, and Cerletti and Bini extended the use of ECT to treat patients with depression and bipolar disorder as well as schizophrenia. Some in the medical community were receptive to this approach because physicians were already using a variety of chemicals to produce **seizures** in patients. Unfortunately, many of their patients died or had severe injuries because the strength of the convulsions could not be well controlled.

Cerletti's reasoning about an association between epilepsy and immunity from schizophrenia was incorrect, as was his theory that ECT works by causing the brain to release what he called "vitalizing" chemicals that cure the symptoms of mental illness. He attempted to prove this theory by injecting patients with a liquid suspension that contained particles of electroshocked pigs' brains. Although this treatment apparently helped to relieve the symptoms of some of Cerletti's patients, it never caught on.

In the 1940s and 1950s, the treatment was considered controversial. As ECT became more widely used, many members of the general public and some in the psychiatric profession were opposed to its use. To them it seemed barbaric. ECT joined **psychosurgery** as one of the most intensely distrusted psychiatric and neurological practices. Many people were frightened simply because ECT was called "shock treatment." Many assumed the procedure would be painful; others thought it was a form of electrocution; and still others believed it would cause brain damage. Unfavorable publicity in newspapers, magazines, and movies added to these fears. Indeed, up through the 1960s, doctors and nurses did not usually explain either ECT or other forms of psychiatric treatment to patients and their families. Moreover, many critics had good reasons for opposing the procedure before it was refined. Neither anesthesia nor muscle relaxants were used in the early days of ECT. As a result, patients had violent seizures, and even though they did not remember them, the thought of the procedure itself seemed frightening. Even more unfortunately, this crude early version of ECT was applied sometimes to patients who could never have benefited from ECT under any conditions.

As the procedures used with ECT became more refined, psychiatrists found that ECT could be an effective treatment for schizophrenia, depression, and bipolar disorder. The use of ECT, however, was phased out when antipsychotic and antidepressant drugs were introduced during the 1950s and 1960s. The psychiatric community reintroduced ECT several years later when patients who did not respond to the new drugs stimulated a search by mental health professionals for effective and, if necessary, non-drug treatments. While the new psychotropic medications provided relief for untold thousands of patients who suffered greatly from their illnesses and would otherwise have been condemned to mental hospitals, the drugs unfortunately produced a number of side effects, some irreversible. Another drawback is that some medications do not have a noticeable effect on the patient's mood for 2–6 weeks. During this time, the patient may be at risk for suicide. In addition, there are patients who do not respond to any medications or have severe allergic reactions to them.

ECT in contemporary practice

ECT is performed in both inpatient and outpatient facilities in specially equipped rooms with oxygen, suction, and cardiopulmonary resuscitation equipment readily available to deal with the rare emergency. A team of healthcare professionals, including a **psychiatrist**, an anesthesiologist, a respiratory therapist, and other assistants, is present throughout the entire procedure.

Administration of ECT

ECT is performed while the patient is unconscious. Unconsciousness is induced by a short-acting barbiturate such as methohexital (Brevital Sodium) or another appropriate anesthetic drug. The drug is given intravenously. To prevent patients from harming themselves during the convulsions or seizures induced by ECT, they are given succinylcholine (Anectine) or a similar drug that temporarily paralyzes the muscles. Because the patients' muscles are relaxed, the seizures does not produce any violent contractions of the limbs and torso. Instead, patients lie quietly on the operating table. One of the patient's hands or feet, however, is tied off with a tourniquet before the muscle relaxant is given. The tourniquet prevents the muscles in this limb from being paralyzed like the muscles in other parts of the patient's body. The hand or foot is used to monitor muscle movement induced by the electrical current applied to the brain.

A breathing tube is then inserted into the unconscious patient's airway and a rubber mouthpiece is inserted into the mouth to prevent the person from biting down on teeth or tongue during the electrically induced convulsion. As the current is applied, brain activity is monitored using **electroencephalography**. These brain wave tracings tell the medical team exactly how long the seizure lasts. The contraction of muscles in the arm or leg not affected by the muscle relaxant also provides an indication of the seizure's duration.

The electrodes for ECT may be placed on both sides of the head (bilaterally) or on one side only (unilaterally). Physicians often use bilateral electrode placement during the first week or so of treatments. An electric current is passed through the brain by means of a machine specifically designed for this purpose. The usual dose of electricity is 70–150 volts for 0.1–0.5 seconds. In the first stage of the seizure (tonic phase), the muscles in the body that have not been paralyzed by medication contract for a period of 5–15 seconds. This is followed by the second stage of the seizure (clonic phase) that is characterized by twitching movements, usually visible only in the toes or in a nonparalyzed arm or leg. These are caused by alternating contraction and relaxation of these same muscles. This stage lasts approximately 10–60 seconds. The physician in charge will try to induce a seizure that lasts between 30 seconds and two minutes. If the first application of electricity fails to produce a seizure lasting at least 25 seconds, another attempt is made 60 seconds later. The session is stopped if the patient has no seizures after three attempts. The entire procedure lasts about 30 minutes.

Unilateral placement of the electrodes, usually on the right side of the patient's head because it is on the side opposite the memory and learning areas of the brain, appears to produce fewer side effects. Another method of administration that is gaining favor is the administration of the electric current in several short bursts rather than a single constant high dose. Like unilateral electrode placement, the "brief pulse" approach to ECT produces fewer side effects.

The absence of seizures is most commonly caused either by the patient's physical condition at the time of treatment or by the individual nature of human responses to drugs and other treatment procedures. Just as there are some patients who do not respond to one type of antidepressant medication but do respond to others, some patients do not respond to ECT.

The total number of ECT treatments that will be given depends on such factors as the patient's age, **diagnosis**, the history of illness, family support, and response to therapy. Treatments are normally given every other day at a rate of two to three per week. The ECT treatments are stopped when the patient's psychiatric symptoms show significant signs of improvement. Depending on the patient's condition, this improvement may happen in a few weeks or, rarely, over a six-month period. In most cases, patients with depression require 6–12 ECT sessions. Only rarely is ECT treatment extended beyond six months. In such infrequent cases, treatments are decreased from two to four per week after the first month to one treatment every month or so.

No one knows for certain why ECT is effective. Because the treatment involves passing an electric

KEY TERMS

Catatonia—A syndrome associated with schizophrenia in which the patient may be stupefied and nearly immobile, holding rigid poses for hours and ignoring external stimuli. At the other extreme, the patient may exhibit extreme hyperactivity.

Hippocampus—A structure in the medial temporal lobe of the brain associated with memory consolidation and spatial navigation.

Neurogenesis—The development of new nerve cells in the brain, whether before birth or during adulthood.

Psychosis—A general psychiatric term for a condition in which the patient loses touch with reality. It is marked by such symptoms as hallucinations, delusions, personality changes, and disordered thinking.

Somatization disorder—A disorder in which patients seek medical treatment for a variety of vague physical ailments with no discernible organic cause. It is usually thought to result from the patient's expressing emotional distress through physical complaints.

current through the brain, which is electrically excitable tissue, it is not surprising that ECT has been shown to affect many neurotransmitter systems. **Neurotransmitters** are chemical messengers in the nervous system that carry signals from nerve cell to nerve cell. The neurotransmitters affected by ECT include **dopamine**, norepinephrine, **serotonin**, and gamma-aminobutyric acid (GABA). A newer theory about the effectiveness of ECT is that it stimulates the growth of new nerve cells in the hippocampus, the part of the brain associated with long-term memory formation and consolidation. This process is known as hippocampal neurogenesis.

Benefits

A majority of patients given ECT notice improvements in their symptoms after two or three treatments, although full improvement typically takes longer. Overall, ECT is a safe procedure. There is no convincing evidence of long-term harmful effects from ECT.

Precautions

Precautions include taking a complete medication history and screening patients for heart problems or other disorders that may contraindicate the use of general anesthesia or of ECT itself.

If an ECT-induced seizure lasts too long (more than two minutes) during the procedure, physicians will control it with an intravenous infusion of an anticonvulsant drug, usually **diazepam** (Valium).

Preparation

Patients and their relatives are typically prepared for ECT by viewing a videotape that explains both the procedure and the risks involved. The physician then answers any questions these individuals might have, and the patient is asked to sign an informed consent form. This form gives the doctor and the hospital legal permission to administer the treatment. Informed consent is a requirement for ECT treatment in the United States and the United Kingdom.

After the form has been signed, the doctor performs a complete physical examination and orders a number of tests that can help identify any potential problem. These tests may include a chest x ray, electrocardiogram (EKG), CT scan, urinalysis, spinal x ray, electroencephalogram (EEG), and complete blood count (CBC).

Some medications, such as lithium and a class of **antidepressants** known as **monoamine oxidase inhibitors (MAOIs)**, should be discontinued for some time before ECT administration. Patients are instructed not to eat or drink for at least eight hours prior to the procedure to reduce the possibility of vomiting and choking. During the procedure itself, the members of the healthcare team closely monitor the patient's vital signs, including blood pressure, heart rate, and oxygen content.

Aftercare

The patient is moved to a recovery area after an ECT treatment. Vital signs are recorded every five minutes until the patient is fully awake, which may take 15–30 minutes. The patient may experience some initial confusion, but this feeling usually disappears in a matter of minutes. The patient may complain of headache, muscle pain, or back pain, which can be relieved by aspirin or another mild medication.

Following successful ECT treatments, patients with bipolar disorder may be given maintenance doses of lithium. Similarly, patients with depression may be given antidepressant drugs. These medications are intended to reduce the chance of **relapse** or the recurrence of symptoms. Some studies have estimated that approximately one-third to one-half of patients treated with ECT relapse within 12 months of treatment. After three years, this figure may increase to two-thirds. Follow-up care

QUESTIONS TO ASK YOUR DOCTOR

- What is your opinion of ECT as a treatment for depression? For other mental disorders?
- Have you ever referred a patient to a psychiatrist for ECT? If so, did the patient find ECT beneficial?
- What is the risk of memory loss with ECT?
- In your opinion, why is ECT still controversial?

with medications for bipolar disorder or depression can reduce the relapse rate in the year following ECT treatment from 50% to 20%. Some patients might relapse because they do not respond well to the medications they take after their ECT sessions are completed. In some cases, patients who relapse may have severe forms of depression that are especially difficult to treat by any method.

Risks

Recent advances in medical technology have substantially reduced the complications associated with ECT. According to the NIMH, the most common side effects of contemporary ECT are headache, nausea, pain in the jaw, and mild muscle aches. Because ECT increases heart rate and raises blood pressure, persons at high risk of having complications following ECT include those with a recent heart attack, uncontrolled high blood pressure, brain tumors, and previous spinal injuries.

One of the most common side effects of ECT is memory loss. Patients may be unable to recall events that occurred before and after treatment. Elderly patients, for example, may become increasingly confused and forgetful as the treatments continue. In a minority of individuals, memory loss may last for months. For the majority of patients, however, recent memories return in a few days or weeks. Both unilateral electrode placement and the use of brief pulses of electricity rather than a continual high dose have been found to reduce memory loss.

Research and general acceptance

Research in the effectiveness of ECT and different methods of administering it is ongoing. The procedure has its own specialty journal, the *Journal of ECT*, in its twenty-seventh year of publication as of 2011. In the early 2000s, the **National Institute of Mental Health** (NIMH) supported the formation of the Consortium for Research in ECT (CORE), a group of five medical centers across the United States that conduct studies of the effectiveness of ECT in treating mental disorders and ways to manage its side effects. Between 2004 and 2011, the consortium published ten major papers about the therapy, comparing it to pharmacologic treatment and also investigating different methods of administering ECT.

There were 54 **clinical trials** of ECT under way in 2011 investigating its effectiveness as a treatment for depression, schizophrenia, posttraumatic stress disorder, **somatization disorder**, and bipolar disorder. Some of the trials involved ECT as an adjunctive therapy for patients receiving medications while others were studying its effectiveness in preventing relapse. One study was investigating the comparative benefits of four different ways to administer ECT to depressed patients (right unilateral ECT at high dose; ultra-brief pulse width ECT; bilateral ECT at moderate dose; and traditional pulse width ECT). Three other studies were investigating ketamine as an anesthetic for patients receiving ECT.

Training and certification

While some medical schools in the United States allow third- and fourth-year medical students to learn how to give ECT under supervision, most trainees are residents in psychiatry. Some residency programs in psychiatry now require residents to receive both didactic (classroom) and hands-on training in ECT, and to demonstrate competency in administering ECT before graduating from the program.

Resources

BOOKS

Fink, Max. *Electroconvulsive Therapy: A Guide for Professionals and Their Patients*. New York: Oxford University Press, 2009.

Higgins, Edmund S., and Mark S. George. *Brain Stimulation Therapies for Clinicians*. Washington, DC: American Psychiatric Publishing, 2009.

Mankad, Mehul V., et al. *Clinical Manual of Electroconvulsive Therapy*. Washington, DC: American Psychiatric Publishing, 2010.

Shorter, Edward, and David Healy. *Shock Therapy: A History of Electroconvulsive Treatment in Mental Illness*. New Brunswick, NJ: Rutgers University Press, 2007.

PERIODICALS

Bolwig, T.G. "How Does Electroconvulsive Therapy Work? Theories on Its Mechanism." *Canadian Journal of Psychiatry* 56 (2011): 13–18.

England, M.L., et al. "Catatonia in Psychotic Patients: Clinical Features and Treatment Response." *Journal of Neuropsychiatry and Clinical Neurosciences* 23 (2011): 223–26.

Gahr, M., et al. "Somatization Disorder Treated with Electroconvulsive Therapy." *Journal of ECT* 27 (September 2011): 266–67.

Gosselink, M.J., et al. "Successful Electroconvulsive Therapy in a 95-Year-Old Man with a Cardiac Pacemaker: A Case Report." *American Journal of Geriatric Psychiatry* 19 (2011): 678–79.

Nahas, Z., and B.S. Anderson. "Brain Stimulation Therapies for Mood Disorders: The Continued Necessity of Electroconvulsive Therapy." *Journal of the American Psychiatric Nurses Association* 17 (2011): 214–16.

Petrides, G., et al. "Seizure Threshold in a Large Sample: Implications for Stimulus Dosing Strategies in Bilateral Electroconvulsive Therapy: A Report from CORE." *Journal of ECT* 25 (2009): 232–37.

Rasmussen, K.G. "Some Considerations in Choosing Electroconvulsive Therapy Versus Transcranial Magnetic Stimulation for Depression." *Journal of ECT* 27 (2011): 51–54.

Rasmussen, K.G., et al. "Is Baseline Medication Resistance Associated with Potential for Relapse after Successful Remission of a Depressive Episode with ECT? Data from the Consortium for Research on Electroconvulsive Therapy (CORE)." *Journal of Clinical Psychiatry* 70 (2009): 232–37.

Sienaert, P. "What We Have Learned about Electroconvulsive Therapy and Its Relevance for the Practising Psychiatrist." *Canadian Journal of Psychiatry* 56 (2011): 5–12.

Smith, G.E., et al. "A Randomized Controlled Trial Comparing the Memory Effects of Continuation Electroconvulsive Therapy Versus Continuation Pharmacotherapy: Results from the Consortium for Research in ECT (CORE) Study." *Journal of Clinical Psychiatry* 71 (2010): 185–93.

Tess, A.V., and Smetana, G.W. "Medical Evaluation of Patients Undergoing Electroconvulsive Therapy." *New England Journal of Medicine* 360, no. 14 (April 2, 2009): 1437–1444.

Tominaga, K., et al. "Symptom Predictors of Response to Electroconvulsive Therapy in Older Patients with Treatment-resistant Depression." *International Journal of General Medicine* 4 (2011): 515–19.

OTHER

Mayo Clinic. "Video: Electroconvulsive Therapy (ECT)." http://www.mayoclinic.com/health/electroconvulsive-therapy/MM00606 (accessed September 25, 2011).

WEBSITES

"Brain Stimulation Therapies." National Institute of Mental Health.http://www.nimh.nih.gov/health/topics/brain-stimulation-therapies/brain-stimulation-therapies.shtml (accessed October 14, 2011).

"Electroconvulsive Therapy (ECT)." Mayo Clinic. July 9, 2010. http://www.mayoclinic.com/health/electroconvulsive-therapy/MY00129 (accessed October 14, 2011).

"Practice Guideline for the Treatment of Patients with Major Depressive Disorder." American Psychiatric Association. November 2010. http://www.psychiatryonline.com/pracGuide/pracGuideTopic_7.aspx (accessed October 14, 2011).

ORGANIZATIONS

American Psychiatric Association, 1000 Wilson Blvd., Ste. 1825, Arlington, VA, 22209-3901, (703) 907-7300, apa@psych.org, http://www.psych.org.

National Institute of Mental Health, 6001 Executive Blvd., Rm. 8184, MSC 9663, Bethesda, MD, 20892-9663, (301) 433-4513; TTY: (301) 443-8431, Fax: (301) 443-4279, (866) 615-6464; TTY: (866) 415-8051, nimhinfo@nih.gov, http://www.nimh.nih.gov.

National Institute of Neurological Disorders and Stroke, PO Box 5801, Bethesda, MD, 20824, (301) 496-5751; TTY: (301) 468-5981, (800) 352-9424, http://www.ninds.nih.gov.

Dean A. Haycock, PhD
Ruth A. Wienclaw, PhD
Rebecca J. Frey, PhD

Electroencephalography

Definition

Electroencephalography (EEG), also know as **brain** wave test, is a neurological test that measures and records electrical activity in the brain over time.

Purpose

The EEG is a key tool in the **diagnosis** and management of epilepsy and other seizure disorders. It is also used to assist in the diagnosis of brain damage and diseases such as **stroke**, brain tumors, encephalitis, intellectual disabilities, and **sleep disorders**, and to determine brain status and brain death.

Description

Brain function is associated with electrical activity, which is always accompanied by an electrical field. This field consists of two parts, the electrical field and the magnetic field, and is called an electromagnetic field. The electroencephalogram records electrical field activity through the use of surface electrodes.

Prior to the recording session, a nurse or technologist attaches approximately 16–21 electrodes to a person's scalp using an electrically conductive, washable paste. The electrodes are placed on the head in a standard

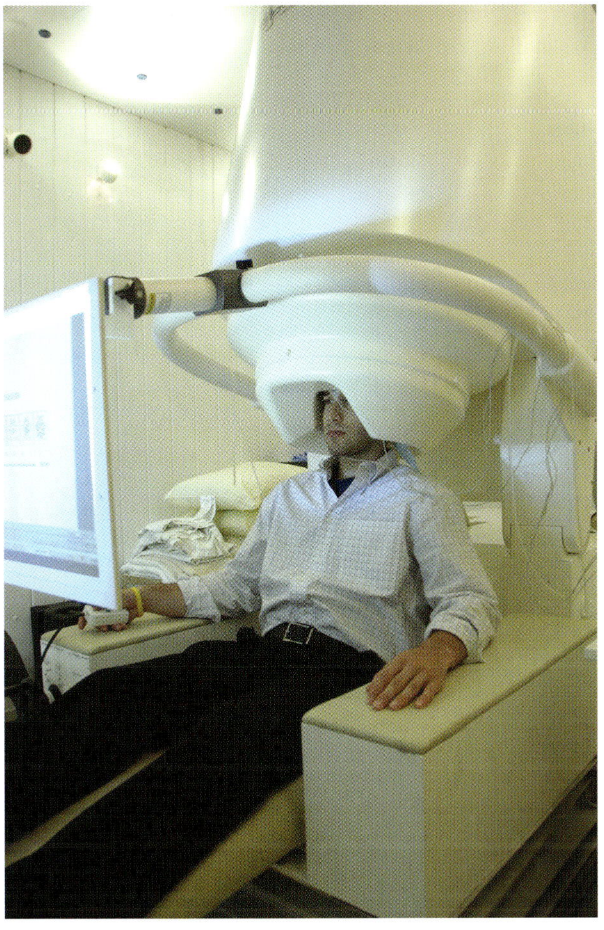

A male patient undergoes magnetoencephalography (MEG). *(U.S. National Institute of Mental Health)*

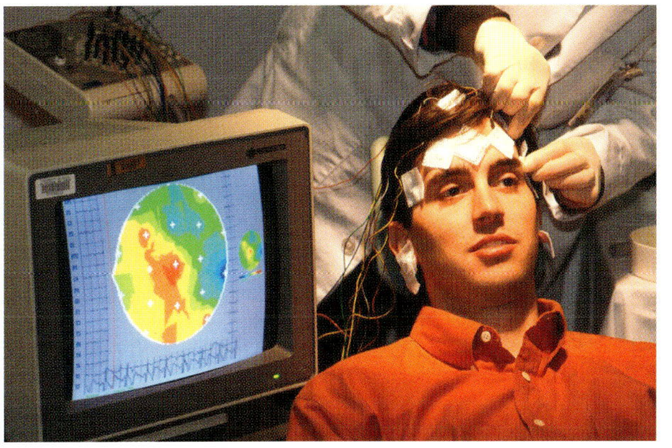

An EEG lab measures the brain waves of a subject. *(© Richard T. Nowitz/Photo Researchers, Inc.)*

pattern based on head circumference measurements. Depending on the purpose for the EEG, implantable, or invasive, electrodes are occasionally used. Implantable electrodes include sphenoidal electrodes, which are fine wires inserted under the zygomatic arch, or cheekbone. Depth electrodes, or subdural strip electrodes, are surgically implanted into the brain and are used to localize a seizure focus in preparation for epilepsy surgery. Once in place, even implantable electrodes do not cause pain. The electrodes are used to measure the electrical activity in various regions of the brain over the course of the test period.

For the test, a person lies on a bed, padded table, or comfortable chair and is asked to relax and remain still while measurements are being taken. An EEG usually takes no more than one hour, although long-term monitoring is often used for diagnosis of seizure disorders. During the test procedure, a person may be asked to breathe slowly or quickly. Visual stimuli such as flashing lights or a patterned board may be used to stimulate certain types of brain activity. Throughout the procedure, the EEG unit makes a continuous graphic record of the person's brain activity, or brain waves, on a long strip of recording paper or computer screen. This graphic record is called an electroencephalogram. If the display is computerized, the test may be called a digital EEG, or dEEG.

The sleep EEG uses the same equipment and procedures as a regular EEG. Persons undergoing a sleep EEG are encouraged to fall asleep completely rather than just relax. They are typically provided a bed and a quiet room conducive to sleep. A sleep EEG lasts up to three hours, or up to eight or nine hours if it is a night's sleep.

In an ambulatory EEG, individuals are hooked up to a portable cassette recorder. They then go about normal activities and take normal rest and sleep for a period of up to 24 hours. During this period, individuals and their family members record any symptoms or abnormal behaviors, which can later be correlated with the EEG to see if they represent **seizures**.

An extension of the EEG technique, called quantitative EEG (qEEG), involves manipulating the EEG signals with a computer using the fast Fourier transform algorithm. The result is then best displayed using a colored gray scale transposed onto a schematic map of the head to form a topographic image. The brain map produced in this technique is a vivid illustration of electrical activity in the brain. This technique also has the ability to compare the similarity of the signals between different electrodes, a measurement known as spectral coherence. Studies have shown the value of this measurement in diagnosis of **Alzheimer's disease** and mild closed-head injuries. The technique can also identify areas of the brain having abnormally slow

KEY TERMS

Encephalitis—Inflammation of the brain.

Epilepsy—A neurological disorder characterized by recurrent seizures with or without a loss of consciousness.

Fast Fourier transform (FFT)—A mathematical process used in EEG analysis to investigate the composition of an EEG signal.

Occipital bone—Bone that forms the back part of the skull.

Sphenoidal electrodes—Fine wire electrodes that are implanted under the cheek bones, used to measure temporal seizures.

Subdural electrodes—Strip electrodes that are placed under dura mater (the outermost, toughest, and most fibrous of the three membranes [meninges] covering the brain and spinal cord). They are used to locate foci of epileptic seizures prior to epilepsy surgery.

Zygomatic arch—Cheekbone. A quadrilateral bone forming the prominence of the cheek. It articulates (touches or moves) with the frontal, sphenoid, maxillary, and temporal bones.

activity when the data are both mapped and compared to known normal values. The result is then known as a statistical or significance probability map (SPM). This allows differentiation between early **dementia** (increased slowing) or otherwise uncomplicated **depression** (no slowing). The quantitative EEG is also known by the acronym BEAM (brain electrical activity mapping).

Magnetoencephalography

Magnetoencephalography, a supplement to EEG, also uses an electroencephalogram to measure the patient's electrical field. Every electrical current generates a magnetic field. The magnetic field is detected by an instrument called a biomagnetometer and recorded as a magnetoencephalograph (MEG). The information provided by the MEG is entirely different from that provided by **computed tomography** (CT), topographic encephalography, or **magnetic resonance imaging** (MRI)—imaging instruments that provide still, structural, and anatomical information. Using MEG, the brain can be observed "in action," rather than just being viewed as a still image. The information recorded by the MEG provides important supplemental information to that recorded by the encephalogram, and when used together, they both provide a much more complete and comprehensive idea of cerebral events.

Magnetoencephalography has been used to map the sensory and motor cortices of the brain, determine the organization of the auditory center of the brain, and study cognitive functions such as speech, memory, attention, and consciousness. This information is critical for neurosurgical planning, such as the removal of brain lesions. Thus, preoperative MEG is valuable in planning the surgical treatment of tumors and malformations. MEG can provide surgeons with real-time computer-generated images of deep-seated lesions that are essential before surgery.

Preparation

An EEG is generally performed as one test in a series of neurological evaluations. Rarely does the EEG form the sole basis for a particular diagnosis.

Full instructions should be given to individuals receiving an EEG when they schedule their test. Typically, individuals taking medications that affect the central nervous system, such as anticonvulsants, stimulants, or **antidepressants**, are told to discontinue their prescription for a short time prior to the test (usually one to two days). However, such requests should be cleared with the treating physician. EEG test candidates may be asked to avoid food and beverages that contain caffeine, a central nervous system stimulant. They may also be asked to arrive for the test with clean hair that is free of styling products to make attachment of the electrodes easier.

Individuals undergoing a sleep EEG may be asked to remain awake the night before their test. They may be given a sedative prior to the test to induce sleep.

Aftercare

If an individual has suspended regular medication for the test, the EEG nurse or technician should advise as to when to begin taking it again.

Risks

The primary risk of EEG is the production of a seizure in a patient with epilepsy. This may result from the temporary discontinuation of anticonvulsant medication or from the provocation of a seizure by an epileptogenic stimulus such as flashing lights or deep breathing. Although the provocation of a seizure may serve to substantiate the diagnosis, all patients with the potential for seizures should be carefully monitored to avoid injury in case a seizure does result.

QUESTIONS TO ASK THE DOCTOR

- Will I experience any side effects after the EEG is performed?
- What preparations are being made to treat an induced seizure?
- Is the supervising physician appropriately certified to interpret an EEG?

Results

In reading and interpreting brain wave patterns, a neurologist or other physician will evaluate the type of brain waves and the symmetry, location, and consistency of brain wave patterns. Brain wave response to certain stimuli presented during the EEG test (such as flashing lights or noise) will also be evaluated.

The rate, height, and length of brain waves vary depending on the part of the brain being studied, and every individual has a unique and characteristic brain-wave pattern. Age and state of consciousness also cause changes in wave patterns. Several wave patterns have been identified:

- Alpha waves—Most of the recorded waves in a normal adult's EEG are the occipital alpha waves, which are best obtained from the back of the head when the subject is awake but resting quietly with eyes closed. These waves, occurring typically in a pattern of 8–13 hertz (cycles per second), are blocked by excitement or by opening the eyes. Abnormal alpha patterns include the presence of alpha rhythms in a newborn, which can signify seizure activity.
- Beta waves—Obtained from the central and frontal parts of the brain, beta waves are closely related to the sensory-motor parts of the brain and are also blocked by opening the eyes. Their frequency is in the range of 13–30 hertz. Marked asymmetry in beta rhythms suggests a structural lesion on the side lacking the beta waves. Beta waves are also commonly measured over skull lesions, such as fractures or burr holes, in activity known as a breach rhythm.
- Delta waves—Delta waves are irregular, slow waves of less than 4 hertz that are normally found in deep sleep and in infants and young children. They indicate an abnormality in an awake adult. Intermittent delta rhythms are also an indication of damage of the relays between the deep gray matter and the cortex of the brain.
- Theta waves—Characterized by rhythmic, slow waves of 4–7 hertz, theta waves usually only occur during sleep. The presence of theta waves in awake adults may indicate an abnormality.

EEG readings of patients with epilepsy or other seizure disorders display bursts, or spikes, of electrical activity. In focal epilepsy, spikes are restricted to one hemisphere of the brain. If spikes are generalized to both hemispheres of the brain, multifocal epilepsy may be present. The EEG can be used to localize the region of the brain where the abnormal electrical activity is occurring. This is most easily accomplished using a recording method, or montage, called an average reference montage. With this type of recording, the signal from each electrode is compared to the average signal from all the electrodes. The negative amplitude (upward movement, by convention) of the spike is observed for the different channels, or inputs, from the various electrodes. The negative deflection will be greatest as recorded by the electrode that is closest in location to the origin of the abnormal activity. The spike will be present but of reduced amplitude as the electrodes move farther away from the site producing the spike. Electrodes distant from the site will not record the spike occurrence.

Diagnostic brain-wave patterns of other disorders vary widely. In general, disease typically increases slow activity, such as theta or delta waves, but decreases fast activity, such as alpha and beta waves. The appearance of excess theta waves (4–8 hertz) may indicate brain injury. Brain-wave patterns in patients with brain disease, intellectual disabilities, and brain injury show overall slowing. A trained medical specialist should interpret EEG results in the context of the patient's medical history and other pertinent medical test results.

Resources

BOOKS

Daube, J.R., and R. Devin. *Clinical Neurophysiology*. 3rd ed. New York: Oxford University Press, 2009.

Ebersole, J.S., and T.A. Pedley. *Current Practice of Clinical Electroencephalography*. 3rd ed. Philadelphia: Lippincott Williams & Wilkins, 2003.

Misulism, Karl E., and T.C. Head. *Essentials of Clinical Neurophysiology*. 3rd ed. London: Butterworth-Heinemann, 2002.

Rowan, A.J., and E. Tolunsky. *Primer of EEG*. London: Elsevier, 2003.

PERIODICALS

Coburn, Kerry L., et al. "The Value of Quantitative Electroencephalography in Clinical Psychiatry: A Report by the Committee on Research of the American Neuropsychiatric Association." *Journal of Neuropsychiatry & Clinical Neurosciences* 18, no. 4 (November 2006): 460–500.

Frith, Chris D. "The Value of Brain Imaging in the Study of Development and Its Disorders." *Journal of Child Psychology and Psychiatry* 47, no. 10 (November 2006): 979–82.

Hurley, Robin A., Ronald Fisher, and Katherine H. Taber. "Windows to the Brain—Sudden Onset Panic: Epileptic Aura or Panic Disorder?" *Journal of Neuropsychiatry & Clinical Neurosciences* 18, no. 4 (November 2006): 436–43.

Knowlton, Robert C., et al. "Magnetic Source Imaging Versus Intracranial Electroencephalogram in Epilepsy Surgery: A Prospective Study." *Annals of Neurology* 59, no. 5 (May 2006): 835–42.

O'Sullivan, S.S., et al. "The Role of the Standard EEG in Clinical Psychiatry." *Human Psychopharmacology: Clinical and Experimental* 21, no. 4 (June 2006): 265–71.

WEBSITES

KidsHealth.org. "EEG (Electroencephalography)." September 2008. http://kidshealth.org/parent/system/medical/eeg.html (accessed October 5, 2011).

ORGANIZATIONS

American Association of Neuromuscular and Electrodiagnostic Medicine, 2621 Superior Drive NW, Rochester, MN, 55901, (507) 288-0100, aanem@aanem.org, http://www.aamnem.org.

American Board of Registration for Electroencephalographic Technologists, 2509 West Iles Ave., Suite 102, Springfield, IL, 62704, (217) 726-7980, Fax: (217) 726-7989, abreteo@att.net, http://www.abret.org.

American Society of Electroneurodiagnostic Technologists, 402 East Bannister Rd., Suite A, Kansas City, MO, 64131-3019, (816) 931-1120, Fax: (816) 931-1145, info@aset.org, http://www.aset.org.

Epilepsy Foundation, 8301 Professional Place, Landover, MD, 20785, (800) 332-1000, Fax: (301) 577-2684, http://www.epilepsyfoundation.org.

L. Fleming Fallon, Jr., MD, DrPH
Laura Jean Cataldo, RN, EdD
Brenda W. Lerner

Enabling behaviors *see* **Addiction**

Encopresis

Definition

Encopresis is an elimination disorder that involves repeatedly having bowel movements in inappropriate places after the age when bowel control is normally expected. Encopresis is also called "soiling" or "fecal incontinence."

Demographics

Encopresis occurs in 1%–3% of children from ages four to seven years and is seen more often in boys than in girls. The frequency of encopresis appears to be independent of social class, and there is no evidence that it runs in families.

Description

By four years of age, most children are toilet trained for bowel movements. After that age, if inappropriate bowel movements occur regularly over a period of several months a child may be diagnosed with encopresis. Encopresis can be intentional or unintentional. Intentional soiling is associated with several psychiatric disorders. Involuntary or unintentional soiling is often the result of constipation.

Causes and symptoms

The only symptom of encopresis is that a person has bowel movements in inappropriate places, such as in clothing or on the floor. This soiling is not caused by taking laxatives or other medications and is not due to a disability or physical defect in the bowel. There are two main types of encopresis, and they have different causes.

Involuntary encopresis

With involuntary encopresis, a person has no control over elimination of feces from the bowel. The feces is semi-soft to almost liquid, and it leaks into clothing without the person making any effort to expel it. Leakage usually occurs during the day when the person is active and ranges from infrequent to almost continuous.

Involuntary soiling usually results from constipation. A hard mass of feces develops in the large intestine and is not completely expelled during a regular bowel movement in the toilet. This mass then stretches the large intestine out of shape, allowing liquid feces behind it to leak out. Up to 95% of encopresis is involuntary.

Although involuntary encopresis, called by the **American Psychiatric Association** (APA) encopresis with constipation and overflow incontinence, is caused by constipation, the constipation may be the result of psychological factors. Experiencing a stressful life event, harsh toilet training, toilet fear, or emotionally disturbing events can cause a child to withhold bowel movements or become constipated. Children separated from their parents during World War II were reported to have shown a high incidence of encopresis, indicating that psychological factors play a role in this disorder.

Voluntary encopresis

A person with voluntary encopresis has control over when and where bowel movements occur and chooses to have them in inappropriate places. Constipation is not a factor, and the feces is usually a normal consistency. Often feces is smeared in an obvious place, although sometimes it is hidden around the house. The APA classifies voluntary encopresis as encopresis without constipation and overflow incontinence.

In young children, voluntary encopresis may represent a power struggle between the child and the caregiver doing the toilet training. In older children, voluntary encopresis is often associated with **oppositional defiant disorder** (ODD), **conduct disorder**, **sexual abuse**, or high levels of psychological stressors.

Diagnosis

To receive an APA **diagnosis** of encopresis, as listed in the ***Diagnostic and Statistical Manual of Mental Disorders*** (*DSM*), a child must have a bowel movement, either intentional or accidental, in an inappropriate place at least once a month for a minimum of three months. In addition, the child must be at least four years old, either chronologically or developmentally, and the soiling cannot be caused by illness, medical conditions (e.g., chronic diarrhea, spina bifida, or anal stenosis), medications or substances, or disabilities. However, it may be caused by constipation.

Treatment

Involuntary encopresis is treated by addressing the cause of the constipation and establishing soft, pain-free stools. This can include:

- increasing the amount of liquids a child drinks
- adding high-fiber foods to the diet
- short-term use of laxatives or stool softeners
- emptying the large intestine by using an enema
- establishing regular bowel habits

Once the constipation is resolved, involuntary encopresis normally stops.

Treatment of voluntary encopresis depends on the cause. When voluntary encopresis results from a power struggle between child and adult, it is treated with **behavior modification**. In addition to taking steps to ensure a soft, pain-free stool, the adult should make toileting a pleasant, pressure-free activity. Some experts suggest transferring the initiative for toileting to the child instead of constantly asking him or her to use the toilet. Others recommend toileting at scheduled times, but without pressure to perform. In either case, success should be praised and failure treated in a matter-of-fact manner. If opposition to using the toilet continues, the family may be referred to a child **psychiatrist** or a pediatric **psychologist**.

With older children who smear or hide feces, voluntary encopresis is usually a symptom of another more serious disorder. When children are successfully treated for the underlying disorder with psychiatric interventions, behavior modification, and education, the encopresis is often resolved.

KEY TERMS

Feces—Waste products eliminated from the large intestine; excrement.

Incontinence—The inability to control the release of urine or feces.

Laxative—Substance or medication that encourages a bowel movement.

Stools—Feces; bowel movements.

Prognosis

Because 80%–95% of encopresis is related to constipation, the success rate in resolving involuntary encopresis is high, although it may take time to establish good bowel habits and eliminate a reoccurrence of constipation. The success rate is also good for younger children in a power struggle with adults over toileting, although the results may be slow. The prognosis for older children with associated behavioral disorders is less promising and depends more on the success of resolving those problems than on direct treatment of the symptoms of encopresis.

Prevention

Power struggles during toilet training that lead to encopresis can be reduced by waiting until the child is developmentally ready and interested in using the toilet. Toilet training undertaken kindly, calmly, and with realistic expectations is most likely to lead to success. Successes should be rewarded and failures accepted. Once toilet training has been established, encopresis can be reduced by developing regular bowel habits and encouraging a healthy, high-fiber diet.

Resources

BOOKS

American Psychiatric Association. *Diagnostic and Statistical Manual of Mental Disorders*. 4th ed., text rev. Washington, DC: American Psychiatric Publishing, 2000.

Sadock, Benjamin J., and Virginia A. Sadock, eds. *Comprehensive Textbook of Psychiatry*. Vol. 2. 7th ed. Philadelphia: Lippincott Williams and Wilkins, 2000.

PERIODICALS

Catto-Smith, Anthony G. "Constipation and Toileting Issues in Children." *Medical Journal of Australia* 182, no. 5 (2005): 242–46. Available online at http://www.mja.com.au/public/issues/182_05_070305/cat10379_fm.html (accessed November 9, 2011).

Coehlo, Deborah Padgett. "Encopresis: A Medical and Family Approach." *Pediatric Nursing* 37, no. 3 (May–June 2011): 107–13.

Friman, Patrick C., Kristi L. Hofstadter, and Kevin M. Jones. "A Biobehavioral Approach to the Treatment of Functional Encopresis in Children." *The Journal of Early and Intensive Behavioral Intervention* 3, no. 3 (Fall 2006): 263–72.

von Gontard, Alexander. "Elimination Disorders: A Critical Comment on DSM-5 Proposals." *European Child & Adolescent Psychiatry* 20, no. 2 (February 2011): 83–88.

OTHER

University of Michigan Health System. "Functional Constipation and Soiling in Children: Guidelines for Clinical Care." September 2008. http://cme.med.umich.edu/pdf/guideline/peds08.pdf (accessed October 5, 2011).

ORGANIZATIONS

American Academy of Child and Adolescent Psychiatry, 3615 Wisconsin Ave. NW, Washington, DC, 20016-3007, (202) 966-7300, Fax: (202) 966-2891, http://aacap.org.

American Psychiatric Association, 1000 Wilson Blvd., Suite 1825, Arlington, VA, 22209-3901, (703) 907-7300, apa@psych.org, http://www.psych.org.

Tish Davidson, AM
Emily Jane Willingham, PhD

Endep *see* **Amitriptyline**

Energy therapies

Definition

Energy therapies is a collective term used to refer to a variety of alternative and complementary treatments based on the use, modification, or manipulation of energy fields. Most energy therapies presuppose or accept the theory that matter and energy are not exclusive opposites, but that matter is simply a denser form of energy that is more easily perceived by the senses. Some energy therapies are associated with systems of traditional Indian or Chinese medicine that are thousands of years old; others draw upon contemporary scientific theories. Energy therapies can be divided for purposes of discussion into two groups—those that utilize energy fields located in, affecting, or emanating from the human body (biofield therapies); and those that use electromagnetic fields in unconventional ways. In addition, there are energy therapies that combine biofield therapy with some aspects of bodywork—Breema, polarity therapy, and qigong are examples of this combined approach.

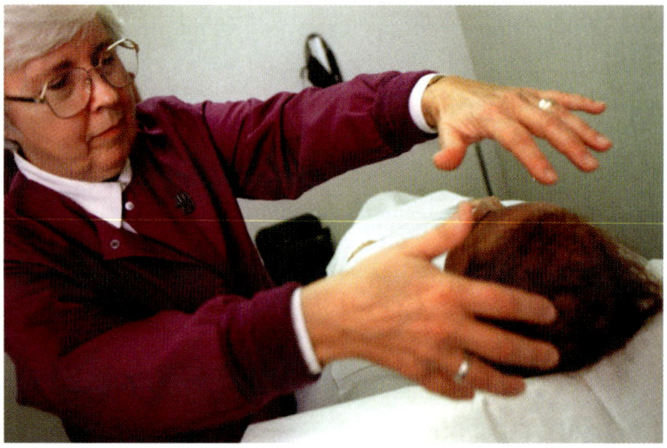

A woman receives healing touch therapy, a type of energy therapy. *(© Susan Tusa/KRT/newscom)*

Purpose

The purpose of energy therapies can be broadly defined as the healing of mental or physical disorders by rebalancing the energy fields in the human body or by drawing upon spiritual energies or forces for such healing. Some energy therapies include internal detoxification or release of trauma-related memories as additional purposes.

Description

Energy therapies vary widely in their understanding of qualifications to be a healer. Some have credentialing or training programs; others do not. Some practitioners of energy therapy believe that all or most people have the capacity to be healers; others regard the ability to use or direct healing energies as a gift or charism that is given only to people who are "chosen" or unusually spiritual.

Although energy therapies are often associated with either Eastern or so-called "New Age" belief systems, most do not expect people in need of healing to give up mainstream Western religious practice or allopathic medical/psychiatric treatments.

Therapeutic touch

Therapeutic touch, or TT, is a form of energy therapy that developed in the United States. It is a noninvasive method of healing derived from an ancient laying-on of hands technique. In TT, practitioners alter the patient's energy field through a transfer of energy from their hands to the patient. Therapeutic touch was developed in 1972 by Dora Kunz, a psychic healer, and Dolores Krieger, a professor of nursing at New York University. The principle behind TT is restoration of balance or harmony to the human energy field, or aura, that is thought to extend several inches to several feet from the body. When illness occurs, it creates a disturbance or blockage in the vital energy field. The TT practitioner uses her/his hands to discern the blockage or disturbance. Although the technique is called "therapeutic touch," there is generally no touching of the client's physical body, only his or her energetic body or field. TT is usually performed on fully clothed patients who are either lying down on a flat surface or sitting up in a chair.

A therapeutic touch session consists of five steps or phases. The first step is a period of **meditation** on the practitioner's part, to become spiritually centered and energized for the task of healing. The second step is assessment or discernment of the energy imbalances in the patient's aura. In this step, the TT practitioner holds his or her hands about 2–3 in. (5–7 cm) above the patient's body and moves them in long, sweeping strokes from the patient's head downward to the feet. The practitioner may feel a sense of warmth, heaviness, tingling, or similar cues, as they are known in TT. The cues are thought to reveal the location of the energy disturbances or imbalances. In the third step, known as the unruffling process, the practitioner removes the energy disturbances with downward sweeping movements. In the fourth step, the practitioner serves as a channel for the transfer of universal energy to the patient. The fifth step consists of smoothing the patient's energy field and restoring a symmetrical pattern of energy flow. After the treatment, the patient rests for 10–15 minutes.

Although therapeutic touch has become a popular alternative or complementary approach in some schools of nursing in the United States and Canada, acceptance by the mainstream medical community varies. Many hospitals permit nurses and staff to perform TT on patients at no extra charge. On the other hand, therapeutic touch became national news in April 1998 when an elementary-school student carried out research for a science project that questioned its claims. Twenty-one TT practitioners with experience ranging from one to 27 years were blindfolded and asked to identify whether the investigator's hand was closer to their right hand or their left. Placement of the investigator's hand was determined by flipping a coin. The TT practitioners were able to identify the correct hand in only 123 (44%) of 280 trials, a figure that could result from random chance alone. Debate about the merits of TT filled the editorial pages of the *Journal of the American Medical Association* for nearly a year after the news reports, and continues to this day.

Qigong

Qigong is a form of Chinese energy therapy that is usually considered a martial art by most Westerners. It is better understood as an ancient Chinese system of postures, exercises, breathing techniques and meditations. Its techniques are designed to improve and enhance the body's *qi*. According to traditional Chinese philosophy and medicine, qi is the fundamental life energy responsible for human health and vitality. Qi travels through the body along channels called meridians. There are 12 main meridians in humans. Each major body organ has qi associated with it, and each organ interacts with particular emotions on the mental level. Qigong techniques are designed to improve the balance and flow of energy throughout the meridians, and to increase the overall quantity and volume of a person's qi.

In the context of energy therapy, qigong is sometimes divided into internal and external qigong. Internal qigong refers to a person's practice of qigong exercises to maintain his or her own health and vitality. Some qigong master teachers are renowned for their skills in external qigong, in which the energy from one person is passed on to another for healing. Chinese hospitals use medical qigong along with herbs, **acupuncture** and other techniques of traditional Chinese medicine. In these hospitals, qigong healers use external qigong and also design specific internal qigong exercises for the patients' health problems.

Reiki

Reiki is a holistic alternative therapy based on Eastern concepts of energy flow and the seven chakras (energy centers) in the human body. Reiki was formulated by a Japanese teacher, Mikao Usui, around 1890, based on Vajrayana (Tibetan) Buddhism, but incorporates meditation techniques, beliefs, and symbols that are considerably older. It is distinctive among energy therapies in its emphasis on self-healing, its spiritual principles, and its accreditation of healers through a system of initiation. Reiki practitioners participate in the healing of emotional and spiritual as well as physical pain through the transmission of universal life energy, called "rei-ki" in Japanese. It is believed that ki flows throughout the universe, but that Reiki connects humans in a more direct way to the universal source. The U.S. Army unveiled a program in 2009 to investigate energy therapies such as Reiki to treat **brain** injuries and **post-traumatic stress disorder** in troops returning home from war. Various other studies are also underway in the United States and Canada, some examining the efficacy of the therapy in coping with pain and anxiety.

Although Reiki involves human touch, it is not massage therapy. The patient lies on a table fully clothed except for shoes while the practitioner places her or his hands over the parts of the body and the chakras in sequence. The hands are held palms downward with the fingers and thumbs extended. If the person is in pain or cannot turn over, the practitioner may touch only the affected part(s). Silence or music appropriate for meditation is considered essential to the treatment. Reiki healers practice daily self-healing, in which they place their hands in traditional positions on their own bodies They may use touch, or distant/non-touch.

Reiki healers are initiated into three levels of practice through attunements, which are ceremonies in which teachers transmit the hand positions and "sacred" symbols. Reiki I healers learn the basic hand positions and can practice direct physical, emotional or mental healing on themselves and others. Reiki II healers are taught the symbols that empower them to do distance or absentee healing. In Reiki III the healer makes a commitment to become a master teacher and do spiritual healing.

Polarity therapy

Polarity therapy, which is sometimes called polarity balancing, is a biofield therapy that resembles Reiki in its emphasis on energy flow, human touch, and the energy centers (chakras) in the human body. Polarity therapy was developed by Dr. Randolph Stone (1890-1981), an American chiropractor and naturopath. It integrates bodywork with diet, yoga-based **exercise**, and self-awareness techniques to release energy blockages in the patient's body, mind, or feelings. Polarity theory divides the body into three horizontal and four vertical zones (right, left, front, and back), each having a positive, negative, or neutral charge. Energy currents in the zones are correlated with five energy centers in the body corresponding to the five elements (ether, air, fire, water, and earth) of Ayurvedic medicine.

Polarity therapy can be done one-on-one or with a group of practitioners working on the patient. The therapist as well as the patient removes shoes. The patient lies fully dressed except for shoes on a massage table or bed, or on the floor. The practitioner takes the patient's history, checks reflexes and touches body parts to determine energy blocks. Polarity therapy uses three levels of touch: no touch (hands held above the body, touching only the energy fields); light touch; and a deep, massaging touch. The therapist balances energy currents in the patient's body by placing his or her "plus" hand on "negative" body parts and vice versa. Polarity therapy involves rocking the patient's body and holding the head as well as more usual massage techniques. It takes about four polarity sessions to treat most conditions, with each session lasting about an hour. After a course of treatment, the polarity practitioner usually suggests drinking plenty of liquids for one to two weeks together with other dietary changes as part of a general internal cleansing or detoxification program. Polarity **yoga** (stretching exercises) is prescribed for the patient's regular workouts at home.

Breema

Breema is a form of body movement energy therapy that combines elements of bodywork, yoga, chiropractic, and New Age philosophy. Breema began in California in 1980. Its founder is Dr. Jon Schreiber, a graduate of Palmer College of Chiropractic. The Breema Health and Wellness Center was opened in Oakland, California, in 1981. The principles of Breema are intended to free people from the conceptual body, defined as "the ideas and images of our body that we carry in our mind." The aim of Breema "is to increase vitality, not to fight sickness, and to create an atmosphere which allows the body to move toward a natural state of balance." A person receiving a Breema treatment works with an instructor or practitioner through a series of individualized exercises on a padded floor. The instructors and practitioners are certified by the Breema Center in Oakland.

Decrystallization is an important part of Breema therapy. According to Breema, decrystallization is a process in which the body is helped to release deeply held, or "crystallized," patterns of chronic discomfort, tension, or emotional pain. As the body releases its crystallizations, its "core energetic patterns" are balanced and realigned. A decrystallization program consists of one or more Breema treatments per week for a year. It includes a set of personalized self-Breema exercises.

Electromagnetic therapies

Electromagnetic therapies cover a variety of treatments that use a source of physical energy outside the body—most often magnets or electromagnetic field stimulation—to treat a range of musculoskeletal disorders. Some forms of magnetic therapy, such as bracelets, gloves, shoe inserts, and similar items containing small magnets meant to be worn near the affected body part, can be self-administered. This form of magnetic therapy has become quite popular among professional athletes and "weekend warriors" to relieve soreness in joints and muscles from over exercise. At present there are two hypothetical explanations of the effectiveness of magnetic therapy. One theory maintains that the magnets stimulate nerve endings in the skin surface to release endorphins, which are pain-relieving chemicals produced by the body in response to **stress** or injury. According to the second hypothesis, the magnets attract certain ions (electrically charged molecules) in the blood, which serves to increase the blood flow in that area of the body. The increased blood flow then relieves the tissue swelling and other side effects of over-exercise that cause pain.

Other forms of electromagnetic therapy require special equipment and cannot be self-administered. These forms of treatment are most commonly used by naturopathic practitioners. One form, called **transcranial magnetic stimulation**, is used in the treatment of **depression**. Another form, called pulsed electromagnetic field stimulation, has been shown to be effective in the treatment of osteoarthritis.

Precautions

In general, persons who are interested in Breema, qigong, or any form of energy therapy that involves vigorous physical exercise or bodywork should seek the advice of a qualified medical practitioner before starting such a program. This precaution is particularly important for persons with chronic heart or lung disease, persons recovering from surgery or acute illness, or persons with arthritis or other disorders that affect the muscles and joints.

Some forms of energy therapy may produce unexpected or startling psychological reactions. For example, a type of psychospiritual energy referred to as Kundalini in Indian yoga sometimes produces experiences of spiritual crisis that may be interpreted by mainstream psychiatrists as symptoms of **schizophrenia** or another psychotic disorder. Practitioners of Reiki healing have reported instances of patients feeling tingling sensations, "spaciness," an "out of body" sensation, sudden warmth, or similar experiences. As a rule, people in treatment for any mental condition or disorder should consult their therapist before beginning any form of energy treatment. This precaution is particularly important for patients diagnosed with post-traumatic stress disorder or a dissociative disorder, and for those who are easily hypnotized. It is also a good idea to find out as much as possible about the background and basic beliefs associated with a specific energy therapy, including the training or credentialing of its practitioners.

KEY TERMS

Aura—An energy field that is thought to emanate from the human body and to be visible to people with special psychic or spiritual powers.

Ayurvedic medicine—The traditional medical system of India. Ayurvedic treatments include diet, exercises, herbal treatments, meditation, massage, breathing techniques, and exposure to sunlight.

Biofield therapies—A subgroup of energy therapies that make use of energy fields (biofields) thought to exist within or emanate from the human body. Biofield therapies include such approaches as Reiki, therapeutic touch, qigong, and polarity balancing.

Bodywork—Any technique involving hands-on massage or manipulation of the body.

Chakra—One of the seven major energy centers in the body, according to traditional Indian yoga.

Endorphins—A group of peptide compounds released by the body in response to stress or traumatic injury. Endorphins react with opiate receptors in the brain to reduce or relieve pain.

Kundalini—In Indian yoga, a vital force or energy at the base of the spine that is activated or released by certain yoga postures or breathing techniques. This release is called the "awakening" of the kundalini. Some Westerners have had kundalini experiences that were diagnosed as psychotic episodes or symptoms of schizophrenia.

Meridians—In traditional Chinese medicine, a network of pathways or channels that convey qi, or vital energy, through the body.

Qi—The traditional Chinese term for vital energy or the life force. The word is also spelled "ki" or "chi" in English translations of Japanese and Chinese medical books.

Preparation

Most forms of energy therapy require little preparation on the patient's part except for the wearing of loose and comfortable clothes. Patients are asked to remove jewelry before a polarity balancing treatment and to remove eyeglasses and shoes prior to Reiki treatment. Qigong should not be practiced on either a full or a completely empty stomach.

Aftercare

Aftercare for therapeutic touch and Reiki usually involves a few moments of quiet rest to maximize the benefits of treatment. Aftercare for polarity therapy includes increased fluid intake for one to two weeks and other dietary adjustments that may be recommended by the practitioner.

Risks

There are no known risks associated with therapeutic touch or polarity balancing. In using Reiki, precautions should be taken with clients diagnosed with schizophrenia, **psychosis**, dissociative disorder, manic/depressive (bipolar) or borderline personality. The risk of physical injury from the exercises involved in Breema or qigong are minimal for patients who have consulted their primary physician beforehand and are working with a qualified instructor.

Mild headache has been reported as a side effect of transcranial magnetic stimulation. No side effects have been associated with self-administered magnetic therapy.

Results

Normal results for energy therapies include increased physical vitality, lowered blood pressure, a sense of calm or relaxation, improved sleep at night, and a strengthened immune system. Some persons report pain relief and speeded-up healing of wounds from magnetic therapy, Reiki, and qigong.

Abnormal results from energy therapies can include physical injury, severe headache, dizziness, depressed mood, or increased anxiety.

Resources

BOOKS

Collinge, William. *Subtle Energy: Awakening to the Unseen Forces in Our Lives*. New York: Warner Books, Inc., 1998.

Krieger, Dolores. *Accepting Your Power to Heal: The Personal Practice of Therapeutic Touch*. New York: Bear and Company, 1993.

Mitchell, Karyn. *Reiki: A Torch in Daylight*. St. Charles, IL: Mind Rivers Publications, 1994.

Pelletier, Kenneth R. "Spirituality and Healing: As Above … So Below." In *The Best Alternative Medicine*. New York: Touchstone, 2002.

Sovatsky, Stuart. "Kundalini Awakening: Breakdown or Breakthrough?" In *Living Yoga: A Comprehensive Guide for Daily Life,* edited by George Feuerstein and Stephan Bodian. New York: Penguin Books, 1993.

Stein, Diane. *All Women Are Healers: A Comprehensive Guide to Natural Healing*. Freedom, CA: The Crossing Press, 1990.

Stein, Diane. *Essential Reiki: A Complete Guide to an Ancient Healing Art*. Freedom, CA: The Crossing Press, Inc., 1995.

Svoboda, Robert, and Arnie Lade. *Tao and Dharma: Chinese Medicine and Ayurveda*. Twin Lakes, WI: Lotus Press, 1995.

OTHER

U.S. National Center for Complementary and Alternative Medicine. "Major Domains of Complementary and Alternative Medicine, Appendix 1," in *Expanding Horizons of Healthcare: Five-Year Strategic Plan 2001–2005*. http://nccam.nih.gov/about/plans/fiveyear/fiveyear.pdf (accessed October 11, 2011).

ORGANIZATIONS

American Association of Naturopathic Physicians, 4435 Wisconsin Ave., NW Ste. 403, Washington, DC, 20016, (202) 237-8150, Fax: (202) 237-8152, (866) 538-2267, http://www.naturopathic.org.

American Polarity Therapy Association, 122 N. Elm St., Ste. 512, Greensboro, NC, 27401, (336) 574-1121, Fax: (336) 574-1151, aptaoffices@polaritytherapy.org, http://www.polaritytherapy.org.

International Society for the Study of Subtle Energies and Energy Medicine, 2770 Arapahoe Rd., Ste. 132, Lafayette, CO, 80026, (303) 425-4625, Fax: (866) 269-0972, http://www.issseem.org.

National Center for Complementary and Alternative Medicine, NCCAM Clearinghouse, PO Box 7923, Gaithersburg, MD, 20898, (888) 644-6226, Fax: (866) 464-3616, info@nccam.nih.gov, http://www.nccam.nih.gov.

Qigong Human Life Research Foundation, PO Box 5327, Cleveland, OH, 44101,

Therapeutic Touch International Association, PO Box 419, Craryville, NY, 12521, (518) 325-1185, Fax: (509) 693-3537, nhpai@therapeutic-touch.org, http://www.therapeutic-touch.org.

Rebecca J. Frey, PhD

Enuresis

Definition

Enuresis, more commonly called bed-wetting, is an elimination disorder that involves the voluntary or involuntary release of urine into bedding, clothing, or other inappropriate places. In adults, loss of bladder control is often referred to as urinary incontinence rather than enuresis; it is frequently found in patients with late-stage **Alzheimer's disease** or other forms of **dementia**.

Demographics

Enuresis is a problem of the young and is twice as common in boys as in girls. At age five, about 7% of boys and 3% of girls have enuresis. This number declines steadily in older children; by age 18, only about 1% of adolescents experience enuresis. Studies done in several countries suggest that there is no apparent cultural influence on the incidence of enuresis in children. On the other hand, the disorder does appear to run in families; children with one parent who wet the bed as a child are five to seven times more likely to have enuresis than children whose parents did not have the disorder in childhood.

Description

Enuresis is a condition that has been described since 1500 B.C. People with enuresis wet the bed or release urine at other inappropriate times. Release of urine at night (nocturnal enuresis) is much more common than daytime, or diurnal, wetting. Enuresis commonly affects young children and is involuntary. Many cases of enuresis cease as the child matures, although some children need behavioral or physiological treatment in order to remain dry.

There are two main types of enuresis in children. Primary enuresis occurs when a child has never established bladder control. Secondary enuresis occurs when a person has established bladder control for a period of six months, then relapses and begins wetting. To be diagnosed with enuresis, a person must be at least five years old or have reached a developmental age of five years. Below this age, problems with bladder control are considered normal.

Causes and symptoms

Enuresis occurs when a person urinates in inappropriate places or at inappropriate times. The *Diagnostic and Statistical Manual of Mental Disorders (DSM)* does not distinguish between those who wet the bed involuntarily and those who voluntarily release urine. Increasingly, however, research findings suggest that voluntary and involuntary enuresis have different causes.

Enuresis in children

Involuntary enuresis is much more common than voluntary enuresis. Involuntary enuresis may be categorized as either primary or secondary. Primary enuresis occurs when young children lack bladder control from infancy. Most of these children have urine control problems only during sleep; they do not consciously, intentionally, or maliciously wet the bed. Research suggests that children who are nighttime-only bed wetters may have a nervous system that is slow to process the feeling of a full bladder. Consequently, these children do not wake up in time to relieve themselves. In other cases, the child's enuresis may be related to a sleep disorder.

Children with diurnal enuresis wet only during the day. There appear to be two types of daytime wetters. One group seems to have difficulty controlling the urge to urinate. The other group consciously delays urinating until they lose control. Some children have both diurnal and nocturnal enuresis.

Several studies have investigated the association of primary enuresis and psychiatric or behavior problems. The results suggest that primary nocturnal enuresis is not caused by psychological disorders. Bed-wetting runs in families, however, and there is strong evidence of a genetic component to involuntary enuresis.

A small number of children have abnormalities in the anatomical structure of their kidney or bladder that interfere with bladder control, but normally the cause is not the physical structure of the urinary system. A few children appear to have to have a lower-than-normal ability to concentrate urine, due to low levels of antidiuretic hormone (ADH). This hormone helps to regulate fluid balance in the body. Large amounts of dilute urine cause the bladder to overflow at night.

Secondary enuresis occurs when a child has stayed dry day and night for at least six months, then returns to wetting. Secondary enuresis usually occurs at night. Many studies have been done to determine if there is a psychological component to enuresis. Researchers have found that secondary enuresis is more likely to occur after a child has experienced a stressful life event such as the birth of a sibling, divorce or death of a parent, or moving to a new house.

Unlike involuntary enuresis, voluntary enuresis is not common. It is associated with such psychiatric disorders as **oppositional defiant disorder** and is substantially different from ordinary nighttime bed-wetting. Voluntary enuresis is always secondary.

Enuresis in adults

Enuresis or urinary incontinence in elderly adults may be caused by loss of independent control of body functions resulting from dementia, bladder infections, uncontrolled diabetes, side effects of medications, or weakened bladder muscles. Urinary incontinence in adults is managed by treatment of the underlying medical condition, if one is present, or by the use of adult briefs with disposable liners.

Diagnosis

Enuresis is most often diagnosed in children because the parents express concern to the child's doctor. The pediatrician or family physician will give the child a physical examination to rule out medical conditions that may be causing the problem, including structural abnormalities in the child's urinary tract. The doctor may also rule out a sleep disorder as a possible cause. In many cases the pediatrician can reassure the child's parents and give them helpful advice.

According to the **American Psychiatric Association**, making a **diagnosis** of enuresis requires that a child must have reached the chronological or developmental age of five. Inappropriate urination must occur at least twice a week for three months, or the frequency of inappropriate urination must cause significant distress and interfere with the child's school and/or social life. Finally, the behavior cannot be caused exclusively by a medical condition or as a side effect of medication.

Treatment

Treatment for enuresis is not always necessary. About 15% of children who have enuresis outgrow it each year after age six. When treatment is desired, a physician will rule out obvious physical causes of enuresis through a physical examination and medical history. Several different treatment options are then available.

Traditional

BEHAVIOR MODIFICATION. **Behavior modification** is often the treatment of choice for enuresis. It is inexpensive and has a success rate of about 75%. The child's bedding includes a special pad with a sensor that rings a bell when the pad becomes wet. The bell wakes the child, who then gets up and goes to the bathroom to finish emptying his bladder. Over time, the child becomes conditioned to waking up when the bladder feels full.

Once this response is learned, some children continue to wake themselves without help from the alarm, while others are able to sleep all night and remain dry. A less expensive behavioral technique involves setting an alarm clock to wake the child every night after a few hours of sleep, until the child learns to wake up spontaneously. In trials, this method was as effective as the pad-and-alarm system. A newer technique involves an ultrasound monitor worn on the child's pajamas. The monitor can sense bladder size, and sets off an alarm once the bladder reaches a predetermined level of fullness. This technique avoids having to change wet bed pads.

Other behavior modifications that can be used alone or with the pad-and-alarm system include:

- restricting liquids starting several hours before bedtime
- waking the child up in the night to use the bathroom
- teaching urinary retention techniques
- giving the child positive reinforcement for dry nights and being sympathetic and understanding about wet nights

PSYCHOTHERAPY. Primary enuresis does not require **psychotherapy**. Secondary enuresis, however, is often successfully treated with therapy. The goal of the treatment is to resolve the underlying stressful event that has caused a **relapse** into bed-wetting. Unlike children with involuntary enuresis, children who intentionally urinate in inappropriate places often have other serious psychiatric disorders. Voluntary enuresis is usually a symptom of another disorder. Therapy to treat the underlying disorder is essential to resolving the enuresis.

Drugs

There are two main drugs for treating enuresis. **Imipramine**, a tricyclic antidepressant, has been used since the early 1960s. It appears to work in up to 60% of cases, although relapse occurs in about 50% of successful treatments. Desmopressin acetate (DDAVP), which acts as an antidiuretic, has been widely used to treat enuresis since the 1990s. It is available as a nasal spray or tablet and can effective in up to 65% of cases. Relapse rates with DDAVP can be as high as 80%.

Alternative

Some success in treating bed-wetting has been reported using hypnosis. When hypnosis works, the results are seen within four to six sessions. **Acupuncture** and massage have also been used to treat enuresis, with inconclusive results.

Prognosis

Enuresis is a disorder that most children outgrow. The short-term success rate with drug treatments is even higher than with behavioral therapy. Drugs do not, however, eliminate the enuresis. Many children who take drugs to control their bed-wetting relapse when the drugs are stopped.

Prevention

Although enuresis cannot be prevented, one side effect of the disorder is the shame and social embarrassment it causes. Children who wet themselves may avoid sleepovers, camp, and other activities where their bed-wetting will become obvious. Loss of these opportunities can cause a loss of self-esteem, social isolation, and adjustment problems. A kind, low-key approach to enuresis helps to prevent these problems.

KEY TERMS

Bladder—A muscular sac in the lower abdomen that holds urine until it is discharged from the body.

Elimination—The medical term for expelling waste from the body.

Primary enuresis—Bed-wetting in a child who has not yet developed bladder control.

Secondary enuresis—Bed-wetting in a child who has established bladder control but has begun to wet the bed again, usually as the result of emotional stress.

Urinary incontinence—A term that is sometimes used for enuresis in adults. Urinary incontinence is often found in patients with late-stage Alzheimer's disease or other adult-onset dementias.

Urinary system—The kidney, urethra, bladder, and associated organs that process urine and eliminate it from the body.

Resources

BOOKS

American Psychiatric Association. *Diagnostic and Statistical Manual of Mental Disorders*. 4th ed., text rev. Washington, DC: American Psychiatric Publishing, 2000.

Mace, Nancy L., and Peter V. Rabins. *The 36-Hour Day*. 5th ed. Baltimore, MD: Johns Hopkins University Press, 2011.

Maizels, Max, Diane Rosenbaum, and Barbara Keating. *Getting Dry: How to Help Your Child Overcome Bed-wetting*. Boston: Harvard Common Press, 1999.

Sadock, Benjamin J., and Virginia A. Sadock, eds. *Comprehensive Textbook of Psychiatry*. Vol. 2. 7th ed. Philadelphia: Lippincott Williams and Wilkins, 2000.

PERIODICALS

Mikkelsen, Edwin J. "Enuresis and Encopresis: Ten Years of Progress." *Journal of the American Academy of Child and Adolescent Psychiatry* 40, no. 10 (October 2001): 1146–58.

WEBSITES

American Academy of Child & Adolescent Psychiatry (AACAP). "Bedwetting." AACAP Facts For Families Pamphlet, Number 18. Washington, DC: American Academy of Child & Adolescent Psychiatry, December 2011. Available online at http://aacap.org/page.ww?name=Bedwetting&section=Facts+for+Families (accessed December 10, 2011).

MedlinePlus. "Enuresis." U.S. National Library of Medicine. National Institutes of Health. http://www.nlm.nih.gov/medlineplus/ency/article/001556.htm (accessed October 6, 2011).

National Guideline Clearinghouse. "Nocturnal Enuresis: The Management of Bedwetting in Children and Young People." U.S. Agency for Health Care Research and Quality. 2011. http://www.guideline.gov/content.aspx?id=25680&search=enuresis (accessed October 6, 2011).

National Kidney and Urologic Diseases Information Clearinghouse. "Urinary Incontinence in Children." U.S. National Institute of Diabetes and Digestive and Kidney Diseases. September 2010. http://kidney.niddk.nih.gov/kudiseases/pubs/uichildren/index.aspx (accessed October 6, 2011).

National Kidney Foundation. "Bedwetting." 2001. http://www.kidney.org/patients/bw/index.cfm (accessed October 6 2011).

ORGANIZATIONS

American Academy of Child and Adolescent Psychiatry, 3615 Wisconsin Ave. NW, Washington, DC, 20016-3007, (202) 966-7300, Fax: (202) 966-2891, http://aacap.org.

National Association for Continence, PO Box 1019, Charleston, SC, 29402-1019, (800) 252-3337, http://www.nafc.org.

National Kidney Foundation, 30 East 33rd Street, New York, NY, 10016, (800) 622-9010, http://www.kidney.org.

Tish Davidson, AM
Emily Jane Willingham, PhD

Epigenetics

Definition

Epigenetics refers to the paradigm for explaining mental health, emphasizing how environmental factors affect the expression of genetic predispositions. In psychology, three approaches have evolved defining epigenetics. The first approach stresses that the interaction of genetics and environment is more important than either individual influence. The second approach emphasizes that all human development is shaped by experience while still following a biological blueprint. The third approach emphasizes that any genetic trait can be "switched on" or "switched off" by specific environmental factors. All three approaches are based on the belief that the cause of every mental disorder has a genetic predisposition and an environmental activator.

Description

Across its short history, psychology has sought to explain any mental health phenomenon as the effect of either genetics or experiences. The Freudian model, which was popular in the early twentieth century, emphasized that an adult's personality is determined by early childhood experience. This idea led to the conclusion that all psychological disorders are caused by traumatic disruptions in the healthy development. More advanced research demonstrated that there is a strong genetic influence on personality traits. Also on the genetic side, the medical model of psychopathology suggests that disorders can be solved by finding the right drug to resolve the disorder. The study of genetic influences on development and mental health has appeared to be most suitable for scientific study. Still, many have come to accept that a person's fate or destiny is not determined by genetics or biology.

The interaction approach

The classical debate over whether genetics or environment has more influence has been termed "nature versus nurture" with various theories taking one side or the other. While most practitioners have accepted the influence of both, the evolution of psychological theory has seen the emergence of theories emphasizing either extreme. Contemplating the extremes has led to the conclusion that the two influences interact in such a way that it is difficult to identify the individual influence of either. The term for the genetic predisposition for a trait is the *genotype.* The actual expression of the trait is the *phenotype.* What the genotype goes through to become the phenotype is the interaction with environmental influences, ranging from diet to maternal care.

With advances in genetic studies, identification of those disorders with strong genetic influences started to emerge. However, these studies could not explain why the genetic influence was not absolute. For example, **schizophrenia** has a high genetic influence. If an identical twin has schizophrenia, there is a strong (but not absolute) probability that his or her twin will also become schizophrenic. Since identical twins share the same genetic foundation, if there is a genetic cause to a disorder, the percentage of twins sharing a disorder should be 100%. The genetic influence hypothesis cannot explain why a good proportion of identical twins do not become schizophrenic when their twins develop schizophrenia. Similarly, the experiential influence hypothesis for such disorders as **post-traumatic stress disorder** (PTSD) cannot explain the individual differences in the intensity and endurance of PTSD among victims sharing the same experience.

In 1999, an important study took place over three different research sites illustrating that genetics have been overly emphasized as influences for personality traits, temperament, and psychological disorders. Researchers John C. Crabbe, Douglas Wahlstein, and Bruce C. Dudek assured that each site had the same set of mice with eight different strains. The mice of the same strains were virtually identical. The three sites created the exact same environmental and living conditions. The goal of the study was to standardize methods for testing various genetic traits. However, the surprise findings were that for most of the assessed tasks, there was little genetic influence on results. If genetics had a strong influence, the performance of the genetically similar mice should be the same. This was not found overall, only for a few individual tasks.

The developmental approach

Developmental **psychologist** Erik Erikson was the first theorist to use the term *epigenetics* to describe the process of development. Erikson saw epigenetic influences as biological age-related social skills that emerged to meet the demands of the social environment. Most development theorists see a similar phenomenon in other aspects of development.

An important contribution to healthy development is establishing attachment in infancy. Attachment is established through the primary caregiver—usually the mother—constantly meeting the infant's needs with a goal of the child learning trust. This lesson of trust stays with the child throughout childhood into maturity. Children who have established a secure attachment with their primary caregiver (usually the mother) feel that the world is manageable and that they have a place in it. Establishing attachment can be thwarted by anxiety in the mother or a nervous temperament in the child. Attachment has been studied in mice and rhesus monkeys.

In the animal studies, researchers looked at how upbringing affected temperament. For example, in mice, **stress** reactivity is a genetic trait that affects how the mother takes care of her young. The mice grow up with the tendency to stress based on genetic influence and early experience. However, if the genetically stressed mice are raised by a genetically calm mother, they grow up to tolerate stress and to later be calm mothers themselves. Generations later, the anxious gene was still present, but the mice acted the same as the genetically calm mice. Regardless of the genetic disposition, the early experiences set a pattern for life, which could be passed on to the next generation.

There were similar findings with rhesus monkeys. Grown rhesus monkeys can change temperament patterns depending on community influences, but they will revert back to the inborn pattern if community influences are altered. However, genetically influenced emotions can be changed for life if the baby monkey is raised by a calm mother in the first six months of life.

The lasting effects of highly reactive temperament and early maternal deprivation have also been studied with rhesus monkeys. When rhesus monkeys suffer maternal deprivation in their early years, there is no measurable negative influence on later life. The one key difference is if the rhesus monkey was born with a highly reactive temperament. Those affected have faulty neuroendocrine systems from infancy that interfere with their growth and metabolism. In later life, these monkeys demonstrated abnormal behavioral and emotional reactions.

Among humans, parenting can provide a point of interaction between heredity and environment. In studies, resilient children growing up in a stressful environment appear to be unaffected by negative influences if they had a good attachment with their mothers in the first 12 to 18 months of life. Studies of the genetic influence of schizophrenia found that adopted children with a genetic predisposition for the disorder tend to avoid the disorder if they are adopted into a supportive family. In the cases where the adopted family was dysfunctional, the genetic predisposition was more likely to arise.

It is the hope of epigenetic studies that unwanted traits, temperaments, and disorders can be "treated" by environmental influences. Changing the environment and enhancing parental support in the early years may counter genetic tendencies. Such research expectations have led scientists to accept that although a person may possess a genetic predisposition for a disorder, whether this predisposition is manifested or not may depend on environmental circumstances. Even where there is an extremely negative environmental condition, the effects may be modified by early childhood influences such as resiliency.

The geneticist approach

A more narrow use of the term *epigenetics* comes from geneticists who investigate why the human genome cannot explain all psychological phenomena. This approach relates to the other two but focuses on how specific environmental factors can interfere with the normal expression of a particular gene while not changing the underlying DNA. Since the beginning of the twentieth century, genetic researchers have recognized that gene function could be altered by agents that did not upset the normal sequence of the gene. More recent discoveries of geneticists have long-range implications of enhancing human achievement and more immediate implications of solving mental disorders.

A breakthrough study in genetics was conducted in recent years by Randy Jirtle with a strain of mice known as agouti mice. These mice carried a specific maladaptive gene that gave them a yellow color as they grew. The gene also interfered with the mice's natural inclination to stop eating when full. Some other traits of this gene left the mice vulnerable to diabetes and cancer. The study focused on how to offset the bad conditions of this gene as early in life as possible. The researchers were testing the theoretical assumption that the gene could be "switched off" through changing the diet of the mother before and during the period of conception. The diet was rich in methyl, a biological compound naturally occurring in many foods. The methyl compound is a known agent in gene imprinting. The process of introducing it into the gene is known as DNA methylation.

By feeding the mother this diet, the researchers were able to prevent the agouti gene from expressing itself in the offspring. The important finding was that the gene

KEY TERMS

Attachment—The bond developed between an infant and the primary caregiver within the first 12 to 18 months of life and expected to have lifelong effects.

DNA methylation—The imprinting process of introducing methyl into a gene, suppressing its usual function.

Environmental influence—Any component of the cause of a behavior or condition that is perceived to be developed from experience.

Genetic influence—Any component of the cause of a behavior or condition that is inherited biologically from parents.

Neuroendocrine system—The part of the autonomic nervous system responsible for growth and hormonal regulation.

Paradigm—The commonly accepted foundations among a group of similar theories, usually derived from a philosophy, including assumptions, terminology, measurements and expectations.

Phenylketonuria (PKU)—An enzyme deficiency present at birth that disrupts metabolism and causes brain damage. If left untreated, the disease progresses into intellectual disability.

Post-traumatic stress disorder (PTSD)—A psychological reaction that continues long after a highly stressful event and is characterized by depression, anxiety, flashbacks, and nightmares.

Schizophrenia—A severe mental illness in which a person has difficulty distinguishing what is real from what is not real. It is often characterized by hallucinations, delusions, and withdrawal from people and social activities.

was still present in later generations but still switched off, even with no dietary change in the later parents. Such a finding challenged the long-existing premise that any environmental influence on the expression of genes would not be found in future generations. Any gene whose expression was modified in one generation was presumed to be changed back with every new generation. Many other studies have reached similar conclusions that epigenetic effects can be passed from one generation to the next. However, while the change can happen quickly in one generation, the effects can be reversed in subsequent generations.

The basis for understanding this genetic manipulation lies in the well-researched area of gene imprinting. Scientists have known for a long time that naturally occurring environmental agents can suppress one or both of a gene's alleles. Each gene consists of two alleles that normally work together unless one is damaged or switched off. If one allele is damaged, the healthy one is expressed. Research has shown that, at times, environmental agents might switch off the healthy allele, allowing the damaged one to express itself as a threat to physical or mental health. What imprinting research has yet to show, but strongly implies, is that the healthy allele might be enhanced through epigenetic agents. The work of genetic researchers is to induce imprinting by manipulating genes or their alleles to promote greater mental and physical health.

There are several organizations working to promote epigenetic research at this genetic level. These include the National Institute of Environmental Health Sciences, Johns Hopkins University Center for Epigenetics in Common Human Disease, the European Human Epigenome Project, and the Epigenome Network of Excellence. Most of these include research with an emphasis on mental health, but the emphasis is usually small.

Disorders susceptible to epigenetic research and treatment

Phenylketonuria (PKU) was once a major source of **intellectual disability** in young children. It was first discovered in the middle 1930s, but the appropriate treatment was not developed until the late 1950s. The treatment consists of a diet without a common amino acid known as phenylketone. The crisis of PKU was a clear case of a genetic deficiency rearranged by an environmental **intervention**. Without the special diet, a child who inherited PKU would be intellectually disabled by his or her first birthday. With the special diet, the child can be expected to lead a relatively normal life.

Schizophrenia is an inherited disorder that is still not fully understood. However, accurate tests are being developed to recognize its genetic markers. It is known that there are more instances of schizophrenia in urban than in rural settings and in industrial nations than in nonindustrial nations. Therefore, environmental changes may reduce the chance of schizophrenia expressing itself when the genetic markers are present. Family setting can influence the onset of schizophrenia, with dysfunctional families having a greater occurrence than supportive families among those genetically predisposed. Researchers are working not only to identify the genetic marker but also to investigate its response to methylation or other imprinting manipulations.

Attachment disorders are another area of interest for researchers developing epigenetic therapy. These evolve from a faulty or incomplete attachment between an infant and the mother or primary caregiver. Infants with attachment disorder grow up to display inappropriate emotions, antisocial behaviors, and inconsistent moods. Although the development of attachment appears to be clearly in the "nurture" side, it can be influenced by the infant's inborn temperament. The results can also have an effect on the neuroendocrine and cognitive systems. The occurrence of attachment disorders may be reduced through parenting classes that teach new parents the importance of the behaviors that foster attachment.

Resources

BOOKS

Durand, V. Mark, and David H. Barlow. *Essentials of Abnormal Psychology,* 5th ed. Mason, OH: Wadsworth, Cengage Learning, 2009.

Allis, C. David, Thomas Jenuwein, and Danny Reinberg, eds. *Epigenetics*. Cold Spring Harbor, NY: Cold Spring Harbor Laboratory Press, 2009.

PERIODICALS

Albert, Paul R. "Epigenetics in Mental Illness: Hope or Hype?" *Journal of Psychiatry and Neuroscience* 35, no. 6 (November 2010): 366. http://dx.doi.org/10.1503/jpn.100148 (accessed September 16, 2011).

Cloud, John. "Why Your DNA Isn't Your Destiny." *TIME* 175, no. 2 (January 18, 2010). http://www.time.com/time/magazine/article/0,9171,1952313,00.html (accessed September 16, 2011).

Stahl, Stephen M. "Epigenetic Hypotheses of Schizophrenia." *Psychopharmacology Educational Updates* 6, no. 8 (August 2010).

———. "Essential Psychopharmastahlogy: Fooling Mother Nature: Epigenetics and Novel Treatments for Psychiatric Disorders." *Psychopharmacology Educational Updates* 6, no. 11 (November 2010).

Weinhold, Bob. "Epigenetics: The Science of Change." *Environmental Health Perspective* 114 (March 1, 2006): 160–67. http://dx.doi.org/10.1289/ehp.114-a160 (accessed August 24, 2011).

WEBSITES

Genetic Science Learning Center, University of Utah. "Epigenetics and the Human Brain." http://learn.genetics.utah.edu/content/epigenetics/brain (accessed September 16, 2011).

Marlow, Sally. "Epigenetics in Psychiatric Disorders: A Guide for Beginners." *BioNews* 549 (March 15, 2010). http://www.bionews.org.uk/page_55848.asp (accessed September 16, 2011).

NOVA. "Epigenetics." PBS video (13:02 min.) Aired July 24, 2007. http://www.pbs.org/wgbh/nova/body/epigenetics.html (accessed September 16, 2011).

ORGANIZATIONS

Johns Hopkins University Center for Epigenetics in Common Human Disease, 855 N Wolfe St., Baltimore, MD, 21205, (410) 614-3489, http://www.hopkinsmedicine.org/epigenetics.

National Institute of Environmental Health Sciences, 111 T. W. Alexander Dr., Research Triangle Park, NC, 27709, (919) 541-0049, webcenter@niehs.nih.gov, http://www.niehs.nih.gov.

Ray F. Brogan, PhD

Epilepsy *see* **Seizures**

Epinephrine *see* **Adrenaline**

Erectile dysfunction

Definition

Erectile dysfunction (ED) is the consistent inability to achieve or maintain a penile erection that is sufficient for satisfactory sexual intercourse.

Demographics

It is estimated that 15–30 million American men suffer from some degree of ED. Of these, 10–20 million have severe ED, resulting in the complete inability to attain or maintain a penile erection. However, ED is believed to be underreported, underdiagnosed, and undertreated due to its perceived **stigma**. In a survey of general medical practice, less than 12% of men with ED reported having received treatment. Thus, the actual incidence of ED may be much higher than most estimates.

The incidence of ED increases with age, along with the incidence of chronic disorders and conditions that are commonly associated with ED, including diabetes, hypertension, and cardiovascular disease. It is estimated that 26% of men in their 50s, 40% of men in their 60s, and 77% of men 75 and older have some degree of ED. The number of American men with ED is estimated to increase by nearly 10 million by 2025, and the worldwide incidence is projected to be more than 320 million.

Description

Although most men experience occasional transient impotence, usually associated with **fatigue**, anger, **depression**, or other stressful emotions, erectile dysfunction is the consistent inability to achieve or maintain an erection. The term "impotence" is now rarely used because of its association with weakness and powerlessness.

Penile erection occurs when the penis becomes engorged with blood. The anatomical compartments—the two corpora cavernosa and the corpus spongiosum—can be distended with up to seven times the normal amount of blood. Along with the relaxation of the penile muscles, this distention results in an erection.

The sequence of events resulting in penile erection is complex. Erection is usually initiated by sexual arousal stimuli in the **brain** as a result of visual, auditory, or olfactory sensations or erotic thoughts. Tactile (touch) sensations of the penis, acting through the spinal cord, play a similar role. Sexual arousal results in the release of nitric oxide from specialized cells. Nitric oxide causes the formation of cyclic glutamine monophosphate (cGMP), which is responsible for dilating the blood vessels of the penis and relaxing the penile muscles, enabling increased blood flow and erection. Compression of the dilated blood vessels against the firm outer lining of the penis prevents the blood from escaping and perpetuates the erection. The enzyme called phosphodiesterase-5 (PDE5) causes the breakdown of cGMP and, in association with nerves from the sympathetic nervous system, enables the penis to return to its flaccid relaxed state. Any defect in this complex cascade of events can result in ED.

Sex is an important quality-of-life issue for adults of all ages, and ED usually results in a reduced quality of life. Many affected men experience depression, distress, and relationship difficulties as a result of ED. Despite this fact, men with ED often fail to seek help. Reasons for this failure include:

- patient ignorance of the availability of safe and effective ED therapies
- inadequate information from physicians about the timing of medications, the need for preliminary sexual arousal, and other factors
- marital discord and lack of partner support
- concerns about invasiveness, adverse effects, discomfort, inconvenience, and cost of therapies
- high rates of discontinuation of therapy due to inadequate responses and adverse effects

ED can occur as part of several mental disorders recognized by the mental health professional's manual, the ***Diagnostic and Statistical Manual of Mental Disorders*** (*DSM*). ED is listed as erectile disorder and is classified by the *DSM* as a sexual dysfunction. ED can also be a symptom of other disorders, such as sexual dysfunction due to a general medical condition or substance-induced sexual dysfunction.

Risk factors

ED is frequently associated with vascular conditions such as hypertension and coronary artery heart disease and may even serve as a marker for the detection of cardiovascular disorders. Additionally, ED is associated with depression that is distinct from the reactive depression that it may cause. Lifestyle factors—such as obesity, physical inactivity, cigarette smoking, and excessive intake of alcohol—are also risk factors for ED.

Causes and symptoms

Because of the complicated nature of the human sexual response and the complex physiology of penile erection and relaxation, it is often difficult or impossible to determine the precise cause of ED in individual cases. Normal erectile function requires the coordination of vascular, neurologic, hormonal, and psychological components, and any condition that interferes with one or more of these processes can result in ED. Multiple factors frequently contribute to ED.

Although the incidence of ED increases with age, it is no longer regarded as an inevitable consequence of aging. Likewise, whereas most cases of ED were once considered primarily psychological and/or psychiatric in origin, it is now recognized that organic, nonpsychological factors play a much more significant role, with physical causes underlying at least 80% of cases. However, significant psychological and social factors, such as guilt, depression, anxiety, tension, or marital discord, are often present in addition to one or more of the following physical components:

- Diabetes mellitus is the single most common cause of ED, resulting from a combination of nerve and blood vessel damage. As many as 50% of male diabetics have ED.
- Hardening of the arteries (arteriosclerosis) is the most common vascular (circulation-related) cause of ED. Diseases of the aorta or the arteries supplying the pelvis and penis or damage to arteries from trauma, surgery, or irradiation can cause ED. Surgery involving the prostate gland may affect both arteries and nerves.
- A variety of diseases and factors can influence penile circulation. For example, Peyronie's disease, characterized by fibrous tissue and bending of the penis, limits the expandability of penile tissues and prevents the venous compression that retains blood in the penis. Arteriosclerotic plaque, injury to the inner lining blood vessels from trauma, surgery, or irradiation, or aortic occlusion (blockage in a main artery leading out of the heart) can compromise penile blood flow and prevent erection.
- Neurological causes of ED include diseases of the brain and spinal cord, such as Alzheimer's disease or multiple sclerosis, respectively.
- Hormonal or endocrine causes of ED are uncommon, although deficient testicular function and low circulating levels of the male sex hormone testosterone can result in erectile dysfunction. These are referred to as

KEY TERMS

Arteriosclerosis—A thickening and hardening of the walls of the arteries with loss of elasticity.

Corpora cavernosa—The pair of columns of erectile tissue on either side of the penis that, together with the corpus spongiosum, produce an erection when filled with blood.

Corpus spongiosum—The column of erectile tissue in the penis that contains the urethra.

Dopamine—A chemical in brain tissue that transmits nerve impulses (a neurotransmitter) and helps to regulate movement and emotions.

Hypertension—Abnormally high arterial blood pressure, which if left untreated can lead to heart disease and stroke.

Hypogonadism—Functional incompetence of the male gonads, with impaired production of hormones and sperm cells.

Nitric oxide (NO)—A regulator of various bodily processes, including penile erection.

Phosphodiesterase-5 (PDE5)—An enzyme that is involved in the loss of penile erection.

Prolactin—A hormone produced by the pituitary gland.

Prostate—The walnut-shaped gland that surrounds the urethra at the neck of the bladder in males and supplies fluid for semen.

Testosterone—The primary male sex hormone.

Urethra—The tube in the penis that discharges urine from the bladder to the outside of the body.

hypogonadism and can be due to congenital abnormalities or testicular disease.

- Various classes of medications can cause ED, although not all drugs within a class have the same effect. For example, some antidepressants are associated with ED, whereas the antidepressant trazodone (Desyrel) tends to prolong penile erection. Some high blood pressure medications, central nervous system medications such as methyldopa for Parkinson's disease, sedatives or tranquilizers such as barbiturates, and antianxiety medications such as diazepam (Valium) can also cause ED.
- Tobacco, alcohol, and illicit drugs, including heroin, can cause ED.
- Psychological factor, including stress, fatigue, depression, guilt, low self-esteem, or negative feelings for or by a sexual partner, can precipitate ED. Depressive symptoms or difficulty coping with anger can be particularly detrimental.

Although the primary ED symptom is the inability to attain or maintain an adequate erection for completed sexual activity, patterns of ED vary. Some men are unable to attain any erection. Others cannot maintain an erection adequate for penetration. Some men lose their erection during sexual intercourse. Others experience an erection only upon awakening or during masturbation.

Diagnosis

Diagnosis requires several different processes, including examination and tests.

Examination

Taking thorough medical, psychosocial (both psychological and social), and sexual histories are an essential first step in the diagnosis of ED. A general medical history can indicate the existence of ED-associated conditions such as high blood pressure, diabetes, or arteriosclerosis, as well as medications that may contribute to ED and any history of **substance abuse**. A psychosocial history includes current sexual practices, the existence of stresses or performance anxiety, and any special circumstances under which ED occurs. The sexual partner's participation in the psychosocial history can be beneficial. The sexual history helps distinguish ED from other abnormalities in sexual function, such as ejaculatory and orgasmic disturbances or loss of sexual desire. The patient's sexual history includes:

- the frequency and duration of sexual intercourse
- the degree and quality of penile erections
- nocturnal erections
- the success or failure of penetration
- any sexual dysfunction of the partner, such as painful intercourse (dyspareunia) or vaginal dryness

Self-administered questionnaires can assist in the evaluation of sexual function. The International Index of Erectile Function (IIEF) is the most widely used.

A routine physical examination is conducted with special emphasis on the genitourinary, circulatory, and neurologic systems. The physician may look for evidence of hypogonadism or congenital conditions causing defective testicular function. The genitalia are examined for testicular size and consistency and penile deformities. A rectal examination can evaluate the size and consistency of the prostate gland and certain muscular reflexes. Vital signs such as blood pressure and pulse are measured.

Tests

Blood tests and/or other assessments for high blood cholesterol, hypertension, coronary artery heart disease, and depression may be performed, since ED can be a marker or symptom of such disorders. Blood levels of the hormones testosterone and prolactin may be measured.

Procedures

A self-test is available for ED. Pharmacological testing involves the injection of a small amount of an agent, such as 10 micrograms of alprostadil (prostaglandin E1), that produces an erection in a patient with normal erectile function. Nocturnal studies are used to identify erectile dysfunction due to organic causes. Patients are monitored in a sleep laboratory for nocturnal erections, since men with physiologically normal erectile function have erections during sleep. Duplex Doppler ultrasonography provides information about arterial and venous blood flow.

Treatment

Various treatments are available and often combined for ED. These may include counseling, surgically implanted prostheses, and alternative remedies.

Traditional

Treatment for ED often involves a combination of therapies. Most men with ED benefit from counseling, which may be individual **psychotherapy**, psychosexual counseling, or **couples therapy**.

Various types of vacuum pumps are available for increasing penile blood flow. A constriction ring around the base of the penis traps the blood and maintains the erection.

Various types of penile prostheses can be surgically inserted into the penis to produce erections. In rare cases, surgery may be used to correct a defect that interferes with penile erection.

Drugs

PDE5 inhibitors are the most common drug treatment for ED. These relax the muscles in the penis to increase penile blood flow and produce an erection. This class of drugs includes sildenafil (Viagra), vardenafil (Levitra), and tadalafil (Cialis). Because they can cause a sudden drop in blood pressure, these drugs should not be used by men who take nitroglycerin for heart problems. PDE5 inhibitors also have been associated with an increased risk for a rare condition called nonarteritic ischemic optic neuropathy, which can lead to sudden vision loss.

Intracavernous injection therapy (ICIT) is the injection of penile structures with the drugs alprostadil (Caverject), papaverine (Pavabid), or phentolamine, which promote blood flow. Alprostadil can also be inserted into the urethra to increase blood flow and relax muscles. Alpha-adrenergic blockers target adrenergic receptors in smooth muscles, causing the blood vessels to dilate more easily. Apomorphine is a morphine derivative that targets **dopamine** receptors to facilitate erections. Rarely, hormone treatments are used to treat ED. Finally, in some cases, the adjustment of prescription or over-the-counter medications is required, if these are interfering with erectile function.

Alternative

Some alternative remedies are suggested for treating ED, but results are conflicting, and none have proven to be clinically effective. These include:

- dehydroepiandrosterone (DHEA)
- ginkgo
- ginseng
- L-arginine
- yohimbe
- epimedium (called horny goat weed among other common names)
- zinc
- pomegranate juice, supplements, or seeds
- folic acid and vitamin E in combination with Viagra

Home remedies

A first step in ED treatment is the alteration or elimination of modifiable risk factors or causes, including smoking, obesity, and substance or alcohol abuse. Exercising can also have a beneficial effect on ED.

QUESTIONS TO ASK YOUR DOCTOR

- What might be causing my ED?
- Are there lifestyle changes that I can make that might reduce my ED?
- What treatment options do you recommend and why?
- What is my prognosis?

Prognosis

A better understanding of ED, combined with new, more effective therapies, has markedly improved the prognosis. It is estimated that at least 65% of all ED cases can be treated successfully. The modification of risk factors, such as physical inactivity, smoking, excessive alcohol intake, certain medications, and obesity, improve the prognosis. A 2010 study found that 30% of obese men with ED had improved function following weight loss. However, other risk factors, including aging and conditions such as diabetes or pelvic surgery affecting nerves, negatively impact the prognosis. ED appears to be a strong risk factor for cardiovascular disease, as well as for death from all causes.

Prevention

ED sometimes can be prevented in at-risk patients with medications for high blood pressure and other ED-associated conditions. Various lifestyle changes, including quitting smoking, losing weight, and avoiding alcohol and other substance abuse, can help prevent ED.

Resources

BOOKS

Blum, Ralph, and Mark Scholz. *Invasion of the Prostate Snatchers: No More Unnecessary Biopsies, Radical Treatment or Loss of Sexual Potency.* New York: Other Press, 2010.

Ellsworth, Pamela, and Bob Stanley. *100 Questions & Answers About Erectile Dysfunction*, 2nd ed. Sudbury, MA: Jones & Bartlett, 2008.

McVary, Kevin T. *Contemporary Treatment of Erectile Dysfunction: A Clinical Guide.* Totowa, NJ: Humana, 2010.

Morgentaler, Abraham. *Testosterone for Life: Revitalize Your Vitality, Sex Drive, Muscle Mass & Overall Health.* New York: McGraw-Hill, 2009.

Price, Joan. *Naked at Our Age: Talking Out Loud About Senior Sex.* Berkeley, CA: Seal Press, 2011.

Steidle, Christopher P., Janet Casperson, and John J. Mulcahy. *Sex and the Heart: Erectile Dysfunction's Link to Cardiovascular Disease.* Omaha, NE: Addicus Books, 2009.

Zaslau, Stanley. *Dx/Rx: Sexual Dysfunction in Men and Women.* Sudbury, MA: Jones & Bartlett Learning, 2011.

PERIODICALS

Heidelbaugh, Joel J. "Management of Erectile Dysfunction." *American Family Physician* 81, no. 3 (February 1, 2010): 305–12.

Katz, Alan, and Anne Katz. "Erectile Dysfunction." *Canadian Medical Association Journal* 56 (September 1, 2010): 898–903.

WEBSITES

"Erectile Dysfunction." American Diabetes Association. http://www.diabetes.org/living-with-diabetes/complications/mens-health/sexual-health/erectile-dysfunction.html (accessed July 26, 2011).

"Erectile Dysfunction." MedlinePlus. http://www.nlm.nih.gov/medlineplus/erectiledysfunction.html (accessed July 26, 2011).

"Erectile Dysfunction." National Institute of Digestive and Kidney Diseases. Last modified September 2, 2010. http://kidney.niddk.nih.gov/kudiseases/pubs/ED (accessed July 26, 2011).

"Erection Self-Test." MedlinePlus. http://www.nlm.nih.gov/medlineplus/ency/article/003339.htm (accessed July 26, 2011).

ORGANIZATIONS

American Diabetes Association, 1710 N Beauregard St., Alexandria, VA, 22311, (800) 342-2383, http://www.diabetes.org.

American Urological Association, 1000 Corporate Blvd., Linthicum, MD, 21090, (410) 689-3700, (866) 746-4282, Fax: (410) 689 3800, aua@AUAnet.org, http://www.auanet.org.

National Kidney and Urologic Diseases Information Clearinghouse, 3 Information Way, Bethesda, MD, 20892-3580, (703) 738-4929, (800) 891-5390, Fax: (703) 738-4929, nkudic@info.niddk.nih.gov, http://kidney.niddk.nih.gov.

Ralph Myerson, MD
Stephanie Watson
Margaret Alic, PhD

Escitalopram

Definition

Escitalopram (Lexapro) is a medication that belongs to the drug class called **selective serotonin reuptake inhibitors (SSRIs)**. Selective serotonin reuptake inhibitors are a group of medications used to treat clinical **depression**, anxiety, and other psychiatric disorders. They specifically act on a chemical called **serotonin**, a type of **brain** neurotransmitter that is involved in normal brain function and can affect the physiological state of clinical depression.

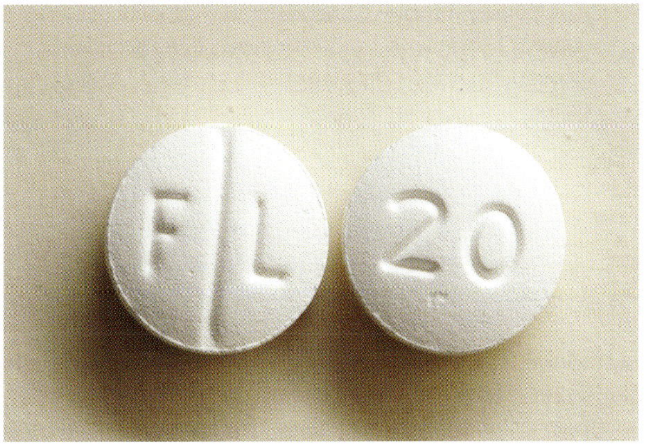

Lexapro (escitalopram), 20 mg. *(© Custom Medical Stock Photo, Inc. Reproduced by permission.)*

Purpose

SSRIs such as escitalopram can be used to treat a broad range of mood and **stress** related psychiatric illnesses. They are mainly used to treat clinical depression and **anxiety disorders**, including **generalized anxiety disorder** (GAD), **panic disorder**, post-traumatic stress syndrome (PTSD), **premenstrual syndrome** disorders (PMS), stress related irritable bowel syndrome, **social phobia**, and the eating disorder **bulimia nervosa**. Choice of agent and whether they are used alone or in combination with other drugs depends on the medical disorder and individual health parameters. Escitalopram specifically is most often used for major depression and generalized anxiety disorder.

Description

Selective serotonin reuptake inhibitors like escitalopram have a therapeutic mechanism of action that is focused on the modulation of the natural body chemical serotonin. Serotonin is a type of neurotransmitter in the brain, specifically a chemical that neurons use to signal one another in complex pathways for brain functioning. **Neurotransmitters** like serotonin bind to chemical receptors on the surface of neurons (brain cells). Once bound to a receptor they affect physiological processes. The receptors activate a sequence of cellular events known as a chemical cascade or signaling pathway. Neurotransmitter signaling pathways are responsible for many normal brain functions. During the signaling process, neurotransmitters such as serotonin travel from one neuron to the next. These chemicals need to cross a short space between the end of one neuron and the beginning of the next neuron known as the synapse or synaptic space. Serotonin is released from the end of neuron one, crosses the synaptic space and binds to a specific receptor for serotonin on the surface of the next neuron (neuron two). Any extra serotonin that is left in the synaptic space is taken back up by neuron one in a process known as reuptake. The more serotonin is allowed to remain in the synaptic space, the more will eventually be allowed to bind to receptors on neuron two and participate in the signaling process. SSRIs such as escitalopram decrease the reuptake of serotonin by neuron one, allowing more serotonin to be present in the synapse and, therefore, more serotonin signaling to occur. It is believed that a decrease in serotonin signaling contributes to illness such as depression and anxiety disorders. SSRIs help by increasing serotonin signaling, with little effect on the synaptic levels of other neurotransmitters.

Whether a patient is going to benefit from an SSRI such as escitalopram may have a genetic component. Individual response to each SSRI varies greatly, and these drugs tend to require several weeks to take effect. The initial trial of **SSRIs** such as escitalopram can be difficult because the side effects begin right away while the beneficial effect takes up to two weeks to develop. Generally, escitalopram is attempted for four to six weeks before concluding it will not have an effect and switching to another agent. If there is an effect but the healthcare provider judges it could be improved, the dose is often increased as the patient is able to tolerate.

Recommended dosage

SSRIs such as escitalopram are taken as oral medications. The dosage varies depending on the individual patient response to the medication regarding its effectiveness, and the individual patient response to the medication regarding side effects. Some people naturally require a higher dose of escitalopram in order to achieve the desired effect. Other patients require a lower dose either for effect or because they quickly develop side effects that are not tolerable.

Escitalopram used for **major depressive disorder** or generalized anxiety disorder is dosed at 10–20 mg daily. Patients generally start at the 10 mg dose and gradually work their way up to the dose needed for effect after a week at the 10 mg dose. Children ages 12 to 17 may be given a trial of 10 mg per day of escitalopram under select circumstances with careful medical supervision. The dose may be increased to 20 mg after three weeks at a lower dose in some circumstances. The elderly are usually kept at a lower dose of 10 mg, due to their increased sensitivity to these medications and their side effects. The maximum dose that may be used is 20 mg per day in other adults. However, the maximum dose may be lower for some patients depending on the development of side effects and the individual ability to tolerate them. Slowly increasing the dose helps with minimizing side effects, and some side effects become lessened with continued use. All SSRIs such as escitalopram need to be slowly tapered off if discontinued, to avoid a discontinuation withdrawal syndrome.

Precautions

SSRIs such as escitalopram have many negative side effects. It usually takes several weeks of medication for the treatment effects to occur, while the undesirable side effects may occur at the onset of treatment. When an SSRI such as escitalopram is prescribed for a patient with a disease like major depression, this time lapse in beneficial versus adverse effects may be difficult for patient **compliance** with treatment. The classic description is a patient who is already feeling depressed takes an SSRI then experiences side effects and so feels worse, all while being told that the patient will eventually get better. This situation can be frustrating for patients with depression. Fortunately, SSRIs like escitalopram do help many people and have fewer overall side effects than some older medications used for the same purpose. Great benefit may be gained if a patient is able to get past the first couple weeks of treatment. Escitalopram is generally tried for four to six weeks to determine whether it is the appropriate agent for a patient. It takes some time to determine whether a particular SSRI like escitalopram will eventually be effective for an individual. Having one SSRI fail in treatment for an individual patient does not mean that another SSRI will not work for that person. Sometimes multiple drugs need to be attempted under physician care before the proper treatment is found for a patient.

When a patient discontinues escitalopram, the dose needs to be tapered down slowly. SSRIs have little to no abuse potential. However, if an SSRI is abruptly discontinued without tapering, there may be symptoms of withdrawal known as SSRI discontinuation syndrome. Withdrawal symptoms of this syndrome may include flu-like symptoms, anxiety, agitation, vivid or bizarre dreams, **insomnia**, nausea, vomiting, diarrhea, sense of imbalance, chills, **fatigue**, dizziness, headache, and other sensory disturbances. Discontinuation syndrome may be avoided completely if the dose of escitalopram is properly tapered down over time.

KEY TERMS

Bipolar disorder—Psychiatric mood disorder characterized by periods of manic behavior that may alternate with periods of depression, also known as manic depressive disorder.

Cytochrome P450 (CYP450)—Enzymes present in the liver that metabolize drugs.

Irritable bowel syndrome—Disorder involving dysfunction of the GI tract that may include symptoms of constipation, diarrhea, or both.

Monoamine oxidase inhibitors (MAOIs)—Type of antidepressant medication that affects various kinds of neurotransmitters including serotonin.

Neurotransmitter—A chemical messenger that travels through the body and acts in the nervous system. Neurotransmitter signaling is responsible for a wide range of bodily processes and is often the target of medications involving the brain and cardiovascular system.

Neurotransmitter receptor—A physical recipient for chemicals called neurotransmitters. Receptors sit on the surface of cells that make up body tissues, and once bound to the neurotransmitter, they initiate the chemical signaling pathway associated with neurotransmitters.

Nonsteroidal anti-inflammatory drugs (NSAIDs)—A class of pain relief medications that also decreases inflammation, such as ibuprofen (Advil), naproxen (Aleve), and acetylsalicylic acid (Aspirin).

Post-traumatic stress syndrome (PTSD)—Psychiatric disorder in which the patient experiences persistent disturbing anxiety based symptoms after experiencing a traumatic event.

Priapism—Medical condition in which the penis is painfully engorged with blood over long periods of time, usually due to medication use and may constitute a medical emergency.

Serotonin—A type of neurotransmitter involved in regulation of the blood vessels, brain processes, and disease states such as depression.

Serotonin syndrome—A potentially life-threatening drug reaction involving an excess of the neurotransmitter serotonin, usually occurring when too many medications that increase serotonin are taken together such as antimigraine triptans and certain antidepressants.

Social phobia—Psychiatric disorder involving excessive fear and anxiety due to social situations with other people.

Synapse—Physical space between neurons that allows the passage of neurotransmitters for chemical signaling pathways.

Escitalopram is not approved for use in children younger than 12 years of age. Children and adults up to age 24 are at risk for developing suicidal thoughts and aggressive behavior when taking **antidepressants**, including escitalopram. Persons of any age should be monitored for worsening depression or suicidal behavior when taking antidepressant drugs. If a patient goes from depressed and unmotivated to depressed and highly motivated in the first few weeks of treatment, it may increase the risk of harmful behavior.

If used during pregnancy, SSRIs such as escitalopram cross the placenta and may affect the fetus. SSRI use during the third trimester of pregnancy is associated with some newborn medical problems. Potential effects on the newborn include respiratory problems, gastrointestinal problems, **seizures**, and feeding problems. SSRIs such as escitalopram may also cause a withdrawal syndrome in newborn babies known as neonatal abstinence syndrome. Symptoms of neonatal abstinence syndrome in a newborn include irritability, physical agitation and restlessness, tremors, increased breathing rate, nasal congestion, nausea, vomiting, and diarrhea. Symptoms usually end by two weeks of age and are most commonly caused by maternal use of **fluoxetine** and **paroxetine** SSRIs, less commonly with escitalopram.

Escitalopram overdose may result in a condition known as **serotonin syndrome**, also called serotonin toxicity, serotonin poisoning, and serotonin storm. Serotonin overdose may be caused by taking multiple drugs that increase the amount of serotonin signaling in the body. While chemical signaling pathways are a part of normal brain function, over-activation can be dangerous. Drugs that increase serotonin signaling may do so by increasing the amount of serotonin available to bind to and activate receptors or by directly activating serotonin receptors. These drugs can cause serotonin overdose if used at the same time or in time periods too close together. Symptoms of serotonin overdose may range from mild to life-threatening, depending on the individual situation. Symptoms may include high blood pressure, high fever, nausea, diarrhea, headache, sweating, increased heart rate, tremor, muscle twitching, **delirium**, shock, coma, and death.

Escitalopram and other SSRIs are discouraged from use in patients with **bipolar disorder**, as they can induce a state of mania in these individuals. There are selective conditions under which a doctor may prescribe SSRIs to a bipolar patient for a short period of time under careful monitoring. The risk of gastrointestinal bleeding may be increased when escitalopram is combined with nonsteroidal anti-inflammatory drugs (NSAIDs) such as ibuprofen (Motrin), aspirin (Bayer, Excedrin), and naproxen sodium (Aleve).

Side effects

SSRIs such as escitalopram are known for having fewer side effects than other types of antidepressant medications, which is one reason why they tend to be the drug of choice in treatment of depression. However, as with all medication, escitalopram does have side effects. Common side effects of escitalopram include nausea, headache, dizziness, constipation, sexual dysfunction, diarrhea, sweating, dry mouth, shakiness, loss of appetite, weight loss, rash, and insomnia. Rare but serious potential side effects include mania, worsened depression and suicidality (especially in the pediatric population), pediatric growth suppression in younger age groups, seizures, serotonin syndrome, discontinuation syndrome, electrolyte imbalances, hypoglycemia, abnormal bleeding, priapism, and glaucoma.

Interactions

Patients should make their doctor aware of all medications and supplements they are taking before using SSRIs like escitalopram. Using alcohol while taking escitalopram can create toxic reactions in the body, and alcohol should be avoided while taking this drug. The use of the herb **St. John's wort** or yohimbe while taking escitalopram may also cause toxicity.

Switching drug treatment for an individual patient from an MAOI to an SSRI may require a waiting period of up to two weeks between drugs. Switching from an SSRI to an MAOI may require a waiting period of up to five weeks duration. Another example of a medication that has additive serotonin effects with escitalopram or other SSRIs is sumatriptan (Imitrex). Sumatriptan is a drug used to treat migraine headaches and acts directly on serotonin receptors in the brain to activate their serotonin signaling pathway. The combination of an SSRI increasing the amount of serotonin available to activate serotonin receptor signaling pathways, and sumatriptan directly activating serotonin receptor signaling pathways, may produce undesirable side effects or overdose. Other drugs that cannot be combined with escitalopram due to risk of serotonin syndrome are the antibiotic linezolid and the drug methylene blue used in some blood-related illnesses.

SSRIs such as escitalopram may inhibit metabolic enzymes in the liver known as cytochrome P450s (CYP450). By inhibiting specific subtypes of CYP450, escitalopram may dangerously increase the levels of other drugs in the body that would have otherwise been metabolized by the CYP450. Escitalopram may increase the potency and side effects of the drugs warfarin, digoxin, beta blocker cardiac drugs such as metoprolol, **benzodiazepines** such as **diazepam** (Valium), antipsychotics such as **haloperidol** and **clozapine**, and certain anti-seizure drugs such as phenytoin. Drugs that may cause toxicity with escitalopram include diuretics (water pills), sleep aids like **zolpidem** (Ambien), diet pills such as sibutramine (Meridia), and mood stabilizers such as lithium. Escitalopram cannot be combined with the antipsychotic medications **pimozide** (Orap) or **thioridazine** (Mellaril) due to dangerous cardiac complications. Escitalopram may not be appropriate for use or may require careful monitoring in patients with liver or kidney impairment, electrolyte imbalances, or seizure disorders.

QUESTIONS TO ASK YOUR DOCTOR

- Can I take the full dose right away or do I need to slowly increase the dose?
- Can I stop taking the medication right away or do I need to slowly decrease the dose?
- When should I eat in reference to taking this medication?
- What time of day should I take this medication?
- How long should I take this medication before I am reassessed?
- Will this medication interact with any of my other prescription medications?
- Are there any over-the-counter medications I should not take with this medicine?
- What are the side effects I should watch for?
- Can I drink alcoholic beverages in the same time frame as taking this medication?

Resources

BOOKS

Brunton, Laurence L., et al. *Goodman and Gilman's The Pharmacological Basis of Therapeutics.* 12th ed. New York: McGraw Hill Medical, 2011.

Stargrove, Mitchell Bebel, et al. *Herb, Nutrient, and Drug Interactions: Clinical Implications and Therapeutic Strategies.* St. Louis: Mosby, 2007.

ORGANIZATIONS

American College of Neuropsychopharmacology, 5034-A Thoroughbred Lane, Brentwood, TN, 37027, (615) 324-2360, Fax: (615) 523-1715, acnp@acnp.org, http://www.acnp.org/default.aspx.

American Psychiatric Association, 1000 Wilson Blvd., Ste. 1825, Arlington, VA, 22209-3901, (703) 907-7300, apa@psych.org, http://www.psych.org.

American Society for Clinical Pharmacology and Therapeutics, 528 N Washington St., Alexandria, VA, 22314, (703) 836-6981, info@ascpt.org, http://www.ascpt.org.

Mental Health America, 2000 N Beauregard St., 6th Fl., Alexandria, VA, 22311, (703) 684-7722, (800) 969-6642, Fax: (703) 684-5968, http://www.nmha.org.

Maria Eve Basile, PhD

Eskalith *see* **Lithium carbonate**

Estazolam

Definition

Estazolam is a sedative-hypnotic drug belonging to the class of drugs known as **benzodiazepines**. It is sold in the United States under the names ProSom and Sedarest.

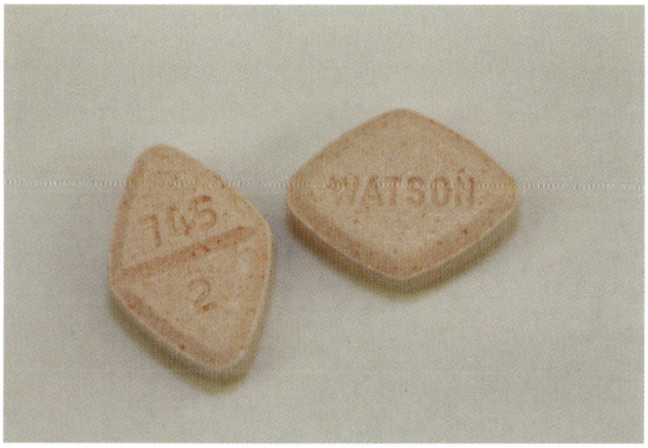

Estazolam, 2 mg. *(© Custom Medical Stock Photo, Inc. Reproduced by permission.)*

Purpose

Estazolam is used as a short-term treatment for **insomnia**. Given at bedtime, estazolam can help patients who have trouble falling asleep, staying asleep, or who have unwanted early morning awakening.

Description

Estazolam belongs to a group of drugs called benzodiazepines. Benzodiazepines are sedative-hypnotic drugs that help to relieve nervousness, tension, and other anxiety symptoms by slowing the central nervous system. To do this, they block the effects of a specific chemical involved in the transmission of nerve impulses in the **brain**, decreasing the excitement level of the nerve cells.

Estazolam, like other benzodiazepines, can be habit-forming and can cause tolerance. Tolerance occurs when a given dosage has less and less effect when the drug is taken over a long time. Therefore, estazolam is recommended only for short-term use.

Estazolam is available in 1 mg and 2 mg tablets, for oral use.

Recommended dosage

Adults are usually prescribed a single 1–2 mg dose of estazolam to be taken at bedtime. The elderly (over age 60) or people with serious health problems require much smaller doses, and are usually started at 0.5 mg at bedtime.

Precautions

Care must be taken when prescribing this medication to anyone with decreased liver or kidney functioning; the elderly; those with a history of **substance abuse**, **depression**, respiratory depression (such as asthma, chronic obstructive pulmonary disease, chronic bronchitis, or other chronic respiratory diseases); narrow-angle glaucoma; or known sleep apnea. People with these health conditions should discuss the risks and benefits of using estazolam with their doctor before starting treatment.

Pregnant women should not use estazolam, because it causes damage to the developing fetus. Because estazolam shows up in breast milk, women who are breast-feeding should not take this drug.

Because estazolam is a nervous system and respiratory depressant, it should not be taken with other such depressants, such as alcohol or other **sedatives**, sleeping pills, or tranquilizers. Furthermore, patients should not drive, operate dangerous machinery, or engage in hazardous activities until the drug's effects have worn off.

Suddenly discontinuing estazolam after several weeks of use may cause uncomfortable symptoms of

KEY TERMS

Benzodiazepines—A group of central nervous system depressants used to relieve anxiety or to induce sleep.

Delusion—A false belief that is resistant to reason or contrary to actual fact.

Depressant—Something that slows down functioning.

Glaucoma—A group of eye diseases characterized by increased pressure within the eye significant enough to damage eye tissue and structures. If untreated, glaucoma results in blindness.

Hallucinations—False sensory perceptions. A person experiencing a hallucination may "hear" sounds or ""see" people or objects that are not really present. Hallucinations can also affect the senses of smell, touch, and taste.

Sleep apnea—Short periods where a person stops breathing during sleep. Breathing restarts spontaneously, however, this condition can lead a lack of oxygen in the body.

withdrawal. Patients should discuss with their doctor how to discontinue estazolam use gradually to avoid such symptoms.

Side effects

The most common side effects of estazolam include sleepiness, slowness of movement, dizziness, and difficulty with coordination.

Less common side effects include anxiety, confusion, depression, memory loss for events occurring after the drug is taken, increased heart rate, and pounding or irregular heartbeat.

Rare side effects include confused thinking, disorientation, **delusions**, irritability, agitation, hallucinations, **seizures**, bizarre and/or aggressive behavior, a drop in blood pressure, weak muscles, skin rash or itching, sores in mouth or throat, fever and chills, difficulty sleeping, odd body and/or eye movements, unusual bruising or easy bleeding, severe **fatigue** or weakness, and yellow eyes or skin (jaundice).

Interactions

Cimetidine (Tagamet), **disulfiram** (Antabuse), and erythromycin (an antibiotic) may increase estazolam's sedative effects.

Rifampin may decrease the effects of estazolam.

Resources

BOOKS

Preston, John D., John H. O'Neal, and Mary C. Talaga. *Handbook of Clinical Psychopharmacology for Therapists*. 5th ed. Oakland, CA: New Harbinger Publications, 2008.

PERIODICALS

Rosenberg, Russell P. "Sleep Maintenance Insomnia: Strengths and Weaknesses of Current Pharmacologic Therapies." *Annals of Clinical Psychiatry* 18, no. 1 (January–March 2006): 49–56.

Rosalyn Carson-DeWitt, MD
Ruth A. Wienclaw, PhD

Etiology of mental illness *see* **Origin of mental illnesses**

Evening primrose oil

Definition

Evening primrose oil is a dietary supplement derived from the seeds of the evening primrose plant, *Oenothera biennis*. Its Latin name is derived from the Greek word for wine, reflecting the folk belief that the plant could relieve the symptoms of a hangover. Other names for the plant are tree primrose and sundrop. Native Americans used the leaves and bark of evening primrose as a sedative and astringent; it was given for stomach and liver complaints as well as disorders of the female reproductive system. More recently, the discovery of antioxidant and other properties of the seed oil has

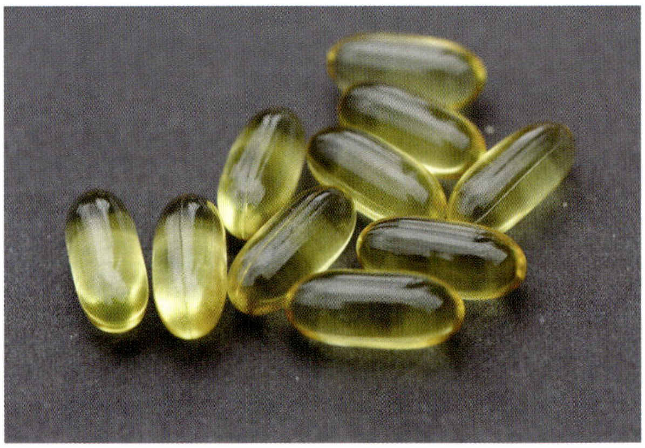

Evening primrose capsules. *(© mitzy/Shutterstock.com)*

focused research on its usefulness in treating a range of diseases and disorders.

Purpose

Evening primrose oil is used by contemporary naturopaths and other alternative practitioners to relieve the discomfort of symptoms associated with PMS, eczema, sunburn, fibrocystic breast disease, arthritis, diabetes, and osteoporosis. However, evening primrose oil has shown little clinical effectiveness in treating most of these conditions, with the best results in treating breast pain and osteoporosis. Some practitioners believe that the supplement can help alleviate symptoms of PMS, **Alzheimer's disease**, and **attention deficit hyperactivity disorder (ADHD)**, but this has not yet been proven in **clinical trials**.

Description

Evening primrose oil is obtained from the seeds of the plant by pressing. The oil can be taken directly as a liquid or in the form of capsules. Evening primrose oil is considered a good source of essential fatty acids (EFAs), predominately Omega 6. EFAs are called essential fatty acids because the human body cannot produce them; they must be obtained from the diet. EFAs maintain the function of cell membranes, regulate pain and inflammation, prevent blood clots, regulate blood pressure and cholesterol levels, and help to produce hormone-like substances known as prostaglandins. Prostaglandins function as inflammation mediators in the short-term regulation of glands and other body organs. It is thought that evening primrose oil relieves symptoms of PMS by preferentially stimulating anti-inflammatory prostaglandins.

Under normal conditions, the body uses an EFA called linoleic acid to produce a compound called gamma linoleic acid, or GLA. Evening primrose oil contains both linoleic acid (74%) and GLA (9%), making it the most familiar and popular source of GLA. The other compounds contained in evening primrose oil are oleic acid (11%) and palmitic acid (6%).

Recommended dosage

Evening primrose oil can be obtained in health food stores in either liquid or capsule form; topical preparations are also available for treating skin conditions. The best quality supplements are organic and cold-pressed, not oxidized by heating. Doses should be stored it in the refrigerator, and standard dosage varies according to the condition being treated.

All parts of the evening primrose plant are safe to eat. The roots can be boiled and eaten like parsnips. The seeds were roasted and used as a coffee substitute when food rationing was in effect during World War II.

KEY TERMS

Antioxidant—Substance that protects the body from damaging reactive oxygen molecules in the body. These reactive oxygen molecules can come from inside the body or from environmental pollution and are thought to play a role in the aging process and the development of degenerative disease.

Astringent—A substance or compound that causes contraction or constriction of soft tissue.

Prostaglandins—A group of unsaturated fatty acids involved in the contraction of smooth muscle, control of inflammation, and many other body processes.

Precautions

Evening primrose oil should not be given to patients with epilepsy, and only after a consultation with a physician should it be given to children.

Side effects

Evening primrose oil has not been reported as having toxic or severe side effects. Some patients, however, have reported nausea, headache, and softening of the stools. Bruising due to damage of the blood platelet function is also possible.

Interactions

Experts in pharmacology advise against using evening primrose oil with phenytoin (Dilantin) or other anticonvulsant medications, as the oil may lower the threshold for **seizures**. No other significant drug interactions have been reported, but persons taking evening primrose oil or any other supplement should alert their physicians to avoid any potential complications.

Resources

BOOKS

Murray, Michael, and Joseph Pizzorno. *Encyclopedia of Natural Medicine*. New York: Three Rivers Press, 1997.

Pelletier, Kenneth R. "Naturopathic Medicine: 'Do No Harm'." In *The Best Alternative Medicine*. New York: Touchstone, 2002.

PERIODICALS

Belch, Jill, and Alexander Hill. "Evening Primrose Oil and Borage Oil in Rheumatologic Conditions." *American Journal of Clinical Nutrition* 71, no. 1 (January 2000): 352S–6S.

Birch, A.E., et al. "Antioxidant Properties of Evening Primrose Seed Extracts." *Journal of Agricultural and Food Chemistry* 49, no. 9 (September 2001): 4502–4507.

Donohue, Maureen. "Evening Primrose Oil May Ease PMS Symptoms." *OB/GYN News* (April 1, 2000).

Dove, D., and P. Johnson. "Oral Evening Primrose Oil: Its Effect on Length of Pregnancy and Selected Intrapartum Outcomes in Low-Risk Nulliparous Women." *Journal of Nurse-Midwifery* 44, no. 3 (May–June 1999): 320–324.

Horowitz, S. "Combining Supplements and Prescription Drugs: What Your Patients Need to Know." *Alternative Complementary Therapy* 6, no. 4 (August 2000): 177–183.

Hudson, Tori. "Evening Primrose Oil." *Townsend Letter for Doctors and Patients* (January 1, 2001): 7.

Miller, Lucinda G. "Herbal Medicinals." *Archives of Internal Medicine* 158 (1998) 2200–11. Available online at http://archinte.ama-assn.org/cgi/content/full/158/20/2200 (accessed November 9, 2011).

Yoon, S., J. Lee, and S. Lee. "The Therapeutic Effect of Evening Primrose Oil in Atopic Dermatitis Patients with Dry Scaly Skin Lesions is Associated with the Normalization of Serum Gamma-Interferon Levels." *Skin Pharmacology and Applied Skin Physiology* 15, no. 1 (January–February 2002) 20–25.

Rebecca J. Frey, PhD

Executive function

Definition

Executive function describes a set of cognitive abilities that control and regulate other abilities and behaviors. Executive functions are necessary for goal-directed behavior. They include the ability to initiate and stop actions, to monitor and change behavior as needed, and to plan future behavior when faced with novel tasks and situations. Executive functions allow individuals to anticipate outcomes and adapt to changing situations. The ability to form concepts and think abstractly are often considered components of executive function.

Description

As the name implies, executive functions are high-level abilities that influence more basic abilities like attention, memory and motor skills. For this reason, they can be difficult to assess directly. Many of the tests used to measure other abilities, particularly those that look at more complex aspects of these abilities, can be used to evaluate executive functions. For example, a person with executive function deficits may perform well on tests of basic attention, such as those that simply ask the individual to look at a computer screen and respond when a particular shape appears, but have trouble with tasks that require divided or alternating attention, such as giving a different response depending on the stimulus presented. Verbal fluency tests that ask people to say a number of words in a certain period of time can also reveal problems with executive function. One commonly used test asks individuals to name as many animals or as many words beginning with a particular letter as they can in one minute. A person with executive function deficits may find the animal naming task simple, but struggle to name words beginning with a particular letter, since this task requires people to organize concepts in a novel way. Executive functions also influence memory abilities by allowing people to employ strategies that can help them remember information. Other tests are designed to assess cognitive function more directly. Such tests may present a fairly simple task but without instructions on how to complete it. Executive functions allow most people to figure out the task demand through trial and error and change strategies as needed.

Executive functions are important for successful adaptation and performance in real-life situations. They allow people to initiate and complete tasks and to persevere in the face of challenges. Because the environment can be unpredictable, executive functions are vital to human ability to recognize the significance of unexpected situations and to quickly make alternative plans when unusual events arise and interfere with normal routines. In this way, executive function contributes to success in work and school and allows people to deal effectively with the stresses of daily life. Executive functions also enable people to inhibit inappropriate behaviors. People with poor executive functions often have problems interacting with other people since they may say or do things that are bizarre or offensive to others. Most people experience impulses to do or say things that could get them in trouble, such as making a sexually explicit comment to a stranger, commenting negatively on someone's appearance, or insulting an authority figure like a boss or police officer; but most people have no trouble suppressing these urges. When executive functions are impaired, however, these urges may not be suppressed. Executive functions are an important component of our ability to fit in socially.

Executive function deficits are associated with a number of psychiatric and developmental disorders,

KEY TERMS

Autism—A developmental disability that appears early in life, in which normal brain development is disrupted and social and communication skills are retarded, sometimes severely.

Cognitive—Pertaining to the mental processes of memory, perception, judgment, and reasoning.

Cortex—Region in the brain where sensation and perception are processed and integrated into thoughts, memories, and abilities; also where actions are planned and initiated.

Dementia—A group of symptoms (syndrome) associated with a progressive loss of memory and other intellectual functions that is serious enough to interfere with a person's ability to perform the tasks of daily life. Dementia impairs memory, alters personality, leads to deterioration in personal grooming, impairs reasoning ability, and causes disorientation.

Executive—Pertaining to supervision, planning, and carrying out duties or actions.

Frontal lobes—A region of the brain that influences higher mental functions often associated with intelligence, such as the ability to foresee the consequences of actions, planning, comprehension, and mood.

Schizophrenia—A severe mental illness in which a person has difficulty distinguishing what is real from what is not real. It is often characterized by hallucinations, delusions, language and communication disturbances, and withdrawal from people and social activities.

Tourette syndrome—Neurological disorder characterized by multiple involuntary movements and uncontrollable vocalizations called tics that come and go over years, usually beginning in childhood and becoming chronic. Sometimes the tics include inappropriate language.

including **obsessive-compulsive disorder**, Tourette syndrome, **depression**, **schizophrenia**, **attention deficit hyperactivity disorder**, and **autism**. Executive function deficits also appear to play a role in antisocial behavior. Chronic heavy users of drugs and alcohol show impairments on tests of executive function. Some of these deficits appear to result from heavy substance use, but there is also evidence suggesting that problems with executive functions may contribute to the development of substance use disorders.

Because executive functions govern so many lower-level abilities, there is some controversy about their physiological basis. Nevertheless, most people who study these abilities agree that the frontal lobes of the **brain** play a major role in executive function. The frontal lobes are the large portions of the brain cortex that lie near the front of the brain. The cortex is the site in the brain where lower level processes like sensation and perception are processed and integrated into thoughts, memories and abilities, and actions are planned and initiated. People with frontal lobe injuries have difficulty with the higher level processing that underlies executive functions. Because of its complexity, the frontal cortex develops more slowly than other parts of the brain, and not surprisingly, many executive functions do not fully develop until adolescence. Some executive functions also appear to decline in old age, and some executive function deficits may be useful in early detection of mild **dementia**.

Resources

BOOKS

Lezak, Muriel Deutsch, et al. *Neuropsychological Assessment*. 3rd ed. New York: Oxford University Press, 2011.

Lichter, David G., and Jeffrey L. Cummings. *Frontal-subcortical Circuits in Psychiatric and Neurological Disorders*. New York: The Guilford Press, 2001.

PERIODICALS

Anderson, Vicki A., et al. "Development of Executive Functions Through Late Childhood and Adolescence in an Australian Sample." *Developmental Neuropsychology* 20, no. 1 (2001): 385–406.

Bryan, Janet, and Mary A. Luszcz. "Measurement of Executive Function: Considerations for Detecting Adult Age Differences." *Journal of Clinical and Experimental Neuropsychology* 22, no. 1 (February 2000): 40–55.

Morgan, Alex B., and Scott O. Lilienfeld. "A Meta-analytic Review of the Relation Between Antisocial Behavior and Neuropsychological Measures of Executive Function." *Clinical Psychology Review* 20, no. 1 (2000): 113–136.

Nathan, Joanna, et al. "The Role of Tests of Frontal Executive Function in the Detection of Mild Dementia." *International Journal of Geriatric Psychiatry* 16, no. 1 (2001): 18–26.

Ready, Rebecca E., Laura Stierman, and Jane S. Paulsen. "Ecological Validity of Neuropsychological and Personality Measures of Executive Functions." *The Clinical Neuropsychologist* 15, no. 3 (2001): 314–323.

Wecker, Nancy S., et al. "Age Effects on Executive Ability." *Neuropsychology* 14, no. 3 (July 2000): 409–414.

ORGANIZATIONS

American Psychological Association, 750 1st Street NE, Washington, DC, 20002-4242, (202) 336-5500; TDD/TTY: (202) 336-6123, (800) 374-2721, http://www.apa.org.

International Neuropsychological Society, 700 Ackerman Rd., Ste. 625, Columbus, OH, 43202, (614) 263-4200, Fax: (614) 263-4366, http://www.the-ins.org.

National Academy of Neuropsychology, 7555 East Hampden Ave., Ste. 525, Denver, CO, 80231, (303) 691-3694, Fax: (303) 691-5983, office@nanonline.org, http://nanonline.org.

Danielle Barry, MS

Exelon *see* **Rivastigmine**

Exercise and mental health

Definition

Exercise directly benefits mental health, in addition to the benefits of exercise-derived improvements in physical health.

Purpose

Exercise helps relieve tension, anxiety, **stress**, anger, and **depression**, and helps enhance a person's general sense of well-being. Exercise and improved physical fitness help build self-confidence, promote positive **body image** and self-esteem, and contribute to a positive outlook. Sports and other physical activities provide an emotional release from anxieties and frustrations. Exercise increases energy levels and mental alertness and improves sleep, all of which contribute to good mental health. Exercising outdoors in the sunlight—so-called "green" activities—can help overcome **seasonal affective disorder** (SAD) or the "winter blues." Many people find exercise to be an enjoyable form of relaxation and an opportunity for socializing. This can be especially important for patients dealing with isolation and loneliness due to a mental health condition.

Over the long term, regular exercise benefits physical health, which contributes to improved mental health. Weight gain is both a common cause and a common result of depression and other mental health problems. Weight gain can also be a side effect of some medications used to treat mental disorders. Exercise can slow or halt weight gain. It can also relieve stress and tension that can otherwise lead to overeating. Aging often has a negative impact on mental health; however, physical activity can help seniors continue to enjoy activities and remain independent—both important contributors to good mental health.

For many people, the effects of exercise on mental health go beyond improving mood and preventing "the blues." Research and clinical experience indicate that exercise can be an effective treatment for more serious mental disorders, including severe depression, **anxiety disorders**, substance dependence, and even **schizophrenia**. Physicians and psychologists commonly prescribe exercise for a range of mental health conditions, in place of or in addition to medications and counseling or **psychotherapy**. Some research suggests that the effects of exercise on mild depression may be longer lasting than the effects of **antidepressants**.

Whereas studies have consistently demonstrated that exercise can benefit mental health, the reverse also appears to be true: the lack of regular exercise is associated with symptoms of depression and anxiety.

Demographics

Approximately 26% of Americans and 20% of Canadians will experience a mental illness at some point in their lives. According to the **National Institute of Mental Health**, more than 4% of Americans have a serious mental illness, including about 6% of females and nearly 8% of young adults between the ages of 18 and 25. Among Americans over age 65, 14% have significant depressive symptoms. Men over age 75 have the highest overall **suicide** rate. Serious mental illness is somewhat more common among Caucasians than among African Americans, Hispanics, and Asian Americans. Mixed-race Americans have the highest rates of serious mental illness.

Regular physical activity is important for the mental health of most people. With the increase in sedentary employment and entertainment via television, video games, and the Internet, activity levels have decreased in recent decades among all age groups. During the same period, the incidence of mental health disorders has risen sharply. Although some of this increase is attributable to greater awareness of mental health issues and improved diagnoses, reduced activity levels may share some of the blame.

Any condition that limits physical activity can have a negative impact on mental health. Physical illnesses and conditions—such as arthritis, cardiovascular disease, **stroke**, cancer, and HIV/AIDS—are often accompanied by depression or other mental problems. Anxiety, fear, or stress can be secondary to such conditions, resulting from concern about the future or restriction of normal activities. Other times, a disease, physical condition, or medication used to treat a condition directly causes depression or other mental problems. For instance, depression is the most common psychiatric **diagnosis** among HIV/AIDS patients, especially women. In addition to causing anxiety and fear, HIV/AIDS and HIV-related medications can contribute directly to depression.

Description

Origins

During the 1970s and 1980s, clinicians began to realize that people who exercised regularly were less likely to experience depression and were less likely to become depressed in the future. A trial conducted in 1999 demonstrated that an aerobic exercise plan was as effective in treating depressed adults as the antidepressant **sertraline** (Zoloft), a drug that earned its manufacturer more than $3 billion annually before its patent expired in 2006. Most subsequent studies have confirmed that regular aerobic exercise can be as effective as medication for treating depression and preventing the recurrence of depressive symptoms.

Effects of exercise

Regular exercise has positive emotional, psychological, and physical effects. Exercise relaxes the mind and body. Physical activity provides a positive means of coping with stress, anxiety, sadness, and depression. It provides a distraction that can break cycles of negative thinking that increase anxiety and depression. In contrast, trying to wait out a depression or attempting to cope with drugs or alcohol often makes symptoms worse. Exercise also can improve self-esteem and self-confidence through a sense of achievement and improved body image and by encouraging social interaction.

Exercise may relieve muscle tension, burn off stress hormones, and increase blood flow to the **brain**. It may lower immune system chemicals that can worsen depression. Exercise also increases body temperature, which may have a calming effect.

Neuroscientists are beginning to understand the ways in which exercise alters brain chemistry. Exercise stimulates the production of endorphins—so-called pleasure hormones that improve mood and relieve stress. It appears that exercise functions in much the same way as antidepressant medications, by regulating the **neurotransmitters serotonin** and norepinephrine. Over a period of several weeks, regular exercise appears to turn on specific genes that increase the levels of galanin in the brain. Galanin is a neurotransmitter that reduces the body's stress response by regulating norepinephrine. This means that new stimuli or negative events—such as a parking ticket or missed appointment—have less effect on emotions.

Exercise also may have a direct effect on nerve cells in the hippocampus—a part of the brain involved in the regulation of mood and responses to antidepressants. In animals, exercise increases the production of brain-derived neurotrophic factor (BDNF), which is necessary for the growth and maintenance of brain cells and can relieve depressive symptoms in humans. Studies in animal models of human depression have found that exercise-induced symptom alleviation depends on the growth of new adult neurons in the brain and may involve the enhanced activity of a nerve growth factor.

Exercise as treatment

Exercise has several advantages as a mental health treatment. It is usually viewed in a positive light, without the **stigma** that is sometimes still associated with medication or psychotherapy. The mood-enhancing effects of exercise are quickly apparent—much faster than the physical benefits of exercise. This immediate effect encourages more exercise. This is particularly important for people who have depression, which is associated with a chronic lack of motivation. Unlike other treatments for mental disorders, exercise provides significant physical health benefits, is inexpensive or free, and is without the side effects that occur with many medications.

Experts generally recommend at least 30 minutes of moderate-intensity aerobic exercise—such as walking—at least five times per week, or 30 minutes of high-intensity aerobic exercise at least three times per week. These are similar to physical fitness recommendations. As little as 30–45 minutes of walking three times per week has been associated with a reduction or alleviation of depressive symptoms. Even small increments of exercise—climbing stairs, walking the dog, or gardening for 10–15 minutes at a time—can have a significant effect. However, more vigorous exercise, such as running or playing a sport, may work faster. Anaerobic exercise, such as weightlifting, may have many of the same mental health benefits as aerobic exercise. Some types of exercise—such as **yoga**, pilates, and tai chi—are geared specifically toward improving mental as well as physical health.

Preparation

Sedentary individuals and those with health problems should always consult their physician before embarking on a new exercise program. Physicians or mental health professionals can prescribe exercise regimens that take into account pain, physical limitations, and mobility issues. It is important to start slowly, gradually increasing exercise intensity and duration as strength and stamina improve.

Regardless of apparent mental health benefits, sticking with an exercise program is a challenge for many people. It is important to choose activities that are both appropriate and enjoyable. Exercise should be

KEY TERMS

Aerobic exercise—Activity that increases the body's requirement for oxygen, thereby increasing respiration and heart rate.

Antidepressant—A drug used to prevent or treat depression.

Anxiety disorder—A group of disorders characterized by anxiety, including panic disorder and post-traumatic stress disorder (PTSD).

Brain-derived neurotrophic factor (BDNF)—A brain protein that helps maintain nerves and promotes the growth of new nerve cells (neurons).

Depression—A mental condition of extreme sadness and loss of interest in life, including problems with appetite, sleep, concentration, and daily functioning; severe depression can lead to suicide attempts.

Eating disorders—Conditions, such as anorexia nervosa and bulimia nervosa, that are characterized by abnormal attitudes toward food, altered appetite control, unhealthy eating habits, and sometimes compulsive exercise; particularly common in young women.

Endorphins—A class of peptides in the brain that are produced during exercise and bind to opiate receptors, resulting in pleasant feelings and pain relief.

Galanin—A neurotransmitter with roles in various physiological processes, including regulation of the stress response.

Hippocampus—A part of the brain that is involved in forming, storing, and processing memory, and in regulating mood.

Hormone—A substance, such as a protein, that is produced in one part of the body and travels through the bloodstream to affect another part of the body.

Neurotransmitter—A chemical—such as norepinephrine or serotonin—that transmits impulses across synapses between nerves.

Norepinephrine—Noradrenaline; a neurotransmitter in the sympathetic nervous system and some parts of the central nervous system, as well as a blood-pressure-raising (vasoconstricting) adrenal hormone.

Pilates—An exercise regimen specifically designed to improve overall physiological and mental functioning.

Schizophrenia—A psychotic disorder characterized by loss of contact with one's environment, deterioration of everyday functioning, and personality disintegration.

Serotonin—A neurotransmitter located primarily in the brain, blood serum, and stomach.

Stroke—A sudden diminishing or loss of consciousness, sensation, or voluntary movement, due to the rupture or obstruction of a blood vessel in the brain.

Tai chi—An ancient Chinese discipline involving controlled movements specifically designed to improve physical and mental well-being.

something to look forward to each day. Goals should be reasonable and achievable, so as not to set oneself up for failure. Some people prefer to exercise at home, out of self-consciousness or financial considerations. Others find that exercising with companions, such as in a gym or group class setting, is more motivating.

Precautions

Although exercise can ease symptoms of anxiety, depression, or another mental disorder, it is not necessarily a substitute for psychotherapy, medication, or other treatment. Appropriate activities and intensity levels should be chosen in consultation with a physician, to avoid the risk of injury.

Compulsive exercise is sometimes a symptom of a mental health disorder, particularly eating disorders such as **anorexia nervosa** or **bulimia nervosa**. People with anorexia may exercise compulsively to lose weight inappropriately. Those with bulimia, which is characterized by episodes of uncontrollable binge eating, may engage in compulsive exercise to prevent weight gain from overeating.

Results

As little as 30 minutes or less of moderate-intensity exercise that raises the heart rate can result in noticeable mood enhancement and anxiety reduction. Many studies have shown that routine exercise can be as effective as medication at relieving depressive symptoms. However, some research suggests that psychological responses to exercise have a genetic component. A large, long-term study of identical twins, published in 2008, found that twins who exercised more had no fewer anxious or depressive symptoms than their identical siblings who

QUESTIONS TO ASK YOUR DOCTOR

- How would I benefit from an exercise program?
- Could exercise replace my antidepressant medication?
- What type of exercise do you recommend?
- How much exercise should I get?

exercised less. It is possible that some types of exercise have more effect on mental health in some people than in others. It is also unclear whether exercise is as effective for treating severe depression as it is for treating mild to moderate depression.

Research and general acceptance

The relationship between mental health and exercise is an area of active research. Studies have extended the mental health benefits of exercise to patients with schizophrenia and schizophrenia-like illnesses, **bipolar disorder**, major depression, and other mental disorders. Exercise has been found to relieve depressive symptoms in adult stroke patients and stroke patients who exercise are much less likely to report depressive symptoms. Studies published in 2010 reported that the amount of exercise by undergraduate students correlated positively with their ratings on mental health scales and that just five minutes of outdoor or "green" activity—walking or gardening—has noticeable mental health benefits, including improved mood and self-esteem. A study published in 2011 found conclusive evidence that tai chi improves mental health in seniors, as well as providing general health benefits and reducing the risk of falls.

A study published in 2010, involving more than 40,000 Norwegians, reported that those who engaged in even small amounts of light, regular exercise were less likely to have depressive symptoms, as long as it was leisure-time exercise rather than physical activity at work. Socializing during exercise was an important beneficial factor. Those who were not active during their free time were almost twice as likely to have depressive symptoms. Exercise intensity did not appear to influence the results.

Schools and hospitals are increasingly using yoga to help children relax and focus and to improve behavior, self-esteem, and academic performance, as well as physical health. Some schools use yoga before statewide tests to help children relax and concentrate. Over the long term, yoga has been found to reduce aggression and improve emotional balance in children. It appears to be particularly helpful for children with special needs, as well as those with eating and mood disorders and **autism**.

Resources

BOOKS

Amen, Daniel G. *Magnificent Mind at Any Age: Natural Ways to Unleash Your Brain's Maximum Potential.* New York: Harmony, 2009.

Carless, David, and Kitrina Douglas. *Sport and Physical Activity for Mental Health.* Ames, IA: Wiley-Blackwell, 2010.

Emmons, Henry. *The Chemistry of Calm: A Powerful, Drug-Free Plan to Quiet Your Fears and Overcome Your Anxiety.* New York: Simon & Schuster, 2010.

Friedman, Peach. *Diary of an Exercise Addict: A Memoir.* Guilford, CT: GPP Life, 2009.

Kemper, Kathi. *Mental Health, Naturally: The Family Guide to Holistic Care for a Healthy Mind and Body.* Elk Grove Village, IL: American Academy of Pediatrics, 2010.

Larsen, Laura. *Fitness and Exercise Sourcebook.* 4th ed. Detroit: Omnigraphics, 2011.

Otto, Michael W., and Jasper A.J. Smits. *Exercise for Mood and Anxiety Disorders: Workbook.* New York: Oxford University Press, 2009.

PERIODICALS

Blue, Laurie. "Is Exercise the Best Drug for Depression?" *Time Health*, June 19, 2010. http://www.time.com/time/health/article/0,8599,1998021,00.html (accessed July 18, 2011).

Dang, Michelle T. "Walking Away the Blues: Exercise for Depression in Older Adults." *Nursing* 40, no. 11 (November 2010): 33.

Demissie, Zewditu, et al., "Physical Activity and Depressive Symptoms Among Pregnant Women: The PIN3 Study." *Women's Mental Health* 14, no. 2 (April 2011): 145–57.

Harvey, William J., et al. "Physical Activity, Leisure, and Health for Persons with Mental Illness." *Palaestra* 25, no. 2 (2010): 36–41.

Lister, Sam. "Lift Your Mood with a Little Leisure-Time Exercise; But Exertion at Work 'Makes No Difference.'" *Times (London)* (November 1, 2010): 17.

Lowry, C.A., S.L. Lightman, and D.J. Nutt. "That Warm Fuzzy Feeling: Brain Serotonergic Neurons and the Regulation of Emotion." *Journal of Psychopharmacology* 23, no. 4 (June 2009): 392–400.

Tyson, Philip, et al. "Physical Activity and Mental Health in a Student Population." *Journal of Mental Health* 19, no. 6 (December 2010): 492–99.

Van Citters, Aricca D., et al. "A Pilot Evaluation of the In SHAPE Individualized Health Promotion Intervention for Adults with Mental Illness." *Community Mental Health Journal* 46, no. 6 (December 2010): 540–52.

WEBSITES

Cassels, Caroline. "Exercise Beneficial for Physical and Mental Health Outcomes in Schizophrenia." Medscape Medical

News. May 12, 2010. http://www.medscape.com/viewarticle/721652 (accessed July 18, 2011).

Mayo Clinic Staff. "Depression and Anxiety: Exercise Eases Symptoms." MayoClinic.com October 23, 2009. http://www.mayoclinic.com/health/depression-and-exercise/MH00043 (accessed July 18, 2011).

National Institute of Mental Health. "Novel Model of Depression from Social Defeat Shows Restorative Power of Exercise." Science Update. April 13, 2010. http://www.nimh.nih.gov/science-news/2010/novel-model-of-depression-from-social-defeat-shows-restorative-power-of-exercise.shtml (accessed July 18, 2011).

National Institute of Mental Health. "Stress-Defeating Effects of Exercise Traced to Emotional Brain Circuit." Science Update. June 9, 2011. http://www.nimh.nih.gov/science-news/2011/stress-defeating-effects-of-exercise-traced-to-emotional-brain-circuit.shtml (accessed July 18, 2011).

Preidt, Robert. "Tai Chi Prevents Falls, Boosts Mental Health in Seniors: Study." *HealthDay*. May 17, 2011. http://www.nlm.nih.gov/medlineplus/news/fullstory_112150.html (accessed July 17, 2011).

ORGANIZATIONS

Mental Health America, 2000 North Beauregard Street, 6th Floor, Alexandria, VA, 22311, (703) 684-7722, Fax: (703) 684-5968, (800) 969-6642, infoctr@mentalhealthamerica.net, http://www.mentalhealthamerica.net.

National Institute on Aging, Building 31, Room 5C27, 31 Center Drive, MSC 2292, Bethesda, MD, 20892, (301) 496-1752, Fax: (301) 496-1072, (800) 222-2225, http://www.nia.nih.gov.

National Institute of Mental Health, Science Writing, Press, and Dissemination Branch, 6001 Executive Boulevard, Room 8184, MSC 9663, Bethesda, MD, 20892-9663, (301) 443-4513, Fax: (301) 443-4279, (866) 615-6464, nimhinfo@nih.gov, http://www.nimh.nih.gov.

Margaret Alic, PhD

Exhibitionism

Definition

Exhibitionism is a mental disorder characterized by a **compulsion** to display one's genitals to an unsuspecting stranger. The term *paraphilia* is derived from two Greek words meaning "outside of" and "friendship-love."

In the United States and Canada, the slang term "flasher" is often used for exhibitionists.

Demographics

The incidence of exhibitionism in the general population is difficult to estimate because persons with this disorder do not usually seek counseling by their own free will. Exhibitionism is one of the three most common sexual offenses in police records (the other two are **voyeurism** and **pedophilia**). It is rarely diagnosed in general mental health clinics, but most professionals believe that it is probably underdiagnosed and underreported.

In terms of the technical definition of exhibitionism, almost all reported cases involve males. A number of mental health professionals, however, have noted that gender bias may be built into the standard definition. Some women engage in a form of exhibitionism by undressing in front of windows as if they are encouraging someone to watch them. In addition, wearing the low-cut gowns favored by some models and actresses have been described as socially sanctioned exhibitionism.

Although the stereotype of an exhibitionist is a "dirty old man in a raincoat," most males arrested for exhibitionism are in their late teens or early twenties. The disorder appears to have its onset before age 18. Like most **paraphilias**, exhibitionism is rarely found in men over 50 years of age.

In the United States most exhibitionists are Caucasian males. About half of exhibitionists are married.

Description

The ***Diagnostic and Statistical Manual of Mental Disorders***, also known as the *DSM-IV-TR,* classifies exhibitionism under the heading of the paraphilias, a subcategory of sexual and gender identity disorders. The paraphilias are a group of mental disorders marked by **obsession** with unusual sexual practices or with sexual activity involving nonconsenting or inappropriate partners (e.g., children or animals).

Exhibitionism is described in the *DSM-IV-TR,* as the exposure of one's genitals to a stranger, usually with no intention of further sexual activity with the other person. For this reason, the term exhibitionism is sometimes grouped together with voyeurism, (peeping, or watching an unsuspecting person or people, usually strangers, undressing or engaging in sexual activity) as a "hands-off" paraphilia. This contrasts with the "hands-on disorders" that involve physical contact with other persons. Some exhibitionists are aware of a conscious desire to shock or upset their target; while others fantasize that the target will become sexually aroused by their display. In some cases, the exhibitionist masturbates while exposing himself (or while fantasizing that he is exposing himself) to the other person.

Changes proposed for the fifth edition of the *DSM* (*DSM-5*, 2013) include renaming exhibitionism to exhibitionistic disorder.

Causes and symptoms

Causes

Several theories have been proposed regarding the origins of exhibitionism, although none are considered conclusive. They include:

- Biological theories. These generally hold that testosterone, the hormone that influences the sexual drive in both men and women, increases the susceptibility of males to develop deviant sexual behaviors. Some medications used to treat exhibitionists are given to lower the patients' testosterone levels.
- Learning theories. Several studies have shown that emotional abuse in childhood and family dysfunction are both significant risk factors in the development of exhibitionism. A Swedish survey (Sweden is globally recognized for its excellent health data survey system) found that exhibitionism is associated with psychological problems, although whether the problems precipitate the behavior or vice versa was not identified. This same study found no association between exhibitionistic behavior and a history of sexual abuse.
- Psychoanalytical theories. These are based on an unsubstantiated assumption that male gender identity requires the male child's separation from his mother psychologically so that he does not identify with her as a member of the same sex, the way a girl does. It is thought that exhibitionists regard their mothers as rejecting them on the basis of their different genitals. Therefore, they grow up with the desire to force women to accept them by making women look at their genitals.
- Head trauma. There are a small number of documented cases of men becoming exhibitionists following traumatic brain injury (TBI) without previous histories of alcohol abuse or sexual offenses.
- A childhood history of attention deficit hyperactivity disorder (ADHD). The reason for the connection is not yet known, but researchers at Harvard have discovered that patients with multiple paraphilias have a much greater likelihood of having had ADHD as children than patients with only one paraphilia.

Some psychiatrists disagree about whether exhibitionism should be considered a disorder of impulse control or whether it falls within the spectrum of obsessive-compulsive disorders (OCDs). Recent studies suggest that there is an obsessive-compulsive element to these behaviors, and some papers now describe these behaviors in a category of compulsive-impulsive sexual behaviors. Single case studies have suggested some effectiveness of drugs used to treat **bipolar disorder** in treating exhibitionistic behaviors, implying a potential link also to bipolar disorders. People who exhibit pedophilia, which is also characterized as a paraphilia, have abnormalities in **brain imaging studies** that are similar to those observed in imaging studies of people with **obsessive-compulsive disorder**. Disruption of **dopamine** and **serotonin** (both nerve signaling molecules) pathways is implicated in many of these disorders.

Symptoms

One expert in the field of treating paraphilias has suggested classifying the symptoms of exhibitionism according to level of severity, based on criteria from the *DSM-III-R* (1987):

- Mild. The person has recurrent fantasies of exposing himself, but has rarely or never acted on them.
- Moderate. The person has occasionally exposed himself (three targets or fewer) and has difficulty controlling urges to do so.
- Severe. The person has exposed himself to more than three people and has serious problems with control.
- A fourth level of severity, catastrophic, would not be found in exhibitionists without other paraphilias. This level denotes the presence of sadistic fantasies which, if acted upon, would result in severe injury or death to the victim.

Because exhibitionism is a hands-off paraphilia, it rarely rises above the level of moderate severity in the absence of other paraphilias.

Diagnosis

Diagnosis of exhibitionism is complicated by several factors. For example, most persons with the disorder come to therapy because of court orders. Some are motivated by fear of discovery by employers or family members, and a minority of exhibitionists enter therapy because their wife or girlfriend is distressed by the disorder. Emotional attitudes toward the disorder vary; some men maintain that the only problem they have with exhibitionism is society's disapproval of it; others, however, feel intensely guilty and anxious.

A second complication of diagnosing exhibitionism is the high rate of comorbidity among the paraphilias as a group and between the paraphilias as a group and other mental disorders. In other words, a patient in treatment for exhibitionism is highly likely to engage in other forms of deviant sexual behavior and to have **depression** (an anxiety or substance-abuse disorder). In addition, many patients with paraphilias do not cooperate with physicians, who may have considerable difficulty making an accurate diagnosis of other disorders that may also exist.

A diagnosis of exhibitionism follows a somewhat different pattern from the standard procedures for diagnosing most mental disorders. A thorough workup in a clinic for specialized treatment of sexual disorders includes the following components:

- A psychiatric evaluation and mental status examination to diagnose concurrent psychiatric and medical conditions, and to rule out schizophrenia, post-traumatic stress disorder (PTSD), intellectual disabilities, and depression.
- A neurologic examination to rule out head trauma, seizures, or other abnormalities of brain structure and function, followed by a computed tomography (CT) scan or magnetic resonance imaging (MRI), if needed.
- Blood and urine tests for substance abuse and sexually transmitted diseases, including an HIV screen.
- Assessment of sexual behaviors. This includes creation of a sex hormone profile and responses to questionnaires. The questionnaires are intended to measure cognitive distortions regarding rape and other forms of coercion, pedophilia, aggression, and impulsivity.

Treatment

Exhibitionism is usually treated with a combination of **psychotherapy**, medications, and adjunctive treatments.

Psychotherapy

Several different types of psychotherapy have been found helpful in treating exhibitionism:

- Cognitive-behavioral therapy (CBT). This approach is generally regarded as the most effective form of psychotherapy for exhibitionism. Patients are encouraged to recognize the irrational justifications that they offer for their behavior, and to alter other distorted thinking patterns.
- Orgasmic reconditioning. In this technique, the patient is conditioned to replace fantasies of exposing himself with fantasies of more acceptable sexual behavior while masturbating.
- Group therapy. This form of therapy is used to get patients past the denial frequently associated with paraphilias, and as a form of relapse prevention.
- Twelve-step groups for sexual addicts. Exhibitionists who feel guilty and anxious about their behavior are often helped by the social support and emphasis on healthy spirituality found in these groups, as well as by the cognitive restructuring that is built into the twelve steps.
- Couples therapy or family therapy. This approach is particularly helpful for patients who are married and whose marriages and family ties have been strained by their disorder.

Medications

There are several different classes of drugs used to treat the patient with exhibitionism and the other paraphilias. However, one difficulty in evaluating the comparative efficacy of different medications should be noted: ethical limitation. Double-blind placebo-controlled studies of medication treatment of sexually deviant men raises the ethical question of the possibility of **relapse** in the subjects who receive the placebo. Withholding a potentially effective drug in circumstances that might lead to physical or psychological injury to a third party is difficult to justify.

Medications are often the only form of treatment for patients with exhibitionism that can suppress deviant behaviors. The categories of drugs used to treat exhibitionism are as follows:

- Selective serotonin reuptake inhibitors (SSRIs). The SSRIs show promise in treating the paraphilias, as well as depression and other mood disorders. It has been found that decreased levels of serotonin in the brain result in an increased sex drive. The SSRIs are appropriate for patients with mild- or moderate-level paraphilias; these patients include the majority of exhibitionists.
- Hormones, their mimics, and their antagonists. The three classes of medications most often used to treat paraphilias are hormones, particularly the synthetic medroxyprogesterone acetate, or MPA; luteinizing hormone-releasing hormone (LHRH) agonists (mimics), which include such drugs as triptorelin (Trelstar), leuprolide acetate, and goserelin acetate; and antiandrogens, which block the uptake and metabolism of testosterone as well as reducing blood levels of this hormone. In particular, these drugs with antiandrogenic effects (interfering with the action of the body's androgenic hormones) have shown some effectiveness.

Surgery

Surgical castration, which involves removal of the testes, is effective in significantly reducing levels of

KEY TERMS

Castration—Desexing a person or animal by surgical removal of the testes (in males) or ovaries (in females). Castration is sometimes offered as a treatment option to violent rapists and pedophiles who are repeat offenders.

Comorbidity—Association or presence of two or more mental disorders in the same patient. A disorder that is said to have a high degree of comorbidity is likely to occur in patients diagnosed with other disorders that may share or reinforce some of its symptoms.

Denial—A psychological defense mechanism that reduces anxiety by excluding recognition of an addiction or similar problem from the conscious mind.

Double-blind placebo-controlled study—A study in which patients are divided into two groups—those who will receive a medication, and those who will receive a placebo (a pill that looks like the medication but has no active ingredients). Neither the patients nor their physicians know which pill any specific patient is receiving.

Paraphilias—A group of mental disorders that is characterized by recurrent intense sexual urges and sexually arousing fantasies generally involving (1) nonhuman objects, (2) the suffering or humiliation of oneself or one's partner (not merely simulated), or (3) children or other nonconsenting persons.

Placebo—An inactive substance or preparation used as a control in experiments with human subjects to test the effectiveness of a medication.

Recidivism—A tendency to return to a previously treated activity, or repeated relapse into criminal or deviant behavior.

Serotonin—A chemical produced by the brain that functions as a neurotransmitter. Low serotonin levels are associated with the paraphilias as well as with mood disorders. Medications known as selective serotonin reuptake inhibitors (SSRIs) can be used to treat exhibitionism and other paraphilias.

Voyeurism—A paraphilia that involves watching unsuspecting people, usually strangers, undress or engage in sexual activity.

testosterone in blood plasma. This form of treatment for paraphilias, however, is generally reserved for more serious offenders than exhibitionists (violent rapists and pedophiles with a history of repeated offenses, for example).

Other treatment methods

Another treatment method that is often offered to people with exhibition disorder is **social skills training**. It is thought that some men develop paraphilias partially because they do not know how to form healthy relationships, whether sexual or nonsexual, with other people. Although social skills training is not considered a substitute for medications or psychotherapy, it appears to be a useful adjunctive treatment for exhibitionism disorder.

Prognosis

The prognosis for people with exhibition disorder depends on a number of factors, including the age of onset, the reasons for the patient's referral to psychiatric care, degree of cooperation with the therapist, and comorbidity with other paraphilias or other mental disorders. For some patients, exhibitionism is a temporary disorder related to sexual experimentation during their adolescence. For others, however, it is a lifelong problem with potentially serious legal, interpersonal, financial, educational, and occupational consequences. People with exhibition disorder have the highest recidivism rate of all the paraphilias; between 20% and 50% of men arrested for exhibitionism are rearrested within two years.

People with exhibitionism disorder are at risk for lifetime employment problems if they acquire a police record. The Americans with Disabilities Act (ADA), enacted by Congress in 1990 to protect workers against discrimination on grounds of mental impairment or physical disability, does not protect persons with paraphilias. People with exhibitionism disorder were specifically excluded by Congress from the provisions of the ADA, along with voyeurs and persons with other sexual behavior disorders.

Prevention

One important preventive strategy includes the funding of programs for the treatment of paraphilias in adolescents. According to one expert in the field, males in this age group have not been studied and are undertreated, yet it is known that paraphilias are usually established before age 18. Recognition of paraphilias in adolescents and treatment for those at risk would lower the risk of recidivism. A second important preventive approach is early recognition and appropriate treatment of people who have committed **child abuse**.

Resources

BOOKS

American Psychiatric Association. *Diagnostic and Statistical Manual of Mental Disorders*. 4th ed., text rev. Washington, DC: American Psychiatric Publishing, 2000.

Carnes, Patrick. *Out of the Shadows: Understanding Sexual Addiction*. 3rd ed. Center City, MN: Hazelden Publishing, 2001.

"Exhibitionism." In *The Merck Manual of Diagnosis and Therapy*, edited by Robert S. Porter and Justin L. Kaplan. 19th ed. Whitehouse Station, NJ: Merck Research Laboratories, 2011.

Kasl, Charlotte D. *Women, Sex, and Addiction*. New York: Harper and Row, 1990.

PERIODICALS

Abouesh, A., and A. Clayton. "Compulsive Voyeurism and Exhibitionism: A Clinical Response to Paroxetine." *Archives of Sexual Behavior* 28, no. 1 (February 1999): 23–30.

Bradford, John M.W. "The Treatment of Sexual Deviation Using a Pharmacological Approach." *The Journal of Sex Research* 37 (August 1, 2000): 485–92.

Carnes, P., and J.P. Schneider. "Recognition and Management of Addictive Sexual Disorders: Guide for the Primary Care Clinician." *Lippincotts Primary Care Practitioner* 4, no. 3 (May–June 2000): 302–18.

de Silva, W. P. "Sexual Variations." *British Medical Journal* 318 (March 6, 1999): 654. Available online at http://www.bmj.com/content/318/7184/654.full (accessed November 9, 2011).

Kafka, Martin P., and J. Hennen. "Psychostimulant Augmentation During Treatment with Selective Serotonin Reuptake Inhibitors in Men with Paraphilias and Paraphilia-Related Disorders: A Case Series." *Journal of Clinical Psychiatry* 61, no. 9 (September 2000): 664–70.

Langstrom, Niklas, and Michael C. Seto. Exhibitionistic and Voyeuristic Behavior in a Swedish National Population Survey." *Archives of Sexual Behavior* 35, no. 4 (2006): 427–35.

Lee, J.K., et al. "Developmental Risk Factors for Sexual Offending." *Child Abuse and Neglect: The International Journal* 26, no. 1 (January 2002): 73–92.

Marazziti, Donatella, and Bernardo Dell. 'Osso. "Topiramate Plus Citalopram in the Treatment of Compulsive-Impulsive Sexual Behaviors." *Clinical Practice in Epidemiology in Mental Health* 2 (May 2006): 9. Available online at http://www.cpementalhealth.com/content/2/1/9 (accessed November 9, 2011).

Schiffer, Boris, et al. "Structural Brain Abnormalities in the Frontostriatal System and Cerebellum in Pedophilia." *Journal of Psychiatric Research* 41, no. 9 (2007) 753–62.

Schober, Justine M., Peter M. Byrne, and Phyllis J. Kuhn. "Leuprolide Acetate is a Familiar Drug that May Modify Sex-Offender Behavior: The Urologist's Role." *BJU International* 97, no. 4 (April 2006) 684–86.

Simpson, G., A. Blaszczynski, and A. Hodgkinson. "Sex Offending as a Psychosocial Sequela of Traumatic Brain Injury." *Journal of Head Trauma and Rehabilitation* 14, no. 6 (December 1999): 567–80.

Sonnenberg, Stephen P. "Mental Disabilities in the Workplace." *Workforce* 79 (June 2000): 632. Available online at http://findarticles.com/p/articles/mi_m0FXS/is_6_79/ai_63256161 (accessed November 9, 2011).

WEBSITES

Miller, John L. "Paraphilias." @athealth.com. December 30, 2010. Available online at http://www.athealth.com/Consumer/disorders/Paraphilias.html (accessed October 6, 2011).

ORGANIZATIONS

Augustine Fellowship, Sex and Love Addicts Anonymous, PO Box 119, New Town Branch, Boston, MA, 02258, (617) 332-1845.

National Association on Sexual Addiction Problems, 22937 Arlington Ave., Ste. 201, Torrance, CA, 90501, (213) 546-3103.

Rebecca Frey, PhD
Emily Jane Willingham, PhD

Exposure treatment

Definition

Exposure treatment is a technique that is widely used in **cognitive-behavioral therapy** (CBT) to help patients systematically confront a feared stimulus in a live or virtual environment or in the imagination. Through repeated exposure to the stimulus, patients are helped to nullify fears and increase self-efficacy. Exposure treatment is also called exposure therapy.

Purpose

Exposure treatment is used for a variety of **anxiety disorders**, and it has also recently been extended to the treatment of substance-related disorders. Generally, exposure treatment involves presenting patients with anxiety-producing stimulus for a long enough time to decrease the intensity of their emotional reactions. As a result, the feared situation or object no longer makes the patients anxious. Exposure treatment can be carried out in real situations, which is called in vivo exposure, or it can be done through imagination, which is called imaginal exposure. More recently, exposure treatment has been extended to include the use of computer-based virtual environments.

The category of imaginal exposure includes **systematic desensitization**, in which patients imagine certain aspects of the feared object or situation combined with relaxation. Graded or graduated exposure refers to exposing the patients to the feared situation in a gradual manner. Flooding refers to exposing patients to the anxiety-provoking or feared situation all at once and keeping them in it until the anxiety and fear subside. There are several variations in the delivery of exposure treatment: patient-directed exposure instructions or self-exposure; therapist-assisted exposure; group exposure; and exposure with response prevention.

The basic purpose of exposure treatment is to decrease a person's anxious and fearful reactions (emotions, thoughts, or physical sensations) through repeated exposures to anxiety-producing material. This reduction of the patient's anxiety response is known as habituation. A related purpose of exposure treatment is to eliminate the anxious or fearful response altogether so that patients can face the feared situation repeatedly without experiencing anxiety or fear. This elimination of the anxiety response is known as extinction.

Description

Exposure treatment usually begins with making lists or hierarchies of situations that make the patients anxious or fearful. The situations are ranked on a scale of zero (representing the situation producing the least anxiety) to ten (representing the situation of highest anxiety). In addition, patients are usually asked to rate their level of anxiety in each situation on a scale from zero (no anxiety or discomfort) to 100 (extreme anxiety and discomfort). This scale is called the subjective units of distress scale (SUDS). Patients may be asked to provide SUDS ratings at regular intervals (for example every five minutes) during exposure treatment.

Methods of delivering exposure treatment

PATIENT-DIRECTED EXPOSURE. Patient-directed exposure is the simplest variation of exposure treatment. After patients make their hierarchy lists with their therapist, they are instructed to move through the situations on the hierarchy at their own rates. Patients start with the lowest anxiety situation on the list, and keep a journal of their experiences. They continue the patient-directed exposure on a daily basis until their fears and anxieties have decreased. For example, if patients are afraid of leaving the house, the first item on the hierarchy might be to stand outside the front door for a certain period of time. After they are able to perform this action without feeling anxious, they would move to the next item on the hierarchy, which might be walking to the end of the driveway. Treatment would proceed in this way until the patients have completed all the items on the hierarchy. During therapy sessions, the therapist reviews their journal, gives them positive feedback for any progress that they have made, and discusses any obstacles that they encountered during exposures to the feared situation.

THERAPIST-ASSISTED EXPOSURE. In this form of exposure treatment, therapists go with patients to the feared location or situation and provides on-the-spot coaching to help them manage their anxieties. Therapists may challenge their patients to experience the maximum amount of anxiety. In prolonged in vivo exposure, therapists and patients stay in the situation as long as it takes for the anxiety to decrease. For example, they might remain in a crowded shopping mall for four or more hours. The therapists also explore the thoughts of patients during this exposure to confront any irrational ways of thinking.

GROUP EXPOSURE. In group exposure, self-exposure and practice are combined with group education and discussion of experiences during exposure to feared situations. These sessions may last as long as three hours and include 30 minutes of education, time for individual exposure practice, and 45 minutes of discussion. Group sessions may be scheduled on a daily basis for 10–14 days.

Exposure treatment for specific anxiety disorders

AGORAPHOBIA. Many research studies have shown that graded exposure treatment is effective for **agoraphobia**. Long-term studies have shown that improvement can be maintained for as long as seven years. Exposure treatment for agoraphobia is best conducted in vivo, in the actual feared situation, such as entering a packed subway car. Exposure treatment for agoraphobia is likely to be more effective when the patient's spouse or friend is involved, perhaps because of the support a companion can offer the patient during practice sessions.

PANIC DISORDER. Exposure treatment is the central component of cognitive-behavioral treatment for **panic disorder**. Treatment for this disorder involves identifying patients' specific fears within their experiences of panic, such as fears of being sick, of losing control, and of embarrassment. Once these fears are identified, patients are instructed to expose themselves to situations in which the fearful thoughts arise (such as walking away from a safe person or place). The rationale behind this instruction is that enduring the anxiety associated with the situation will accustom patients to the situation itself, so that over time the anxiety will diminish or disappear. In this way, patients discover that the feared consequences do not happen in real life.

In some patients, physical symptoms of panic lead to fears about the experience of panic itself. Fears related to the physical symptoms associated with panic can be targeted for treatment by inducing the bodily sensations that mimic those experienced during panic attacks. This technique is called interoceptive exposure. Patients are asked to induce the feared sensations in a number of ways. For example, patients may spin in a revolving chair to induce dizziness or run up the stairs to induce increased heart rate and shortness of breath. They are then instructed to notice what the symptoms feel like, and allow them to remain without doing anything to control them. With repeated exposure, patients learn that the bodily sensations do not signal harm or danger, and need not be feared. Patients are taught such strategies as muscle relaxation and slow breathing to control anxiety before, during, and after the exposure.

Interoceptive exposure treatment for panic usually begins with practice sessions in a therapist's office. Patients may be instructed to practice at home and then practice in a less "safe" environment, such as their work setting or a nearby park. The next step is the addition of the physical activities that naturally produce the feared symptoms. Situational or in vivo exposure would then be introduced for patients with agoraphobia combined with panic disorder. Patients would be instructed to go back into situations that they have been avoiding, such as elevators or busy railroad terminals. If patients develop symptoms of anxiety, they are instructed to use the techniques for controlling anxiety that were previously learned.

The effectiveness of exposure treatment for decreasing panic attacks and avoidance has been well demonstrated. In research studies, 50–90% of patients experience relief from symptoms.

SPECIFIC PHOBIA AND SOCIAL PHOBIA. Graded exposure is used most often to treat specific or simple phobias. In graded exposure, patients approach the feared object or situation by degrees. For example, those afraid of swimming in the ocean might begin by looking at photographs of the ocean, then watching movies of people swimming, then going to the beach and walking along the water's edge, and then working up to a full swim in the ocean. Graded exposure can be done through patient-directed instruction or therapist-assisted exposure. Research studies indicate that most patients respond quickly to graded exposure treatment, and that the benefits of treatment are well maintained.

Treatment for **social phobia** usually combines exposure treatment with cognitive restructuring. This combination seems to help prevent a recurrence of symptoms. In general, studies of exposure treatment for social phobia have shown that it leads to a reduction of symptoms. Since cognitive restructuring is usually combined with exposure, it is unclear which component is responsible for patients' improvement, but there is some indication that exposure alone may be sufficient.

Exposure treatment can be more difficult to arrange for treating social phobia, however, because patients have less control over social situations, which are unpredictable by their nature and can unexpectedly become more intense and anxiety-provoking. Furthermore, social exchanges usually last only a short time; therefore, they may not provide the length of exposure that patients need.

OBSESSIVE-COMPULSIVE DISORDER. The most common nonmedication treatment for **obsessive-compulsive disorder** (OCD) is exposure to the feared or anxiety-producing situation plus response prevention (preventing the patient from performing a compulsive behavior, such as hand washing after exposure to something thought to be contaminated). This form of treatment also uses a hierarchy, and begins with the easiest situation and gradually moves to more difficult situations. Research has shown that exposure to contamination situations leads to a decrease in fears of contamination, but does not lead to changes in the compulsive behavior. In a similar fashion, the response prevention component leads to a decrease in compulsive behavior, but does not affect the patient's fears of contamination. Since each form of treatment affects different OCD symptoms, a combination of exposure and response prevention is more effective than either modality by itself. Exposure combined with response prevention also appears to be effective for treating children and adolescents with OCD.

Prolonged continuous exposure is better than short, interrupted periods of exposure in treating people with OCD. On average, exposure treatment of people with OCD requires 90-minute sessions, although the frequency of sessions varies. Some studies have shown good results with 15 daily treatments spread over a period of three weeks. This intensive treatment format may be best suited for cases that are more severe and complex, as in patients with **depression** as well as OCD. Patients who are less severely affected and are highly motivated may benefit from sessions once or twice a week. Treatment may include both therapist-assisted exposure and self-exposure as homework between sessions. Imaginal exposure may be useful for addressing fears that are hard to incorporate into in vivo exposure, such as fears of a loved one's death. Patients usually prefer gradual exposure to the most distressing situations in their hierarchy; however, gradual exposure does not appear to be more effective than flooding or immediate exposure to the situation.

POST-TRAUMATIC STRESS DISORDER. Exposure treatment has been used successfully in the therapy of **post-traumatic stress disorder** (PTSD) resulting from such traumatic experiences as combat, sexual assault, and motor vehicle accidents. Research studies have reported encouraging results for exposure treatment in reducing PTSD or PTSD symptoms in children, adolescents, and adults. Intrusive symptoms of PTSD, such as nightmares and flashbacks, may be reduced by having patients relive the emotional aspects of the **trauma** in a safe, therapeutic environment. It may take 10–15 exposure sessions to decrease the negative physical sensations associated with PTSD. These sessions may range from one to two hours in length and may occur once or twice a week. Relaxation techniques are usually included before and after exposure. The exposure may be therapist-assisted or patient-directed.

A recent study showed that imaginal exposure and cognitive treatment are equally effective in reducing symptoms associated with chronic or severe PTSD, but that neither brought about complete improvement. In addition, more patients treated with exposure worsened over the course of treatment than patients treated with cognitive approaches. This finding may have been related to the fact that the patients receiving exposure treatment had less frequent sessions with long periods of time between sessions. Some patients diagnosed with PTSD, however, do not seem to benefit from exposure therapy. They may have difficulty tolerating exposure, or have difficulty imagining, visualizing, or describing their traumatic experiences. The use of cognitive therapy to help the patient focus on thoughts may be a useful adjunctive treatment, or serve as an alternative to exposure treatment.

Many people who have experienced sexual assault or rape meet the criteria for PTSD defined in the ***Diagnostic and Statistical Manual of Mental Disorders***, fourth edition, text revision (*DSM-IV-TR*). They may reexperience the traumatic event, avoid items or places associated with the trauma, and have increased levels of physical arousal. Exposure treatment in these cases involves using either imaginal or in vivo exposure to reduce anxiety and any tendencies to avoid aspects of the situation that produce anxiety (also known as avoidance behavior). Verbal description of the event (imaginal exposure) is critical for recovery, although it usually feels painful and threatening to patients. It is important that the patients' verbal descriptions of the traumatic events, along with their expressions of thoughts and feelings related to it, occur as early in the treatment process as possible, to minimize long-term suffering.

Prolonged exposure is the most effective nonmedical treatment for reducing traumatic memories related to PTSD. It combines flooding with systematic desensitization. The goal is to expose patients using both imaginal and in vivo exposure techniques in order to reduce avoidance behaviors and fears. Prolonged exposure may occur over nine to 12 90-minute sessions. During the imaginal exposure phase of treatment, patients are asked to describe the details of the traumatic experiences repeatedly, in the present tense. Patients use the SUDS scale to monitor levels of fear and anxiety. The in vivo component occurs outside a therapist's office; this component involves having clients expose themselves to cues in the environment that they have been avoiding—for example, the place where the motor vehicle accident or rape occurred. Patients are instructed to stay in the fear-producing situation for at least 45 minutes, or until their anxiety levels have gone down significantly on the SUDS rating scale. Often patients will use a coach or someone who will stay with them at the beginning of in vivo practice. The coach's role gradually decreases over time as the patients experience less anxiety.

Recent innovations in exposure treatment

VIRTUAL REALITY EXPOSURE TREATMENT. Virtual reality is a technique that allows people to participate actively in a computer-generated (or virtual) scenario or environment. The participants have a sense of being present in the virtual environment. Virtual reality uses a device mounted on the participant's head that shows computer graphics and visual displays in real time, and tracks the person's body movements. Some forms of virtual reality also allow participants to hold a second device in their hands that enables them to interact more fully with the virtual environment, such as opening a car door.

Virtual reality has been proposed as a new way of conducting exposure therapy because it can provide a sense of being present in a feared situation. Virtual reality exposure may be useful for treating such phobias as fear of heights, flying, or driving, as well as for treating PTSD. This method appears to have several advantages over standard exposure therapy. First, virtual reality may offer patients a greater sense of control because they can instantly turn the device on and off or change its level of intensity. Second, virtual reality protects patients from harm or social embarrassment during their practice sessions. Third, it can be implemented regardless of the patient's ability to imagine or to remain with prolonged imaginal exposure. These proposed advantages of virtual reality over standard exposure therapy have yet to be tested, however.

Some studies have been conducted using virtual reality in the treatment of patients with fear of heights and fear of flying, and in a sample of Vietnam veterans diagnosed with PTSD. These studies of virtual reality exposure therapy have limitations in terms of study design and small sample size, but their positive results suggest that virtual reality exposure therapy deserves further investigation.

CUE EXPOSURE TREATMENT FOR ALCOHOL DEPENDENCE. Cue exposure is a relatively new approach to treating substance-related disorders. It is designed to re-create real-life situations in safe therapeutic environments that expose patients repeatedly to alcohol-related cues, such as the sight or smell of alcohol. It is thought that this repeated exposure to cues, plus prevention of the usual response (drinking alcohol) will reduce and possibly eliminate urges experienced in reaction to the cues.

People diagnosed with alcohol dependence face a number of alcohol-related cues in their environments, including moods associated with previous drinking patterns; people, places, times, and objects associated with the pleasurable effects of alcohol; and the sight or smell of alcoholic beverages. Exposure to these cues increases the patient's risk of **relapse**, because the cues can interfere with a person's use of coping skills to resist the urge to drink. The purpose of cue exposure is to teach patients coping skills for responding to these urges. It is thought that people who practice coping skills in the presence of cues will find the coping skills strengthened, along with the conviction that they can respond effectively when confronted by similar cues in real-life situations.

There are various approaches to cue exposure. The choice of cues is usually based on treatment philosophy and goals, which may require abstinence from alcohol or permit moderate drinking. In abstinence-only programs, patients may be exposed to actual alcohol cues and/or imagined high-risk situations. This imaginal exposure is useful for dealing with cues and circumstances that cannot be reproduced in treatment settings, such as fights. Patients learn and practice urge-specific coping skills. While patients may learn to cope successfully with one cue (e.g., the smell of alcohol), the urge to drink may reappear in response to another cue, such as seeing a friend with whom they used to go to bars. Patients would then learn how to manage this particular cue. This program may take six to eight individual or group sessions and may occur on an inpatient or outpatient basis. Often patients remain in the treatment setting for several hours after the exposure to ensure that any lasting urges are safely managed with a therapist's help.

More specifically, cue exposure focuses on the aspect of alcohol consumption that produces the strongest urge. Patients would report each change in their level of urgency, using a scale of zero to 10 that resembles the SUDS scale. The urge to drink usually peaks after one to five minutes. When the desire for a drink arises, patients are instructed to focus on the cue to see what happens to their desire. In most cases the urge subsides within 15 minutes, which is often different from what the patients expected. In later sessions, the patients are instructed when the urge peaks to imagine using the coping skills that they recently learned. Patients may also be instructed to imagine being in high-risk situations and using the coping skills. Some examples of these coping skills include telling oneself that the urge will go away, picturing the negative consequences of drinking alcohol, and thinking of the positive consequences of staying sober.

Although there has been little research on cue exposure, available studies show positive outcomes in terms of decreasing the patients' consumption of alcohol. There have been, however, few outcome studies comparing cue exposure treatment to other treatment approaches. It may be hard to separate the benefits of exposure from the benefits of coping skills training. In any event, cue exposure treatment is a promising approach that deserves further study to determine if either component alone is sufficient or if a combination of the two is more effective.

Precautions

Exposure treatment is generally a safe treatment method; however, some patients may find that the level of anxiety that occurs during treatment sessions is higher than they can handle. Some studies of exposure treatment have reported a high dropout rate, perhaps because the method itself produces anxiety. In addition, exposure treatment is not effective for all patients; after treatment, some continue to experience anxiety symptoms.

Results

Progress in exposure therapy is often slow in the beginning, and occasional setbacks are to be expected. As patients gain experience with various anxiety-producing

KEY TERMS

Cognitive restructuring—An approach to psychotherapy that focuses on helping patients examine distorted patterns of perceiving and thinking in order to change their emotional responses to people and situations.

Cue—Any behavior or event in a person's environment that serves to stimulate a particular response. For example, the smell of liquor may be a cue for some people to pour themselves a drink.

Desensitization—The reduction or elimination of an overly intense reaction to a cue by controlled repeated exposures to the cue.

Extinction—The elimination or removal of a person's reaction to a cue as a result of exposure treatment.

Flooding—A type of exposure treatment in which patients are exposed to anxiety-provoking or feared situations all at once and kept in it until the anxiety and fear subside.

Habituation—The reduction of a person's emotional or behavioral reaction to a cue by repeated or prolonged exposure.

Hierarchy—In exposure therapy, a list of feared items or situations, ranked from least fearsome to most fearsome.

In vivo—A Latin phrase that means "in life." In modeling and exposure therapies, it refers to practicing new behaviors in a real setting, as distinct from using imagery or imagined settings.

Interoceptive—Referring to stimuli or sensations that arise inside the body. In interoceptive exposure treatment, patients are asked to exercise or perform other actions that produce feared internal physical sensations.

Modality—The medical term for a method of treatment.

Subjective units of distress (SUDS) scale—A scale used by patients during exposure treatment to rate their levels of fear and anxiety with numbers from zero to 100.

Virtual reality—A realistic simulation of an environment, produced by a computer system using interactive hardware and software.

situations, their rates of progress may increase. While flooding can produce positive results more quickly than graded exposure, it is rarely used because of the high level of discomfort associated with it.

Resources

BOOKS

American Psychiatric Association. *Practice Guidelines for the Treatment of Psychiatric Disorders: Compendium 2006*. Washington, DC: American Psychiatric Publishing, 2006.

Richard, David C. S., and Dean Lauterbach, eds. *Handbook of Exposure Therapies*. San Diego, CA: Academic Press, 2006.

Rosqvist, Johan. *Exposure Treatments for Anxiety Disorders: A Practioner's Guide to Concepts, Methods, and Evidence-Based Practice*. New York: Routledge, 2005.

VandenBos, Gary R. ed. *APA Dictionary of Psychology*. Washington, DC: American Psychological Association, 2006.

PERIODICALS

Bornas, Xavier, Miquel Tortella-Feliu, and Jordi Llabrés. "Do All Treatments Work for Flight Phobia? Computer-Assisted Exposure Versus a Brief Multicomponent Non-exposure Treatment." *Psychotherapy Research* 16, no. 1 (January 2006): 41–50.

Conklin, Cynthia A. "Environments as Cues to Smoke: Implications for Human Extinction-Based Research and Treatment." *Experimental and Clinical Psychopharmacology* 14, no. 1 (February 2006): 12–9.

Cottraux, Jean. "Recent Developments in Research and Treatment for Social Phobia (Social Anxiety Disorder)." *Current Opinion in Psychiatry* 18, no. 1 (January 2005): 51–54.

Massad, Phillip M., and Timothy L. Hulsey. "Exposure Therapy Renewed." *Journal of Psychotherapy Integration* 16, no. 4 (December 2006): 417–-28.

Thewissen, Roy, et al. "Renewal of Cue-Elicited Urge to Smoke: Implications for Cue Exposure Treatment." *Behaviour Research and Therapy* 44, no. 10 (October 2006): 1441–49.

Vansteenwegen, Debora, et al. "Verbal, Behavioural and Physiological Assessment of the Generalization of Exposure-Based Fear Reduction in a Spider-Anxious Population." *Behaviour Research and Therapy* 45, no. 2 (February 2007): 291–300.

Wilhelm, Frank H., et al. "Mechanisms of Virtual Reality Exposure Therapy: The Role of the Behavioral Activation and Behavioral Inhibition Systems." *Applied Psychophysiology and Biofeedback* 30, no. 3 (September 2005): 271–84.

Joneis Thomas, PhD
Ruth A. Wienclaw, PhD

Expressive language disorder

Definition

Expressive language disorder occurs when an individual has problems expressing himself or herself using spoken language.

Demographics

Expressive language disorder is a relatively common childhood disorder. Language delays occur in 10%–15% of children under age three, and in 3%–7% of school-age children. Expressive language disorder is more common in boys than in girls: studies suggest that developmental expressive language disorder occurs two to five times more often in boys. The developmental form of the disorder is far more common than the acquired type.

Description

Expressive language disorder is generally a childhood disorder. There are two types of expressive language disorder: the developmental type and the acquired type. Developmental expressive language disorder does not have a known cause and generally appears at the time a child is learning to talk. Acquired expressive language disorder is caused by damage to the **brain**. It occurs suddenly after events such as **stroke** or traumatic head injury. The acquired type can occur at any age.

Causes and symptoms

Causes

There is no clearly identified cause of developmental expressive language disorder. Research is ongoing to determine which biological or environmental factors may be the cause. Acquired expressive language disorder is caused by damage to the brain. Damage can be sustained during a stroke, or as the result of traumatic head injury, **seizures**, or other medical conditions. The way in which acquired expressive language disorder manifests itself depends on which parts of the brain are injured and how badly they are damaged.

Symptoms

Expressive language disorder is characterized by a child having difficulty with self-expression using speech. The signs and symptoms vary drastically from child to child. The child does not have problems with the pronunciation of words, as occurs in **phonological disorder**. The child does have problems putting sentences together coherently, using proper grammar, recalling the appropriate word to use, or other similar problems. A child with expressive language disorder cannot communicate thoughts, needs, or wants at the same level or with the same complexity as peers and often has a smaller vocabulary compared to peers.

Children with expressive language disorder have the same ability to understand speech as their peers and have the same level of intelligence. A child with this disorder may understand words but be unable to use the same words in sentences. The child may understand complex spoken sentences and be able to carry out intricate instructions, although unable to form complex sentences.

There are many different ways in which expressive language disorder can manifest itself. Some children do not properly use pronouns, or leave out functional words such as "is" or "the." Other children cannot recall words that they want to use in the sentence and substitute general words such as "thing" or "stuff." Some children cannot organize their sentences so that the sentences are easy to understand. These children do comprehend the material they are trying to express—they just cannot create the appropriate sentences with which to express their thoughts.

Diagnosis

To diagnose expressive language disorder, children must be performing below their peers at tasks that require communication in the form of speech. This can be hard to determine because it must be shown that an individual understands the material but cannot express that comprehension. Nonverbal tests must be used in addition to tests that require spoken answers. Hearing should also be evaluated because children who do not hear well may have problems putting together sentences in a way that is similar to children with expressive language disorder. In children who are mildly hearing-impaired, the problem can often be resolved by using hearing aids to enhance the child's hearing. Also, children who speak a language other than the dominant language of their society (e.g., English in the United States) in the home should be tested in that language if possible. The child's ability to communicate in English may be the problem, not the child's ability to communicate in general.

The ***Diagnostic and Statistical Manual of Mental Disorders***, fourth edition, text revision (*DSM-IV-TR*), states that there are four general criteria for diagnosing expressive language disorder. The first is that the child communicates using speech at a level that is less developed than expected for his or her intelligence and ability to understand spoken language. The problem with communication using speech must create difficulties for the child in everyday life or in achieving goals. The child must understand what is being said at a level that is age-appropriate, or at a developmental level consistent with the child's age. Otherwise the diagnoses should be **mixed receptive-expressive language disorder**. If the child has intellectual disabilities, poor hearing, or other problems, the difficulties with speech must be greater than is generally associated with disabilities of the child.

Treatment

There are two types of treatment used for expressive language disorder. The first involves the child working one-on-one with a speech therapist on a regular schedule and practicing speech and communication skills. The second type of treatment involves the child's parents and teachers working together to incorporate spoken language that the child needs into everyday activities and play. Both of these treatment can be effective and are often used together.

Prognosis

The developmental form of expressive language disorder generally has a good prognosis. Most children develop normal or nearly normal language skills by high school. In some cases, minor problems with expressive language may never resolve. The acquired type of expressive language disorder has a prognosis that depends on the nature and location of the brain injury. Some people get their language skills back over days or months. For others it takes years, and some people never fully recover expressive language function.

Prevention

There is no known way to prevent developmental expressive language disorder. Because acquired language disorder is caused by damage to the brain, anything that would help to prevent brain damage may help to prevent that type of the disorder. This can include things ranging from lowering cholesterol to preventing stroke to wearing a bicycle helmet to prevent **traumatic brain injury**.

Resources

BOOKS

American Psychiatric Association. *Diagnostic and Statistical Manual of Mental Disorders*. 4th ed., text rev. Washington, DC: American Psychiatric Publishing, 2000.

Sadock, Benjamin J., and Virginia A. Sadock, eds. *Comprehensive Textbook of Psychiatry*. Vol. 2. 7th ed. Philadelphia: Lippincott Williams and Wilkins, 2000.

PERIODICALS

Roberts, Joanne E., Richard M. Rosenfeld, and Susan A. Zeisel. "Otitis Media and Speech and Language: A Meta-Analysis of Prospective Studies." *Pediatrics* 113, no. 3 (March 2004): 238–48.

Stein, Martin T., ed. "Expressive Language Delay in a Toddler." *Journal of Developmental & Behavioral Pediatrics* 22, no. 2 (April 2001): S99–S103.

WEBSITES

MedlinePlus. "Language Disorder—Children." U.S. National Library of Medicine, National Institutes of Health. 2006. http://www.nlm.nih.gov/medlineplus/ency/article/001545.htm (accessed October 6, 2011).

ORGANIZATIONS

American Academy of Pediatrics, 141 Northwest Point Blvd., Elk Grove Village, IL, 60007-1098, (847) 434-4000, Fax: (847) 434-8000, http://www.aap.org.

American Psychological Association, 750 1st Street NE, Washington, DC, 20002-4242, (202) 336-5500; TDD/TTY: (202) 336-6123, (800) 374-2721, http://www.apa.org.

American Speech-Language-Hearing Association, 2200 Research Blvd., Rockville, MD, 20785, (301) 296-5700, http://www.asha.org.

Tish Davidson, AM
Emily Jane Willingham, PhD

F

Factitious disorder

Definition

Factitious disorder (FD) is an umbrella category that covers a group of mental disturbances in which patients intentionally act physically or mentally ill without obvious benefits. According to one estimate, the unnecessary tests and waste of other medical resources caused by FD cost the United States $40 million per year. The term factitious comes from a Latin word that means artificial or contrived.

The ***Diagnostic and Statistical Manual of Mental Disorders,*** fourth edition, text revision (*DSM-IV-TR*) distinguishes FD from **malingering**, which is defined as pretending illness when the individual has a clear motive—usually for economic benefit or to avoid legal trouble.

FD is sometimes referred to as hospital **addiction**, pathomimia, or polysurgical addiction. Variant names for individuals with FD include hospital vagrants, hospital hoboes, peregrinating patients, problem patients, and professional patients.

Demographics

The demographics of FD vary considerably across the different subtypes. Most individuals with the predominantly psychological subtype of FD are males with a history of hospitalizations beginning in late adolescence; few of these people, however, are older than 45. For nonchronic FD with predominantly physical symptoms, women outnumber men by a 3:1 ratio. Most of these women are between 20 and 40 years of age. Individuals with Munchausen syndrome are mostly middle-aged males who are unmarried and estranged from their families. Mothers involved in MSBP are usually married, educated, middle-class women in their early 20s.

Little is known about the rates of various sub-categories of FD in different racial or ethnic groups. The prevalence of FD worldwide is not known. In the United States, some experts think that FD is underdiagnosed because hospital personnel often fail to spot the deceptions that are symptomatic of the disorder. In addition, people with this disorder tend to migrate from one medical facility to another, making tracking difficult. It is also not clear which subtypes of FD are most common. Most observers in developed countries agree, however, that the prevalence of factitious physical symptoms is much higher than the prevalence of factitious psychological symptoms. A large teaching hospital in Toronto reported that 10 of 1,288 patients referred to a consultation service had FD (0.8%). The National Institute for Allergy and Infectious Disease reported that 9.3% of patients referred for fevers of unknown origin had FD. A clinic in Australia found that 1.5% of infants brought in for serious illness by parents were cases of Munchausen syndrome by proxy.

Description

Cases of FD are referenced in the medical literature as early as the second century A.D. by Galen, a famous Roman physician. The term factitious is derived from a book by an English physician named Gavin, published in 1843, entitled *On Feigned and Factitious Diseases*. The modern study of FD, however, began with a 1951 article in *Lancet* by a British **psychiatrist**, Richard Asher, who also coined the term Munchausen's syndrome to describe a chronic subtype of FD. The name Munchausen comes from an eighteenth-century German baron whose stories of his military exploits were published with substantial embellishments. In 1977, the first case of FD with primarily psychological symptoms was reported. FD was recognized as a formal diagnostic category by *DSM-III* in 1980.

DSM-IV-TR defines FD as having three major subtypes: FD with predominantly psychological signs and symptoms; FD with predominantly physical signs and symptoms; and FD with combined psychological and physical signs and symptoms. A fourth syndrome, known as Ganser syndrome, has been classified in the past as a form of FD, although *DSM-IV-TR* groups it with the **dissociative disorders**.

DSM-IV-TR specifies three criteria for FD:

- the patient is intentionally producing or pretending to have physical or psychological symptoms or signs of illness
- the patient's motivation is to assume the role of a sick person
- there are no external motives (as in malingering) that explain the behavior

Psychological FD

FD with predominantly psychological signs and symptoms is listed by *DSM-IV-TR* as the first subcategory of the disorder. It is characterized by the individual feigning psychological symptoms.

Some researchers have suggested adding the following criteria for this subtype of FD.

- The symptoms are inconsistent, changing markedly from day to day and from one hospitalization to the next.
- The changes are influenced by the environment (as when the patient feels observed by others) rather than by the treatment.
- The patient's symptoms are unusual or unbelievable.
- The patient has a large number of symptoms that belong to several different psychiatric disorders.

Physical FD

FD with predominantly physical signs and symptoms is the most familiar to medical personnel. Chronic FD of this type is often referred to as Munchausen's syndrome. The most common ways of pretending illness are: presenting a factitious history (claiming to have had a seizure that never happened); combining a factitious history with external agents that mimic the symptoms of disease (adding blood from a finger prick to a urine sample); or combining a factitious history with maneuvers that produce a genuine medical condition (taking a psychoactive drug to produce psychiatric symptoms). In most cases, these patients sign out of the hospital when they are confronted by staff with proof of their pretending, usually in the form of a laboratory report. Many individuals with Munchausen's syndrome move from hospital to hospital, seeking treatment, and thus are known commonly as "hospital hoboes."

FD with mixed symptoms

FD in this category is characterized by a mix of psychological and physical signs and symptoms.

FD not otherwise specified

FD not otherwise specified is a category that *DSM-IV-TR* included to cover a bizarre subtype in which one person fabricates misleading information about another's health or induces actual symptoms of illness in the other person. First described in 1977 by an American pediatrician, this syndrome is known as Munchausen syndrome by proxy (MSBP) and almost always involves a parent (usually the mother) and child. MSBP is now understood as a form of **child abuse** involving premeditation rather than impulsive acting out. Many pediatricians in the United States believe that MSBP is underdiagnosed.

Ganser syndrome

Ganser syndrome is a rare disorder (with about a 100 documented cases worldwide) that has been variously categorized as a FD or a dissociative disorder. It is named for a German psychiatrist named Sigbert Ganser, who first described it in 1898 from an examination of male prisoners who were thought to be psychotic. Ganser syndrome is used to describe dissociative symptoms and the pretending of **psychosis** that occur in forensic settings.

There are four symptoms regarded as diagnostic of Ganser syndrome:

- *Vorbeireden*: A German word that means "talking beside the point," it refers to a type of approximate answer to an examiner's questions that may appear silly but usually indicates that the patient understands the question. If the examiner asks how many legs a dog has, the patient may answer, "five."
- Clouding of consciousness: The patient is drowsy or inattentive.
- Conversion symptoms: These are physical symptoms produced by unconscious psychological issues rather than diagnosable medical causes. A common conversion symptom is temporary paralysis of an arm or leg.
- Hallucinations.

Virtual FD

Although virtual FD does not appear as a heading in any present diagnostic manual, it is a phenomenon that has appeared with increasing frequency with the rise of Internet usage. The growing use of the personal computer has affected presentations of FD in two important ways. First, computers allow people with sufficient technical skills to access medical records from hospital databases and to cut and paste changes into their own records to falsify their medical histories. Second, computers allow people to enter Internet chat rooms for people with serious illnesses and pretend to be patients with that illness to obtain attention and sympathy. "Munchausen by Internet" can have devastating effects on chat groups, destroying trust when the hoax is exposed.

Causes and symptoms

Causes

The causes of FD, whether physical or psychiatric, are difficult to determine because these patients are often lost to follow-up when they sign out of the hospital. **Magnetic resonance imaging** (MRI) has detected abnormalities in the **brain** structure of some patients with chronic FD, suggesting that there may be biological or **genetic factors** associated with the disorder. Positron-emission tomography (**PET**) scans of patients diagnosed with Ganser syndrome have also revealed brain abnormalities. The results of EEG (**electroencephalography**) studies of these patients are nonspecific.

Several different psychodynamic explanations have been proposed for FD. These include:

- Patients with FD are trying to reenact unresolved childhood issues with parents.
- They have underlying problems with masochism.
- They need to be the center of attention and feel important.
- They need to receive care and nurturance.
- They are bothered by feelings of vulnerability.
- Deceiving a physician allows them to feel superior to an authority figure.

There are several known risk factors for FD, including:

- the presence of other mental or physical disorders in childhood that resulted in considerable medical attention
- a history of significant past relationships with doctors, or of grudges against them
- present diagnosis of borderline, narcissistic, or antisocial personality disorder

Symptoms

SYMPTOMS OF FACTITIOUS DISORDER IN ADULTS OR ADOLESCENTS. Reasons for suspecting FD include:

- The individual's history is vague and inconsistent, or the individual has a long medical record with many admissions at different hospitals in different cities.
- The patient has an unusual knowledge of medical terminology or describes the illness as if reciting a textbook description of it.
- The patient is employed in a medical or hospital-related occupation.
- *Pseudologia fantastica,* a Latin phrase for "uncontrollable lying," is a condition in which the individual provides fantastic descriptions of events that never took place.
- The patient visits emergency rooms at times such as holidays or late Friday afternoons when experienced staff are not usually present and obtaining old medical records is difficult.
- The patient has few visitors even though claiming to be an important person.
- The patient is unusually accepting of surgery or uncomfortable diagnostic procedures.
- The patient's behavior is controlling, attention-seeking, hostile, or disruptive.
- Symptoms are present only when the patient is being watched.
- The patient is abusing substances, particularly prescription painkillers or tranquilizers.
- The course of the "illness" fluctuates, or complications develop with unusual speed.
- The patient has multiple surgical scars, a so-called "gridiron abdomen," or evidence of self-inflicted wounds or injuries.

SYMPTOMS OF MUNCHAUSEN SYNDROME BY PROXY. Factors that suggest a **diagnosis** of MSBP include:

- The patient is a young child; the average age of patients with MSBP is 40 months.
- There is a history of long hospitalizations and frequent emergency room visits.
- Siblings have histories of MSBP, failure to thrive, or death in early childhood from an unexplained illness.
- The mother is employed in a health care profession.
- The mother has been diagnosed with depression or histrionic or borderline personality disorder.
- There is significant dysfunction in the family.

Diagnosis

Diagnosis of FD is usually based on a combination of laboratory findings and the gradual exclusion of other possible diagnoses. In the case of MSBP, the **abuse** is often discovered through covert video surveillance.

The most important differential diagnoses, when FD is suspected, are malingering, **conversion disorder**, or another genuine psychiatric disorder.

Treatment

Medications

Medications have not proved helpful in treating FD by itself, although they may be prescribed for symptoms of anxiety or **depression** if the individual also meets criteria for an anxiety or mood disorder.

Psychotherapy

Knowledge of the comparative effectiveness of different psychotherapeutic approaches is limited by the fact that few people diagnosed with FD remain in long-term treatment. In many cases, however, the factitious disorder improves or resolves if the individual receives appropriate therapy for a comorbid psychiatric disorder. Ganser syndrome usually resolves completely with supportive **psychotherapy**.

One approach that has proven helpful in confronting patients with an examiner's suspicions is a supportive manner that focuses on the individual's emotional distress as the source of the illness rather than on the anger or righteous indignation of hospital staff. Although most individuals with FD refuse psychiatric treatment when it is offered, those who accept it appear to benefit most from supportive rather than insight-oriented therapy.

Family therapy is often beneficial in helping family members understand the individual's behavior and need for attention.

KEY TERMS

Conversion disorder—A type of somatoform disorder in which unconscious psychological conflicts or other factors take the form of physical symptoms that are produced unintentionally. Conversion disorder is part of the differential diagnosis of factitious disorder.

Forensic—Pertaining to courtroom procedure or evidence used in courts of law.

Ganser syndrome—A rare subtype of factitious disorder accompanied by dissociative symptoms. It is most often seen in male patients under severe stress in prison or courtroom settings.

Gridiron abdomen—An abdomen with a network of parallel scars from repeated surgical operations.

Malingering—Knowingly pretending to be physically or mentally ill to avoid some unpleasant duty or responsibility, or for economic benefit.

Masochism—A mental disorder in which people obtain sexual satisfaction through pain or humiliation inflicted by themselves or by another person. The term is sometimes used more generally to refer to a tendency to find pleasure in submissiveness or self-denial.

Legal considerations

In dealing with cases of Munchausen syndrome by proxy, physicians and hospital staff should seek appropriate legal advice. Although covert video surveillance of parents suspected of MSBP is highly effective (between 56% and 92%) in exposing the fraud, it may also be considered grounds for a lawsuit by the parents on argument of entrapment. Hospitals can usually satisfy legal concerns by posting signs stating that they use hidden video monitoring.

All 50 states presently require hospital staff and physicians to notify law enforcement authorities when MSBP is suspected, and to take steps to protect the child. Protection usually includes removing the child from the home, but it should also include an evaluation of the child's sibling(s) and long-term monitoring of the family. Criminal prosecution of one or both parents may also be necessary.

Prognosis

The prognosis of FD varies by subcategory. Males diagnosed with the psychological subtype of FD are generally considered to have the worst prognosis. **Self-mutilation** and **suicide** attempts are common in these individuals. The prognosis for Munchausen's syndrome is also poor; the statistics for recurrent episodes and successful suicides range between 30% and 70%. These individuals do not usually respond to psychotherapy. The prognosis for non-chronic FD in women is variable; some of these patients accept treatment and do quite well. This subcategory of FD, however, often resolves itself after the patient turns 40. MSBP involves considerable risks for the child; 9%–10% of these cases end in the child's death.

Ganser syndrome is the one subtype of FD with a good prognosis. Almost all patients recover within days of the diagnosis, especially if the **stress** that precipitated the syndrome is resolved.

Prevention

FD is not sufficiently well understood to allow for effective preventive strategies—apart from protection of child patients and their siblings in cases of MSBP.

Resources

BOOKS

American Psychiatric Association. *Diagnostic and Statistical Manual of Mental Disorders*. 4th ed., text rev. Washington, DC: American Psychiatric Publishing, 2000.

Eisendrath, Stuart J. "Psychiatric Disorders." *Current Medical Diagnosis & Treatment 2011*, edited by Lawrence M. Tierney, Jr., et al. New York: McGraw-Hill, 2010.

"Psychiatry in Medicine." In *The Merck Manual of Diagnosis and Therapy*, edited by Robert S. Porter and Justin L. Kaplan. 19th ed. Whitehouse Station, NJ: Merck Sharp & Dohme Corp., 2011.

PERIODICALS

Andersen, H.S., D. Sestoft, and T. Lillebaek. "Ganser Syndrome After Solitary Confinement in Prison: A Short Review and a Case Report." *Norwegian Journal of Psychiatry* 55, no. 3 (2001): 199–201.

Feldman, Marc D., and Charles V. Ford. "Liejacking." *Journal of the American Medical Association* 271, no. 2 (May 25, 1994): 1574.

Libow, Judith A. "Child and Adolescent Illness Falsification." *Pediatrics* 105, no. 2 (February 1, 2000): 336–342.

McEwen, Donna R., BSN. "Recognizing Munchausen's Syndrome." *AORN Journal* 67, no. 2 (February 1998): 440–42. Available online at http://findarticles.com/p/articles/mi_m0FSL/is_n2_v67/ai_20651296 (accessed November 9, 2011).

Paulk, David. "Munchausen Syndrome by Proxy." *Clinician Reviews* 11 (August 2001): 783–91.

Russo, Francine. "Cybersickness: Muchausen by internet Breeds a Generation of Fakers." *The Village Voice* June 26, 2001. Available online at http://www.villagevoice.com/2001-06-26/news/cybersickness/1 (accessed November 9, 2011).

Snyder, S.L., M.S. Buchsbaum, and R.C. Krishna. "Unusual Visual Symptoms and Ganser-Like State Due to Cerebral Injury: A Case Study Using (18) F-Deoxyglucose Positron Emission Tomography." *Behavioral Neurology* 11, no. 1 (1998): 51–54.

Stern, Theodore A. "Is Your Patient Faking?" *Medical Economics* 81, no. 23 (December 2004) 60–63.

Szoke, Andrei, and Didier Boillet. "Factitious Disorder with Psychological Signs and Symptoms: Case Reports and Proposals for Improving Diagnosis." *Psychiatry On-Line*, 1999. http://www.priory.com/psych/factitious.htm (accessed November 9, 2011).

Worley, Courtney B., Marc D. Feldman, and James C. Hamilton. "The Case of Factitious Disorder Versus Malingering." *Psychiatric Times* 26, no. 11 (October 30, 2009).

WEBSITES

Cleveland Clinic. "An Overview of Factitious Disorders." November 11, 2008. http://my.clevelandclinic.org/disorders/Factitious_Disorders/hic_An_Overview_of_Factitious_Disorders.aspx (accessed October 6, 2011).

Elwyn, Todd S. "Factitious Disorder." Medscape Reference. 2006. http://emedicine.medscape.com/article/291304-overview (accessed October 6, 2011).

ORGANIZATIONS

American Academy of Child and Adolescent Psychiatry, 3615 Wisconsin Ave. NW, Washington, DC, 20016-3007, (202) 966-7300, Fax: (202) 966-2891, http://aacap.org.

Munchausen by Proxy Survivors Network, PO Box 806177, Saint Clair Shores, MI, 48080, http://www.mbpsnetwork.com.

Rebecca Frey, PhD
Emily Jane Willingham, PhD

False belief of pregnancy *see* **Pseudocyesis**

Familial British dementia *see* **Dementia**

Family education

Definition

Family education or "psychoeducation" is the ongoing process of educating family members about a serious mental illness, or psychological disturbance, in order to improve their coping skills and their ability to help a relative affected by the illness. It may also involve helping family members learn more about how to treat such mental illnesses, along with those physical ailments that may also be present. One of the goals of family education is to help family members and patients better understand and deal with the illness so that the best possible situation can be attained, with a minimum risk of relapses.

Purpose

When someone is diagnosed with a chronic illness, such as diabetes or heart disease, efforts are typically made by his or her doctor not only to educate the individual directly affected by the illness, but to educate and involve his/her family in treatment and care. Historically, this has not been the case with severe mental illnesses such as **schizophrenia**, major **depression** and **anxiety disorders**, **bipolar disorder**, **schizoaffective disorder**, eating disorders, or **personality disorders**.

Historically, most mental health professionals did not educate families about what to expect or how to care for their loved one. In fact, for much of the twentieth century it was believed that mental illness was caused by overly strict or overly permissive parenting styles and, consequently, families were often unfairly blamed for causing these disorders. Mothers were labeled schizophrenogenic, and even well-meaning clinicians tried to keep them and other family members at a distance. Gregory Bateson's "double-bind" theory of the time suggested that contradictory messages and communications by parents were the root cause of the problem. Because of these ideas and the **diagnosis**, the only recourse for most families was to go to public libraries to read and learn as much as they could on their own.

Over the last 25 years, however, advances in genetics, neuroscience, and imaging techniques have provided new evidence that severe mental illnesses are neurobiological in origin. With this scientific knowledge has come greater awareness and understanding that these are "no-fault" **brain** illnesses, and that neither families nor patients should be blamed. Rather, they both should receive the necessary information and support to help them better cope with these complex disorders.

Description

In the United States and elsewhere, the large majority of individuals with severe mental illness live with their families and depend on them for housing, financial assistance, advocacy, and support. For this reason, families require knowledge and skills to actively help their relative benefit from treatment, avoid **relapse**, and achieve recovery. Specifically, family caregivers require information about the illness and its symptoms, including:

- how to better communicate with their family member and professionals the pros and cons of different treatment options, medications and their therapeutic uses and their adverse side effects, signs of relapse, availability of community services and supports
- how to access benefits and entitlements
- how to handle crises or bizarre and troubling behaviors

Because living with an individual with a serious mental disorder can be very stressful, family education must also focus on teaching families about the importance of taking care of themselves.

The National Alliance on Mental Illness (NAMI) is an umbrella organization of more than 1,100 local support and advocacy groups in 50 states. The organization comprises families and individuals affected by serious mental illness who come together for family education, mutual support, and advocacy. Through conferences, **support groups**, and newsletters, family members have opportunities to educate one another and exchange experiences. NAMI has also made great inroads in teaching mental health professionals about the importance of educating family members and involving them in plans for the patient's treatment and rehabilitation. On a more formal level, NAMI has sponsored the Family-to-Family Program, a 12-week free education course that has been attended by over 115,000 family members in more than 42 states. Taught by family volunteers, this is the first peer program in family education in the United States.

Family education is slowly becoming an integral part of treatment, as the practice guidelines for professionals have begun to recommend its use. Families are also utilizing a new generation of books about mental illness—some written by professionals, and others written by, and for, family members. Families are also increasingly using the Internet to learn more about mental disorders.

Family education for parents of children and adolescents

Because major mental illnesses tend to occur in adolescence or early adulthood, most family interventions focus on parents of adult children. However, any parent of a younger child with an emotional or behavioral disturbance can testify to the extraordinary challenges involved in coordinating care. For this reason, more public and private agencies are beginning to provide training, information, education, and financial assistance to family members of children and adolescents with emotional disturbances. The results of research about family education interventions for parents of children

KEY TERMS

Bipolar disorder—A type of mood disorder characterized by one or more episodes of abnormally high energy levels that may or not be accompanied by depression.

Depression—A psychiatric disorder involving feelings of hopelessness and symptoms of fatigue, sleeplessness, suicidal tendencies, and poor concentration.

Eating disorders—A number of medical conditions characterized by abnormal eating habits that can involve either the lack, or the excessive intake, of food and results in physical and/or emotional stress. Two types of eating disorders include anorexia nervosa and bulimia nervosa.

Mental disorder—A psychiatric disorder of mental faculties.

Schizophrenia—A mental disorder involving degraded thinking and emotions.

QUESTIONS TO ASK YOUR DOCTOR

- Will family education help me and my family?
- What should I do if family education does not solve our problems?
- Is there a local organization that can help? A national one?
- Do you recommend any professionals that can help?
- Will my health insurance pay for any of the expenses?
- Do you recommend any books to read? Can I find information on the Internet?

with serious emotional disturbances are just beginning to emerge. Some research suggests that family participation improves service delivery and patient outcomes for this group. In a randomized controlled trial of the training of 200 parents who did or did not receive training, while there were no significant effects on child's mental health status, those family members who were trained showed significant knowledge enhancement and increased effectiveness.

Preparation

To prepare for family education in response to a mental health problem of someone in the family, the first step may be to talk with the family doctor or another trusted health care professional. Many local and national organizations, such as the National Alliance on Mental Illness, the National Family Caregivers Association, the **National Institute of Mental Health**, and Mental Health America, can be of service.

Aftercare

Family education is a process that, once implemented, is continued on a regular basis to provide the best health results for the patient and the best outcome for the caregiver.

Risks

Even with the implementation of family education, the risk of mental relapses is still present. However, with better education, both caregiver and patient should be better equipped to deal with such problems.

Results

Recent research has provided evidence that family education and support leads to improved patient outcomes. For example, **family psychoeducation** provided by mental health professionals has such a compelling research base that it is considered a practice based on the findings of real-life studies of family education and support.

Another type of therapy discussed in the scientific literature has been used in China and India. The family consultation model uses individualized, private consultations between the family and a trained consultant to assist the family on an as-needed basis.

Resources

BOOKS

Lefley, Harriet P. *Family Psychoeducation for Serious Mental Illness*. New York: Oxford University Press, 2009.

Torrey, E. Fuller. *Surviving Schizophrenia: A Manual for Families, Consumers and Providers*. New York: Collins, 2006.

Substance Abuse and Mental Health Services Administration, Center for Mental Health Services. *Family Psychoeducation*. Rockville, MD: U.S. Department of Health and Human Services, 2009.

Walsh, Joseph. *Psychoeducation in Mental Health*. Chicago: Lyceum, 2010.

PERIODICALS

Archie, Suzanne, et.al. "Psychotic Disorders Clinic and First-Episode Psychosis: A Program Evaluation." *Canadian Journal of Psychiatry* 50.1 (January 2005): 46–51.

Dunbar, Sandra B., et.al. "Family Education and Support Interventions in Heart Failure. A Pilot Study." *Nursing Research* 54.3 (May–June 2005): 158–66.

Edelman, Perry, Daniel Kuhn, Bradley R. Fulton, and Gregory A. Kyrouac. "Information and Service Needs of Persons With Alzheimer's Disease and Their Family Caregivers Living in Rural Communities." *American Journal of Alzheimer's Disease and Other Dementias* 21.4 (August–September 2006): 226–33.

Murray-Swank, Aaron B., Alicia Lucksted, Deborah R. Medoff, Ye Yang, Karen Wohlheiter, and Lisa B. Dixon. "Religiosity, Psychosocial Adjustment, and Subjective Burden of Persons Who Care for Those With Mental Illness." *Psychiatric Services* 57.3 (March 2006): 361–65.

WEBSITES

"Basic Facts on Family Psychoeducation." National Alliance of Mental Illness. (August 2003). http://www.nami.org/Template.cfm?Section=About_Treatments_and_Supports&template=/ContentManagement/ContentDisplay.cfm&ContentID=9546 (accessed December 3, 2010).

"Mental Health: A Report of the Surgeon General." U.S. Department of Health and Human Services. http://www.surgeongeneral.gov/library/mentalhealth/home.html (accessed December 3, 2010).

"Schizophrenia." National Institute of Mental Health. (November 29, 2010). http://www.nimh.nih.gov/health/topics/schizophrenia/index.shtml (accessed December 3, 2010).

ORGANIZATIONS

Mental Health America, 2000 N. Beauregard St., 6th Fl., Alexandria, VA, 22311, (703) 684-7722, (800) 969-6642, Fax: (703) 684-5968, http://www1.nmha.org.

National Alliance on Mental Illness, 3803 N Fairfax Dr., Ste. 100, Arlington, VA, 22203, (703) 524-7600, http://www.nami.org.

National Family Caregivers Association, 10400 Connecticut Ave., Ste. 500, Kensington, MD, 20895-3944, (301) 942-6430, (800) 896-3650, Fax: (301) 942-2302, info@thefamilycaregiver.org, http://www.nfcacares.org.

National Institute of Mental Health, 6001 Executive Blvd., Rm. 8184, MSC 9663, Bethesda, MD, 20892-9663, (301) 433-4513; TTY: (301) 443-8431, Fax: (301) 443-4279, (866) 615-6464; TTY: (866) 415-8051, nimhinfo@nih.gov, http://www.nimh.nih.gov.

Irene S. Levine, PhD
Ruth A. Wienclaw, PhD

Family psychoeducation

Definition

Psychoeducation is an educational approach used to help people with severe psychological problems learn to cope with their problems. When family members are included in this education, it is called family psychoeducation. Thus, family psychoeducation is a method for training families under the direction of mental health professionals, so that family members with psychiatric disorders can recover and maintain psychological health. Family psychoeducation has been shown to improve patient outcomes for people with **schizophrenia**, bipolar disorders, **personality disorders**, **depression**, **anxiety disorders**, eating disorders (such as **anorexia nervosa**), and other major mental illnesses.

Purpose

The goal of family psychoeducation is to prevent patients with severe mental illnesses from relapsing, and to promote their re-entry into their home communities, with particular regard for their social and occupational functioning. To achieve this goal, family psychoeducation programs seek to provide families with the information they need about mental illness and give them the coping skills to deal with their family members' psychiatric disorders.

One associated goal of family psychoeducation is to provide support for the patients' families. Families experience many burdens (financial, social, and psychological) in serving as long-term caregivers for their loved ones. Although the primary focus of family psychoeducation groups is improved patient outcomes, one essential intermediate goal is to promote the well-being of the family.

Description

There are several different models of family psychoeducation. Although they include many common elements, these different models are: single- and multiple-family groups; mixed groups that include family members and consumers (patients); groups of varying duration ranging from nine months to more than five years; and groups that focus on patients and families at different phases in the illness. Family psychoeducation programs have been studied extensively and refined by a number of researchers, including Drs. Ian Falloon, Gerald Hogarty, William McFarlane, and Lisa Dixon. For example, the late Dr. Falloon was one of the first psychiatrists to suggest that families should be involved in the treatment of schizophrenia.

The evidence suggests that multiple-family groups, which bring together several patients and their families, lead to better outcomes than single-family psychoeducation groups. The origins of multiple-family **group therapy** go back as far as 1960, when these groups were first assembled to solve ward-management problems in a psychiatric hospital. Lasting a minimum of nine months, the programs provided their participants with information about mental illness, its symptoms and treatment; medication and its side effects; how to communicate with a person with mental illness; and techniques for **crisis intervention** and mutual problem solving.

Dr. Dixon, who is a professor of psychology at the University of Maryland, recently outlined the characteristics of successful family psychoeducation programs.

- The programs consider schizophrenia an illness like any other.
- They are led by mental health professionals.
- They are part of a total treatment plan that includes medication.
- Families are treated as partners rather than patients.
- The programs focus primarily on patient outcomes, and secondarily on family outcomes.
- The programs differ from traditional family therapy in that they do not treat families as part of the problem; they see them as part of the solution.

It is also important that **family education** programs take into account the phase of the patient's illness, the life cycle of both the patient and the family, and the family's cultural context.

Family-to-Family program

The National Alliance on Mental Illness coordinates the Family-to-Family (FTF) Education Program. It is a 12-week course free that is to family caregivers of individuals with severe mental illness. The highly structured, standardized classes are offered in hundreds of communities in the United States, along with several places in Canada, Puerto Rico, and Mexico. Over the years, over 115,000 family members have attended the course. They learn from volunteers who are trained family counselors and, specifically, people who have previously provided (or are currently providing) care to mentally ill family members or loved ones. These instructors provide course materials and instruction to all participants. Some of the topics included within the course include:

- schizophrenia
- major depression
- bipolar disorder (manic depression)
- panic disorder
- obsessive-compulsive disorder
- borderline personality disorder
- brain disorders
- addictive disorders.

Side effects, effective treatment plans, medication strategies, research into **brain** disorders, dealing with mental illness (including problem solving, listening techniques, and communication techniques) are some of the subjects taught during the course. Special attention is given to the emotions and problems that caregivers deal with while caring for mentally ill individuals. The instructors also provide information on advocacy initiatives and local support services. At the end of the course, participants who succeed in all aspects of the course are certified as graduates of the Family-to-Family Education Program.

In 2005, Dixon and colleagues at the University of Maryland were provided a four-year National Alliance on Mental Illness (NAMI) grant to study the effectiveness of the Family-to-Family Education Program. Although ample research has shown that families provide major benefits to adults with serious mental illnesses, little is known about the educational programs and **support groups** that help these family members care for mentally ill relatives. Consequently, Dixon headed a $2.2 million study to determine whether the NAMI Family-to-Family Education Program is effective at providing information and guidance so family members can properly care for mentally ill relatives or loved ones.

Dr. Dixon, the principal investigator on the study, comments on how important it is to provide effective care to mentally ill people and to make sure that caregivers to such people can do the best job possible. Dixon posits that the stresses of mental illness on a family and/or loved one can be so extreme that they put the relationship at risk. As a result of a compromised relationship due to all the difficulties including disrupted family roles and financial strain, the patient's well-being is disrupted.

The study used the Family to Family Education Program that was in operation in five Maryland counties. In all, 318 participants were involved in the study, with about half of them randomly assigned either to immediately enroll in the class or to wait at least three months before another class became available (the control group). All participants (whether they took the class or not) were evaluated (interviewed) before the class started and after it was completed three months later with respect to such topics as (1) problem-focused coping, (2) emotion-focused coping, (3) subjective illness burden, and (4) distress. In other words, the control group had not taken the class at the time of both interviews, but its members were to take the class after the study was completed. The researchers were particularly interested in what benefits accrued from the class that were able to help caregivers provide better care to their mentally ill patients.

The results of the study were published in the journal *Psychiatric Services* under the title "Outcomes of a Randomized Study of a Peer-Taught Family-to-Family Education Program for Mental Illness." The June 2011 article, headed by Dixon, stated that FTF participants had "significantly greater improvement" than the control group in problem-focused coping with respect to empowerment and illness knowledge. The researchers also reported that the FTF participants, but not the members of the control group, had significantly better "emotion-focused coping" when measured by increased acceptances of mental illness of their family members. The FTF participants also had reduced distress and improved "problem-focused coping" when compared with the control group.

However, the researchers found no difference between the two groups with respect to "subjective illness burden." The authors concluded, "This study provides evidence that FTF is effective for enhancing coping and empowerment of families of persons with mental illness, although not for reducing subjective burden. Other benefits for problem solving and reducing distress are suggested but require replication."

Precautions

Precautions should be used when selecting a family psychoeducation program. Make sure that its primary goal is the well-being of the patient, with the secondary goal being the welfare of the family member(s). The program should be conducted by a qualified mental health professional. For the most part, the program is usually offered as part of a comprehensive clinical treatment plan for the mentally ill person. As such, it is incorporated within a medically approved treatment plan. Most family psychoeducation programs last from one to three years, and they are usually conducted based on a specific **diagnosis**.

Preparation

Preparation for family psychoeducation is not necessary. However, it is always wise to learn as much about a subject before delving into it. Therefore, the more knowledge gained in family psychoeducation, the better prepared one will be once involved with its methods.

Aftercare

Family psychoeducation is often a long-term method for treating mental illness. Whether formal treatment is active or not, the use of its techniques within the family setting is necessary and recommended for the continued well-being of the patient (and to avoid relapses) and his or her family members.

Complications

Patients can become overwhelmed with the involvement necessary within family psychoeducation. Consequently, participants and professionals should use caution when treating patients, especially if they are dealing with schizophrenia. It is also wise to realistically describe the situation to all participating members, especially concerning the patient's chances of recovery and the process of treatment. However, it is likely best to minimize any details that may overly **stress** members who are already especially emotional and anxious about the situation. Family psychoeducation experts see information received by the patient in small amounts as much more beneficial than large amounts at any given time.

Results

A large body of evidence supports the use of family psychoeducation as a best practice for young adults with schizophrenia and their families. Because of this compelling evidence, researchers at the University of Maryland, as part of the Schizophrenia Patient Outcomes Research Team (PORT), identified family psychoeducation as an evidence-based practice that should be offered to all families. This and other research studies have shown reduced rates of **relapse** and lower rates of **hospitalization** among patients and families involved in these programs. Other outcomes included increased rates of patient participation in **vocational rehabilitation** programs and employment, decreased costs of care, and improved well-being of family members.

A meta-analysis of 16 individual studies published in 1999 in the *Journal of Mental Health* found that family interventions of fewer than 10 sessions have no effect on the reduction of family burden. Controlled studies in the 2000s continued to support the effectiveness of single- and multiple-family interventions for **bipolar disorder**, major depression, **obsessive-compulsive disorder**, anorexia nervosa, and **borderline personality disorder**. In addition, studies of family psychoeducation have been conducted with a Hispanic population in Los Angeles, California, and outside the United States in China, Norway, and the Netherlands.

Further studies of family psychoeducation were ongoing in the 2010s. For instance, in 2011, a study performed in the Czech Republic was published in the journal *Biomedical Papers*. The article "Psychoeducation for Psychotic Patients" was authored by Drs. Jan Prasko, Kristyna Vrbova, Klara Latalova, and Barbora Mainerova, all of Palacky University in Olomouc, in the Czech Republic. The study looked at psychoeducation

KEY TERMS

Anorexia nervosa—An eating disorder highlighted by a person's denial of a healthy body weight, distortion of their outward appearance, and steadfast refusal to eat much food for a fear that they may gain weight.

Bipolar disorder—A mood disorder characterized by abnormally high energy levels and moodiness, usually without depression.

Depression—A psychiatric disorder involving feelings of hopelessness and symptoms of fatigue, sleeplessness, suicidal tendencies, and poor concentration.

Schizophrenia—A mental disorder involving distorted thinking and emotions.

QUESTIONS TO ASK YOUR DOCTOR

- Do you know how effective family psychoeducation could be for our family?
- Are there any underlying concerns that need to be addressed or corrected before we proceed with family psychoeducation?
- Will our family health insurance cover the training method?
- Will we need family psychoeducation for a short or long time?
- What will happen if it is stopped?

programs given in hospital settings with regard to schizophrenia patients recently discharged from the hospital. They found that the benefits of psychoeducation (those that are provided by the family) continue for up to seven years after leaving the hospital. The authors concluded that the perception of patients is that the program was beneficial and provided better understanding of their lives.

Unfortunately, putting family psychoeducation into effect in clinical settings has not kept pace with research. The Schizophrenia Patient Outcomes Research Team (PORT) study found that only 31% of patients studied reported that their families received information about their illness. One recent strategy to expand these programs includes integrating family psychoeducation into **assertive community treatment** (ACT) programs.

Parental concerns

When children are involved, parents should feel confident that family psychoeducation will better prepare them to respond to all of the problems associated with psychiatric disorders of children.

See also Case management

Resources

BOOKS

Bray, James H., and Mark Stanton, editors. *The Wiley-Blackwell Handbook of Family Psychology.* Chichester, UK: Wiley-Blackwell, 2009.

Gladding, Samuel T. *Family Therapy: History, Theory, and Practice.* Boston: Pearson, 2011.

Hughes, Daniel A. *Attachment Focused Family Therapy Workbook.* New York: W.W. Norton, 2011.

Nichols, Michael P. *The Essentials of Family Therapy.* Boston: Allyn & Bacon, 2011.

Sexton, Thomas L. *Functional Family Therapy in Clinical Practice: An Evidence-Based Treatment Model for Working with Troubled Adolescents.* New York, Routledge, 2011.

Torrey, E. Fuller. *Surviving Schizophrenia: A Manual for Families, Consumers and Providers,* 5th ed. New York: Collins, 2006.

VandenBos, Gary R., editor. *APA Dictionary of Psychology.* Washington, DC: American Psychological Association, 2007.

WEBSITES

Dixon, Lisa B., et al. "Outcomes of a Randomized Study of a Peer-Taught Family-to-Family Education Program for Mental Illness." Psychiatric Services. (June 2011). http://psychservices.psychiatryonline.org/cgi/content/abstract/62/6/591 (accessed August 24, 2011).

"Family to Family Education Program." National Alliance on Mental Illness. http://www.nami.org/template.cfm?Section=Family-to-Family (accessed August 24, 2011).

"Family Psychoeducation vs. Family-to-Family Education Program (FFEP)." National Alliance on Mental Illness. http://www.nami.org/Content/NavigationMenu/Inform_Yourself/About_Mental_Illness/About_Treatments_and_Supports/Family_Psychoeducation.htm (accessed August 24, 2011).

"Lisa B. Dixon M.D." University of Maryland Medical Center. http://medschool.umaryland.edu/facultyresearchprofile/viewprofile.aspx?id=719 (accessed August 24, 2011).

"Pioneer Psychiatrist Brought Families In." New Zealand Herald. (July 22, 2006). http://www.nzherald.co.nz/nz/news/article.cfm?c_id=1&objectid=10392461 (accessed August 24, 2011).

"Schizophrenia." National Alliance on Mental Illness. (February 2007). http://www.nami.org/Template.cfm?Section=By_Illness&template=/ContentManagement/ContentDisplay.cfm&ContentID=7416 (accessed August 24, 2011).

"University of Maryland Gets 4-Year NIMH Grant to Study the Effectiveness of NAMI's Family-to-Family Education Program." National Alliance on Mental Illness. (October 1, 2005). http://www.nami.org/Template.cfm?Section=Family-to-Family&template=/ContentManagement/ContentDisplay.cfm&ContentID=89938 (accessed August 24, 2011).

ORGANIZATIONS

American Psychiatric Association, 1000 Wilson Boulevard, Suite 1825, Arlington, VA, 22209-3901, (703) 907-7300, apa@psych.org, http://www.psych.org

American Psychological Association, 750 First Street, N.E., Washington, DC, 20002, (202) 336-5500, (800) 374-2721, http://www.apa.org

National Alliance on Mental Illness, 3803 North Fairfax Drive, Suite 100, Arlington, VA, 22203, (703) 524-7600, Fax: (703) 524-9094, (800) 950-6264, http://www.nami.org

National Institute of Mental Health, 6001 Executive Boulevard, Room 8184, MSC 9663, Bethesda, MD, 20892-9663, (301) 443-4513, Fax: (301) 443-4279, (866) 615-6464, nimhinfo@nih.gov, http://www.nimh.nih.gov

Irene S. Levine, PhD
Ruth A. Wienclaw, PhD
William A. Atkins, B.B., B.S., M.B.A.

Family therapy

Definition

Family therapy is a form of **psychotherapy** that involves all the members of a nuclear or extended family. It may be conducted by a pair or team of therapists, often a man and a woman in order to treat gender-related issues or to serve as role models for family members. Although some forms of family therapy are based on behavioral or psychodynamic principles, the most widespread form is based on family systems theory. This approach regards the family as a whole, as the unit of treatment, and emphasizes such factors as relationships and communication patterns rather than traits or symptoms in individual members.

Purpose

The purpose of family therapy is to improve relationships between family members and improve behavior patterns of the family as a whole or of subgroups within the family.

Family therapy is often recommended when:

- A family member has schizophrenia or another severe psychosis; the goal in these cases is to help other family members understand the disorder and adjust to the psychological changes that may be occurring in the patient.
- Problems cross generational boundaries, such as when parents share a home with grandparents or children are being raised by grandparents.
- Families deviate from social norms (unmarried parents, gay couples rearing children, etc.). These families may or may not have internal problems, but could be troubled by outside perceptions.
- Family members come from mixed racial, cultural, or religious backgrounds.
- One member is being scapegoated, or their treatment in individual therapy is being undermined.
- The identified patient's problems seem inextricably tied to problems with other family members.
- A blended (i.e., step) family is having adjustment difficulties.

Most family therapists presuppose an average level of intelligence and education on the part of adult members of the family.

Precautions

Some families are not considered suitable candidates for family therapy. They include:

- families in which one, or both, of the parents is psychotic or has been diagnosed with antisocial or paranoid personality disorder
- families whose cultural or religious values are opposed to, or suspicious of, psychotherapy
- families with members who cannot participate in treatment sessions because of physical illness or similar limitations
- families with members who have very rigid personality structures (family members might be at risk for an emotional or psychological crisis)
- families whose members cannot or will not be able to meet regularly for treatment
- families that are unstable or on the verge of breakup

Description

Family therapy tends to be a short-term treatment, usually several months in length, with a focus on resolving specific problems such as eating disorders, difficulties with school, or adjustments to **bereavement** or geographical relocation. It is not normally used for long-term or intensive restructuring of families with severe dysfunctions.

Family therapy is becoming an increasingly common form of treatment as changes in American society are reflected in family structures. It has led to two further developments: couple's therapy, which treats relationship problems between marriage partners or homosexual couples, and the extension of family therapy to religious communities or other groups that resemble families.

In family-therapy sessions, all members of the family and all therapists (if there is more than one) are present at most sessions. The therapists seek to analyze the process of family interaction and communication as a whole and do not take sides with specific members. They may make occasional comments or remarks intended to help family members become more conscious of patterns or structures that had been previously taken for granted. Family therapists who work as a team also model new behaviors for the family through their interactions with each other during sessions.

Family therapy is based on family-systems theory, an approach that considers the family a living organism more than the sum of its individual members. Family therapy uses systems theory to evaluate family members in terms of their position or role within the system. Problems are treated by changing the way the system works rather than trying to "fix" a specific member. Family systems theory is based on several major concepts.

The identified patient

The identified patient (IP) is the family member with the symptom that has brought the family into treatment. The concept of the IP is used by family therapists to keep the family from scapegoating the IP or using him or her as a way of avoiding problems in the rest of the system.

Homeostasis (balance)

The concept of homeostasis presumes that the family system seeks to maintain its customary organization and functioning over time and tends to resist change. The family therapist can use the concept of homeostasis to explain why a certain family symptom has surfaced at a given time, why a specific member has become the IP, and what is likely to happen when the family begins to change.

The extended family field

The extended family field refers to the nuclear family, plus the network of grandparents and other members of the extended family. This concept is used to explain the intergenerational transmission of attitudes, problems, behaviors, and other issues.

Differentiation

Differentiation refers to the ability of each family member to maintain his or her own sense of self while remaining emotionally connected to the family. The capacity to allow members to differentiate is one mark of a healthy family.

Triangular relationships

Family systems theory maintains that emotional relationships in families are usually triangular. Whenever any two persons in the family system have problems with each other, they will "triangle in" a third member as a way of stabilizing their own relationship. The triangles in a family system usually interlock in a way that maintains family homeostasis. Common family triangles include a child and his or her parents; two children and one parent; a parent, a child, and a grandparent; three siblings; or a husband, wife, and an in-law.

Origins

Family therapy is a relatively recent development in psychotherapy. It began shortly after World War II, when doctors treating patients with **schizophrenia** noticed that the patients' families communicated in disturbed ways. The doctors also found that the patients' symptoms rose or fell according to the level of tension between their parents. These observations led to considering a family as an organism or system with its own internal rules, patterns of functioning, and tendency to resist change. The therapists started to treat the families of their patients as whole units rather than focusing on the hospitalized member. They found that in many cases the family member with schizophrenia improved when the "patient" was the entire family system. (This should not be misunderstood to mean that schizophrenia is caused by family problems, although family problems may worsen the condition.) This approach of involving the entire family in the treatment plan and therapy was then applied to families dealing with problems or conditions other than schizophrenia.

Benefits

Results vary, but in good circumstances, the benefits of family therapy include greater insight, increased differentiation of individual family members, improved communication within the family, loosening of previously automatic behavior patterns, and resolution of the problem that led the family to seek treatment.

Preparation

Families are often referred to a specialist in family therapy by a pediatrician or other primary care provider. (Some estimates suggest that as many as 50% of pediatric office visits concern developmental problems in children that are affecting their families.) Physicians may use symptom checklists or psychological screeners to assess a family's need for therapy.

Family therapists may be psychiatrists, clinical psychologists, or other professionals certified by a specialty board in marriage and family therapy. They will usually evaluate a family for treatment by scheduling a series of interviews with members of the immediate family, including young children, and significant or symptomatic members of the extended family. This process allows the therapist(s) to find out how each member of the family sees the problem and provides an initial impression of the

KEY TERMS

Blended family—A family formed by the remarriage of a divorced or widowed parent. It includes a new husband and wife, plus some or all of their children from previous marriages.

Differentiation—The ability to retain one's identity within a family system while maintaining emotional connections with the other members.

Extended family field—A person's family of origin plus grandparents, in-laws, and other relatives.

Family systems theory—An approach to treatment that emphasizes the interdependency of family members rather than focusing on individuals in isolation from the family. This theory underlies the most influential forms of contemporary family therapy.

Genogram—A family tree diagram that represents the names, birth order, sex, and relationships of the members of a family. Therapists use genograms to detect recurrent patterns in the family history and to help the members understand their problems.

Homeostasis—The tendency of a family system to maintain internal stability and resist change.

Identified patient (IP)—The family member whose symptom has emerged or is most obvious.

Nuclear family—The basic family unit, consisting of father, mother, and their biological children.

Scapegoating—The emergence of behavioral problems in one family member, usually the identified patient, who is often punished for problems within the entire family.

Triangling—A process in which two family members diminish the tension between them by drawing in a third member.

family's functioning. Family therapists typically look for the level and types of emotions expressed, patterns of dominance and submission, the roles played by family members, communication styles, and the existence of emotional triangles. They will also note whether these patterns are rigid or relatively flexible.

Preparation also usually includes drawing a genogram—a diagram that depicts significant persons and events in the family's history. Genograms also include annotations about the medical history and major personality traits of each member. Genograms help in uncovering intergenerational patterns of behavior, marriage choices, family alliances and conflicts, the existence of family secrets, and other information that sheds light on the family's present situation.

Risks

There are no major risks involved in receiving family therapy, especially if family members seek therapy with honesty, openness, and a willingness to change. However, some changes that result from the therapy may be seen as risks, such as the possible unsettling of rigid personality defenses in individuals, or the unsettling of couple relationships that had been fragile before the beginning of therapy, for example.

Training and certification

Family therapy can be and is usually provided by clinical **social workers** or licensed therapists known as marriage and family therapists. Many of these therapists have postgraduate degrees and often become credentialed by the American Association for Marriage and Family Therapy (AAMFT).

Resources

BOOKS

Clark, R. Barkley. "Psychosocial Aspects of Pediatrics & Psychiatric Disorders: Psychosocial Assessment of Children & Families." In *Current Pediatric Diagnosis & Treatment,* by William W. Hay Jr., et al. 17th ed. New York: McGraw-Hill Medical, 2004.

Gurman A.S., et al. Family Therapy and Couple Therapy. In *Comprehensive Textbook of Psychiatry,* by B.J. Sadock et al. Philadelphia, PA.: Lippincott Williams & Wilkins, 2009.

ORGANIZATIONS

American Association for Marriage and Family Therapy (AAMFT), 112 South Alfred Street, Alexandria, VA, 22314-3061, (703) 838-9808, Fax: (703) 838-9805, http://www.aamft.org.

Rebecca J. Frey, PhD
Karl Finley

Fanapt *see* **Iloperidone**

Fatigue

Definition

Fatigue may be defined as a subjective state in which one feels tired or exhausted, and in which the capacity for normal work or activity is reduced. There is, however, no commonly accepted definition of fatigue when it is considered in the context of health and illness.

Demographics

Fatigue is a common experience. It is one of the top ten symptoms that people mention when they visit the doctor. Some people, however, are at higher risk for developing fatigue. For example, the risk for women is about 1.5 times the risk for men, and the risk for people who do not exercise is twice that of active people. Some researchers question whether women really are at higher risk: they are more likely than men to go to the doctor with health problems, and men are less likely to admit feeling fatigued. Other risk factors include obesity, smoking, use of alcohol, high stress levels, **depression**, anxiety, and low blood pressure. Having low blood pressure is usually considered desirable in the United States but is regarded as a treatable condition in other countries. Low blood pressure or postural hypotension (sudden lowering of blood pressure caused by standing up) may cause fatigue, dizziness, or fainting.

Description

Fatigue is sometimes described as being primary or secondary. Primary fatigue is a symptom of a disease or mental disorder and may be part of a cluster of such symptoms as pain, fever, or nausea. As the disease or disorder progresses, however, the fatigue may be intensified by the patient's worsening condition, other disease symptoms, or surgical or medical treatment. This subsequent fatigue is called secondary.

A person's experience of fatigue depends on a variety of factors. These factors include culture, personality, the physical environment (light, noise, vibration), availability of social support through networks of family members and friends, the nature of a particular fatiguing disease or disorder, and the type and duration of work or **exercise**. For example, the experience of fatigue associated with disease will be different for someone who is clinically depressed, socially isolated, and out of shape compared to another person who is not depressed, has many friends, and is aerobically fit.

Fatigue is sometimes characterized as normal or abnormal. For example, the feeling of tiredness or even exhaustion after exercising is a normal response and is relieved by resting; many people report that the experience of ordinary tiredness after exercise is pleasant. Moreover, this type of fatigue is called acute because the onset is sudden and the desired activity level returns after resting. On the other hand, there is a kind of fatigue that is not perceived as ordinary and that may develop insidiously over time. This type of fatigue is unpleasant or seriously distressing and is not resolved by rest. Fatigue of this nature is abnormal and referred to as chronic.

Some researchers regard fatigue as a defense mechanism that promotes the effective regulation of energy expenditures. According to this theory, when people feel tired, they take steps to avoid further **stress** (physical or emotional) by resting or by avoiding the stressor. They are then conserving energy. Because chronic fatigue is not normal, however, it is an important symptom of some mental disorders, a variety of physical diseases with known etiologies (causes), and some medical conditions that have no biological markers although they are recognizable syndromes (patterns of symptoms and signs).

Physical sources of fatigue

DISEASE. There are many diseases and disorders in which fatigue is a major symptom. These include cancer, cardiovascular disease, emphysema, multiple sclerosis, rheumatic arthritis, systemic lupus erythematosus, HIV/AIDS, infectious mononucleosis, chronic fatigue syndrome, and fibromyalgia. The reasons for the fatigue, however, vary according to the organ system or body function affected by the disease.

FIBROMYALGIA AND CHRONIC FATIGUE SYNDROME. Fibromyalgia (also known as myofascial syndrome or fibrositis) is a syndrome characterized by pain and achiness in muscles, tendons, and ligaments. There are 18 locations on the body where patients typically feel sore. These locations include areas on the lower back and along the spine, neck, and thighs. A diagnostic criterion for fibromyalgia (FM) is that at least 11 of the 18 sites are painful. In addition to pain, people with FM may experience **sleep disorders**, fatigue, anxiety, and irritable bowel syndrome. Experts have suggested that FM and chronic fatigue syndrome (CFS) are manifestations of the same pain and fatigue syndrome. The care that patients receive for FM or CFS depends in large measure on whether they were referred to a rheumatologist (a doctor who specializes in treating diseases of the joints and muscles), neurologist, or **psychiatrist**.

PAIN. When pain is severe enough, it may disrupt sleep and lead to the development of sleep disorders such as insomnia or hypersomnia. Insomnia is the term for having difficulty falling and/or staying asleep. Hypersomnia refers to excessive sleeping. In general, disrupted sleep is not restorative; people wake up feeling tired, and as a result their pain is worsened and they may become depressed. Furthermore, pain may interfere with movement or lead to too much bed rest, resulting in deconditioning. Sometimes pain leads to social isolation because the person cannot cope with the physical effort involved in maintaining social relationships, or because family members are unsympathetic or resentful of the ill or injured person's reduced capacity for work or participation in family life. All of these factors worsen pain, contributing to further sleep disruption, fatigue, and depression.

SLEEP DISORDERS. There are a variety of sleep disorders that cause fatigue, including insomnia, hypersomnia, sleep apnea, and restless legs syndrome. For example, hypersomnia may be the result of brain abnormalities caused by viral infections. Researchers studying the aftermath of infectious mononucleosis proposed that exposure to viral infections might change brain function with the effect of minimizing restorative sleep; hence, some people developed hypersomnia. Another common disorder is sleep apnea, in which the patient's breathing stops for at least ten seconds, usually more than 20 times per hour. Snoring is common. People may experience choking and then wake up gasping for air; they may develop daytime hypersomnia to compensate. Sleep apnea is associated with aging, weight gain, and depression. It is also a risk factor for stroke and myocardial infarctions. Restless legs syndrome is a condition in which very uncomfortable sensations in the patient's legs cause them to move and wake up from sleep, or keep them from falling asleep. All of these disorders reduce the quality of a person's sleep and are associated with fatigue.

Psychological disorders

While fatigue may be caused by many organic diseases and medical conditions, it is a chief complaint for several mental disorders, including **generalized anxiety disorder** and clinical depression. Moreover, mental disorders may coexist with physical disease. When there is considerable symptom overlap, the differential **diagnosis** of fatigue is especially difficult.

DEPRESSION. In the fourth edition of the ***Diagnostic and Statistical Manual of Mental Disorders*** (*DSM-IV*), the presence of depressed mood or sadness, or loss of pleasure in life, is an important diagnostic criterion for depression. Daily fatigue, lack of energy, **insomnia**, and **hypersomnia** are indicators of a depressed mood. The symptoms of depression overlap with those of CFS; for example, some researchers report that 89% of people with depression are fatigued, as compared to 86–100% of people with CFS. The experience of fatigue, however, seems to be more disabling with CFS than with depression. Another difference between CFS and depression concerns the onset of the disorder. Most patients with CFS experience a sudden or acute onset, whereas depression may develop over a period of weeks or months. Also, while both types of patients experience sleep disorders, CFS patients tend to have difficulty falling asleep, whereas depressed patients tend to wake early in the morning. It is possible for CFS and depression to be comorbidities.

Some researchers believe that there is a link between depression, fatigue, and exposure to too much REM sleep. There are five distinct phases in human sleep. The first two are characterized by light sleep; the second two by a deep restorative sleep called slow-wave sleep; and the last by rapid eye movement or REM sleep. Most dreams occur during REM sleep. Throughout the night, the intervals of REM sleep increase and usually peak around 8:30 A.M. A **sleep deprivation** treatment for depression involves reducing the patient's amount of REM sleep by waking him or her around 6:00 A.M. Researchers think that some fatigue associated with disease may be a form of mild depression and that reducing the amount of REM sleep will reduce fatigue by moderating depression.

GENERALIZED ANXIETY DISORDER. People are diagnosed as having generalized anxiety disorder (GAD) if they experience overwhelming worry or apprehension that persists, usually daily, for at least six months, and if they also experience some of the following symptoms: unusual tiredness, restlessness and irritability, problems with concentration, muscle tension, and disrupted sleep. Stressful life events such as divorce, unemployment, illness, or being the victim of a violent crime are associated with GAD, as is a history of psychiatric problems. Some evidence suggests that women who have been exposed to danger are at risk of developing GAD; women who suffer loss are at risk of developing depression; and women who experience danger and loss are at risk of developing a mix of both GAD and depression.

While the symptoms of CFS and GAD overlap, the disorders have different primary complaints. Patients with CFS complain primarily of tiredness, whereas people with GAD describe being excessively worried. In general, some researchers believe that anxiety contributes to fatigue by disrupting rest and restorative sleep.

STRESS. When someone experiences ongoing pain and stress, organ systems and functional processes eventually break down. These include cardiovascular, digestive, and respiratory systems, as well as the efficient elimination of body wastes. According to the American Psychiatric Association, various chronic diseases are related to stress, including rheumatoid arthritis, cardiac angina, and secondary dysmenorrhea (painful menstruation).

Managing fatigue

The management of fatigue depends in large measure on its causes and the person's experience of it.

KEY TERMS

Biological marker—An indicator or characteristic trait of a disease that facilitates differential diagnosis (the process of distinguishing one disorder from other, similar disorders).

Deconditioning—Loss of physical strength or stamina resulting from bed rest or lack of exercise.

Electrolytes—Substances or elements that dissociate into electrically charged particles (ions) when dissolved in the blood. The electrolytes in human blood include potassium, magnesium, and chloride.

Stress—A physical and psychological response that results from being exposed to a demand or pressure.

Syndrome—A group of symptoms that together characterize a disease or disorder.

For example, if fatigue is acute and normal, the person will recover from feeling tired after exertion by resting. In cases of fatigue associated with influenza or other infectious illnesses, the person will feel energy return as they recover from the illness. When fatigue is chronic and abnormal, however, the doctor will tailor a treatment program to the patient's needs. There are a variety of approaches that include:

- Aerobic exercise. Physical activity increases fitness and counteracts depression.
- Hydration (adding water). Water improves muscle turgor or tension and helps to carry electrolytes.
- Improving sleep patterns. The patient's sleep may be more restful when its timing and duration are controlled.
- Pharmacotherapy (treatment with medications). The patient may be given various medications to treat physical diseases or mental disorders, to control pain, or to manage sleeping patterns.
- Psychotherapy. There are several different treatment approaches that help patients manage stress, understand the motives that govern their behavior, or change maladaptive ideas and negative thinking patterns.
- Physical therapy. This form of treatment helps patients improve or manage functional impairments or disabilities.

In addition to seeking professional help, people can understand and manage fatigue by joining appropriate **self-help groups**, reading informative books, seeking information from clearinghouses on the Internet, and visiting websites maintained by national organizations for various diseases.

Resources

BOOKS

Glaus, A. *Fatigue in Patients with Cancer: Analysis and Assessment.* Thesis published in Recent Results in Cancer Research, 145:I–XI, 1–172. Berlin, Germany: Springer-Verlag, 1998.

Hubbard, John R., and Edward A. Workman, eds. *Handbook of Stress Medicine: An Organ System Approach.* Boca Raton, FL: CRC Press, 1998.

Natelson, Benjamin H. *Facing and Fighting Fatigue: A Practical Approach.* New Haven, CT: Yale University Press, 1998.

Porter, Robert S., and Justin L. Kaplan, eds. *The Merck Manual of Diagnosis and Therapy.* 19th ed. Whitehouse Station, NJ: Merck Research Laboratories, 2011.

Winningham, Maryl L., and Margaret Barton-Burke, eds. *Fatigue in Cancer: A Multidimensional Approach.* Sudbury, MA: Jones and Bartlett Publishers, 2000.

PERIODICALS

Natelson, Benjamin H. "Chronic Fatigue Syndrome." *Journal of the American Medical Association* 285, no. 20 (May 23–30 2001): 2557–59.

WEBSITES

Davis, Caralyn. "What's In a Name: Fibro vs. CFS." Arthritis Foundation. http://forum.psychlinks.ca/fibromyalgia-and-chronic-fatigue/16865-whats-in-a-name-fms-vs-cfs.html (accessed October 7, 2011).

U.S. Centers for Disease Control. "Chronic Fatigue Syndrome." http://www.cdc.gov/cfs (accessed October 7, 2011).

ORGANIZATIONS

National Chronic Fatigue Syndrome and Fibromyalgia Association, PO Box 18426, Kansas City, MO, 64133, (816) 737-1343, http://www.ncfsfa.org.

Tanja Bekhuis, PhD
Emily Jane Willingham, PhD

Feeding disorder of infancy or early childhood

Definition

Feeding Disorder of Infancy or Early Childhood (FDIEC) is characterized by the failure of an infant or young child under six years of age to eat sufficient food and a well-balanced assortment of nutritious foods to order to gain weight and grow normally over a period of one month or more. The disorder can also be characterized by the loss of a significant amount of weight over one month. Feeding disorder is similar to failure to thrive, except that no medical or physiological condition can explain the low food intake or lack of growth.

The ***Diagnostic and Statistical Manual of Mental Disorders***, the guidelines used by medical professionals to diagnose mental disorders, was being updated as of 2012. Proposed changes for the fifth edition include changing the name of feeding disorder of infancy or early childhood to avoidant/restrictive food intake disorder (ARFID). The change encompasses a greater age range than just infancy to early childhood. It will cover individuals who do not eat enough or show little interest in feeding or eating, individuals who accept only a limited diet in relation to sensory features, and individuals whose food refusal is related to aversive experience. The revised version (fifth edition, or *DSM-5*) is scheduled to be available in May 2013.

Demographics

Although minor feeding problems are common in infancy and childhood—parents and caregivers report that 25% to 40% of infants and children have such problems as vomiting, colic, and slow eater or picky eater—true feeding disorder of infancy or early childhood is estimated to occur in 1% to 3% of infants and children. Children separated from their families or living in conditions of poverty or **stress** are at greater risk for contracting the disorder. Mental illness in a parent, or **child abuse** or **neglect**, may also increase the risk of the child developing a feeding disorder. Infants and children with developmental disorders and those born prematurely are also at higher risk of having a feeding disorder.

Description

Infants and children with a feeding disorder fail to grow adequately, or even lose weight with no underlying medical explanation. They do not eat enough energy or nutrients to support growth and do not eat a broad variety of foods from the major groupings of foods. Consequently, they may become irritable or apathetic. Eventually, such children may develop more slowly, physically and mentally. Severe cases of FDIEC that continue into adolescence may cause such children to feel socially isolated. Factors that contribute to development of a feeding disorder include lack of nurturing, failure to read the child's hunger and satiety cues accurately, poverty, or parental mental illness. Successful treatment involves dietary, behavioral, social, and/or psychological **intervention** by a multidisciplinary team of health professionals.

According to the *DSM-5*, an eating or feeding disturbance can be associated with one or more of the following:

- substantial weight loss, failure to gain weight, or halting growth
- extensive deficiency in nutrition
- dependence on external feeding sources
- distinct interference with psychosocial functioning

Causes and symptoms

Causes

Although the cause of feeding disorder of infancy or early childhood is unknown, it can result from many different factors. Some of these factors include poverty; inappropriate parent-child interactions such as failure to read the child's hunger cues or forcing food when the child is not hungry; and lack of proper dietary information. Lack of nurturing and/or parental aggression, anger, or **apathy** can make eating a negative experience for the child, increasing the risk of feeding disorders.

Such disorders are usually diagnosed when the infant or young child is seen by a caregiver or a doctor to be malnourished. After dismissing various medical conditions that could be causing the problem, such as intellectual disability or congenital heart disease, a **diagnosis** of FDIEC is made.

Feeding disorders are more common in infants and children who are born prematurely, had a low birth weight, or who are developmentally delayed. Many medical (or physiological) causes can contribute to eating difficulties, eating aversions, or failure to thrive. These causes include:

- diseases of the central nervous system
- metabolic diseases
- sensory defects
- anatomical abnormalities, such as cleft palate
- muscular disorders, such as cerebral palsy
- heart disease
- gastrointestinal diseases, such as Crohn's disease

To meet criteria for a true feeding disorder of infancy or childhood, these medical conditions must be ruled out.

Symptoms

Because the child or infant with a feeding disorder is not consuming enough energy, vitamins, or minerals to support normal growth, symptoms resemble those seen in malnourished or starving children. The infant or child

KEY TERMS

Cleft palate—A failure of the two sides of the palate within the mouth to meet during fetal development.

Colic—Excessive crying and irritability in babies, which may be caused by numerous problems such as stomach discomfort.

Gastrostomy—A surgical opening into the stomach.

Nasogastric intubation—A process in which a tube is inserted down the throat and into the stomach.

may be irritable, difficult to console, apathetic, withdrawn, and unresponsive. They may have constipation, along with bouts of excessive crying and sleepiness. Children with such disorders may also have tantrums at meals, refuse to eat certain groups of food, or refuse to eat any types of solid or liquid foods.

Children with FDIEC may have physical ailments, such as difficulties accepting or swallowing certain types of foods. They may choke or gag when given food. Such children might also have oral motor and sensory problems. Delays in development, as well as growth, can occur. In general, the younger the child, the greater the risk of developmental delays associated with the feeding disorder.

Laboratory abnormalities may also be associated with the disorder. Blood tests may reveal a low level of protein or hemoglobin in the blood. Hemoglobin is an iron-containing substance in blood that carries oxygen to body cells.

Diagnosis

Between 25% and 35% of children experience minor feeding problems. In infants born prematurely, 40% to 70% experience some type of feeding problem. For a child to be diagnosed with feeding disorder of infancy or early childhood, the disorder must be severe enough to affect growth for a significant period of time. Generally, growth failure is considered to be below the fifth percentile of weight and height.

Diagnosis for feeding disorders begins with an attempt to identify any medical illnesses that might contribute to the problem. The doctor will examine the historical record for height, weight, and head circumference of the child. Medical imaging devices and laboratory studies may be used to complete the examination.

Feeding disorder of infancy of early childhood is diagnosed if all four of the following criteria are present:

- failure to eat adequately over one month or more, with resultant weight loss or failure to gain weight.
- inadequate eating and lack of growth not explained by any general medical or physiological condition, such as gastrointestinal problems, nervous system abnormalities, or anatomical deformations.
- the feeding disorder cannot be better explained by lack of food or by another mental disorder, such as rumination disorder.
- the inadequate eating and weight loss or failure to gain weight occurs before the age of six years.

If feeding behavior or weight gain improves when another person feeds and cares for the child, the existence of a true feeding disorder, rather than some underlying medical condition, is more likely.

Treatment

Successful treatment of feeding disorders requires a multidisciplinary team approach to assess the child's needs and to provide recommendations and education to improve feeding skills, behavior, and nutrient intake. The multidisciplinary team for treatment of feeding disorders in childhood usually includes physicians specializing in problems of the gastrointestinal tract or of the ear, nose, and throat; a dietitian, a **psychologist**, a speech pathologist, and an occupational therapist. Support from **social workers** and physicians in related areas of medicine is also helpful.

An initial evaluation should focus on feeding history, including detailed information on type and timing of food intake, feeding position, meal duration, energy and nutrient intake, and behavioral and parental factors that influence the feeding experience. Actual observation of a feeding session can give valuable insight into the cause of the feeding disorder and appropriate treatments. A medical examination should also be conducted to rule out any potential medical problems or physical causes of the feeding disorder.

After a thorough history is taken and assessment completed, dietary and behavioral therapy is started. The goal of diet therapy is to gradually increase energy and nutrient intake as tolerated by the child to allow for catch-up growth. Depending on the diet history, energy and nutrient content of the diet may be kept lower initially to avoid vomiting and diarrhea. As the infant or child is able to tolerate more food and liquids, energy and nutrient intake is slowly increased over a period of one to two weeks, or more. Eventually, the diet should provide about 50% more than normal nutritional needs of infants

QUESTIONS TO ASK YOUR DOCTOR

- How can we best treat my child's feeding disorder?
- Why did this happen to my child?
- How serious is my child's feeding disorder?
- Could a medical or psychological problem cause my child's feeding disorder?
- How do you diagnose a feeding disorder?

or children of similar age and size. Vitamin and mineral supplements may also be given to correct for any deficiencies unable to be corrected with diet.

Behavioral therapy can help the parent and child overcome conditioned feeding problems and food aversions. Parents must be educated to accurately recognize their child's hunger and satiety cues and to promote a pleasant, positive feeding environment. Changing the texture of foods, the pace and timing of feedings, the position of the body, and even feeding utensils can help the child to overcome aversions to eating. Issues that may contribute to the feeding disorder, such as poverty, abuse, or parental mental illness, must be addressed. Physical and psychosocial problems are also treated to correct any problems that these may be producing within the child.

For extreme cases, a stay in the hospital or other such medical facility may be recommended. In other cases, surgical procedures may be necessary, such as gastrostomy or nasogastric intubation. Gastrostomy is an external surgical opening made into the stomach for such purposes as nutritional support. Nasogastric intubation involves the insertion of a plastic tube through the nose and throat and into the stomach.

Prognosis

If left untreated, infants and children with feeding disorders can have permanent physical, mental, and behavioral damage. However, most children with feeding disorders show significant improvements after treatment, particularly if the child and parent receive intensive nutritional, psychological, and social intervention. Improvement is normally gradual over time. Although it can be fully eliminated with proper treatment, such feeding and eating disorders can lead to permanent and serious mental and physical problems. Such problems can be minimized with early treatment.

Prevention

Providing balanced, age-appropriate foods at regular intervals—for example, three meals and two or three snacks daily for toddlers—can help to establish healthy eating patterns. If a child is allowed to fill up on soft drinks, juice, chips, or other snack prior to meals, appetite for other, more nutritious foods will decrease.

Positive infant and childhood feeding experiences require the child to communicate hunger and satiety effectively, and the parent or caregiver to interpret these signals accurately. This set of events requires a nurturing environment and an attentive, caring adult. Efforts should be made to establish feeding as a positive, pleasant experience. Further, forcing a child to eat or punishing a child for not eating should be avoided.

Resources

BOOKS

American Psychiatric Association. *Diagnostic and Statistical manual of Mental Disorders.* 4th edition, text revised. Washington, DC: American Psychiatric Association, 2000.

Beers, Mark H., et al. *The Merck Manual of Diagnosis and Therapy.* Whitehouse Station, NJ: Merck Research Laboratories, 2006.

Kleinman, Ronald E., editor. *Pediatric Nutrition Handbook.* Elk Grove Village, IL: American Academy of Pediatrics, 2009.

Rakel, Robert E., editor. *Textbook of Family Medicine.* Philadelphia: Saunders/Elsevier, 2007.

Samour, Patricia Queen, and Kathy King, editors. *Pediatric Nutrition.* Sudbury, MA: Jones & Bartlett, 2012.

Sullivan, Peter B., editor. *Feeding and Nutrition in Children with Neurodevelopmental Disability.* London: Mac Keith Press, 2009.

WEBSITES

American Psychiatric Association. "Avoidant/Restrictive Food Intake Disorder." *DSM-5* Development. http://www.dsm5.org/ProposedRevisions/Pages/proposedrevision.aspx?rid=110 (accessed May 23, 2011).

Kennedy Krieger Institute. "Feeding Disorders." http://www.kennedykrieger.org/kki_diag.jsp?pid=1084 (accessed May 23, 2011).

MedlinePlus. "Feeding Disorder of Infancy or Early Childhood." U.S. National Library of Medicine and National Institutes of Health. August 8, 2009. http://www.nlm.nih.gov/medlineplus/ency/article/001540.htm (accessed May 23, 2011).

University of Maryland Medical Center. "Feeding Disorder of Infancy or Early Childhood—Overview." August 2, 2009. http://www.umm.edu/ency/article/001540.htm (accessed May 23, 2011).

ORGANIZATIONS

American Academy of Child and Adolescent Psychiatry, 3615 Wisconsin Avenue, NW, Washington, DC, 20016-3007, (202) 966-7300, Fax: (202) 966-2891, http://www.aacap.org.

American Psychiatric Association, 1000 Wilson Boulevard, Suite 1825, Arlington, VA, 22209-3901, (703) 907-7300, apa@psych.org, http://www.psych.org.

American Psychological Association, 750 First Street, NE, Washington, DC, 20002-4242, (202) 336-5500, (800) 374-2721, http://www.apa.org.

Nancy Gustafson, M.S., R.D., F.A.D.A., E.L.S.
William Atkins, BB, BS, MBA

Female orgasmic disorder

Definition

Female orgasmic disorder (FOD) is the persistent or recurrent inability of a woman to achieve orgasm (climax or sexual release) despite adequate sexual arousal and stimulation. FOD is also known as orgasmic dysfunction or anorgasmia and used to be called inhibited sexual orgasm.

Demographics

The inability to achieve orgasm, discontent with the quality of orgasms, and the ability to achieve orgasm only with a particular type of sexual stimulation are very common sexual complaints among women. It has been suggested that 33%–50% of all women are dissatisfied with the frequencies of their orgasms and that fewer than one third of women consistently experience orgasm with sexual activity. However, FOD applies to the 10% 15% of women have never experienced an orgasm, regardless of the situation or stimulation, and to women who can no longer achieve an orgasm. The occasional failure to reach orgasm or dependence on a particular type of stimulation is not the same as FOD. Women who have never experienced orgasm are more likely to be unmarried, young, and/or sexually inexperienced. FOD has also been associated with menopause and aging, although many women find that their orgasms increase with age.

Description

When a woman becomes sexually excited, the blood vessels in the pelvic region expand, allowing more blood to flow to the genitals—the same process that occurs when men become sexually excited. This effusion is followed by seepage of fluid into the vagina to provide lubrication before and during intercourse. These events are called the lubrication-swelling response.

Body tension and blood flow to the pelvic region continue to build as sexual stimulation increases, either by direct pressure on the clitoris or pressure on the walls of the vagina and cervix. This tension builds as blood flow increases. When tension is released, involuntary, rhythmic contractions of the pelvic floor muscles and possibly the vagina and uterus occur, accompanied by a feeling of intense physical pleasure; this release is called an orgasm. The contractions carry blood away from the genital area and back into general circulation.

The exact physiological mechanisms of the female orgasm are not well understood. Women do not necessarily experience orgasms in the same way, and an individual woman may experience orgasms differently at various times and in different situations. Orgasms vary in intensity, length, and the number of contractions, and, unlike men, women can have multiple orgasms in a short period of time. Some 50%–80% of women experience orgasm only through direct clitoral stimulation. Mature, more sexually experienced women may find it easier to have orgasms than younger or sexually inexperienced women.

Women with FOD still experience sexual arousal and lubrication. However, as body tension builds, they have extreme difficulty or are completely unable to reach climax and release the tension. This can lead to frustration and unfulfilling sexual experiences for both partners, as well as anger, frustration, and other relationship problems. FOD often occurs in conjunction with other **sexual dysfunctions**.

According to the American Psychiatric Association's *Diagnostic and Statistical Manual of Mental Disorders*, the *DSM*, a **diagnosis** of FOD requires that the anorgasmia cannot be solely due to physiological problems nor a symptom of another major mental health disorder. However, FOD can be caused by a combination of physiological and psychological difficulties. To receive a diagnosis of FOD, the condition also must cause personal distress or relationship problems.

FOD is most often a primary or lifelong condition in which women never achieve orgasm with any type of stimulation, including self-stimulation (masturbation), direct stimulation of the clitoris by a partner, or vaginal intercourse. Secondary or acquired FOD affects women who have experienced orgasm at least once in the past, but have lost the ability following an illness or emotional **trauma** or as a side effect of surgery or medication. Acquired FOD is often temporary. Anorgasmia may also be classified as general, meaning that orgasm is never achieved under any circumstances or with any partner, or as situational, meaning that orgasm is only achieved under certain circumstances or with certain types of sexual activity.

Risk factors

Recent studies of twins suggest that genes and heredity play a large role in the development of FOD. A history of sexual or physical **abuse** is also a risk factor for FOD.

Causes and symptoms

FOD is characterized by a woman's inability to achieve orgasm, by extreme difficulty in regularly reaching climax, or by having only unsatisfying orgasms. Some women often come close to orgasm but never reach it. FOD can be caused by psychological factors or by a combination of psychological and physiological factors.

Psychological causes of FOD include:

- feelings of isolation, disconnection, or boredom during sex
- shyness or embarrassment
- performance anxiety or sexual activity that is overly goal-oriented, with excessive pressure to achieve orgasm
- past sexual or physical abuse, rape, incest, or other traumatic sexual experiences
- emotional abuse
- fear of pregnancy
- fear of rejection
- fear of loss of control during orgasm
- self-image problems
- relationship problems
- life stresses, such as financial worries, job loss, or divorce
- guilt or negative feelings toward sex or sexual pleasure—attitudes that are usually learned in childhood or adolescence
- religious or cultural beliefs about sex
- other mental health disorders, such as major depression

Various prescription and over-the-counter medications can cause anorgasmia. These include:

- antidepressants called selective serotonin reuptake inhibitors (SSRIs), such as fluoxetine (Prozac), paroxetine (Paxil), and sertraline (Zoloft)
- antianxiety drugs such as Xanax
- sedatives such as Halcion
- narcotics
- antihistamines
- blood-pressure medications
- chemotherapy drugs

Other physiological causes of FOD include:

- inadequate sexual stimulation and the inability to discuss or explore more stimulating sexual techniques
- lower estrogen levels during and after menopause, which reduce lubrication and require greater stimulation for relaxing and promoting blood flow to the clitoris and vagina
- other normal aging processes
- smoking, alcohol, or other substance abuse
- hormonal disorders and chronic illnesses that affect general health and sexual interest
- damage to the blood vessels of the pelvic region
- conditions that affect or damage pelvic nerves, including pelvic surgery, multiple sclerosis, diabetes, neurological disease, or spinal cord injury
- pelvic floor prolapse—a loosening of the muscles that support internal pelvic organs
- removal of the clitoris (female genital mutilation), a cultural practice in much of Africa and some regions of the Middle East and Asia

Diagnosis

FOD is often self-diagnosed. However, a woman who has never had an orgasm may not realize what is missing in her sexual experience without diagnosis by a physician, women's healthcare specialist, **psychiatrist**, **psychologist**, or sex therapist.

Examination

Diagnosis of FOD includes a complete physical exam and medical, psychological, and sexual histories. The clinician or therapist helps determine whether the problem is primary or acquired and general or situational. FOD sometimes occurs in conjunction with **sexual aversion disorder** and/or **female sexual arousal disorder**, complicating the diagnosis. A diagnosis of FOD requires that:

- Orgasms occur less frequently than would be expected based on the patient's age, sexual experience, and level of sexual stimulation.
- The absence of orgasm results in emotional distress or relationship difficulties.
- The cause is psychological or a combination of psychological and physical factors.
- The absence of orgasm is not a symptom of another psychological disorder, such as depression.

Tests

Blood tests may be performed to measure the levels of estrogen and testosterone.

Treatment

Treatment of FOD requires addressing any underlying physiological causes, psychological factors such as **depression**, and lifestyle factors such as **substance abuse**. Medications may require adjustment. Any associated sexual dysfunctions, such as lack of interest in sex or painful intercourse, must also be addressed. FOD is commonly treated with education, counseling, **cognitive-behavioral therapy**, **psychotherapy**, and/or sex therapy.

Traditional

Psychotherapy or counseling can be effective for treating psychological causes of FOD, especially those causes that are rooted in **sexual abuse**, past sexual or emotional experiences, or cultural taboos. **Couples therapy** may be used to resolve relationship issues that have either caused or resulted from FOD. These processes require time and a joint commitment by couples.

Sex therapists have specialized training for assisting individuals and couples in overcoming sexual dysfunctions. Sex therapy may include:

- directed exercises for increasing stimulation and decreasing inhibitions
- techniques for relaxation, sexual exploration, and direct clitoral stimulation
- encouragement of masturbation, either by self-stimulation or with a vibrator
- Kegel exercises for enhancing sexual response
- communication training and relationship enhancement for couples
- desensitization, or learning to halt responses that are preventing orgasm, particularly in women with severe sexual anxiety

Drugs

Estrogen or a combination of estrogen and progesterone may be used to treat FOD in menopausal women and others with low hormone levels. FOD is sometimes treated with methyltestosterone, a synthetic form of the male sex hormone testosterone, although this practice is controversial and can have various side effects. Testosterone appears to be most effective for women with low testosterone levels resulting from surgical removal of the ovaries.

Alternative

Zestra is a botanical massage oil that warms the clitoris and may increase sexual arousal and orgasm. L-arginine, available in various nutritional supplements and topical applications, may relax the blood vessels and increase blood flow to the genital area, especially the clitoris; however, these assertions have not yet been well studied.

KEY TERMS

Cervix—The neck or narrow lower end of a woman's uterus.

Clitoris—The most sensitive area of the external genitals. Stimulation of the clitoris causes most women to reach orgasm.

Uterus—The hollow muscular sac in which a fetus develops; sometimes called the womb.

Vagina—The part of the female reproductive system that opens to the exterior of the body and into which the penis is inserted during sexual intercourse.

Home remedies

One of the most important factors in overcoming FOD is open and honest communication between partners about sexuality and sexual techniques. Erotic books or videos may help initiate such conversations. Sometimes focusing on clitoral stimulation is all that is needed to overcome FOD. Experimenting with different sexual positions may improve clitoral stimulation. Using a vibrator during sex can also help trigger orgasms.

Many women have found that Kegel exercises which involve the repetitive contraction and relaxation of the pelvic floor muscles, can improve both the frequency and intensity of orgasmic experiences. Repeatedly stopping and starting a urine stream identifies the muscles to be exercised, working up to five sets of ten contractions per day. The longer the contractions are held, the more benefit may result.

Prognosis

FOD can often be successfully treated with a combination of psychotherapy and guided sexual exercises. However, women should not expect to always achieve orgasm in every situation, nor should they expect to always be satisfied with the strength and quality of their climax. Women whose FOD is not due to an identifiable condition or disorder may be more difficult to treat. Couples often need to work through relationship issues that have either resulted from or caused the FOD before they see improvement. Unresolved FOD usually results in a decline in sexual desire and can create resentment and conflict within relationships.

Prevention

Although there is no sure way to prevent FOD, reducing life factors that cause **stress** can be effective. Healthy attitudes toward sex and education about sexual stimulation and responses can help prevent FOD. Seeking counseling or psychotherapy for past trauma or relationship issues can help minimize FOD and other sexual dysfunction problems.

Resources

BOOKS

American Psychiatric Association. *Diagnostic and Statistical Manual of Mental Disorders*. 4th ed., text rev. Washington, DC: American Psychiatric Publishing, 2000.

Komisaruk, Barry. R., et al. *The Orgasm Answer Guide*. Baltimore: Johns Hopkins University Press, 2009.

McCabe, Marita P. "Anorgasmia in Women." In *Systemic Sex Therapy* edited by Katherine M. Hertlein, Gerald R. Weeks, and Nancy Gambescia. New York: Routledge, 2008.

PERIODICALS

Frank, J. E., et al. "Diagnosis and Treatment of Female Sexual Dysfunction." *American Family Physician* 77, no. 5 (March 1, 2008): 635–642. Available online at http://www.aafp.org/afp/2008/0301/p635.html (accessed November 9, 2011).

Graham, Cynthia A. "The *DSM* Diagnostic Criteria for Female Orgasmic Disorder." *Archives of Sexual Behavior* 39, no. 2 (April 2010): 256–270. http://www.dsm5.org/Documents/Sex%20and%20GID%20Lit%20Reviews/SD/GRAHAM.FSAD.DSM.pdf (accessed November 9, 2011).

WEBSITES

Discovery Fit & Health. "Female Orgasmic Disorder: 'I'm Not Able to Climax'." http://health.discovery.com/centers/sex/articles/orgasmic.html (accessed October 7, 2011).

Mayo Clinic. "Anorgasmia." December 23, 2009. http://www.mayoclinic.com/health/anorgasmia/DS01051/METHOD=print (accessed October 7, 2011).

Mayo Clinic. "Female Sexual Dysfunction." April 24, 2010. http://www.mayoclinic.com/health/female-sexual-dysfunction/DS00701 (accessed October 7, 2011).

MedlinePlus. "Orgasmic Dysfunction." U.S. National Library of Medicine, National Institutes of Health. June 5, 2010. http://www.nlm.nih.gov/medlineplus/ency/article/001953.htm (accessed October 7, 2011).

MedlinePlus. "Sexual Problems in Women." U.S. National Library of Medicine, National Institutes of Health. May 2011. http://www.nlm.nih.gov/medlineplus/femalesexualdysfunction.html (accessed October 7, 2011).

ORGANIZATIONS

American Association of Sexuality Educators, Counselors, and Therapists, 1444 I St. NW, Ste. 700, Washington, DC, 20005, (202) 449-1099, Fax: (202) 216-9646, info@aasect.org, http://www.aasect.org.

American College of Obstetricians and Gynecologists, PO Box 96920, Washington, DC, 20090-6920, (202) 638-5577, http://www.acog.org.

U.S. Department of Health and Human Services, Office on Women's Health, 200 Independence Ave., SW, Washington, DC, 20201, (800) 994-9662; TDD: (888) 220-5446, http://www.womenshealth.gov.

Tish Davidson, AM
Emily Jane Willingham, PhD
Margaret Alic, PhD

Female sexual arousal disorder

Definition

Female sexual arousal disorder (FSAD) refers to the persistent or recurrent inability of a woman to achieve or maintain an adequate lubrication-swelling response during sexual activity, despite sexual desire. FSAD stems from both physiological and psychological factors, and it often results in avoidance of sex, painful intercourse, and sexual tension in relationships.

Demographics

FSAD is common in older women due to decreased hormone production after menopause and medical conditions associated with aging. However, because FSAD often occurs in combination with other female **sexual dysfunctions** and can be difficult to distinguish, and because women are often reluctant to seek help for FSAD, it is difficult to determine its incidence. There is also disagreement within the medical community concerning the exact demarcations of the various female sexual dysfunctions. One published review of the medical literature found that 22%–43% of women experience some form of sexual dysfunction. Another study found that about 20% of women have problems with sexual lubrication.

Description

FSAD results from a woman's inability to undergo lubrication and swelling in response to sexual desire and stimulation. This lack of response interferes with sexual desire and satisfying intercourse.

William Masters and Virginia Johnson—the first researchers to extensively examine the physical components of human sexuality—identified four stages of

ALFRED KINSEY (1894–1956)

Alfred Kinsey became a household name in the 1950s with his groundbreaking research on the sexual mores of American women and men. His two major texts, *Sexual Behavior in the Human Male* (1948) and *Sexual Behavior in the Human Female* (1953), opened the way for research into human sexuality.

During the 1940s, Kinsey embarked on a large-scale study of the sexual habits of men and women. Initially, his resources were limited, and he used his own money to hire staff and pay expenses. In 1943, he received a $23,000 grant from the Rockefeller Foundation that enabled him to hire additional employees and expand his efforts. Chief among his staff were colleagues W.B. Pomeroy, Paul Gebhard, and Clyde Martin. The funding legitimized his research, which evolved into the Institute for Sex Research of Indiana University, where Kinsey taught.

Kinsey and his colleagues at the Institute for Sex Research at Indiana University conducted thousands of interviews with men and women about their sexual habits. The 804-page *Sexual Behavior in the Human Male* sold 185,000 copies in its first year and became a *New York Times* bestseller. The work was scientifically based and nonjudgmental, with frank descriptions of biological functions. Although early polls indicated that most Americans were relieved to have an honest and open airing of human sexual practices, there was a tremendous backlash from conservative and religious organizations. *Sexual Behavior in the Human Female* caused an even greater stir. Its more controversial findings included the low incidence of female frigidity, high rates of premarital and extramarital sex, the rapidness of erotic responses, and a detailed discussion of clitoral versus vaginal orgasm. As sales of the book reached 250,000 in the United States alone, Kinsey's methods and motives came under scrutiny. Evangelist Billy Graham stated: "It is impossible to estimate the damage this book will do to the already deteriorating morals of America." The notoriety and resulting conflicts caused Kinsey's research funding to be revoked, and for the remainder of his life he struggled to find support for his work. On August 25, 1956, at the age of 62, Kinsey died of pneumonia and heart complications.

sexual response: excitement, plateau, climax or orgasm, and resolution. More recent models have included emotional aspects of arousal. One model identifies three stages: desire, arousal, and orgasm. FSAD affects the excitement or arousal stage.

The first physiological change in the female body upon becoming aroused or sexually excited is the expansion of the blood vessels in the pelvic region, allowing more blood to flow to the lower abdomen and genitals. Some women experience this as a feeling of fullness in the pelvis, and either consciously or involuntarily contract the muscles in the genital area. The increased blood flow normally results in transudation—the seepage of fluid through the walls of the blood vessels—in this case into the vagina to provide lubrication before and during intercourse. Vaginal lubrication can occur very rapidly, within one minute, and is often very noticeable by the woman and her partner. The increase in blood flow also expands the upper portion of the vagina, the uterus, and the cervix. The lower third of the vagina, the labia, and the area around the clitoris swell and may tingle. The breasts also swell slightly. Together these physiological changes constitute the lubrication-swelling response, designed to facilitate entry of the penis into the vagina.

With FSAD the lubrication-swelling response is either absent or is not maintained through the completion of sexual activity. The lack of arousal and lubrication can result in painful intercourse (**dyspareunia**), emotional distress, and/or relationship problems. FSAD can be lifelong or acquired and generalized or situation-specific.

Causes and symptoms

The major symptom of FSAD is insufficient transudation, often resulting in painful and unsatisfactory intercourse. In addition to vaginal dryness, there is a lack of swelling, tingling, or throbbing in the genital region. Generalized FSAD occurs with different partners and in many different situations, whereas situation-specific FSAD occurs only with certain partners or under particular circumstances. FSAD can be caused by psychological factors or a combination of psychological and physiological factors. Whereas some women have never had a normal lubrication-swelling response, others develop FSAD from physiological changes, such as illness or emotional **trauma**, or as a side effect of surgery, radiation therapy for cancer, or a medication. Physiologically based FSAD can lead to psychological problems that reinforce the disorder.

Arousal disorder that primarily affects the genitals can result from low estrogen or testosterone levels during and after menopause, as well as from vaginal or bladder infections, or changes in the skin around the vulva. Other physiological causes of FSAD include:

- insufficient sexual stimulation
- irritation from contraceptive creams or foams
- smoking, which decreases blood flow throughout the body
- illicit drug use
- lower levels of sex hormones due to breast-feeding
- medical conditions that cause changes in hormone levels, including thyroid disorders, adrenal gland disorders, or removal of the ovaries
- side effects of medications such as antidepressants, antipsychotics, sedatives, high–blood pressure drugs (antihypertensives), or birth control pills or other hormone-containing medications
- reduced blood flow due to damaged blood vessels in the pelvic region, often from an injury or medical conditions such as coronary artery disease, high blood pressure, or diabetes
- damage to nerves in the pelvic area, as from diabetes or multiple sclerosis

Psychological causes of FSAD include:

- fear or anxiety around sex
- chronic mild depression (dysthymia)
- emotional stress
- low self-esteem
- past sexual abuse
- emotional abuse
- bereavement
- self-image problems
- relationship problems
- other mental health disorders, including major depression, posttraumatic stress disorder, or obsessive-compulsive disorder

Diagnosis

Since most women occasionally experience difficulties with sexual arousal, a **diagnosis** of FSAD requires that the lack of lubrication-swelling response is persistent or has occurred intermittently over an extended period and causes emotional distress or relationship difficulties. The ***Diagnostic and Statistical Manual of Mental Disorders*** (*DSM*) requires that FSAD be caused by psychological factors alone or a combination of psychological and physiological factors. Under these criteria, arousal disorder caused by physiological factors alone, such as injury, illness, or menopause, is diagnosed as sexual dysfunction due to a general medical condition. Arousal disorder caused by medication or **substance abuse** alone is diagnosed as substance-induced sexual dysfunction. Arousal difficulties that are symptoms of a major psychological disorder, such as **depression**, or that result from inadequate sexual stimulation are not considered to be FSAD.

Examination

FSAD is usually diagnosed after a woman reports sexual difficulties to her gynecologist, family doctor, psychotherapist, or sex therapist. The physician will take complete medical, psychological, and sexual histories, including a list of medications and details about sexual symptoms. A physical examination, including a gynecological/pelvic exam, will be performed.

Tests

Blood and urine tests may be performed to rule out undiagnosed diabetes or other medical conditions. Hormone levels in the blood may be measured.

Treatment

FSAD treatment requires addressing underlying physiological and psychological causes. When there are physical causes, the root problem or disease is treated. Forms of treatment include therapy, medication, and at-home techniques.

Traditional

Psychotherapy, either as individual or **couples therapy**, addresses emotions, communication, relationship problems, and problem-solving strategies. Sex therapy focuses primarily on the sexual dysfunction. Many couples experiencing sexual dysfunction develop relationship problems and can benefit from traditional psychotherapy even after sexual arousal difficulties are resolved.

The U.S. Food and Drug Administration (FDA) has approved one medical device for treating FSAD. The Eros-Clinical Therapy Device (Eros-CTD) is a small vacuum pump that fits over the clitoral area and exerts a gentle sucking action that stimulates blood flow. In **clinical trials** the device has proved safe and effective for increasing blood flow, sensation, and vaginal lubrication.

Drugs

Sometimes medications, such as the type or timing of an antidepressant, can be adjusted. Poor lubrication related to decreasing hormone levels associated with menopause can often be successfully treated with some forms of hormone replacement therapy (HRT), such as estrogen or testosterone. Nonprescription lubricating gels and hormone creams can supplement a woman's natural lubricant. These are especially useful for pre- and postmenopausal women and for those with occasional arousal difficulties.

Research is focusing on new drugs that increase blood flow to the female genitals, thereby improving lubrication. Some of these drugs are aimed at increasing nitric oxide levels, similar to the drug sildenafil (Viagra) for men.

Alternative

A type of **meditation** called mindfulness, which promotes increased awareness and acceptance, has been found to be helpful in treating FSAD, at least when practiced in the context of **group therapy**.

Home remedies

Home remedies for FSAD include:

- Kegel exercises that increase blood flow to the vulvar and vaginal tissues
- relaxation techniques
- aerobic exercise
- changing the circumstances and settings of sexual activity
- sexual activities other than vaginal intercourse
- exploring sexual techniques that increase stimulation
- experimenting with a vibrator, fantasies, or erotic movies
- couples-focusing exercises to enhance intimacy, lessen anxiety, and increase arousal

Prognosis

Because FSAD has multiple causes, individual response to treatment varies widely. Difficulties with lubrication related to menopause generally have a good prognosis. Stress-related difficulties with arousal typically resolve when the stressor is no longer present. Couples may need to work through relationship issues that have either resulted from or caused the sexual dysfunction before they see an improvement in sexual arousal. This process takes time and a joint commitment to problem solving.

KEY TERMS

Adrenal gland—A small organ located above each kidney that produces hormones related to the sex drive.

Cervix—The neck or narrow lower end of a woman's uterus.

Clitoris—The most sensitive area of the external genitals. Stimulation of the clitoris causes most women to reach orgasm.

Labia—The outside folds of tissue that surround the clitoris and the opening of the urethra in women.

Menopause—A period of decreasing hormonal activity in women, when ovulation stops and conception is no longer possible.

Pelvis—The basin-like cavity in the human body below the abdomen, enclosed by a framework of four bones.

Penis—The external male sex organ.

Thyroid—A gland in the neck that produces the hormone thyroxine, which is responsible for regulating metabolic activity in the body. Supplemental synthetic thyroid hormone is available as pills taken daily when the thyroid fails to produce enough hormone.

Uterus—The hollow muscular sac in which a fetus develops; sometimes called the womb.

Vagina—The part of the female reproductive system that opens to the exterior of the body and into which the penis is inserted during sexual intercourse.

Prevention

There is no sure way to prevent FSAD. Eating a healthy, well-balanced diet, getting enough rest, having regular gynecological checkups, and seeking counseling or psychotherapy when problems begin to appear in a relationship can help minimize sexual arousal problems. Aerobic **exercise** and not smoking also can help prevent FSAD.

Resources

BOOKS

American Psychiatric Association. *Diagnostic and Statistical Manual of Mental Disorders*. 4th ed., text rev. Washington, DC: American Psychiatric Publishing, 2000.

Clinton, Tim, and Laaser, Mark. *The Quick-Reference Guide to Sexuality and Relationship Counseling*. Grand Rapids, MI: Baker Books, 2010.

Rowland, David, and Luca Incrocci. *Handbook of Sexual and Gender Identity Disorders*. Hoboken, NJ: John Wiley & Sons, 2008.

PERIODICALS

Brotto, Lori A., Julia R. Heiman, and Deborah L. Tolman. "Narratives of Desire in Mid-Age Women With and Without Arousal Difficulties." *Journal of Sex Research* 46, no. 5 (September 2009): 387–399.

Graham, Cynthia A. "The *DSM* Diagnostic Criteria for Female Sexual Arousal Disorder." *Archives of Sexual Behavior* 39, no. 2 (April 2010): 240.–55. http://www.dsm5.org/Documents/Sex%20and%20GID%20Lit%20Reviews/SD/GRAHAM.FSAD.DSM.pdf (accessed November 9, 2011).

"Study Explores Possibility of a Female Viagra." *HealthDay*, April 14, 2010.

WEBSITES

Basson, Rosemary. "Overview of Sexual Dysfunction in Women." *The Merck Manual Home Health Handbook for Patients & Caregivers*. November 2008. http://www.merckmanuals.com/home/womens_health_issues/sexual_dysfunction_in_women/overview_of_sexual_dysfunction_in_women.html?qt=female sexual arousal disorder&alt=shl (accessed October 7, 2011).

Family.org. "Sexual Dysfunction in Women." August 2010. http://familydoctor.org/familydoctor/en/diseases-conditions/sexual-dysfunction-women.html (accessed October 7, 2011).

Mayo Clinic staff. "Female Sexual Dysfunction." MayoClinic.com. http://www.mayoclinic.com/health/female-sexual-dysfunction/DS00701 (accessed October 7, 2011).

MedlinePlus. "Sexual Problems Overview." U.S. National Library of Medicine, National Institutes of Health. September 11, 2010. http://www.nlm.nih.gov/medlineplus/ency/article/001951.htm (accessed October 7, 2011).

———. "Sexual Problems in Women." U.S. National Library of Medicine, National Institutes of Health. May 2011. http://www.nlm.nih.gov/medlineplus/femalesexualdysfunction.html (accessed October 7, 2011).

ORGANIZATIONS

American Academy of Family Physicians, 11400 Tomahawk Creek Pkwy., Leawood, KS, 66211-2672, (913) 906-6000, (800) 274-2237, Fax: (913) 906-6075, contactcenter@aafp.org, http://www.aafp.org.

American Association of Sexuality Educators, Counselors, and Therapists, 1444 I Street NW, Suite 700, Washington, DC, 20005, (202) 449-1099, Fax: (202) 216-9646, info@aasect.org, http://www.aasect.org.

American College of Obstetricians and Gynecologists, PO Box 96920, Washington, DC, 20090-6920, (202) 638-5577, http://www.acog.org.

Tish Davidson, AM
Emily Jane Willingham, PhD
Margaret Alic, PhD

Fetal alcohol syndrome

Definition

Fetal alcohol syndrome (FAS) is a pattern of birth defects, learning, and behavioral problems affecting individuals whose mothers drank alcohol during pregnancy. It is the most severe of a range of disorders represented by the term fetal alcohol spectrum disorder (FASD).

Demographics

The occurrence of FAS/FASD is independent of race, ethnicity, or gender of the individual. Individuals from different genetic backgrounds exposed to similar amounts of alcohol during pregnancy may show different symptoms of FAS. The reported rates of FAS vary widely among different populations studied depending on the degree of **alcohol use** within the population and the monitoring methods used. Studies by the Centers for Disease Control (CDC) show that FAS occurs in 0.2 to 1.5 per 1,000 live births in different areas of the United States. FASDs are believed to occur approximately three times as often as FAS.

Description

FAS/FASD is caused by exposure of a developing fetus to alcohol. FASD is used to describe individuals with some, but not all, of the features of FAS. Other terms used to describe specific types of FASD are alcohol-related neurodevelopmental disorder (ARND) and alcohol-related birth defects (ARBD).

Standard test scores of children with fetal alcohol spectrum disorders (FASD) and fetal alcohol syndrome (FAS)

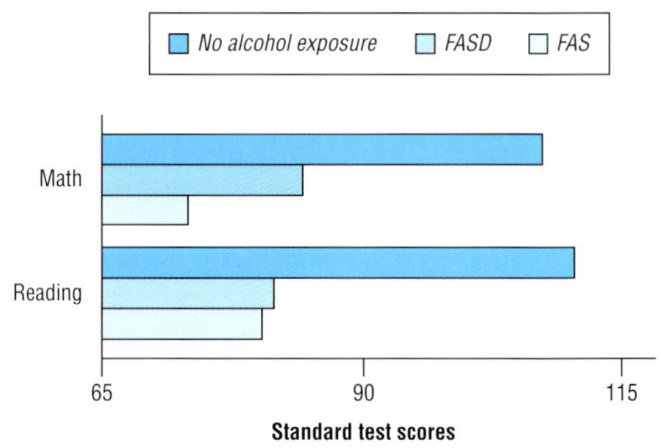

SOURCE: National Organization on Fetal Alcohol Syndrome.

(Graph by PreMediaGlobal. © 2012 Cengage Learning.)

FAS is the most common preventable cause of intellectual disabilities. This condition was first recognized and reported in the medical literature in 1968 in France and in 1973 in the United States. Alcohol is a teratogen, the term used for any drug, chemical, maternal disease, or other environmental exposure that can cause birth defects or functional impairment in a developing fetus. Some features of FAS that may be present at birth include low birth weight, prematurity, and microcephaly. Characteristic facial features may be present at birth or may become more obvious over time. Signs of **brain** damage include delays in development, behavioral abnormalities, and intellectual disabilities, but affected individuals exhibit a wide range of abilities and disabilities.

Fetal alcohol syndrome is one of the conditions being recommended for inclusion in the ***Diagnostic and Statistical Manual of Mental Disorders*** *(DSM-5*, 2013).

FAS is a life-long condition. It is not curable and has serious long-term consequences. Learning, behavioral, and emotional problems are common in adolescents and adults with FAS/FASD.

Risk factors

The only risk factor for a child to develop FAS is the consumption of alcohol by a women who is pregnant. There is no known amount of alcohol use that is safe during pregnancy, nor is there a particular stage of pregnancy during which alcohol use is safe.

Causes and symptoms

Causes

The only cause of FAS is maternal use of alcohol during pregnancy. FAS is not a genetic or inherited disorder. Alcohol drunk by the mother freely crosses the placenta and damages the developing fetus. Alcohol use by the father cannot cause FAS. Not all offspring who are exposed to alcohol during pregnancy have signs or symptoms of FAS; individuals of different genetic backgrounds may be more or less susceptible to the damage that alcohol can cause. The amount of alcohol, stage of development of the fetus, and the pattern of alcohol use create the range of symptoms that encompass FASD.

Symptoms

Classic features of FAS include short stature, low birth weight, poor weight gain, microcephaly, and a characteristic pattern of abnormal facial features. These facial features in infants and children may include small eye openings (measured from inner corner to outer corner), epicanthal folds (folds of tissue at the inner corner of the eye), small or short nose, low or flat nasal bridge, smooth or poorly developed philtrum (the area of the upper lip above the colored part of the lip and below the nose), thin upper lip, and small chin. Some of these features are nonspecific, meaning they can occur in other conditions, or be appropriate for age, racial, or family background.

Other major and minor birth defects that have been reported to occur in conjunction with FAS/FASD include cleft palate, congenital heart defects, strabismus, hearing loss, defects of the spine and joints, alteration of the hand creases, small fingernails, and toenails. Since FAS was first described in infants and children, the **diagnosis** is sometimes more difficult to recognize in older adolescents and adults. Short stature and microcephaly remain common features, but weight may normalize, and the individual may actually become overweight for his/her height. The chin and nose grow proportionately more than the middle part of the face, and dental crowding may become a problem. The small eye openings and the appearance of the upper lip and philtrum may continue to be characteristic. Pubertal changes typically occur at the normal time.

Newborns with FAS may have difficulty nursing due to a poor sucking response, have irregular sleep-wake cycles, decreased or increased muscle tone, **seizures** or tremors. Delays in achieving developmental milestones such as rolling over, crawling, walking, and talking may become apparent in infancy. Behavior and learning difficulties typical in the preschool or early school years include poor attention span, hyperactivity, poor motor skills, and slow language development. **Attention deficit hyperactivity disorder (ADHD)** is often associated with FASD. Learning or intellectual disabilities may be diagnosed during this time.

During middle school and high school years the behavioral difficulties and learning difficulties can be significant. Memory problems, poor judgment, difficulties with daily living skills, difficulties with abstract reasoning skills, and poor social skills are often apparent by this time. It is important to note that animal and human studies have shown that neurologic and behavioral abnormalities can be present without characteristic facial features. These individuals may not be identified as having FAS, but may fulfill criteria for alcohol-related neurodevelopmental disorder (ARND).

FASD continues to affect individuals into adulthood. One study looked atFAS adults and found that about 95% had mental health problems, 82% lacked the ability to live independently, 70% had problems staying employed, 60% had been in trouble with the law, and 50% of men and 70% of women were alcohol or drug abusers.

Another long-term study found that the average IQ of the group of adolescents and adults with FAS in the study was 68 (70 is lower limit of the normal range). However, the range of IQ was quite large, ranging from a low of 20 (severely disabled) to a high of 105 (normal). Academic abilities and social skills were also below normal levels. The average achievement levels for reading, spelling, and arithmetic were fourth grade, third grade, and second grade, respectively. The Vineland Adaptive Behavior Scale was used to measure adaptive functioning in these individuals. The composite score for this group showed functioning at the level of a seven-year-old. Daily living skills were at a level of nine years, and social skills were at the level of a six-year-old.

Diagnosis

In 1996, the Institute of Medicine suggested a five-level system to describe the birth defects, learning problems, and behavioral difficulties in offspring of women who drank alcohol during pregnancy. This system contains criteria including confirmation of maternal alcohol exposure, characteristic facial features, growth problems, learning and behavioral problems, and birth defects known to be associated with prenatal alcohol exposure.

FAS is a clinical diagnosis, meaning that there is no blood, x ray or psychological test that can be performed to confirm the suspected diagnosis. The diagnosis is made based on the history of maternal alcohol use, and detailed physical examination for the characteristic major and minor birth defects and characteristic facial features. It is often helpful to examine siblings and parents of an individual suspected of having FAS, either in person or by photographs, to determine whether findings on the examination might be familial, of if other siblings may also be affected. Sometimes, genetic tests are performed to rule out other conditions that may present with developmental delay or birth defects. Individuals with developmental delay, birth defects, or other unusual features are often referred to a clinical geneticist, developmental pediatrician, or neurologist for evaluation and diagnosis of FAS. Psychoeducational testing to determine IQ and/or the presence of learning disabilities may also be part of the evaluation process.

Treatment

There is no cure for FAS. The disorder is irreversible. Nothing can change the physical features or brain damage associated with maternal alcohol use during the pregnancy. Children should have psychoeducational evaluation to help plan appropriate educational interventions. Common associated diagnoses such **ADHD**, **depression**, or anxiety can be recognized and treated. The disabilities that present during childhood persist into adult life. However, some of the behavioral problems mentioned above may be avoided or lessened by early and correct diagnosis, better understanding of the life-long complications of FAS, and **intervention**. The goal of treatment is to help the individual affected by FAS become as independent and successful in school, employment, and social relationships as possible.

QUESTIONS TO ASK YOUR DOCTOR

- I drank alcohol before I knew I was pregnant. How might this affect my baby?
- How soon can you evaluate the degree to which my baby has been affected by my use of alcohol?
- I am a heavy drinker. Can you refer me to a program to help me control my drinking while I am pregnant?
- My baby was born with FAS. What kind of social services are available to our family?

Prognosis

The prognosis for FAS/FASD depends on the severity of birth defects and the brain damage present at birth. Miscarriage, stillbirth, or death in the first few weeks of life may be outcomes in very severe cases. Generally individuals with FAS have a long list of mental health problems and associated social difficulties: alcohol and drug problems, inappropriate sexual behavior, problems with employment, trouble with the law, inability to live independently, and often confinement in prison, drug or alcohol treatment centers, or psychiatric institutions.

Some of the factors that have been found to reduce the risk of learning and behavioral disabilities in FAS individuals include diagnosis before the age of six years, stable and nurturing home environments, never having experienced personal violence, and referral and eligibility for disability services. Some physical birth defects associated with FAS are treatable with surgery. The long-term data help in understanding the difficulties that individuals with FAS encounter throughout their lifetime and can help families, caregivers, and professionals provide the care, supervision, education and treatment geared toward their special needs.

KEY TERMS

Alcohol—An organic chemical and the active agent in beer, wine, and liquor; chemically known as ethanol.

Alcoholism—Chronic and compulsive use of alcohol that interferes with everyday life.

Binge drinking—The practice of drinking alcoholic beverages to the point of intoxication.

Fetus—The stage of development between embryo and newborn.

Intellectual disability—Characterized by persistently slow learning and below normal intelligence.

Prenatal exposure—Coming in contact with a fetus during pregnancy.

Teratogen—An agent or chemical that causes a birth defect.

Prevention

FAS and FASD are completely preventable by avoiding all use of alcohol while pregnant. Prevention efforts include public education efforts aimed at the entire population, not just women of child bearing age, appropriate treatment for women with high-risk drinking habits, and increased recognition and knowledge about FAS/FASD by professionals, parents, and caregivers.

Resources

BOOKS

Golden, Janet. *Message in a Bottle: The Making of Fetal Alcohol Syndrome*. Cambridge, MA: Harvard University Press, 2005.

Kulp, Jodee, and Liz Kulp. *The Best I Can Be: Living with Fetal Alcohol Syndrome—Effects*. Brooklyn Park, MN: Better Endings New Beginnings, 2006.

Lawryk, Liz. *Finding Perspective: Raising Successful Children Affected by Fetal Alcohol Spectrum Disorders*. Bragg Creek, AB (Canada): OBD Triage Institute, 2005.

Soby, Jeanette M. *Prenatal Exposure to Drugs/Alcohol: Characteristics and Educational Implications of Fetal Alcohol Syndrome and Cocaine/Polydrug Effects*, 2nd ed. Springfield, IL: Charles C Thomas Publishing Ltd, 2006.

PERIODICALS

Franklin, L., et al. "Children With Fetal Alcohol Spectrum Disorders: Problem Behaviors and Sensory Processing." *American Journal of Occupational Therapy* 62, no. 3 (May –June 2008): 265–273.

Green, J. H. "Fetal Alcohol Spectrum Disorders: Understanding the Effects of Prenatal Alcohol Exposure and Supporting Students." *Journal of School Health* 77, no. 3 (March 2007): 103–108.

WEBSITES

Keith Vaux, ed. "Fetal Alcohol Syndrome." Medscape Reference, October 20, 2006. http://emedicine.medscape.com/article/974016-overview (accessed October 7, 2011).

MedlinePlus. "Fetal Alcohol Syndrome." U.S. National library of Medicine, National Institutes of Health. September 5, 2011. http://www.nlm.nih.gov/medlineplus/fetalalcoholsyndrome.html (accessed October 7, 2011).

U.S. Centers for Disease Control and Prevention. "Fetal Alcohol Spectrum Disorders (FASDs)." August 11, 2011. http://www.cdc.gov/ncbddd/fasd/index.html (accessed October 7, 2011).

ORGANIZATIONS

Fetal Alcohol Spectrum Disorders Center for Excellence, 2101 Gaither Rd., Suite 600, Rockville, MD, 20850, (866) 786-7327, fasdcenter@samhsa.hhs.gov, http://www.fascenter.samhsa.gov.

Fetal Alcohol Syndrome (FAS) World Canada, 2448 Hamilton Rd., Bright's Grove, ON, N0N 1C0, (519) 869-8026, http://www.faslink.org.

March of Dimes Foundation, 1275 Mamaroneck Ave., White Plains, NY, 10605, (914) 997-4488, http://www.marchofdimes.com.

National Institute on Alcohol Abuse and Alcoholism, 5635 Fishers Lane, MSC 9304, Bethesda, MD, 20892-9304, http://www.niaaa.nih.gov.

National Organization on Fetal Alcohol Syndrome, 1200 Eton Court NW, 3rd Floor, Washington, DC, 20007, (202) 785-4585, Fax: (202) 466-6456, information@nofas.org, http://www.nofas.org.

Laurie Heron Seaver, M.D.
Tish Davidson, A.M.

Fetishism

Definition

Fetishism is a form of paraphilia, a disorder characterized by recurrent intense sexual urges and sexually arousing fantasies generally involving nonhuman objects, the suffering or humiliation of oneself or one's partner (not merely simulated), or children or other nonconsenting persons. The essential feature of fetishism is recurrent intense sexual urges and sexually arousing fantasies involving specific objects. While any object may become a fetish in the psychological sense, the distinguishing feature is its connection with sex or sexual gratification. A **diagnosis** of fetishism is made only if an individual has acted on these urges, is markedly distressed by them, or if the fetish object is required for gratification.

For some people with a paraphilia such as fetishism, paraphilic fantasies or stimuli may be necessary for erotic arousal and are always included in sexual activity, or the presence of the fetish object may occur only episodically. For example, the fetish object may only be necessary for arousal during periods of **stress**, and at other times the person can function sexually without the fetish or stimuli related to the fetish.

Demographics

How many people have a fetish and the extent the fetish influences their lives and sexual activities are not accurately known. In some rare instances, people with fetishes may enter the legal system as a result of their fetishes, and those cases may be counted or tracked.

Paraphilias such as fetishism are uncommon among females, but some cases have been reported. Females may attach erotic thoughts to specific objects such as items of clothing or pets, but these are uncommon elements in sexual activity. Virtually no information is available on family patterns.

Description

A fetish is a form of paraphilia, and in fetishism, the affected person has created a strong association between an object and sexual pleasure or gratification. A fetish is not simply a pleasant memory—it is a dominant component of most sexual situations. Most fetishes are objects or body parts. Common fetishes involve items of clothing, stuffed animals, or other nonsexual objects. Body fetishes may involve breasts, legs, buttocks, or genitals.

A person with a fetish often spends significant amounts of time thinking about the object of the fetish. Further, the object is intimately related to sexual pleasure or gratification. In the extreme, the presence of the fetish object is required for sexual release and gratification.

Causes and symptoms

Causes

The cause of the association between an object and sexual arousal may be adolescent curiosity or a random association between the object and feelings of sexual pleasure. A random association may be innocent or unappreciated for its sexual content when it initially occurs. For example, a male may enjoy the texture or tactile sensation of female undergarments or stockings. At first, the pleasurable sensation occurs randomly, and then, in time and with experience, the behavior of using female undergarments or stockings as part of sexual activity is reinforced, and the association between the garments and the sexual arousal is made. A person with a fetish may not be able to pinpoint exactly when his or her fetish began. A fetish may be related to activities associated with **sexual abuse**.

Symptoms

Early symptoms for a fetish involve touching the object of desire. The amount of time spent thinking about the fetish object may increase. Over time, the importance of the fetish object expands. In the extreme, it becomes a requirement for achieving sexual pleasure and gratification.

Diagnosis

A diagnosis of a paraphilia involving a fetish is most commonly made by taking a detailed history or by direct observation. According to the ***Diagnostic and Statistical Manual of Mental Disorders*** (the fourth edition, text revision, or *DSM-IV-TR*), the person must have experienced the fantasies or urges centered on a nonliving object or objects for at least six months. In addition, these fantasies, urges, or behaviors must meet the criterion of causing significant distress or impairment in the person's ability to function socially or at work, or in other important environments. Last, the fetish cannot be solely focused on female clothing used in cross-dressing (which falls into the classification of transvestic fetishism) or on sex-aid devices that promote tactile genital stimulation, such as vibrators.

The fifth edition of the *Diagnostic and Statistical Manual of Mental Disorders* (*DSM-5*, 2013) proposes changing the condition fetish to fetishistic disorder.

Treatment

In the earliest stages of behavior therapy, fetishes were narrowly viewed as attractions to inappropriate objects. Aversive stimuli such as shocks were administered to persons undergoing therapy. This approach was not successful. People with fetishes have also been behaviorally treated by orgasmic reorientation, which attempts to help them develop sexual responses to culturally appropriate stimuli that have been otherwise neutral. This therapy has had only limited success.

Most persons who have a fetish never seek treatment from professionals. Many can achieve sexual gratification in culturally appropriate situations. In recent years, American society has developed more tolerance for persons with fetishes than in the past, thus further reducing the already minimal demand for professional treatment.

KEY TERM

Paraphilia—A disorder that is characterized by recurrent intense sexual urges and sexually arousing fantasies generally involving (1) nonhuman objects, (2) the suffering or humiliation of oneself or one's partner (not merely simulated), or (3) children or other nonconsenting persons.

Prognosis

The prognosis for eliminating a fetish is poor because fetishism is generally chronic. Most cases in which treatment has been demanded as a condition of continuing a marriage have not been successful. Most fetishes are relatively harmless in that they usually do not involve other persons or endanger the person with the fetish. Persons with a fetish rarely involve nonconsenting partners.

The personal prognosis for a person with a fetish is good if the fetish and related activities do not impact others or place the person with the fetish in physical danger.

Prevention

Most experts agree that providing gender-appropriate guidance in a culturally appropriate situation will prevent the formation of a fetish. The origin of some fetishes may be random associations between a particular object or situation and sexual gratification. There is no way to predict such an association.

Resources

BOOKS

American Psychiatric Association. *Diagnostic and Statistical Manual of Mental Disorders*. 4th ed., text rev. Washington, DC: American Psychiatric Publishing, 2000.

Gelder, Michael, Paul Harrison, and Philip Cowen. *Shorter Oxford Textbook of Psychiatry*. 5th ed. New York: Oxford University Press, 2006.

Wilson, Josephine F. *Biological Foundations of Human Behavior*. Farmington Hills, MI: Cengage Learning, 2002.

PERIODICALS

Chalkley, A.J., and G.E. Powell. "The Clinical Description of Forty-Eight Cases of Sexual Fetishism." *British Journal of Psychiatry* 142 (1983): 292–95.

FitzGerald, W. A. "Explaining the Variety of Human Sexuality." *Medical Hypotheses* 55, no. 5 (November 2000): 435–39.

Nersessian E. "A Cat as Fetish: a Contribution to the Theory of Fetishism." *International Journal of Psychoanalysis* 79 (1998): 713–25.

Reed, G. S. "The Analyst's Interpretation as Fetish." *Journal of the American Psychoanalytical Association* 45, no. 4 (1997): 1153–81.

Weiss, J. "Bondage Fantasies and Beating Fantasies." *Psychoanalytic Quarterly* 67, no. 4 (October 1998): 626–44.

Wise, T.N., and R.C. Kalyanam. "Amputee Fetishism and Genital Mutilation: Case Report and Literature Review." *Journal of Sexual and Marital Therapy* 26, no. 4 (October–December 2000): 339–44.

ORGANIZATIONS

American Psychiatric Association, 1000 Wilson Blvd., Ste. 1825, Arlington, VA, 22209-3901, (703) 907-7300, apa@psych.org, http://www.psych.org.

American Psychological Association, 750 1st Street NE, Washington, DC, 20002-4242, (202) 336-5500; TDD/TTY: (202) 336-6123, (800) 374-2721, http://www.apa.org.

L. Fleming Fallon, Jr., MD, Dr. P.H.
Emily Jane Willingham, PhD

Figure drawings

Definition

Figure drawings are projective diagnostic techniques in which an individual is instructed to draw a person, an object, or a situation so that cognitive, interpersonal, or psychological functioning can be assessed.

Purpose

A projective test is one in which a test taker responds to or provides ambiguous, abstract, or unstructured stimuli, often in the form of pictures or drawings. While other projective tests, such as the Rorschach Technique and **Thematic Apperception Test**, ask the test taker to interpret existing pictures, figure drawing tests require the test taker to create the pictures themselves. In most cases, figure drawing tests are given to children. This is because it is a simple, manageable task that children can relate to and enjoy.

Some figure drawing tests are primarily measures of cognitive abilities or cognitive development. In these tests, there is a consideration of how well a child draws and the content of a child's drawing. In some tests, the child's self-image is considered through the use of the drawings. In other figure drawing tests, interpersonal relationships are assessed by having the child draw a family or some other situation in which more than one person is present. Some tests are used for the evaluation of **child abuse**. Other tests involve personality interpretation through drawings of objects, such as a tree or a house, as well as people. Finally, some figure drawing tests are used as part of the diagnostic procedure for specific types of psychological or neuropsychological impairment, such as central nervous system dysfunction or intellectual disability.

Precautions

Despite the flexibility in administration and interpretation of figure drawings, these tests require skilled and trained administrators familiar with both the theory behind the tests and the structure of the tests themselves. Interpretations should be made with caution and the limitations of projective tests should be considered. It is generally a good idea to use projective tests as part of an overall test battery. There is little professional support for the use of figure drawing, so the examples that follow should be interpreted with caution.

Description

The Draw-A-Man Test, developed by Goodenough in 1926 was the first formal figure drawing test. It was used to estimate a child's cognitive and intellectual abilities reflected in the drawing's quality. The test was later revised by Harris in 1963 as the Goodenough Harris Drawing Test (GHDT), which included a detailed scoring system and allowed for drawings of men, women, and the self. The scoring system primarily reflected the way in which the child is maturing cognitively. The GHDT is appropriate for children between the ages of 3 and 17, although it has been found to be most useful for children between 3 and 10.

The Draw-A-Person test (DAP) was developed by Machover in 1948 and used figure drawings in a more projective way, focusing on how the drawings reflected the anxieties, impulses, self-esteem, and personality of the test taker. In this test, children are first asked to draw a picture of a person. Then, they are asked to draw a picture of a person of the sex opposite of the first drawing. Sometimes, children are also asked to draw a picture of the self and/or family members. Then, they are asked a series of questions about themselves and the drawings. These questions can be about the mood, the ambitions, and the good and bad qualities of the people in the drawings. The pictures and the questions on the DAP are meant to elicit information about the child's anxieties, impulses, and overall personality. The DAP is the most frequently used figure drawing test today. A scoring system appropriate for adults was developed in 1993 by Mitchel, Trent, and McArthur.

In 1992, Naglieri and his colleagues created a more specific scoring system for figure drawing tests called the Draw-A-Person: Screening Procedure of Emotional Disturbance (DAP:SPED), based on a large standardization sample. This scoring method includes 55 items rated by the test administrator and based on the child's drawings and responses to questions. The DAP:SPED is appropriate for children aged six to 17. It is often used as a screening method for children who may be having difficulties with regard to social adjustment and require further evaluation.

The House-Tree-Person (HTP) test, created by Buck in 1948, provides a measure of a self-perception and attitudes by requiring the test taker to draw a house, a tree, and a person. The picture of the house is supposed to conjure the child's feelings toward his or her family. The picture of the tree is supposed to elicit feelings of strength or weakness. The picture of the person, as with other figure drawing tests, elicits information regarding the child's self-concept. The HTP, though mostly given to children and adolescents, is appropriate for anyone over the age of three.

The Kinetic Family Drawing technique (KFD), developed in 1970 by Burns and Kaufman, requires the test taker to draw a picture of his or her entire family. Children are asked to draw a picture of their family, including themselves, "doing something." This picture is meant to elicit the child's attitudes toward his or her family and the overall family dynamics. The KFD is sometimes interpreted as part of an evaluation of child **abuse**.

The Kinetic School Drawing technique (KSD), developed in 1974 by Prout and Phillips, requires the child to draw a picture of himself or herself, a teacher, and one or more classmates. This picture is meant to elicit the child's attitudes toward people at school and his or her functioning in the school environment.

Results

As with all projective measures, scoring on figure drawing tests is more subjective. Specific scoring systems, such as the DAP:SPED can be used to provide more objective information. Most figure drawing tests have some sort of objective scoring system; however, the instructions given to the child, the questions asked by the test administrator, and the interpretations the administrator makes of the drawings are flexible and this makes it difficult to compare results between children, even on the same measure. Also, many clinicians choose not to rely on the scoring systems and rely entirely on their own intuitive judgments regarding their interpretation of picture content.

KEY TERMS

Projective test—A psychological test in which the test taker responds to or provides ambiguous, abstract, or unstructured stimuli, often in the form of pictures or drawings.

Reliability—The ability of a test to yield consistent, repeatable results.

Standardization—The administration of a test to a sample group of people for the purpose of establishing scoring norms. The DAP:SPED structured scoring system was standardized using a sample of over 2,300 children and adolescents.

Validity—The ability of a test to measure accurately what it claims to measure.

Figure drawings are often interpreted with regard to appropriate cognitive development. Naglieri's DAP: SPED scoring system includes a consideration of what features in a drawing are appropriate for children of various ages. For example, five-year old children are expected to make fairly basic drawings of people, consisting of a head, eyes, nose, mouth, body, arms, and legs. An 11-year-old, on the other hand is expected to have more details in the picture, such as a more defined neck, clothes, and arms in a particular direction.

Sometimes, figure drawings are assessed with regard to self image. Children often projective themselves in the drawings. For example, females with **body image** concerns may reflect these concerns in their drawings. Victims of **sexual abuse** may stress sexual characteristics in their drawings.

Psychological, neuropsychological, or emotional dysfunction can also be considered in figure drawing interpretation. This type of interpretation is often done with figure drawings made by adults. For example, a person who omits or distorts body parts may have emotional impairment. Excessive detail with regard to the sexual nature of the drawing may indicate sexual maladjustment.

Family dynamics are also interpreted through figure drawings. For example, in the Kinetic Family Drawing test, a picture where family members are in separate rooms may indicate isolation or a lack of interaction between family members.

Figure drawings are also interpreted with regard to child abuse. In 1994, Von Hutton developed a scoring system for both the HTP and DAP focusing on indicators of child abuse that may be present in drawings. The drawing of the family in the KFD test may also provide indicators of abuse.

There has been much debate over the overall reliability and validity of figure drawing tests (and projective tests in general). For example, when structured scoring systems are used, the DAP has been found to be a reliable measure, especially for cognitive development in children. However, with regard to specific personality characteristics, self-image issues, or personality dysfunctions, there has been relatively little support for the use of figure drawings.

Resources

BOOKS

Groth-Marnat, Gary. *Handbook of Psychological Assessment*. 5th ed. New York: John Wiley and Sons, 2009.

Kline, Paul. *The Handbook of Psychological Testing*. New York: Routledge, 1999.

Reynolds, Cecil R. *Comprehensive Clinical Psychology, Volume 4: Assessment*. Amsterdam: Elsevier, 1998.

Ali Fahmy, Ph.D.

5-HTP

Definition

5-HTP is the acronym for 5-hydroxytryptophan, also called 5-hydroxy-L-tryptophan. 5-HTP is found primarily in the **brain** and is a by-product of tryptophan, an amino acid found in foods. Tryptophan is an essential amino acid—it cannot be made by the body and must be obtained from food, particularly proteins. In the liver and brain, 5-HTP is converted to an important monoamine neurotransmitter called

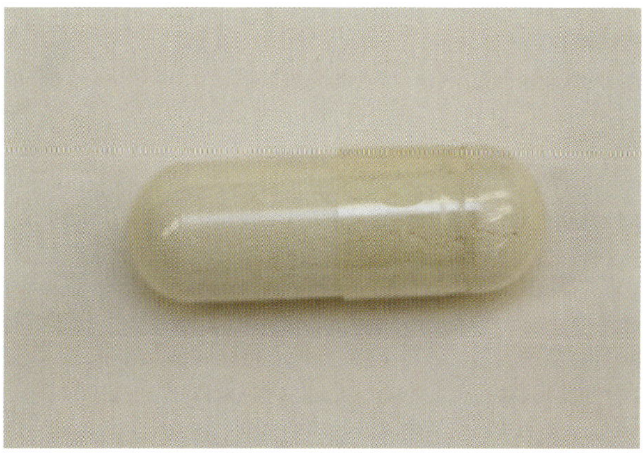

5-HTP supplement. *(© Custom Medical Stock Photo, Inc. Reproduced by permission.)*

serotonin. **Neurotransmitters** are chemical messengers that transmit signals between neurons (nerve cells), coordinating different functions within the body.

Purpose

Because it is converted to serotonin in the body, resulting in higher serotonin levels in the brain, 5-HTP is used to help treat or prevent conditions associated with low levels of serotonin. Serotonin, also called 5-hydroxytryptamine or 5-HT, plays an important role in controlling behavior and moods. It influences many normal brain activities and also regulates the activity of other neurotransmitters. Having adequate levels of serotonin instills a feeling of relaxation, calm, and mild euphoria (extreme happiness). Low levels of serotonin, known as serotonin deficiency syndrome, can lead to **depression**, anxiety, irritability, and **insomnia**.

Other conditions associated with low levels of serotonin include:

- attention deficit hyperactivity disorder (ADHD)
- bulimia
- epilepsy
- fibromyalgia
- headaches
- hyperactivity
- obesity
- obsessive compulsive disorder (OCD)
- panic attacks
- premenstrual syndrome (PMS)
- schizophrenia
- seasonal affective disorder (SAD)

5-HTP is an antioxidant; antioxidants protect the body from damage caused by substances called free radicals (unstable, toxic molecules). In this role, 5-HTP may help slow the aging process and protect the body from illness. Because serotonin is used to make melatonin, taking 5-HTP may help achieve some of the same benefits as melatonin, such as treating jet lag, depression, and insomnia. In treating insomnia, 5-HTP is thought to increase the length of rapid eye movement (REM) sleep, improving overall sleep quality. There is some evidence that 5-HTP can replenish the supply of the pain-relieving molecules called endorphins. Studies have shown that low levels of endorphins are associated with chronic **fatigue** syndrome, fibromyalgia, **stress**, and depression. In addition, 5-HTP affects other neurotransmitters, including norepinephrine and **dopamine**.

Description

In clinical studies, 5-HTP has been proven effective in the treatment of depression and fibromyalgia. Much of the clinical research with 5-HTP focused on the treatment of depression. In 15 separate studies, 5-HTP was tested on a total of 511 patients with different kinds of depression. Over half (56%) of these patients had significant improvement in depression while taking 5-HTP. The compound was found to be as effective as the selective serotonin reuptake inhibitor (SSRI) **fluvoxamine** and the tricyclic **antidepressants** clomipramine and **imipramine**. Many of these studies used relatively high doses ranging from 50–3,250 mg daily.

Three clinical studies found that 5-HTP can significantly improve the pain, anxiety, morning stiffness, and fatigue associated with fibromyalgia. The doses ranged from 300–400 mg daily. In one study, 5-HTP treatment was as effective as a tricyclic antidepressant (**amitriptyline**) and as **monoamine oxidase inhibitors** (MAOI; pargyline or **phenelzine**).

5-HTP may also be useful in treating carbohydrate cravings and binge eating, obesity, insomnia, anxiety, and panic disorders, but further research is needed, as results have been mixed. Three clinical studies found that 5-HTP use led to decreased intake of food and subsequent weight loss in obese patients. The dose used in one study was 900 mg daily, which initially caused nausea in 80% of the patients. In studies done on treating panic disorders, use of 5-HTP instilled patients with a sense of relief.

Although 5-HTP may be a useful alternative to conventional antidepressant drugs, one study indicated that it may be of no value for patients who have failed to respond to traditional drugs. In this study, patients who failed to respond to tricyclic antidepressants were treated with either 5-HTP or a monoamine oxidase inhibitor (MAO–I). Half of the patients improved with the MAOI treatment, while none showed any benefit from 5-HTP treatment.

Recommended dosage

The 5-HTP preparation available commercially is isolated from the seed of an African plant called *Griffonia simplicifolia*. It is available as an enteric coated tablet, which does not break down until it reaches the intestine.

The recommended starting dose for headaches, weight loss, depression, and fibromyalgia is 50 mg three times daily. It can be taken with food, though for weight loss it should be taken 20 minutes before eating. If the supplement is not effective after two weeks, the dose may be increased to 100 mg three times daily, but only with the recommendation of a physician. Insomnia is treated

KEY TERMS

Eosinophilia myalgia syndrome (EMS)—A chronic, painful disease of the immune system that causes joint pain, fatigue, shortness of breath, and swelling of the arms and legs. EMS can be fatal.

Monoamine oxidase inhibitor (MAOI)—An antidepressant drug that prevents the breakdown of monoamine neurotransmitters (such as serotonin) in the gaps between nerve cells. Nardil and Parnate are common MAOI brands.

Neurotransmitter—A chemical messenger that transmits signals between nerve cells.

Selective serotonin reuptake inhibitor (SSRI)—A family of antidepressant drugs that block the reabsorption of serotonin by nerve cells; common brand names include Prozac, Zoloft, and Paxil.

Serotonin syndrome—A syndrome characterized by agitation, confusion, delirium, and perspiration, which is caused by high levels of serotonin in the brain.

Tricyclic antidepressant—A group of antidepressant drugs that all have three rings in their chemical structure. Their mechanism of action is not fully understood, but they appear to extend the duration of action of some neurohormones, including serotonin and norepinephrine. They have also been used to treat some forms of chronic pain. Common brand names are Aventyl, Elavil, Surmontil, and Vivactil.

with 25 mg (which may be increased to 100 mg after a few days) taken 30–45 minutes before bedtime.

Precautions

A very small number of persons taking 5-HTP developed eosinophilia myalgia syndrome (EMS), a potentially fatal condition characterized by blood abnormalities and muscle tenderness and pain. In 1989, a contaminant was found in L-tryptophan that was linked to the development of EMS in some users, and the L-tryptophan supplements were subsequently banned by the U.S. Food and Drug Administration. A similar contaminant (peak X) was found in 5-HTP products produced by six different manufacturers. The 5-HTP contaminant was not at levels high enough to cause illness, so it is not known whether the development of EMS in persons taking 5-HTP is caused by a contaminant or by the drug itself. Excessive doses of 5-HTP may lead to toxic levels of peak X, and until the cause of EMS is determined, 5-HTP is considered unsafe.

Pregnant women should not take 5-HTP because there are no clinical studies on the effects of the supplement on the fetus or newborn. Persons with **Down syndrome** should also not take 5-HTP due to risk of **seizures**; in one study of patients with Down syndrome, 15% of participants suffered seizures after long-term 5-HTP use.

Side effects

Side effects associated with 5-HTP are rare but may include headaches, mild stomachaches, nausea, nasal congestion, and constipation. There are anecdotal reports that taking high doses of 5-HTP causes nightmares or vivid dreams. Side effects may be minimized by starting with a low dose of 5-HTP and taking it with food.

Interactions

5-HTP should not be used with other antidepressant drugs. 5-HTP and antidepressant drugs both work to increase serotonin levels in the brain, and too much serotonin can lead to **serotonin syndrome**, a potentially life threatening condition. Other drugs or supplements that may prove harmful in combination with 5-HTP include carbidopa (Lodosyn), dextromethorphan (Robitussin DM and others), meperidine (Demerol), pentazocine (Talwin), tramadol (Ultram), and **St. John's wort**.

Resources

PERIODICALS

Halford, Jason C.G., et al. "Serotonin (5-HT) Drugs: Effects on Appetite Expression and Use for the Treatment of Obesity." *Current Drug Targets* (March 2005): 201–213.

Keithahn, Christian, and Alexander Lerch. "5-Hydroxytryptophan Is a More Potent in Vitro Hydroxyl Radical Scavenger than Melatonin or Vitamin C." *Journal of Pineal Research* (January 2005): 62–66.

WEBSITES

MedlinePlus. "5-HTP." U.S. National Library of Medicine, National Institutes of Health. http://www.nlm.nih.gov/medlineplus/druginfo/natural/794.html (accessed September 20, 2011).

University of Maryland Medical Center. "5-Hydroxytryptophan (5-HTP)." http://www.umm.edu/altmed/articles/5-htp–000283.htm (accessed September 20, 2011).

University of Michigan Health System. "5-HTP." http://www.uofmhealth.org/health-library/hn-2793000www.uofmhealth.org/health-library/hn-2793000 (accessed September 20, 2011).

Belinda Rowland
Samuel Uretsky, Pharm.D.
David Edward Newton, Ed.D.

Flooding *see* **Exposure treatment**

Fluoxetine

Definition

Fluoxetine is an antidepressant of the type known as **selective serotonin reuptake inhibitors** (SSRI). It is sold in the United States under the brand names Prozac and Sarafem.

Purpose

Fluoxetine is used to treat **depression**, **premenstrual syndrome**, bulimia, and **obsessive-compulsive disorder**.

Description

Serotonin is a neurotransmitter—a **brain** chemical that carries nerve impulses from one nerve cell to another. Researchers think that depression and certain other mental disorders may be caused, in part, because there is not enough serotonin being released and transmitted in the brain. Like the other SSRI **antidepressants**, **fluvoxamine** (Luvox), **sertraline** (Zoloft), and **paroxetine** (Paxil), fluoxetine increases the level of brain serotonin (also known as 5-HT). Increased serotonin levels in the brain may be beneficial in patients with obsessive-compulsive disorder, alcoholism, certain types of headaches, **post-traumatic stress disorder** (PTSD), premenstrual tension and mood swings, and **panic disorder**.

Fluoxetine was the first of the class of antidepressants called **SSRIs** to be approved for use in the United States. In 2000, fluoxetine was approved by the Food and Drug Administration (FDA) for use in treating **premenstrual dysphoric disorder**.

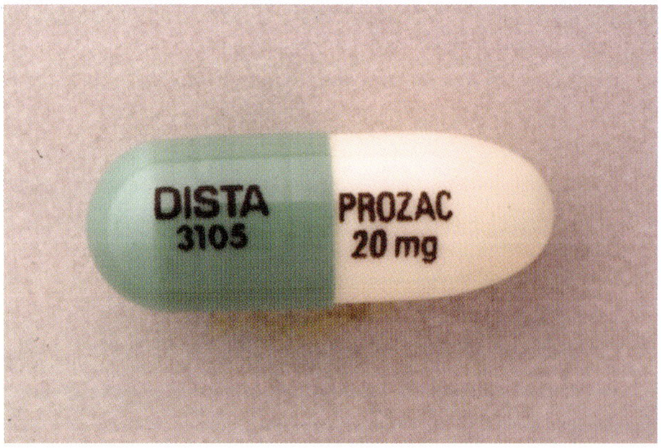

Prozac (fluoxetine hydrochloride). *(© Custom Medical Stock Photo, Inc. Reproduced by permission.)*

The benefits of fluoxetine develop slowly over a period of several weeks. Patients should be aware of this and continue to take the drug as directed, even if they feel no immediate improvement.

Fluoxetine (marketed as Prozac) is available in 10, 20, and 40 mg capsules, 10 mg tablets, and in a liquid solution with 20 mg of active drug per 5 mL. Prozac Weekly capsules are a time-release formula containing 90 mg of active drug. Sarafem is available in 10 and 20 mg capsules.

Recommended dosage

Fluoxetine therapy in adults is started as a single 20 mg dose, initially taken in the morning. Depending on the patient's response after four to six weeks of therapy, this dose can be increased up to a total of 80 mg per day. Doses over 20 mg per day can be given as equally divided morning and afternoon doses.

Precautions

Fluoxetine use should not be stopped abruptly. Patients taking fluoxetine should be monitored closely for **insomnia**, anxiety, mania, significant weight loss, **seizures**, and thoughts of **suicide**. Like other SSRIs, fluoxetine carries a warning regarding use in children and adults up to 24 years of age, who are at an increased risk of developing suicidal thoughts while taking the drug. Caution should also be exercised when prescribing fluoxetine to patients with impaired liver or kidney function, the elderly (over age 60), children, individuals with known manic-depressive disorder or a history of seizures, people with diabetes, and individuals expressing ideas of committing suicide.

Individuals should not take **monoamine oxidase inhibitors (MAOIs)** during fluoxetine therapy and should wait before beginning fluoxetine therapy. If so, they likely will need to wait before taking fluoxetine. Patients should wait at least five weeks after stopping fluoxetine therapy before taking **MAOIs**.

Care should be taken to weigh the risks and benefits of this drug in women who are, or wish to become, pregnant, as well as those who are breastfeeding.

People with diabetes should monitor their blood or urine sugar more carefully, since fluoxetine can affect blood sugar.

Until an individual understands the effects that fluoxetine may have, he or she should avoid driving, operating dangerous machinery, or participating in hazardous activities. Alcohol should not be used while taking fluoxetine.

Side effects

Common side effects include:

- decreased sexual drive
- restlessness
- difficulty sitting still
- skin rash, hives, and itching

Less common side effects include fever and/or chills and pain in joints or muscles.

Rare side effects include:

- pain or enlargement of breasts and/or abnormal milk production in women
- seizures
- fast heart rate
- irregular heartbeats
- red or purple spots on the skin
- low blood sugar and its symptoms (anxiety, chills, cold sweats, confusion, difficulty concentrating, drowsiness, excess hunger, rapid heart rate, headache, shakiness or unsteadiness, severe fatigue)
- low blood sodium and its symptoms (confusion, seizures, drowsiness, dry mouth, severe thirst, decreased energy)
- serotonin syndrome (usually at least three of the following: diarrhea, fever, sweatiness, mood or behavior changes, overactive reflexes, fast heart rate, restlessness, shivering or shaking)
- excitability, agitation, irritability
- pressured talking
- difficulty breathing
- odd body or facial movements

Interactions

Fluoxetine interacts with many other medications. People who may be starting this drug should review the other medications they are taking with their physician and pharmacist for possible interactions. Patients should always inform all of their healthcare providers, including dentists, that they are taking fluoxetine.

When taken with fluoxetine, blood levels of the following drugs may increase:

- benzodiazepines
- beta blockers
- carbamazepine
- dextromethorphan
- haloperidol
- atorvastatin
- lovastatin
- simvastatin
- phenytoin
- tricyclic antidepressants

The following drugs may increase the risk of **serotonin syndrome**: dexfenfluramine, fenfluramine, and tryptophan.

When **buspirone** is taken with fluoxetine, the therapeutic effect of buspirone may be impaired.

Low blood sodium may occur when fluoxetine is taken along with diuretics.

Increased risk of mania and high blood pressure occurs when selegiline is taken along with fluoxetine.

Severe, fatal reactions have occurred when fluoxetine is given along with MAOIs.

KEY TERMS

Diabetes—A disease in which sugar is not metabolized properly. People with diabetes need to monitor their blood or urine sugar carefully if they are taking fluoxetine, because this drug affects blood sugar.

Monoamine oxidase inhibitor (MAOI)—An older class of antidepressants.

Serotonin—A brain chemical that carries nerve impulses from one nerve cell to another.

Resources

BOOKS

Preston, John D., John H. O'Neal, and Mary C. Talaga. *Handbook of Clinical Psychopharmacology for Therapists*. 4th ed. Oakland, CA: New Harbinger, 2004.

PERIODICALS

Anderson, Shawanda W., and Marvin B. Booker. "Cognitive Behavioral Therapy Versus Psychosurgery for Refractory Obsessive-Compulsive Disorder." *Journal of Neuropsychiatry and Clinical Neurosciences* 18, no. 1 (Winter 2006): 129.

Denninger, John W., et al. "Somatic Symptoms in Outpatients with Major Depressive Disorder Treated with Fluoxetine." *Psychosomatics: Journal of Consultation Liaison Psychiatry* 47, no. 4 (July/August 2006): 348–52.

Fava, Maurizio, et al. "Eszopiclone Co-Administered with Fluoxetine in Patients with Insomnia Coexisting with Major Depressive Disorder." *Biological Psychiatry* 59, no. 11 (June 2006): 1052–60.

Hammad, Tarek A., Thomas Laughren, and Judith Racoosin. "Suicidality in Pediatric Patients Treated with Antidepressant Drugs." *Archives of General Psychiatry* 63, no. 3 (March 2006): 332–39.

Kratochvil, Christopher J., et al. "Selecting an Antidepressant for the Treatment of Pediatric Depression." *Journal of the American Academy of Child and Adolescent Psychiatry* 45, no. 3 (March 2006): 371–73.

Lam, Raymond W., et al. "The Can-SAD Study: A Randomized Controlled Trial of the Effectiveness of Light Therapy and Fluoxetine in Patients with Winter Seasonal Affective Disorder." *American Journal of Psychiatry* 163, no. 5 (May 2006): 805–12.

Martenyi, Ferenc, and Victoria Soldatenkova. "Fluoxetine in the Acute Treatment and Relapse Prevention of Combat-Related Post-traumatic Stress Disorder: Analysis of the Veteran Group of a Placebo-Controlled, Randomized Clinical Trial." *European Neuropsychopharmacology* 16, no. 5 (July 2006): 340–49.

McGrath, Patrick J., et al. "Predictors of Relapse in a Prospective Study of Fluoxetine Treatment of Major Depression." *American Journal of Psychiatry* 163, no. 9 (September 2006): 1542–48.

Moreno, Carmen, Ansley M. Roche, and Laurence L. Greenhill. "Pharmacotherapy of Child and Adolescent Depression." *Child and Adolescent Psychiatric Clinics of North America* 15, no. 4 (October 2006): 977–98.

Mowla, Arash, Ahmad Ghanizadeh, and Azadeh Pani. "A Comparison of the Effects of Fluoxetine and Nortriptyline on the Symptoms of Major Depressive Disorder." *Journal of Clinical Psychopharmacology* 26, no. 2 (April 2006): 209–11.

Mulder, Roger T., et al. "Six Months of Treatment for Depression: Outcome and Predictors of the Course of Illness." *American Journal of Psychiatry* 163, no. 1 (January 2006): 95–100.

Nemeroff, Charles B., and Michael E. Thase. "A Double-Blind, Placebo-Controlled Comparison of Venlafaxine and Fluoxetine Treatment in Depressed Outpatients." *Journal of Psychiatric Research* 41, no. 3–4 (April–June 2007): 351–59.

Pinto-Meza, Alejandra, et al. "Gender Differences in Response to Antidepressant Treatment Prescribed in Primary Care. Does Menopause Make a Difference?" *Journal of Affective Disorders* 93, no. 1–3 (July 2006): 53–60.

Pollack, Mark H., et al. "Olanzapine Augmentation of Fluoxetine for Refractory Generalized Anxiety Disorder: A Placebo Controlled Study." *Biological Psychiatry* 59, no. 3 (February 2006): 211–15.

Schreiber, Shaul, and Chaim G. Pick. "From Selective to Highly Selective SSRIs: A Comparison of the Antinociceptive Properties of Fluoxetine, Fluvoxamine, Citalopram, and Escitalopram." *European Neuropsychopharmacology* 16, no. 6 (August 2006): 464–68.

Serrano-Blanco, A., et al. "Effectiveness and Cost-Effectiveness of Antidepressant Treatment in Primary Health Care: A Six-Month Randomised Study Comparing Fluoxetine to Imipramine." *Journal of Affective Disorders* 91, no. 2–3 (Aprril 2006): 153–63.

Taravosh-Lahn, Kereshmeh Christel Bastida, and Yvon Delville. "Differential Responsiveness to Fluoxetine During Puberty." *Behavioral Neuroscience* 120, no. 5 (October 2006): 1084–92.

Taylor, Bonnie P., et al. "Psychomotor Slowing as a Predictor of Fluoxetine Nonresponse in Depressed Outpatients." *American Journal of Psychiatry* 163, no. 1 (January 2006): 73–78.

Tiihonen, Jari, et al. "Antidepressants and the Risk of Suicide, Attempted Suicide, and Overall Mortality in a Nationwide Cohort." *Archives of General Psychiatry* 63, no. 12 (December 2006): 1358–67.

Vasa, Roma A., Anthony R. Carlino, and Daniel S. Pine. "Pharmacotherapy of Depressed Children and Adolescents: Current Issues and Potential Directions." *Biological Psychiatry* 59, no. 11 (June 2006): 1021–28.

ORGANIZATIONS

American Psychiatric Association, 1000 Wilson Blvd., Ste. 1825, Arlington, VA, 22209-3901, (703) 907-7300, apa@psych.org, http://www.psych.org.

National Alliance on Mental Illness, 2107 Wilson Blvd., Ste. 300, Arlington, VA, 22201-3042, Fax: (703) 524-9094, (800) 950-6264, http://www.nami.org.

National Institute of Mental Health, 6001 Executive Blvd., Rm. 8184, MSC 9663, Bethesda, MD, 20892-9663, (301) 433-4513; TTY: (301) 443-8431, Fax: (301) 443-4279, (866) 615-6464; TTY: (866) 415-8051, nimhinfo@nih.gov, http://www.nimh.nih.gov.

Rosalyn Carson-DeWitt, MD
Ruth A. Wienclaw, PhD

Fluphenazine

Definition

Fluphenazine is a phenothiazine antipsychotic sold in the United States under the brand names Permitil and Prolixin. It is also available under its generic name.

Purpose

Fluphenazine is used to treat **schizophrenia** and symptoms of psychotic disorders such as **delusions**, hallucinations, and agitation.

Description

Fluphenazine is one of many drugs in the group called the phenothiazines. Phenothiazines work by inhibiting the actions of the **brain** chemicals **dopamine** and norepinephrine, which are overproduced in individuals with **psychosis**.

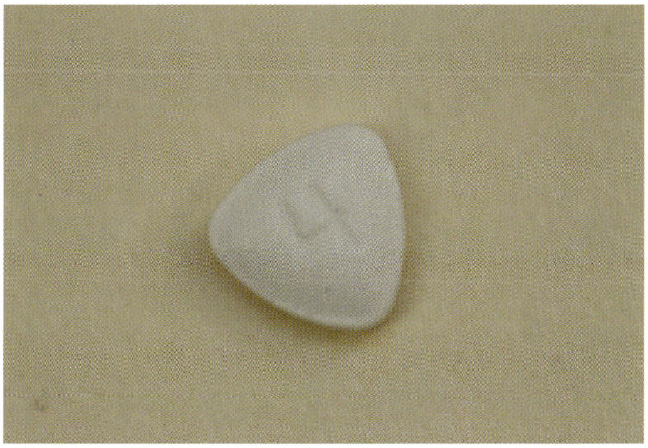

Fluphenazine, 1 mg. *(© Custom Medical Stock Photo, Inc. Reproduced by permission.)*

Fluphenazine is available in 1 mg, 2.5 mg, 5 mg, and 10 mg tablets, a liquid concentrate containing 5 mg/mL, a rapid-onset injectable form containing 2.5 mg/mL, and a long-acting injectable form containing 25 mg/mL.

Recommended dosage

In children over age 16 and in adults, fluphenazine is usually given in oral dosages ranging from 0.5–10 mg daily. The total dosage is usually divided and taken two to four times throughout the day. The dosage is typically reduced at a gradual pace over time to a range between 1 mg and 5 mg. Older adults usually receive lower doses that begin in the range of 1.0–2.5 mg per day. In children under age 16, the usual range is 0.25–3.5 mg per day divided into several doses. Maximum dosage is normally 10 mg per day for this age group.

This drug is also available by injection. In adults, injections into the muscle range from 1.25 to 10 mg per day divided into several doses. A long-acting injectable form can also be administered to patients who have been stabilized on the drug. The dose for the long-acting preparation ranges from 12.5 to 25 mg given every one to four weeks in adults. The dosage for children is lower in all cases.

Precautions

Though fluphenazine treats symptoms similar to those seen in **dementia**, it is not approved by the U.S. Food and Drug Administration (FDA) for this use. Elderly patients taking fluphenazine for dementia-related psychosis are at an increased risk of death.

People with a history of **depression**, lung problems, heart disease, glaucoma, **seizures**, and kidney disease should take fluphenazine only after careful evaluation by their physician. In addition, those undergoing alcohol withdrawal and those who have received **electroconvulsive therapy** should take this drug with great caution and close physician supervision after discussing the risks and benefits with their doctor. Those over age 60 and children under age 12 should take fluphenazine only after a thorough assessment by their physician. Pregnant women should use fluphenazine with great caution.

Fluphenazine may cause drowsiness. People who take this drug should not drive, operate heavy machinery, or perform other hazardous tasks requiring mental alertness until they see how the drug affects them. People taking fluphenazine should avoid significant exposure to sunlight, as the drug may cause people to sunburn more easily. This drug can sometimes change the color of urine to a pinkish or reddish-brown color. Fluphenazine use can make people more susceptible to heat and increase the risk of heatstroke. People taking fluphenazine should get up slowly after being in a reclining position because of potential dizziness.

Side effects

Relatively common side effects that accompany fluphenazine include:

- drowsiness
- dizziness
- rash
- dry mouth
- insomnia
- fatigue
- muscular weakness
- anorexia
- blurred vision
- some loss of muscular control
- amenorrhea (lack of menstruation) in women

Dystonia (difficulty walking or moving) may occur with fluphenazine use. This condition may subside in 24 to 48 hours even when the person continues taking the drug and usually disappears when fluphenazine is discontinued.

Fluphenazine use may lead to the development of symptoms that resemble Parkinson's disease. These symptoms may include a tight or mask-like expression on the face, drooling, tremors, "pill-rolling" motions in the fingers, cogwheel rigidity (abnormal rigidity in muscles characterized by jerky movements when the muscle is passively stretched), and a shuffling gait. Taking anti-Parkinson drugs **benztropine** mesylate or **trihexyphenidyl** hydrochloride along with the fluphenazine usually controls these symptoms.

KEY TERMS

Neuroleptic malignant syndrome—A complicated and potentially fatal condition characterized by muscle rigidity; high fever; alterations in mental status; and cardiac symptoms such as irregular pulse or blood pressure, sweating, tachycardia (fast heartbeat), and arrhythmias (irregular heartbeat).

Phenothiazines—Works by inhibiting the actions of the brain chemicals dopamine and norepinephrine, which are overproduced in individuals with psychosis.

Tardive dyskinesia—A syndrome consisting of involuntary, uncoordinated movements that may appear late in therapy and may not disappear even after the drug is stopped.

Fluphenazine has the potential to produce a serious side effect called **tardive dyskinesia**. This syndrome consists of involuntary, uncoordinated movements that may appear late in therapy and may not disappear even after the drug is stopped. Tardive dyskinesia involves involuntary movements of the tongue, jaw, mouth or face or other groups of skeletal muscles. The incidence of tardive dyskinesia increases with increasing age and with increasing dosage of fluphenazine. Women are at greater risk than men for developing tardive dyskinesia. There is no known effective treatment for tardive dyskinesia, although gradual (but rarely complete) improvement may occur over a long period.

An occasionally reported side effect of fluphenazine is **neuroleptic malignant syndrome**. This is a complicated and potentially fatal condition characterized by muscle rigidity; high fever; alterations in mental status; and cardiac symptoms such as irregular pulse or blood pressure, sweating, tachycardia (fast heartbeat), and arrhythmias (irregular heartbeat). People who think they may be experiencing any side effects from this or any other medication should tell their physician immediately.

Interactions

Barbiturates and the blood pressure drugs known as **beta blockers** can decrease the level of fluphenazine in the blood. Bromocriptine, a drug used for Parkinson's disease, also lowers the level of fluphenazine in the blood. Conversely, antimalarial drugs can increase the level of fluphenazine in the blood.

The combination of fluphenazine with the drugs known as cyclic **antidepressants** lowers the concentrations of both drugs in the blood. Fluphenazine inhibits the blood pressure-lowering effects of the drug called guanadrel. Levodopa, a drug given to patients with Parkinson's disease, is less effective when combined with fluphenazine. The combination of fluphenazine with meperidine can cause very low blood pressure and significant depression of the central nervous system. The use of the muscle relaxant, orphenadrine, can lower the effective levels of fluphenazine in the blood.

Resources

BOOKS

Ananth, Jambur. "Mode of Action of Antipsychotic Agents." *Trends in Schizophrenia Research,* edited by Mary V. Lang, 151–91. Hauppauge, NY: Nova Biomedical Books, 2005.

Consumer Reports Staff. *Consumer Reports Complete Drug Reference.* 2002 ed. Denver: Micromedex Thomson Healthcare, 2001.

Ellsworth, Allan J., et al. *Mosby's Medical Drug Reference.* 2001–2002 ed. St. Louis: Mosby, 2001.

Preston, John D., John H. O'Neal, and Mary C. Talaga. *Handbook of Clinical Psychopharmacology for Therapists.* 6th ed. Oakland, CA: New Harbinger, 2010.

Shanahan, James F., and Christie Naglieri, eds. *Goodman & Gilman's The Pharmacological Basis of Therapeutics.* 12th ed. New York: McGraw-Hill, 2011.

PERIODICALS

Bhagar, Harpriya A., and Alan D. Schmetzer. "The Conventional Long-Acting Antipsychotics." *Annals of the American Psychotherapy Association* 9, no. 1 (Spring 2006): 26–27.

Conley, Robert R., et al. "Risperidone, Quetiapine, and Fluphenazine in the Treatment of Patients with Therapy-Refractory Schizophrenia." *Clinical Neuropharmacology* 28, no. 4 (July/August 2005): 163–68.

Kelly, Deanna L., and Robert R. Conley. "Thyroid Function in Treatment-Resistant Schizophrenia Patients Treated with Quetiapine, Risperidone, or Fluphenazine." *Journal of Clinical Psychiatry* 66, no. 1 (January 2005): 80–84.

———. "A Randomized Double-Blind 12-Week Study of Quetiapine, Risperidone or Fluphenazine on Sexual Functioning in People with Schizophrenia." *Psychoneuroendocrinology* 31, no. 3 (April 2006): 340–46.

Stöllberger, Claudia, Johannes O. Huber, and Josef Finsterer. "Antipsychotic Drugs and QT Prolongation." *International Clinical Psychopharmacology* 20, no. 5 (September 2005): 243–51.

ORGANIZATIONS

American Psychiatric Association, 1000 Wilson Blvd., Ste. 1825, Arlington, VA, 22209-3901, (703) 907-7300, apa@psych.org, http://www.psych.org.

National Alliance on Mental Illness, 2107 Wilson Blvd., Ste. 300, Arlington, VA, 22201-3042, Fax: (703) 524-9094, (800) 950-6264, http://www.nami.org.

National Institute of Mental Health, 6001 Executive Blvd., Rm. 8184, MSC 9663, Bethesda, MD, 20892-9663, (301) 433-4513; TTY: (301) 443-8431, Fax: (301) 443-4279, (866) 615-6464; TTY: (866) 415-8051, nimhinfo@nih.gov, http://www.nimh.nih.gov.

Mark Mitchell, MD
Ruth A. Wienclaw, PhD

Flurazepam

Definition

Flurazepam is a benzodiazepine hypnotic (sleeping medication) that is given by mouth. It is sold in the United States under the brand name of Dalmane, but is also manufactured and sold by several companies under its generic name.

Purpose

Flurazepam is used for the short-term treatment of **insomnia**, a sleep disorder characterized by difficulty in falling or staying asleep.

Description

Flurazepam decreases the time it takes the patient to fall asleep and reduces the number of nighttime awakenings. Flurazepam is a member of a class of drugs called **benzodiazepines**. Such drugs are prescribed to reduce anxiety, relax the skeletal muscles, and induce sleep; other benzodiazepine hypnotics include **temazepam** (Restoril), **triazolam** (Halcion), **quazepam** (Doral), and **estazolam** (ProSom). Benzodiazepines work by enhancing the effects of a naturally occurring chemical in the body called gamma-aminobutyric acid (GABA). GABA is a neurotransmitter, a chemical that helps to conduct nerve impulses across the tiny gaps between nerve cells. GABA works to lower the level of activity in the central nervous system, promoting muscle relaxation, sedation, and sleep. It also plays a role in preventing seizure activity.

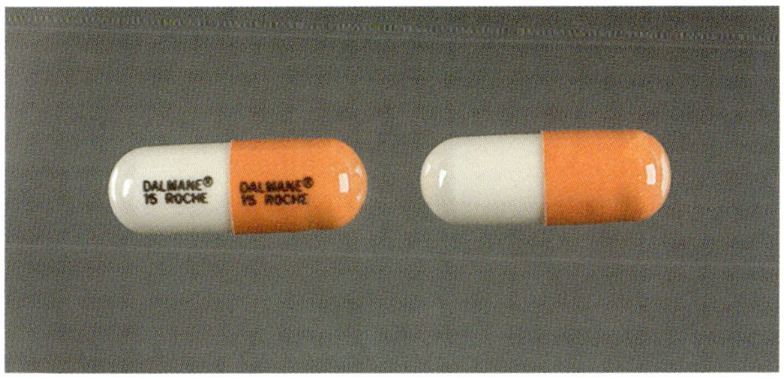

Dalmane (flurazepam), 15 mg. *(U.S. Drug Enforcement Administration)*

Flurazepam is available in 15 mg and 30 mg capsules.

Recommended dosage

The usual dose of flurazepam is 15–30 mg taken by mouth at bedtime. Older or physically weakened patients are usually given the lower dose. Children younger than 15 and women who are pregnant or nursing a baby should not be given flurazepam. In addition, the drug should not be used for longer than four weeks.

Precautions

Because flurazepam is used to help people fall asleep, it should only be taken when the patient is preparing for a full night's sleep (7 to 8 hours). Some patients taking sleep medications have engaged in sleep-related behaviors, including eating, talking, and even driving while asleep, with no recollection of the events. Some of the flurazepam is metabolized (broken down) in the body to form another compound called desalkylflurazepam, which remains in the body for a longer period of time and can cause next-day drowsiness. This kind of hangover effect is most common in people who are taking flurazepam on a daily basis. People who are taking flurazepam may not be able to safely operate machinery or drive a car the next day and should avoid these activities until they learn how the medication affects them.

Patients who take flurazepam for several days or weeks may experience a reaction called rebound insomnia when they stop taking the drug. When a person takes a medication for sleep on a regular basis, the body adjusts to the presence of the drug and tries to counteract the effects of the medication. As a result, when the person stops taking the sleeping medication, the body will take a few nights to return to its normal condition. During this period of readjustment, the person may experience a few sleepless hours each night.

Elderly patients who are taking flurazepam should be monitored for signs of dizziness or loss of coordination. They are at increased risk of falling if they wake up and get out of bed during the night to get a drink of water or use the bathroom.

Side effects

There is a risk of severe allergic reaction upon taking a sleep medication for the first time. Some people experience dizziness, daytime drowsiness, and loss of

KEY TERMS

Benzodiazepines—A group of central nervous system depressants used to relieve anxiety or to induce sleep.

Central nervous system depressant—Any drug that lowers the level of stimulation or excitement in the central nervous system.

Central nervous system stimulant—Any drug that raises the level of activity in the central nervous system.

Gamma-aminobutyric acid (GABA)—A neurotransmitter that helps to lower or reduce the level of excitement in the nerves, leading to muscle relaxation, calmness, sleep, and the prevention of seizures.

Hypnotic—A type of medication that induces sleep.

Metabolism—The group of biochemical processes within the body that release energy in support of life.

Neurotransmitter—A chemical in the brain that transmits messages between neurons, or nerve cells.

Rebound effect—A physical reaction to stopping a medication characterized by the reappearance of the symptom that the medication was given to suppress. For example, people who stop taking flurazepam may experience rebound insomnia.

coordination while they are taking flurazepam. Less common side effects include blurred vision, nausea and vomiting, diarrhea or constipation, nightmares, **depression**, and memory loss or **amnesia**.

Interactions

The effects of flurazepam may be intensified by alcoholic beverages or other central nervous system depressants, such as **sedatives** or antihistamines (allergy medications). These substances should be avoided when taking flurazepam. In addition, flurazepam may interact with antiseizure medications.

Resources

BOOKS

American Society of Health-System Pharmacists. *AHFS Drug Information 2008*. Bethesda, MD: American Society of Health-System Pharmacists, 2008.

Preston, John D., John H. O'Neal, and Mary C. Talaga. *Handbook of Clinical Psychopharmacology for Therapists*. 5th ed. Oakland, CA: New Harbinger Publications, 2008.

PERIODICALS

Blin, Olivier, et al. "A Double-Blind, Placebo- and Flurazepam-Controlled Investigation of the Residual Psychomotor and Cognitive Effects of Modified Release Zolpidem in Young Healthy Volunteers." *Journal of Clinical Psychopharmacology* 26, no. 3 (June 2006): 284–89.

Rosenberg, Russell P. "Sleep Maintenance Insomnia: Strengths and Weaknesses of Current Pharmacologic Therapies." *Annals of Clinical Psychiatry* 18, no. 1 (January–March 2006): 49–56.

Rowlett, James K., et al. "Anti-Conflict Effects of Benzodiazepines in Rhesus Monkeys: Relationship with Therapeutic Doses in Humans and Role of GABA-Sub(A) Receptors." *Psychopharmacology* 184, no. 2 (January 2006): 201–11.

Tamblyn, Robyn, et al. "A 5-Year Prospective Assessment of the Risk Associated with Individual Benzodiazepines and Doses in New Elderly Users." *Journal of the American Geriatrics Society* 53, no. 2 (February 2005): 233–41.

Thomas, Sandra P. "From the Editor—Caution Urged in Prescribing Psychotropic Drugs for Older Patients." *Issues in Mental Health Nursing* 26, no. 4 (May 2005): 357–58.

Jack Raber, Pharm.D.
Ruth A. Wienclaw, PhD

Fluvoxamine

Definition

Fluvoxamine is an antidepressant of the type known as **selective serotonin reuptake inhibitors** (SSRI). It is marketed in the United States under the brand name Luvox.

Purpose

Fluvoxamine is used to treat **obsessive-compulsive disorder** (OCD). It was the first SSRI to be approved by the U. S. Food and Drug Administration (FDA) for treating OCD in children, adolescents, and adults. It may also be prescribed off-label for treating **depression**, but it is not approved by the FDA for this purpose.

Description

Serotonin is a **brain** chemical that carries nerve impulses from one nerve cell to another. Researchers think that depression and certain other mental disorders may be caused, in part, by there not being enough serotonin

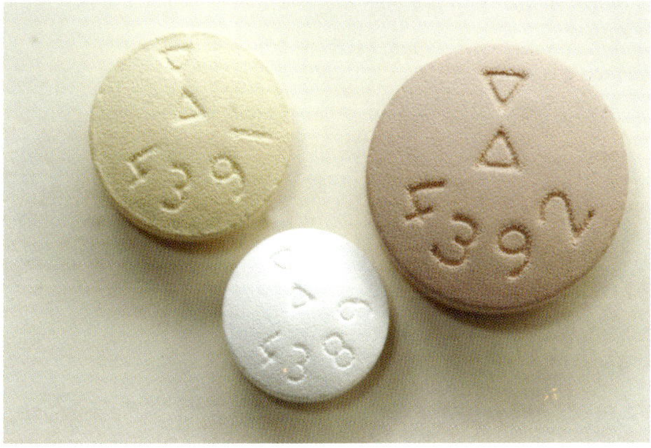

Fluvoxamine, 25, 50, and 100 mg. *(© Custom Medical Stock Photo, Inc. Reproduced by permission.)*

released and transmitted in the brain. Like the other SSRI **antidepressants**, **fluoxetine** (Prozac), **sertraline** (Zoloft), and **paroxetine** (Paxil), fluvoxamine increases the level of brain serotonin (also known as 5-HT). Increased serotonin levels in the brain may be beneficial in patients with OCD, alcoholism, certain types of headaches, **post-traumatic stress disorder** (PTSD), premenstrual tension and mood swings, and **panic disorder**.

Fluvoxamine was approved for use in adults in 1993. In 1997, the FDA approved this medication for the treatment of OCD in children and adolescents.

Fluvoxamine is available in 25, 50 and 100 mg tablets.

Recommended dosage

Fluvoxamine therapy in adults is started as a single 50 mg dose taken at bedtime. Based on the patient's response to the medication, the dosage can be increased by 50 mg every four to seven days, until maximum benefit is achieved. Maximum dosage is 300 mg per day. Dosage over 100 mg per day should be given as equally divided morning and afternoon doses.

Fluvoxamine therapy in children is started as a single 25 mg dose, initially taken at bedtime. Based on the patient's response to the medication, the dosage can be increased by 25 mg every four to seven days, until maximum benefit is achieved. Maximum dosage in children is 200 mg per day. Dosage over 100 mg per day should be given as equally divided morning and afternoon doses.

Precautions

Patients taking fluvoxamine should be monitored closely for the onset of mania, **seizures**, thoughts of **suicide**, and skin problems (including itching, hives, and rashes).

People with impaired liver function, **bipolar disorder** (manic depression), a history of seizures, or individuals contemplating suicide should take fluvoxamine only under close physician supervision.

A group of serious side effects, called **serotonin syndrome**, has resulted from the combination of SSRI drugs such as fluvoxamine and members of another class of antidepressants known as **monoamine oxidase inhibitors (MAOIs)**. Serotonin syndrome usually consists of at least three of the following symptoms:

- diarrhea
- fever
- extreme perspiration
- mood or behavior changes
- overactive reflexes
- fast heart rate
- restlessness
- shivering or shaking

Because of this risk, fluvoxamine should never be taken in combination with **MAOIs**. People taking any MAOI, for example, **phenelzine** sulfate (Nardil) or **tranylcypromine** sulfate (Parnate), should stop the MAOI inhibitor and wait at least 14 days before starting fluvoxamine or any other antidepressant. The same holds true when discontinuing fluvoxamine before starting an MAOI.

Physicians and their patients should weigh the risks and benefits of this drug for women who are or wish to become pregnant, as well as for women who are breastfeeding.

Until patients understand the effects that fluvoxamine may have on them, they should avoid driving, operating dangerous machinery, or participating in hazardous activities.

Like other **SSRIs**, fluvoxamine carries a warning regarding use in children and young people up to 24 years of age, who may be at risk for increased suicidal thoughts and actions during treatment, especially during the first few months. Persons with a personal history or family history of bipolar disorder or who have previously attempted or considered suicide are also at increased risk.

People should not use alcohol while taking fluvoxamine. Fluvoxamine treatment should not be abruptly discontinued.

Side effects

Common side effects of fluvoxamine therapy include decreased sex drive and diminished sexual performance.

Less common side effects of fluvoxamine therapy are changes in mood, behavior, or thinking; difficulty breathing; difficulty urinating; and twitches or uncontrollable movements of the face or body.

Rare side effects include:

- difficulty moving
- blurred vision
- clumsiness or problems with balance
- seizures
- difficulty moving the eyes
- increased uncontrollable movements of the body or face
- changes in the menstrual period
- redness or irritation of the eyes or skin
- peeling, itching, or burning sensation of the skin
- sore throat
- fever, and/or chills
- easy bruising
- nosebleeds
- in women, abnormal milk production

People may also experience symptoms of serotonin syndrome, which usually consists of at least three of the following:

- restlessness
- overexcitement
- irritability
- confusion
- diarrhea
- fever
- overactive reflexes
- difficulty with coordination
- uncontrollable shivering or shaking
- trembling or twitching

Interactions

Fluvoxamine interacts with a long list of other medications. Individuals who are starting this drug should review the other medications they are taking with their physician and pharmacist for possible interactions. Patients should always inform all their healthcare providers, including dentists, that they are taking fluvoxamine.

KEY TERMS

Off-label—The use of a prescription medication to treat conditions outside the indications approved by the Food and Drug Administration (FDA). It is legal for physicians to administer these drugs, but it is not legal for pharmaceutical companies to advertise drugs for off-label uses.

Serotonin—A brain chemical that carries nerve impulses from one nerve cell to another.

Serotonin syndrome—A condition that results from the combination of SSRI drugs such as fluvoxamine and members of another class of antidepressants known as monoamine oxidase inhibitors (MAOIs).

When taken together with fluvoxamine, the effect of the following drugs may be enhanced: **benzodiazepines**, **beta blockers**, **clozapine**, antiseizure drugs phenytoin and **carbamazepine**, tricyclic antidepressants, **pimozide**, and cholesterol-lowering drugs such as atorvastatin, lovastatin, and simvastatin.

The diet pills dexfenfluramine and fenfluramine may increase the incidence of serotonin syndrome when taken with fluvoxamine.

When **buspirone** is given with fluvoxamine, the therapeutic effect of buspirone may be decreased and the risk of seizures increased.

Increased risk of mania and high blood pressure occurs with selegiline.

Severe, fatal reactions mentioned above have occurred when fluvoxamine is given along with MAOIs.

Fluvoxamine given with warfarin (a blood thinner) may increase the possibility of bleeding.

Resources

BOOKS

Preston, John D., John H. O'Neal, and Mary C. Talaga. *Handbook of Clinical Psychopharmacology for Therapists.* 6th ed. Oakland, CA: New Harbinger, 2010.

PERIODICALS

Albers, Lawrence J., et al. "Low-Dose Fluvoxamine as an Adjunct to Reduce Olanzapine Therapeutic Dose Requirements: A Prospective Dose-Adjusted Drug Interaction Strategy." *Journal of Clinical Psychopharmacology* 25, no. 2 (April 2005): 170–74.

Erzegovesi, Stefano, et al. "Low-Dose Risperidone Augmentation of Fluvoxamine Treatment in Obsessive-Compulsive Disorder: A Double-Blind, Placebo-Controlled Study." *European Neuropsychopharmacology* 15, no. 1 (January 2005): 69–74.

Ginsburg, Golda S., Mark A. Riddle, and Mark Davies. "Somatic Symptoms in Children and Adolescents with Anxiety Disorders." *Journal of the American Academy of Child and Adolescent Psychiatry* 45, no. 10 (October 2006): 1179–87.

Husted, David S., et al. "Effect of Comorbid Tics on a Clinically Meaningful Response to 8-Week Open-Label Trial of Fluoxetine in Obsessive-Compulsive Disorder." *Journal of Psychiatric Research* 41, no. 3–4 (April–June 2007): 332–37.

Irons, Jane. "Fluvoxamine in the Treatment of Anxiety Disorders." *Neuropsychiatric Disease and Treatment* 1, no. 4 (2005): 289–99.

Mandelli, Laura, et al. "Improvement of Cognitive Functioning in Mood Disorder Patients with Depressive Symptomatic Recovery During Treatment: An Exploratory Analysis." *Psychiatry and Clinical Neurosciences* 60, no. 5 (October 2006): 598–604.

Morishita, Shigeru, and Seizaburo Arita. "Clinical Characteristics as Predictors of Response to Fluvoxamine, Paroxetine, and Milnacipran in Patients with Depression." *Current Psychiatry Reviews* 1, no. 3 (November 2005): 319–24.

———. "Treatment of Bipolar II Depression with Milnacipran, Fluvoxamine, Paroxetine, or Maprotiline." *International Medical Journal* 12, no. 4 (Dec. 2005): 283–85.

O'Connor, K.P., et al. "Cognitive Behaviour Therapy and Medication in the Treatment of Obsessive-Compulsive Disorder." *Acta Psychiatrica Scandinavica* 113, no. 5 (May 2006): 408–19.

Preskorn, Sheldon H., et al. "The Potential for Clinically Significant Drug-Drug Interactions Involving the CYP 2D6 System: Effects with Fluoxetine and Paroxetine Versus Sertraline." *Journal of Psychiatric Practice* 13, no. 1 (January 2007): 5–12.

Schreiber, Shaul, and Chaim G. Pick. "From Selective to Highly Selective SSRIs: A Comparison of the Antinociceptive Properties of Fluoxetine, Fluvoxamine, Citalopram and Escitalopram." *European Neuropsychopharmacology* 16, no. 6 (August 2006): 464–68.

Van Oppen, Patricia, et al. "Cognitive Therapy and Exposure in Vivo Alone and in Combination With Fluvoxamine in Obsessive-Compulsive Disorder: A 5-Year Follow-Up." *Journal of Clinical Psychiatry* 66, no. 11 (November 2005): 1415–22.

Yoshimura, Reiji, et al. "Successful Treatment for Obsessive-Compulsive Disorder with Addition of Low-Dose Risperidone to Fluvoxamine: Implications for Plasma Levels of Catecholamine Metabolites and Serum Brain-Derived Neurotrophic Factor Levels." *Psychiatry and Clinical Neurosciences* 60, no. 3 (June 2006): 389–93.

ORGANIZATIONS

American Psychiatric Association, 1000 Wilson Blvd., Ste. 1825, Arlington, VA, 22209-3901, (703) 907-7300, apa@psych.org, http://www.psych.org.

National Alliance on Mental Illness, 2107 Wilson Blvd., Ste. 300, Arlington, VA, 22201-3042, Fax: (703) 524-9094, (800) 950-6264, http://www.nami.org.

National Institute of Mental Health, 6001 Executive Blvd., Rm. 8184, MSC 9663, Bethesda, MD, 20892-9663, (301) 433-4513; TTY: (301) 443-8431, Fax: (301) 443-4279, (866) 615-6464; TTY: (866) 415-8051, nimhinfo@nih.gov, http://www.nimh.nih.gov.

Rosalyn Carson-DeWitt, MD
Ruth A. Wienclaw, PhD

Focalin, Focalin XR *see* **Dexmethylphenidate**

Folie á deux *see* **Shared psychotic disorder**

Folstein mini-mental state examination *see* **Mini-mental state examination**

Frontal lobe dementias *see* **Dementia**

Frontotemporal dementia *see* **Pick's disease**

Frotteurism

Definition

Frotteurism is a disorder in which a person derives sexual pleasure or gratification from rubbing, especially the genitals, against another person, usually in a crowd. The person being rubbed is a victim. Frotteurism is a paraphilia, a disorder that is characterized by recurrent intense sexual urges and sexually arousing fantasies generally involving objects, the suffering or humiliation of oneself or one's partner (not merely simulated), or children or other nonconsenting people.

Demographics

Males are much more likely to engage in frotteurism than females. Females are the most common victims of frotteurism. Most acts of frotteurism are performed by people between 15 to 25 years of age. After the age of 25, the acts decline.

Description

The primary focus of frotteurism is touching or rubbing one's genitals against the clothing or body of a nonconsenting person. This behavior most often occurs in situations that allow rapid escape. The frottage (the act of rubbing against the other person) is most commonly practiced in crowded places such as malls, elevators, on busy sidewalks, and on public transportation vehicles.

The most commonly practiced form of frotteurism is rubbing one's genitals against the victim's thighs or buttocks. A common alternative is to rub one's hands over the victim's genitals or breasts.

Most people who engage in frotteurism (sometimes called frotteurs) usually fantasize that they have an exclusive and caring relationship with their victims during the moment of contact. However, once contact is made and broken, the person committing the act realizes that escape is important to avoid prosecution.

KEY TERMS

Frottage—The act of touching or rubbing against the body or genitals of a nonconsenting individual.

Paraphilia—A disorder that is characterized by recurrent intense sexual urges and sexually arousing fantasies generally involving (1) nonhuman objects, (2) the suffering or humiliation of oneself or one's partner (not merely simulated), or (3) children or other nonconsenting people.

Causes and symptoms

Causes

There is no scientific consensus concerning the cause of frotteurism. Most experts attribute the behavior to an initially random or accidental touching of another's genitals that the person finds sexually exciting. Successive repetitions of the act tend to reinforce and perpetuate the behavior.

Symptoms

For the disorder to be clinically diagnosed, the symptoms must meet the diagnostic criteria as listed in the professional's handbook, the ***Diagnostic and Statistical Manual of Mental Disorders.*** These symptoms include:

- experiencing recurrent, intense, or sexually arousing fantasies, sexual urges, or behaviors that involve touching and rubbing against a nonconsenting person
- acting on these sexual urges, or the fantasies or urges cause significant distress to the individual or are disruptive to his everyday functioning

Diagnosis

Most people with frotteurism never seek professional help, but people with the disorder may come into the mental health system as a result of a court order. The **diagnosis** is established in an interview between the person accused of frotteurism and the mental health professional (a **psychiatrist** or a **psychologist**, for example). In the interview, the individual acknowledges that touching others is a preferred or exclusive means of sexual gratification. Because this acknowledgment can bring criminal charges, the disorder is underdiagnosed and its prevalence is largely unknown. In some cases, other people besides the accused may be interviewed, including observers or the victim.

Treatment

For treatment to be successful, the patient must want to modify existing patterns of behavior. This initial step is difficult for most people with this disorder to take.

Behavior therapy is commonly used to try to treat frotteurism. The patient must learn to control the impulse to touch nonconsenting victims. One pharmacological therapy that has been tried with some success in people who engage in frotteurism and other **paraphilias** is leuprolide. The action of this drug ultimately results in suppression of testosterone production, with the effect of reducing sexual urges.

Frotteurism is a criminal act in many jurisdictions. It is usually classified as a misdemeanor. As a result, legal penalties are often minor. It is also not easy to prosecute people who are charged with frotteurism because intent to touch is difficult to prove. In their defense statements, the accused often claim that the contact was accidental.

Prognosis

The prognosis for eliminating frotteurism is poor as most people who engage in the behavior have no desire to change it. Because frotteurism involves nonconsenting partners and is against the law in many jurisdictions, the possibility of embarrassment may deter some individuals.

Prevention

Most experts agree that providing guidance as to behavior that is culturally acceptable will prevent the development of a paraphilia such as frotteurism. The origin of some instances of frotteurism may be a truly accidental contact that becomes associated with sexual gratification. There is no way to predict when such an association will occur.

Resources

BOOKS

American Psychiatric Association. *Diagnostic and Statistical Manual of Mental Disorders*. 4th ed., text rev. Washington, DC: American Psychiatric Publishing, 2000.

Gelder, Michael, Paul Harrison, and Philip Cowen. *Shorter Oxford Textbook of Psychiatry*. 5th ed. New York: Oxford University Press, 2006.

Kohut, John J., and Roland Sweet. *Real Sex: Titillating but True Tales of Bizarre Fetishes, Strange Compulsions, and Just Plain Weird Stuff*. New York: Penguin Group, 2000.

Wilson, Josephine F. *Biological Foundations of Human Behavior*. Farmington Hills, MI: Cengage Learning, 2002.

PERIODICALS

Eiguer, A. "Cynicism: Its Function in the Perversions." *International Journal of Psychoanalysis* 80, no. 4 (1999): 671–84.

Rosler, A., and E. Witztum. "Pharmacotherapy of Paraphilias in the Next Millennium." *Behavioral Sciences & the Law* 18, no. 1 (January/February 2000): 43–56.

Schober, Justine M., Peter M. Byrne, and Phyllis J. Kuhn. "Leuprolide Acetate is a Familiar Drug that May Modify Sex-Offender Behavior: The Urologist's Role." *BJU International* 97, no. 4 (April 2006) 684–86.

Seelig, B.J., and L.S. Rosof. "Normal and Pathological Altruism." *Journal of the American Psychoanalytic Association* 49, no. 3 (2001): 933–59.

ORGANIZATIONS

American Psychiatric Association, 1000 Wilson Blvd., Ste. 1825, Arlington, VA, 22209-3901, (703) 907-7300, apa@psych.org, http://www.psych.org.

American Psychological Association, 750 1st St. NE, Washington, DC, 20002-4242, (202) 336-5500; TDD/TTY: (202) 336-6123, (800) 374-2721, http://www.apa.org.

L.Fleming Fallon, Jr., MD, Dr.P.H.
Emily Jane Willingham, PhD

Fugue *see* **Dissociative fugue**

G

Gabapentin

Definition

Gabapentin is an antiseizure medication. It is sold in the United States under the trade name Neurontin.

Purpose

Gabapentin is used in combination with other antiseizure (anticonvulsant) drugs to manage partial **seizures** with or without generalization in individuals over the age of 12. Gabapentin can also be used to treat partial seizures in children between the ages of 3 and 12. Off-label uses (legal uses not approved by the U.S. Food and Drug Administration [FDA]) include treatment of severe, chronic pain caused by nerve damage, such as occurs in shingles, diabetic neuropathy, multiple sclerosis, or post-herpetic neuralgia. Gabapentin was previously studied in the treatment of **bipolar disorder** but did not show any effectiveness in **clinical trials**.

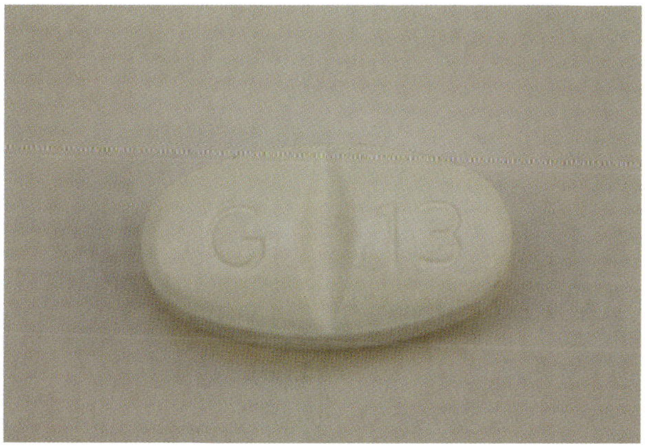

Gabapentin, 800 mg. *(© Custom Medical Stock Photo, Inc. Reproduced by permission.)*

Description

Brain cells normally transmit nerve impulses from one cell to another by secreting chemicals known as **neurotransmitters**. Gabapentin is chemically related to a naturally occurring neurotransmitter called GABA (gamma-amino butyric acid). The actual mechanism of action by which gabapentin acts in the brain to control seizures and treat pain is not known, although it appears to alter the action of nerve cells.

Gabapentin was approved for use in the United States in 1993. A liquid formulation was approved for use in 2000. Use in children ages 3 to 12 was also approved by the FDA in 2000.

Gabapentin is available in 100, 300, and 400 mg capsules; in 600 and 800 mg tablets; and in a liquid solution containing 250 mg per 5 mL.

Recommended dosage

For epilepsy

People over the age of 12 can begin with an initial does of 300 mg three times a day, which can be gradually increased as necessary, usually to no more than 1,800 mg daily. For children ages 3 to 12, the dose is based on body weight, initially 10–15 mg per kilogram per day in three separate doses. The physician may choose to increase this dose as necessary. For a child under the age of 3, the decision about use and dosage will be made by the doctor. For older adults, the maximum daily dose does not usually exceed 600 mg three times a day.

For pain

This dosing involves a gradual increase, with an initial does of 300 mg on the first day, followed by 300 mg twice on the second day, and 300 mg three times on day three. A physician may increase this dose to a maximum daily dose of 1,800 mg.

Precautions

Women who are breast-feeding and people with decreased kidney functioning should discuss the risks and benefits of this drug with their physician. Women who are or wish to become pregnant will also require a careful assessment of the risks and benefits of gabapentin.

Patients should not suddenly discontinue gabapentin, which can result in an increased risk of seizures. If the medication needs to be discontinued, the dosage should be reduced gradually over a week.

Until an individual understands the effects that gabapentin may have, he or she should avoid driving, operating dangerous machinery, or participating in hazardous activities. Alcohol should be avoided while taking gabapentin.

Some patients taking gabapentin have shown changes in their mental health, including the development of suicidal thoughts and behavior. If patients taking gabapentin exhibit any changes in mood or behavior they (or their caregivers) should contact their physician.

Side effects

Multiple side effects often occur when a patient starts taking gabapentin. While these side effects usually go away on their own, if they last or are particularly troublesome, the patient should consult a doctor. More common side effects that occur when first starting to take gabapentin include blurred or double vision; muscle weakness or pain; swollen hands, feet, or legs; trembling or shaking; increased **fatigue** or weakness; unsteadiness; clumsiness; and uncontrollable back-and-forth eye movements or eye rolling. Less common side effects include back pain, constipation, decreased sexual drive, diarrhea, dry mouth and eyes, frequent urination, headache, indigestion, low blood pressure, nausea, ringing in the ears, runny nose, slurred speech, difficulty thinking and sleeping, weight gain, twitching, nausea and/or vomiting, weakness, **depression**, irritability, other mood changes or changes in thinking, and decreased memory. Rare side effects include pain in the lower back or side, difficulty urinating, fever and/or chills, cough, or hoarseness.

Children under age 12 who have the following more common side effects should see a doctor immediately: aggressive behavior, irritability, anxiety, difficulty concentrating and paying attention, crying, depression, mood swings, increased emotionality, hyperactivity, and suspiciousness or distrust.

KEY TERMS

Diabetic neuropathy—A condition in which the nerve endings, particularly in the legs and feet, become less sensitive. Minor injuries, such as blisters or callouses, are not felt and can thus become infected and become more serious problems.

Multiple sclerosis—A disease characterized by patches of hardened tissue in the brain or spinal cord, paralysis, and/or muscle tremors.

Neuralgia—Pain that extends along the course of a nerve.

Neurotransmitter—A chemical in the brain that transmits messages between neurons, or nerve cells.

Interactions

Antacids can decrease gabapentin levels in the blood. They should be taken at least two hours before taking gabapentin.

Resources

BOOKS

Ellsworth, Allan J., et al. *Mosby's Medical Drug Reference*. St. Louis, MO: Mosby, 2007.

PERIODICALS

Vieta, Eduard, et al. "A Double-Blind, Randomized Placebo-Controlled, Prophylaxis Study of Adjunctive Gabapentin for Bipolar Disorder." *Journal of Clinical Psychiatry* 67, no. 3 (March 2006): 473–77.

WEBSITES

MedlinePlus. "Gabapentin." National Library of Medicine, National Institutes of Health. September 22, 2011. http://www.nlm.nih.gov/medlineplus/druginfo/meds/a694007.html (accessed October 7, 2011).

Rosalyn Carson-DeWitt, MD
Emily Jane Willingham, PhD

Galantamine

Definition

Galantamine belongs to a class of drugs called acetylcholinesterase inhibitors. In the United States, galantamine is sold under the brand name Razadyne (formerly Reminyl).

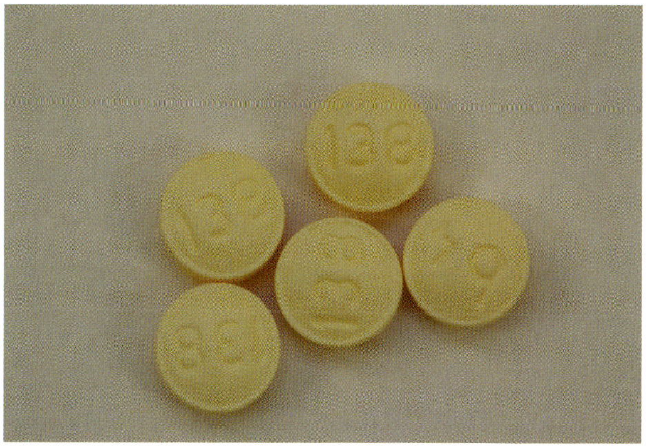

Galantamine, 4 mg. *(© Custom Medical Stock Photo, Inc. Reproduced by permission.)*

KEY TERMS

Acetylcholine—A naturally occurring chemical in the body that transmits nerve impulses from cell to cell. Acetylcholine causes blood vessels to dilate, lowers blood pressure, and slows the heartbeat. Central nervous system well-being is dependent on a balance among the neurotransmitters acetylcholine, dopamine, serotonin, and norepinephrine.

Acetylcholinesterase—The chemical responsible for the breakdown of acetylcholine.

Parkinson's disease—A disease of the nervous system most common in people over age 60, characterized by a shuffling gait, trembling of the fingers and hands, and muscle stiffness.

Purpose

Galantamine is used to treat the symptoms of **Alzheimer's disease** (AD).

Description

Alzheimer's disease develops when **brain** cells, called neurons, undergo an early death. Though AD cannot be cured, it is thought that the premature death of these neurons may be prevented or slowed if stimulated by a brain chemical called acetylcholine. Acetylcholine is recycled by an enzyme called acetylcholinesterase. Galantamine works by inhibiting this enzyme. The inhibition of acetylcholinesterase increases the concentration of available acetylcholine.

Galantamine has only been studied and is only used, in patients with mild-to-moderate AD according to the Alzheimer's Disease Assessment Scale. It is not used in patients with severe AD.

Galantamine is available in 4 mg, 8 mg, and 12 mg tablets.

Recommended dosage

The recommended initial dose of galantamine in adults is 4 mg twice daily. After a minimum of four weeks of treatment with galantamine, the dosage may be increased to 8 mg twice daily. Further increases to 12 mg twice daily should be initiated only after a minimum of four weeks at the previous dose.

Increased side effects associated with higher doses may prevent the increase in dose in some patients. Patients with moderate liver or kidney problems should not exceed 16 mg of galantamine daily.

Precautions

Galantamine should not be used in patients with severe liver or kidney problems. Since there are no well-controlled studies for the use of galantamine in pregnancy, galantamine should only be used if the potential benefits justify the potential risks to the fetus.

Patients who are undergoing anesthesia or bladder or gastrointestinal surgery should take galantamine only after a discussion with their physician. Patients with gastrointestinal problems should be closely monitored if it is decided that they should take galantamine. Galantamine should also be used under close physician supervision in patients who have Parkinson's disease, severe asthma, or chronic obstructive pulmonary disease. Because galantamine may slow down the heart, patients with any heart conditions, and especially patients taking other medications that slow down the heart, should be evaluated before taking galantamine.

Side effects

The most common side effects reported with the use of galantamine are nausea, vomiting, diarrhea, loss of appetite, and abdominal pain. These occur most often during dosage escalation. The average duration of nausea is five to seven days. Side effects tend to be less frequent if the patient is taking a total daily dosage of 16 mg. Eleven percent of patients receiving 24 mg daily lose weight, while 6% of patients receiving 16 mg daily experience weight loss.

Other common side effects include dizziness, headache, tremors, **fatigue**, **depression**, agitation, irritation, and **insomnia**. These side effects have a higher incidence and severity if higher doses are used. If side effects become severe, the dosage should be adjusted downward under physician supervision.

Interactions

There is currently little data regarding potential drug interactions with galantamine. Medications that are known to increase levels of galantamine in the body include cimetidine, erythromycin, ketoconazole, and **paroxetine**.

Resources

PERIODICALS

Ancoli-Israel, Sonia, et al. "Effects of Galantamine Versus Donepezil on Sleep in Patients with Mild to Moderate Alzheimer Disease and Their Caregivers: A Double-Blind, Head-To-Head, Randomized Pilot Study." *Alzheimer Disease & Associated Disorders* 19, no. 4 (October/December 2005): 240–45.

Biederman, Joseph, et al. "A Double-Blind Comparison of Galantamine Hydrogen Bromide and Placebo in Adults with Attention-Deficit/Hyperactivity Disorder: A Pilot Study." *Journal of Clinical Psychopharmacology* 26, no. 2 (April 2006): 163–66.

Brodaty, Henry, et al. "Galantamine Prolonged-Release Formulation in the Treatment of Mild to Moderate Alzheimer's Disease." *Dementia and Geriatric Cognitive Disorders* 20, no. 2–3 (August 2005): 120–32.

Harry, Robin D. J., and Konstantine K. Zakzanis. "A Comparison of Donepezil and Galantamine in the treatment of Cognitive Symptoms of Alzheimer's Disease: A Meta-Analysis." *Human Psychopharmacology: Clinical and Experimental* 20, no. 3 (April 2005): 183–87.

Koontz, Jennifer, and Andrius Baskys. "Effects of Galantamine on Working Memory and Global Functioning in Patients with Mild Cognitive Impairment: A Double-Blind Placebo-Controlled Study." *American Journal of Alzheimer's Disease and Other Dementias* 20, no. 5 (September/October 2005): 295–302.

López-Pousa, S., et al. "Differential Efficacy of Treatment with Acetylcholinesterase Inhibitors in Patients with Mild and Moderate Alzheimer's Disease Over a 6-Month Period." *Dementia and Geriatric Cognitive Disorders* 19, no. 4 (March 2005): 189–95.

Ochoa, Enrique L. M. "Galantamine May Improve Attention and Speech in Schizophrenia." *Human Psychopharmacology: Clinical and Experimental* 21, no. 2 (March 2006): 127–28.

Robinson, Dean M., and Greg L. Plosker. "Galantamine Extended Release in Alzheimer's Disease: Profile Report." *Drugs and Aging* 23, no. 10 (2006): 839–42.

Rockwood, Kenneth, et al. "Attainment of Treatment Goals by People with Alzheimer's Disease Receiving Galantamine: A Randomized Controlled Trial." *Canadian Medical Association Journal* 174, no. 8 (April 11, 2006): 1099–1105.

Schubert, Max H., Keith A. Young, and Paul B. Hicks. "Galantamine Improves Cognition in Schizophrenic Patients Stabilized on Risperidone." *Biological Psychiatry* 60, no. 6 (September 2006): 530–33.

Takeda, A., et al. "A Systematic Review of the Clinical Effectiveness of Donepezil, Rivastigmine and Galantamine on Cognition, Quality of Life and Adverse Events in Alzheimer's Disease." *International Journal of Geriatric Psychiatry* 21, no. 1 (January 2006): 17–28.

WEBSITES

Ortho-McNeil Neurologics, Inc. "Full U.S. Prescribing Information for Razadyne." http://www.razadyneer360.com/full-prescribing-information.html (accessed October 7, 2011).

Ajna Hamidovic, Pharm.D.
Ruth A. Wienclaw, PhD

Gambling disorder

Definition

Gambling disorder (GD), sometimes also called pathological gambling disorder, occurs when a person gambles compulsively to such an extent that the wagering has a severe negative effect on his or her job or career, relationships, mental health, or other important aspects of life. The person may continue to gamble even after they have developed social, economic, interpersonal, or legal problems as a result of the gambling.

The related medical term "ludomania" is defined as a progressive urge to gamble, one that eventually becomes a gambling disorder characterized by frequent, uncontrollable episodes of compulsive gambling. Medical professionals can **diagnosis** clinical pathological

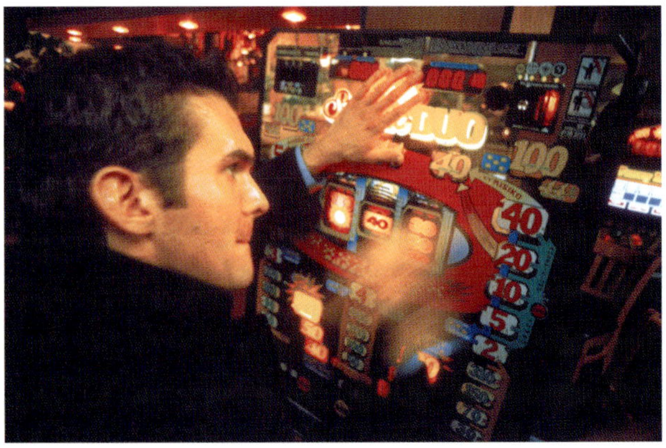

A man plays a slot machine in a casino. *(© Mika/Corbis)*

gambling when the patient meets certain criteria. Such problem gambling is considered an impulse control disorder in medicine.

Demographics

About twice as many males as females in the United States are diagnosed with gambling disorder. Relatively few women, however, are in treatment programs for the disorder, probably because of the greater social **stigma** attached to women who gamble. As a rule, men diagnosed with gambling disorder began gambling as teenagers, whereas women tend to start compulsive gambling at a later age and develop a gambling problem faster than men. In addition, women are developing a gambling disorder at rates that are up to 25% higher than are men. Gambling disorder also tends to be more common in minority groups and in people of a lower socioeconomic status. About 25% of people diagnosed as pathological gamblers had a parent with the disorder. People who smoke tobacco or abuse alcohol are more likely to have GD than people who do not use these substances.

As much as 5% of the general population in the United States may meet criteria for gambling disorder at some point in their lives. In some countries, such as Australia, the number is thought to be as high as 7%.

Description

Gambling disorder is characterized by uncontrollable gambling well beyond the point of a social or recreational activity, such that the gambling has a major disruptive effect on the gambler's life. People who are pathological gamblers may lose their life savings and may even commit crimes (e.g., stealing, embezzling, or forging checks) to get money for their "habit." Relationships and jobs may also be lost as a result of the disorder.

Gambling disorder is sometimes considered as an example of a process, or behavioral, **addiction**, which is as distinct from an addiction to such substances as food, drugs, tobacco, or alcohol. In process addictions, the characteristic "rush" or "high" comes from the series of steps or actions that are involved in the addictive behavior. With gambling, the "high" may be stimulated by the social atmosphere or group setting of the casino, race track, or bingo hall as well as by the excitement of risk-taking. Some gamblers have a "lucky" outfit, item of clothing, or accessory that they wear or take along when gambling; sometimes putting on the outfit or item in question is enough to start the "rush."

People with gambling disorder may engage in many different types of gambling activities. These may include games of chance that are found in casinos, such as slot machines, card games, and roulette. Many of these games are now available on the Internet, the chief difference being that the bettor uses a credit card instead of cash or chips. Other gambling activities may include the state lottery, horse or dog racing, or bingo. The person may place bets on the outcome of an election, baseball or football games, or even the weather on a particular day. Pathological gambling usually develops slowly; people tend to begin with acceptable levels of social or recreational gambling and slowly progress to pathological gambling. In most cases the disorder develops slowly over a period of years; however, there are cases of patients who gambled socially for decades and then began to gamble compulsively under the impact of a major life stressor, such as divorce or being laid off from work.

The **American Psychiatric Association**, through its upcoming *Diagnostic and Statistical Manual of Mental Disorders 5* (*DSM-5*), has proposed to reclassify gambling disorder from the category Impulse-Control Disorders Not Elsewhere Classified to the category Substance-Related Disorders, which will be renamed Addiction and Related Disorders. The revised version (*DSM-5*) of the ***Diagnostic and Statistical Manual of Mental Disorders*** is scheduled to be available in 2013.

Causes and symptoms

Causes

Gambling disorder is considered a **brain** disease similar to other disorders of addiction, like alcohol or drug addiction. The primary mechanism underlying the development and persistence of pathological gambling is the brain's dopamine-based reward system, which is thought to underlie many disorders of addiction or impulse control. The central pathway involved is the mesolimbic pathway of **dopamine** signaling. This pathway exhibits alterations in dopamine levels or signaling in response to some substances; and a similar dopamine response is thought by medical professionals to underlie process addictions, including pathological gambling. The key feature in the brain involved in this process is the nucleus accumbens.

There also are significant psychological factors that may contribute to excessive gambling, often associated with the common comorbidities of pathological gambling, including **depression** and substance use disorder. People who are pathological gamblers may use gambling as an emotional escape from depression; this pattern appears more often in females with the disorder than in males. Some people who are pathological gamblers seek the mood alteration associated with gambling—specifically the excitement and energy that they find in the activity—more than the money involved. In other words, the person with the disorder is reinforced by an emotional "high" rather than by the money itself. Some researchers have found that males diagnosed with gambling disorder were more likely to have been diagnosed with **attention deficit hyperactivity disorder (ADHD)** as children than males in the general population. Other researchers have described compulsive gamblers in general as highly competitive people who are restless and easily bored. People with this disorder exhibit many features in common with those who have substance use disorder, including the urge to engage in the behavior, mounting tension before engaging in the behavior, relief or euphoria during the behavior, a return of the urge, and the presence of external cues that may trigger the behavior.

Other theories about the causes of gambling disorder emphasize cognitive distortions rather than mood problems. Pathological gambling has been associated with dysfunctional thinking patterns; many people with this disorder are highly superstitious or believe that they can control the outcome of events when they are gambling. Many people diagnosed with the disorder also have distorted beliefs about money, tending to see it at the same time as the source of all their problems and the answer to all their problems.

One social change that has been linked with the rise in the number of adults diagnosed with gambling disorder in the United States is the increased availability of legalized gambling. Some studies show that proximity to a casino is associated with increased rates of pathological gambling in a population. However, other studies show the opposite. For instance, a 2008 study in the journal *Psychology of Addictive Behaviors* found that the rates of pathological gambling were not higher near a casino when compared to rates away from such establishments. The study did find, however, that participation and monetary expenditures in gambling establishments were higher the closer in distance individuals were to gambling places.

Symptoms

The symptoms of pathological gambling include preoccupation with gambling activity, often to the extent of interfering with the person's occupational or social functioning. The person often cannot control the gambling behavior, continuing to place bets or go to casinos in spite of attempts to cut back or stop. One common behavior in persons with gambling disorder is "chasing," which refers to betting larger sums of money or taking greater risks in order to undo or make up for previous losses. The person may also lie about his or her gambling or engage in such antisocial behaviors as stealing, credit card fraud, check forgery, embezzling from an employer, or similar dishonest behaviors in order to obtain more money for gambling.

KEY TERMS

Dopamine—A chemical neurotransmitting compound found in the brain that is a precursor of epinephrine.

Functional magnetic resonance imaging—A special type of magnetic resonance imaging (MRI) scan that measures changes in blood flow and blood oxygenation within the body; often abbreviated fMRI.

Histrionic—Relating to being very dramatic or excessive in behavior.

Narcissistic—Relating to a personality disorder in which an individual overestimates his or her own abilities or appearance, such as an extraordinary ability to win at gambling.

Nucleus accumbens—Abbreviated NAcc and also known as accumbens nucleus, is a part of the brain reward system, located in the limbic system, that processes information related to motivation and reward.

Opioid antagonist—A type of receptor antagonist (drug) that acts on opioid receptors.

Pathological—Uncontrollable in nature; relating to disease.

Diagnosis

Pathological gambling disorder is more likely to be diagnosed when the affected person's spouse or family becomes concerned than to be self-reported. **Denial** is common among persons with the disorder. The professional handbook, the *Diagnostic and Statistical Manual of Mental Disorders*, fourth edition, text revision (*DSM-IV-TR*) specifies that the patient must have at least five of the following symptoms to meet criteria for the disorder:

- thinks about gambling all the time
- uses larger and larger amounts of money when gambling
- has tried to stop gambling but failed
- is moody or cranky when trying to stop gambling
- uses gambling as a way to escape problems
- keeps gambling to try to make back money that had previously been lost ("chasing")

- lies about the extent of gambling
- has tried to make money for gambling by engaging in illegal or immoral behavior
- has problems at work or home caused by the gambling
- relies on other people to get him or her out of financial problems caused by the gambling.

Gambling disorder is distinguished from social gambling, in which the person is typically socializing with friends, gambling for a limited period of time, and gambling with a limited sum of money that they can afford to lose. GD is also distinguished from professional gambling, in which participants limit their risks, and discipline their behaviors. Lastly, gambling disorder must be distinguished from a **manic episode**; in most cases, the distinguishing feature of the disorder is that the manic-like behavior disappears after the person leaves the gambling setting, and that other symptoms of a manic episode, such as euphoria, irritability, and sleeplessness, are not present.

Treatment

There are a number of different treatments for gambling disorder. **Psychodynamic psychotherapy** attempts to uncover any underlying psychological factors that trigger the gambling. For people who are gambling to escape, such as those who are depressed, this approach may be very successful. Treating any **substance abuse** problems that may coexist with the pathological gambling can also be helpful. Other types of treatments involve behavioral techniques used to teach relaxation and avoidance of stimuli associated with gambling. **Aversion therapy** appears to be successful in treating pathological gambling disorder in highly motivated patients with some insight into the problem, but is not helpful for patients who are less educated or resistant to behavioral methods of treatment.

Gamblers Anonymous (GA) is a twelve-step program modeled after Alcoholics Anonymous (AA). The gambler's admission that she or he does have a gambling problem, and a willingness to go to meetings are considered the first steps in treating gambling disorder. Looking realistically at what gambling has done to a person's life and a willingness to work hard to stop gambling are also important parts of GA. People involved in this program are expected to attend meetings regularly, make amends for wrongs that their gambling has caused, and find a sponsor (usually of the same gender) to help them through the program. GA also expects people who stop gambling to understand that they probably will never be able to gamble again socially, just as recovering alcoholics cannot drink socially.

Pharmacological treatments for pathological gambling and other process addictions are still being developed and explored. In studies reported thus far, the most effective pharmaceutical treatment has been opioid antagonists, such as **naltrexone** (Depade, ReVia) or nalmefene (Revex), possibly because of their effects on opioid pathways that interact with dopamine signaling pathways in the brain reward system. Treatment may also target co-morbidities of pathological gambling, such as using **selective serotonin reuptake inhibitors (SSRIs)** if mood disorder or **obsessive-compulsive disorder** is present.

Doctors at the University of California at Los Angeles (UCLA), are treating gambling disorders as a brain disease. The amount and severity of gambling disorder in California is increasing annually. Consequently, the state provided $15 million for three years, beginning around 2011, to fund treatment programs for California citizens with a gambling disorder. Dr. Timothy Fong, the codirector of the UCLA Gambling Studies Program, works with the state's Office of Problem Gambling to design, develop, and evaluate treatment programs for gambling disorder. Part of the state funding for gambling disorder is to certify nearly 300 mental health therapists in the treatment of gambling problems.

Prognosis

There are very few statistics on the number of people successfully treated for gambling disorder. It is estimated that one-third of all people with gambling disorder can recover from the disease without treatment. However, that still leaves two-thirds who do not recover. In fact, as many as two out of three people who begin treatment (medication, therapy, or both) for gambling disorder drop out before its completion. Consequently, the negative effects of gambling disorder often leave their lives, and their family, in ruin. It is estimated that $5 billion is spent annually on gambling in the United States. However, during each of those years, people with a gambling disorder are estimated to have accrued tens to hundreds of thousands of dollars in debt.

Besides financial problems, people with gambling disorders suffer from a multitude of mental problems, such as an increased risk of causing domestic violence and **child abuse**. The mental problems are not reserved to the problem gamblers. Children of gamblers with problems are at increased risk from suffering behavioral problems, depression, and substance abuse.

Treatment for any underlying psychological disorders or substance abuse can be very helpful. Sometimes **family therapy** is recommended. Some types of relaxation or behavioral therapy can also be helpful. Gamblers Anonymous can help in many cases, although the program has a high dropout and recurrence rate, and there are few studies that fully analyze the benefits or efficacy of the program. For many people, a combination of more than one of these approaches may be most effective. Even when a person has successfully stopped compulsive gambling, it is unlikely that he or she will ever be able to gamble socially again, or even spend time in places where he or she once gambled.

The Institute for Research on Gambling Disorders announced that five new research projects were awarded in 2010 for the study of gambling disorders. The grants, which totaled $380,466, were awarded by the National Center for Responsible Gaming to researchers at Duke University (North Carolina), Southern Illinois University, the University of Florida, the University of Minnesota, and the University of Missouri.

The research studies were in the grant areas called Exploration Grants, Seed Grants, and Large Grants. The Exploration Grants involve evaluating the risk difference of online gambling versus non-Internet based gambling. A virtual Internet site will be built to simulate online gambling. Subjects will be divided into a pathological gambling group and a control group. Using functional **magnetic resonance imaging** (fMRI) scans, the researchers from the University of Florida will research the neurological activity in the brain when excessive gambling is involved.

Duke University researchers were granted a Seed Grant to test the hypothesis that whether "someone makes a risky or safe choice depends not simply on preferences, but on the strategies they use to acquire and integrate new information." The study will provide further information on the reasons why some people make risky decisions while gambling. Another Seed Grant was awarded to scientists at Southern Illinois University to use fMRI to examine the brain activity of "disordered gamblers" before and after undergoing acceptance and commitment therapy, which is a new therapy being developed to help treat gambling disorders.

Researchers at the University of Missouri were awarded a Large Grant of $172,500 to test whether college students report more or less gambling when they are provided information about their own behaviors while gambling (in what is called "personalized feedback-only intervention"). In addition, University of Minnesota scientists will study the various factors, such as race and gender, which distinguish recreational gamblers and pathological gamblers. They will also study factors that may be responsible for turning recreational gamblers into problem gamblers. This study will use data from the National Epidemiologic Survey on Alcohol and Related Conditions.

In addition, a research study performed in Australia has shown that nearly one in five problem gamblers (17%) has attempted **suicide**. Their statistics are based on patients entering the emergency department at the Alfred hospital in Prahran, Victoria, Australia. The report concluded that this rate of suicide among problem gamblers is about 20 times the rate in a normal population without gambling problems. Commenting on the results of the Australian report, state gaming minister Tony Robinson stated that "one of the underlying drivers of problem gambling is a pre-existing mental health condition."

QUESTIONS TO ASK YOUR DOCTOR

- Am I addicted to gambling?
- Where can I find more information on gambling disorder?
- I can't afford treatment. Will my medical insurance pay for it?
- Do I have an underlying mental illness that is causing me to have gambling disorder?
- How do I stop gambling?
- What type of medicine do you recommend?
- What type of treatment is best for me?

Prevention

Prevention of pathological gambling disorder is very difficult because it is impossible to predict when someone will react to gambling in a way that leads to compulsive gambling. If, however, a person begins to feel that he or she may have a problem, immediate treatment can prevent the development of a disorder that affects all areas of life and may have legal as well as economic consequences. Given the role of proximity to available gambling in the development of the disorder, this factor may be a target in prevention.

Resources

BOOKS

Adamec, Christine. *Pathological Gambling.* New York: Chelsea House, 2011.

Diagnostic and Statistical Manual of Mental Disorders 4th ed., text rev. American Psychiatric Association. Washington D.C.: American Psychiatric Association, 2000.

Haugen, David, and Susan Musser, editors. *Gambling*. Detroit: Greenhaven Press, 2007.

Orford, Jim. *An Unsafe Bet?: The Dangerous Rise of Gambling and the Debate We Should be Having*. Chichester, U.K.: Wiley-Blackwell, 2011

Plante, Thomas G., editor. *Mental Disorders of the New Millennium*. Westport, CT: Praeger, 2006.

Sadock, Benjamin J., Virginia A. Sadock, and Pedro Ruiz, editors. *Kaplan & Sadock' Comprehensive Textbook of Psychiatry*. Philadelphia: Wolters Kluwer Health/Lippincott Williams & Wilkins, 2009.

PERIODICALS

Grant, Jon E., JD, MD, M.P.H., Judson A. Brewer, MD, Ph.D., and Marc N. Potenza, MD, Ph.D. "The Neurobiology of substance and behavioral addictions." *CNS Spectrums* 11 (2006): 924–30.

Hagan, Kate. "Gambling Linked to One in Five Suicidal Patients." *The Age*, (April 21, 2010). http://www.theage.com.au/national/gambling-linked-to-one-in-five-suicidal-patients-20100420-srri.html (accessed May 26, 2011).

Lee, Cynthia. "Doctors Treat Gambling Addiction as Brain Disease." *UCLA Today*, (January 10, 2011). http://www.today.ucla.edu/portal/ut/gambling-addicts-suffer-from-brain-190668.aspx (accessed May 26, 2011).

Lobo, Daniela, S.S., and James L. Kennedy. "The genetics of gambling and behavioral addictions." *CNS Spectrums* 11 (2006): 931–9.

Sevigny S., R. Ladouceur, C. Jacques, and M. Cantinotti. "Links between casino proximity and gambling participation, expenditure, and pathology." *Psychology of Addictive Behaviors* 22, no. 2 (June 2008) 295–301.

WEBSITES

Dryden-Edwards, Roxanne, and William C. Shiel Jr. "Gambling Addiction (Compulsive or Pathological Gambling)." MedicineNet.com. http://www.medicinenet.com/gambling_addiction/article.htm (accessed May 26, 2011).

MedlinePlus. "Pathological Gambling." U.S. Library of Medicine, National Institutes of Health. February 18, 2010. http://www.nlm.nih.gov/medlineplus/ency/article/001520.htm (accessed May 26, 2011).

Reilly, Christine. "NCRG Awarded $380,466 in Research Grants in 2010." Institute on Research for Gambling Disorders. (January 2011). http://www.gamblingdisorders.org/issues-insights/ncrg-awarded-380466-research-grants-2010 (accessed May 26, 2011).

ORGANIZATIONS

Gamblers Anonymous, PO Box 17173, Los Angeles, CA, 90017, (213) 386-8789, Fax: (213) 386-0030, http://www.gamblersanonymous.org.

Institute for Research on Gambling Disorders, 900 Cummings Center, Suite 418-U, Beverly, MA, 01915, (978) 338-6610, Fax: (978) 522-8452, info@gamblingdisorders.org, http://www.gamblingdisorders.org.

National Alliance on Mental Illness, 3803 North Fairfax Drive, Suite 100, Arlington, VA, 22203, (703) 524-7600, Fax: (703) 524-9094, http://www.nami.org.

National Institute of Mental Health, 6001 Executive Boulevard, Room 8184, MSC 9663, Bethesda, MD, 20892-9663, (301) 443-4513, (866) 615-6464, Fax: (301) 443-4279, nimhinfo@nih.gov, http://www.nimh.nih.gov.

Tish Davidson, A.M.
Emily Jane Willingham, Ph.D.
William A. Atkins

Ganser's syndrome

Definition

Ganser's syndrome is a rare disorder in which the individual simulates a psychotic illness or dissociated state. The individual's actions are presumed to be the result of unconscious efforts to escape from an intolerable situation, most typically in psychiatric institutions or prisons. The most common feature of Ganser's syndrome is the giving of approximate answers to questions (e.g., 5 + 3 = 7).

Description

Although this disorder was previously classified as a **factitious disorder**, the **American Psychiatric Association** has redefined Ganser's syndrome and placed it in the category called "Dissociative Disorder Not Otherwise Specified." Sometimes called "the syndrome of approximate answers," Ganser's syndrome is most often seen in male prisoners. In the past, this was so much the case that early clinicians called the syndrome prison **psychosis**, despite the fact that it is not a true psychosis. (Psychosis is characterized by a radical change in personality and a distorted sense of reality.) The disorder has also been referred to as hysterical pseudodementia, due to the resemblance of responses to those of demented patients. However, data on the prevalence of the syndrome and on links within families have not been gathered and analyzed.

Ganser's syndrome is usually sudden in onset and, like **malingering**, seems to arise in response to an opportunity for personal gain or the avoidance of some responsibility. The patient will offer nearly correct replies when asked questions about facts of common knowledge, such as the number of days in a year, the number of months in a year, subtracting 7 from 100, the product of 4 times 5, etc. To such questions, the patient may respond by stating that there are 360 days in a year, 11 months in a year, 94 for the result of subtracting 7 from 100, and that 21 is the product of 4 times 5. These

> **KEY TERMS**
>
> **Factitious disorder**—A type of mental disturbance in which patients intentionally act physically or mentally ill without obvious benefits. It is distinguished from malingering by the absence of an obvious motive, and from conversion disorder by intentional production of symptoms.
>
> **Malingering**—Knowingly pretending to be physically or mentally ill to avoid some unpleasant duty or responsibility, or for economic benefit.

persons appear to have no difficulty in understanding questions asked, but appear to provide incorrect answers deliberately.

This syndrome is seen in conjunction with a preexisting severe personality disorder. However, unless the patient is willing to admit to the manufactured nature of the symptoms, or unless there is conclusive objective evidence contradicting the syndrome, determining whether the patient has a true disorder may be impossible. As with its sudden onset, disappearance of the symptoms can be just as fast. However, symptoms can also appear to worsen if the patient believes someone is watching. When reviewing a case of Ganser's syndrome, the clinician must consider factitious disorder and malingering as alternative diagnoses.

Resources

BOOKS

American Psychiatric Association. *Diagnostic and Statistical Manual of Mental Disorders*. 4th ed., text rev. Washington, DC: American Psychiatric Publishing, 2000.

Enoch, M. David, and Hadrian N. Ball. *Uncommon Psychiatric Syndromes*. New York: Oxford University Press, 2001.

VandenBos, Gary R. ed. *APA Dictionary of Psychology*. Washington, DC: American Psychological Association, 2006.

PERIODICALS

Levenson, James L. "Somatoform Disorders: A Medicolegal Guide." *Journal of Psychosomatic Research* 59, no. 5 (November 2005): 349.

Merckelbach, Harald, et al. "Detecting Malingering of Ganser-Like Symptoms with Tests: A Case Study." *Psychiatry and Clinical Neurosciences* 60, no. 5 (October 2006): 636–38. Available online at http://onlinelibrary.wiley.com/doi/10.1111/j.1440-1819.2006.01571.x/full (accessed November 9, 2011).

Jack H. Booth, PsyD
Ruth A. Wienclaw, PhD

Gender dysphoria *see* **Gender identity disorder**

Gender identity disorder

Definition

Gender identity disorder (GID) as defined by the fourth edition of the ***Diagnostic and Statistical Manual of Mental Disorders*** (*DSM-IV*), is a condition characterized by a persistent feeling of discomfort or inappropriateness concerning one's anatomic sex. The disorder typically begins in childhood with gender identity disconnects and is manifested in adolescence or adulthood by a person dressing in clothing associated with the desired gender (cross-dressing), as opposed to one's birth gender, and exhibiting other behaviors associated with the self-perceived sex identity. In extreme cases, persons with gender identity disorder may seek sexual reassignment surgery (SRS), also known as a "sex-change" operation.

Proposals for the forthcoming fifth edition of *DSM* (*DSM-5*) in 2013 include changing the name of GID to gender dysphoria, eliminating the term "disorder" and dividing the condition into two subgroups on the basis of age. The proposed names for the condition are "Gender dysphoria in children" and "Gender dysphoria in adolescents or adults." The English word *dysphoria* comes from two Greek words meaning "hard" or "difficult" and "to bear" or "to carry," and refers to a chronic or persistent mood of sadness or generalized unease or discomfort. The reader should note that dysphoria is a general term for a condition that can be experienced as a result of **bereavement** or everyday **stress** as well as being a feature of gender issues, **depression**, and some **anxiety disorders**.

The remainder of this entry will discuss the changes in definition and diagnostic criteria proposed for *DSM-5* alongside the present understanding of GID. The major changes proposed for *DSM-5* were based on the desire to remove the **stigma** of mental illness associated with the term "disorder" and to acknowledge the distinction between gender dysphoria related to a disorder of sex development (DSD) and gender dysphoria in a person without a DSD. "Disorder of sexual development" is the preferred term for disorders in which a genetic mutation or hormonal imbalance leads to ambiguous genitalia at birth or other abnormalities of sexual development. The baby's genitalia may appear as normally female, ambiguous, or male but with a very small penis (micropenis). DSDs are sometimes called "intersex conditions."

Demographics

Gender identity disorder/dysphoria is thought to be more prevalent in males than in females. *DSM-IV* estimates that 1 in every 30,000 males and 1 in every 100,000 females in European and North American countries seeks sexual reassignment surgery (SRS). Other researchers note, however, that these figures do not include people who experience a conflict between their biological sex and their perception of themselves as members of the opposite sex but who choose not to seek surgical treatment. Other figures that have been given are 1 in every 10,000 males and 1 in every 30,000 females. Reliable estimates of prevalence for either males or females, however, were not available as of 2011.

Description

Gender identity disorder/dysphoria is a distressing condition to those who have it. It is especially difficult to cope with because it remains unresolved unless and until sexual reassignment surgery has been performed. Most people with this disorder grow up feeling rejected and out of place. **Suicide** attempts and **substance abuse** are common. Most adolescents and adults with the disorder eventually attempt to pass or live as members of the opposite sex.

Gender identity disorder/dysphoria may be as old as humanity. Cultural anthropologists and other scientists have observed a number of cross-gender behaviors in classical and Hindu mythology, Western and Asian classical history, and in many late nineteenth- and early twentieth-century preliterate cultures, including several Native American tribes. This consistent record across cultures and time lends support to the notion that the disorder may be, at least in part, biological in origin. Not all behavioral scientists share this hypothesis, however.

Behavioral experimentation, particularly when a child is young, is considered normal. As they grow, children will often experiment with a variety of gender role behaviors as they learn to make the fine distinctions between masculine and feminine role expectations of the society in which they live. Some young boys occasionally exhibit behaviors that Western culture has traditionally labeled as feminine. Examples of these behaviors include wearing a dress, using cosmetics, or playing with dolls.

In a similar manner, some young girls will occasionally assume masculine roles during play. An example of this behavior includes pretending to be the father when playing house. Some girls temporarily adopt a cluster of masculine behaviors. These youngsters are often designated as tomboys. Most experts agree that such temporary or episodic adopting of behaviors opposite to one's gender is normal and usually constitute learning experiences in the acquisition of normal sex role socialization.

In cases that are considered pathological, however, children deviate from the typical model of exploring masculine and feminine behaviors. Such children develop inflexible, compulsive, persistent, and rigidly stereotyped patterns. On one extreme are boys who become excessively masculine. The opposite extreme is seen in effeminate boys who reject their masculinity and rigidly insist that they are really girls or that they want to become mothers and bear children.

Boys with these traits frequently avoid playing with other boys, dress in female clothing, play predominantly with girls, try out cosmetics and wigs, and display stereotypically feminine gait, arm movements, and body gestures. Although much less common, some girls may similarly reject traditionally feminine roles and mannerisms in favor of masculine characteristics, including a refusal to urinate sitting down. Professional **intervention** is required for both extremes of gender role behavior.

Gender identity disorder/dysphoria is different from transvestitism or **transvestic fetishism**. Transvestic **fetishism** is classified as a paraphilia or type of sexual behavior in which a person derives sexual excitement from behavior that is unusual, extreme, or criminal. Transvestic fetishism refers to deriving sexual excitement from wearing clothing and accessories associated with the opposite sex in one's particular society, as distinguished from wearing such clothing for a theatrical performance or costume party. It is a paraphilia found primarily in males; there were no cases in the English-language medical literature as of 2011 of women becoming sexually excited by wearing men's clothing. Transvestic fetishism is not necessarily associated with gender identity disorder/dysphoria, as most men who engage in transvestic fetishism are content with their assigned sex.

Adults with gender identity disorder sometimes live their lives as members of the opposite sex. They often cross-dress and prefer to be seen in public as a member of the other sex. Some people with the disorder seek gender reassignment surgery.

Persons with gender identity disorder frequently state that they were born the wrong sex. They may describe their sexual organs as being ugly and may refrain from touching their genitalia. People with gender identity disorder may also try to hide their secondary sex characteristics. For instance, males may try to shave off or pluck their body hair. Many men elect to take estrogens in an effort to enlarge their breasts. Females may try to hide their breasts by binding them. There is a growing movement among people who consider themselves transgendered to demand that the condition not be viewed or classified as a disorder but as part of a spectrum of sexual development; the proposed changes in *DSM-5* reflect this demand.

Causes and symptoms

Causes

There was no consensus as of 2011 regarding the causes of gender identity disorder/dysphoria. Various theories have been proposed, such as:

- childhood sexual abuse or traumatic injury to the genitals
- homosexual orientation
- genetic mutations
- variations in brain structure
- variations in brain function
- prenatal exposure to androgens (male sex hormones), the lack of such exposure, or fetal insensitivity to androgens

The sex of a human baby is determined by chromosomes. Males have a Y chromosome and one X chromosome, while females have two X chromosomes. The Y chromosome carries a gene known as the "testis-determining factor." This gene sets off a developmental pathway that is typically male, resulting in testicular development and development of secondary sexual structures that are male, including a penis and scrotum and differentiation in the fetal **brain**. Embryos lacking the testis-determining factor usually develop as females. The newly formed testes are responsible for releasing the hormones that continue the fetus on a male developmental pathway.

These prenatal events provide the biological basis for gender identity disorder. Hormone levels must be appropriate for male development during the appropriate developmental windows for typical male development to occur. In addition, the cellular pathways that recognize the signals the hormones send must also be in place. Changes in hormone levels from the norm or exposure to environmental compounds that behave like hormones in the fetus can alter male development, resulting in a feminized fetus if this alteration ends in inhibition of typical male development.

Disruptions of hormone signaling may arise from a variety of sources, including a disorder in the mother's endocrine system, maternal stress, maternal medications, and some environmental endocrine-active substances.

Postmortem studies conducted on male-to-female transsexuals, non-transsexual men, and non-transsexual women show a significant difference in sex-specific brain structures. Studies have shown that in male-to-female transsexuals, for example, brain structures look like those of nontransgendered women. These studies indicate that one's sense of gender resides in the brain and that it may be biochemically determined. One hypothesis underlying the link between gonadal sex and the sex of the brain is the organization-activation hypothesis. According to this hypothesis, the hormones that organize the body as masculine (result in the formation of a penis rather than a clitoris) also organize the brain as masculine. At puberty, hormones activate the brain for gender-specific sex behavior. In some cases, there may be a disconnect between gonadal development and the brain's sexual development.

In addition to biological factors, such environmental conditions as socialization are thought by some to contribute to gender identity disorder. Social learning theory, for example, proposes that a combination of

KEY TERMS

Cross-dressing—Wearing clothes and other accessories associated with the opposite sex in one's particular society.

Disorder of sex development (DSD)—The term that is increasingly preferred for an atypical pattern of chromosomal, genital, or gonadal development. It is also known as "disorder of sex differentiation."

Dysphoria—A persistent mood of sadness, discomfort, or general unease. The English word comes from two Greek words meaning "difficult" or "hard" and "to bear."

Eunuch—A castrated male, often one castrated at an early age with noticeable hormonal consequences.

Gender dysphoria—Persistent personal discomfort with one's present gender.

Intersex—A term that is sometimes used to refer to having a sexual anatomy that is not standard for either a male or a female. It covers a number of different conditions but is considered a convenient umbrella term for discussing disorders of sex development.

Paraphilia—A type of sexual behavior in which a person derives sexual excitement from behavior that is unusual, extreme, or criminal.

Stigma—Any personal attribute that causes a person to be socially shamed, avoided, or discredited. Mental disorders are a common cause of stigma.

Transvestic fetishism—A condition in which a person is sexually aroused by wearing the clothing of the other sex (as distinct from cross-dressing for a theater role or costume party).

observational learning and different levels and forms of **reinforcement** by parents, family, and friends determine a child's sense of gender, which in turn leads to what society considers appropriate or inappropriate behavior. Recent research, however, suggests that even when people who are transgendered or born with ambiguous genitalia are reared based on their assigned sex, they still retain their perceived sexual identity.

Diagnosis

While a patient with gender issues may begin by consulting a family doctor, referral to a mental health professional is needed to make a formal **diagnosis** of gender identity disorder. In most cases, the professional will be either a **psychiatrist** or a clinical **psychologist**. He or she begins by taking a careful personal history of the patient and obtaining the age of the patient, and determines whether the patient's sexual attraction is to males, females, both, or neither. Laboratory tests are neither available nor required to make a diagnosis of gender identity disorder.

Patients and their families may wish to visit clinics that specialize in assessment of gender identity/dysphoria issues. Two of these facilities are listed under Resources below.

Examination

It is very important not to overlook a physical illness, such as a tumor that might mimic or contribute to a psychological disorder. If there is any question that a physical problem might be the underlying cause of an apparent gender identity disorder, a mental health professional should recommend a complete physical examination by a medical doctor. The patient may be referred to an endocrinologist, a physician who specializes in diagnosing and treating disorders of the glands that produce sex hormones, to determine whether a hormonal imbalance is a factor in the patient's condition.

Tests

Urine and blood samples are taken to rule out previously undiagnosed hormonal disorders. In a few cases, the patient may be given an x ray or other **imaging studies** to rule out abnormalities of, or injuries to, the brain.

DSM-IV criteria for gender identity disorder

Diagnosis of a psychiatric disorder or condition according to *DSM* requires the psychiatrist or psychologist to determine whether the patient meets a set of criteria defined by the manual. The *DSM-IV* criteria requires that:

- The person feels a strong and persistent cross-gender identification.
- The person experiences persistent discomfort with his or her sex or a sense of inappropriateness in the gender role of one's birth sex.
- The disturbance is not concurrent with a physical intersex condition.
- The disturbance causes clinically significant distress or impairment in social, occupational, or other important areas of functioning.

In children with a persistent cross-gender identification, the disturbance is manifested by four (or more) of the following:

- Repeatedly stating a desire to be, or insistence that he or she is, a member of the other sex.
- Strong preference for wearing clothes of the opposite gender. In boys, displaying a preference for cross-dressing or simulating female attire; in girls, insistence on wearing only stereotypically masculine clothing.
- Displaying strong and persistent preferences for cross-sex roles in make-believe play or experiencing persistent fantasies of being a member of the other sex.
- Having an intense desire to participate in the games and pastimes that are stereotypical of the other sex.
- Exhibiting a strong preference for playmates of the other sex.

Among adolescents and adults, the disturbance is manifested by symptoms such as a stated desire to become a member of the other sex, frequent passing as a person of the other sex, a desire to live or be treated as the other sex, or the conviction that he or she has the typical feelings and reactions of the other sex. These characteristics cannot be merely from a desire for any perceived cultural advantages of being the other sex.

Among children that feel a discomfort regarding his or her gender, the disturbance is manifested by any of the following:

- Among boys, asserting that his penis or testes are disgusting or will disappear, asserting that it would be better not to have a penis, or having an aversion toward rough-and-tumble play and rejecting male stereotypical toys, games, and activities.
- Among girls, rejecting the gender-typical practice of urinating in a sitting position, asserting that she has or will grow a penis, or stating that she does not want to grow breasts or menstruate, or having a marked aversion toward normative feminine clothing.

Among adolescents and adults, the disturbance is manifested by symptoms such as preoccupation with getting rid of primary and secondary sex characteristics (e.g., request for hormones, surgery, or other procedures to alter sexual characteristics to simulate the other sex) or a belief that he or she was born the wrong sex.

DSM-5 criteria for gender dysphoria

The proposed criteria for gender dysphoria have been updated several times since the change in name for the condition was suggested, and may change again with the publication of *DSM-5*. The following criteria were posted in May 2011:

IN CHILDREN. There are two subtypes specified of gender dysphoria in children: a) with a disorder of sex development; and b) without a disorder of sex development.

- Criterion A: A marked incongruence between one's experienced/expressed gender and assigned gender, of at least 6 months duration, as manifested by at least 6 of the following indicators, including the first: 1. a strong desire to be of the other gender or an insistence that he or she is the other gender (or some alternative gender different from one's assigned gender); 2. in boys, a strong preference for cross-dressing or simulating female attire; in girls, a strong preference for wearing only typical masculine clothing and a strong resistance to the wearing of typical feminine clothing; 3. a strong preference for cross-gender roles in make-believe or fantasy play; 4. a strong preference for the toys, games, or activities typical of the other gender; 5. a strong preference for playmates of the other gender; 6. in boys, a strong rejection of typically masculine toys, games, and activities and a strong avoidance of rough-and-tumble play; in girls, a strong rejection of typically feminine toys, games, and activities; 7. a strong dislike of one's sexual anatomy; 8. a strong desire for the primary and/or secondary sex characteristics that match one's experienced gender
- Criterion B: the condition is associated with clinically significant distress or impairment in social, occupational, or other important areas of functioning, or with a significantly increased risk of suffering, such as distress or disability.

IN ADOLESCENTS AND ADULTS. As with children, *DSM-5* specifies two subtypes of gender dysphoria in adolescents and adults: with or without a disorder of sex development.

- Criterion A: A marked incongruence between one's experienced/expressed gender and assigned gender, of at least 6 months duration, as manifested by two or more of the following indicators: 1. a marked incongruence between one's experienced/expressed gender and primary and/or secondary sex characteristics (or, in young adolescents, the anticipated secondary sex characteristics); 2. a strong desire to be rid of one's primary and/or secondary sex characteristics because of a marked incongruence with one's experienced/expressed gender (or, in young adolescents, a desire to prevent the development of the anticipated secondary sex characteristics); 3. a strong desire for the primary and/or secondary sex characteristics of the other gender; 4. a strong desire to be of the other gender (or some alternative gender different from one's assigned gender); 5. a strong desire to be treated as the other gender (or some alternative gender different from one's assigned gender); 6. a strong conviction that one has the typical feelings and reactions of the other gender (or some alternative gender different from one's assigned gender).
- Criterion B: same as Criterion B for children.

MALE-TO-EUNUCH GENDER DYSPHORIA. Some researchers have suggested that *DSM-5* add a new category of gender dysphoria known as male-to-eunuch gender dysphoria. This category would include males who do not identify with either their birth sex or with a female gender identity. They seek castration as a way to align their bodies with their brain sex. It was estimated that there were between 7,000 and 10,000 voluntary eunuchs in Canada and the United States in 2011. *DSM-5* had not incorporated male-to-eunuch gender identity disorder in its list of proposed revisions as of 2011; it had, however, listed the condition under the heading of "Conditions Proposed by Outside Sources."

Treatment

Psychotherapy

One common form of treatment for gender identity disorder is **psychotherapy**. The initial aim of treatment is to help individuals function in their biologic sex roles to the greatest degree possible. The World Professional Association for Transgender Health, which has formulated and published its own *Standards of Care* manual for working with transgendered people, does not support psychotherapy designed to convert a transgendered person from their own personal perception of their sex.

Sexual reassignment

Adults who have had severe gender identity disorder for many years sometimes request reassignment of their sex, or sex-change surgery. Before undertaking such surgery, they usually undergo hormone therapy to suppress same-sex characteristics and to accentuate other-sex characteristics. For instance, the female hormone estrogen is given to males to make breasts grow, reduce facial hair, and widen hips. The male hormone testosterone is administered to females to suppress menstruation, deepen the voice, and increase body hair. Following the hormone treatments, preoperative candidates are usually required to live in the cross-gender role for at least a year before surgery is performed. This period is known as "real-life experience" or RLE.

Adults seeking sexual reassignment should be screened for medical conditions that can be worsened by cross-sex hormone therapy. These conditions include heart disease, breast cancer, liver disease, migraine headaches, and blood disorders. There are two goals of hormone therapy in adult transsexuals: reduce the secondary sex characteristics of the patient's biological sex; and supply the individual with the hormones of the desired sex. Adults should also be counseled about the possibility of permanent infertility if they choose to proceed with sex reassignment. In addition, males seeking reassignment as women should be warned that hormone treatment is likely to lower their sex drive, while women seeking reassignment as men are likely to find their sex drive increased by hormone therapy. In terms of cost, hormone therapy costs between $25 and $200 per month.

Transsexuals in any country must also attend to a number of legal concerns, ranging from changing their name and sex on documents ranging from birth certificates (permitted in some states in the United States) and Social Security registration to driver's licenses, bank accounts, passports, voter registration forms, and the like.

Prognosis

If gender identity disorder/dysphoria in a child persists into adolescence, it tends to be chronic in nature. There may be periods of remission. However, adoption of characteristics and activities typical for one's birth sex is unlikely to occur.

Most individuals with gender identity disorder require and appreciate support from several sources. Families, as well as the person with the disorder, need and appreciate both information and support. Local and national **support groups** and informational services exist, and health care providers and mental health professionals can provide referrals.

There is some disagreement regarding the post-treatment satisfaction of people who have undergone sexual reassignment surgery. Early surveys indicated that only 1% regretted their transition; however, other surveys have reported that between 8% and 14% regret their change, and that a few persons have re-transitioned to their original gender. In terms of adjustment after SRS, heterosexual transsexuals have poorer outcomes than homosexual transsexuals; older persons and effeminate homosexuals have poorer outcomes; and male-to-female transsexuals have poorer outcomes than female-to-male. In general, satisfactory results are reported in 87% of male-to-female and 97% of female-to-male SRS patients.

QUESTIONS TO ASK YOUR DOCTOR

- Have you ever treated a patient with gender issues? A patient who has had sexual reassignment hormone therapy or surgery?
- Should I be concerned about a small child's wishes to change his or her sex?
- How can I tell whether my child has a gender identity disorder or is just going through a phase?
- If my child is diagnosed with gender dysphoria, what are the chances that it will resolve by the teen years?
- What is your opinion of sex reassignment surgery?

Prevention

There is no known way to prevent gender identity disorder/dysphoria because there are several possible causes of the condition that are not completely understood.

Resources

BOOKS

American Psychiatric Association. *Diagnostic and Statistical Manual*. 4th ed., text rev. Washington, DC: American Psychiatric Association, 2000.

Balon, Richard, and Robert Taylor Segraves, eds. *Clinical Manual of Sexual Disorders*. Washington, DC: American Psychiatric Publishing, 2009.

Bamberg-Smith, Barbara A. *The Psychology of Sex and Gender*. Boston: Pearson/Allyn and Bacon, 2007.

Bockting, Walter O., and Joshua Goldberg, eds. *Guidelines for Transgender Care*. Binghamton, NY: Haworth Medical Press, 2006.

Einstein, Gillian, ed. *Sex and the Brain*. Cambridge, MA: MIT Press, 2007.

Shrage, Laurie J., ed. *"You've Changed": Sex Reassignment and Personal Identity*. New York: Oxford University Press, 2009.

PERIODICALS

Cohen-Kettenis, P.T., and F. Pfäfflin. "The DSM Diagnostic Criteria for Gender Identity Disorder in Adolescents and Adults." *Archives of Sexual Behavior* 39 (April 2010): 499–513.

Hoshiai, M., et al. "Psychiatric Comorbidity among Patients with Gender Identity Disorder." *Psychiatry and Clinical Neurosciences* 64 (October 2010): 514–519.

Lawrence, A.A. "Proposed Revisions to Gender Identity Disorder Diagnoses in the DSM-5." *Archives of Sexual Behavior* 39 (December 2010): 1253–1260.

Paap, M.C., et al. "Assessing the Utility of Diagnostic Criteria: A Multisite Study on Gender Identity Disorder." *Journal of Sexual Medicine* 8 (January 2011): 180–190.

Roberts, L.F., et al. "A Passion for Castration: Characterizing Men Who Are Fascinated with Castration, But Have Not Been Castrated." *Journal of Sexual Medicine* 5 (July 2008): 1669–1680.

Selvaggi, G., and J. Bellringer. "Gender Reassignment Surgery: An Overview." *Nature Reviews. Urology* 8 (May 2011): 274–282.

WEBSITES

American Psychiatric Association. DSM-5 Development. "Conditions Proposed by Outside Sources." http://www.dsm5.org/PROPOSEDREVISIONS/Pages/ConditionsProposedbyOutsideSources.aspx (accessed May 22, 2011).

American Psychiatric Association. DSM-5 Development. "P 00 Gender Dysphoria in Children." http://www.dsm5.org/ProposedRevisions/Pages/proposedrevision.aspx?rid=192 (accessed May 19, 2011).

American Psychiatric Association. DSM-5 Development. "P 01 Gender Dysphoria in Adolescents or Adults." http://www.dsm5.org/ProposedRevisions/Pages/proposedrevision.aspx?rid=482 (accessed May 19, 2011).

MedlinePlus. "Gender Identity Disorder." http://www.nlm.nih.gov/medlineplus/ency/article/001527.htm (accessed May 19, 2011).

Medscape. "Sexual and Gender Identity Disorders." http://emedicine.medscape.com/article/293890-overview (accessed May 19, 2011).

World Professional Association for Transgender Health (WPATH). "Standards of Care for Gender Identity Disorders." http://www.wpath.org/documents2/socv6.pdf (accessed May 20, 2011).

ORGANIZATIONS

American Association of Sexuality Educators, Counselors, and Therapists (AASECT), 1444 I Street NW, Suite 700, Washington, DC, United States 20005, (202) 449-1099, Fax: (202) 216-9646, info@aasect.org, http://www.aasect.org

Endocrine Society, 8401 Connecticut Ave., Suite 900, Chevy Chase, MD, United States 20815, (301) 941-0200, Fax: (301) 941-0259, (888) 363-6274, http://www.endo-society.org

The Johns Hopkins Hospital, Sexual Behaviors Consultation Unit, 600 North Wolfe Street, Meyer 144, Baltimore, MD, United States 21287, (410) 583-1661, Fax: (410)583-2693, http://www.hopkinsmedicine.org/psychiatry/specialty_areas/sexual_behaviors

University of Minnesota Clinic, Center for Sexual Health, 1300 South 2nd Street, Minneapolis, MN, United States 55454, (612) 624-7821, http://www.fm.umn.edu/phs/clinic/home.html

World Professional Association for Transgender Health (WPATH) [formerly the Harry Benjamin International Gender Dysphoria Association (HBIGDA)], 1300 South Second Street, Suite 180, Minneapolis, MN, United States 55454, [no telephone number given], wpath@wpath.org, http://www.wpath.org

L. Fleming Fallon, Jr., M.D., Dr. P.H.
Rebecca J. Frey, Ph.D.

Gender issues in mental health

Defining gender

In the social sciences, the concept of gender means much more than biological sex. It refers to socially constructed expectations regarding the ways in which people should think and behave, depending on their sexual classification. These stereotypical expectations are commonly referred to as "gender roles." Attitudes toward gender roles are thought to result from complex

Characteristic	Percentage of women		Percentage of men
Classify stress as an 8 or higher on a 10-point scale	28%	vs.	20%
Experienced increasing stress over the last 5 years	49%	vs.	39%
Primary sources of stress	Money (79%) and economy (68%)	vs.	Work (76%)
Preferred forms of stress relief	Reading (57%)	vs.	Listening to music (52%)
Eat as a form of stress relief	31%	vs.	21%
Choose unhealthy foods because of stress	49%	vs.	30%
Experience stress headaches	41%	vs.	30%
Experience upset stomach/ indigestion caused by stress	32%	vs.	21%
Do nothing to manage stress	4%	vs.	9%

SOURCE: American Psychological Association.

Differences in causes and effects of stress between men and women. *(Table by PreMediaGlobal. © 2012 Cengage Learning.)*

interactions among societal, cultural, familial, religious, ethnic, and political influences.

Gender affects many aspects of life, including access to resources, methods of coping with **stress**, styles of interacting with others, self-evaluation, spirituality, and expectations of others. These are all factors that can influence mental health either positively or negatively. Psychological gender studies seek to better understand the relationship between gender and mental health in order to reduce risk factors and improve treatment methods.

Traditional gender roles in many Western societies identify masculinity as having power and being in control in emotional situations, in the workplace, and in sexual relationships. Acceptable male behaviors in this traditional construct include competitiveness, independence, assertiveness, ambition, confidence, toughness, anger, and even violence (to varying degrees). Men are expected to avoid characteristics considered feminine, such as emotional expressiveness, vulnerability (weakness, helplessness, insecurity, worry), and intimacy (especially showing affection to other males).

Traditional femininity is defined as being nurturing, supportive, and assigning high priority to one's relationships. Women are expected to be emotionally expressive, dependent, passive, cooperative, warm, and accepting of subordinate status in marriage and employment. Competitiveness, assertiveness, anger, and violence are viewed as unfeminine and are not generally tolerated as acceptable female behavior, although competitiveness is becoming more widely accepted as appropriate for female athletes and political leaders.

Theories of gender

Differences in gender roles have existed throughout history. Evolutionary theorists attribute these differences to the physiological characteristics of men and women that prescribed their best function for survival of the species. In primitive societies, men adopted the roles of hunting and protecting their families because of their physical strength. Women's ability to bear and nurse children led them to adopt the roles of nurturing young, as well as the less physically dependent roles of gathering and preparing food. These gender-dependent labor roles continued into the period of written human history, when people began to live in cities and form the earliest civilized societies.

In the nineteenth century, the industrial movement marked a prominent division of labor into public and private domains. Men began leaving home to work, whereas women worked within the home. Previously, both men and women frequently engaged in comparably respected, productive activities on their homestead. When men began working in the public domain, they acquired money, which was transferable for goods or services. Women's work, on the other hand, was not transferable. Men's relative economic independence contributed to their power and influence, while women were reduced to an image of frailty and emotionality deemed appropriate only for domestic tasks and child rearing.

Sigmund Freud's psychoanalytic theory of human development, which emerged from Freud's late nineteenth-century European setting and medical training, reflected an attitude of male superiority. Freud asserted that as children, boys recognize they are superior to girls when they discover the difference in their genitals, and that girls, on the other hand, equate their lack of a penis with inferiority. According to Freud, this feeling of inferiority causes girls to idolize and desire their fathers, resulting in passivity, masochistic tendencies, jealousy, and vanity, all seen by Freud as feminine characteristics.

Other developmental theorists rejected Freud's notions. Eric Erikson (in 1950) and Lawrence Kohlberg (in 1969) theorized that all humans begin as dependent on caregivers and gradually mature into independent and autonomous beings. Such theories, however, still favored men because independence has historically been considered a masculine trait. By such a standard, men would consistently achieve greater levels of maturity than females.

Nancy Chodorow's object-relations theory (in 1978) favored neither sex. She proposed that children develop according to interactions with their primary caregivers, who tend to be mothers. Mothers, according to her theory, identify with girls to a greater extent, fostering an ability to form rich interpersonal relationships, as well as dependency traits. Mothers push boys toward independence, helping them to adjust to the male-dominated work environment but rendering them unaccustomed to emotional connection. Chodorow's theory suggests both strengths and weaknesses inherent in male and female development, with neither deemed superior.

Around that same time (1974), Sandra Bem advocated for androgyny, or high levels of both masculinity and femininity, as the key to mental health. Bem constructed the Bem Sex Role Inventory (BSRI), a 60-item questionnaire that measures 20 feminine, 20 masculine, and 20 neutral traits. It classifies subjects as masculine, feminine, androgynous, or undifferentiated. Bem maintains that gender roles are primarily cognitive; that is, that people spontaneously sort attitudes and behaviors into masculine and feminine categories according to the models their culture provides. Sex-typed individuals score highly on the dimension corresponding to their gender while rejecting the characteristics of the other gender. Androgynous individuals score high on both masculine and feminine traits, and typically use situational examples to explain their behavior. Bem concluded that androgyny is a particular way of processing information and that individuals who are androgynous are those who do not use sex-role related cognitive frameworks to guide their information processing.

In the 1980s, such psychologists as Carol Gilligan sought to build respect for stereotypically feminine traits. They introduced the notion that women function according to an ethic of care and relatedness that is not inferior to men's, just different. In 1985, Daniel Stern's developmental theory favored traditional femininity, suggesting that humans start out as unconnected to others and gradually form more complex interpersonal connections as they mature.

The process of learning gender roles is known as "socialization." Children learn which behaviors are acceptable or not acceptable for their sex by observing other people. They may also be shamed by caregivers or peers when they violate gender-role expectations. As a result, gender roles usually become an internal guide for behavior early in childhood. Current studies focus on the ways in which extreme notions of masculinity or femininity affect mental health, and the social processes that shape one's concept of maleness or femaleness.

Psychological and behavioral androgyny are less of a problem in North America and Europe because of widespread changes in society, particularly the entrance of women in large numbers into the military, politics, law, medicine, the ministry, and other occupations that were partly or completely closed to them before World War II. Another factor that has influenced social attitudes toward androgyny is androgynous parenting, a trend in childrearing in which a child's mother and father share equally and relatively interchangeably in parenting responsibilities.

In terms of choices made after adolescence, most young people whose career interests or lifestyle preferences fall outside stereotypical gender roles may more easily find welcoming and supportive communities than they might have before the 1960s. There is also some evidence that older adults with androgynous gender roles enjoy better health and satisfaction with their lives than those who adhere to traditional gender roles. On the other hand, people who grow up within families that recently emigrated from countries still marked by rigid gender roles and stereotypes may find the greater acceptance of androgyny in the West disorienting and upsetting.

Gender-role conflict

According to some researchers, the concepts of masculinity and femininity may simply be sets of personality traits that can be exhibited by either sex, and there may be no true gender differences, although this conclusion is controversial. Individuals vary in degree of adherence to gender roles, resulting in large amounts of behavioral variation within the sexes and potentially less variation between them. However, some scholars maintain that there are specific gender-related traits, including gender bias in mental illness.

Although attitudes toward gender roles are now much more flexible, different cultures retain varying degrees of expectations regarding male and female behavior. Individuals may personally disregard gender expectations, but society may disapprove of their behavior and impose external social consequences. On the other hand, individuals may feel internal shame if they experience emotions or desires characteristic of the opposite sex. In some cultures in which a person's social role is emphasized over individualism, the failure to fulfill that role in ways considered traditionally appropriate can lead to feelings of shame as well. Gender-role conflict, or gender-role stress, results when people feel a discrepancy between how they believe they should act based on gender-role expectations learned in childhood, and how they actually think, feel, or behave. If these discrepancies are unresolved, gender-role conflict contributes to poor mental health.

Gender-role complications

A person's attitude toward the roles associated with his or her gender can be complicated by a number of factors, ranging from having a nonstandard sexual anatomy to bisexual or homosexual orientation to unhappiness with one's biological sex (gender dysphoria).

Sexual orientation

Gay men, lesbians, and bisexuals can experience gender-role conflict as well as heterosexual people. Some studies of gay men indicate that effeminate gays are stigmatized inside as well as outside the gay community, and that they have a higher level of mental health problems than gay men who conform more closely to male gender norms. In addition, same-sex partnerships are complicated by the same gender stereotypes that cause stress in male/female relationships. While research does not support the commonplace belief that gay or lesbian couples organize their relationships around traditional gender roles, with one partner being the "butch" (the "man") and the other being the "femme" (the "woman"), such couples are still often troubled by power struggles and domestic violence. In addition to internal conflict about gender roles, bisexuals suffer the additional complication of being distrusted by both homosexual and heterosexual partners; homosexual **support groups** may reject them if they reveal their heterosexual side; heterosexuals may reject them if they reveal their homosexual feelings.

Disorders of sexual development

Disorders of sexual development (DSDs) is an umbrella term for a group of conditions in which a person has a congenital (present at birth) abnormality or atypical combination of features that make it difficult to determine sex. The abnormalities may be chromosomal, genital, or gonadal. It is estimated that about 1%–1.7% of human infants are born with some degree of sexual ambiguity and that between 0.1% and 0.2% are sexually ambiguous enough to require the attention of a medical specialist. Some doctors prefer the term *intersex* to DSD.

In general, parents are more likely to be concerned about a child with ambiguous genitalia than about other intersex conditions that may not be apparent at birth. The most important consideration is to determine the cause of the ambiguous genitalia. The usual tests that are performed include a karyogram to determine the child's karyotype; this diagram of the chromosomes in a cell is usually made from a white blood cell. Other tests include blood and urine samples to evaluate the levels of sex hormones in the blood, and x-ray or ultrasound studies to clarify the structure of the child's internal sex organs.

The nest step is gender assignment. The doctor may suggest the gender, depending on the baby's genetic sex, the anatomy of the internal sex organs, and the possibility of future reproduction. Depending on the cause of the DSD, treatment may include hormone therapy or surgery. The therapy plan should always include psychological counseling for both the child and the parents, particularly because the child may wish to identify with the other sex when he or she is older.

Gender-free childrearing

One recent complication in gender issues related to mental health is whether it is either possible or desirable to raise a child without an assigned gender identity. This question was discussed intensively in the spring of 2011 when a couple in Canada made headlines with their announcement that they were keeping their third child's sex a secret from everyone except their two older children. The baby's name, Storm, was deliberately chosen to be gender-neutral. Child psychologists are divided on whether the parents' decision is likely to create problems for Storm as she or he grows older. The same division among experts surfaced in 2009 when a Swedish couple had a child they named Pop; they told a Swedish newspaper that "the decision [to give the baby a gender-free name] stemmed from a feminist philosophy that gender is a social construction." It will take a number of years to evaluate whether these experiments in gender-free childrearing are successful, and if so, what defines their "success."

Gender dysphoria

"Gender dysphoria" is the proposed name change for **gender identity disorder** (GID) as defined by the fourth edition of the ***Diagnostic and Statistical Manual of Mental Disorders*** (*DSM-IV*). GID is a condition characterized by a persistent feeling of discomfort or inappropriateness concerning one's anatomic sex. The disorder typically begins in childhood with rejection of or discomfort with one's birth gender and is manifested in adolescence or adulthood by a person dressing in clothing associated with the desired gender (cross-dressing) and exhibiting other behaviors associated with the self-perceived sex identity. In extreme cases, persons with gender identity disorder may seek sexual reassignment surgery (SRS), also known as a "sex-change" operation.

Proposals for the forthcoming fifth edition of the *DSM* (*DSM-5*) in 2013 include changing the name of GID to "Gender Dysphoria," thus eliminating the term "disorder," and dividing the condition into two sub-groups on the basis of age. The proposed names for the condition are "Gender dysphoria in children" and "Gender dysphoria in adolescents or adults." The English word *dysphoria* comes from two Greek words meaning "hard" or "difficult" and "to bear" or "to carry," and refers to a chronic or persistent mood of sadness or generalized unease or discomfort. Most people with this disorder grow up feeling rejected and out of place. **Suicide** attempts and **substance abuse** are common. Most adolescents and adults with the disorder eventually attempt to "pass" or live as members of the opposite sex.

Women's issues

Typical stressors

Women are often expected to occupy a number of roles at the same time: wife, mother, homemaker, employee, or caregiver to an elderly parent. Meeting the demands of so many roles simultaneously leads to stressful situations in which choices must be prioritized.

Women often must choose whether to pursue or further a career versus whether to devote more time to home and family.

Many women prefer to work outside the home because it gives them a greater sense of life satisfaction. For other women, such as those who run single-parent households, employment is not an optionit is a necessity. Compared with men, women frequently have jobs with less autonomy or creativity, which decreases their level of job satisfaction. Women may also have more difficulty being accepted in the workplace because of hierarchical structures preferring men. Documentation repeatedly shows that women's salaries are lower than those of men in comparable positions; women tend to be paid less even when performing the same jobs as men.

When women do choose or are required to work outside the home, they continue to perform the bulk of household duties as well. Sarah Rosenfield reported that, compared to men, women perform 66% more of the domestic work, sleep a half hour less per night, and perform an extra month of work each year. Needless to say, increased workloads and decreased attention to rest and relaxation are stressful and pose obstacles to women's mental health.

Divorce results in more severe consequences for women who choose or are able to stay home in deference to child rearing. Such women depend on marriage for financial security. Such domestic skills as child care and housecleaning are not highly valued by society and thus are poorly compensated in terms of money. Women who have never been employed and then experience divorce often have few options for securing adequate income.

Although women's ability to form meaningful relationships is a buffer against stress, it can also be a source of stress. Caring about another person can be stressful when that person is not doing well physically or emotionally. Many families take for granted that the female members care for sick children or for elderly parents who are no longer self-sufficient. As a result, many women in their forties or fifties are caught between the needs of their college-age offspring and the needs of dependent parents or in-laws. Interpersonal conflicts resulting from these heavy burdens may cause stress or lower self-esteem; a Canadian study reported in 2011 that women caregivers are still more likely to suffer **depression** or post-traumatic stress than men placed in a caregiver role. Women may also view unsuccessful relationships as representing failure on their part to fulfill such traditional feminine qualities as nurturance, warmth, and empathy.

Additional sources of stress common to women include victimization, assertiveness, and physical unattractiveness. Victimization is a constant concern due to the power differential between men and women. Assertiveness may be stressful for women who have had little experience in competitive situations. Physical unattractiveness may cause some women who adhere to unrealistic standards of feminine beauty to experience shame. Women considered unattractive may also experience discrimination in the workplace or in admission to higher education. In addition, the double standard of aging in contemporary society means that all women will eventually have to cope with the **stigma** of the putative unattractiveness associated with aging.

Typical coping strategies

Studies suggest that women typically react to stress by seeking social support, expressing feelings, or using distraction. These strategies might include praying, worrying, venting, getting advice, or engaging in behaviors that are not related to the problem at all (including such antisocial behaviors as drinking alcohol). Seeking social support and distraction are considered avoidant coping strategies because they do not focus on solving or overcoming a problem, only on alleviating the stress associated with the problem. Research is inconclusive regarding whether men or women are more likely to use problem solving, which is considered an active coping strategy.

Typical patterns of psychopathology

Women are more likely than men to experience internalizing disorders. Primary symptoms of internalizing disorders involve negative inner emotions as opposed to outward negative behavior. Depression (both mild and severe) and anxiety (generalized or free-floating anxiety, phobias, and panic attacks) are internalizing disorders common to women. Symptoms include sadness; a sense of loss, helplessness, or hopelessness; doubt about one's ability to handle problems; high levels of worry or nervousness; poor self-esteem; guilt, self-reproach, and self-blame; decreased energy, motivation, interest in life, or concentration; and problems with sleep or appetite. Women also are more likely than men to have eating disorders, and although incidence of **bipolar disorder** is similar between men and women, women manifest rapid cycling more often and have longer depressive episodes.

Men's issues

Typical stressors

Situations that typically produce stress for men are those that challenge their self-identity and cause them to feel inadequate. If their identity closely matches a

KEY TERMS

Androgyny—The condition of having the characteristics of both a man and a woman, or not being clearly identified as male or female. The English word is a combination of two Greek words meaning "(adult) man" and "woman." Androgyny may refer to a person's physical characteristics, to psychological characteristics, or to behavior.

Bem Sex Role Inventory (BSRI)—A 60-item self-administered test that researchers often use to measure psychological androgyny in test subjects. It was devised in 1971 by Sandra Bem.

Congenital—Present at birth.

Disorder of sex development (DSD)—The term that is increasingly preferred for an atypical pattern of chromosomal, genital, or gonadal development. It is also known as disorder of sex differentiation.

Externalizing disorders—Disorders in which a person acts out inner turmoil or conflict on the external environment. The three major characteristics of externalizing disorders are disruptive, hyperactive, and aggressive behaviors.

Gender dysphoria—Persistent personal discomfort with one's present biological sex.

Genitals—The reproductive organs in either sex, especially the external reproductive organs.

Gonad—The organ that makes gametes (germ cells). The gonads in males are called "testicles" and produce sperm; those in females are called "ovaries" and produce eggs.

Internalizing disorders—Disorders related to issues within the self; depression and the anxiety disorders are two common types of internalizing disorders.

Intersex—A term that is sometimes used to refer to having a sexual anatomy that is not standard for either a male or a female. It covers a number of different conditions but is considered a convenient umbrella term for discussing disorders of sex development.

Karyotype—The number and appearance of a complete set of chromosomes in a species or an individual organism. The arrangement of microphotographs of the chromosomes in a standard photographic format is called a "karyogram."

Socialization—The process through which a person learns his or her roles in society. It includes the society's customs, traditions, and professional roles as well as gender roles.

traditional male role, they will experience stress in situations requiring subordination to women or emotional expressiveness. They will also experience stress if they feel they are not meeting expectations for superior physical strength, intellect, or sexual performance. Research indicates that men who strictly adhere to extreme gender roles are at higher risk for mental disorders. They are also at greater risk of dying from undiagnosed cancer, heart disease, and other physical disorders due to reluctance to consult a doctor when symptoms first appear.

Certain cultures are thought to adhere more strictly to traditional male gender roles. In a study by Jose Abreu and colleagues, Latin American men were identified as adopting the most exaggerated form of masculinity, followed by European Americans, and then African Americans. The Latino image of masculinity is often referred to as *machismo* and includes such qualities as concern for personal honor, virility, physical strength, heavy drinking, toughness, aggression, risk taking, authoritarianism, and self-centeredness. African American males are also thought to have a unique image of masculinity; however, Abreu's study showed that African Americans are more egalitarian in terms of gender roles than European Americans.

Typical coping strategies

Men may respond to stress by putting on a tough image, keeping their feelings inside, releasing stress through such activities as sports, actively attempting to solve the problem, denying the problem, abusing drugs or alcohol, or otherwise attempting to control the problem. As stated previously, research is inconclusive regarding whether males or females use problem-solving strategies more often. This type of coping strategy, however, has more frequently been attributed to males. Problem solving is seen as an active coping strategy, which is more effective than such avoidant strategies as **denial**, abuse of drugs or alcohol, or refusal to talk about problems.

Typical patterns of psychopathology

Men are more likely than women to experience externalizing disorders. Externalizing disorders are characterized by symptoms involving negative outward behavior as opposed to internal negative emotions. Such externalizing disorders as substance abuse (both drugs and alcohol) and antisocial behavior (such as anger, hostility, aggression, violence, or stealing) are common to men. Substance abuse results in such negative physical and social consequences as hallucinations, blackouts, physical dependency, job loss, divorce, arrest, organ and **brain** damage, and financial debt. Antisocial behavior impairs interpersonal relationships and can also result in negative consequences in other areas of life, such as run-ins with the criminal justice system.

Men are not exempt from such internalizing disorders as anxiety and depression. In fact, one study found that high levels of masculinity appear to be related to depression in males. Some researchers feel that men's abuse of substances could be considered the male version of depression. Because male gender roles discourage admitting vulnerability, men may resort to substance abuse as a way of covering their feelings.

Men who adhere to rigid gender roles are also at a disadvantage in interpersonal relationships, especially intimate relationships. They may avoid emotional expressiveness or may behave in domineering and hostile ways. These behaviors increase their risk of social isolation, disconnection from nurturance, and participation in unhealthy relationships.

Mental health

Research indicates that, overall, neither men nor women are at greater risk for developing mental disorders as such. Being male or female may indicate susceptibility to certain types of disorders, however. Neither masculinity nor femininity is uniformly positive; both gender identifications have strengths and weaknesses. For example, femininity appears to be protective against antisocial behaviors and substance abuse but is associated with high levels of avoidant coping strategies and low levels of achievement. Masculinity appears to be protective against depression but is high in antisocial behavior and substance abuse.

Information about gender roles has implications for treatment. Women might not seek treatment because of a lack of such resources as money, transportation, or time away from child-care duties. A treatment center that is sensitive to women's issues should seek to provide these resources in order to facilitate access to treatment. Men, on the other hand, might not seek treatment because it is incongruent with their image of masculinity. Therapists may need to offer men less threatening forms of treatment, such as those that focus on cognitive problem solving rather than on emotions.

The focus of therapy may differ according to one's gender issues. Therapists should recognize the potential for shame and defensiveness when exploring gender norms. Externalizing behaviors may point to underlying hidden shame. For women, the importance placed on various roles in their lives and how closely those roles are tied to their self-identity is relevant. Men may be encouraged to connect to the spiritual aspects of their being and to consider less stringent views of masculinity. Therapists should also consider the associated influences of generation, culture, class, occupation, and educational level when exploring gender-role issues. Men often are entering therapy under duress, as the result of a court order or a spousal ultimatum and may begin the therapeutic process from a perspective of defensiveness. In addition, men's reluctance to discuss their emotions means that less is known about their responses to mental health crises than is known about women's responses. A number of researchers maintain that further study of men's experience of mental distress is needed.

Taking either masculine or feminine qualities to an extreme and to the exclusion of the other appears to be detrimental. A non-traditional gender-role orientation would combine the best of both genders: a social focus (reciprocally supportive relationships and a balance between interests of self and others) and active coping strategies.

Flexibility in using coping strategies is also important. Active, problem-focused coping strategies help to change the situation that is causing the problem. Avoidant or emotion-focused coping strategies manage or reduce emotional distress. Avoidant and emotion-focused strategies may be helpful for the immediate crisis but should be used in combination with more active strategies for complete problem resolution.

QUESTIONS TO ASK YOUR DOCTOR

- Have you ever treated a patient with gender dysphoria?
- Can you recommend a support group for men (or women)?
- Can you recommend any treatments to help me deal with stress?
- Where can I learn more about gender issues?

Resources

BOOKS

American Psychiatric Association. *Diagnostic and Statistical Manual of Mental Disorders*. 4th ed., Text rev. Washington, DC: American Psychiatric Association, 2000.

Balon, Richard, and Robert Taylor Segraves, eds. *Clinical Manual of Sexual Disorders*. Washington, DC: American Psychiatric Publishing, 2009.

Bem, Sandra L. *An Unconventional Family*. New Haven, CT: Yale University Press, 1998.

Denmark, Florence L., and Michele A. Paludi, eds. *Psychology of Women: A Handbook of Issues and Theories*, 2nd ed. Westport, CT: Praeger, 2008.

Firestein, Beth A. *Becoming Visible: Counseling Bisexuals across the Lifespan*. New York: Columbia University Press, 2007.

Gilligan, Carol. *In a Different Voice: Psychological Theory and Women's Development.* Cambridge, MA: Harvard University Press, 1982.

Kimmel, Michael S., and Michael A. Messner. *Men's Lives*, 7th ed. Boston, MA: Pearson Allyn and Bacon, 2007.

Miller, Karen, ed. *Male and Female Roles*. Detroit, MI: Greenhaven Press, 2010.

PERIODICALS

Andermann, L. "Culture and the Social Construction of Gender: Mapping the Intersection with Mental Health." *International Review of Psychiatry* 22 (May 2010): 501–512.

Bianchi, F.T., et al. "Partner Selection among Latino Immigrant Men Who Have Sex with Men." *Archives of Sexual Behavior* 39 (December 2010): 1321–1330.

Brennan, D.J., et al. "Men's Sexual Orientation and Health in Canada." *Canadian Journal of Public Health* 101 (May-June 2010): 255–58.

Gale-Ross, R., et al. "Gender Role, Life Satisfaction, and Wellness: Androgyny in a Southwestern Ontario Sample." *Canadian Journal of Aging* 28 (June 2009): 135–46.

Gannon, K., et al. "Re-constructing Masculinity following Radical Prostatectomy for Prostate Cancer." *Aging Male* 13 (December 2010): 258–264.

Kertzner, R.M., et al. "Social and Psychological Well-being in Lesbians, Gay Men, and Bisexuals: The Effects of Race, Gender, Age, and Sexual Identity." *American Journal of Orthopsychiatry* 79 (October 2009): 500–510.

Lawrence, A.A. "Proposed Revisions to Gender Identity Disorder Diagnoses in the DSM-5." *Archives of Sexual Behavior* 39 (December 2010): 1253–1260.

Loughrey, M. "Just How Male Are Male Nurses?" *Journal of Clinical Nursing* 17 (May 2008): 1327–34.

Peate, I. "The Mental Health of Men and Boys: An Overview." *British Journal of Nursing* 19 (October 28-November 10, 2010): 1231–1235.

Ridge, D., et al. "Understanding How Men Experience, Express and Cope with Mental Distress: Where Next?" *Sociology of Health and Illness* 33 (January 2011): 145–159.

Sánchez, F. J., et al. "Reported Effects of Masculine Ideals on Gay Men." *Psychology of Men and Masculinity* 10 (January 2009): 73–87.

Schneider, M., et al. "Differences on Psychosocial Outcomes between Male and Female Caregivers of Children with Life-limiting Illnesses." *Journal of Pediatric Nursing* 26 (June 2011): 186–199.

WEBSITES

American Association for Marriage and Family Therapy (AAMFT). "Therapeutic Issues for Same-sex Couples: Gender Roles." http://www.aamft.org/imis15/Content/Consumer_Updates/Therapeutic_Issues_for_Same-sex_Couples.aspx (accessed May 29, 2011).

American Psychiatric Association. DSM-5 Development. "P 00 Gender Dysphoria in Children." http://www.dsm5.org/ProposedRevisions/Pages/proposedrevision.aspx?rid=192 (accessed May 19, 2011).

American Psychiatric Association. DSM-5 Development. "P 01 Gender Dysphoria in Adolescents or Adults." http://www.dsm5.org/ProposedRevisions/Pages/proposedrevision.aspx?rid=482 (accessed May 19, 2011).

Domestic Violence in Gay Couples. "Choosing to Abuse: Gender Roles." http://www.psychpage.com/gay/library/gay_lesbian_violence/choosing_gender.html (accessed May 29, 2011).

Medscape. "Sexual and Gender Identity Disorders." http://emedicine.medscape.com/article/293890-overview (accessed May 19, 2011).

San Diego Union-Tribune. "Couple's Gender Secret for Baby Touches Off Debate." http://www.signonsandiego.com/news/2011/may/27/couples-gender-secret-for-baby-touches-off-debate (accessed May 27, 2011).

ORGANIZATIONS

American Association for Marriage and Family Therapy (AAMFT), 112 South Alfred Street, Alexandria, VA, United States 22314-3061, (703) 838-9808, Fax: (703) 838-9805, http://www.aamft.org/iMIS15/AAMFT

American Association of Sexuality Educators, Counselors, and Therapists (AASECT), 1444 I Street NW, Suite 700, Washington, DC, United States 20005, (202) 449-1099, Fax: (202) 216-9646, info@aasect.org, http://www.aasect.org

Society for the Psychological Study of Men and Masculinity (Division 51), American Psychological Association, 750 First St. NE, Washington, DC, United States 20002-4242, (202) 216-7602, Fax: (202) 218-3599, kcooke@apa.org, http://www.apa.org/about/division/div51.aspx

University of Minnesota Clinic, Center for Sexual Health, 1300 South 2nd Street, Minneapolis, MN, United States 55454, (612) 624-7821, http://www.fm.umn.edu/phs/clinic/home.html

Wellesley Centers for Women (WCW), Wellesley College, 106 Central Street, Wellesley, MA, United States 02481-8203, (781) 283-2500, wcw@wellesley.edu, http://www.wcwonline.org

Sandra L. Friedrich, M.A.
Emily Jane Willingham, Ph.D.
Rebecca J. Frey, Ph.D.

Generalized anxiety disorder

Definition

Generalized anxiety disorder (GAD) is a disorder characterized by excessive worry and anxiety concerning a number of events and activities. This anxiety is accompanied by such symptoms as restlessness, **fatigue**, inability to concentrate, muscle tension, or disturbed sleep. Individuals with this disorder experience symptoms on most days for a period of at least six months, and find the symptoms difficult to control.

Demographics

The **National Institute of Mental Health** (NIMH) estimates that approximately 6.8 million Americans have GAD. Further it is estimated that twice as many women as men develop GAD. One study that used the *DSM-III-R* criteria concluded that 5% of the United States population, or one person in every 20, will develop GAD at some point.

Some psychiatrists think that generalized anxiety disorder is overdiagnosed in both adults and children. One reason for this possibility is that diagnostic screening tests used by primary care physicians for mental disorders produce a large number of false positives for GAD. One study of the PRIME-MD, a screening instrument for mental disorders frequently used in primary care practices, found that 7 of 10 patients met the criteria for GAD. In-depth follow-up interviews with the patients, however, revealed that only a third of the GAD diagnoses could be confirmed.

Description

Generalized anxiety disorder is characterized by persistent worry that is excessive and that patients find hard to control. Common worries associated with generalized anxiety disorder include work responsibilities, money, health, safety, car repairs, and household chores. Unlike people with phobias or post-traumatic disorders, people with GAD do not have their worries provoked by specific triggers; they may worry about almost anything having to do with ordinary life. It is not unusual for patients diagnosed with GAD to shift the focus of their anxiety from one issue to another as their daily circumstances change. For example, people with GAD may start worrying about finances when several bills arrive in the mail, and then fret about the state of their health when they notice that one of the bills is for health insurance. Later in the day they may read a newspaper article that moves the focus of the worry to a third concern.

Patients usually recognize that their worry is out of proportion in its duration or intensity to the actual likelihood or impact of the feared situation or event. For example, a husband or wife may worry about an accident happening to a spouse who commutes to work by train, even though the worried partner knows objectively that rail travel is much safer than automobile travel on major highways. The anxiety levels of patients with GAD may rise and fall somewhat over a period of weeks or months but tend to become chronic problems. The disorder typically becomes worse during stressful periods in the patient's life.

The ***Diagnostic and Statistical Manual of Mental Disorders,*** fourth edition, text revision (*DSM-IV-TR*) specifies interference with work, family life, social activities, or other areas of functioning as a criterion for generalized anxiety disorder. This may be accompanied by such physical symptoms as **insomnia**, sore muscles, headaches, and digestive upsets. According to the *DSM-IV-TR,* adult patients must experience three symptoms out of a list of six (restlessness, being easily fatigued, having difficulty concentrating, being irritable, high levels of muscle tension, and sleep disturbances) in order to be diagnosed with the disorder.

Patients diagnosed with GAD have a high rate of concurrent mental disorders, particularly major **depression** disorder, other **anxiety disorders**, or a **substance abuse** disorder. They also frequently have or develop such stress-related physical illnesses and conditions as tension headaches, irritable bowel syndrome (IBS), temporomandibular joint dysfunction (TMJ), bruxism (grinding of the teeth during sleep), and hypertension. In addition, GAD often intensifies the discomfort or complications associated with arthritis, diabetes, and other chronic disorders. Patients with GAD are more likely to seek help from a primary care physician than a **psychiatrist**; they are also more likely than patients with other disorders to make frequent medical appointments, to undergo extensive or repeated diagnostic testing, to describe their health as poor, and to smoke tobacco or abuse other substances. In addition, patients with anxiety disorders have higher rates of mortality from all causes than people who are less anxious.

In many cases, it is difficult for the patient's doctor to determine whether the anxiety preceded the physical condition or followed it; sometimes people develop generalized anxiety disorder after being diagnosed with a chronic organic health problem. In other instances, the wear and tear on the body caused by persistent and recurrent worrying leads to physical diseases and disorders. There is an overall "vicious circle" quality to the relationship between GAD and other disorders, whether mental or organic.

Children diagnosed with GAD have much the same anxiety symptoms as adults. The mother of a six-year-old boy with the disorder told his pediatrician that her son "acted like a little man" rather than a typical first-grader. He would worry about such matters as arriving on time for school field trips, whether the family had enough money for immediate needs, whether his friends would get hurt climbing on the playground jungle gym, whether there was enough gas in the tank of the family car, and similar concerns. The little boy had these worries in spite of the fact that his family was stable and happy and had no serious financial or other problems.

GAD often has an insidious onset that begins relatively early in life, although it can be precipitated by a sudden crisis at any age above six or seven years. The idea that GAD often begins in the childhood years even though the symptoms may not become clearly noticeable until late adolescence or the early adult years is gaining acceptance. About half of all patients diagnosed with the disorder report that their worrying began in childhood or their teenage years. Many will say that they cannot remember a time in their lives when they were not worried about something. This type of persistent anxiety can be regarded as part of a person's temperament, or inborn disposition; it is sometimes called trait anxiety. It is not unusual, however, for people to develop the disorder in their early adult years or even later in reaction to chronic **stress** or anxiety-producing situations. For example, there are instances of people developing GAD after several years of taking care of a relative with **dementia**, living with domestic violence, or living in close contact with a friend or relative with **borderline personality disorder**.

The specific worries of people with GAD may be influenced by their ethnic background or culture. The *DSM-IV-TR* cited an observation that being punctual is a common concern of patients with GAD that reflects the value that Western countries place on using time as efficiently as possible. One study of worry in college students from different ethnic backgrounds found that Caucasian and African American students tended to worry a variable amount about a wider range of concerns, whereas Asian Americans tended to worry more intensely about a smaller number of issues. Another study found that a community sample of older Puerto Ricans with GAD overlapped with a culture-specific syndrome called *ataque de nervios,* which resembles **panic disorder** but has features of other anxiety disorders as well as dissociative symptoms. (People experience dissociative symptoms when their perception of reality is temporarily altered—they may feel as if they were in a trance, or that they were observing activity around them instead of participating.) Further research is needed regarding the relationship between people's ethnic backgrounds and their outward expression of anxiety symptoms.

Causes and symptoms

Causes

The causes of generalized anxiety disorder appear to be a mixture of genetic and environmental factors. It has been known for some years that the disorder runs in families. Twin studies as well as the ongoing mapping of the human genome point to a genetic factor in the development of GAD. The role of the family environment (social **modeling**) in an individual's susceptibility to GAD is uncertain. Social modeling, the process of learning behavioral and emotional response patterns from observing one's parents or other adults, appears to be a more important factor for women than for men.

Another factor in the development of GAD is social expectations related to gender roles. Research findings indicate that women have higher levels of emotional distress and lower quality of life than men. The higher incidence of GAD in women has been linked to the diffuse yet comprehensive expectations of women as caregivers. Many women assume responsibility for the well-being and safety of other family members in addition to holding jobs or completing graduate or professional school. The global character of these responsibilities as well as their unrelenting nature has been described as a mirror image of the persistent but nonspecific anxiety associated with GAD.

Socioeconomic status may also contribute to generalized anxiety. One British study found that GAD is more closely associated with an accumulation of minor stressors than with any demographic factors. People of lower socioeconomic status, however, have fewer resources for dealing with minor stressors and so appear to be at greater risk for generalized anxiety.

An additional factor may be the patient's level of muscle tension. Several studies have found that patients diagnosed with GAD tend to respond to physiological stress in a rigid, stereotyped manner. Their autonomic reactions (reactions in the part of the nervous system that governs involuntary bodily functions) are similar to those of people without GAD, but their muscular tension shows a significant increase. It is not yet known, however, whether this level of muscle tension is a cause or an effect of GAD.

Symptoms

The symptomatology of GAD has changed somewhat over time with redefinitions of the disorder in successive editions of the *DSM.* The first edition of the *DSM* and the *DSM-II* did not make a sharp distinction between generalized anxiety disorder and panic disorder. After specific treatments were developed for panic disorder, GAD was introduced in the *DSM-III* as an anxiety disorder without panic attacks or symptoms of major depression. This definition proved to be unreliable. As a result, the *DSM-IV* constructed its definition of GAD around the psychological symptoms of the disorder (excessive worrying) rather than the physical (muscle tension) or autonomic symptoms of anxiety. The *DSM-IV-TR* continued that emphasis, and no changes or revisions have been suggested for the *DSM-5*.

According to the *DSM-IV-TR,* the symptoms of GAD are:

- excessive anxiety and worry about a number of events or activities occurring more days than not for at least six months
- worry that cannot be controlled
- worry that is associated with several symptoms such as restlessness, fatigue, irritability, or muscle tension
- worry that causes distress or impairment in relationships, at work, or at school

In addition, to meet the diagnostic criteria for GAD, the content or focus of the worry cannot change the **diagnosis** from GAD to another anxiety disorder such as panic disorder, **social phobia**, or **obsessive-compulsive disorder**, and the anxiety cannot be caused by a substance (a drug or a medication).

One categorization of GAD symptoms that some psychiatrists use in addition to the *DSM* framework consists of three symptom clusters:

- symptoms related to high levels of physiological arousal: muscle tension, irritability, fatigue, restlessness, insomnia
- symptoms related to distorted thinking processes: poor concentration, unrealistic assessment of problems, recurrent worrying
- symptoms associated with poor coping strategies: procrastination, avoidance, inadequate problem-solving skills

Diagnosis

Diagnosis of GAD, particularly in primary care settings, is complicated by several factors. One is the high level of comorbidity (co-occurrence) between GAD and other mental or physical disorders. Another is the considerable overlap between anxiety disorders and depression. Some practitioners believe that depression and GAD may not be separate disorders after all, because studies have repeatedly confirmed the existence and common occurrence of a "mixed" anxiety/depression syndrome.

Evaluating patients for generalized anxiety disorder includes the following steps:

- Patient interview. The doctor will ask the patients to describe the anxiety, and will note whether it is acute (lasting hours to weeks) or persistent (lasting from months to years). If the patients describe a recent stressful event, the doctor will evaluate them for "double anxiety," which refers to acute anxiety added to underlying persistent anxiety. The doctor may also give the patients a diagnostic questionnaire to evaluate the presence of anxiety disorders. The Hamilton Anxiety Scale is a commonly used instrument to assess anxiety disorders in general. The Generalized Anxiety Disorder Questionnaire for *DSM-IV* (GAD-Q-IV) is a more recent diagnostic tool, and is specific to GAD.
- Medical evaluation. Nonpsychiatric disorders that are known to cause anxiety (hyperthyroidism, Cushing's disease, mitral valve prolapse, carcinoid syndrome, and pheochromocytoma) must be ruled out, as well as certain medications (steroids, digoxin, thyroxine, theophylline, and selective serotonin reuptake inhibitors) that may also cause anxiety as a side effect. Patients should be asked about their use of herbal preparations as well.
- Substance abuse evaluation. Because anxiety is a common symptom of substance abuse and withdrawal syndrome, doctors will ask about patients' use of caffeine, nicotine, alcohol, and other common substances (including prescription medications) that may be abused.
- Evaluation for other psychiatric disorders. This step is necessary because of the frequent overlap between GAD and depression or between GAD and other anxiety disorders.

In some instances the doctor will consult the patient's family for additional information about the onset of the patient's anxiety symptoms, dietary habits, etc.

Treatment

There are several treatment types that have been found effective in treating people with GAD. Most patients with the disorder are treated with a combination of medications and **psychotherapy**.

Medications

Pharmacologic therapy is usually prescribed for patients whose anxiety is severe enough to interfere with daily functioning. Several different groups of medications have been used to treat generalized anxiety disorder.

These medications include the following:

- Benzodiazepines. This group of tranquilizers does not decrease worry, but lowers anxiety by decreasing muscle tension and hypervigilance. They are often prescribed for patients with double anxiety because they act very quickly. The benzodiazepines, however, have several disadvantages: they are unsuitable for long-term therapy because they can cause dependence, and GAD is a long-term disorder; they cannot be given to patients who abuse alcohol; and they cause short-term memory loss and difficulty in concentration. One British study found that benzodiazepines significantly increased a patient's risk of involvement in a traffic accident.

- Buspirone (BuSpar). Buspirone appears to be as effective as benzodiazepines and antidepressants in controlling anxiety symptoms. It is slower to take effect (about two–three weeks), but has fewer side effects. In addition, it treats the worry associated with GAD rather than the muscle tension.
- Tricyclic antidepressants. Imipramine (Tofranil), nortriptyline (Pamelor), and desipramine (Norpramin) have been given to patients with GAD. They have, however, some problematic side effects: imipramine has been associated with disturbances in heart rhythm, and the other tricyclics often cause drowsiness, dry mouth, constipation, and confusion. They increase the patient's risk of falls and other accidents.
- Selective serotonin reuptake inhibitors (SSRIs). Paroxetine (Paxil), one of the SSRIs, was approved by the U.S. Food and Drug Administration (FDA) in 2001 as a treatment for GAD. Venlafaxine (Effexor) appears to be particularly beneficial to patients with a mixed anxiety/depression syndrome; it is the first drug to be labeled by the FDA as an antidepressant as well as an anxiolytic. Venlafaxine is also effective in treating patients with GAD whose symptoms are primarily somatic (manifesting as physical symptoms or bodily complaints).

Psychotherapy

Some studies have found cognitive therapy to be superior to medications and **psychodynamic psychotherapy** in treating GAD, but other researchers disagree with these findings. As a rule, patients with GAD who have **personality disorders**, who are living with chronic social stress (e.g., caring for a parent with **Alzheimer's disease**), or who do not trust psychotherapeutic approaches require treatment with medications. The greatest benefit of cognitive therapy is its effectiveness in helping patients with the disorder to learn more realistic ways to appraise their problems and to use better problem-solving techniques.

Family therapy is recommended insofar as family members can be helpful in offering patients a different perspective on their problems. They can also help patients practice new approaches to problem solving.

KEY TERMS

Anxiolytic—A preparation or substance given to relieve anxiety; a tranquilizer.

Ataque de nervios—A culture-specific anxiety syndrome found among some Latin American groups in the United States and in Latin America. It resembles panic disorder in some respects but also includes dissociative symptoms, and frequently occurs in response to stressful events.

Autonomic nervous system—The part of the nervous system that governs the heart, involuntary muscles, and glands.

Double anxiety—Acute anxiety from a recent stressful event combined with underlying persistent anxiety associated with generalized anxiety disorder.

Free-floating—A term used in psychiatry to describe anxiety that is unfocused or lacking an apparent cause or object.

Insidious—Proceeding gradually and inconspicuously but with serious effect.

Social modeling—A process of learning behavioral and emotional response patterns from observing one's parents or other adults. Some researchers think that social modeling plays a part in the development of generalized anxiety disorder in women.

Temperament—A person's natural disposition or inborn combination of mental and emotional traits.

Temporomandibular joint dysfunction—A condition resulting in pain in the head, face, and jaw. Muscle tension or abnormalities of the bones in the area of the hinged joint (the temporomandibular joint) between the lower jaw and the temporal bone are usually the cause.

Trait anxiety—A type of persistent anxiety found in some patients with generalized anxiety disorder. Trait anxiety is regarded as a feature (trait) of a person's temperament.

Twin study—Research studies that use pairs of twins to study the effects of heredity and environment on behavior or other characteristics.

Alternative and complementary therapies

Several alternative and complementary therapies have been found helpful in treating patients with generalized anxiety disorder. These include **hypnotherapy**, **music therapy**, Ayurvedic medicine, **yoga**, religious practice, and guided imagery **meditation**.

Biofeedback and relaxation techniques are also recommended for patients with GAD in order to lower physiologic arousal. In addition, massage therapy, hydrotherapy, shiatsu, and **acupuncture** have been reported to relieve muscle spasms or soreness associated with GAD.

One herbal remedy that has been used in **clinical trials** for treating GAD is **passionflower** (*Passiflora incarnata*). One team of researchers found that passionflower extract was as effective as **oxazepam** (Serax) in relieving anxiety symptoms in a group of 36 outpatients diagnosed with GAD according to *DSM-IV* criteria. In addition, the passionflower extract did not impair the subjects' job performance as frequently or as severely as the oxazepam.

Prognosis

Generalized anxiety disorder is generally regarded as a long-term condition that may become a lifelong problem. Patients frequently find their symptoms resurfacing or getting worse during stressful periods in their lives. It is rare for patients with GAD to recover spontaneously.

Prevention

The best preventive strategy, given the early onset of GAD, is the modeling of realistic assessment of stressful events by parents, and the teaching of effective coping strategies to their children.

Resources

BOOKS

American Psychiatric Association. *Diagnostic and Statistical Manual of Mental Disorders*. 4th ed., text rev. Washington, DC: American Psychiatric Publishing, 2000.

Dugas, Michel J., and Melisa Robichaud. *Cognitive-Behavioral Treatment for Generalized Anxiety Disorder: From Science to Practice*. New York: Brunner-Routledge, 2006.

Heimberg, Richard G., Cynthia L. Turk, and Douglas S. Mennin, eds. *Generalized Anxiety Disorder: Advances in Research and Practice*. New York: The Guilford Press, 2004.

Nutt, David J., Karl Rickels, and Dan J. Stein. *Generalized Anxiety Disorder: Symptomatology, Pathogenesis and Management*. Oxford: Informa Healthcare, 2002.

Pelletier, Kenneth R. "CAM Therapies for Specific Conditions: Anxiety." In *The Best Alternative Medicine*. Part II. New York: Touchstone, 2007.

Rygh, Jayne L., and William C. Sanderson. *Treating Generalized Anxiety Disorder: Evidence-Based Strategies, Tools, and Techniques*. New York: The Guilford Press, 2004.

PERIODICALS

Allgulander, Christer. "Generalized Anxiety Disorder: What Are We Missing?" *European Neuropsychopharmacology* 16, Suppl. 2 (July 2006): S101–S108.

Allgulander, Christer, Ioana Florea, and Anna K. Trap Huusom. "Prevention of Relapse in Generalized Anxiety Disorder by Escitalopram Treatment." *International Journal of Neuropsychopharmacology* 9, no. 5 (October 2006): 495–505.

Angst, Jules, et al. "Varying Temporal Criteria for Generalized Anxiety Disorder: Prevalence and Clinical Characteristics in a Young Age Cohort." *Psychological Medicine* 36, no. 9 (September 2006): 1283–92.

Baldwin, David S., Anna Karina Trap Huusom, and Eli Maehlum. "Escitalopram and Paroxetine in the Treatment of Generalised Anxiety Disorder: Randomised, Placebo-Controlled, Double-Blind Study." *British Journal of Psychiatry* 189, no. 3 (September 2006): 264–72. Available online at http://bjp.rcpsych.org/content/189/3/264.full (accessed November 9, 2011).

Connor, Kathryn M., Victoria Payne, and Jonathan R. T. Davidson. "Kava in Generalized Anxiety Disorder: Three Placebo-Controlled Trials." *International Clinical Psychopharmacology* 21, no. 5 (September 2006): 249–53.

Goldston, David B., et al. "Reading Problems, Psychiatric Disorders, and Functional Impairment from Mid- to Late Adolescence." *Journal of the American Academy of Child & Adolescent Psychiatry* 46, no. 1 (January 2007): 25–32.

Gosselin, Patrick, et al. "Benzodiazepine Discontinuation Among Adults With GAD: A Randomized Trial of Cognitive-Behavioral Therapy." *Journal of Consulting and Clinical Psychology* 74, no. 5 (October 2006): 908–19.

Hoge, Elizabeth A., et al. "Cross-Cultural Differences in Somatic Presentation in Patients with Generalized Anxiety Disorder." *Journal of Nervous & Mental Disease* 194, no. 12 (December 2006): 962–66.

Kim, Tae-Suk, et al. "Comparison of Venlafaxine Extended Release Versus Paroxetine for Treatment of Patients with Generalized Anxiety Disorder." *Psychiatry and Clinical Neurosciences* 60, no. 3 (June 2006): 347–51.

Kopecek, Miloslav, Pavel Mohr, and Tomas Novak. "Sedative Effects of Low-Dose Risperidone in GAD Patients and Risk of Drug Interactions." *Journal of Clinical Psychiatry* 67, no. 8 (August 2006): 1308–1309.

Labrecque, Joane, et al. "Cognitive-Behavioral Therapy for Comorbid Generalized Anxiety Disorder and Panic Disorder With Agoraphobia." *Behavior Modification* 30, no. 4 (July 2006): 383–410.

Lyddon, William J. "Review: Generalized Anxiety Disorder: Advances in Research and Practice." *Journal of Cognitive Psychotherapy* 20, no. 4 (December 2006): 463–64.

Mennin, Douglas S. "Emotion Regulation Therapy: An Integrative Approach to Treatment-Resistant Anxiety Disorders." *Journal of Contemporary Psychotherapy* 36, no. 2 (June 2006): 95–105.

Montgomery, Stuart A., et al. "Efficacy and Safety of Pregabalin in the Treatment of Generalized Anxiety Disorder: A 6-Week, Multicenter, Randomized, Double-Blind, Placebo-Controlled Comparison of Pregabalin and Venlafaxine." *Journal of Clinical Psychiatry* 67, no. 5 (May 2006): 771–82.

Nutt, David, et al. "Generalized Anxiety Disorder: A Comorbid Disease." *European Neuropsychopharmacology* 16, Suppl. 2 (July 2006): S109–S118.

Skopp, Nancy A., et al. "Investigation of Cognitive Behavior Therapy." *American Journal of Geriatric Psychiatry* 14, no. 3 (March 2006): 292.

Weems, Carl F., et al. "Predisaster Trait Anxiety and Negative Affect Predict Posttraumatic Stress in Youths After Hurricane Katrina." *Journal of Consulting and Clinical Psychology* 75, no. 1 (February 2007): 154–59. http://cretscmhd.psych.ucla.edu/nola/Volunteer/EmpiricalStudies/Predisaster%20trait%20anxiety%20and%20negative%20affect%20predict%20posttraumatic%20stress%20in%20youths%20after%20hurricane%20katrina.pdf (accessed November 9, 2011).

WEBSITES

U.S. National Institute of Mental Health. "Anxiety Disorders." http://www.nimh.nih.gov/anxiety/anxiety.cfm (accessed October 8, 2011).

———. "Generalized Anxiety Disorder." October 6, 2011. http://www.nimh.nih.gov/health/topics/generalized-anxiety-disorder-gad/index.shtml (accessed October 8, 2011).

ORGANIZATIONS

American Psychiatric Association, 1000 Wilson Blvd., Suite 1825, Arlington, VA, 22209-3901, (703) 907-7300, apa@psych.org, http://www.psych.org.

Anxiety Disorders Association of America, 8730 Georgia Ave., Suite 600, Silver Spring, MD, 20910, (240) 485-1001, Fax: (240) 485-1035, http://www.adaa.org.

Mental Health America, 2000 North Beauregard Street, 6th Floor, Alexandria, VA, 22311, (703) 684-7722, (800) 969-6642, Fax: (703) 684-5968, http://www1.nmha.org.

National Alliance on Mental Illness, 3803 North Fairfax Drive, Suite 100, Arlington, VA, 22203, (703) 524-7600, Fax: (703) 524-9094, http://www.nami.org.

National Institute of Mental Health, 6001 Executive Blvd., Room 8184, MSC 9663, Bethesda, MD, 20892-9663, (301) 433-4513; TTY: (301) 443-8431, (866) 615-6464; TTY: (866) 415-8051, Fax: (301) 443-4279, nimhinfo@nih.gov, http://www.nimh.nih.gov.

Rebecca J. Frey, PhD
Ruth A. Wienclaw, PhD

Genetic factors and mental disorders

Definition

Genetic factors play an important role in the etiology (causes) of many mental disorders. In 1990, the Human Genome Project began mapping the entire sequence of human DNA. Completed in 2003, the project has had great implications for psychiatric **diagnosis** and treatment.

Description

Genes appear to influence the development of mental disorders in three major ways:

1. They may govern the organic causes of such disorders as Alzheimer's disease (AD) and schizophrenia.
2. They may be responsible for abnormalities in a person's development before or after birth.
3. They may influence a person's susceptibility to anxiety, depression, personality disorders, and substance abuse disorders.

The two most important examples of mental disorders caused by organic changes or abnormalities in the **brain** are late-onset AD and **schizophrenia**. Both disorders are polygenic, which means that their expression is determined by more than one gene.

Disorders with genetic components

SCHIZOPHRENIA. Researchers have known for many years that first-degree biological relatives of patients with schizophrenia have a greater risk of developing the disorder than the general population. The identical twin of a person with schizophrenia has a 40%–50% risk of developing the disorder.

LATE-ONSET AD. Late-onset AD is another polygenic disorder. It has been known since 1993 that a specific form of a gene for apolipoprotein E (apoE4) on human chromosome 19 is a genetic risk factor for late-onset AD. People who inherited the gene from one parent have a 50% chance of developing AD and a 90% chance if they inherited the gene from both parents. They are also likely to develop AD earlier in life. One of the remaining puzzles about this particular gene, however, is that it is not a consistent marker for AD. In other words, some people who have the apoE4 gene do not develop AD, and some who do not have the gene do develop the disorder.

There are two other forms of AD, early-onset AD and familial AD (FAD), which have different patterns of genetic transmission. Early-onset AD is caused by a defect in one of three genes known as APP, presenilin-1, and presenilin-2, found on human chromosomes 21, 14, and 1, respectively. Early-onset AD is also associated with **Down syndrome**, in that persons with trisomy 21 (three forms of human chromosome 21 instead of two) often develop this form of AD. The brains of people with Down syndrome age prematurely, so those who develop early-onset AD are often only in their late 40s or early 50s when the symptoms of the disease first appear. FAD appears to be related to abnormal genes on human chromosomes 21 and 14.

FRAGILE X SYNDROME. Fragile X syndrome is the most common inherited form of **intellectual disability** and should be considered in the differential diagnosis of any child with developmental delays, signs of intellectual disability, or learning difficulties. The syndrome is caused by a large expansion of a cytosine-guanine-guanine (CGG) repeat, which interferes with normal protein transcription from a gene called the FMR1 gene on the X chromosome. Since males have only one X chromosome, they are more severely affected than females who have a normal FMR1 gene on their second X chromosome. In both genders, there is a correlation between the length of the expansion mutation and the severity of the syndrome.

In addition to developmental disorders of childhood, expansion mutations, such as the one found in Fragile X syndrome, may also be involved in other psychiatric disorders. Clinicians had noticed as early as 1910 that some disorders produce a more severe phenotype or occur at earlier and earlier ages in each successive generation of an affected family. This phenomenon is known as anticipation, but its biological basis was not understood until recently. It is now known that triplet repeats that are long enough to cause disorders are unstable and tend to grow longer from generation to generation. Anticipation has been found in some families affected by **bipolar disorder** and schizophrenia, and some researchers think that it may also be present in some forms of **autism**.

POST-TRAUMATIC SYNDROMES. Researchers have found that some persons are more vulnerable than others to developing dissociative and anxiety-related symptoms following a traumatic experience. Vulnerability to **trauma** is affected by such inherited factors as temperament as well as by family or cultural influences; shy or introverted persons are at greater risk for developing **post-traumatic stress disorder** (PTSD) than their extroverted or outgoing peers. In addition, twin studies indicate that certain abnormalities in brain hormone levels and brain structure are inherited, and that these increase a person's susceptibility to developing **acute stress disorder** (ASD) or PTSD following exposure to trauma.

ANXIETY DISORDERS. It has been known for some time that **anxiety disorders** run in families. Recent twin studies as well as the human genome mapping point to a genetic factor in the development of **generalized anxiety disorder** (GAD). Research has also confirmed earlier hypotheses that there is a genetic component to **agoraphobia**, and that it can be separated from susceptibility to **panic disorder** (PD). Panic disorder was found to be associated with two loci, one on human chromosome 1 and the other on chromosome 11q. Researchers have concluded that agoraphobia and PD are common, heritable anxiety disorders that share some but not all of their genetic loci for susceptibility.

Behavioral phenotypes

Although medical professionals are familiar with the physical phenotypes associated with genetic disorders, the notion of behavioral phenotypes is still controversial. A behavioral phenotype is the characteristic set of behaviors found in patients with a genetic disorder. Behavioral phenotypes include patterns of language usage, cognitive development, and social adjustment as well as behavioral problems. It is important for psychiatrists who treat children and adolescents to understand behavioral phenotypes, because they are better able to identify problem behaviors as part of a genetic syndrome and refer children to a geneticist for an accurate diagnosis.

Examples of behavioral phenotypes are those associated with Down, Prader-Willi, and Williams syndromes. Children with Down syndrome have an increased risk of developing early-onset AD. They are usually quiet and good-tempered, but may also be hyperactive and impulsive. Their behavioral phenotype includes delayed language development and moderate to severe intellectual disability.

Children with Prader-Willi syndrome are often quiet in childhood but develop stubborn, aggressive, or impulsive patterns of behavior as they grow older. They are typically obsessed with food, frequently **hoarding** it, stealing it, or stealing money to buy food. The onset of their overeating is often associated with temper tantrums and other behavioral problems. About 50% of children diagnosed with Prader-Willi syndrome meet the criteria for **obsessive-compulsive disorder** (OCD).

Williams syndrome is a genetic disorder that results from a deletion of locus 23 on chromosome 7q11. Children with this syndrome often have an "elf-like" face with short upturned noses and small chins. Their behavioral phenotype includes talkativeness, friendliness, and a willingness to follow strangers. They are also hyperactive and easily distracted from tasks. The personality profile of children with Williams syndrome is so distinctive that many are diagnosed on the basis of behavioral rather than physical characteristics.

BEHAVIORAL TRAITS. There has been considerable controversy in the past decade concerning the mapping of genetic loci associated with specific human behaviors, as distinct from behavioral phenotypes related to developmental disorders. Research into the genetic component of human behavior is currently conducted with an awareness of the social and political implications of any potential results. Given contemporary concerns about the misuse of findings related to biological race or sex, investigators are usually careful to acknowledge the importance of environmental as well as genetic factors.

Genetic epidemiology

Genetic epidemiology is the branch of medicine that investigates the incidence and prevalence of genetic disorders in specific populations. Researchers in this field make use of specific types of studies to assess the relative importance of genetic and environmental factors in families with a history of inherited disorders.

TWIN STUDIES. Twin studies are based on the assumption that twins reared in the same family share a common environment. Monozygotic (identical) twins have all their genes in common, whereas dizygotic (fraternal) twins share only half their genes. If a certain disorder appears more frequently in monozygotic twins of affected persons than in dizygotic twins, one may assume that the difference is due to genetic factors rather than the family environment. Some phenotypes show clear differences between identical and fraternal twins, including schizophrenia, childhood autism, **attention deficit hyperactivity disorder (ADHD)**, unipolar **depression**, manic depressive disorder, and cognitive abilities as measured by IQ tests.

Twin studies have proved to be particularly important in genetic research into autism. Until the early 1970s, autism was thought to develop as a result of negative parental interaction. The first small-scale twin study of children with autism was done in 1977, and its findings showed that there was a significant difference between monozygotic and dizygotic twin pairs with regard to the appearance of the disorder in siblings. More importantly, the study showed that the similarities within monozygotic pairs of twins included a range of social and cognitive disabilities, not just the autism itself. This finding implied that the phenotype of autism was broader than the older diagnostic categories assumed. In the 1970s and 1980s, advances in cytogenetic techniques led to the discovery that autism was associated with several different chromosomal abnormalities, including the defect that produces fragile X syndrome. A much larger British twin study done in 1995 confirmed earlier findings in the United States: a monozygotic twin of a child diagnosed with autism was 12 times more likely to have the disorder than a dizygotic twin (60% versus 5%). Secondly, the British study confirmed the hypothesis that the genetic risk of autism extends to a broader phenotype; over 90% of the monozygotic twin pairs in the British study shared social and intellectual disabilities similar to those found in patients with autism, but less severe. The causes of autism are not yet known, but research continues to support the hypothesis that there is a genetic component.

FAMILY STUDIES. Family studies are important tools for evaluating environmental effects on children with genetic disorders—and also for evaluating the impact of the disorder on the family environment. Family studies have indicated that families may develop problems in response to a child's illness that may also affect the child's prognosis for recovery.

Family factors fall into three categories: shared genetic material, shared environment, and nonshared environment. These three categories are complicated, however, by the fact that genetic as well as environmental factors affect interactions between parents and children. For example, a parent's behavior toward a child diagnosed with depression is partly shaped by the parent's genetic vulnerability to depression.

In general, much of the impact of a family's environment on a child with a mental disorder is due to nonshared rather than shared interactions. A clinical research measurement called expressed emotion (EE), originally developed to study young adults with schizophrenia, is now used to study families with younger children with mental disorders. EE measures three primary aspects of family members' attitudes toward the child with the illness: criticism, hostility, and emotional over-involvement. A growing number of research studies indicate that EE is a good predictor of the outcome of the child's illness; high EE is a marker of a more difficult course of the disorder and a poorer prognosis.

Clinical applications of genetics in psychiatry

Recent advances in genetics have affected the practice of psychiatry in several ways:

- Genetic counseling is recommended when a couple has already produced a child with intellectual disability, dysmorphic (malformed) features, or developmental delays; when either parent is suspected or known to have a genetic disorder; when the mother is

KEY TERMS

Agoraphobia—An intense fear of being trapped in a crowded, open, or public space where it may be hard to escape, combined with the dread of having a panic attack.

Anxiety—Can be experienced as a troubled feeling, a sense of dread, fear of the future, or distress over a possible threat to a person's physical or mental well-being.

Attention deficit hyperactivity disorder (ADHD)—A developmental disorder characterized by distractibility, hyperactivity, impulsive behaviors, and the inability to remain focused on tasks or activities.

Autism—A severe developmental disorder that usually begins before three years of age and affects a child's social as well as intellectual development.

Body dysmorphic disorder—A psychiatric disorder marked by preoccupation with an imagined physical defect.

Chromosome—A microscopic thread–like structure found within each cell of the body and consists of a complex of proteins and DNA. Humans have 46 chromosomes arranged into 23 pairs. Changes in either the total number of chromosomes or their shape and size (structure) may lead to physical or mental abnormalities.

Depression—A mental state characterized by feelings of sadness, despair, and discouragement.

Differential diagnosis—Comparing and contrasting the signs, symptoms, and laboratory findings of two or more diseases to determine which is causing the patient's condition.

Heritability—The effects of differences in genetics (among the population) in producing differences in behavior.

Obsessive-compulsive disorder—An anxiety disorder in which people cannot prevent themselves from dwelling on unwanted thoughts, acting on urges, or performing repetitious rituals, such as washing their hands or checking to make sure they turned off the lights.

Phenotypes—Observable traits or characteristics.

Prader-Willi syndrome—An uncommon genetic disorder that causes a constant feeling of hunger.

Schizophrenia—A major mental illness marked by psychotic symptoms, including hallucinations, delusions, and severe disruptions in thinking.

Seizure—A convulsion, or uncontrolled discharge of nerve cells that may spread to other cells throughout the brain.

Somatoform disorder—A category of psychiatric disorder characterized by physical complaints that appear to be medical in origin but that cannot be explained in terms of a physical disease, the results of substance abuse, or by another mental disorder.

Substance abuse—Illicit, inaccurate, or recreational use of either prescription or illegal drugs. Alcohol can also be abused as a substance but has its own category, alcohol abuse.

over 35; when there is a family history of a genetic disorder, especially if several members are affected; or if the mother has been exposed during pregnancy to drugs or environmental toxins known to cause birth defects. Genetic counselors do not try to control the couple's decision about a present or future pregnancy; rather, they offer information about the disorder, including treatment options as well as the risk of recurrence. They discuss possible reproductive choices available to the couple and help them adjust to caring for a child who is already affected.

- Preliminary studies of patients with schizophrenia indicate that DNA testing of the gene for a specific serotonin receptor can predict the patient's response to antipsychotic drugs. In the near future, researchers hope to devise genetic tests that will measure patients' responsiveness to specific antidepressant and antianxiety medications. Such tests would greatly simplify the present process of trial-and-error prescribing of drugs for psychiatric disorders.
- Nosology is the branch of psychiatry that deals with the classification of mental disorders. Some current diagnostic labels, including autism and attention deficit hyperactivity disorder, may represent groups of related syndromes rather than a single diagnostic entity. In other instances, genetic studies may lead to eventual reclassification of certain disorders. For example, body dysmorphic disorder, previously considered a somatoform disorder, has been proposed to be reclassified as an obsessive-compulsive disorder in the fifth edition of the *Diagnostic and Statistical Manual of Mental Disorders*, the handbook used by medical professionals in diagnosing mental disorders.

Research and advances in genetics and mental disorders

Geneticist Jonathan Sebat, chief of the Beyster Center for Molecular Genomics of Neuropsychiatric Diseases at the University of California, San Diego, has led studies linking variations in the genetic code (the number of gene copies within the genome) to mental illness. He has demonstrated that certain gene copies within the genome are an underlying factor in autism, schizophrenia, and bipolar disorder. Clinicians at the Beyster Center continue work in this field with the hope that research findings will enable the development of diagnostic and screening tests for psychiatric disease. Sebat and his team of clinicians (which include psychiatrists, cellular scientists, disease biologists and molecular scientists), continue to lead the way in research and advances to further understand the role of genetic factors in mental disorders.

The ongoing search for genes related to psychiatric symptoms and disorders is, however, complicated by several factors:

- Psychiatric diagnosis relies on a doctor's human judgment and evaluation of a patient's behavior or appearance to a greater degree than diagnosis in other fields of medicine. For example, there are no blood or urine tests for schizophrenia or a personality disorder. Diagnostic questionnaires for mental disorders are helpful in trimming the list of possible diagnoses but do not have the same degree of precision or objectivity as laboratory findings.
- Mental disorders almost always involve more than one gene. Studies have shown that one mental disorder can be caused by different genes on different chromosomes in different populations. For example, one study in the late 1980s found two genes on two different chromosomes among two populations that caused manic depression. Studies of schizophrenia done in the late 1980s and early 1990s revealed the same finding—different genes on different chromosomes produced schizophrenia in different populations. It now appears that specific mental disorders are related to different sets of genes that vary across family and ethnic groups.
- Genes associated with mental disorders do not always show the same degree of penetrance, which is defined as the frequency with which a gene produces its effects in a specific group of people. Penetrance is expressed as a percentage. For example, a gene for manic depression may have 20% penetrance, which means that 20% of the members of the family being studied are at risk of developing the disorder.
- Genetic factors in mental disorders interact with a person's family and cultural environment. For example, a person who has a gene associated with susceptibility to alcohol abuse may not develop the disorder if he or she grows up in a family that teaches effective ways to cope with stress and responsible attitudes toward drinking.

Ethical concerns

As the number of tests available for determining genetic markers for mental disorders continues to increase, ethical issues are being debated. These concerns include:

- Regulation of genetic testing—some companies have started to market tests for the apoE4 Alzheimer's gene even though the present benefits of such testing are not clear. The U.S. Department of Health and Human Services has established an advisory committee to study the question of government regulation of genetic testing.
- Confidentiality—the fear of losing health insurance is a major barrier to the acceptance of genetic testing in the general population. Many people do not trust hospitals or research laboratories to keep test results confidential.
- Discrimination—some people are concerned that genetic findings could be used to deny college or graduate school admission to persons at risk for certain disorders, or to restrict their access to employment opportunities.

Resources

BOOKS

American Psychiatric Association. *Diagnostic and Statistical Manual of Mental Disorders.* 4th ed., text rev. Washington, DC. American Psychiatric Association, 2000.

Bennett, Robin L. *The Practical Guide to the Genetic Family History.* 2nd ed. New York: Wiley-Blackwell, 2010.

Dodge, Kenneth A., and Michael Rutter, eds. *Gene-Environment Interactions in Developmental Psychopathology.* New York: The Guilford Press, 2011.

Fusar-Poli, Paolo, Stefan J. Borgwardt, and Phillip McGuire, eds. *Vulnerability to Psychosis: From Neurosciences to Psychopathology.* New York: Psychology Press, 2011.

Leigh, Hoyle. *Genes, Memes, Culture, and Mental Illness.* New York: Springer, 2010.

Peay, Holly Landrum, and Jehannine Claire Austin. *How to Talk with Families About Genetics and Psychiatric Illness.* New York: W. W. Norton & Company, 2011.

PERIODICALS

Boomsma, Dorret I., et al. "Longitudinal Stability of the CBCL-Juvenile Bipolar Disorder Phenotype: A Study in Dutch Twins." *Biological Psychiatry* 60, no. 9 (2006): 912–20.

Douthit, Kathryn Z. "The Convergence of Counseling and Psychiatric Genetics: An Essential Role for Counselors." *Journal of Counseling & Development* 84, no. 1 (2006): 16–28.

Durston, Sarah, et al. "Activation in Ventral Prefrontal Cortex Is Sensitive to Genetic Vulnerability for Attention-Deficit Hyperactivity Disorder." *Biological Psychiatry* 60, no. 10 (2006): 1062–70.

Farmer, Anne, Amanda Elkin, and Peter McGuffin. "The Genetics of Bipolar Affective Disorder." *Current Opinion in Psychiatry* 20, no. 1 (2007): 8–12.

Giménez-Llort, L., et al. "Modeling Behavioral and Neuronal Symptoms of Alzheimer's Disease in Mice: A Role for Intraneuronal Amyloid." *Neuroscience & Biobehavioral Reviews* 1, no. 1 (2007): 125–47.

Harris, Julie Aitken, Philip A. Vernon, and Kerry L. Jang. "Rated Personality and Measured Intelligence in Young Twin Children." *Personality and Individual Differences* 42, no. 1 (2007): 75–86.

Hollingworth, P. "Genome-Wide Association Study of Alzheimer's Disease with Psychotic Symptoms." *Molecular Psychiatry* (October 18, 2011) [e-pub ahead of print]. http://dx.doi.org/10.1038/mp.2011.125 (accessed November 4, 2011).

Hurd, Yasmin L. "Perspectives on Current Directions in the Neurobiology of Addiction Disorders Relevant to Genetic Risk Factors." *CNS Spectrums* 11, no. 11 (2006): 855–62.

Nierenberg, Andrew A., et al. "Family History of Mood Disorder and Characteristics of Major Depressive Disorder: A STAR*D (Sequenced Treatment Alternatives to Relieve Depression) Study." *Journal of Psychiatric Research* 41, no. 3–4 (2007): 214–21.

O'Tuathaigh, Colm M. P., et al. "Susceptibility Genes for Schizophrenia: Characterisation of Mutant Mouse Models at the Level of Phenotypic Behaviour." *Neuroscience & Biobehavioral Reviews* 31, no. 1 (2007): 60–78.

Potter, Alexandra S., Paul A. Newhouse, and David J. Bucci. "Central Nicotinic Cholinergic Systems: A Role in the Cognitive Dysfunction in Attention-Deficit/Hyperactivity Disorder?" *Behavioural Brain Research* 175, no. 2 (2006): 201–11.

State, M. W., and P. Levitt. "The Conundrums of Understanding Genetic Risks for Autism Spectrum Disorders." *Nature Neuroscience* (October 30, 2011) [e-pub ahead of print]. http://dx.doi.org/10.1038/nn.2924 (accessed November 4, 2011).

Taylor, Warren D., David C. Steffens, and K. Ranga Krishnan. "Psychiatric Disease in the Twenty-First Century: The Case for Subcortical Ischemic Depression." *Biological Psychiatry* 60, no. 12 (2006): 1299–1303.

WEBSITES

"Genetics Home Reference." U.S. National Library of Medicine, National Institutes of Health. http://ghr.nlm.nih.gov (accessed November 4, 2011).

"Human Genome Project Information." U.S. Department of Energy Office of Science, Office of Biological and Environmental Research. http://www.ornl.gov/sci/techresources/Human_Genome/home.shtml (accessed November 4, 2011).

ORGANIZATIONS

International Society of Psychiatric Genetics (ISPG), 5034-A Thoroughbred Lane, Brentwood, TN, 37027, (202) 336-5500, http://www.apa.org/index.aspx.

National Human Genome Research Institute, Building 31, Room 4B09, 31 Center Drive, MSC 2152, 9000 Rockville Pike, Bethesda, MD, 20892, (301) 402-0911, Fax: (301) 402-2218, http://www.genome.gov.

National Institute of Mental Health, 6001 Executive Blvd., Rm. 8184, MSC 9663, Bethesda, MD, 20892-9663, (301) 433-4513; TTY: (301) 443-8431, Fax: (301) 443-4279, (866) 615-6464; TTY: (866) 415-8051, nimhinfo@nih.gov, http://www.nimh.nih.gov.

Rebecca J. Frey, Ph.D.
Ruth Wineclaw, Ph.D.
Laura Jean Cataldo, RN, Ed.D.

Gen-XENE *see* **Clorazepate**

Geodon *see* **Ziprasidone**

Geriatric Depression Scale

Definition

The Geriatric **Depression** Scale (GDS) is a 30-item self-report assessment designed specifically to identify depression in the elderly. It is generally recommended as a routine part of a comprehensive geriatric assessment. A short version of the GDS containing 15 questions has been developed. The GDS is also available in a number of languages other than English.

Purpose

Depression is widespread among the elderly, affecting one in six patients treated in general medical practice and an even higher percentage of those in hospitals and nursing homes. Older people have the highest **suicide** rate of any group, and many medical problems common to older people may be related to, or intensified by, a depressive disorder. Recognition of the prevalence of depression among older people prompted the development of the geriatric depression scale in 1982-83. Yes/no responses are thought to be more easily used than the graduated responses found on other standard assessment scales such as the **Beck Depression Inventory**, the Hamilton rating scale for depression, or the Zung self-rating depression scale.

While it is not found in the ***Diagnostic and Statistical Manual of Mental Disorders*** (*DSM-IV-TR*)

Geriatric Depression Scale

1. Are you basically satisfied with your life? YES **NO**
2. Have you dropped many of your activities and interests? **YES** NO
3. Do you feel that your life is empty? **YES** NO
4. Do you often get bored? **YES** NO
5. Are you hopeful about the future? YES **NO**
6. Are you bothered by thoughts you can't get out of your head? **YES** NO
7. Are you in good spirits most of the time? YES **NO**
8. Are you afraid that something bad is going to happen to you? **YES** NO
9. Do you feel happy most of the time? YES **NO**
10. Do you often feel helpless? **YES** NO
11. Do you often get restless and fidgety? **YES** NO
12. Do you prefer to stay at home, rather than going out and doing new things? **YES** NO
13. Do you frequently worry about the future? **YES** NO
14. Do you feel you have more problems with memory than most? **YES** NO
15. Do you think it is wonderful to be alive now? YES **NO**
16. Do you often feel downhearted and blue? **YES** NO
17. Do you feel pretty worthless the way you are now? **YES** NO
18. Do you worry a lot about the past? **YES** NO
19. Do you find life very exciting? YES **NO**
20. Is it hard for you to get started on new projects? **YES** NO
21. Do you feel full of energy? YES **NO**
22. Do you feel that your situation is hopeless? **YES** NO
23. Do you think that most people are better off than you are? **YES** NO
24. Do you frequently get upset over little things? **YES** NO
25. Do you frequently feel like crying? **YES** NO
26. Do you have trouble concentrating? **YES** NO
27. Do you enjoy getting up in the morning? YES **NO**
28. Do you prefer to avoid social gatherings? **YES** NO
29. Is it easy for you to make decisions? YES **NO**
30. Is your mind as clear as it used to be? YES **NO**

Scoring is based on one point for each bolded answer.
Normal: 0–9
Mild depression: 10–19
Severe depression: 20–30

SOURCE: Stanford/VA Aging Clinical Research Center (ACRC).

(Table by PreMediaGlobal. © 2012 Cengage Learning.)

produced by the **American Psychiatric Association**, the GDS is widely recommended for clinical use and is included as a routine part of a comprehensive geriatric assessment. It is also increasingly being used in research on depression in the elderly.

Description

The Geriatric Depression Scale is a self-report assessment developed in 1982 by J.A. Yesavitch and colleagues. Depression scales are either interviewer-administered or by means of self-report. A self-report assessment is easier and quicker to administer, though an interviewer-administered test is generally more sensitive and specific—another reason for using more than one tool to obtain an accurate **diagnosis**. The items may be answered yes or no, which is thought to be simpler than scales that use a five-category response set. One point is assigned to each answer and corresponds to a scoring grid. A score of 10 or 11 or lower is the usual threshold to separate depressed from nondepressed patients.

Yesavitch and his coworkers chose 100 statements that they determined were related to seven common characteristics of depression in later life. These included:

- somatic concern
- lowered affect (affect is the outward expression of emotion)
- cognitive impairment
- feelings of discrimination
- impaired motivation
- lack of future orientation
- lack of self-esteem

The best 30 items were selected after administration of the 100 items to 46 depressed and normal elders. Those items were then administered to 20 elders without depression and 51 who were in treatment for depression. The test was 84% sensitive and 95% specific for a depression diagnosis. Repeated studies have demonstrated the value of GDS.

Examples of the questions in the GDS include:

- Are you basically satisfied with your life?
- Have you dropped many of your activities and interests?
- Are you hopeful about the future?
- Do you often get restless and fidgety?
- Do you frequently get upset over little things?
- Do you enjoy getting up in the morning?

A time frame should be specified for administration of the test, for example, "Answer these questions by thinking of how you've felt the past two weeks."

Precautions

The Geriatric diagnosis of clinical depression should not be made on the GDS results alone. Although the test has well-established reliability and validity, responses should be considered in conjunction with other results from a comprehensive diagnostic work-up.

There is some controversy over whether the GDS is reliable for depression screening in individuals with mild or moderate **dementia**. Several studies have shown good agreement with observer ratings of depression, whether or not the patient had dementia. However, persons with dementia may deny symptoms of depression. It also appears that less educated people are more likely to score in the depressed range on the GDS 15-item short form. These caveats notwithstanding, the GDS can be usefully applied in general medical settings in combination with other clinical assessments,

KEY TERMS

Low affect—Severe lack of interest and emotions; emotional numbness.

Somatic concern—Excessive concern about the body, particularly in relation to illness.

observation, and interviews with elder patient and their families.

Both symptom pattern and symptom severity must be considered when trying to identify depression. These dimensions are taken into account in the development of symptom scales and, while clinical judgment takes priority, a scale such as the GDS can help in identifying persons with depression, whether they are making satisfactory progress with treatment, or when they may need further assessment or referral.

Results

A scoring grid accompanies the GDS. One point is given for each respondent's answer that matches those on the grid. For example, the grid response to "Are you basically satisfied with your life?" is "no." If the elderly person responds in the negative one point is scored; if the response is "yes," then no point is scored. For the 30-item assessment, a score of 0–9 is considered normal; 10–19 indicates mild depression, and a score over 20 is suggestive of severe depression. The maximum number of points that can be scored is 30.

Resources

BOOKS

Gallo, Joseph J., et al. *Handbook of Geriatric Assessment*. 4th ed. Burlington, MA: Jones & Bartlett Publishers, 2005.

Sadavoy, Joel, et al., eds. *Comprehensive Review of Geriatric Psychiatry-II*. 3rd ed. New York: W.W. Norton & Company, 2004.

PERIODICALS

Reynolds, Charles F. III, and David J. Kupfer. "Depression and Aging: A Look to the Future." *Psychiatric Services* 50 (September 1999): 1167–1172.

Wancata, J., et al. "The Criterion Validity of the Geriatric Depression Scale: A Systematic Review." *Acta Psychiatrica Scandanavica* 114, no. 6 (December 2006) 398–410.

ORGANIZATIONS

American Association for Geriatric Psychiatry, 7910 Woodmont Ave., Ste. 1050, Bethesda, MD, 20814-3004, (301) 654-7850, Fax: (301) 654-4137, http://www.AAGPonline.org.

Judy Leaver, MA

Gestalt therapy

Definition

Gestalt therapy is a form of **psychotherapy** that helps the client focus on the here and now rather than on the past. Gestalt therapy stresses the development of client self-awareness and personal responsibility.

Purpose

The goal of Gestalt therapy is to raise clients' awareness regarding how they function in their environment; with family, at work or school, and with friends. The focus of therapy is more on what is happening (the moment-to-moment process) than what is being discussed (the content). Awareness is being alert to the most important events in one's life and environment with full sensorimotor, emotional, cognitive, and energy support. Support is defined as anything that makes contact with or withdrawal from the environment possible, including energy, body support, breathing, information, concern for others, and language, for example.

In therapy, clients become aware of what they are doing, how they are doing it, and how they can change themselves, and at the same time, they learn to accept and value themselves. According to this approach, individuals define, develop, and learn about themselves in relationship to others, and they are constantly changing.

Gestalt therapy is "unpredictable" in that the therapist and client follow moment-to-moment experience and neither knows exactly where this will take them. Gestalt therapy is complex and intuitive, but it is based on the following principles:

- Holism. Gestalt therapy takes into account the whole person including thoughts, feelings, behavior, body sensations, and dreams. The focus is on integration, that is, how the many parts of the person fit together, and how the client makes contact (interacts) with the environment.
- Field theory. According to this theory, everything is related, in flux, interrelated, and in process. The therapist focuses on how the client makes contact with the environment (family, work, school, friends, authority figures).
- The figure-formation process describes how individuals organize or manipulate their environment from moment to moment.
- Organismic self-regulation is the creative adjustment the organism (person) makes in relation to the environment. The person's equilibrium with his or her environment is "disturbed" by the emergence of a

client need, sensation, or interest and is related to the figure-formation process in that the need of the person organizes the field. For example, if an individual wants coffee, this coffee need is what comes out of the diffuse background and becomes "figural" (comes to the forefront of the client's environment or field) and when the individual enters a room, the figural will be related to the coffee need. The therapist is interested in what is figural for a person because it may provide insight into the person's need(s).

- The Now. The concept of the here and now is what is being done, thought, and felt at the moment, and not in the past or the future.
- Unfinished business is defined as the unexpressed feelings that are associated with distinct memories and fantasies. These feelings may be resentment, rage, hatred, pain, anxiety, grief, guilt, and/or abandonment that are not fully experienced in awareness and linger on in the background. The feelings are carried into the present life and cause preoccupations, compulsive behaviors, wariness, and other self-defeating behaviors. Unfinished business will persist until the person faces and deals with these denied or alienated feelings.

The current practice of Gestalt therapy includes treatment of a wide range of problems and has been successfully used to address a wide range of "psychosomatic" disorders including migraine, ulcerative colitis, and spastic neck and back. Therapists work with couples and families, and with individuals who have difficulties coping with authority figures. In addition, Gestalt therapy has been used for brief **crisis intervention**, to help persons with post-traumatic stress disorders, alcohol and drug abuse, **depression**, or **anxiety disorders**; with adults in a poverty program; with seriously mentally ill individuals with psychotic disorders; and those with borderline **personality disorders**.

Description

The relationship between the therapist and the client is the most important aspect of psychotherapy in Gestalt therapy. In Gestalt therapy, the interaction between therapist and client is an ever-changing dialogue marked by straightforward caring, warmth, acceptance, and self-responsibility. There are four characteristics of dialogue:

- inclusion, in which the therapist puts him- or herself, as much as is possible, into the experience of the client. The therapist does not judge, analyze, or interpret what he or she observes.
- presence refers to the therapist expressing his or her observations, preferences, feelings, personal experience, and thoughts to the client.
- commitment to dialogue allows a feeling of connection, or contact, between the therapist and the client.
- dialogue is active and can be nonverbal as well as verbal. It can be dancing, song, words, or any modality that expresses and moves the energy between the therapist and the client.

Gestalt therapy holds the view that people are endlessly remaking or discovering themselves; therefore, individuals are always in constant transformation. The therapist's approach is to help clients: increase or deepen their awareness of themselves and their relationships with others, by attending and engaging with the client; to explore the client's experience; and to describe what is perceived. All techniques used within the therapeutic relationship help clients to work through and move beyond painful emotional blocks. This allows the client to explore new behavior, first in the context of the therapeutic relationship and then, as appropriate, in the outside world.

The therapeutic process begins at the first contact between client and therapist. Assessment and screening are usually done as part of the ongoing relationship with the client and not as a separate period of diagnostic testing and history taking. Assessment information is obtained by beginning the therapeutic work and includes the client's willingness and support for work in the Gestalt therapy framework, the match between the client and the therapist, diagnostic and personality information, the decision regarding the frequency of sessions, the need for adjunctive treatment (such as day treatment or **biofeedback** training), and the need for medication and medical consultation.

Gestalt therapists now make use of the traditional diagnostic categories to obtain necessary information to help patients with serious mental illnesses (such as psychotic disorders and borderline disorders) and because of administrative and insurance reimbursement procedures. Despite these changes, it is believed that Gestalt therapy assessment techniques will continue to be varied since Gestalt therapists draw on other therapeutic systems.

In therapy, the Gestalt therapist is active and sessions are lively and characterized by warmth, acceptance, caring, and self-responsibility and promote direct experiencing of a situation or event rather than passively talking about the event. Events recalled from the past are explored and felt in the here and now of the therapy session. Clients receive input from the therapists in many ways: they can see and hear the therapists react; the therapists can tell them how they are seen and what is seen; therapists may share their own feelings and reveal personal information about themselves; and therapists can discuss how client awareness is limited by how the client and therapist interact with or engage each other—that is, make contact.

The Gestalt therapist has a wide range of active interventions (cognitive and behavioral) at his or her disposal and may use any techniques or methods as long as they are (a) aimed toward increasing awareness, (b) arise out of the dialogue and the therapist's perception of what is going on with the client (sensing, feeling, thinking) in the immediate therapy session, and (c) within the parameters of ethical practice.

Exercises and experiments

Many therapeutic interventions called exercises and experiments have been developed to enhance awareness and bring about client change. Exercises are defined as ready-made techniques that are sometimes used to evoke certain emotions (such as the expression of anger) in clients. Experiments, on the other hand, grow out of the immediate interaction (dialogue) between client and therapist. They are spontaneous, one-of-a-kind, and relevant to a particular moment and the particular development of an emerging issue such as the client's reports of a need, dream, fantasy, and body awareness. Experiments are done with full participation and collaboration with clients and are designed to expand clients' awareness and to help them to try out new ways of behaving rather than to achieve a particular result. These experiments may take many forms. According to Gerald Corey, some are: "imagining a threatening future event; setting up a dialogue between a client and some significant person in his and her life; dramatizing the memory of a painful event; reliving a particularly profound early experience in the present; assuming the identity of one's mother or father through role-playing; focusing on gestures, posture, and other nonverbal signs of inner expression; carrying on a dialogue between two conflicting aspects within the person."

While participating in experiments, clients actually experience the feelings associated with their conflicts or issues. Experiments are tailored to each individual client and used in a timely manner; they are to be carried out in a context that offers safety and support while encouraging the client to risk trying out new behavior. The Gestalt therapy focus is on the entire person and all parts—verbal and nonverbal behaviors, emotional feelings—all are attended to.

Gestalt therapists are said to rely on spontaneity, inventiveness, "present-centeredness," and a range of possible therapeutic encounters, interactions that lead to exercises, and experiments are potentially infinite but can be categorized as follows.

USING STATEMENTS AND QUESTIONS TO FOCUS AWARENESS. Many interventions have to do with simply asking what the client is aware of experiencing or asking simple and direct questions as, "What are you feeling?" and "What are you thinking?" The client may be instructed to start a sentence with "Now, I am aware ..." or asked to repeat a behavior, as in, "Please wring your hands together again." A frequent technique is to follow the client's awareness report with the instruction, "Stay with it!" or "Feel it out!"

CLIENT'S VERBAL BEHAVIOR OR LANGUAGE. Awareness can be enhanced and emphasized through the client's verbal behavior or language since client speech patterns are considered to be an expression of their feelings, thoughts, and attitudes. Some aspects of language that might indicate the clients' avoidance of strong emotions or of self-responsibility are the general pronouns such as "it" and "you." Clients are instructed to substitute, when appropriate, the personal pronoun "I" for these pronouns to assume a sense of responsibility for his or her feelings or thoughts (ownership). Sometimes clients may be asked to change their questions into direct statements in order to assume responsibility for what they say. Other examples of helping clients to be more in control using language are to have them omit qualifiers and disclaimers such as "maybe," "perhaps," or "I guess" from their language patterns. This changes ambivalent and weak statements into more clear and direct statements; to substitute "I won't" for "I can't" because often "can't" gives the feeling of being unable to do something. It may be more accurate to say "I won't" meaning "I choose not to do this for any of various reasons," or use the word, "want" instead of "need" which is considered an indication of urgency and anxiety, and is less accurate. Other changes might be to change "should" and "ought" to "I choose to" or "I want to" increasing the clients' power and control of their lives.

NONVERBAL BEHAVIOR. Awareness can also be enhanced by focusing on nonverbal behavior and may include any technique that makes the clients more aware of their body functioning or helps them to be see how they can use their bodies to support excitement, awareness, and contact. The parts of the body that therapists may attend to include the mouth, jaw, eyes, nose, neck, shoulders, arms, hands, torso, legs, and feet, or the entire body. The therapist, for example, may point out to and explore with the client how he or she is smiling while at the same time expressing anger.

SELF-DIALOGUE. Self-dialogue by clients is an **intervention** used by Gestalt therapists that allows clients to get in touch with feelings that they may be unaware of and, therefore, increase the integration of different parts of clients that do not match or conflicts in clients. Examples of some common conflicts include: "the parent inside versus the child inside," "the responsible one versus the impulsive one," "the puritanical side versus the sexual side," "the good side versus the bad side," "the aggressive self versus the passive self," "the autonomous side versus the resentful side," and "the hard worker versus the goof-off." The client is assisted in accepting and learning to live with his or her polarities and not necessarily getting rid of any one part or trait.

The client is engaged in the self-dialogue by using what is called the empty-chair technique. Using two chairs, the client is asked to take one role (the parent inside, for example) in one chair and then play the other role (the child inside) in the second chair. As the client changes roles and the dialogue continues between both sides of the client he or she moves back and forth between the two chairs. Other examples of situations in which dialogues can be used, according to Corey, include "one part of the body versus the other (one hand versus the other), between a client and another person, or between the self and object such as a building or an accomplishment."

ENACTMENT AND DRAMATIZATION. Enactment increases awareness through the dramatizing of some part of the client's existence by asking him or her to put his or her feelings or thoughts into action, such as instructing the client to "Say it to the person" (when in **group therapy**), or to role-play using the empty chair technique. Exaggeration is a form of enactment in which clients are instructed to exaggerate a feeling, thought, or movement in order to provide more intensity of feelings. Enactment can be therapeutic and give rise to creativity.

GUIDED FANTASY. Guided fantasy (visualization) is a technique some clients are able to use more effectively than using enactment to bring an experience into the here and now. Clients are asked to close their eyes and, with the guidance of the therapist, slowly imagine a scene of the past or future event. More and more details are used to describe the event with all senses and thoughts.

DREAM WORK. Dream work is most important in Gestalt therapy. Working with clients' dreams requires developing a list of all the details of the dream, remembering each person, event, and mood in it and then becoming each of these parts through role-playing and inventing dialogue. Each part of the dream is thought to represent the clients' own contradictory and inconsistent sides. Dialogue between these opposing sides leads clients toward gradual insight into the range of their feelings and important themes in their lives.

AWARENESS OF SELF AND OTHERS. An example of how this technique is used by the Gestalt therapist would be asking the client to "become" another person such as asking the client to be his mother and say what his mother would say if the client came in at 2:00 A.M. This provides more insight for the client rather just asking what the client thinks his mother would say if he came home at 2:00 A.M.

AVOIDANCE BEHAVIORS. Awareness of and the reintegration the client's avoidance behaviors are assisted by the interventions used to increase and enhance awareness of feelings, thoughts, and behaviors.

HOMEWORK. Homework assignments between therapy sessions may include asking clients to write dialogues between parts of themselves or between parts of their bodies, gather information, or do other tasks that are related to and fit with what is going on in the therapy process. Homework may become more difficult as the awareness develops.

Therapy sessions are generally scheduled once a week and individual therapy is often combined with group therapy, marital or **family therapy**, movement therapy, **meditation**, or biofeedback training. Sessions can be scheduled anywhere from once every other week to five times a week and depends on how long the client can go between sessions without loss of continuity or relapsing. Meetings less frequent than once a week are thought to diminish the intensity of the therapy unless the client attends a weekly group with the same therapist. More than twice a week is not usually indicated except with clients who have psychotic disorders, and is contraindicated with those who have a **borderline personality disorder**.

Weekly group therapy may vary from one and one-half hours to three hours in length, with the average length being two hours. A typical group is composed of ten members and usually balanced between males and females. Any age is thought to be appropriate for Gestalt therapy. There are groups for children as well.

Gestalt therapy is considered to have a greater range of styles and modalities than any other therapeutic system, and is practiced in individual therapy, groups, workshops, couples, families, with children, and in agencies such as clinics, family service agencies, hospitals, private practice, growth centers. According to Corey, "The therapeutic style of therapists in each modality vary drastically on many dimensions including degree and type of structure; quantity and quality of techniques used; frequency of sessions, abrasiveness and ease of relating, focus on body, cognitions, feelings; interpersonal contact; knowledge of work within psychodynamic themes; and degree of personal encountering."

Risks

Gestalt therapy is considered to have pioneered the development of many useful and creative innovations in psychotherapy theory and practice. However, there is some concern regarding the abuse of power by the therapist, as well as the high-intensity interaction involved. Therapists who use other techniques can become enchanted with using the techniques of Gestalt therapy without having the appropriate training in Gestalt therapy theory. Gestalt therapists are very active and directive within the therapy session and, therefore, care must be taken that they have characteristics that include sensitivity, timing, inventiveness, empathy, and respect for the client. These characteristics, are dependent on the skill, training, experience, ethics, and judgment of the therapist. In addition, the intensity of the therapy might not be suitable for all patients, and even disruptive for some, despite the competence of the therapist.

Results

Gestalt therapists expect that as a result of their involvement in the Gestalt process clients will: have increased awareness of themselves; assume ownership of their experience rather than making others responsible for what they are thinking, feeling, or doing; develop skills and acquire values that will allow them to satisfy their needs without violating the rights of others; become aware of all their senses (smelling, tasting, touching, hearing, and seeing); accept responsibility for their actions and the resulting consequences; move from expectations for external support toward internal self-support; to be able to ask for and get help from others and be able to give to others.

Resources

BOOKS

Blom, Rinda. *The Handbook of Gestalt Play Therapy: Practical Guidelines for Child Therapists*. London: Jessica Kingsley Publishers, 2006.

Corey, Gerald. "Gestalt Therapy." *Theory and Practice of Counseling and Psychotherapy*. 8th ed. Belmont, CA: Thomson/Brooks/Cole, 2008.

O'Leary, Eleanor. "Breathing and Awareness: The Integrating Mechanisms of Cognitive-Behavioural Gestalt Therapy in Working with Cardiac Patients." In *New Approaches to Integration in Psychotherapy*, edited by Eleanor O'Leary and Mike Murphy. New York: Taylor and Francis, 2006.

VandenBos, Gary R. ed. *APA Dictionary of Psychology*. Washington, DC: American Psychological Association, 2006.

Woldt, Ansel L., and Sarah M. Toman. *Gestalt Therapy: History, Theory, and Practice*. Thousand Oaks, CA: Sage, 2005.

PERIODICALS

Bowman, Deborah, and Tricia A. Leakey. "The Power of Gestalt Therapy in Accessing the Transpersonal: Working with Physical Difference and Disability." *Gestalt Review* 10, no. 1 (2006): 42–59.

Kitzler, Richard. "The Ontology of Action: A Place on Which to Stand for Modern Gestalt Therapy Theory." *International Gestalt Journal* 29, no. 1 (Spring 2006): 43–100.

Wheeler, Gordon. "New Directions in Gestalt Theory and Practice: Psychology and Psychotherapy in the Age of Complexity." In *Co-Creating the Field: Intention and Practice in the Age of Complexity*, edited by Deborah Ullman and Gordon Wheeler. New York: Gestalt Press, June 2009.

Williams, Lynn. "Spirituality and Gestalt: A Gestalt-Transpersonal Perspective." *Gestalt Review* 10, no. 1 (2006): 6–21.

WEBSITES

Miller, Michael Vincent. "Elegiac Reflections on Isadore From." http://www.gestalt.org/from.htm (accessed October 30, 2011).

ORGANIZATIONS

American Psychological Association, 750 1st Street NE, Washington, DC, 20002-4242, (202) 336-5500; TDD/TTY: (202) 336-6123, (800) 374-2721, http://www.apa.org.

Association for the Advancement of Gestalt Therapy, http://www.aagt.org.

Mental Health America, 2000 N. Beauregard Street, 6th Floor, Alexandria, VA, 22311, (703) 684-7722, (800) 969-6642, Fax: (703) 684-5968, http://www1.nmha.org.

National Institute of Mental Health, 6001 Executive Blvd., Room 8184, MSC 9663, Bethesda, MD, 20892-9663, (301) 433-4513; TTY: (301) 443-8431, Fax: (301) 443-4279, (866) 615-6464; TTY: (866) 415-8051, nimhinfo@nih.gov, http://www.nimh.nih.gov.

Janice Van Buren, PhD
Ruth A. Wienclaw, PhD

Ginkgo biloba

Definition

Ginkgo biloba is an herbal dietary supplement made from the leaves of the tree *Ginkgo biloba*. Having been used for thousands of years as a home remedy for various ailments, ginkgo biloba is still used for many medical conditions. Although yet to be medically verified, ginkgo biloba has shown evidence that is also is effective in the treatment of mental illnesses such as **dementia** (including **Alzheimer's disease**), **depression**, and anxiety.

Purpose

Ginkgo biloba, generically called ginkgo and sometimes called *bai guo*, has been used in Traditional

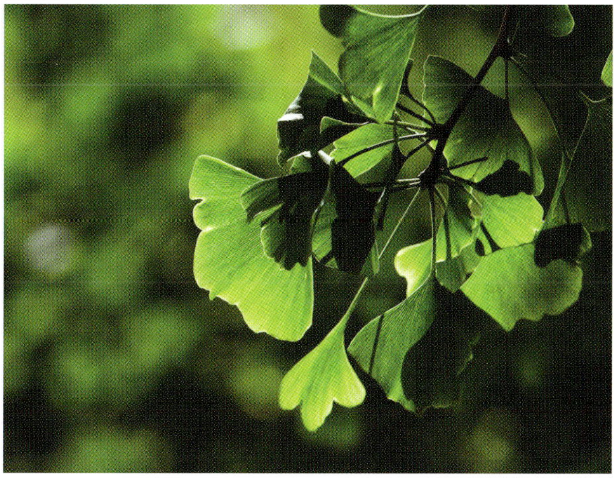

Ginkgo biloba leaves. *(© iStockPhoto.com/Ma Sai)*

Chinese Medicine (TCM) for about 5,000 years to treat memory loss and mood, nerve, circulatory and many other health problems. It often is combined with **ginseng** to boost memory, improve the quality of life, and increase a sense of well-being. The effectiveness of some TCM uses of ginkgo, such as relieving pain caused by clogged arteries in the leg (claudication), treating Alzheimer's disease, and improving blood flow to the **brain** have been evaluated in well-designed studies and are generally accepted by practitioners of conventional medicine. Many other TCM uses of ginkgo biloba are currently being investigated, including those for mental illnesses.

Description

Ginkgo biloba is the last existing member of an ancient family of trees. The fossil record shows that ginkgo trees existed 200 million years ago. *Ginkgo biloba* is native to China, Japan, and Korea. The tree was introduced to North America in the 1700s. Ginkgo trees grow to a height of 65–115 ft (20–35 m). They are extremely resistant to disease and insect damage and can live for several hundred years. Female trees produce bad-smelling fruit-like bodies the size of an apricot that contain seeds. Herbal practitioners sometimes use the seeds in treatment. The much cleaner male ginkgo is a popular tree for urban landscaping.

The fan-shaped leaves of the ginkgo are used for medicinal purposes. About 20 different compounds have been identified in ginkgo leaves, but the medically active ingredients appear to be flavonoids and terpenoids. Flavonoids are antioxidants that help lower the level of free radicals in the body. Terpenoids are thought to protect nerves from damage, reduce inflammation, and decrease blood clotting.

In the United States, *Ginkgo biloba* is cultivated, and the leaves are harvested and dried, then often used to make a standardized extract that contains 24–25% flavonoids and 6% terpenoids. U.S. law does not require the standardization of dietary supplements, so consumers should read all labels carefully. Ginkgo biloba is often sold as capsules and tablets. Dry and liquid ginkgo extract is added to other herbal remedies as well as teas, energy or health bars, and similar products. An injectable form of ginkgo biloba extract that was available in Europe has been withdrawn from the market because of adverse side effects. Most well-designed studies have been done using a total of 80–240 mg of 50:1 standardized extract divided into two or three doses daily and taken by mouth.

Regulation of ginkgo biloba sales

Ginkgo biloba is one of the top-selling herbal remedies in the United States and is even more popular in Europe. Under the 1994 Dietary Supplement Health and Education Act (DSHEA), the U.S. Food and Drug Administration (FDA) regulates the sale of ginkgo biloba as a dietary supplement. At the time the act was passed, legislators felt that supplements did not need to be regulated as rigorously as prescription and over-the-counter drugs used in conventional medicine because many dietary supplements such as ginkgo biloba come from natural sources and have been used for hundreds of years by practitioners of complementary and alternative medicine (CAM).

The DSHEA regulates ginkgo biloba in the same way that food is regulated. Like food manufacturers, manufacturers of herbal products containing ginkgo biloba do not have to prove that they are either safe or effective before they can be sold to the public. This differs from conventional pharmaceutical drugs, which must undergo extensive human testing to prove their safety and effectiveness before they can be marketed. Also unlike conventional drugs, the label for a dietary supplement such as ginkgo biloba does not have to contain any statements about possible side effects. All herbal supplements sold in the United States must show the scientific name of the herb on the label.

Health claims

Ginkgo biloba is one of the most promising traditional herbs investigated by Western medicine. The National Center for Complementary and Alternative Medicine (NCCAM), a government organization within the National Institutes of Health (NIH), is sponsoring **clinical trials** to determine safety and effectiveness of ginkgo biloba as a treatment for more than a dozen diseases and disorders. Individuals interested in participating in a clinical trial at no charge can find a list of open trials at http://www.clinicaltrials.gov.

Some health claims for ginkgo biloba have already been evaluated in large, well-controlled studies that satisfy the proof of safety and effectiveness demanded by conventional medicine. Several mental disorders are included on the effectiveness of ginkgo biloba.

DEMENTIAS AND ALZHEIMER'S DISEASE. There is good evidence that ginkgo biloba can cause short-term improvement in mental function in people with Alzheimer's disease (AD). In a well-designed study, ginkgo biloba was as effective as the prescription drug **donepezil** (Aricept) in slowing the development of dementia in people with mild to moderate Alzheimer's. Ginkgo biloba has also been shown to be effective in improving blood flow to the brain and in treating certain other dementias. The effect of ginkgo biloba on memory in healthy young adults and in people with age-related memory impairment is inconsistent but strong enough to continue to study the effects of the herb in these populations.

However, the National Institutes of Health (NIH) recently funded a comprehensive study—the largest clinical trial on the use of ginkgo biloba for dementia—which ran for eight years. Completed in 2008, 3,069 people aged 75 years and older participated in the study. These people, from four clinical sites, had either normal cognition or mild cognitive impairment. The study was called the "Ginkgo biloba for the Evaluation of Memory (GEM) Study."

These researchers, led by Dr. Steven T. DeKosky of the School of Medicine at the University of Virginia (Charlottesville), found that ginkgo biloba at a dose of 120 mg twice per day was not effective in lowering the incidence rate of dementia nor Alzheimer's disease in these older adults within the United States. The U.S. researchers recommended that further large studies be performed on older adults with respect to the use of ginkgo biloba.

Ginkgo biloba has been shown to be effective with multi-infarct dementia (MID), another type of dementia. Scientific studies have shown that ginkgo biloba was as effective as acetylcholinesterase inhibitor (AChEI) drugs, such as donepezil (Aricept) for the treatment of MID, along with early-stage AD. However, researchers continue to recommend that further studies be performed to compare established drugs with ginkgo biloba.

Age-associated memory impairment (AAMI) is a problem with some older adults, and it is believed to be part of the normal aging process. Most symptoms of AAMI only mildly interfere with daily functions of such individuals. Some researchers contend that AAMI is an early sign of AD or MID. The use of ginkgo biloba has been shown to help with controlling these AAMI symptoms. Some studies show small improvement in memory and other brain function in older adults taking ginkgo biloba. Generally, though, further research is necessary to ensure that such studies are valid.

CEREBRAL INSUFFICIENCY. Cerebral insufficiency is a condition that involves such symptoms as confusion, forgetfulness, **fatigue**, dizziness, depression, anxiety, and decreased physical capabilities. Scientists contend that it is caused by a decreased flow of blood within the brain due to blocked blood vessels. Recent research has shown that ginkgo biloba can help to reduce the severity of such symptoms. However, medical researchers are performing further studies to validate these initial studies.

DEPRESSION AND SEASON AFFECTIVE DISORDER. Some researchers have suggested that ginkgo biloba is useful in treating such mental conditions as depression and **seasonal affective disorder** (SAD), what is sometimes called "winter depression." Some studies of the elderly show minor improvement in the symptoms of depression and SAD with the use of ginkgo biloba. Further studies need to be accomplished to evaluate these health claims.

SCHIZOPHRENIA. Ginkgo biloba has antioxidant properties that have been shown to help in the treatment of **schizophrenia**. Early studies show positive results, although sufficient evidence has yet to be collected to verify this claim.

QUALITY OF LIFE. Ginkgo biloba has been shown to help in providing a better quality of life for people with mental illnesses and other medical conditions. Although ginkgo biloba has helped in such patients, further research is necessary before a clear conclusion can be reached.

Recommended dosage

The recommended dosage of ginkgo biloba is based on research performed on the herbal supplement. Because herbs and supplements, including ginkgo biloba, are neither evaluated nor approved by the U.S. Food and Drug Administration (FDA) concerning their effectiveness, purity, and safety, individual companies may manufacturer them in differing concentrations per product. (As mentioned earlier, the FDA only regulates the sale of ginkgo biloba as a dietary supplement through the DSHEA.) Consequently, these dosages should be used only as basic guidelines. Consult with a trusted medical professional, such as a family doctor or pharmacist, before taking ginkgo biloba.

For adults 18 years or older, 80–240 mg within a 50-to-1 standardized leaf extract have been studied for recommended daily use. Such doses can be taken by mouth two to three times a day. Ginkgo biloba also comes in teabag form, with bags usually containing 30 mg of ginkgo. Concentrated amounts of ginkgo biloba often come in 3–6 mL of 40 mg per mL of leaf extract; with a daily input of three doses. Ginkgo biloba also comes within fortified foods.

For children under the age of 18 years, sufficient medical research has not been performed to make any recommended dosages of ginkgo biloba.

Precautions

Ginkgo biloba seeds contain toxins that can cause vomiting, **seizures**, loss of consciousness, and death, especially in young children. Ginkgo biloba seeds are not safe for anyone, and they should be avoided.

Extracts of the leaf of *Ginkgo biloba* are generally safe and cause few side effects when taken at recommended doses for up to six months. People who are planning to have surgery should stop taking ginkgo biloba at least two days before their operation because of the risk of increased bleeding. The safety of ginkgo biloba in children and pregnant and breastfeeding women is still being studied.

Interactions

Ginkgo biloba is generally well tolerated by most people. However, it has blood-thinning properties and is likely to increase the blood-thinning and anticoagulant effects of medicines such as warfarin (Coumadin), clopidogrel (Plavix), aspirin, and nonsteroidal anti-inflammatory drugs (e.g., Advil, Motrin). Individuals taking these drugs should not begin taking ginkgo biloba without consulting their health care provider. People preparing for dental or surgical procedures should not take ginkgo biloba, and they should get more specific information from the attending physician as to when to temporarily stop taking the herbal supplement.

Ginkgo biloba may also interact with monoamine oxidase inhibitors (MAOIs) used to treat certain kinds of depression and mental illness. Examples of MAOIs include **isocarboxazid** (Marplan), **phenelzine** (Nardil), and **tranylcypromine** (Parnate). Individuals taking MAOIs along with ginkgo biloba may experience increased effects from the drug.

KEY TERMS

Alzheimer's disease—The most common type of dementia that usually occurs late in life and involves confusion, irritability, mood swings, language problems, short-term memory loss, and general decline of the senses.

Dementia—A medical condition that involves the progressive deterioration of intellectual and cognitive function, such as memory.

Diabetes—A medical disorder that involves the production of excessive urine; medically called *diabetes mellitus*; type 1 diabetes (juvenile diabetes) involves failure of body to produce insulin, while type 2 diabetes (adult onset diabetes) involves the body's cells failing to use insulin properly.

Monoamine oxidase—Also called L-monoamine oxidase (MAO), a family of enzymes that catalyze the oxidation of monoamines.

Schizophrenia—A psychiatric disorder with symptoms of self withdrawal, emotional instability, and reality detachment.

Some reports suggest that ginkgo biloba lowers blood sugar levels. Individuals who are taking insulin or other medications that also lower blood sugar, and those with type 2 diabetes, should consult their health care provider before starting to take ginkgo biloba.

Complications

Serious side effects of ginkgo biloba are rare. The most common mild side effects are headache, dizziness, nausea, diarrhea, increased restlessness, and racing heart. Increased bleeding may occur. Allergic reactions to ginkgo are possible but uncommon. In severe rare cases, the skin blisters and sloughs off, a condition called Stevens-Johnson syndrome. People who are allergic to sumac, mango rind, cashews, poison oak, and poison ivy are at slightly higher risk to have an allergic reaction to ginkgo biloba. Ginkgo biloba is not recommended during pregnancy and breastfeeding, due to lack of reliable medical information.

Parental concerns

Parents should be aware that a safe dose of many herbal supplements has not been established for children. Accidental overdose may occur if children are give adult herbal supplements.

QUESTIONS TO ASK YOUR DOCTOR

- Should I try ginkgo biloba?
- What dose would be appropriate for me to take?
- Are there any foods I should avoid?
- Where can I learn reliable information about ginkgo biloba?

Resources

BOOKS

Dasgupta, Amitava, and Catherine A. Hammett-Stabler, editors. *Herbal Supplements: Efficacy, Toxicity, Interactions with Western Drugs, and Effects on Clinical Laboratory Tests.* Hoboken, NJ: Wiley, 2011.

Fragakis, Allison. *The Health Professional's Guide to Popular Dietary Supplements* Chicago: American Dietetic Association, 2007

Hsu, Elisabeth, and Stephen Harris, editors. *Plants, Health and Healing: On the Interface of Ethnobotany and Medical Anthropology.* New York: Berghahn, 2010.

PDR for Herbal Medicines. Montvale, NJ: Thompson, 2007.

Peilin, Sun, editor. *The Treatment of Pain with Chinese Herbs and Acupuncture.* Edinburgh: Elsevier Churchill Livingstone, 2011.

Sutton, Amy L, editor. *Complementary and Alternative Medicine Sourcebook.* Detroit: Omnigraphics, 2010.

Tracy, Timothy S. and Richard L. Kingston, eds. *Herbal Products: Toxicology and Clinical Pharmacology.* Totowa, NJ, Humana Press, 2007.

Wildman, Robert E. C., editor. *Handbook of Nutraceuticals and Functional Foods,* 2nd ed. Boca Raton, FL: CRC/Taylor & Francis, 2007.

PERIODICALS

Akhondzadeh, S. and S. H. Abbasi. "Herbal Medicine in the Treatment of Alzheimer's Disease." *American Journal of Alzheimer's Disease and Other Dementias* 21, no. 2 (Mar-April 2006):113–8.

Dugoua, J. J., et al. "Safety and Efficacy of Ginkgo (Ginkgo biloba) During Pregnancy and Lactation." *Canadian Journal of Clinical Pharmacology* 13, no. 3 (Fall, 2006): e277–84. http://www.cjcp.ca/pdf/CJCP05-037_e277e284F.pdf

Mazza, M., et al., "Ginkgo Biloba and Donepezil: A Comparison in the Treatment of Alzheimer's dementia in a Randomized Placebo-Controlled Double-blind Study." *European Journal of Neurology* 13, no. 9 (September 2006):981–5.

Oh, S. M. and K. H. Chung. "Antiestrogenic Activities of Ginkgo Biloba Extracts." *Steroid Biochemistry and Molecular Biology* 100, nos. 4–5 (August 2006):167–76.

WEBSITES

"Ginkgo." MedlinePlus. October 21, 2011. http://www.nlm.nih.gov/medlineplus/druginfo/natural/333.html (accessed January 13, 2012).

"Ginkgo Biloba." Maryland Medical Center Programs Center for Integrative Medicine. http://www.umm.edu/altmed/articles/ginkgo-biloba-000247.htm (accessed January 13, 2012).

"Ginkgo (Ginkgo Biloba)." Mayo Clinic. April 1, 2011. http://www.mayoclinic.com/health/ginkgo-biloba/NS_patient-ginkgo (accessed July 5, 2011).

"Ginkgo Biloba for the Evaluation of Memory (GEM) Study." National Institutes of Health. March 11, 2011. http://nccam.nih.gov/research/results/gems/qa.htm (accessed July 5, 2011).

"Ginkgo Evaluation of Memory (GEM) Study Fails To Show Benefit in Preventing Dementia in the Elderly." National Center for Complementary and Alternative Medicine. (November 18, 2008). http://nccam.nih.gov/news/2008/111808.htm (accessed July 5, 2011).

ORGANIZATIONS

American Association of Acupuncture and Oriental Medicine, PO Box 162340, Sacramento, CA, 95816, Fax: 1(916) 443-4766, (866) 455-7999, http://www.aaaomonline.org

American Botanical Council, PO Box 14435, Austin, TX, 78723, 1(512) 926-4900, Fax: 1(512) 926-2345, (800) 373-7105, http://abc.herbalgram.org

National Center for Complementary and Alternative Medicine Clearinghouse, PO Box 7923, Gaithersburg, MD, 20898, Fax: 1(866) 464-3616, (888) 644-6226, info@nccam.nih.gov, http://nccam.nih.gov

National Certification Commission for Acupuncture and Oriental Medicine, 76 South Laura St., Suite 1290, Jacksonville, FL, 32202, 1(904) 598-1005, Fax: 1(904) 598-5001, http://www.nccaom.org

Natural Standard, One Davis Square, Somerville, MA, 02144, 1(617) 591-3300, Fax: 1(617) 591-3399, questions@naturalstandard.com, http://naturalstandard.com

Office of Dietary Supplements, Natonal Institutes of Health, 6100 Executive Blvd., Room 3B01, MSC 7517, Bethesda, MD, 20892-7517, 1(301) 435-2920, Fax: 1(301) 480-1845, ods@nih.gov, http://ods.od.nih.gov.

Tish Davidson, A.M.
William Atkins, B.B., B.S., M.B.A.

Ginseng

Definition

Ginseng refers to two closely related herbs of the genus *Panax*. Asian ginseng (*P. ginseng*) and American ginseng (*P. quinquefolius*) have traditionally been used for healing for many centuries. Asian ginseng is also known as Korean

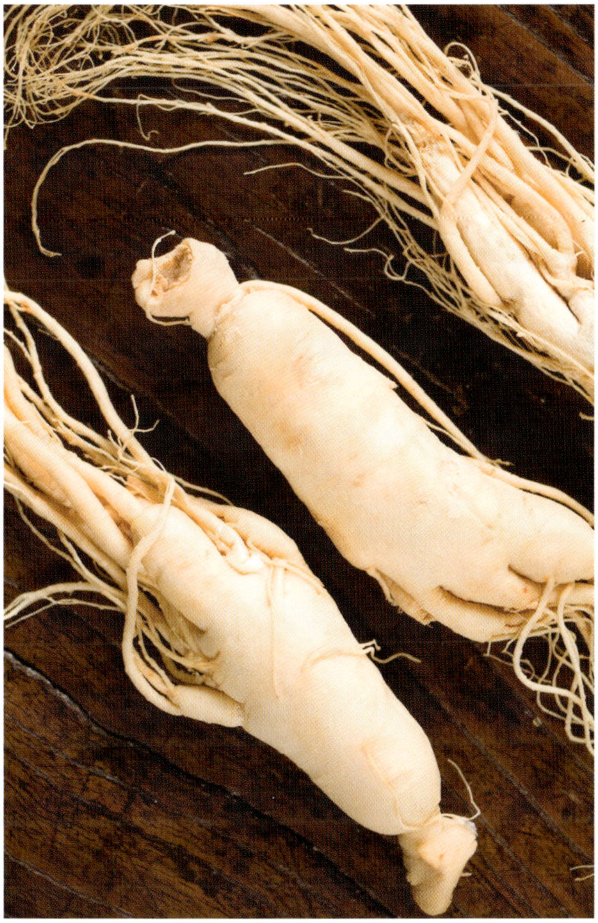

Ginseng root. *(© iStockPhoto.com/Yungshu Chao)*

red ginseng, Chinese ginseng, Japanese ginseng, ginseng radix, ninjin, sang, and ren shen. American ginseng is also known as Canadian ginseng, North American ginseng, Ontario ginseng, Wisconsin ginseng, red berry, sang, and ren shen. Siberian ginseng (*Eleutherococcus senticosus*) is a plant with different properties that belongs to a completely different genus. Ginseng in this entry refers only to Asian and American ginseng of the genus *Panax*.

Purpose

Ginseng has been used for over 2,000 years in Traditional Chinese Medicine (TCM) to boost energy, hasten recovery from illness or injury, reduce **stress**, improve mental and physical performance (including sexual performance) and treat several dozen different infections, gastrointestinal disorders, circulatory problems, and conditions as diverse as burns, cancers, diabetes, migraine headaches, and weight loss. The genus name *Panax* means "heal all," and herbalists consider ginseng to be an almost universal remedy. Most of these traditional uses of ginseng have not yet been substantiated by conventional medicine; however, encouraging results from some well-designed, controlled human studies strongly suggest that ginseng may improve mental performance, especially concerning mental illnesses, and may have other health benefits.

Description

Ginseng is a perennial herb that grows in cool, damp, shady forests. Asian ginseng is native to Northern China, and today it is grown as a cash crop in China, Korea, Japan, and Russia. American ginseng once grew wild from the Appalachian Mountains to Minnesota. Today, it is cultivated mainly in Wisconsin and in the Canadian provinces of Ontario and British Columbia. Most cultivated ginseng from North America is exported to Asia. In both Asia and North America, wild ginseng is threatened with extinction from over-harvesting. In the United States, a government permit is usually required to export wild ginseng. High-quality wild ginseng is very expensive. Illegal harvesting of wild ginseng from public lands is an ongoing law enforcement problem for the U.S. Fish and Wildlife Service.

Ginseng is a slow-growing plant that reaches a height of 12–30 in. (30.5–76.2 cm) and produces red berries. Only the root is used for medicinal purposes. Ginseng is difficult to cultivate. Plants must grow four to six years before the roots can be harvested. Ginseng roots are forked and twisted, looking somewhat like a miniature human body. They are occasionally used fresh but more often are dried and ground or powdered. The root can be soaked to make an extract or tincture. Ground ginseng can be added to tea, and powered ginseng is often placed into capsules. Ginseng extract can be added to products as diverse as chewing gum and soft drinks. In addition, ginseng is sold under dozens of different brand names. It is often found in multi-herb remedies sold under a huge variety of names. The active ingredients of ginseng are thought to be more than 20 compounds called "ginsenosides." Some manufacturers standardize the amount of ginsengosides in their product, while others do not. Standardized products usually contain at least 4 ginsenosides.

Regulation of ginseng sales

In the United States, ginseng is regulated by the Food and Drug Administration (FDA) as a dietary supplement under the 1994 Dietary Supplement Health and Education Act (DSHEA). When the act was passed, legislators felt that these supplements did not need to be regulated as rigorously as prescription and over-the-counter drugs used in conventional medicine, because many dietary supplements such as ginseng come from natural sources and have been used for hundreds of years by practitioners of complementary and alternative medicine (CAM).

The DSHEA regulates ginseng in the same way that food is regulated. Like food manufacturers, manufacturers of herbal products containing ginseng do not have to prove that they are either safe or effective before they can be sold to the public. This differs from conventional pharmaceutical drugs, which must undergo extensive human testing to prove their safety and effectiveness before they can be marketed. Also unlike conventional drugs, the label for a dietary supplement such as ginseng does not have to contain any statements about possible side effects. All herbal supplements sold in the United States must show the scientific name of the herb on the label. Consumers should look for ginseng of the *Panax* variety. Sometimes less-expensive herbs such as Siberian "ginseng" are substituted for true ginseng.

Health claims

Dozens of health claims are made for ginseng, many based on traditional or folk use of the herb. These claims are difficult to substantiate in ways that satisfy conventional medicine, for several reasons, including:

- The amount and strength of ginseng in dietary supplements is not standardized, and a wide range of doses are used in different studies.
- Ginseng is often one of several herbs contained in herbal remedies, making it difficult to tell whether the effects are due to ginseng or another herb.
- Many studies performed on ginseng are poorly designed, so it is impossible to show a direct link between cause and effect, or they are poorly reported, making analysis of the results difficult.
- Many rigorous and well-designed human studies have a small sample size.
- Many studies are sponsored by ginseng growers, manufacturers, or importers who have a financial interest in obtaining positive results.

Despite these drawbacks, there is sufficient scientific evidence that ginseng does provides health benefits. Consequently, the National Center for Complementary and Alternative Medicine (NCCAM), a government organization within the National Institutes of Health (NIH), is sponsoring **clinical trials** to determine safety and effectiveness of ginseng as a treatment for several diseases and disorders, some involving mental conditions. Individuals interested in participating in a clinical trial at no charge can find a list of open trials at http://www.clinicaltrials.gov.

Some health claims for ginseng appear more promising than others. There is good evidence that ginseng can cause short-term improvement in mental performance in both healthy young adults and ill elderly adults. Not enough information is available to determine whether long-term gains also occur, but the results have been promising enough that ginseng is being studied in patients with **Alzheimer's disease** and other dementias. Along with improved mental performance, some studies have shown that ginseng improves the sense of well-being and quality of life. Results of these studies are mixed, with some finding improvements, and others finding no change. The situation is complicated by the fact that different studies define and measure "well-being" and "quality of life" in different ways. In general, people with the worst quality of life report the most improvement.

Many other health claims are made for herbal mixtures that contain ginseng. These claims are extremely difficult to evaluate because of the number of variables, including the strength of the mixture, the effects of the different herbs, and potential interactions among other herbs. Until much more is known about the chemical properties and active ingredients of common medicinal herbs, it will be almost impossible to evaluate these mixtures in a way that satisfies the demands of conventional medicine.

MEMORY. A combination of *Panax* ginseng and ginkgo leaf extract seems to help improve thinking, mathematical skills, and reaction times in middle-age people who are otherwise healthy. Because memory problems could be an early sign of **dementia**, further studies are being pursued to learn more about a potential relationship between ginseng and memory.

ERECTILE DYSFUNCTION. Ginseng has been found to help male impotence, what is often called erectile dysfunction (ED). Taking *Panax* ginseng orally (by mouth) seems to improve sexual function in men with ED. Early studies are being supplemented with further research to validate these initial results.

PREMATURE EJACULATION. Some men have problems during sexual activity that involve **premature ejaculation**. When a *Panax* ginseng-based cream is applied to the skin of the penis, better control of the sexual organism is possible, which helps with premature ejaculation.

Recommended dosage

Always consult with a medical professional before taking ginseng. The recommended dosage should be stated clearly on the package. Use the recommended dosage from the package unless a doctor, pharmacist, or other health care provider states otherwise. If the package does not contain dosage information, do not use it. Different formulations of ginseng are safer than are others. The safest forms are extracts, tinctures, and solids. Always use the same formulation; do not mix forms, because such a practice may cause an accidental overdose. Fluid retention, muscle tension, sleeplessness, or swelling can be signs of an overdose.

According to medical research, when used for **erectile dysfunction**, use approximately 900 mg orally three times daily. For premature ejaculation, a cream containing *Panax* ginseng and other ingredients should be applied to the skin of the penis about one hour before sexual intercourse. Wash the cream off before having intercourse.

Precautions

Ginseng is generally safe and causes few side effects when taken at recommended doses. The generally recommended dose is 100–200 mg of standardized ginseng extract containing 4% ginsenosides once or twice daily. The safety of ginseng in children and pregnant and breastfeeding women has not been studied. Pregnant and breastfeeding women should be aware that some tinctures of ginseng contain high levels of alcohol. Some herbalists recommend that individuals take ginseng for two to three weeks and then take a break of one to two weeks before beginning the herb again.

Independent laboratory analyses have repeatedly found that many products labeled as ginseng contain little or none of the herb. True ginseng is expensive, and unscrupulous manufacturers often substitute low-cost herbs for ginseng. Another problem is that some ginseng products have been found to be contaminated with pesticides, toxins, or other dangerous chemicals that can cause serious side effects. Always purchase ginseng from reputable retailers.

When using ginseng to help with erectile dysfunction, use caution if diabetic. The herb may cause blood sugar levels to decrease. In addition, in a small number of cases, ginseng has been found to cause mania when used together with some **antidepressants**.

Consult with a doctor before considering ginseng if the following conditions are present (or medicines are being taken to treat them): bleeding or blood clotting disorder, high blood pressure, heart disease, or diabetes. In addition, before starting ginseng make sure the doctor is aware of any medicines or herbal supplements being taken, and whether medical conditions, such as plant allergies, are present.

Giving ginseng to infants or children has sometimes lead to serious medical problems and even death from poisoning. It is not known whether ginseng is safe for older children. To be safe, do not give ginseng to any child or adolescent, regardless of age.

Interactions

Ginseng appears to interact with blood-thinning and anti-coagulant medicines such as dalteparin (Fragmin), ticlopidine (Ticlid), cilostazol (Pletal), enoxaparin (Lovenox), heparin, warfarin (Coumadin), clopidogrel (Plavix), aspirin, and nonsteroidal anti-inflammatory drugs (e.g. Advil, Motrin). Individuals taking these drugs should not begin taking ginseng without consulting their health care provider.

Because ginseng lowers blood sugar levels, individuals who are taking insulin or other medications that also lower blood sugar, and those with type 2 diabetes, should be monitored for low blood sugar if they begin taking ginseng. Adjustments in the other medications by the attending physician may be needed.

Ginseng may also interact with **monoamine oxidase inhibitors (MAOIs)** used to treat certain kinds of **depression** and mental illness. Ginseng stimulates the body, as do many of these **MAOIs**. Using them together can use an excessive amount of stimulation, which can lead to restlessness, **insomnia**, anxiousness, and headaches. Examples of MAOIs include **isocarboxazid** (Marplan), **phenelzine** (Nardil) and **tranylcypromine** (Parnate). Individuals taking MAOIs with ginseng may also develop tremors and mania.

Immunosuppressants, those that solve medical problems by reducing the efficiency in which the immune system works, can adversely interact with

KEY TERMS

Alzheimer's disease—The most common type of dementia that usually occurs late in life, involving confusion, irritability, mood swings, language problems, short-term memory loss, and general decline of the senses.

Dementia—A medical condition that involves the progressive deterioration of intellectual and cognitive function, such as memory.

Diabetes—A medical disorder that involves the production of excessive urine; medically called diabetes mellitus; type 1 diabetes (juvenile diabetes) involves failure of the body to produce insulin, while type 2 diabetes (adult onset diabetes) involves the body's cells failing to use insulin properly.

Monoamine oxidase inhibitor—Also called L-monoamine oxidase inhibitor (MAOI), a family of enzymes that catalyze the oxidation of monoamines.

Schizophrenia—A psychiatric disorder with symptoms of self withdrawal, emotional instability, and reality detachment.

ginseng. Ginseng increases the immune system, so taking it with immunosuppressants can cause these medicines to work less effectively. Some immunosuppressant drugs include: azathioprine (Imuran), basiliximab (Simulect), cyclosporine (Neoral), daclizumab (Zenapax), muromonab-CD3 (OKT3), mycophenolate (CellCept), tacrolimus (FK506), sirolimus (Rapamune), prednisone (Deltasone), and corticosteroids (glucocorticoids).

Preliminary evidence suggests that ginseng may interact with certain blood pressure and heart medications, such as digoxin (Lanoxin), a medication used to treat congestive heart failure. The herb may also interfere with the way the liver processes other drugs and herbs. Before beginning to take a supplement containing ginseng, individuals should review their current medications with their health care provider to determine any possible interactions.

Ginseng has been reported to interact with caffeine to cause overstimulation and insomnia in some people. During the day, the two together may cause a person to feel nervous or jittery; it may also cause the heart to beat faster than normal and one's blood pressure to increase. It is not recommended to take coffee, tea, cola, or other drinks or foods containing caffeine together with ginseng. Other stimulant drugs can also cause similar problems. Some of these include diethylpropion (Tenuate), epinephrine, phentermine (Ionamin), and pseudoephedrine (Sudafed).

Other herbs may also adversely react with ginseng. Bitter orange may increase the risk of an irregular heartbeat. Any substance that contains ephedra, such as country mallow, can produce an irregular heartbeat, so using it with ginseng can increase the problem. Herbs that lower blood sugar, such as bitter melon, ginger, goat's rue, fenugreek, kudzu, willow bark, and others, can lower such levels even more when taken with ginseng. Avoid such substances.

Complications

Serious side effects of ginseng are rare. The most common complications are increased restlessness, insomnia, nausea, diarrhea, and rash. Allergic reactions are possible but uncommon. Difficulty breathing; swelling (narrowing) of the throat; or swelling of the lips, tongue, or face may also occur due to a serious allergic reaction. Some of the more serious side effects reported are thought to be the result of contamination with pesticides, heavy metals, or other chemicals rather than side effects caused by ginseng.

High doses of ginseng can increase certain symptoms of **schizophrenia**. Some of the more common symptoms that can be worsened are problems with sleeping at night and feelings of agitation or irritability during the day. Consult with a doctor before taking ginseng if schizophrenia is present.

QUESTIONS TO ASK YOUR DOCTOR

- Should I try ginseng?
- What dose would be appropriate for me to take?
- Are there any foods I should avoid?
- Where is a reliable place to buy ginseng?
- Where can I find reliable information about ginseng?

Contemporary Chinese practitioners recognize a condition known as "ginseng abuse syndrome," caused by taking ginseng incorrectly or excessively. The symptoms of ginseng abuse syndrome include heart palpitations, heaviness in the chest, high blood pressure, dizziness, insomnia, agitation, restlessness, nausea, vomiting, abdominal pain and/or bloating, diarrhea, possible upper digestive tract bleeding, edema, and a red skin rash that is most noticeable on the face. Western herbalists recommend that anyone taking ginseng who develops these symptoms should stop taking the herb at once and contact a licensed practitioner of TCM to determine whether ginseng abuse is the cause of the problem.

Resources

BOOKS

Dasgupta, Amitava, and Catherine A. Hammett-Stabler, editors. *Herbal Supplements: Efficacy, Toxicity, Interactions with Western Drugs, and Effects on Clinical Laboratory Tests.* Hoboken, NJ: Wiley, 2011.

Fragakis, Allison. *The Health Professional's Guide to Popular Dietary Supplements* Chicago: American Dietetic Association, 2007.

Hsu, Elisabeth, and Stephen Harris, editors. *Plants, Health and Healing: On the Interface of Ethnobotany and Medical Anthropology.* New York: Berghahn, 2010.

Johanssen, Kristin. *Ginseng Dreams: The Secret World of America's Most Valuable Plant.* Lexington, KY: University Press of Kentucky, 2006.

PDR for Herbal Medicines. Montvale, NJ: Thompson, 2007.

Peilin, Sun, editor. *The Treatment of Pain with Chinese Herbs and Acupuncture.* Edinburgh: Elsevier Churchill Livingstone, 2011.

Sutton, Amy L, editor. *Complementary and Alternative Medicine Sourcebook.* Detroit: Omnigraphics, 2010.

Taylor, David. *Ginseng, the Divine Root: The Curious History of the Plant That Captivated the World.* Chapel Hill, NC: Algonquin Books of Chapel Hill, 2006.

Tracy, Timothy S. and Richard L. Kingston, eds. *Herbal Products: Toxicology and Clinical Pharmacology.* Totowa, NJ, Humana Press, 2007.

Wildman, Robert E. C., editor. *Handbook of Nutraceuticals and Functional Foods,* 2nd edition. Boca Raton, FL: CRC/ Taylor & Francis, 2007.

WEBSITES

Ginseng. American Cancer Society. (November 28, 2008). http://www.cancer.org/Treatment/TreatmentsandSideEffects/ComplementaryandAlternativeMedicine/HerbsVitaminsandMinerals/ginseng?sitearea=eto (accessed July 6, 2011).

Ginseng. National Center for Complimentary and Alternative Medicine. (April 1, 2011). http://nccam.nih.gov/health/asianginseng (accessed July 6, 2011).

Ginseng, Panax. MedlinePlus. (April 22, 2011). http://www.nlm.nih.gov/medlineplus/druginfo/natural/1000.html (accessed July 5, 2011).

ORGANIZATIONS

American Association of Acupuncture and Oriental Medicine, PO Box 162340, Sacramento, CA, 95816, Fax: 1(916) 443-4766, (866) 455-7999, http://www.aaaomonline.org

American Botanical Council, PO Box 14435, Austin, TX, 78723, 1(512) 926-4900, Fax: 1(512) 926-2345, (800) 373-7105, http://abc.herbalgram.org

National Center for Complementary and Alternative Medicine Clearinghouse, PO Box 7923, Gaithersburg, MD, 20898, Fax: 1(866) 464-3616, (888) 644-6226, info@nccam.nih.gov, http://nccam.nih.gov

National Certification Commission for Acupuncture and Oriental Medicine, 76 South Laura St., Suite 1290, Jacksonville, FL, 32202, 1(904) 598-1005, Fax: 1(904) 598-5001, http://www.nccaom.org

Natural Standard, One Davis Square, Somerville, MA, 02144, 1(617) 591-3300, Fax: 1(617) 591-3399, questions@naturalstandard.com, http://naturalstandard.com

Office of Dietary Supplements, National Institutes of Health, 6100 Executive Blvd., Room 3B01, MSC 7517, Bethesda, MD, 20892-7517, 1(301) 435-2920, Fax: 1(301) 480-1845, ods@nih.gov, http://ods.od.nih.gov.

Tish Davidson, A.M.
William Atkins, B.B., B.S., M.B.A.

Grief

Definition

Grief, which is also known as **bereavement**, is a term used to describe the intense and painful emotions experienced when someone or something a person cares about either dies or is lost. The emotional pain from losing a loved one, whether it is a spouse, child, parent, sibling, friend, or pet, can be the most severe suffering a person must endure. At its most intense, grief can dominate every facet of a person's life, making the carrying out of ordinary responsibilities impossible. Loss and subsequent grief, however, are an inevitable part of life. Painful as it is, grief is a normal response to loss and generally resolves with the passage of time.

KEY TERMS

Anxiety—An overwhelming sense of apprehension and fear; can be experienced as a troubled feeling, a sense of dread, fear of the future, or distress over a possible threat to a person's physical or mental well-being.

Depression—A mental condition characterized by feelings of sadness, despair, and discouragement.

Stressor—A stimulus, or event, that provokes a stress response in an organism. Stressors can be categorized as acute or chronic, and as external or internal to the organism.

Description

Grief is usually characterized by psychological numbness, tearfulness, physical feelings of emptiness in the pit of the stomach, weak knees, shortness of breath, a tendency to sigh deeply, a sense of unreality, and overall emotional distress. Anxiety and longing may alternate with **depression** and despair. **Insomnia** and loss of appetite are common. Initially, people often feel a lack of extreme emotion and may be immune to sensory stimuli; they may find it difficult to accept their loss. Numbness is followed by shock as reality begins to penetrate.

There is generally a disorganization of normal behavior patterns that may make it impossible for a bereaved person to return to work immediately or to take social initiatives. Such acute symptoms usually begin to subside after several months, with emotional balance typically regained within a year. Studies using instruments developed to measure symptoms of grief and bereavement demonstrate wide individual variations in specific symptoms and their intensity. Long after the immediate period of mourning, bereaved persons may continue to feel upset, empty, or tearful. In addition, further losses, additional stressors, or dates of such important anniversaries as a wedding, birthday, or the date of death can reactivate the acute symptoms of grief.

ELISABETH KÜBLER–ROSS (1926–2004)

Swiss-born psychiatrist Elisabeth Kübler–Ross dedicated her career to a topic that had previously been avoided by many physicians and mental health care professionals—the psychological state of the dying. In her counseling of and research on dying patients, Kübler–Ross determined that individuals go through five distinct mental stages when confronted with death, a discovery that has helped other counselors provide more appropriate advice and treatment to grieving clients. Her ideas have been presented to the public in a number of popular texts, including her groundbreaking 1969 work, *On Death and Dying*. She also supported hospice and palliative care, and offered instruction and treatment at the seminars and healing centers she ran for the terminally ill and their caretakers. Her career ended with controversy, but the five stages of grief, also referred to as the Kübler–Ross model, are well known in psychiatric medicine.

Dimensions of grief

Grief and mourning are important life experiences in that they permit a bereaved person to accept the reality of loss and begin to find ways of filling the resultant emptiness. Loss is a significant part of the aging process and can contribute to emotional problems in older people. The impact of loss and resulting grief and mourning is not limited to the death of a loved one. It is also present to a lesser extent in the loss of physical acuity and agility and the loss of social status as a result of retirement and/or growing older.

Unfortunately, people in the United States do not generally receive cultural support for the losses they experience and the need to mourn those losses. Unlike other cultures with specific rituals for grief and mourning, there is often subtle but insistent pressure on Americans—particularly males—to move forward with resumption of regular activities. Onlookers may try to divert the mourner's attention to other topics or discourage crying or talking about the loved one. These responses suggest that grief is not healthy or that it should be minimized or avoided. If the grief is associated with the loss of a pet, the person may be shamed for grieving because "it was just an animal." Women who have had a pregnancy ended by miscarriage also encounter responses that minimize or trivialize the loss of their expected child. Social insensitivity may drive the mourner to grieve in secret or feel guilty because of continued intense feelings of loss.

Stages of grief

Elisabeth Kübler–Ross, a **psychiatrist** who studied death and dying, identified five stages of acceptance in the process of dying. While her work initially referred to the person who is dying, the five stages are also applied to people who are grieving a loss. The stages are sometimes collapsed into three, but the general grieving process includes these components:

- Shock/denial. This stage comprises the initial period after receiving news of the loss. The affected person may say, "There must be a mistake," "This can't be true," or similar expressions of disbelief. People often describe feeling numb or cold in this stage.
- Bargaining. This stage represents an attempt to persuade God or a higher power to change the reality of loss in exchange for improved behavior or some sacrifice on the part of the bereaved person. The mourner may offer, for example, to take better care of their relationship with the loved one if God will bring the loved one back.
- Anger. This emotion may be directed toward the medical establishment, family members, a higher power, or even the person who has died.
- Depression. In this stage, the person's body begins to absorb the reality of the loss. The bereaved person may be unable to eat, sleep, or talk normally with people. They may have episodes of spontaneous crying and such physical symptoms as nausea, headaches, chills, or trembling.
- Acceptance. This is the phase in which the mourner comes to terms with the loss and begins to look ahead once more. Energy returns and the bereaved person is able to reconnect with others, engage in enjoyable activities, and make plans for the future.

There is, however, no "normal" pattern for grief; it is a highly variable experience. People pass through the stages outlined by Kübler–Ross at their own rate, depending on the significance of the loss, previous losses they've experienced, individual resiliency, presence of a support system, and permission to grieve from those around them. Grieving is not a linear process. There is movement back and forth between the stages until acceptance is reached. Occasionally, a person may remain "stuck" in one stage, particularly anger or depression, and may benefit from professional help in order to move on. Remaining in one of the stages indefinitely can create emotional and occupational difficulties.

Bereavement and marriage

Studies show that some widowed people have hallucinations or **delusions** of contact with the lost spouse that may last for years. These hallucinations are more likely to occur in people who were happily married. The most common **hallucination** reported is a sense of the dead spouse's presence. Others report seeing, hearing, or being touched by or spoken to by the spouse.

The interplay of grief and marital quality has led to research findings that contradict earlier widespread beliefs. A 2000 study by Deborah Carr and her colleagues found that anxiety was greater in those who had been highly dependent on their spouses than in those who were less dependent. People who had been in conflicted relationships reported lower levels of yearning for the spouse than those who had enjoyed high levels of marital closeness. Women who had relied on their husbands to do the driving and perform other similar tasks had much higher levels of yearning than men who depended on their wives. This finding contradicts the common belief that grief is more severe if the marriage was conflicted, suggesting a more complex relationship between bereavement and characteristics of the marriage.

Another suggestion of the complex relationship between bereavement and marriage is reflected in studies of sudden and anticipated loss among older widowed people. The sudden death of a spouse was associated with slightly higher levels of yearning among women, but significantly lower yearning among men. Forewarning of the death (extended illness, advancing age) did not affect depression, anger, shock or overall grief 6 or 18 months after the loss. Prolonged forewarning was associated with increased anxiety at 6- and 18-month follow-up interviews after the death.

Grief and mourning may also occur when the loss of a partner occurs through divorce or the end of a dating relationship. Some researchers think that moving to the stage of acceptance is more difficult in such cases because the partner can still be contacted, especially if there are children involved. Seeing a former partner involved in a new relationship can cause the partner mourning the loss to reexperience acute symptoms of grief. Some research evidence suggests that grief related to the breakup of an intimate relationship is more intense for the individual who was left behind than for the person who ended the relationship.

Grieving may be particularly prolonged and intense when certain unexpected losses occur that are outside the ordinary progression of life events. The loss of a parent before a child reaches adulthood or a parent's loss of a child inflict deep emotional wounds for an extended period of time. Similarly, the loss of a loved one to murder, terrorism, or other acts of intentional violence can be harder to bear than death resulting from natural causes or accidents. Death from **suicide** complicates grief by adding possible feelings of shame, blame, or guilt, or unanswered questions as to the deceased's reasons, to the other painful emotions associated with bereavement. The opportunity to fully grieve such significant losses, however, enables survivors to move forward despite the magnitude of their loss.

QUESTIONS TO ASK YOUR DOCTOR

- What counseling options do you recommend for me?
- Can you recommend any support groups for me and my family?

Resources

BOOKS

Burns, Donna M. *When Kids Are Grieving: Addressing Grief and Loss in School*. Thousand Oaks, CA: Corwin Press, 2010.

Coor, C.A., and D.E. Balk, eds. *Handbook of Adolescent Death and Bereavement*.New York: Springer Publishing Co., Inc., 2004.

Harris, Maxine, Ph.D. *The Loss That Is Forever: The Lifelong Impact of the Early Death of a Mother or Father*. New York: Plume, 1996.

James, John W., and Russell Friedman. *The Grief Recovery Handbook,* 20th Anniversary ed. New York, NY: William Morrow Paperbacks, 2009.

Kübler–Ross, Elizabeth, and David Kessler. *Life Lessons*. New York: Scribner. 2001.

Manfred, Erica. *He's History, You're Not: Surviving Divorce After 40*. Guilford, CT: GPP Life, 2009.

Noel, Brook., and Pamela D. Blair. *I Wasn't Ready to Say Goodbye: Surviving, Coping and Healing After the Sudden Death of a Loved One*. Naperville, IL: Sourcebooks, 2008.

Segal, Daniel L., Sara Honn Qualls, and Michael A. Smyer. *Aging and Mental Health*. 2nd ed. New York, NY: Wiley-Blackwell, 2010.

PERIODICALS

Carr, Deborah, et al. "Marital Quality and Psychological Adjustment to Widowhood Among Older Adults." *Journals of Gerontology Series B: Psychological Sciences and Social Sciences* 55, no. 4 (2000): S197–S207.

Carr, Deborah, et al. "Psychological Adjustment to Sudden and Anticipated Spousal Loss Among Older Widowed Persons." *Journals of Gerontology Series B: Psychological Sciences and Social Sciences* 56B, no. 4 (2001): S237-S248. Available online at http://www.cloc.isr.umich.edu/papers/carr2001_jogss.pdf (accessed November 9, 2011).

Zisook, S., et al. "Bereavement, Complicated Grief, and DSM, Part 2: complicated Grief." *Journal of clinical Psychiatry* 71, no. 8 (August 2010): 1097–8 (accessed October 30, 2011).

Zisook, S., R. A. Devaul, and M. A. Click Jr. "Measuring Symptoms of Grief and Bereavement." *American Journal of Psychiatry* 139 (1982): 1590–1593.

ORGANIZATIONS

The Compassionate Friends, PO Box 3696, Oak Brook, IL, 60522, (877) 969-0010, Fax: (630) 990-0246, (630) 990-0010, http://www.compassionatefriends.org.

GROWW (Grief Recovery Online [founded by] Widows and Widowers), 11877 Douglas Rd., #102-PMB101, Alpharetta, GA, 30005, http://www.groww.org.

SHARE Pregnancy and Infant Loss Support, 402 Jackson Street, St. Charles, MO, 63301, (800) 821-6819; (636) 947-6164, Fax: (636) 947-7486, http://www.nationalshare.org.

Widowed Persons Service, 4211 Clyde Park, SW, Unit C, Wyoming, MI, 49509, (616) 538-0101, director@wpsgr.org, http://www.wpsgr.org.

Judy Leaver, MA
Laura Jean Cataldo, RN, Ed.D.

Grief counseling

Definition

Grief counseling refers to a specific form of therapy, or a focus in general counseling with the goal of helping the individual grieve and address personal loss in a healthy manner. Grief counseling is offered individually by psychologists, clergy, counselors or **social workers**, in groups led by professionals, as well as informal **support groups** offered by churches, community groups, or organizations devoted to helping individuals grieve specific losses.

Purpose

The purpose of grief counseling is to help individuals work through the feelings, thoughts, and memories associated with the loss of a loved one. Although grieving can occur for other types of loss as well (such as loss of goals, ideals, and relationships), grief counseling is generally directed toward positive adjustment following loss after the death of a loved one.

Specific tasks of grief counseling include emotional expression about the loss (which can include a wide range of feelings), accepting the loss, adjusting to life after the loss, and coping with the changes within oneself and the world after the loss. Typical feelings experienced by individuals, and addressed in grief counseling, include sadness, anxiety, anger, loneliness, guilt, relief, isolation, confusion, or numbness. Behavioral changes may also be noticed, such as being disorganized, feeling tired, having trouble concentrating, sleep problems, appetite changes, vivid dreams, or daydreaming about the deceased.

Grief counseling helps the individual recognize normal aspects of the grieving or mourning process, cope with the pain associated with the loss, feel supported through the anxiety surrounding life changes that may follow the loss, and develop strategies for seeking support and self-care.

KEY TERMS

Anxiety—Can be experienced as a troubled feeling, a sense of dread, fear of the future, or distress over a possible threat to a person's physical or mental well-being.

Behavioral—Means related to the way a person acts.

Psychological—Refers to mental processes, including thoughts, feelings, and emotions.

Psychologist—A mental health professional who can do psychological testing and provide mental health counseling.

Description

Grief counseling helps the individual work through the feelings associated with the loss of another, accept that loss, determine how life can go on without that person, and consolidate memories in order to be able to move forward. Grief counseling also provides information about the normal grieving process, to help individuals understand that many of the symptoms and changes they are experiencing are a normal, temporary reaction to loss. For some individuals, the primary focus of grief counseling is to help identify ways to express feelings about the loss that the person has been unable to express on his or her own. Individuals who seek grief counseling may be experiencing an emotional numbness, or a residual shock in reaction to the loss, and need assistance to return to a normal life. In those cases, grief counseling will focus on helping the individual get in touch with those feelings and become more active in ones daily routine.

For some people, grieving may initially be so extreme that physical and psychological symptoms may be experienced, while other people appear to experience no symptoms whatsoever. Activities of daily living may feel overwhelming to an individual who has experienced a loss. In these cases, grief counseling may focus on specific coping skills to help the individual resume some normalcy in his or her daily routine. For example, if sleep patterns are disrupted, grief counseling may include consultation with the individual's physician to assist with temporary strategies to increase sleep. If the individual is having trouble getting to work on time, behavioral strategies may be used as an interim measure to help the person return to aspects of normal daily life.

Additional work in grief counseling may involve identifying ways to let go or say good–bye if the individual has not been able to do so successfully. Therapeutic letters may be a helpful mechanism to express thoughts that were not conveyed prior to the death. Dreams are frequently experienced by survivors, and these can be a focus in grief counseling as well. The dreams can often be consoling and as well, a way of consolidating the memories about the deceased.

Precautions

Grieving is a normal life process—an adjustment reaction to a loss. Grief counseling is meant to facilitate that normal process. No specific precautions are warranted. However, there are certain circumstances in which complications to the normal grieving process may occur. These circumstances may involve the loss of a child, or the loss of a loved one due to an accident or homicide, for example.

In these cases of complicated grieving, more extreme responses to the loss may be observed, depending on the individual's capacity for coping, personal resiliency, and support system. For example, if the individual feels isolated, he may be at greater risk for severe depressive symptoms or a **suicide** attempt. Alternatively, if the survivors feel rage or anger over the loss, there may be a risk of harm to others.

Preparation

No specific preparation is required by the participant; however, a need for grief counseling is indicated by prolonged symptoms (such as crying spells, preoccupation with the deceased, lack of motivation, or suicidal thoughts), and the severity of personal distress over the loss. A patient seeking grief counseling would most likely undergo a clinical evaluation by a therapist, before the grief counseling began, so that the therapist could understand the patient's personal history and goals for treatment.

QUESTIONS TO ASK YOUR DOCTOR OR COUNSELOR

- What counseling options do you recommend for me?
- Are there medications to help me with my grief? If so, what are they and should I take a medication?
- What kind of changes can I expect to see with the medication you have prescribed for me?
- What are the side effects associated with the medication you have prescribed for me?
- Can you recommend any counseling or support groups for me and my family?

Aftercare

Aftercare is usually provided through informal support systems, which may include family and friends, as well as support groups.

Risks

A slight risk exists regarding treatment of complicated grief. Such circumstances include chronic, prolonged grieving or unexpected loss (particularly due to a violent accident, suicide, homicide, or the death of a child). These factors complicate the grieving process due to the unexpected, sometimes violent nature of the loss, that feels inconsistent with expectations and desires for loved ones. In these cases, an initial adverse effect may be seen from participation in treatment, due to the increased focus on the loss. This reaction improves over time, as adjustment is facilitated. Two other factors impacting individual adjustment include the type of relationship the individual had with the deceased, and the resiliency of the individual.

Results

Normal results from grief counseling include being able to move on with one's life, recognizing and accepting the physical loss of the individual, and being able to bridge that loss with positive memories of the deceased. Successful coping will be characterized by a return to normal routines, although some symptoms may be experienced periodically throughout the year or on dates of important anniversaries such as a wedding, birthday, or the date of the loss.

Abnormal results would include an unsuccessful outcome of prolonged grief, exhibited by continued preoccupation with the loss of the individual, crying spells, and depressive symptoms being the most likely complications. Some disruption of the daily routine would persist, and there may be extreme emotional responses, that could include no apparent reaction to difficulty containing feelings. Other complications include "unfinished business," or feelings of unresolved issues with the deceased. Sometimes the feelings of unresolved issues can be as simple as wishing they had communicated their love and affection for the person the last time they saw them, or may be as complicated as unresolved feelings about a history of **abuse** by the deceased.

Resources

BOOKS

Burns, Donna M. *When Kids Are Grieving: Addressing Grief and Loss in School.* Thousand Oaks, CA: Corwin Press, 2010.

Coor, C.A., and D.E. Balk, eds. *Handbook of Adolescent Death and Bereavement.*New York, NY: Springer Publishing Co., Inc., 2004.

James, John W., and Russell Friedman. *The Grief Recovery Handbook,* 20th Anniversary ed. New York, NY: Harper Paperbacks, 2009.

Jeffreys, J. Shep. *Helping Grieving People - When Tears Are Not Enough: A Handbook for Care Providers,* 2nd ed. New York, NY: Routledge, 2011.

Kübler–Ross, Elizabeth, and David Kessler. *Life Lessons.* New York: Simon and Schuster and the Elizabeth Kübler–Ross Family Partnership, Ltd. 2001.

Meier, Scott T., and Susan R. Davis. *The Elements of Counseling,* 7th ed. Belmont, CA: Brooks Cole, 2010.

Noel, Brook, and Pamela D. Blair. *I Wasn't Ready to Say Goodbye: Surviving, Coping and Healing After the Sudden Death of a Loved One.* Naperville, IL: Sourcebooks, 2008.

ORGANIZATIONS

The Compassionate Friends, Inc, PO Box 3696, Oak Brook, IL, 60522, http://www.compassionatefriends.org/home.aspx.

GROWW (Grief Recovery Online [founded by] Widows & Widowers), 11877 Douglas Rd., #102-PMB101, Alpharetta, GA, 30005, http://www.groww.org.

SHARE Pregnancy and Infant Loss Support, 402 Jackson Street, St. Charles, MO, 63301, (800) 821-6819, Fax: (636) 947-7486, http://www.nationalshare.org.

SIDS Alliance, 1314 Bedford Ave., Ste. 230, Baltimore, MD, 21208, (800) 221-SIDS, http://www.sidsalliance.org.

Widowed Persons Service, AARP, 601 E. St. NW, Washington, DC, 20049, (202) 434-2260, http://www.aarp.org/relationships/grief-loss/info-2005/newly_widowed.html.

Deanna Pledge, Ph.D.
Laura Jean Cataldo, RN, Ed.D.

Group homes

Definition

Group homes are small, residential facilities located within a community and designed to serve children or adults with chronic disabilities. These homes usually have six or fewer occupants and are staffed 24 hours a day by trained caregivers.

Description

Most group homes are standard, single-family houses, purchased by group home administrators and adapted to meet the needs of the residents. Except for any adaptive features such as wheelchair ramps, group homes are virtually indistinguishable from other homes in the surrounding neighborhood. Group homes may be located in neighborhoods of any socioeconomic status.

Residents of group homes usually have some type of chronic mental disorder that impairs their ability to live independently. Many residents also have physical disabilities such as impairments of vision communication, or ambulation. These individuals require continual assistance to complete daily living and self-care tasks. Some also require supervision due to behavior that may be dangerous to self or others, such as aggression or a tendency to run away.

Although most group homes provide long-term care, some residents eventually acquire the necessary skills to move to more independent living situations. Group homes for children are usually temporary placements, providing care until a foster family can be secured. Others may return to their natural families. Occasionally, halfway homes for people recently released from prison or discharged from a **substance abuse** program may also

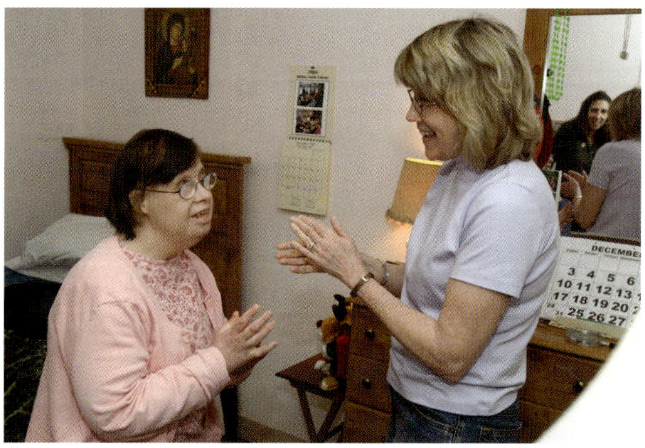

A woman with Down syndrome is visited by her sister at a group home. *(© Ellen B. Senisi/Photo Researchers, Inc.)*

be referred to as group homes. These types of group homes are also transitory in nature.

History and mission

The development of group homes occurred in response to the **deinstitutionalization** movement of the 1960s and 1970s. As psychiatric hospitals closed, discharged individuals needed places to live. Group homes were designed to provide care in the least restrictive environment and to integrate individuals with disabilities into the community, reducing **stigma** and improving quality of life. The environment of a group home was intended to simulate typical family life as much as possible.

Since the passage of the **Community Mental Health** Centers Act in 1963, grants have been available to group homes. State and federal funds such as the Medicaid Home and Community-Based Waiver continue to support the majority of group homes. However, some homes operate on donations from private citizens or civic and religious organizations. Most group homes are owned by private rather than governmental organizations, and can be either nonprofit or for-profit organizations. Group homes are considered more cost effective compared to institutional care. Unfortunately, the number of available group homes has not always matched need, resulting in **homelessness** or rehospitalization for some individuals.

One of the goals of group home living is to increase the independence of residents. Group home staff members teach residents daily living and self-care skills, providing as little assistance as possible. Daily living skills include meal preparation, laundry, housecleaning, home maintenance, money management, and appropriate social interactions. Self-care skills include bathing or showering, dressing, toileting, eating, and taking prescribed medications.

Staff also assure that residents receive necessary services from community service providers, including medical care, physical therapy, occupational therapy, vocational training, education, and mental health services. Most group home residents are assigned a case manager from a community mental health center or other government agency who oversees their care. Case managers review group home documentation regarding skills learned and services received, and make recommendations for adjustments in care.

NIMBY

Unfortunately, group homes have received much opposition from communities. NIMBY (acronym for "not in my backyard") describes the common reaction of community residents when they discover that a group home is targeted for their neighborhood. Current research suggests that protests frequently involve concerns over personal security, declining property values, or a generalized threat to the neighborhood's quality. Some researchers believe that prejudiced attitudes such as ignorance, fear, and distrust are the true reasons for protest.

Usually, neighborhood opposition is unsuccessful due to provisions of the Fair Housing Act of 1968. However, such opposition can be detrimental to the goal of integrating residents into the community. The NIMBY principal is also a concern because as deinstitutionalization continues, the need for additional group homes increases. Statistics show that between 1987 and 1999, the use of group homes serving individuals with developmental disabilities and containing six residents or less increased by 240%.

Social service workers are constantly looking for ways to address NIMBY. Some research has suggested that community concerns decrease with time as community members become familiar with group home residents. Studies have shown that opposition can be decreased by providing advanced notice of plans for a group home, as well as adequate information and discussion about expectations.

Factors affecting group home success

Initially, many people were skeptical about the adequacy of group home care compared to psychiatric hospitals or other institutions. Over the past 25 years, many studies have examined the impact of group home care on residents. These studies have consistently shown increases in adaptive behavior, productivity, community integration, and level of independence.

Risks involved in successfully transitioning an individual to a group home include psychological deterioration such as severe cognitive or physical impairments, physical deterioration that includes being nonambulatory, or mortality issues such as being age 70 or older.

Before considering group home placement—especially for those in the high risk category—extensive planning should be conducted. A complete assessment plan of the individual's needs should specify which agency will be responsible for meeting medical needs, particularly in the event of a crisis. The individual's strengths should be incorporated into the plan whenever possible. For example, if a supportive family is an identified strength, the preferred group home should be close in proximity to facilitate family visits.

KEY TERMS

Ambulation—Ability to walk.

Case manager—A professional who designs and monitors implementation of comprehensive care plans (i.e., services addressing medical, financial, housing, psychiatric, vocational, social needs) for individuals seeking mental health or social services.

Community mental health centers—Organizations that manage and deliver a comprehensive range of mental health services, education, and outreach to residents of a given community.

Community Mental Health Centers Act of 1963—Federal legislation providing grants for the operation of community mental health centers and related services.

Deinstitutionalization—The process of moving people out of mental hospitals into treatment programs or halfway houses in local communities. With this movement, the responsibility for care shifted from large (often governmental) agencies to families and community organizations.

Fair Housing Act of 1968—Federal legislation regarding access to housing that prohibits discrimination based on race, color, national origin, sex, religion, disability, or familial status.

Least restrictive environment—Refers to care options that involve the least amount of restraint and the greatest degree of independence possible, while still meeting the individual's needs and maintaining safety.

Medicaid Home and Community Based-Waiver—Legislation regarding the use of Medicaid funds for care services; allows certain federal requirements to be bypassed so that states can use the funds more flexibly for accessing home- and community-based services rather than using hospitals or intermediate-care facilities.

NIMBY phenomenon—Acronym for Not In My Backyard, describing the common opposition displayed by citizens toward the placement of group homes or other social service facilities in their neighborhoods.

Non-ambulatory—Unable to walk.

Other factors that contribute to group home success are a small staff-to-resident ratio, well-trained staff, and a home-like atmosphere. As with any type of organization, some group homes are better run than others. A careful investigation into a home's procedures is recommended. Research suggests that individuals with severe cognitive impairments often experience a period of disorientation, and may need additional support or supervision for the first few months while adjusting to their new surroundings. Preplacement visits and discussion can reduce anxiety for the future resident.

Resources

BOOKS

Robinson, Julia W., and Travis Thompson. "Stigma and Architecture." In *Enabling Environments: Measuring the Impact of Environment on Disability and Rehabilitation,* edited by Edward Steinfeld and G. Scott Danford. New York: Kluwer Academic/Plenum Publishers, 1999.

Udell, Leslie. "Supports in Small Group Home Settings." In *Dementia, Aging, and Intellectual Disabilities: A Handbook,* edited by Matthew P. Janicki and Arthur J. Dalton. Philadelphia: Brunner/Mazel, Inc. (Routledge), 1999.

PERIODICALS

Anderson, Lynda, Robert Prouty, and K. Charlie Lakin. "Parallels in Size of Residential Settings and Use of Medicaid-Financed Programs." *Mental Retardation* 38, no. 5 (2000): 468–471.

Ducharme, Joseph M., Larry Williams, Anne Cummings, Pina Murray, and Terry Spencer. "General Case Quasi-Pyramidal Staff Training to Promote Generalization of Teaching Skills in Supervisory and Direct-Care Staff." *Behavior Modification* 25, no. 2 (April 2001): 233–254.

"The Impact of Deinstitutionalization on the Seriously and Persistently Mentally Ill Elderly: A One-Year Follow-Up." *Abstracts in Social Gerontology* 45, no. 2 (June 2002): 157–301.

Kim, Dong Soo. "Another Look at the NIMBY Phenomenon." *Health & Social Work* 25, no. 2 (May 2000): 146–148.

Piat, Myra. "The NIMBY Phenomenon: Community Residents' Concerns About Housing for Deinstitutionalized People." *Health & Social Work* 25, no. 2 (May 2000): 127–38.

Spreat, Scott, and James W. Conroy. "Community Placement for Persons with Significant Cognitive Challenges: An Outcome Analysis." *Brief Report Number 13 of a Series on the Well Being of People with Developmetnal Disabilities in Oklahoma* February 2000. Available online at http://www.outcomeanalysis.com/DL/pubs/okr13.pdf (accessed November 9, 2011).

Whittaker, James K. "The Future of Residential Group Care." *Child Welfare* 79, no. 1 (January–February 2000): 59–74.

ORGANIZATIONS

The Arc National Headquarters, 1660 L Street, NW, Ste. 301, Washington, DC, 20036, (202) 534-3700, Fax: (202) 534-3731, info@thearc.org, http://www.thearc.org.

Child Welfare League of America, 1726 M Street NW, Ste. 500, Washington, DC, 20036, (202) 688-4200, Fax: (202) 833-1689, http://www.cwla.org.

National Institute of Mental Health, 6001 Executive Blvd., Room 8184, MSC 9663, Bethesda, MD, 20892-9663, (301) 433-4513; TTY: (301) 443-8431, Fax: (301) 443-4279, (866) 615-6464; TTY: (866) 415-8051, nimhinfo@nih.gov, http://www.nimh.nih.gov.

Office of Fair Housing and Equal Opportunity, Department of Housing and Urban Development, 451 Seventh Street, SW, Washington, DC, 20410, http://portal.hud.gov/hudportal/HUD?src=/program_offices/fair_housing_equal_opp.

Sandra L. Friedrich, MA

Group therapy

Definition

Group therapy is a form of psychosocial treatment where a small group of patients meet regularly to talk, interact, and discuss problems with each other and the group leader (therapist).

Purpose

Group therapy attempts to give individuals a safe and comfortable place where they can work out problems and emotional issues. Patients gain insight into their own thoughts and behavior, and offer suggestions and support to others. In addition, patients who have a difficult time with interpersonal relationships can benefit from the social interactions that are a basic part of the group therapy experience.

Precautions

Patients who are suicidal, homicidal, psychotic, or in the midst of a major acute crisis are typically not referred for group therapy until their behavior and emotional state have stabilized. Depending on their level of functioning, cognitively impaired patients (like patients with organic **brain** disease or a **traumatic brain injury**) may also be unsuitable for group therapy **intervention**. Some patients with sociopathic traits are not suitable for most groups.

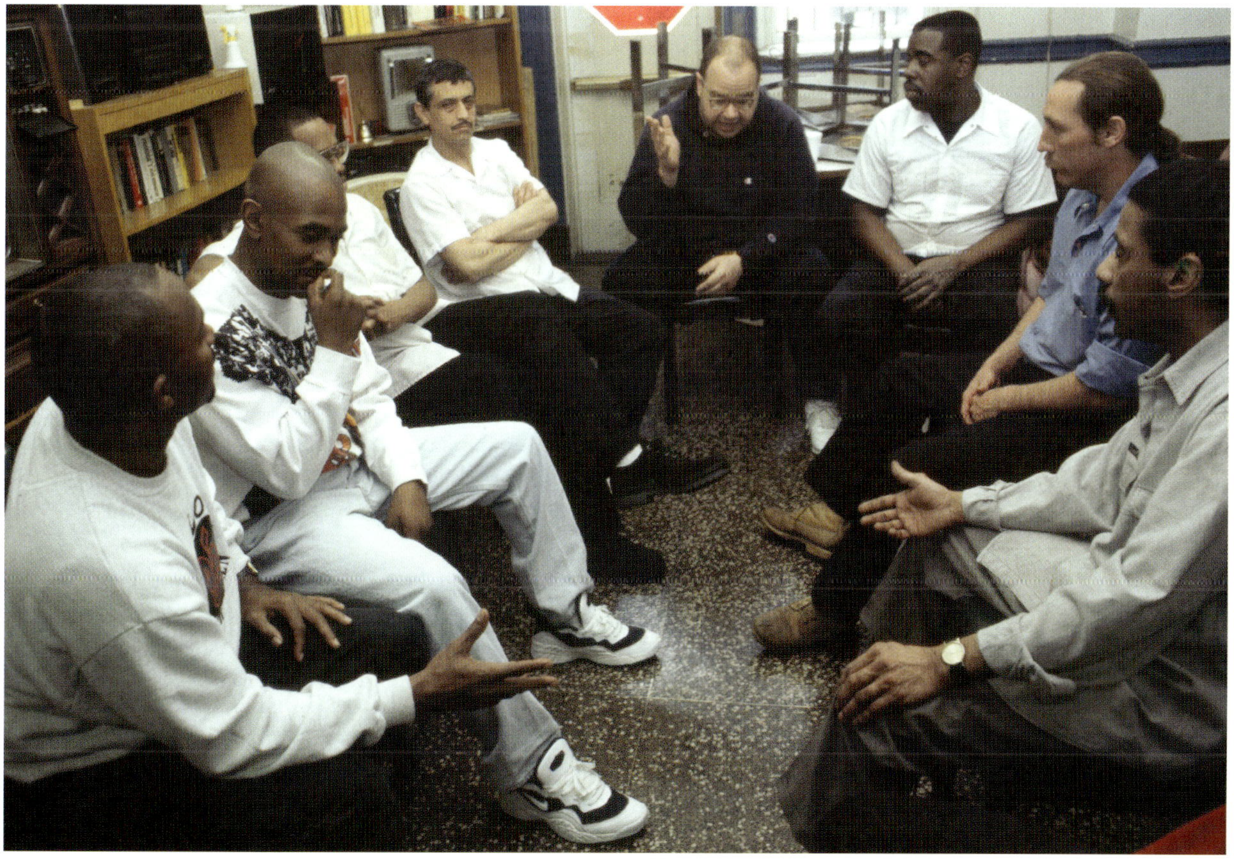

A group of men attend a substance abuse therapy session. *(© David Grossman/Photo Researchers, Inc.)*

Description

A **psychologist**, **psychiatrist**, social worker, or other healthcare professional typically arranges and conducts group therapy sessions. In some therapy groups, two co-therapists share the responsibility of group leadership. Patients are selected on the basis of what they might gain from group therapy interaction and what they can contribute to the group as a whole.

Therapy groups may be homogeneous or heterogeneous. Homogeneous groups have members with similar diagnostic backgrounds (for example, they may all suffer from **depression**). Heterogeneous groups have a mix of individuals with different emotional issues. The number of group members varies widely, but is typically no more than 12. Groups may be time limited (with a predetermined number of sessions) or indefinite (where the group determines when therapy ends). Membership may be closed or open to new members once sessions begin.

The number of sessions in group therapy depends on the makeup, goals, and setting of the group. For example, a therapy group that is part of a **substance abuse** program to rehabilitate inpatients would be called short-term group therapy. This term is used because, as patients, the group members will only be in the hospital for a relatively short period of time. Long-term therapy groups may meet for six months, a year, or longer. The therapeutic approach used in therapy depends on the focus of the group and the psychological training of the therapist. Some common techniques include psychodynamic, cognitive-behavioral, and **Gestalt therapy**.

In a group therapy session, group members are encouraged to openly and honestly discuss the issues that brought them to therapy. They try to help other group members by offering their own suggestions, insights, and empathy regarding their problems. There are no definite rules for group therapy, only that members participate to the best of their ability. However, most therapy groups do have some basic ground rules that are usually discussed during the first session. Patients are asked not to share what goes on in therapy sessions with anyone outside of the group. This protects the confidentiality of the other members. They may also be asked not to see other group members socially outside of therapy because of the harmful effect it might have on the dynamics of the group.

The therapist's main task is to guide the group in self-discovery. Depending on the goals of the group and the training and style of the therapist, he or she may lead the group interaction or allow the group to take their own direction. Typically, the group leader does some of both, providing direction when the group gets off track while letting them set their own agenda. The therapist may guide the group by simply reinforcing the positive behaviors they engage in. For example, if a group member shows empathy to another member, or offers a constructive suggestion, the therapist will point this out and explain the value of these actions to the group. In almost all group therapy situations, the therapist will attempt to emphasize the common traits among group members so that members can gain a sense of group identity. Group members realize that others share the same issues they do.

The main benefit group therapy may have over individual **psychotherapy** is that some patients behave and react more like themselves in a group setting than they would one-on-one with a therapist. The group therapy patient gains a certain sense of identity and social acceptance from their membership in the group. Suddenly, they are not alone. They are surrounded by others who have the same anxieties and emotional issues that they have. Seeing how others deal with these issues may give them new solutions to their problems. Feedback from group members also offers them a unique insight into their own behavior, and the group provides a safe forum in which to practice new behaviors. Lastly, by helping others in the group work through their problems, group therapy members can gain more self-esteem. Group therapy may also simulate family experiences of patients and will allow family dynamic issues to emerge.

Self-help groups like Alcoholics Anonymous and Weight Watchers fall outside of the psychotherapy realm. These self-help groups do offer many of the same benefits of social support, identity, and belonging that make group therapy effective for many. Self-help group members meet to discuss a common area of concern (like alcoholism, eating disorders, **bereavement**, parenting). Group sessions are not run by a therapist, but by a nonprofessional leader, group member, or the group as a whole. Self-help groups are sometimes used in addition to psychotherapy or regular group therapy.

Preparation

Patients are typically referred for group therapy by a psychologist or psychiatrist. Some patients may need individual therapy first. Before group sessions begin, the therapist leading the session may conduct a short intake interview with the patient to determine if the group is right for the patient. This interview will also allow the therapist to determine if the addition of the patient will benefit the group. The patient may be given some preliminary information on the group before sessions begin. This may include guidelines for success (like being open, listening to others, taking risks), rules of the group (like maintaining confidentiality), and educational information on what group therapy is about.

Aftercare

The end of long-term group therapy may cause feelings of **grief**, loss, abandonment, anger, or rejection in some members. The group therapist will attempt to foster a sense of closure by encouraging members to explore their feelings and use newly acquired coping techniques to deal with them. Working through this termination phase of group therapy is an important part of the treatment process.

Risks

Some very fragile patients may not be able to tolerate aggressive or hostile comments from group members. Patients who have trouble communicating in group situations may be at risk for dropping out of group therapy. If no one comments on their silence or makes an attempt to interact with them, they may begin to feel even more isolated and alone instead of identifying with the group. Therefore, the therapist usually attempts to encourage silent members to participate early on in treatment.

Results

Studies have shown that both group and individual psychotherapy benefit about 85% of the patients that participate in them. Optimally, patients gain a better understanding of themselves, and perhaps a stronger set of interpersonal and coping skills through the group therapy process. Some patients may continue therapy after group therapy ends, either individually or in another group setting.

Resources

BOOKS

Bieling, Peter J., Randi E. McCabe, and Martin M. Antony. *Cognitive-Behavioral Therapy in Groups*. New York: Guilford Press, 2006.

Yalom, Irvin D., and Molyn Leszcz. *Theory and Practice of Group Psychotherapy*. 5th ed. New York: Basic Books, 2005.

ORGANIZATIONS

American Psychiatric Association, 1000 Wilson Blvd., Suite 1825, Arlington, VA, 22209-3901, (703) 907-7300, apa@psych.org, http://www.psych.org.

American Psychological Association, 750 1st Street NE, Washington, DC, 20002-4242, (202) 336-5500; TDD/TTY: (202) 336-6123, (800) 374-2721, http://www.apa.org.

Paula Anne Ford-Martin
brenda w. lerner

Guanfacine

Definition

Guanfacine is a medication that inhibits the neurological signaling chemical norepinephrine. Norepinephrine is a type of neurotransmitter involved in normal **brain** function and has an effect on blood pressure, mood, concentration, and impulse control. Guanfacine helps regulate norepinephrine levels in the body and is used in treating high blood pressure, **attention deficit hyperactivity disorder (ADHD)**, and anxiety.

Purpose

Guanfacine is used to treat some of the symptoms of **ADHD** and anxiety, although it is not one of the main drugs used to treat anxiety. It works by regulating actions of the sympathetic nervous system, resulting in decreased blood pressure, reduced anxiety, improved concentration, and control of impulsive behavior and other stressful emotions present with both anxiety and ADHD.

Description

Guanfacine affects the natural body chemical norepinephrine. Norepinephrine is a type of neurotransmitter in the nervous system, a chemical that neurons use to signal one another in complex pathways for normal brain and body functioning. **Neurotransmitters** bind to chemical receptors on the surface of neurons (brain cells) and blood vessels. Once bound to a receptor they affect physiological processes. Neurotransmitter signaling pathways are responsible for many regulatory processes, including blood pressure and neuronal signaling that affects mood, concentration, and impulse control. Drugs such as guanfacine block

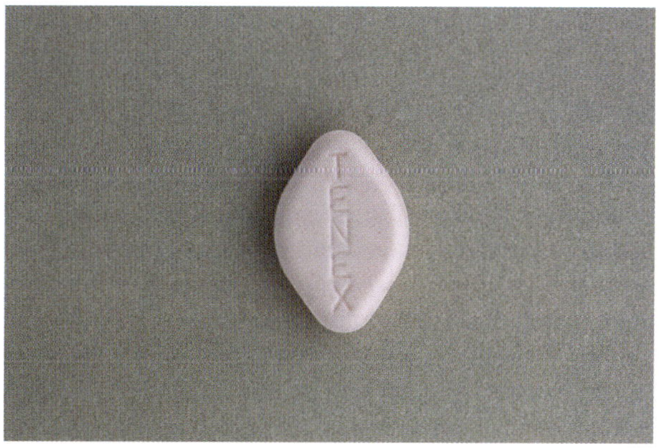

Tenex (guanfacine), 1 mg. *(© Custom Medical Stock Photo, Inc. Reproduced by permission.)*

the receptors for norepinephrine, resulting in more of the chemical left in the brain. This affects areas of the brain involving judgment, response to external stimuli, emotional responses, mental focus, sleep, and impulse control.

Recommended dosage

Guanfacine is given in pill form, and doses are taken at bedtime. The dose chosen depends on the disorder being treated, the patient's age, individual patient response to the medication regarding its effectiveness, and individual patient response to the medication regarding side effects. The dose of guanfacine in adults for treating high blood pressure or anxiety is 1–3 mg taken once per day, as needed to control symptoms. Patients are dosed at the lowest possible effective dose to avoid the development of adverse side effects. Slowly increasing the dose over time helps with minimizing side effects.

Guanfacine used in children for ADHD is dosed based on weight, and the dose is gradually increased over time. For example, children who weigh between 60 and 90 lb (27–40.5 kg) are usually started at a dose of 0.5 mg at bedtime. The dose is increased by 0.5 mg per day per week up to 1.5 mg per day if needed. If higher doses are required for improvement, after two weeks at the 1.5 mg-per-day dosing, the dose is increased to 2 mg per day. Doses are lowered if side effects become intolerable. If guanfacine is discontinued, it is tapered off gradually to avoid nervous system instability.

Precautions

Guanfacine may not be appropriate for use or may require caution in patients with kidney or liver dysfunction, some types of heart disease or recent heart attack, or elderly patients. Kidney and liver function as well as blood pressure may be monitored while taking guanfacine. When a patient discontinues the use of guanfacine, the dose needs to be tapered down slowly. If guanfacine is abruptly discontinued, there may be side effects such as rebound high blood pressure and anxiety. Rare but serious side effects of guanfacine may include sudden loss of consciousness or abnormally low heart rate. Guanfacine is classified as category B for pregnancy. Category B drugs have not been studied in humans during pregnancy, so fetal harm is possible, but it is unlikely. The safety of guanfacine use during breastfeeding is unknown, and so its use is not recommended.

Side effects

Sensitivity to guanfacine varies between patients, and some patients may find lower doses are more than their body system can tolerate. Common side effects of guanfacine are dry mouth, drowsiness, dizziness, constipation, **fatigue**, weakness, headache, and sexual dysfunction. Side effects of abrupt discontinuation of guanfacine include anxiety, restlessness, and increased blood pressure.

KEY TERMS

Neurotransmitter—A chemical messenger that travels through the body and acts in the nervous system. Neurotransmitter signaling is responsible for a wide range of bodily processes and is often the target of medications involving the brain and cardiovascular system.

Neurotransmitter receptor—A physical recipient for chemicals called neurotransmitters. Receptors sit on the surface of cells that make up body tissues, and once bound to the neurotransmitter, they initiate the chemical signaling pathway associated with neurotransmitters.

Norepinephrine—A type of neurotransmitter involved in regulation of concentration, impulse control, judgment, mood, attention span, psychostimulation, and disease states such as ADHD and depression.

Sympathetic nervous system—Part of the nervous system that increases heart rate and blood pressure, sweating, pupil dilation, and mental stress arousal.

Interactions

Patients should make their doctor aware of all medications and supplements they are taking before using guanfacine. Using alcohol while taking guanfacine may create toxic reactions in the body and should be avoided. Drugs that affect the liver, including the antidepressant **mirtazapine**, may affect the metabolism of guanfacine, resulting in too much or too little of the drug in the body. This could lead to increased side effects or even toxic doses. Likewise, guanfacine may affect the metabolism of other drugs, leading to greater or lower doses than therapeutically desired.

Guanfacine should not be used at the same time as **antidepressants** called **monoamine oxidase inhibitors (MAOIs)**. Use of these medications in the same time period may cause a high blood pressure crisis, which can be severe and life-threatening. Switching between drug treatment with an MAOI to guanfacine may require a

> **QUESTIONS TO ASK YOUR DOCTOR**
>
> - Can I take the full dose right away or do I need to slowly increase the dose up to the full amount?
> - Can I stop taking the medication right away or do I need to slowly decrease the dose in order to go off the medication?
> - Should I eat before taking this medication?
> - Will this medication interact with any of my other prescription medications? Over-the-counter drugs? Herbal supplements?
> - What side effects indicate that I have taken too much of this medication?
> - Can I drink alcoholic beverages when I am taking this medication?

waiting period of up to several weeks between drugs. Other drugs that cannot be combined with guanfacine due to risk of high blood pressure include the antibiotic linezolid. Some medications interact with guanfacine to cause additive adverse effects of abnormally low blood pressure, such as the muscle relaxant tizanidine. Sedative drugs also should not be used with guanfacine due to additive effects. Blood pressure medications such as atenolol have antagonistic, or opposing, effects with guanfacine and should not be used in the same time period. Guanfacine should not be used with the herbal supplement yohimbe, as the combination may decrease the efficacy of guanfacine.

Resources

BOOKS

Brunton, Laurence, et al. *Goodman and Gilman's the Pharmacological Basis of Therapeutics*. 12th ed. New York: McGraw Hill Medical, 2011.

Zorumski, Charles F., and Eugene H. Rubin. *Psychiatry and Clinical Neuroscience: A Primer*. New York: Oxford University Press, 2011.

PERIODICALS

Connor, D. F., et al. "Effects of Guanfacine Extended Release on Oppositional Symptoms in Children Aged 6–12 Years with Attention-Deficit Hyperactivity Disorder and Oppositional Symptoms: A Randomized, Double-Blind, Placebo-Controlled Trial." *CNS Drugs* 24, no. 9 (2010): 755–68.

WEBSITES

PubMed Health. "Guanfacine." U.S. National Library of Medicine. http://www.ncbi.nlm.nih.gov/pubmedhealth/PMH0000057 (accessed November 12, 2011).

ORGANIZATIONS

American College of Neuropsychopharmacology, 5034-A Thoroughbred Lane, Brentwood, TN, 37027, (615) 324-2360, Fax: (615) 523-1715, acnp@acnp.org, http://www.acnp.org/default.aspx.

Children and Adults with Attention Deficit/Hyperactivity Disorder, 8181 Professional Place, Ste. 150, Landover, MD, 20785, (301) 306-7070, (800) 233-4050, Fax: (301) 306-7090, http://www.chadd.org.

Mental Health America, 2000 N Beauregard St., 6th Fl., Alexandria, VA, 22311, (703) 684-7722, (800) 969-6642, Fax: (703) 684-5968, http://www.nmha.org.

U.S. Food and Drug Administration, 10903 New Hampshire Ave., Silver Spring, MD, 20993-0002, (888) INFO-FDA (463-6332), http://www.fda.gov.

Maria Eve Basile, PhD

Guided imagery therapy

Definition

Guided imagery therapy (GIT) is a cognitive-behavioral technique in which a client is guided in imagining a relaxing scene or series of experiences, and then in learning to retrieve such images at a later time. As a traditional mind-body technique, it offers ways to concentrate on an image or images in order to influence physical and emotional states. Guided imagery therapy is based on the connections between the emotional control center in the **brain** and the autonomic nervous system, immune system, and endocrine system. The patient produces such remembered images without actually seeing them with the eyes.

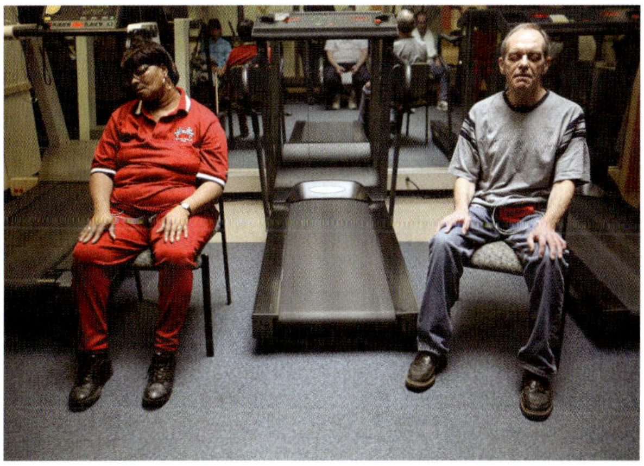

A group of patients in rehabilitation for substance abuse participate in guided imagery therapy. *(© Lisa Dejong/The Plain Dealer/Landov)*

The Academy for Guided Imagery classifies guided imagery therapy into three parts: **stress reduction** and relaxation; active visualization or directed imagery (to improve performance or behavior, or to influence outcomes); and receptive imagery (to provide conscious images to deal with symptoms, illnesses, or other problems).

GIT has been shown to be an effective form of mental-health therapy for such stress-related conditions as **insomnia**, anxiety, migraine headaches, **depression**, breathing rate, and high blood pressure. It is also effective for reducing the symptoms for such non-stress-related conditions as skin rashes (including hives and allergies), irritable bowel syndrome, rheumatoid arthritis, asthma, and Crohn's disease. Guided imagery therapy has also been found to be useful to reduce some side effects of cancer.

Purpose

Numerous clinical observations suggest that an individual visualizing an imagined scene reacts as though it were actually occurring; therefore, "induced" images can have a profound effect on behavior and a marked improvement on mental health. The usefulness of guided imagery techniques has been shown to be effective in helping individuals learn or modify behaviors such as:

- learning to relax
- changing or controlling negative emotions in response to a particular situation, event (e.g., loss of a job), or belief
- preparing for changes they are likely to face in the future (e.g., children leaving home, a parent moving)
- eliminating or reducing undesirable behaviors (e.g., smoking, excessive eating)
- increasing effective pain management
- coping with difficult situations (e.g., an unpleasant boss)
- learning new and desirable behaviors (e.g., assertiveness)
- becoming more motivated (e.g., doing homework between therapy sessions)
- learning from behavior in an earlier situation (e.g., a temper tantrum) in order to feel less shame or guilt
- experimenting with ways to manage stressful or anxiety-producing situations (e.g., giving a presentation in public) by mentally rehearsing the needed behavior(s)

Guided imagery techniques have been applied to—and found to be effective or show promise with—a variety of populations, including individuals with:

- phobias (including agoraphobia, social phobia, and specific phobias)
- mild to moderate depression
- generalized anxiety disorders
- post-traumatic stress disorder
- obsessive-compulsive disorder
- sexual difficulties
- habit disorders
- chronic fatigue syndrome
- children's behavioral disorders
- stuttering
- acute and chronic pain (and other physical disorders)

Guided imagery has also contributed to the achievement of skills and overcoming anxiety in normal life situations that include learning or improving motor skills, test-taking, and public speaking. In addition, visualization and imagery, along with other behavioral techniques, have been applied to the fields of business, industry, child rearing, education, behavioral medicine, and sports.

Demographics

Guided imagery therapy can be conducted on anyone who is willing to participate this form of mental-health therapy and willing to make improvements in psychological problems within their lives. It is not limited by age, race, ethnic background, socioeconomic condition, or other such factors—only on a person' willingness to participate.

Description

Imagery techniques have been combined with a wide range of behavioral and cognitive procedures and treatment methods of some psychotherapeutic approaches, including **behavior modification**, cognitive processing therapy, cognitive-behavior therapy, rational-emotive therapy, multimodal therapy, and **hypnotherapy**. Combinations of treatment methods among these approaches lead to the following general uses of imagery:

- antifuture shock imagery (preparing for a feared future event)
- positive imagery (using pleasant scenes for relaxation training)
- aversive imagery (using an unpleasant image to help eliminate or reduce undesirable behavior)
- associated imagery (using imagery to track unpleasant feelings)
- coping imagery (using images to rehearse to reach a behavioral goal or manage a situation)

- "step-up" technique (exaggerating a feared situation and using imagery to cope with it)

An assessment of the individual's presenting problems is an essential part of treatment, both at the beginning of therapy and throughout the entire process. This is to ensure that the therapist has sufficient understanding of the client's situation and **diagnosis** of the problem(s). The assessment generally covers a variety of areas, such as developmental history (including family, education, employment, and social relationships), past traumatic experiences, specific psychological symptoms, medical and psychiatric treatments, and client goals. Often, clients have several problems, and both the therapist and the client work together on prioritizing specific treatment goals.

Following the assessment, the therapist will present a general rationale for the use of imagery. The therapist might explain that the client will learn techniques in which he or she imagines they or another person are performing a particular behavior. To enhance visualization, it is important to involve all senses in the image. For example, if the client is to be walking down a busy street, he or she is encouraged to imagine hearing sounds from traffic and other people, smell exhaust fumes from buses and aromas from a nearby bakery, and observe body movements and wind in the face. It is stressed to the client that the most critical aspect of imagining is the feeling of actually experiencing the scene—of being in it rather than just seeing oneself in it.

Both the therapist and the client construct a relaxing scene by discussing exactly what the client finds pleasant. It is better if the client chooses all images (positive or negative) and the therapist trains the client to visualize the selected images as vividly as possible.

Once a pleasant scene is decided upon, the client is asked to assume a relaxed position and with closed eyes, if this is comfortable, before being guided in visualization. One common beginning instruction may be: "Imagine you are lying on a warm, sandy beach." The therapist continues to guide the relaxation by saying such phrases as: "Notice the texture of the sand and the color of the sky. Focus on the sounds you hear, and the smells...." The client is asked to practice the image at home between sessions. A tape of the guided imagery in the familiar voice of the therapist can be helpful to some clients in practicing at home.

During visualization, clients are given permission to take control if they need to by changing the image or stopping the activity completely. To help clients maintain control of the image, the therapist may also say to the client, "Take as long as you need to relax," and "Do whatever you need to do in order to feel safe." This empowers clients in using such techniques.

KEY TERMS

Depression—A psychiatric disorder involving feelings of hopelessness and symptoms of fatigue, sleeplessness, suicidal tendencies, and poor concentration.

Generalized anxiety disorder—An anxiety disorder characterized by daily irrational worry that is often also excessive and uncontrolled.

Length of treatment

Treatments using behavioral techniques tend to be relatively brief. However, many factors determine the length of therapy. Generally, treatment takes longer if target behaviors are more numerous and more difficult to specify. Some types of treatments require more sessions than others. For example, techniques using imagery require more sessions than treatments in which the client is exposed to the actual feared situations in real life.

Other factors that determine the length of treatment are the types of presenting disorders, the client's willingness to do homework, how long the client has had the problem, client financial resources, and whether there are supportive family members and friends. The therapist's style and experience may also affect the length of therapy. Clients may be seen several times a week at the start of therapy and then once weekly for several months, and every other month for follow-up for a few more months.

Precautions

The practitioner of guided imagery therapy should use caution when attempting such therapy on someone who is hesitant to use it for personal, religious, spiritual, or other such reasons.

Guided imagery is not used in isolation but as a part of a therapeutic formulation and is appropriate for a range of problems and disorders. It is, however, thought that some techniques—such as imagery used in rational-emotive therapy—can trigger high levels of anxiety in some clients. Therefore, caution should be taken when using these techniques if clients have the following conditions:

- asthma attacks triggered by stress or anxiety
- seizures triggered by stress or anxiety
- cardiac condition or related conditions
- depression with suicidal ideation

- emotional excitability and disturbances
- pregnancy
- severe psychiatric disorders

In these instances, other strategies and techniques that do not trigger high levels of anxiety, such as relaxation exercises or coping imagery, should be considered. When working with clients with these conditions, the therapist should be in consultation with their medical provider.

Preparations

People who perform guided imagery therapy on themselves will be guided with instructions provided by self-help books, CDs, and DVDs. When used under the guidance of a licensed practitioner, no preparations are necessary or advised.

Aftercare

Guided imagery techniques have been taken from behavior therapy and are used by different psychological theories and systems of counseling and **psychotherapy**, including **cognitive-behavioral therapy**. Research has shown these techniques to be effective when applied to specific problems.

Results

Depending on the combination of visualization and imagery techniques used, the therapeutic approach, and client problem(s), it is expected that clients will have positive changes. Specifically, it is normal to have positive changes in specifically defined target behaviors. There should also be a reduction in biases or distortions in thinking, resulting in more effective functioning that, in turn, leads to more positive feelings, behavior, and thinking; and fewer emotional disturbances, more effective coping skills, decreased self-defeating behaviors, and less tension.

Risks

There are no known major risks associated with the technique called guided imagery therapy. Potential risks could occur if it is used to replace traditional therapies, however, but under no circumstances should this be done. Guided imagery therapy always should be used in conjunction with such traditional practices.

Research and general acceptance

Guided imagery therapy is accepted as effective therapy within the realm of **mind-body medicine**. It is well suited to be used with other alternative therapies, such as massage and other such touch therapies and various types of psychotherapy when behavioral improvements are desired.

QUESTIONS TO ASK YOUR DOCTOR

- How likely will guided imagery therapy help me?
- Can you help me find literature to provide more information about the therapy?
- What are some of the best resources on guided imagery therapy?
- How do I find a professional to conduct guided imagery therapy?
- Do you recommend any websites that can help?

Training and certification

The Academy for Guided Imagery (AGI) provides a Professional Certification Training Program in Interactive Guided Imagerysm (IGIsm). According to the AGI, only those individuals certified through the AGI may represent themselves as practicing IGIsm. Licensed psychologists can conduct guided imagery therapy.

Resources

BOOKS

Austad, Carol Shaw. *Counseling and Psychotherapy Today: Theory, Practice, and Research.* Boston: McGraw-Hill Higher Education, 2009.

Feltham, Colin, and Ian E. Horton, editors. *The SAGE Handbook of Counseling and Psychotherapy.* London: Sage, 2006.

Kazantzis, Nikolaos, Mark A. Reinecke, and Arthur Freeman, editors. *Cognitive and Behavioral Theories in Clinical Practice.* New York: Guilford Press, 2010.

WEBSITES

Mayo Clinic staff. "Enhance Healing Through Guided Imagery." MayoClinic.com. January 2, 2008. http://www.mayoclinic.org/news2008-mchi/4403.html (accessed May 23, 2011).

ORGANIZATIONS

Academy for Guided Imagery, 10780 Santa Monica Boulevard, Los Angeles, CA, 90025, (800) 726-2070, Fax: (800) 727-2070, info@acadhi.com, http://acadgi.com.

American Psychiatric Association, 1000 Wilson Boulevard, Suite 1825, Arlington, VA, 22209-3901, (703) 907-7300, apa@psych.org, http://www.psych.org.

American Psychological Association, 750 First Street, NE, Washington, DC, 20002-4242, (202) 336-5500, (800) 374-2721, http://www.apa.org.

Anxiety Disorders Association of America, 8730 Georgia Avenue, Silver Spring, MD, 20910, (240) 485-1001, http://www.adaa.org.

Mental Health America, 2000 North Beauregard Street, Sixth Floor, Alexandria, VA, 22311, (703) 684-7722, (800) 969-6642, Fax: (703) 684-5968, http://www.nmha.org.

National Institute of Mental Health, 6001 Executive Boulevard, Room 8184, MSC 9663, Bethesda, MD, 20892-9663, (301) 443-4513, (866) 615-6464, Fax: (301) 443-4279, http://www.nimh.nih.gov.

Janice Van Buren, PhD
William Atkins

H

Halcion *see* **Triazolam**

Haldol *see* **Haloperidol**

Hallucination

Definition

A hallucination is a sensory perception without a source in the external world. The English word "hallucination" comes from the Latin verb *hallucinari*, which means "to wander in the mind." Hallucinations can affect any of the senses, although certain diseases or disorders are associated with specific types of hallucinations.

It is important to distinguish between hallucinations and illusions or **delusions**, as the terms are often confused in conversation and popular journalism. A hallucination is a distorted sensory experience that appears to be a perception of something real even though it is *not* caused by an external stimulus. For example, some elderly people who have been recently bereaved may have hallucinations in which they "see" the dead loved one. An illusion, by contrast, is a mistaken or false interpretation of a real sensory experience, as when a traveler in the desert sees what looks like a pool of water, but in fact is a mirage caused by the refraction of light as it passes through layers of air of different densities. The bluish-colored light is a real sensory stimulus, but mistaking it for water is an illusion. A delusion is a false belief that a person maintains in spite of evidence to the contrary and in spite of proof that other members of their culture do not share the belief. For example, some people insist that they have seen flying saucers or unidentified flying objects (UFOs) even though the objects they have filmed or photographed can be shown to be ordinary aircraft, weather balloons, satellites, etc.

Demographics

The demographics of hallucinations vary depending on their cause; however, many researchers think that they are underreported for several reasons:

- Fear of being thought "crazy" or mentally ill.
- Gaps in research. For example, some types of hallucinations are associated with disorders that primarily affect the elderly, who are often underrepresented in health surveys.
- Fear of being reported to law enforcement for illegal drug use.

There is no evidence that hallucinations occur more frequently in some racial or ethnic groups than in others. In addition, gender does not appear to make a difference. The demographics of hallucinations associated with some specific age groups, conditions, or disorders are as follows:

- Children. Hallucinations are rare in children below the age of eight. About 40% of children diagnosed with schizophrenia, however, have visual or auditory hallucinations.
- Eye disorders. About 14% of patients treated in eye clinics for glaucoma or age-related macular degeneration report visual hallucinations.
- Alzheimer's disease (AD). About 40%–50% of patients diagnosed with AD develop hallucinations in the later stages of the disease.
- Drug use. According to the 2010 National Survey on Drug Use and Health, 14.8% of persons living in the United States have used hallucinogens in their lifetime, with LSD being the most popular (9.2%), followed by MDMA, or Ecstasy (6.3%). The highest rate of hallucinogen abuse is found in males between the ages of 18 and 25.
- Normal sleep/wake cycles. Sleep researchers in Great Britain and the United States have reported that 30%–37% of adults experience hypnagogic hallucinations, which occur during the passage from wakefulness

into sleep, while about 10%–12% report hypnopompic hallucinations, which occur as a person awakens. Hallucinations related to ordinary sleeping and waking are not considered an indication of a mental or physical disorder.

- Migraine headaches. About 10% of patients diagnosed with migraine headaches experience visual hallucinations prior to the onset of an acute attack.
- Adult-onset schizophrenia. According to the National Institute of Mental Health (NIMH), about 75% of adults diagnosed with schizophrenia experience hallucinations, most commonly auditory or visual. The auditory hallucinations may be command hallucinations, in which the person hears voices ordering him or her to do something.
- Temporal lobe epilepsy (TLE). About 80% of patients diagnosed with TLE report gustatory and olfactory hallucinations as well as auditory and visual hallucinations.
- Narcolepsy. Frequent hypnagogic hallucinations are considered one of four classic symptoms of narcolepsy and are experienced by 60% of patients diagnosed with the disorder.
- Post-traumatic stress disorder (PTSD). Studies of combat veterans diagnosed with PTSD have found that 50%–65% have experienced auditory hallucinations. Visual, olfactory, and haptic hallucinations have been reported by survivors of rape and childhood sexual abuse.

Description

It would be difficult to describe a "typical" hallucination, as these experiences vary considerably in length of time, quality, and sense or senses affected. Some hallucinations last only a few seconds; however, some people diagnosed with Charles Bonnet syndrome (CBS) have reported visual hallucinations lasting over several days, while people who have taken certain drugs have experienced hallucinations involving colors, sounds, and smells lasting for hours. Albert Hoffman, the Swiss chemist who first synthesized lysergic acid diethylamide (LSD), experienced nine hours of hallucinations after taking a small amount of the drug in 1943. In 1896, the American neurologist S. Weir Mitchell published an account of the six hours of hallucinations that followed his experimental swallowing of peyote buttons.

There is not always a close connection between the cause of a person's hallucinations and the emotional response to them. One study of patients diagnosed with CBS found that 30% of the patients were upset by their hallucinations, while 13% found them amusing or pleasant. The environment in which LSD and other **hallucinogens** are taken may affect an individual's psychological constitution and personal reactions. The writer Peter Matthiessen, for example, noted that his 1960s experiences with LSD "were magic shows, mysterious, enthralling," while his wife ". . . freaked out; that is the drug term, and there is no better. . . . [H]er armor had cracked, and all the night winds of the world went howling through." Indeed, like Mathiessen's wife, and in contrast to those for whom hallucinogens prove amusing, most patients with **narcolepsy**, alcoholic hallucinosis, or post-traumatic disorders find their hallucinations frightening.

Causes

Though there are many known causes of hallucinations, the neurological mechanism behind their origin is not yet known. Researchers have identified some factors in the context of specific disorders, and have proposed various hypotheses to explain hallucinations in others, but there does not appear to be a single causal factor that accounts for hallucinations in all people who experience them.

Sleep deprivation

Research subjects who have undergone **sleep deprivation** experiments typically begin to hallucinate after 72–96 hours without sleep. It is thought that these hallucinations result from the malfunctioning of nerve cells within the prefrontal cortex of the **brain**. This area of the brain is associated with judgment, impulse control, attention, and visual association, and is refreshed during the early stages of sleep. When a person is sleep-deprived, the nerve cells in the prefrontal cortex must work harder than usual without an opportunity to recover. The hallucinations that develop on the third day of wakefulness are thought to be hypnagogic hallucinations that occur during "microsleeps," or short periods of light sleep lasting about one to ten seconds.

Post-traumatic memory formation

Hallucinations in **trauma** survivors are caused by abnormal patterns of memory formation during the traumatic experience. In normal situations, memories are formed from sensory data, organized in a part of the brain known as the hippocampus, and integrated with previous memories in the frontal cortex. People then "make sense" of their memories through the use of language, which helps them to describe their experiences to others and to themselves. In traumatic situations, however, bits and pieces of memory are stored in the amygdala, an almond-shaped structure in the brain that ordinarily attaches emotional significance to memories, without being integrated by the hippocampus and interpreted in the frontal cortex. In addition, the region of the brain that governs speech (Broca's area) often shuts down under extreme **stress**. The result is that memories of the traumatic event remain in the amygdala as a chaotic wordless jumble of physical sensations or sensory images that can re-emerge as hallucinations during stressful situations at later points in the patient's life.

Irritative hallucinations

In 1973, a British researcher named Cogan categorized hallucinations into two major groups that he called "irritative" and "release" hallucinations. Irritative hallucinations result from abnormal electrical discharges in the brain, and are associated with such disorders as migraine headaches and epilepsy. Brain tumors and traumatic damage to the brain are other possible causes of abnormal electrical activity manifesting as visual hallucinations.

Hallucinations have also been reported with a number of infectious diseases that affect the brain, including bacterial meningitis, rabies, herpes virus infections, Lyme disease, HIV infection, toxoplasmosis, Jakob-Creuzfeldt disease, and late-stage syphilis.

Release hallucinations

Release hallucinations are most common in people with impaired eyesight or hearing. They are produced by the spontaneous activity of nerve cells in the visual or auditory cortex of the brain in the absence of actual sensory data from the eyes or ears. These experiences differ from the hallucinations of **schizophrenia** in that those patients experiencing release hallucinations are often able to recognize them as unreal. Release hallucinations are also more elaborate and usually longer in duration than irritative hallucinations. The visual hallucinations of patients with CBS are an example of release hallucinations.

Neurotransmitter imbalances

Neurotransmitters are chemicals produced by the body that carry electrical impulses across the gaps (synapses) between adjoining nerve cells. Some neurotransmitters inhibit the transmission of nerve impulses, while others excite or intensify them. Hallucinations in some conditions or disorders result from imbalances among these various chemicals.

NARCOLEPSY. Narcolepsy is a disorder characterized by uncontrollable brief episodes of sleep, frequent hypnagogic or hypnopompic hallucinations, and sleep paralysis. Between 1999 and 2000, researchers discovered that people with narcolepsy have a much lower than normal number of hypocretin neurons, which are nerve cells in the hypothalamus that secrete a neurotransmitter known as hypocretin. Low levels of this chemical are thought to be responsible for the daytime sleepiness and hallucinations of narcolepsy.

PRESCRIPTION MEDICATIONS. Hallucinations have been reported as side effects of such drugs as ketamine (Ketalar), which is sometimes used as an anesthetic but has also been used illegally to commit date rape; **paroxetine** (Paxil), an SSRI antidepressant; **mirtazapine** (Remeron), a serotonin-specific antidepressant; and **zolpidem** (Ambien), a sleep medication. Ketamine prevents brain cells from taking up glutamate, a neurotransmitter that governs perception of pain and of one's relationship to the environment. Paroxetine alters the balance between the neurotransmitters **serotonin** and acetylcholine.

Hallucinations in patients with **Alzheimer's disease** are thought to be a side effect of treatment with neuroleptics (antipsychotic medications), although they may also result from inadequate blood flow in certain regions of the brain. The antiretroviral drugs used to treat HIV infection may also produce hallucinations in some patients.

HALLUCINOGENS AND DRUGS OF ABUSE. Like the hallucinations caused by prescription drugs, hallucinations caused by drugs of abuse result from disruption of the normal balance of neurotransmitters in the brain. Hallucinations in **cocaine** and amphetamine users, for example, are associated with the overproduction of **dopamine**, a neurotransmitter associated with arousal and motor excitability. LSD appears to produce hallucinations by blocking the action of the neurotransmitters serotonin (particularly serotonin-2) and norepinephrine. Phencyclidine (PCP) acts like ketamine in producing hallucinations by blocking the reception of glutamate.

People who have used LSD sometimes experience flashbacks, which are spontaneous recurrences of the hallucinations and other distorted perceptions caused by the drug. Some doctors refer to this condition as hallucinogen persisting perception disorder, or HPPD.

There are two types of alcohol withdrawal syndromes characterized by hallucinations. Alcoholic hallucinosis typically occurs after abrupt withdrawal from alcohol after a long period of excessive drinking. The patient hears threatening or accusing voices rather than "seeing things," and his or her consciousness is otherwise normal. **Delirium** tremens (DTs), on the other hand, is a

KEY TERMS

Amygdala—An almond-shaped brain structure in the limbic system that is activated in stressful situations to trigger the emotion of fear. Hallucinations related to post-traumatic stress are thought to be caused by the activation of memory traces in the amygdala that have not been integrated and modified by other parts of the brain.

Auditory—Pertaining to the sense of hearing.

Charles Bonnet syndrome (CBS)—A disorder characterized by visual hallucinations following a sudden age-related deterioration in a person's vision, most commonly glaucoma or macular degeneration. CBS is named for a Swiss doctor who first described it in his visually impaired grandfather in 1780.

Command hallucination—A type of auditory hallucination in which the person hears voices ordering him or her to perform a specific act.

Corollary discharge—A mechanism in the brain that allows one to distinguish between self-generated and external stimuli or perceptions.

Delusion—A false belief that a person maintains in spite of obvious proof or evidence to the contrary.

Flashback—A vivid sensory or emotional experience that happens independently of the initial event or experience. Flashbacks resulting from the use of LSD are sometimes referred to as hallucinogen persisting perception disorder, or HPPD.

Gustatory—Pertaining to the sense of taste.

Hallucinogen—A drug or other substance that induces hallucinations.

Haptic—Pertaining to the sense of touch; sometimes called tactile hallucinations.

Hippocampus—A part of the brain that is involved in memory formation and learning. The hippocampus is shaped like a curved ridge and belongs to an organ system called the limbic system.

Hypnagogic—Pertaining to drowsiness; refers to hallucinations that occur as a person falls asleep.

Hypnopompic—Persisting after sleep; refers to hallucinations that occur as a person awakens.

Illusion—A false interpretation of a real sensory image or impression.

Irritative hallucinations—Hallucinations caused by abnormal electrical activity in the brain.

Lysergic acid diethylamide (LSD)—The first synthetic hallucinogen, discovered in 1938.

Neuroleptic—Another name for an antipsychotic medication.

Neurotransmitters—Chemicals that carry nerve impulses from one nerve cell to another.

Olfactory—Pertaining to the sense of smell.

Psychosis—A severe mental disorder characterized by loss of contact with reality. Hallucinations are associated with such psychotic disorders as schizophrenia and brief psychotic disorder.

Release hallucinations—Hallucinations that develop after partial loss of sight or hearing, and represent images or sounds formed from memory traces rather than present sensory input. They are called "release" hallucinations because they would ordinarily be blocked by incoming sensory data.

withdrawal syndrome that begins several days after drinking stops. A patient with the DTs is disoriented, confused, depressed, feverish, and sweating heavily as well as hallucinating, and the hallucinations are usually visual.

MOOD DISORDERS. Visual hallucinations occasionally occur in patients diagnosed with **depression**, particularly the elderly. These hallucinations are thought to result from low levels of the neurotransmitter serotonin. The hallucinations that occur in patients with Parkinson's disease appear to result from a combination of medication side effects, depressed mood, and impaired eyesight.

Schizophrenia

The auditory hallucinations associated with schizophrenia may be the end result of a combination of factors. These hallucinations have sometimes been attributed to unusually high levels of the neurotransmitter dopamine in the patient's brain. Other researchers have noted abnormal patterns of brain activity in patients with schizophrenia. In particular, these patients suffer from dysfunction of a mechanism known as corollary discharge, which allows people to distinguish between stimuli outside the self and internal intentions and thoughts. Electroencephalograms (EEGs) of patients with schizophrenia that were taken while the patients were talking showed that corollary discharges from the frontal cortex of the brain (where thoughts are produced) failed to inform the auditory cortex (where sounds are interpreted) that the talking was self-generated. This failure would lead the patients to interpret internal speech as coming from external sources, thus producing auditory hallucinations. In addition, the brains of patients with schizophrenia appear to suffer tissue loss in certain regions. In early 2004, some German researchers reported a direct correlation between the severity of auditory hallucinations in patients with schizophrenia and the amount of brain tissue that had been lost from the primary auditory cortex.

Diagnosis

The differential **diagnosis** of hallucinations can be complicated, but in most cases taking the patient's medical history will help the doctor narrow the list of possible diagnoses. If the patient has been taken to a hospital emergency room, the doctor may ask those who accompanied the patient for information. The doctor may also need to perform a medical evaluation before a psychiatric assessment of the hallucinations can be made. The medical evaluation may include laboratory tests and **imaging studies** as well as a physical examination, depending on the patient's other symptoms. If it is suspected that the patient is suffering from delirium, **dementia**, or a psychotic disorder, the doctor may assess the patient's mental status by using a standard instrument known as the mini-mental status examination (MMSE) or the Folstein (after the clinician who devised it). The MMSE yields a total score based on the patient's appearance, mood, cognitive skills, thought content, judgment, and speech patterns. A score of 20 or lower usually indicates delirium, dementia, schizophrenia, or severe depression.

Hallucinations in elderly patients may require specialized evaluation because of the possibility of overlapping causes. The American Association for Geriatric Psychiatry lists hallucinations as an indication for consulting a geriatric **psychiatrist**. In addition, elderly patients should be routinely screened for visual or hearing impairments.

Treatment

Hallucinations are treated with regard to the underlying disorder. Depending on the disorder, treatment may involve antipsychotic, anticonvulsant, or antidepressant medications; **psychotherapy**; brain or ear surgery; or therapy for drug dependence. Hallucinations related to normal sleeping and waking are not a cause for concern.

Prognosis

The prognosis of hallucinations depends on the underlying cause or disorder.

Resources

BOOKS

American Psychiatric Association. *Diagnostic and Statistical Manual of Mental Disorders*. 4th ed., text rev. Washington, DC: American Psychiatric Publishing, 2000.

Beers, Mark H. "Behavior Disorders in Dementia." In *The Merck Manual of Geriatrics*, edited by Mark H. Beers and Robert Berkow. Whitehouse Station, NJ: Merck Research Laboratories, 2002.

"Drug Use and Dependence." In *The Merck Manual of Diagnosis and Therapy*, edited by Robert S. Porter and Justin L. Kaplan. 19th ed. Whitehouse Station, NJ: Merck Research Laboratories, 2011.

"Fungi—Infecting and Hallucinating." In *Who Goes First? The Story of Self-Experimentation in Medicine*, by Lawrence K. Altman. Berkeley, CA: University of California Press, 1998.

"Psychiatric Emergencies." In *The Merck Manual of Diagnosis and Therapy*, edited by Robert S. Porter and Justin L. Kaplan. Whitehouse Station, NJ: Merck Research Laboratories, 2011.

"Schizophrenia and Related Disorders." In *The Merck Manual of Diagnosis and Therapy*, edited by Robert S. Porter and Justin L. Kaplan. Whitehouse Station, NJ: Merck Research Laboratories, 2011.

PERIODICALS

Braun, Claude M. J., et al. "Brain Modules of Hallucination: An Analysis of Multiple Patients with Brain Lesions." *Journal of Psychiatry and Neuroscience* 28, no. 6 (November 2003): 432–439.

Ford, J. M., and D. H. Mathalon. "Electrophysiological Evidence of Corollary Discharge Dysfunction in Schizophrenia During Talking and Thinking." *Journal of Psychiatric Research* 38, no. 1 (January 2004): 37–46.

Gaser, C., et al. "Neuroanatomy of 'Hearing Voices': A Frontotemporal Brain Structural Abnormality Associated with Auditory Hallucinations in Schizophrenia." *Cerebral Cortex* 14, no. 1 (January 2004): 91–96.

Gleason, Ondria C. "Delirium." *American Family Physician* 67, no. 5 (March 1, 2003): 1027–1034. http://www.aafp.org/afp/2003/0301/p1027.html (accessed November 9, 2011).

Ohayon, M.M. "Prevalence of Hallucinations and Their Pathological Associations in the General Population." *Psychiatry Research* 97, no. 2–3 (December 27, 2000): 153–164.

Pelak, V.S., and G.T. Liu. "Visual Hallucinations." *Current Treatment Options in Neurology* 6, no. 1 (January 2004): 75–83.

Rovner, Barry R. "The Charles Bonnet Syndrome: Visual Hallucinations Caused by Vision Impairment."

Geriatrics 57, no. 8 (June 2002): 45–46. Available online at http://geriatrics.modernmedicine.com/geriatrics/data/articlestandard/geriatrics/232002/21083/article.pdf (accessed November 9, 2011).

Schneider, L. S., and K. S. Dagerman. "Psychosis of Alzheimer's Disease: Clinical Characteristics and History." *Journal of Psychiatric Research* 38, no. 1 (January 2004): 105–111.

Tsai, M.J., Y.B. Huang, and P. C. Wu. "A Novel Clinical Pattern of Visual Hallucination After Zolpidem Use." *Journal of Toxicology: Clinical Toxicology* 41, no. 6 (June 2003): 869–872.

WEBSITES

Cameron, Scott, and Michael Richards. "Hallucinogens." Medscape Reference. Updated June 23, 2011. http://emedicine.medscape.com/article/293752-overview (accessed October 8, 2011).

Chuang, Linda, and Nancy Forman. "Mental Disorders Secondary to General Medical Conditions." Medscape Reference. http://emedicine.medscape.com/article/294131-overview (accessed October 8, 2011).

U.S. National Institute on Drug Abuse. "Research Report: Hallucinogens and Dissociative Drugs." NIH Publication No. 01-4209. http://www.nida.nih.gov/PDF/RRHalluc.pdf (accessed October 8, 2011).

U.S. National Institute of Mental Health. "Schizophrenia." NIH Publication No. 09-3517. September 22, 2011. http://www.nimh.nih.gov/publicat/schizoph.cfm (accessed October 8, 2011).

ORGANIZATIONS

American Academy of Neurology, 1080 Montreal Ave., St. Paul, MN, 55116, (651) 695-2717, (800) 879-1960, Fax: (651) 879-2791, memberservices@aan.com, http://www.aan.com.

American Association for Geriatric Psychiatry, 7910 Woodmont Ave., Ste. 1050, Bethesda, MD, 20814-3004, (301) 654-7850, Fax: (301) 654-4137, http://www.AAGPonline.org.

American Psychiatric Association, 1000 Wilson Blvd., Ste. 1825, Arlington, VA, 22209-3901, (703) 907-7300, apa@psych.org, http://www.psych.org.

National Institute of Mental Health, 6001 Executive Blvd., Room 8184, MSC 9663, Bethesda, MD, 20892-9663, (301) 433-4513; TTY: (301) 443-8431 Fax: (301) 443-4279, (866) 615-6464; TTY: (866) 415-8051, nimhinfo@nih.gov, http://www.nimh.nih.gov.

National Schizophrenia Foundation, 403 Seymour Ave., Ste. 202, Lansing, MI, 48933, (517) 485-7168, Fax: (517) 485-7180, (800) 482-9534, inquiries@nsfoundation.org, http://www.schizophrenia.com.

National Sleep Foundation, 1010 N Glebe Rd., Ste. 310, Arlington, VA, 22201, (703) 243-1697, nsf@sleepfoundation.org, http://www.sleepfoundation.org.

Rebecca Frey, PhD

Hallucinogens and related disorders

Definition

Hallucinogens are a chemically diverse group of drugs that cause changes in a person's thought processes, perceptions of the physical world, and sense of time passing. They can be found naturally in some plants and can be synthesized in the laboratory. Most hallucinogens are abused as recreational drugs. Hallucinogens are also called psychedelic drugs.

Demographics

Hallucinogen use, excluding MDMA, peaked in the United States in the late 1960s as part of the counterculture movement. It then gradually declined until the early 1990s, when it increased. The 2010 U.S. National Survey on Drug Use and Health reported 1.2 million persons had used hallucinogens in the past month, with 695,000 persons taking MDMA, or ecstasy.

Description

Use of hallucinogens is at least as old as civilization. Many cultures have recorded eating certain plants specifically to induce visions or alter the perception of reality. These hallucinations were often part of a religious

Number of emergency department visits involving ecstasy, 2004–2008

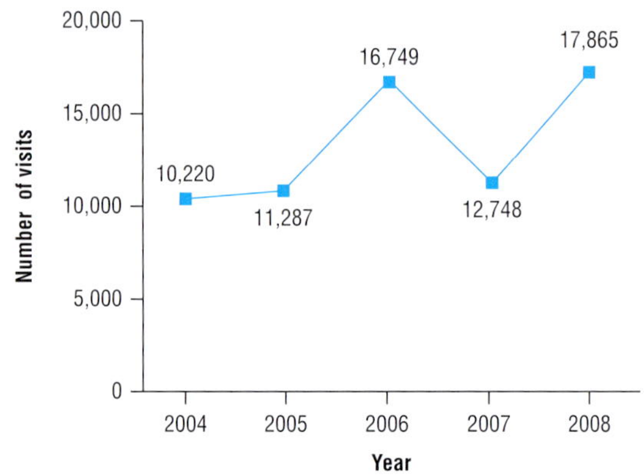

SOURCE: Substance Abuse and Mental Health Services Administration, Center for Behavioral Health Statistics and Quality, "Emergency Department Visits Involving Ecstasy," *The DAWN Report* (March 24, 2011).

Available online at http://oas.samhsa.gov/2k11/DAWN027/Ecstasy.htm. *(Graph by PreMediaGlobal. © 2012 Cengage Learning.)*

or prophetic experience. Shamans in Siberia were known to eat the hallucinogenic mushroom *Amanita muscaria*. The ancient Greeks and the Vikings also used naturally occurring plant hallucinogens. Peyote, a spineless cactus native to the southwestern United States and Mexico, was used by native peoples, including the Aztecs, to produce visions.

Although several hundred plants are known to contain compounds that cause hallucinations, most hallucinogens are synthesized in illegal laboratories for delivery as street drugs. The best known hallucinogens are lysergic acid diethylamide (LSD), mescaline, psilocybin, and MDMA (**ecstasy**). Phencyclidine (PCP, angel dust) can produce hallucinations, as can **amphetamines** and marijuana, but these drugs are considered dissociative drugs, rather than hallucinogens, and act by a different pathway from classic hallucinogens. Dextromorphan, the main ingredient in many cough medicines, has become popular among some populations because of the PCP-like hallucinations it produces. In addition, new designer drugs that are chemical variants of classic hallucinogens are apt to appear on the street at any time. One drug that only recently was added to Schedule I of the 1970 Controlled Substances Act (the classification for many other "hard" drugs with no known therapeutic value) is 5-methoxy-N, N-diisopropyltryptamine (5-MeO-DIPT), a drug derived from the chemical tryptamine that is more commonly known as "Foxy" or "Foxy Methoxy." A related hallucinogen, dimethyltryptamine, occurs naturally in plants in the Amazon but is now synthesized in labs. This drug, more commonly known as DMT, can be a powerful hallucinogen.

Although the various hallucinogens produce similar physical and psychological effects, they are a diverse group of compounds. However, all hallucinogens appear to affect the **brain** in similar ways. While the mechanism of action of hallucinogens is not completely understood, researchers have shown that these drugs bind with one type of **serotonin** receptor ($5\text{-}HT_2$) in the brain.

Serotonin is a neurotransmitter that facilitates transmission of nerve impulses in the brain and is associated with feelings of well-being, as well as many physiological responses. When a hallucinogenic compound binds with serotonin receptors, serotonin is blocked from those receptor sites, and nerve transmission is altered. There is an increase in free (unbound) serotonin in the brain. The result is a distortion of the senses of sight, sound, and touch, disorientation in time and space, and alterations of mood. In the case of hallucinogen intoxication, however, a person is not normally delirious, unconscious, or dissociated. He or she is aware that these changes in perception are caused by the hallucinogen.

LSD

LSD was first synthesized by Albert Hoffman for a pharmaceutical company in Germany in 1938 while he was searching for a headache remedy. Hoffman discovered the hallucinogenic properties of LSD accidentally in 1943. The drug became popular with the counterculture youth of the mid-1960s when its sense-altering properties were reputed to offer a window into enhanced creativity and self-awareness. LSD also occurs naturally in morning glory seeds.

Pure LSD is a white, odorless, crystalline powder that dissolves easily in water, although contaminants can cause it to range in color from yellow to dark brown. LSD was listed as a Schedule I drug under the Controlled Substance Act of 1970, meaning that it has no medical or legal uses and has a high potential for abuse. LSD is not easy to manufacture in a home laboratory, and some of its ingredients are controlled substances that are difficult to obtain. However, LSD is very potent, and a small amount can produce a large number of doses.

On the street, LSD is sold in several forms. Microdots are tiny pills smaller than a pinhead. Windowpane is liquid LSD applied to thin squares of gelatin. Liquid LSD can also be sprayed on sugar cubes. The most common street form of the drug is liquid LSD sprayed onto blotter paper and dried. The paper, often printed with colorful or psychedelic pictures, is divided into tiny squares, each square being one dose. Liquid LSD can also be sprayed on the back of a postage stamp and licked off. Street names for the drug include "acid," "yellow sunshine," "windowpane," "cid," "doses," "trips," and "boomers."

Mescaline

Mescaline is a naturally occurring plant hallucinogen. Its primary source is the cactus *Lophophora williamsii*. This cactus is native to the southwestern United States and Mexico. The light blue-green plant is spineless and has a crown called a "peyote button." This button contains mescaline and can be eaten or made into a bitter tea. Mescaline is also the active ingredient of at least ten other cacti of the genus *Trichocereus* that are native to parts of South America.

Mescaline was first isolated in 1897 by the German chemist Arthur Heffter and first synthesized in the laboratory in 1919. Some experiments were done with the drug to determine whether it was medically useful, but no medical uses were found. However, peyote is culturally significant. It has been used for centuries as part of religious celebrations and vision quests of Native Americans. The Native American Church, which fuses elements of Christianity with indigenous practices, has long used peyote as part of its religious practices.

In 1970, mescaline was listed as a Schedule I drug under the Controlled Substances Act. However, that same year, the state of Texas legalized peyote for use in Native American religious ceremonies. In 1995, a federal law was passed making peyote legal (but only for this use) in all 50 states.

Psilocybin

Psilocybin is the active ingredient in what are known on the street as "magic mushrooms," "shrooms," "mushies," or "Mexican mushrooms." There are several species of mushrooms that contain psilocybin, including *Psilocybe mexicana, P. muscorumi,* and *Stropharia cubensis*. These mushrooms grow in most moderate, moist climates.

Psilocybin-containing mushrooms are usually cooked and eaten (they have a bitter taste) or dried and boiled to make a tea. Although psilocybin can be made synthetically in the laboratory, there is no street market for synthetic psilocybin, and virtually all the drug comes from cultivated mushrooms. In the United States, it is legal to possess psilocybin-containing mushrooms, but it is illegal to traffic in them, and psilocybin and psilocyn (another psychoactive drug found in small quantities in these mushrooms) are both Schedule I drugs.

MDMA

MDMA, short for 3,4-methylenedioxymethamphetamine, and better known as "ecstasy," "XTC," "E," "X," or "Adam," has become an increasingly popular club drug since the 1980s. The hallucinogenically active portion of the drug is chemically similar to mescaline, while its stimulant portion is similar to **methamphetamine**. MDMA was first synthesized in 1912 by a German pharmaceutical company looking for a new compound that would stop bleeding. The company patented the drug but never did anything with it. A closely related drug, methylenedioxyamphetimine, or MDA, was tested by a pharmaceutical company as an appetite suppressant in the 1950s, but its use was discontinued when it was discovered to have hallucinogenic properties. In the 1960s, MDA was a popular drug of abuse in some large cities such as San Francisco.

During the early 1980s, therapists experimented with MDMA, which was legal at the time, as a way to help patients open up and become more empathetic. Recreational use soon followed, and it was declared an illegal Schedule I drug in 1985. For about a year between 1987 and 1988, the drug was again legal as the result of court challenges, but it permanently joined other Schedule I hallucinogens in March 1988.

MDMA is a popular club drug often associated with all-night raves or dance parties. The drug, sold in tablets, is attractive because it combines stimulant effects that allow ravers to dance for hours with a feeling of empathy, reduced anxiety, reduced inhibitions, and euphoria. Some authorities consider MDA and MDMA to be stimulant-hallucinogens and do not group them with classic hallucinogens such as LSD, but research indicates that MDA and MDMA affect the brain in the same way as classic hallucinogens. The **American Psychiatric Association** considers MDMA to be a drug that can cause hallucinogen-related disorders.

PMMA

PMMA (para-Methoxymethamphetamine) is a hallucinogen with effects similar to MDMA, causing rapid heartbeat, high blood pressure, **seizures**, kidney failure, hyperthermia, hallucinations, and death. The compound in PMMA is often found in MDMA, making the substance even more potent and potentially fatal.

Salvia

Salvia (*Salvia divinorum*) is known by many other names, including "Sally D," "Magic Mint," "Shepherdess Herb," "Ska Maria Pastora," "Diviners Sage," and "Sage of the Seers." Originating in Mexico, the drug is a perennial herb in the mint family. It grows in clusters up to three feet high with green leaves and white and purple flowers. Salvia is a potent psychoactive drug containing a chemical called salvinorin A, causing hallucinations noted to be up to five times more potent than the drug LSD. It is thought to act on opioid receptors of the brain, causing both physical and visual impairment and hallucinogenic effects. It is sold in the form of leaves, seeds, and extract and can be chewed or smoked when used. Salvia is not regulated by the federal government, but many states are creating legislation to ban the cultivation and sale of this plant.

Some hallucinogens (such as Salvia), act on opioid receptors of the brain, which like many narcotics, affect perceived levels of physical pain. As such, their use in the future may be implicated as therapeutic agents in pain control. Research and attention to legislation regarding intent for this use are ongoing.

Jimson weed

Jimson weed (*Datura stramonium*) is an herb producing fragrant flowers with a trumpet–like appearance. It grows as a bush in warm climates, and the seeds and leaves of the plant are poisonous and potentially fatal. Also known as "Devils Trumpet," "Devils Weed," "Moonflower," "Thorn Apple," and "Locoweed," jimson weed induces hallucinations, and users are often unaware of its toxicity. Effects include **delirium**, hallucinations, **amnesia**, and violent behavior; symptoms of overdose include seizure, coma, and respiratory arrest. Ingestion of the plant requires emergency treatment and **hospitalization**, as symptoms may last for up to three days.

Causes and symptoms

Hallucinogens are attractive to recreational drug users for a number of reasons:

- They are minimally addictive and there are no physical withdrawal symptoms upon stopping use.
- They produce few serious or debilitating physical side effects.
- They do not usually produce a delusional state, excessive stupor, or excessive stimulation.
- They are easily and cheaply available.
- They produce a high that gives the illusion of increasing creativity, empathy, or self-awareness.
- Deaths from overdoses are rare.

Despite their perceived harmlessness, strong hallucinogens such as LSD can cause frightening and anxiety-evoking emotional experiences, known as "bad trips." Flashbacks, where the sensations experienced while under the influence of a drug recur uncontrollably without drug use, can occur for months after a single drug use. During hallucinogen intoxication, reality may be so altered that a person may endanger himself by believing he is capable of feats such as flying off buildings. Hallucinogens also may induce or cause a worsening of latent psychiatric disorders such as anxiety, **depression**, and **psychosis**. Hallucinogens can also cause **paranoia**, long-term memory loss, personality changes (especially if there is a latent psychiatric disorder), and psychological drug dependence.

Psychological symptoms

Hallucinogens work primarily on the perception of reality. They usually do not create true hallucinations, which are imagined visions or sounds (voices heard in the head, for example) in the absence of any corresponding reality. Instead, classic hallucinogens alter the perception of something that is physically present. A face may appear to "melt" or colors may become brighter, move, and change shape. Sounds may be "seen," rather than heard.

More than with other drugs, the mental state of the hallucinogen user and the environment in which the drug is taken influence the user's experience. LSD, especially, is known for symptoms that range from mellowness and psychedelic visions ("good trips") to anxiety and panic attacks ("bad trips"). Previous good experiences with a drug do not guarantee continued good experiences. People with a history of psychiatric disorders are more likely to experience harmful reactions, as are those who are given the drug without their knowledge.

Normally, mescaline and psilocybin produce uniformly milder symptoms than LSD. During a single drug experience, the user can experience a range of symptoms. Mood can shift from happy to sad or pleasant to frightening and back again several times. Some symptoms occur primarily with MDMA, as indicated. Psychological symptoms of hallucinogen intoxication include:

- distortion of sight, sound, and touch
- confusion of the senses—sounds are "seen" or vision is "heard"
- disorientation in time and space
- delusions of physical invulnerability (especially with LSD)
- paranoia
- unreliable judgment and increased risk taking
- anxiety attacks
- flashbacks after the drug has been cleared from the body
- blissful calm or mellowness
- reduced inhibitions
- increased empathy (MDMA)
- elation or euphoria
- impaired concentration and motivation
- long-term memory loss
- personality changes, especially if there is a latent psychiatric disorder
- psychological drug dependence

Physical symptoms

Although the primary effects of hallucinogens are on perceptions, some physical effects do occur. Physical symptoms include:

- increased blood pressure
- increased heart rate
- nausea and vomiting (especially with psilocybin and mescaline)
- blurred vision, which can last after the drug has worn off
- poor coordination
- enlarged pupils
- sweating
- diarrhea (plant hallucinogens)
- restlessness
- muscle cramping (especially clenched jaws with MDMA)
- dehydration (MDMA)

KEY TERMS

Anxiety—Can be experienced as a troubled feeling, a sense of dread, fear of the future, or distress over a possible threat to a person's physical or mental well-being.

Depression—A mental state characterized by feelings of sadness, despair, and discouragement.

Ecstasy—Best known of the so-called designer amphetamines, also known as MDMA. It produces both stimulant and hallucinogenic effects.

Hallucinations—To hear, see, or otherwise sense things that are not real.Hallucinations can result from nervous system abnormalities, mental disorders, or the use of certain drugs.

Methamphetamine—The most common illegally produced amphetamine.

Panic attack—A period of intense fear or discomfort with a feeling of doom and a desire to escape. The person may shake, sweat, be short of breath, and experience chest pain.

Serotonin—A widely distributed neurotransmitter that is found in blood platelets, the lining of the digestive tract, and the brain, and that works in combination with norepinephrine. It causes very powerful contractions of smooth muscle, and is associated with mood, attention, emotions, and sleep. Low levels of serotonin are associated with depression. Large amounts of serotonin are released after ingestion of MDMA.

- serious increase in body temperature, leading to seizures (MDMA)

Diagnosis

Although not all experts agree, the **diagnosis** of mental disorders recognizes two hallucinogen-related disorders: hallucinogen dependence and hallucinogen abuse. Hallucinogen dependence is the continued use of hallucinogens even when the substances cause the affected individual significant problems, or when the individual knows of adverse effects (memory impairment while intoxicated, anxiety attacks, flashbacks) but continues to use the substances anyway. "Craving" hallucinogens after not using them for a period of time has been reported. Hallucinogen abuse is repeated use of hallucinogens even after they have caused the user impairment that undermines his or her ability to fulfill obligations at work, school, or home, but the use is usually not as frequent as it is among dependent users. In addition to these two disorders, the American Psychiatric Association recognizes eight hallucinogen-induced disorders. These are:

- hallucinogen intoxication
- hallucinogen persistent perception disorder (flashbacks)
- hallucinogen intoxication delirium
- hallucinogen-induced psychotic disorder with delusions
- hallucinogen-induced psychotic disorder with hallucinations
- hallucinogen-induced mood disorder
- hallucinogen-induced anxiety disorder
- hallucinogen-related disorder not otherwise specified

Hallucinogen dependence and abuse are normally diagnosed from reports by the patient (or person accompanying the patient) of use of a hallucinogenic drug. Active hallucinations and accompanying physical symptoms can confirm the diagnosis but need not be present. Routine drug screening does not detect LSD in the blood or urine, although specialized laboratory methods can detect the drug. Hallucinogen dependence differs from other drug dependence in that there are no withdrawal symptoms when the drug is stopped, and the extent of tolerance (needing a higher and higher dose to achieve the same effect) appears minimal.

The fifth edition of the ***Diagnostic and Statistical Manual of Mental Disorders***, also known as the *DSM-5*, is due for publication in May 2013. This edition may include proposed changes and revisions to some current diagnostic criteria for psychiatric diagnoses, including combining "Hallucinogen Abuse" and "Hallucinogen Dependence" into the single diagnosis of "Hallucinogen Use Disorder."

Hallucinogen intoxication is diagnosed based on psychological changes, perceptual changes, and physical symptoms that are typical of hallucinogen use. These changes must not be caused by a general medical condition, other **substance abuse**, or another mental disorder.

Hallucinogen persisting perception disorder, better known as "flashbacks," occur after hallucinogen use followed by a period of lucidity. Flashbacks may occur weeks or months after the drug was used and may occur after a single use or many uses.

To be diagnosed as a psychiatric disorder, flashbacks must cause significant distress or interfere with daily life activities. They can come on suddenly with no warning or be triggered by specific environments. Flashbacks may include emotional symptoms, seeing colors, geometric forms, or, most commonly, persistence of trails of light across the visual field. They may last for months. Flashbacks are most strongly associated with LSD.

Hallucinogen intoxication delirium is rare unless the hallucinogen is contaminated by another drug or chemical such as strychnine. In hallucinogen intoxication, the patient is still grounded in reality and recognizes that the experiences of altered perception are due to using a hallucinogen. In hallucinogen intoxication delirium, the patient is no longer grounded in reality. Hallucinogen-induced psychotic disorders are similar in that the patient loses touch with reality. Psychotic states can occur immediately after using the drug, or days or months later.

Hallucinogen-induced mood disorder and hallucinogen-induced anxiety disorder are somewhat controversial, as hallucinogen use may uncover latent or pre-existing anxiety or mood disorders rather than being the cause of them. However, it does appear that MDMA use can cause major depression.

Treatment

Acute treatment is aimed at preventing the patient from harming himself or anyone else. Since most people experiencing hallucinogen intoxication remain in touch with reality, "talking down" or offering reassurance and support that emphasizes that the disturbing sensations, anxiety, **panic attack**, or paranoia will pass as the drug wears off is often helpful. Patients are kept in a calm, pleasant, but lighted environment and are encouraged to move around while being helped to remain oriented to reality. Occasionally, drugs such as **lorazepam** are given for anxiety. Complications in treatment occur when the hallucinogen has been contaminated with other street drugs or chemicals. The greatest life-threatening risk is associated with MDMA, in which users may develop dangerously high body temperatures. Reducing the patient's temperature is an essential acute treatment.

Treatment for long-term effects of hallucinogen use involves long-term **psychotherapy** after drug use has stopped. Many people find 12-step programs or group support helpful. In addition, underlying psychiatric disorders must be addressed.

Prognosis

Because hallucinogens are not physically addictive, many people are able to stop using these drugs successfully.

QUESTIONS TO ASK YOUR DOCTOR

- What risks are associated with hallucinogen use?
- What symptoms are associated with hallucinogen dependence?
- Does having hallucinogen dependence and abuse put me at risk for other health conditions?
- Can you recommend any treatment and support groups for me?

However, users may be haunted by chronic problems such as flashbacks or mood and **anxiety disorders** either brought about or worsened by use of hallucinogens. It is difficult to predict who will have long-term complications and who will not.

Prevention

Hallucinogen use is difficult to prevent, because these drugs have a false reputation for being nonaddictive and harmless. Drug education and social outlets that provide people with a sense of self-worth are the best ways to prevent hallucinogen and other substance abuse.

Resources

BOOKS

American Psychiatric Association. *Diagnostic and Statistical Manual of Mental Disorders,* 4th ed., Text rev. Washington, DC: American Psychiatric Association, 2000.

American Psychological Association. *Publication Manual of the American Psychological Association,* 6th ed. Washington, DC: American Psychological Association, 2009.

Erickson, Carlton K, Ph.D. *Addiction Essentials: The Go-To Guide for Clinicians and Patients.* New York, NY: W. W. Norton & Company, 2011.

Galanter, Marc, and Herbert D. Kleber, eds. *Textbook of Substance Abuse Treatment,* 2nd ed. Washington, DC: American Psychiatric Press, Inc., 2008.

Holland, Julie, ed. *Ecstasy: The Complete Guide.*Kindle edition. Rochester, Vermont: Park Street Press, 2010.

North, Carol, and Sean Yutzy. *Goodwin and Guze's Psychiatric Diagnosis.* New York, NY: Oxford University Press, 2010.

Sadock, Benjamin J., Virginia Alcott Sadock, and Pedro Ruiz, eds. *Kaplan and Sadock's Comprehensive Textbook of Psychiatry,* 2nd ed. New York, NY: Lippincott Williams & Wilkins, 2009.

WEBSITES

National Institute on Drug Abuse. "NIDA InfoFacts: Hallucinogens—LSD, Peyote, Psilocybin, and PCP." http://drugabuse.gov/infofacts/hallucinogens.html (accessed November 14, 2011).

U.S. Drug Enforcement Administration. "Hallucinogens." http://www.justice.gov/dea/concern/hallucinogens.html (accessed November 14, 2011).

ORGANIZATIONS

American Psychological Association, 750 First Street NE, Washington, DC, 20003, (202) 336-5500, http://www.apa.org/index.aspx.

National Institute on Drug Abuse, 6001 Executive Blvd., Rm. 5213, Bethesda, MD, 20892, (301) 442-1124; Spanish: (240) 221-4007, information@nida.nih.gov, http://www.nida.nih.gov.

The Partnership at Drugfree.org, 352 Park Ave. South, 9th Fl., New York, NY, 10010, (212) 922-1560, http://www.drugfree.org.

Substance Abuse and Mental Health Services Administration, 1 Choke Cherry Rd., Rockville, MD, 20857, (877) SAMHSA-7 (726-4727), (800) TTY: 487-4889, Fax: (240) 221-4292, SAMHSAInfo@samhsa.hhs.gov, http://www.samhsa.gov.

Tish Davidson, A.M.
Emily Jane Willingham, Ph.D.
Laura Jean Cataldo, RN, Ed.D.

Haloperidol

Definition

Haloperidol is a major tranquilizer. It is used to treat psychoses, symptoms of **dementia**, **Tourette syndrome**, and certain serious behavioral disorders in children. In the United States it is sold under the brand name Haldol.

Purpose

Haloperidol is used in the management of symptoms in people requiring long-term antipsychotic therapy. It is also used for controlling tics and inappropriate vocalizations associated with Tourette syndrome in children and adults.

In children, haloperidol is occasionally used to treat severe behavior problems such as combativeness and extreme outbursts that occur without immediate provocation. Occasionally it is used for short-term treatment of children who display excessive motor activity with accompanying difficulty in attention, aggression, impulse control, mood changes, and coping with frustration.

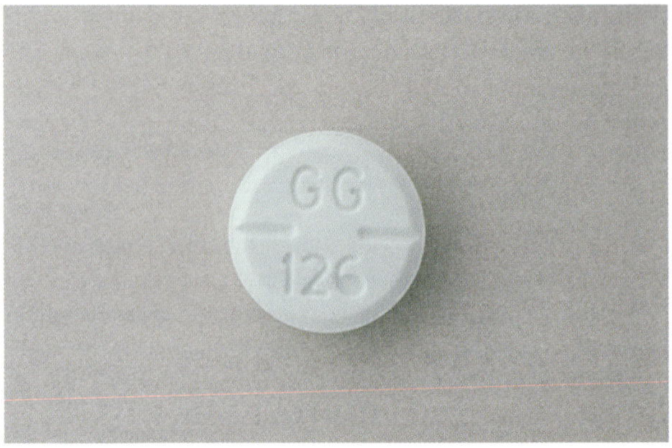

Haloperidol, 10 mg. *(© Custom Medical Stock Photo, Inc. Reproduced by permission.)*

Haloperidol is used only after **psychotherapy** and other medications have been tried and are found to be unsuccessful.

Description

Haloperidol is a major tranquilizer. It is used to control symptoms of psychotic disorders. It can be administered as a pill or by intramuscular injection (a shot).

The precise way in which haloperidol helps control symptoms associated with psychoses or dementia had as of 2011 not been clearly established.

A 2011 study published in *The Lancet* found that haloperidol and two other antipsychotic drugs, **risperidone** and **olanzapine**, better treated the mania associated with **bipolar disorder** than traditional mood stabilizers. The study included 16,000 participants over a 30-year period. Haloperidol treated manic episodes more successfully than ten other drugs, but it was not effective in managing **depression**, a key component of bipolar disorder.

Recommended dosage

For adults, the recommended initial dosage of haloperidol is 0.5–5.0 mg taken two or three times each day. The initial dosage depends on the severity of the symptoms in the person being treated. All people taking haloperidol must be carefully monitored to establish an individualized dosage. Physicians have found a great variability in the amount of haloperidol required to control symptoms.

Children require smaller dosages of haloperidol than do adults. The recommended initial dosage of haloperidol for controlling psychotic symptoms in children is

0.5–2.0 mg taken two or three times each day. The recommended dosage for controlling symptoms of Tourette syndrome and other nonpsychotic disorders is between 0.075 mg and 0.05 mg daily per 2.2 pounds (1 kilogram) of body weight. The total dosage is usually divided into two or three administrations per day. The goal of therapy is to use the smallest amount of haloperidol that will control symptoms. Children under age three should not be given this drug.

Precautions

Haloperidol may cause hypotension (low blood pressure). For this reason people with heart and blood pressure problems should be carefully monitored while taking the drug. Haloperidol carries a risk of causing fatal heart arrhythmias and increases the possibility of having **seizures**. People with a history of seizures or who are taking anticonvulsants (medication to control seizures) should take lower dosages of haloperidol and be closely monitored by a physician until a safe dosage is established. Haloperidol also interferes with the action of the anticoagulant (blood thinning) drug phenindione.

Women who are pregnant, wanting to become pregnant, or are breastfeeding should consult with their doctor before taking haloperidol. Haloperidol may cause extrapyramidal symptoms (EPS) and signs of withdrawal in newborns, especially if the drug was taken during the last trimester of the mother's pregnancy. The primary symptoms of EPS are involuntary movements, such as tremor, contractions, and other motions. Signs of withdrawal include increased agitation, respiratory problems, and trouble feeding. Haloperidol also travels through the breast milk of lactating mothers.

Haloperidol may increase the action of central nervous system depressants such as anesthetics, alcohol, and opiates (some pain killers and sleeping pills). It may also decrease the time required to change from mania to depression among people with bipolar (manic-depressive) disorder.

Like other antipsychotic medications, haloperidol carries a warning regarding use in elderly people with dementia, who suffer from an increased risk of death during treatment with these agents. The drug is not approved by the U.S. Food and Drug Administration (FDA) for use in treating behavior problems related to senile dementia.

Side effects

Haloperidol has the potential to produce a serious side effect called **tardive dyskinesia**. This syndrome consists of involuntary, uncoordinated movements that may not disappear or may only partially improve after the drug is stopped. Tardive dyskinesia involves involuntary movements of the tongue, jaw, mouth, face, or other groups of skeletal muscles. These side effects may appear after people have stopped taking haloperidol. The chance of developing tardive dyskinesia increases with increasing age and dosage of haloperidol. Women are at greater risk than men for developing tardive dyskinesia. There is no known effective treatment for tardive dyskinesia, although gradual (but rarely complete) improvement may occur over a long period.

Haloperidol use may lead to the development of symptoms that resemble Parkinson's disease, but that are not caused by Parkinson's. These symptoms may include a taut or mask-like expression on the face, drooling, tremors, pill-rolling motions in the hands, cogwheel rigidity (abnormal rigidity in muscles characterized by jerky movements when the muscle is passively stretched), and a shuffling gait. Taking the anti-Parkinson's drugs **benztropine** mesylate or **trihexyphenidyl** hydrochloride along with haloperidol helps to control these symptoms. Medication to control parkinsonian symptoms may have to be continued after haloperidol is stopped because the drugs are eliminated at different rates from the body.

Other side effects of haloperidol include:

- anxiety
- restlessness
- agitation
- insomnia
- headache
- euphoria
- drowsiness
- depression
- confusion
- dizziness
- seizures

Unwanted or unexpected effects associated with the use of haloperidol have been reported for virtually all organ systems in the body. Although numerous, such side effects are relatively uncommon.

Interactions

The simultaneous use of haloperidol and lithium, a common treatment for bipolar (manic-depressive) disorder, has been associated with encephalopathic syndrome. People with this syndrome have symptoms

KEY TERMS

Bipolar disorder—A mood disorder marked by alternating episodes of extremely low mood (depression) and exuberant highs (mania), also known as manic-depressive disorder.

Extrapyramidal symptoms (EPS)—A group of side effects associated with antipsychotic medications. EPS includes Parkinson-like symptoms, akathisia (restless leg syndrome), dystonia, and tardive dyskinesia.

of weakness, lethargy, fever, confusion, and high levels of white blood cells.

Haloperidol may increase the effect of central nervous system depressants such as anesthetics, opiates, and alcohol.

Resources

BOOKS

Foreman, John C., and Torben Johansen. *Textbook of Receptor Pharmacology*. 2nd ed. Boca Raton, FL: CRC Press, 2002.

Page, Clive P., and Michael Murphy. *Integrated Pharmacology*. St. Louis: Mosby-Year Book, 2002.

Von Boxtel, Chris J., et al. *Handbook of Clinical Psychopharmacology for Therapists*. 4th ed. Oakland, CA: New Harbinger Publications, 2004.

PERIODICALS

Akhondzadeh, Shahin, et al. "Allopurinol as an Adjunct to Lithium and Haloperidol for Treatment of Patients with Acute Mania: A Double-Blind, Randomized, Placebo-Controlled Trial." *Bipolar Disorders* 8, no. 5, part 1 (October 2006): 485–89.

Aziz, Mohamed, et al. "Remission of Positive and Negative Symptoms in Refractory Schizophrenia with a Combination of Haloperidol and Quetiapine: Two Case Studies." *Journal of Psychiatric Practice* 12, no. 5 (September 2006): 332–36.

Cipriani, Andrea. "Comparative Efficacy and Acceptability of Antimanic Drugs in Acute Mania: A Multiple-treatments Meta-analysis." *The Lancet* (August 17, 2011). Available online at http://www.bioportfolio.com/news/article/772923/articles-Comparative-Efficacy-And-Acceptability-Of-Antimanic-Drugs-In-Acute-Mania.html (accessed August 25, 2011).

Dunn, Michael J., and Simon Killcross. "Clozapine but Not Haloperidol Treatment Reverses Sub-Chronic Phencyclidine-Induced Disruption of Conditional Discrimination Performance." *Behavioural Brain Research* 175, no. 2 (December 2006): 271–77.

Emsley, Robin, Jonathan Rabinowitz, and Rossella Medori. "Remission in Early Psychosis: Rates, Predictors, and Clinical and Functional Outcome Correlates." *Schizophrenia Research* 89, no. 1–3 (January 2007): 129–39.

Green, A.I., et al. "Olanzapine and Haloperidol in First Episode Psychosis: Two-Year Data." *Schizophrenia Research* 86, no. 1–3 (September 2006): 234–43.

Morrens, Manuel, et al. "Psychomotor and Memory Effects of Haloperidol, Olanzapine, and Paroxetine in Healthy Subjects after Short-Term Administration." *Journal of Clinical Psychopharmacology* 27, no. 1 (February 2007): 15–21.

Nasrallah, Henry A., Martin Brecher, and Björn Paulsson. "Placebo-Level Incidence of Extrapyramidal Symptoms (EPS) with Quetiapine in Controlled Studies of Patients with Bipolar Mania." *Bipolar Disorders* 8, no. 5, part 1 (October 2006): 467–74.

Woodward, Neil D., et al. "A Meta-analysis of Cognitive Change with Haloperidol in Clinical Trials of Atypical Antipsychotics: Dose Effects and Comparison to Practice Effects." *Schizophrenia Research* 89, no. 1–3 (January 2007): 211–24.

Zhang, Xiang Yang, et al. "The Effects of Ginkgo Biloba Extract Added to Haloperidol on Peripheral T Cell Subsets in Drug-Free Schizophrenia: A Double-Blind, Placebo-Controlled Trial." *Psychopharmacology* 188, no. 1 (September 2006): 12–17.

ORGANIZATIONS

American Academy of Clinical Toxicology, 6728 Old McLean Village Dr., McLean, VA, 22101, (703) 556-9222, Fax: (703) 556-8729, admin@clintox.org, http://www.clintox.org.

American Academy of Family Physicians, 11400 Tomahawk Creek Pkwy., Leawood, KS, 66211-2672, (913) 906-6000, (800) 274-2237, Fax: (913) 906-6075, contactcenter@aafp.org, http://www.aafp.org.

American Medical Association, 515 N State St., Chicago, IL, 60610, (312) 464-5000, (800) 621-8335, http://www.amaassn.org.

American Psychiatric Association, 1000 Wilson Blvd., Ste. 1825, Arlington, VA, 22209-3901, (703) 907-7300, apa@psych.org, http://www.psych.org.

American Society for Clinical Pharmacology and Therapeutics, 528 N Washington St., Alexandria, VA, 22314, (703) 836-6981, info@ascpt.org, http://www.ascpt.org.

American Society for Pharmacology and Experimental Therapeutics, 9650 Rockville Pike, Bethesda, MD, 20814-3995, (301) 634-7060, http://www.aspet.org.

L. Fleming Fallon, Jr., MD, DrPH
Ruth A. Wienclaw, PhD

Halstead-Reitan Battery

Definition

The Halstead-Reitan Neuropsychological Test Battery (HRNB) is a fixed set of tests used to evaluate **brain** and nervous system functioning in individuals aged 15 years and older. Children's versions are the Halstead Neuropsychological Test Battery for Older Children (ages nine to 14 years) and the Reitan Indiana Neuropsychological Test Battery (ages five to eight years). The set of tests includes those used to measure abstract thoughts, imperception, language, memory, motor dexterity, and sensory-motor integration. The time to complete the HRNB is reported to vary widely among individuals.

Purpose

Neuropsychological functioning refers to the ability of the nervous system and brain to process and interpret information received through the senses. The Halstead-Reitan evaluates a wide range of nervous system and brain functions, including visual, auditory, and tactual input; verbal communication; spatial and sequential perception; the ability to analyze information, form mental concepts, and make judgments; motor output; and attention, concentration, and memory.

The Halstead-Reitan is typically used to evaluate individuals with suspected brain damage, including the extent, location, and nature of the damage. The battery provides useful information regarding the cause of damage (for example, closed head injury, alcohol abuse, **Alzheimer's disease**, **stroke**), which part of the brain is damaged, whether the damage occurred during child hood development, and whether the damage is getting worse, staying the same, or getting better. Information regarding the severity of impairment and areas of personal strengths can be used to develop plans for rehabilitation or care.

Description

Dr. Ward Halstead and Dr. Ralph M. Reitan were the developers of the Halstead-Reitan Battery. Based on studies of patients with neurologic impairments at the University of Chicago, Halstead recognized the need for an evaluation of brain functioning that was more extensive than intelligence testing. He began experimenting with psychological tests that might help identify types and severity of brain damage through observation of a person's behavior in various tasks involving neuropsychological abilities. Initially he chose a set of ten tests; all but three are in the current Halstead-Reitan Battery.

Ralph Reitan, one of Halstead's students, contributed to the battery by researching the tests' ability to identify neurological problems. In a remarkable study, Reitan diagnosed 8,000 patients using only their test results—without meeting the patients or knowing anything about their background. This provided strong support for the battery's effectiveness. Reitan, who is now associated with the Reitan Neuropsychological Laboratory in Tucson, Arizona, adapted the original battery by including additional tests.

The Halstead-Reitan has been researched more than any other neuropsychological test battery. Research continues to support its ability to accurately detect impairment in a large range of neuropsychological functions.

Category Test (CT)

A series of 208 pictures consisting of geometric figures are presented, sorted in groups according to some underlying principle, which the test subject is asked to determine. For each picture, individuals are asked to decide which of four principles they believe is represented and to press a key that corresponds to the number of choice. If they chose correctly, a chime sounds. If they chose incorrectly, a buzzer sounds. The pictures are presented in seven subtests.

The key to this test is that one principle, or common characteristic, underlies each subtest. The numbers 1, 2, 3, and 4 represent the possible principles. If individuals are able to recognize the correct principle in one picture, they will respond correctly for the remaining pictures in that subtest. The next subtest may have the same or a different underlying principle, and individuals must again try to determine that principle using the feedback of the chime and buzzer. The last subtest contains two underlying principles. The test takes approximately one hour to complete, but individuals with severe brain damage may take as long as two hours.

The Category Test is considered the battery's most effective test for detecting brain damage, but does not help determine where the problem is occurring in the brain. The test evaluates abstraction ability, or the ability to draw specific conclusions from general information. Related abilities are solving complex and unique problems, and learning from experience. Children's versions consist of 80 items and five subtests for young children, and 168 items and six subtests for older children.

Scoring involves recording the number of errors. Based on traditional scoring using cutoff values (cutoff scores are scores that indicate the borderline between normal and impaired functioning), scores above 41 are considered indicative of brain impairment for ages 15 to 45 years. For ages 46 years and older, scores above 46 indicate impairment. Reitan has suggested a cutoff of 50 or 51 errors. Recommended cutoffs also vary depending on age and education level.

Tactual Performance Test (TPT)

A form board containing ten cutout shapes, and ten wooden blocks matching those shapes are placed in front of a blindfolded individual. Individuals are then instructed to use only their dominant hand to place the blocks in their appropriate space on the form board. The same procedure is repeated using only the nondominant hand, and then using both hands. Finally, the form board and blocks are removed, followed by the blindfold. From memory, individuals are asked to draw the form board and the shapes in their proper locations. The test usually takes anywhere from 15 to 50 minutes to complete. There is a time limit of 15 minutes for each trial, or each performance segment.

Other names for this test are the Form Board Test and the Seguin-Goddard Formboard. It evaluates sensory ability, memory for shapes and spatial location, motor functions, and the brain's ability to transfer information between its two hemispheres. In addition to simple detection of brain damage, this test also helps determine the side of the brain where damage may have occurred. For children under the age of 15 years, only six shapes are used.

Scoring involves recording the time to complete each of the three blindfolded trials and the total time for all trials combined (time score), the number of shapes recalled (memory score), and the number of shapes drawn in their correct locations (localization score). Generally, the trial for the nondominant hand should be 20% to 30% faster than the trial for the dominant hand, due to the benefit of practice. If the nondominant hand is slower than the dominant hand or more than 30% faster than the dominant hand, brain damage is possible. However, some people without brain damage do not exhibit this typical improvement rate. Injuries of the arms, shoulders, or hands can also affect performance. Scores should be adjusted depending on education level and may vary depending on age.

Trail Making Test (TM)

This test consists of two parts. Part A is a page with 25 numbered circles randomly arranged. Individuals are instructed to draw lines between the circles in increasing sequential order until they reach the circle labeled "End." Part B is a page with circles containing the letters A through L and 13 numbered circles intermixed and randomly arranged. Individuals are instructed to connect the circles by drawing lines alternating between numbers and letters in sequential order, until they reach the circle labeled "End." If individuals make mistakes, the mistakes are quickly brought to their attention, and they continue from the last correct circle. The test takes approximately 5 to 10 minutes to complete.

This test was originally known as Partington's Pathways, or the Divided Attention Test, which was part of the Army Individual Test Battery. The test evaluates information-processing speed, visual-scanning ability, integration of visual and motor functions, letter and number recognition and sequencing, and the ability to maintain two different trains of thought. The test can be administered orally if an individual is incapable of writing. The Color Trails Test, designed for children and individuals of different cultures, uses colors instead of numbers and letters.

Scoring is based on the time it takes to complete each part. Errors naturally increase the total time. Some have argued that the time taken to alert individuals of errors may vary depending on the person giving the test. For adults, scores above 40 seconds for Part A and 91 seconds for Part B have traditionally indicated brain impairment. Current research discourages the use of such traditional cutoffs, preferring ranges depending on age, education, and gender. For example, one study reported that for ages 15 to 19 years, the average time to complete Part A was 25.7 seconds and the time to complete Part B was 49.8 seconds. For ages 80 to 85 years, however, the average time to complete Part A was 60.7 seconds and the time to complete Part B was 152.2 seconds. This demonstrates the importance of considering other variables when scoring.

Finger Tapping Test (FTT)

Individuals place their dominant hand palm down, fingers extended, with the index finger resting on a lever that is attached to a counting device. Individuals are instructed to tap their index finger as quickly as possible for ten seconds, keeping the hand and arm stationary. This trial is repeated five to ten times, until the examiner has collected counts for five consecutive trials that are within five taps of each other. Before starting the test, individuals are given a practice session. They are also given brief rests between each 10-second trial, and one- to two-minute rests after every third trial. This entire procedure is repeated with the nondominant hand. The test takes approximately 10 minutes to complete.

This test is also called the Finger Oscillation Test and the Finger Tapper. The children's version uses an electronic tapper instead of a manual one, which was difficult for children to operate. The test measures motor speed and helps determine particular areas of the brain that may be damaged. Scoring involves using the five accepted trials to calculate an average number of taps per trial for each hand. In general, the dominant hand should perform 10% better than the nondominant hand. Yet this is not always the case, especially with left-handed individuals. Men and younger people tend to perform better than women and older people. Interpretation should also consider education level, intelligence, **fatigue**, general weakness or lack of coordination, **depression**, and injuries to the shoulders, arms, or hands. This test should only be interpreted in combination with other tests in the battery.

Rhythm Test (RT)

Thirty pairs of tape-recorded, nonverbal sounds are presented. For each pair, individuals decide if the two sounds are the same or different, marking "S" or "D" respectively on their answer sheets. The pairs are grouped into three subtests. This test is also called the Seashore Rhythm Test, and is based on the Seashore Tests of Musical Ability. It evaluates auditory attention and concentration, and the ability to discriminate between nonverbal sounds. The test helps detect brain damage, but not the location of damage. Adequate hearing and visual abilities are needed to take this test. Scoring is based on the number of correct items, with higher scores indicating less damage or good recovery. Scores should be interpreted along with information from other tests. Some researchers consider this test unreliable and simplistic. The children's version does not include this test.

Speech Sounds Perception Test (SSPT)

Sixty tape-recorded nonsense syllables containing the sound "ee" (for example, "meer" and "weem") are presented. After each syllable, individuals underline, from a set of four written syllables, the spelling that represents the syllable they heard. This test evaluates auditory attention and concentration and the ability to discriminate between verbal sounds. It provides some information regarding specific areas of brain damage, and may also indicate attention deficits or hearing loss. Scoring and interpretation are similar to that used for the Rhythm Test. The children's version contains fewer syllable choices.

Reitan-Indiana Aphasia Screening Test

Aphasia is the loss of ability to understand or use written or spoken language, due to brain damage or deterioration. In this test, individuals are presented with a variety of questions and tasks that would be easy for someone without impairment. Examples of test items include verbally naming pictures, writing the name of a picture without saying the name aloud, reading printed material of increasing length, repeating words stated by the examiner, simple arithmetic problems, drawing shapes without lifting the pencil, and placing one hand to an area on the opposite side of the body.

This test is a modification of the Halstead-Wepman Aphasia Screening Test. It evaluates language-related difficulties, right/left confusion, and nonverbal tasks. A typical scoring procedure is not used because this is a screening test; its purpose is to detect possible signs of aphasia that may require further evaluation. Subtle language deficits may not be detected.

Reitan-Klove Sensory-Perceptual Examination

This test detects whether individuals are unable to perceive stimulation on one side of the body when both sides are stimulated simultaneously. It has tactile, auditory, and visual components involving the ability to (a) specify whether touch, sound, or visible movement is occurring on the right, left, or both sides of the body; (b) recall numbers assigned to particular fingers (the examiner assigns numbers by touching each finger and stating the number with the individual's eyes closed); (c) identify numbers "written" on fingertips while eyes are closed; and (d) identify the shape of a wooden block placed in one hand by pointing to its shape on a form board with the opposite hand.

Ancillary tests

In addition to the core tests, examiners may choose to administer other tests based on the difficulties that individuals experience. Tests commonly used in combination with the Halstead-Reitan Battery include the Grip Strength Test (or Strength Of Grip Test [SOGT]), the Grooved Pegboard Test, and the Reitan-Klove Lateral Dominance Examination. The SOGT uses a hand dynamometer to measure the strength of both hands, where one hand is considered the dominant hand and the other the nondominant one. The Reitan Klove Lateral Dominance Examination measures preferences for right versus left in activities involving the arms, eyes, feet, hands, and legs.

Still other tests commonly used with the HRNB are the Wechsler Memory Scale, the California Verbal Learning Test, the Buschke Selective Reminding Test, the Rey Auditory Verbal Memory Test, the Rey Complex Figure Test, the Test of Memory and Learning, the **Wide Range Achievement Test**, the **Minnesota Multiphasic Personality Inventory**, and the Wechsler Adult Intelligence Scale or **Wechsler Intelligence Scales** for Children. Some of these tests expand on these measures of functioning in the latest revision of the battery.

Preparation

Preparation for the Halstead-Reitan Neuropsychological Test Battery is not necessary for participants nor is it recommended by professionals.

Precautions

Because of its complexity, the Halstead-Reitan requires administration by a professional examiner and interpretation by a trained **psychologist**. Test results are affected by the examinee's age, education level, intellectual ability, and—to some extent—gender or ethnicity, which should always be taken into account.

Because the Halstead-Reitan is a fixed battery of tests, some unnecessary information may be gathered or some important information may be missed. Overall, the battery requires five to six hours to complete, involving considerable patience, stamina, and cost. The battery has also been criticized for not including specific tests of memory; rather, memory is evaluated within the context of other tests.

Results

Interpretation of the Halstead-Reitan involves analysis of various factors:

- Overall performance on the battery. The Halstead Impairment Index (HII) and the General Neuropsychological Deficit Scale (GNDS) are commonly used to obtain an overall score, although the latest revision now facilitates calculation of a global deficit score that reflects the number and severity of deficits or impairments and incorporates more test measures than were used in previous versions. This summary score weighs deficits more heavily than strengths, which reduces the chance that better performance on a few components of the test will hide impairments. The HII is calculated by counting the total number of tests in the impaired range, and dividing that number by the total tests administered, resulting in a decimal between zero and one (0.0–0.2: normal functioning; 0.3–0.4: mild impairment; 0.5–0.7: moderate impairment; and 0.8–1.0: severe impairment). The GNDS is calculated by assigning a value between zero and four to 42 variables contained in the tests, then summing those values (0–25: normal functioning; 26–40: mild impairment; 41–67: moderate impairment; and 68 and higher: severe impairment).
- Performance on individual tests. Each test must be interpreted in relation to other tests in the battery. Significant poor performance on one test may be due to various factors. However, if a pattern of poor performance occurs on three or more tests, or if significant discrepancies occur on two or more tests, impairment is likely.
- Indications of lateralization and localization. This refers to the particular region of the brain that is damaged. Performance on sensory and motor tasks provides the necessary clues.

The tests within the HRNB have been shown to be effective at differentiating between the brains of normal individuals and those with brain damage. One combined score, called the Halstead Impairment Index, is used for final analysis of its results.

With the test information, a psychologist can diagnose the type of condition present, predict the course of the impairment (staying the same, getting better, or getting worse), and make recommendations regarding treatment, care, or rehabilitation.

In 2004, a revision in the norms used to make determinations about results on the battery was published. This revision includes corrections based on ethnicity in addition to age, gender, and education. The results can be adjusted to demographic components, including African American or Caucasian ethnicity. Also updated is the global deficit score, which reflects the severity and number of deficits on more test measures than previously assessed. The sample used to determine the norms for this 2004 revision also was larger, including more than 1,000 adults, ages 20 to 85 years, for most test endpoints. The revision also has expanded measures of psychological functioning, including Wechsler scores.

QUESTIONS TO ASK YOUR DOCTOR

- Will the HRNB be able to tell specifically what has caused the brain damage?
- Do you know of a psychologist or other professional trained in administering the HRNB?
- Will health insurance cover the test?

See also Executive function; Luria-Nebraska Inventory; Mini-Mental State Exam; Neuropsychological Status Exam; Neuropsychological testing; Psychological assessment and diagnosis

Resources

BOOKS

Goldstein, Laura H., and Jane E. McNeil, editors. *Clinical Neuropsychology: A Practical Guide to Assessment and Management for Clinicians.* Chichester, UK: Wiley, 2004.

Hersen, Michel, and Alan M. Gross, editors. *Handbook of Clinical Psychology.* Hoboken, NJ: J. Wiley & Sons, 2008.

Horton, Jr., Arthur MacNeill, and Danny Wedding, editors. *The Neuropsychology Handbook.* New York City: Springer Publishing, 2008.

Lezak, Muriel D., et al. *Neuropsychological Assessment.* Oxford: Oxford University Press, 2004.

Poreh, Amir M., editor. *The Quantified Process Approach to Neuropsychological Assessment.* New York City: Taylor & Francis, 2006.

Strauss, Esther, Elisabeth M. S. Sherman, and Otfied Spreen. *A Compendium of Neuropsychological Tests: Administration, Norms, and Commentary.* Oxford: Oxford University Press, 2006.

Uzzell, Barbara P., Marcel O. Pontón, and Alfredo Ardila, editors. *International Handbook of Cross-cultural Neuropsychology.* Mahwah, NJ: Lawrence Erlbaum, 2007.

OTHER

"The Halstead-Reitan Neuropsychological Test Battery for Adults: Theoretical, Methodological and Validational Bases." Ralph M. Reitan and Deborah Wolfson, Reitan Neuropsychological Laboratory. http://www.reitanlabs.com/PDFFiles/halstead-reitan%20battery.pdf (accessed December 6, 2011).

WEBSITES

"Halstead-Reitan Neuropsychological Test Battery." Center for Psychological Studies, Nova Southeastern University. http://www.cps.nova.edu/~cpphelp/HRNTB.html (accessed December 6, 2011).

"Revised Comprehensive Norms for an Expanded Halstead-Reitan Battery: Demographically Adjusted Neuropsychological Norms for African American and Caucasian Adults (HRB)." National Alliance of Mental Illness. http://www4.parinc.com/Products/Product.aspx?ProductID=RCNAAC (accessed December 6, 2011).

ORGANIZATIONS

American Psychiatric Association, 1000 Wilson Boulevard, Suite 1825, Arlington, VA, 22209-3901, (703) 907-7300, apa@psych.org, http://www.psych.org.

American Psychological Association, 750 First St., NE, Washington, DC, 20002, (202) 336-5500, (800) 374-2721, http://www.apa.org.

International Neuropsychological Society, 700 Ackerman Road, Suite 625, Columbus, OH, 43202, (614) 263-4200, Fax: (614) 263-4366, http://www.the-ins.org.

National Institute of Mental Health, 6001 Executive Boulevard, Room 8184, MSC 9663, Bethesda, MD, 20892-9663, (301) 443-4513, (866) 615-6464, Fax: (301) 443-4279, nimhinfo@nih.gov, http://www.nimh.nih.gov.

Sandra L. Friedrich, MA
Emily Jane Willingham, PhD

Hamilton Anxiety Scale

Definition

The Hamilton Anxiety Scale (HAS, HAM-A, or HAMA) is a 14-item test measuring the severity of anxiety symptoms developed by German-born-British **psychologist** Max Hamilton (1912–1988) in 1959. It is also sometimes called the Hamilton Anxiety Rating Scale (HARS). The test is administered in an interview format. It measures the severity of anxiety, including anxious mood, fears, abnormal behavior, **insomnia**, and somatic complaints at the time of the interview. It measures many of the features of **generalized anxiety disorder** (GAD), along with accessing its severity, although the test was developed before the medical term was defined. It takes about 15 to 20 minutes to administer the test.

Purpose

The HAS is used to assess the severity of anxiety symptoms present in children and adults. It is also used as an outcome measure when assessing the impact of antianxiety medications, therapies, and treatments and is a standard measure of anxiety used in evaluations of psychotropic drugs. The HAS can be administered prior to medication being started and then again during follow-up visits, so that medication dosage can be changed in part based on the patient's test score.

The HAS provides measures of overall anxiety, psychic anxiety (mental agitation and psychological distress), and somatic anxiety (physical complaints related to anxiety). Hamilton developed the HAS to be appropriate for adults and children; although it is most often used for younger adults, there has been support for the test's use with older adults as well. Hamilton also developed the widely used **Hamilton Depression Scale** (HDS) to measure symptoms of **depression**.

Hamilton developed the scale by using the statistical technique of factor analysis. With this

Hamilton Anxiety Rating Scale (HAM-A)

Code: 0 = Not present, 1 = Mild, 2 = Moderate, 3 = Severe, 4 = Very severe

1 Anxious mood	0 1 2 3 4
Worries, anticipation of the worst, fearful anticipation, irritability	
2 Tension	0 1 2 3 4
Feelings of tension, fatigability, startle response, moved to tears easily, trembling, feelings of restlessness, inability to relax	
3 Fears	0 1 2 3 4
Of dark, of strangers, of being left alone, of animals, of traffic, of crowds	
4 Insomnia	0 1 2 3 4
Difficulty in falling asleep, broken sleep, unsatisfying sleep and fatigue on waking, dreams, nightmares, night terrors	
5 Intellectual	0 1 2 3 4
Difficulty in concentration, poor memory	
6 Depressed mood	0 1 2 3 4
Loss of interest, lack of pleasure in hobbies, depression, early waking, diurnal swing	
7 Somatic (muscular)	0 1 2 3 4
Pains and aches, twitching, stiffness, myoclonic jerks, grinding of teeth, unsteady voice, increased muscular tone	
8 Somatic (sensory)	0 1 2 3 4
Tinnitus, blurring of vision, hot and cold flushes, feelings of weakness, pricking sensation	
9 Cardiovascular symptoms	0 1 2 3 4
Tachycardia, palpitations, pain in chest, throbbing of vessels, fainting feelings, missing beat	
10 Respiratory symptoms	0 1 2 3 4
Pressure or constriction in chest, choking feelings, sighing, dyspnea	
11 Gastrointestinal symptoms	0 1 2 3 4
Difficulty in swallowing, wind abdominal pain, burning sensations, abdominal fullness, nausea, vomiting, borborygmi, looseness of bowels, loss of weight, constipation	
12 Genitourinary symptoms	0 1 2 3 4
Frequency of micturition, urgency of micturition, amenorrhea, menorrhagia, development of frigidity, premature ejaculation, loss of libido, impotence	
13 Autonomic symptoms	0 1 2 3 4
Dry mouth, flushing, pallor, tendency to sweat, giddiness, tension headache, raising of hair	
14 Behavior at interview	0 1 2 3 4
Fidgeting, restlessness or pacing, tremor of hands, furrowed brow, strained face, sighing or rapid respiration, facial pallor, swallowing, etc.	

(Table by PreMediaGlobal. © 2012 Cengage Learning.)

method, he generated a set of symptoms related to anxiety and further determined which symptoms related to psychic anxiety and which related to somatic anxiety. Its major use is as a pharmacotherapy or **psychotherapy** tool, rather than as one used for **diagnosis** or screening.

Description

The HAS is administered by an interviewer who asks a semi-structured series of questions related to symptoms of anxiety. The interviewer then rates the individuals on a five-point scale for each of the 14 items. Seven of the items specifically address psychic anxiety, and the remaining seven items address somatic anxiety. For example, one item specifically addresses fears related to anxiety, another addresses insomnia and sleeping difficulties related to anxiety, and still another item addresses respiratory symptoms related to anxiety.

The seven items rated by the HAS as being psychic symptoms include:

- anxious mood (worries, anticipates the worst, negative attitude)
- heightened fears (various types of fears including fear of strangers, fear of being alone, fear of the dark)
- depressed mood (insomnia, lack of interest in activities and life in general)
- behavior at interview (pacing, tremors, anxiousness, uneasiness during interview process)
- intellectual (loss of concentration, poor memory)
- feelings of tension (restless, easily emotional, frequent bursts of crying, trembling)
- cardiovascular symptoms (chest pains, feelings of lightheadedness and fainting)

The seven items rated by the HAS as being somatic symptoms include:

- somatic complaints (muscular pain)
- gastrointestinal symptoms (weight loss, vomiting, nausea)
- autonomic symptoms (sweaty, pallor, dry mouth)
- insomnia (difficulties falling asleep and staying asleep, having frequent nightmares when asleep)
- somatic complaints (sensory such as blurred vision, tinnitus)
- respiratory symptoms (chest pressure, feeling of choking, shortness of breath)
- genitourinary symptoms (impotence, urgency to urinate, dysmenorrhea)

KEY TERMS

Dysmenorrhea—Painful menstruation.

Psychic—Relating to the mind rather than the body.

Somatic—Relating to the body, rather than the mind.

Tinnitus—Consistent noise in ear.

Preparation

It is not necessary for the individual to prepare for the test.

Risks

The test has been criticized on the grounds that it does not always discriminate between people with anxiety symptoms and those with depressive symptoms (people with depression also score fairly high on the HAS).

Precautions

Because the HAS is administered and rated by the interviewer, there is some subjectivity when it comes to interpretation and scoring. Interviewer bias can affect the results. For this reason, some people prefer self-report measures where scores are completely based on the interviewee's responses.

Results

For the 14 items, the values on the scale range from zero to four: zero means that there is no anxiety (none present), one indicates mild anxiety, two indicates moderate anxiety, three indicates severe anxiety, and four indicates very severe or grossly disabling anxiety. The total anxiety score ranges from 0 to 56. The seven psychic anxiety items elicit a psychic anxiety score that ranges from 0 to 28. The remaining seven items yield a somatic anxiety score that also ranges from 0 to 28. A total score of 17 or less indicates mild anxiety, 18–24 indicates moderate anxiety, and 25 or higher indicates severe anxiety.

One reason that the HAS is widely used is that reliability studies have shown that it measures anxiety symptoms in a fairly consistent way. The measure's validity has also been supported by research.

While there is a tendency for depressed people to also score high on the HAS, some researchers have suggested that anxiety and depression are so closely linked that people can easily score high on measures of both types of symptoms.

The paper and pencil version of this test is in the public domain, meaning that it can easily be found on the Internet for people who are interested in reviewing it. There is also a computer-administered version for use in a computerized, telephone-based interview. This version uses voice recognition to take answers to the respondent's questions. The computerized "interviewer" can even interact in a programmed way with the respondent. A study has indicated that some respondents feel more comfortable answering the questions when they are administered in the telephone format compared to the in-person format.

QUESTIONS TO ASK YOUR DOCTOR

- Do I need to find an administrator who is knowledgeable at administering the Hamilton Anxiety Scale?
- Should I take the test over the Internet or the telephone rather than in an interview format?
- Will the HAS tell me what type of medicine I need (if any), and the amount I will need to take?
- Where can I learn more about the HAS?
- Are there other tests that I can take to help verify its conclusion? Do I need such extra tests to re-verify?

Resources

BOOKS

Baer, Lee, and Mark A. Blais, eds. *Handbook of Clinical Rating Scales and Assessment in Psychiatry and Mental Health.* New York: Humana Press, 2010.

Boyer, Bret A., and M. Indira Paharia. *Comprehensive Handbook of Clinical Health Psychology.* Hoboken, NJ: John Wiley & Sons, 2008.

Maruish, Mark R., ed. *The Use of Psychological Testing for Treatment Planning and Outcomes Assessment.* Mahwah, NJ: Lawrence Erlbaum Associates, 2004.

Rush Jr., A. John, Michael B. First, and Deborah Blacker, eds. *Handbook of Psychiatric Measures.* Washington, DC: American Psychiatric, 2008.

OTHER

"Hamilton Anxiety Test (HAM-A)." Assessment Psychology Online. http://www.assessmentpsychology.com/HAM-A.pdf (accessed December 6, 2010).

WEBSITES

"Hamilton Anxiety Scale (HAMA)—IVR Version." Healthcare Technology Systems. http://www.healthtechsys.com/ivr/assess/ivrhama.html (accessed December 6, 2010).

Ali Fahmy, PhD
Emily Jane Willingham, PhD

Hamilton Depression Scale

Definition

The Hamilton Depression Scale (HDS, HAMD, or HAM-D) is a multiple-choice questionnaire test measuring the severity, and the change, of depressive symptoms in individuals, often those who have already been diagnosed as having a depressive disorder. HDS was originally developed by German-born-British **psychologist** Max Hamilton (1912–1988) in 1960, and revised in 1967, 1969, and 1980. It is sometimes known as the Hamilton Rating Scale for Depression (HRSD) or the Hamilton Depression Rating Scale (HDRS). The test is composed of questions that relate to symptoms common to **depression** such as anxiety, **insomnia**, mood, agitation, and weight loss. The HDS is considered one of the most common clinician-administered tests used to rate the severity of depression and its symptoms. The test takes from 20 to 30 minutes to administer.

Purpose

The HDS is used to assess the severity of depressive symptoms present in both children and adults. It is often used as an outcome measure of depression in evaluations of antidepressant psychotropic medications and is a standard measure of depression used in research of the effectiveness of depression therapies and treatments. It can be administered prior to medication being started and then again during follow-up visits, so that medication dosage can be changed in part based on the patient's test score. The HDS is often used as the standard against which other measures of depression are validated. There is a computerized version available intended for administration by telephone using a voice-recognition system and a computerized "interviewer."

The HDS was developed as a measure of depressive symptoms that could be used in conjunction with clinical interviews with depressed in-hospital patients. Hamilton also designed the Hamilton Depression Inventory (HDI), a self-report measure for adults consistent with his theoretical formulation of depression in the HDS, and the **Hamilton Anxiety Scale** (HAS), an interviewer-rated test measuring the severity of anxiety symptoms.

Description

Depending on the version used, an interviewer can provide ratings for a test with 17 items ($HDRS_{17}$) or 24 items ($HDRS_{24}$). In addition to the items on the 17-item scale, the 24-item scale addresses daytime-only symptoms, helplessness, hopelessness, worthlessness, obsessional symptoms, and paranoid feelings. A 21-item version ($HDRS_{21}$) has also been used for evaluations. Along with the patient interview answers, other information can be used in formulating ratings, such as information gathered from family, friends, and patient records. Hamilton devised the test as an easy-going interview process by keeping its questions informal and general.

Examples of items for which interviewers must give ratings include overall depression, guilt, **suicide**, insomnia, problems related to work, psychomotor disabilities, agitation, anxiety, gastrointestinal and other physical symptoms, loss of libido, **hypochondriasis**, loss of insight, and loss of weight. For the overall rating of depression, for example, Hamilton believed one should look for feelings of hopelessness and gloominess, pessimism regarding the future, and a tendency to cry. For the rating of suicide, an interviewer should look for suicidal ideas and thoughts, as well as information regarding suicide attempts.

For the 17 item HDRS, the following items are included:

- depressed mood (such feelings as helplessness, hopelessness, sadness, worthlessness)
- feelings of guilt
- suicide
- insomnia: early in the night
- insomnia: middle of the night
- insomnia: early in the morning
- work and activities
- intellectual disabilities (such as slowness of thinking and talking, degraded ability to concentrate, decreased motor activity)
- agitation
- anxiety psychic
- anxiety somatic (physiological concomitants of anxiety)—gastrointestinal (dry mouth, gas, indigestion, diarrhea, cramps, belching), cardiovascular (palpitations, headaches), respiratory (hyperventilation, sighing), urinary frequency, sweating
- somatic symptoms—gastrointestinal
- general somatic symptoms
- genital symptoms (such as loss of libido, menstrual disturbances)
- hypochondriasis
- loss of weight
- insight

Hamilton Depression Rating Scale (HDRS)

1 Depressed mood (*sadness, hopeless, helpless, worthless*)

0 Absent.
1 These feeling states indicated only on questioning.
2 These feeling states spontaneously reported verbally.
3 Communicates feeling states nonverbally (e.g., through facial expression, posture, voice and tendency to weep).
4 Patient reports virtually only these feeling states in his/her spontaneous verbal and nonverbal communication.

2 Feelings of guilt

0 Absent.
1 Self reproach, feels he/she has let people down.
2 Ideas of guilt or rumination over past errors or sinful deeds.
3 Present illness is a punishment. Delusions of guilt.
4 Hears accusatory or denunciatory voices and/or experiences threatening visual hallucinations.

3 Suicide

0 Absent.
1 Feels life is not worth living.
2 Wishes he/she were dead or any thoughts of possible death to self.
3 Ideas or gestures of suicide.
4 Attempts at suicide (any serious attempt rate 4).

4 Insomnia: Early in the night

0 No difficulty falling asleep.
1 Complains of occasional difficulty falling asleep (e.g., more than 1/2 hour).
2 Complains of nightly difficulty falling asleep.

5 Insomnia: Middle of the night

0 No difficulty.
1 Patient complains of being restless and disturbed during the night.
2 Waking during the night—any getting out of bed rates 2 (except for purposes of voiding).

6 Insomnia: Early hours of the morning

0 No difficulty.
1 Waking in early hours of the morning but goes back to sleep.
2 Unable to fall asleep again if he/she gets out of bed.

7 Work and activities

0 No difficulty.
1 Thoughts and feelings of incapacity, fatigue or weakness related to activities, work or hobbies.
2 Loss of interest in activity, hobbies or work—either directly reported by the patient or indirect in listlessness, indecision and vacillation (feels he/she has to push self to work or activities).
3 Decrease in actual time spent in activities or decrease in productivity. Rate 3 if the patient does not spend at least three hours a day in activities (job or hobbies) excluding routine chores.
4 Stopped working because of present illness. Rate 4 if patient engages in no activities except routine chores, or if patient fails to perform routine chores unassisted.

8 Retardation (slowness of thought and speech, impaired ability to concentrate, decreased motor activity)

0 Normal speech and thought
1 Slight retardation during the interview.
2 Obvious retardation during the interview.
3 Interview difficult.
4 Complete stupor.

9 Agitation

0 None.
1 Fidgetiness.
2 Playing with hands, hair, etc.
3 Moving about, can't sit still.
4 Hand wringing, nail biting, hair-pulling, biting of lips.

10 Anxiety psychic

0 No difficulty.
1 Subjective tension and irritability.
2 Worrying about minor matters.
3 Apprehensive attitude apparent in face or speech.
4 Fears expressed without questioning.

11 Anxiety somatic (physiological concomitants of anxiety) such as: gastrointestinal (dry mouth, wind, indigestion, diarrhea, cramps, belching), cardiovascular (palpitations, headaches), respiratory (hyperventilation, sighing), urinary frequency, sweating

0 Absent.
1 Mild.
2 Moderate.
3 Severe.
4 Incapacitating.

12 Somatic symptoms gastrointestinal

0 None.
1 Loss of appetite but eating without staff encouragement. Heavy feelings in abdomen.
2 Difficulty eating without staff urging. Requests or requires laxatives or medication for bowels or medication for gastrointestinal symptoms.

13 General somatic symptoms

0 None.
1 Heaviness in limbs, back or head. Backaches, headaches, muscle aches. Loss of energy and fatigability.
2 Any clear-cut symptom rates 2.

14 Genital symptoms (symptoms such as loss of libido, menstrual disturbances)

0 Absent.
1 Mild.
2 Severe.

15 Hypochondriasis

0 Not present.
1 Self-absorption (bodily).
2 Preoccupation with health.
3 Frequent complaints, requests for help, etc.
4 Hypochondriacal delusions.

16 Loss of weight (***rate either a or b***)

a) According to the patient:	**b) According to weekly measurements:**
0 No weight loss.	0 Less than 1 lb weight loss in week.
1 Probable weight loss associated with present illness.	1 Greater than 1 lb weight loss in week.
2 Definite (according to patient) weight loss.	2 Greater than 2 lb weight loss in week.
3 Not assessed.	3 Not assessed.

17 Insight

0 Acknowledges being depressed and ill.
1 Acknowledges illness but attributes cause to bad food, climate, overwork, virus, need for rest, etc.
2 Denies being ill at all.

(Table by PreMediaGlobal. © 2012 Cengage Learning.)

For the 17 items, a "cue" is provided with a position of 0 through 2, 0 through 3, or 0 through 4, depending on the individual cue. For instance, for the item called agitation, 0 represents none; 1, fidgetiness; 2, playing with hands, hair; 3, moving about, unable to sit still; and 4, hand wringing, nail biting, hair-pulling, lip biting. The administrator chooses the cue that best represents the state of the person. Scoring varies depending on the number of items present. For the HDRS17, a score from 0 to 7 indicates a normal range, while a score of 20 or higher indicates at least moderate severity for depression.

The HDS has also been translated into numerous languages, including French, German, Italian, Thai, and Turkish. In addition, an Interactive Voice Response version (IVR) is also available, as is a **Seasonal Affective Disorder** version (SIGH-SAD) and a Structured Interview Version (HDS-SIV). Various lengths, besides the three already mentioned, are also available including HDRS-6 (6 items), HDRS-7 (7 items), HDRS-8 (8 items), and HDRS-29 (29 items),

The HDS is sometimes used in parallel with the one or more of the following tests: the **Beck Depression Inventory**, the Inventory of Depressive Symptomatology, the Montgomery-Asberg Depression Rating Scale, the Raskin Depression Rating Scale, the Quick Inventory of Depressive Symptomatology the Wechsler Depression Rating Scale, and the Zung Self-Rating Depression Scale.

KEY TERMS

Depression—A psychiatric disorder involving feelings of hopelessness and symptoms of fatigue, sleeplessness, suicidal tendencies, and poor concentration.

Hypochondriasis—Also called hypochondria, an excessive preoccupation with health, especially with having an impression of having a serious disease without any medical evidence.

Libido—Emotions relating to sex drive.

Psychic—Relating to the mind rather than the body.

Somatic—Relating to the body, rather than the mind.

Preparation

It is not necessary to prepare for the HDS, nor is any preparation required of medical professionals.

Risks

The test has been criticized on the grounds that it does not adequately identify depression. However, it remains one of the most widely used tests for depression.

Precautions

Some symptoms related to depression, such as self-esteem and self-deprecation, are not explicitly included in the HDS items. Also, because anxiety is specifically asked about on the HDS, it is not always possible to separate symptoms related to anxiety from symptoms related to depression.

Because the HDS is administered and rated by the interviewer, there is some subjectivity when it comes to interpretation and scoring. Interviewer bias can affect the results. For this reason, some people prefer self-report measures where scores are completely based on the interviewee's responses.

Results

In the 17-item version, which is most commonly used, nine of the items are scored on a five-point scale, ranging from zero to four. A score of zero represents an absence of the depressive symptom being measured, a score of one indicates doubt concerning the presence of the symptom, a score of two shows mild to moderate symptoms, a score of three describes moderate to severe symptoms, and a score of four represents the presence of extreme symptoms. The remaining seven items are scored on a three-point scale, from zero to two, with zero representing absence of symptom, one indicating that the symptom is present to a mild or moderate degree, and two showing clear presence of symptoms; while the last item is scored on a two-point scale, with zero representing absence of symptom, one indicating that the symptom is mild, and two showing that it is severe.

For the 17-item version, scores can range from 0 to 54. One formulation suggests that scores between zero and six indicate a person who is typical and lacks morbidity with regard to depression; scores between seven and 17 indicate mild depression; scores between 18 and 24 indicate moderate depression; and scores over 24 indicate severe depression.

There has been evidence to support the reliability and validity of the HDS. The scale correlates highly with other clinician-rated and self-report measures of depression.

Resources

BOOKS

Baer, Lee, and Mark A. Blais, editors. *Handbook of Clinical Rating Scales and Assessment in Psychiatry and Mental Health.* New York: Humana Press, 2010.

QUESTIONS TO ASK YOUR DOCTOR

- Do I need to find an administrator who is knowledgeable at administering the Hamilton Depression Scale? If so, do you have recommendations?
- Can I take the test in any other format than with an interviewer?
- Will the HDS tell me what type of medicine I need (if any), and the amount I will need to take?
- Where can I learn more about the HDS?
- Are there other tests that I can take to help verify its conclusion? Do I need such extra tests to re-verify? Which ones do you recommend for me?

Boyer, Bret A., and M. Indira Paharia. *Comprehensive Handbook of Clinical Health Psychology.* Hoboken, NJ: John Wiley & Sons, 2008.

Maruish, Mark R., ed. *The Use of Psychological Testing for Treatment Planning and Outcomes Assessment.* Mahwah, NJ: Lawrence Erlbaum Associates, 2004.

Nezu, Arthur, George F. Ronan, and Elizabeth A. Meadows, eds. *Practitioner's Guide to Empirically Based Measures of Depression.* New York City: Springer Publishing Company, 2006.

Rush Jr., A. John, Michael B. First, and Deborah Blacker, eds. *Handbook of Psychiatric Measures.* Washington, DC: American Psychiatric, 2008.

VandenBos, Gary R., ed. *APA Dictionary of Psychology.* Washington, DC: American Psychological Association, 2007.

OTHER

"Description of the Hamilton Depression Rating Scale (HAMD) and the Montgomery-Asberg Depression Rating Scale (MADRS)." U.S. Food and Drug Administration. http://www.fda.gov/ohrms/dockets/AC/07/briefing/2007-4273b1_04-DescriptionofMADRSHAMDDepressionR(1).pdf (accessed December 7, 2010).

"Hamilton Depression Rating Scale For Depression." UMass Health Net, University of Massachusetts Medical Center. http://healthnet.umassmed.edu/mhealth/HAMD.pdf (accessed December 7, 2010).

"Hamilton Depression Rating Scale (HDRS)." Servier. http://www.servier.com/App_Download/Neurosciences/Echelles/HDRS.pdf (accessed December 7, 2010).

Ali Fahmy, PhD
Emily Jane Willingham, PhD

Hare Psychopathy Checklist

Definition

The Hare Psychopathy Checklist-Revised (PCL-R) is a psychodiagnostic tool used to rate a person's psychopathic or antisocial tendencies. Psychopaths are people who prey ruthlessly on others using charm, deceit, violence or other methods that allow them to get what they want. The symptoms of psychopathy include lack of a conscience or sense of guilt, lack of empathy; egocentricity, pathological lying, repeated violations of social norms, disregard for the law, shallow emotions, and a history of victimizing others. It also predicts the potential risk for repeat criminal offenders and, on the other hand, the probability for rehabilitation.

Purpose

The PCL-R is used for diagnosing psychopathy in individuals for clinical, legal or research purposes. Developed in the early 1990s, the test was originally designed to identify the degree of a person's psychopathic tendencies. Because psychopaths, however, are often repeat offenders who commit sexual assaults or other violent crimes again and again, the PCL-R is now finding use in the courtroom and in institutions as an indicator of the potential risk posed by subjects or prisoners. The results of the examination have been used in forensic settings as a factor in deciding the length and type of prison sentences and the treatment subjects should or should not receive.

Originally designed to assess people accused or convicted of crimes, the PCL-R consists of a 20-item symptom rating scale that allows qualified examiners to compare a subject's degree of psychopathy with that of a prototypical psychopath. It is accepted by many in the field as the best method for determining the presence and extent of psychopathy in a person.

The Hare checklist is still used to diagnose members of the original population for which it was developed—adult males in prisons, criminal psychiatric hospitals, and awaiting psychiatric evaluations or trial in other correctional and detention facilities. Recent experience suggests that the PCL-R may also be used effectively to diagnose sex offenders as well as female and adolescent offenders.

Description

The Psychopathy Checklist (PCL) and the Psychopathy Checklist Revised were both developed by Canadian researcher and criminal **psychologist** Robert D. Hare (1934–), who is a professor emeritus of the University of British Columbia. The PCL-R contains two parts, a semi-structured interview and a review of the subject's file records and history. During the evaluation, the clinician, usually a psychologist or other such professional, scores 20 items that measure central elements of the psychopathic character. The items cover the nature of the subject's interpersonal relationships; his or her affective or emotional involvement; responses to other people and to situations; evidence of social deviance; and lifestyle. The material thus covers two key aspects that help define the psychopath: selfish and unfeeling victimization of other people, and an unstable and antisocial lifestyle.

The twenty traits assessed by the PCL-R score are:

- glib and superficial charm
- grandiose (exaggeratedly high) estimation of self
- need for stimulation
- pathological lying
- cunning and manipulativeness
- lack of remorse or guilt
- shallow affect (superficial emotional responsiveness)
- callousness and lack of empathy
- parasitic lifestyle
- poor behavioral controls
- sexual promiscuity
- early behavior problems
- lack of realistic long-term goals
- impulsivity
- irresponsibility
- failure to accept responsibility for own actions
- many short-term marital relationships
- juvenile delinquency
- revocation of conditional release
- criminal versatility

The interview portion of the evaluation covers the subject's background, including such items as work and educational history, marital and family status, and criminal background. Because psychopaths lie frequently and easily, the information they provide must be confirmed by a review of the documents in the subject's case history.

The PCL-R (1991 edition) is available in many languages, including Bulgarian, Dutch, Finnish, French, German, Korean, Portuguese (Brazilian), and Spanish (Chilean and European). The PCL-R (second edition) is available in Hebrew, Japanese, and Swedish.

KEY TERMS

Psychopath—A person inflicted with psychopathy.

Psychopathy—A serious personality disorder characterized by antisocial, aggressive, and violent behavior and thoughts, along with a lack of empathy for ones actions.

Preparation

Preparation is not desired nor recommended.

Risks

Dr. Hare considers the results of the test to be highly dependent on the skill of a qualified and experienced clinician. Therefore, Hare requires that the test be tightly controlled, with proper licensing. The administrator is required to be registered with the local state or provincial registration body and have experience with forensic populations. Consequently, Hare receives a royalty on each use of the test. However, under such tight conditions, the results of the test are regarded as highly reliable.

Precautions

Diagnosing someone as a psychopath is a very serious step. It has important implications for a person and for his or her associates in family, clinical, and forensic settings. Therefore, the test must be administered by professionals who have been specifically trained in its use and who have a wide-ranging and up-to-date familiarity with studies of psychopathy.

Professionals who administer the diagnostic examination should have advanced degrees (medical doctor [MD], doctor of philosophy [PhD], or doctor of education [DEd] in a medical, behavioral, or social science field); and registered with a reputable organization that oversees psychiatric or psychological testing and diagnostic procedures. Other recommendations include experience working with convicted or accused criminals or several years of some other related on-the-job training. Because the results are used so often in legal cases, those who administer the test should be qualified to serve as expert witnesses in the courtroom. It is also a good idea, if possible, for two experts to independently test a subject with the PCL-R. The final rating would then be determined by averaging their scores.

Many studies conducted in North America and Europe attest to the value of the PCL-R for evaluating a person's degree of psychopathic traits and, in many cases, for predicting the likelihood of future violent behavior. Some critics, however, are more skeptical about its value.

QUESTIONS TO ASK YOUR DOCTOR

- Will the PCL-R be able to accurately identify psychopathy?
- Do you know a trained and qualified professional to administer the PCL-R?
- Should a second test by another administrator be used to verify the result?

Results

When properly completed by a qualified professional, the PCL-R provides a total score that indicates how closely the test subject matches the "perfect" score that a classic or prototypical psychopath would rate. Each of the twenty items is given a score of 0 (does not apply), 1 (applies somewhat), or 2 (completely applies) based on how well it applies to the subject being tested. A prototypical psychopath would receive a maximum score of 40, while someone with a complete absence of psychopathic traits or tendencies would receive a score of zero. A score of 30 or above qualifies a person for a **diagnosis** of psychopathy. People without criminal backgrounds normally score around 5. Many non-psychopathic criminal offenders score around 22.

The PCL-R has a demonstrated record of reliability and validity among researchers and clinicians. In 2007, a legal controversy arose between two researchers and the PCL-R developer when a paper was about to be published by the **American Psychological Association** concerning the PCL-R.

Three years later, *The New York Times* reported that American researcher Jennifer L. Skeem, from the University of California, Irvine, and Scottish researcher David J. Cooke, from Glasgow Caledonian University, stated the "… checklist was increasingly being mistaken for a complete definition of psychopathy—a broader personality construct that includes deceitfulness, impulsivity and recklessness, though not always aggression or illegal acts." Dr. Hare countered that the test emphasizes "problematic, not antisocial or criminal, behavior."

The paper was published in the June 2010 issue of the journal *Psychological Assessment,* along with a rebuttal from Dr. Hare and a return response from Drs. Skeem and Cooke. The PCL-R is considered by the international scientific community to be one of several forensic psychology tests used for the assessment of psychopathy.

See also Antisocial personality disorder; Sexual sadism

Resources

BOOKS

Babiak, Paul, and Robert D. Hare. *Snakes in Suits: When Psychopaths Go to Work.* New York: Collins Business, 2007.

Fitzgerald, Michael. *Young, Violent and Dangerous to Know.* New York: Nova Science, 2010.

Kantor, Martin. *The Psychopathy of Everyday Life: How Antisocial Personality Disorder Affects All of Us.* Westport, CT: Praeger Publishers, 2006.

Simon, Robert I. *Bad Men Do What Good Men Dream: A Forensic Psychiatrist Illuminates the Darker Side of Human Behavior.* Washington, DC: American Psychiatric, 2008.

Stout, Martha. *The Sociopath Next Door: The Ruthless Versus the Rest of Us.* New York: Broadway Books, 2006.

PERIODICALS

Carey, Benedict. "Academic Battle Delays Publication by 3 Years." *New York Times*, June 11, 2010. http://www.nytimes.com/2010/06/12/health/12psych.html?_r=1 (accessed December 7, 2011).

WEBSITES

"Dr. Robert Hare's Page for the Study of Psychopaths." Hare, Robert D. http://www.hare.org (accessed December 7, 2010).

"Is Criminal Behavior a Central Component of Psychopathy? Conceptual Directions for Resolving the Debate." J.L. Skeem and D.J. Cooke, NCBI. http://www.ncbi.nlm.nih.gov/pubmed/20528069 (accessed December 12, 2010).

"PCL—R™: 2nd Ed. Hare Psychopathy Checklist—Revised: 2nd Edition." Multi-Health Systems. http://www.mhs.com/product.aspx?gr=saf&prod=pcl-r2&id=overview (accessed December 7, 2010).

"Psychopathy Scales: PCL-R." Hare.org. http://www.hare.org/scales/pclr.html (accessed December 7, 2010).

Dean Haycock, PhD

HCR-20 *see* **Historical, Clinical, Risk Management-20**

Health maintenance organization *see* **Managed care**

Historical, Clinical, Risk Management-20 (HCR-20)

Definition

The Historical, Clinical, Risk Management-20 (HCR-20) is an assessment tool that helps mental health professionals estimate a person's probability of violence. It is frequently used in such areas as civil psychiatric, forensic psychiatric, and prison institutional and community settings. The HCR-20 is considered a type of a Structured Professional Judgment (SPJ) risk assessment instrument. The current version of the HCR-20 is version 2. As of December 2011, version 3 was considered "near final," but additional information on its publication was not available. The HCR-20 (version 2) is authored by Christopher D. Webster, Kevin S. Douglas, Derek Eaves, and Stephen D. Hart.

Purpose

The HCR-20's results help mental health professionals make structured clinical decisions about the best treatment and management strategies for potentially violent, mentally disordered individuals, including parolees, forensic mental health patients, and others. For example, if an individual is standing trial for a violent offense, a judge might order that assessments (such as the HCR-20, as well as others) be performed. The results of the evaluation could be used to determine the person's future potential for violence, how the court should proceed, and which kind of facility the person might require. As such, the HCR-20 helps to formulate treatment and management strategies that reduce the risk of violent behaviors in such individuals.

Description

The HCR-20 is an assessment tool. It consists of a list of 20 probing questions about the person being evaluated for violence. The clinician gathers qualitative information about the person being assessed, guided by the HCR-20, and the results are used to make treatment decisions.

The HCR-20 provides significantly improved valid predictions over previous testing methods. Earlier testing methods tended to be more subjective, less focused, and based on the loosely supported judgment of test administrators, or on comparing characteristics of the person being tested with base rates of violent behavior in populations with similar characteristics. The HCR-20 extends the methods of earlier tests and supplements them with a review of dynamic variables, such as **stress** and lack of personal support—both factors important to the person's future adjustment. This review adds to the accuracy of the HCR-20 and increases its practicality.

Available in more than a dozen languages, the HCR-20 has been adopted by numerous criminal justice, forensic, and mental health agencies in Europe, Asia, and North America for the purpose of providing risk assessment and management decisions.

The HCR-20 consists of three main areas: historical, clinical, and risk management. It takes its name (HCR-20) from these three scales and the total number of items (20). The HCR-20 domains are coded with a rating of 0 (not present), 1 (possible/less serious), or 3 (definite/serious).

Historical area

To rate historical areas, the test administrator must do an exhaustive review of background documents, interview people who know the person being assessed, and complete the **Hare Psychopathy Checklist**, another useful assessment. The historical (H) area is considered by many to anchor the full assessment. It includes ten domains or scales (H1 through H10):

- previous violence (H1)
- young age at first violent incident (H2)
- relationship instability (H3)
- employment problems (H4)
- substance use problems (H5)
- major mental illness (H6), such as schizophrenia or bipolar disorder
- psychopathy (H7), which can be defined as personality traits that deviate from social norms, such as manipulating and exploiting others for personal gain
- early maladjustment (H8), or exposure to family and social disruptions during childhood that may have led to coping problems (e.g., abuse, divorce)
- personality disorder (H9), such as paranoia
- prior supervision failure (H10), such as failure to respond to clinical supervision or treatment in the past or refusal to take medications or attend therapy sessions (noncompliance)

Clinical area

The rating of the clinical area requires a clinical interview between the person being assessed and the mental health professional. The professional will apply his or her judgment to the patient's responses. The clinical area (C) consists of five domains or scales (C1 through C5):

- lack of insight (C1), or difficulty understanding cause and effect; for example, people with poor insight might not understand why they do what they do and why their actions matter
- negative attitudes (C2)
- active symptoms of major mental illness (C3)
- impulsivity (C4)
- unresponsiveness to treatment (C5)

KEY TERMS

Psychopath—A person inflicted with psychopathy.

Psychopathy—A serious personality disorder characterized by antisocial, aggressive, and violent behavior and thoughts, along with a lack of empathy for one's actions.

Risk management

The third area, risk management (R), includes five domains or scales (R1 through R5) and assesses the following risks:

- [the person's] plans lack feasibility (R1)
- exposure to destabilizers (R2); family or social supports are missing, or alcohol and drugs are available
- lack of personal support (R3)
- noncompliance with remediation attempts (R4); refusal to attend counseling sessions or take medications
- stress (R5)

Preparation

Preparation is not desired nor recommended by medical professionals.

Precautions

When possible, the test administrator should use supplemental test measures and investigate any unique patterns of violence and its triggers in the person's history. The HCR-20 is not meant to be administered just once; the nature of risk assessment requires ongoing reassessment as circumstances change. Final interpretation of HCR-20 results should be in the context of several factors, including the reason for the person's test referral, base rates of violence in populations with similar characteristics, and assessment of future risks in the person's environment.

A professional trained in conducting individual assessments and in the study of violence should administer the HCR-20. The test administrator should have a background in using assessment tests or should consult a mental health professional. The HCR-20 is not intended to be a stand-alone measure, and it does not cover all risk factors.

Results

The HCR-20 does not allow for a definite prediction of violence. Predictions based on the HCR-20 are estimates of the likelihood of violence and should be presented in terms of low, moderate, or high probability of violence. Probability levels should be considered conditional, given short- and long-term time frames, and should be considered in relation to any relevant factors the individual may encounter. These factors include situations and states of being that may dispose a person to violence or help insulate them against it. Consideration of such factors can aid in reporting the type and extent of risk presented by a person and in selecting **intervention** strategies intended to reduce the probability that an individual will demonstrate violence. These strategies when taken as a whole are called a risk management plan.

Ultimately, HCR-20 results are intended to provide information for decision-makers, so that criminal and mental health–related decisions can be based on the best available estimates of risk of violence. Drs. Kevin Douglas and Laura Guy, both from Simon Fraser University, state, "... the HCR-20 is an attempt to merge science and practice by offering an instrument that can be integrated into clinical practice but also is empirically based and testable."

Resources

BOOKS

Webster, Christopher et. al. *HCR-20: Assessing Risk for Violence, Version 2*. Burnaby, British Columbia, Canada: Mental Health, Law, and Policy Institute, Simon Fraser University, 1997.

OTHER

Douglas, Kevin S., and Laura S. Guy. HCR-20 Violence Risk Assessment Scheme: Overview and Annotated Bibliography. January 12, 2006. http://www.cvp.se/publications/downloadables/hcr-20-bibliography-12jan2005.pdf (accessed October 8, 2011).

WEBSITES

Douglas, Kevin S., LLB, PhD. "HCR-20" http://kdouglas.wordpress.com/hcr-20 (accessed October 8, 2011).

Geoffrey G. Grimm, PhD, LPC

Histrionic personality disorder

Definition

Histrionic personality disorder, often abbreviated as HPD, is a type of personality disorder in which affected individuals display enduring patterns of attention-seeking and excessively dramatic behaviors beginning in early adulthood and present across a broad range of situations.

Individuals with HPD are highly emotional, charming, energetic, manipulative, seductive, impulsive, erratic, and demanding.

Mental health professionals use the ***Diagnostic and Statistical Manual of Mental Disorders*** (*DSM*) to diagnose mental disorders. The 2000 edition of this manual (the fourth edition, text revision, also called the *DSM-IV-TR*) classifies HPD as a personality disorder. More specifically, HPD is classified as a Cluster B (dramatic, emotional, or erratic) personality disorder. Cluster B includes the histrionic, antisocial, borderline, and narcissistic **personality disorders**.

Demographics

General United States population

The prevalence of HPD in the general population is estimated to be approximately 2%-3%.

High-risk populations

Individuals who have experienced pervasive **trauma** during childhood have been shown to be at a greater risk for developing HPD as well as for developing other personality disorders.

Cross-cultural issues

HPD may be diagnosed more frequently in Hispanic and Latin American cultures and less frequently in Asian cultures. Further research is needed on the effects of culture on the symptoms of HPD.

Gender issues

Clinicians tend to diagnose HPD more frequently in females; however, when structured assessments are used to diagnose HPD, clinicians report approximately equal prevalence rates for men and women. In considering the prevalence of HPD, it is important to recognize that gender role stereotypes may influence the behavioral display of HPD and that women and men may display HPD symptoms differently.

Diagnosis

The **diagnosis** of HPD is complicated because it may seem like many other disorders, and also because it commonly occurs simultaneously with other personality disorders. The 1994 version of the *DSM* introduced the criterion of suggestibility and the criterion of overestimation of intimacy in relationships to further refine the diagnostic criteria set of HPD, so that it could be more easily recognizable. Prior to assigning a diagnosis of HPD, clinicians need to evaluate whether the traits evident of HPD cause significant distress. (The *DSM-IV-TR* requires that the symptoms cause significant distress in order to be considered a disorder.) The diagnosis of HPD is frequently made on the basis of an individual's history and results from unstructured and semistructured interviews.

Time of onset/symptom duration

Some psychoanalysts propose that the determinants of HPD date back to early childhood. The pattern of craving attention and displaying dramatic behavior for individuals with HPD begins by early adulthood. Symptoms can last a lifetime, but may decrease or change their form with age.

Individual variations in HPD

Some classification systems distinguish between different types of individuals with HPD: patients with appeasing HPD and patients with disingenuous HPD. Individuals with appeasing HPD have personalities with histrionic, dependent, and obsessive-compulsive components. Individuals with disingenuous HPD possess personality traits that are classified as histrionic and antisocial. Studies have shown that relationships exist between somatic behaviors and women with HPD and between antisocial behaviors and men with HPD.

Dual diagnoses

HPD has been associated with alcoholism and with higher rates of **somatization disorder**, **conversion disorder**, and **major depressive disorder**. Personality disorders such as borderline, narcissistic, antisocial, and dependent can occur with HPD.

Differential diagnosis

Differential diagnosis is the process of distinguishing one mental disorder from other similar disorders. For example, at times, it is difficult to distinguish between HPD and **borderline personality disorder**. **Suicide** attempts, identity diffusion, and numerous chaotic relationships occur less frequently, however, with people diagnosed with HPD. Another example of overlap can occur between people with HPD and **dependent personality disorder**. Patients with HPD and dependent personality disorder share high dependency needs, but only dependent personality disorder is linked to high levels of self-attributed dependency needs. Whereas patients with HPD tend to be active and seductive, individuals with dependent personality disorder tend to be subservient in their demeanor.

Psychological measures

Self-report inventories and projective tests can also be used to help clinicians diagnose HPD. The Minnesota

Multiphasic Personality Inventory-2 (MMPI-2) and the Millon Clinical Multiaxial Inventory-III (MCMI-III) are self-report inventories with extensive empirical support. Results of intelligence examinations for individuals with HPD may indicate a lack of perseverance on arithmetic or on tasks that require concentration.

Description

HPD has a unique position among the personality disorders because it is the only one explicitly connected to a patient's physical appearance. Researchers have found that HPD appears primarily in men and women with above-average physical appearances. Some research has suggested that the connection between HPD and physical appearance holds for women rather than for men. Both women and men with HPD express a strong need to be the center of attention. Individuals with HPD exaggerate, throw temper tantrums, and cry if they are not the center of attention. Patients with HPD are naive and gullible and have a low frustration threshold and strong dependency needs.

Cognitive style can be defined as a way in which individuals work with and solve cognitive tasks such as reasoning, learning, thinking, understanding, making decisions, and using memory. The cognitive style of individuals with HPD is superficial and lacks detail. In their interpersonal relationships, individuals with HPD use dramatization with the goal of impressing others. The enduring pattern of their insincere and stormy relationships leads to impairment in social and occupational areas.

Causes and symptoms

Causes

There is a lack of research on the causes of HPD. Even though the causes for the disorder are not definitively known, it is thought that HPD may be caused by biological, developmental, cognitive, and social factors.

NEUROCHEMICAL/PHYSIOLOGICAL CAUSES. Studies show that patients with HPD have highly responsive noradrenergic systems, the mechanisms surrounding the release of a neurotransmitter called norepinephrine. **Neurotransmitters** are chemicals that communicate impulses from one nerve cell to another in the **brain**, and these impulses dictate behavior. The tendency toward an excessively emotional reaction to rejection, common among patients with HPD, may be attributed to a malfunction in a group of neurotransmitters called catecholamines. Norepinephrine belongs to this group of neurotransmitters.

DEVELOPMENTAL CAUSES. Most psychoanalysts agree that a traumatic childhood can contribute to the development of HPD.

Defense mechanisms are sets of systematic, unconscious methods that people develop to cope with conflict and to reduce anxiety. According to Freud, all people use defense mechanisms, but different people use different types of defense mechanisms. Individuals with HPD differ in the severity of the maladaptive defense mechanisms they use. Patients with more severe cases of HPD may use the following defense mechanisms:

- Repression. Repression is the most basic defense mechanism. When patients' thoughts produce anxiety or are unacceptable to them, they use repression to bar the unacceptable thoughts or impulses from consciousness.
- Denial. Patients who use denial may say that a prior problem no longer exists, suggesting that their competence has increased; however, others may note that there is no change in the patients' behaviors.
- Dissociation. When patients with HPD use the defense mechanism of dissociation, they may display two or more personalities. These two or more personalities exist in one individual without integration.

Patients with less severe cases of HPD tend to employ the following defenses:

- Displacement. Displacement occurs when patients shift an affect from one idea to another. For example, a man with HPD may feel angry at work because the boss did not consider him to be the center of attention. The patient may displace his anger onto his wife rather than becoming angry with his boss.
- Rationalization. Rationalization occurs when individuals explain their behaviors so that they appear to be acceptable to others.

BIOSOCIAL LEARNING CAUSES. A biosocial model in psychology asserts that social and biological factors contribute to the development of personality. Biosocial learning models of HPD suggest that individuals may acquire HPD from inconsistent interpersonal **reinforcement** offered by parents. Proponents of biosocial learning models indicate that individuals with HPD have learned to get what they want from others by drawing attention to themselves.

PERSONAL VARIABLES. Researchers have found some connections between the age of individuals with HPD and the behavior displayed by these individuals. The symptoms of HPD are long-lasting; however, histrionic character traits that are exhibited may change with age. For example, research suggests that young adults employ seductiveness more often than older ones. To impress others, older adults with HPD may shift their strategy from sexual seductiveness to a paternal or maternal seductiveness. Some histrionic symptoms such as attention-seeking, however, may become more apparent as individuals with HPD age.

Symptoms

The *DSM-IV-TR* lists eight symptoms that form the diagnostic criteria for HPD:

- Center of attention: Patients with HPD experience discomfort when they are not the center of attention.
- Sexually seductive: Patients with HPD display inappropriate sexually seductive or provocative behaviors toward others.
- Shifting emotions: The expression of emotions of patients with HPD tends to be shallow and to shift rapidly.
- Physical appearance: Individuals with HPD consistently employ physical appearance to gain attention for themselves.
- Speech style: The speech style of patients with HPD lacks detail. Individuals with HPD tend to generalize, and when these individuals speak, they aim to please and impress.
- Dramatic behaviors: Patients with HPD display self-dramatization and exaggerate their emotions.
- Suggestibility: Other individuals or circumstances can easily influence patients with HPD.
- Overestimation of intimacy: Patients with HPD overestimate the level of intimacy in a relationship.

Treatment

Psychodynamic therapy

HPD, like other personality disorders, may require several years of therapy and may affect individuals throughout their lives. Some professionals believe that psychoanalytic therapy is a treatment of choice for people with HPD because it helps patients become aware of their own feelings. Long-term psychodynamic therapy needs to target the underlying conflicts of individuals with HPD and to assist patients in decreasing their emotional reactivity. Therapists work with thematic material related to intimacy and recall. Individuals with HPD may have difficulty recalling because of their tendency to repress material.

Cognitive-behavioral therapy

Cognitive therapy is a treatment directed at reducing the dysfunctional thoughts of individuals with HPD. Such thoughts include themes about not being able to take care of oneself. Cognitive therapy for people with HPD focuses on a shift from global, suggestible thinking to a more methodical, systematic, and structured focus on problems. Cognitive-behavioral training in relaxation for individuals with HPD emphasizes challenging automatic thoughts about inferiority and not being able to handle one's life. **Cognitive-behavioral therapy** teaches individuals with HPD to identify automatic thoughts, to work on impulsive behavior, and to develop better problem-solving skills. Behavioral therapists employ **assertiveness training** to assist individuals with HPD to learn to cope using their own resources. Behavioral therapists use response cost to decrease the excessively dramatic behaviors of these individuals. Response cost is a behavioral technique that involves removing a stimulus from an individual's environment so that the response that directly precedes the removal is weakened. Behavioral therapy for HPD includes techniques such as **modeling** and behavioral rehearsal to teach patients about the effect of their theatrical behavior on others in a work setting.

Group therapy

Group therapy is suggested to assist individuals with HPD to work on interpersonal relationships. Psychodrama techniques or group role-playing can assist individuals with HPD to practice problems at work and to learn to decrease the display of excessively dramatic behaviors. Using role-playing, individuals with HPD can explore interpersonal relationships and outcomes to understand better the process associated with different scenarios. Group therapists need to monitor the group because individuals with HPD tend to take over and dominate others.

Family therapy

To teach assertion rather than avoidance of conflict, family therapists need to direct individuals with HPD to speak directly to other family members. **Family therapy** can support family members to meet their own needs without supporting the histrionic behavior of the individual with HPD who uses dramatic crises to keep the family closely connected. Family therapists employ behavioral contracts to support assertive behaviors rather than temper tantrums.

Medications

Pharmacotherapy is not a treatment of choice for individuals with HPD unless HPD occurs with another disorder. For example, if HPD occurs with **depression**, **antidepressants** may be prescribed. Medication needs to be monitored for abuse.

Alternative therapies

Meditation has been used to assist extroverted patients with HPD to relax and to focus on their own

KEY TERMS

Behavioral contracts—A behavioral contract is a written agreement that defines the behaviors to be performed and the consequences of the specified behaviors.

Biosocial—A biosocial model in psychology asserts that social and biological factors contribute toward the development of personality.

Catecholamine—A group of neurotransmitters synthesized from the amino acid tyrosine and released by the hypothalamic-pituitary-adrenal system in the brain, in response to acute stress. The catecholamines include dopamine, serotonin, norepinephrine, and epinephrine.

Cognitive style—A way in which individuals work with and perform cognitive tasks such as reasoning, learning, thinking, understanding, making decisions, and using memory.

Differential diagnosis—The process of distinguishing one disorder from other similar disorders.

Disingenuous—Insincere, deceitful, dishonest.

Dissociation—A reaction to trauma in which the mind splits off certain aspects of the traumatic event from conscious awareness. Dissociation can affect the patient's memory, sense of reality, and sense of identity.

Etiology—The cause or origin of a disease or disorder. The word is also used to refer to the study of the causes of disease.

Histrionic—Theatrical.

Identity diffusion—A character formation that is scattered or spread around rather than an identity that becomes solidified or consolidated.

Noradrenergic—Acts similarly to norepinephrine or noradrenaline.

Oral phase—The first of Freud's psychosexual stages of development in which satisfaction is focused on the mouth and lips. During this stage sucking and eating are the primary means of gratification.

Personality disorder—A personality disorder is a maladaptive pattern of behavior, affect, and/or cognitive style displayed in a broad range of settings. The pattern deviates from the accepted norms of the individual's culture and can occur over a lifetime.

Response cost—A behavioral technique that involves removing a stimulus from an individual's environment so that the response that directly precedes the removal is weakened. In a token economy system, response cost is a form of punishment involving loss of tokens due to inappropriate behavior, which consequently results in decreased ability to purchase backup reinforcers.

Somatic—Relating to the body or to the physical.

inner feelings. Some therapists employ hypnosis to assist individuals with HPD to relax when they experience a fast heart rate or palpitations during an expression of excessively dramatic, emotional, and excitable behavior.

Prognosis

The personality characteristics of individuals with HPD are long-lasting. Individuals with HPD use medical services frequently, but they usually do not stay in psychotherapeutic treatment long enough to make changes. They tend to set vague goals and to move toward something more exciting. Treatment for HPD can take a minimum of one to three years and tends to take longer than treatment for disorders that are not personality disorders, such as anxiety or mood disorders. Suicidal tendencies are common in people with HPD and should always be taken seriously.

As individuals with HPD age, they display fewer symptoms. Some research suggests that the difference between older and younger individuals may be attributed to the fact that older individuals have less energy.

Research indicates that a relationship exists between poor treatment outcomes and premature termination from treatment for individuals with Cluster B personality disorders. Some researchers suggest that studies that link HPD to continuation in treatment need to consider the connection between overestimates of intimacy and premature termination from therapy.

Prevention

Early diagnosis can assist patients and family members to recognize the pervasive pattern of reactive emotion among individuals with HPD. Educating people, particularly mental health professionals, about the enduring character traits of individuals with HPD may prevent some cases of mild histrionic behavior from developing into full-blown cases of maladaptive HPD.

Further research in prevention needs to investigate the relationship between variables such as age, gender, culture, and ethnicity in people with HPD.

Resources

BOOKS

American Psychiatric Association. *Diagnostic and Statistical Manual of Mental Disorders*. 4th ed., text rev. Washington, DC: American Psychiatric Publishing, 2000.

Bockian, Neil, and Arthur E. Jongsma, Jr. *The Personality Disorders Treatment Planner*. New York: Wiley, 2001.

Bornstein, Robert F., and Iris L. Malka. "Dependent and Histrionic Personality Disorders." In *Oxford Textbook of Psychopathology*, edited by Theodore Millon and Paul H. Blaney. New York: Oxford University Press, 2008.

Widiger, Thomas A., and Robert F. Bornstein. "Histrionic, Narcissistic, and Dependent Personality Disorders." In *Comprehensive Handbook of Psychopathology,* edited by Patricia B. Sutker and Henry E. Adams. 3rd ed. New York: Springer Science, 2004.

PERIODICALS

Bornstein, Robert F. "Histrionic Personality Disorder, Physical Attractiveness, and Social Adjustment." *Journal of Psychopathology and Behavioral Assessment* 21, no. 1 (March 1999): 79–94.

Bornstein, Robert F. "Implicit and Self-Attributed Dependency Needs in Dependent and Histrionic Personality Disorders." *Journal of Personality Assessment* 71, no. 1 (August 1998): 1–14.

Hilsenroth, Mark J., et al. "The Effects of DSM-IV Cluster B Personality Disorder Symptoms on the Termination and Continuation of Psychotherapy." *Psychotherapy* 35, no. 2 (Summer 1998): 163–76.

ORGANIZATIONS

American Psychiatric Association, 1000 Wilson Blvd., Ste. 1825, Arlington, VA, 22209-3901, (703) 907-7300, apa@psych.org, http://www.psych.org.

American Psychological Association, 750 1st Street NE, Washington, DC, 20002-4242, (202) 336-5500; TDD/TTY: (202) 336-6123, (800) 374-2721, http://www.apa.org.

Judy Koenigsberg, PhD
Emily Jane Willingham, PhD

HMO *see* **Managed care**

Hoarding

Definition

Hoarding is a behavior that leads to the accumulation of objects or pets in the household to the point that the items or animals interfere with daily life and prevent the hoarder's living space from being used for its intended purposes. In some cases, the clutter may pose safety or health hazards. The modern English word *hoard* comes from an Old English or Germanic word meaning "to cover" or "to conceal." Compulsive hoarding is also known as "pathological hoarding" or "disposophobia."

Demographics

Psychiatrists estimate that between 2% and 5% of the adult population in the United States and Canada are compulsive hoarders, with about 4,000 cases of animal hoarding involving up to 250,000 reported animals each year in North America. It is possible that the actual rate of hoarding disorder is higher, as researchers only began to study hoarding in the 1980s, which means that relatively little is known about it in comparison to such disorders as **depression** or **panic disorder**. In addition, many hoarders never seek help for their condition because they do not see it as a problem. Researchers think that hoarding is more prevalent among older adults, although it typically begins in late childhood or adolescence and becomes progressively worse as the person grows older. There are relatively few cases of late-onset hoarding.

There is no indication that race or ethnicity is a factor in hoarding. Women typically begin hoarding at earlier ages than men, but men are more likely than women to become hoarders. With regard to content, clothes, books, and newspapers or magazines are the most commonly hoarded items, but almost any imaginable object can be hoarded. Other commonly hoarded objects include empty boxes and deli containers, junk mail, and craft items.

Description

Hoarding behavior is a combination of three factors: inability to discard unnecessary items, accumulation of a large number of possessions, and difficulty organizing living space. The working group of psychiatrists specializing in **obsessive-compulsive disorder** (OCD) and related disorders for the fifth edition of the ***Diagnostic and Statistical Manual of Mental Disorders*** (*DSM-5*) has proposed adding hoarding disorder to the new edition on the grounds that hoarding differs from OCD in several significant respects, and that inclusion of the disorder would draw greater public awareness.

Hoarding is a complex disorder in that each of the three factors may develop in different ways in different people.

Tendency to accumulate many items:

- Many hoarders are also compulsive shoppers, and may purchase multiples of each item rather than only one.

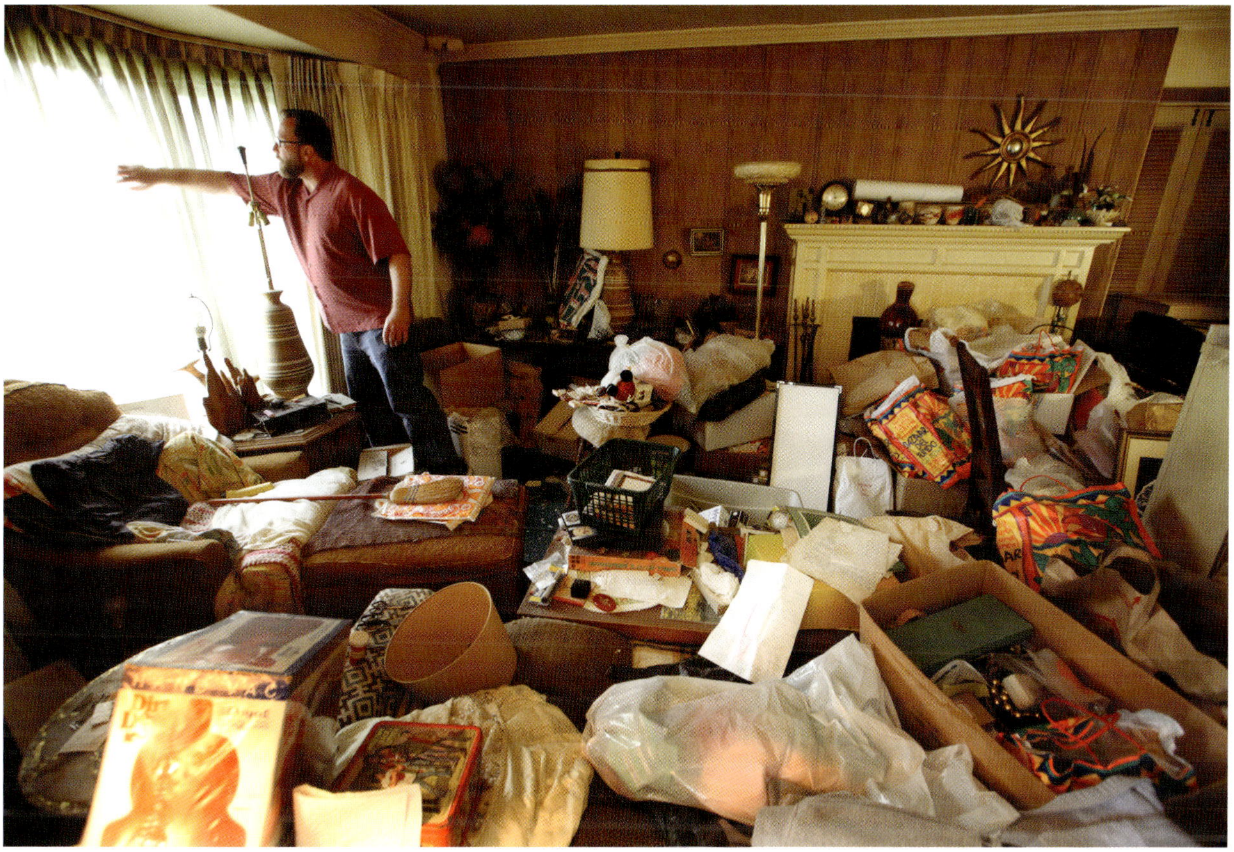

A man prepares to clean out the home of his recently deceased mother, who suffered from hoarding disorder. *(© Sandy Huffaker/Corbis News/Corbis)*

Male hoarders appear to favor such items as hardware, automotive equipment, and electronic gadgets, while women are more likely to purchase jewelry and cosmetics. Both sexes are equally likely to buy clothing, shoes, compact discs, and household items on their shopping sprees.

- About 50% of hoarders report excessive collecting of free items.
- Excessive collecting can also occur without effort, as when the hoarder accumulates boxes or packing material from mail-order purchases.

Difficulty discarding unneeded or useless items:

- Hoarders find it emotionally difficult to throw away, give away, sell, or recycle unused items.
- The most frequent reasons hoarders give for holding on to their possessions are thrift; not wanting to lose the informational content of such items as books, records, magazines; sentimental or emotional attachment to the item; and liking the way the object looks or feels.
- In some cases, the hoarder has tried to clean out the clutter but finds the process so time-consuming that he or she gives up.

Disorganization:

- Many hoarders have difficulty organizing their possessions because they are easily distracted or have problems with information processing (classifying their possessions in order to create and organize storage spaces for them).
- It is not uncommon for hoarders simply to move piles of items from one location to another without effective reorganization.

Researchers who have studied hoarding note that it is different from collecting items of interest to an individual or having some clutter in the home. Collectors usually keep their valued items well organized and often group them in attractive or informative arrangements that others with the same hobby or interest can enjoy. By contrast, hoarders rarely organize their acquisitions. With regard to clutter, having a desk, attic, basement, closet, or other limited part of the house that is cluttered is not by itself evidence of hoarding. It is when the clutter results from excessive acquisition and refusal to discard items, overflows into all living areas, blocks exits, and otherwise interferes with daily activities that it becomes a sign of hoarding.

Hoarding associated with obsessive-compulsive disorder

When hoarding first became a topic of interest to psychiatrists in the 1980s, it was thought to be a subtype of obsessive-compulsive disorder (OCD), an anxiety disorder characterized by intrusive thoughts that produce anxiety (obsessions) accompanied by repetitive behaviors intended to relieve the anxiety (compulsions). Many psychiatrists maintain, however, that most cases of hoarding are not associated with OCD, because the hoarder shows no signs of anxiety and genuinely enjoys his or her possessions. Unlike people with OCD, who recognize that their obsessions and compulsions are abnormal, most hoarders consider their behavior normal and acceptable. The minority of hoarding cases identified with OCD have the following four characteristics:

- Throwing away the item(s) is linked to fear of contamination (from touching the object), fear of catastrophe from discarding the object, or fear of incompleteness (loss of symmetry).
- The hoarder derives no pleasure from the hoarded objects.
- The hoarder has no sentimental attachment to the hoarded items.
- Excessive acquisition is rare in cases of OCD hoarding.

Hoarding in older adults

Hoarding among seniors is increasingly regarded as a serious public health concern as well as a danger to the elderly themselves. First, it is now known that hoarding is more common among older adults than among younger ones; this finding is interesting given the fact that the only other psychiatric disorder that is known to worsen with increasing age is **dementia**. It is not yet known whether hoarding in the elderly is an early indication of dementia or whether dementia follows an earlier history of hoarding.

Hoarding can cause health problems for seniors, given that many suffer from physical as well as cognitive impairments. One study of elderly hoarders found that 45% could not get to their refrigerators because of clutter, 42% could not use their kitchen sink, 42% could not reach their bathtub, 20% could not use their bathroom sink, and 10% could not use their toilet. The space occupied by hoarded items increases the senior's risk of falls, fires, rodent infestation due to unsanitary conditions, and malnutrition resulting from inability to store and prepare food properly. Some seniors on fixed incomes also report **financial stress** from making unnecessary purchases, having to pay for self-storage units, or having to pay housing fines.

Animal hoarding

Animal hoarding was first defined as follows by a research consortium established at Tufts University in 1997:

- The hoarder has more than the typical number of companion animals (cats, dogs, rabbits, hamsters, and birds); however, there are also cases of people hoarding farm animals, wild animals (raccoons, wolves), and exotic animals (snakes, alligators, tigers).
- The hoarder fails to provide even minimal standards of food and water, cleanliness, shelter, and veterinary care. This neglect often results in the animals' illness and death from starvation, spread of infectious disease, and untreated injuries.
- The hoarder is in denial of his or her inability to provide for the animals as well as the effects of that failure on the animals, the house, and other human occupants of the building.
- The hoarder persists in accumulating more animals in spite of failure to care for those already in his or her possession.

Almost any type of animal can be hoarded, although cats appear to be the species most commonly hoarded because they are small, easy to obtain, and easily concealed. Most animal hoarders concentrate on only one species, although there are also many cases of hoarders found with several animal species in their households. It is not known whether there are any psychological factors that influence a hoarder's preference for a particular animal species. Animal hoarders are found among men as well as women, and among medical and veterinary professionals as well as persons with lower levels of education.

Animal hoarding is a type of hoarding behavior that differs from the hoarding of inanimate objects in several important respects. Animal hoarders are usually more disturbed emotionally and have much less insight into their disorder than persons who hoard objects. Their hoarding behavior causes genuine suffering to the animals, many of whom end up being euthanized when the hoarding is discovered, because of advanced infectious disease, malnutrition, or behavior problems caused by the overcrowding. Animal hoarding also presents a considerable public health problem associated with the transmission of zoonoses, a group of infectious viral, bacterial, parasitic, fungal, or prion diseases that can be transmitted from animals to humans or from humans to animals. In addition, animal hoarders are more likely than hoarders of objects to come in contact with the criminal justice system, because most states have stiff legal penalties for animal cruelty; Illinois and Hawaii explicitly mention hoarding as a form of animal cruelty in their relevant legislation.

There is little agreement among psychiatrists as to the best model for explaining animal hoarding. Some consider it an **addiction** similar to a substance addiction, others regard it as a form of OCD, still others think it is best explained as an attachment disorder, and a fourth group regards it as a **delusional disorder** (a disorder in which the person is out of touch with reality).

Risk factors

Risk factors for hoarding disorder include:

- Age. Hoarding seems to begin in late childhood or early adolescence and gets worse during adulthood. School-age children often begin by hoarding such items as broken toys, pens and pencils, old school papers, or old clocks and other small appliances. The disorder becomes more noticeable in adults in their 20s and 30s and a serious problem in those in their 40s and 50s.
- Family history. People who have a family member who is a hoarder are much more likely to become hoarders themselves.
- Traumatic experiences. Such events as death of a loved one (including a pet), divorce, eviction, or losing treasured possessions in a fire or earthquake appear to trigger hoarding in some people.
- Alcohol abuse. About 50% of hoarders have a history of alcoholism.
- Social isolation. This risk factor appears to work in both directions; some people withdraw from human companionship because they are hoarders, whereas others report that they turned to hoarding because they were lonely.

Causes and symptoms

Causes

The causes of hoarding are unclear; however, the disorder is known to run in families, so it is possible that a combination of **genetic factors** and family upbringing contributes to the disorder. A 2007 study published in the *American Journal of Psychiatry* postulated that a region in chromosome 14 might link to the development of compulsive hoarding in families with OCD, but further research is needed.

Another theory maintains that hoarders have different patterns of **brain** activation; namely, that the parts of the brain that control such functions as focusing attention, making decisions, and organizing operate differently in hoarders. One **psychologist** has noted that hoarders pay much more attention to the unusual details of an object (its color, shape, and texture) rather than its use, and that they tend to identify their sense of an object's location visually or spatially (for example, "it's six inches down from the top in the pile of papers on the desk in the back bedroom") rather than by category (for example, "bills to be paid"). Another psychological characteristic that differentiates hoarders of objects from other people is a tendency to humanize their possessions; that is, they attribute human-like qualities to the objects and feel genuine **grief** at the thought of parting with them. Hoarders also form emotional attachments to a wider variety of objects than people who don't hoard.

Symptoms

The symptoms of hoarding include:

- large amounts of clutter in the home or office that make it difficult to move around easily, get work done, or use furniture or appliances
- losing money, bills, or other important items in the clutter
- feeling overwhelmed by the sheer volume of possessions
- being unable to stop taking free items from restaurants or displays
- purchasing multiples of items in order to stock up or because the item is a bargain
- refusing to let repair people into the home
- not inviting friends or family to the home because of embarrassment about the clutter

Diagnosis

There are no laboratory or imaging tests that can diagnose hoarding disorder. The **American Psychiatric Association** (APA) has proposed the following criteria for hoarding disorder to be included in *DSM-5*:

- Criterion A: The person is persistently unable to discard or part with possessions, without regard to the value others place on those items.
- Criterion B: The difficulty arises from strong urges to save items and/or emotional distress at the thought of discarding them.
- Criterion C: The items accumulate to the point that the intended use of the living space or workplace is no longer possible (or the living space is uncluttered only because of the intervention of family members or other third parties).
- Criterion D: The symptoms cause clinically significant distress or impairment in the person's social, occupational, or academic functioning, including maintaining

KEY TERMS

Attachment disorder—A general term used to describe emotional and behavioral problems in children or adults resulting from a failure to form healthy attachments in early childhood to parents or other primary caregivers.

Delusional disorder—A mental illness characterized by the presence of nonbizarre delusions in the absence of other mood or psychotic symptoms. "Nonbizarre" means that the delusion is about a situation that could occur in real life, such as being followed or losing a loved one. In the case of an animal hoarder, the delusion would be that the animals would die or be euthanized if the hoarder did not house them.

Semi-structured interview—A type of psychiatric interview in which the interviewer can ask new questions in the course of the interview, depending on the interviewee's answers to previous questions.

Zoonosis (plural, zoonoses)—Any contagious disease that can be transmitted from nonhuman animals to humans or from humans to nonhuman animals. Zoonoses include viral, bacterial, parasitic, fungal, and prion diseases.

a safe environment for the person and others in the household.

- Criterion E: The hoarding symptoms are not due to a general medical condition (e.g., brain injury, heart disease).
- Criterion F: The hoarding symptoms are not restricted to the symptoms of another mental disorder (e.g., lack of energy in major depression, delusions in schizophrenia, loss of cognitive abilities in dementia)

The proposal also includes two specifiers. The first concerns excessive acquisition; that is, the symptoms "are accompanied by excessive collecting or buying or stealing of items that are not needed or for which there is no available space." The second qualifier concerns the person's degree of insight into their condition, which the **psychiatrist** can rate as "good or fair," "poor," or "absent."

Tests

There are several pencil-and-paper tests that people can take to evaluate whether they have a hoarding disorder. One is the Saving Inventory Revised (SIR), which is a 23-item scale that measures three dimensions of hoarding: excessive acquisition, difficulty discarding, and clutter. Another test is the Hoarding Rating Scale (HRS), which is a five-item semi-structured interview. The URLs for the PDF versions of these two tests are included in the Websites section of the Resources.

Treatment

Treatment of hoarding disorder is a subject of ongoing research. With regard to medications, it was the discovery that hoarders do not respond to the medications usually prescribed for OCD that led researchers to suggest that hoarding is a distinctive disorder rather than a subtype of OCD. While some psychiatrists think that **selective serotonin reuptake inhibitors (SSRIs)** are directly beneficial in treating hoarding, most specialists believe that SSRIs are primarily useful in treating the anxiety or depression associated with hoarding rather than the disorder itself.

Individualized **cognitive-behavioral therapy** (CBT) has been found to be helpful in patients who hoard inanimate objects. The reason for tailoring the specific interventions to each patient is that hoarders vary widely in the types of items they hoard and their reasons for hoarding. CBT for hoarding involves a combination of motivational training (giving the person a reason to stop hoarding), skills training (how to organize possessions and living space), and behavioral experiments (e.g., going shopping without buying anything, or throwing away a specific item) designed to help the person revise their thoughts and feelings about their possessions.

Group therapy is another approach that works well for hoarders. First, it breaks down their social isolation and feelings of shame about the condition of their homes. Second, group therapy helps increase motivation as the group's members swap tips about organization skills, cleaning up clutter, and the like. Third, group therapy lowers the depression and anxiety that many hoarders feel. Internet-based **support groups**, including some for adult sons and daughters of hoarders, are reported to be effective in maintaining the benefits of CBT.

Professional organizers may also be able to help patients with hoarding disorder develop and strengthen organizational skills. Professional organizers can help clients establish systems (e.g., filing) for maintaining organization and teach clients to prioritize activities, which may help persons with hoarding disorder feel more in control of their actions.

Treatment of animal hoarders is much more difficult than therapy for hoarders of objects. As noted above, animal hoarders are usually more seriously disturbed than

QUESTIONS TO ASK YOUR DOCTOR

- Do you have special expertise in helping people with hoarding disorders?
- What are my treatment options?
- What is your opinion of CBT as a treatment for hoarding disorder?
- Will my family be involved in treatment in any way?

other hoarders, and their rate of **relapse** is close to 100% even after receiving fines or prison sentences for animal **abuse**. There was no established effective therapy for animal hoarding as of 2011, although some observers think that placing animal hoarders under extended probation with regular visits from a probation officer would be more effective than a prison term to prevent reoffending.

There were two **clinical trials** that focused solely on hoarding in 2011 (as opposed to including hoarding as a symptom of OCD). One trial was investigating the use of **methylphenidate** ER (Daytrana) as a pharmacological treatment for hoarding, and the other was testing the effectiveness of **cognitive remediation** and **exposure treatment**.

Prognosis

The prognosis of hoarding disorder depends on the person's motivation to change and such other factors as involvement with the legal system. Individualized CBT is reported to be effective in about 70% to 80% of patients. In general, hoarders of animals have a considerably worse prognosis than hoarders of objects.

Prevention

There is no known way to prevent hoarding disorder.

Resources

BOOKS

Antony, Martin M., and Murray B. Stein, eds. *Oxford Handbook of Anxiety and Related Disorders*. New York: Oxford University Press, 2009.

Arluke, Arnold, and Celeste Killeen. *Inside Animal Hoarding: The Case of Barbara Erickson and Her 552 Dogs*. West Lafayette, IN: Purdue University Press, 2009.

Frost, Randy O., and Gail Steketee. *Stuff: Compulsive Hoarding and the Meaning of Things*. Boston, MA: Houghton Mifflin Harcourt, 2010.

Sholl, Jessie. *Dirty Secret: A Daughter Comes Clean about Her Mother's Compulsive Hoarding*. New York: Gallery Books, 2011.

Tolin, David F., Randy O. Frost, and Gail Steketee. *Buried in Treasures: Help for Compulsive Acquiring, Saving, and Hoarding*. New York: Oxford University Press, 2007.

PERIODICALS

Kurutz, Steven. "Children of Hoarders on Leaving the Cluttered Nest." *New York Times*, May 12, 2011. http://www.nytimes.com/2011/05/12/garden/children-of-hoarders-on-leaving-the-cluttered-nest.html?_r=2&hpw=&pagewanted=all (accessed August 3, 2011).

Lambros, Valerie. "Hoarding Disorder Can Have Dangerous Ramifications." *NIH Record*, January 21, 2011. http://nihrecord.od.nih.gov/newsletters/2011/01_21_2011/story1.htm (accessed July 17, 2011).

Mackin, R.S., et al. "Cognitive Functioning in Individuals with Severe Compulsive Hoarding Behaviors and Late Life Depression." *International Journal of Geriatric Psychiatry* 26 (March 2011): 314–321.

Mataix-Cois, D., et al. "Testing the Validity and Acceptability of the Diagnostic Criteria for Hoarding Disorder: a DSM-5 Survey." *Psychological Medicine* 13 (May 2011): 1–10.

Morgan, Kim. "Getting Help to Overcome a Hoarding Disorder." *Houston Chronicle*, March 16, 2010. http://www.chron.com/disp/story.mpl/life/main/6915900.html (accessed July 17, 2011).

Samuels, Jack, et al. "Significant Linkage to Compulsive Hoarding on Chromosome 14 in Families With Obsessive-Compulsive Disorder: Results From the OCD Collaborative Genetics Study." *American Journal of Psychiatry* 164 (March 2007): 493–99. http://dx.doi.org/10.1176/appi.ajp.164.3.493 (accessed September 14, 2011).

Saxena, S. "Pharmacotherapy of Compulsive Hoarding." *Journal of Clinical Psychology* 67 (May 2011): 477–484.

Steketee, G., and D.F. Tolin. "Cognitive-Behavioral Therapy for Hoarding in the Context of Contamination Fears." *Journal of Clinical Psychology* 67 (May 2011): 485–496.

Storch, E.A., et al. "Compulsive Hoarding in Children." *Journal of Clinical Psychology* 67 (May 2011): 507–516.

Timpano, K.R., et al. "The Epidemiology of the Proposed DSM-5 Hoarding Disorder: Exploration of the Acquisition Specifier, Associated Features, and Distress." *Journal of Clinical Psychiatry* 72 (June 2011): 780–786.

Tolin, D.F. and A. Villavicencio. "Inattention, but not OCD, Predicts the Core Features of Hoarding Disorder." *Behaviour Research and Therapy* 49 (February 2011): 120–125.

Wick, J.Y. and G.R. Zanni. "Helping Those with Hoarding Behaviors." *Consultant Pharmacist* 26 (July 2011): 458–467.

OTHER

International OCD Foundation Hoarding Center. "Hoarding Rating Scale (HRS)." http://www.ocfoundation.org/uploadedFiles/Hoarding/Resources/Hoarding%20Rating%20Scale%20with%20interpret.pdf (accessed July 17, 2011).

———. "Saving Inventory Revised (SIR)." http://www.ocfoundation.org/uploadedFiles/Hoarding/Resources/SI-R%28ModifiedFormat%29.pdf (accessed July 17, 2011).

WEBSITES

"About Hoarding." International OCD Foundation Hoarding Center. http://www.ocfoundation.org/hoarding/about.aspx (accessed July 17, 2011).

American Psychiatric Association. "F 02 Hoarding Disorder." DSM-5 Development. http://www.dsm5.org/proposedrevision/pages/proposedrevision.aspx?rid=398 (accessed July 17, 2011).

"Animal Hoarding." American Society for the Prevention of Cruelty to Animals (ASPCA). http://www.aspca.org/aspca-nyc/animal-rescuers/animal-hoarding.aspx (accessed July 17, 2011).

Children of Hoarders: Awareness, Understanding, and Support for COH. http://childrenofhoarders.com/wordpress (accessed July 18, 2011).

"Common Questions about Animal Hoarding." Hoarding of Animals Research Consortium (HARC). http://www.tufts.edu/vet/hoarding/abthoard.htm (accessed July 17, 2011).

Johns Hopkins Health Alerts. "Hoarding: From Cluttered to Clinical." Johns Hopkins Medicine. http://www.johnshopkinshealthalerts.com/alerts/depression_anxiety/hoarding_3826-1.html (accessed July 17, 2011).

Mayo Clinic staff. "Hoarding." MayoClinic.com. http://www.mayoclinic.com/health/hoarding/DS00966 (accessed July 17, 2011).

National Public Radio. "Hoarding: When Too Much 'Stuff' Causes Grief." *Fresh Air from WHYY* [radio program]. http://www.npr.org/templates/story/story.php?storyId=126386317 (accessed September 14, 2011).

Song, Anna, and KATU Web Staff. "Living Landfill: A Portrait of Hoarding Disorder." *KOMO News*, April 28, 2007. http://www.komonews.com/news/local/7224116.html (accessed July 17, 2011).

ORGANIZATIONS

American Psychiatric Association, 1000 Wilson Boulevard, Suite 1825, Arlington, VA, 22209-3901, (703) 907-7300, apa@psych.org, http://www.psych.org.

American Society for the Prevention of Cruelty to Animals (ASPCA), 424 E. 92nd Street, New York, NY, 10128-6804, (212) 876-7700, http://www.aspca.org.

Hoarding of Animals Research Consortium (HARC), c/o Gary Patronek, Animal Rescue League of Boston, 10 Chandler Street, Boston, MA, 02116, (617) 426-9170, Fax: (617) 426-3028, cfapp@tufts.edu, http://www.tufts.edu/vet/hoarding.

International OCD Foundation Hoarding Center, PO Box 961029, Boston, MA, 02196, (617) 973-5801, Fax: (617) 973-5803, info@ocfoundation.org, http://www.ocfoundation.org/hoarding.

Rebecca J. Frey, Ph.D.

Homelessness

Definition

In the United States, definitions of homelessness help determine who can receive shelter and assistance from certain health and social service providers. The Stewart McKinney Homeless Assistance Act of 1987 defines a homeless person as any individual who lacks housing, including an individual whose primary residence during the night is a supervised public or private facility that provides temporary living accommodations, or an individual who is a resident in transitional housing. More specifically, this means that a homeless person is any individual who lacks fixed, regular, and adequate nighttime residence, and an individual who has a primary nighttime residence that is either (i) a supervised temporary living shelter (including transitional housing for the mentally ill), (ii) an institution that provides temporary residence for individuals intended to be institutionalized, or (iii) a place not designed for, or ordinarily used as, a regular sleeping accommodation for human beings.

In addition, the U.S. Department of Housing and Urban Development (HUD) defines chronic homelessness as "an unaccompanied disabled individual who has been continuously homeless for over one year."

Demographics

Methods for estimating the size of the homeless population are evolving and sometimes contested, and are complicated by varying definitions of homelessness. The U.S. Census, while attempting to identify the number of people who are homeless and who use particular types of homeless services, has complex and service-based definitions of homelessness. It also has recognized its limited abilities to define and enumerate the homeless (it is after all a national household survey). In 2000, the Census Bureau defined the Emergency and Transitional Shelter (E&TS) population by surveying people who used a sample of homeless services. They counted homeless people in emergency shelters for adults, runaway youth shelters, shelters for abused women and their children, soup kitchens, and certain outdoor locations. Technically, however, homeless people may reside in "E&TS," in foster care, in jails and prisons, in **group homes**, in worker dorms, non-sheltered in the outdoors, doubled up with families or friends, or temporarily in Census-recognized households. According to the National Coalition for the Homeless, while counting the number of people who use services such as shelters and soup kitchens can yield important information about services, applying these numbers toward estimating numbers of homeless people can result in underestimates of homelessness.

Further complicating the issue of counting homeless people is the fact that in many cases, homelessness is a temporary condition. Because of this fact, some researchers advocate a method of counting all the people who are homeless in a given week or, alternatively, over a given period. However, the numbers of people who find housing and the number of people who newly find themselves homeless fluctuate over time. In contrast, people with mental illness or **substance abuse** problems tend to be chronically without homes—it is difficult for many of these people to find permanent housing. Thus, while these two time-oriented methods of counting homeless can be useful, they, too, have statistical problems—they can overestimate the numbers of homeless people.

According to the 2010 Census, the number of people utilizing emergency shelters and transitional housing was 424,042. However, this figure does not include homeless adults not using such services, sampling error, or some groups outside of the sampled jurisdictions.

Another estimate of homelessness, in a 2007 report by the National Alliance to End Homelessness, estimated that 744,313 people were homeless in 2005. Forty-four percent of those people were unsheltered, and 56% were sheltered. Forty-one percent of the homeless were families.

According to the National Law Center on Homelessness and Poverty, about 3.5 million people (of these about 1.35 million children) are likely to experience homelessness at least once in any given year. This statistic is much higher than the other ones, based on its more relaxed definition of homelessness.

The large variation among these estimates illustrates that, as the National Coalition for the Homeless states, "By its very nature, homelessness is impossible to measure with 100% accuracy."

Description

Homelessness is an acute version of residential instability, which can be compared or contrasted with definitions of poverty. Thus the term "homeless" may also be extended to include people who have nowhere to go and are at imminent risk of losing housing through eviction or institutional discharge. Some definitions of homelessness further specify the duration of time without regular and adequate residence, or the types of temporary living shelter or institutions that are not fixed residences. People who live without alternatives in overcrowded or unhealthy housing conditions may be at risk of homelessness. Worldwide, national, and cultural groups may have variable, and often different, definitions of homelessness, different terms for the condition of being without housing, and different definitions of adequate housing. For all of these reasons, related both to methods of counting and varying definitions, estimating the size of the homeless population is extremely difficult.

The history of homelessness is intertwined with the history of poverty in the United States. Poverty has always been problematic for humanitarian reasons and because it conflicts with the ideal of prosperity for all. Social welfare, based on individualistic ideas of the deserving and undeserving poor, has improved society but not eliminated persistent poverty or homelessness. The 1960s war on poverty was a widely shared value but, in the 1980s, concern about homelessness was confounded by moral evaluations of individual behaviors. While many in the United States have been poor or come from poor families, fewer have experienced homelessness. Therefore, the collective understanding of homelessness in the United States is limited in ways that the understanding of poverty is not.

Homeless adults are poor and have high rates of unmet need for health care. This is in part because poverty is associated with higher risk and rates of illness, particularly mental illnesses including substance abuse. Homeless people experience disproportionate rates and symptoms of mental health disorders, including substance-abuse disorders and dual diagnoses. For these reasons, large portions of federally funded homeless services are medical services, and homeless people are often viewed according to their present or past medical classifications.

Studies researching the incidence, distribution, and control of a disease in a population (known as epidemiological studies) find that between one-third and one-half of homeless people have mental health disorders, and approximately two-thirds have either a mental health or substance-abuse disorder. People with severe mental illness are likewise more likely to become homeless particularly when the disorder is co-morbid (co-occurring) with substance abuse. For this reason, changes in rates of homelessness are often associated with changes in mental health care and **hospitalization** policies.

Mental illnesses compound the vulnerability and needs of homeless adults, as reported by the Surgeon General. Psychiatric disorders exacerbate many types of problems, including housing instability, morbidity (disease), and mortality (death). Psychiatric disorders and lack of stable living conditions complicate general health care for homeless adults.

Causes and consequences

Causes

People with mental illness are at higher risk for becoming homeless due to challenges associated with **deinstitutionalization** and transition planning, and both poverty and disability associated with mental illness.

Social research has studied the causes and consequences of homelessness, surveying homeless people, examining entrances into homelessness, exits from homelessness, and effects of homelessness on health and well-being. Promising explanations for increasing rates of homelessness in the 1980s have included mental disability and illness, lack of social support through jobs and marriage, increased use of drugs and alcohol, and the erosion of low-income housing in urban areas. These explanations mirror the processes of deinstitutionalization in mental health policy, unemployment, **addiction** and abuse, and urban decay. In other words, a direct correlation can be demonstrated between policies and trends, and the rates of homelessness. As deinstitutionalization occurred, for example, the number of mentally ill people without homes increased.

Consequences

Consequences of homelessness include the exacerbation of problems that may have caused homelessness. Homeless people have reduced access to housing, jobs, health care, and basic needs like food and clothing. Isolation and lack of social support are well-documented aspects of homelessness, particularly for homeless people living with mental health or substance abuse disorders. Homeless women and men have been found to have significantly less family support than never-homeless women and men. Disaffiliation from family often limits opportunities for recovery and prevention.

Treatment

Whatever the underlying reason for homelessness (such as poor health, be it mental or physical), two forms of treatment include employment and housing. A person living in a sheltered dwelling is better protected against the myriad causes of homelessness than is a person who is without shelter. People who were previously homeless, but are now living in a home, have a much better chance to recover from the underlying cause(s) of their homelessness.

Treating the underlying causes and eliminating (or managing) them is the first step back to employment and eventually to permanent housing. Private and public projects contribute to the treatment of homelessness, including better education and training of such individuals within the workforce. For instance, case-management programs for the homeless, such as **assertive community treatment** (ACT), can help to ensure that such programs are more effective.

KEY TERMS

Assertive community treatment—An approach to mental health services within a small population that helps individuals manage their mental illness with respect to themselves, family members, work associates, and the community at large.

Epidemiological—The study of the origin, cause, and transmission of diseases.

Mentally ill—A person with a psychiatric disorder of mental faculties.

Psychiatric disorders—Any behavioral or psychological symptoms that impair basic bodily functions and increase one's risk of death and disability.

Prognosis

Homelessness is both a form of poverty and an acute condition of residential instability. Homelessness is compounded by behavioral problems, mental health policy changes, disparities in health and health care, racial inequalities, fluctuations in affordable housing, and lack of social support.

Homelessness in context

Overly individualistic views and explanations of homelessness do not reflect its multiple causes and effects. Like all groups, homeless people are diverse, experiencing and exiting homelessness for a myriad of reasons. Services for homeless adults likewise reflect a variety of needs and experiences. Nonetheless, homelessness remains a national and international concern, particularly in urban areas, for the twenty-first century.

Prevention

Homelessness can be minimized, and in some instances prevented, with the use of effective strategies within homeless service agencies and among individualized efforts. For instance, in 2002, the U.S. Department of Housing and Urban Development (HUD), the Department of Health and Human Services (HHS), and Veterans Affairs (VA) began a combined effort to reduce chronic homelessness in the United States. The grant-funded program provides access by homeless persons to health and social services, along with employment programs. The program guarantees that at least 30% of the grant money goes to providing permanent housing to the homeless.

Homeless service agencies

Services for homeless people can be divided into those providing medical care (including mental health care), those providing housing, and those providing other basic needs. Publicly funded agencies provide the majority of medical care, especially primary and mental health care. Public and private organizations share the responsibilities of providing shelter and housing services, through both large federal programs and smaller need- and faith-based programs. Private agencies deliver most other daily needs to homeless people, through food pantries, soup kitchens, and other charities. Limited data exist on vocational services for homeless adults.

Title VI of the McKinney Homeless Assistance Act of 1987 created the Health Care for the Homeless (HCH) program, authorizing federal funds for primary and mental health care to homeless people. Title VI authorizes several programs to provide an HCH program, a **Community Mental Health** Services block grant program, and two demonstration programs providing mental health and alcohol and drug abuse treatment services to homeless people. HCH funds support providers who offer mental health, **case management**, and health education services, as well as substance-abuse treatment. In 1987, 109 grants were made for homeless health services with $46 million. In 1992, the Act was amended to include homeless and at-risk children, creating a medical home and source of health insurance for young people. In 2010, Congress appropriated $171 million for grants for health care for the homeless. The HCH program is the largest single effort to address the medical needs of the homeless. Each year, the HCH Program serves around 600,000 clients in the United States. To be an HCH service agency requires cultural and linguistic competencies, compassionate community outreach, and providers who reflect the community they serve.

The federal Center for Mental Health Services oversees the Projects for Assistance in Transition from Homelessness (PATH) grant program. The program provides state funds in support services to individuals who are homeless or at risk of becoming homeless, and to those who have serious mental illnesses. These funds amounted to more than $52 million allocated to 463 providers in 2005. States contract with local agencies and nonprofit organizations to provide an array of services, including outreach, support services, a limited set of housing services, and mental health treatment.

QUESTIONS TO ASK YOUR DOCTOR

- What programs are available locally for homelessness?
- Where can medical care be found?
- Where is temporary housing available?
- Is affordable permanent housing available?
- What employment-assistance problems are available?
- What support groups area found in the area?

There are several obstacles or barriers in providing health care to homeless people. First, homeless or persistently poor people may be concerned about their work and sustenance, devaluing their own medical needs. Alienation and **depression** among the homeless can also be an obstacle to providing care. There can be mutual communication problems between providers and patients. Providers may lack cultural understanding that would ease work with homeless clients. Finally, lack of preventive maintenance of medical care by the homeless may result in expensive and extensive needs for care, including hospital care, which may stress the capacities of certain service providers.

How to help the homeless mentally ill

There are many ways that the public can support community and federal efforts to help homeless people living with mental illness. Some strategies include:

- Support collective public and private efforts to build homes, and provide health care for people with unmet medical needs.
- Become educated about the challenges faced by homeless and mentally ill people in American society.
- Stop the practice of equating people in poverty and with illness with their medical conditions, instead of recognizing them as human beings. Succeeding in this step could open doors for recovery of health and housing without demeaning the humanity of people in need.

Recently, the federal government approved the American Recovery and Reinvestment Act of 2009, which allocated $1.5 billion for a Homelessness Prevention and Rapid Re-Housing Program (HPRP), and the Homeless Emergency Assistance and Rapid Transition to Housing (HEARTH) Act, which reauthorizes the HUD Homeless Assistance programs.

Resources

BOOKS

Cloke, Paul, Jon May, and Sarah Johnsen. *Swept Up Lives?* Chichester, West Sussex: Wiley-Blackwell, 2010.

Daly, Gerald. *Homeless.* New York City: Routledge, 2005.

Doak, Melissa J. *Social Welfare: Fighting Poverty and Homelessness.* Detroit: Gale Cengage Living, 2010.

Ellen, Ingrid Gould, and Brendan O'Flaherty, editors. *How to House the Homeless* New York City: Russell Sage Foundation, 2010.

Hartmann, Robert Hartmann, editor. *Homelessness in America.* Westport, CT: Praeger, 2008.

OTHER

"Health Care and Homelessness." National Coalition for the Homeless. May 27, 2009. http://www.nationalhomeless.org/factsheets/Health.pdf (accessed December 12, 2011).

WEBSITES

"Chronic Homelessness." U.S. Department of Housing and Urban Development. July 2009. http://www.hud.gov/offices/cpd/homeless/chronic.cfm (accessed December 12, 2011).

"Homeless Emergency and Rapid Transition to Housing (HEARTH) Act." U.S. Department of Housing and Urban Development. http://www.hudhre.info/hearth (accessed December 12, 2011).

"Homelessness Prevention and Rapid Re-Housing Program." U.S. Department of Housing and Urban Development. http://www.hudhre.info/HPRP (accessed December 12, 2011).

"How Many People Experience Homelessness?" National Coalition for the Homeless. July 2009. http://www.nationalhomeless.org/factsheets/How_Many.html (accessed December 12, 2011).

ORGANIZATIONS

National Alliance on Mental Illness, 3803 North Fairfax Drive, Suite 100, Arlington, VA, 22203, (703) 524-7600, (800) 950-6264, Fax: (703) 524-9094, http://www.nami.org.

National Coalition for the Homeless, 2201 P Street, NW, Washington, DC, 20037, (202) 462-4822, Fax: (202) 462-4823, info@nationalhomeless.org, http://www.nationalhomeless.org.

National Coalition for Homeless Veterans, 333 1/2 Pennsylvania Ave., SE, Washington, DC, 20003-1148, (202) 546-1969, (800) 838-4357, Fax: (202) 546-2063, info@nchv.org, http://www.nchv.org.

National Health Care for the Homeless Council, PO Box 60427, Nashville, TN, 37206-0427, (615) 226-2292, Fax: (615) 226-1656, http://www.nhchc.org.

National Institute of Mental Health, 6001 Executive Boulevard, Room 8184, MSC 9663, Bethesda, MD, 20892-9663, (301) 443-4513, (866) 615-6464, Fax: (301) 443-4279, nimhinfo@nih.gov, http://www.nimh.nih.gov.

Substance Abuse and Mental Health Services Administration, 1 Choke Cherry Road, Rockville, MD, 20857, (877) 726-4727, Fax: (240) 221-4292, http://www.samhsa.gov.

U.S. Department of Housing and Urban Development, 451 7th Street SW, Washington, DC, 20410, (202) 708-1112, http://www.hud.gov.

Michael Polgar, PhD
Stephanie N. Watson

Hospitalization

Definition

Hospitalization, or inpatient care, is the admission to the hospital or other such medical healthcare facility for the treatment of various types of mental illness. For someone with disorders such as **depression** or **bipolar disorder**, a stay in the hospital can help to stabilize the condition for eventually better mental health. However, hospitalization is the most restrictive form of treatment for a psychiatric disorder, addictive disorder, or someone with more than one **diagnosis**. Whether treatment is voluntary or involuntary, the patient relinquishes the freedom to move about and, once admitted, becomes subject to the rules and schedule of a treatment environment.

The use of hospitalization is necessary in cases where individuals are in imminent danger of harming themselves or others or have made **suicide** attempts. Crisis stabilization, **behavior modification**, supervised **substance abuse**, **detoxification**, and medication management are compelling reasons to consider hospitalization. People having hallucinations, **delusions**, thoughts of hurting oneself or others, feelings of exhaustion or depression, or problems with alcohol or substance abuse may need to consider hospitalization. Those people who have not slept or eaten for days due to psychiatric or medical illness, have tried outpatient treatment without an improvement in their lives, or need to make major changes in an existing treatment or medicine are other candidates for hospitalization.

Ideally, hospitalization is at one end of a comprehensive continuum of services for people needing treatment for behavioral problems. It is generally viewed as a last resort after other, less restrictive forms of treatment have failed.

Purpose

For a person to be admitted to a hospital, a medical doctor (in the case of mental health, most often a **psychiatrist**) must "admit" the patient or approve the patient's request to be admitted. Although hospitalization may be considered a drastic treatment **intervention**, it can be essential in keeping people safe, helping monitor and adjust medications, treating medication side effects, supervising alcohol and/or drug detoxification, and stabilizing a patient after an acute psychiatric episode.

Before an individual is hospitalized, an evaluation and a diagnosis must be made by a medical professional. This is required in order for the patient to receive maximum insurance coverage and to receive the most appropriate treatment.

Demographics

Anyone may need the services of a hospital to receive a comprehensive array of medical services to overcome a mental problem. A hospital is an appropriate place to receive those services because a group of trained professionals is associated with all hospitals in the United States. As such, it is a safe and effective way to treat mental illness or other related problems and to learn how to cope with its symptoms. A hospital is also an appropriate place to eliminate stresses that may be contributing to mental problems.

Hospitalization statistics

The U.S. Centers for Disease Control and Prevention (CSC), in its *National Hospital Discharge Survey: 2007 Summary*, states that the number of discharges with mental disorders from hospitals numbered 2.4 million. In addition, the average length of stay within a hospital for inpatient mental-health care was 7.1 days.

The U.S. Department of Health and Human Services (HHS) ranked the principal diagnosis of various mental illnesses according to the number of discharges from hospitals in the United States. In 2009, HHS found that the top five mental illnesses (and the number of hospital discharges) were for: mood disorders (873,176), **schizophrenia** and other psychotic disorders (419,395), alcohol-related disorders (268,093), substance-related disorders (240,837), and **delirium**, **dementia**, and amnestic and other cognitive disorders (133,460).

In 2006, according to the **Substance Abuse and Mental Health Services Administration**, 1,850,000 patients received inpatient treatment in the United States for substance abuse, with 816,000 patients in hospitals, and 934,000 in inpatient treatment centers.

The U.S. government is transferring some mental health patients from federally supported hospitals to outpatient facilities supported by local communities. In a similar move, various states across the United States are doing likewise with their state-sponsored hospitals. Such moves are a response to large financial woes that the federal government and many state governments are currently dealing with because of recessionary conditions in the United States. These community-based treatment facilities have become the focus for treatment of mental health cases in the United States, both at the federal and state levels. Due to overcrowding in many hospitals and the closing of others, private providers are also being contracted to supply services to mental health patients.

Description

Most hospital rooms are similar to basic hotel rooms and are generally large enough for two people. In the case of public hospitals, the rooms may be larger and may contain more beds. Men and women are in separate wings or on separate floors. If a treatment program is housed in a medical hospital, it may cover one or more floors. If one admits oneself into the facility, then one can also sign out within two to seven days (depending on specific state laws) unless the medical staff feels the person has the potential to do harm to one's self or others. If someone else admits the patient, then the patient cannot release himself or herself. In all cases, patients have the right to be explained the treatments planned for them.

Although there is wide variation in the quality of the physical surroundings and the resources available, most inpatient facilities are highly regimented. Patients get up, go to bed, eat, and take medication (if indicated) on a regular schedule. Times are set to awaken in the morning, and eat breakfast, lunch, and dinner. Days are filled with scheduled activities such as individual, family, or **group therapy**, expressive and occupational therapies, psychoeducation, recreation, and, in the case of children or adolescents, several hours of school. Several different doctors on staff and other mental health professionals (e. g., nurses, **social workers**) at the hospital, besides the admitting doctor, may visit to conduct interviews, monitor status, and check on medications.

Most hospital inpatient programs are based on a therapeutic milieu, which means that all the people involved in the patient's care and all the activities are designed to have a therapeutic function for the patient. For example, direct care workers are not simply aides; they are supportive of the patient and provide valuable feedback to the physician, **psychologist**, and social worker about the patient's conduct and progress.

Hospitalization for mental illness may necessitate that the person being admitted to the hospital be confined to a locked section. For the safety of the patient, all personal items, such as jewelry, watches, and cell phones, may be taken away and stored in a secure location. Items that have

Number of certified U.S. psychiatric hospitals and intermediate care facilities for persons with intellectual disabilities (ICF/ID), by state: selected years, 1995–2009

	Psychiatric hospitals				ICF/ID			
	1995	2000	2007	2009	1995	2000	2007	2009
United States	**689**	**515**	**486**	**502**	**7,106**	**6,767**	**6,443**	**6,437**
Alabama	10	9	10	11	8	8	6	5
Alaska	3	2	2	2	6	0	0	0
Arizona	11	8	7	7	12	11	12	12
Arkansas	9	9	9	8	40	40	41	41
California	64	39	31	33	687	1,043	1,151	1,171
Colorado	9	6	7	9	7	3	3	3
Connecticut	10	8	7	6	145	122	118	114
Delaware	3	3	4	4	6	2	2	2
District of Columbia	2	3	3	3	122	130	110	85
Florida	43	26	21	24	110	108	105	102
Georgia	28	15	13	15	12	13	11	9
Hawaii	1	1	1	1	15	22	18	18
Idaho	6	5	5	5	48	66	65	66
Illinois	19	17	14	14	315	317	313	310
Indiana	30	21	20	22	578	574	530	547
Iowa	4	4	4	4	116	127	139	139
Kansas	10	5	4	4	47	42	30	32
Kentucky	13	12	11	11	9	12	9	12
Louisiana	40	17	35	37	454	473	528	548
Maine	4	4	4	4	42	28	20	17
Maryland	14	11	9	9	5	5	4	4
Massachusetts	18	18	16	15	8	7	6	6
Michigan	15	10	10	10	503	2	1	1
Minnesota	6	7	6	7	348	270	218	218
Mississippi	4	2	5	5	12	13	14	14
Missouri	17	15	14	14	26	18	18	18
Montana	2	2	2	2	3	2	1	1
Nebraska	5	4	4	3	4	4	4	3
Nevada	5	4	5	6	14	20	9	9
New Hampshire	3	2	2	2	7	1	1	1
New Jersey	14	16	16	17	10	9	9	8
New Mexico	6	3	2	2	32	43	42	42
New York	35	35	29	28	892	749	581	568
North Carolina	15	11	9	10	320	333	332	332
North Dakota	1	3	3	3	65	66	67	66
Ohio	19	16	16	15	416	461	435	426
Oklahoma	18	12	10	10	37	54	88	84
Oregon	4	4	2	3	2	1	1	1
Pennsylvania	31	26	23	24	252	232	202	200
Rhode Island	3	3	2	2	55	20	5	5
South Carolina	9	7	8	8	174	157	89	89
South Dakota	2	1	1	1	10	4	1	1
Tennessee	16	12	10	11	74	83	83	86
Texas	52	30	34	36	879	915	868	867
Utah	7	4	3	3	14	14	15	15
Vermont	2	2	1	1	6	2	2	1
Virginia	19	17	10	9	20	19	35	39
Washington	4	5	5	5	28	17	14	14
West Virginia	5	4	4	4	63	62	66	67
Wisconsin	17	13	11	11	44	41	19	16
Wyoming	2	2	2	2	4	2	2	2

Data are based on a census of certified facilities.

SOURCE: National Center for Health Statistics, *Health, United States, 2010: With Special Feature on Death and Dying*, Hyattsville, MD: U.S. Department of Health and Human Services, 2011.

Report available online at http://www.cdc.gov/nchs/hus.htm. *(Table by PreMediaGlobal.*

KEY TERMS

Bipolar disorder—A disorder characterized by the psychological symptom of extreme mood swings from euphoria mania ("highs") to serious depression ("lows").

Dementia—A progressive deteriorating disease that causes degradation of the intellectual (cognitive) facilities of the brain, such as memory; however, often without problems in other brain functions such as controlling the senses.

Depression—A disorder that presents psychiatric symptoms such as dejection, hopelessness, lack of concentration, sleeplessness, and sometimes suicidal thoughts.

Psychiatrist—A medical doctor trained to treat people with psychiatric disorders.

Psychologist—A professional with an advanced graduate degree (master's or doctorate), trained to study psychological behavior and provide therapeutic services.

Schizophrenia—A disorder relating to psychiatric symptoms relating to emotional instability, self-withdrawal, and inability to comprehend reality.

the potential to harm the patient, such as sharp objects, may also be taken away. In other cases, the person may have more leeway with respect to their ability to move about within the facility and having personal items.

Precautions

In the public mental health system, less-restrictive forms of treatment other than hospitalization are strongly recommended first. In the late 1960s, the patients' rights movement led to reforms governing **involuntary hospitalization**. Today, the criteria for admission, particularly in the case of involuntary hospitalization, are extremely narrow, reflecting a strong reluctance in the United States to infringe on any person's liberty. The unintended consequences of this public policy are often observed in the numbers of people with mental illnesses who are homeless. So long as they are not posing a danger to themselves or others, they are likely to remain outside the traditional treatment system.

Hospitalization has long been negatively characterized in the media, contributing to the **stigma** of seeking inpatient treatment, even when it is voluntary. Scenes from the 1975 movie *One Flew Over the Cuckoo's Nest* have defined the worst in psychiatric hospital treatment. Such conditions cannot exist long in today's more sophisticated mental health, consumer-focused environment. A reputable facility will be accredited by the Joint Commission on Accreditation of Health Care Organizations, or by a similar governing body, which usually assures a minimum level of service. Most hospitals now have a Patient Advocate, usually an attorney who is on-site daily, or accessible by telephone, and whose job is to investigate complaints and protect patients' rights. In addition, a federal law mandates that every state have a Protection and Advocacy Agency to handle complaints of abuse in hospitals. Although the effectiveness of these agencies varies from state to state, they can be helpful in explaining the rights of hospitalized patients. Some states have also implemented ombudsman programs to address patient complaints and to help people negotiate the mental health system.

Treatment facilities may be locked or unlocked. A locked unit will have tighter security to protect patient privacy and to keep patients from running away. In most cases when patients are voluntarily admitted, they may leave treatment at any time, invoking the right to do so against medical advice.

In the past, patients were often not part of their own treatment planning process. The rise of the patients' rights movement has led to more active patient involvement in all phases of treatment. They have the right to refuse certain forms of treatment. Most hospitals now have a clearly posted Patient's Bill of Rights and may also have a patient's council or other body to represent their interests and recommend changes to the inpatient environment.

Confidentiality is paramount in a hospital setting, and medical professionals are bound by laws to safeguard patient confidentiality. Group therapy rules generally stress the importance of keeping members and the content of group sessions confidential.

Preparation

Even voluntary hospitalization can be overwhelming and anxiety-provoking. As a result, hospital staff will closely observe patients when they are first admitted. If the patients were admitted because of a suicide attempt or a violent episode, a "suicide watch" may be set up with more intensive staffing or in a room that can be monitored easily by nursing staff.

As patients adjust to the hospital routine, more privileges and freedom will be made available. For example, patients may earn privileges or rewards like outings with staff, a weekend pass to go home for a visit, or some other positive consequence if they follow hospital rules and engage in therapeutic activities.

QUESTIONS TO ASK YOUR DOCTOR

- What can I expect during the treatment process?
- What can I do if I reject a particular treatment?
- Do I have to tell my family and friends?
- What happens if I do not get better in the hospital?
- Will my insurance pay for all of it? What is covered, and what is not covered? What happens if I do not have health insurance?

An interdisciplinary treatment team made up of a psychiatrist, psychologist, social worker, nurse, direct care worker (sometimes called a "psychiatric technician" or "mental health worker"), and an expressive therapist usually oversees the care of patients while they are in the hospital. Treatment goals are developed by the team with patient input, and with discharge as a major objective.

Aftercare

Optimally, inpatient treatment prepares patients to cope with the realities of life outside the hospital. Emphasis is placed on how patients will behave differently in order to remain healthy and avoid future hospitalizations. During the discharge phase, patients may be scheduled for outpatient therapy and informed about various medications. Patients often experience anxiety at the thought of leaving the hospital, and this apprehension is addressed in therapy sessions as discharge nears.

In the past, a patient might be admitted to a hospital for a minimum of 30 days. Today's rising health care costs and the prevalence of **managed care** have led to dramatically reduced hospital stays. An optimal outcome under these conditions is medication adjustment, monitoring, and the beginning of stabilization. Studies are continuing to be funded to determine whether shortened stays ultimately lead to more frequent hospitalizations later on.

Risks

Many risks are present whenever facing mental illness. Medical professions are trained to assess the risks that individual patients may pose to themselves and others. For the patient, it is best to abide by the rules during hospitalization and expect that a positive result will occur during the stay. Trained medical personnel are on call 24-hours a day, seven days a week, to treat mental patients confined to a hospital setting.

Resources

BOOKS

Desai, Abhilash K., and George T. Grossberg. *Psychiatric Consultation in Long-term Care: A Guide for Health Care Professionals.* Baltimore: Johns Hopkins University Press, 2010.

Harrison, Anthony, and Chris Hart, editors. *Mental Health Care for Nurses: Applying Mental Health Skills in the General Hospital.* Oxford: Blackwell, 2006.

Jarvis, Carolyn. *Physical Examination and Health Assessment.* St. Louis: Elsevier/Saunders, 2012.

Whittington, Richard, and Caroline Logan, editors. *Self-harm and Violence: Towards Best Practice in Managing Risk in Mental Health Services.* Chichester, U.K.: Wiley-Blackwell, 2011.

PERIODICALS

Link, Bruce, Dorothy M. Castille, and Jennifer Stuber. "Stigma and Coercion in the Context of Outpatient Treatment for People with Mental Illnesses." *Social Science and Medicine* 67 (April 30, 2008): 409–19. http://www.psychodyssey.net/wp-content/uploads/2010/11/Stigma-and-coercion-in-the-context-of-outpatient-treatment-for-people-with-mental-illness.pdf (accessed May 24, 2011).

OTHER

"Understanding Hospitalization for Mental Health." Depression and Bipolar Support Alliance. http://www.dbsalliance.org/pdfs/patienthospitalization.pdf (accessed May 23, 2011).

WEBSITES

Centers for Disease Control and Prevention (CDC). "Mental Health." (October 27, 2010). http://www.cdc.gov/nchs/fastats/mental.htm (accessed May 23, 2011).

———. "Mental Health Organizations by State." http://www.cdc.gov/mentalhealth/state_orgs.htm (accessed May 24, 2011).

Mental Health America. "Mental Illness and the Family: Is Hospitalization Necessary." http://www.nmha.org/go/information/get-info/mi-and-the-family/is-hospitalization-necessary (accessed May 23, 2011).

ORGANIZATIONS

American Psychiatric Association, 1000 Wilson Boulevard, Suite 1825, Arlington, VA, 22209-3901, (703) 907-7300, apa@psych.org, http://www.psych.org.

American Psychological Association, 750 First Street, N.E., Washington, DC, 20002-4242, (202) 336-5500, (800) 374-2721, http://www.apa.org.

Anxiety Disorders Association of America, 8730 Georgia Avenue, Silver Spring, MD, 20910, (240) 485-1001, http://www.adaa.org.

Depression and Bipolar Support Alliance, 730 North Franklin Street, Suite 501, Chicago, IL, 60654-7225, (312) 642-7243, (800) 826-3632, http://www.dbsalliance.org.

Mental Health America, 2000 North Beauregard Street, Sixth Floor, Alexandria, VA, 22311, (703) 684-7722, (800) 969-6642, Fax: (703) 684-5968, http://www.nmha.org.

National Institute of Mental Health, 6001 Executive Boulevard, Room 8184, MSC 9663, Bethesda, MD, 20892-9663, (301) 443-4513, (866) 615-6464, Fax: (301) 443-4279, http://www.nimh.nih.gov.

Substance Abuse and Mental Health Services Administration, 1 Choke Cherry Rd., Rockville, MD, 20857, (877) SAMHSA-7, http://www.samhsa.gov/index.aspx.

Judy Leaver, MA
Emily Jane Willingham, Ph.D.
William A. Atkins

House-tree-person test

Definition

The house-tree-person (HTP) test is a projective personality test, a type of examination in which the test taker responds to or provides ambiguous, abstract, or unstructured stimuli (often in the form of pictures or drawings). In the HTP test, which was developed by American clinical **psychologist** John N. Buck (1906–1983), the test taker is asked to separately draw houses, trees, and persons (as well as possible), and these freehand drawings provide a measure of self-perceptions and attitudes for the administrator. The test also reveals areas of concern or conflict within the individual. As with other projective tests, it has flexible and subjective administration and interpretation.

Purpose

The primary purpose of the HTP is to measure aspects of a person's personality (inner self), along with their outlook to his/her environment and what the person thinks is important, all through interpretation of drawings and responses to questions. It is also sometimes intended as part of an assessment of **brain** damage or overall neurological functioning. It is often used with children and those with limited vocabulary because few words are needed to complete the test. The test is also useful for people with limited intelligence or education or with limited or deprived cultural backgrounds, and those that do not speak English, are mute, or are shy and withdrawn. However, the HTP test is difficult for people with motor-derived problems such as people with strokes and muscular or neurological disabilities.

It is also used with children who have been sexually abused. Such children are often hesitant to verbally state their feelings. However, they will indirectly expose their feelings during the completion of the HTP test. The test can be valuable at helping to provide discrete information on the problems hidden within the child and the unconscious aspects of their personality.

The HTP was developed in 1948 by Mr. Buck, and later updated in 1969 by Buck and American psychologist Emanuel F. Hammer. (Hammer had earlier used the test as a way to compare normal people with sex offenders.) Tests requiring human **figure drawings** were already being utilized as projective personality tests. Buck believed that drawings of houses and trees could also provide relevant information about the functioning of an individual's personality.

Description

The HTP was originally developed to measure intelligence from aspects of the Goodenough scale (also called the Draw-A-Man test), which was designed to measure intellectual function. Today, it is similar to the Draw-A-Person (DAP) test, which is an adoption of the Draw-A-Man test. Buck felt that personality characteristics would be described through art; specifically, that unconscious problems would surface through the drawing of objects. It can be given to anyone over the age of three years. Because the HTP test requires test takers to draw pictures, it is often directed toward children and adolescents. It is also often helpful with individuals suspected of having brain damage or other neurological impairment. The test takes an average of 150 minutes (2.5 hours) to complete; it may take less time with normally functioning adults and much more time with neurologically impaired individuals.

A quantitative scoring system was developed by Buck to provide a measure of interpretation to the drawings. Basic levels of intelligence and personality characteristics were provided and classified in groups. After the drawings are completed, the administrator normally asks sixty questions. The drawings are basically used to interpret associations with home and general lifestyle, families (intrafamilial relationships), home life (including children), parents and children, and married adults.

During the first phase of the test, test takers are asked to use a crayon and white paper to draw pictures, respectively, of a house, a tree, and a person. Each drawing is performed on a separate piece of paper and the test taker is asked to draw each as accurately as possible. Upon completion of the drawings, the test taker is asked questions about the drawings. Buck created sixty questions, which can be asked by examiners. Examiners can also create their own questions or ask unscripted follow-up questions. For example, with reference to the house, Buck wrote questions such as, "Is it a happy house?" and "What is the house made of?" Regarding the tree, questions include, "About how old is that tree?" and "Is the tree alive?" Concerning the person, questions include, "Is that person happy?" and "How does that person feel?"

During the second phase of the test, test takers are asked to draw the same pictures on white paper with a pencil. The questions that follow this phase are similar to the ones in the first phase. Some examiners give only one of the two phases, choosing a crayon, a pencil, or some other writing instrument. In some instances a pencil drawing is first drawn, which is later filled in with different colored crayons.

The way the pictures are drawn reflect characteristics of the individual. The administrator sees a depressed person when few details and faint lines are drawn in any image. The characteristics of drawn lines are important: whether they are long or short, bold or slight, straight or crooked, many or few breaks all tell a story. For instance, bold lines are the sign of an outgoing individual. Generally, the house figure reflects the test taker's home life and family relationships, the tree figure reveals the test taker's experiences, and the person figure discerns the relationships between the test taker and people other than his/her family.

Specifically, if the branches of the tree are upward and/or outward, then the individual is said to be one who strives for achievement. A trunk symbolizes inner strength (ego). In another instance, the head of a person drawn in profile with the body forward shows someone who avoids social conflicts. A house with the ground sloping downward and away is likely to be perceived as a person who, for instance, has feelings of isolation and helplessness when in stressful situations. An overly large roof on a house can represent **schizophrenia**. The windows, doors, and other features of the house all help to define the inner person.

Questions asked by the administrator also reveal much about the test taker. When the question is asked, "Is the tree alive?" and the answer is "No," then such an answer may reveal a maladjusted attitude.

One variation of test administration involves asking the individual to draw two separate persons, one of each sex. Another variation is to have test takers put all the drawings on one page. The specific drawing of the house, tree, and person in each drawing provides the administrator with an assessment of different aspects of the test taker (drawer), and how the individual feels about him or herself.

KEY TERMS

Neurological—Referring to neurology, which is the study of the nervous system.

Qualitative—Relating to quality.

Quantitative—Relating to quantities.

Psychodiagnostic—Various methods used to find abnormal or maladjusted behavior in individuals.

Preparation

There is no need to prepare for the HTP test.

Risks

Because the administration of the test is mostly subjective, scoring and interpreting of the HTP is difficult. Biases may be introduced if a trained administrator is not used.

Precautions

Anyone administering the HTP must be properly trained. The test publishers provide a very detailed 350-page administration and scoring manual. In any case, the administrator should be very cautious as to not to make incorrect assumptions or interpretations.

Parental concerns

The test is easy to administer and does not take much time to complete. In addition, children find it fun to draw pictures, so the HTP test is a simple way for parents to learn more about their children, and to find out whether they are having problems. However, the results of the test can be biased based on the administrator. A well-trained administrator is needed to remove or, at least, minimize the chance of biases creeping into the scoring process. Overall, the NTP test is one of the most widely used projective personality tests used. It is popular with professionals because it yields much clinical information about the patient, while being easy and non-threatening to administer. It is often the first of a battery of psychodiagnostic tests used to assess personality in individuals, especially those that are culturally

QUESTIONS TO ASK YOUR DOCTOR

- What other tests should be performed in addition to the HTP test?
- Do you know of a well-trained administrator for the test?
- Should we be concerned with the subjective nature of interpretation and scoring for the test?
- Will health insurance cover the test?

isolated, educationally deprived, developmentally disabled, and/or non-English speaking.

Results

The HTP is scored in both an objective quantitative manner and a subjective qualitative manner. The quantitative scoring scheme involves analyzing the details of drawings to arrive at a general assessment of intelligence, using a scoring method devised by the test creators. Research has shown this assessment of intelligence correlates highly with other **intelligence tests** such as the Wechsler Adult Intelligence Scale (WAIS).

The primary use of the HTP, however, is related to the qualitative scoring scheme in which the test administrator subjectively analyzes the drawings and the responses to questions in a way that assesses the test taker's personality. For example, a very small house might indicate rejection of one's home life. A tree that has a slender trunk but has large expansive branches might indicate a need for satisfaction. A drawing of a person that has a lot of detail in the face might indicate a need to present oneself in an acceptable social light.

Other methods of interpretation focus on the function of various parts in each of the drawings. In the house drawing, the roof might represent one's intellectual side, the walls might represent the test taker's degree of ego strength, and the doors and windows might represent the individual's relation to the outside world. In the tree drawing, the branches might indicate the test taker's relation to the outside world and the trunk might indicate inner strength.

As with other subjectively scored personality tests, there is little support for its reliability and validity. Individual HTP signs do not correspond to single meanings (and can point to various interpretations); only a series of similar signs can point to a specific problem or concern. Therefore, its interpretation is highly subjective, and its conclusion may be entirely inappropriate. However, there is some evidence that the HTP can differentiate people with specific types of brain damage. More specifically, it has been shown to be effective when looking at the brain damage present in schizophrenic patients.

Resources

BOOKS

Boyer, Bret A., and M. Indira Paharia, eds. *Comprehensive Handbook of Clinical Health Psychology.* Hoboken, NJ: John Wiley and Sons, 2008.

Boyle, Gregory J., Gerald Matthews and Donald H. Saklofske, eds. *The SAGE Handbook of Personality Theory and Assessment* Los Angeles: SAGE, 2008.

Groth-Marnat, Gary. *Handbook of Psychological Assessment.* 4th edition. Hoboken, NJ: John Wiley and Sons, 2003.

Hersen, Michel, ed. *Comprehensive Handbook of Psychological Assessment.* Hoboken, NJ: John Wiley and Sons, 2004.

Kellerman, Henry, and Anthony Burry. *Handbook of Psychodiagnostic Testing: Analysis of Personality in the Psychological Report.* New York: Springer, 2007.

Leeming, David A., Kathryn Madden and Stanton Marlan, eds. *Encyclopedia of Psychology and Religion.* New York: Springer, 2010.

PERIODICALS

"Hammer, Emanuel F., PhD." *New York Times*, May 22, 2005. http://query.nytimes.com/gst/fullpage.html?res=9C0DE5D91F30F931A15756C0A9639C8B63 (accessed December 13, 2011).

Rowe, F. B., W. D. Crews, Jr., and F. W. Finger. "John N. Buck (1906–1983): Did He Practically Establish Clinical Psychology in Virginia?" *Journal of Clinical Psychology* 49, no. 3 (1993): 428–34.

OTHER

Fallahi, Carolyn, R. "The House-Tree-Person Test." Department of Psychology, Central Connecticut State University. http://www.psychology.ccsu.edu/fallahic/HTP%20Outline.ppt#256,1,The House-Tree-Person Test (accessed December 13, 2011).

WEBSITES

Deffenbaugh, Anne M. "The House-Tree-Person Test with Kids Who Have Been Sexually Abused." Education Resources Information Center (ERIC). 2003. http://www.eric.ed.gov/ERICWebPortal/search/detailmini.jsp?_nfpb=true&_&ERICExtSearch_SearchValue_0=ED482760&ERICExtSearch_SearchType_0=no&accno=ED482760 (accessed December 13, 2011).

"House-Tree-Person (H-T-P) Projective Drawing Technique." Western Psychological Services. http://portal.wpspublish.

com/portal/page?_pageid=53,70613&_dad=portal&_schema=PORTAL (accessed December 13, 2011).

Ali Fahmy, PhD

Hypericum *see* **St. John's wort**

Hyperkinetic disorder (HKD) *see* **Attention deficit hyperactivity disorder**

Hypersomnia

Definition

Hypersomnia refers to a group of related disorders that involve excessive daytime sleepiness (EDS). The name of the condition comes from two Greek words that mean "more than normal" and "sleep."

Demographics

There is some disagreement among researchers regarding the prevalence of hypersomnia in the general population because of the lack of clear biological markers for the disorder and the lack of precise diagnostic criteria. On the one hand, general surveys of adults in Canada and the United States report rates of EDS in 0.5%–5% of respondents. On the other hand, the National Sleep Foundation (NSF) reports that as many as 40% of adults have some symptoms of hypersomnia from time to time. In a poll taken by the NSF in 2000, 20% of the respondents reported a level of daytime sleepiness sufficient to interfere with work and other activities. Hypersomnia is the single most common symptom among people who seek help from sleep clinics and accounts for 5%–10% of these patients.

Description

The categorization of excessive daytime sleepiness is not completely clear. In 1966, an American physician William Dement, widely considered the founder of sleep medicine as a medical subspecialty, introduced a distinction between **narcolepsy** and a condition of excessive sleepiness that lacks the symptoms of rapid-onset rapid eye movement (REM) sleep, cataplexy, and sleep paralysis. The International Classification of Sleep Disorders has defined this second condition—primary or idiopathic hypersomnia—as "a disorder of presumed central nervous system (CNS) cause that is associated with excessive sleepiness consisting of prolonged sleep episodes of non-rapid eye movement (NREM) sleep." The fourth edition of the ***Diagnostic and Statistical Manual of Mental Disorders*** (*DSM-IV*) defines primary hypersomnia as excessive daytime sleepiness without narcolepsy or the associated features of other sleep disorders. Changes proposed for the fifth edition of *DSM* (*DSM-5*), due for publication in 2013, include renaming the disorder as "Primary Hypersomnia/Narcolepsy without Cataplexy."

In contrast to narcolepsy, which has well-defined characteristic symptoms, primary or idiopathic hypersomnia is less precisely characterized. Some observers distinguish between a form of primary hypersomnia in which the patient has isolated episodes of EDS without abnormal nighttime awakening and a form in which the patient sleeps for an abnormally long period of time at night (longer than nine hours) and suffers from sleep drunkenness on awaking.

A third but rare condition known as **Kleine-Levin syndrome** (KLS), sometimes called Sleeping Beauty syndrome, is also classified as primary hypersomnia of central origin because it is thought to be caused by some type of systemic disorder (possibly an autoimmune disorder) even though its cause was not fully understood as of 2011. KLS is characterized by periods of sleep lasting up to 20 or more hours a day in episodes that last for several weeks. In addition, people with KLS are often irritable, sometimes to the point of violence. They may be sexually uninhibited (hypersexual) and make indiscriminate sexual advances. There may also be some confusion, depressed mood, and memory deficits. People with Kleine-Levin syndrome often eat uncontrollably and rapidly gain weight, unlike people with other forms of hypersomnia. This form of recurrent hypersomnia is very rare. The disorder, which most often starts in adolescence, generally resolves by the early adult years. The male/female ratio in KLS is 4:1.

Hypersomnia associated with certain medical or psychiatric conditions is classified as secondary hypersomnia. Such conditions include:

- sleep disorders, including sleep-related breathing disorders, sleep-related movement disorders, and circadian rhythm sleep disorders
- sleep deprivation
- mood disorders, particularly depression
- drugs of abuse and some classes of prescription medications
- head trauma
- cancer
- stroke
- encephalitis
- some inflammatory conditions

Risk factors

Risk factors for primary hypersomnia include a family history of the disorder and a history of viral illnesses—particularly Guillain-Barré syndrome, viral hepatitis, mononucleosis, and atypical viral pneumonia. With the exception of KLS, sex is not known to be a risk factor for primary hypersomnia. The onset of primary hypersomnia occurs most commonly in adolescents; it is rare for onset of the disorder to occur in adults over 30. There is no indication that race or ethnicity is a risk factor for primary hypersomnia.

Risk factors for secondary hypersomnia include:

- being a shift worker
- history of alcoholism or drug abuse
- history of head injury or multiple sclerosis
- treatment with prescription drugs associated with daytime sleepiness, including antipsychotics, antihistamines, antidepressants, benzodiazepine tranquilizers, antiepileptic drugs, muscle relaxants, barbiturates, and drugs given to treat nausea or diarrhea
- being diagnosed with obstructive sleep apnea or circadian sleep disorder
- obesity

Causes and symptoms

The cause of primary hypersomnia is not yet known, although some researchers think that it may be associated with malfunctions of the norepinephrine system. Norepinephrine is a neurotransmitter released by specialized neurons in the locus coeruleus, a structure located in the brainstem. Norepinephrine plays a role in the ability to pay attention and focus as well as in the fight-or-flight reaction to **stress**. No genetic or environmental causes of primary hypersomnia had been identified as of 2011.

The symptoms of primary hypersomnia typically include long periods of sleep (as long as 12 hours) with daytime naps that are not refreshing followed by sleep drunkenness on awaking. Patients with primary hypersomnia may fall asleep at work or in class, during meals or conversations with others, or even while driving or operating machinery. They are typically difficult to awaken from daytime naps. Other symptoms may include headaches, trouble thinking clearly, general lack of energy, **depression**, anxiety, fainting episodes, automatic behavior, and orthostatic hypotension (sudden drop in blood pressure when standing upright suddenly after being in a sitting or lying position).

KEY TERMS

Automatic behavior—Activity that a person with narcolepsy can carry out while partially awake but is not conscious of at the time and cannot recall afterward.

Cataplexy—A sudden episode of muscle weakness triggered by emotions. The muscle weakness may cause the person's knees to buckle or the head to drop. In severe cases, the patient may become paralyzed for a few seconds to minutes.

Hypersomnolence—Excessive daytime sleepiness in spite of sufficient nighttime sleep.

Hypothalamus—A part of the forebrain that controls heartbeat, body temperature, thirst, hunger, body temperature and pressure, blood sugar levels, and other functions.

Idiopathic—Arising spontaneously or from an unknown or obscure cause.

Obstructive sleep apnea—A disorder caused by obstruction of the upper airway during sleep and characterized by repeated pauses in breathing during sleep despite efforts to breathe.

Rapid eye movement (REM) sleep—The phase of a sleep cycle in which dreaming occurs; it is characterized by rapid eye movements.

Sleep cycle—A period of NREM sleep followed by a shorter phase of REM sleep. Most adults have four to six sleep cycles per night.

Sleep drunkenness—A condition associated with primary hypersomnia in which the person has an abnormally prolonged period of transition from sleep to wakefulness; is disoriented, drowsy, and uncoordinated; and may behave in an excited or violent fashion.

Sleep paralysis—An abnormal episode of sleep in which the patient cannot move for a few minutes, usually occurring on falling asleep or waking up. It is often found in patients with narcolepsy.

Diagnosis

The **diagnosis** of primary hypersomnia involves a process of exclusion. The editors of *DSM-5* have proposed the following five criteria for Primary Hypersomnia/Narcolepsy without Cataplexy:

- The patient's chief complaint is either unexplained hypersomnia and/or hypersomnolence (sleepiness in spite of sufficient sleep at night), for at least 3 months, occurring three or more times per week. The proposed criterion defines hypersomnia as "a prolonged nocturnal sleep episode or daily sleep amounts" greater than 9 hours per day; and hypersomnolence as "excessive daytime sleepiness with recurrent daytime naps or lapses into sleep that occurs daily or almost daily over at least the last 3 months (when the patient is untreated) and daily sleep amounts greater than 6 hours."

- The patient's periods of sleep are either unrefreshing or last so long that the person's social, academic, or occupational functioning is impaired.
- The hypersomnia is not better accounted for by insomnia or by another sleep disorder, and cannot be accounted for by sleep deprivation or inadequate amounts of sleep.
- The hypersomnia does not occur exclusively during the course of another medical or psychiatric disorder but may occur together with such a disorder.
- The hypersomnia is not caused directly by a medication or drug of abuse.

Examination

Careful history-taking during an office examination is useful in ruling out secondary hypersomnia associated with medications, shift work, drug or alcohol abuse, or jet lag related to frequent travel. The patient may be referred to a neurologist to rule out traumatic head injury, **brain** tumors, or such diseases as encephalitis, or to a **psychiatrist** to be evaluated for a mood or anxiety disorder. Obese patients may require evaluation for obstructive sleep apnea.

Tests

Paper-and-pencil tests that can be given during an office examination include the Epworth Sleepiness Scale, or ESS, which was developed in Australia in the early 1990s. A score of 12 or higher on the ESS suggests hypersomnia. Another questionnaire that can be used in the office is the Stanford Sleepiness Scale (SSS).

Patients may be given tests of motor coordination and complex reaction time, particularly if they have reported falling asleep while driving or if they are employed in occupations that involve driving or operating complex machinery (including train conductors, truckers, airline pilots, and taxicab and school bus drivers). Some states require doctors to report patients who fail to comply with treatment for excessive daytime sleepiness.

Patients with hypersomnia are also evaluated in a sleep laboratory with two tests known as the multiple sleep latency test (MSLT) and the maintenance of wakefulness test (MWT). These tests measure the amount of time that it takes for the patient to fall asleep and the person's ability to stay awake for a certain period of time. Falling asleep in less than 10 minutes on the MSLT is considered an indication of hypersomnia. Unlike patients with narcolepsy, however, patients with hypersomnia have normal REM sleep latency and fewer than 2 sleep-onset REM periods during the test. The MSLT can also be used to rule out obstructive sleep apnea.

Laboratory tests include a complete blood cell count, a test of thyroid function, and (in some cases) a drug screen to rule out a substance-induced sleep disorder. The patient may also be given a CT scan to rule out multiple sclerosis or another neurological disorder, or an electroencephalogram (EEG), a test that measures the electrical activity of the brain.

Treatment

Treatment depends on whether the hypersomnia is primary or secondary. Secondary hypersomnia associated with obstructive sleep apnea can be treated with the use of a continuous positive air pressure (CPAP) machine during sleep. Hypersomnia associated with prescription medications can be treated by discontinuing the drug or switching the patient to a similar medication that is less likely to cause drowsiness.

Drugs

Patients with primary hypersomnia can be treated with such stimulant drugs as modafinil, sodium oxybate, amphetamine, **methamphetamine**, **dextroamphetamine**, **methylphenidate**, and selegiline. Other drugs used to treat hypersomnia include **clonidine**, levodopa, bromocriptine, **antidepressants**, and **monoamine oxidase inhibitors**.

Relatively little research has been done on primary hypersomnia, and the American Academy of Sleep Medicine (AASM) has called for further work in this area. There were only two **clinical trials** under way as of 2011 of other drugs for the treatment of primary hypersomnia. One drug was flumazenil (Anexate), a drug developed in the 1980s to reverse the effects of benzodiazepine tranquilizers. The other drug was clarithromycin (Crixan, Clarac), a macrolide antibiotic used to treat tonsillitis, acute sinusitis, and severe pneumonia. Both studies were being conducted at Emory University in Georgia.

Psychotherapy and lifestyle changes

The AASM recommends **cognitive-behavioral therapy** and changing the patient's daily schedule to

QUESTIONS TO ASK YOUR DOCTOR

- What is the difference between narcolepsy and primary hypersomnia?
- How can I tell whether my sleepiness is a response to sleep deprivation or a symptom of hypersomnia?
- What is your opinion of stimulants as a treatment for hypersomnia?
- I have a relative who has been diagnosed with primary hypersomnia. What should I know about the disorder in order to be helpful to him/her?
- Have you ever treated a patient who was diagnosed with primary hypersomnia?
- Do you think there will ever be a cure for the disorder?

allow for daytime naps, because stimulant drugs are not a substitute for sleep. Other recommended lifestyle changes include avoiding late-night work and social activities that interfere with an early bedtime, along with avoidance of alcohol and caffeinated beverages.

Education of patients and their family about the nature of the disorder is vital. It is not unusual for patients with primary hypersomnia to be misjudged by others as lazy or incompetent. Patients generally function better when their friends, family members, and employers or workplace colleagues are helped to understand the disorder and the available treatments for it.

Prognosis

The prognosis of secondary hypersomnia is generally better than that of primary hypersomnia. Although primary hypersomnia is not fatal by itself, it can result in fatal accidents. Primary hypersomnia typically continues indefinitely; it is a lifelong disorder and may cause severe disruption of the patient's education, employment, and social relationships. There are no known cases of spontaneous remission.

Prevention

There is no known way to prevent primary hypersomnia, because the causes of the disorder are not yet understood.

Resources

BOOKS

American Psychiatric Association. *Diagnostic and Statistical Manual of Mental Disorders,* 4th ed., Text rev. Washington, DC: American Psychiatric Association, 2000.

Benca, Ruth M. *Sleep Disorders: The Clinician's Guide to Diagnosis and Management.* Oxford: Oxford University Press, 2011.

Silvestri, Rosalia, ed. *Sleep Disorders in Neurology.* Hauppauge, NY: Nova Science, 2011.

Wilson, Sue, and David Nutt. *Sleep Disorders.* New York: Oxford University Press, 2008.

PERIODICALS

Ali, M., et al. "Idiopathic Hypersomnia: Clinical Features and Response to Treatment." *Journal of Clinical Sleep Medicine* 15 (2009): 562–68.

Bassetti, C.L., et al. "Cerebrospinal Fluid Histamine Levels Are Decreased in Patients with Narcolepsy and Excessive Daytime Sleepiness of Other Origin." *Journal of Sleep Research* 19 (2010): 620–23.

Janácková, S., et al. "Idiopathic Hypersomnia: A Report of Three Adolescent-onset Cases in a Two-generation Family." *Journal of Child Neurology* 26 (2011): 522–25.

Kotagal, S. "Hypersomnia in Children: Interface with Psychiatric Disorders." *Child and Adolescent Psychiatric Clinics of North America* 18 (2009): 967–77.

Lavault, S., et al. "Benefit and Risk of Modafinil in Idiopathic Hypersomnia vs. Narcolepsy with Cataplexy." *Sleep Medicine* 12 (2011): 550–56.

Pizza, F., et al. "Different Sleep Onset Criteria at the Multiple Sleep Latency Test (MSLT): An Additional Marker to Differentiate Central Nervous System (CNS) Hypersomnias." *Journal of Sleep Research* 20 (2011): 250–56.

Quinnell, T.G., and I.E. Smith. "Narcolepsy, Idiopathic Hypersomnolence and Related Conditions." *Clinical Medicine* 11 (2011): 282–86.

Vernet, C., et al. "Subjective Symptoms in Idiopathic Hypersomnia: Beyond Excessive Sleepiness." *Journal of Sleep Research* 19 (2010): 525–34.

WEBSITES

"Extreme Sleepiness." National Sleep Foundation. http://www.sleepfoundation.org/article/sleep-related-problems/idiopathic-hypersomnia-and-sleep (accessed October 14, 2011).

"Hypersomnia Information Page." National Institute of Neurological Disorders and Stroke. Last updated June 23, 2008. http://www.ninds.nih.gov/disorders/hypersomnia/hypersomnia.htm (accessed October 14, 2011).

"M 01 Primary Hypersomnia/Narcolepsy without Cataplexy." American Psychiatric Association. DSM-5 Development. http://www.dsm5.org/ProposedRevision/Pages/proposedrevision.aspx?rid=66 (accessed October 14, 2011).

Pagel, J.F. "Excessive Daytime Sleepiness." *American Family Physician* 79 (2009): 391–96. http://www.aafp.org/afp/2009/0301/p391.html (accessed September 20, 2011).

"Primary Hypersomnia." Medscape. Last updated February 3, 2011. http://emedicine.medscape.com/article/291699-overview (accessed October 14, 2011).

"Sleep and Hypersomnia." WebMD. Last reviewed March 3, 2010. http://www.webmd.com/sleep-disorders/guide/hypersomnia (accessed October 14, 2011).

ORGANIZATIONS

American Academy of Sleep Medicine, 2510 N Frontage Rd., Darien, IL, 60561, (630) 737-9700, Fax: (630) 737-9790, inquiries@assmnet.org, http://www.aasmnet.org.

American Psychiatric Association, 1000 Wilson Blvd., Ste. 1825, Arlington, VA, 22209-3901, (703) 907-7300, apa@psych.org, http://www.psych.org.

National Institute of Mental Health, 6001 Executive Blvd., Rm. 8184, MSC 9663, Bethesda, MD, 20892-9663, (301) 433-4513; TTY: (301) 443-8431, Fax: (301) 443-4279, (866) 615-6464; TTY: (866) 415-8051, nimhinfo@nih.gov, http://www.nimh.nih.gov.

National Institute of Neurological Disorders and Stroke, PO Box 5801, Bethesda, MD, 20824, (301) 496-5751; TTY: (301) 468-5981, (800) 352-9424, http://www.ninds.nih.gov.

Tish Davidson, AM
Emily Jane Willingham, PhD
Rebecca J. Frey, PhD

Hypnotherapy

Definition

Hypnotherapy is the use of hypnosis as part of psychological or psychiatric treatment. Hypnotherapy may be used in short-term **psychotherapy** to help alleviate symptoms or as part of a long-term plan of psychotherapeutic **intervention** for personality change. Hypnotherapy may use any one or a combination of techniques administered by a trained professional who induces a hypnotic state in the patient and then presents therapeutic suggestions.

Purpose

Hypnosis, when used in conjunction with proven therapeutic procedures, can be a highly effective form of treatment for many mental, psychosomatic, and physical disorders. For example, through the use of regressive techniques, an adult patient may mentally travel back to a point in youth that was particularly troublesome, allowing the healing of old emotional wounds. Another patient can be led to understand that emotional pain has been converted to physical pain, and that the pain can be eliminated once the source has been addressed. Hypnotherapy can also be used to help persons with chronic pain to control the pain without use of medications. There are a number of techniques for correcting dysfunctional behaviors such as self-destructive habits, **anxiety disorders**, and even managing side effects of various medical treatments and procedures.

Hypnotherapy has been used to stop self-destructive and addictive habits like smoking. It has also been used to curb overeaters' urge to eat, to stem the disruptive actions of tics, cure **insomnia**, stop bed-wetting, and minimize anxiety. Excessive **stress** can be generated from any number of sources and can be the springboard for anxiety. Some of the more prominent sources of anxiety and stress for which people seek hypnotherapy are: public speaking, test taking, and job stress. Hypnotherapy also works well for other anxiety disorders such as phobias and has proven to be an effective treatment for mild to moderate **depression**. In one study, hypnotherapy was used in conjunction with traditional

MILTON ERICKSON (1901–1980)

Erickson rose to prominence during the 1940s and 1950s as a pioneer in the medical, dental, and psychotherapeutic uses of hypnosis. He was considered the world's leading authority on the subject of hypnotherapy and was instrumental in establishing worldwide recognition and acceptance of hypnosis as a valid and effective therapeutic technique. He was frequently consulted by doctors and scientists, including anthropologist Margaret Mead, and during the 1950s he collaborated with author Aldous Huxley on research on hypnosis and other states of consciousness.

Erickson practiced psychiatry in Massachusetts and Michigan before moving to Arizona in the late 1940s. He was confined to a wheelchair following a bout with polio but continued to conduct teaching seminars from his Phoenix home. Erickson's teaching style was similar to his psychotherapeutic method—distraction by verbal communication and other forms of indirection disrupted the conscious set, providing access to the subject's unconscious mind. His orientation was eclectic, drawing on the widest range of schools of personality theory for the most useful elements of each. Erickson's books on the subject of hypnotherapy are geared toward health professionals and are, according to a *Psychology Today* reviewer, "written in a style ... as original and personal as [Erickson's] technique."

cognitive therapy to assist persons who had severe aversion to needles. The treatment was necessary, because it was essential that each participant receive periodic medical injections. However, the participants would have become noncompliant without the adjunct intervention of hypnotherapy. In another case, involving care for terminally ill cancer patients, it was concluded that hypnotherapy was more effective at enhancing quality of life and relieving anxiety and depressive symptoms, when compared to others who received traditional care.

Precautions

Confusion can occur when one seeks a hypnotherapist as a result of the various titles, certifications, and licenses in the field. Many states do not regulate the title "hypnotist" or "hypnotherapist," so care must be exercised when selecting someone to see. As a rule, it is best to consult a professional in the field of mental health or medicine, although alternative sources for hypnosis are available. Care must also be taken by the therapist to ensure adequate training and sufficient experience for rendering this specialized service. The therapist must be well-grounded in a psychotherapeutic approach before undertaking the use of hypnotherapy. Professionals should not attempt hypnotherapy with any disorder for which they would not use traditional therapeutic approaches. The patient seeking hypnotherapy is reminded that unskilled or amateur hypnotists can cause harm and should not be consulted for the purpose of implementing positive change in an individual's life. The detrimental effects of being subjected to amateur or inadequately trained persons can be severe and long lasting.

Description

In order to understand hypnotherapy, it is necessary to understand the underlying concepts of hypnosis. A brief review of the history of hypnosis, description of hypnosis, and modern techniques follows.

History of hypnosis

It appears that hypnosis, under other names, has been used since the beginning of time. In fact, it has been insinuated that the earliest description of hypnosis may be portrayed in the Old Testament and in the Talmud. There is also evidence of hypnosis in ancient Egypt, some 3,000 years ago. However, the man credited with the development of what has become modern hypnosis is Friedrich Anton Mesmer. An Austrian physician, Friedrich Anton Mesmer one day watched a magician on a street in Paris demonstrate that he could have spectators do his bidding by touching them with magnets. Fascinated by the demonstration, Mesmer believed the magnets had power of their own and from this belief developed his theory of "animal magnetism." He also believed that good health depended on having correct magnetic flow and that the direction of one's magnetic flow could easily be reversed. He further believed that he could direct this magnetic flow into inanimate objects, which could then be used for the good health of others. The term "mesmerism" came to be applied to his mystical workings. He experienced much success in helping the people of Paris as well as visitors who came from other countries, upon hearing of his powers. Later he was completely discredited by a special commission of the French Academy appointed by the king, resulting in Mesmer's departure from France. Two of the more famous members of the French Academy at the time were chairman of the commission Benjamin Franklin, American ambassador to France, and Dr. Guillotine, the inventor of the execution device.

Later, around 1840, a patient in the office of Scottish physician James Braid accidentally entered a state of trance while waiting for an eye examination. Braid, aware of the disfavor of mesmerism and animal magnetism coined the term "hypnosis," and thus began the serious study of this altered state of awareness.

What is hypnosis?

It is far easier to describe what hypnosis is not than to describe what it is. For example, it is not one person controlling the mind of another. The patient is not unconscious and does not lose control of his or her faculties. People will not do things under hypnosis that they would be unwilling to do otherwise. The person being hypnotized is always in control. The hypnotized person decides how deep the trance will be, what suggestions will be accepted, and when to awaken. Therefore, a hypnotized person cannot be forever "lost" if the therapist should fall dead during an induction or while the patient is deep in trance.

Hypnosis is first and foremost a self-accepted journey away from the reality of the moment. Although the trance state is often referred to as if the patient is asleep, nothing could be further from the truth. The patient is fully awake at all times. The hypnotic subject is simply in a heightened, more receptive state of mind. This fact is proven with inductions called open-eye techniques, where the patient keeps his/her eyes open during the hypnotherapy. Full and deep trance is still achievable.

Trance is commonplace. People fall into trances many times without even being aware that it has happened. Examples of this include reaching the destination of a morning commute, but not recalling the passing of familiar landmarks; daydreaming while sitting in a college classroom; or that anxiety-free state achieved just before going to sleep. The difference between these altered states and clinically used hypnotherapy is that a professionally trained person is involved in helping the patient achieve the trance, which can be done in many ways.

A typical hypnotherapy session has the patient seated comfortably with their feet on the floor and palms on their lap. Of course, the patient could choose to lie down if that option is available and if that will meet the patient's expectation of hypnosis. The therapist can even set the stage for a favorable outcome by asking questions like, "Would you prefer to undergo hypnosis in this chair or on the sofa?" Once patients makes the choice, they are in effect agreeing to undergo hypnosis. Depending on the approach used by the therapist, the next events can vary, but generally will involve some form of relaxing the patient. Suggestions will lead the patient to an increasingly relaxed state. The therapist may wish to confirm the depth of trance by performing tests with the patient. For example, the therapist may suggest that when the eyes close that they will become locked and cannot be opened. The therapist then checks for this by having patients try to open their eyes. Following a successful trial showing the patient's inability to open the eyes, the therapist might then further relax them by using deepening techniques. Deepening techniques will vary for each patient and depend largely on whether the patient represents information through auditory, visual, or kinesthetic means. If the patient is more affected by auditory suggestions, the therapist would use comments such as "You hear the gentle patter of rain on the roof;" or, "The sound of the ocean waves allow you to relax more and more." For the visual person, the therapist might use statements such as, "You see the beautiful placid lake, with trees bending slightly with the breeze." Finally, with the kinesthetic person phrases like, "You feel the warm sun and gentle breeze on your skin," could be used. It is important for the therapist to know if the patient has difficulty with the idea of floating or descending because these sensations are sometimes used to enhance the experience for the patient. However, if the patient has a fear of heights or develops a feeling of oppression with the thought of traveling downward and going deeper and deeper, suggestions implying the unwanted or feared phenomenon will not be taken and can thwart the attempt.

Modern techniques

In order for a hypnotherapist to convey positive suggestions for change, the patient must be in a receptive state. The state is called trance and the method of achieving a trance is through induction. Induction techniques are many and varied and involve the therapist offering suggestions that the patient follows. The formerly common "your eyes are getting heavy" suggestion may still exist, but other more reliable and acceptable (to the patient) forms of induction have come to the forefront. The artful hypnotherapist is always aware of the present condition of the patient and uses this information to lead him/her down the path of induction. In its lighter stages, trance can be noted by the relaxation of muscles. At this point, hands can levitate when given the suggestion, and paresthesia, a feeling of numbness, can be induced. In a medium trance, a patient can be led to experience partial or complete **amnesia**, or failure to recall events of the induction after the fact. A deep trance opens the patient to powerful auditory, visual, or kinesthetic experiences. The phenomenon of time distortion is experienced most profoundly at this level. Patients may believe they have been away briefly, and may react with disbelief when told they were away much longer. Although some work can be done in lighter states of trance, the best circumstance for implementing change is when the patient reaches a deep trance state. At this level, the patient is focused inwardly and is more receptive to positive suggestions for change. This is also the point at which the therapist can invoke posthypnotic suggestions, or instructions given to the patient so he/she will perform some act or experience some particular sensation following awakening from the trance. These suggestions, if accepted by the patient, can be formed to make foods or cigarettes taste bad, or to delay impulses, curb hunger, or eliminate pain, for example. However, it should be noted that posthypnotic suggestions given to a person which run counter to the person's value system, or are not something they are likely to do under ordinary circumstances, will not be accepted and therefore not implemented.

Neuro-Linguistic Programming (NLP) is the name given to a series of models and techniques used to enhance the therapist's ability to do hypnotherapy. NLP consists of a number of models, with a series of techniques based on those models. Sensory acuity and physiology is one model whose premise is that a person's thought processes change their physiological state. People recognize such a physiological change when startled. The body receives a great dose of **adrenaline**, the heart beats faster, the scare may be verbalized by shouting, and the startled person may sweat. Sensory acuity (i.e., being attuned to changes occurring in another person) will strengthen communication to a person in ways over and above simple verbal cues, therefore making the therapist more effective. A second model of NLP deals with representational systems. The idea behind this model is that different people represent knowledge in different sensory styles. In other words, an individual's language reveals that person's mode of representation. There are three basic modes of representation: auditory, visual, and kinesthetic. The same information will be expressed differently by each type. For example, the auditory person might say, "That sounds good to me," the visual person might offer, "I see it the same way," and the kinesthetic person would say, "I'm comfortable with it too."

Preparation

Before people subject themselves to hypnotherapy they are advised to learn as much about the process and about the chosen therapist as is necessary to feel comfortable. Rapport and trust are two key factors. Therapists should be open and willing to answer all questions regarding qualifications, expertise, and methods used. A well-qualified professional will not undertake the use of hypnosis without interviewing the patient to ascertain their level of understanding of the process. This is very important for two reasons. First, it allows the patient the opportunity to have questions answered and to develop some rapport with the therapist. Second, it is important for the therapist to know the patient's expectations since meeting these expectations will enhance the likelihood of success.

Aftercare

Depending on the purpose of the hypnotherapy (e.g., **smoking cessation**, weight loss, improvement in public speaking, or addressing some deep emotional turmoil), follow-up may be advisable. When trying to eradicate unwanted habits, it is good practice to revisit the therapist, based upon a date prearranged between the therapist and the patient, to report progress and, if necessary, to obtain secondary hypnotherapy to reinforce progress made.

Risks

One obvious risk to patients is the insufficiently trained therapist. The inadequately trained therapist can cause harm and distort the normally pleasant experience of hypnotherapy. A second risk for patients is the unscrupulous practitioner who may be both inadequately trained and may have some hidden agenda. These rare individuals are capable of causing great harm to the patient and to the profession. As mentioned above, the patient should carefully scrutinize their chosen therapist before submitting themselves to this dynamic form of therapy.

Results

The result of hypnotherapy is overwhelmingly positive and effective. Countless success stories exist attesting to the benefits of this technique. Many people have stopped smoking, lost weight, managed pain, remembered forgotten information, stopped other addictions, or improved their health and well-being through its use.

Abnormal results can occur in instances where amateurs, who know the fundamentals of hypnosis, entice friends to become their experimental subjects. Their lack of full understanding can lead to immediate consequences, which can linger for some time after the event. If, for example, the amateur plants the suggestion that the subject is being bitten by mosquitoes, the subject would naturally scratch where the bites were perceived. When awakened from the trance, if the amateur forgets to remove the suggestion, the subject will continue the behavior. Left unchecked, the behavior could land the subject in a physician's office in an attempt to stop the itching and scratching cycle. If the physician is astute enough to question the genesis of the behavior and hypnosis is used to remove the suggestion, the subjects may experience long-term negative emotional distress and anger once they understand exactly what happened. The lack of full understanding, complete training, and supervised experience on the part of the amateur places the subject at risk.

Resources

BOOKS

Barabasz, Arreed, and John G. Watkins. *Hypnotherapeutic Techniques*. 2nd ed. New York: Routledge, 2004.

Flemons, Douglas. *Of One Mind: The Logic of Hypnosis, the Practice of Therapy*. New York: W. W. Norton, 2002.

Hawkins, Peter J. *Hypnosis and Stress: A Guide for Clinicians*. New York: Wiley, 2006.

Lynn, Steven Jay, and Irving Kirsch. *Essentials of Clinical Hypnosis: An Evidence Based Approach*. Washington, DC: American Psychological Association, 2006.

Spiegel, Herbert, and David Spiegel. *Trance and Treatment: Clinical Uses of Hypnosis*. 2nd ed. Washington, DC: American Psychiatric Association, 2004.

Yapko, M.D, ed. *Hypnosis and Treating Depression*. New York: Routledge, 2006.

Zarren, Jordan I., and Bruce N. Eimer. *Brief Cognitive Hypnosis: Facilitating the Change of Dysfunctional Behavior*. New York: Springer Publishing, 2002.

PERIODICALS

Bamford, Candy. "A Multifaceted Approach to the Treatment of Phantom Limb Pain Using Hypnosis." *Contemporary Hypnosis* 23, no. 3 (August 2006): 115–26.

Bryant, Richard A., et al. "Hypnotherapy and Cognitive Behaviour Therapy of Acute Stress Disorder: A 3-Year Follow-Up." *Behaviour Research and Therapy* 44, no. 9 (September 2006): 1331–35.

Gay, Marie-Claire. "Effectiveness of Hypnosis in Reducing Mild Essential Hypertension: A One-Year Follow-Up." *International Journal of Clinical and Experimental Hypnosis* 55, no. 1 (January 2007): 67–83.

Kihslinger, Daun, and Marty Sapp. "Hypnosis and Diabetes: Applications for Children, Adolescents, and Adults." *Australian Journal of Clinical Hypnotherapy and Hypnosis* 27, no. 1 (Fall 2006): 19–27.

Kraft, Tom, and David Kraft. "The Place of Hypnosis in Psychiatry: Its Applications in Treating Anxiety Disorders and Sleep Disturbances." *Australian Journal of Clinical and Experimental Hypnosis* 34, no. 2 (November 2006): 187–203.

Mende, Matthias. "The Special Effects of Hypnosis and Hypnotherapy: A Contribution to an Ecological Model of Therapeutic Change." *International Journal of Clinical and Experimental Hypnosis* 54, no. 2 (April 2006): 167–85.

Uccheddu, Ornella Manca, and Antonello Viola. "Descriptive Survey of Therapeutic Alliance in Hypnotherapy." *European Journal of Clinical Hypnosis* 7, no. 1 (2006): 10–25.

ORGANIZATIONS

American Society of Clinical Hypnosis, 140 N. Bloomingdale Rd., Bloomingdale, IL, 60108, (630) 980-4740, Fax: (630) 351-8490, info@asch.net, http://www.asch.net.

Society for Clinical and Experimental Hypnosis, PO Box 252, Southborough, MA, 01772, (508) 598-5553, Fax: (866) 397-1839, info@sceh.us.

Jack H. Booth, PsyD
Ruth A. Wienclaw, PhD

Hypnotics *see* **Sedatives and related disorders**

Hypoactive sexual desire disorder

Definition

Hypoactive sexual desire disorder (HSDD) is defined as the persistent or recurrent extreme aversion to, absence of, and avoidance of all, or almost all, genital sexual contact with a sexual partner. Synonyms for HSDD include sexual aversion, inhibited sexual desire, sexual **apathy**, and sexual anorexia. HSDD is not rare, occurring in both sexes. It is the most common of all female sexual disorders, occurring in at least 20% of women in the United States.

Description

The affected person has a low level of sexual interest and desire that is manifested by a failure to initiate or be responsive to a partner's initiation of sexual activity. HSD becomes a diagnosable disorder when it causes marked distress or interpersonal instability, according to the ***Diagnostic and Statistical Manual of Mental Disorders***, fourth edition, text revision (also known as the *DSM-IV-TR*), the handbook used by mental health professionals to diagnose mental disorders. HSDD may be either situational (solely oriented against one partner), or it may be general, in which case there is a lack of sexual interest in anyone. In the extreme form of HSDD, the patient not only lacks sexual desire, but may also find sex to be repulsive, revolting and distasteful. Phobic or panic responses may be present in extreme cases of HSD. HSDD may be the result of either physical or emotional factors.

Causes and symptoms

Causes

PRIMARY HSD. HSDD may be a primary condition in which the patient has never felt much sexual desire or interest, or it may have occurred secondarily when the patient formerly had sexual desire, but no longer has interest. If lifelong or primary, HSDD may be the consequence of sexual **trauma** such as incest, **sexual abuse**, or rape. In the absence of sexual trauma, there is often a repressive family attitude concerning sex that is sometimes enhanced by rigid religious training. A third possibility is that initial attempts at sexual intercourse resulted in pain or sexual failure. Rarely, HSDD in both males and females may result from insufficient levels of the male sex hormone, testosterone.

ACQUIRED HSD. Acquired, situational HSDD in the adult is commonly associated with boredom in the relationship with the sexual partner. **Depression**, the use of psychoactive or antihypertensive medications, and hormonal deficiencies may contribute to the problem. HSDD may also result from impairment of sexual function, particularly **erectile dysfunction** on the part of the male, or **vaginismus** on the part of the female. Vaginismus is defined as a conditioned voluntary contraction or spasm of the lower vaginal muscles resulting from an unconscious desire to prevent vaginal penetration. An incompatibility in sexual interest between the sexual partners may result in relative HSDD in the less sexually active member. This usually occurs in the presence of a sexually demanding partner.

PAINFUL INTERCOURSE. Painful intercourse (**dyspareunia**) is more common in women than in men, but may be a deterrent to genital sexual activity in both sexes. The causes are usually physical in nature and related to an infection of the prostate gland, urethra, or testes. Occasionally, an allergic reaction to a spermicidal preparation or condom may interfere with sexual intercourse. Painful erections may be a consequence of

Peyronie's disease, which is characterized by fibrotic changes in the shaft of the penis that prevent attainment of a normal erection. In the female, dyspareunia may be caused by vaginismus or local urogenital trauma or inflammatory conditions such as hymenal tears, labial lacerations, urethral bruising, or inflammatory conditions of the labial or vaginal glands.

PRIAPISM. Priapism is the occurrence of any persistent erection of more than four hours duration occurring in the absence of sexual stimulation. It is not associated with sexual excitement and the erection does not subside after ejaculation. Priapism can occur at any age, but clusters of occurrence are common between the ages of five and 10 years and between the ages of 20 and 50. In children, priapism is commonly associated with leukemia and sickle cell disease, or occurs secondary to trauma. The most common cause in adults is the intrapenile injection of agents to correct erectile dysfunction. Priapism may also occur secondary to the use of psychotropic drugs, such as **chlorpromazine** and prazosin. The pain accompanying priapism may be a cause of HSDD.

PROLACTINOMA. A rare but important cause of HSDD is a functioning prolactin-secreting tumor of the pituitary gland, a prolactinoma. Men with this condition typically state that they can achieve an erection, but that they have no interest in sexual relations. In the female, prolactinomas are associated with galactorrhea (lactation in the absence of pregnancy), amenorrhea, symptoms of estrogen deficiency and dyspareunia. Although prolactinomas are benign tumors, they can cause visual disturbances by enlarging and causing pressure on the optic nerves within the confines of the *sella turcica,* the location of the pituitary gland at the base of the **diagnosis** is confirmed by the finding of high levels of circulating prolactin in the blood. Enlargement of the pituitary gland area may be detected by the use of **magnetic resonance imaging** (MRI) or computerized axial tomography (CAT) scanning, also called **computed tomography**.

DELAYED SEXUAL MATURATION. Delayed sexual maturation is a potential cause of HSDD. It is present in boys if there is no testicular enlargement by age 13-and-a-half or if there are more than five years between the initial and complete growth of the genitalia. In girls, delayed sexual maturation is characterized by a lack of breast enlargement by age 13, or by a period greater than five years between the beginning of breast growth and the onset of menstruation. Delayed puberty may be the result of familial constitutional disorders, genetic defects such as Turner's syndrome in females and Klinefelter's syndrome in males, central nervous system disorders such as pituitary conditions that interfere with the secretion of gonadotropic hormones, and chronic illnesses such as diabetes mellitus, chronic renal failure, and cystic fibrosis.

SEXUAL ANHEDONIA. Sexual anhedonia is a rare variant of HSDD seen in the male, in which the patient experiences erection and ejaculation, but no pleasure from orgasm. The cause is attributed to penile anesthesia, due to psychogenic factors occurring in an hysterical or obsessive person. Psychiatric referral is indicated unless there is evidence of spinal cord injury or peripheral neuropathy. Loss of tactile sensation of the penis is unlikely to be organic in cause unless there is associated anesthetic areas in the vicinity of the anus or scrotum.

Symptoms

The HSDD patient complains of a lack of interest in sex even under circumstances that are ordinarily erotic in nature, such as pornography. Sexual activity is infrequent and eventually is absent, often resulting in serious marital discord. HSDD may be selective and focused against a specific sexual partner. When boredom with the usual sexual partner is the cause and frequency of sex with the usual partner decreases, real or fantasized sexual desire toward others may be normal or even increased.

If the cause of HSD falls into a detectable category such as abnormalities of the genitalia, or is due to a related condition such as a prolactinoma, chronic renal disease, diabetes mellitus, genetic disorder, or is familial in nature, the patient will manifest the signs and symptoms of the comorbid (co-occurring) condition. It is important to identify such causes, as their presence will usually dictate appropriate therapy.

Treatment

Currently, there is no approved drug or pharmacological treatment for HSDD and **psychotherapy** has proved to be only minimally effective. A primary goal of therapy is aimed at removal of the underlying cause of HSDD. The choice of medical therapy or behavioral or dynamic psychotherapy depends on the cause. If the cause is related to a medical condition, therapy is directed toward the cure or amelioration of that condition. Examples include cure or amelioration of underlying comorbid conditions such as genitourinary infections, improvement in diabetic control, avoidance of **substance abuse** and of medications that may be potentially responsible.

Therapy should also be directed towards other accompanying sexual disorders such as erectile dysfunction, which may be contributory. In cases where insufficient testosterone is suspected as a possible cause, serum androgen levels should be tested. A testosterone level less than 300 ng/dL in males and less than 10 ng/dL

KEY TERMS

Comorbid—Having another disorder or condition simultaneously.

Dyspareunia—Painful sexual intercourse.

Galactorrhea—Lactation occurring in the absence of pregnancy.

Hypogonadism—Abnormally decreased gonad function with retardation of sexual development.

Priapism—Painful involuntary penile erection persisting in excess of four hours.

Prolactin—A hormone that stimulates milk production and breast development.

Vaginismus—An involuntary tightening of the vaginal muscles that makes sexual intercourse painful, difficult, or impossible.

in females indicates a need for supplemental replacement therapy. If the cause is deemed to be of an interpersonal nature, **couples therapy** may be beneficial, in which case the support and understanding of the sexual partner is essential. Tricyclic **antidepressants** (TCAs) or **monoamine oxidase inhibitors (MAOIs)** may help in the treatment of accompanying depression or panic symptoms.

A recent study has reported that almost a third of nondepressed women with HSDD responded favorably to therapy with sustained release tablets of **bupropion** hydrochloride. The responders noted significant increases in the number of sexual arousals, sexual fantasies, and in the desire to engage in sexual activities. Bupropion hydrochloride (Wellbutrin) is currently approved by the FDA for the treatment of depression. Its favorable action on HSDD may be attributable to its enhancement of certain **neurotransmitters** that affect sexual desire, principally norepinephrine and **dopamine**.

Prognosis

The prognosis for HSDD depends primarily on the underlying cause or causes. In certain medical conditions, the prognosis for development, or recovery of sexual interest, is good. Examples include therapy of hypogonadism with testosterone, or the appropriate treatment of a prolactin-secreting pituitary tumor. On the other hand, in certain genetic defects such as Turner's syndrome and Klinefelter's syndrome, attainment of sexual function is impossible. By far, however, the vast majority of HSDD cases are situational in nature, usually relating to dissatisfaction or loss of interest in the sexual partner. In cases of marital discord, significant assistance may be obtained by counseling given by a health professional trained in the field. Cases of dissatisfaction by both partners often do not respond to such therapy, and frequently culminate in separation, finding a new sexual partner, and divorce.

Prevention

Unfortunately, it is difficult or impossible to predict the occurrence of HSDD in situational cases that comprise the majority of patients. The patience, understanding and support of the sexual partner is essential in those cases of HSDD in which the cause is temporary or transient. Some therapists recommend a period of abstinence from genital sex and have emphasized the value of a period of concentration on non-genital sex in the treatment of HSD.

Resources

BOOKS

Carnes, Patrick, and Joseph Moriarity. *Sexual Anorexia: Overcoming Sexual Self-Hatred.* Center City, MN: Hazelden Press, 1997.

Hawton, Keith. *Sex Therapy: A Practical Guide.* New York: Oxford University Press, 1985.

Lue, Tom F., et al. *Atlas of Clinical Urology: Impotence and Infertility, Volume I.* New York: Current Medicine Group, 1999.

Porter, Robert S., and Justin L. Kaplan, eds. *The Merck Manual of Diagnosis and Therapy.* 19th ed. Whitehouse Station, NJ: Merck Research Laboratories, 2011.

PERIODICALS

Brauer, M. "Attentional and Affective Processing of Sexual Stimuli in Women with Hypoactive Sexual Desire Disorder." *Archives of Sexual Behavior* (September 3, 2011) [e-pub ahead of print]. http://dx.doi.org/10.1007/s10508-011-9820-7 (accessed December 18, 2011).

Fabre, L. F., and L. C. Smith. "The Effect of Major Depression on Sexual Function in Women." *Journal of Sexual Medicine* (August 30, 2011) [e-pub ahead of print]. http://dx.doi.org/10.1111/j.1743-6109.2011.02445.x (accessed December 18, 2011).

Kingsberg, S. "Hypoactive Sexual Desire Disorder: When is Low Sexual Desire a Sexual Dysfunction?" *Journal of Sexual Medicine* 7, no. 8 (2010): 2907–8.

Ralph Myerson, MD

Hypochondriasis

Definition

Hypochondriasis is a mental disorder in which the individual is preoccupied with the thought of having a serious physical disease based on the incorrect or exaggerated interpretation of physical symptoms. This preoccupation continues for at least six months and interferes with the individual's social and occupational functioning even in the face of medical evidence to the contrary. Hypochondriasis is considered a somatoform disorder.

Demographics

According to the *DSM-IV-TR*, hypochondriasis affects 1%–5% of the general population in the United States. The rates of the disorder are higher among clinical outpatients, between 2% and 7%. One recent study suggests that full-blown hypochondriasis is fairly rare, although lesser degrees of worry about illness are more common, affecting as many as 6% of people in a community sample.

Hypochondriasis can appear at any age, although it frequently begins in early adulthood. Men and women appear to equally develop the disorder. The *DSM-IV-TR* notes that people from some cultures may appear to have fears of illness that resemble hypochondriasis, but are in fact influenced by beliefs that are traditional in their culture.

Description

The primary feature of hypochondriasis is excessive fear of having a serious disease. This fear is not relieved when a medical examination finds no evidence of disease. People with hypochondriasis are often able to acknowledge that their fears are unrealistic, but this intellectual realization is not enough to reduce their **diagnosis** of hypochondriasis, preoccupation with fear of disease must cause a great deal of distress or interfere with a person's ability to perform important activities, such as work, school activities, or family and social responsibilities. Hypochondriasis is included in the category of **somatoform disorders** in the ***Diagnostic and Statistical Manual of Mental Disorders*** (*DSM-IV-TR*), which is the reference handbook that clinicians use to guide the diagnosis of mental disorders. Some experts, however, have argued that hypochondriasis shares many features with **obsessive-compulsive disorder** or **panic disorder** and would be more appropriately classified with the **anxiety disorders**.

The fears of a person with hypochondriasis may be focused on the possibility of a single illness, but more often they include a number of possible conditions. The focus of the fears may shift over time as a person notices a new symptom or learns about an unfamiliar disease. The fears appear to develop in response to minor physical abnormalities, like **fatigue**, aching muscles, a mild cough, or a small sore. People with hypochondriasis may also interpret normal sensations as signs of disease. For instance, an occasional change in heart rate or a feeling of dizziness upon standing up will lead a person with hypochondriasis to fears of heart disease or **stroke**. Sometimes hypochondriacal fears develop after the death of a friend or family member, or in response to reading an article or seeing a television program about a disease. Fear of illness can also increase in response to **stress**.

Individuals with hypochondriasis visit physicians frequently; and when told there is nothing physically wrong, they are likely to seek a second opinion since their fears are not soothed. Their apparent distrust of their physicians' opinions can cause tensions in doctor-patient relationships, leading to the patient's further dissatisfaction with health-care providers. Physicians who regularly see a patient with hypochondriasis may become skeptical about any reported symptom, increasing the danger that a real illness may be overlooked. People with hypochondriasis also run the risk of undergoing unnecessary medical tests or receiving unneeded medications. Although they are usually not physically disabled, they may take frequent sick days from work, or annoy friends and family with constant conversation or complaints about illness, reducing their ability to function effectively in some aspects of life.

Causes and symptoms

Causes

The causes behind the development of hypochondriasis are not known, but there are several theories regarding its origin.

AMPLIFICATION OF SENSORY EXPERIENCE. One theory suggests that people with hypochondriasis are highly sensitive to physical sensations. They are more likely than most people to pay close attention to sensations within their bodies (heart rate, minor noises in the digestive tract, the amount or taste of saliva in the mouth, etc.), which magnifies their experience of these feelings. While many people fail to notice minor discomfort as they go about their regular activities, the individual with hypochondriasis pays constant attention to inner sensations and becomes alarmed when these sensations vary in any way. This heightened scrutiny may actually increase the intensity of the sensations, and the intensity of the experience fuels fears that the sensations signal an underlying illness. Once the fears are aroused, preoccupation with the symptom increases, further enhancing the intensity of sensations. The tendency to amplify may be either temporary or chronic; it may also be influenced by situational factors, which helps to explain why hypochondriacal fears are made worse by stress or by events that appear to justify concerns about illness. Some researchers have observed that heightened sensitivity to internal sensations is also a feature of panic disorder, and have suggested that there may be an overlap between the two disorders.

DISTORTED INTERPRETATION OF SYMPTOMS. Another theory points to the centrality of dysfunctional thinking in hypochondriasis. According to this theory, the internal physical sensations of the person with hypochondriasis are not necessarily more intense than those of most people. Instead, people with hypochondriasis are prone to make catastrophic misinterpretations of their physical symptoms. They are pessimistic about the state of their physical health and overestimate their chances of falling ill. Hypochondriasis thus represents a cognitive bias; whereas most people assume they are healthy unless there is clear evidence of disease, the person with hypochondriasis assumes he or she is sick unless given a clean bill of health. Research suggests that people with hypochondriasis make more realistic estimations of their risk of disease than most people, and in fact underestimate their risk of illness. People without hypochondriasis underestimate their risk even more. Some studies indicate that people with hypochondriasis are more likely to have had frequent or serious illnesses as children, which may explain the development of a negative cognitive bias in interpreting physical sensations or symptoms.

Symptoms

The primary symptom of hypochondriasis is preoccupation with fears of serious physical illness or injury. The fears of persons with hypochondriasis have an obsessive quality; they find thoughts about illness intrusive and difficult to dismiss, even when they recognize that their fears are unrealistic. In order to relieve the anxiety that arises from their thoughts, people with hypochondriasis may act on their fears by talking about their symptoms, by seeking information about feared diseases in books or on the Internet, or by "doctor-shopping," going from one specialist to another for consultations. Others may deal with their fears through avoidance, staying away from anything that might remind them of illness or death. Persons with hypochondriasis vary in their insight into their disorder. Some recognize themselves as "hypochondriacs," but have anxiety in spite of their recognition. Others are unable to see that their concerns are unreasonable or exaggerated.

Diagnosis

Hypochondriasis is most likely to be diagnosed when one of the doctors consulted by the patient considers the patient's preoccupation with physical symptoms and concerns excessive or problematic. After giving the patient a thorough physical examination to rule out a general medical condition, the doctor will usually give him or her a psychological test that screens for anxiety or **depression** as well as hypochondriasis. If the results suggest a diagnosis of hypochondriasis, the patient should be referred for **psychotherapy**. It is important to note, however, that patients with hypochondriasis usually resist the notion that their core problem is psychological. A successful referral to psychotherapy is much more likely if the patient's medical practitioner has been able to relate well to the patient and work gradually toward the notion that psychological problems might be related to fears of physical illness.

Specific approaches that have been found useful by primary care doctors in bringing psychological issues to the patient's attention in nonthreatening ways include the following:

- Drawing connections between the patient's current physical symptoms and recent setbacks or upsetting incidents in the patient's life. For example, the patient may come in with health worries within a few days of having a problem in other areas of life, such as their car needing repairs, a quarrel with a family member, an overdue bill, etc.
- Asking the patient to keep a careful diary of his or her symptoms and other occurrences. This diary may be useful in guiding the patient to see patterns in his or her worries about health.
- Scheduling the patient for regular but short appointments. It is also better to see the patient briefly than to prescribe medications in place of an appointment, because many patients with hypochondriasis abuse medications.
- Conducting routine screening tests during a yearly physical for patients with hypochondriasis, while discouraging them from scheduling extra appointments each time they notice a minor physical problem.
- Maintaining a realistic but optimistic tone in conversations with the patient. He or she may wish to talk to the patient about health-related fears and clarify the differences between normal internal body sensations and serious symptoms.

In order to receive a *DSM-IV-TR* diagnosis of hypochondriasis, a person must meet all six of the following criteria:

- The person must be preoccupied with the notion or fear of having a serious disease. This preoccupation is based on misinterpretation of physical symptoms or sensations.

- Appropriate medical evaluation and reassurance that there is no illness present do not eliminate the preoccupation.
- The belief or fear of illness must not be of delusional intensity. Delusional health fears are more likely to be bizarre in nature—for instance, the belief that one's skin emits a foul odor or that food is rotting in one's intestines. The preoccupations must not be limited to a concern about appearance; excessive concerns that focus solely on defects in appearance would receive a diagnosis of body dysmorphic disorder.
- The preoccupation must have lasted for at least six months.
- The person's preoccupation with illness must not simply be part of the presentation of another disorder, including generalized anxiety disorder, obsessive-compulsive disorder, panic disorder, separation anxiety, major depressive episode, or another somatoform disorder.

The *DSM-IV-TR* also differentiates between hypochondriasis with and without poor insight. Poor insight is specified when the patient does not recognize that his or her concerns are excessive or unreasonable.

DSM-5

Proposed changes for the fifth edition of the *DSM* (*DSM-5*, 2013) include changing the diagnosis of hypochondriasis to illness anxiety disorder. Aspects of hypochondriasis are also proposed to be subsumed, along with somatization disorder, undifferentiated somatoform disorder, and pain disorder, into the diagnosis of complex somatic symptom disorder.

Treatment

Traditionally, hypochondriasis has been considered difficult to treat. In the last few years, however, cognitive and behavioral treatments have demonstrated effectiveness in reducing the symptoms of the disorder.

Cognitive therapy

The goal of cognitive therapy for hypochondriasis is to guide patients to the recognition that their chief problem is fear of illness, rather than vulnerability to illness. Patients are asked to monitor worries and to evaluate how realistic and reasonable they are. Therapists encourage patients to consider alternative explanations for the physical signs they normally interpret as disease symptoms. Behavioral experiments are also employed in an effort to change the patient's habitual thoughts. For instance, a patient may be told to focus intently on a specific physical sensation and monitor increases in anxiety. Another behavioral assignment might ask the patient to suppress urges to talk about health-related worries with family members, then observe their anxiety level. Most people with hypochondriasis believe that their anxiety will escalate until they release it by seeking reassurance from others. In fact, anxiety usually crests and subsides in a matter of minutes. Cognitive therapy effectively reduces many symptoms of the disorder, and many improvements persist up to a year after treatment ends.

KEY TERMS

Comorbid psychopathology—The presence of other mental disorders in a patient together with the disorder that is the immediate focus of therapy.

Somatoform disorders—A group of psychiatric disorders in the *DSM-IV-TR* classification that are characterized by the patient's concern with external physical symptoms or complaints. Hypochondriasis is classified as a somatoform disorder.

BEHAVIORAL STRESS MANAGEMENT. One study compared cognitive therapy to behavioral **stress management**. This second form of therapy focuses on the notion that stress contributes to excessive worry about health. Patients were asked to identify stressors in their lives and taught stress management techniques to help them cope with these stressors. The researchers taught the patients relaxation techniques and problem-solving skills, and the patients practiced these techniques in and out of sessions. Although this treatment did not focus directly on hypochondriacal worries, it was helpful in reducing symptoms. At the end of the study, behavioral stress management appeared to be less effective than cognitive therapy in treating hypochondriasis, but a follow-up a year later found that the results of two therapies were comparable.

EXPOSURE AND RESPONSE PREVENTION. This therapy begins by asking patients to make a list of their hypochondriacal behaviors, such as checking body sensations, seeking reassurance from physicians or friends, and avoiding reminders of illness. Behavioral assignments are then developed. Patients who frequently monitor their physical sensations or seek reassurance are asked not to do so, and to allow themselves to experience the anxiety that accompanies suppression of these behaviors. Patients practice exposing themselves to anxiety until it becomes manageable, gradually reducing hypochondriacal behaviors in the process. In a study comparing exposure and response prevention to cognitive therapy, both therapies produced clinically significant results. Although cognitive therapy focuses more on thoughts and exposure therapy more on behaviors, both appear to be effective in reducing both dysfunctional thoughts and behaviors.

Prognosis

Untreated hypochondriasis tends to be a chronic disorder, although the intensity of the patient's symptoms may vary over time. The *DSM-IV-TR* notes that the following factors are associated with a better prognosis: the symptoms develop quickly, are relatively mild, are associated with an actual medical condition, and are not associated with comorbid psychopathology or benefits derived from being ill.

Prevention

Hypochondriasis may be difficult to prevent in a health-conscious society, in which people are constantly exposed to messages reminding them to seek regular medical screenings for a variety of illnesses, and telling them in detail about the illnesses of celebrities and high-ranking political figures. Trendy new diagnostic techniques like full-body MRIs may encourage people with hypochondriasis to seek unnecessary and expensive medical consultations. Referring patients with suspected hypochondriasis to psychotherapy may also help to reduce their overuse of medical services.

Resources

BOOKS

American Psychiatric Association. *Diagnostic and Statistical Manual of Mental Disorders*. 4th ed., text rev. Washington, DC: American Psychiatric Publishing, 2000.

Asmundson, Gordon J. G., Steven Taylor, and Brian J. Cox, eds. *Health Anxiety: Hypochondriasis and Related Disorders*. New York: John Wiley and Sons, 2002.

Maj, Mario, et al., eds. *Somatoform Disorders,* WPA Series, Evidence and Experience in Psychiatry, Volume 9. New York: John Wiley and Sons, 2005.

VandenBos, Gary R. ed. *APA Dictionary of Psychology*. Washington, DC: American Psychological Association, 2006.

Walker, John R., and Patricia Furer. "Treatment of Hypochondriasis and Psychogenic Movement Disorders: Focus on Cognitive-Behavior Therapy." In *Psychogenic Movement Disorders: Neurology and Neuropsychiatry*. edited by Mark Hallett et al. Philadelphia: Lippincott Williams and Wilkins Publishers, 2005.

PERIODICALS

Abramowitz, Jonathan S. "Hypochondriasis: Conceptualization, Treatment, and Relationship to Obsessive Compulsive Disorder." *Annals of Clinical Psychiatry* 17, no. 4 (October–December 2005): 211–17.

Asmundson, Gordon J. G., Steven Taylor, and Michael J. Coons. "Current Directions in the Treatment of Hypochondriasis." *Journal of Cognitive Psychotherapy* 19, no. 3 (Fall 2005): 285–304.

Avia, M.D., and M. A. Ruiz. "Recommendations for the Treatment of Hypochondriac Patients." *Journal of Contemporary Psychotherapy* 35, no. 3 (October 2005): 301–13.

Bleichhardt, Gaby, Barbara Timmer, and Winfried Rief. "Hypochondriasis Among Patients with Multiple Somatoform Symptoms—Psychopathology and Outcome of a Cognitive-Behavioral Therapy." *Journal of Contemporary Psychotherapy* 35, no. 3 (October 2005): 239–49.

Furer, Patricia, and John R. Walker. "Treatment of Hypochondriasis with Exposure." *Journal of Contemporary Psychotherapy* 35, no. 3 (October 2005): 251–67.

Martínez, M. Pilar, and Cristina Botella. "An Exploratory Study of the Efficacy of a Cognitive-Behavioral Treatment for Hypochondriasis Using Different Measures of Change." *Psychotherapy Research* 15, no. 4 (October 2005): 392–408.

Monopoli, John. "Managing Hypochondriasis in Elderly Clients." *Journal of Contemporary Psychotherapy* 35, no. 3 (October 2005): 285–300.

Noyes, Russell Jr., et al. "Distinguishing Between Hypochondriasis and Somatization Disorder: A Review of the Existing Literature." *Psychotherapy and Psychosomatics* 75, no. 5 (August 2006): 270–81.

Starcevic, Vladan. "Fear of Death in Hypochondriasis: Bodily Threat and Its Treatment Implications." *Journal of Contemporary Psychotherapy* 35, no. 3 (October 2005): 227–37.

Stuart, Scott, and Russell Noyes Jr. "Treating Hypochondriasis with Interpersonal Psychotherapy." *Journal of Contemporary Psychotherapy* 35, no. 3 (Fall 2005): 269–83.

Danielle Barry, MS
Ruth A. Wienclaw, PhD

Hypomania

Definition

A hypomanic episode is a distinct period of time that lasts at least four days during which the individual's mood is consistently elevated, expansive, or irritable and is distinct from his or her usual nondepressed mood. Hypomanic episodes are characteristic of bipolar II disorder as well as features of **cyclothymic disorder**. They may also occur as a transitional phase from euthymia (feeling of well-being often associated with individuals with **bipolar disorder** when they are not having a manic or a depressive episode) to mania in cases of bipolar I disorder.

Demographics

Hypomanic episodes associated with bipolar II disorder have the same demographics as that disorder.

Hypomanic episodes can affect both adults and younger patients. In younger patients and adolescents, hypomania may be associated with such behaviors as school truancy, antisocial behavior, failure in school, or **substance abuse**.

Cultural differences can affect the experience and communication of the symptoms of hypomanic disorder, with different cultures interpreting such symptoms as irritability or inflated self-esteem in various ways. Some cultures and subcultures, for example, value such aspects of hypomania as decreased need for sleep, racing thoughts, or increased goal orientation as positive qualities of a productive individual, and do not regard them negatively.

Description

Hypomanic episodes usually begin suddenly with the symptoms rapidly increasing over the course of a day or two. A hypomanic episode may last anywhere from four days to several months, although some clinicians are beginning to argue that hypomanic episodes may be as short as two days in duration. However, because such research is based on the self-reports of patients (who tend not to be aware of their symptoms at first), there is not widespread agreement about this change in diagnostic criteria.

Causes and symptoms

Hypomania is not a disorder in and of itself. The causes of hypomania vary depending on whether it is a characteristic of bipolar I disorder, bipolar II disorder, or cyclothymic disorder.

During a hypomanic episode, the individual's mood is consistently elevated, expansive, or irritable and distinct from his or her usual nondepressed mood. During this period, the individual must also display at least three of the following symptoms (or four if he or she is only irritable) to be diagnosed as hypomanic:

- inflated sense of self-esteem
- decreased need for sleep
- increased talkativeness or need to talk
- racing thoughts or flight of ideas
- easily distracted
- increased goal-oriented activity
- excessive involvement in pleasurable but high-risk activities (for example, buying sprees, sexual indiscretions, foolish investments)

In hypomania, these symptoms are associated with a clear change from the individual's normal behavior and are readily observable by others. Hypomanic symptoms, however, are not severe enough to noticeably affect the individual's functioning at work or in social situations, nor does their presence require **hospitalization**. To be classified as hypomanic, the individual's symptoms cannot contain psychotic features or be due to the direct physiological effects of a substance (such as drug abuse or medication) or a general medical condition (for example, hyperthyroidism).

Diagnosis

It is important to distinguish hypomania from euthymia in patients who are not used to a nondepressed mood state. In addition, although the two have the same list of diagnostic symptoms, hypomanic episodes are different from manic episodes. Hypomanic symptoms are less severe than manic symptoms and do not cause marked impairment of social or occupational functioning. However, approximately 5% to 15% of individuals experiencing hypomanic episodes will eventually develop a **manic episode**.

Many of the warning signs of a hypomanic episode such as increased goal-oriented behavior can also be normal and appropriate given the situation. Sometimes a patient's good mood is just that. Some of the signs of a normal good mood that could distinguish it from hypomania include:

- ability to enjoy reading for a significant period of time without becoming bored
- ability to listen more than talk in a social setting
- no need to do something risky just to shake things up
- ability to complete tasks without repeatedly being distracted
- experience of appropriate anxiety about demands of life such as responsibilities, deadlines, and financial obligations
- ability to enjoy times of peace and quiet
- ability to sleep well at night for an appropriate period of time
- ability to accept well-meaning, constructive criticism without undue irritation

Treatment

Cognitive-behavioral therapy

Cognitive-behavioral therapy (CBT) is regularly used to help patients test how realistic their thought processes and resultant behaviors are. The goal of such reality testing is to help patients weigh the facts more carefully than they would otherwise do and to seek the insights of others before acting on their beliefs. This approach can help patients be more independent in controlling their lives.

One of the tools used in CBT to assist patients in controlling their impulses during hypomanic episodes is keeping a daily journal of their thoughts. Such daily thought records are a structured method to help patients do a reality check on their thinking and actions. For example, patients can look for situations in which they overestimate their capabilities, rely on luck, underestimate risks, minimize problems, or overvalue immediate gratification.

Patients with hypomanic episodes can also be taught to test the validity of their thoughts and beliefs by consulting trusted others. By talking things through with a trusted and objective person, a patient in a hypomanic episode can be helped to test the reality of his or her thoughts and beliefs.

Another method that can help hypomanic patients test reality is to have them rate the relative risks of the options that they are considering by listing the productive potential and destructive risks of their alternatives. If patients are unable to think of examples of destructive risks for their plans, the therapist or other objective outsider can help by giving them examples and helping them to develop their own list of potential risks. Similarly, lists can be made of the benefit to others versus the cost to oneself or the benefit to oneself versus the cost to others.

Patients can also be helped to more realistically evaluate their thoughts and plans through role playing or playing "devil's advocate." Such techniques can be used to do a hypothetical trial run to see what possible consequences might be incurred if an unreasonable risk is taken.

To help reduce impulsivity and recklessness in hypomanic patients, psychotherapists use various different techniques. One technique is to institute a "wait 48 hours before acting" rule to help the patient avoid spur-of-the-moment reckless actions. It is also sometimes helpful for the patient to try to foresee the possible negative consequences of their proposed actions through imagery by describing the bad things that could happen if they took their proposed course of action. Because hypomanic patients are often overly active, it is sometimes also helpful to have them schedule their activities to help them focus their attention on what is important so that they do not become overextended. Hypomanic patients can also be taught listening skills that can help them focus and break the vicious circle of constant activity and to listen to others. Similarly, patients can be taught anticipatory problem-solving skills that help them recognize the symptoms of a building hypomanic episode and to reduce the stressors that put them at risk. It is also helpful for hypomanic patients to minimize or completely avoid situations that are apt to trigger a hypomanic episode such as daredevil hobbies, exaggerated acts of generosity or intimacy with relative strangers, unsupervised expenditures of large amounts of money, or situations that require the use of a lethal weapon. Hypomanic patients can also be taught to help control or adjust their moods through relaxation techniques and breathing control exercises.

KEY TERMS

Bipolar II disorder—One of a group of mood disorders in which the individual has one or more major depressive episodes and at least one hypomanic episode.

Cognitive-behavioral therapy (CBT)—A form of psychotherapy used to help patients modify their behavior by testing their thought processes.

Cyclothymic disorder—A mood disorder in which hypomanic episodes and depressive episodes both occur over the course of at least two years during which time symptom-free periods last no more than two months.

Euthymia—A feeling of well-being often associated with individuals with bipolar disorder when they are not having a manic or a depressive episode.

Mania—Excitement, overactivity, and inappropriate physical and mental restlessness, often accompanied by impaired judgment.

Psychotic—Behavior characteristic of any of a number of severe mental disorders in which the accuracy of perceptions and thoughts is incorrectly evaluated despite evidence to the contrary, affecting the individual's interaction with external reality.

Role playing—A technique used in psychotherapy in which the patient acts out a situation to test attitudes, relationships, actions, and their potential consequences.

Biological treatments

In addition to CBT approaches in controlling hypomanic episodes, several biologic management strategies may help patients. These include:

- optimizing the dose of mood stabilizer or antimanic medication
- encouraging good sleep practices

- discontinuing antidepressants
- including lorazepam or clonazepam (1–6 mg/day) as clinically indicated
- including mood stabilizers such as lithium, divalproex, or carbamazepine in the treatment regimen as appropriate

In most cases, such biologic treatments can be used on an outpatient basis.

Prevention

There are a number of warning signs of hypomania. If patients can be taught to recognize such early warning signs, they have a better chance of using various techniques to help lessen the possibility of acting out and the negative consequences of inappropriate actions that may be associated with hypomania. Attending to such warning signs also can give patients and their doctors more time to adjust medications or arrange for greater supervision to reduce the potential harm from inappropriate behavior.

Some of the typical early warning signs of an impending hypomanic episode include:

- disruption in sleep patterns (for example, decreased subjective need for sleep)
- decrease in anxiety without cause (such as ignoring a deadline or less concern about owing money)
- high levels of optimism without appropriate sound planning and problem-solving (for example, belief that everything will turn out all right even though nothing has been done to make that a reality)
- increased desire to be with others along with relatively poor listening skills (for example, talking at length to someone who is obviously anxious to leave)
- decreased mental concentration (such as difficulty following through or becoming more disorganized than usual)
- increased libido to the point where it affects other areas of life (for example, dressing more provocatively than usual, or inappropriate talk of or joking about sex)
- increased goal-directed behavior to the point where the individual appears driven

According to CBT, if the patient can be taught to recognize the signs of an impending hypomanic episode early enough, he or she will have the time necessary to put into practice the various techniques already discussed to help avoid the negative consequences of potential risky actions.

Resources

BOOKS

American Psychiatric Association. *Diagnostic and Statistical Manual of Mental Disorders*. 4th ed., text rev. Washington, DC: American Psychiatric Publishing, 2000.

Newman, Cory F., et al. *Bipolar Disorder: A Cognitive Therapy Approach*. Washington, DC: American Psychological Association, 2001.

VandenBos, Gary R. ed. *APA Dictionary of Psychology*. Washington, DC: American Psychological Association, 2006.

Yatham, Lakshmi N., and Mario Maj. *Bipolar Disorder: A Clinicianís Guide to Biological Treatments.* New York: John Wiley and Sons, 2010.

PERIODICALS

Akiskal, Hagop S., and Franco Benazzi. "The DSM-IV and ICD-10 Categories of Recurrent [Major] Depressive and Bipolar II Disorders: Evidence that They Lie on a Dimensional Spectrum." *Journal of Affective Disorders* 92, no. 1 (May 2006): 45–54.

Bauer, Michael, et al. "Self-Reported Data from Patients with Bipolar Disorder: Impact on Minimum Episode Length for Hypomania." *Journal of Affective Disorders* 96, no. 1–2 (November 2006): 101–105.

Benazzi, Franco, and Hagop Akiskal. "The Duration of Hypomania in Bipolar-II Disorder in Private Practice: Methodology and Validation." *Journal of Affective Disorders* 96, no. 3 (2006): 189–96.

Mansell, Warren. "The Hypomanic Attitudes and Positive Predictions Inventory (HAPPI): A Pilot Study to Select Cognitions that Are Elevated in Individuals with Bipolar Disorder Compared to Non-Clinical Controls." *Behavioural and Cognitive Psychotherapy* 34, no. 4 (2006): 1–10.

Utsumi, Takeshi, et al. "Clinical Features of Soft Bipolarity in Major Depressive Inpatients." *Psychiatry and Clinical Neurosciences* 60, no. 5 (October 2006): 611–15.

Ruth A. Wienclaw, PhD

Hypomanic episode *see* **Manic episode**

I

Illusion of doubles *see* **Capgras syndrome**

Illusion of false recognition *see* **Capgras syndrome**

Iloperidone

Definition

Iloperidone (Fanapt) is a medication used in the treatment of **schizophrenia**. Iloperidone belongs to a class of drugs known as atypical antipsychotics, which specifically act on two natural body chemicals, **serotonin** and **dopamine**. These chemicals are types of **neurotransmitters** involved in normal **brain** function and can affect the state of **psychosis** and other symptoms of schizophrenia. Iloperidone acts as a neurotransmitter blocker, inhibiting the effects of serotonin and dopamine at their chemical receptors.

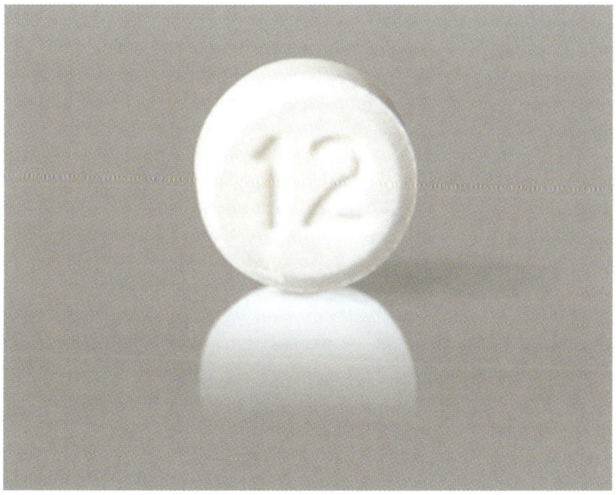

Iloperidone (Fanapt). *(Novartis Pharmaceuticals Corp.)*

Purpose

Iloperidone is an antipsychotic medication. It is in the drug class known as atypical antipsychotics, which have less adverse effects involving **medication-induced movement disorders** than older antipsychotic compounds. The choice of using iloperidone alone or in combination with other drugs in the treatment of schizophrenia depends on the response of the patient to the medication and his or her individual health parameters.

Description

Iloperidone works by inhibiting the absorption of serotonin and norepinephrine in the brain. Since the causes of schizophrenia involve the overactivity of neurotransmitters in some areas of the brain and underactivity in others, antipsychotics such as iloperidone do not completely treat the disorder. The symptoms of schizophrenia known as **positive symptoms**, such as psychosis, are best treated with iloperidone. The cognitive and **negative symptoms** such as withdrawal and difficulty with reasoning are not as well addressed with iloperidone, though the drug has more impact on these types of symptoms than the older and more traditional antipsychotics.

Recommended dosage

Iloperidone is taken as an oral medication. The available doses are 1, 2, 4, 6, 8, 10, and 12 mg pills. The dose is started low and gradually increased to the most effective dose that does not cause intolerable side effects. The first day a patient may take 1 mg twice a day, then 2 mg twice a day on the second day, and then 4 mg per day as needed. The maximum dose is 24 mg per day. If side effects develop or if other drugs are used in combination with iloperidone, the dose may be decreased. Side effects impacting the immune system may make a lower dose or discontinuation of the drug necessary. Some types of severe liver disease may require modification of the dose.

Precautions

Iloperidone is an atypical antipsychotic medication, a class that was developed for the purpose of avoiding some of the side effects often seen with older antipsychotic medications. As a class, these medications cause far fewer movement disorders than older medications, but they still have the potential to cause some disturbing movement-related effects. Patients taking iloperidone must be monitored for the development of movement disorders as well as stiffness, mental status changes, and increased temperature associated with the dangerous **neuroleptic malignant syndrome**. However, iloperidone is less likely to cause these disorders than many other types of antipsychotic medications. Patients taking iloperidone must have their immune system function monitored via periodic blood tests, as the drug can cause dangerous decreases in white blood cells. High blood sugar may also develop, especially in patients at risk for diabetes. Blood sugar is measured before initiating iloperidone dosing, then monitored periodically. Iloperidone carries a risk of low blood pressure and possible temporary loss of consciousness, especially in older or dehydrated patients rising quickly from a lying down position.

Iloperidone and other antipsychotic drugs are associated with an increased risk of death when used in elderly patients with **dementia**. In June 2008, the U.S. Food and Drug Administration (FDA) announced a requirement for manufacturers of iloperidone (and other antipsychotic drugs) to add a warning label to their packaging stating this risk. The reason for the increase was unclear in studies, but most deaths were found to be related to either cardiovascular complications or complications associated with infection. Iloperidone is not approved by the FDA for the treatment of behavior problems in older adults with dementia, and patients in this category (or caregivers of patients in this category) should discuss the risks of taking the drug with their physician.

Iloperidone may not be appropriate for use or may require caution in patients with certain heart abnormalities or disease, liver dysfunction, history of **stroke** or seizure, diabetes, immune dysfunction, patients who are dehydrated, and the elderly. Iloperidone is classified as category C for pregnancy, which means that either there are no adequate human or animal studies or that adverse fetal effects were found in animal studies but there is no available human data. The decision to use category C drugs in pregnancy is generally based on weighing the critical needs of the mother against the risk to the fetus. Other lower category agents are used whenever possible. The safety of iloperidone use during breast-feeding is unknown and so its use is not recommended.

KEY TERMS

Cognitive—Associated with thinking, learning, perception, awareness, and judgment.

Dopamine—A type of neurotransmitter involved in regulation of concentration, impulse control, judgment, mood, attention span, psychostimulation, and disease states such as addiction, and depression.

Insomnia—Disorder involving disturbance of sleep.

Neuroleptic malignant syndrome—Dangerous reaction to antipsychotic medications that involves temperature instability, muscular rigidity, and altered mental status.

Neurotransmitter—A chemical messenger that travels through the body and acts in the nervous system. Neurotransmitter signaling is responsible for a wide range of bodily processes and is often the target of medications involving the brain and cardiovascular system.

Neurotransmitter receptor—A physical recipient for chemicals called neurotransmitters. Receptors sit on the surface of cells that make up body tissues, and once bound to the neurotransmitter, they initiate the chemical signaling pathway associated with neurotransmitters.

Prolactin—Hormone responsible for endocrine function, including lactation.

Psychosis—Loss of contact with reality that may involve false beliefs or hallucinations.

Schizophrenia—Severe psychiatric illness involving the disintegration of thought processes and sometimes including hallucinations.

Serotonin—A type of neurotransmitter involved in regulation of the blood vessels, brain processes, and disease states such as depression.

Side effects

Atypical antipsychotics such as iloperidone are known for having fewer movement related side effects than other types of older antipsychotic medications that act on neurotransmitter receptors in different parts of the brain. This is one reason why as a general class they tend to be the drug of choice in treatment of schizophrenia. However, as with all medication, antipsychotics such as iloperidone do have side effects. Sensitivity to iloperidone varies among patients, and some patients may find

QUESTIONS TO ASK YOUR DOCTOR

- Can I take the full dose right away or do I need to slowly increase the dose up to the full amount?
- Can I stop taking the medication right away or do I need to slowly decrease the dose in order to go off the medication?
- Should I eat before taking this medication?
- Will this medication interact with any of my other prescription medications?
- Are there any over-the-counter medications I should not take with this medicine?
- Will this medicine interact with any of my herbal supplements?
- What side effects indicate that I have taken too much of this medication?
- Can I drink alcoholic beverages when I am taking this medication?

lower doses are more than their body system can tolerate. Common side effects of iloperidone include dizziness, dry mouth, abdominal pain, nausea, diarrhea, weight gain, **fatigue**, increased heart rate, nasal congestion, anxiety, joint pain, sore throat, upper respiratory infections, sexual dysfunction, blurred vision, tremor, rash, and alterations in liver enzymes. Antipsychotics such as iloperidone that act to antagonize dopamine receptors may cause an increase in prolactin, the hormone that causes lactation in women and impotence in men. Low blood pressure or a drop in blood pressure upon standing may result in loss of consciousness. Elderly patients may also be particularly sensitive to sedation, low blood pressure, and other side effects. Rare but serious potential side effects include severe movement disorders, high blood sugar or overt diabetes, stroke, severe difficulty swallowing, dangerous changes in heart rhythm, **seizures**, and changes in blood cells including anemia and decreased immune function. A rare but dangerous possible side effect is neuroleptic malignant syndrome, a reaction involving very high body temperature, altered mental status, and muscular rigidity.

Interactions

Patients should make their doctor aware of all medications and supplements they are taking before using iloperidone. Using alcohol while taking iloperidone may create toxic reactions in the body and should be avoided. Drugs that affect the liver may affect the metabolism of iloperidone, resulting in too much or too little of the drug in the body. This could lead to increased side effects or even toxic doses. Likewise, iloperidone may affect the metabolism of other drugs, leading to greater or lower doses than therapeutically desired.

Many drugs may cause toxicity when used with iloperidone due to additive effects affecting heart rhythm. Drugs that cause these additive effects include the heart medications dronedarone and amiodarone, the chemotherapeutic toremifene, the antibiotics azithromycin and ciprofloxacin, the antifungal fluconazole, the antinausea drug ondansetron, and antipsychotics such as **pimozide**, among many others. The drug bromocriptine used in various neurological and endocrine disorders may cause dangerously low blood pressure when used with iloperidone. Sedative drugs such as codeine and herbal supplements such as calendula, capsicum, kava, and lemon balm may cause additive effects of severe sedation in patients using iloperidone. The herbal supplement Siberian **ginseng** causes antagonizing effects and decreases the effectiveness of iloperidone, as well as exacerbating many psychiatric conditions.

Resources

BOOKS

Brunton, Laurence, et al. *Goodman and Gilman's the Pharmacological Basis of Therapeutics*. 12th ed. New York: McGraw Hill Medical, 2011.

Torrey, E. Fuller. *Surviving Schizophrenia: A Manual for Patients, Family and Providers*. New York: HarperCollins, 2001.

PERIODICALS

Crabtree, B. L., and J. Montgomery. "Iloperidone for the Management of Adults with Schizophrenia." *Clinical Therapeutics* 33, no. 3 (2011): 330–45.

WEBSITES

PubMed Health. "Iloperidone." U.S. National Library of Medicine. http://www.ncbi.nlm.nih.gov/pubmedhealth/PMH0000504 (accessed November 12, 2011).

ORGANIZATIONS

American Society for Clinical Pharmacology and Therapeutics, 528 N Washington St., Alexandria, VA, 22314, (703) 836-6981, info@ascpt.org, http://www.ascpt.org.

National Institute of Mental Health, 6001 Executive Blvd., Rm. 8184, MSC 9663, Bethesda, MD, 20892-9663, (301) 433-4513; TTY: (301) 443-8431, Fax: (301) 443-4279, (866) 615-6464; TTY: (866) 415-8051, nimhinfo@nih.gov, http://www.nimh.nih.gov.

U.S. Food and Drug Administration, 10903 New Hampshire Ave., Silver Spring, MD, 20993-0002, (888) INFO-FDA (463-6332), http://www.fda.gov.

Maria Eve Basile, PhD

Imaginal desensitization *see* **Exposure treatment**

Imaginal exposure *see* **Exposure treatment**

Imaging studies

Definition

Imaging studies are medical tests performed with a variety of techniques that produce pictures of the inside of a patient's body.

Purpose

Imaging studies, also called medical imaging, provide images of parts of the body in order for medical professionals, such as surgeons and family doctors, to diagnose diseases, identify broken bones, and examine the functionality of organs, tissues, and other portions of the body.

Description

Imaging tests are performed using sound waves, radioactive particles, magnetic fields, or x rays that are detected and converted into images after passing through body tissues. Dyes are sometimes used as contrasting agents with x-ray tests so that organs or tissues not seen with conventional x rays can be enhanced. The operating principle of the various techniques is based on the fact that rays and particles interact differently with various types of tissues, especially when abnormalities are present. In this way, the interior of the body can be visualized, and pictures are provided of normal structure and functioning as well as of abnormalities. In the fields pertaining to mental health, including psychology and psychiatry, imaging is often used to help rule out other health problems that could be causing symptoms. Once a **diagnosis** has been established, various imaging techniques may help to confirm the diagnosis and also serve as a way to study the disorder. The imaging techniques may shed new light on the way the disorder affects the **brain**, so that new treatment methods can be implemented. Imaging techniques for psychiatric illnesses are used more in research than in treatment and diagnosis in the clinical setting.

Computed tomography (CT)

Computed tomography (CT), or computed axial tomography (CAT), scans show a cross-section of a part of the body, such as the brain. In this technique, a thin beam of x-ray radiation is used to produce a series of two-dimensional exposures detected at different angles. The exposures are fed into a computer that overlaps them, yielding a single three-dimensional image, such as around a single axis of rotation, analogous to a slice of the organ or body part being scanned. A dye is often injected into the patient to improve contrast and obtain images that are clearer than images obtained solely with x rays. The latest CT equipment allows data to be processed by a computer in various planes, not only in axial (along the axis of the body) or transverse (perpendicular to the body axis) planes.

Around 72 million CT scans were performed in the United States in 2007. Now, in the second decade of the twenty-first century, even more such scans are annually produced in the country and in many parts of the world. The technology's popularity is based on its ability to supplement the use of long-used traditional x rays and diagnosis sonography. CT scans are frequently used to scan the head, lungs, pulmonary arteries, heart, abdomen, pelvis, and extremities. In addition, its popularity is rapidly increasing as CT scans are used more frequently in preventative medicine, such as with people at high risk for colon cancer or heart disease. Further, full-body CT scans are offered at select hospitals and other medical facilities around the United States.

Magnetic resonance imaging (MRI)

Magnetic resonance imaging (MRI) scans also produce cross-sectional images of the body using powerful magnetic fields instead of ionizing radiation. MRI uses a cylinder housing a magnet that will induce the required magnetic field. The patient lies on a platform inside the scanner. The magnetic field aligns nuclei of atoms, such as hydrogen atoms, present in the tissue being scanned in a given direction—what is called magnetization. Following a burst of radio-frequency radiation, the atoms flip back to their original orientation, producing a rotating magnetic field that is detectable by the scanning device. The emitting signals are fed into a computer for conversion into a two-dimensional (2-D) or three-dimensional (3-D) image. When 3-D images are needed, the magnetic field gradients can force nuclei of atoms at various locations to rotate at different speeds. The resulting data allows for 3-D images. Dyes can also be injected into patients to produce clearer images.

Also called nuclear magnetic resonance imaging (NMRI), MRI provides for a clear contrast among the various soft tissues of the body. Consequently, MRI scans are especially useful for such areas of the body as the brain, heart, and muscles. These scans can detect cancer in the body when other types of scans, such as CT scans, cannot.

FUNCTIONAL MAGNETIC RESONANCE IMAGING (FMRI). Functional magnetic resonance imaging (fMRI) scans are a special type of MRI scans. They are used to measure changes in blood flow and blood oxygenation—what are called hemodynamic responses—within the body. Because changes in blood flow and blood oxygenation are related to constantly changing neurological activity in the brain and spinal column, it can be effectively used to detect problems within these highly important regions of the human body.

INTRAOPERATIVE MAGNETIC RESONANCE IMAGING. Intraoperative magnetic resonance imaging (iMRI) scans, another specialized form of MRI scans, are used to view images of the brain while brain surgery is being performed. In other words, intraoperative imaging allows surgeons to see changes taking place within the body, such as the brain, while surgery is progressing. A subset of interventional MRI scanning (MRI scans that generally allow minimally invasive procedures to observe progress being made), iMRI allows surgeons to find the best approach—for example, to remove tumors from the brain without damaging other parts. At the end of the surgery, the iMRI scans also reassure the surgeon that the entire tumor was removed from the brain, and that the surgery was a success. This confirmation prevents the surgical team from having to re-enter the brain a second time, thus making it much more efficient for the medical team and safer for the patient.

Magnetoencephalography

Magnetoencephalography (MEG) is a noninvasive technique that measures magnetic fields produced by neuron activity in the brain. The field measurements provide information about where in the brain the recorded activity is located. MEG is often used in conjunction with other scans, since it produces information about locales (coordinates) that then need to be mapped against an image of the brain.

MEG is primarily used to detect the origin of epileptic **seizures** in the brain. It is also being used to research other disorders, including **schizophrenia**, **dementia**, and **post-traumatic stress disorder**. The advantage of MEG compared to other scans is that it provides information almost instantaneously, offering clinicians a real-time picture of brain activity. It also is very accurate in terms of spatial location. However, MEG is expensive and therefore not as readily available as other types of imaging studies.

Positron emission tomography (PET)

Positron emission tomography (PET) is a non-invasive scanning/imaging technique that utilizes small amounts of radioactive positrons (positively charged particles; also called antielectrons) to visualize body function and metabolism. The **PET** scan uses a special camera and tracer (such as glucose with an added radioactive chemical) to take images of organs and tissues within the body. The camera records the position of the tracer, and the resulting data are then sent to a computer for analysis.

PET scans are especially useful for brain-imaging studies. They are often used to illustrate the differences between brains of people without mental disorders and brains of people with mental disorders. For example, because PET scans can detect brain activity, PET scans of the brains of depressed and nondepressed persons can show researchers where brain activity is decreased in depressed patients. Similar scans have been taken of brains affected by schizophrenia or **Alzheimer's disease**. Such research can help scientists discover new ways to treat these disorders.

Single photon emission computerized tomography (SPECT)

Single photon emission computerized tomography (SPECT) scans are used in research and in diagnosing brain disorders such as Alzheimer's disease and Parkinson's disease. As with PET scans, SPECT scans use gamma-ray-emitting radioisotopes (radioactive isotopes) as a way to produce images of active brain regions. A radioactive tracer is injected into the brain. Because the radioactive tracer does not spread out in the brain, lasts up to one minute, and can be injected at any time, it is especially useful for scanning the brains of epileptic patients because the scan can be taken after an epileptic seizure has passed.

KEY TERMS

Electromagnetic radiation—Radiation including gamma rays, x rays, ultraviolet light, visible light, infrared radiation, microwaves, and radio waves.

Magnetic field—A region around a magnetized body or a current-carrying circuit in which a magnetic force can be detected.

Photon—The smallest amount of electromagnetic radiation that possesses both particle and wave properties.

Positron—The antimatter form of an electron, with the same mass as an electron but with an opposite electrical charge.

SPECT research is ongoing in the early twenty-first century as a way to evaluate patients with various types of seizures, including epileptic seizures, before having surgical procedures. For instance, the Children's Hospital of Pittsburgh, through its Epilepsy Monitoring Unit, regularly performs SPECT scans on children with epilepsy in order to detect changes in blood flow in their brains before epilepsy surgery is performed.

Preparation

The amount of preparation, if any, for the different types of imaging studies is dependent on the type of study being used. Preparation instructions are in place for each type of imaging procedure. Check with the attending medical team or the referring physician before having any scan to determine what type of preparation is necessary. It is important to follow preparatory instructions strictly because failure to do so could result in the session being cancelled or rescheduled.

General guidelines include wearing comfortable clothing, preferably garments that will keep one warm in examination rooms that are usually cool. Avoid wearing jewelry and clothes with metal zippers or other such accessories that could interfere with the operation of the scanning devices. Generally, patients should not eat or have any liquids, except water, for at least four hours before the scheduled scan. Limit the amount of sugar and caffeine for one day before the examination. Drink plenty of water before the scanning session in order to avoid dehydration. These instructions may vary, depending on the type of scan. In addition, most scans require that strenuous physical activity, such as jogging, lifting heavy objects, and bicycling, be avoided for 24 hours before the scan.

Aftercare

A normal schedule and level of activity can be resumed after the scan is complete. One may drink plenty of water or other fluids throughout the rest of the day. Eating a normal amount of food throughout the rest of the day is also recommended.

Risks

When electromagnetic radiation, such as x rays, is used for imaging studies, there is risk from radiation exposure. Exposure to radiation has been linked to cancer, although its exact relationship with respect to imaging studies has yet to be determined. Research is ongoing to determine this link in more detail. Thus, many medical professionals try to reduce the number of scans used on an individual and, when possible, on the duration of each individual scan. Reducing the duration of scans on children is also widely thought to reduce their risks for cancer, although scientific studies have yet to prove such a relationship.

Recently, several scientific studies have suggested a link between cancer and excessive exposure to radiation in such imaging scans. Consequently, under international guidelines set up for anyone using imaging scans, it is assumed that any radiation dose, even a tiny one, poses a health risk to the patient. International consensus states that any radiation exposure through imaging studies provides a very small risk of inducing cancer into the patient.

QUESTIONS TO ASK YOUR DOCTOR

- Will I need to have someone stay with me during the imaging study? Will this person need to drive me home?
- What special precautions should be taken with a child?
- Should I expect any side effects?
- How many scans is it safe to receive in any one year? How far apart should they be spaced?

Results

The images produced during these scans are normally sent to the attending physician. Make an appointment with this medical professional to discuss the results of the scan.

Resources

BOOKS

Armstrong, Peter, Martin L. Wastie, and Andrea G. Rockall. *Diagnostic Imaging*. Chichester, U.K.: Wiley-Blackwell, 2009.

Seeram, Euclid. *Computed Tomography: Physical Principles, Clinical Applications and Quality Control.* St. Louis: Saunders/Elsevier, 2009.

Valk, Peter P., et al., editors. *Positron Emission Tomography: Clinical Practice.* London: Springer, 2006.

Westbrook, Catherine. *Handbook of MRI Techniques.* Chichester, U.K.: Wiley-Blackwell, 2008.

WEBSITES

"Alzheimer's Disease and Dementia." Alzheimer Society of British Columbia. http://www.alzheimerbc.org/Alzheimer-s-Disease-and-Dementia.aspx (accessed May 25, 2011).

"Intraoperative Magnetic Resonance Imaging (iMRI)." Mayo Clinic. http://www.mayoclinic.org/intraoperative-mri (accessed May 24, 2011).

"Parkinson's Disease." PubMed Health, U.S. National Library of Medicine. (May 6, 2011). http://www.ncbi.nlm.nih.gov/pubmedhealth/PMH0001762 (accessed May 25, 2011).

"Single Photon Emission Computed Tomography (SPECT)." Children's Hospital of Pittsburgh. (October 19, 2010). http://www.chp.edu/CHP/single+photon+emission+computed+tomography+(spect) (accessed May 24, 2011).

ORGANIZATIONS

National Institute of Biomedical Imaging and Bioengineering, 31 Center Dr., 1C14, Bethesda, MD, 20892-8859, (301) 469-8859, http://www.nibib.gov.

Monique Laberge, Ph.D.
William Atkins, BB, BS, MBA

Imipramine

Definition

Imipramine is a tricyclic antidepressant. It is sold under the brand name Tofranil in the United States.

Purpose

Imipramine is used to relieve symptoms of **depression**. It is also used in the treatment of **enuresis** (bed-wetting) in people between the ages of 6 and 25.

Description

Imipramine hydrochloride was the first tricyclic antidepressant to be discovered. Tricyclic **antidepressants** act to change the balance of naturally occurring chemicals in the **brain** that regulate the transmission of nerve impulses between cells. Mental well-being is partially dependent on maintaining a correct balance of these brain chemicals. Imipramine is thought to act primarily by increasing the concentration of norepinephrine and **serotonin** (both chemicals that stimulate nerve cells) and, to a lesser extent, by blocking the action of another brain chemical, acetylcholine. Imipramine shares most of the properties of other tricyclic antidepressants, such as **amitriptyline**, **amoxapine**, **clomipramine**, **desipramine**, **nortriptyline**, **protriptyline**, and **trimipramine**.

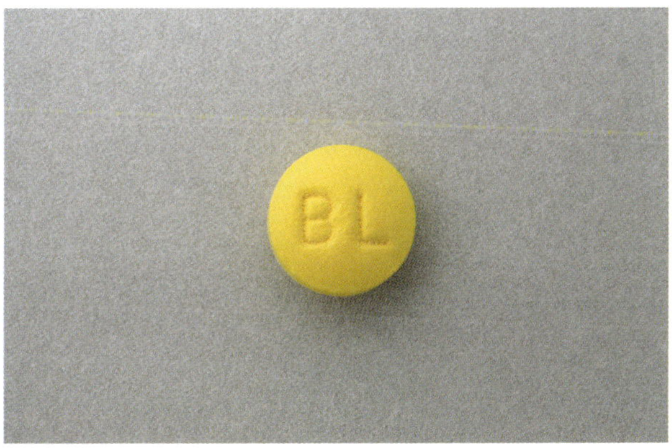

Imipramine, 10 mg. *(© Custom Medical Stock Photo, Inc. Reproduced by permission.)*

The therapeutic effects of imipramine, like other antidepressants, appear slowly. Maximum benefit is often not evident for two to three weeks after starting the drug. People taking imipramine should be aware of this and continue taking the drug as directed even if they do not see immediate improvement.

Recommended dosage

Imipramine is usually started with a total dosage of up to 100 mg per day divided into several smaller doses. This is generally increased to a total of 200 mg per day divided into several doses. Total dosages for patients who are not hospitalized should be no more than 200 mg per day. The recommended maximum dosage for the drug for all patients is 250–300 mg per day. Before dosages greater than 200 mg per day are taken, an electrocardiogram (ECG) should be done. This should be repeated at regular intervals until a steady-state dosage is reached. Lower dosages are recommended for adolescents and older people (over age 60). The lowest dosage that controls symptoms of depression should be used.

Imipramine should be withdrawn gradually, rather than abruptly discontinued. This will help reduce the possibility of a **relapse** into depression.

Precautions

Some studies have shown that children and adults up to age 24 are at an increased risk of developing suicidal thoughts or behaviors when taking antidepressants, including imipramine. Any patient taking imipramine should be closely monitored for signs of worsening depression or other risk factors including panic attacks, difficulty falling asleep, irritability, planning to engage in self-harm or to attempt **suicide**, or abnormal excitement. Any signs that a persons is considering self-harm or suicide warrants an immediate call to the doctor. The risk of suicide may also be increased when imipramine is taken in overdose or combined with alcohol.

Like all tricyclic antidepressants, imipramine should be used cautiously and with close physician supervision in patients, especially the elderly, with benign prostatic hypertrophy, urinary retention, and glaucoma, especially angle-closure glaucoma (the most severe form). Before starting treatment, people with these conditions should discuss the relative risks and benefits of treatment with their doctors to help determine if imipramine is the right antidepressant for them.

A common problem with tricyclic antidepressants is sedation (drowsiness, lack of physical and mental alertness). This side effect is especially noticeable early in therapy. In most patients, sedation decreases or disappears entirely with time, but until then patients taking imipramine should not perform hazardous activities requiring mental alertness or coordination. The sedative effect is increased when imipramine is taken with other central nervous system depressants, such as alcoholic beverages, sleeping medications, other **sedatives**, or antihistamines, and combinations of imipramine with any of these substances should be avoided.

Imipramine may increase heart rate and stress on the heart. It may be dangerous for people with cardiovascular disease, especially those who have recently had a heart attack, to take this drug or other antidepressants in the same pharmacological class. Older people and people with a history of heart disease may develop heart arrhythmias (irregular heartbeat), heart conduction abnormalities, congestive heart failure, heart attack, abnormally rapid heart rates, and strokes. Changes in blood pressure have also been reported.

Manic episodes and the emergence of symptoms of preexisting psychotic states have been reported when imipramine therapy is started.

Patients undergoing surgery should stop taking imipramine at least two weeks before their procedure (if possible), to avoid adverse interactions with the anesthesia.

Side effects

Imipramine shares side effects common to all tricyclic antidepressants. The most frequent of these are dry mouth, constipation, urinary retention, increased heart rate, sedation, irritability, dizziness, and decreased coordination. As with most side effects associated with tricyclic antidepressants, the intensity is highest at the beginning of therapy and tends to decrease with continued use.

Confusion, disorientation, **delusions**, **insomnia**, and anxiety have been reported as side effects in a small percentage of people taking imipramine, as have problems associated with the skin (loss of sensation, numbness and tingling, rashes, spots, itching, and puffiness), **seizures**, ringing in the ears, nausea, vomiting, loss of appetite, diarrhea, and abdominal cramping.

Dry mouth, if severe to the point of causing difficulty speaking or swallowing, may be managed by dosage reduction or temporary discontinuation of the drug. Patients may also chew sugarless gum or suck on sugarless candy in order to increase the flow of saliva. Some artificial saliva products may provide temporary relief.

Interactions

Methylphenidate may increase the effects of imipramine. This is usually avoided by reducing the dosage of imipramine.

Imipramine may increase the depressant action of alcohol. For this reason, people taking imipramine should not drink alcoholic beverages.

Dangerously high blood pressure has resulted from the combination of tricyclic antidepressants, such as imipramine, and members of another class of antidepressants known as **monoamine oxidase inhibitors (MAOIs)**. Patients taking imipramine should not take **MAOIs** (or vice versa). Patients taking any MAOIs, such as Nardil (**phenelzine** sulfate) or Parnate (**tranylcypromine** sulfate), should stop taking the drug and wait at least 14 days before starting treatment with imipramine or any other tricyclic antidepressant. The same holds true when discontinuing imipramine and starting an MAOI.

The sedative effects of imipramine are increased by other central nervous system depressants such as alcohol, sedatives, sleeping medications, or medications used for other mental disorders such as **schizophrenia**. The anticholinergic (drying out) effects of imipramine are additive with other anticholinergic drugs such as **benztropine**, **biperiden**, **trihexyphenidyl**, and antihistamines.

Resources

BOOKS

Adams, Michael, and Norman Holland. *Core Concepts in Pharmacology*. 3rd ed. Upper Saddle River, NJ: 2010.

Foreman, John C., and Torben Johansen. *Textbook of Receptor Pharmacology*. 2nd ed. Boca Raton, FL: CRC Press, 2002.

Page, Clive P., et al. *Integrated Pharmacology*. 3rd ed. St. Louis, MO: Elsevier, 2006.

Von Boxtel, Chris J., Budiono Santoso, and I. Ralph Edwards, eds. *Drug Benefits and Risks: International Textbook of Clinical Pharmacology*. New York: John Wiley and Sons, 2001.

PERIODICALS

Jain A. K., N. S. Thomas, and R. Panchagnula. "Transdermal Drug Delivery of Imipramine Hydrochloride. I. Effect of Terpenes." *Journal of Controlled Release* 79, no. 1–3; (February 19, 2002): 93–101.

Juarez-Olguin, Hugo, et al. "Clinical Evidence of an Interaction Between Imipramine and Acetylsalicylic Acid on Protein Binding in Depressed Patients." *Clinical Neuropharma cology* 25, no. 1 (2002): 32–36.

OTHER

U.S. Food and Drug Administration. "Class Suicidality Labeling Language for Antidepressants." http://www.accessdata.fda.gov/drugsatfda_docs/label/2005/20152s035lbl.pdf (accessed October 9, 2011).

WEBSITES

Daily Med. "Tofranil (imipramine hydrochloride) Injection, Solution (Geigy Pharmaceuticals)." U.S. National Library of Medicine, National Institutes of Health. http://dailymed.nlm.nih.gov/dailymed/drugInfo.cfm?id=2039 (accessed October 9, 2011).

MedlinePlus. "Imipramine." U.S. National Library of Medicine, National Institutes of Health. September 22, 2011. http://www.nlm.nih.gov/medlineplus/druginfo/medmaster/a682389.html (accessed October 9, 2011).

ORGANIZATIONS

American Academy of Clinical Toxicology, 6728 Old McLean Village Drive, McLean, VA, 22101, (703) 556-9222, Fax: (703) 556-8729, admin@clintox.org, http://www.clintox.org.

American Academy of Family Physicians, 11400 Tomahawk Creek Parkway, Leawood, KS, 66211-2672, (913) 906-6000, (800) 274-2237, Fax: (913) 906-6075, contactcenter@aafp.org, http://www.aafp.org.

American Psychiatric Association, 1000 Wilson Blvd., Ste. 1825, Arlington, VA, 22209-3901, (703) 907-7300, apa@psych.org, http://www.psych.org.

American Society for Clinical Pharmacology and Therapeutics, 528 North Washington Street, Alexandria, VA, 22314, (703) 836-6981, http://www.ascpt.org.

American Society for Pharmacology and Experimental Therapeutics, 9650 Rockville Pike, Bethesda, MD, 20814-3995, (301) 634-7060, Fax: (301) 634-7061, http://www.aspet.org.

U.S. Food and Drug Administration, 10903 New Hampshire Ave., Silver Spring, MD, 20993-0002, (888) INFO-FDA (463-6332), http://www.fda.gov.

L. Fleming Fallon, Jr., M.D, Dr. P.H.
Emily Jane Willingham, PhD

Impulse control disorders

Definition

Impulse control disorders are characterized by an individual's inability to resist the impulse to perform an action that is harmful to one's self or others. This condition is a relatively new class of **personality disorders**. Medical researchers surmise that at the root of the problem, the afflicted person desires small, short term pleasures or gains—often performed impulsively and without the ability to resist such behaviors—over the likelihood of much larger, long–term loses. Some of the most common types of these disorders are **intermittent explosive disorder**, **kleptomania**, **pyromania**, compulsive **gambling disorder**, and **trichotillomania**.

Demographics

Such disorders are found in both genders of the population. They usually begin to appear in children in and around the ages of seven to 15 years of age.

Description

All of these impulse control disorders involve the loss or lack of control in certain specific situations. The hallmark of these disorders is the individual's inability to stop impulses that may cause harm to themselves or others. Affected individuals often feel anxiety or tension in considering these behaviors. This anxiety or tension is relieved or diminished once the action is performed.

Intermittent explosive disorder (IED) is more common among males, and involves repeated and aggressive, violet outbursts that lead to assaults on others or destruction of property. These outbursts, often only ten to twenty minutes in duration, are unprovoked or seem to be out of proportion to the event that precedes them. Afterwards, such people often feel remorse and regret from such actions. The outbursts may happen in several separate incidents over a few hours or days or may occur as one or more every so many weeks or months. Examples of intermittent explosive disorder commonly found in daily life include **road rage** and domestic violence and **abuse**.

Kleptomania is more common among females, and involves the theft of objects that are seemingly worthless. The act of stealing relieves tension and anxiety, and increases personal gratification during the act. Once the act is accomplished, individuals feel relieved of their tensions. In addition, they do not steal for the sense of monetary gain. The actual stealing is not preplanned, and the concept of punishment for the crime does not occur to these individuals, although they are aware that what they are doing is wrong. The people afflicted with kleptomania are often very ashamed of their actions afterwards, but are unable to stop themselves and oftentimes unwilling to seek medical or psychological help.

Pyromania is more common among males, and involves setting fires in order to feel pleasure and relieve tension. It is classified by the deliberate setting of fires more than once. Pyromaniacs do not start fires for the same reasons as do arsonists. They are not looking for revenge, monetary gain, or political reasons, only feelings of relief or gratification. They do not start fires as direct part of criminal behavior or due to hallucinations (such as with drug use). The individual exhibits a fascination and attraction to fire and any objects associated with it. Pyromanics often direct their actions toward fire stations and other buildings associated with fire control and prevention.

Pathological gambling occurs in roughly 1%–3% of the population, and involves excessive (compulsive) gambling despite heavy monetary losses. This disorder typically begins in youth, and affected individuals are often competitive, easily bored, restless, and generous. Their losses actually act as a motivating factor in continuing gambling in order to recoup some of what was lost. Pathological gamblers often use lies, theft, and fraud to continue their compulsive gambling habit. They often gamble more during periods of high **stress** or anxiety in order to counter their feelings. Often they gamble for the excitement and not for the money. However, many of them lose large amounts of money, making them more anxious and, in turn, more likely to place larger and riskier bets.

Trichotillomania, also commonly called hair–pulling disorder, involves the uncontrollable, nearly continuous pulling of hair from one's own scalp, face, or other areas of the body, and is more common in females. It often begins in childhood, and is often associated with major **depression** or **attention deficit hyperactivity disorder** (ADHD). There is an increased sense of tension before pulling the hair that is relieved once it is pulled out. Recurrent pulling out of one's hair may result in noticeable hair loss. It can be a mild problem for some people and in others, quite devastating. For all of them, the disorder is very emotional, especially when large amounts of hair are pulled from visible parts of the body, such as from the head. Affected individuals can undergo significant distress and impaired social, occupational, and functional behavior.

Causes and symptoms

The exact causes of impulse control disorders were not fully understood as of 2011. Individuals who have had serious head injuries, however, can be at a higher risk for developing impulse control disorders, as are those with epilepsy.

Some cases of impulse control disorders appear to be side effects of general medical conditions. Several groups of researchers have noted that some older adults with Parkinson's disease become compulsive gamblers as the disease progresses. It is thought that this gambling behavior is a side effect of dopaminergic drugs, as it does not respond to standard treatments for compulsive gambling but only to changes in the patient's medication. A study performed in 2007, headed by a medical researcher from the U.S. National Institute of Neurological Disorders and **Stroke**, found that pathological gamblers who received **dopamine** agonists developed Parkinson's disease at a younger age than those without the disorder. Those with the disorder also scored lower on an impulsivity scale than did other people.

Another medical condition that is associated with impulse control disorders is carcinoid syndrome. In one group of 20 patients with the syndrome, 75% met *DSM–IV* diagnostic criteria for one or another impulse control disorder. The researchers attribute the connection to the high levels of **serotonin** (a neurotransmitter) produced by carcinoid tumors.

The cause of intermittent explosive disorder may be due to environmental, genetic, or biological factors, but the exact cause is still undetermined.

Numerous symptoms of intermittent explosive disorder are:

- irritability
- rage and anger
- tingling
- increased energy
- tremors and palpitations
- tightness of the chest
- headache or pressure in or about the head

The cause of kleptomania is not known for sure in the medical community. Some researchers have suggested that certain chemicals in the **brain** may be linked to the condition. However, additional research is needed before a determination of the cause of the disorder can be announced.

Some of the symptoms of kleptomania are:

- strong urges to steal even though the items are not needed
- tension and anxiety leading up to the act of stealing
- feelings of pleasure and satisfaction while in the act of the theft
- feelings of guilt, embarrassment, and shame afterwards

Although not known for sure, genetic and environmental factors are considered to be possible causes for pathological gambling. Certain natural occurring chemicals in the brain, such as dopamine, norepinephrine, and serotonin indicate possible associations with the disorder. Sometimes, medications taken (external to the disorder) may bring on the disorder. Serious injuries, such as brain **trauma**, can also contribute to pathological gambling.

Several symptoms of pathological gambling are:

- extreme excitement from taking large gambling bets
- being preoccupied with gambling
- increasing the number and/or amount of gambling bets
- showing more interest in gambling than other personal and professional interests
- lying about gambling
- feelings of remorse and guilt after gambling
- large debts and financial problems; also, some legal difficulties may develop
- problems holding onto job and career, and difficulties coping with family responsibilities

For trichotillomania, mutations in the gene SLITRK1 have been associated with the disorder. Tourette syndrome—a syndrome characterized by unusual movements and sounds—is also linked to the disorder. Problems with natural chemicals in the brain, such as dopamine and serotonin, are suggested as a possible cause of trichotillomania.

Symptoms of trichotillomania include:

- bald or patchy spots on the scalp or other parts of the body
- excessive playing with hair or pulled–out hair, including chewing of hair
- thin or missing eyebrows and eyelashes
- pulling hair across the face, especially the lips

Diagnosis

A **diagnosis** of any of these impulse control disorders can be made only after other medical and psychiatric disorders that may cause the same symptoms have been ruled out. Once this is done a medical professional analyzes the physical and mental problems apparent to the patient.

In addition, many doctors administer questionnaires or similar psychiatric screeners as part of the differential diagnosis. Two instruments that were devised in the early 2000s to specifically target impulsive behavior are the Gambling Urge Scale (GUS) and the Lifetime History of Impulsive Behaviors (LHIB) Interview.

For instance, in a medical diagnosis of pathological gambling, five or more of the following symptoms must be present:

- a preoccupation with gambling
- a need to gamble with more money to achieve the thrill of winning
- repeated attempts to control or stop gambling
- irritability or restlessness due to repeated attempts of control
- gambling as an escape from stress
- lying to cover up gambling
- conducting illegal activities, such as embezzling or fraud, to finance gambling
- losing a job or personal relationship due to gambling
- borrowing money to fund gambling

KEY TERMS

Carcinoid syndrome—The pattern of symptoms (often including asthma and diarrhea) associated with carcinoid tumors of the digestive tract or lungs.

Compulsive gambling disorder—An impulse control disorder in which an individual cannot resist gambling despite repeated losses.

Intermittent explosive disorder—A personality disorder in which an individual is prone to intermittent explosive episodes of aggression during which he or she causes bodily harm or destroys property.

Kleptomania—An impulse control disorder characterized by stealing objects that are of little or no value.

Pyromania—An impulse control disorder in which one sets fires.

Trichotillomania—An impulse or compulsion to pull out one's own hair.

Treatment

A combination of psychological counseling and medication are the preferred treatments for impulse control disorders. For kleptomania, pyromania, and trichotillomania, **behavior modification** is usually the treatment of choice. Children with trichotillomania are often helped by antidepressant medication. For pathological gambling, treatment usually involves an adaptation of the model set forth by Alcoholics Anonymous. Individuals are counseled with the goal of eventual responding to appropriate social limits. In the case of intermittent explosive disorder, anger management and medication may be used in extreme cases of aggression.

Prognosis

These disorders can usually be controlled with medication, although the medication may need to be continued long–term to help prevent further aggressive outbursts. Long–term counseling is usually necessary as well. **Support groups** and meetings may also help these individuals.

The prognosis for intermittent explosive disorder, kleptomania, and pyromania is fair. Little is known about the prognosis for trichotillomania, and studies have shown that the condition can disappear for long periods (months to years) without any psychological counseling. For pathological gambling, the prognosis varies greatly from person to person. While total cure for this condition is unlikely, much like alcoholism, long periods of abstinence or continuous abstinence are possible.

Prevention

There are no known preventive treatments or measures for impulse control disorders.

Resources

BOOKS

Aboujaoude, Elias, and Lorrin M. Koran. *Impulse Control Disorders*. New York: Cambridge University Press, 2010.

Grant, Jon E. *Impulse Control Disorders: A Clinician's Guide to Understanding and Treating Behavioral Addictions*. New York: W. W. Norton, 2008.

Hollander, Eris, and Dan J. Stein, eds. *Clinical Manual of Impulse–Control Disorders*. Arlington, VA: American Psychiatric Publishing, 2005.

WEBSITES

Mayo Clinic. "Compulsive Gambling" January 19, 2011. http://www.mayoclinic.com/health/compulsive–gambling/DS00443 (accessed October 9, 2011).

Mayo Clinic. "Intermittent Explosive Disorder." June 10, 2010. http://www.mayoclinic.com/health/intermittent-explosive-disorder/DS00730 (accessed October 9, 2011).

Mayo Clinic. "Kleptomania." October 5, 2011. http://www.mayoclinic.com/health/kleptomania/DS01034 (accessed October 9, 2011).

Mayo Clinic. "Trichotillomania." January 19, 2011. http://www.mayoclinic.com/health/trichotillomania/DS00895 (accessed October 9, 2011).

ScienceDaily. "Characteristics of Increased Risk For Compulsive Gambling Linked To Parkinson's Disease Medications." February 15, 2007. http://www.sciencedaily.com/releases/2007/02/070212184152.htm (accessed October 9, 2011).

ORGANIZATIONS

American Psychiatric Association, 1000 Wilson Blvd., Suite 1825, Arlington, VA, 22209-3901, (703) 907-7300, apa@psych.org, http://www.psych.org.

Gamblers Anonymous International Service Office, PO Box 17173, Los Angeles, CA, 90017, (626) 960-3500, isomain@gamblersanonymous.org, http://www.gamblersanonymous.org.

National Institute of Mental Health, 6001 Executive Blvd., Room 8184, MSC 9663, Bethesda, MD, 20892-9663, (301) 433-4513; TTY: (301) 443-8431, (866) 615-6464; TTY: (866) 415-8051, Fax: (301) 443-4279, nimhinfo@nih.gov, http://www.nimh.nih.gov.

Trichotillomania Learning Center, Inc, 207 McPherson St., Suite H, Santa Cruz, CA, 95060-5863, (831) 457-1004, Fax: (831) 426-4383, info@trich.org, http://www.trich.org.

Liz Meszaros
Rebecca Frey, PhD

Inderal *see* **Propranolol**

Informed consent

Definition

Informed consent is a legal document in all 50 U. S. states, prepared as an agreement for treatment, non-treatment, or for an invasive procedure that requires physicians to disclose the benefits, risks, and alternatives to the treatment, non-treatment, or procedure. It is the method by which a fully informed, rational patient may be involved in the choices about his or her health. Informed consent applies to mental health practitioners (psychiatrists, psychologists, etc.) in their treatment with their clients in generally the same way as physicians with their patients.

Description

Informed consent stems from the legal and ethical right the patient has to decide what is done to his or her body, and from the mental health provider's ethical duty to ensure that the patient is involved in decisions about his or her own health care. The process of ensuring informed consent for treatment involves five elements. All involve information exchange between doctor and patient and are a part of patient education. First, in words the patient can understand, the therapist must convey three things: (1) the details of a treatment or procedure, (2) its potential benefits and serious risks, and (3) any feasible alternatives. The patient should be presented with information on the most likely outcomes of treatment. Next, the practitioner must evaluate whether or not the person has understood what has been said, must ascertain that the risks have been accepted, and that the patient is giving consent to proceed with the treatment with full knowledge and forethought. Finally, the patient must sign the consent form, which documents in generic format the major points of consideration. The only exception to this is securing informed consent during extreme emergencies. It is critical that the patient receive enough information on which to base his or her informed consent, and that the consent is wholly voluntary and has not been forced in any way.

Anyone suffering from an illness, anticipating surgery, or undergoing treatment for a disease is under a great deal of **stress** and anxiety. It may be natural for a patient to be confused or indecisive. When the attending physician has serious doubts about the patient's understanding of the **intervention** and its risks, the patient may be referred for a psychiatric consultation. This is strictly a precaution to ensure that the patient understands what has been explained; declining to be treated or operated on does not necessarily mean the person is incompetent. It could mean that the person is exercising the right to make his or her own healthcare decisions.

Consent is generally not assumed or considered to be implied except in emergency cases where a patient's life is in danger, no prior wishes have been expressed, and a family member or guardian is not present to give consent. Furthermore, a person must possess the mental faculties to understand and give consent; people who are intellectually disabled, intoxicated, or otherwise impaired may not be legally able to consent to treatment.

According to the "Ethical Principles of Psychologists" and "Code of Conduct" designed by the **American Psychological Association**, informed consent also applies when conducting research involving human subjects prior to their participation. Participants in the study should be informed in understandable language to three main points. First, the participant should be informed about the nature of the research. Secondly, participants should be informed that their participation is completely voluntary and that they are free to withdraw from or not participate in the study at any time. Consent must be made without pressure being put on the participant to engage in the study. Finally, the potential consequences of participating or withdrawing should be presented to the participant. This includes risks, discomfort, and limitations of confidentiality.

With regard to either therapy treatment or research participation, another member of the healthcare/research team may obtain the signed informed consent with the assurance that the provider has satisfied the requirements of informed consent.

The actual informed consent form is to document the process and protect the provider and the hospital. Legally, it is proof of what has been covered and the patient agrees to the procedure, risks, benefits and options. The informed consent process is in place for the protection of the patient. It also serves to ensure that everything is discussed with the patient: all of the options, all of the common risks, the worst case scenario, and other similar situations.

Origins

There is a theory that the practice of acquiring informed consent is rooted in the post–World War II Nuremberg Trials. Following the war crimes tribunal in 1949, as a result of the Karl Brandt case, 10 standards were put forth regarding physician's requirements for experimentation on human subjects. This established a new standard of ethical medical behavior for the post–World War II human rights age, and the concept of voluntary informed consent was established. A number of rules accompanied voluntary informed consent within the realms of research. It could only be requested for experimentation for the gain of society, for the potential acquisition of knowledge of the pathology, and for studies performed that avoided physical and mental suffering to the fullest extent possible.

Benefits

There are advantages to the informed consent process. First, it can be empowering to the patient to understand that he/she plays an important role in their own treatment. They are encouraged to be active participants in the treatment process and know their options well enough to make the best treatment decisions for themselves. This also shifts the responsibility to patients to work with the therapist towards their mental health goals possibly increasing self-confidence and autonomy, and decreasing dependence on the therapist.

Precautions

A crucial component of informed consent is that the person signing it is competent or able to make a rational decision and meaningfully give consent. This situation gets more complicated when working with people who are unable to understand what has been explained or are unable to make a reasonable decision about their health care. According to the "Code of Conduct" for psychologists designed by the American Psychological Association, if this is the case, informed permission from a "legally authorized person" should then be sought, if that is a legal alternative. The ethical guidelines are more stringent than legal guidelines in many states, where the informed consent of the parent or guardian is all that is required, whether or not the professional has attempted to explain the procedure to the client.

Although it is necessary to present the procedure or treatment formally to the patient, there is concern that this process could hurt the therapeutic relationship between the client and therapist. For example, if an informed consent is too detailed, it could frighten a new client who may be hesitant about therapy to begin with. In addition, informing patients about the risks of treatment might scare them into refusing it when the risks of non-treatment are even greater.

There are undoubtedly many issues regarding informed consent. As modern society continues to be litigious, the courts and/or government may take on a more active role in deciding the extent to which patients must be informed of treatments, procedures, and **clinical trials** in which they voluntarily become enrolled. Therefore, healthcare providers must become more educated as to what needs to be conveyed to patients, and to what extent.

Resources

BOOKS

Berg, Jessica W., et al. *Informed Consent: Legal Theory and Clinical Practice*. 2nd ed. New York: Oxford University Press, 2001.

PERIODICALS

Caplan, Arthur L. "Ethical Issues Surrounding Forced, Mandated, or Coerced Treatment." *Journal of Substance Abuse Treatment* 31, no. 2, September 2006: 117–20.

Dunn, Laura B., et al. "Assessing Decisional Capacity for Clinical Research or Treatment: A Review of Instruments." *American Journal of Psychiatry* 163, no. 8, August 2006: 1323–34.

Fallon, April. "Informed Consent in the Practice of Group Psychotherapy." *International Journal of Group Psychotherapy* 56, no. 4 (2006): 431–53.

Jackson, Grace E. "Mental Health Screening in Schools: Essentials of Informed Consent." *Ethical Human Psychology and Psychiatry* 8, no. 3, Fall–Winter 2006: 217–24.

WEBSITES

CRICO/RMF.com "Risk Management Issues: Improved Informed Consent." http://www.rmf.harvard.edu/patient-safety-strategies/informed-consent/index.aspx (accessed October 9, 2011).

National Organization of Circumcision Information Resource Centers. "Informed Consent." January 16, 2010. http://www.nocirc.org/consent (accessed October 9, 2011).

University of Washington. "Informed Consent." April 11, 2008. http://depts.washington.edu/bioethx/topics/consent.html (accessed October 9, 2011).

U.S. National Cancer Institute. "A Guide to Understanding Informed Consent." http://www.cancer.gov/clinicaltrials/patientsafety/informed-consent-guide/page1 (accessed October 31, 2011).

Yale University School of Medicine. "Informed Consent." http://www.yalemedicalgroup.org/stw/Page.asp?PageID=STW027361 (accessed October 31, 2011).

Jenifer P. Marom, Ph.D.

Inhalants and related disorders

Definition

The inhalants are a class of drugs that include a broad range of chemicals found in hundreds of different products. Many inhalants are readily available to the general population. These chemicals include volatile solvents (liquids that vaporize at room temperature) and aerosols (sprays that contain solvents and propellants). Examples include glue, gasoline, paint thinner, hair spray, lighter fluid, spray paint, nail polish remover, correction fluid, rubber cement, felt-tip marker fluids, vegetable sprays, and certain cleaners such as spot removers, computer keyboard cleaner, and carburetor cleaner. The inhalants share a common route of administration—that is, they are all drawn into the body by breathing. They are usually taken either by breathing in the vapors directly from a container (sniffing); by inhaling fumes from substances placed in a bag (bagging); or by inhaling the substance from a cloth soaked in it (huffing). Inhalants take effect very quickly because they get into the bloodstream rapidly via the lungs. The high from inhalants is usually brief, so that users often take inhalants repeatedly over several hours.

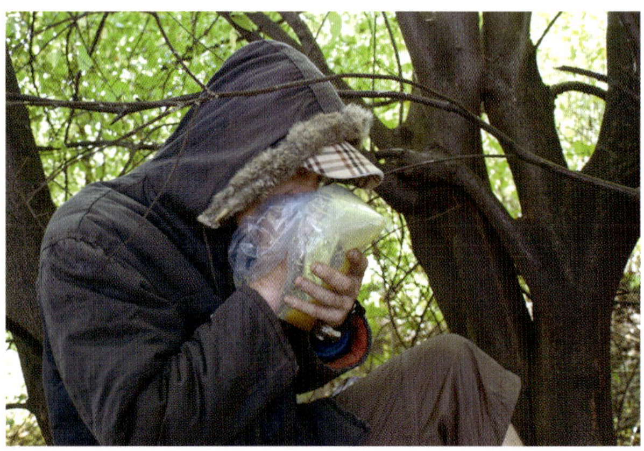

A teenager huffs glue. *(© Mark Harvey/Alamy)*

This pattern of use can be dangerous, leading to unconsciousness or even death.

The latest revision of the manual that is used by mental health professionals to diagnose mental disorders is the ***Diagnostic and Statistical Manual of Mental Disorders*** published in 2000 (also known as *DSM-IV-TR*). It lists inhalant dependence and inhalant abuse as substance use disorders. In addition, the inhalant-induced disorder of inhalant intoxication is listed in the substance-related disorders section as well. Inhalant withdrawal is not listed in the *DSM-IV-TR,* because it is not clear that there is a "clinically significant" withdrawal syndrome. In addition, withdrawal is not included as a symptom of inhalant dependence, whereas withdrawal is a symptom of dependence for all other substances.

The fifth edition of the *Diagnostic and Statistical Manual of Mental Disorders,* also known as the *DSM-5,* is due for publication in May 2013. This edition may include proposed changes and revisions to some current diagnostic criteria for psychiatric diagnoses, including combining inhalant abuse and inhalant dependence into a single diagnosis of inhalant use disorder.

Anesthetic gases (such as nitrous oxide, chloroform, or ether) and nitrites (including amyl or butyl nitrite) are not included under inhalant-related disorders in the *DSM-IV-TR,* because they have slightly different intoxication syndromes. Problems with the use of these substances are to be diagnosed under "other substance-related disorders." There is, however, a significant degree of overlap between the symptoms of disorders related to inhalants and these other substances.

Inhalant dependence

Inhalant dependence, or **addiction**, is essentially a syndrome in which a person continues to use inhalants in spite of significant problems caused by, or made worse by, the use of these substances. People who use inhalants heavily may develop tolerance to the drug, which indicates that they are physically dependent on it.

Inhalant abuse

Inhalant abuse is a less serious condition than inhalant dependence; in most cases, it does not involve physical dependence on the drug. Inhalant abuse refers essentially to significant negative consequences from the recurrent use of inhalants.

Inhalant intoxication

When a person uses enough of an inhalant, they will get high from it. The symptoms of intoxication differ slightly, depending on the type of inhalant, the amount used, and other factors. There is, however, a predictable set of symptoms of inhalant intoxication. When too much of the substance is taken, an individual can overdose.

Demographics

Inhalants are some of the few substances more commonly used by younger children rather than older ones. It has been estimated that 10%–20% of youths aged 12–17 have tried inhalants. About 6% of the United States population admits to having tried inhalants prior to fourth grade. The peak time for inhalant use appears to be between the seventh and ninth grades. Inhalants are sometimes referred to as gateway drugs, meaning they are some of the first drugs that people try before moving on to such other substances as alcohol, marijuana, and **cocaine**. Only a small proportion of those who have used inhalants would meet diagnostic criteria for dependence or abuse.

Males generally use inhalants more frequently than females. However, a National Household Survey on Drug Abuse has shown no gender differences in rates of inhalant use in youths between the ages of 12 and 17. Children younger than 12 and adults who use inhalants, however, are more likely to be male.

A Monitoring The Future (MTF) survey reports that African American children consistently show lower rates of inhalant abuse than youth of other ethnic populations, however, individuals from both rural and urban environments abuse inhalants.

According to a 2008 National Survey on Drug Use and Health (NSDUH) study, 729,000 persons aged 12 or older used inhalants for the first time within the past 12 months, 70% of whom were under the age of 18. In a 2009 report, 2.1 million Americans age 12 and older had abused inhalants. In fact, as of 2011, the **Substance Abuse and Mental Health Services Administration** (SAMHSA) viewed inhalant abuse as a multi–generational problem.

Description

Inhalant dependence

Dependence on inhalants involves problems related to the use of inhalants. It is often difficult for a person to stop using the inhalants despite these problems. Individuals dependent on inhalants may use these chemicals several times per week or every day. They may have problems with unemployment or with family relationships, and/or such physical problems as kidney or liver damage caused by the use of inhalants.

Inhalant abuse

People who abuse inhalants typically use them less frequently than those who are dependent on them. Despite less frequent use, however, a person with inhalant abuse suffers negative consequences. For example, the use of inhalants may contribute to poor grades or school truancy.

Inhalant intoxication

Intoxication from inhalants occurs rapidly (usually within five minutes) and lasts for a short period of time (from 5–30 minutes). Inhalants typically have a depressant effect on the central nervous system, similar to the effects of alcohol; and produce feelings of euphoria (feeling good), excitement, dizziness, and slurred speech. In addition, persons intoxicated by inhalants may feel as if they are floating, or may feel a sense of increased power. Severe intoxication from inhalants can cause coma or even death.

Causes and symptoms

Causes

Because inhalants are readily available and inexpensive, they are often used by children (ages 6–16) and the poor. Factors that are associated with inhalant use include poverty, a history of childhood abuse, poor grades, and dropping out of school. The last two factors may simply be results of inhalant use, however, rather than its causes.

The use of inhalants is highly likely to be influenced by peers. Inhalants are often used in group settings. The solitary consumption of inhalants is associated with heavy, prolonged use; it may indicate that the person has a more serious problem with these substances.

Symptoms

INHALANT DEPENDENCE. The *DSM-IV-TR* specifies that three or more of the following symptoms must occur at any time during a 12-month period (and cause significant impairment or distress) in order to meet diagnostic criteria for inhalant dependence:

- Tolerance. The individual either must use increasingly higher amounts of the drug over time in order to achieve the same effect, or finds that the same amount of the drug has much less of an effect over time than before. After using inhalants regularly for a while, people may find that they need to use at least 50% more than the amount they started with in order to get the same effect.
- Loss of control. The person either repeatedly uses a larger quantity of inhalant than planned or uses the inhalant over a longer period of time than planned. For instance, someone may begin using inhalants on school days, after initially limiting their use to weekends.
- Inability to stop using. The person has either unsuccessfully attempted to cut down or stop using the inhalants, or has a persistent desire to stop using. Users may find that despite efforts to stop using inhalants on school days, they cannot stop.
- Time. The affected person spends large amounts of time obtaining inhalants, using them, being under the influence of inhalants, and recovering from their effects. Obtaining the inhalants might not take up much time because they are readily available for little money, but the person may use them repeatedly for hours each day.
- Interference with activities. The affected person either gives up or reduces the amount of time involved in recreational activities, social activities, and/or occupational activities because of the use of inhalants. The person may use inhalants instead of playing sports, spending time with friends, or going to work.
- Harm to self. The person continues to use inhalants in spite of developing either a physical (liver damage or heart problems, for example) or psychological problem (such as depression or memory problems) that is caused by, or made worse by, the use of inhalants.

INHALANT ABUSE. The *DSM-IV-TR* specifies that one or more of the following symptoms must occur at any time during a 12-month period (and cause significant impairment or distress) in order to meet diagnostic criteria for inhalant abuse:

- Interference with role fulfillment. The person's use of inhalants frequently interferes with his or her ability to fulfill obligations at work, home, or school. People may find they are unable to do chores or pay attention in school because they are under the influence of inhalants.
- Danger to self. The person repeatedly uses inhalants in situations in which their influence may be physically hazardous (while driving a car, for example).
- Legal problems. The person has recurrent legal problems related to using inhalants (such as arrests for assaults while under the influence of inhalants).
- Social problems. The person continues to use inhalants despite repeated interpersonal or relationship problems caused by, or made worse by, the use of inhalants. For example, the affected person may get into arguments related to inhalant use.

KEY TERMS

Addiction—A strong physical or psychological dependence on a physical substance.

Inhalant—A substance a person can sniff, or inhale, to get high.

Stupor—A state of sluggishness or impaired consciousness.

Syndrome—A group or pattern of symptoms or signs that occur together.

INHALANT INTOXICATION. The *DSM-IV-TR* specifies that the following symptoms must be present in order to meet diagnostic criteria for inhalant intoxication:

- Use. The person recently intentionally used an inhalant.
- Personality changes. The person experiences significant behavioral or psychological changes during or shortly after use of an inhalant. These changes may include spoiling for a fight, assaultiveness, poor judgment, apathy ("don't care" attitude), or impaired functioning socially or at work or school.
- Inhalant-specific intoxication syndrome. Two or more of the following symptoms occur during or shortly after inhalant use or exposure: dizziness, involuntary side-to-side eye movements (nystagmus), loss of coordination, slurred speech, unsteady gait (difficulty walking), lethargy (fatigue), slowed reflexes, psychomotor retardation (moving slowly), tremor (shaking), generalized muscle weakness, blurred vision or double vision, stupor or coma, and euphoria (a giddy sensation of happiness or well-being).

Diagnosis

People rarely seek treatment on their own for inhalant dependence or abuse. In some cases, the child or adolescent is taken to a doctor by a parent or other relative who is concerned about personality changes, a chemical odor on the child's breath, or other signs of inhalant abuse. The parent may also have discovered empty containers of the inhaled substance in the child's room or elsewhere in the house. In other cases, the child's or adolescent's use of inhalants is diagnosed during a medical interview, when he or she is taken to a hospital emergency room after overdosing on the inhalant or being injured in an accident related to inhalant use. Although inhalants can be detected in blood or urine samples, laboratory tests might not always confirm the **diagnosis**, because the inhalants do not remain in the system very long.

Inhalant dependence

Other substance use disorders are commonly seen among people diagnosed with inhalant dependence. The use of inhalants is usually secondary to the use of other substances; however, only occasionally are inhalants a person's primary drug of choice.

Inhalant abuse

The use of other substances is not uncommon among people who abuse inhalants.

Inhalant intoxication

Intoxication from the use of such other substances as alcohol, **sedatives**, hypnotics (medications to induce sleep), and anxiolytics (tranquilizers) can resemble intoxication caused by inhalants. Furthermore, people under the influence of inhalants may experience hallucinations (typically auditory, visual, or tactile), other perceptual disturbances (such as illusions), or **delusions** (believing they can fly, for example).

Treatment

Inhalant dependence and abuse

Chronic inhalant users are difficult to treat because they often have many serious personal and social problems. They also have difficulty staying away from inhalants; **relapse** rates are high. Treatment usually takes a long time and involves enlisting the support of the person's family, changing the friendship network if the individual uses with others, teaching coping skills, and increasing self-esteem.

Inhalant intoxication

Inhalant intoxication is often treated in a hospital emergency room when the affected person begins to suffer serious psychological (such as hallucinations or delusions) or medical consequences (such as difficulty breathing, headache, nausea, vomiting) from inhalant use. The most serious medical risk from inhalant use is sudden sniffing death. A person using inhalants, especially if they are using the substance repeatedly in a single, prolonged session, may start to have a rapid and irregular heartbeat or severe difficulty breathing, followed by heart failure and death. Sudden sniffing death can occur within minutes. In addition, inhalant use can cause permanent damage to the **brain**, lungs, kidneys, muscles, and heart. The vapors themselves cause damage, but there are also dangerously high levels of copper, **zinc**, and heavy metals in many inhalants.

People who use inhalants may also be treated for injuries sustained while under the influence of inhalants or while using them. For example, individuals intoxicated by inhalants may fall and injure themselves, or they may drive while intoxicated and have an accident. People who use inhalants may also die from, or require treatment for, burns because many inhalants are highly flammable. They may also need emergency treatment for suffocation from inhaling with a plastic bag over the head or for choking on inhaled vomit.

Prognosis

Inhalant dependence and abuse

The course of inhalant abuse and dependence differs somewhat, depending on the affected person's age. Younger children who are dependent on or abuse inhalants use them regularly, especially on weekends and after school. As children get older, they often stop using inhalants. They may stop substance use altogether, or they may move on to other substances. Adults who abuse or are dependent on inhalants may use inhalants regularly for years. They may also frequently "binge" on inhalants (i.e., use them much more frequently for shorter periods of time). This pattern of use can go on for years.

The use of inhalants and subsequent dependence on the substance occurs among people who do not have access to other drugs or are otherwise isolated (such as prison inmates). Also, as with other substance use disorders, people who have greater access to inhalants are more likely to develop dependence on them. This group of people may include workers in industrial settings with ready access to inhalants.

Prevention

Comprehensive prevention programs that involve families, schools, communities, and the media (such as television) can be effective in reducing **substance abuse**. The recurring theme in these programs is to stay away from drugs in the first place. Avoiding drugs altogether is the primary method of ensuring that one does not develop a substance use disorder.

Parents can help prevent the misuse of inhalants by educating their children about the negative effects of inhalant use. Teachers and parents can help prevent inhalant abuse and dependence by recognizing the signs of inhalant use. Signs include chemical odors on the child's breath or clothes, slurred speech, a drunken or disoriented appearance, nausea or lack of appetite, and inattentiveness and lack of coordination.

QUESTIONS TO ASK YOUR DOCTOR

- What risks are associated with abuse of inhalants?
- What symptoms are associated with inhalant dependence?
- Does having inhalant dependence and abuse put me at risk for other health conditions?
- Can you recommend any treatment and support groups for me?

Resources

BOOKS

American Psychiatric Association. *Diagnostic and Statistical Manual of Mental Disorders,* 4th ed., Text rev. Washington, DC: American Psychiatric Association, 2000.

American Psychological Association. *Publication Manual of the American Psychological Association,*6th ed. Washington, DC: American Psychological Association, 2009.

Erickson, Carlton K, Ph.D. *Addiction Essentials: The Go-To Guide for Clinicians and Patients.*New York, NY: W. W. Norton & Company, 2011.

Galanter, Marc, and Herbert D. Kleber, eds. *Textbook of Substance Abuse Treatment,* 2nd ed. Washington, DC: American Psychiatric Press, Inc., 2008.

Sadock, Benjamin J., MD., Virginia Alcott Sadock, MD., and Pedro Ruiz, MD., eds. *Kaplan and Sadock's Comprehensive Textbook of Psychiatry,* 2nd ed. New York, NY: Lippincott Williams & Wilkins, 2009.

ORGANIZATIONS

National Clearinghouse on Alcohol and Drug Information, PO Box 2345, Rockville, MD, 20847, (877) SAMHSA-7; Hablamos español: (877) 767-8432; TDD: (800) 487-4889, Fax: (240) 221-4292, http://ncadi.samhsa.gov.

National Institute on Drug Abuse, 6001 Executive Blvd., Rm. 5213, Bethesda, MD, 20892, (301) 442-1124; Spanish: (240) 221-4007, information@nida.nih.gov, http://www.nida.nih.gov.

The Partnership at Drugfree.org, 352 Park Ave. S, 9th Floor, New York, NY, 10010, (212) 922-1560, Fax: (212) 922-1570, http://www.drugfree.org.

Substance Abuse and Mental Health Services Administration, 1 Choke Cherry Rd., Rockville, MD, 20857, (877) SAMHSA-7 (726-4727), (800) TTY: 487-4889, Fax: (240) 221-4292, SAMHSAInfo@samhsa.hhs.gov, http://www.samhsa.gov.

Jennifer Hahn, Ph.D.
Laura Jean Cataldo, RN, Ed.D.

Inkblot test *see* **Rorschach inkblot test**

Insomnia

Definition

Insomnia is the inability to obtain an adequate amount or quality of sleep. The difficulty may be in falling asleep, remaining asleep, or waking up too early, or a combination of all three. Sleeplessness is a symptom that may be caused by physical or mental conditions or circumstances, including a general medical condition or psychiatric disorder.

Demographics

The U.S. Centers for Disease Control and Prevention estimates that between 50 and 70 million Americans are affected by some type of sleep disorder, and nearly half of the U.S. population reports at least occasional sleeping problems. Accurate data is difficult to gather, as many people misperceive how much sleep they actually get and how many times they normally wake up during the night. It is generally thought, however, that women are more likely than men to suffer from insomnia. As people age, they are also more likely to experience insomnia, as are people who are generally nervous or tense. According to the National Sleep Foundation (NSF), people who are divorced, widowed, or separated are more likely to experience insomnia than married couples, and insomnia is more frequently reported by persons with a lower socioeconomic status.

Anti-insomnia drugs

Brand name (generic name)	Possible side effects
Ambien (zolpidem tartrate)	Daytime drowsiness, dizziness, headache, muscle or joint pain, tremors
Dalmane (flurazepam hydrochloride)	Decreased coordination, irritability, lightheadedness, pain
Doral (quazepam)	Daytime drowsiness, dizziness, dry mouth, headache
Halcion (triazolam)	Chest pain, decreased coordination, memory impairment
Lunesta (eszopiclone)	Daytime drowsiness, decreased libido, heartburn, nausea, pain
ProSom (estazolam)	Dizziness, headache, nausea, sleep inertia (grogginess), weakness
Restoril (temazepam)	Dizziness, fatigue, headache, nausea, sleep inertia
Sonata (zaleplon)	Change in vision, decreased coordination, loss of appetite, numbness or tingling

(Table by PreMediaGlobal. Reproduced by permission of Gale, a part of Cengage Learning.)

Description

Insomnia is classified both by its nightly symptoms and its duration. Sleep-onset insomnia refers to difficulty falling asleep; maintenance insomnia refers to waking frequently during the night or waking early. Insomnia is also classified in relation to the number of sleepless nights. Short-term insomnia, also called transient or acute insomnia, is a common occurrence and usually lasts only a few days. Long-term, or chronic, insomnia lasts more than three to four weeks. Insomnia can also be classified as either primary or secondary. Primary insomnia is a disorder that cannot be attributed to another condition or disorder, whereas secondary insomnia can be traced back to a source. Possible sources of secondary insomnia include a medical condition; the use of medications, alcohol, or other substances; or a mental disorder such as severe **depression**.

Sleep is essential for mental and physical restoration. Chronic insomnia increases the risk for personal injury and error because of the **fatigue** and delayed reflexes experienced due to lack of sleep. Chronic insomnia can also lead to mood disorders such as depression. On average, adults require approximately 7–8 hours of sleep each night, teenagers need about 9 hours per night, and infants need 16 to 18 hours of sleep each day to function properly and maintain health.

Not all disruptions in the normal pattern of sleeping and waking are considered insomnia. Such factors as jet lag, unusually high levels of **stress**, changing work shifts, or other drastic changes in the person's routine can all lead to sleep problems. Unless the problems are ongoing and severe enough that they are causing distress for the person in important areas of life, he or she is not considered to have insomnia.

Stages of sleep

Sleep consists of two separate states that constantly cycle: rapid eye movement (REM), the stage in which most dreaming occurs, and non-REM (NREM). Four stages of sleep take place during NREM: stage I, when the person passes from relaxed wakefulness; stage II, an early stage of light sleep; and stages III and IV, which are increasing degrees of deep sleep. Most stage IV sleep (also called delta sleep) occurs in the first several hours of sleep. A period of REM sleep normally follows a period of NREM sleep.

Causes and symptoms

Causes

Sleeplessness or insomnia can have many causes, including physical conditions (such as sleep apnea), mental conditions (such as depression), shift work schedules with irregular hours, or experiencing a traumatic event. In the days immediately following the terrorist attacks on September 11, 2001, 47% of Americans rated their sleep as "poor" or "fair," according to NSF's "2002 Sleep in America" poll. In comparison, 27% of poll participants rated sleep as poor or fair for most nights of that year.

Transient insomnia is often caused by a temporary situation in a person's life such as an argument with a loved one, a brief medical illness, or jet lag. When the situation is resolved or the precipitating factor disappears, the condition goes away, usually without medical treatment. Side effects of prescription drugs such as asthma medicines, **steroids**, and **antidepressants** may include insomnia, and it may also be a side effect of over-the-counter products such as nasal decongestants or appetite suppressants.

Chronic insomnia usually has different causes, and there may be more than one factor contributing to sleeplessness. Causes of insomnia include:

- a medical condition or its treatment, including sleep apnea, diabetes, arthritis, a heart condition, and asthma
- use of substances such as caffeine, alcohol, and nicotine
- psychiatric conditions such as mood or anxiety disorders
- stress or depression, such as sadness caused by the loss of a loved one or a job
- a change in work shift
- a work schedule with nontraditional hours, such as those worked by medical professionals, truck drivers, the military, and persons employed by 24-hour businesses
- sleep-disordered breathing, such as snoring
- periodic jerky leg movements (*nocturnal myoclonus*) that occur just as the individual is falling asleep
- restless legs syndrome, which involves the urge to move the legs and may also include feelings of tingling or cramping
- repeated nightmares or panic attacks during sleep

Excessive worrying about whether or not a person will be able to fall asleep may also cause insomnia. The concern creates so much anxiety that the individual's bedtime rituals and behavior actually trigger insomnia, a condition called psychophysiological insomnia.

Symptoms

People with insomnia are unable to achieve a good night's sleep and wake up feeling tired. They may have difficulty falling asleep or may be able to fall asleep without a problem but wake up in the early hours of the morning. The person is then either unable to go back to sleep or drifts into a restless, unsatisfying sleep. Insomnia is a common condition in the elderly and persons suffering from depression. Sometimes sleep patterns are reversed and the individual has difficulty staying awake during the day and takes frequent naps, with the sleep at night being fitful and frequently interrupted.

The lack of restful sleep may result in daytime symptoms of **sleep deprivation**, including a lack of concentration, headaches, anxiety, irritability, fatigue, delayed reflexes, and gastrointestinal symptoms. Lack of sleep has also been associated with an increase in appetite, which can lead to weight gain.

Diagnosis

Insomnia is a disorder that is usually self-reported; that is, patients usually bring up the subject of sleep problems with their doctors rather than the doctor suggesting the **diagnosis**. There are no laboratory tests for insomnia, but the doctor may review a patient's health history or order tests to determine if a medical condition is causing the insomnia. The physician may ask if the patient is depressed, in pain, under stress, working irregular schedules, or taking any medications. The physician may also suggest keeping a sleep diary, in which the patient notes details such as the time they went to bed, the time(s) at which they got up during the night, their activities before bed, use of caffeine, etc. If the patient has a bed partner, information can be obtained about whether the patient snores or is restless during sleep. This information, together with a medical history and physical examination, can help confirm the doctor's assessment and uncover specific factors related to the insomnia.

Insomnia is included in the ***Diagnostic and Statistical Manual of Mental Disorders***, fourth edition, text revised (*DSM-IV-TR*), the guidelines used by medical professionals in diagnosing mental disorders. In order to meet the *DSM-IV-TR* criteria for primary insomnia, a person must experience the symptoms for at least a month, and the symptoms must cause them distress or reduce their ability to function successfully. The symptoms cannot be caused by a different sleep disorder or medical condition or be a side effect of medications or **substance abuse**, though insomnia may be comorbid with (occur together with) other psychiatric disorders, including mania, depression, and **anxiety disorders**.

A fifth edition of the *DSM* (*DSM-5*) is expected to publish in 2013. Proposed revisions to the diagnostic criteria for insomnia include adding the requirement that the sleep difficulty must occur at least three nights per week. Patients should also report at least one daytime impairment related to the loss of sleep.

Treatment

Treatments for insomnia include treating any physical or mental conditions contributing to the sleeplessness, as well as exploring changes in lifestyle that may improve the situation (such as changing work schedules). Behavioral and educational therapies, such as **cognitive-behavioral therapy**, are usually tried first, because they do not have side effects and cannot create a chemical dependence the way some sleep medications can. In seeking treatment, patients may wish to consult a sleep clinic or a doctor who specializes in the treatment of **sleep disorders** as well as their family doctor. Treatment using a combination of approaches is usually most effective.

Traditional

Behavioral and lifestyle changes may help patients overcome sleeplessness. Patients should try to go to bed only when sleepy and use the bedroom only for sleep; activities such as reading, watching television, or snacking should take place elsewhere. Maintaining a comfortable bedroom temperature, reducing noise, and eliminating light may also help. If a person is unable to fall asleep, he or she can go into another room and do some quiet activity such as reading and return to bed when sleepy. Setting an alarm and getting up every morning at the same time, no matter how long a person has slept, may help to establish a regular sleep-wake pattern. Naps during the day should be avoided, but if absolutely necessary, a 30-minute nap early in the afternoon may not interfere with sleep at night.

Sleep-restriction therapy is a technique that restricts the time in bed to the actual time spent sleeping. This approach allows a slight sleep debt to build up, increasing the individual's ability to fall asleep and stay asleep. If a patient sleeps five hours a night, the time in bed is limited to 5–5.5 hours. The time in bed is gradually increased in small segments, with the individual rising at the same time each morning; at least 85% of the time in bed must be spent sleeping.

Drugs

A physician may determine that drug therapy is necessary to treat insomnia. Drugs may be prescribed if the patient is undergoing a crisis or if insomnia persists after a patient has made lifestyle changes. However, drug therapy is regarded as a short-term remedy, not a solution.

Conventional medications given for insomnia include **sedatives**, tranquilizers, and **antianxiety drugs**. All require a doctor's prescription and may be habit-forming. Medications may lose effectiveness over time and can reduce alertness during the day. The medications should be taken up to four times daily or as directed for approximately three to four weeks. The dose will vary with the physician, patient, and medication. If insomnia is related to depression, then an antidepressant medication may be helpful.

Drugs prescribed for improving sleep are called hypnotics. Hypnotics include **benzodiazepines** that are prescribed for anxiety and insomnia. Benzodiazepines commonly prescribed for insomnia include **triazolam** (Halcion), **temazepam** (Restoril), **lorazepam** (Ativan), **alprazolam** (Xanax), **flurazepam** (Dalmane), and **oxazepam** (Serax). Other drugs that may be prescribed include **zolpidem** (Ambien), ramelteon (Rozerem), and eszopiclone (Lunesta). In clinical studies, ramelteon has shown no evidence of potential for abuse, dependence, or withdrawal. Both ramelteon and eszopiclone are approved for long-term use by prescription only.

Over-the-counter sleep products include Nytol, Sominex, Unisom Nightime Tablets, and Tylenol PM. While these products are usually not addictive, some experts believe they are not very effective in sustaining stage IV sleep and can affect the quality of sleep, resulting in daytime drowsiness.

Alternative

Alternative treatments may be used in treating both the symptom of insomnia and its underlying causes. Much treatment is centered on herbal remedies, but as the U.S. Food and Drug Administration does not regulate the safety or efficacy of these treatments, consumers should be cautious when using herbal supplements. Persons interested in herbal supplements should consult with their healthcare provider or complementary medicine practitioner before taking any herbal remedies. This is especially important because some remedies such as melatonin interact with other herbals like **valerian** and prescription medicines.

VALERIAN. Valerian is one of the herbs most commonly used to treat insomnia. In **clinical trials**, people who took valerian fell asleep more quickly and experienced improved slumber. Because of the herb's sedative properties, valerian is used to treat both insomnia and anxiety. Valerian is sold commercially in the form of capsules, extracts, and teas. The capsule or extract dosage ranges from 300 to 600 mg; teas may consist of a mixture of herbs with sedative properties, such as valerian, **chamomile**, hops, lemon balm, **passionflower**, or **St. John's wort**. As a sleep aid, it should be taken shortly before bedtime. People who have trouble falling asleep may see results quickly. It could take from two weeks to a month before a person with chronic insomnia experiences improved sleep.

MELATONIN. Melatonin is a natural hormone that is secreted from the brain's pineal gland. The gland regulates a person's biological clock, particularly day and night cycles. Supplement melatonin is available to help promote sleep and regulate sleep cycles. Melatonin is generally used as a jet lag remedy and may also help establish sleep patterns for shift workers. It has also been successful in clinical trials in treating sleep problems in children with **autism** and **intellectual disability** disorders and in persons who are blind. While melatonin may help people fall asleep more quickly, studies indicate limited success when used for treating insomnia. Melatonin is available in pill form; long-term effects of taking it are not known.

MIND AND BODY RELAXATION. Incorporating relaxation techniques into bedtime rituals may help a person go to sleep faster and improve the quality of sleep. Relaxation techniques are safe and may be effective in reducing sleeplessness. Suggestions include learning to substitute pleasant thoughts for unpleasant ones (imagery training) to help reduce worrying, or listening to recordings that combine the sounds of nature with soft relaxing music. **Meditation**, prayer, and breathing exercises may also be effective.

AROMATHERAPY AND HYDROTHERAPY. **Aromatherapy** promotes relaxation through the use of essential oils, the aromatic extracts of plants. Essential oils may be used for a soothing bath; applied to the face, neck, shoulders, and pillow; or diffused in air. Dream pillows, also known as sleep pillows, are pillows with an opening to insert essential oils, so that scents such as chamomile or **lavender** can be smelled while the person attempts to sleep. Hydrotherapy incorporated with aromatherapy consists of a warm bath scented with essential oils, such as rose, lavender, or marjoram. Valerian may also be added to bath water. Taking a warm bath before bed is thought to naturally reduce the body's temperature, which prepares the body for sleep.

LIGHT THERAPY. **Light therapy** may help some patients with insomnia, particularly those affected by repeatedly waking in the morning rather than having difficulty falling asleep at night. During a light therapy session, the patient sits in front of a light box for a specified period of time. The rays of the light box mimic those of the sun, helping to reset the patient's biological clock. Light therapy is traditionally used in treating **seasonal affective disorder**, a depressive condition caused by the loss of sunlight during winter months.

QUESTIONS TO ASK YOUR DOCTOR

- Why can't I sleep through the night?
- What can I do to help fall asleep and prevent waking up during the night?
- Is it okay for me to take sleeping pills?
- Will I be able to enjoy sleep again?

MASSAGE THERAPY. Massage therapy promotes relaxation by relaxing tense muscles throughout the body. It is especially helpful for restless leg syndrome. A massage once a week by a registered massage therapist may help the individual relieve any stress that is causing sleeplessness.

NUTRITION AND DIETARY THERAPIES. Persons with insomnia should avoid alcohol and caffeine products, which may disrupt the sleep-wake cycle. Eating a healthy diet rich in calcium, magnesium, and the B vitamins, or taking nutritional supplements, may also be beneficial in treating insomnia.

Prognosis

Insomnia can be successfully treated in most adults, although any underlying illness will require treatment in order to correct the related insomnia. Sleep apnea, one possible medical cause of insomnia, is a potentially serious disorder related to breathing difficulties and chronic lung conditions that can be fatal if not treated.

Untreated insomnia has potentially serious consequences, including an increased risk of motor vehicle accidents, impaired school or job performance, and a high rate of absenteeism from work. Though insomnia can be treated, patients who have had insomnia once are at an increased risk for recurrent insomnia.

Prevention

Prevention of insomnia centers around the promotion of a healthy lifestyle. A balance of rest, recreation, and **exercise** in combination with **stress management**, regular physical examinations, and a healthy diet can do much to reduce the risk. Walking is also recommended. However, exercise should be done at least three hours before bedtime, to avoid a stimulating effect. Exercise,

KEY TERMS

Mood disorder—A group of mental disorders involving a disturbance of mood, along with either a full or partial excessively happy (manic) or extremely sad (depressive) syndrome not caused by any other physical or mental disorder. Mood refers to a prolonged emotion.

Sleep apnea—A condition in which a person stops breathing while asleep. These periods can last up to a minute or more and can occur many times each hour. In order to start breathing again, the person must become semi-awake. The episodes are not remembered, but the following day the person feels tired and sleepy. If severe, sleep apnea can cause other medical problems.

Sleep disorder—Any condition that interferes with sleep.

relaxation, and **nutrition** should be considered ongoing preventive measures.

Resources

BOOKS

American Psychiatric Association. *Diagnostic and Statistical Manual of Mental Disorders*. 4th ed., text rev. Washington, DC: American Psychiatric Association, 2000.

Currie, Shawn R. "Sleep Dysfunction." *Clinicians's Handbook of Adult Behavioral Assessment*, edited by Michel Hersen. San Diego, CA: Elsevier Academic Press, 2006: 401–30.

Lee-Chiong, Teofilo L., ed. *Sleep: A Comprehensive Handbook*. New York: Wiley-Liss, 2006.

Mayo Clinic Book of Alternative Medicine. New York: Time Inc. Home Entertainment, 2007.

PERIODICALS

Irwin, Michael R., and Cole, Jason C. "Comparative Meta-Analysis of Behavioral Interventions for Insomnia and Their Efficacy in Middle-Aged Adults and in Older Adults 55+ Years of Age." *Health Psychology* 25, no. 1 (2006): 3–14.

Jansson, Markus, and Steven J. Linton. "The Role of Anxiety and Depression in the Development of Insomnia: Cross-Sectional and Prospective Analyses." *Psychology and Health* 21, no. 3 (2006): 383–97.

———. "Psychosocial Work Stressors in the Development and Maintenance of Insomnia: A Prospective Study." *Journal of Occupational Health Psychology* 11, no. 3 (2006): 241–48.

Lack, Leon, Helen Wright, Kristyn Kemp, and Samantha Gibb. "The Treatment of Early-Morning Awakening Insomnia with 2 Evenings of Bright Light." *SLEEP* 28, no. 5 (2005): 616–23.

Lande, R. G., and C. Gragnani. "Nonpharmacologic Approaches to the Management of Insomnia." *Journal of the American Osteopathic Association* 110, no. 12 (2010): 695–701.

Manber, Rachel, and Allison Harvey. "Historical Perspective and Future Directions in Cognitive Behavioral Therapy for Insomnia and Behavioral Sleep Medicine." *Clinical Psychology Review* 25, no. 5 (2005): 535–38.

Smith, Michael T., and Michael L. Perlis. "Who is a Candidate for Cognitive-Behavioral Therapy for Insomnia?" *Health Psychology* 25, no. 1 (2006): 15–19.

WEBSITES

American Psychiatric Association. "Insomnia." DSM5.org. http://www.dsm5.org/ProposedRevision/Pages/proposedrevision.aspx?rid=65 (accessed September 18, 2011).

Johns Hopkins Health Alert. "Q & As on Insomnia." John Hopkins Medicine. http://www.johnshopkinshealthalerts.com/alerts/depression_anxiety/JohnsHopkinsDepressionAnxietyHealthAlert_799-1.html (accessed November 2, 2011).

Johnston, Smith L., III. "Societal and Workplace Consequences of Insomnia, Sleepiness, and Fatigue." Medscape Education (September 29, 2005). http://www.medscape.org/viewarticle/513572_1 (accessed November 2, 2011).

Mayo Clinic staff. "Insomnia." MayoClinic.com. http://www.mayoclinic.com/health/insomnia/DS00187 (accessed November 2, 2011).

National Sleep Foundation. "Diet, Exercise, and Sleep." http://www.sleepfoundation.org/article/sleep-topics/diet-exercise-and-sleep (accessed November 2, 2011).

ORGANIZATIONS

American Academy of Sleep Medicine, 2510 N Frontage Rd., Darien, IL, 60561, (630) 737-9700, Fax: (630) 737-9790, inquiries@assmnet.org, http://www.aasmnet.org.

American Sleep Association, 614 South 8th St., Ste. 282, Philadelphia, PA, 19147, (443) 593-2285, sleep@1sleep.com, http://www.sleepassociation.org.

National Sleep Foundation, 1010 N. Glebe Rd., Suite 310, Arlington, VA, 22201, (703) 243-1697, http://www.sleepfoundation.org.

L. Lee Culvert
Laura Jean Cataldo, RN, EdD
Heidi Splete

Intake evaluation *see* **Psychological assessment and diagnosis**

Intellectual disability

Definition

Intellectual disability or intellectual developmental disorder (IDD), referred to as intellectual disability in the fourth edition of the ***Diagnostic and Statistical Manual***

Persons under age 18 receiving special education or early intervention services in the United States, by selected characteristics, 2010

Selected characteristic	Number of persons receiving special education or early intervention services	Percentage of total persons under age 18[†]
Total	**5,162,000**	**6.9%**
Gender		
Male	3,465,000	9.1%
Female	1,697,000	4.7%
Age		
Under 12 years	3,177,000	6.3%
12–17 years	1,985,000	8.2%
Race		
White	3,922,000	7.0%
Black or African American	862,000	7.8%
American Indian or Alaska Native	54,000	7.0%
Asian	105,000	3.1%
Native Hawaiian or other Pacific Islander	*19,000	*11.2%
Two or more races	200,000	7.0%

[†]Total number of persons under age 18 years = 74,625,000.
*Estimates preceded by an asterisk have a relative standard error of greater than 30% and less than or equal to 50% and should be used with caution, as they do not meet standards of reliability or precision.

SOURCE: National Center for Health Statistics, Centers for Disease Control and Prevention, "Summary Health Statistics for the U.S. Population: National Health Interview Survey, 2010," *Vital and Health Statistics* 10, no. 251 (December 2011).

(Table by PreMediaGlobal. © 2012 Cengage Learning.)

of Mental Disorders (*DSM-IV*), is a developmental disability that first appears in children under the age of 18. It is defined as a level of intellectual functioning (as measured by standard **intelligence tests**) that is well below average and results in significant limitations in daily living skills (adaptive functioning). The forthcoming edition of the *Diagnostic and Statistical Manual of Mental Disorders* (*DSM-5*, 2013) proposes to rename intellectual disability as intellectual developmental disorder (IDD) and define it as "a disorder that includes both a current intellectual deficit and a deficit in adaptive functioning with onset during the developmental period."

IDD is therefore not a mental illness in the usual sense but rather a disorder defined in order to identify groups of people who need social support and special educational services to carry out tasks of everyday living. On October 5, 2010, "Rosa's Law" went into effect in the United States. Named for a child with IDD living in Maryland, the law requires federal agencies to remove the terms mentally retarded or mental retardation from official documents and replace them with "individual with an intellectual disability" and "intellectual disability."

Demographics

The prevalence of intellectual disability in North America is a subject of heated debate. It is thought to be between 1% and 3% depending upon the population, methods of assessment, and criteria of assessment that are used. Many people believe that the actual prevalence is probably closer to 1%, and that the 3% figure is based on misleading mortality rates; cases that are diagnosed in early infancy; and the instability of the **diagnosis** across the age span. If the 1% figure is accepted, however, it means that about 3 million people with intellectual disability live in the United States. The three most common causes of intellectual disability, accounting for about 30% of cases, are **Down syndrome**, fragile X syndrome, and **fetal alcohol syndrome**. Males are more likely than females to have an intellectual disability in a 1.5:1 ratio, primarily because of the association with fragile X.

Description

Intellectual developmental disorder begins in childhood or adolescence before the age of 18. In most cases, it persists throughout adult life. A diagnosis of IDD is made if an individual has an intellectual functioning level well below average, as well as significant limitations in two or more adaptive skill areas. Intellectual functioning level is defined by standardized tests that measure the ability to reason in terms of mental age (intelligence quotient or IQ). Intellectual disability is generally defined as an IQ score below 70–75. Adaptive skills is a term that refers to skills needed for daily life. Such skills include the ability to produce and understand language (communication); practical skills needed for activities of daily living (ADLs); use of community resources; health, safety, leisure, self-care, and social skills; self-direction; functional academic skills (reading, writing, and arithmetic); and job-related skills.

In general, children with intellectual and developmental impairments reach such developmental milestones as walking and talking much later than children in the general population. Symptoms of intellectual disability may appear at birth or later in childhood. The child's age at onset depends on the suspected cause of the disability. Some people with a mild intellectual disability might not be diagnosed before entering preschool or kindergarten. These children typically have difficulties with social, communication, and functional academic skills. Children who have a neurological disorder or illness such as encephalitis or meningitis may suddenly show signs of cognitive impairment and adaptive difficulties.

DSM-IV categories

The level of impairment varies in severity. The *Diagnostic and Statistical Manual of Mental Disorders*, fourth edition, text revision (*DSM-IV-TR*), the diagnostic standard for mental health care professionals in the United States, classifies four different degrees of intellectual disability: mild, moderate, severe, and profound. These categories are based on the person's level of functioning. The reader should note, however, that *DSM-5* has proposed changes in the categories of severity of IDD. The *DSM-5* website states as of mid-2011 that "Recommendations for severity criteria for this disorder are forthcoming." The present *DSM-IV* categories of severity are as follows:

- Mild intellectual disability: Approximately 85% of people who fall into the *DSM-IV* categories of intellectual disability are in the mild category. Their IQ scores range from 50 to 70, and they can often learn academic skills up to about the sixth-grade level. They can become fairly self-sufficient and in some cases live independently with community and social support.
- Moderate intellectual disability: About 10% of people with intellectual disability are considered moderately disabled. People in this category have IQ scores ranging from 35 to 55. They can carry out work and self-care tasks with moderate supervision. They typically acquire communication skills in childhood and are able to live and function successfully within the community in such supervised environments as group homes.
- Severe intellectual disability: About 3–4% of people with intellectual disability are classified as severe. People in this category have IQ scores of 20 to 40. They may master very basic self-care skills and some communication skills. Many people with this level of impairment can live in a group home.
- Profound intellectual disability: Only 1–2% of people with intellectual disability are classified as profoundly disabled, meaning that they have IQ scores under 20 to 25. They may be able to develop basic self-care and communication skills with appropriate support and training. Their disability is often caused by an accompanying neurological disorder. People with profound intellectual disability need high levels of structure and supervision.

Reasons for changes in DSM-5

The primary reason given by the authors of *DSM-5* for changing the name of the disorder is greater consistency with international opinion and the position of the American Association on Intellectual and Developmental Disabilities (AAIDD). This organization, formerly known as the American Association on Mental Retardation, or AAMR, has developed a widely accepted diagnostic classification system for intellectual disability. In this system, intellectual disability is defined in terms of the environment and context in which the person functions. The AAIDD offers five assumptions that are necessary for defining the presence of an intellectual disability. First, a mental health practitioner must consider the limitations of functioning in a community environmental context, including the person's age group and culture. Second, cultural and linguistic differences and differences in behavioral, sensory, and other factors should be considered. Third, strengths should be given consideration along with weaknesses. Fourth, the purpose of identifying limitations is to determine what supports the person needs. The fifth assumption is that when the appropriate supports are available, the quality of life and functional ability of a person with an intellectual disability will improve. The AAIDD has pushed for changing the name of the disorder because of the **stigma** associated with the term mental retardation.

Other reasons for the proposed changes in *DSM-5* include the need to exclude inaccurate testing as a factor in evaluating persons for IDD; the use of factor analysis to provide greater accuracy in measuring a person's adaptive functioning; and the need for greater accuracy in measuring a person's overall level of functioning. The basic cutoff point (an IQ of 70 or below) will remain unchanged.

Causes and symptoms

Causes

The cause of IDD cannot be identified in about 40% of cases. The following sections discuss known biological and environmental factors that can cause IDD.

GENETIC FACTORS. Hereditary factors are the most common single cause of IDD and are involved in about 30% of cases. The disorder may be caused by an inherited genetic abnormality, such as fragile X syndrome. Fragile X, a defect in the X chromosome in which a repeated group of letters in the DNA sequence reaches a certain threshold number that results in impairment, is the most common inherited cause of IDD. Such single-gene disorders as phenylketonuria (PKU) and other inborn errors of metabolism may also cause IDD if they are not discovered and treated early, although testing of infants for PKU is required at birth, and problems associated with this disorder can be avoided through dietary measures. Abnormalities in chromosome number can also be the cause of IDD. The presence of an extra chromosome 18 (trisomy 18) or chromosome 21 (trisomy 21 or Down syndrome) will result in some level of intellectual disability. In addition, there may be only a partial extra chromosome as a result of accidents at the cellular level, which sometimes results in milder forms of IDD compared to complete trisomies.

PRENATAL AND PERINATAL ILLNESSES AND ISSUES. Fetal alcohol syndrome (FAS) affects one in 3,000 children in Western countries. It is caused when mothers drink heavily during the first twelve weeks (trimester) of pregnancy. Some studies have shown that even moderate **alcohol use** during pregnancy may cause learning disabilities in children. Drug abuse and cigarette smoking during pregnancy have also been linked to intellectual disability.

Maternal infections and such illnesses as glandular disorders, rubella, toxoplasmosis, and cytomegalovirus (CMV) infection can result in IDD in the child, among many other problems, if the developing fetus is exposed. When the mother has high blood pressure (hypertension) or develops toxemia (also called pregnancy-induced hypertension or preeclampsia) during pregnancy, the flow of oxygen to the fetus may in some cases be reduced, potentially resulting in **brain** damage and IDD.

Birth defects that cause physical deformities of the head, brain, and central nervous system frequently cause IDD. A neural tube defect, for example, is a birth defect in which the neural tube that forms the spinal cord does not close completely. This defect, which occurs with varying levels of severity, may cause children to develop an accumulation of cerebrospinal fluid inside the skull (hydrocephalus). The pressure on the brain resulting from hydrocephalus can lead to changes that cause learning impairment.

CHILDHOOD ILLNESSES AND INJURIES. Hyperthyroidism, whooping cough, chicken pox, measles, and Hib disease (a bacterial infection caused by *Haemophilus influenzae* type B) may cause intellectual disability if they are not treated adequately. An infection of the membrane covering the brain (meningitis) or an inflammation of the brain itself (encephalitis) can cause swelling that in turn may cause brain damage and IDD. **Traumatic brain injury** caused by a blow to the head or by violent shaking of the upper body (shaken baby syndrome) may also cause brain damage and IDD in children.

ENVIRONMENTAL FACTORS. Neglected infants who are not provided with the mental and physical stimulation required for normal development may suffer irreversible learning impairment. Children who live in poverty and/or suffer from malnutrition, unhealthy living conditions, abuse, and improper or inadequate medical care are at higher risk. Exposure to lead or mercury can also cause IDD. Many children have developed **lead poisoning** from eating the flaking lead-based paint often found in older buildings.

KEY TERMS

Activities of daily living (ADLs)—A general term for routine activities of self-care (e.g., brushing teeth, dressing oneself, bathing) and functioning independently (e.g., managing money, preparing meals, cleaning house)

Adaptive functioning—A term used to describe a person's having the intellectual, social, and practical skills needed to live independently.

Cytogenetics—The branch of genetics concerned with the structure and function of the individual cell, particularly its chromosome content.

Stigma—Any personal attribute that causes a person to be socially shamed, avoided, or discredited. Mental disorders are a common cause of stigma.

Symptoms

Low IQ scores and limitations in adaptive skills are the hallmarks of IDD, as is failure to reach normal developmental milestones. Aggression, self-injury, and mood disorders are sometimes associated with the disability. The severity of the symptoms and the age at which they first appear depend on the cause. Children with IDD reach developmental milestones significantly later than expected, if at all. If the disorder is caused by chromosomal or other genetic disorders, it is often apparent from infancy. If IDD is caused by childhood illnesses or injuries, learning and adaptive skills that were once easy may suddenly become difficult or impossible to master.

Diagnosis

Examination

If IDD is suspected, a comprehensive physical examination and medical history should be done immediately to discover any organic cause of symptoms. Such conditions as hyperthyroidism and PKU are treatable if discovered early enough when the progression of IDD can be stopped and, in some cases, partially reversed. If a neurological cause, such as brain injury or epilepsy, is suspected, the child may be referred to a neurologist or neuropsychologist for testing.

A complete medical, family, social, and educational history is compiled from existing medical and school records (if applicable) and from interviews with parents.

Tests

In many cases of mild IDD, the disorder is not identified until the child starts school. Schoolchildren are given intelligence tests to measure their learning abilities and intellectual functioning. Such tests include the Stanford-Binet Intelligence Scale, the **Wechsler Intelligence Scales**, the Wechsler Preschool and Primary Scale of Intelligence, and the **Kaufman Assessment Battery for Children**. For infants, the Bayley Scales of Infant Development may be used to assess motor, language, and problem-solving skills. Interviews with parents or other caregivers are used to assess the child's daily living, muscle control, communication, and social skills. The Woodcock-Johnson Scales of Independent Behavior and the Vineland Adaptive Behavior Scales (VABS) are frequently used to evaluate these skills.

Procedures

Recent advances in cytogenetics and microscopy have made the detection of chromosomal abnormalities after birth much more accurate. To investigate the possibility of a genetic disorder, the doctor will obtain a sample of cells from the child's blood or skin. The cells are cultured in the laboratory and prepared for examination under a microscope by one of several purification, preservation, and staining techniques. Analysis of the chromosomes in the cell must be done by a board-certified specialist in cytogenetics.

In addition, amniocentesis (often called amnio) can be performed on fetal cells found in the amniotic fluid in the early second trimester of pregnancy. A sample of the amniotic fluid that surrounds a fetus in the womb is collected through a pregnant woman's abdomen using a needle and syringe. Tests performed on fetal cells found in the amniotic fluid can reveal the presence of Down syndrome as well as many types of genetic disorders. Amniocentesis is recommended for women who will be older than 35 on their due date.

One alternative to amniocentesis now in general use is chorionic villus sampling (CVS), which can be performed as early as the eighth week of pregnancy. CVS can be riskier and is more expensive. The procedure involves the removal of a small piece of placenta tissue (chorionic villi) from the uterus during early pregnancy to screen the baby for genetic defects.

Treatment

Federal legislation entitles children with intellectual impairments and developmental disabilities to free testing and appropriate, individualized education and skills training within the school system from ages three to 21. For children under the age of three, many states have established early **intervention** programs that assess children, make recommendations, and begin treatment programs. Many day schools are available to help train children with developmental and intellectual impairments in skills such as bathing and feeding themselves. Extracurricular activities and social programs are also important in helping children and adolescents who have developmental and intellectual impairments gain self-esteem. Special interventions (usually some form of behavioral therapy) may be needed for children with IDD who have problems with aggression.

Training in independent living and job skills is often begun in late adolescence or early adulthood. The level of training depends on the degree of impairment. People with mild levels of functional and intellectual impairment can often learn the skills needed to live independently and hold outside jobs. People with a great level of impairment may require supervised community living in **group homes** or other residential settings.

Family therapy can help relatives of people with intellectual disabilities develop coping skills. It can also help parents deal with feelings of guilt or anger. A supportive and warm home environment is essential to help people with intellectual disabilities reach their full potential.

QUESTIONS TO ASK YOUR DOCTOR

- What options are available for treating intellectual disabilities?
- What tests would you recommend to diagnose the condition?
- What are the differences between intellectual disabilities and learning problems like dyslexia?
- Have you ever evaluated a child for an intellectual disability disorder?

Prognosis

People with mild to moderate intellectual disability are frequently able to achieve some self-sufficiency and to lead happy and fulfilling lives. To reach these goals, they need appropriate and consistent educational, community, social, family, and vocational supports. The outlook is less promising for those with severe to profound disability. Studies have shown that these people have a shortened life expectancy. The diseases that are usually associated with severe IDD may cause a shorter life span. People with Down syndrome will develop the brain changes that characterize **Alzheimer's disease** in later life and may develop the clinical symptoms of this disease as well. One additional complication in assessing the future health status and life expectancy of children with IDD is their unequal access to high-quality health care.

Prevention

Immunization against diseases such as measles and Hib prevents many of the illnesses that can cause IDD. In addition, all children should undergo routine developmental screening as part of their pediatric care. Screening is particularly critical for those children who may be neglected or undernourished or may live in disease-producing conditions. Newborn screening and immediate treatment for PKU and hyperthyroidism can usually catch these disorders early enough to prevent adverse intellectual and developmental effects.

Good prenatal care can also be preventive. Pregnant women should be educated about the risks of alcohol and drug consumption and the need to maintain good **nutrition** during pregnancy. Tests such as an ultrasonography can determine whether a fetus is developing normally.

Resources

BOOKS

American Psychiatric Association. *Diagnostic and Statistical Manual of Mental Disorders.* 4th ed., text rev. Washington, DC: American Psychiatric Press, 2000.

Burack, Jacob A., et al., eds. *The Oxford Handbook of Intellectual Disability and Development*, 2nd ed. New York: Oxford University Press, 2011.

Knight, Samantha J.L., ed. *Genetics of Mental Retardation: An Overview Encompassing Learning Disability and Intellectual Disability.* New York: Karger, 2010.

Schalock, Robert L., James F. Gardner, and Valerie J. Bradley. *Quality of Life for People with Intellectual and Other Developmental Disabilities: Applications across Individuals, Organizations, Communities, and Systems.* Washington, DC: American Association on Intellectual and Developmental Disabilities, 2007.

PERIODICALS

Brosnan, J., and O. Healy. "A Review of Behavioral Interventions for the Treatment of Aggression in Individuals with Developmental Disabilities." *Research in Developmental Disabilities* 32 (March-April 2011): 437–446.

Gray-Stanley, J.A., and N. Muramatsu. "Work Stress, Burnout, and Social and Personal Resources among Direct Care Workers." *Research in Developmental Disabilities* 32 (May-June 2011): 1065–1074.

McLaughlin, M. R. "Speech and Language Delay in Children." *American Family Physician* 83 (May 15, 2011): 1183–1188.

Prince, E., and H. Ring. "Causes of Learning Disability and Epilepsy: A Review." *Current Opinion in Neurology* 24 (April 2011): 154–158.

Schalock, R.L., et al. "Evidence-based Practices in the Field of Intellectual and Developmental Disabilities: An International Consensus Approach."*Evaluation and Program Planning* 34 (August 2011): 273–282.

Schieve, L.A., et al. "Risk for Cognitive Deficit in a Population-based Sample of U.S. Children with Autism Spectrum Disorders: Variation by Perinatal Health Factors." *Disability and Health Journal* 3 (July 2010): 202–212.

Shaffer, L.G., and B.A. Bejjani. "Development of New Postnatal Diagnostic Methods for Chromosome Disorders." *Seminars in Fetal and Neonatal Medicine* 16 (April 2011): 114–118.

Ward, R.L., et al. "Uncovering Health Care Inequalities among Adults with Intellectual and Developmental Disabilities." *Health and Social Work* 35 (November 2010): 280–290.

WEBSITES

American Association on Intellectual and Developmental Disabilities (AAIDD). "Definition of Intellectual Disability." http://www.aaidd.org/content_100.cfm?navID=21 (accessed May 18, 2011).

American Psychiatric Association. *DSM-5* Development. "A 00 Intellectual Developmental Disorder." http://www.dsm5.org/proposedrevision/pages/proposedrevision.aspx?rid=384# (accessed May 18, 2011).

Medscape. "Pediatric Mental Retardation." http://emedicine.medscape.com/article/289117-overview (accessed May 18, 2011).

National Dissemination Center for Children with Disabilities (NICHCY). NICHCY Disability Fact Sheet #8. "Intellectual Disability." http://nichcy.org/disability/specific/intellectual (accessed May 18, 2011).

ORGANIZATIONS

American Association on Intellectual and Developmental Disabilities (AAIDD), 501 3rd St., NW, Ste. 200, Washington, DC, United States 20001, (202) 387-1968, Fax: (202) 387-2193, (800) 424-3688, http://www.aaidd.org

The Arc, 1660 L St. NW, Ste. 301, Washington, DC, United States 20036, (202) 534-3700, Fax: (202) 534-3731, (800) 433-5255, info@thearc.org, http://www.thearc.org

National Dissemination Center for Children with Disabilities (NICHCY) (formerly National Information Center for Children and Youth and Disabilities), 1825 Connecticut Ave. NW, Ste. 700, Washington, DC, United States 20009, (202) 884-8200, Fax: (202) 884-8441, (800) 695-0285, nichcy@aed.org, http://nichcy.org

President's Committee for People with Intellectual Disabilities (AAIDD), Aerospace Center, Ste. 210, 370 L'Enfant Promenade SW, Washington, DC, United States 20447, (202) 619-0634, Fax: (202) 205-9519, (800) 424-3688, http://www.acf.hhs.gov/programs/pcpid.

Paula Anne Ford-Martin, M.S.
Emily Jane Willingham, Ph.D.
Rebecca J. Frey, Ph.D.

Intelligence tests

Definition

Intelligence tests are psychological tests that are designed to measure a variety mental functions, such as reasoning, comprehension, and judgment.

Purpose

The goal of intelligence tests is to obtain an idea of the person's intellectual potential. The tests center around a set of stimuli designed to yield a score based on the test maker's model of what makes up intelligence. Intelligence tests are often given as a part of a battery of tests.

Description

When taking an intelligence test, a person can expect to do a variety of tasks. These tasks may include having to answer questions that are asked verbally, doing mathematical problems, and doing a variety of tasks that require eye hand coordination. Some tasks may be timed and require the person to work as quickly as possible. Typically, most questions and tasks start out easy and progressively get more difficult. It is unusual for anyone to know the answer to all of the questions or be able to complete all of the tasks. If a person is unsure of an answer, guessing is usually allowed.

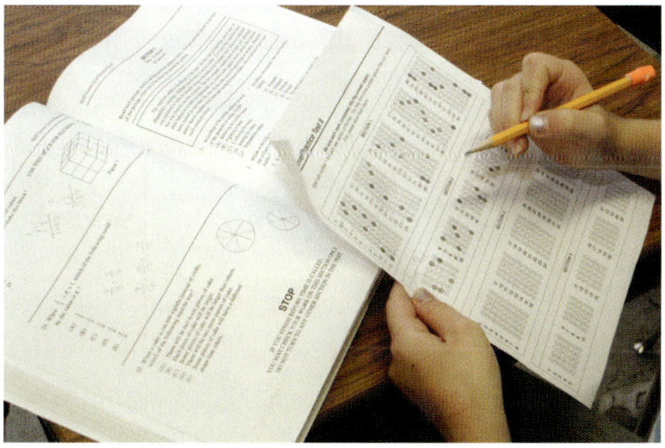

A student checks their work during an SSAT camp. *(© Jen Hulshizer/Star Ledger/Corbis)*

The four most commonly used intelligence tests are:

- Stanford-Binet Intelligence Scales
- Wechsler-Adult Intelligence Scale
- Wechsler Intelligence Scale for Children
- Wechsler Primary & Preschool Scale of Intelligence

In general, intelligence tests measure a wide variety of human behaviors better than any other measure that has been developed. They allow professionals to have a uniform way of comparing a person's performance with that of other people who are similar in age. These tests also provide information on cultural and biological differences among people.

Intelligence tests are excellent predictors of academic achievement and provide an outline of a person's mental strengths and weaknesses. Many times the scores have revealed talents in people that have led to an improvement in their educational opportunities. Teacher, parents, and psychologists are able to devise individual curriculum that matches a person's level of development and expectations.

Some researchers argue that intelligence tests have serious shortcomings. For example, many intelligence tests produce a single intelligence score. This single score is often inadequate in explaining the multidimensional aspects of intelligence. Another problem with a single score is the fact that individuals with similar intelligence test scores can vary greatly in their expression of these talents. It is important to know the person's performance on the various subtests that make up the overall intelligence test score. Knowing the performance on these various scales can influence the understanding of a person's abilities and how these abilities are expressed. For example, two people may have identical scores on intelligence tests, but one person may have obtained the score because of strong verbal skills while the other may have obtained the score because of strong skills in perceiving and organizing various tasks.

Furthermore, intelligence tests only measure a sample of behaviors or situations in which intelligent behavior is revealed. For instance, some intelligence tests do not measure a person's everyday functioning, social knowledge, mechanical skills, and/or creativity. Along with this, the formats of many intelligence tests do not capture the complexity and immediacy of real-life situations. Therefore, intelligence tests have been criticized for their limited ability to predict non-test or nonacademic intellectual abilities. Since intelligence test scores can be influenced by a variety of different experiences and behaviors, they should not be considered a perfect indicator of a person's intellectual potential.

Precautions

There are many different types of intelligence tests and they all do not measure the same abilities. Although the tests often have aspects that are related with each other, we should not expect that scores of one intelligence test measuring a single factor will be similar to scores on another intelligence test measuring a variety of factors. Also, when determining whether or not to use an intelligence test, a person should make sure that the test has been adequately developed and has solid research to show its reliability and validity. Additionally, psychometric testing requires a clinically trained examiner, therefore, the test should only be administered and interpreted by a trained professional.

A central criticism of intelligence tests is that psychologists and educators use these tests to distribute the limited resources of our society. These test results are used to provide rewards such as special classes for gifted students, admission to college, and employment. Those who do not qualify for these resources based on intelligence test scores may feel angry and denied opportunities for success. Unfortunately, intelligence test scores have not only become associated with a person's ability to perform certain tasks, but with self-worth.

Many people are under the false assumption that intelligence tests measure a person's inborn or biological intelligence. Intelligence tests are based on an individual's interaction with the environment and never exclusively measure inborn intelligence. Intelligence tests have been associated with categorizing and stereotyping people. Additionally, knowledge of one's performance on an intelligence test may affect a person's aspirations and motivation to obtain goals. Intelligence tests can be culturally biased against certain minority groups.

Results

The person's raw scores on an intelligence test are typically converted to standard scores. The standard scores allow the examiner to compare the individual's score to other people who have taken the test. Additionally, by converting raw scores to standard scores the examiner has uniform scores and can more easily compare an individual's performance on one test with the individual's performance on another test. Depending on the intelligence test that is used, a variety of scores can be obtained. Most intelligence tests generate an overall intelligence quotient or IQ. As previously noted, it is valuable to know how a person performs on the various tasks that make up the test. This can influence the interpretation of the test and what the IQ means. The average of score for most intelligence tests is 100.

Resources

BOOKS

Kaufman, Alan, S., and Elizabeth O. Lichtenberger. *Assessing Adolescent and Adult Intelligence*. 3rd ed. New York: Wiley, 2005.

Matarazzo, J. D. *Wechsler's Measurement and Appraisal of Adult Intelligence*. 5th ed. New York: Oxford University Press, 1972.

Sattler, Jerome M. "Issues Related to the Measurement and Change of Intelligence." In *Assessment of Children: Cognitive Applications*. 4th ed. San Diego: Jerome M. Sattler, Publisher, Inc., 2001.

Sattler, Jerome M., and Lisa Weyandt. "Specific Learning Disabilities." In *Assessment of Children: Behavioral and Clinical Applications,* by Jerome M. Sattler. 4th ed. San Diego: Jerome M. Sattler, Publisher, Inc., 2002.

Keith Beard, Psy.D.

Intermittent explosive disorder

Definition

Intermittent explosive disorder (IED) is characterized by impulsive acts of aggression, as contrasted with planned violent or aggressive acts. The aggressive episodes may take the form of spells or attacks, with symptoms beginning minutes to hours before the actual acting-out. Other names for IED include rage attacks, anger attacks, and episodic dyscontrol.

Demographics

IED is apparently more common than originally thought. Current research suggests that as many as 16 million Americans may suffer from this disorder. Most studies, however, indicate that it occurs more frequently in males. The most common age of onset is the period from late childhood through the early 20s. The onset of the disorder is frequently abrupt, with no warning period. Close to 82% of patients with IED are often diagnosed with at least one other disorder—particularly **personality disorders**, substance-abuse (especially alcohol abuse) disorders, and neurological disorders.

Description

Intermittent explosive disorder was originally described by the eminent French **psychiatrist** Esquirol as a "partial insanity" related to senseless impulsive acts. Esquirol termed this disorder *monomanies* *instinctives*, or *instinctual monomanias*. These apparently unmotivated acts were thought to result from instinctual or involuntary impulses, or from impulses related to ideological obsessions.

People with intermittent explosive disorder have a problem with controlling their temper. In addition, their violent behavior is out of proportion to the incident or event that triggered the outburst. Impulsive acts of aggression, however, are not unique to intermittent explosive disorder. Impulsive aggression can be present in many psychological and nonpsychological disorders. The diagnosis of intermittent explosive disorder (IED) is essentially a diagnosis of exclusion, meaning that it is given only after other disorders have been ruled out as causes of impulsive aggression.

Patients diagnosed with IED usually feel a sense of arousal or tension before an outburst, and relief of tension after the aggressive act. Patients with IED believe that their aggressive behaviors are justified; however, they feel genuinely upset, regretful, remorseful, bewildered or embarrassed by their impulsive and aggressive behavior.

IED is often grouped with **impulse control disorders**. Recent research, however, suggests an association with **bipolar disorder**, although the exact nature of this association is unclear. Some studies have suggested that some children who have IED are mistakenly diagnosed with bipolar disorder; other studies suggest that IED and Bipolar disorder may lie along the same continuum, may represent different stops along a common trajectory, or may be common comorbid conditions.

Causes and symptoms

Causes

Recent findings suggest that IED may result from abnormalities in the areas of the **brain** that regulate behavioral arousal and inhibition. Research indicates that impulsive aggression is related to abnormal brain mechanisms in a system that inhibits motor (muscular movement) activity, called the *serotoninergic system*. This system is directed by a neurotransmitter called *serotonin* that regulates behavioral inhibition (control of behavior). Some studies have correlated IED with abnormalities on both sides of the front portion of the brain. These localized areas in the front of the brain appear to be involved in information processing and controlling movement, both of which are unbalanced in persons diagnosed with IED. Studies using **positron emission tomography (PET)** scanning have found lower levels of brain glucose (sugar) metabolism in patients who act in impulsively aggressive ways.

Another study based on data from electroencephalograms (EEGs) of 326 children and adolescents treated in a psychiatric clinic found that 46% of the youths who manifested explosive behavior had unusual high-amplitude brain wave forms. The researchers concluded that a significant subgroup of people with IED may be predisposed to explosive behavior by an inborn characteristic of their central nervous system. In sum, there is a substantial amount of convincing evidence that IED has biological causes, at least in some people diagnosed with the disorder.

Other clinicians attribute IED to cognitive distortions. According to cognitive therapists, persons with IED have a set of strongly negative beliefs about other people, often resulting from harsh punishments inflicted by the parents. The child grows up believing that others "have it in for him" and that violence is the best way to restore damaged self-esteem. He or she may also have observed one or both parents, older siblings, or other relatives acting out in explosively violent ways. In short, people who develop IED have learned, usually in their family of origin, to believe that certain acts or attitudes on the part of other people justify aggressive attacks on them.

Although gender roles are not a cause of IED to the same extent as biological and familial factors, some researchers regard them as helping to explain why most people diagnosed with IED are males. According to this theory, men have greater permission from society to act violently and impulsively than women do. They therefore have less reason to control their aggressive impulses. Women who act explosively, on the other hand, would be considered unfeminine as well as unfriendly or dangerous.

Symptoms

IED is characterized by violent behaviors that are impulsive as well as assaultive. One example involved a man who felt insulted by another customer in a neighborhood bar during a conversation that had lasted for several minutes. Instead of finding out whether the other customer intended his remark to be insulting, or answering the insult verbally, the man impulsively punched the other customer in the mouth. Within a few minutes, however, he felt ashamed of his violent act. As this example indicates, the urge to commit the impulsive aggressive act may occur from minutes to hours before acting out and is characterized by the buildup of tension. After the outburst, the IED patient experiences a sense of relief from the tension. While many patients with IED blame someone else for causing their violent outbursts, they also express remorse and guilt for their actions.

Diagnosis

As mentioned, IED is essentially a diagnosis of exclusion. Patients who are eventually diagnosed with IED may come to the attention of a psychiatrist or other mental health professional by several different routes. Some patients with IED, often adult males who have assaulted their wives and are trying to save their marriages, are aware that their outbursts are not normal and seek treatment to control them. Younger males with IED are more likely to be referred for diagnosis and treatment by school authorities or the juvenile justice system, or brought to the doctor by concerned parents.

A psychiatrist who is evaluating a patient for IED would first take a complete medical and psychiatric history. Depending on the contents of the patient's history, the doctor would give the patient a physical examination to rule out head **trauma**, epilepsy, and other general medical conditions that may cause violent behavior. If the patient appears to be intoxicated by a drug of abuse, or suffering symptoms of withdrawal, the doctor may order a toxicology screen of the patient's blood or urine. Specific substances that are known to be associated with violent outbursts include phencyclidine (PCP or angel dust), alcohol, and **cocaine**. The doctor will also give the patient a **mental status examination** and a test to screen for neurological damage. If necessary, a neurologist may be consulted, and **imaging studies** performed of the patient's brain.

If the physical findings and laboratory test results are normal, the doctor may evaluate the patient for personality disorders, usually by administering diagnostic questionnaires. The patient may be given a diagnosis of antisocial or **borderline personality disorder** in addition to a diagnosis of IED.

In some cases, the doctor may need to rule out **malingering**, particularly if the patient has been referred for evaluation by a court order and is trying to evade legal responsibility for his behavior.

Treatment

Some adult patients with IED appear to benefit from cognitive therapy. A team of researchers at the University of Pennsylvania found that cognitive approaches that challenged the patients' negative views of the world and of other people were effective in reducing the intensity as well as the frequency of violent episodes. With regard to gender roles, many of the men reported that they were helped by rethinking manliness in terms of self-control rather than as something to be proved by hitting someone else or damaging property.

Several medications have been used for treating IED. These include **carbamazepine** (Tegretol), an anti-seizure medication; **propranolol** (Inderal), a heart medication that controls blood pressure and irregular heart rhythms; and lithium, a drug used to treat bipolar type II manic-depressive disorder. The success of treatment with lithium and other mood-stabilizing medications is consistent with findings that patients with IED have a high lifetime rate of bipolar disorder.

Prognosis

Little research has been done on patients with IED, although one study did find that such patients have a high lifetime rate of comorbid (co-occurring) bipolar disorder. In some persons IED decreases in severity or resolves completely as the person grows older. In others, the disorder appears to be chronic.

Prevention

As of 2011, preventive strategies included educating young people in parenting skills and teaching children skills related to self-control. Self-control can be practiced like many other skills, and people can improve their present level of self-control with appropriate coaching and practice.

Resources

BOOKS

American Psychiatric Association. *Diagnostic and Statistical Manual of Mental Disorders*. 4th ed., text rev. Washington, DC: American Psychiatric Association, 2000.

Dombrowski, Stefan, Karen L. Gischlar, and Martin Mrazik. *Assessing and Treating Low Incidence/High Severity Psychological Disorders of Childhood*. New York: Springer, 2011.

Grant, Jon E. *Impulse Control Disorders: A Clinician's Guide to Understanding and Treating Behavioral Addictions*. New York: W. W. Norton & Company, 2008.

Stern, Theodore A., Jerrold F. Rosenbaum, Maurizio Fava, Joseph Biederman, and Scott L. Rauch. *Massachusetts General Hospital Comprehensive Clinical Psychiatry*. Philadelphia: Mosby Elsevier, 2008.

PERIODICALS

Ahmed, A. "Latent Structure of Intermittent Explosive Disorder in an Epidemiological Sample." *Journal of Psychiatric Research* 44, no. 10 (2010): 663–72.

Coccaro, E.F. "A Family History Study of Intermittent Explosive Disorder." *Journal of Psychiatric Research* 44, no. 15 (2010): 1101–15.

———. "Intermittent Explosive Disorder: Development of Integrated Research Criteria for Diagnostic and Statistical Manual of Mental Disorders, Fifth Edition." *Comprehensive Psychiatry* 52, no. 2 (2011): 119–25.

WEBSITES

Harvard Medical School. "Treating Intermittent Explosive Disorder." *Harvard Mental Health Letter* (April 2011). http://www.health.harvard.edu/newsletters/Harvard_Mental_Health_Letter/2011/April/treating-intermittent-explosive-disorder (accessed September 7, 2011).

Laith Farid Gulli, M.D.
Bilal Nasser, M.D.

Internet addiction disorder

Definition

Internet **addiction** disorder (IAD) refers to the problematic use of the Internet, including the various aspects of its technology, such as electronic mail (email) and the World Wide Web. It is also known as problematic computer use, pathological computer use, and Internet overuse. The reader should note that Internet addiction disorder is not listed in the mental health professional's handbook, the ***Diagnostic and Statistical Manual of Mental Disorders***, fourth edition, text revision (2000), also called the *DSM*, possibly because the name of the disorder was originally proposed as a satirical spoof by a New York City **psychiatrist** in 1995. Internet addiction has, however, been formally recognized as a disorder by the **American Psychological Association**.

Although some psychiatrists have recommended adding diagnostic criteria for IAD to the forthcoming edition of the *DSM*, known as *DSM-5*, the disorder was not listed among the proposed additions to the manual in mid-2011. Much of the debate focuses on whether IAD is a distinctive disorder or whether it is simply an instance of a new technology being used to support other addictions. For example, there are gambling casinos on the Internet that could reinforce a person's pre-existing gambling addiction. Similarly, someone addicted to shopping could transfer their addiction from the local mall to online stores or such auction sites as eBay. Persons addicted to certain forms of sexual behavior can visit pornography sites on the Internet or use chat rooms as a way to meet others who might be willing to participate in those forms of behavior. The consensus seems to be that most, if not all, persons with IAD fall into established diagnostic categories.

Demographics

In the past, people reported to have an Internet addiction disorder were stereotyped as young, introverted, socially awkward, computer-oriented males. While this stereotype may have been true in the past, the availability of computers and the increased ease of access to the Internet are quickly challenging this notion. As a result, problematic Internet use can be found worldwide in any age group, social class, racial or ethnic group, level of education and income, and gender. One researcher in the Boston area estimates that between 6% and 10% of people who surf the Web suffer from some type of Internet dependency; and the American Academy of Pediatrics (AAP) estimates that between 8% and 12% of American children and adolescents have IAD. One reason for ongoing debate about the demographics of IAD, however, is that the disorder appears to have subtypes (described more fully in the next section) with different subpopulations.

Description

In some respects, addictive use of the Internet resembles other so-called process addictions, in which a person is addicted to an activity or behavior (including gambling, shopping, or certain sexual behaviors) rather than a substance (mood-altering drugs, tobacco, food, etc.). People who develop problems with their Internet use may start off using the Internet on a casual basis and then progress to using the technology in dysfunctional ways.

Some researchers maintain that there are several distinctive types of IAD rather than a single disorder:

- Online gaming. There are reported instances of people falling dead from exhaustion after several days of uninterrupted Internet gaming, although no one knows for certain how often such extreme cases arise.
- Internet pornography. This is a large subgroup; over 60% of people seeking treatment for IAD claim they are involved with online sexual activities that they consider inappropriate. People in this subgroup are more likely than others with IAD to have a substance abuse disorder.
- Online shopping. Most researchers consider online shopping addiction to be an extension of compulsive shopping in brick-and-mortar stores rather than a distinctive disorder, although some consider addiction to online auction sites like eBay to be a separate subtype.
- Email and texting.
- Social media. Social media is a general term for both Web-based and mobile technologies that facilitate

social (rather than business or academic) interaction online. It was estimated that as of 2011, about 22% of all online use in the United States involved social networking sites.

- Blogging. Blogging is a word derived from "weblog," a personal website maintained by an individual or group, with regular additions of commentary, descriptions of events, or personal videos. Most blogs are set up to allow comments from readers, which make a form of social media in many cases.

Many people believe that spending large amounts of time on the Internet is a core feature of the disorder. The amount of time by itself, however, is not as important a factor as the ways in which the person's Internet use is interfering with their daily functioning. Use of the Internet may interfere with social life, school work, or job-related tasks at work. In addition, cases have been reported of persons entering Internet chat rooms for people with serious illnesses or disorders, and pretending to be a patient with that disorder in order to get attention or sympathy. Treatment options often mirror those for other addictions. Although only a limited amount of research has been done on this disorder, the treatments that have been used appear to be effective.

One newer concern about IAD is the growing use of portable or handheld devices that can access the Internet, such as tablet PCs, smartphones, and other devices connected to the Internet via wireless networks. In 2008, mobile access to the Internet exceeded desktop computer-based access for the first time, and the popularity of mobile devices continues to rise. While these devices have much to offer users who need Web access in situations where a desktop computer is unavailable, they also allow others to spend excessive time on the Internet outside their houses or offices.

Risk factors

The most commonly identified risk factors for IAD include age between 12 and 25; pre-existing mood disorders; **diagnosis** of **attention deficit hyperactivity disorder (ADHD)** or **obsessive-compulsive disorder** (OCD); a history of **process addiction**; and a history of drug or alcohol abuse.

Gender is a risk factor for some forms of IAD. Most online gaming and pornography addicts are males, while women are at slightly greater risk for online shopping addiction. There is some evidence that male online shopping addicts are often unrecognized, because they tend to purchase different types of items (e.g., hardware, automotive equipment, and electronic devices or gadgets) from those favored by women (e.g., clothing, jewelry, and cosmetics).

Causes and symptoms

Causes

No one knows what causes a person to be addicted to the Internet, but there are several factors that have been proposed as contributing to Internet addiction. One theory concerns the mood-altering potential of behaviors related to process addictions. Just as a person addicted to shopping may feel a "rush" or pleasurable change in mood from the series of actions related to a spending spree-checking one's credit cards, driving to the mall, going into one's favorite store, etc.-the person with an Internet addiction may feel a similar rush from booting up their computer and going to their favorite websites. In other words, some researchers think that there are chemical changes that occur in the body when someone is engaging in an addictive behavior. Furthermore, from a biological standpoint, there may be a combination of genes that make a person more susceptible to addictive behaviors, just as researchers have located genes that affect a person's susceptibility to alcohol.

In addition to having features of a process addiction, Internet use might be reinforced by pleasurable thoughts and feelings that occur while the person is using the Internet. Although researchers in the field of addiction studies question the concept of an addictive personality as such, it is possible that someone who has one addiction may be prone to become addicted to other substances or activities, including Internet use. People with such other mental disorders or symptoms as **depression**, feelings of isolation, **stress**, or anxiety, may self-medicate by using the Internet in the same way that some people use alcohol or drugs of abuse to self-medicate the symptoms of their mental disorder. Still another theory is that Internet overuse is akin to dissociation in that it allows a person to compartmentalize difficulties in their present life and escape from reality into an online virtual world.

From a social or interpersonal standpoint, there may be familial factors prompting use of the Internet. For example, a person might "surf the Web" to escape family conflict. Another possibility is that social or peer dynamics might prompt excessive Internet use. Some affected persons may lack the social skills that would enable them to meet people in person rather than online. Peer behavior might also encourage Internet use if all of one's friends are using it. **Modeling** may play a role-users can witness and experience how others engage in Internet use and then replicate that behavior. The interactive aspects of the Internet, such as chat rooms, email, and interactive games like Multi-User Dungeons and Dragons (MUDS), seem to be more likely to lead to Internet addiction than purely solitary web surfing.

Symptoms

The most noticeable symptom of Internet addiction is excessive time devoted to Internet use. A person might have difficulty cutting down on his or her online time even when they are threatened with poor grades or loss of a job. There have been cases reported of college students failing courses because they would not take time off from Internet use to attend classes. Other symptoms of addiction may include lack of sleep; **fatigue**; declining grades or poor job performance; **apathy**; and racing thoughts. There may also be a decreased investment in social relationships and activities. A person may lie about how much time was spent online or deny that they have a problem. They may be irritable when offline or angry toward anyone who questions their time on the Internet.

Some pediatricians attribute an increase in depression among adolescents to the widespread popularity of social media. The term Facebook depression has been coined to describe the low self-esteem and mood disorders among some vulnerable adolescents induced by spending hours on Facebook and similar social networking sites. The researchers attribute Facebook depression to the way in which the medium facilitates constant comparisons of the self to other, presumably more popular, peers, and the common practice of posting negative or sarcastic comments on someone else's Facebook page.

Diagnosis

As previously noted, Internet addiction disorder has not yet been added as an official diagnosis to the *DSM*. The following, however, is a set of criteria for Internet addiction that has been proposed by addiction researchers. The criteria are based on the diagnostic standards for pathological gambling.

The patient must meet all of the following criteria:

- Preoccupation with the Internet (thinks about previous online activity or is anticipating the next online session)
- The need to spend longer and longer periods of time online in order to feel satisfied
- Unsuccessful efforts to control, cut back, or stop Internet use.
- Restlessness, moodiness, depression, or irritability when attempting to cut down or stop Internet use.
- Repeatedly staying online longer than originally intended.

The person must meet at least one of the following criteria:

- Jeopardized or risked the loss of a significant relationship, job, educational or career opportunity because of Internet use.
- Lied to family members, a therapist, or others to conceal the extent of involvement with the Internet.
- Uses the Internet as a way of escaping from problems or of relieving an unpleasant mood (such as feelings of helplessness, guilt, anxiety, or depression).

Examination

There are no physical symptoms unique to IAD that can be detected during a standard physical examination.

Tests

There are no laboratory or imaging tests that can detect IAD. A set of self-tests for such specific problems as online pornography, online gaming, online auction addiction, online gambling, and general Internet addiction are available at http://www.netaddiction.com/

KEY TERMS

Blogging—Creating and maintaining an online personal website, in most cases allowing readers to add comments. The term comes from the word weblog, or online diary.

Dissociation—A condition in which a person's thoughts, emotions, sensations, or memories become compartmentalized, usually as a result of a severe emotional trauma.

Facebook depression—A term used to describe an adolescent mood disorder associated with low self-esteem and depressed mood triggered by excessive concern with online social media.

Process addiction—A term used to describe addiction to an activity or behavior rather than a mood-altering chemical. It is also known as behavioral addiction or non-substance-related addiction.

Social media—A general term for both Web-based and mobile technologies that facilitate social (as distinct from commercial or academic) interaction online.

index.php?option=com_content&view=article&id=64&Itemid=88.

Two psychological inventories administered by mental health professionals, the Internet Addiction Test (IAT) and the Internet-Related Problem Scale (IRPS) were still undergoing clinical evaluation as of 2011.

Treatment

Traditional

Since Internet addiction disorder is a relatively new phenomenon, there is little research on the effectiveness of treatment procedures. It may be unrealistic to have a person completely end all Internet use. As our society becomes more and more dependent on computers for business transactions, educational programs, entertainment, and access to information as well as interpersonal communication, it will be difficult for a computer-literate person to avoid using the Internet. Learning how to use the Internet in moderation is often the main objective in therapy, in a way analogous to the way that people with eating disorders need to come to terms with food. Many of the procedures that have been used to treat Internet addiction have been modeled after other addiction treatment programs and **support groups**, particularly twelve-step groups.

Psychological interventions may include such approaches as changing the environment to alter associations that have been made with Internet use, or decrease the **reinforcement** received from excessive Internet use. Psychological interventions such as **cognitive-behavioral therapy** may also help the person identify thoughts and feelings that trigger their use of the Internet. Interpersonal interventions may include such approaches as **social skills training** or coaching in communication skills. Family and couple therapy may be indicated if the user is turning to the Internet to escape from problems in these areas of life. There is also a residential treatment program called ReSTART, which opened in the Pacific Northwest in 2009. The on-site program lasts 45 days and includes intensive individualized assessment as well as individual and **group therapy**.

Relapsing into an addictive behavior is common for anyone dealing with addiction disorders. Recognizing and preparing for **relapse** is often a part of the treatment process. Identifying situations that would trigger excessive Internet use and generating ways to deal with these situations can greatly reduce the possibility of total relapse. One option that works for some people is the installation of individualized content-control software on their computer; the software can be customized to block access to the types of websites that are most problematic for that person.

> **QUESTIONS TO ASK YOUR DOCTOR**
>
> - How can I tell whether I am becoming addicted to Internet use?
> - How can I tell whether another family member or friend has IAD?
> - Do you consider IAD a distinctive disorder or simply a technological variant of other disorders?
> - What treatment would you recommend for someone concerned about excessive Internet use?
> - What is your opinion of content-control software as a form of self-treatment?

Drugs

If a person's Internet addiction disorder has a biological dimension, then medication such as an antidepressant or antianxiety drug may help him or her with these aspects of the addiction. There were no medications as of 2011 that specifically targeted IAD. One clinical trial completed in 2008 of **escitalopram** (Lexapro), an SSRI antidepressant, as a treatment for IAD found no difference between subjects who took the drug and those given a placebo. There were no new **clinical trials** for treatments for IAD as of 2011.

Prognosis

Although extensive studies have not yet been done, treatment appears to be effective in maintaining and changing the behavior of people drawn to excessive use of the Internet. If the disorder is left untreated, the person may experience an increased amount of conflict in his or her relationships. Excessive Internet use may jeopardize a person's employment or academic standing. In addition, such physical problems as fatigue, carpal tunnel syndrome, back pain, and eyestrain may develop.

Prevention

If a person knows that he or she has difficulty with other forms of addictive behavior, they should be cautious in exploring the types of applications that are used on the Internet. In addition, it is important for people to engage in social activities outside the Internet. One recommendation for parents of adolescents is to teach them about the proper uses and limitations of Facebook and other social networking sites as well as showing them how to make friends in everyday life. Finally, mental health workers should investigate ways to participate in the implementation of new technology rather than waiting for its aftereffects.

Resources

BOOKS

McQuade, Samuel C., et al., eds. *Internet Addiction and Online Gaming*. New York: Chelsea House, 2011.

Price, Hannah O., ed. *Internet Addiction*. Hauppauge, NY: Nova Science Publishers, 2010.

Young, Kimberley, and Cristiano Nabuco de Abreu, eds. *Internet Addiction: A Handbook and Guide to Evaluation and Treatment*. Hoboken, NJ: John Wiley and Sons, 2010.

PERIODICALS

Bernardi, S., and S. Pallanti. "Internet Addiction: A Descriptive Clinical Study Focusing on Comorbidities and Dissociative Symptoms." *Comprehensive Psychiatry* 50 (November-December 2009): 510-516.

Dell'Osso, B., et al. "Escitalopram in the Treatment of Impulsive-compulsive Internet Usage Disorder: An Open-label Trial Followed by a Double-blind Discontinuation Phase." *Journal of Clinical Psychiatry* 69 (March 2008): 452–456.

Dong, G., et al. "Precursor or Sequela: Pathological Disorders in People with Internet Addiction Disorder." *PLoS One* 6 (February 16, 2011): e14703.

Gentile, D.A., et al. "Pathological Video Game Use among Youths: A Two-year Longitudinal Study." *Pediatrics* 127 (February 2011): e319–e329.

Stieger, S., and C. Burger. "Implicit and Explicit Self-esteem in the Context of Internet Addiction." *Cyberpsychology, Behavior and Social Networking* 13 (December 2010): 681–688.

Waldron, Heather. "Internet Addiction a Real Problem for U.S. Kids." *AAP News* 31 (May 2010): 26,

Widyanto, L., et al. "A Psychometric Comparison of the Internet Addiction Test, the Internet-Related Problem Scale, and Self-diagnosis." *Cyberpsychology, Behavior and Social Networking* 14 (March 2011): 141–149.

WEBSITES

Laurance, Jeremy. "Addicted! Scientists Show How Internet Dependency Alters the Human Brain." *The Independent UK*, January 12, 2012. http://www.independent.co.uk/news/science/addicted-scientists-show-how-internet-dependency-alters-the-human-brain-6288344.html (accessed January 12, 2012).

MSNBC.com. "Docs Warn about Teens and 'Facebook Depression.'" http://www.msnbc.msn.com/id/42298789/ns/health-mental_health (accessed May 10, 2011).

ReSTART. "Behavioral Addictions FAQs." http://www.netaddictionrecovery.com/the-problem/behavioral-addiction-faq.html (accessed May 10, 2011).

ORGANIZATIONS

American Academy of Pediatrics (AAP), 141 Northwest Point Boulevard, Elk Grove Village, IL, United States 60007-1098, (847) 434-4000, Fax: (847) 434-8000, http://www.aap.org/default.htm

American Psychiatric Association, 1000 Wilson Boulevard, Suite 1825, Arlington, VA, United States 22209-3901, (703) 907-7300, apa@psych.org http://www.psych.org

Center for Online Addiction, PO Box 72, Bradford, PA, United States 16701, (814) 451-2405, Fax: (814) 368-9560, http://www.netaddiction.com

ReSTART, 1001 290th Ave. SE, Fall City, WA, United States 98024-7403, (425) 417-1715, (800) 682-6934, restart@netaddictionrecovery.com, http://www.netaddictionrecovery.com

Keith Beard, Psy.D.
Rebecca J. Frey, Ph.D.

Internet-based therapy

Definition

Internet-based therapy is a form of **psychotherapy** conducted over the Internet rather than in face-to-face sessions. Therapeutic sessions may be conducted using instant messaging, chat rooms, or email messages. Internet-based therapy is also called online therapy or e-therapy.

Internet-based therapy is sometimes classified together with telephone therapy and videoconferencing as remote therapy, as all three forms depend on remote communication technologies. A number of online therapy providers, in fact, offer telephone-based therapy as well as email and online live chat therapy.

Purpose

The purpose of Internet-based therapy is to provide psychological help to persons who either cannot get to a physical office for reasons of disability, geographical isolation, or reluctance to be seen visiting a therapist, or who simply prefer electronic to face-to-face communication.

Description

Online therapy can take several different forms, depending on whether the client chooses live online chat/telephone, webcam, or email sessions. One common practice of online therapists is to ask potential clients to complete an online form in which the client provides basic personal information and a description of their problem or reason for seeking counseling. With e-mail sessions, the client fills out the online pre-session form and sends it by a special secure email service, and the therapist replies within one or two business days. Live online chat can begin as soon as the client fills out the pre-session form. For telephone counseling, the client provides the remote therapist with a telephone number and time to call, and the therapist will call at the scheduled time.

Clients are expected to pay in advance, usually via credit card or PayPal. Some online therapists stipulate that all prepaid sessions must be used within six months of purchase.

Online therapy is recommended only for non-emergency mental health services; most online therapy websites state that their services are not appropriate for persons who are suicidal, suffering from **psychosis**, or having an acute psychiatric crisis. In addition, most will not accept patients under age 18.

Benefits

As the Information Age progresses, more and more services are becoming available over the Internet. We can buy not only books online but also electronics, clothes, and even groceries. In the business world, the requirement and expense of traveling to in-person meetings are often negated by the ability to teleconference. College degrees no longer need to be earned in the classroom but can be acquired in the comfort of one's own home at one's own pace. The wait for a technician on a manufacturer's help line is often replaced by the ability to search the company's database on one's own or to engage in online chat with the same technician to whom one once spoke. Even for medical problems, one can often chat with a physician or nurse practitioner by email rather than going to the office; this service is known as telemedicine.

There is little wonder, therefore, that there is a demand for psychological services over the Internet. Chatting with one's therapist online is more private than going to an office and waiting in an open waiting room. For those in rural areas where access to a therapist is exceedingly difficult, the Internet can provide a convenient alternative for getting the help that one needs.

There are pros and cons to both sides of the issue of online versus face-to-face therapy. First, communicating through email, online chat, or instant messages has the same drawbacks of any written-only communication: Such nonverbal cues as tone of voice, facial expression, and body language are missing, making interpretation of the message more problematic than in a face-to-face situation. On the other hand, the relative anonymity of online interactions make such therapeutic relationships more attractive to those who would hesitate to go into a therapist's office for fear of being found out by others, fear of embarrassment, or unwillingness or inability to get to the office. In addition, online therapy tends to be less expensive than in-office therapy, a consideration for many clients.

There are, of course, some things that cannot be done over the Internet. For example, psychologists and psychiatrists use a variety of tools and techniques to diagnose mental disorders so that they can prescribe the appropriate course of treatment. Some of the tools used in **diagnosis** include such psychometric instruments as the **Minnesota Multiphasic Personality Inventory** (MMPI), such projective instruments as the Rorschach test or the **Thematic Apperception Test** (TAT), and diagnostic interviews. The various tests and instruments used in diagnosis should ethically be given only by a credentialed professional in a controlled situation and cannot be given across the Internet where there is no control over who will see the test; how long the client takes to answer the questions; or even whether it was the client or someone else who took the test. In addition, it would be extremely difficult to diagnose a patient's problem without a face-to-face meeting for a diagnostic interview.

Research into the effectiveness of online therapy is only beginning. However, a number of disorders have been successfully treated electronically. For example, Internet-based therapy has been successful in the treatment of **panic disorder**, **social phobia**, child adjustment after **traumatic brain injury**, and complicated **grief**, among others. It is also recommended for treatment of **agoraphobia**, an anxiety disorder in which people are afraid of wide-open spaces, uncontrolled social situations, and crowds; many are unable to leave their homes without suffering a **panic attack**.

KEY TERMS

Agoraphobia—An anxiety disorder characterized by fear of crowds, open spaces, and/or locations or situations that trigger panic attacks.

Remote therapy—A general term for therapy delivered by electronic communication technologies; it includes Internet-based therapy along with telephone therapy and videoconferencing.

Precautions

As with any service provided over the Internet, one must be an informed consumer not only before choosing an e-therapist, but even before deciding to use Internet-based therapy itself. Because Internet-based therapy is an emerging field, there are still many issues to be resolved. Obviously, one must check the professional credentials of a therapist to make sure that he or she is licensed and must determine whether one is choosing a therapist for online or in-office therapy. In addition, it is unclear at this time whether it is legal for a therapist licensed in one state to treat a patient in another state. Choosing a therapist in one's own state makes this issue irrelevant but requires research.

Client/therapist confidentiality is important in any therapeutic relationship. When choosing an online provider of psychological services, one must be certain not only that the therapist subscribes to a professional code of ethics but also that any information, including personal data about the client, is kept confidential and not sold to, or shared with, third parties. Similarly, it is important to check that the website used in online therapy is secure and that conversations, instant messages, and email transmissions between client and therapist are not recorded on the site's secured host computer.

A statement of ethical principles for conducting online therapy is available on the website of the International Society for Mental Health Online (ISMHO). These principles were officially adopted in 2000. It is important to remember that anything sent over the Internet may be subject to being unlawfully sought out by others and that there is an inherent risk to such communication even on secured servers.

Preparation

As noted above, preparation for online counseling requires the client to complete an online form with contact information and a description of the reason for seeking counseling. The client is also asked to choose the preferred method of contact with the therapist (telephone, email, online chat, or webcam) and to pay in advance for one or more sessions. Preparation should also include researching the therapist's company and/or credentials before making contact.

Risks

Potential risks include technical difficulties with Internet or telephone communication and breaches of security by hackers.

QUESTIONS TO ASK YOUR DOCTOR

- What is your opinion of Internet-based therapy? Of other forms of remote therapy?
- Have you ever referred a patient to an online therapist?
- Have any of your patients mentioned consulting an online therapist? If so, what were their experiences?

Research and general acceptance

Internet-based therapy shows promise for helping people who could not or would not otherwise engage in a therapeutic relationship. This potential is beginning to be tested in research. However, much of this research also recommends that Internet-based therapy be used in conjunction with face-to-face sessions. There are still many technical, logistical, and ethical questions to be answered regarding how the Internet best can be used for therapy. Most insurance companies will not provide reimbursement for therapy conducted over the Internet.

As of early 2011, there were 130 **clinical trials** of Internet-based therapy under way. Some are trials of **cognitive-behavioral therapy** or other specific approaches; other trials are comparing online therapy with face-to-face therapy for specific problems or disorders, including **smoking cessation**, **depression**, social anxiety, panic disorder, and grief disorder. Still other trials are evaluating the effectiveness of Internet-based counseling for patients suffering from chronic physical conditions with an emotional dimension, such as cancer, chronic pain syndromes, **brain** injury, or congestive heart failure.

Training and certification

Online therapists are expected to meet the same educational and state licensure requirements as office- or clinic-based therapists. They may be psychiatrists, clinical or counseling psychologists, **social workers**, marriage and family therapists, or psychiatric nurses. Most have doctoral degrees (M.D., Ph.D., or Psy.D.), with the remainder having master's degrees in psychology, social work, or nursing. There is one professional organization specifically for online therapists, the International Society for Mental Health Online (ISMHO), which was formed in 1997.

Resources

BOOKS

Hsiung, Robert C., ed. *E-therapy: Case Studies, Guiding Principles, and the Clinical Potential of the Internet*. New York: Norton, 2002.

Kraus, Ron, ed. *Online Counseling: A Handbook for Mental Health Professionals*, 2nd ed. Amsterdam, The Netherlands: Elsevier, 2011.

Rochlen, Aaron B. *Applying Counseling Theories: An Online Case-based Approach*. Upper Saddle River, NJ: Pearson/ Merrill Prentice Hall, 2007.

PERIODICALS

Bee, P.E., et al. "Psychotherapy Mediated by Remote Communication Technologies: A Meta-analytic Review." *BMC Psychiatry* 8 (July 2008):

Bockling, C.L., et al. "Disrupting the Rhythm of Depression Using Mobile Cognitive Therapy for Recurrent Depression: Randomized Controlled Trial Design and Protocol." *BMC Psychiatry* 14 (January 2011): 12.

Buhrman, M., et al. "Guided Internet-based Cognitive Behavioural Treatment for Chronic Back Pain Reduces Pain Catastrophizing: A Randomized Controlled Trial." *Journal of Rehabilitation Medicine* 43 (May 2011): 500–505.

Carlbring, P., et al. "Individually-tailored, Internet-based Treatment for Anxiety Disorders: A Randomized Controlled Trial." *Behaviour Research and Therapy* 49 (January 2011): 18–24.

Gainsbury, S., and A. Blaszczynski. "A Systematic Review of Internet-based Therapy for the Treatment of Addictions." *Clinical Psychology Review* 31 (April 2011): 490–498.

Hedman, E., et al. "Internet-Based Cognitive Behavior Therapy vs. Cognitive Behavioral Group Therapy for Social Anxiety Disorder: A Randomized Controlled Non-inferiority Trial." *PLoS One* 6 (March 25, 2011): e18001.

Lampe, L.A. "Internet-based Therapy: Too Good to be True?" *Australian and New Zealand Journal of Psychiatry* 45 (April 2011): 342–343.

Warmerdam, L., et al. "Cost-utility and Cost-effectiveness of Internet-based Treatment for Adults with Depressive Symptoms: Randomized Trial."*Journal of Medical Internet Research* 12 (December 19, 2010): e53.

WEBSITES

eTherapistsonline.com. "About Online Counseling." http://www.etherapistsonline.com/therapy/about.htm (accessed May 11, 2011).

International Society for Mental Health Online (ISMHO). "Suggested Principles for the Online Provision of Mental Health Services." https://www.ismho.org/suggestions.asp#principles (accessed May 11, 2011).

ORGANIZATIONS

Find a Therapist, Inc, 6942 E Lomita, Mesa, AZ, United States 85209, (480) 325-8330, Fax: (480) 396-3213, (866) 450-3463, http://www.etherapistsonline.com

International Society for Mental Health Online (ISMHO), [online contact only] https://www.ismho.org/contact.asp, https://www.ismho.org/home.asp

MyTherapyNet, 22425 Ventura Blvd., Suite 350, Woodland Hills, CA, United States 91364, Fax: (800) 931-9956, (800) 931-9956, customerservice@mytherapynet.com, https://www.mytherapynet.com

Ruth A. Wienclaw, Ph.D.
Rebecca J. Frey, Ph.D.

Interpersonal therapy

Definition

Interpersonal therapy (IPT) is a short-term supportive **psychotherapy** that focuses on the connection between interactions between people and the development of a person's psychiatric symptoms.

Purpose

Interpersonal therapy was initially developed to treat adult **depression**. It has since been applied to the treatment of depression in adolescents, the elderly, and people with Human Immunodeficiency Virus (HIV) infection. There is an IPT conjoint (couple) therapy for people whose marital disputes contribute to depressive episodes. IPT has also been modified for the treatment of a number of disorders, including **substance abuse**; bulimia and **anorexia nervosa**; **bipolar disorder**; and dysthymia. Research is underway to determine the efficacy of IPT in the treatment of patients with **panic disorder** or **borderline personality disorder**; depressed caregivers of patients with traumatic **brain** injuries; depressed pregnant women; and people suffering from protracted **bereavement**.

Interpersonal therapy is a descendant of psychodynamic therapy, itself derived from **psychoanalysis**, with its emphasis on the unconscious and childhood experiences. Symptoms and personal difficulties are regarded as arising from deep, unresolved personality or character problems. **Psychodynamic psychotherapy** is a long-term method of treatment, with in-depth exploration of past family relationships as they were perceived during the client's infancy, childhood, and adolescence.

There are seven types of interventions that are commonly used in IPT, many of which reflect the influence of psychodynamic psychotherapy: a focus on clients' emotions; an exploration of clients' resistance to treatment; discussion of patterns in clients' relationships and experiences; taking a detailed past history; an emphasis on clients' current interpersonal experiences;

exploration of the therapist/client relationship; and the identification of clients' wishes and fantasies. IPT is, however, distinctive for its brevity and its treatment focus. IPT emphasizes the ways in which a person's current relationships and social context cause or maintain symptoms rather than exploring the deep-seated sources of the symptoms. Its goals are rapid symptom reduction and improved social adjustment. A frequent byproduct of IPT treatment is more satisfying relationships in the present.

IPT has the following goals in the treatment of depression: to diagnose depression explicitly; to educate the client about depression, its causes, and the various treatments available for it; to identify the interpersonal context of depression as it relates to symptom development; and to develop strategies for the client to follow in coping with the depression. Because interpersonal therapy is a short-term approach, the therapist addresses only one or two problem areas in the client's current functioning. In the early sessions, the therapist and client determine which areas would be most helpful in reducing the client's symptoms. The remaining sessions are then organized toward resolving these agreed-upon problem areas. This time-limited framework distinguishes IPT from therapies that are open-ended in their exploration. The targeted approach of IPT has demonstrated rapid improvement for patients with problems ranging from mild situational depression to severe depression with a recent history of **suicide** attempts.

Interpersonal therapy has been outlined in a manual by Klerman and Weissman, which ensures some standardization in the training of interpersonal therapists and their practice. Because of this standardized training format, IPT is not usually combined with other talk therapies. Treatment with IPT, however, is often combined with drug therapy, particularly when the client suffers from such mood disorders as depression, dysthymia, or bipolar disorder.

Precautions

Training programs in interpersonal therapy are still not widely available, so that many practicing therapists base their work on the manual alone without additional supervision. It is unclear whether reading the manual alone is sufficient to provide an acceptable standard of care.

While interpersonal therapy has been adapted for use with substance abusers, it has not demonstrated its effectiveness with this group of patients. Researchers studying patients addicted to opiates or **cocaine** found little benefit to incorporating IPT into the standard recovery programs. These findings suggest that another treatment method that offers greater structure and direction would be more successful with these patients.

Description

Since the interpersonal therapy model was developed for the treatment of depression and then modified for use with other populations and mental disorders, an understanding of IPT's approach to depression is crucial. Interpersonal therapists focus on the functional role of depression rather than on its etiology or cause; and they look at the ways in which problematic interactions develop when a person becomes depressed. The IPT framework considers clinical depression as having three components: the development of symptoms that arise from biological, genetic and/or psychodynamic processes; social interactions with other people, which are learned over the course of one's life; and personality, made up of the more enduring traits and behaviors that may predispose a person to depressive symptoms. IPT intervenes at the levels of symptom formation and social functioning, and does not attempt to alter aspects of the client's personality.

Subtypes of IPT

Interpersonal therapy offers two possible treatment plans for persons with depressive disorders. The first plan treats the acute episode of depression by eliminating the current depressive symptoms. This approach requires intervening while the person is in the midst of a depression. The acute phase of treatment typically lasts 2–4 months with weekly sessions. Many clients terminate treatment at that point, after their symptoms have subsided. Maintenance treatment (IPT-M) is the second treatment plan and is much less commonly utilized than acute treatment. IPT-M is a longer-term therapy based on the principles of interpersonal therapy but with the aim of preventing or reducing the frequency of further depressive episodes. Some clients choose IPT-M after the acute treatment phase. IPT-M can extend over a period of 2–3 years, with therapy sessions once a month.

Psychoeducation in IPT

Treatment with IPT is based on the premise that depression occurs in a social and interpersonal context that must be understood for improvement to occur. In the first session, the psychiatric history includes a review of the client's current social functioning and current close relationships, their patterns and their mutual expectations. Changes in relationships prior to the onset of symptoms are clarified, such as the death of a loved one, a child leaving home, or worsening marital conflict.

IPT is psychoeducational in nature to some degree. It involves teaching the client about the nature of depression and the ways that it manifests in his or her life and relationships. In the initial sessions, depressive symptoms are reviewed in detail, and the accurate naming of the problem is essential. The therapist then explains depression and its treatment and may explain to the client that he or she has adopted the "sick role." The concept of the "sick role" is derived from the work of a sociologist named Talcott Parsons, and is based on the notion that illness is not merely a condition but a social role that affects the attitudes and behaviors of the client and those around him or her. Over time, the client comes to see that the sick role has increasingly come to govern his or her social interactions.

Identification of problem areas

The techniques of IPT were developed to manage four basic interpersonal problem areas: unresolved **grief**; role transitions; interpersonal role disputes (often marital disputes); and interpersonal deficits (deficiencies). In the early sessions, the interpersonal therapist and the client attempt to determine which of these four problems is most closely associated with the onset of the current depressive episode. Therapy is then organized to help the client deal with the interpersonal difficulties in the primary problem area. The coping strategies that the client is encouraged to discover and employ in daily life are tailored to his or her individual situation.

UNRESOLVED GRIEF. In normal bereavement, a person experiences symptoms such as sadness, disturbed sleep, and difficulty functioning but these usually resolve in 2–4 months. Unresolved grief in depressed people is usually either delayed grief that has been postponed and then experienced long after the loss; or distorted grief, in which there is no felt emotion of sadness but there may be nonemotional symptoms, often physical. If unresolved grief is identified as the primary issue, the goals of treatment are to facilitate the mourning process. Successful therapy will help the client re-establish interests and relationships that can begin to fill the void of what has been lost.

ROLE DISPUTES. Interpersonal role disputes occur when the client and at least one other significant person have differing expectations of their relationship. The IPT therapist focuses on these disputes if they seem stalled or repetitious, or offer little hope of improvement. The treatment goals include helping the client identify the nature of the dispute; decide on a plan of action; and begin to modify unsatisfying patterns, reassess expectations of the relationship, or both. The therapist does not direct the client to one particular resolution of difficulties and should not attempt to preserve unworkable relationships.

ROLE TRANSITIONS. Depression associated with role transitions occurs when a person has difficulty coping with life changes that require new roles. These may be such transitions as retirement, a career change, moving, or leaving home. People who are clinically depressed are most likely to experience role changes as losses rather than opportunities. The loss may be obvious, as when a marriage ends, or more subtle, as the loss of freedom people experience after the birth of a child. Therapy is terminated when a client has given up the old role; expressed the accompanying feelings of guilt, anger, and loss; acquired new skills; and developed a new social network around the new role.

INTERPERSONAL DEFICITS. Interpersonal deficits are the focus of treatment when the client has a history of inadequate or unsupportive interpersonal relationships. The client may never have established lasting or intimate relationships as an adult, and may experience a sense of inadequacy, lack of self-assertion, and guilt about expressing anger. Generally, clients with a history of extreme social isolation come to therapy with more severe emotional disturbances. The goal of treatment is to reduce the client's social isolation. Instead of focusing on current relationships, IPT therapy in this area focuses on the client's past relationships; the present relationship with the therapist; and ways to form new relationships.

IPT in special populations

ELDERLY CLIENTS. In translating the IPT model of depression to work with different populations, the core principles and problem areas remain essentially the same, with some modifications. In working with the elderly, IPT sessions may be shorter to allow for decreased energy levels, and dependency issues may be more prominent. In addition, the therapist may work with an elderly client toward tolerating rather than eliminating long-standing role disputes.

CLIENTS WITH HIV INFECTION. In IPT with HIV-positive clients, particular attention is paid to the clients' unique set of psychosocial stressors: the **stigma** of the disease; the effects of being gay (if applicable); dealing with family members who may isolate themselves; and coping with the medical consequences of the disease.

ADOLESCENTS. In IPT with adolescents, the therapist addresses such common developmental issues as separation from parents; the client's authority in relationship to parents; the development of new interpersonal relationships; first experiences of the death of a relative or friend; peer pressure; and single-parent families. Adolescents are seen weekly for 12 weeks with once-weekly additional phone contact between therapist and client for the first four weeks of treatment. The parents are interviewed in the initial session to get a comprehensive history of the adolescent's symptoms, and to educate the parents as well as the young person about depression and possible treatments, including a discussion of the need for medication. The therapist refrains from giving advice when working with adolescents, and will primarily use supportive listening, while assessing the client for evidence of suicidal thoughts or problems with school attendance. So far, research does not support the efficacy of antidepressant medication in treating adolescents, though most clinicians will give some younger clients a trial of medication if it appears to offer relief.

CLIENTS WITH SUBSTANCE ABUSE DISORDERS. While IPT has not yet demonstrated its efficacy in the field of substance abuse recovery, a version of IPT has been developed for use with substance abusers. The two goals are to help the client stop or cut down on drug use; and to help the client develop better strategies for dealing with the social and interpersonal consequences of drug use. To meet these goals, the client must accept the need to stop; take steps to manage impulsiveness; and recognize the social contexts of drug purchase and use. **Relapse** is viewed as the rule rather than the exception in treating substance abuse disorders, and the therapist avoids treating the client in a punitive or disapproving manner when it occurs. Instead, the therapist reminds the client of the fact that staying away from drugs is the client's decision.

CLIENTS WITH EATING DISORDERS. IPT has been extended to the treatment of eating disorders. The IPT therapist does not focus directly on the symptoms of the disorder, but rather, allows for identification of problem areas that have contributed to the emergence of the disorder over time. IPT appears to be useful in treating clients with bulimia whose symptoms are maintained by interpersonal issues, including social anxiety; sensitivity to conflict and rejection; and difficulty managing negative emotions. IPT is helpful in bringing the problems underlying the bingeing and purging to the surface, such as conflict avoidance; difficulties with role expectations; confusion regarding needs for closeness and distance; and deficiencies in solving social problems. IPT also helps people with bulimia to regulate the emotional states that maintain the bulimic behavior.

Anorexia nervosa also appears to be responsive to treatment with IPT. Research indicates that there is a connection between interpersonal and family dysfunction and the development of anorexia nervosa. Therapists disagree as to whether interpersonal dysfunction causes or is caused by anorexia. IPT has been helpful because it is not concerned with the origin but rather seeks to improve the client's interpersonal functioning and thereby decreasing symptoms. IPT's four categories of grief, interpersonal disputes, interpersonal deficits, and role transitions correspond to the core issues of clients with anorexia. **Social phobia** is another disorder that responds well to IPT therapy.

KEY TERMS

Bereavement—The emotional experience of loss after the death of a friend or relative.

Bingeing—An excessive amount of food consumed in a short period of time. Usually, while a person binge eats, he or she feels disconnected from reality, and feels unable to stop. The bingeing may temporarily relieve depression or anxiety, but after the binge, the person usually feels guilty and depressed.

Dysthymia—Depression of low intensity.

Dysthymic disorder—A mood disorder that is less severe than depression but usually more chronic.

Etiology—The cause or origin of a disease or disorder. The word is also used to refer to the study of the causes of disease.

Psychosocial—A term that refers to the emotional and social aspects of psychological disorders.

Purging—Inappropriate actions taken to prevent weight gain, often after bingeing, including self-induced vomiting or the misuse of laxatives, diuretics, enemas, or other medications.

Remission—In the course of an illness or disorder, a period of time when symptoms are absent.

Role—The set of customary or expected behavior patterns associated with a particular position or function in society. For example, a person's role as mother is associated with one set of expected behaviors, and her role as a worker with a very different set.

Role transition—Life changes that require an alteration in one's social or occupational status or self-image.

Stigma—A mark or characteristic trait of a disease or defect; by extension, a cause for reproach or a stain on one's reputation. Such sexually transmitted diseases as HIV infection carry a severe social stigma.

Supportive—An approach to psychotherapy that seeks to encourage the patient or offer emotional support to him or her, as distinct from insight-oriented or exploratory approaches to treatment.

Aftercare

Interpersonal therapy as a maintenance approach (IPT-M) could be viewed as aftercare for clients suffering from depression. It is designed as a preventive measure by focusing on the period after the acute depression has passed. Typically, once the client is in remission and is symptom-free, he or she takes on more responsibilities and has increased social contact. These changes can lead to increased **stress** and greater vulnerability to another episode of depression. IPT-M enables clients to reduce the stresses associated with remission and thereby lower the risk of recurrence. The goal of maintenance therapy is to keep the client at his or her current level of functioning. Research has shown that for clients with a history of recurrent depression, total prevention is unlikely, but that maintenance therapy may delay a recurrence.

In general, long-term maintenance psychotherapy by itself is not recommended unless there are such reasons as pregnancy or severe side effects that prevent the client from being treated with medication. IPT-M does, however, seem to be particularly helpful with certain groups of patients, either alone or in combination with medication. Women appear to benefit, due to the importance of social environment and social relations in female gender roles; the effects of the menstrual cycle on symptoms; and complications related to victimization by rape, incest, or battering. IPT is also useful for elderly clients who can't take **antidepressants** due to intolerable side effects or such medical conditions as autoimmune disorders, cardiovascular disorders, diabetes, or other general medical conditions.

Results

The expected outcomes of interpersonal therapy are a reduction or the elimination of symptoms and improved interpersonal functioning. There will also be a greater understanding of the presenting symptoms and ways to prevent their recurrence. For example, in the case of depression, a person will have been educated about the nature of depression; what it looks like for him or her; and the interpersonal triggers of a depressive episode. A person will also leave therapy with strategies for minimizing triggers and for resolving future depressive episodes more effectively. While interpersonal therapy focuses on the present, it can also improve the client's future through increased awareness of preventive measures and strengthened coping skills.

Research has shown that IPT requires clients' commitment to therapy prior to starting the treatment. If clients are resistant to an educational approach, the results of IPT are generally poor. It has been found that when people do not accept IPT's methods and approach at the outset; they are unlikely to be convinced over the course of therapy and they receive little benefit from treatment. IPT clients appear to do better in therapy if they have confidence in their therapist; therefore, if the initial fit between therapist and client is not good, therapy will often be unsuccessful. A client should listen to his or her instincts early in treatment, and either seek out another interpersonal therapist or find a therapist who uses a different approach—such as **cognitive-behavioral therapy**, which was also developed specifically for the treatment of depression.

Resources

BOOKS

American Psychiatric Association. *Diagnostic and Statistical Manual of Mental Disorders*. 4th ed., text rev. Washington, DC: American Psychiatric Publishing, 2000.

Klerman, Gerald L., et al. *Interpersonal Psychotherapy of Depression*. New York: Basic Books, Inc., 1984.

Klerman, Gerald L. and Myrna M. Weissman, eds. *New Applications of Interpersonal Psychotherapy*. Washington, DC: American Psychiatric Press, Inc., 1993.

Mufson, Laura, et al. *Interpersonal Psychotherapy for Depressed Adolescents*. 2nd ed. New York: Guilford Press, 2004.

PERIODICALS

Apple, Robin F. "Interpersonal Therapy for Bulimia Nervosa." *Journal of Clinical Psychology* 55, no. 6 (June 1999): 715–725.

Barkham, Michael, and Gillian E. Hardy. "Counselling and Interpersonal Therapies for Depression: Towards Securing an Evidence-base." *British Medical Bulletin* 57, no. 1 (2001): 115–132.

Frank, Ellen, and Michael E. Thase. "Natural History and Preventative (sic) Treatment of Recurrent Mood Disorders." *Annual Reviews Medicine* 50 (1999): 453–468.

House, Allan, D. M. "Brief Psychodynamic Interpersonal Therapy After Deliberate Self-poisoning Reduced Suicidal Ideation and Deliberate Self-harm." *Evidence Based Mental Health* 5, no. 1 (February 2002): 14.

McIntosh, Virginia V., et al. "Interpersonal Psychotherapy for Anorexia Nervosa." *International Journal of Eating Disorders* 27, no. 2 (March 2000): 125–139.

Mufson, Laura, et al. "Efficacy of Interpersonal Psychotherapy for Depressed Adolescents." *Archives of General Psychiatry* 56, no. 6 (June 1999): 573–579. Available online at http://archpsyc.ama-assn.org/cgi/reprint/56/6/573.pdf (accessed November 9, 2011).

Weissman, Myrna M., and John C. Markowitz. "Interpersonal Psychotherapy: Current Status." *Archives of General Psychiatry* 51, no. 8 (August 1994): 599–606.

ORGANIZATIONS

International Society for Interpersonal Psychotherapy, University of Iowa, Department of Psychiatry, 1-293 Medical Education Building, Iowa City, IA, 52242, (391) 353-4230, Fax: (391) 353-3003, scott-stuart@uiowa.edu, http://interpersonalpsychotherapy.org.

Holly Scherstuhl, M.Ed.

Intervention

Definition

A standard dictionary defines intervention as an influencing force or act that occurs in order to modify a given state of affairs. In the context of behavioral health, an intervention may be any outside process that has the effect of modifying an individual's behavior, cognition, or emotional state. For example, a person experiencing **stress** symptoms may find a variety of interventions effective in bringing relief. Deep breathing, vigorous **exercise**, talking with a therapist or counselor, taking an antianxiety medication, or a combination of these activities are all interventions designed to modify the symptoms and potentially the causes of stress-related discomfort.

The term is also used to describe a specific process designed to break through **denial** on the part of persons with serious addictive disorders. Interventions in this sense of the word involve carefully orchestrated confrontations in which friends, family members, and (in many cases) employers confront the person with the negative impact and consequences of his or her **addiction**. The goal of an intervention is to bring the addicted person to acknowledge that he or she suffers from a disorder and agree to treatment. This goal, however, is not always realized.

Description

There is no one-size-fits-all-intervention for behavioral health disorders. Recent research advances and greater understanding of behavioral health problems have provided an expanded range of treatments that promise better outcomes than those available in the past. For people who overcome the barriers of **stigma**, discrimination, and limited access, there is a broad variety of helpful interventions from which to choose. Both personal preference and the severity of discomfort may influence the choice of talk therapy, the use of medications, participation in self-help or **support groups**, or even inpatient treatment. In most cases, a combination of different interventions has proven to be most effective. As a result, many therapists tend to be eclectic in their practice and use a combination of approaches to in order to be as effective as possible with a wide variety of people.

Psychotherapy or talk therapy involves face-to-face meetings with a therapist who may specialize in a certain approach to treatment, and may include:

- Psychoanalysis is the oldest form of talk therapy. It is a long-term form of treatment intended to uncover a person's subconscious motivations and early patterns in order to resolve present issues.
- Behavioral therapy is designed to change thinking patterns and behavior. Exposure therapy is a subtype of behavioral therapy that is useful in treating obsessive-compulsive disorder and post-traumatic stress disorder. The client is deliberately exposed to stimuli that trigger the painful thoughts or feelings under carefully controlled conditions that include support from the therapist. The individual is then taught techniques to avoid performing the compulsive behaviors or to work through the traumatic event.
- Cognitive therapy seeks to identify and correct dysfunctional thinking patterns that lead to troublesome feelings or behavior.
- Family therapy includes discussion and problem-solving sessions that include all members of the family.
- Group therapy takes place in a small group with the guidance of a therapist. The focus is on individual issues; group members assist each other in problem solving.
- Movement, art, and music therapists use these forms of creative expression to help people deal with strong emotions that are less easily handled in a talk therapy format.

Drug therapy involves the use of prescribed medications to treat the symptoms of certain mental or emotional disorders. It is important for patients to be aware of possible side effects of the medications; to inform the doctor of all other medications and alternative remedies that they are taking; and to have their blood, blood pressure, or other vital signs monitored regularly by the prescribing physician.

Electroconvulsive therapy (ECT) is used to treat **depression** and a few other specific conditions that have not responded to other interventions. It involves a controlled series of electric shocks to certain areas of the **brain**. It has been proven effective for some people despite the fact that it continues to be controversial. Patients should be fully aware of the side effects of ECT and assure themselves that the professional has been properly trained to administer ECT.

Psychosocial treatments may include **talk therapy** and medication in combination with social and vocational training to assist people recovering from severe mental illnesses. Psychosocial interventions may also include education about the illness itself, techniques for managing its symptoms, and ways in which friends and family members can help.

Psychoeducation is a word used to describe the process of teaching people about their illness, its treatment, and early warning signs of **relapse**, so that they can seek treatment before the illness worsens.

Psychoeducation may also include learning about coping strategies, problem solving, and preparation of a crisis plan in the event of a relapse or future episode.

Self-help and support groups are another form of intervention that has become increasingly common in recent years. They exist for almost all disorders and are often based on the basic principles and values of the Alcoholics Anonymous movement founded in the 1930s. Although they are not led by professionals, these groups may be therapeutic because members give one another ongoing support and assistance. Group members share frustrations and successes, recommendations about specialists and community resources, and helpful tips about recovery. They also share friendship and hope for themselves, their loved ones, and others in the group. Unqualified acceptance by other people can be a powerful intervention for people recovering from a mental illness or addictive disorder.

A common question about interventions concerns sources of help or further information. Many communities have a local hotline number that provides referrals and resources, or a mental health association that can direct callers to appropriate clinics, agencies, or groups. Helping resources may include the following:

- A community mental health center, usually a part of the state's department of mental health.
- Local mental health organizations.
- Family physicians.
- Clergy or spiritual counselors.
- Family service agencies, including charities and family or social services sponsored by various churches, synagogues, or other religious groups.
- High school or college guidance counselors.
- Marriage and family counselors.
- Child guidance counselors.
- Accredited psychiatric hospitals.
- Hotlines, crisis centers, and emergency rooms.

There are several categories of mental health professionals who have been specially trained to provide a range of interventions to relieve suffering, treat specific symptoms, or improve overall mental health. Competent professionals are licensed or certified by a particular specialty board or state licensing body. Their credentials imply a certain level of education, training, experience, and subscription to a code of ethics. Mental health professionals include:

- Psychiatrists. Medical doctors with specialized training in the diagnosis and treatment of behavioral and emotional illnesses. They are qualified to prescribe medications. They may also specialize in certain fields within psychiatry, such as child/adolescent or geriatric psychiatry.
- Psychologists. Professional counselors with a doctoral degree (PhD or PsyD) and two or more years of supervised work experience. They are trained to make diagnoses, administer and interpret psychological tests, and provide individual, family and group therapy.
- Clinical social workers. Professionals with a master's degree in social work from an accredited graduate program. They are trained to make diagnoses and provide individual, family and group therapy.
- Licensed professional counselors and mental health counselors. Professionals with a master's degree with supervised work experience and are trained to make diagnoses and provide individual, family and group therapy.
- Certified alcohol and drug abuse counselors. Professionals with specialized training in the treatment of alcohol and drug abuse. They are able to diagnose and provide counseling to individuals, families and groups.
- Nurse psychotherapists. Registered nurses (RNs) with specialized training in psychiatric and mental health nursing. They can diagnose disorders and provide counseling to individuals, families and groups.
- Marital and family therapists. Counselors with a master's or doctor's degree with specialized training in marital and family therapy. They are also trained to diagnose and provide individual, family and group counseling.
- Pastoral counselors. Ordained clergy with advanced training and certification in Level II clinical pastoral education as well as the master's degree in theology (M. Div.) required by most American denominations for ordination. In addition to offering psychological counseling to individuals, families and groups, pastoral counselors have been trained to offer spiritual and sacramental ministry to those who request it.

Resources

WEBSITES

Mental Health America. "When a Parent has a Mental Illness: Interventions and Services for Families." http://www.nmha.org/go/information/get-info/strengthening-families/when-a-parent-has-a-mental-illness-interventions-and-services-for-families (accessed November 14, 2011).

ORGANIZATIONS

American Psychological Association, 750 1st St. NE, Washington, DC, 20002-4242, (202) 336-5500; TDD/TTY: (202) 336-6123, (800) 374-2721, http://www.apa.org.

Mental Health America, 2000 N. Beauregard St., 6th Fl., Alexandria, VA, 22311, (703) 684-7722,

(800) 969-6642, Fax: (703) 684-5968, http://www1.nmha.org.

National Alliance on Mental Illness, 3803 N Fairfax Dr., Ste. 100, Arlington, VA, 22203, (703) 524-7600, http://www.nami.org.

National Mental Health Consumers' Self-Help Clearinghouse, 1211 Chestnut St., Ste. 1207, Philadelphia, PA, 19107, (215) 751-1810, Fax: (215) 636-6312, info@mhselfhelp.org, http://www.mhselfhelp.org.

Substance Abuse and Mental Health Services Administration, 1 Choke Cherry Rd., Rockville, MD, 20857, (877) SAMHSA-7 (726-4727); TTY: (800) 487-4889, Fax: (240) 221-4292, SAMHSAInfo@samhsa.hhs.gov, http://www.samhsa.gov.

Judy Leaver, M.A.

Intuniv *see* **Guanfacine**

Invega *see* **Paliperidone**

Involuntary hospitalization

Definition

Involuntary hospitalization is a legal procedure used to require individuals with mental health disorders to receive inpatient treatment without their consent. The legal justifications vary from state to state but are generally based on a determination that a person is imminently dangerous to self or others, is gravely disabled, or needs immediate care and treatment but is unable to request it. Involuntary hospitalization is considered a controversial course of action and is generally a last resort used in dealing with persons who are either unable to use proper judgment or insight in deciding to accept or refuse treatment or who are considered a danger to themselves or others.

Purpose

The historical justification of civil commitment laws in the United States is based on two primary powers and responsibilities of government. First, governments are responsible for protecting each citizen from injury by another. This power of protection is commonly called police powers. The second power, known as *parens patriae* (Latin for "parent of the nation"), is based on the government's responsibility to care for disabled citizens. A person with a significant mental illness may be civilly committed, or involuntarily hospitalized, under either of these powers. It is understood that the purpose of civil commitment is protecting the safety of the public or of the person with mental illness.

As of 2011, 38 states permitted some type of involuntary commitment procedure (outpatient or inpatient civil commitment), while 34 states (all 38 states except Alabama, Pennsylvania, Virginia, and Wyoming) allowed police pickup or emergency hospitalization. Federal law does not specifically address involuntary commitment or hospitalization of U.S. citizens, so state procedures, and the length of involuntary confinement, vary widely. Most require proof of dangerousness, which can be interpreted in ambiguous ways but generally means that danger is imminent or provable. Confinement usually requires a court hearing within 24 to 72 hours after the emergency commitment procedure to assure due process, or that the individual's rights are met.

Beyond safety issues, mental health professionals have thought that proper psychiatric treatment, even when administered against a person's wishes, is preferable to the continued worsening of a serious mental illness. There is some question currently about the effectiveness of forced treatment in the legal and mental health communities. Involuntary treatment is considered by many patients' rights advocates and mental health consumers to be an oxymoron (a figure of speech that appears contradictory), in that it may protect public safety at the expense of rights of the person with a mental illness. Other public interest groups, such as the Treatment Advocacy Center, support involuntary commitment, arguing that the consequences of non-treatment are far more severe.

Description

Involuntary hospitalization is a complex process because of legal requirements that have been put in place to protect citizens from being hospitalized because of a family quarrel or similar interpersonal issue. In the nineteenth century, for example, it was commonplace for husbands who wanted to end a marriage to have wives hospitalized against their will, or for parents to commit "disobedient" children. At present, however, most states require the person who thinks someone else should be hospitalized to call 911 or their local police department. The procedure thereafter varies from state to state, but in many cases, the department will send a patrol team to answer the call. If the person who has made the call is in the same location as the person needing treatment, one officer will usually talk to the caller in one room while another talks to the person in question. The officers may also interview family members, neighbors, bystanders, or others who may know the affected person or have witnessed their behavior. The police officers will compare their evaluations of the situation, and in most jurisdictions, the officers can then make one of three decisions: decide that the person who made the call has misjudged the situation (for example, the other person may be intoxicated); decide that the affected person is mentally ill but not necessarily dangerous; or take the affected person to the nearest hospital emergency room. They may ask the person who called to accompany them to the hospital. In some states, however, the officers themselves must witness the affected person attempting to harm him- or herself or someone else before they can take him or her to the emergency room.

In the emergency room, the **psychiatrist** on duty will evaluate the affected person for dangerousness as well as the presence of mental illness. He or she will interview the police officers and anyone who accompanied them as well as the affected person. If the affected person has been receiving treatment for a mental disorder, the psychiatrist will usually contact the therapist. In some cases, the affected person will need a medical evaluation, including assessment for **substance abuse** or withdrawal, before the doctor can proceed with a psychiatric assessment. The psychiatric assessment will be thorough, and documented as completely as possible; laboratory tests will be ordered if necessary. When the assessment is complete, the doctor is legally required to decide in favor of the least restrictive environment to which the patient can be safely discharged for continued care.

If the doctor decides that the person is dangerous but not mentally ill, he or she may turn the person back over to law enforcement if necessary. If the person has threatened **suicide** but the psychiatrist does not consider the threat to be legitimate, then he or she may allow the patient to leave the emergency room after assessment. A decision to hospitalize a person involuntarily is based on three considerations: loss of emotional control, clear evidence of a psychotic disorder, or evidence of impulsivity with serious thoughts, threats, or plans to harm self or others. Persons with severe disabilities who are unable to care for themselves or make decisions regarding their treatment may also be candidates for involuntary hospitalization. The affected person is often reassessed the next day to confirm any initial findings. Most states stipulate that the affected person is entitled to a hearing before a judge who specializes in **mental health law** within 72 hours of hospitalization; the judge can order the person released if he or she thinks the person is not dangerous.

Precautions

The use of involuntary hospitalization or any other form of forced treatment is highly controversial, with citizen advocacy groups, mental health professionals, and the general public taking different sides on the topic. In addition, legal advocates and the courts take very seriously the denial of a person's liberty. Involuntary hospitalization is one of the most extreme examples of denial of liberty in a democratic society.

Advocates against involuntary hospitalization argue that forced treatment is indicative of a failed treatment system. People with an intensely personal stake in such a decision may see the necessity of forced treatment to prevent harm to the person with an illness or to others. Some advocates believe that if involuntary **intervention** is enforced, only custodial care should be provided. There is great concern that a person who has been civilly committed to a treatment facility will also receive such forced treatment as strong antipsychotic medications or **electroconvulsive therapy** (ECT). The issue of a person's ability to exercise **informed consent** about his or her treatment is also an area of concern. In addition, there may be worry that inpatient treatment will add to the **stigma** of being diagnosed with a mental illness. One research study found that persons who had been hospitalized (voluntarily or involuntarily) for treatment of a mental illness were even more likely to suffer discrimination in the job market than those who had received only outpatient treatment.

On the other hand, there are patients who claim that an incident of involuntary hospitalization in their own treatment history may not only have saved their lives, but also enabled them to receive treatment at a time when they were not capable of making a decision to do so. Family members sometimes consider involuntary hospitalization their only recourse to prevent worsening of a severe and debilitating mental illness, contact with the criminal justice system, or the devastation and dangers of **homelessness**.

Most persons involved in the mental health community believe that an adequately funded, community-based continuum of care and treatment would drastically reduce the number of cases in which involuntary treatment of any kind is necessary. The use of psychiatric **advance directives** may have an effect on the use of involuntary treatment as well. A psychiatric advance directive is a clearly written statement of an individual's psychiatric treatment preferences or instructions, somewhat like a living will for medical conditions. Psychiatric advance directives have not yet been tested in the court system but are widely endorsed throughout the mental health community as an alternative to involuntary treatment.

Controversy

A number of factors in the early 1980s led to a trend toward declining use of involuntary hospitalization for people with significant mental illnesses. The development and effectiveness of a range of new medications meant that treatment in general was more successful. The continued move toward **deinstitutionalization**, or moving people out of hospitals and into community-based treatments, contributed as well. Treating people in hospitals is inherently expensive and was being viewed as less effective, compared to more innovative and less costly forms of treatment in smaller community programs. A continuing concern about civil liberties led to closer court scrutiny, the right to a hearing and legal counsel, and laws establishing a person's rights to the least restrictive form of treatment.

Recently, however, after a number of tragic and highly publicized violent incidents involving people with severe untreated mental illness, there appears to be a trend toward modification of the criteria required for involuntary hospitalization, court-ordered treatment, and outpatient commitment. Those who advocate liberalizing the process would like a person's previous mental health history to be included in the court's consideration and the standard of dangerousness to be broadened.

For instance, the Virginia Tech shootings that occurred on April 16, 2007, on the campus of Virginia Polytechnic Institute and State University at Blacksburg, Virginia, have caused the state to re-evaluate its requirements for imminent danger in order to commit a person. During the incident, Seung-Hui Cho killed 32 people and wounded another 25 before committing suicide. Cho had previously been diagnosed with severe anxiety disorder. The imminent danger was clarified to eliminate much of the ambiguity within its definition as to whether to involuntarily commit a person that could cause serious physical harm to others or to him- or herself. In 2008, the state of Virginia updated its laws so that people with mental problems now have an easier process to go through in order to get help. Improvements were made to the procedures and criteria for involuntary commitment proceedings, emergency custody orders, temporary detention orders, and other such measures within the commitment process.

In 2011, Jared Lee Loughner attempted to assassinate Arizona Congresswoman Gabrielle Giffords, severely wounding Giffords and killing six others. Prior to the shooting, Loughner's mental health was questioned by his college professors and peers, resulting in his being suspended from school after producing disturbing videos and consistently displaying erratic behavior. If he had wanted to return to school, Loughner would have had to undergo a mental health evaluation, which he did not seek; questions remain as to whether or not forcing treatment could have prevented the events that followed. Still, it's important to remember that the cases of Cho and Loughner are extreme examples and cannot be used as representative of all individuals with mental disorders or all individuals placed under involuntary hospitalization.

KEY TERMS

Electroconvulsive therapy—Treatment involving the use of a small electric current through the brain, which produces an electric shock and results in a seizure.

Mental illness—Any psychiatric disorder that causes unusual (atypical) behavior.

Psychotic disorder—Any psychiatric disorder involving the loss of sense of with reality including symptoms such as hallucinations, delusions, and incoherence; types of such disorder include schizophrenia or mania.

Stigma—A mark or characteristic trait of a disease or disorder generally perceived as negative by society (regardless of fact).

Variances in state laws

The enforcement and breadth of involuntary hospitalization vary depending on state law. Arizona has one of the least restrictive laws in the country, dictating that the state government can place anyone in involuntary hospitalization who is determined to be "persistently or acutely disabled." Other states, such as Nevada, have much more restrictive laws. Before the state of Nevada is able to confine anyone against his or her wishes, it has to demonstrate that the person is a threat to him- or herself or to others. Likewise, in Connecticut, a person can be committed when the person has "psychiatric disabilities and is dangerous to himself or herself or others or gravely disabled."

In North Carolina, the state modified its law (HB 243—Mental Health/Law Enforcement Custody, North Carolina Statutory Changes for Involuntary Commitment) on October 1, 2009, for the involuntary commitment of its citizens for mental health treatment. The amended statute now "allows for termination of the proceedings by the interim facility if the patient no longer warrants commitment or has not been placed in a 24-hour facility within 7 days." The improvement to the law was enacted to clarify what should happen when a person is taken to an emergency department for involuntary commitment when that person is deemed a danger to self or others but is unable to be placed into a state institution.

Preparation

People who are concerned about the mental health of a family member, roommate, or friend are advised to gather information about the legal requirements for involuntary hospitalization in their state ahead of time, because it is not easy to think clearly when someone is acting in a bizarre or frightening manner. It is also a good idea to write down the name and telephone number of the affected person's therapist (if they have one) and the names of any medications that the person is taking.

Results

In the middle part of the twentieth century, the goal of involuntary hospitalization emphasized the rights of the individual—it was generally very difficult to commit someone against his or her will. However, in the later part of that century and now in the first quarter of the twenty-first century, many such laws are being modified to expand the legitimate ways that states can commit someone to a mental institution. Balancing individual rights and the safety of the general population is not an easy task, and for this and other reasons, the right to involuntarily commit someone to a mental hospital continues to be the subject of debate.

Resources

BOOKS

Bloch, Sidney, and Stephen A. Green. *Psychiatric Ethics*. Oxford: Oxford University Press, 2009.

Casher, Michael I., and Joshua D. Bess. *Manual of Inpatient Psychiatry*. New York: Cambridge University Press, 2010.

Kallert, Thomas W., Juan E. Mezzich, and John Monahan, eds. *Coercive Treatment in Psychiatry*. Hoboken, NJ: John Wiley & Sons, 2011.

Kemp, Donna R. *Mental Health in America: A Reference Handbook*. Santa Barbara, CA: ABC-CLIO, 2007.

Ovsiew, Fred, and Richard L. Munich, eds. *Principles of Inpatient Psychiatry*. Philadelphia: Lippincott Williams & Wilkins, 2009.

Ryan, Patrick, and Barry J. Coughlan. *Aging and Older Adult Mental Health: Issues and Implications for Practice*. Hove, UK: Routledge, 2011.

Wahl, Otto F. *Telling Is Risky Business: Mental Health Consumers Confront Stigma*. New Brunswick, NJ: Rutgers University Press, 1999.

PERIODICALS

Abramowitz, M. Z., et al. "Attitudes among Medical and Law Students toward Decision-Making in Regard to Involuntary Psychiatric Hospitalization." *International Journal of Law and Psychiatry* 34, no. 5 (2011): 368–73.

Katsakou, C, et al. "Psychiatric Patients' Views on Why Their Involuntary Hospitalisation was Right or Wrong: A Qualitative Study." *Social Psychiatry and Psychiatric Epidemiology* (August 24, 2011) [e-pub ahead of print]. http://dx.doi.org/10.1007/s00127-011-0427-z (accessed November 4, 2011).

O'Donoghue, B. "Perceptions of Involuntary Admission and Risk of Subsequent Readmission at One-Year Follow-Up: The Influence of Insight and Recovery Style." *Journal of Mental Health* (UK) 20, no. 3 (2011): 249–59.

Russell, B. J. "How Research Ethics' Protections can Contribute to Public Policy: The Case of Community Treatment Orders." *International Journal of Law and Psychiatry* 34, no. 5 (2011): 349–53.

OTHER

Lee, Megan. "HB 243—Mental Health/Law Enforcement Custody: North Carolina Statutory Changes for Involuntary Commitment" (October 1, 2009). North Carolina American Society for Healthcare Risk Management. http://www.nc-ashrm.org/pdfs/HB_243.pdf (accessed July 14, 2011).

WEBSITES

Join Together staff. "Laws About Involuntary Commitment for Substance Abuse Vary Widely among States." DrugFree.org. http://www.drugfree.org/join-together/addiction/laws-about-involuntary-commitment-for-substance-abuse-vary-widely-among-states (accessed July 14, 2011).

Longstreth, Andrew. "Before Tucson Rampage, a Powerful Law Went Unused." Reuters Legal (January 13, 2011). http://www.reuters.com/article/2011/01/13/us-usa-shooting-law-idUSTRE70C6JQ20110113 (accessed July 14, 2011).

Virginia Department of Behavioral Health and Development Services. "Mental Health Law Reform." Virginia.gov. http://www.dbhds.virginia.gov/OMH-MHReform.htm (accessed July 14, 2011).

ORGANIZATIONS

Mental Health America, 2000 N Beauregard St., 6th Fl., Alexandria, VA, 22311, (703) 684-7722, (800) 969-6642, Fax: (703) 684-5968, http://www.nmha.org.

National Alliance on Mental Illness, 3803 North Fairfax Dr., Ste. 100, Arlington, VA, 22203, (703) 524-7600, Fax: (703) 524-9094, http://www.nami.org.

National Mental Health Consumers' Self-Help Clearinghouse, 1211 Chestnut St., Ste. 1207, Philadelphia, PA, 19107, (215) 751-1810, Fax: (215) 636-6312, (800) 553-4539, info@mhselfhelp.org, http://mhselfhelp.org.

Treatment Advocacy Center, 200 N. Glebe Rd., Ste. 730, Arlington, VA, 22203, (703) 294-6001, Fax: (703) 294-6010, info@treatmentadvocacycenter.org, http://www.treatmentadvocacycenter.org.

Judy Leaver, MA
William Atkins, BB, BS, MBA

Isocarboxazid

Definition

Isocarboxazid (brand name Marplan) is an older-generation antidepressant drug.

Purpose

It is used to treat symptoms associated with **major depressive disorder**. Major depressive disorder refers to a long-lasting bout of depressed mood that is severe enough to interfere with basic life activities like work, relationships, sleeping, and eating. Feelings of self-worth, interest, motivation, and pleasure are typically absent while worthlessness, emptiness, being overwhelmed, and sadness are often reported.

Isocarboxazid is used for long-term maintenance of major **depression** and may be most useful for patients whose depression has atypical features. Unless effectiveness has already been established for a particular patient, isocarboxazid would not be the first drug of choice. Its use is limited to those patients who do not respond to first-line **antidepressants** and who are amenable to close supervision. Isocarboxazid's status as a drug of last resort (as is the case with other drugs in its class) is due to its potentially dangerous side effects and the dietary restrictions taking it requires.

The safety of isocarboxazid in children has not been established.

Description

Isocarboxazid belongs to the class of antidepressants known as **monoamine oxidase inhibitors (MAOIs)**. The **MAOIs** inhibit the function of an enzyme in the body called monoamine oxidase; that enzyme breaks down monoamine neurotransmitters—namely **serotonin**, **dopamine**, and norepinephrine. Under normal conditions, monoamine oxidase halts the action of these **neurotransmitters**. With MAOIs, the neurotransmitters last longer and accumulate, and their action is enhanced. It is this enhancement of neurotransmitter action that is thought to contribute to isocarboxazid's therapeutic efficacy.

There are two types of monoamine oxidases; they are denoted MAO-A and MAO-B. Isocarboxazid acts on both types, as do other nonselective **monoamine oxidase inhibitors** such as **phenelzine** and tranylcypromine.

Monoamine oxidase inhibitors do not elevate mood in non-depressed people. In depressed patients, they are used when other, first-line antidepressants are ineffective.

KEY TERMS

Antidepressant—A medication taken to alleviate clinical depression.

Dopamine—A chemical messenger in the brain that regulates reward and movement.

Hypertensive crisis—A precipitous rise in high blood pressure that can lead to brain hemorrhage or heart failure.

Major depressive disorder—A clinical psychiatric diagnosis of chronic depressed mood that interferes with normal life activities.

Monoamine oxidase inhibitors (MAOIs)—A class of antidepressant drugs that work by enhancing the neurotransmitters dopamine, norepinephrine, and serotonin in the brain.

Neurotransmitters—Chemical messengers that transmit signals between nerves.

Norepinephrine—A chemical messenger in the brain that regulates arousal and attention.

Serotonin—A chemical messenger in the brain that regulates arousal and mood.

Recommended dosage

Isocarboxazid is taken orally. As is the case with most antidepressant drugs, patients are started at one dose and medication is gradually increased to a so-called maintenance dose to achieve the best outcome. For isocarboxazid, the starting dose is 10 mg, twice a day. Whereas dosage can vary widely in individual patients, a typical progression would be to increase the dose gradually to 15–30 mg twice a day as a maintenance dose. Because of the delayed therapeutic response, at least one to two weeks should pass before increasing the dose.

Precautions

Patients taking isocarboxazid must be warned about food interactions. Foods like aged cheese, beer, and red wine contain tyramine and in concert with MAOIs can result in hypertensive crisis. Other foods high in tyramine (or dopamine itself) are bananas, fava beans, figs, raisins, yogurt, sour cream, soy sauce, pickled herring, caviar, liver, and tenderized meats; these foods should not be consumed when taking isocarboxazid.

Hypertensive crisis can also occur with certain drug interactions. Monoamine oxidase inhibitors should not be taken with asthma drugs, cold and allergy medications, or diet drugs. Patients taking isocarboxazid should inform their doctors and dentists to avoid being administered a contraindicated medication.

Isocarboxazid use may negatively interact with certain health conditions. It should not be used in patients with cardiovascular disease, cerebrovascular disease, or liver disease, and great caution should be used if there is poor kidney function or a history of **seizures**.

Worsening of depression and risk of **suicide** are relevant to isocarboxazid, as they are to all antidepressant drugs. The risk is especially high during the lag time until therapeutic efficacy can be achieved. Close monitoring of patients for the first four weeks of treatment is advised.

Children and adults up to age 24 are at an increased risk of developing suicidal thoughts and behavior when taking antidepressants, including isocarboxazid. Patients of any age taking isocarboxazid should be monitored for signs of worsening depression or changes in behavior.

Side effects

Isocarboxazid, like the other MAOIs, can cause a variety of side effects apart from food interactions. Common side effects include dizziness and fainting associated with low blood pressure when standing up (orthostatic hypotension), sexual dysfunction, anxiety, headache, nausea, sleep disturbances, edema, constipation, and weight gain. Serious but less common side effects include hepatic damage.

Interactions

A patient should not take isocarboxazid at the same time as other antidepressants. Two to five weeks of wash-out time must pass before switching from a non-MAOI antidepressant drug to isocarboxazid.

The following drugs should not be taken with MAOIs: Stimulants like amphetamine, **methylphenidate**, and epinephrine; dopaminergic drugs like levodopa, L-tryptophan, and phenylalanine; over-the-counter cold and allergy medications like pseudoephedrine and dextromethorphan; diet drugs like ephedrine and phenylpropanolamine; and analgesics like meperidine.

Resources

BOOKS

Charney, Dennis S., and Charles B. Nemeroff. *The Peace of Mind Prescription: An Authoritative Guide to Finding the Most Effective Treatment for Anxiety and Depression.* New York: Mariner Books, 2006.

"Depressive Disorders." In *The Merck Manual of Diagnosis and Therapy*, edited by Robert S. Porter and Justin L. Kaplan. 19th ed. Whitehouse Station, NJ: Merck, 2011.

"Major Depressive Disorder: A Quick Reference Guide." In *Quick Reference to the American Psychiatric Association Practice Guidelines for the Treatment of Psychiatric Disorders: Compendium 2006/Edition 1.* Arlington, VA: American Psychiatric Publishing, 2006.

"Monoamine Oxidase Inhibitors." In *AHFS Drug Information* Bethesda, MD: American Society of Health-System Pharmacists, 2012.

Morrison, Andrew L. *The Antidepressant Sourcebook: A User's Guide for Patients and Families.*New York: Doubleday, 1999.

Jill U. Adams

J

Jet lag *see* **Circadian rhythm sleep disorder**

Journal therapy

Definition

Journal therapy is the purposeful and intentional use of a written record of personal thoughts or feelings to promote growth and psychological healing. It is often used as an adjunct to **psychotherapy** and recovery programs. Healthcare practitioners maintain that written expression fills a very important role in the therapeutic process by providing a mechanism of emotional expression in circumstances in which interpersonal expression is not possible or viable.

Purpose

People have kept journals and diaries to record dreams, memories, and thoughts since ancient times. Emotional expression has also long held a central role in the study and practice of psychology. Throughout history, psychologists have advocated the expression of emotions as essential for good mental and physical health. Since the early 1980s, interest in this topic has resulted in numerous research studies investigating the health benefits of expressive writing.

Description

Journal writing and other forms of writing therapy are based on the premise that the mind and the body are inseparably joined in the healing process. Although there are many methods of conducting journal writing therapy, the therapist often instructs the participant to write about a distressing or traumatic event or thought in one or more sessions.

KEY TERMS

Art therapy—The use of art to assess and treat an individual's development, abilities, personality, interests, concerns, or conflicts.

Psychodynamic—The scientific study of mental or conditional forces developing especially in early childhood and their effect on behavior and mental states.

Although researchers are uncertain about exactly how writing about traumas produces improvements in psychological well-being, some traumatic **stress** researchers believe that ordinary memories are qualitatively different from traumatic memories. Traumatic memories are more emotional and perceptual in nature. The memory is stored as a sensory perception, obsessional thought, or behavioral reenactment. It is associated with persistent, intrusive, and distressing symptoms, including avoidance and intense anxiety that result in observed psychological and biological dysfunction. Thus, one goal in treating traumatic memories is to find a means of processing them.

A narrative that becomes more focused and coherent over a number of writing sessions is often associated with increased improvement, according to several research studies. The memories become deconditioned and restructured into a personal, integrated narrative. Changes in psychological well-being after writing therapy may result from cognitive shifts about the **trauma** either during or after the writing process.

Benefits

Journal writing produces a number of benefits in healthy people. It enhances creativity, helps cope with stress, and provides a written record of memorable life experiences. Likewise, some researchers have found that journal writing has a number of psychological and physical health benefits for people who are ill.

Aside from a reduction in physical symptoms of disease, the psychological benefits include reconciling emotional conflicts, fostering self-awareness, managing behavior, solving problems, reducing anxiety, aiding reality orientation, and increasing self-esteem. Writing therapy has been used as an effective treatment for people with developmental, medical, educational, social, or psychological impairments and is practiced in mental health, rehabilitation, medical, educational, and forensic institutions. Populations of all ages, races, and ethnic backgrounds are served by writing therapy in individual, couple, family, and **group therapy** formats.

The therapeutic use of expressive writing allows individuals to confront topics that may be difficult to address verbally, which alleviates the constraints or inhibitions associated with not talking about the event. The psychological drain of prolonged inhibition is believed to cause or exacerbate stress-related disease processes. Some researchers have found that emotional expression facilitates cognitive processing of traumatic memories, which can help lead to positive emotional and physiological changes. Specifically, written emotional expression is believed to promote integration and understanding of the event(s), thereby reducing the negative emotions associated with the memories.

Precautions

It is advisable that journal therapy be conducted only by a licensed health professional, such as a certified **art therapy** practitioner or trained **psychologist** or **psychiatrist**. While journal writing classes available to the public may perform a variety of useful functions, these classes are not intended to provide psychological therapy. In journal therapy, the participant may, for example, uncover potentially traumatic, repressed, or painful memories. Therefore, a trained health professional may be necessary to supervise the process and treat these symptoms as they arise.

Preparation

In a healthcare setting, the participant often prepares for journal writing by receiving a set of instructions from the therapist. The therapist will explain the length and focus of the writing session or sessions. Other instructions may include directions about how to write, such as in a stream-of-consciousness fashion, without censorship or concern about grammar or style.

Research & general acceptance

Therapeutic writing became an increasingly popular topic in the late twentieth century, not only among trained healthcare professionals, but also among self-improvement speakers without medical training. Seminars, workshops, and Internet sites purportedly offering therapy though expressive writing sprang up around the nation and gained some popular acceptance. Despite the large body of research indicating that writing confers benefits on healthy people, the topic of writing therapy's affects on diseased individuals has not received a great deal of research attention. Although increasingly used by healthcare professionals as an adjunct to various therapeutic approaches, the practice has been criticized by some members of the healthcare community. Many researchers are skeptical of reports that so much measurable improvement in health status can occur in just a few brief writing sessions.

In the United Kingdom, the focus of journal therapy is on descriptive accounts and psychodynamic explanations for subjective improvements in the health status of participants. In the United States, on the other hand, the focus is on formal scientific research aimed at validating the impact of brief, highly standardized writing exercises on physical measures of illness. The research demonstrates that although physical measures of illness may change, the reasons for the change are not always clear.

Journal therapy is not a replacement for medical therapy or other forms of psychotherapy. It is generally accepted as a adjunct therapy that can help relieve stress and allow individuals to communicate feelings and emotions that may be difficult to verbalize.

QUESTIONS TO ASK YOUR DOCTOR

- Is journal therapy a good choice for me or my loved one?
- Can you recommend a therapist trained in journal therapy?
- What other mental or physical health treatments might be beneficial to me in addition to journal therapy?

Training & certification

Although journal therapy is often provided by certified instructors who receive variable amounts of training, journal therapy is best administered by a licensed psychologist (who may also be an art therapist) or psychiatrist.

Educational, professional, and ethical standards for art therapists who conduct writing therapy are regulated by the American Art Therapy Association. The American Art Therapy Credentials Board (ATCB), an independent organization, grants postgraduate supervised experience. A registered art therapist who successfully completes the written examination administered by the ATCB qualifies as Board Certified (ATR-BC), a credential requiring maintenance through continuing education credits.

Resources

BOOKS

Kapitan, Lynn. *An Introduction to Art Therapy Research.* New York: Routledge, 2010.

Penn, Peggy. *Joined Imaginations: Writing and Language in Therapy.* Chagrin Falls, OH: Taos Institute Publications, 2009.

Wadeson, Harriet. *Art Psychotherapy.* 2nd ed. Hoboken, NJ: John Wiley and Sons, 2010.

PERIODICALS

van Emmerik, Arnold, J.H. Kamphuis, and P.M.G. Emmelkamp. "Treating Acute Stress Disorder and Posttraumatic Stress Disorder with Cognitive Behavioral Therapy or Structured Writing Therapy: A Randomized Controlled Trial." *Psychotherapy and Psychosomatics* (2008) 77, no. 2, 93–100.

ORGANIZATIONS

American Art Therapy Association, 225 North Fairfax Street, Alexandria, VA, 22314, info@arttherapy.org, http://www.americanarttherapyassociation.org.

Art Therapy Credentials Board, 3 Terrace Way, Greensboro, NC, 27403-3660, (336) 482-2856, (877) 213-2822, Fax: (336) 482-2852, atcb@nbcc.org, http://www.atcb.org.

Genevieve Slomski
Tish Davidson, AM

Juvenile bipolar disorder

Definition

Juvenile **bipolar disorder** (also called manic-depressive illness) is a chronic condition characterized by repeated swings in mood between mania (a state of elation and high energy) and **depression**. Early-onset bipolar disorder is manic depression that appears very early in life. Historically it was thought that children could not suffer the mood swings of mania or depression, but recent research has revealed that bipolar disorder (or early temperamental features of it) can occur in very young children and that it is much more common than previously thought. This finding has sparked some controversy and some concern that the disorder is being overdiagnosed. As a result of further investigation into this controversy, a new classification has been suggested, for the fifth edition of the ***Diagnostic and Statistical Manual of Mental Disorders*** (*DSM-5*), due to publish in 2013. The new diagnosis, **disruptive mood dysregulation disorder** (DMDD), will not replace juvenile bipolar disorder but may allow more precise **diagnosis** of that entity and may also allow for improved treatment of children with bipolar disorder and children who have DMDD.

Although children with bipolar disorder have not been well studied, the condition is believed to occur as frequently as it does in adults, and it can affect children more severely, affecting about 1% of all adolescents between ages 14 and 18. Adults typically experience abnormally intense moods for weeks or months at a time, but children can have rapid shifts of mood that commonly cycle many times within the day. This cycling pattern is called ultra-ultra rapid or ultradian cycling, and it is most often associated with low arousal states in the mornings followed by afternoons and evenings of increased energy. Bipolar disorder is often hard to diagnose in children, because its symptoms are difficult to distinguish from those of other mental disorders. If left untreated, bipolar disorder can significantly affect a child's relationships, overall functioning, and school performance. It also can lead to violence, drug and **alcohol use**, and **suicide** attempts.

Demographics

The lifetime prevalence of bipolar disorder is between 1% and 3%. However, considering borderline cases, the rate may be as high as 6%. Some research suggests that as many as 1% of children may have bipolar disorder. Although the condition affects males and females equally, in children under 13 the cases are predominantly male.

Description

Juvenile bipolar disorder is a mental condition characterized by repeated episodes of depression, mania, or both symptoms. The child may experience extreme shifts in mood and behavior. For a child to be diagnosed with bipolar disorder, the condition must be severe enough to disrupt the child's normal functioning.

The fourth edition (revised text) of the ***Diagnostic and Statistical Manual of Mental Disorders*** (*DSM-IV-TR*) identifies three types of bipolar mood episodes (these episodes were defined for adults, not children):

- Manic episodes: an elevated or irritable mood that lasts for a period of at least one week

- Hypomanic episodes: a distinct period of persistently elevated, expansive, or irritable mood that lasts for at least four days
- Mixed episodes: increased energy and agitation, coupled with feelings of sadness and worthlessness

Three major subtypes of bipolar disorder exist—bipolar I disorder (BP-I), bipolar II disorder (BP-II), and bipolar disorder not otherwise specified (BP-NOS). The *DSM-IV-TR* defines these bipolar disorder subtypes as follows:

- BP-I: the occurrence of a manic or mixed episode that lasts for at least one week
- BP-II: alternating depressive and hypomanic episodes
- BP-NOS: cases that do not meet the full criteria for the other two bipolar disorder subtypes but that involve an elevated or irritable mood, plus two or three bipolar symptoms (difficulty concentrating, sleep changes, and so on) that are severe enough to interfere with functioning

Evidence exists that juvenile bipolar disorder is a different and more severe form than adult-onset bipolar disorder. The child may cycle more rapidly from emotional highs (elation) to lows (anger and irritability). Bipolar disorder often can coexist with other emotional and behavioral problems, such as **attention deficit hyperactivity disorder (ADHD)**, **conduct disorder** (CD), **schizophrenia**, and **anxiety disorders**.

Controversy surrounds the increasing incidence of juvenile bipolar disorder diagnoses. There are both clinicians and parents who feel that difficult children are often saddled unnecessarily with this diagnosis, which exposes children to the risks and potential side effects of the serious medications used to treat the disorder.

Causes and symptoms

Bipolar disorder has a strong genetic component. Studies suggest that the children or siblings of bipolar individuals have a four-to-six-fold increased risk of developing the disorder. Environmental factors, such as child maltreatment, also may play a role in the development of the condition.

Symptoms of bipolar disorder can be divided into two categories—manic symptoms and depressive symptoms. Children with bipolar disorder may swing through cycles of these two different types of emotions. Manic symptoms include:

- extreme shifts in mood, from anger to euphoria
- bursts of rage
- irritability
- increased energy
- over-inflated sense of self-esteem, grandiose behavior
- decreased need for sleep, without any apparent drowsiness during the day
- lack of attention, moving quickly from one topic or task to the next
- increased sexuality inappropriate to age
- agitation
- willingness to engage in risky behaviors

Depressive symptoms are at the opposite end of the mood spectrum. They include:

- persistent sadness (this can include unexplained crying episodes, reclusiveness, and increased sensitivity)
- decreased energy
- low self-esteem
- sleepiness and increased desire to sleep
- difficulty concentrating
- lack of interest in school and other activities
- persistent thoughts of death or suicide
- unexplained aches and pains
- alcohol or drug use

Children and adolescents with bipolar disorder may have difficulty regulating between these two types of moods. They may have explosive outbursts of anger lasting anywhere from a few minutes to a few hours, followed by periods of extreme happiness. Whereas adults can take months to cycle between mania and depression, children can cycle within weeks or even days, so they are more often symptomatic.

It is sometimes difficult to distinguish manic symptoms with those of ADHD, because hyperactivity and irritability can be hallmarks of both conditions, and both often occur simultaneously. Research suggests that more than half of children and adolescents with bipolar disorder also have ADHD. To distinguish bipolar disorder from ADHD, doctors look for symptoms that are unique to bipolar disorder, such as elated mood, decreased sleep, and grandiose behavior.

Diagnosis

Children with symptoms of bipolar disorder should see a **psychologist** or **psychiatrist** for evaluation, especially if a first-degree family member has a history of the condition. Evaluation is also important in children who are taking stimulant medications for ADHD and who are experiencing manic symptoms as a result. Children with bipolar disorder should be carefully monitored for associated problems, such as **substance abuse**, developmental delays, and suicide.

Diagnosis of children with bipolar disorder is often challenging because the condition can present with other mental disorders, such as depression, and because symptoms (such as boasting and elation) can be difficult to distinguish from other childhood disorders and normal childhood emotions. Doctors often use *DSM-IV* guidelines to diagnose children with bipolar disorder, but these were developed for adults, and the symptoms can differ.

Assessment should include personal and family histories of depression and mood disorders, and identification of mood changes. Diagnostic interviews and questionnaires, such as the diagnostic interview for children and adolescents-revised (DICA-R), the Diagnostic Interview Schedule for Children (DISC), and the Kiddie Schedule for Affective Disorders and Schizophrenia for School-Age Children (K-SADS), can be useful for diagnosis. Clinical rating scales, such as the Mania Rating Scale, can help doctors initially identify illness severity and later assess the effects of treatment on the child's symptoms.

When diagnosing mania episodes, 2005 treatment guidelines from the Academy of Child and Adolescent Psychiatry (AACAP) suggest that doctors use Frequency, Intensity, Number, and Duration (FIND) as a guide:

- Frequency: symptoms occur most days of the week
- Intensity: symptoms are severe enough to cause extreme disturbance in one area of a child's life or moderate disturbance in two areas
- Number: symptoms occur three to four times per day
- Duration: symptoms last for four hours a day (not necessarily contiguous)

Treatment

Most treatment recommendations for children with bipolar disorder are made based on adult research data, because little research has been done on the safety and efficacy of mood stabilizing medications in children. Doctors typically use two types of drugs to treat children with bipolar disorder: mood stabilizers (lithium, divalproex, **carbamazepine**, valproate) and atypical antipsychotics (**olanzapine**, **quetiapine**, **risperidone**). These drugs have only been approved by the U.S. Food and Drug Administration for bipolar disorder in adults, with the exception of lithium, which has been approved for children age 12 and older.

The AACAP panel recommends that doctors treat their patients with medication for a minimum of four to six weeks and reassess if there is a lack of response. Doctors should carefully monitor their patients who are taking these medications because of the risks of side effects. According to the AACAP practice parameters, doctors should consider effectiveness, phase of illness, tolerability, and patient history of medication response, among other factors, when prescribing these medications. Atypical antipsychotics can cause marked weight gain in some children, which can lead to heart problems and diabetes later in life. They have also been linked to a rare but serious condition called **tardive dyskinesia**, which is characterized by abnormal movements.

Drugs used to treat other mental health conditions, such as **antidepressants** for depression and stimulant medications used to treat ADHD, may lead to manic symptoms. If a child becomes manic while taking antidepressants or stimulants, the child may require treatment for bipolar disorder.

Some children with bipolar disorder may benefit from a combination of medication and **psychotherapy**, including **cognitive-behavioral therapy**, which teaches children how to recognize and cope with the emotions that are leading to their condition.

Prognosis

Children with bipolar disorder will typically require ongoing treatment with medication to prevent a **relapse**, and some will require a lifetime of treatment. Even with medication, bipolar disorder can be chronic, with symptoms persisting for many months or even years. In adolescents, bipolar disorder tends to be more chronic and treatment-resistant than it is in adults. The rate of relapse in young people can be greater than 50%.

Prevention

Although the initial onset of bipolar disorder is not preventable, there are strategies to help avoid a relapse. The family of the bipolar child can learn ways to identify relapse symptoms and how to avoid factors that may trigger relapse (such as substance abuse, **stress**, medication noncompliance, or **sleep deprivation**). Families also may be taught communication skills to improve their interpersonal relationships.

Resources

BOOKS

American Psychiatric Association. *Diagnostic and Statistical Manual of Mental Disorders,* 4th ed., text rev. Washington, DC: American Psychiatric Association, 2000.

Faedda, Gianni L., and Nancy B. Austin. *Parenting a Bipolar Child: What to Do and Why*. Oakland, CA: New Harbinger, 2006.

Lombardo, Gregory T. *Understanding the Mind of Your Bipolar Child: The Complete Guide to the Development, Treatment, and Parenting of Children with Bipolar Disorder*. New York: St. Martin's Press, 2006.

Mash, Eric J., and Russell A. Barkley, eds. *Treatment of Childhood Disorders,* 3rd ed. New York: Guilford Press, 2006.

PERIODICALS

Carlson, G. "The Concept of Bipolar Disorder in Children: A History of the Bipolar Controversy." *Child and Adolescent Psychiatry Clinics of North America* 18 (April 1, 2009): 257–71.

Schapir, L. "Bipolar Disorder and Severe Mood Dysregulation in Children and Adolescents." *Harefuah* 147 (June 1, 2008): 526–31.

Stringaris, A. "Irritability in Children and Adolescents: A Challenge for DSM-5." *European Child and Adolescent Psychiatry* 20 (February 1, 2011): 61–66.

ORGANIZATIONS

Child & Adolescent Bipolar Foundation, 820 Davis St., Ste. 520, Evanston, IL, 60201, (847) 492-8510, info@thebalancedmind.org, http://www.thebalancedmind.org.

Depression and Bipolar Support Alliance, 730 N Franklin St., Ste. 501, Chicago, IL, 60654-7225, (800) 826-3632, http://www.dbsalliance.org.

Mental Health America, 2000 N Beauregard St., 6th Fl., Alexandria, VA, 22311, (800) 969-6642, http://www.nmha.org.

National Alliance on Mental Illness, 2107 Wilson Blvd., Ste. 300, Arlington, VA, 22201-3042, Fax: (703) 524-9094, (800) 950-6264, http://www.nami.org.

National Institute of Mental Health, 6001 Executive Blvd., Rm. 8184, MSC 9663, Bethesda, MD, 20892-9663, (301) 433-4513; TTY: (301) 443-8431, Fax: (301) 443-4279, (866) 615-6464; TTY: (866) 415-8051, nimhinfo@nih.gov, http://www.nimh.nih.gov.

Stephanie N. Watson

Juvenile depression

Definition

A **diagnosis** of **depression** is made when the feelings of sadness are severe enough to disrupt the child's daily life. Significant depression also can interfere with a child's development and can potentially lead to alcohol or drug use or **suicide**. Children who experience depression are more likely to be depressed as adults.

Demographics

Approximately 1% to 2% of children and 5% of adolescents experience symptoms of depression, and 3% to 5% of young people have major depressive disorder. The incidence of depression is lower in young children and rises after puberty. In childhood, the rates of depression are about equal in boys and girls, but in adolescence, girls are more than twice as likely to be depressed as boys, possibly due to hormonal changes that occur during puberty. Additionally, girls tend to have an internal locus of control, which is related to self-blame versus the external locus of control experienced by many adolescent males.

Prevalence of major depressive episodes (MDE) in adolescents

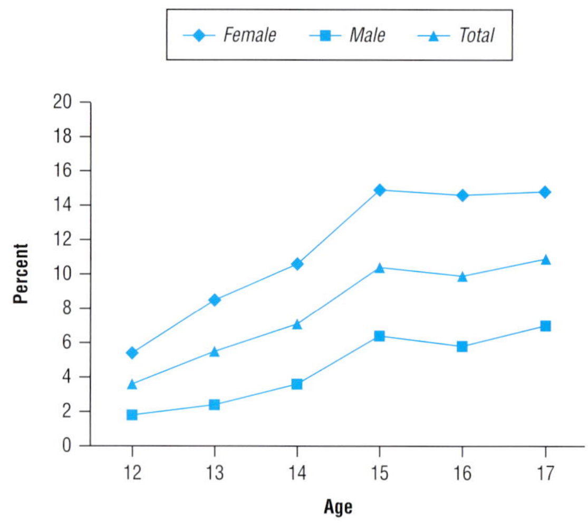

SOURCE: Substance Abuse and Mental Health Services Administration, Center for Behavioral Health Statistics and Quality, "Major Depressive Episode and Treatment among Adolescents: 2009," *The NSDUH Report* (April 28, 2011).

Percentage of adolescents who have experienced an MDE during the past year, by gender. Data available online at http://oas.samhsa.gov/2k11/009/AdolescentDepression.htm. *(Graph by PreMediaGlobal. © 2012 Cengage Learning.)*

One in eight adolescents may suffer from depression; in fact, depression is the most common mental disease in United States for this age group. Studies show that 10–15% of teenagers have already experienced traumatic feelings of depression at some time of their life.

About two-thirds of children with depression have a concurrent mental disorder and thus are at higher risk for developing depression again after receiving treatment. Children with depression have a two- to fourfold increased risk of being depressed as adults. Nearly three-quarters of children and adolescents with depressive disorders do not receive appropriate treatment.

Description

Research has indicated that rates of depression have risen in children and adolescents during the last few decades, although the reason for this rise is unclear. Just as in adults, depression in children can range in severity.

Major depressive disorder is the most severe form of depression. The ***Diagnostic and Statistical Manual***

of Mental Disorders, fourth edition, text revised (*DSM-IV TR*), defines a major depressive episode as five or more symptoms (which can include depressed mood or irritability most of the day, markedly diminished interest in activities, significant weight loss without dieting, **insomnia** or **hypersomnia** nearly every day, agitation, **fatigue**, feelings of worthlessness or guilt, diminished ability to think or concentrate, and recurrent thoughts of death or suicide) within a two-week period.

Dysthymic disorder is a milder, but chronic, form of depression that persists for at least one year in children (episodes last between two and three years). It is characterized by symptoms of depression or irritability, as well as appetite changes, difficulty sleeping, low self-esteem, fatigue, poor concentration, or feelings of hopelessness. Dysthymia can interfere with a child's relationships, schoolwork, and self-esteem.

Causes and symptoms

Although in some cases depression stems from a life event, in other situations it arises without apparent cause.

Causes

Doctors are unsure about the underlying causes of depression, but the problem may arise from neurotransmitter abnormalities in the **brain**. Changes in the prefrontal cortex have been noted in childhood depression, and hormones also seem to play a role.

Depression has both genetic and social components. The condition runs in families, and there is evidence that a child is more likely to develop depression if his or her parent is depressed. Studies have indicated that identical twins, who share the same genes, are about three times more likely to both have major depressive disorder than are fraternal twins, who share fewer of the same genes. It also is possible that growing up with a parent who is depressed makes a child more prone to duplicating the behavior. Negative parenting tactics (such as rejection and lack of nurturing) also can influence the development of depression.

Stressful experiences, such as the death of a loved one, moving to a new city, living in poverty, or suffering sexual or physical **abuse**, can trigger depression, especially in children who are already vulnerable due to inherited factors. Depression can be distinguished from normal sadness during these experiences because its duration is disproportionate to the event.

In some cases, a medical condition, such as cancer, infectious mononucleosis, anemia, thyroid disease, or vitamin deficiency, can trigger depression. Some medications, such as isotretinoin (Accutane), may also lead to depressive symptoms. Depression stemming from illness or medication is referred to as secondary depressive mood disorder.

Symptoms

A child who is experiencing depression may have uncontrollable feelings of sadness. He or she may lose interest in friends, school, and activities. Other symptoms of depression include:

- Feelings of worthlessness or hopelessness
- Crying for no apparent reason
- Change in appetite
- Weight loss or gain
- Disrupted or prolonged sleep
- Lack of energy
- Difficulty concentrating
- Irritable, aggressive, or hostile behaviors
- Aches and pains that have no known medical cause (this is particularly common in children under age seven, who are less able to articulate their emotions)
- Alcohol or drug use
- Suicidal thoughts or actions

Depression often occurs together with other mental disorders, including **anxiety disorders**, **attention deficit hyperactivity disorder**, **substance abuse** disorder, and **oppositional defiant disorder**.

Diagnosis

Diagnosing depression may begin with the child's primary care doctor, who can make a referral to a child **psychiatrist** or **psychologist** if necessary. The doctor will typically start a depression evaluation by interviewing the child and his or her parents. The assessment may include a physical history and examination to rule out any conditions that can cause depression, such as thyroid disorders.

To diagnose depression, doctors sometimes used questionnaires or scales. The **Children's Depression Inventory** (CDI) is commonly used to diagnose children ages 7 to 17 years old. The results of this inventory are represented as a t-score. A t-score of greater than 20 on the long form or greater than 7 on the short form indicates a diagnosis of clinical depression.

Because patients with depression are at greater risk for attempting suicide (major depression increases the suicide risk 12-fold), doctors should assess the child's suicide risk during the initial visit.

QUESTIONS TO ASK YOUR DOCTOR

- What are the indications that my child may suffer from juvenile depression?
- What diagnostic tests are needed for a thorough assessment?
- What treatment options do you recommend for my child?
- What kind of changes can I expect to see with the medications you have prescribed for my child?
- What are the side effects associated with the medications you have prescribed for my child?
- Should we see a specialist? If so, what kind of specialist should I contact?
- Does having depression put my child at risk for other health conditions?
- What tests or evaluation techniques will you perform to see whether treatment has been beneficial for my child?
- What symptoms or adverse effects are important enough that I should seek immediate treatment?
- Can you recommend an organization that will provide me with additional information about juvenile depression?
- Can you recommend any support groups for me and my family?

Treatment

Treatment methods for children with depression include therapy and medication. Therapy may be conducted individually, in groups, or with the child's family. **Cognitive-behavioral therapy** (CBT) is the most thoroughly studied treatment for childhood depression, and research indicates that it is effective for treating mild to moderate depression. CBT involves changing the negative or distorted thoughts that are leading to the depression, and improving the child's coping skills. The therapist can help the child deal with **grief** and more appropriately handle his or her emotions, as well as educate the parents about developing healthier communication strategies and familial relationships. **Interpersonal therapy** (IPT), which is based on the belief that depression is triggered by interpersonal disputes, has also been shown to positively influence depressive symptoms in children and adolescents.

Some newer complementary approaches may be helpful to children with mild depression, including **music therapy**, pet therapy, **dance therapy**, guided imagery, and **yoga**.

In moderate to severe cases of depression, doctors may prescribe antidepressant medications called **selective serotonin reuptake inhibitors (SSRIs)**, such as **fluoxetine** (Sarafem) and **paroxetine** (Paxil). As of 2011, fluoxetine was the only SSRI approved by the U.S. Food and Drug Administration for treating depression in children 8 to 17 years of age. **SSRIs** work by restoring the correct balance of **serotonin** in the brain. However, because **antidepressants** have been linked to an increased risk of suicidal thoughts and behaviors in children and adolescents (the packaging of SSRIs carries a black-box warning regarding this risk), doctors should carefully monitor their young patients for any signs of suicidal tendencies during treatment. Due to their high risk of side effects and lack of effectiveness in a younger population, tricyclic antidepressants such as **imipramine** (Tofranil) are not recommended for children and adolescents.

The recommended treatment duration for children experiencing their first episode of depression is at least six months. Medication should be tapered off over a period of one to two months to prevent symptoms of withdrawal. Subsequent depressive episodes require at least one year of treatment, and children who have had more than three episodes should be treated indefinitely. More severe cases of depression may require a combination of medication and **psychotherapy**. Patients with treatment-resistant depression may require additional medication, such as lithium, as well as extended CBT.

Children or adolescents who are exhibiting suicidal behaviors may be hospitalized until it has been determined that they are no longer a danger to themselves.

Prognosis

Research indicates that starting treatment early can improve the outcomes for children and adolescents with depression. Children usually recover sooner from major depressive episodes than adults. In most cases, children will recover from an initial depressive episode within one to two years, even if they have not been treated in some cases. However, children who have had at least one depressive episode face an increased risk of recurrence during adolescence and adulthood.

Prevention

Although little research exists on the prevention of depression in children, there is some evidence that CBT can prevent the onset of major depression in children

KEY TERMS

Anxiety—Can be experienced as a troubled feeling, a sense of dread, fear of the future, or distress over a possible threat to a person's physical or mental well-being.

Attention deficit hyperactivity disorder (ADHD)—A developmental disorder characterized by distractibility, hyperactivity, impulsive behaviors, and the inability to remain focused on tasks or activities.

Cognitive-behavioral therapy—Psychotherapy technique designed to help people change their attitudes, perceptions, and patterns of thinking.

Insomnia—Waking in the middle of the night and having difficulty returning to sleep, or waking too early in the morning.

Serotonin—A chemical messenger in the brain thought to play a role in mood regulation.

with depressive symptoms and/or anxiety disorders. Family dynamics also can have an impact on the development of depression. A stable, loving, and communicative family can decrease a child's vulnerability to the condition. Parents can help prevent potential problems by identifying depression earlier, when the treatment success odds are greatest. Early identification of depression involves looking for the warning signs, which may be more subtle in children than they are in adults. For example, a depressed child may appear bored, overly tired, withdrawn, or irritable. Children with depression also may experience aches and pains that are not associated with any obvious medical condition.

Resources

BOOKS

American Psychiatric Association. *Diagnostic and Statistical Manual of Mental Disorders.* 4th ed., Text rev. Washington, DC: American Psychiatric Association, 2000.

American Psychological Association. *Publication Manual of the American Psychological Association*, 6th ed. Washington, DC: American Psychological Association, 2009.

Gillberg, Christopher, Richard Harrington, and Hans-Christoph Steinhausen, eds. *A Clinician's Handbook of Child and Adolescent Psychiatry*. Cambridge: Cambridge University Press, 2011.

Jongsma, Arthur E., Jr., L. Mark Peterson, and William P. McInnis. *The Child Psychotherapy Treatment Planner.* 4th ed. Hoboken, NJ: John Wiley & Sons, 2009.

North, Carol, and Sean Yutzy. *Goodwin and Guze's Psychiatric Diagnosis.*New York, NY: Oxford University Press, 2010.

WEBSITES

U.S. National Institute of Mental Health. "Combination Treatment Most Effective in Adolescents with Depression." http://www.nimh.nih.gov/science-news/2004/combination-treatment-most-effective-in-adolescents-with-depression.shtml (accessed November 14, 2011).

ORGANIZATIONS

American Academy of Child and Adolescent Psychiatry, 3615 Wisconsin Ave. NW, Washington, DC, 20016-3007, (202) 966-7300, Fax: (202) 966-2891, http://aacap.org.

American Academy of Pediatrics (AAP), 141 Northwest Point Blvd., Elk Grove Village, IL, 60009-0927, (847) 434-4000, http://www.aap.org.

American Psychological Association, 750 First Street NE, Washington, DC, 20003, (202) 336-5500, http://www.apa.org/index.aspx.

Eunice Kennedy Shriver National Institute of Child Health and Human Development (NICHD), Bldg 31, Room 2A32, MSC 2425, 31 Center Drive, Bethesda, MD, 20892, (800) 370-2943; TTY: (888) 320-6942, Fax: (866) 760-5947, NICHDInformationResourceCenter@mail.nih.gov, http://www.nichd.nih.gov.

Families for Depression Awareness, 395 Totten Pond Road, Ste. 404, Waltham, MA, 02451, (781) 890-0220, Fax: (781) 890-2411, http://www.familyaware.org.

Mental Health America, 2000 N. Beauregard Street, 6th Floor, Alexandria, VA, 22311, (703) 684-7722, (800) 969-6642, Fax: (703) 684-5968, http://www1.nmha.org.

National Alliance on Mental Illness (NAMI), Colonial Place Three, 2107 Wilson Blvd., Suite 300, Arlington, VA, 22201, (703) 524-7600, (800) 950-NAMI (6264), Fax: (703) 524-9094, http://www.nami.org/Hometemplate.cfm.

National Institute of Mental Health (NIMH), 6001 Executive Boulevard, Room 8184, MSC 9663, Bethesda, MD, 20892, (301) 443-4513, (866) 615-6464, Fax: (301) 443-4279, nimhinfo@nih.gov, http://www.nimh.nih.gov/index.shtml.

Stephanie N. Watson
Laura Jean Cataldo, RN, Ed.D.

K

Kaufman Adolescent and Adult Intelligence Test

Definition

The Kaufman Adolescent and Adult Intelligence Test (KAIT) is an individually administered general intelligence test appropriate for adolescents and adults aged 11 to over 85 years. The multi-subtest is considered a battery of neuropsychological, vocational, and clinical tasks, what is called a psychoeducational evaluation. The KAIT requires reasoning and planning abilities, which makes it an interesting and challenging test for anyone to take.

Purpose

The KAIT is intended to measure both fluid and crystallized intelligence. Fluid intelligence refers to abilities such as problem solving and reasoning, and it is generally thought not to be influenced by one's cultural experience or education. Crystallized intelligence refers to acquired knowledge, and it is thought to be influenced by one's cultural experience and education.

The KAIT was developed by American psychologists Alan S. Kaufman (1944–) and Nadeen L. Kaufman (1945–), a husband and wife team, as a method of measuring intelligence assuming broader definitions of fluid and crystallized abilities than assumed by other measures. In addition, they wanted a test based on theories that accounted for developmental changes in intelligence, such as the Cattell-Horn model of fluid/crystallized intelligence. Although the Kaufmans had earlier designed a test for younger children, the **Kaufman Assessment Battery for Children** (K-ABC), they did not consider the KAIT to be an extension of this test. They believed that the developmental and neuropsychological changes specific to adults and adolescents warranted a different testing approach than did the changes relevant to younger children. Thus, a different approach was used when developing the KAIT, although the K-ABC was also based somewhat on the split between fluid and crystallized intelligence.

Theoretically, the KAIT is most influenced by J.L. Horn and Raymond B. Cattell's formulation of the distinction between fluid and crystallized intelligence, sometimes referred to as Gf-Gc theory. Gf refers to general fluid abilities and Gc refers to general crystallized abilities. The KAIT is also influenced by Piaget's theory of cognitive development, specifically the formal operations stage experienced in adolescence. During this stage, adolescents begin to perform complex mental operations and are better able to transform and manipulate information. Another theoretical influence of the KAIT is Luria's theory of planning ability. This theory attempted to explain developmental changes occurring in early adolescence that influence decision making and problem solving.

Description

The KAIT includes two components, a core battery and an expanded battery. The core battery consists of a fluid scale (Fluid IQ, which is short for intelligence quotient), a crystallized scale (Crystallized IQ), composite scale (Composite IQ), and six subtests, and takes about one hour (58 to 73 minutes) to complete. The expanded battery includes the core battery elements as well as four additional subtests and takes about 1.5 hours (83 to 102 minutes) to complete.

The tests for fluid intelligence use paired-associative learning and deductive reasoning. The test taker must use inductive reasoning and deductive reasoning to complete the assignments. The following core battery subtests are related to fluid intelligence (general fluid scale, Gf):

- logical steps, a test of sequential reasoning (visual and oral statements are presented, and the test taker uses logic to solve problems)
- mystery codes, a test measuring induction (test taker must solve a code used to identify a set of pictures, and then uses that code on a new set of pictures)

- rebus learning, a test of long-term memory (a word or concept is learned as provided by a picture representing the word [a rebus], and the test taker reads phrases and sentences composed of these rebuses)

The tests for crystallized intelligence use measures of lexical (word) knowledge and listening abilities. The test taker must synthesize and integrate the provided materials, along with memory, to complete the tasks. The following core battery subtests are related to crystallized intelligence (general crystallized scale, Gc):

- definitions: a test of word knowledge and language development (two sets of word clues are presented, and the test taker provides a word with two different meanings that fits both clues)
- double meanings: a measure of language comprehension (two clues are provided, a word with some letters missing and an oral clue about the meaning of the word, and the test taker responds with the word)
- auditory comprehension: a test of listening ability (test taker listens to a recording or words spoken by the administrator and answers questions about the story)

The expanded battery (measures of delayed recall) also includes:

- memory for block designs, a measure of visual processing related to fluid intelligence (test taker briefly looks at a printed design and builds the design using six cubes and a formboard)
- famous faces, a test of cultural knowledge related to crystallized intelligence (test taker names people of current or historical notoriety based on their picture and verbal clues)
- auditory delayed recall (test taker answers questions about news stories during the administration of auditory comprehension, within crystallized intelligence)
- rebus delayed recall, the two delayed recall subtests provide a general measure of delayed memory (test taker reads phrases and sentences composed of rebuses earlier learned during rebus learning, within fluid intelligence)

There is also an optional supplemental **mental status examination** included in the KAIT battery. The ten items within the mental status measure attention and orientation in time and space. This subtest is only given to examinees with possible mental impairment.

One strength of the KAIT is that most of the subtests are presented in both visual and auditory formats. This gives test takers more variety and allows for measurement of intelligence in different contexts. Also, the test was designed in a way to keep test takers active and engaged.

KEY TERMS

IQ—The acronym for intelligence quotient, or a score derived from one of several standardized tests for intelligence.

Lexical—Relating to individual words that make up a language.

Neuropsychological—Relating to neuropsychology, or the branch of neurology that studies behavior disorders such as memory loss, speech impairment, epilepsy, and others.

Rebus—A puzzle in which syllables of words and names are represented by pictures of objects that sound similar or by letters.

In contrast to other adult-specific or adolescent-specific **intelligence tests**, the KAIT is appropriate for a wider age range. This allows for more accurate tracking of intelligence changes between adolescence and adulthood.

Preparation

Preparation for the Kaufman Adolescent and Adult Intelligence Test is not needed nor necessary.

Precautions

There are very specific rules governing administration of the test that must be adhered to for scoring to be accurate. Thus, administrators must be properly trained to administer the KAIT. Specifically, for all subtests there is a discontinue rule, instructing administrators when to stop administering test items.

The KAIT is not appropriate for children younger than 11 years. A test more appropriate for younger children, such as the K-ABC, should be given instead. The K-ABC is appropriate for children up to the age of 12 years, 6 months, so there is some overlap between the two tests, specifically for children between the ages of 11 and 12 years, 6 months.

Parental concerns

When children take the KAIT, parents should be comforted that it is considered highly reliable and valid, consistently measured, and widely used throughout the professional psychological community for assessment of intelligence.

Results

The KAIT yields several different kinds of scores, including raw scores, scaled scores, and intelligent quotient (IQ) scores. Raw scores and scaled scores are calculated for each subtest (6 for the core battery; 10 for the expanded battery). Raw scores are calculated first, and simply refer to the number of points achieved by the examinee on a particular subtest. Raw scores are converted to scaled scores to ease comparison between subtests and between examinees. The subtest scaled scores are standardized to have a mean of 10 and a standard deviation of 3.

Three IQ scores are obtained: composite intelligence, fluid intelligence, and crystallized intelligence. The IQ scores have a mean of 100 and a standard deviation of 15. The fluid intelligence IQ score is based on the sum of the three fluid intelligence subtests (logical steps, mystery codes, and rebus learning). The crystallized intelligence IQ score is based on the sum of the three crystallized intelligence subtests (definitions, double meanings, and auditory comprehension). The composite intelligence IQ score is based on all six core subtests. The expanded battery subtests are not utilized when computing the three IQ scores.

The KAIS was normalized on a sample of 2,000 people, aged 11 to over 85 years, taken from a representative population within the United States, based on gender, race/ethnic group, and socioeconomic status (of adults or parents, in the case of children). Thirteen age levels composed the group, with at least 125 individuals in each level. Overall, the KAIT has high reliability and validity. Studies have indicated that in relation to other general intelligence tests, the crystallized, fluid, and composite IQ scores are accurately and consistently measured. Data looking at trends related to age show that average subtest and IQ scores are fairly consistent across the age range in which the KAIT is administered.

The KAIT yields IQ scores in a relatively wide range, from much lower than average intelligence to much higher than average intelligence. Because of this, the KAIT is often used as an assessment of individuals with exceptional abilities, such as gifted children.

There have been factor analysis studies comparing the KAIT to the widely used **Wechsler Intelligence Scales** (the Wechsler Intelligence Scale for Children and the Wechsler Adult Intelligence Scale). The KAIT crystallized IQ has been shown to measure abilities similar to those measured by the Wechsler scales' verbal intelligence factor. However, the KAIT Fluid IQ has been shown to measure abilities considerably different from those measured by the Wechsler performance factor, which is thought to be a measure of fluid intelligence.

QUESTIONS TO ASK YOUR DOCTOR

- Do you know of a properly trained administrator for the KAIT?
- Should another test for intelligence be administered in parallel with the KAIT?
- Will my health insurance cover the test?

See also Stanford-Binet intelligence scales

Resources

BOOKS

Boyer, Bret A., and M. Indira Paharia, eds. *Comprehensive Handbook of Clinical Health Psychology*. Hoboken, NJ: John Wiley and Sons, 2008.

Groth-Marnat, Gary. *Handbook of Psychological Assessment*. 4th ed. Hoboken, NJ: John Wiley and Sons, 2003.

Hersen, Michel, ed. *Comprehensive Handbook of Psychological Assessment*. Hoboken, NJ: John Wiley and Sons, 2004.

Kellerman, Henry, and Anthony Burry. *Handbook of Psychodiagnostic Testing: Analysis of Personality in the Psychological Report*. New York: Springer, 2007.

Leeming, David A., Kathryn Madden and Stanton Marlan, eds. *Encyclopedia of Psychology and Religion*. New York: Springer, 2010.

WEBSITES

"Alan S. Kaufman, PhD, and Nadeen L. Kaufman, EdD" [biography]. McGraw-Hill Higher Education. http://www.mhhe.com/mayfieldpub/psychtesting/profiles/karfmann.htm (accessed December 15, 2011).

"Author Bios: Alan S. Kaufman, PhD, and Nadeen L. Kaufman, EdD." Pearson. http://pearsonassessments.com/pai/ca/research/resources/authors/Alan_Nadeen_Kaufman (accessed December 15, 2011).

"Kaufman Adolescent and Adult Intelligence Test (KAIT)." Pearson. http://pearsonassessments.com/HAIWEB/Cultures/en-us/Productdetail.htm?Pid=PAa3650&Mode=summary (accessed December 15, 2011).

"Kaufman Adolescent and Adult Intelligence Test." Nova Southeastern University. http://www.cps.nova.edu/~cpphelp/KAIT.html (accessed December 15, 2011).

Ali Fahmy, Ph.D.

Kaufman Assessment Battery for Children

Definition

The Kaufman Assessment Battery for Children (K-ABC) is a standardized, psychological diagnostic test that assesses cognitive ability (intelligence measured through an intelligence quotient, or IQ) and achievement in children. The original K-ABC was geared to children aged 2 years and 6 months to 12 years and 6 months. The first edition published in 1983 by American psychologists Alan S. Kaufman (1944–) and Nadeen L. Kaufman (1945–) was revised in 2002 (second edition: KABC-II) by the husband-and-wife team to expand its age range (to cover children ages 2.5 to 18 years) and enhance its usefulness. In addition, new subtests were added and existing subtests updated. The KABC-II (referred to as the K-ABC) has a dual theoretical foundation: the Luria neuropsychological model and the Cattell/Horn/Carroll (CHC) model.

Purpose

The K-ABC was developed specifically to evaluate preschoolers, minority groups, and children with learning disabilities and various other disabilities. It is used to provide educational planning and placement, neurological assessment, and research. The assessment is to be administered in a school or clinical setting and is intended for use with English-speaking, bilingual, or nonverbal children. There is also a Spanish edition for use with children whose primary language is Spanish.

Description

Administration of the K-ABC core battery takes between 25 and 55 minutes when the Luria model is administered and between 35 and 70 minutes when the CHC model is used. The Luria model is generally administered for children with "mainstream" cultural and language knowledge and background. The CHC model, which excludes verbal testing, is used for "non-mainstream" children. The older the child, the longer the test generally takes to administer. It is comprised of four global test scores that include:

- sequential processing scales (Gsm), in which the child solves problems involving sequences, such as arranging objects in a series, and completes tasks involving short-term memory, such as recalling numbers or objects in sequence
- simultaneous processing scales (Gv), in which the child solves complex problems involving (1) face recognition, (2) partially complete picture identification, (3) design reproduction with use of rubber triangles, (4) picture selection that completes another picture, (5) picture selection that is similar to another picture, (6) picture location recall, and (7) picture arrangement based on logical order
- achievement scales, in which the child answers questions based on facts learned about famous people and places, mathematics, and story characters
- mental processing composite, a combination of the sequential processing scales and the simultaneous processing scales

There is an additional nonverbal scale that allows applicable subtests to be administered through gestures to hearing impaired, speech/language impaired, or children who do not speak English.

The test consists of 16 subtests—10 mental processing subtests and 6 achievement subtests. Not all subtests are administered to each age group, and only 3 subtests are administered to all age groups. Children ages 2 years, 6 months are given 7 subtests, and the number of subtests given increase with the child's age. For any one child, a maximum of 13 subtests are administered. Children from age 7 years to 12 years, 6 months are given 13 subtests.

The sequential processing scales primarily measure short-term memory and consists of subtests that measure problem-solving skills where the emphasis is on following a sequence or order. The child solves tasks by arranging items in serial or sequential order including reproducing hand taps on a table or recalling numbers that were presented. It also contains a subtest that measures a child's ability to recall objects in the correct order as presented by the examiner.

The simultaneous processing scales examine problem-solving skills that involve several processes at once.

KEY TERMS

IQ—The acronym for intelligence quotient, or a score derived from one of several standardized tests for intelligence.

Neuropsychological—Relating to neuropsychology, or the branch of neurology that studies behavior disorders such as memory loss, speech impairment, epilepsy, and others.

Psychometric—The branch of psychology that deals with the measurement of mental capacities, traits, and processes.

The scales use seven subtests: facial recognition, identification of objects or scenes in a partially completed picture, reproduction of a presented design by using rubber triangles, selecting a picture that completes or is similar to another picture, memory for location of pictures presented on a page, and arrangement of pictures in meaningful order.

The achievement scales measure achievement and focus on applied skills and facts that were learned through the school or home environment. The subtests are expressive vocabulary; ability to name fictional characters, famous persons, and well-known places; mathematical skills; ability to solve riddles; readings and decoding skills; and reading and comprehension skills.

The sequential and simultaneous processing scales are combined to comprise the mental processing composite. This composite measures intelligence on the K-ABC and concentrates on the child's ability to solve unfamiliar problems simultaneously and sequentially. The simultaneous processing scales have a greater impact on the mental processing composite score than do the sequential processing scales. The mental processing composite score is considered the global estimate of a child's level of intellectual functioning.

Preparation

Preparation for the Kaufman Assessment Battery for Children is not needed nor necessary.

Risks

The K-ABC is especially useful in providing information about nonverbal intellectual abilities. However, it has been criticized for not focusing on measures of verbal intelligence in the mental processing composite score, which measures intelligence. Additionally, researchers, who claim the two terms are misleading, have questioned the separation of intelligence and achievement scores. For example, many subtests in the achievement composite are in fact measures of intelligence rather than achievement (knowledge acquired through school and/or home environment). The K-ABC should be used with caution as the primary instrument for identifying the intellectual abilities of children.

Precautions

Administration and interpretation of results (as with all psychometric testing) requires a competent examiner who is trained in psychology and individual intellectual assessment—preferably a **psychologist**.

QUESTIONS TO ASK YOUR DOCTOR

- Do you know of a properly trained administrator for the K-ABC?
- What other test(s) for intelligence could be administered in parallel with the K-ABC? Which ones are best to be taken with the K-ABC?
- Should my child take the Lucia model or the CHC model of the test?
- Where can I learn more about the K-ABC?
- Will my health insurance cover the test?

Results

The K-ABC is a standardized test, which means that a large sample of children in the 2 years, 6 months to 12 years, 6 months age range was administered the examination as a means of developing test norms. Children in the sample were representative of the population of the United States based on age, gender, race or ethnic group, geographic region, community size, parental education, and educational placement (normal versus special classes). From this sample, norms were established.

Based on these norms, the global scales on the K-ABC each have a mean or average score of 100 and a standard deviation of 15. For this test, as with most measures of intelligence, a score of 100 is in the normal or average range. The standard deviation indicates how far above or below the norm a child's score is. For example, a score of 85 is one standard deviation below the norm score of 100.

Test scores provide an estimate of the level at which a child is functioning based on a combination of many different subtests or measures of skills. A trained psychologist is needed to evaluate and interpret the results, determine strengths and weaknesses, and make overall recommendations based on the findings and behavioral observations.

Parental concerns

When children take the K-ABC, parents should be comforted that it is considered highly reliable and valid, consistently measured, and widely used throughout the professional community for assessment of intelligence. However, the K-ABC primarily evaluates nonverbal intelligence, so it is limited with respect to measuring verbal intelligence. In addition, only a trained administrator should interpret the scores of the test.

Professionals advise that the K-ABC should not be used as the primary test, or as the only test, to assess intelligence in children. The K-ABC should be used in parallel with other appropriate intelligence and achievement tests, such as the Wechsler Intelligence Scale for Children.

Resources

BOOKS

Boyer, Bret A., and M. Indira Paharia, eds. *Comprehensive Handbook of Clinical Health Psychology*. Hoboken, NJ: John Wiley and Sons, 2008.

Groth-Marnat, Gary. *Handbook of Psychological Assessment*. 4th ed. Hoboken, NJ: John Wiley and Sons, 2003.

Hersen, Michel, ed. *Comprehensive Handbook of Psychological Assessment*. Hoboken, NJ: John Wiley and Sons, 2004.

Kellerman, Henry, and Anthony Burry. *Handbook of Psychodiagnostic Testing: Analysis of Personality in the Psychological Report*. New York: Springer, 2007.

Leeming, David A., Kathryn Madden and Stanton Marlan, eds. *Encyclopedia of Psychology and Religion*. New York: Springer, 2010.

Sattler, Jerome M. *Assessment of Children: Cognitive Foundations*. San Diego, CA: J.M. Sattler, 2008.

WEBSITES

"Alan S. Kaufman, PhD, and Nadeen L. Kaufman, EdD" [biography]. McGraw-Hill Higher Education. http://www.mhhe.com/mayfieldpub/psychtesting/profiles/karfmann.htm (accessed December 15, 2011).

"Author Bios: lan S. Kaufman, PhD, and Nadeen L. Kaufman, EdD." Pearson. http://pearsonassessments.com/pai/ca/research/resources/authors/Alan_Nadeen_Kaufman (accessed December 15, 2011).

"Kaufman Assessment Battery for Children." Nova Southeastern University. http://www.cps.nova.edu/~cpphelp/KABC.html (accessed December 16, 2011).

"Kaufman Assessment Battery for Children, Second Edition (KABC-II)." Pearson. http://psychcorp.pearsonassessments.com/HAIWEB/Cultures/en-us/Productdetail.htm?Pid=PAa21000&Mode=summary (accessed December 16, 2011).

ORGANIZATIONS

American Psychiatric Association, 1000 Wilson Blvd., Ste. 1825, Arlington, VA, 22209-3901, (703) 907-7300, apa@psych.org, http://www.psych.org.

American Psychological Association, 750 1st St. NE, Washington, DC, 20002-4242, (202) 336-5500; TDD/TTY: (202) 336-6123, (800) 374-2721, http://www.apa.org.

National Association of School Psychologists, 4340 East West Highway, Ste. 402, Bethesda, MD, 20002, (301) 657-0270, (800) 331-5277, Fax: (301) 657-0275, http://www.nasponline.org.

See also Intelligence tests; Luria-Nebraska Neuropsychological Battery

Jenifer P. Marom, Ph.D.

Kaufman Short Neurological Assessment Procedure

Definition

The Kaufman Short Neurological Procedure, often abbreviated as K-SNAP, is a brief test of mental functioning appropriate for adolescents and adults between the ages of 11 and 85 years. It is administered on an individual basis, and measures mental functioning at varying levels of cognitive complexity as well as addressing possible neurological damage.

Purpose

The K-SNAP is intended as a short measure of mental functioning and is sometimes preferable to other longer mental status and intelligence (IQ) examinations. Compared to the **Kaufman Adolescent and Adult Intelligence Test** (KAIT), which is given to people in the same age range and takes over an hour to complete, the K-SNAP takes only 20 to 30 minutes. The K-SNAP provides a measure of general mental status, as well as addressing specific mental abilities. It also allows for assessment of damage to the nervous system.

The K-SNAP was developed by American psychologists Alan S. Kaufman (1944–) and Nadeen L. Kaufman (1945–). Other Kaufman tests include the KAIT and the **Kaufman Assessment Battery for Children** (K-ABC). The Kaufmans based their tests on Horn and Cattell's formulation of the distinction between fluid and crystallized intelligence, sometimes referred to as the Gf-Gc Theory. Gf refers to such general fluid abilities as problem solving and reasoning. Fluid intelligence is thought not to be influenced by a person's cultural experience and education. Gc refers to such general crystallized abilities as acquired knowledge. Crystallized intelligence, unlike fluid intelligence, is thought to be shaped by a person's cultural experience and education.

Because the K-SNAP provides a measure of possible neurological impairment, it is often preferable to other measures of mental status and intelligence. If the doctor suspects that a patient may have a disorder of the nervous system, the doctor can use the K-SNAP as a short initial assessment. Depending on the results of the K-SNAP, the doctor can give more specific tests.

Description

The K-SNAP consists of four subtests administered in the following order of complexity: Mental Status, Gestalt Closure, Number Recall, and Four-Letter Words. Each subtest contains between 10 and 25 items.

The Mental Status subtest assesses the test taker's alertness, attentiveness, and orientation to the environment. In this subtest, the examiner asks the examinee to answer verbal questions. It is the easiest and shortest of the four subtests, containing only 10 items.

The Gestalt Closure subtest provides an assessment of visual closure and simultaneous processing. In this subtest, the examinee is shown partially completed inkblot pictures and is asked to name the objects in the pictures.

The Number Recall subtest assesses sequential processing and short-term auditory memory. In this subtest, the examiner recites series of numbers and the examinee repeats the numbers.

The Four-Letter Words subtest measures the test taker's ability to solve problems and make plans. In this subtest, the examinee is asked to guess a secret word by analyzing a series of four-letter words that provide clues to the answer. It is the most complex of the subtests.

The K-SNAP is a relatively easy test to administer. Except for the Mental Status subtest, the test items are presented on an easel, which is visually appealing to many test takers. Also, because the test is brief and includes a variety of tasks, the test takers often find the test engaging and interesting.

The K-SNAP is considered to be useful in evaluating elderly people, especially with regard to decline in fluid intelligence. The Mental Status subtest can also detect possible age-related impairment in mental functioning.

Compared to other neurological and cognitive assessments, there are smaller than usual differences in K-SNAP performance between African American and Caucasian individuals, especially with regard to fluid intelligence. This cultural neutrality makes the K-SNAP a preferred method for testing African Americans.

Preparation

Preparation for the Kaufman Short Neurological Assessment Procedure is not needed nor necessary.

KEY TERMS

Cognitive—Relating to thoughts and the acquisition of knowledge.

IQ—The acronym for intelligence quotient, or a score derived from one of several standardized tests for intelligence.

Neurological—Relating to neurology, or the branch of medicine dealing with the function and structure of the nervous system, along with its associated diseases and disorders.

Standard deviation—A statistical measure of dispersion; that is, how much a set of values differ from an arithmetic mean.

Risks

One should be careful when using the results of the K-SNAP to assess neurological impairment. It should be used as a supplement to other more extensive and more specific measures of neuropsychological functioning.

Precautions

The K-SNAP is primarily a test of mental and neuropsychological functioning. Although it measures cognitive skills, it should not be used to measure someone's overall intelligence.

Parental concerns

The K-SNAP is suitable for parents and children because it is a short and easy test to take, while still providing a good cognitive evaluation. It is also used as part of a more comprehensive assessment. The K-SNAP is frequently used as the first step in such evaluations, especially within correctional, medical, and psychological facilities.

Results

The K-SNAP was normalized on a representative sample of 2,000 people in the United States. All people were selected to eliminate cultural biases. The procedure yields several scores, including raw scores, scaled scores, a composite score, and an impairment index. Interpretation of the results are based on age-based normative scores or are evaluated from an eight-point impairment index, which is used to determine whether further testing is needed. Raw scores and scaled scores are calculated for each of the four subtests. Raw scores are calculated first; they refer simply to the number of points that the examinee scored on a particular subtest. The raw scores are converted to scaled scores to simplify comparisons between the subtests and between examinees. The subtest scaled scores are standardized to have a mean of 10 and a standard deviation of three.

One composite score is obtained on the K-SNAP. The composite score has a mean of 100 and a standard deviation of 15 and is based on the scores of the four subtests.

The results of the Mental Status subtest are primarily of interest when working with middle-aged or elderly people, as well as people with neurological or cognitive impairments. Most people find the Mental Status subtest very easy, and they get most, if not all, of the items correct.

Some of the interpretation of the K-SNAP involves comparisons of performance on tasks of varying complexity. For example, Gestalt Closure is considered a less complex task than Number Recall. Someone who performs better on the more difficult Number Recall subtest may exhibit some kind of **brain** dysfunction. On the other hand, that person may simply prefer sequential processing tasks.

An impairment index is also calculated and provides an objective measure of cognitive and neurological impairment. The impairment index is based on the following four factors: the K-SNAP composite score; the test taker's performance on the Mental Status subtest; the difference between the scaled scores on the Number Recall and Gestalt Closure subtests; and the difference between the actual composite score and the predicted composite score based on the test taker's level of education. These four factors determine whether a more comprehensive assessment of impairment is necessary. For example, if an examinee has a composite score below 70, a low score on the Mental Status subtest, a large difference in performance in the Number Recall and Gestalt Closure subtests, and a difference of at least 24 points between the predicted and actual composite scores, there may be indications of impairment. One example of such impairment is damage to one hemisphere of the brain.

Overall, the K-SNAP has above-average to good reliability. As a **mental status examination**, it has been shown to have good validity as well. There have been no studies, however, demonstrating the K-SNAP's validity as a measure of neuropsychological impairment. Because the K-SNAP is based on similar theories and on the same standardization sample as other Kaufman tests, such as the KAIT, interpretation across the range of Kaufman tests is easier than comparing results from the K-SNAP to results from tests designed by other persons.

QUESTIONS TO ASK YOUR DOCTOR

- Do you know of a properly trained administrator for the K-SNAP?
- What other test(s) for intelligence could be administered after completing the K-SNAP?
- Should my child take other tests for a better overall assessment of his/her condition?
- Where can I learn more about the K-SNAP?
- Will health insurance cover the test?

Resources

BOOKS

Boyer, Bret A., and M. Indira Paharia, eds. *Comprehensive Handbook of Clinical Health Psychology.* Hoboken, NJ: John Wiley and Sons, 2008.

Groth-Marnat, Gary. *Handbook of Psychological Assessment.* 4th edition. Hoboken, NJ: John Wiley and Sons, 2003.

Hersen, Michel, ed. *Comprehensive Handbook of Psychological Assessment.* Hoboken, NJ: John Wiley and Sons, 2004.

Kellerman, Henry, and Anthony Burry. *Handbook of Psychodiagnostic Testing: Analysis of Personality in the Psychological Report.* New York: Springer, 2007.

Leeming, David A., Kathryn Madden and Stanton Marlan, eds. *Encyclopedia of Psychology and Religion.* New York: Springer, 2010.

Sattler, Jerome M. *Assessment of Children: Cognitive Foundations.* San Diego, CA: J.M. Sattler, 2008.

WEBSITES

"Alan S. Kaufman, PhD, and Nadeen L. Kaufman, EdD." McGraw-Hill Higher Education. http://www.mhhe.com/mayfieldpub/psychtesting/profiles/karfmann.htm (accessed December 15, 2010).

"Alan S. Kaufman, PhD, and Nadeen L. Kaufman, EdD." Pearson. http://pearsonassessments.com/pai/ca/research/resources/authors/Alan_Nadeen_Kaufman (accessed December 15, 2010).

"Kaufman Short Neuropsychological Assessment Procedure (K-SNAP)." Pearson. http://www.pearsonassessments.com/HAIWEB/Cultures/en-us/Productdetail.htm?Pid=paa3560&Mode=summary (accessed December 16, 2010).

ORGANIZATIONS

American Psychiatric Association, 1000 Wilson Blvd., Ste. 1825, Arlington, VA, 22209-3901, (703) 907-7300, apa@psych.org, http://www.psych.org.

American Psychological Association, 750 1st St. NE, Washington, DC, 20002-4242, (202) 336-5500; TDD/TTY: (202) 336-6123, (800) 374-2721, http://www.apa.org.

Ali Fahmy, Ph.D.

Kava kava

Definition

Kava kava is a dioecious shrub native to the Pacific islands. Its botanical name is *Piper methysticum*; it is a member of the Piperaceae, or pepper, family. It is also known as asava pepper or intoxicating pepper. The narcotic drink made from the roots of this shrub is also called kava kava. Kava kava has been widely recommended in recent years as a mild tranquilizer due to its painkilling properties. However, kava kava has been the subject of official safety warnings from the U.S. Food and Drug Administration (FDA) and its counterparts in Canada, France, Germany, Switzerland, and Spain; kava kava is considered "possibly unsafe" by the U.S. National Institutes of Health.

Purpose

The German Commission E, a panel of physicians and pharmacists that reviews the safety and efficacy of herbal preparations, at one time approved the use of kava kava as a nonprescription dietary supplement for the relief of nervous anxiety, **stress**, and restlessness. That approval was withdrawn in the fall of 2001 due to the risks associated with the substance. Kava kava has, however, shown effectiveness in **clinical trials** in treating anxiety and in reducing withdrawal symptoms of patients taking **benzodiazepines**.

In addition to relief of stress and anxiety, kava kava has also been used for **insomnia**, sore or stiff muscles, toothache or sore gums, **attention deficit hyperactivity disorder**, menstrual cramps, uncontrolled epilepsy, and jet lag; however, none of these uses have been proven in clinical trials, either due to unsuccessful results or a lack of evidence.

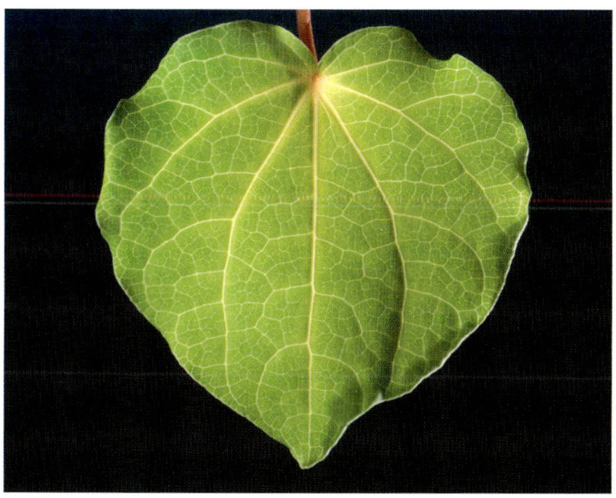

Kava Kava leaf. *(© bildagentur-online.com/th-foto/Alamy)*

Description

The beverage form of kava kava was traditionally prepared in the Pacific Islands by chewing the roots of the kava plant and spitting them into a bowl. The active compounds, known as kavalactones and kavapyrones, are found primarily in the root of the plant and are activated by human saliva. Contemporary Pacific Islanders prepare kava kava by pounding or grinding the roots and mixing them with coconut milk or water. Modern Western manufacturers use alcohol or acetate in making liquid kava preparations. Kava kava is also available in capsule, tablet, powdered, or crushed forms. Experts in herbal medicine recommended the use of kava preparations standardized to contain 70% kavalactones.

Kavalactones are chemicals that affect the **brain** in the same way as benzodiazepines, such as valium, which are sometimes prescribed for **depression**, anxiety, or **sleep disorders**. Kavalactones also have anesthetic properties that can cause the tongue or gums to feel numb. Kavapyrones are chemicals that have anticonvulsant and muscle relaxant properties.

Origins

Captain James Cook is credited with introducing kava kava to Europeans when he visited the South Pacific in 1773. Previously, the inhabitants of the Pacific Islands used kava kava as a ceremonial beverage. It was consumed at weddings, funerals, and birth rituals, and it was offered to honored guests. Kava kava was also drunk as part of healing rituals. The first commercial products containing kava kava were offered to European consumers around 1860.

Recommended dosage

Kava kava should never be given to children, particularly in view of recent health warnings concerning adults.

The usual dose of kava kava that has been recommended to relieve stress or insomnia in adults is 2–4 g of the plant boiled in water, up to three times daily. Alternately, 60–600 mg of kavalactones in a standardized formula could be taken per day.

Precautions

Kava kava has been linked to several cases of severe liver problems, including hepatitis, cirrhosis, and liver failure. Further studies need to be conducted to investigate whether kava kava was truly the cause of liver complications. Until more is known, the U.S. government considers kava kava to be potentially unsafe and advises against its use. If kava kava is used, it should

KEY TERMS

Dioecious—A category of plants that reproduce sexually but have male and female reproductive organs on different individuals.

Kavalactones—Medically active compounds in kava root that act as local anesthetics in the mouth and as minor tranquilizers.

Kavapyrones—Compounds in kava root that act as muscle relaxants and anticonvulsants.

not be used by pregnant or lactating women, as it might adversely affect the fetus or infant. Because of its effects on the central nervous system, persons should not take kava kava prior to driving or operating heavy machinery, and patients undergoing surgery should stop taking kava kava two weeks prior to their procedure. Kava kava may worsen any existing depression and should not be taken by persons with a history of depression.

Side effects

Before reports of liver damage, most side effects from kava kava concerned relatively minor problems, such as numbness in the mouth, headaches, mild dizziness, or skin rashes. In the nineteenth-century, missionaries to the Pacific Islands noted that people who drank large quantities of kava kava developed yellowish scaly skin. A recent study found the same side effect in test subjects who took 100 times the recommended dose of the plant. Kava kava also appears to produce psychological side effects in some patients. A team of Spanish physicians reported that beverages containing kava kava may cause anxiety, depression, and insomnia. In addition, kava kava may cause tremors severe enough to be mistaken for symptoms of Parkinson's disease.

Interactions

Kava kava has been shown to interact adversely with alcoholic beverages and with several categories of prescription medications. It increases the effect of **barbiturates** and other psychoactive medications; in one case study, a patient who took kava kava together with **alprazolam** (a benzodiazepine used to treat anxiety) went into a coma. It may produce dizziness and other unpleasant side effects if taken together with phenothiazines (used to treat **schizophrenia**). Kava kava has also been reported to reduce the effectiveness of levodopa, a drug used in the treatment of Parkinson's disease. To avoid potential reactions with prescription medications, people should inform their physician if they are taking kava kava or any other supplement.

Resources

BOOKS

Cass, Hyla, and Terrence McNally. *Kava: Nature's Answer to Stress, Anxiety, and Insomnia*. Prima Lifestyles, Inc., 1998.

Schulz, V., R. Hänsel, and V. Tyler. *Rational Phytotherapy: A Physician's Guide to Herbal Medicine*. 5th ed. Transl. by T.C. Telger. New York, NY: Springer, 2011.

PERIODICALS

Almeida, J. C., and E. W. Grimsley. "Coma from the Health Food Store: Interaction Between Kava and Alprazolam." *Annals of Internal Medicine* 125, no. 11 (1996): 940–941.

Ballesteros, S., et al. "Severe Adverse Effect Associated with Kava-Kava." *Journal of Toxicology: Clinical Toxicology* 39 (April 2001): 312.

Beltman, W., et al. "An Overview of Contemporary Herbal Drugs Used in the Netherlands." *Journal of Toxicology: Clinical Toxicology* 38 (March 2000): 174.

"France Is Latest to Pull Kava Kava Products." *Nutraceuticals International* (February 2002).

Humbertson, C. L., J. Akhtar, and E. P. Krenzelok. "Acute Hepatitis Induced by Kava Kava, an Herbal Product Derived from *Piper methysticum*." *Journal of Toxicology: Clinical Toxicology* 39 (August 2001): 549.

Kubetin, Sally Koch. "FDA Investigating Kava Kava." *OBGYN News* 37 (February 1, 2002): 29. Available online at http://findarticles.com/p/articles/mi_m0CYD/is_3_37/ai_82879244 (accessed November 9, 2011).

WEBSITES

MedlinePlus."Kava." U.S. National Library of Medicine, National Institutes of Health. http://www.nlm.nih.gov/medlineplus/druginfo/natural/872.html (accessed November 14, 2011).

U.S. Food and Drug Administration. "Kava (Piper methysticum) Dear Healthcare Professional Letter" MedWatch: The FDA Safety and Adverse Event Reporting Program. December 2001. http://www.fda.gov/Safety/MedWatch/SafetyInformation/SafetyAlertsforHumanMedicalProducts/ucm174452.htm (accessed October 9, 2011).

ORGANIZATIONS

American Botanical Council, 6200 Manor Rd., Austin, TX, 78723, (512) 926-4900, (800) 373-7105, Fax: (512) 926-2345, abc@herbalgram.org, http://www.herbalgram.org.

National Center for Complementary and Alternative Medicine, 9000 Rockville Pike, Bethesda, MD, 20892, (888) 644-6226, http://nccam.nih.gov.

NIH Office of Dietary Supplements, 6100 Executive Blvd., Room 3B01, MSC 7517, Bethesda, MD, 20892-7517, (301) 435-2920, Fax: (301) 480-1845, ods@nih.gov, http://www.odp.od.nih.gov.

Rebecca J. Frey, Ph.D.

Kleine-Levin syndrome

Definition

Kleine-Levin syndrome (also known as KLS) is a rare disorder. The most prevalent characteristic of the syndrome is recurring periods of excessive drowsiness and sleep (up to 20 hours per day) that can last weeks.

Demographics

Kleine-Levine syndrome is more common in adolescent males with a 3:1 ratio to females. Approximately 15% of the reported cases in the United States are people with Jewish origins. Age at onset is usually in the late teens and average age at onset is about 16.9 years, with a range from 4 to 82 years. About 81% of cases start in the preteen and teen years. Although it occurs more often in males, symptoms may be worse or the disease longer lasting in females.

Description

Kleine-Levin Syndrome is listed as a "rare disease" by the Office of Rare Diseases of the National Institutes of Health. KLS was first described in 1862 and is considered extremely rare. In addition to excessive drowsiness, an episode of KLS can also involve hypersexuality and compulsive behaviors, including compulsive eating. It usually first manifests in adolescence and appears to lessen and resolve on its own with age. Although cognitive and behavioral disturbances, including transient confusion and memory deficits, can accompany the disorder, there appear to be no lasting, permanent effects. In addition to other manifestations, KLS can be accompanied by mood disorders and an extreme irritability that translates into violent behaviors in atypical cases.

The average number of episodes of KLS among cases is seven, each lasting a median 10 days about every 3.5 months. The median length of time a person experiences the syndrome is eight years, although this time is longer in women and in people who experience less frequent episodes in their first year following onset.

Causes and symptoms

Causes

Most studies suggest that KLS is related to the hypothalamus, the organ in the **brain** that governs appetite, sleep, and hormone cycles, among other things. Researchers have failed to identify specific causes of KLS, although there are some apparent associations between events preceding the first episode of the disorder and its manifestation. The majority of cases are isolated, meaning that they do not appear to have a heritable basis.

Because many people with KLS experienced a viral illness just prior to their first episode, some experts propose that the causative agent is a type of viral or post-autoimmune encephalitis that affects the hypothalamus. Reported infections included tonsillitis, nonspecific flu-like fever, upper respiratory tract infection, and gastroenteritis. One study revealed that three of four autopsied patients with KLS had signs of inflammatory encephalitis in the hypothalamus.

Despite the suggested involvement of the hypothalamus, no association has been found clinically between a KLS episode and changes in hypothalamic hormones, cerebrospinal fluid, or other neurological signs. Similarly, in spite of symptoms such as hypersexuality, there have been no identified related changes in sex steroid hormones. One clinical association with KLS that has been found in 70% of patients is a nonspecific slowing of background brain activity on electroencephalogram testing. All **magnetic resonance imaging** (MRI) and CAT scan imaging of the brain in KLS cases have been normal.

KLS can occur as the primary disease, with onset in the teen years, or it can occur secondary to another disease or health problem, such as multiple sclerosis or brain **trauma**. Although fewer cases of secondary KLS occur compared to primary KLS, patients with secondary KLS may experience much longer and more frequent episodes.

Symptoms

Symptoms of a Kleine-Levin episode can last weeks or even months. In addition to **hypersomnia** (excessive sleepiness), symptoms can include excessive eating without regard to content or quantity, extreme irritability, disorientation and confusion, low energy or no energy, hypersensitivity to noise, disconnection from reality, and

KEY TERMS

Hypersexuality—A clinically significant level of desire to engage in sexual behaviors.

Hypersomnia—Excessive sleepiness.

Hypothalamus—The hypothalamus is part of the brain that links the nervous and endocrine systems and also governs emotion, sexual activity, body temperature, hunger, thirst, and sleep cycles.

blurred vision. A person experiencing a KLS episode may also report hallucinations. The abnormally uninhibited sex drive associated with some KLS episodes occurs more frequently in males and manifests in ways that can be alarming: those affected may expose themselves and make unwanted sexual advances. The disorder is episodic, and affected people behave normally between episodes. Intervals between episodes can sometimes last years.

Although an episode can come on without much warning, there are sometimes prodromal (pre-occurrence) signs that a KLS event is impending, especially a feeling of sudden, overwhelming tiredness. The excessive drowsiness of a KLS episode precludes normal participation in activities. In spite of the hypersomnia, a person experiencing a KLS episode is still able to wake to eat or void.

There may be some **depression** or **amnesia** after an attack. Depression can accompany KLS and an episode of KLS can occur with a recurring episode of depression. About half of patients report a depressive mood in conjunction with a KLS event.

Diagnosis

According to one source, diagnosing KLS is an difficult process and can result in an average delay of four years before a patient receives the correct **diagnosis**.

Treatment

No definitive treatment for KLS exists, and response to current treatments can be limited. A clinician can try to address the excessive sleepiness using orally administered stimulants (**amphetamines**, **methylphenidate**, modafinil). Because there are crossover characteristics between KLS and other mood disorders, lithium or **carbamazepine** are sometimes prescribed, and lithium appears to have some beneficial effect on **relapse** rates in a little less than half of the cases.

Prognosis

Excluding quality-of-life issues, KLS is a benign disorder that usually improves or resolves with age without permanent effects on intellect or physical function.

Prevention

Because the causes of KLS are undefined, prevention measures have not been identified.

Resources

PERIODICALS

Arnulf, I., et al. "Kleine-Levin Syndrome: A Systematic Review of 186 Cases in the Literature." *Brain* 128, no. 12 (2006): 2763–2776. Available online at http://brain.oxfordjournals.org/content/128/12/2763.full (accessed November 9, 2011).

WEBSITES

National Institute of Neurological Disorders and Stroke. "NINDS Kleine-Levin Syndrome Information Page." U.S. National Institutes of Health. http://www.ninds.nih.gov/disorders/kleine_levin/kleine_levin.htm (accessed November 14, 2011).

ORGANIZATIONS

Kleine-Levin Syndrome Foundation, PO Box 5382, San Jose, CA, 95150-5382, (408) 265-1099, Fax: (408) 269-2131, facts@klsfoundation.org, http://www.klsfoundation.org.

National Institute of Neurological Disorders and Stroke, PO Box 5801, Bethesda, MD, 20824, (301) 496-5751; TTY: (301) 468-5981, (800) 352-9424, http://www.ninds.nih.gov.

National Organization for Rare Disorders, 55 Kenosia Ave., PO Box 1968, Danbury, CT, 06813-1968, (203) 744-0100, Fax: (203) 798-2291, (800) 999-6673, http://www.rarediseases.org.

National Sleep Foundation, 1010 N Glebe Rd., Ste. 310, Arlington, VA, 22201, (703) 243-1697, nsf@sleepfoundation.org, http://www.sleepfoundation.org.

Emily Jane Willingham, Ph.D.

Kleptomania

Definition

Kleptomania is an impulse control disorder characterized by a recurrent failure to resist stealing.

Demographics

Studies suggest that 0.6% of the general population may have this disorder and that it is more common in females. In patients who have histories of **obsessive-compulsive disorder**, some studies suggest a 7% correlation with kleptomania. Other studies have reported a particularly high (65%) correlation of kleptomania in patients with bulimia.

Description

Kleptomania is a complex disorder characterized by repeated, failed attempts to stop stealing. It is often seen in patients who are chemically dependent or who have a coexisting mood, anxiety, or eating disorder. Other coexisting mental disorders may include major **depression**, panic attacks, **social phobia**, **anorexia nervosa**, **bulimia nervosa**, **substance abuse**, and obsessive-compulsive disorder. People with this disorder have an overwhelming urge to steal and get a thrill from doing so. The recurrent act of stealing may be restricted to specific objects and settings, but the affected person may or may not describe these special preferences. People with this disorder usually exhibit guilt after the theft.

Detection of kleptomania, even by close family members, is difficult and the disorder often proceeds undetected. There may be preferred objects and environments where theft occurs. One theory proposes that the thrill of stealing helps to alleviate symptoms in persons who are clinically depressed.

Causes and symptoms

Causes

The cause of kleptomania is unknown, although it may have a genetic component and may be transmitted among first-degree relatives. There also seems to be a strong propensity for kleptomania to coexist with obsessive-compulsive disorder, bulimia nervosa, and clinical depression.

Symptoms

The handbook used by mental health professionals to diagnose mental disorders is the *Diagnostic and Statistical Manual of Mental Disorders*. Published by the **American Psychiatric Association**, the *DSM* contains diagnostic criteria and research findings for mental disorders. It is the primary reference for mental health professionals in the United States. The 2000 edition of this manual (fourth edition, text revision), known as the *DSM-IV-TR*, lists five diagnostic criteria for kleptomania:

- Repeated theft of objects that are unnecessary for either personal use or monetary value.
- Increasing tension immediately before the theft.
- Pleasure or relief upon committing the theft.
- The theft is not motivated by anger or vengeance, and is not caused by a delusion or hallucination.
- The behavior is not better accounted for by a conduct disorder, manic episode, or antisocial personality disorder.

Diagnosis

Diagnosing kleptomania is usually difficult since patients do not seek medical help for this complaint, and it may not be detected by initial psychological assessments. The disorder is often diagnosed when patients seek help for another reason, such as depression, bulimia, or for feeling emotionally unstable (labile) or unhappy in general (dysphoric). Initial psychological evaluations may detect a history of poor parenting, relationship conflicts, or acute stressors—abrupt occurrences that cause **stress**, such as moving from one home to another. The recurrent act of stealing may be restricted to specific objects and settings, but the patient may or may not describe these special preferences.

KEY TERMS

Anorexia nervosa—An eating disorder characterized by an intense fear of weight gain accompanied by a distorted perception of one's own underweight body.

Bulimia nervosa—An eating disorder characterized by binges in which large amounts of food are consumed, followed by forced vomiting.

Cognitive-behavioral therapy—An approach to psychotherapy that emphasizes the correction of distorted thinking patterns and changing one's behaviors accordingly.

Obsessive-compulsive disorder—Disorder in which the affected individual has an obsession (such as a fear of contamination, or thoughts he or she doesn't like to have and can't control) and feels compelled to perform a certain act to neutralize the obsession (such as repeated handwashing).

Panic disorder—An anxiety disorder in which an individual experiences sudden, debilitating attacks of intense fear.

Phobia—Irrational fear of places, things, or situations that lead to avoidance.

Rational emotive therapy—A form of psychotherapy developed by Albert Ellis and other psychotherapists based on the theory that emotional response is based on the subjective interpretation of events, not on the events themselves.

Treatment

Once the disorder is suspected and verified by an extensive psychological interview, therapy is normally directed towards impulse control, as well as any accompanying mental disorder(s). **Relapse prevention** strategies, with a clear understanding of specific triggers, should be stressed. Treatment may include psychotherapies such as **cognitive-behavioral therapy** and **rational emotive therapy**. Recent studies have indicated that **fluoxetine** (Prozac) and **naltrexone** (Revia) may also be helpful.

Prognosis

Not much solid information is known about this disorder. Since it is not usually the presenting problem or chief complaint, it is frequently not even diagnosed. There are some case reports that document treatment success with antidepressant medications, although as with almost all psychological disorders, the outcomes vary.

Prevention

There is little evidence concerning prevention. A healthy upbringing, positive intimate relationships, and management of acutely stressful situations may lower the incidence of kleptomania and coexisting disorders.

Resources

BOOKS

Tasman, Allan, et al., eds. *Psychiatry*. 3rd ed. New York: Wiley and Sons, 2008.

Laith Farid Gulli, M.D.

Klonopin *see* **Clonazepam**

K-SNAP *see* **Kaufman Short Neurological Assessment Procedure**

L

Laboratory tests *see* **Imaging studies**

Lamictal *see* **Lamotrigine**

Lamotrigine

Definition

Lamotrigine is an anticonvulsant drug commonly used to prevent **seizures**. In the United States, lamotrigine is available under the trade name of Lamictal.

Purpose

Lamotrigine is used to prevent seizures in individuals with seizure disorders. It is also used as a mood stabilizer in people with **bipolar disorder**.

Description

The U.S. Food and Drug Administration (FDA) approved Lamotrigine in 1994. This drug appears to suppress the activity of neurons (nerve cells) in the **brain**. By stabilizing neurons, lamotrigine prevents seizure activity and may also stabilize abnormal mood swings.

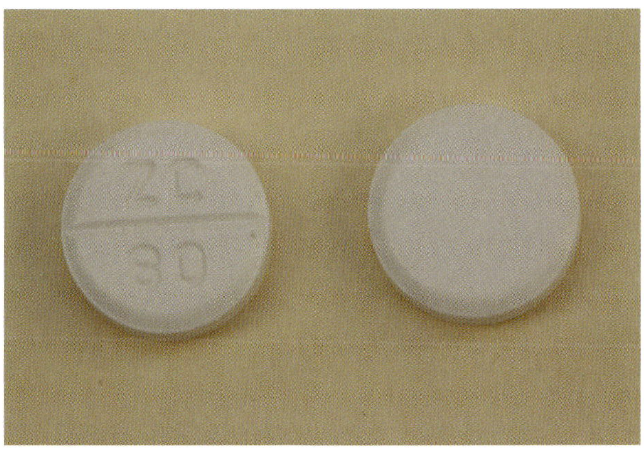

Lamotrigine, 100 mg. *(© Custom Medical Stock Photo, Inc. Reproduced by permission.)*

Lamotrigine is available as both oral and chewable tablets. It is broken down in the liver.

Recommended dosage

The dosage of lamotrigine varies depending upon the age and weight of the patient, other medications that the patient is taking, and whether the patient has heart, liver, or kidney disease. It is common for patients to start with a low dosage of lamotrigine. The dosage is then increased slowly over several weeks to help prevent side effects. The dosage may be adjusted frequently by the prescribing physician.

A common dose for an adult who takes no other medications and has no other diseases is 150–250 mg taken twice daily.

Precautions

A serious and permanently disfiguring rash may occur as a result of lamotrigine. The rash, which is symptom of a systemic reaction to the drug, may be fatal. If a rash occurs, a doctor should be contacted immediately, and the drug should be stopped. People who have experienced any kind of rash while taking lamotrigine should never take the drug again.

Lamotrigine should be used under physician supervision. In persons with heart, kidney, or liver disease, lamotrigine should only be used if the patient and physician determine that the benefits outweigh the risks. The dosage is usually reduced in these individuals. Lamotrigine has also been associated with the risks of developing aseptic meningitis or blood disorders.

Side effects

Side effects that occur in more than 10% of people taking lamotrigine include headache, dizziness, unsteadiness while walking, blurred vision, double vision, nausea, cold-like symptoms such as runny noses or sore throats, and infections.

Although relatively rare, any rash that develops while taking lamotrigine should be evaluated by a healthcare professional, since life-threatening rashes may occur.

Other side effects include confusion, impaired memory, **sleep disorders**, nonspecific pain all over the body, and disruption of menstrual cycles.

Interactions

Some drugs can decrease the levels of lamotrigine in the body. This may make the drug less effective; examples include **carbamazepine**, phenobarbital, primidone, phenytoin, and **valproic acid**. Valproic acid and its close relative, **divalproex sodium**, have also been reported to increase lamotrigine levels in some people, which could increase the side effects of the drug. When lamotrigine and valproic acid or divalproex sodium are used together, there is a greater chance that a serious rash may develop. Very specific dosage guidelines must be followed when these two drugs are used at the same time.

Lamotrigine may increase the levels of carbamazepine in the body, increasing adverse effects associated with carbamazepine.

An increased risk of certain side effects may occur if lamotrigine is used with drugs, such as methotrexate, that inhibit folic acid synthesis.

Resources

BOOKS

Ellsworth, Allan J., et al., eds. *Mosby's Medical Drug Reference.* St. Louis, MO: Mosby, Inc., 1999.

Facts and Comparisons Staff. *Drug Facts and Comparisons.* 6th ed. Saint Louis: Facts and Comparisons; Philadelphia: Lippincott Williams and Wilkins, 2002.

Kelly Karpa, RPh, Ph.D.

Late-life depression

Definition

Late-life depression is **depression** occurring in older individuals. Although often associated with the **stress** and physical problems attendant with advancing age, depression is not a normal part of the aging process.

Demographics

The percentage of Americans 65 years old and older who have clinical depression is significantly greater than for the general population. Whereas approximately 1% of Americans are clinically depressed, nearly 16% of those 65 years of age and older meet the criteria for clinical depression. Similarly, suicide rates for older adults are disproportionately high, particularly for white males.

A **diagnosis** of major depressive disorder is more likely in elderly patients who are also medically ill, older than 70 years of age, and hospitalized or institutionalized. Depression in the elderly is more common when there is a history of depression earlier in life, chronic physical illness, **brain** disease, alcohol abuse, or stressful life events. Elderly women are more likely to become depressed than are elderly men, and single seniors are more likely to become depressed than are those who are married. It has been estimated that as many as 15% of widowed adults will have a serious depression for a year or more after the death of their spouse.

Subsyndromal depression (depression that is clinically significant but does not meet the criteria for major depressive disorder) is more common than major depressive disorder in elderly adults. It is estimated that 15% to 50% of older adults with subsyndromal depression will develop major depressive disorder within two years. Approximately 30% of nursing home residents have subsyndromal depression. As with major depressive disorder, elders with subsyndromal depression tend to be female.

Description

Depression in the aging and the aged is a major public health problem. Many who suffer from late-life depression go undiagnosed. The insidious nature of depression in the elderly is that its symptoms are often obfuscated in the context of the multiple physical problems of many elderly people. As the body ages, it becomes less able to respond to stress and is at increased risk for disease. Disabilities resulting from external factors such as stress, **trauma**, chronic diseases, lifestyle limitations, financial factors, and isolation may accelerate the process, resulting in the symptoms we think of as defining old age. Depression, however, is not a normal part of aging, nor is it inevitable.

The symptoms of late-life depression can be the same as they are for other depressive disorders in younger people, such as **major depressive disorder**, a **bipolar disorder**, or subsyndromal depression. The individual may experience a profound and persistent feeling of sadness or despair or lose interest in things that were once pleasurable (anhedonia). Late-life depression can also exhibit itself in less obvious ways, including sleep disturbance, change in appetite, or disturbed mental functioning. In extreme cases, late-life depression can lead to **suicide**. Depression in late life, however, is treatable.

Late-life depression has a serious association with high rates of suicide. About 16% of all suicides occur in adults over age 65. These statistics suggest that late-life depression is a potentially life-threatening disorder; healthcare providers should maintain a low threshold of suspicion of this disorder in dysthymic older patients, in order to avoid missing the opportunity to intervene effectively.

Causes and symptoms

As opposed to younger individuals, older adults are more likely to have a medical condition in addition to depression. A number of medical conditions have commonly been associated with depression in the elderly. These include:

- coronary artery disease (high blood pressure, history of heart attack, coronary artery bypass surgery, congestive heart failure)
- neurologic disorders (stroke, Alzheimer's disease, Parkinson's disease, Lou Gehrig's disease, multiple sclerosis, Binswanger's disease, senile dementia)
- metabolic disturbances (diabetes, hypoglycemia, hypothyroidism, hyperthyroidism, hyperparathyroidism, Addison's disease)
- cancer (particularly of the pancreas)
- other medical conditions (chronic obstructive pulmonary disease, rheumatoid arthritis, chronic pain, sexual dysfunction, renal dialysis, chronic constipation, viral pneumonia, hepatitis, influenza)

In addition, a number of medications routinely taken by elderly patients may cause depression. These include:

- cardiovascular drugs (clonidine, digitalis, guanethidine, hydralazine, methyldopa, procainamide, propranolol, reserpine, thiazide diuretics)
- chemotherapeutics (6-azauridine, asparaginase, azathioprine, bleomycin, cisplatin, cyclophosphamide, doxorubicin, mithramycin)
- antiparkinsonian drugs (amantadine, bromocriptine, levodopa)
- antipsychotic drugs (fluphenazine, haloperidol)
- sedatives and antianxiety drugs (barbiturates, benzodiazepines, chloral hydrate, ethanol)
- anticonvulsants (carbamazepine, ethosuximide, phenobarbital, phenytoin, primidone)
- anti-inflammatory/anti-infective agents (ampicillin, cycloserine, dapsone, ethambutol, griseofulvin, isoniazid, metoclopramide, metronidazole, nalidixic acid, nitrofurantoin, nonsteroidal anti-inflammatory drugs [NSAIDs], penicillin G procaine, streptomycin, sulfonamides, tetracycline)
- stimulants (amphetamines, caffeine, cocaine, methylphenidate)
- hormones (adrenocorticotropin, anabolic steroids, glucocorticoids, oral contraceptives)
- other medications (choline, cimetidine, disulfiram, lecithin, methysergide, phenylephrine, physostigmine, ranitidine, vinblastine, vincristine)

Because of concurrent medical problems and lowered expectations for functionality, elderly patients with depression are often undiagnosed. In addition, elderly patients often are reluctant to speak about psychological symptoms and consider depression to be a normal response to the aging process. Depressed older people may not report being depressed because they have no hope that anyone will intervene. These factors can make diagnosis difficult.

Depression in older adults does not necessarily present with the same symptoms as in the younger population. Common symptoms in older people that can signify a problem with depression include:

- Unexplained physical complaints—older adults are often reluctant to discuss psychological symptoms, and as a result, symptoms of depression may be expressed in terms of a physical rather than a psychological complaint. For example, depression in older adults is often characterized by physical complaints for which no medical cause can be found, or by physical symptoms that are out of proportion to the underlying medical illness.
- Hopelessness or helplessness—in older adults, it is hopelessness, rather than sadness, that tends to be associated with thoughts of suicide. Statements such as "I wish I were dead already," "I wish I would fall asleep and not wake up," or "what's the use in trying" are cause for immediate concern and should be responded to with psychological assessment rather than platitudes or meaningless assurances that everything is all right. Talk of suicide—even in jest—should always be taken seriously
- Anxiety and worries—older adults often experience general feelings of worry and tension not associated with specific anxiety or panic disorders. Statements of anxiety and worry in older adults often are signs of depression in addition to, or instead of, an anxiety

disorder. Treatment for an anxiety disorder, however, will not treat any underlying depression.

- Memory complaints—depressed older adults may complain about memory loss with or without objective signs of cognitive impairment. Particularly when no demonstrable memory problems can be discerned by simple tests, it is important that the patient also be assessed for depression and treated accordingly.
- Loss of feeling of pleasure (anhedonia)—one common symptom of depression in older adults is the inability to experience pleasure from life and daily events. Expressions of anhedonia might include no longer deriving enjoyment from being with grandchildren; not wanting to read, listen to music, or participate in hobbies once found enjoyable; or feeling estranged from God or no longer being comforted by religion. Although it might seem that being less active and involved in life is a response to illness or decreased abilities associated with aging, research suggests that depression might, in fact, contribute to heart disease, diabetes, and arthritis.
- Slowed movement—"slowing down" is often associated with old age. However, things such as stooped posture, slowed movements, or slowed speech may also be signs of depression. In particular, depression associated with vascular disease is often expressed in such symptoms.
- Irritability—depression in older adults may also be expressed by excessive or easily provoked anger, annoyance, or impatience. Symptoms of irritability include fussiness, whining, or fretfulness even in the face of comforting. When such a pattern is persistent, assessment for depression should be considered.
- Lack of interest in personal care—depressed older adults may believe that they are "not worth the trouble" and fail to follow instructions for taking medications or dietary guidelines as a result. Similarly, depressed older adults may display such symptoms as lack of care about personal appearance—including not getting dressed, bathing, or performing other hygiene activities. Individuals displaying such symptoms should be assessed for depression.
- Other symptoms—sleep disturbance, decreased appetite, weight loss, difficulty concentrating, and fatigue are all common symptoms of late-life depression.

Diagnosis

According to the ***Diagnostic and Statistical Manual of Mental Disorders*** (*DSM-IV-TR*) of the **American Psychiatric Association**, there are nine criteria for major depressive disorder:

- depressed mood
- sleep disturbance
- lack of interest or pleasure in activities
- guilt and feelings of worthlessness
- lack of energy
- loss of concentration and difficult making decisions
- anorexia or weight loss
- psychomotor agitation or delay
- suicidal ideation (thoughts of suicide)

A diagnosis of depression requires at least five of these criteria to be present nearly every day during a two-week period, or a score of 10 or more on the **Beck Depression Inventory** (BDI) or on the **Geriatric Depression Scale**.

Significant depression in older adults does not always meet the criteria for a *DSM-IV-TR* diagnosis of depression. As a result, although depression occurs more frequently in older adults than in the general population, it often goes undiagnosed in seniors. In addition to, or instead of, the classic diagnostic symptoms, older adults may exhibit other symptoms that should be considered when diagnosing depression in older adults.

Screening of an elderly patient for depression should include an electrocardiogram (ECG), urinalysis, general blood chemistry screen, complete blood count, and determination of the levels of thyroid-stimulating hormone, vitamin B12, folate, and medication in the blood.

Treatment

Depression in elderly patients may be treated with medication and/or **psychotherapy** (including **talk therapy** and behavior therapy). Research has shown that a combination of the two treatment options is more effective than the use of medication or therapy alone. Although improvement may be seen as early as two weeks, the full effect of therapy may not be observable for several months. If the patient is having a major depressive episode, recovery may take from 6 to 12 months. This means that therapy for older adults is typically needed for longer periods of time than for the general population.

Medication for depression is generally well tolerated in older adults. Drugs used in treating depression in older adults include **selective serotonin reuptake inhibitors (SSRIs)** (**sertraline**, **fluoxetine**, **paroxetine**, **fluvoxamine**, **citalopram**, **escitalopram**), secondary tricyclic **antidepressants** (**nortriptyline**, **protriptyline**, **desipramine**, **amoxapine**), tertiary tricyclic antidepressants (**amitriptyline**, **imipramine**, **doxepin**, **trimipramine**, **clomipramine**), **monoamine oxidase inhibitors (MAOIs)** (**phenelzine**, **tranylcypromine**), and other antidepressants (**maprotiline**, **bupropion**, **trazodone**, **venlafaxine**, **nefazodone**, **mirtazapine**). As with any medication, the patient should be monitored closely to determine how well he or she is reacting to the medication. If adverse reactions occur, another medication can be tried.

Prognosis

The general prognosis for recovery from depression in older adults is good, although recovery may take longer for older adults than for the general population.

Prevention

Increasingly, it is recognized that although it is imperative to diagnose and treat depression in late life, it is equally important to prevent late-life depression in the first place. Researchers are currently investigating several models of prevention. These focus on individuals at high risk for depression in late life, including those with diseases that often occur with depression.

There are a number of steps that can be taken to help prevent depression. Eating a balanced diet and keeping regular meal times is important, particularly if one has problems with insulin or blood sugar levels. Getting regular **exercise** also helps stave off depression. If one's depression has a seasonal component, taking walks in the morning sunshine or using a light box can also help. Maintaining a regular sleep pattern is also helpful, as is avoiding drugs and alcohol. Those seniors living alone should also make an effort to widen their social support network. Research has found that making friends at a senior center is an excellent way to do this. Steps that can be taken by those who have been diagnosed and are being treated for depression include: continuing to take any antidepressant medications as prescribed until directed to stop by one's physician, and continuing with therapy even after the medications have been stopped.

Researchers are continuing to investigate depression prevention for older adults in the hope that this too-common and undiagnosed disorder can be not only successfully treated, but also prevented in the first place.

Resources

BOOKS

American Psychiatric Association. *Diagnostic and Statistical Manual of Mental Disorders*. 4th ed., text rev. Washington, DC: American Psychiatric Association, 2000.

Baldwin, Robert C., and Jane Garner. "Anxiety and Depression in Women in Old Age." In *Mood and Anxiety Disorders in Women*, edited by David J. Castle, Jayashri Kulkarni, and Kathryn M. Abel. New York: Cambridge University Press, 2006. 242–66.

Ellison, James E., and Sumer K. Verma, eds. *Depression in Later Life: A Multidisciplinary Psychiatric Approach*. London: Informa Healthcare, 2003.

Hinrichsen, Gregory A., and Kathleen F. Clougherty. *Interpersonal Psychotherapy for Depressed Older Adults*. Washington, DC: American Psychological Association, 2006.

Karel, Michele J., Suzann Ogland-Hand, and Margaret Gatz. *Assessing and Treating Late-Life Depression*. New York: Basic Books, 2002.

Roose, Steven P., and Harold A. Sackeim. *Late-Life Depression*. New York: Oxford University Press, 2004.

VandenBos, Gary R., ed. *APA Dictionary of Psychology*. Washington, DC: American Psychological Association, 2007.

PERIODICALS

Aday, Ronald H., Gayle C. Kehoe, and Lori A. Farney. "Impact of Senior Center Friendships on Aging Women Who Live Alone." *Journal of Women and Aging* 18, no. 1 (2006): 57–73.

Akpaffiong, M. J., Mark E. Kunik, and Melanie Wilson-Lawson. "Antidepressant-Associated Side Effects in Older Adult Depressed Patients." *Geriatrics* 63, no. 4 (2008): 18–23.

Beaudreau, Sherry A., and Ruth O'Hara. "The Association of Anxiety and Depressive Symptoms with Cognitive Performance in Community-Dwelling Older Adults." *Psychology and Aging* 24, no. 2 (2009): 507–12.

Braun, Ursula K., Mark E. Kunik, and Catherine Pham. "Recognizing and Managing Depression at End of Life." *Geriatrics* 63, no. 6 (2008): 25–27.

Brenes, G. A., et al. "Treatment of Minor Depression in Older Adults: A Pilot Study Comparing Sertraline and Exercise." *Aging & Mental Health* 11, no. 1 (2007): 61–68.

Carter, Janet, Joanne Rodda, and Zuzana Walker. "Depression in Older Adults." *British Medical Journal* 343, no. 7825 (2011): 683+.

Elderkin-Thompson, et al. "Executive Dysfunction and Memory in Older Patients with Major and Minor Depression." *Archives of Clinical Neuropsychology* 21, no. 7 (2006): 669–76.

Hinton, Ladson, Mark Zweifach, Sabine Oishi, Lingqi Tang, and Jürgen Unützer. "Gender Disparities in the Treatment of Late-Life Depression: Qualitative and Quantitative Findings from the IMPACT Trial." *American Journal of Geriatric Psychiatry* 14, no. 10 (2006): 884–92.

Holley, Caitlin, Stanley A. Murrell, and Benjamin T. Mast. "Psychosocial and Vascular Risk Factors for Depression in the Elderly." *American Journal of Geriatric Psychiatry* 14, no. 1 (2006): 84–90.

Karp, Jordan F., et al. "Preventing Depression in Older Adults." *Clinical Neuropsychiatry: Journal of Treatment Evaluation* 3, no. 1 (2006): 69–80. http://www.clinicalneuropsychiatry.org/pdf/07_Karp.pdf (accessed November 9, 2011).

Schoevers, Robert A., et al. "Prevention of Late-Life Depression in Primary Care: Do We Know Where to Begin?" *American Journal of Psychiatry* 163, no. 9 (2006): 1611–21.

Smit, Filip, Agnieska Ederveen, Pim Cuijpers, Dorly Deeg, Aartjan Beekman. "Opportunities for Cost-effective Prevention of Late-Life Depression: An Epidemiological Approach." *Archives of General Psychiatry* 63, no. 3 (2006): 290–96.

Szanto, Katalin, Benoit H. Mulsant, Patricia R. Houck, Mary Amanda Dew, Alexandre Dombrovski, Bruce G. Pollock, and Charles F. Reynolds III. "Emergence, Persistence, and Resolution of Suicidal Ideation During Treatment of Depression in Old Age." *Journal of Affective Disorders* 98, no. 1–2 (2007): 153–61.

Vaishnavi, Sandeep, and Warren D. Taylor. "Neuroimaging in Late-Life Depression." *International Review of Psychiatry* 18, no. 5 (2006): 443–51.

von Gunten, Armin, Panteleimon Giannakopoulos, and René Duc. "Cognitive and Demographic Determinants of Dementia in Depressed Patients with Subjective Memory Complaints." *European Neurology* 54, no. 3 (2005): 154–58.

Wilby, Frances. "Depression and Social Networks in Community Dwelling Elders: A Descriptive Study." *Journal of Gerontological Social Work* 43, no. 3 (2011): 246–59. http://dx.doi.org/10.1080/01634372.2010.540074 (accessed December 15, 2011).

Yang, Yang. "How Does Functional Disability Affect Depressive Symptoms in Late Life? The Role of Perceived Social Support and Psychological Resources." *Journal of Health and Social Behavior* 47, no. 4 (2006): 355–72.

ORGANIZATIONS

American Association for Geriatric Psychiatry, 7910 Woodmont Ave., Ste. 1050, Bethesda, MD, 20814-3004, (301) 654-7850, Fax: (301) 654-4137, http://www.AAGPonline.org.

American Psychiatric Association, 1000 Wilson Blvd., Ste. 1825, Arlington, VA, 22209-3901, (703) 907-7300, apa@psych.org, http://www.psych.org.

American Psychological Association, 750 1st Street NE, Washington, DC, 20002-4242, (202) 336-5500; TDD/TTY: (202) 336-6123, (800) 374-2721, http://www.apa.org.

Depression and Bipolar Support Alliance, 730 N Franklin Street, Ste. 501, Chicago, IL, 60654-7225, (800) 826-3632, Fax: (312) 642-7243, http://www.dbsalliance.org.

Fuqua Center for Late-Life Depression, Wesley Woods Health Center, 4th Floor, 1841 Clifton Rd. NE, Atlanta, GA, 30329, (404) 728-6948, http://www.fuquacenter.org.

Geriatric Mental Health Foundation, 7910 Woodmont Ave., Ste. 1050, Bethesda, MD, 20814, (301) 654-7850, Fax: (301) 654-4137, web@GMHFonline.org, http://www.gmhfonline.org.

National Alliance on Mental Illness, 3803 N Fairfax Drive, Ste. 100, Arlington, VA, 22203, (703) 524-7600, http://www.nami.org.

Ruth A. Wienclaw, PhD

Lavender

Definition

Lavender is the shrub-like aromatic plant, *Lavandula officinalis*, sometimes called *Lavandula vera* or true lavender.

Purpose

Lavender is a mild sedative and antispasmodic. The essential oil derived from lavender is used in **aromatherapy** to treat anxiety, difficulty sleeping, nervousness, and restlessness. Other preparations of the plant are taken internally to treat sleep disturbances, stomach complaints, loss of appetite, and as a general tonic.

Description

Lavender is a shrubby evergreen bush that grows to about 3 feet (1 m) tall and 4 feet (1.4 m) in diameter. The plant produces aromatic spiky flowers from June to September. An essential oil used for healing and in perfume is extracted from the flowers just before they open.

Lavender is native to the Mediterranean region and is cultivated in temperate regions across the world. There are many species and subspecies. The preferred lavender for medicinal use is *L. officinalis* or true lavender. In Europe lavender has been used as a healing herb for centuries. It was a prominent component of smelling salts popular with women in the late 1800s.

Lavender is used both externally and internally in healing. Externally the essential oil is used in aromatherapy as a relaxant and to improve mood. Aromatherapy can be facilitated through massage, used in the bath, placed in potpourri jars, and burned in specially designed oil burners. Lavender is also used to

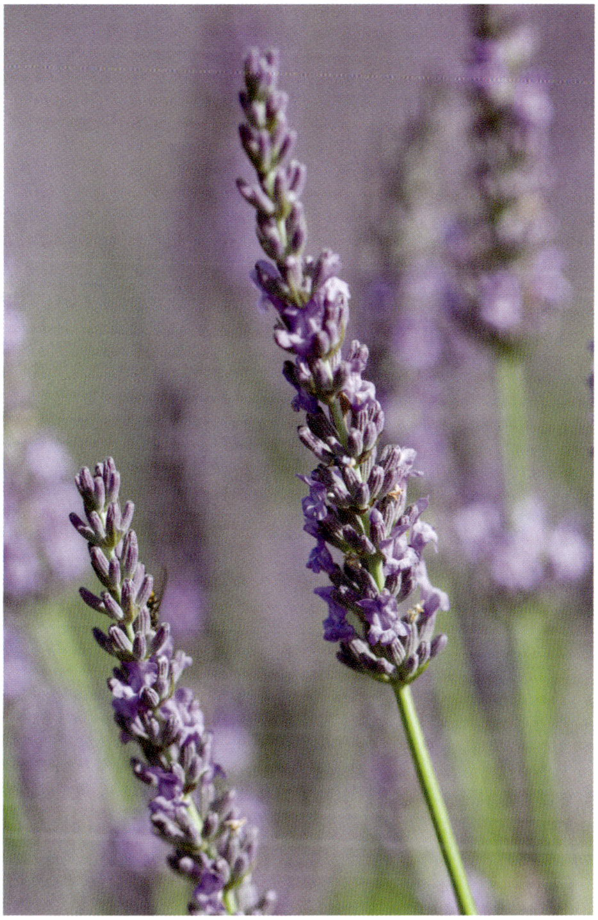

Lavender plant. *(© Iurii Konoval/Shutterstock.com)*

treat **fatigue**, restlessness, nervousness, and difficulty sleeping. Pillows stuffed with lavender have been used as a sleep aid in Europe for many years. Lavender oil applied to the forehead and temples is said to ease headache.

Researchers have isolated the active compounds in lavender. The most important of these is an aromatic volatile oil. Lavender also contains small amounts of coumarins, compounds that dilate (open up) the blood vessels and help control spasms. Some modern scientific research supports the claim that lavender is effective as a mild sedative and a calming agent. In one Japanese study, people exposed to the odor of lavender were found to show less mental **stress** and more alertness than those not exposed to the fragrance when evaluated by psychological tests. In a peer-reviewed British study, when the sleeping room was perfumed with lavender, elderly nursing home residents with **insomnia** slept as well as they did when they took sleeping pills and better than they did when they were given neither sleeping pills nor exposed to lavender fragrance.

Other external uses of the essential oil of lavender are as an antiseptic to disinfect wounds. When used on wounds, lavender oil often is combined with other essential oil extracts to enhance its antiseptic and dehydrating properties. Lavender oil added to bathwater is believed to stimulate the circulation.

Taken internally as a tea made from lavender flowers or as a few drops of lavender oil on a sugar cube, this herb is used as a mild sedative and antispasmodic. The German Federal Health Agency's Commission E established to independently review and evaluate scientific literature and case studies pertaining to medicinal plants has approved the use of lavender tea or lavender oil on a sugar cube to treat restlessness and insomnia. Despite conflicting scientific claims, this organization has also endorsed the internal use of lavender for stomach upsets, loss of appetite, and excess gas. Animal research confirms that lavender oil has an antispasmodic effect on smooth muscle of the intestine and uterus. These results have not been confirmed in humans.

Recommended dosage

Lavender tea is made by steeping 1 to 2 teaspoons of flowers per cup of boiling water. One cup of tea can be drunk three times a day. Alternatively, 1 to 4 drops of lavender oil can be placed on a sugar cube and eaten once a day. Externally, a few drops of oil can be added to bath water or rubbed on the temples to treat headache. Like any herbal product, the strength of the active ingredients can vary from batch to batch, making it difficult to determine exact dosages.

Precautions

The use of lavender, either alone or in combination with other herbs, is not regulated by the U.S. Food and Drug Administration. Unlike pharmaceuticals, herbal and dietary supplements are not subjected to rigorous scientific testing to prove their claims of safety and effectiveness. The strength of active ingredients varies from manufacturer to manufacturer, and the label may not accurately reflect the contents.

Particular problems with lavender oil revolve around substitution of oil from species of lavender other than *Lavandula officinalis*, the preferred medicinal lavender. Most often true lavender oil is adulterated with less expensive lavadin oil. Lavadin oil comes from other species of lavender. It has a pleasant lavender odor, but its chemical compositions, and thus its healing actions, are different from true lavender oil. People purchasing lavender oil or tonics containing lavender should be alert to substitutions.

KEY TERM

Antispasmodic—A medication or preparation given to relieve muscle or digestive cramps.

Side effects

When used in the recommended dosage, lavender is not considered harmful. Some people have reported developing contact dermatitis (a rash) when lavender oil is used directly on the skin.

Interactions

There are no studies on interactions of lavender with conventional pharmaceuticals. Traditionally lavender has been used in combination with other herbs such as tea oil and lemon balm without adverse interactions.

Resources

BOOKS

Peirce, Andrea. *The American Pharmaceutical Association Practical Guide to Natural Medicines*. New York: William Morrow and Company, 1999.

Thomson Healthcare. *PDR for Herbal Medicines*. 4th ed. Montvale, NJ: Thomson Reuters, 2007.

Weiner, Michael, and Janet Weiner. *Herbs that Heal:Prescription for Herbal Healing*. Mill Valley, CA: Quantum Books, 1999.

WEBSITES

Brett, Jennifer. "Lavender: Herbal Remedies." Discovery Fit & Health. http://health.howstuffworks.com/wellness/natural-medicine/herbal-remedies/lavender-herbal-remedies.htm (accessed October 22, 2011).

Tish Davidson, A.M.

Lead poisoning

Definition

Lead poisoning occurs when a person swallows, absorbs, or inhales lead in any form. The result can be damaging to the **brain**, nerves, and many other parts of the body. Acute lead poisoning, which is somewhat rare, occurs when a relatively large amount of lead is taken into the body over a short period of time. Chronic lead poisoning—a common problem in children—occurs when small amounts of lead are taken in over a longer period. The U.S. Centers for Disease Control and Prevention (CDC) defines childhood lead poisoning as a whole-blood lead concentration equal to or greater than 10 micrograms/dL.

Description

Lead can damage almost every system in the human body, and it can also cause high blood pressure (hypertension). It is particularly harmful to the developing brain of fetuses and young children. The higher the level of lead in a child's blood, and the longer this elevated level lasts, the greater the chance of ill effects. Over the long term, lead poisoning in a child can lead to learning disabilities, behavioral problems, and **intellectual disability**. At very high levels, lead poisoning can cause **seizures**, coma, and even death. Most deaths are among males (74%), African Americans (67%), adults over the age of 45 (76%), and Southerners (70%).

About one out of every six children in the United States has a high level of lead in the blood, according to the Agency for Toxic Substances and Disease Registry. Many of these children are exposed to lead through peeling paint in older homes. Others are exposed through dust or soil that has been contaminated by old paint or past emissions of leaded gasoline. Since children between the ages of 12–36 months are apt to put things in their mouths, they are more likely than older children to ingest lead. Pregnant women who come into contact with lead can pass it along to the fetus.

More than 80% of American homes built before 1978 have lead-based paint in them, according to the CDC. The older the home, the more likely it is to contain lead paint and have higher concentrations of lead in the paint. Some homes also have lead in the water pipes or plumbing. People may have lead in the paint, dust, or soil around their homes or in their drinking water without knowing it, since lead can't be seen, smelled, or tasted. Because lead doesn't break down naturally, it can continue to cause problems until it is removed.

Lead poisoning and the broad issue of dangerously high levels of lead in common consumer products is an increasing concern. In 2008, the Consumer Product Safety Improvement Act was introduced, which placed new regulations on the levels of lead in consumer products.

Causes and symptoms

Before scientists knew how harmful it could be, lead was widely used in paint, gasoline, water pipes, and many other products. Today house paint is almost lead free, gasoline is unleaded, and household plumbing is no longer made with lead materials. Still, remnants of the old hazards remain. Sources of lead exposure include:

- Lead-based paint. This is the most common source of exposure to large amounts of lead among preschoolers. Children may eat paint chips from older homes that have fallen into disrepair. They may also chew on painted surfaces such as windowsills. In addition, paint may be disturbed during remodeling.
- Dust and soil. These can be contaminated with lead from old paint or past emissions of leaded gasoline. In addition, pollution from operating or abandoned industrial sites and smelters can find its way into the soil, resulting in soil contamination.
- Drinking water. Exposure may come from lead water pipes, found in many homes built before 1930. Even newer copper pipes may have lead solder. Also, some new homes have brass faucets and fittings that can leach lead.
- Jobs and hobbies. A number of activities can expose participants to lead. These include making pottery or stained glass, refinishing furniture, doing home repairs, and using indoor firing ranges. When adults take part in such activities, they may inadvertently expose children to lead residue that is on their clothing or on scrap materials.
- Food. Imported food cans often have lead solder. Lead may also be found in leaded crystal glassware and some imported ceramic or old ceramic dishes (e.g., ceramic dishes from Mexico). A 2003 study of cases of lead poisoning in pregnant women found that 70% of the patients were Hispanics, most of whom had absorbed the lead from their pottery. In addition, food may be contaminated by lead in the water or soil.
- Folk medicines. Certain folk medicines (for example, alarcon, alkohl, azarcon, bali goli, coral, ghasard, greta, liga, pay-loo-ah, and rueda) and traditional cosmetics (kohl, for example) contain large amounts of lead.
- Moonshine whiskey. Lead poisoning from drinking illegally distilled liquor is a cause of death among adults in the southern United States.
- Gunshot wounds. Toxic amounts of lead can be absorbed from bullets or bullet fragments that remain in the body after emergency surgery.

Chronic lead poisoning

New evidence suggests that lead may be harmful to children even at low levels that were once thought to be safe, and the risk of damage rises as blood levels of lead increase. The symptoms of chronic lead poisoning take time to develop. Children can appear healthy despite having high levels of lead in their blood. Over time, though, problems such as the following may arise:

- learning disabilities
- hyperactivity
- intellectual disability
- slowed growth
- hearing loss
- headaches

Certain **genetic factors** increase the harmful effects of lead poisoning in susceptible children; however, these factors are not completely understood.

Lead poisoning is also harmful to adults, in whom it can cause high blood pressure, digestive problems, nerve disorders, memory loss, and muscle and joint pain. In addition, it can lead to difficulties during pregnancy, as well as cause reproductive problems in men and women.

More recently, chronic exposure to lead in the environment has been found to speed up the progression of kidney disorders in patients without diabetes.

Acute lead poisoning

Acute lead poisoning, while less common, shows up more quickly and can be fatal. Symptoms such as the following may occur:

- severe abdominal pain
- diarrhea
- nausea and vomiting
- weakness of the limbs
- seizures
- coma

Diagnosis

A high level of lead in the blood can be detected with a simple blood test. In fact, testing is the only way to know for sure if children without symptoms have been exposed to lead, since they can appear healthy even as long-term damage occurs. The CDC recommends testing all children at 12 months of age and, if possible, again at 24 months. Testing should start at 6 months for children at risk for lead poisoning. Based on these test results and a child's risk factors, the doctor will then decide whether further testing is needed and how often. In some states, more frequent testing is required by law.

Children at risk

Children with an increased risk of lead poisoning include those who:

- live in or regularly visit a house built before 1978 in which chipped or peeling paint is present
- live in or regularly visit a house that was built before 1978 where remodeling is planned or underway
- have a brother or sister, housemate, or playmate that has been diagnosed with lead poisoning
- have the habit of eating dirt or have been diagnosed with pica
- live with an adult whose job or hobby involves exposure to lead
- live near an active lead smelter, battery-recycling plant, or other industry that can create lead pollution

Adults at risk

Testing is also important for adults whose job or hobby puts them at risk for lead poisoning. This includes people who take part in the following activities:

- glazed pottery or stained glass making
- furniture refinishing
- home renovation
- target shooting at indoor firing ranges
- battery reclamation
- precious metal refining
- radiator repair
- art restoration

Treatment

The first step in treating lead poisoning is to avoid further contact with lead. For adults, this usually means making changes at work or in hobbies. For children, it means finding and removing sources of lead in the home. In most states, the public health department can help assess the home and identify lead sources.

If the problem is lead paint, a professional with special training should remove it. Removal of lead paint is not a do-it-yourself project. Scraping or sanding lead paint creates large amounts of dust that can poison people in the home. This dust can stay around long after the work is completed. In addition, heating lead paint can release lead into the air. For these reasons, lead paint should only be removed by someone who knows how to do the job safely and has the equipment to clean up thoroughly. Occupants, especially children and pregnant women, should leave the home until the cleanup is finished.

KEY TERMS

Chelation therapy—Treatment with chemicals that bind to a poisonous metal and help the body pass it in urine at a faster rate.

Pica—An abnormal appetite or craving for non-food items, often such substances as chalk, clay, dirt, laundry starch, or charcoal.

Medical professionals should take all necessary steps to remove bullets or bullet fragments from patients with gunshot injuries.

Chelation therapy

If blood levels of lead are high enough, the doctor may also prescribe chelation therapy. This refers to treatment with chemicals that bind to the lead and help the body pass it in urine at a faster rate. There are four chemical agents that may be used for this purpose, either alone or in combination. Edetate calcium disodium (EDTA calcium) and dimercaprol (BAL) are given through an intravenous line or in shots, while succimer (Chemet) and penicillamine (Cuprimine, Depen) are taken by mouth. (Although many doctors prescribe penicillamine for lead poisoning, this use of the drug has not been approved by the U.S. Food and Drug Administration.)

Alternative treatment

Changes in diet are no substitute for medical treatment. However, getting enough calcium, **zinc**, and protein may help reduce the amount of lead the body absorbs. Iron is also important, since people who are deficient in this nutrient absorb more lead. Garlic and thiamine, a B-complex vitamin, have been used to treat lead poisoning in animals. However, their usefulness in humans for this purpose has not been proved. Nutritional, botanical, and homeopathic medicines can be administered once the source is removed to help correct any imbalances brought on by lead toxicity.

Prognosis

If acute lead poisoning reaches the stage of seizures and coma, there is a high risk of death. Even if the person survives, there is a good chance of permanent brain damage. The long-term effects of lower levels of lead can also be permanent and severe. However, if chronic lead poisoning is caught early, these negative effects can be limited by reducing future exposure to lead and getting proper medical treatment.

Prevention

Many cases of lead poisoning can be prevented. These steps can help:

- Keep the areas where children play as clean and dust-free as possible.
- Wash pacifiers and bottles when they fall to the floor, and wash stuffed animals and toys often.
- Make sure children wash their hands before meals and at bedtime.
- Mop floors and wipe windowsills and other chewable surfaces, such as cribs, with a damp cloth or mild soap solution.
- Plant bushes next to an older home with painted exterior walls to keep children at a distance.
- Plant grass or another ground cover in soil that is likely to be contaminated, such as soil around a home built before 1960 or located near a major highway.
- Have household tap water tested to find out if it contains lead.
- Use only water from the cold-water tap for drinking, cooking, and making baby formula, since hot water is likely to contain higher levels of lead.
- If the cold water hasn't been used for six hours or more, run it for several seconds, until it becomes as cold as it will get, before using it for drinking or cooking. The more time water has been sitting in the pipes, the more lead it may contain.
- If you work with lead in your job or hobby, change your clothes before you go home.
- Do not store food in open cans, especially imported cans.
- Do not store or serve food in pottery meant for decorative use.

Resources

BOOKS

Legge, Thomas M. *Lead Poisoning and Lead Absorption: The Symptoms, Pathology and Prevention*. Whitefish, MT: Kessinger Publishing, 2007.

PERIODICALS

Lanphear, Bruce P. "The Conquest of Lead Poisoning: A Pyrrhic Victory." *Environmental Health Perspectives* 115 (October 2007): A484–A485.

Parham, Marti. "Toy Recalls & Lead Poisoning: What Parents Need to Know." *Jet*. (September 24, 2007).

Pekkanen, John. "Poisonous Predator: Lead Is Gone from Gasoline and Paint but Continues to Pose Danger to Kids, Particularly in Older Neighborhoods." *Children's Voice Magazine* 16:4 (July–August 2007): 26(5).

Sharmer, L., K. Northrup-Snyder, and W. Juan. "Newly Recognized Pathways of Exposure to Lead in the Middle-Income Home." *Journal of Environmental Health* 70, no. 3, (October 2007): 15–9.

Sloviter, Vikki. "Lead, Lead, Everywhere, What's A Parent to Do?" *Pediatrics for Parents*. (August 2007).

Warniment, Crista. "Lead Poisoning in Children—What Parents Should Know." *Pediatrics for Parents*. (January 1, 2011).

ORGANIZATIONS

Childhood Lead Poisoning Prevention Branch, Centers for Disease Control and Prevention, 1600 Clifton Rd., Atlanta, GA, 30333, (800) 232-4636; TTY: (888) 232-6348, cdcinfo@cdc.gov, http://www.cdc.gov/nceh/lead.

Consumer Product Safety Commission, 4330 East West Highway, Bethesda, MD, 20814, (301) 504-7923, http://www.cpsc.gov.

National Lead Information Center, 422 South Clinton Ave., Rochester, NY, 14620, (1-800) 424-5323, Fax: (585) 232-3111, http://www.epa.gov.

National Safety Council, 1121 Spring Lake Drive, Itasca, IL, 60143-3201, (630) 285-1121, (800) 621-7615, Fax: (630) 285-1315, customerservice@nsc.org, http://www.nsc.org.

Linda Wasmer Smith
Ken R. Wells

Learning disorders

Definition

Learning disorders (LDs), or learning disabilities, are disorders that cause problems in speaking, listening, reading, writing, or mathematical ability in children and adults of average to above-average intelligence. These difficulties significantly interfere with academic achievement or daily living.

In the United States and Canada, LDs are considered to be neurological disorders and reflect problems with information processing in the **brain**. They are not considered to be automatic indications of low intelligence. The Learning Disabilities Association of America (LDA) states, "Learning disabilities should not be confused with learning problems which are primarily the result of visual, hearing, or motor disabilities; of intellectual disability; of emotional disturbance; or of environmental, cultural or economic disadvantages." In the United Kingdom, by contrast, the term "learning disability" is usually associated with low intelligence as well as with specific difficulties with reading, language use, mathematical calculations, or other aspects of learning.

The forthcoming fifth edition of the ***Diagnostic and Statistical Manual of Mental Disorders***, due for publication in 2013, defines four learning disorders, grouped under the general heading of neurodevelopmental disorders. The four learning disorders to be included in the *DSM-5* are:

- learning disorder
- dyslexia (reading disorder)
- dyscalculia (mathematics disorder)
- disorder of written expression

Demographics

Exact statistics for the number of people in the United States and Canada with LDs are difficult to obtain, as many of these disorders go undiagnosed. The National Center for Learning Disabilities states that 15 million children, adolescents, and adults in the United States have learning disorders, with 2.6 million school children involved in special education programs as of 2011. Other sources estimate that LDs occur in approximately 5% to 10% of the North American population. According to the National Institute of Neurological Disorders and Stroke (NINDS), between 8% and 10% of American youngsters below 18 years of age have some type of learning disability.

Between 50% and 70% of LDs are classified as dyslexia; the remaining 30% to 50% fall under the categories of **disorder of written expression**, dyscalculia, or atypical LD. One estimate for disorder of written expression is 6% of the school-age population in Canada and the United States, with another 6% diagnosed with dyscalculia. The statistics can be confusing, however, because it is possible for someone to have more than one learning disorder; in one study, 56% of children with a **reading disorder** also showed poor mathematics achievement, and 43% of children with a mathematical learning disorder showed poor reading skills.

LDs are more common in males than females by a 2:1 or 4:1 ratio. Children with LDs have an increased risk for emotional-behavioral problems and comorbidity; 50% of the 1.6 million children with **attention deficit hyperactivity disorder (ADHD)** have an LD. Approximately 2% to 8% of elementary school children have dyslexia. Speech disorder occurs in approximately 10% of children younger than eight years of age. ADHD is a comorbid condition that occurs in approximately four million school-aged children; 20% of them are unable to focus their attention on required tasks in school and at home.

Dyslexia rates in the United States do not show any racial or ethnic differences.

U.S. children (ages 3–17) thought to have a learning disability[1], by selected characteristics: 2010

	Number of children interviewed[2]	Number of children with a learning disability	Percent
Total (age adjusted)	**61,655**	**4,838**	**7.9%**
Gender			
Male	31,519	2,917	9.3%
Female	30,137	1,921	6.4%
Age			
3–4 years	8,443	267	3.2%
5–11 years	28,666	2,291	8.0%
12–17 years	24,546	2,280	9.3%
Race			
One race	59,155	4,598	7.8%
White	46,607	3,532	7.6%
Black or African American	9,106	904	10.0%
American Indian or Alaska Native	541	*57	*10.2%
Asian	2,746	95	3.5%
Native Hawaiian or other Pacific Islander	155	†	†
Two or more races	2,500	240	9.3%
Black or African American and white	1,082	142	11.5%
American Indian or Alaska Native and white	425	*40	*10.6%

[1]Based on the question, "Has a representative from a school or a health professional ever told you that [child's name] had a learning disability?"
[2]All numbers in thousands
*Estimates preceded by an asterisk had a relative standard error between 30% and 50% and should be used with caution, as they do not meet standards of reliability or precision.
†Estimates had a relative standard error greater than 50% and were not included.

SOURCE: National Center for Health Statistics, U.S. Centers for Disease Control and Prevention, "Summary Health Statistics for U.S. Children: National Health Interview Survey, 2010," *Vital and Health Statistics* 10, no. 250 (December 2011).

(Table by PreMediaGlobal. © 2012 Cengage Learning.)

Some LDs are more common in North America than in other parts of the world. The incidence of dyscalculia among American children is higher than in Japanese, German, or French children.

Description

A learning disability, or specific developmental disorder, is a disorder that inhibits or interferes with the skills of learning; that is, people's abilities to store, process, or produce information. Under federal law, public schools in the United States consider a child to be learning disabled if his or her level of academic achievement is two or more years below the standard for age and IQ level. The term *learning disorder* was first used in the 1960s to describe learning difficulties in

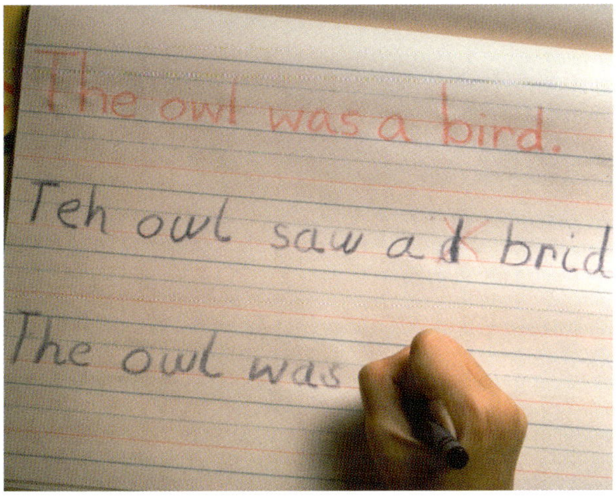
The owl was a bird.
Teh owl saw a brid
The owl was

A learning disorder makes reading and writing a challenge. *(© Will & Deni McIntyre/Science Source/Photo Researchers, Inc.)*

individuals of at least average intelligence whose academic achievement lagged significantly behind their expected potential. It was assumed that some type of central nervous dysfunction was responsible for the discrepancy.

It is important to note that although learning disorders can be classified into subtypes, they are actually a group of disorders with varying characteristics. In addition, there are wide variations in the severity and development of LDs that are unique to each individual diagnosed with a learning disorder. Some experts in the field classify LDs by the specific type of mental processing difficulty that the affected person has rather than whether it appears in reading, writing, or mathematics. Processing difficulties can be identified as affecting input, integration, memory, and output. Any of these processing difficulties could affect a person's ability to read, write, or perform mathematical calculations.

- Input refers to a person's ability to take in information through the senses; for example, to distinguish between similarly shaped letters or similar sounds in spoken language.
- Integration refers to a person's ability to make sense of inputs; that is, to place information obtained through the senses in a logical sequence, organize the information, and make sense of it.
- Memory refers to a person's ability to store information in their short-term, long-term, or working memory so that they can retrieve the information when it is needed.
- Output refers to the person's ability to express what has been integrated and stored, either through language or through motor activity like writing, drawing, or making gestures.

Risk factors

Risk factors for learning disorders include a range of factors that can affect the structure of the brain, its functioning, or both. Some are congenital (present at birth), while others have to do with genetic influences and the family environment. Known risk factors include:

- Fetal alcohol syndrome.
- Prenatal exposure to the mother's cigarette smoking or use of cocaine.
- Family history of learning disorders. LDs are known to run in families. According to the Institute for Behavioral Genetics at the University of Colorado, there is a 36% to 45% heritability of reading disorders in some families.
- History of delayed early language development.
- Being diagnosed with ADHD. Many pediatricians recommend that all children with ADHD should be screened for learning disorders.
- Male sex. Some doctors attribute the higher rate of LDs in boys to abnormally high levels of the male sex hormone testosterone during fetal development, particularly between the sixteenth and twenty-fourth weeks of pregnancy.

Causes and symptoms

The causes of learning disorders are not completely understood. While certain areas of the brain are definitely known to be associated with dyslexia, the structural or functional causes of other learning disorders are still being researched. The Colorado Learning Disabilities Research Center (CLDRC) was conducting five separate research projects as of 2011 involving pairs of identical twins in which at least one twin had either an LD or ADHD. DNA analysis of the twins and their parents was being conducted as well as measurements of the affected twin's response to treatment. The CLDRC researchers were hoping to discover whether there are definite **genetic factors** involved in learning disorders, and whether reading disabilities represent a single syndrome or a group of disorders with several subtypes.

Dyslexia

Modern research techniques have demonstrated that dyslexia is the result of brain deficits in processing sound units and sound-symbol relationships. The cause of dyslexia has been identified as variations in the right temporoparietal-occipital region of the brain, specifically in structures known as the "angular gyrus" and "corpus callosum." The angular gyrus is involved in mathematical as well as language skills, which may explain the connection between dyslexia and dyscalculia. In addition, the left temporo-occipital region, which is active during the automatic perception and processing of visually presented words in skilled readers, is implicated in reading problems. Activity in this region is necessary for rapid perception of word forms.

Genetic studies have identified 8 genetic defects associated with dyslexia as of 2011, with another 20 genetic conditions characterized by normal intelligence combined with reading difficulties in those affected. In addition, the heritability of dyslexia may be higher than 50%, especially in a disorder with a focal deficit in phonologic processing (phonologic dyslexia). Family studies indicate that dyslexia is found in clusters in families and probably reflects an autosomal dominant mode of transmission. Some genetic investigations have identified possible genes for dyslexia located on chromosomes 6 and 15; as of 2011, there were 14 genes identified as candidates.

Most people diagnosed with dyslexia have average or higher intelligence. Persons with dyslexia often have trouble spelling. Affected individuals have difficulty with phonologic processing, which means that they have deficits in identifying and manipulating individual sounds (phonemes) within larger sound units (morphemes and words). The symptoms of dyslexia usually appear before the early school grades. Patients cannot translate a visual stimulus (letters) into a meaningful blend of sounds. Reading is slower and more mechanical, even with treatment. The increased concentration required during reading can impair the person's ability to pay attention. A somewhat less common cause of dyslexia is visualization-comprehension deficits. Persons with visualization-comprehension weakness often exhibit difficulty visualizing what is being read.

KEY TERMS

CAPD—Central auditory processing disorder, the inability to differentiate, recognize, or understand sounds; hearing and intelligence are normal.

Comorbidity—The presence of one or more diseases or disorders in addition to a primary disease or disorder.

Dyscalculia—Difficulty in performing mathematical computations. It is also called "mathematical learning disorder."

Dysgraphia—A writing disorder characterized by illegible handwriting.

Dyslexia—Unexpected difficulty learning to read despite adequate intelligence, motivation, and educational opportunities.

Incidence—A measurement of the risk of developing a specific disease or disorder within a given time period in a specific population.

IQ—Intelligence quotient, or a measure of the intelligence of an individual based on the results of a written test.

Morpheme—The smallest meaningful speech sound.

Motivational therapy—An approach to treatment for learning disorders that emphasizes problem-solving skills, the ability to set and attain goals, and ways to counteract negative thinking and poor self-image.

Phoneme—The smallest detectable sound within a spoken word.

Phonics—A system to teach reading by teaching the speech sounds associated with single letters, letter combinations, and syllables.

Response to intervention (RTI)—An approach to diagnosis of learning disorders based on a child's response (or lack of response) to early interventions with learning problems.

Dyscalculia

The cause of dyscalculia is thought to be a nonverbal weakness. There may be deficits visualizing and visually organizing mathematical concepts and manipulations; one recently proposed theory holds that children with dyscalculia are less precise in working with the approximate number system (an intuitive "number sense" of the comparative magnitude and relationships among numbers). Some researchers have identified as many as 16 separate skills required in learning mathematics, including memorizing facts (such as the multiplication tables); recalling those facts; understanding details; mastering procedures that must be carried out in a particular sequence (such as solving a problem in plane geometry); recognizing patterns; and accumulating knowledge over time. Mathematics is a cumulative discipline that requires students to build on what they have learned in lower grades. Some persons diagnosed with dyscalculia may have short-term or working memory deficits that can interfere with processing mathematical calculations. In addition, children who also have dyslexia will have considerable difficulty with the word problems that are a staple of mathematics instruction in the middle and upper grades. Last, some children have difficulty with mathematics because they are afraid of the subject. The child's anxiety may be related either to difficulty acquiring specific mathematical skills or to fear of humiliation in class.

The symptoms of dyscalculia vary but are usually apparent during the early grade-school years. Some children may show weakness in one particular area, such as counting, but perform adequately in other areas of mathematics. Patients can exhibit either great difficulty or complete inability (known as "acalculia") to perform mathematical calculations.

Disorder of written expression

The causes of disorder of written expression (DWE) were unknown as of 2011. It is relatively unusual for this disorder to appear by itself without dyslexia, dyscalculia, or both. In some persons, DWE may be due to deficits in visual-motor integration and motor coordination. Most causes of DWE occur because there are deficits in the brain concerning information translation from auditory-oral modality to visual-written modality. DWE is usually diagnosed around the time the child is in second or third grade.

Patients with DWE often exhibit spelling deficits that include problems with punctuation, grammar, and development of written ideas. Writing samples from affected persons are typically brief, simple, and difficult to comprehend because of the large number of errors in grammar and punctuation. Patients with visual-motor deficits write with so much care that they often lose track of ideas and thoughts. If motor coordination is the only cause of the problem, then the person's symptoms may be classified more appropriately as a motor skills disorder, not a DWE. The symptoms of DWE are not usually apparent until the third or fourth grade, when written academic work demands the development of ideas.

Diagnosis

In order to meet the criteria established by the **American Psychiatric Association** (APA) for these various diagnoses, the child's skills in these areas must be significantly below those of his or her peers on standardized tests (taking age, schooling, and level of intelligence into account), and the disorders must significantly interfere with academic achievement and/or daily living. **Diagnosis** can be a complex process, however, because there is no universal agreement concerning the magnitude of discrepancy between test scores. There is no consensus concerning which test scores should be analyzed to obtain a statistical analysis of discrepancy. Tests should be administered to establish that low intelligence alone is not the cause of underachievement.

A newer approach to diagnosis is known as response to intervention or RTI. RTI is a treatment model intended to identify children at risk for an LD at an early point, before they meet the full *DSM* criteria for a learning disorder. It is considered an alternative to the discrepancy model for evaluating children with learning difficulties, which has sometimes been criticized as the "wait-to-fail" model. RTI is characterized by early **intervention**, frequent progress measurement, and increasingly intensive research-based instructional interventions for children who continue to have difficulties in learning. Children who respond to early intervention will not require further interventions. Those who do not respond adequately to regular classroom instruction and a more intensive intervention are considered nonresponders. These students can then be referred for further educational assistance through special education programs. One drawback to RTI, however, is that the early interventions must be competently carried out; otherwise, children may be evaluated as nonresponders to treatment and as having a learning disorder when the real cause is poor instruction. Another criticism of RTI is that it is a covert form of school budget management that functions to limit access to expensive special education services by delaying the diagnosis of children who need them.

Examination

A child thought to have a learning disorder should undergo a complete medical examination to rule out an eye disorder, hearing loss, or other organic cause. If a medical problem is not found, a psychoeducational assessment should be performed by a **psychologist**, **psychiatrist**, neurologist, neuropsychologist, or learning specialist. A complete medical, family, social, and educational history is compiled from existing medical and school records and from interviews with the child and the child's parents and teachers. In the case of children suspected of having DWE, it is important to evaluate the child's posture, handedness, pencil grip, and other traits to rule out possible problems related to slow motor development or other physical disorders affecting the hand and wrist.

Tests

A series of written and verbal tests are given to the child to evaluate his or her cognitive and intellectual functioning. Commonly used tests include the Wechsler

Intelligence Scale for Children (WISC-III), the Woodcock-Johnson Psychoeducational Battery, the Peabody Individual Achievement Test-Revised (PIAT-R), and the California Verbal Learning Test (CVLT). Specific tests used to evaluate disorders of written expression include the Test of Early Written Language, for children between 3 and 11 years of age; the Test of Written Language, for children between 7 and 18 years of age; and the Test of Written Spelling, for children between the ages of 6 and 18 years. Federal legislation mandates that all these tests be given free of charge within the public school system.

Treatment

Treatment for a learning disorder is highly individualized. It depends on the specific disorder, the age of the person at the time of diagnosis, the severity of the disorder, the presence of ADHD or other comorbidity, and the assumed underlying cause. For example, people with central auditory processing disorder (CAPD), a common underlying cause of some learning disorders that is centered on a person's inability to process heard language correctly, may undergo therapy with a speech-language pathologist. Other experts may use different kinds of auditory therapies to improve the person's ability to process heard language.

Once a learning disorder has been diagnosed, an individual education plan (IEP) is developed for the child in question. IEPs are based on psychoeducational test findings. They provide for annual testing to measure a child's progress. Students with learning disorders may receive special instruction within a regular general education class, or they may be taught in a special education or learning center for a portion of the day.

Traditional

The treatment team for a child diagnosed with an LD typically includes school counselors, education specialists, specialists in learning disorders, school psychologists, or clinical psychologists with advanced clinical training in administration and interpretation of psychological tests, or psychometrics. Tests for achievement and intelligence should be administered and interpreted by a clinical psychologist or school psychologist. Only a duly licensed or certified clinical or school psychologist can administer the recommended psychological tests. A full written report of results and interpretation of results is typically prepared and submitted to concerned persons.

DYSLEXIA. Common strategies for the treatment of dyslexia focus first on improving a child's recognition of the sounds of letters and language through phonics training. Later strategies focus on comprehension, retention, and study skills. Treatment for affected persons involves intensive tutoring to develop phonologic processing and fluent word reading with treatment objectives that emphasize comprehension. There are several treatment approaches (the Gillingham-Stillman Approach, the Fernald-Keller Approach, or the Lindamood-Bell Reading Program) that provide intensive phonic practice and phonic associations with sensory integration or mnemonic strategies to remember letter-sound blends and relationships.

It is important for parents of a child diagnosed with dyslexia to understand that the disorder is not related to the visual system but is caused by defects in the development of the language processing areas of the brain. Thus, bifocals, eye muscle exercises, or other forms of visual training will not help children with dyslexia.

DYSCALCULIA. Treatment for dyscalculia can vary widely because the disorder may have a variety of causes and presentations, particularly if the child also has dyslexia or ADHD. The treatment program is typically highly individualized. Flash cards and practice drills can help children to memorize simple mathematical operations such as multiplication tables. Dyscalculia due to visual-organization deficits can be treated with visualization techniques to improve math-related skills. Instruction for students with mathematical disorders also emphasizes such real-world uses of mathematics as balancing a checkbook or comparing prices.

Children with dyscalculia may be helped by motivational therapy and investigation of the role of anxiety or phobia in their difficulties with mathematics. New approaches to treatment for dyscalculia are being researched, because the disorder is not yet understood as well as dyslexia or disorders or written expression. There was one clinical study under way as of 2011 investigating transcranial stimulation as a potential treatment for dyscalculia.

DISORDER OF WRITTEN EXPRESSION. There are several treatment plans for DWE, including: writing in more natural environments, for example, keeping a diary and making lists; writing notes and outlines before writing prose; and talking-to-writing progression, which involves the affected child dictating while another person writes down what is dictated. As this latter treatment progresses, the roles are gradually reversed until the child is able to dictate and write without assistance. Treatment continues with dictation made more quiet and discreet until the child is independently thinking and writing. Treatment interventions for atypical LDs involve objectives to expand on the child's strengths and to provide additional experience and practice in nonverbal weakness areas. Students with disorders of written expression are often encouraged to keep journals and to write on a computer keyboard instead of using a pencil; however, most experts maintain that children with DWE should use computers and other assistive technology to complement handwritten exercises rather than relying on them to eliminate handwriting completely.

Other forms of therapy that benefit children with DWE are coaching in basic study skills; the use of child-friendly templates (outlines) to help children structure and sequence their thoughts and ideas before writing their story or essay; and teaching children to think of writing as a process with five parts based on the word "POWER," which stands for "plan, organize, write, edit, and revise." Motivational therapy, which teaches children problem-solving strategies, goal setting, and modifying or eliminating negative beliefs that interfere with academic achievement, is also helpful to those diagnosed with DWE.

Drugs

There are no medications that can treat or cure learning disorders. Some medications, such as stimulants or **antidepressants**, may be prescribed for children with ADHD, **depression**, or other comorbid disorders. These drugs may be effective in helping the child learn by enhancing his or her ability to pay attention and concentrate in school, or in coping with anxiety or depression associated with the LD.

Alternative

There are no alternative therapies that claim to cure learning disorders; however, nutritional therapy and some forms of **relaxation therapy** may be helpful to children and adults during mainstream treatment. Some older children or adolescents may also benefit from **meditation**, which helps in focusing the mind and learning to shut out distractions.

Prognosis

The prognosis for learning disorders depends in part on early diagnosis. However, learning disabilities do persist across the lifespan. The prognosis is highly individualized; some persons with more than one LD, or with an LD in addition to ADHD, may fail to complete high school; the high-school dropout rate for children with learning disabilities is almost 40%. On the other hand, some people diagnosed with LDs may have a single isolated disability that has little effect on their day-to-day functioning.

Children with learning disabilities that go undiagnosed or are improperly treated might never achieve functional literacy. They often develop serious behavioral problems as a result of their frustration with school; in addition, their learning problems are often stressful for other family members and may strain family relationships. The keys to helping these students reach their fullest potential are early detection and the implementation of an appropriate individualized education plan. The prognosis is good for a large percentage of children with reading disorders that are identified and treated early. Learning disorders continue into adulthood, but with proper educational and vocational training, an individual can complete college and pursue a challenging career. Studies of the occupational choices of adults with dyslexia indicate that they do particularly well in such people-oriented professions and occupations as nursing or sales.

QUESTIONS TO ASK YOUR DOCTOR

- How can I tell whether my child has an LD?
- Some of my relatives have been diagnosed with dyslexia. Does that mean that my child will have a reading disorder, too?
- Why are boys more likely to develop LDs than girls?
- What is your opinion of RTI as an approach to learning disorders?
- What are the chances that a child diagnosed with an LD will have a second LD or ADHD?

Prevention

Some learning disorders are potentially preventable if women of childbearing age avoid alcohol, **cocaine**, and tobacco during pregnancy. However, LDs related to heredity and structural abnormalities of the brain are not preventable.

Resources

BOOKS

Burack, Jacob A., et al., eds. *The Oxford Handbook of Intellectual Disability and Development*, 2nd ed. New York: Oxford University Press, 2011.

Goldstein, Sam, Jack A. Naglieri, and Melissa DeVries, eds. *Learning and Attention Disorders in Adolescence and*

Adulthood: Assessment and Treatment, 2nd ed. Hoboken, NJ: John Wiley and Sons, 2011.

Hoover, John J. *Differentiating Learning Differences from Disabilities: Meeting Diverse Needs through Multi-tiered Response to Intervention*. Upper Saddle River, NJ: Pearson, 2009.

Parks, Peggy J. *Learning Disabilities*. San Diego, CA: ReferencePoint Press, 2010.

Pennington, Bruce Franklin. *Diagnosing Learning Disorders: A Neuropsychological Framework*, 2nd ed. New York: Guilford Press, 2009.

PERIODICALS

Annett, M. "Dyslexia and Handedness: Developmental Phonological and Surface Dyslexias Are Associated with Different Biases for Handedness."*Perceptual and Motor Skills* 112 (April 2011): 417–425.

Butterworth, B., et al. "Dyscalculia: From Brain to Education." *Science* 332 (May 27, 2011): 1049–1053.

Duff, F.J., and P.J. Clarke. "Practitioner Review: Reading Disorders: What Are the Effective Interventions and How Should They Be Implemented and Evaluated?" *Journal of Child Psychology and Psychiatry, and Allied Disciplines* 52 (January 2011): 3–12.

Kupfer, D.J., and D.A. Regier. "Neuroscience, Clinical Evidence, and the Future of Psychiatric Classification in DSM-5." *American Journal of Psychiatry* 168 (July 2011): 672–674.

Mazzocco, M.M., et al. "Impaired Acuity of the Approximate Number System Underlies Mathematical Learning Disability (Dyscalculia)." *Child Development* 82 (July-August 2011): 1224–1237.

Miller, B., and P. McCardle. "Moving Closer to a Public Health Model of Language and Learning Disabilities: The Role of Genetics and the Search for Etiologies." *Behavior Genetics* 41 (January 2011): 1–5.

Miller, C.A. "Auditory Processing Theories of Language Disorders: Past, Present, and Future." *Language, Speech, and Hearing Services in Schools* 42 (July 2011): 309–319.

Poelmans, G., et al. "A Theoretical Molecular Network for Dyslexia: Integrating Available Genetic Findings." *Molecular Psychiatry* 16 (April 2011): 365–82.

Willcutt, E.G., et al. "Understanding the Complex Etiologies of Developmental Disorders: Behavioral and Molecular Genetic Approaches." *Journal of Developmental and Behavioral Pediatrics* 31 (September 2010): 533–544.

WEBSITES

American Psychiatric Association. DSM-5 Development. "Neurodevelopmental Disorders." http://www.dsm5.org/proposedrevision/pages/neurodevelopmentaldisorders.aspx (accessed September 26, 2011).

International Dyslexia Association (IDA). "Frequently Asked Questions about Dyslexia." http://www.interdys.org/FAQ.htm (accessed September 27, 2011).

Learning Disabilities Association of America (LDA). "LD Basics." http://www.ldaamerica.org/aboutld/parents/ld_basics/index.asp (accessed September 27, 2011).

Medscape. "Learning Disorder, Mathematics." http://emedicine.medscape.com/article/915176-overview (accessed September 28, 2011).

Medscape. "Learning Disorder, Written Expression." http://emedicine.medscape.com/article/1835883-overview (accessed September 28, 2011).

Medscape. "Reading Learning Disorder." http://emedicine.medscape.com/article/1835801-overview (accessed September 27, 2011).

National Center for Learning Disabilities (NCLD). "LD Explained." http://www.ncld.org/ld-basics/ld-explained (accessed September 27, 2011).

National Institute of Neurological Disorders and Stroke (NINDS). "Learning Disabilities Information Page." http://www.ninds.nih.gov/disorders/learningdisabilities/learningdisabilities.htm (accessed September 27, 2011).

Nemours. "Learning Disabilities." TeensHealth.org. http://teenshealth.org/teen/diseases_conditions/learning/learning_disabilities.html (accessed January 12, 2012).

ORGANIZATIONS

American Psychiatric Association (APA), 1000 Wilson Boulevard, Suite 1825, Arlington, VA, 22209-3901, (703) 907-7300, apa@psych.org, http://www.psych.org.

American Speech-Language-Hearing Association (ASHA), 2200 Research Boulevard, Rockville, MD, 20850-3289, (301) 296-5700, Fax: (301) 296-8580, (800) 638-8255, http://www.asha.org.

Colorado Learning Disabilities Research Center (CLDRC), Institute for Behavioral Genetics, 1480 30th St., Boulder, CO, 80303, (303) 492-7362, Fax: (303) 492-8063, info@ibg.colorado.edu, http://ibgwww.colorado.edu/cldrc.

International Dyslexia Association (IDA), 40 York Rd., 4th Floor, Baltimore, MD, 21204, (410) 296-0232, Fax: (410) 321-5069, http://www.interdys.org ContactUs.htm, http://www.interdys.org.

Learning Disabilities Association of America (LDA), 4156 Library Road, Pittsburgh, PA, 15234–1349, (412) 341-1515, Fax: (412) 344-0224, http://www.ldanatl.org/contact/contact.cfm, http://www.ldanatl.org.

National Center for Learning Disabilities (NCLD), 381 Park Avenue South, Suite 1401, New York, NY, 10016, (212) 545-7510, Fax: (212) 545-9665, (888) 575-7373, ncld@ncld.org, http://www.ncld.org.

National Institute on Deafness and Other Communication Disorders (NIDCD) Information Clearinghouse, 1 Communication Avenue, Bethesda, MD, 20892-3456, Fax: (301) 770-8977, (800) 241-1044, nidcdinfo@ nidcd.nih.gov, http://www.nidcd.nih.gov.

National Institute of Neurological Disorders and Stroke (NINDS), PO Box 5801, Bethesda, MD, 20824, (301) 496-5751, (800) 352-9424, http://www.ninds.nih.gov.

Emily Jane Willingham, Ph.D.
Rebecca J. Frey, Ph.D.

Lexapro *see* **Escitalopram**
Librax *see* **Chlordiazepoxide**
Librium *see* **Chlordiazepoxide**
Lidone *see* **Molindone**

Light therapy

Definition

Light therapy, or phototherapy, is the administration of doses of bright light in order to treat a variety of sleep and mood disorders. It is most commonly used to reregulate the body's internal clock and relieve **depression**.

Purpose

Light therapy is most often prescribed to treat **seasonal affective disorder**, a form of depression resulting from shortened daylight hours in northern latitudes from the late fall to the early spring. It is also occasionally employed to treat such sleep-related disorders as **insomnia** and jet lag. Recently, light therapy has also been found effective in the treatment of nonseasonal forms of depression, including the depressive symptoms of **bipolar disorder**. One study found that bright light reduced depressive symptoms 12%–35% more than a placebo treatment in 9 out of 10 randomized controlled trials.

When used to treat SAD or other forms of depression, light therapy has several advantages over prescription **antidepressants**. Light therapy tends to work faster than medications, alleviating depressive symptoms within 2 to 14 days after beginning light therapy as opposed to an average of 4 to 6 weeks with medication. And unlike antidepressants, which can cause a variety of side effects from nausea to concentration problems, light therapy is extremely well tolerated. Some side effects are possible with light but are generally not serious enough to cause discontinuation of the therapy.

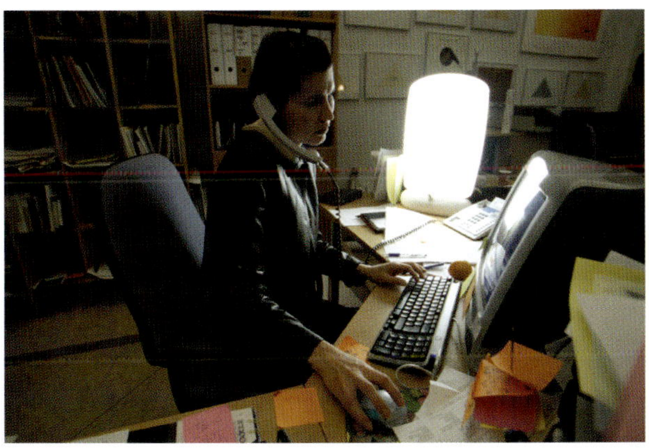

A woman uses a sun lamp to treat seasonal affective disorder. *(© Jochem Wijnands/Picture Contact BV/Alamy)*

There are several other different applications for light therapy, including:

- Full-spectrum/UV light therapy for disorders of the skin. A subtype of light therapy that is often prescribed to treat skin diseases, rashes, and jaundice.
- Cold laser therapy. The treatment involves focusing very low-intensity beams of laser light on the skin and is used in laser acupuncture to treat a myriad of symptoms and illnesses, including pain, stress, and tendinitis.
- Colored light therapy. In colored light therapy, different colored filters are applied over a light source to achieve specific therapeutic effects. The colored light is then focused on the patient, either with a floodlight which covers the patient with the colored light, or with a beam of light that is focused on the area of the illness.
- Back-of-the-knee light therapy. According to a 1998 study published in the journal *Science*, the area behind the human knee known as the popliteal region contains photoreceptors that can help to adjust the body's circadian rhythms. The authors of the study found that they could manipulate circadian rhythms by focusing a bright light on the popliteal region. Further studies are underway to determine the efficacy of this treatment on disorders such as SAD, although there have been cases of treating pain with this method.

Description

Light therapy is generally administered at home. The most commonly used light therapy equipment is a portable lighting device known as a light box. The light box may be a full-spectrum box, in which the lighting element contains all wavelengths of light found in natural light (including UV rays), or it may be a bright light box, in which the lighting element emits non-UV white light. The box may be mounted upright to a wall or slanted down toward a table.

The patient sits in front of the box for a prescribed period of time (anywhere from 15 minutes to several hours). For patients just starting on the therapy, initial sessions are usually only 10–15 minutes in length. Some patients with SAD undergo light therapy sessions two or three times a day, others only once. The time of day and number of times treatment is administered depends on the physical needs and lifestyle of the individual patient. If

> ### KEY TERMS
>
> **Dawn simulation**—A form of light therapy in which the patient is exposed while asleep to gradually brightening white light over a period of an hour and a half.
>
> **Lux**—The International System (IS) unit for measuring illumination, equal to one lumen per square meter.
>
> **Neurotransmitter**—A chemical in the brain that transmits messages between neurons, or nerve cells.
>
> **Seasonal affective disorder (SAD)**—A mood disorder characterized by depression, weight gain, and sleepiness during the winter months. An estimated 4%–6% of the population of Canada and the northern United States suffers from SAD.
>
> **Serotonin**—A neurotransmitter that is involved in mood disorders.

light therapy has been prescribed for the treatment of SAD, it typically begins in the fall and continues throughout the winter and possibly into the early spring. Patients with a long-standing history of SAD are usually able to establish a timetable or pattern to their depressive symptoms and can initiate treatment accordingly before symptoms begin.

The light from a slanted light box is designed to focus on the table it sits upon, so patients may look down to read or do other sedentary activities during therapy. Patients using an upright light box must face the light source and should glance toward the box occasionally without staring directly into the light. The light sources in these light boxes typically range from 2,500–10,000 lux (in contrast, average indoor lighting is 300–500 lux; a sunny summer day is about 100,000 lux).

Patients can purchase their own light boxes for a few hundred dollars, or they may be able to rent them from a healthcare provider or healthcare supply company. Renting gives patients the opportunity to have a trial run of the therapy before making the investment in a light box. Recently, several new light box products have become available, in addition to the traditional boxes. Dawn simulators are lighting devices or fixtures that are programmed to turn on gradually, from dim to bright light, to simulate the sunrise. They are sometimes prescribed for individuals who have difficulty getting up in the morning due to SAD symptoms. Another device known as a light visor is designed to give an individual more mobility during treatment. The visor is a lighting apparatus that is worn like a sun visor around the crown of the head. Patients with any history of eye problems should consult their healthcare professional before attempting to use a light visor.

Precautions

Patients with eye problems should see an ophthalmologist regularly both before and during light therapy. Because UV rays are emitted by the light box, patients taking photosensitizing medications should consult with their healthcare provider before beginning treatment. In addition, patients with medical conditions that make them sensitive to UV rays should also be seen by a healthcare professional before starting phototherapy.

Patients beginning light therapy for SAD may need to adjust the length, frequency, and timing of their phototherapy sessions in order to achieve the maximum benefits. Patients should keep their healthcare provider informed of their progress and the status of their depressive symptoms. Occasionally, additional treatment measures for depression (e.g., antidepressants, herbal remedies, **psychotherapy**) may be recommended as an adjunct, or companion, treatment to light therapy.

Preparation

Full-spectrum light boxes do emit UV rays, so patients with sun-sensitive skin should apply sunscreen before sitting in front of the box for an extended period of time.

Risks

Some patients undergoing light therapy treatments report side effects of eyestrain, headaches, insomnia, **fatigue**, sunburn, and dry eyes and nose. Most of these effects can be managed by adjusting the timing and duration of the light therapy sessions. A strong sunblock and eye and nose drops can alleviate the others. Long-term studies have shown no negative effects to eye function of individuals undergoing light therapy treatment.

A small percentage of light therapy patients may experience **hypomania**, a feeling of exaggerated, hyperelevated mood. Again, adjusting the length and frequency of treatment sessions can usually manage this side effect.

Research and general acceptance

Light therapy is widely accepted by both traditional and complementary medicine as an effective treatment for SAD. The exact mechanisms by which the treatment

QUESTIONS TO ASK YOUR DOCTOR

- Can I use phototherapy while I am taking antidepressants?
- Has bright-light phototherapy been proven to be effective in easing symptoms of seasonal affective disorder?
- What is the correct way to use the lights?

works are not known, but the bright light employed in light therapy may help readjust the body's circadian rhythms, or internal clock. Other popular theories are that light triggers the production of **serotonin**, a neurotransmitter believed to be associated with depressive disorders, or that it influences the body's production of melatonin, a hormone related to circadian rhythms. A recent British study suggests that dawn simulation, in which the patient is exposed to white light of gradually increasing brightness (peaking at 250 lux after 90 min), may be even more effective in treating depression than exposure to bright light. Dawn simulation is typically started around 4:30 or 5 A.M., while the patient is still asleep.

Training and certification

Psychiatrists, psychologists, and other mental healthcare professional prescribe light therapy treatment for SAD. There are also Holistic healthcare professionals and light therapists who specialize in this treatment; in some states, these professionals require a license, so individuals should check with their state board of health to ensure their practitioner has the proper credentials.

Resources

BOOKS

Lam, Raymond W., and Edwin M. Tam. *A Clinician's Guide to Using Light Therapy*. Cambridge: Cambridge University Press, 2009.

Rosenthal, N.E. *Winter Blues: Everything You Need to Know to Beat Seasonal Affective Disorder*. New York: Guilford Press, 2006.

PERIODICALS

Even, C., et al. "Efficacy of Light Therapy in Nonseasonal Depression: A Systematic Review." *Journal of Affective Disorders* 108 (May 2008): 11–23.

Lurie, S.J., et al. "Seasonal Affective Disorder." *American Family Physician* 74 (November 1, 2006): 1521–24.

Sit, D., et al. "Light Therapy for Bipolar Disorder: A Case Series in Women." *Bipolar Disorders* 9, no. 8 (2007): 918–27.

ORGANIZATIONS

National Depressive and Manic Depressive Association, 730 Franklin Street, Suite 501, Chicago, IL, 60610, (800) 826-3632, http://www.ndmda.org.

Society for Light Treatment and Biological Rhythms, 824 Howard Ave., New Haven, CT, 60610.sltbrinfo@gmail.com, http://www.sltbr.org.

Paula Ford-Martin
Rebecca J. Frey, PhD
Heidi Splete

Limbic system *see* **Brain**

Lisdexamfetamine

Definition

Lisdexamfetamine (sold under the brand name Vyvanse) is a medication used to treat **attention deficit hyperactivity disorder (ADHD)**. It belongs to the class of drugs known as central nervous system (CNS) stimulants and acts on the neurological signaling chemicals norepinephrine and **dopamine**. Norepinephrine and dopamine are types of neurotransmitter involved in normal **brain** function and have an effect on mood, concentration, and impulse control.

Purpose

Lisdexamfetamine is used to treat some of the symptoms of **ADHD** in both adults and children six years old and older. It is a CNS stimulant that improves memory, concentration, and impulse control, and belongs

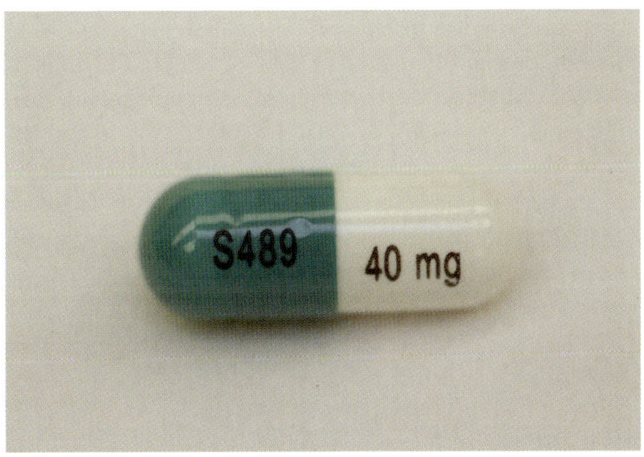

Vyvanse (lisdexamfetamine), 40 mg. *(© Custom Medical Stock Photo, Inc. Reproduced by permission.)*

to the category of drug that remains the mainstay of ADHD therapy. Lisdexamfetamine acts as a prodrug, meaning that the chemical compound present in the swallowed pill is metabolized and altered to another, active drug, once inside the body. Lisdexamfetamine is the inactive prodrug for the active compound **dextroamphetamine**, a compound that acts to treat ADHD. The prodrug compound is used in treatment because this formulation is thought to extend the period of time the drug is effective. The active compound only starts working as the prodrug is metabolized, creating a longer lasting effect. Proper metabolism to the active stimulant requires absorption to the bloodstream from the gastrointestinal (GI) tract and metabolism by the liver. This means no stimulant effect would be gained from injecting the drug directly into the bloodstream, bypassing the GI route that accesses the liver. The required route of administration as well as the delay to metabolism and time of effect also decreases the potential for abuse compared to other types of stimulant medication. The extended effective time mainly removes the need for re-dosing through the school or work day. It is used for patients for whom this is a priority.

Description

After it is taken, lisdexamfetamine is converted to the active compound dextroamphetamine within the body, which has a therapeutic mechanism of action focused on the natural body chemicals norepinephrine and dopamine. Norepinephrine and dopamine are types of neurotransmitter in the nervous system, chemicals that neurons use to signal to one another for normal brain and body functioning. **Neurotransmitters** bind to chemical receptors on the surface of neurons (brain cells). Once bound to a receptor, they affect physiological processes, including mood, concentration, and impulse control. Neurotransmitter reuptake inhibitors such as dextroamphetamine (lisdexamfetamine) decrease the absorption of norepinephrine and dopamine by neuron one, allowing more of the neurotransmitters to be present in the brain. It is believed that a decrease of norepinephrine and dopamine contributes to ADHD. When dextroamphetamine increases the amounts of norepinephrine and dopamine left in the brain, it has an impact on the areas of the brain that involve attention span, judgment, response to external stimuli, memory, motor function, mental focus, and impulse control.

Recommended dosage

Lisdexamfetamine is given as an oral medication in pill form, taken once each morning. It is available in doses that range from 20 to 70 mg. Patients are frequently reassessed for the need for treatment, as drugs for ADHD are avoided unless absolutely necessary. The dose chosen depends on individual patient response to the medication regarding its effectiveness, and individual patient response to the medication regarding side effects. Patients are dosed at the lowest possible effective dose to avoid the development of adverse side effects. Slowly increasing the dose helps with minimizing side effects. The usual dose of lisdexamfetamine in both adults and children six years old and older is 30 mg taken once a day. The dose is increased by 10 or 20 mg increments every week for a maximum of 70 mg a day as needed. Doses are lowered if side effects become intolerable.

Precautions

Lisdexamfetamine reactions vary from patient to patient, with some patients more sensitive to the medication and the development of side effects. Higher doses increase the risk of adverse events, hence the lowest dose possible is used for treatment. Clinicians weigh the potential for benefit with lisdexamfetamine treatment against the potential undesirable outcomes when making treatment decisions.

Lisdexamfetamine has a high potential for abuse and should never be used for longer time periods or at higher doses than prescribed. Patients are often given “drug holidays”—for example, when school is over for the summer—during which they forgo medication to avoid the development of adverse effects. Caution is used in patients with a history of **substance abuse**. Lisdexamfetamine causes a withdrawal syndrome when stopped abruptly and needs to be tapered off.

There is an association between ADHD and **Tourette syndrome**. Patients with Tourette syndrome typically have involuntary movements or vocalizations known as tics. Patients who have Tourette syndrome with ADHD may find that the stimulant medications used to treat ADHD worsen their tics. Caution must be used in treating patients with motor tics, Tourette syndrome, or a family history of the disorder. Lisdexamfetamine may not be appropriate for use in these patients. Rare but serious reactions include severe elevations in blood pressure, heart arrhythmias, heart attack, **stroke**, **seizures**, toxic skin reactions, and sudden death. Some patients develop increased aggressiveness, **psychosis**, mania, or suicidality in the first weeks of use. Children are especially at risk for these behavioral side effects. Patients taking lisdexamfetamine are monitored closely for behavioral changes, especially when starting treatment or after dose changes. Growth retardation may occur with prolonged use.

Lisdexamfetamine may be contraindicated or may require caution in use in patients with high blood pressure, blood vessel disease, heart rhythm abnormalities, heart

KEY TERMS

Bipolar disorder—Psychiatric mood disorder characterized by periods of manic behavior that may alternate with periods of depression, also known as manic depressive disorder.

Dopamine—A type of neurotransmitter involved in regulation of concentration, impulse control, judgment, mood, attention span, psychostimulation, and disease states such as addiction, ADHD, and depression.

Glaucoma—Condition involving increased pressure within the eye that may cause damage and blindness.

Mania—Physiological state of hyperactivity experienced by patients with certain psychiatric illnesses involving inappropriate elevated mood, pressured speech, poor judgment, and sometimes psychotic episodes superimposed on the state of mania.

Monoamine oxidase inhibitors (MAOIs)—Type of antidepressant medication that affects various kinds of neurotransmitters including serotonin.

Neurotransmitter—One of a group of chemicals secreted by a nerve cell (neuron) to carry a chemical message to another nerve cell, often as a way of transmitting a nerve impulse. Examples of neurotransmitters include acetylcholine, dopamine, serotonin, and norepinephrine.

Norepinephrine—A type of neurotransmitter involved in regulation of concentration, impulse control, judgment, mood, attention span, psychostimulation, and disease states such as ADHD and depression.

Prodrug—The inactive form of a drug that is metabolized into an active compound inside the body.

Tic—Involuntary movements (such as twitching or facial grimacing) or vocalizations (such as throat clearing or barking) associated with Tourette syndrome.

Tourette syndrome—An inherited neuropsychiatric disorder characterized by the development of both motor and vocal tics. The tics are preceded by a feeling of tension or urgency in the affected individual until the tic behavior is performed and relieves the perceived feeling of tension.

conditions or structural abnormalities, certain thyroid disorders, liver function impairment or liver disease, kidney function impairment, or glaucoma. Lisdexamfetamine may lower seizure threshold in some patients and may not be appropriate for use in patients with seizure disorder. Cardiac function, heart rate, and blood pressure may be monitored while taking lisdexamfetamine. Lisdexamfetamine is discouraged from use in patients with **bipolar disorder**, as it is more likely to induce a state of mania in these individuals than in those without bipolar disorder. Lisdexamfetamine is classified as category C for pregnancy, which means either there are no adequate human or animal studies; or that adverse fetal effects were found in animal studies, but there is no available human data. The decision whether to use category C drugs in pregnancy is generally based on weighing the critical needs of the mother against the risk to the fetus. Other lower category agents are used whenever possible. There are data that suggest lisdexamfetamine is considered unsafe for use during breastfeeding.

Side effects

Lisdexamfetamine has many side effects in addition to the intended treatment effect. Sensitivity to lisdexamfetamine varies between patients, and some patients may find even lower doses are more than their body system can tolerate. Common reactions include rash, fever, sweating, dizziness, **insomnia**, anxiety, restlessness, mood swings, abdominal pain, nausea and vomiting, decreased appetite, weight loss, changes in blood pressure, tremor, dry mouth, diarrhea, tic exacerbation, shortness of breath, and visual disturbances.

Interactions

Patients should make their doctor aware of all medications and supplements they are taking before using lisdexamfetamine. Using alcohol while taking lisdexamfetamine may create toxic reactions in the body and should be avoided. Patients taking drugs that affect the liver may alter the metabolism of lisdexamfetamine, resulting in too little or too much of the drug in the body. Other drugs may also cause serious effects when used in combination with lisdexamfetamine, such as serious heart rhythm abnormalities, excess nervous system stimulation, or blood pressure changes. Such medica-tions and substances include caffeine, marijuana derivatives, the obesity drug sibutramine, some migraine medications such as ergotamines, and decongestants such as phenylephrine.

QUESTIONS TO ASK YOUR DOCTOR

- Can I take the full dose right away or do I need to slowly increase the dose?
- Can I stop taking the medication right away or do I need to slowly decrease the dose?
- Should I eat when taking this medication?
- What time of day should I take this medication?
- How long should I take this medication before I am reassessed?
- Will this medication interact with any of my other prescription medications? Over-the-counter drugs?
- What are the side effects I should watch for?
- Can I drink alcoholic beverages in the same time frame as taking this medication?

Use of the antipsychotic **pimozide** with lisdexamfetamine increases the risk of motor tics as a side effect of medication. Use of certain other antipsychotics such as **fluphenazine** increase risk of psychosis. Antacids and the glaucoma and diuretic drug acetazolamide decrease the excretion of lisdexamfetamine and its metabolites from the body and may cause toxic levels. Many **antidepressants** interact with lisdexamfetamine, as well. The antidepressant **bupropion** increases the risk of seizures when used with lisdexamfetamine, and **venlafaxine** may cause greater than expected weight loss when used with lisdexamfetamine. A class of antidepressants known as **monoamine oxidase inhibitors (MAOIs)** increase the amount of norepinephrine and dopamine released into the brain and should not be used concurrently with lisdexamfetamine or its metabolites, as the combination may cause overstimulation of the central nervous system and toxicity. A patient switching from an MAOI to lisdexamfetamine will need to stop taking the MAOI for at least two weeks before starting treatment with lisdexamfetamine (and vice versa). Many herbal supplements also interact with lisdexamfetamine and may cause toxicity, including green tea and **ginseng**.

Resources

BOOKS

Brunton, Laurence L., et al. *Goodman and Gilman's The Pharmacological Basis of Therapeutics*. 12th ed. New York: McGraw Hill Medical, 2011.

Stargrove, Mitchell Bebel, et al. *Herb, Nutrient, and Drug Interactions: Clinical Implications and Therapeutic Strategies*. St. Louis: Mosby, 2007.

ORGANIZATIONS

American College of Neuropsychopharmacology, 5034-A Thoroughbred Lane, Brentwood, TN, 37027, (615) 324-2360, Fax: (615) 523-1715, acnp@acnp.org, http://www.acnp.org/default.aspx.

American Psychiatric Association, 1000 Wilson Blvd., Ste. 1825, Arlington, VA, 22209-3901, (703) 907-7300, apa@psych.org, http://www.psych.org.

American Society for Clinical Pharmacology and Therapeutics, 528 N Washington St., Alexandria, VA, 22314, (703) 836-6981, info@ascpt.org, http://www.ascpt.org.

Mental Health America, 2000 N Beauregard St., 6th Fl., Alexandria, VA, 22311, (703) 684-7722, (800) 969-6642, Fax: (703) 684-5968, http://www.nmha.org.

Maria Eve Basile, PhD

Lithium carbonate

Definition

Lithium is a naturally occurring element that is classified as an antimanic drug. It is available in the United States under the brand names Eskalith, Lithonate, Lithane, Lithotabs, and Lithobid. It is also sold under its generic name.

Purpose

Lithium is commonly used to treat mania and bipolar **depression** (manic depression). Less commonly, lithium is used to treat certain mood disorders, such as

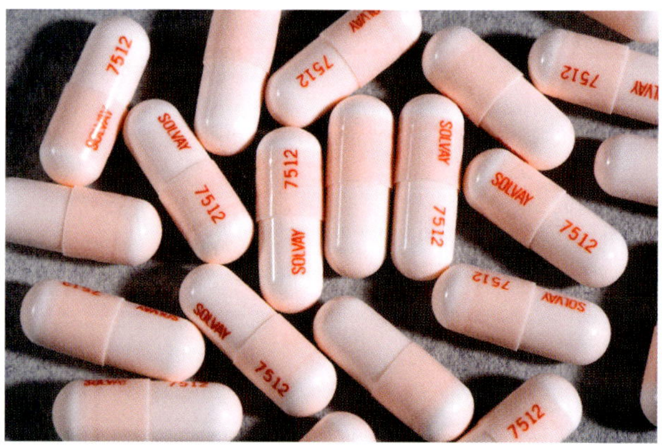

Lithium carbonate. *(© Phil Degginger/Alamy)*

schizoaffective disorder and aggressive behavior and emotional instability in adults and children. Rarely is lithium taken to treat depression in the absence of mania. When this is the case, it is usually taken in addition to other antidepressant medications.

Description

Lithium was first noted as a possible treatment for depression in the 1880s, and in the 1950s it was seen to improve the symptoms of bipolar disease. The way lithium works in the body is unclear, but its therapeutic benefits are probably related to its effects on electrolytes such as sodium, potassium, magnesium, and calcium. Lithium is taken either as lithium carbonate tablets or capsules or as lithium citrate syrup.

The therapeutic effects of lithium may appear slowly. Maximum benefit is often not evident for at least two weeks after starting the drug. People taking lithium should be aware of this and should continue taking the drug as directed even if they do not see immediate changes in mood.

Lithium is available in 300 mg tablets and capsules, 300 mg and 450 mg sustained-release tablets, and a syrup containing approximately 300 mg per teaspoonful.

Recommended dosage

Depending on the patient's medical needs, age, weight, and kidney function, doses of lithium can range from 600 to 2,400 mg per day, although most patients will be stabilized on 600 to 1,200 mg per day. Patients who require large amounts of lithium often benefit from the addition of another antimanic drug, which may allow the dose of lithium to be lowered.

Generally, lithium is taken two or three times daily. However, the entire dose may be taken at once if the physician believes that a single-dose program will increase patient **compliance**. The single-dose schedule is especially helpful for people who are forgetful and may skip doses on a multiple-dose schedule. Additionally, evidence indicates that once-daily doses are associated with fewer side effects.

More than with any other drugs used in the treatment of mental disorders, it is essential to maintain lithium blood levels within a certain narrow range to derive the maximum therapeutic benefit while minimizing serious negative side effects. It is important that patients have their blood levels of lithium measured at regular intervals.

Precautions

Because lithium intoxication may be serious and even life-threatening, blood concentrations of lithium should be measured weekly during the first four weeks of therapy and less often after that.

Patients taking lithium should have their thyroid function monitored and should maintain an adequate sodium (salt) and water balance. Lithium should not be used, or should be used only with very close physician supervision, in patients with kidney impairment, heart disease, and other conditions that affect sodium balance. Dosage reduction or complete discontinuation may be necessary during infection, diarrhea, vomiting, or a prolonged fast. Patients who are pregnant, breast-feeding, over age 60, or taking diuretics ("water" pills) should discuss the risks and benefits of lithium treatment with their doctors before beginning therapy. Lithium should be discontinued 24 hours before a major surgery, but it may be continued normally for minor surgical procedures.

Side effects

Tremor is the most common neurological side effect. Lithium tremor is an irregular, nonrhythmic twitching of the arms and legs that is variable in both intensity and frequency. Lithium-induced tremors occur in approximately half of people taking this medication. The chance of tremors decreases if the dose is reduced. Acute lithium toxicity (poisoning) can result in neurological side effects, ranging from confusion and coordination impairment, to coma, **seizures**, and death. Other neurological side effects associated with lithium therapy include lethargy, memory impairment, difficulty finding words, and loss of creativity.

About 30% to 35% of patients experience excessive thirst and urination, usually due to the inability of the kidneys to retain water and sodium. However, lithium is not known to cause kidney damage.

Lithium inhibits the synthesis of thyroid hormone. About 10% to 20% of patients treated with lithium develop some degree of thyroid insufficiency, but they usually do not require supplementation with thyroid hormone tablets.

Gastrointestinal side effects include loss of appetite, nausea, vomiting, diarrhea, and stomach pain. Weight gain is another common side effect for patients receiving long-term treatment. Changes in saliva flow and enlargement of the salivary glands may occur. An increase in tooth cavities and the need for dental care among patients taking lithium has been reported.

Skin reactions to lithium are common but usually can be managed without discontinuing lithium therapy. Lithium may worsen folliculitis (inflammation of hair follicles), psoriasis, and acne. Thinning of the hair may occur, and, less commonly, hair loss may be experienced. Swollen feet are an uncommon side effect that responds to dose reduction.

Electrocardiographic abnormalities may occur with lithium therapy, but significant cardiovascular effects are uncommon except as the result of deliberate or accidental overdose.

A mild-to-moderate increase in the number of white blood cells is a frequent side effect of lithium use. Conversely, lithium may slow the formation of red blood cells and cause anemia.

Increased risk of fetal cardiovascular disease may be associated with the use of lithium during pregnancy, especially during the first trimester (first three months). For this reason, pregnant women should discontinue lithium use until the second or third trimester and should receive alternative treatments for their mania.

Interactions

Patients taking lithium should always be concerned that other medications they are taking may adversely interact with it; patients should consult their physician or pharmacists about these interactions. The following list represents just some of the medications that lithium may interact with to either (a) increase or decrease the effectiveness of the lithium or (b) increase or decrease the effectiveness of the other drug:

- angiotensin-converting enzyme inhibitors such as captopril, lisinopril, or enalapril
- nonsteroidal anti-inflammatory drugs such as ibuprofen or naprosyn
- diuretics (water pills) such as hydrochlorothiazide, furosemide, or ethacrynic acid
- asthma drugs such as theophylline and aminophylline
- anticonvulsants such as phenytoin and carbamazepine
- calcium channel blockers such as verapamil or diltiazem
- muscle relaxants such as methocarbamol, carisoprodol, and cyclobenzaprine
- metronidazole, a commonly prescribed antibiotic used to treat infections
- antidiabetic therapy
- amiodarone, an antiarrhythmic drug
- antacids containing sodium bicarbonate
- antidepressants

Resources

BOOKS

American Society of Health-System Pharmacists. *AHFS Drug Information 2002.* Bethesda: American Society of Health-System Pharmacists, 2002.

Preston, John D., John H. O'Neal, and Mary C. Talaga. *Handbook of Clinical Psychopharmacology for Therapists.* 4th ed. Oakland, CA: New Harbinger Publications, 2004.

PERIODICALS

Baldessarini, Ross J., Maurizio Pompili, and Leonardo Tondo. "Suicide in Bipolar Disorder: Risks and Management." *CNS Spectrums* 11, no. 6 (June 2006): 465–71.

Baldessarini, Ross J., et al. "Decreased Risk of Suicides and Attempts During Long-Term Lithium Treatment: A Meta-Analytic Review." *Bipolar Disorders* 8, no. 5, part 2 (Oct. 2006): 625–39.

De Fruyt, Jürgen, and Koen Demyttenaere. "Bipolar (Spectrum) Disorder and Mood Stabilization: Standing at the Crossroads?" *Psychotherapy and Psychosomatics* 76, no. 2 (Jan. 2007): 77–88.

El-Mallakh, Rif, et al. "Bipolar II Disorder: Current and Future Treatment Options." *Annals of Clinical Psychiatry* 18, no. 4 (Oct.–Dec). 2006: 259–66.

Eyer, Florian, et al. "Lithium Poisoning: Pharmacokinetics and Clearance During Different Therapeutic Measures." *Journal of Clinical Psychopharmacology* 26, no. 3 (June 2006): 325–30.

Gonzalez-Pinto, Ana, et al. "Suicidal Risk in Bipolar I Disorder Patients and Adherence to Long-Term Lithium Treatment." *Bipolar Disorders* 8, no. 5, part 2 (Oct. 2006): 618–24.

Kellner, Charles H., et al. "Continuation Electroconvulsive Therapy vs Pharmacotherapy for Relapse Prevention in Major Depression." *Archives of General Psychiatry* 63, no. 12 (Dec. 2006): 1337–44.

Livingstone, Callum, and Hagen Rampes. "Lithium: A Review of Its Metabolic Adverse Effects." *Journal of Psychopharmacology* 20, no. 3 (May 2006): 347–55.

McElroy, Susan L., et al. "Antidepressants and Suicidal Behavior in Bipolar Disorder." *Bipolar Disorders* 8, no. 5, part 2 (Oct. 2006): 596–617.

Ozcan, Mehmet Erkan, Geetha Shivakumar, and Trisha Suppes. "Treating Rapid Cycling Bipolar Disorder with Novel Medications." *Current Psychiatry Reviews* 2, no. 3 (Aug. 2006): 361–69.

Patel, Nick C., et al. "Lithium Treatment Effects on Myo-Inositol in Adolescents with Bipolar Depression." *Biological Psychiatry* 60, no. 9 (Nov. 2006): 998–1004.

Singh, Jaskaran B., and Carlos A. Zarate, Jr. "Pharmacological Treatment of Psychiatric Comorbidity in Bipolar Disorder: A Review of Controlled Trials." *Bipolar Disorders* 8, no. 6 (Dec. 2006): 696–709.

Jack H. Raber, Pharm.D.
Ruth A. Wienclaw, PhD

Lithobid *see* **Lithium carbonate**

Lithonate *see* **Lithium carbonate**

Lithotabs *see* **Lithium carbonate**

Living wills *see* **Advance directives**

Lobotomy *see* **Psychosurgery**

Lorazepam

Definition

Lorazepam, a mild tranquilizer in the class of drugs known as **benzodiazepines**, is sold in the United States under the brand names Alzapam, Ativan, or Loraz. It is also available generically.

Purpose

Lorazepam is used for management of anxiety, nausea and vomiting, **insomnia**, and **seizures** (the injectable form). It is also used prior to surgery to produce sedation, sleepiness, drowsiness, relief of anxiety, and a decreased ability to recall the events surrounding the surgery.

Description

Lorazepam is a member of the benzodiazepine family. Benzodiazepines primarily work by enhancing the function of a certain naturally occurring **brain** chemical, gamma-aminobutyric acid (GABA), which is responsible for inhibiting the transmission of nervous impulses in the brain and spinal cord. At the same time, the enhancement of GABA in the brain decreases symptoms associated with anxiety. Lorazepam differs from drugs such as **diazepam** (Valium) and **chlordiazepoxide** (Librium) in that it is shorter-acting and does not accumulate in the body after repeated doses.

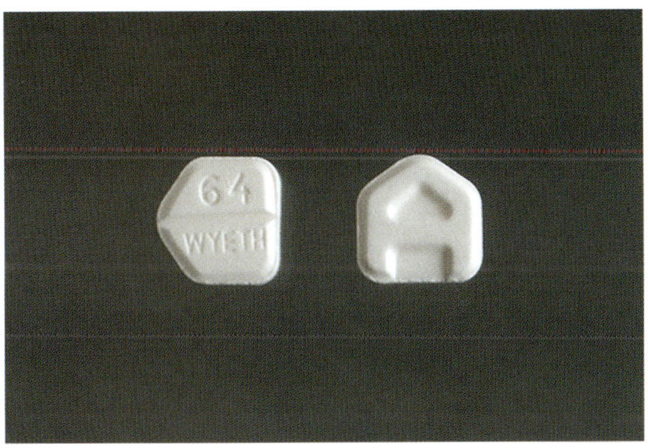

Ativan (lorazepam), 5 mg. *(U.S. Drug Enforcement Administration)*

Lorazepam is available in 0.5 mg, 1 mg, and 2 mg tablets and in an injectable form.

Recommended dosage

Lorazepam is taken several times daily by mouth, or injected, to treat anxiety. Dosage ranges from 1–2 mg taken either every 12 or every eight hours. The maximum daily total dosage for anxiety is 10 mg given in two to three divided doses. For sleep, patients may take from 2 to 4 mg at bedtime. Doses taken before surgery range from 2.5 to 5 mg.

Between 0.5 mg and 1 mg of lorazepam may be taken every six to eight hours to help control treatment-related nausea and vomiting (nausea and vomiting that occur as a side effect of a drug or medical treatment). Two mg of lorazepam are often given half an hour before chemotherapy to help prevent stomach upset. An additional 2 mg may be taken every four hours as needed.

The usual dose to treat seizures is 4 mg given intravenously (through a vein). This dose may be increased to 8 mg in patients who do not respond to the 4 mg dose.

Precautions

Lorazepam, like other drugs of this type, can cause physical and psychological dependence. Patients should not increase the dose or frequency of this drug on their own, nor should they suddenly stop taking this medication. Instead, when stopping the drug, the dosage should gradually be decreased, and then discontinued. If the drug is stopped abruptly, patients may experience agitation, irritability, difficulty sleeping, convulsions, and other withdrawal symptoms.

Patients who are allergic to benzodiazepines should not take lorazepam. Those with narrow-angle glaucoma, pre-existing **depression** of the central nervous system, severe uncontrolled pain, or severe low blood pressure should not take lorazepam. This drug should be used with caution in patients with a history of drug abuse. Children under age 12 should not take lorazepam. Children between the ages of 12 and 18 may take the drug by mouth but not intravenously. Pregnant women and those trying to become pregnant should not take lorazepam. This drug has been associated with damage to the developing fetus when taken during the first three months of pregnancy. Patients taking this drug should not breastfeed. Lorazepam has also been associated with the risk of developing anterograde **amnesia**.

Side effects

Drowsiness and sleepiness are common and expected effects of lorazepam. Patients should not drive,

KEY TERMS

Anterograde amnesia—The inability to form new memories.

Benzodiazepines—A class of drugs that have a hypnotic and sedative action, used mainly as tranquilizers to control symptoms of anxiety.

operate machinery, or perform hazardous activities that require mental alertness until they have a sense of how lorazepam will affect their alertness. Patients over age 50 may experience deeper and longer sedation after taking lorazepam. These effects may subside with continued use or dosage reduction.

The effects of an injection may impair performance and driving ability for 24–48 hours. The impairment may last longer in older patients and those taking other central nervous system depressants, such as some pain medication.

Lorazepam may also make patients feel dizzy, weak, unsteady, or clumsy. Less frequently, they may feel depressed, disoriented, nauseous, or agitated while taking this drug. Other side effects include headache, difficulty sleeping, rash, yellowing eyes, vision changes, and hallucinations. Redness and pain may occur at the injection site.

Patients may experience high or low blood pressure and difficulty in breathing after an injection of lorazepam. Nausea, vomiting, dry mouth, and constipation may also occur. The patient's sex drive may decrease, but this side effect is reversible once the drug is stopped. Patients should alert their physician to confusion, depression, excitation, nightmares, impaired coordination, changes in personality, changes in urinary pattern, chest pain, heart palpitations, or any other side effects.

Interactions

Alcohol and other central nervous system depressants can increase the drowsiness associated with this drug. Some over-the-counter medications depress the central nervous system. The herbal remedies **kava kava** and **valerian** may increase the effects of lorazepam. Patients should check with their doctors before starting any new medications while taking lorazepam. People should not drink alcoholic beverages when taking lorazepam and for 24–48 hours before receiving an injection prior to surgery.

Resources

BOOKS

Lacy, Charles F. *Drug Information Handbook with International Trade Names Index.* Hudson, OH: Lexi-Comp, Inc. 2011.

Preston, John D., John H. O'Neal, and Mary C. Talaga. *Handbook of Clinical Psychopharmacology for Therapists.* 5th ed. Oakland, CA: New Harbinger Publications, 2008.

PERIODICALS

Giersch, Anne, et al. "Impairment of Contrast Sensitivity in Long-Term Lorazepam Users." *Psychopharmacology* 186, no. 4 (July 2006): 594–600.

Hung, Yi-Yung, and Tiao-Lai Huang. "Lorazepam and Diazepam Rapidly Relieve Catatonic Features in Major Depression." *Clinical Neuropharmacology* 29, no. 3 (May–June 2006): 144–47.

Izaute, M., and E. Bacon. "Effects of the Amnesic Drug Lorazepam on Complete and Partial Information Retrieval and Monitoring Accuracy." *Psychopharmacology* 188, no. 4 (November 2006): 472–81.

Kamboj, Sunjeev K., and H. Valerie Curran. "Neutral and Emotional Episodic Memory: Global Impairment After Lorazepam or Scopolamine." *Psychopharmacology* 188, no. 4 (November 2006): 482–88.

Pomara, Nunzio, et al. "Dose-Dependent Retrograde Facilitation of Verbal Memory in Healthy Elderly After Acute Oral Lorazepam Administration." *Psychopharmacology* 185, no. 4 (May 2006): 487–94.

Verster, Joris C., Dieuwke S. Veldhuijzen, and Edmund R. Volkerts. "Is It Safe to Drive a Car When Treated with Anxiolytics? Evidence from On-the-Road Driving Studies During Normal Traffic." *Current Psychiatry Reviews* 1, no. 2 (June 2005): 215–25.

Yacoub, Adee, and Andrew Francis. "Neuroleptic Malignant Syndrome Induced by Atypical Neuroleptics and Responsive to Lorazepam." *Neuropsychiatric Disease and Treatment* 2, no. 2 (February 2006): 235–40.

Debra Wood, RN
Ajna Hamidovic, Pharm.D.
Ruth A. Wienclaw, PhD

Loss *see* **Bereavement; Grief**

Loxapine

Definition

Loxapine is a prescription-only drug used to treat serious mental, nervous, and emotional disorders. Loxapine is sold under the brand name Loxitane in the United States. It is also available in generic form.

Purpose

Loxapine is used to treat a variety of mental disorders including anxiety, mania, **depression**, and psychotic disorders.

KEY TERMS

Extrapyramidal symptoms—A group of side effects associated with antipsychotic medications and characterized by involuntary muscle movements, including contraction and tremor.

Mania—A mood disorder in which a person experiences prolonged elation or irritability characterized by overactivity that can lead to exhaustion and medical emergencies.

Description

Loxapine is in the class of drugs known as *antipsychotic agents*. The exact mode of action of loxapine has not been precisely determined, but this drug has a tranquilizing effect on patients with anxiety, mania, and other psychotic disorders. It is known that loxapine reduces the amount of **dopamine** transmitted within the **brain**. Loxapine is available in 5, 10, 25, and 50 mg tablets.

Recommended dosage

Loxapine is available in oral solution, capsules, tablets, and injectable form. The typical starting dose for adults and children over the age of 16 years is 10 mg given two to four times daily. The maximum range after the initial period is between 60 mg and 100 mg given two to four times daily. After a period of time, the dose is usually lowered to 20–60 mg per day, given in divided doses. Injections are usually given only during the initial phase and are delivered into muscle (IM) in doses ranging from 12.5 mg to 50 mg every four to six hours until a desired level of response is reached. Then, the patient is usually put on the oral (PO) form for maintenance therapy. Guidelines for use in people under the age of 16 have not been established.

Precautions

People taking loxapine should not stop taking this medication suddenly. The dosage should be gradually decreased over time. Loxapine should not be combined with other agents that depress the central nervous system, such as antihistamines, alcohol, tranquilizers, sleeping medications, and seizure medications. Loxapine can cause the skin to become more sensitive to the sun. People taking this drug should use sunscreen with a skin protection factor (SPF) greater than 15.

Loxapine is typically not administered to people who are in a severe drug-induced state or a coma. People with a history of **seizures**, heart disease, prostate enlargement, glaucoma, or chronic obstructive pulmonary disorder should receive loxapine only after careful evaluation. Guidelines for use in children under the age of 16 years have not been established. Loxapine should not be used by women who are pregnant, trying to become pregnant, or breast-feeding. Babies born to mothers who took loxapine during pregnancy may develop extrapyramidal symptoms (EPS) and withdrawal symptoms, including agitation, trouble breathing, and difficulty feeding.

Like other antipsychotic medications, loxapine carries a warning regarding use in elderly people with **dementia**, who suffer from an increased risk of death during treatment. The reason for the increase was unclear in studies, but most deaths were found to be related to either cardiovascular complications or complications associated with infection. Loxapine is not approved by the U.S. Food and Drug Administration for the treatment of behavior problems in older adults with dementia.

Side effects

Rare side effects, which must be reported immediately to a doctor, include seizures, breathing difficulties, irregular heartbeat, significant changes in blood pressure, increased sweating, severe stiffness, extreme weakness, and unusually pale skin. Patients who experience these symptoms should stop using the medication immediately, as these symptoms are considered emergencies. More common, but less serious, side effects include uncontrolled movement of the arms or legs, lip smacking, unusual movements of the tongue, puffing of the cheeks, and uncontrolled chewing movements. These symptoms should also be reported to a doctor immediately.

More common, and even less serious, side effects include difficulty in speaking or swallowing, restlessness, stiffness of arms and legs, trembling, and loss of balance. These symptoms also need to be reported to a doctor. Less common, and not especially significant, side effects include urination problems, muscle spasms, skin rash, and severe constipation. Rare, and not particularly serious, side effects include uncontrolled twisting and movement of the neck, fever, sore throat, unusual bleeding, yellowing of the eyes or skin, and changes in facial expression.

Overdose symptoms include significant drowsiness, severe dizziness, significant breathing difficulties, severe weakness, trembling muscles, and severe uncontrolled movements.

Interactions

Loxapine should not be combined with anticholinergic drugs because of the potential of decreased antipsychotic effects. Loxapine should not be combined with bromocriptine, because the combination can decrease the effectiveness of bromocriptine in patients with pituitary tumors. The combination of loxapine with lithium significantly increases the toxicity of both drugs. Likewise, loxapine and **lorazepam** should not be combined, because the combination of the two has produced very low blood pressure, severe drowsiness, and respiratory depression in rare cases.

Resources

BOOKS

Consumer Reports and American Society of Health-System Pharmacists. *Consumer Reports Complete Drug Reference.* Yonkers, NY: Consumers Reports, 2009.

Ellsworth, Allan J., et al. *Mosby's Medical Drug Reference.* St. Louis, MO: Mosby, 2007.

Preston, John D., John H. O'Neal, and Mary C. Talaga. *Handbook of Clinical Psychopharmacology for Therapists.* 5th ed. Oakland, CA: New Harbinger Publications, 2008.

PERIODICALS

Bourin, Michel, Olivier Lambert, and Bernard Guitton. "Treatment of Acute Mania—From Clinical Trials to Recommendations for Clinical Practice." *Human Psychopharmacology: Clinical and Experimental* 20, no. 1 (January 2005): 15–26.

Janowsky, David S., et al. "Minimally Effective Doses of Conventional Antipsychotic Medications Used to Treat Aggression, Self-Injurious and Destructive Behaviors in Mentally Retarded Adults." *Journal of Clinical Psychopharmacology* 25, no. 1 (February 2005): 19–25.

Reinblatt, Shauna P., et al. "Advanced Pediatric Psychopharmacology: Loxapine Treatment in an Autistic Child with Aggressive Behavior: Therapeutic Challenges." *Journal of Child and Adolescent Psychopharmacology* 16, no. 5 (October 2006): 639–43.

Mark Mitchell, MD
Ruth A. Wienclaw, PhD

Loxitane *see* **Loxapine**

LSD *see* **Hallucinogens and related disorders**

Ludiomil *see* **Maprotiline**

Luria-Nebraska Neuropsychological Battery

Definition

The Luria-Nebraska Neuropsychological Battery, also known as LNNB or Luria-Nebraska Battery, is a standardized test battery used in the screening and evaluation of neuropsychologically impaired individuals.

Purpose

The LNNB was developed in an attempt to combine the qualitative techniques of some neuropsychological tests with the quantitative techniques of other tests. However, the scoring system that most clinicians use is primarily quantitative. The battery measures specific neuropsychological functioning in several areas including motor skills, language abilities, intellectual abilities, nonverbal auditory skills, and visual-spatial skills.

The battery is used by clinicians as a screening tool to determine whether a significant **brain** injury is present or to learn more about known brain injuries. It is also used to determine what the patient is or is not able to do with regard to neuropsychological functioning. For example, the LNNB may be used to determine which intellectual or cognitive tasks a patient may or may not be able to complete. The battery can also be used to arrive at underlying causes of a patient's behavior. More specifically, information regarding the location and nature of the brain injury or dysfunction causing a patient's problems is collected.

The LNNB is also used to help distinguish between brain damage and functional mental disorders such as **schizophrenia**. In addition, within the category of schizophrenia, the battery can be used to help distinguish between patients with normal neuropsychological functioning and those with clear deficits. Besides its specifically clinical use, the battery is sometimes used for legal purposes—the presence or severity of a brain injury may be measured as part of an evaluation used in the court system.

Description

The LNNB is based on the work of Alexander Romanovich Luria (1902–1977), a Soviet neuropsychologist and developmental **psychologist** who performed pioneering theoretical and clinical work with regard to brain function. Luria believed in a primarily qualitative approach to assessment and was opposed to standardization. He did not believe that neuropsychological functioning could be measured quantitatively. Thus, although his name is part of the test itself, his contribution to the LNNB is entirely theoretical. Also, the LNNB is based, in part, on Luria's Neuropsychological Investigation, a measure developed by Danish neuropsychologist Anne-Lise Christensen in 1975. This test included items asked by Luria in his clinical interviews, some of which are used in the LNNB.

The battery, written in 1981 by Charles J. Golden, Arnold D. Purisch, and Thomas A. Hammeke, is designed for people aged 15 years and older and takes between 90 and 150 minutes (1.5 to 2.5 hours) to complete. It has also been shown effective for children 13 and 14 years of age. The battery can be administered in one session or a series of shorter sessions.

Two equivalent forms are available. Form I consists of 269 items and Form II has 279 items. Though both yield similar information, Form II contains improved stimulus cards, which are easier to read than those contained on Form I. In addition, Form II contains an additional scale, the intermediate memory scale, which allows better assessment of memory. Form I is hand scored or computer scored, while Form II is only computer scored. Both contain the following 11 clinical scales:

- reading
- writing
- arithmetic
- visual functions
- memory
- expressive language
- receptive language (speech)
- motor functions
- rhythm
- tactile functions
- intellectual processes

Scores for five summary scales can also be calculated: pathognomonic, right hemisphere, left hemisphere, profile elevation, and impairment. A children's version of the battery, called the Luria-Nebraska Neuropsychological Battery for Children (LNNB-C), appropriate for children aged 8 to 12 years, is also available.

In addition, there are two optional scales, spelling and motor writing. Eight localization scales are also available. These are:

- left frontal
- left sensorimotor
- left parietal-occipital
- left temporal
- right frontal
- right sensorimotor
- right parietal-occipital
- right temporal

Also included are 28 factor scales, which deal with specific sensory and cognitive functions.

KEY TERMS

Frontal—Relating to the forehead (the anterior part of the roof of the brain case).

Neuropsychological—Relating to neuropsychology, or the branch of neurology that studies behavior disorders such as memory loss, speech impairment, epilepsy, and others.

Parietal-occipital—Relating to the parietal and occipital bones or lobes.

Schizophrenia—A mental disorder involving degraded thinking and emotions.

Sensorimotor—Relating to sensory and motor coordination of the nervous system.

Temporal—Relating to the temples.

Preparation

Preparation for the Luria-Nebraska Neuropsychological Battery is not needed nor necessary.

Risks

Risks are inherent in the administration of the LNNB. Because of the length of the test and complexity in interpretation, the examiner (administrator) must be competent and properly trained.

Precautions

Test administration can be difficult or frustrating because many patients undergoing testing have brain damage. The LNNB is portable, so the test can be taken to the patient if he or she is unable to travel to the administration site.

Results

The probability of brain damage is assessed by comparing an individual's score on each of the battery's 11 clinical scales to a critical level appropriate for that person's age and education level. For example, if a person has five to seven scores above the critical level, they most likely have some sign of neurological impairment. Eight or more scores above the critical level indicate a clear history of neurological disorder.

The battery has been criticized by researchers on the grounds that it overestimates the degree of neuropsychological impairment. In other cases, it has failed to detect neuropsychological problems. Also, the intellectual processes scale has not been found to correspond well

QUESTIONS TO ASK YOUR DOCTOR

- Do you know of a properly trained administrator for the LNNB?
- Should another test, or several tests, be administered in parallel with the LNNB?
- Where can I learn more about the test?
- Will health insurance cover the LNNB?

to other measures of intelligence, such as the Wechsler Adult Intelligence Scale (WAIS).

Other research, however, has found it to be a useful measure. It has been found as effective as the **Halstead-Reitan Battery** in distinguishing between individuals with brain damage and individuals without brain damage with psychiatric problems. Part of the inconsistencies in opinion regarding the LNNB may be due to the specific nature of the population being tested by the battery and the difficulties in administration and scoring that some clinicians experience.

American neurologist Arnold D. Purisch reports in a well-researched paper within the journal *NeuroRehabilitation* (2001) about both sides of this issue. Dr. Purisch states, "The major criticisms related to the belief that the qualitative and quantitative approaches could not be fused, that the scales were too heterogeneous to produce meaningful scores, that the battery suffered from significant limitations in sampling of neuropsychological skills, and that it had questionable sensitivity to brain dysfunction." Purisch goes on to state, "These criticisms generally reflected an unawareness of the interpretive process and theory underlying the LNNB, and have been largely negated by a large empirical literature that has evolved over many years."

Resources

BOOKS

Barnovitz, Mary Ann L.C., and Pria Joglekar. *Medical Psychiatry: The Quick Reference.* Philadelphia: Wolters Kluwer Health/Lippincott Williams & Wilkins, 2008.

Golden, Charles J. *Luria-Nebraska Neuropsychological Battery: Adult Form, Screening Test.* Los Angeles: Western Psychological Services, 1987.

Groth-Marnat, Gary. *Handbook of Psychological Assessment.* 4th edition. Hoboken, NJ: John Wiley, 2003.

Gutman, Sharon A., and Alison B. Schonfeld. *Screening Adult Neurologic Populations: A Step-by-Step Instruction Manual.* Bethasda, MD: AOTA Press, 2009.

Hebben, Nancy, and William Milberg. *Essentials of Neuropsychological Assessment.* Hoboken, NJ: John Wiley, 2009.

Hersen, Michel, ed. *Comprehensive Handbook of Psychological Assessment.* Hoboken, NJ: John Wiley, 2004.

Kellerman, Henry, and Anthony Burry. *Handbook of Psychodiagnostic Testing: Analysis of Personality in the Psychological Report.* New York: Springer, 2007.

Leeming, David A., Kathryn Madden, and Stanton Marlan, eds. *Encyclopedia of Psychology and Religion.* New York: Springer, 2010.

Lezak, Muriel D. *Neuropsychological Assessment.* New York: Oxford University Press, 2004.

Riccio, Cynthia A., Jeremy R. Sullivan and Morris J. Cohen. *Neuropsychological Assessment and Intervention for Children and Adolescent Disorders.* Hoboken, NJ: John Wiley, 2010.

WEBSITES

"Luria-Nebraska Neuropsychological Battery (LNNB)." Western Psychological Services. http://portal.wpspublish.com/portal/page?_pageid=53,69305&_dad=portal&_schema=PORTAL (accessed December 17, 2010).

"Misconceptions about the Luria-Nebraska Neuropsychological Battery." NeuroRehabilitation, IOS Press. http://iospress.metapress.com/content/6yyy8w0l4r44674h (accessed December 17, 2010).

ORGANIZATIONS

American Psychiatric Association, 1000 Wilson Blvd., Ste. 1825, Arlington, VA, 22209-3901, (703) 907-7300, apa@psych.org, http://www.psych.org.

American Psychological Association, 750 1st St. NE, Washington, DC, 20002-4242, (202) 336-5500; TDD/TTY: (202) 336-6123, (800) 374-2721, http://www.apa.org.

See also Intelligence tests; Kaufman Assessment Battery for Children; Kaufman Short Neuropsychological Assessment; Neuropsychological testing

Ali Fahmy, Ph.D.

Luvox *see* **Fluvoxamine**

The GALE ENCYCLOPEDIA *of* MENTAL HEALTH

THIRD EDITION

The GALE ENCYCLOPEDIA of MENTAL HEALTH

THIRD EDITION

VOLUME

2

M–Z
ORGANIZATIONS
GLOSSARY
INDEX

KRISTIN KEY, EDITOR

GALE
CENGAGE Learning

Detroit • New York • San Francisco • New Haven, Conn • Waterville, Maine • London

GALE
CENGAGE Learning

Gale Encyclopedia of Mental Health, Third Edition

Project Editor: Kristin Key

Editorial: Tara Atterberry, Donna Batten, Jacqueline Longe, Kristin Mallegg, Brigham Narins, Joseph Palmisano, Bob Romaniuk, Alejandro Valtierra

Product Manager: Anne Marie Sumner

Editorial Support Services: Andrea Lopeman

Indexing Services: Laurie Andriot

Rights Acquisition and Management: Margaret Chamberlain-Gaston

Composition: Evi Abou-El-Seoud

Manufacturing: Wendy Blurton

Imaging: John Watkins

Product Design: Kristine Julien

LIBRARY OF CONGRESS CATALOGING-IN-PUBLICATION DATA

The Gale encyclopedia of mental health / Kristin Key, editor. -- 3rd ed.
p. cm.
Summary: "Alphabetically arranged encyclopedia (500 entries) that covers a wide variety of disorders, treatments, tests, and therapies, focused specifically on topics in mental health"– Provided by publisher.
Includes bibliographical references and index.
ISBN 978-1-4144-9012-0 (hardback) -- ISBN 978-1-4144-9013-7 (vol. 1) – ISBN 978-1-4144-9014-4 (vol. 2)
1. Psychiatry–Encyclopedias. 2. Mental illness–Encyclopedias.
I. Key, Kristin. II. Title: Encyclopedia of mental health.
RC437.G36 2012
616.89003–dc23

2011049279

Gale
27500 Drake Rd.
Farmington Hills, MI, 48331-3535

ISBN-13: 978-1-4144-9012-0 (set) ISBN-10: 1-4144-9012-7 (set)
ISBN-13: 978-1-4144-9013-7 (vol. 1) ISBN-10: 1-4144-9013-5 (vol. 1)
ISBN-13: 978-1-4144-9014-4 (vol. 2) ISBN-10: 1-4144-9014-3 (vol. 2)

This title is also available as an e-book.
ISBN-13: 978-1-4144-9015-1 ISBN-10: 1-4144-9015-1
Contact your Gale, a part of Cengage Learning sales representative for ordering information.

Printed in China
1 2 3 4 5 6 7 16 15 14 13 12

CONTENTS

ALPHABETICAL LIST OF ENTRIES

Q

R

S

T

U

V

W

Y

Z

PLEASE READ—IMPORTANT INFORMATION

The *Gale Encyclopedia of Mental Health, Third Edition* is a health reference product designed to inform and educate readers about mental health, mental disorders, and psychiatry. Gale, Cengage Learning believes the product to be comprehensive, but not necessarily definitive. It is intended to supplement, not replace, consultation with a physician or other healthcare practitioner. While Gale, Cengage Learning has made substantial efforts to provide information that is accurate, comprehensive, and up-to-date, Gale, Cengage Learning makes no representations or warranties of any kind, including without limitation, warranties of merchantability or fitness for a particular purpose, nor does it guarantee the accuracy, comprehensiveness, or timeliness of the information contained in this product. Readers should be aware that the universe of medical knowledge is constantly growing and changing, and that differences of opinion exist among authorities. Readers are also advised to seek professional diagnosis and treatment for any medical condition, and to discuss information obtained from this book with their healthcare provider.

INTRODUCTION

The *Gale Encyclopedia of Mental Health* is a valuable source of information on mental health. The *Encyclopedia* provides in-depth coverage of specific disorders recognized by the American Psychiatric Association in its *Diagnostic and Statistical Manual of Mental Disorders* (*DSM*), as well as other mental health conditions, diagnostic procedures and techniques, therapies, psychiatric medications, alternative treatments, legal concerns, and related topics.

SCOPE

The *Gale Encyclopedia of Mental Health* includes 500 entries on disorders, drugs, tests, and treatments. The *Encyclopedia* minimizes medical jargon and uses language that any reader can understand while still providing thorough coverage, making this text useful to consumers and students alike.

Entries follow a standardized format that provides information at a glance. Categories include:

Disorders and conditions

- Definition
- Demographics
- Description
- Causes and symptoms
- Diagnosis
- Treatment
- Prognosis
- Prevention

Drugs and herbs

- Definition
- Purpose
- Description
- Recommended dosage
- Precautions
- Side effects
- Interactions

Tests and procedures

- Definition
- Purpose
- Description
- Preparation
- Aftercare
- Risks
- Results

Treatments and therapies

- Definition
- Purpose
- Demographics
- Description
- Preparation
- Aftercare
- Risks

Other areas of discussion include Origins, Benefits, Research and general acceptance, and Training and certification, when applicable.

INCLUSION CRITERIA

A preliminary list of mental disorders and related topics was compiled from a wide variety of sources, including professional medical guides and textbooks as well as consumer guides and encyclopedias. An advisory board of professionals from a variety of healthcare fields, including psychology, psychiatry, pharmacy, and social work, evaluated the topics and made suggestions for updates and inclusion. The final selections were determined by Gale editors in conjunction with the advisory board.

ABOUT THE CONTRIBUTORS

The essays in this *Encyclopedia* were written by experienced medical writers, including physicians, pharmacists, and psychologists. All essays were reviewed by advisors to ensure that they are appropriate, up-to-date, and accurate.

HOW TO USE THIS BOOK

The *Gale Encyclopedia of Mental Health* has been designed with ready reference in mind.

- Straight **alphabetical arrangement** of topics allows users to locate information quickly.
- **Bold-faced terms** within entries direct the reader to related articles.
- **Cross-references** placed throughout the *Encyclopedia* direct readers to primary entries from alternate names, drug brand names, and related topics.
- Lists of **key terms** are provided where appropriate to define unfamiliar terms or concepts. A **glossary** of key terms is also included at the back of Volume 2.
- New to this edition, **Questions to Ask Your Doctor** sidebars provide sample questions that patients can ask their physicians.
- **Biographies** of key people recognized for their important work in the field of mental health are profiled in entry sidebars.
- **Resources** at the end of every entry direct readers to additional sources of information on a topic.
- Valuable **contact information** for organizations and support groups is included with each entry and compiled in the back of Volume 2.
- A comprehensive **general index** guides readers to all topics mentioned in the text.

GRAPHICS

The *Gale Encyclopedia of Mental Health* contains 240 color photographs, illustrations, charts, and tables.

ADVISORY BOARD

Several experts in mental health have provided invaluable assistance in the formulation of this encyclopedia, from defining the scope of coverage to reviewing individual entries for accuracy and accessibility. We would like to express our sincere thanks and appreciation for all of their contributions.

CONTRIBUTORS

Margaret Alic, PhD
Science Writer
Eastsound, WA

William Atkins
Medical Writer
Pekin, IL

Maria Eve Basile, PhD
Medical Writer
Roselle, NJ

Rosalyn Carson-DeWitt, MD
Medical Writer
Durham, NC

Laura Jean Cataldo, RN, EdD
Medical Writer
Myersville, MD

L. Lee Culvert
Medical Writer
Alna, ME

Tish Davidson, AM
Medical Writer
Fremont, CA

L. Fleming Fallon Jr., MD, DrPH
Professor of Public Health
Bowling Green University
Bowling Green, OH

Paula Ford-Martin
Medical Writer
Warwick, RI

Rebecca J. Frey, PhD
Research and Administrative Associate
East Rock Institute
New Haven, CT

Sandra L. Friedrich, MA
Science Writer
Clinical Psychology
Chicago, IL

Gary Gilles, MA
Medical Writer
Wauconda, IL

Clare Hanrahan
Medical Writer
Asheville, NC

Kelly Karpa, RPh, PhD
Assistant Professor
Department of Pharmacology
Pennsylvania State University College of Medicine
Hershey, PA

Monique Laberge, PhD
Research Associate
Department of Biochemistry and Biophysics
McGill University
Montreal, Quebec, Canada

Judy Leaver, MA
Behavioral Health Writer and Consultant
Washington, DC

Brenda Wilmoth Lerner, RN
Medical Editor and Writer
Montrose, AL

Mark A. Mitchell, MD
Medical Writer
Seattle, WA

Teresa G. Odle
Medical Writer
Albuquerque, NM

Jack Raber, PharmD
Principal
Clinipharm Services
Seal Beach, CA

Joan Schonbeck, RN
Medical Writer
Massachusetts Department of Mental Health
Marlborough, MA

Genevieve Slomski, PhD
Medical Writer
New Britain, CT

Heidi Splete
Freelance Writer
Washington, DC

Deanna M. Swartout-Corbeil, RN
Medical Writer
Thompsons Station, TN

Samuel Uretsky, PharmD
Medical Writer
Wantagh, NY

Ken R. Wells
Freelance Writer
Laguna Hills, CA

Emily Willingham, PhD
Freelance Writer
Austin, TX

M

Magnetic resonance imaging

Definition

Magnetic resonance imaging (MRI), also referred to as "nuclear magnetic resonance imaging" (NMRI), is one of the most versatile medical imaging technologies currently available for the scanning of the human body. With the use of MRI, doctors can obtain highly refined images (scans) of the body's interior, specifically the nuclei of atoms inside the body, without surgery. By using strong magnets and pulses of radio waves to manipulate the natural magnetic properties in the body, this technique makes higher-quality images of organs and soft tissues than those of other scanning technologies. MRI is particularly useful for imaging the **brain** and spine as well as the soft tissues of joints and the interior structure of bones. The entire body is visible to the technique. Because the technique does not use ionizing radiation, MRI poses no known major health risks.

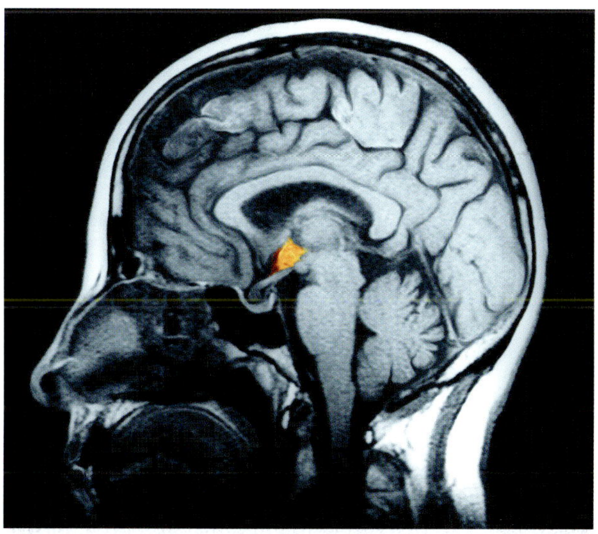

A magnetic resonance imaging (MRI) scan of the human brain; the hypothalamus is highlighted in orange.
(© Phototake. All rights reserved.)

Purpose

The scientific principle behind MRI, which is also called "nuclear magnetic resonance" (NMR), was discovered independently in 1946 by Swiss physicist Felix Bloch (1905–1983) and American physicist Edward Purcell (1912–1997). In 1952, they were awarded the Nobel Prize in Physics for "their development of new ways and methods for nuclear magnetic precision measurements." Then, in 1971, American-Armenian inventor Raymond Damadian (1936–) developed the first Magnetic Resonance (MR) scanning machine that could be used safety on humans based on the principle of NMR. Damadian showed that magnetic resonance could be applied to the scanning of tissues within the human body. The first MRI image was published in 1973 and the first studies on humans were performed in 1977. In 2003, American chemist Paul Lauterbur (1929–2007) and English physicist Peter Mansfield (1933–) won the Nobel Prize in Physiology or Medicine for "their discoveries concerning magnetic resonance imaging."

The latest additions to MRI technology are magnetic resonance angiography (MRA), magnetic resonance spectroscopy (MRS), functional magnetic resonance imaging (fMRI), interventional magnetic resonance imaging (iMRI), and diffusion tensor imaging (DTI). MRA was developed to study blood flow, while MRS can identify the chemical composition of diseased tissue and produce color images of brain function. The specialized form of MRI called fMRI was developed to measure the change in blood flow as related to neurological activity in the brain and spinal column, while iMRI is used to perform interventional radiology procedures (that is, to produce images during minimally invasive procedures). DTI scans, sometimes also called "diffusion MRI scans," are used to measure water flow within the tissues of the brain.

The many advantages of MRI include:

- Detail. MRI creates precise images of the body based on the varying proportions of magnetic elements in different tissues. Minor fluctuations in chemical composition can be determined. MRI images have greater natural contrast than standard x rays, computed tomography scan (CT scan), or ultrasound, all of which depend on the differing physical properties of tissues. This sensitivity lets MRI distinguish fine variations in tissues deep within the body. It also is particularly useful for spotting and distinguishing diseased tissues (tumors and other lesions) early in their development. Often, doctors prescribe an MRI scan to more fully investigate earlier findings of the other imaging techniques.
- Scope. The entire body can be scanned, from head to toe and from the skin to the deepest recesses of the brain. Moreover, MRI scans are not obstructed by bone, gas, or body waste, which can hinder other imaging techniques. (Although the scans can be degraded by motion such as breathing, heartbeat, and normal bowel activity.) The MRI process produces cross-sectional images of the body that are as sharp in the middle as on the edges, even of the brain through the skull. A close series of these two-dimensional (2D) images can provide a three-dimensional (3D) view of a targeted area.
- Safety. MRI does not depend on potentially harmful ionizing radiation, as do standard x-ray and CT scans. There are no known risks specific to the procedure, other than for people who might have metal objects in their bodies.

MRI is being used increasingly during surgical operations, particularly those involving very small structures in the head and neck, as well as for preoperative assessment and planning. Intraoperative MRIs (iMRIs) have shown themselves to be safe as well as feasible, and to improve the surgeon's ability to remove the entire tumor or other abnormality. They are valuable because an image can be produced during the procedure so that, for instance, a missed portion of tumor can be removed immediately, during the initial surgery, rather than having to return for a second procedure.

Given all the advantages, doctors would undoubtedly prescribe MRI as frequently as ultrasound scanning, but the MRI process is complex and costly. The process requires large, expensive, and complicated equipment; a highly trained operator; and a doctor specializing in radiology. Generally, MRI is prescribed only when serious symptoms and/or negative results from other tests indicate a need. Many times, another test is appropriate for the type of **diagnosis** needed.

Doctors may prescribe an MRI scan of different areas of the body. Some of these different areas include:

- Brain and head. MRI technology was developed because of the need for brain imaging. It is one of only a few imaging tools that can see through bone (such as the skull). Consequently, it can deliver high-quality pictures of the brain's delicate soft tissue structures. MRI may be needed for patients with symptoms of a brain tumor, stroke, or infection (like meningitis). MRI also may be needed when cognitive and/or psychological symptoms suggest brain disease (like Alzheimer's disease or Huntington's disease, or multiple sclerosis), or when a developmental or intellectual disability suggests a birth defect. MRI can also provide pictures of the sinuses and other areas of the head beneath the face. Recent refinements in MRI technology may make this form of diagnostic imaging even more useful in evaluating patients with brain cancer, stroke, or epilepsy and can be used as an aid in diagnosing schizophrenia. In particular, a new 3D approach to MRI imaging, "known as diffusion tensor imaging" (DTI), or sometimes as "diffusion magnetic resonance imaging" (dMRI, or diffusion MRI), measures the flow of water within brain tissue, allowing the radiologist to tell where the normal flow of fluid is disrupted and to distinguish more clearly between cancerous and normal brain tissue. The introduction of DTI has led to a technique known as "fiber tracking," which allows the neurosurgeon to tell whether a space-occupying brain tumor has damaged or displaced the nerve pathways in the white matter of the brain. This information, in turn, improves the surgeon's accuracy during the actual operation.
- Spine. Spinal problems can create a host of seemingly unrelated symptoms. MRI is particularly useful for identifying and evaluating degenerated or herniated spinal discs. It can also be used to determine the condition of nerve tissue within the spinal cord.
- Joint. MRI scanning is most commonly used to diagnose and assess joint problems. MRI can provide clear images of the bone, cartilage, ligament, and tendon that comprise a joint. MRI can be used to diagnose joint injuries due to sports, advancing age, or arthritis. MRI can also be used to diagnose shoulder problems, like a torn rotator cuff. MRI can also detect the presence of an otherwise hidden tumor or infection in a joint and can be used to diagnose the nature of developmental joint abnormalities in children.
- Skeleton. The properties of MRI that allow it to see through the skull also allow it to view the inside of bones. It can be used to detect bone cancer, inspect the marrow for leukemia and other diseases, assess bone loss (osteoporosis), and examine complex fractures.

- The rest of the body. While CT and ultrasound satisfy most chest, abdominal, and general body imaging needs, MRI may be needed in certain circumstances to provide better pictures or when repeated scanning is required. The progress of some therapies, like liver cancer therapy, needs to be monitored, and the effect of repeated x-ray exposure is a concern.

Description

In essence, MRI produces a map of hydrogen distribution in the body. Hydrogen (chemical symbol H) is the simplest element known, the most abundant in biological tissue, and one that can be magnetized. It will align itself within a strong magnetic field, like the needle of a compass. The Earth's magnetic field is not strong enough to keep a person's hydrogen atoms pointing in the same direction, but the superconducting magnet of an MRI machine can. This comprises the "magnetic" part of MRI.

Once a patient's hydrogen atoms have been aligned in the magnet, pulses of very specific radio wave frequencies are used to knock them back out of alignment. The hydrogen atoms alternately absorb and emit radio wave energy, vibrating back and forth between their resting (magnetized) state and their agitated (radio pulse) state. This comprises the "resonance" part of MRI.

The MRI equipment records the duration, strength, and source location of the signals emitted by the atoms as they relax, and translates the data into an image on a monitor. This relates to the "imaging" part of MRI. The state of hydrogen in diseased tissue differs from healthy tissue of the same type, making MRI particularly good at identifying tumors and other lesions. In some cases, chemical agents such as gadolinium can be injected to improve the contrast between healthy and diseased tissue.

A single MRI exposure produces a two-dimensional (2D) image of a slice through the entire target area. A series of these image slices closely spaced (usually less than half an inch) makes a virtual three-dimensional (3D) view of the area.

Magnetic resonance spectroscopy (MRS) is a specialized type of MRI, slightly different from MRI because MRS uses a continuous band of radio wave frequencies to excite hydrogen atoms in a variety of chemical compounds other than water. These compounds absorb and emit radio energy at characteristic frequencies, or spectra, which can be used to identify them. Generally, a color image is created by assigning a color to each distinctive spectral emission. This comprises the "spectroscopy" part of MRS. Thus, MRS measures biochemical information about the tissues of the body, while MRI only provides structural information about these tissues. MRS is quite new, and it is available in only a few research centers as a way to perform theoretical research and, in some cases, limited studies on humans. However, it is clear to the medical community that MRS has the potential to greatly improve the diagnosis and treatment of diseases.

Doctors primarily use MRS to study the brain and disorders, like epilepsy, **Alzheimer's disease**, brain tumors, and the effects of drugs on brain growth and metabolism. The technique is also useful in evaluating metabolic disorders of the muscles and nervous system.

Magnetic resonance angiography (MRA) is another variation on standard MRI. MRA, like other types of angiography, looks specifically at fluid flow within the blood (vascular) system, but does so without the injection of dyes or radioactive tracers. Standard MRI cannot make a good picture of flowing blood, but MRA uses specific radio pulse sequences to capture usable signals. The technique is generally used in combination with MRI to obtain images that show both vascular structure and flow within the brain and head in cases of **stroke**, or when a blood clot or aneurysm is suspected.

Regardless of the exact type of MRI planned, or area of the body targeted, the procedure involved is basically the same and occurs in a special MRI suite. The patient usually lies on a narrow table and is made as comfortable as possible. Transmitters are positioned on the body, and the cushioned table that the patient is lying on moves into a long tube that houses the magnet. The tube is as long as an average adult lying down, and it is narrow and open at both ends. Once the area to be examined has been properly positioned, a radio pulse is applied. Then a two-dimensional image corresponding to one slice through the area is made. The table then moves a fraction of an inch, and the next image is made. Each image exposure takes several seconds and the entire examination will last anywhere from 30 to 90 minutes. During this time, the patient is not allowed to move. If the patient moves during the scan, the picture will not be clear.

An open MRI scanner is less restrictive and is usually open on two or three sides. Although this type of machine accommodates larger or claustrophobic persons with greater ease, high-field or "closed" MRI machines usually generate more accurate and detailed images. The stand-up type of open MRI generates images of the spine, allowing the physician to evaluate images made in the weight-bearing state.

Depending on the area to be imaged, the radio-wave transmitters will be positioned in different locations. Some of these different locations include:

- For the head and neck, a helmet-like hat is worn.
- For the spine, chest, and abdomen, the patient lies on the transmitters.

KEY TERMS

Angiography—Any of the different methods for investigating the condition of blood vessels, usually via a combination of radiological imaging and injections of chemical tracing and contrasting agents.

Diffusion tensor imaging (DTI)—A refinement of magnetic resonance imaging that allows the doctor to measure the flow of water and track the pathways of white matter in the brain. It can detect abnormalities in the brain that do not show up on standard MRI scans.

Gadolinium—A very rare metallic element useful for its sensitivity to electromagnetic resonance, among other things. Traces of it can be injected into the body to enhance the MRI pictures.

Hydrogen—The simplest, most common element known in the universe. It is composed of a single electron (negatively charged particle) circling a nucleus consisting of a single proton (positively charged particle). It is the nuclear proton of this element that makes MRI possible by reacting resonantly to radio waves while aligned in a magnetic field.

Ionizing radiation—Electromagnetic radiation that can damage living tissue by disrupting and destroying individual cells. All types of nuclear decay radiation (including x rays) are potentially ionizing. Radio waves do not damage organic tissues they pass through.

Magnetic field—The three-dimensional area surrounding a magnet, in which its force is active. During MRI, the patient's body is permeated by the force field of a superconducting magnet.

Radio waves—Electromagnetic energy of the frequency range corresponding to that used in radio communications, usually 10,000 cycles per second to 300 billion cycles per second. Radio waves are the same as visible light, x rays, and all other types of electromagnetic radiation but are of a higher frequency.

- For the knee, shoulder, or other joint, the transmitters are applied directly to the joint.

Additional probes will monitor vital signs (like pulse or respiration).

The process is very noisy and confining. The patient hears a thumping sound for the duration of the procedure. Since the procedure is noisy, music or videos may be offered as a distraction for the patient. Some patients become anxious or panic because they are in the small, enclosed tube. This is why vital signs are monitored and the patient and medical team can communicate between each other. If the chest or abdomen are to be imaged, the patient will be asked to hold his/her breath as each exposure is made. Other instructions may be given to the patient, as needed. In many cases, an MRI operator, who is not a doctor, will perform the entire examination. However, the supervising radiologist should be available to consult as necessary during the exam and will view and interpret the results later.

Preparation

In some cases (such as for MRI brain scanning or an MRA), a chemical designed to increase image contrast may be given by the radiologist immediately before the exam. If a patient suffers from anxiety or claustrophobia, drugs may be given to help the patient relax.

The patient must remove all metal objects (e.g., watches, jewelry, eye glasses, hair clips). Any magnetized objects (like credit and bank machine cards) should be kept far away from the MRI equipment because they can be erased. Patients may not bring their wallet or keys into the MRI machine. The patient may be asked to wear clothing without metal snaps, buckles, or zippers, unless a medical gown is worn during the procedure. The patient may be asked to remove any hair spray, hair gel, or cosmetics that may interfere with the scan.

Aftercare

No aftercare is necessary unless the patient received medication or had a reaction to a contrast agent. Normally, patients can immediately return to their daily activities. If the examination reveals a serious condition that requires more testing and/or treatment, appropriate information and counseling will be needed.

Risks

MRI poses no known major health risks to the patient and produces no physical side effects. The potential effects of MRI on an unborn baby are not well known. Any woman who is, or may be, pregnant, should carefully discuss this issue with her doctor and radiologist before undergoing a scan. The most common problems are minor bleeding and bruising at the site of contrast injection. Since neither are reportable events, morbidity can only be estimated. Occasionally, an unknown allergy to seafood is discovered after injecting contrast. No deaths have been reported from MRI tests.

QUESTIONS TO ASK YOUR DOCTOR

- How long will the examination take?
- I have metal in my body from a prior surgery. Can I still have an MRI?
- Is MRI the best option for visualizing my condition?
- Should I expect any side effects?
- How long will it take to receive my results?

MRI scanning should not be used when there is the potential for an interaction between the strong MRI magnet and metal objects that might be imbedded in a patient's body. The force of magnetic attraction on certain types of metal objects (including surgical steel) could move them within the body and cause serious injury. Metal may be imbedded in a person's body for several reasons. Some of these reasons include:

- Medical. People with implanted cardiac pacemakers, metal aneurysm clips, or who have had broken bones repaired with metal pins, screws, rods, or plates must tell their radiologist prior to having an MRI scan. In some cases (like a metal rod in a reconstructed leg) the difficulty may be overcome.
- Injury. Patients must tell their doctors if they have bullet fragments or other metal pieces in their body from old wounds. The suspected presence of metal, whether from an old or recent wound, should be confirmed before scanning.
- Occupational. People with significant work exposure to metal particles (working with a metal grinder, for example) should discuss this with their doctor and radiologist. The patient may need pre-scan testing—usually a single, regular x ray of the eyes to see whether any metal is present.

Chemical agents designed to improve the picture and/or allow for the imaging of blood or other fluid flow during MRA may be injected. In rare cases, patients may be allergic to or intolerant of these agents, and these patients should not receive them. If these chemical agents are to be used, patients should discuss any concerns they have with their doctor and radiologist.

The potential side effects of magnetic and electric fields on human health remain a source of debate. In particular, the possible effects on an unborn baby are not well known. Any woman who is, or may be, pregnant should carefully discuss this issue with her doctor and radiologist before undergoing a scan.

As with all medical imaging techniques, being excessively overweight (obese) greatly interferes with the quality of MRI.

Results

A normal MRI, MRA, or MRS result will show the patient's physical condition to fall within normal ranges for the target area scanned. Generally, MRI is prescribed only when serious symptoms and/or negative results from other tests indicate a need. There often exists strong evidence of a condition that the scan is designed to detect and assess. Thus, the results will often be abnormal, confirming the earlier diagnosis. At that point, further testing and appropriate medical treatment are needed. For example, if the MRI indicates the presence of a brain tumor, an MRS may be prescribed to determine the type of tumor so that aggressive treatment can begin immediately without the need for a surgical biopsy.

Resources

BOOKS

Armstrong, Peter, Martin L. Wastie, and Andrea G. Rockall. *Diagnostic Imaging*. Chichester, U.K.: Wiley-Blackwell, 2009.

Culbreth, L. J., and C. Watson. *Magnetic Resonance Imaging Technology*. New York: Cambridge University Press, 2007.

Kastler, B. *Understanding MRI*. 2nd ed. Berlin: Springer-Verlag, 2008.

McRobbie, D. W., E. A. Moore, M. J. Graves, and M. R. Prince. *MRI from Picture to Proton*. 2nd ed. New York: Cambridge University Press, 2007.

Weishaupt, D., V. D. Koechli, and B. Marincek. *How does MRI work?: An Introduction to the Physics and Function of Magnetic Resonance Imaging*. 2nd ed. Berlin: Springer-Verlag, 2008.

Westbrook, Catherine. *Handbook of MRI Techniques*. Chichester, U.K.: Wiley-Blackwell, 2008.

PERIODICALS

Hara, H., T. Akisue, T. Fujimoto, et al. "Magnetic Resonance Imaging of Medullary Bone Infarction in the Early Stage." *Clinical Imaging* 32, no. 2 (2008): 147–151.

Rumboldt, Z. "Imaging of Topographic Viral CNS Infections." *Neuroimaging Clinics of North America* 18, no. 1 (2002): 85–92.

Wada, R., and W. Kucharczyk. "Prion Infections of the Brain." *Neuroimaging Clinics of North America* 18, no. 1 (2008): 183–191.

Zhao, W., J. H. Choi, G. R. Hon, and M. A. Vannan. "Left Ventricular Relaxation." *Heart Failure Clinics* 4, no. 1 (2008): 37–46.

WEBSITES

"Intraoperative Magnetic Resonance Imaging (iMRI)." Mayo Clinic. http://www.mayoclinic.org/intraoperative-mri (accessed May 24, 2011).

MedlinePlus. "MRI." U.S. National Library of Medicine, National Institutes of Health. http://www.nlm.nih.gov/medlineplus/ency/article/003335.htm (accessed May 25, 2011).

———. "MRI scans." http://www.nlm.nih.gov/medlineplus/mriscans.html (accessed May 25, 2011).

ORGANIZATIONS

American College of Radiology, 1891 Preston White Dr., Reston, VA, 20191, (703) 648-8900, http://www.acr.org.

National Institute of Biomedical Imaging and Bioengineering, 31 Center Dr., 1C14, Bethesda, MD, 20892-8859, (301) 469-8859, http://www.nibib.gov.

Kurt Richard Sternlof
Rosalyn Carson-DeWitt, MD
Brenda W. Lerner
William A. Atkins

Magnetic seizure therapy

Definition

Magnetic seizure therapy (MST) is a newer form of convulsive therapy that was under development between the late 1990s and 2011. Many older forms of convulsive therapy use direct electric shocks; however, MST uses rapidly alternating strong magnetic fields to induce **seizures**. In addition to MST, convulsive therapies include **electroconvulsive therapy** (ECT), **transcranial magnetic stimulation** (TMS), deep **brain** stimulation, and **vagus nerve stimulation**.

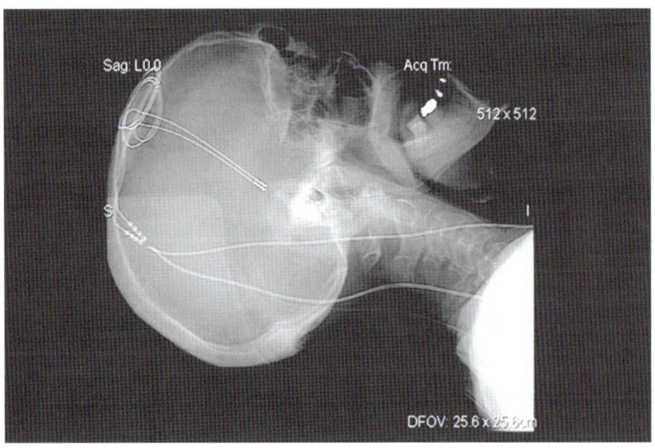

A lateral x ray of a patient's brain, showing the electrodes used in deep brain stimulation. *(© Medical Body Scans/ Photo Researchers, Inc.)*

Purpose

Convulsive therapies, also called electrotherapies and electrical brain stimulations, generally induce a seizure, or convulsion, in a patient to provide improvement in mental illnesses, the chief among them being major **depression**. MST is one of these convulsive therapies. However, it was developed as a safer and more effective form of convulsive therapies.

Description

Therapeutic magnetic seizure induction, the process of MST, was first performed in Bern, Switzerland, in May 2000. Numerous controlled studies on psychiatric patients were performed after that. Although the results of these studies show promise, researchers continue to investigate the effectiveness and safety of MST. As of 2011, MST was not yet considered an established convulsive therapy in the United States.

During MST, the patient is under a general anesthesia. The process involves a generator that produces multiple short bursts of electricity at a frequency of 50 to 100 hertz (Hz). This creates powerful magnetic fields within a wire coil shaped like a figure eight and attached to a paddle. A technician places the coil/paddle directly onto a patient's forehead, near the forehead, or directly onto the scalp. Because the magnetic fields are not absorbed or scattered by the skull, lower frequency current than in ECT is sufficient; thus, MST is safer than ECT because it uses less electricity.

The magnetic fields reach down about one inch (2.5 cm) into the skull to produce electrical current affecting brain cells directly under the coil. These currents do not reach into areas beneath the cortex. However, researchers are working to increase the distance reached to affect deeper-lying brain regions for greater positive results. The risks associated with MST are smaller than those associated with ECT, but they include the standard risks associated with anesthetics. Additionally, memory loss and disruption of concentration and thinking are shorter and less severe.

The oldest convulsive therapy, ECT, has been the standard treatment for medication-resistant major depression since about 1940. However, ECT sends electricity to the brain and requires general anesthesia and muscle relaxants, subjecting patients to these drugs' associated risks. ECT causes memory loss for events close to the event of therapy and prior to therapy, and this memory does not return to all patients. To avoid the larger risks of anesthesia, muscle relaxants, and memory loss, researchers developed alternative convulsive therapies. A novel alternative, MST shows the most promise and was developed from TMS, which does not induce seizures at its generated electrical frequencies of 0.3 to 20 Hz.

TMS generates lower frequencies than required by ECT, so seizures do not occur. TMS is also focused and more localized to avoid the larger brain areas accessed by ECT. As a result, TMS avoids memory loss. TMS does not require general anesthesia, so those associated risks do not exist. Magnetic seizure therapy comprises TMS administered at higher frequencies to induce seizures, at 50 to 100 Hz, but MST uses magnetic fields instead of electricity, and these fields act directly on the brain. The skull does not absorb or scatter the magnetic fields, making MST more efficient than ECT. MST promises greater safety and diminished cognitive side effects over ECT.

Uses for depression, bipolar disorder, and schizophrenia

MST provides positive outcomes in treatment for a number of mental disorders. While the primary illness treated with MST is the same as for ECT, major depression, MST is also successful in cases of **schizophrenia**, bipolar depression, and bipolar mania. In 2005, Mitchell and Loo studied the safety and effectiveness of repetitive MST. They examined meta-analyses and individual patient reports and found that repetitive MST may be most effective in younger patients with no psychotic features and in depression that is not of the longest duration.

Further, they found that some depression occurring in **bipolar disorder** responds better to repetitive MST than do unipolar depressions (those not part of a bipolar syndrome). The majority of depressed patients receiving repetitive MST do not suffer any side effects or only slight discomfort in the stimulated scalp nerves and muscles or an occasional light headache. Sachdev, Loo, Mitchell, and Mahli found in 2005 that repetitive MST produces significant positive outcomes in patients having the deficit syndrome of schizophrenia, which includes lack of talking, emotion, and motivation. This pilot investigation confirmed the existing research regarding MST as a successful treatment for schizophrenia.

Other applications

Harvard Medical School and Stanford University reported that over 30 ongoing controlled studies examining MST in the United States between October 2005 and late 2011 showed positive outcomes. These studies looked at MST as a treatment for mental illnesses and medical conditions having a mental health component. As of 2011, these included major depression, schizophrenia, **schizoaffective disorder**, bipolar disorder, **post-traumatic stress disorder** (PTSD), obsessive compulsive disorder (OCD), Tourette syndrome, Parkinson's disease, **stroke**, and cerebral palsy. Additional applications may be found in future research.

Benefits

Sarah H. Lisanby, a professor of clinical psychiatry at Columbia University and the director of the Division of Brain Stimulation and Therapeutic Modulation at the New York State Psychiatric Institute, found that patients were able to remember their own names, current setting, current date, and current location much more quickly after receiving MST than after undergoing ECT. In fact, MST produced only two minutes of memory loss, while ECT caused memory loss for 13 minutes. MST also caused fewer problems with concentration. In task completion, patients finished a simple task in four minutes after receiving ECT, but in only two minutes after MST, and these differences were significant. Lisanby, who is also the leader of the Transcranial Magnetic Stimulation Unit in the fMRI (functional **magnetic resonance imaging**) Research Center at Columbia University, believes that most depressive patients can improve with TMS and without induced seizures but that some depressed patients may need to undergo a seizure to improve and can benefit more from MST, because it offers fewer and smaller side effects than does ECT. Ongoing research may confirm these findings.

Precautions

MST has been a subject of debate since its inception. Its supporters report numerous well-documented successes, while its detractors insist that long-term patient improvement is possible only through seizures induced by ECT. However, researchers have found that MST seizures do not produce the large and intense side effects of ECT. MST produces fewer and shorter disruptions of memory, concentration, and orientation. Overall, MST may be safer and more efficient than ECT, produce fewer side effects, and perhaps reduce treatment costs.

There is debate on whether MST is more effective than TMS. According to the February 23, 2007, issue of the *Harvard Mental Health Letter,* 40% of medication-resistant depression cases improve with TMS, which does not induce any seizures. TMS may also reduce the time needed for psychiatric drugs to work. TMS may provide some improvement for **obsessive-compulsive disorder** (OCD), but as of 2011, the FDA had not yet approved any repetitive transcranial magnetic stimulation device for treatment purposes other than depression.

Preparation

Preparation for magnetic seizure therapy is not necessary.

Aftercare

After MST is used on a patient, the individual is carefully monitored for side effects of the procedure and other possible complications. Although generally perceived as safer than other convulsive therapies, MST is still not without medical risks.

Risks

As with any medical procedure, risks are present. The risks associated with MST are smaller than those associated with ECT. The standard risk is one involving the use of anesthetics. In addition, memory loss and disruption of concentration and thinking can occur but are usually much less than with ECT.

Results

MST has been viewed as useful in nonhuman primates and in humans with depression. Preliminary results with MST show that induced seizures are more focused, result in less overlap into hippocampal and deep brain structures, and produce less side effects than those seizures induced with ECT.

Research & general acceptance

In a 2006 meta-analysis, researchers Loo, Schweitzer, and Pratt found that recent advances and alternative technical approaches have developed in ECT. They examined recent **clinical trials**, case reports, and research updates in ECT's best practices and completed/ongoing research. Loo, Schweitzer, and Pratt found an increasing use of a number of alternative electrode placements useful in ECT, several variations in stimulus configurations, and two altogether new approaches that are successful. These new approaches are MST and focal electrical stimulation. The researchers decided that MST may promise success and safety in treating a variety of mental illnesses but needs further research. Their conclusion confirms the findings of the meta-analysis of Stanford and colleagues in 2005 that includes 69 separate sources and was as of 2011 approved for continuing education credit learning among physicians and researchers.

KEY TERMS

Anesthesia—A drug that induces loss of sensitivity to pain to all or part of a body.

Bipolar depression—The medical condition involving depression with the presence of at least one manic episode.

Bipolar mania—A mental disorder involving manic episodes frequently with depression.

Convulsion—Uncontrollable motions of limbs of the body or the body itself.

Cortex—The outer layer of the cerebrum in the brain.

Depression—A psychiatric disorder involving feelings of hopelessness and symptoms of fatigue, sleeplessness, suicidal tendencies, and poor concentration.

Hertz—A unit of frequency equal to one cycle per second.

Magnetic field—A region or space that is surrounded by a magnetized body or a current-carrying circuit.

Schizophrenia—A mental disorder involving degraded thinking and emotions, often with auditory hallucinations.

In addition to these findings, as of 2011, Lisanby was researching two distinct forms of MST. One of these uses a wire coil to focus seizures in the prefrontal cortex of the brain. The other form uses a coil to stimulate a broader brain area. This research is part of a wider study of MST effects compared with ECT effects in ongoing research at New York State Psychiatric Institute. Lisanby believes that MST can provide fewer side effects and better results than ECT for individuals with depression and a range of other mental illnesses.

In 2010, a clinical study was conducted in the University Hospital at Bonn, Germany. The investigators conducted a single center, clinical pilot efficacy study. Its goal is to show that magnetic seizure therapy can be effective as an add-on therapy for the treatment of refractory major depression as assessed by the Hamilton Depression Rating Scale.

The study's results showed that magnetic seizure therapy produced similar outcomes when compared to electroconvulsive therapy for the treatment of resistant depression. However, the recovery times from the procedures for MST were much faster than for ECT. In addition, fewer cognitive side effects were seen with the

QUESTIONS TO ASK YOUR DOCTOR

- Is MST my best option?
- What are the risks with MST?
- Do the benefits outweigh the risks?

MST. The results of the study were reported at the annual meeting of the European College of Neuropsychopharmacology. The MST device used for the study was the MagPro MST.

The first commercial MST device was developed by MagVenture, a company headquartered in Denmark. As of December 2010, the MagPro MST was considered the most powerful MST device yet to be developed, being about twice as powerful as other such devices. It was shown to be an effective and reliable device for inducing seizures. Earlier devices were not considered reliable for inducing seizures. Sarah Kayser, of the University Hospital and one of the authors of the German study, noted in an interview with *Clinical Psychiatry News* that the MagPro MST was "much smaller and easier to work with" than older devices, which were "large and unwieldy with multiple components."

Resources

BOOKS

Boyer, Bret A., and M. Indira Paharia, eds. *Comprehensive Handbook of Clinical Health Psychology*. Hoboken, NJ: John Wiley and Sons, 2008.

The Duke Encyclopedia of New Medicine: Conventional and Alternative Medicine for All Ages. London: Rodale, 2006.

Fink, Max. *Electroconvulsive Therapy: A Guide for Professionals and Their Patients*. Oxford: Oxford University Press, 2009.

Lisanby, Sarah H., ed. *Brain Stimulation in Psychiatric Treatment*. Washington, DC: American Psychiatric, 2004.

PERIODICALS

Avery, David H., et al. "A Controlled Study of Repetitive Transcranial Magnetic Stimulation in Medication-Resistant Major Depression." *Biological Psychiatry* 59, no. 2 (2006): 187–94.

Harvard Medical School. "Electroconvulsive Therapy." *Harvard Mental Health Letter* 23, no. 8 (2007): 1–3.

Helwick, Caroline. "Magnetic Seizure Therapy Matches ECT for Depression." *Clinical Psychiatry News* 38, no. 10 (October 1, 2010): 1–2.

Lisanby, Sarah H., A. Peterchev, M. A. Marcolin, and F. Padberg, eds. "Transcranial Brain Stimulation for Treatment of Psychiatric Disorders: Magnetic Seizure Therapy for the Treatment of Depression." *Advances in Biological Psychiatry* 23 (2007): 155–71. (DOI: 10.1159/000101036).

Loo, Colleen K, and Philip B. Mitchell. "A Review of the Efficacy of Transcranial Magnetic Stimulation (TMS) Treatment for Depression, and Current and Future Strategies to Optimize Efficacy." *Journal of Affective Disorders* 88, no. 3 (2005): 255–67.

Loo, Colleen K., Isaac Schweitzer, and Chris Pratt. "Recent Advances in Optimizing Electroconvulsive Therapy." *Australian and New Zealand Journal of Psychiatry* 40, no. 8 (2006): 632–38.

Mitchell, Philip B., and Colleen K. Loo. "Transcranial Magnetic Stimulation for Depression." *Australian and New Zealand Journal of Psychiatry* 40, no. 5 (2006): 406–13.

Sachdev, Perminder, Colleen K. Loo, Philip B. Mitchell, and Gin Malhi. "Transcranial Magnetic Stimulation for the Deficit Syndrome of Schizophrenia: A Pilot Investigation." *Psychiatry and Clinical Neurosciences* 5, no. 3 (2005): 354–57.

Stanford, Arielle D., et al. "Magnetic Seizure Therapy and Other Convulsive Therapies." *Primary Psychiatry* 12, no. 10 (2005): 44–50.

ORGANIZATIONS

American Psychiatric Association, 1000 Wilson Blvd., Ste. 1825, Arlington, VA, 22209-3901, (703) 907-7300, apa@psych.org, http://www.psych.org.

Association for Convulsive Therapy, 5454 Wisconsin Ave., Chevy Chase, MD, 20815, (301) 951-7220, http://www.act-ect.org/act/index.php

New York State Psychiatric Institute, Columbia University Medical Center, 1051 Riverside Dr., New York City, NY, 10032, (212) 543-6000, http://www.nyspi.org.

Patty Inglish, MS

Magnetoencephalogram *see* **Electroencephalography**

Major depressive disorder

Definition

Major depressive disorder (MDD) is a condition characterized by a long-lasting depressed mood or marked loss of interest or pleasure (anhedonia) in all or nearly all activities. Children and adolescents with MDD may be irritable instead of sad. These symptoms, along with others described below, must be sufficiently severe to interfere significantly with the patient's daily functioning.

Demographics

According to Mental Health America, depression affects more than 21 million Americans and is the leading cause of disability within this population for persons aged 15–44. Recent research indicates that 4.9% of the population of the United States meets the diagnostic criteria for MDD at any given time, but 17.1% will experience at least one episode of the disorder at some point during their lives. While the disorder may affect people at any age, it is most commonly diagnosed in young adults in their twenties. For reasons that are not well understood, women are twice as likely to develop MDD as are men; prior to puberty, however, MDD is about equally common in girls and boys. Adolescence is a high-risk period for MDD; while suicide may result from impulsive behavior under **stress** rather than from MDD, it is noteworthy that about 14% of all teenage deaths are due to suicide. The figures for gay and lesbian youth indicate that as many as 20%–35% make suicide attempts. Other risk factors include Hispanic ethnicity; younger age at onset; lower levels of education or income; and being separated or divorced.

Depression appears to have become a more common disorder over the past century. Epidemiologists studying the incidence of depression across time compared groups of people born between 1917 and 1936, between 1937 and 1952, and between 1953 and 1966. Their results indicated that the rate of depression increased progressively from one generation to the next. While no single explanation for the rise in depressive disorders emerged, some researchers have suggested that the breakdown of social support networks caused by higher rates of family disruption and greater social mobility may be important contributing factors.

Description

Major depressive disorder is a serious mental disorder that profoundly affects an individual's quality of life. Unlike normal **bereavement** or an occasional episode of "the blues," MDD causes a lengthy period of gloom and hopelessness and may rob the sufferer of the ability to take pleasure in activities or relationships that were previously enjoyable. In some cases, depressive episodes seem to be triggered by an obviously painful event, but MDD may also develop without a specific stressor. Research indicates that an initial episode of **depression** is likely to be a response to a specific stimulus, but later episodes are progressively more likely to start without a triggering event. A person suffering major depression finds job-related and other responsibilities, such as parenting, to be burdensome and carries them out only with great effort. Mental efficiency and memory are affected, causing even simple tasks to be tiring and irritating. Sexual interest dwindles; many people with MDD become withdrawn and avoid any type of social activity. Even the ability to enjoy a good meal or a sound night's sleep is frequently lost; many depressed people report a chronic sense of malaise (general discomfort or unease). For some, the pain and suffering accompanying MDD become so unendurable that **suicide** is viewed as the only option; MDD has the highest mortality rate of any mental disorder.

Major depressive disorder may be limited to a single episode of depression; more commonly, it may become a chronic condition with many episodes of depressed mood. Other symptoms that may develop include psychotic symptoms (e.g., bizarre thoughts, including delusional beliefs and hallucinations); **catatonia**; postpartum onset (sometimes accompanied by psychotic symptoms); and **seasonal affective disorder**, or SAD.

Such conditions as **postpartum depression** and seasonal affective disorder accompany MDD only under certain circumstances. Postpartum depression begins within four weeks of giving birth. Women with this disorder experience labile mood (frequent drastic mood changes). They may feel helpless and unable to care adequately for their infant, or they may be completely uninterested in the child. The symptoms of postpartum depression are much more severe than those of the relatively common "new baby blues," which affect up to 70% of new mothers. The presence of psychotic symptoms in the mother, too many ruminations (obsessive thoughts), or **delusions** about the infant are associated with a heightened risk of serious harm to the child. The symptoms of postpartum depression are usually attributed to fluctuations in the woman's hormone levels and the emotional impact of bearing a child. The condition is especially likely to occur in women who were highly anxious during pregnancy or had a previous history of mood disorder. SAD is also more common in women than in men; in this case, symptoms of MDD typically begin in fall and winter, especially in northern latitudes in the United States and Canada. Exposure to natural light is limited during the winter in these areas, but the symptoms of SAD typically improve during the spring and summer.

Causes and symptoms

Causes

Because MDD is a relatively common mental disorder, researchers have performed a range of studies to identify possible underlying causes. Three types of causes are commonly identified: intrapsychic, environmental, and biological.

INTRAPSYCHIC. Since Sigmund Freud attributed the development of mental disorders to intrapsychic (occurring inside the mind) conflicts occurring during early childhood, a sizeable number of theorists have suggested that MDD results from a tendency to internalize negative events. Cognitive behavioral treatment models assume that a person's interpretation of situations is responsible for the development of depression rather than the events themselves. Some people blame themselves for negative experiences while attributing positive outcomes to external sources; they may tend to feel guilty, undeserving, and eventually depressed. For example, they may think of their present job as something they obtained by a stroke of good luck; at the same time, they may regard being laid off as something they brought on themselves. When these patterns of thought become habitual, they lead to a style of coping characterized by a view of oneself as worthless, ineffectual, and inferior. In some cases, people pick up these patterns of thinking from their parents or other family members.

Another theory regarding intrapsychic causes attributes depression to so-called "learned helplessness." This theory grew out of research studies on animal learning, comparing dogs that were able to escape from mild electric shocks to dogs that could not escape. The researchers discovered that the dogs who could not escape the mild shocks became passive; later, when they were put in a situation in which they could escape the shocks, they made no attempt to do so but simply lay on their stomachs and whimpered. The animals had, in short, learned to be helpless; they had learned during the first part of the experiment that nothing they had done had any effect on the shocks. Applied to human beings, this theory holds that people tend to become depressed when they have had long-term experiences of helplessness—as would be the case for abused children. Later, when the children have become adults, they do not see themselves as grownups with some control over their lives; they continue to react to setbacks or losses with the same feelings of helplessness that they had as children, and they become depressed.

ENVIRONMENTAL. Environmental theories of the etiology (causation) of MDD emphasize the role of external events in triggering depression. According to this perspective, people become depressed primarily due to unfortunate circumstances that are difficult to change. In some cases, these misfortunes may include environmental disasters or personal losses, but such other factors as low socioeconomic status, oppression associated with one's sex or race, or unpleasant or frustrating relationships are also thought to contribute to depression.

BIOLOGICAL. Ancient medicine alleged that one's state of mind was related to the presence of specific "humors," or fluids, in the body, and various theories have emerged since the eighteenth century regarding possible constitutional factors that affect mood. In recent years, researchers have found numerous abnormalities in the neuroendocrine systems, **neurotransmitters**, and neuroanatomy of the brains of both children and adults with MDD, as well as strong evidence for **genetic factors** in MDD.

Levels of cortisol, a hormone associated with the human "fight-or-flight" response, have long been studied as possible biological markers for depression. In many adults, cortisol levels rise when the person is acutely depressed, and they return to normal when the depression passes. Research findings have been inconsistent regarding cortisol levels in children and adolescents, although there is some evidence that higher levels of cortisol secretion are associated with more severe depressive symptoms and with a higher likelihood of recurrence. However, cortisol levels are not considered reliable enough to be useful in diagnosing MDD.

Another biological factor that has been studied in humans involves changes in the levels of neurotransmitters, which are chemicals that conduct nerve impulses across the tiny gaps between nerve cells. Variations in the levels of certain neurotransmitters have been researched for many years due to their importance in the brain's limbic system, which is the center of emotions and has many important pathways to other parts of the **brain**. In depression, the system that regulates a neurotransmitter called "serotonin" does not function properly. A group of medications known as "serotonin specific reuptake inhibitors," or "SSRIs," are believed to be effective in relieving depression because they prevent **serotonin** from being taken back up too quickly by receptors in the brain.

Differences in the anatomical structure of the brains of children and adults with MDD have suggested several possible explanations for its development. In particular, the prefrontal cortex has been thought to play a role, on the basis of findings in stroke patients with damage to the prefrontal area of the brain, and in children and adults with MDD. Researchers found that stroke patients experienced more severe depression if their stroke occurred closer to the frontal lobe of the brain. Similarly, people with MDD have been found to have decreased frontal lobe volume. Studies of depressed children and adults included subjects who were currently depressed as well as those with a history of depression who were in remission, which suggests that abnormalities in the frontal lobe may be a structural marker of depression. Other neurological studies have reported lower levels of electrical activity in the left frontal cortex among depressed subjects (including the infants of depressed mothers), compared to persons who are not depressed.

Researchers have also been interested in the relationship of genetic factors to depression. It has been known for many years that depression tends to run in families. Convincing evidence of the heritability of depression has been obtained by comparing identical twins (who have identical genetic inheritances) with fraternal twins; these studies have consistently found a higher likelihood of depression between identical than between fraternal twins. Other data indicate that people with a higher genetic risk of depression are more likely to become depressed following a stressful event than are people with fewer genetic risk factors.

Symptoms

The core symptom of major depression is a sad mood that does not go away. While most people have occasional days when they feel out of sorts, persons with MDD experience low feelings that build gradually over a period of days or weeks. They are usually not able to "snap out of it," even when something positive happens. In some cases, the symptoms are preceded by an obvious loss or painful event, such as divorce or a death in the family, but the disorder may also appear to begin "out of the blue." People with MDD often appear sad, irritable, and easily moved to tears. They may sleep poorly and complain of vague physical aches and pains; experience sexual difficulties or loss of interest in sex; drop out of social activities; and come across to others as unhappy or lacking in energy. Some people with MDD may deny that they feel depressed, but they lose their enthusiasm for hobbies or work they once found enjoyable and rewarding. Children and adolescents present with many of these same characteristics, but they may often appear easily frustrated and cranky instead of sad. The symptoms of MDD can be summarized as follows:

- disturbed mood (sad, hopeless, discouraged, "down in the dumps") during most of the day
- loss of interest or pleasure in activities
- change in appetite nearly every day, leading either to weight gain or to loss of 5% of body weight; in children, may appear as a failure to make normal weight gains related to growth
- insomnia (waking in the middle of the night and having difficulty returning to sleep, or waking too early in the morning) or hypersomnia (sleeping much more than normal)
- psychomotor retardation (slowed thinking, speech, body movements) or agitation (inability to sit still, hand-wringing, pulling at clothing, skin, or other objects) that is apparent to others
- sense of worthlessness or unreasonable guilt over minor failings
- problems with clear thinking, concentration, and decision-making
- recurrent thoughts of death or suicide, or making a suicide attempt

KEY TERMS

Anxiety—Can be experienced as a troubled feeling, a sense of dread, fear of the future, or distress over a possible threat to a person's physical or mental well-being.

Cognitive-behavioral therapy—Psychotherapy technique designed to help people change their attitudes, perceptions, and patterns of thinking.

Electroconvulsive therapy (ECT)—Therapy for mood disorders that involves passing electrical current through the brain in order to create a brief convulsion.

Insomnia—Waking in the middle of the night and having difficulty returning to sleep, or waking too early in the morning.

Serotonin—A chemical messenger in the brain, thought to play a role in mood regulation. Low levels of serotonin are associated with depression.

Diagnosis

While many people go through sad or elated moods from time to time, people with major depressive disorder suffer from severe or prolonged mood states that disrupt their daily functioning. Major depressive disorder may be diagnosed when a person visits their family doctor with concerns about their mood, changes in appetite or sleeping patterns, and similar symptoms. Doctors in family practice, in fact, are more likely to be consulted by patients with depression than doctors in any other medical specialty. In addition, a large proportion of people discuss depressed feelings with their clergyperson, who has typically been trained (in the mainstream Christian and Jewish communities) to recognize the signs of depression and to encourage the person to see their doctor. In some cases, a concerned spouse or other family member may take the patient to the doctor.

The **diagnosis** of MDD involves a constellation of symptoms in addition to depressed mood. After taking a careful history, including asking the patient about his or her sleeping patterns, appetite, sex drive, and mood, the doctor will give the patient a physical examination to rule out other possible causes of the symptoms. Certain other disorders may resemble MDD, including cognitive dysfunction caused by the direct effects of a substance (a drug of abuse, medication, or toxic chemical); various medical conditions (e.g., an underactive thyroid gland; strokes; or early stages of **dementia**), or other mental disorders. Such stressful life events as normal bereavement may also produce behaviors similar to those associated with MDD; while a bereaved person may appear to have many of the characteristics of MDD, the disorder would not be diagnosed unless the symptoms continued for more than two months or were extreme in some way. As part of the diagnostic interview, the doctor may give the patient a brief screening questionnaire, such as the **Beck Depression Inventory**, in order to obtain a clearer picture of the symptoms. In addition to interviewing the patient, the doctor may talk to family members or others who can provide information that the patient may forget, deny, or consider unimportant.

The diagnosis of MDD is complicated by the fact that people with MDD frequently suffer from other mental illnesses at the same time, including **anxiety disorders**, **substance abuse** problems, and **personality disorders**. Given that the patient's symptoms may vary according to age, sex, and stage of the illness, some clinicians have suggested that MDD may actually be a collection or group of disorders with a small number of underlying core symptoms rather than a single entity.

The diagnosis of a person with MDD may also include certain specifiers, including the severity and chronicity of the disorder, the presence of psychotic features (delusions or hallucinations); catatonia (remaining motionless for long periods of time, and other peculiarities of posture, movement, or speech); melancholia (depressed mood that is worse in the morning; early-morning wakening; psychomotor retardation or agitation, significant weight loss; or inappropriate guilt); and information regarding postpartum status. If the depression is currently in remission, this fact is also commonly listed as a diagnostic specifier.

DSM

Major depressive disorder is included as a mood disorder in the fourth edition of the ***Diagnostic and Statistical Manual of Mental Disorders*** (*DSM-IV*), the clinical guideline used by medical professionals in diagnosing mental disorders. The fifth edition of the *DSM* (*DSM-5*) is due for publication in May 2013. Proposed changes for the fifth edition include reclassifying mood disorders as depressive disorders and removing the so-called "grief exclusion," which does not consider bereavement or **grief** as a criteria for major depression. The reasoning behind the removal is that research does not support the separation of loss of a loved one from other stressors; however, the proposal has been met with controversy.

Treatment

Because MDD can have a devastating impact on a person's life, the importance of effective treatment cannot be overestimated. Treatment strategies have evolved over the years, according to researchers' varying opinions of the underlying causes of depression, but the outpouring of interest in MDD allows treatment providers to select from a variety of tested approaches.

Psychotherapy

Cognitive psychotherapies for depression are based on the belief that depressed people perceive themselves and the world in unrealistically negative ways. Considerable research has been done regarding the cognitive dimension of depression; for example, studies find that depressed people pay more attention to negative events than to positive ones, and that dwelling on unpleasant experiences prolongs and worsens depressive episodes. Cognitive therapists help patients identify the automatic thoughts that lead them to anticipate poor outcomes or to interpret neutral events in negative ways. The patient is also encouraged to challenge negative thoughts by comparing his or her expectations of events with actual outcomes.

Evidence that poor interpersonal relationships may heighten vulnerability to depression, along with findings that depressed adults and depressed children tend to provoke negative reactions from other people, has prompted the use of **social skills training** as a form of treatment. In this type of therapy, patients are trained to recognize actions and attitudes that annoy or distance other people, and to replace these behaviors with more appropriate ones. Social skills training may be particularly helpful to depressed persons who tend to isolate themselves and have lost confidence in their ability to develop healthy relationships. This treatment model promotes the idea that depression is likely to lift when the patient becomes adept at making new friends and establishing rewarding social supports.

Psychodynamic psychotherapy is often effective in treating patients with MDD whose depression is related to unresolved issues from the past, particularly abuse or other painful childhood experiences. The growth of insight into one's emotional patterns, as well as the supportive aspects of this form of therapy, offer considerable relief from emotional pain to many patients.

Medications

The use of medications in the treatment of depression began in the late 1950s with the successful introduction of tricyclic **antidepressants** and MAO inhibitors. Treatment of depression with medications has greatly increased since the advent of **selective serotonin reuptake inhibitors (SSRIs)** such as **fluoxetine** (Prozac) or **sertraline** (Zoloft). While these medications are no more effective than their predecessors, they have fewer side effects and are much safer for patients who may be likely to overdose. Selecting the optimal antidepressant medication is not always a straightforward process, however, and the patient may have to try out various drugs for a period of weeks or months before finding one that is effective for him or her. In addition, while the **SSRIs** have comparatively few side effects, such complaints as loss of sexual interest or functioning, nervousness, headaches, gastrointestinal complaints, drowsiness, and **insomnia** can be significant obstacles to the patient's taking the medication as directed.

More recently, **Quetiapine** (Seroquel and Seroquel XR), once used for treatment of **schizophrenia** and **bipolar disorder**, may be used together with other antidepressant medications to treat major depressive disorder in adults who did not have an adequate response to antidepressant therapy.

Other mainstream approaches

The use of **electroconvulsive therapy** (ECT), initially introduced in the 1930s, was virtually abandoned as a treatment for MDD for many years, largely as a result of the effectiveness and convenience of psychotropic (mind-altering) medications. Since the 1980s, however, interest in the procedure has renewed; in 1990, the **American Psychiatric Association** published new guidelines for the use of ECT. Despite media portrayals of ECT as an outdated and cruel form of treatment that causes considerable pain, in actuality the patient is given a sedative, and the electrical stimulation is calibrated precisely to produce the maximum therapeutic effects. ECT may be the first line of treatment when a patient cannot tolerate the customary medications or is at high risk of harming himself or herself; but it is more commonly used with patients who fail to respond to drug treatment. In terms of effectiveness, however, ECT actually outperforms medications even among patients who are helped by antidepressants, as well as those who are resistant to drug treatment.

The use of phototherapy (**light therapy**) has proven to be the treatment of choice for patients diagnosed with seasonal affective disorder. Although the reasons for the effectiveness of phototherapy are not yet clear, treatment involves exposing the eyes to bright (2500 lux) light for several minutes a day. Currently, however, there is little evidence to suggest that phototherapy is useful in the treatment of other types of MDD.

Alternative and complementary treatments

The National Center for Complementary and Alternative Medicine (NCCAM) is conducting an ongoing series of clinical tests of alternative and complementary treatments for depression. Those that have been shown to reduce symptoms of depression and compare favorably with conventional treatments include **acupuncture**; Ayurvedic medicine; **meditation**; and a therapeutic diet designed to be free of caffeine and refined sugar.

Herbal preparations are common alternative treatments for depression; in fact, a NCCAM study found that depression is the single most common reason for people in the United States to purchase herbal remedies. Some, such as St. John's wort, have been used in Europe for decades. The German Commission E, which regulates government approval of herbal preparations in German-speaking Europe, recently approved the use of Ginkgo biloba extract as a treatment for depression. The most important caution is that persons who are using herbal remedies, whether to treat depression or other conditions, should always tell their doctor what they are taking, how much, and how often. This warning is crucial because some herbal preparations that are safe in themselves can interact with prescription medications. In particular, **St. John's wort** has been reported to cause interactions with fluoxetine (Prozac).

Some complementary approaches appear to be helpful to persons with depression because they offer pleasurable experiences for the senses or lift the person's spirit. These include **aromatherapy**; **music therapy**; pet therapy; humor; therapeutic massage; and **yoga**.

Prognosis

Major depression is increasingly viewed as a chronic condition for many people. Left untreated, a depressive episode may last four months or longer, regardless of the age of onset. While most people recover fully from a given depressive episode, eventual recurrence is common. Long-term studies of people with MDD indicate that about 60% of patients who have one episode of depression will have a second episode; with each succeeding episode, the chances of a subsequent episode increase (persons having a third episode stand a 90% chance of having a fourth). Between depressive episodes, the patient's mood may return to a nondepressed state (in about two-thirds of the cases) or continue to show some degree of impairment (one-third of cases). Patients who recover only partially between episodes appear to be at especially high risk of recurrence.

QUESTIONS TO ASK YOUR DOCTOR

- What are the indications that I may have major depressive disorder?
- What physical and psychological diagnostic tests are needed for a thorough assessment?
- What treatment options do you recommend for me?
- What kind of changes can I expect to see with the medications you have prescribed for me?
- What are the side effects associated with the medications you have prescribed for me?
- Will medications for major depressive disorder interact with my current medications?
- What tests or evaluation techniques will you perform to see whether treatment has been beneficial for me?
- Should I see a specialist? If so, what kind of specialist should I contact?
- Does having major depressive disorder put me at risk for other health conditions?
- What tests or evaluation techniques will you perform to see whether treatment has been beneficial for my child?
- What symptoms or adverse effects are important enough that I should seek immediate treatment?
- Can you recommend an organization that will provide me with additional information about major depressive disorder?
- Can you recommend any support groups for me and my family?

Community studies indicate that about 60% of the people diagnosed with MDD are greatly improved or fully recovered by one year after diagnosis. A very severe initial episode of depression, the presence of a coexisting **dysthymic disorder**, or the existence of a serious medical condition are associated with a poorer prognosis.

Prevention

While programs specifically aimed at preventing MDD are not widespread, early interventions with children to address some of the issues related to depression have met with success. In particular, social skills training has been found to reduce symptoms of depression, perhaps by enabling children to develop the kinds of social supports and friendships that promote good mental health. Cognitive behavioral techniques that teach people to challenge dysfunctional thought patterns, such as the tendency to deny responsibility for good outcomes and to feel overly responsible for negative events, has been found to successfully reduce the rates of depressive symptoms in children and college students. In addition, psychoeducational work with parents having mood disorders has been effective in improving the adjustment of their children. Long-term follow-up of such approaches is incomplete, but these studies support the possibility that improved individual and family functioning may help to lower rates of depression in the future.

As the factors that increase an individual's vulnerability to depression become better understood, effective strategies for early **intervention** and possible prevention become possible. Brief therapies that target such symptoms as maladaptive thought patterns or interpersonal problems may lower the risk of serious mood disturbances. Knowledge of the mental health implications of natural or humanly caused disasters has already resulted in much improved mental health services to communities in need. It is realistic to expect that appropriate treatment will become more available and accessible to people experiencing less dramatic setbacks to their ability to function in the future.

Resources

BOOKS

American Psychiatric Association. *Diagnostic and Statistical Manual of Mental Disorders.* 4th ed., Text rev. Washington, DC: American Psychiatric Association, 2000.

American Psychological Association. *Publication Manual of the American Psychological Association,* 6th ed. Washington, DC: American Psychological Association, 2009.

Baldwin, Robert. *Depression in Later Life.* New York: Oxford University Press, 2010.

Gillberg, Christopher, Richard Harrington, and Hans-Christoph Steinhausen, eds. *A Clinician's Handbook of Child and Adolescent Psychiatry.* Cambridge: Cambridge University Press, 2011.

Graham, George. *The Disordered Mind: An Introduction to Philosophy of Mind and Mental Illness.* New York: Routledge, 2010.

Jongsma, Arthur E., Jr., L. Mark Peterson, and William P. McInnis. *The Child Psychotherapy Treatment Planner.* 4th ed. Hoboken, NJ: John Wiley & Sons, 2009.

North, Carol, and Sean Yutzy. *Goodwin and Guze's Psychiatric Diagnosis.* New York, NY: Oxford University Press, 2010.

O'Connor, Richard. *Undoing Depression: What Therapy Doesn't Teach You and Medication Can't Give You,* 2nd ed. New York: Little, Brown and Company, 2010.

Pelletier, Kenneth R., MD. *The Best Alternative Medicine* Kindle Edition, Part II, "CAM Therapies for Specific Conditions: Depression." Lady Lake, FL: Fireside, 2010.

Virani, Adil S., et al., eds. *Clinical Handbook of Psychotropic Drugs,* 19th ed. Cambridge, MA: Hogrefe Publishing, 2011.

PERIODICALS

Brodaty, H., et al. "A 25-year Longitudinal Comparison Study of the Outcome of Depression." Psychological Medicine 31 (2001): 1347-1358.

Nolan, Carla L., et al. "Prefrontal Cortical Volume in Childhood-Onset Major Depression." Archives of General Psychiatry 59 (2002): 173-175.

Nuland, Sherwin B., M.D. "The Uncertain Art: Lightning on My Mind." The American Scholar 71 (Spring 2002): 127-131.

Rush, A.J., et al. "Combining Medications to Enhance Depression Outcomes (CO-MED): Acute and Long-Term Outcomes of a Single-Blind Randomized Study." *American Journal of Psychiatry* 168 (2011): 689–701.

ORGANIZATIONS

American Academy of Child and Adolescent Psychiatry, 3615 Wisconsin Avenue NW, Washington, DC, 20016-3007, (202) 966-7300, Fax: (202) 966-2891, http://www.aacap.org.

American Psychological Association, 750 First Street NE, Washington, DC, 20003, (202) 336-5500, http://www.apa.org/index.aspx.

Depression and Bipolar Support Alliance (DBSA), 730 N. Franklin St., Ste. 501, Chicago, IL, 60654, (800) 826-3632, Fax: (312) 642-7243, http://www.dbsalliance.org.

Families for Depression Awareness, 395 Totten Pond Rd., Suite 404, Waltham, MA, 02451, (781) 890-0220, Fax: (781) 890-2411, http://www.familyaware.org.

Mental Health America, 2000 N. Beauregard Street, 6th Floor, Alexandria, VA, 22311, (703) 684-7722, (800) 969-6642, Fax: (703) 684-5968, http://www1.nmha.org.

National Alliance on Mental Illness (NAMI), Colonial Place Three, 2107 Wilson Blvd., Suite 300, Arlington, VA, 22201, (703) 524-7600, (800) 950-NAMI (6264), Fax: (703) 524-9094, http://www.nami.org/Hometemplate.cfm.

National Institute of Mental Health (NIMH), 6001 Executive Boulevard, Room 8184, MSC 9663, Bethesda, MD, 20892, (301) 443-4513, (866) 615-6464, Fax: (301) 443-4279, nimhinfo@nih.gov, http://www.nimh.nih.gov/index.shtml.

Jane A. Fitzgerald, Ph.D.
Laura Jean Cataldo, RN, Ed.D.

Male erectile disorder *see* **Erectile dysfunction**

Male orgasmic disorder

Definition

Male orgasmic disorder may be defined as a persistent or recurrent inability to achieve orgasm despite lengthy sexual contact or while participating in sexual intercourse.

The mental health professional's handbook, the *Diagnostic and Statistical Manual of Mental Disorders (DSM-IV-TR),* includes this disorder among the **sexual dysfunctions**, along with **premature ejaculation**, **dyspareunia**, and others.

Demographics

Male orgasmic disorder is found in all races and ethnic groups. In the case of the lifelong type of the disorder, manifestations will occur around the age of puberty. In certain genetic hypogonadism disorders, such as Klinefelter's syndrome, certain bodily signs and symptoms may alert the physician. Similarly, in associated thyroid, testicular and pituitary abnormalities, there may be other manifestations of the underlying disorder. In the acquired type of male orgasmic disorder, the patient will have had the previous experience of normal sexual function. In these cases, it is usually a situational factor that precipitates the disorder.

Description

The individual affected by male orgasmic disorder is unable to experience an orgasm following a normal sexual excitement phase. The affected man may regularly experience delays in orgasm or may be unable to experience orgasm altogether.

Normal orgasm

It is important to this discussion to understand the characteristics of a "normal" orgasm. The sensation of orgasm in the male includes emission followed by ejaculation. The term emission refers to a sensation of impending ejaculation produced by contractions of the prostate gland, seminal vesicles, and urethra accompanied by generalized muscular tension, perineal contractions, and involuntary pelvic thrusting. Orgasm is followed by a period of resolution characterized by feelings of well-being and generalized muscular relaxation. During this phase, men may be unable to respond to further sexual stimulation, erection, and orgasm for a variable period of time.

It is also important to distinguish orgasm from ejaculation, although in most instances they occur almost simultaneously. Orgasm is a peak emotional and physical experience, whereas ejaculation is simply a reflex action occurring at the lower portion of the spinal cord and resulting in ejection of semen. Some men have been able to recognize the separation of the two processes, enabling them to experience multiple orgasms without the occurrence of ejaculation. Once ejaculation takes place, a period of recovery time is required prior to a subsequent orgasm.

The sensation of orgasm differs between individuals, and individual orgasms may differ in the same individual. All orgasms share certain characteristics in common including rhythmic body and pelvic contractions, elevation of the heart rate, systemic hypertension, hyperventilation, and muscle tension, followed by the sudden release of tension.

The physiological mechanism of normal orgasm

The cycle of sexual response is under the control of a balanced interplay between the two major nervous systems, the sympathetic and the parasympathetic. In general, the sympathetic nervous system prompts action whereas the parasympathetic system's main action is recovery and calming. In order for a penis to become erect, its smooth muscles are relaxed and it becomes congested with blood vessels. This process is mediated by a complex cascade of humoral, neurological, and circulatory events in which the parasympathetic nervous system plays a key role. Orgasm and ejaculation and subsequent relaxation of the penis are predominantly functions of the sympathetic nervous system.

Thus, whereas emission is a balanced interplay between the parasympathetic and sympathetic nervous systems, orgasm and ejaculation are predominantly under the control of the sympathetic nervous system. The mechanisms of this system may be blocked by impaired function of the **brain** or of the hormonal, circulatory, and neurological systems. Additionally, certain medications may block these actions.

Abnormalities affecting the process of orgasm

Abnormalities in these processes may be "primary" or "secondary." Primary abnormalities are of lifelong duration with effective sexual performance never having been experienced. Secondary abnormalities are acquired after a period of normal function. If an orgasmic problem only occurs under a particular set of circumstances, or only with certain sexual partners, the condition is considered to be "situational" rather than "generalized" (occurring regardless of the circumstances or partner). The defect in sexual function may be total or partial.

The evidence strongly suggests that orgasm has more to do with the brain than with the body. Electrode stimulation of certain parts of the brain will produce sexual pleasure similar to that produced by physical stimulation. The fact that orgasm occurs during sleep is supportive of this concept.

Causes and symptoms

Causes

The cause of male orgasmic disorders may be organic (related to a condition in the body), but, in most cases, is of psychological origin. It is important for the physician to make every effort to find an underlying cause because the therapy and prognosis depend upon it. A detailed history (including an interview with the sexual partner, if feasible), a general physical examination, the performance of certain laboratory and, in some cases, special tests, are important in the investigation of the underlying cause of the male orgasmic disorder.

Organic causes of male orgasmic disorder include the following:

- hypogonadism, in which the testes do not produce enough testosterone
- thyroid disorders (both hyperthyroidism—too much thyroid hormone—and hypothyroidism, or abnormally low levels of thyroid hormone)
- pituitary conditions (Cushing's syndrome, excessive production of the hormone that induces lactation called prolactin)
- diseases that affect the nervous system, such as strokes, multiple sclerosis, diabetic neuropathy, spinal cord injuries
- surgery affecting the prostate and other pelvic organs
- diseases of the penis
- substance abuse, including alcohol
- certain medications, including: the phenothiazines (antipsychotics such as chlorpromazine [Thorazine] or trifluoperazine [Stelazine]); certain medications used to treat high blood pressure, including the thiazides (such as triamterene [Dyazide] or spironolactone [Aldactone]) and beta blockers (such as propranolol [Inderal]); and tricyclic antidepressants such as doxepin (Sinequan) and protriptyline (Vivactil)

The most common causes of male orgasmic disorder are psychological in nature. The responsible psychological mechanisms may be "intrinsic" (due to basic internal factors), or "extrinsic" (due to external or environmental factors).

Intrinsic psychological factors that may cause male orgasmic disorder include:

- depression
- feelings of guilt, anger, fear, low self-esteem, and anxiety

- fear of getting the partner pregnant or of contracting a sexually-transmitted disease or HIV

Extrinsic psychological factors that may cause male orgasmic disorder include:

- living under conditions that cause undue stress
- unsatisfactory relationship with sexual partner
- past history of traumatic sexual encounters such as sexual abuse, rape, or incest
- having been raised in an atmosphere of strict sexual taboos

Environmental factors may interfere with sexual functioning. There may be no safe, private place in which the patient can exercise sexual activity or he may be too fatigued from other activities to participate sexually. The difficulties in striving for "safe sex" and the psychological effects that may result from homosexuality may also interfere with sexual function.

Symptoms

In order to be diagnosed with male orgasmic disorder, the following symptoms must be present according to the *DSM-IV-TR*:

- Persistent or recurrent delay in, or absence of, orgasm following a normal sexual excitement phase during sexual activity that the clinician judges to be adequate. The affected man's age is considered, as well.
- As with all of the sexual dysfunctions, the manual states that the dysfunction must cause the affected man "distress or interpersonal difficulty." According to the *DSM-IV-TR,* the orgasmic dysfunction cannot be better accounted for by another disorder (except another sexual disorder), and cannot be due exclusively to the direct effects of **substance abuse**, a medication, or a general medical condition. This entry, however, discusses the full scope of male orgasmic difficulties, and so discusses general medical conditions and medications as well as psychological factors.

In addition to specific symptoms involving sexual function (inability or delay in reaching orgasm after sufficient stimulation), most patients complain of anxiety, guilt, shame and frustration, and many develop bodily complaints on a psychological basis. Although sexual dysfunction usually occurs during sexual activity with a partner, the clinician should inquire about sexual function during masturbation. If problems occur during masturbation, the problem probably has nothing to do with the sexual partner.

The physician should differentiate male orgasmic disorder from other sexual disorders such as retarded or delayed ejaculation and retrograde ejaculation. In both of these conditions, orgasm occurs but is delayed or, in the case of retrograde ejaculation, occurs in a retrograde direction (into the bladder).

Diagnosis

The **diagnosis** is usually readily made on the basis of the patient's history and the presence of the *DSM-IV-TR* diagnostic criteria. Male orgasmic disorder may be part of a complex of sexual malfunctioning that may include **erectile dysfunction**, abnormalities in ejaculation (such as premature ejaculation or retrograde ejaculation), and **hypoactive sexual desire disorder**.

In order to differentiate between the various potential disorders, the physician may request laboratory tests and/or may perform further diagnostic evaluations. Blood plasma levels of testosterone are of help in diagnosing hypogonadism. A number of tests of thyroid, pituitary and adrenal function are available to diagnose hormonal abnormalities of those glands. A test for nocturnal penile erections may be performed to diagnose erectile dysfunction.

Treatment

If an extrinsic mechanism is discovered as the cause of the orgasmic disorder, steps should be taken to eliminate or ameliorate the problem. An example would be substance or alcohol abuse or the use of certain provocative medications. In the case of antihypertensives, for example, a number of equally effective agents are available if the one in current use is suspect. Therapy should be directed toward improvement of concurrent conditions such as diabetes that may be having an adverse effect on sexual function. Environmental factors that interfere with sexual activity should be corrected.

In the majority of cases, **psychotherapy** will be suggested even in those cases where psychological factors are secondary rather than the primary mechanism for the disorder. Such treatment should be rendered by therapists with special training in the disorders of sexual function and who can tactfully evaluate the sexual compatibility of the patient and his partner. Treatment usually requires the support of the sexual partner in improving both the psychological as well as the physical aspects of the problem. A step-wise program of partner stimulation of the patient to initially ejaculate outside the vagina, then at the vaginal labia, and finally inside the vagina may be helpful.

Prognosis

The prognosis of the patient with male orgasmic syndrome is dependent on whether the condition is lifelong or acquired and the condition's causes. Prognosis

KEY TERMS

Antihypertensive—An agent used in the treatment of hypertension (high blood pressure).

Diabetes mellitus—A chronic disease affecting the metabolism of carbohydrates that is caused by insufficient production of insulin in the body.

Diabetic neuropathy—Condition existing in people with diabetes in which the nerves at the extremities, especially the feet, are less sensitive to touch and injury.

Humoral—A term describing a hormonal substance secreted by an endocrine gland (such as the thyroid).

Perineal—An anatomical area located between the external genitals and the anus.

Phenothiazine—A class of drugs widely used in the treatment of psychosis.

Prostate gland—The gland at the base of a male's urethra that produces a component of semen.

Retroperitoneal—The anatomical area between the peritoneum (lining of the abdominal cavity) and the muscular and connective tissues of the abdominal wall.

Seminal fluid—Fluid composed of semen from the testes and prostatic secretions.

Seminal vesicles—Sac-like structures bordering the male urethra and serving as storage depots for the seminal fluid.

Urethra The tubular passage conducting urine from the bladder to the exterior. In the male, the urethra traverses the penis.

is best when it can be demonstrated that the condition is related to some extrinsic or environmental factor that can be corrected or ameliorated. The prognosis is also favorable in those cases that are due to a remedial organic condition such as a thyroid disorder or hypogonadism. The prognosis is guarded when the disorder is found to be secondary to a deep-seated and chronic psychological or actual psychiatric problem that, in itself, carries an unfavorable prognosis.

Prevention

There are no definitive steps that can be taken to prevent the onset of the male orgasmic disorder. Prompt recognition of the syndrome is important so that appropriate therapy can be attempted as early as possible. As with many chronic conditions, the longer the condition exists, the more difficult therapy becomes.

Resources

BOOKS

American Psychiatric Association. *Diagnostic and Statistical Manual of Mental Disorders.* 4th ed., text rev. Washington, DC: American Psychiatric Publishing, 2000.

Lue, Tom F., et al. *Atlas of Clinical Urology: Impotence and Infertility, Volume I.* New York: Current Medicine Group, 1999.

Masters, William, and Virginia Johnson. *Masters and Johnson on Sex and Human Loving.* New York: Little, Brown, 1988.

Steidle, Christopher P. *The Impotence Source Book.* New York: McGraw-Hill, 1999.

Ralph Myerson, M.D.

Malingering

Definition

In the context of medicine, malingering is the act of intentionally feigning or exaggerating physical or psychological symptoms for motives involving personal or financial gain. Various examples of malingering include fabricating mental or physical disorders in order to avoid school, work, or military service; or to obtain financial compensation, avoid criminal prosecution, or obtain narcotics and other drugs.

Demographics

Malingering can occur within any individual all over the world. Because it is often impossible to determine who is malingering and who is not, it is very difficult to statistically measure how frequently malingering occurs. When not detected and allowed to persist in society, malingering places enormous financial burdens on the health care system. According to the Texas Department of Insurance, fraud that includes malingering costs the U.S. insurance industry approximately $150 billion each year.

Description

People may feign physical or psychological illness for any number of reasons. Faked illness may get them out of work, military duty, or criminal prosecution. It can also help them obtain financial compensation through insurance claims, lawsuits, or workers' compensation.

Feigned symptoms may also be a way of getting a doctor to prescribe certain drugs.

According to the **American Psychiatric Association**, patients who malinger are different from people who invent symptoms for sympathy (**factitious disorder**). Patients who malinger clearly have something tangible to gain. People with factitious disorder appear to have a need to play the "sick" role. They may feign illness for attention or sympathy.

Malingering may take the form of complaints of chronic whiplash pain from automobile accidents. Whiplash claims are controversial. Although some people clearly do suffer from whiplash injury, others may be exaggerating the pain for insurance claims or lawsuits. Some intriguing scientific studies have shown that chronic whiplash pain after automobile accidents is almost nonexistent in countries where the legal systems do not encourage personal injury lawsuits or financial settlements. As specifically related to mental illness, the tendency is to fake more common disorders such as **major depressive disorder**, **post-traumatic stress disorder**, and **panic disorder** with **agoraphobia**. Generalized symptoms, such as headaches, dizziness, low back pain, stomach pain, etc., are easily manufactured, and x rays, **magnetic resonance imaging** (MRIs), or CAT scans (computed axial tomography) are unable to determine a physical cause.

The concept that fakers use less severe symptoms to escape detection was validated in 2001 in a research study. Individuals were asked to fake mental illnesses in such a way as to avoid detection by sophisticated psychological tests. All or portions of the following tests were employed in the research: the Structured Inventory of Malingered Symptomatology, the Psychopathic Personality Inventory, the M-Test, and the **Trauma** Symptom Inventory. Slightly over 11% of the 540 research participants successfully avoided detection and were diagnosed with real disorders instead of with malingering. Questionnaires completed by those who successfully faked symptoms showed that they avoided detection by endorsing fewer actual symptoms, staying away from unduly strange or bizarre symptoms, and responding based upon personal experience.

Although ordinarily an intended fraud, malingering may serve an adaptive purpose under circumstances of duress, such as while being held captive. Faking an illness at such a time may allow a person to avoid cooperating with their captors or to avoid punishment.

Causes and symptoms

People malinger for personal gain. Motivation is always external, and the malingering may be used to:

- evade hard or dangerous situations, punishment, or responsibility
- gain rewards such as free income, a source for drugs, sanctuary from police, or free hospital care
- avenge a monetary loss, legal ruling, or job termination

Mental health practitioners become alert to the possibility of malingering when circumstances exist that might help promote such a facade. The symptoms may vary but generally are similar to symptoms involving chronic **fatigue** syndrome or chronic pain—those for which objective tests such as x rays cannot find any physical cause.

Many dishonest methods are used by individuals feigning symptoms of malingering. Some of these include harming oneself, trying to convince medical professionals one has a disease after learning about its details (such as symptoms) in medical textbooks, taking drugs that provoke certain symptoms common in some diseases, performing excess **exercise** to induce muscle strain or other physical types of ailments, and overdosing on drugs.

Diagnosis

Malingering may be suspected when:

- a patient is referred for examination by an attorney
- the onset of illness coincides with a large financial incentive, such as a new disability policy
- objective medical tests do not confirm the patient's complaints
- the patient does not cooperate with the diagnostic work-up or prescribed treatment
- the patient has antisocial attitudes and behaviors (antisocial personality)

The **diagnosis** of malingering is a challenge for doctors. On the one hand, the doctor does not want to overlook a treatable disease. On the other hand, he or she does not want to continue ordering tests and treatments if the symptoms are faked. Malingering is difficult to distinguish from certain legitimate **personality disorders**, such as factitious disorder or post-traumatic stress disorder. In legal cases, malingering patients may be referred to a **psychiatrist**. Psychiatrists use certain written tests to try to determine whether the patient is faking the symptoms.

Treatment

The ***Diagnostic and Statistical Manual of Mental Disorders*** (*DSM*) does not recognize malingering as a

KEY TERMS

Antisocial personality—A personality characterized by attitudes and behaviors at odds with society's customs and moral standards, including illegal acts.

Factitious diseases—Conditions in which symptoms are deliberately manufactured by patients in order to gain attention and sympathy. Patients with factitious diseases do not fake symptoms for obvious financial gain or to evade the legal system.

Post-traumatic stress disorder (PTSD)—A disorder that occurs among survivors of severe environmental stress such as a tornado, an airplane crash, or military combat. Symptoms include anxiety, insomnia, flashbacks, and nightmares. Patients with PTSD are unnecessarily vigilant; they may experience survivor guilt, and they sometimes cannot concentrate or experience joy.

legitimate disorder, so no structured treatment regimen exists. Patients who are purposefully faking symptoms for gain do not want to be cured. Often, the malingering patient fails to report any improvement with treatment, and the doctor may try many treatments without success. Possible treatments may include **cognitive-behavioral therapy**, **psychotherapy**, **family therapy**, or other such types of psychological treatments.

Prognosis

If the person malingering accepts his or her malady, then treatment can be positively received, and the malingering can be minimized or even eliminated. However, if the person does not wish to admit to malingering, treatment is often difficult and lengthy and ends without resolution. Treatment of malingers by the medical profession has found that most patients do not accept psychiatric help. The person will go to another medical facility where their symptoms and medical history are not known, and they are free to once again pursue their acts of malingering. The recovery of malingers who do not accept and acknowledge their problem is rarely accomplished.

Resources

BOOKS

Dell, Paul F., and John A. O'Neil, eds. *Dissociation and the Dissociative Disorders: DSM-V and Beyond*. New York: Routledge, 2009.

Morgan, Joel E., and Jerry J. Sweet, eds. *Neuropsychology of Malingering Casebook*. New York: Psychology Press, 2008.

Rogers, Richard, ed. *Clinical Assessment of Malingering and Deception*. New York: Guilford Press, 2008.

ORGANIZATIONS

American Psychiatric Association, 1000 Wilson Blvd., Ste 1825, Arlington, VA, 22209-3901, (703) 907-7300, apa@psych.org, http://www.psych.org.

Robert Scott Dinsmoor
Jack H. Booth, Psy.D.

Managed care

Definition

Managed care is a generic term used primarily in the United States for various healthcare payment systems that attempt to contain unnecessary costs by controlling the type and level of services provided. An organization that uses managed care is often called a managed care organization, which is abbreviated MCO. Health maintenance organization (HMO) is a term that is often used synonymously with managed care, but HMOs are actually a particular type of managed care organization. Two other managed-care systems are the preferred provided organization (PPO) and the point-of-service (POS).

Purpose

Healthcare reform has been an increasingly urgent concern in the United States over the past 45 years. Until recently, the primary source of health care coverage was indemnity insurance, which pays or reimburses the cost of medical services in the event of a person's illness or injury. Indemnity insurance gives health-care providers few reasons to use less expensive forms of treatment—the insurance companies generally pay for any treatment deemed necessary by a physician. Presumably, this type of system encourages providers to overuse expensive, unnecessary treatments and diagnostic procedures. Patient co-pays and deductibles attempt to limit excessive use of medical services. However, costs continue to rise, resulting in insurance companies' frequently raising premium prices.

The primary intent of managed care is to reduce healthcare costs. Emphasis is placed on preventive care and early **intervention**, rather than care provided after an illness or injury has occurred. The responsibility of limiting services is placed on the service provider rather than the consumer. This limitation is achieved by (a) "gatekeeper" policies that require individuals to get referrals for specialized treatment from their primary

Sources of health insurance among persons 18 or older who received mental health treatment* in the past year: 2005–2009

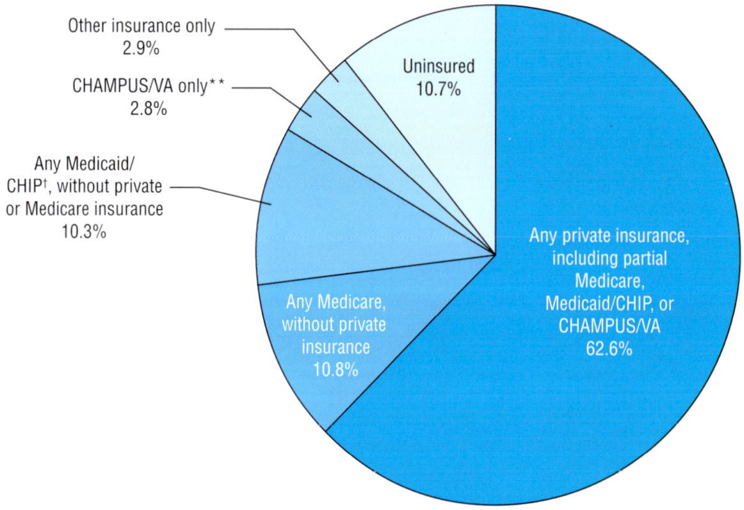

Note: Percentages do not add to 100 percent due to rounding.
*Inpatient care or outpatient care for problems with emotions, nerves, or mental health; does not include treatment for drug or alcohol use.
**Civilian Health and Medical Program of the Uniformed Services (CHAMPUS)/Department of Veterans Affairs (VA)
†Children's Health Insurance Program (CHIP)

SOURCE: Center for Behavioral Health Statistics and Quality, Substance Abuse and Mental Health Services Administration (SAMHSA), "Sources of Payment for Mental Health Treatment for Adults," *The NSUDH Report*, July 7, 2011.

Report available online at http://oas.samhsa.gov/2k11/025/WEB_SR_025.htm. *(Chart by PreMediaGlobal. © 2012 Cengage Learning.)*

physicians; (b) financial incentives (either bonuses or withholding money) for providers to restrict services and contain costs; (c) guidelines requiring adherence by providers at the cost of being dropped from the plan for noncompliance; and (d) review of services by the managed care organization and denial of payment if services are considered unnecessary.

Description

Health maintenance organizations have been in existence in the United States since the late 1800s. In the 1950s, however, the federal government began to encourage the development of HMOs. In 1973, the Health Maintenance Organization Act was passed, and in 1978, a Congressional amendment increased federal aid for HMO development. From 1980 to 1989, U.S. enrollment in HMOs increased from 9 million to 36 million. By 1990, 95% of private insurance companies used some form of managed care. In the 1990s, managed care was incorporated into Medicare and Medicaid plans as well. In the early 2010s, managed care is present in many private health benefit programs. However, although managed care is a mainstay in health care in the United States, it continues to generate controversy because it has not been able to, in most cases, control the costs of medical care in the country. In addition, some critics point out that the quality of medical care has not improved since the introduction of managed care. Such issues were expected to persist in second decade of the twenty-first century.

Managed care organizations frequently contract with a group or panel of healthcare providers. HMOs, preferred provider organizations (PPOs), and point of service (POSs) are examples of these types of contracts. In a health maintenance organization (HMO), the organization enters into a contract with various health-care providers to form a provider network. The providers, such as physicians, hospitals, and other healthcare organizations, under contract to the HMO, provide services to its members at reduced rates in exchange for benefits provided by the HMO, such as the ability to bring in new patients. Members must use the providers in the network in order to receive a reduced rate for services. Each member usually selects a primary care physician (PCP). This PCP, often a family doctor, coordinates all aspects of the patient's care. Because of this role, the patient must see the PCP before being referred to a specialist. These restrictions, along with others, define the HMO plan, but also make it one of the most cost-effective for the patients.

In a preferred provided organization (PPO), the PPO also enters into contracts with healthcare providers to form a provider network. However, in a PPO, a PCP is not used, and members may use any medical professional, within or outside of the network. However, if members use in-network providers, then the costs are less than if an out-of-network provider is used. Although less restrictive than an HMO, the PPO tends to cost more.

The point-of-service (POS) plans are a custom mixture of the HMO and PPO styles. Often members choose which option—HMO or PPO—they wish to use. The POS plan has a provider network that is under contract. A PCP is requested but such coordinators are not required of members. However, if a PCP is not used, then costs are higher. The POS plans usually offer more flexibility than HMOs but may often cost less than PPOs.

Individuals insured under these arrangements may receive care only from providers on the panel. These providers are expected to deliver services according to specific stipulations. Payment is often subject to utilization review, in which delivery of medical services is scrutinized to determine whether the services are necessary. The review may occur with each episode of treatment or may be ongoing by a case manager. If the managed care organization thinks that the services were unnecessary, payment is denied.

Payment arrangements between managed care organizations and care providers are often made in advance. Capitation payment systems are typically used with large healthcare facilities that serve many people. The healthcare provider receives a set amount of money each month based on the number of individuals covered by the plan. The provider may or may not serve that many people in one month. Capitation systems provide a steady, reliable cash flow but involve some economic risk because the services provided may exceed the dollar amount allotted. Another type of payment system uses case rates. The provider receives a predetermined amount of money per individual on a case-by-case basis. The amount of money reflects the estimated service costs to treat the individual patient's condition. Again, the provider takes the risk that unanticipated services will be required.

In the past, mental health services, including **substance abuse** treatment, were routinely excluded from managed care plans. In the 1970s, some mental health care coverage was required in order to meet federal qualifications. Carve-out plans, developed in the 1990s, essentially create a separate managed care plan for mental health services. Mental health services tend to be covered at a lower rate than general health services and, during times of economic troubles, have also been cut back more severely. From 1988 to 1997, mental healthcare spending decreased by 54%, which reflects cutbacks nearly seven times higher than those for general healthcare benefits.

KEY TERMS

Health maintenance organization—A healthcare organization that provides managed-care group health insurance, in which members pay a stated amount on a regular basis and in response receive medical care from participating physicians, hospitals, and other providers.

Medicaid—A federal program in the United States that pays for the medical expenses of people who are unable to pay for most or all of their own medical expenses due to a disability.

Medicare—A federal health insurance program in the United States that provides medical care and hospital treatment for people over a certain age (usually 65 years).

Point-of-service—A healthcare organization that provides managed-care group health insurance and has characteristics of both health maintenance organizations (HMOs) and preferred provider organizations (PPOs).

Preferred provider organization—A healthcare organization that provides managed-care, group health insurance and is a group of doctors, hospitals, and other providers who have contracted with an insurer or administrator to provide health care at reduced rates for its clients.

Mental healthcare providers are also subjected to higher levels of utilization review than medical care providers. As mental healthcare services become more popular in managed care packages, issues have developed. For instance, in the first two decades of the twenty-first century, mental health therapists under managed care systems often are overburdened with paperwork required by HMOs and other such plans. In addition, more sensitive information about patients is required by managed care plans in order to be reimbursed, which does not bode well for the highly secure relationships set up by these patients and clients.

Preparation

People interested in getting medical insurance need to discuss all possible managed care plans with a knowledgeable person within each managed care organization being considered. In addition, they ought to discuss with a trusted medical doctor or other medical professional any concerns or questions that they may have before starting such a plan, during the enrollment process, and while they are members. If they intend to switch plans, they may also wish to find out whether their current physicians participate in the plans they are considering.

Risks

Mental health services within managed care can involve some risks. One risk is the reduced amount of confidentiality for the patient. The relationship between doctor and patient was confidential. However, patients and doctors dealing with managed care organizations are often at odds on this point, as these companies require specific information be sent for evaluation and consideration before they decide to pay on claims. The records of clients, once the property of the doctor and the patient, become the property of the managed care organization. The Health Insurance Portability and Accountability Act of 1996 established some safeguards protecting patient information, but if patients are deemed a possible danger to themselves or others, protected confidential health information may be released.

Ethical concerns

Managed care has been in some respects successful in fulfilling its primary purpose of lowering healthcare costs in the United States. Statistics show decreases in the use of inpatient care and accompanying overall reduction in costs. Many observers, however, argue that the quality of care has suffered as a result. Individuals have fewer choices regarding the locations where they can receive treatment. If a managed care organization closes, individuals under that plan must switch to other care providers under a new plan, which can disrupt ongoing treatment. Care providers often feel that their clients are denied essential care in favor of saving money. Many employers are disillusioned because they face increasing disability claims due to employees having received inadequate treatment for illnesses or injuries. In addition to disability claims, inadequate treatment results in hidden costs to employers in terms of lost productivity.

Another factor in decreased quality of care involves conflicting loyalties for healthcare providers. On the one hand, providers want to ensure quality care for their clients. On the other hand, they are encouraged to provide the least amount of care possible in order to receive financial benefits. Just as dishonest practice was suspected in conjunction with indemnity insurance, managed care creates the potential for inappropriately addressing patients' needs based on monetary concerns. Ultimately, the managed care organization has the right to deny or limit access to a treatment or service, but patients have the right to appeal any care decisions with which they disagree.

QUESTIONS TO ASK YOUR DOCTOR

- What managed care plan is best for me?
- Does my particular health situation mean one plan may be better than another?
- Where can I learn more about my local options for managed care?
- What managed care plans does this office accept?

Future directions

Due to growing popular discontent with managed care organizations, many critics believe that the system will not continue in its current state. Few people, however, expect managed care to completely disappear and indemnity plans to rise to their former prominence. Changes are expected to occur as managed care programs begin competing among themselves. Cost and efficiency will no longer be the main selling point; quality of services will take precedence. Some suggest that along with new systems of managed care and continuing systems of indemnity plans, healthcare providers may even organize and offer services directly to employers, thus eliminating the middle people. This development would be beneficial to all involved: employers would pay less, providers would be better compensated, and clients would receive better care.

Mental health parity—the equivalent treatment of mental illnesses with physical conditions—has improved in the twenty-first century in the United States. In 1996, the U.S. Congress passed the Mental Health Parity Act (MHPA). The law required that issuers of group health plans—those with over 50 employees—could not set the annual and lifetime dollar limits of mental health benefits any lower than the related limits for other services such as medical and surgical benefits. However, the issuers of such plans bypassed the act's requirements by imposing restrictions on the maximum number of provider visits or on the maximum number of days that could be covered under inpatient psychiatric **hospitalization**.

In 2008, a rider attached to the Troubled Asset Relief Program (TARP), which was sponsored by Senator Paul Wellstone (D-MN), amended the MHPA. The rider closed the loopholes in the 1996 bill by prohibiting all group health plans that offered mental health coverage from instituting any types of maximum limits on co-payments, co-insurance, number of visits, or number of days covered for mental-health related hospital visits. The amended law states any medical insurance that includes mental health coverage must include all mental health conditions listed in the latest edition of the American Psychiatric Association's *Diagnostic and Statistical Manual of Mental Disorders*. According to proponents of the legislation, the improved MHPA will make treatment of mental health benefits equivalent with traditional medical health benefits.

Resources

BOOKS

Codd, R. Trent, III. *Destructive Trends in Mental Health: The Well-Intentioned Path to Harm.* New York: Routledge, 2005.

Foster, Joan, and Antonia Murphy. *Psychological Therapies in Primary Care: Setting Up a Managed Care Service.* London: Karnac, 2005.

Scheid, Teresa L. *Tie a Knot and Hang On: Providing Mental Health Care in a Turbulent Environment.* Hawthorne, NY: Aldine de Gruyter, 2004.

PERIODICALS

Addis, Michael E., et al. "Effectiveness of Cognitive-Behavioral Treatment for Panic Disorder versus Treatment as Usual in a Managed Care Setting: 2-Year Follow-Up." *Journal of Consulting and Clinical Psychology* 74, no. 2 (April 2006): 377–85.

Angelo, Ellen Josephine. "Accountable Care Organizations: Are They the Right Answer?" *Nursing Management* 42, no. 2 (February 2011): 20–24.

Beattie, Martha, Patricia McDaniel, and Jason Bond. "Public Sector Managed Care: A Comparative Evaluation of Substance Abuse Treatment in Three Counties." *Addiction* 101, no. 6 (June 2006): 857–72.

Bobbitt, Bruce L. "The Importance of Professional Psychology: A View from Managed Care." *Professional Psychology: Research and Practice* 37, no. 6 (December 2006): 590–97.

Busch, Alisa B., et al. "Schizophrenia, Co-Occurring Substance Use Disorders and Quality of Care: The Differential Effect of a Managed Behavioral Health Care Carve-Out." *Administration and Policy in Mental Health and Mental Health Services Research* 33, no. 3 (May 2006): 388–97.

Cohen, Julie, Jeanne Marecek, and Jane Gillham. "Is Three a Crowd? Clients, Clinicians, and Managed Care." *American Journal of Orthopsychiatry* 76, no. 2 (April 2006): 251–59.

Kilbourne, Amy M., et al. "Management of Mental Disorders in VA Primary Care Practices." *Adminstration and Policy in Mental Health and Mental Health Services Research* 33, no. 2 (March 2006): 208–14.

Liang, Su-Ying, Kathryn A. Phillips, and Jennifer S. Haas. "Measuring Managed Care and Its Environment Using National Surveys: A Review and Assessment." *Medical Care Research and Review* 63, no. 6 (December 2006): 9S–36S.

McLaughlin, Trent P., et al. "Overlap of Anxiety and Depression in a Managed Care Population: Prevalence and Association with Resource Utilization." *Journal of Clinical Psychiatry* 67, no. 8 (August 2006): 1187–93.

Pear, Robert. "House Approves Bill on Mental Health Parity." *The New York Times*, March 6, 2008. http://www.nytimes.com/2008/03/06/washington/06health.html (accessed September 8, 2011).

Raghavan, Ramesh, et al. "Effects of Medicaid Managed Care Policies on Mental Health Service Use Among a National Probability Sample of Children in the Child Welfare System." *Children and Youth Services Review* 28, no. 12 (December 2006): 1482–96.

WEBSITES

MedlinePlus. "Managed Care." U.S. National Library of Medicine, National Institutes of Health. Last updated December 1, 2010. http://www.nlm.nih.gov/medlineplus/managedcare.html (accessed September 8, 2011).

National Conference of State Legislatures. "State Laws Mandating or Regulating State Mental Health Benefits." http://www.ncsl.org/default.aspx?tabid=14352 (accessed November 14, 2011).

Office of the Assistant Secretary for Planning and Evaluation. "Glossary of Managed Care Terms." U.S. Department of Health and Human Services. http://aspe.hhs.gov/Progsys/forum/mcobib.htm (accessed September 8, 2011).

Office for Civil Rights. "Understanding Health Information Privacy." U.S. Department of Health and Human Services. http://www.hhs.gov/ocr/privacy/hipaa/understanding/index.html (accessed September 8, 2011).

ORGANIZATIONS

America's Health Insurance Plans, 601 Pennsylvania Ave., NW, South Building, Ste. 500, Washington, DC, 20004, (202) 778-3200, Fax: (202) 331-7487, ahip@ahip.org, http://www.ahip.org/default.aspx.

Centers for Medicare & Medicaid Services, 7500 Security Blvd., Baltimore, MD, 21244-1850, (800) 633-4223, http://www.medicare.gov.

Sandra L. Friedrich, MA
Ruth A. Wienclaw, PhD
William A. Atkins

Mania *see* **Manic episode**

Manic depression *see* **Bipolar disorder**

Manic episode

Definition

A manic episode is an abnormally elated mental state characterized by feelings of euphoria, lack of inhibitions, racing thoughts, diminished need for sleep, talkativeness, risk taking, and irritability. In extreme cases, mania can induce hallucinations and other psychotic symptoms.

Description

A person experiencing a manic episode shows persistent and often inappropriate enthusiasm. The affected person may demonstrate unusual behaviors such as taking on new projects for which he or she is ill suited, engaging strangers in detailed conversations, and acting without concern for the consequences of personal actions. Less commonly, a person may be abnormally irritable during a manic episode. On average, manic episodes begin before age 25.

Individuals experiencing a manic episode often have feelings of self-importance, elation, talkativeness, sociability, and a desire to initiate goal-oriented activities, coupled with the less desirable characteristics of irritability, impatience, impulsiveness, hyperactivity, and a decreased need for sleep. (**Hypomania** is a term applied to a condition resembling mania. It is characterized by persistent or elevated expansive mood, hyperactivity, inflated self-esteem, etc., but of less intensity than mania.) Severe mania may have psychotic components.

KEY TERMS

Bipolar disorder—Formerly called manic–depressive disorder. A mood disorder characterized alternating periods of overconfidence and activity (manic highs) and depressive lows.

Hypomania—A less severe form of elevated mood state that is a characteristic of bipolar type II disorder.

Mixed mania—A mental state in which symptoms of both depression and mania occur simultaneously.

Psychiatrist—A medical doctor who has completed specialized training in the diagnosis and treatment of mental illness. Psychiatrists can diagnose mental illnesses, provide mental health counseling, and prescribe medications.

Psychologist—A mental health professional who treats mental and behavioral disorders by support and insight to encourage healthy behavior patterns and personality growth. Psychologists also study the brain, behavior, emotions, and learning.

Psychotherapy—The treatment of mental and behavioral disorders by support and insight to encourage healthy behavior patterns and personality growth.

Causes and symptoms

Manic episodes typically occur as a symptom of **bipolar disorder**, a mood disorder characterized by both manic and depressive episodes. Mania can also be induced by the use or abuse of stimulant drugs, such as **cocaine** and **amphetamines**.

The *Diagnostic and Statistical Manual of Mental Disorders,* fourth edition (*DSM–IV*), the diagnostic standard for mental health professionals in the United States, describes a manic episode as an abnormally elevated mood lasting at least one week (and present for the majority of the time during that week) that is distinguished by at least three of the following symptoms:

- inflated self–esteem
- decreased need for sleep
- increased talkativeness
- racing thoughts
- distractibility
- increase in goal-directed activity
- excessive involvement in activities that have a high potential for negative consequences (e.g., risky sexual behavior or irresponsible spending)

If the mood of the patient is irritable and not elevated, four of these symptoms are required.

Many of these symptoms are also present in a hypomanic episode. A hypomanic episode is similar to a manic episode, but the symptoms may be experienced to a lesser extent. The main differences between a manic and hypomanic episode are the following:

- A hypomanic episode may only last four days, whereas a manic episode, by definition, lasts one week.
- In a manic episode, psychotic features (hallucinations and delusions) may be present, but in a hypomanic episode, they cannot be.
- A manic episode significantly impairs the affected person's functions, but a hypomanic episode does not.

Both of these kinds of episodes may be seen in patients with bipolar disorder.

Diagnosis

In addition to observable symptoms, to qualify as a manic episode the *DSM* also states that the change in behavior must be either severe enough to disrupt normal functioning at work or at home or to require **hospitalization** to avoid harm to self or others; alternately, the patient may show signs of **psychosis**. Also, the cause of

KAY REDFIELD JAMISON (1946–)

Kay Redfield Jamison is a psychologist and educator who is considered an authority on manic-depressive illness. Her volume *Manic-Depressive Illness*, compiled with Frederick K. Goodwin, is regarded as a key contribution to the study of manic-depressive illness, a biochemical disorder which results in periods of mania alternating with bouts of depression. The book encompasses a range of issues and subjects, including diagnosis, clinical studies, psychological ramifications, and patho-physiological elements. Larry S. Goldman, reviewing the work in the *New England Journal of Medicine*, acknowledged Jamison and Goodwin as "two highly regarded senior clinicians and researchers" and proclaimed their book "thorough and most readable." Goldman concluded, "It is hard to imagine a clinician working with patients with the illness . . . or a researcher in any part of the field of mood disorders who should not have this tour de force available."

Jamison followed *Manic-Depressive Illness* with *Touched with Fire: Manic-Depressive Illness and the Creative Temperament*, a detailed account of the ties between artistic sensibilities and manic-depressive illness. While conceding that not all artists are manic-depressive, Jamison argues that a significant association exists between the artistic and manic-depressive temperaments. There is, for example, a high rate of suicide among both types. In her analysis, Jamison incorporates scientific and medical data, including diagnostic methods and genetic information, and she applies this data to a host of creative individuals, including the composer Robert Schumann, the painter Vincent Van Gogh, and such American writers as Ernest Hemingway, John Berryman, and Hart Crane. Jamison notes that many of the creative individuals considered in *Touched with Fire* had little recourse to any suitable psycho-medical care.

In 1995 Jamison published *An Unquiet Mind*, a memoir of her own experiences with manic depression. In this volume Jamison recounts her extreme moodiness as a child and relates her first exhilarating experience of mania when she was in her mid-teens. She notes that mania and depression sometimes exist simultaneously. It is during these periods, when the depths of despair are coupled with the impulsiveness characteristic of mania, that sufferers, according to Jamison, are more likely to consider suicide. Jamison discloses in *An Unquiet Mind* that she attempted to take her own life, and she credits psychotherapy with helping her realize greater acceptance and stability.

the episode cannot be attributed to side effects from drug abuse, medication, medical treatment, or a medical condition.

Mania is usually diagnosed and treated by a **psychiatrist** and/or a **psychologist** in an outpatient setting. However, most severely manic patients require hospitalization. In addition to an interview, several clinical inventories or scales may be used to assess the patient's mental status and determine the presence and severity of mania. An assessment commonly includes the Young Mania Rating Scale (YMRS). The Mini–Mental State Examination (MMSE) may also be given to screen out other illnesses such as **dementia**.

Treatment

Mania is treated primarily with drugs. The following mood-stabilizing agents are commonly prescribed to regulate manic episodes:

- Lithium (Cibalith-S, Eskalith, Lithane) is one of the oldest and most frequently prescribed drugs available for the treatment of mania. Because the drug takes four to seven days to reach a therapeutic level in the bloodstream, it is sometimes prescribed in conjunction with neuroleptics (antipsychotic drugs) and/or benzodiazepines (tranquilizers) to provide more immediate relief of mania.
- Carbamazepine (Tegretol, Atretol) is an anticonvulsant drug usually prescribed in conjunction with other mood-stabilizing agents. The drug is often used to treat bipolar patients who have not responded well to lithium therapy.
- Valproate (divalproex sodium, or Depakote; valproic acid, or Depakene) is an anticonvulsant drug prescribed alone or in combination with carbamazepine and/or lithium. For patients experiencing "mixed mania," or mania with features of depression, valproate is preferred over lithium.

Clozapine (Clozaril) is an atypical antipsychotic medication used to control manic episodes in patients who have not responded to typical mood-stabilizing agents. The drug has also been a useful preventative treatment in some bipolar patients. Other new anticonvulsants (**lamotrigine**, **gabapentin**) are being investigated for treatment of mania and bipolar disorder.

Prognosis

Patients experiencing mania as a result of bipolar disorder require long-term care to prevent recurrence; bipolar disorder is a chronic condition that requires lifelong observation and treatment after **diagnosis**. Data show that almost 90% of patients who experience one manic episode will go on to have another.

Prevention

Mania as a result of bipolar disorder can only be prevented through ongoing pharmacologic treatment. Patient education in the form of therapy or **self-help groups** is crucial for training patients to recognize signs of mania and to take an active part in their treatment program. **Psychotherapy** is an important adjunctive treatment for patients with bipolar disorder.

Resources

BOOKS

Borch-Jacobsen, Mikkel. *Making Minds and Madness: From Hysteria to Depression*. New York, NY: Cambridge University Press, 2009.

Graham, George. *The Disordered Mind: An Introduction to Philosophy of Mind and Mental Illness*. New York: Routledge, 2010.

North, Carol, and Sean Yutzy. *Goodwin and Guze's Psychiatric Diagnosis*. New York, NY: Oxford University Press, 2010.

Shams, M.D.K. *Human Relation and Personified Relational Disorders*. Raleigh, NC: lulu.com, 2009.

ORGANIZATIONS

American Academy of Child and Adolescent Psychiatry, 3615 Wisconsin Ave. NW, Washington, DC, 20016-3007, (202) 966-7300, Fax: (202) 966-2891, http://aacap.org.

American Psychiatric Association, 1000 Wilson Blvd., Ste. 1825, Arlington, VA, 22209-3901, (703) 907-7300, apa@psych.org, http://www.psych.org.

American Psychological Association, 750 1st St. NE, Washington, DC, 20002-4242, (202) 336-5500; TDD/TTY: (202) 336-6123, (800) 374-2721, http://www.apa.org.

Mental Health America, 2000 North Beauregard St., 6th Floor, Alexandria, VA, 22311, (703) 684-7722, (800) 969-6642, Fax: (703) 684-5968, http://www1.nmha.org.

National Alliance on Mental Illness, 3803 North Fairfax Dr., Ste. 100, Arlington, VA, 22203, (703) 524-7600, Fax: (703) 524-9094, http://www.nami.org.

National Institute of Mental Health, 6001 Executive Blvd., Room 8184, MSC 9663, Bethesda, MD, 20892-9663, (301) 433-4513; TTY: (301) 443-8431, (866) 615-6464; TTY: (866) 415-8051, Fax: (301) 443-4279, nimhinfo@nih.gov, http://www.nimh.nih.gov.

Paula Anne Ford-Martin
Laura Jean Cataldo, RN, Ed.D.

Maprotiline

Definition

Maprotiline is an antidepressant. It is a member of the tetracyclic antidepressant family of compounds and is administered orally. In the United States, it is sold under the trade name Ludiomil.

Purpose

Maprotiline is an antidepressant intended for use by people with depressive **neurosis** and **bipolar disorder**. It is also occasionally used for the relief of anxiety associated with **depression**.

Description

Maprotiline elevates mood. The precise pharmacological mode of action is not fully understood but it is thought to inhibit the absorption of the neurotransmitter norepinephrine at nerve endings in the **brain**. It is prescribed in 25, 50, and 75 mg tablets.

Recommended dosage

The recommended initial dosage of maprotiline is typically 75 mg, given by mouth in three 25 mg administrations, although some patients may start with an initial dose of 25 mg. The initial dosage should be maintained for at least two weeks. Therapeutic results may be observed in three to seven days. Typically, initial administration may have to be continued for two to three weeks before results are observed.

The recommended total dosage is 150 mg per day. Dosage should be increased 25 mg at a time. The maximum daily dosage for people with severe depression is 225 mg.

Precautions

The use of antidepressant drugs, including maprotiline, in children and adults up to age 24 has been linked to an increased risk of suicidal thoughts and behavior. Patients of any age taking maprotiline should be monitored for signs of worsening depression or changes in behavior. The drug may lower the threshold for a **manic episode** among people with bipolar disorders and should be used only with caution and under close supervision in those patients.

Maprotiline may promote seizure activity. Of all the cyclic **antidepressants**, maprotiline probably causes the highest incidence of **seizures** and has thus fallen out of favor with most psychiatrists. Also for this reason, it should not be combined with other neuroleptics (antipsychotics) that can also cause seizures. Maprotiline should be used with caution in persons with heart disease or certain heart conditions. The drug increases the effect of alcohol and should not be taken with products containing alcohol or **barbiturates**. People taking **monoamine oxidase inhibitors (MAOIs)**, such as **tranylcypromine** (Parnate) and **phenelzine** (Nardil), should not take maprotiline.

Side effects

The most commonly reported side effect of maprotiline is dry mouth. Slightly more than one person in five (22%) experiences this effect. Approximately 16% of users experience drowsiness, 8% report dizziness, and 6% report nervousness and constipation. Other less common reported side effects include anxiety, agitation, **insomnia**, blurred vision, tremor, weakness, **fatigue**, nausea, and headache with blurred vision. Other rare side effects are similar to those experienced by people who use tricyclic antidepressants. These include abnormally high or low blood pressure, tachycardia, and syncope. Hallucinations, disorientation, and mania have been reported, as have vomiting, diarrhea, and gastric distress.

Interactions

Maprotiline should be discontinued or reduced in dosage prior to surgery due to the potential for interactions with anesthetic agents. The drugs cimetidine and **fluoxetine** reduce the elimination of maprotiline, resulting in too much of the drug in the body, which can be dangerous. Conversely, barbiturates and phenytoin increase the elimination of maprotiline, leaving too little of the drug in the body and reducing its therapeutic effects. Cardiovascular toxicity has been reported when maprotiline is used simultaneously with thyroid-replacement medications such as levothyroxine, and maprotiline blocks the pharmacological effect of guanethidine. An increased risk of seizures has been reported with the simultaneous use of physostigmine and maprotiline, and a similar effect has been observed when maprotiline is taken simultaneously with phenothiazine compounds; concurrent use should be avoided.

KEY TERMS

Barbiturates—A class of medications (including Seconal and Nembutal) that causes sedation and drowsiness. They may be prescribed legally, but may also be used as drugs of abuse.

Bipolar disorder—An mental condition characterized by periods of intense elation, energy, and activity (mania) followed by periods of inactivity and depression.

Guanethidine—An antihypertensive drug used to treat high blood pressure.

Hallucination—A false sensory perception. A person experiencing a hallucination may "hear" sounds or "see" people or objects that are not really present. Hallucinations can also affect the senses of smell, touch, and taste.

Manic—Referring to mania, a state characterized by excessive activity, excitement, or emotion.

Monoamine oxidase inhibitors—A group of antidepressant drugs that decrease the activity of monoamine oxidase, a neurotransmitter found in the brain that affects mood.

Norepinephrine—A neurotransmitter in the brain that acts to constrict blood vessels and raise blood pressure. It works in combination with serotonin.

Physostigmine—A short-acting drug that enhances levels of a substance (acetylcholine) between neurons in the brain.

Syncope—A brief lapse of consciousness caused by a temporarily insufficient flow of blood to the brain.

Tachycardia—A pulse rate above 100 beats per minute.

Resources

BOOKS

Foreman, John C., and Torben Johansen. *Textbook of Receptor Pharmacology*. 2nd ed. Boca Raton, FL: CRC Press, 2002.

Page, Clive P., et al. *Integrated Pharmacology*. 3rd ed. St. Louis, MO: Elsevier, 2006.

Preston, John D., John H. O'Neal, and Mary C. Talaga. *Handbook of Clinical Psychopharmacology for Therapists*. 5th ed. Oakland, CA: New Harbinger Publications, 2008.

PERIODICALS

Arenas, M. Carmen, et al. "Are the Effects of the Antidepressants Amitriptyline, Maprotiline, and Fluoxetine on

Inhibitory Avoidance State-Dependent?” *Behavioural Brain Research* 166, no. 1 (January 2006): 150–58.

Mayers, Andrew G., and David S. Baldwin. “Antidepressants and Their Effect on Sleep.” *Human Psychopharmacology: Clinical and Experimental* 20, no. 8 (December 2005): 533–59.

Rambelomanana, S., et al. “Antidepressants: General Practitioners’ Opinions and Clinical Practice.” *Acta Psychiatrica Scandinavica* 113, no. 6 (June 2006): 460–67.

WEBSITES

PubMed Health. “Maprotiline.” U.S. National Library of Medicine. http://www.ncbi.nlm.nih.gov/pubmedhealth/PMH0000597 (accessed November 12, 2011).

ORGANIZATIONS

American Academy of Clinical Toxicology, 6728 Old McLean Village Dr., McLean, VA, 22101, (703) 556-9222, Fax: (703) 556-8729, admin@clintox.org, http://www.clintox.org.

American Academy of Family Physicians, 11400 Tomahawk Creek Parkway, Leawood, KS, 66211-2672, (913) 906-6000, (800) 274-2237, Fax: (913) 906-6075, contactcenter@aafp.org, http://www.aafp.org.

American Medical Association, 515 N State St., Chicago, IL, 60610, (312) 464-5000, (800) 621-8335, http://www.ama-assn.org.

American Psychiatric Association, 1000 Wilson Blvd., Ste. 1825, Arlington, VA, 22209-3901, (703) 907-7300, apa@psych.org, http://www.psych.org.

American Society for Clinical Pharmacology and Therapeutics, 528 North Washington St., Alexandria, VA, 22314, (703) 836-6981, http://www.ascpt.org.

American Society for Pharmacology and Experimental Therapeutics, 9650 Rockville Pike, Bethesda, MD, 20814-3995, (301) 634-7060, Fax: (301) 634-7061, http://www.aspet.org.

L. Fleming Fallon, Jr., MD, DrPH
Ruth A. Wienclaw, PhD

Marijuana *see* **Cannabis and related disorders**

Marital therapy *see* **Marriage counseling**

Marriage counseling

Definition

Marriage counseling is a type of **psychotherapy** for a married couple or established partners that tries to resolve problems in the relationship. Typically, two people attend counseling sessions together to discuss specific issues; however, in some cases only one partner works within the sessions. It may also be called marital therapy, couple therapy, or relationship counseling.

Before the late twentieth century, close friends, family members, or religious leaders primarily performed marriage counseling. Since then, the guidance most often comes from psychiatrists, psychologists, **social workers**, and marriage/family counselors. With the use of such professionals, certifications and regulations have been established to guide and control these activities. One of the most commonly accepted credentials comes from the American Association for Marriage and **Family Therapy**.

Purpose

Marriage counseling provides help to couples, whether they are married or not, and whether the pair are heterosexual or homosexual. It is based on research showing that individuals and their problems are best handled within the context of their relationships. Marriage counselors are trained in psychotherapy and family systems, and focus on understanding their clients’ symptoms and the way their interactions contribute to problems in the relationship.

Various issues are discussed in marriage counseling. Some of the more critical issues addressed include:

- infidelity issues
- sexual problems
- financial difficulties
- physical disabilities
- mental illnesses
- anger management problems
- domestic abuse
- alcohol/substance abuse
- communications difficulties
- interactions with children and other family members

The goal of marital and family therapists is to improve relationships between marital partners or family members, or to help with the dissolution of a difficult relationship with minimum harm to all.

Description

Marriage counseling is usually a short-term therapy that may take only a few sessions to work out problems in the relationship. Longer-term counseling may also occur, with a range of sessions usually from 12 to 24 in number. Typically, marriage counselors ask questions about the couple’s roles, patterns, rules, goals, and beliefs. Therapy often begins as the couple analyzes the good and bad aspects of the relationship. The marriage counselor then works with the couple to help them understand that, in most cases, both partners are contributing to problems in the relationship. Various techniques are employed, such as active listening, role-playing, **behavior modification**, and changing expectations concerning the behaviors of others. They are taught techniques to modify their own behaviors, or taught how to more readily accept the behaviors of others. When this is understood, the two can then learn to change how they interact with each other to solve problems. The partners may be encouraged to draw up a contract in which each partner describes the behavior he or she will be trying to maintain. Sometimes counseling is also provided for the entire family, not just for a couple.

Marriage is not a requirement for two people to get help from a marriage counselor. Any one person wishing to improve his or her relationships can acquire help with behavioral problems, relationship issues, or with mental or emotional disorders. Marriage counselors also offer treatment (pre-marital therapy) for couples before they get married to help them understand potential problem areas. A third type of marriage counseling involves post-marital therapy, in which divorcing couples who share children seek help in working out their differences. Couples in the midst of a divorce find that marriage therapy during separation can help them find a common ground as they negotiate interpersonal issues and child custody.

Choosing a therapist

A marriage counselor is trained to use different types of therapy in work with individuals, couples, and groups.

When looking for a marriage counselor, a couple should find out the counselor's training and educational background, professional associations, such as the AAMFT, and state licensure, and whether the person has experience in treating particular kinds of problem. Marital and family therapists receive training in three areas:

- Academic program. A person must earn a master's degree with an emphasis in marital and family therapy from an accredited academic institution. Most programs of study are 48 semester credit hours in length. The curriculum must include theoretical as well as practical training. Specific areas of competency, such as human sexuality, assessing victims of child abuse, and substance abuse, must be embedded in the curriculum. Students must receive 30 hours of directly supervised counseling and an additional 150 hours of directed counseling practice.
- Supervised clinical experience. Prior to becoming eligible to sit for a licensing exam, candidates must complete a total of approximately 3,000 hours of supervised counseling experiences. The 3,000 hours may include activities related to personal psychotherapy, supervision, direct counseling experience, professional enrichment experiences, and maintaining records. Some (approximately one-quarter) of these hours may be included in the graduate degree training curriculum. All of the clinical experiences are closely supervised.
- Licensing examination. The examination has written and oral components. A license to practice is granted with the successful passage of both parts of the exam. A minimum of 36 hours of continuing education training must be completed every two years as a requirement for relicensing.

The American Association for Marriage and Family Therapy (AAMFT) is a professional organization that offers training and nationally recognized accreditation. Patients should also ask questions concerning fees, insurance coverage, and anything else they want to know before committing to therapy sessions.

Results

Marriage counseling helps couples learn to deal more effectively with problems and can help prevent small problems from becoming serious. Research shows that marriage counseling, when effective, tends to improve a person's physical as well as mental health, in addition to improving the relationship.

Resources

BOOKS

Clinton, Tim, and John Trent. *The Quick-Reference Guide to Marriage and Family Counseling*. Grand Rapids, MI: Baker Books, 2009.

Davis, Rebecca L. *More Perfect Unions: The American Search for Marital Bliss*. Cambridge, MA: Harvard University Press, 2010.

Yount, David. *Making a Success of Marriage: Planning for Happily Ever After*. Lanham, MD: Rowman and Littlefield, 2010.

WEBSITES

Mayo Clinic staff. "Marriage Counseling." MayoClinic.com. http://www.mayoclinic.com/health/marriage-counseling/MY00839 (accessed October 22, 2011).

ORGANIZATIONS

American Association for Marriage and Family Therapy, 112 South Alfred St., Alexandria, VA, 22314-3061, (703) 838-9808, Fax: (703) 838-9805, http://www.aamft.org.

American Psychological Association, 750 1st St. NE, Washington, DC, 20002-4242, (202) 336-5500; TDD/TTY: (202) 336-6123, (800) 374-2721, http://www.apa.org.

Carol A. Turkington

Masochism *see* **Sexual masochism**

Massage *see* **Bodywork therapies**

Mathematics disorder

Definition

Mathematics disorder, formerly called developmental arithmetic disorder, developmental acalculia, or dyscalculia, is a learning disorder in which a person's mathematical ability is substantially below the level normally expected based on his or her individual's age, intelligence, life experiences, educational background, and physical impairments. This disability affects the ability to do calculations as well as the ability to understand word problems and mathematical concepts.

Demographics

The number of children with mathematics disorder is not entirely clear. The fourth edition of the **Diagnostic and Statistical Manual of Mental Disorders** (*DSM-IV*), which is the basic manual consulted by mental health professionals in assessing the presence of mental disorders, indicates that about 1% of school age children have mathematics disorder. Other studies, however, have found higher rates of arithmetical dysfunction in children. Likewise, some studies find no gender difference in the prevalence of mathematics disorder, while others find that girls are more likely to be affected. Mathematics disorder, like other learning disabilities, however, does appear to run in families, suggesting the existence of a genetic component to the disorder.

Description

Mathematics disorder was first described as a developmental disorder in 1937. Since then, it has come to encompass a number of distinct types of mathematical deficiencies. These include:

- difficulty reading and writing numbers
- difficulty aligning numbers in order to do calculations
- inability to perform calculations
- inability to comprehend word problems

The range and number of mathematical difficulties that have been documented suggests that there are several different causes for mathematics disorder. In addition, several known physical conditions cause mathematics disorder. Turner syndrome and fragile X syndrome, both genetic disorders that affect girls, are associated with difficulty in mathematics. Injury to certain parts of the **brain** can also cause inability to perform calculations. These conditions appear to be independent of other causes of mathematics disorder. Mathematics disorder is often associated with other **learning disorders** involving reading and language, although it may also exist independently in children whose reading and language skills are average or above average.

Causes and symptoms

The causes of mathematics disorder are not understood. Different manifestations of the disorder may have different causes. Symptoms of the disorder, however, can be grouped into four categories: language symptoms; recognition or perceptual symptoms; mathematical symptoms; and attention symptoms.

People with language symptoms have trouble naming mathematical terms; understanding word problems; or understanding such mathematical concepts as "greater than" or "less than." People with recognition symptoms have difficulty reading numbers and such operational signs as the plus or minus signs, or aligning numbers properly in order to perform accurate calculations. Mathematical symptoms include deficiencies in the ability to count; to memorize such basic arithmetical data as the multiplication tables; or to follow a sequence of steps in problem solving. Attention symptoms are related to failures in copying numbers and ignoring operational signs. Sometimes these failures are the result of a person's carelessness. At other times, however, they appear to result from a lack of understanding of the factors or operations involved in solving the problem.

In practical terms, parents and teachers may see the following signs of mathematics disorder in a child's schoolwork:

- problems counting
- difficulty memorizing multiplication tables
- inability to grasp the difference between such operations as addition and subtraction
- poor computational skills; many errors in simple arithmetic
- slowness in performing calculations
- difficulty arranging numbers in order (from smallest to largest, for example)
- inability to grasp information on graphs
- difficulty copying numbers or problems
- inability to grasp the concept of place value
- inability align two or three digit numbers to do calculations
- difficulty understanding word problems
- inability to understand mathematical symbols

These symptoms must be evaluated in light of the person's age, intelligence, educational experience, exposure to mathematics learning activities, and general cultural and life experience. The person's mathematical ability must fall substantially below the level of others with similar characteristics. In most cases several of these symptoms are present simultaneously.

Diagnosis

Mathematics disorder is not usually diagnosed before a child is in the second or third grade because of the variability with which children acquire mathematical fluency. Many bright children manage to get through to fourth- or fifth-grade level in mathematics by using memorization and calculation tricks (such as counting on fingers or performing repeated addition as a substitute for multiplication) before their disability becomes apparent. Requests for testing usually originate with a teacher or parent who has observed several symptoms of the disorder.

To receive a **diagnosis** of mathematics disorder according to the criteria established by the **American Psychiatric Association**, a child must show substantially lower than expected ability in mathematics based on his or her age, intelligence, and background. In addition, the child's deficiencies must cause significant interference with academic progress or daily living skills.

In addition to an interview with a child **psychiatrist** or other mental health professional, the child's mathematical ability may be evaluated with such individually administered diagnostic tests as the Enright Diagnostic Test of Mathematics, or with curriculum-based assessments. If the results of testing suggest mathematics disorder, such other causes of difficulty as poor vision or hearing, intellectual disability, or lack of fluency in the language of instruction, are ruled out. The child's educational history and exposure to opportunities for learning mathematics are also taken into account. On the basis of this information, a qualified examiner can make the diagnosis of mathematics disorder.

Treatment

Children who receive a diagnosis of mathematics disorder are eligible for an individual education plan (IEP) that details specific accommodations to learning. Because of the wide variety of problems found under the diagnosis of mathematics disorder, plans vary considerably. Generally, instruction emphasizes basic mathematical concepts, while teaching children problem solving skills and ways to eliminate distractions and extraneous information. Concrete, hands-on instruction is more successful than abstract or theoretical instruction. IEPs also address other language or reading disabilities that affect a child's ability to learn mathematics.

KEY TERMS

Individual education plan (IEP)—A plan of instruction drawn up for an individual student who is having specific difficulties with mathematics, reading, or other skills necessary to progress beyond elementary school.

Prognosis

Progress in overcoming mathematics disorder depends on the specific type of difficulties that the child has with mathematics; the learning resources available; and the child's determination to work on overcoming the disorder. Some children work through their disability, while others continue to have trouble with mathematics throughout life. Children who continue to suffer from mathematics disorder may develop low self-esteem and social problems related to their lack of academic achievement. Later in life they may be more likely to drop out of school and find themselves shut out of jobs or occupations that require the ability to perform basic mathematical calculations.

Prevention

There is no known way to prevent mathematics disorder.

Resources

BOOKS

American Psychiatric Association. *Diagnostic and Statistical Manual of Mental Disorders*. 4th ed., text rev. Washington, DC: American Psychiatric Publishing, 2000.

Sadock, Benjamin J., and Virginia A. Sadock, eds. *Comprehensive Textbook of Psychiatry*. Vol. 2. 7th ed. Philadelphia: Lippincott Williams and Wilkins, 2000.

PERIODICALS

Jordan, Nancy, and Laurie B. Hanich. "Mathematical Thinking in Second-Grade Children with Different Forms of LD." *Journal of Learning Disabilities* 33, no. 6 (November 2000): 567–578.

ORGANIZATIONS

Learning Disabilities Association of America, 4156 Library Rd., Pittsburgh, PA, 15234-1349, (412) 341-1515, http://www.ldanatl.org.

National Center for Learning Disabilities, 381 Park Ave. South, Ste. 1401, New York, NY, 10016, (212) 545-7510, Fax: (212) 545-9665, (888) 575-7373, http://www.ncld.org.

Tish Davidson, A.M.

Matrix model

Definition

The Matrix model of **substance abuse** treatment is a multifaceted treatment program designed to help substance abusers stop drug and **alcohol use** and maintain their sobriety through education and monitoring.

Purpose

The Matrix model, while originally designed as a therapeutic approach to treating abuse of such stimulants as **cocaine** and methamphetamines, has subsequently been applied to the treatment of opiate and alcohol abuse.

The Matrix model treatment system was created in the 1980s when cocaine abuse became rampant among members of the middle and upper-middle classes. The Matrix Institute on Addictions is a nonprofit organization based in California. Founded in 1984 to develop the program that became the Matrix model of substance abuse treatment, the Institute itself has several southern California locations. Other private treatment programs are also using the Matrix model, which has the distinct advantage over some treatment programs of having complete and established written treatment protocols as well as a growing body of research supporting its efficacy.

Prior to the early 1980s, cocaine and **methamphetamine** (MA) treatment programs generally followed one of two courses: community-based outpatient drug treatment programs for low-income users, or high-cost, private inpatient institutional treatment programs for those who could afford them. When middle-income drug abuse became epidemic, there was a need for an effective outpatient program that could address the needs of thousands of drug abusers who were neither wealthy nor living on the street.

The 28-day hospital-based treatment programs typically formulated for private health-care treatment of alcoholism were not seen as useful for cocaine users, who rarely needed inpatient programs. Similarly, **psychotherapy** alone has not been universally effective in helping people stop cocaine use or in preventing **relapse**. The Matrix model was designed to treat drug abuse using multiple modalities in as cost-efficient a manner as possible. Its underlying concept was to serve as an outpatient based on a reputable, evaluable protocol. Beginning with cocaine abuse, the Matrix model was extended to cover methamphetamines and other stimulant abuse treatment. Development and subsequent research on the Matrix model has been funded by grants from the National Institute on Drug Abuse, the Center for Substance Abuse Treatment, the **Substance Abuse and Mental Health Services Administration**, and the U.S. Department of Health and Human Services.

Description

The developers of the Matrix model, rather than engaging in the defense of a single theory, used strategies based on several practical approaches that had been shown to work in drug treatment. By using a matrix design rather than a single methodology, the program designers targeted the multiple factors affecting an individual's chances for recovery. Social influences, education for patient and family members, cognitive-behavioral techniques, **support groups**, individual sessions, and urine and breath testing were all included in the treatment model. The goal of this model was to help stimulant abusers 1) stop their drug use, 2) stay in treatment, 3) learn about issues critical to **addiction** and relapse, 4) receive direction and support from a trained therapist, 5) educate family members affected by the patient's addiction, 6) introduce self-help programs to the addicted persons for continued support and 7) continue monitoring with urine testing. The program lasts 16 weeks, and the program administrators conducted several studies to measure the efficacy of the Matrix model for different users, under different conditions and compared to other treatment methods.

The Matrix model recognizes several factors needed for an effective and lasting treatment. The therapeutic relationship, although not as intensive as traditional psychological therapy (only three 45-minute sessions are scheduled over 16 weeks) is used for engaging the patient in a way that will encourage continued participation and engagement in the program. Although the original program consisted of a greater number of individual sessions, they were soon abandoned in favor of additional group sessions, making the program more cost-effective without reducing its efficacy.

Dissemination of information, by way of patient group meetings, helps individuals understand the physiological and psychological effects of drug use. Family-systems theory has shown that, even in cases where change is in the best interest of the family and the patient, family members consciously and unconsciously resist the efforts of any one member who attempts to change. Education of family members in a group setting helps to educate everyone involved, reducing the risk of family dynamics sabotaging the recovery of the patient.

Planning is considered a vital part of **relapse prevention**: patients are taught to schedule their days to stay busy as well as to think about the ways their daily schedule might contribute to sobriety or relapse. Used as a part of the outpatient treatment program, planning promotes positive activity and helps prevent relapse; it is also needed after a patient has completed the program and needs to rebuild a life in which daily activities are not based on drug-addictive behaviors.

Timing is recognized as an important factor in the process of recovery: education sessions are scheduled so as not to interfere with the early stages of treatment, when patients are detoxifying and cannot comprehend much information beyond their own discomfort and shame. As their recovery continues, the program provides more complex information in a set of standardized lectures. Educating patients is part of a cognitive-behavioral approach that teaches them to notice, challenge, and change irrational or unhelpful thought processes, replacing old habits of thought with more productive and positive ones.

Co-occurring dependency is so common in addiction that no comprehensive treatment program should address a single addiction. The Matrix program recognizes that stimulant users often also use alcohol and marijuana. Program research shows significantly greater relapse rates for people who continue using other drugs. Patients are expected to quit all drugs and alcohol. As part of the Matrix model, breath testing and urinalysis address the possibility that some patients may continue drug or alcohol use, and reveal that this contingency needs to be addressed. Urinalysis and breath testing were made part of the Matrix treatment primarily as a way to validate patients in their recovery as well as providing an early warning of difficulty. Testing works with scheduling and other program components to let patients take responsibility for their recovery. There is room in the approach for response to relapse during treatment, and physiological tests will reveal temporary defeat, whereas patients sometimes cannot.

Although one could argue that the Matrix model is focused primarily on relapse prevention, particular coping skills and behaviors are taught to patients to help them identify situations that may test their sobriety. Called "relapse prevention," these established techniques are part of the program and provide social support. In leading relapse-prevention groups, staff members may also be alerted to patients whose behavior in the group may signal a potential relapse.

Aftercare

A vital component of the Matrix model is the recognition that 12-step programs are widely useful for people in aftercare. Substance abuse treatment is notably more effective when patients have resources for maintaining a drug-free lifestyle after leaving treatment. 12-step meetings are held at the Matrix treatment centers, attended by patients who are advancing in their treatment. The Matrix developers realized that some patients would opt out of 12-step meetings because of their format and emphasis on embracing a higher power and spiritual authority: the Matrix program addresses potential resistance by helping patients find ways to reconcile their personal beliefs with the structure of Alcoholics Anonymous, Narcotics Anonymous, or other self-help programs. This serves several purposes. Patients who might otherwise avoid such meetings after leaving the program may choose instead to attend, increasing their chances of maintaining a drug-free lifestyle; patients learn the format and 12-step "rules" while still in a more fully supportive milieu; and patients have a structured system to enter after leaving the program.

KEY TERMS

Drug abuse—When an individual's repeated use of controlled substances, prescription or over-the-counter drugs, or alcohol causes damage to their health, thought processes, relationships, or functioning at work or school, they can be said to be practicing drug abuse. Using a substance for purposes other than which it is intended (such as inhaling gasoline fumes recreationally) can also be considered drug abuse.

Matrix—In statistics, variables that may influence a particular outcome are placed into a grid, either in columns or in rows. Statistical calculations can be performed that assign different weights to each variable, and the differential weighting of variables can be seen to affect the outcome. In the Matrix model of drug abuse, the variables that affect a positive outcome (such as behavioral techniques, family education or urinalysis testing) are all considered as important parts of a unified treatment plan.

Results

The overall expectation of this therapeutic **intervention** is that patients will leave the program drug free and with enough internal and external resources to maintain a life free of drugs and alcohol. Research comparing the Matrix model to other treatment approaches has found that patients who complete the Matrix treatment programs have statistically higher abstinence rates and lower positive results on drug tests than patients who participate in traditional 28-day in-hospital programs.

Resources

BOOKS

Sorensen, James L., et al., eds. *Drug Abuse Treatment Through Collaboration: Practice and Research Partnerships That Work.* Washington, DC: American Psychological Association, 2003.

PERIODICALS

Obert, Jeanne L., et al. "The Matrix Model of Outpatient Stimulant Abuse Treatment." *Journal of Psychoactive Drugs* 32, no. 2 (April–June 2000): 157–64.

"Program Helps Patients Reduce, Discontinue Methamphetamine Use." *The Brown University Digest of Addiction Theory and Application* 21, no. 4 (April 2002): 1–3.

ORGANIZATIONS

National Institute on Drug Abuse, 6001 Executive Blvd., Rm. 5213, Bethesda, MD, 20892, (301) 442-1124; Spanish: (240) 221-4007, information@nida.nih.gov, http://www.nida.nih.gov.

Matrix Institute on Addictions, http://www.matrixinstitute.org.

Lorena S. Covington, MA

MDMA *see* **Ecstasy**

Medication-induced movement disorders

Definition

Medication-induced movement disorder occurs due to treatment with antipsychotic medications. Most medication-induced **movement disorders** are caused by medications that block the action of **dopamine**, a neurotransmitter that allows communication between two neurons to take place and that is necessary for coordination of movements of different parts of the body. When the receptor where dopamine is supposed to bind is blocked, certain movement-related side effects occur. All of the medications that block dopamine receptors are called neuroleptics.

Neuroleptics include both conventional or typical antipsychotic agents, such as **chlorpromazine** (Thorazine), **haloperidol** (Haldol), and **fluphenazine** (Prolixin), as well as the newer, or atypical, antipsychotic agents such as **clozapine** (Clozaril), **risperidone** (Risperdal), **olanzapine** (Zyprexa), and **quetiapine** (Seroquel). In general, the newer, atypical antipsychotics appear to have a lower likelihood to cause movement disorders than the older, typical medications. Other neuroleptics include certain drugs used in the treatment of physical symptoms such as nausea, and include

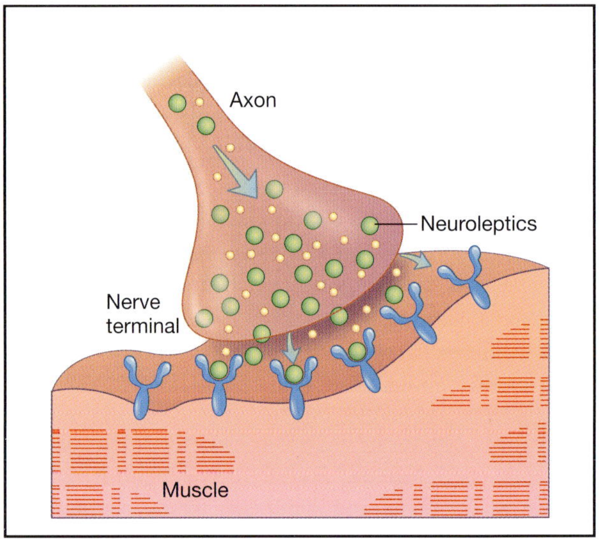

Neuroleptic medications block the action of dopamine, a neurotransmitter that helps coordinate movement. When dopamine cannot reach its receptors (blue channels blocked by neuroleptics), movement-related side effects may occur, including tremor and rigidity. *(Illustration by Electronic Illustrators Group. © 2012 Cengage Learning.)*

prochlorperazine, promethazine, and metoclopramide, as well as **amoxapine** (Asendin), which is marketed as an antidepressant.

There are other medications, however, that do not block dopamine action but still cause movement disorders. They are not referred to as neuroleptics, and they include **lithium carbonate**, **valproic acid** and a class of drugs called **selective serotonin reuptake inhibitors (SSRIs)**. The disorder caused by these medications is called medication-induced postural tremor.

All of the disorders caused by neuroleptics, which include antipsychotics and other medications that block dopamine, as well as disorders caused by non-neuroleptic medications, are collectively referred to as medication-induced movement disorders.

Demographics

Neuroleptic-induced acute dystonia occurs most commonly in young males. It is far less likely to occur with the new medications known as atypical neuroleptic medications, such as clozapine, risperidone, olanzapine, and quetiapine. The possibility of neuroleptic-induced acute dystonia occurring with these atypical medications is less than 5%. The possibility of this side effect occurring with the conventional or typical neuroleptics is about 15%–20%. The incidence is inversely correlated with age, meaning that younger persons are more likely to experience dystonia.

Neuroleptic-induced Parkinsonism is directly correlated with age. This means that older patients are more likely to experience this effect. It occurs in about 30% of patients. Neuroleptic-induced acute akathisia is not related to age and occurs in about 20% of patients being treated with neuroleptics.

The incidence of neuroleptic-induced tardive dyskinesia is related to total lifetime of treatment with antipsychotics. The cumulative incidence is about 5% per year of therapy. This essentially means that there is a 50% chance of developing tardive dyskinesia with 10 years of treatment with neuroleptics.

The incidence of neuroleptic malignant syndrome is about 0.5%. This condition is fatal in about 20% to 30% of cases.

Most available information on medication-induced postural tremor is about lithium-induced tremor. The prevalence of this condition is about 40%.

Description

Neuroleptics

Medication-induced movement disorders caused by neuroleptics are divided into three time periods. The early-onset type, which usually occurs within the first seven days of treatment with neuroleptics, is known as neuroleptic-induced acute dystonia. Neuroleptic-induced acute dystonia is characterized by abnormal contractions of various muscle groups resulting in spasm and/or twisting of the head, neck, jaw, lips, tongue, and eye muscles as well as abnormal movements and postures of the limbs and the trunk.

The intermediate-onset types of movement disorders associated with the use of neuroleptics usually develop within the first three months of treatment. They are known as neuroleptic-induced Parkinsonism and neuroleptic-induced akathisia. Neuroleptic-induced Parkinsonism is associated with difficulty initiating movements. Once movements are initiated, they are very slow. Other characteristics of neuroleptic-induced Parkinsonism are tremor and rigidity in muscles. Neuroleptic-induced akathisia is associated with uncontrollable restlessness that may involve compulsive foot tapping, pacing, and a sense of inner tension.

The late-onset type of neuroleptic-related movement disorder is known as neuroleptic-induced **tardive dyskinesia** and the onset is usually seen many months to years after starting the neuroleptic treatment. Neuroleptic-induced tardive dyskinesia involves grotesque, repetitive, and involuntary movements. They are usually seen in the mouth and face.

A movement disorder that can occur at any time during the course of neuroleptic treatment is known as **neuroleptic malignant syndrome**. It is a serious condition and is characterized by changes in consciousness, ranging from agitation to coma. The patient may experience high fever and increases in blood pressure and heart rate, as well as severe muscular rigidity.

Non-neuroleptics

All of the medication-induced movement disorders are related to the use of neuroleptic medications. However, other drugs, such as lithium, valproic acid, isoproterenol, amphetamine, and theophylline, as well as a class of drugs known as tricyclic **antidepressants**, may also cause a movement disorder that is mainly characterized by postural tremor, a rhythmic alteration in movement. Lithium-induced tremor may take the form of twitching in the arms and legs.

Causes and symptoms

Causes

Neuroleptic-induced movement disorders are caused because the actions of dopamine are blocked. Dopamine is a neurotransmitter necessary for coordination of movements of different parts of the body.

Other medications, which are not classified as neuroleptics, block the action of other **neurotransmitters** as well as dopamine. However, because they essentially block the action of dopamine, they cause similar unwanted effects associated with movements.

Symptoms

Neuroleptic-induced acute dystonia is associated with primarily abnormal postures and muscular spasms. They are usually characterized by abnormal positioning of the head and neck in relation to the body; spasms of the jaw muscles; impaired swallowing, speaking, or breathing; thickened or slurred speech due to a slow movement of the tongue; tongue protrusion or tongue dysfunction; eyes deviated up, down, or sideways; and abnormal positioning of the limbs or trunk. Patients experience pain and cramps in the affected muscles. In addition, many patients experiencing dystonia due to the neuroleptic treatment also experience fear and anxiety. This is especially present in patients who are not aware of the possibility of developing dystonia and who mistakenly associate these side effects as part of their mental illness.

Neuroleptic-induced Parkinsonism includes rigidity, tremor, and bradykinesia (slow movements). The tremor is a rhythmic, three- to six-cycle-per-second motion that is present at rest. The tremor can affect the limbs, head, mouth, or lips. Rigidity signifies the degree of tension present in the muscle. It can be either continuous or intermittent in the affected limbs or joints. Bradykinesia includes decreased arm movements related to walking, as well as difficulty initiating movement. Drooling may occur due to a decrease in pharyngeal motor activity. People experiencing neuroleptic-induced akathisia usually feel anxious, agitated, and unable to relax. They also may pace, rock while sitting and standing, and often rapidly alternate between sitting and standing.

Neuroleptic-induced tardive dyskinesia manifests itself in involuntary movements of the tongue, jaw, trunk, or extremities. It occurs most commonly in patients who have taken older antipsychotic medications for many years, although the condition may appear earlier than that (after one year of treatment with neuroleptics, or even earlier than that, especially in elderly people). The movements can be rapid and jerky, slow and continual, or rhythmic in nature. Over three-fourths of the individuals with neuroleptic-induced tardive dyskinesia have abnormal movements of the face and the mouth. This may include licking, sucking, or smacking of the lips; chewing movements; jaw deviations; grimacing, grunting, and other peculiar sounds; or brow furrowing. About one-half of patients with tardive dyskinesia have abnormal limb movements, while about one-quarter have disposition of the trunk.

The basic features of neuroleptic malignant syndrome is the development of high fever and severe muscle rigidity. These can be accompanied by tremor, changes in level of consciousness ranging from confusion to coma, and increased heart rate and blood pressure. The fever can be mildly elevated (99–100°F) or severe (106°F). Neuroleptic malignant syndrome can be fatal in some cases, while it is relatively benign in others. There are no known predictors of neuroleptic malignant syndrome. However, it usually develops four weeks after starting neuroleptics, and about two-thirds of cases develop within the first week of treatment. A very small number of patients develop neuroleptic malignant syndrome many months after taking the neuroleptic.

Medication-induced postural tremor is characterized by a regular, rhythmic oscillation of hands and fingers, head, mouth, or tongue. The frequency of the tremor ranges from 8 to 12 cycles per second. These are most easily observed when the affected part is in a sustained position (for example if hands are outstretched or the mouth is held open).

Diagnosis

People taking antipsychotic medications and other medications that block dopamine action must be regularly evaluated by a physician to monitor for medication-induced movement disorders. In order for these conditions to be officially diagnosed, certain criteria must be met.

Neuroleptic-induced acute dystonia must have one or more of the following developed in association with the use of neuroleptics: abnormal positioning of the head and neck in relation to the body; spasms of the jaw muscles; impaired swallowing; thickened or slurred speech; tongue protrusion or dysfunction; eyes deviated up, down, or sideways; or abnormal positioning of limbs or trunk. These symptoms need to have developed within seven days of starting the neuroleptic medication. Moreover, the symptoms cannot be associated with an underlying mental disorder, and they cannot be due to a medication other than a neuroleptic. Dystonia due to neuroleptics needs to be distinguished from dystonia due to neuroleptic malignant syndrome.

Neuroleptic-induced Parkinsonism needs to have the triad of symptoms described above which include tremor, rigidity, and bradykinesia (slow movements). These symptoms cannot be related to a non-neuroleptic medication, or a psychiatric condition, such as Parkinson's disease, Wilson's disease, neuroleptic malignant syndrome, or substance withdrawal. Neuroleptic-induced akathisia is due to the use of a neuroleptic and not to anxiety, substance withdrawal, or psychotic agitation. At least one of the symptoms of fidgety movements or swinging the legs, rocking from foot to foot while standing, pacing to relieve restlessness, or inability to sit and stand needs to be present. These symptoms must have developed within four weeks of initiating the therapy with neuroleptics.

Neuroleptic-induced tardive dyskinesia needs to include involuntary movements over a period of at least four weeks that manifest themselves as rapid and jerky, slow and continual, or rhythmic movements. The exposure to neuroleptics needs to be for at least three months, and the symptoms cannot be due to a neurologic condition, such as Huntington's disease, Wilson's disease, Sydenham's (rheumatic) chorea, systemic lupus, or hyperthyroidism.

Neuroleptic malignant syndrome must include severe muscle rigidity and elevated temperature as well as at least two of the following symptoms: sweating, difficulty swallowing, tremor, incontinence, changes in level of consciousness, mutism, increased heart rate, elevated blood pressure, or laboratory evidence of muscle injury. These symptoms cannot be due to another substance or a medical condition, such as viral encephalitis, or mood disorder with catatonic features.

The criteria for diagnosing medication-induced postural tremor includes a development of tremor associated with the use of a medication other than a neuroleptic. The tremor cannot be due to a non-medication condition that was present prior to starting the medication and cannot continue to be present following discontinuation of the medication. These criteria are helpful in distinguishing the tremor due to medication use from the tremor due to anxiety, alcohol withdrawal, **stress**, or **fatigue**. The tremor must have a frequency between 8 and 12 cycles per second, and the tremor must not be caused by neuroleptic-induced Parkinsonism.

Treatment

In an attempt to prevent acute dystonia from developing, physicians may prescribe a preventive medication along with the antipsychotic. Once neuroleptic-induced acute dystonia has appeared, however, there are several treatment options. A medication called **benztropine** in doses ranging from 1 mg to 8 mg is effective in reducing symptoms associated with dystonia. Most patients take 2 mg twice daily for seven days for prevention of dystonia at the time they are starting neuroleptic treatment. When benztropine therapy is initiated, the dose is slowly increased. Moreover, when discontinuing the treatment with benztropine, the dose should be slowly decreased to prevent the nausea and vomiting associated with abrupt withdrawal. Another medication that may be useful in treating neuroleptic-induced acute dystonia is called **trihexyphenidyl**. The doses can vary from 10 mg to 45 mg daily. Younger patients may respond better to the treatment with trihexyphenidyl because they can tolerate higher doses. The third pharmacological option is **diphenhydramine** (Benadryl). This medication can be taken for the period dystonic symptoms last. Another option may include switching the patient to one of the newer antipsychotics, such as clozapine, risperidone, or olanzapine, since each of these has a low incidence of causing dystonia.

There are a couple of ways to treat intermediate-onset movement disorders due to neuroleptics. **Amantadine** is a medication that is approved by the United States Food and Drug Administration for the treatment of Parkinsonian symptoms. Another helpful medication called **propranolol** comes from a class of drugs called **beta blockers**. Propranolol has been reported effective in the treatment of akathisia. The doses that are effective range from 20 mg to 100 mg daily. The response to propranolol is usually seen within the 24 hours of administration. Switching the patient to a newer or atypical antipsychotic, such as clozapine, or decreasing the dose of the current antipsychotic sometimes helps the condition.

There are no effective treatments for tardive dyskinesia once it develops. Tardive dyskinesia is associated and strongly correlated with the cumulative dose of the antipsychotic during years of treatment. Hence, the key to tardive dyskinesia is prevention. If possible, a newer medication, such as clozapine or risperidone, which have only a few case reports of tardive dyskinesia, should be used whenever possible. In many cases, if tardive dyskinesia is noticed early in a regular check-up with the physician, and if the medication causing the condition is stopped, the symptoms of tardive dyskinesia will subside. If the symptoms continue after the antipsychotic has been discontinued, the situation becomes difficult. Treatment will most likely involve movement disorder specialists and may or may not be successful. The medications reserpine and levodopa may be helpful for some patients.

The most common medications used to treat neuroleptic malignant syndrome are dantrolene, (a muscle relaxant that helps with the fever), bromocriptine, and amantadine.

In order to reduce medication-induced postural tremor, the lowest possible dose of the psychiatric drug should be used. Moreover, a medication from the beta blockers, such as propranolol, can be used to help with the symptoms.

Prognosis

The prognoses for the early- and intermediate-onset of movement disorders are very good, especially with the option of switching the patient to a newer antipsychotic such as clozapine.

The prognosis for the late-onset disorder called tardive dyskinesia is very poor. Once the condition occurs, it is essentially irreversible and is very difficult to treat.

Neuroleptic malignant syndrome is a serious condition. It is deadly in about 20%–30% of patients. Those who survive have a good chance of recovering.

Medication-induced postural tremor is very well-controlled with propranolol, and hence the prognosis is good while the patient is being treated with the medication causing the movement disorder.

Prevention

To prevent acute dystonia, some physicians prescribe benztropine diphenhydramine, or other medications that treat dystonia at the outset of treatment with an older antipsychotic.

KEY TERMS

Dystonia—A neurological disorder characterized by involuntary muscle spasms. The spasms can cause a painful twisting of the body and difficulty walking or moving.

Hyperthyroidism—Condition resulting from the thyroid glands secreting excessive thyroid hormone, causing increased basal metabolic rate, and causing an increased need for food to meet the demand of the metabolic activity; generally, however, weight loss results.

Neuroleptic—Another name for antipsychotic medications, such as haloperidol (Haldol) and chlorpromazine (Thorazine).

Neuroleptic-induced acute dystonia—A severe form of the neurological movement disorder caused by the use of neuroleptic drugs.

Neuroleptic-induced akathisia—Refers to the disorder characterized by a physical restlessness (the inability to sit still, for example), and manifested by excessive voluntary movements, as a result of the use of neuroleptic drugs; research indicates it is likely the most common of neuroleptic-induced movement disorders.

Neuroleptic-induced Parkinsonism—Symptoms similar to Parkinson's disease that may appear in people taking neuroleptic (antipsychotic) medications. These symptoms include tremors in muscles and a shuffling gait.

Neuroleptic-induced tardive dyskinesia—A potentially irreversible neurological disorder caused by the use of antipsychotic/neuroleptic medications, with symptoms involving uncontrollable movement of various body parts.

Neuroleptic malignant syndrome—An unusual but potentially serious complication that develops in some patients who have been treated with antipsychotic medications. NMS is characterized by changes in blood pressure, altered states of consciousness, rigid muscles, and fever. Untreated NMS can result in coma and death.

Postural tremor—A continuous quiver that affects body posture and movement.

SLE (Systemic Lupus Erythematosus)—An autoimmune disease that leads to inflammation and damage to various body tissues and parts, including joints, skin, kidneys, heart, lungs, blood vessels, and brain.

Sydenham's chorea—A serious manifestation of acute rheumatic fever that commonly occurs in children ages 7 through 14, peaking at age 8. This disease of the central nervous system is characterized by emotional instability, purposeless movements, and muscular weakness. At its peak in the 1950s it occurred in nearly 50% of the acute rheumatic fever cases, but by 2002 had subsided to a degree of less than 10% of the acute cases.

The most important component of neuroleptic-induced tardive dyskinesia is prevention. If conventional antipsychotics are used, the drug use, drug dose, and the duration of use therefore should be minimized.

In order to avoid medication-induced postural tremor, patients should limit the amount of caffeine consumption. Also, in order to minimize the amount of daytime tremor they should take the psychiatric drug at bedtime.

Resources

BOOKS

American Psychiatric Association. *Diagnostic and Statistical Manual of Mental Disorders*. 4th ed., text rev. Washington, DC: American Psychiatric Publishing, 2000.

Brunton, Laurence, Bruce Chabner, and Bjorn Knollman. *Goodman & Gilman's The Pharmacological Basis of Therapeutics*. 12th ed. New York: McGraw-Hill, 2010.

Lacy, Charles F. *Drug Information Handbook with International Trade Names Index*. Hudson, OH: Lexi-Comp, Inc. 2011.

Sadock, Benjamin J., and Virginia A. Sadock, eds. *Comprehensive Textbook of Psychiatry*. Vol. 2. 7th ed. Philadelphia: Lippincott Williams and Wilkins, 2000.

PERIODICALS

Heaton, Robert, et al. "Stability and Course of Neuropsychological Deficits in Schizophrenia." *Archives of General Psychiatry*. 58, no. 1 (2001): 24–32.

Littrell, Kimberly. "Marked Reduction of Tardive Dyskinesia With Olanzapine." *Archives of General Psychiatry*. 55, no. 3 (March 1998): 398–403.

ORGANIZATIONS

American Psychiatric Association, 1000 Wilson Blvd., Ste. 1825, Arlington, VA, 22209-3901, (703) 907-7300, apa@psych.org, http://www.psych.org.

American Thyroid Association, 6066 Leesburg Pike, Ste. 550, Falls Church, VA, 22041, (703) 998-8890, Fax: (703) 998-8893, thyroid@thyroid.org, http://www.thyroid.org.

Canadian Movement Disorder Group, affiliate of Canadian Congress of Neurological Sciences, 709 7015 Macleod Trail SW, Calgary, AB, CanadaT2H 2K6, http://www.cmdg.org.

We Move, 5731 Mosholu Ave., Bronx, NY, 10471. wemove@wemove.org, http://www.wemove.org.

Ajna Hamidovic, Pharm.D.

Meditation

Definition

Meditation or contemplation involves focusing the mind upon a sound, phrase, prayer, object, visualized image, breath, ritualized movement, or consciousness in order to increase awareness of the present moment, promote relaxation, reduce **stress**, and enhance personal or spiritual growth. The term refers to a group of widely different types of practices all generally founded within, or related to, ancient religious or spiritual traditions. Since the mid-twentieth century, interest in alternative treatments such as meditation has increased for the treatment and management of mental illnesses. As a part of complementary and alternative medicine, meditation is not considered a part of conventional medicine. However, it is often used with conventional medical treatment.

Purpose

Originally, meditation techniques were intended to develop spiritual understanding, awareness, and direct experience of ultimate reality. Many religious traditions developed meditative practices. These include the contemplative practices of Christian religious orders, the Buddhist practice of sitting meditation, and the whirling movements of the Sufi dervishes. Although distinct from each other, the practices share common aspects, such as using specific postures and practicing focused concentration. Today, meditation is used for both religious and secular purposes. Secular goals include:

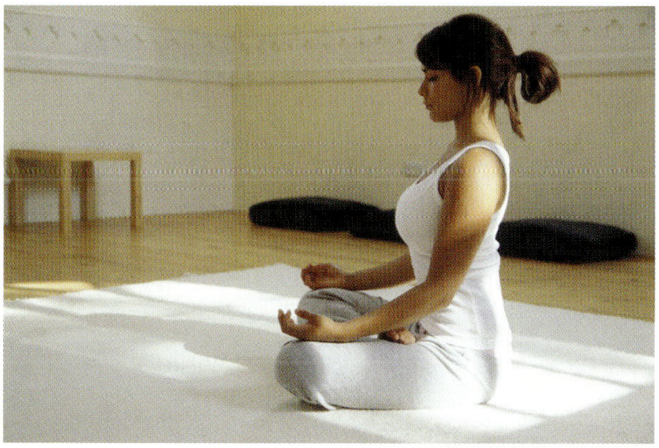

A young woman practices meditation. *(© Angela Hampton Picture Library/Alamy)*

- increased physical relaxation
- decreased stress and anxiety and reduced pain
- reduced depression
- reduced insomnia
- increased calmness
- enriched serenity
- enhanced mental consciousness
- improved psychological balance
- improved coping skills in handling physical problems and illness
- reduced physical or emotional symptoms involving chronic illnesses, such as heart disease, cancer, and human immunodeficiency virus/acquired immune deficiency syndrome (HIV/AIDS)
- improved overall health and well-being

Meditation is used in the treatment of both physiological and psychological problems. However, medical researchers do not completely understand what changes when people meditate and whether such changes help to influence positively the user's health. However, as Western medical practitioners began to consider the mind's role in health and disease, interest increased in the use of meditation in medicine. Meditative practices are increasingly offered in medical clinics and hospitals as a tool for improving health and quality of life. Meditation has been used as the primary therapy for treating certain diseases; as an additional therapy in a comprehensive treatment plan; and as a means of improving the quality of life of people with debilitating, chronic, or terminal illnesses. Medical research is ongoing regarding the applicability of meditation within traditional medicine, including how meditation works to counter diseases and conditions.

Demographics

Meditation techniques have been practiced for millennia. Although meditation is an important spiritual practice in many religious and spiritual traditions, it can be practiced by anyone regardless of their religious or cultural background to relieve stress and pain. As reported by the U.S. National Center for Complimentary and Alternative Medicine, a 2007 American study that followed 23,393 adults found that 9.4% of them had used meditation in the past year, compared to a similar study performed in 2002 that showed 7.6% of the respondents had used meditation over the past year.

Description

Meditation refers to such specific techniques and approaches as concentration meditation, relaxation response, transcendental meditation, mantra meditation, mindfulness meditation, and Zen Buddhist meditation. Many of these techniques originated in ancient Asian religions and spiritual traditions, such as Buddhism. Although meditation practices continue within religious communities, they also are used in secular settings to promote health and well-being. Meditation can be performed while sitting or lying quietly or while moving.

Sitting meditation is done in an upright seated position, either in a chair or cross-legged on a cushion on the floor. The spine is straight yet relaxed. Sometimes the eyes are closed; sometimes individuals gaze into the distance or at a specific object. Depending on the type of meditation, meditators may concentrate on the breath as it is inhaled and exhaled; they may count their inhalations or repeat a sound or chant. Meditators may visualize a certain image or focus on the center of the body. They may consciously remain open to all sensory experience and note with detachment the flow of thoughts that occur to them. They may also perform stylized ritual movements with their hands.

Movement meditation can be spontaneous or choreographed. Movement meditation is particularly helpful for those people who find it difficult to remain still.

Generally speaking, there are two types of meditation: concentration meditation and mindfulness meditation. Concentration meditation practices involve focusing attention on a single object. Objects of meditation can include the breath; an inner or external image; a movement pattern (as in tai chi or **yoga**); or a sound, word, or phrase that is repeated silently as a mantra. The purpose of concentrative practices is to train one's attention or develop concentration. When thoughts or emotions arise, the meditator gently directs the mind back to the original object of concentration.

Mindfulness meditation practices involve becoming aware of the entire field of attention. The meditator is instructed to be aware of all thoughts, feelings, perceptions, or sensations as they arise in each moment. Mindfulness meditation practices are enhanced by the meditator's ability to focus and quiet the mind. Many meditation practices are a blend of these two forms.

In treating physiological conditions, three types of meditation have been used: (1) transcendental meditation (TM); (2) relaxation response, an approach developed by American cardiologist Herbert Benson (1935–); and (3) mindfulness meditation, specifically the program of mindfulness-based **stress reduction** (MBSR) developed by American molecular biologist Jon Kabat-Zinn (1944–).

Transcendental meditation

Transcendental meditation (TM) has its origins in the Vedic tradition of India and was introduced to the West by Maharishi Mahesh Yogi (1914–2008). TM gained worldwide attention in the 1960s when the rock-and-roll group The Beatles was trained in the technique. It is one of the most widely practiced forms of meditation in the West. In TM, the meditator sits with closed eyes and concentrates on a single syllable or word (mantra) for 20 minutes at a time, twice a day. When thoughts or feelings arise, the attention is brought back to the mantra. According to American **psychologist** Charles N. Alexander, an important TM researcher and professor at Maharishi International University, "During TM, ordinary waking mental activity is said to settle down, until even the subtlest thought is transcended and a completely unified wholeness of awareness ... is experienced. In this silent, self-referential state of pure wakefulness, consciousness is fully awake to itself alone." TM supporters believe that TM practices are more beneficial than other meditation practices.

Frequently, medical studies of TM have focused on such topics as mental health, **addiction**, rehabilitation, and cognition. A study published in 2006, which was funded by the U.S. National Institutes of Health, found that TM may help to prevent health problems caused by environmental and psychosocial stresses in a variety of people from different ethnic backgrounds. Researchers from the Institute for Natural Medicine and Prevention at Maharishi University of Management in Fairfield, Iowa, looked at how TM and Maharishi consciousness-based health care affects blood pressure, psychosocial stress, surrogate markers for atherosclerotic cardiovascular disease (CVD), and mortality. They concluded that TM could "include enhanced resistance to physiological and psychological stress and improvements in homeostatic and self-repair processes" and "may offer clinical and cost effectiveness advantages for health care, particularly in preventive cardiology."

Relaxation response

The relaxation response involves a similar form of mental focusing. One of the first Western doctors to conduct research on the effects of meditation, Benson developed this approach after observing the health benefits of a state of bodily calm he calls "the relaxation response." In order to elicit this response in the body, Benson teaches patients to focus on the repetition of a word, sound, prayer, phrase, or movement activity (including swimming, jogging, yoga, and even knitting) for 10 to 20 minutes at a time, twice a day. Patients are also taught not to pay attention to distracting thoughts and to return their focus to the original repetition when rising thoughts seem to distract them. The individual chooses the focused repetition. Instead of repeating a prescribed Sanskrit term, the meditator chooses something that is personally meaningful, such as a phrase from a prayer.

Mindfulness meditation

Mindfulness meditation derives from traditional Buddhist meditation practices. Jon Kabat-Zinn (1944–) has been instrumental in bringing this form of meditation into medical settings. In formal mindfulness practice, the meditator sits with eyes closed, focusing the attention on the sensations and movement of the breath for approximately 45 to 60 minutes at a time, at least once a day. Informal mindfulness practice involves bringing awareness to every activity in daily life. Wandering thoughts or distracting feelings are simply noticed without resistance or reaction. The essence of mindfulness meditation is not what one focuses on but rather the quality of awareness the meditator brings to each moment. It is practiced by bringing attention to the experiences of breathing in and out, concentrating on this action while focusing one's mind on the experience itself—all the while not reacting or judging what is being experienced.

According to Kabat-Zinn, in his book *Mind/Body Medicine*, "It is this investigative, discerning observation of whatever comes up in the present moment that is the hallmark of mindfulness and differentiates it most from other forms of meditation. The goal of mindfulness is for you to be more aware, more in touch with life and whatever is happening in your own body and mind at the time it is happening—that is, the present moment." The mindfulness-based stress reduction (MBSR) program, which Kabat-Zinn first established at the University of Massachusetts Medical School, consists of a series of complementary-medicine classes involving meditation, movement, and group process. There are over 200 MBSR programs offered in healthcare settings around the world.

Meditation is not considered a medical procedure or **intervention** by most insurers. Many patients pay directly for meditation training. Frequently, religious groups or meditation centers offer meditation instruction free of charge or for a nominal donation. Hospitals may offer MBSR classes at a reduced rate for their patients and a slightly higher rate for the general public.

Benefits

Meditation benefits people with or without acute medical illness or stress. People who meditate frequently have been shown to feel less anxiety and **depression**. They also report that they experience more enjoyment and appreciation of life and that their relationships with others are improved. Meditation produces a state of deep relaxation and a sense of balance or equanimity. According to physician Michael J. Baime, director of the UPenn Program for Mindfulness at the University of Pennsylvania Health System, "Meditation cultivates an emotional stability that allows the meditator to experience intense emotions fully while simultaneously maintaining perspective on them." Out of this experience of emotional stability, one may gain greater insight and understanding about one's thoughts, feelings, and actions. This insight in turn offers the possibility to feel more confident and in control of life. Meditation facilitates a greater sense of calm, empathy, and acceptance of oneself and others.

Meditation can be used with other forms of medical treatment and is an important complementary therapy for both the treatment and prevention of many stress-related conditions. Regular meditation can reduce the number of symptoms experienced by patients with a wide range of illnesses and disorders. Based upon clinical evidence, as well as theoretical understanding, meditation is considered to be one of the better therapies for **panic disorder**, **generalized anxiety disorder**, substance dependence and abuse, ulcers, colitis, chronic pain, psoriasis, and **dysthymic disorder**. It is considered a valuable adjunctive therapy for moderate hypertension (high blood pressure), prevention of cardiac arrest (heart attack), prevention of atherosclerosis (hardening of arteries), arthritis (including fibromyalgia), cancer, **insomnia**, migraine, and prevention of **stroke**.

Meditation may also be a valuable complementary therapy for allergies and asthma because of the role stress plays in these conditions. Meditative practices have been reported to improve function or reduce symptoms in patients with some neurological disorders as well. These include people with Parkinson's disease, people who experience **fatigue** with multiple sclerosis, and people with epilepsy who are resistant to standard treatment.

Overall, health organizations such as the National Institutes of Health view meditation and similar forms of relaxation as ways to improve health and quality of life and to lower healthcare costs. Many physicians, nurses, and occupational therapists in the United States accept meditation as a beneficial adjunct to conventional medical or surgical treatments.

KEY TERMS

Dervish—A member of the Sufi order, in which the practice of meditation involves whirling ecstatic dance.

Mantra—A sacred word or formula repeated over and over to concentrate the mind.

Transcendental meditation—A meditation technique based on Hindu practices that involves the repetition of a mantra.

A March 18, 2011, article in the *New York Times* highlighted the popularity that transcendental meditation in the United States. The article concentrated on the effect that various celebrities, such as Russell Brand, Susan Sarandon, and Martin Scorsese, have had on the TM movement. In addition, the article "Look Who's Meditating Now" noted that many research studies show the positive effects of daily TM for the "mind, body and behavior." The *New York Times* article also mentioned the large number of studies funded by the U.S. National Institutes of Health. Such studies have investigated the effects of meditation on such medical conditions as hypertension (high blood pressure), atherosclerosis, and the risk of cardiac events (such as heart attacks, strokes, and congestive heart failure).

In the early 2000s, numerous studies were funded by the U.S. National Center for Complementary and Alternative Medicine (NCCAM). These studies indicated the benefits of meditation for certain medical conditions, such as "Meditation May Make Information Processing In the Brain More Efficient" (June 2007); "Meditation May Increase Empathy" (March 2008); "Mantram Instruction May Help HIV-Positive Individuals Handle Stress" (January 2009); "Transcendental Meditation Helps Young Adults Cope with Stress" (December 2009); and "Mindfulness Meditation Is Associated with Structural Changes in the Brain" (January 2011).

With respect to stress, which in some cases is seen as a precursor to various mental illnesses, the December 2009 study found that TM helped college students reduce psychological stress and cope more effectively with school-related responsibilities. The group of students with the highest likelihood of developing hypertension (high blood pressure) were found to decrease their blood pressure level when they practiced TM on a regular basis. A NCCAM article stated that "This could be good news for the many students experiencing academic, financial, and social pressures that can lead to psychological distress—especially in light of evidence that college-age people with even slightly elevated blood pressure are three times more likely to develop hypertension within 30 years."

It is important to note that independent systematic reviews of these studies do not necessarily agree with their findings.

Preparation

People who want to meditate usually make the following preparations:

- Find a quiet location that contains few distractions.
- Assume a comfortable posture, one that may involving sitting, lying down, or standing, as specified by the meditation technique being used.
- Focus attention on a specified object, sense perception, word or phrase (a mantra), or movement of breath.
- Allow distractions to come and go without concern, calmly returning attention to the chosen point of focus after each disruption.

Risks

Meditation appears to be safe for most people. There are, however, case reports and studies noting some adverse effects, such as **depersonalization**, or a sense of being detached from one's experiences. To an extent, this is a goal of meditation, but the effect may progress to the extreme and feel unpleasant or alarming. In one particular study, 33%–50% of the people participating in long silent meditation retreats (two weeks to three months) reported increased tension, anxiety, confusion, and depression. However, most of these same people also reported positive effects from their meditation practice. Kabat-Zinn notes that these studies fail to differentiate between serious psychiatric disturbances and normal emotional mood swings. These studies do suggest, however, that meditation may not be recommended for people with psychotic disorders, severe depression, and other severe **personality disorders** unless they are also receiving psychological or medical treatment.

Research & general acceptance

The scientific study of the physiological effects of meditation began in the early 1960s. Certain studies indicated that meditation affects metabolism, the endocrine system, the central nervous system, and the autonomic nervous system. In one study, three advanced practitioners of Tibetan Buddhist meditation practices demonstrated the ability to increase "inner heat" as much as 61%. During a different meditative practice, they were able to dramatically slow down the rate at which their bodies consumed oxygen. Preliminary research shows that mindfulness meditation is associated with increased levels of melatonin.

Despite the inherent difficulties in designing research studies, there is significant evidence of the medical benefits of meditation. Meditation is particularly effective as a treatment for chronic pain. Studies have shown meditation reduces symptoms of pain and pain-related drug use. In a 1986 four-year follow-up study conducted by Kabat-Zinn and his colleagues, the majority of patients in an MBSR program reported "moderate to great improvement" in pain as a result of participation in the program. Later studies supported his findings, including a 2011 study published in the *Journal of Neuroscience* that found meditation to be as effective—and in some cases more effective—than pain medications.

Research also suggests that meditation is effective in the treatment of chemical dependency. Numerous studies show that TM is helpful in **smoking cessation** programs and programs for drug and alcohol abuse.

Studies suggest that meditation is helpful in reducing symptoms of anxiety and in treating anxiety-related disorders. Furthermore, a study of patients with psoriasis showed that those practicing mindfulness meditation had more rapid clearing of their skin condition, with standard ultraviolet (UV) light treatment, than the control subjects. Another study found that meditation decreased the symptoms of fibromyalgia; over half of the patients reported significant improvement. Research by a group of ophthalmologists indicated that nearly 60% of a group of patients being treated for glaucoma found meditation helpful in coping with their eye disorder. In addition, meditation was one of several **stress management** techniques used in a small study of men with HIV. The study showed improvements in the T-cell counts (a group of white blood cells that play a key role in immunity) of the men, as well as in several psychological measures of well-being.

Training & certification

There is no program of certification or licensing for instructors who wish to teach meditation as a medical therapy. Meditation teachers within a particular religious tradition usually have extensive experience and expertise with faith questions and religious practices but may not have been trained to work with medical patients. Different programs have varied requirements for someone to teach meditation. In order to be recognized as an instructor of TM, one must receive extensive training. The Center for Mindfulness in Medicine, Health Care and Society at the University of Massachusetts Medical Center offers training and workshops for health professionals and others interested in teaching mindfulness-based stress reduction. The center does not, however, certify that someone is qualified to teach meditation. The University of Pennsylvania Program for Stress Management suggests that individuals have at least 10 years of personal experience with the practice of mindfulness meditation before receiving additional instruction to teach meditation. Teachers are also expected to spend at least two weeks each year in intensive meditation retreats.

QUESTIONS TO ASK YOUR DOCTOR

- How do you think meditation may benefit me?
- What other treatment options do you recommend for me?
- Will meditation interfere with my current medications?
- Is there an exercise regimen you would recommend to help me cope with my condition?
- What symptoms or behaviors are important enough that I should seek immediate treatment?

Resources

BOOKS

Bear, Marina. *The Little Book of Meditation: A Guide to Stress-Free Living*. Berkeley, CA: SLG, 2009.

Chopra, Deepak. *Reinventing the Body, Resurrecting the Soul: How to Create a New You.* New York: Harmony, 2009.

Liebler, Nancy, and Sandra Moss. *Healing Depression the Mind-Body Way: Creating Happiness with Meditation, Yoga, and Ayurveda.* Hoboken, NJ: Wiley, 2009.

McNally, Lama Christie. *The Tibetan Book of Meditation.* New York: Doubleday Religion, 2009.

PERIODICALS

Alecksander, Irina. "Look Who's Meditating Now." *New York Times,* March 18, 2011. http://www.nytimes.com/2011/03/20/fashion/20TM.html?_r=1 (accessed August 14, 2011).

Kabat-Zinn, J., L. Lipworth, R. Burney, and W. Sellers, "Four Year Follow-up of a Meditation-based Program for the Self-regulation of Chronic Pain: Treatment Outcomes and Compliance." *Clinical Journal of Pain* 2, no. 3 (1986):159–73.

Zeidan, Fadel. "Brain Mechanisms Supporting the Modulation of Pain by Mindfulness Meditation." *Journal of Neuroscience* 31, no. 14 (2011): 5540–48.

WEBSITES

"Meditation: An Introduction." National Center for Complementary and Alternative Medicine. Last updated June 2010. http://nccam.nih.gov/health/meditation/overview.htm#research (accessed August 14, 2011).

"Research Results for Meditation." National Center for Complementary and Alternative Medicine. Last modified February 24, 2011. http://nccam.nih.gov/research/results/topics/index.php?title=Meditation (accessed August 14, 2011).

Schneider, Robert H., et al. "Cardiovascular Disease Prevention and Health Promotion with the Transcendental Meditation Program and Maharishi Consciousness-based Health Care." National Institutes of Health. http://www.ncbi.nlm.nih.gov/pmc/articles/PMC2267926 (accessed August 14, 2011).

"Transcendental Meditation Helps Young Adults Cope with Stress." National Center for Complementary and Alternative Medicine, December 7, 2009. http://nccam.nih.gov/research/results/spotlight/051410.htm (accessed August 14, 2011).

"What Is Mindfulness-Based Stress Reduction?" Mindful Living Programs. http://www.mindfullivingprograms.com/whatMBSR.php (accessed August 14, 2011).

ORGANIZATIONS

Benson-Henry for Mind Body Medicine, 151 Merrimac St., 4th Fl., Boston, MA, 02114, (617) 643-6090, Fax: (617) 643-6077, mindbody@partners.org, http://www.massgeneral.org/bhi.

Center for Mindfulness in Medicine, Health Care and Society, 55 Lake Ave. N, Worcester, MA, 01655, (508) 856-2656, mindfulness@umassmed.edu, http://www.umassmed.edu/cfm/home/index.aspx.

Insight Meditation Society, 1230 Pleasant St., Barre, MA, 01005, (978) 355-4378, http://www.dharma.org.

Linda Chrisman
Rebecca J. Frey, PhD
Laura Jean Cataldo, RN, EdD
William A. Atkins, BB, BS, MBA

Mellaril *see* **Thioridazine**

Memantine

Purpose

Memantine HCl (trade name Namenda) is an N-methyl-D-aspartate (NMDA) receptor antagonist used to treat moderate to severe **Alzheimer's disease** (AD).

Description

A recent theory concerning the mechanism underlying AD is that abnormal glutamate activity in the **brain** causes overexcitation of NMDA receptors, which may play a role in the development and progression of AD. Memantine is a NMDA-receptor antagonist, which hypothetically allows the continued physiological activation of NMDA receptors for continued learning and memory. However, memantine does not appear to prevent or slow the degeneration of brain cells in patients with AD.

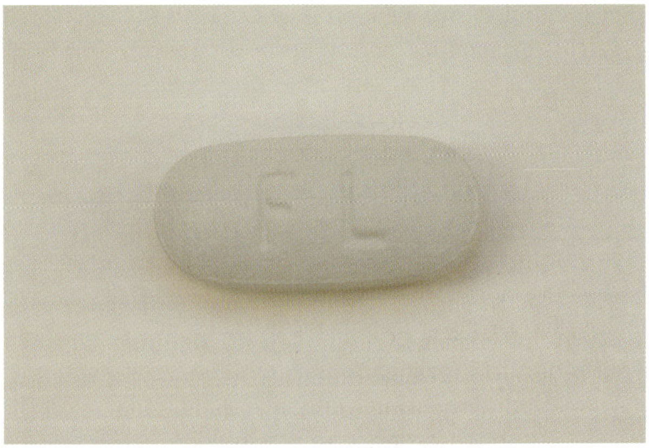

Namenda (memantine), 10 mg. *(© Custom Medical Stock Photo, Inc. Reproduced by permission.)*

Randomized, double-blind, placebo-controlled **clinical trials** of memantine have demonstrated significant improvement of day-to-day functioning in moderate to severe AD.

Recommended dosage

Memantine is available in tablet form, or as an oral solution for patients who have difficulty swallowing tablets. Typically, patients are gradually put on memantine by taking 5 mg once a day for the first week, 5 mg twice a day for the second week (10 mg total per day), and 10 mg in the morning and 5 mg in the evening for the third week (15 mg total per day). After that, the maintenance dosage of memantine is 10 mg twice a day (20 mg total per day). Memantine can be taken with or without food.

Precautions

Clinical trials of memantine found it to be safe and well tolerated. However, anyone with a known hypersensitivity to memantine HCl or any of the inert substances used as a vehicle for the drug should not take memantine. The dosage of memantine should be reduced for patients with severe kidney impairment.

Side effects

No significant difference has been found between patients taking memantine and patients taking a placebo

KEY TERMS

Alzheimer's disease—Alzheimer's disease (AD) is a progressive neurologic disease in which dementia results from the degeneration of brain cells through the formation of senile plaques and neurofibrillary tangles. AD is the most common cause of dementia.

Clinical trial—A controlled scientific experiment designed to investigate the effectiveness of a drug or treatment in curing or lessening the symptoms of a disease or disorder.

Control group—A group in a research study that does not receive the experimental treatment. For example, in an experiment testing the effectiveness of a new drug, the control group might receive the current drug of choice while the experimental group receives the new drug under investigation.

Double-blind study—A research study in which neither the participants nor the professional giving them the drug or treatment know whether they are receiving the experimental treatment or a placebo or control treatment.

Placebo—A preparation without pharmacological effect that is given in place of a drug in clinical trials to determine the effectiveness of the drug under study; a "sugar pill."

Randomization—The process of randomly assigning participants in an experiment to the various conditions (that is, experimental and control groups) so that each individual has an equal chance of being assigned to any of the groups. Randomization helps ensure that each of the groups is roughly the same and that the results are due to the treatment, not to the makeup of the groups.

in vital signs, electrocardiogram values, or laboratory values (serum chemistry, hematology, and urinalysis). The most common adverse reactions to memantine are:

- dizziness
- confusion
- headache
- constipation
- agitation
- falling
- accidental injury

Compared with a placebo, memantine showed a lower level of gastrointestinal side effects (such as constipation, diarrhea, vomiting, or nausea).

Interactions

Studies have revealed that the use of memantine in combination therapy with **donepezil**, a cholinesterase inhibitor, is frequently more effective than the use of donepezil alone in the treatment of moderate to severe AD. Using memantine and donepezil in combination therapy does not affect the actions of either drug. Memantine has been shown to be both safe and effective in such combination therapy.

Studies on memantine have shown low potential for negative interaction with other drugs.

Resources

BOOKS

Burns, Alistair, and Bengt Winblad, eds. *Severe Dementia*. New York: John Wiley & Sons, 2006.

VandenBos, Gary R. ed. *APA Dictionary of Psychology*. Washington, DC: American Psychological Association, 2006.

PERIODICALS

Alexopoulos, G. S., et al. "Treatment of Dementia and Its Behavioral Disturbances." *Postgraduate Medicine* (January 2005): 1–111.

Cummings, Jeffrey L., et al. "Behavioral Effects of Memantine in Alzheimer Disease Patients Receiving Donepezil Treatment." *Neurology* 67, no. 1 (July 2006): 57–63.

Danysz, W., et al. "Neuroprotective and Symptomalogical Action of Memantine Relevant for Alzheimer's Disease." *Neurotoxicity Research* 2 (2000): 85–98.

Doody, R. S. "Refining Treatment Guidelines in Alzheimer's Disease." *Geriatrics* Suppl. (June 2005): 14–20.

Doraiswamy, P. M. "Non-Cholinergic Strategies for Treating and Preventing Alzheimer's Disease." *CNS Drugs* 16, no. 12 (2002): 811–24.

Fox, Chris, et al. "Memantine Combined with an Acetyl Cholinesterase Inhibitor—Hope for the Future?" *Neuropsychiatric Disease and Treatment* 2, no. 2 (2006): 121–25.

Hartmann, S., and H. J. Möbius. "Tolerability of Memantine in Combination with Cholinesterase Inhibitors in Dementia Therapy." *International Clinical Psychopharmacology* 18 (March 2003): 81–85.

Maidment, Ian, et al. "Drug Treatment for Alzheimer's Disease: The Way Forward." *International Journal of Geriatric Psychiatry* 21, no. 1 (2006): 6–8.

Orgogozo, J. M., et al. "Efficacy and Safety of Memantine in Patients with Mild to Moderate Vascular Dementia." *Stroke* 33, no. 7 (July 2002): 1834–39.

Reisberg, B., et al. "Memantine in Moderate-to-Severe Alzheimer's Disease." *New England Journal of Medicine* 348, no. 14 (2003): 1333–41.

Schneider, Lon S., Karen S. Dagerman, Julian P.T. Higgins, and Rupert McShane. "Lack of Evidence for the Efficacy of Memantine in Mild Alzheimer Disease." *Archives of Neurology* 68, no. 8 (2011): 991–998. http://archneur.ama assn.org/cgi/content/short/archneurol.2011.69 (accessed November 14, 2011).

Tariot, Pierre N., et al. "Memantine Treatment in Patients with Moderate to Severe Alzheimer Disease Already Receiving Donepezil: A Randomized Controlled Trial." *Journal of the American Medical Association* 291, no. 3 (January 21, 2004): 317–24. Available online at http://jama.ama-assn.org/content/291/3/317.full (accessed November 9, 2011).

Xiong, G., and P. M. Doraiswamy. "Combination Drug Therapy for Alzheimer's Disease: What Is Evidence-Based, and What Is Not?" *Geriatrics* 60, no. 6 (2005): 22–26.

WEBSITES

Forest Laboratories, Inc. "Namenda." http://www.namenda.com (accessed October 22, 2011.

Ruth A. Wienclaw, PhD

Men's mental health *see* **Gender issues in mental health**

Mental health courts

Definition

Mental health courts are used to divert criminal offenders with mental health problems from serving sentences in penitentiaries to fulfilling community-based treatment programs combined with court supervision. Because many prisons and jails are overcrowded, the goal of these programs is to help individuals with mental illnesses move forward with their recovery while preserving public safety. Some mental health courts hear felony cases, but most only hear misdemeanor cases. All mental health courts are voluntary. People with mental illnesses that have committed a crime have a choice of prison or program participation.

Qualifying mental illness for the Mental Health Courts Program is defined by law as: "a diagnosable mental, behavioral, or emotional disorder (A) of sufficient duration to meet diagnostic criteria within the most recent edition of the ***Diagnostic and Statistical Manual of Mental Disorders***, published by the **American Psychiatric Association**; and (B) that has resulted in functional impairment that substantially interferes with or limits one or more major life activities."

Purpose

The Mental Health Courts Program was established by an act of the U.S. Congress in 2000 to address the particular needs of mentally ill or intellectually disabled defendants. The traditional criminal court system in the United States is designed to process individuals who have been charged with crimes, but it does not account for special considerations, such as mental illness. Mental health courts provide defendants with mental illnesses, who have primarily committed misdemeanor and nonviolent crimes, with supervised treatment in order to reduce the number of incarcerated people with mental illness and to prevent those who have a mental illness from continually cycling through the court system. Those who successfully complete the program avoid prolonged incarceration and may have their charges dismissed.

Demographics

Approximately 1.5 million persons with mental illness are processed by the criminal justice system per year. The National Alliance on Mentally Illness estimates that as many as 40% of mentally ill individuals will encounter the criminal justice system at some point in their lives. Research finds that mentally ill inmates are at greater risk for assault and **suicide** than are other inmates.

Description

Before mental health courts were established, persons with mental illness who broke the law were not differentiated from other criminals. Because of this, the prison population contained about twice as many inmates with mental illness as those in state mental hospitals. In prison, the conditions of mentally ill inmates generally worsened over time, as they often did not receive proper medications or treatment. The criminal justice system had neglected these people, and ignored their mental state. However, their plight was eventually realized, in part due to overcrowding within the prison system, and steps were taken to remedy the situation, resulting in the creation of mental health courts.

After the mental health court system was established, persons with mental illnesses who were being processed through the criminal justice system were eligible to be sent to treatment programs instead of to jail or prison (providing they met the program's eligibility requirements). During their participation in the court program, after being processed through a mental health court, patients are provided treatment and support based on the underlying problems, especially their mental health conditions, that have led to their involvement with the criminal justice system. Time spent within the program is dependent on the terms and conditions of release decided by ongoing mental health assessments.

The mental health court system includes judges, prosecutors, defense attorneys, and other court personnel.

KEY TERMS

Criminal justice system—The system instituted by federal, state, and local governments to control and deter crime and to punish persons who violate laws.

Felony—A serious crime, such as murder, which is much more serious then a minor crime and much more severely punished than a misdemeanor crime, punishable by at least one year in prison.

Misdemeanor—A minor crime, such as petit larceny (petty theft), which is punishable by not more than one year in prison.

All have an interest or expertise in helping persons with mental illness or **substance abuse** disorders. There are approximately 175 mental health courts operating in the United States, and the program is administered by the Bureau of Justice Assistance and the **Substance Abuse and Mental Health Services Administration**.

The Justice and Mental Health Collaboration Program (JMHCP), a grant program that promotes public safety by facilitating collaboration among the criminal justice, juvenile justice, mental health treatment, and substance abuse systems, increases access to treatment for people with mental illnesses who are inside the criminal justice system by funding grants for mental health courts and similar programs. It was authorized by the Mentally Ill Offender Treatment and Crime Reduction Act of 2004 and is administrated by the Bureau of Justice Assistance (BJA), a division of the Office of Justice Programs.

Origins

In the 1980s, judges, attorneys, and jail officials, realizing that there were a large percentage of persons with mental illness being processed through the criminal justice system, began to call for more specific court-related treatment programs for these individuals. At that time, Judge Evan Dee Goodman, of the Marion Municipal Court in Indianapolis, Indiana, helped to establish a court to deal with mental health cases, which involved psychiatric treatment of criminals arrested on minor charges. The court was terminated in the early 1990s, but is still considered an early version of what came to be called the mental health court system.

In 1997, the first recognized mental health court opened in Broward County, Florida. Three years later, Congress passed the America's Law Enforcement and Mental Health Project Act to relieve the burden on the criminal justice system and on corrective institutions, and to provide individuals with the tools they need to stay out of the criminal justice system. In 2001, the first mental health court for juveniles began operations in Santa Clara, California.

Mental health courts were modeled after drug courts, which since 1989 have been providing drug treatment to addicts who are convicted of crimes. Individuals who complete drug court-mandated programs are eligible to have their criminal charges reduced or dismissed.

Process

Mental health courts generally take between 15 and 375 cases each year, a small percentage of defendants with mental illness. They try individuals with mental illness separately from other cases. Mental health courts vary in the kinds of mental health diagnoses and criminal charges they will accept, how the court monitors a defendant's treatment, and the kinds of pleas an individual can make. In the past, mental health courts would only accept people who were charged with nonviolent offenses, such as trespassing or vandalism. Today, some mental health courts will accept those who have committed more violent crimes, including assault and robbery, but these individuals often require additional supervision.

Although the process can vary from court to court, generally a defendant is referred to a mental health court. Referrals can come from a number of individuals, including family members, law enforcement officials, or judges. Defendants who are too violent or disturbed to appear in court may first be referred to a crisis center for stabilization.

In most mental health courts, defendants are required to plead "guilty" or "no contest" to qualify for treatment (referred to as the post-adjudication model). The defendant then receives a psychiatric evaluation, and, if deemed stable enough and eligible to stand trial in the mental health court, the judge will defer to the treatment decisions of mental health professionals. Mental health professionals under the direction of the court implement the treatment plan, which may include inpatient or outpatient counseling, housing placement, education, vocational training, job placement, health care, and rehabilitation for substance abuse, as needed.

During the treatment period, the patient must return to the court periodically for assessments. When a defendant successfully completes the treatment program, his or her case is considered resolved. Sometimes the charges will be reduced, and sometimes the case will be dismissed. Defendants who do not successfully complete the program are returned to a regular court for another trial, and they may have to face jail time if convicted.

Pros and cons

PROS. For the individuals and communities they serve, as well as for the criminal justice system in general, mental health courts offer several advantages over traditional courts:

- They improve the outcomes for people with mental illness by helping them obtain treatment.
- They lower recidivism rates for people with mental illness who enter the criminal justice system.
- They free jail cells for more serious offenders.
- They are considered a more cost-effective method than correctional institutions to treat defendants with mental illness.

CONS. The program has its critics, however. Some of the arguments against mental health courts, regardless of legitimacy, are as follows:

- They further stigmatize mental illness.
- They provide incentives to mentally ill individuals to commit crimes so that they can receive treatment.
- They could lead police to arrest people with mental illness just to get them into treatment.
- They divert resources used for mental illness treatment from the general community to those with criminal records.

Other arguments question the requirement of a guilty plea, claiming that some individuals with mental illness may not have the ability to make an informed decision. However, only persons deemed competent enough to stand trial are eligible for mental health courts, and participation is completely voluntary.

Results

Although there is little research available to confirm the effectiveness of mental health courts in general, there have been studies conducted on individual mental health courts that suggest positive outcomes. Research overall indicates that participants in mental health courts are less likely to return to jail and generally spend fewer days in jail than those who are processed through the regular court system.

A 1999 study presented at the symposium "Mental Health Courts: Promises and Limitations" followed offenders with mental illness who had spent an average of 18 days in mental hospitals and 85 days in jail in one year. The following year, while on Alaska's mental health court program, they spent only three days in mental hospitals and 16 days in jail. In 2001, in a Pittsburgh, Pennsylvania, mental health court, only 10% of 223 participants were arrested for a second time after completing their treatment programs.

A study conducted in the Broward County, Florida, mental health court and published in the July 2005 *Psychiatric Services* found that mentally ill defendants had greater access to treatment than they otherwise would have had, and they spent an average of 75% fewer days in jail compared to those who went through the traditional court system.

The August 2006 *Harvard Mental Health Letter* mentions a study conducted in California that found that offenders processed in a mental health court who were rearrested were generally charged with technical violations of parole rather than new crimes. Another California study of a mental health court in San Francisco, conducted in 2007, found that participants who had followed a treatment program for 18 months were 26% less likely to commit new crimes and 55% less likely to commit new violent crimes, compared to individuals with mental illness who had served the same amount of time in a county jail.

A study published in the February 2011 issue of *Archives of General Psychiatry* looked at outcomes of four mental health courts in California, Indiana, and Minnesota. The study found that mental health courts lowered subsequent arrest rates for persons completing treatment programs as part of these courts. In addition, the researchers, headed by Dr. Henry J. Steadman of Policy Research Associates (Delmar, New York), found that the time period during which individuals with serious psychiatric illnesses were incarcerated was also shortened after going through mental health court programs.

However, not all of the research has been positive. A study published in the July 2005 *Psychiatric Services* found a disproportionate balance of gender and ethnic groups represented in the mental health courts. Women and Caucasians in the study were more likely to be referred to mental health courts than were men and other ethnic groups, even though the majority of prison inmates are male (90%–94%) and minorities (63%). That study also found that participants in one mental health court had no significant improvement in clinical symptoms, compared to those who went through the general court system.

Resources

BOOKS

Frank, Richard, and Thomas G. McGuire. *Mental Health Treatment and Criminal Justice Outcomes*. Cambridge, MA: National Bureau of Economic Research, 2010.

Gideon, Lior, and Hung-En Sung, eds. *Rethinking Corrections: Rehabilitation, Reentry, and Reintegration*. Los Angeles: SAGE, 2011.

Johnson, Sandra J. *Assertive Community Treatment: Evidence-Based Practice or Managed Recovery*. New Brunswick, NJ: Transaction, 2011.

Rogers, Richard, and Daniel W. Shuman. *Fundamentals of Forensic Practice: Mental Health and Criminal Law*. New York: Springer, 2005.

Scott, Charles L., ed. *Handbook of Correctional Mental Health*. Washington, DC: American Psychiatric Publishing, 2010.

PERIODICALS

Schwartz, Emma. "Mental Health Courts." *U.S. World News and World Report* (February 7, 2008). http://www.usnews.com/news/national/articles/2008/02/07/mental-health-courts (accessed October 24, 2011).

Steadman, Henry J. "Effect of Mental Health Courts on Arrests and Jail Days: A Multisite Study." *Archives of General Psychiatry* 62, no. 2 (2011): 167–72.

OTHER

Almquist, Lauren, and Elizabeth Dodd. *Mental Health Courts: A Guide To Research-Informed Policy And Practice*. New York: Council of State Governments Justice Center, 2009. http://www.ojp.usdoj.gov/BJA/pdf/CSG_MHC_Research.pdf (accessed October 24, 2011).

Thompson, Michael, Fred Osher, and Denise Tomasini-Joshi. *Improving Responses to People with Mental Illnesses: The Essential Elements of a Mental Health Court*. New York: Council of State Governments Justice Center, 2007. http://www.ojp.usdoj.gov/BJA/pdf/MHC_Essential_Elements.pdf (accessed October 24, 2011).

WEBSITES

Bureau of Justice Assistance. "Mental Health Courts Program." Office of Justice Programs. http://www.ojp.usdoj.gov/BJA/grant/mentalhealth.html (accessed October 24, 2011).

Mental Health America. "Position Statement 53: Mental Health Courts." http://www.nmha.org/go/position-statements/53 (accessed October 24, 2011).

ORGANIZATIONS

Bureau of Justice Assistance, 810 Seventh St. NW, 4th Fl., Washington, DC, 20531, (202) 616-6500, (866) 859-2687, Fax: (202) 305-1367, http://www.ojp.usdoj.gov/BJA/index.html.

Council of State Governments Justice Center, 100 Wall St., 20th Fl., New York, NY, 10005, (212) 482-2320, http://www.justicecenter.csg.org.

National Alliance on Mental Illness, 3803 North Fairfax Drive, Ste. 100, Arlington, VA, 22203, (703) 524-7600, Fax: (703) 524-9094, http://www.nami.org.

National Council for Community Behavioral Healthcare, 1701 K St. NW, Ste. 400, Washington, DC, 20006, (202) 684-7457, Fax: (202) 386-9391, communications@thenationalcouncil.org, http://www.thenationalcouncil.org.

National Institute of Mental Health, 6001 Executive Blvd., Rm. 8184, MSC 9663, Bethesda, MD, 20892-9663, (301) 433-4513; TTY: (301) 443-8431, (866) 615-6464; TTY: (866) 415-8051, Fax: (301) 443-4279, nimhinfo@nih.gov, http://www.nimh.nih.gov.

Stephanie N. Watson
William A. Atkins

Mental health law

Definition

Mental health law is the body of laws and legal standards applied when considering the civil rights of a person with mental illness as defined by law. Key emphases include the areas of involuntary commitment and criminal justice.

Description

Mental health law is involved in the consideration of many issues, including:

- whether a person can be committed against his or her will
- what society's responsibility should be in treating individuals with mental disorders
- whether a mental disorder can serve as evidence that a crime did not involve criminal intent, and if so, at what severity

In legal terms, the concept of mental illness describes a person who is perceived to have impaired thoughts and emotions that may lead to the person being a threat to him/herself or others. The legal concept of mental illness is different from that of a therapist diagnosing a mental disorder. A clinically diagnosed psychological disorder is characterized by identifiable symptoms, clear origins, and recommended treatments. The constantly changing legal concept of mental illness is understandably broader, because it is influenced by societal concerns and the attempt to establish well-accepted criteria of what rights and responsibilities should be afforded someone with a mental illness has proven controversial.

Declaring someone mentally ill can serve as legal grounds for involuntary commitment in a mental hospital or institution. Mental illness also may serve as grounds for avoiding prosecution for a crime if the accused is deemed unable to discern right from wrong or to otherwise conform his or her behavior to societal standards. However, not everyone who demonstrates abnormal behavior has a mental disorder. Even persons with mental disorders have the right to choose their own lifestyle, unless it poses a danger to themselves or others.

Origins

The history of mental health law includes the parallel developments of humane treatment of persons with mental disabilities, respect for people with such disabilities, and recognition of the diminished reasoning ability of some accused criminals. These developments stemmed from an increased awareness of mental illness as a disease, reducing the mystery previously associated with it.

The theory of a biological basis for mental illness dates to ancient times. However, the most common treatments prior to the fifteenth century involved "mystical interventions." While the supernatural approach was gradually rejected over the next few centuries, treatments for mental health disorders were often odd and based upon unproven conjectures.

In the late 1800s, a cure for syphilis unexpectedly brought about the end of hallucinations and **delusions** in those infected. Many took this as a sign that all mental illnesses had a physical basis. A disease model for the cure of mental illness grew in acceptance. John Grey led the movement to make mental hospitals more comfortable and humane. Around the same time, Dorothea Dix worked to raise awareness of "mental hygiene," a humane approach to treating those with mental disabilities by encouraging social interaction.

In England, the M'Naghten rule was developed in response to the controversy that arose when members of a jury acquitted a murderer whom they believed acted out of insanity. To ensure a legal precedent in future cases of this sort, the M'Naghten rule emphasized that such a verdict could only apply if the accused was not aware of reality or the wrongness of his or her actions while committing the crime. This standard was later amended to allow the jury to decide whether the rules applied in each specific trial. The M'Naghten rule was the accepted standard in the United States until 1964, when the case of *Durham v. United States* (214 F.2d 862 (D.C. Cir. 1954)) brought about an analysis that developed new rules.

The Durham rule held that the accused was not guilty if the criminal act was the result of a mental illness or deficiency. This standard at first appeared to be more specific than the M'Naghten rule. However, it proved inadequate, because most mental health professionals could not agree on whether the behavior leading to a crime was the symptom of mental illness. Recognition of the inadequacies of the M'Naghten rule and the Durham rule led the legal profession to reexamine the insanity defense.

The movements for humane treatment of those with mental disabilities developed a focus of treating the person as someone of personal worth. The logical outgrowth of this focus was that, as individuals, persons with mental disabilities were entitled to rights, responsibilities, and privileges. Although it took until the modern era for these attitudes to take root, they originated in the teachings of reformers such as Benjamin Rush, Dorothea Dix, and John Grey. Laws respecting the rights of those with mental disabilities include establishing standards for involuntary commitment, least restrictive environment, and patient privacy.

The insanity defense

The limitation of the M'Naghten rule and the Durham rule led to a professional discussion of how to legally protect people who commit criminal acts while mentally disabled. If a driver is delusional and unaware of pedestrians, his or her actions could hurt or kill one of those pedestrians. However, because there is no criminal intent, the driver should not be punished. The legal question becomes how to distinguish both the effect of mental illness and the lack of criminal intent.

An American Law Institute committee addressed this question in 1962. Taking the position that punishment should deter crime, the American Law Institute suggested that treating the mental disorder would be more likely to deter future crime than would punishing the individual. Their standards focused on mental illness that prevented the person from understanding the wrongness of his or her actions, or from conforming to the requirements of the law. The American Law Institute also noted that mental illness did not apply to any abnormal trait resulting in repeated criminal or antisocial behavior. This seemingly limited the defense; however, another component of the American Law Institute's conclusions, the concept of diminished capacity, broadened the defense in a significant way. Diminished capacity holds that there is no criminal intent if the accused cannot understand the nature of his or her behavior due to mental illness. Diminished capacity made the standards of the M'Naghten rule more liberal and open-ended for the defendants to plea and the juries to decide. As a result, many states accepted diminished capacity as a foundation for the plea, "not guilty by reason of insanity."

This plea or jury finding has been controversial in recent decades due to several high-profile cases that shocked the general public. One case was that of John Hinckley, who attempted to assassinate President Ronald Reagan. Hinckley was found not guilty by reason of insanity. The idea that a would-be presidential assassin could escape punishment enraged many people. As a result, Congress passed the Insanity Defense Law, which moved the standards closer to the M'Naghten rule. The goal of the Insanity Defense Law was to make the insanity plea more difficult to apply.

A few years before Hinckley, another high-profile case was tried in San Francisco. Dan White, a resigned city supervisor, murdered Mayor George Moscone and Supervisor Harvey Milk. At White's trial, he successfully argued that he had suffered diminished capacity at the time of the shootings. The charge of murder was reduced to manslaughter, and he was out of prison in five years. The public outrage led to California eliminating its diminished capacity law, requiring stricter standards for an insanity plea.

The case of Andrea Yates also received much media attention. Yates murdered her five children in the summer of 2001 after years of suffering from clinical **depression** and **psychosis**. In her first trial, the jury could not accept that she did not know the wrongness of her actions, despite her history of mental illness. After a second trial, she was found not guilty by reason of insanity. One important result of Andrea Yates's first trial was the demonstration that a jury could distinguish between delusional thought and moral reasoning.

These cases have led people to protest the insanity plea, because they think it is misused more often than it serves justice. However, the reality is more sobering. A 1994 study by Silver, Cirincione, and Steadman found that random interviewees overestimated by two times the percentage of felonies acquitted by the insanity plea. The public's perception of how many felons attempt an insanity plea was also overestimated by forty times in this study. Further, the estimation of felons being released after a successful insanity plea was consistently higher on the survey than in reality, no matter how the question was qualified.

The "not guilty by reason of insanity" verdict is an awkward decision for many juries, as demonstrated by the Andrea Yates' case. Yates's second verdict was essentially "guilty, but with mental illness." This "guilty, but with mental illness" verdict has been advocated in cases where the jury feels that the accused should receive a prison sentence but urges that they receive treatment for their mental illness as well. Yates's guilty verdict was overturned on the condition that she would be admitted to a mental hospital until she was cured of her mental illness, but she is not expected to leave the mental hospital. Advocates of the "guilty, but with mental illness" verdict feel that if an accused person is cured of the mental disorder, he or she should still serve the remainder of his or her prison sentence.

Involuntary commitment

One key issue in mental health law is the involuntary commitment of people with mental disorders. Most societies feel a responsibility to help those who are unable to take care of themselves. The noble goal of asylums and mental hospitals throughout history has been to ensure that those with mental disabilities are cared for in ways that will reduce their symptoms and enhance their well-being. A lesser historical goal has been to remove these individuals from the daily life of the community. When reformers worked to ensure that the noble goal was met, the asylums tended to become overcrowded and therefore ineffective. Since their institution, many people have abused the asylums as a means of sending away troublesome family members. These considerations perennially raise the question, when is involuntary commitment appropriate for those with mental disabilities?

After the fall of the Soviet Union, many Americans were shocked to learn that political dissidents in the Soviet Union were routinely locked up and declared mentally ill based on their having disagreed with the government. However, similar situations have occurred in the United States. Many people with no diagnosed mental disabilities have been placed in mental hospitals indefinitely. When the Willowbrook hospital, maintained by the state of New York, was investigated in 1972, some of the inmates were found to have no symptoms of mental or developmental disability. Several had cerebral palsy and could not communicate effectively. Others had so little education in their youth that they appeared to have an intellectual disability but could have adapted to adult life had they not been confined. There was no sign of regular professional treatment for any disability. Unfortunately, such problems were found in many mental hospitals across the country.

In the 1970s, the case of Kenneth Donaldson drew the attention of the U.S. Supreme Court. Donaldson was held against his will at the Florida State Hospital for 15 years. During this time, he was diagnosed as paranoid schizophrenic, but the evidence was weak, and there was no follow-up **diagnosis**. During his year of confinement, he received no substantial treatment. In 1972, the Supreme Court ruled that a person's mental disability is not a sufficient reason for involuntary commitment. The decision stated that the government cannot commit someone when he or she is capable of self-care or is able to maintain an independent lifestyle with the willing support of concerned individuals, such as family members or friends. In 1979, the Court clarified the decision and stated that even if the person's quality of life could be improved through involuntary commitment, the state could not lock up a mentally ill person who was not dangerous. The state had to demonstrate that the person was dangerous to himself or others.

Consequently, a person who does need services or treatment for mental illness has a right to refuse them. The perceived effect has been that persons with severe mental disabilities who are not receiving treatment will most likely become involved in the legal system, a trend that has come to be known as the "criminalization of those with mental disabilities."

The Supreme Court rulings did not undermine the legal notion of *parens patriae*, which is the accepted idea that the state can become involved in a person's life to protect him or her from self-harm or **neglect**, even against the person's will. Many people with mental disabilities who might be well served by commitment live on the streets with no identifiable home. Their relatives argue that these homeless people do not understand how they are placing themselves at risk by refusing treatment. The National Alliance on Mental Illness represents such relatives in an effort to allow involuntary commitment out of concern for the individual. Homeless individuals with mental illness fit the description of someone who cannot independently take care of him/herself. Most civil commitment laws justify involuntary commitment in such cases.

KEY TERMS

Civil commitment—The involuntary confinement of those who cannot care for themselves.

Criminalization—The de facto societal trend over several decades of sending people with mental disabilities to jails and prisons instead of to institutions.

Deinstitutionalization—The movement to close ineffective, costly institutions with the goal of better serving people with mental disabilities in their homes and communities.

Diminished capacity—The inability of a person to understand the nature of his or her behavior when committing a criminal act.

Insanity defense—The common term for the defense that an accused person makes to argue against his or her actions having criminal intent because of an underlying mental illness.

Parens patriae—The legal concept by which the state has the responsibility to protect those with mental disabilities from self-harm.

Deinstitutionalization

A combination of overcrowding in the mental hospitals and Supreme Court decisions led to a movement of **deinstitutionalization** in the 1970s and early 1980s. The goal of this movement was to reduce the number of persons living in institutions by helping the residents live on their own outside the institution. The goal to close down the institutions was founded on many assumptions, some truer than others. One truth was that many of the institutions were inefficient, callous, and expensive to run. Many mental health advocates felt that the mentally disabled would be better served in a family environment, a group home, or a community-based treatment program.

One misconception behind deinstitutionalization was that new medications could reduce the need for institutions. In some conditions, this may hold true, so long as patients remember to take their medications regularly. However, not all conditions are treatable with medication, and some of the most successful treatments rely on a combination of medication and behavioral therapies. Also, without consistent monitoring, individuals can stop taking their medication and return to a state of disability.

Least restrictive environment

Least restrictive environment is a component of deinstitutionalization and maintains that persons with mental or developmental disabilities should receive services in the setting that most encourages the person's independence. This usually means living in facilities for those with severe disabilities. However, the facilities are expected to teach and encourage self-care, as well as foster dignity and self-respect among the residents. A person who can live independently with some monitoring could, for example, live in a group home with access to 24-hour support. The staff also should recognize the need for the individuals to make as many of their own decisions as they can reasonably handle. States that apply the concept of least restrictive environment tend to better balance the issues of serving those with disabilities without compromising their rights.

Resources

BOOKS

Durand, V. Mark, and David H. Barlow. *Essentials of Abnormal Psychology*. Belmont, CA: Wadsworth, Cengage Learning, 2010.

Erickson, Patricia E., and Stephen K. Erickson. *Crime, Punishment, and Mental Illness: Law and the Behavioral Sciences in Conflict*. New Brunswick, NJ: Rutgers University Press, 2008.

Gostin, Lawrence, et al., eds. *Principles of Mental Health Law and Policy*. New York: Oxford University Press, 2010.

Meyer, Robert G., and Christopher M. Weaver. *Law and Mental Health: A Case-Based Approach*. New York: The Guilford Press, 2005.

PERIODICALS

Atkinson, J. A., and Reilly, J. "The Recent History of Concepts of 'Dangerousness' in Mental Health Law in the UK." *History and Philosophy of Psychology* 13, no. 1 (2011): 45–51.

Bonnie, Richard J., et al. "Mental Health System Transformation after the Virginia Tech Tragedy." *Health Affairs* 28, no. 3 (2009): 793–803.

Taylor, Steven J. "Caught in the Continuum: A Critical Analysis of the Principle of the Least Restrictive Environment." *Research and Practice for Persons with Severe Disabilities* 29, no. 4 (2004).

WEBSITES

Mental Health America. "Position Statement 57: In Support of the Insanity Defense." http://www.nmha.org/go/position-statements/57 (accessed October 24, 2011).

World Health Organization. "Mental Health, Human Rights and Legislation." http://www.who.int/mental_health/policy/legislation/policy/en (accessed October 24, 2011).

ORGANIZATIONS

The Bazelon Center for Mental Health Law, 1101 15th Street NW, Suite 1212, Washington, DC, 20005, (202) 467-5730, info@bazelon.org, http://www.bazelon.org.

National Alliance on Mental Illness, 3803 N Fairfax Dr., Ste. 100, Arlington, VA, 22203, (703) 524-7600, (800) 950-NAMI (6264), http://www.nami.org.

Ray F. Brogan, PhD

Mental health and violence

Definition

As media reports of violent crimes committed by mentally ill persons are prominently featured worldwide, many people have come to associate mental illness with violence and aggression. Research shows that mentally ill persons receiving treatment are no more likely to display violence or aggression against others than people without mental illness, unless **substance abuse** is involved. Substance abuse raises the risk of violent behavior for persons both with and without mental illness. A major study published in 2009 revealed that although persons with mental illness were more likely to be a victim of violence than to commit a violent act, most people still regard people with mental illness as potentially dangerous. This misguided perception contributes to the isolation of persons with serious mental illness and for some helps potentiate a lack of integration into society.

Demographics

Mental illness happens to people in all societies regardless of gender, age, socioeconomic status, or location. According to the World Health Organization (WHO), more than 450 million people, or about 7% of the world's population, have a mental illness at any given time. When including mild **depression** or **anxiety disorders**, this estimate is likely lower than the actual prevalence of mental illness. In the United States and Western Europe, for example, about 25% of the adult population, or one in four adults, is estimated to have a diagnosable mental illness within any given year.

Serious mental illness, defined as any mental disorder that limits participation in the main activities of living including self-care, productive work, or communication with others, occurs much less frequently, or in about 5% of adults in the United States. The U.S. National Institutes of Health reports that females are more likely to be diagnosed with serious mental illness than males, and the peak prevalence of serious mental illness occurs in the 18–25 age group. It is among the seriously mentally ill group that most acts of violence committed by persons with mental illness occur, although this number is small. When a person with severe mental illness is in a period of **psychosis** (out of touch with reality and likely experiencing hallucinations or **delusions**), they are about three times more likely to be violent than when their illness is stabilized with treatment. Nevertheless, persons with serious mental illness are much more likely to harm themselves than to harm others.

Description

Aggression or violence does have a small correlation with **schizophrenia**, **post-traumatic stress disorder**, and **borderline personality disorder** when the disease remains untreated. Schizophrenia is a chronic **brain** disorder that affects about 1% of the population. People with schizophrenia tend to interpret reality and everyday stimuli in an abnormal fashion. Thinking and communication is sometimes disordered, and hallucinations can be present, as well as delusions and **paranoia**. Schizophrenia tends to be a long-term condition and affected persons rely on medication and supportive therapy to cope with symptoms and maintain daily function in life's activities. In the unlikely event that an untreated person with schizophrenia becomes aggressive toward others, the aggression is usually committed at home and is usually focused toward family members or friends.

Post-traumatic stress disorder (PTSD) is a form of anxiety disorder that stems from the physical and psychological reactions of witnessing a traumatic or dangerous event. When it is in danger, the body releases stress hormones that initiate the "fight-or-flight" response, shunting blood to the major muscle groups, heightening senses, and allowing the body it's best chance to perform in a manner that will survive the threatening situation. In PTSD, the body reacts to everyday stimuli by the same method as if it was still experiencing the danger. A person with PTSD can experience anger and difficulty concentrating or sleeping, can become preoccupied with frightening thoughts, and can experience physical sensations such as a racing heart while they relive the danger during flashbacks. When PTSD is accompanied by depression and left untreated, it can be associated with an increase in aggression or violence toward a domestic partner or rarely toward others. Relationship violence in PTSD has been linked to both men and women with PTSD.

Persons with borderline personality disorder (BPD) experience reoccurring patterns of disordered and unstable mood and self-image. They have difficulty maintaining close relationships; their feelings are intense but also include frequent and marked shifts. People with borderline personality disorder may function highly in an environment such as work or school by manipulating others, but can have difficulty forming attachments. A person with BPD is likely to be impulsive, impatient, and to display anger as in a temper tantrum, or, alternatively, to display brooding and antipathy. Trusting others is difficult. When following impulses, some people with BPD resort to excessive spending, gambling, or substance abuse. Depression and feelings of inadequacy often accompany BPD, as well as fears of abandonment and, occasionally, brief periods of psychosis can occur. Although the vast majority of people with BPD are not violent or criminals, the condition has been linked with criminality and episodes of violent behavior. People with BPD are also more likely to harm themselves than to harm others.

Causes and symptoms

Violent behavior is not a symptom of mental illness. Severe mental illness can include symptoms such as delusions and hallucinations that seem real and are frightening to a person with disordered thoughts. These may be heightened by perceived threats if a person is experiencing paranoia. When a person experiences these symptoms during a period of psychosis, he or she could possibly become aggressive, only because they are afraid and misunderstanding what is happening around them. When a person with PTSD feels the physical symptoms that accompany a sense of danger, he or she could also misinterpret what is happening and react with aggression.

KEY TERMS

Delusion—A fixed and irrational belief.

Hallucination—An unreal perception involving any of the senses that appears real to the person experiencing the hallucination.

Paranoia—An unwarranted sense of suspicion or being persecuted.

Psychosis—A state of impaired, disorganized thought that does not include recognizing reality.

Aggression or violence associated with BPD is usually the result of impulsivity.

Mental illness can happen to anyone and is most likely due to a complex combination of genetic and environmental factors that trigger chemistry changes in the brain. Genetic vulnerabilities likely set the stage for mental illness, which can be potentiated by environmental stressors such as experiencing **neglect**, abuse, violence, or traumatic events. Scientists are also studying the potential roles of vitamin deficiencies, brain injury, complications during birth, drug abuse, and certain infections in the development of mental illness.

Diagnosis

Diagnosis of a serious mental disorder is most often made by a **psychiatrist**, a physician specializing in mental health, mental illness, and brain chemistry. Criteria for each psychiatric diagnosis is set forth in a standard called the ***Diagnostic and Statistical Manual of Mental Disorders***, currently in its fourth edition (with the fifth due for publication in 2013). Psychiatrists usually diagnose a psychiatric disorder based upon observation and conversation with their patient, although physical examination, image studies, and lab work can also provide relevant information to support a diagnosis. When a person has a serious mental illness, physicians or therapists routinely assess the potential for self-harm or aggression toward others as part of the overall treatment plan.

Treatment

Treatment for serious mental illness usually involves both psychotropic medicines and **cognitive-behavioral therapy**. Medicines help maintain a balanced mood and reduce the hallucinations and other troubling symptoms of mental illness. This does not cure the mental illness, but it allows the person to better function and to gain the most value from additional therapy. Cognitive-behavioral therapy (**talk therapy**) examines the particular feelings and perceptions that interfere with a person's ability to function in society with a normal sense of self and their environment. Therapists help the person with mental illness to recognize their maladaptive thoughts and to examine their validity, and then to cope with them by adopting alternative thoughts. For most people with severe mental illness, these therapies can be delivered in an outpatient setting. Temporary inpatient care helps during a period of psychosis or acute crisis. Key to reducing or eliminating periods of psychosis is continued medication and therapy and rapid access to a healthcare provider when symptoms increase.

Prognosis

Serious mental illnesses are treatable conditions, and most people experience relief from symptoms and a better quality of life as long as treatment continues. When mental illness is treated and there is no concurrent abuse of drugs or alcohol, then a person with mental illness is no more likely to commit a violent act than the general population. In fact, the majority of violence in the United States is committed by young males aged 18–30, with drugs or alcohol often a contributing factor. Only 1 in 200 persons with schizophrenia is likely to seriously injure someone else over the course of a lifetime, and he or she is many times more likely to commit **suicide** than to seriously harm someone else.

Prevention

Identifying mental illness as early as possible and receiving effective treatment is key to preventing violence among people with serious mental illness. This is particularly important during the first episode of illness, as it sets a pattern for recognizing dealing with the illness in a positive rather than aggressive manner. Treating any substance abuse problems concurrently with the mental illness is also a top priority to help prevent violence. When a rare violent tragedy occurs with a link to mental illness, it is a likely indication that something is wrong with the individual's treatment (or lack of treatment), or even the mental health care system as a whole. Quick access to mental health care and follow up remains a challenge for public health officials. Ideally, a person with serious mental illness would have rapid access to therapy and medications that lasts for as long as they need it.

Since the 2007 shootings at Virginia Tech university in Blacksburg, Virginia, that were carried out by a student diagnosed with a severe mental illness, universities, workplaces, and other and institutions across the United States have taken action to recognize and help members of their communities with mental illness that could be feeling stress or in crisis. Along with rapid communication systems via e-mail or text, counselors are often on call around the clock to enable rapid **intervention**. National and state governments are also re-examining some aspects of privacy laws that currently allow persons diagnosed with severe mental illness to fall between the cracks of the healthcare system regarding follow up. Any change in these laws will be carefully considered in order to balance the privacy rights of the individual with their need for access to continuing treatment.

Removing the **stigma** from mental illness is also important to helping persons with severe mental illness integrate into their communities without fear of persecution. When media outlets sensationalize the rare violent acts made by persons with mental illness, the public tends to distance themselves from people with mental illness and perpetuate inaccurate stereotypes. As the public begins to recognize that people with mental illness are more often the victim of violence, not the perpetrators of violence, mental illness will no longer be considered the first explanation for aggressive or violent behavior.

Resources

BOOKS

Empie, Kristine M. *Workplace Violence and Mental Illness.* New York: LFB Scholarly, 2003.

McFarlane, Alexander C., G. D. Schrader, and C. Bookless. *The Prevalence of Victimization and Violent Behavior in the Seriously Mentally Ill.* Canberra: Australian Institute of Criminology, 2005.

Serper, Mark R., and Andrea J. Bergman. *Psychotic Violence, Methods, Motives, Madness.* Madison, CT: Psychosocial Press, 2003.

Yakeley, Jessica. *Working with Violence: A Contemporary Psychoanalytic Approach.* Basingstoke, UK: Palgrave Macmillan, 2010.

PERIODICALS

American Psychiatric Association. *American Psychiatric Association Fact Sheet: Violence and Mental Illness.* Washington, DC: American Psychiatric Association, 1994.

Corrigan, P. W., A. C. Watson, A. C. Warpinski, and G. Gracia. "Implications of Educating the Public on Mental Illness, Violence, and Stigma." *Psychiatric Services* 55, no. 5 (2004): 577–80.

Douglas, K.S., S. D. Hart, and L. S. Guy. "Psychosis as a Risk Factor for Violence to Others: A Meta-Analysis." *Psychological Bulletin* 135, no. 5 (2009): 679–706.

Friedman, Richard A. "Mental Illness and Violence: How Strong is the Link?" *New England Journal of Medicine* 355, no. 20 (2006): 2064–66.

Langan, J. "Challenging Assumptions About Risk Factors and the Role of Screening for Violence Risk in the Field of

Mental Health." *Health, Risk and Society* 12, no. 2 (2010): 85–100.

Volavka J., and J. Swanson. "Violent Behavior in Mental Illness: the Role of Substance Abuse." *JAMA: the Journal of the American Medical Association* 304, no. 5 (2010): 563–64.

OTHER

Gonzales, Alberto R., Michael O. Leavitt, and Margaret Spellings. "Report to the President on Issues Raised by the Virginia Tech Tragedy." U.S. Department of Health and Human Services. http://www.hhs.gov/vtreport.pdf (accessed February 7, 2011).

"Violence and Mental Illness: Unpacking the Myths." Canadian Mental Health Association. http://www.cmha.bc.ca/files/3-violence_myths.pdf (accessed February 7, 2011).

WEBSITES

National Institute of Mental Health. "New Factors Identified for Predicting Violence in Schizophrenia." Science Update. July 18, 2006. http://www.nimh.nih.gov/science-news/2006/new-factors-identified-for-predicting-violence-in-schizophrenia.shtml (accessed February 7, 2011).

SANE Australia. "Violence and Mental Illness." http://www.sane.org/information/factsheets-podcasts/209-violence-and-mental-illness (accessed February 7, 2011).

Trudeau, Michelle. "Researchers Investigate Aggressive Students' Mental Health." *Morning Edition*, NPR (National Public Radio). http://www.npr.org/templates/story/story.php?storyId=5642298 (accessed February 7, 2011).

Brenda Wilmoth Lerner, RN

Mental retardation *see* **Intellectual disability**

Mental status examination

Definition

A mental status examination (MSE) is an assessment of a patient's level of cognitive (knowledge-related) ability, appearance, emotional mood, and speech and thought patterns at the time of evaluation. It is one part of a full neurologic (nervous system) examination and includes the examiner's observations about the patient's attitude and cooperativeness as well as the patient's answers to specific questions. The most commonly used MSE is the Folstein Mini-Mental Status Examination (MMSE), developed in 1975.

Purpose

The purpose of a mental status examination is to assess the presence and extent of a person's mental impairment. The cognitive functions that are measured during the MSE include the person's sense of time, place, and personal identity; memory; speech; general intellectual level; mathematical ability; insight or judgment; and reasoning or problem-solving ability. Complete MSEs are most commonly given to elderly people and to other patients being evaluated for **dementia** (including AIDS-related dementia). Dementia is an overall decline in a person's intellectual function—including difficulties with language, simple calculations, planning or decision-making, and motor (muscular movement) skills, as well as loss of memory. The MSE is an important part of the differential **diagnosis** of dementia and other psychiatric symptoms or disorders. The MSE results may suggest specific areas for further testing or specific types of required tests. A mental status examination can also be given repeatedly to monitor or document changes in a patient's condition.

Description

The MMSE of Folstein evaluates five areas of mental status, namely, orientation, registration, attention and calculation, recall, and language. A complete MSE is more comprehensive and evaluates the following ten areas of functioning:

- Appearance. The examiner notes the person's age, race, sex, civil status, and overall appearance. These features are significant because poor personal hygiene or grooming may reflect a loss of interest in self-care or physical inability to bathe or dress oneself.
- Movement and behavior. The examiner observes the person's gait (manner of walking), posture, coordination, eye contact, facial expressions, and similar behaviors. Problems with walking or coordination may reflect a disorder of the central nervous system.
- Affect. Affect refers to a person's outwardly observable emotional reactions. It may include either a lack of emotional response to an event or an overreaction.
- Mood. Mood refers to the underlying emotional "atmosphere" or tone of the person's answers.
- Speech. The examiner evaluates the volume of the person's voice, the rate or speed of speech, the length of answers to questions, the appropriateness and clarity of the answers, and similar characteristics.
- Thought content. The examiner assesses what the patient is saying for indications of hallucinations, delusions, obsessions, symptoms of dissociation, or thoughts of suicide. Dissociation refers to the splitting off of certain memories or mental processes from conscious awareness. Dissociative symptoms include feelings of unreality, depersonalization, and confusion about one's identity.

- Thought process. Thought process refers to the logical connections between thoughts and their relevance to the main thread of conversation. Irrelevant detail, repeated words and phrases, interrupted thinking (thought blocking), and loose, illogical connections between thoughts, may be signs of a thought disorder.
- Cognition. Cognition refers to the act or condition of knowing. The evaluation assesses the person's orientation (ability to locate himself or herself) with regard to time, place, and personal identity; long- and short-term memory; ability to perform simple arithmetic (counting backward by threes or sevens); general intellectual level or fund of knowledge (identifying the last five presidents, or similar questions); ability to think abstractly (explaining a proverb); ability to name specified objects and read or write complete sentences; ability to understand and perform a task (showing the examiner how to comb one's hair or throw a ball); ability to draw a simple map or copy a design or geometrical figure; ability to distinguish between right and left.
- Judgment. The examiner asks the person what he or she would do about a common-sense problem, such as running out of a prescription medication.
- Insight. Insight refers to a person's ability to recognize a problem and understand its nature and severity.

The length of time required for an MSE depends on the patient's condition. It may take as little as five minutes to examine a healthy person. Patients with speech problems or intellectual impairments, dementia, or other organic **brain** disorders may require 15 or 20 minutes. The examiner may choose to spend more time on certain portions of the MSE and less time on others, depending on the patient's condition and answers.

Preparation

Preparation for an MSE includes a careful medical and psychiatric history of the patient. The history helps the examiner to interpret the patient's appearance and answers with greater accuracy, because some physical illnesses may produce psychiatric symptoms or require medications that influence the patient's mood or attentiveness. The psychiatric history should include a family history as well as the patient's personal history of development, behavior patterns, and previous treatment for mental disorders (if any). Symptoms of dissociation, for example, often point to a history of childhood **abuse**, rape, or other severe emotional traumas in adult life. The examiner should also include information about the patient's occupation, level of education, marital status, and right- or left-handedness. Information about occupation and education helps in evaluating the patient's use of language, extent of memory loss, reasoning ability, and similar functions. Handedness is important in determining which half of the patient's brain is involved in writing, picking up a pencil, or other similar tasks that he or she may be asked to perform during the examination.

KEY TERMS

Aphasia—The loss of the ability to speak, or to understand written or spoken language. A person who cannot speak or understand language is said to be aphasic.

Cognition—The mental activities associated with thinking, learning, and memory.

Coma—A state of prolonged unconsciousness in which a person cannot respond to spoken commands or mildly painful physical stimuli.

Delusion—A belief that is resistant to reason or contrary to actual fact. Common delusions include delusions of persecution, delusions about one's importance (sometimes called delusions of grandeur), or delusions of being controlled by others.

Dementia—A decline in a person's level of intellectual functioning. Dementia includes memory loss as well as difficulties with language, simple calculations, planning or decision-making, and motor (muscular movement) skills.

Differential diagnosis—Comparing and contrasting the signs, symptoms, and laboratory findings of two or more diseases to determine which is causing the patient's condition.

Dissociation—The splitting off of certain mental processes from conscious awareness. Specific symptoms of dissociation include feelings of unreality, depersonalization, and confusion about one's identity.

Hallucination—A sensory experience, usually involving either sight or hearing, of something that does not exist outside the mind.

Illusion—A false visual perception of an object that others perceive correctly. A common example is the number of sightings of "UFOs" that turn out to be airplanes or weather balloons.

Obsession—Domination of thoughts or feelings by a persistent idea, desire, or image.

Organic brain disorder—An organic brain disorder refers to impaired brain function due to damage or deterioration of brain tissue.

Aftercare

Depending on the examiner's specific observations, the patient may be given additional tests for follow-up. These tests might include blood or urine samples to test for drug or alcohol abuse, anemia, diabetes, disorders of the liver or kidneys, vitamin or thyroid deficiencies, medication side effects, syphilis, or AIDS. Brain imaging (CT, MRI, or **PET** scans) may be used to look for signs of **seizures**, strokes, head **trauma**, brain tumors, or other evidence of damage to specific parts of the brain. A spinal tap may be performed if the doctor thinks the patient may have an infection of the central nervous system.

Precautions

An MSE cannot be given to a patient who cannot pay attention to the examiner, such as may be the case with a patient who is in a coma or unconscious, completely unable to speak (aphasic), or not fluent in the language of the examiner.

Results

Normal results for a mental status examination depend to some extent on the patient's history, level of education, and recent life events. For example, a depressed mood is appropriate in the context of a recent death or other sad event in the patient's family but inappropriate in the context of a recent pay raise. Speech patterns are often influenced by racial or ethnic background as well as by occupation or schooling. In general, however, the absence of obvious **delusions**, hallucinations, or thought disorders together with the presence of insight, good judgment, and socially appropriate appearance and behavior are considered normal results. A normal numerical score for the MMSE is between 28 and 30.

Abnormal results for a mental status examination include:

- any evidence of organic brain damage
- evidence of thought disorders
- a mood or affect that is clearly inappropriate to its context
- thoughts of suicide
- disturbed speech patterns
- dissociative symptoms
- delusions or hallucinations

A score below 27 on the MMSE usually indicates an organic brain disorder.

Resources

BOOKS

McPhee, Stephen, and Maxine Papadakis. *Current Medical Diagnosis and Treatment, 2010*. 49th ed. New York: McGraw-Hill Medical, 2009.

Porter, Robert S., and Justin L. Kaplan, eds. *The Merck Manual of Diagnosis and Therapy*. 19th ed. Whitehouse Station, NJ: Merck Research Laboratories, 2011.

Rebecca J. Frey, PhD

Mesoridazine

Definition

Mesoridazine is a member of the phenothiazine family of drugs (drugs that reduce the action of the neurotransmitter **dopamine** in the **brain**) and is sold under the brand name Serentil in the United States.

Purpose

Mesoridazine is effective in the treatment of **schizophrenia**, alcoholism, psychoneuroses (disorders of the brain), and organic brain disorders (disorders caused by temporary brain dysfunction or permanent brain damage).

Description

When used for the treatment of schizophrenia, mesoridazine reduces symptoms of emotional withdrawal, anxiety, tension, hallucinations, reduced **affect**, and **paranoia** (suspiciousness). It is often useful in persons for whom other tranquilizers are ineffective. In treating organic brain syndrome, mesoridazine effectively manages hyperactivity and difficult behaviors associated with mental deficiency. Mesoridazine relieves anxiety, nausea, vomiting, tension, and **depression** when used to treat alcoholism. It does not have side effects that affect liver function. It relieves similar symptoms when used to treat persons with psychoneurotic disorders.

Mesoridazine can be taken by mouth or given by intramuscular injection. It is supplied as 25 mg/mL in injection form, and tablets are supplied in 10, 25, 50, and 100 mg strengths.

Recommended dosage

The usual dosage used for treating schizophrenia is 50–400 mg per day and is usually administered three

KEY TERMS

Anxiety—An emotion that can be experienced as a troubled feeling, sense of dread, fear of the future, or distress over a possible threat to a person's physical or mental well-being.

Depression—A mental state characterized by feelings of sadness, despair, discouragement, and low energy, often with overeating and/or over-sleeping.

Dopamine—A chemical in brain tissue that serves as a neurotransmitter (transmitter of nerve impulses) and helps to regulate movement and emotions.

Hallucinations—To hear, see, or otherwise sense things that are not real. Hallucinations can result from nervous system abnormalities, mental disorders, or the use of certain drugs.

Insomnia—The inability to fall asleep or remain asleep.

Schizophrenia—A major mental illness marked by psychotic symptoms, including hallucinations, delusions, and severe disruptions in thinking.

times per day. It is begun at a low level and slowly increased until an adequate therapeutic effect is achieved. For persons with organic brain syndrome, an optimum dosage is 75–300 mg per day, administered in three equal amounts. The optimum dosage for persons being treated for alcoholism is 50–300 mg per day, administered in three doses. The usual dosage range for persons with psychoneuroses is 30–150 mg per day, administered in three equal amounts.

Precautions

Before taking mesoridazine, patients should read the accompanying medication guide. Mesoridazine has the potential to produce a serious syndrome called **tardive dyskinesia**. This syndrome consists of involuntary, uncoordinated movements (especially of the tongue, jaw, mouth, or face). It usually develops either late in the course of treatment or after medication has been discontinued and is potentially irreversible. Symptoms similar to those experienced by people with Parkinson's disease have been linked with the administration of mesoridazine. Mesoridazine is inappropriate for use with central nervous system depression, and it should not be administered to persons in a coma.

QUESTIONS TO ASK YOUR DOCTOR

- What kind of changes can I expect to see or feel with this medication?
- Does it matter what time of day I take this medication? If so, what is the recommendation?
- Should I take this medication with or without food?
- What are the side effects associated with this medication?
- Will this medication interact or interfere with other medications I am currently taking?
- What symptoms or adverse effects are important enough that I should seek immediate treatment?

Side effects

A serious and relatively common side effect of mesoridazine is tardive dyskinesia, a potentially irreversible syndrome for which there is no known effective treatment. The chances of developing tardive dyskinesia increase with both increasing dosage and increasing patient age.

The most common side effects of mesoridazine are drowsiness and low blood pressure and are most frequently reported in persons given relatively high dosages. Side effects also tend to appear relatively early in treatment. Mesoridazine tends to have a remarkably low incidence of side effects compared to other phenothiazine compounds. However, as mentioned, Parkinson-like symptoms have been linked with the administration of mesoridazine. These include restlessness and akathisia (agitation) and dystonia (difficulty walking or moving). These are generally controlled with **benztropine** mesylate or **trihexyphenidyl** hydrochloride.

Other known side effects include:

- anxiety
- restlessness
- agitation
- insomnia
- headache
- euphoria
- drowsiness
- depression
- confusion
- dizziness

Unwanted or unexpected effects associated with the use of mesoridazine have been reported for virtually all organ systems in the body. Although numerous, such side effects are relatively uncommon. An occasionally reported side effect is **neuroleptic malignant syndrome**, a complicated and potentially fatal condition characterized by muscle rigidity, high fever, alterations in mental status, and cardiac symptoms such as irregular pulse or blood pressure, sweating, tachycardia and arrhythmias.

Interactions

Mesoridazine increases the effect of drugs and substances that depress the central nervous system. This class of drugs includes anesthetics, opiates, **barbiturates**, atropine, and alcohol.

Resources

BOOKS

Albers, Lawrence J., Rhoda K. Hahn, and Christopher Reist. *Handbook of Psychiatric Drugs.* Laguna Hills, CA: Current Clinical Strategies, 2010.

American Society of Health-System Pharmacists. *AHFS Drug Information 2011.* Bethesda, MD: ASHP, 2011.

Graham, George. *The Disordered Mind: An Introduction to Philosophy of Mind and Mental Illness.* New York: Routledge, 2010.

Holland, Leland Norman, and Michael Patrick Adams. *Core Concepts in Pharmacology.* 3rd ed. New York: Prentice Hall, 2011.

North, Carol, and Sean Yutzy. *Goodwin and Guze's Psychiatric Diagnosis.* New York: Oxford University Press, 2010.

Preston, John D., John H. O'Neal, and Mary C. Talaga. *Handbook of Clinical Psychopharmacology for Therapists.* 6th ed. Oakland, CA: New Harbinger, 2010.

PERIODICALS

Dallaire, S. "Thioridazine (Mellaril) and Mesoridazine (Serentil): Prolongation of the QTc Interval." *Canadian Medical Association Journal* 164, no. 1 (2001): 91–95.

Nelson, J.C. "Diagnosing and Treating Depression in the Elderly." *Journal of Clinical Psychiatry* 62, Supp. 24 (2001): 18–22.

Ray, W.A., S. Meredith, P.B. Thapa, K.G. Meador, K. Hall, and K.T. Murray. "Antipsychotics and the Risk of Sudden Cardiac Death." *Archives of General Psychiatry* 58, no. 12 (2001): 1161–67.

Varvel A., E. Vann, E. Wise, D. Philibin, and H. Porter. "Effects of Antipsychotic Drugs on Operant Responding After Acute and Repeated Administration." *Psychopharmacology (Berlin)* 160, no. 2 (2002): 182–91.

ORGANIZATIONS

American Academy of Clinical Toxicology, 6728 Old McLean Village Dr., McLean, VA, 22101, (703) 556-9222, Fax: (703) 556-8729, admin@clintox.org, http://www.clintox.org.

American Academy of Family Physicians, 11400 Tomahawk Creek Pkwy., Leawood, KS, 66211-2672, (913) 906-6000, (800) 274-2237, Fax: (913) 906-6075, contactcenter@aafp.org, http://www.aafp.org.

American Psychiatric Association, 1000 Wilson Blvd., Ste. 1825, Arlington, VA, 22209-3901, (703) 907-7300, apa@psych.org, http://www.psych.org.

American Psychological Association, 750 1st St. NE, Washington, DC, 20002-4242, (202) 336-5500; TDD/TTY: (202) 336-6123, (800) 374-2721, http://www.apa.org.

American Society for Clinical Pharmacology and Therapeutics, 528 N Washington St., Alexandria, VA, 22314, (703) 836-6981, info@ascpt.org, http://www.ascpt.org.

National Alliance on Mental Illness, 2107 Wilson Blvd., Ste. 300, Arlington, VA, 22201-3042, Fax: (703) 524-9094, (800) 950-6264, http://www.nami.org.

National Institute of Mental Health, 6001 Executive Blvd., Rm. 8184, MSC 9663, Bethesda, MD, 20892-9663, (301) 433-4513; TTY: (301) 443-8431, Fax: (301) 443-4279, (866) 615-6464; TTY: (866) 415-8051, nimhinfo@nih.gov, http://www.nimh.nih.gov.

U.S. Food and Drug Administration, 10903 New Hampshire Ave., Silver Spring, MD, 20993-0002, (888) INFO-FDA (463-6332), http://www.fda.gov.

L. Fleming Fallon, Jr., MD, DrPH
Laura Jean Cataldo, RN, EdD

Methadone

Definition

Methadone is classified as an opioid (an analgesic that is used for severe pain). In the United States, methadone is also known as dolophine, methenex and methadose.

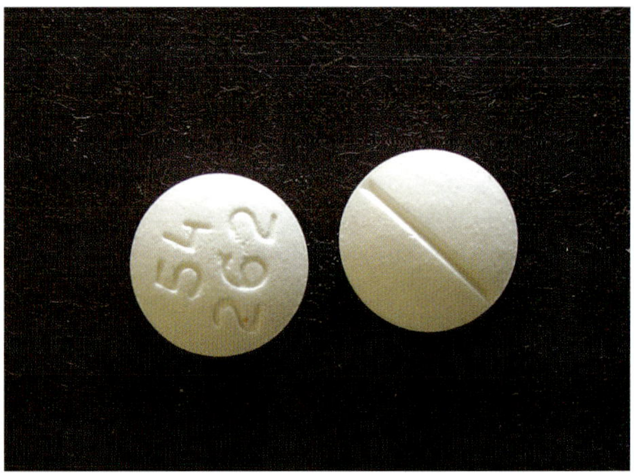

Methadone, 30 mg. *(© Custom Medical Stock Photo, Inc. Reproduced by permission.)*

Purpose

Methadone is used in the long-term maintenance treatment of narcotic **addiction**. Both heroin and methadone are **opioids**; as such, methadone and heroin bind to the same places in the **brain**. Methadone, however, is the opioid of choice for the treatment of narcotic addiction since it is longer lasting and patients do not experience the "high" associated with the drug of abuse. In opioid maintenance therapy, a person addicted to heroin receives methadone instead of heroin. Essentially, the person is switched from an opioid that gives a "high" to an opioid that does not. The dose of methadone may then be decreased over time so that the person can overcome his or her opioid addiction without experiencing withdrawal symptoms, or, after a person has received methadone for a period of time, he or she may choose to go through **detoxification** with **clonidine**. In the United States, methadone treatment is associated with a significant reduction in predatory crime, improvement in socially acceptable behavior and psychological well-being.

Methadone may also be prescribed for pain relief, but in these cases, the physician must note this use on the prescription.

Description

Methadone has been used successfully to treat narcotic addiction for over twenty years in the United States. Methadone is the only FDA-approved agent in its class for the maintenance treatment of narcotic addiction.

Methadone for maintenance treatment is dispensed in methadone clinics. The program needs to be registered with the Drug Enforcement Administration. For admission to methadone treatment in clinical programs, federal standards mandate a minimum of one year of opiate addiction as well as current evidence of addiction. Pregnant, opiate-addicted females can be admitted with less than a one-year history and AIDS patients are routinely accepted. New patients must report daily, take medication under observation, and participate in recommended psychosocial treatments.

Some studies have shown that more than 50% of patients in methadone clinics do not abuse drugs in the first month of treatment. After 10 months, however, the success rate drops to approximately 20%. Moreover, major **depression** is a powerful predictor of **relapse** in methadone treatment. If the patient has dual addictions (alcoholism along with the heroin addiction, for example), management of the other addiction increases the success rate of the methadone therapy. Proper psychiatric and psychological treatment can considerably improve methadone treatment outcome.

In the cases of pregnant women who are addicted to heroin, detoxification (discontinuing the opioid altogether) is associated with a high rate of spontaneous abortions in the first trimester and premature delivery in the third trimester. Therefore, pregnant women can be in methadone maintenance programs if they are at risk of returning to drug dependence. These women should receive the lowest effective dose, receive appropriate prenatal care, and be warned about risks of returning to drug abuse, as well as the dangers associated with withdrawal effects of methadone. Methadone is associated with lower birth weights and smaller head circumference, but it has never been shown that this has any impact on the infants' further development.

Methadone is available in 5, 10, and 40 mg tablets and a solution.

Recommended dosage

The initial dose of methadone is 20 mg daily with additional 10 mg given four to eight hours later. After achieving initial dosing of about 40 mg daily, the dose should be increased since there is evidence that the relapse rate is significantly lower in patients on 80-100 mg daily rather than 40-50 mg daily. The stabilization to maintenance dosing requires one to three months.

The minimum effective dose is 60 mg daily. Patients on lower maintenance doses have recently been studied and have shown shorter treatment retention and have continued heroin use. If patients are stable on methadone for six months or longer, their methadone dose should not be increased by 33% or more, as this sudden increase in dose is associated with an increase in craving for the drugs that were previously abused. Some heroin patients need to be on doses up to 180 mg daily to provide adequate maintenance and to prevent relapse.

Precautions

Methadone should not be used in patients who have had hypersensitivity to methadone. Patients who experience an allergic reaction to other opioids, which may include a generalized rash or shortness of breath, such as morphine, hydromorphone, oxymorphone, or codeine may try methadone. They are less likely to develop the same reaction since methadone has a different chemical structure. Methadone should be administered carefully in patients with pre-existing respiratory problems, history of bowel obstruction, glaucoma, renal problems, and hyperthyroidism.

As stated, pregnant women can be in methadone maintenance programs if they are at risk of returning to drug dependence. Methadone is associated with smaller birth weights and smaller head circumference.

Intentional or accidental overdose of methadone can lead to unconsciousness, coma, or death. The signs of methadone overdose include confusion, difficulty speaking, **seizures**, severe nervousness or restlessness, severe dizziness, severe drowsiness, and/or slow or troubled breathing. These symptoms are increased by alcohol or other central nervous system (CNS) depressants. Anyone who feels that he or she, or someone else, may have overdosed on methadone, or a combination of methadone and other central nervous system depressants, should seek emergency medical attention for that person at once.

Side effects

Most adverse effects of methadone are mild and seen only in the beginning of therapy. Initially patients may develop sedation and analgesia. It takes about four to six weeks for tolerance to these effects to develop. Tolerance to constipation and sweating may take longer to develop.

A few patients who are on larger doses of methadone may experience respiratory problems. These patients also may experience unwanted cardiac effects.

A small number of patients report a decrease in libido, impotence, and premature, delayed, or failed ejaculation. There are a few reports of occasional menstrual irregularities in female patients on methadone.

Interactions

Life-threatening interactions with other drugs have not been identified. One of the initial side effects of methadone could include dizziness and sedation, and these effects are worsened if the patient is also taking other narcotics, **benzodiazepines**, or is consuming alcohol.

Methadone magnifies the effects of alcohol and other central nervous system depressants, such as antihistamines, cold medicines, **sedatives**, tranquilizers, other prescription and over-the-counter (OTC) pain medications, **barbiturates**, seizure medications, muscle relaxants, and certain anesthetics including some dental anesthetics. Alcohol and other central nervous system depressants should not be taken or consumed while methadone is being taken.

Monoamine oxidase inhibitors (MAOIs), such as Parnate (**tranylcypromine**) and Nardil (**phenelzine**), should be avoided by people taking methadone. Medications like **naltrexone** and naloxone should never be used concurrently with methadone. People must stop taking methadone for 7 to 10 days before starting naltrexone or naloxone.

See also Alcohol and related disorders; Disease concept of chemical dependency; Opioids and related disorders

Resources

BOOKS

Albers, Lawrence J., Rhoda K. Hahn, and Christopher Reist. *Handbook of Psychiatric Drugs. 2001–2002*. Laguna Hills, CA: Current Clinical Strategies Publishing, 2008.

Kay, Jerald, Allan Tasman, and Jeffrey A. Lieberman. *Psychiatry: Behavioral Science and Clinical Essentials*. Philadelphia: W.B. Saunders Company, 2000.

PERIODICALS

Curran, Valarie H. "Additional Methadone Increases Craving for Heroin: A Double-Blind, Placebo-Controlled Study of Chronic Opiate Users Receiving Methadone Substitution Treatment." *Addiction* 94, no. 5 (May 1999): 665–74.

Strain, Eric. "Moderate-vs High-Dose Methadone in the Treatment of Opioid Dependence." *Journal of the American Medical Association* 281, no. 11 (1999): 1000–1005.

Ajna Hamidovic, Pharm.D.

Methamphetamine

Definition

Methamphetamine, or meth, is an addictive central nervous system (CNS) stimulant. The U.S. Drug Enforcement Administration (DEA) lists methamphetamine as a Schedule II drug, which means it has high abuse potential but some medical value. Because of this abuse potential, prescriptions for methamphetamine

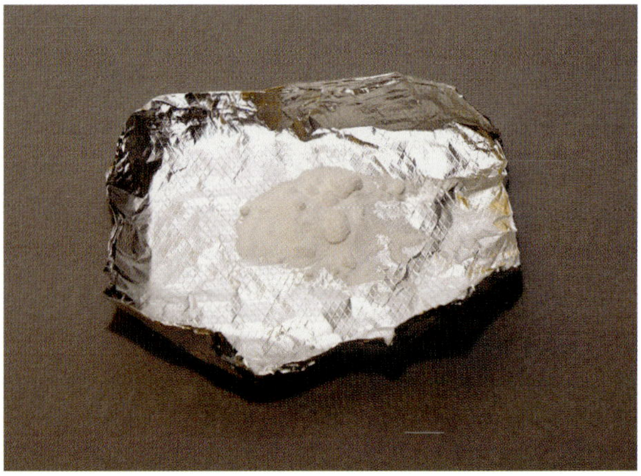

Methamphetamine in powder form. *(U.S. Drug Enforcement Administration)*

Methamphetamine
Short-term effects: • Increased alertness • Rapid and irregular heartbeat • Rise in blood pressure and body temperature
Long-term effects: • Anxiety and feelings of confusion • Dental problems • Increased risk of contracting diseases such as HIV/AIDS and hepatitis • Insomnia • Mood disturbances • Violent behavior
In 2010, 353,000 Americans aged 12 and older had abused methamphetamine at least once in the past month.
SOURCE: National Institutes of Health, National Institute on Drug Abuse, "Methamphetamine." Available online at: http://www.drugabuse.gov/drugpages/methamphetamine.html; also Substance Abuse and Mental Health Services Administration, *Results from the 2010 National Survey on Drug Use and Health.* Available online at: http://www.oas.samhsa.gov/NSDUH/2k10NSDUH/2k10Results.htm.

(Table by PreMediaGlobal. © 2012 Cengage Learning.)

cannot be refilled. It goes by the street names of ice, crystal, crystal meth, speed, crank, and glass.

Demographics

The national Monitoring the Future survey of 2008 found that in 2007 about 1.3 million Americans had used methamphetamine, a decrease from 1.9 million in 2006. This survey found that 2.3% of eighth graders, 2.4% of 10th graders, and 2.8% of twelfth graders had tried methamphetamine at some time in their lives.

In the United States, methamphetamine use peaks in white men 30–40 years old; however, according to the 2010 *National Survey on Drug Use and Health*, the average age of first use in 2010 was 18.8 years. Methamphetamine use is highest in the western U.S. states. Internationally, methamphetamine use is highest in Eastern Europe and Southeast Asia.

Methamphetamine is produced illegally in many countries, including the United States, and it can be synthesized with readily available materials. The drug's misuse is deemed to be a major social problem.

Purpose

Methamphetamine was first synthesized in Japan in 1919 and was used as a drug therapy in asthma inhalers in the 1930s. **Amphetamines** of all kinds were used during World War II by both sides to increase alertness and prolong wakefulness of military troops. After the war, the government developed stricter regulations for the manufacture and use of amphetamines, but the drugs remained popular among people who wanted to stay awake for long periods (e.g., students, long-haul truckers) and were commonly used by people who wanted to lose weight. In 1970, more restrictions were put on methamphetamine, and it was branded as a Schedule II drug. Despite the dangers, methamphetamine remains a popular drug of abuse.

Description

Methamphetamine is similar to other CNS stimulants, such as amphetamine (its parent drug), **methylphenidate**, and **cocaine**, in that it stimulates **dopamine** reward pathways in the **brain**. Consistent with its stimulant profile, methamphetamine causes increased activity and talkativeness, decreased appetite and **fatigue**, and a general sense of well being. Compared to amphetamine, methamphetamine is more potent and longer lasting, and it has more harmful effects on the brain. In animals, a single high dose of methamphetamine has been shown to damage nerve terminals in the dopamine-containing regions of the brain.

Methamphetamine is a white, odorless, bitter-tasting crystalline powder that easily dissolves in water or alcohol. Misuse occurs in many forms, as methamphetamine can be smoked, snorted, injected, or taken orally. When smoked or injected, methamphetamine enters the brain rapidly and immediately produces an intense but short-lived rush that many abusers find extremely pleasurable. Snorting or oral ingestion produces euphoria—a feeling of being high—within minutes. As with other abused stimulants, methamphetamine is most often used in a binge-and-crash pattern. A "run" of repeated doses may be continued over the course of days (binge) before stopping (crash). Exhaustion occurs with repeated use of methamphetamine, involving intense fatigue and need for sleep after the stimulation phase.

Recommended dosage

Approved medical indications for the drug are the sleep disorder **narcolepsy**, **attention deficit hyperactivity disorder** (**ADHD**), and extreme obesity, but in each case methamphetamine is a second-line drug at best and is used only after other, less harmful drugs have failed.

The prescription drug (brand name Desoxyn) comes in the form of a small white tablet, which is orally ingested. Dosing begins at 5 mg once or twice a day and

KEY TERMS

Central nervous system (CNS)—Part of the nervous system consisting of the brain, cranial nerves, and spinal cord. The brain is the center of higher processes, such as thought and emotion, and is responsible for the coordination and control of bodily activities and the interpretation of information from the senses. The cranial nerves and spinal cord link the brain to the peripheral nervous system, that is, the nerves present in the rest of body.

Dopamine—A neurochemical made in the brain that is involved in many brain activities, including movement and emotion.

Hallucination—A false or distorted perception of objects, sounds, or events that seems real. Hallucinations usually result from drugs or mental disorders.

Psychosis—A serious mental disorder characterized by defective or lost contact with reality often with hallucinations or delusions.

Relapse—A recurrence of symptoms after a period of improvement or recovery.

Tolerance—The requirement for higher doses of a substance or more frequent engagement in an activity to achieve the same effect.

is increased weekly until the lowest effective dose is attained. Desoxyn should not be taken with other stimulants (including caffeine and decongestants) or antidepressant drugs (especially **monoamine oxidase inhibitors** [MAOIs], but also tricyclic **antidepressants**). Desoxyn should not be taken by patients with glaucoma, cardiovascular disease (including hypertension and arteriosclerosis), or hyperthyroidism.

Precautions

Short-term effects of methamphetamine relate to its stimulation of the brain and the cardiovascular system. Euphoria and rush, alertness, increased physical activity, and decreased sleep and appetite occur from an increase in available dopamine in the brain. Any or all of these effects can lead to compulsive use of the drug. Methamphetamine causes rapid heart beat (tachycardia), increased respiration, and increased blood pressure (hypertension), and with very high doses, increased body temperature (hyperthermia) and convulsions can occur.

QUESTIONS TO ASK YOUR DOCTOR

- How can I tell if someone in my family is using methamphetamine?
- What type of therapy do you recommend for methamphetamine users?
- Can you recommend a treatment center for methamphetamine addiction?
- Will my insurance pay for this treatment?
- What should I tell my friends and family about my family member's methamphetamine problem?
- What should I say to my family member whom I suspect of using methamphetamine?

Chronic use of methamphetamine can result in two hallmark features of **addiction**: tolerance and dependence. Tolerance to the euphoric effects in particular can prompt abusers to take higher or more frequent doses of the drug. Withdrawal symptoms in chronic users include **depression**, anxiety, fatigue, and an intense craving for the drug. Users who inject methamphetamine risk contracting life-threatening viruses such as HIV and hepatitis through the use of dirty needles.

Addiction is a complex disorder, and prospects for individual addicts vary widely. Chronic methamphetamine use causes changes in brain and mental functions. While some effects are reversible, others are long lasting and possibly permanent. Relapses are common, and cravings may continue for a long time after drug use has stopped.

Side effects

With repeated use, methamphetamine can cause anxiety, **insomnia**, mood disturbances, confusion, hallucinations, **psychosis**, and violent behavior. Psychotic features sometimes emerge, such as **paranoia**, hallucinations, and **delusions**, and can last well after methamphetamine use has stopped. **Stroke** and weight loss are other long-term effects.

Treatment

For acute intoxication accompanied by psychosis, patients may be calmed by reassurance and a quiet setting, but sometimes antipsychotic drugs or **sedatives** are administered. Substances that prevent absorption from the gastrointestinal tract (e.g., activated charcoal) may be used if the drug was taken orally. Additional care is given as needed (e.g., keeping the airways open, treatment of **seizures**). Individual with methamphetamine intoxication may be violent, agitated, and a danger to themselves and others.

The most effective treatment for methamphetamine addiction is cognitive-behavioral **intervention** such as counseling but may also include **family education**, drug testing, and group support in a twelve-step program. The goal of these modalities is to modify the patient's thinking, expectations, and behaviors to increase coping skills in the face of stressors. Contingent management is a promising behavioral intervention, in which incentives are provided in exchange for staying clean and for participating in treatment. Residential programs/therapeutic communities may be helpful, particularly in more severe cases.

Antidepressant drugs such as **bupropion** (Wellbutrin) can be a useful treatment aid, but as of 2011, there were no FDA-approved medications specifically for the treatment of stimulant addiction.

Resources

BOOKS

Lee, Steven J. *Overcoming Crystal Meth Addiction: An Essential Guide to Getting Clean.* New York: Marlowe, 2006.

Weisheit, Ralph A., and William White. *Methamphetamine: Its History, Pharmacology, and Treatment.* Center City, MN: Hazelden, 2009.

WEBSITES

"Methamphetamine." MedlinePlus, September 11, 2010. http://www.nlm.nih.gov/medlineplus/methamphetamine.html (accessed August 14, 2011).

"NIDA InfoFacts: Methamphetamine." National Institute on Drug Abuse, March 2010. http://www.drugabuse.gov/infofacts/methamphetamine.html (accessed August 14, 2011).

Richards, John R. "Toxicity, Methamphetamine." Medscape. http://emedicine.medscape.com/article/820918-overview (accessed August 14, 2011).

Volkow, Nora D. "Methamphetamine Abuse and Addiction." National Institute on Drug Abuse, 2006. http://www.nida.nih.gov/ResearchReports/methamph/methamph.html (accessed August 14, 2011).

ORGANIZATIONS

National Clearinghouse on Alcohol and Drug Information, PO Box 2345, Rockville, MD, 20847, (877) SAMHSA-7; Spanish: (877) 767-8432; TDD: (800) 487-4889, Fax: (240) 221-4292, http://ncadi.samhsa.gov.

National Council on Alcoholism and Drug Dependence Inc., 244 E 58th St., 4th Fl., New York, NY, 10022, (212) 269-7797, (800) NCA-CALL, Fax: (212) 269-7510, national@ncadd.org, http://www.ncadd.org.

The Partnership at Drugfree.org, 352 Park Ave. S., 9th Fl., New York, NY, 10010, (212) 922-1560, Fax: (212) 922-1570, http://www.drugfree.org.

Jill U. Adams
Tish Davidson, AM

Methylphenidate

Definition

Methylphenidate is a mild, central nervous system stimulant. In the United States, the drug is sold under the brand name Ritalin.

Purpose

Methylphenidate is used primarily in the treatment of **attention deficit hyperactivity disorder (ADHD)** in children and adults. It also may be used to treat **narcolepsy**, a sleep disorder. In rare cases, it is used to decrease sedation and lethargy from opioid pain medications and to help improve the mood of a terminally ill person suffering from **depression**.

Description

The mode of action for methylphenidate is not fully understood. It presumably activates the **brain** stem arousal system and cortex to produce a stimulant effect. The brain stem arousal system increases levels of electrical activity in the brain. The effect of methylphenidate is to produce increased alertness and, although

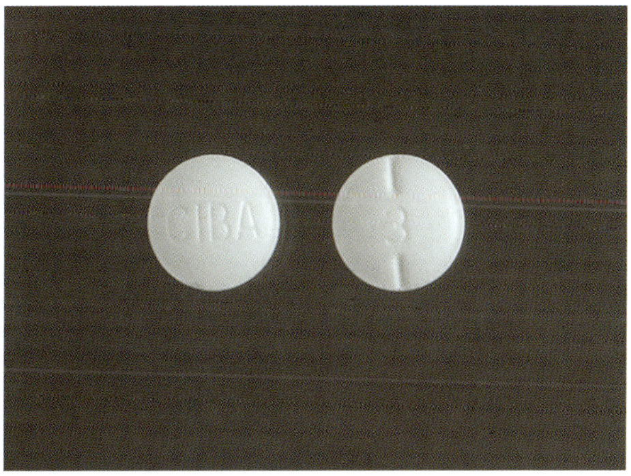

Methylphenidate (Ritalin), 10 mg. *(U.S. Drug Enforcement Administration)*

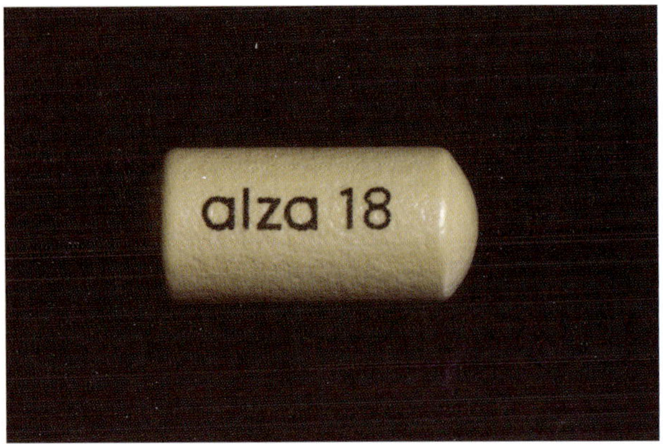

Concerta (methylphenidate). *(© Custom Medical Stock Photo, Inc. Reproduced by permission.)*

children with **ADHD** are overactive and have decreased attention spans, in these children, methylphenidate actually decreases motor restlessness and increases attention span.

Methylphenidate is offered in various forms of administration:

- oral solution and chewable tablets (Methylin, Ritalin)
- extended release (Metadate ER, Metadate CD, Ritalin SR)
- long acting (Concerta, Ritalin LA)
- patch (Daytrana)

Tablets are available in 5, 10, and 20 mg strengths; an extended release form is available as a 20 mg tablet; a long acting form is available in 10, 20, 30, and 40 mg strengths; and the patch is available in 10, 15, 20, and 30 mg strengths.

Recommended dosage

The recommended dosage of methylphenidate is determined by trial and error based on individual responses. Methylphenidate is usually administered in two or three separate doses each day, preferably 45 minutes before a meal. For children with ADHD, the initial recommended dosage is 5 mg twice daily before breakfast and lunch, increased by 5–10 mg per week to a maximum of 60 mg per day. The average total dosage is 20–30 mg per day, although 10–60 mg is not uncommon. For narcolepsy in adults, the recommended dose is 5–20 mg two to three times a day, taken 30–45 minutes before meals.

The drug should be taken exactly as directed. Methylphenidate can become habit forming if taken in greater amounts or for longer periods than necessary. Individuals should take the last dose of the day before 6 P.M. to decrease sleep difficulties. The tablet should not be broken or crushed, as doing so changes the time for absorption. If the normal time of administration is missed, persons should take the drug as soon as possible. However, two tablets should not be taken at the same time.

KEY TERMS

Anxiety—An emotion that can be experienced as a troubled feeling, sense of dread, fear of the future, or distress over a possible threat to a person's physical or mental well-being.

Attention deficit hyperactivity disorder (ADHD)—A developmental disorder characterized by distractibility, hyperactivity, impulsive behaviors, and the inability to remain focused on tasks or activities.

Depression—A mental state characterized by feelings of sadness, despair, discouragement, and low energy, often with oversleeping and/or overeating.

Hallucinations—Perceptions without external stimulus. Hallucinations can result from nervous system abnormalities, mental disorders, or the use of certain drugs.

Tourette syndrome—An abnormal condition that causes uncontrollable facial grimaces and tics and arm and shoulder movements. Tourette syndrome is perhaps best known for uncontrollable vocal tics that include grunts, shouts, and use of obscene language (coprolalia).

Precautions

Methylphenidate has a great potential to produce physical and mental dependence. Administration should not be stopped abruptly. Such action can cause withdrawal symptoms, including depression, paranoid feelings, thoughts of **suicide**, anxiety, agitation, and sleep disturbances. Methylphenidate should not be given to persons with extreme anxiety, tension, agitation, severe depression, mental or emotional instability, or a history of alcohol or drug abuse. It is not indicated for use by those with **Tourette syndrome**, people with **tic disorders**, glaucoma, or certain mental-health conditions. The drug should be used cautiously in persons with high blood pressure, those with a history of **seizures**, and women who are breastfeeding. Methylphenidate is not typically ordered for women during their childbearing years unless the physician determines that the benefits outweigh the risks.

QUESTIONS TO ASK YOUR DOCTOR

- What kind of changes can I expect to see or feel with this medication?
- Does it matter what time of day I take this medication? If so, what is the recommendation?
- Should I take this medication with or without food?
- What are the side effects associated with this medication?
- Will this medication interact or interfere with other medications I am currently taking?
- What symptoms or adverse effects are important enough that I should seek immediate treatment?

Methylphenidate should not be ordered for children younger than six years of age as its safety has not been determined in this age group. People should not drive or operate machinery or appliances until they understand how this drug affects them. They should not drive if they become lightheaded or dizzy. Methylphenidate may cause irregularities in the composition of the blood and produce changes in liver function. People taking methylphenidate should receive regular blood tests.

Side effects

The most common side effects are nervousness, difficulties with sleep, tachycardia, and increased blood pressure. Reducing the dose or changing the time the drug is taken may reduce some side effects. Affected persons should discuss any adverse reactions with their healthcare professional. Individuals taking methylphenidate should receive regular blood pressure and pulse checks. Methylphenidate also may cause dizziness, irritability, vision changes, drowsiness, and a poor appetite. Less common side effects include chest pain, palpitations, joint pain, skin rash, and uncontrolled movements or speech. Side effects may also include a rapid or irregular heartbeat, stomach upset, nausea, headache, blood in the urine or stool, muscle cramps, red dots on the skin, or bruises. At higher dosages or with long-term use, people may experience weight loss or mental changes such as confusion, false beliefs, mood changes, hallucinations, or feelings that they or their environment are not real.

Interactions

Several drugs may interact adversely with methylphenidate, including anticoagulants and drugs to prevent seizures, combat depression, and treat high blood pressure. The dosages of these drugs may be reduced when taken simultaneously with methylphenidate.

Resources

BOOKS

Albers, Lawrence J., Rhoda K. Hahn, and Christopher Reist. *Handbook of Psychiatric Drugs.* Laguna Hills, CA: Current Clinical Strategies, 2010.

American Society of Health-System Pharmacists. *AHFS Drug Information 2011.* Bethesda, MD: ASHP, 2011.

Barkley, Russell A. *Taking Charge of ADHD: The Complete, Authoritative Guide for Parents.* Rev. ed. New York: Guilford Press, 2000.

Chandler, Chris. *The Science of ADHD: A Guide for Parents and Professionals.* New York: Wiley-Blackwell, 2011.

Graham, George. *The Disordered Mind: An Introduction to Philosophy of Mind and Mental Illness.* New York: Routledge, 2010.

Holland, Leland Norman, and Michael Patrick Adams. *Core Concepts in Pharmacology.* 3rd ed. New York: Prentice Hall, 2011.

North, Carol, and Sean Yutzy. *Goodwin and Guze's Psychiatric Diagnosis.* New York: Oxford University Press, 2010.

Preston, John D., John H. O'Neal, and Mary C. Talaga. *Handbook of Clinical Psychopharmacology for Therapists.* 6th ed. Oakland, CA: New Harbinger, 2010.

PERIODICALS

Miller, A.R., C.E. Lalonde, K.M. McGrail, and R.W. Armstrong. "Prescription of Methylphenidate to Children and Youth, 1990–1996." *Canadian Medical Journal* 165, no. 11 (2001): 1489–94.

Perring C. "Medicating Children: The Case of Ritalin." *Bioethics* 11, no. 3–4 (1997): 228–40.

Sund, A.M., and P. Zeiner. "Does Extended Medication with Amphetamine or Methylphenidate Reduce Growth in Hyperactive Children?" *Norwegian Journal of Psychiatry* 56, no. 1 (2002): 53–57.

ORGANIZATIONS

American Academy of Clinical Toxicology, 6728 Old McLean Village Dr., McLean, VA, 22101, (703) 556-9222, Fax: (703) 556-8729, admin@clintox.org, http://www.clintox.org.

American Academy of Family Physicians, 11400 Tomahawk Creek Pkwy., Leawood, KS, 66211-2672, (913) 906-6000, (800) 274-2237, Fax: (913) 906-6075, contactcenter@aafp.org, http://www.aafp.org.

American Neurological Association, 5841 Cedar Lake Rd., Ste. 204, Minneapolis, MN, 55416, (952) 545-6284, ana@llmsi.com, http://www.aneuroa.org.

American Psychiatric Association, 1000 Wilson Blvd., Ste. 1825, Arlington, VA, 22209-3901, (703) 907-7300, apa@psych.org, http://www.psych.org.

American Psychological Association, 750 1st St., NE, Washington, DC, 20002-4242, (202) 336-5500; TDD/TTY: (202) 336-6123, (800) 374-2721, http://www.apa.org.

American Society for Clinical Pharmacology and Therapeutics, 528 N Washington St., Alexandria, VA, 22314, (703) 836-6981, info@ascpt.org, http://www.ascpt.org.

National Institute of Mental Health, 6001 Executive Blvd., Rm. 8184, MSC 9663, Bethesda, MD, 20892-9663, (301) 433-4513; TTY: (301) 443-8431, (866) 615-6464; TTY: (866) 415-8051, Fax: (301) 443-4279, nimhinfo@nih.gov, http://www.nimh.nih.gov.

L. Fleming Fallon, Jr., MD, DrPH
Laura Jean Cataldo, RN, EdD

Military mental health

Definition

Military health care, or military medicine, is not recognized as a specialty by the American Board of Medical Specialties (ABMS); nonetheless, it is a distinctive category of medical and psychiatric practice. In the twenty-first century, military medicine involves routine health care (including mental health care) for military personnel and their dependents, but it also includes battlefield treatment and evacuation, disease prevention, disaster relief, health care for military personnel in such extreme environments as deserts and the polar regions, and research in these fields—including mental health research. Aerospace medicine and undersea medicine are newer subspecialties that have developed within the larger field of military medicine.

Military suicide rates

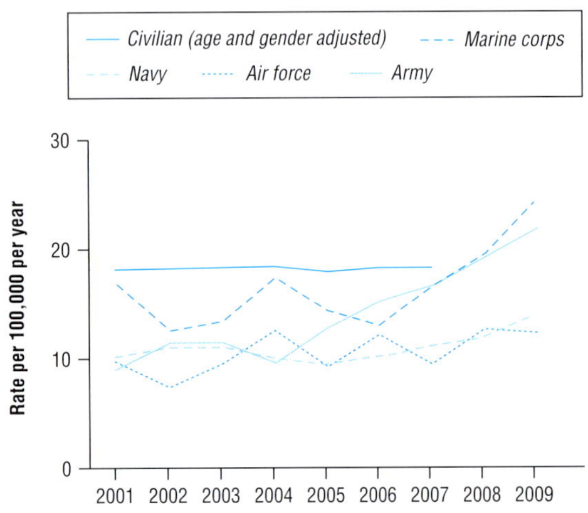

SOURCE: U. S. Army, "Health Promotion, Risk Reduction, Suicide Prevention Report (HP/RR/SP)," 2010.

(Graph by PreMediaGlobal. © 2012 Cengage Learning.)

Military physicians are often stationed with the troops they serve, and they must be acquainted with unusual diseases, traumatic injuries, and psychological stressors that are rarely encountered in civilian settings. The Borden Institute of the U.S. Army Medical Department was founded in 1987 to publish textbooks of military medicine on topics ranging from chemical warfare and health care in harsh environments to preventive medicine and medical ethics. As of 2011, the Institute had published 20 separate textbooks; volumes 5 and 6 are titled *Military Psychiatry* and *War Psychiatry*, respectively.

Veterans' health care in the United States dates back to the Revolutionary War, when the first federal military hospital, Hand Hospital, was opened in Pittsburgh in 1778. Contemporary veterans' health care includes a range of different services, from post-deployment counseling and routine medical checkups to inpatient medical and mental health care, including hospice care. The Department of Veterans Affairs (VA) system is currently divided into 21 geographical regions known as Veterans Integrated Service Networks or VISNs. These regions include both VA hospitals and Vet Centers, which are run by the Veterans Health Administration (VHA), and community-based outpatient clinics staffed by civilian physicians who work in partnership with the VA.

Demographics

U.S. military personnel on active duty are under the care of the Military Health System (MHS), which covers approximately 9.5 million beneficiaries, including the families of active duty personnel as well as retirees and their families. The MHS has about 137,000 employees and an annual budget of $42 billion; it operates 65 hospitals, 412 clinics, and 414 dental clinics at facilities across the United States and around the world, as well as facilities in overseas combat theater operations. The health benefits program for active duty personnel, their dependents, and retirees using civilian healthcare providers is known as TRICARE.

The MHS also operates the Uniformed Services University of the Health Sciences (USU), a graduate university established in Bethesda, Maryland, in 1972 that includes a medical school, dental school, school of nursing, and graduate school in the biomedical sciences offering PhD and DPH degrees. USU had about 850 students enrolled in all its graduate programs as of 2011.

Veterans are eligible for benefits from the Veterans Benefits Administration (VBA), depending on their

Demographic characteristics of Operation Iraqi Freedom (Iraq) and Operation Enduring Freedom (Afghanistan and surrounding regions) veterans newly utilizing VA healthcare services between October 7, 2001, and March 31, 2007, followed until March 31, 2008, by mental health category

Characteristic	Total veterans	Veterans with no mental health diagnosis		Veterans diagnosed with mental health disorders other than PTSD*		Veterans diagnosed with PTSD*	
Total	249,440	157,844		37,868		53,728	
Age group							
15–24	75,715	45,726	(60.4%)	11,859	(15.7%)	18,130	(24.0%)
25–29	65,117	39,734	(61.0%)	10,415	(16.0%)	14,968	(23.0%)
30–39	54,123	33,942	(62.7%)	8,085	(14.9%)	12,096	(22.4%)
40–49	44,059	31,239	(70.9%)	5,869	(13.3%)	6,951	(15.8%)
50–59	9,906	6,815	(68.8%)	1,568	(15.8%)	1,523	(15.4%)
60+	505	374	(74.1%)	71	(14.1%)	60	(11.9%)
Gender							
Male	217,793	137,779	(63.3%)	31,936	(14.7%)	48,078	(22.1%)
Female	31,610	20,032	(63.4%)	5,929	(18.8%)	5,649	(17.9%)
Race/ethnicity							
White	166,509	105,484	(63.4%)	25,113	(15.1%)	35,912	(21.6%)
Black	41,700	26,320	(63.1%)	6,234	(15.0%)	9,146	(21.9%)
Hispanic	27,384	16,837	(61.5%)	4,613	(16.9%)	5,934	(21.7%)
Other	13,847	9,203	(66.5%)	1,908	(13.8%)	2,736	(19.8%)
Marital status							
Married	92,128	52,706	(57.2%)	15,131	(16.4%)	24,291	(26.4%)
Never married	87,565	50,671	(57.9%)	16,137	(18.4%)	20,757	(23.7%)
Divorced, widowed, or separated	22,725	11,119	(48.9%)	4,796	(21.1%)	6,810	(30.0%)
Active duty or reserve							
Active duty	125,836	78,986	(62.8%)	18,949	(15.1%)	27,901	(22.2%)
National Guard/Reserve	123,604	78,858	(63.8%)	18,919	(15.3%)	25,827	(20.9%)
Military rank							
Enlisted (e.g., private, corporal, sergeant)	231,673	143,428	(61.9%)	36,170	(15.6%)	52,075	(22.5%)
Officer (e.g., lieutenant, colonel, general)	17,767	14,416	(81.1%)	1,698	(9.6%)	1,653	(9.3%)
Military branch							
U.S. Army	163,335	97,561	(59.7%)	24,991	(15.3%)	40,783	(25.0%)
U.S. Air Force	28,684	23,093	(80.5%)	3,855	(13.4%)	1,736	(6.0%)
U.S. Marine Corps	30,483	17,631	(57.8%)	4,123	(13.5%)	8,729	(28.6%)
U.S. Navy/Coast Guard	26,938	19,559	(72.6%)	4,899	(18.2%)	2,480	(9.2%)
Multiple deployments							
Yes	78,645	48,832	(62.1%)	11,193	(14.2%)	18,620	(23.7%)
No	170,795	109,012	(63.8%)	26,675	(15.6%)	35,108	(20.6%)
Main VA facility type**							
Medical center	195,133	124,341	(63.7%)	29,597	(15.2%)	41,195	(21.1%)
Outpatient clinic	52,277	31,656	(60.6%)	8,156	(15.6%)	12,465	(23.8%)
Distance to closest VA facility							
Less than 25 miles	130,474	83,934	(64.3%)	20,094	(15.4%)	26,446	(20.3%)
More than 25 miles	117,146	72,779	(62.1%)	17,500	(14.9%)	26,866	(22.9%)

*Post-traumatic stress syndrome
**Veterans Affairs
Notes: Variables may contain missing data; therefore, numbers within each category may not equate to the total number of participants.
PTSD was the most common mental health diagnosis in the study population (21.5%), followed by depression (18.3%), adjustment disorder (11.1%), anxiety disorder (10.6%), substance use disorder (8.4%), and alcohol use disorder (7.3%).

SOURCE: Cohen, Beth E., Kris Gima, Daniel Bertenthal, Sue Kim, Charles R. Marmar and Karen H. Seal. "Mental Health Diagnoses and Utilization of VA Non-Mental Health Medical Services Among Returning Iraq and Afghanistan Veterans." *Journal of General Internal Medicine* 25, no. 1 (January 2010): 18–24.

membership in one of eight priority groups. Those retired from long-term military service, those with service-related injuries or conditions, and those awarded the Purple Heart are in the higher-priority groups. Veterans without service-related conditions are eligible for treatment on the basis of financial need. In 2010, there were one million veterans receiving disability benefits, most of them from the period of the Vietnam War (early 1960s–1973).

Description

Historical background

Military medicine and veterans' benefits both originated with Augustus Caesar (63 B.C.–14 A.D.), the first emperor of Rome. Augustus reorganized the Roman army, putting it on a professional footing and creating the first dedicated medical corps in military history. He established a medical school for the training of army physicians (who were responsible for veterinary care for the army's horses and pack animals as well as surgery and medical care for the soldiers), who had to pass detailed course work and examinations to be allowed to join the army. Other innovations were the formation of special groups of soldiers tasked with retrieving the wounded from the battlefield; construction of permanent hospitals (*valetudinaria*) within the army's fortified camps, with special isolation rooms for soldiers with infectious diseases; and the establishment of medical specialties within the army medical corps.

The Civil War was also the first war to bring veterans' mental health issues to the attention of doctors. Jacob Mendez da Costa (1833–1900), a professor at Jefferson Medical College in Philadelphia, identified a disorder that he called the "irritable heart," an anxiety disorder that he observed in Civil War veterans, characterized by breathlessness, panicky feelings, and chest pains on mild exertion. It was sometimes called "soldier's heart" in World War I. Although da Costa's syndrome was not the same as what is now called *post-traumatic stress disorder* (PTSD), recent historical studies of Civil War veterans' health records indicate that many of these men also met contemporary criteria for PTSD. Those at greatest risk were men younger than 18 at the time of service and those who served in units with higher-than-average casualty rates. In addition, doctors and nurses who treated combat casualties developed PTSD even when they were not on the battlefield themselves. Walt Whitman (1819–1892), the famous poet, served as a nurse in a military hospital in Washington, DC between 1862 and 1865; his diary records such symptoms of PTSD as flashbacks, nightmares, **insomnia**, startle reactions, and nausea after his periods on duty.

Mental health issues in the military

Post-traumatic stress disorder

Post-traumatic stress disorder, or PTSD, was not formally introduced as a psychiatric diagnostic category until the third edition of the ***Diagnostic and Statistical Manual of Mental Disorders*** (*DSM-III*) in 1980, although it has doubtless affected civilians as well as combat veterans for millennia. The earliest recorded case of it concerns an uninjured Athenian hoplite (citizen-soldier) who became blind from emotional shock after witnessing the death of a comrade during the Battle of Marathon in 490 B.C. It is helpful to keep in mind in this context that psychiatry itself is a relatively young medical specialty; Sigmund Freud was a boy of five at the outbreak of the Civil War in 1861.

The notion of evaluating soldiers in combat situations for psychiatric as well as physical symptoms originated in the British army on the Western Front during World War I (1914–1918) when infantrymen in the trenches began to develop what was then called "shell shock"—a combat **stress** reaction marked by indecision, disorientation, inability to set priorities, and a blank and unfocused expression colloquially known as the "thousand-yard stare," a sign of dissociation. During World War II (1939–1945), the condition was generally called "combat fatigue" or "traumatic war neurosis," terms that are now obsolete. It was not until the Vietnam War that studies of combat veterans eventually produced the current definition of PTSD. The **diagnosis** was not applied to civilian survivors of traumatic incidents until the 1980s.

Demographics for PTSD for American veterans of different wars are difficult to estimate because of changing definitions of combat stress reactions as well as differences among branches of the service and the theaters in which they operated. The overall lifetime rate of PTSD for World War II veterans is estimated at 25%, with rates in the Army and Marine Corps higher than in the Navy, Coast Guard, or Air Force (called the "Army Air Corps" before 1947). For World War II veterans who had been prisoners of war, the rate of PTSD was three times higher (36%) for POW veterans of the Pacific Theater than for those taken prisoner in Europe (12%); traumatic memories persisted as long as 65 years after the experience of captivity. The lifetime rate for Vietnam veterans is estimated at 31% for men and 27% for women; for veterans of the Gulf War, from 9% to 24%; for veterans of Operation Iraqi Freedom (OIF) and Operation Enduring Freedom (OEF), 10% to 18%. For purposes of comparison, the lifetime rate of PTSD in the general population is 7% to 8%. Risk factors for PTSD in OIF/OEF veterans include lower service rank, single marital status, female gender, Hispanic ethnicity, longer deployment time, **traumatic brain injury**, family problems at home, prior history of childhood **trauma**, and lower level of education.

The VA established the National Center for PTSD in 1989 to perform research and education on the understanding, treatment, and prevention of PTSD. Although the Center does not provide direct clinical care for veterans with PTSD, it educates both military and civilian physicians about the disorder, maintains a research database called PILOTS (Published International Literature on Traumatic Stress), and has a website with numerous pages about various aspects of PTSD, ranging from self-assessment and self-help to women's issues, post-deployment syndrome, and special programs for Native American, Hispanic, and African American veterans.

Gulf War syndrome

Gulf War syndrome (GWS) is a condition reported by some veterans of the 1991 Gulf War marked by chronic **fatigue**; headaches; memory problems; disturbed sleep; and digestive, skin, muscle, and joint disorders. GWS is a controversial diagnosis because of the wide variety of symptoms claimed as its characteristic features and because of the lack of a standardized definition of the syndrome. A report issued by the Institute of Medicine (IOM) in 2006 concluded, "Although veterans of the first Gulf War report significantly more symptoms of illness than soldiers of the same period who were not deployed, studies have found no cluster of symptoms that constitute a syndrome unique to Gulf War veterans." One reason given for the existence of a distinct syndrome was exposure to a combination of chemicals and contaminants never previously encountered in a war zone. These included bromide pills given to protect troops from the effects of nerve agents, depleted uranium munitions, and anthrax and botulinum vaccines. Another environmental hazard was toxic smoke from hundreds of burning oil wells.

About 700,000 American men and women served in the Gulf War in 1991; about 30% of them have registered with the database set up by the American Legion to track illnesses related to the war. Studies conducted by the Institute of Medicine and the National Academy of Sciences (NAS) in 2005 and 2006 surveyed 19,000 veterans of the Gulf War. Other medical reports by doctors in the field covered an additional 80,000 soldiers. What seems clear is that the medical symptoms of GWS cannot be explained as PTSD. While some veterans of the Gulf War did develop PTSD, a second IOM report in 2010 concluded that "the excess of unexplained medical symptoms reported by deployed Gulf war veterans cannot be reliably ascribed to any known psychiatric disorder." The medical symptoms are now generally described as multisystem illness, or MSI.

Post-deployment syndrome

Post-deployment syndrome (PDS) is sometimes used to describe a combination of PTSD, **depression**, **generalized anxiety disorder** (GAD), chronic pain, and traumatic **brain** injury (TBI) lasting longer than three to six months. It is a condition diagnosed primarily in veterans of the conflicts in Iraq and Afghanistan rather than earlier wars. Research into PDS was ongoing as of 2011, with a focus on finding effective treatments.

Women's issues

Women have served in frontline combat at least occasionally since the nineteenth century. According to diaries from the period and government records, about 750 women successfully disguised themselves as men and served in both Union and Confederate armies during the Civil War. Russian women served in combat in both World War I (the "Women's Battalion of Death" numbered about 2,000 soldiers in 1917) and World War II (about 800,000 women served as snipers, tank crew members, machine gunners, and pilots during the course of the war). Although American women generally served in support roles during earlier conflicts, as of 2011 they were the fastest growing group of veterans. Women currently account for 11% of all OIF/OEF veterans.

The VA has identified four particular stressors for women in the military: combat missions, military sexual trauma or MST (defined as "any kind of unwanted sexual attention includ[ing] insulting sexual comments, unwanted sexual advances, or even sexual assault"), feeling alone or unsupported in newly formed military units, and concern about children or elderly parents at home. There is evidence that sexual harassment and assault are more common in wartime than in peacetime military duty. A study of MST during the Gulf War reported high rates of sexual assault (7%), physical sexual harassment (33%), and verbal sexual harassment (66%). In another study, 23% of female users of VA healthcare reported experiencing at least one sexual assault while in the military.

One reason that MST is so debilitating is that the military places a very high value on unit cohesion; thus, reporting sexual harassment or assault perpetrated by another member of the unit is considered taboo. Male victims of MST have a higher rate of PTSD (65%) than females (45%), partly because the male gender role causes many men to feel intense shame about their

KEY TERMS

Combat stress reaction—A general term for mental health symptoms that include depression, fatigue, dissociative symptoms, difficulty focusing, and irritability. It is not identical to PTSD but may be a precursor of it. The condition was sometimes referred to as "combat fatigue" in World War II.

Dissociation—A psychological mechanism in which the mind splits off certain aspects of a traumatic event from conscious awareness. Dissociation can affect the patient's memory, sense of reality, and sense of identity. Dissociative symptoms are commonly experienced by persons with PTSD.

Post-deployment syndrome (PDS)—A term developed recently to describe a constellation of mental disorders found in veterans of the conflicts in Iraq and Afghanistan. PDS includes PTSD, generalized anxiety disorder, major depression, chronic pain, and traumatic brain injury.

Resilience—In psychiatry, the ability of a person to respond positively to, or bounce back from, trauma or hardship. Resilience is considered a process of interaction between the person and his or her environment rather than a one-time action.

Syndrome—A group of signs or symptoms that occur together and characterize or define a particular disease or disorder.

Triage—A process for determining the order and priority of emergency treatment for injured people (civilians or military personnel); the order and priority of emergency transport; and/or the injured person's transport destination.

victimization, making them less likely to seek professional help.

Traumatic brain injury

Traumatic brain injury (TBI) refers to a type of closed-head injury resulting from a blow or jolt to the head; it can result from whiplash injuries as well as a motor vehicle accident, blast, or fall. TBIs can be evaluated as mild, moderate, or severe, depending on whether the person was knocked out and how long they were unconscious. In a mild TBI, the person either does not lose consciousness at all or is unconscious for 30 minutes or less. In a moderate TBI, the person is unconscious for longer than 30 minutes but less than six hours. Unconsciousness lasting longer than six hours indicates a severe TBI.

One of the difficulties of diagnosing a TBI is that some of the emotional and cognitive symptoms overlap with those of PTSD. TBI symptoms may include trouble with concentration, acting without thinking, memory loss, difficulty translating thoughts into words, anger, anxiety, depression, or changes in personality. It is important to make sure that someone who has suffered a TBI together with (or instead of) PTSD receives the proper treatment. People with TBIs should not receive certain types of medications, including several classes of antidepressant drugs, which may aggravate some symptoms of the TBI, such as vertigo. Other drugs that should be avoided include those that may make the patient more susceptible to **seizures** (e.g., **bupropion**) or drugs that may cause confusion (e.g., **benzodiazepines**, lithium).

TBIs are of particular concern to current military and VA doctors because the rate of such injuries is higher (22%) in veterans of Iraq and Afghanistan than in Vietnam veterans (12%). The major causes of TBIs in recent veterans are blasts, motor vehicle accidents, and gunshot wounds. Because many veterans with TBIs have coexisting PTSD or **substance abuse** disorders, they typically take longer than civilians to recover from these head injuries. Veterans with TBIs are also almost twice as likely to attempt **suicide** than veterans who did not suffer such injuries.

Suicide

Statistics kept since World War I indicate that American combat veterans are twice as likely to die from suicide than male adults in the general population. In 2011, the VA reported that there were, on average, 950 suicide attempts each month among veterans receiving some type of VA treatment. Seven percent of these attempts were successful; 11% of attempters were expected to try again within the next nine months. The number of veterans' suicides between 2005 and 2009—1,100—exceeded that of the number of military personnel killed in Afghanistan since 2001.

Access to health care is an important factor in suicide prevention among veterans. Only 8 million of the 23 million veterans in the United States are currently registered with the Department of Veteran Affairs. The data indicate that for veterans between the ages of 18 and 29, the suicide rate is lower for those receiving VA health care than for those who do not seek help. The VA's suicide hotline (800-273-8255, press 1) receives about 10,000 calls per month from current and former service members. One major area of concern is the rising risk of suicide among OIF and OEF veterans. In 2009, there were 1,621 suicide attempts by men and 247 by women veterans of these conflicts, with 94 men and 4 women dying. As in the civilian population, women veterans attempt suicide more often than men, but men are more often successful, mostly because they are more likely to use firearms.

In 2011, the NIMH and the U.S. Army announced the beginning of a suicide-prevention study known as the Army Study to Assess Risk and Resilience in Servicemembers, or the Army STARRS program. The largest study ever conducted to assess mental health issues among military personnel, the Army STARRS program will run through 2014. The study has four separate components: an investigation of historical data, evaluation of new soldiers, an All-Army study, and a health outcomes investigation. Participation is voluntary.

QUESTIONS TO ASK YOUR DOCTOR

- Have you ever practiced medicine in a military setting?
- Have you ever treated military personnel on active duty?
- What do you consider the distinctive features of military medicine and health care for veterans?
- Have you ever diagnosed or treated a veteran with PTSD?
- Is there a VA health care facility in the area?

Military mental health services

Statistics indicate that almost half of the 1 million service personnel deployed to Iraq or Afghanistan between 2002 and 2009 sought some form of health care from the VA. Of that fraction, 48% (about 221,000 persons) were diagnosed with mental health issues, including depression and **anxiety disorders** other than PTSD. Treatment is available for veterans at all VA hospitals, Vet Centers, and community clinics working in partnership with the VA.

As of 2011, there were over 200 specialized treatment programs for PTSD within the VA system, covering veterans from World War II and all later conflicts. Several types of therapy are offered, including individualized assessment and **psychotherapy**, medications, **family therapy**, and **group therapy** (including anger management, combat support, and groups for veterans of specific conflicts). Programs range from intensive residential or inpatient treatment programs lasting 28–90 days in day clinics, walk-in community-based clinics, and Vet Center group therapy programs staffed by veterans. A special 60-day residential PTSD program for women veterans, the National Women's Trauma Recovery Program (WTRP), is run by the center in Menlo Park, California.

The National Center for PTSD also has a menu of self-help options on its website, ranging from mindfulness practice and recommendations for a healthy lifestyle to an iPhone app called PTSD Coach that helps users recognize and manage symptoms of PTSD.

According to the VA, there are a number of reasons why veterans are often reluctant to seek help for mental health issues:

- They do not want to be seen as weak.
- They are concerned about privacy.
- They would rather rely on family and friends.
- They are concerned about possible side effects of medications.
- They do not think treatment will help them.
- They have problems with access to treatment, in terms of cost or geographical location.
- If they are still actively serving, they are concerned about losing future promotions.

As of 2011, there were 322 **clinical trials** under way in the general area of mental health care for veterans. Studies include investigations of various types of psychotherapy and other interventions for PTSD, telephone case monitoring and outreach for World War II veterans as well as younger veterans, Internet- and smartphone-based psychotherapy for rural veterans, suicide-prevention programs, special studies of women veterans, trials of various medications for Gulf War veterans with multisystem illness, and investigations of programs for post-deployment reintegration into civilian life.

Resources

BOOKS

Bradley, Matthew H., ed. *Veterans' Benefits and Care.* Hauppauge, NY: Nova Science Publishers, 2009.

Cifu, David X., and Cory Blake. *Overcoming Post-deployment Syndrome: A Six-Step Mission to Health.* New York: Demos Health, 2011.

Gabriel, Richard A. *Man and Wound in the Ancient World: A History of Military Medicine from Sumer to the Fall of Constantinople.* Washington, DC: Potomac Books, 2012.

McCallum, Jack E. *Military Medicine: From Ancient Times to the 21st Century.* Santa Barbara, CA: ABC-CLIO, 2008.

Rice, Gary H. *A Sketch of Military Medicine in Canada, 1867–2009.* Carleton Place, ON: GEHR Pub. of Mississippi Mills, 2009.

Ritchie, Elspeth Cameron, ed. *Combat and Operational Behavioral Health*. Falls Church, VA: Office of The Surgeon General, United States Army, 2011.

PERIODICALS

Brenner, L.A., et al. "Suicide and Traumatic Brain Injury Among Individuals Seeking Veterans Health Administration Services." *Journal of Head Trauma Rehabilitation* 26 (July–August 2011): 257–64.

Cohen, Beth E., et al. "Mental Health Diagnoses and Utilization of VA Non-Mental Health Medical Services Among Returning Iraq and Afghanistan Veterans." *Journal of General Internal Medicine* 25, no. 1 (2010): 18–24.

Hoge, C.W., et al. "Combat Duty in Iraq and Afghanistan, Mental Health Problems and Barriers to Care." *U.S. Army Medical Department Journal* (July–September 2008): 7–17.

Hsu, David. "Walt Whitman: An American Civil War Nurse Who Witnessed the Advent of Modern American Medicine." *Archives of Environmental and Occupational Health* 65 (October–December 2010): 238–239. http://www.tandfonline.com/doi/pdf/10.1080/19338244.2010.524510 (accessed August 2, 2011).

Jones, E. "Shell Shock at Maghull and the Maudsley: Models of Psychological Medicine in the UK." *Journal of the History of Medicine and Allied Sciences* 65 (July 2010): 368–95.

Kang, H.K., et al. "Health of US Veterans of 1991 Gulf War: A Follow-up Survey in 10 Years." *Journal of Occupational and Environmental Health* 51 (April 2009): 401–10.

Khardis, A., et al. "Posttraumatic Stress, Family Adjustment, and Treatment Preferences among National Guard Soldiers Deployed to OEF/OIF." *Military Medicine* 176 (February 2011): 126–31.

Liberman, Moishe, et al. "The History of Trauma Care Systems from Homer to Telemedicine." *McGill Journal of Medicine* 7, no. 2 (2004). http://www.med.mcgill.ca/mjm/issues/v07n02/feature_rev/feature_rev.htm (accessed August 2, 2011).

Max, Jill. "Medicine and the Military." *Yale Medicine*, Spring 2011. http://www.med.yale.edu/external/pubs/ym_sp11/feature2_military.html (accessed August 1, 2011).

Maze, Rick. "18 Veterans Commit Suicide Each Day." *Army Times*, April 22, 2010. http://www.armytimes.com/news/2010/04/military_veterans_suicide_042210w (accessed August 5, 2011).

Pizarro, Judith, et al. "Physical and Mental Health Costs of Traumatic War Experiences among Civil War Veterans." *Archives of General Psychiatry* 63 (February 2006): 193–200. http://archpsyc.ama-assn.org/cgi/reprint/63/2/193 (accessed August 2, 2011).

Rintamaki, L.S., et al. "Persistence of Traumatic Memories in World War II Prisoners of War." *Journal of the American Geriatrics Society* 57 (December 2009): 2257–62.

Sher, L., and R. Yehuda. "Preventing Suicide among Returning Combat Veterans: A Moral Imperative." *Military Medicine* 176 (June 2011): 601–2.

Street, A.E., et al. "A New Generation of Women Veterans: Stressors Faced by Women Deployed to Iraq and Afghanistan." *Clinical Psychology Review* 29 (December 2009): 685–94.

Wells, T.S., et al. "Mental Health Impact of the Iraq and Afghanistan Conflicts: A Review of US Research, Service Provision, and Programmatic Responses." *International Review of Psychiatry* 23 (April 2011): 144–52.

OTHER

U.S. Army. *Army Health Promotion, Risk Reduction, Suicide Prevention Report 2010.* http://csf.army.mil/downloads/HP-RR-SPReport2010.pdf (accessed November 14, 2011).

WEBSITES

American Psychiatric Association. "Healthy Minds, Healthy Lives: Military." http://www.healthyminds.org/more-info-for/military.aspx (accessed January 5, 2012).

Army STARRS Home Page. http://www.armystarrs.org (accessed August 11, 2011).

Cifu, David, and Cory Blake. "Post-Deployment Syndrome: The Illness of War." BrainLineMilitary.org. http://www.brainlinemilitary.org/content/2011/03/post-deployment-syndrome-the-illness-of-war.html (accessed August 4, 2011).

DoD Live. "Improving the Care of Female Veterans." http://www.dodlive.mil/index.php/2011/07/improving-the-care-of-female-veterans (accessed August 3, 2011).

Military Pathways. "Military Mental Health Screening Program." http://www.militarymentalhealth.org/Welcome.aspx (accessed January 5, 2012).

National Center for PTSD. "Issues Specific to Women." http://www.ptsd.va.gov/public/pages/fslist-specific-women.asp (accessed August 3, 2011).

National Center for PTSD. "PTSD Overview" (includes "Understanding PTSD" Flash player module). http://www.ptsd.va.gov/public/pages/fslist-ptsd-overview.asp (accessed August 3, 2011).

National Center for PTSD. "Return from War." http://www.ptsd.va.gov/public/reintegration/guides-rwz.asp (accessed December 10, 2011).

National Center for PTSD. "Traumatic Brain Injury and PTSD." http://www.ptsd.va.gov/public/pages/traumatic_brain_injury_and_ptsd.asp (accessed August 4, 2011).

U.S. Army Medical Department. "Army Behavioral Health." http://www.behavioralhealth.army.mil (accessed January 5, 2012).

ORGANIZATIONS

Borden Institute, 1546 Porter St., Ste. 207, Fort Detrick, MD, United States 21702, (301) 619-3470, Fax: (301) 619-3471, bordeninfo@amedd.army.mil, http://www.bordeninstitute.army.mil/index.html.

National Center for PTSD, 810 Vermont Avenue NW, Washington, DC, United States 20420, (802) 296-6300, ncptsd@va.gov, http://www.ptsd.va.gov/index.asp.

Uniformed Services University of the Health Sciences (USU), 4301 Jones Bridge Rd., Bethesda, MD, United States 20814, (301) 295-1219, (800) 515-5257, Fax: (301) 295-3757, http://www.usuhs.mil.

U.S. Department of Veterans Affairs (VA), 810 Vermont Avenue NW, Washington, DC, United States 20420, (800) 827-1000; Mental health crisis line: (800) 273-8255 (press 1), http://www.va.gov.

Rebecca J. Frey, Ph.D.

Mind-body medicine

Definition

Mind-body medicine, also known as behavioral medicine, is the field of medicine concerned with the ways that the mind and emotions influence the body and physical health.

Purpose

Mind-body therapies have shown promise in treating cancer, heart disease, hypertension, asthma, and mental illness. They have been used as effective complementary therapies alongside such conventional treatments as surgery and chemotherapy. Mind-body therapies have also been shown to increase quality of life, reduce pain, and improve symptoms for people with chronic diseases and health conditions. They may also help control and reverse certain diseases, particularly those that are stress-related. By reducing **stress**, mind-body therapies may even prevent many diseases. Another benefit of mind-body therapies is that they pose very little risk. Some are inexpensive, and most have few side effects.

Description

Origins

There was a time not long ago when Western medicine believed that health depended solely upon the physical mechanisms of the body—that is, that a person is made up only of physical and chemical reactions that can be measured and manipulated scientifically. The notion that the mind and body live in separate compartments, so to speak, goes back to certain philosophers of classical antiquity. This concept of mind-body separation was also present in such religious groups as the Gnostics and some sects on the fringes of medieval Christianity. The scientific version of this split between mind and body is generally traced back to the seventeenth-century French philosopher Rene Descartes, whose thinking aided the development of science. It has taken a lot of time and research, three centuries after Descartes, for mainstream medicine to begin to accept that the mind plays a role in health and disease.

The idea that the mind and body interact is not new, however. It can be traced to the Wisdom literature in the Old Testament and to Hippocrates, the father of Western medicine. The ancient Hebrews attributed some physical illnesses to **grief** or anger. Hippocrates believed that health depends upon a balance of the body, mind and environment, and that disease is caused by imbalances in these areas. As modern science progressed, the mind and emotions became neglected, since researchers found it difficult to measure and quantify mental states with the scientific methods and equipment that were so highly valued.

Modern mind-body relationships become apparent

In the early 1900s, Harvard physiologist Walter Cannon coined the term "fight-or-flight response" for the body's reaction to threats, a response that causes increases in heart rate, blood pressure, blood sugar, muscle tension and respiration. During the 1950s, Hans Selye of McGill University pioneered research in what he called stress. Selye determined that the fight-or-flight response could be triggered by psychological factors as well as by physical threats. Stress includes having fight-or-flight reactions in situations where there is no immediate threat except mental perceptions and worries. Stress is not necessarily negative, except when people fail to cope with it effectively. Selye's work laid the groundwork for researchers to determine that stress and reactions to it play an integral role in health and disease.

Other mind-body relationships became apparent to medical researchers. The so-called placebo effect has been studied by doctors and psychologists for years. In clinical experiments, people who are given inert substances made to look like medicines, such as sugar pills, sometimes experience the same improvements as those patients who are given real medications. It is estimated that nearly one out of every three patients improves with medication simply because of the placebo effect and not because of the drug itself. Researchers have also noted that some conditions and illnesses have no physical explanations. Doctors termed these conditions psychosomatic illnesses, as they seem to be caused by the psyche, or mind.

Researchers then theorized that certain personality types are susceptible to particular conditions. For instance, "Type A" personalities tend to be aggressive, ambitious, and always rushed. They tend to cope with stress by getting angry and upset. Researchers have found that these personalities are more prone to heart disease, high blood pressure, and other stress-related conditions. "Type B" personalities are those who cope with stressful situations with communication and balance instead of anger and aggression, and have been found to be less prone to stress-related conditions. Researchers have added a "Type C" personality, who tends to suppress emotions and has trouble with self-expression. Some clinicians have proposed a link between suppressed emotions and the development of cancer.

In the 1970s, Dr. Herbert Benson at Harvard Medical School discovered what he called the "relaxation response." Benson observed that trained **yoga** specialists (yogis) could control bodily functions that had previously been believed to be autonomic, or beyond the control of the mind. During **meditation**, these yogis could reduce their heart rates, blood pressure, metabolism, body temperature, and other physiological processes to surprising levels. Other people who were then taught meditation were able to reach deep states of relaxation and calmness. This relaxation response, as Benson termed it, is essentially the opposite of the fight-or-flight response. The relaxation response reduces blood pressure, respiration, heart rate, oxygen consumption, muscle tension, and other bodily processes that are elevated by stress. Researchers soon began to theorize that if stress could have harmful effects on health, then the relaxation response might have the opposite effect. It was not long before the Harvard Mind-Body Medical Institute was founded, and other major medical clinics followed by integrating mind-body practices and studies into their health programs. A new field opened up in academic medicine called psychoneuroimmunology (PNI), which is the study of how the mind and nervous system affect the immune system. Studies have since shown that the mind and emotions play roles in many diseases, including cancer, diabetes, heart disease, gastrointestinal problems, and asthma.

In the past few decades, researchers have begun to unravel the complex ways in which the mind and body interact. Many findings have demonstrated that the mind and body are intimately interconnected. Medical science has shown that the nervous system works closely with the immune system, systems that were at one time believed to be separate. Nerve endings have been found that connect directly to important components of the immune system called lymph nodes. This connection demonstrates that there is a physical link between the mind and the immune system. Studies have also shown that thoughts and emotions alone can influence the activity of immune system cells.

Methods

There are many alternative techniques that draw upon the interconnections between mind and body. These include **art therapy**, **assertiveness training**, autogenic training, bioenergetics, **biofeedback**, breath therapy, guided imagery, **dance therapy** and movement therapy, dreamwork, **Gestalt therapy**, **group therapy**, hypnosis, meditation, mindfulness training, Jungian **psychoanalysis**, postural integration, prayer and faith healing, progressive relaxation, psychodrama, **psychotherapy**, Reichian therapy, **support groups**, and yoga. Some of the most widely used techniques are meditation, mindfulness training, biofeedback, breath therapy, hypnosis, guided imagery, and movement therapies.

Meditation

There are many forms of meditation, but they all have the same goal, which is to calm and focus the mind. As beginning meditators find out, however, calming and clearing the mind of thoughts and worries is easier said than done. When performed on a regular basis, meditation is an efficient way of promoting the relaxation response. Meditation is used to ease the physical discomfort of many health problems, including stress-related conditions, chronic pain, panic disorders, and tension headaches.

Meditation can be practiced anywhere, but a quiet and peaceful setting is recommended. Persons should sit up straight or lie in a comfortable position. Breathing during meditation should be deep, calm, and slow. The meditator may concentrate on the breath or on a still object such as a flower or candle flame. The meditator often may repeat a soft sound, word, or phrase, known as a mantra. Mantras can be affirmative statements, prayers, or humming sounds. The goal of the meditator is to concentrate deeply in order to reduce the amount of thinking, and to calm the worries and thoughts that typically fill the mind. When thoughts or distractions arise, the meditator should allow them to pass without directing attention toward them.

Meditation is usually practiced twice a day, for 20 minutes at a time, preferably at consistent times to develop discipline. It can be learned from books or tapes, but instruction is widely available and recommended, as beginners can find properly meditating and quieting the mind to be difficult at first.

Mindfulness training

This form of mental discipline was made popular by Dr. Jon Kabat-Zinn, a **psychologist** at the University of Massachusetts Medical Center, who has written some popular books on mind-body medicine. Kabat-Zinn uses mindfulness training to help patients deal with chronic illnesses and pain. Mindfulness training is also good for stress-related conditions and persons undergoing difficult

KEY TERMS

Behavioral medicine—The branch of medicine that studies mind-body relationships.

Fight-or-flight response—The body's reaction to threats.

Mantra—A sacred word or formula repeated over and over to concentrate the mind.

Placebo—A pharmacologically inactive substance disguised as a real medication.

Psychoneuroimmunology—The study of the relationships among mind, nervous system, and immune response.

Psychosomatic—A type of physical illness caused by mental factors.

Relaxation response—The calming of bodily responses through relaxation techniques.

Vipassana—A Buddhist meditative practice that emphasizes deep attentiveness to the present moment.

treatments like surgery or chemotherapy. Practitioners of mindfulness claim it helps them experience more pleasure and less stress in their everyday activities.

Mindfulness training originated from a Buddhist practice called *vipassana*. Its basic idea is that deep awareness of the present moment is the essential discipline. Lack of awareness and attention can lead to stress and bad health habits. To be mindful is to participate fully in whatever one is doing at the present moment, whether reading, walking, working, eating, exercising, relaxing, etc. When a person pays full attention to the present moment without judgment, then worries about the past and future tend to disappear, and stress levels are also significantly reduced.

Mindfulness training teaches that painful situations and emotions should be experienced with full attention as well, which helps people to confront and accept them. Mindfulness training uses techniques like the body scan, in which the patient focuses full attention on each part of the body in succession. This technique helps people become more aware of their bodies and learn to control their reactions to stress, change, and illness.

Biofeedback

Biofeedback uses special instruments that measure and display heart rate, perspiration, muscle tension, **brain** wave activity, body temperature, respiratory patterns, and other indicators of stress and physiological activity. Patients can observe their measurements and learn to consciously control functions that were previously unconsciously controlled. Biofeedback also helps people learn how to initiate the relaxation response quickly and effectively.

Biofeedback is used to treat hypertension, stress-related headaches, migraine headaches, **attention deficit hyperactivity disorder**, and diabetes. Biofeedback is used often in physical therapy to rehabilitate damaged nerves and muscles. It is also an approved treatment for a vascular disorder called Raynaud's syndrome. Patients with this syndrome experience blanching and numbness in their hands and feet in response to cold or emotional stress.

Breath therapy

Breath therapy works on the premise that breathing plays a central role in the body and mind. People who are under stress tend to breathe rapidly and shallowly, whereas slow and deep breathing has been shown to reduce stress and promote the relaxation response. In Ayurvedic medicine and traditional Chinese medicine, the breath is considered the most important metabolic function. In yoga, there is a science of breathing techniques known as pranayama, which is designed to reduce stress and promote health.

Breath therapy is often used in conjunction with meditation and other mind-body techniques. It can be learned from books and tapes or from a yoga or mind-body specialist. It is an inexpensive treatment, and once learned can be practiced easily anywhere.

Hypnosis

Hypnosis is deeply focused attention that brings about a trance state that is somewhere between waking and sleeping. During hypnosis, the mind is very open to suggestion. Mental imagery is often used in conjunction with hypnosis to maximize positive thinking and healing.

Hypnosis, or **hypnotherapy**, is used to reduce stress, anxiety, and pain, and help patients suffering from chronic diseases. It is also used to assist people in overcoming bad health habits and addictions to **nicotine**, alcohol and drugs. Some dentists use hypnosis to help patients relax during dental procedures. Research continues to show the benefits of hypnosis. Hypnosis is best performed by trained hypnotherapists, who can teach techniques of self-hypnosis to the patient.

Guided imagery

This technique uses the imagination to stimulate healing responses in the body, as studies have shown that the imagination can cause the same activity in the brain and immune system as real events. Patients are taught to imagine places or situations in which they have felt happy, healthy, or safe. Patients can also focus on images that increase confidence, reduce stress, and promote healing. Mental imaging techniques are also used in conjunction with many other mind-body techniques like meditation and hypnosis, as it is an efficient means of promoting positive mental attitudes. Mental imaging techniques can be learned from books, audiotapes, videos, and from professional therapists and teachers.

Movement therapy

Movement routines, such as dance therapy, have been shown to have a significant mind-body element. In these therapies, which also include martial arts, yoga, and tai chi, strict routines of physical movements are designed to involve high levels of mental concentration and awareness of the body. Movement therapies are good for people who have trouble sitting still for meditation and are an excellent way of improving physical strength and mental health at the same time.

Precautions

Mind-body practices are safe and have few side effects. They should not, however, be relied upon solely when other medical care is required. Consumers should seek reliable and properly trained practitioners, particularly in those practices and states for which certification is not required by law.

Costs can vary widely for mind-body treatments, depending on the type and the medical training of the practitioner. Consumers should be aware of their insurance provisions, in case their provider does not cover mind-body treatments.

Research & general acceptance

Because of its increasing acceptance by mainstream medicine, mind-body medicine has been the subject of intense research. Studies have shed new light on everything from the minute interactions of the immune and nervous systems to the effective results of individual therapies like meditation and guided imagery. Other studies have indicated relationships between stress and disease. Some eye-opening results have been observed as well, such as studies that have shown that cancer and heart disease patients utilizing mind-body techniques had significantly longer survival rates on average than those patients who did not use mind-body therapies. Despite increasingly proven benefits to mind–body medicine, few health plans pay for the treatments.

QUESTIONS TO ASK YOUR DOCTOR

- How can I benefit from mind-body treatment?
- Is it beneficial to integrate mind-body techniques with my conventional medicines or other therapies?
- What specific practices or treatments would you recommended for me?

Resources

BOOKS

Harrington, Anne. *The Cure Within: A History of Mind-Body Medicine*. New York: W.W. Norton & Co, 2009.

Mayo Clinic. *Mayo Clinic Book of Alternative Medicine: The New Approach to Using the Best of Natural Therapies and Conventional Medicine*. New York: Time Inc. Home Entertainment, 2007.

Rotan, Leo W., and Veronika Ospina-Kammerer. *MindBody Medicine: Foundations and Practical Applications*. New York: Taylor & Francis Ltd., 2007.

PERIODICALS

Vaucher, Andrea R., "Doctor's Orders: Cross Your Legs and Say 'Om'." *Los Angeles Times* (October 29, 2007).

Wang, Chenchen, Jean Paul Collett, and Joseph Lau. "The Effect of Tai Chi on Health Outcomes in Patients With Chronic Conditions A Systematic Review." *Archives Internal Medicine* 164 (2004): 493–501.

OTHER

U.S. National Center for Complementary and Alternative Medicine. "Mind-Body Medicine: An Overview." National Institutes of Health. August 2005. http://www.qigonginstitute.org/html/papers/NCCAMmindbody.pdf (accessed November 9, 2011).

ORGANIZATIONS

Academy for Guided Imagery, 10780 Santa Monica Boulevard, Los Angeles, CA, 90025, (800) 726-2070, Fax: (800) 727-2070, info@acadhi.com, http://acadgi.com.

American Society of Clinical Hypnosis, 140 N. Bloomingdale Rd., Bloomingdale, IL, 60108, (630) 980-4740, Fax: (630) 351-8490, http://www.asch.net.

Biofeedback Certification International Alliance, 10200 W 44th Ave., Ste. 304, Wheatridge, CO, 80033, (303) 420-2902, http://www.bcia.org/i4a/pages/index.cfm?pageid=1.

Center for Mind Body Medicine, http://www.cmbm.org.

National Center for Complementary and Alternative Medicine, 9000 Rockville Pike, Bethesda, MD, 20892, info@nccam.nih.gov, http://nccam.nih.gov.

Vipassana Meditation Center, PO Box 24, Shelbourne Falls, MA, 01370, (413) 625-2160, http://www.dhamma.org/en/schedules/schdhara.shtml.

Douglas Dupler
Teresa G. Odle
Brenda W. Lerner

Mini-mental state examination

Definition

The mini-mental state examination, which is also known as the MMSE, standardized MMSE, SMMSE, or the Folstein, is a brief examination consisting of 11 questions, scored with a maximum of 30 points, intended to evaluate an adult patient's level of cognitive functioning, specifically looking for **brain** impairment with respect to **dementia**, such as **Alzheimer's disease**. The test was introduced in 1975 by Marshall Folstein and colleagues and designed for use with elderly patients who are able to cooperate at an optimum level with an examiner for only a brief period, perhaps no more than a few minutes. It tests for cognitive function by assessing attention and calculation, language abilities, orientation, visual-spatial ability, and word recall.

Purpose

The MMSE concentrates on the cognitive aspects of mental functioning, excluding questions about the patient's mood or such abnormal experiences as dissociation. It is used most often to evaluate older adults for **delirium** or dementia. The MMSE can be used to detect the severity of cognitive impairment, to measure decline in cognitive function, to follow the course of the patient's illness, and to monitor responses to treatment. In the early 2000s, it was professionally approved as a measurement of a patient's ability to complete an advance directive, or so-called living will.

The test has been used in research as a screener in epidemiological studies for disorders that affect cognition and to monitor changes in subjects' cognition during **clinical trials**. In 2001, the MMSE was recommended by a special panel of experts for use as a screener in evaluating cognitive function in depressed patients. It has also been used to measure the effects of **acupuncture** in improving mood and some cognitive skills in patients with Alzheimer's disease.

The MMSE evaluates six areas of cognitive function: orientation, attention, immediate recall, short-term recall, language, and the ability to follow simple verbal and written commands. In addition, it provides a total score allowing the examiner to place the patient on a scale of cognitive function. It correlates well with a standard measure of cognition in adults, the Wechsler Adult Intelligence Scale (WAIS). In contrast to the Wechsler, which takes about an hour or more to administer, the MMSE can be completed in ten minutes or less.

Description

The mini-mental state examination identifies serious mental functions, including arithmetic, memory, and orientation. It screens for cognitive impairment in individuals from 18 to 100 years of age. The test is divided into two sections, together taking from 10 to 15 minutes to administer. The first part requires vocal responses to the examiner's questions. The patient is asked to repeat a short phrase after the examiner; to count backward from 100 by 7s; to name the current president of the United States (in Great Britain, the names of the queen and her four children); and similar brief items. It tests the patient's orientation, memory, and attention. The maximum score on this section is 21.

In the second part of the examination, the patient is asked to follow verbal and written instructions, write a sentence spontaneously, and copy a complex geometric figure similar to a Bender-Gestalt figure—a series of nine designs each on separate cards given the test taker who is asked to reproduce them on blank paper. The sentence item usually asks the patient to explain the meaning of a simple proverb such as "People who live in glass houses shouldn't throw stones." The maximum score for the second section is 9. Patients with vision problems can be assisted with large writing. The MMSE is not timed.

The eight categories (and their descriptions and maximum number of points) of the MMSE are:

- orientation to time (questions asked about time, such as "What time is it?"; 5 maximum points)
- orientation to place (questions asked about location, such as "What floor are we on in this building?"; 5 maximum points)
- registration (asked to repeat whatever is stated; 3 maximum points)
- attention and calculation (asked to spell words backwards, count backwards by seven; 5 maximum points)
- recall (asked to recall three words that were previously requested to be remembered; 3 maximum points)
- language (asked to name objects, such as pencil or watch; 2 maximum points)

- repetition (asked to speak back a phrase; 1 maximum point)
- complex commands (asked to draw figures and other various tasks; 6 maximum points)

Little information is available on allowances made in scoring the MMSE for patients whose first language is not English or who have difficulty with standard spoken English. However, in 2010, the Psychological Assessment Resources (PAR), the publisher of the test, released MMSE in a second edition (MMSE-2), with translations in Chinese (simplified), Dutch, French, German, Hindi, Italian, Russian, Spanish (Latin America), Spanish (Europe), and Spanish (United States). This second edition is authored by Marshal F. Folstein and Susan E. Folstein.

The MMSE-2 is similar to the first edition, with the basic structure and scoring retained and problems in the first edition corrected. In addition, some wording for the registration/recall and repetition tasks was changed slightly so that translations could be made. The comprehensive task was also altered to make it easier for persons with physical disabilities.

The second edition MMSE was normalized from a sample of over 1,500 people with either Alzheimer's disease or subcortical dementia. Reliability and validity was established with the use of this normative sample.

Several new features were added to the MMSE-2, including a brief version (BV) of the MMSE-2. The MMSE-2 BV is used when a fast cognitive screening test is required. Administration of the BV takes about five minutes. In addition, an expanded version (EV) of the MMSE-2 is also offered. The 90-item MMSE-2 EV expands on the scoring of the MMSE-2 by increasing the (scoring) sensitivity to individuals with less severe cognitive problems. As such, the expanded version includes two new tasks: story memory (which is an immediate recall of a short story) and processing speed (a symbol-digit coding task). The EV takes about 20 minutes to administer.

The MMSE-2 correlates well with the digit span forward and digit span backward subtests of the Wechsler Memory Scale, third edition; the digit symbol and block design subtests of the Wechsler Adult Intelligence Scale, revised; the Category Naming Test; the Boston Naming Test; the Trail Making Test; the Judgment of Line Orientation; the Stroop Color and Word Test; and the Hopkins Verbal Learning Test, revised.

Preparation

Preparation for the MMSE is neither necessary nor required.

KEY TERMS

Alzheimer's disease—A type of dementia that involves brain disease and progressive degradation of the brain, which involves memory loss and an eventual inability to think and function.

Cognitive—Relating to thoughts and the acquisition of knowledge.

Dementia—The progressive deterioration of intellectual functions, such as memory, within the brain. A type of dementia is Alzheimer's disease.

Schizophrenia—A mental disorder involving degraded thinking and emotions.

Aftercare

There is no aftercare as such for the person who takes this test, but test results are useful to medical professionals and caregivers. The MMSE is used primarily as a valid and reliable way to screen for Alzheimer's disease. Although it is not meant to be used solely as a screening device for such dementia, it can be used as a beginning test to identify persons without the disease. It is also used as a means to chart the course of cognitive declines over time. Consequently, it is a useful way to document a person's response to treatment in the past and to prescribe treatment in the future.

Risks

There is no risk to individuals taking this test. The MMSE should not be used as the sole criterion for assessment during differential **diagnosis** of psychiatric disorders, as there are many disorders and conditions that affect cognitive functioning. The results of the MMSE should be interpreted in the context of the patient's history, a full **mental status examination**, a physical examination, and laboratory findings, if any.

A patient's score on the MMSE must be interpreted according to his or her age and educational level. Scores range from 0 to 30. Whereas the median score is 29 for persons 18–24 years of age, it is 25 for those who are 80 years or older. The median score is 22 for persons with a fourth-grade education or less; 26 for those who completed the eighth grade; and 29 for those who completed high school or college. A complete table within the MMSE Pocket Norms Guide is available for interpreting MMSE scores according to the patient's reference groups for age and education level. Scores of 25 or higher are generally regarded as normal (without cognitive impairment), whereas scores of between 10 and

QUESTIONS TO ASK YOUR DOCTOR

- Do I need to find a qualified health care professional who is knowledgeable at administering the MMSE? If so, who do you recommend?
- Will the MMSE results indicate what treatment is needed?
- Where can I learn more about the MMSE?
- What are the best tests that can be taken to help verify the MMSE's conclusion? Which ones do you recommend?

19 indicate moderate cognitive impairment, and scores of less than 10 indicate severe impairment. It is possible to earn a high score but still have strong cognitive problems.

Precautions

The MMSE should be administered and scored only by a qualified healthcare professional, such as a **psychologist**, physician, or nurse.

Results

The maximum total score on the basic MMSE is 30. As a rule, scores of 20 or lower indicate delirium, dementia, **schizophrenia**, or a mood disorder. Normal subjects and those with a primary diagnosis of personality disorder score close to the median for their age and education level.

The MMSE-2 adds to the original MMSE by allowing for more precise evaluations of individuals with less severe forms of cognitive impairment, such as subcortical dementia. However, the second edition is generally equivalent to the original one, with the addition of the brief version and the expanded version. In fact, administrators can switch between the editions without altering longitudinal data and without changing scoring.

Resources

BOOKS

Barnovitz, Mary Ann, and Pria Joglekar. *Medical Psychiatry: The Quick Reference.* Philadelphia: Wolters Kluwer Health/Lippincott Williams & Wilkins, 2008.

Groth-Marnat, Gary. *Handbook of Psychological Assessment,* 5th ed. Hoboken, NJ: John Wiley and Sons, 2009.

Hersen, Michel, ed. *Industrial and Organizational Assessment.* Vol. 4 of *Comprehensive Handbook of Psychological Assessment.* Edited by Jay C. Thomas. Hoboken, NJ: John Wiley and Sons, 2004.

Kellerman, Henry, and Anthony Burry. *Handbook of Psychodiagnostic Testing: Analysis of Personality in the Psychological Report,* 4th ed. New York City: Springer, 2010.

Leeming, David A., Kathryn Madden, and Stanton Marlan, eds. *Encyclopedia of Psychology and Religion.* New York City: Springer, 2011.

Lezak, Muriel D., Diane B. Howieson, and David W. Loring. *Neuropsychological Assessment,* 4th ed. New York: Oxford University Press, 2004.

McPhee, Stephen J., and Maxine A. Papadakis, eds. *Current Medical Diagnosis & Treatment 2011.* New York City: McGraw-Hill Medial, 2011.

WEBSITES

"Mini-Mental® State Examination, 2nd Edition." PAR: Creating Connections, Changing Lives. http://www4.parinc.com/Products/Product.aspx?ProductID=MMSE-2 (accessed July 27, 2011).

ORGANIZATIONS

American Psychiatric Association, 1000 Wilson Blvd., Ste. 1825, Arlington, VA, 22209-3901, (703) 907-7300, apa@psych.org, http://www.psych.org.

American Psychological Association, 750 1st St. NE, Washington, DC, 20002, (202) 336-5500, (800) 374-2721, http://www.apa.org.

National Institute of Neurological Disorders and Stroke, PO Box 5801, Bethesda, MD, 20892, (301) 496-5751, (800) 352-9424, http://www.ninds.nih.gov.

Rebecca J. Frey, PhD

Minnesota Multiphasic Personality Inventory

Definition

The Minnesota Multiphasic Personality Inventory, known as the MMPI, and its revised second edition (MMPI-2) are **psychological assessment** instruments used to gather information on the personalities, attitudes, and mental health of persons aged 18 and older to aid in clinical **diagnosis**. The test identifies mental illness and abnormal behavior by evaluating personality traits of the test taker. It is one of the most widely used personality inventory tests used in psychology, especially in the area of mental health.

Purpose

The results of the MMPI-2 allow the test administrator to make inferences about the client's typical behaviors and way of thinking. The clinician evaluates the test taker's personal characteristics by comparing the test taker's answers to those given by various psychiatric and nonpsychiatric comparison groups. By analyzing the test taker's patterns of response to the test items, the examiner is able to draw some tentative conclusions about the client's level of adaptation, behavioral characteristics, and personality traits. The outcomes help the examiner to determine the test taker's severity of impairment, outlook on life, approaches to problem solving, typical mood states, likely diagnoses, and potential problems in treatment. The MMPI-2 is used in a wide range of settings for a variety of procedures. The inventory is often used as part of inpatient psychiatric assessments, differential diagnosis, and outpatient evaluations. In addition, the instrument is often used by expert witnesses in forensic settings as part of an evaluation of a defendant's mental health, particularly in criminal cases. The MMPI has also been used to evaluate candidates for employment in some fields, and in educational counseling.

The MMPI-2 is preferred to the older MMPI because of its larger and more representative community comparison group (also referred to as the "normative" group). The original version of the MMPI is no longer available from the publisher, although some institutions continue to use old copies of it.

Description

The MMPI-2 is composed of 567 true/false items. It can be administered using a printed test booklet and an answer sheet filled in by hand, or by responding to the items on a computer. For the person with limited reading skills or the visually impaired respondent, the MMPI-2 items are available on audiotape. Although the MMPI-2 is frequently referred to as a test, it is not an academic test with "right" and "wrong" answers. Personality inventories like the MMPI-2 are intended to discover what the respondent is like as a person. A number of areas are "tapped into" by the MMPI-2 to answer such questions as: "Who is this person and how would he or she typically feel, think, and behave? What psychological problems and issues are relevant to this person?" Associations between patterns of answers to test items and particular traits or behaviors have been discovered through personality research conducted with the MMPI-2. The inventory items are not arranged into topics or areas on the test. The areas of personality that are measured are interspersed in a somewhat random fashion throughout the MMPI-2 booklet. Some examples of true-or-false statements similar to those on the MMPI-2 are:

- "I wake up with a headache almost every day."
- "I certainly feel worthless sometimes."
- "I have had peculiar and disturbing experiences that most other people have not had."
- "I would like to do the work of a choir director."

The MMPI-2 is intended for use with adults over age 18; a similar test, the MMPI-A, is designed for use with adolescents. The publisher produces the MMPI-2 in English and Spanish versions. The test has also been translated into Dutch-Flemish, two French dialects (France and Canada), German, Hebrew, Hmong, Italian, and three Spanish dialects (for Spain, Mexico, or the United States).

Origins

From the 1940s to the 1980s, the original MMPI was the most widely used and most intensely researched psychological assessment instrument in the United States and worldwide. American **psychologist** Starke R. Hathaway (1903–1984) and American neuropsychiatrist J. Charnley McKinley (1891–1950), both from the University of Minnesota (Minneapolis-St. Paul), developed the MMPI in the late 1930s, and it was first published in 1940. The MMPI utilized a process called empirical keying, which was an innovation. Most assessment tools prior to the MMPI used questions or tasks that were merely assumed by the test designer to realistically assess the behaviors under question. The empirical keying process was radically different. To develop empirical keying, the creators of the original MMPI wrote a wide range of true-or-false statements, many of which did not directly target typical psychiatric topics. Research was then conducted with groups of psychiatric inpatients, hospital visitors, college students and medical inpatients, who took the MMPI in order to determine which test items reliably differentiated the psychiatric patients from the others. The test developers also evaluated the items that reliably distinguished groups of patients with a particular diagnosis from the remaining pool of psychiatric patient respondents; these items were grouped into subsets referred to as clinical scales.

An additional innovation in the original MMPI was the presence of validity scales embedded in the test questions. These sets of items, scattered randomly throughout the MMPI-2, allow the examiner to assess whether the respondent answered questions in an open and honest manner, or tried to exaggerate or conceal information. One means of checking for distortions in responding to the instrument is asking whether the test taker refused to admit to some less-than-ideal actions that most people probably engage in and will admit to doing. An example of this type of question would be (true or false) "If I could sneak into the county fair or an amusement park without paying, I would." Another type of validity check that assesses honesty in responses is whether the client admits to participating in far more unusual behaviors and actions than were admitted to by both the psychiatric comparison group and the general community sample. The validity scales also identify whether the test taker responded inconsistently or randomly.

The MMPI-2, which has demonstrated continuity and comparability with its predecessor, was published in 1989. The revised version was based on a much larger and more racially and culturally diverse normative community comparison group than the original version. Also, more in-depth and stringent research on the qualities and behaviors associated with different patterns of scores allows improved accuracy in predicting test-respondents' traits and behaviors from their test results.

Three years later, in 1992, the MMPI-A was first published, with A standing for Adolescent. The most recent revision, published in 2006, consists of 478 items within 12 test categories; a short form consisting of 350 items is also available. The MMPI-A, administered individually or within a group, targets adolescents 14 to 18 years of age.

In 2003, the MMPI-2-RF (Restructured Form) was introduced. The MMPI-2-RF consists of 338 items and cites itself as being an alternative to, not a replacement for, the MMPI-2. The most recent revision was published in 2008 by Pearson Assessments.

Scoring

The clinical scales within the MMPI-2 are designed to measure common diagnoses. They include:

- Scale 1 (Hypochondriasis [Hs] Scale) measures bodily symptoms as perceived by the person with regards to their health and health issues. It contains 32 items.
- Scale 2 (Depression [D] Scale) measures a person's symptoms with regard to depression. It contains 57 items.
- Scale 3 (Hysteria [Hy] Scale) measures the emotional ity of a person, along with their perception of vulnerability and their awareness of such problems. It contains 60 items.
- Scale 4 (Psychopathic Deviate [Pd] Scale) measures the amount of control that a person wants in life, the amount of anger resulting from lack of control in one's life, and the amount of disrespect for the rules of society. It contains 50 items.
- Scale 5 (Masculinity/Femininity [MF] Scale) measures how men and women compare with masculine and feminine (respectively) interests and behaviors of stereotypical characters. It contains 56 items.
- Scale 6 (Paranoia [Pa] Scale) measures a person's level of trust, suspiciousness, and sensitivity to such emotions. It contains 40 items.
- Scale 7 (Psychasthenia [Pt] Scale) measures levels and tendencies of anxiety, worry, doubts, and obsessiveness. It contains 48 items.
- Scale 8 (Schizophrenia [Sc] Scale) measures the unusual cognitive, perceptual, and emotional experiences of a person. It contains 78 items.
- Scale 9 (Mania [Ma] Scale) measures a person's level of energy. It contains 46 items.
- Scale 0 (Social Introversion [Si] Scale) measures the level at which a person enjoys and is comfortable around other people. It contains 69 items.

Specific conditions or syndromes that the test can help identify include **depression**, **hypochondriasis**, hysteria, **paranoia**, and **schizophrenia**. Raw scores based on deviations from standard responses are entered on personality profile forms to obtain the individual results. There is also a validity scale to thwart attempts to "fake" the test. Because the MMPI-2 is a complex test whose results can sometimes be ambiguous (and/or skewed by various factors), professionals tend to be cautious in interpreting it, often preferring broad descriptions to specific psychiatric diagnoses, unless these are supported by further testing and observable behavior. A fifth-grade reading level is required in order to take the test. However, a tape-recorded version is available for those with limited literacy, visual impairments, or other problems.

Risks

Although the MMPI-2 may be administered by trained clerical staff or by computer, for best results the examiner should meet the test taker before giving the test in order to establish the context and reassure the client. Most importantly, the test responses should be interpreted only by a qualified mental health professional with postgraduate education in psychological assessment and specialized training in the use of the MMPI-2. While computer-generated narrative reports are available and can be a useful tool, they should be evaluated (and edited if needed) by the on-site professional to individualize the reported results. Computer scoring and hypothesis generation is complex, and only reputable software programs should be used.

Although the MMPI-2 may yield extensive information about the client, it is not a replacement for a clinical interview. The clinical interview helps the test

KEY TERMS

Battery—A number of separate items (such as tests) used together. In psychology, a group or series of tests given with a common purpose, such as personality assessment or measurement of intelligence.

Biopsychosocial history—A history of significant past and current experiences that influence client behaviors, including medical, educational, employment, and interpersonal experiences. Alcohol or drug use and involvement with the legal system are also assessed in a biopsychosocial history.

Empirical—Verified by actual experience or by scientific experimentation.

Forensic—Pertaining to courtroom procedure or evidence used in courts of law.

Hypothesis—An assumption, proposition, or educated guess that can be tested empirically.

Personality inventory—A type of psychological test that is designed to assess a client's major personality traits, behavioral patterns, coping styles, and similar characteristics. The MMPI-2 is an example of a personality inventory.

Psychological assessment—A process of gathering and synthesizing information about a person's psychological makeup and history for a specific purpose, which may be educational, diagnostic, or forensic.

Scale—A subset of test items from a multi-item test.

administrator to develop conclusions that best apply to the client from the many hypotheses generated from test results. Furthermore, important aspects of the client's behaviors may emerge in an interview that were not reflected in the test results. For similar reasons, the test results should not be interpreted until the clinician has obtained a biopsychosocial history from the client.

The MMPI-2 should be administered as part of a battery, or group, of tests rather than as an isolated assessment measure. A comprehensive assessment of a person will typically include the Rorschach; the **Thematic Apperception Test** (TAT) or the Sentence Completion Test; and the Wechsler Adult Intelligence Scale, Revised (WAIS-R) or similar test of cognitive functioning, as well as the MMPI-2.

The test has been criticized in the past as being too personal when asking many of its questions, with topics pertaining to a person's sex life, religious beliefs, and political viewpoints. Lawsuits attempting to protect the privacy of individuals and the fairness of employment practices have been brought against individuals and organizations that use the test.

Results

The true/false items are organized after scoring into validity, clinical, and content scales. The inventory may be scored manually or by computer. After scoring, the configuration of the test taker's scale scores is marked on a profile form that contrasts each client's responses to results obtained by the representative community comparison group. The clinician is able to compare a respondent's choices to those of a large normative comparison group as well as to the results derived from earlier MMPI and MMPI-2 studies. The clinician forms inferences about the client by analyzing his or her response patterns on the validity, clinical and content scales, using published guidebooks to the MMPI-2. These texts are based on results obtained from over 10,000 MMPI/MMPI-2 research studies.

In addition to the standard validity, clinical, and content scales, numerous additional scales for the MMPI have been created for special purposes over the years by researchers. These special supplementary scale scores are often incorporated into the examiner's interpretation of the test results. Commonly used supplementary scales include the MacAndrews Revised Alcoholism Scale, the Addiction Potential Scale, and the Anxiety Scale. The clinician may also choose to obtain computerized reporting, which yields behavioral hypotheses about the respondent, using scoring and interpretation algorithms applied to a commercial database.

Resources

BOOKS

Andrade, Heidi L., and Gregory J. Cizek, eds. *Handbook of Formative Assessment*. New York: Routledge, 2009.

Butcher, James N., and Carolyn L. Williams. *Essentials of MMPI2 and MMPIA Interpretation*. 2nd ed. Minneapolis: University of Minnesota Press, 2000.

Butcher, J. N., et al. *MMPI-2: Manual for Administration, Scoring and Interpretation*. Revised. Minneapolis: University of Minnesota Press, 2001.

Drummond, Robert J., and Karen Jones. *Assessment Procedures for Counselors and Helping Professionals*. 7th ed. Boston: Pearson, 2010.

Frick, Paul J., Christopher T. Barry, and Randy W. Kamphaus. *Clinical Assessment of Child and Adolescent Personality and Behavior*. 3rd ed. New York: Springer, 2010.

Graham, John R. *MMPI-2: Assessing Personality and Psychopathology*. 5th ed. New York: Oxford University Press, 2011.

Graham, John R., Yossef S. Ben-Porath, and John L. McNulty. *MMPI-2: Correlates for Outpatient Community Mental*

Health Settings. Minneapolis: University of Minnesota Press, 1999.

Green, Susan K., and Robert L. Johnson. *Assessment is Essential*. Boston: McGraw-Hill, 2009.

Kaufman, James C. *Intelligent Testing: Integrating Psychological Theory and Clinical Practice*. Cambridge, UK: Cambridge University Press, 2009.

Spies, Robert A., Janet F. Carlson, and Kurt F. Geisinger. *The Eighteenth Mental Measurements Yearbook*. Buros Center for Testing, 2010.

PERIODICALS

Bennett, Drake. "Against Types." *Boston Globe*, September 12, 2004. http://www.boston.com/news/globe/ideas/articles/2004/09/12/against_types (accessed October 22, 2011).

Butcher, James N. "MMPI-2/MMPI-A Research Project: Research and Clinical Applications," University of Minnesota. http://www1.umn.edu/mmpi (accessed October 22, 2011).

"Dr. Starke R. Hathaway, 80; Invented Psychological Test." *The New York Times*, July 5, 1984. http://www.nytimes.com/1984/07/05/obituaries/dr-starke-r-hathaway-80-invented-psychological-test.html (accessed October 22, 2011).

McNulty, J.L., J.R. Graham, and Y. S. Ben-Porath. "An Empirical Examination of the Correlates of Well-defined and Not Defined MMPI-2 Codetypes." *Journal of Personality Assessment* 71, no. 3 (1998): 393–410.

Paul, Annie Murphy. "Invasion of the Minnesota Normals." *The Believer*, (August 2004), http://www.believermag.com/issues/200408/?read=article_paul (accessed October 22, 2011).

Deborah Rosch Eifert, Ph.D.
William Arthur Atkins

Mirtazapine

Definition

Mirtazapine is most commonly used to treat **depression**. Mirtazapine is available in the United States under the trade names of Remeron and Remeron SolTab.

Mirtazapine, sold under the trade name Remeron, is taken by mouth and swallowed whole. Remeron SolTabs should be allowed to dissolve in the mouth. No water is needed when taking the SolTabs, since these tablets disintegrate in saliva and are not swallowed whole.

Purpose

Mirtazapine is best known for treating depression. However, it may also be used for treating anxiety or to make people drowsy just before surgery.

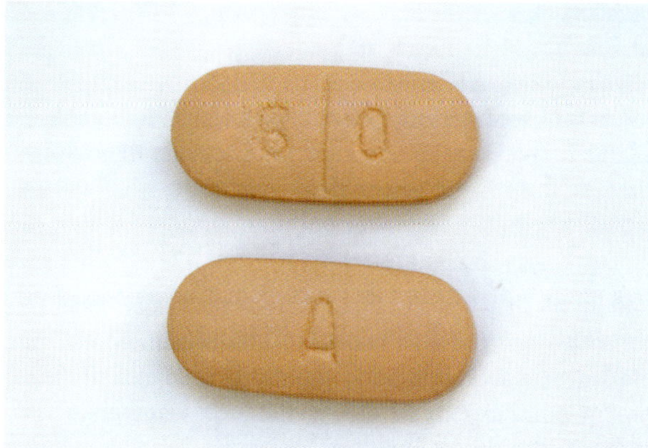

Mirtazapine, 30 mg. *(© Custom Medical Stock Photo, Inc. Reproduced by permission.)*

Description

Mirtazapine is usually thought of as an antidepressant, that is, a drug that alleviates symptoms of depression. Approved by the Federal Drug Administration (FDA) in 1996, it is believed to alter the activities of some chemicals in the **brain** and, in this way, reduce chemical imbalances responsible for causing depression and anxiety. As with all **antidepressants**, it may take several weeks of treatment before full beneficial effects are seen. Mirtazapine is broken down by the liver and eliminated from the body mostly by the kidneys. It is supplied in 15, 30, and 45 mg tablets.

Recommended dosage

The recommended initial dose of mirtazapine in 15 mg taken at bedtime. The dose may be increased in 15 mg increments every one or two weeks as needed until symptoms of depression or anxiety resolve. Typical doses range between 15 and 45 mg. Dosages above 45 mg per day are not recommended. Elderly people or those with liver or kidney disease should use mirtazapine carefully, since they may be more sensitive to some of the drug's side effects.

Precautions

Mirtazapine may cause weight gain and may increase cholesterol levels and should be used carefully in overweight individuals and those with high cholesterol levels. If symptoms of fever, sore throat, or irritation in the mouth occur, a healthcare provider should be notified. Rarely, mirtazapine may lower blood counts, causing people to be at an increased risk of serious complications, including infections. In theory, mirtazapine may increase the tendency for **seizures**. As a result, it should be used carefully in people with epilepsy or

KEY TERMS

Anxiety—An emotion that can be experienced as a troubled feeling, sense of dread, fear of the future, or distress over a possible threat to a person's physical or mental well-being.

Depression—A mental state characterized by feelings of sadness, despair, discouragement, low energy, often with oversleeping and/or overeating.

Monoamine oxidase inhibitors (MAOIs)—A class of antidepressants used to treat certain types of depression. Monoamine oxidase inhibitors are especially useful in treating people whose depression is combined with other problems such as anxiety, panic attacks, phobias, or the desire to sleep too much.

Seizure—A convulsion, or uncontrolled discharge of nerve cells that may spread to other cells throughout the brain.

other seizure disorders. Mirtazapine may alter moods or cause mania. It should be used carefully in people with a history of mania. Mirtazapine may alter liver function and should be used cautiously by those with a history of liver disease. If abdominal pain, yellowing of the skin or eyes, darkening of urine, or itching occurs, a healthcare provider should be notified immediately.

More than 50% of individuals using mirtazapine report feeling sleepier than normal and 7% feel dizzy. As a result, people taking mirtazapine should not participate in activities that require mental alertness, such as driving, until they know how the drug will affect them. Because there is an increased likelihood of **suicide** in depressed individuals, close supervision of those at high risk for suicide attempts using this drug is recommended. Children and young people up to age 24 are particularly affected, especially during the early stages of treatment. Mirtazapine is not recommended in pregnant or breast-feeding women. Use of the medicine should not be abruptly stopped, as withdrawal symptoms may occur.

Side effects

The most common side effects that cause people to stop taking mirtazapine are sleepiness and nausea. Other common side effects are dizziness, increased appetite, and weight gain. Less common adverse effects are weakness and muscle aches, flu-like symptoms, low blood-cell counts, high cholesterol, back pain, chest pain, rapid heartbeats, dry mouth, constipation, water retention, difficulty sleeping, nightmares, abnormal thoughts, vision disturbances, ringing in the ears, abnormal taste in the mouth, tremor, confusion, upset stomach, and increased urination.

QUESTIONS TO ASK YOUR DOCTOR

- What kind of changes can I expect to see or feel with this medication?
- Does it matter what time of day I take this medication? If so, what is the recommendation?
- Should I take this medication with or without food?
- What are the side effects associated with this medication?
- Will this medication interact or interfere with other medications I am currently taking?
- What symptoms or adverse effects are important enough that I should seek immediate treatment?

Interactions

Use of mirtazapine with **monoamine oxidase inhibitors (MAOIs),** such as Parnate (**tranylcypromine**) and Nardil (**phenelzine**), is prohibited due to the potential for high fever, muscle stiffness, sudden muscle spasms, rapid changes in heart rate and blood pressure, and the possibility of death. In fact, there should be a lapse of at least 14 days between taking an MAOI and taking mirtazapine (and vice versa).

Because mirtazapine may cause drowsiness, it should be used carefully with other medications that also make people prone to sleepiness, such as antidepressants, antipsychotics, antihistamines, antianxiety agents, and alcohol. Increased sleepiness has been reported when mirtazapine was used with both alcohol and the antianxiety drug **diazepam**.

Resources

BOOKS

Albers, Lawrence J., Rhoda K. Hahn, and Christopher Reist. *Handbook of Psychiatric Drugs.* Laguna Hills, CA: Current Clinical Strategies, 2010.

American Society of Health-System Pharmacists. *AHFS Drug Information 2011.* Bethesda, MD: ASHP, 2011.

Graham, George. *The Disordered Mind: An Introduction to Philosophy of Mind and Mental Illness.* New York: Routledge, 2010.

Holland, Leland Norman, and Michael Patrick Adams. *Core Concepts in Pharmacology*. 3rd ed. New York: Prentice Hall, 2011.

North, Carol, and Sean Yutzy. *Goodwin and Guze's Psychiatric Diagnosis*. New York: Oxford University Press, 2010.

Preston, John D., John H. O'Neal, and Mary C. Talaga. *Handbook of Clinical Psychopharmacology for Therapists*, 6th ed. Oakland, CA: New Harbinger, 2010.

ORGANIZATIONS

American Academy of Clinical Toxicology, 6728 Old McLean Village Dr., McLean, VA, 22101, (703) 556-9222, Fax: (703) 556-8729, admin@clintox.org, http://www.clintox.org.

American Psychiatric Association, 1000 Wilson Blvd., Ste. 1825, Arlington, VA, 22209-3901, (703) 907-7300, apa@psych.org, http://www.psych.org.

American Psychological Association, 750 1st St. NE, Washington, DC, 20002-4242, (202) 336-5500; TDD/TTY: (202) 336-6123, (800) 374-2721, http://www.apa.org.

American Society for Clinical Pharmacology and Therapeutics, 528 N Washington St., Alexandria, VA, 22314, (703) 836-6981, info@ascpt.org, http://www.ascpt.org.

Depression and Bipolar Support Alliance, 730 N Franklin St., Ste. 501, Chicago, IL, 60654, (800) 826-3632, Fax: (312) 642-7243, http://www.dbsalliance.org.

National Alliance on Mental Illness, 2107 Wilson Blvd., Ste. 300, Arlington, VA, 22201-3042, Fax: (703) 524-9094, (800) 950-6264, http://www.nami.org.

National Institute of Mental Health, 6001 Executive Blvd., Rm. 8184, MSC 9663, Bethesda, MD, 20892-9663, (301) 433-4513; TTY: (301) 443-8431, Fax: (301) 443-4279, (866) 615-6464; TTY: (866) 415-8051, nimhinfo@nih.gov, http://www.nimh.nih.gov.

U.S. Food and Drug Administration, 10903 New Hampshire Ave., Silver Spring, MD, 20993-0002, (888) INFO-FDA (463-6332), http://www.fda.gov.

Kelly Karpa, RPh, PhD.
Laura Jean Cataldo, RN, EdD

Mixed episode

Definition

A mixed episode is a discrete period during which a person experiences nearly daily fluctuations in mood that qualify for diagnoses of **manic episode** and major depressive episode. Over the course of at least one week, the mood of a person experiencing a mixed episode will rapidly change between abnormal happiness or euphoria and sadness or irritability.

Description

To qualify for a **diagnosis** of mixed episode, symptoms must be severe enough to interfere with an individual's ability to carry out daily routines at work or home, or to require **hospitalization**. Males may be more susceptible to this condition than females. Young people and those more than 60 years of age with **bipolar disorder** may be more prone to mixed episodes than others. A manic episode or a major depressive episode is more likely to turn into a mixed episode than vice versa. Manic episodes can also appear in an individual who does not suffer from these or other disturbances. If the episode can be attributed to side effects related to any medical treatment, medical condition, medication, or drugs of abuse, it is not classified as a mixed episode.

See also Depression

Dean A. Haycock, Ph.D.

Mixed receptive-expressive language disorder

Definition

Mixed receptive-expressive language disorder is diagnosed when a child has problems expressing him- or herself using spoken language and also has problems understanding what people say to him or her.

Demographics

Mixed receptive-expressive language disorder is diagnosed in about 5% of preschool-age children and 3% of children in school. It is less common than expressive language disorder. Children who have mixed receptive-expressive language disorder are more likely to have other disorders as well. Between 40% and 60% of preschoolers who have this disorder may also have phonological disorder (difficulty forming sounds). **Reading disorder** is linked to as many as half the children with mixed receptive-expressive language disorder who are of school age. Children with mixed receptive-expressive language disorder are also more likely to have psychiatric disorders, especially attention deficit disorder (ADD); it is estimated that 30%–60% of children with mixed receptive-expressive language disorder also have ADD. Children from families with a history of language disorders are more likely to have this or other language disorders.

Description

Mixed receptive-expressive language disorder is generally a disorder of childhood. There are two types of mixed receptive-expressive language disorder: developmental and acquired. Developmental mixed receptive-expressive language disorder does not have a known cause and normally appears at the time that a child is learning to talk. Acquired mixed receptive-expressive language disorder is caused by direct damage to the **brain**. It occurs suddenly after such events as a **stroke** or traumatic head injury. The acquired type can occur at any age.

Causes and symptoms

Causes

There is no known cause of developmental mixed receptive-expressive language disorder. Researchers are conducting ongoing studies to determine whether biological or environmental factors may be involved. The acquired form of the disorder results from direct damage to the brain. Damage can be sustained during a stroke, or as the result of traumatic head injury, **seizures**, or other medical conditions. The specific symptoms of the acquired form of the disorder generally depend on the parts of the patient's brain that have been injured and the severity of the damage.

Symptoms

The signs and symptoms of mixed receptive-expressive language disorder are for the most part the same as the symptoms of **expressive language disorder**. The disorder has signs and symptoms that vary considerably from child to child. In general, mixed receptive-expressive language disorder is characterized by a child's difficulty with spoken communication. The child does not have problems with the pronunciation of words, which is found in **phonological disorder**. The child does, however, have problems constructing coherent sentences, using proper grammar, recalling words, or similar communication problems. A child with mixed receptive-expressive language disorder is not able to communicate thoughts, needs, or wants at the same level or with the same complexity as his or her peers. In addition, the child often has a smaller vocabulary than his or her peers.

Children with mixed receptive-expressive language disorder also have significant problems understanding what other people are saying to them. This lack of comprehension may result in inappropriate responses or failure to follow directions. Some people think these children are being deliberately stubborn or obnoxious, but this is not the case. They simply do not understand what is being said. Some children with this disorder have problems understanding such specific types of terms as abstract nouns, complex sentences, or spatial terms.

Diagnosis

The **diagnosis** would be expressive language disorder. If the child is intellectually disabled, hard of hearing, or has other physical problems, the difficulties with speech must be greater than generally occurs with the other disabilities the child may have in order for the child to be diagnosed with this disorder.

The disorder is usually diagnosed in children because a parent or teacher expresses concern about the child's problems with spoken communication. The child's pediatrician may give the child a physical examination to rule out such medical problems as hearing loss. Specific testing for mixed expressive-receptive language disorder requires the examiner to demonstrate that the child not only communicates less well than expected, but also understands speech less well. It can be hard, however, to determine what a child understands. As a result, most examiners will use nonverbal tests in addition to tests that require spoken questions and answers in order to assess the child's condition as accurately as possible. In children who are mildly hearing-impaired, the problem can often be corrected by using hearing aids. Children who speak a language other than English (or the dominant language of their society) at home should be tested in that language if possible. In some cases, the child's ability to understand and communicate in English is the problem, not his or her competence with spoken language in general.

Treatment

Mixed receptive-expressive language disorder should be treated as soon as it is identified. Early **intervention** is the key to a successful outcome. Treatment involves teachers, siblings, parents, and anyone else who interacts regularly with the child. Regularly scheduled one-on-one treatment that focuses on specific language skills can also be effective, especially when combined with a more general approach involving family members and caregivers. Teaching children with this disorder specific communication skills so they can interact with their peers is important, as problems in this area may lead to later social isolation, **depression**, or behavioral problems. Children who are diagnosed early and taught reading skills may benefit especially, because problems with reading are often associated with mixed receptive-expressive language disorder and can cause serious long-term academic problems. There is little information comparing different treatment methods; often several are tried in combination.

KEY TERMS

Phonological disorder—A developmental disorder of childhood in which the child fails to use speech sounds that are appropriate for his or her age level and native language or dialect.

Prognosis

The developmental form of mixed receptive-expressive language disorder is less likely to resolve well than the developmental form of expressive language disorder. Most children with the disorder continue to have problems with language skills. They develop them at a much slower rate than their peers, which puts them at a growing disadvantage throughout their educational career. Some persons diagnosed with the disorder as children have significant problems with expressing themselves and understanding others in adult life.

The prognosis of the acquired type of mixed receptive-expressive language disorder depends on the nature and location of the brain injury. Some people get their language skills back over days or months. For others it takes years, and some people never fully recover expressive language function or the ability to understand speech.

Prevention

Because the causes of developmental mixed receptive-expressive language disorder are unclear, there are no specific ways to prevent it. A healthy diet during pregnancy and regular prenatal care are always recommended. Because the acquired form of the disorder is caused by damage to the brain, anything that helps to prevent brain damage may offer protection against that form of the disorder. Preventive measures include such precautions as lowering blood cholesterol levels, which may help to prevent stroke, or wearing bicycle helmets or automobile seat belts to prevent traumatic head injury.

Resources

BOOKS

American Psychiatric Association. *Diagnostic and Statistical Manual of Mental Disorders*. 4th ed., text rev. Washington, DC: American Psychiatric Publishing, 2000.

Sadock, Benjamin J., and Virginia A. Sadock, eds. *Comprehensive Textbook of Psychiatry*. Vol. 2. 7th ed. Philadelphia: Lippincott Williams and Wilkins, 2000.

PERIODICALS

Stein, Martin T., ed. "Expressive Language Delay in a Toddler." *Journal of Developmental & Behavioral Pediatrics* 22, no. 2 (April 2001): S99–S103.

ORGANIZATIONS

American Academy of Pediatrics, 141 Northwest Point Blvd., Elk Grove Village, IL, 60007-1098, (847) 434-4000, Fax: (847) 434-8000, http://www.aap.org.

American Psychological Association, 750 1st Street NE, Washington, DC, 20002-4242, (202) 336-5500, TDD/TTY: (202) 336-6123, (800) 374-2721, http://www.apa.org.

American Speech-Language-Hearing Association, 2200 Research Blvd., Rockville, MD, 20785, (301) 296-5700, http://www.asha.org.

Tish Davidson, A.M.

MMPI *see* **Minnesota Multiphasic Personality Inventory**

MMSE *see* **Mini-mental state examination**

Moban *see* **Molindone**

Modeling

Definition

Modeling, which is also called observational learning or imitation, is a behaviorally based procedure that involves the use of live or symbolic models to demonstrate a particular behavior, thought, or attitude that a client may want to acquire or change. Modeling is sometimes called vicarious learning, because the client need not actually perform the behavior in order to learn it.

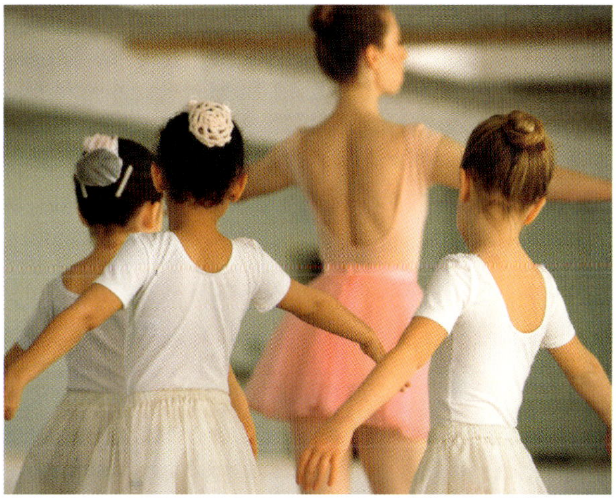

One method of learning is modeling, or imitating another person to learn a skill, as is done in dance classes. *(© ImageState/Alamy)*

Purpose

Modeling therapy is based on social learning theory. This theory emphasizes the importance of learning that is derived from observing and imitating role models, and learning about rewards and punishments that follow behavior. The technique has been used to eliminate unwanted behaviors, reduce excessive fears, facilitate learning of social behaviors, and many more. Modeling may be used either to strengthen or to weaken previously learned behaviors.

Modeling has been used effectively to treat individuals with **anxiety disorders**; **post-traumatic stress disorder**; **specific phobias**; **obsessive-compulsive disorder**; eating disorders; **attention deficit hyperactivity disorder**; and **conduct disorder**. It has also been used successfully in helping individuals acquire such social skills as public speaking or assertiveness. The effectiveness of modeling has led to its use in behavioral treatment of persons with **substance abuse** disorders, who frequently lack important behavioral skills. These persons may lack assertiveness, including the ability to say "no"; in addition, they may have thought patterns that make them more susceptible to substance abuse.

Modeling when used alone has been shown to be effective for short-term learning. It is, however, insufficient for long-lasting behavior change if the target behavior does not produce rewards that sustain it. Modeling works well when it is combined with role-play and **reinforcement**. These three components are used in a sequence of modeling, role-play, and reinforcement. Role-play is defined as practice or behavioral rehearsal of a skill to be used later in real-life situations. Reinforcement is defined as rewarding the model's performance or the client's performance of the newly acquired skill in practice or in real-life situations.

Several factors increase the effectiveness of modeling therapy in changing behaviors. Modeling effects have been shown to be more powerful when:

- The model is highly skilled in enacting the behavior; is likable or admirable; is friendly; is the same sex and age; and is rewarded immediately for the performance of the particular behavior.
- The target behavior is clearly demonstrated with very few unnecessary details; is presented from the least to the most difficult level of behavior; and several different models are used to perform the same behavior(s).

Description

Types of modeling

Therapy begins with an assessment of the client's presenting problem(s). The assessment usually covers several areas of life, including developmental history (the client's family background, education, employment, social relationships); past traumatic experiences; medical and psychiatric history; and an outline of the client's goals. The client works with the therapist to list specific treatment goals; to determine the target behavior(s) to be learned or changed; and to develop a clear picture of what the behavior(s) will look like. The therapist then explains the rationale and concepts of the treatment. He or she also considers any negative consequences that may arise as the client makes changes in his or her behavior.

The client then observes the model enacting the desired behavior. Some models may demonstrate poor or inadequate behaviors as well as those that are effective. This contrast helps the client to identify ineffective behaviors as well as desired ones. Modeling can be done in several different ways, including live modeling, symbolic modeling, participant modeling, or covert modeling.

Live modeling refers to watching a real person, usually the therapist, perform the desired behavior the client has chosen to learn. For example, the therapist might model good telephone manners for a client who wants a job in a field that requires frequent telephone contact with customers.

Symbolic modeling includes filmed or videotaped models demonstrating the desired behavior. Other examples of symbolic models include photographs, picture books, and plays. A common example of symbolic modeling is a book for children about going to the hospital, intended to reduce a child's anxiety about hospitals and operations. With child clients, cartoon figures or puppets can be used as the models. Self-modeling is another form of symbolic modeling in which clients are videotaped performing the target behavior. The video is than replayed and clients can observe their behaviors and how they appear to others. For example, public speaking is one of the most common feared situations in the general adult population. A law student who is afraid of having to present arguments in a courtroom might be videotaped speaking to classmates who are role-playing the judge and members of the jury. The student can then review the videotape and work on his or her speech problems or other aspects of the performance that he or she would like to change.

In participant modeling, the therapist models anxiety-evoking behaviors for the client, and then prompts the client to engage in the behavior. The client first watches as the therapist approaches the feared object, and then approaches the object in steps or stages with the therapist's encouragement and support. This type of modeling is often used in the treatment of specific phobias. For example, a person who is afraid of dogs might be asked to watch the therapist touch or pet a dog, or perhaps accompany the therapist on a brief walk with a dog. Then, with the therapist's encouragement, the client might begin by touching or holding a stuffed dog, then watching a live dog from a distance, then perhaps walking a small dog on a leash, and eventually by degrees touching and petting a live dog.

In covert modeling, clients are asked to use their imagination, visualizing a particular behavior as the therapist describes the imaginary situation in detail. For example, a child may be asked to imagine one of his or her favorite cartoon characters interacting appropriately with other characters. An adult client is asked to imagine an admired person in his or her life performing a behavior that the client wishes to learn. For example, a person may greatly admire their mother for the way she handled the challenges of coming to the United States from another country. If the client is worried about the challenge of a new situation in their own life (changing careers, having their first child, etc.), the therapist may ask them to imagine how their mother would approach the new situation, and then imagine themselves acting with their mother's courage and wisdom.

Models in any of these forms may be presented as either a coping or a mastery model. The coping model is shown as initially fearful or incompetent and then is shown as gradually becoming comfortable and competent performing the feared behavior. A coping model might show a small child who is afraid of swimming in the ocean, for example. The little boy or girl watches smaller children having fun playing in the waves along the edge of the shore. Gradually the child moves closer and closer to the water and finally follows a child his or her age into the surf. The mastery model shows no fear and is competent from the beginning of the demonstration. Coping models are considered more appropriate for reducing fear because they look more like the client, who will probably make mistakes and have some setbacks when trying the new behavior.

Having the model speak his or her thoughts aloud is more effective than having a model who does not verbalize. As the models speak, they show the client how to think through a particular problem or situation. A common example of this type of modeling is sports or cooking instruction. A golf or tennis pro who is trying to teach a beginner how to hold and swing the club or racquet will often talk as they demonstrate the correct stance and body movements. Similarly, a master chef will often talk to students in a cooking class while he or she is cutting the ingredients for a dish, preparing a sauce, kneading dough, or doing other necessary tasks. The model's talking while performing an action also engages the client's sense of hearing, taste, or smell as well as sight. Multisensory involvement enhances the client's learning.

Role-playing

Role-playing is a technique that allows the client opportunities to imitate the modeled behaviors, which strengthens what has been learned. Role-play can be defined as practice or behavior rehearsal; it allows the client to receive feedback about the practice as well as encouraging the use of the newly learned skill in real-life situations. For example, a group of people who are trying to learn social skills might practice the skills needed for a job interview or for dealing with a minor problem (returning a defective item to a store, asking someone for directions, etc.). Role-play can also be used for modeling, in that the therapist may role-play certain situations with clients. During practice, the therapist frequently coaches, prompts, and shapes the client's enactment of the behavior so the rehearsals come increasingly close to the desired behavior.

Feedback and social reinforcement of the client's performance in the practice phase is an important motivator for behavior change. Feedback may take the form of praise, approval, or encouragement, or it may be corrective, with concrete suggestions for improving the performance. Suggestions are followed by additional practice. Such tangible reinforcements as money, food, candy, or tokens have been used with young children and chronic psychiatric patients. The therapist may teach the client how to use self-reinforcement; that is, using self-praise after performing the desired behavior. The purpose of reinforcement is to shift the client's performance concerns from external evaluation by others to internal evaluation of their own efforts.

Modeling in group settings

Modeling has been shown to be effective in such group programs as **social skills training** and **assertiveness training** as well as in individual therapy. The general approach to both social skills training and assertiveness training is the incorporation of the modeling, role-play, and reinforcement sequence. After assessment of each group member's presenting problem, each member is asked to keep a diary of what happened when the situation occurred during the week. Group members develop goals for dealing with their individual situations, and each person determines how he or she can meet these goals. Modeling is done with either the therapist or other group members role-playing how to deal effectively with a particular problem situation.

Length of treatment

While modeling therapy is a relatively short-term approach to behavioral change, some therapeutic techniques take longer than others. Imagery, for example, requires more sessions than in vivo (real-life) treatments.

In vivo work that takes place outside the therapist's office would require longer time periods for each session. Other considerations include the nature of the client's problem; the client's willingness to do homework; the client's financial resources; and the presence and extent of the client's support network. The therapist's length of experience and personal style also affect the length of therapy.

There are, however, guidelines of treatment length for some disorders. Treatment of obsessive-compulsive disorder may require five weekly sessions for approximately three weeks, with weekly follow-up sessions for several months. Depressive disorders may require 3–6 months, with the client experiencing short-term relief after 3–4 weeks of treatment. General anxiety disorder may also take several months of weekly sessions. The length of treatment depends on the ability to define and assess the target behaviors. Clients may meet with the therapist several times a week at the beginning of treatment; then weekly for several months; then monthly for follow-up sessions that may become fewer in number or spaced more widely until therapy is terminated.

Results

Modeling or observational learning is effective as a method of learning such behaviors as self-assertion, self-disclosure, helping others, empathic behaviors, moral judgment, and many other interpersonal skills. Modeling is also effective in eliminating or reducing such undesirable behaviors as uncontrolled aggression, smoking, weight problems, and single phobias.

The expected outcome is that clients will be able to use their new behaviors outside the treatment setting in real-life situations. This result is called transfer of training, generalization, or maintenance. Homework is the most frequently used technique for transfer of training. Homework may represent a contractual agreement between the therapist and the client in which the client gives a report on his or her progress at each meeting.

To ensure that generalization occurs and that clients will use their new skills, several "transfer enhancers" are used to increase the likelihood of successful transfer of training. Transfer enhancers include:

- Giving clients appropriate rationales and concepts, rules, or strategies for using skills properly.
- Giving clients ample opportunity to practice new skills correctly and successfully.
- Making the treatment setting as much like the real-life situation as possible.
- Giving clients opportunities to practice their new skills in a variety of physical and interpersonal settings.
- Giving clients adequate external social reinforcement and encouraging internal self-reinforcement as they use their skills successfully in real life.

Resources

BOOKS

Braswell, Lauren, and Philip C. Kendall. "Cognitive-Behavioral Therapy with Youth." In *Handbook of Cognitive Behavioral Therapies,* edited by Keith S. Dobson. 2nd ed. New York: The Guilford Press. 2001.

Jinks, Gordon. "Specific Strategies and Techniques." In *Handbook of Counselling and Psychotherapy,* edited by Colin Feltham and Ian Horton. Thousand Oaks, CA: Sage Publications, 2006.

Sharf, Richard S. "Behavior Therapy." Chapter 8 in *Theories of Psychotherapy and Counseling: Concepts and Cases.* 5th ed. Farmington Hills, MI: Cengage Learning, 2012.

ORGANIZATIONS

American Psychological Association, 750 1st Street NE, Washington, DC, 20002-4242, (202) 336-5500, TDD/TTY: (202) 336-6123, (800) 374-2721, http://www.apa.org.

Association for Behavioral and Cognitive Therapies, 305 Seventh Ave., 16th Floor, New York, NY, 10001-6008, (212) 647-1890, Fax: (212) 647-1865, http://www.abct.org.

Mental Health America, 2000 N. Beauregard Street, 6th Floor, Alexandria, VA, 22311, (703) 684-7722, (800) 969-6642, Fax: (703) 684-5968, http://www1.nmha.org.

National Institute of Mental Health, 6001 Executive Blvd., Room 8184, MSC 9663, Bethesda, MD, 20892-9663, (301) 433-4513, TTY: (301) 443-8431, Fax: (301) 443-4279, (866) 615-6464, TTY: (866) 415-8051, nimhinfo@nih.gov, http://www.nimh.nih.gov.

Janice Van Buren, Ph.D.

Molindone

Definition

Molindone is an antipsychotic previously sold under the trade name Moban. In early 2010, the supplier of molindone ceased production on the drug, and by June of the same year, it was no longer available in the United States.

Purpose

Molindone was used to treat psychotic symptoms assosiated with **depression**, mania, or **schizophrenia**.

KEY TERMS

Depression—A mental state characterized by feelings of sadness, despair, discouragement, low energy, and often oversleeping and/or overeating.

Dopamine—A chemical in brain tissue that serves to transmit nerve impulses (is a neurotransmitter) and helps to regulate movement and emotions.

Extrapyramidal symptoms—A group of side effects associated with antipsychotic medications and characterized by involuntary muscle movements, including contraction and tremor.

Hallucinations—A perception without external stimulus. Hallucinations can result from nervous system abnormalities, mental disorders, or the use of certain drugs.

Mania—An abnormal elevation in mood. The individual may appear excessively cheerful and talkative, have grandiose ideas, and may sleep less. Sometimes the elevation in mood is marked by irritability and hostility rather than cheerfulness. Those experiencing mania may seem to be in a frenzy and often will make poor, bizarre, or dangerous choices in their personal and professional lives.

Schizophrenia—A major mental illness marked by psychotic symptoms, including hallucinations, delusions, and severe disruptions in thinking.

Description

Molindone was taken orally and was rapidly absorbed and metabolized. Peak levels were reached within 90 minutes of taking the medication, and its effect lasted 24 to 36 hours. Molindone was available in 5, 10, 25, and 100 mg tablets.

Recommended dosage

The dosage of molindone was adjusted to the lowest level needed to control symptoms. The usual initial dosage was 50 to 75 mg per day. This might have been increased to 100 mg per day three to four days after beginning treatment. A maximal dosage of 225 mg per day was sometimes required.

Precautions

Prolonged or chronic administration of molindone increased the probability of developing **tardive dyskinesia**, a condition characterized by involuntary, uncoordinated movements involving the head, neck, trunk, feet, and hands. Examples of the movements involving the face and head include wormlike movement of the tongue, grimacing, chewing, and lip smacking. Tardive dyskinesia usually disappears once the affected person stops taking the associated medication, but sometimes it is irreversible.

Persons in a coma or experiencing central nervous system depression from alcohol, **barbiturates**, or narcotics were not prescribed molindone.

Drowsiness was often reported by people using molindone. For that reason, persons using molindone were advised not to operate machinery or drive automobiles.

Molindone caused the level of prolactin (a hormone that initiates lactation) in the blood to rise. This was a potential problem for persons with a personal or family history of breast cancer, as the increase could lead to the initiation of breast cancer. For this reason, the benefits of the drug were carefully evaluated before it was administered to persons at risk for breast cancer.

Molindone was associated with an increased risk of death when used in elderly patients with **dementia**. In June 2008, the U.S. Food and Drug Administration (FDA) announced a requirement for manufacturers of molindone (and other antipsychotic drugs) to add a warning label to their packaging stating this risk. The reason for the increase was unclear in studies, but most deaths were found to be related to either cardiovascular complications or complications associated with infection. Molindone was not approved by the FDA for the treatment of behavior problems in older adults with dementia.

In July 2009, the FDA made safety labeling changes to the warnings section for this drug to include information stating that occurrences of leukopenia, neutropenia, and agranulocytosis (issues relating to blood cells) had been reported with the use of molindone. The FDA cautioned that users of this medication should be monitored for signs of infection and also be monitored frequently for changes in blood count values.

Babies born to mothers who took molindone during pregnancy were likely to develop extrapyramidal symptoms (EPS) and withdrawal symptoms, including agitation, trouble breathing, and difficulty feeding. Breastfeeding was not recommended while taking the drug.

Side effects

Molindone had the potential to produce tardive dyskinesia. This syndrome consisting of involuntary, uncoordinated movements is potentially irreversible. The incidence of tardive dyskinesia was higher with increasing age and with increasing dosage of molindone. Tardive dyskinesia is more likely to occur after a long period of taking antipsychotic drugs, such as molindone, but it may also appear after such drug use has been discontinued. Females are at greater risk than males for developing tardive dyskinesia. Involuntary movements of the tongue, jaw, mouth, or face characterize tardive dyskinesia. These may be accompanied by involuntary movements of the arms, legs, and trunk. There is no known effective treatment for tardive dyskinesia.

Parkinson-like symptoms were also linked with the administration of molindone. These included restlessness and agitation (akathisia) and difficulty walking or moving (dystonia). These were generally controlled with **benztropine** mesylate or **trihexyphenidyl** hydrochloride.

An occasionally reported side effect of molindone was **neuroleptic malignant syndrome**, a complicated and potentially fatal condition characterized by muscle rigidity, high fever, alterations in mental status, and cardiac symptoms, including irregular pulse or blood pressure, sweating, tachycardia, or arrhythmias. This condition is considered a medical emergency.

Interactions

Molindone increased the effect of central nervous system depressants (drugs and substances that depress the central nervous system). This class of drugs includes anesthetics, opiates, barbiturates, atropine, and alcohol.

Molindone interfered with the absorption of phenytoin and tetracyclines.

Resources

BOOKS

Albers, Lawrence J., Rhoda K. Hahn, and Christopher Reist. *Handbook of Psychiatric Drugs.* Laguna Hills, CA: Current Clinical Strategies, 2010.

American Society of Health-System Pharmacists. *AHFS Drug Information 2011.* Bethesda, MD: ASHP, 2011.

Graham, George. *The Disordered Mind: An Introduction to Philosophy of Mind and Mental Illness.* New York: Routledge, 2010.

Holland, Leland Norman, and Michael Patrick Adams. *Core Concepts in Pharmacology.* 3rd ed. New York: Prentice Hall, 2011.

North, Carol, and Sean Yutzy. *Goodwin and Guze's Psychiatric Diagnosis.* New York: Oxford University Press, 2010.

Preston, John D., John H. O'Neal, and Mary C. Talaga. *Handbook of Clinical Psychopharmacology for Therapists.* 6th ed. Oakland, CA: New Harbinger, 2010.

PERIODICALS

Bagnall A., et al. "Molindone for Schizophrenia and Severe Mental Illness." *Cochrane Database Systematic Review* no. 2 (2000): CD002083.

Dhaware, B.S., et al. "Effects of Amantadine on Modification of Dopamine-Dependent Behaviours by Molindone." *Indian Journal of Medical Science* 54, no. 8 (2000): 321–24.

Glazer, W.M. "Expected Incidence of Tardive Dyskinesia Associated with Atypical Antipsychotics." *Journal of Clinical Psychiatry* 61, Supp. 4 (2000): 21–26.

ORGANIZATIONS

U.S. Food and Drug Administration, 10903 New Hampshire Ave., Silver Spring, MD, 20993-0002, (888) INFO-FDA (463-6332), http://www.fda.gov.

L. Fleming Fallon, Jr., MD, DrPH
Laura Jean Cataldo, RN, EdD

Monoamine oxidase inhibitors (MAOIs)

Definition

Monoamine oxidase inhibitors (MAOIs) are a class of **antidepressants** most often used to treat atypical **depression**. MAOIs carry the risk of dangerous interactions with certain foods, so they are prescribed only after other antidepressants prove ineffective.

Purpose

The mood-altering effects of MAOIs were initially discovered in the 1940s during efforts to use the first MAOI as a treatment for tuberculosis. The drug was ineffectual against tuberculosis, but the patients taking it reported enhanced mood. Based on these results, MAOIs were used in the 1950s in **clinical trials** for patients with depression. It was discovered that the drugs' common property was inhibition of monoamine oxidase (also called MAO), an enzyme that breaks down mood-regulating **neurotransmitters**, including **dopamine**, **serotonin**, and norepinephrine and epinephrine (also known as noradrenaline and **adrenaline**). By inhibiting the enzyme that breaks down these chemicals, MAOIs allow these neurotransmitters to persist and exert their mood-enhancing effects longer. One class of MAOIs also has recently been developed as a therapy for Parkinson's symptoms.

MAOIs were in widespread use from the 1960s through the 1980s, but fell out of favor as newer drugs with fewer potentially severe side effects and interactions came on the market.

Description

MAOIs can be divided into two main groups. The first group encompasses the nonselective, systemic, irreversible MAOIs and includes **phenelzine** (Nardil), **isocarboxazid** (Marplan), and **tranylcypromine** (Parnate), which are approved by the U.S. Food and Drug Administration for treatment of depression. They are considered nonselective because they target both types of MAOs: MAO-A and MAO-B. Their action is called "irreversible" because they bind the enzyme so strongly that even after a person stops taking them, two or three weeks must pass before the effects of the drugs subside.

The second group consists of the selective inhibitors, which inhibit either MAO-A or MAO-B, as the name implies. Those that inhibit MAO-A, including moclobemide (Aurorix, Manerix) and brofaromine (Consonar), are also known as RIMAS (reversible inhibitors of MAO-A). The use of a selective inhibitor can help prevent some of the food-drug interactions associated with the nonselective inhibitors. RIMAS are not approved for use in the United States.

The other drugs in the second group are inhibitors of MAO-B. These drugs, which include selegiline (Eldepryl) and rasagiline (Azilect), are not used orally for treatment of depression but instead are used in very low doses for treatment of Parkinson's symptoms. Because low dopamine levels are associated with Parkinson's symptoms, and these drugs block the MAO that breaks down dopamine, their effect of increasing dopamine levels has proved beneficial. At higher dosages, however, these MAO-B–inhibiting drugs become nonselective inhibitors, targeting both MAO-A and MAO-B and exerting antidepressant effects. In addition to their potential use in Parkinson's treatment, these MAO-B inhibitors hold promise as therapies for **attention deficit hyperactivity disorder**, stimulant abuse, and **smoking cessation**.

A low-dose, transdermal selegiline patch (Emsam) is also approved by the FDA for treatment of depression.

Recommended dosage

Dosages of MAOIs vary depending on the specific drug. Most are taken orally, but selegiline has been tested in the form of a transdermal patch that lessens exposure in the gastrointestinal tract, preventing some of the food-drug interactions associated with MAOIs.

Nonselective MAOIs

All of the nonselective MAOIs are taken as oral tablets. Isocarboxazid is started at 10 mg taken twice per day. The healthcare provider may gradually increase the dose, but the recommended maximum is no more than 60 mg/day. The adult dose of phenelzine is based on body weight; initially, it is 0.45 mg/lb (1 mg/kg) per day to a maximum dose of no more than 90 mg/day. For older adults, the initial dose is 15 mg in the morning; this dose can be increased, but to no more than 60 mg/day. Tranylcypromine is initially dosed at 30 mg per day and may be increased up to 60 mg/day. In older adults, the regimen is 2.5–5 mg/day to start. This dosage can be increased as needed, but usually to no more than 45 mg/day. For patients younger than 16, the dose should be determined by the practicing physician for all three drugs.

Selective MAOIs

The transdermal selegiline patch is available in three sizes that deliver 6, 9, or 12 mg/day through the skin. It should be applied to dry skin on the upper torso (below the neck and above the waist), upper thigh, or outer surface of the arm every 24 hours. Oral selegiline should not be used at daily doses exceeding 10 mg per day, and this dose should be split into two doses of 5 mg each, taken at breakfast and lunch. Exceeding the 10 mg limit can shift the drug's activity into nonselective inhibition, precipitating food interactions. Oral selegiline is usually taken in conjunction with dopamine-boosting drugs, such as levodopa (also called L-dopa), although it also appears to be effective when used alone. The oral dose for rasagiline is 1 mg once daily if taken alone. If taken in conjunction with levodopa, the recommended starting dose is 0.5 mg once a day, which can be increased to 1 mg a day if necessary.

Precautions

For the nonselective MAOIs (isocarboxazid, phenelzine, tranylcypromine), certain foods should be avoided. These include foods high in tyramine, a chemical found in foods that have been fermented or aged, including cheeses, fava beans, yeast- or meat-based extracts, meat that has been smoked or pickled, some kinds of sausages (e.g., pepperoni or salami), sauerkraut, and overripe fruit. The patient's healthcare provider should supply anyone prescribed these MAOIs with a list of foods to avoid, and patients should also avoid alcohol and large amounts of caffeine.

For people using the selegiline patch with the lowest level of delivery (6 mg/day) or taking oral selegiline at low doses for Parkinson's disease, dietary adjustment is not indicated; however, people using the 9 or 12 mg/day patches should observe dietary restrictions to avoid foods containing tyramine, like those required for the nonselective MAOIs.

In clinical trials, MAOI antidepressants increased the risk of suicidal thinking and behavior in children and adolescents with psychiatric disorders, including major depressive disorder. The average risk in pediatric trials for patients taking these drugs was twice that of patients taking placebo (4% vs. 2%, respectively).

People taking MAOIs must be sure to let their healthcare provider know if they are taking any other medications or drugs, especially the following:

- other antidepressant medications, such as fluoxetine (Prozac) or sertraline (Zoloft)
- some anticonvulsants, such as carbamazepine (Equetro) and oxcarbazepine (Trileptal)
- opioids, such as meperidine (Demerol)
- dextromethorphan, a component of many cough suppressant medications
- decongestants or appetite suppressants containing ephedrine, pseudoephedrine, phenylephrine, or phenylpropanolamine
- antihypertensive medications
- ciprofloxacin (Cipro)
- stimulants, especially amphetamines
- asthma medication
- insulin or antidiabetic medication
- cocaine
- tryptophan as a supplement or as a sleep aid
- St. John's wort

People taking MAOIs must also tell their healthcare provider of any other medical problems, especially alcohol abuse, chest pain, headaches, asthma, diabetes, kidney disease, epilepsy, heart or blood vessel disease, recent heart attack or stroke, high blood pressure, mental illness or a history of mental illness, Parkinson's disease, or hyperthyroidism.

There is an increased risk of birth defects when the nonselective MAOIs are taken during the first three months of pregnancy. Selegiline is classified as a pregnancy category C drug. This category indicates that animal reproduction studies showed an adverse effect on the fetus but there is no sufficient data in humans; however, potential benefits may outweigh potential risks for pregnant women in some cases. Tranylcypromine passes into the breast milk, but the status of the other two nonselective MAOIs is unknown. Selegiline passes into the milk of rodents, but it is unknown whether or not it passes into human breast milk. No studies on rasagiline in human breast milk have been done.

Even after a patient has stopped taking an MAOI, he or she must continue to exercise precautions for at least two weeks due to the time lapse between the end of treatment and the cessation of the drug's effects in the body.

Side effects

A person taking MAOIs must watch for symptoms of very high blood pressure. These include chest pain, enlarged pupils, fast or slow heartbeat, sensitivity to light, increased sweating, nausea or vomiting, and stiff or sore neck. Other potential side effects include dizziness or lightheadedness (can be common), headache, drowsiness, sleep disturbances, **fatigue**, weakness, and tremors. Gastrointestinal side effects can include either constipation or diarrhea and dry mouth. A person taking an MAOI may experience weight gain or, in the case of selegiline, weight loss. A sudden drop in blood pressure with a change in posture is possible, as is swelling in the feet or lower legs. Some people have reported sexual disturbances, including impotence or an inability to experience orgasm. Urinary changes may include decreased fluid volume or more frequent urination.

The only commonly reported side effect for the selegiline patch as of 2011 was an occasional skin reaction at the application site. A less common side effect was lightheadedness related to low blood pressure.

Interactions

One important role of MAO is breaking down tyramine, the compound in foods that have undergone aging or fermentation. Normally, because MAO is active, consuming these foods does not result in much tyramine entering the system. However, when an MAOI interferes with the activity of MAO, tyramine from these foods does enter the system and can elicit what has been called the "cheese reaction" (related to the association of tyramine with aged cheeses). This response can be life-threatening because of tyramine's effects on heart rate and blood pressure; the cheese reaction can produce a severe spike in blood pressure, leading to a hypertensive crisis. For this reason, people taking nonselective MAOIs must avoid foods that contain tyramine and continue this avoidance for at least two weeks after they stop taking the drug. People on the lowest dose (6 mg) of the selegiline patch do not need to exercise any tyramine-related dietary modifications. Users of MAOIs also will be advised about limiting tryptophan consumption, especially in the form of supplements.

Many drugs should not be taken with MAOIs, especially other antidepressants, anticonvulsants, **opioids**, dextromethorphan, decongestants, and **amphetamines**.

Patients using MAOIs should be sure to tell their doctor of any other drugs that they are taking.

Resources

PERIODICALS

Amsterdam, Jay D., and J. Alexander Bodkin. "Selegiline Transdermal System in the Prevention of Relapse of Major Depressive Disorder. A 52-week, Double-blind, Placebo-substitution, Parallel-group Clinical Trial." *Journal of Clinical Psychopharmacology* 26, no. 6 (2006): 579–586.

Howland, Robert H. "MAOI Antidepressant Drugs." *Journal of Psychosocial Nursing* 44, no. 6 (2006): 9–12.

Youdim, Moussa B.H., Dale Edmondson, and Keith F. Tipton. "The Therapeutic Potential of Monoamine Oxidase Inhibitors." *Nature Reviews Neuroscience* 7, no. 4 (2006): 295–309.

WEBSITES

Drugs.com. "Eldepryl Capsules." http://www.drugs.com/pro/eldepryl-capsules.html (accessed October 22, 2011).

Drugs.com. "Nardil" http://www.drugs.com/pro/nardil.html (accessed October 22, 2011.

Mayo Clinic staff. "Depression (major depression): Monoamine Oxidase Inhibitors (MAOIs)." MayoClinic.com. http://www.mayoclinic.com/health/maois/MH00072 (accessed October 22, 2011).

U.S. Food and Drug Administration. "FDA Approves Emsam (selegiline) as First Drug Patch for Depression." FDA News Release. February 28, 2006. http://www.fda.gov/NewsEvents/Newsroom/PressAnnouncements/2006/ucm108607.htm (accessed October 22, 2011).

ORGANIZATIONS

American Parkinson Disease Association, Inc, 135 Parkinson Ave., Staten Island, NY, 10305, (718) 981-8001, Fax: (718) 981-4399, apda@apdaparkinson.org, http://www.apdaparkinson.com.

American Psychiatric Association, 1000 Wilson Blvd., Ste. 1825, Arlington, VA, 22209-3901, (703) 907-7300, apa@psych.org, http://www.psych.org.

Emily Jane Willingham, Ph.D.

Mood disorders *see* **Bipolar disorder; Depression and depressive disorders**

Mourning *see* **Bereavement; Grief**

Movement disorders

Definition

Movement disorders are a group of diseases and syndromes affecting the ability to produce and control movement.

Description

Although it seems simple and effortless, normal movement in fact requires an astonishingly complex system of control. Disruption of any portion of this system can cause a person to produce movements that are too weak, too forceful, too uncoordinated, or too poorly controlled for the task at hand. Unwanted movements may occur at rest. Intentional movement may become impossible. Such conditions are called movement disorders.

Abnormal movements themselves are symptoms of underlying disorders. In some cases, the abnormal movements are the only symptoms. Disorders causing abnormal movements include:

- Parkinson's disease
- parkinsonism caused by drugs or poisons
- Parkinson-plus syndromes (progressive supranuclear palsy, multiple system atrophy, and cortical-basal ganglionic degeneration)
- Huntington's disease
- Wilson's disease
- inherited ataxias (Friedreich's ataxia, Machado-Joseph disease, and spinocerebellar ataxias)
- Tourette syndrome and other tic disorders
- essential tremor
- restless leg syndrome
- dystonia
- stroke
- cerebral palsy
- encephalopathies
- intoxication
- poisoning by carbon monoxide, cyanide, methanol, or manganese

Causes and symptoms

Causes

Movement is produced and coordinated by several interacting **brain** centers, including the motor cortex, the cerebellum, and a group of structures in the inner portions of the brain called the basal ganglia. Sensory information provides critical input on the current position and velocity of body parts, and spinal nerve cells (neurons) help prevent opposing muscle groups from contracting at the same time.

To understand how movement disorders occur, it is helpful to consider a normal voluntary movement, such as reaching to touch a nearby object with the right index finger. To accomplish the desired movement, the arm

KEY TERMS

Botulinum toxin—Any of a group of potent bacterial toxins or poisons produced by different strains of the bacterium *Clostridium botulinum*. The toxins cause muscle paralysis, and thus force the relaxation of a muscle in spasm.

Cerebral palsy—A movement disorder caused by a permanent brain defect or injury present at birth or shortly after. It is frequently associated with premature birth. Cerebral palsy is not progressive.

Computed tomography (CT)—An imaging technique in which cross-sectional x rays of the body are compiled to create a three-dimensional image of the body's internal structures.

Encephalopathy—An abnormality in the structure or function of tissues of the brain.

Essential tremor—An uncontrollable (involuntary) shaking of the hands, head, and face. Also called familial tremor because it is sometimes inherited, it can begin in the teens or in middle age. The exact cause is not known.

Fetal tissue transplantation—A method of treating Parkinson's and other neurological diseases by grafting brain cells from human fetuses onto the basal ganglia. Human adults cannot grow new brain cells but developing fetuses can. Grafting fetal tissue stimulates the growth of new brain cells in affected adult brains.

Hereditary ataxia—One of a group of hereditary degenerative diseases of the spinal cord or cerebellum. These diseases cause tremor, spasm, and wasting of muscle.

Huntington's disease—A rare hereditary condition that causes progressive chorea and mental deterioration that ends in dementia. Huntington's symptoms usually appear in patients in their 40s. There is no effective treatment.

Levodopa (L-dopa)—A substance used in the treatment of Parkinson's disease. Levodopa can cross the blood-brain barrier that protects the brain. Once in the brain, it is converted to dopamine and thus can replace the dopamine lost in Parkinson's disease.

must be lifted and extended. The hand must be held out to align with the forearm, and the forefinger must be extended while the other fingers remain flexed.

THE MOTOR CORTEX. Voluntary motor commands begin in the motor cortex located on the outer, wrinkled surface of the brain. Movement of the right arm is begun by the left motor cortex, which generates a large volley of signals to the involved muscles. These electrical signals pass along upper motor neurons through the midbrain to the spinal cord. Within the spinal cord, they connect to lower motor neurons, which convey the signals out of the spinal cord to the surface of the muscles involved. Electrical stimulation of the muscles causes contraction, and the force of contraction pulling on the skeleton causes movement of the arm, hand, and fingers. Damage to or death of any of the neurons along this path causes weakness or paralysis of the affected muscles.

ANTAGONISTIC MUSCLE PAIRS. Movement is also supported by opposing, or antagonistic, muscle pairs. Contraction of the biceps muscle, located on the top of the upper arm, pulls on the forearm to flex the elbow and bend the arm. Contraction of the triceps, located on the opposite side, extends the elbow and straightens the arm. Within the spine, these muscles are normally wired so that willed (voluntary) contraction of one is automatically accompanied by blocking of the other. The command to contract the biceps provokes another command within the spine to prevent contraction of the triceps. In this way, these antagonist muscles are kept from resisting one another. Spinal cord or brain injury can damage this control system and cause involuntary simultaneous contraction and spasticity, an increase in resistance to movement during motion.

THE CEREBELLUM. Once the movement of the arm is initiated, sensory information is needed to guide the finger to its precise destination. In addition to sight, the most important source of information comes from the "position sense" provided by the many sensory neurons located within the limbs (proprioception). Proprioception is the response that allows a person to touch the nose with the finger even with the eyes closed. The balance organs in the ears provide important information about posture. Both postural and proprioceptive information are processed by a structure at the rear of the brain called the cerebellum. The cerebellum sends out electrical signals to modify movements as they progress, "sculpting" the barrage of voluntary commands into a tightly controlled, constantly evolving pattern. Cerebellar disorders cause inability to control the force, fine positioning, and speed of movements (ataxia). Disorders of the cerebellum may also impair the ability to judge distance so that a person under- or overreaches the target (dysmetria). Tremor

Magnetic resonance imaging (MRI)—An imaging technique that uses a large circular magnet and radio waves to generate signals from atoms in the body. These signals are used to construct images of internal structures.

Parkinson's disease—A slowly progressive disease that destroys nerve cells in the basal ganglia and thus causes loss of dopamine, a chemical that aids in transmission of nerve signals (neurotransmitter). Parkinson's is characterized by shaking in resting muscles, a stooping posture, slurred speech, muscular stiffness, and weakness.

Positron emission tomography (PET)—A diagnostic technique in which computer-assisted x rays are used to track a radioactive substance inside a patient's body. PET can be used to study the biochemical activity of the brain.

Progressive supranuclear palsy—A rare disease that gradually destroys nerve cells in the parts of the brain that control eye movements, breathing, and muscle coordination. The loss of nerve cells causes palsy, or paralysis, that slowly gets worse as the disease progresses. The palsy affects ability to move the eyes, relax the muscles, and control balance.

Restless legs syndrome—A condition that causes an annoying feeling of tiredness, uneasiness, and itching deep within the muscle of the leg. It is accompanied by twitching and sometimes pain. The only relief is in walking or moving the legs.

Tourette syndrome—An abnormal condition that causes uncontrollable facial grimaces and tics and arm and shoulder movements. Tourette syndrome is perhaps best known for uncontrollable vocal tics that include grunts, shouts, and use of obscene language (coprolalia).

Wilson's disease—An inborn defect of copper metabolism in which free copper may be deposited in a variety of areas of the body. Deposits in the brain can cause tremor and other symptoms of Parkinson's disease.

during voluntary movements can also result from cerebellar damage.

THE BASAL GANGLIA. Both the cerebellum and the motor cortex send information to a set of structures deep within the brain that help control involuntary components of movement (basal ganglia). The basal ganglia send output messages to the motor cortex, helping to initiate movements, regulate repetitive or patterned movements, and control muscle tone.

Circuits within the basal ganglia are complex. Within this structure, some groups of cells begin the action of other basal ganglia components and some groups of cells block the action. These complicated feedback circuits are not entirely understood. Disruptions of these circuits are known to cause several distinct movement disorders. A portion of the basal ganglia called the substantia nigra sends electrical signals that block output from another structure called the subthalamic nucleus. The subthalamic nucleus sends signals to the globus pallidus, which in turn blocks the thalamic nuclei. Finally, the thalamic nuclei send signals to the motor cortex. The substantia nigra, then, begins movement and the globus pallidus blocks it.

This complicated circuit can be disrupted at several points. For instance, loss of substantia nigra cells, as in Parkinson's disease, increases blocking of the thalamic nuclei, preventing them from sending signals to the motor cortex. The result is a loss of movement (motor activity), a characteristic of Parkinson's.

In contrast, cell loss in early Huntington's disease decreases blocking of signals from the thalamic nuclei, causing more cortex stimulation and stronger but uncontrolled movements.

Disruptions in other portions of the basal ganglia are thought to cause tics, tremors, dystonia, and a variety of other movement disorders, although the exact mechanisms are not well understood.

Some movement disorders, including Huntington's disease and inherited ataxias, are caused by inherited genetic defects. Some diseases that cause sustained muscle contraction limited to a particular muscle group (focal dystonia) are inherited, but others are caused by **trauma**. The cause of most cases of Parkinson's disease is unknown, although genes have been found for some familial forms.

Symptoms

Movement disorders are usually broken down into two types of movement: hyperkinetic movement and hypokinetic movement. Hyperkinetic movement disorders are characterized by a significant and excessive amount of motor activity. This type also includes cases where there is a significant amount of abnormal involuntary movement. Hypokinetic movement disorders are those in which there is an abnormally reduced amount of intentional motor activity.

Hyperkinetic movement disorders are characterized by two types of behavior: rhythmical and irregular. Tremor is a rhythmic movement that is further divided into three forms: rest, postural, and intention. Rest tremor is most prominent when an individual is at rest and decreases with voluntary activity. Postural tremor occurs when an individual attempts to support a position against gravity (such as holding an arm outstretched). Intention tremor occurs during voluntary movement toward a specific target.

Irregular involuntary movements are classified by their speed and site of occurrence. Tics are rapid irregular movements that are controlled with voluntary effort. The types of rapid irregular movements that cannot be controlled voluntarily are called chorea, hemiballismus, and myoclonus. Chorea is a rapid, jerking movement that most often affects the face or limbs. Hemiballismus is the sudden and extreme swinging of a limb. Myoclonus is a rapid, irregular movement that usually occurs for a short period of time. It usually occurs when the person is at rest, and it often affects more than one area of the body at a time.

One of the most well-known hyperkinetic movement disorders is Huntington's disease, characterized by chorea-type movements. This disease is inherited and usually develops between 30 and 50 years of age. Persons with this condition have progressive **dementia**, and the condition eventually causes death. Children of persons with Huntington's disease have a 50% chance of developing the condition. **Stereotypic movement disorder** is characterized by repetitive behaviors that meet no functional need such as hand waving; rocking; head banging; mouthing of objects; or biting, picking, or hitting oneself. These behaviors interfere with normal activities and are not caused by **substance abuse** or a general medical condition.

The symptoms of hypokinetic movement disorders include a rigid, stone-like face; decreased limb motion during walking; and stiff turning movements. These features are classified as bradykinesia, while akinesia is the absence of purposeful movement. The most common type of hypokinetic movement disorder is Parkinson's disease, caused by the loss of neurons containing **dopamine** in the area of the brain called the substantia nigra pars compacta. The loss of these neurons is a part of the alteration of vital motor circuits in the brain that leads to a slowing of intentional movements.

Diagnosis

Diagnosis of movement disorders requires a careful medical history and a thorough physical and neurological examination. Brain **imaging studies** are usually performed. Imaging techniques include **computed tomography** scan (CT scan), **positron emission tomography (PET)**, or **magnetic resonance imaging** (MRI) scans. Routine blood and urine analyses are performed. A lumbar puncture (spinal tap) may be necessary. Video recording of the abnormal movement is often used to analyze movement patterns and to track progress of the disorder and its treatment. Genetic testing is available for some forms of movement disorders.

Treatment

Treatment of a movement disorder begins with determining its cause. Physical and occupational therapy may help make up for lost control and strength. Drug therapy can help compensate for some imbalances of the basal ganglionic circuit. For instance, levodopa (L-dopa) or related compounds can substitute for lost dopamine-producing cells in Parkinson's disease. Conversely, blocking normal dopamine action is a possible treatment in some hyperkinetic disorders, including tics. Oral medications can also help reduce overall muscle tone. Local injections of botulinum toxin can selectively weaken overactive muscles in dystonia and spasticity. Destruction of peripheral nerves through injection of phenol can reduce spasticity. All of these treatments may have some side effects.

Surgical destruction or inactivation of basal ganglionic circuits has proven effective for Parkinson's disease and is being tested for other movement disorders. Transplantation of fetal cells into the basal ganglia has produced mixed results in Parkinson's disease.

Prognosis

The prognosis for a patient with a movement disorder depends on the specific disorder.

Prevention

Prevention depends on the specific disorder.

See also Medication-induced movement disorders

Resources

BOOKS

Chaudhuri, Ray, K., and William Ondo. *Movement Disorders in Clinical Practice.* New York: Springer, 2010.

Newell, Lori A. *The Book of Exercise and Yoga for Those with Parkinson's Disease: Using Movement and Meditation to Manage Symptoms.* Charleston, SC: CreateSpace, 2010.

Truong, Daniel D., Mayank Pathak, and Karen Frei. *Living Well with Dystonia: A Patient Guide.* New York: Demos Health, 2010.

Wyborny, Sheila. *Tourette Syndrome.* Farmington Hills, MI. Gale, Cengage Learning, 2011.

ORGANIZATIONS

American Academy of Neurology, 1080 Montreal Ave., St. Paul, MN, 55116, (651) 695-2717, (800) 879-1960, Fax: (651) 879-2791, memberservices@aan.com, http://www.aan.com.

American Physical Therapy Association, 1111 North Fairfax St., Alexandria, VA, 22314-1488, (703) 684-APTA (2782), TDD: (703) 683-6748, (800) 999-APTA (2782), http://www.apta.org.

The Movement Disorder Society, 555 East Wells St., Ste. 1100, Milwaukee, WI, 53202-3823, (414) 276-2145, http://www.movementdisorders.org.

Worldwide Education and Awareness for Movement Disorders, One Gustave L. Levy Pl., PO Box 1052, New York, NY, 10029, (800) 437-6683, http://www.wemove.org.

Richard Robinson
Laura Jean Cataldo, RN, Ed.D.

Movement therapies *see* **Bodywork therapies**

MRI *see* **Magnetic resonance imaging**

Multi-infarct dementia *see* **Vascular dementia**

Multiple personality disorder *see* **Dissociative identity disorder**

Multisystemic therapy

Definition

Multisystemic therapy (MST) is an intensive family- and community-based treatment program designed to make positive changes in the various social systems (home, school, community, peer) that contribute to the serious antisocial behaviors of children and adolescents who are at risk for out-of-home placement. These out-of-home placements might include foster care, **group homes**, residential care, correctional facilities, or **hospitalization**.

Purpose

MST operates with the fundamental assumption that parents, guardians, or those who have primary caregiving responsibilities to children, have the most important influence in changing problem behaviors in children and adolescents. The primary goals of MST are to:

- develop in parents or caregivers the capacity to manage future difficulties
- reduce juvenile criminal activity
- reduce other types of antisocial behaviors, such as drug abuse
- achieve these outcomes at a cost savings by decreasing rates of incarceration and other out-of-home placements

MST was created approximately 30 years ago as an intensive family- and community-based treatment program to focus on juvenile offenders presenting with serious antisocial behaviors and who were at risk for out-of-home placement. The program has been shown to be effective with targeted populations that include inner-city delinquents, violent and chronic juvenile offenders, juvenile offenders who abuse or are dependent on substances and also have psychiatric disorders, adolescent sex offenders, and abusive and neglectful parents. A more recent focus of MST has been to treat youths who present with psychiatric emergencies, such as suicidal ideation, homicidal ideation, **psychosis**, or threat of harm to self or others due to mental illness. The results are promising and indicate that MST is an effective alternative to psychiatric hospitalization. Some treatment conditions and interventions were modified to take care of this new population, including developing a crisis plan during the initial family assessment and adding child and adolescent psychiatrists, psychiatric residents, and crisis caseworkers to the MST treatment team. Supervision by the treatment team was increased from weekly to daily meetings. Caseloads of MST therapists were reduced from five to three families, increasing the intensity of the **intervention**. When some adolescents were hospitalized for safety, the MST staff maintained clinical responsibility for the adolescent who was insulated from the usual activities due to inpatient care.

MST is licensed by MST Services, Inc., through the Medical University of South Carolina.

Description

MST programs are usually housed in community-based mental health organizations with a focus that is more rehabilitative than punitive. The program staff creates strong working relationships with referral sources, such as persons within the juvenile justice system and the family court. They work closely with deputy juvenile officers, social welfare workers, teachers, and guidance counselors to obtain the perspectives of multiple systems or "stakeholders" who have the common goal of improving children, adolescent, and family treatment. Each youth referred to the program is assigned to an MST therapist who designs individualized interventions in accordance, with the nine MST treatment principles, thereby addressing individual needs of the youth and his or her specific environment.

MST is a time-limited (four to six months) intensive therapeutic program that provides services in the family's home, at other locations (school, neighborhoods), or wherever the family feels most comfortable. After the initial sessions, the family members who attend sessions with the therapist will vary depending on the nature of the particular problem being discussed. For example, children are not included in sessions addressing intimate marital issues between parents or dealing with poor parental discipline, so as not to undermine parental authority.

Characteristics of the MST model such as availability of the MST staff (24 hours a day, seven days a week), flexible scheduling, and delivery of services in the home—all provide safety for the family, prevent violence, foster a joint working relationship between therapist and family, provide the family with easier access to needed services, increase the likelihood that the family will stay in treatment, and help the family maintain changes in behaviors. The MST staff are full-time practitioners, and they wear pagers, carry cellular telephones, and work in teams of three. They can provide intensive services because of small caseloads and have multiple contacts with the family during the week, sometimes even daily. They stay as long as required and at times most convenient to the family, including weekends, evenings, and holidays. Services provided by staff at unusual times (10 P.M. to 8 A.M.) are discouraged, except in emergencies. The development of an informal support system in which the family can call on a friend or relative at crucial times is part of the treatment goals. Families have less contact with the therapist as they get closer to being discharged from treatment.

MST is designed to be a flexible intervention to provide highly individualized treatment to families. Specific treatment techniques or therapies are used as a part of MST interventions. These include parent-behavior training, structural **family therapy**, and strategic family and **cognitive-behavioral therapy**. In addition, some biological influences, such as **depression** and depressive disorders, may be identified, and psychotropic medications are integrated into treatment. This model does not support one method for obtaining successful changes in behaviors; however, there are nine guiding principles of treatment:

- The primary purpose of assessment is to understand the fit between the identified problems and their broader systemic context. At the initial visit with the family, the staff begins to assess the family's strengths; capabilities; needs; problems; environmental support systems; and transactions with social systems, such as peers, extended family, friends, teachers, parental workplace, referral resources, and neighbors. The therapist and family work together to identify and prioritize problems to be targeted for change, determine interventions, and develop a treatment plan. The assessment is conducted in a manner that empowers family members by encouraging them to define their problems, needs, strengths, and—except in matters of imminent safety—set their priorities. The assessment is gradually updated until the family has reached its goals and is functioning independently.
- Therapeutic contacts emphasize the positive and should use systemic strengths as levers for change. MST is a strength-based treatment program and adherence to this principle decreases negativity among family members, builds positive expectations and hope, identifies strengths, and decreases therapist and family frustrations by emphasizing problem solving. It also builds the caregiver's confidence. The therapist develops and maintains the focus on the strength of the family and positive thinking through the use of positive language, teaching, and the technique of reframing negative thoughts and beliefs; the liberal use of positive rewards for appropriate behaviors; using a problem-solving stance rather than one of failure and seeing barriers as challenges; and identifying and using what the family does well.
- Interventions are designed to promote responsible behavior and decrease irresponsible behavior among family members. The therapist assists parents and youths in behaving in a responsible manner across a variety of domains. Parental duties include providing support, guidance, and discipline; expressing love and nurturance; protection; advocacy; and meeting basic physical needs. The primary responsibilities of the child and adolescent include complying with family and societal rules, attending school and putting forth reasonable effort, helping around the house, and not harming self or others. Therapists will spend a great deal of time throughout the treatment process enhancing, developing, and maintaining the responsible behaviors of parents through praise and support. Other family members who become engaged in the treatment process are also encouraged by the therapist to reinforce responsible parental behaviors that will help maintain these behaviors when treatment ends. It has been noted that when parents increase their responsibilities, there is almost always improvement in the child's behavior. Parental

abdication of responsibilities may be caused by factors such as mental illness or the lack of necessary parenting skills. Interventions are designed to address these influences. For children and adolescents, positive reinforcement and discipline are used to increase responsible behaviors and decrease irresponsible behaviors. Parents are encouraged to clearly outline their expectations for compliance and punishments for noncompliance before putting them into action. For example, the child should know ahead of time that missing curfew will result in being grounded for a week. Parents are also taught to praise often for compliant behaviors.

- Interventions are focused on the present and action oriented, targeting specific and well-defined problems. Due to time limitations of the MST model, family members are required to work intensely to solve often long-standing problems. Once information has been gathered and assessed, therapist and family jointly formalize problem and goals into a treatment plan. The plan specifies which changes in what behavior or skill will be achieved by whom, by what method or action, and in what period of time within the limits of the program. The treatment plan contains the family's ultimate aims that are to be accomplished by the end of the treatment period, and intermediate goals or incremental steps needed to reach the overarching goals. These intermediate goals are measurable and time-limited, and the interventions chosen are those that have been determined to have the most immediate and powerful impact on the problem behavior. The therapist assists families in meeting their specific goals by helping them focus their time, energy, and resources on their assignments. Also, the expected outcome of each intervention is described in observable and measurable terms before the treatment plan is put into action. This aids the MST staff and the family in determining whether the interventions are effective or if alternatives are needed.
- Interventions should target sequences of behavior within and between multiple systems that maintain the identified problem. For example, if an ineffective parenting style (permissive, authoritarian, neglectful) is identified as a factor in influencing the problem behavior, it will be targeted for an intervention. However, if the parents are having marital difficulties that lead to disagreements in child-rearing practices, and these difficulties are sustaining the poor parenting style, the marital issues will be the focus of an additional intervention. The family may also have some practical or concrete needs (housing, heat, transportation) that are affecting parental discipline, and these may require interventions across the family–community support system.
- Interventions are developmentally appropriate and fit the needs of the youth. The nature of the intervention should take into account the age and maturity of the child or adolescent and the caregiver. It is noted that, for children and young adolescents, interventions aimed at increasing parental control are the most appropriate. Such interventions might include introducing systematic monitoring, reward, and discipline systems. For an older adolescent, interventions would most likely focus on preparing the youth for entry into the adult world, such as increasing his or her social maturity. Other interventions may be needed to overcome obstacles to independent living, such as having the teenager participate in GED classes or enter a vocational training school. The developmental stage of the caregiver is also important to consider. For example, grandparents may not have the physical or emotional health to become primary caregivers but may be able to assist parents in other ways, such as helping with homework or sitting with the youth after school for a few hours.
- Interventions are designed to require daily or weekly effort by family members. This leads to a more rapid decrease in the problem behavior and current and continuous evaluation of whether the intervention is working and producing the expected results. For example, if a parent sits near the child while he is doing homework, he or she can gauge the child's progress toward the anticipated goal of better school performance. This design also allows family members to experience immediate success and obtain positive feedback.
- Intervention effectiveness is evaluated continuously from multiple perspectives with providers assuming accountability for overcoming barriers to successful outcomes. Before intervention is implemented the therapist is required to document anticipated outcomes for each intervention by describing the observable and measurable goals of treatment. This information is used to assess the successes achieved or barriers encountered and to assess the impact of the intervention. The MST staff may also be in daily contact with teachers and administrators, deputy juvenile officers, and welfare professionals who provide feedback regarding whether the interventions across systems are successful in changing behaviors.
- Interventions are designed to promote treatment generalization and long-term maintenance of therapeutic change by empowering caregivers to address family members' needs across multiple systemic contexts. The MST therapist, the MST team, and the provider agency are responsible for engaging the family in treatment, making services for the family easier to obtain, and achieving positive outcomes for the child or adolescent and the family in every case. The program's achievement of

KEY TERMS

Psychotropic medication—Medication that has an effect on the mind, brain, behavior, perceptions, or emotions. Psychotropic medications are used to treat mental illnesses because they affect a patient's moods and perceptions.

Punitive—Concerned with, or directed toward, punishment.

Rehabilitative—To restore; to put back into good condition.

successful goals and maintenance of behavior change is due to staff adherence to the treatment model. Research has demonstrated that strong adherence correlates to strong case outcomes. The key to the success of the model is intensive and ongoing staff training. Clinical staff training includes five days of orientation training, weekly supervision with an MST expert, and quarterly booster training. On-site supervisors are also intensively trained to ensure that the MST staff adhere to the MST model.

Results

At the end of MST treatment, parents are provided with the resources needed to parent effectively and maintain better family structure and cohesion. Specifically, parents:

- are able to systematically monitor the behavior of their child or adolescent
- have learned to use appropriate reward and discipline measures to maintain new behavioral changes
- can communicate more effectively with each other and their children
- can advocate for their children and themselves across social systems (e.g., school, social services)
- can problem-solve daily conflicts
- can maintain positive relations with natural social supports such as extended family, friends, and church members
- are able to maintain a positive working relationship with school personnel
- have learned strategies to monitor and promote the child's or adolescent's school performance and/or vocational functioning

Other outcomes to be expected have to do with the youth's relationships with peers and his or her performance in school. Specifically, it is expected that the child or adolescent has decreased his or her association with delinquent and/or drug-using peers; has increased his or her relationships with positive peers and engages in positive activities through after-school activities, organized athletics, or volunteer or paid activities; has better school performance; and has had no days, or fewer days, requiring out-of-home placement.

Resources

BOOKS

Henggeler, Scott W., et al. *Multisystemic Therapy for Antisocial Behavior in Children and Adolescents*. New York: Guilford Press, 2009.

Swenson, Cynthia Cupit, et al. *Multisystemic Therapy and Neighborhood Partnerships: Reducing Adolescent Violence and Substance Abuse*. New York: Guilford Press, 2009.

PERIODICALS

Cox, Kathleen F. "Examining the Role of Social Network Intervention as an Integral Component of Community-Based, Family-Focused Practice." *Journal of Child and Family Studies* 14, no. 3 (September 2005): 443–54.

Ellis, Deborah A., et al. "Multisystemic Therapy for Adolescents With Poorly Controlled Type I Diabetes: Stability of Treatment Effects in a Randomized Controlled Trial." *Journal of Consulting and Clinical Psychology* 75, no. 1 (February 2007): 168–74.

Littell, Julia H. "Lessons from a Systematic Review of Effects of Multisystemic Therapy." *Children and Youth Services Review* 27, no. 4 (April 2005): 445–63.

Schaeffer, Cindy M., and Charles M. Borduin. "Long-Term Follow-Up to a Randomized Clinical Trial of Multisystemic Therapy With Serious and Violent Juvenile Offenders." *Journal of Consulting and Clinical Psychology* 73, no. 3 (June 2005): 445–53.

Schoenwald, Sonja K., Elizabeth J. Letourneau, and Colleen Halliday-Boykins. "Predicting Therapist Adherence to a Transported Family-Based Treatment for Youth." *Journal of Clinical Child and Adolescent Psychology* 34, no. 4 (December 2005): 658–70.

Timmons-Mitchell, Jane, et al. "An Independent Effectiveness Trial of Multisystemic Therapy With Juvenile Justice Youth." *Journal of Clinical Child and Adolescent Psychology* 35, no. 2 (June 2006): 227–36.

ORGANIZATIONS

National Institute of Mental Health, 6001 Executive Blvd., Room 8184, MSC 9663, Bethesda, MD, 20892-9663, (301) 433-4513; TTY: (301) 443-8431, Fax: (301) 443-4279, (866) 615-6464; TTY: (866) 415-8051, nimhinfo@nih.gov, http://www.nimh.nih.gov.

Office of Juvenile Justice and Delinquency Prevention, 810 Seventh St. NW, Washington, DC, 20531, (202) 307-5911, http://www.ojjdp.gov.

Janice VanBuren, PhD
Ruth A. Wienclaw, PhD

Munchausen syndrome *see* **Factitious disorder**

Music therapy

Definition

Music therapy is a technique of complementary medicine that uses music prescribed in a skilled manner by trained therapists. Programs are designed to help patients overcome physical, emotional, intellectual, and social challenges. Applications range from improving the well-being of geriatric patients in nursing homes to lowering the **stress** level and pain of women in labor. Music therapy is used in many settings, including schools, rehabilitation centers, hospitals, hospices, nursing homes, community centers, and sometimes even in the home.

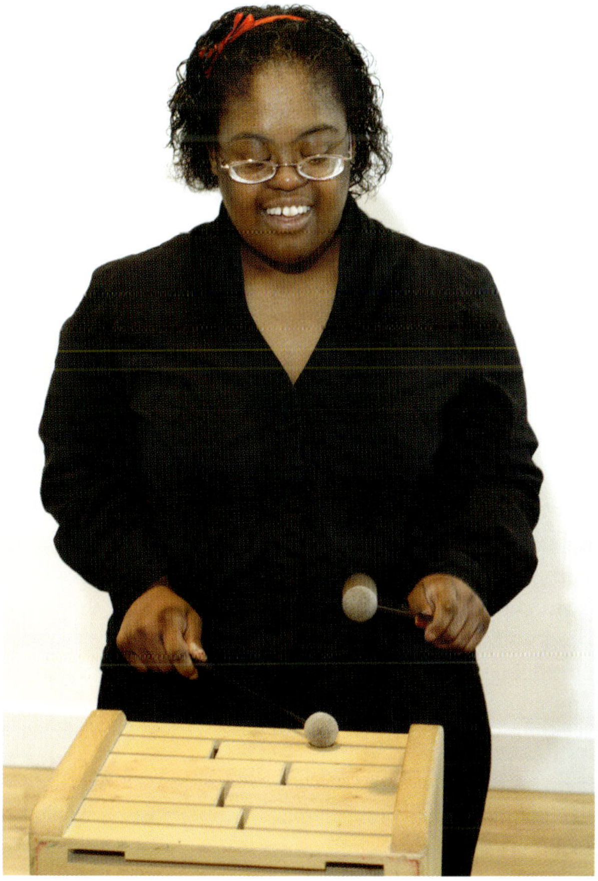

A woman plays the xylophone during a music therapy session for persons with learning disabilities. *(© Paula Solloway/Alamy)*

Purpose

Music can be beneficial for everyone. Although it can be used therapeutically for people who have physical, emotional, social, or cognitive deficits, even those who are healthy can use music to relax, reduce stress, improve mood, or to accompany **exercise**. There are no potentially harmful or toxic effects. Music therapists help their patients achieve a number of goals through music, including improvement of communication, academic strengths, attention span, and motor skills. They may also assist with behavioral therapy and pain management.

Description

Music has been used throughout human history to express and affect human emotion. In biblical accounts, King Saul was reportedly soothed by David's harp music, and the ancient Greeks expressed views about music having healing effects as well. Many cultures are steeped in musical traditions. It can change mood, have stimulant or sedative effects, and alter physiologic processes such as heart rate and breathing. The apparent health benefits of music to patients in Veterans Administration hospitals following World War II led to it being studied and formalized as a complementary healing practice. Musicians were hired to continue working in the hospitals. Degrees in music therapy became available in the late 1940s, and in 1950, the first professional association of music therapists was formed in the United States. The National Association of Music Therapy merged with the American Association of Music Therapy in 1998 to become the American Music Therapy Association.

Benefits

Brain function physically changes in response to music. The rhythm can guide the body into breathing in slower, deeper patterns that have a calming effect. Heart rate and blood pressure are also responsive to various types of music. The speed of the heartbeat tends to speed or slow depending on the volume and speed of the auditory stimulus. Louder and faster sounds tend to raise both heart rate and blood pressure; slower, softer, and more regular tones produce the opposite result. Music can also relieve muscle tension and improve motor skills. It is often used to help rebuild physical patterning skills in rehabilitation clinics. Levels of endorphins, natural pain relievers, are increased and levels of stress hormones are decreased in individuals while they listen to music. This latter effect may partially explain the ability of music to improve immune function. A study at Michigan State University showed that even 15 minutes of exposure to music can increase interleukin-1 levels, a consequence which also heightens immunity.

Mental effects

Depending on the type and style of sound, music can either sharpen mental acuity or assist in relaxation. Memory and learning can be enhanced, and this effect has been used with good results in children with learning disabilities. This effect may also be partially due to increased concentration that many people have while listening to music. Better productivity is another outcome of an improved ability to concentrate. The term "Mozart effect" was coined after a study showed that college students performed better on math problems when they were listening to classical music.

Emotional effects

The ability of music to influence human emotion is well known and is used extensively by moviemakers. A variety of musical moods may be used to create feelings of calm, tension, excitement, or romance. Lullabies have long been popular for soothing babies as they fall asleep. Music can also be used to express emotion nonverbally, which can be a valuable therapeutic tool in some settings.

Goals

Music is used to form a relationship between the therapist and the patient. The music therapist sets goals on an individual basis, depending on the reasons for treatment, and selects specific activities and exercises to help the patient progress. Objectives may include development of communication, cognitive, motor, emotional, and social skills. Some of the techniques used to achieve this are singing, listening, instrumental music, composition, creative movement, guided imagery, and other methods as appropriate. Other disciplines may be integrated as well, such as dance, art, and psychology. Patients may develop musical abilities as a result of therapy, but this is not a major concern. The primary aim is to improve patients' ability to function.

Techniques

Learning to play an instrument is an excellent activity for developing motor skills in individuals with developmental delays, brain injuries, or other motor impairment. It is also an exercise in impulse control and group cooperation. Creative movement is another activity that can help to improve coordination, as well as strength, balance, and gait. Improvisation facilitates the nonverbal expression of emotion. It encourages socialization and communication about feelings as well. Singing develops articulation, rhythm, and breath control. Remembering lyrics and melody is an exercise in sequencing for **stroke** victims and others who may be intellectually impaired. Composition of words and music is one avenue available to assist patients in working through fears and negative feelings. Listening is an excellent way to practice attending and remembering. It may also make patients aware of memories and emotions that need to be acknowledged and perhaps talked about. Singing and discussion are related methods, which are used with some patients to encourage dialogue. Guided imagery and music (GIM) is a popular technique developed by music therapist Helen Bonny. Listening to music is used as a path to invoke emotions, pictures, and symbols from patients. This is a bridge to the exploration and expression of feelings.

KEY TERMS

Adjunctive—Describes a form of treatment that is not strictly necessary to a therapy regimen but is helpful. Music therapy is an example of an adjunctive form of treatment.

Entrainment—The patterning of body processes and movements to the rhythm of music.

Physiologic—Describes the physiology, particularly normal, healthy, physical functioning.

Music and children

The sensory stimulation and playful nature of music can help to develop children's ability to express emotion, communicate, and develop rhythmic movement. Some evidence shows that speech and language skills can be improved through the stimulation of both hemispheres of the brain. Just as with adults, appropriately selected music can decrease stress, anxiety, and pain among children. Music therapy in a hospital environment with those who are sick, preparing for surgery, or recovering postoperatively is appropriate and beneficial. Children can also experience improved self-esteem through musical activities that allow them to succeed.

Newborns may enjoy even greater benefits from music. Premature infants experience more rapid weight gain and an earlier discharge from the hospital than their peers who are not exposed to music. There is also anecdotal evidence of improved cognitive function in premature infants from listening to music.

Music and rehabilitation

Patients with brain damage from stroke, **traumatic brain injury**, or other neurologic conditions have been shown to exhibit significant improvement as a result of music therapy. This is theorized to be partially the result of entrainment, which is the synchronization of movement with the rhythm of the music. Consistent practice leads to gains in motor skill ability and efficiency. Cognitive processes and language skills often benefit from appropriate musical **intervention**.

Music therapy has also shown effectiveness in rehabilitating the hearing of children and adults who have had cochlear implant surgery to treat impaired hearing. Young children who have never heard sounds face a lengthy rehabilitation in order to learn how to interpret sound and form speech. Music therapy can serve as a bridge between nonverbal communication and the new sounds that toddlers are hearing and processing into language. In older adults with cochlear implants, music therapy can offer relaxation to minimize distortion among new sounds and cues to remembering old sounds. Individualized music therapy is also used to reduce noise levels in people with tinnitus, or ringing in the ears.

Music and the elderly

The geriatric population can be prone to anxiety and **depression**, particularly in nursing home residents. Chronic diseases causing pain are also not uncommon in this setting. Music is an excellent outlet to provide enjoyment, relaxation, relief from pain, and an opportunity to socialize and reminisce about music that has had special importance to individuals. It can have a striking effect on patients with **Alzheimer's disease**, even sometimes allowing them to focus and become more responsive for a time. Music has also been observed to decrease the agitation that is so common with this disease. One study shows that elderly people who play a musical instrument are more physically and emotionally fit as they age than their nonmusical peers are.

Music and psychiatric disorders

Music can be an effective tool for treating the mentally or emotionally ill. **Autism** is one disorder that has been particularly researched. Music therapy has enabled some autistic children to relate to others and have improved learning skills. **Substance abuse**, **schizophrenia**, **paranoia**, and disorders of personality, anxiety, and affect have all benefited from music therapy. In these groups, participation and social interaction are promoted through music. Reality orientation is improved. Patients are helped to develop coping skills, reduce stress, and express their feelings.

In the treatment of psychotic disorders, however, the benefits of music therapy appear to be limited. One study of patients diagnosed with schizophrenia or schizoaffective **psychosis** found that while music therapy improved the patients' social relationships, these benefits were relatively short-lived.

Music and hospice care

Pain, anxiety, and depression are major concerns with patients who are terminally ill, whether they are in hospice or not. Music can provide some relief from pain, through the release of endorphins and the promotion of relaxation. It can also provide an opportunity for the patient to reminisce and talk about the fears that are associated with death and dying. Music may help regulate the rapid breathing of a patient who is anxious and soothe the mind. The Chalice of Repose project, headquartered at St. Patrick Hospital in Missoula, Montana, is one organization that attends to and nurtures critical patients through the use of music in a practice called music-thanatology, developed by Therese Schroeder-Sheker. Practitioners in this program work to relieve suffering through music prescribed for the individual patient.

Music and childbirth

Research has proven that women require less pharmaceutical pain relief during labor if they make use of music. Listening to music that is familiar and associated with positive imagery is the most helpful. During early labor, music promotes relaxation. Maternal movement is helpful to get the baby into a proper birthing position and dilate the cervix. Enjoying some "music to move by" can encourage the mother to stay active for as long as possible during labor. The rhythmic auditory stimulation may also prompt the body to release endorphins, which are a natural form of pain relief. Many women select different styles of music for each stage of labor, with a more intense or faster-moving piece as the natural accompaniment to the more difficult parts of labor. Instrumental music is often preferred.

The benefits of music therapy during childbirth have also been shown to apply to other surgical procedures. Women who have listened to music tapes during gynecologic surgery have more restful sleep following the procedure and less postoperative soreness.

Precautions

Patients making use of music therapy should not discontinue medications or therapies prescribed by other health providers without prior consultation.

Research and general acceptance

There is little disagreement among physicians that music can be of some benefit for patients, although the extent of its effects on physical well-being remains a matter of debate among members of the medical community. Acceptance of music therapy as an adjunctive treatment modality is increasing, however, due to the growing diversity of patient populations receiving music therapy. Research has shown that listening to music can decrease anxiety, pain, and recovery time. There is also evidence supporting its use for the specific subpopulations discussed. A therapist referral can be made through the AMTA.

Training and certification

Music therapists are themselves often talented musicians; they also study the ways in which music can be applied to specific groups and circumstances. Coursework includes classes in music history and performance, behavioral science, and education. The American Music Therapy Association dictates what classes must be included in order for a music therapy program to be certified. There are approximately 70 colleges with approved curricula. A six-month internship follows the completion of the formal music therapy program, and graduates are then able to take a national board exam to gain certification.

There are about 5,000 board certified music therapists in the United States. The field is growing rapidly as an increasing number of both inpatient and outpatient healthcare settings incorporate music therapy into their treatment modalities.

Resources

BOOKS

Boxill, Edith Hillman, and Kristen M. Chase. *Music Therapy for Developmental Disabilities*. Austin, Tex: Pro-Ed, Inc. 2007.

Nordoff, Paul, and Clive Robbins. *Creative Music Therapy: A Guide to Fostering Clinical Musicianship*. 2nd ed. Gilsum, N.H.: Barcelona Publishers, 2007.

Oldfield, Amelia, and Claire Flower. *Music Therapy with Children and Their Families*. Gateshead, UK: Athenaeum Press, 2008.

Sacks, Oliver W. *Musicophilia: Tales of Music and the Brain*. New York: Alfred A. Knopf, 2007.

Sekeles, Chava. *Music Therapy: Death and Grief*. Gilsum, NH: Barcelona Publishers, 2007.

Serlin, Ilene A. *Whole Person Healthcare*. Praeger Perspectives. Westport, CT: Praeger, 2007.

PERIODICALS

Avers, Laura, Ambika Mathur, and Deepak Kamat. "Music Therapy in Pediatrics." *Clinical Pediatrics*. 46, no. 7 (October 2007): 575–579.

Lite, Jordan. "Sonic Health Boost: Music Therapy Can Fight Pain and Disease." *Prevention*. (January 2008): 53–57.

Parker, A.B., "Music Therapy Clarifications." *Journal of Psychosocial Nursing and Mental Health Services* 47, no. 4 (April 2009): 15.

Romo, R., and L. Gifford. "A Cost-Benefit Analysis of Music Therapy in a Home Hospice." *Nursing Economics*. (November–December 2007): 34.

Talwar, N., et al. "Music Therapy for In-Patients with Schizophrenia: Exploratory Randomized Controlled Trial." *The British Journal of Psychiatry: the Journal of Mental Science*. 189 (2006): 405–9.

ORGANIZATIONS

American Music Therapy Association, 8455 Colesville Rd., Suite 1000, Silver Spring, MD, 20910, (301) 589-3300, Fax: (301) 589-5175, http://www.musictherapy.org.

Judith Turner
Rebecca J. Frey, PhD
Brenda W. Lerner

Mutual support *see* **Support groups**

N

Naltrexone

Definition

Naltrexone is classified as a pure opiate antagonist. It is sold in the United States under the brand names ReVia and Depade and is also manufactured and sold under its generic name.

Purpose

Naltrexone is used as part of medically supervised **behavior modification** programs to help patients who have stopped taking narcotics or alcohol to continue to abstain from opiates or alcohol.

Description

Opiates are a group of drugs that are either derived from opium (e.g., morphine, hydromorphone, oxymorphone, heroin, codeine, hydrocodone, oxycodone) or chemically resemble these opium derivatives (such as meperidine). They are commonly referred to as narcotics. Some opiates have medically valid uses, while others are recreational drugs of abuse. All are physically addictive.

The drug naltrexone is an opiate antagonist. This means that it blocks and reverses the physical effects of drugs such as morphine, hydromorphone, oxymorphone, heroin, meperidine, codeine, hydrocodone, oxycodone and other drugs classified as narcotics. When given to patients who have been successfully treated for opiate **addiction**, it not only decreases cravings for these types of drugs, it also helps patients who use opiates while taking naltrexone to avoid experiencing the euphoria associated with their use. In these two ways, naltrexone helps prevent re-addiction to opiates.

Chemically, naltrexone is not an alcohol antagonist. However, when it is used in combination with behavior modification in a person recovering from alcoholism, naltrexone decreases the craving for alcohol. This helps patients to prevent a return to **alcohol use** or decreases the severity of **relapse** by reducing the amount of alcohol consumed during the relapse or decreasing the length of the relapse.

Naltrexone is available in 50 mg oral tablets.

Recommended dosage

After successful **detoxification** from opiates, people who used them will receive a test dose of 25 mg of naltrexone, then be observed for one hour for symptoms of opiate withdrawal. If no problems occur after this test dose, another 25 mg test dose is administered.

Getting such people to comply with treatment for opiate addiction is the single most important aspect in maintaining an opiate-free state. Different schedules for taking naltrexone have been developed to help meet the needs of individuals complying with taking the drug. Following successful initiation of therapy, naltrexone may be administered in one of the following ways:

- 50 mg daily, Monday through Friday, and 100 mg on Saturday
- 100 mg every other day
- 150 mg every third day
- 100 mg on Monday and Wednesday and 150 mg on Friday
- 150 mg on Monday and 200 mg on Thursday

The duration of treatment with naltrexone for people with opiate dependence varies with patient need, although most patients will require at least six months of treatment.

The usual dose of naltrexone for alcohol dependence is 50 mg daily, although a few patients may require only 25 mg daily. The proper duration of therapy is not known, as studies of the use of naltrexone in people with alcohol dependence did not go beyond 12 weeks.

KEY TERMS

Antagonist—A substance whose actions counteract the effects of or work in the opposite way from another chemical or drug.

Opiates—A class of drugs that is either derived from opium (i.e., morphine, hydromorphone, oxymorphone, heroin, codeine, hydrocodone, oxycodone) or resembles these opium derivatives (such as meperidine) and is commonly referred to as narcotics.

Precautions

In a very small number of patients, naltrexone may be toxic and cause damage to the liver. Before starting naltrexone and throughout treatment, patients should receive monthly liver function tests to assess the drug's effect on the liver.

Patients should be free of all opiates for seven to ten days before starting naltrexone. Naltrexone may cause opiate withdrawal symptoms in people whose bodies are not free from opiates. Patients should be observed for opiate withdrawal immediately following the first dose of the drug.

Patients may have a false sense of security that the presence of naltrexone in their system makes them immune from the effects of opiates. In actuality, patients are more sensitive to the effects of opiates when taking naltrexone, and patients receiving naltrexone who continue to use or receive opiates should be monitored for signs and symptoms of opiate overdose.

Side effects

The following represents the most common side effects associated with naltrexone:

- nausea, vomiting, diarrhea, cramps
- headache, insomnia, anxiety, irritability, depression, dizziness
- joint and muscle pain
- rash

Interactions

Because naltrexone is an opiate antagonist, opiate derivatives that are used medicinally in treating coughs, diarrhea, and pain may no longer be effective.

The combination of naltrexone and **disulfiram**, a drug that is also used for alcohol abuse, may cause increased liver toxicity and liver damage. This combination should be avoided unless, in consultation with a physician, it is decided that the potential benefits of this combination outweigh the risks.

See also Opioids and related disorders

Resources

BOOKS

American Society of Health-System Pharmacists. *AHFS Drug Information 2008.* Bethesda, MD: American Society of Health-System Pharmacists, 2008.

Preston, John D., John H. O'Neal, and Mary C. Talaga. *Handbook of Clinical Psychopharmacology for Therapists.* 5th ed. Oakland, CA: New Harbinger Publications, 2008.

PERIODICALS

Anton, Raymond F., et al. "Combined Pharmacotherapies and Behavioral Interventions for Alcohol Dependence: The COMBINE Study: A Randomized Controlled Trial." *Journal of the American Medical Association* 295, no. 17 (May 2006): 2003–17.

Armeli, Stephen, et al. "The Effects of Naltrexone on Alcohol Consumption and Affect Reactivity to Daily Interpersonal Events Among Heavy Drinkers." *Experimental and Clinical Psychopharmacology* 14, no. 2 (May 2006): 199–208.

Comer, Sandra D., et al. "Injectable, Sustained-Release Naltrexone for the Treatment of Opioid Dependence: A Randomized, Placebo-Controlled Trial." *Archives of General Psychiatry* 63, no. 2 (February 2006): 210–18.

Johansson, Björn Axel, Mats Berglund, and Anna Lindgren. "Efficacy of Maintenance Treatment with Naltrexone for Opioid Dependence: A Meta-Analytical Review." *Addiction* 101, no. 4 (April 2006): 491–503.

Morley, Kirsten C., et al. "Naltrexone Versus Acamprosate in the Treatment of Alcohol Dependence: A Multi-Centre, Randomized, Double-Blind, Placebo-Controlled Trial." *Addiction* 101, no. 10 (October 2006): 1451–62.

Nunes, Edward V., et al. "Behavioral Therapy to Augment Oral Naltrexone for Opioid Dependence: A Ceiling on Effectiveness?" *American Journal of Drug and Alcohol Abuse* 32, no. 4 (2006): 503–17.

O'Brien, Charles, and James W. Cornish. "Naltrexone for Probationers and Parolees." *Journal of Substance Abuse Treatment* 31, no. 2 (September 2006): 107–11.

Petrakis, Ismene L.,et al. "Naltrexone and Disulfiram in Patients with Alcohol Dependence and Comorbid Post-Traumatic Stress Disorder." *Biological Psychiatry* 60, no. 7 (October 2006): 777–83.

Pettinati, Helen M., et al. "The Status of Naltrexone in the Treatment of Alcohol Dependence: Specific Effects on Heavy Drinking." *Journal of Clinical Psychopharmacology* 26, no. 6 (December 2006): 610–25.

Rohsenow, Damaris J., et al. "High-Dose Transdermal Nicotine and Naltrexone: Effects on Nicotine Withdrawal, Urges, Smoking, and Effects of Smoking." *Experimental and*

Clinical Psychopharmacology 15, no. 1 (February 2007): 81–92.

Roozen, Hendrik G., et al. "A Systematic Review of the Effectiveness of Naltrexone in the Maintenance Treatment of Opioid and Alcohol Dependence." *European Neuropsychopharmacology* 16, no. 5 (July 2006): 311–23.

Sullivan, Maria A., et al. "Predictors of Retention in Naltrexone Maintenance for Opioid Dependence: Analysis of a Stage I Trial." *The American Journal on Addictions* 15, no. 2 (March–April 2006): 150–59.

Jack Raber, Pharm. D.
Ruth A. Wienclaw, PhD

Narcissistic personality disorder

Definition

Narcissistic personality disorder (NPD) is included in the ***Diagnostic and Statistical Manual of Mental Disorders*** (*DSM*), a handbook that mental health professionals use to diagnose mental disorders, as one of several **personality disorders**. As a group, these disorders are described in the revised fourth edition (*DSM-IV-TR*) as "enduring pattern[s] of inner experience and behavior" that are sufficiently rigid and deep-seated to bring a person into repeated conflicts with his or her social and occupational environment. *DSM-IV-TR* specifies that these dysfunctional patterns must be regarded as nonconforming or deviant by the person's culture, and cause significant emotional pain and/or difficulties in relationships and occupational performance.

To meet the **diagnosis** of a personality disorder, the patient's problematic behaviors must appear in two or more of the following areas:

- perception and interpretation of the self and other people
- intensity and duration of feelings and their appropriateness to situations
- relationships with others
- ability to control impulses

It is important to note that all the personality disorders are considered to have their onset in late adolescence or early adulthood. Doctors rarely give a diagnosis of personality disorder to children on the grounds that children's personalities are still in process of formation and may change considerably by the time they are in their late teens.

NPD is defined more specifically as a pattern of grandiosity (exaggerated claims to talents, importance, or specialness) in the patient's private fantasies or outward behavior; a need for constant admiration from others; and a lack of empathy for others. The term *narcissistic* is derived from an ancient Greek legend, the story of Echo and Narcissus. According to the legend, Echo was a woodland nymph who fell in love with Narcissus, who was an uncommonly handsome but also uncommonly vain young man. He contemptuously rejected her expressions of love. She pined away and died. The god Apollo was angered by Narcissus' pride and self-satisfaction, and condemned him to die without ever knowing human love. One day, Narcissus was feeling thirsty, saw a pool of clear water nearby, and knelt beside it in order to dip his hands in the water and drink. He saw his face reflected on the surface of the water and fell in love with the reflection. Unable to win a response from the image in the water, Narcissus eventually died beside the pool.

Havelock Ellis, a British **psychologist**, first used the story of Echo and Narcissus in 1898 as a capsule summary of pathological self-absorption. The words *narcissist* and *narcissistic* have been part of the vocabulary of psychology and psychiatry ever since. They have, however, been the subjects of several controversies. In order to understand NPD, the reader may find it helpful to have an outline of the different theories about narcissism in human beings, its relation to other psychiatric disorders, and its connections to the wider culture. NPD is unique among the *DSM-IV-TR* personality disorders in that it has been made into a symbol of the problems and discontents of contemporary Western culture as a whole.

Demographics

DSM-IV-TR states that 2% to 16% of the clinical population and slightly less than 1% of the general population of the United States suffers from NPD. Between 50% and 75% of those diagnosed with NPD are males. Little is known about the prevalence of NPD across racial and ethnic groups.

Gender issues

The high preponderance of male patients in studies of narcissism has prompted researchers to explore the effects of gender roles on this particular personality disorder. Some have speculated that the gender imbalance in NPD results from society's disapproval of self-centered and exploitative behavior in women, who are typically socialized to nurture, please, and generally focus their attention on others. Others have remarked that the imbalance is more apparent than real, and that it reflects a basically sexist definition of narcissism. These researchers suggest that definitions of the disorder should be rewritten in future editions of *DSM* to account for ways in which narcissistic personality traits manifest differently in men and in women.

Professional and leadership positions

One important aspect of NPD that should be noted is that it does not prevent people from occupying, as well as aspiring to, positions of power, wealth, and prestige. Many people with NPD, as Kernberg's classification makes clear, are sufficiently talented to secure the credentials of success. In addition, narcissists' preoccupation with a well-packaged exterior means that they often develop an attractive and persuasive social manner. Many high-functioning narcissists are well liked by casual acquaintances and business associates who never get close enough to notice the emptiness or anger underneath the polished surface.

Unfortunately, narcissists in positions of high visibility or power—particularly in the so-called helping professions (medicine, education, and the ministry)—often do great harm to others. In recent years a number of books and articles have been published within the religious, medical, and business communities regarding the problems caused by professionals with NPD. One **psychiatrist** noted in a lecture on substance abuse among physicians that NPD is one of the three most common psychiatric diagnoses among physicians in court-mandated substance abuse programs. A psychologist who serves as a consultant in the evaluation of seminary students and ordained clergy has remarked that the proportion of narcissists in the clergy has risen dramatically since the 1960s. Researchers in the field of business organization and management styles have compiled data on the human and economic costs of executives with undiagnosed NPD.

Description

A good place to begin a discussion of the different theories about narcissism is with the observation that NPD exists as a diagnostic category only in *DSM-IV-TR*, which is an American diagnostic manual. The *International Statistical Classification of Diseases and Related Health Problems, Tenth Revision* (*ICD-10*, the European equivalent of *DSM*) lists only eight personality disorders. What *DSM-IV-TR* defines as narcissistic personality disorder, *ICD-10* lumps together with "eccentric, impulsive-type, immature, passive-aggressive, and psychoneurotic personality disorders."

DSM-IV-TR specifies nine diagnostic criteria for NPD. For the clinician to make the diagnosis, an individual must fit five or more of the following descriptions:

- He or she has a grandiose sense of self-importance (exaggerates accomplishments and demands to be considered superior without real evidence of achievement).
- He or she lives in a dream world of exceptional success, power, beauty, genius, or "perfect" love.
- He or she thinks of him-or herself as "special" or privileged, and that he or she can only be understood by other special or high-status people.
- He or she demands excessive amounts of praise or admiration from others.
- He or she feels entitled to automatic deference, compliance, or favorable treatment from others.
- He or she is exploitative towards others and takes advantage of them.
- He or she lacks empathy and does not recognize or identify with others' feelings.
- He or she is frequently envious of others or thinks that they are envious of him or her.
- He or she "has an attitude" or frequently acts in haughty or arrogant ways.

In addition to these criteria, *DSM-IV-TR* groups NPD together with three other personality disorders in its so-called Cluster B. These four disorders are grouped together on the basis of symptom similarities, insofar as patients with these disorders appear to others as overly emotional, unstable, or self-dramatizing. The other three disorders in Cluster B are antisocial, borderline, and histrionic personality disorders.

The *DSM-IV-TR* clustering system does not mean that all patients can be fitted neatly into one of the three clusters. It is possible for patients to have symptoms of more than one personality disorder or to have symptoms from different clusters. In addition, patients diagnosed with any personality disorder may also meet the criteria for mood, **substance abuse**, or other disorders.

Subtypes of NPD

AGE GROUP SUBTYPES. Ever since the 1950s, when psychiatrists began to notice an increase in the number of their patients that had narcissistic disorders, they have made attempts to define these disorders more precisely. NPD was introduced as a new diagnostic category in *DSM-III*, which was published in 1980. Prior to *DSM-III*, narcissism was a recognized phenomenon but not an official diagnosis. At that time, NPD was considered virtually untreatable because people who suffer from it rarely enter or remain in treatment; typically, they regard themselves as superior to their therapist, and they see their problems as caused by other people's "stupidity" or "lack of appreciation." More recently, however, some psychiatrists have proposed dividing narcissistic patients into two subcategories based roughly on age: those who suffer from the stable form of NPD described by

DSM-IV-TR, and younger adults whose narcissism is often corrected by life experiences.

This age group distinction represents an ongoing controversy about the nature of NPD—whether it is fundamentally a character disorder, or whether it is a matter of learned behavior that can be unlearned. Therapists who incline toward the first viewpoint are usually pessimistic about the results of treatment for patients with NPD.

PERSONALITY SUBTYPES. Other psychiatrists have noted that patients who meet the *DSM-IV-TR* criteria for NPD reflect different clusters of traits within the *DSM-IV-TR* list. One expert in the field of NPD has suggested the following subcategories of narcissistic personalities:

- Craving narcissists. These are people who feel emotionally needy and undernourished, and may well appear clingy or demanding to those around them.
- Paranoid narcissists. This type of narcissist feels intense contempt for him- or herself, but projects it outward onto others. Paranoid narcissists frequently drive other people away from them by hypercritical and jealous comments and behaviors.
- Manipulative narcissists. These people enjoy "putting something over" on others, obtaining their feelings of superiority by lying to and manipulating them.
- Phallic narcissists. Almost all narcissists in this subgroup are male. They tend to be aggressive, athletic, and exhibitionistic; they enjoy showing off their bodies, clothes, and overall "manliness."

Causes and symptoms

Causes

At present there are two major theories about the origin and nature of NPD. One theory regards NPD as a form of arrested psychological development while the other regards it as a young child's defense against psychological pain. The two perspectives have been identified with two major figures in psychoanalytic thought, Heinz Kohut and Otto Kernberg respectively.

Both theories about NPD go back to Sigmund Freud's pioneering work *On Narcissism,* published in 1914. In this essay, Freud introduced a distinction which has been retained by almost all later writers—namely, the distinction between primary and secondary narcissism. Freud thought that all human infants pass through a phase of primary narcissism, in which they assume they are the center of their universe. This phase ends when the baby is forced by the realities of life to recognize that it does not control its parents (or other caregivers) but is in fact entirely dependent on them. In normal circumstances, the baby gives up its fantasy of being all-powerful and becomes emotionally attached to its parents rather than itself. What Freud defined as secondary narcissism is a pathological condition in which the infant does not invest its emotions in its parents but rather redirects them back to itself. He thought that secondary narcissism developed in what he termed the pre-Oedipal phase of childhood; that is, before the age of three. From a Freudian perspective, then, narcissistic disorders originate in very early childhood development, and this early origin is thought to explain why they are so difficult to treat in later life.

CAUSES IN THE FAMILY OF ORIGIN. Kohut and Kernberg agree with Freud in tracing the roots of NPD to disturbances in the patient's family of origin—specifically, to problems in the parent-child relationship before the child turned three. Where they disagree is in their accounts of the nature of these problems. According to Kohut, the child grows out of primary narcissism through opportunities to be mirrored by (i.e., gain approval from) his or her parents and to idealize them, acquiring a more realistic sense of self and a set of personal ideals and values through these two processes. On the other hand, if the parents fail to provide appropriate opportunities for idealization and mirroring, the child remains "stuck" at a developmental stage in which his or her sense of self remains grandiose and unrealistic while at the same time he or she remains dependent on approval from others for self-esteem.

In contrast, Kernberg views NPD as rooted in the child's defense against a cold and unempathetic parent, usually the mother. Emotionally hungry and angry at the depriving parents, the child withdraws into a part of the self that the parents value, whether looks, intellectual ability, or some other skill or talent. This part of the self becomes hyperinflated and grandiose. Any perceived weaknesses are "split off" into a hidden part of the self. Splitting gives rise to a lifelong tendency to swing between extremes of grandiosity and feelings of emptiness and worthlessness.

In both accounts, the child emerges into adult life with a history of unsatisfactory relationships with others. The adult narcissist possesses a grandiose view of the self but has a conflict-ridden psychological dependence on others. At present, however, psychiatrists do not agree in their description of the central defect in NPD; some think that the problem is primarily emotional while others regard it as the result of distorted cognition, or knowing. Some maintain that the person with NPD has an "empty" or hungry sense of self while others argue that the narcissist has a "disorganized" self. Still others regard the core problem as the narcissist's inability to test reality and construct an accurate view of him- or herself.

MACROSOCIAL CAUSES. One dimension of NPD that must be taken into account is its social and historical context. Psychiatrists became interested in narcissism shortly after World War II (1939–45), when the older practitioners in the field noticed that their patient population had changed. Instead of seeing patients who suffered from obsessions and compulsions related to a harsh and punishing superego (the part of the psyche that internalizes the standards and moral demands of one's parents and culture), the psychiatrists were treating more patients with character disorders related to a weak sense of self. Instead of having a judgmental and overactive conscience, these patients had a weak or nonexistent code of morals. They were very different from the patients that Freud had treated, described, and analyzed. The younger generation of psychiatrists then began to interpret their patients' character disorders in terms of narcissism.

In the 1960s historians and social critics drew the attention of the general public to narcissism as a metaphorical description of Western culture in general. These writers saw several parallels between trends in the larger society and the personality traits of people diagnosed with narcissistic disorders. In short, they argued that the advanced industrial societies of Europe and the United States were contributing to the development of narcissistic disorders in individuals in a number of respects. Some of the trends they noted include the following:

- The mass media's preoccupation with "lifestyles of the rich and famous" rather than with ordinary or average people.
- Social approval of open displays of money, status, or accomplishments ("if you've got it, flaunt it") rather than modesty and self-restraint.
- Preference for a leadership style that emphasizes the leader's outward appearance and personality rather than his or her inner beliefs and values.
- The growth of large corporations and government bureaucracies that favor a managerial style based on "impression management" rather than objective measurements of performance.
- Social trends that encourage parents to be self-centered and to resent their children's legitimate needs.
- The weakening of churches, synagogues, and other religious or social institutions that traditionally helped children to see themselves as members of a community rather than as isolated individuals.

Although discussion continues about the location and forms of narcissism in the larger society, no one now denies that personality disorders both reflect and influence the culture in which they arise. Family therapists are now reporting on the treatment of families in which the children are replicating the narcissistic disorders of their parents.

Symptoms

Most observers regard grandiosity as the most important single trait of a narcissistic personality. It is important to note that grandiosity implies more than boasting or prideful display as such—it signifies self-aggrandizement that is not borne out by reality. For example, a person who claims that he or she was the most valuable player on a college athletic team may be telling the truth about their undergraduate sports record. Their claim may be bad manners but is not grandiosity. On the other hand, someone who makes the same claim but had an undistinguished record or never even made the team is being grandiose. Grandiosity in NPD is related to some of the diagnostic criteria listed by *DSM-IV-TR*, such as demanding special favors from others or choosing friends and associates on the basis of prestige and high status rather than personal qualities. In addition, grandiosity complicates diagnostic assessment of narcissists because it frequently leads to lying and misrepresentation of one's past history and present accomplishments.

Other symptoms of NPD include:

- a history of intense but short-term relationships with others; inability to make or sustain genuinely intimate relationships
- a tendency to be attracted to leadership or high-profile positions or occupations
- a pattern of alternating between unrealistic idealization of others and equally unrealistic devaluation of them
- assessment of others in terms of usefulness
- a need to be the center of attention or admiration in a working group or social situation
- hypersensitivity to criticism, however mild, or rejection from others
- an unstable view of the self that fluctuates between extremes of self-praise and self-contempt
- preoccupation with outward appearance, "image," or public opinion rather than inner reality
- painful emotions based on shame (dislike of who one is) rather than guilt (regret for what one has done)

People diagnosed with NPD represent a range of levels of functioning. Otto Kernberg has described three levels of narcissistic impairment. At the top are those who are talented or gifted enough to attract all the admiration and attention that they want; these people may never enter therapy because they don't feel the need. On the second level are those who function satisfactorily in their jobs but seek professional help because they cannot form healthy relationships or because they feel generally bored and aimless. Narcissists on the lowest level have frequently been diagnosed with another mental disorder and/or have gotten into trouble with the law. They often have severe difficulties with anxiety and with controlling their impulses.

Diagnosis

The diagnosis of NPD is complicated by a number of factors.

Complications of diagnosis

NPD is difficult to diagnose for several reasons. First, some people with NPD function sufficiently well that they do not come to the attention of therapists. Second, narcissists are prone to lie about themselves; thus it may take a long time for a therapist to notice discrepancies between a patient's version of his or her life and information gained from others or from public records. Third, many traits and behaviors associated with NPD may be attributed to other mental disorders. Low-functioning narcissists are often diagnosed as having **borderline personality disorder** (BPD), particularly if they are female; if they are male, they may be diagnosed as having **antisocial personality disorder** (ASPD). If the person with NPD has a substance abuse disorder, some of their narcissistic behaviors may be written off to the mood-altering substance. More recently, some psychiatrists have pointed to a tendency to confuse narcissistic behaviors in people with NPD who have had a traumatic experience with full-blown **post-traumatic stress disorder** (PTSD). Given the lack of clarity in the differential diagnosis of NPD, some therapists are calling for a fundamental revision of *DSM-IV-TR* definitions of the personality disorders.

An additional complication is posed by economic considerations. The coming of **managed care** has meant that third-party payers (insurance companies) prefer short-term **psychotherapy** that concentrates on a patient's acute problems rather than on underlying chronic issues. Since narcissists are reluctant to trust others or form genuine interpersonal bonds, there is a strong possibility that many therapists do not recognize NPD in patients that they are treating for only a few weeks or months.

Diagnostic interviews

Diagnosis of NPD is usually made on the basis of several sources of information: the patient's history and self-description, information from family members and others, and the results of diagnostic questionnaires. One questionnaire that is often used in the process of differential diagnosis is the Structured Clinical Interview for *DSM-III-R* Disorders, known as the SCID-II.

The most common diagnostic instrument used for narcissistic NPD is the Narcissistic Personality Inventory (NPI). First published by Robert R. Raskin and Calvin S. Hall in 1979, the NPI consists of 223 items consisting of paired statements, one reflecting narcissistic traits and the other nonnarcissistic. Subjects are required to choose one of the two items. The NPI is widely used in research as well as diagnostic assessment.

Treatment

Treatment for NPD focuses primarily on psychotherapy, though medications may be used to alleviate symptoms associated with other disorders.

Medication

There are no medications used specifically for the treatment of NPD. Patients with NPD who are also depressed or anxious may be given drugs for relief of those symptoms. There are anecdotal reports in the medical literature that the **selective serotonin reuptake inhibitors**, or **SSRIs**, which are frequently prescribed for **depression**, may reinforce narcissistic grandiosity and lack of empathy with others.

Psychotherapy

Several different approaches to individual therapy have been tried with NPD patients, ranging from classical **psychoanalysis** and Adlerian therapy to rational-emotive approaches and **Gestalt therapy**. The consensus that has emerged is that therapists should set modest goals for treatment with NPD patients. Most of them cannot form a sufficiently deep bond with a therapist to allow healing of early-childhood injuries. In addition, the tendency of these patients to criticize and devalue their therapists (as well as other authority figures) makes it difficult for therapists to work with them.

An additional factor that complicates psychotherapy with NPD patients is the lack of agreement among psychiatrists about the causes and course of the disorder. Other types of therapy that may be tried include **cognitive-behavioral therapy**, **family therapy**, and **group therapy**.

KEY TERMS

Grandiosity—Exaggerated and unrealistic self-importance; inflated self-assessment. Grandiosity is considered one of the core characteristics of persons diagnosed with NPD.

Macrosocial—Pertaining to the wider society, as distinct from such smaller social groupings as families, neighborhoods, etc.

Narcissistic Personality Inventory (NPI)—The most widely used English-language diagnostic instrument for narcissistic personality disorder. Based on the *DSM-III* criteria for NPD, the NPI is frequently used in research studies as well as patient assessment.

Primary narcissism—Sigmund Freud's term for a normal phase in early childhood development in which the infant has not yet learned to distinguish between itself and its world, and sees other people and things in its environment as extensions of itself.

Projection—A psychological process in which a person unconsciously attributes unacceptable feelings to someone else. Narcissists often project their envy onto other people, claiming that the person in question is envious of them.

Splitting—A psychological process that occurs during the childhood of a person with NPD, in which the child separates aspects of him- or herself that the parents value from those that they disregard.

Superego—According to Freud, the part of the mind that represents traditional parental and societal values. The superego is the source of guilt feelings.

Hospitalization

Low-functioning patients with NPD may require inpatient treatment, particularly those with severe self-harming behaviors or lack of impulse control. Hospital treatment, however, appears to be most helpful when it is focused on the immediate crisis and its symptoms rather than the patient's underlying long-term difficulties.

Prognosis

The prognosis for younger persons with narcissistic disorders is hopeful to the extent that the disturbances reflect a simple lack of life experience. The outlook for long-standing NPD, however, is largely negative. Some narcissists are able, particularly as they approach their midlife years, to accept their own limitations and those of others, to resolve their problems with envy, and to accept their own mortality. Most patients with NPD, on the other hand, become increasingly depressed as they grow older within a youth-oriented culture and lose their looks and overall vitality. The retirement years are especially painful for patients with NPD because they must yield their positions in the working world to the next generation. In addition, they do not have the network of intimate family ties and friendships that sustain most older people.

Prevention

The best hope for prevention of NPD lies with parents and other caregivers who are close to children during the early preschool years. Parents must be able to demonstrate empathy in their interactions with the child and with each other. They must also be able to show that they love their children for who they are, not for their appearance or their achievements. And they must focus their parenting efforts on meeting the child's changing needs as he or she matures, rather than demanding that the child meet their needs for status, comfort, or convenience.

Resources

BOOKS

American Psychiatric Association. *Diagnostic and Statistical Manual of Mental Disorders*. 4th ed., text rev. Washington, DC: American Psychiatric Publishing, 2000.

Capps, Donald. *The Depleted Self: Sin in a Narcissistic Age*. Minneapolis: Augsberg Fortress Press, 1993.

Goodman, Cynthia Lechan, and Barbara Leff. *The Everything Guide to Narcissistic Personality Disorder*. Avon, MA: Adams Media, 2012.

Lowen, Alexander. *Narcissism: Denial of the True Self*. New York: Touchstone, 1985.

World Health Organization (WHO). *The ICD-10 Classification of Mental and Behavioural Disorders*. Geneva: WHO, 1993.

PERIODICALS

Billingham, Robert E., et al. "Narcissistic Injury and Sexual Victimization Among Women College Students." *College Student Journal* 33 (September 1999): 62–70.

Coid, J.W. "Aetiological Risk Factors for Personality Disorders." *British Journal of Psychiatry* 174 (June 1999): 530–538.

Karterud, S., et al. "Validity Aspects of the Diagnostic and Statistical Manual of Mental Disorders, Fourth Edition, Narcissistic Personality Disorder Construct." *Comprehensive Psychiatry* 52, no. 5 (2011): 517–26.

Raskin, R.N., and C.S. Hall. "A Narcissistic Personality Inventory." *Psychological Reports* 45, no. 2 (October 1979): 590.

Ritter, K., et al. "Lack of Empathy in Patients with Narcissistic Personality Disorder." *Psychiatry Research* 187, nos. 1–2 (2011): 241–47.

Ronningstam, E. "Narcissistic Personality Disorder in DSM-V—In Support of Retaining a Significant Diagnosis." *Journal of Personality Disorders* 25, no. 2 (2011): 248–59.

Tschanz, Brian T. "Gender Differences in the Study of Narcissism: A Multi-Sample Analysis of the Narcissistic Personality Inventory." *Sex Roles: A Journal of Research* 38 (May 1998): 209 216.

ORGANIZATIONS

American Psychiatric Association, 1000 Wilson Blvd., Ste. 1825, Arlington, VA, 22209-3901, (703) 907-7300, apa@psych.org, http://www.psych.org.

National Institute of Mental Health, 6001 Executive Blvd., Room 8184, MSC 9663, Bethesda, MD, 20892-9663, (301) 433-4513; TTY: (301) 443-8431, Fax: (301) 443-4279, (866) 615-6464; TTY: (866) 415-8051, nimhinfo@nih.gov, http://www.nimh.nih.gov.

Rebecca J. Frey, Ph.D.

Narcolepsy

Definition

Narcolepsy is a neurological disorder caused by the brain's inability to regulate normal sleep/wake cycles. It is marked by excessive daytime sleepiness, uncontrollable sleep attacks, and cataplexy (a sudden loss of muscle tone, usually lasting up to half an hour). It was first described and named in 1880 by a French physician, Jean-Baptiste-Édouard Gélineau (1828–1906). Gélineau derived the name for the disease from two Greek words that mean "numbness" and "seizure."

Demographics

As of 2011, narcolepsy was the second leading cause of excessive daytime sleepiness diagnosed by sleep centers in North America after obstructive sleep apnea. The rate of narcolepsy in the general population varies widely around the world: in Israel, for example, only about one person per 500,000 is diagnosed with narcolepsy, whereas the rate in Japan is one person in every 600. In the United States, narcolepsy affects about one person in every 2,000–3,000; it is slightly more common among African Americans than among members of other races. According to the National Institute of Neurological Disorders and Stroke (NINDS), there may be cases of the disease that are undiagnosed because they lack the symptom of cataplexy.

Narcolepsy is slightly more common in men than in women; the male/female ratio is 1.64:1. It is not thought to be inherited; however, about 10% of Americans with narcolepsy have a relative with the condition, but this percentage is low compared to other disorders that are known to be purely genetic in origin. Most cases of narcolepsy are sporadic, which means that they occur at random as isolated instances without evidence of contagious transmission or genetic inheritance.

Description

Narcolepsy can affect people in any age group but may not be diagnosed for as long as 10 to 15 years after onset. It can be a disabling condition. Because people with narcolepsy can fall asleep in the daytime in the middle of other activities, including eating, driving, or operating heavy equipment, they can be involved in serious accidents. People with untreated narcolepsy are involved in automobile accidents roughly 10 times more often than the general population. Children or adolescents with narcolepsy can fall behind in school or be judged as lazy even though they are of normal or even superior intelligence.

Having narcolepsy does not mean that people with the disorder sleep more than other people. The disorder is better understood as a disturbance of the normal boundaries between sleeping and waking rather than simply sleeping too much. A normal adult who sleeps for about 8 hours has 4–6 sleep cycles during that time. A sleep cycle is a period of a type of sleep called non-rapid eye movement (NREM) sleep followed by a period of rapid eye movement (REM) sleep. REM sleep is characterized by increased **brain** activity, rapid movement of the eyes below the lids, and sleep paralysis. Individuals who say that they were having a dream when they woke up have been awakened from REM sleep. In normal adults, a sleep cycle is about 100–110 minutes long, 80–100 minutes of NREM sleep followed by 10–20 minutes of REM sleep.

In narcolepsy, however, individuals' sleep cycles do not follow this normal pattern. Instead, individuals falls into REM sleep very shortly after falling asleep. In addition, the short periods of sleep that they have during the daytime are REM sleep. This abnormal entry into REM sleep helps to explain such symptoms of narcolepsy as sleep paralysis and cataplexy.

Risk factors

While there are clusters of cases of narcolepsy in some families, genetics is not a major risk factor. Some researchers believe that **trauma**, immune system dysfunction, hormonal imbalances, and emotional **stress** are possible triggers for the appearance of the disorder, although the associations were not clear enough as of 2011 to identify these conditions as definite risk factors.

Narcolepsy

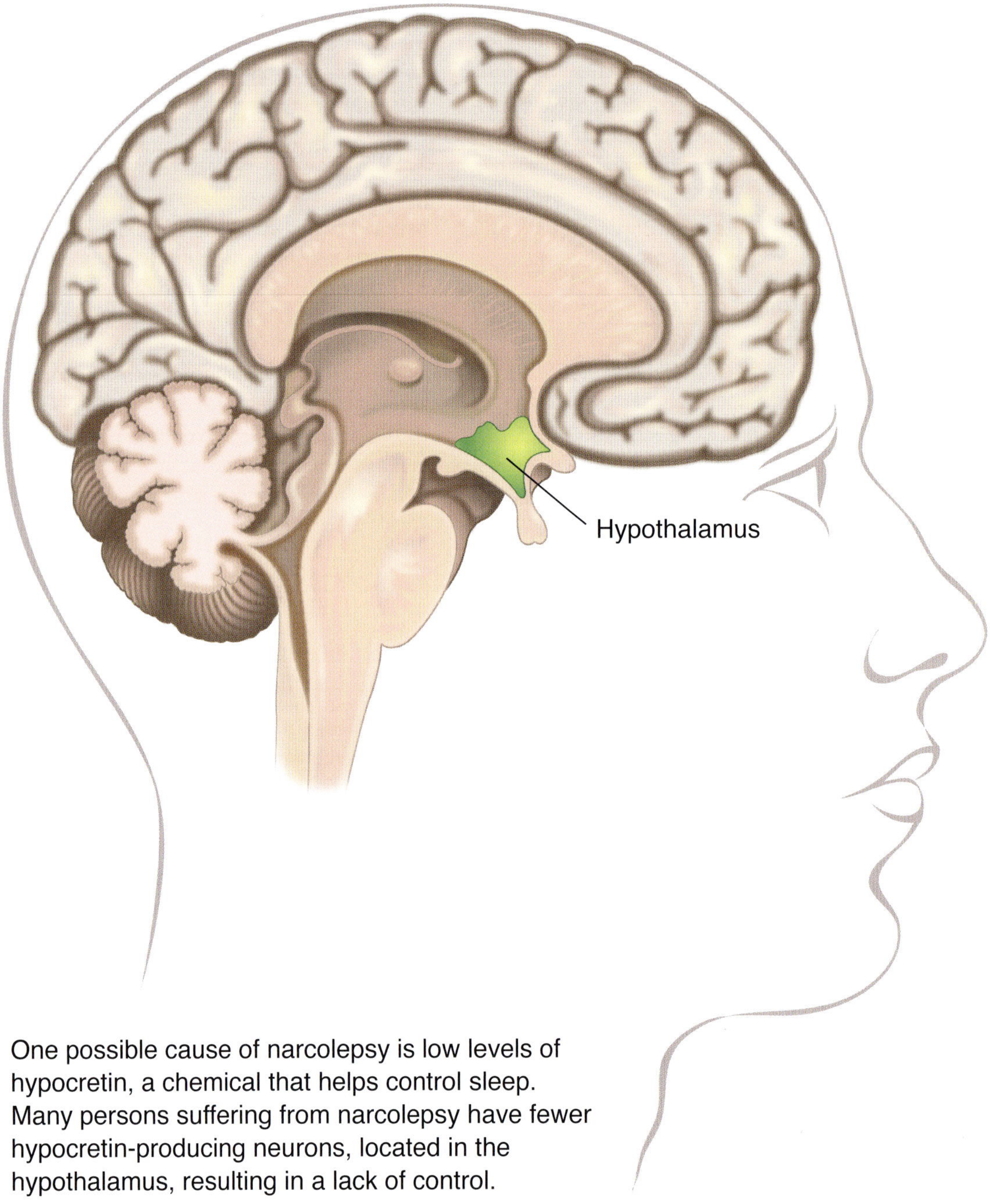

One possible cause of narcolepsy is low levels of hypocretin, a chemical that helps control sleep. Many persons suffering from narcolepsy have fewer hypocretin-producing neurons, located in the hypothalamus, resulting in a lack of control.

(Illustration by Electronic Illustrators Group. Reproduced by permission of Gale, a part of Cengage Learning.)

Causes and symptoms

Causes

The cause of narcolepsy was unclear as of 2011, but it is thought to be a combination of genetic, neurotransmitter, and hormonal factors. Some progress has been made since the late 1990s in identifying two pieces of the puzzle. The first is a connection between narcolepsy and changes in a set of genes on chromosome 6 called the HLA complex. The HLA gene family provides instructions for making a group of related proteins known as the human leukocyte antigen (HLA) complex. The HLA complex helps the immune system distinguish the body's own proteins from proteins made by foreign invaders such as viruses and bacteria. From 88% to 98% of patients affected by narcolepsy have been shown to be

HLA DQB1*0602 positive. This allele (form of gene) strongly increases the susceptibility for cataplexy although 41% of patients without cataplexy are carriers. DRB1 and DQB1 genes have been sequenced in narcolepsy patients, but no mutation has been identified. This suggests that these genes strongly confer susceptibility to narcolepsy without their function being defective. Researchers accordingly think that non-HLA genes may also be involved in susceptibility to narcolepsy.

It is thought that changes in the HLA genes may be linked to the loss of cells in the brain that secrete the hypocretins (also called orexins), two closely related hormones secreted by a small group of cells in the hypothalamus that regulate the sleep/wake cycle. In fact, one of the proposed changes in the fifth edition of the ***Diagnostic and Statistical Manual of Mental Disorders*** (*DSM-5*) is to list the disorder as Narcolepsy/Hypocretin Deficiency. Researchers do not yet know exactly what causes the loss of the brain cells that make the hypocretins. Because the HLA complex has been linked to other autoimmune disorders, however, some doctors think that narcolepsy may be an autoimmune disease. Experiments conducted at Stanford University School of Medicine in 2009 offer some support for this hypothesis. Other researchers think that the hypocretin-producing cells may be damaged by some type of infection, but this theory had not been proven as of 2011.

The third piece of the puzzle is abnormal neurotransmitter function. Some studies of narcolepsy in dogs indicate that abnormally low levels of the neurotransmitter acetylcholine are associated with cataplexy.

Symptoms

Narcolepsy in adults has four primary symptoms known as the narcoleptic tetrad (children, however, rarely have all four):

- Excessive daytime sleepiness (EDS). This symptom may take the form of microsleeps of a few seconds, a long-lasting feeling of drowsiness, or daytime episodes of sleep lasting half an hour or longer.
- Cataplexy. Cataplexy refers to a sudden loss of muscle tone that may result in slurred speech, sagging of the facial muscles, general muscle weakness, inability to hold up the head, buckling of the knees, or loss of strength in the arms. Cataplexy is often triggered by strong emotions, whether positive feelings such as laughter or pleasant surprise or negative emotions such as fear, shock, or anger. Cataplexy can last from a few seconds to as long as 30 minutes. Individuals are awake and alert during an episode of cataplexy even though they may appear unconscious to others.
- Hypnagogic hallucinations. "Hypnagogic" refers to the period of partial alertness that people have when they are waking up or falling asleep. People with narcolepsy experience vivid and sometimes frightening dreams when they are half awake, and they may mistake these dreams for reality.
- Sleep paralysis. Sleep paralysis refers to a temporary inability to move or speak while falling asleep or waking up. These episodes last only one or two minutes and do not affect everyone with narcolepsy, but they can be frightening to patients who do have them.

Other symptoms experienced by some people with narcolepsy are automatic behavior, in which individuals talk to others or perform a routine task such as sorting laundry or making a cup of coffee without conscious awareness or later memory of their action or conversation. People with narcolepsy may also suffer from episodes of **insomnia** or have sleep disturbances in which they thrash about in bed at night or act out their dreams by screaming or waving their arms. Sudden weight gain leading to obesity also occurs in many patients after the symptoms of narcolepsy appear.

Diagnosis

The **diagnosis** of narcolepsy is often delayed because its symptoms resemble those of other disorders such as **depression**, seizure disorders, simple lack of sleep, or even illegal drug use. About 50% of American adults diagnosed with the disorder report that they first noticed its symptoms when they were teenagers. Most cases of narcolepsy first appear in people between the ages of 10 and 25 years, but the disorder has been diagnosed in children as young as three and in adults over 50.

Examination

A routine office physical examination is usually unrevealing, although the patient may be referred to a neurologist to rule out a brain tumor or some other structural abnormality of the brain. The diagnosis of narcolepsy is based on a combination of the patient's history, the results of a screening questionnaire, and overnight testing in a sleep laboratory. The screening questionnaire that is used most commonly is the Epworth Sleepiness Scale, or ESS, which was developed in Australia in the early 1990s. The patient may also be asked to keep a sleep diary for one or two weeks and wear a device called an actigraph, which resembles a wrist watch and measures the person's sleep.

Tests

Imaging tests are not useful in diagnosing narcolepsy. The tests most commonly used to evaluate a

KEY TERMS

Automatic behavior—Activity that a person with narcolepsy can carry out while partially awake but is not conscious of at the time and cannot recall afterward.

Cataplexy—A sudden episode of muscle weakness triggered by emotions. The muscle weakness may cause the person's knees to buckle or the head to drop. In severe cases, the patient may become paralyzed for a few seconds to minutes.

Eugeroic—A type of medication that promotes wakefulness.

Excessive daytime sleepiness (EDS)—A persistent sense of mental cloudiness, a lack of energy, a depressed mood, or extreme state of exhaustion.

Hypnagogic hallucinations—Auditory or visual hallucinations that occur while falling asleep.

Hypocretins—A pair of closely related neuropeptide hormones that promote wakefulness, secreted by a small group of cells in the hypothalamus. The hypocretins are also called orexins and are identified as hypocretin-1 (orexin-A) and hypocretin-2 (orexin-B).

Hypothalamus—A part of the forebrain that controls heartbeat, body temperature, thirst, hunger, body temperature and pressure, blood sugar levels, and other functions.

Microsleep—A brief episode of sleep lasting from a fraction of a second to 30 seconds. It may result from sleep deprivation, sleep apnea, or oxygen deprivation as well as from narcolepsy.

Non-rapid eye movement (NREM) sleep—The first phase of a sleep cycle, in which there is little or no eye movement.

Off-label—Referring to the use of a prescription medication for an unapproved reason to use it, an unapproved age group, or an unapproved dosage level.

Orexins—Another name for the hypocretins.

Rapid eye movement (REM) sleep—The phase of a sleep cycle in which dreaming occurs; characterized by rapid eye movements.

Sleep cycle—A period of NREM sleep followed by a shorter phase of REM sleep. Most adults have 4–6 sleep cycles per night.

Sleep paralysis—An abnormal episode of sleep in which the patient cannot move for a few minutes, usually occurring on falling asleep or waking up. It is often found in patients with narcolepsy.

person for narcolepsy are sleep tests performed in a specially designed laboratory. The patient will usually be tested overnight in a medical center equipped with a polysomnograph. The polysomnograph is a machine that measures the electrical activity of the heart and brain, breathing, and eye movement while the patient is sleeping. Another sleep test is the multiple sleep latency test or MSLT. The patient is given a chance to sleep every two hours during normal waking time. Observations are made of the time taken to reach various stages of sleep. The MSLT measures the degree of the patient's daytime sleepiness and also detects how soon REM sleep begins.

Another test that may be done in the hospital is a lumbar puncture (spinal tap), which is performed to obtain a sample of the patient's cerebrospinal fluid (CSF). The sample can be tested for its hypocretin level, to determine whether the patient's hypocretin level is abnormally low. DSM-5 specifies a hypocretin level lower than one-third of the normal reference value as one of the diagnostic criteria of narcolepsy. If the diagnosis is uncertain, a genetic blood test can reveal the existence of certain substances in people who have a tendency to develop narcolepsy. Positive test results suggest but do not prove the existence of narcolepsy.

Treatment

There is no cure for narcolepsy. Treatment is multimodal, involving a combination of medications, lifestyle changes, and **psychotherapy**. There were no surgical treatments for narcolepsy as of 2011.

Drugs

Medications given to treat narcolepsy must be tailored to the individual patient because most have side effects, and patients may tolerate some drugs in a given class better than others. Amphetamine-like stimulant drugs are often prescribed to control drowsiness and EDS attacks. Patients who do not like taking high doses of stimulants may choose to take smaller doses and manage their lifestyles, such as by napping every couple of hours, to relieve daytime sleepiness. **Antidepressants**, including **venlafaxine**, **imipramine**, **duloxetine**, and **fluoxetine**, are often effective in treating symptoms of abnormal REM sleep. In 2002, the FDA approved Xyrem (sodium oxybate or gamma hydroxybutyrate, also known as GHB) for treating people with narcolepsy who experience episodes of cataplexy.

Modafinil (brand name Provigil) belongs to a class of stimulants known as eugeroics, which have been used to treat narcolepsy in the United States since the late 1990s. Eugeroic stimulants enhance alertness without many of the physical side effects or potential for dependence or abuse commonly associated with **amphetamines**. Another eugeroic approved by the FDA to treat narcolepsy is armodafinil (Nuvigil), which has fewer side effects than modafinil. It is important, however, for persons taking stimulant medications to notify their employer, because the drugs may show up during pre-employment urine tests. With the discovery of the gene associated with narcolepsy, researchers are hopeful that other treatments can be designed to relieve the symptoms of the disorder.

There were no drugs approved by the FDA as of 2011 to treat narcolepsy in children. In most cases children are treated with lower dosages of drugs approved to treat adults. This type of drug usage (in this case, using a medication for an unapproved age group) is known as off-label prescribing.

Newer drug treatments for narcolepsy include thyrotropin-releasing hormone (TRH), histamine agonists, immunotherapy and hypocretin replacement therapies.

Lifestyle adjustments

Lifestyle changes recommended for patients with narcolepsy include:

- Getting enough sleep at night. Patients are advised to go to bed and get up at the same time every day rather than changing their sleeping schedule frequently.
- Taking scheduled short naps at intervals during waking hours. This practice helps to reduce daytime sleepiness.
- Avoiding the use of alcohol and tobacco. These substances can make it harder to sleep at night.
- Getting regular exercise. Physical exercise 4–5 hours before bedtime helps many people with narcolepsy sleep better. Children in particular benefit from regular sports activities or other forms of exercise.
- Being careful to avoid driving when tired or sleepy.
- Joining a narcolepsy support group. Finding understanding and support from others with the same disorder is particularly helpful to patients who may have waited years to be diagnosed and suffered the loss of jobs, relationships, or educational opportunities in the meantime.

QUESTIONS TO ASK YOUR DOCTOR

- What can be done to control excessive sleepiness during the day?
- What medications can help control symptoms?
- How efficient is sodium oxybate for treatment of cataplexy?
- What are the side effects of the medications you have prescribed for me?
- What lifestyle adjustments can help me cope with the disorder?
- What are some of the newer treatments for narcolepsy?
- Have you ever treated a patient with narcolepsy?

Prognosis

Narcolepsy is not a degenerative disease, and patients do not develop other neurologic symptoms. People with narcolepsy can expect to live normal life spans (barring accidents). Narcolepsy can, however, interfere with a person's ability to work, play, drive, and perform other daily activities. Early diagnosis is important because the impact of the disorder on a person's education, employment, relationships, and self-esteem can be severe. According to one study, 24% of adults with narcolepsy had to quit working and 18% had been fired from their jobs because of their disease. In severe cases, the disorder prevents people from living a normal life, leading to depression and a loss of independence.

Prevention

There is no known way to prevent narcolepsy, because its causes are not yet understood.

Resources

BOOKS

Baumann, Christian R., ed. *Narcolepsy*. New York: Springer, 2011.

Benca, Ruth M. *Sleep Disorders: The Clinician's Guide to Diagnosis and Management*. Oxford: Oxford University Press, 2011.

Santos, Guillermo, and Lautar Villalba, eds. *Narcolepsy: Symptoms, Causes, and Diagnosis*. New York: Nova Science, 2010.

PERIODICALS

Bogan, R.K. "Armodafinil in the Treatment of Excessive Sleepiness." *Expert Opinion on Pharmacotherapy* 11 (2010): 993–1002.

Cao, M. "Advances in Narcolepsy." *Medical Clinics of North America* 94 (2010): 541–55.

Cao, M., and C. Guilleminault. "Hypocretin and Its Emerging Role as a Target for Treatment of Sleep Disorders." *Current Neurology and Neuroscience Reports* 11 (2011): 227–34.

Golicki, D., et al. "Modafinil for Narcolepsy: Systematic Review and Meta-analysis." *Medical Science Monitor* 16 (2010): RA177–RA186.

Hauw, J.J., et al. "Neuropathology of Sleep Disorders: A Review." *Journal of Neuropathology and Experimental Neurology* 70 (2011): 243–52.

Pack, A.I., and G.W. Pien. "Update on Sleep and Its Disorders." *Annual Review of Medicine* 62 (2011): 447–60.

Raizen, D.M., and M.N. Wu. "Genome-wide Association Studies of Sleep Disorders." *Chest* 139 (2011): 446–52.

Siegel, J.M. "REM Sleep: A Biological and Psychological Paradox." *Sleep Medicine Reviews* 15 (2011): 139–42.

Smolensky, M.H., et al. "Sleep Disorders, Medical Conditions, and Road Accident Risk." *Accident Analysis and Prevention* 43 (2011): 533–48.

Sullivan, S.S. "Narcolepsy in Adolescents." *Adolescent Medicine: State of the Art Reviews* 21 (2010): 542–55.

Zaharna, M., et al. "Expert Opinion on Pharmacotherapy of Narcolepsy." *Expert Opinion on Pharmacotherapy* 11 (J2010): 1633–45.

WEBSITES

American Psychiatric Association. DSM-5 Development. "M 03 Narcolepsy/Hypocretin Deficiency." http://www.dsm5.org/ProposedRevision/Pages/proposedrevision.aspx?rid=196# (accessed October 27, 2011).

Mayo Clinic. " Narcolepsy." http://www.mayoclinic.com/health/narcolepsy/DS00345 (accessed October 27, 2011).

Medscape. "Narcolepsy." http://emedicine.medscape.com/article/1188433-overview (accessed October 27, 2011).

Narcolepsy Network. " About Narcolepsy." http://www.narcolepsynetwork.org/about-narcolepsy (accessed October 27, 2011).

National Institute of Neurological Disorders and Stroke (NINDS). " Narcolepsy Fact Sheet." http://www.ninds.nih.gov/disorders/narcolepsy/detail_narcolepsy.htm (accessed October 27, 2011).

National Sleep Foundation. "Narcolepsy and Sleep." http://www.sleepfoundation.org/article/sleep-related-problems/narcolepsy-and-sleep (accessed October 27, 2011).

Stanford University School of Medicine Center for Narcolepsy. "About Narcolepsy." http://med.stanford.edu/school/Psychiatry/narcolepsy/symptoms.html (accessed October 27, 2011).

Stanford University School of Medicine Center for Narcolepsy. "Movies of Narcolepsy/Cataplexy." This is a page with links to seven film clips of narcolepsy or cataplexy in dogs, fish, and mice as well as humans. http://med.stanford.edu/school/Psychiatry/narcolepsy/moviedog.html (accessed October 27, 2011).

ORGANIZATIONS

American Academy of Neurology, 1080 Montreal Ave., St. Paul, MN, 55116, (651) 695-2717, Fax: (651) 695-2791, (800) 879-1960, http://www.aan.com.

American Academy of Sleep Medicine, 2510 North Frontage Rd., Darien, IL, 60561, (630) 737-9700, Fax: (630) 737-9790, inquiries@aasmnet.org, http://www.aasmnet.org.

Narcolepsy Network, 110 Ripple Lane, North Kingstown, RI, 02852, (401) 667-2523, Fax: (401) 633-6567, (888) 292-6522, narnet@narcolepsynetwork.org, http://www.narcolepsynetwork.org.

National Institute of Mental Health, 6001 Executive Blvd., Rm. 8184, MSC 9663, Bethesda, MD, 20892-9663, (301) 443-4513, Fax: (301) 443-4279, (866) 615-6464, nimhinfo@nih.gov, http://www.nimh.nih.gov/index.shtml.

National Institute of Neurological Disorders and Stroke, PO Box 5801, Bethesda, MD, 20824, (301) 496-5751, (800) 352-9424, http://www.ninds.nih.gov.

National Sleep Foundation, 1010 N. Glebe Rd., Ste. 310, Arlington, VA, 22201, (703) 243-1697, nsf@sleepfoun dation.org, http://www.sleepfoundation.org.

Stanford University School of Medicine Center for Narcolepsy, 450 Broadway St., Pavilion B, 2nd Fl., Redwood City, CA, 94063, (650) 725-6517 Fax: (650) 725-4913, http://med.stanford.edu/school/Psychiatry/narcolepsy.

Michelle Lee Brandt
Rebecca J. Frey, PhD
Monique Laberge, PhD

Nardil *see* **Phenelzine**

National Institute of Mental Health

Definition

The National Institute of Mental Health (NIMH) is the U.S. government agency that conducts and supports research on mental illness and mental health. The NIMH is a component of the National Institutes of Health (NIH) and was one of the first four institutes created. Proposed by the National Mental Health Act in 1946, the institute was formally established in 1949. Specific areas of research include the **brain**, behavior, and mental health services.

Purpose

The NIMH is dedicated to improving the mental health of the American people, fostering better understanding, **diagnosis**, treatment, rehabilitation, and prevention of mental and brain disorders. The NIMH's mission is "to transform the understanding and treatment of mental illnesses through basic and clinical research, paving the way for prevention, recovery, and cure."

Description

In order to carry out its mission, the NIMH supports research by awarding more than 2,000 research grants to scientists working in universities or other research facilities. Grants support the study of all aspects of mental illness, from biological to social, and they also help identify specific areas where research is needed. The NIMH also supports a large in-house research program, consisting of more than 500 scientists, that studies the causes of and new treatments for mental illnesses. In addition, the NIMH collects and disseminates statistical information to scientists and researchers, conducts training and career development programs, supports small business research programs, sponsors **clinical trials**, and prepares and distributes a wide variety of educational materials.

Among the key areas of research interest for NIMH are neuroscience and behavioral science, including sciences basic to the understanding of the anatomical and chemical basis of brain disorders, and the most prevalent mental disorders and their causes and prevention, such as **schizophrenia**, mood disorders, **anxiety disorders**, eating disorders, and **Alzheimer's disease**. Specific outside research divisions include the Division of Neuroscience and Basic Behavioral Science (DNBBS), the Division of Adult Translational Research and Treatment Development (DATR), the Division of Developmental Translational Research (DDTR), the Division of AIDS Research (DAR), and the Division of Services and **Intervention** Research (DSIR). Additional research efforts include the NIMH Professional Coalition for Research Progress and the NIMH Alliance for Research Progress.

The NIMH operates under the Office of the NIMH Director. Outside of the five research divisions, additional divisions include the Division of Extramural Activities (DEA) and the Division of Intramural Research Programs (DIRP). Advisory boards and groups include the National Advisory Mental Health Council (NAMHC), peer review committees, a board of scientific counselors (BSC), and the NIMH Outreach Partnership Program, which focuses on improving access to mental health information within communities.

Professional publications

The National Institute of Mental Health communicates current research, diagnosis and treatment information to professionals and the public through conferences, symposia and meetings, and works closely with professional and voluntary organizations and other federal agencies. The institute produces a number of publications, including booklets, brochures, and fact sheets, available in both English and Spanish. The NIMH also produces videos and podcasts on mental health topics, which are available on the NIMH website at: http://www.nimh.nih.gov/news/index.shtml.

ORGANIZATIONS

National Institute of Mental Health, 6001 Executive Blvd., Rm. 8184, MSC 9663, Bethesda, MD, 20892-9663, (301) 433-4513; TTY: (301) 443-8431, (866) 615-6464; TTY: (866) 415-8051, Fax: (301) 443-4279, nimhinfo@nih.gov, http://www.nimh.nih.gov.

Navane *see* **Thiothixene**

Nefazodone

Definition

Nefazodone is a prescription drug commonly used to treat **depression**. Nefazodone was available in the United States under the trade name of Serzone, but its maker is no longer marketing it under that name. It is still available in the United States as generic brands.

Purpose

Nefazodone is considered an antidepressant and is best known for treating depression. It may be used to treat **major depressive disorder**, **dysthymic disorder**, and the depressed phase of **bipolar disorder**. As with all **antidepressants**, it may take several weeks before full beneficial effects are seen.

Description

Nefazodone was approved by the U.S. Food and Drug Administration (FDA) in 1994. It is believed to increase the amounts of some chemicals in the **brain**. By altering the activities of specific brain chemicals, nefazodone may reduce the chemical imbalances responsible for causing depression.

The drug is available as tablets in several different strengths, including 50, 100, 150, 200, and 250 mg tablets.

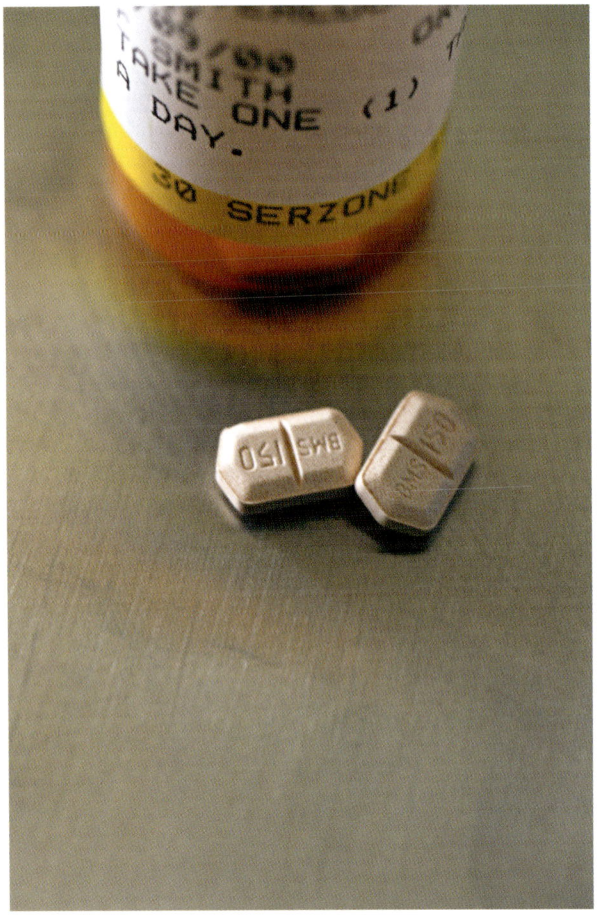

Serzone (nefazodone). *(© Michelle Del Guercio/Photo Researchers, Inc.)*

Nefazodone is broken down by the liver.

Recommended dosage

For most people, the recommended initial dose of nefazodone is 100 mg taken by mouth twice daily. The dose may be increased in 100- or 200 mg increments once a week. Most commonly, final dosages range between 300–600 mg taken by mouth each day.

It is recommended that the initial dose of nefazodone be lowered to 50 mg twice daily for individuals over age 65 or with debilitations, because these individuals may be more sensitive to some of the drug's side effects.

Precautions

Patients should read the medication guide before starting treatment with nefazodone. The drug has been associated with liver failure, which has led the FDA to add a warning to its label, advising of this possibility. People who exhibit symptoms that include yellowing skin or eyes, dark urine, or stomach pain should contact a doctor immediately.

In addition, antidepressants have been associated with an increased risk of patients harming or killing themselves. The FDA has advised that this drug should not be administered to children under the age of 18. If it is prescribed for a child or adolescent, caregivers should watch the patient carefully for signs of intention to commit self-harm or attempt **suicide**. These symptoms can develop suddenly and include new or worsening depression, talk about self-harm or suicide, agitation, panic attacks, aggression, and changes in sleep patterns.

People who have a history of epilepsy or other seizure disorders, heart attack, **stroke**, high blood pressure, or mania may require close physician supervision while taking nefazodone. Nefazodone may increase the tendency to have **seizures**, and it should be used carefully by people with epilepsy or other seizure disorders. Nefazodone may lower blood pressure. This effect may be most noticeable when rising suddenly from a lying or sitting position. People with a history of heart attack or stroke, those taking medications for high blood pressure, or people who are dehydrated may be most sensitive to this effect and may feel dizzy or faint when standing up suddenly. Nefazodone may alter moods or cause mania, so patients with a history of mania should use nefazodone with caution.

In rare situations, men taking nefazodone may experience longlasting, painful erections. If this occurs, a health care provider should be notified immediately.

Because there is an increased likelihood of suicide in individuals with depression, close supervision of those at high risk for suicide attempts is recommended. Nefazodone is not recommended for women who are pregnant or breast-feeding.

Side effects

The most common side effects that cause people to stop taking nefazodone are dizziness, difficulty sleeping, weakness, or agitation. Other common adverse effects include sleepiness, dry mouth, nausea, constipation, blurred vision, and confusion.

Less common adverse effects associated with nefazodone are headache, flu-like symptoms, low blood pressure, itching, rash, upset stomach, fluid retention, muscle aches, thirst, memory impairment, nerve pain, nightmares, difficulty walking, ringing in the ears, urinary difficulties, breast pain, or vaginal irritation.

It has recently been discovered that in rare situations, nefazodone causes liver failure. If nausea, stomach pains, yellowing of the skin or eyes, itching, or darkening of urine occurs while taking nefazodone, a health care professional should be consulted immediately.

Interactions

Use of nefazodone with antidepressants referred to as **monoamine oxidase inhibitors (MAOIs)** is strongly discouraged due to the potential for high fever, muscle stiffness, sudden muscle spasms, rapid changes in heart rate and blood pressure, and the possibility of death. In fact, there should be a lapse of at least 14 days between taking a monoamine oxidase inhibitor and nefazodone, or at least seven days should pass if switching from nefazodone to an MAOI. Some examples of **MAOIs** include **phenelzine** (Nardil) and **tranylcypromine** (Parnate).

Some other drugs such as **trazodone** (Desyrel) and sibutramine may also interact with nefazodone and cause a syndrome characterized by irritability, muscle stiffness, shivering, muscle spasms, and altered consciousness. If nefazodone is used with **buspirone** (BuSpar), the dosage of buspirone should be lowered to prevent adverse effects. Additionally, when nefazodone is used in combination with digoxin (Lanoxin), frequent monitoring of blood levels of digoxin is recommended to prevent toxicity.

Nefazodone should not be used with the drugs **triazolam** (Halcion) and **alprazolam** (Xanax), because the side effects of these drugs are likely to increase. Use of nefazodone should also be avoided with **carbamazepine** (Tegretol), because nefazodone is likely to lose its effectiveness.

It is best to avoid using nefazodone with **pimozide** (Orap) due to an increased tendency for severe and potentially life-threatening irregular heartbeats.

When used with gemfibrozil or other drugs that lower cholesterol levels, the risk of muscle pain and weakness may be increased.

Because nefazodone may cause drowsiness, it should be used carefully with other medications that also make people prone to sleepiness such as antidepressants, antipsychotics, antihistamines, and alcohol.

Resources

BOOKS

Ellsworth, Allan J., et al. *Mosby's Medical Drug Reference*. St. Louis: Mosby, 2007.

Wolters Kluwer Health. *Drug Facts and Comparisons 2012*. 66th ed. St. Louis: Lippincott, Williams & Wilkins, 2011.

PERIODICALS

Ahmad, Syed Rizwanuddin. "Adverse Drug Event Monitoring at the Food and Drug Administration: Your Report Can Make a Difference." *Journal of General Internal Medicine* 18:1 (January 2003): 47–60. http://www.pubmedcentral.nih.gov/articlerender.fcgi?artid=1494803 (accessed October 23, 2011).

WEBSITES

Drugs.com. "Serzone" http://www.drugs.com/pro/serzone.html (accessed October 23, 2011).

MedlinePlus. "Nefazodone." U.S. National Library of Medicine, National Institutes of Health. 2011. http://www.nlm.nih.gov/medlineplus/druginfo/medmaster/a695005.html (accessed October 23, 2011).

U.S. Food and Drug Administration. "Determination That SERZONE (Nefazodone Hydrochloride) Was Not Withdrawn from Sale for Reasons of Safety or Effectiveness." *Federal Register*. October 26, 2004. http://www.federalregister.gov/articles/2004/10/26/04-23857/determination-that-serzone-nefazodone-hydrochloride-was-not-withdrawn-from-sale-for-reasons-of (accessed October 23, 2011).

U.S. Food and Drug Administration. "Nefazodone hydrochloride Information. FDA Alert: Suicidal Thoughts or Actions in Children and Adults." 2011. http://www.fda.gov/Drugs/DrugSafety/PostmarketDrugSafetyInformationforPatientsandProviders/ucm108105.htm (accessed October 23, 2011).

Kelly Karpa, RPh, PhD
Emily Jane Willingham, PhD

Negative symptoms

Definition

Negative symptoms are thoughts, feelings, or behaviors normally present which are absent or diminished in a person with a mental disorder.

Description

Examples of negative symptoms are social withdrawal, **apathy** (decreased motivation), poverty of speech (brief replies), inability to experience pleasure (anhedonia), limited emotional expression, or defects in attention control. The term "negative symptoms" is specifically used for describing **schizophrenia**, but sometimes used more generally in reference to disorders such as **depression** or **dementia**. These symptoms may be associated with altered brainwave activity or **brain** damage. They can be more difficult to diagnose than **positive symptoms** (hallucinations, **delusions**, bizarre behavior, or formal thought disorder) because they represent a lesser degree of normal, desirable activity rather than the presence of undesirable or bizarre behavior. Side effects of certain medications, demoralization (loss of positive emotions like hope or confidence usually as the result of situations where one feels powerless), or a lack of stimulation in one's environment can also cause negative symptoms, so these possibilities must be ruled out before attributing the symptoms to a disorder.

Sandra L. Friedrich, M.A.

Neglect

Definition

Neglect occurs when a parent or other primary caretaker chooses not to fulfill their obligations to care for, provide for, or adequately supervise and monitor the activities of their child. Parental and caregiving obligations include the physical, emotional, and educational well-being of the child. Thus, neglect can also occur when the parent or caretaker does not seek adequate medical or dental care for the child. Another definition of neglect is when the parental figure does not provide sufficient food, clothing, or shelter.

Parents are also expected to provide for the emotional needs of the child. Thus, neglect can occur when parents abandon the child, or simply have no time to spend with the child, in essence leaving the child to raise himself. If the child is actually left without supervision, this certainly constitutes neglect as well.

The final feature of neglect includes educational neglect, which often occurs when one child is responsible for other children in the family. Shifting the responsibility of caring for younger children to another child in the family prevents the caregiving child from participating in age-appropriate activities such as attending school. This is a relatively common situation that makes it difficult for the oldest—and perhaps all of the children—to attend school. Parental responsibility includes providing adequate guidance and supervision for the children to regularly attend school. Truancy is not only a problem for children, but may be part of the picture of neglect as well.

Effects of neglect

Consequences of neglect are generally cumulative, and often negatively affect the child's development. For example, poor **nutrition** has negative consequences on the child's physical and psychological development. If proper nutrients are not available at critical growth periods, the child's development will not follow the normal and usual pattern. Common physical and psychological reactions to neglect include stunted growth, chronic medical problems, inadequate bone and muscle growth, and lack of neurological development that negatively affects normal **brain** functioning and information processing. Processing problems may often make it difficult for children to understand directions, may negatively impact the child's ability to understand social relationships, or may make completion of some academic tasks impossible without assistance or **intervention** from others. Lack of adequate medical care may result in long-term health problems or impairments such as hearing loss from untreated ear infections.

Long-term mental health effects of neglect are inconsistent. Effects of neglect can range from chronic **depression** to difficulty with relationships; however, not all adults neglected as children will suffer from these results. Some individuals are more resilient than others and are able to move beyond the emotional neglect they may have experienced. Characteristics of resilient individuals include an optimistic or hopeful outlook on life, and feeling challenged rather than defeated by problems.

Factors associated with neglect

Although each family's situation is unique with regard to stressors and characteristics that might precipitate neglect, there are some general factors that have been associated with neglect of a child. These factors include characteristics of the parental figure and socioeconomic status.

Parental figures who neglect may have been neglected or abused themselves. There is a tendency for parental figures that neglect their children to have low self-esteem, poor impulse control, and to experience anxiety or depression. Other factors associated with neglect often include inadequate information about child development, including age-appropriate expectations of what children may be able to do. The parents may also feel overwhelmed by parenting responsibilities and feel negatively about the child's demands on them. Such parents may never have fully adopted the role of parent or the caregiving the parental role requires. Internal pressures often push the caregivers to take care of their own needs (perhaps inappropriately), while ignoring the needs of the child. **Substance abuse** is often associated with neglect, particularly for those parents who are more self-absorbed and focused on their needs rather than their child's. This characteristic is also consistent with the findings of other studies indicating that some neglectful parents have an inability to be empathic, or to understand the feelings and needs of others.

Although **abuse** may occur across all levels of income and education, neglect is more often associated with severe levels of poverty and lower educational level. The external stressors may feel more extreme in single parent families as well, leading to neglectful behavior. Even in families where the parent is attempting to provide for the children, absence due to multiple work demands may lead to a neglectful situation. Families that are disorganized and socially isolated are more likely to neglect the children in their care.

Unlike victims of abuse, there are few consistent characteristics associated with victims of neglect. Retrospective studies of adults neglected as children indicate that females are slightly less resilient to neglect than men.

Prevalence

The number of children nationwide who are harmed or endangered by neglect is greater than any type of abuse. Neglect is consistently reported in more than half of the substantiated reports of mistreatment handled by the authorities.

Prevention and treatment

Interventions are usually aimed at two levels: community prevention efforts and individual parenting skills. A community-based program that actually combines the two facets of intervention is the "Parents as Teachers" program, which is available through many local school districts throughout the nation and is free of charge. Benefits of the program include its accessibility—parents simply need to call for the free service—and the in-home interventions provided by the program. Although the program is not part of the social service network of agencies, the fact that workers go into the home replicates that aspect of caseworker interventions. The simple act of having a paraprofessional in one's home can reduce the likelihood of neglect. Specific interventions that further reduce the likelihood of neglect include focusing on the parent-child relationship, reviewing appropriate expectations for the child's behavior (based on child development principles), and teaching basic parenting skills.

Other treatment options are generally more formal, and may be initiated by a call from a mandated reporter with concerns about neglect. Mandated reporters include physicians, teachers, and counselors. Any of these professionals may make the initial call if neglect is suspected. Concerned individuals may also call social services to report suspected neglect. In these cases of forced treatment, parents may be less willing participants in treatment efforts aimed at behavioral change for themselves and their families. In other instances, the parent or child may already be in treatment, and the focus on reducing neglectful behaviors may be incorporated into the existing treatment relationship. Factors to focus on in formal treatment aimed at reducing the likelihood of neglect may include specific parenting skills, home visits to allow monitoring of the relationship, as well as other individual needs such as substance abuse treatment, or empathy skill training.

Treatment efforts for the child should include family counseling aimed at communication skills and appropriate expression of affection and emotion within the family. Assertiveness skills training may be helpful for older adolescents in asking for their perceived needs.

Resources

BOOKS

McKenry, P. C., S. J. Price, and C. A. Price eds. *Families & Change*. 4th ed. Thousand Oaks, CA: Sage Publications, 2009.

PERIODICALS

English, D. J. "The Extent and Consequences of Child Maltreatment." *The Future of Children* 8, no. 1 (Spring 1998): 39–53.

Horwitz, A. V., et al. "The Impact of Childhood Abuse and Neglect on Adult Mental Health: A Prospective Study." *Journal of Health & Social Behavior* 42, no. 2 (June 2001): 184–201.

Deanna Pledge, Ph.D.

Neurocognitive disorders *see* **Alzheimer's disease; Delirium; Dementia; Traumatic brain injury; Vascular dementia**

Neuroleptic malignant syndrome

Definition

Neuroleptic malignant syndrome (NMS) is a rare but potentially fatal condition that can occur in people who take neuroleptic medication to treat **schizophrenia**, mania, **delusional disorder**, and other types of mental illnesses. There is evidence that sympathetic nervous system activation or dysfunction may be significantly associated with the underlying pathogenesis of NMS. NMS, which is characterized by motor dysfunction, extremely high fever, and changes in consciousness, is most commonly associated with older generation typical neuroleptics such as **haloperidol** (Haldol) and **chlorpromazine** (Largactil). However, the newer, atypical antipsychotic agents, such as **clozapine** (Clozaril), risperidone (Risperdal), and **olanzapine** (Zyprexa), also have been associated with NMS symptoms. NMS additionally has been reported in patients with Parkinson's disease who have had their medications (such as levodopa) rapidly withdrawn.

Non-neuroleptic agents associated with NMS block central **dopamine** pathways and include metoclopramide (Reglan), lithium, and **amoxapine** (Asendin). The syndrome also shares features with malignant hyperthermia and the **serotonin syndrome**.

Demographics

Neuroleptic malignant syndrome occurs in between 0.02% and 2.44% of people who are treated with neuroleptic medications, although there is no universal agreement on this statistic. The mortality rate with NMS is between 5% and 11.6%, also with no complete consensus on this figure. Mortality from the condition has declined over the years (down from 20% to 30%) but remains significant. Death generally results after respiratory failure, diffuse intravascular coagulation (DIC), cardiovascular collapse, myoglobinuric renal failure, and arrhythmias. There is a predilection toward males but none associated with age. There is a 2:1 male-to-female ratio, which is thought to occur because men are treated with neuroleptic agents more frequently than women.

Description

NMS is believed to be related to the dopaminergic system. Dopamine is a neurotransmitter that transmits messages between nerve cells in the **brain**. It regulates mood, emotion, motivation, and movement. Neuroleptic antipsychotic drugs act as antagonists at dopamine receptors, meaning that they block the receptors, thereby preventing dopamine from attaching to the receptors and causing its response from the decreased availability of dopamine itself. Sometimes, blocking these receptors can result in **movement disorders** and difficulty regulating body heat, both of which are symptoms associated with NMS. NMS typically begins within the first two to four weeks after a patient starts taking antipsychotic medications or is put on a higher dose of the medication, although symptoms may manifest sooner or much later.

Risk factors

A variety of factors may increase an individual's risk of developing this condition, including:

- High environmental temperatures
- Dehydration
- Agitation or catatonia in a patient
- High initial dose or rapid dose increase of neuroleptic, and use of high-potency or intramuscular, long-acting (depot) preparations
- Simultaneous use of more than one causative agent
- Sudden discontinuation of medications for Parkinson disease
- Past history of organic brain syndromes, depression, or bipolar disorder
- Past episode of neuromuscular malignant syndrome (risk of recurrence may be as high as 30%)

Causes and symptoms

Causes

Although researchers have identified several risk factors for NMS, the precise cause is unknown. **Genetic factors** may play a role, however, and NMS has been reported to run in families. Researchers have identified alterations or deletions to the CYP2D6 genes in people with NMS. Changes to these genes may affect the way neuroleptics are metabolized by the liver, resulting in higher blood concentrations.

Symptoms

The **diagnosis** is confirmed, but not excluded, when the following are observed:

- Recent treatment with neuroleptics within the past one to four weeks
- Hypothermia (above 38°C)
- Muscular rigidity
- Exclusion of other drug-induced, system, or neuropsychiatric illness
- At least five of the following: Change in mental status; Tachycardia (abnormally rapid heartbeat); Hypertension or hypotension; Diaphoresis or sialorrhea; Leukocytosis; Tremor; Incontinence; Increased creatine phosphokinase (CPK) or urinary myoglobin; and Metabolic acidosis

Diagnosis

Early diagnosis of NMS is essential to prevent fatality. Physicians begin by ruling out conditions with similar symptoms. Laboratory studies include a complete blood count; urine myoglobin; CPK; arterial blood gas; liver function tests; blood cultures; serum and urine toxic screening for **cocaine**, **amphetamines**, and other gents; blood urea nitrogen; and calcium and phosphate levels. Blood tests of patients with NMS reveal high levels of creatine kinase, a muscle enzyme, as well as abnormally

KEY TERMS

Atypical antipsychotic—A class of newer generation antipsychotic medications that are used to treat schizophrenia and other psychotic disorders.

Dopamine—A neurotransmitter in the brain that helps regulate emotion and movement.

Dopamine agonist—A drug that binds to dopamine receptors and produces effects that are similar to dopamine.

Dopamine antagonist—A substance that binds to dopamine receptors, preventing dopamine from binding and triggering its response.

Electroencephalogram—A diagnostic technique that measures electrical activity in the brain.

Neuroleptic drugs—The class of drugs used to treat schizophrenia, mania, and other types of mental disorders.

Parkinson's disease—A degenerative condition of the central nervous system that results in reduced dopamine production, leading to symptoms such as tremors, muscle rigidity, and difficulty with balance and coordination.

high levels of leukocytes (white blood cells). An electroencephalogram (EEG), which measures electrical activity in the brain, will show a slowing of brain function. Chest radiography is performed to rule out aspiration pneumonia. A lumbar puncture, sometimes with a preceding CT scan, is performed to diagnose meningitis in patients who have high fever and altered mental status.

Treatment

Because little research has been done on NMS, treatment guidelines are limited. The first line of treatment is to discontinue the medication that is believed to be causing the condition, exclude other medical conditions, begin aggressive supportive care, and administrate pharmacotherapies, such as **benzodiazepines** (**diazepam**), muscle relaxants, and dopamine agonists (bromocriptine), which can be used to control symptoms. After the medication is stopped, most patients will improve within two weeks, although symptoms may persist for as long as several months. Doctors typically recommend waiting for at least two weeks after the patient's symptoms have improved before restarting antipsychotic medications, to prevent a **relapse** of NMS. After that period, atypical antipsychotic medications are preferred over the older generation antipsychotic drugs, because they are associated with a lower risk of NMS.

Patients should be carefully monitored while recovering from NMS. Doctors will check the patient's creatine kinase levels, as well as his or her overall health, and will ensure that the patient receives adequate **nutrition** and hydration and does not progress to kidney failure.

Prognosis

With early diagnosis and treatment, mortality from NMS can be prevented. However, because the condition can recur at any time, patients must be monitored over the long term.

Prevention

The only way to entirely prevent NMS is to avoid the use of neuroleptic drugs. But because NMS is rare, and because many patients rely on these drugs for the treatment of mental disorders, avoiding these drugs is neither practical nor feasible in many cases. However, using the newer atypical antipsychotics and/or lowering the dose may reduce the risk of NMS.

Resources

BOOKS

Brunton, Laurence, Bruce Chabner, and Bjorn Knollman. *Goodman & Gilman's The Pharmacological Basis of Therapeutics* 12th ed. New York: McGraw-Hill, 2010.

Caroff, Stanley N., et al. *Neuroleptic Malignant Syndrome and Related Conditions*. 2d ed. Arlington, VA: American Psychiatric Publishing, 2003.

Kring, Ann M., Gerald C. Davison, John M. Neale, and Sheri L. Johnson. *Abnormal Psychology*. 11th ed. Hoboken, NJ: John Wiley & Sons, 2009.

Meyer, Jerrold S., and Linda F. Quenzer. *Psychopharmacology: Drugs, the Brain and Behavior*. Sunderland, MA: Sinauer Associates, Inc., 2005.

ORGANIZATIONS

Mental Health America, 2000 N Beauregard Street, 6th Floor, Alexandria, VA, 22311, (703) 684-7722, (800) 969-6642, Fax: (703) 684-5968, http://www.nmha.org.

National Institute of Mental Health, 6001 Executive Blvd., Room 8184, MSC 9663, Bethesda, MD, 20892-9663, (301) 433-4513; TTY: (301) 443-8431, Fax: (301) 443-4279, (866) 615-6464; TTY: (866) 415-8051, nimhinfo@nih.gov, http://www.nimh.nih.gov.

National Parkinson Foundation, Inc, 1501 NW 9th Ave./Bob Hope Rd., Miami, FL, 33136-1494, (305) 243-6666, Fax: (305) 243-6073, (800) 327-4545, contact@parkinson.org, http://www.parkinson.org.

Neuroleptic Malignant Syndrome Information Service, Box 1069, Sherburne, NY, 13460-1069, (607) 674-7920, Fax: (607) 674-7910, info@nmsis.org, http://www.nmsis.org.

Stephanie N. Watson

Neurolinguistic programming *see* **Hypnotherapy**

Neurontin *see* **Gabapentin**

Neuropsychiatry

Definition

Neuropsychiatry is an integrative, collaborative discipline that deals with the psychiatric aspects of neurological disease. The terms "neuropsychiatry" and "behavioral neurology" are frequently used interchangeably.

Purpose

Patients who may benefit from the services of a neuropsychiatrist are those who have a known neurological disease accompanied by cognitive, emotional, or behavioral deficits, as well as patients who have comorbid psychiatric and neurologic disorders. A neuropsychiatrist may be called upon to consult when a patient exhibits psychiatric symptoms that are unresponsive to the usual treatment approaches, and the differential **diagnosis** extends to a neurological cause, with secondary psychiatric manifestations. Examples of conditions that may be responsive to a neuropsychiatric approach include epilepsy, head injury, **attention deficit hyperactivity disorder**, **dementia**, **tardive dyskinesia**, atypical spells, and irritability.

Description

Neuropsychiatry lies in the interface between the disciplines of neurology and psychiatry. For many centuries, neurology and psychiatry formed a single unified field. Even in the late nineteenth century, many medical practitioners and researchers, such as Sigmund Freud, Jean-Martin Charcot, and Eugen Bleuler, did not distinguish between the study of the mind and the **brain**. In the twentieth century, however, neurology and psychiatry became separate, distinct disciplines. Neurology focused on disorders, such as **stroke**, multiple sclerosis, and Parkinson's disease, that were clearly characterized by disease of, or damage to, the brain and resulted in behavioral and cognitive problems as well as somatic symptoms related to movement and sensation. Psychiatry, on the other hand, concerned itself with behavioral, cognitive, personality, and emotional disorders, such as **depression**, **schizophrenia**, and **anxiety disorders**. Initially, these conditions were not typically seen as problems related to sensory or motor dysfunction, and consequently revealed few or no pathologic symptoms during standard neurologic examinations.

> **KEY TERMS**
>
> **Differential diagnosis**—Comparing and contrasting the signs, symptoms, and laboratory findings of two or more diseases to determine which is causing the patient's condition.
>
> **Tardive dyskinesia**—Involuntary movements of the face and/or body, a side effect of the long-term use of some older antipsychotic drugs.

The impetus for a change in this divide between neurology and psychiatry has come from the advances made in neuroscience during the second half of the twentieth century. With advances in the understanding of the underlying biology of psychiatric disorders, it has become difficult to draw a clear line between the mind and the brain, or the psychological and physical manifestations of a disease. Because of these advances, scientists and clinicians are now able to assess the structure and functioning of the brain in new ways. Many new techniques developed in the latter half of the twentieth century and the beginning of the twenty-first century have shown that behavioral, emotional, and cognitive disorders are often accompanied by physical changes in the brain. For example, **magnetic resonance imaging** studies have revealed structural abnormalities in the brains of patients who suffer from schizophrenia, and functional magnetic resonance imaging and **positron emission tomography** techniques have demonstrated that brain function is abnormal in such patients. Researchers and clinicians are also now more cognizant of the fact that disorders that were traditionally in the domain of neurology, such as Parkinson's disease, are often accompanied by emotional and cognitive symptoms like depression and even dementia.

In addition, treatments that target the brain, such as pharmacotherapy, **transcranial magnetic stimulation**, **vagus nerve stimulation** and deep brain stimulation are being used or are being investigated for their potential to alleviate disorders that have traditionally been considered psychiatric, such as depression and **obsessive-compulsive disorder**. Disorders that are currently recognized as being within the purview of neuropsychiatry include, but are not limited to, neurocognitive disorders, drug-induced **movement disorders**, Tourette syndrome, stroke and head injury, chronic **fatigue** syndrome, Parkinson's disease, attention deficit hyperactivity disorder, and dementia.

Territorial struggles between psychiatry and neurol ogy continue. Modern neuropsychiatry, which has emerged only in the last two decades, is still a discipline with ill-defined boundaries, frequently competitive with both psychiatry and neurology. Training programs in neuropsychiatry are still being developed, but a number of schools have instituted neuropsychiatry programs, including the University of South Carolina, Dartmouh, and the University of Pennsylvania.

Resources

BOOKS

Goldstein, Gerald, Theresa M. Incagnoli, and Antonio E. Puente, eds. *Contemporary Neurobehavioral Syndromes.* New York: Psychology Press, 2011.

Rhawn, Joseph. *Neuropsychology, Neuropsychiatry, and Behavioral Neurology.* Critical Issues in Neuropsychology. New York: Plenum Press, 2010.

Williamson, Peter, and John Allman. *The Human Illnesses: Neuropsychiatric Disorders and the Nature of the Human Brain.* New York: Oxford University Press, 2011.

Yudofsky, Stuart C., and Robert E. Hales. *Essentials of Neuropsychiatry and Behavioral Neurosciences.* Arlington, VA: American Psychiatric Publishing, 2010.

PERIODICALS

Aybek, Selma, Richard Kanaan, and Anthony S. David. "The Neuropsychiatry of Conversion Disorder." *Current Opinion in Psychiatry* 21, no. 3 (2008): 275–80.

Elvevåg, B., and D.R. Weinberger. " Introduction: Genes, Cognition and Neuropsychiatry." *Cognitive Neuropsychiatry* 14, nos. 4–5 (2009): 261–75.

Vaishnavi, Sandeep, et al. "Behavioral Neurology and Neuropsychiatry Fellowship Training: The Johns Hopkins Model." *Journal of Neuropsychiatry and Clinical Neuroscience* 21 (Summer 2009): 335–41. http://dx.doi.org/10.1176/appi.neuropsych.21.3.335 (accessed September 7, 2011).

Yudofsky, Stuart C., ed. *The Journal of Neuropsychiatry and Clinical Neurosciences.* American Neuropsychiatric Association. http://neuro.psychiatryonline.org/index.dtl (accessed September 7, 2011).

ORGANIZATIONS

American Neuropsychiatric Association, 700 Ackerman Road, Suite 625, Columbus, OH, 43202, (614) 447-2077, anpa@osu.edu, http://www.anpaonline.org/home.php.

International Neuropsychiatric Association, INA Secretariat Office Neuropsychiatric Institute Euroa Centre, The Prince of Wales Hospital, Barker St., Randwick, NSW 2031, Australia, 61293823816, Fax: 61293823774, angie.russell@unsw.edu.au, http://www.inawebsite.org.

Ruvanee Pietersz Vilhauer, PhD
Rosalyn Carson-DeWitt

Neuropsychological testing

Definition

Clinical neuropsychology is a field with historical origins in both psychology and neurology. The primary activity of neuropsychologists is assessment of **brain** functioning through structured and systematic behavioral observation. Neuropsychological tests are designed specifically to examine a variety of cognitive abilities, including speed of information processing, attention, memory, language, and executive functions, which are necessary for goal-directed behavior. Such scientifically validated tests are administered generally to individuals to evaluate brain functions. These tests cover a wide range of mental processes from simple motor performance to complex problem solving and reasoning.

By testing a range of cognitive abilities and examining patterns of performance in different cognitive areas, neuropsychologists can make inferences about underlying brain function, including its structure and pathway. Consequently, neuropsychological testing is a primary way that neuropsychologists and other scientists assess neuropsychological function in humans.

Purpose

Neuropsychological testing is an important component of the assessment and treatment of **traumatic brain injury**, attention deficits, developmental milestone failures (in children), **dementia**, neurological conditions, psychiatric disorders, drug or alcohol abuse, and other such problems. Neuropsychological testing is also an important tool for examining the effects of toxic substances and medical conditions on brain functioning.

Testing helps to assess such functions as working memory and attention, short-term and long-term memory, processing speed, reasoning and problem-solving ability, ability to understand and express language, visual-spatial organization, visual-motor coordination, and planning and organizational abilities.

Description

Neuropsychological testing is based on psychometric theory. A sample from a general population (control group) is used as the foundation for scoring, with individual scores compared to the normalized sample.

Origins

As early as the seventeenth century, scientists theorized about associations between regions of the brain and specific functions. French philosopher René

KEY TERMS

Dementia—The progressive deterioration of intellectual functions, such as memory, within the brain. Alzheimer's disease is a type of dementia.

Psychiatric—Relating to psychiatry.

Psychometric—A branch of psychology that deals with measurement of mental capacities, processes, and traits.

Visual-motor—The ability to coordinate vision and bodily movements.

Visual-spatial—The ability to manipulate multidimensional figures mentally.

Descartes (1596–1650) believed the human soul could be localized to a specific brain structure, the pineal gland. In the eighteenth century, Austrian physiologist Franz Joseph Gall (1758–1828) advocated the theory that specific mental qualities such as spirituality or aggression were governed by discrete parts of the brain. In contrast, French physiologist Marie Jean Pierre Flourens (1794–1867) contended that the brain was an integrated system that governed cognitive functioning in a holistic manner.

Later discoveries indicated that brain function is both localized and integrated. French physician Pierre Paul Broca (1824–1880) and German physician Karl Wernicke (1848–1905) furthered understanding of localization and integration of function when they reported the loss of language abilities in patients with lesions to two regions in the left hemisphere of the brain.

The modern field of neuropsychology emerged in the twentieth century, combining theories based on anatomical observations of neurology with the techniques of psychology, including objective observation of behavior and the use of statistical analysis to differentiate functional abilities and define impairment. Soviet neuropsychologist Alexander Romanovich Luria (1902–1977) played a major role in defining neuropsychology as it is practiced today. Luria formulated two principal goals of neuropsychology: to localize brain lesions and analyze psychological activities arising from brain function through behavioral observation.

American neuropsychologist Ralph M. Reitan later emphasized the importance of using standardized psychometric tests to guide systematic observations of brain-behavior relationships. Specifically, Dr. Reitan and Dr. Ward Halstead co-developed the Halstead-Reitan Battery—one of many neuropsychological tests used commonly in the twenty-first century—which is used to evaluate brain and nervous system function in individuals 15 years of age and older.

Applications

Before the introduction of neuroimaging techniques such as **computed tomography** (CT), **magnetic resonance imaging** (MRI), **electroencephalography** (EEG), and **positron emission tomography (PET)**, neuropsychological testing was the only way for clinicians to evaluate the condition of the living brain. These neuroimaging techniques allow for the observation of brain lesions or structural abnormalities in living patients. Today, neuropsychological testing and neuroimaging techniques are used together to determine which part of the brain is affected in a given patient.

Neuropsychological tests can identify syndromes associated with problems in a particular area of the brain. For instance, a patient who performs well on tests of attention, memory, and language, but poorly on tests that require visual spatial skills, such as copying a complex geometric figure or making designs with colored blocks, may have dysfunction in the right parietal lobe, the region of the brain involved in complex processing of visual information. When a patient complains of problems with verbal communication after a **stroke**, separate tests that examine production and comprehension of language help neuropsychologists identify the location of the stroke in the left hemisphere. Neuropsychological tests can also be used as screening tests to see whether more extensive diagnostic evaluation is appropriate. Neuropsychological screening of elderly people complaining of memory problems can help identify those at risk for dementia versus those experiencing normal age-related memory loss.

As neuropsychological testing came to play a less vital role in localization of brain dysfunction, clinical neuropsychologists found new uses for their skills and knowledge. By clarifying which cognitive abilities are impaired or preserved in patients with brain injury or illness, neuropsychologists can predict how well individuals will respond to different forms of treatment or rehabilitation. Although patterns of test scores illustrate profiles of cognitive strength and weakness, neuropsychologists can also learn a great deal about patients by observing how they approach a particular test. For example, two patients can complete a test in very different ways yet obtain similar scores. One patient may work slowly and methodically, without making errors, while another rushes through the test, making several errors, but quickly correcting them. Some individuals persevere despite repeated failure on a series of test items, while others refuse to continue after a few failures. These differences might not be apparent in test scores but can help clinicians choose among rehabilitation and treatment approaches.

Performance on neuropsychological tests is usually evaluated through comparison to the average performance of large samples of normal individuals. Most tests include tables of these normal scores, often divided into groups based on demographic variables, like age and education, that appear to affect cognitive functioning. This allows individuals to be compared to appropriate peers.

Evaluation

The typical neuropsychological examination evaluates sensation and perception, gross and fine motor skills, basic and complex attention, visual spatial skills, receptive and productive language abilities, recall and recognition memory, and executive functions such as cognitive flexibility and abstraction. Motivation and personality are often assessed as well, particularly when clients are seeking financial compensation for injuries, or cognitive complaints are not typical of the associated injury or illness.

Test methods

Some neuropsychologists prefer to use fixed test batteries, like the **Halstead-Reitan Battery** or the Luria-Nebraska Battery, for all patients. These batteries include tests of a wide range of cognitive functions, and those who advocate their use believe that all functions must be assessed in each patient in order to avoid diagnostic bias or failure to detect subtle problems. The more common approach today, however, is to use a flexible battery based on hypotheses generated through a clinical interview, observation of the patient, and review of medical records.

While the flexible approach to neuropsychological testing is more prone to bias, it has the advantage of preventing unnecessary testing. Since patients often find neuropsychological testing stressful and fatiguing, and these factors can negatively influence performance, advocates of the flexible battery approach argue that tailoring test batteries to particular patients can provide more accurate information. Moreover, because insurance companies generally have a fixed amount for reimbursement of psychological testing, a more focused approach may assist in payment for testing services.

Numerous neuropsychological tests are available. Some of the more popular ones include (in alphabetical order):

- Ammons Quick Test
- Beck Depression Inventory and Beck Anxiety Inventory
- Clinical Dementia Rating
- Cognitive Assessment Screening Instrument
- Continuous Performance Task
- Finger Tapping Test
- Halstead-Reitan Battery
- Kaufman Assessment Battery for Children
- Luria-Nebraska Battery
- Minnesota Multiphasic Personality Inventory
- Repeatable Battery for the Assessment of Neuropsychological Status
- Rorschach Projective Technique
- Shipley Institute of Living Scale
- Test of Memory and Learning
- Wechsler Adult Intelligence Scale and Wechsler Intelligence Scale for Children
- Wide Range Achievement Test
- Wonderlic Personnel Test
- Word Memory Test

QUESTIONS TO ASK YOUR DOCTOR

- Which test(s) do you recommend in this specific instance?
- Where can I learn more about neuropsychological testing?
- How can I know whether the administrator of any particular test is qualified?
- How can I determine the credentials of the neuropsychologist?
- What happens if the various tests taken come up with different conclusions?

Risks

Neuropsychological testing runs the risk of being biased if a trained and experienced administrator is not used. Therefore, neuropsychological testing should be carried out by a licensed **psychologist** trained in neuropsychology. When qualified personnel are used to collect behavioral, cognitive, language, and executive functioning skills, such data can lead to an accurate **diagnosis** of the individual.

Results

The results of neuropsychological testing are used as a primary way to assess neuropsychological function in humans. Testing includes scores, behavior observations, distinct and consistent patterns, and clinical history, which are all used in combination to provide a final assessment of individuals. Results in neuropsychological testing can be affected due to an individual's age, education, gender, and cultural background.

Different tests may differ based on validity, reliability, sensitivity, and specificity. Validity refers to the degree by which a test measures what it intended to measure. Reliability refers to the consistency and accuracy of the test; that is, how well scores remain consistent when extraneous variables are present (such as illness or injury). Sensitivity refers to the ability of the test to measure abnormalities, while specificity refers to the ability of the test to distinguish individuals with a specific abnormality from other individuals without such abnormality or with other types of abnormalities.

Resources

BOOKS

Feifer, Steven G., and Gurmal Rattan, editors. *Emotional Disorders: A Neuropsychological, Psychopharmacological, and Educational Perspective.* Middletown, MD: School Neuropsych Press, 2009.

Gorske, Tad T. and Steven R. Smith. *Collaborative Therapeutic Neuropsychological Assessment.* New York: Springer, 2009.

Grant, Igor, and Kenneth M. Adams, editors. *Neuropsychological Assessment of Neuropsychiatric and Neuromedical Disorders.* Oxford: Oxford University Press, 2009.

Hebben, Nancy, and William Millberg. *Essentials of Neuropsychological Assessment.* Hoboken, NJ: John Wiley and Sons, 2009.

Lezak, Muriel Deutsh, et al. *Neuropsychological Assessment.* Oxford: Oxford University Press, 2004.

Mitrushina, Maura N., et al. *Handbook of Normative Data for Neuropsychological Assessment.* New York: Oxford University Press, 2005.

Spreen, Otfried, Esther Strauss, and Elisabeth M. S. Sherman. *A Compendium of Neuropsychological Tests: Administration, Norms, and Commentary.* Oxford: Oxford University Press, 2006.

Walsh, Kevin, and David Darby. *Walsh's Neuropsychology: A Clinical Approach.* Edinburgh: Elsevier Churchill Livingstone, 2005.

ORGANIZATIONS

American Psychiatric Association, 1000 Wilson Boulevard, Suite 1825, Arlington, VA, 22209-3901, (703) 907-7300, apa@psych.org, http://www.psych.org.

American Psychological Association, 750 First Street NE, Washington, DC, 20002, (202) 336-5500, (800) 374-2721, http://www.apa.org.

International Neuropsychological Society, 700 Ackerman Road, Suite 625, Columbus, OH, 43202, (614) 263-4200, Fax: (614) 263-4366, http://www.the-ins.org.

National Academy of Neuropsychology, 7555 East Hampden Avenue, Suite 525, Denver, CO, 80231, (303) 691-3694, Fax: (303) 691-5983, office@nanonline.org, http://nanonline.org.

Danielle Barry, M.S.

Neurosis

Definition

Neurosis is a term generally used to describe a nonpsychotic mental illness which triggers feelings of distress and anxiety and impairs functioning.

Description

Origins

The word *neurosis* means "nerve disorder," and was first coined in the late eighteenth century by William Cullen, a Scottish physician. Cullen's concept of neurosis encompassed those nervous disorders and symptoms that do not have a clear organic cause. Sigmund Freud later used the term *anxiety neurosis* to describe mental illness or distress with extreme anxiety as a defining feature.

There is a difference of opinion over the clinical use of the term neurosis today. It is not generally used as a diagnostic category by American psychologists and psychiatrists any longer, and was removed from the American Psychiatric Association's ***Diagnostic and Statistical Manual of Mental Disorders*** in 1980 with the publication of the third edition (it last appeared as a diagnostic category in *DSM-II*). Some professionals use the term to describe anxious symptoms and associated behavior, or to describe the range of mental illnesses outside of the psychotic disorders (such as **schizophrenia**, **delusional disorder**). Others, particularly psychoanalysts (psychiatrists and psychologists who follow a psychoanalytical model of treatment, as popularized by Freud and Carl Jung), use the term neurosis to describe the internal process itself (called an unconscious conflict) that triggers the anxiety characteristic.

Categories

The neurotic disorders are distinct from psychotic disorders in that the individual with neurotic symptoms has a firm grip on reality, and the psychotic patient does not. Before their reclassification, there were several major traditional categories of psychological neuroses, including:

KAREN HORNEY (1885–1952)

The German-born American psychoanalyst Karen Danielsen Horney was a pioneer of neo-Freudianism. She believed that every human being has an innate drive toward self-realization and that neurosis is essentially a process obstructing this healthy development.

Horney focused on the central position of conflict and solutions to conflict in neurosis in *Our Inner Conflicts* (1945). She saw the neurotic child feeling helpless and isolated in a potentially hostile world, seeking a feeling of safety in compulsive moves toward, against, and away from others. Each of these moves came to constitute comprehensive philosophies of life and patterns of interpersonal relating. The conflict between these opposed moves she called the basic conflict and recognized that it required the individual to resort to means for restoring a sense of inner unity. These means she called the neurotic solutions.

Neurosis and Human Growth (1950) was Horney's definitive work, in which she placed her concept of healthy development in the foreground. She viewed the real self as the core of the individual, the source of inherent, constructive, evolutionary forces which under favorable circumstances grow and unfold in a dynamic process of self-realization. She presented "a morality of evolution," in which she viewed as moral all that enhances self-realization and as immoral all that hinders it. The most serious obstacle to healthy growth was the neurotic solution, which she called self-idealization, the attempt to see and to mold oneself into a glorified, idealized, illusory image with strivings for superiority, power, perfection, and vindictive triumph over others. This search for glory inevitably leads the individual to move away from himself (alienation) and against himself (self-hate). "At war with himself," his suffering increases, his relationships with others are further impaired, and the self-perpetuating neurotic cycle continues.

anxiety neurosis, depressive neurosis, obsessive-compulsive neurosis, somatization, **post-traumatic stress disorder**, and compensation neurosis—not a true neurosis, but a form of **malingering**, or feigning psychological symptoms for monetary or other personal gain.

Resources

BOOKS

American Psychiatric Association. *Diagnostic and Statistical Manual of Mental Disorders*. 4th ed., text rev. Washington, DC: American Psychiatric Publishing, 2000.

Fenichel, Otto M., and Leo Rangell. *The Psychoanalytic Theory of Neurosis: 50th Anniversary Edition*. New York: W.W. Norton and Son. 1995.

Paula Ford-Martin, M.S.

Neurotic excoriation *see* **Dermatillomania**

Neurotransmitters

Definition

Neurotransmitters are chemicals located and released in the **brain** to allow an impulse from one nerve cell to pass to another nerve cell.

Description

Approximately 50 neurotransmitters have been identified. There are billions of nerve cells located in the brain, which do not directly touch each other. Nerve cells communicate messages by secreting neurotransmitters. Neurotransmitters can excite or inhibit neurons (nerve cells). Common neurotransmitters include:

- Acetylcholine: Acetylcholine is particularly important in the stimulation of muscle tissue. After stimulation, acetylcholine degrades to acetate and choline, which are absorbed back into the first neuron to form another acetylcholine molecule. The poison curare blocks transmission of acetylcholine. Some nerve gases inhibit the breakdown of acetylcholine, producing a continuous stimulation of the receptor cells and spasms of muscles such as the heart.
- Aspartate: An amino acid that stimulates neurons in the central nervous system, particularly those that transfer information to the area of the brain called the cerebrum.
- Dopamine: Dopamine facilitates critical brain functions and, when unusual quantities are present, abnormal dopamine neurotransmission may play a role in Parkinson's disease, certain addictions, and schizophrenia.
- Epinephrine (adrenaline) and norepinephrine: These compounds are secreted principally from the adrenal gland. Secretion causes an increased heart rate and the

enhanced production of glucose as a ready energy source (the fight-or-flight response).

- Gamma aminobutyric acid (GABA): An inhibitory neurotransmitter, GABA is associated with anxiety disorder and mood disorders.
- Insulin: A peptide secreted by the pancreas that stimulates other cells to absorb glucose.
- Oxytocin: A short protein (peptide) that is released within the brain, ovary, and testes. The compound stimulates the release of milk by mammary glands, contractions during birth, and maternal behavior.
- Serotonin: Synthesized from the amino acid tryptophan, serotonin is assumed to play a biochemical role in mood and mood disorders, including anxiety, depression, and bipolar disorder.
- Somatostatin: Another peptide, which is inhibitory to the secretion of growth hormone from the pituitary gland, of insulin, and of a variety of gastrointestinal hormones involved with nutrient absorption.

Mechanism of impulse transmission

Each neurotransmitter can directly or indirectly influence neurons in a specific portion of the brain, thereby affecting behavior. A nerve impulse travels through a nerve in a long, slender cellular structure called an axon, and it eventually reaches a structure called the presynaptic membrane, which contains neurotransmitters to be released in a free space called the synaptic cleft. Freely flowing neurotransmitter molecules are picked up by receptors (structures that appear on cellular surfaces and fit together with molecules like a lock and key) located in a structure called the postsynaptic membrane of another nearby neuron. Once the neurotransmitter is picked up by receptors in the postsynaptic membrane, the molecule is internalized in the neuron and the impulse continues. This process of nerve cell communication is extremely rapid.

Once the neurotransmitter is released from the neurotransmitter vesicles of the presynaptic membrane, the normal movement of molecules should be directed to receptor sites located on the postsynaptic membrane. However, in certain disease states, the flow of the neurotransmitter is defective. For example, in **depression**, the flow of the inhibitory neurotransmitter **serotonin** is defective, and molecules flow back to their originating site (the presynaptic membrane) instead of to receptors on the postsynaptic membrane that will transmit the impulse to a nearby neuron.

The mechanism of action and localization of neurotransmitters in the brain has provided valuable information concerning the cause of many mental disorders, including clinical depression and chemical dependency, and in researching medications that allow normal flow and movement of neurotransmitter molecules.

Neurotransmitters, mental disorders, and medications

SCHIZOPHRENIA. Impairment of dopamine-containing neurons in the brain is implicated in **schizophrenia**, a mental disease marked by disturbances in thinking and emotional reactions. Medications that block **dopamine** receptors in the brain, such as **chlorpromazine** and **clozapine**, have been used to alleviate the symptoms and help patients return to a normal social setting.

DEPRESSION. In depression, there appears to be abnormal excess or inhibition of signals that control mood, thoughts, pain, and other sensations. Depression is treated with **antidepressants** that affect norepinephrine and serotonin in the brain. The antidepressants help correct the abnormal neurotransmitter activity. **Fluoxetine** (Prozac) is a selective serotonin reuptake inhibitor (SSRI) that appears to establish the level of serotonin required to function at a normal level. As the name implies, the drug inhibits the re-uptake of serotonin neurotransmitter from synaptic gaps, thus increasing neurotransmitter action. In the brain, then, the increased serotonin activity alleviates depressive symptoms.

ALZHEIMER'S DISEASE. **Alzheimer's disease** is characterized by memory loss and the eventual inability for self-care. The disease seems to be caused by a loss of cells that secrete acetylcholine in the basal forebrain (region of brain that is the control center for sensory and associative information processing and motor activities). Some medications to alleviate the symptoms have been developed, but at present there is no known treatment for the disease.

GENERALIZED ANXIETY DISORDER. People with **generalized anxiety disorder** (GAD) experience excessive worry that causes problems at work and in the maintenance of daily responsibilities. Evidence suggests that GAD involves several neurotransmitter systems in the brain, including norepinephrine and serotonin.

ATTENTION DEFICIT HYPERACTIVITY DISORDER. People affected by **attention deficit hyperactivity disorder (ADHD)** experience difficulties in the areas of attention, overactivity, impulse control, and distractibility. Research shows that dopamine and norepinephrine imbalances are strongly implicated in causing **ADHD**.

OTHERS. Substantial research evidence suggests a correlation of neurotransmitter imbalance with other mental disorders, including **borderline personality disorder**, **schizotypal personality disorder**, **avoidant personality disorder**, **social phobia**, **histrionic personality disorder**, and **somatization disorder**.

DRUG ADDICTIONS. **Cocaine** and crack cocaine are psychostimulants that affect neurons containing dopamine in the areas of the brain known as the limbic and frontal cortex. When cocaine is used, it generates a feeling of confidence and power. However, when large amounts are taken, people "crash" and suffer from physical and emotional exhaustion as well as depression.

Opiates, such as heroin and morphine, appear to mimic naturally occurring peptide substances in the brain that act as neurotransmitters with opiate activity called endorphins. Natural endorphins of the brain act to kill pain, cause sensations of pleasure, and cause sleepiness. Endorphins released with extensive aerobic **exercise**, for example, are responsible for the "rush" that long-distance runners experience. It is believed that morphine and heroin combine with the endorphin receptors in the brain, resulting in reduced natural endorphin production. As a result, the drugs are needed to replace the naturally produced endorphins and **addiction** occurs. Attempts to counteract the effects of the drugs involve using medications that mimic them, such as nalorphine, naloxone, and **naltrexone**.

One of the depressant drugs in widest use, alcohol, is believed to cause its effects by interacting with the GABA receptor. Initially anxiety is controlled, but greater amounts reduce muscle control and delay reaction time due to impaired thinking.

Resources

BOOKS

Stern, T.A., et al. *Massachusetts General Hospital Comprehensive Clinical Psychiatry,* 1st ed. Philadelphia: Mosby Elsevier, 2008.

ORGANIZATIONS

American Academy of Neurology, 1080 Montreal Ave., St. Paul, MN, 55116, (651) 695-2717, (800) 879-1960, Fax: (651) 879-2791, memberservices@aan.com, http://www.aan.com.

American Medical Association, 515 N State St., Chicago, IL, 60610, (312) 464-5000, (800) 621-8335, http://www.amaassn.org.

American Neurological Association, 5841 Cedar Lake Rd., Ste. 204, Minneapolis, MN, 55416, (952) 545-6284, ana@llmsi.com, http://www.aneuroa.org.

National Institutes of Health, 9000 Rockville Pike, Bethesda, MD, 20892, (301) 496-4000; TTY: (301) 402-9612, http://www.nih.gov.

National Institute of Neurological Disorders and Stroke (NINDS), PO Box 5801, Bethesda, MD, 20824, (301) 496-5751; TTY: (301) 468-5981, (800) 352-9424, http://www.ninds.nih.gov.

Laith Farid Gulli, MD
Mary Finley

Nicotine and related disorders

Definition

Nicotine is the main psychoactive ingredient in tobacco. It is a physically and psychologically addictive drug. Nicotine is the most influential dependence-producing drug in the United States and worldwide, and its use is associated with many serious health risks.

Demographics

Although the prevalence of smoking has gradually decreased in the United States and many other industrialized countries since the 1970s, the use of tobacco products is rapidly increasing in developing nations, where approximately 80% of current smokers live. Younger populations may be particularly vulnerable. For example, a CDC survey from 2003 found that almost 42% of teenaged boys in one city in Mali were cigarette smokers. The World Health Organization currently attributes more than five million deaths per year globally to tobacco use among the estimated one billion smokers worldwide, a death total expected to increase to eight million by 2030. Another 600,000 deaths occur in nonsmokers as a result of exposure to secondhand smoke. Use of tobacco products in developing countries is of particular concern, because these countries often lack adequate healthcare resources to treat smoking-related diseases, let alone support **smoking cessation** programs.

In the United States, men are more likely to smoke than women (33.7% to 21.5%). In developing countries, male smokers outnumber women smokers, but among adolescent populations, girls and boys are becoming more equal in their rates of smoking. In the United States, people who smoke tend to have less formal education than those who do not, with the lowest smoking rates in persons with college degrees. At least 50% of patients diagnosed with psychiatric problems are smokers, while more than three-quarters of those who abuse other substances also smoke.

According to the National Survey on Drug Use and Health, from 1997 to 2010, smoking among U.S. middle- and high-school students had declined after increasing dramatically in the 1990s. Smoking is most prevalent among adults aged 18 to 25, with an estimated 40.8% of all smokers falling within this age group. Among different ethnic groups, the highest rates of smoking resided in American Indian or Alaskan Native populations (35.8%), followed by persons who were two or more races (32%), Caucasians (29.5%), and African Americans (27.3%).

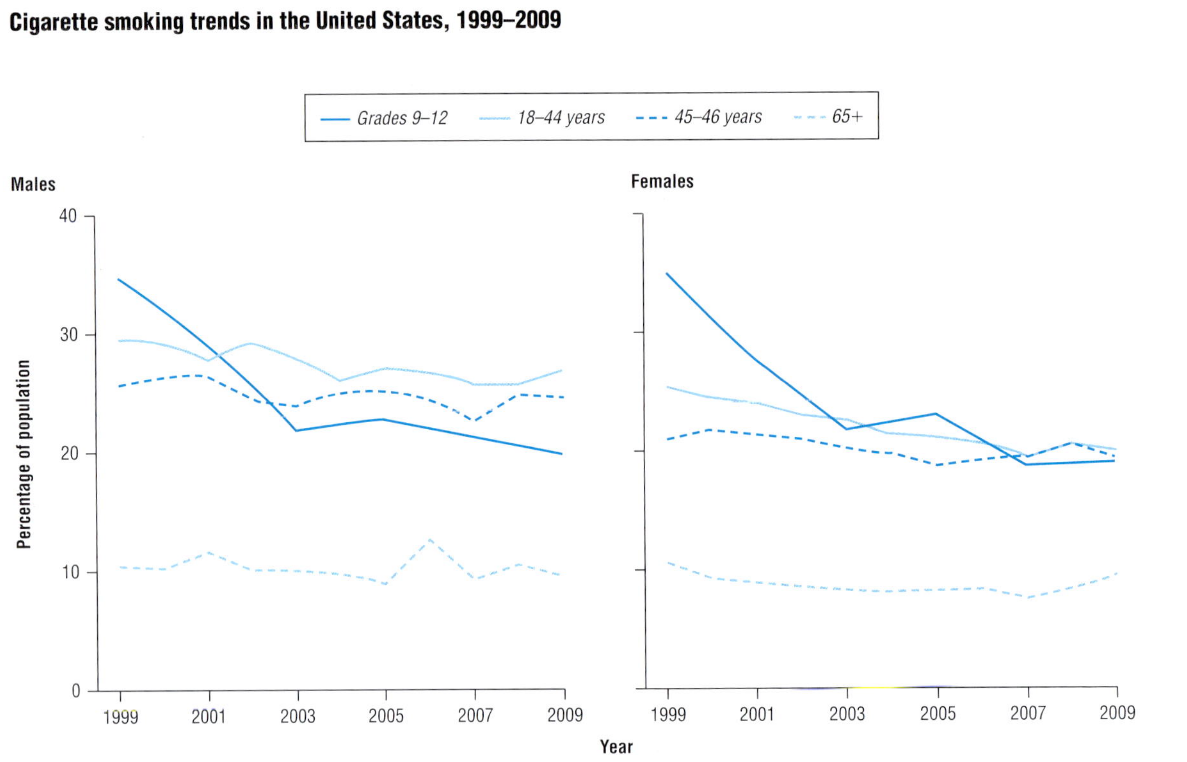

SOURCE: National Center for Health Statistics, *Health, United States, 2010: With Special Feature on Death and Dying* (Hyattsville, MD: U.S. Department of Health and Human Services, 2011).

Report available online at http://www.cdc.gov/nchs/hus.htm. *(Graphs by PreMediaGlobal. © 2012 Cengage Learning.)*

Recent research suggests that there may be a genetic component to nicotine dependence, just as there is for alcohol dependence. Studies show that girls (but not boys) whose mothers smoked during pregnancy are four times more likely to smoke than those whose mothers were tobacco-free during pregnancy. Other research suggests that the absence of a certain enzyme in the body protects the body against nicotine dependence.

Description

Nicotine is the most addictive and psychoactive chemical in tobacco, a plant native to North America. Early European explorers learned to smoke its leaves from indigenous peoples who had been using tobacco for hundreds of years. They took tobacco back to Europe, where it became immensely popular. Tobacco became a major source of income for the American colonies and later for the United States. Advances in cigarette-making technology caused a boom in cigarette smoking in the early 1900s. Before the early twentieth century, most people who used tobacco used pipes, cigars, or chewing tobacco.

In the 1950s, researchers began to link cigarette smoking to certain respiratory diseases and cancers. In 1964, the Surgeon General of the United States issued the first health report on smoking. Cigarette smoking peaked in the United States in the 1960s, then began to decline as health concerns about tobacco increased. In 1971, cigarette advertising was banned from television, although tobacco products are still advertised in other media today. There were about 69.6 million adult smokers in the United States in 2010, and approximately 2.4 million people had smoked their first cigarette in the previous month. Most active smokers are addicted to nicotine.

Pure nicotine is a colorless liquid that turns brown and smells like tobacco when exposed to air. Nicotine can be absorbed through the skin, the lining of the mouth and nose, and the moist tissues lining the lungs. Cigarettes are the most efficient nicotine delivery system. Once tobacco smoke is inhaled, nicotine reaches the **brain** in less than 15 seconds. Because people who smoke pipes and cigars do not inhale, they absorb nicotine more slowly. Nicotine in chewing tobacco and snuff is absorbed through the mucous membranes lining the mouth and nasal passages. There are also several "hard snuff" and other new tobacco products being produced and marketed as alternative to traditional

KEY TERMS

Cold turkey—A slang term for stopping the use of nicotine (or any other addictive drug) suddenly and completely.

Dopamine—A chemical in brain tissue that serves to transmit nerve impulses and helps to regulate movement and emotions.

Epinephrine—Also known as adrenaline, the hormone secreted by the adrenal glands in response to stress.

Neurotransmitter—One of a group of chemicals secreted by a nerve cell (neuron) to carry a chemical message to another nerve cell, often as a way of transmitting a nerve impulse. Examples of neurotransmitters include acetylcholine, dopamine, serotonin, and norepinephrine.

Plaque—A sticky cholesterol-containing substance that builds up on the walls of blood vessels, reducing or blocking blood flow.

Tolerance—A progressive decrease in the effectiveness of a drug with long-term use, requiring higher doses to achieve the desired effect.

Withdrawal—Symptoms experienced by a person who has become physically dependent on a drug, experienced when the drug use is discontinued.

tobacco products. At least one study of the nicotine content of these products has found that some have lower levels of nicotine than regular tobacco products, but others contain comparable levels.

Causes and symptoms

How nicotine works

Nicotine is the main addictive drug among the 4,000 compounds found in tobacco smoke. Other substances in smoke as tar and carbon monoxide present documented health hazards, but they are not addictive and do not cause cravings or withdrawal symptoms to the extent that nicotine does. Neuroimaging technology has shown that levels of monoamine oxidase, the enzyme responsible for boosting mood-enhancing molecule levels in the brain, increase in response to smoking, even though nicotine does not affect levels of this enzyme. Thus, some other compound in cigarette smoke must be acting to exert this effect. In addition, a compound in cigarette smoke called acetaldehyde may contribute to tobacco **addiction** and may have a stronger effect in adolescents.

Nicotine is both a stimulant and a sedative. It is a psychoactive drug, meaning that it works in the brain, alters brain chemistry, and changes mood. Once tobacco smoke is inhaled, nicotine passes rapidly through the linings of the lungs and into the blood. It quickly circulates to the brain where it stimulates release of **dopamine**, a neurotransmitter (nerve signaling molecule) that affects mood. Drugs that elicit an increase in dopamine influence the brain's "reward" pathway, causing the user to turn again to the drug for another pleasurable, rewarding dopamine response. This release accounts for the pleasurable sensation that most smokers feel almost as soon as they light a cigarette. Nicotine also decreases anger and increases the efficiency of a person's performance on long, dull tasks.

As nicotine affects the brain, it also stimulates the adrenal glands. The adrenal glands are small, pea-sized organs located above each kidney that really act as two different endocrine organs. The adrenal gland produces several hormones in the medulla, or inner layer, including epinephrine, also called **adrenaline**. Under normal circumstances, adrenaline is released in response to **stress** or a perceived threat. It is sometimes called the "fight or flight" hormone, because it prepares the body for action. When adrenaline is released, blood pressure, heart rate, blood flow, and oxygen use increase. Glucose, a simple form of sugar used by the body, floods the body to provide extra energy to muscles. The overall effect of the release of the stress hormones is strain on the cardiovascular (heart and blood vessels) system. This response to stress produces inflammation in the blood vessels that ultimately results in buildup of plaque, which can block the vessels and cause **stroke** or heart attack.

Most people begin smoking between the ages of 12 and 20. Few people start smoking as adults over 21. Adolescents who smoke tend to begin as casual smokers, out of rebellion or a perceived need for social acceptance. Dependence on nicotine develops rapidly, however; one study suggests that 85%–90% of adolescents who smoke four or more cigarettes become regular smokers. Nicotine is addictive, so being tobacco-free soon feels uncomfortable for users. In addition, smokers quickly develop tolerance to nicotine. Tolerance is a condition that occurs when the body needs a larger and larger dose of a substance to produce the same effect. For smokers, tolerance to nicotine means more frequent and more rapid smoking. Soon most smokers develop physical withdrawal symptoms when they try to stop smoking. Users of other forms of tobacco experience the same effects; however, the delivery of nicotine is slower and the effects may not be as pronounced.

Nicotine dependence

In addition to the physical dependence caused by the actions of nicotine on the brain, there is a strong psychological component to the dependency of most users of tobacco products, especially cigarette smokers. Most people who start smoking or using smokeless tobacco products do so because of social factors. These include:

- desire to fit in with peers
- acceptance by family members who use tobacco
- rebelliousness
- association of tobacco products with maturity and sophistication
- positive response to tobacco advertising

Such personal factors as mental illness (**depression**, anxiety, **schizophrenia**, or alcoholism), the need to reduce stress and anxiety, or a desire to avoid weight gain also influence people to start smoking. Once smoking has become a habit, whether physical addiction occurs or not, psychological factors play a significant role in a person's continuing to smoke. People who want to stop smoking may be discouraged from doing so because:

- they live or work with people who smoke and who are not supportive of their quitting
- they believe they are incapable of quitting
- they perceive no health benefits to quitting
- they have tried to quit before and failed
- they associate cigarettes with specific pleasurable activities or social situations that they are not willing to give up
- they fear gaining weight

Successful smoking cessation programs must treat both the physical and psychological aspects of nicotine addiction.

Nicotine withdrawal

The **American Psychiatric Association** first recognized nicotine dependence and nicotine withdrawal as serious psychological problems in 1980. Today nicotine is considered an addictive drug, although a common and legalized one.

Quitting nicotine can be difficult. Among people who try, between 75% and 80% **relapse** within six months. Because of this rate, research has found that smoking cessation programs that last longer than six months can greatly enhance quit rates, achieving rates as high as 50% at one year. Combining a nicotine-withdrawal product with a behavioral-modification or support program has produced the greatest success rates.

The combination of physiological and psychological factors make withdrawal from nicotine very difficult. Symptoms of nicotine withdrawal include:

- irritability
- restlessness
- increased anger or frustration
- sleep disturbances
- inability to concentrate
- increased appetite or desire for sweets
- depression
- anxiety
- constant thoughts about smoking
- cravings for cigarettes
- decreased heart rate
- coughing

Withdrawal symptoms are usually more pronounced in smokers than in those who use smokeless tobacco products, and heavy smokers tend to have more symptoms than light smokers when they try to stop smoking. People with depression, schizophrenia, alcoholism, or mood disorders may find it especially difficult to quit, as nicotine offers temporary relief for some of the symptoms of these disorders.

Symptoms of nicotine withdrawal begin rapidly and peak within one to three days. Withdrawal symptoms generally last three to four weeks, but a significant number of smokers have withdrawal symptoms lasting longer than one month. Some people have strong cravings for tobacco that last for months, even though the physical addiction to nicotine is gone. These cravings often occur in settings in which the person formerly smoked, such as at a party, while driving, or after a meal. Researchers believe that much of this extended craving is psychological.

Diagnosis

Smokers usually self-diagnose their nicotine dependence and nicotine withdrawal. Such questionnaires as the Fagerstrom Test for Nicotine Dependence (FTND), a short six-item assessment of cigarette use, help to determine the level of tobacco dependence. Physicians and mental health professionals are less concerned with **diagnosis**, which is usually straightforward, than with determining the physical and psychological factors in each patient that must be addressed for successful smoking cessation.

The ***Diagnostic and Statistical Manual of Mental Disorders***, the handbook used by medical professionals in diagnosing mental health conditions, recognizes two smoking-related disorders: tobacco use disorder and tobacco withdrawal disorder. The criteria for diagnosing a tobacco use disorder is the same for any **substance abuse** disorder. Specific criteria include experiencing symptoms of tolerance or withdrawal, unsuccessful attempts at quitting, and smoking for longer or more often than was originally intended. Criteria for tobacco withdrawal include experiencing withdrawal symptoms within 24 hours after quitting (or reducing intake).

Treatment

Most people do not decide to stop smoking all of the sudden. Instead, they go through several preparatory stages before taking action. First is the precontemplation stage, in which the smoker does not even consider quitting. Precontemplation is followed by the contemplation stage, in which the smoker thinks about quitting, but takes no action. Contemplation eventually turns to preparation, often when counselors or family members encourage or urge the smoker to quit. Now the smoker starts making plans to quit soon. Finally the smoker arrives at the point of taking action.

Having decided to stop smoking, a person has many choices of programs and approaches. When mental health professionals are involved in smoking cessation efforts, one of their first jobs is to identify the physical and psychological factors that keep the person smoking. This identification helps to direct the smoker to the most appropriate type of program. Assessment examines the frequency of the person's smoking, his or her social and emotional attachment to cigarettes, commitment to change, available support system, and barriers to change. These conditions vary from person to person, which is why some smoking cessation programs work for one person and not another.

Medications

Before 1984, there were no medications to help smokers quit. In that year, a nicotine chewing gum (Nicorette) was approved by the U.S. Food and Drug Administration (FDA) as a prescription drug for smoking cessation. In 1996, it became available without prescription. Nicorette was the first of several medications used for nicotine replacement therapy, intended to gradually reduce nicotine dependence to prevent or reduce withdrawal symptoms. This approach, called tapering, is used in withdrawal of other addictive drugs. Studies indicate that people using these replacement therapies do not become addicted to them.

Nicotine gum comes in two strengths, 2 mg and 4 mg. Lozenges (Commit, Nicorette lozenge) are also available in the same doses. As the gum is chewed, nicotine is released and absorbed through the lining of the mouth. Over a 6- to 12-week period, the amount and strength of gum chewed can be decreased until the smoker is weaned away from his or her dependence on nicotine. People trying to quit smoking are instructed to use the gum when they feel a craving. Products with caffeine may limit nicotine absorption and should be avoided in a window of time around the gum "dose." Some people may not like the taste of the gum, and other common side effects include burning mouth and sore jaw. Pregnant or lactating women and persons with heart problems, diabetes, or ulcers should consult with a doctor before beginning any nicotine-replacement product.

Nicotine transdermal patches have been available without prescription since 1996. They are marketed under several brand names, including Habitrol, Nicoderm, NicoDerm CQ, Prostep, and Nicotrol. All but Nicotrol are 24-hour patches; Nicotrol is a 16-hour patch designed to be removed at night. The patches are worn on the skin between the neck and the waist and provide a steady delivery of nicotine through the skin. Patches like Nicoderm come in varying strengths, and after several weeks, users can move down to a patch that delivers a lower dose. With the Nicotrol patch, a user simply ceases use after six weeks. Some people using the 24-hour patches experience sleep disturbances, and a few develop mild skin irritations, but generally side effects are few. Doctors recommend not smoking while using the patch.

Two other nicotine delivery devices are available by prescription only. One is a nicotine nasal spray. It has the advantage of delivering nicotine rapidly, just as a cigarette does, but it delivers a much lower dose than a cigarette. Treatment with nasal spray usually lasts four to six weeks. Side effects include cold-like symptoms (runny nose, sneezing, etc.). A nicotine inhaler is also available that delivers nicotine through the tissues of the mouth. A major advantage of the inhaler is that it provides an alternative to having a cigarette in one's hands while still delivering nicotine. It delivers less nicotine in cold weather (under 50°F). Recommendations for both the spray and the inhaler are that they be used at least hourly at first.

Prescription drugs outside of nicotine replacement therapy have been approved for the treatment of nicotine dependence. The first-approved drug was **bupropion** (Zyban), an antidepressant that acts to cut down withdrawal symptoms. This drug may be used in combination with a nicotine-replacement therapy and behavioral therapy.

A newer drug is varenicline (Chantix), which was developed to help people stop smoking. This drug acts directly on the proteins in the brain that recognize and bind nicotine. Interfering with their action not only stops the brain from sending the pleasurable message of nicotine but also reduces the feelings of nicotine withdrawal. Some studies indicate that this drug can double a person's chances of quitting smoking. Side effects of this drug can include headache, nausea, vomiting, sleep problems, gas, and changes in taste sensation.

Other drugs used in some smoking cessation programs include **nortriptyline** (Pamelor), a tricyclic antidepressant, and **clonidine** (Catapres), a high blood pressure medication. Side effects of these drugs include dry mouth and drowsiness. Both of these drugs are second-line treatments (used only when other treatments have shown no results) and are considered off-label uses (not approved by the FDA for this purpose).

Behavioral treatments

Behavioral treatments are used to help smokers learn to recognize and avoid specific situations that trigger desire for a cigarette. They also help the smoker learn to substitute other activities for smoking. Behavioral treatments are almost always combined with smoker education, and they usually involve forming a support network of other smokers who are trying to quit.

Behavioral treatments often take place in **support groups** either in person or online. They are most effective when combined with nicotine reduction therapy. Other supportive techniques include the use of rewards for achieving certain goals and contracts to clarify and reinforce the goals. Aversive techniques include asking the smoker to inhale the tobacco smoke deeply and repeatedly to the point of nausea, so that smoking is no longer associated with pleasurable sensations. Overall, quit rates are highest when **behavior modification** is combined with nicotine replacement therapy and tapering. Behavior modification once was conducted in person, but with the advent of a telephonic and virtual world on the Internet, behavioral approaches are also available via mail, telephone, and the Web for greater access and flexibility. The U.S. Department of Health and Human Services sponsors a toll-free number for people who want to quit: 800-QUIT-NOW (800-784-8669). This number serves as the point of contact for smokers who want information and help.

Alternative treatments

Many alternative therapies have been tried to help smokers withdraw from nicotine. Hypnosis has proved helpful in some cases, but has not been tested in controlled **clinical trials**. **Acupuncture**, relaxation techniques, restricted environmental stimulation therapy (REST, a combination of relaxation and hypnosis techniques), special **diets**, and herbal supplements have all been used to help people stop smoking. Of these alternative techniques, clinical studies of REST showed substantial promise in helping people stop smoking permanently.

Prognosis

Smoking is a major health risk associated with nicotine dependence, with approximately 50% of long-term smokers dying from smoking-related diseases, according to the FDA. It is the top cause of preventable death in the United States and kills an estimated 443,000 U.S. citizens each year—more than alcohol, illegal drug, homicide, **suicide**, car accidents, and HIV rates combined. Of those 443,000, about 40% will die from cancer, 35% from heart disease and stroke, and 25% from lung disease. Most lung cancers, the leading cause of cancer death in the United States, are linked to smoking, and smoking is linked to about one-third of all cancer deaths. Smoking also causes such other lung problems as chronic bronchitis and emphysema, as well as worsening the symptoms of asthma. Other cancers associated with smoking include cancers of the mouth, esophagus, stomach, kidney, colon, and bladder. Smoking accounts for a large percentage of cardiovascular deaths and significantly increases the risk of heart disease, heart attack, stroke, and aneurysm. Women who smoke during pregnancy have more miscarriages, premature babies, and low–birth weight babies than nonsmokers. In addition, there is an increased risk that a child born to a mother who smokes will die of sudden infant death syndrome (SIDS), making smoking an avoidable factor in this tragic occurrence. Secondhand smoke also endangers the health of nonsmokers in the smoker's family or workplace. Although most of these effects are not caused directly by nicotine, it is the dependence on nicotine that keeps people smoking.

Even though it is difficult for smokers to break their chemical and psychological dependence on nicotine, most of the negative health effects of smoking are reduced or reversed after quitting. Therefore, it is worth trying to quit smoking at any age, regardless of the length of time a person has had the habit.

Mental health problems

Persons with mental health problems, such as depression, anxiety, and schizophrenia, are two to three times more likely to smoke than persons without these conditions. However, smoking has also been associated with the risk of developing mental health problems, which has prompted some researchers to wonder whether smoking is a causal factor in mental illnesses or just prevalent due to effects of nicotine. However, a study published in the *Archives of General Psychiatry* in 2010 suggested that tobacco smoke may have some implications in the development of mental illness. The study focused on the impact of secondhand smoke on individuals and found that nonsmokers were 1.5 times more likely to develop mental health problems if regularly exposed to secondhand smoke. A similar study focused on children, published in the *Archives of Pediatrics & Adolescent Medicine*, found that children exposed to secondhand smoke were more likely to develop behavioral problems such as **attention deficit hyperactivity disorder (ADHD)**. Neither study is definitive of smoking's impact on mental health, and further research is needed, but along with the varied and severe physiological effects of smoking, there is risk of a negative psychological impact, as well.

Prevention

The best way to avoid nicotine dependence and withdrawal is to avoid the use of tobacco products. In September 2012, the FDA will start requiring all cigarette manufacturers to display large, pictographic warning labels on cigarette packaging to deter consumers from purchasing cigarettes. The labels feature images focused on the negative effects of smoking, such as damaged lungs, oral cancer, children affected by secondhand smoke, and even a deceased person. The goal of the new labels is to both help current smokers quit smoking and to prevent others from starting smoking. The images are available on the FDA website: http://www.fda.gov/TobaccoProducts/Labeling/CigaretteWarningLabels/default.htm.

Resources

BOOKS

Bock, Gregory, and Jamie Goode, eds. *Understanding Nicotine and Tobacco Addiction: Novartis Foundation Symposium, 275*. Chichester, UK: John Wiley & Sons, 2006.

Cooper, Grant. *Never Smoke Again: The Top 10 Ways to Stop Smoking Now & Forever*. Garden City Park, NY: Square One Publishers, 2007.

Henningfield, Jack E., Edythe D. London, and Sakire Pogun. *Nicotine Psychopharmacology*. Berlin: Springer, 2009.

Miller, Michael W. *Brain Development: Normal Processes and the Effects of Alcohol and Nicotine*. Oxford: Oxford University Press, 2006.

Naff, Clay Farris. *Nicotine and Tobacco*. San Diego: ReferencePoint Press, Inc, 2007.

PERIODICALS

Berrettini W. "Nicotine Addiction." *The American Journal of Psychiatry* 165 (September 2008): 1089–92.

Caggiula A.R., et al. "The Role of Nicotine in Smoking: a Dual-reinforcement Model." *Nebraska Symposium on Motivation* 55 (2009): 91–109.

DiFranza, J.R. "Hooked From the First Cigarette." *Scientific American*. 298 (April 21, 2008): 82–7.

Glasser, I. "Letters: Nicotine Anonymous May Benefit Nicotine-Dependent Individuals." *American Journal of Public Health*. 100, no. 2 (February 2010): 196.

Oncken C., et al. "Nicotine Gum for Pregnant Smokers: A Randomized Controlled Trial." *Obstetrics and Gynecology*. 112, no. 4 (2008): 859–67.

WEBSITES

Nicotine Anonymous. http://www.nicotine-anonymous.org (accessed October 23, 2011).

Smokefree.gov. "Quit Smoking Today." http://www.smokefree.gov (accessed October 23, 2011).

ORGANIZATIONS

American Cancer Society, 250 Williams Street NW, Atlanta, GA, 30303, http://www.cancer.org.

American Lung Association, 1301 Pennsylvannia Ave. NW, Suite 800, Washington, DC, 20004, (202) 785-3355, Fax: (202) 452-1805, info@lungusa.org, http://www.lungusa.org.

Tish Davidson, AM
Emily Jane Willingham, PhD
Brenda W. Lerner

Nightmare disorder

Definition

Nightmare disorder, which is also called dream anxiety disorder, is characterized by the occurrence of repeated dreams during which the sleeper feels threatened and frightened. The sense of fear causes the person to awake.

Demographics

The actual percentage of people that suffer from nightmare disorder is not known, as many people do not seek treatment for it. There are, however, estimates of the proportion of the population that experience occasional nightmares. Many children suffer from nightmares that concern their parents. Estimates on the number of children who have recurrent nightmares range from 10%–50%. In children, however, nightmares are not usually associated with psychiatric illness.

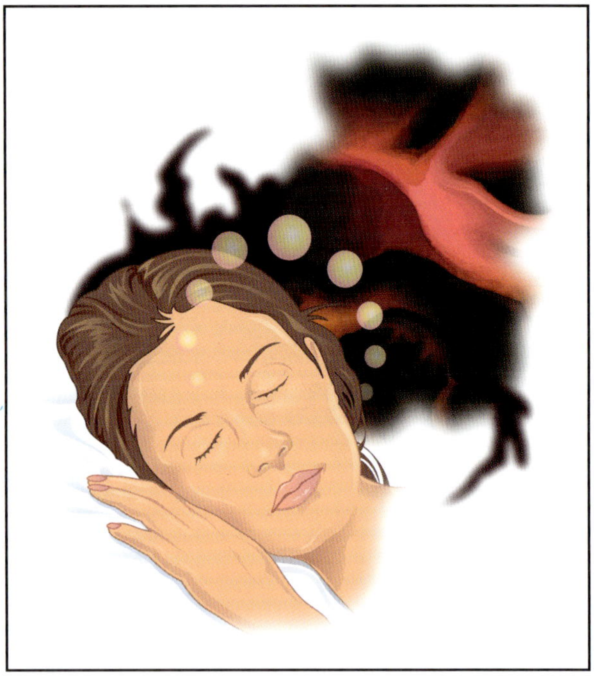

Nightmares can be caused by psychological traumas or stress and anxiety. *(Illustration by Electronic Illustrators Group. © 2012 Cengage Learning.)*

The number of children experiencing nightmares decreases as they get older. More than 3% of young adults have frequent nightmares, but only about 1% of mature adults experience nightmares once or twice a week. Half of the adults in the United States who experience regular nightmares have diagnosable psychiatric illnesses. Women are estimated to have nightmares two to four times more frequently than men. There is some uncertainty as to whether this figure reflects an actual difference between the sexes in the frequency of nightmares, or whether women are simply more likely than men to report nightmares. Nightmares typically decrease in frequency as people grow older.

Description

Nightmares are dreams that cause intense fear. These dreams are often complex and fairly long. During the dream the sleeper usually encounters or experiences a threat to their life or safety. Nightmares are also reported that do not involve physical danger but threaten the dreamer's pride or integrity.

As the dream progresses, the threat to the person usually increases, as does their sense of fear. Waking usually occurs just as the threat or danger reaches its climax. It is often difficult for a person to return to sleep after waking from a nightmare. Nightmares usually occur during the second half of the night's sleep.

Causes and symptoms

During the course of a nightmare the sleeper may moan, talk, or move slightly, although these signs do not always appear. The person wakes completely from the nightmare with a profound sense of fear. Waking is usually accompanied by increased heart rate, sweating, and other symptoms of anxiety or fear. Once fully awake, the person usually has a good recall of the dream and what made it so frightening. Because of the physical symptoms of anxiety and because clarity is achieved immediately upon waking, returning to sleep after a nightmare is often difficult. The vividness of the recall and the prominence of the dream images in the person's mind can also make it difficult to calm down and return to sleep.

Sometimes people may avoid going to sleep after a particularly intense nightmare because of the fear of having another bad dream. In addition, people may have problems falling asleep if they are experiencing anxiety caused by the fear of having nightmares. As a result, these people may have the signs and symptoms associated with mild **sleep deprivation**, such as decreased mental clarity, problems paying attention, excessive daytime sleepiness, irritability, or mild **depression**.

The causes of nightmares are not known for certain. Adults who have nightmares on a regular basis constitute a small minority of the American population. About half of these people are thought to suffer from psychiatric disorders that cause nightmares. Nightmares may also be triggered by major psychological traumas, such as those experienced by patients with **post-traumatic stress disorder**. For most patients who do not have an underlying mental disorder, the nightmares are attributed to **stress**. Nightmares that occur on an irregular and occasional basis are usually attributed to life stressors and associated anxiety.

Some researchers think that artistic or creative people are at greater risk for nightmares, as are people who are generally sensitive. These people are considered to have well-developed imaginations and are more sensitive to environmental and social factors.

Nightmares can be a side effect of some medications or drugs of abuse, including drugs given for high blood pressure; levodopa and other drugs given to treat Parkinson's disease; **amphetamines**, **cocaine**, and other stimulants; and some **antidepressants**. Withdrawal from alcohol and other medications can also sometimes cause nightmares.

Diagnosis

A **diagnosis** of nightmare disorder is usually made because the person reports the problem to their family physician or a **psychiatrist**. There are no laboratory tests for nightmare disorder, although the doctor may give the patient a physical examination to rule out any medical conditions that may be causing anxiety or stress.

Nightmares are characterized by awakening with a sense of fear, a clear recollection of the dream, and the physical symptoms of anxiety. Nightmares can occur during nighttime sleep or daytime naps. A patient experiencing nightmares must meet the criteria listed in the *Diagnostic and Statistical Manual of Mental Disorders* (*DSM*) to be diagnosed with nightmare disorder. The manual, which provides guidelines used by the **American Psychiatric Association** for diagnosing psychiatric disturbances, lists four distinct criteria:

- The patient must experience repeated awakenings from frightening or disturbing dreams.
- When the patient awakes, he or she must wake fully and be aware of his or her surroundings.
- The nightmares or the resulting loss of sleep must cause the patient distress in important areas of his or her life.
- The nightmares cannot be directly attributed to another mental disorder or be the direct effects of medications, substance abuse, or a medical condition.

Nightmare disorder can be confused with **sleep terror disorder**. Both disorders are characterized by an arousal during sleep when the patient shows symptoms of anxiety or fear. During a nightmare, the patient may move slightly or moan but does not generally display dramatic or active symptoms. After a nightmare, the patient becomes fully awake and is aware of his or her surroundings. Sleep terror, however, is characterized by a partial arousal from sleep during an episode, in which the patient is generally nonresponsive. Their own cries and screams usually cause them to wake. Patients do not remember either the sleep terror episode or what caused the fear, whereas patients who have nightmares remember them with great clarity and often in considerable detail. Such symptoms of fear or anxiety as increased heart rate, dilated pupils, and sweating are not as dramatic in patients with nightmare disorder as they are in patients experiencing sleep terrors.

Treatment

Nightmares that are associated with a psychiatric disorder are managed by treating the underlying disorder. For patients without psychiatric disorders, psychological counseling to deal with any recurring themes in the nightmares may be helpful. Children may not require treatment for nightmares unless the dreams are causing significant distress, as nightmares generally resolve as children mature.

KEY TERMS

Dream anxiety disorder—Another name for nightmare disorder.

Sleep terror disorder—A sleep disorder that is distinguished from nightmare disorder by the intensity of associated anxiety symptoms, the absence of complete wakefulness, and the person's difficulty recalling the episode.

Because stress is thought to be the most common cause of nightmares, **stress reduction** techniques may prove to be effective complementary treatments. Typical relaxation techniques such as **yoga**, **meditation**, or **exercise** may be helpful. **Psychotherapy** can be an effective way to identify major stressors in the person's life and to explore ways in which they may be reduced or eliminated.

Prognosis

Nightmare disorder can be a lifelong disorder. A general improvement in symptoms often takes place, however, as the patient gets older. Treatment for any underlying psychological disorders can be very successful.

Resources

BOOKS

Aldrich, Michael S. *Sleep Medicine*. New York: Oxford University Press, 1999.

American Psychiatric Association. *Diagnostic and Statistical Manual of Mental Disorders*, 4th ed., text rev. Washington, DC: American Psychiatric Publishing, 2000.

Chokroverty, Sudhansu. *Sleep Disorders Medicine: Basic Science, Technical Considerations, and Clinical Aspects*. 3rd ed. Philadelphia: Saunders Elsevier, 2009.

Sadock, Benjamin J., and Virginia A. Sadock, eds. *Comprehensive Textbook of Psychiatry*. Vol. 2. 7th ed. Philadelphia: Lippincott Williams and Wilkins, 2000.

PERIODICALS

Krakow, Barry, et al. "Imagery Rehearsal Therapy for Chronic Nightmares in Sexual Assault Survivors with Posttraumatic Stress Disorder." *Journal of the American Medical Association* 286, no. 5 (August 2001) 537–45.

ORGANIZATIONS

American Academy of Sleep Medicine, 2510 N Frontage Rd., Darien, IL, 60561, (630) 737-9700, Fax: (630) 737-9790, inquiries@assmnet.org, http://www.aasmnet.org.

National Sleep Foundation, 1010 North Glebe Rd., Suite 310, Arlington, VA, 22201, (703) 243-1697, nsf@sleepfoundation.org, http://www.sleepfoundation.org.

Tish Davidson, A.M.

NIMH *see* **National Institute of Mental Health**

NLP *see* **Hypnotherapy**

Norepinephrine *see* **Adrenaline**

Norpramin *see* **Desipramine**

Nortriptyline

Definition

Nortriptyline is a tricyclic antidepressant. It is sold in the United States under the brand names Aventyl and Pamelor, and is also available under its generic name.

Purpose

Nortriptyline is used to relieve symptoms of **depression**. The drug is more effective for endogenous depression than for other forms of depression. Endogenous depression is depression arising from metabolic changes within a person, such as chemical or hormonal imbalances. Nortriptyline is also used to treat premenstrual depression, **panic disorder**, chronic pain, and some skin conditions. In addition, nortriptyline is being investigated for the treatment of **nicotine** dependence.

Description

Tricyclic **antidepressants** act to change the balance of naturally occurring chemicals in the **brain** that regulate the transmission of nerve impulses between cells. The precise way in which nortriptyline elevates mood is not fully understood. The drug inhibits the activity of **neurotransmitters** such as acetylcholine, histamine, and 5-hydroxytryptamine. Studies have indicated that nortriptyline interferes with the release, transport, and storage of catecholamines, another group of chemicals involved in nerve impulse transmission.

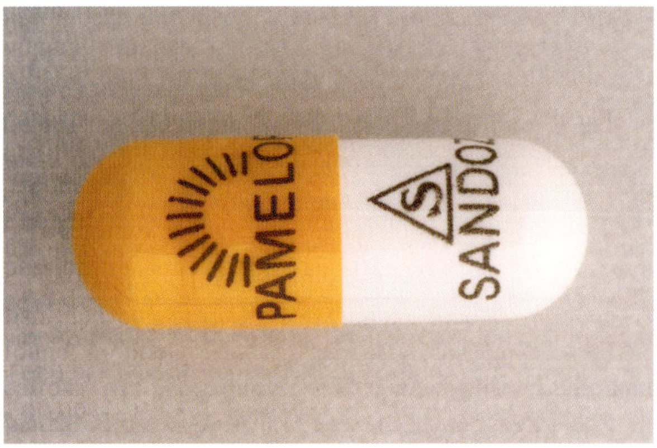

Pamelor (nortriptyline hydrochloride). *(© Custom Medical Stock Photo, Inc. Reproduced by permission.)*

Recommended dosage

As with any antidepressant, the dose of nortriptyline must be carefully adjusted by the physician to produce the desired therapeutic effect. Nortriptyline is available in 10, 25, 50, and 75 mg capsules, as well as in a 10 mg/5mL solution. The usual dosage for nortriptyline is 25 mg given three or four times each day. The optimum total dose of the drug is 50–150 mg daily. Total dosage in excess of 150 mg is not recommended. The recommended dose for older adults (over age 60) and adolescents is 30–50 mg per day. Nortriptyline is not recommended for use by children.

The therapeutic effects of nortriptyline, like other tricyclic antidepressants, appear slowly. Maximum benefit is often not evident for two to three weeks after starting the drug. People taking nortriptyline should be aware of this and continue taking the drug as directed even if they do not see immediate improvement.

Once symptoms of depression have been controlled, the lowest dosage that maintains the effect should be taken. People who take 100 mg or more of nortriptyline per day should have their blood tested periodically for nortriptyline concentrations. The results of these tests will show whether the dose is appropriate, too high, or too low.

Precautions

Like all tricyclic antidepressants, nortriptyline should be used cautiously and with close physician supervision in people, especially the elderly, who have benign prostatic hypertrophy, urinary retention, and glaucoma, especially angle-closure glaucoma (the most severe form). Before starting treatment, people with these conditions should discuss the relative risks and benefits of treatment with their doctors to help determine if nortriptyline is the right antidepressant for them.

Children and adults up to age 24 taking antidepressant drugs, including nortriptyline, are at increased risk for developing suicidal thoughts and actions. Patients of any age taking nortriptyline should be monitored for signs of worsening depression or changes in behavior.

Nortriptyline may increase the possibility of having **seizures**. Patients should tell their physicians if they have a history of seizures, including seizures brought on by the abuse of drugs or alcohol. These people should use nortriptyline only with caution and be closely monitored by their physicians.

When used by people with **schizophrenia**, nortriptyline may worsen **psychosis**, increase hostility in some patients, or activate other symptoms that had not previously been expressed. When used by people with **bipolar disorder**, symptoms of mania may be magnified. Patients with a history of **suicide** attempts, thoughts of suicide, or drug overdose should be monitored carefully when using nortriptyline. Nortriptyline can either increase or decrease blood sugar levels, depending on the patients and their medical conditions. Nortriptyline should be used with great caution when patients are receiving **electroconvulsive therapy**.

Nortriptyline may increase heart rate and cause irregular heartbeat. It may also raise or lower blood pressure. It may be dangerous for people with cardiovascular disease, especially those who have recently had a heart attack, to take this drug or other antidepressants in the same pharmacological class. In rare cases in which patients with cardiovascular disease must receive nortriptyline, they should be monitored closely for cardiac rhythm disturbances and signs of cardiac **stress** or damage.

A common problem with tricyclic antidepressants such as nortriptyline is sedation (drowsiness and lack of physical or mental alertness). This side effect is especially noticeable early in therapy. In most patients, sedation decreases or disappears entirely with time, but until then patients taking nortriptyline should not perform hazardous activities requiring mental alertness or coordination. The sedative effect is increased when nortriptyline is taken with other central nervous system depressants, such as alcoholic beverages, sleeping medications, other **sedatives**, or antihistamines. It may be dangerous to take nortriptyline in combination with these substances.

KEY TERMS

Acetylcholine—A naturally occurring chemical in the body that transmits nerve impulses from cell to cell. Generally, it has opposite effects from dopamine and norepinephrine; it causes blood vessels to dilate, lowers blood pressure, and slows the heartbeat. Central nervous system well-being is dependent on a balance among acetylcholine, dopamine, serotonin, and norepinephrine.

Benign prostate hypertrophy—Enlargement of the prostate gland.

Bipolar syndrome—An abnormal mental condition characterized by periods of intense elation, energy, and activity followed by periods of inactivity and depression.

Catecholamine—A group of neurotransmitters synthesized from the amino acid tyrosine and released by the hypothalamic-pituitary-adrenal system in the brain in response to acute stress. The catecholamines include dopamine, serotonin, norepinephrine, and epinephrine.

Endogenous depression—Depression arising from causes within a person, such as chemical or hormonal imbalances.

Manic—Referring to mania, a state characterized by excessive activity, excitement, or emotion.

Neurotransmitter—A chemical in the brain that transmits messages between neurons, or nerve cells.

Side effects

Nortriptyline shares side effects common to all tricyclic antidepressants. The most frequent of these are dry mouth, constipation, urinary retention, increased heart rate, sedation, irritability, dizziness, and decreased coordination. As with most side effects associated with tricyclic antidepressants, the intensity is highest at the beginning of therapy and tends to decrease with continued use.

Dry mouth, if severe to the point of causing difficulty speaking or swallowing, may be managed by dosage reduction or temporary discontinuation of the drug. Patients may also chew sugarless gum or suck on sugarless candy in order to increase the flow of saliva. Some artificial saliva products may give temporary relief.

Men with prostate enlargement who take nortriptyline may be especially likely to have problems with urinary retention. Symptoms include having difficulty starting a urine flow and more difficulty than usual passing urine. In most cases, urinary retention is managed with dose reduction or by switching to another type of antidepressant.

Problems associated with the skin (loss of sensation, numbness and tingling, rashes, spots, itching, and puffiness), seizures, and ringing in the ears have also been reported. Nausea, vomiting, loss of appetite, diarrhea, and abdominal cramping are associated with nortriptyline usage. Skin rash, sensitivity to sunlight, and itching have been linked to nortriptyline use. People who think they may be experiencing any side effects from this or any other medication should talk to their physicians.

Interactions

Dangerously high blood pressure has resulted from the combination of tricyclic antidepressants, such as nortriptyline, and members of another class of antidepressants known as **monoamine oxidase inhibitors**

(MAOIs). Because of this, nortriptyline should never be taken in combination with **MAOIs**. Patients taking any MAOIs, for example **phenelzine** (Nardil) or **tranylcypromine** (Parnate), should stop taking the MAOI and wait at least 14 days before starting nortriptyline or any other tricyclic antidepressant. The same holds true when discontinuing nortriptyline and starting an MAOI.

Cimetidine (Tagamet) may slow the elimination of nortriptyline, thus increasing the amount of nortriptyline in the body, which can result in toxic levels or increased side effects. Quinidine also raises the circulating levels of the drug, requiring a decrease in the dosage of nortriptyline.

The sedative effects of nortriptyline are increased by other central nervous system depressants such as alcohol, sedatives, sleeping medications, or medications used for other mental disorders such as schizophrenia. The symptoms of increased heart rate, blurred vision, and difficulty urinating are increased when nortriptyline is taken with other drugs such as **benztropine**, **biperiden**, **trihexyphenidyl**, and antihistamines.

Resources

BOOKS

Foreman, John C., and Torben Johansen. *Textbook of Receptor Pharmacology*. 2nd ed. Boca Raton, FL: CRC Press, 2002.

Hall, Sharon M. "Tricyclic Antidepressants in the Treatment of Nicotine Dependence." In *Medication Treatments for Nicotine Dependence,* edited by Tony P. George. Boca Raton, FL: CRC Press, 2007.

Page, Clive P., et al. *Integrated Pharmacology*. 3rd ed. St. Louis: Elsevier, 2006.

Preston, John D., John H. O'Neal, and Mary C. Talaga. *Handbook of Clinical Psychopharmacology for Therapists*. 5th ed. Oakland, CA: New Harbinger Publications, 2008.

PERIODICALS

Foulds, Jonathan, et al. "Developments in Pharmacotherapy for Tobacco Dependence: Past, Present and Future." *Drug and Alcohol Review* 25, no. 1 (January 2006): 59–71.

Hensley, Paula L. "A Review of Bereavement-Related Depression and Complicated Grief." *Psychiatric Annals* 36, no. 9 (September 2006): 619–26.

Hughes, John R., Lindsay F. Stead, and Tim Lancaster. "Nortriptyline for Smoking Cessation: A Review." *Nicotine & Tobacco Research* 7, no. 4 (August 2005): 491–99.

Mulder, Roger T., et al. "Six Months of Treatment for Depression: Outcome and Predictors of the Course of Illness." *American Journal of Psychiatry* 163, no. 1 (January 2006): 95–100.

Shelton, Richard C., et al. "Olanzapine/Fluoxetine Combination for Treatment-Resistant Depression: A Controlled Study of SSRI and Nortriptyline Resistance." *Journal of Clinical Psychiatry* 66, no. 10 (October 2005): 1289–97.

Szanto, Katalin, et al. "Emergence, Persistence, and Resolution of Suicidal Ideation During Treatment of Depression in Old Age." *Journal of Affective Disorders* 98, no. 1–2 (February 2007): 153–61.

Wagena, E. J., P. Knipschild, and M. P. A. Zeegers. "Should Nortriptyline Be Used as a First-Line Aid to Help Smokers Quit? Results from a Systematic Review and Meta-Analysis." *Addiction* 100. no. 3 (March 2005): 317–26.

Wisner, Katherine L., et al. "Postpartum Depression: A Randomized Trial of Sertraline Versus Nortriptyline." *Journal of Clinical Psychopharmacology* 26, no. 4 (August 2006): 353–60.

ORGANIZATIONS

American Medical Association, 515 N State Street, Chicago, IL, 60610, (312) 464-5000, (800) 621-8335, http://www.ama-assn.org.

American Psychiatric Association, 1000 Wilson Blvd., Ste. 1825, Arlington, VA, 22209-3901, (703) 907-7300, apa@psych.org, http://www.psych.org.

American Society for Clinical Pharmacology and Therapeutics, 528 North Washington Street, Alexandria, VA, 22314, (703) 836-6981, http://www.ascpt.org.

American Society for Pharmacology and Experimental Therapeutics, 9650 Rockville Pike, Bethesda, MD, 20814-3995, (301) 634-7060, Fax: (301) 634-7061, http://www.aspet.org.

L. Fleming Fallon, Jr., MD, Dr.P.H.
Ruth A. Wienclaw, PhD

Nutrition counseling

Definition

Nutrition counseling is an ongoing process in which a health professional, usually a registered dietitian, works with an individual to assess his or her usual dietary intake and identify areas where change is needed. The nutrition counselor provides information, educational materials, support, and follow-up to help the individual make and maintain the needed dietary changes.

Purpose

The goal of nutrition counseling is to help a person make and maintain dietary changes. For a person with a mental disorder, dietary change may be needed to promote healthier eating, to adopt a therapeutic diet, or to avoid nutrient-drug interactions. Nutrition counseling is an integral part of treatment for persons with eating disorders or chemical dependencies. Persons taking certain drugs, such as **monoamine oxidase inhibitors**, used to treat

depression and **anxiety disorders**, need to follow a tyramine-controlled diet to avoid dietary interference with their medication. Many drugs used to treat mental disorders can cause weight gain or loss, so persons taking these drugs may also benefit from nutrition counseling.

The nutrition counselor and individual work together to assess current eating patterns and identify areas where change is needed. Registered dietitians have met certain education and experience standards and are well qualified to provide nutrition counseling, but nurses, physicians, and health educators also provide nutrition counseling.

Description

Assessing dietary habits

Nutrition counseling usually begins with an interview in which the counselor asks questions about a person's typical food intake. Nutrition counselors use different methods to assess typical food intake.

The 24-hour recall method is a listing of all the foods and beverages a person consumed within the previous 24-hour period. The nutrition counselor may ask a person to recall the first thing he or she ate or drank the previous morning. The counselor then records the estimated amounts of all the foods and beverages the person consumed the rest of the day. The 24-hour food recall can be used to provide an estimate of energy and nutrient intake. However, people tend to over- or underestimate intake of certain foods, and food intake on one day may not accurately represent typical food intake.

A food frequency questionnaire can sometimes provide a more accurate picture of a person's typical eating patterns. The nutrition counselor may ask the client how often he or she consumes certain food groups. For example, the counselor may ask a person how many servings of dairy products, fruits, vegetables, grains and cereals, meats, or fats he or she consumes in a typical day, week, or month.

Daily food records are also useful in assessing food intake. An individual keeps a written record of the amounts of all foods and beverages consumed over a given period of time. The nutrition counselor can then use the food records to analyze actual energy and nutrient intake. Three-day food records kept over two weekdays and one weekend day are often used.

Assessing body weight

Nutrition counselors may assess an individual's body weight by comparing his or her weight to various weight-for-height tables. A rough rule of thumb for determining a woman's ideal body weight is to allow 100 lb (45 kg) for the first 5 ft (1.5 m) of height plus 5 lb (2.3 kg) for every additional inch. A man is allowed 106 lb (48 kg) for the first 5 ft (1.5 m) of height plus 6 lb (2.7 kg) for every additional inch. However, this guide does not take into account a person's frame size.

Body mass index, or BMI, is another indicator used to assess body weight. BMI is calculated as weight in kilograms divided by height in meters squared. A BMI of 20 to 25 is considered normal weight, a BMI of less than 20 is considered underweight, and a BMI of greater than 25 is considered overweight.

Identifying changes needed

The initial dietary assessment and interview provide the basis for identifying behaviors that need to be changed. Sometimes a person already has a good idea of what dietary changes are needed, but may require help making the changes. Other times the nutrition counselor can help educate a person on the health effects of different dietary choices. The nutrition counselor and client work together to identify areas where change is needed, prioritize changes, and problem-solve as to how to make the changes.

Making dietary change is a gradual process. An individual may start with one or two easier dietary changes the first few weeks and gradually make additional or more difficult changes over several weeks or months. For example, an easy change for a person might be switching from 2% to skim milk, or taking time for a quick yogurt or granola bar in the morning instead of skipping breakfast. More difficult changes might be learning to replace high-fat meat choices with leaner ones, or including more servings of vegetables daily.

In making dietary changes, each individual's situation and background must be carefully considered. Factors that affect food decisions include an individual's ethnic background, religion, group affiliation, socioeconomic status, and world view.

Identifying barriers to change

Once the needed changes have been identified, the client and nutrition counselor think through potential problems that may arise. For example, changing eating behaviors may mean involving others, purchasing different foods, planning ahead for social events, or bringing special foods to work. Some common barriers to changing eating habits include:

- inconvenience
- social gatherings
- food preferences
- lack of knowledge or time
- cost

Setting goals

The nutrition counselor and client set behavior-oriented goals together. Goals should focus on the behaviors needed to achieve the desired dietary change, not on an absolute value, such as achieving a certain body weight. For a person working to prevent weight gain associated with certain medications, for example, his or her goals might be to increase the amount of fruits, vegetables, and whole grains consumed each day. Such changes would help prevent weight gain while placing the emphasis on needed behaviors rather than on actual weight.

Finding support

Family members are encouraged to attend nutrition counseling sessions with the client, especially if they share responsibility for food selection and preparation. Although the individual must make food choices and take responsibility for dietary changes, having the support and understanding of family and friends makes success more likely.

Maintaining changes

The challenge for the nutrition client lies not in making the initial dietary changes, but in maintaining them over the long term. Self-monitoring, realistic expectations, and continued follow-up can help a person maintain dietary changes.

Self-monitoring involves regularly checking eating habits against desired goals and keeping track of eating behaviors. Keeping a food diary on a daily or periodic basis helps the individual be more aware of his or her eating behaviors and provides a ready tool to analyze eating habits. Sometimes a simplified checklist to assure adequate intake of different food groups may be used.

Individuals and nutrition counselors should not expect perfect dietary compliance—slips inevitably occur. The goal is to keep small slips, such as eating a few extra cookies, from becoming big slips, like total abandonment of dietary change. The counselor can help the client identify situations that may lead to **relapse** and plan ways to handle the situations ahead of time.

Nutrition counseling is an ongoing process that can take months or years. In follow-up nutrition counseling sessions, the individual and counselor analyze food records together and problem-solve behaviors that are especially difficult to change. Follow-up counseling also allows the opportunity to reevaluate goals and strategies for achieving those goals.

KEY TERMS

Body mass index, or BMI—A measure of body fat, calculated as weight in kilograms over the square of height in meters.

Food frequency questionnaire—A listing of how often a person consumes foods from certain food groups in a given period of time.

Registered dietitian—A person who has met certain education and experience standards and is well-qualified to provide nutrition counseling.

Twenty-four-hour recall—A listing of the type and amount of all foods and beverages consumed by a person in a 24-hour period.

Resources

BOOKS

American Dietetic Association. *Manual of Clinical Dietetics*. 6th ed. Chicago: American Dietetic Association, 2000.

Hammond, Kathleen A. "Dietary and Clinical Assessment." In *Krause's Food Nutrition, and Diet Therapy*, by L. Kathleen Mahan, Sylvia Escott-Stump, and Janice L. Raymond. Philadelphia: W.B. Saunders Company, 2011.

Hunt, Paula. "Dietary Counseling." In *Essentials of Human Nutrition*, by Jim Mann and A. Stewart Truswell. Oxford: Oxford University Press, 1998.

Mitchell, Mary Kay. *Nutrition Across the Life Span*. Long Grove, IL: Waveland Press, 2008.

PERIODICALS

Harris-Davis, E., and B. Haughton. "Model for Multicultural Nutrition Counseling Competencies." *Journal of the American Dietetic Association* 100, no. 10 (2000): 1178–85.

ORGANIZATIONS

American Dietetic Association, 120 South Riverside Plaza, Ste. 2000, Chicago, IL, 60606, (312) 899-0040, (800) 877-1600, http://www.eatright.org.

Nancy Gustafson, M.S., R.D., F.A.D.A., E.L.S.

Nutrition and mental health

Introduction and overview

A person's food intake affects mood, behavior, and **brain** function. A hungry person may feel irritable and restless, whereas a person who has just eaten a meal may feel calm and satisfied. A sleepy person may feel more productive after a cup of coffee and a light snack. A person who has consistently eaten less food or energy than needed over a long period of time may be apathetic and moody.

Nutrition and the brain

The human brain has high energy and nutrient needs. Changes in energy or nutrient intake can alter both brain chemistry and the functioning of nerves in the brain. Intake of energy and several different nutrients affect levels of chemicals in the brain called **neurotransmitters**. Neurotransmitters transmit nerve impulses from one nerve cell to another, and they influence mood, sleep patterns, and thinking. Deficiencies or excesses of certain vitamins or minerals can damage nerves in the brain, causing changes in memory, limiting problem-solving ability, and impairing brain function.

Nutrition and mental health

Mental health can be influenced by several nutritional factors, including: overall energy intake, intake of the energy-containing nutrients (proteins, carbohydrates, and fats), alcohol intake, and intake of vitamins and minerals. Often deficiencies of multiple nutrients, rather than a single nutrient, are responsible for changes in brain functioning.

In the United States and other developed countries, alcoholism is often responsible for nutritional deficiencies that affect mental functioning. Diseases can also cause nutritional deficiencies by affecting absorption of nutrients into the body or increasing nutritional requirements. Poverty, ignorance, and fad **diets** also contribute to nutritional deficiencies.

Energy intake and mental health

Energy, often referred to as the calorie content of a food, is derived from the carbohydrate, protein, fat, and alcohol found in foods and beverages. Although vitamins and minerals are essential to the body, they provide no energy. The human brain is metabolically very active and uses about 20%–30% of a person's energy intake at rest. Individuals who do not eat adequate calories from food to meet their energy requirements will experience changes in mental functioning. Simply skipping breakfast is associated with lower fluency and problem-solving ability, especially in individuals who are already slightly malnourished. A hungry person may also experience lack of energy or motivation.

Chronic hunger and energy deprivation profoundly affect mood and responsiveness. The body responds to energy deprivation by shutting or slowing down nonessential functions and altering activity levels, hormonal levels, oxygen and nutrient transport, the body's ability to fight infection, and many other bodily functions that directly or indirectly affect brain function. People with a consistently low energy intake often feel apathetic, sad, or hopeless.

Developing fetuses and young infants are particularly susceptible to brain damage from malnutrition. The

KEY TERMS

Antioxidant—A substance that works to counteract the damage done to human tissue by the breakdown of fatty acids. Dietary antioxidants include beta-carotene and vitamins C and E as well as selenium.

Depression—A mental state characterized by feelings of sadness, despair, and discouragement.

Dopamine—A chemical in brain tissue that serves to transmit nerve impulses (a neurotransmitter) and helps to regulate movement and emotions.

Fat-soluble vitamin—A vitamin that dissolves in, and can be stored in, body fat or the liver.

Hormone—A chemical messenger that is produced by one type of cell and travels through the bloodstream to change the metabolism of a different type of cell.

Mineral—An inorganic substance found in the earth that is necessary in small quantities for the body to maintain health. Examples: zinc, copper, iron.

Neurotransmitter—One of a group of chemicals secreted by a nerve cell (neuron) to carry a chemical message to another nerve cell, often as a way of transmitting a nerve impulse. Examples of neurotransmitters include acetylcholine, dopamine, serotonin, and norepinephrine.

Norepinephrine—A hormone released by nerve cells and the adrenal medulla that causes constriction of blood vessels. Norepinephrine also functions as a neurotransmitter.

Serotonin—A widely distributed neurotransmitter that is found in blood platelets, the lining of the digestive tract, and the brain, and that works in combination with norepinephrine. It causes very powerful contractions of smooth muscle and is associated with mood, attention, emotions, and sleep. Low levels of serotonin are associated with depression.

extent of the damage depends on the timing of the energy deprivation in relation to stage of development. Malnutrition early in life has been associated with below-normal intelligence, and functional and cognitive defects.

Carbohydrates and mental health

Carbohydrates include starches, naturally occurring and refined sugars, and dietary fiber. Foods rich in starches and dietary fiber include grain products like breads, rice, pasta, and cereals, especially whole-grain products; fruits; and vegetables, especially starchy vegetables like potatoes. Foods rich in refined sugars include cakes, cookies, desserts, candy, and soft drinks.

Carbohydrates significantly affect mood and behavior. Eating a meal high in carbohydrates triggers release of a hormone called insulin in the body. Insulin helps let blood sugar into cells, where it can be used for energy, but it also has other effects in the body. As insulin levels rise, more tryptophan enters the brain. Tryptophan is an amino acid, or a building block of protein, that affects levels of neurotransmitters in the brain. As more tryptophan enters the brain, more of the neurotransmitter **serotonin** is produced. Higher serotonin levels in the brain enhance mood and have a sedating effect, promoting sleepiness. This effect is partly responsible for the drowsiness some people experience after a large meal.

Some researchers and many parents claim that a high sugar intake causes hyperactivity in children. Although carefully controlled studies do not support this conclusion, high sugar intake is associated with dental problems. Further, foods high in refined sugars are often low in other nutrients, making it prudent to limit their use.

Proteins and mental health

Proteins are made up of amino acids linked together in various sequences and amounts. The human body can manufacture some of the amino acids, but there are eight essential amino acids that must be supplied in the diet. A complete or high-quality protein contains all eight of the essential amino acids in the amounts needed by the body. Foods rich in high-quality protein include meats, milk and other dairy products, and eggs. Dried beans and peas, grains, and nuts and seeds also contain protein, although the protein in these plant foods may be low in one or more essential amino acid. Generally, combining any two types of plant protein foods together will yield a complete, high-quality protein. For example, a peanut butter and jelly sandwich combines grain protein from the bread with nut protein from the peanut butter to yield a complete protein. A bean and corn dish, such as refried beans in a corn tortilla, combines bean and grain protein for another complete protein combination.

Protein intake and intake of individual amino acids can affect brain functioning and mental health. Many of the neurotransmitters in the brain are made from amino acids. The neurotransmitter **dopamine** is made from the amino acid tyrosine. The neurotransmitter serotonin is made from the amino acid tryptophan. If the needed amino acid is not available, levels of that particular neurotransmitter in the brain will fall, and brain functioning and mood will be affected. For example, if there is a lack of tryptophan in the body, not enough serotonin will be produced, and low brain levels of serotonin are associated with low mood and even aggression in some individuals. Likewise, some diseases can cause a buildup of certain amino acids in the blood, leading to brain damage and mental defects. For example, a buildup of the amino acid phenylalanine in individuals with a disease called phenylketonuria (PKU) can cause brain damage and **intellectual disability**. States require testing of newborns for the presence of this metabolic disorder.

Fats and mental health

Dietary intake of fats may also play a role in regulating mood and brain function. Dietary fats are found in both animal and plant foods. Meats, regular-fat dairy products, butter, margarine, and plant oils are high in fats. In terms of health, some of these fats are considered "good fats," and some are considered "bad fats." The "good fats" are unsaturated (the fat's carbon chain is not completely filled in every spot with a hydrogen) and polyunsaturated fats. Some "good" fats, such as olive oil, have been shown to offer some protection against heart disease and some cancers. The "bad fats" include saturated fats (all hydrogen spots are full) and trans fats (also called "partially hydrogenated" fats or oils), which have achieved recent notoriety for their apparent role in reducing levels of HDL cholesterol (the "good" cholesterol). The "bad" fats are considered to increase a person's risk of heart disease and other diseases.

Although numerous studies clearly document the benefits of a cholesterol-lowering diet for the reduction of heart disease risk, some studies suggest that reducing fat and cholesterol in the diet may deplete brain serotonin levels, causing mood changes, anger, and aggressive behavior. Some low-carbohydrate diets, such as the "South Beach Diet," have achieved popularity in part because of their link with beneficial changes in cholesterol levels.

Other studies have looked at the effects of a particular kind of fat, the omega-3 fatty acids found in fish oils, and brain functioning. Although a few studies suggest that omega-3 fatty acids are helpful with bipolar affective disorder and **stress**, results are inconclusive.

High levels of saturated fat in the diet contribute to atherosclerosis, or clogging of the arteries. Atherosclerosis can decrease blood flow to the brain, impairing brain functioning. If blood flow to the brain is blocked, a **stroke** occurs.

Alcohol and mental health

A high alcohol intake can interfere with normal sleep patterns and thus can affect mood. Alcoholism is one of the most common causes of nutritional deficiencies in developed countries. Alcoholic beverages provide energy but virtually no vitamins or minerals. A person who consumes large amounts of alcohol will meet their energy needs but not their vitamin and mineral needs. In addition, extra amounts of certain vitamins are needed to break down alcohol in the body, further contributing to nutrient deficiencies.

Vitamins and mental health

Thiamin

Thiamin is a B vitamin found in enriched grain products, pork, legumes, nuts, seeds, and organ meats. It is intricately involved with metabolizing glucose, or blood sugar, in the body. Glucose is the brain's primary energy source. Thiamin is also needed to make several neurotransmitters.

Alcoholism is often associated with thiamine deficiency. Alcohol interferes with thiamin metabolism in the body, and diets high in alcohol are often deficient in vitamins and minerals. Individuals with a thiamin deficiency can develop **Wernicke-Korsakoff syndrome**, which is characterized by confusion, mental changes, abnormal eye movements, and unsteadiness that can progress to severe memory loss.

Vitamin B-12

Vitamin B-12 is found only in foods of animal origin, like milk, meat, or eggs. Strict vegans who consume no animal-based foods need to supplement their diet with vitamin B-12 to meet the body's need for this nutrient.

Vitamin B-12 is needed to maintain the outer coating, called the myelin sheath, on nerve cells. Inadequate myelin results in nerve damage and impaired brain function. Vitamin B-12 deficiency can go undetected in individuals for years, but it eventually causes low blood iron, irreversible nerve damage, **dementia**, and brain atrophy.

Folic acid

Folic acid is another B vitamin found in foods such as liver, yeast, asparagus, fried beans and peas, wheat, broccoli, and some nuts. Many grain products are also fortified with folic acid. In the United States, alcoholism is a common cause of folic acid deficiency.

Folic acid is involved in protein metabolism in the body and in the metabolism of some amino acids, particularly the amino acid methionine. When folic acid levels in the body are low, methionine cannot be metabolized properly, and levels of another chemical, homocysteine, build up in the blood. High blood homocysteine levels increase the risk of heart disease and stroke.

Even modest folic acid deficiency in women causes an increased risk of neural tube defects, such as spina bifida, in developing fetuses. Folic acid deficiency also increases the risk of stroke. Some studies suggest that folic acid deficiency leads to a range of mental disorders, including **depression**, but this concept remains controversial. Folic acid deficiency can lower levels of serotonin in the brain.

Niacin

The B vitamin niacin is found in enriched grains, meat, fish, wheat bran, asparagus, and peanuts. The body can also make niacin from the essential amino acid tryptophan, which is found in high-quality animal protein foods like meat and milk. Niacin deficiency used to be common in the southern United States, but is now common only in countries such as India and China.

Niacin is involved in releasing energy in the body from carbohydrates, proteins, and fats. A deficiency of niacin produces many mental symptoms such as irritability, headaches, loss of memory, inability to sleep, and emotional instability. Severe niacin deficiency progresses to a condition called pellagra, which is characterized by the four D's: dermatitis (a rash resembling a sunburn), diarrhea, dementia, and ultimately, death. The mental symptoms in pellagra can progress to **psychosis**, **delirium**, coma, and death.

Vitamin B-6

Vitamin B-6, also known as pyridoxine, is found in many plant and animal foods, including chicken, fish, pork, whole-wheat products, brown rice, and some fruits and vegetables. In healthy individuals, deficiency of vitamin B-6 is rare, but certain drugs, including some antidepressant drugs, can induce vitamin B-6 deficiency.

Vitamin B-6 is needed by the body to produce most of the brain's neurotransmitters. It is also involved in hormone production. Although rare, vitamin B-6 deficiency is characterized by mental changes such as **fatigue**, nervousness, irritability, depression, **insomnia**, dizziness, and nerve changes. These mental changes are related to the body's decreased ability to manufacture neurotransmitters with vitamin B-6 deficiency.

Just as vitamin B-6 deficiency causes mental changes, so does excess of vitamin B-6. Vitamin B-6 supplements are used by many individuals for a variety of conditions, including carpal tunnel syndrome, **premenstrual syndrome**, and fibrocystic breast disease. Doses of 500 mg per day or more can cause nerve damage, dizziness, sensory loss, and numbness.

Vitamin E

Vitamin E is a fat-soluble vitamin that is found in plant oils, green leafy vegetables, and fortified breakfast cereals. Vitamin E deficiency is very rare, except in disorders that impair absorption of fat-soluble vitamins into the body, such as cystic fibrosis and liver diseases.

Vitamin E deficiency causes changes in red blood cells and nerve tissues. It progresses to dizziness, vision changes, muscle weakness, and sensory changes. If left untreated, the nerve damage from vitamin E deficiency can be irreversible. Because it is an antioxidant, vitamin E has also been studied for treatment of neurological conditions such as Parkinson's and **Alzheimer's disease**. Vitamin E and other antioxidants, such as vitamin C, had shown some promise in treating Alzheimer's, but larger analyses have found no beneficial effect of vitamin E supplements and have in fact identified a greater association between vitamin E supplementation and death from any cause in Alzheimer's patients. This far, vitamin E has shown no effects in slowing the progression of Parkinson's disease, and the only antioxidant that exhibits even minor effectiveness is coenzyme Q10.

Vitamin A

Vitamin A is a fat-soluble vitamin found in meats, fish, and eggs. A form of vitamin A, beta-carotene, is found in orange and green leafy vegetables such as carrots, yellow squash, and spinach. Headache and increased pressure in the head are associated with both deficient and excess vitamin A intake. Among other effects, excess vitamin A intake can cause fatigue, irritability, and loss of appetite. Generally, doses must exceed 25,000 international units of vitamin A over several months to develop such symptoms.

Minerals and mental health

Iron

Iron is a trace mineral that is essential for formation of hemoglobin, the substance that carries oxygen to cells throughout the body. Iron is found in meat, poultry, and fish. Another form of iron that is not as well absorbed as the form in animal foods is found in whole or enriched grains, green leafy vegetables, dried beans and peas, and dried fruits. Consuming a food rich in vitamin C, such as orange juice, at the same time as an iron-containing plant food will enhance iron absorption from the food.

Iron deficiency eventually leads to anemia, with insufficient oxygen reaching the brain. The anemia can cause fatigue and impair mental functioning. Iron deficiency during the first two years of life can lead to permanent brain damage.

Magnesium

The mineral magnesium is found in green leafy vegetables, whole grains, nuts, seeds, and bananas. In areas with hard water, the water may provide a significant amount of magnesium. In addition to its involvement in bone structure, magnesium aids in the transmission of nerve impulses.

Magnesium deficiency can cause restlessness, nervousness, muscular twitching, and unsteadiness. Acute magnesium deficiency can progress to **apathy**, delirium, convulsions, coma, and death.

Manganese

Manganese is a trace mineral found in whole grains and nuts, and to a lesser extent, fruits and vegetables. It is involved in carbohydrate metabolism and brain functioning. Although very rare, manganese deficiency can cause abnormalities in brain function. Miners of manganese in South America have developed manganese toxicity called "manganese madness," with neurological symptoms similar to Parkinson's disease.

Copper

The richest sources of the trace mineral copper in the diet are organ meats, seafood, nuts, seeds, whole-grain breads and cereals, and chocolate. In addition to other functions, copper is involved in iron metabolism in the body and in brain functioning. Deficiency of copper causes anemia, with inadequate oxygen delivery to the brain and other organs. Copper deficiency also impairs

QUESTIONS TO ASK YOUR DOCTOR

- How can I tell if I am getting the right nutrients?
- How do the nutritional choices I make impact my physical and mental health?
- What dietary changes would you recommend for me?
- What tests or evaluation techniques can you perform to see whether my nutritional choices promote a healthy condition?
- Are there foods I should avoid because of the medications I am taking?
- What physical symptoms or behaviors are important enough that I should seek immediate treatment?

brain functioning and immune system response, including changes in certain chemical receptors in the brain and lowered levels of neurotransmitters.

Zinc

The trace mineral **zinc** is found in red meats, liver, eggs, dairy products, vegetables, and some seafood. Among other functions, zinc is involved in maintaining cell membranes and protecting cells from damage. Zinc deficiency can cause neurological impairment, influencing appetite, taste, smell, and vision. It has also been associated with apathy, irritability, jitteriness, and fatigue.

Selenium

Good sources of the trace mineral selenium include seafood, liver, and eggs. Grains and seeds can also be good sources of selenium, depending on the selenium content of the soil they are grown in. Selenium is needed for the synthesis of some hormones and helps protect cell membranes from damage.

Although selenium deficiency is very rare, selenium toxicity has occurred in regions of the world with high selenium soil content. Selenium toxicity causes nervous system changes, fatigue, and irritability.

Increasing interest in the role of nutrition and mental health

Only within the last 100 years have the scientific and medical communities documented the benefits that good nutrition has on physical and mental health. The medical community recognizes that a proper diet is an important factor in maintaining good physical and mental health, and in preventing and managing many diseases.

According to some studies some mental disorders may be triggered by deficiencies of certain nutrients. For instance, the rates of depression are low in countries where people eat a lot of fish, while the rate of depression steadily rises in the United States as Americans eat increasingly more processed food and less fresh fish and vegetables containing omega-3 fats. In one study, 53% of bipolar patients on placebo (olive oil) became ill again within four months, while none of the patients who were given 9.6 g daily of omega-3 fatty acids (as fish oil) did. Furthermore, a 25% decrease in schizophrenic symptoms was observed in patients receiving eicosapentaenoic acid (EPA), one of the omega-3 fatty acids contained in fish oil.

Balanced nutrition plays a role in preventing coronary heart disease, osteoporosis, weakness, diabetes, obesity, and some mental disorders. In addition to good nutrition, a well–balanced **exercise** program can improve general health, build endurance, and slow many of the effects of aging. The benefits of good nutrition have been shown not only to improve physical health but also to enhance emotional well–being.

Resources

BOOKS

Benton, David., ed. *Lifetime Nutritional Influences on Cognition, Behaviour and Psychiatric Illness.* Philadelphia: Woodhead Publishing, 2011.

Katz, David L., M.D., M.P.H. *Nutrition in Clinical Practice.* New York: Lippincott, Williams, and Wilkins, 2008.

North, Carol, and Sean Yutzy. *Goodwin and Guze's Psychiatric Diagnosis.* New York: Oxford University Press, 2010.

Null, Gary, Ph.D. *The Food-Mood Connection: Nutritional and Environmental Approaches to Mental Health and Physical Wellbeing,* Kindle Edition. New York: Seven Stories Press, 2011.

Sharon, Michael, MD. *Nutrient A-Z: A User's Guide to Foods, Herbs, Vitamins, Minerals & Supplements*, 4th ed. New York: Carlton Publishing Group, 2009.

Shils, Maurice E. *Modern Nutrition in Health and Disease,* 11th ed. New York: Williams and Wilkins, 2012.

Smith, Pamela Wartian, M.D. *What You Must Know About Vitamins, Minerals, Herbs, & More: Choosing the Nutrients That Are Right for You.* Garden City Park, NY: Square One Publishers, Inc., 2008.

PERIODICALS

Boothby, Lisa A., and Paul L. Doering. "Vitamin C and vitamin E for Alzheimer's disase." *The Annals of Pharmacotherapy* 39(2005): 2073–2080.

Golomb, Beatric A., Michael H. Criqui, Halbert White, and Joel E. Dimsdale. "Conceptual foundations of the UCSF statin study." *Archives of Internal Medicine* 164 (2004):153–162.

Lakhan, Shaheen E., and Karen F. Vieira. "Nutritional Therapies for Mental Disorders." *Nutrition Journal* 7, no. 2 (2008). http://dx.doi.org/10.1186/1475-2891-7-2 (accessed November 7, 2011).

Lichtenstein, Alice H. "Dietary fat, carbohydrate, and protein: effects on plasma lipoprotein patterns." *Journal of Lipid Research* 47(2006): 1661–1667.

Parker, Gordon, Gibson, Neville A., Brotchie, Heather, Heruc, Gabriella, Rees, Anne-Marie, and Hadzi-Pavlovic, Dusan. "Omega-3 fatty acids and mood disorders." *American Journal of Psychiatry* 163 (2006): 969–978.

Weber, Cynthia A., and Michael E. Ernst. "Antioxidants, supplements, and Parkinson's disease." *The Annals of Pharmacotherapy* 40(2006): 935–938.

Young, Simon N. "Clinical Nutrition: 3. The Fuzzy Boundary Between Nutrition and Psychopharmacology." *Canadian Medical Association Journal* 166 (2002): 205–209.

WEBSITES

American Academy of Family Physicians. "Nutrition and Mental Health." FamilyDoctor.org. http://familydoctor.org/familydoctor/en/prevention-wellness/emotional-well-being/mental-health/nutrition-and-mental-health.html (accessed November 7, 2011).

ORGANIZATIONS

American Academy of Family Physicians, 11400 Tomahawk Creek Pkwy., Leawood, KS, 66211-2672, (913) 906-6000, (800) 274-2237, Fax: (913) 906-6075, contactcenter@aafp.org, http://www.aafp.org.

American Dietetic Association, 120 South Riverside Plaza, Ste. 2000, Chicago, IL, 60606, (312) 899-0040, (800) 877-1600, http://www.eatright.org.

American Psychiatric Association, 1000 Wilson Blvd., Ste. 1825, Arlington, VA, 22209-3901, (703) 907-7300, apa@psych.org, http://www.psych.org.

Mental Health America, 2000 N. Beauregard Street, 6th Floor, Alexandria, VA, 22311, (703) 684-7722, (800) 969-6642, Fax: (703) 684-5968, http://www1.nmha.org.

National Alliance on Mental Illness (NAMI), Colonial Place Three, 2107 Wilson Blvd., Suite 300, Arlington, VA, 22201, (703) 524-7600, (800) 950-NAMI (6264) Fax: (703) 524-9094, http://www.nami.org/Hometemplate.cfm.

National Institute of Mental Health (NIMH), 6001 Executive Boulevard, Room 8184, MSC 9663, Bethesda, MD, 20892, (301) 443-4513, (866) 615-6464, Fax: (301) 443-4279, nimhinfo@nih.gov, http://www.nimh.nih.gov/index.shtml.

U.S. Food and Drug Administration (FDA), 10903 New Hampshire Ave., Silver Spring, MD, 20993, (888) 463-6332, http://www.fda.gov.

Tish Davidson, A.M.
Nancy Gustafson, M.S., R.D., F.A.D.A., E.L.S.
Laura Jean Cataldo, RN, Ed.D.

O

Obsession

Definition

An obsession is an unwelcome, uncontrollable, and persistent idea, thought, image, or emotion that a person can not help thinking even though it creates significant distress or anxiety.

Description

Obsessive ideas seem unnatural or alien to those who have them, but are nevertheless recognized as originating from the person's own thoughts—they are not seen as **delusions** sent or controlled by an outside party.

Typical obsessions include fear of contamination as from doorknobs or handshakes, worry about leaving things in their proper order, persistent doubts about one's responsible behavior, scary images involving violent acts, and images of sexual acts. People with obsessions may find themselves acting in compulsive ways in largely futile attempts to relieve the anxiety associated with their persistent, unpleasant thoughts. Others suffering from obsessions may try very hard to control or ignore them. It is important to note that legitimate worries about daily concerns—paying bills, studying for exams, keeping a job, interpersonal relationships—are not obsessions. Although they can occasionally be carried to obsessive lengths, these concerns can change with circumstances and, in most cases be controlled, with planning, effort, and action. Obsessions relate to problems that most people would consider far removed from normal, daily events and concerns.

Dean A. Haycock, Ph.D.

Obsessive-compulsive disorder

Definition

Obsessive-compulsive disorder (OCD) is classified as an anxiety disorder marked by the recurrence of intrusive or disturbing thoughts, impulses, images, or ideas (obsessions) accompanied by repeated attempts to suppress these thoughts through the performance of certain irrational and ritualistic behaviors or mental acts (compulsions). The obsessions and compulsions take up large amounts of the patient's time (an hour or longer every day) and usually cause significant emotional distress for the patient and difficulties in patient's relationships with others.

OCD should not be confused with **obsessive-compulsive personality disorder** even though the two disorders have similar names. Obsessive-compulsive

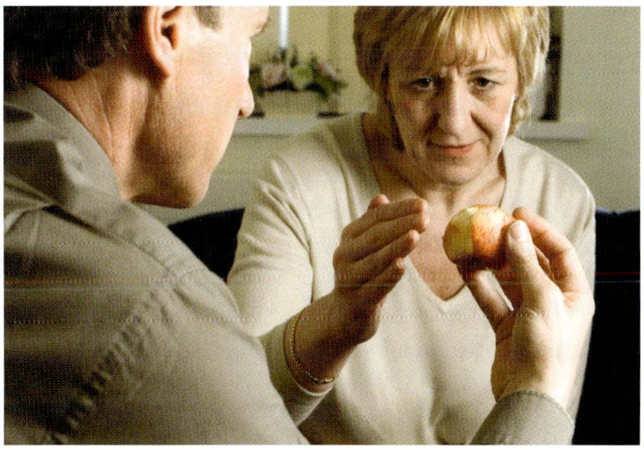

A woman undergoes therapy for obsessive-compulsive disorder (OCD). *(© Phototake. All rights reserved.)*

personality disorder is not characterized by the presence of obsessions and compulsions; rather, it is a lifelong pattern of insistence on control, orderliness, and perfection that begins no later than the early adult years. It is possible, however, for a person to have both disorders.

Demographics

Although descriptions of patients with OCD have been reported since the fifteenth century in religious and medical literature, the condition was widely assumed to be rare until very recently. Epidemiological research since 1980 has now identified OCD as the fourth most common psychiatric illness, after phobias, substance use disorders, and major depressive disorders. OCD is at present classified as a form of anxiety disorder, but current studies indicate that it results from a combination of psychological, neurobiological, genetic, and environmental causes.

According to some estimates, 1 adult in every 50 in North America currently has OCD, and 2 out of 50 have had it at some point in their lives. According to the International OCD foundation, 2–3 million adults in the United States have OCD. It is likely, however, that the disorder is underdiagnosed because many people who suffer from it are embarrassed by their symptoms and often skilled at hiding them from others.

OCD can begin at any age, including childhood; in fact, between one-third and one-half of adults diagnosed with the disorder say that their symptoms began in childhood. The most common age for the emergence of symptoms is between 10 and 24 years, with slightly more women than men being diagnosed with OCD. Childhood OCD is more common in males, and the sex ratio does not favor females until adulthood. People with OCD appear to be less likely to marry than persons diagnosed with other types of mental disorders.

OCD is equally common in all races and ethnic groups in the United States, although patients' specific obsessions are sometimes influenced by their cultural background. For example, fears of violating religious practices or beliefs are reported to be more common among Roman Catholics and Orthodox Jews than among Protestants. Worldwide, cross-cultural studies of OCD indicate that while the incidence of the disorder seems to be about the same in most countries, the symptoms are often shaped by the patient's culture of origin. For example, a patient from a Western country may have a contamination **obsession** that is focused on germs, whereas a patient from India may fear contamination by touching a person from a lower social caste.

Males and females are equally likely to develop OCD; however, males are more likely to begin showing symptoms in childhood and adolescence, and females are more likely to develop symptoms in their early twenties.

Description

OCD is sometimes described as a malfunction of the brain's information processing system. Everyone has upsetting thoughts or impulses from time to time—such as the urge to shout dirty words in public or thinking about hitting someone—but most people are able to let go of these things and not worry about them. A person with OCD, however, gets stuck on the thoughts or impulses and cannot put them aside. These thoughts or impulses are called obsessions. The person who has them may think that he or she is "going crazy" or will not be able to keep from acting on the thoughts. To cope with the anxiety, the person with OCD engages in repetitive behaviors or mental acts to undo, counteract, or control the obsessions. These behaviors are called compulsions.

Common obsessions include fears of contamination by germs or dirt; fear that one has harmed someone; thoughts of violence or of killing a pet or family member; worrying about thoughts that violate one's religious beliefs; and fear of performing sexual acts that the person dislikes. Common compulsions include repeated hand washing or bathing; checking doors or car windows over and over to be sure they are locked; counting objects; insisting that personal possessions like clothes in a closet or items on a desk be arranged "just so"; touching objects in a specific sequence; and **hoarding** items that are not needed.

It is important to recognize that people with OCD are distressed by these behaviors and usually realize that they do not make sense. Compulsions may consume several hours of the patient's day, interfering with work, school, family life, and other activities. They can also be harmful to health; there are instances of people damaging their skin by frequent hand washing or taking long showers. Unlike people with **substance abuse** or eating disorders, people with OCD do not find their rituals pleasurable or satisfying; they are done only to manage their fears.

Studies of families with OCD members indicate that the particular expression of OCD symptoms may be affected by the responses of other people. Families with a high level of tolerance for the symptoms are more likely to have members with more extreme or elaborate symptoms. Problems often occur when the OCD member's obsessions and rituals begin to control the entire family. For example, other family members may find themselves running late for appointments because the OCD member insists on completing their obsessional ritual before they will get in the car.

Risk factors

Known risk factors for OCD include:

- a family history of OCD
- a history of head trauma

- being diagnosed with Tourette syndrome or attention deficit hyperactivity disorder (ADHD)
- a high level of intelligence and education
- higher socioeconomic status
- a pre-existing anxiety disorder, particularly PTSD, phobias, or social anxiety disorder
- high levels of long-term environmental stress

Causes and symptoms

There are various causes and symptoms for obsessive-compulsive disorder.

Causes

At one time it was thought that OCD was caused by childrearing practices that made the person anxious. Such compulsions as repeated washing or checking door locks were explained as rituals intended to please parents who were overly concerned with cleanliness or safety. In the early part of the twentieth century, Sigmund Freud theorized that OCD symptoms were caused by punitive, rigid toilet-training that led to internalized conflicts. This type of psychological explanation is no longer considered useful.

There are several more recent theories about the possible causes of OCD:

- Genetic: It is known that having other family members with OCD increases a person's risk of developing the disorder. Childhood-onset OCD appears to run in families more than adult-onset OCD and is more likely to be associated with tic disorders. Twin studies indicate that monozygotic, or identical twins, are more likely to share the disorder than dizygotic, or fraternal twins. The concordance (match) rate between identical twins is not 100%, however, which suggests that the occurrence of OCD is affected by environmental as well as genetic factors. In addition, it is the general nature of OCD that seems to run in families rather than the specific symptoms; thus, one family member who is affected by the disorder may have a compulsion about washing and cleaning while another is a compulsive counter. Although two genes have been linked to OCD, one discovered in 1994 and the other in 2007, researchers have not yet been able to prove that either or both cause the disorder.
- Abnormally low levels of serotonin in the brain: Serotonin is a chemical produced by the brain that regulates mood, appetite, sleep, and memory. Serotonin affects the efficiency of communication between the front part of the brain (the cortex) and structures that lie deeper in the brain known as the basal ganglia. Dysfunction in the serotonergic system occurs in certain other mental illnesses, including major depression. OCD appears to have a number of features in common with the so-called obsessive-compulsive spectrum disorders, which include Tourette syndrome, Sydenham's chorea, eating disorders, trichotillomania, and delusional disorders. One piece of evidence that supports the serotonin theory is that patients with OCD who are given a type of antidepressant that makes more serotonin available to brain cells obtain some relief from their symptoms. These antidepressants are called selective serotonin reuptake inhibitors, or SSRIs.
- Differences in brain structure: Researchers who have used magnetic resonance imaging (MRI) to map the regions of the brain have found that patients diagnosed with OCD had significantly less white matter in their brains than did normal control subjects. Other studies using positron emission tomography (PET) scanning indicate that OCD patients have patterns of brain activity that differ from those of people without mental illness or with some other mental illness. These findings suggest that there is a widely distributed brain abnormality in OCD.
- Infections: OCD in children has sometimes been attributed to a complication of strep throat. This theory holds that the affected child's body produces antibodies against the strep throat bacteria. The disorders were sometimes referred to as pediatric autoimmune neuropsychiatric disorders associated with streptococcal infections (PANDAS). It was thought that antibodies in the child's blood cross-react with structures in the basal ganglia, producing or worsening the symptoms of OCD or tic disorders. However, this theory is no longer as widely accepted as it was in the 1990s; it is now controversial and considered unproven.

Symptoms

The symptoms of OCD should not be confused with the ability to focus on detail or to check one's work that is sometimes labeled "compulsive" in everyday life. This type of attentiveness is an important factor in academic achievement and in doing well in such fields that require close attention to detail as accounting, medicine, or engineering. By contrast, the symptoms of OCD are serious enough to interfere with the person's daily functioning. Historical examples of OCD include a medieval Englishman named William of Oseney, who spent twelve hours per day reading religious books in order to be at peace with God, and Freud's Rat Man, a patient who had repeated dreams of cursing Freud and covering him with dung. While the Rat Man was ashamed of these impulses and had no explanation for them, he could not control them.

More recent accounts of OCD symptoms include those of a young man who compulsively touched every electrical outlet as he passed, washed his hands several times an hour, and returned home repeatedly to check that the doors and windows were locked. Another account describes a firefighter who was worried that he had throat cancer. He spent three hours a day examining his throat in the mirror, feeling his lymph nodes, and asking his wife if his throat appeared normal.

More common obsessions and compulsions are described below.

CONTAMINATION. People with contamination obsessions are usually preoccupied with a fear of dirt or germs. They may avoid leaving home or allowing visitors to come inside in order to prevent contact with dirt or germs. Some people with contamination obsessions may wear gloves, coats, or even masks if they are forced to leave their house for some reason. Obsessions with contamination may also include abnormal fears of such environmental toxins as lead, asbestos, or radon.

Washing compulsions are commonly associated with contamination obsessions. For example, a person concerned about contamination from the outside may shower and launder all clothing immediately upon coming home. The **compulsion** may be triggered by direct contact with the feared object, but in many cases, even being in its general vicinity may stir up intense anxiety and a strong need to engage in a washing compulsion. The late Howard Hughes exhibited this kind of washing compulsion; he would even burn his clothing after finding out that he had been in the same room with a sick person. Another man who was afraid of contamination could not take even a short walk down the street without experiencing a compulsion to disinfect the soles of his shoes, launder all his clothing, and wash his hands until they were raw after he returned to his apartment.

Washing compulsions may not always be caused by a fear of germs. That is, a need for perfection or for symmetry may also lead to unnecessary washing. In such cases, the individual may be concerned about being perfectly clean or feel that he cannot leave the shower until his left foot has been washed exactly as many times as his right foot. Other people with washing compulsions may be unable to tolerate feeling sweaty or otherwise not clean.

OBSESSIONAL DOUBTING. Obsessional doubting refers to the fear of having failed to perform some task adequately and that dire consequences will follow as a result. Although individuals with this symptom may try to suppress the worrisome thoughts or images, they usually experiences a rising anxiety which then leads to a compulsion to check the task. For example, they may worry about forgetting to lock the door or turn off the gas burner on the stove and spend hours checking these things before leaving home. In one instance, a man was unable to throw away old grocery bags because he feared he might have left something valuable inside one of them. Immediately after looking into an empty bag, he would again have the thought, "What if I missed something in there?" In many cases, no amount of checking is sufficient to dispel the maddening sense of doubt.

NEED FOR SYMMETRY. Persons suffering from an obsession about symmetry often report feeling acutely uncomfortable unless they perform certain tasks in a symmetrical or balanced manner. Thus, crossing one's legs to the right must be followed by crossing legs to the left; scratching one side of the head must be followed by scratching the other; tapping the wall with a knuckle on the right hand must be followed by tapping with one on the left, and so on. Sometimes the person may have a thought or idea associated with the compulsion, such as a fear that a loved one will be harmed if the action is not balanced, but often there is no clearly defined fear, only a strong sense of unease.

AGGRESSIVE AND SEXUAL OBSESSIONS. Aggressive and sexual obsessions are often particularly horrifying to those who experience them. For some people, obsessive fears of committing a terrible act in the future compete with fears that they may already have done something awful in the past. Compulsions to constantly check and confess cause such individuals to admit to evildoing in which they had no part, a phenomenon familiar to law enforcement following highly publicized crimes. These obsessions often involve violent or graphic imagery that is upsetting and disgusting to the person, such as rape, physical assault, or even murder. One case study concerned a young woman who constantly checked the news to reassure herself that she had not murdered anyone that day; she felt deeply upset by unsolved murder cases. A middle-aged man repeatedly confessed to having molested a woman at work, despite no evidence of such an action ever occurring in his workplace.

SYMPTOMS IN CHILDREN. Obsessions and compulsions in children are often focused on germs and fears of contamination. Other common obsessions include fears of harm coming to self or others, fears of causing harm to another person, obsessions about symmetry, and excessive moralizing or religiosity. Global warming is an increasingly common focus of such obsessive moralizing in the twenty-first century.

Childhood compulsions frequently include washing, repeating, checking, touching, counting, ordering, and

KEY TERMS

Basal ganglia—A group of masses of gray matter located in the cerebral hemispheres of the brain that control movement as well as some aspects of emotion and cognition.

Behavioral therapy—An approach to treatment that focuses on extinguishing undesirable behavior and replacing it with desired behavior.

Cognitive-behavioral therapy (CBT)—An approach to psychotherapy that emphasizes the correction of distorted thinking patterns and changing one's behaviors accordingly.

Compulsion—A repeated behavior or mental act carried out to control or neutralize obsessions.

Neurotransmitter—A chemical in the brain that transmits messages between neurons, or nerve cells.

Obsession—A recurrent, distressing, intrusive thought, image, or impulse.

Selective serotonin reuptake inhibitors (SSRIs)—A group of antidepressants that works by increasing the amount of serotonin available to nerve cells in the brain.

Serotonin—A brain chemical that influences mood, anger, anxiety, body temperature, and appetite.

Sydenham's chorea—A serious manifestation of acute rheumatic fever that commonly occurs in children ages 7 through 14, peaking at age 8. This disease of the central nervous system is characterized by emotional instability, purposeless movements, and muscular weakness.

Tic—A sudden involuntary behavior that is difficult or impossible for the person to suppress. Tics may be either motor (related to movement) or vocal, and may become more pronounced under stress.

Trichotillomania—A disorder marked by repeated pulling and tugging of one's hair, usually resulting in noticeable hair loss on the scalp or elsewhere on the body.

arranging. Younger children are less likely to have full-blown anxiety-producing obsessions, but they often report a sense of relief or strong satisfaction (a "just right" feeling) from completing certain ritualized behaviors. Since children are particularly skillful in disguising their OCD symptoms from adults, they may effectively hide their disorder from parents and teachers for years.

Unusual behaviors in children that may be signs of OCD include:

- Avoidance of scissors or other sharp objects. A child may be obsessed with fears of hurting herself or others.
- Chronic lateness or dawdling. The child may be performing checking rituals (e.g., repeatedly making sure all her school supplies are in her bookbag).
- Daydreaming or preoccupation. The child may be counting or performing balancing rituals mentally.
- Spending long periods of time in the bathroom. The child may have a handwashing compulsion.
- Schoolwork handed in late or papers with holes erased in them. The child may be repeatedly checking and correcting her work.

For both children and adults, the symptoms of OCD wax and wane in severity; the specific content of obsessions and compulsions may change over time. The disorder, however, very seldom goes away by itself without treatment. People with OCD in all age groups typically find that their symptoms worsen during major life changes or following highly stressful events.

Diagnosis

The **diagnosis** of OCD is often delayed because patients are often ashamed of their symptoms and skilled at hiding them. It has been estimated that it takes an average of 17 years from the time that a patient's symptoms begin for that person to be diagnosed correctly and receive treatment for OCD. Another reason for the delay is that a person with OCD often has other disorders, including substance abuse disorders, **bipolar disorder**, **panic disorder**, or **depression**, and the OCD symptoms may be attributed to the other disorders. In children, OCD is sometimes misdiagnosed as **autism** or **Tourette syndrome**.

The diagnosis of OCD may also be complicated because of the number of other conditions that resemble it. For example, major depression may be associated with self-perceptions of being guilty, bad, or worthless, which are excessive and unreasonable. Similarly, eating disorders often include bizarre thoughts about size and weight, ritualized eating habits, or the hoarding of food. Delusional disorders may entail unusual beliefs or behaviors, as do such other mental disorders as **trichotillomania**, **hypochondriasis**, the **paraphilias**, and substance use disorders. Thus, accurate diagnosis of OCD depends on the careful analysis of many variables to determine whether the apparent obsessions and compulsions might be better accounted for by some other disorder or to the direct effects of a substance or a medical condition.

In addition, OCD may coexist with other mental disorders, most commonly depression. It has been estimated that about 34% of patients diagnosed with OCD are depressed at the time of diagnosis and that 65% will develop depression at some point in their lives.

Examination

Persons who are thought to have OCD are given a complete **mental status examination**. They are evaluated for memory, disturbances of mood and emotions, the presence of hallucinations or **delusions**, the risk of **suicide** or homicide, and judgment (whether the persons have insight into their symptoms). They should also be evaluated for the presence of Tourette syndrome or other **tic disorders**, as these comorbid diagnoses may influence treatment decisions.

The presence of hair loss, eczema, or scabs or scratches on the skin caused by compulsive washing, trichotillomania, or picking at the skin may be additional evidence for the diagnosis of OCD. There may not, however, be any physical evidence of the disorder.

Tests

There are no laboratory tests for OCD. The primary care doctor will refer the patient to a **psychiatrist** or **psychologist** for a specialized interview. The diagnosis is based on a combination of the patient's symptom history and their answers to a diagnostic questionnaire. The questionnaire most often used is the Yale-Brown Obsessive Compulsive Scale (Y-BOCS). The Y-BOCS has 10 items, five for obsessions and five for compulsions. The questions evaluate the time consumed by symptoms, the extent to which they interfere with functioning, how much they distress the patient, and what the patient has done to try to control the symptoms.

Treatment

There are various treatments for obsessive-compulsive disorder.

Traditional

Treatment for OCD is usually based on a combination of medications and **psychotherapy**.

PSYCHOTHERAPY. Behavioral treatments using the technique of exposure and response prevention (ERP; sometimes called exposure and ritual prevention) are particularly effective in treating OCD. In this form of therapy, the patient and therapist draw up a list, or hierarchy, of the patient's obsessive and compulsive symptoms. The symptoms are arranged in order from least to most upsetting. The patient is then systematically exposed to the anxiety-producing thoughts or behaviors, beginning with the least upsetting. The patient is asked to endure the feared event or image without engaging in the compulsion normally used to lower anxiety. For example, a person with a contamination obsession might be asked to touch a series of increasingly dirty objects without washing their hands. In this way, the patient learns to tolerate the feared object, reducing both worrisome obsessions and anxiety-reducing compulsions. About 75%–80% of patients respond well to exposure and response prevention, with very significant reductions in symptoms.

Other types of psychotherapy have met with mixed results. **Psychodynamic psychotherapy** is helpful to some patients who are concerned about the relationships between their upbringing and the specific features of their OCD symptoms. Cognitive-behavioral psychotherapy may be valuable in helping the patient to become more comfortable with the prospect of exposure and prevention treatments, as well as helping to identify the role that the patient's particular symptoms may play in his or her own life, and what effects family members may have on the maintenance and continuation of OCD symptoms. Cognitive-behavioral psychotherapy is not intended to replace exposure and response prevention but may be a helpful addition to it. The combination of medication and CBT has been shown to be a particularly helpful form of therapy for OCD.

SURGERY. A very small number of patients with severe OCD that does not respond to medications or ERP are treated surgically. The surgeon makes a small cut in a part of the **brain** called the cingulate bundle. This technique produces significant benefits for about 30% of patients who receive the operation. It is considered a treatment of last resort for OCD.

Researchers are studying the effectiveness of newer drugs in treating OCD as well as deep brain stimulation or DBS. In DBS, thin wires are implanted in the parts of the brain that have been linked to OCD symptoms. A battery-powered stimulator sends electrical pulses to the brain at regular intervals in order to interfere with the activity of the nerve cells in the target areas. DBS has already been used to treat Parkinson's disease and is considered an experimental treatment for Tourette syndrome.

In addition to DBS, current **clinical trials** are also exploring the application of **transcranial magnetic stimulation** (TMS) for OCD as a noninvasive treatment approach. In TMS, weak electric currents are induced in brain tissue by rapidly changing magnetic fields. The

QUESTIONS TO ASK YOUR DOCTOR

- What are the warning signs of OCD?
- I have a close relative with OCD. What are the chances that my child will develop the disorder?
- What treatments do you recommend?

Food and Drug Administration (FDA) approved a TMS device called NeuroStar for use in adults in the United States in October 2008.

Drugs

The medications usually prescribed to treat OCD are the **selective serotonin reuptake inhibitors** or **SSRIs**. These drugs work by increasing the amount of **serotonin** available to some of the nerve endings in the brain. Some patients also benefit from the tricyclic antidepressant **clomipramine**.

It is important, however, to know that the SSRIs must be prescribed with care in treating children and adolescents with OCD. Young patients and adults up to age 24 taking antidepressants for **major depressive disorder** have been found to be at increased risk for developing suicidal thoughts and actions. The risk appears to be reduced in patients taking SSRIs for OCD, but all patients taking SSRIs should be monitored for changes in behavior or worsening depression. According to a 2009 article published in the journal American Family Physician, about 15% of persons with OCD make at least one suicide attempt.

Alternative

Because OCD sometimes responds to selective serotonin reuptake inhibitors (SSRI) **antidepressants**, herbalists believe a botanical medicine called **St. John's wort** (*Hypericum perforatum*) might have some beneficial effect as well. Known popularly as "Nature's Prozac," St. John's wort is prescribed by herbalists for the treatment of anxiety and depression. They believe that this herb affects brain levels of serotonin in the same way that SSRI antidepressants do. Herbalists recommend a dose of 300 mg, three times per day. In about one out of 400 people, St. John's wort (like Prozac) may initially increase the level of anxiety. Homeopathic constitutional therapy can help rebalance the patient's mental, emotional, and physical well-being, allowing the behaviors of OCD to abate over time.

Other alternative treatments for OCD are intended to lower the patient's anxiety level; some are thought to diminish the compulsions themselves. Alternative recommendations include the following:

- Bach flower remedies, such as white chestnut for obsessive thoughts and repetitive thinking.
- Traditional Chinese medicine (TCM), specifically a mixture of bupleurum and dong quai, to strengthen the spleen and regulate the liver. (In TCM, obsessive-compulsive disorder is explained as liver stagnation and a weak spleen.)
- Aromatherapy; a mixture of lavender, rosemary, and valerian is thought to promote for relaxation.
- Yoga; yogis in India developed a special technique of yogic breathing specifically for OCD. The specific yogic technique for treating OCD requires blocking the right nostril with the tip of the thumb; slow deep inspiration through the left nostril; holding the breath; and slow complete expiration through the left nostril. This is followed by a long breath-holding out period.
- Schuessler tissue salts; for OCD, specific doses of *Ferrum phosphorica* and tablets of *Kali phosphorica* are recommended daily.
- Massage therapy, with special emphasis on loosening the muscles in the neck, back, and shoulders.

Prognosis

The prognosis of OCD varies from person to person. The disorder rarely goes away on its own. Few OCD patients become completely symptom-free, but about 70% of patients benefit from treatment; however, symptoms may increase and decrease in a cyclical pattern over time. About 15% of patients get steadily worse over time even with treatment and may eventually become unable to function.

Prevention

There is no known way to prevent OCD; however, early diagnosis and prompt treatment can help to prevent the patient's symptoms from getting worse.

Resources

BOOKS

Cobert, Josiane, and Barton Cobert. *100 Questions and Answers about Your Child's Obsessive Compulsive Disorder*. Sudbury, MA: Jones and Bartlett, 2010.

Deane, Ruth. *Washing My Life Away: Surviving Obsessive-Compulsive Disorder*. Philadelphia: Jessica Kingsley, 2005.

Hyman, Bruce M., and Cherry Pedrick. *Obsessive-Compulsive Disorder*. Minneapolis, MN: Twenty-First Century Books, 2009.

Starcevic, Vladan. *Anxiety Disorders in Adults: A Clinical Guide*, 2nd ed. New York: Oxford University Press, 2009.

PERIODICALS

D'Alessandro, T.M. "Factors Influencing the Onset of Childhood Obsessive-Compulsive Disorder." *Pediatric Nursing* 35 (January-February 2009): 43–46.

Fenske, Jill N., and Thomas L. Schwenk. "Obsessive-Compulsive Disorder: Diagnosis and Management." *American Family Physician* 80, no. 3 (2009): 239–245. http://www.aafp.org/afp/2009/0801/p239.html#afp20090801p239-b3 (accessed January 11, 2012).

Huyser, C., et al. "Paediatric Obsessive-Compulsive Disorder, a Neurodevelopmental Disorder? Evidence from Neuroimaging." *Neuroscience and Biobehavioral Reviews* 33 (June 2009): 818–30.

Leckman, J.F., et al. "Symptom Dimensions and Subtypes of Obsessive-Compulsive Disorder: A Developmental Perspective." *Dialogues in Clinical Neuroscience* 11 (2009): 21–33.

Schläpfer, T.E., and B.H. Bewernick. "Deep Brain Stimulation for Psychiatric Disorders—State of the Art." *Advances and Technical Standards in Neurosurgery* 34 (2009): 37–57.

Shulman, S.T. "Pediatric Autoimmune Neuropsychiatric Disorders Associated with Streptococci (PANDAS): Update." *Current Opinion in Pediatrics* 21 (February 2009): 127–30.

WEBSITES

"Obsessive-Compulsive Disorder." National Alliance on Mental Illness. Last modified May 2003. http://www.nami.org/Template.cfm?Section=By_Illness&Template=/TaggedPage/TaggedPageDisplay.cfm&TPLID=54&ContentID=23035 (accessed September 16, 2011).

"Obsessive-Compulsive Disorder (OCD)." National Institute of Mental Health. http://www.nimh.nih.gov/health/topics/obsessive-compulsive-disorder-ocd/index.shtml (accessed September 16, 2011).

"Obsessive-Compulsive Disorder: What It Is and How to Treat It." American Academy of Family Physicians. Last modified May 2010. http://familydoctor.org/online/famdocen/home/common/mentalhealth/anxiety/133.html (accessed September 16, 2011).

ORGANIZATIONS

American Psychiatric Association, 1000 Wilson Blvd., Ste. 1825, Arlington, VA, 22209-3901, (703) 907-7300, apa@psych.org, http://www.psych.org.

Anxiety Disorders Association of America, 8730 Georgia Ave., Silver Spring, MD, 20910, (240) 485-1001, Fax: (240) 485-1035, http://www.adaa.org.

National Alliance on Mental Illness, 2107 Wilson Blvd., Ste. 300, Arlington, VA, 22201-3042, Fax: (703) 524-9094, (800) 950-6264, http://www.nami.org.

National Institute of Mental Health, 6001 Executive Blvd., Rm. 8184, MSC 9663, Bethesda, MD, 20892-9663, (301) 433-4513; TTY: (301) 443-8431, Fax: (301) 443-4279, (866) 615-6464; TTY: (866) 415-8051, nimhinfo@nih.gov, http://www.nimh.nih.gov.

Obsessive Compulsive Foundation, PO Box 961029, Boston, MA, 02196, (617) 973-5801, http://www.ocfoundation.org.

Jane A. Fitzgerald
Rebecca J. Frey, PhD

Obsessive-compulsive personality disorder

Definition

Obsessive-compulsive personality disorder (OCPD) is a type of personality disorder marked by rigidity, control, perfectionism, and an overconcern with work at the expense of close interpersonal relationships. Persons with this disorder often have trouble relaxing because they are preoccupied with details, rules, and productivity. They are often perceived by others as stubborn, stingy, self-righteous, and uncooperative.

Obsessive-compulsive personality disorder is included in the ***Diagnostic and Statistical Manual of Mental Disorders** (DSM)*, a handbook used by medical professionals in diagnosing mental disorders. Personality disorders are defined by the DSM as causing significant impairments in relations with the self (sense of identity) and others. The World Health Organization's *International Classification of Diseases* (ICD), which is the European counterpart of the *DSM*, refers to OCPD as "anankastic personality disorder."

It is important to distinguish between OCPD and **obsessive-compulsive disorder** (OCD), which is an anxiety disorder characterized by the presence of intrusive or disturbing thoughts, impulses, images or ideas (obsessions), accompanied by repeated attempts to suppress these thoughts through the performance of irrational and ritualistic behaviors or mental acts (compulsions). It is unusual but possible, however, for a patient to suffer from both disorders, especially in extreme cases of **hoarding** behavior. In some reported cases of animal hoarding, the people involved appear to have symptoms of both OCD and OCPD.

Demographics

Obsessive-compulsive personality disorder is estimated to occur in about 1% of the population, although rates of 3–10% are reported among psychiatric outpatients. The disorder is usually diagnosed in late adolescence or young adulthood. In the United States, OCPD occurs almost twice as often in men as in women.

Some researchers attribute this disproportion to gender stereotyping, in that men have greater permission from general Western culture to act in stubborn, withholding, and controlling ways.

Description

People suffering from OCPD have careful rules and procedures for conducting many aspects of their everyday lives. While their goal is to accomplish things in a careful, orderly manner, their desire for perfection and insistence on going "by the book" often overrides their ability to complete a task. For example, one patient with OCPD was so preoccupied with finding a mislaid shopping list that he took much more time searching for it than it would have taken him to rewrite the list from memory. This type of inflexibility typically extends to interpersonal relationships. People with OCPD are known for being highly controlling and bossy toward other people, especially subordinates. They will often insist that there is one and only one right way (their way) to fold laundry, cut grass, drive a car, or write a report. In addition, they are so insistent on following rules that they cannot allow for what most people would consider legitimate exceptions. Their attitudes toward their own superiors or supervisors depend on whether they respect these authorities. People with OCPD are often unusually courteous to superiors that they respect, but resistant to or contemptuous of those they do not respect.

While work environments may reward their conscientiousness and attention to detail, people with OCPD do not show much spontaneity or imagination. They may feel paralyzed when immediate action is necessary; they feel overwhelmed by trying to make decisions without concrete guidelines. They expect colleagues to stick to detailed rules and procedures, and often perform poorly in jobs that require flexibility and the ability to compromise. Even when people with OCPD are behind schedule, they are uncomfortable delegating work to others because the others may not do the job "properly." People with OCPD often get so lost in the finer points of a task that they cannot see the larger picture; they are frequently described as "unable to see the forest for the trees." They are often highly anxious in situations without clearly defined rules because such situations arouse their fears of making a mistake and being punished for it. An additional feature of this personality disorder is stinginess or miserliness, frequently combined with an inability to throw out worn-out or useless items. This characteristic has sometimes been described as "pack rat" behavior.

People diagnosed with OCPD come across to others as difficult and demanding. Their rigid expectations of others are also applied to themselves, however; they tend to be intolerant of their own short-comings. Such persons feel bound to present a consistent facade of propriety and control. They feel uncomfortable with expressions of tender feelings and tend to avoid relatives or colleagues who are more emotionally expressive. This strict and ungenerous approach to life limits their ability to relax; they are seldom if ever able to release their needs for control. Even recreational activities frequently become another form of work. A person with OCPD, for example, may turn a tennis game into an opportunity to perfect his or her backhand rather than simply enjoying the **exercise**, the weather, or the companionship of the other players. Many OCPD sufferers bring office work along on vacations in order to avoid "wasting time," and feel a sense of relief upon returning to the structure of their work environment. Not surprisingly, this combination of traits strains their interpersonal relationships and can lead to a lonely existence.

Causes and symptoms

Causes

No single specific cause of OCPD has been identified. Since the early days of Freudian **psychoanalysis**, however, faulty parenting has been viewed as a major factor in the development of personality disorders. Current studies have tended to support the importance of early life experiences, finding that healthy emotional development largely depends on two important variables: parental warmth and appropriate responsiveness to the child's needs. When these qualities are present, the child feels secure and appropriately valued. By contrast, many people with personality disorders did not have parents who were emotionally warm toward them. Patients with OCPD often recall their parents as being emotionally withholding and either overprotective or overcontrolling. One researcher has noted that people with OCPD appear to have been punished by their parents for every transgression of a rule, no matter how minor, and rewarded for almost nothing. As a result, the child is unable to safely develop or express a sense of joy, spontaneity, or independent thought; and begins to develop the symptoms of OCPD as a strategy for avoiding punishment. Children with this type of upbringing are also likely to choke down the anger they feel toward their parents; they may be outwardly obedient and polite to authority figures, but at the same time treat younger children or those they regard as their inferiors harshly.

Genetic contributions to OCPD have not been well documented. Cultural influences may, however, play a part in the development of OCPD. That is, cultures that are highly authoritarian and rule-bound may encourage child-rearing practices that contribute to the development of OCPD. On the other hand, simply because a culture is comparatively strict or has a strong work ethic does not mean it is necessarily unhealthful. In Japanese societies, for example, excessive devotion to work, restricted emotional expression, and moral scrupulosity are highly valued characteristics that are rewarded within that culture. Similarly, certain religions and professions require exactness and careful attention to rules in their members; the military is one example. OCPD is not diagnosed in persons who are simply behaving in accordance with such outside expectations as military regulations or the rule of a religious order. Appropriate evaluation of persons from other cultures requires close examination in order to differentiate people who are merely following culturally prescribed patterns from people whose behaviors are excessive even by the standards of their own culture.

Symptoms

The symptoms of OCPD include a pervasive overconcern with mental, emotional, and behavioral control of the self and others. Excessive conscientiousness means that people with this disorder are generally poor problem-solvers and have trouble making decisions; as a result, they are frequently highly inefficient. Their need for control is easily upset by schedule changes or minor unexpected events. While many people have some of the following characteristics, a person who meets the *DSM-IV-TR* criteria for OCPD must display at least four of them:

- Preoccupation with details, rules, lists, order, organization, or schedules to the point at which the major goal of the activity is lost.
- Excessive concern for perfection in small details that interferes with the completion of projects.
- Dedication to work and productivity that shuts out friendships and leisure-time activities, when the long hours of work cannot be explained by financial necessity.
- Excessive moral rigidity and inflexibility in matters of ethics and values that cannot be accounted for by the standards of the person's religion or culture.
- Hoarding things, or saving worn-out or useless objects even when they have no sentimental or likely monetary value.
- Insistence that tasks be completed according to one's personal preferences.
- Stinginess with the self and others.
- Excessive rigidity and obstinacy.

Diagnosis

It is relatively unusual for OCPD to be diagnosed as the patient's primary reason for making an appointment with their doctor. In many cases the person with OCPD is unaware of the discomfort that his or her stubbornness and rigidity cause other people, precisely because these traits usually enable them to get their way with others. They are more likely to enter therapy because of other issues. **Diagnosis** of OCPD depends on careful observation and appropriate assessment of the individual's behavior; the person must not only give evidence of the attitudes and behaviors associated with OCPD, but these must be severe enough to interfere with their occupational and interpersonal functioning.

The differential diagnosis will include distinguishing between obsessive-compulsive disorder (OCD) and OCPD. A person who has obsessions and compulsions that they experience as alien and irrational is more likely to be suffering from OCD, whereas the person who feels perfectly comfortable with self-imposed systems of extensive rules and procedures for mopping the kitchen floor probably has OCPD. In addition, the thoughts and behaviors that are found in OCD are seldom relevant to real-life problems; by contrast, people with OCPD are preoccupied primarily with managing (however inefficiently) the various tasks they encounter in their daily lives.

Some features of OCPD may occur in other personality disorders. For example, a person with a **narcissistic personality disorder** may be preoccupied with perfection and be critical and stingy toward others; narcissists are usually generous with themselves, however, while people with OCPD are self-critical and reluctant to spend money even on themselves. Likewise, a person with **schizoid personality disorder**, who lacks a fundamental capacity for intimacy, may resemble someone with OCPD in being formal and detached in dealing with others. The difference here is that a person with OCPD, while awkward in emotional situations, is able to experience caring and may long for close relationships. Certain medical conditions may also mimic OCPD, but are distinct in that the onset of the symptoms is directly related to the illness. Certain behaviors related to **substance abuse** may also be mistaken for symptoms of OCPD, especially if the substance problem is unrecognized.

As described earlier, diagnosis may also be complicated by the fact that behaviors similar to OCPD may be normal variants within a given culture, occupation, or religion; however, in order to fulfill criteria for the personality disorder, the behaviors must be sufficiently severe as to impair the patient's functioning.

Treatment

Psychotherapy

Psychotherapeutic approaches to the treatment of OCPD have found insight-oriented psychodynamic techniques and **cognitive-behavioral therapy** to be helpful for many patients. This choice of effective approaches stands in contrast to the limitations of traditional forms of **psychotherapy** with most patients diagnosed with OCD. Learning to find satisfaction in life through close relationships and recreational outlets, instead of only through work-related activities, can greatly enrich the OCPD patient's quality of life. Specific training in relaxation techniques may help patients diagnosed with OCPD who have the so-called "Type A" characteristics of competitiveness and time urgency as well as preoccupation with work.

It is difficult, however, for a psychotherapist to develop a therapeutic alliance with a person with OCPD. The patient comes into therapy with a powerful need to control the situation and the therapist; a reluctance to trust others; and a tendency to doubt or question almost everything about the therapy situation. The therapist must be alert to the patient's defenses against genuine change and work to gain a level of commitment to the therapeutic process. Without this commitment, the therapist may be fooled into thinking that therapy has been successful when, in fact, the patient is simply being superficially compliant.

Medications

For many years, medications for OCPD and other personality disorders were thought to be ineffective since they did not affect the underlying causes of the disorder. More recent studies, however, indicate that treatment with specific drugs may be a useful adjunct (help) to psychotherapy. In particular, the medications known as **selective serotonin reuptake inhibitors (SSRIs)** appear to help the OCPD patient with his or her rigidity and compulsiveness, even when the patient did not show signs of pre-existing **depression**. Medication can also help the patient to think more clearly and make decisions better and faster without being so distracted by minor details. While symptom control may not "cure" the underlying personality disorder, medication does enable some OCPD patients to function with less distress.

Prognosis

Individuals with OCPD often experience a moderate level of professional success, but relationships with a spouse or children may be strained due to their combination of emotional detachment and controlling behaviors. In addition, people with OCPD often do not attain the level of professional achievement that might be predicted for their talents and abilities because their rigidity and stubbornness make them poor "team players" or supervisors. Although there are few large-scale outcome studies of treatments for OCPD, existing reports suggest that these patients do benefit from psychotherapy to help them understand the emotional issues underlying their controlling behaviors and to teach them how to relax. Since OCPD sufferers, unlike people with OCD, usually view their compulsive behaviors as voluntary, they are better able to consider change, especially as they come to fully recognize the personal and interpersonal costs of their disorder.

KEY TERMS

Anankastic personality disorder—The European term for obsessive-compulsive personality disorder.

Compulsion—A strong impulse to perform an act, particularly one that is irrational or contrary to one's will.

Obsession—A persistent image, idea, or desire that dominates a person's thoughts or feelings.

Therapeutic alliance—The technical term for the cooperative relationship between therapist and patient that is considered essential for successful psychotherapy.

Prevention

Most theories attribute the development of OCPD to early life experiences, including a lack of parental warmth; parental overcontrol and rigidity, and few rewards for spontaneous emotional expression. Little work has been done, however, in identifying preventive strategies.

Resources

BOOKS

Alarcon, Renato D., Edward F. Foulks, and Mark Vakkur. *Personality Disorders and Culture*. New York: John Wiley and Sons, 1998.

Baer, Lee. "Personality Disorders in Obsessive-Compulsive Disorder." In *Obsessive-Compulsive Disorders: Practical Management*, by Michael Jenike, Lee Baer, and William E. Minichiello. 3rd ed. St. Louis: Mosby, 1998.

Jenike, Michael. "Psychotherapy of Obsessive-Compulsive Personality." In *Obsessive-Compulsive Personality Disorders: Practical Management*, edited by Michael Jenike,

Lee Baer, and William E. Minichiello. 3rd ed. St. Louis: Mosby, 1998.

Kay, Jerald, Allen Tasman, and Jeffery Liberman. "Obsessive-Compulsive Disorder." In *Psychiatry: Behavioral Science and Clinical Essentials*, edited by Michael Jenike, Lee Baer, and William Minichiello. Philadelphia: W.B. Saunders, 2000.

Millon, Theodore. *Personality-Guided Therapy*. New York: John Wiley and Sons, 1999.

World Health Organization (WHO). *The ICD-10 Classification of Mental and Behavioural Disorders*. Geneva: WHO, 1993.

PERIODICALS

Barber, Jacques P., et al. "Alliance Predicts Patients' Outcome Beyond In-Treatment change in Symptoms." *Journal of Consulting and Clinical Psychology* 68, no. 6 (December 2000); 1027–1032.

Nordahl, Hans M., and Tore C. Stiles. "Perceptions of Parental Bonding in Patients with Various Personality Disorders, Lifetime Depressive Disorders, and Healthy Controls." *Journal of Personality Disorders* 11, no. 4 (1997): 391–402.

Samuels, Jack, et al. "Personality Disorders and Normal Personality Dimensions in Obsessive-Compulsive Disorder." *British Journal of Psychiatry* 177 (2000) 457–462.

Zaider, Talia, Jeffrey G. Johnson, and Sarah J. Cockell. "Psychiatric Comorbidity Associated with Eating Disorder Symptomatology Among Adolescents in the Community." *International Journal of Eating Disorders* 28, no. 1 (July 2000): 58–67.

ORGANIZATIONS

Anxiety Disorders Association of America, 8730 Georgia Ave., Silver Spring, MD, 20910, (240) 485-1001, Fax: (240) 485-1035, http://www.adaa.org.

Freedom From Fear, 308 Seaview Ave., Staten Island, NY, 10305, (718) 351-1717, help@freedomfromfear.org, http://www.freedomfromfear.org.

Jane A. Fitzgerald, Ph.D.

Olanzapine

Definition

Olanzapine is classified as an atypical antipsychotic drug. It is available in the United States under the brand names Zyprexa and Zyprexa Zydis.

Purpose

Olanzapine is used to treat **schizophrenia** and to control manic episodes of **bipolar disorder**. It may be prescribed off-label to treat symptoms of **dementia** related to **Alzheimer's disease** but is not approved by the U.S. Food and Drug Administration (FDA) for this purpose.

Description

Olanzapine is thought to modify the actions of several chemicals in the **brain**. Olanzapine is chemically related to another atypical antipsychotic agent, **clozapine**, but differs both chemically and pharmacologically from the earlier phenothiazine antipsychotics.

Olanzapine is available as 2.5 mg, 5 mg, 7.5 mg, 10 mg, 15 mg, and 20 mg tablets that can be swallowed (Zyprexa) and 5 mg, 10 mg, 15 mg, and 20 mg tablets that disintegrate when placed under the tongue (Zyprexa Zydis). Olanzapine is broken down by the liver.

A new, long-acting injection form of olanzapine is also available to treat schizophrenia, which obviates some of the issues of medication adherence that often complicate treatment. This form maintains therapeutic levels for 2–4 weeks.

Recommended dosage

Recently, the effectiveness of olanzapine was evaluated in the Clinical Antipsychotic Trials of **Intervention** Effectiveness (**CATIE**) Schizophrenia Study. This study evaluated the effectiveness and side effects of atypical antipsychotics, including olanzapine, in comparison to a conventional antipsychotic drug in the treatment of schizophrenia.

The study found that the conventional antipsychotic generally was equally effective and tolerated as well as the newer, more expensive, atypical antipsychotic medications. Of the atypical antipsychotics, olanzapine performed somewhat better than the other drugs being investigated. Patients taking this drug were less likely to be hospitalized for psychotic **relapse** and tended to stay on their medication longer. However, patients on olanzapine also tended to gain significant weight and experience other metabolic changes associated with diabetes than did patients taking the other drugs in the study.

Olanzapine and another atypical, **risperidone**, tended to be better tolerated than the other atypical antipsychotics investigated, although only 35% of participants on olanzapine were able to continue taking it throughout the entire 18 months of the study. Participants who stopped taking their antipsychotic medication in Phase 1 because it was not adequately controlling their symptoms were more likely to stay on their medication if they were switched to olanzapine or risperidone rather than to **quetiapine** or **ziprasidone**. There was no difference among the four medications

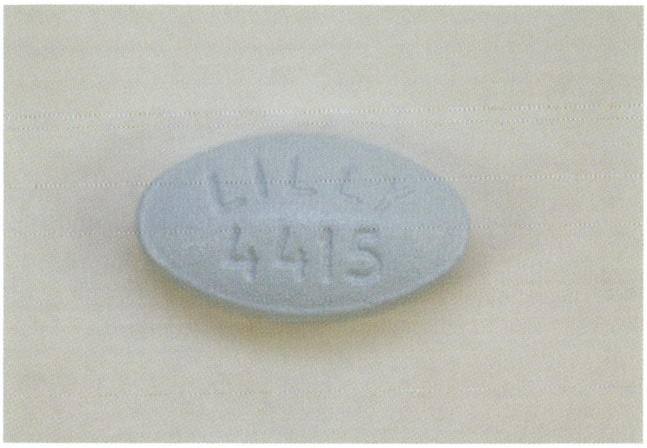

Zyprexa (olanzapine), 15 mg. *(© Custom Medical Stock Photo, Inc. Reproduced by permission.)*

tested in Phase 2, however, for participants who had stopped taking their Phase 1 medication because they experienced adverse side effects.

In Phase 2 of the study, the drug clozapine was more effective in controlling symptoms than the other atypical antipsychotics under evaluation. For patients whose symptoms were not well controlled on clozapine, olanzapine and risperidone tended to be more effective than the drugs ziprasidone or quetiapine.

The dosage of olanzapine varies depending upon the reason for its use. When used to treat schizophrenia, 5–10 mg is the typical starting dosage. If dosage adjustments are needed, increases are made in 5 mg increments once a week. When treating schizophrenia, a total daily dosage of 10–15 mg is usually effective. When olanzapine is used to treat acute manic episodes, initial doses of olanzapine are often 10–15 mg, and 20 mg per day may be needed for maximum effect. The safety of doses greater than 20 mg per day has not been determined.

Olanzapine is eliminated from the body more quickly in young people than in older (over age 60) individuals, in men more quickly than in women, and in smokers more quickly than in nonsmokers. Dosage adjustments may be needed based upon individual patient characteristics.

Precautions

Caution should be used in patients with heart disease because the drug may cause blood pressure to fall too low, resulting in dizziness, rapid heartbeats, or fainting. Olanzapine should be used carefully in people with known seizure disorders since olanzapine may alter properties of the brain, making **seizures** occur more easily. People with liver disease should have their liver function monitored regularly while taking olanzapine. Women who are pregnant or breast-feeding should not take olanzapine. Babies born to mothers who took olanzapine during pregnancy may develop extrapyramidal symptoms (EPS) and withdrawal symptoms, including agitation, trouble breathing, and difficulty feeding. People with phenylketonuria, a disorder in which the body is unable to metabolize a protein called phenylalanine, should avoid olanzapine disintegrating tablets, because this form of the drug contains phenylalanine. Olanzapine has also been associated with the risk of developing a blood disorder.

Like other antipsychotic medications, olanzapine carries a warning regarding use in elderly people with dementia, who suffer from an increased risk of death during treatment with these agents. The reason for the increase was unclear in studies, but most deaths were found to be related to either cardiovascular complications or complications associated with infection. Olanzapine is not approved by the FDA for the treatment of behavior problems in older adults with dementia.

Side effects

Side effects that occur in more than 5% of patients taking olanzapine include involuntary movements, weakness, dizziness, extreme drowsiness, nonviolent objectionable behavior, constipation, weight gain, dry mouth, low blood pressure, stomach upset, increased appetite, cold-like symptoms, or fever.

Other side effects that are possible include rash, body aches and pains, elevated liver enzymes, vision abnormalities, chest pain, or rapid heartbeats.

Olanzapine has the potential to produce a serious side effect called **tardive dyskinesia**. This syndrome consists of involuntary, uncoordinated movements that may appear late in therapy and that may not disappear even after the drug is stopped. Tardive dyskinesia involves involuntary movements of the tongue, jaw, mouth, face, or other groups of skeletal muscles. The incidence of tardive dyskinesia increases with increasing age and with increasing dosage of olanzapine. Women are at greater risk than men for developing tardive dyskinesia. There is no known effective treatment for tardive dyskinesia, although gradual (but rarely complete) improvement may occur over a long period.

An occasionally reported side effect of olanzapine is **neuroleptic malignant syndrome**. This is a complicated and potentially fatal condition characterized by muscle rigidity, high fever, alterations in mental status, and cardiac symptoms such as irregular pulse or blood pressure, sweating, tachycardia (fast heartbeat), and arrhythmias (irregular heartbeat).

KEY TERMS

Extrapyramidal symptoms—A group of side effects associated with antipsychotic medications and characterized by involuntary muscle movements, including contraction and tremor.

Off-label use—Drugs in the United States are approved by the Food and Drug Administration (FDA) for specific uses based on the results of clinical trials. However, it is legal for physicians to administer these drugs for other "off-label" uses. It is not legal for pharmaceutical companies to advertise drugs for off-label uses.

Interactions

Any drug that causes drowsiness may lead to decreased mental alertness and impaired motor skills when taken with olanzapine. Some examples include alcohol, **antidepressants** such as **imipramine** (Tofranil) or **paroxetine** (Paxil), antipsychotics such as **thioridazine** (Mellaril), and some antihistamines. Because olanzapine may lower blood pressure, it may reduce blood pressure to dangerously low levels if taken with drugs that are used to treat high blood pressure. **Carbamazepine** (Tegretol), a drug commonly used to treat seizures, may decrease the effectiveness of olanzapine.

Resources

BOOKS

Physicians' Desk Reference 2011. 66th ed. Montvale, NJ: PDR Network, 2011.

Preston, John D., John H. O'Neal, and Mary C. Talaga. *Handbook of Clinical Psychopharmacology for Therapists*. 5th ed. Oakland, CA: New Harbinger Publications, 2008.

Wolters Kluwer Health. *Drug Facts and Comparisons 2012*. 66th ed. St. Louis: Lippincott, Williams & Wilkins, 2011.

PERIODICALS

Casey, Daniel E. "Implications of the CATIE Trial on Treatment: Extrapyramidal Symptoms." *CNS Spectrums* 11, no. 7, Supp. 7 (July 2006): 25–31.

Gentile, Salvatore. "Extrapyramidal Adverse Events Associated with Atypical Antipsychotic Treatment of Bipolar Disorder." *Journal of Clinical Psychopharmacology* 27, no. 1 (February 2007): 35–45.

Glick, Ira D. "Understanding the Results of CATIE in the Context of the Field." *CNS Spectrums* 11, no. 7, Supp. 7 (July 2006): 40–47.

Haro, Josep Maria, et al. "Remission and Relapse in the Outpatient Care of Schizophrenia: Three-Year Results from the Schizophrenia Outpatient Health Outcomes Study." *Journal of Clinical Psychopharmacology* 26, no. 6 (December 2006): 571–78.

Harvey, Philip D., Christopher R. Bowie, and Antony Loebel. "Neuropsychological Normalization with Long-Term Atypical Antipsychotic Treatment: Results of a Six-Month Randomized, Double-Blind Comparison of Ziprasidone vs. Olanzapine." *Journal of Neuropsychiatry & Clinical Neurosciences* 18, no. 1 (February 2006): 54–63.

Jarema, Marek. "Atypical Antipsychotics in the Treatment of Mood Disorders." *Current Opinion in Psychiatry* 20, no. 1 (January 2007): 23–29.

Kinon, Bruce J., et al. "Randomized, Double-Blind 6-Month Comparison of Olanzapine and Quetiapine in Patients with Schizophrenia or Schizoaffective Disorder with Prominent Negative Symptoms and Poor Functioning." *Journal of Clinical Psychopharmacology* 26, no. 5 (October 2006): 453–61.

Lieberman, Jeffrey A., et al. "Effectiveness of Antipsychotic Drugs in Patients with Chronic Schizophrenia." *New England Journal of Medicine* 353, no. 12 (September 2005): 1209–23.

Lipkovich, I., et al. "Predictors of Risk for Relapse in Patients with Schizophrenia or Schizoaffective Disorder During Olanzapine Drug Therapy." *Journal of Psychiatric Research* 41, no. 3–4 (April–June 2007): 305–10.

McCue, Robert E., et al. "Comparative Effectiveness of Second-Generation Antipsychotics and Haloperidol in Acute Schizophrenia." *British Journal of Psychiatry* 189 (November 2006): 433–40.

McEvoy, Joseph P., et al. "Effectiveness of Clozapine Versus Olanzapine, Quetiapine, and Risperidone in Patients with Chronic Schizophrenia Who Did Not Respond to Prior Atypical Antipsychotic Treatment." *American Journal of Psychiatry* 163, no. 4 (April 2006): 600–10.

Meltzer, Herbert Y., and William V. Bobo. "Interpreting the Efficacy Findings in the CATIE Study: What Clinicians Should Know." *CNS Spectrums* 11, Supp. 7 (July 2006): 14–24.

Morrens, Manuel, et al. "Psychomotor and Memory Effects of Haloperidol, Olanzapine, and Paroxetine in Healthy Subjects After Short-Term Administration." *Journal of Clinical Psychopharmacology* 27, no. 1 (February 2007): 15–21.

Nasrallah, Henry A. "Metabolic Findings From the CATIE Trial and Their Relation to Tolerability." *CNS Spectrums* 11, no. 7, Supp. 7 (July 2006): 32–39.

Schneider, Lon S., et al. "Effectiveness of Atypical Antipsychotic Drugs in Patients with Alzheimer's Disease." *New England Journal of Medicine* 355, no. 15 (October 2006): 1525–38.

Stroup, T. Scott, et al. "Effectiveness of Olanzapine, Quetiapine, Risperidone, and Ziprasidone in Patients with Chronic Schizophrenia Following Discontinuation of a Previous Atypical Antipsychotic." *American Journal of Psychiatry* 163, no. 4 (April 2006): 611–22.

Kelly Karpa, R.Ph., PhD
Ruth A. Wienclaw, PhD

Opioids and related disorders

Definition

Opioids are a class of drugs that include both natural and synthetic substances. The natural opioids (referred to as "opiates") include opium and morphine. Heroin, the most abused opioid, is synthesized from opium. Other synthetics (only made in laboratories) and commonly prescribed for pain, such as cough suppressants, or as anti-diarrhea agents, include codeine, oxycodone (OxyContin), meperidine (Demerol), fentanyl (Sublimaze), hydromorphone (Dilaudid), **methadone**, and propoxyphene (Darvon). Heroin is usually injected, either intravenously (into a vein) or subcutaneously (under the skin), but it can be smoked or used intra-nasally (i.e., "snorted"). Other opioids are either injected or taken orally.

The manual that is used by mental health professionals to diagnose mental disorders is the ***Diagnostic and Statistical Manual of Mental Disorders***. The latest edition of this manual was published in 2000 and is also known as the *DSM-IV-TR*. It lists opioid dependence and opioid abuse as substance use disorders. In addition, the opioid-induced disorders of opioid intoxication and opioid withdrawal are listed in the substance-related disorders section as well.

The fifth edition of the *Diagnostic and Statistical Manual of Mental Disorders,* also known as the *DSM-5*, is due for publication in May 2013. Proposed changes and revisions to the criteria for psychiatric diagnoses include combining the diagnoses of opioid abuse and opioid dependence into the single diagnosis of opioid use disorder. (The previous diagnoses of opioid intoxication and opioid withdrawal will be retained.)

Opioid dependence

Opioid dependence, or **addiction**, is essentially a syndrome in which a person continues to use opioids in spite of significant problems caused by, or made worse by, the use of opioids. Typically, individuals with opioid dependence are physically dependent on the drug as evidenced by tolerance and/or withdrawal.

Opioid abuse

Opioid abuse is less severe than opioid dependence and typically does not involve physical dependence on the drug. Opioid abuse is essentially repeated significant negative consequences of using opioids recurrently.

Opioid intoxication

When an individual uses a sufficient amount of an opioid, they will get "high" from the drug. Some people, however, have negative experiences when they use an opioid. When too much of an opioid is taken, an individual can overdose.

Opioid withdrawal

Individuals who use opioids on a regular basis, even if only for a few days, may develop a tolerance to the drug and experience physiological and psychological symptoms when they stop using it. The "abstinence syndrome" related to opioids is very similar to a bad case of influenza (or the "flu").

Classes of narcotics

Narcotics of natural origin

Codeine
Morphine
Opium
Thebaine

Semi-synthetic narcotics

Heroin
Hydrocodone
Hydromorphone
Oxycodone

Synthetic narcotics

Butorphanol
Dextropropoxyphene
Fentanyl
Meperidine
Pentazocine

Narcotics treatment drugs

Buprenorphine
LAAM
Methadone

SOURCE: U.S. Department of Justice, Drug Enforcement Administration, *Drugs of Abuse*, "Chapter 4: Narcotics." Available online at: http://www.justice.gov/dea/pubs/abuse/4-narc.htm (accessed August 19, 2010).

(Table by PreMediaGlobal. © 2012 Cengage Learning.)

Description

Opioid dependence

Dependence on opioids involves significant physiological and psychological changes, which make it extremely difficult for an individual to stop using them. Recurrent use of opioids causes actual changes in how the **brain** functions. An individual who is addicted to opioids cannot simply just stop using, despite significant negative consequences related to their use. Marital difficulties, including divorce, unemployment, and drug-related legal problems, are often associated with opioid dependence. People who are dependent on opioids often plan their day around obtaining and using opioids.

Opioid abuse

People who abuse opioids typically use them less frequently than those who are dependent on them. However, despite less frequent use, an individual with opioid abuse can suffer negative consequences. For example, while intoxicated on opioids, an individual may get arrested for their behavior.

Opioid intoxication

An individual who uses opioids typically experiences drowsiness ("nodding off"), mood changes, a feeling of heaviness, dry mouth, itching, and slurred speech. Individuals who use heroin intravenously describe an intense euphoria (or "rush"), a floating feeling, and total indifference to pain. Symptoms of intoxication usually last several hours. Severe intoxication from an overdose of opioids is life-threatening because breathing may stop.

Opioid withdrawal

Tolerance to opioids occurs quickly. Regular users of opioids take doses that would kill someone who has never used before. After regular use, the human body adapts to the regular presence of the drug, and the person feels "normal" only when they have opioids in their system. Therefore, when an opioid-dependent individual stops using opioids abruptly, he or she will experience withdrawal symptoms. Withdrawal symptoms from heroin usually begin six to eight hours after last use and peak after two days. Acute withdrawal typically lasts no more than seven to ten days, but some symptoms of withdrawal (such as craving, **insomnia**, anxiety, or lack of interest) can last six months or longer. Although withdrawal is very uncomfortable, it is not life-threatening unless there is an underlying medical condition, such as heart disease. In addition to physical withdrawal, "psychological withdrawal" often occurs. The individual who is dependent on opioids has difficulty imagining living without the drug, since they were dependent on it to function. This is similar to how someone who is addicted to **nicotine** may feel after giving up cigarettes.

Causes and symptoms

Causes

There are no clear-cut causes of drug use other than the initial choice to use the drug. This decision to use may be highly influenced by peer group. Typically, the age of first use of heroin is about 16, but it has been dropping in recent years.

Certain social and behavioral characteristics, however, are more commonly seen among individuals who become dependent on opioids than those who do not. For instance, many heroin users come from families in which one or more family members use alcohol or drugs excessively or have mental disorders (such as **antisocial personality disorder**). Often heroin users have had health problems early in life, behavioral problems beginning in childhood, low self-confidence, and anti-authoritarian views.

Among opioid-dependent adolescents, a "heroin behavior syndrome" has sometimes been described. This syndrome consists of **depression** (often with anxiety symptoms), impulsiveness, fear of failure, low self-esteem, low frustration tolerance, limited coping skills, and relationships based primarily on mutual drug use.

Symptoms

OPIOID DEPENDENCE. The *DSM-IV-TR* specifies that three or more of the following symptoms must occur at any time during a 12-month period (and cause significant impairment or distress) in order to meet diagnostic criteria for opioid dependence:

- Tolerance: The individual either has to use increasingly higher amounts of the drug over time in order to achieve the same drug effect or finds that the same amount of the drug has much less of an effect over time than before.
- Withdrawal: The individual either experiences the characteristic abstinence syndrome (i.e., opioid-specific withdrawal) or uses opioids or similar-acting drugs in order to avoid or relieve withdrawal symptoms.
- Loss of control: The individual either repeatedly uses more opioids than planned or uses the opioids over longer periods of time than planned.
- Inability to stop using: The individual has either unsuccessfully attempted to cut down or stop using the opioids or has a persistent desire to stop using.
- Time: The individual spends a lot of time obtaining opioids, getting money to buy opioids, using opioids, being under the influence of opioids, and recovering from the effects of opioids.
- Interference with activities: The individual either gives up or reduces the amount of time involved in recreational activities, social activities, and/or occupational activities.
- Harm to self: The individual continues to use opioids despite having either a physical or psychological

problem (e.g., depression) that is caused or made worse by the opioid use.

OPIOID ABUSE. The *DSM-IV-TR* specifies that one or more of the following symptoms must occur at any time during a 12-month period (and cause significant impairment or distress) in order to meet diagnostic criteria for opioid abuse:

- Interference with role fulfillment: The individual's use of opioids repeatedly interferes with the ability to fulfill obligations at work, home, or school.
- Danger to self: The individual repeatedly uses opioids in situations in which it may be physically hazardous (e.g., while driving a car).
- Legal problems: The individual has recurrent opioid-related legal problems (e.g., arrests for possession of narcotics).
- Social problems: The individual continues to use opioids despite repeated interpersonal or relationship problems caused by, or made worse by, the use of opioids.

OPIOID INTOXICATION. The *DSM-IV-TR* specifies that the following symptoms must be present in order to meet diagnostic criteria for opioid intoxication:

- Use: The individual recently used an opioid.
- Changes: The individual experiences significant behavioral or psychological changes during, or shortly after, use of an opioid. These changes may include euphoria initially, followed by slowed movements or agitation, impaired judgment, apathy (a "don't care attitude"), dysphoric mood (e.g., depression), or impaired functioning socially or at work.
- Opioid-specific intoxication syndrome: The pupils in the eyes get smaller. In addition, drowsiness or coma, slurred speech, and/or impaired memory or attention during, or shortly after, opioid use occur.

OPIOID WITHDRAWAL. The *DSM-IV-TR* specifies that the following symptoms must be present in order to meet diagnostic criteria for opioid withdrawal:

- Abstinence: Either the individual has stopped using (or has reduced the amount of) opioids, or an opioid antagonist (i.e., a drug, such as naloxone, that blocks the action of opioids) has been administered.
- Opioid-specific withdrawal syndrome: Three or more symptoms develop after abstinence. These symptoms include dysphoric (negative) mood, nausea or vomiting, muscle aches, runny nose or watery eyes, dilated pupils, goosebumps or sweating, diarrhea, yawning, fever, and insomnia.
- Impairment or distress: The withdrawal symptoms must cause significant distress to the individual or impairment in functioning (socially, at work, or any other important area).
- Not due to other disorder: The withdrawal symptoms cannot be due to a medical condition or other mental disorder.

KEY TERMS

Amphetamines—A group of powerful and highly addictive substances that stimulate the central nervous system. Amphetamines may be prescribed for various medical conditions but are often purchased illicitly and abused.

Anxiety—Can be experienced as a troubled feeling, a sense of dread, fear of the future, or distress over a possible threat to a person's physical or mental well-being.

Depression—A mental state characterized by feelings of sadness, despair, and discouragement.

Demographics

There are at least 600,000 individuals with opioid dependence living in the United States. It has been estimated that almost 1% of the population has met criteria for opioid dependence or abuse at some time in their lives.

In the late 1800s and early 1900s, individuals who were dependent on opioids were primarily white and from middle socioeconomic groups. However, since the 1920s, minorities and those from lower socioeconomic groups have been overrepresented among those with opioid dependence. It appears that availability of opioids and subcultural factors are key in opioid use. Therefore, medical professionals (who have access to opioids) are at higher risk for developing opioid-related disorders.

Males are more commonly affected by opioid disorders than females—they are three to four times more likely than females to be dependent on opioids. Age also is a factor in opioid dependence. There is a tendency for rates of dependence to decrease beginning at 40 years of age. Problems associated with opioid use are usually first seen in the teens and 20s.

Diagnosis

Diagnosis of opioid-related disorders are based on patient interviews and observations of symptoms, including signs of withdrawal, such as dilated pupils, watery eyes, frequent yawning, and anxiety.

Opioid dependence

Other mental disorders are common among individuals with opioid dependence. It has been estimated that 90% of those with opioid dependence have one or more other mental disorders. Depression (usually either major depression or substance-induced mood disorder) is the most common disorder. Opioid-dependent individuals frequently report suicidal ideation (thoughts) and insomnia. Other substance-use disorders (such as alcoholism), **anxiety disorders**, antisocial personality disorder, **post-traumatic stress disorder**, and a history of **conduct disorder** are also fairly common.

Opioid intoxication

Intoxication on other substances, such as alcohol, **sedatives**, hypnotics, and anxiolytics, can resemble intoxication on opioids. Furthermore, dilated pupils can be seen in hallucinogen intoxication, amphetamine intoxication, and **cocaine** intoxication.

Opioid withdrawal

The restlessness and anxiety seen in opioid withdrawal are also seen in withdrawal from sedatives, hypnotics, and anxiolytics.

Treatment

Opioid dependence

Because opioid-related disorders are complex, multiple treatment approaches are often necessary. Generally, the more treatment (e.g., a combination of medication, individual therapy, and **self-help groups**), and the longer the treatment (i.e., at least three months), the better the outcomes. There are a wide variety of treatment options, both inpatient or residential and outpatient:

- Methadone maintenance treatment. Methadone is a long-acting opioid that is generally administered in an outpatient setting (a methadone maintenance clinic). The methadone prevents the individual from experiencing opioid withdrawal, reduces opioid craving, and enables the individual to have access to other services (such as individual counseling, medical services, and HIV-prevention education). A proper dose of methadone also prevents the individual from getting "high" from heroin. Methadone maintenance therapy can decrease criminal activity, decrease HIV-risk behaviors, and increase stability of employment. Low-dose methadone maintenance treatment is preferable for pregnant individuals who would otherwise use illicit opioids. One longer-acting alternative to methadone is LAAM (levo-alphacetylmethadol). Individuals receiving the proper doses of LAAM only need to take it three times per week, instead of every day as with methadone.
- Opioid antagonist treatment. An opioid antagonist is a medication that blocks the effects of opioids. Treatment with an antagonist, usually naltrexone (Trexan), typically takes place on an outpatient basis following an inpatient medical detoxification from opioids. The effects of taking any opioids are blocked by the naltrexone and prevent the individual from getting "high," thereby discouraging individuals from seeking opioids. By itself, this treatment is suitable for individuals who are highly motivated to discontinue opioid use. However, antagonists can be used in addition to other treatment modalities or with individuals who have been abstinent for some time but fear a relapse.
- Opioid agonist-antagonist treatment. An opioid agonist is a drug that has an action similar to morphine. Buprenorphine (Buprenex) is an example of an opioid agonist-antagonist, which means it acts as both an agonist (having some morphine-like action) and antagonist (blocking the effects of additional opioids). Buprenorphine has been shown to reduce opioid use effectively. It is also being studied for opioid detoxification.
- Outpatient drug-free treatment. These are outpatient treatment approaches that do not include medications. There are a number of different types of programs ranging from simple drug education to intensive outpatient programs that offer most of the services of an inpatient setting. Some programs may specialize in treating specific groups of people who are opioid-dependent (e.g., those with co-occurring mental disorders).
- Residential or inpatient treatment. These include inpatient rehabilitation programs (usually seven to 30 days in length) and long-term residential programs (e.g., therapeutic communities). Rehabilitation programs provide an inpatient atmosphere following detoxification and usually offer individual and group counseling as well as medical services. Therapeutic communities are designed to be more than six months long and are highly structured. The primary focus is on resocializing the individual to a drug-free and crime-free lifestyle.
- Individualized drug counseling. Individual counseling is often a part of a methadone maintenance program or inpatient rehabilitation program. The primary focus is on helping the individual learn strategies to reduce or stop their opioid use and learn coping mechanisms to maintain abstinence. Twelve-step participation is encouraged, and referrals for medical, psychiatric, employment, or other services are made as necessary.
- Supportive-expressive psychotherapy. This type of individual psychotherapy may be a part of a

methadone maintenance program or offered alone. The focus of this type of therapy is to help individuals feel comfortable talking about themselves, work on relationship issues, and solve problems without resorting to opioids or other drugs.

- Self-help groups. Narcotics Anonymous (NA) is a twelve-step group based on the same model as Alcoholics Anonymous. This self-help group can provide social support to an individual in the process of reducing or stopping opioid use. Participation in NA is often encouraged or is a required component of other types of treatment for opioid dependence. Nar-Anon is a group for family members and friends of opioid-dependent individuals.
- Alternative therapies. Hypnosis, guided imagery, biofeedback, massage, and acupuncture have all been studied as adjunctive treatments for opioid dependence, but none has been proven to be effective.

Opioid abuse

Most of the treatments for opioid dependence would be appropriate for opioid abuse except methadone maintenance and opioid antagonist treatment.

Opioid intoxication

An opioid antagonist, naloxone (Narcan), can be administered to reverse the effects of acute intoxication or overdose on most opioids.

Opioid withdrawal

Opioid withdrawal can be treated on either an inpatient basis (**detoxification**) or an outpatient basis (methadone detoxification):

- Inpatient detoxification program. Typically, this would be from three to seven days. The withdrawal can be medically managed. Clonidine can be administered to help reduce some symptoms of withdrawal.
- Outpatient methadone detoxification. Methadone would be substituted for the illicit opioid, and the dose would be gradually reduced. Detoxification from methadone is easier (i.e., the symptoms are less severe) than from heroin. However, the withdrawal or abstinence syndrome also lasts longer. Clonidine may also be administered during the methadone detoxification to help reduce withdrawal symptoms.

Prognosis

Opioid dependence

Recovering from opioid dependence is a long, difficult process. Typically, multiple treatment attempts are required. Relapsing, or returning to opioids, is not uncommon even after many years of abstinence. Brief periods of abstinence are common.

Inpatient detoxification from opioids alone, without additional treatment, does not appear to have any effect on opioid use. However, other treatments have been shown to reduce opioid use, decrease illegal activity, decrease rates of HIV-infection, reduce rates of death, and increase rates of employment. Benefits are greatest for those who remain in treatment longer and participate in many different types of treatment (e.g., individual and group counseling in addition to methadone maintenance).

Risk Evaluation and Mitigation Strategy

In February 2009, the U.S. Food and Drug Administration (FDA) announced that it had contacted the manufacturers of opioid pain medications (including fentanyl, morphine, and oxycodone), with plans requiring them to employ a risk evaluation and mitigation strategy (REMS) to ensure that the benefits of these drugs outweigh the risks. The authority for the FDA to require REMS comes from the FDA Amendments Act of 2007 (FDAAA).

The rationale for REMS is that opioid drugs are of benefit when used properly and are a needed component of pain management for specific patient populations; however, these drugs impose serious risks when they are used improperly. Therefore, there is a need for guidelines to be put into place in order to prevent abuse, misuse (intentional or unintentional), and accidental overdose of these drugs. To improve the safe use of these drugs, changes would include new warning labels, risk–management plans, and direct communications to prescribers and patients.

The FDA will require REMS from manufacturers to ensure that the benefits of a drug product outweigh its risks and to establish measures to ensure safe use of these

QUESTIONS TO ASK YOUR DOCTOR

- What risks are associated with opioid use and opioid abuse?
- What symptoms are associated with opioid dependence?
- Do opioid dependence and abuse put me at risk for other health conditions?
- Can you recommend any treatment and support groups for me?

drugs. Establishing REMS will purport to demonstrate a balance between access to the medications and measures to manage and reduce their risks.

Plans and final recommendations to finalize REMS are ongoing. For more information, visit the FDA's website at: http://www.fda.gov/Drugs/DrugSafety/InformationbyDrugClass/ucm163647.htm.

Prevention

The best single thing an individual can do to prevent opioid-related disorders is to never use illicit opioids such as heroin. Opioids are powerfully addicting, especially if used intravenously. The risk of becoming dependent on appropriately prescribed opioids, however, is generally low except for individuals who already have a substance use disorder.

On a larger scale, comprehensive prevention programs that utilize family, schools, communities, and the media can be effective in reducing **substance abuse**. The recurring theme in these programs is not to use drugs in the first place.

Resources

BOOKS

American Psychiatric Association. *Diagnostic and Statistical Manual of Mental Disorders*. 4th ed., text rev. Washington, DC: American Psychiatric Association, 2000.

American Psychological Association. *Publication Manual of the American Psychological Association*. 6th ed. Washington, DC: American Psychological Association, 2009.

Erickson, Carlton K., Ph.D. *Addiction Essentials: The Go-To Guide for Clinicians and Patients*. New York: W. W. Norton & Company, 2011.

Galanter, Marc, and Herbert D. Kleber, eds. *Textbook of Substance Abuse Treatment*. 2nd ed. Washington, DC: American Psychiatric Press, Inc., 2008.

North, Carol, and Sean Yutzy. *Goodwin and Guze's Psychiatric Diagnosis*. New York: Oxford University Press, 2010.

Sadock, Benjamin J., Virginia Alcott Sadock, and Pedro Ruiz, eds. *Kaplan and Sadock's Comprehensive Textbook of Psychiatry,* 2nd ed. New York: Lippincott Williams & Wilkins, 2009.

WEBSITES

National Institute on Drug Abuse. "Prescription Drugs: Abuse and Addiction." U.S. National Institutes of Health. http://drugabuse.gov/ResearchReports/Prescription/prescription2.html

ORGANIZATIONS

American Psychological Association, 750 First Street NE, Washington, DC, 20003, (202) 336-5500, http://www.apa.org/index.aspx.

National Institute on Drug Abuse, 6001 Executive Blvd., Rm. 5213, Bethesda, MD, 20892, (301) 442-1124; Spanish: (240) 221-4007, information@nida.nih.gov, http://www.nida.nih.gov.

The Partnership at Drugfree.org, 352 Park Avenue South, 9th Floor, New York, NY, 10010, (212) 922-1560, (855) DRUGFREE (378-4373; helpline), Fax: (212) 922-1570, webmail@drugfree.org, http://www.drugfree.org.

Substance Abuse and Mental Health Services Administration Referral Resource, 1 Choke Cherry Rd., Rockville, MD, 20857, (877) SAMHSA-7 (726-4727), (800) TTY: 487-4889, Fax: (240) 221-4292, SAMHSAInfo@samhsa.hhs.gov, http://www.samhsa.gov.

Jennifer Hahn, Ph.D.
Laura Jean Cataldo, RN, Ed.D.

Oppositional defiant disorder

Definition

Oppositional defiant disorder (ODD) is a disorder found primarily in children and adolescents. It is characterized by negative, disobedient, or defiant behavior that is worse than the normal "testing" behavior most children display from time to time. Most children go through periods of being difficult, particularly during the period from 18 months to three years, and later during adolescence. These difficult periods are part of the normal developmental process of gaining a stronger sense of individuality and separating from parents. ODD, however, is defiant behavior that lasts longer and is more severe than normal individuation behavior, but is not so extreme that it involves violation of social rules or the rights of others.

The mental health professional's handbook, ***Diagnostic and Statistical Manual of Mental Disorders***, fourth edition, text revision (*DSM-IV-TR*), classifies ODD as a disruptive behavior disorder.

Demographics

Oppositional defiant disorder is thought to occur in about 6% of all children and teenagers in the United States, with a range from 2%–16%. It is more common in families of lower socioeconomic status. Boys are more likely to have ODD than are girls. However, in older children, its occurrence is approximately equal with respect to gender. In one study, 8% of children from low-income families were diagnosed with ODD. The disorder is often apparent by the time a child is about six years old. The *Merck Manual* reports that ODD usually develops by the age of eight years. Boys tend to be diagnosed with this disorder more often than girls in the preteen years, but it is equally common in males and females by adolescence.

It is estimated that about one-third of children who have **attention deficit hyperactivity disorder (ADHD)** also have ODD. Children who have ODD are also often diagnosed with anxiety or **depression**.

Description

Children who have ODD are often disobedient. They are easily angered and may seem to be angry much of the time. Very young children with the disorder will throw temper tantrums that last for 30 minutes or longer, over seemingly trivial matters.

In addition, the child with ODD often starts arguments and will not give up. Winning the argument seems to be very important to a child with this disorder. Even if the youth knows that he or she will lose a privilege or otherwise be punished for continuing the tantrum or argument, he or she is unable to stop. Attempting to reason with such a child often backfires, because the child perceives rational discussion as a continuation of the argument.

Most children with ODD, however, do not perceive themselves as being argumentative or difficult. It is usual for such children to blame all of their problems on others. Such children can also be perfectionists and have a strong sense of justice regarding violations of what they consider correct behavior. They are impatient and intolerant of others. They are more likely to argue verbally with other children than to get into physical fights.

Older children or adolescents with ODD may try to provoke others by being deliberately annoying or critical. For example, a teenager may criticize an adult's way or speaking or dressing. This oppositional behavior is usually directed at an authority figure, such as a parent, coach, or teacher. Youths diagnosed with ODD, however, can also be bullies who use their language skills to taunt and abuse other children.

In May 2013, the **American Psychiatric Association** is due to publish the new edition of the *DSM*. Named *DSM-5*, the ADHD and Disruptive Behavior Disorders Work Group, which is co-chaired by Drs. David Shaffer and F. Xavier Castellanos, is working on proposed revisions to ODD, along with other disruptive disorders. According to the group, the definition of ODD is proposed to be: "A persistent pattern of angry and irritable mood along with defiant and vindictive behavior as evidenced by four (or more) of the following symptoms being displayed with one or more persons other than siblings.":

- Angry/Irritable Mood: (1) Loses temper; (2) Is touchy or easily annoyed by others; (3) Is angry and resentful.
- Defiant/Headstrong Behavior: (4) Argues with adults; (5) Actively defies or refuses to comply with adults' requests or rules; (6) Deliberately annoys people; (7) Blames others for his or her mistakes or misbehavior.
- Vindictiveness: (8) Has been spiteful or vindictive at least twice within the past six months.

The members of the Work Group also make the following statement that is under consideration: "The persistence and frequency of these behaviors should be used to distinguish a behavior that is within normal limits from a behavior that is symptomatic to determine if they should be considered a symptom of the disorder. For children under 5 years of age, the behavior must occur on most days for a period of at least six months unless otherwise noted (see symptom #8). For individuals 5 years or older, the behavior must occur at least once per week for at least six months, unless otherwise noted (see symptom #8). While these frequency criteria provide a minimal level of frequency to define symptoms, other factors should also be considered such as whether the frequency and intensity of the behaviors are non-normative given the person's developmental level, gender, and culture."

The following two statements are also under consideration: "The disturbance in behavior causes clinically significant impairment in social, educational, or vocational activities." and "The behaviors may be confined to only one setting or in more severe cases present in multiple settings."

Causes and symptoms

Causes

The exact cause of ODD is not known for certain within the medical community. However, three causes are thought to contribute to the disorder: biological, genetic, and environmental. Based on previous medical studies, problems found in the **brain**, whether occurring at birth or due to injuries suffered later in life, have been associated with serious psychological problems in children. Abnormalities in the prefrontal cortex of the brain, along with damaged neurotransmitter function in the dopaminergic, noradrenergic, and serotonergic systems, all seem to contribute to ODD. Lower-than-normal cortisol and higher-than-normal testosterone levels are other factors genetically associated with the presence of ODD. In addition, an existing mental illness, such as depression or an anxiety disorder, is thought to add to the risk of developing ODD later in life.

KEY TERMS

Antisocial personality disorder—A psychological condition in which a person appears to be unaware of, or indifferent to, the feelings of others and to normal social rules and standards.

Attention deficit hyperactivity disorder—A disorder that usually begins in childhood and is characterized by an inability to focus on tasks, sit still, and control impulses.

Depression—A disorder that is characterized by such symptoms as feelings of hopelessness, lack of energy, sleeplessness, and, sometimes, thoughts of suicide.

Disruptive behavior disorder—A broader term that includes two similar disorders: oppositional defiant disorder, and conduct disorder.

Genetics are likely to be a factor, meaning that ODD could be an inherited medical disorder. Children and teenagers with close family members who have mental illnesses, such as **anxiety disorders**, mood disorders, and **personality disorders**, are at increased risk of developing ODD. In addition, the environment surrounding a child or teen may increase their risk of ODD. Such environmental factors include **substance abuse**, exposure to toxins, poor **nutrition**, dysfunctional family life, and inconsistent discipline at home or at school.

All three factors—biology, genetics, and environment—could be directly the result of family life. Specifically, ODD has been called a problem of families, not of individuals. It occurs in families in which some or all of the following factors are present:

- Limits set by parents are too harsh or too lax, or an inconsistent mix of both.
- Family life lacks clear structure; rules, limits, and discipline are uncertain or inconsistently applied.
- At least one parent models oppositional behavior in his or her own interactions with others. For example, the mother or father may get into frequent disputes with neighbors, store clerks, other family members, in front of the child.
- At least one parent is emotionally or physically unavailable to the child due to emotional problems of the parent (such as depression); separation or divorce; or work hours.

The defiant behavior may be an attempt by the child to feel safe or to gain control. It may also represent an attempt to get attention from an unresponsive parent.

There may be a genetic factor involved in ODD; the disorder often seems to run in families. However, this pattern may reflect behavior learned from previous generations rather than the effects of a gene or genes for the disorder.

Symptoms

According to *DSM-IV-TR*, a **diagnosis** of ODD may be given to children who meet the following criteria, provided that the behavior occurs more frequently than usual, compared to children of the same age and developmental level.

A pattern of negativistic, hostile, and defiant behavior lasting at least six months, during which four (or more) of the following are present. The child:

- often loses his or her temper
- frequently argues with adults
- often disregards adults' requests or rules
- deliberately tries to provoke people
- frequently blames others for his or her mistakes or misbehavior
- is often easily irritated by others
- is often angry and resentful
- is often spiteful.

In order to make the diagnosis of oppositional defiant disorder, the behavioral disturbances must cause significant impairment in the child's social, academic, or occupational functioning, and the behaviors must not occur exclusively during the course of a psychotic or mood disorder. In addition, the child must not meet criteria for **conduct disorder**, which is a more serious behavioral disorder. If the youth is 18 years or older, he or she must not meet criteria for **antisocial personality disorder**.

Diagnosis

Oppositional defiant disorder is diagnosed when the child's difficult behavior lasts longer than six months. There is no standard test for diagnosing ODD. A full medical checkup may be done to ensure that there is no medical problem causing the child's behavior. The medical examination is followed by a psychological evaluation of the child, which involves an interview with a mental health professional. The mental health professional may also interview the child's parents and teachers. Psychological tests are sometimes given to the child to rule out other disorders.

Evaluation for ODD includes ruling out a more disruptive behavioral disorder known as *conduct disorder* (CD). CD is similar to ODD but also includes physical aggression toward others, such as fighting or deliberately trying to hurt another person. Children with CD also frequently break laws or violate the rights of others (for example, by stealing). They tend to be more covert than children with ODD, lying and keeping some of their unacceptable behavior secret.

The diagnosis of ODD may specify its degree of severity as mild, moderate, or severe.

Treatment

Treatment of ODD focuses on both the child and the parents. The goals of treatment include helping the child to feel protected and safe and to teach him or her appropriate behavior. Parents may need to learn how to set appropriate limits with a child and how to deal with a child who acts out. They may also need to learn how to teach and reinforce desired behavior.

Parents may also need help with problems that may be distancing them from the child. Such problems can include alcoholism or drug dependency, depression, or financial difficulties. In some cases, legal or economic assistance may be necessary. For example, a single mother may need legal help to obtain child support from the child's father so that she will not need to work two jobs and can stay at home in the evenings with the child.

The specific treatment for ODD is determined by the medical professional, based on many factors, including age, severity of symptoms, and the child's ability to participate in, and deal with, the various therapies. Treatment is usually one or more of the following: behavioral therapy, contingency management, cognitive therapy, **parent management training**, **group therapy**, and medication.

Behavioral therapy

Behavioral therapy is usually effective in treating ODD. It focuses on changing specific behaviors, not on analyzing the history of the behaviors or the very early years of the child's life. The theory behind behavioral therapy is that a person can learn a different set of behaviors to replace those that are causing problems. As the person obtains better results from the new behavior, he or she will want to continue that behavior instead of reverting to the old one. To give an example, the child's parents may be asked to identify behaviors that usually start an argument. They are then shown ways to stop or change those behaviors in order to prevent arguments.

Contingency management

Contingency management techniques may be included in behavioral therapy. The child and the parents may be helped to draw up contracts that identify unwanted behaviors and spell out consequences. For example, the child may lose a privilege or part of his or her allowance every time he or she throws a temper tantrum. These contracts can include steps or stages—for example, lowering the punishment if the child begins an argument but manages to stop arguing within a set period of time. The same contract may also specify rewards for desired behavior. For example, if the child has gone for a full week without acting out, he or she may get to choose which movie the family sees that weekend. These contracts may be shared with the child's teachers.

The parents are encouraged to acknowledge good or nonproblematic behavior as much as possible. Attention or praise from the parent when the child is behaving well can reinforce his or her sense that the parent is aware of the child even when he or she is not acting out.

Cognitive therapy

Cognitive therapy may be helpful for older children, adolescents, and parents. In cognitive therapy, the person is guided to greater awareness of problematic thoughts and feelings in certain situations. The therapist can then suggest a way of thinking about the problem that would lead to behaviors that are more likely to bring the person what they want or need. For example, a girl may be helped to see that much of her anger derives from feeling that no one cares about her, but that her angry behavior is the source of her problem because it pushes people away.

Parent management training

Parent management training (PMT) is used as an avenue to train families to better deal with their child with ODD. The PMT has been shown to be effective toward reducing, or even eliminating, negative interactions between parents and children. Training with PMT involves teaching parents to change their behaviors, which indirectly changes the behavior of their children. PMT concentrates on increasing positive attention (such as non-aversive punishment) to the ODD child, while eliminating negative attention. For example, parents are taught not to reinforce disruptive or deviant behaviors with negative attention (such as aversive punishments). In addition, parents are taught to spend more time with their OCD child in order to identify their positive behaviors more easily so they can positively reinforce such actions.

Group therapy

ODD can be treated with group therapy, in which behaviors and reactions are modeled in a classroom setting with other ODD children. Real-life situations are set up in which the children act out situations that promote empathy, listening, and effective problem solving. Often, parents attend with other parents for a combined meeting.

Intervention early in the life of a child is more effective than waiting for the child to grow out of it or intervening later in life. In younger children, combined treatment in which parents attend group therapy sessions while the children go to other meetings has consistently resulted in the best results. Group therapy for adolescents with ODD is most beneficial when it is well organized, structured, and focused on developing the skills of effective problem solving, empathy, and listening.

Medication

Although behavioral therapies are the cornerstone of treatment for ODD, medication may also be helpful in some cases. Children who have concurrent ADHD may need medical treatment to control their impulsivity and extend their attention span. Children who are anxious or depressed may also be helped by appropriate medications.

Prognosis

Treatment for ODD is usually a long-term commitment. Seek help from a qualified medical professional as early as possible in order to provide the best results for a child. It may take a year or more of treatment to notice improvement. It is important for families to continue with treatment even if immediate results are not apparent.

If ODD is not treated, or if treatment is abandoned, the child has a higher likelihood of developing conduct disorder, which is a more serious mental illness. The risk of developing conduct disorder is lower in children who are only mildly defiant. It is higher in children who are more defiant and in children who also have ADHD. In adults, conduct disorder is called antisocial personality disorder (ASD).

Children who have untreated ODD are also at risk for developing passive-aggressive behaviors as adults. Persons with passive-aggressive characteristics tend to see themselves as victims and blame others for their problems.

However, when ODD is identified early and properly, the results of the treatment are usually very effective.

Prevention

Prevention of ODD begins with good parenting. If at all possible, families and the caregivers they encounter should be on the lookout for any problem that may prevent parents from giving children the structure and attention they need.

QUESTIONS TO ASK YOUR DOCTOR

- What treatment options do you recommend for our child?
- In what way do you think medication will benefit my child with ODD?
- What is our first step to treating ODD in my child?
- What can we do as parents to help our child?
- Where can we learn more about ODD?
- How can my child's school help his or her treatment?
- Are there any support groups that could help us understand ODD?

Early identification of ODD and ADHD is necessary to obtain help for the child and family as soon as possible. The earlier ODD is identified and treated, the more likely the child will be able to develop healthy patterns of relating to others.

Resources

BOOKS

American Psychiatric Association. *Diagnostic and Statistical Manual of Mental Disorders*. 4th edition, text revised. Washington, DC: American Psychiatric Association Publishing. 2000.

Beers, Mark H. *Merck Manual of Diagnosis and Therapy*. Rahway: Merck, 2011.

Black, Donald W., and Nancy C. Andreasen. *Introductory Textbook of Psychiatry*. Washington D.C.: American Psychiatric Publishing, 2006.

Corcoran, Jacqueline. *Mental Health Treatment for Children and Adolescents*. Oxford: Oxford University Press, 2011.

Leeming, David A., Kathryn Madden, and Stanton Marlan, editors. *Encyclopedia of Psychology and Religion*. New York: Springer, 2010.

Matthys, Walter, and John E. Lochman. *Oppositional Defiant Disorder and Conduct Disorder in Childhood*. Chichester: Wiley-Blackwell, 2010.

Morrison, James. *DSM-IV Made Easy: The Clinician's Guide to Diagnosis*. New York: Guilford Press, 2006.

Sadock, Benjamin J. *Kaplan & Sadock's Pocket Handbook of Clinical Psychiatry*. Philadelphia: Wolters Kluwer Health/ Lippincott Williams & Wilkins, 2010.

WEBSITES

Helping Children and Youth With Conduct Disorder and Oppositional Defiant Disorder: Systems of Care. U.S. Substance Abuse and Mental Health Services Administration. (January 2006). http://store.samhsa.gov/product/

Helping-Children-and-Youth-With-Conduct-Disorder-and-Oppositional-Defiant-Disorder-Systems-of-Care/SMA06-4200 (accessed July 4, 2011).

Oppositional Defiant Disorder. eMedicine. (February 8, 2008). http://emedicine.medscape.com/article/918095-overview#aw2aab6b2 (accessed July 15, 2011).

Oppositional Defiant Disorder. HealthyPlace.com. (January 2, 2009). httphttp://www.healthyplace.com/other-info/psychiatric-disorder-definitions/oppositional-defiant-disorder/menu-id-71 (accessed July 15, 2011).

Oppositional Defiant Disorder. WebMD. http://www.webmd.com/mental-health/oppositional-defiant-disorder (accessed July 15, 2011).

Q 00 Oppositional Defiant Disorder. American Psychiatric Association. (2010). http://www.dsm5.org/ProposedRevisions/Pages/proposedrevision.aspx?rid=106 (accessed July 15, 2011).

ORGANIZATIONS

American Academy of Child and Adolescent Psychiatry, 3615 Wisconsin Avenue, N.W., Washington, DC, 20016-3007, 1(202) 966-7300, Fax: 1(202) 966-2891, http://aacap.org.

American Psychiatric Association, 1000 Wilson Boulevard, Suite 1825, Arlington, VA, 22209, 1(703) 907-7300, apa@psych.org, http://www.psych.org.

Federation of Families for Children's Mental Health, 9605 Medical Center Drive, Rockville, MD, 20850, 1(240) 403-1901, Fax: 1(240) 403-1909, ffcmh@ffcmh.org, http://ffcmh.org.

Mental Health America, 2000 N. Beauregard Street, 6th Floor, Alexandria, VA, 22311, 1(703) 684-7722, Fax: 1(703) 684-5968, (800) 969-6642, http://www1.nmha.org.

National Alliance on Mental Illness, 3803 North Fairfax Drive, Suite 100, Arlington, VA, 22203, 1(703) 524-7600, Fax: 1 (703) 524-9094, http://www.nami.org.

National Institute of Mental Health, 6001 Executive Boulevard, Room 8184, MSC 9663, Bethesda, MD, 20892-9663, 1 (301) 443-4513, Fax: 1(301) 443-4279, (866) 615-6464, nimhinfo@nih.gov, http://www.nimh.nih.gov.

Jody Bower, M.S.W.
William Atkins, B.B., B.S., M.B.A.

Orap *see* **Pimozide**

Origin of mental illnesses

Historical background

Mental illness in the ancient world

Over the history of the healing arts, there has been a succession of theories regarding the root causes of mental illness. Early writings from such ancient civilizations as those of Greece, India, and Egypt focused on demonic possession as the cause. This concept eventually disappeared only to resurface again in the Middle Ages in Europe, along with inadequate treatment of the mentally ill. Demons or "foul spirits" were believed to attach themselves to individuals and make them depressed ("poor-spirited") or "mad." The word *mad* became an early synonym for **psychosis**. Unfortunately, the "possessed" included people with seizure disorders as well as others suffering from what are now known to be medical disorders. Few genuinely helpful treatments were available to relieve the suffering of the mentally ill.

The Hippocratic tradition

Hippocrates, a Greek physician who lived around 400 B.C. and is regarded as the source of the Hippocratic Oath taken by modern physicians, first introduced the concept of disturbed physiology (organic processes or functions) as the basis for all illnesses, mental or otherwise. Hippocrates did not describe disturbances of the nervous system as we do today, in terms of a chemical imbalance or a low level of **neurotransmitters** (the chemical messengers sent between **brain** cells). Instead, he used the notion of an imbalance of "humors." Humors were defined as bodily fluids influenced by the environment, the weather, foods, and other external factors, producing various imbalances in a person's state of health. Hippocrates' theory was an early version of the idea that physiological disturbances or body chemistry might play a role in the development of mental illness. Most importantly, perhaps, Hippocrates' concept placed mental illness on the same footing as other medical disorders by highlighting the belief that the mentally ill are genuinely suffering, and therefore need to be treated like other sick persons rather than as moral degenerates. Sadly, modern society has not fully overcome the tendency to stigmatize persons with mental disorders. Hippocrates' perspective, however, meant that someone with **depression** or **schizophrenia** could be viewed as being in a state of disease just like a diabetic or someone with high blood pressure.

The nineteenth century

Toward the end of the nineteenth century, several European neurologists began actively investigating the causes of mental illness. Chief among them, and destined to change forever the understanding of mental illness, was Sigmund Freud. Although psychology and psychiatry have advanced considerably since Freud, his explorations were revolutionary. Freud introduced the concepts of the unconscious and the ego to modern thought, and reintroduced the ancient art of dream

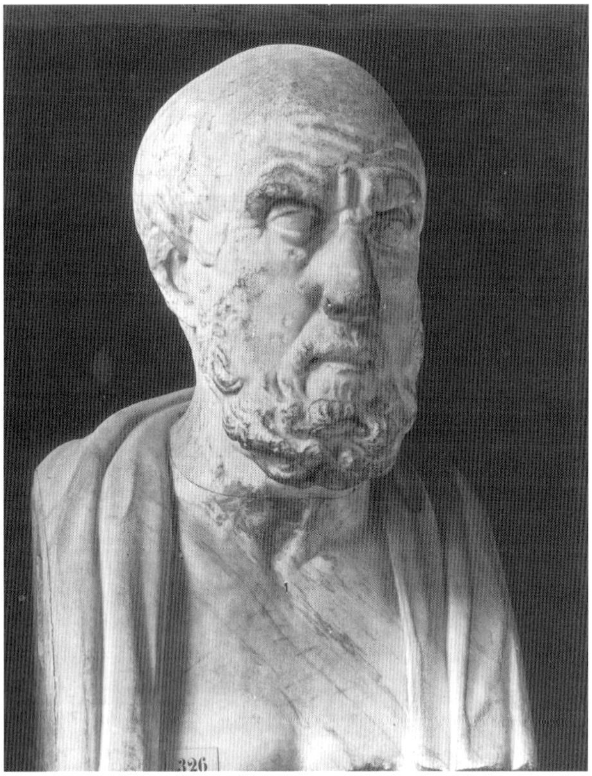

A bust of Hippocrates. *(© The Art Gallery Collection/Alamy)*

interpretation, but from a psychological standpoint. Freud also regarded human psychological states as an energy system in which blockages in the flow of thought (repression or suppression, for example) would result in disease or illness, expressed as mental or emotional loss of balance. He introduced the notion of a "talking cure"; through the use of **talk therapy** alone, many patients would improve. This method of treatment is still used today, although the technique of talk therapy itself has undergone further development. Freud's early advances in understanding the mind, however, awaited further anatomical and biochemical discoveries of the structures and functions of the human brain. As a result, early psychiatry (from two Greek words, *psyche*, meaning "soul" or "mind" and *iatros*, meaning "physician") split into two competing traditions, one that followed Freud in emphasizing thoughts, emotions and dreams as keys to the healing of mental disorders, and another that looked for clues to these disorders in the tissues of the brain.

In the first half of the twentieth century, psychiatry was advanced by the discovery of medications that helped to alleviate depression, mania, and psychosis. As often occurs in the history of medicine, physicians stumbled upon solutions before they understood the mechanisms that made the treatment work. Later studies began to reveal that certain patients responded to medications that increased certain neurotransmitters. Drugs that increased the levels of the neurotransmitters norepinephrine and **serotonin** seemed to help depressed patients. Similarly, medications that blocked the transmission of **dopamine**, another neurotransmitter, provided relief for patients suffering from hallucinations and **paranoia**. These insights have led to the present emphasis on the biochemistry of the human brain. If, however, the biochemical model becomes the only view of mental health, modern psychiatry risks becoming "mindless." Clearly, a unified theory is needed to understand all the factors that contribute to mental disorders, and to do justice to the complexity of each human being. Understanding all the factors that lead to a disease state has much to do with an adequate treatment response.

Nature and nurture

One attempt to unify the varied theories regarding the origin of mental illness is called simply the "nature versus nurture" theory. It is really the nature *and* nurture theory, however, as it establishes the importance of two forces in the development of mental illness. For example, "nature" refers to biological factors that produce a tendency or predisposition to develop certain diseases. For instance, parents who have high blood pressure have offspring who have a higher probability of developing the same condition. If, on the other hand, these offspring learn to eat properly, **exercise**, and live in a relatively peaceful home, for instance, they may be able to avoid the expression of high blood pressure that runs in their family. This example illustrates the impact that a person's environment may have on the development of physical disease. Researchers believe the same holds true for mental illnesses. For example, researchers know that patients with schizophrenia who return to a family environment in which there is a high level of expressed emotion, such as critical and angry remarks, have more frequent psychotic episodes that require **hospitalization**. Thus, it appears that the interaction between the biological and psychological dimensions of a person and his or her environment determines the likelihood of expressing a mental illness, or perhaps any illness whatsoever. There is, however, no accurate prediction or test that will determine whether a specific person will develop a certain mental illness, even if many members of his or her family are positive for that disease.

Conversely, a child with minimal genetic predisposition to mental illness may develop mental illness if he or she is traumatized in any number of ways, such as being raised in a non-nurturing or a physically, mentally, or emotionally abusive household. As of now, scientists do not know why some people become mentally ill while others do not. Much research remains to be done; although theories abound, the precise etiology or origin of all mental illnesses remains uncertain.

CARL JUNG (1875–1961)

Carl Gustav Jung was born in Kesswil, Switzerland, on July 26, 1875, to a Protestant clergyman who moved his family to Basel when Jung was four. While growing up, Jung exhibited an interest in many diverse areas of study but finally decided to pursue medicine at the University of Basel and the University of Zurich, earning his degree in 1902. He also studied psychology in Paris. In 1903, Jung married Emma Rauschenbach, his companion and collaborator. The couple had five children.

Jung's professional career began in 1900 at the University of Zurich, where he worked as an assistant to Eugene Blueler in the psychiatric clinic. During his internship, he and some co-workers used an experiment that revealed groups of ideas in the unconscious psyche, which he named "complexes." Jung sent his publication *Studies in Word Association* (1904) to Sigmund Freud after finding his own beliefs confirmed by Freud's work. Jung and Freud became friends and collaborators until 1913, when Jung's ideas began to conflict with Freud's. During the time following this split, Jung published *Two Essays on Analytical Psychology* (1916, 1917) and *Psychological Types* (1921). Jung's later work developed from the concepts in his *Two Essays* publication, and he became known as a founder of modern depth psychology.

In 1944, Jung gave up his psychological practice and his explorations after he suffered a severe heart attack. Jung received honorary doctorates from numerous universities, and in 1948 he founded the C. G. Jung Institute in Zurich. He became a controversial figure in his later years because of his association with Nazi sympathizers, his interest in such subjects as alchemy and flying saucers (he wrote a book about the latter in 1959), and revelations of his extramarital affairs with several of his patients. Jung died on June 6, 1961.

Current theories about the origin of mental disorders

Biological theories

GENETIC FACTORS. Genetics is, at this time, an important area of research for psychiatric disorders. For example, a specific gene has been associated with **bipolar disorder** (also known as "manic-depressive disorder"), but unfortunately, the switch that controls the expression of the disorder is still unknown. It is currently thought that many genes go into the expression or non-expression of any human characteristic, such as a facial feature or a certain aspect of mental health. Research done on identical twins has provided strong support for a genetic component in the development of schizophrenia. For instance, the average person in the United States has a 1% chance of developing schizophrenia, while the identical twin of a person diagnosed with schizophrenia has a 50% chance, even if he or she has been reared by adoptive parents. Other researchers who are studying schizophrenia have found that during embryonic development, there are nerve cells that do not migrate to their proper position in the brain. On the other hand, none of the genetic or embryological findings can account for the rare, but occasional, recoveries from schizophrenia, indicating that biology alone does not determine the occurrence of mental disorders.

Dementias are also noted to run in families, but most of these disorders cannot be predicted with any certainty for the following generation. Only one dementing disorder, Huntington's chorea, which is really a movement disorder with a psychiatric component, appears to be determined by a single gene. **Dementia** of the Alzheimer's type does seem to have a familial pattern, but again, the expression of the disease in any specific individual is not predictable at this time. Scientists believe that similar statements can be made for many mental disorders that run in families, such as **obsessive-compulsive disorder** (OCD), eating disorders, depression, anxiety, and **panic disorder**. The roles of the environment and learning behavior in the ultimate expression of genetically predisposed individuals are, however, undisputed.

EPIGENETICS. Epigenetics is a new field of research whose name means "beyond the genome"; it is the study of heritable changes caused by the activation and deactivation of genes without any change in the underlying DNA sequence of the organism. These changes are governed by the epigenome, which is the name given to the group of chemicals in cells that mark or tag the genome (the DNA in the cell) in such a way as to direct its activities.

The epigenome can switch genes on and off in one of two ways. The first way, known as "methylation," involves the attachment of methyl groups (hydrocarbon groups containing one carbon and three hydrogen atoms) to the DNA molecule itself in specific places. Methylation turns genes on and off by affecting the interactions of genes and the proteins they encode. The second process, known as "histone modification," affects DNA indirectly. Histones are proteins that serve as "spools" for winding up the long DNA molecules inside a chromosome. Chemicals in the epigenome can attach themselves to the tails of histones and affect how tightly they "wrap" DNA. Tightly wrapped DNA may result in a gene being silenced, while loosely wrapped DNA may result in the activation of a gene.

While the epigenome can be inherited from parents, it is also flexible over the course of a person's lifetime. Unlike the genome, it can change. The epigenome could be said to represent the intersection between a person's genome and the environment. Diet, emotional **stress**, early life experiences, smoking and drug abuse, prescription medications, environmental pollution, and other factors are known to affect the chemical tags in a person's epigenome. As of 2011, changes in the epigenome had been linked not only to cancer and diabetes, but also to such mental disorders as schizophrenia, substance use disorders, **autism** spectrum disorders, depression, and intellectual disability.

NEUROTRANSMITTER-RELATED CHEMICAL IMBALANCES. This theory of the origin of mental disorders has become the foundation of most psychiatric treatment today. It has legitimated psychiatry by returning it to the world of biological medicine. Diabetes may offer a helpful analogy. In diabetes, a chemical necessary to health (insulin) is missing and can be replaced, essentially restoring the patient's health. In mental illness, the neurotransmitters in the brain may be present in insufficient amounts. These chemicals or transmitters allow communication between nerve cells; as a result, they coordinate information processing throughout the brain. As a person reads, for example, chemical levels rise and fall in response to the letters; the meaning they have; the reader's eye movements, thoughts, reflections and associations; and the feelings the reader may have while reading. Thus, a person's brain chemistry is changed by everything that influences him or her, whether internally or externally. While the discovery of certain neurotransmitters and their roles in mental disorders has led, in turn, to the discovery of effective medications to treat these disorders, it has also resulted in the unfortunate notion that medication is the only method of treatment that is helpful.

Major neurotransmitters identified thus far include acetylcholine, dopamine, epinephrine, norepinephrine, histamine, and serotonin. Serotonin and norepinephrine are most highly implicated in depression, panic disorder and anxiety, as well as OCD. Most of the medications found effective for these disorders are drugs that increase the availability of serotonin and norepinephrine (such as the selective serotonin re-uptake inhibitors, or **SSRIs**). In particular, depression, panic disorder, **anxiety disorders**, and OCD have responded strongly to medications that increase serotonin levels. However, not all people with these disorders respond well to the medications, or they may need a combination of medications and **psychotherapy** to be effectively treated. Medications that block the effects of dopamine in certain parts of the brain are effective in controlling auditory and visual hallucinations as well as paranoia in patients with psychotic disorders.

STRESS-RELATED FACTORS. Stress is something everyone in modern society seems to understand. There are two basic kinds of stress: inner stress from previous traumas or wounds that affect one's present life; and outer stress, or the environmental issues that complicate life on a daily basis, such as work or family problems. The interplay of these two forms of stress affects brain chemistry just as it can affect physical health. Numerous studies have shown that when people are chronically stressed in life, they are vulnerable to depression, anxiety, and other disorders. Seventy percent of the adults in one recent European war situation were found to have depression, which is a normal human response to relentless stress. Researchers currently think that the mechanism that triggers this depression is the depletion of certain neurotransmitters, particularly serotonin and norepinephrine, which may lead to other biochemical imbalances. For instance, most people diagnosed with schizophrenia have their first psychotic episode during such stressful situations as leaving home for college or military service.

Genetic factors may add to a person's susceptibility to mental illness by lowering the body's production of neurotransmitters during difficult life transitions. The same combination of circumstances might affect the development of high blood pressure, diabetes, or ulcers in some families.

GENERAL MEDICAL CONDITIONS. It is important to note that bacterial and viral infections, metabolic illnesses, medications and street drugs can all affect a person's mental status. Insults (injuries) to the brain can cause a person to be disoriented, speak incoherently, have difficulty concentrating, hallucinate, or even act out violently. When clinicians see disorientation and an abrupt change in a person's level of alertness, they refer to the altered mental state as "delirium." **Delirium** is considered a medical emergency because the underlying cause must be identified and treated as quickly as possible. The exact way in which infectious disease and chemical agents change human mental function is unclear and thus might not be visible on **imaging studies**.

The elderly are particularly vulnerable to changes in mental status resulting from apparently minor changes in body chemistry. Fever, dehydration, electrolyte imbalances, and even aspirin or antibiotics can all have an abrupt effect on the mental status of the elderly. Older people are susceptible simply because older brain tissue is more sensitive to the slightest change in metabolism or the presence of toxins.

Certain infectious diseases have severe effects on the brain. One example is HIV/AIDS, in which approximately 70% of patients suffering from full-blown AIDS develop dementia, depression, or delirium. Another sexually transmitted disease (STD) that can end in dementia if untreated is syphilis. Late-stage syphilis, sometimes called "neurosyphilis," might not appear until 4 to 25 years after the initial infection; treatment can halt the progress of the disease at that point but cannot undo damage to the nervous system that has already occurred.

Similarly, at least 50% of patients with multiple sclerosis develop depression from the effects of the disease on brain tissues, not simply as a reaction to knowing that they have MS. Any infectious disease that causes inflammation inside the skull, such as meningitis or encephalitis, will usually result in some change in mental status; fortunately, these changes are usually completely reversible. Other infectious diseases that have been linked to depression and other mental disorders include Lyme disease, toxoplasmosis, and tuberculosis.

Another group of infectious diseases that cause changes in mental status (dementia and eventual death) are the prion diseases, also known as "transmissible spongiform encephalopathies" (TSEs) because of the sponge-like holes they leave in infected brains. Prions are infectious agents that consist of protein in a misfolded form. Prions are distinct from all other infectious materials in that they do not contain any genetic material. Some prion diseases are transmissible among humans or from compatible animal species to humans. These prion diseases, which include kuru and mad cow disease, are classified as zoonoses. Other prion diseases, such as some cases of Creutzfeldt-Jakob disease (CJD), fatal familial **insomnia** (FFI), and Gerstmann-Sträussler-Scheinker disease (GSS), can be inherited; they are caused by a mutation in the *PRNP* gene. Still other cases of prion diseases are sporadic; CJD and FFI sometimes occur in people with no known history of the disease in their family and with no known exposure to infectious materials.

One controversial possible connection between infectious disease and OCD is exemplified by "PANDAS," the acronym for Pediatric Autoimmune Neuropsychiatric Disorder Associated with Group A Streptococcus. Group A streptococcus is an autoimmune disorder thought to cause OCD symptoms (neuropsychiatric symptoms) in children with streptococcal infection of the tonsils and pharynx (more commonly known as strep throat). The neuropsychiatric symptoms are believed to result from an autoimmune reaction, meaning that antibodies made to fight the bacteria mistakenly attack part of the brain, resulting in symptoms of OCD. As of 2011, however, PANDAS had not been validated as a **diagnosis**. The usefulness of the diagnosis has been disputed by some researchers who maintain that this subset of patients does not differ significantly from the remainder of the pediatric population, and that streptococcal infections do not increase the risk of OCD. A study published in early 2011 reported that there was no evidence for a temporal connection between Group A streptococcal infections and **tic disorders** or OCD in children who meet the published PANDAS diagnostic criteria.

Disorders of metabolism can certainly mimic depression, anxiety, and, sometimes, even psychosis. Overproduction of thyroid hormone (thyrotoxicosis) can cause agitation, anxiety, mania and even psychosis; while a lack of thyroid hormone produces symptoms of depression and is routinely checked in patients with depression of recent onset. Imbalances in glucose (sugar) management can result in mood swings and should always be evaluated. Less commonly, malfunctions of the adrenal glands can profoundly affect a person's energy level and mental activity. The role of estrogen in postmenopausal depression has been intensively studied in recent years, but the findings remain inconclusive.

NEUROPATHOLOGY. Neuropathology refers to damage to the brain tissue itself that results in mental illness. The dementias are placed in this category, since the brains of persons diagnosed with dementia exhibit microscopic changes in tissue structure when viewed under a microscope. These changes may ultimately appear on tests such as a CAT scan of the brain. Larger changes are seen with strokes, which result when the blood supply is cut off to a specific area of the brain and causes localized damage. In these instances, a person may have altered speech patterns but retain the ability to think clearly, or vice versa. The losses are somewhat predictable and specific, based on the area of the brain that was affected and the extent of oxygen starvation of the tissue in that region.

Brain tumors and accidental injuries to the head are random in their effects, and the deficits are usually less predictable. Each case must be examined individually. As with strokes, however, the location of the injury or tumor will determine the resulting mental status changes or deficits. Patients suffering **traumatic**

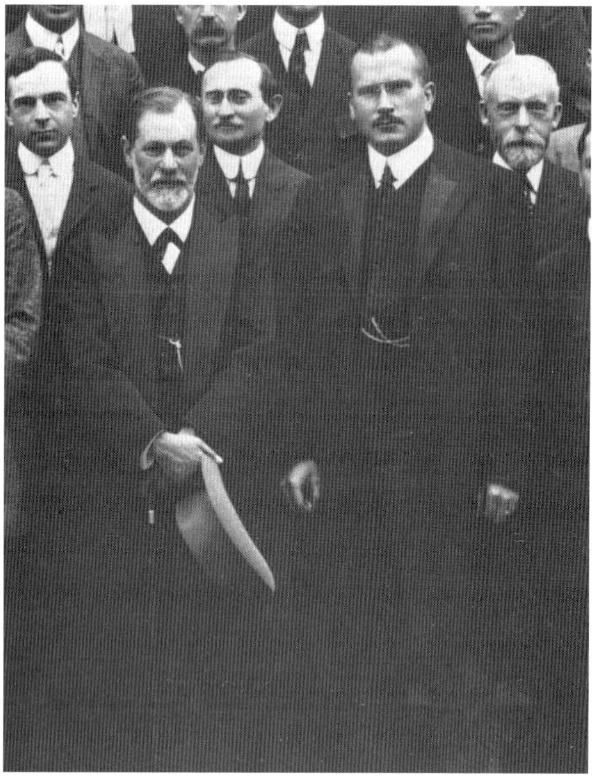

Sigmund Freud (left) with Carl Jung (right). *(© Mary Evans Picture Library/Alamy)*

brain injury (TBI), whether the head wound is closed or penetrating, are at increased risk of mood disorders, personality changes, **substance abuse** disorders, dementia, and psychotic disorders if they survive the accident or criminal attack that caused the wound. The most common causes of TBI in the United States as of 2011 were motor vehicle accidents, falls, and contact sports.

Pancreatic and certain colon cancers are particularly interesting for psychiatrists. These tumors are frequently accompanied by depression even though they are located in organs that are far removed from the brain. Long-term studies of cancer survivors have reported high rates of depression and anxiety as well as cognitive limitations in these persons even though they have been cured of their cancers. More research is needed on the relationship between mood disorders and certain illnesses; it is possible that the tumor releases, into the bloodstream, compounds that have depressive effects or that depression results from the psychological issues of dealing with a serious medical illness.

NUTRITIONAL FACTORS. There is no doubt that poor **nutrition** leads to mental imbalances. While few people in the United States are truly starving or completely depleted nutritionally, instances of mental disorders related to malnutrition still occur in this country. The B vitamins are essential for mental clarity and stability. Insufficient amounts of the B vitamins, which include thiamin, nicotinamide, pyridoxine, and B, can result in confusion, irritability, insomnia, depression, and, in extreme cases, psychosis. The body does not store these vitamins, so persons should monitor their daily intake to ensure a sufficient supply. Tryptophan is an amino acid and supplement that is a building block for serotonin, the neurotransmitter that has been found to be essential in treating depression, anxiety, panic, and OCD, among others. Tryptophan is so important nutritionally that studies have shown that its absence in the diet will result in depression even when the person is taking a prescription antidepressant to increase the availability of serotonin.

Psychological/interpersonal theories

PSYCHODYNAMIC THEORIES. Freud certainly opened the doors for humans to understand themselves in terms of psychology, or the notion that how one thinks and feels affects one's view of the world. He also found that simple conversation could help some very sick people out of depressions and other mental disorders. His work essentially demonstrated that extreme inner conflicts can become a source of mental illness. These extreme internal conflicts can occur, for instance, when one loves another deeply but also feels that that person is hurting them or limiting their development in some way. If the person who is causing pain or hindering growth is a parent or other powerful figure, these intense feelings can be hidden away or repressed. Also, a lack of honesty about reality can lead to any number of illnesses. For instance, feelings of anger and powerlessness, if unrecognized, may place the person at risk for developing aggressive behaviors or depression if insights and appropriate coping skills are not gained. These psychological disharmonies, if ignored, can lead to disease if they are sufficiently intense or associated with central relationships in the person's life.

Freud's view of psychological conflicts as rooted in sexual repression was questioned by Jung, a **psychiatrist** and protégé of Freud, who believed that people's lives are affected by deep spiritual forces that he called "archetypes." Jung's work centered on psychological imbalances stemming from spiritual distress. There were other theorists after Freud, such as Alfred Adler, who regarded power as the central motivating force of human personality, or Melanie Klein, who emphasized the significance of envy.

Following the Second World War, behavioral and cognitive theories have emphasized the role of learning in the development of mental disorders. Children growing up in an abusive home, for example, may be "rewarded" by not being beaten if they learn to be quiet and internalize everything. This internalized state may be a precursor of full-blown depression in later years. Unconscious assumptions based on early experiences may spill over into other situations later in life. As another example, children may learn to be "good" for their parents or society by taking on careers they don't like or belief systems that don't fit them, all for approval by the perceived higher authority.

Cognitive approaches to therapy maintain that people construct their view of the world from beliefs and feelings based on deeper assumptions about their own competencies. Depression, for instance, would be seen as a spiral downward into negative self-talk and feelings of inadequacy. Re-examining these negative assumptions then breaks the cycle based on erroneous thinking (cognition) that is causing the depression, anxiety, or aberrant behavior. Studies have shown that three months of cognitive therapy are as effective as medication in the treatment of depression. This finding clearly shows that talk therapy does change the chemistry of the brain.

TRAUMA-RELATED FACTORS. Psychological traumas are events that are outside the experience of everyday life, although the exact definition of a traumatic experience may vary from person to person, country to country, and century to century. Traumas in early life, such as sexual or physical abuse, can lead to mood disorders and contribute to the development of **personality disorders**. Horrendous early traumas involving torture of a child, other people, or animals, may result in **dissociative identity disorder**, formerly called "multiple personality disorder." Dissociation is a self-protective mechanism for separating conscious awareness from repeated traumas. It has sometimes been described as self-hypnosis, but most clinicians believe that it is not under the patient's control, at least initially.

In later life, such severe traumas as war, rape, natural disasters, or any similar event can lead to psychiatric difficulties. **Post-traumatic stress disorder** (PTSD) is a well-known condition that affects war veterans. Extreme **trauma** causes the brain to record impressions in a way that is different from ordinary formation of memories. These disjointed impressions may re-emerge as flashbacks months or years after the traumatic experience. Chronic and repetitive trauma, exemplified by intermittent abuse or hostage situations, can lead to a chronic form of PTSD as well.

One subcategory of psychiatric disorders that occur in response to traumatic shock is termed "fugue states." Fugue states are poorly understood but can be described as conditions of total memory loss after witnessing an overwhelmingly horrible accident or atrocity. These states of memory loss can last from minutes to years.

SOCIOCULTURAL FACTORS. Some mental disorders are influenced by social values and social interactions shaped by those values. **Anorexia nervosa**, bulimia, and **body dysmorphic disorder** are the most commonly used examples of mental illnesses in this category. With the increased visibility of unnaturally slender women in modern society (as seen everywhere in advertising, television shows, movies, and celebrity fan magazines), doctors have seen a tremendous rise in the occurrence eating disorders. "You can never be too thin or too rich," a saying attributed to the Duchess of Windsor, is a phrase that has many women, and some men, monitoring their every ounce of food intake. The core of the illness is a lack of self-esteem combined with feelings that one's world is out of control. Some clinicians add fear of sexual maturation to this list of psychological causes of eating disorders. The common denominator is that these patients apparently believe they can control their world by controlling their food intake. Although neurotransmitter deficits have been found in patients with bulimia, whose vomiting may actually change their body chemistry, the desire to be thin is the conscious motivating force.

Modern society also values activity over rest, doing over being, thinking over feeling, resulting in many people becoming slaves to work and productivity, and having little respect for their inner life. Many cases of mild stress-related disorders run the risk of developing into full-blown generalized anxiety, panic, and depressive disorders. Mental health requires a reasonable balance between work and activity on the one hand and periods of rest and relaxation on the other.

ALCOHOL AND SUBSTANCE ABUSE. Alcohol is a central nervous system depressant. It plays a prominent role in the development of (at least) depression and is often involved in other mental disorders. In addition, persons who abuse alcohol are at increased risk of mental disorders related to nutritional deficiencies. A lack of thiamin, a B-vitamin, can result in permanent brain damage in the form of severe dementia even at an early age. Persons undergoing withdrawal from alcohol are also at risk for delirium tremens, a serious condition that can result in cardiovascular shock and death.

Street drugs are well known for their effects on young people's mood and behavior. Permanent brain damage may result from the use of some so-called designer drugs. One example is **Ecstasy**, which can cause permanent memory loss and severe depression that responds only slowly to treatment. Street drugs must always be considered as a possible factor in the sudden

KEY TERMS

Biopsychosocial model—An approach to human health that holds that a combination of biological, psychological, and social factors should be taken into account when evaluating a patient rather than physical factors alone.

Dissociation—A condition in which a person's thoughts, emotions, sensations, or memories become compartmentalized, usually as a result of a severe emotional trauma.

Epigenetics—The study of heritable changes in an organism's appearance or gene expression caused by chemical reactions and factors other than changes in the organism's DNA sequences.

Epigenome—The collection of chemical compounds derived from food, medications, and other sources, that mark the genome in ways that affect the DNA in the genome both directly and indirectly.

Genome—The complete set of DNA in a cell.

Histone—A type of protein that serves as a "spool" for wrapping DNA within a chromosome.

Kuru—A prion disease associated with the cannibalism formerly practiced by the Fore people of Papua New Guinea. Its name comes from a word in the Fore language that means "to shake" or "to tremble."

Magnetoencephalography (MEG)—A newer form of brain imaging that captures and records the brain's magnetic fields produced by electrical currents occurring naturally in brain tissue. MEG can identify split-second changes in brain activity.

Methylation—A process in which chemical tags called "methyl groups" (made of one carbon and three hydrogen atoms) attach themselves to a DNA molecule in specific locations, thus affecting the level of a gene's activity.

Neurotransmitter—Any of several chemicals produced in the body that function to convey impulses from nerve cells to target cells.

Prion—An infectious agent consisting of protein in a misfolded form. Its name is a combination of "protein" and "infection."

Sporadic—Occurring at random in persons with no known risk factors or genetic mutations.

Vagus nerve stimulation (VNS)—An experimental treatment for depression that involves implanting a stimulator device which sends electrical impulses at timed intervals to the left vagus nerve.

Zoonosis (plural, zoonoses)—Any disease that can be transmitted from nonhuman animals to humans or from humans to nonhuman animals. Some prion diseases are zoonoses, as are such infectious diseases as toxoplasmosis, Lyme disease, and rabies.

onset of a mental illness in a young person. Moreover, they may precipitate a first psychotic episode in a person with a genetic predisposition to schizophrenia. In this case, the drug is the stressor that reveals the person's dormant susceptibility to the disorder.

Current theory and future directions

The biopsychosocial model of mental illness

All of the above factors are most succinctly summarized in terms of the biopsychosocial model of mental illness. Biological contributions, thoughts and perceptions, social pressures, and environmental stressors, the presence or absence of nurturing and consistency of love, core values, and self-worth, are just a few of the things that contribute to making up the psychological uniqueness of every human being. In addition to the above, researchers are actively examining the role of spirituality in mental health and recovery. No single factor can be said to be the sole cause of mental illness; rather, disorders result from a complex set of forces that act upon each person as an individual. Finding the various elements that contributed to the onset of an illness requires considerable patience from the patient, his or her family, and health professionals. Identifying all factors, if possible, provides the best road map for the healing process.

New directions

In the future, scientists will certainly modify and expand our thought-models about the mind and brain. For example, a new treatment called **transcranial magnetic stimulation** (TMS) is being evaluated as an alternative to electric shock therapy. TMS uses powerful magnets instead of electricity and is delivered to specific areas of the brain. Hence, in the future, scientists must integrate some of the electromagnetic aspects of nature into the mind-brain puzzle. One experimental newer form of TMS is **magnetic seizure therapy** (MST), which resembles TMS in using a magnet to stimulate specific portions of the brain but uses a higher electrical frequency in order to induce a seizure. As of 2011, studies were under way to evaluate the effectiveness of MST as a treatment for depression. Another newer method of direct brain stimulation is **vagus nerve stimulation** (VNS), in which a device implanted under the skin near the shoulder sends electrical impulses to the left vagus nerve, which sends messages to areas in the brain that control sleep and mood. Although the Food and Drug Administration (FDA) approved VNS for the treatment of major depression in 2005, results have been mixed; as of 2011, the treatment was still considered experimental.

New techniques of brain imaging may also lead to a better understanding of the causes of mental illness. **Magnetic resonance imaging** (MRI) has been in use for some years and has led to a range of new specialized forms of MRI that yield new information about the brain's functioning in real time. For example, functional MRI (fMRI) makes use of the different properties of oxygenated and deoxygenated hemoglobin in the blood to produce images of changes in blood flow in the brain associated with neural activity. While fMRI can be used to identify which parts of the brain are activated during performance of certain tasks, it is also extremely sensitive to early signs of **stroke**, thus improving diagnosis of this potentially devastating condition and allowing much earlier treatment. Another new form of brain imaging that is yielding information about the brain's functioning is magnetoencephalography or MEG. MEG maps brain activity by measuring and recording magnetic fields produced by electrical currents occurring naturally in the brain. MEG can capture split-second changes in the brain's functioning. Researchers are currently studying it as a possible tool in the diagnosis of schizophrenia and a way to evaluate the speed of patients' responses to antidepressant medication.

In addition to new forms of neuroimaging, the **National Institute of Mental Health** (NIMH) is researching alternative healing modalities. Prominent among them is **acupuncture**, which has been used to treat depression, anxiety, and panic disorder. Other alternative treatments being studied include the effects of prayer, **meditation**, creative writing, and **yoga**.

Epigenetics offers the potential to evaluate people at risk for certain mental disorders before they occur. For example, the possibility of identifying changes in a person's epigenome resulting from abuse or other forms of trauma in early childhood may lead to strategies to prevent depression in later life, or even to devise treatments that will reverse the chemical changes in the epigenome caused by the abuse. Similarly, changes in the epigenome resulting from drug or alcohol abuse may prove to be reversible, thus opening the way to more effective treatments for **addiction**. Last, the study of the heritability of the chemical tags found on a person's DNA and histones may provide more information about the heritability of mental disorders as well as such diseases as cancer and diabetes.

Deeper exploration of the human condition is both inevitable and desirable. Perhaps researchers will find better answers by asking the question, 'What makes people healthy?' instead of simply looking at what makes us sick. In the end, researchers may find proof of some of the ancient truths taught by spiritual teachers from all traditions, and that the physical changes seen with the naked eye or under a microscope are really just the symptoms, and not the causes, of imbalances.

Resources

BOOKS

American Psychiatric Association. *Diagnostic and Statistical Manual of Mental Disorders*. 4th ed., text rev. Washington, DC: American Psychiatric Association, 2000.

American Psychiatric Association. *Practice Guideline for the Psychiatric Evaluation of Adults*, 2nd ed. Washington, DC: American Psychiatric Association, 2010.

Freeman, Hugh, ed. *A Century of Psychiatry*. St. Louis, MO: Mosby, 1999.

Koch, Jeremias, ed. *Mental Illnesses: Descriptions, Causes, and Treatments*. New York: Nova Science Publishers, 2010.

Susser, Ezra, et al. *Psychiatric Epidemiology: Searching for the Causes of Mental Disorders*. New York: Oxford University Press, 2006.

PERIODICALS

Bale, T.L., et al. "Early Life Programming and Neurodevelopmental Disorders." *Biological Psychiatry* 68 (August 15, 2010): 314–319.

Barak, Y., and D. Aizenberg. "Is Dementia Preventable? Focus on Alzheimer's Disease." *Expert Review of Neurotherapeutics* 10 (November 2010): 1689–1698.

Gannon, P., et al. "Current Understanding of HIV-associated Neurocognitive Disorders Pathogenesis." *Current Opinion in Neurology* 24 (June 2011): 275–283.

Harrington, C.B., et al. "It's Not Over When It's Over: Long-term Symptoms in Cancer Survivors—A Systematic Review." *International Journal of Psychiatry in Medicine* 40 (February 2010): 163–181.

Howland, R.H., et al. "The Emerging Use of Technology for the Treatment of Depression and Other Neuropsychiatric Disorders." *Annals of Clinical Psychiatry* 23 (February 2011): 48–62.

Iwase, S., and Y. Shi. "Histone and DNA Modifications in Mental Retardation." *Progress in Drug Research* 67 (2011): 147–173.

Leckman, J.F., et al. "Streptococcal Upper Respiratory Tract Infections and Exacerbations of Tic and Obsessive-compulsive Symptoms: A Prospective Longitudinal

Study." *Journal of the American Academy of Child and Adolescent Psychiatry* 50 (February 2011): 108–118.

Lee, C.H., et al. "Initially Unrecognized Dementia in a Young Man with Neurosyphilis." *Neurologist* 15 (March 2009): 95–97.

McQuown, S.C., and M.A. Wood. "Epigenetic Regulation in Substance Use Disorders." *Current Psychiatry Reports* 12 (April 2010): 145–153.

Perrin, M., et al. "Critical Periods and the Developmental Origins of Disease: An Epigenetic Perspective of Schizophrenia." *Annals of the New York Academy of Sciences* 1204 (September 2010: Suppl. E8–E13.

Reeves, R.R., and R.L. Panguluri. "Neuropsychiatric Complications of Traumatic Brain Injury." *Journal of Psychosocial Nursing and Mental Health Services* 49 (March 2011): 42–50.

Siekmeier, P.J., and S.M. Stufflebeam. "Patterns of Spontaneous Magnetoencephalographic Activity in Patients with Schizophrenia." *Journal of Clinical Neurophysiology* 27 (June 2010): 179–190.

WEBSITES

Discover Magazine. "The Switches That Can Turn Mental Illness On and Off." http://discovermagazine.com/2010/jun/15-brain-switches-that-can-turn-mental-illness-on-off (accessed June 3, 2011).

National Human Genome Research Institute (NHGRI). "Epigenomics Fact Sheet." http://www.genome.gov/27532724 (accessed June 2, 2011).

National Institute of Mental Health (NIMH). "Brain Basics." http://www.nimh.nih.gov/health/brain-basics/brain-basics.shtml (accessed June 2, 2011).

National Institute of Mental Health (NIMH). "Brain Stimulation Therapies." http://www.nimh.nih.gov/health/topics/brain-stimulation-therapies/brain-stimulation-therapies.shtml (accessed June 2, 2011).

National Institute of Neurological Disorders and Stroke (NINDS). "Traumatic Brain Injury Information Page." http://www.ninds.nih.gov/disorders/tbi/tbi.htm (accessed June 3, 2011).

PBS Nova. "Epigenetics." (13-minute video at link). http://www.pbs.org/wgbh/nova/body/epigenetics.html (accessed May 31, 2011).

University of Utah Genetic Science Learning Center. "Epigenetics and the Human Brain." http://learn.genetics.utah.edu/content/epigenetics/brain (accessed May 31, 2011).

WebMD. "Causes of Mental Illness." http://www.webmd.com/anxiety-panic/mental-health-causes-mental-illness (accessed June 2, 2011).

ORGANIZATIONS

American Psychiatric Association (APA), 1000 Wilson Boulevard, Suite 1825, Arlington, VA, 22209-3901, (703) 907-7300, apa@psych.org, http://www.psych.org

National Human Genome Research Institute (NHGRI), Building 31, Room 4B09, 31 Center Drive, MSC 2152, 9000 Rockville Pike, Bethesda, MD, 20892-2152, (301) 402-0911, Fax: (301) 402-2218, http://www.genome.gov

National Institute of Mental Health (NIMH), 6001 Executive Boulevard, Room 8184, MSC 9663, Bethesda, MD, 20892-9663, (301) 443-4513, Fax: (301) 443-4279, (866) 615-6464, nimhinfo@nih.gov, http://www.nimh.nih.gov/index.shtml

National Institute of Neurological Disorders and Stroke (NINDS), PO Box 5801, Bethesda, MD, 20824, (301) 496-5751, (800) 352-9424, http://www.ninds.nih.gov

Beth A. Bollinger, M.D.
Rebecca J. Frey, Ph.D.

Oxazepam

Definition

Oxazepam is a member of a family of tranquilizers known as **benzodiazepines**. It is sold in the United States under the brand name Serax and in Canada under the brand name Ox-Pam. Generic forms of oxazepam are also available.

Purpose

Oxazepam is prescribed to treat feelings of tension and anxiety. It is also used to calm patients who are suffering from the symptoms of alcohol withdrawal.

Description

Oxazepam slows down certain **brain** functions by blocking specific chemicals that transmit messages among the nerve cells in the brain.

Recommended dosage

The typical starting dose for adults ranges from 5–15 mg per day. The dosage is sometimes increased by

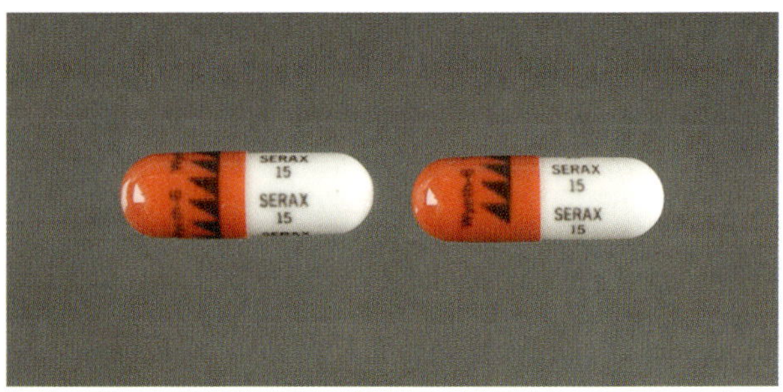

Serax (oxazepam), 15 mg. *(U.S. Drug Enforcement Administration)*

the doctor, but 80 mg is usually the maximum amount prescribed per day. The amount used each day is typically divided into at least two doses. Oxazepam is taken by mouth and is available in tablets and capsules. It can be taken with food if the patient is having side effects in the digestive tract.

Oxazepam is not FDA-approved for use in children under six years. However, in clinical practice, the medication is often used with close physician supervision. The typical starting dose for children aged 2–16 years is 5 mg. The doctor may increase this dose if necessary. Typically, the dose does not exceed 40 mg per day and is given in divided doses. Children under two years of age should receive a dose based on body weight. The doctor must determine whether the child needs the drug, as well as the dosage.

Precautions

The doctor should monitor the patient at regular intervals to ensure that the medicine is not causing troublesome side effects. Monitoring the patient is particularly important if the drug is being taken over a long period of time. Patients should not stop taking oxazepam suddenly, especially if they are taking large doses. The dose should be tapered (gradually decreased), and then stopped. Suddenly discontinuing oxazepam may cause a rebound effect. In a few cases, patients have reported serious withdrawal symptoms when they stopped taking oxazepam, including nausea, vomiting, muscle cramps, and unusual irritability.

Oxazepam should be given with great care to elderly patients; people who are significantly disabled; and people with a history of liver or kidney disease, drug abuse, or breathing problems. Pregnant women should not take oxazepam because of the risk of birth defects in the baby; a woman who becomes pregnant while she is taking the drug should tell her doctor at once. Likewise, nursing mothers should not use oxazepam while they breast feed. Oxazepam and other benzodiazepines should never be combined with alcohol or other drugs that depress (lower the activity of) the central nervous system. Oxazepam and other benzodiazepines may be habit forming and should be used under physician supervision, especially for long-term treatment. Patients who have a history of alcohol abuse, drug abuse, brain disease, mental **depression**, mental illness, sleep apnea, or myasthenia gravis should tell their doctor about their condition. Patients who have been diagnosed with glaucoma or serious psychological disorders should not receive oxazepam. Oxazepam has been associated with the risk of developing anterograde **amnesia**.

KEY TERMS

Anterograde amnesia—The inability to form new memories.

Benzodiazepines—A class of drugs that have a hypnotic and sedative action, used mainly as tranquilizers to control symptoms of anxiety.

Side effects

Rare, but serious, side effects associated with the use of oxazepam include: anxiety, mental depression, reduced memory, and confusion. Even more rare are disorientation, **delusions**, **seizures**, unusually low blood pressure, sleeping difficulties, muscle weakness, and changes in behavior.

Less serious, but more common, side effects include: difficulty talking, dizziness, clumsiness, and drowsiness. Less common, but not particularly serious, side effects include dry mouth, general weakness, headache, mild abdominal pain, constipation, diarrhea, nausea, and vomiting.

When the patient stops taking oxazepam, nervousness, irritability, and sleeping problems are common withdrawal side effects. Less common withdrawal side effects can include confusion, hearing problems, stomach cramps, increased sweating, mental depression, nausea, and vomiting. Rare withdrawal side effects can include seizures, hallucinations, and paranoid ideas.

Interactions

Patients should always inform every health professional that they deal with—doctors, pharmacists, nurses, dentists, and others—about every medication they take. Oxazepam, alcohol, and other medications that cause drowsiness can intensify one another's effects. Some medications that are used to treat viral infections, fungal infections, high blood pressure, and some heart-rhythm problems can increase the effects of oxazepam.

Heavy smoking decreases the effectiveness of oxazepam.

Resources

BOOKS

Brunton, Laurence, Bruce Chabner, and Bjorn Knollman. *Goodman & Gilman's The Pharmacological Basis of Therapeutics* 12th ed. New York: McGraw-Hill, 2010.

Consumer Reports and American Society of Health-System Pharmacists *Consumer Reports Complete Drug Reference.* Yonkers, NY: Consumers Reports, 2009.

Ellsworth, Allan J., et al. *Mosby's Medical Drug Reference*. St. Louis: Mosby, 2007.

Venes, Donald. *Taber's Cyclopedic Medical Dictionary*. 21st ed. Philadelphia: F.A. Davis Company, 2009.

Mark Mitchell, M.D.

Oxcarbazepine

Definition

Oxcarbazepine (Trileptal) belongs to the class of drugs known as anticonvulsants, used to treat seizure disorders. Oxcarbazepine, like other anticonvulsants, works to decrease abnormal neuronal electrical signaling in the **brain**.

Purpose

Oxcarbazepine is used to treat partial **seizures**, which arise from discrete portions of the brain and may cause involuntary movements of a discrete body part such as the fingers. When consciousness is maintained, the seizure is known as a simple partial seizure. When consciousness is lost, the seizure is a complex partial seizure. Oxcarbazepine is used to treat these types of partial seizures in both children and adults. It may be used as monotherapy or in combination with other antiseizure medications.

Description

Oxcarbazepine is an anticonvulsant medication that works by stabilizing abnormal electrical activity in the brain. Brain cells called neurons use electrical signals to communicate with each other as a part of normal functioning. The electrical signals are created through the use of charged molecules called ions, such as sodium and chloride. The surfaces of neurons contain openings that conduct these ions called ion channels. Neurons propagate electrical signals by opening and closing ion channels on their respective surfaces as the signal travels from one neuron to the next. Seizure disorders are not fully understood, but they are known to involve abnormal electrical signaling between neurons. Anticonvulsants help control seizures by stabilizing both the rate and the amount of signaling that occurs. Oxcarbazepine helps by decreasing the amount of sodium signaling and sodium signal propagation that occurs.

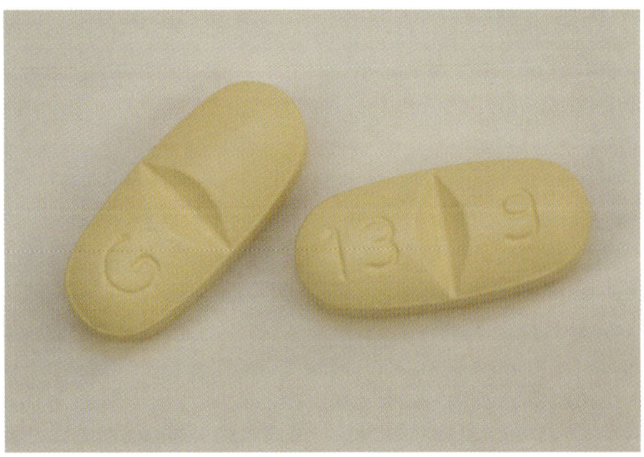

Oxcarbazepine, 60 mg. *(© Custom Medical Stock Photo, Inc. Reproduced by permission.)*

Recommended dosage

Oxcarbazepine is taken as an oral medication. The dosage used varies depending on the medical condition being treated, individual patient response to the medication regarding its effectiveness, and individual patient response to the medication regarding side effects. Some people naturally require a higher dose of oxcarbazepine in order to achieve the desired effect. Other patients require a lower dose either for effect or because they quickly develop side effects that are not tolerable.

Oxcarbazepine used for partial seizures as an adjunct treatment in combination with other anticonvulsants is usually dosed at 600 mg taken twice a day. Patients may start at 300 mg twice daily for the first week of treatment and gradually work their way up to the dose needed for effect. Oxcarbazepine used as monotherapy is started at the same low doses and gradually brought up to 1,200 mg twice a day over a time period of several weeks. Any previous adjunct medications are gradually decreased simultaneously. The maximum dose of oxcarbazepine used is 2,400 mg per day. Children are given lower doses based on their weight, with the same regimen of gradually increasing dosages. Patients are dosed at the lowest possible effective dose to avoid the development of adverse side effects. Slowly increasing the dose helps with minimizing side effects, and some side effects become lessened with continued use. Patients are periodically reassessed to determine whether there is need for continued treatment with oxcarbazepine. All anticonvulsants including oxcarbazepine need to be slowly tapered off if discontinued, to avoid a rebound seizure syndrome.

Precautions

Oxcarbazepine may not be appropriate for use or may require caution in patients with **dementia**, **depression**, past **suicide** attempts, kidney dysfunction, patients

KEY TERMS

Ion—Charged molecule such as sodium or chloride used in neuronal signaling in the brain.

Ion channel—Physical opening on the surface of neurons that allows the passage of charged ions propagating neuronal signaling in the brain.

Monoamine oxidase inhibitors (MAOIs)—Type of antidepressant medication that affects various kinds of neurotransmitters.

who are dehydrated, have diarrhea or electrolyte abnormalities, and those who are elderly. Kidney and liver function, as well as blood electrolytes and behavioral changes, may be monitored while taking oxcarbazepine. Oxcarbazepine may reduce the amount of sodium in the blood to dangerous levels. When a patient discontinues the use of oxcarbazepine, the dose needs to be tapered down slowly. If oxcarbazepine is abruptly discontinued without tapering, there may be an increase in the incidence of seizures.

Oxcarbazepine may lower the effectiveness of birth control pills; persons taking oral contraceptives should use a second form of protection when taking oxcarbazepine. Oxcarbazepine is classified as category C for pregnancy, which means that either there are no adequate human or animal studies or that adverse fetal effects were found in animal studies but there is no available human data. The decision to use category C drugs in pregnancy is generally based on weighing the critical needs of the mother against the risk to the fetus. Other lower category agents are used whenever possible. Oxcarbazepine is also excreted into breast milk; the safety of use when breastfeeding is unknown and thus is not recommended.

Side effects

Sensitivity to oxcarbazepine varies among patients, and some patients may find lower doses are more than their body system can tolerate. Common side effects of oxcarbazepine include nausea, vomiting, abdominal pain, headache, dizziness, **fatigue**, somnolence, confusion, nervousness, impaired concentration, speech, and coordination, vision and gait changes, tremor, electrolyte abnormalities, changes in liver enzymes, skin rash and acne, hair loss, and sensitivity to sunlight. Rare but serious potential side effects include severe and possibly dangerous electrolyte abnormalities; changes in various types of blood cells, including decrease in immune function and severe anemia; toxic and life-threatening skin

QUESTIONS TO ASK YOUR DOCTOR

- Can I take the full dose right away or do I need to slowly increase the dose up to the full amount?
- Can I stop taking the medication right away or do I need to slowly decrease the dose in order to go off the medication?
- Should I eat before taking this medication?
- Will this medication interact with any of my other prescription medications? Over-the-counter drugs? Herbal supplements?
- What side effects should I watch for that tell me I have taken too much of this medication?
- Can I drink alcoholic beverages when taking this medication?

reactions, severe allergic reactions, inflammation of the pancreas, and suicidality.

Interactions

Patients should make their doctor aware of all medications and supplements they are taking before using oxcarbazepine. Using alcohol while taking oxcarbazepine may create toxic reactions in the body and should be avoided. Drugs that affect the liver may alter the metabolism of oxcarbazepine, resulting in too much or too little of the drug in the body. This could lead to increased side effects or even toxic doses. Likewise, oxcarbazepine may affect the metabolism of other drugs, leading to greater or lower doses of those drugs than therapeutically desired. For example, oxcarbazepine may lower levels of antiviral medications such as rilpivirine; other drugs on which oxcarbazepine has this effect are cholesterol medications such as atorvastatin, oral contraceptives, antibiotics such as clarithromycin, and chemotherapeutics such as temsirolimus.

Oxcarbazepine should not be used at the same time as **monoamine oxidase inhibitors (MAOIs)**, a class of antidepressant drugs Use of these medications during the same period may cause a medical condition called **serotonin syndrome**, which can be severe and life-threatening. Symptoms may include high blood pressure, high fever, nausea, diarrhea, headache, sweating, increased heart rate, tremor, muscle twitching, **delirium**, shock, coma, and death. Switching between drug treatment with an MAOI to oxcarbazepine may require a waiting period of up to several weeks between drugs. Other drugs that cannot be combined with oxcarbazepine due to risk of **serotonin** syndrome include the antibiotic linezolid. Oxcarbazepine should not be used with large doses of the herbal supplements ginkgo biloba or **St. John's wort**, as the combination may decrease the efficacy of oxcarbazepine and induce seizures. The herbal supplements evening primrose, **valerian**, and **kava kava** should also be avoided and may induce seizures.

Resources

BOOKS

Brunton, Laurence, et al. *Goodman and Gilman's the Pharmacological Basis of Therapeutics*. 12th ed. New York: McGraw Hill Medical, 2011.

WEBSITES

PubMed Health. "Oxcarbazepine." U.S. National Library of Medicine. http://www.ncbi.nlm.nih.gov/pubmedhealth/PMH0000176 (accessed November 8, 2011).

ORGANIZATIONS

American Association for Clinical Chemistry, 1850 K St. NW, Ste. 625, Washington, DC, 20006, Fax: (202) 887-5093, (800) 892-1400, http://www.aacc.org.

American Society for Clinical Pharmacology and Therapeutics, 528 N Washington St., Alexandria, VA, 22314, (703) 836-6981, info@ascpt.org, http://www.ascpt.org.

U.S. Food and Drug Administration, 10903 New Hampshire Ave., Silver Spring, MD, 20993-0002, (888) INFO-FDA (463-6332), http://www.fda.gov.

Maria Eve Basile, PhD

P

Pain disorder

Definition

Pain disorder is one of several **somatoform disorders** described in the revised fourth edition of the mental health professional's handbook, the ***Diagnostic and Statistical Manual of Mental Disorders*** (*DSM-IV-TR*). The term *somatoform* means that symptoms are physical but are not entirely understood as a consequence of a general medical condition or as a direct effect of a substance, such as a drug. Pain in one or more anatomical sites is the predominant complaint and is severe enough to require medical or therapeutic **intervention**. Pain disorder is classified as a mental disorder because psychological factors play an important role in the onset, severity, worsening, or maintenance of pain.

Demographics

There is very little information regarding rates of pain disorder. A major difficulty is that the diagnostic categories for psychogenic pain disorder in *DSM-III*, somatoform pain disorder in *DSM-III-R*, and pain disorder in *DSM-IV* and *DSM-IV-TR* are not equivalent. Further, many criticize the somatoform disorder group (which includes pain disorder) as being an aggregate of disorders that are not truly distinct from one another. This lack of distinctiveness suggests to some researchers that a more appropriate system of classification should be dimensional rather than categorical. If shared dimensions or characteristics of the several somatoform disorders exist, differences among disorders should be a matter of degree along the possible dimensions, similar to spectrum disorders. The critics of the *DSM* categorical approach would prefer a dimensional or multiaxial system, because when classification systems are improved, the reliability and validity of measures assessing disorders also improve, making better prevalence estimates possible.

Description

In 1994, the International Association for the Study of Pain (IASP) defined pain as an unpleasant sensory or emotional experience arising from real or probable tissue damage. The perception of pain is, in part, a psychological response to noxious stimuli. This definition addresses the complex nature of pain and moves away from the earlier dualistic idea that pain is either psychogenic (of mental origin) or somatogenic (of physical origin). The contemporary view characterizes pain as multidimensional, meaning that the central nervous system, emotions, cognitions (thoughts), and beliefs are simultaneously involved.

When a patient's primary complaint is the experience of pain, and when impairment at home, work, or school causes significant distress, a **diagnosis** of pain disorder may be warranted. The diagnosis is further differentiated by a subtype, which is assigned depending on whether or not the pain is primarily accounted for by psychological factors or in combination with a general medical condition, and whether the pain is acute (less than six months) or chronic (six months or more). The classification of pain states is important since the effectiveness of treatment depends on the aptness of the diagnosis of pain disorder and its type.

DSM-5

Earlier names for this disorder include psychogenic pain disorder and somatoform pain disorder. There is some overlap in the meaning of these terms, but views regarding the nature of pain have been changing and they are, therefore, not equivalent diagnostic categories. Sometimes pain disorder is referred to as somatization, but this is an imprecise term and is easily confused with **somatization disorder**. There is a current discussion about recategorizing somatoform or somatization-spectrum disorders, including pain disorder, for the fifth edition of the *DSM* (*DSM-5*, 2013). Proposed changes as of 2011 subsumed pain disorder

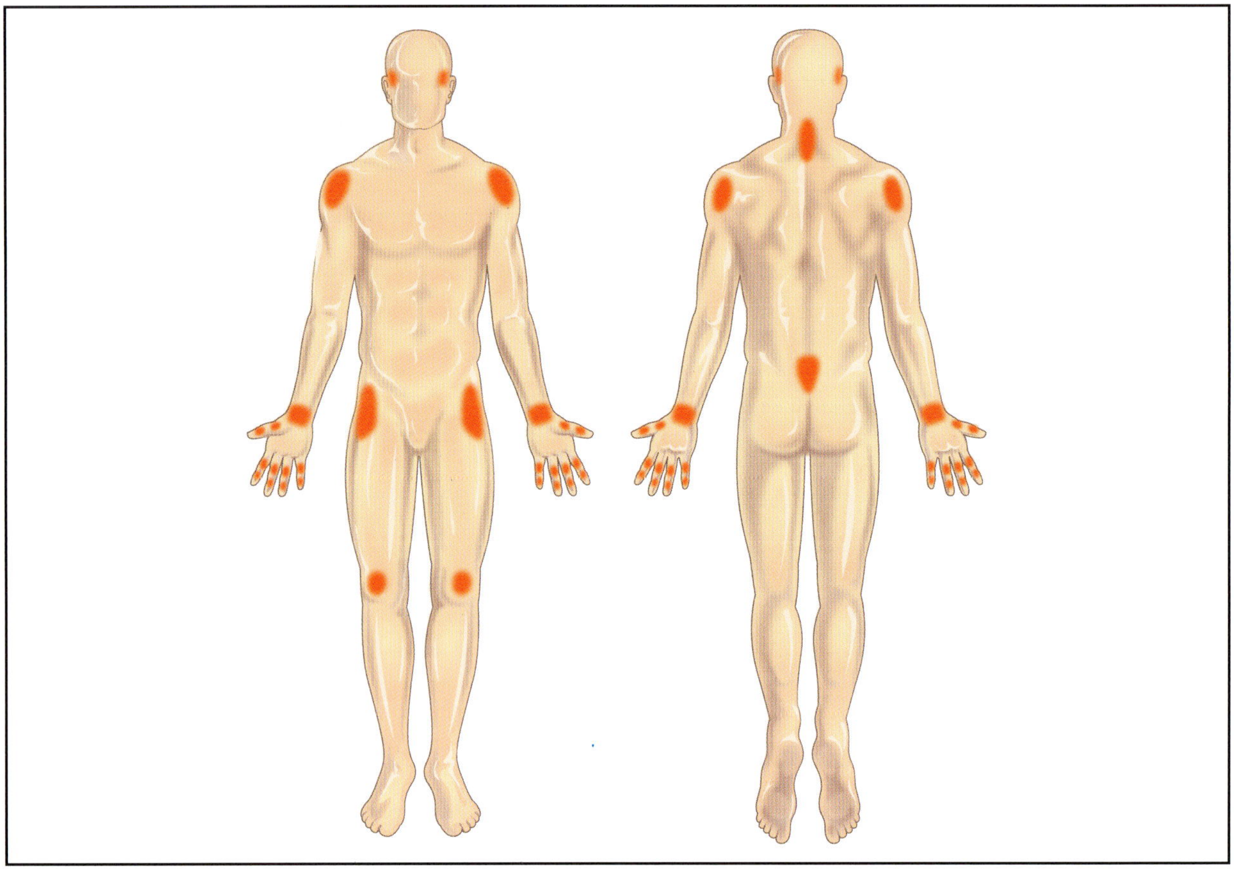

Highlighted areas show common sites of chronic pain. *(Illustration by Electronic Illustrators Group. © 2012 Cengage Learning.)*

into the diagnosis for complex somatic symptom disorder. The reason for the change centers on the complexity of the diagnostic criteria for some of the disorders and the tendency for patients to perceive some of the terms as socially stigmatizing.

Causes and symptoms

Causes

Common sites of pain include the back (especially lower back), head, abdomen, and chest. Causes of pain vary depending on the site; however, in pain disorder, the severity or duration of pain or the degree of associated disability is unexplained by observed medical or psychological problems.

The prevailing biopsychosocial model of mental disorders suggests that multiple causes may be attributed to pain disorder, especially when the pain is chronic. There are four domains of interest when assessing pain:

- The underlying organic problem or medical condition, if there is one. For example, fibromyalgia (a pain syndrome involving fibromuscular tissue), skeletal damage, pathology of an internal organ, migraine headache, and peptic ulcer all have characteristic patterns of pain and a particular set of causes.
- The experience of the pain. The severity, duration, and pattern of pain are important determinants of distress. Uncontrolled or inadequately managed pain is a significant stressor.
- Functional impairment and disability. Pain is exacerbated by loss of meaningful activities or social relationships. Disruption or loss may lead to isolation and resentment or anger, which further increases pain.
- Emotional distress. Depression and anxiety are the most common correlates of pain, especially when the person suffering feels that the pain is unmanageable, or that the future only holds more severe pain and more losses.

A therapist or team of health professionals will weigh the relative causal contributions, assign priorities for therapeutic intervention, and address the several domains in a multimodal fashion. For example, the design of a treatment plan in a pain clinic may involve a physician, psychotherapist, occupational therapist, physical therapist, anesthesiologist, **psychologist**, and nutritionist.

Symptoms

Symptoms vary depending on the site of pain and are treated medically. However, there are common symptoms associated with pain disorder, regardless of the site:

- negative or distorted cognition, such as feeling helpless or hopeless with respect to pain and its management
- inactivity, passivity, and/or disability
- increased pain requiring clinical intervention
- insomnia and fatigue
- disrupted social relationships at home, work, or school
- depression and/or anxiety

Diagnosis

A **psychiatrist** or mental health professional arrives at the diagnosis of pain disorder after considering several questions. An important preliminary question is whether the pain is entirely accounted for by a general medical condition. If so, the diagnosis of pain disorder is ruled out; if not, the psychiatrist considers whether the pain is feigned. If the psychiatrist believes the patient is pretending to be in pain, the patient is diagnosed as **malingering** for external rewards, such as mood-altering drugs, or as having a **factitious disorder** that reflects the patient's need to adopt a sick role. Neither malingering nor factitious disorder is in the somatoform group.

The psychiatrist may employ a variety of methods to assess the severity of pain and the contribution of psychological factors to the experience of pain. These include structured interviews (where the questions asked are standardized), open or unstructured interviews, numerical rating scales, visual analog scales (where the patient makes a mark along a line to indicate severity of pain or selects a face to represent the degree of pain), and instruments such as the McGill Pain Questionnaire or the West Haven-Yale Multidimensional Pain Inventory.

There are several conditions that rule out a diagnosis of pain disorder:

- dyspareunia, or painful sexual intercourse
- somatization disorder, characterized by a long history of pain that began prior to age 30 and involves the gastrointestinal, reproductive, and nervous systems
- conversion disorder, which includes motor or sensory dysfunction in addition to pain
- a mood, anxiety, or psychotic disorder, if any one of these more fully accounts for the pain

This last exclusion rests upon a very subjective opinion. Subjectivity reduces inter-rater reliability and is one of the points raised by critics of the *DSM* category for pain disorder. A final consideration in diagnosing pain disorder is whether the pain is acute or chronic.

Treatment

Depending on whether the pain is acute or chronic, management may involve one or more of the following: pharmacological treatment (medication), **psychotherapy** (individual or group), and family, behavioral, physical, or occupational therapy. If the pain is acute, the primary goal is to relieve the pain. Customary agents include acetaminophen or nonsteroidal anti-inflammatory drugs (NSAIDs). If opioid analgesics are prescribed, they are often combined with NSAIDs so that a lower dose may be used, as **opioids** have strong addictive potential. Psychotherapy is less important for the treatment of acute pain as compared to chronic pain disorder. In comparison, treatment of chronic pain disorder usually requires some sort of psychotherapy in combination with medication.

Antidepressants

Tricyclic **antidepressants** (TCAs) help reduce pain, improve sleep, and strengthen the effects of opioids (such as codeine and oxycodone), as well as treat moderate **depression**. Relief of pain may occur in a few days while lessening of depression may take several weeks. Usually, TCAs for pain are prescribed at doses 33% to 50% lower than when prescribed for depression. TCAs are particularly effective for neuropathic pain, headache, facial pain, fibromyalgia, and arthritis.

Treatment of sleep dysfunction

Pain and depression diminish the restorative quality of sleep. When the cycle of pain, depression, **insomnia**, and **fatigue** is established, it tends to be self-perpetuating. Treatment may include antidepressants, relaxation training, or education regarding good sleep hygiene.

Cognitive-behavioral therapy

Many people who suffer chronic pain experience isolation, distress, frustration, and a loss of confidence regarding their ability to cope; subsequently, they may adopt a passive, helpless style of problem solving. The goal of **cognitive-behavioral therapy** (CBT) is to restore a sense of self-efficacy by educating patients about the pain-and-tension cycle, by teaching them how to actively manage pain and distress, and by informing them about the therapeutic effects of their medications. CBT is time limited, structured, and goal oriented.

KEY TERMS

Acute—Having a sudden onset and lasting a short time.

Biopsychosocial model—A hypothetical explanation for why something occurs that includes biological, psychological, and social causes or correlates.

Chronic—A disease or condition that progresses slowly but persists or reoccurs over time.

Factitious disorder—A disorder in which the physical or psychological symptoms are produced or controlled by the patient.

Inter-rater reliability—The degree to which judgments about a person are consistent among raters or diagnosticians.

Malingering—Pretending to be sick in order to be relieved of an unwanted duty or obtain some other obvious benefit.

Multiaxial—A type of classification system that involves numeric measurement along more than one dimension and is not based on assignment to mutually exclusive categories.

Multimodal—Several types of therapeutic interventions such as heat or ice packs, electrical stimulation, or ultrasound; sometimes refers to a mix of physical and psychological therapies.

Neuropathic—Relating to neural damage.

Pain states—The four-way classification of pain disorder: (1) acute with psychological factors, (2) acute with psychological factors and a general medical condition, (3) chronic with psychological factors, and (4) chronic with psychological factors and a general medical condition.

Somatization—When mental or emotional distress is expressed physically in a way that disrupts body function.

Some tension-reducing techniques include progressive muscle relaxation, visual imagery, hypnosis, and **biofeedback**. Pain diaries are useful for describing daily patterns of pain and for helping the patient identify any activities, emotions, and thoughts that alleviate or worsen pain. Diaries also are useful in evaluating the effectiveness of medication. Patients may be taught pacing techniques or scheduling strategies to restore and maintain meaningful activities.

The cognitive aspect of CBT is based on cognitive-social learning theory. The focus is on helping the patient to restructure his or her ideas about the nature of pain and the possibility of effective self-management. In particular, the patient is taught to identify and then modify negative or distorted thought patterns of helplessness and hopelessness.

Operant conditioning

The principles of operant conditioning are taught to the patient and family members so that activity and non-pain behaviors are reinforced or encouraged. The goal is to eliminate pain behaviors, such as passivity, inactivity, and over-reliance on medication.

Other treatments

Other treatments used in the management of pain include **acupuncture**, transcutaneous electrical nerve stimulation (TENS), trigger point injections, massage, nerve blocks, surgical ablation (removal of a part or pathway), **meditation**, **exercise**, **yoga**, and music and **art therapy**.

Prognosis

The prognosis for total remission of symptoms is good for acute pain disorder but is not as promising for chronic pain disorder. The typical pattern for chronic pain entails occasional flare-ups alternating with periods of low to moderate pain. The prognosis for remission of symptoms is better when patients are able to continue working; unemployment and the attendant isolation, resentment, and inactivity are correlates of a continuing pain disorder. Additionally, if **reinforcement** of pain behavior is in place (for example, financial compensation for continuing disability, an overly solicitous spouse, or abuse of addictive drugs), remission is less likely.

The results of outcome studies comparing pain disorder treatments point to cognitive-behavioral therapy in conjunction with antidepressants as the most continually effective regimen. However, people in chronic pain may respond better to other treatments, and both the patient and the health professional(s) need to work together to find an individualized mix of effective coping strategies.

Prevention

Pain disorder may be prevented by early intervention at the onset of pain or in the early stages of recurring pain. When pain becomes chronic, it is especially important to find help or learn about and implement strategies to manage the distress before inactivity and hopelessness develop. Most patients in pain first contact their primary care physician, who may make a referral to a mental health professional or pain clinic. Many physicians will reassure the patient that a referral for psychological help is not stigmatizing, does not in any way minimize the experience of pain or the medical condition, and does not imply that the physician believes the pain is imaginary. On the contrary, the accepted IASP definition of pain fully recognizes that all pain is, in part, an emotional response to actual damage or to the threat of damage.

Resources

BOOKS

American Psychiatric Association. *Diagnostic and Statistical Manual of Mental Disorders*. 4th ed., text rev. Washington, DC: American Psychiatric Publishing, 2000.

Martin, Ronald L., and Sean H. Yutzy. "Somatoform Disorders." In *Psychiatry*, edited by Allan Tasman, Jerald Kay, and Jeffrey A. Lieberman. 3rd ed. New York: Wiley and Sons, 2008.

Masheb, Robin M., and Robert D. Kerns. "Pain Disorder." In *Effective Brief Therapies: A Clinician's Guide*, edited by Michael Hersen and Maryka Biaggio. San Diego: Academic Press, 2000.

Simon, Gregory E. "Management of Somatoform and Factitious Disorders." In *A Guide to Treatments that Work*, edited by Peter E. Nathan and Jack M. Gorman. New York: Oxford University Press, 1998.

PERIODICALS

King, Steven. "The Classification and Assessment of Pain." *International Review of Psychiatry* 12, no. 2 (2000): 86–90.

Kroenke, Kurt. "Physical Symptom Disorder: A Simpler Diagnostic Category for Somatization-Spectrum Conditions." *Journal of Psychosomatic Research* 60, no. 4 (April 2006): 335–9.

Merskey, Harold. "Pain, Psychogenesis, and Psychiatric Diagnosis." *International Review of Psychiatry* 12, no. 2 (2000): 99–102.

Sunil, Verma, and Rollin M. Gallagher. "Evaluating and Treating Co-morbid Pain and Depression." *International Review of Psychiatry* 12, no. 2 (2000): 103–14.

WEBSITES

MedlinePlus. "Somatoform Pain Disorder." U.S. National Library of Medicine, National Institutes of Health. http://www.nlm.nih.gov/medlineplus/ency/article/000922.htm (accessed October 23, 2011).

ORGANIZATIONS

American Academy of Pain Medicine, 4700 W. Lake, Glenview, IL, 60025, (847) 375-4731, Fax: (847) 375-6477, info@painmed.org, http://www.painmed.org.

American Chronic Pain Association, PO Box 850, Rocklin, CA, 95677, (800) 533-3231, Fax: (916) 632-3208, ACPA@pacbell.net, http://www.theacpa.org.

American Psychiatric Association, 1000 Wilson Blvd., Ste. 1825, Arlington, VA, 22209-3901, (703) 907-7300, apa@psych.org, http://www.psych.org.

Tanja Bekhuis, Ph.D.
Emily Jane Willingham, Ph.D.

Paliperidone

Definition

Paliperidone (sold under the brand name Invega) is a medication used in the treatment of the psychiatric diseases **schizophrenia** and **schizoaffective disorder**. Paliperidone belongs to a class of drugs known as atypical antipsychotics, which specifically act on two natural body chemicals, **serotonin** and **dopamine**. These chemicals are types of **neurotransmitters** involved in normal **brain** function and can affect the **psychosis** and other symptoms of schizophrenia and schizoaffective disorder. Paliperidone acts as a neurotransmitter blocker, inhibiting the effects of serotonin and dopamine.

Purpose

Paliperidone is a type of drug known as an atypical antipsychotic; atypical antipsychotics are thought to have less adverse side effects than older antipsychotic drugs. The decision to use paliperidone alone or in combination with other drugs depends on the particular medical disorder, the response of the patient to the medication, and individual health parameters.

Description

Paliperidone works by inhibiting the absorption of the neurotransmitters serotonin and norepinephrine. Specifically, paliperidone blocks the signaling of these neurotransmitters in the brain by binding their corresponding neurotransmitter receptors. The pathology of schizophrenia is thought to involve the overactivity of neurotransmitter signaling in some areas of the brain and underactivity in others; antipsychotics such as

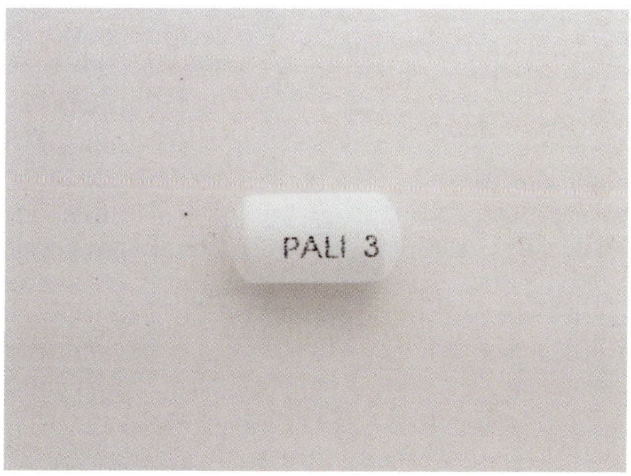

Invega (paliperidone), 3 mg. *(© Custom Medical Stock Photo, Inc. Reproduced by permission.)*

KEY TERMS

Bipolar disorder—Psychiatric mood disorder characterized by periods of manic behavior that may alternate with periods of depression, also known as manic depressive disorder.

Cognitive—Associated with thinking, learning, perception, awareness, and judgment.

Dopamine—A type of neurotransmitter involved in regulation of concentration, impulse control, judgment, mood, attention span, psychostimulation, and disease states such as addiction, and depression.

Insomnia—Disorder involving disturbance of sleep.

Mania—Physiological state of hyperactivity experienced by patients with certain psychiatric illnesses involving inappropriate elevated mood, pressured speech, poor judgment, and sometimes psychotic episodes.

Neuroleptic malignant syndrome—Dangerous reaction to antipsychotic medications that involves temperature instability, muscular rigidity, and altered mental status.

Neuronal signaling—The electrical or chemical pathway by which neurons communicate.

Neurotransmitter—One of a group of chemicals secreted by a nerve cell (neuron) to carry a chemical message to another nerve cell, often as a way of transmitting a nerve impulse. Examples of neurotransmitters include acetylcholine, dopamine, serotonin, and norepinephrine.

Neurotransmitter receptor—A physical recipient for chemicals called neurotransmitters. Receptors sit on the surface of cells that make up body tissues, and once bound to the neurotransmitter, they initiate the chemical signaling pathway associated with neurotransmitters.

Prolactin—Hormone responsible for endocrine function, including lactation.

Psychosis—Loss of contact with reality that may involve false beliefs or hallucinations.

Schizophrenia—Severe psychiatric illness involving the disintegration of thought processes and sometimes including hallucinations.

Serotonin—A type of neurotransmitter involved in regulation of the blood vessels, brain processes, and disease states such as depression.

paliperidone help address the deficits but do not completely treat the disorder. The symptoms of schizophrenia known as **positive symptoms**, such as psychosis, are best treated with paliperidone. The negative and cognitive symptoms such as withdrawal and difficulty reasoning are not as well addressed with paliperidone, but paliperidone has more impact on these types of symptoms than older antipsychotics. Paliperidone is also effective in treating mania, or a mixed state of mood elevation and **depression**.

Recommended dosage

Paliperidone is taken as an oral medication. The available doses are 1.5, 3, 6, and 9 mg pills. The 9 mg dose is an extended release formulation. Patients being treated for schizophrenia are usually started at 6 mg, taken in the morning. The dose is gradually increased to the most effective dose that does not cause intolerable side effects. The daily dose may be increased by 3 mg roughly every 5–7 days. The maximum dose is 12 mg per day. Dosing for schizoaffective disorder is similar. For either disorder, the dose is decreased if the patient has impairment of kidney function or severe liver disease. If side effects develop or if other drugs are to be used in combination with paliperidone, the dose may also be decreased. Side effects impacting the immune system may require a lower dose or complete discontinuation of the drug. Patients are periodically reassessed for the need of treatment.

Precautions

Paliperidone is an atypical antipsychotic medication, a class that was developed for the purpose of avoiding some of the side effects often seen with older, typical antipsychotic medications. As a class, these medications cause fewer **medication-induced movement disorders** than older medications but still have the potential to cause some significant movement-related effects. Patients taking paliperidone must be monitored for the development of **movement disorders** as well as stiffness, mental status changes, and increased temperature associated with a dangerous syndrome known as **neuroleptic malignant syndrome**. However, paliperidone is less likely to cause these disorders than many other types of antipsychotic medications. Patients taking paliperidone must have their immune system function monitored via periodic blood tests, as the drug can cause dangerous decreases in white blood cells. High blood sugar may also develop, especially in patients at risk for diabetes. Blood sugar is measured before initiating paliperidone dosing then monitored periodically. Paliperidone carries a risk of low blood pressure and possible temporary loss of consciousness, especially in older or dehydrated patients rising quickly from a lying down position.

Paliperidone may not be appropriate for use or may require caution in patients with heart abnormalities or disease, liver dysfunction, kidney dysfunction, history of **stroke** or seizure, diabetes, or immune dysfunction; patients who are dehydrated or have diarrhea or electrolyte abnormalities; and the elderly. Paliperidone should not be used in elderly patients to treat symptoms of **dementia**; use of paliperidone for this purpose is not approved by the U.S. Food and Drug Administration, and elderly patients taking paliperidone for dementia-related symptoms are at increased risk of stroke or death.

Paliperidone is classified as category C for pregnancy, which means either there are no adequate human or animal studies or that adverse fetal effects were found in animal studies, but there is no available human data. The decision whether to use category C drugs during pregnancy is generally based on weighing the critical needs of the mother against the risk to the fetus. Other lower category agents are used whenever possible. There are data that suggest paliperidone is considered unsafe for use during breast-feeding, and its use is not recommended.

Side effects

Atypical antipsychotics such as paliperidone are known for having fewer movement-related side effects than other types of older antipsychotic medications that act on neurotransmitter receptors in different parts of the brain. This is one reason why as a general class they tend to be the drug of choice in treatment of schizophrenia or other disorders involving psychosis such as schizoaffective disorder. However, as with all medications, antipsychotics such as paliperidone have side effects. Sensitivity to paliperidone varies between patients, and some patients may find that even lower doses are more than their body system can tolerate. Common side effects of paliperidone include headache, dizziness, dry mouth, cough, nausea, upset stomach, weight gain, **fatigue**, increased heart rate, excess salivation, anxiety, tremor, heart rhythm abnormalities, skin sensitivity to sunlight, and fever. Antipsychotics such as paliperidone that act to antagonize dopamine receptors may cause an increase in prolactin, the hormone that causes lactation in women and impotence in men. Low blood pressure or a drop in blood pressure upon standing may result in loss of consciousness. Rare but serious potential side effects include severe movement disorders, high blood sugar or overt diabetes, stroke, severe difficulty swallowing, dangerous changes in heart rhythm, **seizures**, and changes in blood cells including anemia and decreased immune function. A rare but dangerous possible side effect is neuroleptic malignant syndrome, a reaction involving very high body temperature, altered mental status, and muscular rigidity.

QUESTIONS TO ASK YOUR DOCTOR

- Can I take the full dose right away or do I need to slowly increase the dose up to the full amount?
- Can I stop taking the medication right away or do I need to stop slowly?
- Should I eat before taking this medication?
- Will this medication interact with any of my other prescription medications? Over-the-counter-drugs? Herbal supplements?
- What side effects should I watch for while taking this medication?
- Can I drink alcoholic beverages in the same time frame as taking this medication?

Interactions

Patients should make their doctor aware of all medications and supplements they are taking before using paliperidone. Using alcohol while taking paliperidone may create toxic reactions in the body and should be avoided. Drugs that affect the liver may alter the metabolism of paliperidone, resulting in too little or too much of the drug in the body. This could lead to increased side effects or even toxic doses. Likewise, paliperidone may affect the metabolism of other drugs, leading to greater or lower doses than therapeutically desired.

Many drugs may cause toxicity and adversely affect heart rhythm when used in combination with paliperidone. These drugs include multiple types of heart medications, including dronedarone and amiodarone; the antimalaria drug mefloquine; the chemotherapeutic toremifene; the antifungal drug voriconazole; the antibiotics azithromycin, clarithromycin, and ciprofloxacin; and antipsychotics such as **pimozide** and **ziprasidone**, among many others. The drug bromocriptine used in various neurological and endocrine disorders may cause dangerously low blood pressure when used with paliperidone. Sedative drugs such as codeine and herbal supplements such as calendula, capsicum, kava, and lemon balm may cause additive effects of severe sedation in patients using paliperidone. The herbal supplement Siberian **ginseng** causes antagonizing effects and decreases the effectiveness of paliperidone, as well as exacerbating many psychiatric conditions.

Resources

BOOKS

Brunton, Laurence L., et al. *Goodman and Gilman's The Pharmacological Basis of Therapeutics.* 12th ed. New York: McGraw Hill Medical, 2011.

Stargrove, Mitchell Bebel, et al. *Herb, Nutrient, and Drug Interactions: Clinical Implications and Therapeutic Strategies.* St. Louis: Mosby, 2007.

WEBSITES

PubMed Health. "Paliperidone." U.S. National Library of Medicine. http://www.ncbi.nlm.nih.gov/pubmedhealth/PMH0000356 (accessed November 8, 2011).

ORGANIZATIONS

American College of Neuropsychopharmacology, 5034-A Thoroughbred Lane, Brentwood, TN, 37027, (615) 324-2360, Fax: (615) 523-1715, acnp@acnp.org, http://www.acnp.org/default.aspx.

American Psychiatric Association, 1000 Wilson Blvd., Ste. 1825, Arlington, VA, 22209-3901, (703) 907-7300, apa@psych.org, http://www.psych.org.

American Society for Clinical Pharmacology and Therapeutics, 528 N Washington St., Alexandria, VA, 22314, (703) 836-6981, info@ascpt.org, http://www.ascpt.org.

Mental Health America, 2000 N Beauregard St., 6th Fl., Alexandria, VA, 22311, (703) 684-7722, (800) 969-6642, Fax: (703) 684-5968, http://www.nmha.org.

U.S. Food and Drug Administration, 10903 New Hampshire Ave., Silver Spring, MD, 20993-0002, (888) INFO-FDA (463-6332), http://www.fda.gov.

Maria Eve Basile, PhD

Pamelor *see* **Nortriptyline**

Panic attack

Definition

Panic attacks, the hallmark of **panic disorder**, are discrete episodes of intense anxiety. Panic attacks can also be experienced by people with **anxiety disorders**, mood disorders, substance-related disorders (e.g., **cocaine addiction**), or general medical conditions (e.g., hyperthyroidism).

Description

Panic attacks are intense anxiety experiences that occur suddenly over discrete periods of time, and are characterized by intense apprehension or fearfulness in situations where there is no actual danger. Physical symptoms of a panic attack may include palpitations, difficulty breathing, chest pain or discomfort, choking or smothering sensations, excessive perspiration, or dizziness. Panic attacks often include the fear of going crazy, losing control, or dying. Panic attacks triggered by a specific experience are called situational panic attacks, since a certain situation (e.g., public speaking, driving, shopping in a crowded store) initiates the intense anxiety.

Persons affected with panic attacks usually exhibit a broad range of clinical signs and symptoms that include:

- heart palpitations (accelerated heart rate)
- shaking or trembling
- sweating
- shortness of breath or sensation of feeling smothered or choked
- feeling of tingling
- chest discomfort or pain
- nausea or abdominal distress
- feeling dizzy, light headed, unsteady or faint
- perceptions of being detached from oneself (depersonalization), or a feeling out of touch with reality (derealization)
- chills or hot flashes
- fear of dying
- fear of going crazy or losing control

A person meets the criteria for a panic attack if the symptoms start abruptly, reach a quick peak (usually within 10 minutes), and if the affected individual has at least four symptoms as listed above. In persons who have less than four symptoms during an attack, the disorder is called a limited symptom attack.

It is typical that affected persons who seek treatment usually have one to two attacks a week and in worse periods may have one daily attacks or several within a week.

As stated, panic attacks can be experienced as a result of stimulant chemical usage, such as cocaine. There is evidence to suggest that persons with panic attacks are sensitive to certain chemicals such as caffeine, carbon dioxide, antihistamines, and, in women, progesterone replacement. Exposure to these substances may precipitate an attack.

Resources

BOOKS

Bope, Edward T., and Rick D. Kellerman. *Conn's Current Therapy*. Philadelphia: Elsevier, 2012.

Schmidt, Leonard J., and Brooke Warner. *Panic: Origins, Insight, and Treatment*. Berkeley, CA: North Atlantic Books, 2002.

Starcevic, Vladan. *Anxiety Disorders in Adults: A Clinical Guide*. 2nd ed. New York: Oxford University Press, 2010.

VandenBos, Gary R., ed. *APA Dictionary of Psychology*. Washington, DC: American Psychological Association, 2006.

ORGANIZATIONS

Anxiety Disorders Association of America, 8730 Georgia Ave., Silver Spring, MD, 20910, (240) 485-1001, Fax: (240) 485-1035, http://www.adaa.org.

Laith Farid Gulli, MD
Jean Suvan, BS, RDH

Panic disorder

Definition

Panic disorder is a condition in which a person suffers recurrent panic attacks. Panic attacks are sudden attacks that are not caused by a substance (such as caffeine), medication, or by a medical condition (such as high blood pressure). During the attack, the sufferer may experience sensations such as accelerated or irregular heartbeats, shortness of breath, dizziness, or a fear of losing control. The sudden attack builds quickly (usually within 10 minutes) and is almost paralyzing in its severity. When a **diagnosis** of panic disorder is given, the disorder can be considered one of two different types—panic disorder with or without **agoraphobia**.

Agoraphobia is a fear of being in a place or situation from which escape might be difficult or embarrassing or in which help may not be available in the case of a **panic attack**. It is not clear why some people develop agoraphobia and other people do not. Many people

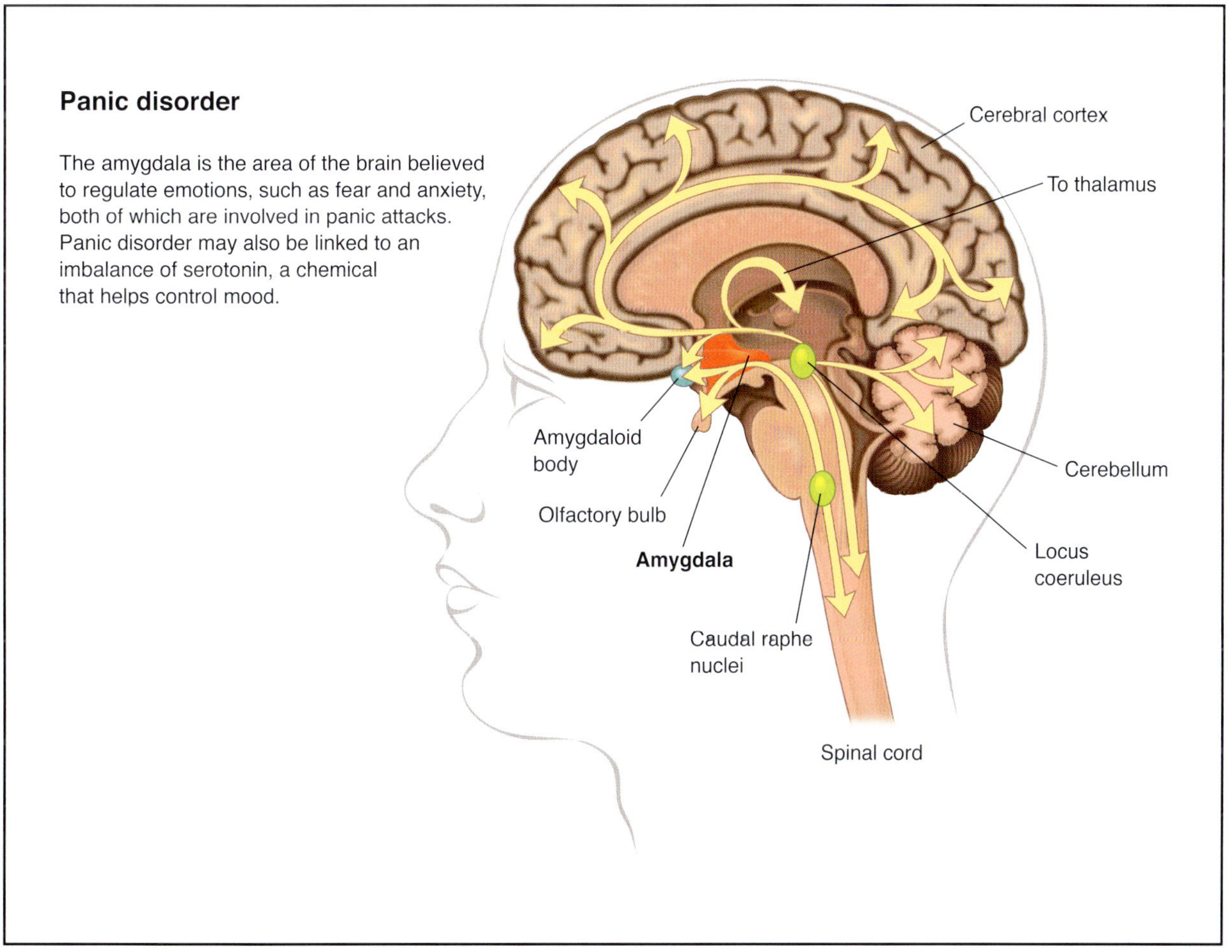

(Illustration by Electronic Illustrators Group. Reproduced by permission of Gale, a part of Cengage Learning.)

may develop their agoraphobia symptoms right after their first attack, but others do not develop agoraphobia until years after their attacks began.

The handbook for mental health professionals (called the ***Diagnostic and Statistical Manual of Mental Disorders***, or the *DSM*) classifies panic disorder with and without agoraphobia as **anxiety disorders**.

Demographics

Factors such as race, gender, and socioeconomic status are important factors in the development of panic disorder. An individual has a 1%–2% chance of developing panic disorder with or without agoraphobia. The symptoms usually begin when individuals are in their early to mid-twenties. Women are twice as likely as men to develop panic attacks regardless of age. The **National Institute of Mental Health** Epidemiologic Catchment Area Study (ECA) shows no significant differences between the races or ethnic groups, although it appears that African American and Hispanic men between the ages of 40 and 50 have lower rates of panic disorder than white men. Panic disorder patients are at increased risk for major **depression** and the development of agoraphobia. According to ECA studies, an individual with panic disorder has a 33% chance of developing agoraphobia. People without panic disorder only have a 5.5% chance of developing agoraphobia. Again, women were found to be more likely to develop agoraphobia than men. Over the course of their lifetime, African Americans were more likely to develop agoraphobia than whites or Hispanics. Agoraphobia is more prevalent among people with less education and lower economic class.

Description

Panic disorder can be difficult to distinguish from other mental illnesses such as major depression, other anxiety disorders, or medical conditions such as heart attacks. Panic attacks differ from general anxiety in that the episodes last for discrete periods of time, and the symptoms that people suffer are more intense. Panic attacks have three types: unexpected, situationally bound, and situationally predisposed. The unexpected attacks occur without warning and without a trigger. The situationally bound attacks happen repeatedly when the person is performing or preparing to perform some activity or even when the person thinks about doing that activity. For example, a person whose panic attacks are triggered by being in crowds can have an attack just by thinking about going to a shopping mall. Situationally predisposed attacks are similar to the situationally bound attacks, except that they do not always occur when the trigger stimulus is encountered. For example, someone who experiences panic attacks while in crowds may sometimes be in crowds and not experience attacks or may experience attacks in noncrowded situations as well.

Panic disorder without agoraphobia

Panic disorder without agoraphobia is defined by the fourth edition of the *DSM* (*DSM-IV-TR*) as a disorder in which patients are plagued by panic attacks that occur repeatedly and without warning. After these attacks, affected individuals worry for one month or more about having more embarrassing attacks and may change their behavior with regard to these attacks. For example, patients may fear that they have a cardiac condition and may quit a job or quit exercising because of the fear. Patients may also worry that they are going to lose control or appear insane to other people. Panic disorder without agoraphobia has a less severe set of symptoms than panic disorder with agoraphobia. Patients without agoraphobia do not become housebound; they suffer panic attacks but do not have significant interference in their level of function and are still able to accomplish their daily activities.

Panic disorder with agoraphobia

People who suffer from panic disorder with agoraphobia may experience their agoraphobia in one of two ways. They may experience sudden, unexpected panic attacks that cause them to fear being in a place where help might not be available, or they may experience sudden panic attacks in specific, known situations and fear those situations or places that may trigger attacks. In either case, the fear of further panic attacks restricts affected individuals' ability to complete activities. For example, people whose attacks are triggered by being in crowds may avoid shopping malls for fear that they will be in a crowd and have a panic attack. Individuals may experience sudden, debilitating panic attacks without a particular trigger, and, as a result, they are afraid to go to a supermarket (or similar place) for fear that a panic attack could occur while they are there and no one would be able to help.

Panic disorder in the DSM-5

The fifth edition of the *DSM* (*DSM-5*), due to publish in May 2013, has proposed recategorizing panic disorders and agoraphobia so that each one becomes a separate diagnosis within the category of anxiety disorders. The **American Psychiatric Association** website describing the planned revisions states that panic attack alone will not warrant a separate diagnosis but that both panic disorder and agoraphobia will be treated as separate entities.

Causes and symptoms

Causes

BIOCHEMICAL/PHYSIOLOGICAL CAUSES. It is extremely difficult to study the **brain** and the underlying causes of psychiatric illness; and understanding the chemistry of the brain is the key to unlocking the mystery of panic disorder. The amygdala is the part of the brain that causes fear and the response to **stress**. It has been implicated as a vital part of anxiety disorders. Sodium lactate, a chemical that the body produces when muscles are fatigued, and carbon dioxide are known to induce panic attacks. These substances are thought to inhibit the release of **neurotransmitters** in the brain, which leads to the panic attacks. One hypothesis is that sodium lactate stimulates the amygdala and causes panic attacks. Another hypothesis is that patients with panic disorder have a hypersensitive internal suffocation alarm. This means that the patients's brain sends the body false signals that not enough oxygen is being received, causing the affected persons to increase their breathing rate. Panic disorder patients have attacks when their overly sensitive alarm goes off unpredictably. Yohimbine, a drug used to treat male sexual dysfunction, stimulates a part of the brain called the locus ceruleus and induces panic symptoms thus pointing to this area of the brain's involvement in panic disorder. Brain neurotransmitters **serotonin** and GABA are suspected to be involved in causing the disorder, as well.

GENETICS. Genetics also plays a pivotal role in the development of panic disorder. Twin studies have demonstrated that there is a higher concordance in identical versus fraternal twins thus supporting the idea that panic disorders are inherited. Family studies have also demonstrated that panic attacks run in families. Relatives of patients with panic disorder are four to 10 times more likely to develop panic disorder. People who develop early onset of panic attacks in their mid-20s are more likely to have relatives who have panic disorder. When relatives of patients with panic disorder are exposed to high levels of carbon dioxide, they have panic attacks. Another hypothesis is that patients with panic disorder who develop agoraphobia have a more severe form of the disease. Current efforts to identify a gene for panic disorder have not been successful.

PERSONAL VARIABLES. There are several themes in the psychology of panic disorder. Research has shown that patients who develop panic disorder have difficulty with anger. They also have difficulty when their job responsibilities are increased (as in the case of a promotion) and are sensitive to loss and separation. People with this disorder often have difficulty getting along with their parents, whom they see as controlling, critical, and demanding, causing the patients to feel inadequate. Early maternal separation is thought to be an underlying cause of panic disorder.

Panic disorder patients also have a pattern of dependency in their interpersonal relationships. As children, people with panic disorder relied on parents to protect them from fear. As a result, they become dependent on their parents and fear detaching from them. They constantly feel as though they are trapped.

There is also an association between **sexual abuse** and patients who have panic attacks. Sixty percent of female patients with panic disorder were sexually abused as children. This explains their difficulty with developing trusting relationships.

Symptoms

PANIC ATTACK. The *DSM-IV-TR* lists thirteen symptoms to meet the criteria for a diagnosis of panic attack. Affected persons must have four or more of these symptoms within ten minutes of the beginning of an attack in order to meet the panic attack criteria:

- bounding or pounding heartbeat or fast heart rate
- sweating
- shaking
- shortness of breath
- feeling of choking
- pains in the chest; many people feel as though they are having a heart attack
- nausea or stomach ache
- feeling dizzy or lightheaded as if they are going to pass out
- feeling of being outside of their body or are detached from reality
- fear that they are out of control or crazy
- fear that they are going to die
- feeling of tingling or numbness
- chills or hot flashes

PANIC DISORDER WITHOUT AGORAPHOBIA. The *DSM-IV-TR* criteria for panic disorder without agoraphobia include:

- recurrent panic attacks (see above) that occur without warning for one month
- persistent worry that panic attacks will recur
- possible change in behavior because of that fear
- no agoraphobia
- not due to a medical condition or substance abuse

- not due other mental illness like specific phobia, social phobia, obsessive-compulsive disorder, separation anxiety disorder, or post-traumatic stress disorder

PANIC DISORDER WITH AGORAPHOBIA. The *DSM-IV-TR* criteria for panic disorder with agoraphobia are the same as panic disorder without agoraphobia, but with the addition of agoraphobia. The symptoms of agoraphobia include fear of being in situations that can trigger panic attacks and avoiding places where attacks have occurred because of the affected persons' fear that they will not be able to leave or will not be able to get help. People with this condition may need to have another person accompany them when going to a place that may trigger anxiety attacks. Sometimes this fear can be so severe that affected individuals become housebound. This fact is important to consider because 15% of the general population can have one spontaneous panic attack without the recurrence of symptoms.

Diagnosis

Differential diagnosis

Differential diagnosis is the process of distinguishing one diagnosis from other, similar diagnoses. Panic disorder can be difficult to distinguish from other anxiety disorders such as specific phobia and **social phobia**. However, in general, specific phobia is cued by a specific trigger or stimulus and social phobia by specific social situations, whereas the panic attacks of panic disorder are completely uncued and unexpected. In certain cases, it may be difficult to distinguish between certain situational phobias and panic disorder with agoraphobia, and mental health professionals must use the *DSM* and professional judgment in these cases. Panic attacks that occur during sleep and wake affected persons up are more characteristic of panic disorder than are the other disorders that include panic attacks. It can be distinguished from **post-traumatic stress disorder** (PTSD), **obsessive-compulsive disorder** (OCD), and **generalized anxiety disorder** (GAD), again by what cues the attacks. In PTSD, thinking about the traumatic event can trigger attacks. In obsessive-compulsive disorder, worries about getting dirty can fuel an attack of anxiety. In generalized anxiety disorder, general worries or concerns can lead to the symptoms of panic. However, in panic disorder, a main component is that the affected individual fears recurrent panic attacks.

Panic attacks can often be difficult to distinguish from other physical problems such as hyperthyroidism, hyperparathyroidism, seizure disorder, and cardiac disease. If patients are middle-aged or older and have other complaints, including dizziness and headaches, their attacks are more likely to be a medical problem and not panic attacks. Panic attacks can also be difficult to distinguish from drug abuse since any drug that stimulates the brain can cause the symptoms. For example, **cocaine**, caffeine, and **amphetamines** can all cause panic attacks. Therefore, individuals must be free of all drugs before a diagnosis of panic disorder can be made. Many patients may attempt to self-medicate with alcohol to try to calm down. Withdrawal from alcohol can lead to worse panic symptoms. Patients may believe that they are reducing symptoms whereas they are actually exacerbating their panic attacks.

Dual diagnosis

Individuals with panic disorders have a high rate of coexisting depression. Patients who have panic disorder have about a 40%–80% chance of developing major depression. In most situations, the panic disorder happens first and the depression comes later. Patients are also at risk for **substance abuse** difficulties as a result of attempts to stop attacks. These attempts may involve the use of alcohol, illicit or unprescribed **sedatives**, or **benzodiazepines** (medications that slow down the central nervous system, having a calming effect). Patients with panic disorder are not at high risk for **suicide** attempts. A recent Harvard-Brown study showed that people with panic disorder with or without agoraphobia are not at risk for suicide unless they have other conditions such as depression or substance abuse.

Psychological measures and diagnostic testing

Currently there is no diagnostic test for panic disorder. Patients who have panic attacks should receive a thorough medical examination to rule out any medical condition. Patients should have baseline blood counts and glucose should be measured. Patients with cardiac symptoms need a cardiac workup and should see their primary medical doctor. Patients who have complaints of dizziness should receive a thorough neurological evaluation. There are several psychological inventories that can help the clinician diagnose panic disorder including the **Beck Depression Inventory** (BDI), Beck Anxiety Inventory (BAI), Specific Fear Inventory, Clinical Anxiety Scale (CAS), and the Clinical Global Inventory (CGI).

Treatment

There are various treatments for panic disorder.

Psychological and social interventions

A psychotherapeutic technique that is critical to the treatment of panic disorder is **cognitive-behavioral**

therapy (CBT). Patients are panic-free within six months in about 80–90% of cases. Some people may experience long-term effects after the treatments have been stopped. About half of the patients say that they have rare attacks even two years after treatment has ended.

New studies reveal that the approach to treating panic disorder should have three aspects: the cognitive, the physiological, and the behavioral. The cognitive techniques try to focus on changing the patient's negative thoughts—such as "I will die if I don't get help." Patient education about symptoms is also critical to the treatment of panic attacks. In one physiological approach, patients are taught breathing techniques in an effort to try to help them lower their heart rate and decrease their anxiety. Repeated exposure to physical symptoms associated with the panic disorder is also a part of treatment. For example, patients may cause themselves to hyperventilate in effort to reproduce the panic symptoms. In behavioral approaches, individuals who experience panic attacks need to be exposed to situations that they may have previously feared. Patients can also be taken to places associated with agoraphobia with the therapist.

Some patients may benefit from **psychodynamic psychotherapy** and **group therapy**. Psychodynamic **psychotherapy** explores thoughts and ideas of the person's subconscious. It takes a longer time to achieve efficacy than cognitive-behavioral therapy, but it can be just as effective for patients with panic disorder. Group therapy is also just as helpful to some patients as CBT. **Support groups** can also be helpful to some patients. It can be very therapeutic and healing for individuals to discuss their problems with someone who has actually experienced the same symptoms. Patients can learn from each other's coping styles.

Medical treatments

Panic disorder patients have a 50–80% chance of responding to treatment, which attempts to block the symptoms of panic attacks. Treating the agoraphobia symptoms is more challenging. Developing some anti-panic regimens that address all symptoms is important. The Food and Drug Administration (FDA) approves only five classes of drugs for treating panic disorder. They are:

- benzodiazepines
- Selective serotonin reuptake inhibitors (SSRIs), which cause a buildup of serotonin. This buildup is thought to cause the antidepressant effect.
- Tricyclic antidepressants (TCAs)
- Monoamine oxidase inhibitors (MAOIs) and reversible MAOIs, which inhibit the breakdown of neurotransmitters in the brain, including dopamine and serotonin
- Atypical antidepressants, including bupropion (Wellbutrin), mirtazapine (Remeron), trazodone (Desyrel), and others

Patients should first be started on a low-dose SSRI and then the dose should be increased slowly. Patients with panic disorder are extremely sensitive to the side effects that many patients experience in the first weeks of antidepressant therapy. Patients should also have a benzodiazepine, such as **clonazepam** (Klonopin) or **alprazolam** (Xanax) in the first weeks of treatment until the antidepressant becomes therapeutic. Most people need the same dose of antidepressant as patients with major depression. About 60% of patients will have improvement in their symptoms while taking an antidepressant and a benzodiazepine. Patients with mitral valve prolapse may benefit from a beta blocker. Patients who have tried an SSRI and after six weeks show no improvement can be switched to another SSRI, benzodiazepine, TCA, MAOI, or **venlafaxine** (Effexor). An SSRI should be stopped if patients have intolerable side effects such as loss of sexual libido, weight gain, or mild form of manic depression. When **SSRIs** are stopped, it is important that the dosage is gradually tapered because patients can suffer symptoms when it is abruptly withdrawn. These symptoms may include confusion, anxiety, and poor sleep.

Alternative therapies

Some alternative therapies for panic disorder are hypnosis, **meditation**, **yoga**, proper **nutrition**, **exercise**, and abdominal breathing techniques that foster relaxation, and visualization. Visualization is imagining oneself in the stressful situation while relaxed so that coping strategies can be discovered. The herb kava has been studied in trials to treat anxiety attacks and has been found to be effective in some **clinical trials**, but it has not been studied intensely enough to determine its benefits and side effects and has been associated with liver toxicity.

Prognosis

Patients with panic disorder have a poor prognosis particularly if untreated. Patients often **relapse** when they attempt to discontinue treatment. However, if patients are compliant and willing to stay in treatment, then the long-term prognosis is good. According to one study, eight years after treatment has been completed, 30–40% of patient were doing better. Only 10–20% of patients were doing poorly. Patients with panic attacks have a relapsing and remitting course that can be worsened by significant stressors such as the death of a spouse or divorce. Cognitive-behavioral therapy has an

80–90% chance that the patient will benefit six months after treatment. Medications have a 50–80% efficacy. If patients are committed to staying in treatment, their prognosis is very favorable.

Prevention

Although panic disorder is not totally preventable, individuals with a strong family history of susceptibility to panic attacks are encouraged to be aware of the symptoms and get treatment early. **Compliance** with treatment is important to the recovery from panic disorder.

Resources

BOOKS

American Psychiatric Association. *Diagnostic and Statistical Manual of Mental Disorders.* 4th ed., text rev. Washington DC: American Psychiatric Publishing, 2000.

Burns, David D. *When Panic Attacks: The New, Drug-Free Anxiety Therapy That Can Change Your Life.* New York: Random House, 2007.

Craske, Michelle G., and David H. Barlow. *Mastery of Your Anxiety and Panic: Therapist Guide.* New York: Oxford University Press, 2007.

Wilson, Reid. *Don't Panic: Taking Control of Anxiety Attacks,* 3rd ed. New York: Harper Collins, 2009.

PERIODICALS

Bednar, F., and D.M. Simeone. "Internet-Based Treatment for Panic Disorder: Does Frequency of Therapist Contact Make a Difference?" *Cognitive Behaviour Therapy* (March 18, 2009): 1–14.

Busch, F.N., et al. "A Study Demonstrating Efficacy of a Psychoanalytic Psychotherapy for Panic Disorder: Implications for Psychoanalytic Research, Theory, and Practice." *Journal of the American Psychoanalytic Association* 57, no. 1 (February 2009): 131–48.

Powers, A., and D. Westen. "Personality Subtypes in Patients with Panic Disorder." *Comprehensive Psychiatry* 50, no. 2 (March–April 2009): 164–72.

Starcevic, V. "Treatment of Panic Disorder: Recent Developments and Current Status." *Expert Review of Neurotherapeutics* 8, no. 8 (August 2008): 1219–32.

Teng, E.G., et al. "When Anxiety Symptoms Masquerade as Medical Symptoms: What Medical Specialists Know about Panic Disorder and Available Psychological Treatments." *Journal of Clinical Psychology in Medical Settings* 15, no. 4 (December 2008): 314–21.

WEBSITES

"Answers to Your Questions About Panic Disorder." APA, April 25, 2009. http://www.apa.org/topics/anxietyqanda.html (accessed September 16, 2011).

"Panic Disorder." NIMH, March 31, 2009. http://www.nimh.nih.gov/health/topics/panic-disorder/index.shtml (accessed September 16, 2011).

"Panic Disorder." MedlinePlus, April 13, 2009. http://www.nlm.nih.gov/medlineplus/panicdisorder.html (accessed September 16, 2011).

"Panic Disorder (Panic Attack)." Anxiety Disorders Association of America. Last modified April 25, 2009. http://www.adaa.org/GettingHelp/AnxietyDisorders/Panicattack.asp (accessed September 16, 2011).

"What Is a Panic Attack?" American Psychiatric Association. Last modified April 25, 2009. http://healthyminds.org/factsheets/LTF-Panic.pdf (accessed September 16, 2011).

"When Fear Overwhelms: Panic Disorder." NIMH. Last modified April 25, 2009. http://www.nimh.nih.gov/health/publications/when-fear-overwhelms-panic-disorder/index.shtml (accessed September 16, 2011).

ORGANIZATIONS

American Psychiatric Association, 1000 Wilson Blvd., Ste. 1825, Arlington, VA, 22209-3901, (703) 907-7300, apa@psych.org, http://www.psych.org.

American Psychological Association, 750 1st St., NE, Washington, DC, 20002-4242, (202) 336-5500; TDD/TTY: (202) 336-6123, (800) 374-2721, http://www.apa.org.

Anxiety Disorders Association of America, 8730 Georgia Ave., Silver Spring, MD, 20910, (240) 485-1001, Fax: (240) 485-1035, http://www.adaa.org.

Mental Health America, 2000 N Beauregard St., 6th Fl., Alexandria, VA, 22311, (800) 969-6642, http://www.nmha.org.

National Institute of Mental Health, 6001 Executive Blvd., Rm. 8184, MSC 9663, Bethesda, MD, 20892-9663, (301) 443-4513; TTY: (301) 443-8431, Fax: (301) 443-4279, (866) 615-6464; TTY: (866) 415-8051, nimhinfo@nih.gov, http://www.nimh.nih.gov.

Susan Hobbs, MD

Paranoia

Definition

Paranoia is a symptom in which an individual feels as if the world is "out to get" him or her. When people are paranoid, they feel as if others are always talking about them behind their backs. Paranoia causes intense feelings of distrust, and can sometimes lead to overt or covert hostility.

Demographics

Paranoia is a very human feeling. Nearly everyone has experienced it at some or another time, to varying degrees. Paranoia exists on a continuum, ranging from a feeling of distrust due to an occasional misinterpretation of cues that can be appropriately dealt with and reinterpreted, to an overarching pattern of actual paranoia that affects every interpersonal interaction.

Some research studies have suggested that 6% of all women and 13% of all men have some chronic level of mistrust towards the motivations of others towards them. Only about 0.5% to 0.25% of men and women can actually be diagnosed with **paranoid personality disorder**, however. It remains interesting to researchers that men are more prone to paranoid traits and mental disorders with paranoid features than are women.

Description

An individual suffering from paranoia feels suspicious, and has a sense that other people want to do him or her harm. As a result, the paranoid individual changes his or her actions in response to a world that is perceived as personally threatening. Objective observers may be quite clear on the fact that no one's words or actions are actually threatening the paranoid individual. The hallmark of paranoia is a feeling of intense distrust and suspiciousness that is not in response to input from anybody or anything in the paranoid individual's environment.

Other symptoms of paranoia may include

- Self-referential thinking: The sense that other people in the world (even complete strangers on the street) are always talking about the paranoid individual.
- Thought broadcasting: The sense that other people can read the paranoid individual's mind.
- Magical thinking: The sense that the paranoid individual can use his or her thoughts to influence other people's thoughts and actions.
- Thought withdrawal: The sense that people are stealing the paranoid individual's thoughts.
- Thought insertion: The sense that people are putting thoughts into the paranoid individual's mind.
- Ideas of reference: The sense that the television and/or radio are specifically addressing the paranoid individual.

Causes and symptoms

Researchers do not understand fully what chemical or physical changes in the **brain** cause paranoia. Paranoia is a prominent symptom that occurs in a variety of different mental disorders, as well as a symptom of certain physical diseases. Furthermore, use of certain drugs or chemicals may cause symptoms of paranoia in an otherwise normal individual.

Paranoia is often manifested as part of the symptom complex of **schizophrenia**. In fact, one of the subtypes of schizophrenia is termed "paranoid schizophrenia," which actually refers to a type of schizophrenia in which the individual is particularly preoccupied with **delusions** in which the world seems to be pitted against him or her. As with other forms of schizophrenia, sufferers often lack contact with reality, and display hallucinations, flat or emotionless **affect**, and disorganized thinking and behavior.

Paranoid personality disorder is diagnosed when an individual does not have other symptoms of schizophrenia, but a personality that is driven by chronic manifestations of paranoia. These individuals are mistrustful, suspicious, and convinced that the world is out to get them.

In order for an individual to be diagnosed with paranoid personality disorder, he or she must display at least four of the following traits:

- chronically suspicious that people are lying or cheating him or her in some way
- frequently preoccupied with whether people are loyal or trustworthy
- cannot confide in others for fear of being betrayed
- misinterprets benign comments or events as being personally threatening
- harbors long-term grudges against others who are perceived as having been threatening or insulting in some way
- sees others' actions and/or words attacking him or her in some way, and therefore goes on the counterattack
- repeatedly assumes that partner or spouse is unfaithful

Paranoia can also occur as a symptom of other neurological diseases. Individuals suffering from the aftereffects of strokes, brain injuries, various types of **dementia** (including **Alzheimer's disease**), Huntington's disease, and Parkinson's disease may manifest paranoia as part of their symptom complex. The paranoia may decrease in intensity when the underlying disease is effectively treated, although since many of these diseases are progressive, the paranoia may worsen over time along with the progression of the disease's other symptoms.

A number of different medications and drugs can cause paranoia. These include corticosteroid medications, H-2 blockers (cimetidine, ranitidine, famotidine), some muscle relaxants (Baclofen), antiviral/anti-Parkinson drugs (**amantadine**), some **amphetamines** (including Ritalin), anti-HIV medications, **antidepressants** (Nardil). Abused drugs that can prompt paranoia include alcohol, **cocaine**, marijuana, **ecstasy** (MDMA), amphetamines (including Ritalin), LSD, and PCP (angel dust). Withdrawal from addictive drugs may also cause symptoms of paranoia.

Treatment

It can be quite challenging to get an individual who is suffering from paranoia to accept treatment. Their paranoid condition makes them distrustful of people's motivations towards them, so that even a medical doctor appears to be a suspicious party. Medications that may be offered are usually looked at with great distrust, and efforts at **psychotherapy** are considered "mind control" by a profoundly paranoid individual.

The first step to be taken when someone is suffering from paranoia is determining whether an easily reversible situation (such as an adverse reaction to a medication) might be causing the paranoia. If so, discontinuing the drug (either immediately or by gradually weaning the dose) might end the symptoms of paranoia.

Patients who have other diseases, such as Alzheimer's disease or other forms of dementia, Huntington's disease, or Parkinson's disease may notice that their paranoid symptoms improve when their general medical condition is treated. The circumstance that can occur as their underlying disease progresses, is that the paranoia may return or worsen over time.

People who are suffering from diagnosable mental conditions such as schizophrenia or paranoid personality disorder may benefit from the use of typical antipsychotic medications, such as **chlorpromazine** or Haldol, or from the newer, atypical antipsychotic medications, such as **clozapine**, **olanzapine**, or **risperidone**.

Cognitive-behavioral therapy (CBT) or other forms of psychotherapy may be helpful for certain people who have paranoia. CBT attempts to make a person more aware of his or her actions and motivations, and tries to help the individual learn to more accurately interpret cues around him or her, in an effort to help the individual change dysfunctional behaviors. Difficulty can enter into a therapeutic relationship with a paranoid individual, due to the level of mistrust and suspicion that is likely to interfere with their ability to participate in this form of treatment.

Support groups can be helpful for some paranoid individuals and are particularly helpful in assisting family members and friends who must learn to live with or care for individuals experiencing paranoia.

Prognosis

It is difficult to predict the prognosis of an individual who has paranoia. If there is an underlying mental illness, such as schizophrenia or paranoid personality disorder, then the paranoia is likely to be a lifelong condition. It may improve with some treatments (remission), only to become exacerbated under other more stressful conditions, or with changes in medication.

Individuals who have symptoms of paranoia as part of another medical condition may also have a waxing-and-waning-course.

When paranoia is caused by the use of a particular drug or medication, it is possible that discontinuing that substance may completely reverse the symptoms of paranoia.

Resources

BOOKS

Tasman, Allan, et al., eds. *Psychiatry*. 3rd ed. New York: Wiley and Sons, 2008.

ORGANIZATIONS

National Alliance on Mental Illness, 3803 N Fairfax Drive, Ste. 100, Arlington, VA, 22203, (703) 524-7600, http://www.nami.org.

National Institute of Mental Health, 6001 Executive Blvd., Room 8184, MSC 9663, Bethesda, MD, 20892-9663, (301) 433-4513; TTY: (301) 443-8431, Fax: (301) 443-4279, (866) 615-6464; TTY: (866) 415-8051 nimhinfo@nih.gov, http://www.nimh.nih.gov.

Rosalyn Carson-DeWitt, M.D.

Paranoid personality disorder

Definition

People with paranoid personality disorder (PPD) have long-term and unwarranted suspicions that other people are hostile, threatening, or demeaning. These beliefs are steadfastly maintained in the absence of any real supporting evidence. The disorder, named after the Greek word for "madness," is one of ten **personality disorders** described in the fourth edition of the ***Diagnostic and Statistical Manual of Mental Disorders*** (*DSM-IV-TR*), the guidebook used by mental health professionals to diagnose mental disorders. Proposed changes for the fifth edition (*DSM-5*) include removing PPD as an individual diagnosis.

Despite the pervasive suspicions they have of others, patients with PPD are not delusional (except in rare, brief instances brought on by **stress**). Most of the time, they are in touch with reality, except for their misinterpretation of others' motives and intentions. PPD patients are not psychotic but their conviction that others are trying to "get them" or humiliate them in some way often leads to hostility and social isolation.

Demographics

As of 2011, it was not yet possible to determine the number of people with PPD with any accuracy. This lack of data might be expected for a disorder that is characterized by extreme suspiciousness. Such patients in many cases avoid voluntary contact with such people as mental health workers who have a certain amount of power over them. There are, nonetheless, some estimates of the prevalence of PPD. According to the *DSM-IV-TR*), between 0.5% and 2.5% of the general population of the United States may have PPD, while 2%–10% of outpatients receiving psychiatric care may be affected. A significant percentage of institutionalized psychiatric patients, between 10% and 30%, might have symptoms that qualify for a **diagnosis** of PPD. Finally, the disorder appears to be more common in men than in women.

There are indications in the scientific literature that relatives of patients with chronic schizophrenia may have a greater chance of developing PPD than people in the general population. Also, the incidence of the disorder may be higher among relatives of patients suffering from another psychotic disorder known as delusional disorder of the persecutory type.

Description

People with PPD do not trust other people. In fact, the central characteristic of people with PPD is a high degree of mistrustfulness and suspicion when interacting with others. Even friendly gestures are often interpreted as being manipulative or malevolent. Whether the patterns of distrust and suspicion begin in childhood or in early adulthood, they quickly come to dominate the lives of those suffering from PPD. Such people are unable or afraid to form close relationships with others.

They suspect strangers, and even people they know, of planning to harm or exploit them when there is no good evidence to support this belief. As a result of their constant concern about the lack of trustworthiness of others, patients with this disorder often have few intimate friends or close human contacts. They do not fit in and they do not make good "team players." Interactions with others are characterized by wariness and not infrequently by hostility. If they marry or become otherwise attached to someone, the relationship is often characterized by pathological jealousy and attempts to control their partner. They often assume their sexual partner is "cheating" on them.

People suffering from PPD are very difficult to deal with. They never seem to let down their defenses. They are always looking for and finding evidence that others are against them. Their fear, and the threats they perceive in the innocent statements and actions of others, often contributes to frequent complaining or unfriendly withdrawal or aloofness. They can be confrontational, aggressive and disputatious. It is not unusual for them to sue people they feel have wronged them. In addition, patients with this disorder are known for their tendency to become violent.

Despite all the unpleasant aspects of a paranoid lifestyle, however, it is still not sufficient to drive many people with PPD to seek therapy. They do not usually walk into a therapist's office on their own. They distrust mental health care providers just as they distrust nearly everyone else. If a life crisis, a family member or the judicial system succeeds in getting a patient with PPD to seek help, therapy is often a challenge. Individual counseling seems to work best but it requires a great deal of patience and skill on the part of the therapist. It is not unusual for patients to leave therapy when they perceive some malicious intent on the therapist's part. If the patient can be persuaded to cooperate—something that is not easy to achieve—low-dose medications are recommended for treating such specific problems as anxiety, but only for limited periods of time.

If a mental health care provider is able to gain the trust of a patient with PPD, it may be possible to help the patient deal with the threats that he or she perceives. The disorder, however, usually lasts a lifetime.

Causes and symptoms

Causes

No one knows what causes paranoid personality disorder, although there are hints that familial factors may influence the development of the disorder in some cases. There seem to be more cases of PPD in families that have one or more members who suffer from such psychotic disorders as **schizophrenia** or **delusional disorder**.

Other possible interpersonal causes have been proposed. For example, some therapists believe that the behavior that characterizes PPD might be learned. They suggest that such behavior might be traced back to childhood experiences. According to this view, children who are exposed to adult anger and rage with no way to predict the outbursts and no way to escape or control them develop paranoid ways of thinking in an effort to cope with the stress. PPD would emerge when this type of thinking becomes part of the individual's personality as adulthood approaches.

Studies of identical (or monozygotic) and fraternal (or dizygotic) twins suggest that **genetic factors** may also play an important role in causing the disorder. Twin studies indicate that genes contribute to the development of childhood personality disorders, including PPD. Furthermore, estimates of the degree of genetic contribution to the development of childhood personality disorders are similar to estimates of the genetic contribution to adult versions of the disorders.

Symptoms

A core symptom of PPD is a generalized distrust of other people. Comments and actions that healthy people would not notice come across as full of insults and threats to someone with the disorder. Yet, generally, patients with PPD remain in touch with reality; they don't have any of the hallucinations or **delusions** seen in patients with psychoses. Nevertheless, their suspicions that others are intent on harming or exploiting them are so pervasive and intense that people with PPD often become very isolated. They thus avoid normal social interactions. And because they feel so insecure in what is a very threatening world for them, patients with PPD are capable of becoming violent. Innocuous comments, harmless jokes and other day-to-day communications are often perceived as insults.

Paranoid suspicions carry over into all realms of life. Those burdened with PPD are frequently convinced that their sexual partners are unfaithful. They may misinterpret compliments offered by employers or coworkers as hidden criticisms or attempts to get them to work harder. Complimenting a person with PPD on their clothing or car, for example, could easily be taken as an attack on their materialism or selfishness.

Because they persistently question the motivations and trustworthiness of others, patients with PPD are not inclined to share intimacies. They fear such information might be used against them. As a result, they become hostile and unfriendly, argumentative or aloof. Their unpleasantness often draws negative responses from those around them. These rebuffs become "proof" in the patient's mind that others are, indeed, hostile to them. They have little insight into the effects of their attitude and behavior on their generally unsuccessful interactions with others. Asked if they might be responsible for negative interactions that fill their lives, people with PPD are likely to place all the blame on others.

A brief summary of the typical symptoms of PPD includes:

- suspiciousness and distrust of others
- questioning hidden motives in others
- feelings of certainty, without justification or proof, that others are intent on harming or exploiting them
- social isolation
- aggressiveness and hostility
- little or no sense of humor

Diagnosis

There were no laboratory tests or **imaging studies** as of 2011 that could be used to confirm a diagnosis of PPD. The diagnosis is usually made on the basis of the doctor's interview with the patient, although the doctor may also give the patient a diagnostic questionnaire.

Diagnostic criteria

Mental health care providers look for at least five distinguishing symptoms in patients who they think might suffer from PPD. The first is a pattern of suspiciousness about, and distrust of, other people when there is no good reason for either. This pattern should be present from at least the time of the patient's early adulthood.

In addition to this symptom that is required in order to make the PPD diagnosis, the patient should have at least four of the following seven symptoms as listed in the *DSM-IV-TR*:

- The unfounded suspicion that people want to deceive, exploit or harm the patient.
- The pervasive belief that others are not worthy of trust or that they are not inclined to or capable of offering loyalty.
- A fear that others will use information against the patient with the intention of harming him or her. This fear is demonstrated by a reluctance to share even harmless personal information with others.
- The interpretation of others' innocent remarks as insulting or demeaning; or the interpretation of neutral events as presenting or conveying a threat.
- A strong tendency not to forgive real or imagined slights and insults. People with PPD nurture grudges for a long time.
- An angry and aggressive response in reply to imagined attacks by others. The counterattack for a perceived insult is often rapid.
- Suspicions, in the absence of any real evidence, that a spouse or sexual partner is not sexually faithful, resulting in such repeated questions as "Where have you been?" "Whom did you see?" and other types of jealous behavior.

Differential diagnosis

Psychiatrists and clinical psychologists should be careful not to confuse PPD with other mental disorders or behaviors that have some symptoms in common with the paranoid personality. For example, it is important to make sure that the patient is not a long-term user of amphetamine or **cocaine**. Chronic abuse of these stimulants can produce paranoid behavior. Also, some prescription medications might produce **paranoia** as a side effect; so it is important to find out what drugs, if any, the patient is taking.

There are other conditions that, if present, would mean a patient with paranoid traits does not have PPD. For example, if the patient has symptoms of schizophrenia, hallucinations or a formal thought disorder, a diagnosis of PPD can't be made. The same is true of fixed delusions, which are not a feature of PPD.

Also, the suspiciousness and other characteristic features of PPD must have been present in the patient for a long time, at least since early adulthood. If the symptoms appeared more recently than that, a person can't be given a diagnosis of this disorder.

There are at least a dozen disorders or other mental health conditions listed in the *DSM-IV-TR* that could be confused with PPD after a superficial interview because they share similar or identical symptoms with PPD. It is important to eliminate the following entities before settling on a diagnosis of PPD: paranoid schizophrenia; **schizotypal personality disorder**; **schizoid personality disorder**; persecutory delusional disorder; mood disorder with psychotic features; symptoms and/or personality changes produced by disease, medical conditions, medication or drugs of abuse; paranoia linked to the development of physical disabilities; and borderline, histrionic, avoidant, antisocial or narcissistic personality disorders.

In some individuals, symptoms of PPD may precede the development of schizophrenia. Should a patient who has been correctly diagnosed with PPD later develop schizophrenia, the *DSM-IV-TR* suggests that the diagnosis on the patient's medical record be changed from "Paranoid Personality Disorder" to "Paranoid Personality Disorder (Premorbid)."

If PPD is removed from the *DSM-5* (2013) as a separate diagnosis, it will still be represented and diagnosed by a combination of core impairments in personality functioning and specific pathological personality traits (such as antagonistic, psychotic).

Treatment

Because they are suspicious and untrusting, patients with PPD are not likely to seek therapy on their own. A particularly disturbing development or life crisis may prompt them to get help. More often, however, the legal system or the patient's relatives order or encourage him or her to seek professional treatment. But even after a patient finally agrees or is forced to seek treatment, the nature of the disorder poses very serious challenges to therapists.

Psychotherapy

The primary approach to treatment for such personality disorders as PPD is **psychotherapy**. The problem is that patients with PPD do not readily offer therapists the trust that is needed for successful treatment. As a result, it has been difficult to gather data that would indicate what kind of psychotherapy would work best. Therapists face the challenge of developing rapport with someone who is, by the nature of his or her personality disorder, distrustful and suspicious; someone who often sees malicious intent in the innocuous actions and statements of others. The patient may actively resist or refuse to cooperate with others who are trying to help.

Mental health workers treating patients with PPD must guard against any show of hostility on their part in response to hostility from the patient, which is a common occurrence in people with this disorder. Instead, clinicians are advised to develop trust by persistently demonstrating a nonjudgmental attitude and a professional desire to assist the patient.

It is usually up to the therapist alone to overcome a patient's resistance. **Group therapy** that includes family members or other psychiatric patients, not surprisingly, isn't useful in the treatment of PPD due to the mistrust people with PPD feel towards others. This characteristic also explains why there are no significant **self-help groups** dedicated to recovery from this disorder. It has been suggested, however, that some people with PPD might join cults or extremist groups whose members might share their suspicions.

To gain the trust of PPD patients, therapists must be careful to hide as little as possible from their patients. This transparency should include note taking; details of administrative tasks concerning the patient; correspondence; and medications. Any indication of what the patient would consider "deception" or covert operation can, and often does, lead the patient to drop out of treatment. Patients with paranoid tendencies often don't have a well-developed sense of humor; those who must interact with people with PPD probably should not make jokes in their presence. Attempts at humor may seem like ridicule to people who feel so easily threatened.

With some patients, the most attainable goal may be to help them to learn to analyze their problems in dealing with other people. This approach amounts to supportive therapy and is preferable to psychotherapeutic approaches that attempt to analyze the patient's motivations and possible sources of paranoid traits. Asking about a patient's past can undermine the treatment of PPD patients. Concentrating on the specific issues that are troubling the patient with PPD is usually the wisest course.

With time and a skilled therapist, the patient with PPD who remains in therapy may develop a measure of

KEY TERMS

Delusion—A false belief that is resistant to reason or contrary to actual fact.

Delusional disorder of the persecutory type—A psychotic disorder characterized by a patient's belief that others are conspiring against him or her.

Hallucination—False sensory perceptions. A person experiencing a hallucination may "hear" sounds or "see" people or objects that are not really present. Hallucinations can also affect the senses of smell, touch, and taste.

Neuroleptic—Another name for the older antipsychotic medications, such as haloperidol (Haldol) and chlorpromazine (Thorazine).

Paranoia—A mental disorder characterized by baseless suspicions or distrust of others, often delusional in intensity.

Paranoid personality—A personality disorder characterized by unwarranted suspicion, jealousy, hypersensitivity, social isolation and a tendency to detect malicious intent in the words and actions of others.

Psychosis—Severe state that is characterized by loss of contact with reality and deterioration in normal social functioning; examples are schizophrenia and paranoia. Psychosis is usually one feature of an over-arching disorder, not a disorder in itself. (Plural: psychoses)

Rapport—A relation of empathy and trust between a therapist and patient.

Schizophrenia—A severe mental illness in which a person has difficulty distinguishing what is real from what is not real. It is often characterized by hallucinations, delusions, language and communication disturbances, and withdrawal from people and social activities.

Supportive—An approach to psychotherapy that seeks to encourage the patient or offer emotional support to him or her, as distinct from insight-oriented or exploratory approaches to treatment.

trust. But as the patient reveals more of his or her paranoid thoughts, the clinician will continue to face the difficult task of balancing the need for objectivity about the paranoid ideas and the maintenance of a good rapport with the patient. The therapist thus walks a tightrope with this type of patient. If the therapist is not straightforward enough, the patient may feel deceived. If the therapist challenges paranoid thoughts too directly, the patient will be threatened and probably drop out of treatment.

Medications

While individual supportive psychotherapy is the treatment of choice for PPD, medications are sometimes used on a limited basis to treat related symptoms. If, for example, the patient is very anxious, **antianxiety drugs** may be prescribed. In addition, during periods of extreme agitation and high stress that produce delusional states, the patient may be given low doses of antipsychotic medications.

Some clinicians have suggested that low doses of neuroleptics should be used in this group of patients; however, medications are not normally part of long-term treatment for PPD. One reason is that no medication has been proven to relieve effectively the long-term symptoms of the disorder, although the **selective serotonin reuptake inhibitors** such as **fluoxetine** (Prozac) have been reported to make patients less angry, irritable and suspicious. **Antidepressants** may even make symptoms worse. A second reason is that people with PPD are suspicious of medications. They fear that others might try to control them through the use of drugs. It can therefore be very difficult to persuade them to take medications unless the potential for relief from another threat, such as extreme anxiety, makes the medications seem relatively appealing. The best use of medication may be for specific complaints, when the patient trusts the therapist enough to ask for relief from particular symptoms.

Prognosis

Paranoid personality disorder is often a chronic, lifelong condition; the long-term prognosis is usually not encouraging. Feelings of paranoia, however, can be controlled to a degree with successful therapy. Unfortunately, many patients suffer the major symptoms of the disorder throughout their lives.

Prevention

With little or no understanding of the cause of PPD, it is not possible to prevent the disorder.

Resources

BOOKS

Allen, Thomas E., et al. *A Primer on Mental Disorders: A Guide for Educators, Families, and Students.* Lantham, MD: Scarecrow Press, 2001.

American Psychiatric Association. *Diagnostic and Statistical Manual of Mental Disorders.* 4th ed., text rev. Washington, DC: American Psychiatric Publishing, 2000.

Frances, Allen, and Michael B. First. *Your Mental Health: A Layman's Guide to the Psychiatrist's Bible*. New York, NY: Scribner, 1998.

"Personality Disorders." In *The Merck Manual of Diagnosis and Therapy*, edited by Robert S. Porter and Justin L. Kaplan. 19th ed. Whitehouse Station, NJ: Merck Research Laboratories, 2011.

Porter, Robert S., and Justin L. Kaplan, eds. *The Merck Manual of Diagnosis and Therapy*. 19th ed. Whitehouse Station, NJ: Merck Research Laboratories, 2011.

Weiner, Alan S. Weiner. *Personality Disorders in Children and Adolescents*. 1st ed. New York, NY: Basic Books, 2000.

PERIODICALS

Coolidge, F.L., L.L. Thede, and K.L. Jang. "Heritability of Personality Disorders in Childhood: A Preliminary Investigation." *Journal of Personality Disorders* 15, no. 1 (February 2001): 33–40.

Webb, C.T., and D.F. Levinson. "Schizotypal and Paranoid Personality Disorder in the Relatives of Patients with Schizophrenia and Affective Disorders: A Review." *Schizophrenia Research* 11, no. 1 (December 1993): 81–92.

WEBSITES

DualDiagnosis.org. "Paranoid Personality Disorder." http://www.dualdiagnosisdrugrehabs.org/116/paranoid-personality-disorder.html (accessed October 24, 2011).

PsychCentral.com. "Paranoid Personality Disorder Treatment." http://psychcentral.com/disorders/sx37t.htm (accessed October 24, 2011).

ORGANIZATIONS

American Psychiatric Association, 1000 Wilson Blvd., Ste. 1825, Arlington, VA, 22209-3901, (703) 907-7300, apa@psych.org, http://www.psych.org.

International Society for the Study of Personality Disorders, University of Michigan Health System, Psychiatry MCHC-6, Box 5295, 1500 East Medical Center Drive, Ann Arbor, MI, 48109-5295, (734) 936-8316, Fax: (734) 936-9761, http://www.isspd.com.

Mental Health America, 2000 N. Beauregard Street, 6th Floor, Alexandria, VA, 22311, (703) 684-7722, (800) 969-6642, Fax: (703) 684-5968, http://www1.nmha.org.

Dean A. Haycock, Ph.D.

Paraphilias

Definition

Paraphilias are sexual feelings or behaviors that may involve sexual partners that are not human, not consenting, or that involve suffering by one or both partners.

Description

According to the ***Diagnostic and Statistical Manual of Mental Disorders*** (known as the *DSM*) fourth edition text revised (*DSM-IV-TR*), the manual used by mental health professionals to diagnose mental disorders, it is not uncommon for an individual to have more than one paraphilia. The *DSM-IV-TR* lists the following paraphilias: **exhibitionism**, **fetishism**, **frotteurism**, **pedophilia**, **sexual masochism**, **sexual sadism**, **transvestic fetishism**, and **voyeurism**. The *DSM-IV-TR* also includes a category for paraphilia not otherwise specified, which is the category for the less common paraphilias, including necrophilia, zoophilia, and others.

Exhibitionism

Exhibitionism is the exposure of genitals to a nonconsenting stranger. In some cases, the individual may also engage in autoeroticism while exposing himself. Generally, no additional contact with the observer is sought; the individual is stimulated sexually by gaining the attention of and startling the observer.

Fetishism

People with this disorder achieve sexual gratification with the use of objects, most commonly women's undergarments, shoes, stockings, or other clothing item.

Frotteurism

Individuals with this disorder are gratified by touching or rubbing a non-consenting person. This behavior often occurs in busy, crowded places, such as on busy streets or on crowded buses or subways.

Pedophilia

Pedophilia involves sexual activity with a child, generally under age 13. The *DSM-IV-TR* describes a criterion that the individual with pedophilia be over 16 years of age and be at least five years older than the child. Individuals with this disorder may be attracted to either males or females or both, although incidents of pedophilic activity are almost twice as likely to be repeated by those individuals attracted to males. Individuals with this disorder develop procedures and strategies for gaining access to and trust of children.

Sexual masochism

Masochism is a term applied to a specific sexual disorder but which also has a broader usage. The sexual disorder involves pleasure and excitement produced by pain, either inflicted by others or by oneself. It usually begins in childhood or adolescence and is chronic. An individual with this disorder achieves gratification by experiencing pain. Masochism is the only paraphilia in which any noticeable number of women participate—about 5% of masochists are female. The term comes from the name of a nineteenth-century Austrian writer, Leopold von Sacher-Masoch, whose novels often included characters who were obsessed with the combination of sex and pain.

In the broader sense, masochism refers to any experience of receiving pleasure or satisfaction from suffering pain. The psychoanalytic view is that masochism is aggression turned inward, onto the self, when a person feels too guilty or is afraid to express it outwardly.

Sexual sadism

A sadistic individual achieves sexual gratification by inflicting pain on another person.

In psychoanalytic theory, sadism is related to the fear of castration, while the behaviorist explanation of sadomasochism (the deviant sexual practice combining sadism and masochism) is that its constituent feelings are physiologically similar to sexual arousal. Separate but parallel descriptions are given for sexual sadism and sexual masochism in the *DSM-IV-TR*. The clinical diagnostic criteria for both are recurrence of the behavior over a period of at least six months, and significant distress or impairment of the ability to function as a result of the behavior or associated urges or fantasies. Either type of behavior may be limited to fantasies (sometimes while one is engaged in outwardly nondeviant sex) or acted out with a consenting partner, a non-consenting partner, or in the case of masochism, alone. Sadomasochism occurs in both males and females, and in both heterosexual and homosexual relationships.

Transvestic fetishism

This disorder is characterized by heterosexual males who dress in women's clothing to achieve a sexual response. The activity may begin in adolescence, and in secret; later, as an adult, the man may dress as a woman completely and in public. Not all men who cross-dress are unhappy with their gender, but some are. In a small minority of men with transvestic fetishism, gender dysphoria (unhappiness with original gender) may emerge, and those men may eventually seek hormonal treatments or surgical sex reassignment to enable them to live permanently as women.

Voyeurism

Voyeurism is a paraphilia in which a person finds sexual excitement in watching unsuspecting people who are nude, undressing, or having sex. Voyeurs are almost always male, and the victims are usually strangers. A voyeur may fantasize about having sex with the victim but almost never actually pursues this. The voyeur may return to watch the same stranger repeatedly, but there is rarely any physical contact.

Voyeurs are popularly known as "peeping Toms," based on the eleventh-century legend of Lady Godiva. According to the story, Tom was a tailor who "peeped" at Lady Godiva as she rode naked through the streets of Coventry, England, in a sacrificial act to get her husband to lower taxes. Tom was struck with blindness for not looking away like everyone else.

Uncommon paraphilias

BESTIALITY. Bestiality is a term that describes sexual feelings or behaviors involving animals. Termed zoophilia by *DSM-IV* this is an uncommon disorder. The disorder does not specify an animal or category of animals; the person with zoophilia may focus sexual feelings on domesticated animals, such as dogs, or farm animals, such as sheep or goats.

NECROPHILIA. Necrophilia is a term that describes sexual feelings or behaviors involving corpses.

Resources

BOOKS

American Psychiatric Association. *Diagnostic and Statistical Manual of Mental Disorders*. 4th ed., text rev. Washington, DC: American Psychiatric Publishing, 2000.

Baumeister, Roy F. *Escaping the Self: Alcoholism, Spirituality, Masochism, and Other Flights from the Burden of Selfhood*. New York: Basic Books, 1993.

Caplan, Paula J. *The Myth of Women's Masochism*. 2nd ed. Toronto: University of Toronto Press, 1993.

Carnes, Patrick. *Out of the Shadows: Understanding Sexual Addiction*. 3rd ed. Center City, MN: Hazelden Publishing, 2001.

PERIODICALS

Guay, D.R. "Drug Treatment of Paraphilic and Nonparaphilic Sexual Disorders." *Clinical Therapeutics* 31, no. 1 (January 2009): 1–31.

WEBSITES

"Paraphilias." The Merck Manual Home Health Handbook. http://www.merckmanuals.com/home/print/mental_health_disorders/sexuality/paraphilias.html (accessed December 12, 2011).

Parental alienation disorder

Definition

Parental alienation disorder (PAD), also called "parental alienation syndrome" (PAS), is a controversial condition that occurs when one parent attempts to negatively affect a child's relationship with the other parent (for instance, in child custody disputes). The specific term "parental alienation syndrome" was coined in 1985 by Richard A. Gardner (1931–2003), a child **psychiatrist**. At that time, Gardner defined PAS as a "disorder that arises primarily in the context of child custody disputes. Its primary manifestation is the child's campaign of denigration against a parent with no justification. It is caused by a combination of a programming (brainwashing) parent's indoctrinations and the child's own contributions to the vilification of the targeted parent."

Demographics

There are no reliable statistics for the prevalence of PAD in North America, although discussions of the subject in the mass media as well as professional medical and legal journals suggest that it is largely limited to middle- and upper middle-class families.

There is little agreement about the gender demographic in alienating versus targeted parents. Gardner himself changed his mind about the gender ratio following his initial publications about PAS. In the mid-1980s, Gardner stated that the mother was the alienator in 90% of parental alienation cases, based on the increase in the number of **child abuse** cases that were reported in the 1980s. He theorized that mothers used allegations of physical or **sexual abuse** to win custody, terminate the father's visitation rights, or punish the ex-husband. By 2002, Gardner acknowledged that men and women were equally likely to be alienators.

Description

There is no universally agreed-upon description of PAD, although it is most often described as when one parent's attempts to sway their child's opinion of the other parent, whether consciously or unconsciously, occur concurrently with the child's own words or actions against the other parent. In severe cases, the child will refuse to interact with the alienated parent. Others, however, prefer to avoid defining the condition as a syndrome or disorder, choosing instead to refer simply to parental alienation (PA) and focus on the alienated child and the family situation that has led to the child's estrangement from the rejected parent.

Parental alienation disorder has been proposed by outside sources for addition to the fifth edition of the ***Diagnostic and Statistical Manual of Mental Disorders*** (*DSM-5*). In 2005, the **American Psychological Association** issued a statement that it would not take a formal stand on the existence of parental alienation syndrome and noted the lack of empirical evidence for PAD. In November 2010, the *DSM-5* working group on childhood and adolescent disorders stated that there is insufficient scientific evidence to justify the inclusion of parental alienation in the new diagnostic manual. In addition, PAD is not recognized as a disorder in the World Health Organization's *International Statistical Classification of Diseases and Related Health Problems*, tenth edition (ICD-10).

Controversy

The classification of PAD as a mental disorder is highly controversial. One reason is that there has been no agreement among psychiatrists, psychologists, family therapists, and other mental health professionals about its definition: whether PAD is a syndrome (a cluster of symptoms that occur together and are characteristic of a specific disease or disorder), a social dynamic, a mental disorder (in the child), or a relational problem (between parent and child). This fourth definition has been suggested by William Bernet as a justification for including parental alienation disorder under the heading of "Other Conditions That May Be a Focus of Clinical Attention" in *DSM-5*. The changing definitions and descriptions of PAD over the 25 years since Gardner first proposed its existence add to confusion in the courtroom as well as controversy among therapists.

Another major area of controversy is the actual prevalence of the disorder. One 2003 study of 215 California children maintained that PAD is likely to be overreported. The attitudes of the children toward their parents varied, but only a few were considered extreme, either negatively or positively. In addition, a large study of allegations of sexual abuse in child custody cases reported that such allegations are very rare and account for only 2% of child custody lawsuits.

Still another area of disagreement is whether PAD occurs only in separating or divorcing families, or whether it can occur in intact families when one parent (or stepparent or grandparent) seeks power over the other by turning the child or children against the targeted parent. Recent supporters of the existence of the syndrome claim that it can be found in families that are not presently involved in separation or divorce proceedings.

Gardner's own career is a significant source of controversy over PAD. In addition to serving as an expert witness for fathers in child custody cases, he held controversial views on **pedophilia** and other aberrant forms of sexual behavior, maintaining that such behaviors contribute to the survival of the species. Gardner stated in a 1992 article that sexual activities between an adult and a child create a "charged-up child" who will welcome sexual experiences at an early age and be more likely to reproduce. In a 1991 article, Gardner argued that Western society is "excessively moralistic and punitive" toward pedophiles. Gardner was also opposed to mandatory reporting of child abuse and lobbied Congress to abolish legally mandated reporting. He committed **suicide** in 2003 when the symptoms of a chronic neurological pain syndrome became worse.

The remaining reason for ongoing controversy over PAD is its use as a litigation strategy in divorce cases. The fathers' rights movement, a collection of organizations that emerged in the 1980s out of the conviction that the legal system discriminates against men in child custody cases, took up Gardner's early publications. Women's groups generally oppose recognizing PAD as a **diagnosis**, claiming that it has been used in courtroom proceedings to remove children from the custody of a qualified parent and to then stigmatize that parent.

KEY TERMS

Alienator—The parent attempting to negatively affect the child's opinion of the other (targeted or alienated) parent.

Ambivalence—A state of having conflicting feelings about the same person or situation at the same time.

Fathers' rights movement—A social movement that emerged in the 1980s in response to what members consider gender bias in favor of women in family law.

Syndrome—A group or cluster of symptoms that occur together and are characteristic of a specific disease or disorder.

Risk factors

Risk factors for the development of parental alienation disorder can include the following actions or behaviors by the alienating parent:

- severe mental disorder
- alcohol or drug abuse
- inability to control anger in the presence of children
- consistently returning the child or children late (more than 30 minutes) following a visit
- making verbal threats to abduct the children
- withholding visits and/or the child refusing to see the targeted parent

Other risk factors include the presence of an intrusive or controlling stepparent or grandparent in the household or any indications that the child is being mentally, physically, or sexually abused.

Causes and symptoms

Causes

The possible causes of parental alienation disorder (in the alienating parent) are identified as:

- unresolved anger toward the divorcing spouse
- unresolved issues with his or her family of origin
- narcissistic or paranoid personality disorder
- being so wrapped up in the child that he or she has no separate identity and regards the child's relationship with the other parent as a threat
- insecurity about his or her parenting skills, and projecting that insecurity onto the other parent
- the influence of a new spouse or domineering and meddlesome grandparents

Symptoms

Gardner listed eight symptoms of parental alienation syndrome in children:

- ongoing denigration of, and hatred toward, the targeted parent
- weak, silly, or frivolous rationalizations of the hateful behavior
- absence of ambivalence (mixed feelings) toward the targeted parent
- maintaining that the decision to reject the targeted parent is his or hers alone (referred to as the "independent thinker phenomenon")
- knee-jerk support of the favored parent
- lack of guilt for treating the rejected parent badly
- using catchphrases or scenarios borrowed from the favored parent
- expanding the rejection of the targeted parent to include his or her extended family and friends

Gardner went on to define three levels of severity of PAS:

- Mild—the child has only six of the eight symptoms; lack of ambivalence and absence of guilt over cruelty to the alienated parent do not appear.
- Moderate—all eight symptoms are present at a moderate intensity.
- Severe—all eight symptoms are present at a high level of severity.

Diagnosis

As of 2011, there were no formally accepted diagnostic criteria for parental alienation disorder, no published and tested assessments or questionnaires to make the diagnosis, and no imaging or laboratory tests to make or confirm the diagnosis. No large-scale controlled studies of the validity and reliability of the concept of parental alienation disorder have yet been conducted. In addition, a survey of 448 mental health and legal professionals reported in 2009 that the respondents were cautious about the applicability of PAD in child custody cases; they were reluctant to support the concept of PAD and did not regard it as meeting admissibility standards for courtroom proceedings.

Bernet proposed the following diagnostic criteria for parental alienation disorder in 2010:

- Criterion A: The child aligns himself or herself with one parent and refuses contact with the alienated parent.
- Criterion B: The child exhibits the first two symptoms listed by Gardner—continuous rejection of the alienated parent, and irrational justifications for the alienation.
- Criterion C: The child manifests two or more of the remaining six symptoms on Gardner's list.
- Criterion D: The "disturbance" lasts for at least two months.
- Criterion E: The "disturbance" causes significant distress or impairment in the child's social, academic, and other areas of functioning.
- Criterion F: The child's refusal to see the rejected parent has no legitimate justification (such as abuse).

Tests

At one point, Gardner published what he called the Sexual Abuse Legitimacy Scale to evaluate children who claimed they had been sexually abused by a parent. The scale was dismissed by child psychologists and psychiatrists and was consequently withdrawn. There was no published and tested diagnostic measure for PAD as of 2011.

Treatment

Gardner's recommendations for treating children with PAD were severe, including complete **denial** of contact between mother and child, and "deprogramming" the child of the belief that he or she has been abused. In some cases, children have become suicidal when forced to live with abusive fathers.

There is no agreement among contemporary therapists who accept the existence of PAD as to what type of therapeutic approach works best with children, nor were there any studies published as of 2011 comparing different forms of **psychotherapy**. There is, however, a general recognition that Gardner's punitive approach is unacceptable and could possibly lead to violation of the civil rights of parents.

Another aspect of treatment for PAD is the financial benefit to therapists if PAD is included in *DSM-5*. Bernet has been quoted as saying that inclusion of PAS in *DSM-5* "would spur insurance coverage, stimulate more systematic research, lend credence to charge of parental alienation in court, and raise the odds that children would get timely treatment." Opponents of inclusion have charged that proponents of the syndrome are looking for a way to expand their practices. A family lawyer in Florida has maintained that much of the current momentum to add PAS to *DSM-5* is monetary; psychologists and other consultants profit from conducting the evaluations and therapies involved in family court disputes.

Prognosis

Gardner stated in the 1980s that PAD inflicted irreparable harm on the children he diagnosed with the syndrome, in that the relationship between the child and the targeted parent could never be re-established. Other mental health professionals who accept the existence of PAD are less pessimistic but still maintain that it has serious long-term effects on children, including **depression**, **substance abuse**, a history of failed relationships and multiple divorces, and alienation from their own children.

Resources

BOOKS

Bernet, William, ed. *Parental Alienation, DSM-5, and ICD-11.* Springfield, IL: Charles C. Thomas, Publisher, 2010.

Brock, Michael G., and Samuel Saks. *Contemporary Issues in Family Law and Mental Health.* Springfield, IL: Charles C. Thomas, Publisher, 2008.

Darnall, Douglas. *Divorce Casualties: Understanding Parental Alienation*, 2nd ed. Lanham, MD: Taylor Publishing Co., 2008.

Gardner, Richard A. *Therapeutic Interventions for Children with Parental Alienation Syndrome.* Cresskill, NJ: Creative Therapeutics, 2001.

PERIODICALS

Baker, Amy J.L. "Parental Alienation Syndrome: The Parent/Child Disconnect." *Social Work Today* 8 (November–December 2008): 26. http://www.socialworktoday.com/archive/102708p26.shtml (accessed July 12, 2011).

Barton, Adriana. "Diagnosing Divorce: Should Parental Alienation Be a Mental Disorder?" *The Globe and Mail* (May 9, 2011). http://www.theglobeandmail.com/life/the-hot-button/diagnosing-divorce-should-parental-alienation-be-a-mental-disorder/article2015939 (accessed July 12, 2011).

Bernet, W. "Parental Alienation Disorder and DSM-V." *American Journal of Family Therapy* 36 (May 2008): 349–66.

Bow, J.N., et al. "Examining Parental Alienation in Child Custody Cases: A Survey of Mental Health and Legal Professionals." *American Journal of Family Therapy* 37 (February 2009): 127–45.

Bruch, C.S. "Parental Alienation Syndrome and Parental Alienation: Getting It Wrong in Child Custody Cases." *Family Law Quarterly* 35 (2001): 527–52.

Farkas, M.M. "An Introduction to Parental Alienation Syndrome." *Journal of Psychosocial Nursing and Mental Health Services* 49 (April 2011): 20–26.

Gardner, R.A. "Denial of the Parental Alienation Syndrome Also Harms Women." *American Journal of Family Therapy* 30 (March 2002): 191–202.

Hoult, J. "The Evidentiary Admissibility of Parental Alienation Syndrome: Science, Law, and Policy." *Children's Legal Rights Journal* 26 (January 2006): 1–61.

Johnston, J.T. "Parental Alignments and Rejection: An Empirical Study of Alienation in Children of Divorce." *Journal of the American Academy of Psychiatry and the Law* 31 (February 2003): 158–70.

Winter, Mary. "Recognizing Parental Alienation Syndrome." *Denver Post*, December 5, 2010. http://www.denverpost.com/opinion/ci_16763836 (accessed July 11, 2011).

OTHER

Bernet, William, and Joseph N. Kenan. "Proposed Text for Parental Alienation Disorder in DSM-5." Lecture presented to the Forensic Mental Health Association of California, March 24, 2011. http://www.fmhac.net/Assets/Documents/2011/Presentations/BernetParental%20Alienation.pdf (accessed July 12, 2011).

WEBSITES

American Psychiatric Association. "Conditions Proposed by Outside Sources." DSM-5 Development. http://www.dsm5.org/ProposedRevisions/Pages/ConditionsProposed-byOutsideSources.aspx (accessed July 12, 2011).

Crary, David. "Is Parental Alienation a Mental Disorder?" MSNBC.com. October 1, 2010. http://www.msnbc.msn.com/id/39463768/ns/health-mental_health (accessed July 11, 2011).

Dallam, Stephanie J. "Dr. Richard Gardner: A Review of His Theories and Opinions on Atypical Sexuality, Pedophilia, and Treatment Issues." Leadership Council on Child Abuse and Interpersonal Violence. http://www.leadershipcouncil.org/1/res/dallam/2.html (accessed July 11, 2011).

———. "The Parental Alienation Syndrome: Is It Scientific?" Leadership Council on Child Abuse and Interpersonal Violence. http://www.leadershipcouncil.org/1/res/dallam/3.html (accessed July 11, 2011).

Lithwick, Dahlia. "Mommy Hates Daddy and You Should Too." Slate.com. May 17, 2011. http://www.slate.com/id/2294831 (accessed July 12, 2011).

Meier, Joan S. "Parental Alienation Syndrome & Parental Alienation: Research Reviews." VAWnet.org (National Online Resource Center on Violence Against Women). http://www.vawnet.org/sexual-violence/summary.php?doc_id=1679&find_type=web_desc_AR (accessed August 4, 2011).

ORGANIZATIONS

American Academy of Psychiatry and the Law (AAPL), One Regency Drive, PO Box 30, Bloomfield, CT, 06002, (860) 242-5450, (800) 331-1389, Fax: (860) 286-0787, http://www.aapl.org/contact.htm, http://www.aapl.org.

American Psychiatric Association, 1000 Wilson Boulevard, Suite 1825, Arlington, VA, 22209-3901, (703) 907-7300, apa@psych.org, http://www.psych.org.

Canadian Symposium for Parental Alienation Syndrome (CS-PAS), 150 Hollidge Blvd., Suite 252, Aurora, Canada ONL4G 8A3, (647) 476-3170, info@cspas.ca, http://cspas.ca.

Leadership Council on Child Abuse and Interpersonal Violence, c/o Joyanna Silberg, Ph.D., 6501 North Charles Street, PO Box 6815, Baltimore, MD, 21285-6815. desk1@leadershipcouncil.org, http://www.leadership-council.org/index.html.

National Council of Juvenile and Family Court Judges (NCJFCJ), PO Box 8970, Reno, NV, 89507, (775) 784-6012, Fax: (775) 784-6628, staff@ncjfcj.org, http://www.ncjfcj.org.

Rebecca J. Frey, Ph.D.

Parent management training

Definition

Parent management training (PMT) is an adjunct to treatment that involves educating and coaching parents to change their child's problem behaviors using principles of learning theory and **behavior modification**.

Purpose

The aim of PMT is to decrease or eliminate a child's disruptive or inappropriate behaviors at home or school and to replace problematic ways of acting with positive interactions with peers, parents and authority figures such as teachers. In order to accomplish this goal, PMT focuses on enhancing parenting skills. The PMT therapist coaches parents in applying strategies such as rewarding positive behavior, and responding to negative behavior by removing rewards or enforcing undesirable consequences (punishments). Although PMT focuses on specific targeted behaviors rather than on the child's **diagnosis**, it has come to be associated with the treatment of certain disorders. PMT is used in treating **oppositional defiant disorder**, **conduct disorder**, **intermittent explosive disorder** (age-inappropriate tantrums), and attention deficit disorder with hyperactivity (**attention deficit hyperactivity disorder**). Antisocial behaviors such as firesetting and truancy can also be addressed through PMT.

Description

In PMT, the therapist conducts initial teaching sessions with the parent(s), giving a short summary of foundational concepts in behavior modification; demonstrating interventions for the parents; and coaching parents in carrying out the techniques of PMT. Early meetings with the therapist focus on training in the principles of behavior modification, response-contingent learning, and ways to apply the techniques. Parents are instructed to concretely and specifically define the behavior(s) to be changed. In addition, they learn how to observe and identify relevant behavior and situational factors, and how to chart or otherwise record the child's behavior. Defining, observing and recording behavior are essential to the success of this method, because when behaviors such as fighting or tantrums are highlighted in concrete, specific ways, techniques of **reinforcement** and punishment can be put to use. Progress or its absence is easier to identify when the description of the behavior is defined with enough clarity to be measurable, and when responses to the PMT interventions are tracked on a chart. After the child's parents grasp the basic interventions as well as when and how to apply them, the techniques that the parents practiced with the therapist can be carried out at home.

Learning theory, which is the conceptual foundation of PMT, deals with the ways in which organisms learn to respond to their environment, and the factors that affect the frequency of a specific behavior. The core of learning theory is the notion that actions increase or decrease in frequency depending on the consequences that occur immediately after the actions. Research in parent-child interactions in families with disruptive, difficult, or defiant children shows that parental responses are often unintentionally reinforcing the unwanted behaviors. PMT trains parents to become more aware of their reactions to a child's behavior. The parents learn to provide attention, praise, and increased affection in reaction to the child's desired behaviors, and to withdraw attention, suspend displays of affection, or withdraw privileges in instances of less desirable behavior.

The most critical element of PMT is offering positive reinforcement for socially appropriate (or at least nondeviant) behaviors. An additional component involves responding to any undesired behaviors by removing rewards or applying punishment. These two types of response to the child must be carried out with great consistency. Consistent responding is important because erratic responses to unwanted behavior can actually cause the behavior to increase in frequency. For instance, if a child consistently throws tantrums in stores, hoping to be given something to end the tantrum, inconsistent parent responses can worsen the situation. If a parent is occasionally determined not to give in, but provides a candy bar or a toy to end the tantrum on other occasions, the child learns either to have more tantrums, or to have more dramatic tantrums. The rise in the number or intensity of tantrums occurs because the child is trying to increase the number of opportunities to obtain that infrequent parental reward for the behavior. Planning responses ahead of time to predefined target behaviors by rewarding desired actions and by withdrawing rewards or applying punishment for undesirable behavior is a fundamental principle of PMT. Consistent consequences, which are contingent on (in response to) the child's behavior, result in behavior change. Parents practice therapeutic ways of responding to their child's behavior in the PMT sessions with the therapist.

Through PMT, parents learn that positive rewards for appropriate behaviors can be offered in a variety of ways. Giving praise, providing extra attention, earning points toward obtaining a reward desired by the child, earning stickers or other small indicators of positive behavior, earning additional privileges, hugging (and other affectionate gestures) are all forms of reward. The technical term for the rewarding of desired behavior is *positive reinforcement*. Positive reinforcement refers to consequences that cause the desired target behavior to increase.

PMT instructs parents to cancel rewards or give punishments when the child behaves in undesirable ways. The removal of rewards usually entails time away from the circumstances and situations in which the child can do desired activities or receive attention. The concept of a "time out" is based on this notion of removal of rewards. Time out from rewards customarily means that the child is removed from people and stimulation for a certain period of time; it can also include loss of privileges.

Punishment in PMT is not necessarily what parents typically refer to as punishment; it most emphatically is *not* the use of physical punishment. A punishment in PMT involves a response to the child's negative behavior by exposing the child to something he or she regards as unpleasant. Examples of punishments might include having to redo the correct behavior so many times that it becomes annoying; verbal reproaches; or

KEY TERMS

Behavior modification—An approach to therapy based on the principles of operant conditioning. Behavior modification seeks to replace undesirable behaviors with preferable behaviors through the use of positive or negative reinforcement.

Positive reinforcement—A procedure or response that rewards a desired behavior.

Response-contingent—An approach to treatment in which rewards or punishments are given in response to a particular behavior to be encouraged or corrected.

Social learning theory—A subset of learning theories based on the concept that human behavior originates in and is affected by the interplay among the person's learned experiences, previous behaviors, and environmental influences.

the military standby—"drop and give me fifty"—having to do pushups or situps or laps around a playing field to the point of discomfort.

The least challenging problems, which have the greatest likelihood of successful change, are tackled first, in hope of giving the family a "success experience." The success experience is a positive reinforcement for the family, increasing the likelihood that they will continue using PMT in efforts to bring about change. In addition, lower-level behavioral problems provide opportunities for parents to become skilled in intervening and to learn consistency in their responses. After the parents have practiced using the skills learned in PMT on the less important problems, more severe issues can be tackled.

In addition to face-to-face sessions with the parents, some PMT therapists make frequent telephone calls to the parents between sessions. The purposes of the calls are to remind parents to continue to be consistent in applying the techniques; to answer questions about the work at home; and to praise the parents' attempts to correct the child's behavior. In addition, ongoing support in sessions and on the telephone helps parents feel less isolated and thus more likely to continue trying to use learning principles in managing their child. Troubleshooting any problems that arise regarding the application of the behavioral techniques is handled over the telephone and in the office sessions.

An additional aspect of learning theory is that rewarding subunits of the ultimately desired behavior can lead to developing more complex new actions. The subunits are finally linked together by changing the ways in which the rewards are given. This process is called "chaining." Sometimes, if the child shows no elements of the desired response, then the desired behavior is demonstrated for the child and subsequent "near hits" or approximations are rewarded. To refine "close but not quite" into the targeted response, rewards are given in a slightly "pickier" manner. Rewarding successive approximations of the desired behavior is also called "shaping."

Risks

The best way to learn to alter parental responses to child behaviors is with the support and assistance of a behavioral health professional (**psychologist**, **psychiatrist**, clinical social worker). Parents often inadvertently reinforce the problem behaviors, and it is difficult for a parent to see objectively the ways in which he or she is unintentionally supporting the defiant or difficult behavior. Furthermore, inappropriate application of such behavioral techniques as those used in PMT can actually make the problem situation worse. Families should seek therapists with valid credentials, skills, training and experience in PMT.

Results

Typically, the parents should notice a decrease in the unwanted behaviors after they implement the techniques learned in PMT at home. Of the various therapies used to treat childhood disorders, PMT is among those most frequently researched. PMT has shown effectiveness in changing children's behavior in very well-designed and rigorous studies. PMT has a greater effect on behavior than many other treatments, including **family therapy** or **play therapy**. Furthermore, the results—improved child behavior and reduction or elimination of undesirable behavior—are sustained over the long term. When a group of children whose families had used PMT were examined one to fourteen years later, they had maintained higher rates of positive behavior and lower levels of problem behavior.

Resources

BOOKS

Hendren, R. L. *Disruptive Behavior Disorders in Children and Adolescents*. Review of Psychiatry Series, Vol. 18, no. 2. Washington, DC: American Psychiatric Press, 1999.

Webster-Stratton, C., and M. Herbert. *Troubled Families—Problem Children: Working with Parents, a Collaborative Process*. Chichester, England: Wiley, 1995.

PERIODICALS

Feldman, Julie, and Alan E. Kazdin. "Parent Management Training for Oppositional and Conduct Problem Children." *Clinical Psychologist* 48, no. 4 (1995): 3–5. Available online at http://www.apa.org/divisions/div12/Rev_Est/pmt_child.html (accessed November 9, 2011).

Golding, Kim. "Parent Management Training as an Intervention to Promote Adequate Parenting." *Clinical Child Psychology and Psychiatry* 5, no. 3 (2000): 357–372.

Kazdin, A. E. "Parent Management Training: Evidence, Outcome and Issues." *Journal of American Academic Child and Adolescent Psychiatry* 36, no. 10 (October 1997): 1349–1356.

ORGANIZATIONS

American Academy of Child and Adolescent Psychiatry, 3615 Wisconsin Ave. NW, Washington, DC, 20016-3007, (202) 966-7300, Fax: (202) 966-2891, http://aacap.org.

Association for Behavioral and Cognitive Therapies, 305 Seventh Ave., 16th Floor, New York, NY, 10001-6008, (212) 647-1890, Fax: (212) 647-1865, http://www.abct.org.

North American Family Institute, 26 Howley Street, Peabody, MA, 01960, (978) 538-0286, Fax: (978) 531-9313, http://www.nafi.com.

Deborah Rosch Eifert, Ph.D

Parnate *see* **Tranylcypromine**

Paroxetine

Definition

Paroxetine is an antidepressant of the type known as **selective serotonin reuptake inhibitors (SSRIs)**. It is sold in the United States under the brand name Paxil.

Purpose

Paroxetine is approved by the U.S. Food and Drug Administration (FDA) for treatment of **depression** and for the following **anxiety disorders**: **obsessive-compulsive disorder**, **panic disorder**, **generalized anxiety disorder**, **post-traumatic stress disorder**, and social anxiety disorder.

Description

Paroxetine increases the amount of **serotonin** (also called "5-HT") available in the **brain**. Serotonin is a neurotransmitter, or chemical in the brain that carries nerve impulses from a sending neuron (nerve cell) to a receiving neuron. The sending neuron releases serotonin into a little gap between neurons, called the synapse. The

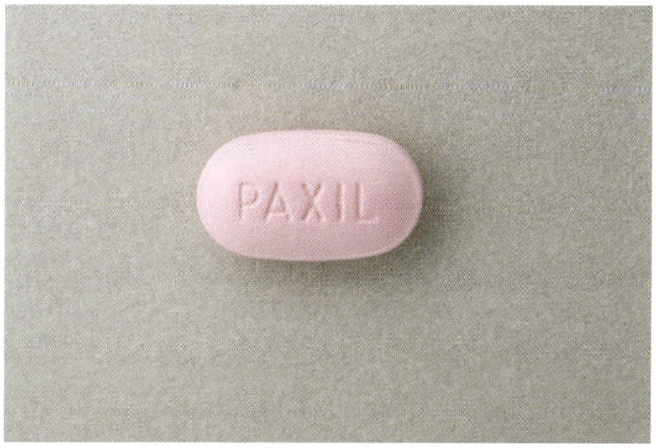

Paxil (paroxetine), 20 mg. *(© Custom Medical Stock Photo, Inc. Reproduced by permission.)*

receiving neuron picks up the serotonin from the synapse, allowing the nerve impulse to continue on its way.

Researchers think that depression and certain other disorders may be caused, in part, because there is not enough available serotonin in the brain. Normally, once a nerve impulse has crossed the synapse, serotonin is reabsorbed by the sending neuron that released it. Once reabsorbed, this serotonin is no longer available and cannot interact with a receiving neuron. Paroxetine blocks the reabsorption, or re-uptake, of serotonin, leaving it available to stimulate receiving neurons. Therefore, paroxetine facilitates the transmission of nerve impulses by increasing available serotonin in the brain and thus increasing its effectiveness.

Paroxetine is an antidepressant that is virtually completely absorbed via oral administration. Food does not reduce its absorption.

The benefits of paroxetine develop slowly over a period of up to four weeks. Patients should be aware of this and continue to take the drug as directed, even if they feel no immediate improvement.

Recommended dosage

The recommended dosage of paroxetine is 20–50 mg per day. The drug should be taken only once per day. An appropriate initial dosage is 20 mg. Dosage changes should not be made more frequently than once per week.

The recommended dosage for older persons or individuals with liver or kidney disease is 10 mg per day. The total dosage for such persons should not exceed 40 mg per day.

Precautions

Paroxetine should never be taken with **monoamine oxidase inhibitors (MAOIs)**.

Paroxetine may lower the threshold for a **manic episode** among people with bipolar (manic-depressive) disorders. For this reason, the drug should be used only with caution and under close supervision in these patients. It may also increase the chance of having a seizure in people with a history of seizure disorders.

The possibility of **suicide** is a component of depression. The minimum number of doses of paroxetine should be dispensed at any one time to minimize the potential for use as a suicide agent.

Hyponatremia (abnormally low concentration of sodium in the blood) has been associated with the use of paroxetine. In all cases, this condition resolved when the drug was discontinued. Most of these instances occurred among older individuals who were also taking diuretics (water pills).

Like other **SSRIs**, paroxetine carries a warning regarding use in children and adults up to the age of 24, who appear to have an increased risk of developing suicidal thoughts or actions while using these agents.

Side effects

Common side effects associated with paroxetine include headache, weakness, chills, malaise, nausea, and sleepiness. Other complaints included dry mouth, dizziness, tremors, constipation, diarrhea, and problems with ejaculation. Adverse reactions to paroxetine have been reported for all organ systems of the body, but all of these side effects are uncommon.

In general, the incidence of side effects increases as the dosage of paroxetine increases.

Interactions

There is the potential for a fatal interaction with another class of antidepressant drugs called monoamine-oxidase inhibitors (**MAOIs**). There have been reports of dangerously elevated body temperature, muscle rigidity, and rapid changes in vital signs, such as heart rate and blood pressure. Mental changes ranging from extreme agitation to **delirium** and coma have also been reported. Because of this, paroxetine should never be taken in combination with MAO inhibitors. Patient taking any MAO inhibitors, for example Nardil (**phenelzine** sulfate) or Parnate (**tranylcypromine** sulfate), should stop the MAO inhibitor then wait at least 14 days before starting paroxetine or any other antidepressant. The same holds true when discontinuing paroxetine and starting an MAO inhibitor.

The combination of paroxetine with the antipsychotic drug **thioridazine** has the potential to cause fatal cardiac arrhythmias (irregular heartbeat). The use of paroxetine in combination with tryptophan may result in unwanted reactions, including agitation, restlessness, and gastrointestinal distress. Paroxetine may also increase the chance of having a seizure in people with a history of seizure disorders. People taking anticonvulsants to control **seizures** should be closely monitored, and a physician may need to adjust the dosage of their seizure medication.

People with **bipolar disorder** are commonly treated with lithium. No interactions between paroxetine and lithium have been reported, nor are there any reported interactions with the common antianxiety drug **diazepam** (Valium).

Phenobarbital at dosages greater than 100 mg per day decreases the bioavailability of paroxetine in some persons. Paroxetine has been reported to increase the systemic bioavailability of procyclidine.

Resources

BOOKS

Adams, Michael, and Norman Holland. *Core Concepts in Pharmacology.* Philadelphia: Lippincott-Raven, 1998.

Foreman, John C., and Torben Johansen. *Textbook of Receptor Pharmacology*. 2nd ed. Boca Raton, FL: CRC Press, 2002.

Von Boxtel, Chris J., Budiono Santoso, and I. Ralph Edwards. *Drug Benefits and Risks: International Textbook of Clinical Pharmacology*. New York: John Wiley and Sons, 2001.

PERIODICALS

Hegeman, J., et al. "Unraveling the Association between SSRI Use and Falls: An Experimental Study of Risk Factors for Accidental Falls in Long-Term Paroxetine Users." *Clinical Neuropharmacology* 34, no. 6 (2011): 210–15.

Tomita, Tetsu, et al. "The Association between Sunshine Duration and Paroxetine Response Time in Patients with Major Depressive Disorder." *Journal of Affective Disorders* (December 6, 2011) [e-pub ahead of print]. http://dx.doi.org/10.1016/j.jad.2011.11.012 (accessed January 6, 2012).

WEBSITES

PubMed Health. "Paroxetine." U.S. National Library of Medicine. http://www.ncbi.nlm.nih.gov/pubmedhealth/PMH0001037 (accessed January 6, 2012).

ORGANIZATIONS

National Institute of Mental Health, 6001 Executive Blvd., Rm. 8184, MSC 9663, Bethesda, MD, 20892-9663, (301) 443-4513; TTY: (301) 443-8431, (866) 615-6464; TTY: (866) 415-8051, Fax: (301) 443-4279, nimhinfo@nih.gov, http://www.nimh.nih.gov.

U.S. Food and Drug Administration, 10903 New Hampshire Ave., Silver Spring, MD, 20993-0002, (888) INFO-FDA (463-6332), http://www.fda.gov.

L. Fleming Fallon, Jr., M.D., Dr.P.H.

Paruresis *see* **Toilet phobia**

Passionflower

Definition

Passionflower (*Passiflora incarnata*) is a vine whose leaves and flowers are widely used in Europe to make a herbal remedy for anxiety and **insomnia**. The plant, which is native to the tropical regions of North America, was first used by the Aztecs of Mexico as a folk remedy for these conditions. Passionflower is also known as maypop, apricot vine, passion vine, and granadilla. It grows as much as 30 ft. (10 m) tall, with a thick, woody stem.

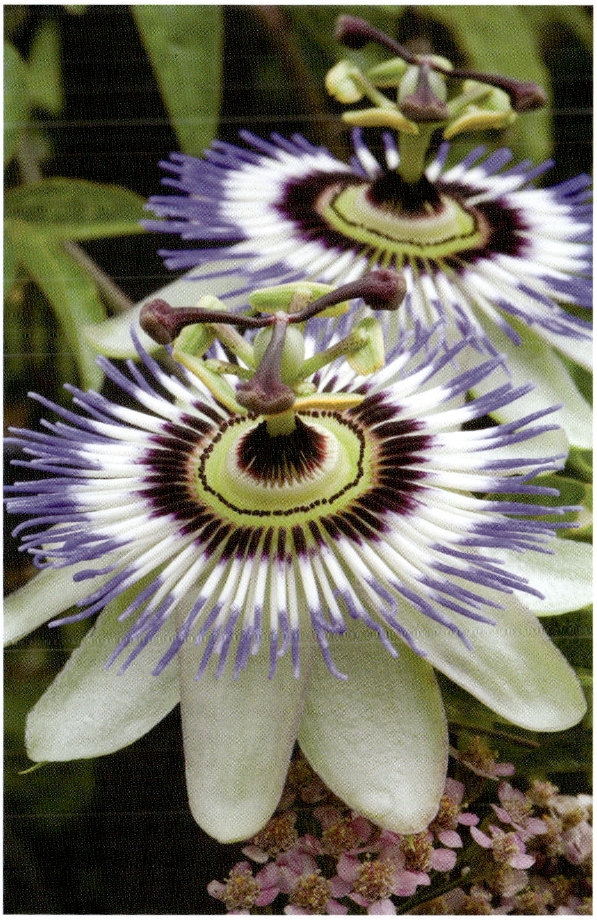

Passionflower plant. *(© iStockPhoto.com/Lidian Neeleman)*

The parts of the plant that grow above the ground are gathered to make passionflower preparations. They may be used either fresh or dried. The most common sources of the passionflower that is used today are India, the West Indies, and the southern United States; the vine can also be grown in Mexico and Latin America.

Purpose

Passionflower is used as a sedative and anxiolytic far more frequently in Great Britain and Europe than in the United States. In Britain, passionflower is the single most common ingredient in herbal **sedatives**, and the German Commission E approved it for use as a tranquilizer. It is also used in homeopathic remedies. In addition to its long-standing uses as a remedy for anxiety and insomnia, passionflower has been shown to be effective in treating narcotic drug withdrawal and adjustment disorder. Passionflower may be recommended for the treatment of gastrointestinal disorders related to anxiety, asthma, tachycardia (an abnormally rapid heartbeat), menstrual cramps, **seizures**, **attention deficit hyperactivity disorder**, and hysteria, but these uses have not yet been proven by **clinical trials**. A topical preparation made from passionflower has been used to treat hemorrhoids.

Description

Passionflower preparations may be made from the flowers, leaves, or shoots of the plant. After the first fruits of the plant have matured, younger shoots growing 12.7–17.8 cm above the ground are harvested and air dried. The plant material is used to prepare infusions, teas, liquid extracts, and tinctures of passionflower. In Europe, passionflower is often combined with lemon balm or **valerian** to make a sedative tea. The standardized formula approved by the German Commission E contains 30% passionflower, 40% valerian root, and 30% lemon balm. Passionflower is also used to make a special sedative tea for children, which typically includes 30% passionflower, 30% lemon balm, 30% **lavender** flower, and 10% **St. John's wort**. Passionflower is sometimes combined with hawthorn to make a remedy for stomach cramps associated with gastritis.

Although passionflower has been shown in animal studies to have sedative and antispasmodic effects, researchers are not yet certain which compounds in the plant have these properties. Passionflower is known to contain flavonoids and a group of alkaloid compounds that include harman, harmine, harmaline, and harmalol. Some researchers have hypothesized that the medicinal effects of passionflower derive from a combination of these substances rather than from any of them in isolation. A recent Swiss study, however, appears to indicate that a flavonoid called chrysin may be the source of passionflower's anxiolytic properties.

Recommended dosage

As the German recipe indicates, passionflower is considered safe for children. Dosages for children should be calculated on the basis of the child's weight. Since most adult dosages of herbal remedies assume an average adult weight of 150 lb. (70 kg), a child weighing 50 lb. (23 kg) can be given one-third of the adult dose.

Recommended adult doses of passionflower are as follows:

- Infusion: 2–5 g of dried herb, up to three times daily
- Fluid extract (1:1 ratio in a solution of 25% alcohol): 0.5–1.0 mL up to three times daily
- Tincture (1:5 ratio in a solution of 45% alcohol): 0.5–2.0 mL up to three times daily

Precautions

Passionflower should not be used in doses higher than the recommended levels. Because it has a sedative effect, it should not be combined with alcoholic beverages or prescription sedatives. Passionflower should not be used by pregnant or lactating women or for children under six months old, and persons undergoing surgery should stop using passionflower at least two weeks before their procedure.

Side effects

Passionflower is considered generally safe when taken short term. Reported possible side effects include confusion, dizziness or vertigo, vasculitis (blood vessel inflammation), and abnormal muscle contraction or movement.

Interactions

The alkaloids found in passionflower, especially harman and harmaline, may increase the effects of a class of prescription **antidepressants** called **monoamine oxidase inhibitors (MAOIs)**. These drugs are most often prescribed for **depression**, panic attacks, and eating disorders. Passionflower may also increase the effects of sedative medications and should not be used in conjunction with either of these drugs.

KEY TERMS

Antispasmodic—A medication or preparation given to relieve muscle or digestive cramps.

Anxiolytic—A preparation or substance given to relieve anxiety; a tranquilizer.

Flavonoids—Plant pigments that have a variety of effects on human physiology. Some of these pigments have anti-inflammatory, anticarcinogenic, and antioxidant effects.

Gastritis—Inflammation of the lining of the stomach.

Infusion—The most potent form of extraction of a herb into water. Infusions are steeped for a longer period of time than teas.

Tincture—An alcohol-based herbal extract prepared by soaking parts of the plant in a mixture of alcohol and water. Established ratios and dilutions are followed.

Resources

BOOKS

Awang, Dennis, V.C. *Tyler's Herbs of Choice*. New York: CRC Press, 2009.

"Western Herbal Medicine: Nature's Green Pharmacy." In *The Best Alternative Medicine*, by Kenneth R. Pelletier. New York: Touchstone, 2002.

PERIODICALS

Zanoli, P., R. Avallone, and M. Baraldi. "Behavioral Characterisation of the Flavonoids Apigenin and Chrysin." *Fitoterapia* 71, Suppl. 1 (2000): S117–S123.

WEBSITES

MedlinePlus. "Passionflower." U.S. National Library of Medicine, National Institutes of Health. http://www.nlm.nih.gov/medlineplus/druginfo/natural/871.html (accessed November 14, 2011).

ORGANIZATIONS

American Botanical Council, 6200 Manor Rd., Austin, TX, 78723, (512) 926-4900, (800) 373-7105, Fax: (512) 926-2345, abc@herbalgram.org, http://www.herbalgram.org.

National Center for Complementary and Alternative Medicine, 9000 Rockville Pike, Bethesda, MD, 20892, (888) 644-6226, http://nccam.nih.gov.

NIH Office of Dietary Supplements, 6100 Executive Blvd., Room 3B01, MSC 7517, Bethesda, MD, 20892-7517, (301) 435-2920, Fax: (301) 480-1845, ods@nih.gov, http://www.odp.od.nih.gov.

Rebecca J. Frey, Ph.D.

Pathological gambling disorder *see* **Gambling disorder**

Paxil *see* **Paroxetine**

Paxipam *see* **Galantamine**

PCP *see* **Phencyclidine and related disorders**

Pedophilia

Definition

Pedophilia is a paraphilia that involves an abnormal interest in children. A paraphilia is a disorder that is characterized by recurrent intense sexual urges and sexually arousing fantasies generally focused on nonhuman objects; the suffering or humiliation of oneself or one's partner (not merely simulated); or animals, children, or other nonconsenting persons. Pedophilia is also a psychosexual disorder in which the fantasy or actual act of engaging in sexual activity with prepubertal children is the preferred or exclusive means of achieving sexual excitement and gratification. It may be directed toward children of the same sex or children of the opposite sex. Some pedophiles are attracted to both boys and girls. Some are attracted only to children, while others are attracted to adults as well as to children.

Pedophilia is defined by mental health professionals as a mental disorder, but the American legal system defines acting on a pedophilic urge as a criminal act.

Demographics

Pedophilia is one of the more common paraphilias; the large worldwide market for child pornography suggests that it is more frequent in the general population than prison statistics would indicate. Together with **voyeurism** and **exhibitionism**, pedophilia is one of the three paraphilias most commonly leading to arrest by the police.

The onset of pedophilia usually occurs during adolescence. Occasional pedophiles begin their activities during middle age but this late onset is uncommon.

The frequency of behavior associated with pedophilia varies with psychosocial **stress**. As the pedophile's stress levels increase, the frequency of his or her acting out generally rises. This manifestation echoes those of a behavioral **addiction**.

Pedophilia is more common among males than among females. In addition, the rate of recidivism for persons with a pedophilic preference for males is approximately twice that of pedophiles who prefer females.

Marital status, socioeconomic level, educational background, and religious observance does not seem to predict pedophilia. Little is known about the incidence of pedophilia in different racial or ethnic groups.

Description

The focus of pedophilia is sexual activity with a child. Many courts interpret this reference to age to mean children under the age of 18. Most mental health professionals, however, confine the definition of pedophilia to sexual activity with prepubescent children, who are generally age 13 or younger. The term *ephebophilia*, derived from the Greek word for "youth," is sometimes used to describe sexual interest in young people in the first stages of puberty.

The sexual behaviors involved in pedophilia cover a range of activities and may or may not involve the use of force. Some pedophiles limit their behaviors to exposing themselves or masturbating in front of the child, or fondling or undressing the child, but without genital contact. Others, however, compel the child to participate in oral sex or full genital intercourse.

The most common overt aspect of pedophilia is an intense interest in children. There is no typical pedophile. Pedophiles may be young or old, male or female, although the great majority are males. Unfortunately, some pedophiles are professionals who are entrusted with educating or maintaining the health and well-being of young persons, while others are entrusted with children to whom they are related by blood or marriage.

Causes and symptoms

Causes

A variety of different theories exist regarding the causes of pedophilia. A few researchers attribute pedophilia, along with the other **paraphilias**, to biology. They hold that testosterone, one of the male sex hormones, predisposes men to develop deviant sexual behaviors. As of 2011, no genes or hereditary factors had been associated with the development of pedophilia.

Pedophilia, as a disorder based in **compulsion** and impulse control, may be related to other disorders associated with obsessive-compulsive and impulsive behaviors. Research, including an imaging study, suggests that abnormalities in an area of the **brain** called the frontal cortex are associated with pedophilia. Other studies have identified similar abnormalities in obsessive-compulsive spectrum disorders. In addition, recent research indicates that pedophilic behavior may be rooted in early disturbances in neurological development, although a clear biological basis for the disorder has not yet been established. Neurotransmitter (nerve signaling molecules) pathways in the brain related to mood regulation have been implicated; these include pathways involving **serotonin** and **dopamine**.

Some experts believe that there is an association between pedophilia and having been sexually abused as a child. Still others think that it derives from the person's interactions with parents during their early years of life. Some researchers attribute pedophilia to arrested emotional development; that is, the pedophile is attracted to children because he or she has never matured psychologically. Some regard pedophilia as the result of a distorted need to dominate a sexual partner. Because children are smaller and usually weaker than adults, they may be regarded as nonthreatening potential partners. This drive for domination is sometimes thought to explain why most pedophiles are males.

Symptoms

A pedophile often seems particularly trustworthy to the children who are potential victims. Potential pedophiles may volunteer their services to athletic teams, Scout troops, or religious or civic organizations that serve youth. In some cases, pedophiles who are attracted to children within their extended family may offer to baby-sit for their relatives. They often have good interpersonal skills with children and can easily gain the children's trust.

Some pedophiles offer rationalizations or excuses that enable them to avoid assuming responsibility for their actions. They may blame the children for being too attractive or sexually provocative. They may also maintain that they are "teaching" the child about "the facts of life" or "love"; this rationalization is frequently offered by pedophiles who have molested children related to them. All these rationalizations may be found in pornography with pedophilic themes.

Diagnosis

According to the ***Diagnostic and Statistical Manual of Mental Disorders,*** fourth edition text revised, the following criteria must be met to establish a **diagnosis** of pedophilia.

- Over a period of at least six months, the affected person must experience recurrent, intense and sexually arousing fantasies, sexual urges or actual behaviors involving sexual activity with a prepubescent child or children aged 13 or younger.
- The fantasies, sexual urges or behaviors must cause clinically significant distress or impairment in social, occupational or other important areas of daily functioning.
- The affected person must be at least age sixteen and be at least five years older than the child or children who are the objects or targets of attention or sexual activity.

A diagnosis of pedophilia cannot be assigned to an individual in late adolescence (age 17 to 19) who is involved in an ongoing sexual relationship with a 12- or 13-year-old person.

In establishing a diagnosis of pedophilia, it is important for a mental health professional to determine if the patient is attracted to males, females or both. It is also important to determine whether incest is a factor in the relationship. Finally, the doctor must determine whether the pedophilia is exclusive or nonexclusive; that is, whether the patient is attracted only to children (exclusive pedophilia) or to adults as well as to children (nonexclusive pedophilia).

One difficulty with the diagnosis of the disorder is that persons with pedophilia rarely seek help voluntarily from mental health professionals. Instead, counseling and treatment is often the result of a court order. An interview that establishes the criteria for diagnosis may be enough to diagnose the condition, or surveillance or Internet records obtained through the criminal investigation may also be used.

An additional complication in diagnosis is that the paraphilias as a group have a high rate of comorbidity with one another and an equally high rate of comorbidity with major **depression**, **anxiety disorders**, and **substance abuse** disorders. A person diagnosed with pedophilia may also meet the criteria for exhibitionism or for a substance abuse or mood disorder.

Treatment

In the earliest stages of **behavior modification** therapy, pedophiles may be narrowly viewed as being attracted to inappropriate persons. Such aversive stimuli as electric shocks have been administered to persons undergoing therapy for pedophilia. This approach has not been very successful.

Types of treatment for pedophilia include **psychotherapy** and medication. Therapy is often undergone for many years but still does not have a high rate of success in inducing persons with pedophilia to change their behavior.

The three classes of medications most often used to treat pedophilia (and other paraphilias) are: hormones, particularly the synthetic medroxyprogesterone acetate (MPA); luteinizing hormone-releasing hormone (LHRH) agonists (mimics), which include such drugs as triptorelin (Trelstar), leuprolide acetate, and goserelin acetate; and antiandrogens, which block the uptake and metabolism of testosterone as well as reducing blood levels of this hormone. In particular, these drugs with antiandrogenic effects (interfering with the action of the body's androgenic hormones) have shown some efficacy in reducing the rate of recidivism. Most clinical studies of these drugs have been done in Germany, where the legal system has allowed their use in treating repeat sexual offenders since the 1970s. Researchers have reported some benefit with leuprolide acetate, for example, finding during a two-year study that none of the pedophiles being administered the drug re-offended.

Surgical castration is sometimes offered as a treatment to pedophiles who are repeat offenders or who have pleaded guilty to violent rape.

Increasingly, pedophiles are being prosecuted under criminal statutes and being sentenced to prison terms. Imprisonment removes them from society for a period of time but does not usually remove their pedophilic tendencies. As of 2011, all U.S. states had a registration and tracking system in place for sexual offenders. Legal challenges to this practice are pending in various jurisdictions.

Prognosis

The prognosis of successfully ending pedophilic habits among persons who practice pedophilia is not favorable. Pedophiles have a high rate of recidivism; that is, they tend to repeat their acts often over time.

The rate of prosecution for pedophiles through the criminal justice system has increased in recent years. Pedophiles are at high risk of being beaten or killed by other prison inmates. For this reason, they must often be kept isolated from other members of a prison population. Knowledge of the likelihood of abuse by prison personnel and inmates is not, however, an effective deterrent for most pedophiles.

Prevention

The main method for preventing pedophilia is avoiding situations that may promote pedophilic acts. Children should never be allowed to be in one-on-one situations with any adult other than their parents or trustworthy family members. Having another youth or adult as an observer provides some security for all concerned.

Children should be taught to yell or run if they are faced with an uncomfortable situation and reassured that it is acceptable to scream or call for help.

KEY TERMS

Castration—Desexing a person or animal by surgical removal of the testes (in males) or ovaries (in females). Castration is sometimes offered as a treatment option to pedophiles who are violent rapists and/or repeat offenders.

Comorbidity—Association or presence of two or more mental disorders in the same patient. A disorder that is said to have a high degree of comorbidity is likely to occur in patients diagnosed with other disorders that may share or reinforce some of its symptoms.

Ephebophilia—Sexual desire on the part of an adult for youths in the early stages of puberty, as distinct from prepubertal children.

Incest—Unlawful sexual contact between persons who are biologically related. Many therapists, however, use the term to refer to inappropriate sexual contact between any members of a family, including stepparents and stepsiblings.

Paraphilia—A disorder that is characterized by recurrent intense sexual urges and sexually arousing fantasies generally involving nonhuman objects, the suffering or humiliation of oneself or one's partner (not merely simulated), or children or other non-consenting persons.

Recidivism—A tendency to return to a previously treated activity, or repeated relapse into criminal or deviant behavior.

Voyeurism—A paraphilia that involves watching unsuspecting people, usually strangers, undress or engage in sexual activity.

Another basis of preventing pedophilia is education. Adults who work with youth should be trained on how to avoid situations that may be construed as promoting pedophilia.

All U.S. states conduct some type of background check on childcare providers, but they do not always check for a history of abuse or neglect. A law proposed in 2011 (Child Care Protection Act of 2011) will, if passed, require more extensive background checking.

The Boy Scouts of America has tried to address the problem of pedophilia by creating a training program that is required for all adults in the organization. All applications for volunteers are reviewed and approved by several persons. Adults and youth are required to use separate facilities on all activities.

Secret meetings and one-on-one interactions between adults and youth are prohibited. This program has received several national awards.

Resources

BOOKS

American Psychiatric Association. *Diagnostic and Statistical Manual of Mental Disorders*. 4th ed., text rev. Washington, DC: American Psychiatric Publishing, 2000.

Gelder, Michael, Paul Harrison, and Philip Cowen. *Shorter Oxford Textbook of Psychiatry*. 5th ed. New York: Oxford University Press, 2006.

Wilson, Josephine F. *Biological Foundations of Human Behavior*. Farmington Hills, MI: Cengage Learning, 2002.

PERIODICALS

Berlin, F. S. "Letters to Editor: Treatments to Change Sexual Orientation." *American Journal of Psychiatry* 157, no. 5 (May 2000): 8–9.

Cohen, L.J., et al. "Impulsive Personality Traits in Male Pedophiles Versus Healthy Controls: Is Pedophilia an Impulsive-Aggressive Disorder?" *Comprehensive Psychiatry* 43, no. 2 (March–April 2002). 127–34.

Hill, S.A. "The Man Who Claimed to Be a Paedophile." *Journal of Medical Ethics* 26, no. 2 (2000): 137–8.

O'Donohue, W., L.G. Regev, and A. Hagstrom. "Problems with the DSM-IV Diagnosis of Pedophilia." *Sexual Abuse* 12, no. 2 (2000): 95–105.

Schiffer, Boris, et al. "Structural Brain Abnormalities in the Frontostriatal System and Cerebellum in Pedophilia." *Journal of Psychiatric Research* 41, no. 9 (2007) 753–62.

Schober, Justine M., Peter M. Byrne, and Phyllis J. Kuhn. "Leuprolide Acetate is a Familiar Drug That May Modify Sex-Offender Behavior: The Urologist's Role." *British Journal of Urology International* 97 (2006): 684–6.

ORGANIZATIONS

American Academy of Family Physicians, 11400 Tomahawk Creek Parkway, Leawood, KS, 66211-2672, (913) 906-6000, (800) 274-2237, Fax: (913) 906-6075, contactcenter@aafp.org, http://www.aafp.org.

American Academy of Pediatrics, 141 Northwest Point Blvd., Elk Grove Village, IL, 60007-1098, (847) 434-4000, Fax: (847) 434-8000, http://www.aap.org.

American Medical Association, 515 N State Street, Chicago, IL, 60610, (312) 464-5000, (800) 621-8335, http://www.ama-assn.org.

American Psychiatric Association, 1000 Wilson Blvd., Ste. 1825, Arlington, VA, 22209-3901, (703) 907-7300, apa@psych.org, http://www.psych.org.

American Psychological Association, 750 1st Street NE, Washington, DC, 20002-4242, (202) 336-5500; TDD/TTY: (202) 336-6123, (800) 374-2721, http://www.apa.org.

L. Fleming Fallon, Jr., MD, Dr. P.H.
Emily Jane Willingham, Ph.D.

Peer groups

Description

Peer groups are an important influence throughout one's life, but they are more critical during the developmental years of childhood and adolescence. There is often controversy about the influence of a peer group versus parental influence, particularly during adolescence. Recent studies show that parents continue to have significant influence, even during adolescence, a reassuring finding for many parents. It appears that the power of the peer group becomes more important when the family relationships are not close or supportive. For example, if the parents work extra jobs and are largely unavailable, their children may turn to their peer group for emotional support. This also occurs when the conflict between parents and children during adolescence, or at any time during a child's development, becomes so great that the child feels pushed away and seeks closeness elsewhere. Most children and adolescents in this situation are not discriminating about the kind of group they join. They will often turn to a group simply because that group accepts them, even if the group is involved in illegal or negative activities. Gang involvement, for example, is a common form of organized—often antisocial—peer interaction. Gangs may be based on ethnicity, sex, and/ or common activity. Most youths who join gangs come from families where drug and **alcohol use**, financial burdens, and broken relationships are common. The need for affiliation or closeness is often greater than the need to "do the right thing" for some adolescents who feel isolated and abandoned by members of their own family. Being part of a gang provides such individuals with acceptance and security not available at home or in other peer groups.

Membership in peer groups

Despite significant gains in diversity training, current studies continue to show that children are less likely to accept those who are different from themselves. The differences can be as obvious as physical impairments, or as subtle as differences in academic motivation. These rigid standards may create an atmosphere of exclusion for some children and adolescents that pushes them toward peer acceptance of any type.

Peer groups offer children and adults alike the opportunity to develop various social skills, such as leadership, sharing or teamwork, and empathy. Peer groups also offer the opportunity to experiment with new

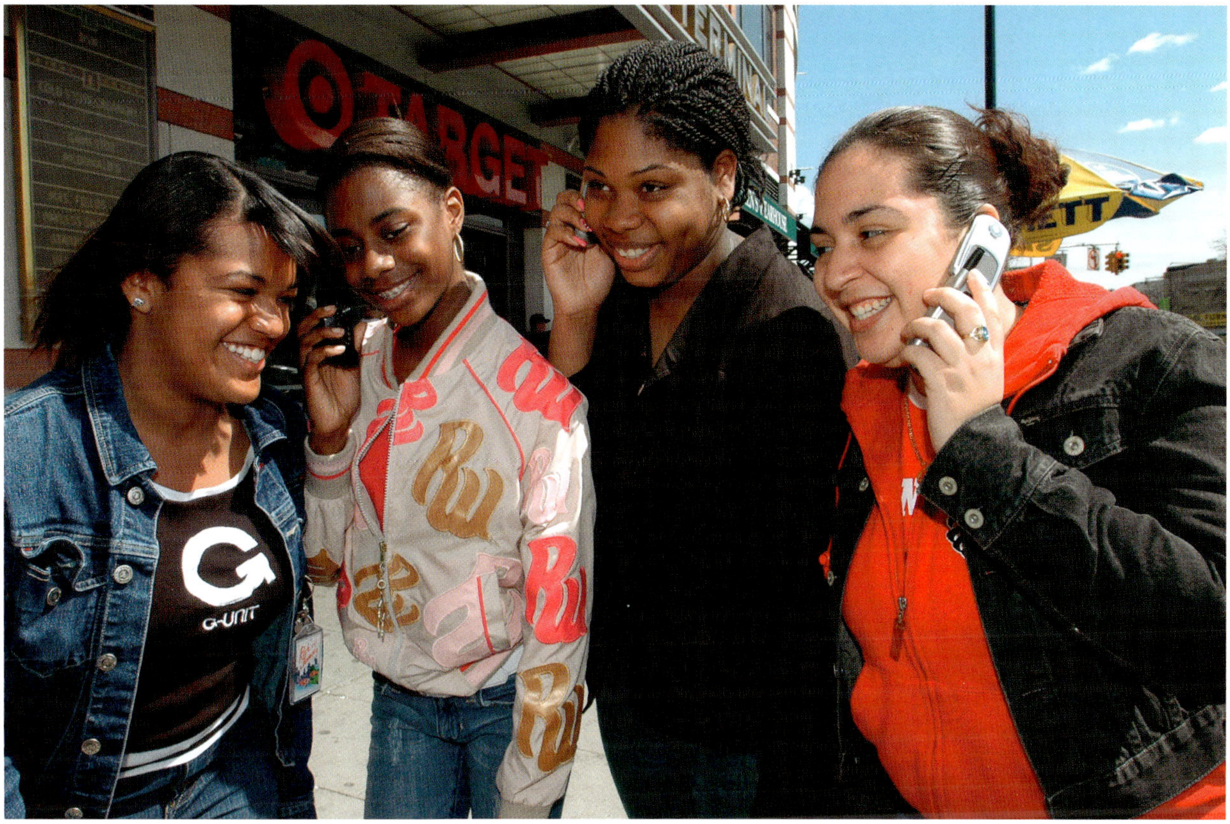

Peer group interaction has immense influence on adolescents. *(© Frances Roberts/Alamy)*

roles and interactions, similar to treatment groups, although they are less structured. It is for this reason that many children and adolescents drift from one group to another as they "find themselves," or work toward formation of their relatively permanent identity.

Aggression in peer groups

Although **bullying** and teasing have long been part of peer group interactions, these negative behaviors have increased over the last decade, resulting in school violence in many instances. As children and adolescents feel marginalized from their peers, anger builds to a point of rage at times. It is at those times that violence erupts within the school or community setting.

Negative peer interactions also occur more frequently following friendships or romantic relationships that have gone sour. The level of harassment that many of these children—often young women—experience is great enough for parents to become involved. In some cases, it may be necessary to move the child to another school district. A potential remediation for these negative interactions includes more active teacher involvement when negative social interactions are observed.

Influence of peer groups

Peer groups can also have a positive influence—a fact many parents have known for years. Studies support parent's perceptions that the influence of friends can have a positive effect on academic motivation and performance. Conversely, experimentation with drugs, drinking, vandalism, and stealing may also be increased by interaction with the peer group.

Interventions

Since schools are often the site of negative peer interactions, school personnel have a unique opportunity for effective **intervention**. Many schools have peer-mediation programs, in which students are encouraged to resolve conflicts on their own without the use of violence or aggression. School counselors also organize groups within the school to handle various problems, including providing **social skills training** and empathy training.

Risks

Peer groups often provide an example for negative and harmful behaviors. Cluster **suicide** is one such

KEY TERMS

Cluster suicide—Refers to the phenomenon of additional suicides being attempted or completed after one suicide has occurred within a small community, such as a group of high school students.

example. When a teen realizes that someone he or she knew has attempted or has committed suicide, the teen may see suicide as a viable option for him- or herself as well. For this reason schools and local media should exercise caution when reporting such tragedies. Care must be taken not to portray the suicide glamorously or mythically.

When parents try to protect their children by telling them to stay away from certain friends, they should realize that sometimes this only encourage them to seek out negative role models. Parents should be supportive of their child and redirect their child's activities to more positive and prosocial peers and events. A trusted adult friend, such as a scout leader or a respected coach, may be an important part of the redirection effort.

As noted, children and adolescents without strong family connections, or at least a positive connection with other adults in their life, face a higher risk of negative influence from peer groups. If the child or adolescent has not been able to form bonds with positive peer groups, it is more likely they will be perceived as distant and different from their peers, making them feel more like outsiders. Lower standards of acceptance often exist in less positive peer groups, making it easier for people to join. Unfortunately, many such groups often engage in self-destructive and antisocial activities.

Resources

BOOKS

Juvonen, J., and S. Graham, eds. *Peer Harassment in School: The Plight of the Vulnerable and Victimized.* New York: The Guilford Press, 2001.

PERIODICALS

Pearl, R., et al. "The Social Integration of Students with Mild Disabilities in General Education Classrooms: Peer Group Membership and Peer-assessed Social Behavior." *Elementary School Journal* 99, no. 2 (November 1998): 167–185.

Ryan, A. M. "The Peer Group as a Context for the Development of Young Adolescent Motivation and Achievement." *Child Develoment* 72, no. 4 (July/August 2001): 1135–1150.

Schwartz, D. "Subtypes of Victims and Aggressors in Children's Peer Groups." *Journal of Abnormal Child Psychology* 28, no. 2 (April 2000): 181–192.

Deanna Pledge, Ph.D.

Pemoline

Definition

Pemoline is classified as a central nervous system (CNS) stimulant. It is no longer available in the United States but was previously sold under the brand names Cylert and PemADD as well as its generic name.

Purpose

Pemoline was used in combination with psychological, educational, and social support for the treatment of people with **attention deficit hyperactivity disorder (ADHD)**.

Description

Pemoline is a central nervous system stimulant that derives at least some of its effects by increasing levels of **dopamine** in the **brain**. Dopamine is one of several **neurotransmitters** in the brain. Neurotransmitters are naturally occurring chemicals that regulate the transmission of nerve impulses from one cell to another. Mental and physical well-being are partially dependent on

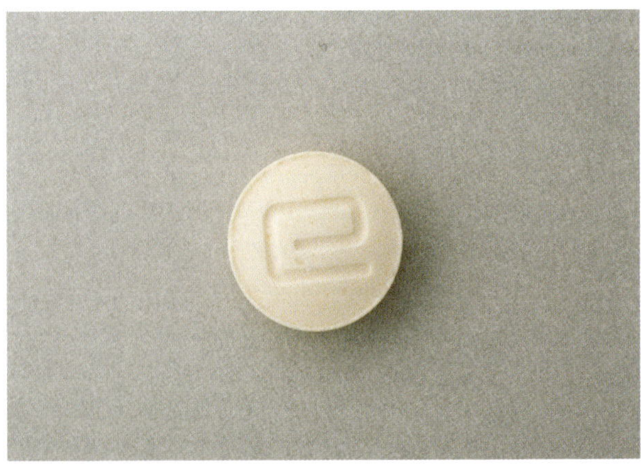

Cylert (pemoline), a drug used to treat attention deficit hyperactivity disorder (ADHD), is no longer available in the United States due to a risk of liver toxicity. *(© Custom Medical Stock Photo, Inc. Reproduced by permission.)*

maintaining the proper balance among the various neurotransmitters in the brain.

Pemoline is similar in its effects to **dextroamphetamine** and **methylphenidate**, two other drugs used to treat **ADHD**, although it is not chemically related to these drugs. The mechanism of action of CNS stimulants in the treatment of ADHD is not totally clear, but likely includes increased mental alertness, decreased mental **fatigue**, and an increased sense of well-being.

Pemoline is no longer manufactured for use, due to its association with potentially life-threatening liver toxicity. Symptoms of liver toxicity range from mild reversible changes in liver function tests to acute liver failure. The risk of liver damage should be weighed against any therapeutic benefit derived from treatment with pemoline.

Resources

BOOKS

American Society of Health-System Pharmacists. *AHFS Drug Information 2002.* Bethesda: American Society of Health-System Pharmacists, 2002.

Preston, John D., John H. O'Neal, and Mary C. Talaga. *Handbook of Clinical Psychopharmacology for Therapists.* 4th ed. Oakland, CA: New Harbinger Publications, 2004.

PERIODICALS

Bonnet, Udo, and Eugen Davids. "A Rare Case of Dependence on Pemoline." *Progress in Neuro-Psychopharmacology & Biological Psychiatry* 30, no. 7 (September 2006): 1340–41.

Krauseneck, Till, and Michael Soyka. "Delusional Parasitosis Associated with Pemoline." *Psychopathology* 38, no. 2 (March–April 2005): 103–4.

Pliszka, Steven R., et al. "The Texas Children's Medication Algorithm Project: Revision of the Algorithm for Pharmacotherapy of Attention-Deficit/Hyperactivity Disorder." *Journal of the American Academy of Child & Adolescent Psychiatry* 45, no. 6 (June 2006): 642–57.

WEBSITES

U.S. Food and Drug Administration. "Information for Healthcare Professionals: Pemoline Tablets and Chewable Tablets (marketed as Cylert)." U.S. Department of Health and Human Services. http://www.fda.gov/Drugs/DrugSafety/PostmarketDrugSafetyInformationforPatientsandProviders/ucm126461.htm (accessed August 18, 2011).

Jack Raber, Pharm.D.
Ruth A. Wienclaw, PhD

Pentobarbital *see* **Barbiturates**

Permitil *see* **Fluphenazine**

Perphenazine

Definition

Perphenazine is a phenothiazine antipsychotic used to treat serious mental disorders. It has also been used to treat severe nausea and vomiting. It is sold in the United States under the brand name Trilafon and is also available under its generic name.

Purpose

Perphenazine is used to treat psychotic disorders and severe nausea and vomiting.

Description

Perphenazine is one of many drugs in the class called phenothiazine derivatives. Phenothiazines work by inhibiting the actions of the **brain** chemicals **dopamine** and norepinephrine, which are overproduced in individuals with **psychosis**. It is a member of the group of "first-generation" antipsychotics, which had fallen out of favor with the advent of the "second-generation" drugs, thought to be more effective and confer fewer side effects. However, a recent study found that perphenazine is as effective as some of the newer drugs and is more cost effective.

Recommended dosage

For the treatment of psychosis, adults usually receive a total of 4 mg to 16 mg taken as tablets in three or four doses daily, up to a maximum of 64 mg each day. There is also a liquid form available to be taken orally. Injections of perphenazine are also available and are typically given in 5 mg doses every 6 hours, up to 15 mg per day. Hospitalized patients can receive up to 30 mg per day in the injectable form of perphenazine.

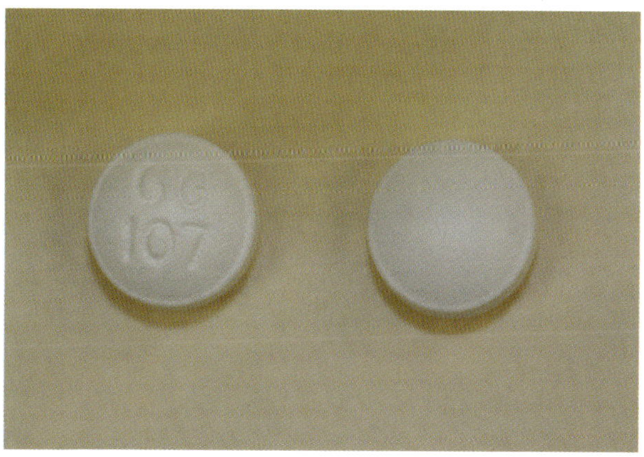

Perphenazine, 4 mg. *(© Custom Medical Stock Photo, Inc. Reproduced by permission.)*

Adult patients with serious nausea and vomiting receive 8 mg to 16 mg per day as tablets, divided into several doses, up to a maximum of 24 mg per day. Injections are typically given in 5 mg to 10 mg doses every 6 hours, up to 15 mg per day in patients who are not confined to bed. Hospitalized patients can receive up to a maximum of 30 mg per day. Intravenous perphenazine can be given to nausea and vomiting patients up to 1 mg every 1 to 2 minutes to a maximum of 5 mg.

The correct dosage of perphenazine must be carefully determined for each patient. Physicians try to find a dose that controls symptoms of the disease without causing intolerable side effects. Dosage guidelines for the treatment of psychosis have not been established for children under the age of 12. In children over age 12, the lowest adult dosage is generally used to treat psychosis. Children with severe nausea and vomiting are usually given 5 mg injections every six hours.

Precautions

Persons who take perphenazine should not stop taking the drug abruptly. Instead, the dose should be decreased gradually, then stopped. People who take perphenazine often develop sunburn easily; sunscreen should be used by persons, especially fair-skinned individuals, taking perphenazine.

Persons who are known to have severe central nervous system **depression** should not take perphenazine or any other drug in its class. In addition, those with a prior history of brain damage, coma, or bone marrow depression should not receive perphenazine without a thorough evaluation by a doctor.

Children under the age of 12, the elderly (over age 65), and those with a history of epilepsy, glaucoma, prostate problems, severe asthma, or other severe breathing problems should receive perphenazine only with great caution and under close supervision of a physician. In addition, persons with a history of heart or blood vessel disease and those with a history of liver or kidney disease should take perphenazine only after a thorough evaluation. Perphenazine should also be used cautiously when taken over a long period. Rarely should perphenazine be taken by pregnant or nursing women; it passes into the breastmilk and can cause drowsiness and adverse side effects in the infant.

Side effects

Serious or life-threatening side effects due to perphenazine are rare. However, if any of these occur, patients should contact their doctors or get immediate medical attention: **seizures**, irregular heartbeat, significant changes in blood pressure, muscle stiffness, weakness, pale skin color, and increased sweating. The treating doctor should be contacted immediately if any of these common side effects develops: rapid movements of the tongue, uncontrolled chewing movement, unusual amounts of lip smacking, and frequent movement of the arms or legs. The treating doctor should be contacted relatively soon if any of the following common side effects develops: reduced balance control, muscle spasms, restlessness, trembling, weakness in the limbs, blurred vision, and decreased night vision.

Less-common side effects that need to be reported to the doctor include severe sunburn, skin rashes, and urination problems. Rare side effects that should be reported to the doctor include abdominal pain, muscle aches, joint aches, fever, chills, muscle weakness, and vomiting. Common, but not serious, side effects include constipation, drowsiness, decreased sweating, mouth dryness, and nasal congestion. Uncommon, and not typically serious, side effects include decreased sexual desire, increased susceptibility to sunburn, menstrual cycle changes, swelling or pain in the breasts, and weight gain.

Perphenazine is not approved for the treatment of psychosis in elderly patients with **dementia**. In 2005, the FDA released a public health advisory warning patients and doctors against using **perphenazine** and other atypical antipsychotics off-label. In studies, these drugs significantly increased the risk of death in older patients with dementia, compared to placebo. Most of the deaths were associated with heart failure or infections such as pneumonia. Atypical antipsychotics also have been associated with an increased risk for **stroke** in elderly patients with dementia-related psychosis.

Interactions

Combining perphenazine with drugs such as the antimalarials amodiaquine, chloroquine, and sulfadoxine-pyrimethamine (Fansidar) can increase the concentrations within the body of these antimalarials.

Perphenazine combined with **barbiturates** tends to lower the concentrations of perphenazine in the body. Combining perphenazine with **clonidine** (Catapress), guanadrel (Hylorel), and guanethidine (Ismelin) can produce dangerously low blood pressure.

Perphenazine should not be combined with alcohol, because alcohol increases the drug's depressive effect on the central nervous system. Perphenazine inhibits the effects of levodopa in Parkinson's patients when the two are combined. Lithium combined with perphenazine lowers the levels of both drugs.

Perphenazine should not be combined with analgesics (pain killers) containing narcotics, because the combination increases depressive effects on the central nervous system. Orphenadrine (Norflex) combined with perphenazine can reduce the beneficial effects of perphenazine.

Resources

BOOKS

Brunton, Laurence, Bruce Chabner, and Bjorn Knollman. *Goodman & Gilman's The Pharmacological Basis of Therapeutics.* 12th ed. New York: McGraw-Hill, 2010.

Consumer Reports and American Society of Health-System Pharmacists. *Consumer Reports Complete Drug Reference.* Yonkers, NY: Consumers Reports, 2009.

Ellsworth, Allan J., et al. *Mosby's Medical Drug Reference.* St. Louis, MO: Mosby, 2007.

Venes, Donald. *Taber's Cyclopedic Medical Dictionary.* 21st ed. Philadelphia: F.A. Davis Company, 2009.

PERIODICALS

Rosenheck, R.A., et al. "Cost-Effectiveness of Second Generation Antipsychotics and Perphenazine in a Randomized Trial of Treatment for Chronic Schizophrenia." *American Journal of Psychiatry* 163 (2006): 2080–89.

WEBSITES

MedlinePlus. "Perphenazine." U.S. National Library of Medicine, National Institutes of Health. http://www.nlm.nih.gov/medlineplus/druginfo/meds/a682165.html (accessed December 19, 2011)

U.S. Food and Drug Administration. "Information on Conventional Antipsychotics." http://www.fda.gov/Drugs/DrugSafety/PostmarketDrugSafetyInformationforPatients andProviders/ucm107211.htm (accessed December 12, 2011).

Mark Mitchell, MD
Emily Jane Willingham, PhD

Personality disorders

Definition

Personality disorders are a group of mental disturbances defined as ongoing patterns of social behavior that are detrimental to those who display them or to others. The behaviors are generally regarded as being inconsistent with cultural norms and may cause significant emotional pain or difficulties in relationships and occupational performance. In addition, the patient usually sees the disorder as being consistent with his or her self-image (ego-syntonic) and may be resistant to change. The ***Diagnostic and Statistical Manual of Mental Disorders*** (*DSM*) defines personality disorders as "impairments in personality functioning, [characterized by] pathological personality traits."

Demographics

Personality disorders have their onset in late adolescence or early adulthood. Doctors rarely give a **diagnosis** of personality disorder to children on the grounds that children's personalities are still in the process of formation and may change considerably by the time they are in their late teens. In retrospect, however, many individuals with personality disorders could be judged to have shown evidence of the problems in childhood.

It is difficult to give close estimates of the percentage of the population that has personality disorders. Patients with certain personality disorders, including antisocial and borderline disorders, are more likely to get into trouble with the law or otherwise attract attention than are patients whose disorders chiefly affect their capacity for intimacy. On the other hand, some patients, such as those with narcissistic or obsessive-compulsive personality disorders, may be outwardly successful because their symptoms are useful within their particular occupations. It has been estimated that about 15% of the general population of the United States has a personality disorder, with higher rates in poor or troubled neighborhoods. The rate of personality disorders among patients in psychiatric treatment is between 30% and 50%. It is possible for patients to have a so-called dual diagnosis; for example, they may have more than one personality disorder, or a personality disorder together with a substance abuse problem.

Description

Persons affected by personality disorders, sometimes called "character disorders," have rigid personality traits and coping styles, are unable to adapt to changing situations, and experience impairment in the following areas:

- perception and interpretation of the self and other people
- intensity and duration of feelings and their appropriateness to situations
- relationships with others
- ability to control impulses

The revised fourth edition of the *Diagnostic and Statistical Manual of Mental Disorders* (*DSM-IV-TR*) specifies ten personality disorders: paranoid, schizoid, schizotypal, antisocial, borderline, histrionic, narcissistic, avoidant, dependent, and obsessive-compulsive. Some psychiatrists propose additional categories, including passive-aggressive personality disorder, characterized by a need to control or punish others through frustrating them or sabotaging plans; cyclothymic personality disorder, characterized by intense mood swings alternating between high spirits and moroseness or gloom; and depressive personality disorder, characterized by a negative and pessimistic approach to life. One criticism of the general category of personality disorders is that it is based on Western notions of uniqueness, as different cultures may have different definitions of normalcy.

Paranoid

Patients with **paranoid personality disorder** are characterized by suspiciousness and a belief that others are out to harm or cheat them. They have problems with intimacy and may join cults or groups with paranoid belief systems. Some are litigious, bringing lawsuits against those they believe have wronged them. Although not ordinarily delusional, these patients may develop psychotic symptoms under severe **stress**. According to a 2007 study performed by Dr. Mark F. Lenzenweger (from the Department of Psychology at State University of New York at Binghamton) and colleagues, an estimated 2.3% of the general population meet the *DSM-IV* criteria for paranoid personality disorder. (The statistics provided by the **National Institute of Mental Health** for personality disorders are sourced from Lenzenweger's study.)

Schizoid

Schizoid patients are perceived by others as "loners" without close family relationships or social contacts. Indeed, they are aloof and really do prefer to be alone. They may appear cold to others because they rarely display strong emotions. They may, however, be successful in occupations that do not require personal interaction. About 4.9% of the general population have this disorder (Lenzenweger et al.); it is slightly more common in men than in women.

Schizotypal

Patients diagnosed as schizotypal are often considered odd or eccentric because they pay little attention to their clothing and sometimes have peculiar speech mannerisms. They are socially isolated and uncomfortable at parties or other social gatherings. In addition, people with **schizotypal personality disorder** often have oddities of thought, including "magical" beliefs or peculiar ideas (for example, a belief in telepathy or unidentified flying objects [UFOs]) that are outside of their cultural norms. About 3.3% of the general population have schizotypal personality disorder (Lenzenweger et al.). It is slightly more common in males. Schizotypal disorder should not be confused with **schizophrenia**, although there is some evidence that the disorders are genetically related.

Antisocial

Patients with **antisocial personality disorder** are sometimes referred to as sociopaths or psychopaths. They are characterized by lying, manipulativeness, and a selfish disregard for the rights of others; some may act impulsively. People with antisocial personality disorder are frequently chemically dependent and sexually promiscuous. An estimated 1% of the general population have antisocial personality disorder (Lenzenweger et al.), and the disorder is much more often diagnosed in men than in women.

Borderline

Patients with **borderline personality disorder** (BPD) are highly unstable, with wide mood swings, a history of intense but stormy relationships, impulsive behavior, and confusion about career goals, personal values, or sexual orientation. These often highly conflictual ideas may correspond to an even deeper confusion about their sense of self (identity). People with BPD frequently cut or burn themselves, or threaten or attempt **suicide**. Many of these patients have histories of severe childhood **abuse** or **neglect**. About 1.6% of the general population have BPD (Lenzenweger et al.), with women diagnosed more often than men.

Histrionic

Patients diagnosed with this disorder impress others as overly emotional, overly dramatic, and hungry for attention. They may be flirtatious or seductive as a way of drawing attention to themselves, yet they are emotionally shallow. Histrionic patients often live in a romantic fantasy world and are easily bored with routine. About 2% to 3% of the population is thought to have this disorder. Although historically the disorder has been more associated with women in clinical settings, there may be bias toward diagnosing women with the **histrionic personality disorder**.

Narcissistic

Narcissistic patients are characterized by self-importance, a craving for admiration, and exploitative attitudes toward others. They have unrealistically inflated views of their talents and accomplishments, and may become extremely angry if they are criticized or outshone by others. Narcissists may be professionally successful but rarely have long-lasting intimate relationships. Fewer than 1% of the population has this disorder; about 75% of those diagnosed with it are male.

Avoidant

Patients with **avoidant personality disorder** are fearful of rejection and shy away from situations or occupations that might expose their supposed inadequacy. They may reject opportunities to develop close relationships because of their fears of criticism or humiliation. Patients with this personality disorder are often diagnosed with **dependent personality disorder** as well. Many also fit the criteria for **social phobia**. Approximately 5.2% of the population have avoidant personality disorder (Lenzenweger et al.).

Dependent

Dependent patients are afraid of being on their own and typically develop submissive or compliant behaviors in order to avoid displeasing people. They are afraid to question authority and often ask others for guidance or direction. Dependent personality disorder is diagnosed more often in women, but it has been suggested that this finding reflects social pressures on women to conform to gender stereotyping or bias on the part of clinicians. About 0.6% of the U.S. population have dependent personality disorder (Lenzenweger et al.).

Obsessive-compulsive

Patients diagnosed with this disorder are preoccupied with keeping order, attaining perfection, and maintaining mental and interpersonal control. They may spend a great deal of time adhering to plans, schedules, or rules from which they will not deviate, even at the expense of openness, flexibility, and efficiency. These patients are often unable to relax and may become "workaholics." They may have problems in employment as well as in intimate relationships because they are very stiff and formal, and insist on doing everything their way. About 2.4% of the population have **obsessive-compulsive personality disorder** (Lenzenweger et al.).

Causes and symptoms

Causes

Personality is formed early in life, during childhood. However, disorders in personality can develop during that time of life, based on two factors: heredity and environment. Heredity is those inherited tendencies that occur because they are passed down from parents to children. There is nothing that can be done to prevent these tendencies (sometimes called a person's temperament) from occurring because they happen naturally—they are within one's genes. However, the experiences that one has in life are due to that person's surrounding environment. They are affected by family, friends, and even complete strangers—along with the situations that are encountered in everyday life.

Personality disorders are thought to result from a bad interface, so to speak, between a child's temperament and character on one hand, and his or her family environment on the other. Temperament can be defined as a person's innate or biologically shaped basic disposition; character is defined as the set of attitudes and behavior patterns that the individual acquires or learns over time. Since children must learn to adapt to their specific families, they may develop personality disorders in the course of struggling to survive psychologically in disturbed or stressful families. For example, nervous or high-strung parents might be unhappy with a baby who is very active and try to restrain him or her at every opportunity. The child might then develop an avoidant personality disorder as the outcome of coping with constant frustration and parental disapproval. As another example, **child abuse** is believed to play a role in shaping borderline personality disorder. One reason that some therapists use the term "developmental damage" instead of "personality disorder" is that it takes the presumed source of the person's problems into account.

Some patients with personality disorders come from families that appear to be stable and healthy. It has been suggested that these patients are biologically hypersensitive to normal family stress. Levels of the **brain** chemical (neurotransmitter) **dopamine** may influence a person's level of novelty-seeking, and **serotonin** levels may influence aggression.

Symptoms

There are many symptoms associated with personality disorder. Generally, they include:

- angry outbursts
- inadequate impulse control
- mistrust and suspicion of others
- need for instant gratification
- problematic relationships
- social isolation
- substance and/or drug abuse
- trouble making friends
- wide and/or frequent mood swings

Diagnosis

A new edition of the *DSM* (*DSM-5*) is due to be published in May 2013. Proposed changes for the *DSM-5* include a reduction of the ten personality disorder types to six:

- antisocial personality disorder (dyssocial personality disorder)
- avoidant personality disorder
- borderline personality disorder
- narcissistic personality disorder
- obsessive-compulsive personality disorder
- schizotypal personality disorder

To account for the disorders that have been removed, a diagnostic category of "Personality Disorder Trait Specified" has been proposed, which accounts for any additional disorders that cause significant impairments in personal and social functioning and that are linked to a specific personality trait:

- negative affectivity, or frequent negative emotions—anxiety, depression, fear, drastic mood swings, paranoia
- detachment, or withdrawal from social interactions—avoidances, depression, lack of joy in social situations
- antagonism, or tendency or desire to hurt others—anger or irritability, manipulation, deceit, aggression
- disinhibition/compulsivity, or impulsive or compulsive behaviors—risk taking, lack of concentration, stubbornness, no sense of responsibility
- psychoticism, or professing "unusual" beliefs—abnormal thoughts, eccentric behavior

The *DSM-5* proposals also include revision of the general diagnosis of *personality disorder,* with the goal of being more specific, being soundly based in clinical observation and experience, and accounting for deviations in cultural norms. The *DSM-IV-TR* criteria defined personality disorder as:

- exhibiting pattern of beliefs and/or behaviors that vary from cultural norms, in the areas (at least two) of cognition, affectivity, interpersonal relations, and impulsivity)
- beliefs/behaviors are inflexible and unaffected by situation or environment
- beliefs/behaviors lead to severe impairment in interpersonal functioning, including social and occupational
- beliefs/behaviors are long-lasting, dating to adolescent/early adulthood
- beliefs/behaviors cannot be attributed to another disorder (physical or mental) or to a substance

By contrast, the proposed *DSM-5* diagnostic criteria require a patient to exhibit all of the following:

- impairments in personal (identity) and interpersonal functioning and relations
- at least one personality trait (negative affectivity, detachment, antagonism, disinhibition/compulsivity, psychoticism)
- consistent behavior, unaffected by situation or environment
- behaviors that are not part of the perceived cultural norm or that are not in line with the individual's level of development
- impairments that are not otherwise explained by substance use or a medical condition

Diagnosis of personality disorders is complicated by the fact that affected persons rarely seek help until they are in serious trouble or until their families (or the law) pressure them to get treatment. The reason for this slowness is that the problematic traits are so deeply entrenched that they seem normal (ego-syntonic) to the patient. Diagnosis of a personality disorder depends, in part, on the patient's age. Although personality disorders originate during the childhood years, they are considered adult disorders. Some patients, in fact, are not diagnosed until late in life because their symptoms had been modified by the demands of their job or by marriage. After retirement or the spouse's death, however, these patients' personality disorders become fully apparent. In general, however, if the onset of the patient's problem is in mid- or late life, the doctor will rule out **substance abuse** or personality change caused by medical or neurological problems before considering the diagnosis of a personality disorder. It is unusual for people to develop personality disorders "out of the blue" in mid-life.

There are no tests that can provide a definitive diagnosis of personality disorder. Most doctors will evaluate a patient on the basis of several sources of information collected over a period of time in order to determine how long the patient has been having difficulties, how many areas of life are affected, and the severity of the dysfunction.

Interviews

The doctor may schedule two or three interviews with the patient, spaced over several weeks or months, in order to rule out an adjustment disorder caused by job loss, **bereavement**, or a similar problem. An office interview allows the doctor to form an impression of the patient's overall personality as well as obtain information about his or her occupation and family.

During the interview, the doctor will note the patient's appearance, tone of voice, body language, eye contact, and other important nonverbal signals, as well as the content of the conversation. In some cases, the doctor may contact other people (family members, employers, close friends) who know the patient well in order to assess the accuracy of the patient's perception of his or her difficulties. It is quite common for people with personality disorders to have distorted views of their situations or to be unaware of the impact of their behavior on others.

Psychological testing

Doctors use psychological testing to help in the diagnosis of a personality disorder. These tests are administered and interpreted by a licensed **psychologist**, and doctors will usually refer patients to specific psychologists for testing.

PERSONALITY INVENTORIES. Personality inventories are tests with true/false or yes/no answers that can be used to compare the patient's scores with those of people with known personality distortions. The single most commonly used test of this type is the **Minnesota Multiphasic Personality Inventory**, or MMPI. Another test that is often used is the Millon Clinical Multiaxial Inventory, or MCMI.

Projective tests are unstructured, meaning that instead of giving one-word answers to questions, the patient is asked to talk at some length about a picture that the psychologist has shown him or her, or to supply an ending for the beginning of a story. Projective tests allow the clinician to assess the patient's patterns of thinking, fantasies, worries or anxieties, moral concerns, values, and habits. Common projective tests include the Rorschach, in which the patient responds to a set of ten inkblots; and the **Thematic Apperception Test** (TAT), in which the patient is shown drawings of people in different situations and then tells a story about the picture.

Treatment

At one time, psychiatrists thought that personality disorders did not respond very well to treatment. This opinion was derived from the notion that human personality is fixed for life once it has been molded in childhood, and from the belief among people with personality disorders that their own views and behaviors are correct, and that others are the ones at fault. More recently, however, doctors have recognized that humans can continue to grow and change throughout life. Most patients with personality disorders are now considered to be treatable, although the degree of improvement may vary depending on the severity and life situation of one's particular personality disorder. The type of treatment recommended depends on the personality characteristics associated with the specific disorder. For the most part, many personality disorders are chronic so treatment is often for an extended period. In addition, a team of medical professionals are often included within the treatment. This professional team may include a primary care provider (such as a family doctor), **psychiatrist**, psychotherapist, pharmacist, and **social workers**. One or more treatments may be needed. These include **hospitalization**, **psychotherapy**, and medications.

Hospitalization

npatient treatment is rarely required for patients with personality disorders. However, in some cases, a personality disorder may be so severe that psychiatric hospitalization is necessary, as may be the case with patients with borderline personality disorder who are threatening suicide or suffering from drug or alcohol withdrawal, or patients with paranoid personality disorder who are having psychotic symptoms. Psychiatric hospitalization is generally recommended only when persons are not able to care for themselves or are in immediate danger of harming themselves or someone else.

Psychotherapy

Psychoanalytic psychotherapy is suggested for patients who can benefit from insight-oriented treatment. These patients typically include those with dependent, obsessive-compulsive, and avoidant personality disorders. Doctors usually recommend individual psychotherapy for narcissistic and borderline patients, but they often refer these patients to therapists with specialized training in these disorders. Psychotherapeutic treatment for personality disorders may take as long as three to five years. It is considered the primary way to treat personality disorders effectively.

Insight-oriented approaches are not recommended for patients with paranoid or antisocial personality disorders. These patients are likely to resent the therapist and see him or her as trying to control or dominate them.

Supportive therapy is regarded as the most helpful form of psychotherapy for patients with **schizoid personality disorder**.

COGNITIVE-BEHAVIORAL THERAPY. Cognitive-behavioral approaches are often recommended for patients with avoidant or dependent personality disorders. Patients in these groups typically have mistaken beliefs about their competence or likableness.

These assumptions can be successfully challenged by cognitive-behavioral methods. More recently, American psychiatrist Aaron T. Beck (1921–), a professor emeritus in the Department of Psychiatry at the University of Pennsylvania, and his coworkers have successfully extended their approach to cognitive therapy to all ten personality disorders as defined by DSM-IV.

GROUP THERAPY. **Group therapy** is frequently useful for patients with schizoid or avoidant personality disorders because it helps them to break out of their social isolation. It has also been recommended for patients with histrionic and antisocial personality disorders. These patients tend to act out, and pressure from peers in group treatment can motivate them to change. Because patients with antisocial personality disorder can destabilize groups that include people with other disorders, it is usually best if these people meet exclusively with others who have APD in homogeneous groups. However, getting patients with personality disorders to commit and participate to group therapy can be difficult.

FAMILY THERAPY. **Family therapy** may be suggested for patients whose personality disorders cause serious problems for members of their families. It is also sometimes recommended for borderline patients from over-involved or possessive families.

DIALECTICAL BEHAVIOR THERAPY. This type of therapy teaches patients to tolerate and better adapt to stress, along with training that helps with the regulation of emotions and the improvement of relationships with others. Dialectical behavior therapy has the most empirical support of any treatment for personality disorders, particularly with individuals with borderline personality disorder.

PSYCHODYNAMIC PSYCHOTHERAPY. This type of psychotherapy helps those in need to be more aware of unconscious thoughts and behaviors. Along with this new insight, the therapy also helps the patient to understand motivations and conflicts in order to live a more normal life.

PSYCHOEDUCATION. Directed at the patient, along with family and friends, this therapy helps all parties concerned to better understand and deal with the mental illness and develop better coping strategies and problem-solving skills.

Medications

Medications may be prescribed for patients with specific personality disorders. The type of medication depends on the disorder. In general, however, patients with personality disorders are helped only moderately by medications.

ANTIPSYCHOTIC DRUGS. Antipsychotic drugs, such as **haloperidol** (Haldol), may be given to patients with paranoid personality disorder if they are having brief psychotic episodes. Patients with borderline or schizotypal personality disorder are sometimes given antipsychotic drugs in low doses; however, the efficacy of these drugs in treating personality disorder is less clear than in schizophrenia.

MOOD STABILIZERS. **Carbamazepine** (Tegretol) is a drug that is commonly used to treat **seizures**, but is also helpful for borderline patients with rage outbursts and similar behavioral problems. Lithium and valproate may also be used as mood stabilizers, especially among people with borderline personality disorder.

ANTIDEPRESSANTS AND ANTIANXIETY MEDICATIONS. Medications in these categories are sometimes prescribed for patients with schizoid personality disorder to help them manage anxiety symptoms while they are in psychotherapy. **Antidepressants** are also commonly used to treat people with borderline personality disorder.

Treatment with medications is not recommended for patients with avoidant, histrionic, dependent, or narcissistic personality disorders. The use of potentially addictive medications should be avoided in people with borderline or antisocial personality disorders. However, some avoidant patients who also have social phobia may benefit from **monoamine oxidase inhibitors** (MAOIs), a particular class of antidepressant.

Prognosis

The prognosis for recovery depends in part on the specific disorder. Although some patients improve as they grow older and have positive experiences in life, personality disorders are generally lifelong disturbances with periods of worsening (exacerbations) and periods of improvement (remissions). Others, particularly schizoid patients, have better prognoses if they are given appropriate treatment. Beck and his coworkers estimate that effective cognitive therapy with patients with personality disorders takes two to three years on average. Patients with paranoid personality disorder are at some risk for developing delusional disorders or schizophrenia.

The personality disorders with the poorest prognoses are the antisocial and the borderline. Borderline patients are at high risk for developing substance abuse disorders or bulimia. About 80% of hospitalized borderline patients attempt suicide at some point during treatment, and about 5% succeed in committing suicide. Borderline patients

KEY TERMS

Character—An individual's set of emotional, cognitive, and behavioral patterns learned and accumulated over time.

Cognitive therapy—A form of psychotherapy that focuses on changing people's patterns of emotional reaction by correcting distorted patterns of thinking and perception.

Developmental damage—A term that some therapists prefer to personality disorder, on the grounds that it is more respectful of the patient's capacity for growth and change.

Ego-syntonic—Consistent with one's sense of self, as opposed to ego-alien or dystonic (foreign to one's sense of self). Ego-syntonic traits typify patients with personality disorders.

Personality—The organized pattern of behaviors and attitudes that makes a human being distinctive. Personality is formed by the ongoing interaction of temperament, character, and environment.

Projective tests—Psychological tests that probe into personality by obtaining open-ended responses to such materials as pictures or stories. Projective tests are often used to evaluate patients with personality disorders.

Rorschach test—A well-known projective test that requires the patient to describe what he or she sees in each of ten inkblots. It is named for the Swiss psychiatrist who invented it.

Temperament—A person's natural or genetically determined disposition.

are also the most likely to sue their mental health professional for malpractice.

Prevention

The most effective preventive strategy for personality disorders is early identification and treatment of children at risk. High-risk groups include abused children, children from troubled families, children with close relatives diagnosed with personality disorders, children of substance abusers, and children who grow up in cults or extremist political groups.

Resources

BOOKS

Dobbert, Duane L. *Understanding Personality Disorders: An Introduction.* Westport, CT: Praeger, 2007.

Graham, George. *The Disordered Mind: An Introduction to Philosophy of Mind and Mental Illness.* New York: Routledge, 2010.

North, Carol, and Sean Yutzy. *Goodwin and Guze's Psychiatric Diagnosis.* New York: Oxford University Press, 2010.

O'Donohue, William, Katherine A. Fowler, and Scott O. Lilienfield. *Personality Disorders: Toward the DSM-V.* Thousand Oaks, CA: Sage Publications, 2007.

PERIODICALS

Hesse, Morten, and Paul Moran. "Screening for Personality Disorder with the Standardised Assessment of Personality: Abbreviated Scale (SAPAS): Further Evidence of Concurrent Validity." *BMC Psychiatry* 10 (January 2010): 10. http://dx.doi.org/10.1186/1471-244X-10-10 (accessed August 31, 2011).

Lenzenweger, Mark F., et al. "DSM-IV Personality Disorders in the National Comorbidity Survey Replication." *Biological Psychiatry* 62, no. 6 (2007): 553–64 http://dx.doi.org/10.1016/j.biopsych.2006.09.019 (accessed August 31, 2011).

Skodol, A.E., et al. "Relationship of Personality Disorders to the Course of Major Depressive Disorder in a Nationally Representative Sample." *American Journal of Psychiatry* 168, no. 3 (2011): 257–64.

OTHER

American Psychiatric Association. "Side By Side Comparison Table of the Criteria for the Personality Disorders." http://www.dsm5.org/Documents/Diagnostic%20Criteria%20for%20Personality%20Disorder%20(Comparison%20of%20DSM-IV%20DSM-5%20old%20DSM-5%20new.pdf (accessed August 31, 2011).

WEBSITES

American Psychiatric Association. "Proposed Revisions: Personality Disorders." DSM-5 Development. http://www.dsm5.org/proposedrevision/Pages/PersonalityDisorders.aspx (accessed August 31, 2011).

Bienenfeld, David. "Personality Disorders." Medscape Reference. (June 14, 2010). http://www.emedicine.com/med/topic3472.htm (accessed August 31, 2011).

Mayo Clinic staff. "Personality Disorders." MayoClinic.com (September 10, 2010). http://www.mayoclinic.com/health/personality-disorders/DS00562 (accessed August 25, 2011).

"Personality Disorders: Statistics." OutOfTheFog.net http://outofthefog.net/Statistics.html#PDPrevalence (accessed August 24, 2011).

ORGANIZATIONS

American Psychiatric Association, 1000 Wilson Boulevard, Suite 1825, Arlington, VA, 22209, (703) 907-7300, apa@psych.org, http://www.psych.org.

Mental Health America, 2000 N. Beauregard Street, 6th Floor, Alexandria, VA, 22311, (703) 684-7722, Fax: (703) 684-5968, (800) 969-6642, http://www1.nmha.org.

National Alliance on Mental Illness, 3803 North Fairfax Drive, Suite 100, Arlington, VA, 22203, (703) 524-7600, Fax: (703) 524-9094, http://www.nami.org.

National Institute of Mental Health, 6001 Executive Boulevard, Room 8184, MSC 9663, Bethesda, MD, 20892-9663, (301) 443-4513, Fax: (301) 443-4279, (866) 615-6464, nimhinfo@nih.gov, http://www.nimh.nih.gov.

Treatment and Research Advancements (National Association for Personality Disorders), 23 Greene Street, New York, NY, 10013, (212) 966-6514, tara4bpd@gmail.com, http://www.tara4bpd.org.

Rebecca J. Frey, Ph.D.
Laura Jean Cataldo, RN, Ed.D.
William A. Atkins, B.B., B.S., M.B.A.

Person-centered therapy

Definition

Person-centered therapy (PCT), also known as "client-centered," "non-directive," or "Rogerian therapy," is an approach to counseling and **psychotherapy** that places much of the responsibility for the treatment process on the "client" (the term preferred over "patient"), with the therapist taking a nondirective role. As such, psychologists and counselors use a non-directive approach to treat their clients.

Purpose

Two primary goals of person-centered therapy are increased self-esteem and greater openness to experience. Some of the related changes that this form of therapy seeks to foster in clients include closer agreement between the client's idealized and actual selves; better self-understanding; lower levels of defensiveness, guilt, and insecurity; more positive and comfortable relationships with others; and an increased capacity to experience and express feelings at the moment they occur.

Description

Developed from the 1930s to the 1950s by American **psychologist** Carl Rogers (1902–1987), client-centered therapy departed from the typically formal, detached role of the therapist emphasized in **psychoanalysis** and other forms of treatment.

Background

Rogers believed that therapy should take place in a supportive environment created by a close personal relationship between client and therapist. Rogers's introduction of the term "client," rather than "patient," expresses his rejection of the traditionally hierarchical relationship between therapist and client and his view of them as equals. In person-centered therapy, the client determines the general direction of therapy, while the therapist seeks to increase the client's insight and self-understanding through informal clarifying questions.

Beginning in the 1960s, person-centered therapy became associated with the human potential movement. This movement, dating back to the beginning of the 1900s, reflected an altered perspective of human nature. Previous psychological theories viewed human beings as inherently selfish and corrupt. For example, Austrian neurologist Sigmund Freud's theory focused on sexual and aggressive tendencies as the primary forces driving human behavior. The human potential movement, by contrast, defined human nature as inherently good. From its perspective, human behavior is motivated by a drive to achieve one's fullest potential.

Self-actualization, a term derived from the human potential movement, is an important concept underlying person-centered therapy. It refers to the tendency of all human beings to move forward, grow, and reach their fullest potential. When humans move toward self-actualization, they are also prosocial; that is, they tend to be concerned for others and behave in honest, dependable, and constructive ways. The concept of self-actualization focuses on human strengths rather than human deficiencies. According to Rogers, self-actualization can be blocked by an unhealthy self-concept (negative or unrealistic attitudes about oneself).

Rogers adopted terms such as "person-centered approach" and "way of being" and began to focus on personal growth and self-actualization. He also pioneered the use of encounter groups, adapting the sensitivity training (T-group) methods developed by German-American psychologist Kurt Lewin (1890–1947) and other researchers at the National Training Laboratories in the 1950s. More recently, two major variations of person-centered therapy have developed: experiential therapy, developed by American psychotherapist Eugene Gendlin in 1979; and process-experiential therapy, developed by Canadian psychologist Leslie Greenberg and colleagues in 1993.

While person-centered therapy is considered one of the major therapeutic approaches, along with psychoanalytic and **cognitive-behavioral therapy**, Rogers's influence is felt in schools of therapy other than his

CARL ROGERS (1902–1987)

Carl Rogers was an American psychotherapist who originated person-centered, nondirective counseling. In 1928, Rogers moved to Rochester, New York, where he began work as a psychologist for the Society for Prevention of Cruelty to Children. In contrast to Teachers College, many colleagues in Rochester emphasized a psychoanalytic approach to behavior. Through the practical and personal experiences in this clinic, however, he began to recognize that the results of both measurement psychologists and psychoanalysts were "never more than superficially effective."

Several incidents in the Rochester clinic helped him "to perceive . . . that it is the client who knows what hurts, what direction to go, what problems are crucial, what experiences have been deeply buried. It began to occur to me that unless I had a need to demonstrate my own cleverness and learning, I would do better to rely upon the client for direction of movement in the therapeutic process." For effective counseling, the psychotherapist, Rogers believed, is "to be genuine and without a facade . . . . and to be empathetic in understanding. As a result the client begins to feel positive and accepting toward himself . . . . his own defenses and facade diminishes . . . . he becomes more open . . . . and he finds that he is free to grow and change in desired directions."

During his lifetime, Rogers published approximately 260 articles and 15 books, which have had a significant influence on the development of psychology in the twentieth century. He was prominent in the human potential movement, and his book on encounter groups had an impressive impact. After the mid-1970s Rogers was especially interested in facilitating groups involving antagonistic factions, whether the hostilities arose out of cultural, racial, religious, or national issues. He facilitated a group from Belfast (Northern Ireland) containing militant Protestants and Catholics from Ireland and the English. He was involved in intercultural groups whose participants came from many nations, including participants from the Eastern European bloc countries. He facilitated black-white groups in South Africa. He was deeply interested in applying the principles of the person-centered approach to international affairs in the interest of world peace. He died in 1987.

own. The concepts and methods he developed are used in an eclectic fashion by many different types of counselors and therapists.

Preparation

Preparing for PCT is as important to the professional therapist as it is to the client.

Process

Rogers believed that the most important factor in successful therapy was not the therapist's skill or training, but rather his or her attitude. Three interrelated attitudes on the part of the therapist are central to the success of person-centered therapy: congruence, unconditional positive regard, and empathy. Congruence refers to the therapist's openness and genuineness—the willingness to relate to clients without hiding behind a professional facade. Therapists who function in this way have all their feelings available to them in therapy sessions and may share significant emotional reactions with their clients. Congruence does *not* mean, however, that therapists disclose their own personal problems to clients in therapy sessions or shift the focus of therapy to themselves in any other way.

Unconditional positive regard means that the therapist accepts the client totally for who he or she is, without evaluating or censoring, and without disapproving of particular feelings, actions, or characteristics. The therapist communicates this attitude to the client by a willingness to listen without interrupting, judging, or giving advice. This attitude of positive regard creates a nonthreatening context in which the client feels free to explore and share painful, hostile, defensive, or abnormal feelings without worrying about personal rejection by the therapist.

The third necessary component of a therapist's attitude is empathy ("accurate empathetic understanding"). The therapist tries to appreciate the client's situation from the client's point of view, showing an emotional understanding of and sensitivity to the client's feelings throughout the therapy session. In other systems of therapy, empathy with the client would be considered a preliminary step to enabling the therapeutic work to proceed; but in person-centered therapy, it actually constitutes a major portion of the therapeutic work itself. One primary way to convey this empathy is by active listening that shows careful and perceptive attention to what the client is saying. In addition to standard techniques, such as eye contact, that are common to any good listener, person-centered therapists employ a special method called "reflection," which consists of paraphrasing and/or summarizing what a client has just said. This technique shows that the therapist is listening carefully and accurately, and gives clients an added opportunity to examine their own thoughts and feelings as they hear them repeated by another person. Generally, clients respond by elaborating further on the thoughts they have just expressed.

According to Rogers, when these three attitudes (congruence, unconditional positive regard, and empathy) are conveyed by a therapist, clients can freely express themselves without having to worry about what the therapist thinks of them. The therapist does not attempt to change the client's thinking in any way. Even negative expressions are validated as legitimate experiences. Because of this nondirective approach, clients can explore the issues that are most important to them—not those considered important by the therapist. Based on the principle of self-actualization, this undirected, uncensored self-exploration allows clients to eventually recognize alternative ways of thinking that will promote personal growth. The therapist merely facilitates self-actualization by providing a climate in which clients can freely engage in focused, in-depth self-exploration.

Applications

Rogers originally developed person-centered therapy in a children's clinic while he was working there; however, person-centered therapy was not intended for a specific age group or subpopulation but has been used to treat a broad range of people. Rogers worked extensively with people with **schizophrenia** later in his career. His therapy has also been applied to persons suffering from **depression**, anxiety, alcohol disorders, cognitive dysfunction, and **personality disorders**. Some therapists argue that person-centered therapy is not effective with nonverbal or poorly educated individuals; others maintain that it can be successfully adapted to any type of person. The person-centered approach can be used in individual, group, or **family therapy**. With young children, it is frequently employed as **play therapy**.

There are no strict guidelines regarding the length or frequency of person-centered therapy. Generally, therapists adhere to a one-hour session once per week. True to the spirit of person-centered therapy, however, scheduling may be adjusted according to the client's expressed needs. The client also decides when to terminate therapy. Termination usually occurs when he or she feels able to better cope with life's difficulties.

KEY TERMS

Depression—A psychiatric disorder involving feelings of hopelessness and symptoms of fatigue, sleeplessness, suicidal tendencies, and poor concentration.

Humanistic therapy—Sometimes also called "humanistic psychology," a perspective that stresses that people are basically good but deviate from that tendency through mental and social problems. It uses a holistic approach that focuses on individual potential and growth, along with self-actualization.

Psychoanalysis—The study of human psychological functioning and behavior.

Schizophrenia—A mental disorder involving degraded thinking and emotions.

Risks

Person-centered therapy has been criticized over the years for its unorthodox style of providing therapy to clients. However, the medical community has proved that it is an effective style of therapy. Clients also view PCT as a widely popular style of treatment.

Results

The expected results of person-centered therapy include:

- improved self-esteem; trust in one's inner feelings and experiences as valuable sources of information for making decisions
- increased ability to learn from (rather than repeat) mistakes
- decreased defensiveness, guilt, and insecurity
- more positive and comfortable relationships with others
- an increased capacity to experience and express feelings at the moment they occur
- openness to new experiences and new ways of thinking about life.

Normal results

Outcome studies of humanistic therapies in general and person-centered therapy in particular indicate that people who have been treated with these approaches maintain stable changes over extended periods of time; that they change substantially compared to untreated

QUESTIONS TO ASK YOUR DOCTOR

- Where can I learn more about person-centered therapy?
- Would person-centered therapy be better for me than traditional therapy?
- Is is helpful to undergo person-centered therapy and traditional therapy at the same time?
- Do you know of any therapists who are trained in person-centered therapy?

persons; and that the changes are roughly comparable to the changes in clients who have been treated by other types of therapy. Humanistic therapies appear to be particularly effective in clients with depression or relationship issues. Person-centered therapy, however, appears to be slightly less effective than other forms of humanistic therapy in which therapists offer more advice to clients and suggest topics to explore.

Abnormal results

If therapy has been unsuccessful, the client will not move in the direction of self-growth and self-acceptance. Instead, he or she may continue to display behaviors that reflect self-defeating attitudes or rigid patterns of thinking.

Several factors may affect the success of person-centered therapy. If an individual is not interested in therapy (for example, he or she was forced to attend therapy), that person might not work well together with the therapist. The skill of the therapist may be another factor. In general, clients tend to overlook occasional therapist failures if a satisfactory relationship has been established. A therapist who continually fails to demonstrate unconditional positive regard, congruence, or empathy cannot effectively use this type of therapy. A third factor is the client's comfort level with nondirective therapy. Some studies have suggested that certain clients may get bored, frustrated, or annoyed with a Rogerian style of therapeutic interaction.

Resources

BOOKS

Cain, David J., ed. *Humanistic Psychotherapies: Handbook of Research and Practice,* Washington, DC: American Psychological Association, 2002.

———. *Person-centered Psychotherapies.* Washington, DC: American Psychological Association, 2010.

———. *Person-centered Therapy Over Time.* Washington, DC: American Psychological Association, 2010.

Purton, Campbell. *Person-centered Therapy: The Focusing-oriented Approach.* Houndmills, Basingstoke, Hampshire: Palgrave Macmillan, 2004.

Rogers, Carl. *Client-Centered Therapy.* Boston: Houghton Mifflin, 1951.

———. *On Becoming a Person.* Boston: Houghton Mifflin, 1961.

———. *A Way of Being.* Boston: Houghton Mifflin, 1980.

Wilkins, Paul. *Person-Centered Therapy: 100 Key Points.* London: Routledge, 2010.

OTHER

Grant, Shelia K. "Person-Centered Therapy." California State University. http://www.csun.edu/~hcpsy002/Psy460_Ch07_Handout_ppt.pdf (accessed December 21, 2010).

ORGANIZATIONS

Association for the Development of the Person-Centered Approach,http://www.adpca.org.

Center for Studies of the Person, 1150 Silverado, Suite 112, La Jolla, CA, 92037, (858) 459-3861, http://www.center-fortheperson.org.

World Association for Person-Centered and Experiential Psychotherapy and Counseling, PO Box 142, Ross-on-Wye, United Kingdom, HR9 9AG, +44 1989 763 901 http://www.pce-world.org.

Sandra L. Friedrich, M.A.

Pervasive developmental disorders

Definition

Pervasive developmental disorders (PDDs) include five different conditions: **Asperger syndrome**, **autism**, **childhood disintegrative disorder** (CDD), pervasive developmental disorder not otherwise specified (PDDNOS), and **Rett syndrome**. The disorders are classified together because of the similarities among them. The three most common shared problems involve communication skills, motor skills, and social skills. Since there are no clear diagnostic boundaries separating these conditions, it is sometimes difficult to distinguish one from the other for diagnostic purposes. Because of this, PDDs (with the exception of Rett syndrome) are sometimes called autism spectrum disorders, meaning that the disorders share symptoms but differ in severity.

Demographics

Asperger syndrome, autism, and childhood disintegrative disorder are four to five times more common in boys, while Rett syndrome has been diagnosed primarily in girls.

All of these disorders are considered rare, though the prevalence of autism has risen in recent years. The U.S. Centers for Disease Control and Prevention estimates that, on average, 1 in 110 children are affected by an autism spectrum disorder, more than those affected by spina bifida, cancer, or **Down syndrome**. The increase in prevalence may be due partly to improved recognition and **diagnosis**.

Description

Asperger syndrome

Children afflicted with Asperger syndrome exhibit difficulties in social relationships and communication. They are reluctant to make eye contact, do not respond to social or emotional contacts, do not initiate play activities with peers, and do not give or receive attention or affection. To receive this diagnosis, an individual must demonstrate normal development of language, thinking, and coping skills. Due to an impaired coordination of muscle movements, children with Asperger syndrome appear to be clumsy. They usually become deeply involved in a select few interests, which tend to occupy most of their time and attention.

Autism

Autism is frequently evident within the first year of life and must be diagnosed before age three. It is associated with moderate intellectual disabilities in three out of four cases. Children with autism generally do not want to be held, rocked, cuddled, or played with. They are unresponsive to affection, show no interest in peers or adults, and have few interests. Other symptoms include avoidance of eye contact, absence of facial expressions, and the use of gestures to express needs. Actions are repetitive, routine, and restricted; rocking, hand and arm flapping, unusual hand and finger movements, and attachment to objects rather than pets and people are common. Speech, play, and other behaviors appear repetitive and without imagination. Children with autism tend to be overactive, aggressive, and self-injurious and do not like changes in routine. They are often highly sensitive to touch, noise, and smells.

Childhood disintegrative disorder

Childhood disintegrative disorder, also called Heller's disease, most often develops between two and ten years of age. Children with CDD develop normally until two to three years of age and then begin to disintegrate rapidly. Signs and symptoms include deterioration of the ability to use and understand language to the point where they are unable to carry on a conversation. This is accompanied by loss of control of the bladder and bowels. Any interest or ability to play and engage in social activities is lost. The behaviors are nearly identical with those of autism. However, childhood disintegrative disorder becomes evident later in life and results in developmental regression, or loss of previously attained skills, whereas autism can be detected as early as the first month of life and results in a failure to progress.

Pervasive developmental disorder not otherwise specified

The term pervasive developmental disorder not otherwise specified (PDDNOS) is also referred to as atypical personality development, atypical PDD, or atypical autism. Individuals with this disorder share some of the same signs and symptoms of autism or related conditions but do not meet all of the criteria for diagnosis for any of the other four syndromes included in PDDs. Because children diagnosed with PDDNOS do not all exhibit the same combination of characteristics, it is difficult to conduct research on this disorder. Limited evidence available suggests that patients are seen by medical professionals later in life than is the case for children with autism, and they are less likely to have intellectual deficits.

Rett syndrome

Rett syndrome was first described in 1966 and is found almost exclusively in girls. In Rett syndrome, the cells in the **brain** experience difficulty in communicating with each other. The growth of the head falls behind the growth of the body, resulting in an **intellectual disability**. These conditions are accompanied by deficits in movement (motor) skills and a loss of interest in social activities. Children with Rett syndrome typically develop normally for 6–18 months (stage one), then development slows down and stops (stage two). Stage three is characterized by a loss of the speech and motor skills already acquired, typically between nine months and three years of age. Stage four begins with a return to learning that will continue across the lifespan but at a very slow rate. Problems with coordination and walking are likely to continue and even worsen. Other conditions that can occur with Rett syndrome are convulsions, constipation, breathing problems, impaired circulation in the feet and legs, and difficulty chewing or swallowing.

Causes and symptoms

Causes

The causes of these disorders are unknown, although brain structure abnormalities, genetic mutation, and alterations in brain function are believed to play a role. Still, no single brain abnormality or location has been connected to a cause. In 2004, scientists reported finding the gene mutation (on gene MECP2) present in 80% of people affected with Rett syndrome. A number of causes have been associated with autism, including genes, environmental factors, and chemical imbalances, but none have been proven. Various neurological conditions, such as convulsions, are commonly found to accompany PDDs.

Symptoms

Because PDDs share similar symptoms, distinctions between conditions must be carefully made to ensure correct diagnosis. Key distinctions are as follows.

PDDNOS:

- impairment of two-way social interaction
- repetitive and predictable behavior patterns and activities

Autism (in addition to the symptoms of PDDNOS):

- severe impairment in communication
- abnormal social interaction and use of language for social communication or imaginative play before age of three
- not better accounted for by another psychiatric disorder

Asperger syndrome (in addition to the symptoms of PDDNOS):

- clinically significant impairment in social, occupational, or other areas of functioning
- no general delay in language
- no delay in cognitive development, self-help skills, or adaptive behavior
- not better accounted for by another pervasive developmental disorder or schizophrenia

Rett syndrome:

- a period of normal development between 6–18 months
- normal head circumference at birth, followed by a slowing of head growth
- intellectual disabilities
- repetitive hand movements

CDD:

- normal development for at least two years
- loss of skills in at least two of the following areas: language, social skills, bowel or bladder control, play, movement skills
- abnormal functioning in at least two of the following areas: social interaction, communication, behavior patterns
- not better accounted for by another PDD or mental illness

KEY TERMS

Hydrotherapy—This term literally means "water treatment" and involves the use of water in physical therapy as well as treatment of physical and emotional illness.

Mutation—A change in a gene. A gene mutation may alter a trait or characteristic of an individual or may manifest as a disease; the mutation can also be transmitted to offspring.

Neurological conditions—A condition that has its origin in some part of the patient's nervous system.

Diagnosis

The diagnosis of a pervasive developmental disorder is made by medical specialists based on a thorough examination of the patient, including observing behavior and gathering information from parents and caregivers.

Treatment

Treatment for children with pervasive developmental disorders is limited. Those who can be enrolled in educational programs will need a highly structured learning environment, a teacher-student ratio of not more than 1:2, and a high level of parental involvement that provides consistent care at home. **Psychotherapy** and **social skills training** may prove helpful to some. There is no specific medication available for treating the core symptoms of any of these disorders, though research is promising. Some psychiatric medications may be helpful in controlling particular behavior difficulties, such as agitation, mood instability, and self-injury. **Music therapy**, massage, and hydrotherapy may exert a calming effect on behavior. Treatment may also include physical and occupational therapy.

Prognosis

In general, the prognosis of all of these conditions is tied to the severity of the illness. The higher the patient's IQ (intelligence quotient) and ability to communicate, the better the prognosis. The prognosis for Asperger syndrome is the most positive, and children with Asperger syndrome are likely to grow up to be functional independent adults, though they will always have problems with social relationships. The prognosis for autism is not as good, though great strides have been made in recent years in its treatment. The prognosis for childhood disintegrative disorder is even less favorable,

QUESTIONS TO ASK YOUR DOCTOR

- What are the indications that my child may have a pervasive developmental disorder?
- What physical and psychiatric diagnostic tests does my child need?
- What treatment options do you recommend for my child?
- What symptoms are important enough that I should seek immediate treatment?
- Can you recommend any support groups for me and my family?

and children with CDD will require intensive and long-term care. Children diagnosed with PDDNOS have a better prognosis, because their initial symptoms are usually milder, their IQ scores are higher, and their language development is stronger.

All persons with PDDs are at greater risk for developing serious mental illness than the general population, and many will always need some level of custodial care. In the past, individuals with PDD were confined to institutions, but many are now able to live in **group homes** or supervised apartments.

Prevention

Until the causes of pervasive developmental disorders are known, it will remain impossible to prevent these conditions.

Resources

BOOKS

American Psychiatric Association. *Diagnostic and Statistical Manual of Mental Disorders*. 4th ed., text rev. Washington, DC: American Psychiatric Association, 2000.

American Psychological Association. *Publication Manual of the American Psychological Association*. 6th ed. Washington, DC: American Psychological Association, 2009.

Coplan, James, MD. *Making Sense of Autistic Spectrum Disorders: Create the Brightest Future for Your Child with the Best Treatment Options*. New York: Bantam, 2010.

Schilling, Shondra, and Curt Schilling. *The Best Kind of Different: Our Family's Journey with Asperger's Syndrome*. New York: HarperCollins, 2010.

Taylor, Paul. *A Beginner's Guide to the Autism Spectrum Disorders: Essential Information for Parents and Professionals*. Philadelphia: Jessica Kingsley Publishers, 2011.

Volkmar, Fred, R., and Lisa A Wiesner. *A Practical Guide to Autism: What Every Parent, Family Member, and Teacher Needs to Know*. Sudbury, MA: Wiley, 2009.

PERIODICALS

Muhle, Rebecca, Stephanie V. Trentacoste, and Isabelle Rapin. "The Genetics of Autism." *Pediatrics* (May 2004): 1389–91.

Tateno, M., et al. "Pervasive Developmental Disorders and Autism Spectrum Disorders: Are These Disorders One and the Same?" *Psychiatric Investigation* 8, no. 1 (2011): 67–70.

Wink, L. K., C. A. Erickson, and C. J. McDougle. "Pharmacologic Treatment of Behavioral Symptoms Associated with Autism and Other Pervasive Developmental Disorders." *Current Treatment Options in Neurology* 12, no. 6 (2010): 529–38.

WEBSITES

National Institute of Mental Health. "Autism Spectrum Disorders (Pervasive Developmental Disorders)." http://mentalhealth.gov/health/publications/autism/complete-index.shtml (accessed November 2, 2011).

Autism Program at Yale. "Information About Pervasive Developmental Disorders (PDD)." Yale School of Medicine. http://medicine.yale.edu/childstudy/autism/information/index.aspx (accessed November 2, 2011).

ORGANIZATIONS

American Academy of Child and Adolescent Psychiatry, 3615 Wisconsin Ave. NW, Washington, DC, 20016-3007, (202) 966-7300, Fax: (202) 966-2891, http://aacap.org.

Autism Society of America, 4340 East-West Hwy, Suite 350, Bethesda, MD, 20814, (301) 657-0881, (800) 3-AUTISM (328-8476), http://www.autism-society.org.

International Rett Syndrome Association, 4600 Devitt Drive, Cincinnati, OH, 45246, (800) 818-7388, Fax: (513) 874-2520, http://www.rettsyndrome.org.

National Organization for Rare Disorders (NORD), PO Box 1968, Danbury, CT, 06813-1968, (203) 744-0100, (800) 999-6673, Fax: (203) 798-2291, orphan@rarediseases.org, http://www.rarediseases.org.

Teresa G. Odle
Donald G. Barstow, RN
Laura Jean Cataldo, RN, EdD

PET *see* **Positron emission tomography**

Phencyclidine and related disorders

Definition

Phencyclidine (PCP) is a street drug known as "angel dust" that causes physiological changes to the nervous and circulatory system, disturbances in thinking and behavior, and can cause hallucinations, psychotic disorder, mood disorder, and anxiety disorder.

Demographics

According to a Drug and Alcohol Services Information System (DASIS) report, in an analysis of PCP admissions, researchers found that 49% of people admitted for a substance-use problem with PCP as the primary substance were African American; another 26% were Hispanic, and 19% were Caucasian. Admissions for PCP as the primary drug were less than 1% of overall admissions for substance-use problems. In addition, admissions for PCP use in the United States were more frequent in the West and Northeast than in the South or Midwest. The average age at admission was 28 years, and most PCP users were male. In terms of education, people admitted for PCP substance-use problems were more likely to have dropped out of high school and less likely to have full-time employment than people admitted for other drugs. However, they were less likely to have an accompanying psychiatric problem than people admitted for other substances.

A study entitled *Monitoring the Future* is conducted every year by the University of Michigan and funded by the National Institute on Drug Abuse (NIDA). The 2007 report revealed that 2.1% of high school seniors had used PCP once, while 0.9% had used PCP at least one time in the previous year. In addition, 21% of high school seniors deemed PCP as *very easy* or *fairly easy* to obtain. The 2009 survey showed that 122,000 Americans age 12 and older had abused PCP at least one time in 2008, and the 2010 report revealed that 1.0% of high school seniors had used PCP at least one time in 2009.

Description

PCP is the best known of several related drugs, including ketamine, cyclohexamine, and dizocilpine. PCP was first synthesized by a pharmaceutical company in the 1950s and sold under the brand names Sernyl and Sernylan until 1967. It was hoped that PCP could be used as a dissociative anesthetic, because it produced a catatonic state in which patients were dissociated from their environment and from pain but not unconscious. Problems with side effects as the drug wore off, including agitated behavior and hallucinations, made PCP unsuitable for medical use. Ketamine (Ketlar, Ketaject) is less potent, has fewer side effects, and is approved for use as a human anesthetic.

PCP became an illicit street drug in the mid-1960s. It was most commonly found in large cities such as New York and San Francisco, and even in the early 2000s, most users lived in urban areas. Into the 1970s, PCP

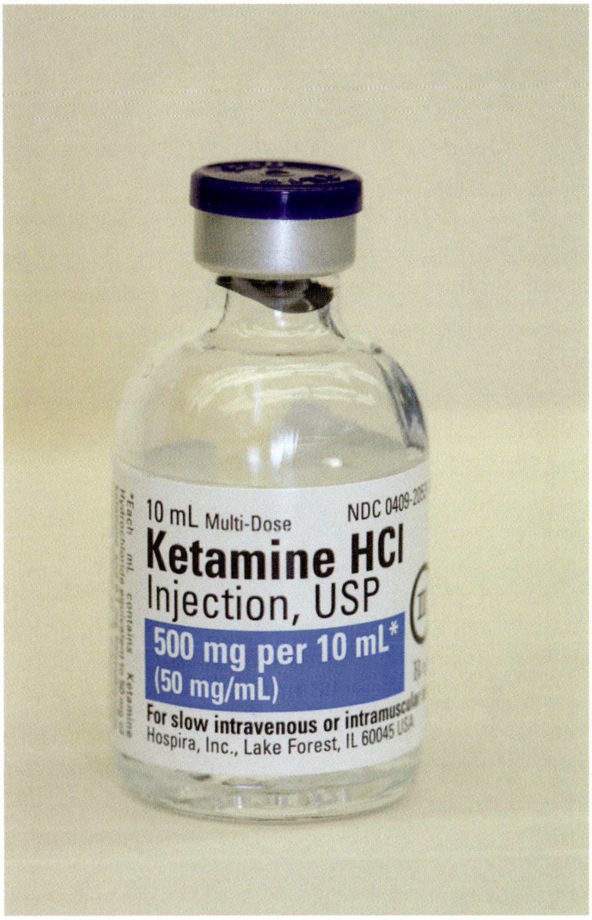

10 mL vial of ketamine; when used illicitly, the liquid is usually evaporated and snorted. *(© Custom Medical Stock Photo, Inc. Reproduced by permission.)*

appeared mainly as a contaminant of other illicit drugs, especially marijuana, and **diagnosis** of PCP use was complicated by the fact that many people did not know they had ingested the drug.

PCP is easy to manufacture and is inexpensive. By the late 1970s, in some urban areas its use equaled that of crack **cocaine**. Use of PCP peaked between 1973 and 1979. After 1980, PCP use declined, although as with many illicit drugs, its popularity increases and decreases in cycles.

People who use PCP exhibit both behavioral and physiological signs. The effects of PCP are erratic, and serious complications can occur at relatively low doses. It is often difficult to distinguish PCP use from the use of other illicit drugs, and many people who use PCP also abuse other substances. According to the *Diagnostic and Statistical Manual of Mental Disorders,* fourth edition, text revision (*DSM-IV-TR*), which presents guidelines used by the **American Psychiatric Association** for diagnosis of mental disorders, phencyclidine can induce mood

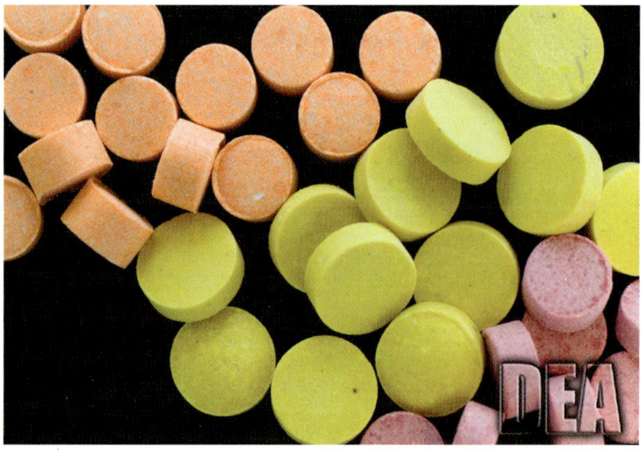

PCP pills. *(U.S. Drug Enforcement Administration)*

disorder, psychotic disorder, and anxiety disorder. These classifications are somewhat controversial and not all are recognized by international psychiatric organizations. Animal studies suggest that both conditions occur, just as they do with many other abused drugs.

PCP is a Schedule II drug under the Controlled Substances Act, which means it has a high potential for abuse and dependence and has severe restrictions for medical use. In its pure form, it is a white powder that dissolves easily in water. Once dissolved, the solution can be sprayed on tobacco or marijuana cigarettes. Less pure forms range from yellowish-tan to brown and can be a sticky mass. On the street PCP has many names, including angel dust, devil dust, tranq, hog, crazy Eddie, rocket fuel, embalming fluid, wack, and ozone. Crack cocaine combined with PCP is sometimes called tragic magic. Marijuana laced with PCP is called love boat, killer weed, or crystal supergrass.

Causes and symptoms

Causes

PCP is easy to manufacture and is inexpensively available on the street in most cities, especially East Coast cities. It can be eaten, smoked, injected, or snorted, and is readily soluble and will cross the skin barrier if in liquid form PCP is spilled on skin or clothing. The most common methods of ingestion are eating and smoking marijuana or tobacco on which liquid PCP has been sprayed. PCP is long-acting. It accumulates in body fat and flashbacks can occur as it is released from fat during **exercise**.

PCP binds to receptors in the **brain** and interferes with the chemical reactions that mediate the transmission of nerve impulses. It is deactivated slowly by the liver and excreted in urine. Although there are no controlled human studies on PCP intoxication, monkeys allowed free use of PCP will dose themselves repeatedly and maintain an almost continuous state of intoxication. They exhibit withdrawal symptoms if their supply of the drug is restricted. PCP is considered to be psychologically and possibly physically addictive in humans.

Symptoms

PCP produces both physiological and psychological symptoms. Effects of the drug are erratic and not always dose-dependent.

Physical symptoms include:

- involuntary rapid movements of the eyes vertically or horizontally
- high blood pressure
- racing heartbeat
- dizziness and shakiness
- drooling
- increased body temperature
- reduced response to pain
- slurred speech
- excessive sensitivity to sound
- lack of muscle coordination
- muscle rigidity or frozen posture
- seizures
- breakdown of muscle and excretion of muscle proteins in urine
- coma
- death

Psychiatric and social symptoms include:

- disordered thinking and confusion
- impaired judgment
- belligerence
- aggressiveness
- agitation
- impulsiveness and unpredictability
- schizophrenic-like psychoses
- hallucinations of sight, sound, or touch
- memory impairment
- difficulty in social-emotional relationships
- chaotic lifestyle, including difficulty functioning at work or school and legal and financial problems

PCP is known for its variability of symptoms, which change both from person to person and from exposure to exposure. In addition, symptoms come and go throughout a period of intoxication that can last 1–2 hours for low-dose exposure to 1–4 days for high-dose exposure. Severity of symptoms is not always related to the size of the dose as measured by blood levels of the drug.

KEY TERMS

Addiction—A strong physical or psychological dependence on a physical substance.

Anxiety—A troubled feeling, a sense of dread, fear of the future, or distress over a possible threat to a person's physical or mental well-being.

Dependence—The adaptation of neurons and other physical processes to the use of a drug, followed by withdrawal symptoms when the drug is removed; physiological and/or psychological addiction.

Hallucinations—Heard, seen, or otherwise sensed perceptions that are not empirically real. Hallucinations can result from nervous system abnormalities, mental disorders, or the use of certain drugs.

Intoxication—The presence of significant problem behaviors or psychological changes following ingestion of a substance.

Schizophrenia—A major mental illness marked by psychotic symptoms, including hallucinations, delusions, and severe disruptions in thinking.

Seizure—A convulsion, or uncontrolled discharge of nerve cells, that may spread to other cells throughout the brain.

Stuporous—A state of sluggishness or impaired consciousness.

Substance abuse—A milder form of addiction than substance dependence. Generally, people who have been diagnosed with substance abuse do not experience the tolerance or withdrawal symptoms—the signs of physiological dependence—that people dependent on a substance experience.

Withdrawal—Symptoms experienced by a person who has become physically dependent on a drug, experienced when the drug use is discontinued.

Three rough phases of intoxication have been established: behavioral toxicity, stuporous stage, and comatose stage. Many users fluctuate between phases, and some have symptoms that do not fit neatly into any phase. In the behavioral toxicity stage, people tend to gaze blankly while their eyes dart horizontally or vertically. Muscle control is poor, and individuals may make repetitive movements, grind their teeth, or grimace. Body temperature, heart rate, and respiration are mildly elevated. Vomiting and drooling may occur.

In the stuporous phase, the eyes are wide open, and individuals appear wide awake but in a stupor. **Seizures** may occur if individuals are stimulated. The eyes may dart in any direction while the gaze remains fixed. Body temperature is increased substantially. Heart and respiration rate are increased by about 25%. Muscles are rigid with twitching.

In the comatose stage, which may last 1–4 days, individuals are in a deep coma. Their pupils are dilated, and their eyes drift. Body temperature is elevated to the point of being life-threatening. The heart rate is dangerously high, increasing to about twice the normal level, and blood pressure is dangerously low. Breathing may stop for brief periods (apnea). There is no response to pain, and individuals sweat heavily. Death is possible, although most deaths from PCP occur in earlier stages through accidents or **suicide**.

Diagnosis

Diagnosis of PCP abuse or dependence is often complicated by the fact that symptoms are variable. Most people who use PCP also use other drugs (74% of users in one survey used at least one other substance), and PCP can be a contaminant in other street drugs or can itself be contaminated with other chemicals. PCP use is also found among people with psychiatric disorders. In many ways, PCP mimics the symptoms of **schizophrenia**.

The American Psychiatric Association describes two classes of PCP disorders: PCP dependence and PCP abuse. In addition, it recognizes seven other PCP-induced psychiatric disorders.

PCP dependence can be difficult to pinpoint because, unlike many other drugs of abuse, PCP does not invariably cause craving in individuals who use it. In addition, although studies of specific populations have identified signs of tolerance or withdrawal, these symptoms have not been clearly categorized for PCP use. Generally, a person with PCP dependence will engage in PCP use several times a day and persist in using it, even when psychological problems (such as anxiety or rage) and/or medical problems (such as high blood pressure or seizures) occur. Aggression has been identified as a key problem for people dependent on PCP. People with psychiatric disorders are more likely to have bad side effects from PCP than those without psychiatric problems. Because PCP is readily stored in fat and released as fat stores are used, adverse effects of PCP dependence can continue for weeks after the drug is discontinued.

People who exhibit signs of PCP abuse may use the drug less often than those with dependence, but they also may experience interference with their ability to fulfill their responsibilities at school, work, or home. In addition, with the impaired judgment associated with PCP use, individuals may engage in dangerous

QUESTIONS TO ASK YOUR DOCTOR

- What risks are associated with PCP abuse?
- What symptoms are associated with PCP dependence?
- Does having PCP dependence and abuse put me at risk for other health conditions?
- Can you recommend any treatment and support groups for me?

behaviors, such as driving a car while under the drug's influence. Use of the drug may trigger trouble in personal relationships or with the law.

Phencyclidine-induced disorders include:

- PCP intoxication with or without perceptual disturbances
- PCP intoxication delirium
- PCP-induced psychotic disorder
- PCP-induced mood disorder
- PCP-induced anxiety disorder
- PCP-induced disorders not otherwise specified

PCP intoxication and **delirium** are diagnosed by a history of recent PCP use, behavioral changes, and physical changes that are not accounted for by any other substance use, medical condition, or psychiatric condition. PCP is present in the blood and urine. With PCP intoxication, individuals may have hallucinations but be aware that these are caused by PCP use.

PCP delirium is diagnosed when individuals exhibit muddled thinking, hostility, bouts of hyperactivity and aggressiveness, and schizophrenic-like symptoms, as well as the more severe physical symptoms listed above. PCP delirium can last for hours or days.

It may be difficult initially to separate PCP intoxication or delirium from other mental disorders, as symptoms may mimic **depression**, schizophrenia, mood disorders, **conduct disorder**, and **antisocial personality disorder**. People with PCP intoxication also have physical and psychological symptoms similar to those that occur with the use of other illicit drugs, complicating diagnosis. A complete physical and psychological history helps rule out these other conditions.

Treatment

People experiencing PCP intoxication or delirium often hurt themselves or others. They are generally kept in an environment in which there is as little stimulation as possible. They are restrained only as much as is necessary to keep them from hurting themselves or others until the level of PCP in their bodies can be reduced. Antipsychotic medications may be used to calm patients in cases of PCP delirium.

There are no quick ways to rid the body of PCP. If the PCP has been eaten, stomach pumping or feeding activated charcoal may help keep the drug from being absorbed into the bloodstream. Physical symptoms such as high body temperature are treated as needed.

Most people recover from PCP intoxication or delirium without major medical complications. Many are habitual users who return to use almost immediately. There are no specific behavioral therapies to treat PCP use. **Antidepressants** are sometimes prescribed. Long-term residential treatment or intensive outpatient treatment along with urine monitoring offer some chance of success. Narcotics Anonymous, a self-help group, may be helpful for some patients.

Prognosis

Relapse and return to PCP use is common, even among people who have experienced severe medical and psychiatric complications from the drug. Because many users also abuse other drugs, their success in renouncing PCP is tied to their successful treatment for other addictions. Successful treatment takes persistence, patience, and a functional support system, all of which many users lack.

Prevention

PCP intoxication and related disorders can be prevented by not using the drug.

Resources

BOOKS

American Psychiatric Association. *Diagnostic and Statistical Manual of Mental Disorders,* 4th ed., text rev. Washington, DC: American Psychiatric Publishing, 2000.

American Psychological Association. *Publication Manual of the American Psychological Association,* 6th ed. Washington, DC: American Psychological Association, 2009.

Doweiko, Harold E. *Concepts of Chemical Dependency,* 8th ed. Belmont, CA: Brooks Cole, 2011.

Erickson, Carlton K. *Addiction Essentials: The Go-To Guide for Clinicians and Patients.* New York: Norton, 2011.

WEBSITES

"The DASIS Report: Characteristics of Primary Phencyclidine (PCP) Admissions: 2001." Drug and Alcohol Services Information System (SAMHSA). May 7, 2004. http://

store.samhsa.gov/product/Characteristics-of-Primary-Phencyclidine-PCP-Admissions-2001/SR019 (accessed October 3, 2011).

"NIDA InfoFacts: PCP (Phencylcidine)." National Institute on Drug Abuse. Last modified June 2009. http://www.nida.nih.gov/Infofacts/PCP.html (accessed October 3, 2011).

ORGANIZATIONS

American Council for Drug Education, 50 Jay St., Brooklyn, NY, 11201, (646) 505-2061, acde@phoenixhouse.org, http://www.acde.org.

American Psychiatric Association, 1000 Wilson Blvd., Ste. 1825, Arlington, VA, 22209-3901, (703) 907-7300, apa@psych.org, http://www.psych.org.

American Psychological Association, 750 1st St. NE, Washington, DC, 20002-4242, (202) 336-5500; TDD/TTY: (202) 336-6123, (800) 374-2721, http://www.apa.org.

American Society for Clinical Pharmacology and Therapeutics, 528 N Washington St., Alexandria, VA, 22314, (703) 836-6981, info@ascpt.org, http://www.ascpt.org.

National Institute on Drug Abuse. National Institutes of Health, 6001 Executive Blvd., Rm. 5213, Bethesda, MD, 20892, (301) 442-1124; Spanish: (240) 221-4007, information@nida.nih.gov, http://www.nida.nih.gov.

Tish Davidson, AM
Emily Jane Willingham, PhD
Laura Jean Cataldo, RN, EdD

Phenelzine

Definition

Phenelzine is classified as a monoamine oxidase inhibitor (MAOI). It is used to treat several types of serious **depression**. In the United States, phenelzine is sold under the brand name Nardil.

Purpose

Phenelzine is used to treat certain types forms of serious depression and severe depression complicated by severe anxiety that do not respond to other antidepressant drugs.

Description

Phenelzine is a member of a class of drugs called **monoamine oxidase inhibitors**. Monoamine oxidase, or MAO, is an enzyme found throughout the body. In the **brain**, MAO breaks down norepinephrine and **serotonin**, two naturally occurring chemicals that are important in maintaining mental well-being and preventing depression. Monoamine oxidase inhibitors such as phenelzine reduce the activity of MAO. Less norepinephrine and serotonin are broken down, so their levels rise. This helps to lift depression.

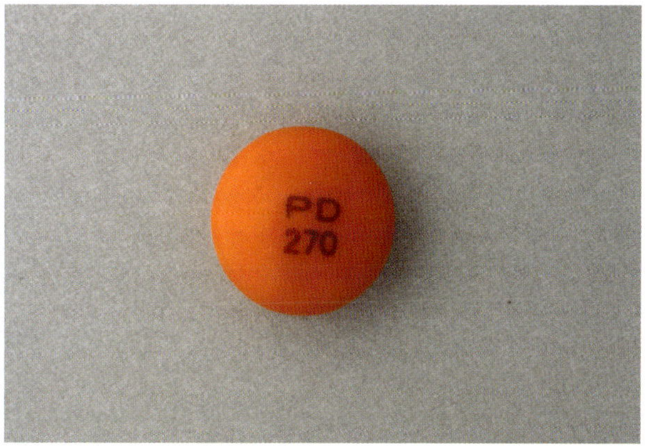

Nardil (phenelzine), 15 mg. *(© Custom Medical Stock Photo, Inc. Reproduced by permission.)*

Phenelzine is effective for treating depression, especially complicated types of depression that have not responded to more traditional **antidepressants**. However, phenelzine also affects the MAO enzyme in many other areas of the body. This accounts for the large number of serious side effects and drug interactions caused by the drug.

Recommended dosage

Adults are usually started on 15 mg of phenelzine three times per day. This dosage can be increased to a maximum of 90 mg per day if lower doses are not effective and if the patient can tolerate the higher dose without excessive side effects. After the maximum benefits are achieved, the dosage is usually lowered over several weeks to the lowest level that is effective. This could be as little as 15 mg daily or every other day.

In general, phenelzine is not recommended for people over the age of 60. When it is used by the elderly, the starting dosage is usually 15 mg taken in the morning. This dose may be gradually increased over time to a maximum of 60 mg. Phenelzine is not approved by the U.S. Food and Drug Administration (FDA) for use in patients younger than 18, and recommended dosage in such cases has not been established.

Phenelzine can be taken with food or on an empty stomach. It should not be taken close to bedtime, because it can interfere with sleep. The benefits of this drug may not become apparent for as long as four to eight weeks. Patients should be aware of this and continue taking the drug as directed even if they do not see an immediate improvement.

Precautions

People with a history of congestive heart failure, high blood pressure, cardiovascular disease, headache, kidney disease, or liver disease should not take phenelzine or, if they do take it, they should be under careful medical supervision and monitoring. Children under the age of 18 and people with a history of low blood pressure, **bipolar disorder**, angina, hyperactivity, diabetes mellitus, **seizures**, suicidal thoughts, and overactive thyroid should discuss the risks and benefits of this drug with their physician, and the decision to use phenelzine should be made on an individual case basis. If these patients receive phenelzine, it should be taken only under the careful supervision of a doctor. Evidence suggests that phenelzine should not be used during pregnancy or while nursing.

Children and adults up to age 24 are at an increased risk of developing suicidal thoughts or actions when taking an antidepressant drug, including phenelzine. Patients of any age taking the drug should be monitored for signs of worsening depression or changes in behavior.

People taking phenelzine should get up slowly from a reclining position to prevent dizziness. Caution should be used when operating heavy machinery or performing hazardous activities that require alertness. Patients preparing to undergo surgery should stop taking phenelzine at least ten days before their procedure.

It is very important for the doctor to determine the lowest dosage of phenelzine that produces benefits. When this dosage is exceeded, side effects and interactions increase substantially. Over-the-counter medications that contain decongestants or dextromethorphan (for example, some cough syrups and cold remedies) should not be taken while using phenelzine. In addition, foods and beverages that contain tyramine should not be eaten while using this medication. These foods include yeast or meat extracts, fermented sausage, overripe fruit, sauerkraut, cheese, and fava beans. Phenelzine should not be used within two weeks of undergoing surgery that requires anesthesia.

Side effects

The enzyme monoamine oxidase regulates functions throughout the body. Phenelzine decreases the activity of monoamine oxidase in all the areas of the body where it exists, not just in the brain. This is why phenelzine is capable of causing a wide variety of side effects in many different organ systems.

The most common and unavoidable side effects associated with phenelzine use are swelling of the feet and ankles, low blood pressure upon arising from a reclining position, and **insomnia** if taken near bedtime. Mild side effects and ones that are not frequent include skin rash, headache, dizziness, confusion, memory impairment, drowsiness, weakness, shakiness, muscle twitching, constipation, indigestion, appetite changes, and dry mouth. Although these side effects are considered mild, they should be reported to the patient's physician.

More serious side effects include hepatitis coupled with jaundice, high blood pressure crisis, excessive nervousness, and changes in heart rate. The high blood pressure crisis involves significantly increased blood pressure, severe headache, heart palpitations, nausea, vomiting, and sweating. These symptoms need immediate medical attention. Sexual function can be affected in both men and women.

Interactions

Phenelzine interacts with a long list of drugs. Some of these interactions can cause death. This section is not a complete list of interactions, but it includes the most serious ones. Patients must make sure that every health care professional who takes care of them (for example, doctors, dentists, podiatrists, optometrists, pharmacists, nurses) knows that they take phenelzine, as well as all of the other prescription, nonprescription, and herbal drugs they take.

All foods and beverages containing tyramine need to be avoided while taking this medication. Coffee, tea, and cola beverages should be restricted to one serving per day. Alcohol should not be used while taking phenelzine, because it can significantly increase blood pressure.

Any type of amphetamine and other stimulant should not be used, because this combination can increase blood pressure to dangerously high levels. Phenelzine should not be combined with other antidepressants, because of increased risk of dangerously high blood pressure and manic episodes. Patients taking phenelzine should stop the drug and wait at least 14 days before starting any other antidepressant. The same holds true when discontinuing another antidepressant and starting phenelzine.

Phenelzine combined with **clomipramine** (Anafranil) can cause death. Diet drugs and decongestants containing compounds such as dextromethorphan should not be combined with phenelzine because of an increased

KEY TERMS

Angina—Severe pain and a feeling of constriction around the heart.

Bipolar disorder—A mood disorder marked by alternating episodes of extremely low mood (depression) and exuberant highs (mania).

Hepatitis—An inflammation of the liver that can be caused by a variety of factors.

Jaundice—A yellowing of the skin caused by excess bilirubin in the blood; a liver disorder.

Tyramine—Intermediate product between the chemicals tyrosine and epinephrine in the body and a substance normally found in many foods. Found especially in protein-rich foods that have been aged or fermented, pickled, or bacterially contaminated, such as cheese, beer, yeast, wine, and chicken liver.

risk of seizures and agitation. Phenelzine can decrease the effectiveness of high blood pressure drugs, such as guanadrel (Hylorel) and guanethidine (Ismelin). Phenelzine combined with the Parkinson's disease drug levodopa (Dopar, Larodopa) can produce severely high blood pressure. Lithium should not be used with phenelzine because of the risk of developing an extremely high fever. Phenelzine can prolong the effects of muscle relaxants and **barbiturates** when either of the two are taken with phenelzine.

Resources

BOOKS

Brunton, Laurence, Bruce Chabner, and Bjorn Knollman. *Goodman & Gilman's The Pharmacological Basis of Therapeutics* 12th ed. New York: McGraw-Hill, 2010.

Consumer Reports and American Society of Health-System Pharmacists. *Consumer Reports Complete Drug Reference.* Yonkers, NY: Consumers Reports, 2009.

Ellsworth, Allan J., et al. *Mosby's Medical Drug Reference.* St. Louis, MO: Mosby, 2007.

Venes, Donald. *Taber's Cyclopedic Medical Dictionary.* 21st ed. Philadelphia: F.A. Davis Company, 2009.

WEBSITES

PubMed Health. "Phenelzine." U.S. National Library of Medicine. http://www.ncbi.nlm.nih.gov/pubmedhealth/PMH0000573 (accessed November 13, 2011).

ORGANIZATIONS

National Institute of Mental Health, 6001 Executive Blvd., Rm. 8184, MSC 9663, Bethesda, MD, 20892-9663, (301) 433-4513; TTY: (301) 443-8431, Fax: (301) 443-4279, (866) 615-6464; TTY: (866) 415-8051 nimhinfo@nih.gov, http://www.nimh.nih.gov.

U.S. Food and Drug Administration, 10903 New Hampshire Ave., Silver Spring, MD, 20993-0002, (888) INFO-FDA (463-6332), http://www.fda.gov.

Mark Mitchell, M.D.

Phobias *see* **Agoraphobia; Social phobia; Specific phobias**

Phonological disorder

Definition

Phonological disorder occurs when a child does not develop the ability to produce some or all sounds necessary for speech that are normally used at his or her age.

Demographics

Phonological disorder of unknown cause is considered significantly more common than phonological disorder that is caused by neurological or structural abnormalities. It has been estimated that 7%–8% children who are five years old have phonological disorder with any cause (developmental phonological disorder). About 7.5% of children between the ages of three and eleven are thought to have development phonological disorder. Phonological disorder is more common in boys than it is in girls. Estimates suggest that two to four times as many boys as girls have the disorder. Children who have phonological disorder are more likely to have other language problems and disorders. Children with one or more family members who have this or similar language disorders are also considered to be more likely to have phonological disorders.

Description

Phonological disorder is sometimes referred to as articulation disorder, developmental articulation disorder, or speech sound production disorder. If there is no known cause, it is sometimes called "developmental phonological disorder." If the cause is known to be of neurological origin, the names "dysarthria" or "dyspraxia" are often used. Phonological disorder is characterized by a child's inability to create speech at a level expected of his or her age group because of an inability to form the necessary sounds.

There are many different levels of severity of phonological disorder. These range from speech that is completely incomprehensible, even to a child's immediate family members, to speech that can be understood by everyone but in which some sounds are slightly mispronounced. Treatment for phonological disorder is important not only for the child's development to be able to form speech sounds, but for other reasons, as well. Children who have problems creating speech sounds may have academic problems in subject areas such as spelling or reading. Also, children who sound different than their peers may find themselves frustrated and ridiculed, and may become less willing to participate in play or classroom activities.

Causes

Phonological disorder is often divided into three categories based on the cause of the disorder. One cause is structural problems, or abnormalities in the areas necessary for speech sound production, such as the tongue or the roof of the mouth. These abnormalities make it difficult for children to produce certain sounds, and in some cases make it impossible for a child to produce the sounds at all. The structural problem causing the phonological disorder generally needs to be treated before the child goes into language therapy. This therapy is especially useful, because in many of these cases correction of the structural problem results in correction of the speech sound problem.

The second category of phonological disorder is problems caused by neurological problems or abnormalities. This category includes problems with the muscles of the mouth that do not allow the child sufficient fine motor control over the muscles to produce all speech sounds.

The third category of phonological disorder is phonological disorder of an unknown cause. This is sometimes called " developmental phonological disorder." Although the cause is not known, there is much speculation. Possible causes include slight **brain** abnormalities, causes rooted in the child's environment, and immature development of the neurological system.

Symptoms

The symptoms of phonological disorder differ significantly depending on the age of the child. It is often difficult to detect this disorder, as the child with phonological disorder develops speech sounds more slowly than his or her peers; generally, however, he or she develops them in the same sequence. Therefore, speech that may be normal for a four-year-old child may be a sign of phonological disorder in a six-year-old.

Nearly all children develop speech sounds in the same sequence. The consonant sounds are grouped into three main groups of eight sounds each: the early eight, the middle eight, and the late eight. The early eight include consonant sounds such as "m," "b," and "p." The middle eight include sounds such as "t," "g," and "chi," and the late eight include more complicated sounds such as "sh," "th," "z," and "zh." Many children do not normally finish mastering the late eight until they are seven or eight years old. As children normally develop speech sound skills, there are some very common mistakes that are made. These include the omission of sounds, (e.g., frequently at the end of words), the distortion of sounds, or the substitution of one sound for another. Often the substitution is of a sound that the child can more easily produce for one that he or she cannot.

Diagnosis

The **diagnosis** for phonologic disorder depends greatly on the age of the child in question. Children who are four years old may have speech production difficulties that show normal development for their age, while children who are eight years old and making the same mistakes may have phonological disorder. In children with phonological disorder, the pattern and order of speech sound acquisition is usually similar to that of normally developing children. However, the speech sound skills develop more slowly, so age is an important factor in determining a diagnosis of phonological disorder. Children with phonological disorder may make the same speech sound mistakes as younger, normally developing children. In some cases, however, children with phonological disorder have demonstrated more instances of omissions, substitutions, and distortions in their speech.

When exploring a diagnosis of phonological disorder, it is generally recommended that a physician check for other possible causes of the signs and symptoms. A child's hearing should be checked, because speech sounds that are not heard well by a child cannot be imitated and learned well. In school-age children, reading comprehension should be checked to discover any other language disorders, which are sometimes present in addition to phonological disorder. Any general developmental delays should also be checked by the physician. It is important to remember that for some children whose mother tongue is one other than English, the problems with speech sounds may result from poor crossover of sounds between the child's languages. When diagnosing a child who a different mother tongue, it is recommended that tests involve the child's first language, as well as English. It must be remembered that in some parts of the country, normal pronunciation of some words is different from pronunciation in other parts of the country. Therefore a child's background and history can be very important in making a diagnosis.

The ***Diagnostic and Statistical Manual of Mental Disorders*** (*DSM-IV-TR*) states that for a diagnosis of phonological disorder to be made, three general criteria must be met. The first criterion is that the child is not developing speech sounds skills considered to be appropriate for his or her age group. Also, this lack of speech sound acquisition must be causing problems for the child at home, at school, or in other important aspects of the child's life. If the child has an intellectual disability, has problems with his or her speech or hearing, or if there is environmental deprivation, a diagnosis of phonological disorder may still be appropriate. The diagnosis can only be made if the lack of speech sounds skill is considered greater than can the child's other problems.

Treatment

Treatment by a speech-language pathologist is generally recommended for children with phonological disorders. The therapy will differ depending on an individual child's needs, but generally takes the form of practicing sounds. Sometimes the child is shown the physical ways that the sound is made, such as where to place the tongue and how to form the lips. Repetition of the difficult sounds with the therapist is an integral part of treatment. There is debate over the way that children with more severe forms of the disorder should be treated. Some therapists believe that the sounds that are learned later in development should be addressed first, even if the child has not developed the more simple sound skills. Other therapists believe that simple sounds should be treated first, as it is easier for children with phonological disorder to master them. One other school of thought is that when the child develops a sense of accomplishment when these sounds are mastered, and he or she will more willingly continue with treatment.

Children who have phonological disorder because of neurological or structural problems that do not allow them to produce some sounds are often helped to find approximate alternatives for the sounds within the range of sounds that they are able to produce.

Prognosis

The prognosis for children with phonological disorder is generally good. For many children, the problem resolves spontaneously. It is reported that in 75% of children with mild or moderate forms of the disorder, and whose problems do not stem from a medical condition, the symptoms resolve before age six. In many other cases, children who receive treatment eventually develop normal or close to normal speech. In some cases, there may be mild effects that last until adulthood, but speech is completely understandable. For children with phonological disorder due to a neurological or structural cause, the outcome generally rests on how well the cause of the problem is treated.

KEY TERMS

Dysarthria—A group of speech disorders caused by disturbances in the strength or coordination of the muscles of the speech mechanism as a result of damage to the brain or nerves. Difficulty talking and speaking.

Dyspraxia—Developmental dyspraxia is an impairment or immaturity of the organization of movement. It is a defect in the way the brain processes information, resulting in messages not being correctly or fully transmitted. The term dyspraxia comes from the word "praxis," meaning "doing" or "acting." Dyspraxia is associated with problems of perception, language, and thought.

Prevention

There is no known way to prevent phonological disorder. A healthy diet during pregnancy and regular prenatal care may help to prevent some of the neurological or structural problems that can result in the disorder.

Resources

BOOKS

American Psychiatric Association. *Diagnostic and Statistical Manual of Mental Disorders*. 4th ed., text rev. Washington, DC: American Psychiatric Publishing, 2000.

Sadock, Benjamin J., and Virginia A. Sadock, eds. *Comprehensive Textbook of Psychiatry*. Vol. 2. 7th ed. Philadelphia: Lippincott Williams and Wilkins, 2000.

PERIODICALS

Rvachew, Susan, and Michele Nowak. "The Effect of Target-Selection Strategy on Phonological Learning." *Journal of Speech, Language, and Hearing Research* 44, no. 3 (June 2001): 610–623.

Weismer, Susan Ellis, et al. "Nonword Repetition Performance in School-age Children With and Without Language Impairment." *Journal of Speech, Language, and Hearing Research* 43, no. 4 (August 2000) 865–878.

ORGANIZATIONS

American Academy of Child and Adolescent Psychiatry, 3615 Wisconsin Ave. NW, Washington, DC, 20016-3007, (202) 966-7300, Fax: (202) 966-2891, http://aacap.org.

American Speech-Language-Hearing Association, 2200 Research Blvd., Rockville, MD, 20785, (301) 296-5700, http://www.asha.org.

American Academy of Pediatrics, 141 Northwest Point Blvd., Elk Grove Village, IL, 60007-1098, (847) 434-4000, Fax: (847) 434-8000, http://www.aap.org.

Tish Davidson, A.M.

Pica

Definition

Pica is a term that refers to cravings for substances that are not foods. Materials consumed by patients with pica include dirt, ice, clay, glue, sand, chalk, beeswax, chewing gum, laundry starch, and hair.

Demographics

Pica tends to taper off as children grow older. The disorder occasionally continues into adolescence but is rarely observed in adults who are not disabled.

Pica is observed more commonly during the second and third years of life and is considered to be developmentally inappropriate in children older than 18–24 months. Research findings indicate that the disorder occurs in 25%–33% of young children and 20% of children in mental health clinics. Among individuals with intellectual disabilities, pica occurs most often in those between the ages of 10–20 years. Among young pregnant women, the onset of pica is frequently associated with a first pregnancy in late adolescence or early adulthood. Although pica usually stops at the end of the pregnancy, it may continue intermittently for years.

Pica usually occurs with equal frequency among males and females. It is relatively uncommon, however, among adolescent and adult males of average intelligence who live in developed countries.

Description

Pica is the craving or ingestion of nonfood items. The cravings found in patients diagnosed with pica may be associated with a nutritional deficiency state, such as iron-deficiency anemia; with pregnancy; or with an intellectual disability or mental illness. The word *pica* is derived from the Latin word for magpie, a species of bird that feeds on whatever it encounters.

According to the ***Diagnostic and Statistical Manual of Mental Disorders*** (*DSM*) which presents guidelines used by the American Psychiatric Association for diagnosis of mental disorders, a **diagnosis** of pica requires that the patient persists in eating nonfood substances for at least one month. The behavior must be inappropriate for the patient's stage of development. Further, it must not be approved or encouraged by the patient's culture.

Causes and symptoms

Causes

The cause of pica is not known. Many hypotheses have been developed to explain the behavior. These have included a variety of such factors as cultural influences, low socioeconomic status, deficiency diseases, and psychological disorders.

Malnutrition is often diagnosed at the same time as pica. A causal link has not been established. Eating clay has been associated with iron deficiency; however, whether decreased iron absorption is caused by eating clay or whether iron deficiency prompts people to eat clay is not known. Some cultural groups are said to teach youngsters to eat clay. Persons with iron deficiency anemia have also been reported to chew on ice cubes. Again, the mechanism or causal link is not known.

Eating paint is most common among children from families of low socioeconomic status. It is often associated with lack of parental supervision. Hunger also may result in pica.

Among persons with intellectual disabilities, pica has been explained as the result of an inability to tell the difference between food and nonfood items. This explanation, however, is not supported by examples of nonfood items that were deliberately selected and eaten by persons with limited mental faculties.

Pica, iron deficiency, and a number of other physiological disturbances in humans have been associated with decreased activity of the **dopamine** system in the **brain**. Dopamine is a neurotransmitter, or chemical that helps to relay the transmission of nerve impulses from one nerve cell to another. This association has led some researchers to think that there may be a connection between abnormally low levels of dopamine in the brain and the development of pica. No specific underlying biochemical disorders have been identified, however.

Risk factors for pica include the following:

- parental/child psychopathology
- family disorganization

- environmental deprivation
- pregnancy
- epilepsy
- brain damage
- intellectual disabilities
- pervasive developmental disorders

Symptoms

Infants and children diagnosed with pica commonly eat paint, plaster, string, hair, and cloth. Older children may eat animal droppings, sand, insects, leaves, pebbles and cigarette butts. Adolescents and adults most often ingest clay or soil.

The symptoms of pica vary with the item ingested:

- Sand or soil is associated with gastric pain and occasional bleeding.
- Chewing ice may cause abnormal wear on teeth.
- Eating clay may cause constipation.
- Swallowing metal objects may lead to bowel perforation.
- Eating fecal material often leads to such infectious diseases as toxocariasis, toxoplasmosis, and trichuriasis.
- Consuming lead can lead to kidney damage and intellectual disabilities.

Diagnosis

Pica is often diagnosed in a hospital emergency room, when the child or adolescent develops symptoms of **lead poisoning**, bowel perforation, or other medical complications caused by the nonfood items that have been swallowed. Laboratory studies may be used to assess these complications. The choice of imaging or laboratory studies depends on the characteristics of the ingested materials and the resultant medical problems.

The examining doctor may order a variety of **imaging studies** in order to identify the ingested materials and treat the gastrointestinal complications of pica. These imaging studies may include the following:

- abdominal x rays
- barium examinations of the upper and lower gastrointestinal (GI) tracts
- upper GI endoscopy to diagnose the formation of bezoars (solid masses formed in the stomach) or to identify associated injuries to the digestive tract

Films and studies may be repeated at regular intervals to track changes in the location of ingested materials.

KEY TERMS

Behavior modification—An approach to therapy based on the principles of operant conditioning. Behavior modification seeks to replace undesirable behaviors with preferable behaviors through the use of positive or negative reinforcement.

Bezoar—A hard ball of hair or vegetable fiber that may develop in the stomach of humans as the result of ingesting nonfood items.

Chelation—A method of treating lead or mercury poisoning by giving medications that remove heavy metals from the bloodstream. The medications that are used are called chelating agents.

Dopamine—A chemical in brain tissue that serves to transmit nerve impulses (is a neurotransmitter) and helps to regulate movement and emotions.

Neurotransmitter—A chemical in the brain that transmits messages between neurons, or nerve cells.

Toxocariasis—Infection with roundworm larvae, commonly transmitted by the feces of dogs and cats.

Toxoplasmosis—A parasitic infection caused by the intracellular protozoan *Toxoplasmosis gondii*. Humans are most commonly infected by swallowing the oocyte form of the parasite in soil (or kitty litter) contaminated by feces from an infected cat; or by swallowing the cyst form of the parasite in raw or undercooked meat.

Trichuriasis—Infection with the larvae of roundworms. These parasites may live for 10–20 years in humans.

Treatment

The most effective strategies for treatment are based on **behavior modification**, but with limited success. Pica associated with a nutritional deficiency often clears up when the missing nutrient is added to the patient's diet.

Few studies have examined the efficacy of drug treatments for pica. Ongoing research, however, is exploring the relationship between pica and abnormally low levels of the neurotransmitter dopamine. This line of research may help to identify new medications for the treatment of pica. There is some evidence that medications used to manage severe behavioral problems in children may be useful in treating coexisting pica.

Lead poisoning resulting from pica may be treated by chelating medications, which are drugs that remove lead or other heavy metals from the bloodstream. The two medications most often given for lead poisoning are dimercaprol, which is also known as BAL or British Anti-Lewisite; and edetate calcium disodium (EDTA). A medical toxicologist (a doctor who specializes in treating poisoning cases) may be consulted regarding children's dosages of these drugs.

In some cases, surgery may be required to remove metal objects from the patient's digestive tract or to repair tissue injuries. It is particularly important to remove any objects made of lead (fishing weights, lead shot, pieces of printer's type, etc.) as quickly as possible because of the danger of lead poisoning.

Prognosis

Pica frequently ends spontaneously in young children and pregnant women. Untreated pica, however, may persist for years, especially in persons with intellectual and developmental disabilities.

Prevention

There is no known way to prevent pica at the present time. Educating people, particularly young couples with children, about healthy nutritional practices is the best preventive strategy.

Resources

BOOKS

American Psychiatric Association. "Pica." In *Diagnostic and Statistical Manual of Mental Disorders*. 4th ed., text rev. Washington, DC: American Psychiatric Association, 2000.

Herrin, Marcia, and Nancy Matsumoto. *The Parent's Guide to Childhood Eating Disorders*. New York: Henry Holt and Company, 2002.

Palmer, Robert L. *Helping People With Eating Disorders: A Clinical Guide to Assessment and Treatment*. New York: John Wiley and Sons, 2000.

Woolsey, Monika M. *Eating Disorders: A Clinical Guide to Counseling and Treatment*. Chicago: American Dietetic Association, 2002.

PERIODICALS

Grewal P., and B. Fitzgerald. "Pica with Learning Disability." *Journal of the Royal Society of Medicine* 95, no. 1 (January 2002): 39–40.

Hamilton S., et al. "Neonatal Lead Poisoning From Maternal Pica Behavior During Pregnancy." *Journal of the National Medical Association* 93, no. 9 (September 2001): 317–319.

Roberts-Harewood M., and S.C. Davies. "Pica in Sickle Cell Disease: 'She Ate the Headboard.'" *Archives of Diseases of Children* 85, no. 6 (2001): 510.

WEBSITES

Eating-Disorder.org. "Pica Eating Disorders." http://www.eating-disorder.org/pica-eating-disorders.html (accessed October 23, 2011).

PubMed Health. "Pica." U.S. National Library of Medicine, National Institutes of Health. February 28, 2010. http://www.ncbi.nlm.nih.gov/pubmedhealth/PMH0002505 (accessed October 23, 2011).

ORGANIZATIONS

American Academy of Family Physicians, 11400 Tomahawk Creek Parkway, Leawood, KS, 66211-2672, (913) 906-6000, (800) 274-2237, Fax: (913) 906-6075, contactcenter@aafp.org, http://www.aafp.org.

American Academy of Pediatrics, 141 Northwest Point Blvd., Elk Grove Village, IL, 60007-1098, (847) 434-4000, Fax: (847) 434-8000, http://www.aap.org.

American College of Physicians, 190 N Independence Mall W, Philadelphia, PA, 19106-1572, (215) 351-2400, (800) 523-1546, http://www.acponline.org.

American Medical Association, 515 N State Street, Chicago, IL, 60610, (312) 464-5000, (800) 621-8335, http://www.ama-assn.org.

L. Fleming Fallon, Jr., M.D., Dr.P.H.

Pick's disease

Definition

Frontotemporal **dementia** (FTD), originally known as Pick's disease, is a rare form of dementia that is associated with shrinking of the frontal and temporal anterior lobes of the **brain**. The name and classification of FTD has been a topic of discussion for over a century. The current designation of the syndrome groups together Pick's disease, primary progressive aphasia, and semantic dementia as FTD. As it is defined today, the symptoms of FTD fall into two clinical patterns that involve either (1) changes in behavior, or (2) problems with language. The first type features behavior that can be either impulsive (disinhibited) or bored and listless (apathetic) and includes inappropriate social behavior; lack of social tact; lack of empathy; distractibility; loss of insight into the behaviors of oneself and others; an increased interest in sex; changes in food preferences; agitation or, conversely, blunted emotions; neglect of personal hygiene; repetitive or compulsive behavior; and decreased energy and motivation. The second type primarily features symptoms of language disturbance, including difficulty making or understanding speech, often in conjunction with the behavioral type's symptoms. Spatial skills and memory remain intact. Although the exact etiology of Pick's diseases is not known, there is a strong genetic component to the disease; FTD often runs in families.

Demographics

Pick's disease is rare, affecting less than 1% of the U.S. population. It accounts for about 2%–5% of all cases of dementia. Although it sometimes appears in younger or older people, it typically begins in middle age, between the ages of 50 and 60 years. The average age of onset is 54 years and it tends to occur more often in women than in men.

Description

Pick's disease was first described by Arnold Pick, a Czechoslovakian physician who was trained in clinical neurology, psychiatry, and neuropathology. In 1892, Pick reported on a 71-year-old man with progressive loss of language and mental deterioration. After the man died, autopsy revealed asymmetrical atrophy of the frontal cortex of the brain. In 1911, Alois Alzheimer confirmed the pattern of atrophy found in brains of patients with Pick's disease. The term Pick's disease was coined by A. Gans in 1922.

The cortical atrophy seen in Pick's disease is different from **Alzheimer's disease**, although there are major overlaps with Alzheimer's presenile dementia. In Pick's disease, shrinkage is greatest in the frontal and temporal lobes. One of the characteristics of Pick's disease is microtubule-associated tau proteins, which are the main cytoskeletal components modified during the neurodegenerative changes associated with this disease. In Alzheimer's disease, any area of the brain may be affected. Abnormalities called Pick bodies and Pick cells (abnormally swollen nerve cells) are also found in the brains of individuals with Pick's disease. Pick bodies are found inside nerve cells and contain the abnormal form of tau protein that is associated with Pick's disease.

Researchers continue to debate how to classify Pick's disease. Today, few researchers use the term Pick's disease, although it is still used by patients, caregivers, and some health practitioners. Currently, Pick's disease is considered to be part of a syndrome that includes not only Pick's disease but also primary progressive aphasia and semantic dementia, which are two related disorders. The syndrome is known as FTD. Some researchers have suggested that some cases of frontotemporal dementia in which Pick bodies or Pick cells are absent may also represent a form of Pick's disease.

Causes and symptoms

The symptoms of Pick's disease vary among individuals, but changes in behavior, emotions, and language are frequently associated with neurological problems related to movement and memory. Behavioral changes include disinhibition, inappropriate behavior, compulsions such as a tendency to overeat or eat a particular kind of food, repetitive behavior, social withdrawal, inability to keep a job, difficulty initiating tasks and following through, difficulty maintaining personal hygiene, and a short attention span. Emotional changes include mood swings, inappropriate mood, lack of concern for the feelings of others, **apathy**, and indifference to behavioral changes. Language changes include decreased ability to read, write, speak, and understand language. Speech difficulties may range from difficulty finding words and diminished vocabulary to a complete inability to speak. Patients also sometimes display echolalia, or a tendency to repeat the words of others. Patients may also experience difficulty with movement and coordination, muscle weakness or rigidity, and progressively worsening memory loss. Urinary incontinence may also occur.

In the early stages of Pick's disease, patients frequently demonstrate personality changes that are manifested as inappropriate behavior. This is in contrast to Alzheimer's disease, which, in its early stages, is characterized mainly by memory loss. As Pick's disease progresses, patients become aphonic and apathetic. They eventually lapse into a vegetative state and become completely disabled. Death occurs because of malnutrition, infections, or general failure of body systems.

Diagnosis

Diagnosing Pick's disease is difficult, because symptoms overlap with those of other disorders, such as Alzheimer's disease and other dementias that affect the frontal lobes of the brain. According to the National Institutes of Health, at the present time, a definitive **diagnosis** can only be made with a brain biopsy, an invasive procedure in which a small sample of brain tissue is surgically removed for examination. Other diagnostic methods are more commonly used, which allow a diagnosis to be made by ruling out other causes of dementia.

Diagnostic procedures include a detailed clinical evaluation to assess personal and family health history, other medical conditions, overall health status, use of prescription or nonprescription drugs, current symptoms, and changes in daily functioning. Blood tests may be done to detect problems in organ function, hormone levels, and vitamin deficiencies. Neurologic exams may be performed to determine which areas of the brain are affected, and can include **electroencephalography** (EEG), computerized tomography (CT) scans, and **magnetic resonance imaging** (MRI) scans. A psychiatric evaluation may be carried out to determine whether the patient suffers from disorders such as **depression**, which can mimic or worsen the symptoms of Pick's disease.

Treatment

There is no cure for Pick's disease, and currently, there are no known medications that slow the progression of the disease. Medications that are used to treat Alzheimer's disease should not be used to treat Pick's disease, because they may increase aggression in patients.

Treatments for Pick's disease are designed to manage its symptoms. **Behavior modification** strategies, which involve rewarding appropriate behavior, may help to decrease unacceptable or dangerous behaviors. Speech therapy may be helpful for increasing language use. Occupational therapy may be used to help patients improve performance of daily living tasks. Encouraging new hobbies may help to relieve boredom in patients and decrease behavior problems.

Disorders that exacerbate confusion, such as heart failure, hypoxia, thyroid disorders, anemia, nutritional deficiencies, infections, and depression, should be treated. Medications that increase confusion, such as anticholinergics, analgesics, cimetidine, central nervous system depressants, and lidocaine, should be stopped if they are not clearly needed. In some cases, medications may be prescribed to treat aggression, agitation, or dangerous behavior.

In the early stages of Pick's disease, legal advice may help families make ethical decisions about caring for a patient.

As the disease progresses, patients may require constant monitoring and care, either at home or in an institutionalized setting. Help from visiting nurses and aides, volunteer workers, and adult protective services may be needed. Families may benefit from counseling, to help them deal with the difficulties of caring for patients. **Support groups** can also be a helpful resource for families.

Prognosis

The prognosis for Pick's disease is poor. It is a rapidly progressing disease. Death commonly occurs between 2 to 10 years after the onset of the disease.

KEY TERMS

Analgesics—Drugs that reduce pain.

Anticholinergics—Drugs that block the action of acetylcholine, a naturally occurring chemical that is involved in communication between nerve cells.

Atrophy—Shrinkage or deterioration.

Cimetidine—A drug that decreases the amount of acid in the stomach. It is used to treat conditions such as ulcers, gastroesophageal reflux disease, and heartburn.

Computerized tomography (CT) scan—An imaging technique in which x rays are taken of the brain from several different angles and combined through a computer to provide an image of the brain.

Electroencephalography (EEG)—A recording of the electric potentials of the brain from electrodes attached to the scalp.

Frontal lobe—A part of the brain that is involved in processes such as muscle movement, speech production, working memory, planning, reasoning, and judgment.

Hypoxia—Oxygen deficiency.

Lidocaine—A local anesthetic.

Magnetic resonance imaging (MRI) scan—An imaging technique in which magnetic fields, radio waves, and computer enhancement are used to create an image of brain structure.

Primary progressive aphasia—A disorder in which there is progressive loss of language skills.

Semantic dementia—A disorder in which there is progressive loss of knowledge about words and word meanings.

Temporal lobe—A part of the brain that is involved in processing auditory and visual information, emotion and motivation, and understanding language.

Prevention

There are currently no known ways of preventing Pick's disease.

Resources

BOOKS

American Psychiatric Association. *Diagnostic and Statistical Manual of Mental Disorders*. 4th ed., text rev. Washington, DC: American Psychiatric Publishing, 2000.

Brookshire, Robert H. *Introduction to Neurogenic Communication Disorders*. 6th ed. St. Louis, MO: Mosby, 2007.

PERIODICALS

Amano, Nanji. "Editorial: Neuropsychiatric Symptoms and Depression in Neurodegenerative Diseases." *Psychogeriatrics* 4, no. 1 (2004): 1–3.

Hardin, Sonya, and Brenda Schooley. "A Story of Pick's Disease: A Rare Form of Dementia." *Journal of Neuroscience Nursing* 34, no. 3 (June 1, 2002): 117–23.

Odawara, T., et al. "Short Report: Alterations of Muscarinic Acetylcholine Receptors in Atypical Pick's Disease without Pick Bodies." *Journal of Neurology, Neurosurgery and Psychiatry* 74, no. 7 (2003): 965–67.

Pearce, J. M. S. "Historical Note: Pick's Disease." *Journal of Neurology, Neurosurgery and Psychiatry* 74, no. 2 (2003): 169.

WEBSITES

MedlinePlus. "Cimetidine." U.S. National Library of Medicine, National Institutes of Health. September 22, 2011. http://www.nlm.nih.gov/medlineplus/druginfo/meds/a682256.html (accessed October 23, 2011).

MedlinePlus. "Pick's Disease." U.S. National Library of Medicine, National Institutes of Health. October 19, 2011. http://www.nlm.nih.gov/medlineplus/print/ency/article/000744.htm (accessed October 23, 2011).

U.S. National Institute of Neurological Disorders and Stroke. "NINDS Frontotemporal Dementia Information Page." January 21, 2011. http://www.ninds.nih.gov/disorders/picks/picks.htm (accessed October 23, 2011).

ORGANIZATIONS

Association for Frontotemporal Degeneration, Radnor Station Building 2, Ste. 320, 290 King of Prussia Rd., Radnor, PA, 19103, (267) 514-7221, (866) 507-7222, http://www.theaftd.org.

National Aphasia Association, 350 Seventh Ave., Ste. 902, New York, NY, 10001, (800) 922-4622, naa@aphasia.org, http://aphasia.org.

National Institute of Neurological Disorders and Stroke (NINDS), PO Box 5801, Bethesda, MD, 20824, (800) 352-9424; or (301) 496-5751; TTY (301) 468-5981, http://www.ninds.nih.gov.

Pick's Disease Support Group, info@pdsg.org.uk, http://www.pdsg.org.uk.

Ruvanee Pietersz Vilhauer, PhD

Pimozide

Definition

Pimozide is an atypical antipsychotic drug used to treat serious motor and verbal tics associated with **Tourette syndrome**. It is sold under the brand name Orap.

KEY TERMS

Dopamine—A chemical in brain tissue that serves to transmit nerve impulses (neurotransmitter) and helps to regulate movement and emotions. Large amounts of dopamine are released following ingestion of amphetamines.

Extrapyramidal symptoms—A group of side effects associated with antipsychotic medications and characterized by involuntary muscle movements, including contraction and tremor.

Schizophrenia—A major mental illness marked by psychotic symptoms, including hallucinations, delusions, and severe disruptions in thinking.

Seizure—A convulsion or uncontrolled discharge of nerve cells that may spread to other cells throughout the brain.

Tourette syndrome—An abnormal condition that causes uncontrollable facial grimaces and tics and arm and shoulder movements. Tourette syndrome is perhaps best known for uncontrollable vocal tics that include grunts, shouts, and use of obscene language (coprolalia).

Purpose

Pimozide is classified as an atypical antipsychotic drug. It is structurally similar to **haloperidol**, which was the first drug to be used in treating Tourette syndrome. Pimozide is most often used to treat symptoms of Tourette syndrome, although it has also been used for treating **schizophrenia**, mania, and other behavioral disorders.

Description

Excess **dopamine** activity in the **brain** is associated with the verbal and physical tics observed in Tourette syndrome. Like haloperidol, pimozide is believed to inhibit the actions of dopamine, a chemical in the brain.

Pimozide is broken down by the liver and eliminated from the body by the kidneys. Because pimozide is associated with health risks, it should not be used for tics that are simply annoying or cosmetic. Pimozide should be used only in patients with severe symptoms after other drug therapy has been tried and failed.

Pimozide is available in 1 mg and 2 mg tablets.

Recommended dosage

The common starting dose of pimozide in adults is 1–2 mg per day. The dose may be increased every other day until 0.2 mg per 2.2 pounds (1 kg) of body weight per day or 10 mg per day is reached, whichever is less. Doses that exceed 0.2 mg per kg per day or 10 mg daily are not recommended.

In children, the usual initial dose is 0.05 mg per 2.2 pounds (1 kg) daily and increased every 3 days to a maximum dose of 0.2 mg per kg (or 10 mg) per day.

Periodically the dosage of pimozide should be reduced to determine if tics are still present. Patients should be maintained on the lowest dose that is effective in treating this disorder.

Precautions

Pimozide is associated with an increased risk of death when used in elderly patients with **dementia**. In June 2008, the U.S. Food and Drug Administration (FDA) announced a requirement for manufacturers of pimozide (and other antipsychotic drugs) to add a warning label to their packaging stating this risk. The reason for the increase was unclear in studies, but most deaths were found to be related to either cardiovascular complications or complications associated with infection. Pimozide is not approved by the FDA for the treatment of behavior problems in older adults with dementia, and patients in this category (or caregivers of patients in this category) should discuss the risks of taking pimozide with their physician.

Pimozide may alter the rhythm of the heart, resulting in potentially fatal heart arrhythmias. As a result, it should be used with caution in people with heart disease, and these patients should be observed carefully while receiving the drug.

Women should not take pimozide while pregnant or breastfeeding. Babies born to mothers who took pimozide during pregnancy may develop extrapyramidal symptoms (EPS) and withdrawal symptoms, including agitation, trouble breathing, and difficulty feeding.

Pimozide may cause extreme drowsiness and should be used carefully by people who need to be mentally alert.

Pimozide should not be used by people with mild tics, by individuals taking stimulants such as **methylphenidate** (Ritalin), **pemoline** (Cylert), or **dextroamphetamine** (Dexedrine) since these drugs may cause tics. It should be used under close physician supervision by people who have a history of seizure disorders, as it may increase the risk and frequency of **seizures**.

Side effects

The most common side effects associated with pimozide are sleepiness, headache, stomach upset, muscle tightness, muscle weakness, difficulty moving, tremor, abnormal behavior, visual disturbances, and impotence.

QUESTIONS TO ASK YOUR DOCTOR

- What kind of changes can I expect to see or feel with this medication?
- Does it matter what time of day I take this medication? If so, what is the recommendation?
- Should I take this medication with or without food?
- What are the side effects associated with this medication?
- Will this medication interact or interfere with other medications I am currently taking?
- What symptoms or adverse effects are important enough that I should seek immediate treatment?

Other side effects that might also occur with pimozide are rapid heart rates or irregular heart rhythms, low blood pressure, constipation, dry mouth and eyes, rash, breast pain, breast milk production, loss of bladder control, or low blood cell counts.

Pimozide use cause symptoms that resemble Parkinson's disease. These symptoms may include a tight or mask-like expression on the face, drooling, tremors, pill-rolling motions in the hands, cogwheel rigidity (abnormal rigidity in muscles characterized by jerky movements when the muscle is passively stretched), and a shuffling gait. Taking anti-Parkinson drugs **benztropine** mesylate or **trihexyphenidyl** hydrochloride along with the pimozide usually controls these symptoms.

Pimozide has the potential to produce a serious side effect called **tardive dyskinesia**. This syndrome consists of involuntary, uncoordinated movements that may appear late in therapy and not disappear even after the drug is stopped. Tardive dyskinesia involves involuntary movements of the tongue, jaw, mouth or face or other groups of skeletal muscles. The incidence of tardive dyskinesia increases with increasing age and with increasing dosage of pimozide. Women are at greater risk than men for developing tardive dyskinesia. There is no known effective treatment for tardive dyskinesia, although gradual (but rarely complete) improvement may occur over a long period.

An occasionally reported side effect of pimozide is **neuroleptic malignant syndrome**, a complicated and potentially fatal condition characterized by muscle rigidity, high fever, alterations in mental status, and cardiac symptoms such as irregular pulse or blood pressure, sweating, tachycardia (fast heartbeat), and arrhythmias (irregular heartbeat). People who think they may be experiencing any side effects from pimozide or any other medication should talk to their physician promptly.

Interactions

If pimozide is used with bethanechol (Urecholine), **clonidine** (Catapress), **fluoxetine** (Prozac), indomethacin (Indocin), meperidine (Demerol), **paroxetine** (Paxil), quinidine, or **trazodone** (Desyrel), the side effects associated with pimozide may be increased.

There is an increased risk of irregular heart rhythms if pimozide is used with other antipsychotics, certain **antidepressants**, some heart drugs, and antibiotics such as erythromycin.

The beneficial effects of pimozide may be reduced if used with bromocriptine (Parlodel), **carbamazepine** (Tegretol), levodopa (Larodopa, Sinemet), lithium, or phenobarbital.

Some antibiotics, antifungals, antidepressants, and drugs used for AIDS may prevent the breakdown of pimozide by the liver and thus increase the amount of pimozide in the body. The combination of pimozide and these classes of drugs should be used cautiously if at all.

Pimozide may increase the sedative effects of other central nervous system depressants such as alcohol, sleeping pills, antihistamines, and antidepressants.

Pimozide should not be taken with grapefruit juice, as it inhibits the metabolism of the drug in the body.

Resources

BOOKS

Albers, Lawrence J., Rhoda K. Hahn, and Christopher Reist. *Handbook of Psychiatric Drugs.* Laguna Hills, CA: Current Clinical Strategies, 2010.

American Society of Health-System Pharmacists. *AHFS Drug Information 2011.* Bethesda, MD: ASHP, 2011.

Graham, George. *The Disordered Mind: An Introduction to Philosophy of Mind and Mental Illness.* New York: Routledge, 2010.

Holland, Leland Norman, and Michael Patrick Adams. *Core Concepts in Pharmacology.* 3rd ed. New York: Prentice Hall, 2011.

North, Carol, and Sean Yutzy. *Goodwin and Guze's Psychiatric Diagnosis.* New York: Oxford University Press, 2010.

Preston, John D., John H. O'Neal, and Mary C. Talaga. *Handbook of Clinical Psychopharmacology for Therapists.* 6th ed. Oakland, CA: New Harbinger, 2010.

ORGANIZATIONS

American Academy of Clinical Toxicology, 6728 Old McLean Village Dr., McLean, VA, 22101, (703) 556-9222, Fax: (703) 556-8729, admin@clintox.org, http://www.clintox.org.

American Academy of Family Physicians, 11400 Tomahawk Creek Pkwy., Leawood, KS, 66211-2672, (913) 906-6000, (800) 274-2237, Fax: (913) 906-6075, contactcenter@aafp.org, http://www.aafp.org.

American Academy of Neurology, 1080 Montreal Ave., St. Paul, MN, 55116, (651) 695-2717, (800) 879-1960, Fax: (651) 879-2791, memberservices@aan.com, http://www.aan.com.

American Neurological Association, 5841 Cedar Lake Rd., Ste. 204, Minneapolis, MN, 55416, (952) 545-6284, ana@llmsi.com, http://www.aneuroa.org.

American Psychiatric Association, 1000 Wilson Blvd., Ste. 1825, Arlington, VA, 22209-3901, (703) 907-7300, apa@psych.org, http://www.psych.org.

American Society for Clinical Pharmacology and Therapeutics, 528 N Washington St., Alexandria, VA, 22314, (703) 836-6981, info@ascpt.org, http://www.ascpt.org.

Mental Health America, 2000 N. Beauregard St., 6th Fl., Alexandria, VA, 22311, (703) 684-7722, (800) 969-6642, Fax: (703) 684-5968, http://www1.nmha.org.

National Institute of Neurological Disorders and Stroke (NINDS), PO Box 5801, Bethesda, MD, 20824, (301) 496-5751; TTY: (301) 468-5981, (800) 352-9424, http://www.ninds.nih.gov.

Kelly Karpa, RPh, PhD
Laura Jean Cataldo, RN, EdD

Play therapy

Definition

Play therapy refers to a method of **psychotherapy** with children in which a therapist uses a child's fantasies and the symbolic meanings of his or her play as a medium for understanding and communication with the child.

Purpose

The aim of play therapy is to decrease those behavioral and emotional difficulties that significantly interfere with a child's normal functioning. Inherent in this aim is improved communication and understanding between the child and his or her parents. Less obvious goals include improved verbal expression, ability for self-observation, improved impulse control, more adaptive ways of coping with anxiety and frustration, and

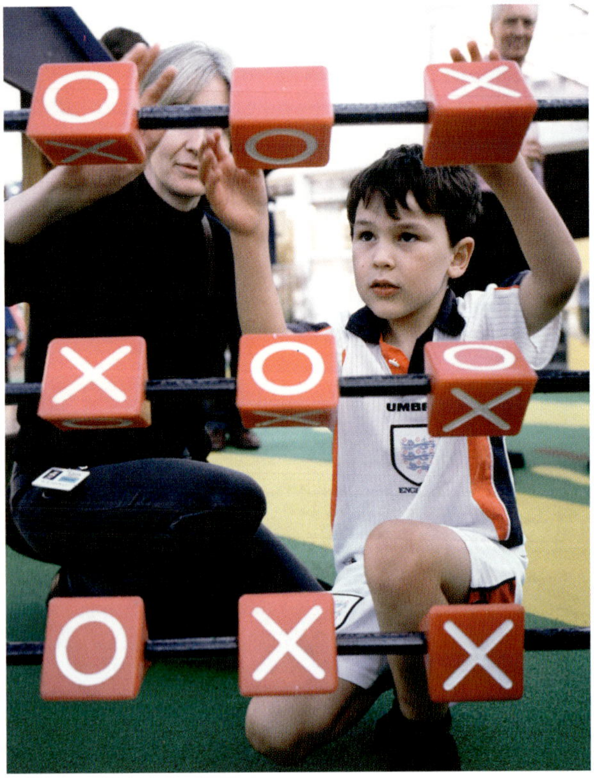

A boy plays in a play area designed to assess children with special needs. *(© James King-Holmes/Photo Researchers, Inc.)*

improved capacity to trust and to relate to others. In this type of treatment, the therapist uses an understanding of cognitive development and the different stages of emotional development as well as the conflicts common to these stages when treating the child.

The use of play therapy relies on the fact that children will process the world in a way that is different from the adult approach. Some researchers describe two stages of function for children at the elementary school level: the "preoperational stage" (ages 2 to 7 years) and the "concrete operations stage" (ages 8 to 11 years). In the preoperational stage, children are still learning how to use language, which employs symbols (words) to mentally represent the things in their world. They tend to have rigid thinking processes, limited only to what is before them, without digging more deeply. Because this results in a lack of true understanding of the world around them, they will provide their own explanations, employing "magical thinking." The child's play, as a result, will increasingly employ imagination and fantasy as he or she ages. Adults who can understand how the play and fantasy translate from a child to an adult world can interpret the child's language.

Play therapy thus relies on the fact that the language of children, especially very young children, is play. Play also serves several other roles for children that can be used in the process of play therapy, including providing a sense of control and a way to develop coping skills. A skilled play therapist will be able to make the most of these factors in using play therapy as a way to translate the child's communications.

Play therapy is used to treat problems that are interfering with the child's normal development. Such difficulties are extreme in degree and have been occurring for many months without resolution. Reasons for treatment include, but are not limited to, temper tantrums, aggressive behavior, nonmedical problems with bowel or bladder control, difficulties with sleeping or having nightmares, and experiencing worries or fears. This type of treatment is also used with children who have experienced sexual or physical **abuse**, **neglect**, the loss of a family member, medical illness, physical injury, or any experience that is traumatic.

At times, children in play therapy will also receive other types of treatment. For instance, youngsters who are unable to control their attention, impulses, tendency to react with violence, or who experience severe anxiety may take medication for these symptoms while participating in play therapy. The play therapy addresses the child's psychological symptoms. Other situations of dual treatment include children with **learning disorders**. These youngsters may receive play therapy to alleviate feelings of low self-esteem, excessive worry, helplessness, and incompetence that are related to their learning problems and academic struggles. In addition, they should receive a special type of tutoring called **cognitive remediation**, which addresses the specific learning issues.

Description

In play therapy, the clinician may meet with the child alone for sessions or with a parent present, and may arrange times to meet with parents separately, depending on the situation. In some forms of play therapy, the therapist may observe the child at play with the parent. The structure of the sessions is maintained in a consistent manner to provide a feeling of safety and stability for the child and parents. Sessions are scheduled for the same day and time each week and occur for the same duration. The frequency of sessions is typically one or two times per week, and meetings with parents occur about two times per month, with some variation. The session length will vary depending on the environment. For example, in private settings, sessions usually last 45 to 50 minutes while in hospitals and mental health clinics the duration is typically 30 minutes. The number of sessions and duration of treatment varies according to the treatment objectives.

MELANIE KLEIN (1882–1960)

The Austrian psychotherapist and child psychologist Melanie Klein developed methods of play technique and play therapy in analyzing and treating child patients. Raised in a Jewish middle-class family, she lacked both the academic background and the medical training usually found in those who choose psychoanalysis for a profession. She was a married woman with children when she began undergoing analysis about 1912. During her analysis she began to observe the behavior of a disturbed child relative and to interpret this behavior in the light of her own psychoanalytic experience. Her analyst, recognizing his patient's aptitude, encouraged her in her efforts at child therapy, a hitherto neglected area.

Originally trained as a Freudian psychoanalyst, Klein made observations and conclusions regarding child behavior that led her to views differing from those held by orthodox Freudian psychoanalysts. She was one of the first to engage in child analysis, beginning in 1920. She evolved a system of play therapy to supplement the usual psychoanalytic procedure, perhaps because the age of her clients indicated more appropriate methods than the exclusively verbal free-association technique then used with adult patients. Gradually she evolved a technique more suitable for probing the deep-layered recesses of the child's mind. By providing the child with small toys representing father, mother, or siblings, she was able to elicit the child's subconscious feelings. Her technique also used the child's free play and spontaneous communications.

Her first paper, "The Development of a Child," was presented to the Budapest Congress of Psychoanalysis in 1919, the year in which she became a member of the Hungarian Psychoanalytic Society. In 1921 she went to the Berlin Psychoanalytic Institute as the first child therapist.In what has been called her second period, beginning in 1934, Klein theorized her previous observations on child behavior, arriving at conceptual conclusions based on them. She then wrote of her earlier findings, on the "depressive position" and the "schizoid-paranoid position," indicating possible ways in which these infancy states relate to psychotic processes in adults.

During the initial meeting with parents, the therapist will want to learn as much as possible about the nature of the child's problems. Parents will be asked for information about the child's developmental, medical, social, and school history, whether or not previous evaluations and interventions were attempted, and the nature of the results. Background information about the parents is also important since it provides the therapist with a larger context from which to understand the child. This process of gathering information may take one to three sessions, depending on the style of the therapist. Some clinicians gather the important aspects of the child's history during the first meeting with parents and will continue to ask relevant questions during subsequent meetings. The clinician also learns important information during the initial sessions with the child.

Sessions with parents are important opportunities to keep the therapist informed about the child's current functioning at home and at school and for the therapist to offer some insight and guidance to parents. At times, the clinician will provide suggestions about parenting techniques and about alternative ways to communicate with their child, and will also serve as a resource for information about child development. Details of child sessions are not routinely discussed with parents. If the child's privacy is maintained, it promotes free expression in the therapist's office and engenders a sense of trust in the therapist. Therapists will, instead, communicate to the parents their understanding of the child's psychological needs or conflicts.

For the purposes of explanation, treatment can be described as occurring in a series of initial, middle, and final stages. The initial phase includes evaluation of the problem and teaching both child and parents about the process of therapy. The middle phase is the period in which the child has become familiar with the treatment process and comfortable with the therapist. The therapist is continuing to evaluate and learn about the child, but has a clearer sense of the youngster's issues and has developed, with the child, a means for the two to communicate. The final phase includes the process of ending treatment and saying goodbye to the therapist.

During the early sessions, the therapist may talk with the child about the reason the youngster was brought in for treatment and explain that the therapist helps make children's problems go away. Youngsters often deny experiencing any problems. It is not necessary for them to acknowledge having any since they may be unable to do so due to normal cognitive and emotional factors or because they are simply not experiencing any problems. The child may be informed about the nature of the sessions, specifically that he or she can say or play or do anything desired while in the office as long as no one gets hurt; what is said and done in the office will be kept private unless the child is in danger of harming himself.

Children communicate their thoughts and feelings through play more naturally than they do through verbal communication. As the child plays, the therapist begins to recognize themes and patterns or ways of using the materials that are important to the child. Over time, the clinician helps the child begin to make meaning out of the play. This is important because the play reflects issues which are important to the child and typically relevant to their difficulties.

When the child's symptoms have subsided for a stable period of time and when functioning is adequate with peers and adults at home, in school, and in extracurricular activities, the focus of treatment will shift away from problems and onto the process of saying goodbye. This last stage is known as the termination phase of treatment and it is reflective of the ongoing change and loss that human beings experience throughout their lives. Since this type of therapy relies heavily on the therapist's relationship with the child and also with parents, ending therapy will signify a change and a loss for all involved, but for the child in particular. In keeping with the therapeutic process of communicating thoughts and feelings, this stage is an opportunity for the child to work through how he or she feels about ending therapy and about leaving the therapist. In addition to allowing for a sense of closure, it also makes it less likely that the youngster will misconstrue the ending of treatment as a rejection by the therapist, which would taint the larger experience of therapy for the child. Parents also need a sense of closure and are usually encouraged to process the treatment experience with the therapist. The therapist also appreciates the opportunity to say goodbye to the parents and child after having become involved in their lives in this important way, and it is often beneficial for parents and children to hear the clinician's thoughts and feelings with regards to ending treatment.

Precautions

Play therapy addresses psychological issues and is not used to alleviate medical or biological problems. Children who are experiencing physical problems should see a physician for a medical evaluation to clarify the nature of the problem and, if necessary, receive the appropriate medical treatment. Likewise, children who experience academic difficulties need to receive a neuropsychological or in-depth psychological evaluation in order to clarify the presence of a biologically based learning disability. In both of these cases, psychological problems may be present in addition to medical ailments and learning disabilities. It is necessary to evaluate and treat both physical and psychological issues. Alternatively, evaluations may show that medical or biological causes are not evident, and this is important information for the parents and therapist.

Preparation

It is recommended that parents explain to the child that they will be going to see a therapist and discuss, if possible, the particular problem and that the therapist is going to teach both parents and child how to make things better. As described earlier, the child may deny even obvious problems, but mainly just needs to agree to meet the therapist and to see what therapy is like.

Aftercare

Children sometimes return to therapy for additional sessions when they experience a setback that cannot be easily resolved.

Results

Normal results include the significant reduction or disappearance of the main problems for which the child was initially seen. The child should also be functioning adequately at home, in school, and with peers, and should be able to participate in and enjoy extracurricular activities.

Sometimes play therapy does not alleviate the child's symptoms. This situation can occur if the child is extremely resistant and refuses to participate in treatment or if the child's ways of coping are so rigidly held that it is not possible for them to learn more adaptive ones.

Resources

BOOKS

Chethik, Morton. *Techniques of Child Therapy*. 2nd ed. New York: The Guilford Press, 2003.

Lovinger, Sophie L. *Child Psychotherapy: From Initial Therapeutic Contact to Termination*. New Jersey: Jason Aronson, 1998.

Webb, Nancy Boyd, ed. *Play Therapy with Children in Crisis*. 3rd ed. New York: The Guilford Press, 2007.

PERIODICALS

Naylor, Angie. "When A Child Plays." *Counselling and Psychotherapy Journal* 16, no. 5 (June 2005): 29–31.

Ray, Dee C., et al. "Play Therapy Practices Among Elementary School Counselors." *Professional School Counseling* 8 (April 2005): 360–65.

ORGANIZATIONS

American Psychological Association, 750 1st Street NE, Washington, DC, 20002-4242, (202) 336-5500; TDD/TTY: (202) 336-6123, (800) 374-2721, http://www.apa.org.

Association for Play Therapy, Inc, 3198 Willow Ave., Ste. 110, Clovis, CA, 93703, (599) 294-2128, Fax: (559) 294-2129, info@a4pt.org, http://www.a4pt.org.

Susan Fine, Psy.D.
Emily Jane Willingham, PhD

PMDD *see* **Premenstrual dysphoric disorder**

PMS *see* **Premenstrual syndrome**

Polysomnography

Definition

Polysomnography is a set of tests performed while a patient sleeps. It is used to diagnose and evaluate **sleep disorders**, and examines at a minimum **brain** wave patterns, the movements of both eyes, and the tone of at least one skeletal muscle.

Purpose

Polysomnography is used to diagnose and evaluate many types of sleep disorders, including disorders of initiating or maintaining sleep (dyssomnias) and disorders during sleep (parasomnias), including medical, psychiatric, and dental disorders that have symptoms during sleep. A relatively common dyssomnia is sleep apnea, a disorder most prevalent in middle-aged and elderly obese men, in which the muscles of the soft palate in the back of the throat relax and close off the airway during sleep. Sleep apnea may cause the patient to snore loudly and gasp for air at night, and to be excessively sleepy and doze off during the day.

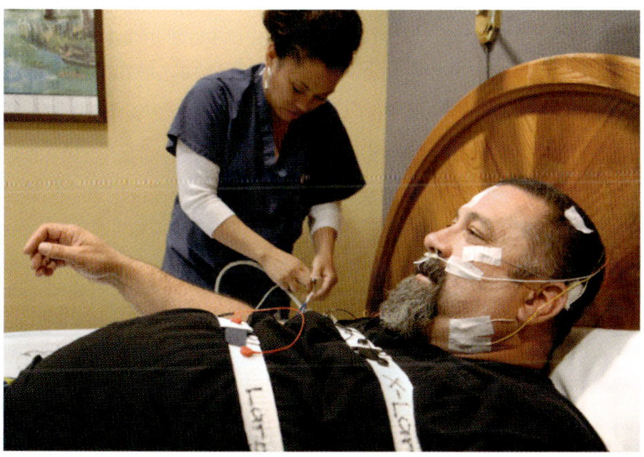

A man prepares to undergo polysomnography at a sleep disorders clinic. *(© Florence Low/MCT/newscom)*

Another dyssomnia often evaluated by polysomnography is **narcolepsy**. Narcoleptics suffer from excessive daytime sleepiness, sudden attacks of muscle weakness (cataplexy), and hallucinations at sleep onset. Some parasomnias that can be detected using polysomnography include disorders of arousal or rapid-eye-movement (REM) sleep problems, such as nightmares. Medical conditions including sleep-related asthma, **depression**, and **panic disorder** can be evaluated. Teeth-grinding (bruxism) or neurological problems such as restless leg syndrome show up during polysomnography. Finally, the tests can also be used to detect or evaluate **seizures** of sleep-related epilepsy that occur in the middle of the night, when the patient and his or her family are unlikely to be aware of them.

Description

Polysomnography is performed during an overnight stay in a sleep laboratory. While the patient sleeps, a wide variety of tests can be performed.

One form of monitoring is **electroencephalography** (EEG), in which electrodes are attached to the patient's scalp in order to record his or her brain wave activity. The electroencephalograph records brain wave activity from different parts of the brain and charts them on a graph. The EEG not only helps doctors establish what stage of sleep the patient is in, but may also detect seizures. Standard tests have at least one central electrode attached to the scalp and one reference electrode attached to the ear. Other electrodes can be added in order to pinpoint the area of the brain where abnormal activity is occurring.

Another form of monitoring is continuous electrooculography (EOG), which records eye movement and is useful in determining when the patient is going through a stage of REM sleep. Both EEG and EOG can be helpful in determining sleep latency (the time that transpires between lights out and the onset of sleep), total sleep time, the time spent in each sleep stage, and the number of arousals from sleep.

The air flow through the patient's nose and mouth is measured by heat-sensitive devices called thermistors. This measurement can help detect episodes of apnea (stopped breathing), or hypopnea (inadequate breathing). Another test, called pulse oximetry, measures the amount of oxygen in the blood and can be used to assess the degree of oxygen starvation during episodes of hypopnea or apnea.

The electrical activity of the patient's heart is also measured using electrocardiography (ECG or EKG). Electrodes are affixed to the patient's chest and pick up electrical activity from various areas of the heart. They help detect cardiac arrhythmias (abnormal heart rhythms), which may occur during periods of sleep apnea. Blood pressure is also measured as episodes of sleep apnea sometimes dangerously elevate blood pressure.

A final standard measurement is the tone of at least one skeletal muscle, often a muscle of the chin (mentalis or submentalis). This is done using electromyography (EMG), which involves placing an electrode on the muscle to record its contractions. If normal, measurements will indicate the general atonia present during REM sleep. Other EMG channels can be placed, particularly on the leg (anterior tibialis), to indicate movement during sleep.

Depending on the suspected disorder, polysomnography can also include sound monitoring to record snoring; video monitoring to document body positions; core body temperature readings; incident light intensities; penile swelling (tumescence); and pressure and pH at various levels of the esophagus.

One test that is often performed in conjunction with polysomnography is a Multiple Sleep Latency Test (MSLT). This test is also performed in a sleep laboratory and involves the recording of the sleep of several naps during the day after the overnight test. The MSLT is particularly important for a complete **diagnosis** of narcolepsy.

Preparation

Patient preparation is necessary to ensure that the night or nights in the sleep laboratory are as close as possible to an unmediated night in the patient's own home. Patients should bring suitable sleepwear and make sure their hair is clean and free from gels or sprays that may interfere with electrode functioning. They should be advised to maintain usual awake-sleep cycles and avoid sleeping pills, alcohol, stimulants, and strenuous **exercise** before the test.

Aftercare

Once the test is over, the monitors are detached from the patient. No special measures need to be taken after polysomnography.

Precautions

The greatest limitation to polysomnography are the differences between the recording conditions and those that are present in the patient's home. The differences between the sleep laboratory and home have the highest effect on the first night of testing. Detection and elimination of this "first night effect" can be accomplished by the rather costly step of recording for multiple nights. Multiple night recordings are also sometimes necessary to obtain information about problems that only appear sporadically.

Results

Standard analysis involves the manual review and scoring of either paper tracings or recordings projected on a computer monitor. Automatic, computer-based systems are becoming more and more common in clinical and research settings.

Overnight parameters such as the times of lights on/off, total time in bed, and total sleep time are factored into the results. The overnight recording is divided into time periods of approximately 30 seconds. The standard EEG, EMG, and EOG recordings are evaluated, and the predominant stage of sleep, according to the manual of Rechtschaffen and Kales, is assigned to the entire time period.

This data is used to calculate total time and relative proportion of the night spent in each of the six stages of sleep, including REM and non-REM. Latencies to REM and slow-wave sleep (SWS) are also recorded.

Special note is made of such neurophysiologic events as epileptic episodes, intrusion of alpha-type brain waves into sleep, or periodic activity of the tibialis anterior. Respiratory activities, including apneic or hypopneic episodes and oxygen saturation, are correlated with sleep stages. Other parameters measured, such as body position, gastroesophageal reflux, bruxism, and penile tumescence, are recorded.

If a sleep apnea syndrome is diagnosed, primarily through a showing of periodic breathing stoppage and effects on the pulse and heart, a trial of continuous positive airway pressure or a trial of an oral appliance may be undertaken, either in a partial-night or second-night polysomnography recording.

Healthcare team roles

Polysomnography is often performed by a specially trained technician called a polysomnographic technologist. Training programs for this position can involve

KEY TERMS

Apnea—A brief suspension or interruption of breathing.

Arrhythmia—Any disturbance in the normal rhythm of the heartbeat.

Bruxism—Habitual, often unconscious, grinding of the teeth.

Hypopnea—Breathing that is too shallow to maintain adequate levels of oxygen in the blood.

Narcolepsy—A disorder characterized by frequent and uncontrollable attacks of deep sleep.

Oximetry—The measurement of blood oxygen levels.

Parameter—A characteristic or factor that is measured during a test of a complex process or activity like sleep.

Parasomnia—A type of sleep disorder characterized by abnormal changes in behavior or body functions during sleep, specific stages of sleep, or the transition between sleeping and waking.

Thermistor—An electrical device whose resistance decreases with rises in temperature.

one- to two-year programs in training as an electrodiagnostic technologist, with additional time for the polysomnography courses. Some typical courses in this area include:

- fundamentals of polysomnography
- sleep disorders
- infant and pediatric polysomnography
- polysomnography instrumentation
- polysomnography recording and monitoring
- polysomnography record scoring

Registration in polysomnography is available from the Board of Registered Polysomnography Technologists. The certification requires passing a written test.

Resources

BOOKS

Misulis, Karl E. "Polysomnography Basics." In *Essentials of Clinical Neurophysiology,* by Karl E. Misulis and T.C. Head. 3rd ed. London: Butterworth-Heinemann, 2002.

PERIODICALS

Grandjean, Cynthia, and Susanne Gibbons. "Assessing Ambulatory Geriatric Sleep Complaints." *The Nurse Practitioner* 25, no. 9 (September 2000): 25, 29–32, 35.

WEBSITES

Armon, Carmel, K.G. Johnson, and Asim Roy. "Polysomnography." Medscape Reference. November 23, 2009. http://www.emedicine.com/neuro/topic566.htm (accessed October 23, 2011).

ORGANIZATIONS

American Association of Sleep Technologists, 2510 North Frontage Rd., Darien, IL, 60561, (630) 737-9704, Fax: (630) 737-9788, AAST@aastweb.org, http://www.aastweb.org.

National Sleep Foundation, 1010 N Glebe Rd., Ste. 310, Arlington, VA, 22201, (703) 243-1697, nsf@sleepfoundation.org, http://www.sleepfoundation.org.

Michelle L. Johnson, M.S., J.D.

Polysubstance dependence

Definition

Polysubstance dependence refers to a type of substance dependence disorder in which an individual uses at least three different classes of substances indiscriminately and does not have a favorite drug that qualifies for dependence on its own.

Demographics

Young adults (between the ages of 18 and 24) have the highest rates of use for all substances. Generally, males tend to be diagnosed with more substance use disorders.

Description

The ***Diagnostic and Statistical Manual of Mental Disorders***, fourth edition, text revision (*DSM-IV-TR*), which presents guidelines used by the American Psychiatric Association for diagnosis of mental disorders, defines polysubstance dependence as repeated use of at least three groups of substances (not including caffeine and nicotine) with no single predominate substance. For example, an individual may use **cocaine**, **sedatives**, and **hallucinogens** indiscriminately (i.e., no single drug predominated or no "drug of choice") for a year or more. The individual may not meet criteria for cocaine dependence, sedative dependence, or hallucinogen dependence, but may meet criteria for polysubstance dependence when all three drugs are considered as a group.

Causes and symptoms

Causes

There is very little documented regarding the causes of polysubstance dependence.

Symptoms

The *DSM-IV-TR* specifies that three or more of the following symptoms must occur at any time during a 12-month period (and cause significant impairment or distress) in order to meet diagnostic criteria for substance dependence:

- Tolerance: The individual either has to use increasingly higher amounts of the drugs over time in order to achieve the same drug effect or finds that the same amount of the drug has much less of an effect over time than before. After using several different drugs regularly for a while, an individual may find they need to use at least 50% more of the amount they began using in order to get the same effect.
- Withdrawal: The individual either experiences withdrawal symptoms when he or she stops using the drugs or the individual uses drugs in order to avoid or relieve withdrawal symptoms.
- Loss of control: The individual either repeatedly uses more drugs than planned or uses the drugs over longer periods of time than planned. For instance, an individual may begin using drugs (any combination of three or more types of drugs) on weekdays in addition to weekends.
- Inability to stop using: The individual has either unsuccessfully attempted to cut down or stop using the drugs or has a persistent desire to stop using. An individual may find that, despite efforts to stop using drugs on weekdays, he or she is unable to do so.
- Time: The individual spends a lot of time obtaining drugs, using drugs, being under the influence of drugs, and recovering from the effects of drugs.
- Interference with activities: The individual either gives up or reduces the amount of time involved in recreational activities, social activities, and/or occupational activities because of the use of drugs. An individual may use drugs instead of engaging in hobbies, spending time with friends, or going to work.
- Harm to self: The individual continues to use drugs despite having either a physical or psychological problem that is caused by or made worse by the use of drugs.

Diagnosis

Individuals who abuse alcohol and other drugs usually meet criteria for **substance abuse** and/or dependence for each individual substance used. Multiple diagnoses are given in this situation (cocaine dependence, hallucinogen dependence, and sedative dependence, for example). Polysubstance dependence is reserved only for those situations when an individual uses multiple substances indiscriminately and meets criteria for dependence on these substances, taken as a whole.

Treatment

There is very little documented regarding the treatment of polysubstance dependence. However, several treatments have been tried. Psychological evaluation and tests may be used to assess the affected individual. The person may be admitted into a hospital or treatment center as an inpatient, and/or he or she may receive **cognitive-behavioral therapy**.

Prognosis

The course of substance dependence varies from short-lived episodes to chronic episodes lasting years. The individual with substance dependence may alternate between periods of heavy use with severe problems, periods of no use at all, and periods of use with few problems.

Prevention

The best single thing an individual can do to prevent polysubstance dependence is to avoid using drugs including alcohol altogether. On a larger scale, comprehensive prevention programs that utilize family, schools, communities, and the media (such as television) can be effective in reducing substance abuse.

Resources

BOOKS

American Psychiatric Association. *Diagnostic and Statistical Manual of Mental Disorders*. 4th ed., text rev. Washington, DC: American Psychiatric Publishing, 2000.

Kaplan, Harold, and Benjamin Sadock, eds. *Synopsis of Psychiatry*. 10th ed. Baltimore: Lippincott Williams & Wilkins, 2007.

Jennifer Hahn, Ph.D.

Positive symptoms

Definition

Positive symptoms are thoughts, behaviors, or sensory perceptions present in a person with a mental disorder, but not present in people in the normal population.

Description

Examples of positive symptoms are hallucinations (seeing, hearing, or smelling things not really there), **delusions** (belief in ideas not based on reality), disorganized speech (loose association between ideas, derailment of sentences, incoherence, illogical statements, excessive detail, and rhyming of words), or bizarre behavior. In other disorders, positive symptoms are primarily associated with **schizophrenia** or **psychosis**.

Sandra L. Friedrich, M.A.

Positron emission tomography (PET)

Definition

Positron emission tomography (PET) is a noninvasive scanning/imaging technique that utilizes small amounts of radioactive positrons (positively charged particles; also called "antielectrons") to visualize body function and metabolism. The PET scan uses a special camera and tracer (such as glucose with an added radioactive chemical) to take images of organs and tissues within the body. The camera records the position of the tracer, and the resulting data are then sent to a computer for analysis.

When higher levels of chemical activity occur in the body, the radioactive chemical within the tracer will accumulate in such areas. These areas show up as brighter spots on a PET scan and are useful for evaluating problems within the body. The resulting image is used to evaluate for body disorders such as cancer, neurological problems, and heart disease, along with the flow of blood and the function of organs. PET scans are especially useful to study **brain** activity in mentally ill patients and how mental illness can change activity within the brain.

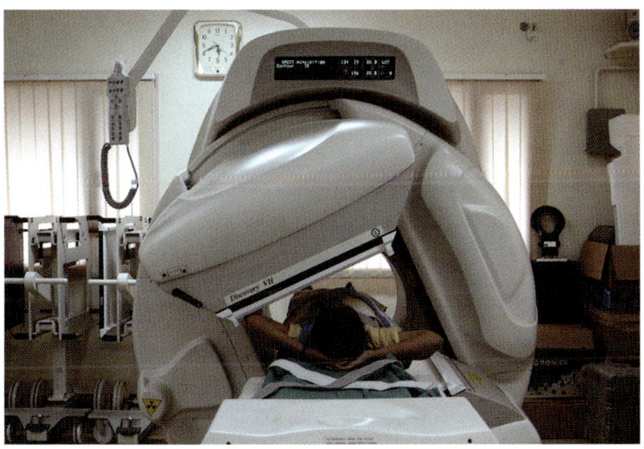

A patient prepares to undergo a positron emission tomography (PET) scan. *(© Dinodia Photos/Alamy)*

Purpose

PET is the fastest-growing nuclear medicine tool in terms of increasing acceptance and applications. It is useful in the **diagnosis**, staging, and treatment of cancer because it provides information that cannot be obtained by other techniques, such as **computed tomography** (CT) and **magnetic resonance imaging** (MRI).

PET scans are performed at medical centers equipped with a small cyclotron. Smaller cyclotrons and increasing availability of certain radiopharmaceuticals are making PET a more widely used imaging modality.

Physicians first used PET to obtain information about brain function, and to study brain activity in various neurological diseases and disorders including **stroke**, epilepsy, **Alzheimer's disease**, Parkinson's disease, and Huntington's disease; and in psychiatric disorders such as **schizophrenia**, **depression**, **obsessive-compulsive disorder** (OCD), **attention deficit hyperactivity disorder (ADHD)**, and **Tourette syndrome**. PET is now used to evaluate patients for types of cancer, including head and neck, brain, lymphoma, melanoma, lung, colorectal, breast, prostate, and esophageal. Cancer is more likely to show up on a PET scan than on a CT or MRI scan.

Because of the clarity of a PET scan, doctors can better see how advanced a cancer is at its place or origin and whether it has spread to other parts of the body. In order to treat cancer, a PET scan is often performed along with a CT or MRI scan. PET also is used to evaluate heart muscle function in patients with coronary artery disease (CAD) or cardiomyopathy. A PET scan is able to determine whether there is poor blood flow to the heart, which is a sign of CAD. If poor blood flow is found, a PET scan also helps to determine the best treatment, for example, coronary artery bypass graft surgery.

PET scans are especially useful for brain-imaging studies. They are often used to illustrate the differences between brains of people without mental disorders and brains of people with mental disorders. For example, because PET scans can detect brain activity (such as blood flow and metabolic activity), PET scans of the brains of depressed and nondepressed persons can show researchers where brain activity is decreased in depressed patients. Similar scans have been taken of brains affected by schizophrenia or Alzheimer's disease. They are also used for people suspected of having amyotrophic lateral sclerosis (ALS), transient ischemic attack (TIA), multiple sclerosis (MS), and other nervous system disorders. Such research can help scientists discover new ways to treat these disorders. Further, once treated, PET scans can tell medical professionals how the activity within specific areas of the brain of mentally ill patients has changed. In psychiatric illness, PET scans are primarily used in research studies rather than as aids to treatment in clinical settings.

Description

While in a nuclear medicine department of a hospital or a specialized PET center, the PET involves injecting a patient with a radiopharmaceutical similar to glucose, a form of sugar. Often fludeoxyglucose (FDG), which contains a radioactive isotope (such as fluorine-18), is used as the trace material. The tracer is a liquid that is placed into the body usually through an intravenous injection into a vein on the arm (or the substance may also be inhaled or swallowed). While the patient lies very still on a table, the tracer moves through the body, collecting at specific organs or tissues. An hour after injection of this tracer, a PET scanner images a specific metabolic function by measuring the concentration and distribution of the tracer throughout the body. The scanner, which is shaped like a doughnut, moves around the patient. The complete test usually takes from one to three hours.

When it enters the body, the tracer courses through the bloodstream to the target organ, where it emits positrons. The positively charged positrons collide with negatively charged electrons, producing gamma rays (a type of electromagnetic radiation). The positrons are absorbed to a different extent by cells varying in their metabolic rate. The gamma rays are detected by photomultiplier-scintillator combinations positioned on opposite sides of the patient. These signals are processed by the computer, and images are generated.

PET scans do not show as much detail as computed tomography (CT) scans or magnetic resonance imaging (MRI) scans. However, PET scans provide an advantage over CT and MRI because they can determine whether a lesion is malignant. The two other modalities provide images of anatomical structures but often cannot provide a determination of malignancy. CT and MRI show structure, while PET shows function. PET has been used in combination with CT and MRI to identify abnormalities with more precision and indicate areas of most active metabolism. This additional information allows for more accurate evaluation of cancer treatment and management.

KEY TERMS

Computed tomography—An imaging technique that produces images of cross-sections of the body using data acquired through x rays directed in various directions through the body and onto a screen.

Magnetic resonance imaging—An imaging technique that produces images of the body's soft tissues with the use of electromagnetic radiation and a strong magnetic field.

Photomultiplier—A device that is designed to be extremely sensitive to electromagnetic radiation, especially within the ultraviolet, visible, and near-infrared ranges of the electromagnetic spectrum.

Positron—A positively charged particle; also called an "antielectron," the antimatter counterpart of the electron.

Radioactive—Relating to radiation emitted by certain substances.

Radiopharmaceutical—A radioactive drug.

Scintillator—A material that exhibits the property of luminescence (also called "scintillation") when it is excited by ionizing radiation.

Precautions

Several precautionary factors may cause the PET scan to be canceled or invalidated. Three of them that might cancel the test are using alcohol, caffeine, or tobacco within 24 hours of the test; using **sedatives** before the test; or taking medicines such as insulin (which can change a body's metabolism). Two conditions that might invalidate the test include not lying still during the test or being too anxious or nervous during the test. In addition, a PET scan may have to be delayed if a patient recently had a biopsy taken from the body, chemotherapy, radiation therapy, or any type of surgery.

Preparation

Before having or scheduling a PET scan, inform the referring doctor about any of the following: diabetes, pregnancy, or breastfeeding. The dosage of any diabetic medicine on the day of the scan may be reduced or eliminated to accommodate the PET procedure. Do not breastfeed for at least one day before having a PET scan. Discuss this with a medical profession before having the test. In addition, tell the referring doctor about any other medicines or herbal remedies being taken. Such substances may be stopped before the PET test. Do not smoke tobacco products, drink caffeinated beverages or foods, or drink alcoholic beverages for at least 24 hours before the test. Do not eat or drink for at least six hours before the test. Discuss the PET scan with the referring doctor or the attending medical team for other such considerations.

Inform the referring doctor if a fear of enclosed spaces is a problem or of any concerns regarding anxiety or **panic attack** while undergoing the test.

During the test, a small prick or sting may be felt at the injection site. When the tracer liquid is inserted into the body, it may initially make the patient feel warm and slightly flushed. In a small number of instances, patients feel sick to their stomach or may develop a headache. Always inform the medical staff if this occurs.

Aftercare

Resume a normal schedule and level of activity after the scan is complete. Drink plenty of water or other fluids throughout the rest of the day to flush the tracer out of the body.

Risks

A consent form may be required to be signed before the test. Discuss any potential risks with the PET scan with the referring physician or other medical professional. Risk of slight damage to cells or tissue is possible, but minimal, from the low levels of radiation used for the test. Most of the radioactive tracer is flushed out of the body within six to 24 hours. The tracer may cause an allergic reaction, but such incidents are rare. The injection site of the tracer may become sore or swell. If so, the medical staff will apply a warm, moist compress and check the area from time to time for any other medical needs. Benefits usually are considered when talking with a medical professional about this test, and whether they outweigh the risks.

Results

The images produced during these scans are normally sent to the attending physician. Make an appointment with this medical professional to discuss the results of the scan. Results normally are available to the doctor within one to two days. A normal result means that blood flow is normal, and organs and tissues examined are operating as they should. With this result, the tracer has flowed through the body in a normal distribution.

An abnormal result means different things depending on the portion of the body scanned. If the heart has been scanned, then a decreased flow of blood into or out of the heart and increased glucose metabolism may indicate that blood vessels are blocked. One possible diagnosis could be the presence of coronary artery disease; however, a medical professional is best to make that determination. If the brain was scanned, and a decreased flow of blood and oxygen and an increased glucose metabolism were found, then epilepsy is one of several possible diagnoses. If only a decreased flow of blood and oxygen was found, then one probable diagnosis is a stroke. On the other hand, if only a decreased glucose metabolism was discovered, then **dementia** could be a possible diagnosis. In all cases, doctors will thoroughly review the results to make a determination as to why this abnormal result occurred. In many cases, further tests will be performed to validate the results of the PET scan.

QUESTIONS TO ASK YOUR DOCTOR

- How long will the examination take?
- What may prevent me from having a PET scan?
- Is PET the best option for visualizing my condition?
- When will the results be provided to me?
- Will I need to have someone with me during the imaging study? Will this person need to drive me home?
- What special precautions should be taken with a child?
- Should I expect any side effects?
- How many scans should I have in any one year? How far apart should they be spaced?

Resources

BOOKS

Armstrong, Peter, Martin L. Wastie, and Andrea G. Rockall. *Diagnostic Imaging.* Chichester, U.K.: Wiley-Blackwell, 2009.

Lin, Eugene, and Abass Alavi. *PET and PET/CT: A Clinical Guide.* New York: Thieme, 2009.

Lynch, T. B., J. Clarke, and G. Cook. *PET/CT in Clinical Practice.* London: Springer-Verlag, 2007.

Valk, Peter P., et al., editors. *Positron Emission Tomography: Clinical Practice.* London: Springer, 2006.

Workman, Ronald B., Jr., et al., editors. *PET/CT: Essentials for Clinical Practice.* New York: Springer Science-Business Media, 2006.

WEBSITES

Neuroimaging and Mental Illness: A Window Into the Brain. National Institute of Mental Health. (October 19, 2010). http://www.nimh.nih.gov/health/publications/neuroimaging-and-mental-illness-a-window-into-the-brain/neuroimaging-and-mental-illness-a-window-into-the-brain.shtml (accessed May 31, 2011).

Positron Emission Tomography (PET) Scan. Mayo Clinic. (May 7, 2011). http://www.mayoclinic.com/health/pet-scan/MY00238 (accessed May 27, 2011).

ORGANIZATIONS

American College of Physicians, 190 North Independence Mall West, Philadelphia, PA, 19106-1572, (215) 351-2400, (800) 523-1546, http://www.acponline.org.

American College of Radiology, 1891 Preston White Drive, Reston, VA, 20191, (703) 648-8900, http://www.acr.org.

American Heart Association, 7272 Greenville Avenue, Dallas, TX, 75231, (800) 242-8721, http://www.americanheart.org.

American Medical Association, 515 N. State Street, Chicago, IL, 60610, (800) 621-8335, http://www.ama-assn.org.

National Cancer Institute, 6116 Executive Boulevard, Suite 300, Bethesda, MD, 20892-8322, (800) 422-6237, http://www.nci.nih.gov.

National Institute of Biomedical Imaging and Bioengineering, 31 Center Dr., 1C14, Bethesda, MD, 20892-8859, (301) 469-8859, http://www.nibib.gov.

Dan Harvey
Lee A. Shratter, MD
Brenda W. Lerner
William A. Atkins

Postpartum depression

Definition

Postpartum **depression** (PPD) is a mood disorder that begins after childbirth and usually lasts at least six weeks.

Demographics

There is a 20% to 30% risk of postpartum depression for women who have had a previous depressive episode not associated with pregnancy. Additionally, there is an increased risk of recurrence in subsequent pregnancies since more than half of patients have more than one episode.

Description

PPD affects approximately 10% to 20% of all childbearing women. The onset of postpartum depression tends to be gradual and may persist for many months or develop into a second bout following a subsequent pregnancy. Mild to moderate cases are sometimes unrecognized by women themselves. Many women feel ashamed and may conceal their difficulties. This is a serious problem that disrupts women's lives and can affect the baby, other children, partners, and other relationships. Levels of depression for fathers can also increase significantly.

Postpartum depression is often divided into two types: early onset and late onset. Early-onset PPD most often seems like the "blues," a mild brief experience during the first days or weeks after birth. During the first week after the birth, up to 80% of mothers experience the "baby blues." This period is usually a time of extra sensitivity; symptoms include tearfulness, irritability, anxiety, and mood changes, which tend to peak between three to five days after childbirth. The symptoms normally disappear within two weeks without requiring specific treatment apart from understanding, support, skills, and practice. Some depression, **fatigue**, and anxiety may fall within the normal range of reactions to giving birth.

Late-onset PPD appears several weeks after birth. It involves slowly growing feelings of sadness, depression, lack of energy, chronic fatigue, inability to sleep, change in appetite, significant weight loss or gain, and difficulty caring for the baby.

Causes and symptoms

The cause of postpartum depression has been extensively studied. Alterations of hormone levels of prolactin, progesterone, estrogen, and cortisol are not significantly different from those of patients who do not suffer from postpartum depression. However, some research indicates a change in a **brain** chemical that controls the release of cortisol.

Research suggests that postpartum depression is unlikely to occur in a patient with an otherwise psychologically uncomplicated pregnancy and past history. There is no association of postpartum depression with marital status, social class, or the number of live children born to the mother. However, there seems to be an increased chance to develop this disorder after pregnancy loss.

Certain characteristics have been associated with increased risk of developing postpartum depression. These risk factors include:

- medical indigence—that is, being in need of health care and not being able to receive it, possibly due to lack of medical insurance
- being younger than 20 years old at time of delivery
- being unmarried
- having been separated from one or both parents in childhood or adolescence
- receiving poor parental support and attention in childhood
- having had limited parental support in adulthood

Edinburgh Postnatal Depression Scale (EPDS)

As you are pregnant or have recently had a baby, we would like to know how you are feeling. Please check the answer that comes closest to how you have felt **IN THE PAST 7 DAYS**, not just how you feel today.

Here is an example, already completed.

I have felt happy:

- ☐ Yes, all the time
- ☒ Yes, most of the time
- ☐ No, not very often
- ☐ No, not at all

This would mean: "I have felt happy most of the time" during the past week. Please complete the other questions in the same way.

In the past 7 days:

1. I have been able to laugh and see the funny side of things
   - ☐ As much as I always could
   - ☐ Not quite so much now
   - ☐ Definitely not so much now
   - ☐ Not at all

2. I have looked forward with enjoyment to things
   - ☐ As much as I ever did
   - ☐ Rather less than I used to
   - ☐ Definitely less than I used to
   - ☐ Hardly at all

*3. I have blamed myself unnecessarily when things went wrong
   - ☐ Yes, most of the time
   - ☐ Yes, some of the time
   - ☐ Not very often
   - ☐ No, never

4. I have been anxious or worried for no good reason
   - ☐ No, not at all
   - ☐ Hardly ever
   - ☐ Yes, sometimes
   - ☐ Yes, very often

*5. I have felt scared or panicky for no very good reason
   - ☐ Yes, quite a lot
   - ☐ Yes, sometimes
   - ☐ No, not much
   - ☐ No, not at all

*6. Things have been getting on top of me
   - ☐ Yes, most of the time I haven't been able to cope at all
   - ☐ Yes, sometimes I haven't been coping as well as usual
   - ☐ No, most of the time I have coped quite well
   - ☐ No, I have been coping as well as ever

*7. I have been so unhappy that I have had difficulty sleeping
   - ☐ Yes, most of the time
   - ☐ Yes, sometimes
   - ☐ Not very often
   - ☐ No, not at all

*8. I have felt sad or miserable
   - ☐ Yes, most of the time
   - ☐ Yes, quite often
   - ☐ Not very often
   - ☐ No, not at all

*9. I have been so unhappy that I have been crying
   - ☐ Yes, most of the time
   - ☐ Yes, quite often
   - ☐ Only occasionally
   - ☐ No, never

*10. The thought of harming myself has occurred to me
   - ☐ Yes, quite often
   - ☐ Sometimes
   - ☐ Hardly ever
   - ☐ Never

SOURCE: Cox, J.L., J.M. Holden, and R. Sagovsky, "Detection of Postnatal Depression: Development of the 10-item Edinburgh Postnatal Depression Scale," *British Journal of Psychiatry* 150 (June 1987): 782–86.

Items with an asterisk are reverse scored (3, 2, 1, 0 instead of 0, 1, 2, 3). *(Table by PreMediaGlobal. © 2012 Cengage Learning.)*

- having a poor relationship with the baby's father
- having economic problem with housing or income
- being dissatisfied with amount of education
- having low self-esteem
- having past or current emotional problem(s)
- having a family history of depression

Experts have not determined for certain what causes postpartum depression. Most likely, it is caused by a combination of factors that vary from person to person. Some researchers think that women are vulnerable to depression at all major turning points in their reproductive cycle, childbirth being only one of these markers. Factors before the baby's birth that are associated with a higher risk of PPD include severe vomiting (hyperemesis), premature labor contractions, and psychiatric disorders in the mother. In addition, new mothers commonly experience some degree of depression during the first weeks after birth. Pregnancy and birth are accompanied by sudden hormonal changes that affect emotions. Additionally, the 24-hour responsibility for a newborn infant requires a major psychological and lifestyle adjustment for most mothers, even after the first child. These physical and emotional stresses are usually accompanied by inadequate rest until the baby's routine stabilizes, so fatigue and depression are not unusual.

KEY TERMS

Hyperemesis—Severe vomiting during pregnancy. Hyperemesis appears to increase a woman's risk of postpartum depression.

Postpartum—Following childbirth.

Studies suggest that the hormone oxytocin in particular may play a role in postpartum depression. Oxytocin is associated with feelings of attachment and bonding. In a study conducted in Switzerland and published in 2011, researchers measured oxytocin levels in 74 healthy pregnant women during the third trimester of pregnancy. Overall, women with lower oxytocin levels during the third trimester were at greater risk for postpartum depression two weeks after delivery. However, more research is needed in larger groups to confirm the findings, and some experts argue that two weeks after delivery is too soon to assess postpartum depression.

In addition to hormonal changes and disrupted sleep, certain cultural expectations appear to place women from those cultures at increased risk of postpartum depression. For example, women who bear daughters in societies with a strong preference for sons are at increased risk of postpartum depression. In other cultures, a strained relationship with the husband's family is a risk factor. In Western countries, domestic violence is associated with a higher rate of PPD.

Experiences of PPD vary considerably but usually include several symptoms.

Feelings:

- persistent low mood
- inadequacy, failure, hopelessness, helplessness
- exhaustion, emptiness, sadness, tearfulness
- guilt, shame, worthlessness
- confusion, anxiety, and panic
- fear for the baby and of the baby
- fear of being alone or going out

Behaviors:

- lack of interest or pleasure in usual activities
- insomnia or excessive sleep, nightmares
- not eating or overeating
- decreased energy and motivation
- withdrawal from social contact
- poor self-care
- inability to cope with routine tasks

Thoughts:

- inability to think clearly and make decisions
- lack of concentration and poor memory
- avoidance of decision making
- fear of being rejected by the partner
- worry about harm or death to partner or baby
- ideas about suicide

Some symptoms may not indicate a severe problem. However, persistent low mood or loss of interest or pleasure in activities, along with four other symptoms occurring together for a period of at least two weeks, indicate clinical depression and require treatment.

There are several important risk factors for postpartum depression:

- stress
- lack of sleep
- poor nutrition
- lack of support from one's partner, family, or friends
- family history of depression
- labor/delivery complications for mother or baby
- premature or postmature delivery
- problems with the baby's health
- separation of mother and baby
- a difficult baby (temperament, feeding, sleeping problems)
- preexisting neurosis or psychosis

Physical and emotional **stress** during delivery in conjunction with great demands for infant care may cause the patient to neglect other family members, increasing the woman's feelings of worthlessness, isolation, and being trapped. Patients may also feel as if they are inadequate mothers, causing them guilt and embarrassment.

Diagnosis

Diagnosis of postpartum depression entails a clinical interview with the patient to assess symptoms. A doctor or other professional healthcare provider may ask the mother about thoughts and feelings and take a detailed personal history. Clinical assessment may be conducted by a **psychologist** or **psychiatrist**, who can determine the risk factors and diagnose the condition. A comprehensive **psychological assessment** interview may reveal a previous depressive cycle or a family history of depression—important risk factors. The most widely used standard for diagnosis is the Edinburgh Postnatal Depression Scale (EPDS), a simple and short

10-question scale. A score of 12 or greater on the EPDS is considered high risk for postpartum depression.

Treatment

Several treatment options exist, including medication, **psychotherapy**, counseling, and group treatment and support strategies. Treatment should begin as soon as the diagnosis is established. One effective treatment combines antidepressant medication and psychotherapy. These types of medication are often effective when used for three to four weeks. Any medication use must be carefully considered if the woman is breastfeeding, but with some medications, continuing breastfeeding is safe. There are many classes of antidepressant medications. The two most commonly prescribed for PPD are **selective serotonin reuptake inhibitors (SSRIs)** such as **citalopram** (Celexa), **escitalopram** (Lexapro), **fluoxetine** (Prozac), **paroxetine** (Paxil, Pexeva), and **sertraline** (Zoloft), and tricyclics, such as **amitriptyline** (Elavil), **desipramine** (Norpramin), **imipramine** (Tofranil), and **nortriptyline** (Aventyl, Pamelor). Nevertheless, medication alone is not sufficient and should always be accompanied by counseling or other support services. Also, many women with postpartum depression feel isolated. It is important for these women to know that they are not alone in their feelings. There are various postpartum depression **support groups** available in local communities, often sponsored by nonprofit organizations or hospitals. Support information is available by contacting postpartum depression organizations. Women can find a local support group by calling the Kristin Brooks Hope Center helpline at (800) 442-4673. Women who have thoughts of **suicide** should immediately call the national toll-free 24-hour suicide hotline at (800) 784-2433.

When medications are combined with psychological therapy, the rates for successful treatment are increased. **Interpersonal therapy** and **cognitive-behavioral therapy** have been found to be effective.

Adjunct therapies such as **acupuncture**, traditional Chinese medicine, **yoga**, **meditation**, and herbs may be helpful for mothers suffering from postpartum depression.

An important part of treating postpartum depression is self-care, which should not be underestimated or ignored.

A new mother can apply at-home strategies to help cope with the stress of becoming a parent, such as:

- valuing her role as a mother and trusting her own judgment
- making each day as simple as possible
- avoiding extra pressures or unnecessary tasks
- trying to involve her partner more in the care of the baby
- discussing with her partner how both can share the household chores and responsibilities
- scheduling frequent outings, such as walks and short visits with friends
- sharing her feelings with her partner or friends
- talking with other mothers to help keep problems in perspective
- trying to sleep or rest when the baby is sleeping
- taking care of personal health and well-being

Exercise, including yoga, can help enhance a new mother's emotional well-being. New mothers should also try to cultivate good sleeping habits and learn to rest when they feel physically or emotionally tired. It is important for a woman to learn to recognize her own warning signs of fatigue and respond to them by taking a break.

QUESTIONS TO ASK YOUR DOCTOR

- How do I know if I have postpartum depression?
- What type of treatment do you recommend for me?
- What symptoms or behaviors are important enough that I should seek immediate treatment?
- Can you recommend any support groups for me and my family?

Prognosis

When a woman has supportive friends and family, mild postpartum depression usually disappears quickly. If depression becomes severe and a mother cannot care for herself and the baby, **hospitalization** may be necessary. Medication, counseling, and support from others usually resolve even severe depression in three to six months. The prognosis for postpartum depression is better if it is detected early during its clinical course and a combination of **SSRIs** and psychotherapy is available and initiated.

Prevention

Mothers should be advised prior to hospital discharge that if the "maternity blues" last longer than two weeks or pose tough difficulties with family interactions, they should call the hospital where their baby was delivered and get a referral for a psychological evaluation. Education concerning risk factors and reduction of these is important. Prophylactic (preventive) use of SSRIs is indicated two to three weeks before delivery to prevent the disorder in a patient with a past history of depression, since recurrence rates are high. Use of medication during pregnancy should always take place under careful medical supervision.

Resources

BOOKS

Beck, Cheryl Tatano, and Jeanne Watson Driscoll. *Postpartum Mood and Anxiety Disorders: A Clinician's Guide.* Sudbury, MA: Jones and Bartlett, 2006.

Poulin, Sandra. *The Mother-to-Mother Postpartum Depression Support Book.* New York: Berkley Trade, 2006.

Shields, Brooke. *Down Came the Rain: My Journey Through Postpartum Depression.* New York: Hyperion Books, 2006.

Subcommittee on Health, U.S. House of Representatives. *Improving Women's Health: Understanding Depression after Pregnancy. (Hearing before the Subcommittee on Health of the Committee on Energy and Commerce, House of Representatives, One Hundred Eighth Congress, Second Session, September 29, 2004.)* Washington, DC: U.S. Government Printing Office, 2005.

Venis, Joyce A., and Suzanne McCloskey. *Postpartum Depression Demystified: An Essential Guide for Understanding the Most Common Complication after Childbirth.* New York: Marlowe, 2007.

PERIODICALS

Barnes, Diana Lynn. "Postpartum Depression: Its Impact on Couples and Marital Satisfaction." *Journal of Systemic Therapies* 25, no. 3 (Fall 2006): 25–42.

Gaby, Alan R. "Fish Oil for Postpartum Depression." *Townsend Letter: The Examiner of Alternative Medicine* (October 2006): 40.

Haslam, Divna M., Kenneth I. Pakenham, and Amanda Smith. "Social Support and Postpartum Depressive Symptomatology: The Mediating Role of Maternal Self-Efficacy." *Infant Mental Health Journal* 27, no. 3 (May–June 2006): 276–91.

Hung, Chich-Hsiu. "The Hung Postpartum Stress Scale." *Journal of Nursing Scholarship* (Spring 2007): 71–75.

Klier, Claudia M., et al. "The Role of Estrogen and Progesterone in Depression after Birth." *Journal of Psychiatric Research* 41, no. 3–4 (April–June 2007): 273–79.

Klotter, Jule. "Exercise and Postpartum Depression." *Townsend Letter: The Examiner of Alternative Medicine* (October 2007): 42–44.

McGinnis, Marianne. "Baby Blues? Get Help Early." *Prevention* (January 2006): 107.

Moehler, E., et al. "Maternal Depressive Symptoms in the Postnatal Period Are Associated with Long-Term Impairment of Mother-Child Bonding." *Archives of Women's Mental Health* 9, no. 5 (September 2006): 273–78.

Nylen, Kimberly J., et al. "Maternal Depression: A Review of Relevant Treatment Approaches for Mothers and Infants." *Infant Mental Health Journal* 27, no. 4 (July/August 2006): 327–43.

Ramashwar, S. "In China, Women Who Give Birth to Girls Face an Increased Risk of Postpartum Depression." *International Family Planning Perspectives* (December 2007): 191–93.

Sharma, Verinder. "A Cautionary Note on the Use of Antidepressants in Postpartum Depression." *Bipolar Disorders* 8, no. 4 (August 2006): 411–14.

Skrundtz, M. "Plasma Oxytocin Concentration During Pregnancy is Associated with Development of Postpartum Depression." *Neuropsychopharmacology* 36, no. 9 (August 2011): 1886–93.

ORGANIZATIONS

Kristin Brooks Hope Center, 615 7th St., NE, Washington, DC, 20002, (202) 536-3200, (800) 442-4673, http://www.hopeline.com.

National Institute of Mental Health, 6001 Executive Blvd., Room 8184, MSC 9663, Bethesda, MD, 20892, (866) 615-6464, http://www.nimh.nih.gov.

Postpartum Support International, PO Box 60931, Santa Barbara, CA, 93160, (805) 967-7636, (800) 944-4773, http://www.postpartum.net.

Laith Farid Gulli, MD
Nicole Mallory, MS, PA-C
Laura Jean Cataldo, RN, EdD
Heidi Splete

Post-traumatic stress disorder

Definition

Post-traumatic **stress** disorder (PTSD) is a complex anxiety disorder that may occur when individuals experience or witness an event perceived as a threat and in which they experience fear, terror, or helplessness. PTSD is sometimes summarized as "a normal reaction to abnormal events." It was first defined as a distinctive disorder in 1980. Originally diagnosed in veterans of the Vietnam War, it is now recognized in civilian survivors of rape or other criminal assaults; natural disasters; plane crashes, train collisions, or industrial explosions; acts of terrorism; **child abuse**; or war.

Demographics

PTSD can develop in almost anyone in any age group exposed to a sufficiently terrifying event or chain of events. The **National Institute of Mental Health**

(NIMH) estimated in 2007 that about 7.7 million adults in the United States have PTSD. One study found that 3.7% of a sample of teenage boys and 6.3% of adolescent girls had PTSD. It is estimated that people's risk of developing PTSD over the course of their life is between 8 and 10%. Women are at greater risk of PTSD following sexual assault or domestic violence, whereas men are at greater risk of developing PTSD following military combat. On average, 30% of soldiers who have been in a war zone develop PTSD. Recent statistics on PTSD in U.S. military personnel returning from Iraq demonstrated that, using more inclusive parameters, between 20.7% and 30.5% of troops suffered from PTSD; using stricter parameters, PTSD was present in 5.6–11.3% of troops.

Traumatic experiences are surprisingly common in the general North American population. More than 10% of the men and 6% of the women in one survey reported experiencing four or more types of **trauma** in their lives. The most frequently mentioned traumas are:

- witnessing someone being badly hurt or killed
- being involved in a fire, flood, earthquake, severe hurricane, or other natural disaster
- being involved in a life-threatening accident (workplace explosion or transportation accident)
- being in military combat

PTSD is more likely to develop in response to an intentional human act of violence or cruelty such as a rape or mugging than as a reaction to an impersonal catastrophe like a flood or hurricane. It is not surprising that the traumatic events most frequently mentioned by men diagnosed with PTSD are rape, combat exposure, childhood **neglect**, and childhood physical **abuse**. For women diagnosed with PTSD, the most common traumas are rape, sexual molestation, physical attack, being threatened with a weapon, and childhood physical abuse.

PTSD can also develop in therapists, rescue workers, or witnesses of a frightening event as well as in those who were directly involved. This process is called vicarious traumatization.

Description

The experience of PTSD has sometimes been described as like being in a horror film that keeps replaying and cannot be shut off. It is common for people with PTSD to feel intense fear and helplessness and to relive the frightening event in nightmares or in their waking hours. Sometimes the memory is triggered by a sound, smell, or image that reminds the sufferer of the traumatic event. These re-experiences of the event are called flashbacks. Persons with PTSD are also likely to be jumpy and easily startled or to go numb emotionally and lose interest in activities they used to enjoy. They may have problems with memory and with getting enough sleep. In some cases they may feel disconnected from the real world or have moments in which their own bodies seem unreal; these symptoms are indications of dissociation, a process in which the mind splits off certain memories or thoughts from conscious awareness. Many people with PTSD turn to alcohol or drugs in order to escape the flashbacks and other symptoms of the disorder, even if only for a few minutes.

Risk factors

Factors that influence the likelihood of a person's developing PTSD include:

- The nature, intensity, and duration of the traumatic experience. For example, someone who just barely escaped from the World Trade Center before the towers collapsed is at greater risk of PTSD than someone who saw the collapse from a distance or on television.
- The person's previous history. People who were abused as children, who were separated from their parents at an early age, or who have a previous history of anxiety or depression are at increased risk of PTSD.
- Genetic factors. Vulnerability to PTSD is known to run in families.
- The availability of social support after the event. People who have no family or friends are more likely to develop PTSD than those who do.

HIGH-RISK POPULATIONS. Some subpopulations in the United States are at greater risk of developing PTSD. The lifetime prevalence of PTSD among persons living in depressed urban areas or on Native American reservations is estimated at 23%. For victims of violent crimes, the estimated rate is 58%.

PTSD also appears to be more common in seniors than in younger people. Thirteen percent of the senior population reports they are affected by PTSD in comparison to 7–10% of the entire population. Reports of **elder abuse** crimes have gone up by 200% since 1986. Also, the incidence of PTSD is known to be higher in Holocaust survivors, war veterans, and cancer or heart surgery survivors, which accounts for a significant portion of older Americans. Of those seniors who are military veterans, there is an increasing number who are isolated and/or in poor health as a result of PTSD.

Children are also susceptible to PTSD and their risk is increased exponentially as their exposure to the event increases. Children experiencing abuse, the death of a parent, or those located in a community suffering a traumatic event can develop PTSD. Two years after the

Oklahoma City bombing of 1995, 16% of children within a 100-mile radius of Oklahoma City with no direct exposure to the bombing had increased symptoms of PTSD. Weak parental response to the event, having a parent suffering from PTSD symptoms, and intensified exposure to the event via the media all increase the possibility of a child's developing PTSD symptoms. In addition, a developmentally inappropriate sexual experience for a child may be considered a traumatic event, even though it may not have actually involved violence or physical injury. Proposed changes to the fifth edition of the ***Diagnostic and Statistical Manual of Mental Disorders*** (*DSM-5*, 2013) include post-traumatic stress disorder in preschool children among its new diagnoses.

MILITARY VETERANS. Studies conducted between 2004 and 2006 with veteran participants from the wars in Iraq and in Afghanistan found a strong correlation between duration of combat exposure and PTSD. Veterans of combat in Iraq reported a higher rate of PTSD than those deployed to Afghanistan because of longer exposure to warfare.

Information about PTSD in veterans of the Vietnam era is derived from the National Vietnam Veterans Readjustment Survey (NVVRS), conducted between 1986 and 1988. The estimated lifetime prevalence of PTSD among American veterans of this war is 30.9% for men and 26.9% for women. An additional 22.5% of the men and 21.2% of the women have been diagnosed with partial PTSD at some point in their lives. The lifetime prevalence of PTSD among veterans of World War II and the Korean War is estimated at 20%.

CROSS-CULTURAL ISSUES. Further research needs to be done on the effects of ethnicity and culture on post-traumatic symptoms. As of the early 2010s, most PTSD research had been done by Western clinicians working with patients from a similar background. Researchers do not yet know whether persons from non-Western societies have the same psychological reactions to specific traumas or whether they develop the same symptom patterns.

PROTECTIVE OR RESILIENCE FACTORS. As important as the question of *who* gets PTSD is also the question of who does *not* get PTSD. Why do some people who are exposed to traumatic events succumb to the long-lasting aftereffects of PTSD, whereas others seem to endure the trauma and successfully move on. Researchers have identified the following resilience factors, which seem to decrease the likelihood that traumatic exposure will lead to PTSD:

- actively seeking support from friends, family, or others following a traumatic incident
- engaging with a formal support group
- maintaining a positive view of personal actions during the course of or in response to the traumatic incident
- implementing a coping strategy
- feeling as if a lesson has been learned from the traumatic event
- not becoming paralyzed with terror; being able to respond and react effectively despite fear

Causes and symptoms

The causes of PTSD are not completely understood. One major question that has not yet been answered is why some people involved in a major disaster develop PTSD and other survivors of the same event do not. For example, a survey of 988 adults living close to the World Trade Center conducted in November 2001 found that only 7% had been diagnosed with PTSD following the events of September 11; the other 93% were anxious and upset, but they did not develop PTSD. Research into this question is ongoing.

Causes

When PTSD was first suggested as a diagnostic category for *DSM-III* in 1980, it was controversial precisely because of the central role of outside stressors as causes of the disorder. Psychiatry has generally emphasized the internal abnormalities of individuals as the source of mental disorders; prior to the 1970s, war veterans, rape victims, and other trauma survivors were often blamed for their symptoms and regarded as cowards, moral weaklings, or masochists. The high rate of psychiatric casualties among Vietnam veterans, however, led to studies conducted by the Veterans Administration. These studies helped to establish PTSD as a legitimate diagnostic entity with a complex set of causes.

BIOCHEMICAL/PHYSIOLOGICAL CAUSES. Present neurobiological research indicates that traumatic events cause lasting changes in the human nervous system, including abnormal levels of secretion of stress hormones. In addition, in PTSD patients, researchers have found changes in the amygdala and the hippocampus—the parts of the **brain** that form links between fear and memory. Experiments with ketamine, a drug that inactivates one of the **neurotransmitters** in the central nervous system, suggest that trauma works in a similar way to damage associative pathways in the brain. **Positron emission tomography (PET)** scans of PTSD patients suggest that trauma affects the parts of the brain that govern speech and language.

SOCIOCULTURAL CAUSES. Studies of specific populations of PTSD patients (combat veterans, survivors of rape or genocide, former political hostages or prisoners, etc.) have shed light on the social and cultural causes of PTSD. In general, societies that are highly authoritarian, glorify violence, or sexualize violence have high rates of PTSD even among civilians.

OCCUPATIONAL FACTORS. Persons whose work exposes them to traumatic events or who treat trauma survivors may develop secondary PTSD (also known as compassion **fatigue** or burnout). These occupations include specialists in emergency medicine, police officers, firefighters, search-and-rescue personnel, psychotherapists, and disaster investigators. The degree of risk for PTSD is related to three factors: the amount and intensity of exposure to the suffering of trauma victims, the worker's degree of empathy and sensitivity, and unresolved issues from the worker's personal history.

PERSONAL VARIABLES. Although the most important causal factor in PTSD is the traumatic event itself, individuals differ in the intensity of their cognitive and emotional responses to trauma; some persons appear to be more vulnerable than others. In some cases, this greater vulnerability is related to temperament or natural disposition, with shy or introverted people being at greater risk. In other cases, the person's vulnerability results from chronic illness, a physical disability, or previous traumatization—particularly abuse in childhood. Studies done by the U.S. Department of Veterans Affairs have found some evidence that race and ethnicity may also play a factor, with veterans belonging to ethnic minority groups at higher risk of experiencing PTSD after combat.

Symptoms

DSM-IV-TR specifies six diagnostic criteria for PTSD:

- Traumatic stressor: The patient has been exposed to a catastrophic event involving actual or threatened death or injury or a threat to the physical integrity of the self or others. During exposure to the trauma, the person's emotional response was marked by intense fear, feelings of helplessness, or horror. In general, stressors caused intentionally by human beings (genocide, rape, torture, abuse) are experienced as more traumatic than accidents, natural disasters, or "acts of God."
- Intrusive symptoms: Patients experience flashbacks, traumatic daydreams, or nightmares, in which they relive the trauma as if it were recurring in the present. Intrusive symptoms result from an abnormal process of memory formation. Traumatic memories have two distinctive characteristics: they can be triggered by stimuli that remind the patient of the traumatic event, or they may have a "frozen" or wordless quality, consisting of images and sensations rather than verbal descriptions.
- Avoidant symptoms: Patients attempt to reduce the possibility of exposure to anything that might trigger memories of the trauma and to minimize their reactions to such memories. This cluster of symptoms includes feeling disconnected from other people, psychic numbing, and avoidance of places, persons, or things associated with the trauma. Patients with PTSD are at increased risk of substance abuse as a form of self-medication to numb painful memories.
- Hyperarousal: Hyperarousal is a condition in which the nervous system is always on "red alert" for the return of danger. This symptom cluster includes hypervigilance, insomnia, difficulty concentrating, general irritability, and an extreme startle response. Some clinicians think that this abnormally intense startle response may be the most characteristic symptom of PTSD.
- Duration of symptoms: The symptoms must persist for at least one month.

KEY TERMS

Benzodiazepines—A class of drugs that have a hypnotic and sedative action, used mainly as tranquilizers to control symptoms of anxiety.

Cognitive-behavioral therapy—A type of psychotherapy used to treat anxiety disorders (including PTSD) that emphasizes behavioral change as well as alteration of negative thought patterns.

Cortisol—A hormone produced by the adrenal glands near the kidneys in response to stress.

Dissociation—The splitting off of certain mental processes from conscious awareness. Many PTSD patients have dissociative symptoms.

Flashback—A temporary reliving of a traumatic event.

Hyperarousal—A state of increased emotional tension and anxiety, often including jitteriness and being easily startled.

Hypervigilance—A condition of abnormally intense watchfulness or wariness. Hypervigilance is one of the most common symptoms of PTSD.

Prevalence—The percentage of a population that is affected by a specific disease at a given time.

Selective serotonin reuptake inhibitors (SSRIs)—A class of antidepressants that works by blocking the reabsorption of serotonin in the brain, raising the levels of serotonin.

Trauma—A severe injury or shock to a person's body or mind.

- Significance: Patients suffer from significant social, interpersonal, or work-related problems as a result of the PTSD symptoms. A common social symptom of PTSD is a feeling of disconnection from other people (including loved ones), from the larger society, and from spiritual, religious, or other significant sources of meaning.

Diagnosis

The **diagnosis** of PTSD is based on the patient's history, including the timing of the traumatic event and the duration of the patient's symptoms.

Examination

Consultation with a mental health professional for diagnosis and a plan of treatment is always advised. Many of the responses to trauma, such as shock, terror, irritability, blame, guilt, **grief**, sadness, emotional numbing, and feelings of helplessness, are natural reactions. For most people, resilience is an overriding factor, and trauma effects diminish within six to sixteen months. It is when these responses continue or become debilitating that PTSD is often diagnosed.

As outlined in *DSM-IV,* the exposure to a traumatic stressor means that an individual experienced, witnessed, or was confronted by an event or events involving death or threat of death, serious injury or the threat of bodily harm to oneself or others. The individual's response must involve intense fear, helplessness, or horror. A two-pronged approach to evaluation is considered the best way to make a valid diagnosis because it can gauge under-reporting or over-reporting of symptoms. The two primary forms are structured interviews and self-report questionnaires. Spouses, partners, and other family members may also be interviewed. Because the evaluation may involve subtle reminders of the trauma in order to gauge a patient's reactions, individuals should ask for a full description of the evaluation process beforehand. Asking what results can be expected from the evaluation is also advised.

A number of structured interview forms have been devised to facilitate the diagnosis of post-traumatic stress disorder:

- Clinician Administered PTSD Scale (CAPS) developed by the National Center for PTSD
- Structured Clinical Interview for DSM (SCID)
- Anxiety Disorders Interview Schedule-Revised (ADIS)
- PTSD-Interview
- Structured Interview for PTSD (SI-PTSD)
- PTSD Symptom Scale Interview (PSS-I)

Self-reporting checklists provide scores to represent the level of stress experienced. Some of the most commonly used checklists are:

- The PTSD Checklist (PCL), which has one list for civilians and one for military personnel and veterans
- Impact of Event Scale-Revised (IES-R)
- Keane PTSD Scale of the MMPI-2
- Mississippi Scale for Combat Related PTSD and the Mississippi Scale for Civilians
- Post Traumatic Diagnostic Scale (PDS)
- Penn Inventory for Post-Traumatic Stress
- Los Angeles Symptom Checklist (LASC)

Tests

There are no laboratory or imaging tests that can detect PTSD, although the doctor may order **imaging studies** of the brain to rule out head injuries or other physical causes of the patient's symptoms.

Treatment

Various treatments are used for post-traumatic stress disorder.

Traditional

Treatment for PTSD usually involves a combination of medications and **psychotherapy**. If patients have started to abuse alcohol or drugs, they must be treated for the **substance abuse** before being treated for PTSD. If they are diagnosed with coexisting **depression**, treatment should focus on the PTSD because its course, biology, and treatment response are different from those associated with major depression. Patients with the disorder are usually treated as outpatients; they are not hospitalized unless they are threatening to commit **suicide** or harm other people.

Mainstream forms of psychotherapy used to treat patients who have already developed PTSD include:

- Cognitive-behavioral therapy. There are two treatment approaches to PTSD included under this heading: exposure therapy, which seeks to desensitize the patient to reminders of the trauma; and anxiety management training, which teaches the patient strategies for reducing anxiety. These strategies may include relaxation training, biofeedback, social skills training, distraction techniques, or cognitive restructuring.
- Psychodynamic psychotherapy. This approach helps the patient recover a sense of self and learn new coping strategies and ways to deal with intense

emotions related to the trauma. Typically, it consists of three phases: establishing a sense of safety for the patient; exploring the trauma itself in depth; helping the patient re-establish connections with family, friends, the wider society, and other sources of meaning.

- Discussion groups or peer-counseling groups. These groups are usually formed for survivors of specific traumas, such as combat, rape/incest, and natural or transportation disasters. They help patients to recognize that other survivors of the shared experience have had the same emotions and reacted to the trauma in similar ways. They appear to be especially beneficial for patients with guilt issues about their behavior during the trauma (e.g., submitting to rape to save one's life or surviving the event when others did not).
- Family therapy. This form of treatment is recommended for PTSD patients whose family life has been affected by the PTSD symptoms.

Drugs

In general, medications are used most often in patients with severe PTSD to treat the intrusive symptoms of the disorder as well as feelings of anxiety and depression. These drugs are usually given as one part of a treatment plan that includes psychotherapy or **group therapy**. As of 2012, no single medication was considered a primary cure for PTSD. The **selective serotonin reuptake inhibitors (SSRIs)** appear to help the core symptoms when given in higher doses for five to eight weeks, while the tricyclic antidepressants (TCAs) or the **monoamine oxidase inhibitors (MAOIs)** are most useful in treating anxiety and depression.

Sleep problems can be lessened with brief treatment with an antianxiety drug, such as a benzodiazepine like **alprazolam** (Xanax), but long-term usage can lead to disturbing side effects, including increased anger, drug tolerance, dependency, and abuse. **Benzodiazepines** are also not given to PTSD patients diagnosed with coexisting drug or alcohol abuse.

Alternative

Relaxation training, which is sometimes called anxiety management training, includes breathing exercises and similar techniques intended to help the patient prevent hyperventilation and relieve the muscle tension associated with the fight-or-flight reaction of anxiety. **Yoga**, aikido, tai chi, and **dance therapy** help patients work with the physical as well as the emotional tensions that either promote anxiety or are created by the anxiety.

Other alternative or complementary therapies are based on physiological and/or energetic understanding of how the trauma is imprinted in the body. These therapies affect a release of stored emotions and resolution of them by working with the body rather than merely talking through the experience. One example of such a therapy is somatic experiencing (SE), developed by Peter Levine. SE is a short-term, biological, body-oriented approach to PTSD or other trauma. This approach heals by emphasizing physiological and emotional responses, without re-traumatizing the person, without placing the person on medication, and without the long hours of conventional therapy.

When used in conjunction with therapies that address the underlying cause of PTSD, relaxation therapies such as hydrotherapy, massage therapy, and **aromatherapy** are useful to some patients in easing PTSD symptoms. Essential oils of **lavender**, **chamomile**, neroli, sweet marjoram, and ylang-ylang are commonly recommended by aromatherapists for stress relief and anxiety reduction.

Some patients benefit from spiritual or religious counseling. Because traumatic experiences often affect patients' spiritual views and beliefs, counseling with a trusted religious or spiritual advisor may be part of a treatment plan. A growing number of pastoral counselors in the major Christian and Jewish bodies in North America have advanced credentials in trauma therapy. Native Americans are often helped to recover from PTSD by participating in traditional tribal rituals for cleansing memories of war and other traumatic events. These rituals may include sweat lodges, prayers and chants, or consultation with a shaman or tribal healer.

Several controversial methods of treatment for PTSD have been introduced since the mid-1980s. Some have been developed by mainstream medical researchers while others are derived from various forms of alternative medicine. These methods are controversial because they do not offer any scientifically validated explanations for their effectiveness. They include:

- Eye Movement Desensitization and Reprocessing (EMDR). This is a technique in which the patient re-imagines the trauma while focusing visually on movements of the therapist's finger. It is claimed that the movements of the patient's eyes reprogram the brain and allow emotional healing.
- Tapas Acupressure Technique (TAT). TAT was developed in 1993 by licensed acupuncturist Tapas Fleming. It is derived from traditional Chinese medicine (TCM), and its practitioners maintain that a large number of acupuncture meridians enter the brain at certain points on the face, especially around the eyes. Pressure on these points is thought to release traumatic stress.

QUESTIONS TO ASK YOUR DOCTOR

- What are my chances of recovering completely from PTSD? How long do you think it might take?
- What medications would you recommend and why?
- What should I do when I have a flashback?
- Can you help me explain my symptoms to my family and friends?

- Thought Field Therapy. This therapy combines the acupuncture meridians of TCM with analysis of the patient's voice over the telephone. The therapist then provides an individualized treatment for the patient.
- Traumatic Incident Reduction. This is a technique in which the patient treats the trauma like a videotape and "runs through" it repeatedly with the therapist until all negative emotions have been discharged.
- Emotional Freedom Techniques (EFT). EFT is similar to TAT in that it uses the body's acupuncture meridians, but it emphasizes the body's entire "energy field" rather than just the face.
- Counting Technique. Developed by a physician, this treatment consists of a preparation phase, a counting phase in which the therapist counts from 1 to 100 while the patient re-imagines the trauma and a review phase. Like Traumatic Incident Reduction, it is intended to reduce the patient's hyperarousal.

Healthcare team roles

It is essential for all treatment team members to know their roles and execute them properly throughout the treatment and recovery phases of this disorder. Depending on whether outpatient or inpatient treatment is being provided, the team leaders may include psychiatrists, psychologists, nursing staff, behavior specialists, physical therapists, and other medical/behavioral staff. In some cases it may be appropriate to include the patient's religious or spiritual advisor as a member of the team.

Prognosis

The prognosis of PTSD is difficult to determine because patients' personalities and the experiences they undergo vary widely. A majority of patients get better, including some who do not receive treatment. One study reported that the average length of PTSD symptoms in patients who get treatment is 32 months, compared to 64 months in patients who are not treated.

Factors that improve a patient's chances for full recovery include prompt treatment, early and ongoing support from family and friends, a high level of functioning before the frightening event, and an absence of alcohol or substance abuse.

About 30% of people with PTSD never recover completely, however. A few commit suicide because their symptoms get worse rather than improving.

Prevention

PTSD is impossible to prevent completely because natural disasters and human acts of violence will continue to occur. In addition, it is not possible to tell beforehand how any given individual will react to a specific type of trauma. Prompt treatment after a traumatic event may lower the survivor's risk of developing severe symptoms.

Resources

BOOKS

American Psychiatric Association. *Diagnostic and Statistical Manual of Mental Disorders*. 4th ed., text rev. Washington, DC: American Psychiatric Publishing, 2000.

Antony, Martin M., and Murray B. Stein, eds. *Oxford Handbook of Anxiety and Related Disorders*. New York: Oxford University Press, 2009.

Bradley, W., et al. *Neurology in Clinical Practice*, 5th ed. Philadelphia: Butterworth-Heinemann, 2008.

Brohl, Kathryn. *Working with Traumatized Children: A Handbook for Healing*, rev. ed. Arlington, VA: CWLA Press, 2007.

Grey, Nick, ed. *A Casebook of Cognitive Therapy for Traumatic Stress Reactions*. New York: Routledge, 2009.

Slone, Laurie B., and Matthew J. Friedman. *After the War Zone: A Practical Guide for Returning Troops and Their Families*. Cambridge, MA: Da Capo Lifelong, 2008.

PERIODICALS

Cohen, J.A., and M.S. Scheeringa. "Post-traumatic Stress Disorder Diagnosis in Children: Challenges and Promises." *Dialogues in Clinical Neuroscience* 11 (2009): 91–99.

Evans, S., et al. "Disability and Posttraumatic Stress Disorder in Disaster Relief Workers Responding to September 11, 2001, World Trade Center Disaster." *Journal of Clinical Psychology* 65 (April 22, 2009): 684–94.

Hamblen, J.L., et al. "Cognitive Behavioral Therapy for Postdisaster Distress: A Community-Based Treatment Program for Survivors of Hurricane Katrina." *Administration and Policy in Mental Health* 36 (May 2009): 206–14.

Smith, T.C., et al. "PTSD Prevalence, Associated Exposures, and Functional Health Outcomes in a Large, Population-

Based Military Cohort." *Public Health Reports* 124 (January-February 2009): 90–102.

WEBSITES

"Helping Children Cope with Violence and Disasters: What Parents Can Do." National Institute of Mental Health. http://www.nimh.nih.gov/health/publications/helping-children-and-adolescents-cope-with-violence-and-disasters-what-parents-can-do/index.shtml (accessed September 16, 2011).

Hope for Recovery: Understanding PTSD [video]. National Center for PTSD. http://www.ncptsd.va.gov/ncmain/ncdocs/videos/emv_hoperecovery_gpv.html (accessed September 16, 2011).

"Post-Traumatic Stress Disorder." National Alliance on Mental Illness. http://www.nami.org/Template.cfm?Section=By_Illness&Template=/TaggedPage/TaggedPageDisplay.cfm&TPLID=54&ContentID=23045 (accessed September 16, 2011).

"What Is PTSD?" National Center for PTSD Fact Sheet. http://www.ncptsd.va.gov/ncmain/ncdocs/fact_shts/fs_what_is_ptsd.html (accessed September 16, 2011).

ORGANIZATIONS

American Academy of Experts in Traumatic Stress, 203 Deer Rd., Ronkonkoma, NY, 11779, (631) 543-2217, Fax: (631) 543-6977, info@aaets.org, http://www.aaets.org.

American Psychiatric Association, 1000 Wilson Blvd., Ste. 1825, Arlington, VA, 22209-3901, (703) 907-7300, apa@psych.org, http://www.psych.org.

Anxiety Disorders Association of America, 8730 Georgia Ave., Silver Spring, MD, 20910, (240) 485-1001, Fax: (240) 485-1035, http://www.adaa.org.

National Alliance on Mental Illness, 2107 Wilson Blvd., Ste. 300, Arlington, VA, 22201-3042, Fax: (703) 524-9094, (800) 950-6264, http://www.nami.org.

National Center for PTSD, U.S. Department of Veterans Affairs, 810 Vermont Ave. NW, Washington, DC, 20420, (802) 296-6300, ncptsd@va.gov, http://www.ncptsd.va.gov.

National Institute of Mental Health, 6001 Executive Blvd., Rm. 8184, MSC 9663, Bethesda, MD, 20892-9663, (301) 433-4513; TTY: (301) 443-8431, Fax: (301) 443-4279, (866) 615-6464; TTY: (866) 415-8051, nimhinfo@nih.gov, http://www.nimh.nih.gov.

Rebecca J. Frey, PhD

Premature ejaculation

Definition

Premature ejaculation (PE) refers to the persistent or recurrent discharge of semen with minimal sexual stimulation before, on, or shortly after penetration; before the person wishes it; and earlier than he expects it.

Description

In making the diagnosis of PE, the clinician must take into account factors that affect the length of time that the man feels sexually excited. These factors include the age of the patient and his partner; the newness of the sexual partner; and the location and recent frequency of sexual activity.

Premature ejaculation that takes place before the man's penis enters the woman's vagina will interfere with conception if the couple is planning a pregnancy. Continued lack of ejaculatory control may lead to sexual dissatisfaction for either or both members of the couple. It may become a source of marital tension, disturbed interpersonal relationships, or eventual separation or divorce.

Failure to respond to treatment for PE and the complications that may result from it should encourage the patient to seek further help from a health provider trained and experienced in treating the problem.

Causes and symptoms

Causes

Premature ejaculation (PE) is a common complaint. The available evidence supports the notion that control and modulation of sexual excitement is learned behavior, and if it has been learned incorrectly or inadequately, it can be relearned. PE is only rarely caused by a physical or structural problem; in these cases it is usually associated with other physical symptoms, usually pain. In rare cases, PE may be associated with a neurological condition; infection of the prostate gland; or urethritis (inflammation of the duct that carries urine and semen to the outside of the body). With the rising prevalence of **substance abuse**, an increasing number of cases of PE are being diagnosed in patients withdrawing from drugs, especially **opioids**.

PE may be of lifelong duration or develop in later life, especially if a difficult interpersonal relationship is one of its causes. Although PE is commonly associated with psychological symptoms, especially performance anxiety and guilt, these symptoms are its consequences rather than its causes. Once PE is firmly established, however, the accompanying psychological factors, especially in combination with sexual overstimulation, may form a self-perpetuating cycle that makes the disorder worse.

Premature ejaculation is common in adolescents where it may be made worse by feelings of sinfulness concerning sexual activity, fear of discovery, fear of making the partner pregnant, fear of contracting a sexually transmitted disease (STD), or performance anxiety. Adults may have similar concerns as well as interpersonal factors related to the sexual partner.

Symptoms

In PE, ejaculation occurs earlier than the patient and/or the couple would like, thus preventing full satisfaction from intercourse, especially on the part of the sexual partner, who frequently fails to attain orgasm. PE is almost invariably accompanied by marked emotional upset and interpersonal difficulties that may add frustration to an already tense situation, which makes the loss of sexual fulfillment even worse. It is also important to differentiate male orgasm from ejaculation. Some men are able to distinguish between the two events and enjoy the pleasurable sensations associated with orgasm apart from the emission of semen, which usually ends the moment of orgasm. In these cases, the partner is capable of achieving her own orgasm and sexual satisfaction.

Diagnosis

The physical examination of a patient who is having problems with PE usually results in normal findings. Abnormal findings are unusual. The best source of information for diagnosing the nature of the problem is the patient's sexual history. On taking the patient's history, the clinician should concentrate on the sexual history, making sure that both partners have adequate and accurate sexual information. Ideally, the sexual partner should participate in the history and is often able to contribute valuable information that the patient himself may be unaware of or unwilling to relate. The female partner should also be examined by a gynecologist in order to ascertain her sexual capabilities and to eliminate the possibility that the size or structure of her genitals is part of the reason for the male's premature ejaculation.

Treatment

Preferably, therapy for PE should be conducted under the supervision of a health professional trained in sexual dysfunction. Both partners must participate responsibly in the therapeutic program. Treatment of PE requires patience, dedication and commitment by both partners, and the therapist must convey this message to both. The first part of therapy requires both partners to avoid intercourse for a period of several weeks. This period of abstinence is helpful in relieving any troublesome performance anxiety on the part of the man that may interfere with therapy.

Behavioral techniques, taught either individually, conjointly, or in groups, are effective in the therapy of PE. A preliminary stage of all treatment is termed "sensate focus" and involves the man's concentration on the process of sexual arousal and orgasm. He should learn each step in the process, most particularly the moment prior to ejaculation. The sexual partner participates in the process, maintaining an awareness of her partner's sensations and how close he is to ejaculating. At this point, two techniques are commonly used:

- The "stop and start" technique. This approach involves sexual stimulation until the man recognizes that he is about to ejaculate. At this time, the stimulation is discontinued for about thirty seconds and then resumed. This sequence of events is repeated until ejaculation is desired by both partners, with stimulation continuing until ejaculation occurs.
- The "squeeze" technique. This approach involves sexual stimulation, usually by the sexual partner, until the man recognizes that he is about to ejaculate. At this time stimulation ceases. The patient or his partner gently squeezes the end of the penis at the junction of the glans penis (tip of the penis) with the shaft. The squeezing is continued for several seconds. Sexual stimulation is withheld for about 30 seconds and then resumed. This sequence of events is repeated by the patient alone or with the assistance of his partner until ejaculation is desired. At this point stimulation is continued until the man ejaculates.

The patient and his partner should be advised against trying any of the many unproven remedies that are available either over the counter or popularized on

KEY TERMS

Abstinence—Refraining from sexual intercourse for a period of time.

Ejaculation—The discharge of semen by the male reproductive organs.

Glans—The tip of the penis.

Orgasm—Another word for sexual climax. In the male, orgasm is usually accompanied by ejaculation but may be experienced as distinct from ejaculation.

Prostate—A muscular gland surrounding the urethra in males at the base of the urinary bladder. The prostate gland secretes the fluid that combines with the male sperm cells to form semen.

Semen—A thick whitish fluid containing sperm, produced by the male reproductive organs.

Urethritis—Inflammation of the urethra, which is the duct that carries urine and (in males) semen to the outside of the body.

the Internet. Certain prescription medications, especially **antidepressants** that produce delayed ejaculation as a side effect, may be useful as therapeutic adjuncts. The use of a class of drugs known as **selective serotonin reuptake inhibitors (SSRIs)** has shown promise in the treatment of premature ejaculation. The SSRIs prolong the time it takes the man to ejaculate by as much as 30 minutes. The SSRIs most commonly used to treat PE are **sertraline** (Zoloft) and **fluoxetine** (Prozac), which are currently approved by the Food and Drug Administration (FDA) for use in treating **depression** and panic attacks. It is important to emphasize that the use of these drugs to treat premature ejaculation is still considered experimental, as the FDA had not approved them for this specific use as of 2011.

Prognosis

In most cases (some observers claim a 95% success rate), the patient is able to control ejaculation through education and practice of the techniques recommended by a health professional. In chronic cases that do not respond to treatment, the PE may be related to a serious psychological or psychiatric condition, including depression or anxiety. Patients in this category may benefit from **psychotherapy**.

See also Male orgasmic disorder

Resources

BOOKS

Lue, Tom F., et al. *Atlas of Clinical Urology: Impotence and Infertility, Volume I*. New York: Current Medicine Group, 1999.

Masters, William, and Virginia Johnson. *Masters and Johnson on Sex and Human Loving*. New York: Little, Brown, 1988.

Steidle, Christopher P. *The Impotence Source Book*. New York: McGraw-Hill, 1999.

Ralph Myerson, M.D.

Premenstrual dysphoric disorder

Definition

Premenstrual dysphoric disorder (PMDD) is a collection of physical and emotional symptoms that occurs 5 to 11 days before a woman's period begins and goes away once menstruation starts. PMDD is a severe form of **premenstrual syndrome** (PMS).

KEY TERMS

Antidepressant—A medication used to relieve the symptoms of clinical depression.

Beta blockers—Class of drug that primarily works by blunting the action of adrenaline, the body's natural fight-or-flight chemical.

Nonsteroidal anti-inflammatory drugs—This class of drugs includes aspirin and ibuprofen, and primarily works by interfering with the formation of prostaglandins, enzymes implicated in pain and inflammation.

Demographics

PMS is estimated to affect 30%–80% of childbearing age. The more severe form of the disorder, PMDD, affects 3–8% of women of childbearing age. Up to 40% of women have PMDD symptoms that are so severe they interfere with their daily activities. Individuals are more at risk if they are in their late 20s and early 40s; have a history of **depression**, alcohol abuse, anxiety/tension, affective lability, or irritability/anger; are overweight; are under **stress**; have a maternal history of the disorder; use significant quantities of caffeine; or do not **exercise**. Clinical studies suggest that more than two million women in the United States may be affected by PMDD.

Description

While PMS is mild or moderate in severity, PMDD is considerably more severe. The symptoms of depressed mood, anxiety, lability, and intense irritability or anger result in significant problems with functioning. Like PMS, menstruation results in resolution of PMDD symptomatology.

Causes and symptoms

Although the actual cause of PMDD is not known, it is believed to be related to hormonal changes that occur before menstruation. The most common symptoms include headache; swelling of ankles, feet, and hands; backache; abdominal cramps; heaviness or pain; bloating and/or gas; muscle spasms; breast tenderness; weight gain; recurrent cold sores; acne; nausea; constipation or diarrhea; food cravings; anxiety or panic; confusion; difficulty concentrating or forgetfulness; poor judgment; and depression.

Diagnosis

PMDD is diagnosed when symptoms occur during the second half of the menstrual cycle (14 days or more after the first day of a woman's period), are absent for about seven days after the period ends, increase in severity as the cycle progresses, go away when the menstrual flow begins or shortly thereafter, and occur for at least three consecutive menstrual cycles. There are no tests to diagnose it. The **diagnosis** of PMDD emphasizes and requires psychologically important mood symptoms.

PMDD was listed in the appendix of the fourth edition of the ***Diagnostic and Statistical Manual of Mental Disorders*** (*DSM-IV*), but it is under consideration for its own listing as a depressive disorder in the forthcoming fifth edition (*DSM-5*), due to be published in 2013. The proposed criteria state that a woman may be diagnosed with PMDD if at least five of the following symptoms occur within a week of the onset of menses, and are minimal or absent by the first week after menses. At least one of the five symptoms must be one of the first four listed to meet the criteria for diagnosis and must be severe enough to interfere with normal work and life activities:

- mood swings, including sudden feelings of sadness or increased sensitivity to rejection
- irritability, anger, or an increase in personal conflicts
- depressed mood, including self-deprecating thoughts or a sense of hopelessness
- anxiety and tension
- reduced interest in activities, such as work, school, or social outings
- trouble concentrating
- fatigue, loss of energy
- change in appetite, including binges or cravings
- changes in sleep patterns
- feeling overwhelmed
- physical symptoms, including breast tenderness or swelling, joint pain, bloating, or weight gain

Treatment

Selective serotonin reuptake inhibitors (**SSRIs**) are used to treat the depressive and anxious symptoms of PMDD. These include **fluoxetine**, **sertraline**, **paroxetine**, **fluvoxamine**, **citalopram**, and **escitalopram**. Additionally, nonsteroidal anti-inflammatory drugs, such as ibuprofen and aspirin, may help with bloating and pain; beta blockers may help with migraines. Women with significant fluid retention (manifested by bloating, breast pain, weight gain) may benefit from the use of diuretics.

In October 2006, the FDA approved the use of the birth control pill YAZ for treating PMDD. YAZ contains a synthetic form of progesterone called drospirenone and estrogen in the form of ethinyl estradiol. Reports indicate that YAZ alleviates both physical and emotional symptoms of PMS and PMDD. In 2011, the FDA issued a safety alert warning that women taking a newer type of birth control containing the progestin hormone drospirenone may be at higher risk for developing potentially deadly blood clots than women taking pills with an older type of progestin hormone.

QUESTIONS TO ASK YOUR DOCTOR

- What types of treatments are available?
- What types of side effects from treatments can I expect? What are your recommendations to help me deal with those side effects?
- Are there any lifestyle changes that I should make? Dietary changes? Changes in activity level?
- What type of diet should I follow? Are there foods I should avoid?

Alternative treatment

Nonpharmaceutical treatments include a variety of lifestyle changes, such as following a healthy diet, exercise, sufficient rest, decreased caffeine and alcohol intake, stress-relief therapies, and possibly alternative therapies such as **aromatherapy**. Certain vitamins and supplements may also help, such as vitamin B6, calcium, magnesium, and vitamin E. Some experts also suggest increasing consumption of vitamin D and omega-3 fatty acids. Certain herbs may also help with symptom relief, including vitex, black cohosh, **valerian**, **kava kava**, and **St. John's wort**.

Prognosis

The prognosis varies for each woman, and is largely dependent on how much work she is willing to do in terms of lifestyle changes. Additionally, planning for PMDD symptoms, joining a support group, and communicating with her spouse and family can help minimize the negative effects of PMDD and its impact on a woman's home and work environments.

Prevention

Some women may find their PMDD disappears periodically. Exercise, stress relief strategies, diet, and nutritional supplements can have the greatest impact in preventing PMDD.

Resources

Katz, V. L., et al. *Comprehensive Gynecology*. 5th ed. St. Louis: Mosby, 2007.

WEBSITES

PubMed Health. "Premenstrual Dysphoric Disorder." U.S. National Library of Medicine. http://www.ncbi.nlm.nih.gov/pubmedhealth/PMH0004461 (accessed November 14, 2011).

ORGANIZATIONS

Office on Women's Health, U.S. Department of Health and Human Services, 200 Independence Ave. SW, Washington, DC, 20201, (800) 994-9662; TDD: (888) 220-5446, http://www.womenshealth.gov.

Heidi Splete

Premenstrual syndrome

Definition

Premenstrual syndrome (PMS) refers to symptoms that occur between ovulation and the onset of menstruation. The symptoms include both physical symptoms, such as breast tenderness, back pain, abdominal cramps, headache, and changes in appetite, as well as psychological symptoms of anxiety, **depression**, and unrest. Severe forms of this syndrome are referred to as **premenstrual dysphoric disorder** (PMDD). These symptoms may be related to hormones and emotional disorders.

Demographics

As many as 80% of women report that they experience some change in mood, behavior, and physical sensations or functioning in the time period before the onset of menses, although most women do not find these changes troubling. PMDD affects about 5% to 8% of women between puberty and menopause. About 10% to 40% of all menstruating women have PMS, which means that they experience symptoms that are marked enough to impair relationships, work, or family life but do not have symptoms that are severe enough to warrant a **diagnosis** of PMDD. Although many researchers list these and similar estimates of the prevalence of PMS, others point out that such estimates may be inaccurate because PMS is not a well-defined condition, and because prevalence estimates are usually derived from women's retrospective reports. Retrospective reports are often flawed because of memory distortions. For example, it is possible that some women who experience symptoms throughout the menstrual cycle misremember them as occurring only in the period prior to menstruation.

PMS can begin at any age after menarche or at the time of the first menstrual period. PMS occurs most often in women who ovulate, but women who do not ovulate may also experience it. For example, it may occur in women around the time of menopause, when women sometimes have menstrual periods, even when they do not ovulate. According to the National Women's Health Information Center, PMS is most common in women who are between their late 20s and early 40s, have at least one child, have a family history of depression, and have suffered from depression in the past. Some scientists have suggested that PMS is more likely to occur in women who eat large amounts of chocolate, or women who drink heavily. Women with PMS typically seek medical help for the condition in their 30s.

Description

In their reproductive years, women normally have fluctuations of various hormones over the course of the menstrual cycle. An average menstrual cycle lasts about 28 days, although a normal cycle can range from 21 to 35 days. Many hormones are released into the blood during the menstrual cycle, including estrogen and progesterone. Fluctuations in hormone levels cause changes in the ovaries and the uterus. On around day 14 of a 28-day cycle, an egg is released from the ovaries, in a process called ovulation. After ovulation, the luteal phase of the menstrual cycle begins. The luteal phase lasts about 14 days in a normal 28-day menstrual cycle. If the egg is not fertilized by a sperm, the lining of the uterus is shed in the process called menstruation. The onset of menstruation, or menses, marks the end of the luteal phase. The characteristic features of PMS are physical and emotional symptoms that start in the luteal phase and disappear soon after the onset of menses.

The cluster of symptoms associated with premenstrual syndrome was first described in the scientific literature in 1931, by R.T. Frank, the chief of obstetrics and gynecology at New York's Mt. Sinai Hospital. The term "premenstrual syndrome" was coined in 1953, in an article written by the English physician Katharina Dalton, who believed that PMS was due to a deficiency of the hormone progesterone.

PMS occurs in the middle of a symptom continuum that ranges from premenstrual molimina, or the normal signs heralding the onset of menses, to severe distress and dysfunction. The large majority of women between the ages of menarche and menopause experience physical, emotional, and/or behavioral changes during the time period before the start of menses, but many of them do not find these changes troubling. Women who experience severe symptoms are considered to have premenstrual dysphoric disorder, or PMDD, which was formerly called late luteal phase dysphoric disorder. The ***Diagnostic and Statistical Manual of Mental Disorders***, fourth edition (*DSM-IV*), describes PMDD as a condition that warrants further study before being granted the status of a specific disorder, but PMDD is used as a diagnostic category. For a woman to be diagnosed as having PMDD, she must have at least 5 of 11 symptoms, which include sadness, tension, mood swings, irritability, reduced interest in usual activities, difficulty concentrating, **fatigue**, appetite and sleep changes, a sense of being overwhelmed, and physical symptoms such as bloating or pain. At least one of the symptoms must be a mood symptom, and symptoms have to be present for most days during the luteal period for most months in the past year. Symptoms must remit shortly after the onset of menses.

Women who experience symptoms that are troubling enough to affect relationships, work, or family life but whose symptoms do not meet the criteria for PMDD are considered to have PMS. PMS is not listed as a psychiatric disorder in the *DSM-IV*. According to the tenth edition of the *International Statistical Classification of Diseases and Related Health Problems, ICD-10*, a diagnosis of PMS can be made even if only one distressing symptom is present. The American College of Obstetricians and Gynecologists guidelines for diagnosing PMS require at least one symptom to be present in the five days preceding the menses for three consecutive menstrual cycles.

Some people criticize the characterization of PMS as a disorder. They point out that PMS is not well defined and that many women experience PMS symptoms. They fear that making PMS into a disorder stigmatizes women in general and makes women subject to negative portrayals in popular culture. Women are described as "PMSing," aggressive, hostile, and crazy, and are the frequent targets of jokes about the effects of the menstrual cycle. The idea that women are strongly influenced by their menstrual cycles can have an impact on their professional lives, even though there is little evidence that PMS impairs task performance. Some people even suggest that the promotion of PMS as a disorder is attributable to a profit motive. They claim that the concept of PMS exists partly because it is financially beneficial for hospitals and clinics to provide treatments for PMS, even though many of these treatments are ineffective or unproved.

Others advocate defining PMS as a disorder. They argue that PMS is a significant burden for many women, and that women with PMS are relieved to have the condition recognized as a real problem, rather than have it be dismissed as the product of an overactive imagination.

Symptoms

Symptom type can vary from menstrual cycle to cycle, as can symptom severity. The PMS symptoms most commonly reported by women are bloating, irritability, and difficulty sleeping. Other symptoms include breast discomfort, headaches, swelling of hands or feet, back pain, joint or muscle aches, fatigue, lapses in memory, decreased interest in sex, angry outbursts, restlessness, difficulty concentrating, confusion, depression, anxiety, social withdrawal, and cravings for sweet or salty foods and caffeine.

Causes

The causes of PMS are unclear. Scientists have put forward many theories to explain the etiology of PMS, including low levels of the hormone progesterone, changes in the ratio of the hormone estrogen to progesterone, increases in the activity of the adrenal gland, too much of the hormone prolactin, decreased endorphins, and too little prostaglandin, among others. Research does not provide consistent support for any of these theories.

However, most scientists do agree that abnormal levels of the neurotransmitter **serotonin**, or abnormal bodily responses to serotonin, may be involved in PMS. The fluctuations of hormones during the menstrual cycle may have an effect on serotonin function, but the details of the mechanisms involved are still unclear. Evidence for the involvement of serotonin in PMS comes from the fact that PMS and PMDD have many symptoms in common with disorders such as depression, which involve abnormalities related to serotonin levels. Also, many women with PMDD and PMS find that symptoms are alleviated when they take **selective serotonin reuptake inhibitors (SSRIs)**, which are antidepressant drugs that increase the levels of serotonin available to nerve cells.

Because there are many different kinds of PMS symptoms and many different etiological theories with partial support, some researchers speculate that there may be more than one form and multiple causes of PMS.

Diagnosis

There are no laboratory tests for diagnosing PMS, because the cause of the condition is unknown. A diagnosis of PMS is typically made only after a woman has kept a record of daily symptoms over the course of the menstrual cycle for at least three months. This allows women to determine whether their symptoms occur only during the luteal phase of the cycle or at other times as well.

A diagnosis of PMDD is given only after ruling out the possibility of a premenstrual increase in the symptoms of another disorder. Some women with general medical conditions such as seizure disorders, endocrine dysfunctions, cancer, systemic lupus erythematosus, anemia, endometriosis, and some kinds of infections may experience higher levels of negative mood and fatigue during the premenstrual period. Some women with psychological disorders, such as depression, **anxiety disorders**, **bulimia nervosa**, substance use problems, and **personality disorders**, may also experience exacerbations of their symptoms during the premenstrual period. These women, however, experience symptoms throughout the menstrual cycle, unlike women with PMS, who only experience symptoms during the luteal phase.

Treatment

Treatments for PMS include lifestyle changes, drug therapy, nutritional supplements, and herbal remedies.

Traditional

Changes in lifestyle, rather than drug therapy, are recommended for women who experience mild PMS. For many women, regular **exercise** alleviates PMS symptoms. One theory suggests that a decrease in endorphin levels in the late luteal phase may result in premenstrual symptoms. Exercise causes endorphins to be released, which may help to alleviate the depressive symptoms that some women with PMS experience. Twenty to thirty minutes of aerobic exercise at least three days a week are recommended.

Because **stress** can exacerbate PMS, taking steps to reduce work and family stress, especially in the premenstrual period, can be helpful. Women who experience PMS may find it helpful to avoid scheduling stressful activities on days when they expect to have symptoms. Dealing with issues at work and within relationships that produce conflict may also be helpful, because achieving a sense of control can reduce stress.

Although some researchers point out that there is no evidence that dietary changes can alleviate PMS, others recommend keeping dietary salt levels low to prevent fluid retention and bloating, and reducing caffeine intake to alleviate breast discomfort and reduce jitteriness.

Drugs

The main pharmacological agents used to treat PMS are **SSRIs**, antianxiety medications, drugs that induce chemical menopause, hormones, and oral contraceptives.

The U.S. Food and Drug Administration (FDA) has approved the use of the SSRIs **fluoxetine** and **sertraline** for the treatment of PMDD. Although the FDA has not approved these drugs for PMS, reports indicate that they are helpful for treating PMS. The dose that is prescribed for PMDD and PMS is typically smaller than that used to treat depression. SSRIs typically take two to four weeks before they begin to have an effect on the symptoms of depression, but they alleviate the symptoms of PMS and PMDD in a much shorter time, usually in one or two days. For depression, intermittent dosing with SSRIs is not usually effective, but for PMS and PMDD SSRIs are effective when taken daily only during the luteal phase of the menstrual cycle.

Studies show that SSRIs are not effective for about 40% of women with PMDD. These results may indicate that hormones and **neurotransmitters** other than serotonin are also implicated in PMDD.

Some practitioners report that **alprazolam** is effective for alleviating the anxiety that some women with PMS experience. Alprazolam is a benzodiazepine drug that is sold under the brand name Xanax. Other reports indicate that alprazolam is not an effective treatment for negative premenstrual mood symptoms and that it can also impair task performance. In addition, the use of alprazolam can lead to **addiction**.

Chemically inducing menopause is an effective way of eliminating PMS and PMDD, but because this treatment has many side effects, it is only used as a last resort. Drugs such as leuprolide, which is sold under the brand name Lupron, are used to induce chemical menopause. Leuprolide is similar to a gonadotropin-releasing hormone, a hormone naturally released by the **brain**. Leuprolide reduces estrogen production by the ovaries. Because low estrogen can lead to problems such as thinning of bones, estrogen is sometimes administered to women who take drugs like Lupron, to reduce side effects such as osteoporosis and hot flashes. However, estrogen add-back therapy is very expensive and may result in the return of PMS symptoms.

In the 1950s, the English physician Katharina Dalton treated many women with PMS by giving them supplements of the hormone progesterone. She reported that progesterone was effective in alleviating symptoms in these women. More recent research in the United States has not confirmed Dalton's results. Despite this, gynecologists still sometimes prescribe progesterone for PMS, because some women report benefits. Natural progesterone, or synthetic progesterone in the form of drugs such as Provera, may be used. Progesterone injections can be given in the form of Depo-Provera, which is a contraceptive. A dose of injected Depo-Provera lasts for three months. It prevents women from getting periods. The drug has a sedative effect on some women and so alleviates premenstrual anxiety. The drug can, however, have negative side effects, including bleeding or spotting, depression, and weight gain.

Some women with PMS find that symptoms are alleviated when they take a low-dose birth control pill, although, for unknown reasons, other women actually have worsening of symptoms when they use oral contraceptives. In October 2006, the FDA approved the use of the birth control pill YAZ for treating PMDD. YAZ contains a synthetic form of progesterone called drospirenone and estrogen in the form of ethinyl estradiol. Reports indicate that YAZ alleviates both physical and emotional symptoms of PMS. In 2011 the FDA issued a safety alert warning that women taking a newer type of birth control containing the progestin hormone drospirenone may be at higher risk for developing potentially deadly blood clots than women taking pills with an older type of progestin hormone.

Alternative

Some health practitioners suggest using nutritional and herbal supplements, selected to treat the primary symptoms experienced, although their effectiveness in alleviating PMS is controversial. Some nutritional supplements and herbs can be toxic or may interact with medications. There are varying dosage recommendations for many of these supplements in the scientific literature. For these reasons, women should consult with their physicians before using such substances.

For fluid retention problems, diuretic therapy with 25 mg of spironolactone twice a day is sometimes recommended. Spironolactone is sold under the trade name Aldactone. Other reports indicate that a spironolactone supplement of 100 mg per day improves both the physical and mood symptoms of PMS. Using a calcium supplement of 1,200–1,500 mg daily also appears to reduce PMS symptoms in some women. Some practitioners recommend using vitamin B6 supplements of 50–100 mg daily, but others recommend a higher dose. Vitamin B6 is a natural diuretic and may help to reduce bloating. Furthermore, vitamin B6 appears to suppress the action of prolactin, which is a hormone that may be involved in PMS. Vitamin B6 may also play a role in the metabolism of serotonin, which appears to be involved in PMS. A Vitamin E supplement of about 400–600 units a day is sometimes suggested for helping to alleviate breast discomfort. Daily supplements of magnesium appear to reduce symptoms related to fluid retention such as weight gain, breast tenderness, swelling of hands and feet, and abdominal bloating. Dose recommendations vary from 200–600 mg daily.

Some practitioners report that women who use **evening primrose oil** find that it occasionally alleviates PMS symptoms, although others report that studies have not demonstrated its effectiveness. Evening primrose is a plant that has a fatty acid essential to the body, called gamma-linoleic acid. Some researchers have speculated that gamma-linoleic acid may help PMS symptoms by raising the levels of prostaglandin in the body. Other oils that contain gamma-linoleic acid are borage oil, black currant oil, and rapeseed oil.

The Mexican wild yam (*Dioscorea villosa*) contains a substance that may be converted to progesterone in the body. Because this substance is readily absorbed through the skin, it can be found as an ingredient in many skin creams. (Some products also have natural progesterone added to them.) Some herbalists believe that these products can have a progesterone-like effect on the body and decrease some of the symptoms of PMS.

KEY TERMS

Adrenal gland—A gland that produces many different hormones, including estrogen, progesterone, and stress hormones.

Anemia—A condition in which red blood cells do not supply enough oxygen to body tissues.

Benzodiazepine—A class of antianxiety drugs.

Bulimia nervosa—An eating disorder in which binge eating is followed by inappropriate and often dangerous efforts to control body weight.

Contraceptive—A method that prevents conception and pregnancy.

Endocrine dysfunction—A problem relating to inadequate or excessive production of hormones.

Endometriosis—A condition in which the tissue that is normally present in the lining of the uterus grows elsewhere in the body.

Endorphin—A neurotransmitter that acts like a natural opiate, relieving pain and producing euphoria.

Gonadotropin-releasing hormone—A hormone produced by the brain that stimulates the pituitary gland to release hormones that trigger ovulation.

Luteal phase—The period of time between ovulation and menstruation.

Menarche—The first menstrual period.

Menopause—The cessation of menstrual periods.

Neurotransmitter—A chemical that sends signals from one nerve cell to another.

Osteoporosis—The thinning of bone and loss of bone density.

Personality disorder—A chronic pattern of behaving and relating to others that causes significant distress and impairs functioning.

Premenstrual molimina—The normal signs that indicate that menses will soon occur.

Prostaglandin—A chemical produced in the body, which is involved in many functions, including blood pressure regulation and inflammation.

Systemic lupus erythematosus—A chronic, inflammatory autoimmune disorder.

The most important way to alter hormone levels may be by eating more phytoestrogens. These plant-derived compounds have an effect similar to estrogen in the body. One of the richest sources of phytoestrogens is soy products, such as tofu. Additionally, many supplements can be found that contain black cohosh (*Cimicifugaracemosa*) or dong quai (*Angelica sinensis*), which are herbs high in phytoestrogens. Red clover (*Trifolium pratense*), alfalfa (*Medicago sativa*), licorice (*Glycyrrhiza glabra*), hops (*Humulus lupulus*), and legumes are also high in phytoestrogens. Increasing the consumption of phytoestrogens is also associated with decreased risks of osteoporosis, cancer, and heart disease.

Many **antidepressants** act by increasing serotonin levels. An alternative means of achieving this is to eat more carbohydrates. For instance, two cups of cereal or a cup of pasta have enough carbohydrates to effectively increase serotonin levels. An herb known as **St. John's wort** (*Hypericum perforatum*) has stood up to scientific trials as an effective antidepressant. As with the standard antidepressants, however, it must be taken continuously and does not show an effect until used for 46 weeks. There are also herbs, such as skullcap (*Scutellaria lateriflora*) and kava (*Piper methysticum*), that can relieve the anxiety and irritability that often accompany depression. An advantage of these herbs is that they can be taken when symptoms occur rather than continually. Chaste tree (*Vitex agnus-castus*) in addition to helping rebalance estrogen and progesterone in the body, also may relieve the anxiety and depression associated with PMS.

The only alternative therapy that has shown clinical promise in reducing symptoms of PMS is calcium. Regular and increased calcium intake appears to alleviate and even prevent PMS symptoms in women; however, the calcium must be ingested from food sources and not from supplements. Evidence for all other nutritional or herbal therapies is conflicting. Patients should always discuss taking supplements with their physicians before beginning treatment.

Prevention

Maintaining a good diet, one low in sugars and fats and high in phytoestrogens and complex carbohydrates, may prevent some of the symptoms of PMS. Women should try to exercise three times a week, keep in generally good health, and maintain a positive self image. Avoidance of caffeine and/or alcohol may help some women. Because PMS is often associated with stress, avoidance of stress or developing better means to deal with stress can be important.

Prognosis

Women who have PMS typically experience symptoms throughout their reproductive years, except during pregnancy. In some women, PMS can become more severe around the time of menopause, in the perimenopausal time period. PMS generally remits after menopause.

Resources

BOOKS

American Psychiatric Association. *Diagnostic and Statistical Manual of Mental Disorders*. 4th ed., text rev. Washington, DC: American Psychiatric Publishing, 2000.

Minkin, Mary Jane, and Carol V. Wright. *The Yale Guide to Women's Reproductive Health From Menarche to Menopause*. New Haven, CT: Yale University Press, 2003.

Ratcliff, Kathryn Strother. *Women and Health: Power, Technology, Inequality and Conflict in a Gendered World*. Upper Saddle River, NJ: Prentice-Hall, 2008.

Speroff, Leon, and Marc A. Fritz. *Clinical Gynecologic Endocrinology and Infertility*. 7th ed. Philadelphia: Lippincott Williams & Wilkins, 2010.

PERIODICALS

Clayton, A.H., et al. "Exploratory Study of Premenstrual Symptoms and Serotonin Variability." *Archives of Women's Mental Health* 9, no. 1 (January 2006): 51–57.

Hudson, Tori. "Premenstrual Syndrome: A Review of Herbal and Nutritional Supplements." *Townsend Letter for Doctors and Patients* 270 (January 2006). 126–31.

Mishell, Daniel R. "Premenstrual Disorders: Epidemiology and Disease Burden." *American Journal of Managed Care* 11, no. 16 Suppl. (2005): S473–79.

Rapkin, Andrea J. "New Treatment Approaches for Premenstrual Disorders." *American Journal of Managed Care* 11, no. 16 Suppl. (December 2005): S480–91.

Strine, Tara W., Daniel P. Chapman, and Indu B. Ahluwalia. "Menstrual-Related Problems and Psychological Distress among Women in the United States." *Journal of Women's Health* 14, no. 4 (May 2005): 316–23.

Yonkers, Kimberly A. "Management Strategies for PMS/PMDD." *Journal of Family Practice* 53, no. 9 (September 2004): SS15–20.

WEBSITES

Drugs.com. "FDA Approves New Indication for YAZ to Treat Emotional and Physical Symptoms of Premenstrual Dysphoric Disorder (PMDD)." October 5, 2006. http://www.drugs.com/news/fda-approves-yaz-emotional-physical-premenstrual-dysphoric-disorder-1929.html (accessed October 23, 2011).

MEDgle Patient GPS.com. "Premenstrual Syndrome." July 24, 2011. http://www.medgle.com/rw/diagnoses/premenstrual+syndrome (accessed October 23, 2011).

ORGANIZATIONS

American College of Obstetricians and Gynecologists, PO Box 96920, Washington, DC, 20090-6920, (202) 638-5577, http://www.acog.org.

The Hormone Foundation, 8401 Connecticut Ave., Ste. 900, Chevy Chase, MD, 20815-5817, (800) 467-6663, Fax: (301) 941-0259, hormone@endo-society.org, http://www.hormone.org.

National Institute of Mental Health, 6001 Executive Blvd., Room 8184, MSC 9663, Bethesda, MD, 20892-9663, (301) 433-4513; TTY: (301) 443-8431, Fax: (301) 443-4279, (866) 615-6464; TTY: (866) 415-8051 nimhinfo@nih.gov, http://www.nimh.nih.gov.

National Women's Health Information Center, 8270 Willow Oaks Corporate Drive, Ste. 101, Fairfax, VA, 22031, (800) 994-9662, http://www.womenshealth.gov.

Ruvanee Pietersz Vilhauer, PhD

Prescription drug abuse

Definition

Prescription drug abuse is the use of medicine prescribed by a doctor in dosages other than the prescribed dosage; for reasons other than the symptoms for which it was prescribed; by a person other than for whom it was prescribed; or as a recreational drug.

Demographics

According to the National Institute on Drug Abuse (NIDA), the abuse of prescription drugs and over-the-counter medications in the United States more than doubled between 1999 and 2009. More than 7 million Americans were abusing prescription drugs in 2010, according to the National Survey on Drug Use and Health.

Prescription drugs are abused most often by adolescents and young adults in their twenties. In youths aged 12–17, girls are more likely than boys to abuse prescription drugs; the rate is about even in adults. In young people, prescription drug abuse often is recreational. In this group, there is a correlation between **alcohol use**, other types of drug abuse, risky sexual behavior, and prescription drug abuse.

Description

The three categories of prescription drugs that are the most abused are opioid pain relievers, central nervous system depressants prescribed as **sedatives** or tranquilizers, and stimulants used to treat **attention deficit hyperactivity disorder (ADHD)**.

Opioids

Opioids are narcotic pain-relieving drugs that block certain receptors in the **brain** and reduce the individual's perception of pain. Morphine, the first medical opioid, is a natural product derived from the sap of the opium poppy. Today most opioid drugs with medical uses are synthetic compounds that act in ways similar to morphine. Commonly prescribed opioids include codeine, hydrocodone (Vicodin),

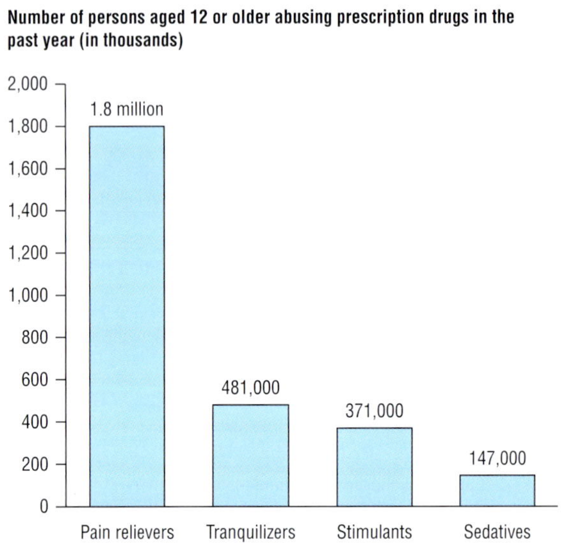

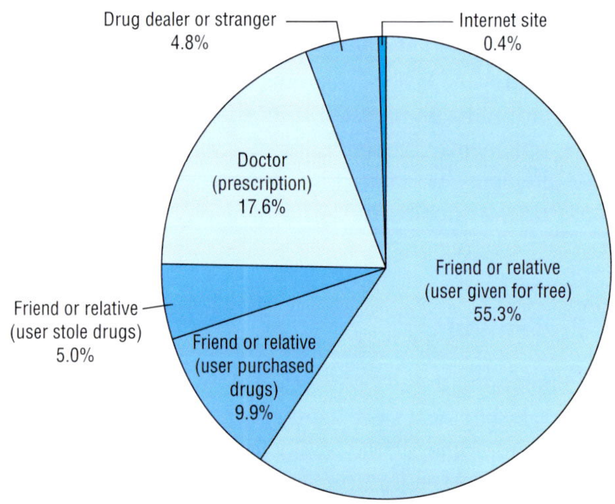

SOURCE: Substance Abuse and Mental Health Services Administration (SAMHSA), Office of Applied Studies, *Results from the 2009 National Survey on Drug Use and Health, Volume I: Summary of National Findings* (September 2010).

Report available online at http://oas.samhsa.gov/NSDUH/2k9NSDUH/2k9Results.htm. *(Graphs by PreMediaGlobal. © 2012 Cengage Learning.)*

methadone, oxycodone (OxyContin), meperidine (Demerol), propoxyphene (Darvon), hydromorphone (Dilaudid), and fentanyl (Fentora). Of these, hydrocodone, oxycodone, and codeine are the most frequently abused. Heroin, another drug in this group, is commonly abused but has no medical use and is never prescribed.

Opioids are very effective in controlling pain. Side effects include drowsiness and constipation. When taken exactly as prescribed, opioids are rarely addictive. When abused, opioids can be physically addictive and tolerance can develop. Large doses can depress breathing and cause death.

In people with a genuine medical need for pain control, abuse can develop by taking a larger or more frequent dose than prescribed. However, most abuse arises from recreational drug use. This is especially true of oxycodone, hydrocodone, and codeine. OxyContin and Vicodin, for example, are tablets that can be crushed into a powder and snorted or dissolved in water and injected. This practice is particularly dangerous as it quickly exposes the abuser to high levels of the drug. Overdoses can be fatal. Codeine usually is taken orally. It is a common component of prescription cough syrups and is found in combination tablets with acetaminophen (e.g., Tylenol with codeine).

Many opioid abusers get their drugs from friends or family members who have had legitimate prescriptions for the drugs but have unused drugs remaining after treatment. Others go prescription shopping, visiting several doctors and claiming severe pain symptoms for which they receive multiple prescriptions for an opioid drug. In some cases, these drugs are bought without a prescription over the Internet from suppliers in countries where a prescription is not required. Opioids also are sold as street drugs.

Central nervous system depressants

Central nervous system (CNS) depressants are prescribed as sedatives and tranquilizers to treat **sleep disorders** and anxiety. Commonly abused drugs in this category include **barbiturates** such as mephobarbital (Mebaral) and sodium phenobarbital (Nebutal); **benzodiazepines** such as **diazepam** (Valium), **alprazolam** (Xanax), and **estazolam** (Prosom), which are used to treat anxiety; and sleep medications such as **zolpidem** (Ambien), **zaleplon** (Sonata), and eszopiclone (Lunesta). Both barbiturates and benzodiazepine have a fairly high potential for physical **addiction**. The newer sleep medications have less potential to be physically addictive.

CNS depressants increase the amount of a neurotransmitter in the brain called gamma-aminobutyric acid (GABA). This produces a feeling of calm and drowsiness, which is what makes these drugs effective in treating anxiety and **insomnia**. CNS depressants usually are taken orally (tablets or capsules) and are sometimes taken to counteract the effect of illicit stimulant drugs. Taken with alcohol, these drugs are especially dangerous, as alcohol also is a CNS depressant. Overdose, especially in combination with alcohol, can be fatal. People who take CNS depressants for a long time and then suddenly stop taking them can have withdrawal symptoms and **seizures**. Many people who abuse CNS depressants get them by prescription shopping or from family and friends.

Stimulants

Stimulant prescription drugs are used to treat **ADHD**, **narcolepsy**, and sometimes **depression** that is unresponsive to other drug therapies. Stimulant drugs increase alertness, attention, and energy. Common stimulant drugs of abuse include **dextroamphetamine** (Dexedrine), **methylphenidate** (Ritalin, Concerta), and the amphetamine Adderall. Prescription stimulants are particularly popular among high school and college students who use them to increase concentration and energy when studying. These drugs also are used to get high.

Although stimulants increase focus and concentration by increasing the level of the neurotransmitter **dopamine** in the brain, they also can have serious side effects including increased blood pressure, irregular heartbeat, increased body temperature, insomnia, irritability, and seizures. Heart failure is possible, especially when these drugs are mixed with antidepressant drugs or over-the-counter cold medications containing decongestants.

Many prescription stimulants are acquired through a legitimate prescription and then abused in the way they are taken. Alternately, people who have no medical need for the drugs buy them from friends with legitimate prescriptions. Ritalin and Adderall abuse are especially common on college campuses. **Amphetamines** also can be bought as street drugs, and in some cases prescription stimulant drugs can be ordered through the Internet from countries where prescriptions are not required.

Causes and symptoms

The number of prescriptions written for common drugs of abuse has undergone an eight-fold increase in the past 20 years. Some experts believe that intensive drug advertising on television and in magazines has encouraged patients to ask their doctors for prescriptions for specific drugs, especially pain medicines and sleep aids. In addition, Internet pharmacies have made it easier to acquire these drugs without a proper medical examination and prescription.

KEY TERMS

Attention deficit hyperactivity disorder (ADHD)—A learning and behavioral disorder characterized by difficulty in sustaining attention, impulsive behavior, and excessive activity.

Central nervous system (CNS)—Part of the nervous system consisting of the brain, cranial nerves, and spinal cord. The brain is the center of higher processes, such as thought and emotion and is responsible for the coordination and control of bodily activities and the interpretation of information from the senses. The cranial nerves and spinal cord link the brain to the peripheral nervous system, which consists of the nerves present in the rest of body.

Dopamine—A neurochemical made in the brain that is involved in many brain activities, including movement and emotion.

Narcolepsy—A disorder in which the individual can fall into a deep sleep without warning.

Narcotic—A drug derived from opium or compounds similar to opium. Such drugs are potent pain relievers and can affect mood and behavior. Long-term use of narcotics can lead to dependence and tolerance.

Neurotransmitter—One of a group of chemicals secreted by a nerve cell (neuron) to carry a chemical message to another nerve cell, often as a way of transmitting a nerve impulse. Examples of neurotransmitters include acetylcholine, dopamine, serotonin, and norepinephrine.

Tolerance—A decrease in sensitivity to a drug. When tolerance occurs, a person must take more and more of the drug to get the same effect.

The reasons people abuse prescription drugs are varied but include:

- an attempt to eliminate pain (opioids)
- to increase concentration and focus (stimulants)
- to treat insomnia (CNS depressants)
- to relieve anxiety (CNS depressants)
- to get high
- because they believe prescription drugs, unlike street drugs, to be safe

Behaviors that suggest prescription drug abuse include:

- stealing or forging prescriptions
- stealing drugs from the medicine cabinets of family or friends
- repeatedly claiming to have lost a prescription so that another must be written
- visiting multiple doctors for the same symptoms and getting prescriptions from each one
- an increase in extreme mood swings
- changes in sleep patterns
- changes in energy level
- increased irritability

Diagnosis

Diagnosis can be difficult. Doctors may become alerted to prescription drug abuse through behaviors such as requesting replacement for "lost" prescriptions or early renewal of prescriptions. In other cases, a family member may suggest prescription drug abuse is occurring. Finally there may be physical signs of drug abuse. These will vary depending on the type of drug being abused.

Examination

A complete medical history, especially a medication history, and a physical examination are the starting point of a diagnosis of prescription drug abuse. Blood and urine tests can identify some drugs of abuse, although they are often more helpful in monitoring progress toward recovery than in making an initial diagnosis. Often, however, the patient or a patient's family member will express concern about prescription drug usage that will initiate a conversation leading to a diagnosis of drug abuse.

Treatment

There are two approaches to treatment: drug therapy and **psychotherapy**. For best results, these therapies often are used together. Treatment must take into account the type of drug used, the length of use, the health status of the individual, abuse of other substances such as alcohol or illicit drugs, the mental health status of the individual, and his or her life circumstances.

No single type of treatment is right for all prescription drug abusers. Physically addicted individuals should be in a supervised **detoxification** program. Serious negative health consequences and withdrawal symptoms may occur if the individual simply stops taking the drug of abuse on his or her own initiative.

Drugs

Of the three major categories of abused prescription drugs, only opioids can be treated with drugs. **Naltrexone** is a medication that blocks the effects of opioids drugs. It is used most often to treat overdoses. Serious physical opioid addiction can be treated with methadone or buprenorphine (Buprenex, Subutex) to relieve withdrawal symptoms and help prevent drug cravings. Methadone is a synthetic opioid that eliminates withdrawal symptoms. It is often used to treat heroin addiction but under some circumstances may used to treat addiction to other opioids. Buprenorphine treatment has not been well studied in relation to prescription drug addiction. Both methadone and buprenorphine are tightly controlled and are not be available from all doctors.

No drug therapy exists to treat CNS depressant addiction or prescription stimulant addiction. Nevertheless, some drugs may be used to help stabilize mood swings during withdrawal. It is especially important that people who are addicted to barbiturates or benzodiazepines be treated in a supervised detoxification program. Use of these drugs must be reduced gradually (tapered) to prevent serious health consequences.

Psychotherapy

Group or individual **cognitive-behavioral therapy** and **family therapy** often are used to treat individuals addicted to any type of drug. Cognitive behavioral therapy helps individuals understand the factors that trigger prescription drug abuse and to replace negative behaviors with positive ones. Family therapy helps families deal with underlying tensions in family relationships and to accept and deal with relapses.

Prognosis

Recovery depends on the type and strength of drug the individual is abusing and the length of time the drug has been abused. Relapses are common. Another problem in treating prescription drug addiction involves exchanging one addictive drug for another—for example, eliminating sedative dependence but replacing it with alcohol dependence. The greatest chance of complete recovery comes with early and intensive treatment, with family involvement or other support.

Prevention

The following tips can help prevent prescription drug abuse:

- Take all drugs in the amount and at the time intervals prescribed.
- Properly discard all unused prescription medicines.
- Do not share prescriptions or use drugs prescribed for another person, even if that person shares the same symptoms.
- Monitor children's or teen's prescription drug use.

Resources

BOOKS

Colvin, Rod. *Overcoming Prescription Drug Addiction: A Guide to Coping and Understanding*. 3rd ed. Omaha, NE: Addicus Books, 2008.

WEBSITES

Mayo Clinic. "Prescription Drug Abuse." June 25, 2010. http://www.mayoclinic.com/print/prescription-drug-abuse/DS01079 (accessed October 23, 2011).

MedlinePlus. "Prescription Drug Abuse." U.S. National Library of Medicine, National Institutes of Health. October 19, 2011. http://www.nlm.nih.gov/medlineplus/prescription drugabuse.html (accessed October 23, 2011).

U.S. National Institute on Drug Abuse. "Prescription Drug Abuse." May 2011. http://drugabuse.gov/tib/prescription.html (accessed October 23, 2011).

U.S. National Institute on Drug Abuse. "Prescription Drugs: Abuse and Addiction." http://www.nida.nih.gov/ResearchReports/Prescription/prescription7.html (accessed October 23, 2011).

ORGANIZATIONS

Drug Enforcement Administration, Mailstop AES, 8701 Morrissette Drive, Springfield, VA, 22152, (800) 882-9539, http://www.justice.gov.

National Council on Alcoholism and Drug Dependence, Inc., 244 East 58th Street, 4th Fl., New York, NY, 10022, (212) 269-7797, Fax: (212) 269-7510, http://www.ncadd.org.

National Institute on Drug Abuse, 6001 Executive Blvd., Room 5213, Bethesda, MD, 20892-9561, http://www.nida.nih.gov.

The Partnership at Drugfree.org, 352 Park Ave. South, 9th Floor, New York, NY, 10010, (212) 922-1560, Fax: (212) 922-1570, http://www.drugfree.org.

Tish Davidson, AM

Presenile dementia *see* **Alzheimer's disease**

Primary hypersomnia *see* **Hypersomnia**

Primary insomnia *see* **Insomnia**

Pristiq *see* **Desvenlafaxine**

Problem-solving skills training *see* **Cognitive problem-solving skills training**

Process addiction

Definition

A process **addiction**, also known as behavioral addiction, is the repetitive occurrence of impulsive behaviors regardless of the negative consequences the behaviors may trigger.

Demographics

Adolescence is a period of critical vulnerability in the development of addiction, for both cultural and neurobiological reasons. Age at onset for kleptomania is not known, but it is usually before adulthood, and two-thirds of people with kleptomania are female. Pyromania is both extremely rare and understudied, and no one has established the range of age at onset. The best-studied process addiction is pathological gambling, and its demographics can vary based on environmental factors, including proximity to a gambling location and exposure to gambling. It is more prevalent among males, and rates can be as high as 8% among adolescents and college-age students. The little research done thus far on Internet addiction suggests that it can affect any age or socioeconomic group.

Description

Process or behavioral addiction became a focus of study in the 1980s and 1990s. Researchers hypothesized that changes wrought in the brain's reward system by certain substances (e.g., **cocaine**) and leading to substance use problems or addiction may also underlie the exercise of dysfunctional, directed behaviors that have negative consequences. In other words, the addictions may differ in nature (a process like gambling versus taking a substance like cocaine), but the end result in the brain/body is the same. To paraphrase one researcher, the **brain** does not care whether or not the reward comes from a chemical stimulus or from an experience.

Many of the behaviors listed in the ***Diagnostic and Statistical Manual of Mental Disorders,*** fourth edition, text revision (also known as the *DSM-IV-TR*) as "Impulsive-Compulsive, Not Elsewhere Classified," may fall under the umbrella of process addiction. An essential feature of an impulse disorder is the inability to resist engaging in an act that can harm the individual or others. For most, if not all, of these disorders, the act or behavior is preceded by a feeling of tension or anticipation. The behavior itself brings on a feeling of pleasure, gratification, or relief, and following the behavior, the person may or not feel regret or self-reproach.

In addition to the impulsive nature of the behaviors, there is also a pattern of behavioral addiction. The features of this group of disorders include the urge to engage in a behavioral sequence that has negative consequences or is counterproductive; a feeling of increasing tension as the execution of the behavior approaches; a resurgence of the urge after a lapse of hours, days, or weeks; and the presence of external cues for the behavior that vary and are specific to a particular behavioral addiction. These patterns are similar to those manifested in substance addiction and can be classified as addictions because they have the same components as substance/chemical addictions, including mood modification, tolerance, withdrawal, and **relapse**.

Among this group of impulsive-compulsive behaviors that may also be classified as behavioral addictions are pathological gambling, **kleptomania**, **pyromania**, **trichotillomania** (recurrent pulling out of one's own hair), compulsive buying, and compulsive sexual behavior. The suite of disorders may also include compulsive Internet/computer use. Of these disorders, pathological gambling has received the most attention and study. These disorders may ultimately be included in a new category in the *DSM-5,* called "Substance and Behavioral Addictions." This category is under review to include pathological gambling, kleptomania, pyromania, and disorders currently listed under "Impulsive-Compulsive Behaviors Not Otherwise Specified," along with compulsive buying and impulsive-compulsive sex behavior.

Causes and symptoms

Causes

Being the child of a person who has an impulsive disorder such as pathological gambling may be a risk factor. Early onset of alcohol or drug use can exacerbate the severity of process addiction, and this pattern also holds true at least for pathological gambling. Adolescence is a critically vulnerable time, primarily because the brain areas affected as addiction develops are immature and susceptible. The immaturity may lead to a greater level of impulsive behaviors.

There have been some genetic links indicated in studies of pathological gambling and compulsive buying.

The mechanism underlying addiction involves disruptions in **serotonin** and **dopamine** signaling and monoamine oxidase (MAO) activity. The MAO gene lies on the X chromosome, which can result in the observed sex differences in some behavioral addiction disorders. Males, who have only one X chromosome, express only the gene their single X chromosome carries; females have two X chromosomes, and having one normal version of MAO on one X chromosome can compensate for having a mutant version on the other chromosome.

Symptoms

Dopamine is a neurotransmitter involved in reward pathways in the brain and in the development or

reinforcement of behaviors. This molecule and its associated proteins have been strongly implicated in **substance abuse** and behavioral addiction. People with process addiction may share many symptoms with people who have substance use disorders, including **depression**, loneliness, social impairment, and distraction.

Some symptoms are specific to a given behavior. For example, in impulsive-compulsive sex behavior, the person may have frequent, intrusive thoughts about sex and engage repeatedly in sex behaviors that may spiral out of their control.

Some criteria have been proposed for considering a behavior an addiction. These include the level of significance certain cues have for the person, the manifestation of withdrawal symptoms, tolerance (i.e., the need to engage in the behavior more or longer for the same effect), relapse, and mood modification. According to the World Health Organization and the **American Psychological Association**, another criterion is loss of control.

Diagnosis

These behaviors, although listed as different disorders in the *DSM-IV-TR,* share a suite of similar diagnostic features. These features include failure to resist the associated impulse (e.g., gambling or stealing), feelings of tension before engaging in the behavior, and a feeling of pleasure or relief when the behavior is being performed.

Comorbidities

The specific behavioral or process addiction of pathological gambling has been associated with high rates of psychiatric comorbidity and mortality, one of many similarities between substance and process addictions. There is a frequent co-occurrence of some behavioral addictions with depression, **suicide** attempts, and anxiety.

Association with substance abuse

There are substantial similarities between a disorder like pathological gambling and substance use disorder, from the comorbidities to personality features, behavioral measures, and neurobiological observations; substance use disorder and behavioral or process addiction often occur together. For example, low serotonin levels have been identified in people with pathological **gambling disorder** and in people with alcohol dependency. There is the phenomenon of "cross priming," in which the development of an addiction to a substance primes an individual's neural circuitry for susceptibility to a process addiction; for example, amphetamine use might prime a person biochemically for developing a gambling problem. Among pathological gamblers, as many as 70% people addicted to gambling are addicted to **nicotine**, 50%–70% have alcohol problems, and up to 40% have problems with abuse of other drugs.

The converse is that people who have substance use disorders can be up to 10 times more likely also to have a pathological gambling problem, and there are similar relationships between substance use disorder and kleptomania or compulsive buying. Compulsive sexual behavior and substance use disorder occur together in 25% and 71% of cases, respectively.

Treatment

As with substance abuse, **denial** can be a key characteristic of the behavior in process addiction, and any treatment begins with recognition and acknowledgment of the problem.

Pharmacologic approaches

The medical establishment is still in the early stages of developing and applying pharmacological treatment for process addiction. **Selective serotonin reuptake inhibitors (SSRIs)** have proven beneficial in some studies, but not in others. More effective, at least for pathological gambling and kleptomania, are opioid antagonists like **naltrexone** and nalmefene. The efficacy of these drugs may result from the interaction of the opioid system with dopamine signaling pathways.

Pharmacological treatments can be based on comorbidities. For example, if **obsessive-compulsive disorder**, depression, or anxiety are present, SSRIs may be effective. Mood stabilizers might be efficacious if **bipolar disorder** is present, and if **attention deficit hyperactivity disorder** (ADHD) is a comorbidity, stimulants or inhibitors of dopamine or noradrenaline reuptake (MAO-B inhibitors) may be beneficial.

Benzodiazepines can actually reduce inhibitions even more but are not recommended except in emergency situations.

Therapeutic approaches

The 12-step programs (e.g., Gamblers Anonymous) are enormously popular and well recognized, but their dropout rates are high and few studies have established their level of effectiveness. Other therapeutic approaches can involve **cognitive-behavioral therapy**, motivational interviewing, or **relapse prevention**, all based on approaches used for substance use disorders. The

KEY TERMS

Dopamine—A neurotransmitter involved in the reward pathways in the brain.

MAO-B inhibitors—Inhibitors of dopamine or noradrenaline reuptake by monoamine oxidase.

SSRI—Selective serotonin reuptake inhibitor.

Trichotillomania—Recurrent pulling out of one's own hair.

therapeutic approach may also need to be disorder specific; for example, for impulsive-compulsive sexual behavior, **couples therapy** may be warranted.

Prognosis

These disorders are considered to be chronic, and relapses in those that have been reasonably well studied, such as pathological gambling, are common. However, at least in the case of pathological gambling, appropriate treatment can help in management of the disorder.

Prevention

Prevention is based on decreased exposure to targets of process addiction; for example, little or no exposure to gambling can be helpful to people at risk. Early **intervention** may also be preventative.

Resources

BOOKS

American Psychiatric Association. *Diagnostic and Statistical Manual of Mental Disorders*. 4th ed., text rev. Washington, DC: American Psychiatric Publishing, 2000.

PERIODICALS

Grant, Jon E., Judson A. Brewer, and Marc N. Potenza. "The Neurobiology of Substance and Behavioral Addictions." *CNS Spectrum* 11, no. 12 (December 2006): 924–930.

Lobo, Daniela S.S., and James L. Kennedy. "The Genetics of Gambling and Behavioral Addictions." *CNS Spectrum* 11, no. 12 (December 2006): 931–939.

Mick, Thomas M., and Eric Hollander. "Impulsive-Compulsive Sexual Behavior." *CNS Spectrum*. 11, no. 12 (December 2006): 944–955.

Pallanti, Stefano. "From Impulse-control Disorders Toward Behavioral Addictions." *CNS Spectrum* 11, no. 12 (December 2006): 921–922.

Pallanti, Stefano, Silvia Bernardi, and Leonardo Quercioli. "The Shorter PROMIS Questionnaire and the Internet Addiction Scale in the Assessment of Multiple Addictions in a High-school Population: Prevalence and Related Disability." *CNS Spectrum* 11, no. 12 (December 2006): 966–974.

WEBSITES

American Psychological Association. "Addictions." http://www.apa.org/topics/addiction/index.aspx (accessed October 24, 2011).

MedlinePlus. "Pathological Gambling." U.S. National Library of Medicine, National Institutes of Health. http://www.nlm.nih.gov/medlineplus/ency/article/001520.htm (accessed October 24, 2011).

ORGANIZATIONS

American Psychiatric Association, 1000 Wilson Blvd., Ste. 1825, Arlington, VA, 22209-3901, (703) 907-7300, apa@psych.org, http://www.psych.org.

Gamblers Anonymous, International Service Office, PO Box 17173, Los Angeles, CA, 90017, (626) 960-3500, Fax: (626) 960-3501, isomain@gamblersanonymous.org, http://www.gamblersanonymous.org.

Sex Addicts Anonymous, ISO of SAA, PO Box 70949, Houston, TX, 77270.info@saa-recovery.org, http://saa-recovery.org.

Emily Jane Willingham, Ph.D.

Program of Assertive Community Treatment (PACT) *see* **Assertive community treatment**

Prolixin *see* **Fluphenazine**

Propranolol

Definition

Propranolol is classified as a beta blocker. It is sold in the United States under the brand name Inderal. When combined with the diuretic, hydrochlorothiazide, it is sold under the brand name Inderide. Propranolol also is

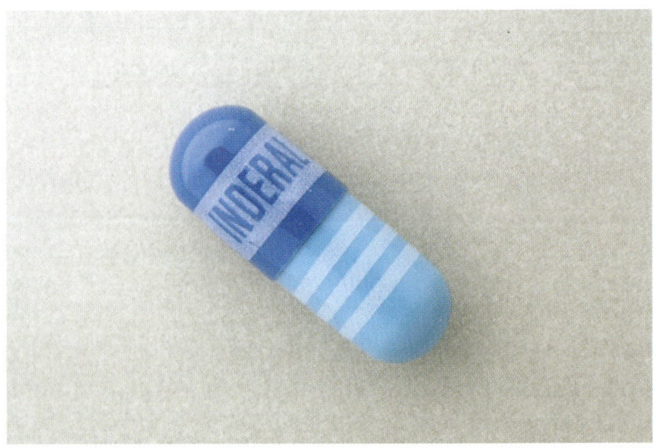

Inderal (propranolol), 120 mg. *(© Custom Medical Stock Photo, Inc. Reproduced by permission.)*

produced as a generic product by a number of generic manufacturers.

Purpose

Propranolol is approved by the U.S. Food and Drug Administration (FDA) for the treatment of hypertension (high blood pressure), angina, certain types of cardiac arrhythmias, certain types of cardiac output diseases, a sympathetic nervous system disorder known as pheochromocytoma, hyperthyroid conditions, heart attack, and tremors of a variety of origins. It is also used in the prevention of migraine headaches and on occasion for the treatment of **medication-induced movement disorders** caused by antipsychotic drugs and certain anxiety states in people suffering from a specific form of **social phobia**. **Beta blockers**, such as propranolol, are not useful for people with general social phobia who are anxious in most social situations; instead, propranolol may be more useful for people who are anxious about specific performance situations, such as presenting a speech before an audience.

Description

Propranolol falls into the broad pharmacologic category known as beta blockers. Beta blockers block specific sites in the central nervous system known as beta-adrenergic receptor sites. When these sites are blocked, heart rate and blood pressure are reduced and patients become less anxious. Because of this, propranolol is useful in treating chest pain, high blood pressure, and excessive nervousness. Unfortunately, propranolol often makes breathing disorders, such as asthma, worse because it tends to constrict breathing passages and sometimes causes fluid to build up in the lungs if it excessively depresses the heart.

In the treatment of anxiety, propranolol is usually not administered on a chronic basis but, rather, prior to stressful events such as public speaking or acting. In the treatment of certain types of tremors, especially tremors secondary to a drug, and **movement disorders** secondary to antipsychotic therapy, propranolol is administered throughout the day in divided doses. Propranolol is available in 10, 20, 40, 60, and 80 mg tablets; in 60, 80, 120, and 160 mg long-acting capsules; and in an injectable form containing 1 mg per mL. It is also combined with the diuretic hydrochlorothiazide in tablets and extended-release capsules.

Recommended dosage

For the treatment of performance anxiety or stage fright, a single dose of 10–40 mg may be administered 20–30 minutes before the event. For the treatment of tremors, especially tremors secondary to lithium, doses range from 20 to 160 mg per day administered in two or three divided doses. For the treatment of movement disorders secondary to antipsychotic drug therapy, doses range from 10 to 30 mg three times daily.

KEY TERMS

Beta blocker—Drugs that block beta-adrenergic receptors on neurons in the central nervous system. When these sites are blocked, heart rate, blood pressure, and anxiety levels decrease.

Brachycardia—Slow heartbeat, defined as a rate of less than 60 beats per minute.

Diuretic—An agent that increases the amount of urine; often used to decrease fluid retention in bodily tissues.

Epinephrine (adrenaline)—The principal blood pressure–raising hormone and a relaxant of the bronchial and intestinal smooth muscles; prescribed to (among other things) stimulate the heart and as a muscle relaxant in bronchial asthma.

Glaucoma—A group of eye diseases characterized by increased pressure within the eye significant enough to damage eye tissue and structures. If untreated, glaucoma results in blindness.

Hypotension—Low blood pressure.

Ischemia—Localized anemia of tissues due to obstructed inflow of blood.

Laryngospasm—Spasms that close the vocal apparatus of the larynx (the organ of voice production).

Neurotransmitter—One of a group of chemicals secreted by a nerve cell (neuron) to carry a chemical message to another nerve cell, often as a way of transmitting a nerve impulse.

Norepinephrine (noradrenaline)—A hormone with similar stimulatory effects to epinephrine but, in contrast to epinephrine, has little effect on cardiac (heart) output and in relaxing smooth muscles.

Raynaud's syndrome—A disorder of the circulatory or vascular system characterized by abnormally cold hands and feet because of constricted blood vessels in these areas.

Thrombocytopenia—A condition involving abnormally low numbers of platelets (blood clotting agents) in the blood; usually associated with hemorrhaging (bleeding).

Precautions

Precautions should be taken when administering propranolol in the following situations:

- liver or renal (kidney) failure
- prior to screening tests for glaucoma
- a history of immediate allergic reaction (known as anaphylaxis) to a beta blocker of any kind

In addition, a person taking propranolol should never suddenly stop taking the drug because of the risk of chest pain or heart attack in some people who do so.

Side effects

The following side effects have been observed with propranolol. Most have been mild and transient and rarely require the withdrawal of therapy:

- cardiovascular: brachycardia, congestive heart failure, hypotension, Raynaud's syndrome
- central nervous system: light-headedness, mental depression, insomnia, vivid dreams, disorientation, memory loss
- gastrointestinal: nausea, vomiting, abdominal pain, cramping, diarrhea, constipation, bowel ischemia
- allergic: fever, rash, laryngospasm, thrombocytopenia
- respiratory: bronchospasm
- hematologic: bone marrow suppression, bleeding under the skin

Interactions

Interactions with drugs that deplete the body of the **neurotransmitters** epinephrine and norepinephrine have been reported with concomitant propranolol. This group includes reserpine and guanethidine. Fainting, hypotension, dizziness, and slow heart rate have occurred under these circumstances. Drugs known as calcium channel blockers may decrease the pumping ability of the heart and lead to the development of cardiac arrhythmias. Nonsteroidal anti-inflammatory agents (e.g., ibuprofen and naproxen) may blunt the blood pressure–lowering effects of propranolol. Aluminum hydroxide antacids greatly reduce the rate of absorption of propranolol, as does alcohol. Interactions have also been reported with the drugs phenytoin, rifampin, phenobarbital, **chlorpromazine**, lidocaine, thyroxin, cimetidine, and theophylline.

Resources

BOOKS

Physicians' Desk Reference 2011. 66th ed. Montvale, NJ: PDR Network, 2011.

Springhouse. *Nursing 2003 Drug Handbook*. Springhouse, PA: Lippincott, Williams and Wilkins, 2002.

Venes, Donald. *Taber's Cyclopedic Medical Dictionary*. 21st ed. Philadelphia: F.A. Davis Company, 2009.

WEBSITES

MedlinePlus. "Propranolol Oral." U.S. National Library of Medicine, National Institutes of Health.http://www.nlm.nih.gov/medlineplus/druginfo/meds/a682607.html (accessed November 13, 2011).

DailyMed. "Inderal La (propranolol hydrochloride) Capsule, Extended Release." U.S. National Library of Medicine, National Institutes of Health. http://dailymed.nlm.nih.gov/dailymed/drugInfo.cfm?id=6143 (accessed October 24, 2011).

ORGANIZATIONS

U.S. Food and Drug Administration, 10903 New Hampshire Ave., Silver Spring, MD, 20993-0002, (888) INFO-FDA (463-6332), http://www.fda.gov.

Ralph Myerson, MD

Emily Jane Willingham, PhD

Prosom *see* **Estazolam**

Protriptyline

Definition

Protriptyline is an oral tricyclic antidepressant. It is sold in the United States under the brand name Vivactil and is also available under its generic name.

Purpose

Protriptyline is used primarily to treat **depression** and to treat the combination of symptoms of anxiety and depression. Like most **antidepressants** of this chemical

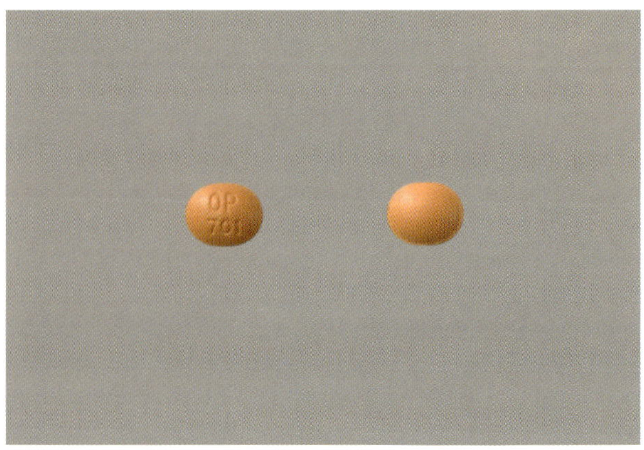

Vivactil (protriptyline). *(Teva Pharmaceuticals USA, Inc.)*

and pharmacological class, protriptyline has also been used in limited numbers of patients to treat **panic disorder**, **obsessive-compulsive disorder**, **attention deficit hyperactivity disorder**, **enuresis** (bed-wetting), eating disorders such as **bulimia nervosa**, **cocaine** dependency, and the depressive phase of **bipolar disorder**; it has also been used to support **smoking cessation** programs. However, not all of these uses are approved by the U.S. Food and Drug Administration (FDA).

Description

Tricyclic antidepressants act to change the balance of naturally occurring chemicals in the **brain** that regulate the transmission of nerve impulses between cells. Protriptyline acts primarily to increase the concentration of norepinephrine and **serotonin** (both chemicals that stimulate nerve cells) and, to a lesser extent, to block the action of another brain chemical, acetylcholine. Protriptyline shares most of the properties of other tricyclic antidepressants, such as **amitriptyline**, **clomipramine**, **desipramine**, **imipramine**, **nortriptyline**, and **trimipramine**. Studies comparing protriptyline with these other drugs have shown that protriptyline is no more or less effective than other antidepressants of its type. Its choice for treatment is as much a function of physician preference as any other factor.

The therapeutic effects of protriptyline, like those of other antidepressants, appear gradually. Maximum benefit is often not evident for at least two weeks after starting the drug. People taking protriptyline should be aware of this and continue taking the drug as directed even if they do not see immediate improvement.

Recommended dosage

As with any antidepressant, protriptyline must be carefully adjusted by the physician to produce the desired therapeutic effect. Protriptyline is available as 5 mg and 10 mg tablets. Doses range from 15 to 40 mg per day and can be taken in one daily dose or divided into up to four doses daily. Some patients with severe depression may require up to 60 mg per day.

In people over age 60, therapy should be initiated at a dose of 5 mg three times a day and increased under supervision of a physician as needed. Patients over age 60 who are taking a daily doses of 20 mg or more should be closely monitored for side effects such as rapid heart rate and urinary retention.

Precautions

Antidepressants have been associated with an increased risk of patients up to age 24 harming themselves or attempting or committing suicide. The FDA has advised that such drugs should not be administered to children under the age of 18. Patients of any age should be monitored carefully for signs of intention to commit self-harm or attempt **suicide** when taking antidepressants. These symptoms can develop suddenly and include new or worsening depression, talk about self-harm or suicide, agitation to panic attacks, aggression, and changes in sleep patterns.

Like all tricyclic antidepressants, protriptyline should be used cautiously and with close physician supervision in people, especially the elderly, who have benign prostatic hypertrophy, urinary retention, and glaucoma, especially angle-closure glaucoma (the most severe form). Before starting treatment, people with these conditions should discuss the relative risks and benefits of treatment with their doctors to help determine if protriptyline is the right antidepressant for them.

A common problem with tricyclic antidepressants is sedation (drowsiness and lack of physical and mental alertness). This side effect is especially noticeable early in therapy. In most patients, sedation decreases or disappears entirely with time, but until then patients taking protriptyline should not perform hazardous activities requiring mental alertness or coordination. The sedative effect is increased when protriptyline is taken with other central nervous system depressants, such as alcoholic beverages, sleeping medications, other **sedatives**, or antihistamines. It may be dangerous to take protriptyline in combination with these substances. Protriptyline may increase the possibility of having **seizures**. Patients should tell their physician if they have a history of seizures, including seizures brought on by the abuse of drugs or alcohol. These people should use protriptyline only with caution and be closely monitored by their physician.

Protriptyline may increase heart rate and stress on the heart. It may be dangerous for people with cardiovascular disease, especially those who have recently had a heart attack, to take this drug or other antidepressants in the same pharmacological class. In rare cases where patients with cardiovascular disease must take protriptyline, they should be monitored closely for cardiac rhythm disturbances and signs of cardiac stress or damage.

Side effects

Protriptyline shares side effects common to all tricyclic antidepressants. The most frequent of these are dry mouth, constipation, urinary retention, increased heart rate, sedation, irritability, dizziness, and decreased coordination. As with most side effects associated with tricyclic antidepressants, the intensity is highest at the

KEY TERMS

Acetylcholine—A naturally occurring chemical in the body that generally produces effects that are the opposite of those produced by dopamine and norepinephrine. Central nervous system well-being is dependent on a balance among acetylcholine, dopamine, serotonin, and norepinephrine.

Anticholinergic—Related to the ability of a drug to block the nervous system chemical acetylcholine. When acetylcholine is blocked, patients often experience dry mouth and skin, increased heart rate, blurred vision, and difficulty urinating. In severe cases, blocking acetylcholine may cloud thinking and cause delirium.

Benign prostate hypertrophy—Enlargement of the prostate gland.

Norepinephrine—A neurotransmitter in the brain that acts to constrict blood vessels and raise blood pressure. It works in combination with serotonin.

Serotonin—A widely distributed neurotransmitter that is found in blood platelets, the lining of the digestive tract, and the brain, and that works in combination with norepinephrine. It causes very powerful contractions of smooth muscle, and is associated with mood, attention, emotions, and sleep. Low levels of serotonin are associated with depression.

beginning of therapy and tends to decrease with continued use.

Dry mouth, if severe to the point of causing difficulty speaking or swallowing, may be managed by dosage reduction or temporary discontinuation of the drug. Patients may also chew sugarless gum or suck on sugarless candy in order to increase the flow of saliva. Some artificial saliva products may give temporary relief.

Men with prostate enlargement who take protriptyline may be especially likely to have problems with urinary retention. Symptoms include having difficulty starting a urine flow and more difficulty than usual passing urine. In most cases, urinary retention is managed with dose reduction or by switching to another type of antidepressant. In extreme cases, patients may require treatment with bethanechol, a drug that reverses this particular side effect. People who think they may be experiencing any side effects from this or any other medication should tell their physicians.

Interactions

Dangerously high blood pressure has resulted from the combination of tricyclic antidepressants, such as protriptyline, and members of another class of antidepressants known as **monoamine oxidase inhibitors** (MAOIs). Because of this, protriptyline should never be taken in combination with MAOIs. Patients taking any MAOIs, for example **phenelzine** (Nardil) or **tranylcypromine** (Parnate), should stop taking the MAOI and wait at least 14 days before starting protriptyline or any other tricyclic antidepressant. The same holds true when discontinuing protriptyline and starting an MAOI.

Protriptyline may decrease the blood pressure–lowering effects of **clonidine**. Patients who take both drugs should be monitored for loss of blood-pressure control, and the dose of clonidine should be increased as needed.

The sedative effects of protriptyline are increased by other central nervous system depressants such as alcohol, sedatives, sleeping medications, or medications used for other mental disorders such as **schizophrenia**. The anticholinergic effects of protriptyline are additive with other anticholinergic drugs such as **benztropine**, **biperiden**, **trihexyphenidyl**, and antihistamines.

Resources

BOOKS

American Society of Health-System Pharmacists. *AHFS Drug Information 2008*. Bethesda, MD: American Society of Health-System Pharmacists, 2008.

DeVane, C. Lindsay, Pharm.D. "Drug Therapy for Mood Disorders." In *Fundamentals of Monitoring Psychoactive Drug Therapy*. Baltimore: Williams and Wilkins, 1990.

WEBSITES

MedlinePlus. "Protriptyline." U.S. National Library of Medicine, National Institutes of Health. http://www.nlm.nih.gov/medlineplus/druginfo/meds/a604025.html (accessed November 13, 2011).

U.S. Food and Drug Administration. "Antidepressant Use in Children, Adolescents, and Adults." http://www.fda.gov/Drugs/DrugSafety/InformationbyDrugClass/ucm096273.htm (accessed October 24, 2011).

U.S. Food and Drug Administration. "Historical Information on Antidepressant Use in Children, Adolescents, and Adults." http://www.fda.gov/Drugs/DrugSafety/InformationbyDrugClass/ucm096293.htm (accessed October 24, 2011).

ORGANIZATIONS

National Institute of Mental Health, 6001 Executive Blvd., Rm. 8184, MSC 9663, Bethesda, MD, 20892-9663, (301) 433-4513; TTY: (301) 443-8431, Fax: (301) 443-4279,

(866) 615-6464; TTY: (866) 415-8051, nimhinfo@nih.gov, http://www.nimh.nih.gov.

U.S. Food and Drug Administration, 10903 New Hampshire Ave., Silver Spring, MD, 20993 0002, (888) INFO-FDA (463-6332), http://www.fda.gov.

Jack Raber, Pharm.D.
Emily Jane Willingham, PhD

Prozac *see* **Fluoxetine**

Pseudocyesis

Definition

Pseudocyesis is the medical term for a false pregnancy. Pseudocyesis can cause many of the signs and symptoms of pregnancy, and often resembles the condition in every way except for the presence of a fetus.

Demographics

The rate of pseudocyesis in the United States has declined significantly in the past century. In the 1940s there was one occurrence for approximately every 250 pregnancies. This rate has since dropped to between one and six occurrences for every 22,000 births. The average age of the affected woman is 33, though cases have been reported for women as young as six-and-a-half and as old as 79. More than two-thirds of women who experience pseudocyesis are married, and about one third have been pregnant at least once. Women who have been victims of incest may be at greater risk for developing pseudocyesis. Although pseudocyesis is overwhelmingly a disorder of females, there have been at least three reported cases of males with it. Pseudocyesis is found in some mammals other than humans, most often cats, dogs, and rabbits. In these animals, researchers have found that prolactin, the hormone that produces mammalian milk, plays a role in the development of the false pregnancy.

Description

Pseudocyesis has been observed and written about since antiquity. Hippocrates set down the first written account around 300 B.C., and recorded 12 different cases of women with the disorder. One of the most famous historical examples is Mary Tudor (1516–1558), Queen of England, who believed twice that she was pregnant when she was not. Some even attribute the violence that gave her the nickname "Bloody Mary" as a reaction to the disappointment of finding out that she was not carrying a child. Other historians believe that the queen's physicians mistook fibroid tumors in her uterus for a pregnancy, as fibroids can enlarge a nonpregnant uterus. She retired to her chambers for 14 months for the first false pregnancy, only to emerge humiliated, without a child. On the second occasion, the cause of her symptoms may have been advanced ovarian cancer, which some medical historians believe eventually killed her.

Pseudocyesis has become increasingly rare in many parts of the world in which accurate pregnancy tests have become widely available. Cultures that place high value on pregnancy, or that make close associations between fertility and a person's worth, still have high rates of the disorder.

Causes and symptoms

Causes

No single theory about the causes of pseudocyesis is universally accepted by mental health professionals. The first theory attributes the false pregnancy to emotional conflict. It is thought that an intense desire to become pregnant, or an intense fear of becoming pregnant, can create internal conflicts and changes in the endocrine system, which may explain some of the symptoms of pseudocyesis. The second theory concerns wish fulfillment. It holds that if a women desires pregnancy badly enough she may interpret minor changes in her body as signs of pregnancy. The third leading theory is the **depression** theory, which maintains that chemical changes in the nervous system associated with some depressive disorders could trigger the symptoms of pseudocyesis.

Symptoms

The symptoms of pseudocyesis are similar to the symptoms of true pregnancy and are often hard to distinguish from the natural signs of pregnancy such as morning sickness, tender breasts, and weight gain. Many health care professionals can be deceived by the symptoms associated with pseudocyesis. Eighteen percent of women with pseudocyesis were at one time diagnosed as pregnant by a medical professional. In some cases the only difference between pregnancy and pseudocyesis is the presence of a fetus.

The sign of pseudocyesis that is common to all cases is that the affected patient is convinced that she is pregnant. Abdominal distension is the most common physical symptom of pseudocyesis, and 63%–97% of women with pseudocyesis experience it. The abdomen expands in the same manner as it does during pregnancy, so that the affected woman looks pregnant. This phenomenon is thought to be caused by buildup of gas, fat, feces, or urine. These symptoms often resolve under general anesthesia, and the woman's abdomen returns to its normal size.

KEY TERMS

Cervix—The neck or narrow lower end of the uterus. Softening of the cervix is one of the signs of pregnancy.

Distension—The condition of being stretched or expanded, as the abdomen of a pregnant woman.

Quickening—A term that refers to the movements or other signs of life of a fetus in the womb.

The second most common physical sign of pseudocyesis is menstrual irregularity (56–98% of women with the disorder experience this). Between 48% and 75% of women are also reported to experience the sensation of fetal movements known as quickening, even though there is no fetus present. Some of the other common signs and symptoms include gastrointestinal symptoms, breast changes or secretions, labor pains, uterine enlargement, and softening of the cervix. One percent of women eventually experience false labor. In addition, some women actually test positive on pregnancy tests.

Treatment

Because pseudocyesis is not known to have a direct underlying physical cause, there are no general recommendations regarding treatment with medications. In some cases, however, the patient may be given medications for such symptoms as the cessation of menstruation. Because most patients with pseudocyesis have underlying psychological problems, they should be referred to a psychotherapist for the treatment of these problems. At the same time, however, it is important for the treating professional not to minimize the reality of the patient's physical symptoms.

The use of ultrasound or other imaging techniques has had the most success is demonstrating to the patient that she is not really pregnant.

Alternative therapies

There have been reports of patients being cured of pseudocyesis by hypnosis, purgatives, massage, **opioids**, or by experiencing "hysterical childbirth" after nine months of symptoms, but few data are available on the effectiveness of these or similar procedures.

Prognosis

Symptoms of pseudocyesis generally last from a few months to a few years. In most cases, symptoms last for a full nine months. Treatments involving **psychotherapy** have high success rates, as they treat the underlying psychological causes of the disorder.

Resources

BOOKS

Knobil, Ernst, and Jimmy D. Neill, eds. *Encyclopedia of Reproduction*. New York: Elsevier, 1998.

Sadock, Benjamin J., and Virginia A. Sadock, eds. *Comprehensive Textbook of Psychiatry*. Vol. 2. 7th ed. Philadelphia: Lippincott Williams and Wilkins, 2000.

PERIODICALS

Aldrich, Knight. "Sixteenth-Century Psychosomatics." *Psychiatric News*. American Psychiatric Association. April 16, 1999. http://www.psychiatricnews.org/pnews/99-04-16/history.html (accessed October 24, 2011).

Hendricks-Matthews, Marybeth K., and Douglas M. Hoy. "Pseudocyesis in an Adolescent Incest Survivor." *Journal of Family Practice* 36, no. 1, (January 1993): 97–104.

Paulman, Paul M., and Abdul Sadat. "Pseudocyesis." *Journal of Family Practice* 30, no. 5, (May 1990): 575–82.

Tish Davidson, A.M.
Emily Jane Willingham, PhD

Psychiatric assessment *see* **Psychological assessment and diagnosis**

Psychiatrist

Definition

A psychiatrist is a physician who specializes in the **diagnosis** and treatment of mental disorders.

Description

Psychiatrists treat patients privately and in hospital settings through a combination of **psychotherapy** and medication. Their training consists of four years of medical school, followed by three or four years of psychiatric residency. Subspecialities usually involve completion of a fellowship that lasts two or more years following the residency. Psychiatrists may receive certification from the American Board of Psychiatry and Neurology (ABPN), which requires two years of clinical experience beyond residency and the successful completion of a written and an oral test. Unlike a medical license, board certification is not legally required to practice psychiatry.

Psychiatrists may practice general psychiatry or choose a specialty, such as child psychiatry, geriatric psychiatry, treatment of **substance abuse**, forensic (legal) psychiatry, emergency psychiatry, intellectual disabilities, community psychiatry, or public health. Some focus their research and clinical work primarily on psychoactive medication, in which case they are referred to as psychopharmacologists. Psychiatrists may be called upon to address numerous social issues, including juvenile delinquency, family and marital dysfunction, legal competency in criminal and financial matters, and treatment of mental and emotional problems among prison inmates and in the military.

Psychiatrists treat the biological, psychological, and social components of mental illness simultaneously. They can investigate whether symptoms of mental disorders have physical causes, such as a hormone imbalance or an adverse reaction to medication, or whether psychological symptoms are contributing to physical conditions, such as cardiovascular problems and high blood pressure. Because they are licensed physicians, psychiatrists—unlike psychologists and psychiatric social workers—can prescribe medication; they are also able to admit patients to the hospital. Other mental health professionals who cannot prescribe medication themselves often establish a professional relationship with a psychiatrist.

Psychiatrists may work in private offices, private psychiatric hospitals, community hospitals, state and federal hospitals, or community mental centers. Often, they combine work in several settings. In addition to their clinical work, psychiatrists often engage in related professional activities, including teaching, research, and administration. The **American Psychiatric Association**, the oldest medical specialty organization in the United States, supports the profession by offering continuing education and research opportunities, keeping members informed about new research and public policy issues, helping to educate the public about mental health issues, and serving as an advocate for people affected by mental illness.

ORGANIZATIONS

American Psychiatric Association, 1000 Wilson Blvd., Ste. 1825, Arlington, VA, 22209-3901, (703) 907-7300, apa@psych.org, http://www.psych.org.

American Board of Psychiatry and Neurology, 2150 E Lake Cook Rd., Ste. 900, Buffalo Grove, IL, 60089, (847) 229-6500, Fax: (847) 229-6600, http://www.abpn.com.

Emily Jane Willingham, PhD

Psychoanalysis

Definition

Psychoanalysis, as a form of therapy, is based on the understanding that human beings are largely unaware of the mental processes that determine their thoughts, feelings, and behavior, and that psychological suffering can be alleviated by making those processes known to the individual. Psychoanalysis is practiced by a trained psychoanalyst, also referred to as an analyst.

Purpose

Primary goals of psychoanalysis include symptom relief, increased self-awareness, and a more objective capacity for self-observation. Other aims might include improved relationships with others and the capacity to live a more deeply satisfying life. Typically, an individual seeks treatment in order to alleviate some difficulty, such as unhappiness in work or love, disturbances in mood or self-esteem, or troubling personality traits. With the exception of those that are physically based, psychoanalysis views such symptoms as related to unconscious mental processes, and because these mental forces are not within the individual's awareness, symptoms cannot be relieved with perseverance or with the help of friends or family. Through a slowly unfolding process, psychoanalysis demonstrates to the individual how unconscious mental processes affect current modes of thinking, feeling and interacting with others. It also demonstrates that these processes can be traced back to early experiences and relationships with caregivers and family members. This kind of insight enables individuals to identify the sources of their, sometimes, troubling thoughts, feelings and behavior and, as a result, gives new meaning to current modes of functioning. Generally, this type of transformation of character takes several years to accomplish due to the intense nature of the process. It requires a sacrifice of time, money, and mental energy. The resulting transformation offers the means for adaptive, enduring changes in personality. These are changes that enable the individual to live a more productive, satisfying, and pleasurable life.

Description

Austrian neurologist Sigmund Freud (1856–1939) originally developed the theory and technique of psychoanalysis in the 1890s. As such, it is sometimes also called Freudian psychology. Freud's ideas are still used in contemporary practice; however, many have been further developed or refined, and some even abandoned.

ERICH FROMM (1900–1980)

Erich Fromm was born in Frankfurt-am-Main, Germany, the son of Naphtali Fromm, a wine merchant, and Rosa Krause. Throughout his career, Fromm strove toward an understanding of human existence based upon the breaking down of barriers—between individuals as well as between schools of thought. In a *Los Angeles Times* obituary of the famous psychologist, a reviewer summarizes: "Fromm's lifelong concern was how people could come to terms with their isolation, insignificance and doubts about life's meaning." As his theories developed over the decades into what would later be collectively labeled "social humanism," he incorporated knowledge and information culled from such diverse fields as Marxist socialism and Freudian psychology. The psychologist used these schools of thought as building blocks for developing original theories that, like his idiosyncratic life, often ran against popular beliefs. As a psychologist, he diverged from the Freudian school, in which the unconscious was the main factor in understanding human actions, by pointing out the importance of the influence of social and economic factors.

Most of Fromm's work was an application of psychoanalysis, sociology philosophy, and religion to the peculiar problems of man in modern industrialize society. In *Escape from Freedom,* he postulated that "modern man, freed from the bonds of pre-individualistic society, which simultaneously gave him security and limited him, has not gained freedom in the positive sense of the realization of his individual self; that is, the expression of his intellectual, emotional and sensuous potentialities. Freedom, though it has brought him independence and rationality, has made him isolated and, thereby, anxious and powerless." This problem, the individual's tenuous relationship to institutions and society, became the core of such later works as *Man for Himself: An Enquiry into the Psychology of Ethics and The Sane Society.*

Fromm's penultimate book, *To Have or To Be?,* presents "the viewpoint and challenge of radical humanistic psychoanalysis," explains Paul Roazen in *Nation.* The volume has been seen as the culmination of Fromm's work at that time and maintains, according to a publisher's note, "that two modes of existence are struggling for the spirit of humankind; the having mode, which concentrates on material possession, acquisitiveness, power, and aggression and is the basis of such universal evils as greed, envy, and violence; and the being mode, which is based in love, in the pleasure of sharing, and in meaningful and productive rather than wasteful activity. Dr. Fromm sees the having mode bringing the world to the brink of psychological and ecological disaster, and he outlines a program for socio-economic change [to] turn the world away from its catastrophic course."

One such post-Freudian theory is called interpersonal psychoanalysis, which was developed primarily by Erich Fromm, Frieda Fromm-Reichmann, and Clara Thompson. It delves into interpersonal interactions; specifically, the way people handle negative emotions, such as anxiety, and their interactions with others as they deal with such emotions.

The theory and technique of psychoanalysis continues to integrate new insights about human development and behavior based on psychoanalytic research and discoveries from related fields. Different schools of psychoanalytic theory have evolved out of the original Freudian one, reflecting a variety of ideas and perspectives.

In psychoanalysis, an individual in treatment is seen four to five times per week for 45- to 50-minute sessions. The individual lies comfortably on a couch while the analyst sits in a chair behind the person, out of view. The person is then asked to say whatever comes into his or her mind. Although this structure varies depending on the theory and style of the analyst, this is the most typical and traditional manner in which sessions are conducted. These conditions are maintained consistently, making it possible for thoughts and feelings to emerge that had once been outside of the person's awareness. The process of free associating, or saying whatever comes to mind, is challenging because people are taught at a young age to keep many ideas and feelings to themselves. When the analyst is out of view, it removes the possibility for eye contact, making it easier to speak spontaneously. Free association is also made easier by the analyst's nonjudgmental attitude—in listening to the individual, in the attention and interest given to seemingly unimportant details, and in the objective and caring attitude with which the analyst understands the individual.

As the person speaks, unconscious sources of present-day difficulties gradually emerge. Specifically, the analyst begins to notice repetitive aspects of behavior. Some of them may include particular subjects about which the person finds it hard to speak, as well as habitual ways in which the person relates to the psychoanalyst. The analyst begins to reveal these to the person in a gradual and thoughtful manner. Sometimes these revelations are accepted as correct and helpful. At other times they are rejected, corrected, or refined.

During the years of an analysis, the individual will grapple with new insights repeatedly, each time comprehending them in new ways. There will be an enhanced emotional and intellectual understanding, in addition to seeing matters from the perspective of different periods of life. As in all worthwhile learning processes, this one includes times of deep satisfaction and great frustration, periods of growth and regression. Overall, the analyst and individual work together to modify debilitating life patterns, to ameliorate troubling symptoms, and to release emotional and intellectual resources bound up in unconscious psychological processes. A transformation will occur eventually, and be one in which the person's understanding of themselves and of others, along with their productivity in work and capacity to love, changes in profound and enduring ways.

Psychoanalysis is used at times with other forms of treatment. Medication may be warranted in selected situations—if an individual suffers from a severe mood disturbance which interferes with his or her capacity to participate in treatment, for example. In general, medication is used as a tool that allows the individual to benefit from the psychoanalytic process; it is an adjunct therapy, while psychoanalysis is the primary curative one. There are also occasions in which psychoanalysis is provided concurrently with **couples therapy** or **family therapy** or with **group therapy**. Treatment recommendations, whether for psychoanalysis alone or in combination with couples, family, or group therapy, are based both on the individual's particular needs and the practice of the treating psychoanalyst.

Finally, psychoanalysis is not only a type of therapy. It is also a theory of human development from infancy to old age, a method for understanding thought processes. It offers a way of thinking about aspects of society and culture such as religion, prejudice, and war.

Benefits

Anyone interested should seek a consultation with a psychoanalyst in order to determine if this treatment is appropriate. People often begin psychoanalysis after having also participated in psychoanalytic **psychotherapy**, which is a less intense form of treatment.

QUESTIONS TO ASK YOUR DOCTOR

- Can I benefit from psychoanalysis?
- Should I use psychoanalysis with other forms of treatment?
- Does my health insurance pay for psychoanalysis?
- How to I find a qualified and experienced psychoanalyst?
- What happens if psychoanalysis does not help me?
- Will I need medication in addition to psychoanalysis? If so, what kind of medicine, and why?

Individuals who are the most suited for psychoanalysis are those who have experienced satisfactions in work, with friends, in marriage, but who nonetheless experience a general dissatisfaction with their life—suffering from long-standing **depression**, anxiety, sexual difficulties, physical symptoms without physical basis, or typically feel isolated or alone. Some people need analysis because their habitual ways of living interfere with experiencing greater pleasure or productivity in life. Individuals need to be psychologically minded with an interest in becoming more self-aware, and a determination to forgo quick symptom relief in favor of a more gradual therapeutic process.

Psychoanalysis is also practiced with children and adolescents, with some variation in technique. Specifically, fantasy play and drawings are used with children in addition to verbal communication. During the treatment of children and young adolescents, parents are consulted on a regular basis so that the analyst can develop a more holistic understanding of the youngster's world. The goal of child and adolescent psychoanalysis is to alleviate symptoms and to remove any obstacles that interfere with normal development.

Precautions

The term "psychoanalyst" can be used by anyone in the psychological profession, so it is important to know the credentials of an analyst prior to beginning treatment.

Preparation

Potential patients should learn more and gain a basic understanding of psychoanalysis before entering such a

KEY TERMS

Depression—A psychiatric disorder involving feelings of hopelessness and symptoms of fatigue, sleeplessness, suicidal tendencies, and poor concentration.

Holistic—Analysis of the entire system, rather than of individual parts.

Psychotic—Relating to psychosis, or a psychiatric disorder characterized by hallucinations, a distorted view of reality, and other such mental problems.

program. In addition, patients with the following general criteria have been shown to have a better chance for success in their treatment:

- ability to relate to the therapist so that an effective relationship can be established
- average intellect, along with a general understanding of psychological theory
- ability to tolerate sadness, disappointment, and other painful/negative emotions
- capacity to separate real and fantasy situations

Risks

The use of psychoanalysis can be a risk to individuals if professionals are not properly trained. In addition, patients suffering from severe depression or psychotic disorders, such as **schizophrenia**, are considered not to be suitable candidates for psychoanalysis. Persons with addictions or dependencies (such as alcohol **addiction** or prescription drug dependency), aggression or **impulse control disorders** (such as **kleptomania**, or compulsive stealing), or acute mental crises (or personal tragedies, for instance, death of family member) should resolve these serious problems before beginning psychoanalysis.

Results

Normal results include symptom relief and an enduring, adaptive change in personality.

Some individuals do not benefit from this in-depth form of treatment. They instead experience increased distress, or do not progress after a sufficient amount of treatment sessions. In these cases, people are typically transitioned to a less intensive form of treatment such as psychoanalytic psychotherapy.

Training and certification

In addition to having received advanced degrees in mental health (psychiatry, psychology, social work), trained psychoanalysts have also graduated from psychoanalytic training institutes. Institute training consists of three parts: course work on psychoanalytic theory and technique; supervised analyses (meaning that the candidate conducts analyses while being supervised by a seasoned psychoanalyst); and, third, candidates undergo a personal psychoanalysis. A personal analysis is considered a vital part of the training, as it enables candidates to learn about their own psychological processes. In turn, the knowledge enhances their capacity to treat others. This type of training program takes a minimum of four years to complete. Psychoanalysts also practice psychoanalytic psychotherapy, a less intensive form of treatment. It relies on the same theory of human development and a similar technique.

Resources

BOOKS

Britzman, Deborah P. *Freud and Education*. New York: Routledge, 2011.

Corsini, Raymond J., and Danny Wedding, eds. *Current Psychotherapies*. Belmont, CA: Brooks/Cole, 2011.

Kandel, Eric. *Psychiatry, Psychoanalysis, and the New Biology of Mind*. Arlington, VA: American Psychiatric Publishing, 2005.

Lichtenberg, Joseph D., Frank M. Lachmann and James L. Fosshage. *Psychoanalysis and Motivational Systems: A New Look*. New York: Routledge, 2011.

Person, Ethel S., Arnold M. Cooper and Glen O. Gabbard, eds. *The American Psychiatric Publishing Textbook of Psychoanalysis*. Arlington, VA: American Psychiatric Publishing, 2005.

WEBSITES

American Psychoanalytic Association. "About Psychoanalysis."http://www.apsa.org/About_Psychoanalysis.aspx (accessed December 22, 2010).

ORGANIZATIONS

American Psychoanalytic Association, 309 E 49th St., New York City, NY, 10017-1601, (212) 752-0450, Fax: (212) 593-0571, http://www.apsa.org.

International Psychoanalytical Association, Woodside Lane, London, United Kingdom, N12 8UD, 44 20 8446 8324, 44 20 8445 4729, ipa@ipa.org.uk, http://www.ipa.org.uk/Public.

National Psychological Association for Psychoanalysis, 40 W 13th St., New York City, NY, 10011, (212) 924-7440, Fax: (212) 989-7543, info@npap.org, http://www.npap.org.

Susan Fine, Psy.D
Stephanie N. Watson

Psychodynamic psychotherapy

Definition

Psychodynamic **psychotherapy**, sometimes also called psychodynamic therapy, is a method of verbal communication used to help a person find relief from emotional pain. It is based on the theories and techniques of **psychoanalysis**. Psychodynamic psychotherapy is similar to psychoanalysis in that it attributes emotional problems to the patient's unconscious motives and conflicts. It differs from classical psychoanalysis, however, in that psychodynamic psychotherapists do not necessarily accept the view of Austrian neurologist Sigmund Freud (1856–1939) that these unconscious motives and conflicts are ultimately sexual in nature. The method also uses the interaction between client and therapist much more than in other forms of therapy. Psychodynamic psychotherapy is used with individual, group, couples, and **family therapy**.

Oftentimes, when people talk about psychotherapy they really mean psychodynamic psychotherapy. Although psychodynamic psychotherapy is the term used by professionals in the field, it is also commonly called client-centered therapy, existential psychotherapy, Gestalt psychotherapy, Group psychotherapy, and many other such terms.

Purpose

The goals of psychodynamic psychotherapy vary depending on the method of treatment, which can be broadly described as either expressive or supportive. Expressive therapy seeks to relieve symptoms through the development of insight, or the slowly developing awareness of feelings and thoughts that were once outside of the person's awareness. Expressive therapy is based on the rationale that difficulties experienced in adult life originate in childhood; that children do not possess the maturity for making effective choices nor the independence to do so; and that methods of adapting developed in childhood may no longer be effective for adapting to the world as an adult. Through guidance from a therapist, the adult becomes aware of present ways of coping that are ineffective, and how they served a purpose in childhood but are no longer relevant. The person learns that he or she now has a range of new options for solving problems and for living in general that are now based on his or her maturity and independence.

In contrast to expressive therapy which is exploratory, supportive therapy remains closer to the surface of the patient's issues. Supportive therapy is an approach that is used to relieve immediate distress; to return the person to his or her previous level of functioning; and to strengthen adaptive ways of coping that the individual already possesses in order to prevent further discomfort. Expressive and supportive methods of treatment are not completely separate categories because elements of supportive therapy are used in expressive treatment and vice versa, depending on the therapeutic need. For instance, if a person in exploratory treatment is experiencing distress, a supportive approach may be used for a period of time in order to help the person feel more stable.

People seek psychodynamic psychotherapy for a variety of reasons that include but are not limited to the following: prolonged sadness; anxiety and **depression**; sexual difficulties; physical symptoms without physical basis; persistent feelings of isolation and loneliness; and the desire to be more successful in work or love. People seek therapy because they have not been able to develop a stable resolution for their difficulties on their own or with the help of friends and family members.

Description

Sessions of psychodynamic psychotherapy may be scheduled from one to three days per week, with greater frequency allowing for more in-depth treatment. The duration of individual sessions varies, but typically lasts for 45 to 50 minutes. It is not usually possible at the outset of treatment to estimate the number of sessions that will be necessary to achieve the person's goals. It is possible, however, for the person to make arrangements for a specific number of sessions.

Psychodynamic psychotherapy begins with a period of evaluation during which the client discusses with the therapist the reasons for seeking treatment. This process gives the therapist the opportunity to learn about the person, to develop an understanding of his or her troubles, and to formulate ideas about how treatment should proceed. This phase of interviewing and learning may take place in one session or over a series of sessions; or it may be done in a less structured manner, depending on the therapist's style. During the initial sessions, such factors as the frequency and length of sessions and the policy for payment will also be discussed. At some point within the first few sessions, the therapist and the individual will come to a mutual understanding of the goals for treatment. After the initial evaluation, sessions will be devoted to the client discussing what is on his or her mind. It is the therapist's job to listen and to help identify patterns of thinking, feeling and interacting that may be contributing to the patient's current struggles. Consequently, the person: (1) becomes more aware of his or her thoughts and feelings; (2) learns how some present ways of coping are no longer adaptive even though they may have been necessary in childhood; and (3) discovers that he or she as an adult has a greatly expanded repertoire of resources and, consequently, can use far more effective ways to deal with problems. Deeper awareness and new insights stimulate psychological growth and change.

Psychodynamic psychotherapy places great importance on the therapeutic dyad, which is a medical term for the relationship between the therapist and the patient. It is within the context of the therapeutic dyad that positive changes in the patient's outlook and behaviors are able to unfold. This relationship is unique because the therapist maintains a uniform, neutral, and accepting stance. Unlike other well-intentioned people in the person's life, the therapist has been trained to listen objectively and without criticism. This therapeutic attitude makes it easier for the person seeking treatment to speak freely and to therefore provide as much information for the therapist to work with as is possible.

Treatment continues until the troubling symptoms have been reduced or alleviated and the person is consistently making use of more adaptive methods of coping with greater insight. For some people, this positive experience inspires them to proceed with further treatment to bring about additional adaptive changes. For others, meeting the initial goals will be sufficient. If so, the focus of sessions turns to issues related to the end of treatment. This final phase of treatment is as important as the beginning and middle stages because it allows the individual to develop insight about his or her therapeutic experience. People need time to clarify how they feel about leaving the therapeutic relationship, and this termination involves identifying and understanding feelings about separation, maturation, loss, and change. The length of time allotted to the termination phase varies with the type of treatment and the needs of the individual.

While many patients benefit from individual psychotherapy alone, some instances call for such additional therapies as family, couples, or **group therapy** in combination with individual treatment. A second treatment modality might be recommended when the patient's progress in individual treatment is highly dependent on relationships with significant others or with interpersonal relationships in general. Psychotropic (mood- or behavior-altering) medication may also be prescribed as an adjunct (help) to treatment in order to manage disturbances in anxiety and depression level, mood, or thinking. Whether additional treatments are recommended is based on the needs of the individual.

KEY TERMS

Anxiety—A psychological state characterized by strong feelings of worry, nervousness, apprehension, or agitation.

Depression—A psychiatric disorder involving feelings of hopelessness and symptoms of fatigue, sleeplessness, suicidal tendencies, and poor concentration.

Psychoanalysis—A form of therapy based on the understanding that human beings are largely unaware of the mental processes that determine their thoughts, feelings, and behavior, and that psychological suffering can be alleviated by making those processes known to the individual.

Preparation

Preparation for psychodynamic psychotherapy is not needed nor necessary. However, a period of introduction is often used before treatment begins so the therapist and patient can get to know each other better and the therapist can evaluate the patient as to the reasons for seeking treatment.

Aftercare

After a course of psychodynamic psychotherapy has ended, the person should, overall, continue to handle difficulties in a more adaptive manner; experience improved interpersonal relationships and productivity at work; and continue to develop new insights into his or her thoughts, feelings and behavior. In supportive treatment, insight and personality change are not the primary goals of treatment; therapist and patient work toward a continuation of general stability in the person's life.

Risks

Like all therapies, psychodynamic psychotherapy may or may not work successfully for the individual. Patients may like or dislike the method, depending on their individual conditions, personalities, and other factors. It does have a very good record for effectiveness for certain mental illness conditions, such as depression and **personality disorders**. However, because of its varied nature with which it is carried out psychodynamic psychotherapy is difficult to assess its actual effectiveness on a quantitative basis.

QUESTIONS TO ASK YOUR DOCTOR

- Do you think psychodynamic psychotherapy is suited to my particular problem?
- Where can I learn more about psychodynamic psychotherapy?
- If I get better with the therapy, are there other therapies that can be used as a "next step" in my recovery?
- Will my health insurance pay for it?
- How will I know when I no longer need therapy?
- What happens if I have a relapse after stopping therapy?

Results

Psychodynamic psychotherapy is considered to be an effective way to treat various types of mental health problems. Dr. Jonathan Shedler, from the University of Colorado, published a paper stating that psychodynamic psychotherapy is "highly effective" based on scientific evidence. The paper, entitled "The Efficacy of Psychodynamic Psychotherapy," was published in 2010 in the journal *American Psychologist* (volume 654, number 2). Shedler concluded in the study that psychodynamic psychotherapy is, at the very least, as effective as other forms of therapy. In addition, Shedler found that psychodynamic psychotherapy is a long-lasting type of therapy for patients, allowing them to lead a much healthier life, without all of the major symptoms, before such therapy was performed.

Resources

BOOKS

O'Donohue, William, Nicholas A. Cummings and Janet L. Cummings, eds. *Becoming a Psychotherapist*. Amsterdam; Boston: Elsevier Academic Press, 2006.

Person, Ethel Spector, Arnold M. Cooper and Glen O. Gabbard, eds. *The American Psychiatric Publishing Textbook of Psychoanalysis*. Washington, DC: American Psychiatric Publishing, 2005.

Prochaska, James O., and John C. Norcross. *Systems of Psychotherapy: A Transtheoretical Analysis*. Belmont, CA: Brooks/Cole, 2010.

WEBSITES

American Psychological Association. "Psychodynamic Psychotherapy Brings Lasting Benefits through Self-Knowledge." http://www.apa.org/news/press/releases/2010/01/psychodynamic-therapy.aspx (accessed December 29, 2010).

ORGANIZATIONS

American Psychiatric Association, 1000 Wilson Blvd., Ste. 1825, Arlington, VA, 22209-3901, (703) 907-7300, apa@psych.org, http://www.psych.org.

American Psychoanalytic Association, 309 East 49th Street, New York City, NY, 10017, (212) 752-0450, Fax: (212) 593-0571, info@aspa.org, http://www.apsa.org.

American Psychological Association, 750 1st St. NE, Washington, DC, 20002-4242, (202) 336-5500; TDD/TTY: (202) 336-6123, (800) 374-2721, http://www.apa.org.

Susan Fine, Psy.D.

Psychogenic excoriation *see* **Dermatillomania**

Psychological assessment and diagnosis

Definition

A psychological assessment is the process of gathering and evaluating data about a patient's symptoms, mental state, behaviors, and background. It is also called a biopsychosocial or psychiatric assessment. The assessment is used to diagnose mental disorders and as a first step in determining appropriate treatment.

Purpose

The purpose of a psychological assessment is to organize and evaluate information about a patient in order to arrive at a **diagnosis** and recommend a course of treatment. Nearly half of all Americans experience some type of mental disorder at some point in their lives, and as many as 60% of physical complaints for which patients seek medical advice result from or are affected by psychological problems, often anxiety or **depression**. The process of assessment and diagnosis is typically initiated by a patient or family member seeking help for a primary complaint or problem that is interfering with daily activities or affecting quality of life. Accurate assessment and diagnosis is critical for the selection of appropriate medication or other treatment plan.

Assessment and diagnosis are used for the following psychological and psychiatric conditions and disorders, among others:

- anxiety
- depression
- psychological trauma
- post-traumatic stress disorder (PTSD)

- dissociative conditions
- personality disorders
- bipolar disorder
- psychosis
- schizophrenia
- chronic pain
- substance abuse
- eating disorders
- sleep disorders
- domestic violence
- dementia
- Alzheimer's disease
- neurological disorders
- traumatic brain injury

Childhood and adolescent conditions and disorders that are subject to assessment and diagnosis include:

- behavior/conduct disorders
- social problems
- emotional disorders
- anxiety
- depression
- acute and chronic neurological conditions
- developmental delays
- dyslexia
- learning disorders and disabilities
- autism spectrum disorders
- attention deficit hyperactivity disorder (ADHD)
- eating disorders

Description

Various physiological diseases, disorders, and conditions—such as diabetes and thyroid and seizure disorders—can contribute to or even mask psychological and mental health conditions and interfere with psychological assessment and diagnosis. Therefore, a thorough physical examination and appropriate medical tests and procedures may need to be performed prior to psychological assessment and diagnosis. A neurological assessment and **brain** imaging also may be required.

Assessment and diagnosis usually involve the direct examination of the patient by a **psychologist** or **psychiatrist**, although in some instances this may not be possible. Increasingly, initial assessment occurs in primary-care settings and is followed by in-depth assessment and diagnosis by a mental health professional. Different diagnoses require different types of assessments. However, assessments usually involve standardized interviews that can assess psychological status or establish a psychiatric diagnosis. Cognitive and/or behavioral assessments may be performed in place of or in addition to a psychological assessment. Psychometric measurements are standardized quantifications of different variables, including personality, emotional status, cognitive functioning, behavior, and academic achievement. The entire process is often referred to as psychological testing.

Structured interview

A biopsychosocial assessment is a standard structured interview that is accepted as an effective diagnostic tool. It includes:

- identifying information
- chief complaint or problem
- history of the current illness or condition
- past medical and psychological history
- personal history
- family history
- substance use and abuse history

The interview opens with general and emotionally neutral questions. These include the patient's name, age, occupation, and marital status. The clinician inquires as to the patient's immediate reasons for seeking help, and the patient is asked to describe the onset of signs and symptoms that comprise the current problem. Information about additional symptoms and any previous mental disorders can assist the clinician in formulating pertinent questions during subsequent sections of the interview.

The patient's medical history may reveal problems—such as thyroid disease, Parkinson's disease, head **trauma**, or brain infections—that could be responsible for current psychological symptoms. The patient is also asked about previous psychological/psychiatric treatments, including hospitalizations, outpatient or **substance abuse** treatments, and medications, and the duration, effectiveness, and outcomes of treatments.

Personal history covers the patient's entire life, beginning with prenatal development. The patient is asked about maternal **nutrition** and drug and **alcohol use** during pregnancy, as well as any maternal abortions or miscarriages, birth trauma, and siblings. The early childhood phase—infancy to three years—may include questions about temperament, developmental milestones (e.g., walking, talking, toilet training), nutrition and feeding, family relationships, behavioral problems, hospitalizations, and separation from caregivers. The middle childhood phase—3 to 11 years—includes pertinent information about education and learning, relationships with peers and family, behavioral problems, and general personality development. Adolescence—12 to 18 years—includes school history, behavioral problems, and sexual development. The adulthood section details the patient's education, sexual history, relationships and/or marriages, peer relationships, occupations, and current circumstances. Family history is also very important, since many mental disorders are inherited or tend to run in families. Family interactions can also affect the manifestation of symptoms.

Substance abuse history delineates the patient's past and current use of alcohol, **nicotine**, caffeine, prescribed medications, and illicit drugs, including **sedatives** and depressants, opiates, **cocaine**, marijuana, and **hallucinogens**. Questions focus on the patient's age at first use, age at last use, period of heaviest use, usage within the past 30 days, and frequency, amounts, and methods of usage. The interviewer takes note of any tolerance, dependence, treatment, medical complications (such as HIV/AIDS), and legal problems (such as driving while impaired) that were associated with substance use or abuse.

Mental status examination

The **mental status examination** (MSE) follows the biopsychosocial history. It includes the clinician's observations of the patient, questions about feelings, and assessments of thought processes, memory, and cognition.

The clinician's observations focus on the patient's appearance, behavior, speech, and affect or emotional state. The patient's general appearance, hygiene, grooming, and attire are noted, as well as behaviors such as abnormal movements, hyperactivity, and eye contact with the interviewer. Fluency, rate, clarity, and tone of speech are all important. They can be indicative of mental state. For example, fast talking may suggest anxiety, as well as speech impairments, oral problems (such as dentures or cleft palate), mania, or intoxication. The patient is questioned about current mood, and affect or emotional state are observed and interpreted by the clinician throughout the interview. Affect is described in standardized terms, such as excitable, flat, inappropriate, or labile (rapidly shifting).

Thought processes—the form and content of thoughts—include basic orientation in time and place, such as the ability to identify oneself and loved ones, the current date, and the route to the medical office. The clinician also observes the connectedness, coherence, and logic of the patient's thoughts and notes any thought disturbances. These include circumstantial thinking (circuitous, persistent storytelling), tangential thinking (irrelevant responses to questions), black/white (extreme) thinking, or impoverished (minimally responsive) thinking, as well as **delusions**, hallucinations, phobias, obsessions, or suicidal or homicidal thoughts.

The MSE includes assessments of cognition, such as attention; awareness; long-, intermediate-, and short-term memory; general knowledge; abstract thinking ability; insight; and judgment. The patient might be asked to spell a word forward and backward, name the current president, read and/or write a passage, compare two objects, or explain the meaning of common sayings.

Pediatric

Special procedures are used for the assessment and diagnosis of children. If possible, assessment and diagnosis should be performed by a pediatrician, child psychologist or psychiatrist, or pediatric neurologist. The assessment is usually carried out in consultation with the child's family. In addition to observations of the child and standardized assessment instruments or structured interviews, discussions involve both the child and the family. The parents must provide a complete medical and family/social history. The child's social, economic, and cultural environment must be taken into consideration.

Preparation

Choosing a qualified mental health practitioner for assessment and diagnosis is important. Depending on the specific problem, it may be appropriate to seek out a specialist in anxiety/depressive disorders, pain management, chemical dependency, or other disorders, or specific types of treatments, such as **cognitive-behavioral therapy** or **hypnotherapy**. Assessment and diagnosis should take place in a private, quiet, nonthreatening environment. The clinician should attempt to make the patient as comfortable as possible. In the case of a language barrier, a competent translator is essential for accurate assessment and diagnosis.

Aftercare

Aftercare is determined by the assessment and diagnosis. It may include additional assessments and tests, perhaps by a specialist, to confirm a diagnosis and determine appropriate treatment. Treatments may include various interventions, psychoactive medications, and/or **psychotherapy**, cognitive-behavioral therapy, **family therapy**, or some other form of counseling. With pediatric assessment and diagnosis, parents should obtain copies of the clinician's notes, assessments, and diagnosis, and

KEY TERMS

Affect—The expression of emotion through such features as facial expressions, hand gestures, and tone of voice. Types of affect include flat (inanimate, no expression), blunted (minimally responsive), inappropriate relative to the context, and labile (abrupt changes in type and intensity of emotion).

Alzheimer's disease—A progressive, neurodegenerative disease characterized by loss of function and death of nerve cells in several areas of the brain, leading to loss of mental functions, such as memory and learning. Alzheimer's disease is the most common cause of dementia.

Assessment—A psychological assessment, usually via a structured interview, to gather information for diagnosing a mental disorder.

Attention deficit hyperactivity disorder (ADHD)—A persistent pattern of inattention, hyperactivity and/or impulsiveness. The pattern is more frequent and severe than is typically observed in people at a similar level of development.

Autism spectrum disorder (ASD)—A range of variable developmental disorders that includes an impaired ability to communicate and form normal social relationships.

Biopsychosocial history—A history of experiences and other factors that influence behaviors, including medical, educational, occupational, and interpersonal histories, as well as any alcohol or drug use or criminal activity.

Bipolar disorder—A recurrent mood disorder, also known as manic-depressive disorder, in which patients have extreme mood swings from depression to mania or a mixture of both.

Cognition—Conscious intellectual activity, including thinking, imagining, reasoning, remembering, and learning.

Delusion—A strongly held false belief, such that the belief that one is being poisoned or has a fatal illness, despite all evidence to the contrary.

Dementia—A group of symptoms (syndrome) associated with chronic progressive impairment of memory, reasoning ability, and other intellectual functions; personality changes; deterioration in personal grooming; disorientation; and sometimes delusions.

Dependence—Physiological or psychological addiction to alcohol or a drug, possibly followed by withdrawal symptoms when use is terminated.

Dissociation—Disconnection from oneself.

Dyslexia—A variable learning disability that is usually characterized by difficulty reading, writing, and spelling. It often runs in families; also called developmental reading disorder (DRD) or specific reading disability.

Eating disorder—A condition characterized by an abnormal attitude toward food, altered appetite control, and unhealthy eating habits.

Hallucinations—False sensory perceptions, for example, hearing sounds or seeing people or objects that are not there. Hallucinations can also affect the senses of smell, touch, and taste.

Phobia—Irrational fear of places, things, or situations, leading to avoidance.

Post-traumatic stress disorder (PTSD)—A psychological response to a highly stressful event, typically characterized by depression, anxiety, flashbacks, nightmares, and avoidance of reminders of the traumatic experience.

Psychometric—Quantitative methods for mental and psychological measurements.

Schizophrenia—A psychotic disorder characterized by loss of contact with one's environment, deterioration of everyday functioning, and personality disintegration.

Tolerance—Progressive decrease in the effectiveness of a drug with long-term use.

ensure that they understand the diagnosis and treatment options.

Risks

The major risk of assessment is a wrong diagnosis. Accurate information gathering and objective note-taking are essential for psychological assessments. However, these can be difficult to obtain if the patient is not forthcoming with information, perhaps out of embarrassment or **denial** of symptoms. For example, although depression is quite common in older people, its assessment and diagnosis can be difficult. Clinical symptoms of depression in the elderly may be very different from those

QUESTIONS TO ASK YOUR DOCTOR

- What type of assessment do you recommend for me?
- Who will perform the assessment?
- What will my assessment involve?
- How long will my assessment take?
- What information will my assessment provide?
- Will I have full access to the assessment report?

in younger individuals. Older people tend to complain of physical rather than psychological symptoms. Symptoms of medical disorders, as well as complications from social isolation and personal loss, can mask signs of depression and other mental disorders. Certain portions of an assessment also are quite subjective. Misperceptions, misunderstandings, or inexperience on the part of the interviewer can lead to misdiagnoses. Improper diagnosis presents the risk of inappropriate treatment.

Results

Complete assessments help establish either a tentative or definitive diagnosis. Based on the assessment and diagnosis, the patient may be declared healthy or referred for psychological therapy or other **intervention** and/or prescribed psychoactive medication.

Resources

BOOKS

Butcher, James Neal, Susan Mineka, and Jill M. Hooley. *Abnormal Psychology*, 14th ed. Boston: Allyn & Bacon, 2010.

Dziegielewski, Sophia F. *DSM-IV-TR in Action*, 2nd ed. Hoboken, NJ: John Wiley & Sons, 2010.

Hersen, Michel, and Alan M. Gross, eds. *Handbook of Clinical Psychology*. Hoboken, NJ: John Wiley & Sons, 2008.

Sue, David, and Diane M. Sue. *Foundations of Counseling and Psychotherapy: Evidence-Based Practices for a Diverse Society*. Hoboken, NJ: John Wiley & Sons, 2008.

PERIODICALS

Jones, Karyn Dayle, Tabitha Young, and Monica Leppma. "Mild Traumatic Brain Injury and Posttraumatic Stress Disorder in Returning Iraq and Afghanistan War Veterans: Implications for Assessment and Diagnosis." *Journal of Counseling and Development* 88, no. 3 (Summer 2010): 372–76.

WEBSITES

"Breaking Ground, Breaking Through: The Strategic Plan for Mood Disorders Research." National Institute of Mental Health. http://www.nimh.nih.gov/about/strategic-planning-reports/breaking-ground-breaking-through–the-strategic-plan-for-mood-disorders-research.pdf (accessed July 24, 2011).

"Psychology Is a Behavioral and Mental Health Profession." American Psychological Association. http://www.apa.org/about/gr/issues/health-care/profession.aspx (accessed July 24, 2011).

"What Parents Should Know About Treatment of Behavioral and Emotional Disorders in Preschool Children." American Psychological Association. http://www.apa.org/pubs/info/brochures/kids-meds.aspx (accessed July 24, 2011).

ORGANIZATIONS

American Psychiatric Association, 1000 Wilson Blvd., Ste. 1825, Arlington, VA, 22209-3901, (703) 907-7300, apa@psych.org, http://www.psych.org.

American Psychological Association, 750 1st St., NE, Washington, DC, 20002-4242, (202) 336-5500, (800) 374-2721, http://www.apa.org.

Mental Health America, 2000 N Beauregard St., 6th Fl., Alexandria, VA, 22311, (703) 684-7722, (800) 969-6642, Fax: (703) 684-5968, http://www.nmha.org.

National Alliance on Mental Illness, 3803 N Fairfax Dr., Ste. 100, Arlington, VA, 22203, (703) 524-7600, (800) 950-6264, Fax: (703) 524-9094, http://www.nami.org.

National Institute of Mental Health, 6001 Executive Blvd., Rm. 8184, MSC 9663, Bethesda, MD, 20892-9663, (301) 443-4513, (866) 615-6464, Fax: (301) 443-4279, nimhinfo@nih.gov, http://www.nimh.nih.gov.

Sidran Institute, PO Box 436, Brooklandville, MD, 21022-0436, (410) 825-8888, Fax: (410) 560-0134, info@sidran.org, http://www.sidran.org.

Laith Farid Gulli, MD
Bilal Nasser, MD
Robert Ramirez
Margaret Alic, PhD

Psychologist

Definition

A psychologist is a social scientist who studies behavior and mental processes, generally in a research or clinical setting.

Description

As psychology has grown and changed throughout history, it has been defined in numerous ways. As early as 400 B.C., the ancient Greeks philosophized about the relationship of personality characteristics to physiological traits. Since then, philosophers have proposed theories to

SIGMUND FREUD (1856–1939)

The work of Sigmund Freud, the Austrian founder of psychoanalysis, marked the beginning of a modern, dynamic psychology by providing the first systematic explanation of the inner mental forces determining human behavior.

Early in his career Sigmund Freud distinguished himself as a histologist, neuropathologist, and clinical neurologist, and in his later life he was acclaimed as a talented writer and essayist. However, his fame is based on his work in expanding man's knowledge of himself through clinical research and corresponding development of theories to explain the new data. He laid the foundations for modern understanding of unconscious mental processes (processes excluded from awareness), neurosis (a type of mental disorder), the sexual life of infants, and the interpretation of dreams. Under his guidance, psychoanalysis became the dominant modern theory of human psychology and a major tool of research, as well as an important method of psychiatric treatment, which currently has thousands of practitioners all over the world. The application of psychoanalytic thinking to the studies of history, anthropology, religion, art, sociology, and education has greatly changed these fields.

Sigmund Freud was born on May 6, 1856, in Freiberg, Moravia (now Czechoslovakia). Sigmund was the first child of his twice-widowed father's third marriage. His mother, Amalia Nathanson, was 19 years old when she married Jacob Freud, aged 39. Sigmund's two stepbrothers from his father's first marriage were approximately the same age as his mother, and his older stepbrother's son, Sigmund's nephew, was his earliest playmate. Thus the boy grew up in an unusual family structure, his mother halfway in age between himself and his father. Though seven younger children were born, Sigmund always remained his mother's favorite. When he was 4, the family moved to Vienna, the capital of the Austro-Hungarian monarchy and one of the great cultural, scientific, and medical centers of Europe. Freud lived in Vienna until a year before his death.

explain human behavior. In the late nineteenth century the emergence of scientific method gave the study of psychology a new focus. In 1879, the first psychological laboratory was opened in Leipzig, Germany, by Wilhelm Wundt, and soon afterward the first experimental studies of memory were published. Wundt was instrumental in establishing psychology as the study of conscious experience, which he viewed as made up of elemental sensations. In addition to the type of psychology practiced by Wundt—which became known as structuralism—other early schools of psychology were functionalism, which led to the development of behaviorism, and Gestalt psychology. The **American Psychological Association** was founded in 1892 with the goals of encouraging research, enhancing professional competence, and disseminating knowledge about the field.

With the ascendance of the Viennese neurologist Sigmund Freud and his method of **psychoanalysis** early in the twentieth century, emphasis shifted from conscious experience to unconscious processes investigated by means of free association and other techniques. According to Freud, behavior and mental processes were the result of mostly unconscious struggles between the drive to satisfy basic instincts, such as sex or aggression, and the limits imposed by society. At the same time that Freud's views were gaining popularity in Europe, an American psychology professor, John B. Watson, was pioneering the behavioral approach, which focuses on observing and measuring external behaviors rather than the internal workings of the mind. B. F. Skinner, who spent decades studying the effects of reward and punishment on behavior, helped maintain the predominance of behaviorism in the United States through the 1950s and 1960s. Since the 1970s, many psychologists have been influenced by the cognitive approach, which is concerned with the relationship of mental processes to behavior. Cognitive psychology focuses on how people take in, perceive, and store information, and how they process and act on that information.

Additional psychological perspectives include the neurobiological approach, focusing on relating behavior to internal processes within the **brain** and nervous system, and the phenomenological approach, which is most concerned with the individual's subjective experience of the world rather than the application of psychological theory to behavior. Although all these approaches differ in their explanations of individual behavior, each contributes an important perspective to the overall psychological understanding of the total human being. Most psychologists apply the principles of various approaches in studying and understanding human nature.

Along with several approaches to psychology there are also numerous, overlapping subfields in which these approaches may be applied. Most subfields can be categorized under one of two major areas of psychology referred to as basic and applied psychology. Basic psychology encompasses the subfields concerned with the advancement of psychological theory and research. Experimental psychology employs laboratory experiments to study basic behavioral processes, including sensation, perception, learning, memory, communication, and motivation, that different species share. Physiological psychology is concerned with the ways in which biology shapes behavior and mental processes, and developmental psychology is concerned with behavioral development over the entire life span. Other subfields include social psychology, quantitative psychology, and the psychology of personality.

Applied psychology is the area of psychology concerned with applying psychological research and theory to problems posed by everyday life. It includes clinical psychology, the largest single field in psychology. Clinical psychologists—who represent 40% of all psychologists are involved in **psychotherapy** and psychological testing. Clinical psychologists are trained in research and often work in university or research settings, studying various aspects of psychology. Like clinical psychologists, counseling psychologists apply psychological principles to diagnose and treat individual emotional and behavioral problems. Other subfields of applied psychology include school psychology, which involves the evaluation and placement of students; educational psychology, which investigates the psychological aspects of the learning process; and industrial and organizational psychology, which study the relationship between people and their jobs. Community psychologists investigate environmental factors that contribute to mental and emotional disorders; health psychologists deal with the psychological aspects of physical illness, investigating the connections between the mind and a person's physical condition; and consumer psychologists study the preferences and buying habits of consumers as well as their reactions to certain advertising.

In response to society's changing needs, new fields of psychology are constantly emerging. One type of specialization, called environmental psychology, focuses on the relationship between people and their physical surroundings. Its areas of inquiry include such issues as the effects of overcrowding and noise on urban dwellers and the effects of building design. Another specialty is forensic psychology, involving the application of psychology to law enforcement and the judicial system. Forensic psychologists may help create personality profiles of criminals, formulate principles for jury selection, or study the problems involved in eyewitness testimony. Yet another emerging area is program evaluation, whose practitioners evaluate the effectiveness and cost efficiency of the programs.

Depending on the nature of their work, psychologists may practice in a variety of settings, including colleges and universities, hospitals and **community mental health** centers, schools, and businesses. A growing number of psychologists work in private practice and may also specialize in multiple subfields. Most psychologists earn a PhD degree in the field, which requires completion of a four- to six-year post-bachelors' degree program offered by a university psychology department. The course of study includes a broad overview of the field, as well as specialization in a particular subfield, and completion of a dissertation and an internship (usually needed only for applied psychology, such as clinical, counseling, and school psychology). Students who intend to practice only applied psychology rather than conduct research have the option of obtaining a Psy.D. degree, which differs in the limited emphasis that is put on research and a dissertation that does not have to be based on an empirical research study.

ORGANIZATIONS

American Psychological Association, 750 1st Street NE, Washington, DC, 20002-4242, (202) 336-5500; TDD/TTY: (202) 336-6123, (800) 374-2721, http://www.apa.org.

Emily Jane Willingham, PhD

Psychopharmacology

Definition

Psychopharmacology is the branch of medicine that investigates the properties and legitimate uses of psychoactive substances and their effects on human thinking, emotions, sensations, and behavior. The name comes from three Greek words meaning "mind" or "soul," "drug," and "study of." Although recreational ("street") drugs also have psychoactive properties, psychopharmacology is primarily concerned with the development and testing of drugs for the treatment of mental disorders or their symptoms. Psychoactive drugs are also known as psychopharmaceuticals or psychotropic drugs.

Psychoactive drugs interact with specific molecules found on the surfaces of cells in the central nervous system known as receptors. The action of a psychopharmaceutical on a receptor is called the drug's pharmacodynamics, while the body's use of the drug (the drug's absorption within the body and its eventual excretion) is called its pharmacokinetics.

Purpose

Psychopharmacology has several purposes, including the research and development of new drugs to treat mental disorders, including drugs derived from natural sources as well as those synthesized in the laboratory; improved understanding of the mechanisms of drug activity in the **brain** and central nervous system; and improved understanding of long-term as well as short-term side effects of psychopharmaceuticals and their interactions with other medications.

Demographics

Psychopharmacology has moved over the past half century into a leading subspecialty of biochemistry, largely on account of the increasing use of medications rather than **psychotherapy** to treat mental disorders. The number of Americans diagnosed with mental disorders has risen dramatically since the 1980s—between 1987 and 2007, the number of Americans receiving supplemental Social Security payments for mental disability rose from 1 in every 184 adults to 1 in every 76, an increase of 250%. The increase in diagnoses of mental illness in children is even more remarkable: a 35-fold increase over the same twenty-year period. A survey conducted by the **National Institute of Mental Health** (NIMH) between 2001 and 2003 reported that 46% of the randomly sampled adults met criteria for at least one of four categories of mental illness at some point in their lives: mood disorders, **anxiety disorders**, impulse-control disorders, and **substance abuse** disorders.

The increases are attributed at least in part to the popularity of psychopharmaceuticals; within ten years after the 1987 introduction of Prozac—the first of the **selective serotonin reuptake inhibitors** (SSRIs)—the number of patients diagnosed with **depression** tripled. As of 2011, 10% of Americans over six years of age were taking antidepressant medications. With regard to antipsychotics, the newer so-called atypical antipsychotics are now the top-selling class of drugs in the United States, ahead of cholesterol-lowering medications. This steep climb in the number of patients taking psychotropic medications in less than three decades is a major reason for the reinvestigation of the effectiveness of these drugs.

Description

Origins

PRESCIENTIFIC USE OF PSYCHOACTIVE SUBSTANCES. The use of psychoactive substances goes back to prehistoric times. Before the rise of scientific biochemistry in the nineteenth century, most psychoactive preparations were derived from plants. Tribal cultures made use of psychedelic mushrooms and cacti (such as the peyote cactus) to induce altered states of consciousness; there is evidence that some of these substances were used as early as 10,000 B.C.E. With the development of agriculture and the formation of settled villages during the New Stone Age (around 9,500 B.C.E.), humans began to make use of cultivated plants for both recreational and medicinal purposes.

Most early human societies discovered alcoholic beverages in the form of fermented products such as wine and beer (distilled liquors such as gin and whiskey were not developed until the seventeenth century). With regard to anesthesia, the painkilling properties of the opium poppy were known to the ancient Sumerians, Egyptians, Indians, Greeks, and Romans. In addition to these plant-derived psychoactive substances, ancient societies in both the East and the West collected and studied herbs for their medicinal properties. While medieval European and Native American herbalists generally favored preparations made from a single plant, traditional Chinese medicine developed complex formulas for medicines that required several different herbs to produce the desired result.

In the sixteenth and seventeenth centuries, European settlement of North America and trade with Turkey introduced two new plants containing psychoactive substances to the West: tobacco and coffee beans. In contrast to alcohol and **opioids**, which are depressants, the **nicotine** in tobacco and the caffeine in coffee are stimulants. Caffeine is the most widely used psychoactive substance in the world, with 85% of American adults consuming coffee on a daily basis.

PSYCHOPHARMACOLOGY IN THE MODERN WORLD. It was not until the establishment of organic chemistry as a subdiscipline within chemistry in the late nineteenth century that modern psychopharmaceuticals were made possible. The discovery of the concept of chemical structure, made independently in 1858 by Friedrich August Kekulé (1829–1896) and Archibald Scott Couper (1831–1892), permitted the synthesis of complex molecules in the laboratory through multistep processes. By the end of the nineteenth century, Bayer AG in Germany patented its brand of acetylsalicylic acid under the name of aspirin. Although many of the new pharmaceutical companies that were formed between the 1890s and the outbreak of World War I in 1914 were primarily interested in creating completely new synthetic compounds, others began to investigate the chemical compounds found in herbs and other natural sources. Many of the most important drugs used in psychiatry in the twentieth century resulted from research into herbal lore, including some compounds that were originally developed to treat infections and were found to change a person's mental state only accidentally.

The use of psychopharmaceuticals to treat mental illness was relatively uncommon before the 1950s. From the 1880s onward, **psychoanalysis**, **psychodynamic psychotherapy**, and other forms of the therapy were the primary methods of treatment; although Freud himself experimented with using **cocaine** to relieve depression in his patients between 1883 and 1887 and used it to regulate his own moods until 1896. In the 1950s, however, the discovery of several classes of anxiolytics, particularly the **barbiturates** and the benzodiazepine tranquilizers, made it possible to treat anxiety disorders with medications, and the tricyclic **antidepressants**, first discovered in the mid-1950s, were soon recommended for the treatment of major depression. The oldest antipsychotic drugs, **chlorpromazine** (Thorazine) and the phenothiazines, were used to treat **schizophrenia** as early as 1952.

The rise of the so-called counterculture in the 1960s, with its use of **hallucinogens** and other street drugs to induce altered states of consciousness, led to some psychiatrists' recommending the use of **cannabis** (marijuana), peyote, and psilocybin as adjuncts to traditional psychotherapy. Lysergic acid diethylamide (LSD), first synthesized by the Swiss chemist Albert Hoffman (1906–2008) in 1938, was first used by psychiatrists in 1947, but controversy over its popularity in the drug culture of the 1960s led to restrictions on its use by mainstream therapists.

The success of the first antipsychotics and the tricyclic antidepressants led to the so-called biological psychiatry movement, based on the notion that mental disorders are fundamentally biological in origin. Biological psychiatrists proposed the chemical imbalance theory of mental disorders, namely that mental illnesses are the end result of too little or too much of neurotransmitters—such as **serotonin**, norepinephrine, or dopamine—in the central nervous system. The shift from the older psychoanalytic theories of mental illness to biological psychiatry was reflected in the third edition of the ***Diagnostic and Statistical Manual of Mental Disorders*** (*DSM-III*), published in 1980.

One major problem with the chemical imbalance theory, however, is that it did not explain the time lag that typically occurs between the biological activity of the first doses of an antidepressant and symptom relief; studies indicated that the neurotransmitter levels in the patient's body began to change within hours, but changes in the patient's mood took weeks. A more recent version of the theory holds that depression and other disorders result from degenerative changes in the neurons (nerve cells) in the central nervous system and/or the loss of functional connections between neurons and that antidepressants work by stimulating the growth of new neurons or repairing their interconnections.

Types of psychoactive drugs

There are seven major classes of psychoactive drugs:

- Antidepressants. These drugs are used to treat major depression and some anxiety disorders. Most of them work by inhibiting the breakdown of serotonin, norepinephrine, or both. The five major types of antidepressants are the monoamine oxidase inhibitors (MAOIs), tricyclic (TCAs) and tetracyclic (TeCAs) antidepressants, selective serotonin reuptake inhibitors (SSRIs), and serotonin-norepinephrine reuptake inhibitors (SNRIs).
- Antipsychotics. These drugs are used to relieve the hallucinations and other psychotic symptoms of schizophrenia. They may also be used to help stabilize moods in patients with bipolar disorder even when no psychotic symptoms are present. The older antipsychotics (also called the typical antipsychotics) were developed in the 1950s and include such drugs as the phenothiazines. Examples of atypical antipsychotics include the drugs risperidone, aripiprazole, and clozapine.
- Anxiolytics and hypnotics. These drugs are prescribed to relieve anxiety. Sometimes called tranquilizers, the anxiolytics include benzodiazepines, some of the SSRIs, barbiturates, and buspirone. Barbiturates are rarely prescribed except as sleeping medications (hypnotics) because of their potential for abuse (including suicide when combined with alcohol). Benzodiazepines are considered safer; they include the drugs diazepam, lorazepam, and chlordiazepoxide. Zolpidem, which is not a benzodiazepine, is frequently prescribed as a hypnotic.
- Depressants. Anxiolytics and antipsychotics are sometimes classified as depressants. Other depressants include ethanol (beverage alcohol), which does not require a prescription, and prescription sedatives, opioid pain relievers (also called narcotics), and anesthetics.
- Hallucinogens. These drugs are generally associated with recreational drug use, but some were being used in clinical trials in 2011 as antianxiety agents. These include LSD, psilocybin, dimethyltryptamine (DMT), and cannabis.

KEY TERMS

Antidepressant—Any of a group of medications given to relieve mood disorders, including anxiety disorders as well as major depression. Antidepressants include monoamine oxidase inhibitors (MAOIs), tricyclic (TCAs) and tetracyclic (TeCAs) antidepressants, selective serotonin reuptake inhibitors (SSRIs), and serotonin-norepinephrine reuptake inhibitors (SNRIs).

Anxiolytic—Any of a group of medications prescribed to relieve anxiety. Also called tranquilizers, anxiolytics include benzodiazepines, some of the selective serotonin reuptake inhibitors (SSRIs), barbiturates, and buspirone.

Attention deficit hyperactivity disorder (ADHD)—A persistent pattern of inattention, hyperactivity, and/or impulsiveness; the pattern is more frequent and severe than is typically observed in people at a similar level of development.

Biological psychiatry—An approach to psychiatry that attributes mental disorders to biochemical or other biological malfunctions of the central nervous system, as distinct from the patient's childhood issues and life history.

Blood-brain barrier—A specialized, semi-permeable layer of cells around the blood vessels in the brain that controls which substances can leave the circulatory system and enter the brain.

Depressant—Any psychoactive substance that lowers the function or activity level of a specific part of the body or brain. Depressants are sometimes referred to as "downers." These include anxiolytics, sedatives, antipsychotics, opioids, and anesthetics as well as nonprescription substances such as alcohol.

Hallucinogen—A drug that distorts sensory perceptions and disturbs emotion, judgment, and memory. Hallucinogens are often used to induce trances, meditation, and dream states.

Hypnotic—A medication that causes sleep.

Narcotic—Another term for an opioid drug.

Opioid—Any of a group of potent pain-relieving drugs derived from the opium poppy or synthesized in the laboratory. Opioids bind to opioid receptors in the brain, spinal cord, and digestive tract.

Pharmacodynamics—The study of the effects of drugs on the human body.

Pharmacokinetics—The study of the absorption, distribution, and elimination of drugs from the body.

Placebo—A pill or liquid given during the study of a drug or dietary supplement that contains no medication or active ingredient, used to test the effectiveness of the drug or supplement in question. Usually study participants do not know if they are receiving the drug or the placebo.

Psychoactive—Referring to any substance that crosses the blood-brain barrier and acts primarily upon the central nervous system, leading to changes in mood, perception, thinking, feeling, or behavior.

Receptor—In biochemistry, a substance (usually a protein) found on the surface of a cell that interacts with specific other molecules, drugs, hormones, or antibodies.

Stimulant—A type of psychoactive substance that increases alertness or wakefulness. Stimulants are sometimes referred to as "uppers."

Tardive dyskinesia—A disorder characterized by involuntary and repetitive body movements that sometimes develops after long-term use of antipsychotic medications.

Tranquilizer—Another name for anxiolytic.

- Mood stabilizers. These drugs are used to treat bipolar disorder, particularly manic episodes. Lithium carbonate, the oldest mood stabilizer, was discovered in 1949. Other mood stabilizers belong to the class of drugs used to treat epilepsy known as anticonvulsants. These drugs include such medications as valproic acid, carbamazepine, and gabapentin.
- Stimulants. Stimulants are among the most widely prescribed psychotropic drugs and are used to treat attention deficit hyperactivity disorder (ADHD), narcolepsy, and occasionally depression that does not respond to other medications. Stimulants can be addictive and are not recommended for patients with substance abuse disorders. Prescription stimulants include such drugs as methylphenidate and various amphetamine compounds.

Benefits

The benefits of psychoactive drugs are a source of considerable controversy. A growing number of psychiatrists prefer to combine prescriptions for psychotropic drugs with cognitive-behavioral or psychodynamic psychotherapy rather than relying on drugs by themselves. One reason for preferring a combined approach is the growing recognition that many mood disorders, as well as other mental health problems, are related to dysfunctional behaviors and not just abnormalities in brain structure or function. Correcting the cognitive distortions that reinforce the behavior is more effective over the long run than suppressing or alleviating symptoms via medication. Psychotropic drugs may, however, be prescribed for short-term symptom relief.

Precautions

There are several precautions that patients should observe before taking any psychotropic drug:

- Have a discussion with the doctor about the drug: its benefits, risks, and possible side effects, and whether other forms of treatment are available
- Inform the doctor of any allergic reactions to any medications of any type, and making sure the doctor has a complete list of all other medications (over-the-counter as well as prescription) that the patient is taking
- Read the instructions that come with the drug carefully and ask the doctor or pharmacist to explain anything that is unclear or hard to understand
- Take the medication only as directed; do not increase or decrease the dose or the frequency of the dose without telling the doctor. It is particularly important not to stop taking the drug without consulting the doctor, as some psychotropic medications (particularly benzodiazepines, opioid pain relievers, and SSRIs) can produce withdrawal syndromes if abruptly discontinued.
- Store the drug at the appropriate temperature and away from sunlight. If there are small children in the household, keep the drug in a locked cabinet or other safe place.
- Do not share the medication with other family members. This precaution is particularly important if anyone in the family has a substance abuse disorder.

Risks

There are a number of risks associated with prescription psychoactive drugs:

- Short-term adverse effects. Psychopharmaceuticals have well-known side effects that range from constipation, drowsiness, fluid retention, and nausea to loss of sexual interest, loss of coordination, skin rashes, and liver disorders. Several studies have shown that a majority of patients taking antidepressants stop using them within a year because of the side effects. Many subjects participating in clinical trials of antidepressants were able to figure out that they were receiving the real drug rather than a placebo because they experienced adverse side effects.
- Long-term adverse effects. Researchers are increasingly aware of the potential for long-term adverse effects of psychoactive medications—effects that may not appear for some years. One of the first long-term adverse effects to appear was tardive dyskinesia, a movement disorder that develops in patients taking the older antipsychotics for long periods of time. More recently, there is evidence that antipsychotics lead to shrinkage of tissue in the prefrontal cortex of the brain and that the extent of shrinkage is in direct proportion to the dosage level and duration of treatment.
- Interactions with alcohol and other medications. Depressant medications in general should not be taken with alcohol, which intensifies their effects. MAOIs have been found to have potentially dangerous interactions with amphetamines, SSRIs, SNRIs, and many other drugs.
- Withdrawal effects. Patients should not stop taking any psychoactive drug without consulting their doctor, as many of these medications can produce withdrawal symptoms if they are suddenly discontinued. SSRIs, opioids, and benzodiazepines can produce symptoms ranging from irritability and anxiety to sensory disturbances and seizures if they are suddenly withdrawn. An important aspect of withdrawal effects is that they are often mistaken for a recurrence of the patient's disorder. The result is that the patient is often put back on the medication that caused the withdrawal effects, usually at a higher dosage.
- Dependence and abuse. Many classes of psychoactive drugs are associated with the risk of dependency and abuse, particularly in long-term users. Amphetamines are not recommended for treatment of persons with a history of substance abuse. Opioid dependency is another well-known problem, particularly addiction to such semi-synthetic opioids as oxycodone.

Research and general acceptance

Recent research has led to a reexamination of the widespread use of psychotropic drugs. One reason is increasing questioning of the chemical imbalance theory of mental illness. As researchers have pointed out, the theory does not account for the fact that neurotransmitter levels have been found to be normal in people with mental disorders prior to treatment. It appears increasingly likely that the theory developed when doctors discovered that psychopharmaceuticals changed the levels of certain **neurotransmitters** in the brain; the doctors then assumed that the mental illness was caused by abnormal levels of neurotransmitters. It is entirely possible that any symptom relief by psychoactive drugs is due to some other method entirely.

Another part of the problem is the recent discovery through the Freedom of Information Act that **clinical trials** of psychotropic drugs that yielded negative results were never published, while those with positive findings received considerable publicity. One researcher discovered that of 42 trials of the six most frequently prescribed antidepressants approved by the U.S. Food and Drug Administration (FDA) between 1987 and 1999, most had negative outcomes. Most trials found that placebos were about 82% as effective as the antidepressants when measured by the **Hamilton Depression Scale**, a widely used instrument. Yet because the few positive trials were widely reported, most doctors as well as patients were convinced that the antidepressants were highly effective.

A major study that failed to show the superiority of antidepressants to placebos was the 2006 Sequenced Treatment Alternatives to Relieve Depression (STAR*D) study of depression. One of the largest clinical trials ever undertaken, the study enrolled 4,041 patients across the United States who were diagnosed as moderately to severely depressed. The results showed that after a year's time, all but 108 of the 4,041 patients had either dropped out of treatment or relapsed—only 3% of the original patient group remained. A researcher who investigated the outcome of the **STAR*D study** stated, "The STAR*D analysis found that the effectiveness of antidepressant therapies was probably even lower than the modest one reported by the study authors with an apparent progressively increasing dropout rate across each study phase."

Clinical Antipsychotic Trials in **Intervention** Effectiveness (**CATIE**), a study of antipsychotic medications that was conducted between 2000 and 2004, found that the older antipsychotics were as effective for many patients as the newer and far more expensive atypical antipsychotics. In addition, it is significant that several follow-up CATIE studies were designed specifically to investigate the side effects of antipsychotic medications, in particular weight gain and a rise in blood cholesterol levels.

One question that arises from the recent reevaluation of psychopharmaceuticals is why the effectiveness of the drugs has been potentially overrated for so long. Several reasons have been proposed:

- The use of medications for mental illness removed much of the stigma previously attached to it. By attributing the symptoms of mental disorders to chemical imbalances in the brain, psychopharmacologists helped to reassure patients (and for children, their parents) that they were not "bad" people or the products of "bad parenting," but simply people with malfunctioning nervous systems.
- The discovery of antibiotics, effective vaccines against many diseases, and other "wonder drugs" in the 1940s and 1950s fostered a general cultural belief that many human problems can be solved by the right drug. Whereas previous generations recognized that some forms of grief and loss are normal responses to life events and will heal with time, people who grew up after the 1960s are more likely to have absorbed the belief that they need an antidepressant (or some other drug) to help them over temporary sadness. They then attribute their improvement after a few months to the pill rather than normal resolution of grief.
- The greater willingness of insurance companies to reimburse patients for medications rather than psychotherapy for mental health issues. With the rise of managed care in the 1980s, it became easier for doctors to simply prescribe psychotropic drugs rather than recommending counseling.
- The rapid increase of direct-to-consumer advertising of drugs on American television after 1998 (with the exception of New Zealand, other countries do not permit such advertising on television). Many of these ads exaggerate the effectiveness of antidepressants, hypnotics, and other psychoactive drugs.
- The placebo effect. The placebo effect refers to improvement in a patient's condition brought about by the patient's expectations of and confidence in an inert substance that is believed to be a drug. In other words, the effectiveness of many psychoactive drugs appears to be largely based on the placebo effect.

One sign that criticisms of the overuse of psychopharmaceuticals are having an effect is the appearance of articles in financial journals advising against investment in the companies that manufacture them. Another indication is reports in general scientific journals that pharmaceutical manufacturers are shutting down research into new drugs for psychiatric disorders.

Resources

BOOKS

Kirsch, Irving. *The Emperor's New Drugs: Exploding the Antidepressant Myth*. New York: Basic Books, 2010.

Lichtblau, Leonard. *Psychopharmacology Demystified*. Clifton Park, NY: Delmar Cengage Learning, 2011.

Sinacola, Richard S., and Timothy Peters-Strickland. *Basic Psychopharmacology for Counselors and Psychotherapists*, 2nd ed. Boston: Pearson, 2012.

Stahl, Stephen M. *Stahl's Essential Psychopharmacology: The Prescriber' s Guide,* 4th ed. New York: Cambridge University Press, 2011.

Whitaker, Robert. *Anatomy of an Epidemic: Magic Bullets, Psychiatric Drugs, and the Astonishing Rise of Mental Illness in America.* New York: Crown, 2010.

PERIODICALS

Alvarez, P.A., and J. Pahissa. "QT Alterations in Psychopharmacology: Proven Candidates and Suspects." *Current Drug Safety* 5 (January 2010): 97–104.

Angell, Marcia. "The Epidemic of Mental Illness: Why?" [part one of a two-part article]. *New York Review of Books* 58, no. 11 (June 23, 2011). http://www.nybooks.com/articles/archives/2011/jun/23/epidemic-mental-illness-why/?pagination=false (accessed September 16, 2011).

———. "The Illusions of Psychiatry." [part two of a two-part article]. *New York Review of Books* 58, no. 12 (July 14, 2011). http://www.nybooks.com/articles/archives/2011/jul/14/illusions-of-psychiatry/?pagination=false (accessed September 16, 2011).

Cressy, Daniel. "Psychopharmacology in Crisis." *Nature News*, June 14, 2011. http://dx.doi.org/10.1038/news.2011.367 (accessed September 16, 2011).

Claessens, S.E., et al. "Development of Individual Differences in Stress Responsiveness: An Overview of Factors Mediating the Outcome of Early Life Experiences." *Psychopharmacology (Berlin)* 214 (March 2011): 141–54.

Pigott, H.E., et al. "Efficacy and Effectiveness of Antidepressants: Current Status of Research." *Psychotherapy and Psychosomatics* 79 (May 2010): 267–79.

Praharaj, S.K., et al. "Sensory Disturbances Associated with Serotonin Reuptake Inhibitors: Brief Review." *Human Psychopharmacology* 25 (April 2010): 216–21.

Pratt, H.D. "Point-counter-point: Psychotherapy in the Age of Pharmacology." *Pediatric Clinics of North America* 58 (February 2011): 1–9.

WEBSITES

Leventhal, Allan M. "What Underlies Psychopharmacology?" *Dissident Voice*, May 4, 2011. http://dissidentvoice.org/2011/05/what-underlies-psychopharmacology (accessed September 16, 2011).

ORGANIZATIONS

American College of Neuropsychopharmacology, 5034-A Thoroughbred Lane, Brentwood, TN, 37027, (615) 324-2360, Fax: (615) 523-1715, acnp@acnp.org, http://www.acnp.org/default.aspx.

American Society for Clinical Pharmacology and Therapeutics, 528 N Washington St., Alexandria, VA, 22314, (703) 836-6981, info@ascpt.org, http://www.ascpt.org.

European College of Neuropsychopharmacology (ECNP), PO Box 85410, Utrecht, Netherlands3508 AK, +31302538567, Fax: +31302538568, secretariat@ecnp.eu, http://www.ecnp.eu.

Rebecca J. Frey, Ph.D.

Psychosis

Definition

Psychosis is a symptom or feature of mental illness typically characterized by radical changes in personality, impaired functioning, and a distorted or nonexistent sense of objective reality.

Description

Patients suffering from psychosis have impaired reality testing; that is, they are unable to distinguish personal subjective experience from the reality of the external world. They experience hallucinations and/or **delusions** that they believe are real, and may behave and communicate in an inappropriate and incoherent fashion. Psychosis may appear as a symptom of a number of mental disorders, including mood and **personality disorders**. It is also the defining feature of **schizophrenia**, **schizophreniform disorder**, **schizoaffective disorder**, **delusional disorder**, and the psychotic disorders (i.e., **brief psychotic disorder**, **shared psychotic disorder**, psychotic disorder due to a general medical condition, and **substance-induced psychotic disorder**).

Causes and symptoms

Psychosis may be caused by the interaction of biological and psychosocial factors, depending on the disorder in which it presents; psychosis can also be caused by purely social factors, with no biological component.

Biological factors that are regarded as contributing to the development of psychosis include genetic abnormalities and substance use. With regard to chromosomal abnormalities, studies indicate that 30% of patients diagnosed with a psychotic disorder have a microdeletion at chromosome 22q11. Another group of researchers has identified the gene G72/G30 at chromosome 13q33.2 as a susceptibility gene for childhood-onset schizophrenia and psychosis not otherwise specified.

With regard to **substance abuse**, several different research groups reported in 2004 that **cannabis** (marijuana) use is a risk factor for the onset of psychosis.

Migration is a social factor that influences people's susceptibility to psychotic disorders. Psychiatrists in Europe have noted the increasing rate of schizophrenia and other psychotic disorders among immigrants to almost all Western European countries. Black immigrants from Africa or the Caribbean appear to be especially vulnerable. The stresses involved in migration include family breakup, the need to adjust to living in large urban areas, and social inequalities in the new country.

Schizophrenia, schizophreniform disorder, and schizoaffective disorder

Psychosis in schizophrenia and perhaps schizophreniform disorder appears to be related to abnormalities in the structure and chemistry of the **brain**, and appears to have strong genetic links, but its course and severity can be altered by social factors such as **stress** or a lack of support within the family. The cause of schizoaffective disorder is less clear cut, but biological factors are also suspected.

Delusional disorder

The exact cause of delusional disorder has not been conclusively determined, but potential causes include heredity, neurological abnormalities, and changes in brain chemistry. Some studies have indicated that delusions are generated by abnormalities in the limbic system, the portion of the brain on the inner edge of the cerebral cortex that is believed to regulate emotions. Delusional disorder is also more likely to develop in persons who are isolated from others in their society by language difficulties and/or cultural differences.

Brief psychotic disorder

Trauma and stress can cause a short-term psychosis (less than a month's duration) known as brief psychotic disorder. Major life-changing events such as the death of a family member or a natural disaster have been known to stimulate brief psychotic disorder in patients with no prior history of mental illness.

Psychotic disorder due to a general medical condition

Psychosis may also be triggered by an organic cause, termed a psychotic disorder due to a general medical condition. Organic sources of psychosis include neurological conditions (for example, epilepsy and cerebrovascular disease), metabolic conditions (for example, porphyria), endocrine conditions (for example, hyper- or hypothyroidism), renal failure, electrolyte imbalance, or autoimmune disorders.

Substance-induced psychotic disorder

Psychosis is also a known side effect of the use, abuse, and withdrawal from certain drugs. So-called recreational drugs, such as hallucinogenics, PCP, **amphetamines**, **cocaine**, marijuana, and alcohol, may cause a psychotic reaction during use or withdrawal. Certain prescription medications such as **steroids**, anticonvulsants, chemotherapeutic agents, and antiparkinsonian medications may also induce psychotic symptoms. Toxic substances such as carbon monoxide have also been reported to cause substance-induced psychotic disorder.

Shared psychotic disorder

Shared psychotic disorder, also known as *folie à deux* or psychosis by association, is a relatively rare delusional disorder involving two (or more) people with close emotional ties. In the West, shared psychosis most commonly develops between two sisters or between husband and wife, while in Japan the most common form involves a parent and a son or daughter. Shared psychosis occasionally involves an entire nuclear family.

Psychosis is characterized by the following symptoms:

- Delusions. Those delusions that occur in schizophrenia and its related forms are typically bizarre (i.e., they could not occur in real life). Delusions occurring in delusional disorder are more plausible, but still patently untrue. In some cases, delusions may be accompanied by feelings of paranoia.
- Hallucinations. Psychotic patients see, hear, smell, taste, or feel things that aren't there. Schizophrenic hallucinations are typically auditory or, less commonly, visual; but psychotic hallucinations can involve any of the five senses.
- Disorganized speech. Psychotic patients, especially those with schizophrenia, often ramble on in incoherent, nonsensical speech patterns.
- Disorganized or catatonic behavior. The catatonic patient reacts inappropriately to his/her environment by either remaining rigid and immobile or by engaging in excessive motor activity. Disorganized behavior is behavior or activity that is inappropriate for the situation, or unpredictable.

Diagnosis

Patients with psychotic symptoms should undergo a thorough physical examination and history to rule out such possible organic causes as **seizures**, **delirium**, or alcohol withdrawal, and such other psychiatric conditions as dissociation or panic attacks. If a psychiatric cause such as schizophrenia is suspected, a mental health professional will typically conduct an interview with the patient and administer one of several clinical inventories, or tests, to evaluate mental status. This assessment takes place in either an outpatient or hospital setting.

Psychotic symptoms and behaviors are considered psychiatric emergencies, and persons showing signs of psychosis are frequently taken by family, friends, or the police to a hospital emergency room. A person diagnosed as psychotic can be legally hospitalized

KEY TERMS

Brief psychotic disorder—An acute, short-term episode of psychosis lasting no longer than one month. This disorder may occur in response to a stressful event.

Delirium—An acute but temporary disturbance of consciousness marked by confusion, difficulty paying attention, delusions, hallucinations, or restlessness. Delirium may be caused by drug intoxication, high fever related to infection, head trauma, brain tumors, kidney or liver failure, or various metabolic disturbances.

Delusional disorder—Individuals with delusional disorder suffer from long-term, complex delusions that fall into one of six categories: persecutory, grandiose, jealous, erotomanic, somatic, or mixed.

Delusions—An unshakable belief in something untrue that cannot be explained by religious or cultural factors. These irrational beliefs defy normal reasoning and remain firm even when overwhelming proof is presented to refute them.

Hallucinations—False or distorted sensory experiences that appear to be real perceptions to the person experiencing them.

Paranoia—An unfounded or exaggerated distrust of others, sometimes reaching delusional proportions.

Porphyria—A disease of the metabolism characterized by skin lesions, urine problems, neurologic disorders, and/or abdominal pain.

Schizoaffective disorder—Schizophrenic symptoms occurring concurrently with a major depressive or manic episode.

Schizophrenia—A debilitating mental illness characterized by delusions, hallucinations, disorganized speech and behavior, and inappropriate or flattened affect (a lack of emotions) that seriously hampers the afflicted individual's social and occupational functioning. Approximately 2 million Americans suffer from schizophrenia.

Schizophreniform disorder—A short-term variation of schizophrenia that has a total duration of one to six months.

Shared psychotic disorder—Also known as *folie à deux,* shared psychotic disorder is an uncommon disorder in which the same delusion is shared by two or more individuals.

Tardive dyskinesia—Involuntary movements of the face and/or body that are a side effect of the long-term use of some older antipsychotic (neuroleptic) drugs. Tardive dyskinesia affects 15%-20% of patients on long-term neuroleptic treatment.

against his or her will, particularly if he or she is violent, threatening to commit **suicide**, or threatening to harm another person. A psychotic person may also be hospitalized if he or she has become malnourished or ill as a result of failure to feed, dress appropriately for the climate, or otherwise take care of him- or herself.

Treatment

Psychosis that is symptomatic of schizophrenia or another psychiatric disorder should be treated by a **psychologist** and/or **psychiatrist**. An appropriate course of medication and/or psychosocial therapy is employed to treat the underlying primary disorder. If the patient is considered to be at risk for harming himself or others, inpatient treatment is usually recommended.

Treatment of shared psychotic disorder involves separating the affected persons from one another as well as using antipsychotic medications and **psychotherapy**.

Antipsychotic medication such as **thioridazine** (Mellaril), **haloperidol** (Haldol), **chlorpromazine** (Thorazine), **clozapine** (Clozaril), sertindole (Serlect), **olanzapine** (Zyprexa), or **risperidone** (Risperdal) is usually prescribed to bring psychotic symptoms under control and into remission. Possible side effects of antipsychotics include dry mouth, drowsiness, muscle stiffness, and **tardive dyskinesia** (involuntary movements of the body). Agranulocytosis, a potentially serious but reversible health condition in which the white blood cells that fight infection in the body are destroyed, is a possible side effect of clozapine. Patients treated with this drug should undergo weekly blood tests to monitor white blood cell counts for the first six months, then every two weeks thereafter.

After an acute psychotic episode has subsided, antipsychotic drug maintenance treatment is typically employed and psychosocial therapy and living and vocational skills training may be attempted.

Prognosis

Prognosis for brief psychotic disorder is quite good; for schizophrenia, less so. Generally, the longer and more severe a psychotic episode, the poorer the prognosis is for the patient. Early **diagnosis** and treatment are critical to improving outcomes for the patient across all psychotic disorders.

Approximately 10% of America's permanently disabled population is comprised of schizophrenic individuals. The mortality rate of schizophrenic individuals is also high—approximately 10% of schizophrenics commit suicide, and 20% attempt it. However, early diagnosis and long-term follow up care can improve the outlook for these patients considerably. Roughly 60% of patients with schizophrenia will show substantial improvement with appropriate treatment.

Resources

BOOKS

Capps, Donald. *Understanding Psychosis: Issues and Challenges for Sufferers, Families, and Friends*. Lanham, MD: Rowman & Littlefield, 2010.

Porter, Robert S., and Justin L. Kaplan, eds. *The Merck Manual of Diagnosis and Therapy*. 19th ed. Whitehouse Station, NJ: Merck Research Laboratories, 2011.

PERIODICALS

Addington, A. M., et al. "Polymorphisms in the 13q33.2 Gene G72/G30 Are Associated with Childhood-Onset Schizophrenia and Psychosis Not Otherwise Specified." *Biological Psychiatry* 55, no. 10 (May 15, 2004): 976–980.

Hutchinson, G., and C. Haasen. "Migration and Schizophrenia: The Challenges for European Psychiatry and Implications for the Future." *Social Psychiatry and Psychiatric Epidemiology* 39, no. 5 (May 2004): 350–357.

Sim, M.G., E. Khong, and G. Hulse. "Cannabis and Psychosis." *Australian Family Physician* 33, no. 4 (April 2004): 229–232.

Tolmac, J., and M. Hodes. "Ethnic Variation among Adolescent Psychiatric In-Patients with Psychotic Disorders." *British Journal of Psychiatry* 184 (May 2004): 428–431.

Verdoux, H., and M. Tournier. "Cannabis Use and Risk of Psychosis: An Etiological Link?" *Epidemiologia e psichiatria sociale* 13, no. 2 (April–June 2004): 113–119.

Williams, N. M., and M. J. Owen. "Genetic Abnormalities of Chromosome 22 and the Development of Psychosis." *Current Psychiatry Reports* 6, no. 3 (June 2004): 176–182.

ORGANIZATIONS

American Psychiatric Association, 1000 Wilson Blvd., Suite 1825, Arlington, VA, 22209-3901, (703) 907-7300, apa@psych.org, http://www.psych.org.

American Psychological Association, 750 1st Street NE, Washington, DC, 20002-4242, (202) 336-5500; TDD/TTY: (202) 336-6123, (800) 374-2721, http://www.apa.org.

National Alliance on Mental Illness, 3803 North Fairfax Drive, Suite 100, Arlington, VA, 22203, (703) 524-7600, Fax: (703) 524-9094, http://www.nami.org.

National Institute of Mental Health, 6001 Executive Blvd., Room 8184, MSC 9663, Bethesda, MD, 20892-9663, (301) 433-4513; TTY: (301) 443-8431, (866) 615-6464; TTY: (866) 415-8051, Fax: (301) 443-4279, nimhinfo@nih.gov, http://www.nimh.nih.gov.

Paula Anne Ford-Martin
Rebecca Frey, PhD

Psychosurgery

Definition

Psychosurgery is the treatment of a psychiatric disorder using surgical techniques to destroy **brain** tissue and is now rarely used.

Purpose

Psychosurgery is considered a last-resort treatment for extreme and debilitating psychiatric disorders.

Description

Early psychosurgery—historical perspective

Brain surgery, a medical practice requiring extraordinary levels of skill and care, may be one of the oldest of all medical procedures. This surprising observation is supported by physical evidence dating back 40,000 years to Neolithic times. Archaeologists have found numerous human skulls showing signs of a procedure called

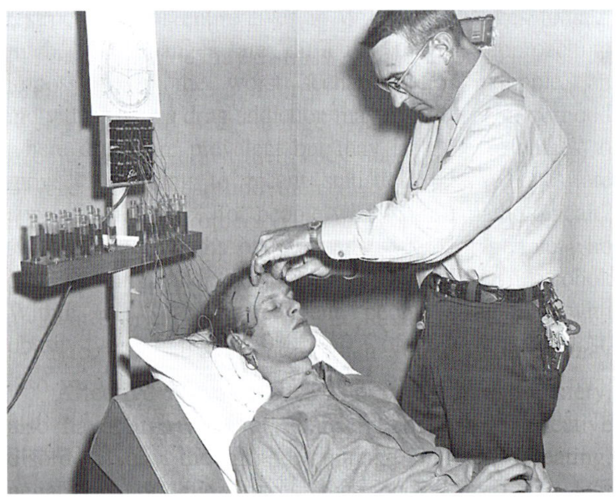

Prisoner at Vacaville Penitentiary in California, 1961, being prepared for a lobotomy. At that time, many psychiatrists believed that criminal behavior was lodged in certain parts of the brain, and lobotomies were frequently practiced on prisoners. *(© Ted Streshinsky/Corbis)*

trepanation or trepanning—an operation in which a hole is cut through the bone that covers the brain (skull) in order to access the brain. A key feature of the wounds found in these ancient skulls is the smoothness and shininess around the edges of the holes. This is a clear sign of new bone growth and evidence that the person whose skull was opened not only survived the operation but lived months or even years afterward while the bone regrew.

Opening a person's skull is a serious procedure, even with today's advanced surgical techniques. The prospect of undergoing the operation in the late Stone Age may appear to us to imply certain death. However, the survival rate of the operation was quite high. Close examination of archeological findings suggests that 75% of those who underwent the procedure lived long enough for new bone to grow around the opening. That number is actually higher than the survival rate for brain surgery during the nineteenth century, when Stone Age trepanned skulls were first identified. Brain surgery during the mid-1860s frequently resulted in infections that killed up to 75% of patients.

Trepanned skulls have been found all over the world, including sites in Peru, China, India, France, and parts of the Middle East and Africa. While trepanning is an effective surgical technique for relieving pressure on the brain caused by bleeding, most archaeologists suspect the operation was carried out in the Stone Age to achieve a different goal. Trepanning, they suspect, was performed to release evil spirits or demons, which the shamans or witch doctors of the time believed produced symptoms of what we know as mental disorders and, perhaps, diseases of the brain. The instruments used in trepanning were likely to have been made of obsidian, a very hard, glass-like, volcanic rock that can hold a very sharp cutting edge. There is also evidence that the end of a wooden stick, hardened by fire and turned back-and-forth rapidly while pressed against the skull may have served as a primitive, but effective, surgical drill.

Neuroscientist and author Elliot Valenstein believes that trepanning did not amount to intentional brain surgery. He quotes from the Latin text by the twelfth-century surgeon Roger of Salerno, who wrote: "For mania and melancholy, the skin of the top of the head should be incised in a cruciate fashion and the skull perforated to allow matter to escape."

A curious example of what might be called pseudo-psychosurgery occurred during the Middle Ages. Some unscrupulous individuals wandered across Europe convincing gullible people that mental disorders were caused by a "stone of madness." To fool others, they faked operating on the brains of mentally ill individuals and, using sleight-of-hand, appeared to produce a real stone from the victim's head, thus "proving" their claim and effecting a "cure." No doubt, these frauds quickly moved on to other towns before their patients showed signs of continuing psychiatric symptoms.

The impetus for developing a radical treatment

Unfortunately, effective treatments for mental illnesses remained unavailable until the second half of the twentieth century. Before then, psychiatric "care" consisted mostly of imprisonment, neglect, restraint, and/or punishment. During the eighteenth century, more humane conditions of confinement were introduced, but effective treatments remained unavailable. Physicians were desperate for treatments that might make it easier to control violent and deranged patients.

By the end of the nineteenth century, researchers became aware of the role played by the frontal cortex—a part of the brain located behind the forehead—in behavior control. They discovered from the results of animal experiments and by observing humans who suffered damage to this part of the brain that the frontal lobes affect emotions and behavior. This bit of knowledge, combined with the development of effective anesthesia, led to the first modern instances of psychosurgery during the 1890s. A Swiss surgeon named Gottlieb Burkhardt deliberately damaged the frontal lobes of six psychiatric patients in hopes of relieving psychiatric symptoms; at least one of his subjects died and the experimental surgery was discontinued amid criticism from other physicians.

Psychosurgery in the twentieth century

PREFRONTAL LEUCOTOMY. In 1900, an Estonian surgeon, Lodivicus Puusepp, picked up where Burkhardt left off. He cut nerve tracks leading from the frontal lobes to other parts of the brain in psychiatric patients, with unimpressive results. A decade later, he injected tissue-destroying chemicals into the frontal lobes of mentally ill patients through holes drilled over the frontal lobes. Although the procedure accomplished little or nothing in the way of therapy, Puusepp remained optimistic about the ability of this procedure to improve the condition of psychiatric patients. Interest in the frontal lobes as a target for treating mental disorders continued on a small scale until the heyday of psychosurgery began in the 1930s.

In 1935, researchers in the United States reported that damaging the frontal lobes and a nearby region of the brain called the prefrontal cortex could pacify a previously aggressive chimpanzee. A Portuguese **psychiatrist**, Antonio Egas Moniz, learned of these results and recruited neurosurgeon Almeida Lima to operate on some humans suffering from severe psychoses. Moniz's aim was to disconnect nerve pathways running from the frontal lobes to a part of the brain called the thalamus, which is located closer to the center of the brain. By cutting these connections, Moniz hypothesized that he could disconnect a neural circuit that ran from the frontal cortex to the thalamus and then to other parts of the brain's surface. He hoped that interrupting this pathway would disrupt the repetitive thoughts that Moniz believed were responsible for psychotic symptoms.

Despite a lack of supportive evidence behind Moniz's theory, it was both accepted and performed by others in his field, likely because psychiatrists were so desperate for a treatment for severe cases of mental illness that they allowed themselves to support the use of a procedure that was unproven and increasingly subject to abuse.

Moniz and Lima called their procedure leucotomy. It involved trepanning the skull, one hole on each side of the head; inserting a wire knife; and cutting the targeted nerve fibers. Results were mixed enough for Moniz to recommend that the procedure be reserved only for the most seriously mentally ill patients for whom no other course of care or treatment worked. Nevertheless, after 1936, use of the technique spread rapidly, with equally unimpressive results overall. With little evidence of effectiveness and facing opposition from many psychiatrists, particularly psychotherapists, the technique would probably have been abandoned were it not for a pair of American physicians who revived the questionable procedure.

THE PREFRONTAL LOBOTOMY. American neurologist Walter Freeman and neurosurgeon James Watts began operating on patients in 1936 and soon began aggressively promoting its effectiveness. Eventually, they overcame doubts expressed by their colleagues who somewhat reluctantly accepted the procedure now referred to as prefrontal lobotomy. In 1946, Freeman simplified Moniz's leucotomy procedure, reducing it to a less complicated, less messy, and less time-consuming operation known as the "ice-pick lobotomy." This allowed Freeman to literally line up patients and, under local anesthesia, tap an ice pick through the thin bone on the roof of their eye sockets. With the ice pick in the brain, Freeman would sweep it back and forth to cut the frontal lobe's connections to the rest of the brain. This in-and-out procedure required no **hospitalization** but many physicians viewed it with alarm. Watts himself refused to cooperate with Freeman after this technique was developed.

Still, in the 1940s, U.S. physicians performed an estimated 20,000 lobotomies. It was equally popular in other countries, where more than 50,000 operations were conducted during the same period. Moniz's warning was forgotten. The procedure was not reserved for the most hopeless cases but instead applied to "difficult" patients, becoming a way to control behavior rather than to relieve symptoms of mental disorder. The abuse often bordered on the criminal. Despite the ethical considerations, Moniz received the 1949 Nobel Prize for Medicine and Physiology for pioneering the procedure.

Critics of the operation began to convince others that there was no scientific proof that lobotomies helped mentally ill patients. It could certainly calm violent patients, but it did so at a terrible cost. As one nurse who recently treated an aged patient who had been lobotomized years before said, "You look in her eyes and you see there is no one there." Victims of the procedure lacked emotions, ambition, social skills, and the ability to plan. The operation was used to control the mentally ill and others, such as uncontrollable children and political dissidents, whose behavior did not conform to society's standards. Arguments against the procedure were powerful: it permanently and severely damaged the brain and often produced unreactive, lifeless individuals whose personalities were forever destroyed. With the introduction of psychotherapeutic drugs—especially **chlorpromazine** (Thorazine)—in the mid-1950s, lobotomies fell out of fashion.

Deep brain stimulation

A surgical procedure called deep brain stimulation (DBS) is currently being used to treat neurological symptoms of Parkinson's disease. DBS is utilized when patients cannot be adequately controlled with medication, and can help treat the neurological symptoms of

KEY TERMS

Computed tomography—An imaging technique in which cross-sectional x rays of the body are compiled to create a three-dimensional image of the body's internal structures; also referred to as CT or CAT scan.

Magnetic resonance imaging (MRI)—An imaging technique that uses a large circular magnet and radio waves to generate signals from atoms in the body. These signals are used to construct images of internal structures.

Psychiatrist—A medical doctor who has completed specialized training in the diagnosis and treatment of mental illness. Psychiatrists can diagnose mental illnesses, provide mental health counseling, and prescribe medications.

Trepanation—An operation in which a hole is cut through the bone that covers the brain (skull) in order to access the brain.

Parkinson's such as tremors, slowed movements, rigidity, and unsteady gait.

DBS involves the surgical implantation of an electrode, an extension wire, and a device called a neurostimulator. The electrode is implanted into the brain through a small opening in the skull, and the extension wire is connected between the electrode to the neurostimulator (a battery operated device similar to a pacemaker), which is implanted under the skin in the collarbone region. Surgeons use **magnetic resonance imaging** (MRI) or **computed tomography** (CT) scans before the procedure to identify the area of the brain that is causing the neurological symptoms. After the device is in place, electrical impulses are sent from the neurostimulator unit and wire system to the brain, where impulses block electrical signals causing the Parkinson's neurological symptoms.

Deep brain stimulation serves to block nerve impulses, but it does not destroy nerve cells or destroy brain tissue, giving it the advantage of being easily programmed or adjusted to the degree of symptoms or being reversed in use altogether. Many patients with Parkinson's disease find they can take fewer medications (reducing the number of medication side effects) when the medications are used in conjunction with DBS. The U.S. Food and Drug Administration (FDA) approved DBS as a treatment for Parkinson's disease in 2002, and it is also being studied for use in treating symptoms of **depression**, obsessive compulsive disorder (OCD), and **Tourette syndrome**. To find out more about medical research studies and these **clinical trials**, visit the U.S. National Institutes of Health website on clinical trials: http://clinicaltrials.gov.

Modern psychosurgery

No one advocates the use of classical lobotomies today as a treatment for mental disorders. Previously, a small minority of neurologists advocated the use of very precise surgical techniques to produce small lesions in defined areas of the brain to treat rare cases of severe mental illness, such as life-threatening depression or incapacitating anxiety or obsessions, but there is little need for such procedures today. Antipsychotic and antidepressant medications are the preferred options for treating mental disorders. Mainstream medicine now classifies psychosurgery as an experimental procedure, and many rules exist to protect patients who might be subjected to it. The majority of mental health professionals believe that psychosurgery is either never justified or should only be considered as a last resort, to be reserved for the most extreme cases of untreatable mental disease when all other therapies have failed and the potential benefits outweigh the risks.

Resources

BOOKS

American Psychiatric Association. *Diagnostic and Statistical Manual of Mental Disorders*. 4th ed., text rev. Washington, DC: American Psychiatric Association, 2000.

American Psychological Association. *Publication Manual of the American Psychological Association*. 6th ed. Washington, DC: American Psychological Association, 2009.

Dowbiggin, Ian. *The Quest for Mental Health: A Tale of Science, Medicine, Scandal, Sorrow, and Mass Society*. New York: Cambridge University Press, 2011.

Kapur, Narinder, ed. *The Paradoxical Brain*. New York: Cambridge University Press, 2011.

Levine, Brian, and Fergus I. M. Craik, eds. *Mind and the Frontal Lobes: Cognition, Behavior, and Brain Imaging*. New York: Oxford University Press, 2011.

Valenstein, Elliot S. *Great and Desperate Cures, The Rise and Decline of Psychosurgery and Other Radical Treatments for Mental Illness*. New York: Basic Books, 1986.

ORGANIZATIONS

American Psychiatric Association, 1000 Wilson Blvd., Ste. 1825, Arlington, VA, 22209-3901, (703) 907-7300, apa@psych.org, http://www.psych.org.

American Psychological Association, 750 1st St. NE, Washington, DC, 20002-4242, (202) 336-5500; TDD/TTY: (202) 336-6123, (800) 374-2721, http://www.apa.org.

Mental Health America, 2000 N. Beauregard St., 6th Fl., Alexandria, VA, 22311, (703) 684-7722, (800) 969-6642, Fax: (703) 684-5968, http://www1.nmha.org.

National Alliance on Mental Illness, 3803 N Fairfax Dr., Ste. 100, Arlington, VA, 22203, (703) 524-7600, http://www.nami.org.

National Institute of Mental Health, 6001 Executive Blvd., Rm. 8184, MSC 9663, Bethesda, MD, 20892-9663, (301) 443-4513; TTY: (301) 443-8431, Fax: (301) 443-4279, (866) 615-6464; TTY: (866) 415-8051, nimhinfo@nih.gov, http://www.nimh.nih.gov.

U.S. National Institutes of Health, 9000 Rockville Pike, Bethesda, MD, 20892, (301) 496-4000; TTY: (301) 402-9612, http://www.nih.gov.

Dean A. Haycock, Ph.D.
Laura Jean Cataldo, RN, Ed.D.

Psychotherapy

Definition

Psychotherapy is the treatment of mental or emotional disorders and adjustment problems through the use of psychological techniques rather than through

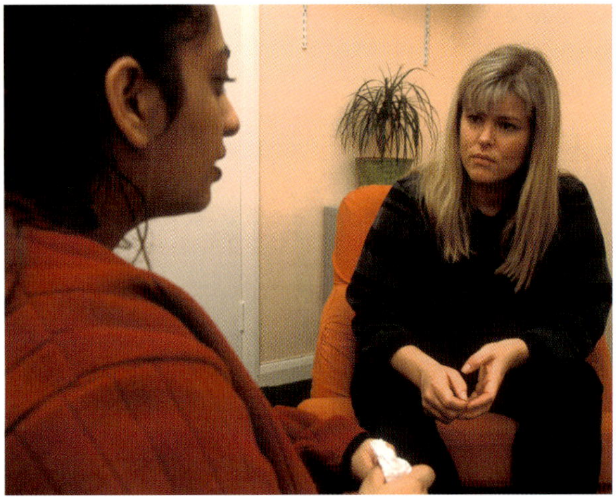

A therapist (on the right) in a counselling session with a patient. *(© Photofusion Picture Library/Alamy)*

physical or biological means. Many different approaches to psychotherapy exist. Each approach applies to a specific situation for individuals. Psychotherapy is often commonly called counseling, therapy, or **talk therapy**.

Purpose

Psychotherapy is used to treat mental health issues and problems that occur in daily life. These issues and problems can include mood disorders (including **depression**), **schizophrenia**, addictions (e.g., alcohol, gambling, sex, drug), **anxiety disorders** (e.g., phobias, panic attacks, **stress**), eating disorders (e.g., bulimia, anorexia), and **personality disorders**.

Outside of diagnosed mental health conditions, psychotherapy can help with conflicts at work, in school, at home, and in other situations, such as dealing with grief after the death of a parent or minimizing aggressive behavior. It is also used to deal with serious health problems, such as cancer, and to learn techniques for coping with painful experiences in the past (such as combat in a war or **child abuse**).

Description

Psychoanalysis, the first modern form of psychotherapy, was called the "talking cure," and the many varieties of therapy practiced today are still characterized by their common dependence on a verbal exchange between the counselor or therapist and the person seeking help. The therapeutic interaction is characterized by mutual trust, with the goal of helping individuals change destructive or unhealthy behaviors, thoughts, and emotions. It is common for experienced therapists to combine several different approaches or techniques. Therapy is terminated when the treatment goals have been met or if the client and/or therapist conclude that it is not working. It can be effective to phase out treatment by gradually reducing the frequency of therapy sessions. Even after regular therapy has ended, the client may return for periodic follow-up and reassessment sessions.

Psychodynamic approach

Freudian psychoanalysis places emphasis on uncovering unconscious motivations and breaking down defenses. Therapy sessions may be scheduled once or even twice a week for a year or more. This type of therapy is appropriate when internal conflicts contribute significantly to a person's problems.

Behavioral techniques

In contrast to the psychodynamic approach, behavior-oriented therapy is geared toward helping people see their problems as learned behaviors that can be modified, without looking for unconscious motivations or hidden meanings. According to the theory behind this approach, once behavior is changed, feelings will change as well. Probably the best-known type of behavioral therapy is **behavior modification**, which focuses on eliminating undesirable habits by providing positive **reinforcement** for the more desirable behaviors.

Another behavioral technique is **systematic desensitization**, in which people are deliberately and gradually exposed to a feared object or experience to help them overcome their fears. A person who is afraid of dogs may first be told to visualize a dog, then be given a stuffed toy dog, then be exposed to a real dog seen at a distance, and eventually be forced to interact with a dog at close range. Relaxation training is another popular form of behavior therapy and is used in systematic desensitization. Through techniques such as deep breathing, visualization, and progressive muscle relaxation, clients learn to control fear and anxiety.

Cognitive methods

Some behavior-oriented therapy methods are used to alter not only overt behavior, but also the thought patterns that drive it. This type of treatment is known as **cognitive-behavioral therapy** (or just cognitive therapy). Its goal is to help people break out of distorted, harmful patterns of thinking and replace them with healthier ones. Common examples of negative thought patterns include: magnifying or minimizing the extent of a problem; "all or nothing" thinking (i.e., a person regards himself or herself as either perfect or worthless); overgeneralization (arriving at broad conclusions based

ALFRED ADLER (1870–1937)

Austrian psychiatrist Alfred Adler founded the school of individual psychology, a comprehensive "science of living." His system emphasizes the uniqueness of the individual and his or her relationships with society. In 1902, Austrian neurologist Sigmund Freud (1856–1939) invited Adler to join a small discussion group, which later became the illustrious Vienna Psychoanalytic Society. Adler was an active member but did not consider himself a pupil or disciple of Freud. He could not agree with Freud's basic assumption that sex was the main determinant of personality, and all that this implied: the dominance of biological factors over the psychological; the push of drives, making for identical, predictable patterns; the part commanding the whole; pleasure-seeking as humans' prime motivation. Whereas Freud tried to explain humans in terms of their similarity to machines and animals, Adler sought to understand and influence humans precisely in terms of what makes them different from machines and animals (concepts and values). This humanistic view characterized all the principles of his theory. Adler's views diverged ever more from those of Freud and, in 1911, he resigned from Freud's circle to formulate and found his own school.

Adler's psychology has been judged the first in a social-science direction. "In addition to regarding an individual's life as a unity, we must also take it together with its context of social relations ... [it] is not capable of doing just as it likes but is constantly confronted with tasks ... inseparably tied up with the logic of man's communal life." Adler specified three main tasks of life: occupation, association with others, and love and marriage. He also referred to them as "social ties," for they all require cooperation for their solution. Humankind's very uniqueness is influenced by relations to others: "The style of the child's life cannot be understood without reference to the persons who look after him."

The therapist's function, according to Adler, is not to treat "mental disease" but to divine the error in the patient's way of life and lead him or her to greater maturity. To this end, Adler introduced a number of diagnostic approaches. Among these, his theory of dreams, the meaning of early childhood recollections, and the role of birth order in the family have become widely known and adopted. The understanding of the patient achieved in this way is not one of depth but of context in the larger whole of his or her total transactions. This is the basis for changing the patient's picture of himself or herself and the world. In addition to this reorganization, Adler wished the patient to appreciate his or her own power of self-determination and have the courage to exercise it. To encourage the patient, the therapist must express a disinterested concern that evokes and fosters feelings of trust and fellowship.

on one incident, for example); and personalization (continually seeing oneself as the cause or focus of events).

In cognitive-behavioral therapy, a therapist may talk to the client, pointing out illogical thought patterns, or may use a variety of techniques, such as thought substitution, in which a frightening or otherwise negative thought is driven out by substituting a pleasant thought in its place. Clients may also be taught to use positive self-talk, a repetition of positive affirmations. Cognitive therapy usually takes a longer amount of time than behavior therapy, as it treats more serious problems.

Couples therapy

Couples therapy focuses on the relationship between two people, typically people who have a romantic or sexual connection. The aim of the therapy is to concentrate on the problems of the relationship and make each partner feel that they have an equal role. The therapy can be administered by either a male or female therapist, but many couples feel that having both a male and female therapist in the session is beneficial, though this practice is not typical.

Family and group therapy

Family therapy has proven effective in treating a number of emotional and adjustment problems. While the client's immediate complaint is the initial focus of attention, the ultimate goal of family therapy is to improve the interaction between all family members and enhance communication and coping skills on a long-term basis (although therapy itself need not cover an extended time period). **Group therapy**, which is often combined with individual therapy, offers the support and companionship of other people experiencing the same or similar problems and issues.

KEY TERMS

Anorexia nervosa—An eating disorder highlighted by a person's denial of a healthy body weight, distortion of their outward appearance, and steadfast refusal to eat much food for a fear that they may gain weight.

Attention deficit hyperactivity disorder (ADHD)—A condition found mostly in children, with primary symptoms of an inability to concentrate, inappropriate behaviors, and impulsiveness.

Cognitive behavioral techniques—A type of therapy used to solve problems concerning dysfunctional behaviors (responses), emotions (feelings), and cognitions (abilities to gather knowledge) through a proven systematic set of procedures.

Cognitive therapy—A type of psychiatric treatment involving the treatment of anxiety and/or depression, which encourages patients to confront their problems in order to improve their behavior.

Depression—A psychiatric disorder involving feelings of hopelessness and symptoms of fatigue, sleeplessness, suicidal tendencies, and poor concentration.

Eating disorders—A number of medical conditions characterized by abnormal eating habits that can involve either the lack, or the excessive intake, of food, which results in physical and/or emotional stress. Two types of eating disorders include anorexia nervosa and bulimia nervosa.

Psychodynamic psychotherapy—A method of verbal communication used to help a person find relief from emotional pain.

Schizophrenia—A mental disorder involving degraded thinking and emotions.

Stress—A physical and psychological response that results from being exposed to a demand or pressure.

Preparation

Preparation for psychotherapy should include discussing the problem first with a family doctor or other medical professional. They can help to provide insight into the problem and make recommendations for further treatment. They also can provide information on which type of psychotherapists to use, based on education, background, expertise, and other valid measures.

Aftercare

After psychotherapy sessions are formally ended, the patient may return to the therapist for periodic check-ups and to make sure a **relapse** is not occurring.

Tests

There are several reasons for performing psychological tests after an individual completes psychotherapy, including court requests, rehabilitation, and learning or emotional problems. For instance, a judge may request a person be tested for use within a court case, such as in custody or accident cases. In addition, school officials may request such a test for a child suspected of having a learning or behavioral problem, such as **attention deficit hyperactivity disorder (ADHD)**.

Risks

Psychotherapists use various techniques within psychotherapy to increase self-awareness, improve behavior and cognition, and develop insights within their patients. Individual, couples, group, and family sessions may be given. Various personal and interpersonal problems are treated during these times. Professional psychotherapists—such as clinical psychologists, mental health counselors, **social workers**, family therapists, and many others—are trained, certified, and licensed to perform such therapies, though abilities vary among individual professionals, as they do in any field.

In addition, such professionals may have certifications and licenses in one or more areas of expertise. For instance, licensed professional counselors (LPCs) may have special certifications in mental health, rehabilitation, and school counseling. Specific approaches and methods, along with specific psychotherapists, may or may not be conducive to all individuals. Consequently, the desired results may not be fulfilled in all cases.

It is important to note that any professional can adopt the title of psychotherapist, even if he or she isn't licensed. When seeking therapy, it is best to inquire as to the practitioner's credentials to assure that they are licensed to conduct therapy.

Although such risks are present in psychotherapy, they are usually minor compared with the problem at the central focus of the therapy. During such therapy, these problems will be identified, so serious and/or painful feelings will often cause discomfort, anxiety, or stress. In addition, the therapist may use exposure therapy, which confronts the patient with their problem and may cause additional stress. For instance, if an individual has a fear of confined spaces, part of the therapy might include riding an elevator with the therapist and, eventually,

QUESTIONS TO ASK YOUR DOCTOR

- How can psychotherapy help me?
- What type of specialist do you recommend I use for psychotherapy?
- Will my health insurance pay for psychotherapy?
- How will I know when psychotherapy sessions are no longer needed?
- Will psychotherapy cure my condition?
- Will I need additional sessions in the future once I complete psychotherapy?

alone. In the end, the successful conclusion of therapy often outweighs any risks.

Results

Results may vary in psychotherapy due to wide approach to the treatment of mental or emotional disorders and adjustment. However, it can be successful with the right psychotherapist and a positive attitude from the patient. Before attending the first session, make goals you wish to attain so they can be discussed with the therapist. In addition, therapy works better when the patient attends all appointments made by the therapist. When attending sessions, the more effort and time expended by the patient, the more likely successful results will be attained. In any case, therapy is a good step for identifying and resolving problems in order to live a healthier and happier life.

Resources

BOOKS

Corey, Gerald. *Theory and Practice of Counseling and Psychotherapy,* 7th ed. Belmont, CA: Thomson/Brooks Cole, 2005.

Corsini, Raymond J., and Danny Wedding. *Current Psychotherapies.* Belmont, CA: Wadsworth, 2007.

Seligman, Linda. *Theories of Counseling and Psychotherapy: Systems, Strategies, and Skills,* 2nd ed. Upper Saddle River, NJ: Prentice Hall, 2005.

Sharf, Richard S. *Theories of Psychotherapy & Counseling: Concepts and Cases.* Belmont, CA: Wadsworth, 2007.

PERIODICALS

Anderson, Rebecca A., and Clare S. Rees. "Group Versus Individual Cognitive-Behavioural Treatment for Obsessive-Compulsive Disorder: A Controlled Trial." *Behaviour Research and Therapy* 45, no. 1 (January 2007): 123–37.

Pepper, Robert. "Too Close for Comfort: The Impact of Dual Relationships on Group Therapy and Group Therapy Training." *International Journal of Group Psychotherapy* 57, no. 1 (January 2007): 13–23.

Powles, William E. "Reflections on 'What is a Group?'" *International Journal of Group Psychotherapy* 57, no. 1 (January 2007): 105–113.

Roback, Howard B., and Randall F. Moore. "On the Ethical Group Psychotherapist." *International Journal of Group Psychotherapy* 57, no. 1 (January 2007): 49–59.

WEBSITES

Mayo Clinic staff. "Psychotherapy." MayoClinic.com. http://www.mayoclinic.com/health/psychotherapy/MY00186 (accessed December 31, 2010).

ORGANIZATIONS

American Psychiatric Association, 1000 Wilson Boulevard, Suite 1825, Arlington, VA, 22209-3901, (703) 907-7300, apa@psych.org, http://www.psych.org.

American Psychoanalytic Association, 309 East 49th Street, New York City, NY, 10017, (212) 752-0450, Fax: (212) 593-0571, info@aspa.org, http://www.apsa.org.

American Psychological Association, 750 First Street, N.E., Washington, DC, 20002, (202) 336-5500, (800) 374-2721, http://www.apa.org.

American Psychotherapy Association, 2750 East Sunshine Street, Springfield, MO, 65804, (417) 823-0173, (800) 205-9165, http://www.americanpsychotherapy.com.

Ruth A. Wienclaw, PhD

Psychotherapy integration

Definition

Psychotherapy integration is defined as an approach to **psychotherapy** that includes a variety of attempts to look beyond the confines of single-school approaches to see what can be learned from other perspectives. It is characterized by openness to various ways of integrating diverse theories and techniques. Psychotherapy integration can be differentiated from an eclectic approach in that an eclectic approach is one in which a therapist chooses interventions because they work (the therapist relies solely on supposed efficacy) without looking for a theoretical basis for using the technique. In contrast, psychotherapy integration attends to the relationship between theory and technique.

Purpose

The purpose of psychotherapy integration is to bring together, or integrate, the different schools of psychotherapy so that the personality of an individual is more comprehensively studied. Specifically, it strives to combine the affective, cognitive, behavioral, and physiological systems of a person's personality.

Description

The term "psychotherapy" integration has been used in several different ways. It has been applied to approaches including common factors, assimilative integration, technical eclecticism, and theoretical integration.

Common factors

"Common factors" refers to aspects of psychotherapy that are present in most, if not all, approaches to therapy. These techniques cut across all theoretical lines and appear in all psychotherapeutic activities. Because the techniques are common to all approaches to psychotherapy, the name has been given to this variety of psychotherapy integration. Examples of some common factors include:

- an established therapeutic alliance between the patient and the therapist
- exposure of the patient to prior difficulties, either in imagination or in reality
- a new corrective emotional experience that allows the patient to experience past problems in new and more benign ways
- expectations by both the therapist and the patient that positive change will result from the treatment
- therapist qualities, such as attention, empathy, and positive regard, that are facilitative of change in treatment
- the provision by the therapist, to the patient, of a reason for the problems that are being experienced.

No matter what kind of therapy is practiced, each of these common factors is present. It is difficult to imagine a treatment that does not begin with the establishment of a constructive and positive therapeutic alliance. The therapist and the patient agree to work together, and they both feel committed to a process of change occurring in the patient. Within every approach to treatment, the exposure of the patient to prior difficulties is present. In some instances, the exposure is in vivo (i.e., occurs in real life), and the patient will be asked directly to confront the source of the difficulties. In many cases, the exposure is verbal and in imagination. However, in every case, the patient must express those difficulties in some manner and, by doing so, re-experiences those difficulties through this exposure.

In successful treatment, the exposure usually is followed by a new corrective emotional experience. The "corrective emotional experience" refers to a situation in which an old difficulty is re-experienced in a new and more positive way. As the patient re-experiences the problem in a new way, that problem can be mastered, and the patient can move on to a more successful adjustment.

Having established a therapeutic alliance, and being exposed to the problem in a new and more positive context, both the therapist and the patient always expect positive change to occur. This faith and hope is a common factor that is an integral part of successful therapy. Without this hope and expectation of change, it is unlikely that the therapist can be helpful, and if the patient does not expect to change, it is unlikely that he or she will experience any positive benefit from the treatment. The therapist must possess some essential qualities, such as paying attention to the patient, being empathic with the patient, and making his or her positive regard for the patient clear in the relationship. Finally, the patient must be provided with a credible reason for the problems that he or she is undergoing. This reason is based in the therapist's theory of personality and change. The same patient going to different therapists may be given different reasons for the same problem. As long as the reason is credible, and the patient has a way to understand what had been incomprehensible, that may be sufficient for change to occur.

Assimilative integration

The second major approach to psychotherapy integration is assimilative integration, an approach in which the therapist has a commitment to one theoretical approach but is also willing to use techniques from other therapeutic approaches.

For example, a therapist may try to understand patients in terms of psychodynamic theory, because he or she finds this most helpful in understanding what is happening in the course of the treatment. However, the therapist may also recognize that there are techniques outside psychodynamic theory that work very well, and these may then be used in the treatment plan. The psychodynamic therapist can occasionally use cognitive-behavioral techniques, such as homework, and may occasionally use humanistic approaches, such as a two-chair technique, but always retains a consistent psychodynamic understanding.

The treatment can take place in a way that is beneficial to the patient and is not bound by the restrictions of the therapist's favorite way to intervene. The patient might not be aware that integration is taking place, but he or she does feel that a consistent approach is being maintained. Most patients are not familiar with theory and therefore do not realize that different techniques are generated by different theoretical understandings, and only are concerned with whether the treatment is helpful or not.

Inherent in psychotherapy integration is the conviction that there is no single approach to therapy that is suitable to every patient. Both in single-school approaches and in psychotherapy integration, the treatment must be suitable for the individual patient. In making the treatment suitable for the individual patient, the therapist must understand the patient, and that establishes a place for theory. Assimilative integration is particularly useful in that theory helps in the understanding of the needs of the patient, but then several different approaches to technique can help to design a treatment that fits that particular understanding. The treatment plan then must undergo continuous revision as the understanding of the patient gets fuller and deeper over the course of the treatment.

Technical eclecticism

Technical eclecticism is a variation of assimilative integration and is most common among those practitioners who refer to themselves as eclectic. In technical eclecticism, the same diversity of techniques is displayed as in assimilative integration, but there is no unifying theoretical understanding that underlies the approach. Rather, the therapist relies on previous experience and on knowledge of the theoretical and research literature to choose interventions that are appropriate for the patient.

The obvious similarity between assimilative integration and technical eclecticism is that both rely on a wide variety of therapeutic techniques, focusing on the welfare of the patient rather than on allegiance to any particular school of psychotherapy. The major difference between the two is that assimilative integration is bound by a unifying theoretical understanding, whereas technical eclecticism is free of theory and relies on the experience of the therapist to determine the appropriate interventions.

Theoretical integration

The fourth approach to psychotherapy integration is called "theoretical integration." This is the most difficult level at which to achieve integration because it requires integrating theoretical concepts from different approaches, and these approaches may differ in their fundamental philosophy about human behavior. Whereas assimilative integration begins with a single theory and brings together techniques from different approaches, theoretical integration tries to bring together those theoretical approaches themselves and then to develop what in physics is referred to as a "grand unified theory." Neither psychotherapists nor physicists have been successful to date in producing a grand unified theory. It is difficult to imagine a theory that really can combine an approach that has one philosophical understanding, with another that has a different philosophical understanding. For example, a psychodynamic approach believes that an early difficulty leads to a pattern of behavior that is repetitive, destructive, and nearly impossible to resolve. In contrast, behavior therapy sees problems as much more amenable to change. This difference may represent a basic incompatibility between the two theories. Therefore, theoretical integration would be faced with the task of integrating a theory about the stability of behavior with a theory about the ready changeability of behavior, and unless this obstacle can be overcome, theoretical integration will not be achieved.

Conclusions

The general point in three of these approaches—common factors, assimilative integration, and theoretical integration—is that there is a clear value to the role of theory in psychotherapy integration, whether the theory concerns the way integration works (theoretical integration), the framework that governs the choice of interventions (assimilative integration), or the organizing principle for understanding the common factors that are present in all psychotherapy. Technical eclecticism is not

KEY TERMS

Cognitive behavioral techniques—A type of therapy that is used to solve problems concerning dysfunctional behaviors (responses), emotions (feelings), and cognitions (abilities to gather knowledge) through a proven systematic set of procedures.

Cognitive therapy—A type of psychiatric treatment involving the treatment of anxiety and/or depression, which encourages patients to confront their problems in order to improve their behavior.

Psychoanalysis—A form of therapy based on the understanding that human beings are largely unaware of the mental processes that determine their thoughts, feelings, and behavior, and that psychological suffering can be alleviated by making those processes known to the individual.

Psychodynamic therapy—Sometimes also called "psychodynamic psychotherapy," it is a method of verbal communication that is used to help a person find relief from emotional pain.

QUESTIONS TO ASK YOUR DOCTOR

- How can psychotherapy integration help me?
- Why will it help?
- What type of specialist do you recommend I use for psychotherapy integration?
- Where can I find more information relating to psychotherapy integration, specifically relating to my condition?
- Will a therapist using psychotherapy integration be better for me rather than a therapist using only one approach to psychotherapy?
- Will my health insurance pay for psychotherapy integration?
- How will I know when psychotherapy integration sessions are no longer needed?
- Will psychotherapy integration cure my condition?
- Will I need additional sessions in the future once completing psychotherapy integration?

concerned with theory, but it does view the benefit of the patient to be of more significance than the adherence to any single theory.

Aftercare

As with any approach to psychotherapy, aftercare is usually necessary even with the most successful of the results.

Risks

About half of therapists mix schools of psychotherapy in their practice, while the other half remain purists. Some controversy exists as to which is better: "purist schools" (those that do not mix the various school of psychotherapy) or "psychotherapy integration schools" (those that do).

Results

For the most part, therapists and patients have benefited from the use of psychotherapy integration, as it allows more flexibility in the therapist to treat patients. In psychotherapy integration, the therapist has the ability to use different approaches based on the specific needs of individual patients. As such, the professional can customize therapy to individual needs. Although usually more complex, psychotherapy integration has more potential to be successful. However, its success is strongly based on the experience and expertise of the therapist, one in which long-term training is especially important.

Resources

BOOKS

Corey, Gerald. *Theory and Practice of Counseling and Psychotherapy,* 7th ed. Belmont, CA: Thomson/Brooks Cole, 2005.

Corsini, Raymond J., and Danny Wedding. *Current Psychotherapies.* Belmont, CA: Wadsworth, 2007.

Gold, Jerold R. *Key Concepts in Psychotherapy Integration.* New York City: Springer, 2006.

Norcross, John C., and Marvin R. Goldfried, editors. *Handbook of Psychotherapy Integration.* New York City: Oxford University Press, 2005.

Scaturo, Douglas. *Clinical Dilemmas In Psychotherapy: A Transtheoretical Approach To Psychotherapy Integration.* Washington, DC: American Psychological Association, 2005.

Seligman, Linda. *Theories of Counseling and Psychotherapy: Systems, Strategies, and Skills,* 2nd ed. Upper Saddle River, NJ: Prentice Hall, 2005.

Sharf, Richard S. *Theories of Psychotherapy & Counseling: Concepts and Cases.* Belmont, CA: Wadsworth, 2007.

Stricker, George. *Psychotherapy Integration.* Washington, DC: American Psychological Association, 2010.

Stricker, George, and Jerold R. Gold, editors. *Comprehensive Handbook of Psychotherapy Integration.* New York City: Spring, 2004.

PERIODICALS

Allen, David M. "Use of Between-Session Homework in Systems-Oriented Individual Psychotherapy." *Journal of Psychotherapy Integration* 16, no. 2 (June 2006): 238–53.

Beitman, Bernard D., and Angela M. Soth. "Activation of Self-Observation: A Core Process Among the Psychotherapies." *Journal of Psychotherapy Integration* 16, no. 4 (December 2006): 383–97.

Brodley, Barbara T. "Client-Initiated Homework in Client-Centered Therapy." *Journal of Psychotherapy Integration* 16, no. 2 (June 2006): 140–61.

Melito, Richard. "Integrating Individual and Family Therapies: A Structural-Developmental Approach." *Journal of Psychotherapy Integration* 16, no. 3 (September 2006): 346–81.

Watson, Jeanne C. "Reconciling Different Voices—Developing as an Integrative Scientist Practitioner." *Journal of Psychotherapy Integration* 16, no. 1 (March 2006): 20–35.

WEBSITES

Mayo Clinic staff. "Psychotherapy." MayoClinic.com. http://www.mayoclinic.com/health/psychotherapy/MY00186 (accessed December 31, 2011).

ORGANIZATIONS

American Psychiatric Association, 1000 Wilson Boulevard, Suite 1825, Arlington, VA, 22209-3901, (703) 907-7300, apa@psych.org, http://www.psych.org.

American Psychoanalytic Association, 309 East 49th Street, New York City, NY, 10017, (212) 752-0450, Fax: (212) 593-0571, info@aspa.org, http://www.apsa.org.

American Psychological Association, 750 First Street, N.E., Washington, DC, 20002, (202) 336-5500, (800) 374-2721, http://www.apa.org.

American Psychotherapy Association, 2750 East Sunshine Street, Springfield, MO, 65804, (417) 823-0173, (800) 205-9165, http://www.americanpsychotherapy.com.

Society for the Exploration of Psychotherapy Integration, geostricker@gmail.com, http://sepiweb.org.

George Stricker, PhD
Ruth A. Wienclaw, PhD

Pyromania

Definition

Pyromania is defined as a pattern of deliberate setting of fires for pleasure or satisfaction derived from the relief of tension experienced before the firesetting. The name of the disorder comes from two Greek words that mean "fire" and "loss of reason" or "madness." The clinician's handbook ***Diagnostic and Statistical Manual of Mental Disorders***, also known as the *DSM*, classifies pyromania as a disorder of impulse control, meaning that a person diagnosed with pyromania fails to resist the impulsive desire to set fires—as opposed to the organized planning of an arsonist or terrorist.

Demographics

The true incidence of pyromania in the general U.S. population remains unknown, but it is considered a rare disorder. Pyromania is diagnosed more frequently in men than in women, and repeated firesetting appears to be more common in children and adolescents than in adult males. In a 2005 review of 600 Finnish male arsonists, led by Finnish **psychiatrist** Nina Lindberg, less than 2% of the arsonists met the *DSM* criteria for pyromania, with the majority attributing alcohol to their firesetting. However, repeated firesetting at the adolescent level is a growing social and economic problem that poses major risks to the health and safety of other people and the protection of their property. In the United States, fires set by children and adolescents are more likely to result in someone's death than any other type of household disaster. The National Fire Protection Association stated that for 2008, fires set by juveniles caused 70 deaths, 910 injuries, and $279 million in property damage.

Some researchers theorize that children and adolescents attracted to firesetting when they are younger "graduate" in adult life to more serious crimes, including serial rape and murder. A number of serial killers, including David Berkowitz, the "Son of Sam" killer, and David Carpenter, the so-called Trailside Killer of the San Francisco Bay area, turned out to have been firesetters in their adolescence. Berkowitz admitted having started more than two thousand fires in Brooklyn-Queens in the early 1970s.

Another hypothesis regarding pyromania in adults is that it is more likely to emerge in the form of workplace violence. The Americans with Disabilities Act (ADA) typically forbids employers to discriminate against workers with mental or physical disabilities as long as they are qualified to perform their job. However, in 1997, the Equal Employment Opportunities Commission (EEOC) excluded pyromania (along with **kleptomania**, compulsive gambling, disorders of sexual behavior, and the use of illegal drugs) from the list of psychiatric conditions for which employers are expected to make "reasonable accommodation." The EEOC's exclusion of pyromania indicates that workers with this disorder are considered a "direct threat" to other people and property that employers are allowed to screen them out during the hiring process.

Description

Pyromania is classified by the *DSM* as an impulse-control disorder, which are disorders characterized by an inability to resist carrying out an action, despite potentially negative or harmful consequences. Some psychiatrists, however, question this classification based on the connection they find between adolescent firesetting and similar behavior in adults. One team of German researchers remarked, "Repeated firesetting, resulting from being fascinated by fire, etc., may be less a disturbance of impulse control but rather the manifestation of a psychoinfantilism, which, supported by alcohol abuse, extends into older age."

Firesetting in children and adolescents

Although most cases of firesetting in the United States involve children or adolescents rather than adults, the *DSM-IV-TR* criteria for pyromania are difficult to apply to this population. Most younger firesetters are diagnosed as having conduct disorders rather than pyromania; significantly, most of the psychiatric literature dealing with this age group speaks of "firesetting" rather than pyromania.

Some observers have attempted to classify children and adolescents who set fires as either pathological or nonpathological. Children in the former group are motivated primarily by curiosity and the desire to experiment with fire. Most are between 5 and 10 years of age and do not understand the dangers of playing with fire, and few have major psychological problems. Those who are considered to be pathological firesetters are further subdivided into five categories, which are not mutually exclusive:

- Firesetting as a cry for help. Children in this category set fires as a way of calling attention to a psychological problem, such as depression, or to an interpersonal problem, including parental separation and divorce or physical and sexual abuse.
- Delinquent firesetters. Firesetters in this category are most likely to be between the ages of 11 and 15. Their firesetting is part of a larger pattern of aggression that may also include vandalism and hate crimes. They are, however, more likely to damage property with their firesetting than to injure people.
- Severely disturbed firesetters. These youths are often diagnosed as either psychotic or paranoid and appear to be reinforced by the sensory aspects of firesetting. Some set fires as part of suicide attempts.
- Cognitively impaired firesetters. This group includes children whose impulse control is damaged by a neurological or medical condition such as fetal alcohol syndrome.
- Sociocultural firesetters. Children in this group are influenced by antisocial adults in their community and set fires in order to win their approval.

Pyromania in adults

Pyromania in adults has a high rate of comorbidity with other disorders, including **substance abuse** disorders, **obsessive-compulsive disorder** (OCD), **anxiety disorders**, and mood disorders. However, few widespread, rigorously controlled studies have been done on adult patients diagnosed with pyromania.

Causes and symptoms

Causes

Most studies of causation regarding pyromania have focused on children and adolescents who set fires. Early studies in the field used the categories of Freudian **psychoanalysis** to explain this behavior. Freud had hypothesized that firesetting represented a regression to a primitive desire to demonstrate power over nature. In addition, some researchers have tried to explain the fact that pyromania is predominantly a male disorder with reference to Freud's notion that fire has a special symbolic relationship to the male sexual urge. A study done in 1940 attributed firesetting to fears of castration in young males, and speculated that adolescents who set fires do so to gain power over adults. The 1940 study is important also because it introduced the notion of an "ego triad" of firesetting, **enuresis** (bed-wetting), and cruelty to animals as a predictor of violent behavior in adult life. Subsequent studies have found that a combination of firesetting and cruelty to animals is a significant predictor of violent behavior in adult life, but that the third member of the triad (bed-wetting) is not.

The causes of firesetting among children and teenagers are complex and not well understood, but theorized causes can be classified as either individual or environmental. Individual factors that may contribute to firesetting include:

- Antisocial behaviors and attitudes. Some adolescent firesetters have also committed other crimes, including forcible rape, nonviolent sexual offenses, and vandalism of property.
- Sensation seeking. Some youths may attracted to firesetting out of boredom or a lack of other forms of recreation.
- Attention seeking. Firesetting may be seen as a way of provoking reactions from parents and other authorities.
- Lack of social skills. Many youths arrested for firesetting are absent significant friendships.
- Lack of fire-safety skills or knowledge of the dangers associated with firesetting.

There are discrepancies between researchers' understanding of individual factors in firesetting and reports from adolescents themselves. One study of 17 teenaged firesetters, 14 males and 3 females, found 6 different self-reported reasons for firesetting: revenge, crime concealment, peer group pressure, accidental firesetting, **denial** of intention, and fascination with fire. The motivations of revenge and crime concealment would exclude these teenagers from being diagnosed with pyromania based on the *DSM* criteria.

Environmental factors that may contribute to adolescent firesetting include:

- Poor supervision on the part of parents or other adults.
- Early learning experiences of watching adults use fire carelessly or inappropriately.
- Parental neglect or lack of emotional involvement.
- Parental psychopathology. Firesetters are significantly more likely to have been physically or sexually abused than children of similar economic or geographic backgrounds. They are also more likely to have witnessed their parents abusing drugs or acting violently.
- Peer pressure. Having peers who smoke or play with fire is a risk factor for a child's setting fires himself.
- Stressful life events. Some children and adolescents resort to firesetting as a way of coping with personal crises or a lack of family support.

Symptoms

Firesetting among children and adolescents and pyromania in adults may be either chronic or episodic; some persons may set fires frequently as a way of relieving

KEY TERMS

Arson—The deliberate setting of fires for criminal purposes, usually to collect insurance money or to cover up evidence of another crime. It is distinguished from pyromania by its connection with planning and forethought rather than failure of impulse control.

Comorbidity—Association or presence of two or more mental disorders in the same patient. A disorder that is said to have a high degree of comorbidity is likely to occur in patients diagnosed with other disorders that may share or reinforce some of its symptoms.

Delusion—A false belief that is resistant to reason or contrary to actual fact. Common delusions include delusions of persecution, delusions of personal importance (sometimes called delusions of grandeur), or delusions of being controlled by others. Pyromania is excluded as a diagnosis if the patient is setting fires on the basis of a delusion.

Kleptomania—A disorder of impulse control characterized by repeated stealing or shoplifting of items that the person does not need.

Spontaneous remission—Recovery from a disease or disorder that cannot be attributed to medical or psychiatric treatments.

tension, while others apparently do so only during periods of unusual **stress** in their lives. Pyromania in adults has also been associated with symptoms of depressed mood, thoughts of **suicide**, repeated conflicts in interpersonal relationships, and poor ability to cope with stress.

Diagnosis

The *DSM* specifies six criteria that must be met for a patient to be diagnosed with pyromania:

- The patient must have set fires deliberately and purposefully on more than one occasion.
- The patient must have experienced feelings of tension or emotional arousal before setting the fires.
- The patient must indicate that he or she is fascinated with, attracted to, or curious about fire and situations surrounding fire (for example, the equipment associated with fire, the uses of fire, or the aftermath of firesetting).
- The patient must experience relief, pleasure, or satisfaction from setting the fire or from witnessing or participating in the aftermath.
- The patient does not have other motives for setting fires, such as financial motives, ideological convictions (such as terrorist or anarchist political beliefs), anger or revenge, the need to cover up another crime, delusions or hallucinations, or impaired judgment resulting from substance abuse, dementia, an intellectual disability, or traumatic brain damage.
- The firesetting cannot be better accounted for by antisocial personality disorder, a conduct disorder, or a manic episode.

Diagnosis of pyromania is complicated by a number of factors; one important factor is the adequacy of the diagnostic category itself. Some psychiatrists are not convinced that the impulse-control disorders should be identified as a separate group, in that problems with self-control are part of the picture in many psychiatric disorders. **Bulimia nervosa**, **borderline personality disorder**, and **antisocial personality disorder** are all defined in part by low levels of self-control but are not considered impulse-control disorders.

Another complication of diagnosis is the lack of experience on the part of mental health professionals in dealing with firesetting. In many cases they are either unaware that the patient is repeatedly setting fires, or they regard the pattern as part of a cluster of antisocial or dysfunctional behaviors.

Treatment

Children and adolescents

Treatment of children and adolescents involved with repeated firesetting appears to be more effective following a case-management approach rather than a medical model, as many young firesetters come from chaotic households. Treatment should begin with a structured interview with the parents as well as the child, in order to evaluate stresses on the family, patterns of supervision and discipline, and similar factors. The next stage in treatment should be tailored to the individual child and his or her home situation. A variety of treatment approaches, including problem-solving skills, anger management, communication skills, aggression replacement training, and cognitive restructuring, may be necessary to address all the emotional and cognitive issues involved in each case.

Adults

Pyromania in adults is considered difficult to treat because of the lack of insight and cooperation on the part of most patients diagnosed with the disorder. Treatment usually consists of a combination of medication—usually one of the **selective serotonin reuptake inhibitors**

(SSRIs), a class of antidepressant drugs—and long-term insight-oriented **psychotherapy**.

Prognosis

The prognosis for recovery from firesetting among children and adolescents depends on the mix of individual and environmental factors involved. Current understanding indicates that children and adolescents who set fires as a cry for help, or who fall into the cognitively impaired or sociocultural categories, benefit the most from therapy and have fairly positive prognoses. The severely disturbed and delinquent types of firesetters have a more guarded outlook.

The prognosis for adults diagnosed with pyromania is generally poor. There are some cases of spontaneous remission among adults, but the rate of spontaneous recovery is not known.

Prevention

Prevention of pyromania requires a broad-based and flexible approach to treatment of children and adolescents who set fires. In addition to better assessments of young people and their families, fire safety education is an important preventive strategy that is often overlooked.

In addition to preventive measures directed specifically at firesetting, recent research into self-control as a general character trait offers hope that it can be taught and practiced like many other human skills. If programs could be developed to improve people's capacity for self-control, they could potentially prevent a wide range of psychiatric disorders.

Resources

BOOKS

American Psychiatric Association. *Diagnostic and Statistical Manual of Mental Disorders*. 4th ed., text rev. Washington, DC: American Psychiatric Publishing, 2000.

Baumeister, Roy F. "Crossing the Line: How Evil Starts." In *Evil: Inside Human Violence and Cruelty,* by Roy F. Baumeister and Aaron Beck. New York: W. H. Freeman and Company, 2001.

Douglas, John, and Mark Olshaker. *Mindhunter: Inside the FBI's Elite Serial Crime Unit*. Audio ed. New York: Simon and Schuster, 2010.

Graham, George. *The Disordered Mind: An Introduction to Philosophy of Mind and Mental Illness*. New York: Routledge, 2010.

McElroy, Susan, and Lesley M. Arnold. "Impulse-Control Disorders." *Treatments of Psychiatric Disorders,* edited by Glen O. Gabbard. 4th ed. Washington, DC: American Psychiatric Publishing, 2007.

North, Carol, and Sean Yutzy. *Goodwin and Guze's Psychiatric Diagnosis*. New York, NY: Oxford University Press, 2010.

PERIODICALS

Evenden, John. "Impulsivity: A Discussion of Clinical and Experimental Findings." *Journal of Psychopharmacology* 13, no. 2 (March 1999): 180–192.

Everall, Ian Paul, and Ann Leconteur. "Firesetting in an Adolescent Boy with Asperger's Syndrome." *British Journal of Psychiatry* 157 (September 1990): 284–287.

Laubichler W., A. Kuhberger, P. Sedlmeier. "'Pyromania' and Arson. A Psychiatric and Criminologic Data Analysis." [in German] *Nervenarzt* 67 (September 1996): 774–780.

Slavkin, Michael L., and Kenneth Fineman. "What Every Professional Who Works with Adolescents Needs to Know About Firesetters." *Adolescence* 35 (Winter 2000): 759–764.

Strayhorn, Joseph M., Jr. "Self-Control: Theory and Research." *Journal of the American Academy of Child and Adolescent Psychiatry* 41, no. 1 (January 2002): 7–16.

Swaffer, Tracey, and Clive R. Hollin. "Adolescent Firesetting: Why Do They Say They Do It?" *Journal of Adolescence* 18, no. 5 (October 1995): 619–624.

Zugelder, Michael T., Steven D. Maurer, and Paul Champagne. "Dangerous Directives? Liability and the Unstable Worker." *Business Horizons* 42, no. 1 (January 1, 1999): 40–48.

WEBSITES

Juvenile Firesetter Intervention Program. "Juvenile Firesetting Statistics." http://www.stopfiresetting.com/florida/Home/JuvenileFiresettingStatistics/tabid/103/Default.aspx (accessed October 24, 2011).

ORGANIZATIONS

American Academy of Child and Adolescent Psychiatry, 3615 Wisconsin Ave. NW, Washington, DC, 20016-3007, (202) 966-7300, Fax: (202) 966-2891, http://aacap.org.

American Psychiatric Association, 1000 Wilson Blvd., Ste. 1825, Arlington, VA, 22209-3901, (703) 907-7300, apa@psych.org, http://www.psych.org.

American Psychological Association, 750 1st Street NE, Washington, DC, 20002-4242, (202) 336-5500; TDD/TTY: (202) 336-6123, (800) 374-2721, http://www.apa.org.

National Alliance for Research on Schizophrenia and Depression, The Brain and Behavior Research Fund, 60 Cutter Mill Rd., Ste. 404, Great Neck, NY, 11021, (516) 829-0091, Fax: (516) 487-6930, info@bbrfoundation.org, http://www.narsad.com.

National Alliance on Mental Illness, 3803 N Fairfax Drive, Ste. 100, Arlington, VA, 22203, (703) 524-7600, http://www.nami.org.

National Institute of Mental Health, 6001 Executive Blvd., Room 8184, MSC 9663, Bethesda, MD, 20892-9663, (301) 433-4513; TTY: (301) 443-8431, Fax: (301) 443-4279, (866) 615-6464; TTY: (866) 415-8051 nimhinfo@nih.gov, http://www.nimh.nih.gov.

Rebecca J. Frey, PhD
Laura Jean Cataldo, RN, EdD

Q

Quazepam

Definition

Quazepam belongs to a class of drugs called **benzodiazepines**. These drugs ease anxiety and slow the central nervous system. In the United States, quazepam is sold under the brand name Doral.

Purpose

Quazepam is approved by the U.S. Food and Drug Administration (FDA) for the treatment of **insomnia**.

Description

Quazepam is unique in its drug properties in two ways. First, some other types of benzodiazepines have an effect called rebound insomnia. This means that the insomnia becomes worse than the original insomnia when the drug is used for extended periods. Quazepam has a minimal tendency to cause rebound insomnia. Second, quazepam is eliminated from the body slowly. This gives quazepam an advantage over certain other medications in the benzodiazepine class, such as **alprazolam** or halazepam, in that patients do not experience early-morning insomnia, since there is still enough medication to induce sleep in the very early morning hours.

Quazepam's sedating effect lasts only for about four weeks of continuous use. The medication is most effective for an intermediate-term treatment of insomnia (two weeks), rather than for a long duration of treatment of more than four weeks. Hence, long-term treatment for insomnia with quazepam should be avoided.

Quazepam comes in 7.5 mg and 15 mg tablets.

Recommended dosage

Effective doses of quazepam for the treatment of insomnia range from 7.5 mg to 30 mg at bedtime. Most patients start by taking 15 mg at bedtime. Adjustments from this dosage can be made as determined by the individual. In some patients, a dosage as low as 7.5 mg is sufficient to reduce insomnia.

Elderly patients (over age 65) should receive a dosage of 7.5 mg, because it takes longer to eliminate the drug from their bodies. Because quazepam is eliminated by the liver, dosage reduction may be necessary in patients with liver problems.

Precautions

Quazepam has an addictive potential when used for too long. Patients can become dependent on quazepam and may experience withdrawal symptoms when they stop taking the drug. Patients preparing to stop treatment with quazepam should gradually decrease the dose over time.

Patients who have a condition known as sleep apnea should not use quazepam. This condition involves episodes of breathing difficulty and oxygen deficiency that occur throughout the night. Patients who are pregnant or who had allergic reactions to quazepam should not take quazepam.

People who need to remain mentally alert, such as those who are driving or operating dangerous machinery, should wait to take quazepam, since it causes drowsiness. Some patients taking sleep aids, including quazepam, have engaged in various behaviors while asleep, such as driving or eating, with no recollection of the events. The sedative effects of quazepam are intensified when the drug is taken with alcohol. It is best not to drink alcoholic beverages while taking quazepam. Patients with compromised respiratory function (breathing problems), as well as patients with a history of drug or alcohol abuse, should be closely monitored during the short-term treatment with quazepam.

Side effects

The effects of quazepam taken at bedtime may last, or hang over, into the next day. This is the most common

KEY TERMS

Benzodiazepines—A group of central nervous system depressants used to relieve anxiety or to induce sleep.

side effect of quazepam. The symptoms of this condition include drowsiness, daytime sleepiness, slurred speech, and mental sluggishness. This effect is dose-related, and seems to occur most frequently in patients taking 30 mg doses. These effects are experienced less commonly with the 15 mg dose, but this dose may not be effective in eliminating insomnia some patients. Some people experience headaches and dizziness when taking quazepam.

A small number of patients experience dry mouth, weight loss, abnormal taste perception, abdominal pain, nausea, vomiting, and either diarrhea or constipation due to quazepam. These effects occur in about 1% to 10% of people taking the drug.

Side effects that occur in less than 1% of patients include skin problems such as rash or skin inflammation, muscle cramps, rigidity, and blurred vision. Patients who experience an allergic reaction (anaphylaxis) or severe facial swelling (angioedema) should contact their physicians immediately.

Interactions

Cimetidine (Tagamet) and ketoconazole increase the levels of quazepam in the body, potentially causing toxicity or increased side effects. Conversely, the drug theophylline decreases the effectiveness of quazepam. **Valerian**, **kava kava**, and alcohol cause increased central nervous system **depression**, which may increase sedation, drowsiness, and slowed reflexes if used while taking quazepam. Patients taking quazepam should not consume any products containing grapefruit, including grapefruit juice, as they may inhibit the absorption of quazepam, resulting in too much of the drug in the body.

Resources

BOOKS

Lacy, Charles F. *Drug Information Handbook with International Trade Names Index.* Hudson, OH: Lexi-Comp, Inc. 2011.

Preston, John D., John H. O'Neal, and Mary C. Talaga. *Handbook of Clinical Psychopharmacology for Therapists.* 5th ed. Oakland, CA: New Harbinger Publications, 2008.

PERIODICALS

Rosenberg, Russell P. "Sleep Maintenance Insomnia: Strengths and Weaknesses of Current Pharmacologic Therapies." *Annals of Clinical Psychiatry* 18, no. 1 (January–March 2006): 49–56.

WEBSITES

U.S. Food and Drug Administration. "FDA Requests Label Change for All Sleep Disorder Drug Products." March 14, 2007. http://www.fda.gov/NewsEvents/Newsroom/PressAnnouncements/2007/ucm108868.htm (accessed November 13, 2011).

ORGANIZATIONS

U.S. Food and Drug Administration, 10903 New Hampshire Ave., Silver Spring, MD, 20993-0002, (888) INFO-FDA (463-6332), http://www.fda.gov.

Ajna Hamidovic, Pharm.D.
Ruth A. Wienclaw, PhD

Quetiapine

Definition

Quetiapine is an atypical antipsychotic drug used to treat symptoms of **schizophrenia**. It works by changing the activity of certain natural substances in the brain. Quetiapine it is available with a prescription under the trade name Seroquel.

Purpose

Quetiapine tablets and extended-release tablets are used to treat the symptoms of schizophrenia, and are used alone or with other medications to treat or prevent episodes of mania or depression in patients with bipolar disorder. The extended-release tablets are also used along with other medication to treat depression. Quetiapine

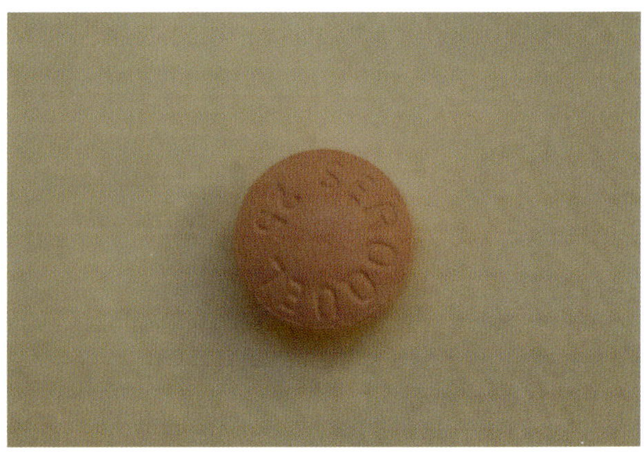

Seroquel (quetiapine), 25 mg. *(© Custom Medical Stock Photo, Inc. Reproduced by permission.)*

may be used as part of a treatment program to treat biopolar and schizophrenia in children.

Description

Quetiapine is thought to modify the actions of several chemicals in the **brain**. It is chemically related to another atypical antipsychotic agent, **clozapine**, but differs from earlier phenothiazine antipsychotics.

The effectiveness of quetiapine was evaluated in the Clinical Antipsychotic Trials of Intervention Effectiveness (**CATIE**) Schizophrenia Study. The study evaluated the effectiveness and side effects of newer antipsychotic drugs (sometimes referred to as "atypical antipsychotics") in comparison to a conventional antipsychotic drug in the treatment of schizophrenia. Contrary to expectations, the study found that the conventional antipsychotic generally was equally effective and tolerated as well as the newer, more expensive, atypical antipsychotic medications.

Only 16% of participants taking quetiapine in the Phase 1 study were able to continue throughout the entire 18 months. Participants who stopped taking their antipsychotic medication in Phase 1 because it was not adequately controlling their symptoms were more likely to stay on their medication if they were switched to **olanzapine** or **risperidone** rather than quetiapine or **ziprasidone**. There were no differences among the four medications tested in Phase 2, however, for participants who had stopped taking their Phase 1 medication because they experienced adverse side effects.

In Phase 2 of the study, the drug clozapine was more effective in controlling symptoms than the other atypical antipsychotics under evaluation. For patients whose symptoms were not well controlled on clozapine, olanzapine and risperidone tended to be more effective than ziprasidone or quetiapine.

Quetiapine is available in 25 mg, 100 mg, and 200 mg tablets.

Recommended dosage

Initially, a dosage of 25 mg should be taken twice a day. Each dose should be increased by 25–50 mg increments every three to four days until achieving a target dose of 300–400 mg per day, administered in two or three divided doses. It is not known whether doses higher than 800 mg per day are safe.

Precautions

Quetiapine is associated with an increased risk of death when used in elderly patients with **dementia**. In June 2008, the U.S. Food and Drug Administration (FDA) announced a requirement for manufacturers of quetiapine (and other antipsychotic drugs) to add a warning label to their packaging stating this risk. The reason for the increase was unclear in studies, but most deaths were found to be related to either cardiovascular complications or complications associated with infection. Quetiapine is not approved by the FDA for the treatment of behavior problems in older adults with dementia, and patients in this category (or caregivers of patients in this category) should discuss with their physician the risks of taking quetiapine.

Children and adolescents up to age 24 are at increased risk of developing suicidal thoughts and actions while taking quetiapine. It should not be taken by women who are pregnant, trying to become pregnant, or breastfeeding. Babies born to mothers who took quetiapine during pregnancy may develop extrapyramidal symptoms (EPS) and withdrawal symptoms, including agitation, trouble breathing, and difficulty feeding.

Caution should be used in patients with heart disease because the drug may cause blood pressure to fall too low, resulting in dizziness, rapid heartbeat, or fainting. Quetiapine users may also be at risk for potentially fatal heart arrhythmias, especially when taken in combination with other drugs that carry the risk of arrhythmia.

Quetiapine may increase cholesterol levels and contribute to the formation of cataracts. Because of this possibility, cholesterol levels should be checked periodically and yearly eye exams should be performed.

Quetiapine may cause liver damage. As a result, patients should notify their health care providers if they experience flu-like symptoms, notice yellowing of their skin or eyes, or experience abdominal pain. Liver function should be assessed periodically. The drug should be used cautiously in people with a history of liver disease or alcoholic cirrhosis. Quetiapine should be also be used carefully by those with a history of seizure disorders, as it may increase the tendency to have **seizures**.

KEY TERMS

Extrapyramidal symptoms—A group of side effects associated with antipsychotic medications and characterized by involuntary muscle movements, including contraction and tremor.

Insomnia—Waking in the middle of the night and having difficulty returning to sleep, or waking too early in the morning.

Seizure—A convulsion, or uncontrolled discharge of nerve cells that may spread to other cells throughout the brain.

Quetiapine may alter the function of the thyroid gland. Those taking supplements for low thyroid function may require dosage adjustments in their thyroid medication.

Quetiapine may cause extreme drowsiness and should be used carefully by people who need to be mentally alert.

Side effects

Relatively common side effects that accompany quetiapine usage include drowsiness, dizziness, rash, dry mouth, **insomnia**, **fatigue**, muscular weakness, anorexia, blurred vision, some loss of muscular control, and amenorrhea (lack of menstruation) in women.

Dystonia (difficulty walking or moving) may occur with quetiapine use. This condition may subside in 24 to 48 hours, even when the person continues taking the drug, and it usually disappears when quetiapine is discontinued.

Quetiapine use may lead to the development of symptoms that resemble Parkinson's disease. These symptoms may include a tight or mask-like expression on the face, drooling, tremors, pill-rolling motions in the hands, cogwheel rigidity (abnormal rigidity in muscles characterized by jerky movements when the muscle is passively stretched), and a shuffling gait. Taking the anti-Parkinson's drugs **benztropine** mesylate or **trihexyphenidyl** hydrochloride along with the quetiapine usually controls these symptoms.

Quetiapine has the potential to produce a serious side effect called **tardive dyskinesia**. This syndrome consists of involuntary, uncoordinated movements that may appear late in therapy and not disappear even after the drug is stopped. Tardive dyskinesia involves involuntary movements of the tongue, jaw, mouth, face, or other groups of skeletal muscles. The incidence of tardive dyskinesia increases with age and with dosage of quetiapine. Women are at greater risk than men for developing tardive dyskinesia. There is no known effective treatment for tardive dyskinesia, although gradual (but rarely complete) improvement may occur over a long period.

One occasionally reported side effect of quetiapine use is **neuroleptic malignant syndrome**. This is a complicated and potentially fatal condition characterized by muscle rigidity, high fever, alterations in mental status, and cardiac symptoms such as irregular pulse or blood pressure, sweating, tachycardia (fast heartbeat), and arrhythmias (irregular heartbeat). People who think they may be experiencing any side effects from this or any other medication should talk to their physicians promptly.

QUESTIONS TO ASK YOUR DOCTOR

- What kind of changes can I expect to see or feel with this medication?
- Does it matter what time of day I take this medication? If so, what is the recommendation?
- Should I take this medication with or without food?
- What are the side effects associated with this medication?
- Will this medication interact or interfere with other medications I am currently taking?
- What symptoms or adverse effects are important enough that I should seek immediate treatment?

Interactions

Quetiapine may be less effective when it is taken with drugs like **carbamazepine** (Tegretol), phenytoin (Dilantin), rifampin (Rifadin), **barbiturates**, **thioridazine** (Mellaril), or corticosteroids, such as prednisolone, methylprednisolone, prednisone, and dexamethasone because these drugs increase the breakdown of quetiapine in the liver, causing lower-than-normal levels of the drug.

Antifungal drugs, such as fluconazole (Diflucan) or ketoconazole (Nizoral), and antibiotics, such as erythromycin or clarithromycin (Biaxin), and cimetidine (Tagamet) may decrease the breakdown of quetiapine in the liver, causing higher-than-normal levels of the drug.

Any drug that causes drowsiness may lead to decreased mental alertness and impaired motor skills when taken with quetiapine. Some examples include alcohol, **antidepressants**, such as **imipramine** (Tofranil) or **paroxetine** (Paxil), antipsychotics, such as thioridazine (Mellaril), and some antihistamines.

Resources

BOOKS

Albers, Lawrence J., MD, Rhoda K. Hahn, MD, and Christopher Reist, MD. *Handbook of Psychiatric Drugs.* Laguna Hills, CA: Current Clinical Strategies Publishing, 2010.

American Society of Health-System Pharmacists. *AHFS Drug Information 2011.* Bethesda: American Society of Health-System Pharmacists, 2011.

Graham, George. *The Disordered Mind: An Introduction to Philosophy of Mind and Mental Illness.*New York, NY: Routledge, 2010.

Holland, Leland Norman, and Michael Patrick Adams. *Core Concepts in Pharmacology,*3rd ed. New York, NY: Prentice Hall, 2011.

North, Carol, and Sean Yutzy. *Goodwin and Guze's Psychiatric Diagnosis.*New York, NY: Oxford University Press, 2010.

Preston, John D., John H. O'Neal, and Mary C. Talaga. *Handbook of Clinical Psychopharmacology for Therapists,* 6th ed. Oakland, CA: New Harbinger Publications, 2011.

PERIODICALS

Casey, Daniel E. "Implications of the CATIE Trial on Treatment: Extrapyramidal Symptoms." *CNS Spectrums* 11. no. 7, Supp. 7 (July 2006): 25–31.

El-Mallakh, Rif, et al. "Bipolar II Disorder: Current and Future Treatment Options." *Annals of Clinical Psychiatry* 18, no. 4 (Oct.–Dec. 2006): 259–66.

Gentile, Salvatore. "Extrapyramidal Adverse Events Associated with Atypical Antipsychotic Treatment of Bipolar Disorder." *Journal of Clinical Psychopharmacology* 27, no. 1 (Feb. 2007): 35–45.

Glick, Ira D. "Understanding the Results of CATIE in the Context of the Field." *CNS Spectrums* 11.7, Supp. 7 (July 2006): 40–47.

Haro, Josep Maria, et al. "Remission and Relapse in the Outpatient Care of Schizophrenia: Three-Year Results from the Schizophrenia Outpatient Health Outcomes Study." *Journal of Clinical Psychopharmacology* 26, no. 6 (Dec. 2006): 571–78.

Jarema, Marek. "Atypical Antipsychotics in the Treatment of Mood Disorders." *Current Opinion in Psychiatry* 20, no. 1 (Jan. 2007): 23–29.

Lieberman, Jeffrey A., et al. "Effectiveness of Antipsychotic Drugs in Patients with Chronic Schizophrenia." *New England Journal of Medicine* 353, no. 12 (Sept. 2005): 1209–23.

McEvoy, Joseph P., et al. "Effectiveness of Clozapine Versus Olanzapine, Quetiapine, and Risperidone in Patients with Chronic Schizophrenia Who Did Not Respond to Prior Atypical Antipsychotic Treatment." *American Journal of Psychiatry* 163, no. 4 (Apr. 2006): 600–10.

Meisenzahl, E.M., et al. "Effects of Treatment with the Atypical Neuroleptic Quetiapine on Working Memory Function: A Functional MRI Follow-Up Investigation." *European Archives of Psychiatry and Clinical Neuroscience* 256, no. 8 (Dec. 2006): 522–31.

Meltzer, Herbert Y., and William V. Bobo. "Interpreting the Efficacy Findings in the CATIE Study: What Clinicians Should Know." *CNS Spectrums* 11, no. 7, Supp. 7 (July 2006): 14–24.

Nasrallah, Henry A. "Metabolic Findings from the CATIE Trial and Their Relation to Tolerability." *CNS Spectrums* 11, no. 7, Supp. 7 (July 2006): 32–39.

Nasrallah, Henry A., Martin Brecher, and Björn Paulsson. "Placebo-Level Incidence of Extrapyramidal Symptoms (EPS) with Quetiapine in Controlled Studies of Patients with Bipolar Mania." *Bipolar Disorders* 8.5, part 1 (Oct. 2006): 467–74.

Pae, Chi-Un, et al. "Adjunctive Risperidone, Olanzapine and Quetiapine for the Treatment of Hospitalized Patients with Bipolar I Disorder: A Retrospective Study." *Progress in Neuro-Psychopharmacology & Biological Psychiatry* 30, no. 7 (Sept. 2006): 1322–25.

Savaskan, Egemen, et al. "Treatment of Behavioural, Cognitive and Circadian Rest-Activity Cycle Disturbances in Alzheimer's Disease: Haloperidol vs. Quetiapine." *International Journal of Neuropsychopharmacology* 9, no. 5 (Oct. 2006): 507–16.

Schneider, Lon S., et al. "Effectiveness of Atypical Antipsychotic Drugs in Patients with Alzheimer's Disease." *New England Journal of Medicine* 355, no. 15 (Oct. 2006): 1525–38.

Stroup, T. Scott, et al. "Effectiveness of Olanzapine, Quetiapine, Risperidone, and Ziprasidone in Patients with Chronic Schizophrenia Following Discontinuation of a Previous Atypical Antipsychotic." *American Journal of Psychiatry* 163, no. 4 (Apr. 2006): 611–22.

Tariot, Pierre N., et al. "Quetiapine Treatment of Psychosis Associated With Dementia: A Double-Blind, Randomized, Placebo-Controlled Clinical Trial." *American Journal of Geriatric Psychiatry* 14, no. 9 (Sept. 2006): 767–76.

Thase, Michael E., et al. "Efficacy of Quetiapine Monotherapy in Bipolar I and II Depression: A Double-Blind, Placebo-Controlled Study (The BOLDER II Study)." *Journal of Clinical Psychopharmacology* 26. no. 6 (Dec. 2006): 600–09.

Weiden, Peter J. "EPS Profiles: The Atypical Antipsychotics Are Not All the Same." *Journal of Psychiatric Practice* 13. no. 1 (Jan. 2007): 13–24.

ORGANIZATIONS

American Psychiatric Association, 1000 Wilson Boulevard, Suite 1825, Arlington, VA, 22209, (703) 907-7300, apa@psych.org, http://www.psych.org.

Mental Health America, 2000 N. Beauregard Street, 6th Floor, Alexandria, VA, 22311, (703) 684-7722, (800) 969-6642, Fax: (703) 684-5968, http://www1.nmha.org.

National Alliance on Mental Illness (NAMI), Colonial Place Three, 2107 Wilson Blvd., Suite 300, Arlington, VA, 22201, (703) 524-7600, (800) 950-NAMI (6264), Fax: (703) 524-9094, http://www.nami.org/Hometemplate.cfm.

National Institute of Mental Health (NIMH), 6001 Executive Boulevard, Room 8184, MSC 9663, Bethesda, MD, 20892, (301) 443-4513, (866) 615-6464, Fax: (301) 443-4279, nimhinfo@nih.gov, http://www.nimh.nih.gov/index.shtml.

U.S. Food and Drug Administration, 10903 New Hampshire Ave., Silver Spring, MD, 20993-0002, (888) INFO-FDA (463-6332), http://www.fda.gov.

Kelly Karpa, R.Ph., Ph.D.
Ruth A. Wienclaw, Ph.D.
Laura Jean Cataldo, RN, Ed.D.

R

Rational behavior therapy *see* **Rational emotive therapy**

Rational emotive therapy

Definition

Rational emotive therapy (RET) is a psychotherapeutic approach that proposes that unrealistic and irrational beliefs cause many emotional problems.

Purpose

RET is a form of **cognitive-behavioral therapy** (CBT). The primary focus of this treatment approach is to suggest changes in thinking that will lead to changes in behavior, thereby alleviating or improving symptoms. The therapy emphasizes changing irrational thinking patterns that cause emotional distress into thoughts that are more reasonable and rational. RET can be used to treat persons affected from disorders such as anxiety, **depression**, and **stress**.

Description

Rational emotive therapy was developed by Albert Ellis (1913–2007) in the mid-1950s. Ellis proposed that people become unhappy and develop self-defeating habits because of unrealistic or faulty beliefs. In Ellis's research reports from 1979 and 1987, he introduced the model that most irrational beliefs originate from three core ideas, each one of which is unrealistic. These three core and unrealistic views include:

1. I must perform well to be approved of by others who are perceived significant
2. You must treat me fairly—if not, then it is horrible and I cannot bear it
3. Conditions must be my way and if not I cannot stand to live in such a terrible and awful world

These irrational thoughts can lead to **grief** and needless suffering.

RET is considered an active therapy. The RET therapist will strive to change irrational beliefs, challenge thinking, and promote rational self-talk. Various strategies are used to achieve these goals, including:

- disputing irrational beliefs (the therapist points out how irrational it would be for a client to believe he or she had to be good at everything to be considered a worthwhile person)
- reframing (presenting situations in a more positive angle)
- problem solving
- role playing
- modeling
- use of humor

The client may also be requested to complete certain exercises at home or to read about the disorder (**bibliotherapy**).

Preparation

Before a client begins RET, he or she may undergo an assessment with the therapist. This assessment is called a biopsychosocial assessment, consisting of a structured interview. The questions and information-gathering during this assessment typically cover areas such as past medical and psychological history, family and social history, sex and drug history, employment and education history, and criminal history. The interview provides information for a **diagnosis** or a tentative diagnosis requiring further testing or consultation.

KEY TERMS

Modeling—A behavioral therapy technique in which a patient first observes and then imitates a desired behavior.

Relapse—A recurrence of symptoms after a period of improvement or recovery.

Aftercare

Aftercare may or may not be indicated. This is usually decided on between the patient and mental health practitioner. Aftercare follow-up may be recommended if the affected person is at risk of **relapse** behaviors.

Precautions

There are no major precautions or risks associated with RET. Persons entering treatment must be willing to change their behaviors that promote **negative symptoms**. There is a possibility that treatment may not benefit the affected person; this possibility becomes more likely for patients who have multiple psychological disorders.

Results

If a patient has success with RET, they will begin to understand the repetitive patterns of irrational thoughts and disruption caused by symptoms. The individual in therapy will develop skills to improve his or her specific problems, resulting in improved self-esteem and the development of a sense that life events change and that outcomes may not always be favorable, with the ability to adapt to or accept these changes. Persons who are unwilling to change and adhere to treatment recommendations may not gain any new beneficial behaviors.

Resources

BOOKS

Coon, D. *Essentials of Psychology*. Florence Grove, KY: Wadsworth, 2002.

ORGANIZATIONS

The Albert Ellis Institute, 45 East 65th Street, New York, NY, 10021, (212) 535-0822, Fax: (212) 249-3582, info@albertellis.org, http://www.rebt.org.

Laith Farid Gulli, MD
Nicole Mallory, MS, PA-C

Reactive attachment disorder of infancy or early childhood

Definition

In reactive attachment disorder (RAD) of infancy or early childhood, the normal healthy bond between infant and parent or caregiver is not established or is broken. Infants normally "bond" or form an emotional attachment, to a parent or other caregiver by the eighth month of life. This includes the child's basic needs for affection, comfort, and nurturing.

From about the second through the eighth month, most infants will respond to attention from a variety of caregivers, if the caregivers are familiar. By the eighth month, however, normal infants have established a strong emotional preference for one or two primary caregivers. They are distressed if separated from these caregivers for even a few hours, even if another familiar person is present. If this bonding process is interfered with, it can have severe emotional and physical consequences for the child. For instance, it can permanently and adversely affect the **brain** of a growing child. Thus, reactive attachment disorder is caused within a child by a history of insufficient care and/or social contact from the child's caregiver, often the parents. This results in the child in never being able to establish caring and loving attachments with others.

Reactive attachment disorder, sometimes called a *post-traumatic disorder,* is considered a severe, but relatively uncommon, disorder that can affect infants and young children well into their adult years by disenabling them from establishing future relationships.

Two internationally based documents are used to classify medical conditions and mental disorders. The *International Statistical Classification of Diseases and Related Health Problems* (ICD), provided for by the World Health Organization, states in its latest version (ICD-10) that the inhibited form of the disorder is called reactive attachment disorder (RAD), while the disinhibited form is called disinhibited attachment disorder (DAD). The ***Diagnostic and Statistical Manual of Mental Disorders*** (*DSM*), published by the **American Psychiatric Association**, does not differentiate between the two in its latest version (*DSM-IV-TR*); however, that may change with the future version (*DSM-5*).

Demographics

The prevalence of reactive attachment disorder has been estimated at 1% of all children under the age of five years. Children orphaned at a young age have a much higher likelihood of this problem. Otherwise, RAD can appear in any infant or young child without favoring any particular gender, racial, or ethnic group, and without regard to any specific socioeconomic level.

Description

In reactive attachment disorder, an infant or young child has not formed an emotional bond with a parent or other caregiver. Somehow an inability of a child to form normal attachments toward a parent, or parents, has occurred. This affects the child's ability to interact normally with others. Such a problem is likely the result of early experiences of **abuse**, **neglect**, or sudden separation from parents, or caregivers, between the ages of six months to three years. It could also result from a lack of communications or responsiveness between child and caregiver or from a change of caregivers during this span of time. Consequently, the child may develop severe emotional and social problems that extend into adulthood. There may be learning problems and physical problems, such as slow growth and failure to develop as expected.

The mental disorder is characterized by prominent actions that are disturbed and inappropriate within the general social context. In its two basic forms, a person with RAD may have a consistent inability to initiate or respond to social interactions, possess an inhibited behavior, and shun attachments to nearly everyone—what is called the "inhibited" form. This form of RAD occurs most likely when a child does not develop any attachments to any caregiver very early in life. In this other major form, what is called "disinhibited," the person is extremely sociable, to a degree that he or she has an unusual closeness or friendliness with strangers. They aggressively seek out attention, frequently ask for help in performing tasks or activities, have inappropriate age-related behaviors, or appear anxious most of the time. This form of RAD is more likely when a child had multiple caregivers early in life or had various caregivers at different points in childhood.

The forthcoming edition of the *Diagnostic and Statistical Manual of Mental Disorders* (*DSM-5*, 2013) proposes to change some features of how it describes reactive attachment disorder by differentiating RAD into two disorders. This division is likely to include the following two designations: reactive attachment disorder of infancy and early childhood, and disinhibited social engagement disorder.

Proposed criteria (as stated by the American Psychiatric Association's *DSM-5* Development website) for Reactive Attachment Disorder of Infancy or Early Childhood include:

- The child must display a pattern of inappropriate (for developmental level) or disturbing attachment behaviors. Behaviors must be present before five years of age. The attachment behaviors must be consistent, and the child's demeanor must exhibit as inhibited or emotionally withdrawn. The child must rarely demonstrate signs of attachment toward parents or other caregivers, such as not seeking comfort when upset or not responding to comfort when offered.
- The child must exhibit persistent social and emotional disturbances as characterized by at least two of the following:
  1. an absence of social or emotional responses in interactions with others
  2. limited or lack of positive affect
  3. unexplained irritability, sadness, or fearfulness during normal (nonthreating) interactions
- The child's symptoms must not meet the criteria for an autism spectrum disorder
- At least one of the following conditions must be present in the household:
  1. child's basic emotional needs are not met by the caregiver
  2. child's basic physical needs are not met by the caregiver
  3. constant changes in or turnover of primary caregiver are present
  4. child is raised in unusual settings
- The child must be at least nine months old.

Proposed criteria (as stated by the American Psychiatric Association's *DSM-5* Development website) for Disinhibited Social Engagement Disorder include:

- The child must regularly interact with strangers and exhibit at least two of the following symptoms:
  1. Reduced or no hesitation in approaching strangers
  2. Lack of boundaries in interpersonal interactions
  3. Failure to check in with caregiver
  4. Willingness or lack of hesitation to go off with strangers
- The child's behavior does not meet the criteria for impulsivity in attention deficit hyperactivity disorder.
- At least one of the following conditions must be present in the household:
  1. child's basic emotional needs are not met by the caregiver

2. child's basic physical and safety needs are not met by the caregiver
3. constant changes in or turnover of primary caregiver are present
4. child is given frequent and harsh punishments

- The child must be at least nine months old.

Causes and symptoms

Causes

An infant does not know how to form an emotional attachment to another person, any more than it knows how to feed or clean itself. Bonding is a necessary developmental step in a baby's growth. It occurs as the infant is cared for, talked to, played with, and comforted consistently. This helps the infant feel as if it knows what will happen every time it sees a certain person. When this process is interfered with, the infant may never learn how to trust or love.

Many things can interfere with the bonding process. Some of these include:

- Loss of parents. The most common cause of reactive attachment disorder is the child being orphaned or put in foster care at a very early age. The infant may receive care from many people or be moved from place to place often. A bond to a single consistent caregiver, therefore, cannot be formed.
- Neglect or impaired care giving. If the infant is not cared for consistently, he or she will not learn to trust. This includes emotional neglect, where the caregivers may keep the baby clean and fed, but do not allow time for play and bonding. Very often, this occurs when the parent or caregiver has a problem that prevents him or her from giving adequate consistent attention to the infant. Such problems include major depression, psychosis, drug or alcohol abuse, intellectual disability, physical illness, and poverty. The parent may also have been a neglected child or may be very young themselves and simply may not know how to parent adequately. A mother may have postpartum depression after the birth of the child, which may prevent her from adequately taking care of the baby.
- Abuse or pain. Even if an infant is getting love and attention some of the time, he or she may not learn to attach itself to a caregiver if it comes to expect pain on occasion from the caregiver. Illness or pain that the caregiver cannot ease can have the same effect.
- Institutional care. Being in the hospital or other such medical facility for a long period during the early formative years of a child can cause a child not to receive the emotional care it needs.
- Poverty. Being in a situation where extreme poverty is rampant in the family providing care to the child, which may result in the child being ignored due to other pressures within the family.

In disrupted families with more than one child, one child may have reactive attachment disorder while others do not. It is not clear what role personality plays in this problem. It is sometimes suggested that the temperament of the child may play a role. Some young children may be more susceptible to **stress** or unpredictable situations than others, even in the same family, which may cause one child to have RAD in a family while another does not. RAD is a disorder that is not well understood. It is not known what precisely causes it in children but research is ongoing.

Symptoms

Infants with this problem often resist being held or touched and do not reach out when others come near. They are often sad-looking, without any smiling, and may look withdrawn and listless. Such infants may also seem sleepy or "slow." They may not seem aware of what is going on around them, and often they do not follow others with the eyes as they move around the room. These infants often do not have an interest in playing with toys or games involving the actions of others. They may be slow to gain weight. On the other hand, some appear to be overly aware and nervous.

Young children may seem withdrawn and passive. They may ignore others or respond to others in odd ways. For instance, they may dismiss comments or gestures that attempt to provoke comfort or caring. Some may seem overly familiar with strangers and touch or cling to people they have just met. They may also act aggressive toward children around their own age. However, they lack empathy for others. Their behavior comes across to others as needy and strange, unlike the normal friendliness of children. They have a general attitude of being awkward or uncomfortable in situations where such behaviors are not common. Such young children may also try to hide feelings of anger or disgust. They may also not ask for help or assistance when such actions are needed.

Other symptoms of reactive attachment disorder in children can include the following:

- inability to learn from mistakes (poor cause-and-effect thinking)
- learning problems or delays in learning

KEY TERMS

Attention deficit hyperactivity disorder (ADHD)—A disorder primarily in children that is characterized by the inability to concentrate, along with hyperactivity and inappropriate and/or impulsive behaviors.

Autistic spectrum disorder—A mental disorder characterized by abnormal behaviors with regard to social interactions and communications, along with obsessive, repetitive behaviors and only limited perceived interests.

Depression—A disorder characterized by persistent feelings of hopelessness, sadness, and dejection, along with the regular inability to sleep and lack of energy; suicidal tendencies are also sometimes present.

Psychosis—A disorder characterized by hallucinations, distorted ideas of reality, delusions, and other symptoms related to schizophrenia and mania.

- impulsive behavior
- abnormal speech patterns
- destructive or cruel behavior

The ICD-10 describes the following for both RAD and DAD:

- markedly disturbed and developmentally inappropriate social relatedness in most contexts
- disturbance is not accounted for solely by developmental delay and does not meet the criteria for pervasive development disorder
- onset before five years of age
- history of significant neglect
- implicit lack of identifiable, preferred attachment figure

Diagnosis

The standard manual for mental health professionals in the United States is the *Diagnostic and Statistical Manual of Mental Disorders*. This manual lists criteria for diagnosing various mental disorders. The most recent edition, the fourth edition text revised is also known as the *DSM-IV-TR*. According to *DSM-IV-TR*, reactive attachment disorder is diagnosed when the following criteria are met:

- Presence of strange and developmentally inappropriate social interactions, beginning before age five years. The child does not respond to or initiate social interactions in a way that would be developmentally appropriate; instead, the child is either inhibited or is disinhibited in his or her interactions. Inhibited reactions may be excessively vigilant, restrained, or ambivalent. (The child may respond to caregivers with a mixture of approach, avoidance, and resistance to comforting, as an example from the manual.) Disinhibited reactions occur in a variety of social interactions, and the child does not discriminate among people he or she chooses as attachment figures. This child will treat near strangers with inappropriate familiarity.
- The child's inappropriate social skills are not due exclusively to developmental delay (as in intellectual disability) and the child's symptoms do not meet criteria for a pervasive developmental disorder.
- The child has received care in which his or her basic needs—either emotional or physical—are often unmet, or in which stable attachments have not been able to form (such as when primary caregivers change often).

An infant is diagnosed as having reactive attachment disorder when he or she fails to show signs of bonding to a parent or caregiver by the age of eight months. Infants normally start to follow the parent or caregiver with their eyes and smile in response to attention by about two months. By about five months, the child should reach out to be picked up and obviously enjoy simple interactive games like "peekaboo."

Treatment

First, the child's safety and physical health must be attended to. A child who is being abused or has been physically neglected may need to be hospitalized for a while. This is done to separate the child from the harmful situation and to take care of any medical problems resulting from neglect or abuse.

The next step is either to make the child's home environment stable or to place the child in a more stable home. Child protective services may be brought in at this point. The home situation must be evaluated, and the parents or caregivers assessed for emotional fitness to care for the child. The parents or caregivers may be given training in proper childcare and emotional nurturing. **Family therapy** may be needed in some cases to help the parents or caregivers and other children in the family.

With a young infant, the parents or caregivers will be encouraged to have a regular schedule for the infant and to spend time each day simply holding and playing with the infant.

Treatment of children who are past infancy is difficult. It is important to find a therapist experienced in the treatment of children with reactive attachment disorder. Most therapists use a mix of techniques, but primarily psychological counseling and parent or caregiver education. The therapist may seek to help the child relive and work through **grief** and anger from a prior **trauma** or loss. Cognitive therapy may be used to help an older child understand and reframe negative thoughts about himself or herself, or about parents or caregivers. If the child is too young to verbalize or think rationally, techniques such as **play therapy** or **art therapy** may be used to help bring out and work through feelings. Behavioral therapy may be used to help guide development of wanted behaviors.

Although reactive attachment disorder is a permanent condition, treatment can help children to develop better and more stable relationships with parents or caregivers than would be possible without treatment.

Prognosis

There has not been much research to date on the course of this problem. It appears that children who are identified and treated early have a better chance of learning how to form appropriate bonds with other people.

Children who are not treated, or who are treated later in life, have a greater chance of having permanent problems relating to other people. Some of these problems include:

- delayed physical and cognitive development and growth
- poor self-esteem and self-image
- immature behavior
- antisocial or delinquent behavior
- relationship problems with both genders
- anger-management problems along with temper-control problems
- eating disorders, along with resulting malnutrition, which can cause further medical disorders
- depression, anxiety
- learning problems
- addiction to alcohol or drugs
- inability to hold a job, unemployment
- sexual problems or inappropriate sexual behaviors

QUESTIONS TO ASK YOUR DOCTOR

- What treatment options are available?
- Is there a cure for RAD?
- What permanent damage can be caused by RAD?
- What is the best prognosis for my child?
- Are there organizations that specialize in RAD? Is so, where can I learn more?
- Will my insurance cover the treatment?

Prevention

Prevention of reactive attachment disorder begins with good parenting. As far as possible, health care providers and families should be on the lookout for any problem that may prevent parents from giving children the structure and attention they need. If a child loses its primary caregivers, a stable environment with consistent attention from one or two caregivers should be provided as soon as possible.

Early identification of reactive attachment disorder is necessary to get help to the child and family as soon as possible. The earlier this problem is identified and treated, the more likely it is that the child will be able to develop healthy patterns of relating to others.

Resources

BOOKS

American Psychiatric Association. *Diagnostic and Statistical Manual of Mental Disorders,* 4th edition, text revision. Washington, DC: American Psychiatric Press, 2000.

Black, Donald, and Nancy C. Andresen. *Introductory Textbook of Psychiatry.* Washington D.C.: American Psychiatric, 2011.

Dulcan, Mina K., editor. *Dulcan's Textbook of Child and Adolescent Psychiatry.* Washington D.C.: American Psychiatric Press, 2010.

Sadock, Benjamin J., Viginia A. Sadock, Pedro Ruiz, et al., editors. *Kaplan & Sadock's Comprehensive Textbook of Psychology.* Philadelphia: Wolters Kluwer Health/Lippincott Williams & Wilkins; 2009.

World Health Organization. *International Statistical Classification of Diseases and Related Health Problems, Tenth Revision (ICD-10).* Geneva: World Health Organization, 1992.

WEBSITES

"Diagnostic and Statistical Manual." American Psychiatric Association. http://www.psych.org/mainmenu/research/dsmiv.aspx (accessed May 27, 2011).

"G 00 Reactive Attachment Disorder." American Psychiatric Association. http://www.dsm5.org/ProposedRevisions/Pages/proposedrevision.aspx?rid=120 (accessed May 27, 2011).

Mayo Clinic staff. "Reactive Attachment Disorder." Mayo Clinic.com. http://www.mayoclinic.com/health/reactive-attachment-disorder/DS00988 (accessed May 27, 2011).

ORGANIZATIONS

American College of Physicians, 190 North Independence Mall West, Philadelphia, PA, 19106-1572, (215) 351-2400, (800) 523-1546, http://www.acponline.org.

American Medical Association, 515 N. State Street, Chicago, IL, 60610, (800) 621-8335, http://www.ama-assn.org.

American Psychiatric Association, 1000 Wilson Boulevard, Suite 1825, Arlington, VA, 22209, (703) 907-7300, (888) 357-7924, apa@psych.org, http://www.psych.org.

Association for Treatment and Training in the Attachment of Children, PO Box 533, Lake Villao, IL, 60046, (847) 453-8224, Fax: (847) 356-7856, questions@attach.org, http://www.attach.org.

Jody Bower, M.S.W.
William Atkins,

Reading disorder

Definition

Reading disorder is a learning disorder that involves significant impairment of reading accuracy, speed, or comprehension to the extent that the impairment interferes with academic achievement or activities of daily life. Also referred to as reading disability, reading difficulty, and dyslexia, reading disorder is the most commonly diagnosed learning disability in the United States. It is defined by the **American Psychiatric Association** (APA) as "reading achievement . . . that falls substantially below that expected given the individual's chronological age, measured intelligence, and age-appropriate education." Reading disorder is distinct from alexia, which is the term for loss of the ability to read caused by **brain** damage from injury or disease. However, neurological studies of alexia have helped researchers better understand reading disabilities.

Demographics

Estimates of the number of people with **learning disorders** range from 2%–15% of the general population. Most research studies give a figure of 5%. About 80% of people with a learning disorder have reading disorder. Other studies suggest that about 4% of school-age children have reading disorder. People with reading disorder are more likely to have a parent or sibling with the disorder.

Originally it was thought that reading disorder affected more boys than girls (in a ratio of 5:1), but later studies found boys to be only slightly more likely than girls to have reading disorder. Incidence estimates are skewed because boys tend to act out more in class and are consequently referred more frequently for special education. **Diagnosis** is complicated by the fact that anywhere from 20%–55% of dyslexics also suffer from **attention deficit hyperactivity disorder (ADHD)**, a behavioral disorder that may aggravate reading problems. In addition, about one-quarter of children with reading disorder have **conduct disorder**. **Oppositional defiant disorder** and **depression** also occur in higher-than-average rates in children with reading disorder. Almost all people with reading disorder have difficulties spelling, and about 80% of them have other language problems.

Description

Reading disorder is a learning disorder characterized by a significant disparity between an individual's general intelligence and his or her reading skills. Learning disorders, formerly called academic skills disorders, are disorders that account for difficulty learning and poor academic performance when low performance cannot be attributed to **intellectual disability**, low intelligence, lack of learning opportunities, or such specific physical problems as vision or hearing deficits. Common learning disabilities include reading disorder, often called dyslexia; **mathematics disorder**; **disorder of written expression**; and some language processing disorders.

Reading disorder was first recognized in the late nineteenth century. It was initially called pure word blindness and then developmental alexia. Starting in the 1960s, educators commonly referred to reading disorder as dyslexia, from the Greek word *dys*, meaning poor or inadequate, and the word *lexis* meaning words or language.

Reading disorder can cause severe problems in reading, and consequently in academic work, even in people with normal intelligence, educational opportunities, motivation to learn to read, and emotional self-control. Reading disorder is different from slowness in learning or intellectual developmental disorder. In reading disorder, there is a significant gap between the expected level of performance and actual achievement. Difficulties in reading can occur on many levels, and reading disorder may have multiple causes that manifest in different ways.

Types of reading disorders

Reading disabilities have been classified as either dyseidetic, dysphonetic, or mixed. Persons with the dyseidetic type are able to sound out individual letters phonetically but have trouble identifying patterns of letters when they are grouped together. Their spelling tends to be phonetic even when incorrect ("laf" for "laugh"). By comparison, dysphonic readers have difficulty relating letters to sounds, so their spelling is chaotic. They are able to recognize words they have memorized but cannot sound out new ones. They may be able to read near the appropriate grade level but are poor spellers. Persons with mixed reading disabilities have both the dyseidetic and dysphonic types of reading disorder.

Risk factors

Risk factors for reading disorders include a concurrent diagnosis of **attention deficit hyperactivity disorder (ADHD)**, a family history of reading disorder, and delayed early language development. About 40% of boys and 20% of girls with a dyslexic parent develop the disorder. Dyslexia is believed to occur equally in all races.

Causes and symptoms

Causes

The causes of reading disorder are not completely understood but are thought to be related to differences in the structure and functioning of the brain, particularly areas of the brain known as the left perisylvian region, the left temporo-occipital region, and the right fronto-parietal cortex. Persons with reading difficulties appear to process information in different parts of the brain from those without reading disorders. Learning to read is a complex task. It requires coordination of the muscles of the eye to follow a line of print, spatial orientation to interpret letters and words, visual memory to retain the meaning of letters and sight words, sequencing ability, a grasp of sentence structure and grammar, and the ability to categorize and analyze. In addition, the brain must integrate visual cues with memory and associate them with specific sounds. The sounds, or phonemes, must then be associated with specific meanings, and for comprehension, the meanings must be retained while a sentence or passage is read. Reading disorder occurs when any of these processes are disrupted. For that reason, the roots of reading disorder have proved difficult to isolate, and may be different in different individuals.

Reading disorder is known to run in families, and a number of genes linked to dyslexia have been identified. Many participate in gene development, and several genetic studies have found gene linkages on chromosomes 1 and 6 that demonstrate heterogeneous (multiple methods of) transmission. **Positron emission tomography (PET)** studies have shown that dyslexics assigned reading tasks show a lower level of activity than children with normal reading skills in a part of the brain known as the left inferior parietal cortex, a region that is necessary for the rapid perception of word forms. Studies using functional **magnetic resonance imaging** (fMRI) pinpointed the left inferior frontal gyrus, the left inferior parietal lobule, and the left middle temporal gyrus as areas of low activation in children with dyslexia given word tests to complete. Another indication that specific areas of the brain are involved in dyslexia comes from case studies of children who have suffered **stroke**. In one study reported in 2006, a six-year-old boy had suffered a stroke affecting the left hemisphere of his brain. He was able to read words that he had learned prior to the stroke, but attempts to read unfamiliar words were unsuccessful until he received special training.

One surprising finding, reported by a team of researchers at Hong Kong University in 2008, is that the part of the brain affected by dyslexia appears to differ according to the child's primary language. The researchers used magnetic resonance imaging (MRI) to compare a group of children whose first language is English with a second group raised to speak Chinese. The scientists found that the English speakers use a different part of the brain when reading from that used by the Chinese students. The difference is apparently related to the fact that English is an alphabetic language whereas Chinese uses symbols to represent words.

Symptoms

Common characteristics of children with reading disorder include:

- difficulty identifying single words
- problems understanding the sounds in words, sound order, or rhymes
- problems with spelling
- transposing letters in words
- omitting or substituting words
- poor reading comprehension
- slow reading speed (oral or silent)

In addition to these symptoms, children with a reading disorder may also struggle with:

- learning to speak
- organizing thoughts and ideas into clear written and spoken language
- memorizing number facts, such as the multiplication tables
- reading quickly enough to understand what is being read—some children with dyslexia read so slowly that they cannot remember the beginning of a sentence by the time they reach the end of it, particularly if it is a long and complicated sentence
- making their way through longer reading assignments
- spelling words correctly
- making rhymes
- learning foreign languages, which involves a basic understanding of grammar and the parts of speech
- performing mathematical calculations correctly
- opposites and directions

Diagnosis

Evaluation of reading ability must be done on an individual basis in order to make a diagnosis of reading disorder and distinguish it from slow learning or low intelligence. Though reading disorder is rarely diagnosed in children before age five or six, because formal instruction in reading does not begin before kindergarten or first grade in most U.S. schools, preschool-age children may exhibit certain problems, such as trouble sounding out words and difficulty memorizing sequence information such as the days of the week, that may foreshadow a reading disability.

Anyone who is suspected of having reading disorder or any other learning disability should have a comprehensive evaluation, including hearing, vision, and intelligence testing. The test should include all areas of learning and learning processes, not just reading. In school-age children, this evaluation often involves a team of educators, educational psychologists, and child psychiatrists.

Examination

The diagnostic process takes several steps. The first step is an office examination by the child's doctor to rule out any disorders of vision or hearing that could interfere with learning. The child may also be referred to a neurologist (a specialist in disorders of the nervous system) for further evaluation to make sure that the child does not have a brain tumor or other physical disease of the brain.

The next step is usually intelligence testing and an evaluation of the child's reading and speaking skills by a qualified expert. This type of evaluation involves testing the child's short-term memory or asking the child to read nonsense words as a test of their ability to link letters and sounds. In addition, the child may be evaluated psychologically to see whether depression, anxiety, or social problems are causing the learning difficulty. The examiner must take into account the child's age, intelligence, educational opportunities, and such cultural factors as whether the language spoken at home is different from the language used in school instruction.

Reading disorder is diagnosed when reading achievement is substantially below what would be expected after taking into account the above factors. To meet the ***Diagnostic and Statistical Manual of Mental Disorders*** *(DSM)* diagnostic criteria for reading disorder, the reading problems must substantially interfere with his or her schoolwork or daily life. If a physical condition is present (for example, intellectual disability or hearing loss), the reading deficit must be in excess of what one would normally associate with the physical disability.

Treatment

Treatment approaches vary from visual stimulation to special **diets** to enhanced reading instruction. However, it is generally agreed that customized education is the only successful remedy, and the American Academy of Ophthalmology, the American Academy of Pediatrics, and the American Association for Pediatric Ophthalmology and Strabismus have issued a policy statement warning against visual treatments and recommending a cross-disciplinary educational approach. After a child's specific difficulties in reading and understanding language have been analyzed by an expert, a treatment program is drawn up tailored to his or her needs. Under the provisions of the Individuals with Disabilities Education Act (IDEA) of 2004, any child with a diagnosed learning disability, including reading disorder or dyslexia, should be eligible for an Individual Education Program (IEP) that provides customized instruction at school designed to address his or her disability.

The first researcher to identify and study dyslexia, Samuel Torrey Orton, developed the core principles of such an approach in the 1920s. The work of three of his followers—teachers Bessie Stillman, Anna Gillingham, and Beth Slingerland—underlies many of the programs in use today, including Project READ, the Wilson Reading System, and programs based on the Herman method. These and other successful programs have three characteristics in common. They are:

- Sound/symbol (phonics)-based. They break words down into their smallest visual components: letters and the sounds associated with them.

KEY TERMS

Digraph—A pair of letters that represents a single speech sound. In English, the *th* in "thumb" and the *ei* in "vein" are examples of digraphs.

Dyslexia—Another term for reading disorder.

Phonics—A method of teaching reading and spelling based on the phonetic interpretation of ordinary spelling.

- Multisensory. Good programs attempt to form and strengthen mental associations among visual, auditory, and kinesthetic channels of stimulation. The student simultaneously sees, feels, and says the sound-symbol association. For example, a student may trace the letter or letter combination with his or her finger while pronouncing a word out loud.
- Highly structured. Remediation begins at the level of the single letter-sound, then works up to digraphs (a pair of letters representing a single speech sound), syllables, and finally words and sentences in a systematic fashion. Repetitive drills and practice serve to form necessary associations between sounds and written symbols.

When ADHD is co-diagnosed with a reading disorder, special care should be taken to identify specific reading problems and to define cognitive as well as behavioral learning objectives.

Psychotherapy

Persons with reading disorders often need and benefit from **psychotherapy** because of possible struggles with low self-esteem associated with their disability. Many persons with reading disorder feel that they are stupid or less capable than they really are, and are likely to drop out of school if they are not diagnosed and treated early.

Prognosis

Many famous and successful people have suffered from reading disorders, including at least two Presidents of the United States. How well a person compensates for this disorder depends on the severity of the impairment and the type of educational remediation that he or she receives. Generally, people who are identified as having a reading disorder before grade three and who receive intensive reading education can do well. There is, however, a great deal of variation among people in intelligence, educational opportunities, and the will to overcome a reading disorder, as well as in the type and severity of the problem. All these factors combine to determine the ultimate outcome of this disorder. The prognosis is usually good if the condition is diagnosed early and the person is enrolled in a good remedial program. Learning disabilities can affect a person's self-esteem, and so support from family, friends, and teachers also help improve the chances of overcoming this disorder. Reading disorders can persist into adult life, but many people with reading disorders are able to achieve personal and professional success.

Prevention

There is no known way to prevent reading disorder. Early **intervention** is the key to preventing the associated symptoms of low self-esteem, lack of interest in school, and poor behavior that often accompany low academic achievement.

Resources

BOOKS

American Psychiatric Association. *Diagnostic and Statistical Manual of Mental Disorders*. 4th ed., text rev. Washington, DC: American Psychiatric Publishing, 2000.

Hulme, Charles, and Margaret J. Snowling. *Developmental Disorders of Language Learning and Cognition*. Malden, MA: Wiley-Blackwell, 2009.

PERIODICALS

Bower, Bruce. "Dyslexia Tied to Disrupted Brain Network." *Science News* 153 (March 7, 1998): 150.

Germano, E., A. Gagliano, and P. Curatolo. "Comorbidity of ADHD and Dyslexia." *Developmental Neuropsychology* 35, no. 5 (September 2010): 475–93.

Matvy, Mike. "A Silicon Bullet for Dyslexia: A New Solution for an Old Problem." *The Exceptional Parent* 30 (November 2000) 52–56.

Waldie, K.E., and M. Hausmann. "Right Fronto-parietal Dysfunction in Children with ADHD and Developmental Dyslexia as Determined by Line Bisection Judgements." *Neuropsychologia* 48, no. 12 (October 2010): 3650–3656.

WEBSITES

Crouch, Eric R., Peter M. Dozier, and Angelo P. Giardino. "Reading Learning Disorder." Medscape Reference. http://emedicine.medscape.com/article/1835801-overview (accessed October 24, 2011).

National Center for Learning Disabilities. "What is Dyslexia?" http://www.ncld.org/ld-basics/ld-aamp-language/reading/dyslexia (accessed October 24, 2011).

U.S. National Institute of Neurological Disorders and Stroke. "NINDS Dyslexia Information Page." http://www.ninds.nih.gov/disorders/dyslexia/dyslexia.htm (accessed October 24, 2011).

ORGANIZATIONS

Learning Disabilities Association of America, 4156 Library Rd., Pittsburgh, PA, 15234-1349, (412) 341-1515, http://www.ldanatl.org.

National Center for Learning Disabilities, 381 Park Ave. South, Ste. 1401, New York, NY, 10016, (212) 545-7510, Fax: (212) 545-9665, (888) 575-7373, http://www.ncld.org.

Tish Davidson, A.M.

Reinforcement

Definition

Reinforcement is an act, process, circumstance, or condition that increases the probability of a person repeating a response. A reinforcer is a stimulus that follows some behavior and increases the probability that the behavior will occur. For example, when teaching a child to clean his room, a parent might reinforce him by giving him a reward for doing so without being reminded. The reward reinforces the desired behavior and increases the probability that the child will clean his room again in the future.

Description

In psychology, reinforcement is associated with two types of conditioning: classical (or Pavlovian) conditioning and operant (or Skinnerian) conditioning. Operant conditioning is frequently used to increase the frequency of a desired response by developing positive associations between it and a stimulus or reinforcer. **Behavior modification** uses the principles of operant conditioning or other learning techniques to improve symptoms or to increase desired behavior.

In operant conditioning (as developed by B. F. Skinner), positive reinforcers are rewards that strengthen a conditioned response after it has occurred, such as feeding a hungry pigeon after it has pecked a key. Negative reinforcers are stimuli that are removed when the desired response has been obtained. For example, when a rat is receiving an electric shock and presses a bar that stops the shock, the shock is a negative reinforcer—it is an aversive stimulus that reinforces the bar-pressing behavior. The application of negative reinforcement may be divided into two types: escape and avoidance conditioning. In escape conditioning, the subject learns to escape an unpleasant or aversive stimulus (a dog jumps over a barrier to escape electric shock). In avoidance conditioning, the subject is presented with a warning stimulus, such as a buzzer, just before the aversive stimulus occurs and learns to act on it in order to avoid the stimulus altogether.

Punishment can be used to decrease unwanted behaviors. Punishment is the application of an aversive stimulus in reaction to a particular behavior. For children, a punishment could be the removal of television privileges when they disobey their parents or teachers. The removal of the privileges follows the undesired behavior and decreases its likelihood of occurring again.

Reinforcement may be administered according to various schedules. A particular behavior may be reinforced every time it occurs, which is referred to as continuous reinforcement. In many cases, however, behaviors are reinforced only some of the time, which is termed partial or intermittent reinforcement. Reinforcement may also be based on the number of responses, or scheduled at particular time intervals. In addition, it may be delivered in regularly or irregularly. These variables combine to produce four basic types of partial reinforcement. In fixed-ratio (FR) schedules, reinforcement is provided following a set number of responses (a factory worker is paid for every garment he assembles). With variable-ratio (VR) schedules, reinforcement is provided after a variable number of responses (a slot machine pays off after varying numbers of attempts). Fixed-interval (FI) schedules provide for reinforcement of the first response made within a given interval since the previous one (contest entrants are not eligible for a prize if they have won one within the past 30 days). Finally, with variable-interval (VI) schedules, first responses are rewarded at varying intervals from the previous one.

Resources

BOOKS

Flora, Stephen Ray. *The Power of Reinforcement*. Albany, NY: State University of New York Press, 2004.

VandenBos, Gary R. ed. *APA Dictionary of Psychology*. Washington, DC: American Psychological Association, 2006.

PERIODICALS

Bogdan, Ryan, and Diego A. Pizzagalli. "Acute Stress Reduces Reward Responsiveness: Implications for Depression." *Biological Psychiatry* 60, no. 10 (November 2006): 1147–54.

Dallery, Jesse, Irene M. Glenn, and Bethany R. Raiff. "An Internet-Based Abstinence Reinforcement Treatment for Cigarette Smoking." *Drug and Alcohol Dependence* 86, no. 2–3 (January 12, 2007): 230–38.

Doran, Neal, Dennis McChargue, and Lee Cohen. "Impulsivity and the Reinforcing Value of Cigarette Smoking." *Addictive Behaviors* 32, no. 1 (January 2007): 90–98.

Fernandez, Melanie A., et al. "The Principles of Extinction and Differential Reinforcement of Other Behaviors in the

Intensive Cognitive-Behavioral Treatment of Primarily Obsessional Pediatric OCD." *Clinical Case Studies* 5, no. 6 (December 2006): 511–21.

Hand, Dennis J., Andrew T. Fox, and Mark P. Reilly. "Response Acquisition With Delayed Reinforcement in a Rodent Model of Attention-Deficit/Hyperactivity Disorder (ADHD)." *Behavioural Brain Research* 175, no. 2 (December 2006): 337–42.

Rieskamp, Jörg. "Positive and Negative Recency Effects in Retirement Savings Decisions." *Journal of Experimental Psychology: Applied* 12, no. 4 (December 2006): 233–50.

Ruth A. Wienclaw, PhD

Relapse and relapse prevention

Definition

In the course of illness, relapse is a return of symptoms after a period of time when no symptoms are present. Any strategies or treatments applied in advance to prevent future symptoms are known as relapse prevention.

Purpose

When people seek help for mental disorders, they receive treatment that, hopefully, reduces or eliminates symptoms. However, once they leave treatment, they may gradually revert to old habits and ways of living. This results in a return of symptoms known as relapse. Relapse prevention aims to teach people strategies that will maintain the wellness skills they learned while in treatment.

Prevention of relapse in mental disorders is crucial, not only because symptoms are detrimental to quality of life, but also because the occurrence of relapse increases chances for future relapses. In addition, with each relapse, symptoms tend to be more severe and have more serious consequences.

Description

Relapse is a concern with any disorder, whether physical or psychological. Cancer is a prime example of a physical condition where relapse is common, either after a short period or many years of remission (being symptom free). Psychological disorders can follow a similar pattern, and certain psychological disorders tend to have a higher rate of relapse than others. Addictive disorders, such as alcohol and drug abuse, smoking, overeating, and pathological gambling, are known for having high levels of relapse. Many addictions involve a lifestyle centered around the addictive behavior. In such cases, individuals must not only discontinue the addictive habit, they must also restructure their entire lives in order for changes to last. Such vast changes are difficult at best, approaching impossible in the worst scenarios. For example, an individual with a drug addiction may live in a neighborhood where drugs are prevalent but may lack the resources to move. According to recent statistics, relapse rates are approximately 33% for people who gamble pathologically (within three months of treatment), 90% for people who quit smoking, and 50% for people who abuse alcohol. Within one year of treatment, people struggling with obesity typically regain 30% to 50% of the weight they lost.

Common early warning signs of relapse

Behavioral changes

- Isolation, avoidance of social situations
- Changes in appetite and/or sleep patterns
- Participation in risky or dangerous behaviors (e.g., alcohol or illicit drug use)
- Increased emotional outbursts, especially when inappropriate for the situation
- Reduced energy levels
- Apathy, loss of motivation
- Disregard for personal hygiene

Cognitive changes

- Lack of concentration
- Loss of memory recall
- Trouble making decisions
- Abnormal thought patterns—racing, slowed, or jumbled
- Constant pessimism and negativity
- Hearing voices
- Thoughts or acts of self-harm
- Excessive dwelling on past events with thoughts of regret

Emotional changes

- Anxiety
- Aggressive behavior
- Depression
- Restlessness
- Increased irritability
- Paranoia

SOURCE: Julie O'Sullivan and Jillian Gilbert, "Early Warning Signs," Inner North Brisbane Mental Health Service, Royal Brisbane Hospital.

Report available online at http://www.health.qld.gov.au/rbwh/docs/early_warning_signs.pdf. *(Table by PreMediaGlobal. © 2012 Cengage Learning.)*

Affective disorders, such as **depression** and anxiety, also have high rates of relapse. People with affective disorders are thought to engage in self-defeating, negative thought patterns that occur more or less automatically. These thought patterns affect behavior, resulting in unproductive or negative consequences. Negative consequences are regarded by such individuals as proof that their original self-defeating thoughts must be correct. The thought-behavior pattern becomes a repetitive cycle, with negative thoughts resulting in negative behavioral outcomes, and consequences of negative behavior encouraging more self-defeating thoughts. This cycle is extremely difficult to break, because it becomes a habitual way of responding to the world that occurs almost without awareness. Relapse rates for depression are reportedly as high as 80%.

Serious psychiatric disorders such as **bipolar disorder** and **schizophrenia** have high rates of relapse, especially when the conditions are not properly treated. According to the World Federation for Mental Health, rates for bipolar disorder are approximately 40%–50% after one year without a **manic episode** and 70%–75% after five years without episode. In patients with schizophrenia, the risk of relapse is reduced to 20% when treated with antipsychotic drugs, compared to 60% taking a placebo. Without continuing treatment, up to 90% of patients relapse within two years, and 80% of patients who discontinue medication after experiencing an episode will relapse.

Relapse among people who commit sex offenses is a constant safety concern for those in the community. However, some statistics show that this population has a very low rate of relapse. A report by Robin J. Wilson and colleagues indicated rates as low as 3.7% to 6.3%. This same report stated that, among various criminal offenses, those who commit sex offenses relapse at lower rates than those who commit general offenses. Other professionals may not necessarily agree with this study, however. Those who commit sex offenses are considered at a higher risk for relapse if they display little insight into the impact of their crime. Those at high risk of committing a sex offense are not typically released back into the community.

For many types of disorders, initial treatment is often effective at eliminating the unwanted behavior. However, these effects are rarely maintained long-term without some type of preventive planning. Results of medications are similar; symptoms are alleviated, but once the medication is discontinued, symptoms return unless the individual has had some type of training in coping with his or her disorder and that training has been effective. There are various forms of relapse prevention training. Most follow a similar pattern with and employ the following common elements:

- Identifying high-risk situations: Symptoms are often initiated by particular times, places, people, or events. For example, a person with agoraphobia is more likely to experience symptoms of panic in a crowded building. An essential key to preventing relapse is to be aware of the specific situations where one feels vulnerable. These situations are called "triggers," because they trigger the onset of symptoms. While people with the same mental disorder may share similar triggers, triggers can also be highly individual. People tend to react—sometimes unknowingly—to negative experiences in their past. For example, a woman who was sexually abused as a child may have negative emotions when in the presence of men who resemble her abuser. Because some triggers occur without conscious awareness, individuals may not know all their triggers. Many prevention programs encourage individuals to closely monitor their behavior, reflecting on situations where symptoms occurred and determining what was happening immediately before the onset of symptoms. With this kind of analysis, a pattern often emerges that gives clues about the trigger.
- Learning alternate ways to respond to high-risk situations: Once triggers have been identified, one must find new ways of coping with those situations. The easiest coping mechanism for high-risk situations is to avoid them altogether. This may include avoiding certain people who have a negative influence or avoiding locations where the symptom is likely to occur. In some instances, avoidance is a good strategy. For example, individuals who abuse alcohol may successfully reduce their risk by avoiding bars or parties. In other instances, avoidance is not possible or advisable. For example, individuals attempting to lose weight may notice that they are more likely to binge at certain times during the day. One cannot avoid a time of day. Rather, by being aware of this trigger, one can purposely engage in alternate activities during that time. Strategies for coping with unavoidable triggers are generally skills that need to be learned and practiced in order to be effective. Strategies include—but are not limited to—discussion of feelings, whether with a friend, counselor, or via a hotline; distraction, such as music, exercise, or engaging in a hobby; refocusing techniques, such as meditation, deep-breathing exercises, progressive muscle relaxation (focusing on each muscle group separately, and routinely tensing then relaxing that muscle), prayer, or journaling; and cognitive restructuring, such as positive affirmation statements (such as, "I am worthwhile"), active problem solving (defining the problem, generating possible solutions, identifying the consequences of those solutions, choosing the best solution), challenging the validity of negative thoughts, or guided imagery (imagining oneself in a different place or handling a situation appropriately).
- Creating a plan for healthy living: Besides being prepared for high-risk situations, relapse prevention also focuses on general principles of mental health that, if followed, greatly reduce the likelihood of symptoms. These include factors such as balanced nutrition, regular exercise, sufficient sleep, health education, reciprocally caring relationships, productive and recreational interests, and spiritual development.

- Developing a support system: Many research studies have demonstrated the importance of social support in maintaining a healthy lifestyle. Individuals who are socially isolated tend to display more symptoms of mental disorders. Conversely, individuals with mental disorders tend to have more difficultly initiating and maintaining relationships due to inappropriate social behavior. For such people, a support system may be nonexistent. Research suggests that support systems are most effective when they are naturally occurring—in other words, when a circle of family and friends who genuinely care about the individual is already in place. However, artificially created support systems are certainly better than none at all. For this reason, relapse prevention programs strive to involve family members and other significant persons in the treatment program. Everyone in the support system should be knowledgeable about the person's goals, what that person is like when he or she is doing well, and warning signs that the person may be on a path toward relapse. The support system agrees on who will take what role in encouraging, confronting, or otherwise caring for that person. Self-help groups such as Alcoholics Anonymous or Moderation Management are often examples of artificially created support systems.
- Preparing for possible relapse: Although the ultimate goal of relapse prevention is to avoid relapse altogether, statistics demonstrate that relapse potential is very real. Individuals need to be aware that, even when exerting their best efforts, they may occasionally experience lapses (one occurrence of a symptom or behavior) or relapses (return to a previous, undesirable level of symptoms or behavior). Acknowledging the potential for relapse is important, because many people consider a lapse or relapse as evidence of personal failure and give up completely. In their widely acclaimed book for professionals, *Motivational Interviewing*, William R. Miller and Stephen Rollnick cite a study by Prochaska and DiClemente that found that smokers typically relapse between three and seven times before quitting for good. From the perspective of Miller and Rollnick, each relapse can be a step closer to full recovery if relapse is used as a learning experience to improve prevention strategies. Although some argue that such a tolerant attitude invites relapse, general consensus is that individuals need to forgive themselves if relapse occurs and then move on. Some prevention programs include designing a crisis plan to be put into effect if a relapse occurs. The crisis plan involves specific actions to be taken by the individual or members of the support system.

These elements are common to all relapse prevention programs, but programs can be further customized to meet the particular characteristics of a disorder. For example, prevention of depression or anxiety may focus on becoming aware of thoughts as passing mental events rather than facts about self or reality. Learning to identify bodily sensations that accompany maladaptive thoughts is also important for preventing depression and anxiety. Addictive disorders concentrate on reactions to social pressure, interpersonal

KEY TERMS

Addictive disorder—A disorder involving repetitive participation in a certain activity, in spite of negative consequences and despite attempts to stop the behavior. Alcohol abuse is an example.

Affective disorder—A disorder involving extreme emotional experience that is not congruent with the environmental circumstances (for example, feeling sad when there is no easily identifiable reason, as in depression).

Cognitive restructuring—An approach to psychotherapy that focuses on helping the patient examine distorted patterns of perceiving and thinking in order to change their emotional responses to people and situations.

Guided imagery—Techniques where individuals actively imagine themselves in a scene (usually a different location, such as a relaxing beach, or a trigger situation where one handles the situation successfully), typically guided by another person describing the scene.

Lapse—A single, isolated occurrence of a symptom or negative behavior.

Positive affirmation statements—Statements repeated to oneself, either aloud or mentally, that reflect attitudes of self-worth.

Progressive muscle relaxation—Relaxation exercises where one slowly tenses and then relaxes each muscle group separately in a systematic order.

Refocusing techniques—Techniques that direct one's attention away from overwhelming, negative thoughts and emotions by focusing on inner peace and managing one issue at a time.

Remission—In the course of an illness or disorder, a period of time when symptoms are absent.

Trigger—Any situation (people, places, times, events, etc.) that causes one to experience a negative emotional reaction, which is often accompanied by a display of symptoms or problematic behavior.

conflicts, and negative emotional states as part of a relapse prevention plan.

Preparation

As with any type of therapeutic treatment, success of relapse prevention programs depend heavily on motivation. If an individual is not interested in making life changes, he or she is not likely to follow a prevention plan. Individuals low in motivation may need to participate in group or individual **psychotherapy** before deciding whether to enter a relapse prevention program.

Aftercare

Aftercare typically consists of participation in **support groups**. For addictions, 12-step groups (such as Alcoholics Anonymous) are most commonly recommended. These types of groups can be attended daily. Support groups exist for other types of mental disorders, and may be run by peers or a professional facilitator. Aftercare groups, usually run in treatment facilities by professional staff, may be used to continue practicing skills and to trouble-shoot problems individuals are experiencing with their prevention plans in everyday life. Aftercare groups usually meet less frequently (once a week or month) and may gradually taper off. Some relapse-prevention programs may use telephone contacts or individual therapy sessions to help individuals continue to use prevention skills effectively.

Results

Successful relapse prevention programs will empower individuals to make choices about how they respond in stressful, high-risk situations (triggers) rather than responding in habitual, unhealthy ways. Individuals should be aware of their personal triggers, use positive strategies for coping with **stress**, practice healthy lifestyle choices, involve others in their efforts, and have a realistic attitude regarding relapse. Use of these prevention skills should reduce symptoms and increase the time span between occurrences of lapses or relapses.

If an individual is unmotivated to make life changes, or a relapse prevention program has been ineffective, that individual will demonstrate few (if any) of the prevention skills learned. The individual will show little improvement in symptomatic or problematic behavior. Periods of remission (symptom-free behavior) will be short and relapses will occur frequently.

Resources

BOOKS

Copeland, Mary Ellen. *Winning Against Relapse: A Workbook of Action Plans for Recurring Health and Emotional Problems*. Oakland, CA: New Harbinger Publications, 1999.

Miller, William R. and Stephen Rollnick. *Motivational Interviewing: Preparing People to Change Addictive Behavior*. New York: Guilford Press, 1991.

PERIODICALS

Brandon, Thomas H., et al. "Preventing Relapse Among Former Smokers: A Comparison of Minimal Interventions Through Telephone and Mail." *Journal of Consulting and Clinical Psychology* 68, no. 1 (February 2000): 103–113.

Carich, Mark S., John F. Newbauer, and Mark H. Stone. "Using Relapse Intervention Strategies to Treat Sexual Offenders." *Journal of Individual Psychology* 57, no. 1 (Spring 2001): 26–36.

Echeburua, Enrique, Javier Fernandez-Montalvo, and Concepcion Baez. "Relapse Prevention in the Treatment of Slot-Machine Pathological Gambling: Long-Term Outcome." *Behavior Therapy* 31, no. 2 (2000): 351–364.

Hartzler, Bryan, and Chris Brownson. "The Utility of Change Models in the Design and Delivery of Thematic Group Interventions: Applications to a Self-Defeating Behaviors Group." *Group Dynamics: Theory, Research, and Practice* 5, no. 3 (September 2001): 191–199.

Monti, Peter M., and Damaris J. Rohsenow. "Coping Skills Training and Cue-Exposure Therapy in the Treatment of Alcoholism." *Alcohol Research and Health* 23, no. 2 (Spring 1999): 107–115.

Perri, Michael G., et al. "Relapse Prevention Training and Problem-Solving Therapy in the Long-Term Management of Obesity." *Journal of Consulting and Clinical Psychology* 69, no. 4 (August 2000): 722–726.

Teasdale, John D., et al. "Prevention of Relapse/Recurrence in Major Depression by Mindfulness-Based Cognitive Therapy." *Journal of Consulting and Clinical Psychology* 68, no. 4 (2000): 615–623.

Wilson, Robin J., et al. "Community-Based Sex Offender Management: Combining Parole Supervision and Treatment to Reduce Recidivism." *Canadian Journal of Criminology* 42, no. 2 (2000): 177–188.

OTHER

World Federation for Mental Health. "Serious Mental Illness: Symptoms, Treatment and Causes of Relapse." http://www.wfmh.org/PDF/KEEPINGCARE/Serious%20Mental%20Illness%20fact%20sheet.pdf (accessed October 11, 2011).

ORGANIZATIONS

National Institute of Mental Health, 6001 Executive Blvd., Room 8184, MSC 9663, Bethesda, MD, 20892-9663, (301) 433-4513; TTY: (301) 443-8431, Fax: (301) 443-4279, (866) 615-6464; TTY: (866) 415-8051, nimhinfo@nih.gov, http://www.nimh.nih.gov.

National Institute on Alcohol Abuse and Alcoholism, 5635 Fishers Lane, MSC 9304, Bethesda, MD, 20892-9304, http://www.niaaa.nih.gov.

National Institute on Drug Abuse, 6001 Executive Blvd., Room 5213, Bethesda, MD, 20892, (301) 442-1124; Spanish: (240) 221-4007, information@nida.nih.gov, http://www.nida.nih.gov.

Sandra L. Friedrich, M.A.

Relaxation therapy

Definition

Relaxation therapy is a broad term used to describe a number of techniques that promote **stress reduction**, the elimination of tension throughout the body, and a calm and peaceful state of mind.

Purpose

Relaxation therapy as a general term includes various forms: transcendental **meditation** (TM), **yoga**, tai chi, qigong, and vipassana (a Buddhist form of meditation meaning insight and also known as mindfulness meditation). Progressive relaxation, a treatment that is designed to rid the body of anxiety and related tension through progressive relaxation of the muscle groups, was first described by Edmund Jacobson in his 1929 book *Progressive Relaxation*. In 1975, Herbert Benson published his groundbreaking work *The Relaxation Response*, which described in detail the stress-reduction mechanism in the body that short-circuits the fight-or-flight response and lowers blood pressure, relieves muscle tension, and controls heart rate. This work gave further credence and legitimacy to the link between mind and body medicine. A number of commonly used relaxation techniques, such as cue-controlled relaxation, are a direct result of Benson's work in this area.

Description

A number of different relaxation methods are available. Some of the most widely taught and most frequently practiced by healthcare providers are progressive relaxation, cue-controlled relaxation, breathing exercises, guided imagery, and **biofeedback**.

Progressive relaxation

Progressive relaxation is performed by first tensing and then relaxing the muscles of the body, one group at a time. Muscle groups can be divided a number of different ways, but a common method is to use the following groupings: (a) hands and arms; (b) head, neck, and shoulders; (c) torso, including chest, stomach and back; and (d) buttocks, thighs, lower legs, and feet. The patient lies or sits in a comfortable position and then starts with the first muscle group, focusing on the feeling of the muscles and the absence or presence of tension. The patient then tenses the first muscle in the group, holds the tension for approximately five seconds, and releases and relaxes for up to 30 seconds. The contrast allows the individual to notice difference between feelings of tension and those of relaxation. The procedure is repeated with the next muscle in the group and so on, until the first group is completed. The patient then starts on the next muscle group.

Progressive relaxation can be guided with verbal cues and scripts, either memorized by the patient or provided on instructional audiotapes. The procedure remains the same, but the individual is prompted on which muscles to flex and relax and given other cues about noticing the difference between the tense and relaxed state. Some individuals may prefer progressive relaxation that is prompted with a tape because it allows them to completely clear their minds and to just follow instructions.

Deep breathing exercises

Individuals under **stress** often experience fast, shallow breathing. This type of breathing, known as chest breathing, can lead to shortness of breath, increased muscle tension, and inadequate oxygenation of blood. Breathing exercises can both improve respiratory function and relieve stress and tension.

Before starting to learn breathing exercises, individuals should first become aware of their breathing patterns. This can be accomplished by placing one hand on the chest and one hand on the abdomen and observing which hand moves further during breathing. If it is the hand placed on the chest, then chest breathing is occurring, and breathing exercises may be beneficial.

Deep breathing exercises are best performed while lying flat on the back, usually on the floor with a mat. The knees are bent, and the body (particularly the mouth, nose, and face) is relaxed. One hand is placed on the chest and one on the abdomen to monitor breathing technique. The individual takes a series of long, deep breaths through the nose, attempting to raise the abdomen instead of the chest. Air is exhaled through the relaxed mouth. Deep breathing can be continued for up to 20 minutes. After the **exercise** is complete, the individual checks again for body tension and relaxation. Once deep breathing techniques have been mastered, an individual can use deep breathing at any time or place as a quick method of relieving tension.

Release-only relaxation

Like progressive relaxation, release-only relaxation focuses on relieving feelings of tension in the muscles.

However, it eliminates the initial use of muscle tensing as practiced in progressive relaxation, focusing instead solely on muscle relaxation. Release-only relaxation is usually recommended as the next step in relaxation therapy after progressive relaxation has been mastered.

In release-only relaxation, breathing is used as a relaxation tool. The individual sits in a comfortable chair and begins to focus on breathing, envisioning tension leaving the body with each exhale. Once deep abdominal breathing is established, the individual begins to focus on releasing tension in each muscle group, until the entire body is completely relaxed.

Cue-controlled relaxation

Cue-controlled relaxation is an abbreviated tension-relief technique that combines elements of release-only relaxation and deep breathing exercises. It uses a cue, such as a word or mental image, to trigger immediate feelings of muscle relaxation. The cue must first be associated with relaxation in the individual's mind. Individuals choose the cue and then use it in breathing and release-only relaxation exercises repeatedly until the cue starts to automatically trigger feelings of relaxation outside the treatment sessions. Cues can be as simple as a given word such as "one" and are frequently used on relaxation audiotapes. They can also be a visual cue, such as a mental image of a white sand beach, a flower-filled meadow, or clear blue sky. Guided imagery also uses visualization exercises to produce feelings of relaxation.

Guided imagery

Guided imagery is a two-part process. The first component involves reaching a state of deep relaxation through breathing and muscle relaxation techniques. During the relaxation phase, individuals close their eyes and focus on the slow in and out of their breath. Instead, individuals might focus on releasing the feelings of tension from their muscles, starting with the toes and working up to the top of the head. Relaxation tapes often feature soft music or tranquil, natural sounds such as rolling waves and chirping birds in order to promote feelings of relaxation.

Once complete relaxation is achieved, the second component of the exercise is the imagery, or visualization, itself. Relaxation imagery involves conjuring pleasant images that rest the mind and body. These may be past experiences or idealized new situations.

The individual may also use mental rehearsal. Mental rehearsal involves imagining a situation or scenario and its ideal outcome. It can be used to reduce anxiety about an upcoming situation, such as childbirth, surgery, or even a critical event such as an important competition or a job interview. Individuals imagine themselves going through each step of the event, visualizing harmony and good will in the whole process and positive outcome.

> **KEY TERMS**
>
> **Qigong**—An exercise practice derived from traditional Chinese medicine and designed to facilitate energy flow throughout the body.
>
> **Tai chi**—A martial art that uses exercise to balance the body's energy flow to the body center in order to promote physical well-being.

Biofeedback

Biofeedback, or applied psychophysiological feedback, is a patient-guided treatment that teaches individuals to manipulate muscle tension through relaxation, visualization, and other cognitive techniques. The term biofeedback refers to the biological signals that are fed back, or returned, to the individual in order for that person to develop the relaxation techniques.

During biofeedback, one or more special sensors are placed on the body. These sensors measure muscle tension, **brain** waves, heart rate, and body temperature, and translate the information into a visual and/or audible readout, such as a paper tracing, a light display, or a series of beeps. While viewing the instantaneous feedback from the biofeedback monitors, the individual begins to recognize what thoughts, fears, and mental images influence physical reactions. By monitoring this relationship between mind and body, the individual can then use thoughts and mental images deliberately to manipulate heart beat, brain wave patterns, body temperature, and other bodily functions, and to reduce feelings of stress. This is achieved through relaxation exercises, mental imagery, and other cognitive therapy techniques.

As the biofeedback response takes place, the individual can actually see or hear the results of the relaxation efforts instantly through the sensor readout on the biofeedback equipment. Once these techniques are learned and the individual is able to recognize the state of relaxation or visualization necessary to alleviate symptoms, the biofeedback equipment itself is no longer needed. The person then has a powerful, self-administered treatment technique for dealing with problem symptoms.

Dozens of other effective therapies promote relaxation, including hypnosis, meditation, yoga, **aromatherapy**, hydrotherapy, tai chi, massage, **art therapy**, and others. Individuals should choose a type of relaxation therapy based on their own interests and lifestyle.

HERBERT BENSON (1935–)

Dr. Herbert Benson, the guru of mind/body medicine, was born in 1935. He graduated from Wesleyan University and the Harvard School of Medicine. He nurtured his interest in mind/body relationships and developed expertise in behavioral medicine and spiritual healing. In his research, Benson straddled the thin line between medicine and religion. He conceived of what he called a three-legged approach to health care: self-care, pharmaceuticals, and medical treatment or surgery. His most significant work was his discovery of the relaxation response, which is the connection between lowered blood pressure and transcendental meditation. He was quoted by Daphne Howland of BeWell.com saying that "[B] elief is one of the most powerful healing tools we have in our therapeutic arsenal."

Benson served as the Mind/Body Institute associate professor of medicine at Harvard School of Medical and worked as the chief of the Division of Behavioral Medicine at the Beth Israel Deaconess Medical Center in Boston, Massachusetts. In 1988 he founded the Mind/Body Medical Institute in Boston, where he served as founding president. He lectured extensively about his work. On November 5, 1997, Benson addressed the Committee on Appropriations of the U.S. House of Representatives and spoke on the topic of "Healing and the Mind." Benson authored scores of scientific papers along with six books pertaining to his years of study, including *The Mind/Body Effect* in 1979, *Relaxation Response* in 1990, and *Timeless Healing: The Power and Biology of Belief* in 1996. Altogether his books sold over four million copies. Among his many honors and awards, Benson received the John Templeton Spirituality and Medicine Curricular Award in 1999.

Benefits

Stress and tension have been linked to numerous ailments, including heart disease, high blood pressure, atherosclerosis, irritable bowel syndrome, ulcers, **anxiety disorders**, **insomnia**, and **substance abuse**. Stress can also trigger a number of distinct physical symptoms, including nausea, headache, hair loss, **fatigue**, and muscle pain. Relaxation therapies have been shown to reduce the incidence and severity of stress-related diseases and disorders in many patients.

Preparations

When considering relaxation therapy to alleviate physical symptoms such as nausea, headache, high blood pressure, fatigue, or gastrointestinal problems, individuals should consult a doctor first to make sure that an underlying disorder or disease is not causing the symptoms. A complete physical examination and comprehensive medical history will be performed, and even if an organic cause for the symptoms is found, relaxation exercises may still be recommended as an adjunct, or complementary, treatment to relieve discomfort.

Relaxation therapy should always take place in a quiet, relaxing atmosphere in which the person has a comfortable place to sit or recline. Some people find that quiet background music improves their relaxation sessions. If an instructional audiotape or videotape is to be used, the appropriate equipment should be available.

The relaxation session, which can last from a few minutes to an hour, should be uninterrupted. Taking the phone off the hook, turning off cell phones, dimming the lights, and asking family members for privacy and silence can ensure a more successful and relaxing session.

Precautions

Most commonly practiced relaxation techniques are completely safe and free of side effects.

Relaxation techniques that involve special exercises or body manipulation such as massage, tai chi, and yoga should be taught or performed by a qualified healthcare professional or instructor. These treatments may not be suitable for individuals with certain health conditions such as arthritis or fibromyalgia. These individuals should consult with their healthcare professional before engaging in such therapies.

Biofeedback may not be recommended in some individuals who use a pacemaker or other implantable electrical devices. These individuals should inform their biofeedback therapist before starting treatments, as certain types of biofeedback sensors have the potential to interfere with implantable devices.

QUESTIONS TO ASK YOUR DOCTOR

- In what way do you think relaxation therapy will benefit me?
- What tests or evaluation techniques will you perform to see if relaxation therapy has been beneficial for me?
- What other treatment options do you recommend for me?
- Will relaxation therapy interfere with my current medications?
- What symptoms or behaviors are important enough that I should seek immediate treatment?

Relaxation therapy may not be suitable for some patients. Patients must be willing to take an active role in the treatment process and to practice techniques learned in treatment at home.

Some relaxation therapies may also be inappropriate for cognitively impaired individuals (e.g., patients with organic brain disease or a **traumatic brain injury**) depending on their level of functioning. Given the wide range of relaxation therapies available, if one type of relaxation treatment is deemed inappropriate for these patients, a suitable alternative can usually be recommended by a qualified healthcare professional.

Side effects

Relaxation therapy can induce sleepiness, and some individuals may fall asleep during a session. Relaxation therapy should not be performed while a person is operating a motor vehicle or in other situations in which full and alert attention is necessary. Other than this, there are no known adverse side effects to relaxation therapy.

Research and general acceptance

Relaxation therapies are generally well-accepted by the medical community for relief of stress and anxiety.

Some research has also indicated that relaxation therapy may be useful for certain physiological conditions. One study, for example, reported results indicating that relaxation therapy reduced the incidence of preterm labor in women at risk for delivering prematurely. It also found that women who discontinued relaxation exercises for whatever reasons delivered earlier and had lower birth-weight babies than those who continued the treatment. Positive benefits of relaxation therapy have also been reported for persons who have high blood pressure. Another study of 90 individuals who had previously experienced a heart attack reported a more favorable long-term outcome among the patients when they underwent both relaxation therapy and exercise training than exercise training alone. In 2006, researchers conducted a study of the therapy's impact on patients with chronic heart failure. For the study, 121 patients were split into control and experimental groups, with the experimental group receiving training in progressive muscle relaxation. The experimental group reported greater reduction in psychological distress compared to the control group. The researchers concluded that the training might be useful as part of a disease-management program for these patients, although further research would be necessary to discover if any other benefits could be attributed to the relaxation therapy.

Not all research supports relaxation therapy as a treatment option. A report published in 2001 reviewed numerous studies of the effectiveness of relaxation therapies on bronchial asthma. The report concluded that "little evidence in its favor has been presented." It noted, however, that healthcare professionals "continue to include relaxation training as a component in the nonpharmacological treatment of asthma."

Training and certification

Relaxation therapy techniques are used by many licensed therapists, counselors, psychologists, psychiatrists, and other healthcare professionals. Many self-help books, audiotapes, and videos are available that give instruction in relaxation techniques.

Resources

BOOKS

Bear, Marina. *The Little Book of Meditation: A Guide to Stress-Free Living*. Berkeley, CA: SLG Books, 2009.

Davis, Martha, E. R. Eshelman, and Matthew McKay. *The Relaxation & Stress Reduction Workbook*, 6th ed. Oakland, CA: New Harbinger Publications, 2009.

Devereux, Charla. *Aromatherapy: The Essence of Well-being (Book-in-a-Box)*. Wilmington, DE: Tower.com, Inc., 2011.

Schenkman, Steven. *Massage Therapy: What It Is and How It Works*. Florence, KY; Cengage Learning, 2009.

PERIODICALS

Yu, Doris. "Abstract 2506: Relaxation Therapy in Patients with Chronic Heart Failure: A Randomized Controlled Trial." *Circulation* 114 (2006): 517.

ORGANIZATIONS

American Psychological Association, 750 1st Street NE, Washington, DC, 20002-4242, (202) 336-5500; TDD/

TTY: (202) 336-6123, (800) 374-2721, http://www.apa.org.

National Association of Holistic Aromatherapy, PO Box 1868, Banner Elk, NC, 28604, (828) 898-6161, Fax: (828) 898-1965, info@naha.org, http://www.naha.org.

Paula Ford-Martin
Laura Jean Cataldo, RN, EdD

Remeron *see* **Mirtazapine**

Respite

Definition

Respite literally means a period of rest or relief. Respite care provides a caregiver temporary relief from the responsibilities of caring for individuals with chronic physical or mental disabilities.

Purpose

Respite was developed in response to the **deinstitutionalization** movement of the 1960s and 1970s. Maintaining individuals in their natural homes rather than placing them in long-term care facilities was viewed as beneficial to the individual, the involved family, and society (in terms of lowered healthcare costs). The primary purpose of respite care is to relieve the **stress** felt by caregivers, enabling them to continue caring for the individual.

Respite care is typically provided for individuals with disorders related to aging (**dementia**, frail health), terminal illnesses, chronic health issues, or developmental disabilities. More recently, children with behavior disorders have also been eligible for respite care. Respite care is usually recreational and does not include therapy or treatment.

Description

Caregivers frequently experience stress in the forms of physical **fatigue**, psychological distress (resentment, frustration, anxiety, guilt, **depression**), and disruption in relations with other family members. The emotional aspects of caring for a family member are often more taxing than the physical demands. Increased caregiver stress may result in health problems such as ulcers, high blood pressure, difficulty sleeping, weight loss or gain, or breathing difficulties. Respite care offers caregivers the opportunity to relax and destress so that they are able to resume their roles.

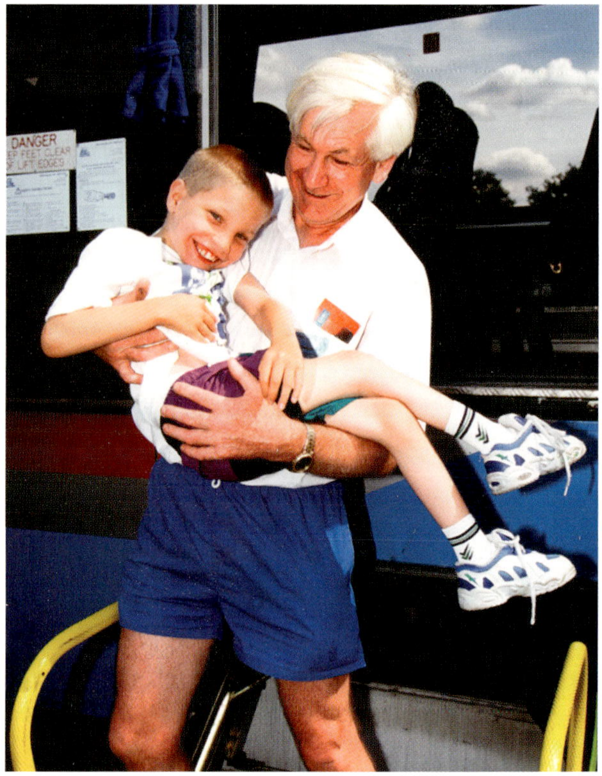

A respite caregiver carries a boy off of a bus after a camping trip for the disabled. *(© Photofusion Picture Library/ Alamy)*

Length of respite care can be anywhere from a few hours to several weeks. Services may be used frequently or infrequently, such as for emergencies, vacations, one day per week or month, weekends, or everyday. A variety of services are available, and the type of service is often closely related to the characteristics of the facility:

- In-home respite services consist of a worker who comes to the family home while the caregiver is away. These services are usually provided by agencies that recruit, screen, and train workers. This type of respite is usually less disruptive to the individual with the disability, provided there is a good match between the worker and the patient. However, concerns over the reliability and trustworthiness of the worker can be an additional source of stress for the caregiver.
- Respite centers are residential facilities specifically designed for respite care. Adult day care programs and respite camps also fall into this category. This type of respite offers more peace of mind to the caregiver and may provide a stimulating environment for the individual with the disability. However, centers usually restrict length of stay and may exclude individuals based on severity of disability.

- Institutional settings sometimes reserve spaces to be used for respite purposes. These include skilled nursing facilities, intermediate care facilities, group homes, senior housing, regular day care or after-school programs for children, and hospitals. Some of these facilities provide higher levels of care but are less "home-like." The individual with the disability may oppose staying in an institutional setting or may fear abandonment.
- Licensed foster care providers can also provide respite services in their homes.

Funding

Costs of respite care present a financial burden to many families. **Community mental health** centers often fund respite services if the individual meets certain criteria, including eligibility for Medicaid. Wraparound programs (also accessed through community mental health centers) for children with emotional or behavioral disorders also pay for respite services. Veteran's Administration hospitals provide respite care at little or no charge if the individual receiving the care is a veteran (but not if the caregiver is a veteran). Private insurance companies rarely pay for respite, and many respite providers do not accept this form of payment. Some respite facilities have sliding-scale fees. Other facilities operate as a co-op, where caregivers work at the facility in exchange for respite services.

In addition, respite agencies may have difficulty recruiting and retaining qualified employees, because limited funding prevents agencies from offering desirable salaries. The high turnover and unavailability of employees may result in delays in service delivery or family dissatisfaction with services. Advocacy for policy changes regarding funding is needed.

Barriers to using respite services

Recent research suggests that families who use respite tend to have higher levels of perceived stress, lower levels of support from others, and fewer resources. In many of these families, the individuals in need of care have more severe disabilities, problem behaviors such as aggression or self-injury, and communication difficulties; are school-aged; and are more dependent for basic needs such as eating, toileting, and dressing.

It has been well documented that many families eligible for respite care never utilize these services. Many caregivers obtain respite in informal ways not offered by respite services. Some researchers have suggested that respite care should be just one form of service available to caregivers, with other possible services including home-delivered meals, transportation assistance, recreational resources, or care skills training. Additional reasons for the non-utilization of respite care include:

- Unfamiliarity. Some families are unaware that such services exist, or may be uncertain about how to access services. This implies a need for improved referral services.
- Funding. Limited funding may prevent some families from receiving services.
- Caregiver qualities. Some caregivers experience guilt or anxiety over allowing someone else to care for their loved one. Being able to maintain one's family independently may be tied to gender roles or cultural

KEY TERMS

Behavior disorders—Disorders characterized by disruptive behaviors such as conduct disorder, oppositional defiant disorder, and attention deficit hyperactivity disorder.

Deinstitutionalization—The process of moving people out of mental hospitals and into treatment programs or halfway houses in local communities. With this movement, the responsibility for care shifted from large (often governmental) agencies to families and community organizations.

Developmental disabilities—Disabilities that are present from birth and that delay or prevent normal development, such as intellectual disability or autism.

Intermediate care facility—An inpatient facility that provides periodic nursing care.

Medicaid—A program jointly funded by state and federal governments that reimburses hospitals and physicians for the care of individuals who cannot pay for their own medical expenses. These individuals may be in low-income households or may have chronic disabilities.

Skilled nursing facility—An inpatient facility that provides 24-hour nursing services to individuals in need of extended care.

Veteran's Administration hospitals—Medical facilities operated by the federal government explicitly for veterans of the U.S. military.

Wraparound programs—A relatively new form of mental health service delivery that strives to accommodate all family members based on self-defined needs, flexibly incorporating both formal and informal community services.

customs. Relatives and friends may assist in caregiving, making formal respite unnecessary.

- Care recipient qualities. Occasionally the individual with the disability is opposed to respite care; he or she may not trust strangers or may refuse to leave home. In other instances, the individual may have special needs, such as certain behaviors or physical care, that are too challenging for the respite provider to address.
- Program qualities. Many researchers believe that respite programs are not adequately meeting the needs of families. In some cases, times that services are offered are inconvenient. Individuals with severe disabilities who pose the most need for services are sometimes excluded.

In 2006, the U.S. Congress introduced the Lifespan Respite Care Program. The program promotes the funding of respite services, in order to benefit overall care. Objectives of the program include expanding and improving the quality of respite care programs, improving the execution of services among programs, and increasing access to programs. As of 2011, 30 states had been granted funds for respite care programs.

Resources

BOOKS

Ownby, Lisa L., et al. *Partners Plus: Families and Caregivers in Partnerships: A Family-Centered Guide to Respite Care*. Washington, DC: Child Development Resources, U.S. Department of Education, Early Education Program for Children with Disabilities, 1999.

Tepper, Lynn M. and John A. Toner, eds. *Respite Care: Programs, Problems, and Solutions*. Philadelphia: The Charles Press, 1993.

PERIODICALS

Chan, Jeffrey B., and Jeff Sigafoos. "A Review of Child and Family Characteristics Related to the Use of Respite Care in Developmental Disability Services." *Child and Youth Care Forum* 29, no. 1 (2000): 27–37.

Chappell, Neena L., R. Colin Reid, and Elizabeth Dow. "Respite Reconsidered: A Typology of Meanings Based on the Caregiver's Point of View." *Journal of Aging Studies* 15, no. 2 (2001): 201–216.

ORGANIZATIONS

ARCH National Respite Network and Resource Center, Chapel Hill Training-Outreach Project, 800 Eastowne Drive, Ste. 105, Chapel Hill, NC, 27514, (919) 490-5577, Fax: (919) 490-4905, http://www.chtop.com.

National Aging Information Center, One Massachusetts Ave. NW, Washington, DC, 20001, (202) 619-0724 Fax: (202) 357-3555, aoainfo@aoa.hhs.gov, http://www.aoa.gov.

National Dissemination Center for Children with Disabilities, 1825 Connecticut Ave NW, Ste. 700, Washington, DC, 20009, (202) 884-8200, Fax: (202) 884-8441, http://www.nichcy.org.

The Arc National Headquarters, 1660 L Street, NW, Ste. 301, Washington, DC, 20036, (202) 534-3700, Fax: (202) 534-3731, info@thearc.org, http://www.thearc.org.

Sandra L. Friedrich, M.A.

Response prevention *see* **Exposure treatment**

Restless legs syndrome

Definition

Restless legs syndrome (RLS) is a neurological disorder characterized by uncomfortable sensations in the legs and, less commonly, the arms. These sensations are exacerbated (heightened) when the person with RLS is at rest. The sensations are described as crawly, tingly, prickly and occasionally painful. They result in a nearly insuppressible urge to move around. Symptoms are often associated with sleep disturbances.

Demographics

As much as 10% of the population of the United States and Europe may suffer from some degree of restless legs syndrome. Fewer cases are indicated in India, Japan and Singapore, suggesting racial or ethnic factors play a role in the disorder. Although the demographics can vary greatly, the majority of people suffering from RLS are female. The age of onset also varies greatly, but the number of people suffering from RLS increases with age. However, many people with RLS report that they had symptoms of the disorder in their childhood. These symptoms were often disregarded as growing pains or hyperactivity. In addition, some evidence suggests that there is a genetic component to RLS and it may run in families.

Description

Restless legs syndrome is a sensory-motor disorder that causes uncomfortable feelings in the legs, especially during periods of inactivity. Some people also report sensations in the arms, but this occurs much more rarely. The sensations occur deep in the legs and are usually described with terms that imply movement such as prickly, creepy-crawly, boring, itching, achy, pulling, tugging and painful. The symptoms result in an irrepressible urge to move the leg and are relieved when the person suffering from RLS voluntarily moves. Symptoms tend to be worse in the evening or at night.

Restless legs syndrome is associated with another disorder called periodic limb movements in sleep (PLMS). It is estimated that four out of five patients with RLS also suffer from PLMS. PLMS is characterized by jerking leg movements while sleeping that may occur as frequently as every 20 seconds. These jerks disrupt sleep by causing continual arousals throughout the night.

People with both RLS and PLMS are prone to abnormal levels of exhaustion during the day because they are unable to sleep properly at night. They may have trouble concentrating at work, at school or during social activities. They may also have mood swings and difficulty with interpersonal relationships. **Depression** and anxiety may also result from the lack of sleep. RLS affects people who want to travel or attend events that require sitting for long periods of time.

KEY TERMS

Anemia—A condition that affects the size and number of red blood cells. It often results from lack of iron or certain B vitamins and may be treated with iron or vitamin supplements.

Insomnia—Trouble sleeping. People who suffer from RLS often lose sleep either because they spend time walking to relieve discomfort or because they have PLMS, which causes them to wake often during the night.

Periodic limb movements in sleep (PLMS)—Random movements of the arms or legs that occur at regular intervals of time during sleep.

Causes and symptoms

Restless legs syndrome is categorized in two ways. Primary RLS occurs in the absence of other medical symptoms, while secondary RLS is usually associated with some other medical disorder. Although the cause of primary RLS is currently unknown, a large amount of research into the cause of RLS is taking place. Researchers at Johns Hopkins University published a study in July 2003 suggesting that iron deficiencies may be related to the disorder. They dissected brains from cadavers of people who suffered from RLS and found that the cells in the midbrain were not receiving enough iron. Other researchers suggest that RLS may be related to a chemical imbalance of the neurotransmitter **dopamine** in the **brain**. There is also evidence that RLS has a genetic component. RLS occurs three to five times more frequently in an immediate family member of someone who has RLS than in the general population. A site on a chromosome that may contain a gene for RLS has been identified by molecular biologists.

In many people, other medical conditions play a role in RLS and the disorder is therefore termed secondary RLS. People with peripheral neuropathies (injury to nerves in the arms and legs) may experience RLS. Such neuropathies may result from diabetes or alcoholism. Other chronic diseases such as kidney disorders and rheumatoid arthritis may result in RLS. Iron deficiencies and blood anemias are often associated with RLS and symptoms of the disease usually decrease once blood iron levels have been corrected. **Attention deficit hyperactivity disorder** (ADHD) has also been implicated in RLS. Pregnant women often suffer from RLS, especially in the third trimester. Some people find that high levels of caffeine intake may result in RLS.

The symptoms of RLS are all associated with unpleasant feelings in the limbs. The words used to describe these feelings are various, but include such adjectives as deep-seated crawling, jittery, tingling, burning, aching, pulling, painful, itchy or prickly. They are usually not described as a muscle cramp or numbness. Most often the sensations occur during periods of inactivity. They are characterized by an urge to get up and move. Such movements include stretching, walking, jogging or simply jiggling the legs. The feelings worsen in the evening.

A variety of symptoms are associated with RLS, but may not be characteristic of every case. Some people with RLS report involuntary arm and leg movements during the night. Others have difficulty falling asleep and are sleepy or fatigued during the day. Many people with RLS have leg discomfort that is not explained by routine medical exams.

Eighty-five percent of RLS patients either have difficulty falling asleep or wake several times during the night, and almost half experience daytime **fatigue** or sleepiness. It is common for the symptoms to be intermittent. They may disappear for several months and then return for no apparent reason. Two thirds of patients report that their symptoms become worse with time. Some older patients claim to have had symptoms since they were in their early 20s, but were not diagnosed until their 50s. Suspected under-diagnosis of RLS may be attributed to the difficulty experienced by patients in describing their symptoms.

Diagnosis

A careful history enables the physician to distinguish RLS from similar types of disorders that cause night time discomfort in the limbs, such as muscle cramps, burning feet syndrome, and damage to nerves that detect sensations or cause movement (polyneuropathy).

The most important tool the doctor has in **diagnosis** is the history obtained from the patient. There are several common medical conditions that are known to either cause or to be closely associated with RLS. The doctor may link the patient's symptoms to one of these conditions, which include anemia, diabetes, disease of the spinal nerve roots (lumbosacral radiculopathy), Parkinson's disease, late-stage pregnancy, kidney failure (uremia), and complications of stomach surgery. In order to identify or eliminate such a primary cause, blood tests may be performed to determine the presence of serum iron, ferritin, folate, vitamin B_{12}, creatinine, and thyroid-stimulating hormones. The physician may also ask if symptoms are present in any close family members, since it is common for RLS to run in families and this type is sometimes more difficult to treat.

In some cases, sleep studies such as **polysomnography** are undertaken to identify the presence of PLMS that are reported to affect 70%–80% of people who suffer from RLS. The patient is often unaware of these movements, since they may not cause him to wake. However, the presence of PLMS with RLS can leave the person more tired, because it interferes with deep sleep. A patient who also displays evidence of some neurologic disease may undergo electromyography (EMG). During EMG, a very small, thin needle is inserted into the muscle and electrical activity of the muscle is recorded. A doctor or technician usually performs this test at a hospital outpatient department.

RLS is under consideration for inclusion in the fifth edition of the ***Diagnostic and Statistical Manual of Mental Disorders*** (*DSM-5*, 2013). The proposed diagnostic criteria describes RLS as the urge to move the legs, accompanied by uncomfortable sensations, and requires the following to be present:

- The sensations start or increase during rest or inactivity.
- The sensations are only partly relieved by moving the legs.
- The sensations are worse in the evening or at night, or they only occur in the evening or at night.

In addition, the above symptoms must be accompanied by at least one of the following conditions

- fatigue
- daytime sleepiness
- problems with concentration, memory, or learning
- mood disturbances
- behavioral problems
- problems at work or school due to lack of sleep
- problems with interpersonal relationships

The *DSM-5* notes that these symptoms should occur despite ample opportunities for sleep.

Treatment

The first step in treatment is to treat existing conditions that are known to be associated with RLS and that will be identified by blood tests. If the patient is anemic, iron (iron sulfate) or vitamin supplements (folate or vitamin B_{12}) will be prescribed. If kidney disease is identified as a cause, treatment of the kidney problem will take priority.

After treating underlying disorders, treatment for restless legs syndrome is generally two-pronged, consisting of making lifestyle changes and using medications to relieve some of the symptoms. Lifestyle changes involve altering the diet, exercising and performing other self-directed activities, and practicing good sleep hygiene. Although the United States Food and Drug Administration has not yet approved any drugs for treating RLS, four classes of pharmaceuticals have been found effective for treating RLS: dopaminergic agents, **benzodiazepines**, **opioids** and anticonvulsants.

Drugs

Dopaminergic agents are the first type of drug prescribed in the treatment of RLS. Most commonly doctors prescribe dopamine-receptor agonists that are used to treat Parkinson's disease such as Mirapex (pramipexole), Permax (pergolide) and Requip (ropinirole). Sinemet (carbidopa/levodopa), which is a drug that adds dopamine to the nervous system, is also commonly prescribed. Sinemet has been used the more frequently than other drugs in treating RLS, but recently a problem known as augmentation has been associated with its use. When augmentation develops, symptoms of RLS will return earlier in the day and increasing the dose will not improve the symptoms.

Antiepileptic drugs are those used for people with **seizures**. These are also useful in the treatment of RLS, and include Neurontin (**gabapentin**), Carbatrol (**carbamazepine**), Keppra (levetiracetam), and Topamax (topiramate).

Benzodiazepines are drugs that sedate and are typically taken before bedtime so that a patient with RLS can sleep more soundly. The most commonly prescribed sedative in RLS is Klonopin (**clonazepam**).

Opioids are synthetic narcotics that relieve pain and cause drowsiness. They are usually taken in the evening. The most commonly used opioids prescribed for RLS include Darvon or Darvocet (propoxyphene), Dolophine (**methadone**), Percocet (oxycodone), Ultram (Tramadol) and Vicodin (hydrocodone). One danger associated with opioids is that they can be addicting.

A few drugs have been found to worsen symptoms of RLS and they should be avoided by patients exhibiting RLS symptoms. These include anti-nausea drugs such as Antivert, Atarax, Compazine and Phenergan. Calcium channel blockers that are often used to treat heart conditions should be avoided. In addition, most anti-depressants tend to exacerbate symptoms of RLS. Finally, antihistamines such as Benadryl have been found to aggravate RLS symptoms in some people.

Home remedies

Simple changes to the diet have proven effective for some people suffering from RLS. Vitamin deficiencies are a common problem in RLA patients. In patients with RLS, most physicians will check the levels of blood serum ferritin, which can indicate low iron storage. If these levels are below 50 mcg/L, then supplemental iron should be added to the diet. Other physicians have found that supplements of vitamin E, folic acid and B vitamins, and magnesium provide relief to symptoms or RLS. Reducing or eliminating caffeine and alcohol consumption has been effective in other patients.

Alternative

It is likely that the best alternative therapy will combine both conventional and alternative approaches. Levodopa may be combined with a therapy that relieves pain, relaxes muscles, or focuses in general on the nervous system and the brain. Any such combined therapy that allows a reduction in dosage of levodopa is advantageous, since this will reduce the likelihood of unacceptable levels of drug side effects. Of course, the physician who prescribes the medication should monitor any combined therapy. Alternative methods may include:

- Acupuncture. Patients who also suffer from rheumatoid arthritis may especially benefit from acupuncture to relieve RLS symptoms. Acupuncture is believed to be effective in arthritis treatment and may also stimulate those parts of the brain that are involved in RLS.
- Homeopathy. Homeopaths believe that disorders of the nervous system are especially important because the brain controls so many other bodily functions. The remedy is tailored to the individual patient and is based on individual symptoms as well as the general symptoms of RLS.
- Reflexology. Reflexologists claim that the brain, head, and spine all respond to indirect massage of specific parts of the feet.
- Nutritional supplements. Supplementation of the diet with vitamin E, calcium, magnesium, and folic acid may be helpful for people with RLS.

Some alternative methods may treat the associated condition that is suspected to cause restless legs. These include:

- Anemia or low ferritin levels. Chinese medicine will emphasize stimulation of the spleen as a means of improving blood circulation and vitamin absorption. Other treatments may include acupuncture and herbal therapies, such as ginseng (*Panax ginseng*) for anemia-related fatigue.
- Late-stage pregnancy. There are few conventional therapies available to pregnant women, since most of the drugs prescribed are not recommended for use during pregnancy. Pregnant women may benefit from alternative techniques that focus on body work, including yoga, reflexology, and acupuncture.

Prognosis

RLS usually does not indicate the onset of other neurological disease. However, it is a lifelong condition for most people. It may remain static, although two-thirds of patients get worse with time. The symptoms usually progress gradually. Treatment with Levodopa is effective in moderate to severe cases that may include significant PLMS. However, this drug produces significant side effects, and continued successful treatment may depend on carefully monitored use of combination drug therapy. The prognosis is usually best if RLS symptoms are recent and can be traced to another treatable condition that is associated with RLS. Some associated conditions are not treatable. In these cases, such as for rheumatoid arthritis, alternative therapies such as **acupuncture** may be helpful.

Prevention

Diet is key in preventing RLS. A preventive diet will include an adequate intake of iron and the B vitamins, especially B_{12} and folic acid. Strict vegetarians should take vitamin supplements to obtain sufficient vitamin B_{12}. Ferrous gluconate may be easier on the digestive system than ferrous sulfate, if iron supplements are prescribed. Some medications may cause symptoms of RLS. Patients should check with their doctor about these possible side effects, especially if symptoms first occur after starting a new medication. Caffeine, alcohol, and **nicotine** use should be minimized or eliminated. Even a hot bath before bed has been shown to prevent symptoms for some sufferers.

Resources

BOOKS

Ferri, Fred, ed. *Ferri's Clinical Advisor 2010*. 1st ed. Philadelphia: Mosby Elsevier, 2009.

Goetz, C.G. *Goetz's Textbook of Clinical Neurology*. 3rd ed. Philadelphia: Saunders, 2007.

Goldman, L., and D. Ausiello, eds. *Cecil Textbook of Internal Medicine*. 23rd ed. Philadelphia: Saunders, 2008.

Rakel, R. *Textbook of Family Medicine 2007*. 7th ed. Philadelphia: Saunders Elsevier, 2009.

Rakel, R. E., and E. T. Bope. *Conn's Current Therapy*. 60th ed. Philadelphia: Saunders Elsevier, 2009.

WEBSITES

American Psychiatric Association. "Restless Legs Syndrome." DSM-5 Development. http://www.dsm5.org/proposedrevision/pages/proposedrevision.aspx?rid=403 (accessed September 11, 2011).

National Institute of Neurological Disease and Stroke. "Restless Legs Syndrome Fact Sheet." U.S. National Institutes of Health. http://www.ninds.nih.gov/disorders/restless_legs/detail_restless_legs.htm (accessed September 11, 2011).

ORGANIZATIONS

Restless Legs Syndrome Foundation, 1904 Banbury Road, Raleigh, NC, 27608-4428, (919) 781-4428, http://www.rls.org.

Ann M. Haren
Heidi Splete

Restoril *see* **Temazepam**

Rett syndrome

Definition

Rett syndrome is a progressive neurological disorder seen almost exclusively in females. The disorder is characterized by an early-onset slowing of the infant's head growth and a reduction in **brain** size by as much as 30%; it is the leading cause of genetically based profound **intellectual disability** in girls. The most common symptoms include decreased speech, cognitive disabilities, severe lack of muscle control, small head size, and unusual hand movements.

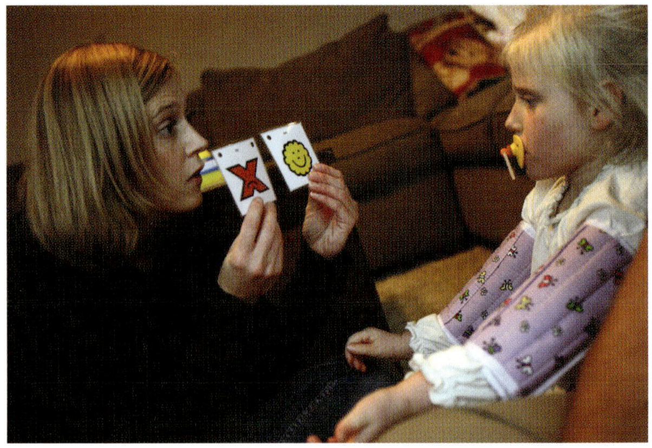

A mother communicates with her daughter by using flash cards; her daughter has Rett syndrome, a neurological disorder that can affect language abilities. *(© Kimberly P. Mitchell/Detroit Free Press/MCT/newscom)*

Demographics

Rett syndrome affects almost only females. Males who carry the same gene mutation gene typically are miscarried before birth or die as infants. Rett syndrome usually is fatal in males because they have a single X chromosome, and the Y chromosome they carry cannot compensate for this mutation on their X chromosome. Females with a mutation in the gene that causes Rett syndrome are able to survive because the presence of the second normal X chromosome partially compensates for the mutation on the other X chromosome. Rett syndrome is believed to affect all ethnic groups and nationalities with an equal frequency of about one case for every 10,000 to 15,000 live female births.

Description

Rett syndrome was first described by an Austrian physician, Andreas Rett, in 1966; prior to 1983, however, little was known about the syndrome because it was quite rare. Although Rett syndrome was thought at first to result from the destruction or degeneration of brain tissue, genetic research has indicated that it is caused by the failure of the infant's brain to develop normally. This developmental failure is caused by a genetic mutation affecting production of a key protein that regulates brain development.

Rett syndrome has a distinctive onset and course. In classic Rett syndrome, which occurs only in girls, the child develops normally during the first 6 to 18 months of life. In many cases, at around the fifth month, head growth slows or stagnates, and the child loses any purposeful hand movements that she had previously developed. Language and motor skills regress rapidly. Purposeful hand use gives way to repetitive hand-washing or hand-wringing gestures. **Seizures** occur in up to 90% of affected girls,

KEY TERMS

Congenital—Refers to a disorder which is present at birth.

Joint contractures—Stiffness of the joints that prevents full extension.

Mutation—A mutation is a change in a gene. Since genes determine how a body is structured and functions, any change in a gene will produce some change in these areas.

Neurological conditions—A condition that has its origin in some part of the patient's nervous system.

Seizure—A convulsion, or uncontrolled discharge of nerve cells that may spread to other cells throughout the brain.

and 50%–80% of children with the disorder will eventually develop epilepsy. Screaming fits and crying are features that arise by age 18 to 24 months. The disorder can also include characteristics of **autism**, tremors, and panic-like attacks. Rett syndrome is associated with severe or profound intellectual disability.

Some atypical forms of Rett syndrome, including congenital, late-onset, and preserved-speech Rett, are now being diagnosed in people formerly diagnosed with other disorders, such as autism or learning disability, who carry the genetic mutation linked to Rett syndrome. Males who have inherited an extra X chromosome and are carrying the mutation, or in whom the gene is mutated very early in their development, can manifest a form of the disorder. The features of this form of Rett may not be as severe in nature, because only some of the person's cells will carry the mutation. Because males normally inherit only one X chromosome, those with the mutation usually have such severe problems at birth that they do not survive into their second year.

Rett syndrome is included in the fourth edition of the *Diagnostic and Statistical Manual of Mental Disorders* (*DSM-IV-TR*), the handbook used by medical professionals in diagnosing mental disorders, as a pervasive developmental disorder of childhood. However, proposed changes for the fifth edition (*DSM-5*) include removing Rett syndrome as a mental health **diagnosis**.

Causes and symptoms

Causes

A genetic mutation on the X chromosome is the cause of Rett syndrome. Because only a single copy of this mutated gene is required to give rise to the disease, it is considered an X-linked, dominant disorder. About 99.5% of cases of the syndrome arise from a new mutation in the egg or sperm cell line of a parent, rather than existing in the body cells of the parent. It is possible to be a carrier of an X chromosome with this mutation without knowing, because most cells in a woman's body shut down one of her two X chromosomes. If most of the cells shut down the X carrying the disease-causing gene, she will not manifest the severe symptoms and may bear children, who have a 50% chance of inheriting the mutation-carrying X chromosome from her. Because Rett syndrome usually is the result of a new mutation, however, multiple cases in a single family are rare, but if a pregnant woman is found to be an unaffected carrier or if the couple has a child with the condition, prenatal testing is available.

The gene that causes Rett syndrome is MECP2, which lies on the long arm of the X chromosome. The protein that it encodes is required for life and is necessary for appropriate brain development. Its job is to turn off certain genes at specific developmental periods and to ensure that the correct form of a particular protein is made. When MECP2 does not function correctly, the development of the brain does not occur in an appropriately regulated manner. The genes with which it interacts are thought to relate to nerve cell signaling, and the protein that MECP2 encodes exists at high levels in normal nerve cells. In its absence, the parts of the brain responsible for emotion, sensation, and movement do not communicate correctly with one another, leaving the brain in a permanently infantile developmental state.

Symptoms

The symptoms of Rett syndrome have been described in terms of four stages in the child's development:

- Stage 1, early onset (6–18 months of age): The early symptoms of Rett syndrome are not always noticeable in Stage 1. The infant may not make eye contact with family members and may not show much interest in toys. She may be considered a "good baby" because she is so calm and quiet. On the other hand, there may be noticeable hand-wringing and slowing of head growth.
- Stage 2, rapid deterioration (1–4 years old): This stage may be either rapid or gradual in onset. The child loses her ability to speak and to make purposeful hand movements. Hand-to-mouth movements may appear, as well as hand-wringing or hand-clapping gestures. These movements may be nearly constant while the child is awake but disappear during sleep. There may

be noticeable episodes of breath holding and hyperventilating (rapid shallow breathing). The child may have trouble sleeping and may become irritable. If she is able to walk, she will start to look unsteady on her feet and may have periods of trembling or shaking. Slowed growth of the head is usually most noticeable during this stage.

- Stage 3, plateau (2–10 years): Motor problems and seizures often appear during this stage. The child's behavior, however, often shows some improvement, with less irritability and crying. She may show greater interest in her surroundings, and her attention span and communication skills often improve. Many patients with Rett syndrome remain in stage 3 for most of their lives.
- Stage 4, late deterioration of motor skills (usually after 10 years of age): In stage 4, patients with Rett syndrome gradually lose their mobility; some stop walking while others have never learned to walk. There is, however, no loss of cognitive or communication skills, and repetitive hand movements may decrease. The spine begins to develop an abnormal sideways curvature (scoliosis), and the patient may develop muscle rigidity. Puberty begins at the same age as in most girls.

Diagnosis

Rett syndrome can be diagnosed based on either the diagnostic criteria established in the *DSM-IV-TR* or based on testing of the MECP2 gene for mutations. Molecular analysis of the MECP2 gene for mutations will correctly identify at least four out of five females who have classic Rett syndrome.

Diagnoses based on *DSM-IV-TR* criteria are made after observation of the child—usually over a period of several hours or days—and interviews with the parents. The diagnosis can be made by a pediatrician or primary care physician, but should be confirmed by a pediatric neurologist (specialist in disorders of the nervous system in children) or developmental pediatrician. After the examiner has excluded the possibility of other developmental disorders, there are six criteria that must be met for a diagnosis of the classic form of Rett syndrome, and a secondary group of supportive criteria that are frequently observed in Rett syndrome patients but are not necessary to make the diagnosis.

The diagnostic criteria for Rett syndrome include the following:

- a period of apparently normal development before 6–18 months of age
- a normal-sized head at birth followed by slowing of head growth between 5 months and 4 years
- severe impairment in the use of language and loss of purposeful hand motion
- repetitive hand movements that include one or more of the following: hand-washing, hand-wringing, or hand-clapping gestures
- shaking of the chest or torso, particularly when the child is agitated or upset
- in children able to walk, an unsteady, stiff-legged, wide-based gait

Supportive criteria

Supportive criteria are criteria that are not essential to the diagnosis of a particular disorder, because some people with the disorder do not have them, but they are present in enough cases to be associated with the diagnosis. Supportive criteria provide strong evidence that a person who exhibits these criteria does in fact have the disorder. The supportive criteria for Rett syndrome do not always appear in young children but are often observed as the child grows older. Supportive criteria for Rett syndrome include:

- dysfunctional breathing, which may include hyperventilation, breath holding, and air swallowing
- abnormal electroencephalogram (EEG) patterns
- seizures
- difficulties in chewing and swallowing
- constipation
- muscle rigidity and joint contracture that increases with age
- scoliosis (curvature of the spine from side to side)
- teeth grinding (bruxism)
- small feet in relation to overall height
- slow overall growth
- loss of body fat and muscle mass
- abnormal sleeping patterns combined with irritability or agitation
- poor circulation in the feet and legs

Variant Rett syndrome

Because genetic testing has revealed some gradations in the manifestation of Rett syndrome, there also is a list of suggested criteria for the variant form of the condition. These include a set of main criteria, of which three symptoms must be met:

- reduction or lack of hand skills
- reduction or complete loss of speech, including infant babble
- presence of stereotyped hand movements
- lost or diminished communication abilities

- slowed head growth from early childhood
- regression that is followed by recovery of interaction.

There are also 11 suggested supportive criteria for the variant form of Rett syndrome, with the dictate that at least 5 symptoms must be present:

- breathing irregularities
- bruxism
- abnormal locomotion
- spinal deformity that results in a hunched appearance (kyphosis) or scoliosis (curvature of the spine)
- loss of muscle in the lower limbs
- feet that are cold, discolored, and small
- sleep disturbances, including nighttime screaming
- unexpected episodes of screaming or laughing
- the appearance of a reduced awareness of pain
- intense eye contact

Treatment

There is no single treatment regimen that is applicable to all patients with Rett syndrome. A suite of therapies that may be useful include speech, occupational, and physical therapy. While these therapies will not cure Rett syndrome, they may help ameliorate some aspects of the disorder. Some patients benefit from medications for muscular rigidity or for specific mood or behavioral problems, such as anxiety or irritability. Because of the increased risk of a potentially deadly irregular heartbeat, females with Rett syndrome should avoid drugs that can exacerbate the problem, including antipsychotics, anesthetics, and some antibiotics. A child **psychiatrist** should be consulted in regard to medications.

Parents of children with Rett syndrome are often helped by supportive therapy groups for parents of children with **pervasive developmental disorders**. Another type of program that is helpful for parents centers on learning skills for coping with the behaviors of children with Rett syndrome. These programs are usually led by a behavioral **psychologist**.

Prognosis

The prognosis for Rett syndrome patients is poor. In most cases, there is a steady loss of cognition and of movement-related, social, and behavioral skills throughout the patient's lifetime, though some patients do make modest developmental gains in adolescence. The average life expectancy of a person with Rett syndrome is estimated to be around age 40. Females with the classic form of Rett syndrome usually live to adulthood, but there is a high incidence of sudden death among this group, possibly because of irregular heartbeat.

Children who have Rett syndrome can and do attend school. Some attend special schools targeting children with their disabilities, while others attend neighborhood schools and participate in the general classroom environment. In the United States, the Individuals with Disabilities Education Act (IDEA) ensures eligibility for early **intervention** services in a Birth-to-Three program if children are diagnosed before the age of three.

Prevention

Because most cases result from new mutations of the MECP2 gene rather than transmission of a defective gene from the parents, there are no known strategies for preventing Rett syndrome. Though genetic testing is available, it is not usually recommended unless another child in the family has the syndrome.

QUESTIONS TO ASK YOUR DOCTOR

- What are the indications that my child may have Rett syndrome?
- What diagnostic tests are needed for a thorough assessment?
- What treatment options do you recommend?
- Should I see a specialist? If so, what kind of specialist should I contact?
- How will I know if treatment has been beneficial?
- What physical limitations do you foresee?
- What associated medical problems does my child have that will need treatment along with Rett syndrome?
- What sort of behaviors can I expect from my child?
- Is my child eligible for any early intervention programs available locally?
- What can we do at home to best help our child?
- What should I tell my other children/relatives/ friends about this disorder?
- Does having Rett syndrome put my child at risk for other health conditions?
- Can you recommend any support groups for me and my family?

Resources

BOOKS

American Psychiatric Association. *Diagnostic and Statistical Manual of Mental Disorders*. 4th ed., text rev. Washington, DC: American Psychiatric Association, 2000.

American Psychological Association. *Publication Manual of the American Psychological Association*. 6th ed. Washington, DC: American Psychological Association, 2009.

Bennett, Robin L. *The Practical Guide to the Genetic Family History*. 2nd ed. New York: Wiley-Blackwell, 2010.

Goldstein, Sam, and Cecil R. Reynolds, eds. *Handbook of Neurodevelopmental and Genetic Disorders in Children*. 2nd ed. New York: The Guilford Press, 2010.

Shannon, Joyce Brennfleck, ed. *Autism and Pervasive Developmental Disorders Sourcebook*. 2nd ed. Detroit: Omnigraphics, 2011.

PERIODICALS

Bradbury, Jane. "Advance Made in Understanding Rett's Syndrome." *Neurology, The Lancet* 4 (2005): 83.

Gura, T. "Gene Defect Linked to Rett Syndrome." *Science* 286 (Oct. 1, 1999): 27.

Jan, M., J. M. Dooley, and K. E. Gordon. "A Male Rett Syndrome Variant: Application of Diagnostic Criteria." *Pediatric Neurology* 20 (1999): 238–40.

Lane, J. B., et al. "Clinical Severity and Quality of Life in Children and Adolescents with Rett Syndrome." *Neurology* (Oct. 19, 2011) [e-pub ahead of print]. http://dx.doi.org/10.1212/WNL.0b013e3182377dd2 (accessed November 2, 2011).

Viola, Angèle, et al. "Metabolic Fingerprints of Altered Brain Growth, Osmoregulation and Neurotransmission in a Rett Syndrome Model." *PLOS [Public Library of Science] ONE* 2, no. 1 (2007): e157. http://dx.doi.org/10.1371/journal.pone.0000157 (accessed November 2, 2011).

WEBSITES

ClinicalTrials.gov. "Rett Syndrome Clinical Trials." U.S. National Institutes of Health. http://clinicaltrials.gov/ct2/results?term=Rett+Syndrome+ (accessed September 26, 2011).

Eunice Kennedy Shriver National Institute of Child Health and Human Development. "Rett Syndrome." U.S. National Institutes of Health. http://www.nichd.nih.gov/health/topics/Rett_Syndrome.cfm (accessed November 2, 2011).

MedlinePlus. "Rett Syndrome." U.S. National Library of Medicine. http://www.nlm.nih.gov/medlineplus/rettsyndrome.html (accessed September 26, 2011).

National Institute of Neurological Disorders and Stroke. "Rett Syndrome Fact Sheet." U.S. National Institutes of Health. http://www.ninds.nih.gov/disorders/rett/detail_rett.htm (accessed September 26, 2011).

ORGANIZATIONS

Angelman, Rett & Prader-Willi Syndromes Consortium (ARPWSC), Rare Diseases Clinical Research Network, University of Alabama at Birmingham, Birmingham, AL, (205) 934-1130, Fax: (205) 975-6330, jlane@uab.edu, http://rarediseasesnetwork.epi.usf.edu/arpwsc.

Genetic Alliance, 4301 Connecticut Ave. NW, Suite 404, Washington, DC, 20008-2369, (202) 966-5557, Fax: (202) 966-8553, info@geneticalliance.org, http://www.geneticalliance.org.

International Rett Syndrome Association, 4600 Devitt Drive, Cincinnati, OH, 45246, (800) 818-7388, Fax: (513) 874-2520, http://www.rettsyndrome.org.

National Institute of Neurological Disorders and Stroke, PO Box 5801, Bethesda, MD, 20824, (301) 496-5751; TTY: (301) 468-5981, (800) 352-9424, http://www.ninds.nih.gov.

National Organization for Rare Disorders (NORD), PO Box 1968, Danbury, CT, 06813-1968, (203) 744-0100, (800) 999-6673, Fax: (203) 798-2291, orphan@rarediseases.org, http://www.rarediseases.org.

Rebecca J. Frey, PhD
Emily Jane. Willingham, PhD
Laura Jean Cataldo, RN, EdD

Revia *see* **Naltrexone**

Reward deficiency syndrome (RDS)

Definition

Reward Deficiency Syndrome, or RDS, is related to a number of mental health disorders, rather than standing alone as a separate and distinct mental illness. The mental illnesses to which RDS is related include a wide range of addictions, compulsive behaviors, and impulsive behaviors.

RDS refers to the breakdown of the reward cascade, and resultant aberrant conduct, due to genetic and environmental influences. RDS is a DNA-related gene and chromosome type of syndrome that interferes with the usual achievement of human physiological drives such as food, water, and sexual reproduction. The A1 (minor) allele of the D2 **dopamine** receptor (DRD2) gene has been shown to be associated with alcoholism, particularly its severe form, as well as with smoking, obesity, and other addictive behaviors.

Addiction is a **brain** disorder that causes the compulsive and continued use of and cravings for substances, regardless of negative consequences. These behaviors are related to neurotransmitter dysregulation, notably that of dopamine and **serotonin**. Addiction, along with **compulsion**, affects the nucleus accumbens, the part of the brain that produces pleasure. Because of its biologic basis, these behaviors are chronic with a propensity toward **relapse**. Addiction/compulsion

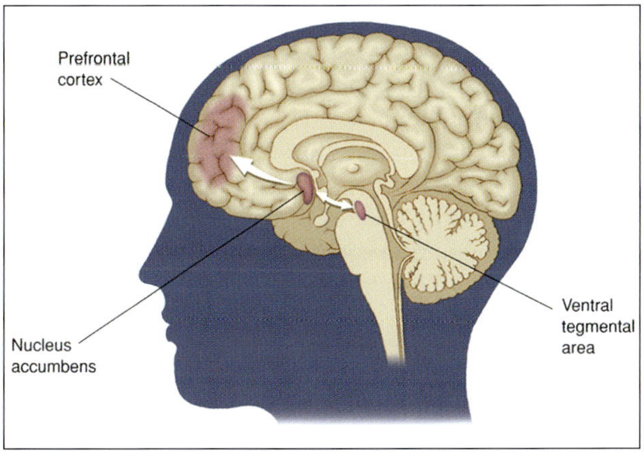

Illustration showing areas of the brain associated with addiction. *(Illustration by Frank Forney. Reproduced by permission of Cengage Learning.)*

causes loss of control over alcohol, **nicotine**, and substance use, so that uncontrollable behaviors occur more quickly as this mental disorder progresses. The name for this particular pattern is Reward Deficiency Syndrome. Defined by pharmacology professor Kenneth Blum in the 1990s, RDS arises in the human genetic units labeled the D2 (dopamine) receptor and the A1 allele. RDS is also linked to such illnesses as **attention deficit hyperactivity disorder** and Tourette syndrome, **conduct disorder**, obesity, gambling, **post-traumatic stress disorder** (PTSD), and **premenstrual syndrome** (PMS).

Demographics

Children of alcohol-addicted or substance-addicted individuals are more highly at risk for developing **alcohol use** and substance use disorders than the general population. Thus, they are more likely to suffer from RDS. There is also evidence of the hereditary nature of some other RDS-related illnesses, especially morbid obesity, attention deficit (ADD/ADHD), and PMS.

Disruptive behavior disorders such as conduct disorder in youth and antisocial personality disorder in adults are related to RDS. The youth-related disorders frequently coexist with substance abuse problems. Other groups that may be affected by RDS are older adults with mood/anxiety disorders who self-medicate in grieving the losses of old age, incarcerated populations, the homeless, and those with eating disorders. Because obesity includes growing proportions of Americans from all demographic classifications in recent decades, and RDS is related to some of these cases, then RDS may affect all demographic designations, but further research is needed to clarify this with certainty.

Description

In the 1950s, researchers experimented placing electrodes into a rat's brain. They discovered that the rat chose pressing a lever attached to the electrodes to provide brain stimulation, even over the basic needs of food and water. This suggested that the implanted brain area is the "pleasure center" of the brain. It contains the nucleus accumbens, a brain structure related to addictions, but also interestingly relevant to processing the rewards of food, sex, and video games (a modern addiction in some individuals). Neurologic reward pathways are very important to human survival, because they provide the drives for pleasure that require eating, love/sex, and reproduction for species survival. These natural rewards facilitate the release of dopamines in both the brain's nucleus accumbens and frontal lobes.

Pharmacologist Kenneth Blum found that individuals with RDS generally possess a specific chromosome sequence in their DNA. This sequence is most often the A1 allele, D2 dopamine receptor. People with this sequence have 20% to 30% fewer D2 reward receptors than in the general population. This makes it more difficult for the pleasure drives to be met, forcing the individuals into high-risk behaviors to gain that fulfillment. In addition, people with the A1 allele are 74% more likely to have one or more of several RDS-related mental illnesses. These illnesses are related to addictions, compulsive behaviors, and impulsive behaviors.

Listed in the 2000 edition of the *Diagnostic and Statistical Manual (DSM-IV)* of the **American Psychiatric Association**, disorders that stem from RDS include alcohol abuse, **substance abuse**, nicotine/tobacco use, compulsive disorder, attention deficit hyperactivity disorder, conduct disorder, **antisocial personality disorder**, obesity, PTSD, and PMS. Such individuals need to stimulate themselves in abundance simply to feel normal. Alcohol and drugs used for stimulation of the pleasure center injures a person's dopamine and endorphin system even more. With each use of drugs or alcohol, the difference between feeling high or even "normal" and being sober becomes larger and larger. Staying sober becomes boring and results in an overarching anxiety and irritability. To alleviate these bad feelings, these individuals often turn back to alcohol and drugs, sometimes overdosing and accidentally or purposefully dying in the process.

Prevalence

It is difficult to estimate the prevalence of RDS among the American population because of its many manifestations. Not only alcohol and substance use disorders but also tobacco/nicotine use, schizoid/avoidant behavior, PTSD, **ADHD**, Tourette syndrome,

KEY TERMS

A1 allele—An allele related to RDS.

A1 D2—A chromosome sequence related to RDS.

Allele—One member of a pair or a series of genes that occupy a specific position on a specific chromosome.

D2—A dopamine receptor.

Dopamine—The neurotransmitter responsible for desire.

Frontal lobes—The large lobes at the front of the brain responsible for reasoning, problem-solving, and logic.

Neurotransmitter—A chemical that relays and amplifies electric signals between brain and central nervous system cells (neurons).

Nucleus accumbens—A structure deep inside and near the center of the brain that makes up a major part of the pathway of pleasure and reward.

Serotonin—The neurotransmitter responsible for satisfaction and inhibition.

aggression, obesity and aberrant weight gain, PMS, and perhaps other mental disorders all fall under the RDS umbrella.

Because the prevalence of **co-occurring disorders** has increased in the last 30 years, the overall prevalence of RDS has also increased, being related to co-occurring disorders (always including substance/alcohol abuse). Further, the co-occurrence of mental illness and substance abuse itself is found in 50% of all individuals suffering from any of the severe mental disorders (SMDs). Therefore, RDS is related to these 50% of cases, possibly a proportion of the other 50% of SMDs, and to the further problems associated with substance and alcohol abuse and impulsive and compulsive behaviors: higher rates of relapse and **hospitalization**, incarceration, violence, **homelessness**, **suicide**, and exposure to infections such as HIV and hepatitis. It is not known how many Americans with obesity and other above-mentioned disorders are RDS-connected, in the absence of genetic testing.

Diagnosis

A thorough multidiscipline assessment is used to establish an individualized treatment plan for alcohol and substance abuse clients and should be used with RDS-related disorders. In addition, it is becoming increasingly important to establish gene involvement via genetic testing. This process begins with a clinical interview of the patient and family, which is vital in recognizing behavior patterns. A number of substance abuse checklists can help determine the presence of a substance abuse disorder. Genetic testing can establish the physical basis for RDS-related disorders. Mental health tests can uncover psychiatric illnesses. These tests include the **Minnesota Multiphasic Personality Inventory** (MMPI), Rorschach inkblot, and other personality and projective tests.

Treatment

Kenneth Blum was awarded U.S. Patent Number 6955873 for *Diagnosis and treatment system for reward deficiency syndrome (RDS) and related behaviors* on October 18, 2005. The diagnostic technique includes four kits for obtaining buccal (inner cheek) swabs for the following primary clusters of disorders: 1) neurotransmitter, tryptophan, and opiate related problems in RDS behaviors, 2) the same problems in relation to weight gain, 3) allele analysis for attention deficit hyperactivity disorder, and 4) substance use disorders (SUDs), obesity, smoking, Tourette syndrome, schizoid/avoidant behavior, aggression, post-traumatic stress disorder (PTSD), and PMS.

In addition to swabs, the **diagnosis** includes the RDS Inventory Scale test, patented under this patent number. Upon analysis of the results of the swab or swabs obtained from a single client, the physician may or may not administer the patented medication formula via injection or oral ingestion for each kit that suggests treatment. Other treatments include a range of psychiatric medications and talking therapies, as well as holistic multidisciplinary techniques traditionally used for RDS-related mental illnesses before genetic testing and Blum's treatment process was established.

Prognosis

Education, prevention, and early diagnosis are all vital to the mental health of individuals who may be at risk for RDS-related disorders. In particular, the earlier that alcohol and substance use disorders can be diagnosed, the better are the chances for successful treatment. Genetic testing for the A1D2 sequence of RDS is available and can be used in early diagnosis in infants and youth.

Resources

PERIODICALS

Baicy, Kate. "Can Food Be Addictive? Insights on Obesity from Neuroimaging and Substance Abuse Treatment and Research." *Nutrition Noteworthy* 7, no. 1 (2005): article 4.

Blum, K., et al. "Genotrimtrade Mark, a DNA-Customized Nutrigenomic Product, Targets Genetic Factors of Obesity: Hypothesizing a Doamine-Glucose Correlation Demonstrating Reward Deficiency Syndrome (RDS)." *Medical Hypotheses* 68, no. 4 (2006): 844–52.

Blum K., et al. "Reward Deficiency Syndrome in Obesity: A Preliminary Cross-Sectional Trial with a Genotrim Variant." *Advances in Therapy* 23, no. 6 (2006):1040–51.

Blum K., et al. "Reward Deficiency Syndrome." *American Scientist* 84, no. 4 (1996): 132–45.

Bowirrat, A., and Oscar-Berman, M. "Relationship between Dopaminergic Neurotransmission, Alcoholism, and Reward Deficiency Syndrome." *American Journal Of Medical Genetics. Part B, Neuropsychiatric Genetics: the Official Publication of the International Society of Psychiatric Genetics* 132, no. 1 (2005): 29–37.

Comings, D. E., et al. "Neurogenetic Interactions and Aberrant Behavioral Co-morbidity of Attention Deficit Hyperactivity Disorder (ADHD): Dispelling Myths." *Theoretical Biology and Medical Modelling* 2, no. 50 (2005): http://www.tbiomed.com/content/pdf/1742-4682-2-50.pdf.

Dick, Danielle M., Richard J. Rose, and Jaakko Kaprio. "The Next Challenge for Psychiatric Genetics: Characterizing the Risk Associated with Identified Genes." *Annals of Clinical Psychiatry* 18, no. 4 (2006): 223–31.

Eisenberg, D. J., et al. "Examining Impulsivity as an Endophenotype Using a Behavioral Approach: A DRD2 TaqI A and DRD4 48-bp VNTR Association Study." *Behavioral and Brain Functions* 3, no. 2 (2007). http://www.behavioralandbrainfunctions.com/content/pdf/1744-9081-3-2.pdf.

Linazaroso, G., N. van Biercom, and A. Lasa. "Hypothesis: Parkinson's Disease, Reward Deficiency Syndrome and Addictive Effects of Levodopa." *Neurlogia* 19, no. 3 (2004):117–27.

Schultz, W. "Behavioral Theories and the Neurophysiology of Reward." *Annual Review of Psychology* 57 (2006): 87–115.

Shaffer, H. J., et al. "Toward a Syndrome Model of Addiction: Multiple Expressions, Common Etiology." *Harvard Review Psychiatry.* 12, no. 6 (2004): 367–74.

Volkow, N. D., et al. "Rain DA D2 Receptors Predict Reinforcing Effects of Stimulants in Humans: Replication Study." *Synapse* 46, no. 2 (2002): 79–82.

Wang, G., N. D. Volkow, P. K. Thanos, and J. S. Fowler. "Similarity Between Obesity and Drug Addiction as Assessed by Neurofunctional Imaging: A Concept Review." *Journal of Addictive Diseases* 23, no. 3 (2004): 39–53.

ORGANIZATIONS

American Psychiatric Association, 1000 Wilson Blvd., Ste. 1825, Arlington, VA, 22209-3901, (703) 907-7300, apa@psych.org, http://www.psych.org.

Patty Inglish, MS

Riluzole

Purpose

Riluzole (brand name Rilutek), a member of the benzothiazole class of drugs, is the only medication that has been proven effective for treating amyotrophic lateral sclerosis (ALS or Lou Gehrig's disease, a degenerative disease that affects neurons in the **brain** and spinal cord). Research indicates that the neuroprotective properties of riluzole might also make it useful for treating **depression**, although it is not approved by the U.S. Food and Drug Administration (FDA) for that purpose.

Description

Riluzole acts on glutamate, an excitatory amino acid neurotransmitter that carries messages to and from nerve cells in the brain. Glutamate is part of the glutamatergic system, which plays a role in memory and information processing. An excess of glutamate is believed to lead to ALS symptoms. Abnormal glutamate levels have also been implicated in depression and other mood disorders. In animal studies, for example, increased glutamate in the brain was associated with feelings of anxiety and fear. Riluzole works by blocking the release of glutamate in the brain. Riluzole also inhibits sodium channels and activates potassium channels leading to alterations in calcium currents. The mechanism responsible for any effect on ALS or depression symptoms may be a combination of an effect on glutamate release and these other effects.

Although **antidepressants** are the mainstay of treatment for mood disorders, studies indicate that about 30% to 40% of patients do not respond to them. Therefore, researchers are investigating new therapeutic agents that are more effective with fewer adverse effects.

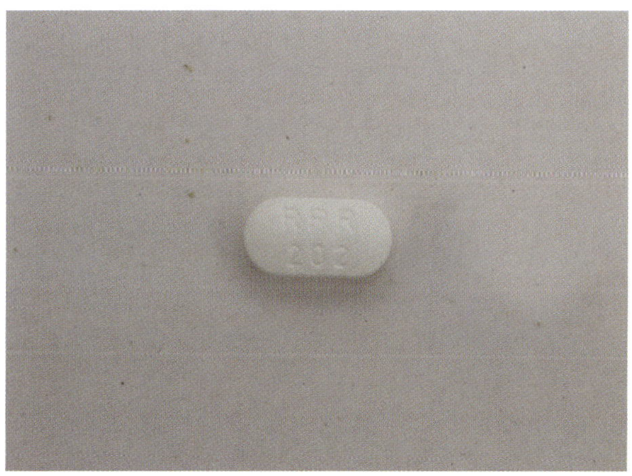

Rilutek (riluzole), 50 mg. *(© Custom Medical Stock Photo, Inc. Reproduced by permission.)*

Preliminary studies have demonstrated the effectiveness of riluzole for treating major depression, **bipolar disorder**, and **generalized anxiety disorder**. A study published in December 2005 in the *American Journal of Psychiatry* found that riluzole was effective in achieving remission in about half of a group of adults who had been diagnosed with generalized anxiety disorder. In a 2004 study that was published in February 2005 in *Biological Psychiatry*, riluzole improved symptoms in patients with treatment-resistant depression (depression that had not responded to antidepressant medications). Riluzole also was well tolerated in these studies.

Researchers say larger, placebo-controlled trials are needed to confirm the results of these preliminary investigations. As of 2011, new research was underway, including controlled studies investigating the potential effects of riluzole on the treatment of bipolar disorder. Research also indicates that riluzole might be effective for the treatment of obsessive-compulsive and panic disorders, but further study is needed.

Recommended dosage

Because riluzole was not yet FDA-approved for treating mood disorders as of 2011, appropriate doses have only been described in research studies. In studies, patients have been given between 50 and 200 mg of riluzole per day.

Precautions

Because riluzole blocks the release of the excitatory neurotransmitter, glutamate, this drug can cause drowsiness. Patients are advised to use caution when driving or operating machinery. Alcohol can increase this side effect, and people who are taking the drug should therefore avoid or use alcohol in moderation. Women who are pregnant, plan to become pregnant, or are breastfeeding should let their doctor know before taking this medication. Smoking cigarettes can decrease the effectiveness of this medication by causing the body to eliminate riluzole more quickly.

People who have liver dysfunction should use caution when taking this drug because it may not metabolize properly. Researchers who have studied the drug recommend that patients who are taking it be monitored for potential liver function problems.

Side effects

The side effects most commonly reported with riluzole include:

- abdominal pain
- constipation
- decreased saliva
- diarrhea
- dizziness
- drowsiness
- dry mouth
- headache
- insomnia
- muscle weakness
- nausea
- vertigo
- vomiting

These symptoms may be lessened by lowering the dose.

Interactions

The following drugs may decrease the rate at which riluzole is eliminated, which could potentially cause a buildup of the drug in the body:

- amitriptyline
- caffeine
- phenactin
- quinolones
- theophylline

KEY TERMS

Amyotrophic lateral sclerosis (ALS or Lou Gehrig's disease)—A degenerative disease that affects nerves of the brain and spinal cord, and results in eventual paralysis.

Bipolar disorder—A brain disorder that causes rapid mood shifts.

Generalized anxiety disorder—A mental disorder characterized by excessive and uncontrollable worry.

Glutamate—An excitatory amino acid neurotransmitter that carries messages to and from nerve cells in the brain.

Glutamatergic system—The neurotransmitter system in the central nervous system that plays a role in memory formation and information processing, and that is believed to play a role in depression and other mood disorders.

Obsessive-compulsive disorder—A disorder marked by persistent thoughts or fears, which lead to the compulsion to repeat a particular task over and over again.

Conversely, the following substances may increase the rate at which riluzole is eliminated from the body, potentially reducing its effectiveness:

- cigarettes
- charcoal-grilled foods
- barbiturates
- rifampicin

Resources

BOOKS

Mondimore, Francis Mark. *Bipolar Disorder: A Guide for Patients and Families*. 2nd ed. Baltimore: The Johns Hopkins University Press, 2006.

Ropper, Allan, MD, and Martin A. Samuels. *Adams and Victor's Principles of Neurology*. 8th ed. New York: The McGraw Hill Companies, 2009.

Swartz, Karen L. *Johns Hopkins White Papers: Depression and Anxiety*. New York: Medletter Associates, 2005.

PERIODICALS

Sanjay, Mathew J., et al. "Open-label Trial of Riluzole in Generalized Anxiety Disorder." *American Journal of Psychiatry*. 162, no. 12 (December 2005): 2379–81.

Zarate, Carlos A. Jr., et al. "An Open-label Trial of the Glutamate-modulating Agent Riluzole in Combination with Lithium for the Treatment of Bipolar Depression." *Biological Psychiatry*. 57, no. 4 (February 15, 2005): 430–32.

Zarate, Carlos Al Jr., et al. "Glutamatergic Modulators: the Future of Treating Mood Disorders?" *Harvard Review of Psychiatry* 18, no. 5 (2010): 293–303.

WEBSITES

Yale School of Medicine. "Depression Treatment Study." Yale Depresion Research Clinic. http://psychiatry.yale.edu/research/programs/clinical_people/trials/sanacora1.aspx (accessed November 13, 2011).

ORGANIZATIONS

American Psychiatric Association, 1000 Wilson Blvd., Ste. 1825, Arlington, VA, 22209-3901, (703) 907-7300, apa@psych.org, http://www.psych.org.

Brain and Behavior Research Foundation, 60 Cutter Mill Rd., Ste. 404, Great Neck, NY, 11021, (516) 829-0091, Fax: (516) 487-6930, http://www.bbrfoundation.org.

National Alliance on Mental Illness, 3803 N Fairfax Drive, Ste. 100, Arlington, VA, 22203, (703) 524-7600, http://www.nami.org.

National Institute of Mental Health, 6001 Executive Blvd., Room 8184, MSC 9663, Bethesda, MD, 20892-9663, (301) 433-4513; TTY: (301) 443-8431, Fax: (301) 443-4279, (866) 615-6464; TTY: (866) 415-8051, nimhinfo@nih.gov, http://www.nimh.nih.gov.

Stephanie N. Watson

Risperdal *see* **Risperidone**

Risperidone

Definition

Risperidone is classified as an atypical antipsychotic drug. It is sold in the United States under the brand name of Risperdal.

Purpose

Risperidone is used for the management of symptoms of psychotic disorders such as **schizophrenia**.

Description

Risperidone is considered an atypical antipsychotic. Atypical antipsychotics are chemically unrelated to the older antipsychotic drugs. Where older antipsychotic drugs primarily inhibit the actions of **dopamine**, a chemical in the **brain**, risperidone may also have some action against another brain chemical, **serotonin**. The proper levels of both dopamine and serotonin are influential in maintaining mental well-being.

One advantage of using risperidone over one of the older antipsychotic drugs is a lower incidence of Parkinsonian-like side effects. These side effects may be sufficiently troublesome, causing patients to discontinue treatment for their schizophrenia. For this reason, patients who have had negative experiences with older antipsychotics may benefit from risperidone. Some patients who showed little improvement with older antipsychotic drugs responded better to risperidone.

Recently, the effectiveness of risperidone was evaluated in the Clinical Antipsychotic Trials of **Intervention** Effectiveness (**CATIE**) Schizophrenia Study. This study evaluated the effectiveness and side

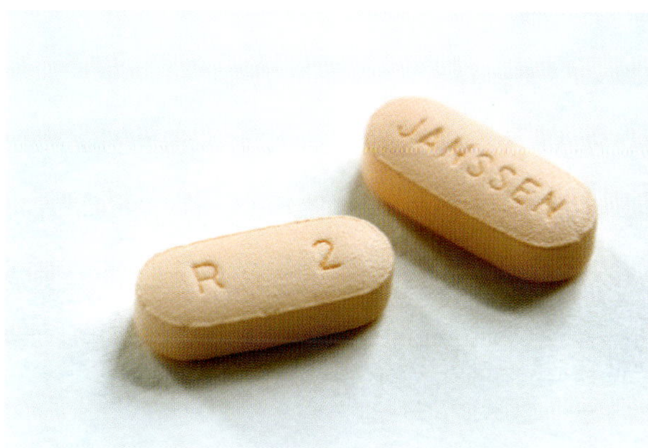

Risperdal (risperidone). *(© Chris Gallagher/Photo Researchers, Inc.)*

effects of atypical antipsychotics, including risperidone, in comparison to a conventional antipsychotic drug in the treatment of schizophrenia.

Contrary to expectations, the study found that the conventional antipsychotic generally was equally effective and tolerated as well as the newer, more expensive, atypical antipsychotic medications. The study showed that risperidone and another atypical, **olanzapine**, tend to be better tolerated than the other atypical antipsychotics investigated, although only 35% of participants on risperidone were able to continue taking it throughout the entire 18 months of the study. Participants who stopped taking an alternate antipsychotic medication in Phase 1 because it was not adequately controlling their symptoms were more likely to stay on their medication if they were switched to risperidone or olanzapine than to the drugs **quetiapine** or **ziprasidone**. There was no difference between the four medications, however, for participants who had stopped because of adverse side effects.

In Phase 2 of the study, the drug **clozapine** was more effective in controlling symptoms than the other atypical antipsychotics. For patients whose symptoms were not well controlled on clozapine, risperidone and olanzapine tended to be more effective than ziprasidone or quetiapine. Of the drugs evaluated, risperidone had the least adverse side effects.

Recommended dosage

Risperidone is available in 0.25 mg, 0.5 mg, 1 mg, 2 mg, 3 mg, and 4 mg tablets and a solution containing 1 mg of drug in each milliliter of solution. For treating psychotic disorders in adults, the usual starting dose of risperidone is 1 mg twice daily. Dosage is increased gradually until a target dose of 3 mg twice daily is reached. Some patients do just as well with a single daily dose (6 mg once a day, for example). There is little clinical evidence to indicate that increasing the daily dose beyond 8 mg offers additional benefit. However, higher doses may contribute to additional side effects. If the dose needs to be adjusted, the changes should be made no more often than once per week.

In older patients (over age 60), starting dosage should not exceed 1 mg daily. Most patients should not take more than 3 mg daily. People with low blood pressure and those who have kidney disease should take a similarly reduced dose.

Precautions

Patients with a history of cardiovascular disease or low blood pressure should take risperidone only after discussing the risks and benefits with their physicians, and then with close physician monitoring. Risperidone may cause abnormal heart rhythm (arrhythmia) that may prove fatal.

Risperidone has occasionally been associated with **seizures**. People with a past history of seizures should discuss with their doctors whether risperidone is the right antipsychotic for them to use.

People taking risperidone should avoid operating a motor vehicle or other dangerous machinery until they see how risperidone affects them.

Some people have trouble regulating their body temperatures while taking risperidone and are at risk of developing malignant hyperthermia. Patients receiving this drug should be aware of this and should avoid extremes in outdoor temperatures.

The use of risperidone and other antipsychotic drugs has been associated with an increased risk of death when used in elderly patients with **dementia**. In studies, these drugs significantly increased death in older patients with dementia, compared to placebo. Most of the deaths were associated with heart failure or infections such as pneumonia. Risperidone has not been approved by the U.S. Food and Drug Administration (FDA) for the treatment of **psychosis** or behavioral problems in elderly patients with dementia.

Women who are pregnant should not take risperidone and should alert their physicians if they become pregnant while on risperidone. Babies born to mothers who took risperidone during pregnancy may develop extrapyramidal symptoms (EPS) and withdrawal symptoms, including agitation, trouble breathing, and difficulty feeding. Breast-feeding is not recommended while taking the drug.

Patients may develop hyperglycemia (high blood sugar) while taking risperidone. People with schizophrenia are more likely to develop diabetes than those without schizophrenia, and taking risperidone increases this risk. Patients should alert their doctors immediately if they experience symptoms of diabetes, including excessive thirst or hunger, frequent urination, blurry vision, or **fatigue**.

Risperidone has been associated with the risk of developing hyperprolactinemia, a blood disorder caused by heightened levels of the hormone prolactin. Symptoms include amenorrhea and lactation in women and breast development and **erectile dysfunction** in men.

Side effects

The most common and bothersome side effect associated with risperidone is decreased blood pressure while standing up (known as "orthostatic hypotension"). This can cause dizziness or fainting. A decrease in blood

KEY TERMS

Amenorrhea—Abnormal cessation of menstruation.

Extrapyramidal symptoms—A group of side effects associated with antipsychotic medications and characterized by involuntary muscle movements, including contraction and tremor.

pressure usually occurs early in therapy, when the proper dose is still being established. It is more common in older patients than in younger ones. Usually this side effect disappears entirely with time. If it continues, the physician may decrease the dose. Meanwhile, people taking risperidone should be aware of this side effect and get up slowly if they have been sitting for an extended time.

The most common nervous system side effects of risperidone include **insomnia**, agitation, anxiety, and headache. Early in therapy, patients may experience an inability to think clearly or perform certain tasks that require mental alertness. High doses of risperidone can cause unwanted sleepiness in about 40% of patients.

Antipsychotic drugs, including risperidone, can cause side effects that are similar to the symptoms of Parkinson's disease, including muscle tremor, difficulty with voluntary movements, and poor muscle tone. They normally disappear if the drug is stopped.

The most common gastrointestinal side effects include nausea, vomiting, constipation, and difficulty digesting food. Risperidone may cause weight gain.

Up to 10% of patients taking risperidone experience rhinitis (runny nose).

Interactions

There is very little information about how risperidone interacts with other drugs. However, because some patients receiving risperidone experience lowered blood pressure while standing, it is expected that other drugs that lower blood pressure may increase the incidence and severity of this side effect when taken with risperidone.

Resources

BOOKS

American Society of Health-System Pharmacists. *AHFS Drug Information 2008.* Bethesda, MD: American Society of Health-System Pharmacists, 2008.

Preston, John D., John H. O'Neal, and Mary C. Talaga. *Handbook of Clinical Psychopharmacology for Therapists*. 5th ed. Oakland, CA: New Harbinger Publications, 2008.

PERIODICALS

Casey, Daniel E. "Implications of the CATIE Trial on Treatment: Extrapyramidal Symptoms." *CNS Spectrums* 11, no. 7, Supp. 7 (July 2006): 25–31.

Gentile, Salvatore. "Extrapyramidal Adverse Events Associated with Atypical Antipsychotic Treatment of Bipolar Disorder." *Journal of Clinical Psychopharmacology* 27, no. 1 (February 2007): 35–45.

Glick, Ira D. "Understanding the Results of CATIE in the Context of the Field." *CNS Spectrums* 11, no. 7, Supp. 7 (July 2006): 40–47.

Haro, Josep Maria et al. "Remission and Relapse in the Outpatient Care of Schizophrenia: Three-Year Results from the Schizophrenia Outpatient Health Outcomes Study." *Journal of Clinical Psychopharmacology* 26, no. 6 (December 2006): 571–78.

Haupt, Martin, Alfonso Cruz-Jentoft, and Dilip Jeste. "Mortality in Elderly Dementia Patients Treated with Risperidone." *Journal of Clinical Psychopharmacology* 26, no. 6 (December 2006): 566–70.

Lieberman, Jeffrey A., et al. "Effectiveness of Antipsychotic Drugs in Patients with Chronic Schizophrenia." *New England Journal of Medicine* 353, no. 12 (September 2005): 1209–23.

Luby, Joan et al. "Risperidone in Preschool Children with Autistic Spectrum Disorders: An Investigation of Safety and Efficacy." *Journal of Child and Adolescent Psychopharmacology* 16, no. 5 (October 2006): 575–87.

McCue, Robert E., et al. "Comparative Effectiveness of Second-Generation Antipsychotics and Haloperidol in Acute Schizophrenia." *British Journal of Psychiatry* 189 (November 2006): 433–40.

Meltzer, Herbert Y., and William V. Bobo. "Interpreting the Efficacy Findings in the CATIE Study: What Clinicians Should Know." *CNS Spectrums* 11, Supp. 7 (July 2006): 14–24.

Nasrallah, Henry A. "Metabolic Findings From the CATIE Trial and Their Relation to Tolerability." *CNS Spectrums* 11, no. 7, Supp. 7 (July 2006): 32–39.

Pandina, Gahan J., Michael G. Aman, and Robert L. Findling. "Risperidone in the Management of Disruptive Behavior Disorders." *Journal of Child and Adolescent Psychopharmacology* 16, no. 4 (August 2006): 379–92.

Savas, Haluk A., et al. "Use of Long-Acting Risperidone in the Treatment of Bipolar Patients." *Journal of Clinical Psychopharmacology* 26, no. 5 (October 2006): 530–31.

Schneider, Lon S., et al. "Effectiveness of Atypical Antipsychotic Drugs in Patients with Alzheimer's Disease." *New England Journal of Medicine* 355, no. 15 (October 2006): 1525–38.

Stroup, T. Scott et al. "Effectiveness of Olanzapine, Quetiapine, Risperidone, and Ziprasidone in Patients with Chronic Schizophrenia Following Discontinuation of a Previous Atypical Antipsychotic." *American Journal of Psychiatry* 163, no. 4 (April 2006): 611–22.

Taylor, David M., Corina Young, and Maxine X. Patel. "Prospective 6-Month Follow-Up of Patients Prescribed Risperidone Long-Acting Injection: Factors Predicting

Favourable Outcome." *International Journal of Neuropsychopharmacology* 9, no. 6 (December 2006): 685–94.

Troost, Pieter W., et al. "Neuropsychological Effects of Risperidone in Children with Pervasive Developmental Disorders: A Blinded Discontinuation Study." *Journal of Child and Adolescent Psychopharmacology* 16, no. 5 (October 2006): 561–73.

Weiden, Peter J. "EPS Profiles: The Atypical Antipsychotics Are Not All the Same." *Journal of Psychiatric Practice* 13, no. 1 (Jan. 2007): 13–24.

Jack Raber, Pharm.D.
Ruth A. Wienclaw, PhD

Ritalin *see* **Methylphenidate**

Rivastigmine

Definition

Rivastigmine is a drug used to treat symptoms of **Alzheimer's disease**. In the United States, rivastigmine is sold as the brand name drug Exelon.

Purpose

Rivastigmine is used to treat symptoms of Alzheimer's disease in individuals with mild to moderate illness. It has also been used to treat **dementia** caused by other conditions such as Lewy body disease or following strokes. The drug may produce mild improvements in symptoms of thinking for a short period of time, but rivastigmine does not cure or stop progression of underlying diseases.

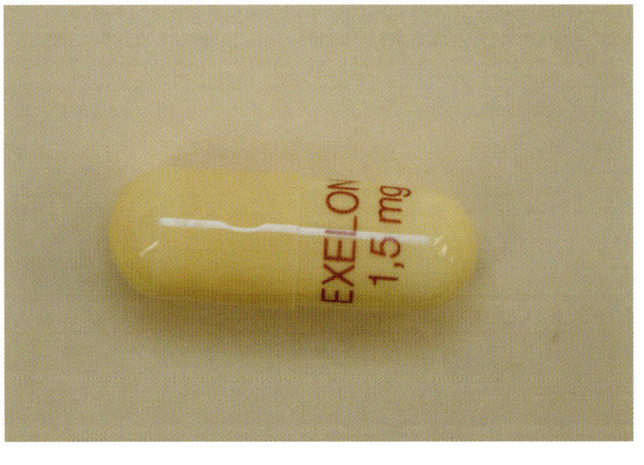

Exelon (rivastigmine), 1.5 mg. *(© Custom Medical Stock Photo, Inc. Reproduced by permission.)*

Description

The U.S. Food and Drug Administration approved rivastigmine in 2000 specifically for treating Alzheimer's disease. In patients with Alzheimer's disease, some cells in specific regions of the **brain** die. Because of this cell death, these brain cells lose their ability to transmit nerve impulses. Brain cells normally transmit nerve impulses to one another by secreting various chemicals known as **neurotransmitters**.

Brain cells that make and secrete a neurotransmitter called acetylcholine are affected early in the course of Alzheimer's disease. Rivastigmine prevents the breakdown of acetylcholine in the brain, thus temporarily increasing its concentration. In doing so, rivastigmine may improve the thinking process by facilitating nerve impulse transmission within the brain.

Rivastigmine is available as capsules in four different strengths and as an oral solution for use by people who have difficulty swallowing. It is also available in a transdermal patch that is applied to the skin. Unlike some other drugs used to treat Alzheimer's disease, rivastigmine is not broken down by the liver. As a result, it may be preferred in the treatment of people with Alzheimer's disease who have liver disease.

Recommended dosage

The initial dosage of rivastigmine is 1.5 mg taken two times per day. If this dose is tolerated without difficulty, the dosage may be increased to 3 mg twice a day after at least two weeks at the lower dosage. Some people are unable to tolerate nausea, vomiting, anorexia, and weight loss that occur with higher dosages. If the drug does not cause significant adverse effects, the dose may be increased to 4.5 mg two times per day, followed by 6 mg two times per day. The dosage should be increased slowly, at two-week intervals. If side effects occur and cannot be tolerated, the drug may be stopped for several doses. When the drug is started again, the same dosage or the next lower dosage may be tried. The maximum daily dosage is 6 mg two times per day.

The patch is applied to dry skin on the back, upper arm, or chest. The patch is left on for 24 hours and then replaced with a new patch. Each new patch should be applied to a new area of skin; the same location should not be used until a two-week period has passed.

Precautions

Rivastigmine may slow heart rates, increase acid in the stomach, make urination difficult, cause breathing difficulties, and may possibly contribute to **seizures**. As a result, it should be used with close physician supervision and monitoring in people with certain heart

KEY TERMS

Acetylcholine—A naturally occurring chemical in the body that transmits nerve impulses from cell to cell. Generally, it has opposite effects from dopamine and norepinephrine; it causes blood vessels to dilate, lowers blood pressure, and slows the heartbeat. Central nervous system well-being is dependent on a balance among acetylcholine, dopamine, serotonin, and norepinephrine.

Dementia—A group of symptoms (syndrome) associated with a progressive loss of memory and other intellectual functions that is serious enough to interfere with a person's ability to perform the tasks of daily life. Dementia impairs memory, alters personality, leads to deterioration in personal grooming, impairs reasoning ability, and causes disorientation.

Lewy body disease—A type of dementia that resembles Alzheimer's disease but progresses more rapidly. Common symptoms include fluctuations in confusion and recurring visual hallucinations. In this disease, abnormal brain cells are distributed throughout the brain.

Neurotransmitter—A chemical in the brain that transmits messages between neurons, or nerve cells.

Placebo—An inactive substance or preparation used as a control in experiments with human subjects to test the effectiveness of a drug or herbal preparation. Some patients may experience a medicinal response or experience side effects to a placebo simply because they have faith in its powers even though it contains no medicine.

conditions, tendencies to stomach ulcers, bladder obstruction, asthma or chronic obstructive pulmonary disease, and a history of seizure disorders.

Individuals taking rivastigmine should be reassessed periodically to determine whether the drug is providing any benefits. If caregivers feel the drug is no longer beneficial, it may be stopped.

Side effects

The most frequent side effects associated with rivastigmine involve stomach upset. Nausea, vomiting, anorexia, heartburn, and weakness occur in more than 5% of people and at twice the rate of people taking placebo pills. Dizziness and headaches also occur in more than 10% of people taking rivastigmine.

Other less common side effects include difficulty sleeping, confusion, **depression**, anxiety, sleepiness, hallucinations, tremors, fainting, aggression, constipation, gas, overwhelming **fatigue**, weight loss, increased sweating, and infections.

Interactions

Drugs such as dicyclomine may inhibit the effects of rivastigmine. Other drugs like bethanechol may possibly increase some of the side effects of rivastigmine. Rivastigmine may interact with some of the drugs used to relax muscles during surgery. The interaction increases the effects of both drugs.

Resources

BOOKS

Tekin, Sibel, and Roger Lane. "Rivastigmine in the Treatment of Dementia Associated with Parkinson's Disease: A Randomized, Double-Blind, Placebo-Controlled Study." In *Progress in Neurotherapeutics and Neuropsychopharmacology,* edited by Jeffrey L. Cummings. New York: Cambridge University Press, 2006.

Wolters Kluwer Health. *Drug Facts and Comparisons 2012.* 66th ed. St. Louis: Lippincott, Williams & Wilkins, 2011.

PERIODICALS

de Tommaso, Marina, et al. "Two Years' Follow-Up of Rivastigmine Treatment in Huntington Disease." *Clinical Neuropharmacology* 30, no. 1 (January–February 2007): 43–46.

Dybicz, Sharon B., et al. "Patterns of Cholinesterase-Inhibitor Use in the Nursing Home Setting: A Retrospective Analysis." *American Journal of Geriatric Pharmacotherapy* 4, no. 2 (June 2006): 154–60.

Eskander, Mariam F., et al. "Rivastigmine Is a Potent Inhibitor of Acetyl- and Butyrylcholinesterase in Alzheimer's Plaques and Tangles." *Brain Research* 1060, no. 1–2 (Oct. 2005): 144–52.

Farlow, Martin R., et al. "Efficacy of Rivastigmine in Alzheimer's Disease Patients with Rapid Disease Progression: Results of a Meta-Analysis." *Dementia and Geriatric Cognitive Disorders* 20, no. 2–3 (August 2005): 192–97.

Guillem, Francois, et al. "Are Cholinergic Enhancers Beneficial for Memory in Schizophrenia? An Event-Related Potentials (ERPs) Study of Rivastigmine Add-On Therapy in a Crossover Trial." *Progress in Neuro-Psychopharmacology & Biological Psychiatry* 30, no. 5 (July 2006): 934–45.

Miyasaki, J.M., et al. "Practice Parameter: Evaluation and Treatment of Depression, Psychosis, and Dementia in Parkinson Disease (an Evidence-Based Review): Report of the Quality Standards Subcommittee of the American Academy of Neurology." *Neurology* 66, no. 7 (April 2006): 996–1002.

Ringman, John M., and Jeffrey L. Cummings. "Current and Emerging Pharmacological Treatment Options for Dementia." *Behavioural Neurology* 17, no. 1 (2006): 5–16.

Rongve, Arvid, and Dag Aarsland. "Management of Parkinson's Disease Dementia: Practical Considerations." *Drugs and Aging* 23, no. 10 (2006): 807–22.

Sharma, Tonmoy, et al. "Cognitive Effects of Adjunctive 24-Weeks Rivastigmine Treatment to Antipsychotics in Schizophrenia: A Randomized, Placebo-Controlled, Double-Blind Investigation." *Schizophrenia Research* 85, no. 1–3 (July 2006): 73–83.

Takeda, A., et al. "A Systematic Review of the Clinical Effectiveness of Donepezil, Rivastigmine and Galantamine on Cognition, Quality of Life and Adverse Events in Alzheimer's Disease." *International Journal of Geriatric Psychiatry* 21, no. 1 (January 2006): 17–28.

WEBSITES

Drugs.com. "Rivastigmine Patch." http://www.drugs.com/cdi/rivastigmine-patch.html (accessed November 13, 2011).

PubMed Health. "Rivastigmine." U.S. National Library of Medicine. http://www.ncbi.nlm.nih.gov/pubmedhealth/PMH0000190 (accessed November 13, 2011).

ORGANIZATIONS

U.S. Food and Drug Administration, 10903 New Hampshire Ave., Silver Spring, MD, 20993-0002, (888) INFO-FDA (463-6332), http://www.fda.gov.

Kelly Karpa, R.Ph.,PhD
Ruth A. Wienclaw, PhD

RLS *see* **Restless legs syndrome**

Road rage

Definition

Road rage is an extreme form of aggressive driving. Road rage is distinguished by its extreme response (often violent or assaultive in nature) and by its intent to harm another individual either physically or psychologically. Road rage is not considered to be a psychiatric disorder.

Demographics

Research indicates that younger drivers tend to be more likely to engage in aggressive and risk-taking driving behaviors, although aggressive driving is observed in all ages. Research does not support the conclusion that males are more aggressive drivers than females.

Description

Although the term "road rage" has been popularized by the media, there is no consensus among researchers over the definition of this term. Aggressive driving—of which road rage is an extreme subset—includes a wide variety of behaviors such as speeding, cutting off another driver in traffic, tailgating, horn honking, and light flashing. Aggressive driving may also include more extreme actions ranging from roadside arguments or rude gestures to even shootings and assaults.

Road rage is differentiated from the more general concept of aggressive driving by both degree and intent. Definitions of road rage often include the concept that the anger is uncontrolled and violent. Road rage is not an isolated phenomenon; similar incidents have been found in the workplace (workplace rage) and airports (airport rage).

Causes and symptoms

There are numerous theories relating to the causes of aggressive driving and road rage. Most of these theories revolve around the concept of driver frustration and anger. It has been hypothesized, for example, that the competitiveness of the driving environment leads to aggressive driving behavior or that aggressive driving is part of a territorial defense reaction.

In some individuals, road rage may be a symptom of **intermittent explosive disorder** (IED). IED is an impulse-control disorder in which the individual acts on his or her impulses in assaultive or destructive ways that are out of proportion to the events or factors that triggered the act. IED is a pattern of aggressive behavior rather than an isolated incident, and is not caused by any other mental disorder, general condition, or chemical substance.

It also has been suggested that road rage can be a result of other underlying causes. These include

Aggressive driving and road rage symptoms

- Thoughts of harassment toward other drivers, whether verbal or physical
- Verbally expressing these thoughts to other passengers in the vehicle
- Disregarding traffic safety rules
- Engaging in aggressive and risky driving behaviors, including:
    - Following other cars too closely
    - Speeding
    - Weaving in and out of traffic
    - Speeding up to beat a traffic light
    - Cutting between vehicles to change lanes
    - Using the horn (excessively)
    - Flashing headlights at oncoming traffic (excessively)
    - Braking abruptly or repeatedly to get other drivers to not follow so closely
    - Passing another driver and then purposely slowing down

SOURCE: Washington State Patrol.

(Table by PreMediaGlobal. © 2012 Cengage Learning.)

social maladjustment, personal maladjustment, and psychopathology.

Diagnosis

For those situations where road rage is caused by IED, diagnostic criteria include:

- discrete episodes where the individual acts out aggressive impulses that result in violent assault or destruction of property
- aggressive response to driving stressors that is excessively disproportionate to the provocation
- absence of other disorders that may cause violent outbursts (e.g., antisocial personality disorder, borderline personality disorder, attention deficit hyperactivity disorder)
- absence of a general medical condition that may express itself in aggressiveness (e.g., head injury, Alzheimer's disease)
- individual is not taking medications with the potential side effect of increased aggressive behavior
- no substance abuse

Diagnosis of road rage is made based on a psychiatric interview to assess mental and behavioral symptoms. For road rage stemming from non-psychiatric causes, driving anger scales and driver's **stress** profiles are also available. Individuals may also be referred for treatment by court mandate.

Treatment

For road rage caused by IED, treatment may be achieved through **cognitive-behavioral therapy** (CBT) and/or psychotropic medication. CBT helps individuals recognize and become aware of the impulses that result in aggressive behavior so that they can control the impulses before they are acted upon. This therapy is typically supplemented by teaching the individuals **stress management** skills.

Road rage not related to IED has been successfully treated with desensitization therapy that helps the individual learn to not react to stimuli that provoke an aggressive response, stress management training including relaxation techniques, and other anger management techniques.

Prognosis

With therapy and proper training, the prognosis for controlling road rage is good.

KEY TERMS

Cognitive behavior therapy (CBT)—A form of psychotherapy that aims to identify and modify the individual's inappropriate behavior as well as the underlying maladaptive thought processes.

Psychotropic drug—A drug that acts on or influences the activity of the mind.

Stressor—An internal or external event, force, or condition that results in physical or psychological stress.

Territorial aggression—The response of aggressively defending a defined space perceived as being threatened by a member of the same species.

Prevention

Prevention of road rage is dependent on helping individuals recognize the symptoms of their anger and teaching them techniques to reduce their stress or control their reaction to stressors.

Resources

BOOKS

American Psychiatric Association. *Diagnostic and Statistical Manual of Mental Disorders*. 4th ed., text rev. Washington, DC: American Psychiatric Publishing, 2000.

Galovski, Tara E. *Road Rage: Assessment and Treatment of the Angry, Aggressive Driver*. Washington, DC: American Psychological Association, 2006.

Garase, Maria L. *Road Rage*. New York: LFB Scholarly Publications, 2006.

VandenBos, Gary R. ed. *APA Dictionary of Psychology*. Washington, DC: American Psychological Association, 2006.

Ruth A. Wienclaw, Ph.D.

Rorschach inkblot test

Definition

The Rorschach inkblot test, also known as the Rorschach Technique, the Rorschach psychodiagnostic test, the Rorschach test, and popularly as simply the "Inkblot Test," is a projective personality assessment based on the test taker's reactions to a series of 10 standardized unstructured images or "inkblots." These inkblots are then psychologically interpreted by

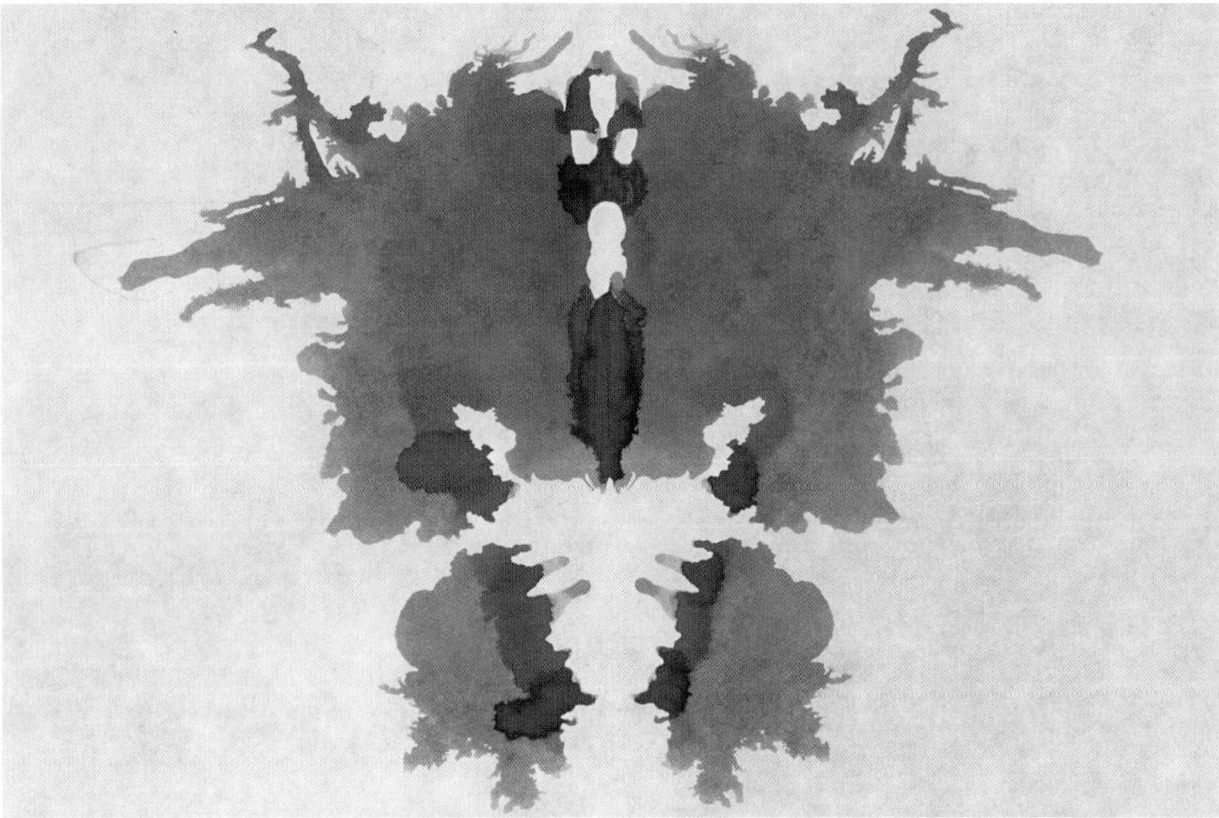

An inkblot picture, such as the ones used in the Rorschach inkblot test. *(© Custom Medical Stock Photo, Inc. Reproduced by permission.)*

psychologists and other trained professionals. As a projective psychological test, the Rorschach test was founded on the hypothesis that subjects will interject their own personalities into neutral appearing images, thus revealing their own personality characteristics, hidden emotions, underlying conflicts, reactions to surroundings and the environment, illogical thought processes, and underpinned motivations.

Purpose

The purpose of the Rorschach test is to examine and **diagnosis** the personality characteristics of people, along with the functioning of their emotions. It is also used expressly to better understand thought disorders in people, especially when such persons are unwilling or unable to openly talk about such problems.

Description

The Rorschach test remains one of the most widely used projective psychological test in the world, although its popularity has declined somewhat over the past several decades. It is often included as one of a series of tests used to assess personality, such as for investigations where forensic assessment is needed and in clinical settings where evaluations of mentally disturbed are required. It is generally administered to adolescents and adults but can be used with children as young as three years of age. It must be administered on an individual basis; group evaluations are not possible.

The Rorschach test is used to assess personality structure and identify emotional problems. The test provides information about a child's thought processes, perceptions, motivations, and attitude toward his or her environment, and it can detect internal and external pressures and conflicts as well as illogical or psychotic thought patterns. It can aid in diagnosing and treating a wide range of psychological problems and psychiatric disorders, including **depression**, **schizophrenia**, and **anxiety disorders**.

The untimed, individually administered test consists of interpreting a series of 10 complicated looking inkblots. The test consists of the test taker being shown inkblots on separate white cards and then being asked a set of standard questions about what he or she sees. The administrator of the test traditionally sits slightly behind the test taker. Five of the ten original inkblots consist entirely of black ink on a white background, while two use black and red ink and three consist of several colors of ink.

The subject observes all of the 10 inkblots, one at a time, in a "free association" phase. Each inkblot is verbally described as to what it resembles. Then the administrator presents all of them again so that the subject has time to make additional responses as to what was originally seen in what is called the "inquiry" phase. The subject is allowed to hold the cards, rotate them, and take other such actions, all of which may add to the final interpretation by the administrator. During this time, the administrator notes all responses and actions by the subject, may ask questions to clarify responses, and maintains a running tabulation of the score.

Responses are tabulated, placed in summary form, and scored according to a set of criteria. Swiss **psychologist** Hermann Rorschach (1884–1922), who pioneered the test in 1921, did not provide a comprehensive scoring system, but many different ones have since been developed. The most thorough and widely used one is the Exner system, which was created by U.S. psychologist John E. Exner Jr. (1928–2006). In 1969 Exner published the book *The Rorschach Systems* and, later, *The Rorschach: A Comprehensive System.* Many consider the Exner system, which was released in 1987, to be the most objective and reliable method of scoring the test, showing especially high reliability among different evaluators. The Exner Comprehensive Rorschach System uses a computer-based scoring system, which includes score summaries and provides possible adjustment and personality descriptions for each subject.

Origins

Dr. Hermann Rorschach was interested in painting and drawing at an early age. By the time he entered graduate school Rorschach was still undecided as to whether to pursue a career in art or science. Although deciding upon science, he incorporated his interest in art within his professional activities; specifically, with his interest in "inkblot pictures" that went back to his childhood experiences.

Rorschach developed his series of inkblots after studying hundreds of introverted and extroverted patients in parallel with a lesser number of normal (control) subjects. Backed with about 10 years of research into using such inkblots to study patients, Rorschach wrote the book *Pscyodiagnostik (Psychodiagnostics)* in 1921, which detailed his studies and research into the use of inkblots to test the personality of people. In the book, he selected 10 specific inkblot cards as the foundation of his test. In 1942, the book was translated into English, and it was published as *Psychodiagnostics: A Diagnostic Test Based on Perception.*

KEY TERMS

Projective psychological test—Any test in psychology that is designed to allow the test subject to respond to ambiguous (those having more than one meaning) stimuli (such as images), which are intended to reveal to the evaluator hidden emotions and personality characteristics of the subject.

Psychodiagnostic—Various methods used to examine and analyze the factors that form human behavior, especially abnormal behavior.

Preparation

Preparation for the test is not necessary nor recommended.

Risks

Though only trained professionals should administer the test and evaluate it afterwards, the subjective nature of the test allows for the possibility of uncertainty in the results. Even though the Exner system is widely used in the scoring of the test, researchers sometimes criticize it for its lack of objectivity, reliability, and validity. Two professionals have the potential for scoring one individual very differently, based on the individual judgments of each person. The test itself is criticized for its inability to accurately assess personality in patients previously exposed to the inkblots.

The test often takes several hours to complete and interpret, which is sometimes seen as a negative for the test.

Results

Overall, the results of the test provide the administrator (evaluator) with information on cognitive and personality characteristics of the subject. Based on the subject's responses and actions, the evaluator should be able to reveal certain underlying characteristics of the individual, such as any conflicts residing within the person and any perceptions that the individual may have of the world or others. Because the evaluator must interpret the responses and actions of the subject, the interpretations of the subject by different evaluators may vary.

The scoring of the Rorschach test is based on several factors, such as the content of the subject's response. The content observed by the subject is usually classified by the evaluator in one of such groupings as humans, animals, nature, clothing, or abstract. A subject seeing a movie star would be grouped under human, while a leaf from a maple tree would be categorized under nature.

However, content alone is not the sole factor used in evaluations. A particular characteristic of the inkblot may determine the response by the subjects. Such a *determinant* includes the shape (or form) of the inkblot, along with subfactors such as color, movement, and shading. For instance, people who see movement (motion) within the inkblots are usually evaluated as introspective or intellectual. Those who see stationary objects in the inkblots are considered more practical by nature.

The Rorschach can be interpreted by the *location* within the inkblot from which the response originated. Location may consist of the entire blot, sections of it, or only specific details within it. Other factors include *popularity* (how common was the response when compared to others) and *originality* (how uncommon was the response).

The final outcome of the test can be affected by the demeanor of the subject, such as if he/she is cooperative or hostile toward the test, and/or the evaluator. These behaviors can influence the evaluator in the final scoring of the test.

The scoring of the Exner system, often considered one of the most reliable ways to score the Rorschach test, uses clusters of Rorschach variables as the centerpiece of its ability to accurately evaluate responses. It also contains a sequential search strategy that forces the evaluator to evaluate in a particular order. The Exner system uses a method that is objective, reliable, and follows a standardized procedure to assure unbiased evaluations.

Resources

BOOKS

Aronow, Edward, Marvin Reznikoff, and Kevin Moreland. *The Rorschach Technique: Perceptual Basics, Content Interpretation, and Applications.* Boston: Allyn and Bacon, 1994.

Drummond, Robert J. *Assessment Procedures for Counselors and Helping Professionals.* Boston: Pearson, 2010.

Frick, Paul J., Christopher T. Barry and Randy W. Kamphaus. *Clinical Assessment of Child and Adolescent Personality and Behavior.* New York: Springer, 2010.

Green, Susan K., and Robert L. Johnson. *Assessment Is Essential.* Boston: McGraw-Hill Higher Education, 2010.

Hart, Diane. *Authentic Assessment: A Handbook for Educators.* Menlo Park, CA: Addison-Wesley, 1994.

Lee, Steven W., ed. *Encyclopedia of School Psychology.* Thousand Oaks, CA: Sage, 2005.

Leichtman, Martin. *The Rorschach: A Developmental Perspective.* Hillsdale, NJ: Analytic Press, 1996.

McAfee, Oralie, and Deborah J. Leong. *Assessing and Guiding Young Children's Development and Learning.* Upper Saddle River, NJ: Pearson, 2011.

McCullough, Virginia E. *Testing and Your Child: What You Should Know about 150 of the Most Common Medical, Educational, and Psychological Tests.* New York: Plume, 1992.

Mindes, Gayle. *Assessing Young Children.* Boston: Pearson, 2011.

Psychodiagnostics: Bibliography. New York: Grune and Stratton, 1954.

Rorschach, Hermann. *Psychodiagnostik.* Bern: Bircher, 1921.

WEBSITES

"Are You Using the Right Assessment Instrument for the Right Child?" State Education Resource Center. http://www.ctserc.org/initiatives/ece/ecetests.shtml (accessed October 4, 2010).

"The Classical Rorschach." Göteborg University. http://www.phil.gu.se/fu/ro.html (accessed October 11, 2010).

Hermann Rorschach Archives and Museum website. http://www.zb.unibe.ch/rorschach/en/index.html (accessed October 11, 2010).

International Society of the Rorschach and Projective Methods website. http://www.rorschach.com (accessed October 11, 2010).

William Arthur Atkins

Rumination disorder

Definition

Rumination disorder may be diagnosed when a person deliberately brings food back up into the mouth and either rechews and reswallows it or spits it out.

Demographics

Rumination disorder occurs primarily in infants. The onset usually occurs before the infant's first birthday. The disorder is also more common in people with intellectual disabilities. The onset of rumination disorder is typically later in persons with intellectual disabilities, and may not appear until puberty or even the early adult years. Rumination disorder is rare and thought to occur more often in males than in females. People who have anorexia or bulimia may begin to ruminate only in adult life. One report found that up to 20% of people with bulimia may ruminate.

Description

Rumination disorder is sometimes called merycism. It is a disorder most commonly found in infants and is associated with intellectual disability. During rumination, previously eaten food is intentionally brought back into the mouth. Sometimes the child spits it out, but in other cases, the food is rechewed and reswallowed. The regurgitation is not caused by a medical condition. In many cases, the child has had an illness associated with vomiting that occurs before the onset of rumination disorder. Rumination has also been observed in severe cases of eating disorders among teenagers as well as adults.

Causes and symptoms

Causes

There is no general agreement on the causes of rumination disorder. In infants, it is thought to be caused by a lack of nurturing or physical contact. The child's rumination may represent an attempt to stimulate or soothe him- or herself. Biological factors are also being explored as possible causes of rumination disorder.

Symptoms

The symptoms of rumination include both the regurgitation of food and, in infants, the effort made to regurgitate that food. In infants, the attempts to bring up food can include putting fingers in the mouth, sucking on the tongue, and arching the back. When food is brought up, the cheeks expand and appear puffed. Sometimes an observer can detect the rechewing; the person often appears to take pleasure in the act. The person's breath may have a foul or sour odor. Some infants, especially those who have just begun ruminating, will expel most or all of the regurgitated food from their mouths. When this expulsion occurs, it is often mistaken for normal infant vomiting. As an infant continues to ruminate, he or she often learns to keep more and more of the regurgitated food in the mouth.

Diagnosis

The ***Diagnostic and Statistical Manual of Mental Disorders***, fourth edition, text revision (*DSM-IV-TR*), which is the standard reference work for mental health professionals, gives only three general criteria for diagnosing rumination disorder. The first is that the person's behavior of deliberately bringing up and rechewing food must have lasted for at least a month. The regurgitation and rechewing must happen after a period of time in which the person did not ruminate. In addition, the rumination cannot result from a medical condition such as esophageal reflux. In addition, the manual specifies that the rumination cannot be associated with anorexia or bulimia.

Rumination disorder may be difficult to diagnose. One reason for this difficulty is that infants or adults who do not expel any of their regurgitated food can often be identified only by a puffing of the cheeks when the food is in the mouth or by an unpleasant breath odor. In addition, because many people and infants who ruminate find the experience a positive and pleasurable one, there are no physical signs of discomfort to bring the disorder to the attention of caretakers or others.

Some experts disagree with the statement of the *Diagnostic and Statistical Manual* that a **diagnosis** of rumination disorder cannot be made if the rumination is associated with anorexia or bulimia. These experts maintain that diagnosing and treating rumination disorder in patients who have other eating disorders is important for the sake of the patient's health.

Treatment

Treatment for rumination disorder depends on the cause of the behavior. Infants who are thought to ruminate because of a lack of affection may be fed by someone other than their mother or father. This person can be a replacement while their parents receive treatment themselves. Other approaches involve therapy and parenting education to create a stronger bond between the parents and the child.

The treatment of adult patients includes giving them chewing gum to use when rumination might normally occur. Other researchers have found that giving adults with intellectual disabilites filling meals may reduce rumination. Treating such eating disorders as anorexia or bulimia frequently helps to resolve the rumination that may be associated with those disorders. **Behavior modification** techniques that help a patient to unlearn the ruminating behavior have also been used.

Prognosis

In many cases rumination that begins in infancy stops on its own. The disorder should be treated, however, because infants with untreated rumination disorder are at risk of malnutrition and death caused by dehydration. Treatments for rumination disorder are generally very effective. Treatment of associated eating disorders in adults is generally regarded as successful.

KEY TERMS

Merycism—Another name for rumination disorder.

Regurgitation—The return of partly digested food from the stomach to the mouth. Regurgitation may be either an intentional act or an involuntary physical reaction.

Ruminate—To chew or rechew regurgitated food.

Prevention

There is no known way to prevent rumination disorder. It is possible, however, that a strong parent-child bond may reduce the possibility of the disorder occurring in infants.

Resources

BOOKS

American Psychiatric Association. *Diagnostic and Statistical Manual of Mental Disorders*. 4th ed., text rev. Washington, DC: American Psychiatric Publishing, 2000.

Sadock, Benjamin J., and Virginia A. Sadock, eds. *Comprehensive Textbook of Psychiatry*. Vol. 2. 7th ed. Philadelphia: Lippincott Williams and Wilkins, 2000.

PERIODICALS

Weakley, Melinda M., Theodore A. Petti, and George Karwisch. "Case Study: Chewing Gum Treatment of Rumination in an Adolescent with an Eating Disorder." *Journal of the American Academy of Child and Adolescent Psychiatry* 36, no. 8 (August 1997): 1124–1128.

ORGANIZATIONS

American Academy of Pediatrics, 141 Northwest Point Blvd., Elk Grove Village, IL, 60007-1098, (847) 434-4000, Fax: (847) 434-8000, http://www.aap.org.

Tish Davidson, A.M.

S

SAD *see* **Seasonal affective disorder**

Sadism *see* **Sexual sadism**

Saffron

Description

Saffron is an herbal preparation harvested from the stigma of the *Crocus sativus* flower. It is dark orange and threadlike in appearance, with a spicy flavor and pungent odor. The plant is grown in India, Spain, France, Italy, the Middle East, and the eastern Mediterranean region.

Purpose

In addition to its culinary uses, saffron is prescribed as an herbal remedy to stimulate the digestive system, ease colic and stomach discomfort, and minimize gas. It is also used as an emmenagogue, to stimulate and promote menstrual flow in women.

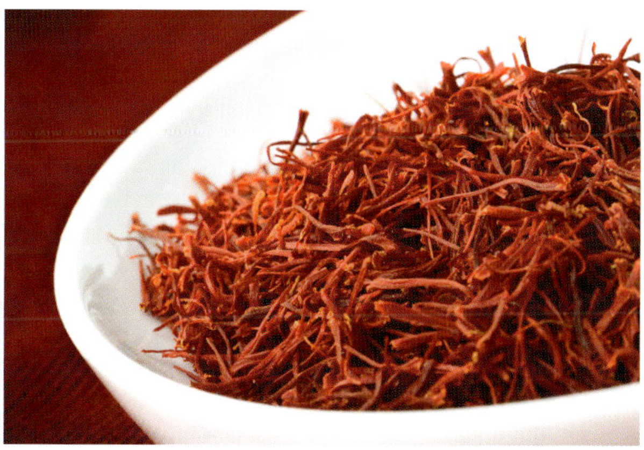

Bowl of saffron. *(© iStockPhoto.com/Dan Bachman)*

Preliminary studies have shown that saffron may also be a useful tool in fighting cancer. According to a 1999 study, use of the herb slowed tumor growth and extended lifespan in female rats. A 2002 study done at Indiana University indicated that saffron may not only be effective in treating certain types of cancer but is significantly less likely to cause birth defects if given to pregnant women than all-trans-retinoic acid (ATRA), the compound most often given to treat these cancers. Saffron may thus be a preferable alternative to treating ATRA-sensitive cancers in women of childbearing age.

A 2004 review of previous research in animal models and with cultured human malignant cell lines concluded that **clinical trials** are warranted to define the possible chemopreventive properties of saffron. A 2006 study at the National Institute of Pediatrics in Mexico concluded that "saffron itself, as well as its carotenoid components, might be used as potential cancer chemopreventive agents."

Additional human studies have indicated that saffron has powerful antioxidant properties; that is, it helps to protect living tissues from free radicals and other harmful effects of oxidation. In Iran and Japan, pharmacology studies in 2000 and 2002 confirmed that saffron extract has an anticonvulsant activity.

Two chemical components of saffron extract, crocetin and crocin, reportedly improved memory and learning skills in learning-impaired rats in a Japanese study published in early 2000. These properties indicate that saffron extract may be a useful treatment for neurodegenerative disorders and related memory impairment.

In 2005 in the *Journal of Ethnopharmacology* researchers reported on the first scientific study to test the effectiveness of saffron as a treatment for symptoms of mild to moderate **depression**. Daily dosages of 30 mg saffron extract (standardized to 0.7 mg of safranal) were compared to 20 mg of **fluoxetine** (Prozac) in 38 people. Participants were aged 18 to 55 years. At the conclusion of the six-week trial, both treatments demonstrated significant improvements in depressive symptoms. There was no significant difference between the herbal treatment and the drug treatment as far as the amount of improvement demonstrated. However, participants who took the saffron extract did not report side effects, such as sexual dysfunction, tremor, or sweating, sometimes attributed to fluoxetine. Symptoms were evaluated with the Hamilton Rating Scale for Depression prior to the study and at intervals of one, two, four, and six weeks.

An Iranian study published in March 2007 revealed that saffron was as effective as fluoxetine (Prozac) in the treatment of depression, noting that both saffron and fluoxetine yielded similar side effects for users of both groups. In fact, scientists at the University of Medical Sciences in Tehran now believe that saffron is as beneficial as fluoxetine in the treatment of mild to moderate depression. In January 2010, the *Journal of Natural Medicines* published findings showing that laboratory mice that were given saffron extracts, exhibited stress-adaptive benefits, supporting beliefs that saffron may be beneficial in treatment for depression.

Saffron has also been found to be beneficial for depression associated with **premenstrual syndrome** (PMS). An Iranian study published in March 2008 determined that women between the age of 20 and 45 reported a significant reduction in their PMS depression. The women (who took 30 mg of saffron a day for two concurrent menstrual cycles) noted relief of these symptoms; however, more research was said to be needed to determine possible negative effects of saffron associated with PMS, before it could be established as a safe and therapeutic treatment regimen for PMS.

As of 2011, saffron was being investigated for the following medicinal uses:

- to help control the effects of mild to moderate Alzheimer's disease
- to help improve mood
- to improve circulation
- to inhibit cancer cell proliferation against breast, liver, pancreatic, and skin cancers

Preparations

Saffron is harvested by drying the orange stigma of the *Crocus sativus* flower over fire. Over 200,000 crocus stigmas must be harvested to produce one pound of saffron. This volume makes the herb extremely expensive, and it is often cut with other substances of a similar color (e.g., marigold) to keep the price down.

Safranal, a terpene aldehyde, is formed during the drying process. It is the component responsible for much of saffron's characteristic fragrance.

KEY TERMS

Antioxidants—Enzymes that bind with free radicals to neutralize their harmful effects.

Crocetin—A reddish-yellow plant pigment found in saffron that has been studied for its anticancer effectiveness.

Decoction—An herbal extract produced by mixing an herb with cold water, bringing the mixture to a boil, and letting it simmer to evaporate the excess water. Decoctions are usually chosen over infusion when the botanical or herb in question is a root, seed, or berry.

Emmenagogue—A medication or substance given to bring on a menstrual period.

Free radicals—Reactive molecules created during cell metabolism that can cause tissue and cell damage like that which occurs in aging and with such disease processes as cancer.

Stigma—The thread-like filament found in the center of a flower where pollen collects.

Tincture—A liquid extract of an herb prepared by steeping the herb in an alcohol and water mixture.

Because saffron is frequently used as a spice to flavor a variety of dishes, particularly in Mediterranean recipes, it can often be purchased by mail order and at gourmet food stores, as well as at health food stores. The herb is usually sold in either powdered form or in its original threadlike stigma form. Saffron is expensive and can cost as much $315 per ounce.

For medicinal purposes, saffron can be taken by mouth in powder, tincture, or liquid form. To make a liquid saffron decoction, mix 6–10 stigmas or strands of saffron in one cup of cold water, bring the mixture to a boil, and then let it simmer. The saffron is then strained out of the decoction, which can be drunk either hot or cold. An average recommended dose of saffron decoction is 0.5–1 cup daily.

Saffron should be stored in an airtight container in a cool location away from bright light to maintain its potency. The herb can be frozen. Properly stored saffron can be used for up to two years. A good measure of the herb's freshness and potency is its odor. If the saffron does not have a noticeable pungent smell, it is probably past its peak.

Precautions

Because saffron can stimulate uterine contractions, pregnant women should never take the herb for medicinal purposes.

QUESTIONS TO ASK YOUR DOCTOR

- In what way do you think saffron will benefit me?
- Will saffron interfere with my current medications?
- What symptoms are important enough that I should seek immediate treatment?

Saffron should always be obtained from a reputable source that observes stringent quality control procedures and industry-accepted good manufacturing practices. Because of its high cost, saffron is sometimes found in adulterated form, so package labeling should be checked carefully for the type and quality of additional ingredients.

Legislation known as the Dietary Supplement Health and Education Act (DSHEA) was passed in 1994 in an effort to standardize the manufacture, labeling, composition, and safety of botanicals and supplements. Botanical supplements are regulated by the FDA; however, they are not required to undergo any approval process before reaching the consumer market and are classified as nutritional supplements rather than drugs.

Side effects

Although there are no known side effects or health hazards associated with recommended dosages of saffron preparations in healthy individuals, people with chronic medical conditions should consult their healthcare professional before taking the herb. In addition, pregnant women should never take saffron, as the herb stimulates uterine contractions and may cause miscarriage.

Despite earlier reports of serious adverse effects from as little as 5 grams of saffron, there is no scientific evidence as to the toxicity of *Crocus sativus*. According to Subhuti Dharmananda, director of the Institute for Traditional Medicine in Portland, Oregon, "all recent research reports indicate that saffron is non-toxic." The so-called meadow saffron *(Colchicum autumnale)* is highly toxic, however, and is sometimes mistaken for the non-toxic medicinal plant *Crocus sativus*.

Interactions

There are no reported negative interactions between saffron and other medications and herbs, but saffron may alter the efficacy of other drugs. Patients should always consult with their physicians before taking any herbs or supplements.

Resources

BOOKS

Awang, Dennis V.C. *Tyler's Herbs of Choice: The Therapeutic Use of Phytomedicinals,* 3rd ed. Boca Raton, FL: CRC Press, 2009.

Barnes, Joanne, et al. *Herbal Medicines (Includes CD-ROM),* 3rd ed. London: Pharmaceutical Press, 2007.

Micozzi, Marc S. *Fundamentals of Complementary and Alternative Medicine.* New York: Saunders, 2010.

Physician's Desk Reference. *PDR for Nonprescription Drugs, Dietary Supplements, and Herbs 2009,* 30th ed. New York: PDR, 2008.

Smith, Pamela Wartian. *What You Must Know About Vitamins, Minerals, Herbs, & More: Choosing the Nutrients That Are Right for You.* Garden City Park, NY: Square One, 2008.

PERIODICALS

Dharmananda, Subhuti. "Saffron: An Anti-Depressant Herb." *Institute for Traditional Medicine* (May 2005). http://www.itmonline.org/articles/saffron/saffron.htm (accessed October 3, 2011).

Noorbala, A.A. "Hydro-alcoholic Extract of Crocus Sativus versus Fluoxetine in the Treatment of Mild to Moderate Depression: A Double-Blind, Randomized Pilot Trial." *Journal of Ethnopharmacology* 97, no. 2 (2005): 281–84.

ORGANIZATIONS

Institute for Traditional Medicine, 2017 SE Hawthorne Blvd., Portland, OR, 97214, (503) 233-4907, http://www.itmonline.org.

National Center for Complementary and Alternative Medicine, 9000 Rockville Pike, Bethesda, MD, 20892, (888) 644-6226, http://nccam.nih.gov.

Office of Dietary Supplements, National Institutes of Health, 6100 Executive Blvd., Rm. 3B01, MSC 7517, Bethesda, MD, 20892-7517, (301) 435-2920, Fax: (301) 480-1845, ods@nih.gov, http://dietary-supplements.info.nih.gov.

Paula Ford-Martin
Laura Jean Cataldo, RN, EdD

Sage

Definition

Common sage is a small, perennial plant or bush with woody stems, aromatic grayish leaves, and white or blue-to-purplish flowers. A member of the Lamiaceae, or mint, family and genus *Salvia*, it is also referred to as garden, meadow, or true sage. More than 750 species of sage exist in Central and South America, Central Asia and the Mediterranean, and Eastern Asia.

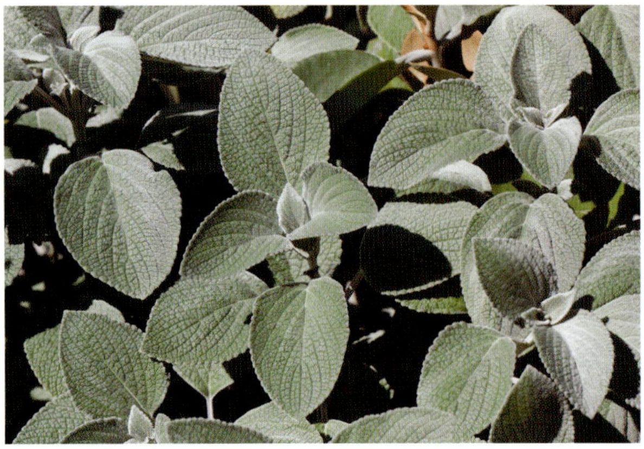

Sage plant. *(© Elliotte Rusty Harold/Shutterstock.com)*

Sage has been used since ancient times for medicinal and culinary purposes; it is commonly used as an herb in poultry stuffing. With regard to mental health, alternative medicine practitioners tout sage as a way to reduce anxiety and other symptoms prevalent in mental disorders.

Purpose

Sage is a celebrated herb long valued for its many uses. The Romans revered the herb as a sacred plant, and the Egyptians used it to treat the plague. Nicholas Culpeper (1616–54), the seventeenth-century herbalist and astrologer, believed sage was under the dominion of the planet Jupiter. Folk belief placed the herb under the influence of Venus, and sage was traditionally used to aid conception. One folk tradition encouraged eating a bit of sage each day during the month of May to assure immortality. Failing to live up to this promise, sage was traditionally planted on graves.

Sage's main constituents are volatile oil, diterpene bitters, thujone, camphor, tannins, triterpenoids, resin, flavonoids, estrogenic substances, saponins, and phenolic acids, including rosmarinic and caffeic acids. The herb purportedly acts as an antiallergen, antibiotic, antiperspirant, antiseptic, antispasmodic, astringent, and carminative.

Sage has been used as a general tonic (a beverage that generally makes one feel better). It is the preferred beverage tea in many cultures, particularly in China, where the root of the species *S. miltiorrhiza*, known as *dan shen*, is used for its soothing and healing qualities.

Description

Sage (*Salvia officinalis*, abbreviated *S. officinalis*) is native to the Mediterranean and naturalized throughout Europe and North America. The genus name is taken from the Latin *salvare,* meaning "to save." The specific name *officinalis* indicates that sage was included on official lists of medicinal herbs.

There are numerous species of sage, but *S. officinalis* is the best known for its medicinal purposes. It often serves as the standard to which other sage species are compared. Other species also noted for medicinal purposes are *S. officinalis purpurascens* ("Purpurea," red or purple common sage), *S. miltiorrhiza* (Chinese sage, red sage), *S. fruticosa* (Greek sage), and *S. lavandulifolia.* (Spanish sage).

Sage thrives in full sun and well-drained soils, growing wild in some areas. It is a hardy, evergreen shrub with a deep taproot and an erect root stalk that produces woody, square, slightly downy, branching stems that may reach a height of 4 feet (1.2 m). The familiar plant has long, light green leaf stalks that bear simple, opposite, lance- or oval-shaped leaves. The strong and pliable leaves are veined, with a velvet-like, somewhat crinkled, texture and may grow to 2 inches (5.1 cm) long in some species. Leaf margins resemble a fine embroidery finish with rounded, minutely toothed edges. They are a gray green on the top and lighter on the underside. The entire plant is strongly aromatic, with a familiar pungency. Fresh leaves are bitter to the taste. Sage blossoms in the middle of summer with small white, blue, or purple flowers.

Among its many virtues, sage has been shown by researchers to help calm the central nervous system and reduce anxiety. Medical research also found that sage helps to enhance mood and improve memory and cognitive skills. Some tout sage as helping to reduce chemical imbalances in the **brain** and thus helping to reduce symptoms commonly associated with Alzheimer's disease (AD), a type of **dementia**. In a 2003 study published in the *Journal of Clinical Pharmacy and Therapeutics*, persons with mild to moderate AD given sage extract for four months experienced improved cognitive functioning. However, further research is needed; the National Center for Complementary and Alternative Medicine (NCCAM) has conducted a trial on the effects of sage on memory and cognitive performance in patients with AD, which was expected to be completed in December 2012.

Recommended dosage

The sage leaf is the medicinal part of the herb. Both the fresh and dried leaves may be used for medicinal purposes. The leaves are harvested when the herb begins to flower in the summer of its second year. The leaves are removed from the woody branches. Then they are spread in a single layer on a tray or screen in a warm, airy, and shady place. Exposure to direct sunlight during the drying process results in a significant loss of the volatile oil. Dried leaves are stored in a dark, airtight container.

KEY TERMS

Central nervous system—The part of the nervous system that includes the brain and spinal cord but excludes the peripheral nerves.

Hypertension—The medical term for high blood pressure.

Thujone—A natural chemical compound found in sage as well as in wormwood and certain other spices. In large quantities it can cause hallucinations and convulsions.

Tonic—A preparation or medicine that invigorates, strengthens, or restores tone to body tissues.

To make an infusion, 1 pint (0.5 L) of nonchlorinated water that has just reached the boiling point is poured over 2–3 teaspoons (0.3–0.5 fl oz) of dried or fresh sage leaves in a glass container. The mixture is covered and steeped for 10–15 minutes. This liquid can be drunk warm or cold, up to 3 cups (25 fl oz) daily.

For improved cognitive functioning with **Alzheimer's disease**, the suggested dose is 0.04 oz. (1 g) of sage extract per day. Patients should always consult with their physicians before starting any treatment, even alternative or complementary treatments, especially if taking concurrent medications.

Tinctures of sage are available commercially. A standard dose is 16–40 drops, up to three times daily.

Precautions

Sage preparations in medicinal doses should not be used during pregnancy and breastfeeding. Pregnant women should avoid sage because of the possibility that the chemical thujone may be present in various species of sage. Increased amounts of thujone can bring on a menstrual period in women. If a woman is pregnant, such an incident will cause a miscarriage. In addition, some research has shown that thujone may reduce the amount of milk for mothers who are breastfeeding a child.

People with epilepsy should not use sage due to the thujone content in the herb. Thujone may trigger convulsions in these people, with its essential oil containing as much as 25% thujone. These essential oils may accumulate in the body, so long-term or high dose use of sage (for more than two weeks at a time) should be avoided.

In addition, in large enough doses, thujone can be poisonous. Consequently, it can cause **seizures** and damage to the liver and nervous systems in anyone taking the chemical. The amount of thujone in sage varies depending on various factors such as growing conditions and time of harvest.

QUESTIONS TO ASK YOUR DOCTOR

- Do you know how effective sage might be for me with regards to my symptoms?
- Are there any underlying medical concerns that need to be addressed or corrected before I take sage?
- Will health insurance cover the use of sage?
- How long may I take sage before noticing any difference?

Diabetics should avoid sage because it can lower their blood sugar levels, which is called hypoglycemia. People with high blood pressure (hypertension) should also avoid sage. Sage can increase blood pressure, which can be dangerous for people already with higher than normal blood pressure. Those allergic to sage or other plants in the mint family should also avoid this herb.

Side effects

There are no adverse side effects when sage is taken in designated therapeutic doses. However, sage may interfere with absorption of iron and other minerals.

Interactions

Various interactions have been reported between sage and prescription medications. Medications used to prevent seizures (anticonvulsants) can interact with sage because both alter the state of certain chemicals in the brain. As such, using both can alter the effectiveness of such medicines. Some antiseizure medicines are **carbamazepine** (Tegretol), **gabapentin** (Neurontin), primidone (Mysoline), and **valproic acid** (Depakene). Sedative medications, which are called central nervous system (CNS) depressants, also interact with sage. When used together they can cause excessive sleepiness and drowsiness. Some sleep aid medicines are **clonazepam** (Klonopin), **lorazepam** (Ativan), and **zolpidem** (Ambien).

Resources

BOOKS

Dasgupta, Amitava, and Catherine A. Hammett-Stabler, eds. *Herbal Supplements: Efficacy, Toxicity, Interactions with Western Drugs and Effects on Clinical Laboratory Tests.* Hoboken, NJ: Wiley, 2011.

PDR for Herbal Medicines. Montvale, NJ: Thomson, 2007.

Tang, Tifan. *Chinese Herbal Medicines: Comparisons and Characteristics.* Edinburgh: Churchill Livingstone/ Elsevier, 2010.

Ulbricht, Catherine E. *Davis's Pocket Guide to Herbs and Supplements.* Philadelphia: F. A. Davis, 2011.

Woods, Michael, and Mary B. Woods. *Ancient Medical Technology: From Herbs to Scalpels.* Minneapolis: Twenty-First Century Books, 2011.

PERIODICALS

Akhondzadeh, S., et al. "*Salvia officinalis* Extract in the Treatment of Patients with Mild to Moderate Alzheimer's Disease: A Double Blind, Randomized and Placebo-controlled Trial." *Journal of Clinical Pharmacy and Therapeutics* 28, no. 1 (2003): 53–59.

WEBSITES

Brett, Jennifer. "Sage: Herbal Remedies." Discovery Health. http://health.howstuffworks.com/wellness/natural-medicine/herbal-remedies/sage-herbal-remedies.htm (accessed September 8, 2011).

National Center for Complementary and Alternative Medicine (NCCAM). "Sage." U.S. National Institutes of Health. http://nccam.nih.gov/health/sage (accessed September 8, 2011).

ORGANIZATIONS

American Botanical Council, 6200 Manor Rd., Austin, TX, 78723, (512) 926-4900, Fax: (512) 926-2345, abc@herbalram.org, http://abc.herbalgram.org.

American Psychiatric Association, 1000 Wilson Blvd., Ste. 1825, Arlington, VA, 22209, (703) 907-7300, apa@psych.org, http://www.psych.org.

National Center for Complementary and Alternative Medicine Clearinghouse, 9000 Rockville Pike, Bethesda, MD, 20892, info@nccam.nih.gov, http://nccam.nih.gov.

Natural Standard, One Davis Sq., Somerville, MA, 02144, (617) 591-3300, Fax: (617) 591-3399, http://naturalstandard.com.

Office of Dietary Supplements, National Institutes of Health, 6100 Executive Blvd., Rm. 3B01, MSC 7517, Rockville, MD, 20892-7517, (301) 435-2920, Fax: (301) 480-1845, ods@nih.gov, http://ods.od.nih.gov.

United States Pharmacopoeia, 12601 Twinbrook Pkwy., Rockville, MD, 20852-1790, (800) 227-8772, http://www.usp.org.

Clare Hanrahan
Rebecca J. Frey, PhD
William A. Atkins, BB, BS, MBA

St. John's wort

Definition

St. John's wort is a perennial, yellow-flowering plant that grows in the wild throughout Europe and is now found also in North America. The plant has been used as a popular herbal folk remedy for centuries, but more recently, practitioners of conventional Western medicine have been exploring its utility for treating **depression** and anxiety.

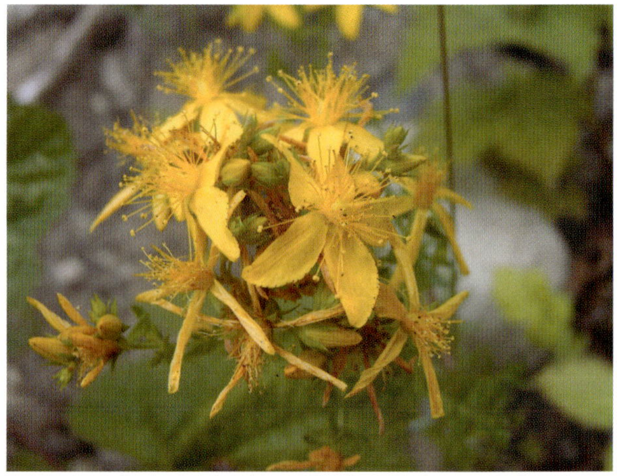

St. John's wort. *(© Jim Dubois/Shutterstock.com)*

Purpose

Writings since the Middle Ages have described using St. John's wort as treatment for inflammation, injuries, burns, muscle pain, anxiety, high blood pressure, stomach problems, fluid retention, **insomnia**, hemorrhoids, cancer, and depression. Research conducted over the last decade of the twentieth century in Europe studied the efficacy of St. John's wort for the treatment of depression and anxiety. Research protocols have been developed in the United States to study the same issues, to determine appropriate dosages, to develop standard formulations, and to define whether it can be used for all forms of depression or only for more mild forms of the condition.

Description

Hypericum perforatum is the most medicinally important species of the Hypericum genus, commonly known as St. John's wort or Klamath weed. There are as many as 400 species in the genus, which belongs to the Clusiaceae family. Native to Europe, St. John's wort is found throughout the world. It thrives in sunny fields, open woods, and gravelly roadsides. Early colonists brought this plant to North America, and it has become naturalized in the eastern United States and California, as well as in Australia, New Zealand, eastern Asia, and South America. St. John's wort has long been one of the most commonly used herbs in the United States, especially among women. The popular use of the herb declined in the late 1990s, however, due in part to research reports that the hypericum in the plant may be

KEY TERMS

Immunosuppressant—Medications that suppress or lower the body's immune system, primarily used to help the body accept a transplanted organ.

Monoamine oxidase inhibitors (MAOIs)—A group of antidepressant drugs that decrease the activity of monoamine oxidase, a neurotransmitter found in the brain that affects mood.

Reserpine—Medication to treat high blood pressure. Brand names include Serpalan, Novoreserpine, and Reserfia.

Theophylline—A medication used to treat asthma. Sold under many brand names, including Aerolate Sr, Respbid, and Theolair.

Warfarin—A medication that helps to prevent the formation of clots in the blood vessels. Sold as Coumadin in the U.S.

less effective in treating depression than previously claimed.

Research has yet to completely explain how St. John's wort affects the **brain** in depression. It is, however, thought to change the balance of chemicals in the brain in much the same way as **selective serotonin reuptake inhibitors (SSRIs)** such as **fluoxetine**, and **monoamine oxidase inhibitors (MAOIs)**, such as **isocarboxazid**. The active ingredients are thought to be compounds called hypericin and pseudohypericin, although researchers are attempting to identify other chemicals that may be involved in the herb's effectiveness.

The leaves and flowers of St. John's wort are both used. St. John's wort is available as pills, capsules, extracts, dried herbs for tea, and oil infusions for skin applications.

St. John's wort has been proven clinically effective in treating mild-to-moderate depression. In 2005, the British Journal of Psychiatry reported on 37 previous scientific studies comparing the clinical benefits to adults with depressive disorders of hypericum in St. John's wort and either a placebo or a standard antidepressant. The trials suggested that St. John's wort extract had "minimal beneficial effects" in treating major depression, but showed "similar beneficial effects" in cases of mild depression as when using a standard antidepressant. St. John's wort also shows promise in treating **somatoform disorders**. Research on its treatment of anxiety and other conditions is conflicting and inconclusive.

Recommended dosage

Because dosages of herbal preparations are not always standardized, it is important to discuss with a knowledgeable practitioner the most reliable form of St. John's wort. Recommendations call for 300–500 mg (of a standardized 0.3% hypericin extract) three times daily. It can take four to six weeks to notice the antidepressant effects of this preparation.

Alternatively, one to two teaspoons of dried St. John's wort can be put into a cup of boiling water and steeped for 10 minutes to make tea. The recommended dose of tea is one to two cups daily. Again, four to six weeks may be necessary in order to notice improvement in symptoms of depression.

Precautions

There are a number of important precautions to observe in using St. John's wort. Pregnant or lactating women should not use the herb at all. Animal studies have linked St. John's wort to lower birth weight, and there are studies showing that breastfed infants whose mothers are using St. John's wort may experience drowsiness or colic.

Persons taking prescription **antidepressants** of any kind should not use St. John's wort at the same time, as the herb may precipitate a health crisis known as **serotonin syndrome**. **Serotonin** syndrome is potentially life threatening; it is characterized by changes in level of consciousness, behavior, and neuromotor functioning as a result of increased levels of the neurotransmitter serotonin in the central nervous system. Drug interactions are the most common cause of serotonin syndrome. Several cases of serotonin syndrome have been reported in patients who were taking St. John's wort by itself or in combination with **SSRIs**, fenfluramine (Pondimin), or **nefazodone** (Serzone). Patients taking **MAOIs** must carefully avoid taking St. John's wort due to serious adverse effects of combining the two.

Depression can be a serious, even life-threatening, condition; therefore, it is imperative that depressed patients using St. John's wort are carefully monitored.

Side effects

People taking St. John's wort may develop one or all of the following side effects:

- skin rash due to sun sensitivity (the most common side effect)
- headache, dizziness, dry mouth, constipation
- abdominal pain, confusion, sleep problems, and high blood pressure (less frequently experienced)

Interactions

Again, a knowledgeable professional should be consulted before St. John's wort is taken to determine the appropriateness of its use and avoid serious interactions. Interactions include:

- A possible decrease in effectiveness of reserpine, warfarin, theophylline, immunosuppressant medications such as cyclosporine, and antiviral drugs such as indinavir.
- Dangerous interactions when used with other antidepressant medicines (especially MAOIs), digoxin, and loperamide.
- Interactions with oral birth control pills. St. John's wort may interfere with the effectiveness of birth control pills, increasing the risk of pregnancy; an alternative form of birth control should be considered while taking St. John's wort. In addition, women taking both birth control pills and St. John's wort may notice bleeding between menstrual periods.

Other drugs with reported interactions include **amphetamines**, asthma **inhalants**, decongestants, diet pills, narcotics, and tryptophan and tyrosine (amino acids). Moreover, anesthesiologists have reported that the herb increases bleeding time in patients under general anesthesia. Patients should always consult a mainstream health practitioner before using St. John's wort and should discontinue taking it at least two weeks prior to major surgery.

See also Depression

Resources

BOOKS

Rister, Robert, and Siegrid Klein. *The Complete German Commission E Monographs: Therapeutic Guide to Herbal Medicines*. Austin, TX: American Botanical Council, 1998.

PERIODICALS

Linde, K., M.M. Berner, and L. Kriston. "St. John's Wort for Depression." *Cochrane Database of Systematic Reviews* 8, no. 4 (October 2008): CD000448.

WEBSITES

U.S. National Center for Complementary and Alternative Medicine. "Questions and Answers: A Trial of St. John's Wort (*Hypericum perforatum*) for the Treatment of Major Depression." http://nccam.nih.gov/news/2002/stjohnswort/q-and-a.htm (accessed October 27, 2011).

U.S. National Center for Complementary and Alternative Medicine. "St. John's Wort and Depression." http://nccam.nih.gov/health/stjohnswort/sjw-and-depression.htm (accessed October 27, 2011).

ORGANIZATIONS

National Center for Complementary and Alternative Medicine, 9000 Rockville Pike, Bethesda, MD, 20892, info@nccam.nih.gov, http://nccam.nih.gov.

Rosalyn Carson-DeWitt, M.D.

SAMe

Definition

SAMe (S-adenosyl-L-methionine, sometimes also written as S-adenosylmethionine) is a naturally occurring chemical compound found throughout the entire body. It is involved in many chemical reactions that are necessary for life. For instance, SAMe helps to maintain cell membranes and make **dopamine**, melatonin, and **serotonin** in the body. It is available as a natural dietary supplement and can be purchased without a prescription (over-the-counter). In mental health, it is used to treat conditions such as **attention deficit hyperactivity disorder (ADHD)** and **depression**.

Purpose

People take supplements of SAMe for many reasons, including to relieve symptoms of heart disease, fibromyalgia, osteoarthritis, bursitis, heart disease, tendonitis, chronic lower back pain, chronic fatigue syndrome (CFS), multiple sclerosis, spinal cord injuries, migraine headaches, **lead poisoning**, liver disease, and Parkinson's disease, as well as to improve intellectual performance.

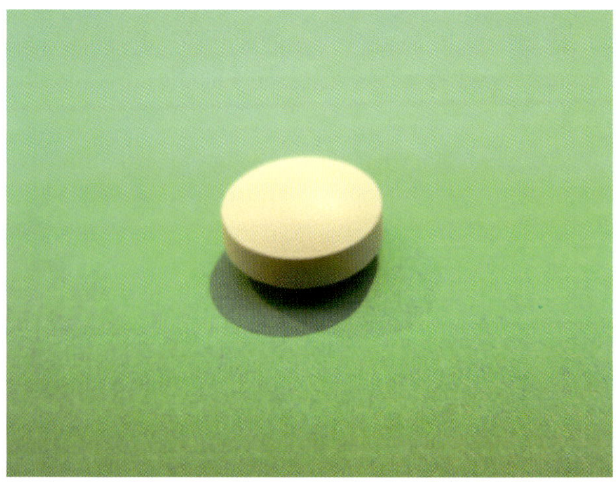

SAMe supplement. *(© Custom Medical Stock Photo, Inc. Reproduced by permission.)*

KEY TERMS

Antioxidant enzyme—An enzyme that can counteract the damaging effects of oxygen in tissues.

Bipolar disorder—Also referred to as manic depression, a mood disorder marked by alternating episodes of extremely low mood (depression) and exuberant highs (mania).

Dopamine—A chemical compound and neurotransmitter, which is a precursor of epinephrine.

Homocysteine—An amino acid with the chemical formula $HSCH_2CH_2CH(NH_2)CO_2H$.

Melatonin—A hormone derived from serotonin that produces changes in the color of the skin.

Serotonin—A chemical that acts as a neurotransmitter, with the formula $C_{10}H_{12}N_2O$.

Within the realm of mental illness, SAMe is used to treat anxiety, depression, **ADHD**, and **dementia**, including Alzheimer's disease. Some evidence suggests that taking SAMe can improve symptoms of depression within two weeks, which is considerably faster than the time it takes for oral antidepressant prescription drugs to work. (Prescription **antidepressants** often take a minimum of two weeks for patients to begin noticing any effect, and many take up to four to six weeks.)

Description

SAMe is a specific form of the amino acid methionine, a substance that, when not metabolized properly, allows homocysteine to build up in the blood. (High levels of homocysteine have been associated with increased risk for cardiovascular disease.) SAMe is also an antioxidant, a substance that protects the body from damaging reactive oxygen molecules. These reactive oxygen molecules can come from inside the body or from environmental pollution and are thought to play a role in the aging process and the development of degenerative disease. In general, SAMe is thought to raise the level of functioning of other amino acids in the body.

Although people use SAMe for many reasons, the best evidence as of 2011 indicated that SAMe may be most effective in relieving symptoms of osteoarthritis. However, it is increasingly used for treating depression. Several studies have indicated that oral SAMe and intravenous SAMe are effective treatments for depression. The studies researching the oral SAMe were mostly small studies of short duration, but they show promise for the use of SAMe in treating depression. Some found that SAMe may almost be as effective as tricyclic antidepressants, traditional medicines used to treat depression. Other research has shown that taking SAMe may be helpful for depression only when prescription antidepressants are not effective. Additional and more extensive studies of SAMe are necessary to validate these results.

Research studies have also been conducted to test the effects of SAMe on ADHD. The conclusions are not definite with respect to SAMe being effective at reducing symptoms of ADHD, as not enough studies have been completed. As of 2011, the medical consensus was that SAMe may possibly reduce symptoms of ADHD; the National Institutes of Health stated that, based on limited research, "SAMe might lessen ADHD symptoms in adults."

Recommended dosage

SAMe can be taken orally or intravenously. Oral administration is more common. When taken by mouth, doses of 400–1,600 mg daily have been suggested based on study results. However, a specific recommended therapeutic dosage had not been established as of 2011.

In treating depression, 200 mg of SAMe has been administered intravenously or intramuscularly for 14 days while simultaneously beginning therapy with prescription antidepressant drugs. If SAMe is used without prescription antidepressants, 200–400 mg per day by intravenous or intramuscular injections has been used. When treating other medical conditions, doses as high as 800 mg daily by injection have been used. Again, intravenous administration is rare in the United States.

Precautions

As a natural supplement, SAMe has not been evaluated by the Food and Drug Administration (FDA). Claims of safety or effectiveness for treating any medical disorder have not been thoroughly studied by any governmental agency, and there is no regulation of natural supplements. This means that potencies and purities may vary between lots or among manufacturers. It is also possible that supplements may not contain the ingredients that are listed on product labels.

SAMe should be used carefully by individuals with a history of **bipolar disorder** since it may aggravate symptoms of mania. When used with prescription antidepressant medications, life-threatening symptoms may occur. It should be used with prescription antidepressant drugs only under close medical supervision. Individuals should not begin taking SAMe until one week or more after stopping an antidepressant medicine, and two weeks or more after taking **phenelzine** (Nardil) or **tranylcypromine** (Parnate).

When users take SAMe by mouth, it may cause stomach upset, including gas, vomiting, diarrhea or soft stool, constipation, and nausea. Although SAMe may cause an upset stomach, it is generally recommended to take on an empty stomach for better absorption. Prospective users ought to ask a doctor to determine what is best in their case. SAMe can also cause dry mouth, headache, mild **insomnia**, anorexia, sweating, increased thirst, blurred vision, restlessness, dizziness, and nervousness. The benefits of the medication may show up within one week; however, it may take as long as four to eight weeks before the full effects are shown. Users should not suddenly discontinue use of SAMe; rather, it is recommended that use be gradually discontinued. In addition, alcohol should not be consumed with SAMe.

Increased anxiety has occurred in people with depression when taking SAMe. Furthermore, a conversion to mania has been reported in those with a history of bipolar disorder. Patients with Parkinson's disease have frequently reported worse symptoms while taking SAMe.

Women who are pregnant or breastfeeding should use extreme caution when using SAMe. Its safety under those situations has not been adequately researched, and the medical community recommends that SAMe not be used by women who are pregnant or breastfeeding.

People scheduled for surgery should stop taking SAMe at least two weeks before surgery because of a heightened risk of complications. Part of this risk involves adverse reactions to the central nervous system when individuals are taking SAMe.

Interactions

Use of SAMe with antidepressant drugs (especially **selective serotonin reuptake inhibitors**, or **SSRIs**) may cause life-threatening symptoms, including agitation, tremors, anxiety, rapid heartbeats, difficulty breathing, diarrhea, shivering, muscle stiffness, and excessive sweating. The combination can also cause insomnia. Use of SAMe with a prescription antidepressant must be approved by a physician, and close medical supervision is required. Medications for depression include **amitriptyline** (Elavil), **clomipramine** (Anafranil), **fluoxetine** (Prozac), **imipramine** (Tofranil), **paroxetine** (Paxil), and **sertraline** (Zoloft).

QUESTIONS TO ASK YOUR DOCTOR

- In what way do you think SAMe will benefit me?
- Will SAMe interfere with my current medications?
- What symptoms or adverse effects are important enough that I should seek immediate treatment?

In addition, **monoamine oxidase inhibitors** (MAOI) drugs also treat depression. Taking SAMe with MAOIs can cause serious symptoms, including anxiety, heart problems, and shivering. Two types of MAOIs are phenelzine (Nardil) and tranylcypromine (Parnate).

People should not take SAMe if they are also taking dextromethorphan (Robitussin DM and others), levodopa (which is used to treat Parkinson's disease), meperidine (Demerol), pentazocine (Talwin), or tramadol (Ultram).

SAMe may offer beneficial drug interactions when used with some medications. More research is needed, but some scientists think that SAMe may protect the liver from damage caused by some drugs, including acetaminophen, alcohol, estrogens, **steroids**, and several other prescription drugs.

SAMe, which increases serotonin in the **brain**, should not be taken with other herbs and supplements that also increase serotonin levels, such as **5-HTP**, Hawaiian baby woodrose, L-tryptophan, and St. John's wort.

Resources

BOOKS

Marian, Mary J., Pamela Williams-Mullen, and Jennifer Muir Bowers. *Integrating Therapeutic and Complementary Nutrition.* Boca Raton, FL: CRC, 2006.

Micozzi, Marc S. *Fundamentals of Complementary and Alternative Medicine.* New York: Saunders, 2010.

Pelletier, Kenneth R. "Western Herbal Medicine: Nature's Green Pharmacy." Chapter 6 in *The Best Alternative Medicine.* New York: Simon and Schuster, 2007.

Physician's Desk Reference. *PDR for Nonprescription Drugs, Dietary Supplements, and Herbs 2009,* 30th ed. New York: PDR, 2008.

Purchon, Nerys. *The Essential Natural Health Bible: The Complete Home Guide to Herbs and Oils, Natural Remedies and Nutrition.* NSW, Australia: Millennium House, 2011.

Therapeutic Research Faculty. *Natural Medicines Comprehensive Database 2007*. Stockton, CA: Natural Medicines Database, 2006.

PERIODICALS

Mischoulon, David, and Maurizio Fava. "Role of S-adenosyl-L-methionine in the Treatment of Depression: A Review of the Evidence." *American Journal of Clinical Nutrition* 76, no. 5 (November 2002): 1158S–61S. http://www.ajcn.org/content/76/5/1158S.full (accessed September 8, 2001).

Nelson, J. Craig. "S-Adenosyl Methionine (SAMe) Augmentation in Major Depressive Disorder." *American Journal of Psychiatry* 167 (August 2010): 889–91.

Rucklidge, J. J., J. Johnstone, and B. J. Kaplan. "Nutrient Supplementation Approaches in the Treatment of ADHD." *Expert Review of Neurotherapeutics* 9, no. 4 (2009): 461–76.

Ryan, Susan, and Karolyn A. Gazella. "Evaluation of S-Adenosyl-L-Methionine (SAMe) as Primary or Adjuvant Treatment of Depression." *Natural Medicine Journal* 3, no. 1 (January 2011): 8–11. http://naturalmedicinejournal.com/article_content.asp?article=9 (accessed September 8, 2011).

WEBSITES

MedlinePlus. "SAMe." National Institutes of Health. Last updated March 5, 2011. http://www.nlm.nih.gov/medlineplus/druginfo/natural/786.html (accessed September 8, 2011).

St. John, Don. "S-Adenosyl-L-Methionine (SAMe)." University of Iowa Hospitals and Clinics. Last updated January 31, 2000. http://www.uihealthcare.com/topics/medicaldepartments/psychiatry/medications/same.html (accessed September 8, 2011).

ORGANIZATIONS

American Botanical Council, 6200 Manor Rd., Austin, TX, 78723, (512) 926-4900, Fax: (512) 926-2345, abc@herbalram.org, http://abc.herbalgram.org.

American Psychiatric Association, 1000 Wilson Blvd., Ste. 1825, Arlington, VA, 22209-3901, (703) 907-7300, apa@psych.org, http://www.psych.org.

National Center for Complementary and Alternative Medicine Clearinghouse, 9000 Rockville Pike, Bethesda, MD, 20892, info@nccam.nih.gov, http://nccam.nih.gov.

Natural Standard, One Davis Square, Somerville, MA, 02144, (617) 591-3300, Fax: (617) 591-3399, http://naturalstandard.com.

Office of Dietary Supplements, National Institutes of Health, 6100 Executive Blvd., Rm. 3B01, MSC 7517, Rockville, MD, 20892-7517, (301) 435-2920, Fax: (301) 480-1845, ods@nih.gov, http://ods.od.nih.gov.

United States Pharmacopoeia, 12601 Twinbrook Pkwy., Rockville, MD, 20852-1790, (800) 227-8772, http://www.usp.org.

Kelly Karpa, RPh, PhD
Laura Jean Cataldo, RN, EdD
William A. Atkins, BB, BS, MBA

SAMSHA *see* **Substance Abuse and Mental Health Services Administration**

Saphris *see* **Asenapine**

Savant syndrome

Definition

Below-normal intelligence combined with a special talent or ability in a specific area.

Demographics

It is estimated that there are about 100 persons worldwide with savant syndrome; about 50 of these would be considered prodigious savants, meaning that their special skill is so outstanding that it would be remarkable even in a non-impaired person.

Description

Children who display savant syndrome have traditionally been referred to as "idiot" or autistic savants, because their IQ is usually between 40 and 70, although some have had IQs as high as 114. The negative connotations of the term "idiot" have led to the disuse of "idiot savant"; because the syndrome is often associated with **autism** or **Asperger syndrome**, the latter term is more frequently heard. Persons with savant syndrome have an exceptional talent or skill in a particular area in spite of their low IQ, such as the ability to process mathematical calculations at a phenomenal speed. These special talents are called "splinter skills." Savant syndrome is not recognized as a medical **diagnosis** and is considered more as a phenomenon that occurs with certain developmental disorders.

Persons with savant syndrome

Well-known persons with savant syndrome include Kim Peek (1951–2009), a man who could recite 12,000 complete books from memory but whose IQ was slightly below average and had motor difficulties. The 1988 movie *Rain Man* is based on Peek's early life. Another well-known person is Hikari Oe (1963–), a Japanese composer with epilepsy, visual impairments, and autism. Alonzo Clemons, an American who lives in Colorado, sculpts animal figures in less than 20 minutes from images of animals that he sees briefly on a television or computer screen, yet he could not tie his shoes or feed himself as a child. Since his debut as a sculptor in 1986, Clemons has been able to live independently in his own apartment and compete in the Special Olympics as a weight lifter.

Causes and symptoms

Persons with savant syndrome have been the subject of much scientific study, although the nature and cause of their seemingly contradictory abilities are not well understood. In addition to its association with autism and Asperger syndrome, savant syndrome has also been reported to develop in some persons who have suffered head injuries, usually those that impair functioning in the left side of the **brain**. Another possibility is that savant syndrome is genetic. Studies of families of children with savant syndrome point to a deletion or other abnormality in the region of chromosome 15q11-13.

Savant syndrome is found more often in males than in females; it affects four to six males for every female. This gender disproportion is explained by the theory that savant syndrome in general is caused by damage to the left hemisphere of the brain being compensated for by neurons in the right hemisphere. In the male fetus, the high levels of circulating testosterone can hinder the growth of neurons in the left hemisphere of the brain, which is slower to develop than the right hemisphere and hence more vulnerable to prenatal influences. CT scans and SPECT imaging of several savants has in fact demonstrated damage to or structural abnormalities in the left hemisphere.

Savant skills occur in a number of different areas, including music, the visual arts, and mathematics. Experts believe that the most common skills demonstrated by savants depend on extraordinary memory. Persons with savant syndrome may be able to memorize extensive amounts of data in such areas as sports statistics, population figures, or historical and biographical data. One particular type of memorization common to persons with savant syndrome is the ability to calculate what day of the week a particular date fell on or will fall on. The first account of savant syndrome was published in a German medical journal in 1783, and described a young man who had this ability. Another type of mathematical skill is lightning calculation. In 1789, the eminent American physician Benjamin Rush described the case of Thomas Fuller, who was of distinctly subnormal intelligence but could calculate with astonishing rapidity. When Rush asked Fuller how many seconds a man had lived who was 70 years, 17 days, and 12 hours old, he took only 90 seconds to come up with the correct answer: 2,210,500,800—even making corrections for the 17 leap years included in the man's life span. Other skills include being able to calculate distances and angles with great precision by sight and being able to accurately gauge the passing of time without a clock or watch.

Prognosis

The prognosis of savant syndrome depends on the extent of the underlying disorder.

Resources

BOOKS

Howe, Michael J. *Fragments of Genius: The Strange Feats of Idiots Savants*. London: Routledge, 1989.

Obler, L.K., and D. Fein, eds. *The Exceptional Brain: Neuropsychology of Talent and Special Abilities.* New York: Guilford Press, 1988.

Treffert, Darold A., MD. *Extraordinary People: Understanding Savant Syndrome*. New York: Backinprint.com, 2006.

PERIODICALS

Fitzgerald, M. "Asperger's Disorder and Mathematicians of Genius." *Journal of Autism and Developmental Disorders* 32, no. 1 (February 2002): 59–60.

Newport, G. "How Do They Do It? Insight on Calendar Skills from an Asperger's Savant." *Journal of Autism and Developmental Disorders* 36 (February 2006): 285–286.

Sacks, Oliver. "A Neurologist's Notebook: Prodigies." *The New Yorker* 70 (January 9, 1995): 44.

Treffert, D.A., and D.D. Christensen. "Inside the Mind of a Savant." *Scientific American* 293 (December 2005): 108–113.

WEBSITES

Treffert, Darold A. "Genius Among Us: Alonzo Clemons." Wisconsin Medical Society. http://www.wisconsinmedicalsociety.org/savant_syndrome/savant_profiles/alonzo_clemons (accessed December 11, 2011).

———. "Islands of Genius." Wisconsin Medical Society. http://www.wisconsinmedicalsociety.org/savant_syndrome/savant_articles/islands (accessed October 26, 2011).

Wisconsin Medical Society. "Savant Syndrome: What's New?" http://www.wisconsinmedicalsociety.org/savant_syndrome/whats_new (accessed October 27, 2011).

ORGANIZATIONS

National Institute of Neurological Disorders and Stroke, PO Box 5801, Bethesda, MD, 20824, (301) 496-5751, TTY: (301) 468-5981, (800) 352-9424, http://www.ninds.nih.gov.

Schizoaffective disorder

Definition

Schizoaffective disorder is a mental illness that involves both psychotic symptoms and conspicuous, long-enduring, severe symptoms of mood disorder. The cluster of symptoms experienced by people with schizoaffective disorder can resemble—at various times in its course—bipolar disorder, major depressive episode with psychotic features, or **schizophrenia**.

Demographics

Because of the imprecise nature of the **diagnosis**, the actual rate of brief schizoaffective disorder in adults is unknown. The proportion of schizoaffective disorder identified in persons undergoing treatment for psychiatric disorders has ranged from 2% to almost 30%, depending on the study cited. More females than males (overall) suffer from schizoaffective disorder. However, similar to gender ratios in clinical **depression** and **bipolar disorder**, it seems that there is a much higher ratio of women to men in the depressive subtype, whereas the bipolar subtype has a more even gender distribution. Thus, the higher ratio of women overall is primarily caused by the concentration of women within the depressive subtype of schizoaffective disorder.

Description

The schizoaffective disorder classification is applied when a mental health patient meets diagnostic criteria for both schizophrenia and an affective (mood) disorder—either depression or bipolar disorder. In patients with schizoaffective disorder, mood and psychotic symptoms occur predominantly simultaneously and the mood disturbance is long-lasting. However, periods of experiencing serious psychotic symptoms without serious mood disturbance are also a definitive feature. In bipolar disorder and depression with psychotic features, psychotic symptoms only occur during an active episode of mania or severe clinical depression. Schizoaffective disorder is characterized by periods during which psychotic symptoms are experienced without simultaneous severe mood changes. If the patient is encountered for the first time during such a period of psychotic symptoms in the absence of mood changes, it can appear that the individual has schizophrenia. However, in a person who has psychotic symptoms, the presence of long-standing severe mood disturbance suggests possible schizoaffective disorder if they also have periods of psychotic symptoms without concurrent mood fluctuations.

Schizoaffective disorder is typically identified by a process of lengthy observation and elimination of another diagnostic alternative over a long course of care. Because of the need for longitudinal observation and collection of a wealth of information before an accurate diagnosis is possible, most people with schizoaffective disorder have borne other diagnostic labels prior to the schizoaffective diagnosis (usually bipolar disorder).

Symptoms of schizoaffective disorder vary considerably from patient to patient. **Delusions**, hallucinations, and evidence of disturbances in thinking—as observed in full-blown schizophrenia—may be seen. Similarly, mood fluctuations, such as those observed in major depression or bipolar disorder, may also be seen. These symptoms tend to appear in distinct episodes that impair the individual's ability to function well in daily life. Between episodes, some patients with schizoaffective disorder remain chronically impaired, while others may do quite well in day-to-day living.

Causes and symptoms

Causes

Because clear identification of schizoaffective disorder has traditionally been challenging, scientists have conducted far less research relating to the disorder than studies relating to schizophrenia or mood disorders. However, there are indications that there is a genetic component to the disorder. Close relatives of people with schizoaffective disorder have higher rates of both schizophrenia and mood disorder. The disorder most typically strikes in early adulthood; in some cases, there appears to be a major trigger, or some form of life **stress**, initiating the occurrence of the symptoms. In cases where an identifiable stressor is involved, the person tends to have a better outcome than when such is not the case. Some evidence suggests that the bipolar form of schizoaffective disorder is more treatable and yields better outcomes than the depressive form. Similarly, some clinicians believe that "schizomanic" patients are fundamentally different from "schizodepressed" types; the former are similar to bipolar patients, while the latter are a very heterogeneous group.

RELATIONSHIP TO PERSONALITY DISORDER. People with **personality disorders** appear to be more susceptible to developing psychotic reactions in response to stress. One aspect of personality disorder is that when life becomes more demanding and difficult than can be tolerated, the individual with personality disorder may lapse into a brief psychotic episode. For some individuals, personality disorder may be a predecessor to the development of schizoaffective disorder. Those with preexisting schizotypal, paranoid, schizoid, and borderline personality disorders may be more vulnerable to developing a schizoaffective disorder than the general population.

Symptoms

PSYCHOTIC SYMPTOMS. Both psychotic symptoms and mood disorder symptoms are experienced by individuals with schizoaffective disorder. In schizoaffective disorder, at least two of the major symptoms of **psychosis** are evident in the patient. Classic psychotic symptoms can occur during mood disturbances as well as in periods without extreme mood changes.

Hallucinations, delusions, and strange bodily movements or lack of movements (catatonic behavior) are all psychotic symptoms that may be observed. Additionally, minimal or peculiar speech, lack of drive to act on one's behalf, bizarre or primitive (socially inappropriate or immature) behavior, or near-absent emotionality are also typical psychotic symptoms that may occur. Of course, not all of the possible psychotic symptoms will occur concurrently in a single person with schizoaffective disorder. Importantly, to meet the criteria for the schizoaffective disorder diagnosis, delusions or hallucinations (the most "prototypical" of the psychotic symptoms) must be observed within a fairly lengthy period of time during which there is no form of mood disturbance.

MOOD DISTURBANCE. An extremely important and challenging aspect of schizoaffective disorder is that mood problems are prominent. Patients with schizoaffective disorder frequently experience depressed mood or mania within days of the appearance of psychotic symptoms. During mood episodes, psychotic features are simultaneously evident. The disruption of mood may be depressive, manic, or take the form of a **mixed episode** (which includes both depressive and manic features). If only depressed mood occurs, the individual is described as having the depressive subtype of schizoaffective disorder. If mixed episodes or manic episodes are noted, the patient is identified as having the bipolar form of schizoaffective disorder.

Diagnosis

The ***Diagnostic and Statistical Manual of Mental Disorders*** (*DSM-IV-TR*), produced by the **American Psychiatric Association**, is used by most mental health professionals in North America and Europe to diagnose mental disorders. The *DSM-IV-TR* provides these major criteria for diagnosing schizoaffective disorder:

- At least two of the following symptoms of psychosis present for at least one month: delusions, hallucinations, disorganized speech (strange, peculiar, difficult to comprehend), disorganized (bizarre or childlike) behavior, catatonic behavior, minimal speech (approaching mutism), lack of drive to act on one's own behalf, and a perceived absence of emotions.
- Delusions or hallucinations have occurred for at least two weeks in the absence of prominent mood symptoms.
- During a "substantial portion" of the period of active illness, the individual meets criteria for one of the following mood disturbances: major depressive episode, manic episode, mixed episode.
- The symptoms are not caused by a biologically active entity, such as drugs, alcohol, adverse reaction to a medication, physical injury, or medical illness.

Even using the *DSM-IV-TR* criteria, identification of schizoaffective disorder remains difficult and relatively subjective. An unusual condition in this set of diagnostic criteria is the need to weigh the relative prominence of the mood symptoms and to identify a period of psychotic symptoms that occurred without significant mood disturbance. In the various other psychotic disorders, frequently a low level of depression accompanies the symptoms. When depressive symptoms are the sole form of mood disturbance, only subjective clinical judgment determines whether there has been sufficient severity or duration of that disturbance to merit the possibility of schizoaffective disorder. An additional complication is the cultural relativity of "psychotic symptoms." If the psychotic-like behaviors shown are expected and valued in the person's culture or religion, and these behaviors occur in a traditionally affirming context such as religious services or **meditation**, then schizoaffective disorder would not be diagnosed.

As stated, schizoaffective disorder is typically identified by a process of lengthy observation and elimination of other diagnostic alternatives over a long course of care. A very thorough history of the patient's entire past experiences of psychiatric symptoms, mental health treatments, and response to different kinds of medications that have been taken, helps in determining whether that individual is suffering from schizoaffective disorder. Information about current and past experiences is collected in interviews with the patient and possibly in discussion with the patient's immediate family. Data also may be gathered from earlier medical records with the patient's consent. In order to examine the sufferer's ability to concentrate, to remember, to understand his or her situation realistically, and to think logically, the clinician may use a semistructured interview called a **mental status examination**. The mental status examination is designed to uncover psychotic or demented thought processes. **Psychological assessment** instruments, such as the MMPI-2, the **Rorschach Inkblot Test**, various mood disorder questionnaires, or structured diagnostic interviews, are sometimes used aid in diagnosis.

Treatment

Atypical, novel, or newer-generation antipsychotic medications are very effective in schizoaffective disorder treatment. Examples of atypical or novel antipsychotic medications include **aripiprazole** (Abilify), **risperidone** (Risperdal), **quetiapine** (Seroquel), and **olanzapine**

(Zyprexa). If the patient's psychotic symptoms are acute and accompanied by agitation, a number of different antipsychotics can be used to terminate the flare-up of acute agitated psychosis. Agitation is a state of frantic activity that is often accompanied by anger or marked fearfulness; when in an agitated state, the patient is more likely to cause harm to self or others. In agitated psychotic states, the antipsychotic agent **haloperidol** (Haldol) is often given as an injection, accompanied by other medications that decrease anxiety and slow behavior (often **lorazepam**, also known as Ativan). At this time, no atypical antipsychotics are available in an injectable formulation. If the patient is not extremely agitated, usually a novel antipsychotic is used, given orally daily for a lengthier period of time.

In some cases, the antipsychotic medication is not sufficient to overcome the mood disturbance component of the disorder, although some antipsychotics have thymoleptic (mood-affecting) qualities. Some of the atypical antipsychotic medications are thought to have antidepressant properties, and olanzapine has U.S. Food and Drug Administration (FDA) approval for the management of acute manic psychosis.

If there is little response to novel antipsychotic monotherapy (treatment with only one medication), an additional compound may be given to target the mood disorder aspect of the illness. The choice of which drug should be added to the medication regimen to decrease mood disorder problems is determined by the subtype of schizoaffective disorder shown by the patient. If the patient experiences the bipolar form, a mood stabilizer is added, often **valproic acid** (Depakote), **carbamazepine** (Tegretol), or lithium (Eskalith or Lithobid). In schizoaffective disorder of the bipolar type, if little response occurs to the usual antipsychotic/mood stabilizer combinations, the mental health patient may be prescribed **clozapine** (Clozaril or other generic formulations), which appears to be both antipsychotic and mood-stabilizing. However, because clozapine has the potential (in a very minute number of cases) to cause lethal alterations in the composition of blood, and because its use requires regular monitoring with recurrent blood testing, it is reserved as a "last-resort" therapy. In cases of the depressive subtype, psychiatrists may prescribe an antidepressant such as **citalopram** (Celexa), **venlafaxine** (Effexor), **paroxetine** (Paxil), or **fluoxetine** (Prozac) as an adjunct to the antipsychotic. In certain cases of depressive subtypes, where medications have been ineffective in resolving the extreme mood or where psychosis is so severe as to be life-threatening, **electroconvulsive therapy** may be utilized. Electroconvulsive therapy has also been shown to be effective in major depressive episode with psychotic features.

KEY TERMS

Catatonic behavior or catatonia—Catatonic behavior or catatonia is a descriptive term that describes both possible extremes related to movement. Catalepsy is the motionless aspect of catatonia—in which a person with catalepsy may remain fixed in the same position for hours on end. Rapid or persistently repeated movements, frequent grimacing and strange facial expressions, and unusual gestures are the opposite end of the catatonia phenomenon, involving an excess or distorted extreme of movement.

Delusion—A false belief that is resistant to reason or contrary to actual fact.

Hallucinations—False sensory perceptions. A person experiencing a hallucination may "hear" sounds or "see" people or objects that are not really present. Hallucinations can also affect the senses of smell, touch, and taste.

Psychosis or psychotic symptoms—Disruptions in perceiving reality, thinking logically, and speaking or behaving in normal fashion. Hallucinations, delusions, catatonic behavior, and peculiar speech are all symptoms of psychosis. In *DSM-IV-TR,* psychosis is usually one feature of an overarching disorder, not a disorder in itself (with the exception of the diagnosis of psychosis not otherwise specified).

Medication is not the only treatment avenue. Supportive **psychotherapy** and psychoeducation is helpful to decrease the patient's fears and to inform the patient about the psychiatric illness. **Cognitive-behavioral therapy** aims to modify the thoughts and behaviors that provoke mood disturbance or prevent full involvement and collaboration in therapy for the mental illness. Psychoeducation and cognitive-behavioral therapy are not effective in lieu of biological therapy, but are enhancing, meaningful components of a "whole-person" approach used in concert with medications for the best possible outcomes.

Prognosis

The prognosis for patients with schizoaffective disorder is largely dependent on the form of the disorder and the presence or absence of a trigger. If a major life event is a prompting stressor, or an unusual traumatic experience preceded the occurrence of the disorder, chances for improvement are higher. If there is not a particular triggering event, or if the schizoaffective disorder occurred in an individual with a premorbid personality disorder, the outcome is less likely to be positive. The bipolar form of the disorder may respond better to treatment than the depressive form. Generally, the earlier the disorder is identified and treated and the fewer lapses from medications, the more positive the outcome.

Prevention

Given that this disorder appears to have a strong genetic or biologic aspect, society-wide prevention approaches are not likely to be fruitful. However, a promising strategy is to educate physicians, psychologists, and **social workers**, as well as people at higher risk for the disorder, about the characteristics and treatability of schizoaffective disorder. Such education of care providers and high-risk individuals would foster early identification and treatment. In schizoaffective disorder, similar to schizophrenia and bipolar disorder, better response is predicted the earlier treatment begins. Because severe stressors theoretically can trigger this disorder (in some cases), strong social support and immediate postcrisis counseling for severe stress could possibly prevent the development of the disorder in some susceptible people.

Resources

BOOKS

American Psychiatric Association. *Diagnostic and Statistical Manual of Mental Disorders*. 4th ed., text rev. Washington, DC: American Psychiatric Publishing, 2000.

Graham, George. *The Disordered Mind: An Introduction to Philosophy of Mind and Mental Illness*. New York: Routledge, 2010.

Murray, William H., ed. *Schizoaffective Disorders: New Research*. Hauppauge, NY: Nova Science Publishers, 2006.

Nemitz, Susan Beth. *Living with Schizoaffective Disorder*. Frederick, MD: PublishAmerica, 2009.

Texas, Nami, and Deborah Colleen Rose, ed. *Diagnosis—Schizophrenia and Schizoaffective Disorder: Visions for Tomorrow—The Basics*. Charleston, SC: CreateSpace, 2009.

PERIODICALS

Lipkovich, I., et al. "Predictors of Risk for Relapse in Patients with Schizophrenia or Schizoaffective Disorder During Olanzapine Drug Therapy." *Journal of Psychiatric Research* 41, no. 3–4 (April–June 2007): 305–10.

Maier, Wolfgang. "Do Schizoaffective Disorders Exist at All?" *Acta Psychiatrica Scandinavica* 113, no. 5 (May 2006): 369–71.

Pinninti, Narsimha, et al. "Severity of Self-Reported Depression in Patients with a Schizoaffective Disorder." *Journal of Psychopathology and Behavioral Assessment* 28, no. 3 (September 2006): 165–70.

Risch, S. Craig, et al. "Donepezil Effects on Mood in Patients with Schizophrenia and Schizoaffective Disorder." *International Journal of Neuropsychopharmacology* 9, no. 5 (October 2006): 603–5.

Simpson, George M., et al. "A 1-Year Double-Blind Study of 2 Doses of Long-Acting Risperidone in Stable Patients with Schizophrenia or Schizoaffective Disorder." *Journal of Clinical Psychiatry* 67, no. 8 (August 2006): 1194–1203.

Strous, Rael D., et al. "Comparison Between Risperidone, Olanzapine, and Clozapine in the Management of Chronic Schizophrenia: A Naturalistic Prospective 12-Week Observational Study." *Human Psychopharmacology: Clinical and Experimental* 21, no. 4 (June 2006): 235–43.

Vollmer-Larsen, A., et al. "Schizoaffective Disorder—The Reliability of Its Clinical Diagnostic Use." *Acta Psychiatrica Scandinavica* 113, no. 5 (May 2006): 402–7.

ORGANIZATIONS

American Psychiatric Association, 1000 Wilson Blvd., Suite 1825, Arlington, VA, 22209-3901, (703) 907-7300, apa@psych.org, http://www.psych.org.

American Psychological Association, 750 1st St. NE, Washington, DC, 20002-4242, (202) 336-5500; TDD/TTY: (202) 336-6123, (800) 374-2721, http://www.apa.org.

Brain and Behavior Research Foundation, 60 Cutter Mill Rd., Suite 404, Great Neck, NY, 11021, (516) 829-0091, Fax: (516) 487-6930, info@bbrfoundation.org, http://www.bbrfoundation.org.

Mental Health America, 2000 North Beauregard St., 6th Fl., Alexandria, VA, 22311, (703) 684-7722, (800) 969-6642, Fax: (703) 684-5968, http://www1.nmha.org.

National Alliance on Mental Illness, 3803 N Fairfax Dr., Suite 100, Arlington, VA, 22203, (703) 524-7600, Fax: (703) 524-9094, http://www.nami.org.

National Institute of Mental Health, 6001 Executive Blvd., Rm. 8184, MSC 9663, Bethesda, MD, 20892-9663, (301) 433-4513; TTY: (301) 443-8431, (866) 615-6464; TTY: (866) 415-8051, Fax: (301) 443-4279, nimhinfo@nih.gov, http://www.nimh.nih.gov.

Deborah Rosch Eifert, PhD
Martha Sajatovic, PhD
Ruth A. Wienclaw, PhD

Schizoid personality disorder

Definition

Schizoid personality disorder is characterized by a persistent withdrawal from social relationships and lack of emotional responsiveness in most situations. Individuals with schizoid personality disorder tend to be consistently emotionally cold, lack tender feelings for others, be indifferent to feelings of others, and are unable to form close relationships with more than two people. Schizoid personality disorder, however, does not include the characteristic patterns of speech, behavior, and thought associated with **schizotypal personality disorder**. Schizoid personality disorder is sometimes referred to as a "pleasure deficiency" because of the seeming inability of the person affected to experience joyful or pleasurable responses to life situations.

Demographics

Of all **personality disorders**, schizoid personality disorder is the least commonly diagnosed personality disorder in the general population. The prevalence is approximately 1%. It is diagnosed slightly more often in males than in females.

Description

People with schizoid personality disorder have little or no interest in developing close interpersonal relationships. They appear aloof, introverted, and prefer being alone. Those who know them often label them as shy or a "loner." They turn inward in an effort to shut out social relationships. It is common for people with schizoid personality disorder to avoid groups of people or appear disinterested in social situations, even when they involve family. They are often perceived by others as socially inept.

A closely related trait is the absence of emotional expression. Others routinely interpret this apparent void of emotion as disinterest, lack of concern, and insensitivity to the needs of others. The person with schizoid personality disorder has particular difficulty expressing anger or hostility. In the absence of any recognizable emotion, the person portrays a dull demeanor and is easily overlooked by others. People with schizoid personality disorder tend to prefer to be viewed as "invisible," which aids their quest to avoid social contact with others.

People with schizoid personality disorder may be able to hold jobs and meet the expectations of employers if the responsibilities do not require more than minimal interpersonal involvement. People with this disorder may be married, but do not develop close intimate relationships with their spouses and typically show no interest in sexual relations. Their speech is typically slow and monotonous with a lethargic demeanor. Because their tendency is to turn inward, they can easily become preoccupied with their own thoughts to the exclusion of what is happening in their environment. Attempts to communicate may drift into tangents or confusing associations. They are also prone to being absentminded.

Causes and symptoms

Causes

The schizoid personality disorder has its roots in the family of the affected person. These families are typically emotionally reserved, have a high degree of formality, and have a communication style that is aloof and impersonal. Parents usually express inadequate amounts of affection to the child and provide insufficient amounts of emotional stimulus. This lack of stimulus during the first year of life is thought to be largely responsible for the person's disinterest in forming close, meaningful relationships later in life.

People with schizoid personality disorder have learned to imitate the style of interpersonal relationships modeled in their families. In this environment, affected people fail to learn basic communication skills that would enable them to develop relationships and interact effectively with others. Their communication is often vague and fragmented, which others find confusing. Many individuals with schizoid personality disorder feel misunderstood by others.

Symptoms

As presented in the *Diagnostic and Statistical Manual of Mental Disorders*. (*DSM-IV-TR*), the following seven diagnostic criteria are assessed in patients who may be diagnosed with schizoid personality disorder:

- Avoids close relationships. People with this disorder show no interest or enjoyment in developing interpersonal relationships; this may also include family members. They perceive themselves as social misfits and believe they can function best when not dependent on anyone except themselves. They rarely date, often do not marry, and have few, if any, friends.
- Prefers solitude. They prefer and choose activities that they can do by themselves without dependence upon or involvement with others. Examples of activities they might choose include mechanical or abstract tasks such as computer or mathematical games.
- Avoids sex. There is typically little or no interest in having a sexual experience with another person. This would include a spouse if the affected person is married.
- Lacks pleasure. There is an absence of pleasure in most activities. A person with schizoid personality disorder seems unable to experience the full range of emotion accessible to most people.
- Lacks close friends. People affected with this disorder typically do not have the social skills necessary to develop meaningful interpersonal relationships. This

results in few ongoing social relationships outside of immediate family members.

- Indifferent to praise or criticism. Neither positive nor negative comments made by others elicit an emotionally expressive reaction. Those with schizoid personality disorder do not appear concerned about what others might think of them. Despite their tendency to turn inward to escape social contact, they practice little introspection.
- Emotional detachment. The emotional style of those with schizoid personality disorder is aloof and perceived by others as distant or "cold." They seem unable or uninterested in expressing empathy and concern for others. Emotions are significantly restricted and most social contacts would describe their personality as very bland, dull, or humorless. The person with schizoid personality disorder rarely picks up on or reciprocates normal communicational cues such as facial expressions, head nods, or smiles.

Diagnosis

The symptoms of schizoid personality disorder may begin in childhood or adolescence, showing as poor peer relationships, a tendency toward self-isolation, and underachievement in school. Children with these tendencies appear socially out of step with peers and often become the object of malicious teasing by their peers, which increases the feelings of isolation and social ineptness they feel.

For a **diagnosis** of schizoid personality disorder to be accurately made, the affected person must exhibit an ongoing avoidance of social relationships and a restricted range of emotion in interpersonal relationships that began by early adulthood. There must also be the presence of at least four of the above-mentioned symptoms.

A common difficulty in diagnosing schizoid personality disorder is distinguishing it from autistic disorder and **Asperger syndrome**, which are characterized by more severe deficits in social skills. Other individuals who would display social habits that might be viewed as "isolating" should not be given the diagnosis of schizoid personality disorder unless the personality traits are inflexible and cause significant obstacles to adequate functioning.

The diagnosis is based on a clinical interview to assess symptomatic behavior. Other assessment tools helpful in diagnosing schizoid personality disorder include:

- Minnesota Multiphasic Personality Inventory (MMPI-2)
- Millon Clinical Multiaxial Inventory (MCMI-II)
- Rorschach Psychodiagnostic Test
- Thematic Apperception Test (TAT)

Treatment

A major goal of treating a patient diagnosed with schizoid personality disorder is to combat the tendencies toward social withdrawal. Strategies should focus on enhancing self-awareness and sensitivity to their relational contacts and environment.

Psychodynamically oriented therapies

A psychodynamic approach would typically not be the first choice of treatment due to the patient's poor ability to explore his or her thoughts, emotions, and behavior. When this treatment is used, it usually centers around building a therapeutic relationship with the patient that can act as a model for use in other relationships.

Cognitive-behavioral therapy

Attempting to cognitively restructure the patient's thoughts can enhance self-insight. Constructive ways of accomplishing this would include concrete assignments such as keeping daily records of problematic behaviors or thoughts. Another helpful method can be teaching social skills through role-playing. This might enable individuals to become more conscious of communication cues given by others and sensitize them to others' needs.

Group therapy

Group therapy may provide patients with a socializing experience that exposes them to feedback from others in a safe, controlled environment. It can also provide a means of learning and practicing social skills in which they are deficient. Since patients usually avoid social contact, timing of group therapy is of particular importance. It is best to first develop a therapeutic relationship between therapist and patient before starting a group therapy treatment.

Family and marital therapy

It is unlikely that a person with schizoid personality disorder will seek **family therapy** or marital therapy. If pursued, it is usually on the initiative of the spouse or other family member. Many people with this disorder do not marry and end up living with and are dependent upon immediate family members. In this case, therapy may be recommended for family members to educate them on aspects of change or ways to facilitate communication. Marital therapy (also called **couples therapy**) may focus on helping the couple to become more involved in each other's lives or improve communication patterns.

KEY TERMS

Asperger syndrome—A condition in which young children experience impaired social interactions and develop limited repetitive patterns of behavior.

Autistic disorder—A developmental disability that appears early in life, in which normal brain development is disrupted and social and communication skills are retarded, sometimes severely.

Millon Clinical Multiaxial Inventory (MCMI-II)—A self-report instrument designed to help clinicians assess *DSM-IV*-related personality disorders and clinical syndromes. It provides insight into 14 personality disorders and 10 clinical syndromes.

Minnesota Multiphasic Personality Inventory (MMPI-2)—A comprehensive assessment tool widely used to diagnose personality disorders.

Rorschach Psychodiagnostic Test—This series of 10 "inkblot" images allows patients to project their interpretations that can be used to diagnose particular disorders.

Thematic Apperception Test (TAT)—A projective test using stories and descriptions of pictures to reveal some of the dominant drives, emotions, sentiments, conflicts, and complexes of a personality.

Medications

Some patients with this disorder show signs of anxiety and **depression** that may prompt the use of medication to counteract these symptoms. In general, to date no definitive medication is used to treat schizoid symptoms.

Prognosis

Because people with schizoid personality disorder seek to be isolated from others, which includes those who might provide treatment, there is only a slight chance that most patients will seek help on their own initiative. Those who do may stop treatment prematurely because of their difficulty maintaining a relationship with the professional or their lack of motivation for change.

If the degree of social impairment is mild, treatment might succeed if its focus is on maintenance of relationships related to the patient's employment. The need for patients to support themselves financially can act as a higher incentive for pursuit of treatment outcomes. Once treatment ends, however, it is highly likely the patient will **relapse** into a lifestyle of social isolation similar to that before treatment.

Prevention

Because schizoid personality disorder originates in the patient's family of origin, the only known preventive measure is a nurturing, emotionally stimulating, and expressive caretaking environment.

Resources

BOOKS

American Psychiatric Association. *Diagnostic and Statistical Manual of Mental Disorders*. 4th ed., text rev. Washington, DC: American Psychiatric Publishing, 2000.

Beck, Aaron T., Arthur Freeman, and Denise D. Davis. *Cognitive Therapy of Personality Disorders*. New York: The Guilford Press, 2006.

Livesley, W. John. *Practical Management of Personality Disorder*. New York: The Guilford Press, 2003.

Millon, Theodore, et al. *Personality Disorders in Modern Life*. 2nd ed. New York: John Wiley and Sons, 2004.

VandenBos, Gary R. ed. *APA Dictionary of Psychology*. Washington, DC: American Psychological Association, 2006.

PERIODICALS

Camisa, Kathryn M., et al. "Personality Traits in Schizophrenia and Related Personality Disorders." *Psychiatry Research* 133, no. 1 (January 2005): 23–33.

Kavaler-Adler, Susan. "Anatomy of Regret: A Developmental View of the Depressive Position and a Critical Turn Toward Love and Creativity in the Transforming Schizoid Personality." *American Journal of Psychoanalysis* 64, no. 1 (March 2004): 39–76.

ORGANIZATIONS

American Psychiatric Association, 1000 Wilson Blvd., Ste. 1825, Arlington, VA, 22209-3901, (703) 907-7300, apa@psych.org, http://www.psych.org.

Gary Gilles, MA
Ruth A. Wienclaw, PhD

Schizophrenia

Definition

Schizophrenia is a disorder or group of disorders whose symptoms include disturbances in thinking, emotional responsiveness, and behavior. The word schizophrenia comes from the Greek roots of *skhizein* ("to split") and *phren* ("mind"). At one time, it was thought that the term schizophrenia was synonymous with a multiple personality disorder (split personality), but this is no longer the case. Generally, this disorder is the most chronic and disabling of the severe mental

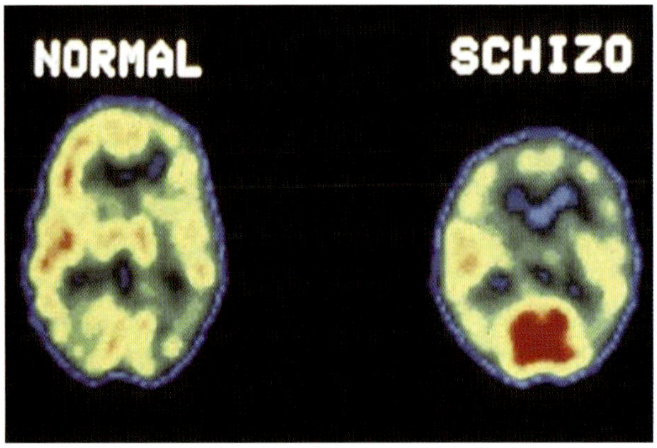

Positron emission tomography (PET) scans comparing a healthy brain (left) with the brain of a person with schizophrenia. *(© Photo Researchers, Inc.)*

disorders and is associated with abnormalities of **brain** structure and function, disorganized speech and behavior, **delusions**, and hallucinations. Schizophrenia is considered a psychotic disorder or a **psychosis**.

Demographics

The World Health Organization (WHO) estimates that schizophrenia affects about 24 million people worldwide. Approximately 2.4–2.7 million Americans are affected by schizophrenia, according to the **National Institute of Mental Health** (NIMH). The incidence of schizophrenia in the United States appears to be uniform across racial and ethnic groups, although there seems to be higher rates within small minority groups in large urban neighborhoods. A study done in the United Kingdom replicated the U.S. findings, with significantly higher rates of schizophrenia among racial minorities living in large cities. The rates of schizophrenia are highest in areas in which these minority groups form the smallest proportion of the local population. The British study included Africans, West Indians of African descent, and Asians.

Schizophrenia is a leading cause of disability around the world; the WHO counts schizophrenia as one of the world's 10 leading causes of disability. Unfortunately, less than half are receiving appropriate and effective care. The situation is worse in developing countries, where about 90% of people with schizophrenia are left untreated. In addition, about 1 in 10 Americans who commit **suicide** have schizophrenia, **depression**, or another mental illness. According to the federal Agency for Healthcare Research and Quality, 70%–80% of people diagnosed with schizophrenia are either unemployed or underemployed (working in jobs well below their actual capabilities). Ten percent of Americans with permanent disabilities have schizophrenia, as well as 20%–30% of the homeless population.

In North America and Western Europe, the gender ratio in schizophrenia is 1.2:1, with males being affected slightly more often than females. There is a significant gender difference in average age at onset; the average for males is between ages 18 and 25 years (late teen years to early 20s), whereas for women there are two peaks: one in the 20s and another in the early 30s. About 15% of all women who develop schizophrenia are diagnosed after age 35. In some women, the first symptoms of the disorder appear postpartum (after giving birth). Many women with schizophrenia are initially misdiagnosed as having depression or **bipolar disorder**, because women with schizophrenia are likely to have more difficulties with emotional regulation than men with the disorder. However, females tend to have higher levels of functioning prior to symptom onset than do males. Although more males acquire schizophrenia in childhood compared to females, this distinction goes away by the time of adolescence with females nearly equal to males in the frequency of the disorder.

In most developed countries, the incidence of schizophrenia appears to be higher among people born in cities than among those born in rural areas. In addition, there appears to be a small generational factor, with the incidence of schizophrenia gradually declining in later-born generations of a family. Paternal age, or the age of the father at conception, may also affect the risk of schizophrenia developing in the offspring, with persons with older fathers being more at risk.

Description

People diagnosed with schizophrenia do not always display the same sets of symptoms; in addition, a given patient's symptoms may change over time. Since the nineteenth century, doctors have recognized different subtypes of the disorder, but no single classification system has gained universal acceptance. Some psychiatrists prefer to speak of schizophrenia as a group or family of disorders ("the schizophrenias") rather than as a single entity.

The symptoms of schizophrenia are usually treatable, but the condition is much more easily treated when diagnosed in its earlier stages and before other functional disabilities arise. Symptoms of schizophrenia can appear at any time after age 6 or 7 years, although onset during adolescence or early adult life is most common. There are a few case studies in the medical literature of schizophrenia in children younger than 5 years, but they are extremely rare. Schizophrenia that appears after age 45 years is considered late-onset schizophrenia, and about 1%–2% of cases are diagnosed in patients over 80 years.

The onset of symptoms in schizophrenia may be either abrupt (sudden) or insidious (gradual). Often, however, the condition goes undetected for two to three years after the onset of diagnosable symptoms, because the symptoms occur in the context of previous cognitive and behavioral problems or diagnoses. In most cases, however, the patient's first psychotic episode is preceded by a prodromal (warning) phase, characterized by a variety of behaviors that may include angry outbursts, withdrawal from social activities, loss of attention to personal hygiene and grooming, anhedonia (loss of enjoyment), and other unusual behaviors. The psychotic episode itself is typically characterized by delusions—false but strongly held beliefs that result from the patient's inability to separate real from unreal events—and hallucinations, which are disturbances of sense perception. Hallucinations can affect any of the senses (sight, smell, taste), but the most common form of **hallucination** in schizophrenia is auditory ("hearing voices"). Autobiographical accounts by people who have recovered from schizophrenia indicate that these hallucinations are frightening and confusing. Patients often find it difficult to concentrate on work, studies, or formerly pleasurable activities because of the constant "static" or "buzz" of hallucinated voices.

There is no "typical" pattern or course of the disorder following the first acute episode. The patient may never have a second psychotic episode; others have occasional episodes over the course of their lives but can lead somewhat normal lives otherwise. About 70% of patients diagnosed with schizophrenia have a second psychotic breakdown within five to seven years after the first one. Some patients remain chronically ill; of these, some remain at a fairly stable level while others grow steadily worse and become severely disabled.

Subtypes of schizophrenia

The revised fourth edition of the ***Diagnostic and Statistical Manual of Mental Disorders*** (*DSM-IV-TR*), the handbook used by medical professionals in diagnosing mental disorders, specifies five subtypes of schizophrenia:

- Paranoid type. The central feature of this subtype is the presence of auditory hallucinations or delusions alongside relatively unaffected mood and cognitive functions. The patient's delusions usually involve persecution, grandiosity, or both. About a third of schizophrenias diagnosed in the United States belong to this subtype.
- Disorganized type. The core features of this subtype include disorganized speech, disorganized behavior, and flat or inappropriate affect. The person may lose the ability to perform most activities of daily living and may also make faces or display other oddities of behavior. This type of schizophrenia was formerly called "hebephrenic" (derived from the Greek word for puberty), because some of the patients' actions resemble adolescent behaviors.
- Catatonic type. Catatonia refers to disturbances of movement, whether remaining motionless for long periods of time or excessive and purposeless movement. The absence of movement may take the form of catalepsy, which is a condition in which the patient's body has a kind of waxy flexibility and can be repositioned by others, but where the patient will not initiate the movement, or negativism, a form of postural rigidity in which the patient resists being moved by others. A catatonic patient may assume bizarre postures or imitate the movements of other people.
- Undifferentiated type. Patients in this subtype have some of the characteristic symptoms of schizophrenia but do not meet the full criteria for the paranoid, disorganized, or catatonic subtypes.
- Residual type. Patients in this category have had at least one psychotic episode and continue to have some negative symptoms of schizophrenia but do not have current psychotic symptoms.

Proposed changes for the fifth edition of the *DSM* (*DSM-5*, 2013) include removing the subtypes from the new edition and changing the classification of schizophrenia to schizophrenia spectrum disorders.

Cultural variables

There appear to be some differences across cultures in the symptoms associated with schizophrenia. The catatonic subtype appears to be more common in non-Western countries than in Europe or North America. Other studies indicate that persons diagnosed with schizophrenia in developing countries have a more acute onset of the disorder but better outcomes than patients in industrialized countries.

Association with violence

The connection between schizophrenia and personal assault or violence deserves mention because it is a major factor in the reactions of family members and the general public to a **diagnosis** of schizophrenia and is responsible for some of the **stigma** associated with the disorder. Many patients report that the popular image of a schizophrenic as "a time bomb waiting to explode" is a source of considerable emotional **stress**.

Risk factors for violence in a patient diagnosed with schizophrenia include male gender, age below 30 years, prediagnosis history of violence, paranoid subtype, nonadherence to medication regimen, **homelessness**, and heavy **substance abuse**. On the other hand, it should be noted that most crimes of violence are committed by

E. FULLER TORREY: SCHIZOPHRENIA RESEARCHER

American psychiatrist E. Fuller Torrey (1937–), who has been especially involved in researching and treating schizophrenia, is the author of numerous works of nonfiction dealing with mental illness. In his first major work, *The Mind Game: Witchdoctors and Psychiatrists,* Torrey compares modern psychiatric practices to those of primitive witchdoctors, and in *The Death of Psychiatry* he alleges that modern psychiatry has misdiagnosed maladjustment as mental illness. In the latter work, Torrey advocates support systems for the socially traumatized and recommends neurological help for the truly unbalanced.

Torrey's other writings include *Why Did You Do That? Rainy Day Games for a Post-Industrial Society*, a game-book in which he counsels readers on the importance of recognizing biological, sociological, and psychological factors in assessing human behavior. He also wrote *Surviving Schizophrenia: A Manual for Families, Consumers, and Providers,* in which he supplements a detailed account of the disease's genetic origin and symptoms with testimony from schizophrenics. The fifth edition of *Surviving Schizophrenia* was published in 2006.

In 1998, Torrey founded the Treatment Advocacy Center, a nonprofit organization focused on the proper treatment of severe mental disorders such as schizophrenia. Torrey also serves as a director of the Stanley Medical Research Institute, which conducts research on schizophrenia and bipolar disorder.

people without a diagnosis of schizophrenia, and people with schizophrenia are more likely to be victims of crimes rather than perpetrators.

Causes and symptoms

Causes

Schizophrenia is considered the end result of a combination of genetic, biochemical, developmental, and environmental factors, some of which are still not completely understood. Schizophrenia is often called a "multifactorially inherited" disease, meaning that many factors play roles in its development. There is no known single cause of the disorder.

Researchers have known for many years that first-degree biological relatives (siblings) of patients with schizophrenia have a 10% risk of developing the disorder, as compared with 1% in the general population. If one parent has schizophrenia, his or her child is 10%–15% more likely to also develop the disorder. In larger families, if multiple siblings have schizophrenia, the risk becomes higher for the remaining siblings to develop schizophrenia. The monozygotic (identical) twin of a person with schizophrenia has a 40%–50% risk of developing the disorder; the fact that this risk is not higher, however, indicates that environmental as well as **genetic factors** may be implicated in the development of schizophrenia.

Some specific regions on certain human chromosomes have been linked to schizophrenia, but no one gene can be identified as the direct cause. Scientists believe that the genetic factors underlying schizophrenia vary across different ethnic groups and that the development is likely the result of more than one genetic mutation, making schizophrenia a polygenic disorder. According to the NIMH, persons with schizophrenia have higher rates of rare mutations; hundreds of genes could be involved in the causation of the disorder.

There is some evidence that schizophrenia may be a type of developmental disorder related to the formation of faulty connections between nerve cells during fetal development. In adolescence, the changes in the brain that normally occur during puberty interact with these connections to trigger the symptoms of the disorder. Other researchers have suggested that a difficult childbirth may result in developmental vulnerabilities that eventually lead to schizophrenia; further research is needed on both of these topics.

In 2002, NIMH researchers demonstrated the existence of a connection between two abnormalities of brain functioning in patients with schizophrenia, with the findings published in the January issue of *Nature Neuroscience*. The researchers used radioactive tracers and **positron emission tomography (PET)** to show that reduced activity in a part of the brain called the prefrontal cortex was associated in the patients but not in the control subjects, with abnormally elevated levels of **dopamine** in the striatum. High levels of dopamine are related to the delusions and hallucinations of psychotic episodes in schizophrenia. These findings suggest that treatment directed at the prefrontal cortex might be more effective than present antipsychotic medications, which essentially target dopamine levels without regard to specific areas of the brain.

Certain environmental factors during pregnancy may also be associated with an increased risk of schizophrenia in the offspring. These include the mother's exposure to starvation or famine, influenza during the second trimester of pregnancy, and Rh incompatibility (which involves the Rh antigen, sometimes also called the Rhesus factor) in a second or third pregnancy. Environmental stressors related to home and family life (e.g., parental death or divorce, family dysfunction) or to separation from the family of origin in late adolescence (e.g., going away to college or military training; marriage) may trigger the onset of schizophrenia in individuals with genetic or psychological vulnerabilities.

Some researchers are investigating a possible connection between schizophrenia and viral infections of the hippocampus, a structure in the brain that is associated with memory formation and the human stress response. It is thought that damage to the hippocampus might account for the sensory disturbances found in schizophrenia. Another line of research related to viral causes of schizophrenia concerns a protein deficiency in the brain. The human genome project, a 13-year project that mapped the complete human genome, found that up to 8% of the genome consists of viruses within the deoxyribonucleic acid (DNA), including the borna virus, which supposedly has an association with schizophrenia. The finding remained controversial as of 2011, as further research studies attempted to verify the claim.

The multifactorial and polygenic etiology (origins or causes) of schizophrenia complicates the search for preventive measures against the disorder. It is possible that the human genome mapping will help identify the specific genes that contribute to susceptibility to schizophrenia. The NIMH has compiled the world's largest registry of families affected by schizophrenia in order to attempt to pinpoint specific genes for further study; the institute estimates that at least 60% of the factors that cause schizophrenia may be due to genetic related susceptibility. The NIMH also sponsors a Prevention Research Initiative to identify points in the development of schizophrenia at which patients could benefit from the application of preventive efforts.

Symptoms

The symptoms of schizophrenia are divided into two major categories: **positive symptoms**, which are defined by the *DSM-IV-TR* as excesses or distortions of normal mental functions, and **negative symptoms**, which represent a loss or reduction of normal functioning. Of the two types, the negative symptoms are more difficult to evaluate, because though they account for much of the morbidity (unhealthiness) associated with schizophrenia, they may be influenced by outside factors, such as a concurrent depression or an unstimulating environment.

POSITIVE SYMPTOMS. The positive symptoms of schizophrenia include four so-called "first-rank" or Schneiderian symptoms, named for a German **psychiatrist** who identified them in 1959:

- Delusions. A delusion is a false belief that is resistant to reason or to confrontation with actual facts. The most common form of delusion in patients with schizophrenia is persecutory; the person believes that others—family members, clinical staff, terrorists, etc.—are "out to get" them. Another common delusion is referential, which means that the person interprets objects or occurrences in the environment (a picture on the wall, a song played on the radio, laughter in the corridor, etc.) as being directed at or referring to them.
- Somatic hallucinations. Somatic hallucinations refer to sensations or perceptions about a person's body that have no known medical cause, such as feeling that snakes are crawling around in the intestines or that the eyes are emitting radioactive rays.
- Auditory hallucinations. Auditory hallucinations consist of hearing voices and are the most common form of hallucination in schizophrenia, although visual, tactile, olfactory, and gustatory hallucinations may also occur. Personal accounts of recovery from schizophrenia often mention "the voices" as one of the most frightening aspects of the disorder.
- Thought insertion or withdrawal. These terms refer to the notion that other beings or forces (God, aliens from outer space, the Central Intelligence Agency [CIA], etc.) can put thoughts or ideas into a person's mind or remove them.

Other positive symptoms of schizophrenia include:

- Disorganized speech and thinking. A person with schizophrenia may ramble from one topic to another (derailment or loose associations), give unrelated answers to questions (tangentiality), or say things that cannot be understood because there is no grammatical structure to the language ("word salad" or incoherence).
- Disorganized behavior. This symptom includes such behaviors as agitation, age-inappropriate silliness, inability to maintain personal hygiene, dressing inappropriately for the weather, sexual self-stimulation in public, shouting at people, etc.
- Catatonic behavior. Catatonic behaviors have been described with regard to the catatonic subtype of

schizophrenia. This particular symptom is sometimes found in other mental disorders.

NEGATIVE SYMPTOMS. The negative symptoms of schizophrenia include:

- Blunted or flattened affect, or the loss of emotional expressiveness. The person's face may be unresponsive or expressionless, and speech may lack vitality or warmth.
- Alogia, sometimes called poverty of speech. The person has little to say and is not able to expand on their statements. A doctor examining the patient must be able to distinguish between alogia and unwillingness to speak.
- Avolition, or a lack of goal-directed activities. They may sit in one location for long periods of time or show little interest in joining group activities.
- Anhedonia, or the loss of one's capacity for enjoyment or pleasure.

COGNITIVE SYMPTOMS. Persons with schizophrenia also display cognitive deficits, or trouble with tasks involving thought, learning, and memory. Cognitive symptoms of schizophrenia include an inability to apply facts or knowledge when making decisions (**executive function**), lack of concentration, and problems with utilizing new knowledge (working memory).

OTHER SYMPTOMS AND CHARACTERISTICS. Some symptoms and features are not considered diagnostic of schizophrenia, but most patients with the disorder display one or more of the following symptoms or characteristics:

- Dissociative symptoms, particularly depersonalization and derealization.
- Anosognosia. This term originally referred to the inability of stroke patients to recognize their physical disabilities, but it is sometimes used to refer to lack of insight in patients with schizophrenia. Anosognosia is associated with higher rates of noncompliance with treatment, a higher risk of repeated psychotic episodes, and a poorer prognosis for recovery; approximately 50% of individuals with schizophrenia display anosognosia, according to the organization Mental Health America.
- High rates of substance abuse disorders. About 50% of patients diagnosed with schizophrenia meet criteria for substance abuse or dependence. While substance abuse does not cause schizophrenia, it can worsen the symptoms of the disorder. Patients may have particularly bad reactions to amphetamines, cocaine, PCP (phencyclidine, commonly called "angel dust") or marijuana. It is thought that patients with schizophrenia are attracted to drugs of abuse as self-medication for some of their symptoms. The most common substance abused by patients with schizophrenia is tobacco; 90% of patients are heavy cigarette smokers, compared to 25%–30% in the general adult population. Smoking is a serious problem for people with schizophrenia because it interferes with the effectiveness of their antipsychotic medications as well as increasing their risk of lung cancer and other respiratory diseases.
- High risk of suicide. About 40% of patients with schizophrenia attempt suicide at least once, and 10% eventually complete the act.
- High rates of obsessive-compulsive disorder and panic disorder.
- Downward drift. Downward drift is a sociological term that refers to having lower levels of educational achievement and/or employment than a person's parents.

People with schizophrenia are also more apt to acquire metabolic syndrome, which is a combination of different medical disorders that together increase the risk of developing diabetes, cardiovascular disease, and other related medical maladies. Also known as insulin resistance syndrome, cardiometabolic syndrome, metabolic syndrome X, and Reaven's syndrome, the condition is brought about by a sedentary lifestyle, poor eating habits, and other related factors. Studies have shown that over 30% of people with schizophrenia are also diagnosed with metabolic syndrome. In addition, about 20%–25% of people in the United States are estimated to have metabolic syndrome, with slightly more women having it than men. The risk of developing metabolic syndrome increases with age. Weight gain may also be a side effect of antipsychotic medications.

Diagnosis

There are no symptoms that are unique to schizophrenia and no single symptom that is a diagnostic hallmark of the disorder. In addition, laboratory tests or **imaging studies** are unable to establish or confirm a diagnosis of schizophrenia. The diagnosis is based on a constellation or group of related symptoms and should be completed by a psychiatrist.

As part of the process of diagnosis, the doctor will take a careful medical history and order laboratory tests of the patient's blood or urine in order to rule out general medical conditions or substance abuse disorders that may be accompanied by disturbed behavior. X rays or other imaging studies of the head may also be ordered. Medical conditions to be ruled out include epilepsy, head **trauma**, brain tumor, Cushing's syndrome, Wilson's disease, Huntington's disease, and encephalitis. Drugs of abuse

Antipsychotic medications

Generic name	Trade name	FDA approved age
aripiprazole	Abilify	10+ for bipolar disorder, manic or mixed episodes; 13–17 for schizophrenia and bipolar disorder
chlorpromazine	Thorazine	18+
clozapine	Clozaril	18+
fluoxetine & olanzapine	Symbyax (Prozac & Zyprexa)	18+ (combination antipsychotic and antidepressant)
fluphenazine	(generic only)	18+
haloperidol	Haldol	3+
iloperidone	Fanapt	18+
loxapine	Loxitane	18+
molindone	Moban	18+
olanzapine	Zyprexa	18+; ages 13–17 as second-line treatment for manic or mixed episodes of bipolar disorder and schizophrenia
paliperidone	Invega	18+
perphenazine	(generic only)	18+
pimozide	Orap	12+ for Tourette syndrome
quetiapine	Seroquel	13+ for schizophrenia; 18+ for bipolar disorder; 10–17 for treatment of manic and mixed episodes of bipolar disorder
risperidone	Risperdal	13+ for schizophrenia; 10+ for bipolar mania and mixed episodes; 5–16 for irritability associated with autism
thioridazine	(generic only)	2+
thiothixene	Navane	18+
trifluoperazine	Stelazine	18+
ziprasidone	Geodon	18+

SOURCE: National Institute of Mental Health.

"Alphabetical List of Medications," available online at: http://www.nimh.nih.gov/health/publications/mental-health-medications/alphabetical-list-of-medications.shtml. *(Table by PreMediaGlobal. © 2012 Cengage Learning.)*

that may cause symptoms resembling schizophrenia include **amphetamines** ("speed"), **cocaine**, and phencyclidine (PCP). In older patients, **dementia** and **delirium** must be ruled out. If the patient has held jobs involving exposure to mercury, polychlorinated biphenyls (PCBs), or other toxic substances, environmental poisoning must also be considered in the differential diagnosis.

The doctor must also rule out other mental disorders that may be accompanied by psychotic symptoms, such as mood disorders; brief psychotic disorders; dissociative disorder not otherwise specified or **dissociative identity disorder**; **delusional disorder**; schizotypal, schizoid, or paranoid **personality disorders**; and **pervasive developmental disorders**. In children, childhood-onset schizophrenia must be distinguished from communication disorders with disorganized speech and from **attention deficit hyperactivity disorder**.

After other organic and mental disorders have been ruled out, it must be determined whether the patient meets the following criteria, as specified by the *DSM*:

- The patient must have two (or more) of the following symptoms during a one-month period: delusions, hallucinations, disorganized speech, disorganized or catatonic behavior, or negative symptoms.
- The patient must exhibit a decline in social, interpersonal, or occupational functioning, including personal hygiene or self-care.
- The symptomatic behavior must last for at least six months.

Treatment

Current treatment of schizophrenia focuses on symptom reduction and **relapse prevention**, since the causes of the disorder have not yet been clearly identified. Unfortunately, not all patients with schizophrenia receive adequate treatment. In addition, many people with schizophrenia do not take their medication, either because they forget, because it does not adequately control their symptoms, because it produces adverse side effects, because they cannot afford it, or because they are not aware of the severity of their condition.

Medications

Antipsychotic medications, namely neuroleptics and atypical antipsychotics, are the primary treatment for schizophrenia. They work to suppress dopamine and **serotonin** activity, respectively, and help to reduce the severity of the positive symptoms. However, they do not help with the negative symptoms or with cognitive problems.

Drug therapy for the disorder is complicated by several factors: the unpredictability of a given patient's response to specific medications, the number of potentially troublesome side effects, the high rate of substance abuse among patients with schizophrenia, and the possibility of drug interactions between antipsychotic medications and **antidepressants** or other medications that may be prescribed for the patient. Therapy is further complicated when patients do not take or do not consistently take their medications. Proper adherence to medication regimens includes always taking the proper dosage within the time frame as determined by the attending medical professional. Medicines may need to be adjusted periodically by the doctor, and the patient should make sure such changes are done without delay.

NEUROLEPTICS. The first antipsychotic medications for schizophrenia were introduced in the 1950s and were known as dopamine antagonists. They are sometimes called neuroleptics and include **haloperidol** (Haldol), **chlorpromazine** (Thorazine), **perphenazine** (Trilafon), and **fluphenazine** (Prolixin). About 40% of patients, however, fail to respond to treatment with these medications. Neuroleptics can control most of the positive symptoms of schizophrenia as well as reduce the frequency and severity of relapses but they have little effect on negative symptoms. In addition, these medications have problematic side effects, ranging from dry mouth, blurry vision, and restlessness (akathisia) to long-term side effects such as **tardive dyskinesia** (TD). TD is a disorder characterized by involuntary movements of the mouth, lips, arms, or legs; it affects about 15%–20% of patients who have been receiving neuroleptic medications over a period of years. Discomfort related to these side effects is one reason why 40% of patients treated with the older antipsychotics do not adhere to their medication regimens.

ATYPICAL ANTIPSYCHOTICS. The atypical antipsychotics, also called second-generation antipsychotics, were introduced in the 1990s. They are sometimes called serotonin dopamine antagonists, or SDAs. These medications include **aripiprazole** (Abilify), **clozapine** (Clozaril), **risperidone** (Risperdal), **quetiapine** (Seroquel), **ziprasidone** (Geodon), and **olanzapine** (Zyprexa). The newer drugs were developed in the hopes that they would be more effective in treating the negative symptoms of schizophrenia and have fewer side effects. Clozapine has been reported to be effective in patients who do not respond to neuroleptics and to reduce the risk of suicide attempts. The atypical antipsychotics, however, do have weight gain as a side effect, and patients taking clozapine must have their blood monitored periodically for signs of agranulocytosis, or a drop in the number of white blood cells.

Prochlorperazine (Buccastem, Compazine, Phenotil, Stemetil, Stemzine), a dopamine receptor antagonist, may be used to treat schizophrenia on a short-term basis when other medicines have not worked effectively. It is not considered to be a first-line treatment for the disorder. The drug works by decreasing abnormal feelings and thoughts within the brain. Prochlorperazine is not approved for the use in treating behavioral problems in older adults with dementia due to an increased risk of death. It should also not be used in anyone younger than two years of age or who weighs less than 20 lb. (9 kg).

The FDA approved lurasidone (Latuda) on October 29, 2010, for the treatment of schizophrenia in adults. **Clinical trials** showed that lurasidone helped to reduce both positive and negative symptoms of schizophrenia. Lurasidone is unique among antipsychotic drugs in that is does not impair learning and memory functions in the patient. The most common side effects in clinical trials included drowsiness or **fatigue**, restlessness, the urge to move (akathisia), nausea, tremors and other abnormal movements, slowed movement, muscle stiffness (Parkinsonism), and agitation. Since lurasidone is a fairly new drug, its general widespread effectiveness and effects of long-term use are not yet known.

The Clinical Antipsychotic Trials of **Intervention** Effectiveness (**CATIE**) Schizophrenia Study was designed to compare the effectiveness of several atypical antipsychotic drugs against the traditional drugs. It was a Phase IV clinical trial funded by the National Institute of Mental Health and coordinated by the University of North Carolina at Chapel Hill. Contrary to expectations, the study found that the new drugs did not perform significantly better than the older drugs. The results of the CATIE study had implications in helping persons with schizophrenia and their physicians make decisions about which other drugs to try, especially when certain medications either did not adequately control symptoms or produced adverse side effects.

OTHER PRESCRIPTION MEDICATIONS. Patients with schizophrenia have a lifetime prevalence of 80% for major depression; others suffer from phobias or other **anxiety disorders**. The doctor may prescribe antidepressants or a short course of **benzodiazepines** along with antipsychotic medications.

Inpatient treatment

Patients with schizophrenia are usually hospitalized during acute psychotic episodes, to prevent harm to themselves or to others and to begin treatment with antipsychotic medications. A patient having a first

KEY TERMS

Attention deficit hyperactivity disorder—A medical condition that primarily occurs within children, which is characterized by the inability to concentrate, along with inappropriate age-related behavior or impulsive behavior.

Brief psychotic disorder—A medical disorder in which the period of psychosis is generally shorter than in other such disorders, is non-reoccurring, and cannot be classified as another related disorder.

Computed tomography—A medical imaging technique in which cross-sectional x rays of the body are compiled to create a three-dimensional image of the body's internal structures.

Delusional disorder—A mental disorder characterized by one or more non-bizarre delusions (such as thinking the police are constantly watching) without the presence of other significant psychopathology.

Dissociative disorder—Medical disorders characterized by disruptions or breakdowns of awareness, identity, memory, and/or perception.

Dissociative identity disorder—Also called multiple personality disorder, a mental condition in which a person displays multiple distinct personalities (alter egos).

DNA (deoxyribonucleic acid)—The hereditary material that makes up genes; influences the development and functioning of the body.

Magnetic resonance imaging—A medical imaging technique that uses electromagnetic radiation, along with a magnetic field, to produce images of the soft tissues within the body, such as the brain and spinal column.

Mood disorder—A medical disorder where a disturbance has occurred in an individual's mood; also called mood affective disorder.

Paranoid personality disorder—A disorder characterized by constant suspicion and mistrust of others.

Pervasive developmental disorder—A disorder involving the lack of development of basic skills of communication and socialization.

Polygenic—A trait or disorder that is determined by several different genes. Most human characteristics, including height, weight, and general body build, are polygenic. Schizophrenia and late-onset AD are considered polygenic disorders.

Positron emission tomography—A medical imaging technique that allows for the scanning of the metabolic activity of the body's organs, which is useful to diagnose cancer, locate brain tumors, and investigate other disorders.

Stigma—A mark or characteristic trait of a disease or disorder generally perceived as negative by society (regardless of fact).

psychotic episode is usually given a **computed tomography** (CT) or **magnetic resonance imaging** (MRI) scan to rule out structural brain disease.

Outpatient treatment

In recent years, patients with schizophrenia who have been stabilized on antipsychotic medications have been given psychosocial therapies of various types to assist them with motivation, self-care, and forming relationships with others. In addition, because many patients have had their education or vocational training interrupted by the onset of the disorder, they may be helped by therapies directed toward improving their social functioning and work skills.

Specific outpatient treatments that have been used in patients with schizophrenia include:

- Rehabilitation programs. These programs may offer vocational counseling, job training, problem-solving and money management skills, use of public transportation, and social skills training.
- Cognitive-behavioral therapy and supportive psychotherapy.
- Family psychoeducation. This approach is intended to help family members understand the patient's illness, cope with the problems it creates for other family members, and minimize stresses that may increase the patient's risk of relapse.
- Self-help groups. These groups provide mutual support for family members as well as patients. They can also serve as advocacy groups for better research and treatment, and to protest social stigma and employment discrimination.
- Support groups.
- Group homes or other care facilities. Persons with schizophrenia may be able to live in a residential facility aimed toward helping persons with psychiatric

QUESTIONS TO ASK YOUR DOCTOR

- What medication do you think will be best for me?
- What other treatment options do you recommend for me?
- What symptoms or behaviors are important enough that I should seek immediate treatment?
- Are there any support groups available for my family?

disorders; the patient is able to maintain a sense of independence but is still receiving treatment and has a support system in place.

Prognosis

According to the NIMH, about 20% of patients with schizophrenia recover the full level of functioning that they had before the onset of the disorder, with 10% achieving significant and lasting improvement and 30%–35% showing some improvement with intermittent relapses and some disabilities. The remaining 30% are severely and permanently incapacitated. Even with some improvements, the 80% who do not achieve full recovery of functioning are left with cognitive or intellectual impairments that can lead to problems when reintegrating into mainstream society. Patients may experience difficulty in school, in the workplace, and in forming healthy relationships with others. The majority (60%–70%) of patients with schizophrenia do not marry or have children, and most have very few friends or social contacts. The impact of these social difficulties as well as the stress caused by the symptoms themselves is reflected in the high suicide rate among patients with schizophrenia—about 10% commit suicide within the first ten years after their diagnosis, a rate that is about 20 times higher than that of the general population.

Factors associated with a good prognosis include relatively good functioning prior to the first psychotic episode, a late or sudden onset of illness, female gender, treatment with antipsychotic medications shortly after onset, good **compliance** with treatment, a family history of mood disorders rather than schizophrenia, minimal cognitive impairment, and a diagnosis of paranoid or nondeficit subtype. Factors associated with a poor prognosis include early age of onset, a low level of prior functioning, delayed treatment, heavy substance abuse, noncompliance with treatment, a family history of schizophrenia, and a diagnosis of disorganized or deficit subtype with many negative symptoms.

Prevention

Schizophrenia cannot be prevented. However, early diagnosis and treatment will help to improve the lives of those afflicted with the disorder. It is especially important to properly diagnose and promptly treat the symptoms of the first episode of schizophrenia. The National Alliance on Mental Illness (NAMI) recently completed the Schizophrenia Patient Outcomes Research (PORT) Team study, which was aimed at determining the most effective treatments for schizophrenia; the results can be found in the *NAMI Consumer and Family Guide to Schizophrenia Treatment.*

Resources

BOOKS

American Psychiatric Association. *Diagnostic and Statistical Manual of Mental Disorders*. 4th ed., text rev. Washington, DC: American Psychiatric Association, 2000.

Beck, Aaron T., et al. *Schizophrenia: Cognitive Therapy, Research, and Therapy*. New York: Guilford Press, 2009.

Beers, Mark H., ed. *Merck Manual of Diagnosis and Therapy*. Rahway, NJ: Merck, 2006.

Lieberman, Jeffrey A., T. Scott Stroup, and Diana O. Perkins, eds. *The American Psychiatric Publishing Textbook of Schizophrenia*. Arlington, VA: American Psychiatric, 2006.

Meyer, Jonathan M., and Henry A. Nasrallah, ed. *Medical Illness and Schizophrenia*. Washington, DC: American Psychiatric, 2009.

Siegel, Steven J., and LaRiena N. Ralph. *Demystifying Schizophrenia for the General Practitioner*. Sudbury, MA: Jones and Bartlett, 2011.

VandenBos, Gary R., ed. *APA Dictionary of Psychology*. Washington, DC: American Psychological Association, 2007.

Williamson, Peter. *Mind, Brain, and Schizophrenia*. Oxford: Oxford University Press, 2006.

PERIODICALS

Meyer-Lindenberg, Andreas. "Reduced Prefrontal Activity Predicts Exaggerated Striatal Dopaminergic Function in Schizophrenia." *Nature Neuroscience* 5, no. 3 (2002): 267–71.

Barrowclough, Christine, et al. "Group Cognitive-Behavioural Therapy for Schizophrenia." *British Journal of Psychiatry* 189, no. 6 (Dec. 2006): 527–32.

Carr, Vaughan J., Terry J. Lewin, and Amanda L. Neil. "What Is the Value of Treating Schizophrenia?" *Australian and New Zealand Journal of Psychiatry* 40, no. 11–12 (Nov. 2006): 963–71.

Gray, Richard, et al. "Adherence Therapy for People with Schizophrenia." *British Journal of Psychiatry* 189, no. 6 (Dec. 2006): 508–14.

Hashimoto, Kenji. "Elevated Glutamine/Glutamate Ratio in Cerebrospinal Fluid of First Episode aAnd Drug Naive Schizophrenic Patients." *BMC Psychiatry* 5, no. 6 (2005).

http://dx.doi.org/10.1186/1471-244X-5-6 (accessed November 5, 2011).

Lawrence, R., T. Bradshaw, and H. Mairs. "Group Cognitive Behavioural Therapy for Schizophrenia: A Systematic Review of the Literature." *Journal of Psychiatric and Mental Health Nursing* 13, no. 6 (Dec. 2006): 673–81.

Lipkovich, I., et al. "Predictors of Risk for Relapse in Patients With Schizophrenia or Schizoaffective Disorder During Olanzapine Drug Therapy." *Journal of Psychiatric Research* 41, no. 3–4 (April–June 2007): 305–10.

Masand, Prakash S., et al. "Polypharmacy in Schizophrenia." *International Journal of Psychiatry in Clinical Practice* 10, no. 4 (Dec. 2006): 258–63.

Yanos, P. T., and R. H. Moos. "Determinants of Functioning and Well-Being Among Individuals With Schizophrenia: An Integrated Model." *Clinical Psychology Review* 27, no. 1 (Jan. 2007): 58–77.

WEBSITES

American Psychiatric Association. "Schizophrenia Spectrum and Other Psychotic Disorders." DSM-5 Development. http://www.dsm5.org/proposedrevision/Pages/SchizophreniaSpectrumandOtherPsychoticDisorders.aspx (accessed July 18, 2011).

"CATIE." University of North Carolina School of Medicine, Department of Psychiatry. http://www.catie.unc.edu (accessed November 5, 2011).

Fox, Stuart. "8 Percent of Human Genome Was Inserted By Virus, and May Cause Schizophrenia." Popular Science (January 7, 2010). http://www.popsci.com/science/article/2010-01/8-percent-human-dna-comes-virus-causes-schizophrenia (accessed July 18, 2011).

MedlinePlus. "Metabolic Syndrome." U.S. National Library of Medicine, National Institutes of Health. http://www.nlm.nih.gov/medlineplus/metabolicsyndrome.html (accessed July 18, 2011).

National Alliance on Mental Illness. "Schizophrenia." http://www.nami.org/Template.cfm?Section=By_Illness&Template=/TaggedPage/TaggedPageDisplay.cfm&TPLID=3&ContentID=10850 (accessed November 5, 2011).

———. "Schizophrenia Patient Outcomes Research Team (PORT)." http://www.nami.org/Template.cfm?Section=eNews_Archive&template=/contentmanagement/contentdisplay.cfm&ContentID=3814 (accessed November 4, 2011).

National Institute of Mental Health. "Clinical Trials: Schizophrenia." http://www.nimh.nih.gov/trials/schizophrenia.shtml (accessed July 18, 2011).

———. "Schizophrenia." http://www.nimh.nih.gov/health/publications/schizophrenia/for-more-information-on-schizophrenia.shtml (accessed July 18, 2011).

Smith, Melinda, and Jeanne Segal. "Schizophrenia Treatment & Recovery." Helpguide.org. http://helpguide.org/mental/schizophrenia_treatment_support.htm (accessed November 5, 2011).

University of Chicago Medical Center. "Schizophrenia." http://www.uchospitals.edu/online-library/content=P00762 (accessed July 18, 2011).

U.S. Food and Drug Administration. "FDA Approves Latuda to Treat Schizophrenia in Adults" (October 28, 2010). http://www.fda.gov/NewsEvents/Newsroom/PressAnnouncements/ucm231512.htm (accessed July 18, 2011).

World Health Organization. "Schizophrenia." http://www.who.int/mental_health/management/schizophrenia/en (accessed July 18, 2011).

ORGANIZATIONS

American Psychiatric Association, 1000 Wilson Blvd., Ste. 1825, Arlington, VA, 22209, (703) 907-7300, apa@psych.org, http://www.psych.org.

Federation of Families for Children's Mental Health, 9605 Medical Center Dr., Rockville, MD, 20850, (240) 403-1901, Fax: (240) 403-1909, ffcmh@ffcmh.org, http://ffcmh.org.

Mental Health America, 2000 N Beauregard St., 6th Fl., Alexandria, VA, 22311, (703) 684-7722, Fax: (703) 684-5968, (800) 969-6642, http://www1.nmha.org.

National Alliance on Mental Illness, 3803 North Fairfax Dr., Ste. 100, Arlington, VA, 22203, (703) 524-7600, Fax: (703) 524-9094, http://www.nami.org.

National Institute of Mental Health, 6001 Executive Blvd., Rm. 8184, MSC 9663, Bethesda, MD, 20892-9663, (301) 443-4513, Fax: (301) 443-4279, (866) 615-6464, nimhinfo@nih.gov, http://www.nimh.nih.gov.

The Stanley Medical Research Institute, Research on Schizophrenia and Bipolar Disorder, info@stanleyresearch.org, http://www.stanleyresearch.org/dnn.

Treatment Advocacy Center, 200 N. Glebe Rd., Ste. 730, Arlington, VA, 22203, (703) 294-6001, Fax: (703) 294-6010, info@treatmentadvocacycenter.org, http://www.treatmentadvocacycenter.org.

Rebecca Frey, PhD
Ruth A. Wienclaw, PhD
William A. Atkins, BB, BS, MBA

Schizophreniform disorder

Definition

Schizophreniform disorder (SFD) is characterized by the same basic features as **diagnosis** is changed to **schizophrenia**.

Demographics

The actual rate of SFD is unknown, mainly because SFD is difficult to measure except in retrospect. In the first few weeks of symptoms, SFD cannot be differentiated from **brief psychotic disorder**. Once the symptoms persist past one month and are identified as SFD, six months or more must pass before one can determine if a mental health consumer had "classic" SFD or was in the early phase of a more chronic mental disorder. Given that a majority of SFD sufferers go on to be diagnosed with schizophrenia, the best inferences about demographics and gender differences in SFD would be drawn from similar information available regarding schizophrenia.

Description

The person experiencing SFD shows at least two psychotic symptoms, which may be either "positive" or "negative." **Positive symptoms** are those that are present but that do not normally occur or which are in excess of what normally occurs. Positive symptoms of **psychosis** include hallucinations, **delusions**, strange bodily movements or frozen movement (catatonic behavior), peculiar speech, and bizarre or primitive (socially inappropriate) behavior. **Negative symptoms** are factors that normally occur but are absent or deficient with the disorder. Various deficiencies in behavior, emotionality, or speech constitute the negative symptoms of psychosis that are observed in some cases of SFD. Negative symptoms of psychosis include avolition, affective flattening, and logia.

Avolition is a lack of effort to act on one's own behalf or to engage in behaviors directed at accomplishing a purpose. Affective flattening or blunted **affect** refers to a decrease or low level of emotion, shown as a wooden quality to one's emotions or a near absence of emotionality. Alogia refers to a disruption in the thought process reflected in the person's speech. One form of alogia is "poverty of speech." Impoverished speech is brief, limited, and terse and generally emerges only in response to questions or prompts rather than flowing spontaneously. An impairment termed "poverty of content" occurs when the information or concepts that the individual is attempting to convey cannot be understood because of limitations in the method of communicating. The meaning behind the phrases is obscured or missing. Typically, in poverty of content, the person's speech, while comprehensible in terms of its orderliness of grammar and vocabulary, does not convey substantial meaning because the phrasing is overly concrete and literal or overly abstract and fanciful.

Among the various positive symptoms of psychosis that can be a part of SFD, delusions are a fairly common. Delusions are strongly held irrational and unrealistic beliefs that are highly resistant to alteration. Even when the person encounters evidence that would invalidate the delusion, the unjustified and improbable belief remains a conviction. Often, delusions are paranoid or persecutory in tone. In these types of delusions, the person is excessively suspicious and continually feels at the mercy of conspirators believed to be determined to cause harm to the sufferer. However, delusions can also take on other overtones. Some delusions are grandiose, while others may involve elaborate love fantasies (erotomanic delusions). Delusions may involve somatic content, or may revolve around extreme and irrational jealousy.

Peculiar or disorganized speech, catatonic behavior, and bizarre or primitive behavior are all additional positive psychotic symptoms that may occur in SFD. Speech disorganization can involve words blended together into incomprehensible statements, also known as "word salad." In some persons disorganized speech takes the form of echolalia, which is the repetition of another person's exact spoken words, restated either immediately after the initial speaker or after a delay of minutes or hours. Catatonic behavior or **catatonia** involves the presence of one of the possible extremes related to movement. Catalepsy is the motionless end of the catatonic spectrum; in catalepsy, a person may remain unmoving in one fixed position for long periods. The opposite end of the catatonia phenomenon is demonstrated in rapid or persistently repeated movements, recurrent grimacing and odd facial expressions, and contorted or strange gestures. Bizarre or primitive behavior in SFD ranges from childlike behaviors in unsuitable circumstances to unusual practices such as **hoarding** refuse items perceived by the sufferer to be valuable, caching food all over the home, or wandering purposelessly through the streets.

Only rarely would all these various psychotic symptoms be observed simultaneously in one person with SFD. Instead, each individual with SFD has a constellation of symptoms, practices, and thought processes that is unique to that person.

Unlike any other diagnoses offered in the ***Diagnostic and Statistical Manual of Mental Disorders*** (*DSM-IV-TR*), the SFD diagnosis always includes an indication of the patient's prognosis—the potential outcome for an individual with a particular illness—based on the features observed and the usual course of the illness. If an individual with SFD has several positive prognostic factors, there is a much higher likelihood of complete recovery without **relapse** into psychosis. Such positive prognostic factors include prominent confusion during the illness, rapid (rather than gradual) development of symptoms during a four-week period, good previous interpersonal and goal-oriented functioning, and lack of negative symptoms of psychosis.

Causes and symptoms

Causes

Several views regarding the causes of the disorder have been put forth by researchers and clinicians.

AN EARLY PHASE OF ANOTHER PSYCHIATRIC DISORDER. A number of follow-up studies have examined the relationship between SFD and other disorders such as schizophrenia, **schizoaffective disorder**, and **bipolar disorder**. The majority of these studies have found that between 50% and 75% of persons with SFD eventually develop schizophrenia. Of those persons with a history of SFD who do not subsequently receive a diagnosis of schizophrenia, only a small portion have no further psychiatric disturbance. The other diagnoses that may be observed in persons formerly diagnosed with SFD are schizoaffective disorder or bipolar I disorder.

The most common subsequent diagnosis is schizophrenia, with the next most common being schizoaffective disorder. Because of the high rate of later schizophrenia in SFD sufferers, many clinicians have come to think of SFD as being an initial phase of schizophrenia. It is impossible to identify, during an episode of SFD, whether any one particular case will improve without any relapse into psychotic symptoms, or if the mental health client is actually in the early phase of schizophrenia or schizoaffective disorder. Follow-up studies indicate that being frequently confused during a period of SFD is often associated with gradual complete recovery.

LENGTHY POSTPARTUM PSYCHOSIS. Intense hormonal changes occurring in childbirth and immediately afterward can result in a short-term psychotic disorder often referred to as "postpartum psychosis." When the psychotic symptoms in this condition persist for more than one month but fewer than six months, an SFD diagnosis may be given.

DIATHESIS AND STRESS. "Diathesis" is a medical term meaning that some element of one's physiology makes one particularly prone to develop an illness if exposed to the right conditions. Diathesis is another way of saying there is a personal predisposition to develop a disorder; the predisposition is biologically based and is genetically acquired (inherited in the person's genes). Temporary psychotic reactions may occur in persons who have the diathesis for psychosis, when the individual is placed under marked **stress**. The stress may result from typical life transition experiences such as moving away from home the first time, being widowed, or getting divorced. In some cases, the stressor is more intense or unusual, such as surviving a natural disaster, wartime service, being taken hostage, or surviving a terrorist attack. When the psychotic responses last less than a month, then this reaction is labeled "brief psychotic disorder." Highly susceptible persons may show psychotic symptoms for longer than one month and might be given the SFD diagnosis. If the psychotic symptoms are purely reactive, when the stressor ceases or more support is available, the individual is likely to return to a nonpsychotic mode of functioning. In persons with a strong diathesis or predisposition, the initial psychotic reaction may "tip over" from the category of a brief reaction into a longer-term, persistent psychiatric disorder. The diathesis-stress model is applied not only to SFD, but also to schizophrenia, schizoaffective disorder, and the most severe forms of mood disorders.

CULTURALLY DEFINED DISORDERS. Many cultures have forms of mental disorder, unique to that culture, that would meet criteria for SFD. In culturally defined disorders, a consistent set of features and presumed causes of the syndrome are localized to that community. Such disorders are termed "culture-bound." Examples of culture-bound syndromes that might meet SFD criteria are "amok" (Malaysia), or "locura" (Latino Americans). Amok is a syndrome characterized by brooding, persecutory delusions, and aggressive actions. Locura involves incoherence, agitation, social dysfunction, erratic behavior, and hallucinations.

Symptoms

The *DSM-IV-TR* provides three major criteria for SFD. First, the patient must display at least two persistent positive or negative symptoms of psychosis (delusions; disorganized speech that is strange, peculiar, or difficult to comprehend; disorganized, bizarre, or childlike behavior; catatonic behavior; hallucinations; or negative symptoms). In addition, the symptoms must be manifest for a limited time (i.e., at least one month, but less than six months). Third, the symptoms must not be attributable to biological influences (e.g., drugs, medication, alcohol, physical illness or injury) or another disorder (e.g., schizoaffective disorder or schizophrenia).

Diagnosis

Despite the clarity of the *DSM-IV-TR* criteria, identification of SFD is less than clear-cut. The emphasis on the length of time that symptoms have been evident and the presence or absence of good prognostic factors make SFD one of the most unusually defined of the *DSM-IV-TR* disorders. While duration of symptoms is the major distinction among brief psychotic disorder, SFD, and schizophrenia, it can be difficult to clearly determine the length of time symptoms have existed. An additional complication is that the cultural context in which the "psychotic symptoms" are experienced determines whether the behaviors are viewed as pathological or acceptable. When psychotic-like behaviors are expected to occur normally as part of the person's culture or religion, and when the behaviors occur in a culturally positive context such as a religious service, SFD would not be diagnosed.

Information about current and past experiences is collected in an interview with the client, and possibly in discussion with the client's family. **Psychological assessment** instruments (e.g., Rorschach technique, **Minnesota Multiphasic Personality Inventory**, and mood disorder questionnaires) or structured diagnostic interviews may also be used to aid in the diagnosis.

In addition, part of defining SFD involves examining possible biological influences on the development of the individual's psychotic symptoms. When the psychotic features result from a physical disease, a reaction to medication, or intoxication with drugs or alcohol, then these symptoms are not considered SFD. Also, if hallucinations, delusions, or other psychotic symptoms are experienced solely during episodes of clinical **depression** or mania, the patient is diagnosed with a mood disorder rather than SFD.

Treatment

The main line of treatment for SFD is antipsychotic medication. These medications are often very effective in treating SFD. Mood-stabilizing drugs similar to those used in bipolar disorder may be used if there is little response to other interventions. Postpartum psychosis is also treated with antipsychotics and, possibly, hormones. Supportive therapy and education about mental illness is often valuable. The most useful interventions in culture-bound syndromes are those that are societally prescribed; for example, a sacred ceremony to ease the restless spirits of deceased ancestors might be a usual method of ending the psychotic-like state, in that particular culture.

Prognosis

For the large number of mental health patients with SFD who are later diagnosed with a more chronic form of mental illness, the prognosis is fairly poor. However, when the condition manifests with prominent confusion during the illness, rapid (rather than gradual) development of symptoms during a four-week period, good previous interpersonal and goal-oriented functioning and lack of negative symptoms of psychosis, a full recovery is much more likely.

Prevention

If the SFD is a persistent postpartum psychosis, a prevention option is to avoid having additional children. The physician may anticipate the postpartum problem and prescribe an antipsychotic medication regimen to begin immediately after delivery as a preventive measure. Although prevention of psychotic disorders is difficult to accomplish, the earlier treatment begins, the better the outcome. Therefore, efforts are more generally focused on early identification of SFD and other psychotic-spectrum disorders.

KEY TERMS

Erotomanic delusions—Erotomanic delusions involve the mistaken conviction that someone is in love with the delusional person. Often, the love object is a public figure of some prominence, such as an actress, rock star, or political figure. David Letterman and Jodie Foster are celebrities who have both been victimized by persons with erotomanic delusions.

Grandiose delusions—Grandiose delusions magnify the person's importance; the delusional person may believe himself or herself to be a famous person, to have magical superpowers, or to be someone in a position of enormous power (such as being the king or president).

Hallucinations—False sensory perceptions. A person experiencing a hallucination may "hear" sounds or "see" people or objects that are not really present. Hallucinations can also affect the senses of smell, touch, and taste.

Psychosis—Severe state that is characterized by loss of contact with reality and deterioration in normal social functioning; examples are schizophrenia and paranoia. Psychosis is usually one feature of an overarching disorder, not a disorder in itself (Plural: psychoses.)

Somatic—Somatic comes from *soma*, the Greek word for body; thus, somatic hallucinations are bodily. Somatic delusions are strongly held but erroneous ideas about the characteristics or functioning of one's body. An example is a mental health client who refuses to eat because of a belief that there is a hole in the stomach that will spill anything consumed into the body cavity, when such is not actually the case.

Resources

BOOKS

American Psychiatric Association. *Diagnostic and Statistical Manual of Mental Disorders*. 4th ed., text rev. Washington, DC: American Psychiatric Publishing, 2000.

Mueser, Kim T. "Family Intervention for Schizophrenia." In *Innovations in Clinical Practice: Focus on Adults,* edited by Leon VandeCreek. Sarasota, FL: Professional Resource Press/Professional Resource Exchange, 2005.

VandenBos, Gary R., ed. *APA Dictionary of Psychology.* Washington, DC: American Psychological Association, 2006.

PERIODICALS

Norman, Ross M.G., et al. "Early Signs in Schizophrenia Spectrum Disorders." *Journal of Nervous and Mental Disease* 193, no. 1 (January 2005): 17–23.

Deborah Rosch Eifert, PhD
Ruth A. Wienclaw, PhD

Schizotypal personality disorder

Definition

Schizotypal personality disorder is a personality disorder characterized by peculiarities of thought, perception, speech, and behavior. Although schizotypal personality disorder is considered a severe disorder, the symptoms are not severe enough to be classified as schizophrenic.

Demographics

Schizotypal personality disorder appears to occur more frequently in individuals who have an immediate family member with **schizophrenia**. The prevalence of schizotypal personality disorder is approximately 3% of the general population and is believed to occur slightly more often in males.

Symptoms that characterize a typical **diagnosis** of schizotypal personality disorder should be evaluated in the context of the individual's cultural situation, particularly those regarding superstitious or religious beliefs and practices. (Some behaviors that Western cultures may view as psychotic are viewed within the range of normal behavior in other cultures.)

Description

Schizotypal personality disorder is characterized by an ongoing pattern in which the affected person distances him- or herself from social and interpersonal relationships. Affected people typically have acute discomfort when put in circumstances where they must relate to others. These individuals are also prone to cognitive and perceptual distortions and a display a variety of eccentric behaviors that others often find confusing. People with schizotypal personality disorder are more comfortable turning inward, away from others, than learning to have meaningful interpersonal relationships. This preferred isolation contributes to distorted perceptions about how interpersonal relationships are supposed to happen. These individuals remain on the periphery of life and often drift from one aimless activity to another with few, if any, meaningful relationships.

A person with schizotypal personality disorder has odd behaviors, and his or her thoughts are typically viewed by others as eccentric, erratic, and bizarre. They are known on occasion to have brief psychotic episodes. Their speech, while coherent, is marked by a focus on trivial detail. Thought processes of people with schizotypal personality disorder include magical thinking, suspiciousness, and illusions. These thought patterns are believed to be the sufferer's unconscious way of coping with social anxiety. To some extent, these behaviors stem from being socially isolated and having a distorted view of appropriate interpersonal relations.

Causes and symptoms

Causes

Schizotypal personality disorder is believed to stem from the affected person's family of origin. Usually the parents of the affected person were emotionally distant, formal, and displayed confusing parental communication. This **modeling** of remote, unaffectionate relationships is then reenacted in the social relationships encountered in the developing years. The social development of people with schizotypal personality disorder shows that many were also regularly humiliated by their parents, siblings, and peers resulting in significant relational mistrust. Many display low self-esteem, along with self-criticism and self-deprecating behavior. This further contributes to a sense that they are socially incapable of having meaningful interpersonal relationships.

Symptoms

The ***Diagnostic and Statistical Manual of Mental Disorders***, the mental health manual, specifies nine diagnostic criteria for schizotypal personality disorder:

- Incorrect interpretations of events. Individuals with schizotypal personality disorder often have difficulty seeing the correct cause and effect of situations and how they affect others. For instance, the schizotypal may misread a simple nonverbal communication cue, such as a frown, as someone being displeased with them, when in reality it may have nothing to do with them. Their perceptions are often distortions of what is really happening externally, but they tend to believe their perceptions more than what others might say or do.

- Odd beliefs or magical thinking. These individuals may be superstitious or preoccupied with the paranormal. They often engage in these behaviors as a desperate means to find some emotional connection with the world they live in. This behavior is seen as a coping mechanism to add meaning in a world devoid of much meaning because of the social isolation these individuals experience.
- Unusual perceptual experiences. These might include having illusions, or attributing a particular event to some mysterious force or person who is not present. Affected people may also feel they have special powers to influence events or predict an event before it happens.
- Odd thinking and speech. People with schizotypal personality disorder may have speech patterns that appear strange in their structure and phrasing. Their ideas are often loosely associated, prone to tangents, or vague in description. Some may verbalize responses by being overly concrete or abstract, and may insert words that serve to confuse rather than clarify a particular situation, yet make sense to the speaker. They are typically unable to have ongoing conversation and tend to talk only about matters that need immediate attention.
- Suspicious or paranoid thoughts. Individuals with schizotypal personality disorder are often suspicious of others and display paranoid tendencies.
- Emotionally inexpressive. Their general social demeanor is to appear aloof and isolated, behaving in a way that communicates they derive little joy from life. Most have an intense fear of being humiliated or rejected, yet repress most of these feelings for protective reasons.
- Eccentric behavior. People with schizotypal personality disorder are often viewed as odd or eccentric due to their unusual mannerisms or unconventional clothing choices. Their personal appearance may look unkempt—they may wear clothes that do not "fit together," clothes that are too small or too large or are noticeably unclean.
- Lack of close friends. Because they lack the skills and confidence to develop meaningful interpersonal relationships, they prefer privacy and isolation. As they withdraw from relationships, they increasingly turn inward to avoid possible social rejection or ridicule. If they do have any ongoing social contact, it is usually restricted to immediate family members.
- Socially anxious. Persons with schizotypal personality disorder are noticeably anxious in social situations, especially with people with whom they are not familiar. They can interact with others when necessary, but prefer to avoid as much interaction as possible because their self-perception is that they do not fit in. Even when exposed to the same group of people over time, their social anxiety does not seem to lessen. In fact, it may progress into distorted perceptions of paranoia involving the people they are in social contact with.

Diagnosis

The symptoms of schizotypal personality disorder may begin showing in childhood or adolescence as a tendency toward solitary pursuit of activities, poor peer relationships, pronounced social anxiety, and underachievement in school. Other symptoms that may be present during the developmental years are hypersensitivity to criticism or correction, unusual use of language, odd thoughts, or bizarre fantasies. Children with these tendencies appear socially out-of-step with peers and often become the object of malicious teasing by their peers, which increases the feelings of isolation and social ineptness they feel. For a diagnosis of schizotypal personality disorder to be accurately made, there must also be the presence of at least four of the nine diagnostic criteria listed by the *Diagnostic and Statistical Manual of Mental Disorders*.

The symptoms of schizotypal personality disorder can sometimes be confused with the symptoms seen in schizophrenia. The bizarre thinking associated with schizotypal personality disorder can be perceived as a psychotic episode and misdiagnosed. While brief psychotic episodes can occur in the patient with schizotypal personality disorder, the **psychosis** is not as pronounced, frequent, or as intense as in schizophrenia. For an accurate diagnosis of schizotypal personality disorder, the symptoms cannot occur exclusively during the course of schizophrenia or other mood disorder that has psychotic features.

Another common difficulty in diagnosing schizotypal personality disorder is distinguishing it from other the schizoid, avoidant, and paranoid **personality disorders**. Some researchers believe that the schizotypal personality disorder is essentially the same as the schizoid disorder, but many feel there are distinguishing characteristics. Schizoids are deficient in their ability to experience emotion, while people with schizotypal personality disorder are more pronounced in their inability to understand human motivation and communication. While **avoidant**

personality disorder has many of the same symptoms as schizotypal personality disorder, the distinguishing symptom in schizotypal is the presence of behavior that is noticeably eccentric. The schizotypal differs from the paranoid by tangential thinking and eccentric behavior.

The diagnosis of schizotypal personality disorder is based on a clinical interview to assess symptomatic behavior. Other assessment tools helpful in confirming the diagnosis of schizotypal personality disorder include:

- Minnesota Multiphasic Personality Inventory (MMPI-2)
- Millon Clinical Multiaxial Inventory (MCMI-II)
- Rorschach Psychodiagnostic Test
- Thematic Apperception Test (TAT)

Treatment

The patient with schizotypal personality disorder finds it difficult to engage in and remain in treatment. For those higher functioning individuals who seek treatment, the goal will be to help them function more effectively in relationships rather than restructuring their personality.

Psychodynamically oriented therapies

A psychodynamic approach will typically seek to build a therapeutically trusting relationship that attempts to counter the mistrust most people with this disorder intrinsically hold. The hope is that some degree of attachment in a therapeutic relationship could be generalized to other relationships. Offering interpretations about the patient's behavior will not typically be helpful. More highly functioning sufferers who have some capacity for empathy and emotional warmth tend to have better outcomes in psychodynamic approaches to treatment.

Cognitive-behavioral therapy

Cognitive approaches will most likely focus on attempting to identify and alter the content of the thoughts of the person with schizotypal personality disorder. Distortions that occur in both perception and thought processes are addressed. An important foundation for this work is the establishment of a trusting therapeutic relationship. This relaxes some of the social anxiety felt in most interpersonal relationships and allows for some exploration of the thought processes. Constructive ways of accomplishing this might include, among others: communication skills training; the use of videotape feedback to help the affected person perceive his or her behavior and appearance objectively; and practical suggestions about personal hygiene and employment.

Interpersonal therapy

Treatment using an interpersonal approach will allow the individual with schizotypal personality disorder to remain relationally distant while he or she "warms up" to the therapist. Gradually the therapist would hope to engage the patient after becoming "safe" through lack of coercion. The goal is to develop trust in order to help the patient gain insight into the distorted and magical thinking that dominates his/her thought process. New self-talk can be introduced to help orient the individual to reality-based experience. The therapist can mirror this objectivity to the patient.

Group therapy

Group therapy may provide the patient with a socializing experience that exposes them to feedback from others in a safe, controlled environment. It is typically recommended only for patients who do not display severe eccentric or paranoid behavior. Most group members would be uncomfortable with these behavioral displays and it would likely prove destructive to the group dynamic.

Family and marital therapy

It is unlikely that a person with **schizoid personality disorder** will seek family or marital therapy. Many patients do not marry and end up living with and being dependent upon first-degree family members. If they do marry they often have problems centered on insensitivity to their partner's feelings or behavior. Marital therapy (**couples therapy**) may focus on helping the couple to become more involved in each other's lives or improve communication patterns.

Medications

There is considerable research on the use of medications for the treatment of schizotypal personality disorder due to its close symptomatic relationship with schizophrenia. Among the most helpful medications are the antipsychotics that have been shown to control symptoms such as illusions and phobic anxiety, among others. **Amoxapine** (trade name Asendin), is a tricyclic antidepressant with antipsychotic properties, and has been effective in improving schizophrenic-like and depressive symptoms in schizotypal patients. Other **antidepressants** such as **fluoxetine** (Prozac) have also been used successfully to reduce symptoms of anxiety, paranoid thinking, and **depression**.

KEY TERMS

Millon Clinical Multiaxial Inventory (MCMI-II)—A self-report instrument designed to help the clinician assess DSM-IV-related personality disorders and clinical syndromes. It provides insight into 14 personality disorders and 10 clinical syndromes.

Minnesota Multiphasic Personality Inventory (MMPI-2)—A comprehensive assessment tool widely used to diagnosed personality disorders.

Rorschach Psychodiagnostic Test—This series of 10 "inkblot" images allows the patient to project their interpretations which can be used to diagnose particular disorders.

Thematic Apperception Test (TAT)—A projective test using stories and descriptions of pictures to reveal some of the dominant drives, emotions, sentiments, conflicts, and complexes of a personality.

Prognosis

The prognosis for the individual with schizotypal personality disorder is poor due to the ingrained nature of the coping mechanisms already in place. Schizotypal patients who depend heavily on family members or others are likely to regress into a state of **apathy** and further isolation. While some measurable gains can be made with mildly affected individuals, most are not able to alter their ingrained ways of perceiving or interpreting reality. When combined with poor social support structure, most will not enter any type of treatment.

Prevention

Since schizotypal personality disorder originates in the patient's family of origin, the only known preventative measure is a nurturing, emotionally stimulating, and expressive environment.

Resources

BOOKS

American Psychiatric Association. *Diagnostic and Statistical Manual of Mental Disorders.* 4th ed., text rev. Washington, DC: American Psychiatric Publishing, 2000.

Millon, Theodore, et al. *Personality Disorders in Modern Life.* 2nd ed. New York: John Wiley and Sons, 2004.

Silverstein, Marshall L. "Descriptive Psychopathology and Theoretical Viewpoints: Schizoid, Schizotypal, and Avoidant Personality Disorders." In *Disorders of the Self: A Personality-Guided Approach.* Washington, DC: American Psychological Association, 2007.

VandenBos, Gary R., ed. *APA Dictionary of Psychology.* Washington, DC: American Psychological Association, 2006.

PERIODICALS

Badcock, Johanna C., and Milan Dragovic. "Schizotypal Personality in Mature Adults." *Personality and Individual Differences* 40, no. 1 (January 2006): 77–85.

Harvey, Philip D., et al. "Dual-Task Information Processing in Schizotypal Personality Disorder: Evidence of Impaired Processing Capacity." *Neuropsychology* 20, no. 4 (July 2006): 453–60.

Raine, Adrian. "Schizotypal Personality: Neurodevelopmental and Psychosocial Trajectories." *Annual Review of Clinical Psychology* 2 (2006): 291–326.

Trotman, Hanan, Amanda McMillan, and Elaine Walker. "Cognitive Function and Symptoms in Adolescents with Schizotypal Personality Disorder." *Schizophrenia Bulletin* 32, no. 3 (July 2006): 489–97.

Wuthrich, Viviana M., and Timothy C. Bates. "Confirmatory Factor Analysis of the Three-Factor Structure of the Schizotypal Personality Questionnaire and Chapman Schizotypy Scales." *Journal of Personality Assessment* 87, no. 3 (2006): 292–304.

ORGANIZATIONS

American Psychiatric Association, 1000 Wilson Blvd., Ste. 1825, Arlington, VA, 22209-3901, (703) 907-7300, apa@psych.org, http://www.psych.org.

Gary Gilles, MA
Ruth A. Wienclaw, PhD

Seasonal affective disorder

Definition

Seasonal affective disorder (SAD) is a mood disorder in which major depressive episodes and/or manic episodes occur at predictable times of the year, with depressive episodes typically occurring during the fall and winter months. The term SAD can also be applied to depressive episodes with a seasonal pattern that do not meet the criteria for **major depressive disorder** or a **bipolar disorder** (i.e., subsyndromal). SAD is also sometimes called seasonal mood disorder and seasonal **depression**.

Demographics

SAD is more likely to occur in higher latitudes where there is less sunlight during the fall and winter

KEY TERMS

Bipolar disorder—Formerly called manic-depressive disorder, a mood disorder characterized alternating periods of overconfidence and activity (manic highs) and depressive lows.

Melatonin—A naturally occurring hormone involved in regulating the body's internal clock.

Phototherapy—Also called light therapy, a therapy in which the patient is exposed to a bright light to compensate for reduced exposure to sunlight.

Serotonin—5-Hydroxytryptamine; a substance that occurs throughout the body with numerous effects, including neurotransmission. Inadequate amounts of serotonin are implicated in some forms of depression and obsessive-compulsive disorder.

months. In addition, younger individuals are at higher risk for seasonal depressive episodes than are older persons. In fact, people who are most at risk for developing SAD are those between the ages of 15 to 55 years. Although 60–90% of individuals with a seasonal component to their depressive disorder are women, it is unclear whether this statistic reflects a gender factor specifically for SAD or merely reflects the underlying risks associated with recurrent major depressive disorder. Cases of SAD have been seen in children and adolescents; however, the disorder usually begins when individuals are in their twenties.

Seasonal affective disorder is believed to be relatively common. It is estimated that up to 6% of the population may experience SAD, and up to 20% of Americans may suffer from a mild version of the symptoms (subsyndromal) associated with SAD. One study conducted in the United States and reported in the *New York Times* at the end of 2007 found that in New Hampshire 9.7% of the state's population is affected by SAD, whereas only 1.4% of the population of Florida is affected.

It is not yet known whether a seasonal pattern is more likely in recurrent major depressive disorder or in bipolar disorders. However, the seasonal pattern is more likely to occur in bipolar I disorder (BID) than in bipolar II disorder (BIID).

Description

According to the ***Diagnostic and Statistical Manual of Mental Disorders*** (DSM), published by the **American Psychiatric Association**, a seasonal pattern can exist with major depressive disorder or with major depressive episodes in bipolar I disorder or bipolar II disorder. To be characterized as a seasonal disorder, the onset and remission of the major depressive episodes must occur at characteristic times of year. In most cases of SAD, major depressive episodes occur in the fall and winter months and remit during the spring and summer. Less frequently, some individuals suffer from predictable major depressive episodes during the summer.

Risk factors

Studies have found that women are more likely to be diagnosed with seasonal affective disorder than men; however, men with the disorder are more likely to have severe symptoms. SAD is believed to have a hereditary component, so having a close family member who has been diagnosed with SAD is a significant risk factor for the disorder. SAD is more likely to be diagnosed in young adults than in older adults. Individuals who live in areas far from the equator (at high latitudes) where the duration of sunlight changes substantially during the year are at higher risk for SAD.

SAD can become worse as time goes by, leading to such problems as suicidal thoughts and behaviors; further withdrawal from social activities and society in general; continuing problems at school, home, or at work; and substance and/or alcohol abuse. Such complications from SAD can be corrected with proper **diagnosis** and treatment.

Causes and symptoms

It is not known with certainty what causes SAD. Many theories concerning the origins of SAD link it to irregularities in an individual's biological rhythms. These are triggered by lengthening or shortening of daylight that occurs with the changing seasons. Among these theories, the phase shift hypothesis (PSH) states that SAD patients become depressed in the fall and winter because the later dawn at this time of year causes circadian rhythms to become out of synchronization with respect to clock time and the body's sleep-wake cycle. Specifically, PSH states that SAD is a result of a mismatch between an individual's circadian rhythms related to the sleep-wake cycle and the biological circadian pacemaker in the hypothalamus of the **brain**.

Another theory connects SAD to the body's melatonin levels. The body produces more melatonin at night than during the day, and it helps people feel sleepy at nighttime. There is also more melatonin in the body during winter, when the days are shorter. Some researchers believe that excessive melatonin release during winter causes feelings of drowsiness or depression.

A third theory connects SAD to reduced **serotonin** levels. Serotonin is a neurotransmitter important for the regulation of mood. Reduced levels of sunlight have been shown to be linked to drops in serotonin levels in the brain, which can cause symptoms of depression.

Common symptoms of SAD include:

- anxiety and depression
- moodiness and irritability
- hopelessness
- lack of energy
- difficulty concentrating and coordinating activities
- excessive sleepiness during the day or abnormally prolonged sleep at night (hypersomnia)
- tendency to overeat (hyperphagia), including weight gain and/or craving for carbohydrates
- significant impairment of social and occupational functioning (e.g., lack of interest in social interactions, increased sensitivity to negative reactions from others, or lack of interest in normally enjoyable activities)

Diagnosis

Four criteria must be met for a major depressive disorder, BID, or BIID to be characterized as seasonal. First, there must be a regular relationship between the onset of the depressive episodes and the time of year. For most cases of SAD, depressive episodes occur during the fall and winter seasons. Second, full remission of the depressive episodes (or a change from depression to mania or **hypomania** in the case of bipolar disorders) must also occur at predictable times of the year. Third, the seasonal cycle of onset and remission of major depressive episodes must have occurred within the last two years without any nonseasonal depressive episodes during that time. Fourth, seasonal episodes of depression must occur significantly more frequently than nonseasonal depressive episodes over the course of the person's lifetime.

Other factors used with the four main criteria when diagnosing SAD are sleeping more than usual, being hungry (especially for carbohydrates), and gaining weight—all during periods of SAD. Having a close relative, such as a parent, sister, or brother, with SAD is also a factor used to diagnose the condition.

QUESTIONS TO ASK YOUR DOCTOR

- Is phototherapy an appropriate treatment for me?
- Would the addition of a medication be likely to improve my symptoms?
- What are the side effects?
- Should I seek treatment before I expect my symptoms to appear next year?
- When should I reduce or stop treatment?

During the diagnosis process, it is important to distinguish SAD from depression caused by other factors that may cause depression such as seasonal unemployment or school schedule. In addition, SAD should be distinguished from the so-called holiday blues, a condition not related to circadian rhythms but to such psychosocial factors as increased obligations, expectations that one should be joyous, or early childhood memories or unresolved childhood conflicts.

Treatment

The goal of treatment for SAD is to alleviate the symptoms associated with the disorder. In most cases, the prescribed treatment regimen needs to be followed for the months in which the SAD occurs and can be stopped during the remainder of the year. Many people with SAD can be treated effectively with **light therapy**, although some people may require other therapies or medications as well.

Traditional

The first-line treatment for seasonal affective disorder is phototherapy, also called light therapy, which exposes the patient to bright artificial light to compensate for reduced sunlight in winter. Light therapy uses a device called a light box that contains a set of fluorescent or incandescent lights in front of a reflector. Typically, the patient sits for 30 minutes next to a 10,000-lux box (which is about 50 times brighter than ordinary indoor light) that produces a bright full-spectrum light. (Lux, sometimes abbreviated lx, is a measurement of luminous power per area.) Various wavelengths of light have been tried for the treatment of SAD, and research continued as of 2011 to determine the best possible methods. Light therapy appears to be safe for most people. However, it may be harmful for those with eye diseases. The most common side effects are vision problems such as eyestrain, headaches, irritability, and **insomnia**. In addition, hypomania (elevated or expansive mood, characterized by hyperactivity and inflated self esteem) may occasionally occur.

Counseling, such as **cognitive-behavioral therapy** (CBT), is also helpful in treating the symptoms of SAD. CBT concentrates on an individual's behavioral patterns and thoughts in order to control the symptoms of any medical condition that includes depression and anxiety, such as SAD. It is also useful in controlling such problems as eating disorders, chronic pain, panic disorders, and chronic **fatigue** syndrome.

Drugs

When a major depressive disorder or a bipolar disorder has seasonal characteristics, it may be treated with antidepressant medication. **Fluoxetine** (Prozac) has shown to be as effective as light therapy in controlled **clinical trials**. In 2006, the U.S. Food and Drug Administration (FDA) approved the prescription medication **bupropion** HCl extended release tablets (Wellbutrin XL) for the prevention of SAD. The effectiveness of Wellbutrin XL has been demonstrated in clinical trials with adults having a history of a major depressive disorder occurring in the fall and winter months. Wellbutrin XL, however, is recommended only for individuals whose SAD symptoms meet the criteria for a major depressive disorder. Other **antidepressants** may also be prescribed for SAD.

Alternative

Medical literature also suggests that the over-the-counter compound melatonin may help to alleviate SAD symptoms. Melatonin is a hormone produced by the pineal gland that helps regulate the body's seasonal changes. Research funded by the **National Institute of Mental Health** suggests that a low dose of synthetic or pharmacy-grade melatonin taken in the evening along with exposure to bright light in the morning may be effective in relieving the symptoms of SAD. However, as of 2011, more research was needed to determine the safety and effectiveness of such treatment.

Home remedies

Cases of SAD that do not meet all the criteria for formal diagnosis (subsyndromal cases) may also be improved with phototherapy. Activities such as getting outdoors in the sunshine in the morning or rearranging one's home or office to maximize exposure to sunlight during the day may help mild SAD symptoms. Although a trip to the tropics or other sunny place is also of help in overcoming the effects of SAD, the problem returns once the individual is again exposed to shortened daylight hours.

Prognosis

For cases of subsyndromal SAD, the prognosis for control of symptoms through phototherapy treatment is good. For cases in which SAD is a seasonal characteristic of a major depressive disorder or bipolar disorder, the prognosis is generally the same as for the underlying disorder.

Prevention

There is no known way to prevent SAD. Spending time during waking hours in direct sunlight may help to prevent or reduce symptoms. If an individual has experienced SAD in the past, a doctor or therapist may recommend beginning treatment before the symptoms are expected to occur to help control the symptoms and to minimize the negative effects of the disorder.

Resources

BOOKS

American Psychiatric Association. *Diagnostic and Statistical Manual of Mental Disorders.* 4th ed., text rev. Washington, DC: American Psychiatric Association, 2000.

Dziegielewski, Sophia F. *DSM-IV-TR in Action.* Hoboken, NJ: John Wiley & Sons, 2010.

Partonen, Timo, and Seithikurippu R. Pandi-Perumal, eds. *Seasonal Affective Disorder: Practice and Research,* 2nd ed. New York: Oxford University Press, 2010.

Rohan, Kelly J. *Coping with the Seasons: A Cognitive-Behavioral Approach to Seasonal Affective Disorder.* New York: Oxford University Press, 2009.

Rosenthal, Norman E. *Winter Blues: Everything You Need to Know to Beat Seasonal Affective Disorder.* New York: Guilford Press, 2006.

Smith, Laura L., and Charles H. Elliott. *Seasonal Affective Disorder for Dummies.* Indianapolis, IN: Wiley, 2007.

PERIODICALS

Friedman, Richard A. "Brought on by Darkness, Disorder Needs Light." *New York Times* (December 18, 2007). http://www.nytimes.com/2007/12/18/health/18mind.html (accessed July 27, 2011).

Gill, Jessica M., and Saligan, Leorey N. "Don't Let SAD Get You Down This Season." *Nurse Practitioner* (December 2008): 22–27.

Rankin, Lisa. "Seasonal Affective Order vs. 'Winter Blues.'" *Ohio Nurses Review* 86, no. 1 (January–February 2011):

16. http://www.ohnurses.org/AM/TemplateRedirect.cfm?template=/CM/ContentDisplay.cfm&ContentID=7841 (accessed August 19, 2011).

Rohan, Kelly J., et al. "Winter Depression Recurrence One Year After Cognitive-Behavioral Therapy, Light Therapy, or Combination Treatment." *Behavior Therapy* (September 2009): 225–38.

WEBSITES

Mayo Clinic staff. "Seasonal Affective Disorder (SAD)." MayoClinic.com. http://www.mayoclinic.com/health/seasonal-affective-disorder/DS00195 (accessed July 27, 2011).

MedlinePlus. "Seasonal Affective Disorder." U.S. National Library of Medicine, National Institutes of Health. http://www.nlm.nih.gov/medlineplus/seasonalaffectivedisorder.html (accessed July 27, 2011).

ORGANIZATIONS

Depression and Bipolar Support Alliance, 730 N Franklin St., Ste. 501, Chicago, IL, 60654-7225, (800) 826-3632, Fax: (312) 642-7234, http://www.dbsalliance.org.

Mental Health America, 2000 N Beauregard St., 6th Fl., Alexandria, VA, 22311, (703) 684-7722, (800) 969-6642, Fax: (703) 684-5968, http://www.nmha.org.

National Institute of Mental Health, 6001 Executive Blvd., Rm. 8184, MSC 9663, Bethesda, MD, 20892-9663, (301) 443-4513. TTY (301) 443-8431, (866) 615-6464, TTY (866) 415-8051, Fax: (301) 443-4279, http://www.nimh.nih.gov.

Ruth A. Wienclaw, PhD
Tish Davidson, AM

Sedatives and related disorders

Definition

Sedatives are drugs that depress the central nervous system and produce a calming effect on the body. They are used to relieve anxiety, agitation, or behavioral excitement. When used improperly, sedatives may lead to symptoms of abuse, dependence, and withdrawal. Sedatives are often referred to as "tranquilizers," and the similar classes of sedatives and hypnotics are sometimes referred to as one group: the "sedative-hypnotics."

Demographics

Many people, including about 90% of those who are hospitalized, are given some type of prescription sedative. Of the people who use sedatives, only a few become dependent. People who become dependent usually fall into three categories. Some are drug addicts who use sedatives along with other street drugs. These are usually young people between the ages of 15 and 25. Others are alcoholics who use sedatives to treat chronic anxiety or sleep problems associated with their alcohol dependence. Still others use sedatives under the direction of a doctor to treat long-term pain, anxiety, or sleeplessness. These people may become dependent by increasing the amount of a sedative they take as tolerance develops, without telling their doctor.

Sedative abuse is not a major **addiction** problem with street drug users. Many people who are dependent on sedatives are middle-aged and middle-class people who start taking the drug for a legitimate medical reason. Women may be more at risk than men for developing sedative dependence. Sedative dependence is the most common type of drug addiction among the elderly. Older people do not clear the drug from their bodies as efficiently as younger people and thus may become dependent on lower, therapeutic doses.

Description

Sedatives and similar drugs are available by prescription and have many medical uses. They are used in conjunction with surgery and are prescribed to treat pain, anxiety, panic attacks, **insomnia**, and, in some cases, convulsions. Most people who take prescription sedatives take them responsibly and benefit from their use. Some people misuse these drugs. They may do so unintentionally by increasing their prescribed dose without medical advice. Intentional abusers buy these drugs on the street for recreational use or get them from friends or family members who have prescriptions. Sedatives are not popular street drugs, and when they are used recreationally it is usually in conjunction with other illicit drugs or alcohol. When taken exactly as prescribed, sedatives rarely create major health risks.

A chemically diverse group of drugs are discussed together in this entry because they all appear to work in the body the same way and produce similar problems of abuse, dependence, intoxication, and withdrawal. These drugs work in the **brain** by increasing the amount of the neurotransmitter gamma-aminobutyric acid (GABA). **Neurotransmitters** help to regulate the speed at which nerve impulses travel. When the amount of GABA increases, the speed of nerve transmissions decreases. Thus, these drugs depress the nervous system and cause reduced pain, sleepiness, reduced anxiety, and muscle relaxation.

The most widely prescribed and best-studied sedatives belong to a group called "benzodiazepines." Prescription **benzodiazepines** and their relatives include **alprazolam** (Xanax), **chlordiazepoxide** (Librium), **clonazepam** (Klonopin), **clorazepate** (Tranxene), **diazepam** (Valium), **estazolam** (ProSom), **flurazepam** (Dalmane), halazepam (Paxipam), **lorazepam**, (Ativan), **oxazepam** (Serax), prazepam (Centrax), **quazepam** (Doral), **temazepam** (Restoril), **triazolam** (Halcion). Other drugs that act in a similar manner include the **barbiturates** amobarbital (Amytal), aprobarbital (Alurate), butabarbital (Butisol), phenobarbital, (Nebutal), and secobarbital, (Seconal). In addition, **chloral hydrate** (Notec), ethchlorvynol (Placidyl), glutehimide (Doriden), meprobamate (Miltown, Equanil, Equagesic, Deprol), and **zolpidem** (Ambien) have similar actions. These are meant for short-term use and may cause chemical dependence with prolonged use.

A class of non-benzodiazepine hypnotics for treatment of insomnia are becoming widely popular in the United States. **Zaleplon** (Sonata), zolpidem (Ambien), and eszopiclone (Lunesta) are three such drugs. **Amnesia** and sleepwalking resulting from use of non-benzodiazepine hypnotics to treat **sleep disorders** have been reported. Charges of driving while intoxicated on these drugs, particularly when the patient does not sleep long enough after taking a dose, are a potentially dangerous consequence.

Causes and symptoms

Sedatives and other drugs in this class are physically and sometimes psychologically addicting. People taking sedatives rapidly develop tolerance for the drugs. Tolerance occurs when a larger and larger dose must be taken to produce the same effect. Because sedatives are physically addicting, people with sedative dependence experience physical withdrawal symptoms when these drugs are discontinued.

Sedative abuse occurs when people misuse these drugs but are not addicted to them. Many people who abuse sedatives also use other illicit drugs. They may use sedatives to come down off a **cocaine** high or to enhance the effect of **methadone**, a heroin substitute.

Sedative dependence occurs when there is a physical addiction, when a person actively seeks sedatives (for example, by going to several doctors and getting multiple prescriptions) and continues to use these drugs despite the fact that they cause interpersonal problems and difficulties meeting the responsibilities of daily life.

Sedative intoxication

Sedative intoxication occurs when a person has recently used one of these drugs and shows certain psychosocial symptoms such as hostility or aggression, swings in mood, poor judgment, inability to function in social settings or at work, or inappropriate sexual behavior. Because sedatives depress the central nervous system, physical symptoms include slurred speech, lack of coordination, inattention, impaired memory or "blackouts" and extreme sluggishness, stupor, or coma. Sedative intoxication can appear very similar to alcohol intoxication in its symptoms. Overdoses can be fatal.

Sedative withdrawal

Physical addiction is the main problem with sedative dependence. Sedative withdrawal is similar to alcohol withdrawal. Symptoms of sedative withdrawal are almost the reverse of the symptoms of sedative intoxication. They include:

- increased heart rate
- faster breathing
- elevated blood pressure
- increased body temperature
- sweating
- shaky hands
- inability to sleep
- anxiety
- nausea
- restlessness

About one-quarter of people undergoing sedative withdrawal have **seizures**. If withdrawal is severe, they may also have visual or auditory hallucinations (sedative withdrawal **delirium**). Often, people who experience these more severe symptoms are using additional drugs.

The timeframe for withdrawal symptoms to appear varies depending on the chemical structure of the drug being taken. Withdrawal symptoms can occur hours or days after stopping use. For example, people withdrawing from Valium might not develop withdrawal symptoms for a week and might not have peak symptoms until the second week. Low-level symptoms can linger even longer. Generally, the longer a person takes a drug, and the higher the dose, the more severe the withdrawal symptoms. It is possible to have withdrawal symptoms when a therapeutically prescribed dose is taken for a long time.

Sedative dependence is thought to be able to induce other mental health disorders, although there is some disagreement in the mental health community about how these disorders are defined and classified. Other disorders

KEY TERMS

Anxiety—Can be experienced as a troubled feeling, a sense of dread, fear of the future, or distress over a possible threat to a person's physical or mental well-being.

Anxiolytic—A drug that relieves anxiety.

Hallucinations—Hearing, seeing, or otherwise sensing things that are not real. Hallucinations can result from nervous system abnormalities, mental disorders, or the use of certain drugs.

Insomnia—Waking in the middle of the night and having difficulty returning to sleep, or waking too early in the morning.

Panic attack—A period of intense fear or discomfort with a feeling of doom and a desire to escape. The person may shake, sweat, be short of breath, and experience chest pain.

Seizure—A convulsion, or uncontrolled discharge of nerve cells that may spread to other cells throughout the brain.

that may result from sedative dependence and withdrawal include:

- sedative-induced persisting dementia
- sedative-induced persisting amnestic disorder
- sedative-induced psychotic disorder (with or without hallucinations)
- sedative-induced mood disorder
- sedative-induced anxiety disorder
- sedative-induced sexual dysfunction
- sedative-induced sleep disorder

Diagnosis

Diagnosis of sedative intoxication is made based on recent use of the drug, presence of the symptoms listed above, and presence of the drug in a blood or urine sample. Without a blood or urine test, sedative intoxication can be difficult to distinguish from alcohol intoxication except for the absence of the odor of alcohol. People experiencing sedative intoxication usually remain grounded in reality. However, if they lose touch with reality, they may be diagnosed as having sedative intoxication delirium.

Diagnosis of sedative withdrawal is based on the symptoms listed above. It can be difficult to distinguish from alcohol withdrawal. Withdrawal may occur with or without hallucinations and delirium. Diagnosis depends on whether a person remains grounded in reality during withdrawal.

Diagnosis of other mental disorders induced by sedative dependence requires that the symptoms be in excess of those usually found with sedative intoxication or withdrawal. They cannot be accounted for by other **substance abuse** or another mental or physical disorder.

The fifth edition of the ***Diagnostic and Statistical Manual of Mental Disorders***, also known as the *DSM-5*, is due for publication in May 2013. This edition may include proposed changes and revisions to some current diagnostic criteria for psychiatric diagnoses, including combining "Substance Abuse" and "Dependence" into a single disorder, thus modifying "Sedative, Hypnotic, or Anxiolytic Abuse" and "Sedative, Hypnotic, or Anxiolytic Dependence" into one diagnosis of "Sedative, Hypnotic, or Anxiolytic Use Disorder."

Treatment

Treatment depends on how large a dose of sedative the patient is taking, the length of time it has been used, and the patient's individual psychological and physical state.

Physiological treatment

Successful treatment of sedative dependence is based on the idea of gradually decreasing the amount of drug the patient uses in order to keep withdrawal symptoms to a manageable level. This is called a "drug taper." The rate of taper depends on the dependency dose of the drug, the length of time the drug has been taken, a person's individual mental and physical response to drug withdrawal, and any complicating factors such as other substance abuse or other physical or mental illness.

For people dependent on a low dose of sedatives, the current level of use is determined, and then the amount of drug is then reduced by 10 to 25%. If withdrawal symptoms are manageable, reduction is continued on a weekly basis. If withdrawal symptoms are too severe, the patient is stabilized at the lowest dose with manageable symptoms until tapering can be restarted. This gradual reduction of use may take weeks, and the rate must be adjusted to the response of each patient individually.

People dependent on high doses of sedatives are usually hospitalized because of the possibility of life-threatening withdrawal symptoms. A blood or urine test is used to determine the current level of usage. The patient is often switched to an equivalent dose of a different sedative or phenobarbital (a barbiturate) to aid

QUESTIONS TO ASK YOUR DOCTOR

- What risks are associated with abuse of sedative medications?
- What symptoms are associated with sedative dependence?
- Does having sedative dependence and abuse put me at risk for other health conditions?
- Can you recommend any treatment and support groups for me?

in withdrawal while controlling withdrawal symptoms. The tapering process begins, but more gradually than with low-dose dependency. Often, other drugs are given to combat some of the withdrawal symptoms.

Psychological treatment

Cognitive-behavioral therapy (CBT) may be used in conjunction with drug tapering. This type of **talk therapy** aims at two things: to educate patients to recognize and cope with the symptoms of anxiety associated with withdrawal, and to help patients change their behavior in ways that promote coping with **stress**. Patients are taught to mentally talk their way through their anxiety and stress. Some people find **support groups** and journal-keeping to be helpful in their recovery. Recovering from dependency is a slow process, best achieved when a person has a good social support system, patience, and persistence.

Prognosis

The people who have the best chance of becoming sedative-free are those who became dependent through taking long-term therapeutic doses. Although stopping any addiction takes time and work, with a properly managed course of treatment, chances of success are good.

People who abuse multiple street drugs must receive treatment for their multiple drug dependencies. Sedative abuse is low on their list of problems, and the chances of their becoming drug-free are low. Alcoholics also have a difficult time withdrawing from sedatives.

Prevention

The best way to prevent sedative-related disorders is to take these drugs only for the exact length of time, and in the exact amount, prescribed by a doctor.

Resources

BOOKS

American Psychiatric Association. *Diagnostic and Statistical Manual of Mental Disorders.* 4th ed., text rev. Washington, DC: American Psychiatric Association, 2000.

American Psychological Association. *Publication Manual of the American Psychological Association.* 6th ed. Washington, DC: American Psychological Association, 2009.

Erickson, Carlton K, PhD. *Addiction Essentials: The Go-To Guide for Clinicians and Patients.* New York: W. W. Norton & Company, 2011.

PERIODICALS

Compton, Wilson M., et al. "Prevalence, Correlates, and Comorbidity of DSM-IV Antisocial Personality Syndromes and Alcohol and Specific Drug Use Disorders in the United States: Results From the National Epidemiologic Survey on Alcohol and Related Conditions." *Journal of Clinical Psychiatry.* 66, no. 6, Jun. 2005: 677–85.

McCabe, Sean Esteban, and Carol J. Boyd. "Sources of Prescription Drugs for Illicit Use." *Addictive Behaviors.* 30, no. 7, Aug. 2005: 1342–50.

McCabe, Sean Esteban, Christian J. Teter, and Carol J. Boyd. "Medical Use, Illicit Use, and Diversion of Abusable Prescription Drugs." *Journal of American College Health* 54, no. 5, Mar.–Apr. 2006: 269–78.

ORGANIZATIONS

American Psychological Association, 750 First St. NE, Washington, DC, 20003, (202) 336-5500, http://www.apa.org/index.aspx.

National Institute on Drug Abuse, 6001 Executive Blvd., Rm. 5213, Bethesda, MD, 20892, (301) 442-1124; Spanish: (240) 221-4007, information@nida.nih.gov, http://www.nida.nih.gov.

The Partnership at Drugfree.org, 352 Park Ave. S, 9th Fl., New York, NY, 10010, (212) 922-1560, (855) DRUG-FREE (378-4373; helpline), Fax: (212) 922-1570, webmail@drugfree.org, http://www.drugfree.org.

Substance Abuse and Mental Health Services Administration Referral Resource, 1 Choke Cherry Rd., Rockville, MD, 20857, (877) SAMHSA-7 (726-4727), (800) TTY: 487-4889, Fax: (240) 221-4292, SAMHSAInfo@samhsa.hhs.gov, http://www.samhsa.gov.

Tish Davidson, A.M.
Laura Jean Cataldo, RN, Ed.D.

Seizures

Definition

A seizure is a sudden change in behavior characterized by changes in sensory perception (sense of feeling) or motor activity (movement) due to an abnormal firing

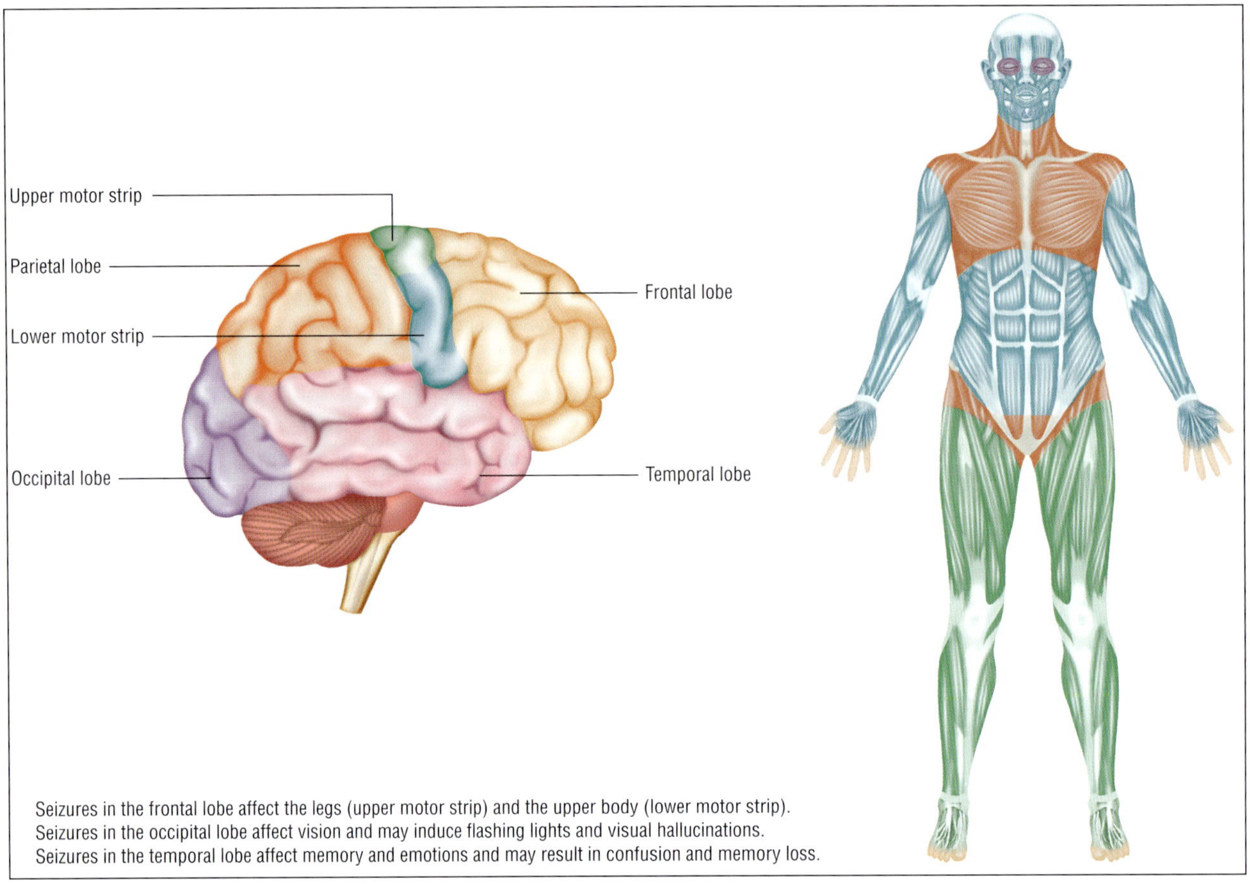

Illustration showing where different types of seizures occur in the brain; the colors of the brain correspond with the body parts affected. *(Illustration by PreMediaGlobal. © 2012 Cengage Learning.)*

of nerve cells in the **brain**. Epilepsy is a condition characterized by recurrent seizures that may include repetitive muscle jerking called convulsions.

Demographics

Epilepsy and seizures affect a reported 3 million—or 1%—of Americans of all ages, although up to 10% of the population may experience at least one seizure during their lives; some of these events are febrile convulsions associated with high fevers in childhood. Every year, about 200,000 new cases are diagnosed and about 300,000 people have their first convulsion. The annual costs of treatment for seizure and epilepsy, in direct and indirect costs, is about $12.5 billion. Men are slightly more likely than women to develop epilepsy, and its prevalence is higher among minority populations in the United States.

Seizures caused by fever have a recurrence rate of 51% if the attack occurred in the first year of life, whereas recurrence rate is decreased to 25% if the seizure took place during the second year. Approximately 88% of children who experience seizures caused by fever in the first two years experience recurrence.

About 45 million people worldwide are affected by epilepsy. The incidence is highest among young children (under age 2) and the elderly (over age 65). High-risk groups include people with a previous history of brain injury or lesions; children with intellectual disabilities, cerebral palsy, or both; patients with **Alzheimer's disease** or stroke; and children with at least one parent who has epilepsy.

Description

Seizure disorders and their classification date back to the earliest medical literature accounts in history. In 1964, the Commission on Classification and Terminology of the International League Against Epilepsy (ILAE) devised the first official classification of seizures, which was revised in 1981 and again in 1989. They then proposed to use a diagnostic scheme of five diagnostic levels or axes, rather than a classification scheme, for characterizing seizures. These axes are (1) the events that occur during the seizure;

Anticonvulsant and mood-stabilizing medications

Generic name	Trade name	FDA approved age
carbamazepine	Tegretol	Any age (for seizures)
divalproex sodium (valproic acid)	Depakote	2+ (for seizures)
gabapentin	Neurontin	18+
lamotrigine	Lamictal	18+
lithium carbonate	Eskalith, Lithobid	12+
lithium citrate	(generic only)	12+
oxcarbazepine	Trileptal	4+
topiramate	Topamax	18+

SOURCE: National Institute of Mental Health. **"Alphabetical List of Medications," available online at: http://www.nimh.nih.gov/health/publications/mental-health-medications/alphabetical-list-of-medications.shtml.** *(Table by PreMediaGlobal. © 2012 Cengage Learning.)*

(2) the type of seizure, chosen from a list that can include where the seizure localizes in the brain and what stimulates it; (3) the type of epileptic syndrome most closely associated with the seizure; (4) the underlying medical or other causes of the syndrome; and (5) the level of impairment the seizure causes. These are proposed recommendations that are still under discussion.

The ILAE classification, meanwhile, is accepted worldwide and is based on electroencephalographic (EEG) studies. Based on this system, seizures can be classified as either focal or generalized. Each of these categories can also be further subdivided.

Focal seizures

A focal (partial) seizure develops when a limited, confined population of nerve cells fire their impulses abnormally on one hemisphere of the brain. (The brain has two portions or cerebral hemispheres—the right and left hemispheres.) Focal seizures are divided into simple or complex based on the level of consciousness (wakefulness) during an attack. Simple partial seizures occur in patients who are conscious, whereas complex partial seizures demonstrate impaired levels of consciousness.

Generalized seizures

A generalized seizure results from initial abnormal firing of brain nerve cells throughout both the left and right hemispheres. Generalized seizures can be classified as follows:

- Tonic-clonic seizures: This is the most common type among all age groups and is categorized into several phases beginning with vague symptoms that appear hours or days before an attack. These seizures are sometimes called grand mal seizures.
- Tonic seizures: These are typically characterized by a sustained nonvibratory contraction of muscles in the legs and arms. Consciousness is also impaired during these episodes.
- Atonic seizures (also called "drop attacks"): These are characterized by sudden, limp posture and a brief period of unconsciousness, and last for one to two seconds.
- Clonic seizures: These are characterized by a rapid loss of consciousness with loss of muscle tone, tonic spasm, and jerks. The muscles become rigid for about 30 seconds during the tonic phase of the seizure and alternately contract and relax during the clonic phase, which lasts 30–60 seconds.
- Absence seizures: These are subdivided into typical and atypical forms based on duration of attack and level of consciousness. Absence (petit mal) seizures generally begin at about the age of four and stop by the time the child becomes an adolescent. They usually begin with a brief loss of consciousness and last 1–10 seconds. People having petit mal seizures become very quiet and may blink, stare blankly, roll their eyes, or move their lips. A petit mal seizure lasts 15–20 seconds. When it ends, individuals resume whatever they were doing before the seizure began, will not remember the seizure, and may not realize that anything unusual happened. Untreated, petit mal seizures can recur as many as 100 times a day and may progress to grand mal seizures.
- Myoclonic seizures: These are characterized by rapid muscular contractions accompanied with jerks in facial and pelvic muscles.

Subcategories are commonly diagnosed based on electroencephalographic (EEG) results. Terminology for classification in infants and newborns is still controversial.

Causes and symptoms

Causes

Simple partial seizures can be caused by congenital abnormalities (abnormalities present at birth), tumor growths, head **trauma**, **stroke**, and infections in the brain or nearby structures. Generalized tonic-clonic seizures are associated with drug and alcohol abuse, and low levels of blood glucose (blood sugar) and sodium. Certain psychiatric medications, antihistamines, and even antibiotics can precipitate tonic-clonic seizures. Absence seizures are implicated with an abnormal imbalance of certain chemicals in the brain that modulate nerve cell activity (one of these **neurotransmitters** is called gamma-aminobutyric acid or GABA, which functions as an inhibitor). Myoclonic seizures are commonly diagnosed in newborns and children.

Symptoms

Symptoms for the different types of seizures are specific.

Partial seizures

SIMPLE PARTIAL SEIZURES. Multiple signs and symptoms may be present during a single simple partial seizure. These symptoms include specific muscles tensing and then alternately contracting and relaxing, speech arrest, vocalizations, and involuntary turning of the eyes or head. There could be changes in vision, hearing, balance, taste, and smell. Additionally, patients with simple partial seizures may have a sensation in the abdomen, sweating, paleness, flushing, hair follicles standing up (piloerection), and dilated pupils (the dark center in the eye enlarges). Seizures with psychological symptoms include thinking disturbances and hallucinations, or illusions of memory, sound, sight, time, and self-image.

COMPLEX PARTIAL SEIZURES. Complex partial seizures often begin with a motionless stare or arrest of activity; this is followed by a series of involuntary movements, speech disturbances, and eye movements.

Generalized seizures

Generalized seizures have a more complex set of signs and symptoms.

TONIC-CLONIC SEIZURES. Tonic-clonic seizures usually have vague prodromal (pre-attack) symptoms that can start hours or days before a seizure. These symptoms include anxiety, mood changes, irritability, weakness, dizziness, lightheadedness, and changes in appetite. The tonic phases may be preceded with brief (lasting only a few seconds in duration) muscle contractions on both sides of affected muscle groups. The tonic phase typically begins with a brief flexing of trunk muscles, upward movement of the eyes, and pupil dilation. Patients usually emit a characteristic vocalization. This sound is caused by contraction of trunk muscles that forces air from the lungs across spasmodic (abnormally tensed) throat muscles. This is followed by a very short period (10–15 seconds) of general muscle relaxation. The clonic phase consists of muscular contractions with alternating periods of no movements (muscle atonia) that gradually increase duration until abnormal muscular contractions stop. Tonic-clonic seizures end in a final generalized spasm. The affected person can lose consciousness during tonic and clonic phases of seizure.

Tonic-clonic seizures can also produce chemical changes in the body. Patients commonly experience lowered carbon dioxide (hypocarbia) due to breathing alterations, increased blood glucose (blood sugar), and an elevated level of a hormone called prolactin. Once affected people regain consciousness, they are usually weak, and have a headache and muscle pain. Tonic-clonic seizures can cause serious medical problems such as trauma to the head and mouth, fractures in the spinal column, pulmonary edema (water in the lungs), aspiration pneumonia (a pneumonia caused by a foreign body being lodged in the lungs), and sudden death. Attacks are generally one minute in duration.

TONIC SEIZURES. Tonic and atonic seizures have distinct differences but are often present in the same patient. Tonic seizures are characterized by nonvibratory muscle contractions, usually involving flexing of arms and relaxing or flexing of legs. The seizure usually lasts less than 10 seconds but may be as long as one minute. Tonic seizures are usually abrupt and patients lose consciousness. Tonic seizures commonly occur during nonrapid eye movement (nonREM) sleep and drowsiness. Tonic seizures that occur during wakeful states commonly produce physical injuries due to abrupt, unexpected falls.

ATONIC SEIZURES. Atonic seizures, also called "drop attacks," are abrupt, with loss of muscle tone lasting one to two seconds, but with rapid recovery. Consciousness is usually impaired. The rapid loss of muscular tone could be limited to head and neck muscles, resulting in head drop, or it may be more extensive involving muscles for balance, causing unexpected falls with physical injury.

CLONIC SEIZURES. Generalized clonic seizures are rare and seen typically in children with elevated fever. These seizures are characterized by a rapid loss of consciousness, decreased muscle tone, and a generalized spasm that is followed by jerky movements.

ABSENCE SEIZURES. Absence seizures are classified as either typical or atypical. The typical absence seizure is characterized by unresponsiveness and behavioral arrest, abnormal muscular movements of the face and eyelids, and lasts less than 10 seconds. In atypical absence seizures, the affected person is generally more conscious, the seizures begin and end more gradually, and do not exceed 10 seconds in duration.

MYOCLONIC SEIZURES. People with myoclonic seizures commonly exhibit rapid muscular contractions. Myoclonic seizures are seen in newborns and children who have either symptomatic or idiopathic (cause is unknown) epilepsy.

Diagnosis

Patients seeking help for seizures should first undergo an EEG that records brain-wave patterns emitted between nerve cells. Electrodes are placed on the head, sometimes for 24 hours, to monitor brain-wave activity and detect both normal and abnormal impulses. **Imaging**

KEY TERMS

Electroencephalograph (EEG)—An instrument that measures the electrical activity of the brain. The EEG traces the electrical activity in the form of wave patterns onto recording paper. Wave patterns that have sudden spikes or sharp waves strongly suggest seizures. An EEG with a seizure-type wave pattern is called an epileptiform EEG.

Hallucination—False sensory perceptions. A person experiencing a hallucination may "hear" sounds or "see" people or objects that are not really present. Hallucinations can also affect the senses of smell, touch, and taste.

Illusion—A misperception or misinterpretation in the presence of a real external stimulus.

studies such as **magnetic resonance imaging** (MRI) and computerized axial tomography (CAT)—that take still "pictures"—are useful in detecting abnormalities in the temporal lobes (parts of the brain associated with hearing) or for helping diagnose tonic-clonic seizures. A complete blood count (CBC) can be helpful in determining whether a seizure is caused by a neurological infection, which is typically accompanied by high fever. If drugs or toxins in the blood are suspected to be the cause of the seizure(s), blood and urine screening tests for these compounds may be necessary.

Antiseizure medication can be altered by many commonly used medications, such as sulfa drugs, erythromycin, warfarin, and cimetidine. Pregnancy may also decrease serum concentration of antiseizure medications; therefore, frequent monitoring and dose adjustments are vital to maintain appropriate blood concentrations of the antiseizure medication—known as the therapeutic blood concentration. Some medications taken during pregnancy could affect the fetus, and women must discuss with their doctors the costs and benefits of any medication taken during pregnancy.

Diagnosis requires a detailed and accurate history, and a physical examination is important because this may help identify neurological or systemic causes. In cases in which a central nervous system (CNS) infection (e.g., meningitis or encephalitis) is suspected, a lumbar puncture (or spinal tap) can help detect an increase in immune cells (white blood cells) that develop to fight the specific infection. (A lumbar puncture involves removing a small amount of cerebrospinal fluid—the fluid that bathes and nourishes the brain and spinal cord—from the spinal chord by syringe.)

Treatment

Treatment is targeted primarily to:

- assist the patient in adjusting psychologically to the diagnosis and in maintaining as normal a lifestyle as possible.
- reduce or eliminate seizure occurrence.
- avoid side effects of long-term drug treatment.

Simple and complex partial seizures respond to drugs such as **carbamazepine**, **valproic acid** (valproate), phenytoin, **gabapentin**, tiagabine, **lamotrigine**, and topiramate. Tonic-clonic seizures tend to respond to valproate, carbamazepine, phenytoin, and lamotrigine. Absence seizures seem to be sensitive to ethosuximide, valproate, and lamotrigine. Myoclonic seizures can be treated with valproate and **clonazepam**. Tonic seizures seem to respond favorably to valproate, felbamate, and clonazepam.

People treated with a class of medications called **barbiturates** (Mysoline, Mebral, phenobarbital) have adverse cognitive (thinking) effects. These cognitive effects can include decreased general intelligence, attention, memory, problem solving, motor speed, and visual motor functions. The drug phenytoin (Dilantin) can adversely affect speed of response, memory, and attention. Other medications used for treatment of seizures do not have substantial cognitive impairment.

Surgical treatment may be considered when medications fail. Advances in medical sciences and techniques have improved methods of identifying the parts of the brain that generate abnormal discharge of nerve impulses. The most common type of surgery is the extratemporal cortical resection. In this procedure, a small part of the brain responsible for causing the seizures is removed. An option of last resort for people with extreme, uncontrollable seizures is functional hemispherectomy, in which communication between the two hemispheres of the brain is severed. Surgical **intervention** may be considered a feasible treatment option if:

- the site of seizures is identifiable and localized.
- surgery can remove the seizure-generating (epileptogenic) area.
- surgical procedure will not cause damage to nearby areas.

Another treatment approach that has been found to reduce seizures in some children is the ketogenic diet. This diet reduces available glucose in the body, forcing the child's body to turn to fat stores for energy. It is a high-fat diet that results in the person getting about 80% of their calories from fat. No one is exactly sure why this diet, which mimics starvation in the body, works to prevent seizures. It also does not work for every child, and the reasons for that also are unclear.

Prognosis

About 30% of patients with severe seizures (starting in early childhood), continue to have attacks and usually never achieve a remission state. In the United States, the prevalence of treatment-resistant seizures is about one to two per 1,000 people. About 60–70% of people achieve a five-year remission within 10 years of initial diagnosis. Approximately half of these patients become seizure-free. Usually the prognosis is better if seizures can be controlled by one medication, the frequency of seizures decreases, and there is a normal EEG and neurological examination prior to medication cessation.

People affected by seizures have increased death rates compared with the general population. Patients who have seizures of unknown cause have an increased chance of dying due to accidents (primarily drowning). Other causes of seizure-associated death include abnormal heart rhythms, water in the lungs, or heart attack.

Prevention

There are no gold-standard recommendations for prevention because seizures can be caused by **genetic factors**, blood abnormalities, many medications, illicit drugs, infection, neurologic conditions, and other systemic diseases. If a person has had a previous attack or has a genetic propensity, care is advised when receiving medical treatment or if diagnosed with an illness correlated with possible seizure development.

Resources

BOOKS

Goetz, Christopher G. *Textbook of Clinical Neurology*. Philadelphia: W. B. Saunders Company, 2003.

Goldman, Lee, and Andrew I. Schafer, eds. *Goldman's Cecil Medicine*, 24th ed. Philadelphia: Elsevier, 2011.

Goroll, Allan H., and Albert G. Mulley. *Primary Care Medicine*. 6th ed. Philadelphia: Lippincott Williams and Wilkins, 2009.

PERIODICALS

Dodrill, C. R., and C. G. Matthew. "The Role of Neuropsychology in the Assessment and Treatment of Persons with Epilepsy." *American Psychologist* 47, no. 9 (September 1992): 1139–42.

ORGANIZATIONS

Epilepsy Foundation, 8301 Professional Pl., Landover, MD, 20785, (800) 332-1000, Fax: (301) 577-2684, http://www.epilepsyfoundation.org.

International League Against Epilepsy, 342 N Main St., West Hartford, CT, 06117-2507, (860) 586-7547, Fax: (860) 586-7550, http://www.ilae-epilepsy.org.

National Institutes of Health, 9000 Rockville Pike, Bethesda, MD, 20892, (301) 496-4000; TTY: (301) 402-9612, http://www.nih.gov.

Laith Farid Gulli, MD
Alfredo Mori, MD, FACEM
Emily Jane Willingham, PhD

Selective mutism

Definition

Selective mutism is a childhood disorder in which a child does not speak in some social situations although he or she is able to talk normally at other times.

Demographics

Selective mutism is generally considered a rare disorder. It is found in about 1% of patients in mental health settings, but it occurs in only about 0.01% of the general United States population. Some researchers maintain, however, that selective mutism occurs more frequently than these data suggest. There may be many unreported cases of selective mutism that resolve with time and require no **intervention**.

In terms of age grouping, selective mutism may appear at the very beginning of a child's social experience or may begin in later childhood. Some cases have been recorded in which selective mutism does not begin until high school. Onset in late adolescence is unusual, however; the most common age of onset for the disorder is the early elementary school years.

Selective mutism is often associated with **social phobia** in adult life. Children with selective mutism disorder may be more likely as adults to have a high level of social anxiety even if they do not meet the diagnostic criteria for social phobia. The disorder appears to run in families Children whose parents are anxious in social settings, were exceptionally timid as children, or suffered from selective mutism themselves in childhood, are at greater risk for developing selective mutism.

Description

Selective mutism was first described in the 1870s, at which time it was called "aphasia voluntaria." This name shows that the absence of speech was considered to lie under the control of the child's will. In 1934 the disorder began to be called selective mutism, a name that still implied purposefulness on the part of the silent child. In the 1994 edition of the ***Diagnostic and Statistical Manual of Mental Disorders*** (*DSM-IV*) the disorder was renamed selective mutism. This name is considered preferable because it suggests that the child is mute only in certain situations, without the implication that the child remains silent on purpose.

Selective mutism is characterized by a child's inability to speak in one or more types of social situation, although the child is developmentally advanced to the point that speech is possible. The child speaks proficiently in at least one setting, most often at home with one or both parents, and sometimes with siblings or extended family members. Some children also speak to certain friends or to adults that are not related to them; but this variant of selective mutism is somewhat less common.

The most common place for children to exhibit mute behavior is in the classroom, so that the disorder is often first noticed by teachers. Because of this characteristic, selective mutism is most frequently diagnosed in children of preschool age through second grade. As the expectation of speech becomes more evident, selective mutism can have more pronounced negative effects on academic performance. Children who do not talk in classroom settings or other social situations because the language of instruction is not their first tongue are not considered to have the disorder of selective mutism.

Causes and symptoms

The symptoms of selective mutism are fairly obvious. The child does not talk in one or more social situations in which speech is commonly expected and would facilitate understanding. Some children with selective mutism do not communicate in any way in certain settings, and act generally shy and withdrawn. The disorder is also often associated with crying, clinging to the parent, and other signs of social anxiety. Other children with the disorder, however, may smile, gesture, nod, and even giggle, although they do not talk.

Consensus regarding the most common causes of selective mutism has changed significantly over time. When the disorder was first studied, and for many years thereafter, it was thought to be caused by severe **trauma** in early childhood. Some of these causative traumas were thought to include rape, molestation, incest, severe physical or emotional **abuse**, and similar experiences. In addition, many researchers attributed selective mutism to family dynamics that included an overprotective mother and an abnormally strict or very distant father. While all of these factors may contribute to selective mutism in certain cases, none of them are considered to be common causes of selective mutism.

Selective mutism is instead frequently attributed to high levels of social anxiety in children and not to traumatic events in their early years. Children with selective mutism have been found to be more timid and shy than most children in social situations; and to exhibit signs of **depression**, **obsessive-compulsive disorder**, and **anxiety disorders**. Some children have been reported to dislike speaking because they are uncomfortable with the sound of their own voice or because they think their voice sounds abnormal.

Many links have also been found between selective mutism and speech development problems. Language reception problems have also been documented in selectively mute children. Although there is no evidence indicating that selective mutism is the direct result of any of these difficulties in language development, possible connections are being explored.

Diagnosis

The criteria for diagnosing selective mutism disorder given by the *Diagnostic and Statistical Manual of Mental Disorders*, fourth edition, text revision (*DSM-IV-TR*) include the failure to speak in some social situations even though the child may talk at other times. This criterion is not met if the child does not speak at all in any situation.

The child's inability to talk must interfere with the achievement of such relevant goals as schoolwork, play with friends, or communication of needs. In addition, the lack of speech must persist for at least one month. The first month of school should not be included in this measurement because many children are shy and unwilling to talk freely until they feel comfortable with their new teacher, classmates, and surroundings.

Furthermore, the child's lack of speech cannot be attributed to unfamiliarity with the language they must use in school or social settings. The **diagnosis** of selective mutism does not apply to children from immigrant families who may not feel comfortable conversing in a second language. Moreover, the child's inability to talk cannot be attributed to **stuttering** or similar speech disorders, which may make the child uncomfortable because they are aware that their speech sounds different from the speech of their peers. The lack of speech also must not be attributable to **schizophrenia**, **autism**, or other mental health disorders.

The disorder of selective mutism is usually noticed first by parents or teachers of affected children. It is often hard for doctors to diagnose selective mutism because it is unlikely that the child in question will talk to them. Therefore it may be difficult for a general practitioner to assess the existence of any underlying language or developmental problems that may be either causing or exacerbating the disorder. Tests that evaluate mental development without verbal responses from the patient may be used successfully to evaluate children with selective mutism.

There are also ways to test the child's speech development in the situations in which he or she does talk. One method involves interviews with the parents or whomever the child does speak to on a regular basis. This method can be fairly subjective, however. It is more useful for the doctor to obtain a tape or video recording of the child talking in a situation in which he or she feels comfortable. The child's hearing should be checked, as speech problems are often related to hearing disorders. Observing the child at play activities or asking him or her to draw pictures offer other effective ways to determine the child's reactions in social situations.

Treatment

A number of different approaches have been used in attempts to treat selective mutism. Recent opinion has moved away from the idea that it is caused by a trauma, and attempts to treat it have followed accordingly. The factors that are most intensively studied at present are underlying anxiety problems. In the few cases in which an underlying trauma is discovered to be the source of the problem, counseling to help treat the underlying problems is recommended. Treatments of any kind are generally found to be more effective when the family of the child is involved in decisions about his or her treatment.

Behavior modification

Selective mutism can be treated by using a **reinforcement** approach. This method gives positive rewards to the child in the form of praise, treats, privileges, or anything else that the child values. In general rewards are given for speech, and withheld for silence. The use of punishments alongside the rewards is not generally recommended because it would place more **stress** on children who are already severely anxious. The positive reinforcement technique is generally found to be at least partially successful in most cases.

Another technique for modifying behavior in children with selective mutism is known as stimulus fading. This technique sets goals of increasing difficulty for the child to meet. For example, the child might be encouraged to start talking by whispering, then work up gradually to talking at full volume. Alternately, the child could start by talking to one person who is not a family member and gradually add names until he or she feels comfortable talking to more than one person at a time. Stimulus fading has been found to be particularly effective when it is used in conjunction with positive reinforcement techniques.

Treatment with medications

In some cases selective mutism is treatable with medication. **Fluoxetine** (Prozac), which is one of the **selective serotonin reuptake inhibitors (SSRIs)** is the drug that has been studied most often as a treatment for selective mutism. Treatment with medication is more successful in younger children. Overall fluoxetine has been found to reduce the symptoms of selective mutism in about three-fourths of children. Other drugs used to treat anxiety and social phobia disorders may also be effective in certain cases.

Prognosis

Selective mutism is considered treatable in that many cases of the disorder are thought to resolve on their own, although treatment can be very effective. There is little information about the long-term outcome of selective mutism. Researchers have noted, however, that while many children with the disorder do show improvement in speech, their anxiety in social situations persists.

KEY TERM

Stimulus fading—A form of behavior modification used to treat children with selective mutism, in which goals of gradually increasing difficulty are set for the child.

Resources

BOOKS

American Psychiatric Association. *Diagnostic and Statistical Manual of Mental Disorders*. 4th ed., text rev. Washington, DC: American Psychiatric Publishing, 2000.

Sadock, Benjamin J., and Virginia A. Sadock, eds. *Comprehensive Textbook of Psychiatry*. Vol. 2. 7th ed. Philadelphia: Lippincott Williams and Wilkins, 2000.

PERIODICALS

Dow, Sara P., et al. "Practical Guidelines for the Assessment and Treatment of Selective Mutism." *Journal of the American Academy of Child and Adolescent Psychiatry* 34, no. 7 (July 1995): 836–847.

Dummit, Steven E. III, et al. "Fluoxetine Treatment of Children with Selective Mutism: An Open Trial." *Journal of the American Academy of Child and Adolescent Psychiatry* 35, no. 5 (May 1996): 615–622.

Joseph, Paul R. "Selective Mutism—The Child Who Doesn't Speak at School." *Pediatrics* 104, no. 2 Part 1 (August 1999): 308–309.

Stein, Martin T., Isabelle Rapin, and Diane Yapko. "Selective Mutism." *Journal of Developmental & Behavioral Pediatrics* 22, no. 2 Suppl. (April 2001): S123.

ORGANIZATIONS

Selective Mutism Group—A Division of Childhood Anxiety Network, Inc, http://www.selectivemutism.org.

Tish Davidson, A.M.

Selective serotonin reuptake inhibitors (SSRIs)

Definition

Selective **serotonin** reuptake inhibitors (SSRIs) are a class of antidepressant medicines that help increase the activity of a chemical in the **brain** called serotonin. They are also called serotonin boosters.

Purpose

Serotonin is a neurotransmitter, which is a substance that helps send messages between nerves in the brain. It is believed that problems with serotonin levels play a role in determining a person's mood and behavior.

SSRIs are used to treat a wide variety of mental disorders, including:

- major depressive disorder
- obsessive-compulsive disorder
- posttraumatic stress disorder (PTSD)
- social and generalized anxiety
- panic disorder
- postmenstrual dysphoric disorder (PMDD)

Sometimes, a health-care provider will prescribe an SSRI for a condition other than the approved ones listed on the drug's label. This is called off-label use. Off-label uses for SSRIs include the treatment of obesity, certain types of irritable bowel syndrome (IBS), and bulimia, an eating disorder. The American Medical Association has reported that SSRI use in persons with **depression** who have had a heart attack reduces the risk of death and repeated heart attacks.

Description

SSRIs act on the central nervous system. They prevent nerve cells in the brain, called receptors, from soaking up serotonin. The action of soaking up, or absorbing, a substance is called reuptake. When serotonin reuptake is blocked, the serotonin has nowhere to go, and the levels of the chemical in the brain increase. SSRIs were released in the U.S. market in 1987. **Fluoxetine** (Prozac) was the first type of SSRI sold in the United States. Ten years later, more than half of Americans receiving outpatient treatment for major depression were prescribed an SSRI.

SSRIs include:

- citalopram (Celexa)
- escitalopram (Lexapro)
- fluoxetine (Prozac)
- fluvoxamine (Luvox)
- paroxetine (Paxil)
- sertraline (Zoloft)

Recommended dosage

SSRIs are taken by mouth. They are available in many different forms. Extended-release (XR) and controlled-release (CR) forms slowly release medicine into the body over several hours. Most SSRIs are taken once a day. The exact dosage needed depends on the specific drug, the person's age, and medical condition being treated. The medicine must be taken regularly for several weeks before an effect is seen. If symptoms continue, a different type of medicine may be prescribed.

Precautions

Pregnant women

Pregnant women should discuss the use and safety of SSRIs with their health care providers. In 2006, the U.S. Food and Drug Administration (FDA) warned that mothers who take SSRIs after the 20th week of pregnancy have an increased risk of giving birth to babies with a serious heart and lung disorder called persistent pulmonary hypertension (PPHN). The FDA classifies a drug according to how it may affect a baby during pregnancy and breastfeeding. Most SSRIs fall into pregnancy category C, which means: 1) no animal and human studies have been done, or 2) animal studies have shown the drugs cause harm to a fetus, but more complete human studies are needed. The SSRI **paroxetine** (Paxil) falls into a higher risk category. The American College of Obstetricians and Gynecologists has recommended that pregnant women avoid taking Paxil. The organization encourages patients and doctors to carefully weigh the possible risk of birth defects against a woman's individual risk of depression during pregnancy.

Children and young adults

Sometimes SSRIs may make depression worse or cause suicidal thoughts or behaviors. A government review of all studies involving antidepressant use among children and adolescents concluded that 4% of those taking SSRIs thought about **suicide** or displayed suicidal behavior. In October 2004, the FDA told the manufacturers of **antidepressants** that they must include a warning on the medicine's label that tells users the drugs have been linked to an increase in suicide in children and young adults. Such an alert is called a "black box warning." According to the FDA, the use of SSRIs among people aged 10 to 19 has risen sharply in recent years. Children and adolescents taking any type of antidepressants should be closely watched for signs of suicidal tendencies, behavior changes, or worsening of depression.

Other medical conditions

SSRIs should be used with caution in people with kidney or liver problems and diabetes, and in women who are producing breast milk (lactating).

Side effects

Side effects depend on the specific type of SSRI, but those most commonly reported are listed below:

Central nervous system

- anxiety
- dizziness
- drowsiness
- headache
- light-headedness
- nervousness
- tremors
- trouble sleeping

KEY TERMS

Metabolism—A series of chemical changes that break down food, medicine, and body tissue.

Monoamine oxidase inhibitor (MAOI)—An older type of antidepressant medicine.

Neurotransmitter—A substance that helps send messages between nerve cells.

Persistent pulmonary hypertension (PPHN)—A life-threatening disorder seen in newborn babies in which blood does not properly enter the lungs.

Tricyclic antidepressant (TCA)—An older group of antidepressants that were introduced in the 1960s. TCAs affect the activity of serotonin and another body chemical called norepinephrine.

Skin

- itching
- rash
- sweating

Gastrointestinal system

- anorexia nervosa (an eating disorder)
- changes in taste
- constipation
- diarrhea
- dry mouth
- indigestion
- nausea and vomiting

Reproductive system

- painful menstruation
- changes in sexual function, such as difficulty becoming aroused or reaching orgasm

Respiratory system

- sore throat
- upper respiratory infections

Other

- increased body temperature
- weakness
- weight loss

Forgetting to take several doses or stopping the drug suddenly can cause symptoms of withdrawal, which may include a flu-like feeling, nausea, headache, dizziness, and tiredness.

Interactions

Taking SSRIs together with other drugs that affect serotonin levels, such as **monoamine oxidase inhibitors (MAOIs)** or tricyclic antidepressants, can lead to a rare but life-threatening drug reaction called "serotonin syndrome." Symptoms of **serotonin syndrome** occur within minutes to hours, and may include high blood pressure, mental status changes, and increased body temperature (hyperthermia).

Taking SSRIs with the herbal remedy **St. John's wort** may also cause this reaction.

SSRIs may slow down the body's metabolism of many other drugs. The following drugs have also been reported to interact with SSRIs and, when taken together, may lead to dangerously high serotonin levels:

- antipsychotics
- benzodiazepines
- beta blockers
- calcium channel blockers
- cocaine
- codeine
- dextromethorphan
- fenfluramine
- levodopa
- pentazocine

Resources

BOOKS

Karch, Amy M. *2012 Lippincott's Nursing Drug Guide.* Baltimore, MD: Lippincott Williams & Wilkins, 2011.

Kasper, Dennis L., et al. *Harrison's Principles of Internal Medicine.* 17th ed. New York, NY: McGraw-Hill, 2008.

Marx, J., R. Hockberger, and R. Walls. *Rosen's Emergency Medicine: Concepts and Clinical Practice.* 7th ed. St. Louis, MO: Mosby, 2010.

ORGANIZATIONS

Mental Health America, 2000 N Beauregard St., 6th Fl., Alexandria, VA, 22311, (703) 684-7722, (800) 969-6642, Fax: (703) 684-5968, http://www.nmha.org.

National Alliance on Mental Illness, 3803 N Fairfax Dr., Ste. 100, Arlington, VA, 22203, (703) 524-7600, http://www.nami.org.

National Institute of Mental Health, 6001 Executive Blvd., Rm. 8184, MSC 9663, Bethesda, MD, 20892-9663, (301) 433-4513, TTY: (301) 443-8431, Fax: (301) 443-4279, (866) 615-6464, TTY: (866) 415-8051, nimhinfo@nih.gov, http://www.nimh.nih.gov.

Kelli Miller Stacy

Self-control strategies

Definition

Self-control strategies are cognitive and behavioral skills used by individuals to maintain self-motivation and achieve personal goals. Initially the skills may be learned from a therapist, text, or self-help book. However, the individual is responsible for using these skills in real-life situations to produce the desired changes.

There are many varieties of self-control strategies. Other terms for self-control strategies are "behavioral self-control training," "cognitive self-regulation," and "self-management techniques." In recent years, the term "self-management" has replaced "self-control," because that term implies changing behavior through sheer willpower. Self-management, on the other hand, involves becoming aware of the natural processes that affect a particular behavior and consciously altering those processes, resulting in the desired behavior change.

Purpose

Most people who decide to use self-control strategies are dissatisfied with a certain aspect of their lives. For example, people may feel they smoke too much, **exercise** too little, or have difficulty controlling anger. Self-control strategies are useful for a wide range of concerns, including medical conditions (such as diabetes, chronic pain, asthma, arthritis, incontinence, or obesity), addictions (such as drug and alcohol abuse, smoking, gambling, or eating disorders), occupational issues (such as study habits, organizational skills, or job productivity), and psychological issues (such as **stress**, anxiety, **depression**, excessive anger, hyperactivity, or **shyness**). If symptoms are severe, self-control strategies may be used in conjunction with other therapies, but they should not be the only form of treatment.

The goal of self-control strategies is to reduce behavioral deficiencies or behavioral excesses. Behavioral deficiencies occur when an individual does not engage in a positive, desirable behavior frequently enough. The result is a missed future benefit. For example, a student who rarely studies might not graduate. Behavioral excesses occur when an individual engages in negative, undesirable behavior too often. This results in a negative consequence. For example, a person who smokes may develop lung cancer.

In the case of behavioral deficiencies, one may fail to engage in a desirable behavior because it does not provide immediate gratification. With behavioral excesses, there is usually some type of immediate gratification and no immediate negative consequence. Self-control strategies help individuals to become aware of their own patterns of behavior and to alter those patterns (usually by creating artificial rewards or punishments) so that the behavior will be more or less likely to occur.

Description

The description of self-control strategies may include the theoretical bases for self-control strategies, the development of a self-control program, and the types of self-control strategies.

Theoretical bases for self-control strategies

Self-control strategies are based primarily on the social cognitive theory of Canadian **psychologist** Albert Bandura (1925–). According to Bandura, one's behavior is influenced by a variety of factors, including one's own thoughts and beliefs, and elements in the environment. Bandura proposed that certain beliefs, self-efficacy, and outcome expectancies are important factors in determining which behaviors an individual will attempt, and how motivated the individual will be when engaging in those behaviors. Self-efficacy is one's belief about how well he or she can perform a given task, regardless of that person's actual ability. Outcome expectancies are what the person believes will happen as a result of engaging in a certain behavior. If self-efficacy and outcome expectancies are inaccurate, the individual may experience behavioral deficits or excesses.

Canadian psychotherapist Donald Meichenbaum developed the idea of self-instructional training, which is a major part of self-control strategies. Meichenbaum believed that learning to control behavior begins in childhood, based on parental instruction. Children eventually control their own behavior by mentally repeating the instructions of their parents. These internal instructions may be positive or negative. Self-instructional training teaches individuals to become aware of their self-statements, evaluate whether these self-statements are helpful or hindering, and replace maladaptive self-statements with adaptive ones.

American psychologist Frederick H. Kanfer (1925–2002) suggested that individuals achieve self-control by using a feedback loop consisting of continuous monitoring, evaluating, and reinforcing of their own behavior. This loop occurs naturally in everyone. However, the loop can be maladaptive if (a) only negative factors are noticed, and positive factors are ignored during the monitoring phase, (b) standards are unrealistic during the evaluation phase, or (c) responsibility is accepted for negative behaviors but not for positive behaviors during the **reinforcement** phase. Self-control strategies help individuals to be aware of these phases and to make the appropriate changes in monitoring, evaluation, and reinforcement.

Development of a self-control program

Self-control strategies are often taught in treatment centers, group or individual therapies, schools, or vocational settings. However, self-control programs may also be designed without the help of a professional, especially if the problem being addressed is not severe. The use of professionals, at least initially, may increase the likelihood that the program will succeed. Following are the necessary steps for creating a self-control program:

- Making a commitment. A plan cannot succeed unless one is committed to following through. Ways of increasing commitment level include listing the benefits of adhering to the program, telling others about one's intentions, posting written reminders of commitments around one's home, putting a significant amount of time and energy into designing the program, and planning ways to deal with obstacles ahead of time.
- Identifying the problem. The behavior in need of change is referred to as the "target behavior" or the "controlled behavior." A precise definition of the target behavior is a crucial first step. This is usually done by keeping detailed records about when, where, and how the behavior occurs, for one to two weeks. The record-keeping should also focus on other competing behaviors that may be interfering with the target behavior. For example, for a person who is trying to cut down on calorie consumption, a competing behavior would be to eat high-calorie snack foods. It is important to note the antecedents and consequences of the target and competing behaviors; in other words, what typically occurs immediately before (antecedents) and after (consequences) these behaviors? The antecedents and consequences are factors that influence the occurrence of the behavior. Sometimes just the process of record-keeping alters the target behavior by increasing the individual's awareness of what he or she is doing.
- Setting a goal. Once the target behavior has been defined, the individual must decide in what way that behavior should be changed. The goal should be specific so that future progress can be measured. This may entail listing circumstances or behaviors that must be present, as well the degree to which they must be present, in order for a goal to be achieved. For example, a goal to "reduce hyperactivity" in a grade-school student is vague. "Remaining in seat for seven

KEY TERMS

Depression—A psychiatric disorder involving feelings of hopelessness and symptoms of fatigue, sleeplessness, suicidal tendencies, and poor concentration.

Eating disorders—A number of medical conditions characterized by abnormal eating habits that can involve either the lack, or the excessive intake, of food, which results in physical and/or emotional stress. Two types of eating disorders include anorexia nervosa and bulimia nervosa.

Hyperactivity—Activities that are unusually active and restless, and without the person having the ability to concentrate for any extended period.

Stress—A physical and psychological response that results from being exposed to a demand or pressure.

out of fourteen half-hour periods daily" is much more specific. Indicating a period in which the goal can realistically be achieved is also recommended. Goals should be realistic. It is better to set a small goal and to progress to bigger goals than to set a big goal and become quickly discouraged.

- Applying self-control strategies. The self-control strategies are known as "controlling behaviors." Choice of strategies will depend on the target behavior. Types of strategies are discussed later.
- Self-monitoring. While using the self-control strategies, one should continue to keep records regarding the occurrence of the target behavior. Keeping written records is essential for determining whether the strategies are effective. If one is gradually meeting the goal requirements, the strategies can be assumed to be effective. If little progress toward the goal is evident, either the strategies are being used incorrectly or the strategies are ineffective and should be changed. Self-monitoring can be done informally (for example, by making notes on an index card) or formally (for example, by using predesigned data sheets). In any case, self-monitoring should gather the necessary information but should not become too lengthy or complex. The individual will lose motivation to continue monitoring if the procedures are overly time-consuming or inconvenient.
- Making revisions as necessary. Based on the information gathered during self-monitoring, the individual decides if changes in the plan are necessary. One advantage of self-control programs is that the individual chooses the strategies that will work best for him or her. This freedom of choice increases the likelihood that the individual will adhere to the program. Therefore, self-control programs should always be flexible and adaptable.

Types of self-control strategies

Self-control strategies can be grouped into three broad categories:

ENVIRONMENTAL STRATEGIES. Environmental strategies involve changing times, places, or situations where one experiences problematic behavior. Examples include:

- changing the group of people with whom one socializes
- avoiding situations or settings where an undesirable behavior is more likely to occur
- changing the time of day for participating in a desirable behavior to a time when one will be more productive or successful.

BEHAVIORAL STRATEGIES. Behavioral strategies involve changing the antecedents or consequences of a behavior. Examples include:

- increasing social support by asking others to work towards the same or a similar goal
- placing visual cues or reminders about goal in one's daily environment
- developing reinforcers (rewards) for engaging in desirable behaviors, or punishers for engaging in undesirable behaviors
- eliminating naturally occurring reinforcers for undesirable behavior
- engaging in alternative, positive behaviors when one is inclined to engage in an undesirable behavior
- creating ways to make a desirable behavior more enjoyable or convenient
- scheduling a specific time to engage in a desirable behavior
- writing a behavioral contract to hold oneself accountable for carrying out the self-control program.

COGNITIVE STRATEGIES. Cognitive strategies involve changing one's thoughts or beliefs about a particular behavior. Examples include:

- using self-instructions to cue oneself about what to do and how to do it
- using self-praise to commend oneself for engaging in a desirable behavior

- thinking about the benefits of reaching one's goal
- imagining oneself successfully achieving a goal or using imagery to distract oneself from engaging in an undesirable behavior
- substituting positive self-statements for unproductive, negative self-statements.

In a therapeutic setting, self-control strategies are usually taught in weekly group sessions over a period of several weeks. The sessions typically include an educational lecture regarding a specific strategy, group discussion of how the strategy should be applied and how to cope with potential obstacles (**relapse prevention**), role-playing or rehearsal of the strategy, a review of the session, and a homework assignment for further practice. Sessions usually focus on one strategy at a time. Preferably, an individual should master one strategy before attempting another. After the series of training sessions are complete, the individual is responsible for implementing the strategies in daily life.

QUESTIONS TO ASK YOUR DOCTOR

- Will self-control strategies help me?
- What should I do if self-control strategies do not solve my problem?
- Should I tell my friends and family before starting a self-control strategy?
- Will this type of training help me with other concerns?
- Is it difficult to use a self-control strategy?
- Should medication be used, too?
- Will related support groups help me?
- How long should I use a self-control strategy?
- Is it very expensive?

Preparation

Individuals must prepare for the use of a self-control strategy because knowledge and skills must be learned in order to produce the desired results.

Aftercare

Relapse is a concern in any therapeutic situation. Current research suggests that individuals are more likely to continue using newly learned self-control strategies if they have periodic follow-up contact with a professional or other designated person. The contact serves at least three purposes: (1) a source of accountability, (2) review of strategy use to ensure proper application, and (3) discussion of problematic situations and development of plans to overcome these situations.

Risks

Self-control strategies are especially prone to short-circuiting of contingencies. This refers to the tendency for individuals to partake of reinforcers at inappropriate occasions, or to avoid punishers designated in their plan. If contingencies are short-circuited, the desired behavior change is unlikely to occur.

Relapse is another risk involved in self-control strategies. Causes of relapse include:

- a poorly defined target behavior (progress cannot be recognized)
- unrealistic or long-term goals without immediate sources of reinforcement
- failure to anticipate and plan for obstacles to goal-achievement
- overreaction to occasional setbacks
- negative self-talk, especially when one feels that goals are not being satisfactorily met
- failure to use desirable or frequent reinforcers
- ineffective consequences for undesirable behavior
- an inaccurate or unnecessarily complex monitoring system.

Results

Results of self-control strategies vary widely based on individual use.

Normal results

Ideally, individuals will use self-control strategies independently in their everyday surroundings to meet their designated goals. They will decrease behavioral deficiencies and excesses, engaging in desirable behaviors more often, or engaging in undesirable behaviors less frequently or not at all.

Abnormal results

If the self-control strategies are ineffective or used improperly, individuals might not show any changes or may show increases in behavioral deficiencies or excesses.

Resources

BOOKS

Dobson, Keith S., ed. *Handbook of Cognitive-Behavioral Therapies.* 3rd ed. New York City: Guilford Press, 2010.

Martin, Garry, and Joseph Pear. *Behavior Modification: What It Is and How to Do It.* 9th ed. Boston: Prentice Education/ Allyn & Bacon, 2011.

Miltenberger, Raymond G. *Behavior Modification: Principles and Procedures.* 4th ed. Belmont, CA: Thomson Wadsworth, 2008.

PERIODICALS

"Frederick H. Kanfer, 76." *Chicago Tribune* (November 16, 2002). http://articles.chicagotribune.com/2002-11-16/news/0211160183_1_psychology-behavior-master-s-and-doctorate-degrees (accessed January 3, 2011).

OTHER

Ove R. Myrseth, Kristian, and Ayelet Fishbach. "Self-Control: A Function of Knowing When and How to Exercise Restraint." Booth School of Business, University of Chicago. http://faculty.chicagobooth.edu/ayelet.fishbach/research/cdir.pdf (accessed January 3, 2011).

WEBSITES

"Donald Meichenbaum, PhD (biography)." Institute for the Advancement of Human Behavior. http://www.iahb.org/html/meichenbaum.html (accessed January 3, 2011).

"Dr. Albert Bandera (biography)." University of Alberta. http://www.psych.ualberta.ca/~gcpws/Bandura/Biography/Bandura_bio1.html (accessed January 3, 2011).

ORGANIZATIONS

American Psychotherapy Association, 2750 East Sunshine St., Springfield, MO, 65804, (417) 823-0173, (800) 205-9165, http://www.americanpsychotherapy.com.

Association for Behavioral Analysis International, 550 West Centre Ave., Ste. 1, Portage, MI, 49024, (269) 492-9310, Fax: (269) 492-9316, http://www.abainternational.org.

Beck Institute for Cognitive Therapy and Research, One Belmont Ave., Ste. 700, Bala Cynwyd, PA, 19004-1610, (610) 664-3020, Fax: (610) 664-4437, beckinst@gim.net, http://www.beckinstitute.org.

Cambridge Center for Behavioral Studies, PO Box 7067, Cummings Center, Ste. 340F, Beverly, MA, 01915, (978) 369-2227, http://www.behavior.org.

Cognitive-Behavioral Therapy Institute, 211 East 43rd St., Ste. 1500, New York City, NY, 10017, (212) 490-3590, http://www.cbtinstitute.com.

See also Behavior modification; Bibliotherapy; Cognitive-behavioral therapy; Cognitive retraining techniques; Guided imagery therapy; Rational emotive therapy; Social skills training

Sandra L. Friedrich, M.A.

Self-harm *see* **Self-mutilation**

Self-help groups

Definition

Self-help groups—also called mutual help or mutual aid groups—are composed of peers who share a similar mental, emotional, or physical problem, or who are interested in a focal issue, such as education or parenting. Historically, people banded together to improve their chances for survival by pooling their social and economic resources; however, contemporary groups are more likely to organize around a theme or problem.

Purpose

Most self-help groups are voluntary, nonprofit associations open to anyone with a similar need or interest; however, spin-off groups also exist to meet the needs of particular types of people; for example, the elderly, women, or specific ethnic groups. Usually, groups are led by peers, have an informal structure, and are free (except for small donations to cover meeting expenses). However, professionals of various kinds lead some self-help groups.

Description

In the past 30 years or so, the number of self-help organizations and groups operating in communities

Substance abuse treatment

In 2010, approximately 4.1 million persons aged 12 or older received treatment for substance abuse.

Locations and methods of treatment included:

Self-help groups	2.3 million treated
Outpatient rehabilitation program	1.7 million
Outpatient mental health center	999,000
Inpatient rehabilitation	986,000
Hospital inpatient	731,000
Private doctor's office	653,000
Hospital emergency room	467,000
Prison or jail	342,000

SOURCE: Substance Abuse and Mental Health Services Administration, Office of Applied Studies, *Results from the 2010 National Survey on Drug Use and Health: Summary of National Findings* (September 2011).

Report available online at http://oas.samhsa.gov/NSDUH/2k10NSDUH/2k10Results.htm. *(Table by PreMediaGlobal. © 2012 Cengage Learning.)*

throughout the United States has risen dramatically; some organizations operate in several countries, primarily in the developed world. One of the reasons for the rapid proliferation of groups focusing on health problems may be the advent of managed health care. For individuals with insurance plans offering limited mental health coverage, self-help groups are an economical way to find emotional and social support.

Self-help groups and therapy

Because of the peer-led, informal, and democratic (as opposed to hierarchical and medical) structure, health professionals consider self-help groups for mental or emotional problems to be an adjunct to therapy. While there are therapeutic aspects associated with participation—principally, intimacy as a result of self-disclosure, personal growth in response to others' role **modeling**, and erosion of **denial** as a result of social confrontation—the primary value of contemporary groups is in the mutual aid offered by members to one another. Although the nature of self-help groups is outside the medical realm, doctors and therapists see participation as a way to improve the outcome related to either ongoing or future formal treatment.

Another issue arguing against considering self-help groups as a type of therapy is that the variety of groups is extensive; groups available may include advocacy groups with a focus on legal or social remedies, groups organized around housing or employment needs, and groups focusing on racial or gender issues. Additionally, the self-help movement shares some characteristics with volunteerism and consumerism. In general, members who persevere have experience with other voluntary organizations and believe in the value of donating time and service; also, members may be thought of as consumers who participate in their own care and who have experience and knowledge of relevant goods and services.

Types of self-help groups

TWELVE-STEP GROUPS. The most popular type of self-help group is based on the 12 steps and 12 traditions of Alcoholics Anonymous (AA), founded in 1935. The 12 steps are a guide to recovery from alcoholism or **addiction**, whereas the 12 traditions are a code of ethics. AA and other 12-step programs are based on the spiritual premise that turning one's life and will over to a personally meaningful "higher power," such as God or Spirit, is the key to recovery. Another essential idea is that sobriety or recovery (not cure) depends on the admission of powerlessness with respect to alcohol or the substance(s) abused. This idea is offensive to critics of 12-step groups, but others believe that this admission accurately reflects the contemporary view of addiction as a disease. Furthermore, people with a familial, genetic vulnerability to addiction are particularly at risk. While some studies suggest that 20% of people suffering from alcoholism will experience remission without benefit of therapy or a 12-step group, most will suffer deteriorating health and dysfunctional, if not ruined, social relationships. In other words, most alcoholics need formal therapy or an informal self-help program to recover. While the dropout rate for AA groups during the first three months is high, alcoholics who persevere have a good chance of attaining and maintaining sobriety or abstinence. This is especially true if the person regularly attends a home group (90 meetings in the first 90 days, slowly diminishing to two or three times per week for years thereafter) and finds an experienced and sympathetic sponsor who also is in recovery.

In addition to AA and its sister organizations, Narcotics Anonymous (NA) and Cocaine Anonymous (CA), a number of 12-step organizations exist for a variety of disorders, including Gamblers Anonymous (GA), Schizophrenics Anonymous (SA), Emotions Anonymous (EA), and Overeaters Anonymous (OA).

HEALTH PROBLEMS AND DISEASES. Self-help organizations also provide support for individuals struggling with the physical and emotional effects of life-threatening or chronic health problems. For example, support exists for people coping with weight management, human immunodeficiency virus/acquired immune deficiency syndrome (HIV/AIDS), multiple sclerosis, muscular dystrophy, cancer, incontinence, and for the families of individuals who suffer from these conditions. Also, support exists for people who share interests or circumstances, such as groups for women who breastfeed (LaLeche League), singles, older adults, and new parents.

Self-help groups for family members of the afflicted person are available, offering support to those whose loved ones may be ill, addicted, or distressed. Family members may unwittingly reinforce illness or addictive behaviors, or may need help coping with the person in distress. Al-Anon, an organization for friends and families of alcoholics, is a companion organization to AA, as is Alateen, a program for teenagers who have been hurt by the alcoholism of significant people in their lives. **Support groups** for caregivers of individuals with life-threatening or terminal illnesses, such as cancer, often meet at treatment centers and hospitals. One popular club for people with cancer, as well as for their friends and family, is Gilda's Club, founded by actor/comedian Gene Wilder

(1933–), Gilda Radner's widower. Gilda Radner (1946–1989), the well-known actress/comedian from *Saturday Night Live*, died at age 42 from ovarian cancer. Gilda's Clubs joined with the Wellness Community to become the Cancer Support Community on June 1, 2011, with clubs all over the world.

ONLINE GROUPS AND CLEARINGHOUSES. A growing trend in the self-help movement is the online support communities, as well as online resource centers and clearinghouses. Chat rooms, bulletin boards, and electronic mailing lists all provide convenient, around-the-clock access to peer support. Many large-scale consumer healthcare websites provide forums for discussions on numerous diseases and disorders, and major online commercial services, such as Google (http://www.google.com/Top/Society/Support_Groups/), provide sites for health care and patient support. In some cases, professionals moderate online groups, although many are exclusively organized and populated by peers. There are self-help groups, such as LaLeche League, that hold some meetings online, often at their own websites.

Features of self-help groups

ACCESSIBILITY. Accessibility and economy are appealing features of self-help groups. Since the groups are free, organizations such as AA and NA are very cost-effective. In addition, meetings are easy to locate through local newspaper announcements, hospitals, health care centers, churches, school counselors, and community agencies. For AA and sister organizations that encourage frequent attendance, hundreds of meetings may be held each week in large metropolitan areas. Furthermore, with the proliferation of online support communities and growth of connectivity to the Internet, self-help groups are becoming as accessible for individuals in rural areas as they are for those in large cities.

ANONYMITY. An important characteristic of 12-step groups is the preservation of anonymity by revealing first names only and by maintaining strict confidentiality of personal details and experiences shared during meetings. Online self-help groups offer even more anonymity since the exchanges are not face-to-face. The virtual anonymity of online experience helps to reduce social discomfort and discrimination, or stereotyping otherwise associated with real-life perceptions of age, disabilities, race, gender, or culture.

SOCIAL SUPPORT AND MUTUAL AID. Self-help groups provide an intact community and a sense of belonging. The social support and mutual aid available in a group may be critical to recovery, rehabilitation, or healthy coping. This is especially true for socially isolated people or people from dysfunctional families, who may have little or no emotional support. Participating in a social network of peers reduces social and emotional isolation and supports healthy behavior. Group members can offer unconditional support and, collectively, are a repository of helpful experiential knowledge.

SELF-ESTEEM AND SELF-EFFICACY. Self-help groups promote self-esteem or self-respect by encouraging reciprocal caring; the concept of self-efficacy, or the belief that one is capable, is promoted by reinforcing appropriate behavior and beliefs and by sharing relevant information regarding the disease or condition. For example, there may be an exchange of information regarding how to cope with failed or disrupted relationships, about what is reasonable to expect from healthcare professionals, about how to manage pain or public embarrassment, about where to go and to whom for a variety of needs. In groups such as AA, self-efficacy also is promoted by sponsors who act as mentors and role models, and by encouraging rotating leadership roles.

INTROSPECTION AND INSIGHT. Introspection, or contemplation, is another fundamental feature of many self-help groups, particularly for groups that follow a 12-step program of recovery. For example, the fourth step of AA states that members make "a searching and fearless moral inventory" of themselves, and the tenth step states that members continue "to take personal inventory" and admit wrongdoing. Introspection is particularly beneficial to individuals who are not entirely aware of the moral repercussions of and motivation for their behavior. In a sense, working through some of the 12 steps resembles the cognitive restructuring learned in **cognitive-behavioral therapy** (CBT), as maladaptive ideas and behaviors are transformed.

SPIRITUAL RECOVERY. The final step in a 12-step program recognizes that recovery entails a spiritual awakening; furthermore, recovering addicts are enjoined to spread the message to others suffering from addiction. Recovery depends on giving up both injurious self-will and denial of maladaptive behavior, and turning to a higher power. Members are urged to seek guidance or inspiration from this higher power. For many addicts, the key to recovery is a spiritually guided movement away from self-centeredness or self-absorption, and a turning towards the "power greater than ourselves" through prayer and **meditation**.

ADVOCACY. Some self-help groups meet to advocate or promote social and legislative remedies with respect to the issue of concern. For example, HIV/AIDS groups have lobbied for improved access to prescription drugs. Groups lobby for reforms by identifying key legislators and policy makers; they submit papers or suggestions for more equitable laws and policies to these key people. They also

KEY TERMS

Anorexia nervosa—An eating disorder highlighted by a person's denial of a healthy body weight, distortion of their outward appearance, and steadfast refusal to eat much food for a fear that they may gain weight.

Cognitive behavioral techniques—A type of therapy that are used to solve problems concerning dysfunctional behaviors (responses), emotions (feelings) and cognitions (abilities to gather knowledge) through a proven systematic set of procedures.

Cognitive therapy—A type of psychiatric treatment involving the treatment of anxiety and/or depression, which encourages patients to confront their problems in order to improve their behavior.

Eating disorders—A number of medical conditions characterized by abnormal eating habits that can involve either the lack, or the excessive intake, of food, which results in physical and/or emotional stress. Two types of eating disorders include anorexia nervosa and bulimia nervosa.

Schizophrenia—A mental disorder involving degraded thinking and emotions.

conduct public education programs (including programs meant to redress the harm of stigmatization). There are groups that advocate for more funds for research and for improved services for people who suffer from one of many diseases or mental disorders. The most important grassroots organization of families and consumers of psychiatric services (former or current patients) is the National Alliance on Mental Illness (NAMI). This organization was founded in 1979, and blends self-help with advocacy efforts for the improvement of research, services, and public awareness of major mental illnesses. Their advocacy efforts target both the federal and state levels.

Preparation

Someone preparing to join a self-help group is advised to learn as much as possible before actually attending a meeting. The more knowledge gained before using a self-help group, the more likely the experience will be positive.

Aftercare

Although individuals may not remain active in self-help groups after recovering from their condition, such groups remain open in aftercare, in case of a **relapse** or other such problems or concerns. For instance, an individual dealing with alcoholism may leave an alcohol rehabilitation program and return to a normal life. However, such sober individuals may return for support activities provided by self-help groups on a periodic basis.

Risks

Risks are always present in self-help groups. However, such help is usually welcomed by individuals needing support from a group so they do not have to deal with their problem alone.

Advocacy versus mutual aid

In some organizations, there is a growing overlap between self-help efforts and community development. Critics maintain that focusing on issues such as crime prevention, affordable housing, and economic development drains time and effort from social support and mutual aid. Nevertheless, some organizations continue to develop both advocacy and support.

Lack of professional involvement

The absence of professional guidance may mean that a member in need of formal **psychotherapy** or treatment may be discouraged from seeking professional help. On the other hand, too much professional involvement in the group may compromise the quality of mutual aid.

The "thirteenth step"

There is a well-known risk associated with attending 12-step groups termed the "thirteenth step." Women new to the groups, especially young women, are at their most vulnerable in the early stages of recovery. Male sexual predators who attend meetings take advantage of the atmosphere of intimacy and mutual trust. To cope with the possibility of sexual exploitation, young females are encouraged to attend meetings with a family member or a trusted adult, and all women are encouraged to find a same-sex sponsor.

Substituting addictions

The early months of a 12-step program are especially difficult. Typically, an addict in early recovery either replaces an addictive substance with a new one, or intensifies his/her concurrent use of another substance.

It is not uncommon for people who are chemically dependent to also have an addictive sexual disorder. (When someone is addicted to sex, there is an intense desire to gratify sexual urges and fantasies or to behave

QUESTIONS TO ASK YOUR DOCTOR

- Will a self-help group help me?
- What should I do if participation in a self-control group does not solve my problem?
- Should I tell my friends and family before starting a self-help group?
- Will this type of training help me with other concerns?
- Is it difficult to be involved with a self-help group?
- Will other related support groups help me in my particular case?
- How long should I be actively involved with a self-help group?
- Is it very expensive?

in ways that cause clinically significant distress; sexual indulgence, often compulsive, is a major disruptive force with respect to social relationships.) In one four-year study of a treatment program, 33% of the chemically addicted patients also were sexually compulsive. Some physicians believe that the predatory "thirteenth step" is evidence of turning from one addiction to another—in this case, addictive sexual disorder.

Members at varying stages of recovery

Another common risk is associated with the varying levels of recovery in a self-help group—that of being actively involved in the abuse of alcohol and/or drugs. Newcomers need to realize that not all members are interested in supporting their recovery, and that people in later stages of recovery may be more reliable. Furthermore, some members are required to attend by disciplinary entities, such as employers or correctional authorities.

Ongoing meetings

One criticism of self-help groups, especially 12-step groups, is that in the eyes of families and friends, members who persevere and attend the meetings seem to become "addicted" to the program. However, physicians who support self-help groups point out that since addiction is a disease, addicts are particularly vulnerable to relapse, and that ongoing involvement with a self-help community surely is better than suffering the recurring misery associated with active addiction.

Alternatives to 12-step groups

For addicts who find the spirituality of 12-step groups offensive and irrational, and who believe that public proclamation of powerlessness at group meetings is demoralizing, alternative groups exist. For example, a well-known organization, Rational Recovery (RR), is based on the cognitive-behavioral principles of American **psychologist** Albert Ellis (1913–2007). RR emphasizes self-reliance, rational thinking as a result of cognitive restructuring, and the development of a new repertoire of behaviors to respond effectively to events that trigger relapse.

Results

Worldwide, self-help groups are becoming increasingly popular. They are effective in providing mutual support and are good resources for finding needed information. However, when searching for an appropriate group prospective members should ask their friends, physicians, and counselors for references, and then visit a few groups before deciding on which one to attend. Also, information clearinghouses on the Internet are a good first step.

See also Co-occurring disorders; Depression; Disease concept of chemical dependency; Gambling disorder; Group therapy; Polysubstance dependence; Substance abuse and related disorders

Resources

BOOKS

Bloch, Douglas. *Healing from Depression: 12 Weeks to a Better Mood (A Body Mind, and Spirit Recovery Program).* Fort Worth, FL: Nicolas-Hays, 2009.

Brown, Louis, and Scott Wituk, ed. *Mental Health Self-Help: Consumer and Family Driven Initiates.* New York City: Springer, 2010.

Dobson, Keith S., ed. *Handbook of Cognitive-Behavioral Therapies.* 3rd ed. New York City: Guilford Press, 2010.

Gottlieb, Richard, ed. *The Complete Directory for People with Chronic Illness: Condition, Descriptions, Associations, Publications, Research Centers, Support Groups, Websites.* Amenia, NY: Grey House, 2009.

Humphreys, Keith. *Circles of Recovery: Self-help Organizations for Addictions.* Cambridge, UK: Cambridge University Press, 2004.

Martin, Garry, and Joseph Pear. *Behavior Modification: What It Is and How to Do It.* 9th ed. Boston: Prentice Education/ Allyn & Bacon, 2011.

Miltenberger, Raymond G. *Behavior Modification: Principles and Procedures.* 4th ed. Belmont, CA: Thomson Wadsworth, 2008.

Schenker, Mark D. *A Clinician's Guide to 12-step Recovery.* New York City: W. W. Norton, 2009.

WEBSITES

"Self-Help Group Sourcebook Online." American Self-Help Group Clearinghouse. http://www.mentalhelp.net/selfhelp (accessed January 4, 2011).

ORGANIZATIONS

Al-Anon/Alateen, 1600 Corporate Landing Pkwy., Virginia Beach, VA, 23454-5617, (757) 563-1600, Fax: (757) 563-1655, http://www.al-anon.alateen.org.

Alcoholics Anonymous, PO Box 459 (11th Fl., 475 Riverside Dr. at W 120th St., New York City, 10115), New York, NY, 10163, (212) 870-3400, http://www.alcoholics-anonymous.org.

American Psychotherapy Association, 2750 E Sunshine St., Springfield, MO, 65804, (417) 823-0173, (800) 205-9165, http://www.americanpsychotherapy.com.

Association for Behavioral Analysis International, 550 W Centre Ave., Ste. 1, Portage, MI, 49024, (269) 492-9310, Fax: (269) 492-9316, http://www.abainternational.org.

Cancer Support Community (formerly Gilda's Club), 1050 17th St. NW, Washington, DC, 20036, (202) 659–9709, Toll Free: (888) 793-9355, Fax: (202) 974-7999, http://cancersupportcommunity.org.

Cocaine Anonymous, 21720 S Wilmington Ave., Ste. 304 or PO Box 492000, Long Beach or Los Angeles, CA, 90810-1641 or 90049-8000, (310) 559-5833, Fax: (310) 559-2554, cawso@ca.org, http://www.ca.org.

Emotions Anonymous, PO Box 4245, St. Paul, MN, 55104-0245, (651) 647-9712, Fax: (651) 647-1593, http://www.emotionsanonymous.org.

Gamblers Anonymous, PO Box 17173, Los Angeles, CA, 90017, (213) 386-8789, Fax: (213) 386-0030, http://www.alcoholics-anonymous.org.

LaLeche League, 957 North Plum Grove Rd., Schaumburg, IL, 60173, (847) 519-7730, (800) LALECHE (525-3243), Fax: (847) 969-0460, http://www.llli.org.

Narcotics Anonymous, PO Box 9999, Van Nuys, CA, 91409, (818) 773-9999, Fax: (818) 700-0700, http://www.na.org.

National Alliance on Mental Illness, 3803 N Fairfax Dr., Ste. 100, Arlington, VA, 22203, (703) 524-7600, (800) 950-NAMI (6264), Fax: (703) 524-9094, http://www.nami.org.

National Mental Health Consumers' Self-Help Clearinghouse, 1211 Chestnut St., Ste. 1207, Philadelphia, PA, 19107, (215) 751-1810, (800) 553-4539, Fax: (215) 636-6312, info@mhselfhelp.org, http://mhselfhelp.org.

Overeaters Anonymous, PO Box 44020 (6075 Zenith Ct. NE), Rio Rancho, NM, 87174-4020 (87144-6424), (505) 891-2664, Fax: (505) 891-4320, http://www.oa.org.

Rational Recovery, Box 800, Lotus, CA, 95651, (530) 621-2667, Fax: (530) 621-4374, https://rational.org/index.php?id=1.

Schizophrenics Anonymous, http://www.schizophrenia.com.

Tanja Bekhuis, Ph.D.
Paula Ford-Martin, M.A.
Stephanie N. Watson

Self-mutilation

Definition

Self-mutilation, a feature of self-harm or self-injury, is defined as intentional injury to one's own body tissues without an accompanying conscious intention to commit **suicide**. Although this behavior can appear similar to a suicide attempt, the phrase "deliberate self harm" is preferred to "suicide attempt" because the reasons and motivation behind self-harm or mutilation are generally quite different from those that underlie attempted suicide. Self-mutilation is considered a coping mechanism, although not a positive one.

Self-mutilation and self-harm are not explicitly listed as disorders in the 2000 edition of the ***Diagnostic and Statistical Manual of Mental Disorders***, also known as the *DSM*, although some clinicians argue that they should be listed under the category of **impulse control disorders**. The 2000 edition (the fourth edition, text revision, also known as *DSM-IV-TR*) mentions self-injury as a symptom or criterion for **diagnosis** of **borderline personality disorder** (BPD); **stereotypic movement disorder**, which can be a comorbidity of **autism** or intellectual disability; and **factitious disorder** (specifically factitious disorder with predominantly physical signs and symptoms), in which the person fakes a physical illness. For example, the self-mutilation behavior in factitious disorder might involve pulling out one's hair or purposely exacerbating a healing wound

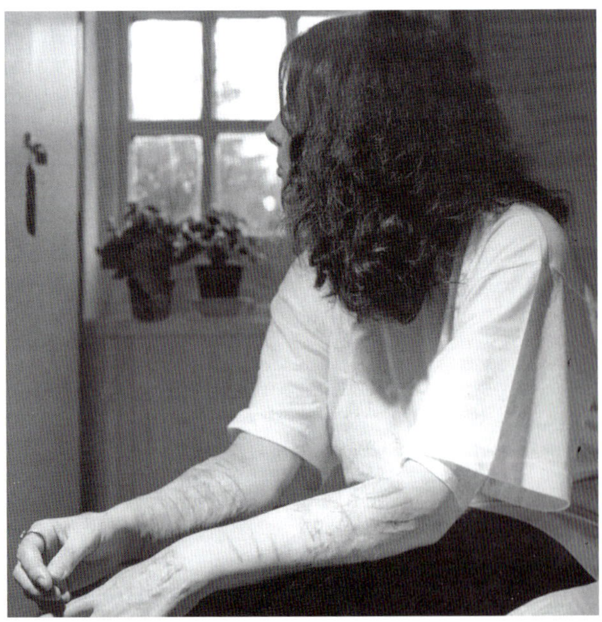

Woman with scars from self-mutilation. *(© Photofusion Picture Library/Alamy)*

to mimic disease symptoms. Self-harm, including self-mutilation, also can be associated with other disorders listed in the *DSM-IV*, including **post-traumatic stress disorder** (PTSD).

Demographics

The incidence of self-harm has received more attention in clinical populations rather than in community or nonclinical groups. Groups at risk of self-harm include depressed adolescents, those experiencing an interpersonal crisis, and those who have done it before. Although reported incidence in the research literature can vary from study to study, there is some overlap. Some studies report a rate of 4% in the general adult population and 21% in the adult clinical population. Adolescents make up the group at greatest risk: In the community, rates have been reported ranging from 14 to 39% of respondents and a range of 14 to 21% among high school students; in adolescent psychiatric inpatient samples, rates are as high as 40 to 61%. Studies have identified self-harm behaviors in 4% of military recruits and 14 to 35% of psychology students at public universities. Research indicates that self-mutilating behavior occurs among nonclinical populations at higher rates than previously thought.

Rates of frequent self-mutilation activity are significantly higher among lesbian and bisexual women, and the behavior was long thought to be more prevalent among females, although recent findings indicate a similar prevalence in both sexes. Although the function of self-mutilation usually differs from the motivations underlying a suicide attempt, one study suggests that 20 to 45% of those who engage in self-harm think about suicide. In addition, someone who experiences one episode of self-harm may be likely to engage in another: As many as 30% of adolescents who report a previous incident of self-harm will do it again.

Description

Self-mutilation can take different forms and have different functions depending on the individual. In some nonpsychiatric subpopulations, self-mutilation is a sanctioned activity; for example, in some adolescents, mutilation of tissues is socially acceptable and done in a group or to gain acceptance from the group. Self-harm or self-mutilation may also accompany cognitive deficits or **psychosis**, and in the most severe expression of the practice can manifest as auto-castration or even self-immolation.

The focus here is self-mutilation that occurs in the absence of cognitive deficits or psychosis. What is known is that this behavior can be a manifestation of anguish that the person cannot otherwise express, or it can be a way for the person to cope with and relieve tension. In some cases, it has been construed as a method of self-punishment. In general, self-mutilation results in so little actual harm to the body that medical professionals and even family members often do not know that the mutilation is taking place. In addition, the person who engages in self-mutilation may go to great lengths to hide the resulting physical signs. The most common forms of self-mutilation are sticking the skin with needles, scratching, or cutting. Other forms of repetitive self-mutilation are punching or slapping the face, burning the skin, and swallowing harmful substances. Matthew Nock has published extensively on studies of self-harm and self-mutilation.

People who engage in self-mutilation often claim that it is accompanied by excitement and that it reduces or relieves such negative feelings as tension, anger, anxiety, **depression**, and loneliness. They also describe it as addictive. Self-mutilating behavior may occur in episodes, with periods of remission, or it may be continuous over a number of years. Characteristics commonly seen in persons with this disorder are perfectionism, dissatisfaction with one's physical appearance, and difficulty controlling and expressing emotions. Repetitive self-mutilation often worsens over time, resulting in increasingly serious forms of injury that may culminate in suicide.

Risk factors

General risk factors for self-mutilation include:

- History of sexual abuse or the death of a parent during childhood
- Parents who are perfectionistic or critical of the child's physical appearance
- Diagnosis of concurrent depression, PTSD, borderline personality disorder, or anxiety disorder
- Female sex
- Age between 12 and 25
- Lesbian or bisexual orientation
- Frequent and excessive use of drugs of abuse or alcohol

There is a correlation between self-harm and suicide attempts, feelings of hopelessness and other symptoms of depression, anxiety, external expectations of perfection, and most often, a history of **abuse**. Risk factors can be classified into two categories: environmental risk factors and individual risk factors. In addition, risk factors from one category can influence those of the other and vice versa.

Environmental risk factors

Some of the most commonly seen environmental risk factors in self-mutilation are associated with abuse experienced in childhood. Most research into the phenomenon of self-harm has focused on **sexual abuse**, but there are some indications that self-harm can also be associated with physical abuse and even emotional abuse, and it is strongly associated with low self-esteem. Almost any discussion about factors directly related to self-harm, however, is theoretical because of the paucity of actual experimental or empirical data.

In what may be a blurring of the distinction between socially sanctioned self-mutilation and the kind of self-mutilation discussed here, another risk factor for engaging in this behavior is awareness that others in one's peer group are doing it. **Substance abuse** also can be a contributing factor, and depression may lead someone to turn to self-mutilation as a coping mechanism. Perfectionism may also be a risk factor. Perfectionism consistently correlates with thoughts and behaviors related to self-injury.

Individual risk factors

The interaction of environmental factors and personal factors arises because of the individual ways in which people respond to environmental risk factors. Researchers have identified alexithymia, which is the inability to express feelings verbally, as an individual risk factor. The importance of this inability to express emotion as a risk factor in self mutilation is underscored by research that suggests that self-harmers who learn to express their feelings verbally decrease their self-harming behavior.

Causes and symptoms

The major cause of self-mutilation is the underlying motivation. Self-injury is closely linked to dysfunctions of emotional expression. For some who self mutilate, the physical pain of cutting or scratching provides a distraction from emotional pain. Others may use self mutilation as a way to punish themselves or relieve a feeling of evil, while for others the practice offers a relief from tension or a way to "feel real" through the physical pain or the visible evidence of physical injury. Causing physical pain to one's body through self mutilation may also provide an outlet for a person who has difficulty communicating emotions like anger or emotional pain. In addition, people who engage in self mutilation may be trying, either consciously or subconsciously, to alter the behavior of someone near them or seek help, although many people who self harm go to great lengths to conceal the signs of the behavior.

KEY TERMS

Borderline personality disorder (BPD)—A pattern of behavior characterized by impulsive acts, intense but chaotic relationships with others, identity problems, and emotional instability.

Comorbidity—The presence of one or more additional diseases or disorders in a patient diagnosed with a primary disorder.

Dissociation—A condition in which a person's thoughts, emotions, sensations, or memories become compartmentalized, usually as a result of a severe emotional trauma.

Impulse control disorders—A group of emotional disorders characterized by the repeated inability to refrain from performing a particular action that is harmful either to oneself or others.

The immediate triggers for self mutilation often center on some kind of interpersonal crisis. A person may have just experienced a separation from a partner, a major confrontation with a parent, or have just run away from home, for example.

The signs that a self-mutilation event has occurred are obvious, but less obvious are the symptoms that one will occur. A recent study found that individuals engaging in self-mutilating behavior usually thought about it for only a few minutes or even less time before completing the act; almost half reported not thinking about it at all before doing it. This association of impulsivity with self-mutilation may be related to the specific characteristics of the population studied, which was a group of adolescents who had previously self-mutilated. High levels of dissociation (a defense mechanism to isolate and protect the psyche from thoughts, emotions, or physical sensations that cause anxiety) may accompany self-mutilating behavior.

There are some signs that may precede an impulsive act of self-mutilation. These signs include trouble with parents, school, partners, or siblings; health problems; trouble with peers, including being bullied; depression; and low self esteem. Again, knowing that others in the peer group are doing it can also be a precipitating factor.

Diagnosis

Many cases of self-mutilation may never come to the attention of a clinician, parent, or caregiver. Often, identified self-mutilation has occurred in the context of a personality disorder, such as BPD. It may also appear as a manifestation of other psychiatric disorders, including substance abuse, **intermittent explosive disorder**, and eating disorders.

Self-mutilation and borderline personality disorder

For a person with BPD, self-mutilating behavior offers relief during a dissociative episode by functioning as an affirmation of the ability to feel or by relieving the person's personal feeling of being bad. Clinical populations with BPD have been the target of most studies focusing on self-harm, and in these populations, emotional vulnerability appears to play an important role in whether an individual will self-harm and in the development of BPD itself. Emotional vulnerability involves two aspects: emotional reactivity (high sensitivity to stimuli) and emotional intensity (extreme reactions to those stimuli). These factors are among the individual characteristics that might interact with environmental factors to elicit self-mutilating behaviors. Persons with BPD may have feel empty or detached to the point of anhedonia, an inability to experience pleasure from things that most people find pleasurable, such as eating good food. In addition, they may exhibit a narrow range of **affect**, the mood that a person displays to others. These signs of emotional inexpressivity may, according to some research, increase the possibility that a person with BPD will engage in self mutilating behavior.

Self-mutilation and suicide

Because self-mutilation can be interpreted as a cry for help, suicide can be a concern for those who become aware that an individual is self mutilating. Research suggests that there is a distinction between the risk of suicide and impulsive self-mutilation compared to self-mutilation that is deliberate and well thought out. Statistically, 20% to 25% of self harmers think about suicide, and the risk of suicide after self-harm ranges from 0.24% to 4.3%. Among the self-harming population, suicide risk factors include being an adolescent male, using a violent method of self-harm, and a history of inpatient treatment at a psychiatric facility. Some other features also are associated with conscious suicidal intent in a person who self-mutilates: self-mutilation performed alone; attempts to hide the behavior; preparations made for death, such as a plan for disposition of effects; or an act of self-harm that was planned considerably in advance (i.e., it was not impulsive).

Proposed diagnostic criteria for DSM-5

The fifth edition of *DSM,* known as *DSM-5,* may contain a new category for self-mutilation, called non-suicidal self injury (NSSI). The proposed criteria for NSSI are as follows:

- The person has on five or more days within the past year engaged in self-injury for purposes of inflicting pain (i.e., not tattooing or body piercing). The person does not intend to commit suicide, and the injury is more severe than minor wound-picking or nail biting.
- The self-injury is associated with at least two of the following four characteristics: negative thoughts preceding the act; a period of preoccupation with self-injury before the act that is difficult to resist; frequent urges to self-injure (which may or may not be acted out); and the self-injury has a purpose (relief from painful feelings or induction of positive feelings).
- The self-injury leads to significant distress or impairment in interpersonal, academic, or other important areas of functioning.
- The behavior is not associated with intoxication, psychosis, or delirium, and cannot be better accounted for by another physical or mental disorder.

The proposed criteria include two subtypes of NSSI, one in which individuals injure themselves fewer than five times per year but think about it often, and one in which the person may have suicidal intent as well as self-injury.

Examination

In some cases, an office examination will disclose physical evidence of self-mutilation, such as needle or burn marks, scars, or bruises. Another clue for the doctor is that the patient is wearing a long-sleeved shirt or long pants in hot weather. The patient may also acknowledge that he or she self-mutilates.

Tests

There are a number of questionnaires and inventories that can be administered in the examiner's office to determine whether the patient meets the criteria for BPD. In addition, a group of therapists in the United Kingdom has evaluated a possible new instrument for self-harming behaviors. There are, however, no laboratory tests (blood or urine samples) that can be used to either diagnose or rule out self-mutilation.

Treatment

Treatment for self-harming behavior tends to be psychological rather than physiological.

Traditional

Psychotherapy treatments for self mutilation include dialectical behavioral therapy, problem-solving therapy, and **cognitive-behavioral therapy**.

DIALECTICAL BEHAVIORAL THERAPY. Dialectical behavioral therapy is a relatively new approach developed by Marsha Linehan at the University of Washington. It focuses on teaching alternative ways to manage emotion and handle distress. The relationship between emotional inexpressivity and self-harm suggests that those who engage in self-mutilating behaviors to express emotions might benefit from a clinical approach involving tutoring in other methods of emotional expression. Dialectical behavioral therapy (DBT), which involves individual therapy and group skills training, was originally developed for individuals with BPD who engage in self-harm, but it is now used for self-harming individuals with a wide variety of other psychological issues, including eating disorders and substance dependence. Research indicates that the approach is helpful in reducing self-harm.

PROBLEM-SOLVING THERAPY. Problem-solving therapy involves developing and rehearsing coping strategies for the situations that may precipitate self harm. The approach can involve the entire family, using structured family interventions over five or six sessions. Focus is on improved cognitive and social skills to facilitate sharing feelings, controlling emotion, and family negotiation. Group treatment can also be a facet of problem-solving therapy. Briefly, this therapeutic approach identifies problems, prioritizes them, defines goals, and establishes and executes a strategy to achieve the goals, addressing any psychological issues that become obstacles along the way.

COGNITIVE-BEHAVIORAL THERAPY. In cases of self-mutilation accompanied by depression, a suggested approach is cognitive-behavioral therapy (CBT), which involves identifying patterns of destructive or negative behaviors or thinking and modifying them to be more realistic and pragmatic.

Other potential treatments for self mutilation in the context of other disorders include treatment for any substance abuse, anger management therapy, or environmental changes.

Drugs

There are no medications specifically indicated for self-injury. The doctor may, however, prescribe **antidepressants** to help the patient cope with strong feelings. The medications most often given to treat self-mutilation are the **selective serotonin reuptake inhibitors (SSRIs)**, which work by increasing the level of **serotonin** in the spaces (synapses) between nerve cells in the central nervous system. The SSRIs include **fluoxetine** (Prozac), **citalopram** (Celexa), **paroxetine** (Paxil), **fluvoxamine** (Luvox), and **sertraline** (Zoloft).

In extreme cases (such as when the patient's self-inflicted injuries are life-threatening), the doctor may recommend inpatient psychiatric treatment. Another option is a day hospital program.

QUESTIONS TO ASK YOUR DOCTOR

- I think my teenager is engaging in self-cutting. What steps should I take to get help?
- Have you ever treated an adolescent who engaged in self-mutilation? What was the outcome?
- What is your opinion of psychotherapeutic approaches to treatment for self-mutilation?
- What is your opinion of medications as treatment for impulse control disorders?

Prognosis

Some studies indicate that following self-harm, some adolescents see improvement in their relationship with their parents. In addition, research suggests that self-harm may result in more support from social networks. In terms of decreasing the incidence of self-harm, self-harmers who learn to express their feelings verbally see a decrease in self-mutilating behaviors.

Prevention

Due to the lack of research on the disorder, self mutilation remains a poorly understood phenomenon, and prevention measures have not been thoroughly explored. In addition, the mixed and varied development pathways that lead to self-harm may complicate efforts at prevention. The risk factors for self-harm are often associated with other pathologies, and an awareness of this association might be a potential aid in targeting prevention.

Specific preventive strategies include helping young people with a history of self-injury to expand their social networks; forming peer counseling groups; and educating adolescents about the effects of the mass media in encouraging self-injury.

Resources

BOOKS

Aboujaoude, Elias, and Lorrin M. Koran. *Impulse Control Disorders*. New York: Cambridge University Press, 2010.

American Psychiatric Association. *Diagnostic and Statistical Manual of Mental Disorders*. 4th ed., text rev. Washington, DC: American Psychiatric Association, 2000.

Black, Donald W., and Nancy C. Andreasen. *Introductory Textbook of Psychiatry.* 5th ed. Arlington, VA: American Psychiatric Publishing, 2011.

Favazza, Armando R. *Bodies under Siege: Self-mutilation, Nonsuicidal Self-injury, and Body Modification in Culture and Psychiatry.* 3rd ed. Baltimore: Johns Hopkins University Press, 2011.

Friedman, Lauri S., ed. *Self-mutilation.* Detroit, MI: Greenhaven Press, 2009.

Nock, Matthew, ed. *Understanding Nonsuicidal Self-Injury: Origins, Assessment, and Treatment.* Arlington, VA: American Psychological Association, 2009.

PERIODICALS

Dawood, A. W. "Medicolegal Aspects of 3 Cases of Bizarre Self-mutilation." *American Journal of Forensic Medicine and Pathology* 32 (March 2011): 35–38.

Evren, C., et al. "Self-mutilative Behaviours in Male Alcohol-dependent Inpatients and Relationship with Posttraumatic Stress Disorder." *Psychiatry Research* 186 (March 30, 2011): 91–96.

Hintikka, J., et al. "Mental Disorders in Self-Cutting Adolescents." *Journal of Adolescent Health* 44 (May 2009): 464–67.

Hulbert, C., and R. Thomas. "Predicting Self-injury in BPD: An Investigation of the Experiential Avoidance Model." *Journal of Personality Disorders* 24 (October 2010): 651–53.

Stein, D. J., et al. "Trichotillomania (Hair Pulling Disorder), Skin Picking Disorder, and Stereotypic Movement Disorder: Toward DSM-V." *Depression and Anxiety* 27 (June 2010): 611–26.

Vrouva, I., et al. "The Risk-taking and Self-harm Inventory for Adolescents: Development and Psychometric Evaluation." *Psychological Assessment* 22 (December 2010): 852–65.

WEBSITES

American Psychiatric Association. *DSM-5 Development.* "V 01 Non-Suicidal Self Injury." http://www.dsm5.org/proposedrevision/pages/proposedrevision.aspx?rid=443 (accessed September 8, 2011).

Massachusetts General Hospital for Children. "Self-Mutilation." http://www.massgeneral.org/children/adolescenthealth/articles/aa_self-mutilation.aspx (accessed September 8, 2011).

Mayo Clinic. "Self-injury/Cutting." http://www.mayoclinic.com/health/self-injury/DS00775 (accessed September 8, 2011).

Smith, Melinda, and Jeanne Segal. "Cutting and Self-Harm." Helpguide.org. August 2011. http://www.helpguide.org/mental/self_injury.htm (accessed September 8, 2011).

ORGANIZATIONS

American Psychiatric Association, 1000 Wilson Blvd., Ste. 1825, Arlington, VA, 22209-3901, (703) 907-7300, apa@psych.org, http://www.psych.org.

National Alliance on Mental Illness, 2107 Wilson Blvd., Ste. 300, Arlington, VA, 22201-3042, Fax: (703) 524-9094, (800) 950-6264, http://www.nami.org.

National Institute of Mental Health, 6001 Executive Blvd., Rm. 8184, MSC 9663, Bethesda, MD, 20892-9663, (301) 433-4513; TTY: (301) 443-8431, Fax: (301) 443-4279, (866) 615-6464; TTY: (866) 415-8051, nimhinfo@nih.gov, http://www.nimh.nih.gov.

Emily Jane Willingham, PhD
Rebecca J. Frey, PhD

Senior mental health

Definition

Senior mental health refers to the mental health of persons over the age of 65, including disorders and other mental health issues that are more common later in life. Senior mental health is a rapidly growing field of research and treatment due to the increased proportion of older adults in the general population worldwide.

Senior mental health issues are currently treated by a recognized subspecialty of psychiatry known as *geriatric psychiatry* or *geropsychiatry.* The American Board of Psychiatry and Neurology, which certifies doctors who choose to specialize in this field, established what was then called an "additional qualification" program for geriatric psychiatry in 1989. In 1997, the American Board of Medical Specialties (ABMS) formally renamed the program "Certification in the Subspecialty of Geriatric Psychiatry." As of 2011, psychiatrists in this subspecialty must complete a one-year fellowship in geriatric psychiatry following a four-year residency in general psychiatry and must pass a lengthy written and oral examination.

Demographics

In the United States, longer life expectancy coupled with the size of the post–World War II "baby boomer" generation (76 million people) means that the number of adults over 65 will swell from 13% of the population in 2000 to 20% by 2030. During the same period, the number of older adults with mental illness is expected to double to 15 million. Adults over the age of 85 are currently the fastest-growing segment of the U.S. population.

Women comprise the majority of older adults in Canada and the United States. At age 65, there are 118 women for every 100 men. At age 85, there are 241 women for every 100 men. The proportion of minorities among older adults is also increasing; minorities are expected to account for 25% of seniors in 2030, up from 16% in 1998.

Specialists maintain that mental illness in general is underreported and underdiagnosed in older adults in North America. Nearly 20% of persons 55 years and older experience mental disorders that are not part of normal aging; the most common of these are mood disorders and cognitive impairment. In particular, the rate of **suicide** among seniors is higher than that of any other age group; the rate of suicide among adults 85 and older is twice the national average. In terms of ethnicity, Caucasian seniors have the highest rate of suicide, followed by Asian Americans, Hispanics, and African Americans.

Description

Mental health care for older adults is complicated by several factors that do not affect younger adults as often. The first factor is physical changes, including the effects of aging on sense perception, particularly hearing, sight, and taste. The loss of keenness of sense perception often means that the elderly do not enjoy certain activities as much as they once did, such as dining out; playing, singing, or listening to music; and painting, drawing, or other forms of art. Other changes that affect older adults' outlook on life include problems with sleep, difficulty coping with change, and increased vulnerability to physical injuries from falls or automobile accidents.

Another factor affecting care is the difficulty of prescribing medications for mood disorders or other mental health issues that will not cause problematic interactions with drugs given to treat the physical disorders prevalent in older adults. These conditions include type 2 diabetes, high blood pressure, arthritis, heart disease, cancer, and Parkinson's disease. The practice of taking many different prescription drugs is called *polypharmacy,* and it is more common among the elderly than in any other segment of the population.

A third factor is the social and geographical isolation of many seniors. Older adults must cope with **bereavement** and **grief** more often than younger people. In addition, the loss of a spouse or friends may make getting to regular appointments for mental health care difficult. There are currently 20 million drivers over the age of 65 on American roads, with this number expected to double by 2020. Many older adults, however, often give up driving based on health conditions, loss of eyesight, or recommendations from law enforcement officers, family members, or primary care physicians. Having to stop driving represents a significant loss of independence for many older adults and can worsen **depression** or other mood disorders, as well as complicating access to mental health care.

The mental health issues that are most common among seniors include **anxiety disorders**, **dementia** and Alzheimer's disease, **late-life depression**, suicide, alcoholism, and **substance abuse**.

Anxiety disorders

It is estimated that 11.4% of adults over age 55 meet criteria for an anxiety disorder each year in the United States and Canada. Worries over health, finances, and maintaining independence are common triggers of anxiety disorders in older adults. In contrast to younger people, however, the most common anxiety disorders in seniors are phobias rather than **panic disorder** or **obsessive-compulsive disorder**. **Generalized anxiety disorder** (GAD) is much more common among younger adults than in seniors, although it may develop in an older adult after he or she is diagnosed with diabetes, heart disease, or another chronic physical disorder.

An increasingly common sign of anxiety among older adults is **hoarding**. While hoarding behavior typically begins in late childhood or adolescence, it usually worsens with age and may reach a critical point in adults over 50.

With regard to treatment, seniors do not respond as well to antianxiety medications as younger people; they usually experience some symptom relief but not the complete elimination of anxiety. Older adults are usually managed on lower doses of these medications than younger patients.

Cognitive impairment

The most common form of dementia among older adults is **Alzheimer's disease** (AD). AD affects about 4.5 million people in the United States alone, and that number is projected to exceed 13 million by the year 2050. It is thought that nearly 10% of all people over age 65, and that up to half of those over age 85 have Alzheimer's disease or another form of dementia. The symptoms of dementia affect about 5% of adults aged 65 to 74 and 40% of those older than 85. About 19 million Americans have a family member with AD or another dementing illness.

Other dementing illnesses that affect older adults include **vascular dementia**, Lewy body dementia, frontotemporal dementia, and dementia associated with HIV infection. Dementia may also accompany Parkinson's disease, Huntington's disease, Creutzfeldt-Jakob disease, and late-stage syphilis. It is possible for a patient to suffer from more than one type of dementia.

KEY TERMS

Dementia—A chronic, global, usually irreversible loss of memory and other aspects of cognition.

Lewy body dementia—A type of dementia characterized by the presence of abnormal sphere-shaped clumps of protein in nerve cells in the brain.

Polypharmacy—The use of a number of different medications by the same patient. Polypharmacy is most common among the elderly and those taking psychiatric medications.

Depression

Depression in older adults is widely misunderstood. On the one hand, there are many aspects of aging, such as bereavement, loss of physical strength, and the appearance or worsening of chronic illness that contribute to "blue" moods or sadness in seniors. However, the assumption that clinical depression is a "normal" or inevitable part of aging is incorrect. The actual rate of major depression in the general population declines with age, although depressive symptoms are more common in older adults. An estimated 6% of Americans aged 65 and older (about two million persons) develop a diagnosable depressive illness each year. Ironically, major depression among seniors is underdiagnosed and undertreated; one study reported that only 11% of depressed seniors in primary care receive adequate antidepressant treatment, with 34% receiving inadequate treatment and 55% receiving no treatment at all.

Major depression in the elderly can be difficult to diagnose because it can mimic the early signs of dementia or Parkinson's disease; it may also coexist with substance abuse disorders or such chronic physical illnesses as thyroid disorders. An older adult with depressive symptoms should be evaluated by a neurologist as well as a geriatric **psychiatrist** to make sure that major depression is adequately diagnosed and treated. One recent development in nonpharmacological treatments of depression in seniors is the growing recognition that cognitive dysfunction needs to be addressed as well as the emotional symptoms of the disorder.

Suicide

As noted above, suicide is a growing problem among older Americans, particularly in men and those over 85 years of age. Research conducted by the **National Institute of Mental Health** (NIMH) indicates that the following additional factors increase a senior's risk of suicide:

- white race; Asian men, Hispanic men, and African American men are less likely to attempt or commit suicide than Caucasians
- a family history of suicide
- a history of previous suicide attempts
- being a frontline combat veteran
- a history of abuse in childhood
- recent stressful events, such as separation or divorce; job loss or financial difficulty; or death of spouse, partner, friend, or pet
- medical illness, especially terminal illness
- pain, particularly chronic, severe, or intractable pain
- loss of mobility or independence
- alcohol or substance abuse, which can weaken impulse control
- presence of a psychiatric illness

More than 90% of Americans, including seniors, who commit suicide have a significant mental illness. Major depression accounts for 60% of all suicides. Other mental disorders that increase the risk of suicide among seniors include **schizophrenia**, alcoholism, substance abuse, **borderline personality disorder**, Huntington's disease, and epilepsy.

Protective factors that lower a senior's risk of suicide include:

- a significant friendship network
- religious faith and practice; older African American women have a particularly low rate of suicide because of their high rate of church membership
- a stable marriage or close-knit extended family
- a strong interest in, or commitment to, a project or cause that brings people together, such as community service, neighborhood associations, book clubs, hobby groups, other activity groups.

Although seniors are less likely to attempt suicide than younger people, according to the National Strategy for Suicide Prevention (NSSP), they are more likely than younger persons to use highly lethal means of suicide. According to a Canadian study, seniors are most likely to use firearms to commit suicide, followed by hanging, self-poisoning, and leaping from heights.

Alcohol and substance abuse

Alcohol and substance abuse are greater problems among seniors than many people recognize. The National Institute on Alcohol Abuse and Alcoholism (NIAAA) estimates that between 2% and 10% of seniors living in the community meet *DSM-IV* criteria for substance dependence or abuse. Another study reported that 6% of seniors are heavy drinkers, which is defined as having two or more drinks per day. These disorders can trigger a number of health-related problems in seniors and worsen those that already exist. Alcohol abuse is four times more common among men than women ages 65 and older.

One major reason for the negative effects of heavy drinking on health in older adults is that the human body metabolizes (i.e., digests and uses) alcohol much less efficiently as it ages; thus, a senior may get drunk on the same amount of alcohol that he or she could drink without noticeable effects when he or she was younger. Studies have shown that a 65-year-old who consumes the same amount of alcohol as a 20-year-old will have a blood alcohol level 20% higher, and a 90-year-old will have a blood alcohol 50% higher. Some of the specific health risks of substance abuse in the elderly are:

- high blood pressure and increased risk of stroke
- increased risk of cancer of the head, neck, or esophagus
- increased risk of cirrhosis of the liver
- increased risk of falls and fall-related injuries, particularly in women; studies indicate that heavy drinking in older women also increases the risk of osteoporosis
- increased risk of malnutrition
- high risk of interactions with prescription drugs that the senior may be taking for other conditions
- decline in cognitive function; some researchers think that alcohol abuse increases a senior's risk of Alzheimer's disease, but further research is needed

Diagnosis of alcohol or substance abuse in the elderly is complicated by several factors. One is that the signs of alcohol or substance dependence are easy to confuse with age-related changes in muscle coordination, cognition, mood, social functioning, and the like. Older alcoholics are also less likely to be noticed if they no longer drive or work outside the home. In addition, about one-third of seniors who abuse alcohol are so-called late-onset drinkers; they are people who did not abuse alcohol when they were younger but have turned to it out of loneliness or bereavement. Late-onset seniors typically have higher levels of education and income than the two-thirds of older substance abusers with previous histories of alcohol or drug dependence.

In contrast to younger adults, seniors are less likely to use illicit "street" drugs, with rates of less than 0.1% of adults over 65. **Prescription drug abuse**, however, is relatively common among seniors, particularly older women.

QUESTIONS TO ASK YOUR DOCTOR

- Can you give me a referral for a geriatric psychiatrist?
- Have you ever treated a caregiver for emotional stress?
- What can I do to avoid mental health conditions associated with aging?
- Can you recommend any support groups for elderly patients?

Caregiver issues

One significant concern in geriatric psychiatry is the **stress** placed on caregivers for the elderly. Many seniors with Alzheimer's disease and other forms of dementia are cared for by family members or friends, at least in the early stages of the disease. As of 2011, almost 25% of U.S. households were providing care for a family member over the age of 50. The average age of these primary caregivers was over 60 years of age, and more than 75% were women. With regard to mental health issues among caregivers for the elderly, studies indicate that 46% meet the criteria for clinical depression; almost half of those caring for a person with Alzheimer's report significant emotional distress. In many cases, geriatric psychiatrists treat the mental health issues of their patient's caregiver(s) as well as their patient's disorders.

Treatment

Most seniors with mental health issues do not receive care from specialists; only about 3% are seen by geriatric psychiatrists. About half of seniors with mental health issues do not consult any physician for help; those who do, usually ask for help from their primary care physician. Seniors in the United States have the lowest rate of mental health care utilization of any adult age group: older adults account for only 7% of all inpatient mental health services, 6% of community-based mental health services, and 9% of private psychiatric care, even though they represent 13% of the population. The reasons given for seniors' underutilization include the **stigma** attached to mental illness, lack of access to mental health services, poor coordination among mental healthcare providers and services for the elderly, lack of funding, transportation difficulties, and a shortage of health care professionals.

Funding for mental health care among seniors comes from a combination of Medicare, Medicaid, private insurance, state and local governments, and block grants awarded and administered by the Center for Mental Health Services of the **Substance Abuse and Mental Health Services Administration** (SAMHSA). Medicare coverage is not comprehensive; as of 2011, it covered only 50% of the cost of mental health services, and it did not cover the cost of prescription medications.

Specialists in the field of geriatric psychiatry are concerned about the growing shortfall of physicians in the field. About 2,500 psychiatrists have been board-certified in geriatric psychiatry since 1990; there were 56 approved fellowship programs in the field as of 2011. The National Institute on Aging (NIA) estimated in 1997 that 4,000 to 5,000 geriatric psychiatrists will be needed by 2030 to keep up with the growth of the elderly population; however, at the present rate of certification, there will be only about 2,700 physicians in the field at that time (allowing for a 3% loss each year due to death and retirement).

With regard to research, there were 179 **clinical trials** in the general field of geriatric psychiatry under way in 2011. Some of these studies are investigating the effectiveness of telemedicine in meeting the mental health needs of seniors, new screeners to detect depression in older adults, **transcranial magnetic stimulation** as a possible treatment for depression, and various treatments for **sleep disorders** in the elderly. Other researchers are studying various drugs for the treatment of Alzheimer's and other types of dementia, ranging from lithium and the atypical antipsychotics ordinarily used to treat schizophrenia to experimental drugs that have not yet been approved by regulatory agencies.

Resources

BOOKS

Agronin, Marc E., and Gabe J. Maletta, eds. *Principles and Practice of Geriatric Psychiatry*. 2nd ed. Philadelphia: Wolters Kluwer Health/Lippincott Williams and Wilkins, 2011.

American Psychiatric Association. *Diagnostic and Statistical Manual of Mental Disorders*. 4th ed., text rev. Washington, DC: American Psychiatric Association, 2000.

Blazer, Dan G., and David C. Steffens, eds. *The American Psychiatric Publishing Textbook of Geriatric Psychiatry*. 4th ed. Washington, DC: American Psychiatric Pub., 2009.

Craft, Edwin, Saul M. Levin, and Richard K. Ehara, eds. *Substance Abuse among Older Adults: Physicians' Guide*. Rockville, MD: U.S. Dept. of Health and Human Services, Substance Abuse and Mental Health Services Administration, Center for Substance Abuse Treatment, 2010.

Halter, Jeffrey B., et al., eds. *Hazzard's Geriatric Medicine and Gerontology*. 6th ed. New York: McGraw Medical, 2006.

PERIODICALS

Alexopoulos, G.S. "Psychotherapy for Late-Life Depression." *Journal of Clinical Psychiatry* 71 (June 2010): e13.

Baldwin, R.C. "Preventing Late-Life Depression: A Clinical Update." *International Psychogeriatrics* 22 (December 2010): 1216–24.

Kalapatapu, R.K., et al. "Alcohol Use Disorders in Geriatrics." *International Journal of Psychiatry in Medicine* 40 (March 2010): 321–37.

Madhusoodanan, S., et al. "Primary Prevention in Geriatric Psychiatry." *Annals of Clinical Psychiatry* 22 (November 2010): 249–61.

Mahgoub, N., et al. "Self-injurious Behavior in the Nursing Home Setting." *International Journal of Geriatric Psychiatry* 26 (January 2011): 27–30.

Milka, M. "Study Details Lingering Effects of Stroke." *Journal of the American Medical Association* 306 (July 13, 2011): 142–43.

Siemens, I., and L. Hazelton. "Communicating with Families of Dementia Patients: Practical Guide to Relieving Caregiver Stress." *Canadian Family Physician* 57 (July 2011): 801–2.

Tartaglia, M.C., et al. "Neuroimaging in Dementia." *Neurotherapeutics* 8 (January 2011): 82–92.

Voaklander, D.C., et al. "Medical Illness, Medication Use and Suicide in Seniors: A Population-Based Case Control." *Journal of Epidemiology and Community Health* 62 (February 2008): 138–46.

Wilkins, V.M., et al. "Late-life Depression with Comorbid Cognitive Impairment and Disability: Nonpharmacological Interventions." *Clinical Interventions in Aging* 15 (November 2010): 323–31.

WEBSITES

American Association for Geriatric Psychiatry (AAGP). "Geriatrics and Mental Health—The Facts." http://www.aagpgpa.org/prof/facts_mh.asp (accessed August 6, 2011).

National Institute of Mental Health (NIMH). "Older Adults: Depression and Suicide Facts." http://www.nimh.nih.gov/health/publications/older-adults-depression-and-suicide-facts-fact-sheet/index.shtml (accessed August 6, 2011).

National Institute of Mental Health (NIMH). "Older Adults and Mental Health." http://www.nimh.nih.gov/health/topics/older-adults-and-mental-health/index.shtml (accessed August 6, 2011).

ORGANIZATIONS

American Association for Geriatric Psychiatry (AAGP), 7910 Woodmont Ave., Ste. 1050, Bethesda, MD, United States 20814-3004, (301) 654-7850, Fax: (301) 654-4137, main@aagponline.org, http://www.aagpgpa.org.

American Geriatrics Society (AGS), 40 Fulton St., 18th Fl., New York, NY, United States 10038, (212) 308-1414, Fax: (212) 832-8646, info.amger@americangeriatrics.org, http://www.americangeriatrics.org.

International Psychogeriatric Association (IPA), 550 Frontage Rd., Ste. 3759, Northfield, IL, United States 60093, (847) 501-3310, Fax: (847) 501-3317, http://www.ipa-online.org.

National Institute on Aging (NIA), Bldg. 31, Rm. 5C27, 31 Center Dr., MSC 2292, Bethesda, MD, United States 20892, (301) 496-1752, Fax: (301) 496-1072, (800) 222-2225, http://www.nia.nih.gov.

National Institute of Mental Health (NIMH), 6001 Executive Blvd., Rm. 8184, MSC 9663, Bethesda, MD, United States 20892-9663, (301) 443-4513, Fax: (301) 443-4279, (866) 615-6464, nimhinfo@nih.gov, http://www.nimh.nih.gov/index.shtml.

Rebecca J. Frey, Ph.D.

Sensory integration disorder

Definition

Sensory integration disorder or dysfunction (SID) is a neurological disorder that results from the brain's inability to integrate certain information received from the body's five basic sensory systems. These sensory systems are responsible for detecting sights, sounds, smell, tastes, temperatures, pain, and the position and movements of the body. The **brain** then forms a combined picture of this information in order for the body to make sense of its surroundings and react to them appropriately. The ongoing relationship between behavior and brain functioning is called sensory integration (SI), a theory that was first pioneered by A. Jean Ayres, Ph.D., OTR in the 1960s.

Description

Sensory experiences include touch, movement, body awareness, sight, sound, smell, taste, and the pull of gravity. Distinguishing between these is the process of sensory integration (SI). While the process of SI occurs automatically and without effort for most, for some the process is inefficient. Extensive effort and attention are required in these individuals for SI to occur, without a guarantee of it being accomplished. When this happens, goals are not easily completed, resulting in sensory integration disorder (SID).

The normal process of SI begins before birth and continues throughout life, with the majority of SI development occurring before the early teenage years. The ability for SI to become more refined and effective coincides with the aging process as it determines how well motor and speech skills, and emotional stability develop. The beginnings of the SI theory by Ayres instigated ongoing research that looks at the crucial foundation it provides for complex learning and behavior throughout life.

Causes and symptoms

The presence of a sensory integration disorder is typically detected in young children. While most children develop SI during the course of ordinary childhood activities, which helps establish such things as the ability for motor planning and adapting to incoming sensations, others' SI ability does not develop as efficiently. When their process is disordered, a variety of problems in learning, development, or behavior become obvious.

Those who have sensory integration dysfunction may be unable to respond to certain sensory information by planning and organizing what needs to be done in an appropriate and automatic manner. This may cause a primitive survival technique called "fright, flight, and fight," or withdrawal response, which originates from the "primitive" brain. This response often appears extreme and inappropriate for the particular situation.

The neurological disorganization resulting in SID occurs in three different ways: the brain does not receive messages due to a disconnection in the neuron cells; sensory messages are received inconsistently; or sensory messages are received consistently, but do not connect properly with other sensory messages. When the brain poorly processes sensory messages, inefficient motor, language, or emotional output is the result.

According to Sensory Integration International (SII), a nonprofit corporation concerned with the impact of sensory integrative problems on people's lives, the following are some signs of sensory integration disorder (SID):

- oversensitivity to touch, movement, sights, or sounds
- underreactivity to touch, movement, sights, or sounds
- tendency to be easily distracted
- social and/or emotional problems
- activity level that is unusually high or unusually low
- physical clumsiness or apparent carelessness
- impulsive, lacking in self-control
- difficulty in making transitions from one situation to another
- inability to unwind or calm self
- poor self concept
- delays in speech, language, or motor skills
- delays in academic achievement

While research indicates that sensory integrative problems are found in up to 70% of children who are considered learning disabled by schools, the problems of sensory integration are not confined to children with learning disabilities. SID transfers through all age groups, as well as intellectual levels and socioeconomic groups. Factors that contribute to SID include: premature birth;

autism and other developmental disorders; learning disabilities; delinquency and **substance abuse** due to learning disabilities; stress-related disorders; and brain injury. Two of the biggest contributing conditions are autism and **attention deficit hyperactivity disorder** (ADHD).

Diagnosis

In order to determine the presence of SID, an evaluation may be conducted by a qualified occupational or physical therapist. An evaluation normally consists of both standardized testing and structured observations of responses to sensory stimulation, posture, balance, coordination, and eye movements. These test results and assessment data, along with information from other professionals and parents, are carefully analyzed by the therapist who then makes recommendations about appropriate treatment.

Treatment

Occupational therapists play a key role in the conventional treatment of SID. By providing sensory integration therapy, occupational therapists are able to supply the vital sensory input and experiences that children with SID need to grow and learn. Also referred to as a "sensory diet," this type of therapy involves a planned and scheduled activity program implemented by an occupational therapist, with each "diet" being designed and developed to meet the needs of the child's nervous system. A sensory diet stimulates the "near" senses (tactile, vestibular, and proprioceptive) with a combination of alerting, organizing, and calming techniques.

Motor skills training methods that normally consist of adaptive physical education, movement education, and gymnastics are often used by occupational and physical therapists. While these are important skills to work on, the sensory integrative approach is vital to treating SID.

The sensory integrative approach is guided by one important aspect—the child's motivation in selection of the activities. By allowing them to be actively involved, and explore activities that provide sensory experiences most beneficial to them, children become more mature and efficient at organizing sensory information.

Alternative treatment

Sensory integration disorder (SID) is treatable with occupational therapy, but some alternative methods are emerging to complement the conventional methods used for SID.

KEY TERMS

Axon—A process of a neuron that conducts impulses away from the cell body. Axons are usually long and straight.

Cortical—Regarding the cortex, or the outer layer of the brain, as distinguished from the inner portion.

Neurotransmission—When a neurotransmitter, or chemical agent released by a particular brain cell, travels across the synapse to act on the target cell to either inhibit or excite it.

Proprioceptive—Pertaining to proprioception, or the awareness of posture, movement, and changes in equilibrium and the knowledge of position, weight, and resistance of objects as they relate to the body.

Tactile—The perception of touch.

Vestibular—Pertaining to the vestibule; regarding the vestibular nerve of the ear which is linked to the ability to hear sounds.

Therapeutic body brushing is often used on children (not infants) who overreact to tactile stimulation. A specific non-scratching surgical brush is used to make firm, brisk movements over most of the body, especially the arms, legs, hands, back and soles of the feet. A technique of deep joint compression follows the brushing. Usually begun by an occupational therapist, the technique is taught to parents who need to complete the process for three to five minutes, six to eight times a day. The time needed for brushing is reduced as the child begins to respond more normally to touch. In order for this therapy to be effective, the correct brush and technique must be used.

A report in 1998 indicated the use of cerebral electrical stimulation (CES) as being helpful to children with conditions such as moderate to severe autistic spectrum disorders, learning disabilities, and sensory integration dysfunction. CES is a modification of Transcutaneous Electrical Nerve Stimulation (TENS) technology that has been used to treat adults with various pain problems, including arthritis and carpal tunnel syndrome. TENS therapy uses a low voltage signal applied to the body through the skin with the goal of replacing painful impressions with a massage-like sensation. A much lower signal is used for CES than that used for traditional TENS, and the electrodes are placed on the scalp or ears. Occupational therapists who have studied the use of CES suggest that CES for children with SID can result in improved brain activity. The device is worn by children at home for 10 minutes at a time, twice per day.

Music therapy helps promote active listening. Hypnosis and **biofeedback** are sometimes used, along with **psychotherapy**, to help those with SID, particularly older patients.

Prognosis

By providing treatment at an early age, sensory integration disorder may be managed successfully. The ultimate goal is for the individual to be better able to interact with his or her environment in a more successful and adaptive way.

Resources

BOOKS

Auer, Christopher, Susan Blumberg, and Lucy Jane Miller. *Parenting a Child with Sensory Processing Disorder: A Family Guide to Understanding and Supporting Your Sensory-Sensitive Child.* Oakland, CA: New Harbinger Publications, 2006.

WEBSITES

Sensory Processing Disorder Foundation. "About SPD." http://www.sinetwork.org/about-sensory-processing-disorder.html (accessed November 14, 2011).

ORGANIZATIONS

Sensory Integration International/The Ayres Clinic, 200 2nd Ave. S, 447, St. Petersburg, FL, 33701-4313, (888) 271-2744.

Sensory Processing Disorder Foundation, 5420 S Quebec St., Ste. 135, Greenwood Village, CO, 80111, (303) 794-1182, Fax: (303) 322-5550, http://www.sinetwork.org.

Beth A. Kapes

Separation anxiety disorder

Definition

Like many childhood concerns, separation anxiety is normal at certain developmental stages. For example, when a child between the ages of 8 and 14 months is separated from her mother or other primary caretaker, she may experience distress. This is normal. However, separation anxiety that occurs at later ages is considered a disorder because it is outside of normal developmental expectations, and because of the intensity of the child's emotional response. Separation anxiety disorder occurs most frequently from the ages of 5 to 7 and from 11 to 14.

Environmental stimuli and internal cues from the child himself interact in the presentation of separation anxiety disorder. Separation anxiety disorder is defined by the primary expression of excessive anxiety that occurs upon the actual or anticipated separation of the child from adult caregivers—most often the parents. Significant problems in daily functioning for the child and parents can result from the disorder. Common fears observed in the presentation of separation anxiety include concerns about the parents' health or well-being (less frequently the child's own health), general catastrophes, natural disasters, or the child becoming lost/separated from the parents. Disrupted sleep, difficulty falling asleep alone, fear of monsters, or nightmares are also commonly experienced by children with separation anxiety disorder.

Family routines, parents' work schedules, and siblings' activities may all be negatively affected by the excessive anxiety and demands of the child with separation anxiety disorder. Family life is often disrupted by efforts to soothe the child. Parents can become stressed themselves as they try to maintain their daily routines and obligations, while attempting to manage their child's anxiety. The family's adjustment is often made more difficult due to the sudden appearance of symptoms.

Demographics

Prevalence estimates of separation anxiety disorder are 4%–5% of the population. Gender differences have not been observed, although girls do present more often with **anxiety disorders** in general. Of those diagnosed with separation anxiety disorder, approximately 75% experience school refusal. The most frequently observed ages for occurrence of separation anxiety disorder are in children ages 5 to 7 years and again from ages 11 to 14 years. It is at these times the children may feel more challenged by the developmental tasks of entering school or beginning puberty.

Description

Children experiencing separation anxiety disorder display significant distress upon separation from the parent or other primary caregiver. Separation anxiety disorder often becomes problematic for families during elementary school, although it can also occur in older or younger children. The child appears fearful because he or she thinks something horrible will happen to the child or parent while they are apart. The child's responses to separation may include crying or becoming angry with the adult in an attempt to manipulate the situation. When thwarted by the adult's appropriate boundaries, expectations, and structure (the child must attend school, for example), the child's distress may become displaced into other maladaptive or negative behaviors. The child may begin to exhibit behavioral problems at school or at home when there has been no previous history of such problems. The child may seek out a new, negative peer group in order to gain attention or avoid separation.

Many children are unable to describe their specific fear. The feelings may seem more general and engulfing, especially to the younger child, making description more difficult and the feelings more overpowering. Children, and even adolescents, may experience difficulty describing their internal thoughts and feelings, which is normal. The ability to self-monitor, or observe one's own behavior or decision-making process, does not develop until late in adolescence for some individuals. When caregivers press the child experiencing separation anxiety for explanations, the feelings of anxiety can actually become more overwhelming. The intensity of the child's emotional response, accompanied by a lack of explanation, can become very frustrating for parents. Children or adolescents with an angry or frustrated parent may create a reasonable explanation for their fears to appease caregivers, and to keep them from leaving. Lying to take the emphasis off their strong feelings may be one of the early behavioral changes that can accompany separation anxiety.

Although exposure to a specific stressor is not required for the development of separation anxiety disorder, in many cases, a specific incident may precipitate the onset of the disorder (the traumatic events of the terrorist attacks against the United States on September 11, 2001, for example). Another common precipitant is the holiday or summer break from school. Some children experience significant difficulty returning to school after a relatively short break, but certainly after summer and holidays.

Causes and symptoms

Causes

- Environmental change. Separation anxiety disorder is often precipitated by change or stress in the child's life and daily routine, such as a move, death or illness of a close relative or pet, starting a new school, a traumatic event, or even a return to school after summer vacation.
- Genetic influence. Evidence suggests a genetic link between separation anxiety disorders in children and a history of panic disorder, anxiety, or depression in their parents. Infants with anxious temperaments may have a predisposition toward later development of anxiety disorders.
- Parent/child attachment. Quality of attachment between children and their parents has also been identified as a factor in separation anxiety disorder. If the child senses emotional distance, the behaviors may be an attempt to draw the parent in more closely. The problematic behaviors can also draw the attention and care of others as well.
- Developmental considerations. Children develop at different rates when compared to each other (boys mature slower than girls, for example). Furthermore, the rate of development within the same person can vary across different types of functioning (for example, a gifted child is advanced intellectually but may be behind developmental expectations for social and emotional areas of functioning). A slower rate of development in the intellectual, social, emotional, or physical arena can foster anxiety within the child, making the separation more difficult.
- Cognitive factors. Children repeatedly worry about what they are afraid of (getting lost or a parent getting hurt, for example). The thought patterns are repeated within the child's mind until his emotions are beyond his control. The child may feel he is unable to think about anything else other than his fears, which contributes to his anxiety and irrational behaviors.
- Behavioral factors. The child or adolescent's crying and clinging behaviors may be developed by the child to cope with the feelings of anxiety associated with certain people, environment, or situations, such as attending school. The behaviors serve to distract attention away from the child's negative feelings, while nurturing the anxiety and fear into a greater part of the child's daily experience. For children, the behavioral component often becomes the mode of expression for the anxiety. The behavior may appear manipulative at times, due to the quick disappearance of symptoms once the threat of separation passes.
- Stress factors and influence. Symptoms of separation anxiety disorder may be exacerbated by a change in routine, illness, lack of adequate rest, a family move, or change in family structure (such as death, divorce, parent illness, birth of a sibling). The child's symptoms may also be affected by a change in caregivers or changes in parents' response to the child in terms of discipline, availability, or daily routine. Even if changes are positive or exciting, the change may feel uncomfortable and precipitate an anxious response in the child.

Symptoms

The *Diagnostic and Statistical Manual of Mental Disorders (DSM-IV-TR)*, a handbook for mental health professionals that aids in **diagnosis**, lists the following criteria for separation anxiety disorder.

- Recurrent excessive distress upon separation. The child may become focused on the separation long before the actual event, or simply at the time of the anticipated separation. The recurrent behavioral pattern does not respond to intervention. The child experiences extreme distress, a highly charged emotional response that is repeated when the child anticipates separation from the caregiver. The child's fears trigger more anxiety and the emotional response intensifies.
- Persistent and excessive worry. The content of the worry may include some type of harm occurring to the child himself or toward the parents, or it may focus on becoming lost or separated indefinitely from the parent or caregiver.
- Repetitive nightmares. The child may experience repeated nightmares with themes of being chased, harmed, or separated from her family. Some fears are age-appropriate, but in separation anxiety disorder, the intensity of the fears becomes overwhelming to the child, leaving little opportunity for the child to control her emotions or behaviors. Although dreams are often a way of exploring and making sense of daily life, children with separation anxiety disorder report nightmares that represent their irrational fears or preoccupation with disaster.
- Complaints of physical symptoms. The child may feign illness (headaches, stomachaches, etc.) to avoid separation, or the child may actually experience nausea upon separation. If allowed to continue, the child may develop psychosomatic symptoms (physical symptoms with a psychological origin) that prevent the child from attending or fully participating in school activities. In these cases, the separation anxiety may develop into a more serious hypochondriacal state in which the child complains of chronic pain, which results in the child getting what she wants (i.e., not attending school).
- Persistent reluctance or refusal to engage in age-appropriate activities. The child may refuse to attend school because of preoccupation about separation from the parent. The child may also experience reluctance to be alone at home or at school without another adult being immediately available. The child may resist sleep without an adult present. The disorder causes significant disruption in the child's daily routine and may decrease the ability to perform previously mastered tasks. The child may appear to have reverted to behaviors from a younger age. The intensity of her emotions blocks the child's ability to communicate her feelings in ways other than through behaviors. Examples include tantrums, hitting, or clinging. Crying is one of the primary behaviors associated with separation anxiety disorder. The crying can become quite intense, making it difficult for the child to regain composure.
- Enmeshment or unusual interest in parents' schedules. The child wants to know all the details of the daily routine, a behavior which minimizes the anxiety the child is feeling.
- Quick resolution of symptoms (upon meeting child's demands). It may be hard for parents to accept the reality of the disorder because the symptoms often disappear quickly when separation does not occur. It is this component that can feel manipulative to those in the child's life.

Diagnosis

The mental health professional will usually make the diagnosis of separation anxiety disorder based on information gathered during an interview process involving the parent(s) and the child. It is usually preferable for the interviews with the parent and child to occur separately; however that may not be possible because of the child's intense anxiety about separation.

As noted, separation anxiety disorder is generally diagnosed by history, including parental report; however, a few measures of general anxiety exist that can be used to supplement the history. These include Pediatric Anxiety Rating Scale, Children's Global Assessment Scale, Children's Anxiety Scale, Screen for Child Anxiety Related Emotional Disorders (SCARED-R), Multi-Dimensional Anxiety Scale for Children, and Achenbach's Child Behavior Checklist.

Duration of disturbance prior to diagnosis is a minimum of four weeks, occurring prior to the age of 18 years.

The disorder is described as "early onset" prior to the age of 6, and is generally not diagnosed after the age of 18. However, some researchers are describing another type of separation anxiety experienced by parents when their adolescents leave home. Readers may recognize this stage of life as the "empty nest syndrome," however, no such formal diagnosis exists for a parental form of separation anxiety.

Treatment

The most effective treatments for separation anxiety disorder involve parents, as well as school personnel when appropriate. Giving the child a sense of safety and security is key to successful treatment. Current treatment methods combine some form of group or individual cognitive behavioral **intervention**. Treatment options include cognitive-behavioral therapy, imagery, modeling, systematic desensitization, positive role models, behavior modification, reminders, distraction and altruism, and medication management.

Cognitive-behavioral therapy

Cognitive-behavioral therapy is a treatment approach designed to alter a person's thoughts, beliefs, and images as a way of changing behavior. In treating a child with separation anxiety disorder, the goal is to help the child label her fears and identify the irrational beliefs and assumptions underlying her fears. By confronting and correcting her false beliefs, a parent can help his or her child become less anxious about separation.

Imagery

With imagery, a child uses his imagination to see himself being successful in a stressful situation. For example, before heading off to school, a child could imagine how he will handle separation from mom. Instead of crying, he sees himself calmly saying goodbye to his mom. The use of positive mental pictures may help diminish some of the child's anxiety and fear before separation actually occurs.

Modeling

Parents and teachers can be helpful in **modeling** appropriate behaviors and coping mechanisms at home and at school. For example, parents can model being relaxed when saying goodbye to their children and other people.

Systematic desensitization

Systematic desensitization is a **behavior modification** technique in which a person is gradually exposed to an anxiety-provoking or fearful object or situation while learning to be relaxed. A child with separation anxiety disorder may be taught to spend longer and longer periods of time at school without a caregiver present by teaching her relaxation techniques for managing her anxiety.

Positive role models

Using positive role models, whether in real life or in books, can also be helpful for children. Reading books about other children successfully separating from their caregiver can give the anxious child the confidence that he can do it, too. Watching his friends calmly separate from their caregivers can also empower the child to do the same.

Behavior modification

Behavior modification uses a system of rewards and reinforcements to change behavior. This method has been shown to be effective in a majority of cases involving children and separation anxiety disorder, even at one-year follow-up.

Reminders

Small items that remind the child of his bond with his parents can sometimes be helpful in managing the child's anxiety. Typical objects could include a smooth stone in the child's pocket, a picture of the family in the child's notebook, or a friendship bracelet. Allowing phone calls or contact throughout the day is generally not effective, as it provides a more direct reminder of the caregiver's absence.

Distraction and altruism

Distraction and altruism is another strategy that can be useful in treating separation anxiety disorder. Helping the child focus on things outside himself can provide a healthy distraction. For instance, the child may be asked to take care of a pet at school. Such distractions from the child's internal thoughts and feelings coupled with a "fun" responsibility can help the child move away from his internal state of anxiety.

Medication management

Medication is helpful in certain cases where the anxiety is so debilitating that the child is unable to participate in other forms of treatment, or go about his daily routine. Medication management most often involves some type of antianxiety or antidepressant drug. Specific classes include the **selective serotonin reuptake inhibitors (SSRIs)** that influence **neurotransmitters** in the **brain** to regulate emotional response. Before any medication is given, however, it is essential that a careful medical and psychiatric evaluation be performed by a trained health professional.

Prognosis

More than 60% of children participating with their parents in cognitive-behavioral treatment are successful in managing their symptoms without medication. Symptoms generally do not re-appear in exactly the same way as the initial presentation; however, the child may have a heightened sensitivity to normal life transitions, such as changing schools. Families can help children cope with these transitions by visiting the new school, meeting teachers, and getting to know some students.

Separation anxiety disorder has a poorer prognosis in environments where threat of physical harm or separation actually exist.

Existence of other conditions, such as **autism**, decrease the likelihood of a positive prognosis. Presence of separation anxiety disorder in childhood is sometimes associated with early onset **panic disorder** in adults.

Studies indicate a lower prevalence of **alcohol use** and suicidal ideation in children or adolescents who

KEY TERM

Neurotransmitter—A chemical in the brain that transmits messages between neurons, or nerve cells.

experience separation anxiety disorder. **Depression** is commonly associated with anxiety disorders. Developing social skills can also be negatively affected by separation anxiety disorder.

Prevention

Prevention can be enhanced through parent effectiveness training that emphasizes the child's positive and successful coping strategies when dealing with separation. Overly anxious parents may need to develop their own support mechanisms and systems to manage their feelings and avoid influencing their children negatively.

Resources

BOOKS

American Psychiatric Association. *Diagnostic and Statistical Manual of Mental Disorders*. 4th ed., text rev. Washington, DC: American Psychiatric Publishing, 2000.

Brandt, Amy. *Benjamin Comes Back*. Transl. by Eida de la Vega. St. Paul, MN: Redleaf Press, 2000.

Penn, Audrey. *The Kissing Hand*. Terre Haute, IN: Tanglewood Press, 2007.

Silverman, W.K. and Andy P. Field, eds. *Anxiety Disorders in Children and Adolescents: Research, Assessment and Intervention*. 2nd ed. New York, NY: Cambridge University Press, 2011.

PERIODICALS

Burke, P., and R.C. Baker. "Is Fluvoxamine Safe and Effective for Treating Anxiety Disorders in Children?" *Journal of Family Practice* 50, no. 8 (August 2001).

Goodwin, R., et al. "Obsessive-Compulsive Disorder and Separation Anxiety Co-morbidity in Early Onset Panic Disorder" *Psychological Medicine* 31, no. 7 (October 2001): 1307–1310.

Kaplow, J.B., et al. "The Prospective Relation between Dimensions of Anxiety and the Initiation of Adolescent Alcohol Use." *Journal of Clinical Child Psychology* 30, no. 3 (September 2001): 316–326.

Kendall, P.C., E.V. Brady, and T. Verduin. "Comorbidity in Childhood Anxiety Disorders and Treatment Outcome." *Journal of the American Academy of Child & Adolescent Psychiatry* 40, no. 7 (July 2001): 787–794.

Muris, P., et al. "The Revised Version of the Screen for Child Anxiety Related Emotional Disorders (SCARED:R)." *British Journal of Clinical Psychology* 40, no. 1 (March 2001): 323–336.

Shortt, A.L., P.M. Barrett, and T.L. Fox. "Evaluating the FRIENDS Program: A Cognitive-Behavioral Group Treatment for Anxious Children and Their Parents." *Journal of Clinical Child Psychology* 30, no. 4 (December 2001): 525–535.

Southam-Gerow, M.A., P.C. Kendall, and V.R. Weersing. "Examining Outcome Variability: Correlates of Treatment Response in a Child and Adolescent Anxiety Clinic." *Journal of Clinical Child Psychology* 30, no. 3 (September 2001): 422–436.

Walkup, J.T., et al. "Fluvoxamine for the Treatment of Anxiety Disorders in Children and Adolescents." *The New England Journal of Medicine* 344, no. 17 (April 2001): 1279–85.

ORGANIZATIONS

American Academy of Child and Adolescent Psychiatry, 3615 Wisconsin Ave. NW, Washington, DC, 20016-3007, (202) 966-7300, Fax: (202) 966-2891, http://aacap.org.

Anxiety Disorders Association of America, 8730 Georgia Ave., Silver Spring, MD, 20910, (240) 485-1001, Fax: (240) 485-1035, http://www.adaa.org.

Deanna Pledge, Ph.D.

Serax *see* **Oxazepam**

Serentil *see* **Mesoridazine**

Seroquel *see* **Quetiapine**

Serotonin

Definition

Serotonin (pronounced ser-oh-TOH-nin) is a monoamine neurotransmitter—one of the chemicals naturally produced in the body that serves to convey nerve impulses across the gaps (synapses) between nerve cells. It is also known as 5-hydroxytryptamine or 5-HT. Monoamine means that a molecule of the neurotransmitter contains a single amino group. The chemical formula of serotonin is $C_{10}H_{12}N_2O$.

Purpose

Serotonin conveys nerve impulses across gaps (synapses) between nerve cells. It controls various functions in the body and various psychological characteristics as well.

Description

In its pure form, serotonin is a white powder that is slightly soluble in water. Serotonin was first discovered in blood in 1948 and was found to act as a

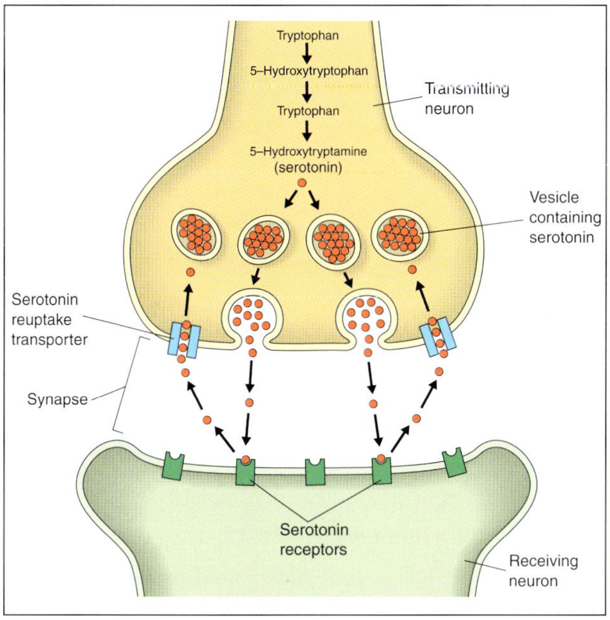

Diagram showing the role of serotonin in neuron (brain cell) communication. *(Illustration by Frank Forney. Reproduced by permission of Cengage Learning.)*

vasoconstrictor, a chemical compound that causes blood vessels to narrow or tighten. Its name comes from a combination of "serum" and "tone." Serotonin is found in a wide variety of plants and animals other than humans; it is an active ingredient in the venom found in stinging nettle plants and wasp, hornet, and scorpion stingers.

As its alternate name suggests, serotonin is derived from tryptophan, an essential amino acid. "Essential" means that the amino acid cannot be synthesized by the organism that needs it and must therefore be part of the organism's diet. Tryptophan is, however, plentiful in many foods, including chocolate, poultry, red meat, oats, dried dates, tofu, papayas, bananas, yogurt, milk, cottage cheese, eggs, sesame, chickpeas, sunflower and pumpkin seeds, peanuts, and fish. Serotonin is synthesized in the body from tryptophan by a short metabolic pathway that involves two enzymes, tryptophan hydroxylase (TPH) and amino acid decarboxylase (DDC). There are two genes in humans that encode TPH, located on chromosomes 11 and 12. The gene in humans that encodes DDC is located on chromosome 7.

Serotonin is synthesized in two different locations in the body, the **brain** and the intestines, and operates along two distinctive pathways depending on its source. About 5–10% of the serotonin in the human body is synthesized by serotonergic neurons (nerve cells) in the brain, where it functions as a neurotransmitter. The serotonin in the central nervous system (CNS) has a variety of functions, including mood regulation, appetite regulation, sexual desire, and sleep. Serotonin in the CNS also has some effect on cognitive functions, including memory, imagination, and learning. The greater part of the body's serotonin (about 90%), however, is secreted by enterochromaffin cells in the lining of the digestive tract. About 80% of the body's serotonin is utilized in the gut or by the smooth muscle tissues of the respiratory and cardiovascular systems, with the remainder stored in the platelets in the bloodstream. The serotonin in the platelets plays a role in the aggregation (clumping) of platelets during the process of blood clotting.

The brain's supply of serotonin is secreted by the raphe nuclei, a collection of nine pairs of neurons located along the length of the brainstem. The lower raphe nuclei have axons (long slender projections that carry nerve impulses away from the cell body) extending into the cerebellum and the spinal cord, while the axons of the upper raphe nuclei extend throughout the remainder of the brain, from the frontal cortex and hypothalamus to the amygdala and the hippocampus. Almost all the 40 million neurons in the human brain are influenced either directly or indirectly by the serotonin secreted by the raphe nuclei.

Serotonin receptors

At least 15 different types of serotonin receptors had been identified as of 2011, grouped into seven families numbered from 5-HT_1 through 5-HT_7. These receptors are protein molecules found on the surfaces of neurons and other cells that receive and respond to serotonin. The serotonin receptors modulate the release of such other **neurotransmitters** as norepinephrine, GABA, acetylcholine, and **dopamine**. They also regulate the release of a number of different hormones, including oxytocin, prolactin, cortisol, vasopressin, and corticotropin.

The serotonin receptors influence a wide variety of biological processes and neurological functions, including sleep, thermoregulation, nausea, vomiting, mood, aggression, anxiety, memory, cognition, learning, and appetite. Some of the specific 5-HT receptors, the locations of their activity, and their functions are as follows:

- 5-HT_{1A}. Active in blood vessels and CNS; affects aggression, anxiety, blood pressure regulation, hunger, memory, imagination, mood, cardiovascular tone, heart rate, respiration, ability to feel pain, sexual behavior, vomiting, temperature regulation, sleep, and addiction
- 5-HT_{1B}. Active in blood vessels and CNS; affects movement (locomotion), aggression, anxiety, blood

pressure regulation, memory, mood, learning, sexual behavior, and addiction

- 5-HT_{1D}. Active in blood vessels and CNS; affects vasoconstriction, movement, and anxiety
- 5-HT_{1F}. Active in CNS and involved in migraine headaches.
- 5-HT_{2A}. Active in the digestive tract, smooth muscles, blood vessels, CNS, peripheral nervous system, and platelets; affects anxiety, blood pressure regulation, temperature regulation, hunger, learning, memory, mood, cognition, sexual behavior, sleep, and addiction
- 5-HT_{2B}. Active in the digestive tract, smooth muscles, blood vessels, CNS, peripheral nervous system, and platelets; affects peristalsis, blood pressure regulation, hunger, anxiety, and sleep.
- 5-HT_{2C}. Active in the digestive tract, smooth muscles, blood vessels, CNS, peripheral nervous system, and platelets; affects anxiety, movement, peristalsis, blood pressure regulation, hunger, mood, sexual behavior, temperature regulation, sleep, and addiction
- 5-HT_3. Active in the digestive tract, CNS, and peripheral nervous system; affects anxiety, peristalsis, vomiting, learning, memory, and addiction
- 5-HT_4. Active in the digestive tract, CNS, and peripheral nervous system; affects breathing, hunger, peristalsis, learning, memory, mood, and anxiety
- 5-HT_{5A}. Active in CNS; affects movement and sleep
- 5-HT_6. Active in CNS; affects cognition, learning, memory, anxiety, and mood
- 5-HT_7. Active in the digestive tract, blood vessels, and CNS; affects blood pressure regulation, breathing, temperature regulation, sleep, memory, mood, and anxiety

The 5-HT receptors are the targets of antipsychotic, antiemetic, antimigraine, and appetite suppressant drugs as well as **antidepressants**, LSD and other **hallucinogens**, and street drugs such as **ecstasy**.

The serotonin transporter

The serotonin transporter, or SERT (also known as 5-HTT), is a monoamine protein that regulates the amount of serotonin in the synapses between neurons. More specifically, it recycles serotonin by conveying (transporting) serotonin from the synaptic space back into the presynaptic neuron, thus ending the activity of the neurotransmitter at the synapse. SERT is the target of many antidepressant drugs, particularly those classified as **selective serotonin reuptake inhibitors**, or **SSRIs**. The SSRIs work by reducing the ability of serotonin to bind to the transporter protein. Changes in the metabolism of the serotonin transporter have been linked to various disorders ranging from **obsessive-compulsive disorder** (OCD), **depression**, and alcoholism to **social phobia** and high blood pressure.

SERT can also be found in platelets in blood serum, where serotonin itself functions as a vasoconstrictor.

SERT is encoded by a gene known as *SLC6A4*, located on chromosome 17 at locus 17q11.1–q12. Variations (polymorphisms) in this gene have been associated with increased susceptibility to depression and **anxiety disorders**. The *SLC6A4* gene has a region known as *5-HTTLPR*, which has two forms: a long form with 16 repeats and a short form with 14 repeats. The short form appears to be associated with a lower rate of gene transcription and a higher risk of anxiety disorders and PTSD in persons with this polymorphism.

Serotonin and mood disorders

Serotonin has been nicknamed the "happiness hormone" because of its association with positive mood. Its role in mood disorders, however, was not completely understood as of 2011. One reason for the ongoing questions is researchers' inability to measure directly the levels of serotonin in the living brain. Although it is thought that low levels of serotonin are associated with depression, the theory has not been proven. While it has been shown that levels of serotonin in the bloodstream are lower in depressed people, no one is certain whether the low levels of serotonin cause depression or whether depression causes blood levels of serotonin to drop.

In addition, it is not yet known how low levels of serotonin activity result in the brain; possible causes include insufficient production of serotonin in the raphe nuclei, too few receptor sites to respond to the serotonin that is produced, a shortage of tryptophan in the body, or inability of the serotonin to reach the HT receptors.

One possible explanation for the association between serotonin and depression focuses on the fact that serotonin boosts the production of new brain cells and that depression—particularly depression caused by stress—suppresses brain cell regeneration. According to this theory, the SSRI antidepressants work by stimulating the growth of new brain cells, which in turn relieves the patient's depressed mood.

Serotonin and antidepressants

A surprising recent finding is the relationship between bone formation or bone loss and serotonin. Serotonin formed in the digestive tract acts like a hormone to inhibit the formation of new bone while serotonin formed in the brain helps to increase bone mass. A related finding is that selective serotonin reuptake inhibitor (SSRI)

KEY TERMS

Agonist—Any chemical that binds to a receptor on a cell surface and stimulates that cell to respond.

Antidepressant—Any of a group of medications given to relieve mood disorders, including anxiety disorders as well as major depression. Antidepressants include monoamine oxidase inhibitors (MAOIs), tricyclic (TCAs) and tetracyclic (TeCAs) antidepressants, selective serotonin reuptake inhibitors (SSRIs), and serotonin-norepinephrine reuptake inhibitors (SNRIs).

Axon—A long, threadlike projection that is part of a nerve cell.

Brainstem—The lowermost portion of the brain, adjoining and continuous with the spinal cord. The brainstem regulates heart and respiratory function, the sleep cycle, and the nerves that convey sensory information to the face and neck.

Enterochromaffin cells—Specialized cells in the thin layer of tissue lining the cavity (lumen) of the digestive tract. Also known as Kulchitsky cells, enterochromaffin cells provide about 90% of the human body's supply of serotonin.

Neurotransmitter—Any of a group of chemicals produced in the body that function to convey impulses from nerve cells (neurons) to target cells. Serotonin is a neurotransmitter.

Peripheral nervous system—The part of the nervous system that lies outside the brain and spinal cord. It connects the central nervous system with sensory organs, muscles, blood vessels, and glands.

Peristalsis—The waves of muscular contraction in the intestines that push the food along during the process of digestion.

Platelet—A small, irregularly shaped cell fragment that plays an important role in blood clotting. Platelets are also called thrombocytes.

Raphe nuclei—A group of nine pairs of compact clusters of nerve cells found in the brainstem that secrete serotonin for use in the brain.

Receptor—In biochemistry, a substance (usually a protein) found on the surface of a cell that interacts with specific other molecules, drugs, hormones, or antibodies.

Serotonin transporter (SERT)—A protein that removes serotonin from the spaces between neurons (synaptic clefts) and thus terminates its action. In effect, SERT recycles serotonin by returning it to the neuron that originally released it (the presynaptic neuron).

Synapse—A connection between a neuron (nerve cell) and another cell (which may be a neuron or another type of cell) that allows the neuron to transmit a chemical or electrical signal to the receiving cell.

Tryptophan—An essential amino acid produced in the body by the action of trypsin (a digestive enzyme) on protein molecules.

Vasoconstrictor—Any substance that causes blood vessels to narrow or tighten. Serotonin is a vasoconstrictor.

antidepressants paradoxically discourage the formation of new bone when given at the dosage levels needed to treat major depression. This finding suggests that the SSRIs should be used with caution in patients with osteoporosis.

Drugs related to serotonin or serotonin receptor regulation

There are several different classes of drugs approved by the Food and Drug Administration (FDA) for use in the United States that work by acting on the serotonin transporter (SERT).

SELECTIVE SEROTONIN REUPTAKE INHIBITORS (SSRIs). There were six drugs in this category approved for the treatment of major depression as of 2011:

- fluoxetine (Prozac)
- sertraline (Zoloft)
- citalopram (Celexa)
- escitalopram (Lexapro)
- paroxetine (Paxil, Pexeva)
- fluoxetine combined with olanzapine, an atypical antipsychotic (Symbyax)

Some SSRIs are available in extended-release (XR) or controlled-release (CR) forms. These formulations allow patients to take the medication only once a day or once a week.

Vilazodone (Viibryd) is a new SSRI approved by the FDA in January 2011 that also acts as a partial receptor agonist. This dual action means that the drug affects the absorption of serotonin by receptors on the postsynaptic neuron as well as limiting the effectiveness of the transporter protein in returning serotonin to the presynaptic neuron. It is thought that vilazodone is less likely than the other SSRIs to produce such side effects as weight gain and sexual problems.

SEROTONIN AND NOREPINEPHRINE REUPTAKE INHIBITORS (SNRIs). There were three SNRIs approved for use in treating major depression as of 2011. These drugs are sometimes referred to as dual reuptake inhibitors:

- venlafaxine (Effexor)
- duloxetine (Cymbalta)
- desvenlafaxine (Pristiq)

Precautions

Serotonin syndrome is an increasingly frequent and potentially life-threatening condition that results from excessive amounts of serotonin in the body. It is most likely to occur when a person takes two drugs that both affect the levels of serotonin that remain in the brain or are released elsewhere in the body. Serotonin syndrome may result from several different drug combinations: a triptan (class of drugs given to relieve migraine headaches) and either an SSRI or an SNRI; a monoamine oxidase inhibitor (MAOI, an older class of antidepressants) and either an SSRI or an SNRI; or a pain reliever (meperidine, fentanyl, or cyclobenzaprine) or dextromethorphan (the active ingredient in many cough medicines) and either an SSRI or an SNRI. Serotonin syndrome has also been reported to occur with street drugs, including **cocaine**, **methamphetamine**, LSD, and ecstasy; herbal supplements, particularly **St. John's wort** and **ginseng**; antinausea drugs, particularly ondansetron and metoclopramide; lithium, a mood stabilizer; linezolid, an antibiotic; and ritonavir, a drug used to treat AIDS.

The symptoms of serotonin syndrome usually appear within minutes or hours (usually about six hours) after taking the drugs. Milder symptoms include diarrhea, shivering, and goose bumps on the skin. The patient may also experience headache, muscle twitching, heavy sweating, restlessness, confusion, rapid heart rate, and high blood pressure. Severe serotonin syndrome can be life-threatening; its symptoms include **seizures**, irregular heartbeat, high fever, and loss of consciousness. The syndrome causes around 125 deaths each year in the United States.

There were no specific tests to diagnose serotonin syndrome as of 2011; the **diagnosis** depends partly on the patient's medication history and partly on the doctor's ruling out other possible diagnoses. A person who notices any of the symptoms of serotonin syndrome shortly after starting a new medication or increasing the dosage of a medication that affects serotonin levels should call the doctor at once or go to the hospital emergency department. If the symptoms are severe or worsening rapidly, it is vital to seek emergency help at once. In the hospital, the patient may be treated with muscle relaxants, **benzodiazepines** to reduce agitation, cyproheptadine to block serotonin production, other drugs to regulate heart rate and blood pressure, and oxygen and intravenous fluids to treat high fever. Patients with very high fever may need to be intubated, given medications that paralyze muscles, and placed on a respirator.

In milder cases, the symptoms of serotonin syndrome usually go away within a day of discontinuing medications that increase serotonin production and/or taking drugs that block serotonin production.

Resources

BOOKS

American Psychiatric Association. *Diagnostic and Statistical Manual of Mental Disorders*. 4th ed., text rev. Washington, DC: American Psychiatric Association, 2000.

Kalueff, Allan V., and Justin L. Laporte, eds. *Experimental Models in Serotonin Transporter Research*. New York: Cambridge University Press, 2010.

Marino, Alessia G., and Ilaria C. Russo, eds. *Serotonin: New Research*. New York: Nova Science, 2009.

Stahl, Stephen M. *Antidepressants*. New York: Cambridge University Press, 2009.

Zorumski, Charles F., and Eugene H. Rubin. *Psychiatry and Clinical Neuroscience: A Primer*. New York: Oxford University Press, 2011.

PERIODICALS

Ables, Adrienne, and Raju Nagubilli. "Prevention, Diagnosis, and Management of Serotonin Syndrome." *American Family Physician* 81 (2010): 1139–42. http://www.aafp.org/afp/2010/0501/p1139.html (accessed October 12, 2011).

Angier, Natalie. "Job Description Grows for Our Utility Hormone." *New York Times*, May 3, 2011. http://www.nytimes.com/2011/05/03/science/03angier.html?_r=1&pagewanted–all (accessed October 12, 2011).

Armbruster, D., et al. "Serotonin Transporter Gene Variation and Stressful Life Events Impact Processing of Fear and Anxiety." *International Journal of Neuropsychopharmacology* 12 (2009): 393–401.

Barton, David A., et al. "Elevated Brain Serotonin Turnover in Patients with Depression: Effect of Genotype and Therapy." *Archives of General Psychiatry* 65, no. 1 (2008): 38–46. http://archpsyc.ama-assn.org/cgi/content/full/65/1/38 (accessed October 12, 2011).

Byrd, L. "Serotonin Syndrome: What Is It? Causes, Recognition, and Management." *Geriatric Nursing* 31 (2010): 387–89.

Ducy, P. "5-HT and Bone Biology." *Current Opinion in Pharmacology* 11 (2011): 34–38.

Khan, A., et al. "A Randomized, Double-blind, Placebo-controlled, 8-week Study of Vilazodone, a Serotonergic

Agent for the Treatment of Major Depressive Disorder." *Journal of Clinical Psychiatry* 72 (2011): 441–47.

Richerson, G.B., and G.F. Buchanan. "The Serotonin Axis: Shared Mechanisms in Seizures, Depression, and SUDEP." *Epilepsia* 52, Suppl. 1 (2011): 28–38.

Wankerl, M., et al. "Current Developments and Controversies: Does the Serotonin Transporter Gene-linked Polymorphic Region (5-HTTLPR) Modulate the Association between Stress and Depression?" *Current Opinion in Psychiatry* 23 (2010): 582–87.

WEBSITES

National Human Genome Research Institute (NHGRI). "Frequently Asked Questions about Pharmacogenomics." National Institutes of Health. http://www.genome.gov/27530645 (accessed October 12, 2011).

"Serotonin Syndrome." MayoClinic.com. http://www.mayoclinic.com/health/serotonin-syndrome/DS00860 (accessed October 12, 2011).

ORGANIZATIONS

American Association for Clinical Chemistry, 1850 K St. NW, Ste. 625, Washington, DC, 20006, Fax: (202) 887-5093, (800) 892-1400, http://www.aacc.org.

American Society for Clinical Pharmacology and Therapeutics, 528 N Washington St., Alexandria, VA, 22314, (703) 836-6981, info@ascpt.org, http://www.ascpt.org.

National Institute of Mental Health, 6001 Executive Blvd., Rm. 8184, MSC 9663, Bethesda, MD, 20892-9663, (301) 433-4513; TTY: (301) 443-8431, Fax: (301) 443-4279, (866) 615-6464; TTY: (866) 415-8051, nimhinfo@nih.gov, http://www.nimh.nih.gov.

Rebecca J. Frey, PhD

Serotonin syndrome

Definition

Serotonin syndrome is a dangerous and potentially life-threatening condition that results from too much of the neurotransmitter serotonin in the body.

Description

Serotonin is a type of neurotransmitter in the nervous system, a chemical that neurons (**brain** cells) use to signal one another in complex pathways for normal brain and body functioning. **Neurotransmitters** such as serotonin bind to chemical receptors on the surface of neurons. Once bound to a receptor, they affect physiological processes. The receptors activate a sequence of cellular events known as a chemical cascade or signaling pathway. Neurotransmitter signaling pathways are responsible for many regulatory processes, including the signaling that affects mood and emotional stability.

It is believed that a decrease in serotonin contributes to illnesses such as **depression** and **anxiety disorders**. Various types of antidepressant medication such as **selective serotonin reuptake inhibitors (SSRIs)** and selective serotonin and norepinephrine reuptake inhibitors (SSNRIs) decrease the absorption of serotonin, resulting in increased levels of serotonin in the body. However, taking some of these **antidepressants** or other medications that increase serotonin at the same time can result in too much serotonin left in the body. Overactivity of serotonin can be dangerous, resulting in serotonin syndrome, also called serotonin toxicity, serotonin poisoning, and serotonin storm.

Causes and symptoms

Causes

Serotonin overdose may be caused by taking multiple drugs that increase the amount of serotonin in the body. Drugs that increase serotonin include **SSRIs**, such as **paroxetine** (Paxil) and **fluoxetine** (Prozac); SSNRIs, such as **duloxetine** (Cymbalta); and antidepressants called **monoamine oxidase inhibitors (MAOIs)**. Other drugs include the antibiotic linezolid and the migraine drug sumatriptan. The combination of any of these drugs increases the amount of serotonin, producing undesirable additive effects or overdose. Other drugs that cannot be combined with these medications due to risk of serotonin syndrome are the antipsychotics **chlorpromazine** and **fluphenazine**, some pain killers such as tramadol, and the herbal supplements yohimbine and **St. John's wort**.

Symptoms

Symptoms of serotonin overdose may range from mild to life-threatening, depending on the individual situation. The intensity of clinical findings seems to correlate with the degree of serotonergic activity, meaning that the more drugs taken, the worse the syndrome. Symptoms may include high blood pressure, high fever, nausea, vomiting, diarrhea, headache, sweating, increased heart rate, tremor, muscle twitching and rigidity, shock, coma, and death. Hyper reflexia are common, especially in the lower extremities. Mental status changes include anxiety, agitated **delirium**, restlessness, and disorientation.

Diagnosis

The **diagnosis** of serotonin syndrome is made based on clinical grounds, as opposed to any diagnostic test. A detailed history and physical exam is necessary for diagnosis. Information regarding the prescription and nonprescription medications, supplements, or illicit drugs the patient is taking is critical. Changes in doses or dose scheduling are also important, including whether extended release preparations are being used. A thorough description of the time of onset and type of symptoms is part of the diagnostic history. Most cases of serotonin syndrome occur within 24 hours of drug overdose, with the first six hours being a common time for onset. Physical exam may demonstrate increased heart rate and blood pressure, increased temperature, and dramatic swings in vital signs. Other physical exam findings include agitation, abnormal eye movements, dilated pupils, tremors, muscle twitching and rigidity, hyper reflexia, flushed skin, dry mucous membranes, and sweating.

The most accurate set of diagnostic criteria for serotonin syndrome is the Hunter Toxicity Criteria Decision Rules. These criteria require the patient to have taken a serotonergic agent and to have one of the following: repeated spontaneous muscular spasms of rhythmic contractions called clonus, inducible clonus plus agitation or sweating, ocular (eye) clonus plus agitation or sweating, tremor with hyper reflexia, severely rigid muscle tone, or high temperature plus inducible or ocular clonus.

Treatment

Serotonin syndrome progresses rapidly and must be treated quickly. The first step in treating the condition is discontinuation of all serotonergic agents. Supportive care is aimed at stabilization and normalization of all vital signs, as well as oxygen and intravenous fluids. Patients may be given **sedatives** such as **diazepam** (Valium) and sometimes short-acting medications for controlling blood pressure and heart rate. These measures are usually sufficient for mild serotonin syndrome.

Patients with more severe illness may require treatment with medications that antagonize or block serotonin signaling. The antidote of choice in these circumstances is cyproheptadine, which blocks serotonin activity and causes sedation. Critically ill patients may even require paralysis and endotracheal intubation with assisted breathing in an intensive care unit. Control of body temperature caused by muscle fasciculation (twitch) is critical for treatment and is accomplished through sedation or paralysis; drugs such as acetaminophen are not used. Once treatment is concluded, the patient is observed for a period to ensure that the illness has subsided and that vital signs are stabilized. Some

KEY TERMS

Clonus—Muscular spasm involving repeated, rhythmic contractions. Clonus may be spontaneous or inducible and may involve major body muscles or eye muscles.

Endotracheal intubation—The insertion of a flexible tube into the trachea for purposes of anesthesia, airway protection, and mechanical lung ventilation.

Monoamine oxidase inhibitors (MAOIs)—Type of antidepressant medication that affects various kinds of neurotransmitters, including serotonin.

Neurotransmitter—One of a group of chemicals secreted by a nerve cell (neuron) to carry a chemical message to another nerve cell, often as a way of transmitting a nerve impulse. Examples of neurotransmitters include acetylcholine, dopamine, serotonin, and norepinephrine.

Neurotransmitter receptor—A physical recipient for chemicals called neurotransmitters. Receptors sit on the surface of cells that make up body tissues, and once bound to the neurotransmitter, they initiate the chemical signaling pathway associated with neurotransmitters.

Selective serotonin norepinephrine reuptake inhibitors (SSNRI)—Drug class that acts to specifically inhibit the reuptake of serotonin and norepinephrine with little effect on other types of neurotransmitters, thereby decreasing side effects associated with broader-acting drugs.

Selective serotonin reuptake inhibitors (SSRI)—Drug class that acts to specifically inhibit the reuptake of serotonin with little effect on other types of neurotransmitters, thereby decreasing side effects associated with broader-acting drugs.

Serotonergic—Related to serotonin.

Serotonin—A type of neurotransmitter involved in regulation of the blood vessels, brain processes, and disease states such as depression.

Serotonin syndrome—A potentially life-threatening drug reaction involving an excess of the neurotransmitter serotonin, usually occurring when too many medications that increase serotonin are taken together.

Synapse—Physical space between neurons that allows the passage of neurotransmitters for chemical signaling pathways.

drugs may cause symptoms for days and require extensive observation. Cardiac activity is monitored continuously. A reassessment of the need for any prescribed serotonergic agents is conducted at the conclusion of treatment.

Prognosis

Prognosis for mild serotonin syndrome is good with proper treatment. For all cases, quick treatment is key to a positive prognosis.

Prevention

Serotonin syndrome is prevented by not taking more than one serotonergic agent at any given time. Patients should follow dosing instructions for all medications exactly as prescribed.

Resources

BOOKS

Brunton, Laurence, et al. *Goodman and Gilman's the Pharmacological Basis of Therapeutics*. 12th ed. New York: McGraw Hill Medical, 2011.

Kalueff, Allan V., and Justin L. Laporte, eds. *Experimental Models in Serotonin Transporter Research*. New York: Cambridge University Press, 2010.

Marino, Alessia G., and Ilaria C. Russo, eds. *Serotonin: New Research*. New York: Nova Science, 2009.

PERIODICALS

Ables, Adrienne, and Raju Nagubilli. "Prevention, Diagnosis, and Management of Serotonin Syndrome." *American Family Physician* 81, no. 9 (2010): 1139–42. http://www.aafp.org/afp/2010/0501/p1139.html (accessed October 12, 2011).

Byrd, L. "Serotonin Syndrome: What Is It? Causes, Recognition, and Management." *Geriatric Nursing* 31, no. 5 (2010): 387–89.

Richerson, G.B., and G.F. Buchanan. "The Serotonin Axis: Shared Mechanisms in Seizures, Depression, and SUDEP." *Epilepsia* 52, Suppl. 1 (2011): 28–38.

WEBSITES

Mayo Clinic staff. "Serotonin Syndrome." MayoClinic.com. http://www.mayoclinic.com/health/serotonin-syndrome/DS00860 (accessed October 12, 2011).

ORGANIZATIONS

American Association for Clinical Chemistry, 1850 K St. NW, Ste. 625, Washington, DC, 20006, Fax: (202) 887-5093, (800) 892-1400, http://www.aacc.org.

American Society for Clinical Pharmacology and Therapeutics, 528 N Washington St., Alexandria, VA, 22314, (703) 836-6981, info@ascpt.org, http://www.ascpt.org.

National Institute of Mental Health, 6001 Executive Blvd., Rm. 8184, MSC 9663, Bethesda, MD, 20892-9663, (301) 433-4513, TTY: (301) 443-8431, Fax: (301) 443-4279, (866) 615-6464, TTY: (866) 415-8051, nimhinfo@nih.gov, http://www.nimh.nih.gov.

Maria Eve Basile, PhD

Sertraline

Definition

Sertraline is an antidepressant that belongs to the class of drugs called **selective serotonin reuptake inhibitors (SSRIs)**. In the United States it is sold under the brand name Zoloft.

Purpose

Sertraline is approved by the U.S. Food and Drug Administration (FDA) for use in adults in treating **major depressive disorder**, **obsessive-compulsive disorder** (OCD), **panic disorder**, **post-traumatic stress disorder** (PTSD), **premenstrual dysphoric disorder** (PMDD), and social anxiety disorder. Sertraline is not approved in persons younger than the age of 24 unless used in the treatment of OCD.

Description

Serotonin is a **brain** chemical that carries nerve impulses from one nerve cell to another. Researchers think that **depression** and certain other mental disorders may be caused, in part, because there is not enough serotonin being released and transmitted in the brain. Like the other SSRI **antidepressants**, **fluvoxamine** (Luvox), **fluoxetine** (Prozac), and **paroxetine** (Paxil), sertraline increases the level of brain serotonin (also

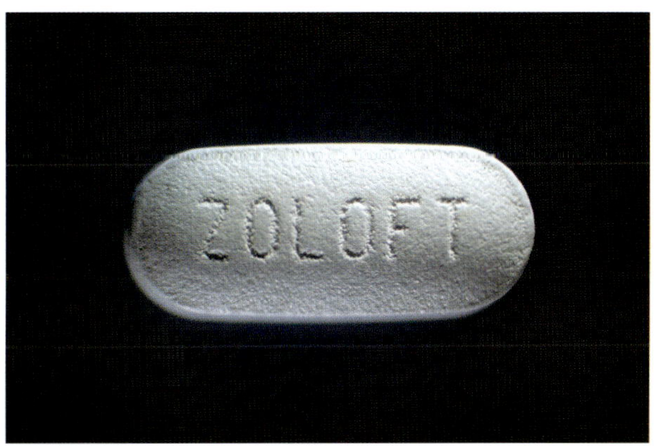

Zoloft (sertraline). *(© Leonard Lessin, FBPA/Photo Researchers, Inc.)*

known as 5-HT). Increased serotonin levels in the brain may be beneficial in patients with obsessive-compulsive disorder, alcoholism, certain types of headaches, post-traumatic **stress** disorder (PTSD), pre-menstrual tension and mood swings, and panic disorder. Sertraline is not more or less effective than the other SSRI drugs although selected characteristics of each drug in this class may offer greater benefits in some patients. Fewer drug interactions have been reported with sertraline, however, than with other medications in the same class.

The benefits of sertraline develop slowly over a period of up to four weeks. Patients should be aware of this and continue to take the drug as directed, even if they feel no immediate improvement.

Controversy still exists regarding the effectiveness of SSRI antidepressants, like sertraline. Some research has shown that other modalities, such as **cognitive-behavioral therapy**, are equally effective.

Sertraline is available in 25 mg, 50 mg and 100 mg tablets, or as a 20 mg per mL solution.

Recommended dosage

The recommended dosage of sertraline depends on the disorder being treated. The initial recommended dosage for depression and obsessive-compulsive disorder is 50 mg daily. This may be increased at intervals of at least one week to the maximum recommended dosage of 200 mg daily. For the treatment of panic disorder and post-traumatic stress disorder, the initial dose is 25 mg once daily. This dosage is increased to 50 mg daily after one week. If there is no therapeutic response, the dosage may be increased to the maximum of 200 mg daily at intervals of at least one week. These dosages may need to be reduced in elderly patients (over age 65) or in people with liver disease.

For the treatment of obsessive-compulsive disorder in the pediatric population, treatment should be initiated at a dose of 25 mg per day in children 6 to 12 years of age and 50 mg per day in children 13 to 17 years of age. Doses may be increased at one-week intervals to a total daily dose of 200 mg.

Precautions

A group of serious side effects, referred to collectively as **serotonin syndrome**, have resulted from the combination of antidepressants such as sertraline and members of another class of antidepressants known as **monoamine oxidase inhibitors (MAOIs)**. Serotonin syndrome usually consists of at least three of the following symptoms: diarrhea, fever, sweatiness, mood or behavior changes, overactive reflexes, fast heart rate, restlessness, shivering or shaking. Because of this, sertraline should never be taken in combination with **MAOIs**. Patient taking any MAOIs—for example, Nardil (**phenelzine** sulfate) or Parnate (**tranylcypromine** sulfate)—should stop the MAOI and wait at least 14 days before starting sertraline or any other antidepressant. The same holds true when discontinuing sertraline and starting an MAOI. Also, people should not take sertraline oral concentrate while using **disulfiram** (Antabuse). Sertraline should never be taken by people who are taking any other SSRI antidepressants.

Children and adults up to age 24 are at an increased risk of developing suicidal thoughts and behaviors when taking sertraline or any other antidepressant drug. Patients of all ages should be monitored for signs of worsening depression or changes in behavior. Sertraline may precipitate a shift to mania in patients with **bipolar disorder**. The drug should be used with cautiously and with close physician supervision by people with a prior history of **seizures**, people who are at an increased risk of bleeding, and those for whom weight loss is undesirable. The risk of bleeding may increase when taking sertraline with medication that thins the blood, including aspirin.

Side effects

More than 5% of patients experience **insomnia**, dizziness, and headache. About 14% of men report delayed ejaculation while 6% report decreased sex drive while taking this drug. In order to reduce these sexual side effects patients can wait for tolerance to develop (this may take up to 12 weeks), reduce the dose, have drug holidays (where the weekend dose is either decreased or skipped), or discuss with their physician using a different antidepressant.

More than 10% of patients report nausea and diarrhea while taking sertraline. Other possible side effects include agitation, anxiety, rash, constipation, vomiting, tremors, or visual difficulty. Although most side effects eventually subside, it may take up to four weeks for people to adjust to the drug.

Interactions

Sertraline interacts with **St. John's wort**, an herbal remedy for depression. The risk of seizures is increased in patients using tramadol and sertraline. Taking sertraline with MAO inhibitors may result in the serious side effects discussed above. Erythromycin, an antibiotic, may inhibit the breakdown of sertraline in the liver and cause increased central nervous system effects such as drowsiness and decreasing of mental alertness. Other antidepressants should not be taken by people using sertraline except in rare cases where prescribed by a physician. If a combination of antidepressants is considered beneficial, a low dose of tricyclic antidepressants (10–25 mg daily) should be used.

Sertraline should not be taken with grapefruit juice as the combination may increase sertraline levels in the body.

Resources

BOOKS

Jacobson, J.L., Jacobson, AM. *Psychiatric Secrets.* 2nd ed. Philadelphia: Hanley & Belfus, 2001.

Stern, T.A., et al. *Massachusetts General Hospital Comprehensive Clinical Psychiatry.* 1st ed. Philadelphia: Mosby Elsevier, 2008.

PERIODICALS

Edwards, Guy. "Systemic Review and Guide to Selection of Selective Serotonin Reuptake Inhibitors." *Drugs.* 57 (1999): 507–33.

Hirschfeld, Robert. "Management of Sexual Side Effects of Antidepressant Therapy." *Journal of Clinical Psychiatry.* 60 (1999): 27–30.

WEBSITES

PubMed Health. "Sertraline." U.S. National Library of Medicine. http://www.ncbi.nlm.nih.gov/pubmedhealth/PMH0001017 (accessed January 9, 2012).

Ajna Hamidovic, Pharm.D.

Serzone *see* **Nefazodone**

Sexual abuse

Definition

Sexual **abuse** in general is the forcing of unwanted sexual contact or behavior by one person on another. It may involve two adults, or an adult and an adolescent or a child. In some jurisdictions, it may also be used to describe the abuse of a younger child by an adolescent or older child. Sexual abuse may or may not involve direct physical contact; it also includes such behaviors as **voyeurism** (peeping), exposing one's genitals, showing pornographic materials to the victim, stalking, sexual harassment online or by telephone, and seductive or sexually explicit remarks or comments.

Unwanted sexual contact that is infrequent, brief in duration, or immediate is called sexual assault. Sexual assault includes not only forcible rape but also any other sexual contact that results from coercion, including being touched, grabbed, fondled or kissed against one's will, or being shown the perpetrator's genitals. Rape is defined as nonconsensual oral, anal, or vaginal penetration of the victim by body parts or objects using force, threats of bodily harm, or by taking advantage of a victim who is incapacitated or otherwise incapable of giving consent. Incapacitation may include mental disability, forced or voluntary intoxication, being a minor, or any other condition defined in law that indicates that the person is unable to give consent.

The seduction of a child through offers of affection or bribes of some kind is also considered sexual assault. Sexual intercourse with a child below the age of consent is defined as statutory rape, while sexual intercourse between two close relatives is called incest. While laws vary somewhat from state to state, sexual assault and rape are generally defined as felonies in most jurisdictions in the United States. Sexual abuse between spouses is considered a form of domestic violence.

Sexual abuse in the workplace, school or college, military facility, or other institutional setting is called sexual harassment or sexual misconduct. It occurs when a person in a position of power or authority compels someone to participate in unwanted sexual activity for fear of job loss, demotion, a failing grade, or a similar penalty.

Demographics

Sexual abuse is increasingly recognized as a cause or trigger of mental health problems in persons of all genders, age groups, and racial and ethnic groups worldwide. The National Crime Victimization Survey reports an average of 280,000 sexual assaults (including rape and attempted rape) each year in the United States. Current estimates indicate that someone is sexually assaulted every two minutes somewhere in North America, and that 1 in 6 women and 1 in 33 men will be the victim of a sexual assault at least once in their lifetimes. According to the Centers for Disease Control and Prevention (CDC), sexual assaults account for 10% of all assault-related visits by women to hospital emergency rooms in North America.

As many as one out of three girls and one out of five boys under age 18 in North America have been sexually abused, according to the U.S. Department of Justice (DOJ). Current estimates of incest and other forms of childhood sexual abuse range from 12% to 40%, depending on settings and population. Most studies have found that among women, approximately 20% report experiencing sexual abuse in childhood. Significant underreporting of abuse occurs because children are too ashamed or afraid to tell anyone or because they think that they will not be believed. Legal procedures for corroborating sexual abuse can also be an impediment.

In recent years, however, increased public awareness of child sexual abuse has resulted in more reporting and more prosecutions.

Rape

More than 100,000 rapes (about 300 episodes every day) are reported in the United States every year. It is thought, however, that many—possibly most—rapes are not reported; according to the American Medical Association, rape is the most underreported violent crime. The Rape, Abuse and Incest National Network (RAINN) estimates that 60% of all rapes are not reported to the police, and that 15 out of every 16 rapists never spend a single day in jail.

Most rapes in North America are committed by males between the ages of 20 and 50. About half of all rapes are committed against females 18 years of age or younger, although rape victims range in age from infants 2 months old to women in their 80s; about 4% of female rape victims are 50 years of age or older. About 50% of rapes involve strangers; the other 50% are committed by men known to their victims. About 5% of rapes involve family members. Forcible rape may involve forcible oral/genital contact or anal rape (sometimes called sodomy) as well as vaginal penetration.

Human trafficking

A growing problem related to the sexual abuse of children is human trafficking, or the commercial sexual exploitation of people. The Trafficking Victims Protection Act, a law passed by Congress in 2000, defines any child under the age of 18 years old who is used for the purpose of exploitation through sexual servitude (prostitution), regardless of the absence of monetary bribes, manipulation, fraud, coercion, threats, force, or violence, as a commercially sexually exploited child and a victim of human trafficking. This means that a child or adolescent does not have to prove that he or she was tricked or forced into prostitution or other forms of sexual exploitation to be considered a victim of human trafficking. According to the DOJ, the average age of entry into prostitution in North America is 12 to 14 years. About 300,000 children in the United States and Canada are thought to be victims of human trafficking each year. The majority are girls, coerced into such activities as stripping, escort services, and posing for pornographic pictures or films as well as prostitution.

Description

Children

Although child sexual abuse can involve violence, it is more likely to involve other forms of coercion. Whereas infants and young children are defenseless, older children may be susceptible to lies, bribes, or threats. Most often they acquiesce to the demands of adults who hold inherent power over them. Abusers may manipulate a child through a process called grooming, which can involve gaining the child's trust, confusing the child about normal forms of "love," preparing the child to accept sexual abuse, and ensuring that the child will not tell others. Grooming can also involve creating a public persona in which the abuser is held in high regard by the child's family and community.

Sexual abuse can overwhelm a child with horror, confusion, disbelief, fear, and shame. Sometimes children become passive in an attempt to dissociate their minds from the physical reality of the abuse. This passivity can be misconstrued as consent. Some children attempt to repress memories of the abuse or rationalize it into insignificance.

Sexual abuse can leave a child emotionally devastated. Even very young children, who may not understand what has happened, are unable to cope with the overstimulation. Children aged five and older may feel caught between loyalty or affection toward their abuser and their knowledge that the sexual activity is wrong. If the abuser is a family member, the child may be afraid of breaking up the family. Some abusers threaten children with withdrawal of love. Children often feel that they are to blame for the abuse and this combination of shame and guilt reinforces the abuser's insistence on secrecy.

Not all forms of child sexual abuse involve adult abusers. Sibling incest is considered the most common form of incest; most cases involve older brothers abusing younger siblings of either sex. Adolescent perpetrators of sibling incest are reported to use violence more frequently and more severely than adult perpetrators; abuse their victims over a longer period of time; are more likely than a father or stepfather to penetrate the victim; and are more likely than a father or stepfather to choose a very young victim.

Adults

Sexual abuse of adults is commonplace worldwide. It includes human trafficking and sexual abuse of incapacitated adults as well as forcible rape, **frotteurism**, and stalking or other nonphysical forms of unwanted sexual advances.

DOMESTIC VIOLENCE. Domestic violence includes sexual violence within families as well as beatings or other forms of physical assault. The term "marital rape" is used to describe nonconsensual intercourse between husband and wife; "intimate partner violence" or IPV is used to refer to sexual violence between former (divorced) spouses, common-law partners, dating partners, or live-in boyfriends or girlfriends. IPV may refer to same-sex as well as opposite-sex violence. Some researchers use the term "family violence" to include sexual violence toward elderly persons living in the household as well as the abuse of children or adolescents.

The CDC estimates that women in the United States experience about 4.8 million intimate-partner related physical assaults and rapes each year, while men are the victims of about 2.9 million intimate-partner related physical assaults per year. About 2,500 people in North America die each year at the hands of intimate partners; 70% are women and 30% are men.

STALKING. Stalking has been recognized in law as a crime only recently. It refers to obsessive and unwanted attention directed by an individual or group to another person. A form of harassment and intimidation, stalking is usually sexual in nature, intended to obtain or force a relationship with someone who is unavailable or unwilling. It can be defined as willful and repeated following, watching and/or harassing of another person. Stalkers may resort to verbal threats or property damage in order to frighten or intimidate the victim. About 3.4 million cases of stalking are reported in the United States each year.

Most cases of stalking involve young adults between the ages of 18 and 24, with 25% of these cases involving cyberstalking, or stalking someone online. Most victims of stalking know the perpetrator(s). According to the DOJ, 43% of male victims report being stalked by a woman, with 41% stalked by another man. Women who are stalked report being stalked by males in 67% of cases, with 24% being stalked by another woman.

Special populations

ELDER ABUSE. Sexual abuse of the elderly is significantly underreported, partly because victims are ashamed and unwilling to speak up, and partly because many people mistakenly believe that older adults are unlikely to be the targets of sexual abuse. In addition, elderly persons suffering from Alzheimer's or another form of **dementia** may be unable to remember the details of the abuse or to report it. A study commissioned by the National Institute of Justice in 2007 reported that:

- Elderly victims of sexual assault are rarely evaluated for psychological aftereffects of the attack.
- The older the victim, the less likely the perpetrator is to be convicted of sexual assault.
- The perpetrator is more likely to be charged with a crime and convicted if the victim shows signs of physical injury.
- Assailants of elderly people living independently are more likely to be charged and convicted than those who attack seniors in assisted living situations.

A study published in the *Journal of the American Geriatrics Society* in 2010 reported that most cases of sexual aggression against elderly people in long-term care facilities are perpetrated by residents rather than staff, and that the most common single cause is hypersexuality associated with dementia. These cases have the potential to cause significant physical injury to the victims as well as emotional distress to perpetrators and victims alike.

ADULTS WITH DEVELOPMENTAL DISABILITIES. People in any age group with developmental disabilities are particularly likely to be abused. One research team estimates that more than 90% of people with developmental disabilities will experience some form of sexual abuse at some time in their lives, while 49% will experience 10 or more abusive incidents. Other studies indicate that 68% of girls and 30% of boys with developmental disabilities are sexually abused before their 18th birthday, yet these crimes go unreported—one attorney in California found that only 4.5% of sexual assaults on the developmentally disabled are reported, compared to 44% for the general population.

According to recent research, 15,000 to 19,000 people with developmental disabilities are raped each year in the United States. A Canadian study reported that 40% of women with disabilities have been assaulted or raped; and that 54% of boys and 50% of girls with hearing disorders have been sexually abused. In most cases, developmentally disabled people are sexually abused by their caregivers, whether paid staff or family members. A study of 162 cases of sexual abuse of disabled people indicated that 28% were perpetrated by direct care staff members, including psychiatrists; 19% were committed by family members; 15.2% by neighbors or family friends; 9.8% by babysitters; and 3% by dates. With regard to gender, 81.7% of the victims were women; 90.8% of the abusers were men.

PRISON RAPE. Prison rape refers to rape of adults committed within prisons. It is used most often to refer to the rape of inmates by other inmates, whether male/male or female/female, but is sometimes used to refer to the rape of inmates by prison staff or the rape of staff members by inmates. Statistics very widely; the most widely accepted estimate is that 1 in 10 male inmates is raped in prison, mostly by fellow prisoners. Another estimate obtained by the FBI is that between 9% and 14% of male inmates are sexually assaulted. For women, the figure is 1 in 40; however, the perpetrators are usually prison staff rather than other inmates.

MILITARY SEXUAL TRAUMA. The U.S. Veterans Administration (VA) defines military sexual **trauma** (MST) as "any kind of unwanted sexual attention includ[ing] insulting sexual comments, unwanted sexual advances, or even sexual assault." Since the 1980s, military sexual trauma (MST) has been increasingly recognized as a mental health issue for servicemen as well as servicewomen on active duty. There is also evidence that sexual harassment and assault are more common in wartime than in peacetime military duty. A study of MST during the Gulf War reported high rates of sexual assault (7%), physical sexual harassment (33%), and verbal sexual harassment (66%). In another study, 23% of female users of VA healthcare reported experiencing at least one sexual assault while in the military.

Male victims of MST have a higher rate of PTSD (65%) than females (45%), partly because the male gender role causes many men to feel intense shame about their victimization, making them less likely to seek professional help. Although male MST is considerably underreported in armies worldwide, the most recent figures for reported cases in the U.S. armed forces are 1.1% of male service members over the course of their military careers, with a range between 0.03% and 12.4%.

Risk factors

Risk factors for sexual abuse include:

- age—both young children and the elderly are at increased risk of sexual abuse because they are perceived as relatively unable to defend themselves
- female sex
- physical or developmental impairments
- homelessness—homeless adolescents of either sex are at high risk of being raped or forced into prostitution within three days of living on the streets
- habitual alcohol or drug abuse—substance abuse increases a person's risk of being assaulted, tricked, or coerced into unprotected voluntary sexual activity, or engaging in prostitution in order to pay for drugs
- African American, Native American, Hispanic, or mixed ethnicity
- imprisonment
- living in overcrowded housing
- war, rioting, the aftermath of a major disaster, or other forms of social breakdown

Causes and symptoms

Causes

Perpetrators of sexual abuse differ in their motivations, degree of psychopathology, past history of trauma, and current mental and physical health status. Some perpetrators of sexual abuse have multiple victims, while others may be obsessed with a single individual—often someone with whom they had or tried to have a relationship. Perpetrators tend to be angry people with a need to control or dominate others, although there are also some offenders who suffer from emotional dependency and neediness, **delusions**, **schizophrenia**, or a narcissistic sense of entitlement to the victim's attention or affection.

Some abusers of adults as well as children suffer from **personality disorders**, **impulse control disorders**, or psychosis. Some abusers of children have a specific psychiatric disorder known as **pedophilia**—sexual attraction to prepubescent children. A related disorder is hebephilia, or sexual attraction to children in the early stages of puberty. This is not to imply, however, that all persons with these conditions engage in sexual abuse, as quite the opposite is true—the majority do not participate in sexual abuse.

Some sexual abuse is situational, such as parents who abuse their children only when they are under the influence of alcohol or drugs or are under severe **stress**, or adults who may not have planned a sexual assault but take advantage of the victim's intoxication, disability, or other form of incapacitation. Prison rape, particularly male/male rape, is often considered a form of situational sexual abuse, as is MST.

Many perpetrators of sexual abuse were themselves abused as children, and may abuse others in adult life as a form of revenge against the parents or other adults who had victimized them. Other perpetrators witnessed family violence and came to regard it as acceptable, or were exposed to cultural beliefs that support or encourage sexual abuse and violence.

Last, there are a few diseases and disorders characterized by hypersexuality (loss of sexual inhibitions and self-control), and people with these conditions may act inappropriately and abusively toward other adults as well as children. These disorders include **Kleine-Levin syndrome**, a rare disorder primarily found in teenage boys; Klüver-Bucy syndrome, another rare behavioral disorder caused by malfunctions in the temporal lobe of the **brain**; **bipolar disorder**; and the side effects of some drugs given to treat Parkinson disease. Researchers disagree, however, as to when hypersexuality should be regarded as a person's primary disorder and when it should be considered a secondary symptom of another disease.

Symptoms

Sexual abuse results in a variety of physical and psychiatric symptoms in survivors that may range from minor injuries to life-threatening conditions.

KEY TERMS

Age of consent—The minimum age at which a person is considered legally competent to consent to sexual acts. It should not be confused with the voting age, driving age, legal drinking age, or marriageable age. In most jurisdictions in the United States, the age of consent is 16 or 18, but it may be set as low as 12 or as high as 21.

Felony—A major crime, such as sexual assault, aggravated assault and battery, grand theft, rape, burglary, arson, and similar acts.

Frotteurism—The practice of rubbing one's pelvis or (for males) erect penis against a nonconsenting person for sexual gratification. It frequently occurs in subway cars or other crowded public places; most perpetrators are strangers to their victims. Frotteurism is considered a form of sexual assault.

Grooming—Deliberately establishing an emotional connection with someone in order to manipulate them psychologically and lower their resistance against sexual activity.

Hebephilia—Sexual attraction on the part of an adult to children in the early stages of puberty.

Human trafficking—Illegal trade in human beings, whether adults or children, for the purposes of reproductive slavery, prostitution, other forms of sexual exploitation, or forced labor.

Hymen—A membrane that partially or completely covers the vaginal opening in females prior to first intercourse.

Hypersexuality—A general term for extremely frequent or suddenly increased sexual urges or activity. It is usually associated with lowered sexual inhibitions.

Incest—Sexual intercourse or inappropriate sexual contact between two people who are too closely related to legally marry.

Pedophilia—A sexual perversion in which children are the preferred sexual object.

Pornography—Sexually explicit pictures, writings, or other material produced for the purpose of sexual arousal.

Sexual assault nurse examiner (SANE)—A nurse with specialized training in the care and forensic examination of victims of sexual assault.

Sodomy—A term that is sometimes used for anal rape.

Stalking—The willful and repeated following, watching and/or harassing of another person, usually with the intent of forcing the victim into a dating or sexual relationship.

Statutory rape—Sexual activity, often coercive, in which one party is below the age of consent.

Syndrome—A group of signs or symptoms that occur together and characterize or define a particular disease or disorder.

Voyeurism—Sexual stimulation by visual means, usually by observing an unsuspecting individual.

PHYSICAL SYMPTOMS. According to the CDC, the physical symptoms of sexual abuse or sexual assault may include one or more of the following:

- unexplained cuts, scratches, and bruises
- unexplained internal injuries, broken bones, or head trauma
- vaginal or rectal bleeding, pain, itching, redness, swelling, or discharge
- painful urination or bowel movements
- difficulty sitting or walking
- rarely, injury to the buttocks, lower abdomen, or extremities
- pregnancy or a sexually transmitted disease (STD), especially in a child under age 14

Many adult survivors of rape experience a variety of physical symptoms ranging from tension headaches and generalized muscle pain to specific symptoms in the parts of the body that were penetrated during the assault. Survivors of oral rape may have a variety of mouth and throat complaints, nausea and vomiting, and bulimia or anorexia, while survivors of vaginal or anal rape may suffer from abdominal cramping, dysmenorrhea, constipation, or diarrhea.

PSYCHIATRIC SYMPTOMS. Almost all survivors of sexual abuse or assault have one or more psychiatric symptoms or full-blown disorders after the abuse, although some symptoms may not appear for months or even years afterward. The symptoms and disorders most commonly experienced by abuse survivors include:

- major depression
- anxiety disorders, including generalized anxiety disorder, panic disorder, and phobias
- sleep disorders

- dissociative disorders, including dissociative identity disorder (formerly known as multiple personality disorder)
- eating and substance abuse disorders
- cutting and other forms of self-injury
- Stockholm syndrome, a group of psychological symptoms that occur in some persons in captive, hostage, or long-term abuse situations, in which the victim develops positive feelings toward the captor or abuser
- suicidal feelings and/or suicide attempts
- borderline personality disorder (BPD)—this disorder is more likely to develop in children who have been sexually abused for long periods of time than in adult survivors
- repeated victimization—some abuse survivors engage in high-risk lifestyles or occasional episodes of risky behavior that increase their chances of being attacked or abused again

RAPE TRAUMA SYNDROME. Rape trauma syndrome (RTS) is a term first coined by Ann Burgess and Lynda Holmstrom in 1974 to describe a complex form of psychological trauma to an adult rape victim (male or female) reflected in disruptions of the survivor's emotional, cognitive, physical, and interpersonal behaviors. RTS is a syndrome with two phases, the first of which is an acute phase that lasts from several days to several weeks after the assault. Survivors react in different ways during the acute phase. Some survivors are expressive, meaning that they show their emotions by crying, yelling, or being openly angry. Others are controlled; they may be completely silent about the rape and go about their daily routines as if nothing has happened. Neither type of response is considered better than the other.

The second phase of RTS is the reorganization phase, in which the survivor tries to recover the sense of safety and ability to trust others that she or he had before the rape. The survivor must cope with intense feelings of guilt and shame as well as fear and anxiety. In some cases the survivor may feel disconnected or dissociated from her or his body. Male survivors are more likely than females to have questions about their sexual identity and orientation; they are also more likely to postpone or avoid treatment. One study of 100 male rape survivors found that the average time interval between the assault and seeking therapy was 16 years.

Diagnosis

The **diagnosis** and examination of victims of sexual abuse or assault is complicated by the involvement of law enforcement as well as the victim's need for medical care. The time limits for evidence collection depend on the specific jurisdiction but usually range from 72 to 120 hours. With adults, it is important to immediately document as many details of the incident or relationship as possible, including the location of the abuse or assault; duration of the abuse or assault; identity of the perpetrator, if known; the number of perpetrators, if more than one; home address or workplace of the assailant, if known; whether a weapon, drugs, or alcohol were involved; and whether the victim washed, showered, or douched after the abuse or assault. In the case of adult women, the doctor will need to obtain the date of the woman's last menstrual period, birth control method, and time of last consensual intercourse.

Some medical centers have specially trained sexual assault nurse examiners, or SANEs; in others, the emergency room physician will conduct the physical examination of the victim and record the findings, including bruises, cuts, the presence of sperm, and other evidence of resistance to the attack. Most hospitals have prepackaged rape kits with the needed equipment and detailed instructions for evidence collection. Careful documentation is vital to protect the victim if the case goes to trial. Maintaining a chain of custody for legal purposes requires the documentation of each transfer of the evidence kit from the time it is opened until it is sealed and placed in a secure area.

In the case of minors, a child who reports sexual abuse or is suspected of having been abused should have a complete physical examination as soon as possible, preferably within 72 hours. An examination is ordered whenever a case of suspected sexual abuse is reported to the police or child protection agency. Medical professionals, teachers, and childcare professionals are required by law to report suspected cases of sexual abuse.

The physician will look for any signs of physical injury or sexual abuse, particularly in the mouth and throat and around the anus and penis or vagina. The hymen—a thin membrane covering the opening to the vagina—may be affected in abused girls. Most children, however, are not physically harmed during sexual abuse; signs of abuse are usually temporary; and the abuse is often not reported or discovered until some time after the last occurrence. Therefore, diagnostic findings from a physical examination of a child are rare.

Psychological evaluation of sexually abused children by a trained professional is essential to determine whether treatment is required. Children are often afraid to talk openly about their abuse and therefore must be made to feel very safe. The assessment includes the child's:

- abuse history and other life stressors, such as frequent moves or personal losses
- current stressors, such as medical problems or learning disabilities
- present emotional state
- coping strategies, such as withdrawal or behavioral symptoms
- strengths, such as creativity or athletic ability
- communication skills
- friendships
- attachments to adults

Tests

Blood and/or urine tests may be performed to check for STDs, including syphilis and HIV. In some cases, a drug screen may be performed as well. Women of childbearing age may be tested for pregnancy.

Imaging tests will be performed in cases of apparent or suspected head trauma, gunshot wounds, or other injuries involving weapons.

The victim's clothing and any sheets on which he or she may have been placed if transported to the emergency room in an ambulance should be kept and carefully folded. Care is needed to preserve cuts, tears, stains, or other damage to the clothing; fibers, hairs, dried blood and other body fluids found on the victim's body; and other trace evidence that may be useful for microscopic or DNA analysis.

Procedures

In adult victims, endoscopic examination of the vagina (in women) or anus (in victims of either sex) may be done, because it allows the doctor or SANE to photograph injuries to the victim's body. About two-thirds of adult rape victims have trauma to the body outside the genital region, including signs of attempted strangulation; bite marks; blunt traumatic injuries to the head, face, torso, or limbs; and penetrating injuries. Many victims also have defensive injuries, including cuts, abrasions, and bruises.

If sexual abuse of a child included physical harm, injuries may be photographed for use in prosecution of the perpetrator. As with adults, serious injuries to a child may require diagnostic imaging procedures.

Treatment

Almost all survivors of sexual abuse or assault benefit from one or more forms of psychotherapy or counseling. While classical **psychoanalysis** is not helpful, the following approaches are recommended:

- insight-oriented psychodynamic psychotherapy, useful for adults who were abused as children and need to understand how the abuse has affected their later life in order to prevent revictimization
- supportive therapy, intended to reinforce the patient's healthy methods of coping with symptoms rather than exploring deeper psychological issues
- group therapy
- cognitive-behavioral therapy, useful in changing the survivor's beliefs about the abuse that may be contributing to depression or anxiety disorders
- family therapy, recommended for survivors whose intimate relationships have been damaged or otherwise affected by the abuse or assault
- pastoral counseling, beneficial for survivors whose religious or spiritual beliefs and practices have been affected by their traumatic experiences

Drugs

Antibiotics are given to reduce the risk of STD transmission. The usual dose for adults includes intramuscular ceftriaxone in a single dose, metronidazole by mouth in a single dose, and either azithromycin by mouth in a single dose or doxycycline by mouth twice a day for seven days.

Adolescent or adult women of childbearing age may be given the option of taking Ovral (an oral contraceptive) to prevent pregnancy if the results of the hospital pregnancy test are negative. The usual dosage is two tablets by mouth at the time of treatment in the emergency room, followed by a second dose of two tablets 12 hours later.

Alternative

Some survivors of sexual abuse and assault report being helped by **acupuncture**, mindful **meditation**, prayer, relaxation techniques, **biofeedback**, massage therapy, **yoga**, tai chi, and other forms of movement therapy. Other survivors find **art therapy**, **music therapy**, and **journal therapy** helpful as ways of dealing with memories of and feelings about the abuse.

Prognosis

Sexual abuse has a high mortality rate as well as contributing to long-term physical and psychiatric problems for survivors. According to a study done in San Francisco, 25% of children exploited for commercial sex required **hospitalization** for suicide attempts, while 52% had been hospitalized for drug overdoses. Another study reported that the average life expectancy of a child prostitute after entry into prostitution is 7 years, with murder and HIV/AIDS as the leading causes of death.

Prevention

Not all forms of sexual abuse and assault are completely preventable, as children do not choose their families of origin (or adoptive families), and adults can be taken by surprise in a number of apparently safe situations. The CDC and RAINN suggest the following tips for avoiding potentially abusive situations:

- Be aware of your surroundings; avoid the use of headphones, text messaging, ear buds, or other devices that may interfere with situational awareness.
- Keep your car in good working order, cell phone charged, and money for a taxi in your pocket or otherwise readily available.
- Trust your instincts about unsafe neighborhoods or suspicious people and avoid them.
- Choose friends and associates wisely; learn to recognize the signs of possessive or otherwise abusive behavior early, before you become too deeply involved.
- Go with a group of friends to social gatherings rather than alone. Take your drink with you as you move about the party rather than leaving it unattended, and never accept a drink from someone you don't know and trust.

Resources

BOOKS

Barnett, Ola, Cindy L. Miller-Perrin, and Robin D. Perrin. *Family Violence across the Lifespan: An Introduction.* 3rd ed. Thousand Oaks, CA: Sage Publications, 2011.

Giordano, Angelo P., Elizabeth M. Datner, and Janice B. Asher, eds. *Sexual Assault: Victimization across the Life Span: A Clinical Guide*. St. Louis, MO: G.W. Medical Pub., 2003.

Itzin, Catherine, Ann Taket, and Sarah Barter-Godfrey, eds. *Domestic and Sexual Violence and Abuse: Tackling the Health and Mental Health Effects*. New York: Routledge, 2010.

Ledray, Linda, Ann Wolbert Burgess, and Angelo P. Giardino, eds. *Medical Response to Adult Sexual Assault: A Resource for Clinicians and Related Professionals.* St. Louis, MO: STM Learning, 2011.

Smyth, Michael A. *Prison Rape: Law, Media, and Meaning*. El Paso, TX: LFB Scholarly Pub., 2011.

PERIODICALS

Allard, C. B. "Military Sexual Trauma Research: A Proposed Agenda." *Journal of Trauma and Dissociation* 12 (March 2011): 324–345.

Belluardo-Crosby, M. "Mental Illness and Problematic Sexual Behaviors. A Review of the Recent Literature." *Journal of Psychosocial Nursing and Mental Health Services* 49 (February 2011): 24–28.

Carlson, B. E., et al. "Sibling Incest: Reports from Forty-One Survivors." *Journal of Child Sexual Abuse* 15 (April 2006): 19–34.

Cook, S. L., et al. "Emerging Issues in the Measurement of Rape Victimization." *Violence against Women* 17 (February 2011): 201–218.

Garrity, S. E. "Sexual Assault Prevention Programs for College-Aged Men: A Critical Evaluation." *Journal of Forensic Nursing* 7 (March 2011): 40–48.

Greenfield, E. A., et al. "Childhood Abuse as a Risk Factor for Sleep Problems in Adulthood: Evidence from a U.S. National Study." *Annals of Behavioral Medicine* 42 (October 2011): 245–256.

Hoyt, T., et al. "Military Sexual Trauma in Men: a Review of Reported Rates." *Journal of Trauma and Dissociation* 12 (March 2011): 244-260.

Keogh, A. "Rape Trauma Syndrome: Time to Open the Floodgates?" *Journal of Forensic and Legal Medicine* 14 (May 2007): 221–224.

Linden, Judith A. "Care of the Adult Patient after Sexual Assault." *New England Journal of Medicine* 365 (September 1, 2011): 834–841. http://www.nejm.org/doi/full/10.1056/NEJMcp1102869 (accessed October 2, 2011).

Rosen, T., et al. "Sexual Aggression between Residents in Nursing Homes: Literature Synthesis of an Underrecognized Problem." *Journal of the American Geriatrics Society* 58 (October 2010): 1970–1979.

OTHER

Centers for Disease Control and Prevention (CDC). "Fact Sheet: Understanding Sexual Violence." http://www.cdc.gov/violenceprevention/pdf/SV_factsheet_2011-a.pdf (accessed October 3, 2011).

———. "Preventing Intimate Partner and Sexual Violence: Program Activities Guide." http://www.cdc.gov/violenceprevention/pdf/IPV-SV_Program_Activities_Guide-a.pdf (accessed October 3, 2011).

Chicago Alliance Against Sexual Exploitation. "Know the Facts: Commercial Sexual Exploitation of Children." http://www.caase.org/ckfinder/userfiles/files/KtF_CSEC.pdf (accessed October 3, 2011).

WEBSITES

Ernoehazy, William, Jr. "Sexual Assault." Medscape Reference. December 3, 2009. http://emedicine.medscape.com/article/806120-overview (accessed September 4, 2011).

Merck Manual for Health Care Professionals Online. "Child Maltreatment: Sexual Abuse." http://www.merckmanuals.com/professional/pediatrics/child_maltreatment/overview_of_child_maltreatment.html#v1106301 (accessed September 4, 2011).

———. "Medical Examination of the Rape Victim." http://www.merckmanuals.com/professional/sec19/ch267/ch267a.html (accessed August 10, 2011).

National Center for PTSD. "Sexual Assault against Women." U.S. Department of Veterans Affairs. http://www.ptsd.va.gov/public/pages/sexual-assault-females.asp (accessed August 3, 2011).

National Institute of Justice (NIJ). "Rape and Sexual Violence." http://www.nij.gov/topics/crime/rape-sexual-violence/welcome.htm (accessed September 5, 2011).

———. "Sexual Abuse of the Elderly." http://www.nij.gov/topics/crime/elder-abuse/sexual-abuse.htm (accessed September 5, 2011).

———. "Stalking." http://www.nij.gov/topics/crime/stalking/welcome.htm (accessed October 1, 2011).

Rape, Abuse and Incest National Network (RAINN). "Effects of Sexual Assault." http://www.rainn.org/get-information/effects-of-sexual-assault (accessed October 1, 2011).

ORGANIZATIONS

American Academy of Child and Adolescent Psychiatry (AACAP), 3615 Wisconsin Ave. NW, Washington, DC, United States 20016-3007, (202) 966-7300, Fax: (202) 966-2891, http://www.aacap.org

American Psychiatric Association (APA), 1000 Wilson Blvd., Ste. 1825, Arlington, VA, United States 22209-3901, (703) 907-7300, apa@psych.org, http://www.psych.org

Centers for Disease Control and Prevention (CDC), 1600 Clifton Rd., Atlanta, GA, United States 30333, (800) 232-4636, cdcinfo@cdc.gov, http://www.cdc.gov.

Child Welfare Information Gateway, Children's Bureau/ACYF, 1250 Maryland Ave. SW, 8th Fl., Washington, DC, United States 20024, (800) 394-3366; Abuse report line: (800) 422-4453, info@childwelfare.gov, http://www.childwelfare.gov.

National Institute of Justice (NIJ), 810 Seventh Street NW, Washington, DC, United States 20531, http://www.nij.gov.

National Sexual Violence Resource Center (NSVRC), 123 North Enola Dr., Enola, PA, United States 17025, (717) 909-0710, Fax: (717) 909-0714, (877) 739-3895, resources@nsvrc.org, http://www.nsvrc.org.

Rape, Abuse and Incest National Network (RAINN), 2000 L St. NW, Ste. 406, Washington, DC, United States 20036, (202) 544-1034, (800) 656-HOPE, info@rainn.org, http://www.rainn.org.

U.S. Department of Veterans Affairs (VA), 810 Vermont Ave. NW, Washington, DC, United States 20420, (800) 827-1000, Mental health crisis line: (800) 273-8255 (press 1), http://www.va.gov.

Rebecca J. Frey, Ph.D.

Sexual addiction

Definition

Psychiatrists do not agree on the exact definition of sexual **addiction**. The general elements of sexual addiction are a compulsive pattern of sexual behavior that arises from distorted thinking; sexual behavior that interferes with personal relationships, work, or other responsibilities; and often sex with multiple partners who are seen as objects to be used rather than people.

Demographics

Because there is no professional agreement on the definition of sexual addiction, the number of people thought to be addicted to sex is unknown. What is known is that sexual addiction is much more common in men than women. People addicted to sex are not necessarily sex offenders, nor are all sexual molesters and rapists addicted to sex. Many persons with sexual addictions have other mental health and impulse control problems contributing to their addictive behaviors.

Description

Although a healthy interest in sex is normal, sexual addiction goes well beyond normal healthy interest. With sexual addiction, thinking about sexual activity and having sex dominate a person's thoughts to a degree that it interferes with his or her healthy personal relationships and activities. According to the organization Sex Addicts Anonymous, this compulsive interest in sex covers a wide range of activities, including:

- compulsive masturbation
- compulsive viewing of pornography
- compulsive phone sex
- multiple affairs outside of an established relationship
- frequent sex with anonymous partners
- multiple one-night stands
- prostitution or using prostitutes
- exhibitionism
- voyeurism
- sexual stalking
- sexual molestation or rape

Causes and symptoms

The cause of sexual addiction is not known. Some researchers have suggested that abnormal **brain** chemistry is responsible. Others suggest that early experiences and childhood **sexual abuse** contribute to the disorder.

KEY TERMS

Bipolar disorder—A mood disorder characterized by alternating periods of excessive energy and activity (mania) and depression.

Dissociation—A psychological mechanism in which the mind splits off certain aspects of a traumatic event from conscious awareness. Dissociation can affect the patient's memory, sense of reality, and sense of identity.

Obsessive-compulsive disorder (OCD)—An anxiety disorder in which a person cannot prevent him- or herself from dwelling on unwanted thoughts, acting on urges, or performing repetitious rituals, such as washing hands repeatedly.

Paraphilia—Recurring strong sexual arousal to fantasies, objects, situations, or individuals that are not considered normal in the individual's culture.

Nevertheless, there is general agreement among psychiatrists that persons with a sexual addiction usually have one or more additional mental health disorders. Where experts disagree is over whether these mental health disorders alone are enough to cause the addictive behavior or whether sexual addiction is a separate disorder present in addition to other psychiatric disorders.

Common psychiatric disorders among individuals exhibiting sexually addictive behavior include:

- obsessive-compulsive disorder (OCD)
- paraphilia
- bipolar disorder
- mania
- impulse control disorders
- substance abuse
- depression
- post traumatic stress disorder (PTSD)

Specific symptoms of sexual addiction vary with the sex act involved—however, a cycle of events appears to be common. In stage one, the individual has some ongoing emotional stressor(s) (e.g., fear, pain, anger, and loneliness). The individual is unable to develop a healthy way to relieve or cope with the stressor(s). As a result, the individual moves on to stage two. In stage two, the individual begins to dissociate and separate thoughts and emotions from contemplated or anticipated actions. It is as if the actions belong to someone else and will have no consequences for the individual. In stage three, the individual moves from thinking about acting on his or her thoughts to actually acting on them. This may mean making obscene phone calls, viewing pornography, or searching for a sexual partner. The action culminates in sexual release, and then there is a period ranging from hours to weeks before the cycle starts again.

Diagnosis

Diagnosis of sexual addiction is difficult, as many sex addicts deny that they have a problem. It is also complicated by the fact that sexual addiction often is associated with other mental health disorders. Sexual addiction is not recognized as a specific diagnosis in the ***Diagnostic and Statistical Manual of Mental Disorders***, fourth edition, text revised (*DSM-IV-TR*), a guidebook produced by the **American Psychiatric Association** (APA) to classify mental disorders. Instead, it is classified as a sexual disorder not otherwise specified (NOS). This designation is intended to be used when other causes for the behavior, such as **impulse control disorders** and **obsessive-compulsive disorder**, have been eliminated.

A fifth edition of the *DSM* (*DSM-5*) is expected to publish in 2013. Within the APA, there has been substantial controversy over whether sexual addiction should be classified as a separate psychiatric disorder. As of 2011, sexual addiction was not a specific diagnosis, but persons with sexual addiction may meet the criteria for hypersexual disorder, a new diagnosis proposed for the *DSM-5*. Hypersexual disorder is characterized by repeated thoughts of and engagement in sexual behaviors, to the extent that the actions significantly interfere with a person's daily life or cause the person distress. The behaviors must not be the result of drug or alcohol use or a psychiatric or medical condition.

Treatment

There are two approaches to treating sexual addiction. Psychiatrists who see the disorder as mainly caused by a compulsive disorder or as a variation on an impulse control disorder may treat the disorder with drugs such as **fluoxetine** (Prozac) or **clomipramine** (Anafranil), along with **psychotherapy**.

Psychiatrists who see sexual addiction as its own disorder are more likely to use psychotherapy to help the individual control addictive behavior. However, unlike addiction to drugs or alcohol, the goal of treating sexual addiction is not complete abstinence from sex, but rather to develop a normal, healthy approach to sex. Psychotherapy for sexual addiction may involve treatment at a residential center or intensive outpatient therapy.

Regardless of where the therapy takes place, the individual should be treated by professionals experienced in dealing with sexual compulsions. Some therapy may involve couples. Often, therapy is supplemented by a 12-step recovery program such as the one designed by Sex Addicts Anonymous. Since many persons addicted to sex have other mental health disorders, such as **substance abuse** or **depression**, these also are treated with drugs and psychotherapy.

Prognosis

Recovery from sexual addiction is difficult. The earlier the addiction is treated (i.e., stage one or two, before thoughts have been translated into actions), the greater the chance for recovery. Most sex addicts, however, do not recognize their disorder in its early stages and thus do not receive early treatment. Often it takes a major life-altering event to propel the sex addicted individual into treatment. Even then, relapses are common. Prognosis is also affected by the success or failure of treatment for other disorders such as substance abuse.

Prevention

Since the causes of sexual addiction are not clear, there is no definitive form of prevention. Recognizing the problem and getting early treatment for stressors can help prevent behaviors from becoming a full-blown sexual addiction.

Resources

BOOKS

Canning, Maureen. *Lust, Anger, and Love: Understanding Sexual Addiction and the Road to Healthy Intimacy.* Naperville, IL: Sourcebooks, 2008.

Steffens, Barbara, and Marsha Means. *Your Sexually Addicted Partner: Ways to Cope and Deal.* Far Hills, NJ: New Horizon Press, 2009.

PERIODICALS

Carnes, P. J., et al. "PATHOS: A Brief Screening Application for Assessing Sexual Addiction." *Journal of Addiction Medicine* (August 3, 2011) [e-pub ahead of print]. http://dx.doi.org/10.1097/ADM.0b013e3182251a28 (accessed November 13, 2011).

Elmore, J. L. "SSRI Reduction of Nonparaphilic Sexual Addiction." *CNS Spectrums* 5, no. 11 (2000): 53–56.

Garcia, F. D., and F. Thibaut. "Sexual Addictions." *American Journal of Drug and Alcohol Abuse* 36, no. 5 (2010): 254–60.

Hook, J. N., et al. "Measuring Sexual Addiction and Compulsivity: A Critical Review of Instruments." 36, no. 3 (2010): 227–60.

Irons, Richard, and Jennifer P. Schneider. "Differential Diagnosis of Addictive Sexual Disorder Using the DSM-IV." In *Sexual Addiction & Compulsivity* 3, (1996): 7–21. http://www.jenniferschneider.com/articles/diagnos.html (accessed October 27, 2011).

WEBSITES

Herkov, Michael. "What Is Sexual Addiction?" PsychCentral.com. 2006. http://psychcentral.com/lib/2006/what-is-sexual-addiction (accessed October 27, 2011).

International Institute for Trauma & Addiction Professionals. "Sexual Addiction Screening Test." SexHelp.com, 2011. http://www.sexhelp.com/sast.cfm (accessed October 27, 2011).

MedicineNet.com. "Sexual Addiction." March 12, 2010. http://www.medicinenet.com/sexual_addiction/article.htm (accessed October 27, 2011).

Morrison, Keith. "Battling Sexual Addiction." MSNBC. February 24, 2004. http://www.msnbc.msn.com/id/4302347/ns/dateline_nbc/t/battling-sexual-addiction (accessed November 13, 2011).

ORGANIZATIONS

American Psychiatric Association, 1000 Wilson Blvd., Ste. 1825, Arlington, VA, 22209-3901, (703) 907-7300, apa@psych.org, http://www.psych.org.

Sex Addicts Anonymous, PO Box 70949, Houston, TX, 77270, (1-800) 477-8191, info@saa-recovery.org, http://www.sexaa.org.

Tish Davidson, AM

Sexual aversion disorder

Definition

Sexual aversion disorder is a disorder characterized by disgust, fear, revulsion, or lack of desire in consensual relationships involving genital contact.

Normal loss of desire

To understand sexual aversion disorder, one should first understand that there are circumstances in which it is normal for people to lose interest in sexual activity. The reader can then compare these situations to the loss of desire associated with serious sexual disorders, including sexual aversion disorder.

There are a number of reasons that people lose interest in sexual intercourse. It is normal to experience a loss of desire during menopause; directly after the birth of a child; before or during menstruation; during recovery from an illness or surgery; and during such major or stressful life changes as death of a loved one, job loss, retirement, or divorce. These are considered normal causes for fluctuations in sexual desire and are generally temporary. Changing roles, such as becoming a parent for the first time or making a career change have also been found to cause loss of desire. Not having enough time for oneself or to be alone with one's partner may also contribute to normal and naturally reversible loss of desire. Loss of privacy resulting from moving a dependent elderly parent into one's home is a common cause of loss of desire in middle-aged couples. **Depression**, **fatigue**, or **stress** also contribute to lessening of sexual interest.

Demographics

Both men and women can experience sexual aversion disorder. It is thought to be more common in women than in men, possibly because women are more likely than men to be victims of rape and other forms of sexual assault. There are relatively few statistics on the number of people with sexual aversion disorder because it is often confused with other disorders, or with the normal fluctuations in desire associated with life stress. Also, many people find sex a difficult subject to discuss even with a physician, so that the number of people who seek help are probably fewer than the number of people with the disorder overall.

Description

Sexual aversion disorder represents a much stronger dislike of and active avoidance of sexual activity than the normal ups and downs in desire described above. Sexual aversion disorder is characterized not only by a lack of desire, but also by fear, revulsion, disgust, or similar emotions when the person with the disorder engages in genital contact with a partner. The aversion may take a number of different forms; it may be related to specific aspects of sexual intercourse, such as the sight of the partner's genitals or the smell of his or her body secretions, but it may include kissing, hugging, and petting, as well as intercourse itself. In some cases the person with sexual aversion disorder avoids any form of sexual contact; others, however, are not upset by kissing and caressing, and are able to proceed normally until genital contact occurs.

There are several subclassifications of sexual aversion disorder. It may be lifelong (always present) or acquired after a traumatic experience; situational (with a specific partner or in a specific set of circumstances) or generalized (occurring with any partner and in all situations). Sexual aversion may be caused by psychological factors or by a combination of physical and psychological factors.

Causes and symptoms

There are a number of causes of sexual aversion disorder. The most common causes are interpersonal problems and traumatic experiences. Interpersonal problems generally cause situation-specific sexual aversion disorder, in which the symptoms occur only with a specific partner or under certain conditions. In such cases underlying tension or discontent with the relationship is often the cause. Reasons for unhappiness with the relationship may include the discovery of marital infidelity; major disagreements over children, money, and family roles; domestic violence; lack of personal hygiene on the partner's side; or similar problems. Interpersonal problems are often the cause if intercourse was once enjoyed but is no longer desired.

Traumatic experiences have also been found to cause sexual aversion disorder, often of the generalized variety. Some possible traumas include rape, incest, molestation, or other forms of **sexual abuse**. The patient then associates intercourse with a painful experience or memory, possibly one that he or she is trying to forget. Sexual aversion disorder may also be caused by religious or cultural teachings that associate sexual activity with excessive feelings of guilt.

The symptoms of sexual aversion disorder can range from mild to severe. Mild symptoms include lack of interest and mild disgust. Severe symptoms can include panic attacks with all the symptoms of such an attack, including dizziness, shortness of breath, intense fear, and rapid heartbeat. People suffering from sexual aversion disorder often go out of their way to avoid situations that could end in sexual contact through any means they can think of, including going to bed at different times from the spouse, spending extra time at work, or trying to make themselves less sexually attractive.

Diagnosis

A **diagnosis** of sexual aversion disorder is usually made when the affected person or his or her partner mentions the problem itself or their dissatisfaction with the relationship to their family physician, gynecologist, or psychotherapist. An important first step in diagnosis is a thorough physical examination, preferably of both partners, to rule out physical causes of the disorder in the affected person, and to rule out a sexually transmitted disease, physical deformity, or lack of personal cleanliness in the partner that may contribute to the affected person's avoidance of sex.

According to the mental health profession's ***Diagnostic and Statistical Manual of Mental Disorders*** (*DSM-IV-TR*) of the **American Psychiatric Association**, to meet criteria for a diagnosis of sexual aversion disorder the patient must not only avoid nearly all genital contact

KEY TERM

Coitus—Sexual intercourse.

with his or her partner but have strong negative feelings about such contact or its possibility. In addition, the problem must be causing serious difficulties and unhappiness either for the patient or for his or her partner. In addition, there must not be any underlying physical causes, such as certain disorders of the circulatory system, skin diseases, medication side effects, or similar problems that could cause a loss of desire. To be diagnosed with sexual aversion disorder, the affected person does not have to avoid all sexual contact, but must indicate that he or she is actively avoiding genital contact.

Many other sexual disorders have signs and symptoms similar to those of sexual aversion disorder, which complicates the differential diagnosis. Sexual aversion disorder is often found in conjunction with other sexual disorders; in some cases several diagnoses are appropriate for one patient.

One disorder similar in many aspects to sexual aversion disorder is hypoactive sexual disorder. Many of the signs, such as avoiding sexual contact in a variety of ways, are similar. The primary difference between the two disorders is that a patient with hypoactive sexual disorder is not interested in sex at all and does not have sexual fantasies of any variety. A patient with sexual aversion disorder, by comparison, may have normal sexual fantasies, and even function normally with some partners, although not with a specific partner. Also, a patient with hyposexual disorder will not enjoy or desire any anticipation in sexual activities including kissing and caressing. Some, though not all, people with sexual aversion disorder do enjoy sexual foreplay until the point of genital contact.

Sexual aversion disorder and hypoactive sexual disorder are both considered to be caused mainly by psychological factors and to manifest psychological symptoms. Another disorder that can have some similar symptoms is **female sexual arousal disorder** (FSAD). FSAD refers to a woman's recurrent inability to achieve or maintain an adequate lubrication-swelling response during sexual activity. Lack of lubrication is a physical problem that may have either physical or psychological causes. Women with FSAD find intercourse uncomfortable or even painful. As a result of the physical discomfort, the woman often will avoid intercourse and sexual activity with her partner that may lead to intercourse. Although FSAD is a disorder with physical symptoms as well as psychological ones, it is easily confused with sexual aversion disorder because it may manifest as a problem of interest or desire.

Treatment

Sexual aversion disorder is not thought to have any commonplace underlying physiological causes. The usual treatment is a course of **psychotherapy** for the psychological condition(s) that may be causing the problem. **Marriage counseling** is often appropriate if the disorder concerns a spouse. Medications can be used to treat some symptoms that may be associated with sexual aversion disorder, such as panic attacks, if they are severe enough to be causing additional distress.

Prognosis

When sexual aversion disorder is addressed as a psychological disorder treatment can be very successful. Psychotherapy to treat the underlying psychological problems can be successful as long as the patient is willing to attend counseling sessions regularly. For sexual aversion disorder that is situational or acquired, psychotherapy for both the patient and his or her partner (**couples therapy**) may help to resolve interpersonal conflicts that may be contributing to the disorder. Panic attacks caused by or associated with the disorder can be treated successfully by medication if the doctor considers this form of treatment necessary.

If sexual aversion disorder is not diagnosed, discussed, or treated, the result may be infidelity, divorce, or chronic unhappiness in the relationship or marriage.

Resources

BOOKS

American Psychiatric Association. *Diagnostic and Statistical Manual of Mental Disorders*. 4th ed., text rev. Washington, DC: American Psychiatric Publishing, 2000.

Sadock, Benjamin J., and Virginia A. Sadock, eds. *Comprehensive Textbook of Psychiatry*. Vol. 2. 7th ed. Philadelphia: Lippincott Williams and Wilkins, 2000.

PERIODICALS

Brotto, L. A. "The DSM Diagnostic Criteria for Sexual Aversion Disorder." *Archives of Sexual Behavior* 39, no. 2 (2010): 271–77.

Fabre, L. F., and L. C. Smith. "The Effect of Major Depression on Sexual Function in Women." *Journal of Sexual Medicine* 9, no. 1 (2012): 231–39.

Kingsberg, S. A., and G. Knudson. "Female Sexual Disorders: Assessment, Diagnosis, and Treatment." CNS Spectrums 16, no. 2 (2011) [e-pub ahead of print]. http://www.cnsspectrums.com/aspx/articledetail.aspx?articleid=3577 (accessed January 9, 2012).

Tish Davidson, A.M.

Sexual deviance *see* **Paraphilias**

Sexual dysfunctions

Definition

Sexual dysfunction disorders, sometimes also called sexual dysfunctions, are problems (malfunctions) that interfere with any stage of normal sexual activity, such as the desire, arousal, initiation, consummation, orgasm, or satisfaction with sex. Such disorders inhibit, or in some cases stop, the individual or the couple from enjoying sexual activity. They may begin early in life or may develop over time after experiencing many years of fulfilling sexual activity. Such sexual dysfunctions, which may be physical and/or psychological in nature, may cause an individual to have a partial or total inability to participate in one or many stages of the sexual act. **Depression**, guilt, and past sexual experiences may contribute to sexual disorders. A physical malady may also be responsible for not being able to enjoy or participate in sex.

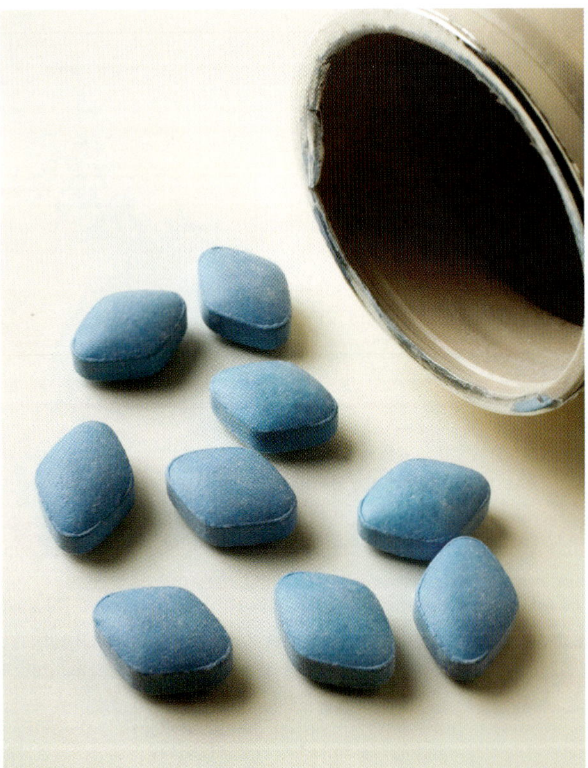

Viagra pills. *(© Garry Gay/Alamy)*

Demographics

Such sexual dysfunction disorders occur in both men and women and are independent of sexual preference or orientation. Such disorders are more common in people who abuse alcohol or drugs, and in those who have chronic medical disorders such as diabetes and degenerative neurological disorders. Psychological problems may cause problems with maintaining relationships, which consequently can cause problems with sex. Couples with an open, honest, and stable relationship are more apt to avoid psychological dysfunction than those without such relationships.

Age is a significant factor in sexual dysfunctions. Most cases appear in people who are in their early adult years, such as beginning around 20 years of age and going throughout their late 30s and early 40s. For women, sexual dysfunction is also more common in women during their perimenopause (transitional period in which a woman's body shifts from regular cycles of ovulation and menstruation to infertility, or menopause) and postmenopause (stage in which menopause is complete).

Description

Probably nowhere in human health do the body and mind interact more than during sex. There are four generally recognized phases of sexual activity, involving both mental and physical responses, which are applicable to both men and women. These phases are in sequence:

- desire or appetite—fantasies or thoughts about sex
- excitement—physical changes to prepare the body for intercourse and accompanying sense of sexual pleasure
- orgasm—physical response that leads to the peak of physical pleasure and release of sexual tension
- resolution—physical relaxation accompanied by a feeling of well-being and satisfaction

Sexual-dysfunction disorders can occur in any of these four phases. Their cause may be physiological or psychological. More than one sexual dysfunction disorder may appear simultaneously. The ***Diagnostic and Statistical Manual of Mental Disorders*** (latest edition *DSM-IV-TR*), produced by the **American Psychiatric Association** and used by most mental health professionals in North America and Europe to diagnose mental disorders, recognizes nine specific sexual dysfunctions:

- Disorders of desire: These interfere with the initiation of sex and include hypoactive sexual desire disorder (low interest in sex, or low libido) and sexual aversion disorder (objections to having the genitals touched). A decreased sexual interest may be caused by a lowered production of estrogen in women or testosterone in both men and women. It also can be caused by the normal aging process, certain medications, stress or depression, fatigue, pregnancy in women and other problems.

- Disorders of excitement or sexual arousal: These are female sexual arousal disorder (when a woman fails to have physiological responses associated with arousal), and male erectile disorder (when a man fails to get an adequate erection, also referred to as erectile dysfunction). Past terms used with such disorders include frigidity in women and impotence in men.
- Disorders of the orgasm phase: These are female orgasmic disorder (when a woman fails to reach orgasm); and male orgasmic disorder (when a man fails to reach orgasm) and premature ejaculation (when a man reaches orgasm too soon).
- Sexual pain disorders (associated with intercourse and orgasm): These disorders are vaginismus (a condition in which the outer part of a woman's vagina causes involuntary spasms that cause pain and interferes with sexual intercourse) and dyspareunia (a condition in which there is pain during intercourse in either men or women, often caused by insufficient lubrication of the vagina in women).

Changes proposed for the fifth edition of the *DSM* (*DSM 5*, 2013) including placing the following disorders within the diagnostic category of Sexual Dysfunctions (previously Sexual and Gender Identity Disorders):

- erectile disorder
- female orgasmic disorder
- delayed ejaculation
- early ejaculation
- sexual interest/arousal disorder in women
- hypoactive sexual desire disorder in men
- genito-pelvis pain/penetration disorder
- substance-induced sexual dysfunction
- sexual dysfunction associated with a known general medical condition
- other specified sexual dysfunction
- unspecified sexual dysfunction

A new category entitled Gender Dysphoria has been proposed to incorporate the remaining disorders previously grouped with the sexual dysfunctions. The members of the American Psychiatric Association working group for the Sexual Dysfunctions chapter are also considering including diagnostic criteria for hypersexual disorder in the appendix.

In addition, medications or illicit drugs may cause substance-induced sexual dysfunction, and sexual dysfunction may be caused by a general medical condition such as diabetes or nerve damage. If the sexual dysfunction falls into none of the above areas, it is classified as sexual dysfunction not otherwise specified.

Causes and symptoms

The causes of sexual dysfunction disorders are varied, as are their symptoms. In general, symptoms prevent the initiation of sex or the completion of the sex act, or they interfere with satisfaction derived from sex. Almost everyone has some problem with sexual functioning or fulfillment at some point in his or her life, but not all problems are considered sexual dysfunction disorders. Sexual satisfaction is very personal and individual, so what may be an annoyance for one couple may be a serious problem for another. However, estimates suggest that roughly one-fourth of the adult population may have a sexual dysfunction disorder. More women than men report having sexual dysfunction disorders, but the difference may be that women are more open and active about seeking help with sexual problems than are men.

Causes

Some physical causes of sexual dysfunctions include:

- enlarged prostate gland
- injuries, such as with the back
- various chronic diseases, such as multiple sclerosis and diabetic neuropathy
- numerous drugs, including alcohol, antihypertensives, anticonvulsants, neuroleptics, antihistamines, narcotics, nicotine, psychotherapeutics, stimulants, and selective serotonin reuptake inhibitors (SSRI) antidepressant drugs
- endocrine disorders (of the adrenal, pituitary, and thyroid)
- organ failure, such as heart and lungs
- hormonal deficiency, such as with estrogen and testosterone
- nerve damage
- decreased blood flow and other such problems
- birth defects, such as abnormalities in the pelvis or the ovaries (in women)
- insufficient vaginal lubrication

Some psychological causes of sexual dysfunctions include such disorders as **bipolar disorder**, depression, epilepsy, and **schizophrenia**. For instance, in bipolar disorder, a person may feel too elated at times, or too depressed at other times, to have or act on sexual desires.

KEY TERMS

Anticonvulsants—Drugs that treat epileptic seizures.

Antihypertensives—Drugs that treat hypertension; that is, high blood pressure.

Kegel exercises—Repetitive contractions to tone the pubococcygeus muscle of the pelvic floor for enhancing sexual response during intercourse or controlling incontinence.

Neuroleptics—Drugs that treat psychosis, such as hallucinations.

Psychotherapeutics—The general term for drugs such as tranquilizers, sedatives, analgesics, and stimulants.

Selective serotonin reuptake inhibitors—Drugs that treat depression, anxiety, and some personality disorders.

Symptoms

Some symptoms of sexual dysfunctions include:

- inability to feel aroused (both men and women)
- lack of interest in sex (both men and women)
- pain with intercourse (both men and women, but more likely in women)
- delay or absence of ejaculation when properly stimulated (men)
- inability to control timing of ejaculation (men)
- inability to get an erection (men)
- inability to keep an erection throughout intercourse (men)
- burning sensation in or around the vulva or in the vagina during sexual contact (women)
- inability to reach orgasm (women)
- inability to relax vaginal muscles (which prevents intercourse) (women)
- inadequate vaginal lubrication before and/or during sexual intercourse (women)
- low libido due to physical or hormonal problems, psychological problems, or relationship problems (women)

Diagnosis

Diagnosis begins when a medical professional conducts a thorough sexual and medical history and often performs a physical examination including laboratory tests. The doctor will conduct tests based on the specific sexual-dysfunction symptoms experienced by the patient.

Treatment

Treatment for sexual dysfunction depends on its cause. It must be individualized based on the cause and the specific dysfunction. Treatment includes physiological treatment, **psychotherapy**, and/or education and communication counseling. Medical causes can be treated, and usually reversed, with medication and/or surgery. Causes from disabilities or physical illnesses can be improved with physical therapy or mechanical aids (such as penile implants). For instance, women can increase blood flow to certain muscles within the pelvic floor, which produce organisms, with the use of Kegel exercises.

Most people can be helped to resolve their problems and improve their sex life. For instance, men can be helped with sildenafil (Viagra), which increases blood flow within the penis, when they have trouble in having an erection. Women can get help, for instance, with lubricating gels, when they are exceptionally dry within the vaginal area. For depression or anxiety associated with sexual dysfunction, **antidepressants** can help to counter the problem in both men and women.

Many behavioral therapies are offered that help with sexual dysfunction. For instance, cognitive behavior therapy offers men with **erectile dysfunction** help to overcome the problem. Therapists teach patients to eliminate distractions during sexual activity and to communicate better with their partner with regard to their special needs. Generally, the sooner the person receives help, the easier the problem is to resolve. Support of a partner is often critical to successful resolution of the problem. The Masters and Johnson treatment strategies have been available since the late 1950s to solve sexual dysfunctions of many types.

Prognosis

People with sexual dysfunction should seek professional medical advice. The probable outcome of such medical advice is generally good for the cases of physical causes. Doctors can successfully diagnose the root of such sexual dysfunction so it can be eliminated or controlled. However, the longer the physical dysfunction is left untreated, the more difficult it is to overcome.

Some types of sexual dysfunction cannot be treated with medical or surgical treatments. These include psychological factors. However, the prognosis for treating these causes is still good for moderate or

QUESTIONS TO ASK YOUR DOCTOR

- What is causing my sexual problem?
- What tests can be done to solve my problem?
- Will a lifestyle change help?
- What type of counseling is advised?
- Are impotence and erectile dysfunction the same thing?
- Could menopause cause my sexual dysfunction?

temporary dysfunction relating to these factors with the use of psychotherapy. Those with more serious or permanent causes are less likely to have positive outcomes. In any case, people with psychological sexual dysfunctions should seek medical attention immediately, such as victims of sexual **trauma** (such as rape or abuse) whose dysfunction is impairing sexual activities. Counseling to overcome such problems is possible if proper help is found in a timely manner.

Some forms of sexual dysfunction can lead to infertility, including: failure to have sexual intercourse, infrequent sexual intercourse, erectile or ejaculatory dysfunction, and **vaginismus** or dyspareunia.

Prevention

Open and informative communications between parents and children about sex, relationships, and health can help prevent or, at least, minimize physiological problems that may develop in the early years of sexual contact. Such information will also help to maximize the chances of having healthy sexual relationships.

Over-the-counter (nonprescription) and prescription medications, which can have adverse consequences with sexual activities, should be discussed with a medical professional if sexual dysfunctions occur. The medical community recommends drinking alcoholic beverages in moderation or avoiding them altogether.

Resources

BOOKS

American Psychiatric Association. *Diagnostic and Statistical Manual of Mental Disorders.* 4th ed., text revised. Washington, DC: American Psychiatric Association, 2000.

Black, Donald W., and Nancy C. Andreasen. *Introductory Textbook of Psychiatry.* Washington, DC: American Psychiatric Pub., 2011.

Braun-Harvey, Douglas. *Sexual Health in Recovery: A Professional Counselor's Manual.* New York: Springer, 2011.

Leiblum, Sandra R., ed. *Treating Sexual Desire Disorders: A Clinical Casebook.* New York: Guilford 2010.

Levine, Stephen B., et al., eds. *Handbook of Clinical Sexuality for Mental Health Professionals.* New York: Routledge, 2010.

Sadock, Benjamin J., and Virginia A. Sadock, eds. *Kaplan & Sadock's Pocket Handbook of Clinical Psychiatry.* Philadelphia: Wolters Lluwer Health/Lippincott Williams & Wilkins, 2010.

Zaslau, Stanley, ed. *Dx/Rx: Sexual Dysfunction in Men and Women.* Sudbury, MA: Jones & Bartlett Learning, 2011.

WEBSITES

American Psychiatric Association. "Sexual Dysfunctions." DSM-5 Development. http://www.dsm5.org/proposedrevision/Pages/SexualDysfunctions.aspx (accessed May 27, 2011).

MedlinePlus. "Female Sexual Dysfunction." April 24, 2010. http://www.mayoclinic.com/health/female-sexual-dysfunction/DS00701 (accessed May 29, 2011).

———. "Sexual Problems Overview." September 11, 2010. http://www.nlm.nih.gov/medlineplus/ency/article/001951.htm (accessed May 29, 2011).

ORGANIZATIONS

American Association of Sexuality Educators, Counselors, and Therapists, 1444 I St. NW, Ste. 700, Washington, DC, 20005, (202) 449-1099, Fax: (202) 216-9646, http://www.aasect.org.

Sexuality Information and Education Council of the United States, 1706 R St. NW, Washington, DC, 20009, (202) 265-2405, Fax: (202) 462-2340, http://www.aasect.org.

Tish Davidson, A.M.

Sexual masochism

Definition

The essential feature of sexual masochism is the feeling of sexual arousal or excitement resulting from receiving pain, suffering, or humiliation. The pain, suffering, or humiliation is real and not imagined and can be physical or psychological in nature. A person with a **diagnosis** of sexual masochism is sometimes called a masochist.

The ***Diagnostic and Statistical Manual of Mental Disorders***, also known as the *DSM*, is used by mental health professionals to diagnose specific mental disorders. In the 2000 edition of this manual (the Fourth Edition Text Revision also known as *DSM-IV-TR*) sexual masochism is one of several **paraphilias**. Paraphilias are intense and recurrent sexually arousing urges, fantasies, or behaviors.

Demographics

Although masochistic sexual fantasies often begin in childhood, the onset of sexual masochism typically occurs during early adulthood. When actual masochistic behavior begins, it will often continue on a chronic course for people with this disorder, especially when no treatment is sought.

Sadomasochism involving consenting partners is not considered rare or unusual in the United States. It often occurs outside of the realm of a mental disorder. More people consider themselves masochistic than sadistic.

Sexual masochism is slightly more prevalent in males than in females.

Death due to hypoxyphilia is a relatively rare phenomenon. Data indicate that less than two people per million in the United States and other countries die from hypoxyphilia.

Description

In addition to the sexual pleasure or excitement derived from receiving pain and humiliation, an individual with sexual masochism often experiences significant impairment or distress in functioning due to masochistic behaviors or fantasies.

With regard to actual masochistic behavior, the person may be receiving the pain, suffering, or humiliation at the hands of another person. This partner may have a diagnosis of **sexual sadism** but this is not necessarily the case. Such behavior involving a partner is sometimes referred to as sadomasochism.

Masochistic acts include being physically restrained through the use of handcuffs, cages, chains, and ropes. Other acts and fantasies related to sexual masochism include receiving punishment or pain by means of paddling, spanking, whipping, burning, beating, electrical shocks, cutting, rape, and mutilation. Psychological humiliation and degradation can also be involved.

Masochistic behavior can also occur in the context of a role-playing fantasy. For example, a sadist can play the role of teacher or master and a masochist can play the role of student or slave.

The person with sexual masochism may also be inflicting the pain or suffering on himself or herself. This can be done through **self-mutilation**, cutting, or burning.

The masochistic acts experienced or fantasized by the person sometimes reflect a sexual or psychological submission on the part of the masochist. These acts can range from relatively safe behaviors to very physically and psychologically dangerous behavior.

The *DSM* lists one particularly dangerous and deadly form of sexual masochism called hypoxyphilia. People with hypoxyphilia experience sexual arousal by being deprived of oxygen. The deprivation can be caused by chest compression, noose, plastic bag, mask, or other means and can be administered by another person or be self-inflicted.

Causes and symptoms

Causes

There is no universally accepted cause or theory explaining the origin of sexual masochism, or sadomasochism in general. However, there are some theories that attempt to explain the presence of sexual paraphilias in general. One theory is based on learning theory that paraphilias originate because inappropriate sexual fantasies are suppressed. Because they are not acted upon initially, the urge to carry out the fantasies increases and when they are finally acted upon, a person is in a state of considerable distress and/or arousal. In the case of sexual masochism, masochistic behavior becomes associated with and inextricably linked to sexual behavior.

There is also a belief that masochistic individuals truly want to be in the dominating role. This causes them to become conflicted and thus submissive to others.

Another theory suggests that people seek out sadomasochistic behavior as a means of escape. They get to act out fantasies and become new and different persons.

Symptoms

Individuals with sexual masochism experience sexual excitement from physically or psychologically receiving pain, suffering, and/or humiliation. They may be receiving the pain, suffering, or humiliation at the hands of another person, who may or may not be a sadist, or they may be administering the pain, suffering, or humiliation themselves.

They experience distressed or impaired functioning because of the masochistic behaviors, urges, and fantasies. This distress or impairment can impact functioning in social, occupational, or other contexts.

Diagnosis

The *DSM* criteria for sexual masochism include recurrent intense sexual fantasies, urges, or behaviors involving real acts in which the individual with the disorder is receiving psychological or physical suffering, pain, and humiliation. The suffering, pain, and humiliation cause the person with sexual masochism to be sexually aroused. The fantasies, urges, or behaviors must be present for at least six months.

The diagnostic criteria also require that the person has experienced significant distress or impairment because of these behaviors, urges, or fantasies. The distress and impairment can be present in social, occupational, or other functioning.

Sexual masochism must be differentiated from normal sexual arousal, behavior, and experimentation. It should also be differentiated from sadomasochistic behavior involving mild pain and/or the simulation of more dangerous pain. When this is the case, a diagnosis of sexual masochism is not necessarily warranted.

Sexual masochism must also be differentiated from self-defeating or self-mutilating behavior that is performed for reasons other than sexual arousal.

Individuals with sexual masochism often have other sexual disorders or paraphilias. Some individuals, especially males, have diagnoses of both sexual sadism and sexual masochism.

Treatment

Behavior therapy is often used to treat paraphilias. This can include management and conditioning of arousal patterns and masturbation. Therapies involving cognitive restructuring and **social skills training** are also utilized.

Medication is also used to reduce fantasies and behavior relating to paraphilias. This is especially true of people who exhibit severely dangerous masochistic behaviors.

Treatment can also be complicated by health problems relating to sexual behavior. Sexually transmitted diseases and other medical problems, especially when the sadomasochistic behavior involves the release of blood, can be present. Also, people participating in hypoxyphilia and other dangerous behaviors can suffer extreme pain and even death.

Prognosis

Because of the chronic course of sexual masochism and the uncertainty of its causes, treatment is often difficult. The fact that many masochistic fantasies are socially unacceptable or unusual leads some people who may have the disorder to not seek or continue treatment.

Treating a paraphilia is often a sensitive subject for many mental health professionals. Severe or difficult cases of sexual masochism should be referred to professionals who have experience treating such cases.

Prevention

Because it is sometimes unclear whether sadomasochistic behavior is within the realm of normal experimentation or indicative of a diagnosis of sexual masochism, prevention is a tricky issue. Often, prevention refers to managing sadomasochistic behavior so it primarily involves only the simulation of severe pain and it always involves consenting partners familiar with each other's limitations.

Also, because fantasies and urges originating in childhood or adolescence may form the basis for sadomasochistic behavior in adulthood, prevention is made difficult. People may be very unwilling to divulge their urges and discuss their sadistic fantasies as part of treatment.

Resources

BOOKS

American Psychiatric Association. *Diagnostic and Statistical Manual of Mental Disorders*. 4th ed., text rev. Washington, DC: American Psychiatric Publishing, 2000.

Baxter, Lewis R. Jr., and Robert O. Friedel, eds. *Current Psychiatric Diagnosis & Treatment*. Philadelphia: Current Medicine, 1999.

Black, Donald W., and Nancy C. Andreasen. *Introductory Textbook of Psychiatry*. 5th ed. Arlington, VA: American Psychiatric Publishing, 2011.

Ebert, Michael H., et al. *Current Diagnosis & Treatment in Psychiatry*. New York: McGraw-Hill, 2008.

Ali Fahmy, Ph.D.

Sexual sadism

Definition

The essential feature of sexual sadism is a feeling of sexual excitement resulting from administering pain, suffering, or humiliation to another person. The pain, suffering, or humiliation inflicted on the other is real; it is not imagined and may be either physical or psychological in nature. A person with a **diagnosis** of sexual sadism is sometimes called a sadist. The name of the disorder is derived from the proper name of the Marquis Donatien de Sade (1740-1814), a French aristocrat who became notorious for writing novels around the theme of inflicting pain as a source of sexual pleasure.

The ***Diagnostic and Statistical Manual of Mental Disorders***, also known as the *DSM*, is used by mental health professionals to give diagnoses of specific mental disorders. In the 2000 edition of this manual, sexual sadism is listed as one of several **paraphilias**. The paraphilias are a group of mental disorders characterized by **obsession** with unusual sexual practices or with sexual activity involving nonconsenting or inappropriate partners (such as children or animals). The paraphilias may include recurrent sexually arousing urges or fantasies as well as actual behaviors.

Demographics

Although sadistic sexual fantasies often begin in the person's childhood, the onset of active sexual sadism typically occurs during early adult life. When actual sadistic behavior begins, it will often continue on a chronic course for people with this disorder, especially if they do not seek help.

Sexual sadism with consenting partners is much more common than with nonconsensual partners. When consenting partners are involved, the sadist and the masochist may be either male or female. When non-consenting partners are involved, the sadist is almost always a male.

Sadomasochism involving consenting partners is not considered rare or unusual in the United States. It often occurs outside of the realm of a mental disorder. Fewer people consider themselves sadistic than masochistic.

Description

In addition to the sexual pleasure or excitement derived from inflicting pain and humiliation on another, a person diagnosed with sexual sadism often experiences significant impairment or distress in functioning due to actual sadistic behaviors or sadistic fantasies.

With regard to actual sadistic behavior, the person receiving the pain, suffering, or humiliation may or may not be a willing partner. Whether or not the partner is consenting, it is the very real suffering they are experiencing that is arousing to the sadist. When the sexual activity is consensual, the behavior is sometimes referred to as sadomasochism. The consenting partner may be given a diagnosis of **sexual masochism**. Like sadism, masochism is a term derived from a proper name; in this instance, from Leopold von Sacher-Masoch (1836-1895), an Austrian novelist who described the disorder in his books.

The sadistic acts performed or fantasized by a person with sadism often reflect a desire for sexual or psychological domination of another person. These acts range from behavior that is not physically harmful although it may be humiliating to the other person (such as being urinated upon), to criminal and potentially deadly behavior. Acts of domination may include restraining or imprisoning the partner through the use of handcuffs, cages, chains, or ropes. Other acts and fantasies related to sexual sadism include paddling, spanking, whipping, burning, beating, administering electrical shocks, biting, urinating or defecating on the other person, cutting, rape, murder, and mutilation.

In extreme cases, sexual sadism can lead to serious injury or death for the other person. According to the *DSM* these catastrophic results are more likely when the paraphilia is diagnosed as severe, and when it is associated with **antisocial personality disorder**, a personality disorder that may include psychotic symptoms.

Causes and symptoms

Causes

There is no universally accepted cause or theory explaining the origin of sexual sadism, or of sadomasochism. Some researchers attempt to explain the presence of sexual paraphilias in general as the result of biological factors. Evidence for this viewpoint comes from abnormal findings from neuropsychological and neurological tests of sex offenders.

Some researchers believe that paraphilias are related to such other problems as **brain** injury, **schizophrenia**, or another mental disorder. Often, people with sexual disorders or symptoms of paraphilia are diagnosed with other mental disorders.

Another theory about paraphilias is derived from learning theory. It suggests that paraphilias develop because the person is required to suppress, or squelch, inappropriate sexual fantasies. Because the fantasies are not acted out initially, the urge to carry them out increases. When the person finally acts upon the fantasies, they are in a state of considerable distress and/or arousal. This theory is not accepted by forensic experts at the Federal Bureau of Investigation (FBI) and other researchers who study sexual offenses. Rather than suppressing fantasies, most people who are eventually arrested for crimes involving sexual sadism begin with milder forms of acting on them and progressing to more harmful ways of acting out. For example, the FBI's database indicates that these people—almost always males—start out by collecting pornographic materials that depict sadistic acts, or they may draw ropes and chains on the photographs of models in swimsuit or lingerie advertisements. They then typically progress to following women at a distance, to hiring a prostitute in order to act out the fantasy, and to asking a girlfriend or other willing partner to cooperate with their fantasy. In other words, the severity of sadistic acts tends to increase over time.

Symptoms

Individuals with sexual sadism derive sexual excitement from physically or psychologically administering pain, suffering, and/or humiliation to another person, who may or may not be a consenting partner.

They may experience distressed or impaired functioning because of the sadistic behaviors or fantasies. This distress or impairment may be due to the fact that the partner is not consenting.

Diagnosis

The diagnosis of sexual sadism is complicated by several factors, beginning with the fact that most persons with the disorder do not enter therapy voluntarily. Some are referred to treatment by a court order. Some are motivated by fear of discovery by employers or family members, and a minority enter therapy because their wife or girl friend is distressed by the disorder. The diagnosis of sexual sadism is based on the results of a psychiatrist's interview with the patient. In some cases a person with sexual sadism may be referred to a specialized clinic for the treatment of sexual disorders. In the clinic, he will be given questionnaires intended to measure the presence and extent of cognitive distortions regarding rape and other forms of coercion, aggression, and impulsivity.

DSM-IV-TR criteria for sexual sadism include recurrent intense sexual fantasies, urges, or behaviors involving real acts in which another person is suffering psychological or physical suffering, pain, and humiliation. The victim's suffering, pain, and humiliation cause the person with sexual sadism to become aroused. The fantasies, urges, or behaviors must be present for at least six months.

The diagnostic criteria also require either that the person has acted on these urges or fantasies with a nonconsenting person, or that the person has experienced noticeable distress or interpersonal problems because of these urges or fantasies.

Sexual sadism must be differentiated from normal sexual arousal, behavior, and experimentation. Some forms of mild aggression, such as "love bites" or scratching, are within the range of normal behavior during sexual intercourse. Sadism should also be differentiated from sadomasochistic behavior that involves only mild pain and/or the simulation of more dangerous pain. When these factors are present, a diagnosis of sexual sadism is not necessarily warranted.

Other mental disorders, such as the psychotic disorders, may include elements of sadism or other paraphilias. For example, patients with psychotic symptoms may perform sadistic acts for reasons other than sexual excitement. In these cases, an additional diagnosis of sexual sadism is not warranted.

Persons diagnosed with sexual sadism may have other sexual disorders or paraphilias. Some individuals, especially males, have diagnoses of both sexual sadism and sexual masochism.

KEY TERMS

Forensic—Pertaining to courtroom procedure or evidence used in courts of law.

Masochism—A mental disorder in which a person obtains sexual satisfaction through pain or humiliation inflicted by the self or by another person. The term is sometimes used more generally to refer to a tendency to find pleasure in submissiveness or self-denial.

Medroxyprogesterone acetate (MPA)—A female hormone that may be prescribed for male patients with sexual sadism or other paraphilias. MPA helps to control sexual urges in men by speeding up the clearance of testosterone from the bloodstream.

Paraphilias—A group of mental disorders that is characterized by recurrent intense sexual urges and sexually arousing fantasies generally involving (1) non-human objects, (2) the suffering or humiliation of oneself or one's partner (not merely simulated), or (3) children or other non-consenting persons.

Sadism—A mental disorder in which sexual arousal and gratification are obtained by inflicting pain or humiliation on another person.

Treatment

Behavior therapy is often used to treat paraphilias. This approach to treatment may include the management and conditioning of arousal patterns and masturbation. Therapies involving cognitive restructuring and **social skills training** are also often utilized.

Medication may be used to reduce fantasies and behavior relating to paraphilias. This form of treatment is especially recommended for people who exhibit sadistic behaviors that are dangerous to others. The medications that may be used include female hormones (most commonly medroxyprogesterone acetate, or MPA), which speed up the clearance of testosterone from the bloodstream; antiandrogen medications, which block the body's uptake of testosterone; and the **selective serotonin reuptake inhibitors**, or **SSRIs**.

Nonconsensual sadistic behavior often leads to problems with the criminal justice system. Issues related to legal problems may impair or delay the patient's treatment. Persons with sexual sadism may be reluctant to seek or continue treatment because they fear being reported to the police or being named in a lawsuit by an unwilling partner.

Treatment of sexual sadism may also be complicated by health problems related to sexual behavior. Sexually transmitted diseases and other medical problems may be present, especially when the sadistic behavior involves the release of blood or other body fluids.

Prognosis

Because of the chronic course of sexual sadism and the uncertainty of its causes, treatment is often difficult. The fact that many sadistic fantasies are socially unacceptable or unusual leads many people who may have the disorder to avoid or drop out of treatment. Treating a paraphilia is often a sensitive subject for many mental health professionals. Severe or difficult cases of sexual sadism should be referred to a specialized clinic for the treatment of sexual disorders or to professionals with experience in treating such cases.

As was noted previously, acts of sexual sadism tend to grow more violent or bizarre over time. As males with the disorder grow older, however, their ability to commit such acts begins to decrease. Sexual sadism is rarely diagnosed in men over 50.

Prevention

Because it is sometimes unclear whether sadomasochistic behavior is within the realm of normal experimentation or indicative of a diagnosis of sexual sadism, prevention is a tricky issue. Often, prevention refers to managing sadistic behavior so it never involves non-consenting individuals and it primarily involves the simulation of pain and not real pain.

Also, because fantasies and urges originating in childhood or adolescence may form the basis for sadomasochistic behavior in adulthood, prevention is difficult. People may be very unwilling to divulge their urges and discuss their sadistic fantasies.

Resources

BOOKS

American Psychiatric Association. *Diagnostic and Statistical Manual of Mental Disorders*. 4th ed., text rev. Washington, DC: American Psychiatric Publishing, 2000.

Baxter, Lewis R. Jr., and Robert O. Friedel, eds. *Current Psychiatric Diagnosis & Treatment*. Philadelphia: Current Medicine, 1999.

Black, Donald W., and Nancy C. Andreasen. *Introductory Textbook of Psychiatry*. 5th ed. Arlington, VA: American Psychiatric Publishing, 2011.

Douglas, John, and Mark Olshaker. *Mindhunter: Inside the FBI's Elite Serial Crime Unit*. Audio ed. New York: Simon and Schuster, 2010.

Ebert, Michael H., et al. *Current Diagnosis & Treatment in Psychiatry*. New York: McGraw-Hill, 2008.

Ali Fahmy, Ph.D.

Sexual Violence Risk-20

Definition

The Sexual Violence Risk-20, also called the SVR-20, is an assessment instrument used by mental health professionals.

Purpose

The SVR-20 provides a structure for reviewing information important in characterizing an individual's risk of committing sexual violence and for targeting plans to manage that risk. The instrument's authors define sexual violence as, "actual, attempted, or threatened sexual contact with a person who is nonconsenting or unable to give consent."

Precautions

SVR-20 results should be finalized and interpreted by a professional who is familiar with the scientific literature on sexual violence, and who is experienced in conducting individual assessments on sexual and violent offenders. The instrument cannot provide new information about past behavior or profile an examinee as a sexually violent offender. Rather, it helps provide a structure to follow in estimating risk of sexual violence under certain circumstances. The instrument should not be used as a stand-alone measure, and predictions derived from its use should be subject to critical review. It is especially important to place results in the contexts of the examinee's personal style, likely environmental conditions, and base rates of sexual violence in other offenders with similar characteristics.

Description

The SVR-20 is a tool that helps guide a professional in conducting a minimally comprehensive assessment of sexual violence risk. The assessment process is based on six principles:

- It is important to gather a depth of information about the examinee's personal, social, occupational, mental health, illegal, and other relevant behavior.
- Information should be gathered using a variety of sources and methods, including (and not limited to) record reviews, interviews, and psychological, physiological, and medical techniques.
- Information should be gathered from the examinee, his or her relatives and acquaintances, the victim(s), professionals who have interacted with the examinee, and any other sources likely to yield useful information.
- The examinee's history and future exposure to risk factors should be considered.
- The examiner should critically weigh the accuracy, credibility, and applicability of the data that has been gathered.
- The risk assessment process should be ongoing, with regular reassessments for many examinees.

The content of the SVR-20 was developed following a comprehensive review of similar instruments and of the scientific literature on risk for sexual violence and reoffense. The SVR-20 materials consist of a reference manual and protocol sheets that are filled out by the examiner. The instrument includes three major sections: Psychosocial Adjustment, Sexual Offenses, and Future Plans. The SVR-20 items are rated as not present, somewhat or possibly present, or clearly present. The overall pattern is used in forming a professional judgment about the person's risk of sexual recidivism (low, medium, or high). It is intended as a qualitative, not as an absolute, measure. However, the scores of no, maybe/sometimes, and yes can be converted into values (0, 1, and 2, respectively), a method that has been validated in a Swedish study. The SVR-20 has proven again and again to be an excellent tool for evaluating recidivism risk.

The Psychosocial Adjustment section includes 11 risk factors: sexual deviation, victim of **child abuse**, psychopathy, major mental illness, substance use problems, suicidal/homicidal ideation, relationship problems, employment problems, past nonsexual violent offenses, past nonviolent offenses, and past supervision failure.

The Sexual Offenses section includes seven risk factors: high-density sex offenses, multiple sex offense types, physical harm to victim(s) in sex offenses, uses weapons or threats of death in sex offenses, escalation in frequency and severity of sex offenses, extreme minimization or **denial** of sex offenses, and attitudes that support or condone sex offenses.

KEY TERMS

High-density sex offenses—Several offenses within a short period of time.

Risk assessment—The process of gathering and interpreting data useful in estimating the probability that an individual will demonstrate sexual violence.

Risk management—Using the results of a risk assessment to tailor intervention strategies intended to reduce the likelihood that an individual will demonstrate sexual violence.

Sexual violence—Actual, attempted, or threatened sexual contact with a person who is nonconsenting or unable to give consent.

The Future Plans section includes two factors: lacks realistic plans and negative attitude toward **intervention**. Aside from factors related to the examinee's thinking and personality, items found in the first and second sections reference fixed or relatively stable characteristics.

The first and third sections are relevant not only to sexual violence, but also to violence in general. There is also an unstructured supplementary section entitled Other Considerations that can be used to describe unique factors relevant to an examinee's probability of risk.

Results

The SVR-20 does not allow for the definite prediction of sexual violence. Prediction of risk is summarized using a rating of low, moderate, or high. Although the instrument's authors did not provide decision-making guidelines for determining the appropriate rating, they did recommend five questions to consider in communicating a "Risk Message" derived from the results:

- What is the likelihood that the individual will engage in sexual violence, if no efforts are made to manage the risk?
- What is the probable nature, frequency, and severity of any future sexual violence?
- Who are the likely victims of any future sexual violence?
- What steps could be taken to manage the individual's risk for sexual violence?
- What circumstances might exacerbate the individual's risk for sexual violence?

Typically, answers to these and other questions are fashioned in the form of a report for those responsible for making decisions about the examinee. Studies have shown that this evaluative measure works to distinguish recidivists who engage in sexual violence from those who engage in general violence.

Resources

BOOKS

Boer, D., et al. *Manual for the Sexual Violence Risk-20.* Burnaby, British Columbia, Canada: The British Columbia Institute Against Family Violence, copublished with the Mental Health, Law, and Policy Institute at Simon Fraser University, 1997.

Laws, D. Richard, and O'Donohue, William T., eds. *Sexual Deviance: Theory, Assessment, and Treatment.* 2nd ed. New York, Guilford Press, 2008.

Marshall, W., D. Laws, and H. Barbaree, eds. *Handbook of Sexual Assault: Issues, Theories, and Treatment of the Offender.* New York: Springer, 1990.

PERIODICALS

Craig, Leam A., Anthony Beech, and Kevin D. Browne. "Cross-Validation of the Risk Matrix 2000 Sexual and Violent Scales." *Journal of Interpersonal Violence* 21 (May 2006): 612–33.

Menzies, R., and C.D. Webster. "Construction and Validation of Risk Assessments in a Six-Year Follow-Up of Forensic Patients: A Tridimensional Analysis." *Journal of Consulting and Clinical Psychology* 63, no. 5 (October 1995): 766–78.

Monahan, J. "Mental Disorder and Violent Behavior." *American Psychologist* 47, no. 4 (April 1992): 511–21.

ORGANIZATIONS

American Psychological Association, 750 1st St. NE, Washington, DC, 20002-4242, (202) 336-5500; TDD/TTY: (202) 336-6123, (800) 374-2721, http://www.apa.org.

Association for the Treatment of Sexual Abusers, 4900 SW Griffith Dr., Ste. 274, Beaverton, OR, 97005, (503) 643-1023, Fax: (503) 643-5084, atsa@atsa.com, http://www.atsa.com.

British Columbia Institute Against Family Violence, 409 Granville St., Ste. 551, Vancouver, BC, CanadaV6C 1T2, (604) 669-7055, (877) 755-7055, resource@bcifv.org, http://www.bcifv.org.

Geoffrey G. Grimm, PhD, LPC
Emily Jane Willingham, PhD

Shared psychotic disorder

Definition

Shared psychotic disorder, a rare and atypical psychotic disorder, occurs when an otherwise healthy person (secondary partner) begins believing the **delusions** of someone with whom they have a close relationship (primary partner) who is suffering from a psychotic disorder with prominent delusions. This disorder is also referred to as "folie á deux."

Shared psychotic disorder is also referred to by other names, such as **psychosis** of association, contagious insanity, infectious insanity, double insanity, and communicated insanity. There have been cases involving multiple persons, the most significant, being a case involving an entire family of 12 people (folie á douze).

Demographics

Given the fact that the preponderance of cases occur within the same family, the theory about the origins of the disorder come from a psychosocial perspective. Approximately 55% of secondary cases of the disorder have first-degree relatives with psychiatric disorders, not including the primary partner. This is not true of individuals with the primary **diagnosis**, as they showed a roughly 35% incidence.

Little data is available to determine the prevalence of shared psychotic disorder. While it has been argued that some cases go undiagnosed, it is nevertheless a rare finding in clinical settings.

Description

In cases of shared psychotic disorder, the primary partner is most often in a position of strong influence over the other person. This allows the primary partner, over time, to erode the defenses of the secondary partner by forcing their strange belief upon him or her. Most of the time, this disorder occurs within a nuclear family. In fact, more than 95% of the cases reported involved people in the same family. Without regard to the number of persons within the family, shared delusions generally involve two people. There is the primary, most often the dominant person, and the secondary or submissive person. This becomes fertile ground for the primary (dominant) partner to press for understanding and belief by others in the family.

Causes and symptoms

Causes

There are several variables that have great influence on the creation of shared psychotic disorder. For example, family isolation, closeness of the relationship to the person with the primary diagnosis, the length of time the relationship has existed, and the existence of a dominant-submissive factor within the relationship. The submissive partner in the relationship may be predisposed to have a mental disorder. Often the submissive partner meets the criteria for **dependent personality disorder**. Nearly 75% of the delusions are of the persecutory type.

An example of shared psychotic disorder involving the delusion of persecution is a 52-year-old married female and her 48-year-old husband with multiple sclerosis who believed that they were being harassed and watched by the Irish Republican Army (IRA). They were hospitalized and both became stable after two weeks on an antipsychotic medication. However, an interesting point in this case is that they were separated for that two-week period. The general consensus has been that, once separated, the submissive partner will let go of the delusion, that it would resolve itself simply due to separation. That did not happen in this case. Both partners had to be treated with proper medications before the delusion resolved.

In a case involving a middle-aged mother and an adolescent daughter, the delusions were multifaceted. The mother held the persecutory belief that someone in her neighborhood was manufacturing illegal drugs of some sort, and that they were periodically spraying something odorless, tasteless, and invisible into the air. The sprayed substance made her and her teenaged daughter "act crazy." Oddly enough, the effects of the spraying began shortly after the husband left for work in the morning and resolved shortly before he returned in the afternoon. The family raised ducks at their home, and the mother and daughter believed that the men making the illegal drugs were using the family ducks "as a food source" to stay near their hideout and avoid detection by police. Finally, mother and daughter also believed that occasional gunshots in their countryside landscape were meant as warnings to prevent anyone from learning about the misdeeds of the drug makers. This case was revealed when the daughter ran away from home, fearing that men with guns were coming to kill them. She was subsequently placed in the care of a child protective services agency. The bizarre stories began to unfold. Both mother and daughter received psychiatric care.

Symptoms

The principal feature of shared psychotic disorder is the unwavering belief by the secondary partner in the dominant partner's delusion. The delusions experienced by both partners in shared psychotic disorder are far less bizarre than those found in schizophrenic patients; they are, therefore, believable. Since these delusions are often within the realm of possibility, it is easier for the dominant partner to impose his/her idea upon the submissive, secondary partner.

KEY TERMS

Delusions—Irrational beliefs that defy normal reasoning, and remain firm even when overwhelming proof is presented to dispute them. Delusions are distinct from culturally or religiously based beliefs that may be seen as untrue by outsiders.

Schizophrenia—A major mental illness marked by psychotic symptoms, including hallucinations, delusions, and severe disruptions in thinking.

Diagnosis

A clinical interview is required to diagnose shared psychotic disorder. There are basically three symptoms required for the determination of the existence of this disorder:

- An otherwise healthy person, in a close relationship with someone who has an established delusion, develops a delusion himself/herself.
- The content of the shared delusion follows exactly or closely resembles that of the established delusion.
- Some other psychotic disorder, such as schizophrenia, is not in place and cannot better account for the delusion manifested by the secondary partner.

Treatment

The treatment approach most recommended is to separate the secondary partner from the source of the delusion. If symptoms have not dissipated within one to two weeks, antipsychotic medications may be required.

Once stabilized, **psychotherapy** should be undertaken with the secondary partner, integrating the dominant partner once he/she has also received medical treatment and is stable.

Prognosis

If the secondary partner is removed from the source of the delusion and proper medical and psychotherapeutic treatment are rendered, the prognosis is good. However, as stated above, the separation alone may not be successful. The secondary partner may require antipsychotic medication. Even after treatment, since

QUESTIONS TO ASK YOUR DOCTOR

- What are the indications that I may have shared psychotic disorder?
- What physical and psychiatric diagnostic tests do I need?
- What treatment options do you recommend for me?
- What kind of changes can I expect to see with the medications you have prescribed for me?
- What are the side effects associated with the medications you have prescribed for me?
- What tests or evaluation techniques will you perform to see if treatment has been beneficial for me?
- What symptoms are important enough that I should seek immediate treatment?
- Can you recommend any support groups for me and my family?

this shared psychotic disorder is primarily found in families, the family members tend to reunite following treatment and release. If family dynamics return to pretreatment modes, a **relapse** could occur. Periodic monitoring by a social services agency is advised for as long as a year following treatment.

Prevention

In an effort to prevent relapse, **family therapy** should also be considered to re-establish the nuclear family and to provide social support to modify old family dynamics. This would favor a new behavioral paradigm. The family cannot afford to continue in isolation as it did in the past and will require support from community agencies.

Resources

BOOKS

American Psychiatric Association. *Diagnostic and Statistical Manual of Mental Disorders.* 4th ed. Washington, DC: American Psychiatric Association, 2000.

Cooper, Rachel. *Classifying Madness: A Philosophical Examination of the Diagnostic and Statistical Manual of Mental Disorders.* New York: Springer, 2010.

Graham, George. *The Disordered Mind: An Introduction to Philosophy of Mind and Mental Illness.* New York: Routledge, 2010.

North, Carol, and Sean Yutzy. *Goodwin and Guze's Psychiatric Diagnosis.* New York: Oxford University Press, 2010.

Sadock, Benjamin J., and Virginia A. Sadock. *Kaplan & Sadock's Synopsis of Psychiatry.* 10th ed. New York: Lippincott, Williams and Wilkins, 2007.

PERIODICALS

Lai, Tony T.S., et al. "Folie á Deux in the Aged: A Case Report." *Clinical Gerontologist* 22 (2001): 113–117.

Malik, Mansoor A., and Serena Condon. "Induced Psychosis (Folie á Deux) Associated with Multiple Sclerosis." *Irish Journal of Psychological Medicine* 17 (2000): 73–77.

Mergui, J., et al. "Shared Obsessive-Compulsive Disorder: Broadening the Concept of Shared Psychotic Disorder." *Australian and New Zealand Journal of Psychiatry* 44, no. 9 (2010): 859–62.

ORGANIZATIONS

American Psychological Association, 750 1st St. NE, Washington, DC, 20002-4242, (202) 336-5500, TDD/TTY: (202) 336-6123, (800) 374-2721, http://www.apa.org.

Mental Health America, 2000 N. Beauregard St., 6th Fl., Alexandria, VA, 22311, (703) 684-7722, (800) 969-6642, Fax: (703) 684-5968, http://www1.nmha.org.

National Alliance on Mental Illness, 3803 N Fairfax Dr., Ste. 100, Arlington, VA, 22203, (703) 524-7600, http://www.nami.org.

National Institute of Mental Health, 6001 Executive Blvd., Rm. 8184, MSC 9663, Bethesda, MD, 20892-9663, (301) 443-4513, TTY: (301) 443-8431, Fax: (301) 443-4279, (866) 615-6464, TTY: (866) 415-8051, nimhinfo@nih.gov, http://www.nimh.nih.gov.

Jack H. Booth, Psy.D.
Laura Jean Cataldo, RN, Ed.D.

Shift work sleep disorder *see* **Circadian rhythm sleep disorder**

Shyness

Definition

Shyness is a personality trait that produces behaviors ranging from feeling uncomfortable at a party to an extreme fear of being watched by others while talking on the telephone.

Description

Shyness affects people of all ages. A toddler might run from strangers and cling to his or her parents. While kindergarten is frightening for many children, some students are anxious about the first day of school until they graduate from college. Job interviews are stressful for people uncomfortable talking about themselves. For some people, feelings of self-worth are related to their careers. Retirement may bring feelings of lower self-esteem.

Shyness is linked to **brain** activity, how a person was raised and other experiences, and the person's reaction to those experiences.

Social phobia

Extreme shyness is sometimes referred to as a **social phobia**. Also known as social anxiety disorder, a social phobia is a psychiatric condition defined as a "marked and persistent fear" of some situations. Social phobia may cause a person to remain unemployed, according to the organization Mental Health America. True social phobia affects about 3% of people.

Introversion

Shyness is different from introversion; a person with introversion enjoys being alone and intentionally avoids situations like parties, whereas a shy person wants to be around people. However, shyness is stronger than the desire to be sociable. The shy person is afraid to go to the party and stays home alone.

Causes and symptoms

Causes

A person's temperament is related to the amygdala, the part of the brain related to emotions and new situations. The amygdala evaluates new situations based on memories of past experiences. If the new situation appears threatening, the amygdala sends a warning signal. The amygdala in a shy person is extremely sensitive and much more active than that of an outgoing person. The increased activity causes the person to withdraw either physically or emotionally. This withdrawal is known as inhibition.

Brain activity is one component of shyness, but environment also plays a role. If a child has outgoing, nurturing parents, he or she is more likely to imitate their behavior. If a child has a teacher that is mocking and critical, the child may develop lifelong fear of the first day of school. A person embarrassed in a job interview could become anxious in future interviews.

Symptoms

At the root of shyness is a feeling of self-consciousness. This may cause the person to blush, tense up, or start sweating. Those are some reactions caused when the brain signals its warning. The person may avoid eye contact, look down, become very quiet, or fumble over words.

Symptoms vary because there are degrees of shyness. A person might be very quiet when meeting new people, but then become talkative when he or she feels comfortable with them. A person who is nervous during job interviews may not be afraid of social gatherings.

Social phobia

Social phobia causes an extreme fear of being humiliated or embarrassed in front of people, according to the NMHA. It may be connected to low self-esteem or feelings of inferiority. A person with social phobia is not fearful in all situations and may feel comfortable around people most of the time. However, social phobias have caused people to drop out of school, avoid making friends, and keep away from other fear-provoking situations. Fears range from speaking in pubic and dating to using public restrooms or writing when other people are present.

According to the NMHA, a person with social phobia may feel that everyone is looking at them, A trivial mistake is regarded as much more serious and blushing is painfully embarrassing. Social phobia is frequently accompanied by **depression** or **substance abuse**.

Diagnosis

In many cases, persons will realize on their own that they are shy and may take steps to overcome their shyness. Adults and youths may buy self-help books or take classes on subjects like overcoming shyness and **assertiveness training**. These classes may be taught by counselors, psychologists, or people with experience conquering shyness. Healthcare providers often schedule these classes. They may be taught in settings ranging from adult schools to social service agencies; costs of the classes will vary.

Children may not know that there are treatment solutions for their shyness. Parents and educators should be alert for symptoms of shyness in younger children. Schools and family resource centers can provide referrals if it appears that counseling will help get their child diagnosed.

Medical diagnosis

Based on the child's circumstances, parents may take their children to see a healthcare provider. Some insurance plans require an appointment with a doctor before a referral to a counselor or a **psychologist** is given. The health professional will conduct an assessment and then recommend treatment.

Children and adults may need medical treatment for social phobia. An adult's **diagnosis** will also include a medical exam to determine if there is a physical cause for symptoms. If a medical cause has been ruled out, the patient will undergo a psychiatric evaluation.

Diagnostic fees and the time allocated for evaluation vary for both shyness and social phobia. Diagnosis could span several hour-long sessions that cover an initial evaluation, personality tests, and a meeting to set therapy goals. Insurance may cover part of the costs.

Treatment

Shyness treatment concentrates on changing behavior so that the person feels more at ease in shyness-provoking situations. The person may be guided by a self-help book or participate in individual or **group therapy**.

Traditional

Books and therapy generally focus on behavioral therapy and **cognitive-behavioral therapy**. One method of behavioral therapy is to expose the person to the situation that triggers fear. This could start with rehearsing a job interview with a friend or making eye contact with a store clerk. Over time, the person may go on interviews to gain experience rather than to be hired. Another person might move from eye contact to attending a social event such as a concert to become more at ease around strangers.

Therapy also focuses on developing skills to cope in new situations. These include taking deep breaths to relax and practicing small talk. Cognitive-therapy helps the person learn how thinking patterns contribute to symptoms, according to NMHA. The person is taught techniques to change those thoughts or to stop symptoms. This association maintains this therapy is very effective for people with social phobias.

Therapy sessions may be led by a licensed marriage and family counselor, a psychologist, or a **psychiatrist**. The cost of group therapy is generally an hourly fee with therapy planned for a set time.

Drugs

Treatment may also include medication. Prescription drugs like **paroxetine** (Paxil) are generally only prescribed to people with social **anxiety disorders**. Paxil is traditionally prescribed for depression and other mood disorders. The patient takes one tablet daily.

Insurance may cover part of the costs of therapy and medicine.

Alternative

Alternative treatments for shyness focus on treating accompanying symptoms like tension and **stress**. **Relaxation therapy** guides the person through a series of actions to relieve tension. The activity starts with deep breathing, and the person progressively focuses on the head and different parts of the body. The exercise may start with the head, neck, shoulders, moving down to the one foot and then the other. Some techniques involve tightly tensing and then releasing each body part. Another method is to concentrate on relaxing each part or imagining that it becomes warm.

Another self-treatment is **aromatherapy**. **Lavender** is a relaxing scent and is available in liquid form as an essential oil. Stress may be relieved by adding lavender oil to a bath. Some people carry the oil with them; if they become anxious, they can dab the oil on a cotton pad and breathe in the lavender to feel calmer.

Prognosis

Shyness may not be permanent. Children often outgrow shyness, and behavioral changes and therapy can help adults with shyness feel more at ease. Furthermore, some aspects of shyness are positive—persons who are shy are frequently good listeners and are empathetic, or aware of others' feelings.

Prevention

Shyness is a personality trait related to a person's biology and experiences. The part of shyness related to the brain cannot be changed. However, parents can provide a nurturing environment and teach children coping skills, which may help to prevent shyness.

To help combat the avoidance symptom caused by shyness, adults may wish to engage in enjoyable hobbies with social components. Recreational activities like walking groups combine physical exercise with the opportunity to socialize. Enrolling in a class at an adult school or community college provides the opportunity to learn and make new friends. Classes like these can boost confidence as a person learns a hands-on skill or discovers that others value her or his opinion.

Resources

WEBSITES

American Psychological Association. "Shyness." http://www.apa.org/topics/shyness/index.aspx (accessed October 27, 2011).

Cooper, Lisa. "Shy Child, Shy Adult." BabyZone.com. http://www.babyzone.com/toddler/toddler_development/social_skills/article/shy-child-shy-adult (accessed October 27, 2011).

KidsHealth.org. "Shyness." http://www.kidshealth.org/teen/your_mind/emotions/shyness.html (accessed October 27, 2011).

ORGANIZATIONS

American Psychological Association, 750 1st Street NE, Washington, DC, 20002-4242, (202) 336-5500, TDD/TTY: (202) 336-6123, (800) 374-2721, http://www.apa.org.

Mental Health America, 2000 North Beauregard St., 6th Fl., Alexandria, VA, 22311, (703) 684-7722, (800) 969-6642, Fax: (703) 684-5968, http://www.nmha.org.

Shyness Research Institute, 4201 Grant Line Rd., New Albany, IN, 47150, (812) 941-2295, Fax: (812) 941-2591, bcarducc@ius.edu, http://www.ius.edu/shyness.

Liz Swain

Simple phobia *see* **Specific phobias**

Sinequan *see* **Doxepin**

Single photon emission computed tomography

Definition

Single photon emission **computed tomography** (SPECT) is a type of imaging study used in nuclear medicine that uses radioactive materials injected through a vein that pass into the **brain** or other organ generating a high-resolution image. SPECT relies on two technologies: computed tomography (CT) and the use of a radioactive material (radionuclide) to label a compound known as a tracer. Tracking the tracer's movement through body tissues, and the rate of its radioactive decay allows the doctor to obtain 3-D images of blood flow in the heart, electrical activity in different areas of the brain, or to scan for tumors or bone disease by using a device called a gamma camera contained within the SPECT machine.

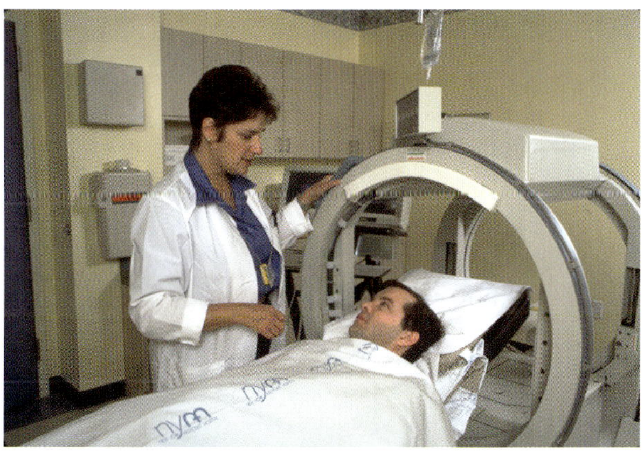

A man prepares to undergo a single photon emission computed tomography (SPECT) scan. *(© David M. Grossman/newscom)*

Purpose

SPECT is used to diagnose head **trauma**, epilepsy, **dementia**, and cerebrovascular disease. Development of a radiotracer called Tc99m (technctium-99) increased the resolution of brain images generated from SPECT. The images yield accurate spatial and contrast resolutions. Other radioactive isotopes used in SPECT are iodine-123, xenon-133, thallium-201, and fluorine-18. The resulting sharp images enable the clinician to visualize tiny structures within the brain or other parts of the body. The accuracy of SPECT images makes it a useful clinical and research tool.

SPECT is used to diagnose the following disease states:

- Cerebrovascular disease or stroke: SPECT is used to detect ischemia (reduced blood flow), determine stroke causes, evaluate transient ischemia, determine prognosis, and monitor treatment.
- Such forms of dementia as Alzheimer's disease: SPECT studies can be used effectively to rule out other medical causes of dementia.
- Head trauma: SPECT is used to detect increased numbers of lesions following the period after head trauma. The high resolution and accurate brain images of SPECT can detect lesions in the brain that are not possible to visualize using other techniques such as positron emission tomography (PET) scanning. SPECT images give important information concerning prognosis (also sometimes called outcome) and treatment of persons affected with head injury.
- Epilepsy: The radioactive material injected before SPECT imaging concentrates at the seizure locus (the region that contains nerve cells that generate an abnormal impulse). This concentration helps identify the location of seizures and assists clinicians concerning management and outcomes.
- Corpus striatum: SPECT allows clinicians to visualize a specific area of the brain called the corpus striatum, which contains the neurotransmitter dopamine. Circuitry in the corpus striatum and interaction with dopamine can help provide valuable information concerning movement disorders, schizophrenia, mood disorders, and hormone diseases (given that hormones require control and regulation from the brain in the pituitary gland and hypothalamus).

SPECT imaging is a sensitive research tool for measuring blood flow through the brain (cerebral blood flow), in persons who have psychological disorder such as **obsessive-compulsive disorder** (higher blood flow) and alcoholism (lower blood flow).

SPECT has also been used in myocardial perfusion imaging (MPI), which is a test done to evaluate patients for coronary artery disease. It is based on the understanding that diseased heart tissue under stress receives less blood than normal heart tissue (myocardium). A special form of technetium-99 known as Tc-sestamibi is injected. The patient's heart is then stressed by either **exercise** or by the administration of a drug, usually dobutamine, adenosine, or dipyridamole. SPECT imaging performed after the stress reveals the distribution of the Tc-sestamibi within the different regions of the heart muscle. The patient is usually asked to return 1–7 days after the stress test for another set of SPECT images taken while the patient is at rest. Doctors then compare the two sets of images. If the images following the stress test are normal, the patient does not have to return for a second SPECT scan.

Other SPECT diagnostic indications and procedures are similar to other **imaging studies**, such as computed tomography, **magnetic resonance imaging**, and **PET**.

Description

In most cases, the SPECT scan requires injecting the patient with a compound containing the radioactive tracer or administering the tracer through an infusion given intravenously in the arm. In some cases, the patient may inhale the tracer through the nose. The patient is then asked to lie quietly in a room for 15–30 minutes while the radioactive tracer is absorbed by the body.

In the second phase of the scan, the patient is positioned by the healthcare team on a table in the room with the SPECT machine. The exact position depends on the part of the patient's body or the organ system that is being investigated. The SPECT machine itself contains a gamma camera, an imaging device that detects gamma rays given off by the radioactive tracer in the patient's body. The SPECT machine rotates around the patient while the gamma camera records a series of two-dimensional images of the patient's body organs. These images are then sent to a computer that produces 3-D images of the organs in question.

Research studies of the brain utilizing SPECT have been conducted to study changes in and the effects of certain brain receptors. Researchers utilize SPECT scans to map brain metabolism and look at blood flow and activity patterns in the brain, helping assess and evaluate brain function.

KEY TERMS

Gamma camera—A device inside the SPECT machine that forms images of the gamma rays emitted by the radionuclides used in tracers in nuclear medicine.

Gamma rays—Extremely short-wavelength electromagnetic radiation released during the process of radioactive decay.

Myocardium—The specialized involuntary muscle tissue found in the walls of the heart.

Nuclear medicine—A branch of medicine that makes use of radioisotopes (also called radionuclides) to evaluate the rate of radioactive decay in diagnosing and treating various diseases.

Prodromal—The early stage or the start of a disease, before specific or characteristic symptoms occur.

Radionuclide—An atom with an unstable nucleus that emits gamma rays during the process of its radioactive decay. Radionuclides, also known as radioisotopes, are used to make the tracers used in SPECT. The most common radionuclides used in SPECT are iodine-123, technetium-99m, xenon-133, thallium-201, and fluorine-18.

Tracer—A substance containing a radioisotope, injected into the body and followed in order to obtain information about various metabolic processes in the body.

Preparation

Patients wear comfortable clothing for a SPECT scan and expect to stay in the hospital for 1–3 hours. They do not need to fast beforehand or omit the medications they usually take.

Aftercare

Aftercare consists of drinking extra fluids to speed the excretion of the radioactive tracer in the urine. The tracer is usually flushed out in the patient's urine within a few hours after the scan. Any remaining tracer is broken down in the body within the next two days.

Risks

SPECT scans are generally safe and well tolerated by most patients. Some people, however, may experience bruising, bleeding, or pain at the point at which the needle was inserted into their vein. A small number of patients have allergic reactions to the radionuclide.

QUESTIONS TO ASK YOUR DOCTOR

- What are the indications that I should have a SPECT scan performed?
- What kind of diagnostic results can be determined with the use of a SPECT scan?
- Should I have other diagnostics tests in addition to a SPECT scan? If so, what other tests should I have?
- How long will SPECT take?
- Is there anything I can do to help rid my body of the radioactive tracer?
- Is there an alternative to this test?
- Will insurance cover SPECT?

Precautions

Women who are pregnant or breastfeeding should not have SPECT scans because the radioactive tracer can be passed to the fetus or the nursing baby. Women of childbearing age may be asked to have a pregnancy test before a SPECT scan.

Resources

BOOKS

Eisenberg, Ronald, and Alexander Margulis. *A Patient's Guide to Medical Imaging*. New York: Oxford University Press, 2011.

Elgazzar, Abdelhamid E. *A Concise Guide to Nuclear Medicine*. New York: Springer, 2011.

Heller, Gary V., April Mann, and Robert C. Hendel, eds. *Nuclear Cardiology: Technical Applications*. New York: McGraw-Hill Medical, 2009.

Levine, Harry III. *Medical Imaging*. Santa Barbara, CA: ABC-CLIO, 2010.

PERIODICALS

Aggarwal, N.R., et al. "Role of Cardiac MRI and Nuclear Imaging in Cardiac Resynchronization Therapy." *Nature Reviews: Cardiology* 6 (December 2009): 759–70.

Alford, R., et al. "Molecular Probes for the In Vivo Imaging of Cancer." *Molecular Biosystems* 5 (November 2009): 1279–91.

Goffin, K., et al. "Neuronuclear Assessment of Patients with Epilepsy." *Seminars in Nuclear Medicine* 38 (July 2008): 227–39.

Heller, G.V., et al. "Recent Advances in Cardiac PET and PET/CT Myocardial Perfusion Imaging." *Journal of Nuclear Cardiology* 16 (November/December 2009): 962–69.

Placantonakis, D.G., and T.H. Schwartz. "Localization in Epilepsy." *Neurologic Clinics* 27 (November 2009): 1015–30.

Salerno, M., and G.A. Beller. "Noninvasive Assessment of Myocardial Perfusion." *Circulation: Cardiovascular Imaging* 2 (September 2009): 412–24.

Stein, P.D., et al. "SPECT in Acute Pulmonary Embolism." *Journal of Nuclear Medicine* 50 (December 2009): 1999–2007.

ORGANIZATIONS

American College of Physicians, 190 N Independence Mall W, Philadelphia, PA, 19106-1572, (215) 351-2400, (800) 523-1546, http://www.acponline.org.

American Heart Association, 7272 Greenville Ave., Dallas, TX, 75231, (800) 242-8721, http://www.americanheart.org.

American Medical Association, 515 N State St., Chicago, IL, 60610, (312) 464-5000, (800) 621-8335, http://www.ama-assn.org.

National Cancer Institute, 6116 Executive Boulevard, Suite 300, Bethesda, MD, 20892, (800) 422-6237, Fax: (301) 402-0601, http://www.nci.nih.gov.

Laith Farid Gulli, MD
Alfredo Mori, MD
Jean Suvan, BSc, RDH
Laura Jean Cataldo, RN, EdD

Skills training *see* **Social skills training**

Skin picking *see* **Dermatillomania**

Sleep deprivation

Definition

Sleep deprivation is an inadequate amount of sleep for a given individual.

Demographics

Sleep deprivation has become so widespread in industrialized societies that daytime drowsiness may no longer seem abnormal. Between 1998 and 2005, the number of American adults who reported getting eight or more hours of sleep on weekday nights fell from 35% to 26%. Driver **fatigue** causes 100,000 accidents and 1,500 deaths annually in the United States.

Sleep deprivation is considered to be a widespread chronic health problem among American teenagers. A 2006 poll found that only 20% of teens got adequate sleep on school nights: by the end of high school they averaged fewer than seven hours, and most teens reported feeling tired during the day.

Recommended hours of sleep, by age group

Infants	
0–2 months	12–18 hours
2–12 months	14–15 hours
Toddlers/Children	
1–3 years	12–14 hours
3–5 years	11–13 hours
5–10 years	10–11 hours
Adolescents	
10–17 years	8.5–9.25 hours
Adults	
18+	7–9 hours

SOURCE: National Sleep Foundation, "How Much Sleep Do We Really Need?"

Available online at http://www.sleepfoundation.org/article/how-sleep-works/how-much-sleep-do-we-really-need. *(Table by PreMediaGlobal. © 2012 Cengage Learning.)*

Although sleep disturbances and disorders do not necessarily result in sleep deprivation, they can contribute to it:

- About half of all people over age 65 suffer frequent sleep disturbances.
- About 60 million Americans suffer from frequent or extended periods of insomnia resulting in sleep deprivation. The incidence of insomnia increases with age, affecting about 40% of women and 30% of men.
- An estimated 18 million Americans have sleep apnea, although it usually goes undiagnosed.
- Restless legs syndrome (RLS) is one of the most common sleep disorders that causes sleep deprivation, especially among older people. RLS is estimated to affect as many as 12 million Americans.
- Narcolepsy—which affects about 250,000 Americans—can cause nighttime insomnia, resulting in sleep deprivation.
- Most people with mental disorders—including depression and schizophrenia—have sleep disturbances that cause sleep deprivation.
- Many blind people have lifelong sleeping problems, including insomnia and a type of permanent jet lag, which can result in sleep deprivation.

Description

Sleeping and wakefulness are controlled by neurotransmitters—chemical messengers in the brain—that act on different sets of nerve cells or neurons. The **neurotransmitters serotonin** and norepinephrine in the brainstem—the connection between the **brain** and the spinal cord—keep parts of the brain active during wakefulness and are switched off during sleep. Also during wakefulness, an important chemical called adenosine builds up in the blood to the point where it eventually causes drowsiness and is broken down during sleep.

Humans normally cycle through five stages of sleep throughout the night, with one complete sleep cycle averaging 90–120 minutes:

- Stage 1 consists of drowsiness, drifting in and out of sleep, and being easily awakened.
- Stage 2 is light sleep, which accounts for about 50% of total sleeping time.
- Stage 3 is deep sleep.
- Stage 4 is slow-wave deep sleep.
- Stages 1, 3, and 4 together account for about 30% of sleeping time.
- Rapid eye movement (REM) sleep accounts for about 20% of total sleep time.

During the first sleep cycles of the night, deep sleep is relatively long and REM sleep short. REM periods gradually increase in length as deep sleep shortens. Towards waking almost all sleep is stages 1, 2, and REM.

Sleep is essential for survival and sleep deprivation can eventually result in death. However, scientists have only recently begun to understand the many functions of sleep. It is required for proper nervous system functioning. Parts of the brain that are involved in emotions, decision-making, and social interactions are less active during sleep. These neurons may need sleep to repair and replenish themselves, and sleep may also be necessary for growing new neurons and for exercising neuronal functions that are less active during wakefulness.

However, other parts of the brain are very active during sleep. During this period of low sensory input, the brain consolidates recently acquired memories. Nerve-signaling patterns that are generated during the day are repeated during deep sleep. REM sleep is required for learning certain mental skills, and sleep may be necessary for encoding memories and learning.

Many cells in the body produce more protein during deep and REM sleep, so sleep may be necessary for replenishing energy and repairing damage in cells throughout the body. Growth hormones in children and young adults are released during deep sleep, and sleep is required for proper immune system function and cytokines—chemicals that fight infection—are produced during sleep.

Sleep requirements

The amount of sleep required to prevent deprivation depends on a variety of factors, especially age and genetics:

- Infants need about 16 hours of sleep out of every 24 hours, with about 50% spent in REM.
- Toddlers need about 14 hours of sleep, which gradually decreases with age to a requirement of slightly over nine hours in teenagers.
- Most adults need 7–8 hours of sleep each night, although individual requirements may vary from 4 to 12 hours per night.
- Researchers have identified a gene called DEC2 that turns off some genes involved in controlling circadian rhythms—the internal clock that regulates the sleep-wake cycle. People with certain mutations in the DEC2 gene require only about six hours of sleep per night.
- Women often need several extra hours of sleep during the first three months of pregnancy.
- Although older people tend to sleep more lightly and for shorter periods, they need about the same amount of total sleep as when they were younger.

For most people, sleep deprivation accumulates as a "sleep debt," which must be made up. The ability to function relatively well—at least for short periods—under conditions of sleep deprivation appears to be genetically determined. Estimates suggest that 10%–15% of people function adequately on little or no sleep, whereas another 10%–15% cannot function at all without sleep. Most people cannot function at all after 48 hours without sleep, nor do humans appear to adapt to sleep deprivation. One study found that subjects who slept only 4–6 hours per night for 14 consecutive nights showed cognitive impairment equivalent to going without sleep for three consecutive days.

Although people may adjust to a sleep-depriving schedule, daily functioning and physical and mental health suffer, as sleep deprivation interferes with concentration, learning, and problem-solving. At least 6 hours of regular sleep are required for peak memory performance, and sleep deprivation is directly linked to memory loss. In addition, sleep deprivation may:

- interfere with work, school, and social interactions
- cause stress
- slow reaction times; sleep-deprived people perform at least as poorly on driving simulators and hand-eye coordination tasks as people who are intoxicated
- disrupt the decision-making machinery of the brain, impairing judgment, increasing risky behaviors, and reducing sensitivity to loss
- increase the risk of falls and accidents
- increase the risk for many health problems, including hypertension, cardiovascular disease, diabetes, obesity, and infections
- increase appetite and inhibit weight loss, even with proper exercise and diet
- increase the effects of alcohol.
- cause sleep paralysis, a rare but frightening condition in which a person temporarily loses the ability to speak or move while falling asleep or waking up

Teenagers require an average of 9.25 hours of sleep per night for brain development, health, and optimal performance. Sleep-deprived teens are at risk for:

- impaired cognitive function and decision-making
- health problems
- poor grades and athletic performance
- emotional and behavioral problems
- depression
- substance abuse
- violence
- automobile accidents

Risk factors

Risk factors for sleep deprivation include:

- anxiety and stress
- careers with long or irregular working hours
- night or shift work
- work requiring long-distance travel
- multiple jobs
- combining full-time work and school
- being a family caregiver

Causes and symptoms

Causes

Sleep deprivation is most often caused by lifestyle choices or the requirements of work, school, or caregiving. Irregular sleep patterns that differ between weekdays and weekends can harm the quality of sleep. A new baby often results in sleep-deprived parents. Teenagers with hectic schedules of school, homework, athletics, after-school activities, jobs, and family and social obligations find themselves without enough hours for quality sleep. Furthermore, hormonal changes in adolescence set most teens' biological clocks on later schedules than those of children and adults. Teens may be wide awake—albeit exhausted—at bedtime but still have to wake up early for school.

Foods and drugs that change the balance of neurotransmitters in the brain can cause sleep deprivation, including caffeinated drinks, such as coffee, and drugs, such as diet pills and decongestants, which stimulate the brain and can cause **insomnia**. Many **antidepressants** suppress REM sleep, and substances such as alcohol and **nicotine** deprive the brain of REM sleep.

KEY TERMS

Adenosine—A nucleoside that plays multiple physiological roles in energy transfer and molecular signaling, as a component of RNA, and as an inhibitory neurotransmitter that promotes sleep.

Apnea—The transient cessation of breathing.

Circadian rhythm—A 24-hour cycle of physiological or behavioral activities.

Cytokines—A class of proteins, including interferons and interleukins, that are released by cells as part of the immune response and as mediators of intercellular communication.

Insomnia—Prolonged or abnormal inability to obtain adequate sleep.

Melatonin—A hormone involved in regulation of circadian rhythms.

Narcolepsy—A condition characterized by brief attacks of deep sleep.

Neurotransmitters—Chemicals that transmit nerve impulses from one nerve cell to another.

REM—Rapid eye movement; a stage of the normal sleep cycle characterized by rapid eye movements, increased forebrain and midbrain activity, and dreaming.

Restless legs syndrome (RLS)—A neurological disorder characterized by aching, burning, or creeping sensations in the legs and an urge to move the legs, often resulting in insomnia.

Changes in regions of the brain and in neurotransmitters can result in sleep deprivation. Sleeping problems in older people may be a normal part of aging or can be related to underlying medical conditions, medications, medical treatments, or sleep-disrupting hospital routines. Anxiety or chronic pain can cause sleep deprivation, which, in turn, can cause **anxiety disorders** or make it harder to cope with pain. Other conditions that can cause sleep deprivation include menopause, vision loss, **attention deficit hyperactivity disorder (ADHD)**, head injury, **stroke**, cancer, and **Alzheimer's disease**.

Sleep disorders may also result in sleep deprivation. There are more than 70 known sleep disorders; the most common include:

- insomnia, which can have various causes—including stress, jet lag, diet, or an underlying medical condition—and almost always affects next-day functioning
- sleep apnea, or disrupted breathing during sleep, which causes frequent awakenings
- RLS, a condition that causes constant leg movement and insomnia and is either inherited or linked to conditions such as pregnancy, anemia, or diabetes
- periodic limb movement disorder (PLMD), which often accompanies RLS and causes repeated awakenings
- narcolepsy, which is characterized by brief attacks of daytime deep sleep and is usually caused by an inherited malfunction in the regulation of sleep-wake cycles

Symptoms of sleep deprivation include:

- difficulty awakening each morning
- daytime drowsiness
- microsleeps—very brief, often unnoticed—periods of sleep during waking hours
- falling asleep during school or work
- need for frequent naps
- routinely falling asleep within five minutes of lying down
- disrupted sleep
- parasomnias—uncontrollable actions during sleep, such as sleepwalking
- headaches
- poor school or work performance
- inability to concentrate
- inability to perform mathematical calculations
- impaired memory
- problems with decision-making
- clumsiness or impaired physical performance
- irritability or mood swings
- paranoia
- confusion
- hallucinations
- decreased consciousness

Although sleep deprivation can be an effective therapy for people with certain types of **depression**, it can cause depression in otherwise healthy people. Sleep deprivation can also trigger manic episodes of agitation and hyperactivity in people with **bipolar disorder** and **seizures** in patients with some types of epilepsy.

Diagnosis

Examination

Sleep deprivation is usually readily diagnosed from the symptoms accompanying the lack of sleep. Underlying medical problems resulting in sleep deprivation may require further diagnoses.

Procedures

Simple devices are available for detecting sleep apnea. Sleep apnea may be diagnosed at a specialized sleep center using **polysomnography** to record brain waves, heartbeat, and breathing for an entire night.

Treatment

Traditional

The usual treatment for sleep deprivation is sleep. Underlying conditions that result in sleep deprivation require more extensive treatments. For example, severe sleep apnea may require a mask—called a continuous positive airway pressure (CPAP) device—to keep the airways open during sleep. Surgery may be required to correct an airway obstruction.

Drugs

Caffeine and other stimulants cannot overcome the effects of severe sleep deprivation. However, various products are available to treat sleep disturbances that can result in sleep deprivation:

- Over-the-counter sleep aids usually contain antihistamines. Although they are sometimes effective, they have side effects, and tolerance can develop after just a few days of use.
- RLS and PLMD are often relieved with drugs that affect the neurotransmitter dopamine.
- Daily melatonin supplements may improve nighttime sleep in blind patients.

The U.S. Food and Drug Administration (FDA) has approved several sleep aids—called **sedatives** or hypnotics—for indefinite use. However, most sleeping pills are usually prescribed only for short-term insomnia, because they usually become ineffective after several weeks of nightly use and may be habit-forming. If sleeping pills are used for too long, they can actually cause insomnia. Some persons taking sleep aids experience next-day grogginess or engage in behaviors during sleep, such as sleep eating or sleep driving. If medical disorder is causing the sleep deprivation, use of sleep aids may mask the underlying condition, and sleep aids may negatively interact with alcohol or other medications. In persons with sleep apnea, sleep aids may prevent them from waking up to breathe.

Alternative

Alternative treatments for insomnia and other sleep disturbances include **cognitive-behavioral therapy** (CBT); hypnosis; melatonin, a hormone derived from the neurotransmitter serotonin; and tryptophan, an amino acid precursor of serotonin.

Herbal remedies for insomnia include lemon balm, **chamomile**, **valerian** root, **kava kava**, **passionflower**, **lavender**, and **St. John's wort**, although the efficacy of such herbs has not been proven. Patients should discuss the use of herbal supplements with their doctor.

Home remedies

Short-term sleep deprivation may require only a night or two of additional sleep. Longer-term sleep deprivation may require a sleep vacation—a few days devoted to sleeping as much as needed. Mild sleep apnea can be treated effectively by weight loss or by not sleeping on one's back.

Prognosis

Sleep deprivation is usually readily reversible with adequate sleep.

Prevention

Sleep deprivation is preventable by getting as much sleep as an individual requires. Sleep deprivation caused by mild insomnia can often be prevented by:

- sleeping on a schedule—going to bed and rising at the same time every day, including weekends
- structuring daily activities
- exercising 20–30 minutes every day, especially 5–6 hours before sleep
- practicing stress management
- avoiding caffeine, nicotine, and alcohol
- relaxing before bed with activities such as reading or a warm bath that become routinely associated with sleep
- avoiding extreme temperatures that prevent falling or staying asleep
- avoiding lying awake in bed for more than 20 minutes since this can cause anxiety
- reading, watching television, listening to music, or performing an activity until drowsy
- sleeping until sunrise or waking with very bright lights to reset one's internal clock each day
- getting an hour of morning sun exposure

Resources

BOOKS

Bellenir, Karen. *Sleep Information for Teens*. Detroit: Omnigraphics, 2008.

Chokroverty, Sudhansu. *100 Questions & Answers About Sleep and Sleep Disorders*. Sudbury, MA: Jones and Bartlett, 2008.

Epstein, Lawrence J., and Steven Mardon. *The Harvard Medical School Guide to a Good Night's Sleep*. New York: McGraw-Hill, 2007.

Mindell, Jodi A. *Sleep Deprived No More: From Pregnancy to Early Motherhood—Helping You & Your Baby Sleep Through the Night*. New York: DeCapo Press, 2007.

PERIODICALS

Bergin, Christi A., and David A. Bergin. "Sleep: The E-ZZZ Intervention." *Educational Leadership* 67, no. 4 (December 2009/January 2010): 44–47.

He, Ying, et al. "The Transcriptional Repressor DEC2 Regulates Sleep Length in Mammals." *Science* 325, no. 5942 (August 14, 2009): 866–870.

Kowalczyk, Liz. "Turns Out, There's No Magic in that Traditional Number Eight When Figuring Out How Many Hours of Shut-Eye You Need." *The Boston Globe* (December 28, 2009): G6.

Liberatore, Stephanie. "Health Wise: December 2009." *The Science Teacher* 76, no. 9 (December 2009): 62–63.

WEBSITES

Helpguide.org. "How to Stop Snoring." August 2011. http://www.helpguide.org/life/snoring.htm (accessed October 27, 2011).

MedlinePlus. "Sleep Disorders." U.S. National Library of Medicine, National Institutes of Health. http://www.nlm.nih.gov/medline plus/tutorials/sleepdisorders/ htm/index.htm (accessed October 27, 2011).

National Sleep Foundation. "Backgrounder: Later School Start Times." http://www.sleepfoundation.org/article/hot-topics/backgrounder-later-school-start-times (accessed October 27, 2011).

U.S. National Institute of Neurological Disorders and Stroke. "Brain Basics: Understanding Sleep." NIH Publication No.06-3440-c. http://www.ninds. nih.gov/disorders/brain_basics/understanding_sleep.htm (accessed October 27, 2011).

ORGANIZATIONS

American Academy of Sleep Medicine, 2510 N Frontage Rd., Darien, IL, 60561, (630) 737-9700, Fax: (630) 737-9790, inquiries@assmnet.org, http://www.aasmnet.org.

National Institute of Neurological Disorders and Stroke, PO Box 5801, Bethesda, MD, 20824, (301) 496-5751, TTY: (301) 468-5981, (800) 352-9424, http://www.ninds.nih.gov.

National Sleep Foundation, 1010 North Glebe Rd., Suite 310, Arlington, VA, 22201, (703) 243-1697, nsf@sleepfoundation.org, http://www.sleepfoundation.org.

Margaret Alic, PhD

Sleep disorders

Definition

Sleep disorders are various syndromes characterized by disturbance in the amount of sleep, quality or timing of sleep, or in behaviors or physiological conditions associated with sleep, which individuals experience. There are about 81 different sleep disorders, according to the second edition of the *International Classification of Sleep Disorders*. To qualify for the **diagnosis** of sleep disorder, the condition must be a persistent problem, cause individuals significant emotional distress, and interfere with their social or occupational functioning.

Because sleep requirements vary from person to person, there is no specific amount of time spent sleeping that can be used as a cutoff to determine whether individuals have a sleep disorder. Some healthy adults need as much as 10 hours of sleep per night, whereas others need as little as five hours.

Demographics

Sleep disorders are a common problem in the general population of North America. Researchers estimate that 20%–40% of adults report difficulty sleeping at some point each year. About one-third of all Americans have a sleep disorder at some point in their lives. Twenty percent of adults say that they have problems with chronic **insomnia**, and 17% consider their sleeping problem to be serious.

As far as is known, sleep disorders are equally common in all racial and ethnic groups in Canada and the United States.

Description

Normal sleep

Although sleep is a basic behavior in animals as well as humans, researchers still do not completely understand all of its functions in maintaining health. Between 1980 and 2010, however, laboratory studies on human volunteers have yielded information about the different types of sleep. Increasing interest in sleep disorders led to the recognition of sleep medicine as a distinct medical subspecialty with its own board certification procedures in 1978. Researchers have learned about the cyclical patterns of different types of sleep and their relationships to breathing, heart rate, **brain** waves, and other physical functions. These measurements are obtained by a technique called **polysomnography**.

There are five stages of normal human sleep. Four stages consist of non-rapid eye movement (NREM) sleep, with unique brain wave patterns and physical changes occurring. Dreaming occurs in the fifth stage, during rapid eye movement (REM) sleep.

- Stage 1 NREM sleep occurs while a person is falling asleep. It represents about 5% of a normal adult's sleep time.
- Stage 2 NREM sleep is the beginning of "true" sleep, when a person's electroencephalogram (EEG) shows distinctive wave forms called sleep spindles and K complexes. About 50% of sleep time is stage 2 REM sleep.
- Stages 3 and 4 NREM sleep, also called delta or slow wave sleep, are the deepest levels of sleep and represent 10–20% of sleep time. They usually occur during the first 30–50% of the sleeping period.
- REM sleep accounts for 20–25% of total sleep time. It usually begins about 90 minutes after the person falls asleep, an important measure called REM latency. It alternates with NREM sleep about every hour and a half throughout the night. REM periods increase in length over the course of the night.

Sleep cycles vary with a person's age. Children and adolescents have longer periods of stage 3 and stage 4 NREM sleep than do middle-aged or elderly adults. Because of this difference, doctors need to take a patient's age into account when evaluating a sleep disorder. Total REM sleep also declines with age.

The average length of nighttime sleep varies among different age groups. Infants typically need about 16 hours of sleep each day, whereas adolescents need about 9 hours. Most adults sleep 7–9 hours a night, although pregnant women may need as many as 10 or 11 hours of sleep. These population averages appear to be constant throughout the world. In temperate climates, however, people often notice that sleep time varies with the seasons. It is not unusual for people in North America and Europe to sleep about 40 minutes longer per night during the winter.

Primary sleep disorders

Sleep disorders are classified based on what causes them. Primary sleep disorders are distinguished from those that are not caused by other mental disorders, prescription medications, **substance abuse**, or medical conditions. The two major categories of primary sleep disorders are the dyssomnias and the parasomnias.

DYSSOMNIAS. Dyssomnias are primary sleep disorders in which the patient suffers from changes in the amount, restfulness, and timing of sleep. The most important dyssomnia is primary insomnia, which is defined as difficulty in falling asleep or remaining asleep that lasts for at least one month. It is estimated that 35% of adults in the United States experience insomnia during any given year, but the number of these adults who are experiencing true primary insomnia is unknown. Primary insomnia can be caused by a traumatic event related to sleep or bedtime, and it is often associated with increased physical or psychological arousal at night. People who experience primary insomnia are often anxious about not being able to sleep. They may then associate all sleep-related things (their bed, bedtime, etc.) with frustration, making the problem worse. They then become more stressed about not sleeping. Primary insomnia usually begins when individuals are young adults or in middle age.

Hypersomnia is a condition marked by excessive sleepiness during normal waking hours. Individuals have either lengthy episodes of daytime sleep or episodes of daytime sleep on a daily basis even though they are sleeping normally at night. In some cases, patients with primary hypersomnia have difficulty waking in the morning and may appear confused or angry. This condition is sometimes called sleep drunkenness and is more common in males. The number of people with primary hypersomnia is unknown, although 5–10% of patients in sleep disorder clinics have the disorder. Primary hypersomnia usually affects young adults between the ages of 15 and 30.

Nocturnal myoclonus and **restless legs syndrome** (RLS) can cause either insomnia or hypersomnia in adults. Patients with nocturnal myoclonus wake up because of cramps or twitches in their calves. These patients feel sleepy the next day. Nocturnal myoclonus is sometimes called periodic limb movement disorder (PLMD). RLS patients have a crawly or aching feeling in their calves that can be relieved by moving or rubbing the legs. RLS often prevents individuals from falling asleep until the early hours of the morning, when the condition is less intense.

Kleine-Levin syndrome is a recurrent form of hypersomnia that affects a person 3–4 times a year. Doctors do not know the cause of this syndrome. It is marked by 2–3 days of sleeping 18–20 hours per day, hypersexual behavior, compulsive eating, and irritability. Men are three times more likely than women to have the syndrome. There is no cure for this disorder.

Narcolepsy is a dyssomnia characterized by recurrent "sleep attacks" that individuals cannot fight. The sleep attacks are about 10–20 minutes long. Individuals feel refreshed by the sleep, but typically feel sleepy again several hours later. Narcolepsy has three major symptoms in addition to sleep attacks: cataplexy, hallucinations, and sleep paralysis. Cataplexy is the sudden loss of muscle tone and stability ("drop attacks"). Hallucinations may occur just before falling asleep (hypnagogic) or right after waking up (hypnopompic) and are associated with an episode of REM sleep. Sleep paralysis occurs during the transition from being asleep to waking up. About 40% of patients with narcolepsy have or have had another mental disorder. Although narcolepsy is often regarded as an adult disorder, it has been reported in children as young as three years of age. Almost 18% of patients with narcolepsy are 10 years old or younger. It is estimated that 0.02–0.16% of the general population suffer from narcolepsy. Men and women are equally affected.

Breathing-related sleep disorders are syndromes in which patients' sleep is interrupted by problems with their breathing. There are three types of breathing-related sleep disorders:

- Obstructive sleep apnea syndrome is the most common form of breathing-related sleep disorder, marked by episodes of blockage in the upper airway during sleep. It is found primarily in obese people. Patients with this disorder typically alternate between periods of snoring or gasping (when their airway is partly open) and periods of silence (when their airway is blocked). Very loud snoring is a clue to this disorder.
- Central sleep apnea syndrome is primarily found in elderly patients with heart or neurological conditions that affect their ability to breathe properly. It is not associated with airway blockage and may be related to brain disease.
- Central alveolar hypoventilation syndrome is found most often in extremely obese people. These individuals' airway is not blocked, but their blood oxygen level is too low.
- Mixed-type sleep apnea syndrome combines symptoms of both obstructive and central sleep apnea.

Circadian rhythm sleep disorders are dyssomnias resulting from a discrepancy between individuals' daily sleep/wake patterns and demands of social activities, shift work, or travel. The term *circadian* comes from a Latin word meaning "daily." There are three circadian rhythm sleep disorders. Delayed sleep phase type is characterized by going to bed and arising later than most people. Jet lag type is caused by travel to a new time zone. Shift work type is caused by shifts in one's work schedule. People who are ordinarily early risers appear to be more vulnerable to jet lag and shift work-related circadian rhythm disorders than people who are "night owls." Some individuals do not fit the pattern of these three disorders and appear to be the opposite of the delayed sleep phase type. These patients have an advanced sleep phase pattern and cannot stay awake in the evening but wake up on their own in the early morning.

PARASOMNIAS. Parasomnias are primary sleep disorders in which the patient's behavior is affected by specific sleep stages or transitions between sleeping and waking. They are sometimes described as disorders of physiological arousal during sleep.

Nightmare disorder is a parasomnia in which individuals are repeatedly awakened from sleep by frightening dreams and are fully alert on awakening. The actual rate of occurrence of nightmare disorder is unknown. Approximately 10–50% of children between three and five years of age have nightmares. They occur during REM sleep, usually in the second half of the night. These children are usually able to remember the content of the nightmare and may be afraid to go back to sleep. More females than males have this disorder, but it is not known whether the sex difference reflects a difference in occurrence or a difference in reporting. Nightmare disorder is most likely to occur in children or adults under severe or traumatic **stress**.

Sleep terror disorder is a parasomnia in which patients awaken screaming or crying. These individuals also have physical signs of arousal, like sweating or shaking. This disorder is sometimes called pavor nocturnus. Unlike nightmares, sleep terrors typically occur in stage 3 or stage 4 NREM sleep during the first third of the night. Individuals may be confused or disoriented for several minutes and cannot recall the content of the dream. They may fall asleep again and not remember the episode the next morning. Sleep terror disorder is most common in children 4–12 years of age and is outgrown in adolescence. It affects about 3% of children. Less than 1% of adults have the disorder. In adults, it usually begins between the ages of 20 and 30. In children, more males than females have the disorder. In adults, men and women are equally affected.

Sleepwalking disorder, which is sometimes called somnambulism, occurs when individuals are capable of complex movements during sleep, including walking. Like sleep terror disorder, sleepwalking occurs during stage 3 and stage 4 NREM sleep during the first part of the night. If individuals are awakened during a sleepwalking episode, they may be disoriented and have no memory of the behavior. In addition to walking around, patients with sleepwalking disorder have been reported to eat, use the bathroom, unlock doors, or talk to others. It is estimated that 10–30% of children have at least one episode of sleepwalking. However, only 1–5% meet the criteria for sleepwalking disorder. The disorder is most common in children 8–12 years of age. It is unusual for sleepwalking to occur for the first time in adults.

KEY TERMS

Apnea—The temporary absence of breathing. Sleep apnea consists of repeated episodes of temporary suspension of breathing during sleep.

Benzodiazepines—A class of sedative drugs used to treat sleep disorders.

Cataplexy—Sudden loss of muscle tone (often causing a person to fall), usually triggered by intense emotion. It is regarded as a diagnostic sign of narcolepsy.

Circadian rhythm—Any body rhythm that recurs in 24-hour cycles. The sleep-wake cycle is an example of a circadian rhythm.

Cognitive-behavioral therapy (CBT)—A type of psychotherapy that helps patients identify and change problematic thoughts and behaviors.

Dyssomnia—A primary sleep disorder in which the patient suffers from changes in the quantity, quality, or timing of sleep.

Electroencephalogram (EEG)—The record obtained by a device that measures electrical impulses in the brain.

Hypersomnia—An abnormal increase of 25% or more in time spent sleeping. Patients usually have excessive daytime sleepiness.

Hypnotic—A medication that makes a person sleep.

Hypopnea—Shallow or excessively slow breathing usually caused by partial closure of the upper airway during sleep, leading to disruption of sleep.

Insomnia—Difficulty in falling asleep or remaining asleep.

Jet lag—A temporary disruption of the body's sleep-wake rhythm following high-speed air travel across several time zones. Jet lag is most severe in people who have crossed eight or more time zones in 24 hours.

Kleine-Levin syndrome—A disorder that occurs primarily in young males, three or four times a year. The syndrome is marked by episodes of hypersomnia, hypersexual behavior, and excessive eating.

Melatonin—A hormone produced by the pineal gland that is associated with sleep and that may be useful in the treatment of some sleep disorders.

Narcolepsy—A lifelong sleep disorder marked by four symptoms: sudden brief sleep attacks, cataplexy, temporary paralysis, and hallucinations. The hallucinations are associated with falling asleep or the transition from sleeping to waking.

Nocturnal myoclonus—A disorder in which the patient is awakened repeatedly during the night by cramps or twitches in the calf muscles; sometimes called periodic limb movement disorder (PLMD).

Non-rapid eye movement (NREM) sleep—A type of sleep that differs from rapid eye movement (REM) sleep. The four stages of NREM sleep account for 75–80% of total sleeping time.

Parasomnia—A primary sleep disorder in which the person's physiology or behaviors are affected by sleep, the sleep stage, or the transition from sleeping to waking.

Pavor nocturnus—Another term for sleep terror disorder.

Polysomnography—Laboratory measurement of a patient's basic physiological processes during sleep. Polysomnography usually measures eye movement, brain waves, and muscular tension.

Primary sleep disorder—A sleep disorder that cannot be attributed to a medical condition, another mental disorder, or prescription medications or other substances.

Rapid eye movement (REM) sleep—A phase of sleep during which the person's eyes move rapidly beneath the lids. It accounts for 20–25% of sleep time. Dreaming occurs during REM sleep.

REM latency—After a person falls asleep, the amount of time it takes for the first onset of REM sleep.

Restless legs syndrome (RLS)—A disorder in which the patient experiences crawling, aching, or other disagreeable sensations in the calves that can be relieved only by movement. RLS is a frequent cause of difficulty falling asleep at night.

Sedative—A medication given to calm agitated patients; sometimes used as a synonym for hypnotic.

Sleep latency—The amount of time that it takes to fall asleep. Sleep latency is measured in minutes and is important in diagnosing depression.

Somnambulism—Another term for sleepwalking.

Unlike sleepwalking, REM sleep behavior disorder occurs later in the night, and individuals can remember what they were dreaming. The physical activities of these individuals are often violent.

Sleep disorders related to other conditions

In addition to the primary sleep disorders, there are three categories of sleep disorders that are caused by or related to substance use or other physical or mental disorders.

SLEEP DISORDERS RELATED TO MENTAL DISORDERS. Many mental disorders, especially **depression** or one of the **anxiety disorders**, can cause sleep disturbances. Psychiatric disorders are the most common cause of chronic insomnia.

SLEEP DISORDERS DUE TO MEDICAL CONDITIONS. Some patients with chronic neurological conditions such as Parkinson's disease or Huntington's disease may develop sleep disorders. Sleep disorders have also been associated with viral encephalitis, brain disease, and hypo- or hyperthyroidism.

SUBSTANCE-INDUCED SLEEP DISORDERS. The use of drugs, alcohol, and caffeine frequently produces disturbances in sleep patterns. Alcohol abuse is associated with insomnia. Individuals may initially feel sleepy after drinking, but they wake up or sleep fitfully during the second half of the night. Alcohol can also increase the severity of breathing-related sleep disorders. With **amphetamines** or **cocaine** use, individuals typically suffer from insomnia during drug use and hypersomnia during drug withdrawal. **Opioids** usually make short-term users sleepy. However, long-term users develop tolerance and may suffer from insomnia.

In addition to alcohol and drugs that are abused, a variety of prescription medications can affect sleep patterns. These medications include antihistamines, corticosteroids, asthma medicines, and drugs that affect the central nervous system.

Sleep disorders in children and adolescents

Pediatricians estimate that 20–30% of children have difficulties with sleep that are serious enough to disturb their families. Although sleepwalking and night terror disorder occur more frequently in children than in adults, children can also suffer from narcolepsy and sleep apnea syndrome.

Risk factors

Risk factors for sleep disorders include:

- Gender. Primary insomnia is more common in women than in men, while obstructive sleep apnea is twice as common in men as in women.
- Age. Older adults are more likely to develop sleep disorders; the rate rises from 5% of adults between 30 and 50 to 30% in those over 50. One reason for the greater risk of sleep disorders in seniors is that they are more likely to have medical conditions that disturb sleep or to be taking medications that cause sleep disruption.
- Employment that requires frequent travel across time zones or frequent changes in work schedules
- Environmental factors, including noise, high altitude, and abnormally hot or cold temperatures
- Smoking. Heavy smokers often wake up after only a few hours of sleep due to nicotine withdrawal.
- High levels of emotional stress, whether job-related or associated with family or personal problems
- Family history of sleep disorders. Sleepwalking is particularly likely to occur in families.
- Having a disease or disorder that causes physical discomfort
- Genetic factors. There is increasing evidence that obstructive sleep apnea, narcolepsy, and restless legs syndrome are associated with susceptibility genes for these disorders, although no specific genes had been identified as of 2011.

Causes and symptoms

The causes of sleep disorders have already been discussed with respect to the classification of these disorders.

The most important symptoms of sleep disorders are insomnia and sleepiness during waking hours. Insomnia is by far the more common of the two symptoms. It covers a number of different patterns of sleep disturbance. These patterns include inability to fall asleep at bedtime, repeated awakening during the night, and/or inability to go back to sleep once awakened.

Diagnosis

Diagnosis of sleep disorders usually requires a psychological history as well as a medical history. The patient's sex and age are useful starting points in assessing the problem. The doctor may also talk to other family members in order to obtain information about the patient's symptoms. The family's observations are particularly important to evaluate sleepwalking, kicking in bed, snoring loudly, or other behaviors that the patient cannot remember.

Examination

With the exception of sleep apnea syndromes, physical examinations are not usually revealing.

Tests

The doctor may order blood or urine tests to determine whether the patient's sleep disorder is associated with anemia, thyroid dysfunction, alcoholism, or opioid abuse. The patient's blood oxygen level may be tested during sleep in order to determine whether sleep apnea or other types of sleep-disordered breathing are involved. Imaging tests are not routinely done for sleep disorders but may be ordered in some cases to rule out brain tumors or other medical conditions.

Sleep logs

Many doctors ask patients to keep a sleep diary or sleep log for a minimum of one to two weeks in order to evaluate the severity and characteristics of the sleep disturbance. The patient records medications taken as well as the length of time spent in bed, the quality of the sleep, and similar information. Some sleep logs are designed to indicate circadian sleep patterns as well as simple duration or restfulness of sleep.

Psychological testing

The doctor may use psychological tests or inventories to evaluate insomnia because it is frequently associated with mood or affective disorders. The **Minnesota Multiphasic Personality Inventory** (MMPI), the Millon Clinical Multiaxial Inventory (MCMI), the **Beck Depression Inventory**, and the Zung Depression Scale are the tests most commonly used in evaluating this symptom.

Self-report tests

The Epworth Sleepiness Scale, a self-rating form developed in Australia, consists of eight questions used to assess daytime sleepiness. Scores range from 0–24, with scores higher than 16 indicating severe daytime sleepiness.

Laboratory sleep studies

If the doctor is considering breathing-related sleep disorders, myoclonus, or narcolepsy as possible diagnoses, the doctor may ask the patient to be tested in a sleep laboratory or at home with portable instruments.

POLYSOMNOGRAPHY. Polysomnography can be used to help diagnose sleep disorders as well as conduct research into sleep. In some cases the patient is tested in a special sleep laboratory. The advantage of this testing is the availability and expertise of trained technologists, but it is expensive. However, portable equipment is available for home recording of certain specific physiological functions.

MULTIPLE SLEEP LATENCY TEST. The multiple sleep latency test (MSLT) is frequently used to measure the severity of the patient's daytime sleepiness. The test measures sleep latency (the speed with which the patient falls asleep) during a series of planned naps during the day. The test also measures the amount of REM sleep that occurs. Two or more episodes of REM sleep under these conditions indicate narcolepsy. This test can also be used to help diagnose primary hypersomnia.

REPEATED TEST OF SUSTAINED WAKEFULNESS. The repeated test of sustained wakefulness (RTSW) measures sleep latency by challenging the patient's ability to stay awake. In the RTSW, the patient is placed in a quiet room with dim lighting and is asked to stay awake. As with the MSLT, the testing pattern is repeated at intervals during the day.

Treatment

Traditional

Treatment for a sleep disorder depends on what is causing the disorder. For example, if major depression is the cause of insomnia, then treatment of the depression with **antidepressants** should resolve the insomnia. In other cases, a change of environment or work schedule may help.

Drugs

Sedative or hypnotic medications are generally recommended only for insomnia related to a temporary stress (such as surgery or **grief**) because of the potential for **addiction** or overdose. In general, these drugs are given for two weeks or less in order to reduce the risk of dependence. **Trazodone**, a sedating antidepressant, is often used for chronic insomnia that does not respond to other treatments. Sleep medications may also cause problems for elderly patients because of possible interactions with their other prescription medications. Among the safer hypnotic agents are **lorazepam**, **temazepam**, and **zolpidem**. **Chloral hydrate** is often preferred for short-term treatment in elderly patients because of its mildness. Short-term treatment is recommended because this drug may be habit forming.

Narcolepsy is treated with such stimulants as **dextroamphetamine** sulfate or **methylphenidate**. Nocturnal myoclonus has been successfully treated with **clonazepam**.

Children with sleep terror disorder or sleepwalking are usually treated with **benzodiazepines** because this type of medication suppresses stage 3 and stage 4 NREM sleep.

If the cause of insomnia is RLS, treatment includes massage, warm baths, and visualization techniques to distract from the discomfort. The only medication approved by the U.S. Food and Drug Administration (FDA) for the treatment of RLS is ropinirole (Requip), although drugs used for the treatment of Parkinson's disease, benzodiazepines, and anticonvulsant medications also may be effective for this disorder.

Psychotherapy

Psychotherapy is recommended for patients with sleep disorders associated with depression or other mental disorders. In many cases the patient's scores on the Beck or Zung inventories will suggest the appropriate direction of treatment.

Cognitive-behavioral therapy (CBT) is a form of psychotherapy that is often recommended for insomnia as a way of breaking the cycle of anxiety about sleep and sleeplessness associated with insomnia. Patients are typically advised to limit the amount of time they spend in bed and to change certain habits that may contribute to the insomnia. For example, some patients are clock watchers who check their bedside clocks frequently to see how little sleep they are getting. They will be advised to put the clock under the bed or in some other location where they cannot see it during the night.

Sleep education

"Sleep hygiene" or sleep education for sleep disorders often includes instructing the patient in methods to enhance sleep. Patients are advised to do the following:

- wait until they are sleepy before going to bed
- avoid using the bedroom for work, reading, or watching television
- get up at the same time every morning no matter how much or how little they have slept
- avoid smoking and avoid drinking liquids with caffeine
- get some physical exercise early in the day every day
- limit fluid intake after dinner; in particular, avoid alcohol because it frequently causes interrupted sleep
- learn to meditate or practice relaxation techniques
- avoid tossing and turning in bed; instead, get up and listen to relaxing music or read

Lifestyle changes

Patients with sleep apnea or hypopnea are encouraged to stop smoking, avoid alcohol or drugs of abuse, and lose weight in order to improve the stability of the upper airway.

In some cases, patients with sleep disorders related to jet lag or shift work may need to change employment or travel patterns. Patients may need to avoid rapid changes in shifts at work.

Children with nightmare disorder may benefit from limits on television or movies. Violent scenes or frightening science fiction stories appear to influence the frequency and intensity of children's nightmares.

Surgery

Although making a surgical opening into the windpipe (a tracheostomy) for sleep apnea or hypopnea in adults is a treatment of last resort, it is occasionally performed if the patient's disorder is life threatening and cannot be treated by other methods. In children and adolescents, surgical removal of the tonsils and adenoids is a fairly common and successful treatment for sleep apnea. Most sleep apnea patients are treated with continuous positive airway pressure (CPAP). Sometimes an oral prosthesis is used for mild sleep apnea.

Alternative

Some alternative approaches may be effective in treating insomnia caused by anxiety or emotional stress. **Meditation** practice, breathing exercises, and **yoga** can break the vicious cycle of sleeplessness, worry about inability to sleep, and further sleeplessness for some people. Yoga can also help some people to relax muscular tension in a direct fashion. The breathing exercises and meditation can keep some patients from obsessing about sleep.

Homeopathic practitioners recommend that people with chronic insomnia see a professional homeopath. They do, however, prescribe specific remedies for at-home treatment of temporary insomnia: *Nux vomica* for alcohol or substance-related insomnia, *Ignatia* for insomnia caused by grief, *Arsenicum* for insomnia caused by fear or anxiety, and *Passiflora* for insomnia related to mental stress.

Melatonin has also been used as an alternative treatment for sleep disorders. Melatonin is produced in the body by the pineal gland at the base of the brain. This substance is thought to be related to the body's circadian rhythms.

Practitioners of Chinese medicine usually treat insomnia as a symptom of excess yang energy. Cinnabar is recommended for chronic nightmares. Either magnetic magnetite or "dragon bones" is recommended for insomnia associated with hysteria or fear. If the insomnia appears to be associated with excess yang energy arising from the liver, the practitioner will give the patient oyster shells. **Acupuncture** treatments can help bring about balance and facilitate sleep.

Dietary changes, such as eliminating stimulant foods (coffee, cola, chocolate) and late-night meals or snacks, can be effective in treating some sleep disorders. Nutritional supplementation with magnesium, as well as botanical medicines that calm the nervous system, can also be helpful. Among the botanical remedies that may be effective for sleep disorders are **valerian** (*Valeriana officinalis*), **passionflower** (*Passiflora incarnata*), and skullcap (*Scutellaria lateriflora*).

Home remedies

Warm milk before bedtime is a classic home remedy for insomnia. It is thought that this treatment works for many people because milk contains tryptophan, an amino acid that increases the brain's production of melatonin.

QUESTIONS TO ASK YOUR DOCTOR

- How do I know if I am experiencing a sleep disorder?
- What diagnostic tests are needed for a thorough assessment?
- What type of sleep disorder do I have?
- Will I need to go to a sleep laboratory?
- Is the sleep problem related to an underlying physical condition?
- Should I consider psychotherapy?
- What type of treatment do you recommend for me?
- Should I see a specialist? If so, what kind of specialist should I contact?
- What symptoms are important enough that I should seek immediate treatment?

Prognosis

The prognosis depends on the specific disorder. Children usually outgrow sleep disorders. Patients with Kleine-Levin syndrome usually get better around age 40. Narcolepsy, however, is a lifelong disorder, although cataplexy can be successfully controlled with medication, and many people find that their symptoms naturally decrease after age 60. The prognosis for sleep disorders related to other conditions depends on successful treatment of the substance abuse, medical condition, or other mental disorder. The prognosis for primary sleep disorders is affected by many things, including the patient's age, sex, occupation, personality characteristics, family circumstances, neighborhood environment, and similar factors.

About 85% of people with insomnia find relief with a combination of sleep hygiene and medication. Although there is no cure for sleep apnea, treatment can reduce the associated risks of high blood pressure and heart disease.

Insomnia and other sleep disorders are not fatal in and of themselves; however, chronic insomnia is associated with an increased risk of depression and **suicide**. In addition, insufficient sleep increases a person's risk of accidents on the road and in the workplace, with the possibility of serious injury or death. Driver **fatigue** is responsible for an estimated 100,000 motor vehicle accidents and 1,500 deaths each year in the United States, according to the National Highway Traffic Safety Administration.

Prevention

Certain sleep disorders, such as insomnia, can sometimes be prevented by practicing good sleep hygiene. Sleep hygiene involves going to bed at a regular time each night and avoiding stimulating activities, smoking, or heavy meals close to bedtime. Sleep apnea may be prevented in some cases by controlling body weight.

Resources

BOOKS

American Academy of Sleep Medicine. *International Classification of Sleep Disorders: Diagnostic and Coding Manual*. 2nd ed. Westchester, IL: AASM, 2005.

American Psychiatric Association. *Diagnostic and Statistical Manual of Mental Disorders*. 4th ed., text rev. Washington, DC: American Psychiatric Association, 2000.

Berry, Richard B. *Fundamentals of Sleep Medicine*. New York: Saunders, 2011.

Chokroverty, Susan, ed. *Sleep Disorders Medicine: Basic Science, Technical Considerations, and Clinical Aspects*. 3rd ed. New York: Saunders, 2009.

Clete, A. Kushida, ed. *Handbook of Sleep Disorders*. 2nd ed. New York: Informa Healthcare, 2008.

Colligan, L.H. *Sleep Disorders*. New York: Marshall Cavendish Benchmark, 2009.

Foldvary-Schaefer, Nancy. *Cleveland Clinic Guide to Sleep Disorders*. New York: Kaplan, 2009.

Jacobs, Gregg D. *Say Good Night to Insomnia*. New York: Holt Paperbacks, 2009.

Kushida, Clete A., ed. *Handbook of Sleep Disorders*. 2nd ed. New York: Informa Healthcare, 2009.

Lee-Chiong, Teofilo L. *Sleep Medicine Essentials*. Hoboken, NJ: Wiley-Blackwell, 2009.

Mindell, Jodi A., and Judith A. Owens. *A Clinical Guide to Pediatric Sleep: Diagnosis and Management of Sleep Problems*. 2nd ed. New York: Lippincott Williams & Wilkins, 2009.

Pollak, Charles, et al. *Encyclopedia of Sleep and Sleep Disorders*. 3rd ed., rev. New York: Facts On File, 2010.

PERIODICALS

Bae, C.J., et al. "The Use of Sleep Studies in Neurologic Practice." *Seminars in Neurology* 29 (September 2009): 305–19.

Billiard, M. "REM Sleep Behavior Disorder and Narcolepsy." *CNS and Neurological Disorders Drug Targets* 8 (August 2009): 264–70.

Caylak, E. "The Genetics of Sleep Disorders in Humans: Narcolepsy, Restless Legs Syndrome, and Obstructive Sleep Apnea Syndrome." *American Journal of Medical Genetics, Part A* 149A (November 2009): 2612–26.

Fetveit, A. "Late-life Insomnia: A Review." *Geriatrics and Gerontology International* 9 (September 2009): 220–34.

Gallicchio, L., and B. Kalesan. "Sleep Duration and Mortality: A Systematic Review and Meta-analysis." *Journal of Sleep Research* 18 (June 2009): 148–58.

Goodday, R. "Diagnosis, Treatment Planning, and Surgical Correction of Obstructive Sleep Apnea." *Journal of Oral and Maxillofacial Surgery* 67 (October 2009): 2183–96.

Gromov, I., and D. Gromov. "Sleep and Substance Use and Abuse in Adolescents." *Child and Adolescent Psychiatry Clinics of North America* 18 (October 2009): 929–46.

Moyer, D.E., et al. "Restless Legs Syndrome: Diagnostic Time-savers, Tx Tips." *Journal of Family Practice* 58 (August 2009): 415–23.

Uhde, T.W., et al. "Anxiety and Sleep Problems: Emerging Concepts and Theoretical Treatment Implications." *Current Psychiatry Reports* 11 (August 2009): 269–76.

WEBSITES

"Can't Sleep? What to Know about Insomnia." National Sleep Foundation. http://www.sleepfoundation.org/article/sleep-related-problems/insomnia-and-sleep (accessed October 4, 2011).

"Insomnia." Mayo Clinic. Last updated January 7, 2011. http://www.mayoclinic.com/health/insomnia/DS00187 (accessed October 4, 2011).

"Kleine-Levin Syndrome Information Page." National Institute of Neurological Disorders and Stroke. Last updated March 12, 2009. http://www.ninds.nih.gov/disorders/kleine_levin/kleine_levin.htm (accessed October 4, 2011).

Lubit, Roy H., et al. "Sleep Disorders." Medscape Reference, May 21, 2009. http://emedicine.medscape.com/article/287104-overview (accessed October 4, 2011).

"Sleepwalking." Mayo Clinic. Last modified August 12, 2011. http://www.mayoclinic.com/health/sleepwalking/DS01009 (accessed October 4, 2011).

"What Is Sleep?" American Sleep Association, May 2007. http://www.sleepassociation.org/index.php?p=whatissleep (accessed October 4, 2011).

ORGANIZATIONS

American Academy of Sleep Medicine, 2510 N Frontage Rd., Darien, IL, 60561, (630) 737-9700, Fax: (630) 737-9790, inquiries@assmnet.org, http://www.aasmnet.org.

American Psychiatric Association, 1000 Wilson Blvd., Ste. 1825, Arlington, VA, 22209-3901, (703) 907-7300, apa@psych.org, http://www.psych.org.

Anxiety Disorders Association of America, 8730 Georgia Ave., Silver Spring, MD, 20910, (240) 485-1001, Fax: (240) 485-1035, http://www.adaa.org.

National Institute of Neurological Disorders and Stroke, PO Box 5801, Bethesda, MD, 20824, (301) 496-5751; TTY: (301) 468-5981, (800) 352-9424, http://www.ninds.nih.gov.

National Sleep Foundation, 1010 N. Glebe Road, Ste. 310, Arlington, VA, 22201, (703) 243-1697, nsf@sleepfoundation.org, http://www.sleepfoundation.org.

Rebecca J. Frey, PhD
Ruth A. Wienclaw, PhD
Laura Jean Cataldo, RN, EdD

Sleep terror disorder

Definition

Sleep terror disorder is defined as repeated temporary arousal from sleep, during which the affected person appears and acts extremely frightened.

Demographics

Sleep terror disorder is much more common in children than it is in adults. It is estimated that approximately 1%–6% of children in the United States experience sleep terror at some point in their childhood. For most children, sleep terrors begin between the ages of 4 and 12. The problem usually disappears during adolescence. Sleep terror disorder appears to be more common in boys than in girls; some studies have reported that preadolescent boys are the group most commonly affected. No figures are available for the rates of the disorder in different racial or ethnic groups.

Sleep terrors in children are not associated with any psychological disorders.

Fewer than 1% of adults have sleep terror disorder. For most adults, sleep terrors begin in their 20s or 30s, although it is possible for someone to suffer from episodes of sleep terror starting from childhood. In the adult population, sleep terrors affect both sexes equally. They are, however, often associated with psychological disorders, most commonly anxiety, personality, or post-traumatic disorders. People who have a family history of sleep terrors or **sleepwalking disorder** are about 10 times more likely to develop sleep terror disorder than those who do not.

Description

Sleep terror disorder is sometimes referred to as *pavor nocturnus* when it occurs in children, and *incubus* when it occurs in adults. Sleep terrors are also sometimes called night terrors, though sleep terror is the preferred term, as episodes can occur during daytime naps as well as at night.

Sleep terror disorder is frequently confused with **nightmare disorder**. The two are similar in the sense that both are related to bad dreams. Nightmare disorder, however, involves a significantly smaller amount of physical movement than does sleep terror. Normally, people experiencing nightmare disorder do not get out of bed, and people experiencing nightmare disorder often have problems going back to sleep because of the nature of their dream. Most people experiencing sleep terrors, however, go back to deep sleep without ever having fully awakened. People experiencing nightmares can generally remember their dreams and some of the events in the dream leading up to their awakening, and they often awake from nightmares just as they are about to experience the most frightening part of a disturbing dream. People experiencing sleep terrors, however, can sometimes recall a sense of profound fear but often do not remember the episode at all.

Causes and symptoms

Causes

The causes of sleep terror are for the most part unknown. Some researchers suggest that sleep terrors are caused by a delay in the maturation of the child's central nervous system. Such factors as **sleep deprivation**, psychological **stress**, and fever may also trigger episodes of sleep terror.

Symptoms

The symptoms of sleep terror are very similar to the physical symptoms of extreme fear. These include rapid heartbeat, sweating, and rapid breathing (hyperventilation). The heart rate can increase up to two to four times the person's regular rate. Sleep terrors cause people to be jolted into motion, often sitting up suddenly in bed. People sometimes scream or cry. The person's facial expression may be fearful.

People experiencing sleep terror are not fully awake. They are nearly impossible to bring to consciousness or comfort, and sometimes respond violently to attempts to console or restrain them. In many cases, once the episode is over the person returns to sleep without ever waking fully. People often do not have any recollection of the episode after later awaking normally, although they may recall a sense of fear.

People experiencing sleep terror disorder sometimes get out of bed and act as if they are fighting or fleeing something. During this time injuries can occur. Cases have been reported of people falling out of windows or falling down stairs during episodes of sleep terror.

Episodes of sleep terror usually occur during the first third of a person's night sleep, although they can occur even during naps taken in the daytime. Although sleep terror episodes resemble nightmares, they usually occur during NREM (non-rapid eye movement) sleep rather than during the normal dreaming of REM (rapid eye movement) sleep. The average sleep terror episode lasts less than 15 minutes. Usually only one episode occurs per night, but in some cases terror episodes occur in clusters. It is unusual for a person to have many episodes in a single night, although upwards of 40 have been

KEY TERMS

Nightmare—A frightening dream that occurs during REM sleep. Nightmares are distinguished from night terrors by the fact that night terrors occur during a different phase of sleep and do not involve dreaming. Children who awaken from nightmares remember them, while children with night terrors often remember nothing about what caused the awakening.

Non-rapid eye movement (NREM) sleep—Stages of sleep during which rapid eye movements do not occur. The majority of sleep consists of the four stages of NREM sleep.

Rapid eye movement (REM) sleep—A stage of sleep during which the sleeper's eyes move back and forth rapidly. Most dreams occur during REM sleep.

reported. Most persons with the disorder have only one occurrence per week, or just a few per month.

Diagnosis

Sleep terror is diagnosed most often in children when parents express concern to the child's pediatrician. A fact sheet from the American Academy of Child and Adolescent Psychiatry suggests that parents consult a child **psychiatrist** if the child has several episodes of sleep terror each night, if the episodes occur every night for weeks at a time, or if the episodes interfere with the child's daytime activities. The **diagnosis** is usually made on the basis of the child's and parents' description of the symptoms. There are no laboratory tests for sleep terror disorder. In adults, the disorder is usually self-reported to the patient's family doctor. Again, the diagnosis is usually based on the patient's description of the symptoms.

The ***Diagnostic and Statistical Manual of Mental Disorders***, the standard reference work used by mental health professionals in diagnosing mental disorders, classifies sleep terror disorder as a disorder of arousal. In order to meet the *DSM* criteria for diagnosis, patients must experience repeated episodes accompanied by fear-related symptoms, such as increased heart rate or sweating; be unable to recall their dreams or the entire episode; and remain asleep during the episode, despite external efforts to awaken them. The episodes must not be attributed to a medical condition or drug use.

Treatment

If sleep terror episodes are infrequent, then treatment may not be necessary as long as the episodes are not interfering significantly with the person's life. Some people may want to rearrange their bedroom furniture to minimize the possibility of hurting themselves or others if they get out of bed during a sleep terror episode. To keep children from becoming overly worried about their sleep terrors, experts suggest that parents avoid placing unnecessary emphasis on the episodes. **Psychotherapy** is often helpful for adults concerned about the specific triggers of sleep terror episodes.

Several different medications have been used to treat sleep terror disorder, with varying degrees of success. One of the most common is **diazepam** (Valium). Diazepam is a hypnotic (sleep-inducing medication) and is thought to be useful in the prevention of sleep terror episodes because it acts as a nervous system depressant. There are many different types of hypnotics, and choosing one for a patient depends on other drugs that the patient may be taking, any medical or psychological conditions, and other health factors. Most studies of medications as treatments for sleep terror disorder have been done on adult patients; there is little information available on the use of medications to treat the disorder in children.

QUESTIONS TO ASK YOUR DOCTOR

- How do I know if I (or my child) am experiencing sleep terror disorder?
- What diagnostic tests are available for a thorough assessment?
- What symptoms are important enough that I should seek immediate treatment?
- What type of treatment do you recommend?
- Should I see a specialist? If so, what kind of specialist should I contact?

Prognosis

In most children, sleep terror disorder resolves before or during adolescence without any treatment. Adults often respond well to diazepam or another hypnotic. Psychotherapy and avoidance of any stressors that may precipitate terror episodes may be helpful as well. Episodes of sleep terrors often decrease with age. This decrease is due to the fact that the amount of slow-wave sleep, the sleep phase during which terror episodes usually occur, declines with age.

Resources

BOOKS

American Psychiatric Association. *Diagnostic and Statistical Manual of Mental Disorders*. 4th ed., text rev. Washington, DC: American Psychiatric Publishing, 2000.

Berry, Richard B. *Fundamentals of Sleep Medicine*. New York, NY: Saunders, 2011.

Chokroverty, Sudhansu. *Sleep Disorders Medicine: Basic Science, Technical Considerations, and Clinical Aspects*. 3rd ed. Philadelphia: Saunders Elsevier, 2009.

Cooper, Rachel. *Classifying Madness: A Philosophical Examination of the Diagnostic and Statistical Manual of Mental Disorders*. New York: Springer, 2010.

Kaplan, Harold, and Benjamin Sadock, eds. *Synopsis of Psychiatry*. 10th ed. Baltimore: Lippincott Williams & Wilkins, 2007.

Kushida, Clete, A., ed. *Handbook of Sleep Disorders*. 2nd ed. New York, NY: Informa Healthcare, 2008.

Lee-Chiong, Teofilo L. *Sleep Medicine Essentials*. Hoboken, NJ: Wiley-Blackwell, 2009.

Mindell, Jodi A., and Judith A. Owens. *A Clinical Guide to Pediatric Sleep: Diagnosis and Management of Sleep Problems*. 2nd ed. New York: Lippincott Williams & Wilkins, 2009.

North, Carol, and Sean Yutzy. *Goodwin and Guze's Psychiatric Diagnosis*. New York, NY: Oxford University Press, 2010.

Pollak, Charles P., Michael Thorpy, and Jan Yager. *The Encyclopedia of Sleep and Sleep Disorders*. New York: Facts on File, 2009.

PERIODICALS

Owens, Judith A., Richard P. Millman, and Anthony Spirito. "Sleep Terrors in a 5-Year-Old Girl." *Pediatrics & Adolescent Medicine* 153, no. 3 (March 1999).

WEBSITES

American Academy of Child & Adolescent Psychiatry (AACAP). "Children's Sleep Problems." AACAP Facts For Families Pamphlet #34. Washington, DC: American Academy of Child & Adolescent Psychiatry, 2004.

ORGANIZATIONS

American Academy of Child and Adolescent Psychiatry, 3615 Wisconsin Ave. NW, Washington, DC, 20016-3007, (202) 966-7300, Fax: (202) 966-2891, http://aacap.org.

American Academy of Sleep Medicine, 2510 N Frontage Rd., Darien, IL, 60561, (630) 737-9700, Fax: (630) 737-9790, inquiries@assmnet.org, http://www.aasmnet.org.

National Sleep Foundation, 1010 N Glebe Rd., Ste. 310, Arlington, VA, 22201, (703) 243-1697, nsf@sleepfoundation.org, http://www.sleepfoundation.org.

Tish Davidson, A.M.
Laura Jean Cataldo, RN, Ed.D.

Sleepwalking disorder

Definition

Sleepwalking disorder, also called somnambulism, is characterized by repeated episodes of motor activity during sleep such as sitting up in bed, rising, and walking around, among others. The person appears to be awake because their eyes are usually open and they can maneuver around objects, but is considered asleep.

Sleepwalking disorder is one of several **sleep disorders** listed in the ***Diagnostic and Statistical Manual of Mental Disorders***, produced by the **American Psychiatric Association** and used by most mental health professionals in North America and Europe to diagnose mental disorders.

Demographics

Sleepwalking can occur at any age but is most common in children, with the first episodes usually between the ages of 4 and 8. The peak of sleepwalking behavior occurs at about 12 years of age. Between 10% and 30% of children have had at least one episode of sleepwalking. Sleepwalking disorder is seen in 1%–17% of children and occurs more frequently in boys. It is more frequently found in children if a close relative also has a history of sleepwalking, In fact, identical twins are more likely to sleepwalk than are other siblings. Adults who sleepwalk typically have a history of sleepwalking that stems back to childhood. Sleepwalking events occur in approximately 1%–7% of adults while sleepwalking disorder occurs in about 0.5%.

Description

Sleepwalking episodes usually occur during the first third of the night during the deepest phase of sleep (delta sleep or slow-wave sleep). The episodes can last anywhere from a few minutes up to one hour, with 5 to 15 minutes being average. Sleepwalkers appear to be awake but are typically unresponsive to individuals who attempt to communicate with them. Persons who sleepwalk typically have no memory or awareness of their actions or movement upon waking. However, sleepwalkers sometimes wake up while sleepwalking, remembering a dream they were having, which was being acted out during their sleepwalking episode. After going back to bed, the person will fall back into a light stage of sleep. The next morning, most sleepwalkers do not remember their sleepwalking activities the night before, although some people have vague recollections of what they did or said.

Activities while sleepwalking can be as simple as walking around and talking. However, sometimes activities can be less routine, such as the woman reported in 2008 in the journal *Sleep Medicine* who turned on her computer, logged in with her username and password, and wrote e-mails to friends inviting them to a party. Other such sleepwalking incidents by people include driving a car, taking knives from a kitchen drawer, playing a musical instrument, feeding pets, washing clothes, dressing, talking on the telephone, moving furniture, walking down the street or around the house, painting, cooking, or eating. Physical violence, abusive speech, and even murder has been reported from sleepwalking incidents.

Sometimes night terrors occur with sleepwalking. The person may seem confused or agitated, or extremely fearful or violent. During such terrors, the person may scream or throw their arms up into the air. Frequently, night terrors have a reoccurring theme, possibly from a frightening incident as a child or one that recently occurred as an adult. Although these episodes resemble nightmares, they usually occur during non-rapid eye movement (NREM) sleep rather than during the normal dreaming of rapid eye movement (REM) sleep. The patient often cannot recall the episode the next morning. They are non-REM dream experiences from which the sleeper never fully awakes and which he or she does not recall upon awakening. This condition mostly occurs in children and can be treated with hypnosis or medication in severe cases.

People who frequently sleepwalk often will feel tired and fatigued the next day. They may feel uneasy or restless, have less concentration, and experience some degree of dysfunction, such as delayed response time. Researchers often describe sleepwalking disorder as sleepwalking once or twice a month. Chronic sleepwalking may occur more frequently and may cause serious problems at home, work, or at school due to lack of restful sleep.

During an episode of sleepwalking, a related disorder may occur. For instance, people with nocturnal sleep-related eating disorder (NS-RED) will eat while sleepwalking. Often, the sleepwalker will walk to the kitchen, make a meal, and eat food while still asleep. Another similar sleep disorder is night eating syndrome (NES), which is characterized by a person eating during the night, while fully awake, because they are fearful that they cannot get back to sleep unless they eat food.

Causes and symptoms

Causes

There appears to be a genetic component for individuals who sleepwalk. The condition is 10 times more likely to occur in close relatives of known sleepwalkers than in the general public. These families also tend to be deep sleepers.

Sleepwalking may also be triggered by fever, which directly affects the nervous system, general illness, **alcohol use**, **sleep deprivation**, irregular or chaotic sleep schedule, and emotional **stress**. Certain drugs can also cause sleepwalking disorder such as neuroleptics (drugs that treat **psychosis**), stimulants (drugs that increase physical and/or mental activities), sedative/hypnotics (drugs that increase sleep or relaxation), **antianxiety drugs** (drugs that reduce anxiety), antiseizure drugs (drugs that reduce the chance of **seizures**), antiarrhythmic heart drugs (drugs that reduce or eliminate irregular heartbeat), and antihistamines (drugs that treat allergies). Hormonal changes that occur during adolescence, menstruation, and pregnancy can be also be triggers for sleepwalking. Sleepwalking episodes are more likely during times of physiological or psychological stress.

Certain medical conditions also increase the likelihood of sleepwalking, such as fever, gastroesophageal reflux (when food re-enters the esophagus from the stomach), night asthma, heart arrhythmias, night seizures (convulsions), obstructive sleep apnea (breathing temporarily stops while sleeping), and psychiatric disorders (such as panic attacks).

Symptoms

The *DSM-IV-TR* (fourth edition, text revised) specifies six diagnostic criteria for sleepwalking disorder:

- Repeated episodes of rising from bed during sleep. These episodes may include sitting up in bed, looking around, and walking, and usually occur during the first third of the night.
- Unresponsive to attempts at communication. During sleepwalking, the person typically has his or her eyes open, with dilated pupils, a blank stare, and does not respond to another's attempts at communication. Affected persons typically are only awakened with great difficulty.
- No recollection of the sleepwalking incident. Upon waking, the person typically has no memory of the sleepwalking events. If the individual does awaken from the sleepwalking episode, they may have a vague memory of the incident. Often, sleepwalkers will return to bed, or fall asleep in another place with no recall of how they got there.
- No impairment of mental activity upon waking. If an individual awakens during a sleepwalking episode, there may be a short period of confusion or disorientation, but there is no impairment of mental activity or behavior.
- Causes significant distress to life situations. Sleepwalking causes significant disruption of social and occupational situations or affects other abilities to function.
- Not due to substance use or abuse. Sleepwalking disorder is not diagnosed if the cause is related to drug abuse, medication, or a general medical condition.

Proposed changes for the fifth edition of the *DSM* (*DSM-5*) include subsuming sleepwalking disorder and **sleep terror disorder** into one **diagnosis** called disorder of arousal. The diagnostic criteria is similar but includes subtypes of sleepwalking, sleep terrors, or confusion upon arousal.

Diagnosis

The line that separates periodic sleepwalking from sleepwalking disorder is not clearly defined. Individuals or families most often seek professional help when the episodes of sleepwalking are violent, pose a risk for injury, or impair the person's ability to function. For a diagnosis of sleepwalking disorder to be made, the person must experience a significant amount of social, occupational, or other impairment related to the sleepwalking problem. Episodes that have a long history extending from childhood through adolescence and especially into adulthood are more likely to be diagnosed with sleepwalking disorder.

Since the individual cannot recall the sleepwalking activity, diagnosis by means of interview is of little benefit, unless it involves someone who has witnessed the sleepwalking behavior. The preferred method for accurate diagnosis is through **polysomnography**. This technique involves hooking electrodes to different locations on the affected person's body to monitor **brain** wave activity, heart rate, breathing, and other vital signs while the individual sleeps. Monitoring brain–wave patterns (via an electroencephalogram) and physiologic responses during sleep can usually give sleep specialists an accurate diagnosis of the condition and determine the effective means of treatment, if any.

Sleepwalking disorder can be difficult to distinguish from sleep terror disorder. In both cases, the individual has motor movement, is difficult to awaken, and does not remember the incident. The primary difference is that sleep terror disorder typically has an initial scream and signs of intense fear and panic associated with the other behaviors.

Treatment

Treatment for sleepwalking is often unnecessary, especially if episodes are infrequent and pose no hazard to the sleepwalker or others. If sleepwalking is recurrent, or daytime **fatigue** is suspected to result from disturbed sleep patterns, polysomnography may be recommended to determine whether some form of treatment may be helpful. If stress appears to trigger sleepwalking events in adults, **stress management**, **biofeedback** training, or relaxation techniques can be beneficial. Hypnosis has been used help sleepwalkers awaken once their feet touch the floor. **Psychotherapy** may help individuals who have underlying psychological issues that could be contributing to sleep problems.

Medications are sometimes used in the more severe cases with adults. Benzodiazepines—antianxiety drugs—such as **alprazolam** (Xanax), **clonazepam** (Klonopin), or **diazepam** (Valium) can be used to help relax muscles, although these may not result in fewer episodes of sleepwalking. A tricyclic antidepressant (TCA) may also be used, such as **amitriptyline** (Elavil), butriptyline (Evadyne), dibenzepin (Noveril), lofepramine (Lomont), metapramine (Timaxel), **nortriptyline** (Aventyl HCl, Pamelor), or **protriptyline** (Vivactil). When medications are used, they are typically prescribed in the lowest dose necessary and only for a limited period. Such drugs will reduce chemical processes within the brain that affect sleep and, consequently, reduce or eliminate sleepwalking. Hypnosis and biofeedback have also been used effectively in the treatment of sleepwalking disorder.

Sedative drugs used to treat sleep disorders may actually cause sleepwalking and other behaviors during sleep, including sleep eating and sleep driving. In 2007, the U.S. Food and Drug Administration required manufacturers of sedative drugs to add a warning label detailing the risks of engaging in sleep behaviors when taking the medications. Such drugs include **zolpidem** (Ambien), **flurazepam** (Dalmane), **triazolam** (Halcion), eszopiclone (Lunesta), **zaleplon** (Sonata), and **temazepam** (Restoril), among others.

KEY TERMS

Electroencephalogram (EEG)—A recording of electrical activity in the brain.

Non-rapid eye movement (NREM) sleep—Stages of sleep during which rapid eye movements do not occur. The majority of sleep consists of the four stages of NREM sleep.

Rapid eye movement (REM) sleep—A stage of sleep during which the sleeper's eyes move back and forth rapidly. Most dreams occur during REM sleep.

Sleep terror (or night terror) disorder—A disorder in which the patient wakes up physically aroused and screaming or crying.

Prognosis

Most cases of sleepwalking subside over time. Sleepwalking in childhood usually disappears without treatment by age 15. If sleepwalking episodes persist into early adulthood, treatment is recommended. With an accurate diagnosis and appropriate treatment, episodes of sleepwalking can be greatly reduced and, in some cases, eliminated. Research into sleepwalking in the 2010s finds that sleepwalking disorder may be based on previous

QUESTIONS TO ASK YOUR DOCTOR

- How do I know if I am experiencing a sleepwalking disorder?
- What role does my family history play in my sleepwalking disorder?
- Could any of the medications I am taking be causing me to sleepwalk?
- What symptoms are important enough that I should seek immediate treatment?
- What diagnostic tests are needed for a thorough assessment?
- What type of treatment do you recommend?
- Should I see a specialist? If so, what kind of specialist should I contact?
- Is there any way I can prevent sleepwalking?
- What safety precautions should I take?

psychiatric issues, and actions performed while sleeping may be dependent on one's past (and not independent, arbitrary activities).

Prevention

Sleepwalking is relatively common and is not cause for concern. The major risk associated with sleepwalking is accidental injury. Persons with sleepwalking disorder should take precautions to block stairways, lock windows, keep floors cleared of harmful objects, etc., before going to sleep at night. Although most sleepwalkers are harmless, their activities can be dangerous to themselves or others. A sleepwalker may become violent if they, for instance, have their path blocked or if they become irritated with their environment. If they are trying to act out a dream or nightmare, they may try to interact with a bystander with aggressive or violent behavior.

If taking certain medications, a medical condition, or exposure to significant stressors are suspected triggers of sleepwalking episodes, a doctor should be consulted for a complete assessment.

Resources

BOOKS

American Psychiatric Association. *Diagnostic and Statistical Manual of Mental Disorders.* 4th ed, text rev. Washington, DC: American Psychiatric Association, 2000.

Berry, Richard B. *Fundamentals of Sleep Medicine.* New York: Saunders, 2011.

Chokroverty, Susan, ed. *Sleep Disorders Medicine: Basic Science, Technical Considerations, and Clinical Aspects.* 3rd ed. New York: Saunders, 2009.

Clete, A. Kushida, ed. *Handbook of Sleep Disorders.* 2nd ed. New York: Informa Healthcare, 2008.

Lee-Chiong, Teofilo L. *Sleep Medicine Essentials.* Hoboken, NJ: Wiley-Blackwell, 2009.

Mindell, Jodi A., and Judith A. Owens. *A Clinical Guide to Pediatric Sleep: Diagnosis and Management of Sleep Problems.* 2nd ed. New York: Lippincott Williams & Wilkins, 2009.

North, Carol, and Sean Yutzy. *Goodwin and Guze's Psychiatric Diagnosis.* New York: Oxford University Press, 2010.

Pollak, Charles P., et al. *A The Encyclopedia of Sleep and Sleep Disorders.* New York: Facts on File, 2009.

PERIODICALS

Dobson, Roger. "Zzz-mail: What Happens When Sleepwalkers Go Online." *The Telegraph* (May 26, 2011). http://www.telegraph.co.uk/news/newstopics/howaboutthat/3743289/Zzz-mail-What-happens-when-sleepwalkers-go-online.html (accessed July 19, 2011).

WEBSITES

American Psychiatry Association. "Sleep-Wake Disorders." DSM-5 Development. http://www.dsm5.org/Proposed-Revision/Pages/Sleep-WakeDisorders.aspx (accessed July 19, 2011).

American Sleep Association. "Sleep Eating." http://www.sleepassociation.org/index.php?p=sleepeating (accessed November 6, 2011).

PubMed Health. "Sleepwalking." U.S. National Library of Medicine. http://www.ncbi.nlm.nih.gov/pubmedhealth/PMH0001811 (accessed November 6, 2011).

U.S. Food and Drug Administration. "FDA Requests Label Change for All Sleep Disorder Drug Products." http://www.fda.gov/NewsEvents/Newsroom/PressAnnouncements/2007/ucm108868.htm (accessed November 6, 2011).

ORGANIZATIONS

American Academy of Child and Adolescent Psychiatry, 3615 Wisconsin Ave. NW, Washington, DC, 20016-3007, (202) 966-7300, Fax: (202) 966-2891, http://www.aacap.org.

American Academy of Sleep Medicine, 2510 N Frontage Rd., Darien, IL, 60561, (630) 737-9700, Fax: (630) 737-9790, http://www.aasmnet.org.

American Medical Association, 515 N State St., Chicago, IL, 60654, (800) 621-8335, http://www.ama-assn.org.

American Psychiatric Association, 1000 Wilson Blvd., Ste. 1825, Arlington, VA, 22209, (703) 907-7300, apa@psych.org, http://www.psych.org.

American Sleep Association, http://www.sleepassociation.org.

Better Sleep Council, 501 Wythe St., Alexandria, VA, 22314-1917, http://www.bettersleep.org.

National Sleep Foundation, 1010 N. Glebe Rd., Ste. 310, Arlington, VA, 22201, (703) 243-1697, nsf@sleepfoundation.org, http://www.sleepfoundation.org.

Gary Gilles, M.A.
Laura Jean Cataldo, RN, EdD.
William A. Atkins, BS

Smoking *see* **Nicotine and related disorders**

Smoking cessation

Definition

Smoking cessation therapy consists of procedures that educate smokers about the dangers of smoking, motivate them to smoking abstinence, and assist them in their endeavors to quit by way of counseling and pharmaceutical interventions.

Purpose

The goal of smoking cessation is to get smokers to stop smoking or to help them when they **relapse**. Because **nicotine addiction** is strong and the cues to smoke are so prevalent, experts on smoking agree that occasional relapse is normal: One estimate is that smokers who eventually quit for good make at least three or four attempts before freeing themselves of the addiction, and approximately 50% of quitters relapse during the first week or two of trying to quit.

Demographics

Smoking is a key factor in lung cancer, heart attack, cerebrovascular disease, and chronic obstructive pulmonary disease (COPD), which are four of the primary causes of death in the United States. About one-third of deaths due to cancer, heart disease, and **stroke** and around 90% of COPD cases are directly attributable to tobacco use. Individuals who smoke after age 35 have a 50% chance of dying from smoking-related causes, and smokers have an average life span that is shorter by 8 to 10 years than nonsmokers.

Smoking-related illness costs the United States between $96 billion a year in healthcare costs, according to the U.S. Centers for Disease Control and Prevention (CDC). An efficacious treatment approach that significantly cuts the numbers of smokers has a great positive impact on the economy, health care, and insurance costs, and the vast social costs generated by the premature death of approximately 443,000 people per year. The Surgeon General's Office, the U.S. Public Health Service, the National Cancer Institute, and many other governmental and nonprofit organizations, as well as private healthcare agencies, have concerned themselves with the importance of smoking cessation, resulting in established guidelines for clinical practice as well as

Symptom	Cause	Duration	Relief
Craving for cigarette	Nicotine craving	Begins in first week and can linger for months	Distract yourself with other activities (e.g., exercise, hobbies, etc.)
Coughing, dry throat, nasal drip	Body ridding itself of mucus in lungs and airways	Several weeks	Drink plenty of fluids, use cough drops
Irritability, impatience	Nicotine craving	2–4 weeks	Exercise, practice relaxation techniques, avoid caffeine
Lack of concentration	Lack of nicotine stimulation	A few weeks	Reduce workload, avoid stress
Fatigue	Lack of nicotine stimulation	2–4 weeks	Practice relaxation techniques, nap
Insomnia	Nicotine craving temporarily reduces deep sleep	2–4 weeks	Avoid caffeine after 6 p.m.
Hunger	Cigarette cravings confused with hunger pangs	Up to several weeks	Drink water or low-calorie drinks, eat low-calorie snacks
Constipation, gas	Intestinal movement decreases with lack of nicotine	1–2 weeks	Drink plenty of fluids, add fiber to diet, exercise

Side effects of nicotine withdrawal and possible remedies. *(Table by PreMediaGlobal. Reproduced by permission of Gale, a part of Cengage Learning.)*

continuing research on which strategies work and which ones do not.

Description

The U.S. Department of Health and Human Services/Public Health Service Guideline *Treating Tobacco Use and Dependence* (updated in 2008), a comprehensive, evidence-based blueprint for smoking cessation, established the necessity for medical practitioners to take a proactive stance in regard to patients' smoking. This article was based on a review of more than 3,000 articles on tobacco addiction that had been published from 1975 to 1994. The guideline was designed to provide clinicians and others with specific information regarding effective cessation treatments, and it advocated the "frank discussion of personal health risks, the benefits of smoking cessation, and available methods to assist in stopping smoking," an approach designed to raise physician concern about smoking, which had generally not been a topic broached with patients until smoking-related diseases developed. The guidelines provide a strategy by which to approach the problem of patient smoking: The "Five A's" model.

The model of the Five A's specifies:

- Ask to systematically identify all tobacco users at every visit.
- Advise smokers to quit smoking.
- Assess the smoker's willingness to stop; if the smoker is not willing, educate as to the "Five R's."
- Assist smokers who are willing to stop smoking. Tests of nicotine dependence help determine effective treatments.
- Arrange follow-up support. Quick follow-up can prevent or curtail early relapse.

One research estimate is that 5% of smokers will stop smoking if their doctor advises them to, and that educating smokers about the health effects of smoking can motivate them to quit in higher numbers. Motivation to stop smoking can be increased by social support and pharmaceutical interventions, and early relapse can be prevented more easily if the smoker has a follow-up appointment within a week of the stated quitting date.

Smoking cessation methods focus on getting smokers into treatment in the first place by targeting resistance and increasing motivation. If patients are not willing to quit, medical personnel are expected to employ the use of guidelines called the "Five R's":

- Relevance. The medical practitioner discusses the relevance of quitting smoking to the particular individual, perhaps targeting health concerns, family health, or the financial impact of smoking.
- Risks. The medical practitioner engages patients in discussion of the health risks of smoking.
- Rewards. The medical practitioner helps patients identify potential rewards, such as saving money (more than $2,000 a year for a pack-a-day habit), a variety of health improvements, raised self-esteem, improved taste and sense of smell, and setting a good example for children.
- Roadblocks. The practitioner and patient discuss the problems that prevent the patient from quitting, and the practitioner attempts to address the patient's concerns (for example, fear of weight gain). By this time, physicians will also educate patients as to the symptoms of nicotine withdrawal. Irritability, increased food cravings, headaches, lack of concentration, urges to use tobacco, and restlessness are some of the symptoms associated with nicotine withdrawal.
- Repetition. The medical practitioner engages patients unwilling to quit in this discussion at every appointment.

In 2002, a study of **managed care** providers revealed that 71% of the responding plans had written their own guidelines for smoking cessation treatment, and a majority stated that their guidelines were based on the Five A's model. Smoking cessation treatment typically involves primary identification of smokers and their willingness to quit, a behavioral treatment component, and provision of pharmacotherapy.

Once the patient has indicated willingness to take part in a smoking cessation program, the prescribed therapy is generally pharmaceutical. Although telephone counseling has been shown to assist smokers in staying off tobacco, with group or individual counseling also showing some usefulness, it is without doubt that nicotine replacement therapy (NRT) or other drugs greatly contribute to smoking abstinence. Researchers have found that use of any of the drugs currently prescribed for nicotine addiction double or even triple the chances that patients will quit smoking.

Pharmacotherapy

There are currently three primary pharmacologic interventions in smoking cessation: nicotine replacement therapy (NRT), **bupropion** (Wellbutrin, Wellbutrin XL, Zyban), and varenicline (Chantix). The three replacement therapies of choice act differently to affect a similar change: Patients manage to quit smoking with significantly less physiologic distress and less chance of relapse than those who use only behavioral strategies or go "cold turkey."

NRT works by replacing the delivery method of nicotine with chewing gum, lozenges, a nicotine patch, nasal spray, or an "inhaler" that actually works by oral absorption, not by inhalation. Nicotine is delivered to the body in doses that decrease over time, allowing users to eventually end their dependence. Side effects of NRT include nausea, flatulence and other digestive problems, and mouth and jaw soreness from chewing the gum; skin irritation at patch sites; rhinitis, sneezing, and watery eyes for the spray; and throat irritation for the inhaler. Patients' previous health issues determine which, if any, of the NRTs will be prescribed. NRT is not prescribed for patients who have suffered a recent heart attack, who have angina or arrhythmia, or for women who are pregnant or nursing.

Bupropion, an antidepressant drug, inhibits the body's reuptake of the **neurotransmitters dopamine** and norepinephrine. Like **selective serotonin reuptake inhibitors (SSRIs)**, another class of antidepressant drugs, bupropion works because it produces higher levels of neurotransmitters in the **brain**, which in turn create enhanced feelings of well-being. Unlike other **SSRIs**, bupropion has some effect on **serotonin** but has its primary effects on dopamine. Originally used as an antidepressant drug, bupropion has been used in smoking cessation both for those suffering solely from nicotine addiction and for those who have concurrent symptoms of **depression**. Bupropion can be used on its own or together with nicotine replacement products. Several studies have indicated that the combination helps more smokers quit than either method by itself. Bupropion is the only antidepressant currently approved by the FDA for use as a smoking cessation product.

Varenicline, a nicotinic receptor partial agonist, works by targeting nicotine receptors in the brain. The drug attaches itself to the nicotine receptors and blocks nicotine from reaching the receptors. This action blocks the pleasurable sensation smokers derive from smoking. Varenicline is available by prescription only.

Two other drugs, **nortriptyline** (Pamelor) and **clonidine** (Catapres), are sometimes used when the primary treatments are unsuccessful. Nortriptyline is a tricyclic antidepressant that acts by increasing levels of norepinephrine. Clonidine is a drug primarily used for treating high blood pressure. Neither drug is approved by the FDA for treating nicotine dependence, and their uses in smoking cessation are considered off-label.

Behavioral therapy

Smoking cessation programs are more effective when patients learn behavioral coping strategies in addition to using drug therapy; however, given the strength of the physical addiction, if only one therapeutic modality is to be used, pharmacotherapy is generally considered the more effective choice. That said, many smokers find comfort in being able to pick up the phone and talk to someone when cravings become unmanageable. In a best-case scenario (and in most of the managed care programs today), patients have access to behavioral, supportive, and drug therapies.

Alternative treatments

Other approaches that have been used to help smokers quit include hypnosis and **acupuncture**. The evidence for the usefulness of hypnosis is largely anecdotal. It appears to be most helpful when used in combination with nicotine replacement products or bupropion. Although acupuncture has been used in Western countries since the 1970s to help people quit smoking, it does not appear to be particularly effective in this regard.

Precautions

Seeing a physician regularly while using smoking cessation drugs is important. The physician will check to make sure the medicine is working as it should and will watch for unwanted side effects.

Some side effects of smoking cessation drugs include:

- nausea
- vomiting
- severe pain in the stomach or abdomen
- severe diarrhea
- severe dizziness
- fainting
- convulsions (seizures)
- low blood pressure
- fast, weak, or irregular heartbeat
- hearing or vision problems
- severe breathing problems
- severe watering of the mouth or drooling
- cold sweat
- severe headache
- confusion
- severe weakness

Bupropion should not be taken by patients with a history of **seizures**, high blood pressure, anorexia, or **bulimia nervosa**, or patients who are also taking monoamine oxidase inhibitor (MAOI) medications. These include such drugs as furazolidone, **isocarboxazid**, and

KEY TERMS

Nicotine—A poisonous chemical usually derived from the tobacco plant, whose affect on the brain begins within seven seconds after it is inhaled. It causes the adrenal glands to secrete epinephrine, a neurotransmitter that causes the user to experience a nearly immediate feeling of euphoria. The neurotransmitter dopamine is also released, increasing the feeling of well-being. Nicotine also elevates blood pressure, causes the release of glucose into the bloodstream, and increases the heart rate and respiration rate. Nicotine, with its near instant but short duration "high," is extremely addictive, and its presence in tobacco products, such as cigarettes, pipe tobacco, and chewing tobacco, becomes even more dangerous due to other carcinogenic ingredients present in those products.

Neurotransmitter—One of a group of chemicals secreted by a nerve cell (neuron) to carry a chemical message to another nerve cell, often as a way of transmitting a nerve impulse. Neurotransmitters affect various sensations in the body, such as pleasure, pain, hunger, and fear. Examples of neurotransmitters include acetylcholine, dopamine, serotonin, and norepinephrine.

Off-label use—Drugs in the United States are approved by the Food and Drug Administration (FDA) for specific uses based on the results of clinical trials. However, it is legal for physicians to administer these drugs for other off-label uses not approved by the FDA. It is not legal for pharmaceutical companies to advertise drugs for off-label uses.

Selective serotonin reuptake inhibitors (SSRIs)—A class of antidepressants that works by blocking the reabsorption of serotonin in brain cells, raising the level of the chemical in the brain.

phenelzine. Bupropion may also interact with phenytoin, **carbamazepine**, and levodopa.

Bupropion and varenicline are associated with serious mental health side effects including depression, agitation, thoughts of **suicide**, hostility, and attempted suicide. These side effects tend to occur shortly after the patient begins to take the medication and typically stop once the patient stops taking the drug. Patients experiencing these symptoms should be closely monitored by a physician until the side effects stop, and individuals with known psychiatric or mental health problems are at particularly high risk.

Aftercare

Aftercare consists of maintenance or relapse interventions such as Nicotine Anonymous, a 12-step program that offers support to those who want to quit cigarettes and quit smoking. Maintenance and relapse can be considered lifelong endeavors because a smoker is either not smoking or has suffered a temporary setback that can be addressed by cycling though the stages again. Some researchers say that most smokers will relapse three or four times before quitting; others estimate it to be closer to ten or fifteen times. Aftercare for smoking, like for all addictions, focuses on supportive services and addressing relapse as quickly as possible.

Resources

PERIODICALS

Anczak, John, and Robert Nogler. "Tobacco Cessation in Primary Care: Maximizing Intervention Strategies." *Clinical Medicine & Research* 1, no. 3 (July 2003): 201–16.

Fiore, Michael C., et al. "Clinical Practice Guideline: Treating Tobacco Use and Dependence: 2008 Update." *U.S. Department of Health and Human Services, Public Health Service* May 2008.

Mallin, Robert. "Smoking Cessation: Integration of Behavioral and Drug Therapies." *American Family Physician* 65, no. 6 (March 2002): 1107–15.

McPhillips-Tangum, Carol, et al. "Addressing Tobacco in Managed Care: Results of the 2002 Survey." *Preventing Chronic Disease* 1, no. 4 (October 2004): 1–11.

Rollins, Gina. "With Smoking Cessation Drugs, Dosage is Key." *American College of Physicians-American Society of Internal Medicine Observer,* April 2002. http://www.acpinternist.org/archives/2002/04/smoking.htm (accessed October 27, 2011).

Wu, Ping, et al. "Effectiveness of Smoking Cessation Therapies: a Systematic Review and Meta-Analysis." *BMC Public Health* (December 2006): 1–16.

WEBSITES

Nicotine Anonymous. http://www.nicotine-anonymous.org (accessed October 27, 2011).

U.S. Centers for Disease Control and Prevention. "Smoking & Tobacco Use: How to Quit." http://www.cdc.gov/tobacco/how2quit.htm (accessed October 27, 2011).

U.S. National Cancer Institute. "Free Help to Quit Smoking." http://www.cancer.gov/cancertopics/smoking (accessed October 27, 2011).

Lorena S. Covington, MA

Social anxiety disorder *see* **Social phobia**

Social communication disorder

Definition

Social communication disorder (SCD) is a new concept proposed for addition to the fifth edition of the ***Diagnostic and Statistical Manual of Mental Disorders*** (*DSM-5*), the guidelines used by medical professionals in diagnosing mental disorders. There is no corresponding disorder in *DSM-IV*. The new criteria are intended to help diagnose children who have unexpected difficulty with pragmatics—the aspect of language skills that concerns the appropriate use of language in social situations—in spite of a relatively normal vocabulary for their age and the ability to form grammatically correct sentences. One additional reason for the new **diagnosis** is to distinguish children with social communication disorder from those diagnosed with **autism** spectrum disorder (ASD). Although children with social communication disorder may share some of the difficulties that children with ASD have in communicating effectively with others, they do not exhibit the repetitive behaviors and limited range of interests found in children with ASD. SCD is proposed to be added as a neurodevelopmental disorder in the category of communication disorders.

Demographics

The demographics of social communication disorder were unknown as of 2011. According to the **National Institute of Mental Health** (NIMH), about one in every 110 eight-year-olds in the United States has an autism spectrum disorder, with boys being four times as likely to be diagnosed with an ASD as girls. The presence of ASD must be completely ruled out before a child can receive the diagnosis of social communication disorder.

Description

To understand the new diagnosis, it is helpful to look at the history of controversy and changes in diagnostic classification that have taken place among child psychiatrists and language specialists since the early 1980s. The controversy concerned whether children with certain types of language impairments belonged to the spectrum of autistic disorders or whether they should be diagnosed as simply having a language disorder that affected their social relationships. The debate began in 1983 with a study by Isabelle Rapin and Doris Allen, professors of neurology and child psychiatry, respectively. Rapin and Allen suggested using the term "semantic pragmatic disorder" (SPD) for children who are excessively talkative, do not seem to fully understand the meaning or words, and lack conversational skills in interacting with others. The word *semantic* refers to the ability to understand the meaning of words and use them correctly, while *pragmatic* refers to practical language skills, namely the ability to understand the rules of conversation, such as knowing what to say and when to say it, taking turns with the conversation partner, and the like. Children with SPD differed from autistic children in that they did not show the full range of symptoms considered characteristic of autism.

The next stage toward the proposed definition of SCD for *DSM-5* was the introduction of the phrase "pragmatic language impairment" (PLI) to describe children whose primary difficulty with social conversation is pragmatic rather than semantic. Whereas a child who has difficulties with the semantics of language may not know the meaning of abstract words (such as "vague" or "freedom"), may have difficulty understanding words referring to emotions (such as "fearful" or "embarrassed"), and often has difficulty with figurative or nonliteral expressions (such as "raining cats and dogs" or "sitting pretty"), the child with PLI has difficulties that typically involve three basic communication skills:

- Using language for different purposes, such as making a request, asking a question, greeting someone, giving information, or promising something.
- Changing the use of language according to the situation or the conversation partner. This aspect of pragmatics includes such skills as talking differently with a baby, another child, or an adult; giving background information to someone unfamiliar with a subject; and talking differently in a classroom compared to home or a playground.
- Following basic rules for polite conversation, such as taking turns, not interrupting the other person, staying on topic, knowing how to change the topic appropriately, knowing how to read such nonverbal signals as body language or facial expression, maintaining appropriate eye contact, and knowing how close to stand to the other person while talking.

The present *DSM-5* proposal for social communication disorder is based on the premise, as stated by the **American Psychiatric Association**, that "pragmatic difficulties (in children) constitute a fundamentally different form of language impairment" and should be distinguished from ASD.

KEY TERMS

Audiologist—A health care professional with special training in testing people for hearing loss or other hearing disorders.

Pragmatic language impairment (PLI)—A term that is used by some researchers as equivalent to social communication disorder. PLI was previously known as *semantic pragmatic disorder* or *SPD*.

Pragmatics—A subfield of linguistics that explores the ways in which context contributes to the meaning of language. In ordinary usage, pragmatics refers to a person's ability to know what is appropriate to say, where and when to say it, and the give-and-take nature of conversation.

Semantics—A subfield of linguistics that focuses on the meaning of words; in ordinary usage, the ability to use words correctly and understand their meanings.

Speech-language pathologist—A professional with special training in the evaluation and treatment of persons with voice, speech, and language disorders.

Risk factors

The risk factors for SCD have not yet been established, because the proposed disorder is considered to be different from ASD.

Causes and symptoms

The causes of SCD were not known as of 2011.

The symptoms of SCD may include the following:

- delayed language development
- difficulty making and maintaining friendships and relationships because of delayed language development
- referring facts to stories and having trouble comprehending jokes, sarcasm, or lies
- communication patterns appearing rude and inconsiderate to others
- talking in long monologues; perhaps telling a story that includes so many details that the listener loses interest
- difficulty extracting the main point of a question or conversation
- frequently missing contextual cues (tone of voice, body language, specific social setting) in a conversation
- difficulty assessing what the other person does or does not already know about the topic of conversation
- little variety in use of language
- difficulty understanding what is socially appropriate (not fitting the criteria for conduct disorder)

Diagnosis

The diagnosis of SCD is complex and difficult. One major problem is that there are no generally accepted assessment tools that are both reliable and practical. Another difficulty is that many children do not fit neatly into any diagnostic category. A child with pragmatic language difficulties may, for example, have 1) only isolated difficulties with pragmatic language skills; 2) both pragmatic and semantic difficulties with language; 3) pragmatic language difficulties together with another disorder on the autism spectrum (such as **Asperger syndrome**); or 4) pragmatic language difficulties together with another disorder that does not belong to the autism spectrum (such as **attention deficit hyperactivity disorder** [ADHD]).

Because of the complexity of diagnosis, a child with symptoms of SCD should be evaluated by a team of specialists, which may include his or her pediatrician, a speech-language pathologist (SLP), an audiologist, a **psychologist**, and possibly the child's teachers, if he or she is of school age.

The proposed *DSM-5* criteria for social communication disorder are as follows:

- Criterion A: The child's language difficulty is one of pragmatics, which affects the child's social relationships and his or her understanding of conversations with others. The child's difficulty cannot be explained on the basis of general cognitive abilities or the child's ability to form sentences and follow the rules of grammar.
- Criterion B: The child's problems with social communication limit his or her ability to function effectively in interpersonal communication, "social participation, academic achievement, or occupational performance, alone or in any combination."
- Criterion C: ASD must be ruled out as a possible diagnosis.
- Criterion D: The symptoms must be present in early childhood, although they may not be fully revealed until the social demands on the child go beyond his or her limited capacities.

No criteria for the severity of social communication disorder had been determined as of 2011.

Examination

In some cases, the child's doctor or a speech-language pathologist may recommend having the child's hearing evaluated to rule out a hearing disorder.

QUESTIONS TO ASK YOUR DOCTOR

- Does my child's problem seem to be one of language only, or are there other areas of concern?
- Would it help my child to see a speech-language pathologist?
- What types of treatment do you suggest?
- How can I help as a parent?
- How can my child's teacher help?

Tests

As of 2011, there were no laboratory or imaging tests being used to diagnose social communication disorder. With regard to psychological tests, there are two instruments that may be used to evaluate a child for ASD. These include the Social Communication Questionnaire (SCQ), which is a 40-item screener for autism spectrum disorder to be filled out by the child's parents. It takes about 10 minutes to complete. Another instrument that was developed in the United Kingdom in 2002 and is more widely used there than in North America is the Diagnostic Interview for Social and Communication Disorders (DISCO). The DISCO is an interview-based instrument for the diagnosis of autism and autism spectrum disorders. It was not clear as of 2011, however, whether either of these tests would be useful in distinguishing between ASD and SCD.

Treatment

Treatment for social communication disorder is highly individualized, as it is for other communication disorders. The therapy is usually conducted by the speech-language pathologist rather than by a pediatrician or other medical doctor. There is no one-size-fits-all approach to treating children with SCD; however, common goals might include helping the child to:

- distinguish between a sincere voice and a sarcastic one, or between a kind voice and a mean or angry one
- recognize and correctly interpret facial expressions and body language
- distinguish between "baby talk" and the kind of language to use with adults
- use verb tenses correctly and distinguish between singular and plural nouns
- take turns in conversations and tell when he or she is going on too long

The SLP may also work with the child's parents or teachers, coaching them on ways to improve the child's communication skills. These may include asking questions or otherwise helping the child to use language for different purposes; taking advantage of everyday situations to practice greetings and farewells, requesting items at the dinner table, and the like; role-playing conversations in which the child pretends to be talking to different people in different situations; and showing the child how important nonverbal signals are in conversation.

Prognosis

The prognosis for SCD depends on the child's overall intelligence and family situation and whether he or she has another medical or mental disorder along with the SCD.

Prevention

There is no known way to prevent social communication disorder, because its causes are not yet understood.

Resources

BOOKS

Bishop, Dorothy V.M., and Laurence B. Leonard. *Speech and Language Impairments in Children: Causes, Characteristics, Intervention and Outcome*. Hove, East Sussex, UK: Psychology Press, 2000.

Damico, Jack S., Nicole Müller, and Martin J. Ball, eds. *Handbook of Language and Speech Disorders*. Malden, MA: Wiley-Blackwell, 2010.

Norbury, Courtney Frazier, J. Bruce Tomblin, and Dorothy V. M. Bishop, eds. *Understanding Developmental Language Disorders in Children*. New York, NY: Psychology Press, 2008.

Rapin I, Allen D. "Developmental Language Disorders: Nosologic Considerations." In *Neuropsychology of Language, Reading, and Spelling*, edited by Ursula Kirk, 155–184. New York: Academic Press, 1982.

PERIODICALS

Freed, J., et al. "Literacy Skills in Primary School-Aged Children with Pragmatic Language Impairment: A Comparison with Children with Specific Language Impairment." *International Journal of Language and Communication Disorders* 46 (May 2011): 334–347.

Van Agt, H., et al. "The Impact on Socio-emotional Development and Quality of Life of Language Impairment in 8-Year-Old Children."*Developmental Medicine and Child Neurology* 53 (January 2011): 81–88.

Wing, L., et al. "The Diagnostic Interview for Social and Communication Disorders: Background, Inter-rater Reliability and Clinical Use." *Journal of Child Psychology and Psychiatry, and Allied Disciplines* 43 (March 2002): 307–325.

WEBSITES

American Psychiatric Association. "A 05 Social Communication Disorder." DSM-5 Development. http://www.dsm5.org/proposedrevision/pages/proposedrevision.aspx?rid=489# (accessed July 19, 2011).

American Speech-Language-Hearing Association (ASHA). "Pragmatic Language Tips." http://www.asha.org/public/speech/development/PragmaticLanguageTips.htm (accessed July 20, 2011).

———. "Social Language Use (Pragmatics)." http://www.asha.org/public/speech/development/pragmatics.htm (accessed July 20, 2011).

Melfi, Renee S. "Communication Disorders." Medscape Reference. http://emedicine.medscape.com/article/317758-overview (accessed July 20, 2011).

National Institute on Deafness and Other Communication Disorders (NIDCD). "Autism and Communication." National Institutes of Health. http://www.nidcd.nih.gov/health/voice/autism.html (accessed July 20, 2011).

National Institute of Mental Health (NIMH). "Autism Spectrum Disorders (Pervasive Developmental Disorders)." National Institutes of Health. http://www.nimh.nih.gov/health/topics/autism-spectrum-disorders-pervasive-developmental-disorders/index.shtml (accessed July 20, 2011).

ORGANIZATIONS

American Psychiatric Association, 1000 Wilson Blvd., Ste. 1825, Arlington, VA, 22209-3901, (703) 907-7300, apa@psych.org, http://www.psych.org.

American Speech-Language-Hearing Association (ASHA), 2200 Research Blvd., Rockville, MD, 20850-3289, (301) 296-5700, (800) 638-8255, Fax: (301) 296-8580, http://www.asha.org.

Callier Center for Communication Disorders, 1966 Inwood Rd., Dallas, TX, 75235, (214) 905-3000, Fax: (214) 905-3022, http://www.utdallas.edu/calliercenter.

I CAN (children's communication charity), 8 Wakley St., London, United Kingdom EC1V 7QE, 011 4420 7(843) 2510, Fax: 011 4420 7(843) 2569, info@ican.org.uk, http://www.ican.org.uk.

National Institute on Deafness and Other Communication Disorders (NIDCD), 31 Center Dr., MSC 2320, Bethesda, MD, 20892-2320, (301) 496-7243, Fax: (301) 402-0018, (800) 241-1044, nidcdinfo@nidcd.nih.gov, http://www.nidcd.nih.gov.

National Institute of Mental Health (NIMH), 6001 Executive Blvd., Rm. 8184, MSC 9663, Bethesda, MD, 20892-9663, (301) 443-4513, Fax: (301) 443-4279, (866) 615-6464, nimhinfo@nih.gov, http://www.nimh.nih.gov/index.shtml.

Rebecca J. Frey, Ph.D.

Social phobia

Definition

According to the handbook used by mental health professionals to diagnose mental disorders, the ***Diagnostic and Statistical Manual of Mental Disorders***, fourth edition, text revision, also known as the *DSM-IV-TR*, social phobia is an anxiety disorder characterized by a strong and persistent fear of social or performance situations in which individuals might feel embarrassment or humiliation. Generalized social phobia refers to a fear of most social interactions combined with fear of most performance situations, such as speaking in public or eating in a restaurant. Persons who are afraid of only one type of performance situation or afraid of only a few rather than most social situations may be described as having nongeneralized, circumscribed, or specific social phobia.

Social phobia, which is also known as social anxiety disorder, is a serious mental health problem in the United States. In any given year, social phobia affects 3.7% of the U.S. population between the ages of 18 and 54, or about 5.3 million people. It is the third most common psychiatric condition after **depression** and alcoholism. Patients diagnosed with social phobia have the highest risk of alcohol abuse of all patients with **anxiety disorders**; in addition, they suffer from worse impairment than patients with major medical illnesses, including congestive heart failure and diabetes.

Demographics

The prevalence of social phobia in the general U.S. population is difficult to evaluate because researchers differ in their estimation of the threshold of "significant interference" with the person's occupational or educational functioning. In addition, different studies have focused on different subtypes of social phobia. One study found that about 20% of the adults surveyed reported high levels of anxiety related to public speaking or other types of public performance, but only 2% indicated sufficient distress to meet the diagnostic criteria of social phobia. Because of these differences in measurement, epidemiological and community-based studies give figures for a lifetime prevalence of social phobia that fall between 3 and 13%.

The types of situations associated with social phobia are different in the general population as contrasted with clinical populations. Surveys of adults in the general population indicate that most people diagnosed with social phobia are afraid of public speaking; only 45% report being afraid of meeting new people or having to talk to strangers. Fears related to eating, drinking, or writing in public, or using a public restroom, are much less common in this group. By contrast, people being treated for social phobia in outpatient clinics are more likely to be afraid of a range of social situations rather than just one. Social phobia accounts for 10–20% of the anxiety disorders diagnosed in patients in outpatient clinics, but it is rarely the reason for hospitalizing a patient.

The same difference between general and clinical populations affects the sex ratios given for social phobia. Community-based studies suggest that social phobia is more common in women, but in most samples of clinical patients, the sex ratio is either 1:1 or males are in the majority. A study of social phobia in prepubertal children found that girls were more likely to verbalize anxiety than boys, but the researchers who observed the children interact with adults and with one another did not observe any behavioral differences between boys and girls. The researchers concluded that the apparently higher rates of social phobia in women may simply reflect women's greater openness about their feelings.

With regard to race, the same study found no statistically significant difference in the incidence of social phobia between Caucasian and African American children. This finding was consistent with a 1995 study that failed to find differences based on race in lists of children's top 10 fears. Further research, however, is necessary in order to determine whether social phobia has different symptom patterns or rates of development in different racial or ethnic groups.

The demographics of social phobia in young children are particularly difficult to determine because of changes in diagnostic categories and criteria in successive editions of *DSM*. Social phobia was introduced as a diagnostic category in *DSM-III*, which was published in 1980. Neither *DSM-III* nor its 1987 revision restricted social phobia to adults, but the disorder was rarely diagnosed in children—most likely because *DSM-III* and *DSM-III-R* listed two diagnoses for children, overanxious disorder and avoidant disorder of childhood, whose symptoms overlapped those of social phobia. Statistics based on *DSM-III-R* criteria for social phobia placed the prevalence of the disorder in children in the general population at about 1%. The revisions of the diagnostic criteria in *DSM-IV*, however, have led to an apparent dramatic increase in the prevalence of social phobia in children. One study done in 1997 reported that 18% of the children in a clinical sample met *DSM-III-R* criteria for social phobia but that 40% of the children in the same sample had social phobia according to *DSM-IV* criteria.

Description

Social phobia varies in its development and initial presentation. In some young people, the disorder grows out of a history of **shyness** or social inhibition. In others, social phobia becomes apparent following a move to a new school or similar developmental challenge. In adults, circumscribed social phobia may be associated with a change of occupation or job promotion, the most common example being the emergence of the disorder with regard to public speaking in a person whose previous jobs did not require them to make presentations or speeches in front of others. The onset of social phobia may be insidious, which means that it gets worse by slow degrees. About one-half of all patients, however, experience a sudden onset of social phobia following a particularly humiliating or frightening experience. For example, in one British case study, the patient's social phobia developed abruptly after her father's sudden death. The patient had had an argument with her father one morning, and he was killed in an accident later in the day. The onset of social phobia almost always occurs in childhood or the midteens; onset after age 25 is unusual. The disorder is often a lifelong problem, although its severity may diminish in adult life.

Adults and adolescents with social phobia, as well as many children with the disorder, have sufficient insight to recognize that their fears are excessive or unwarranted. This factor often adds to their distress and feelings of inferiority.

Social phobia is of major concern to society as a whole for two reasons. One reason is the disorder's very high rate of comorbidity with such other mental health problems as major depression and **substance abuse**. In comparison with patients diagnosed with other anxiety disorders, patients with social phobia have higher averages of concurrent anxiety disorders (1.21 versus 0.45); comorbid depression or other disorders (2.05 versus 1.19); and lifetime disorders (3.11 versus 2.05). The most common comorbid disorders diagnosed in patients with social phobia are major depression (43%); **panic disorder** (33%); **generalized anxiety disorder** (19%); PTSD (36%); alcohol or substance abuse disorder (18%); and attempted **suicide** (23%).

The second reason is the loss to the larger society of the gifts and talents that these patients possess. Social phobia can have a devastating effect on young people's intellectual life and choice of career, causing them to abandon their educations, stay in dead-end jobs, refuse promotions involving travel or relocation, and make similar self-defeating choices because of their fear of classroom participation, job interviews, and other social interactions in educational and workplace settings. One sample of patients diagnosed with social phobia found that almost one-half had failed to finish high school; 70% were in the bottom two quartiles of socioeconomic status (SES); and 22% were on welfare. In addition to their academic and employment-related difficulties, people with social phobia have limited or nonexistent social support networks. They are less likely to marry and start families of their own because of their fear of interpersonal relationships. Many continue to live at home with their parents even as adults or remain in unfulfilling relationships.

Causes and symptoms

Causes

The causes of social phobia appear to be a combination of physical and environmental factors. The symptoms vary among individuals of different ages.

NEUROBIOLOGICAL FACTORS. There is some evidence that social phobia can be inherited. A group of researchers at Yale identified a genetic locus on human chromosome 3 that is linked to **agoraphobia** and two genetic loci on chromosomes 1 and 11q linked to panic disorder. Because social phobia shares some traits with panic disorder, it is likely that there are also genes that govern susceptibility to social phobia. In addition, researchers at the **National Institute of Mental Health** (NIMH) identified a gene in mice that appears to govern fearfulness.

Positron emission tomography (PET) scans of patients diagnosed with social phobia indicate that blood flow is increased in a region of the **brain** (the amygdala) associated with fear responses when the patients are asked to speak in public. In contrast, **PET** scans of control subjects without social phobia show that blood flow during the public speaking exercise is increased in the cerebral cortex, an area of the brain associated with thinking and evaluation rather than emotional arousal. The researchers concluded that patients with social phobia have a different neurochemical response to certain social situations or challenges that activates the limbic system rather than the cerebral cortex.

TEMPERAMENT. A number of researchers have pointed to inborn temperament (natural predisposition) as a broad vulnerability factor in the development of anxiety and mood disorders, including social phobia. More specifically, children who manifest what is known as behavioral inhibition in early infancy are at increased risk for developing more than one anxiety disorder in adult life, particularly if the inhibition remains over time. Behavioral inhibition refers to a group of behaviors that are displayed when the child is confronted with a new situation or unfamiliar people. These behaviors include agitated movement (such as hyperextension), crying, and general irritability, followed by withdrawing, seeking comfort from a familiar person, and stopping what one is doing when one notices the new person or situation. Children of depressed or anxious parents are more likely to develop behavioral inhibition. One study of preadolescent children diagnosed with social phobia reported that many of these children had been identified as behaviorally inhibited in early childhood.

PSYCHOSOCIAL FACTORS. The development of social phobia is also influenced by parent-child interactions in a patient's family of origin. Several studies have found that the children of parents with major depression, whether or not it is comorbid with panic disorder, are at increased risk of developing social phobia. Children of parents with major depression and comorbid panic disorder are at increased risk of developing more than one anxiety disorder. A family pattern of social phobia, however, is stronger for the generalized than for the specific or circumscribed subtype.

It is highly likely that the children of depressed parents may acquire certain attitudes and behaviors from their parents that make them more susceptible to developing social phobia. One study of children with social phobia found that their cognitive assessment of ambiguous situations was strongly negative, not only with regard to the dangerousness of the situation but also in terms of their ability to cope with it. In other words, these children tend to overestimate the threats and dangers in life and to underestimate their strength, intelligence, and other resources for coping. This process of learning from observing the behavior of one's parents or other adults is called social **modeling**.

Still another psychosocial factor related to the development of social phobia in children and adolescents is the general disintegration in the social fabric of the developed countries since World War II. A number of social theorists as well as physicians and therapists have noted that children are exposed more frequently to both real-life and media depictions of aggressive behavior and abrasive language than earlier generations. Children also learn about frightening or unpleasant social realities at earlier and earlier ages. The increased rate of social phobia and school refusal among adolescent girls has been linked to the greater crudity of teasing from boys in junior high and high school. In addition, the fortress mentality reflected in the architecture of high-rise apartment buildings and gated communities for those who can afford them also sends children the message that other people are to be feared. While trends in the larger society may not directly cause social phobia (or other

KEY TERMS

Agoraphobia—Abnormal anxiety regarding public places or situations from which the patient may wish to flee or in which he or she would be helpless in the event of a panic attack.

Panic attack—A time-limited period of intense fear accompanied by physical and cognitive symptoms. Panic attacks may be unexpected or triggered by specific internal or external cues.

mental disorders), they are nonetheless important indirect influences.

Symptoms

The symptoms of social phobia are somewhat different in children and adults, in that the early onset of social phobia typically means that children with the disorder fail to achieve at their predicted level, whereas adults and adolescents show declines from previously achieved levels of functioning.

SYMPTOMS IN CHILDREN. Symptoms of social phobia in children frequently include tantrums, crying, "freezing," clinging to parents or other familiar people, and inhibiting interactions to the point of refusing to talk to others (mutism).

SYMPTOMS IN ADULTS. The symptoms of social phobia in adults include a range of physical signs of anxiety as well as attitudes and behaviors.

- blushing, sweating, nausea, diarrhea, dry mouth, tremors, and other physical indications of anxiety
- difficulties with self-assertion
- extreme sensitivity to criticism, rejection, or negative evaluations
- intense preoccupation with the reactions and responses of others
- heightened fears of being embarrassed or humiliated
- avoidance of the feared situation(s) and anticipatory anxiety

In adults, there is often a "vicious circle" quality to the symptoms, in that the anxiety and symptoms lead to actual or perceived poor performances, which in turn increase the anxiety and avoidance. A common example is performance anxiety related to musical instruments; the person who is afraid of having to play the piano in a recital, for example, may become so anxious that the muscles in the hands become tense, thus producing frequent mistakes in fingering and sound production during the recital performance.

Not all adults with social phobia appear shy or outwardly nervous to other people. Some adults are able to force themselves to attend social events, give public presentations, or interact with others by self-medicating with alcohol or limiting the time period of their interactions. These strategies, however, prevent the underlying fears and disabilities from being addressed.

Diagnosis

The **diagnosis** of social phobia is usually made on the basis of the patient's history and reported symptoms. The doctor may also decide to administer diagnostic questionnaires intended to rule out other phobias, other anxiety disorders, and major depression. In diagnosing a child, the doctor will usually ask the child's parents, teachers, or others who know the child well for their observations.

Children and adolescents

A doctor who is evaluating a child for social phobia must take into account that children do not have the freedom that adults usually have to avoid the situations that frighten them. As a result, they may not be able to explain why they are anxious. It is important to evaluate the child's capacity for social relationships with people that he or she knows; and to assess his or her interactions with peers for indications of social phobia, not only his or her behavior around adults.

A semi-structured interview that a doctor can use to assess social phobia in children is the Anxiety Disorders Interview Schedule for Children (ADIS-C). A newer clinician-administered test is the Liebowitz Social Anxiety Scale for Children and Adolescents (LSAS-CA). Self-report inventories for children include the Child Depression Inventory (CDI), and the Social Phobia and Anxiety Inventory for Children (SPAI-C). Parents can be asked to complete the Child Behavior Checklist (CBL), and teachers may be given the Teacher's Report Form (TRF).

Adults

Diagnostic instruments for assessing social phobia in adults are more problematic. Some general screeners that are used in primary care settings, such as the ***Structured Clinical Interview for DSM-IV*** Screen (SCID-Screen), do include questions related to social phobia but can take as long as 25 minutes to administer. Others, such as the Primary Care Evaluation of Mental Disorders, or Prime-MD, are not specific for social phobia. Instruments designed to measure social phobia by itself, such as the

Fear of Negative Evaluation Scale and the Social Avoidance and Distress Scale, are lengthy and generally more useful for monitoring the progress of therapy. Another clinician-administered interview for social phobia in adults, the Liebowitz Social Anxiety Scale (LSAS), was not in widespread use as of 2011.

Many physicians, however, have found that the addition of a few selected questions to a general screener for mental disorders is helpful in detecting social phobia. One study found that giving patients three specific statements with yes/no answers detected 89% of cases of social phobia:

- Being embarrassed or looking stupid are among my worst fears.
- Fear of embarrassment causes me to avoid doing things or speaking to people.
- I avoid activities in which I am the center of attention.

Treatment

Social phobia responds well to proper treatment; however, patients with social phobia have a distinctive set of barriers to treatment. Unlike persons with some other types of mental disorders, they are unlikely to deny that they have a problem. What researchers have found is that in comparison to persons suffering from other disorders, persons with social phobia are significantly more likely to say that financial problems, uncertainty over where to go for help, and fear of what others might think prevent them from seeking treatment. The researchers concluded that providing better information about community services as well as easing the psychological and financial burdens of patients with social phobia would significantly improve their chances of recovery. Left untreated, social phobia can become a chronic, disabling disorder that increases the patient's risk of suicide.

Medications

About 53% of patients diagnosed with social phobia are treated with medications. Drug treatment has proven beneficial to patients with this disorder; however, no one type of medication appears to be clearly superior to others. Selection of a medication depends on the subtype of the patient's social phobia; the presence of other mental disorders; and the patient's occupation and personal preferences.

Specific medications that are used to treat social phobia include:

- Benzodiazepine tranquilizers. These are often prescribed for patients who need immediate relief from anxiety. They have two major drawbacks, however; they are habit-forming, and they are unsuitable for patients with comorbid alcohol or substance abuse disorders. Benzodiazepines are, however, sometimes prescribed for patients who have a low risk for substance abuse and have not responded to other medications.
- Monoamine oxidase inhibitors (MAOIs). About two-thirds of patients with social phobia show significant improvement when treated with these drugs. MAOIs, however, have the disadvantage of requiring patients to stick to a low-tyramine diet that excludes many popular foods, and requiring them to avoid many over-the-counter cold and cough preparations.
- Selective serotonin reuptake inhibitors (SSRIs). About 50–75% of patients with social phobia benefit from treatment with SSRIs. The SSRIs appear to work best in patients with comorbid major depression or panic disorder. Sertraline (Zoloft) has been recommended for patients with generalized social phobia.
- Beta blockers. These medications, which include propranolol (Inderal), are given to patients with mild to moderate circumscribed performance anxiety to suppress the symptoms of panic. The patient takes the medication on an as-needed basis rather than a standing dosage, for instance, when facing a known trigger event (e.g., flying or speaking publicly). Beta-blockers do not appear to be helpful for patients with generalized social phobia.
- Botulism toxin. In conjunction with SSRIs, Botox is helpful for some patients to control sweating, a symptom of panic that may escalate the phobia.
- Alternative drugs. Anti-convulsant drugs such as gabapentin (Neurontin) and levetiracetam (Keppra) show promise as a treatment for social phobia.

Psychotherapy

The type of **psychotherapy** most commonly recommended for treatment of social phobia is **cognitive-behavioral therapy** (CBT). Mild to moderate cases of social phobia often show considerable improvement with CBT alone; patients with more severe social phobia benefit from a combination of CBT and an appropriate medication. Cognitive-behavioral treatment of adults diagnosed with social phobia usually combines exposure therapy with cognitive restructuring techniques. In exposure therapy, the patient is exposed to small "doses" of the feared situation that are gradually lengthened in time. The chief drawback to exposure therapy for social phobia is that some feared situations are easier to replicate for purposes of treatment than others. Patients who are afraid of public speaking or musical performance can practice performing in front of any group of people

QUESTIONS TO ASK YOUR DOCTOR

- What are the indications that I may have social phobia?
- What physical and psychiatric diagnostic tests do I need?
- What treatment options do you recommend for me?
- What kind of changes can I expect to see with the medications you have prescribed for me?
- What are the side effects associated with the medications you have prescribed for me?
- What tests or evaluation techniques will you perform to see if treatment has been beneficial for me?
- What actions or activities would you recommend for dealing with social phobia?
- What symptoms are important enough that I should seek immediate treatment?
- Can you recommend any support groups for me and my family?

that can be collected to help, but it is not so easy to arrange exposure sessions for a patient who is afraid of interactions with a specific teacher, employer, or supervisor. The other aspect of CBT that is used in treating social phobia in adults is cognitive restructuring. This approach challenges patients to reconsider and then replace the biased cognitions that have led them to overestimate the dangers in social situations and to underestimate his or her own resources for coping with them.

Several trial programs of CBT **group therapy** have been used with adolescents with social phobia. One pilot program situated the group meetings in the school rather than in a clinic, on the grounds that most of the fears of adolescents with social phobia revolve around school activities. Another CBT group for adolescents was conducted in a clinical setting. Both programs included **social skills training** alongside exposure therapy and cognitive restructuring, and both were reported to be moderately successful at one-year follow-up.

Other approaches

Other approaches that have been used to treat social phobia include **family therapy** and relaxation techniques.

Prognosis

The prognosis for recovery from social phobia is good, given early diagnosis and appropriate treatment. The prognosis for persons with untreated social phobia, however, is poor. In most cases, these individuals become long-term underachievers, at high risk for alcoholism, major depression, and suicide.

Prevention

Given that some of the factors implicated in social phobia are neurobiological or genetic, the best preventive strategy is early identification of children with behavioral inhibition and developing techniques for assisting their social development.

Resources

BOOKS

American Psychiatric Association. *Diagnostic and Statistical Manual of Mental Disorders.* 4th ed., text rev. Washington, DC: American Psychiatric Association, 2000.

Cooper, Rachel. *Classifying Madness: A Philosophical Examination of the Diagnostic and Statistical Manual of Mental Disorders.* New York: Springer, 2010.

Graham, George. *The Disordered Mind: An Introduction to Philosophy of Mind and Mental Illness.* New York: Routledge, 2010.

Heimberg, Richard G., et al., eds. *Social Phobia: Diagnosis, Assessment, and Treatment.* New York: Guilford Press, 2006.

Hofmann, Stefan. *Cognitive-Behavior Therapy of Social Phobia: Evidence-Based and Disorder-Specific Treatment Techniques.* Oxford: Routledge, 2007.

North, Carol, and Sean Yutzy. *Goodwin and Guze's Psychiatric Diagnosis.* New York: Oxford University Press, 2010.

Otto, Michal, and Stefan Hofmann, eds. *Avoiding Treatment Failures in the Anxiety Disorders (Series in Anxiety and Related Disorders).* New York: Springer, 2009.

Sadock, Benjamin J., and Virginia A. Sadock. *Kaplan & Sadock's Synopsis of Psychiatry.* 10th ed. New York: Lippincott, Williams and Wilkins, 2007.

Stravynski, Ariel. *Fearing Others: The Nature and Treatment of Social Phobia.* New York: Cambridge University Press, 2007.

PERIODICALS

Andersson, Gerhard, et al. "Internet-Based Self-Help with Therapist Feedback and in Vivo Group Exposure for Social Phobia: A Randomized Controlled Trial." *Journal of Consulting and Clinical Psychology* 74, no. 4 (2006): 677–86.

Black, Donald W. "Efficacy of Combined Pharmacotherapy and Psychotherapy versus Monotherapy in the Treatment of Anxiety Disorders." *CNS Spectrums* 11, no. 10 Suppl. 12 (2006): 29–33.

Smits, Jasper A., et al. "The Efficacy of Videotape Feedback for Enhancing the Effects of Exposure-Based Treatment for

Social Anxiety Disorder: A Controlled Investigation." *Behaviour Research and Therapy* 44, no. 12 (2006): 1773–85.

Voncken, Marisol J., et al. "Hiding Anxiety versus Acknowledgment of Anxiety in Social Interaction: Relationship with Social Anxiety." *Behaviour Research and Therapy* 44, no. 11 (2006): 1673–79.

ORGANIZATIONS

American Psychiatric Association, 1000 Wilson Blvd., Ste. 1825, Arlington, VA, 22209-3901, (703) 907-7300, apa@psych.org, http://www.psych.org.

American Psychological Association, 750 1st St. NE, Washington, DC, 20002-4242, (202) 336-5500, TDD/TTY: (202) 336-6123, (800) 374-2721, http://www.apa.org.

Anxiety Disorders Association of America, 8730 Georgia Ave., Silver Spring, MD, 20910, (240) 485-1001, Fax: (240) 485-1035, http://www.adaa.org.

Association for Behavioral and Cognitive Therapies, 305 7th Ave., 16th Fl., New York, NY, 10001, (212) 647-1890, Fax: (212) 647-1865, (866) 615-6464, http://www.abct.org.

Rebecca J. Frey, PhD
Laura Jean Cataldo, RN, EdD

Social skills training

Definition

Social skills training (SST) is a form of individual or **group therapy** used by teachers, therapists, and trainers to help those who need to learn to overcome inhibition or social ineffectiveness in their interactions with others. SST may use any of a number of techniques, including behavior rehearsal, cognitive rehearsal, and **assertiveness training**.

Purpose

Goals

One major goal of social skills training is to teach persons who may or may not have emotional problems about the verbal as well as nonverbal behaviors involved in social interactions. There are many people who have never been taught such interpersonal skills as making "small talk" in social settings, or the importance of good eye contact during a conversation. In addition, many people have not learned to "read" the many subtle cues contained in social interactions, such as how to tell when someone wants to change the topic of conversation or shift to another activity. Social skills training helps patients learn to interpret these and other social signals so they can determine how to act appropriately in the company of other people in a variety of different situations. SST proceeds on the assumption that when people improve their social skills or change selected behaviors, they will raise their self-esteem and increase the likelihood that others will respond favorably to them. Trainees learn to change their social behavior patterns by practicing selected behaviors in individual or group therapy sessions. Another goal of social skills training is to improve a patient's ability to function in everyday social situations. Social skills training can help patients to work on specific issues—for example, improving one's telephone manners—that interfere with their jobs or daily lives.

Treatment of specific disorders

A person who lacks certain social skills may have great difficulty building a network of supportive friends and acquaintances as he or she grows older, and may become socially isolated. Moreover, one of the consequences of loneliness is an increased risk of developing emotional problems or mental disorders. Social skills training has been shown to be effective in treating patients with a broad range of emotional problems and diagnoses. Some of the disorders treated by social skills trainers include **shyness**; **adjustment disorders**; marital and family conflicts, **anxiety disorders**, **attention deficit hyperactivity disorder**, **social phobia**, alcohol dependence; **depression**; **bipolar disorder**; **schizophrenia**; developmental disabilities; **avoidant personality disorder**; **paranoid personality disorder**; **obsessive-compulsive disorder**; and **schizotypal personality disorder**.

One specific example of the ways in which social skills training can be helpful is its application to alcohol dependence. In treating patients with alcohol dependence, a therapist who is using social skills training focuses on teaching the patients ways to avoid drinking when they go to parties where alcohol is served or when they find themselves in other situations in which others may pressure them to drink.

Another example is the application of social skills training to social phobia or shyness. People who suffer from social phobia or shyness are not ignorant of social cues, but they tend to avoid specific situations in which their limitations might cause them embarrassment. Social skills training can help these patients to improve their communication and social skills so that they will be able to mingle with others or go to job interviews with greater ease and self-confidence. Some studies indicate that the social skills training given to patients with shyness and social phobia can be applied to those with avoidant personality disorder, but more research is needed to differentiate among the particular types of social skills that benefit specific groups of patients, rather than treating social skills as a single entity. When trainers apply social skills training to the treatment of other **personality disorders**, they focus on the specific skills required to handle the issues that emerge with each disorder. For example, in the treatment of **obsessive-compulsive personality disorder** (OCD), social skills trainers focus on helping patients with OCD to deal with heavy responsibilities and **stress**.

People with disabilities in any age group can benefit from social skills training. Several studies demonstrate that children with developmental disabilities can acquire positive social skills with training. Extensive research on the effects of social skills training on children with attention deficit hyperactivity disorder shows that SST programs are effective in reducing these children's experiences of school failure or rejection as well as the aggressiveness and isolation that often develop in them because they have problems relating to others.

SST can be adapted to the treatment of depression with a focus on assertiveness training. Depressed patients often benefit from learning to set limits to others, to obtain satisfaction for their own needs, and to feel more self-confident in social interactions. Research suggests that patients who are depressed because they tend to withdraw from others can benefit from social skills training by learning to increase positive social interactions with others instead of pulling back.

There has been extensive research on the effective use of social skills training for the treatment of schizophrenia, in outpatient clinics as well as inpatient units. SST can be used to help patients with schizophrenia make better eye contact with other people, increase assertiveness, and improve their general conversational skills.

Social skills training with other therapies

Social skills training is often used in combination with other therapies in the treatment of mental disorders. For example, in the treatment of individuals with alcohol dependence, social skills training has been used together with cognitive restructuring and coping skills training. Social skills training has also been integrated with exposure therapy, cognitive restructuring, and medication in the treatment of social phobia. Social skills training has been used within **family therapy** itself in the treatment of marital and family conflicts. Moreover, SST works well together with medication for the treatment of depression. For the treatment of schizophrenia, social skills training has often been combined with pharmacotherapy, family therapy, and assertive **case management**.

Description

Techniques in social skills training

Therapists who use social skills training begin by breaking down complex social behaviors into smaller portions. Next, they arrange these smaller parts in order of difficulty, and gradually introduce them to the patients. For example, a therapist who is helping a patient learn to feel more comfortable at parties might make a list of specific behaviors that belong to the complex behavior called "acting appropriately at a party," such as introducing oneself to others; making conversation with several people at the party rather than just one other guest; keeping one's conversation pleasant and interesting; thanking the host or hostess before leaving; and so on. The patient would then work on one specific behavior at a time rather than trying to learn them all at once.

Such specific techniques as instruction, **modeling**, role-playing, shaping, feedback, and **reinforcement** of positive interactions may be used in SST. For example, instruction may be used to convey the differences among assertive, passive, and aggressive styles of communication. The technique of monitoring may be used to ask patients to increase their eye contact during a conversation. In role-playing exercises, group members have the opportunity to offer feedback to one another about their performances in simulated situations. For example, two members of the group may role-play a situation in which a customer is trying to return a defective purchase to a store. The others can then give feedback about the "customer's" assertiveness or the "clerk's" responses.

Content of social skills training

SST may be used to teach people specific sets of social competencies. A common focus of SST programs is communication skills. A program designed to improve people's skills in this area might include helping them with nonverbal and assertive communication and with making conversation. It might also include conversational skills that are needed in different specific situations; for example, job interviews, informal parties, and dating. The skills might be divided further into such subjects as beginning, holding, and ending conversations, or expressing feelings in appropriate ways.

Another common focus of SST programs involves improving a patient's ability to perceive and act on social cues. Many people have problems communicating with others because they fail to notice or do not understand other people's cues, whether verbal or nonverbal. For example, some children become unpopular with their peers because they force their way into small play groups, when a child who has learned to read social signals would know that the children in the small group do not want someone else to join them, at least not at that moment. Learning to understand another person's spoken or unspoken messages is as important as learning conversational skills. A social skills program may include skills related to the perceptual processing of the conversation of other individuals.

Scheduling

Social skills training may be given as an individual or as a group treatment once or twice a week, or more often depending upon the severity of a patient's disorder and the level of his or her social skills. Generally speaking, children appear to gain more from SST in a peer group setting than in individual therapy. Social skill training groups usually consist of approximately 10 patients, a therapist, and a cotherapist.

Cultural and gender issues

Social skills training programs may be modified somewhat to allow for cultural and gender differences. For example, eye contact is a frequently targeted behavior to be taught during social skills training. In some cultures, however, downcast eyes are a sign of respect rather than an indication of social anxiety or shyness. In addition, girls or women in some cultures may be considered immodest if they look at others, particularly adult males, too directly. These modifications can usually be made without changing the basic format of the SST program.

Generalization or transfer of skills

Current trends in social skills training are aimed at developing training programs that meet the demands of specific roles or situations. This need developed from studies that found that social skills acquired in one setting or situation are not easily generalized or transferred to another setting or situation. To assist patients in using their new skills in real-life situations, trainers use role-playing, teaching, modeling, and practice.

Precautions

Social skills training should rest on an objective assessment of the patient's actual problems in relating to other people.

It is important for therapists who are using SST to move slowly so that the patient is not overwhelmed by trying to change too many behaviors at one time. In addition, social skill trainers should be careful not to intensify the patient's feelings of social incompetence. This caution is particularly important in treating patients with social phobia, who are already worried about others' opinions of them.

One additional precaution is related to the transfer of social skills from the therapy setting to real-life situations. This transfer is called "generalization" or "maintenance." Generalization takes place more readily when the social skills training has a clear focus and the patient is highly motivated to reach a realistic goal. In addition, social skills trainers should be sure that the new skills being taught are suitable for the specific patients involved.

Preparation

Preparation for social skills training requires tact on the therapist's part, as patients with such disorders as

KEY TERMS

Antisocial—Behaving in ways that purposefully disregard the rights of others and break society's rules or laws.

Antisocial behavior—Behavior that differs significantly from the norms of society and is considered harmful to society.

Anxiety disorder—A group of conditions that cause people to feel extreme fear or worry that sometimes is accompanied by symptoms such as dizziness, chest pain, or difficulty sleeping or concentrating.

Attention deficit hyperactivity disorder (ADHD)—A condition that makes it hard for a person to pay attention, sit still, or think before acting.

Obsessive-compulsive disorder (OCD)—A condition that causes people to become trapped in a pattern of repeated, unwanted thoughts, called "obsessions," and a pattern of repetitive behaviors, called "compulsions."

Schizophrenia—A serious mental disorder that causes people to experience hallucinations, delusions, and other confusing thoughts and behaviors, which distort their view of reality.

Social phobia—An anxiety disorder characterized by a strong and persistent fear of social or performance situations in which the patient might feel embarrassment or humiliation.

social phobia or paranoid personality disorder may be discouraged or upset by being told that they need help with their social skills. One possible approach is through reading. The social skills therapist may recommend some self-help books on social skills in preparation for the treatment. Second, the therapist can ease the patient's self-consciousness or embarrassment by explaining that no one has perfect social skills. One additional consideration before starting treatment is the possibility of interference from medication side effects. The therapist will usually ask the patient for a list of all medications that he or she takes regularly.

One of the most critical tasks in preparation for social skills training is the selection of suitable target behaviors. It is often more helpful for the therapist to ask the patient to identify behaviors that he or she would like to change, rather than pointing to problem areas that the therapist has identified. The treatment should consider the patient's particular needs and interests. Whereas social skills training for some patients may include learning assertiveness on the job, training for others may include learning strategies for dating. Therapists can prepare patients for homework by explaining that the homework is the practice of new skills in other settings; and that it is as relevant as the therapy session itself.

Aftercare

Some studies strongly suggest the need for follow-up support after an initial course of social skills training. One study showed that follow-up support doubled the rate of employment for a group of patients with schizophrenia, compared to a group that had no follow–up.

Results

Outcome studies indicate that social skills training has moderate short-term effects but limited long-term effects. SST programs that include social perspective-taking may have greater long-term effects than traditional SST programs based on cognitive-behavioral models. In general, social skills training tends to generalize or transfer to similar contexts rather than to contexts that are not similar to the training. SST programs for patients with developmental disabilities should include programming for generalization so that the patients can transfer their newly acquired skills more effectively to real-life settings. One approach to improving generalization is to situate the training exercises within the patient's work, living, or social environment.

One of the benefits of social skills training programs is flexibility. The treatment can take place either as individual or group therapy, and new trainers can learn the techniques of SST fairly quickly. One additional advantage of SST is that it focuses on teaching skills that can be learned rather than emphasizing the internal or biological determinants of social adequacy. Future research should explore the integration of social skills training with the needs of families from different cultural backgrounds; the relationship between social skills training and different categories of mental disorders; the transfer of skills from therapeutic contexts to daily life; and improving patients' long-term gains from SST.

Resources

BOOKS

Center, Frostig. *The Six Success Factors for Children with Learning Disabilities: Ready-to-Use Activities to Help Kids with LD Succeed in School and in Life.* New York: Jossey-Bass, 2009.

Taffe, Richard. *Social Skills Training with Aggressive-Rejected Children.* Saarbrücken, Germany: Lambert Academic Publishing, 2010.

VandenBos, Gary R., ed. *APA Concise Dictionary of Psychology.* Washington D.C.: American Psychological Association, 2009.

White, Susan Williams, PhD. *Social Skills Training for Children with Asperger Syndrome and High-Functioning Autism.* New York: The Guilford Press, 2011.

PERIODICALS

Chronis, Andrea M., Heather A. Jones, and Veronica L. Raggi. "Evidence-Based Psychosocial Treatments for Children and Adolescents with Attention-Deficit/Hyperactivity Disorder." *Clinical Psychology Review* 26, no. 4 (June 2006): 486–502.

de Boo, Gerly M., and Pier J. M. Prins. "Social Incompetence in Children with ADHD: Possible Moderators and Mediators in Social-Skills Training." *Clinical Psychology Review* 27, no. 1 (January 2007): 78–97.

Fenstermacher, Kevin, Daniel Olympia, and Susan M. Sheridan. "Effectiveness of a Computer-Facilitated Interactive Social Skills Training Program for Boys with Attention Deficit Hyperactivity Disorder." *School Psychology Quarterly* 21, no. 2 (Summer 2006): 197–224.

Gresham, Frank M., Mai Bao Van, and Clayton R. Cook. "Social Skills Training for Teaching Replacement Behaviors: Remediating Acquisition Deficits in At-Risk Students." *Behavioral Disorders* 31, no. 4 (August 2006): 363–77.

Konstantareas, M. Mary. "Social Skills Training in High Functioning Autism and Asperger's Disorder." *Hellenic Journal of Psychology* 3, no. 1 (April 2006) 39–56.

Kopelowicz, Alex, Robert Paul Liberman, and Roberto Zarate. "Recent Advances in Social Skills Training for Schizophrenia." *Schizophrenia Bulletin* 32, Supplement 1, (October 2006): S12–23.

Pfammatter, Mario; Junghan, Ulrich Martin, and Hans Dieter Brenner. "Efficacy of Psychological Therapy in

Schizophrenia: Conclusions From Meta-Analyses." *Schizophrenia Bulletin* 32, Supplement 1, (October 2006): S64–80.

Sim, Leslie, et al. "Effectiveness of a Social Skills Training Program with School Age Children: Transition to the Clinical Setting." *Journal of Child and Family Studies* 15, no. 4 (August 2006): 409–18.

ORGANIZATIONS

American Psychiatric Association, 1000 Wilson Blvd., Ste. 1825, Arlington, VA, 22209-3901, (703) 907-7300, apa@psych.org, http://www.psych.org.

American Psychological Association, 750 1st St. NE, Washington, DC, 20002-4242, (202) 336-5500; TDD/TTY: (202) 336-6123, (800) 374-2721, http://www.apa.org.

Judy Koenigsberg, Ph.D.
Ruth A. Wienclaw, Ph.D.
Laura Jean Cataldo, RN, Ed.D.

Social workers

Definition

A social worker is a helping professional who is distinguished from other human service professionals by a focus on both the individual and his or her environment. Generally, social workers have at least a bachelor's degree from an accredited education program and in most states they must be licensed, certified, or registered. A Master's in Social Work is required for those who provide **psychotherapy** or work in specific settings such as hospitals or nursing homes.

Description

Social workers comprise a profession that had its beginnings in 1889 when Jane Addams founded Hull House and the American settlement house movement in Chicago's West Side. The ethics and values that informed her work became the basis for the social work profession. They include respect for the dignity of human beings, especially those who are vulnerable, an understanding that people are influenced by their environment, and a desire to work for social change that rectifies gross or unjust differences.

The social work profession is broader than most disciplines with regard to the range and types of problems addressed, the settings in which the work takes place, the levels of practice, interventions used, and populations served. It has been observed that social work is defined in its own place in the larger social environment, continuously evolving to respond to and address a changing world. Although several definitions of social work have been provided throughout its history, common to all definitions is the focus on both the individual and the environment, distinguishing it from other helping professions.

Social workers may be engaged in a variety of occupations ranging from hospitals, schools, clinics, police departments, public agencies, court systems to private practices or businesses. They provide the majority of mental health care to persons of all ages in this country, and in rural areas they are often the sole providers of services. In general, they assist people to obtain tangible services; help communities or groups provide or improve social and health services; provide counseling and psychotherapy with individuals, families, and groups; and participate in policy change through legislative processes. The practice of social work requires knowledge of human development and behavior; of social, economic and cultural institutions; and of the interaction of all these factors.

Resources

PERIODICALS

Gibelman, Margaret. "The Search for Identity: Defining Social Work—Past, Present, Future." *Social Work* 44, no. 4 (July 1999).

WEBSITES

National Association of Social Workers. "Choices: Careers in Social Work" (2011). http://www.naswdc.org/pubs/choices/choices.htm (accessed October 27, 2011).

ORGANIZATIONS

National Association of Social Workers, 750 First St. NE, Ste. 700, Washington, DC, 20002-4241, (202) 408-8600, http://www.naswdc.org.

Judy Leaver, M.A.

Sodium amobarbital *see* **Barbiturates**

Sodium pentobarbital *see* **Barbiturates**

Somatization disorder

Definition

Somatization disorder is a psychiatric condition marked by multiple medically unexplained physical, or somatic, symptoms. In order to qualify for the **diagnosis** of somatization disorder, somatic complaints must be serious enough to interfere significantly with a person's ability to perform important activities, such as work, school, or family and social responsibilities, or lead the person experiencing the symptoms to seek medical treatment.

Somatization disorder has long been recognized by psychiatrists and psychologists and was originally called Briquet's syndrome in honor of Paul Briquet, a French physician who first described the disorder in the nineteenth century. It is included in the category of somatic symptom disorders in the ***Diagnostic and Statistical Manual of Mental Disorders***, the professional handbook that aids clinicians in diagnosing mental disorders. Somatic symptom disorders are characterized as disorders with psychological origins that manifest in physical symptoms.

Demographics

According to the *DSM-IV-TR* (fourth edition, text revised), somatization disorder is rare in males in the United States, although higher rates are seen among males from some cultural and ethnic groups. The *DSM-IV-TR* estimates that between 0.2% and 2% of women and less than 0.2% of men suffer from somatization disorder in the United States. Sex ratios may arise from different rates of seeking treatment. However, studies of unexplained somatic symptoms in the general population find less striking differences in rates between men and women. Specific symptoms may vary across cultures. For example, the *DSM-IV-TR* notes that the sensation of worms in the head or ants crawling under the skin are sometimes reported in African and South Asian countries, but rarely seen in North American patients.

Description

Individuals with somatization disorder suffer from a number of vague physical symptoms, involving at least four different physical functions or parts of the body. The physical symptoms that characterize somatization disorder cannot be attributed to medical conditions or to the use of drugs, and individuals with somatization disorder often undergo numerous medical tests (with negative results) before the psychological cause of their distress is identified. Symptoms are often described as burning sensations, pains that move from place to place, strange tastes on the tongue, tingling, or tremors. While many symptoms resemble those associated with genuine diseases, some of the symptoms reported by people with somatization disorder are not. The individual usually visits many different physicians in hopes of finding a treatment but may be met with several different results or diagnoses. This can be dangerous if the patient ends up taking several different medications, which risks harmful drug interactions.

While the physical symptoms of somatization disorder frequently lack medical explanations, they are not fabricated by the patient. A person with somatization disorder has suffered from physical pain, discomfort, and dysfunction for an extended period of time and wishes to identify the cause of their illness and find relief.

Causes and symptoms

Causes

DEFENSE AGAINST PSYCHOLOGICAL DISTRESS. One of the oldest theories about the cause of somatization disorder suggests that it is a way of avoiding psychological distress. Rather than experiencing **depression** or anxiety, some individuals will develop physical symptoms. According to this model, somatization disorder is a defense against psychological pain that allows some people to avoid the **stigma** of a psychiatric diagnosis. While getting the care and nurturing they need from doctors and others who are responsive to their apparent medical illnesses, many patients are encouraged to continue their manipulative behavior.

Many patients described by Sigmund Freud would be diagnosed today with somatization disorder. His patients were usually young women who complained of numerous physical symptoms. In the process of speaking with Freud, they would often recall a number of distressing memories; discussing these memories frequently led to the relief of physical symptoms. These cases formed the foundation of Freud's psychoanalytic treatment. Although this theory offers a plausible explanation for somatization disorder, research indicates that people with multiple physical symptoms are actually more likely to report psychiatric symptoms than those with few physical problems. These findings appear to support a connection between psychological and physical distress, but are inconsistent with the idea that physical symptoms offer a defense against overt psychiatric symptoms.

HEIGHTENED SENSITIVITY. An alternative theory suggests that somatization disorder arises from a heightened sensitivity to internal sensations. People with somatization disorder may be keenly aware of the minor pains and discomforts that most people simply ignore. A similar theory has been offered to account for **panic disorder**. Studies have shown that people with panic disorder are particularly sensitive to internal sensations like breathing rate and heartbeats, which may lead them to react with intense fear to minor internal changes. The physiological or psychological origins of this hypersensitivity to internal sensations and their relevance to somatization disorder are still not well understood.

CATASTROPHIC THINKING. According to this theory, somatization disorder results from negative beliefs and exaggerated fears about the significance of physical sensations. Individuals with somatization disorder are more likely to believe that vague physical symptoms are indicators of serious disease and to seek treatment for them. For instance, someone with somatization disorder may fear that a headache signals a **brain** tumor, or that shortness of breath indicates the onset of asthma. When their doctors can find no medical explanation for the symptoms, the patients may fear that they have a rare disease; they frantically look for specialists who can provide a diagnosis. Anxiety causes them to focus even more intensely on their symptoms, which in turn become more salient and disabling. Many people with somatization disorder reduce or eliminate many activities out of fear that exertion will worsen their symptoms. With fewer activities to distract them from their symptoms, they spend more time worrying about physical problems, resulting in greater distress and disability.

Symptoms

Gastrointestinal (GI) complaints, such as nausea, bloating, diarrhea, and sensitivities to certain foods are common, and at least two different GI symptoms are required for the diagnosis. Sexual or reproductive symptoms, including pain during intercourse, menstrual problems, and **erectile dysfunction** are also necessary features for a diagnosis of somatization disorder. Other frequent symptoms are headaches, pain in the back or joints, difficulty swallowing or speaking, and urinary retention. To qualify for the diagnosis, at least one symptom must resemble a neurological disorder, such as **seizures**, problems with coordination or balance, or paralysis.

Diagnosis

To meet the *DSM-IV-TR* diagnostic criteria for somatization disorder, the patient must have a history of multiple physical complaints that began before age 30 and continued for several years. These symptoms must cause significant impairment to social, occupational, or other areas of functioning or lead the patient to seek medical treatment.

The *DSM-IV-TR* also specifies the following:

- The individual must report a history of pain affecting at least four different parts or functions of the body. Examples include headaches, back, joint, chest or abdominal pain, or pain during menstruation or sexual intercourse.
- A history of at least two gastrointestinal symptoms, such as nausea, bloating, vomiting, diarrhea, or food intolerance must be reported.
- There must be a history of at least one sexual or reproductive symptom, such as lack of interest in sex, problems achieving erection or ejaculation, irregular menstrual periods, excessive menstrual bleeding, or vomiting throughout pregnancy.
- One symptom must mimic a neurological condition. Examples include weakness; paralysis; problems with balance or coordination; seizures; hallucinations; loss of sensations such as touch, seeing, hearing, tasting, or smelling; difficulty swallowing or speaking; or amnesia and loss of consciousness. Pseudo-neurologic symptoms like these are the primary characteristics of another somatoform disorder known as conversion disorder.

If a thorough medical evaluation reveals no evidence of an underlying medical or drug- or medication-induced condition, the diagnosis of somatization disorder is likely. People with genuine medical conditions can qualify for the diagnosis if the level of functional impairment reported is more than would be expected based on medical findings. The symptoms must not be intentionally produced. If the patient is feigning symptoms, a diagnosis of **factitious disorder** or **malingering** would most likely be considered.

DSM-5

Revisions for the fifth edition of the *DSM* (*DSM-5*, 2013) propose subsuming the symptoms of somatization disorder into the diagnosis of complex somatic symptom disorder, which will also include the diagnoses of **hypochondriasis** and **pain disorder**. Proposed criteria include experiencing at least one somatic symptom that significantly interferes with the patient's daily life; excessive occupation with the symptom(s), such as obsessive anxiety or worry over the cause; and occurrence of the symptom(s) for at least six months.

Treatment

Cognitive behavior therapy

Cognitive-behavioral therapy (CBT) for somatization disorder focuses on changing negative patterns of thoughts, feelings, or behaviors that contribute to somatic symptoms. The cognitive component of the treatment focuses on helping patients identify dysfunctional thinking about physical sensations. With practice, patients learn to recognize catastrophic thinking and develop more rational explanations for their feelings. The behavioral component aims to increase activity. Patients with somatization

KEY TERMS

Factitious disorder—A feigned disorder in which the physical or psychological symptoms are controlled or produced by the patient.

Malingering—Pretending to be sick in order to be relieved of an unwanted duty or obtain some other obvious benefit.

disorder have usually reduced their activity levels as a result of discomfort or out of fear that activity will worsen symptoms. CBT patients are instructed to increase activity gradually while avoiding overexertion that could reinforce fears. Other important types of treatment include relaxation training, sleep hygiene, and communication skills training. Preliminary findings suggest that CBT may help reduce distress and discomfort associated with somatic symptoms; however, it has not yet been systematically compared with other forms of therapy.

Medications

Antidepressant medications may help to alleviate symptoms of somatization disorder. According to one study, patients with somatization disorder who took the antidepressant **nefazodone** (Serzone) showed reductions in physical symptoms, increased activity levels, and lower levels of anxiety and depression at the end of treatment.

Prognosis

Untreated somatization disorder is usually a chronic condition, though specific symptoms can come and go and severity may fluctuate over time. Somatization disorder poses a serious problem for society, since many who suffer from it become functionally disabled and unable to work. In addition, patients with unexplained physical symptoms strain already overburdened health-care resources. Unexplained physical symptoms are extremely common among patients visiting general practitioners, with some estimates suggesting that more than two-thirds of general medical patients have symptoms that cannot be explained by medical tests. Fortunately, there is preliminary evidence that **psychotherapy** and medication can effectively reduce symptoms and disability.

Prevention

Greater awareness of somatization disorder, particularly among physicians, can help identify individuals with somatization disorder and deliver appropriate psychological or psychiatric treatments.

Resources

BOOKS

American Psychiatric Association. *Diagnostic and Statistical Manual of Mental Disorders*. 4th ed., text rev. Washington, DC: American Psychiatric Publishing, 2000.

Breuer, Josef, and Sigmund Freud. *Studies on Hysteria*. New York: Basic Books, 2000.

Butcher, James N., and Carolyn L. Williams. *Essentials of MMPI2 and MMPIA Interpretation*. 2nd ed. Minneapolis: University of Minnesota Press, 2000.

PERIODICALS

Allen, Lesley A., et al. "Cognitive Behavior Therapy for Somatization Disorder: A Preliminary Investigation." *Journal of Behaviour Therapy and Experimental Psychiatry* 32, no. 2 (June 2001): 53–62.

Cameron, Oliver G. "Interoception: The Inside Story—A Model for Psychosomatic Process." *Psychosomatic Medicine* 63 (2001): 697–710.

Hotopf, Matthew, Michael Wadsworth, and Simon Wessely. "Is 'Somatisation' a Defense Against the Acknowledgement of Psychiatric Disorder?" *Journal of Psychosomatic Research* 50 (2001): 119–124.

Menza, Matthew, et al. "Treatment of Somatization Disorder with Nefazodone: A Prospective, Open-label Study." *Annals of Clinical Psychiatry* 13, no. 3 (September 2001): 153–158.

Nimnuan, Chaichana, Matthew Hotopf, and Simon Wessely. "Medically Unexplained Symptoms: An Epidemiological Study in Seven Specialties." *Journal of Psychosomatic Research* 51 (2001): 361–367.

Rief, Winifred, Aike Hessel, and Elmar Braehler. "Somatization Symptoms and Hypochondriacal Features in the General Population." *Psychosomatic Medicine* 63 (2001): 595–602.

Danielle Barry, M.S.

Somatoform disorders

Definition

Somatoform disorders are a group of disorders characterized by the occurrence of somatization, a term that describes the expression of psychological or mental difficulties through physical symptoms. Somatization takes a number of forms, ranging from preoccupation with potential or genuine but mild physical problems to the development of actual physical pain, discomfort, or dysfunction. Somatization appears to be fairly common, but a somatoform disorder **diagnosis** is not warranted unless symptoms cause significant distress or disability.

Description

Somatization disorder is characterized by a history of multiple unexplained medical problems or physical complaints beginning prior to age 30. In the nineteenth and early twentieth centuries, somatization disorder was known as Briquet's syndrome or hysteria—a more generic term for such a condition. People with somatization disorder report symptoms affecting multiple organ systems or physical functions, including pain, gastrointestinal distress, sexual problems, and symptoms that mimic neurological disorders. Although medical explanations for their symptoms cannot be identified, individuals with somatization disorder experience genuine physical discomfort and distress. Review of their medical histories will usually reveal visits to a number of medical specialists, and many patients take numerous medications prescribed by different doctors, running the risk of dangerous drug interactions.

DSM-IV-TR

The revised fourth edition of the ***Diagnostic and Statistical Manual of Mental Disorders*** (*DSM-IV-TR*), the professional handbook clinicians use to diagnose mental disorders, describes seven disorders under the category of somatoform disorders. These disorders are somatization disorder, **undifferentiated somatoform disorder**, **conversion disorder**, **pain disorder**, **hypochondriasis**, **body dysmorphic disorder**, and somatoform disorder not otherwise specified.

- Undifferentiated somatoform disorder is similar to somatization disorder but may involve fewer symptoms, have a shorter duration, or begin after the age of 30. Common symptoms include chronic fatigue, loss of appetite, gastrointestinal distress, or problems involving the genitals or urinary tract. This diagnosis is appropriate for patients with symptoms of somatization disorder who do not meet all diagnostic criteria.
- Conversion disorder is marked by unexplained sensory or motor symptoms that resemble those of a neurological or medical illness or injury. Common symptoms include paralysis, loss of sensation, double vision, seizures, inability to speak or swallow, and problems with coordination and balance. Symptoms often reflect a naive understanding of the nervous system, and physicians often detect conversion disorder when symptoms do not make sense anatomically. For instance, a patient may report loss of both touch and pain sensation on one side of the body, when a genuine lesion would result in loss of touch and pain sense on opposite sides of the body. The name conversion disorder reflects a theoretical understanding of the disorder as a symbolic conversion of a psychological conflict into a concrete physical representation. Patients with conversion disorder may not express the level of distress one would expect from someone with a disabling neurological condition. This phenomenon is traditionally called *la belle indifference*.
- The primary feature of pain disorder is physical pain that causes significant distress or disability or leads an individual to seek medical attention. Pain may be medically unexplained, or it may be associated with an identifiable medical condition but manifest more severely than the condition would warrant. Common symptoms include headache, backache, and generalized pain in muscles and joints. Pain disorder can be severely disabling, causing immobility that prevents patients from working, fulfilling family responsibilities, or engaging in social activities. Like patients with somatization disorder, people with pain disorder often have a history of consultations with numerous physicians.
- Hypochondriasis is diagnosed when a person is excessively concerned by fears of having a physical disease or injury. Individuals with hypochondriasis usually do not complain of disabling or painful symptoms. Instead, they tend to overreact to minor physical symptoms or sensations, like rapid heartbeat, sweating, small sores or fatigue. Many people with hypochondriasis develop fears in response to the illness or death of a friend or family member, or after reading about a condition or seeing a feature on television. Hypochondriacal fears can be confined to a single disease or involve a number of different physical concerns. Individuals with hypochondriasis seek frequent reassurance by consulting with physicians or talking about their fears, yet these efforts provide only temporary relief from their fears. Although hypochondriasis is usually not as disabling as somatoform disorders involving the development of actual physical symptoms, it can put stress on relationships or reduce work productivity through time lost to frequent medical appointments and tests.
- Body dysmorphic disorder is characterized by preoccupation with a defect in physical appearance. Often the defect of concern is not apparent to other observers, or if there is a genuine defect, it is far less disfiguring than the patient imagines. Common preoccupations include concerns about the size or shape of the nose, skin blemishes, body or facial hair, hair loss, or "ugly" hands or feet. Individuals with body dysmorphic disorder may be extremely self-conscious, avoiding social situations because they fear

others will notice their physical defects or even make fun of them. They may spend hours examining the imagined defect or avoid mirrors altogether. Time-consuming efforts to hide the defect, such as application of cosmetics or adjustments of clothing or hair, are common. Many people with body dysmorphic disorder undergo procedures like plastic surgery or cosmetic dentistry, but are seldom satisfied with the results.

- Somatoform disorder not otherwise specified is diagnosed when somatoform symptoms are present but criteria for another somatoform disorder are not met. *DSM-IV-TR* includes several examples of symptoms that could merit this diagnosis, including false pregnancy and hypochondriacal fears or unexplained physical symptoms of recent onset or short duration.

DSM-5

There is some disagreement among researchers about the *DSM-IV-TR* somatoform disorders category. Some have argued that hypochondriasis and body dysmorphic disorder are more similar to obsessive compulsive disorder than to other somatoform disorders, while others think hypochondriasis may be more appropriately classified with the **anxiety disorders**. Proposed changes for the fifth edition of the *DSM* (*DSM-5*, 2013) have addressed some of these concerns by reorganizing the category of somatoform disorders under the new name of somatic symptom disorders. If approved, the new category will include seven disorders, with body dysmorphic disorder moved to the category of obsessive-compulsive and related disorders:

- complex somatic symptom disorder (subsumes diagnoses of pain disorder, somatization disorder, undifferentiated somatoform disorder, and some aspects of hypochondriasis)
- simple somatic symptom disorder (includes previous diagnosis of somatoform disorder not otherwise specified)
- illness anxiety disorder (hypochondriasis)
- functional neurological disorder (conversion disorder)
- psychological factors affecting medical condition
- other specified somatic symptom disorder
- unspecified somatic symptom disorder

Resources

BOOKS

American Psychiatric Association. *Diagnostic and Statistical Manual of Mental Disorders*. 4th ed., text rev. Washington, DC: American Psychiatric Publishing, 2000.

Phillips, Katherine A. *The Broken Mirror: Understanding and Treating Body Dysmorphic Disorder*. New York: Oxford University Press, 2005.

Pilowsky, Issy. *Abnormal Illness Behaviour*. Chichester, UK: John Wiley and Sons, 1997.

PERIODICALS

Neziroglu, Fugen, Dean McKay, and Jose A. Yaryura-Tobias. "Overlapping and Distinctive Features of Hypochondriasis and Obsessive-Compulsive Disorder." *Journal of Anxiety Disorders* 14, no. 6 (November–December 2000): 603–614.

Danielle Barry, M.S.

Somnambulism *see* **Sleepwalking disorder**

Somnote *see* **Chloral hydrate**

Sonata *see* **Zaleplon**

Specific phobias

Definition

Specific phobia is a disorder in which the affected individual displays a marked and enduring fear of specific situations or objects. The *Diagnostic and Statistical Manual of Mental Disorders, Fourth Edition Text Revision* (*DSM IV TR*), used by mental health professionals to diagnose mental disorders, classifies specific phobia as a type of anxiety disorder. Formerly, specific phobia was known as simple phobia.

Demographics

Specific phobias are common. The prevalence rates of specific phobia in community samples range from 4–8%. Over the course of a lifetime, the prevalence estimates in community samples range from 7.2–11.3%. Individuals whose family members have specific phobia are at a higher risk for developing this disorder.

There are approximately twice as many women with specific phobia as there are men with this disorder. The specific gender ratio variable varies depending upon the type of specific phobia. Approximately 75–90% of people with the animal, situational, and natural environment triggers are female. Approximately 55–70% of people with the blood-injection-injury subtype are female. For height phobias, there is a reduced ration of women to men, although the phobias are still more common in women. Illness phobias are more common in men.

Description

Specific phobia has a unique position among the **anxiety disorders** in that individuals with this disorder do not experience pervasive anxiety, nor do they seek treatment as readily as individuals with other anxiety disorders. Unlike individuals with other anxiety disorders, individuals with specific phobias experience extreme fear as soon as they encounter a defined situation or object, a phobic stimulus. For example, an individual with a specific phobia of dogs will become extremely anxious when confronting a dog. Individuals with specific phobias experience impairment or a significant amount of anguish. They may lead restricted lifestyles depending upon the phobia trigger. Adults and adolescents with specific phobias recognize that their fear is unreasonable. Children, by contrast, may not recognize that their fear of the phobic stimulus is unreasonable or extreme.

Types of specific phobias include situational, object, and other. Situational specific phobia is diagnosed if an individual's fear is triggered by a defined situation, such as flying, enclosed places, tunnels, driving, bridges, elevators, or using public transportation. Object specific phobias include animal, natural environment, and blood-injection-injury type triggers. Animal type is diagnosed if an individual's fear is triggered by animals or insects. Natural environment type is diagnosed if an individual's fear is cued by storms, water, or heights. Blood-injection-injury type is diagnosed if an individual's fear is cued by seeing an injury or blood or by an injection or other invasive medical treatment. Other type specific phobia is diagnosed if an individual's fear is triggered by other stimuli such as fear of vomiting, choking, becoming ill, falling down if far from a means of physical support, and a child's fears of loud noises or characters in costume.

Researchers have found that the frequency of type for adults in clinical settings, from least to most frequent, is: animal, blood-injection-injury, natural environment, and situational. The most common phobias for community samples, however, are phobias of heights, mice, spiders, and insects.

Causes and symptoms

There are numerous causes for specific phobias, and the symptoms are also numerous.

Causes

The development of a specific phobia may be determined by a variety of factors. Behavioral, cognitive, and social theories of learning and conditioning, psychodynamic models such as the psychoanalytic theory of Freud, physiological studies of the **brain**, family background, and genetic predisposition, variations in sociocultural themes, and **trauma** can influence the development of specific phobia disorder. In some cases, a specific traumatic event triggers the development of a specific phobia; however, in most cases no single underlying cause can be pinpointed.

LEARNING AND CONDITIONING CAUSES. As of 2011, research on phobias focused primarily on information processing, learning, and conditioning themes. Learning to experience fear is the core of a conditioning perspective. Informational and instructional factors can result in the formation of fears. For example, an individual who frequently hears of plane crashes in the news may develop a specific phobia of flying. Research shows that individuals with specific phobias pay more attention to information about danger than do individuals who do not have specific phobias. Vicarious acquisition occurs when an individual witnesses a traumatic event or sees another individual behave with fear when confronting a phobic stimulus. Direct conditioning occurs when an individual is frightened by a phobic stimulus.

A major determinant of specific phobias is conditioning. Association and avoidance are types of conditioning. In association conditioning, a stimulus that was initially neutral begins to trigger an anxiety response. For example, if an individual is driving one day and experiences a strong anxiety response, an association may form between driving and anxiety. Individuals do not become phobic until they begin to avoid. In avoidance conditioning, individuals learn to avoid a stimulus that triggers anxiety. Every time individuals avoid the phobic stimulus, driving, for example, they are rewarded by the relief from anxiety.

TRAUMATIC CAUSES. Another determinant of specific phobias is trauma. For example, individuals who have been attacked by a dog may develop a specific phobia disorder and become conditioned to fear dogs. Individuals who observe others experiencing a trauma also may be more likely to develop specific phobia disorder. For example, individuals who witness people falling from a building may develop a specific phobia disorder of falling from heights. Phobias with a traumatic origin may have a sudden onset and develop rapidly.

PHYSIOLOGICAL CAUSES. Some research has suggested that the high activation of brain pathways that correspond to the cognitive and emotional constituents of anxiety biologically predispose individuals to specific phobias.

GENETIC AND FAMILY CAUSES. Although specific phobia is frequently attributed to environmental causes such as **modeling**, learning by association, and negative **reinforcement**, genetic predisposition can influence this disorder. An individual who has a family member with a specific phobia is at an increased risk for developing this disorder. Some research indicates that the pattern of types is similar within families. For example, a first-degree

KEY TERMS

Agoraphobia—Abnormal anxiety regarding public places or situations from which the individual may feel compelled to flee or in which he or she would be helpless in the event of a panic attack.

Beta blocker—An anti-hypertensive (blood pressure-lowering) drug that limits the activity of epinephrine, a hormone that increases blood pressure.

Cognitive-behavioral therapy—A type of psychotherapy in which people learn to recognize and change negative and self-defeating patterns of thinking and behavior.

Hypochondriasis—An anxiety disorder in which the individual believes real or imagined symptoms are indicative of a serious or life-threatening illness or condition.

Schizophrenia—A severe mental disorder in which a person loses touch with reality and may have illogical thoughts, delusions, hallucinations, behavioral problems and other disturbances.

biological relative of individuals with a situational type phobia is more likely to have a situational phobia. Studies indicate that the blood and injury phobias have strong familial patterns.

SOCIOCULTURAL CAUSES. There is not much information about cultural differences in specific phobias. Phobia content may vary by culture. Fear of a phobic stimulus such as magic or spirits, present in several cultures, is diagnosed as a specific phobia only if the fear is excessive for a particular culture and if the fear triggers major distress or interferes with functioning. Some research indicates that African Americans are more likely than whites to report specific phobias. Some studies show that specific phobias are less common among whites born in the United States and immigrant Mexican Americans than among Mexican Americans born in the United States. Research suggests mixed data with regard to the role of socioeconomic status, with some data associating specific phobia disorder with a lower socioeconomic level.

PERSONAL VARIABLES. Studies suggest a relationship between age and specific phobia. Research indicates some connections between the age of individuals with specific phobias and insight into the extreme quality of their fears. Insight increases with age. Children, unlike adults and adolescents, often do not report feelings of distress about having phobias. Insight into the unreasonable nature of the fear is not required for a **diagnosis** of specific phobia in children. The animal and natural environment types of specific phobia are common and generally transitory in children. Some studies indicate a connection between gender and specific phobia. Research shows that specific phobias from the animal type are more common among women. Some studies suggest, however, that women are more likely to report specific phobias and to seek treatment than men.

Symptoms

DSM-IV-TR delineates seven diagnostic criteria for specific phobia:

- Significant and enduring fear of phobic stimulus: Patients with specific phobia display marked and enduring fear when they encounter a defined situation or object, the phobic stimulus.
- Anxiety response to phobic stimulus: Patients with specific phobia display anxiety as soon as they confront the phobic stimulus. When they confront the phobic stimulus, a defined situation or object, patients with specific phobia may experience a panic attack related to the specific situation. Children may cry, cling, freeze, or have tantrums when they express their anxiety in the face of the phobic stimulus.
- Recognition: Although adolescents and adults realize that their fear is unreasonable and disproportionate to the situation, children may not recognize that their fear is excessive.
- Avoidance: Individuals with specific phobia avoid the phobic stimulus or endure it with deep distress and anxiety.
- Impairment and distress: Individuals with specific phobia display avoidance, distress, and anxious anticipation when they encounter the phobic stimulus. Their avoidance reactions interfere with their daily functioning, or they express significant distress about having a phobia.
- Duration: To diagnose specific phobia in a patient who is under 18 years of age, the duration of the disorder needs to be at least six months.
- Not accounted for by another disorder: A diagnosis of specific phobia is assigned if the phobic avoidance, panic attacks, or anxiety related to the defined situation or object are not better accounted for by other disorders.

Diagnosis

The diagnosis of specific phobia is complicated by factors such as degree of impairment and differential diagnosis, that is, fear caused by another mental disorder.

Although fears of specified situations or objects are common, a diagnosis of specific phobia relies on the degree of impairment.

With regard to differentiating specific phobia types, factors such as the focus of fear and the predictability and timing of the reaction to the phobic stimulus across the specific phobia types can assist clinicians to differentiate. With regard to differentiating specific phobia from other disorders, there are several disorders with similar symptoms. They include **panic disorder** with **agoraphobia**, **social phobia**, **post-traumatic stress disorder**, **obsessive-compulsive disorder**, **hypochondriasis**, **schizophrenia**, and delusional and other psychotic disorders.

Generally, a diagnosis of specific phobia rather than panic disorder is made when there are no spontaneous panic attacks and no fear of panic attacks. It is often difficult to differentiate specific phobia, situational type, from panic disorder with agoraphobia. Specific phobia, situational type, is commonly diagnosed when an individual displays situational avoidance without unexpected and recurrent panic attacks. By contrast, panic disorder with agoraphobia is diagnosed if an individual experiences an initial onset of panic attacks that are not anticipated and subsequently experiences avoidance of several situations considered triggers of panic attacks. Although individuals with specific phobia, unlike individuals with panic disorder with agoraphobia, do not display enduring anxiety, anxious anticipation may occur when confrontation with a phobic stimulus is likely to occur. The *DSM-IV-TR* outlines differentiating factors as to the type and number of panic attacks, the number of avoided contexts, and the focus of the fear. At times, both diagnoses, specific phobia and panic disorder with agoraphobia, need to be assigned.

Psychological measures

Measures used to diagnose specific phobia include behavioral observation, clinical interviews, physiological evaluation, and self-report measures. The behavioral avoidance task (BAT) is a common behavioral observation method used to assess specific phobia. Often the diagnosis of specific phobia is made on the basis of an individual's responses to semistructured interviews, such as the Anxiety Disorders Interview Schedule for *DSM-IV* (ADIS-IV) and the **Structured Clinical Interview for *DSM-IV*** Axis I disorders (SCID-IV). To assist in differential diagnosis between specific phobias and other disorders with similar characteristics, clinicians use the anxiety disorders interview schedule for *DSM-IV* (ADIS-IV). Physiological evaluations usually include heart-rate monitors. Self-report questionnaires include measures such as the subjective units of discomfort/distress scale (SUDS), the most frequently used self-report measure, the fear survey schedule (FSS-III), and the mutilation questionnaire, specifically for measuring fear of the blood type of specific phobia.

Time of onset and symptom duration

Generally, the initial symptoms of specific phobia occur when an individual is a child or a young adolescent. The type of phobia determines the typical age of onset. The blood, animal, and natural environment types typically begin when an individual is a child; however, many new cases of the natural environment type occur when an individual is a young adult. The onset for the height type usually begins in adolescence. The onset age for the situational type often occurs in childhood and peaks in the mid-twenties. There is no specific onset age for phobias with a traumatic origin.

Individual variations in specific phobia

Classification systems distinguish between individuals with different types of specific phobias. The types of specific phobia, situation, object, and other, relate to particular features such as the age, gender, and culture of an individual. Some researchers propose that to distinguish individual differences in treatment planning, it is more helpful to simply name the specific phobia rather than to use the type classification system.

Dual diagnoses

Specific phobia often occurs with other disorders of mood and anxiety and with substance-related disorders. When specific phobias occur with other disorders in clinical contexts, the primary diagnosis is associated with greater distress. The blood-injury-injection type of specific phobia may occur with physical symptoms such as vasovagal fainting, which is characterized by a short heart rate acceleration and blood pressure elevation. Then the heart rate decelerates and the blood pressure drops. Research shows that individuals who have one specific phobia type are more likely to have other phobias of the same type.

Treatment

Specific phobias are highly treatable. They are most effectively treated by psychological rather than pharmaceutical treatments. The primary goal of most treatments of specific phobias is to reduce fear, phobic avoidance, impairment, and distress.

Cognitive-behavioral therapy

Cognitive-behavioral therapy has been effective in treating specific phobias. There has not been much research on the effects of cognitive therapy alone on specific phobias. Cognitive therapists challenge fearful thoughts and replace them with more positive thoughts. Although some studies show that cognitive therapy may assist patients in decreasing anxiety related to their exposure exercises, research indicates that cognitive therapy alone is probably not an effective treatment for specific phobia. Researchers suggest adding panic management strategies, such as cognitive restructuring, to assist with behavioral treatments.

Several studies indicate that real-life desensitization or exposure is the most effective and long-lasting treatment for a broad range of specific phobias. Desensitization includes a process by which individuals unlearn the association between the phobic stimulus and anxiety. Incremental exposure involves the patient's gradual facing of the phobic stimulus through a series of graded steps. Wolpe's imagery desensitization is suggested so that patients with specific phobias can face the fear in imagery before attempting real-life exposure. Unlike many of the other treatments, the treatment gains of real-life exposure are maintained upon follow-up. Some desensitization treatments employ flooding as a useful strategy. When flooding is used, patients maintain a high anxiety level without retreating. Similar to desensitization, flooding can be used both in imagination and in real life encounters. Flooding may not be appropriate for many individuals because it can trigger a higher level of sensitization and fear reinforcement. For real-life exposure, a patient needs to be highly motivated because the treatment may lead to temporary discomfort. Primary reasons for poor **compliance** with cognitive-behavioral treatment include lack of time, anxiety, and low motivation.

Psychodynamic therapy

Psychodynamic therapy, or insight-oriented therapy, assists patients in becoming aware of the symbolic nature of their anxiety and in exploring traumatic past events. Insight-oriented therapy aims to expose and reduce patients' unconscious conflicts, increase patients' understanding of their underlying thoughts, and assist patients in gaining conscious control over their psychological conflicts. In psychodynamic therapy, for example, patients may discover that their anxiety may be connected to aggressive or sexual feelings and thoughts.

Group therapy

There is little research on **group therapy** for specific phobia disorder. Some studies suggest that group treatment has been effective for dental and spider phobias.

Drugs

Little research has been devoted to the relationship between medication and specific phobia. Generally, pharmacotherapy has not been considered a treatment of choice for individuals with specific phobias. **Benzodiazepines** (sedative drugs that slow the central nervous system to ease nervousness and tension) may decrease anxiety the occurs before an individual enters a phobic situation. A low dose of a benzodiazepine, such as **clonazepam** (Klonopin) or **alprazolam** (Xanax), may be indicated to decrease some fear arousal before real-life exposure to a phobic trigger. The reduction of symptoms, however, may interfere with the treatment. Before beginning real-life exposure, an antidepressant, such as **sertraline** (Zoloft) or **paroxetine** (Paxil), may be suggested to increase motivation for undertaking an uncomfortable treatment. **Beta blockers** also can assist individuals to confront the specific phobia.

Alternative therapies

Research shows some benefits for specific phobias with applied relaxation. Relaxation training includes abdominal breathing and muscle relaxation on a regular basis. Studies have indicated that applied muscle tension helps individuals with blood type phobias to avoid fainting. When patients tense their muscles several times they temporarily increase their blood pressure and keep from fainting when they see blood. Similar to real-life exposure, the gains from applied tension are maintained upon follow-up. Other alternative therapies include immersive virtual reality, **hypnotherapy**, eye-movement desensitization and reprocessing (EMDR), and energy balance approaches such as massage and **acupuncture**.

Prognosis

If specific phobias exist in adolescence, they have a greater chance of persisting in early adulthood. Specific phobias that continue into adulthood generally become chronic if they are not treated. Furthermore, there is a greater chance for an individual diagnosed with specific phobia to develop new phobias as a young adult. Phobias contracted during childhood or adolescence that continue into young adulthood remit approximately 20% of the time. Individuals with specific phobias often fail to seek treatment. For those who seek treatment, research suggests that compared to individuals with specific phobias whose fear diminishes slowly during exposure, individuals with specific phobias whose fear diminishes more rapidly have a better prognosis for recovery.

One factor in prognosis is the distinction between fear onset and phobia onset. Individuals with specific phobias of animal, blood, heights, and driving have a fear

QUESTIONS TO ASK YOUR DOCTOR

- Can you recommend a psychotherapist or other mental health professional for me?
- Is there a mental health professional in your practice with experience in treating phobias?
- Are there any support groups for my phobia in this area?
- How can I tell if my phobia is severe enough to require treatment?
- Will my insurance cover treatment for my phobia?

onset nine years earlier than their phobia onset. Some studies have shown that generalized anxiety level, severity of symptoms, and prior experience with the phobic stimulus are factors that have been associated with treatment outcome.

Although most mental health professionals consider specific phobia that begins in childhood to be a benign disorder, it can last for years if left untreated. Some studies indicate, however, that specific phobia does not become worse and usually diminishes as an individual ages. Without treatment, the prognosis is poor for an individual who has multiple phobias.

Prevention

Early detection is a key to assisting individuals with mild cases of specific phobia to seek treatment to prevent the development of full-blown cases of the disorder. Individuals who are at risk for developing specific phobia as well as individuals who already have been diagnosed with specific phobia need to avoid caffeine because caffeine can increase arousal, causing increased anxiety. Further research is needed to discover variables that predict the reason that only certain individuals will develop specific phobias after conditioning or acquiring information that leads to fear.

Resources

BOOKS

Daitch, Carolyn. *Anxiety Disorders: The Go-To Guide for Clients and Therapists.* New York: Norton, 2011.

Doctor, Ronald M., Ada P. Kahn, and Christine Adamec. *The Encyclopedia of Phobias, Fears, and Anxieties,* 3rd ed. New York: Facts on File, 2008.

Korgeski, Gregory P. *The Compete Idiot's Guide to Phobias.* New York: Alpha, 2009.

PERIODICALS

Baker, Aaron, et al. "Does Habituation Matter? Emotional Processing Theory and Exposure Therapy for Acrophobia." *Behaviour Research and Therapy,* 48, no. 11 (November 2010): 1139–43.

Coelho, Carlos M., and Guy Wallis. "Deconstructing Acrophobia: Physiological and Psychological Precursors to Developing a Fear of Heights." *Depression and Anxiety* 27, no. 9 (September 2010): 864–70.

Trumpf, Julia, et al. "Specific Phobia Predicts Psychopathology in Young Women." *Social Psychiatry and Psychiatric Epidemiology,* 45, no. 12 (December 2010): 1161–66.

ORGANIZATIONS

American Psychiatric Association, 1000 Wilson Blvd., Ste. 1825, Arlington, VA, 22209-3901, (703)907-7300, (888) 357-7924, apa@psych.org, http://www.psych.org.

American Psychological Association, 750 1st St. NE, Washington, DC, 20002-4242, (202) 336-5500, (800) 374-2721, apa@psych.org, http://www.apa.org.

Anxiety Disorders Association of America, 8730 Georgia Ave., Ste. 600, Silver Spring, MD, 20910, (240) 485-1001, Fax: (240) 485-1035, information@adaa.org, http://www.adaa.org.

Judy Koenigsberg, PhD
Tish Davidson, AM

SPECT *see* **Single photon emission computed tomography**

Speech-language pathology

Definition

Treatment for the improvement or cure of communication disorders, including speech, language, and swallowing disorders. The term used to describe professionals in this discipline is speech and language pathologist (SLP).

Description

The discipline of speech-language pathology includes professionals that are trained in the techniques, strategies, and interventions designed to improve or correct communication disorders. Communication disorders include disorders of speech, language, and swallowing.

In 2012, there were more than 126,000 speech-language pathologists in the United States certified by the American Speech-Language-Hearing Association (ASHA), and nearly 20,000 audiologists, who often work with speech pathologists to diagnose disorders. Speech disorders

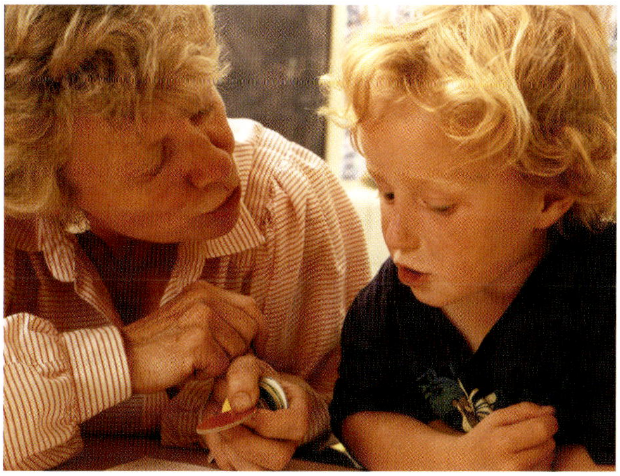

A speech therapist works with a young boy. *(© Hattie Young/ Photo Researchers, Inc.)*

treated by speech-language pathologists include voice disorders (abnormalities in pitch, volume, vocal quality, or resonance or duration of sounds), articulation disorders (problems producing speech sounds), and fluency disorders (impairment in speech fluency, such as **stuttering**). Language disorders include developmental or acquired conditions that lead to difficulties in understanding or producing language. Speech-language pathologists participate in the screening, assessment, and treatment of patients who experience one or a combination of these disorders.

Persons with isolated speech sound disorders are often helped by articulation therapy, in which they practice repeating specific sounds, words, phrases, and sentences. For individuals experiencing voice disorders, a combination of medical and behavioral treatments are often helpful. For stuttering and other fluency disorders, treatment approaches usually help individuals develop techniques to both reduce the severity of stuttering and allow the individual to produce more fluent speech. For all of these therapies, individuals are taught to cope more effectively with their speech in progressively difficult situations, starting with speaking alone to the pathologist and ending with speaking to a group of people. In treating children with developmental language disorders, treatment often focusses on **modeling** and stimulation of correct productions of language. This type of approach may also be useful for adults with language disorders, secondary to a **stroke** or degenerative neurological disorder. For people with severe communication disorders, those due to either a speech or language problem, speech pathologists can assist with alternate means of communication, such as manual signing and computer-synthesized speech. Finally, speech-language pathologists have become increasingly involved with the assessment and treatment of individuals with swallowing disorders, or dysphagia.

The majority of speech-language pathologists work in public schools. They are also found at both residential health care facilities and outpatient clinics that specialize in communication disorders. Finally, speech-language pathologists are often employed at hospitals and universities. Professional training programs in speech-language pathology are offered at both the undergraduate and graduate levels. Undergraduate training may include classes in biology, anatomy, psychology, linguistics, education, and special education. Graduate training, at both the masters and doctoral level, provides much deeper opportunities to study communication disorders and their treatment. To receive the Certificate of Clinical Competence(CCC) in speech-language pathology individuals must hold a master's degree in communications sciences and disorders from a program accredited by the ASHA and complete their Clinical Fellowship Year (CFY).

Resources

ORGANIZATIONS

American Academy of Private Practice in Speech-Language Pathology and Audiology, 7349 Topanga Canyon Blvd., Canoga Park, CA, 91303,

American Speech-Language-Hearing Association, 2200 Research Blvd., Rockville, MD, 20785, (301) 296-5700, http://www.asha.org.

National Black Association for Speech-Language and Hearing, 700 McKnight Park Dr., Ste. 708, Pittsburgh, PA, 15237, (412) 366-1177, Fax: (412) 366-8804, NBASLH@nbaslh.org, http://www.nbaslh.org.

Rodney Gabel, Ph.D.

Speech sound disorder *see* **Phonological disorder**

Speech therapy *see* **Speech-language pathology**

Split personality disorder *see* **Dissociative identity disorder**

Stanford-Binet intelligence scales

Definition

The Stanford-Binet Intelligence Scales is a widely used intelligence test. It is a comprehensive, norm-referenced individually administered examination.

Purpose

The purpose of the Stanford-Binet Intelligence Scales, sometimes also called the Stanford-Binet test or simply the "Stanford-Binet,"is to assess general intelligence and cognitive abilities in children and adults from the ages of 2 to over 85. Specifically, it tests intelligence in four areas: abstract and visual reasoning, quantitative reasoning, short-term memory skills, and verbal reasoning.

Description

Origins

Considered the oldest and most influential intelligence test, the Stanford-Binet Intelligence Scales was devised in 1916 by Stanford University **psychologist** Lewis Terman (1877–1956), using the Binet-Simon model. French psychologist Alfred Binet (1857–1911) created what is considered the first usable intelligence test. Dr. Binet was given this task by the French government for the purpose of developing a method to assess and identify intellectually deficient children so they could be eventually placed in special needs classes.

Later, in 1908 and 1911, Binet and French psychologist Theodore Simon (1872–1961) revised what is today called the Binet-Simon Scale. The test consisted of various activities (such as touching one's ear and drawing objects or figures from memory) that were commonly performed by children at various ages. Binet and Simon selected these activities based on numerous years of observing children as they played and lived their lives. The two psychologists used 50 children—10 children in five age groupings who were considered of average intelligence by their teachers—to validate 30 activities of increasing difficulties.

Although many psychologists and other professionals question some of the test's concepts, such as mental age and intelligence quotient (IQ), the test is still widely used to assess cognitive development, and often to determine placement in special education classes. The Stanford-Binet Intelligence Scales is considered to have introduced the modern era of intelligence testing (or IQ testing) that continues now into the twenty-first century. The scoring of this test is based on the performance of age-related tasks. For example, a five-year-old child, who successfully completed all of the assigned tasks that a normal five-year-old could pass, would be scored as having a mental age that was equivalent to his/her chronological age.

Specifics

Most recently revised in 2003, the Stanford-Binet Intelligence Scales, Revision Five (Stanford-Binet 5, or SB5), can be used with children, from ages two years and older, and adults. Consisting of questions and short tasks arranged from easy to difficult, the Stanford-Binet measures a wide variety of verbal and nonverbal skills. Its structure is divided into four areas (1) hybrid structure, (2) verbal routing test, (3) nonverbal routing test, and (4) verbal and nonverbal age scales.

The abilities measured by the Stanford-Binet 5 include scales involving (1) Full Scale IQ (a comprehensive measure of cognitive ability, is based on the taking of the subtests), (2) two domain scores (nonverbal IQ and verbal IQ), and (3) five factor indexes (both nonverbal and verbal). The five factor indexes include:

- nonverbal fluid reasoning
- verbal fluid reasoning
- nonverbal knowledge
- verbal knowledge
- nonverbal quantitative reasoning
- verbal quantitative reasoning
- nonverbal visual-spatial processing
- verbal visual-spatial processing
- nonverbal working memory
- verbal working memory

Besides the five factor indexes, two special routing subtests—Nonverbal-Fluid Reasoning: Object Series/Matrices; and Verbal-Knowledge: Vocabulary—are also provided—together called the Abbreviated Battery. These two subtests are taken before the Stanford-Binet 5 test. Depending on the scores of these two routing subtests, the administrator may begin the SB5 test at Level 1, 2, 3, 4, or 5.

The SB5 Nonverbal subtests, which require minimal receptive language skills and fine-motor coordination, include:

- Nonverbal Knowledge (Picture Absurdities [Levels 4–6] and Procedural Knowledge [Levels 2–3])
- Nonverbal Quantitative Reasoning [Levels 2–6]
- Nonverbal Visual-Spatial Processing (Form Board [Levels 1–2] and Form Patterns [Levels 3–6])
- Nonverbal Working Memory (Block Span [Levels 2–6] and Delayed Response [Level 1])

The Verbal subtests, which require the reading, speaking and comprehending of age-appropriate English, include:

- Verbal Fluid Reasoning (Early Reasoning [Levels 2–3], Verbal Absurdities [Level 4], and Verbal Analogies [Levels 5–6])
- Verbal Quantitative Reasoning [Levels 2–6]
- Verbal Visual-Spatial Processing (Position and Direction [Levels 2–6])

KEY TERMS

Abstract reasoning—The ability to analyze information and to solve problems.

IQ—The acronym for intelligence quotient.

Quantitative reasoning—The ability to complete mathematical problems and to apply mathematics on a practical level.

Verbal reasoning—The ability to understand and reason using concepts involving words (within a particular language).

- Verbal Working Memory (Memory for Sentences [Levels 2–3] and Last Word [Levels 4–6])

Total testing time of the SB5 is 45 to 75 minutes for the Full Scale IQ Battery, with the time variance depending on the test taker's age and the number of subtests given. About 30 minutes is required to administer the Verbal and Nonverbal IQ scales. The Abbreviated Battery test takes from 15 to 20 minutes to complete.

While the test taker's attitude and behavior during the test are noted, they are not used to determine the result, which is arrived at by converting a single raw score for the entire test to a figure indicating "mental age" (the average age of a child achieving that score). A formula is then used to arrive at the intelligence quotient, or IQ. An IQ of 100 means that the child's chronological and mental ages match. Traditionally, IQ scores of from 90 to 109 are considered average, scores below 70 indicate mental disability, and scores of 140 or above place a child into the "gifted" category.

The Stanford-Binet 5 was standardized using a sample of 4,800 individuals (selected at random from all part of the country) from the U.S. Census taken in 2000. A Stanford-Binet Intelligence Scales for Early Childhood is also available for children two years to seven years, three months. In its fifth edition, the test is also called the Early SBS. Both the Stanford-Net 5 and the Early SBS are published by Riverside Publishing, which is headquartered in Rolling Meadows, Illinois.

Preparation

Preparation for the test is neither needed nor recommended.

Results

The SB5 requires that all administrators be skilled at administering the test. Such skill comes from administering a sufficient number of practice tests to establish a reliable knowledge of the testing procedure. Workshops are often used for the training of personnel used to administer the SB5, as are graduate-level testing courses.

The technical manual provided with the SB5 provides sufficient evidence that the scoring process is reliable. The review of the SB5 by the Mental Measurements Yearbook (MMY), Buros Institute, stated that internal consistency reliability coefficients for the IQ scores were from 0.95 to 0.98, while the coefficients for the five Factor Index scores ranged from 0.90 to 0.92. The MMY review added, ". . . all reliability coefficients were quite high and appropriate for an instrument of this magnitude."

The MMY review concluded with the following summary: "The publication of the newest revision of this well-established test of intelligence continues an almost 100-year-old tradition of evolution and refinement. Despite some technical and statistical limitations (e.g., lower stability for young children and individuals with low cognitive abilities, problematically high correlations with achievement, uncertain factor structure) the SB5 offers important improvements over the previous version of the scale and remains one of the premier instruments for the assessment of cognitive abilities of children, adolescents, and adults."

Resources

BOOKS

Becker, K.A. *History of the Stanford-Binet intelligence scales: Content and psychometrics.* Itasca, IL: Riverside Publishing, 2003.

Binet, Alfred, and Théodore Simon (translated by Elizabeth S. Kite). *The Development of Intelligence in Children (the Binet-Simon Scale).* Baltimore: Williams and Wilkins, 1916.

Drummond, Robert J. *Assessment Procedures for Counselors and Helping Professionals.* Boston: Pearson, 2010.

Green, Susan K., and Robert L. Johnson. *Assessment is Essential.* Boston: McGraw-Hill Higher Education, 2010.

Hart, Diane. *Authentic Assessment: A Handbook for Educators.* Menlo Park, CA: Addison-Wesley, 1994.

McAfee, Oralie, and Deborah J. Leong. *Assessing and Guiding Young Children's Development and Learning.* Upper Saddle River, NJ: Pearson, 2011.

McCullough, Virginia E. *Testing and Your Child: What You Should Know about 150 of the Most Common Medical, Educational, and Psychological Tests.* New York: Plume, 1992.

Mindes, Gayle. *Assessing Young Children.* Boston: Pearson, 2011.

Santrock, John W. *Concept of Intelligence.* New York: McGraw-Hill, 2008.

OTHER

"Stanford-Binet Intelligence Scales, Fifth Edition Assessment Service Bulletin Number 1." Nelson Education, http://www.assess.nelson.com/pdf/sb5-asb1.pdf (accessed October 19, 2010).

WEBSITES

"Alfred Binet." Indiana University. (July 25, 2007), http://www.indiana.edu/~intell/binet.shtml (accessed October 19, 2010).

"Mental Measurements Yearbook, Buros Center for Testing." Buros Institute for Mental Measurements, http://www.unl.edu/buros (accessed October 5, 2010).

"Stanford-Binet Intelligence Scales, Fifth Edition (SB5)." Nelson Education, http://www.assess.nelson.com/test-ind/stan-b5.html (accessed October 19, 2010).

"Stanford-Binet Intelligence Scales for Early Childhood (Early SB5)." Nelson Education, http://www.riversidepublishing.com/products/earlySB5/index.html (accessed October 19, 2010).

William Arthur Atkins

STAR*D study

Definition

The Sequenced Treatment Alternatives to Relieve **Depression** (STAR*D) Study was the largest and longest national trial ever designed to determine which treatments work best in people with **major depressive disorder** (MDD) who have not responded to an antidepressant. MDD is characterized by feelings of persistent sadness, worthlessness, guilt, and lack of interest in daily activities severe enough to interfere with such daily activities.

Purpose

The goal of the study was to help doctors better understand how to treat depression. Previously, the medical literature had provided doctors with little guidance on which treatments to use on their patients who do not respond to initial treatments. The STAR*D study was designed to help doctors learn which treatment plans (including medication dose and duration) are most effective for improving symptoms in patients with chronic depression and have the fewest side effects. The study also may enable doctors to determine how long they should attempt one therapy before moving on to another type of treatment. In addition, STAR*D provided information about the risk of **relapse**, which is defined as the return of depressive symptoms.

Description

The STAR*D study was a seven-year, $35 million-effort funded by the **National Institute of Mental Health** (NIMH) that began in 1999. It involved more than 4,000 participants, ages 18 to 75, with chronic or recurrent major depression. The patients were being or were about to be treated for depressive symptoms at primary care or psychiatric facilities. Major depression is of significant concern to doctors, because it can lead to significant functional impairment and mortality.

To reflect real-life treatment situations, STAR*D was conducted at private practices and public clinics, rather than in universities or other research facilities. In addition, participants were able to choose their own range of treatments. Researchers selected drugs that were the safest, easiest to take, and most commonly used, so the results could immediately be applied to clinical practice.

Researchers

The study was led by Dr. John Rush of the University of Texas Southwestern Medical Center. The following 13 other research centers also participated in the trial:

- Clinical Research Institute—Kansas
- Laureate Psychiatric Hospital & Clinic (Oklahoma)
- Massachusetts General Hospital
- New York State Psychiatric Institute
- Northwestern University (Illinois)
- Oklahoma Tuscaloosa VA Medical Center
- University of California at Los Angeles
- University of California at San Diego
- University of Michigan
- University of North Carolina at Chapel Hill
- University of Pittsburgh
- Vanderbilt University (Tennessee)
- Virginia Commonwealth University

Participants

More than 4,000 participants were initially involved in the study. The average age was 41 years. About 64% of participants were female and 36% were male. About 76% were Caucasian, 18% were African American, 13% were Hispanic, and 6% were of other races.

Participants were either being treated for depression or were entering into treatment at 41 primary care and psychiatric clinics throughout the United States. All of those involved in the study had moderate to severe depression. Seventy-five percent had had two or more depressive episodes in their lifetime. The other 25% were

Treatment choices throughout STAR*D

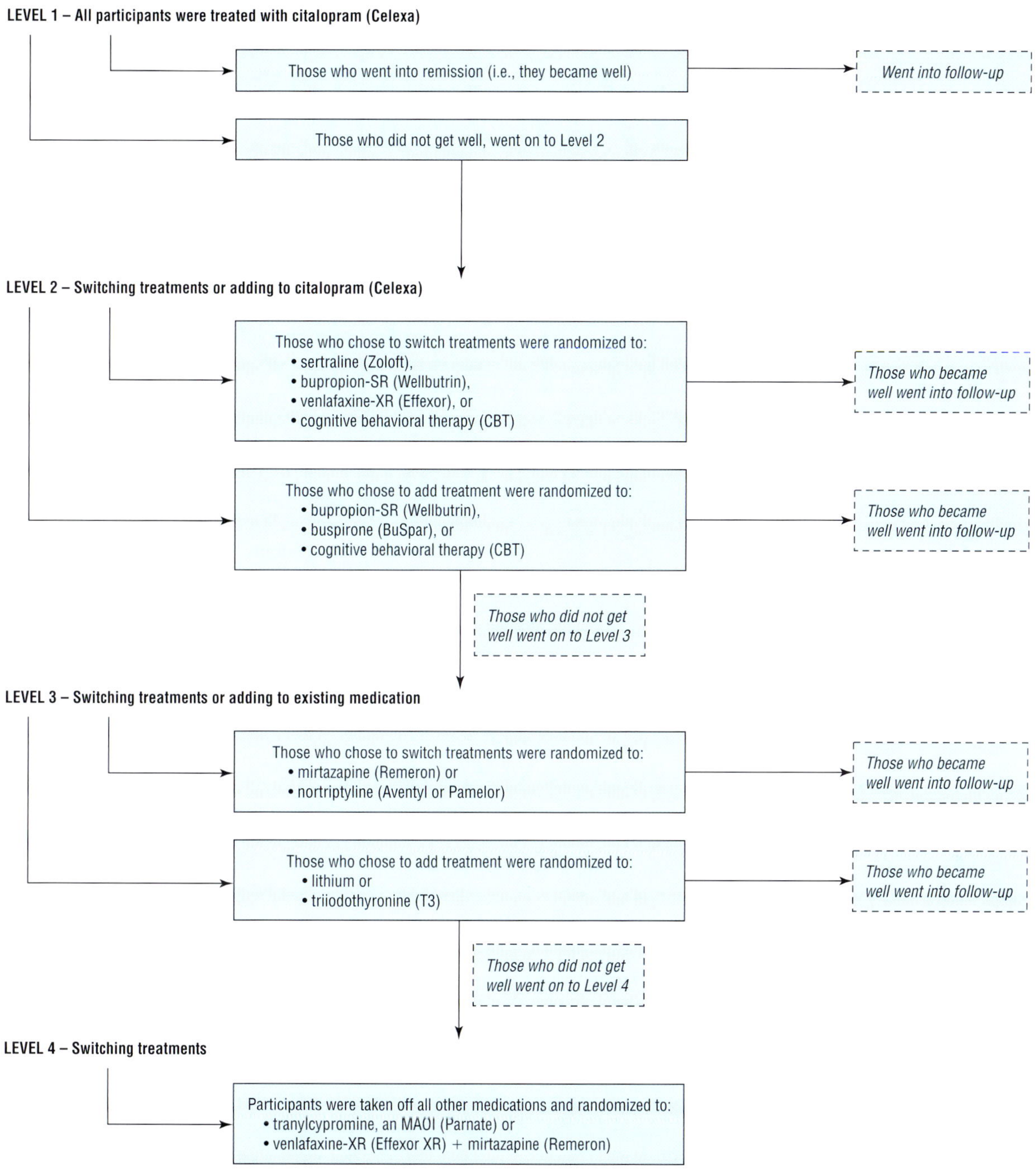

SOURCE: National Institute of Mental Health.

Additional information on the STAR*D study available from the National Institute of Mental Health at http://www.nimh.nih.gov/trials/practical/stard/allmedicationlevels.shtml. *(Diagram by PreMediaGlobal. © 2012 Cengage Learning.)*

currently experiencing an episode of depression that had lasted for at least two years.

The STAR*D study had broader participation than most studies of its kind. However, people with **schizophrenia**, **schizoaffective disorder**, **bipolar disorder**, an eating disorder, **obsessive-compulsive disorder**, or a **substance abuse** problem were not eligible for the study. Also, those who were already participating in **cognitive-behavioral therapy** or who were taking psychotropic medications could not participate.

Out of the 4,041 initial participants who entered Level 1 of STAR∗D, 1,438 progressed to Level 2, 376 entered Level 3, and 108 moved on to Level 4 (see level descriptions below). Participants left the program because they entered remission, or they desired to leave the program because of side effects, or they opted to leave for personal reasons.

Preparation

Participants prepared for the study by first meeting with a trained professional who assessed their condition and, later, with a medical doctor.

Examination: Assessments

At the first visit, participants met with a trained clinical research coordinator (CRC), who did not have knowledge of the treatment they were about to receive or were already receiving. The CRC asked the participants about the following:

- history of depression symptoms
- family history of MDD, bipolar disorder, or alcohol and substance abuse
- duration of current depressive episode
- treatment history for the current depressive episode
- past and current substance abuse
- history of suicide attempts
- current mental illnesses.

The CRC also rated the participants' symptom severity using established psychological scales. Patients completed self-questionnaires to determine their psychiatric disorders and depression score. Participants were later given phone interviews by a computer-based voice response system to ascertain their functioning and quality of life.

At doctor visits, the participants were evaluated for medication effectiveness and side effects. The STAR∗D researchers also evaluated the patients to determine whether a change in dosage was necessary.

Medications

The following medications were used in the STAR*D study:

- bupropion SR (Wellbutrin SR)
- buspirone (BuSpar;)
- citalopram (Celexa)
- lithium (Eskalith, Lithobid)
- mirtazapine (Remeron)
- nortriptyline (Pamelor, Aventyl)
- sertraline (Zoloft)
- tranylcypromine (Parnate)
- triiodothyronine (T3, Cytomel)
- venlafaxine XR (Effexor XR).

Treatments

The treatments used in STAR∗D were the same as those typically used by doctors to treat clinical depression. Participants received only active medications; therefore, placebos were not used.

The study included four treatment levels, each of which could continue for up to 14 weeks. Participants progressed to the next level when their symptoms did not respond to the their current treatment.

The four levels were as follows:

- Level 1: All participants received the antidepressant citalopram (brand name, Celexa). Citalopram is a selective serotonin reuptake inhibitor (SSRI). It works by interfering with the ability of nerve cells in the brain to take up the neurotransmitter, serotonin. This neurotransmitter has been associated with symptoms of depression.
- Level 2: Participants who did not become symptom-free, or who experienced side effects on citalopram, had a choice of seven different treatment options. Four options involved taking either a new medication or engaging in cognitive-behavioral therapy. The other three options added a new medication or cognitive-behavioral therapy to the citalopram participants were already taking. All treatments were randomly chosen from those that the participant had deemed acceptable.
- Level 3: Participants who did not become symptom-free at the previous level were allowed to try one of four other treatment options. They could switch to therapy with either nortriptyline or mirtazapine, or continue taking their current antidepressant along with either lithium or triiodothyronine.
- Level 4: Participants who did not become symptom-free at the previous level were randomly assigned to take either tranylcypromine or a combination of venlafaxine and mirtazapine.

Once participants went into full remission, in which they no longer experienced symptoms of depression, they began a 12-month follow-up process.

Results

The results of the STAR∗D study were published in medical and scientific journals in 2006, including the

KEY TERMS

Bipolar disorder—A mood disorder characterized by abnormally high energy levels and moodiness, usually without depression.

Cognitive-behavioral therapy—A type of therapy used to solve problems concerning dysfunctional behaviors (responses), emotions (feelings) and cognitions (abilities to gather knowledge) through a proven systematic set of procedures.

Cognitive therapy—A type of psychiatric treatment involving the treatment of anxiety and/or depression, which encourages patients to confront their problems in order to improve their behavior.

Depression—A psychiatric disorder involving feelings of hopelessness and symptoms of fatigue, sleeplessness, suicidal tendencies, and poor concentration.

Eating disorders—A number of medical conditions characterized by abnormal eating habits that can involve either the lack, or the excessive intake, of food, which results in physical and/or emotional stress. Two types of eating disorders include anorexia nervosa and bulimia nervosa.

Psychotropic medication—A drug that is used to treat mental disorders.

Schizophrenia—A mental disorder involving degraded thinking and emotions.

Substance abuse—Overuse of a drug or alcohol, which leads to addiction.

American Journal of Psychiatry on November 1, 2006. Outcomes included measures of depressive symptoms, social function, and patient satisfaction.

Researchers found that remission rates were about 37% for participants in Level 1, 31% in Level 2, and 13% in Levels 3 and 4. However, some patients dropped out of the study early.

Overall, the findings suggested that more than half of patients who stayed in treatment for one or two steps will achieve remission. But those patients who do not respond after two different treatment courses have a much lower chance of remission, and a higher risk of relapse.

The results of STAR*D emphasized the need for improved and individualized treatment plans when treating major depression. Research topics prompted by the STAR*D results include learning to predict how patients will respond to treatments and treatment sequences, so as to treat them more effectively, and assessing the use of combination medication therapies earlier in treatment. In 2007, a study based on STAR*D discovered that a slight gene variation predisposed patients to respond to **citalopram**. Using the genetic material of patients who had participated in STAR*D, researchers found that those with the variation (in genes *GRIK4* or *HTR2A*) were 23% more likely to be treated successfully with citalopram.

Resources

BOOKS

Appleton, William S. *The New Antidepressants and Antianxieties.* New York: Plume, 2004.

Beers, Mark H. *The Merck Manual of Medical Information,* 2nd Home Ed. New York: Pocket, 2004.

McCullough, James P. Jr. *Treating Chronic Depression with Disciplined Personal Involvement: Cognitive Behavioral Analysis System of Psychotherapy (CBASP),* first ed. New York: Springer, 2006.

Pettit, Jeremy W., and Thomas E. Joiner.*Chronic Depression: Interpersonal Sources, Therapeutic Solutions.* Washington, DC: American Psychological Association, 2005.

PERIODICALS

Asparouhov, Tihomir, et al. "Growth Modeling with Nonignorable Dropout: Alternative Analyses of the STAR*D Antidepressant Trial." *Psychological Methods* 16, no. 1 (2011): 17.

Fava, Maurizio, et al. "The Impact of Nonclinical Factors on Care Use for Patients with Depression: A STAR*D Report." *CNS Neuroscience & Therapeutics* 15, no. 4 (2009): 320.

Gaynes, B.N., et al. "A Direct Comparison of Presenting Characteristics of Depressed Outpatients from Primary vs. Specialty Care Settings: Preliminary Findings from the STAR*D Clinical Trial." *General Hospital Psychiatry* 27, no. 2 (March–April 2005): 87–96.

Pigott, H. Edmund, et al. "Efficacy and Effectiveness of Antidepressants: Current Status of Research." *Psychotherapy and Psychosomatics* 79, no. 5 (2010): 267–79.

Rush, A.J. "STAR*D: What We Have Learned." *American Journal of Psychiatry* 164 (2007): 201–4.

Rush, A.J., et al. (STAR*D Investigators Group). "Sequenced Treatment Alternatives to Relieve Depression (STAR*D): Rationale and Design." *Controlled Clinical Trials* 25, no. 1 (February 2004): 119–42.

Wisniewski, S.R., et al. "Can Phase III Trial Results and Antidepressant Medications Be Generalized to Clinical Practice? A STAR*D Report." *American Journal of Psychiatry* 166, no. 5 (2009): 599–607.

Young, E.A., et al. "Sex Differences in Response to Citalopram: A STAR*D Report." *Journal of Psychiatric Research* 43 (2009): 503–11.

WEBSITES

"Sequenced Treatment Alternatives to Relieve Depression (STAR*D) Study." National Institute of Mental Health. http://www.nimh.nih.gov/trials/practical/stard/index.shtml (accessed July 21, 2011).

"STAR*D (Sequenced Treatment Alternatives to Relieve Depression)." University of Pittsburgh. http://www.edc.pitt.edu/stard (accessed July 21, 2011).

ORGANIZATIONS

American Psychological Association, 750 1st St. NE, Washington, DC, 20002-4242, (202) 336-5500, TDD/TTY: (202) 336-6123, (800) 374-2721, http://www.apa.org.

National Alliance on Mental Illness, 3803 N Fairfax Dr., Ste. 100, Arlington, VA, 22203, (703) 524-7600, http://www.nami.org.

National Institute of Mental Health, 6001 Executive Blvd., Rm. 8184, MSC 9663, Bethesda, MD, 20892-9663, (301) 433-4513, TTY: (301) 443-8431, Fax: (301) 443-4279, (866) 615-6464, TTY: (866) 415-8051, nimhinfo@nih.gov, http://www.nimh.nih.gov.

Stephanie N. Watson
William Atkins

Stelazine *see* **Trifluoperazine**

STEP-BD study

Definition

The Systematic Treatment Enhancement Program for **Bipolar Disorder** (STEP-BD) was a long-term, outpatient research study conducted within the United States that aimed to find out which treatments, or treatment combinations, are most effective for countering **depression** and mania and for preventing recurrent episodes in people with bipolar disorder.

Purpose

The STEP-BD is one of the largest studies to have evaluated treatments for bipolar disorder. This chronic condition, which is characterized by repeated swings in mood between mania (a state of elation and high energy) and depression, can significantly affect quality of life if not properly treated.

Researchers with the STEP-BD investigated the most effective treatment methods for bipolar episodes (mania and depression), including medication, psychological therapies, and other modalities. The researchers evaluated treatments based on cost-effectiveness, improvements in patients' social functioning and quality of life, and prevention of recurrence. As part of the study, the investigators also looked at the characteristics of patients with bipolar disorder.

Demographics

The study began in September 1998 and ended in September 2005. It included approximately 4,350 participants with bipolar disorder, who were being treated at 20 clinical treatment centers throughout the United States.

Description

The STEP-BD study was a $28-million, seven-year effort funded by the National Institutes of Mental Health (NIMH). Researchers followed 4,360 participants with bipolar disorder to determine which treatments were most effective for mania and depressive episodes, and for preventing recurrence.

The study offered two treatment arms, called pathways—a real-world, non-controlled Best Practice Pathway, and a randomized and controlled Randomized Care Pathway. Participants had the opportunity to join in both pathways. Researchers were able to compare the two pathways to see how the evaluated treatments worked both in clinical and real-world settings.

Best Practice Pathway

In the "Best Practice Pathway," participants were followed by a STEP-BD certified doctor, and all treatment choices were individualized. Everyone enrolled in STEP-BD was able to participate in this pathway. Participants and their doctors worked together to decide on the best treatment plans and to change these plans if needed. In addition, anyone who wished to stay on his or her current treatment upon entering STEP-BD was permitted do so in this pathway. Adolescents and adults aged 15 years or older were eligible to participate in the Best Practice Pathway.

Randomized Care Pathway

Patients ages 18 years or older had the option of entering the "Randomized Care Pathway" portion of the trial. Patients in this pathway remained on their mood-stabilizing medication, but some were also started on another medication or **talk therapy**. The patients were randomly assigned to treatments, and the study was double-blinded, meaning that neither the doctors nor their patients were aware of which treatment was given. (Double-blinding is done to prevent bias among both researchers and patients.) Approximately 1,500 patients were involved in at least one Randomized Care Pathway. Patients remained with the same physician throughout the course of the study.

Researchers

All researchers involved in STEP-BD were specially trained for the project in the treatment of bipolar disorder. The study was coordinated by Massachusetts General Hospital and the University of Pittsburgh School of Medicine.

The following research centers served as clinical sites for the study:

- Baylor College of Medicine (Texas)
- Case Western Reserve University (Ohio)
- Cornell University (New York)
- Howard University (Washington, DC)
- Massachusetts General Hospital
- New York Presbyterian Hospital
- New York University
- Rush-Presbyterian-St. Luke's Medical Center (Illinois; now named the Rush University Medical Center)
- Stanford University (California)
- State University of New York, Buffalo
- University of Arizona
- University of California, San Diego
- University of Colorado
- University of Louisville (Kentucky)
- University of Massachusetts
- University of Missouri
- University of Oklahoma
- University of Pennsylvania
- University of Pittsburgh (Pennsylvania)
- University of Texas, San Antonio

Participants

STEP-BD enrolled 4,360 patients with bipolar disorder in the United States. To enter the study, participants had to be at least 15 years of age and meet the ***Diagnostic and Statistical Manual of Mental Disorders***, fourth edition (*DSM-IV*) criteria for bipolar I disorder, bipolar II disorder, cyclothymia, bipolar disorder not otherwise specified (BD-NOS), or **schizoaffective disorder**, bipolar subtype. The goal of STEP-BD was to evaluate all of the best-practice treatment options used for bipolar disorder: mood-stabilizing medications, **antidepressants**, atypical antipsychotics, and psychosocial interventions—or "talk" therapies—including **cognitive-behavioral therapy**, family-focused therapy, interpersonal and social rhythm therapy, and collaborative care (psychoeducation).

Some of the patients had already been treated for bipolar disorder before entering the study, whereas others had not received prior treatment. Many of the patients had other mental illnesses, such as anxiety or **substance abuse** problems. Doctors evaluated the participants upon entry (baseline) and monitored their progress throughout the study. Patients were considered to be recovering if they had no more than two moderate symptoms for at least one week. They were considered recovered if they had no more than two moderate symptoms for at least eight weeks.

Treatments

Drugs and behavioral therapies were used in the STEP-BD study.

Drugs included:

- lithium (a mood-stabilizing medication)
- valproate (an anticonvulsant medication that has mood-stabilizing effects)
- lamotrigine (a newer anticonvulsant medication)
- risperidone (an atypical antipsychotic medication)
- bupropion (an antidepressant)
- paroxetine (a type of antidepressant called a selective serotonin reuptake inhibitor [SSRI])
- tranylcypromine (a type of antidepressant known as a monoamine oxidase inhibitor [MAOI])
- inositol (a natural substance that acts as a chemical messenger)

Behavioral therapies included:

- cognitive-behavioral therapy
- family-focused therapy
- interpersonal and social rhythms therapy

Preparation

Participants prepared for the study by first meeting with their family doctor and/or STEP-BD certified doctor, who then assessed their condition and later assisted them throughout their treatment within the STEP-BD study.

Results

In addition to evaluating treatment outcomes, the STEP-BD study looked at the coexistence of other mental disorders, types of medications commonly prescribed for bipolar disorder, and recurrence rates, among other areas of study.

The following were some of the research findings to come out of the STEP-BD study:

- Coexistence of other mental disorders: Among a subgroup of the first 500 patients in the STEP-BD study, more than 50% had a lifetime history of anxiety disorder, 38% had a history of alcohol abuse or dependence, and 26% had a history of substance of abuse or dependence.
- Most common existing treatments for bipolar disorder: Researchers looked at the first 500 patients entering the study and found that the majority (72%)were taking mood-stabilizer medications, such as lithium or carbamazepine, when they began STEP-BD. The next most common class of medications taken was antidepressants (40%), followed by anticonvulsants (32%) and antipsychotic agents (31%).
- Treatment-resistant bipolar depression: Researchers tested three different medications, lamotrigine, inositol, and risperidone, on a subgroup of 66 participants with bipolar depression who had not previously responded to treatment. The recovery rate was 24% with lamotrigine, 17% with inositol, and 4.6% with risperidone. The researchers said their results suggested that lamotrigine may be superior to inositol and risperidone for improving symptoms of treatment-resistant bipolar depression.
- The effectiveness of psychotherapy on bipolar disorder: Researchers looked at a subgroup of the first 1,000 people enrolled in the STEP-BD study. About 60% of these patients had at least one psychotherapy session during the first year of the study. Among participants with more severe depressive symptoms at the outset of the study, more frequent psychotherapy sessions were associated with less severe mood symptoms and better functioning. The researchers said that these results suggest that patients with more severe bipolar disorder might benefit from more frequent psychotherapy sessions.
- Bipolar disorder recurrence: In a prospective study of 1,469 STEP-BD participants, more than half of the patients (58%) achieved recovery. However, almost half of those who recovered experienced a recurrence during the two-year follow-up period. Researchers said that these findings indicate that bipolar disorder has a strong likelihood of recurrence.

STEP-BD Acute Depression Medication Trial

The Acute Depression Medication Trial was a part of the STEP-BD. The trial's results were reported online on March 28, 2007, in the *New England Journal of Medicine.* Participants who had originally enrolled in the STEP-BD Best Practice Pathway (BPP), but whose depression had not improved or who had experienced additional depressive episodes while in the study, could opt out of the study with the option of entering the Acute Depression Medication Trial (ADMT).

In all, 366 people (18 years of age or older) participated in the ADMT, a randomized controlled trial that looked at antidepressant medication treatment options for acute depressive episodes. Specifically, researchers wanted to determine whether an antidepressant added to a mood-stabilizing treatment program was more effective at treating bipolar depressive episodes than using a mood-stabilizer drug by itself, and whether a standard antidepressant medication could lead a person from depression to mania.

Within the ADMT, 179 of the participants received up to 26 weeks of one of two antidepressant medications (**paroxetine** or **bupropion**), along with a mood stabilizer, to treat their depression. The other 187 people (the control group) received a placebo (sugar pill), along with a mood stabilizer, for their depression treatment.

KEY TERMS

Bipolar disorder—A mood disorder characterized by abnormally high energy levels and moodiness, usually without depression.

Cognitive behavioral techniques—A type of therapy used to solve problems concerning dysfunctional behaviors (responses), emotions (feelings), and cognitions (abilities to gather knowledge) through a proven systematic set of procedures.

Cognitive therapy—A type of psychiatric treatment involving the treatment of anxiety and/or depression, which encourages patients to confront their problems in order to improve their behavior.

Depression—A psychiatric disorder involving feelings of hopelessness and symptoms of fatigue, sleeplessness, suicidal tendencies, and poor concentration.

Mania—An intense and/or excessive interest for something that leads to a psychiatric disorder characterized by impulsive behavior, excessive physical activities, and other such impulsive actions.

Substance abuse—Overuse of a drug or alcohol, which leads to addiction.

QUESTIONS TO ASK YOUR DOCTOR

- How can the STEP-BD study help me in my problems?
- Where can I learn more about STEP-BD?
- Has more research been performed relating to the STEP-BD?

The group that received the antidepressant medication and a mood stabilizer achieved a 24% "durable recovery," which was defined to be at least eight weeks with no more than two depressive or two manic symptoms. The placebo/mood stabilizer group had a 27% durable recovery rate. The researchers concluded that the antidepressant medication added to a mood stabilizer did not improve the recovery from bipolar depression when compared to using only a mood stabilizer. They also noted that adding an antidepressant to the mood stabilizer did not increase the risk of a person switching from depression to mania or **hypomania**.

The **National Institute of Mental Health** added, "... because study participants tolerated both treatments well—less than 1 percent of participants suffered severe adverse effects—the results indicate that properly administered mood-stabilizing medication is an acceptable first-line treatment for outpatients with bipolar depression."

Resources

BOOKS

Basco, Monica Ramirez, and A. John Rush. *Cognitive Behavioral Therapy for Bipolar Disorder.* 2nd ed. New York: Guilford Press, 2005.

Borch-Jacobsen, Mikkel. *Making Minds and Madness: From Hysteria to Depression.* Cambridge: Cambridge University Press, 2009.

Dziegielewski, Sophia F. *DSM-IV-TR in Action.* Hoboken, NJ: John Wiley & Sons, 2010.

Evans, Dwight L., Dennis S. Charney, and Lydia Lewis. *The Physician's Guide to Depression & Bipolar Disorders.* New York: McGraw-Hill, 2005.

Freeman, Hugh, ed. *A Century of Psychiatry.* St. Louis: Mosby, 1999.

Peterson, David B. *Psychological Aspects of Functioning, Disability, and Health.* New York: Springer, 2011.

Schulte-Markwort, Michael, Kathrin Marutt, and Peter Riedesser, eds. *Cross-walks ICD-10-DSM IV-TR: A Synopsis of Classifications of Mental Disorders.* Cambridge, MA: Hogrefe & Huber, 2003.

Suppes, Trisha, and Ellen B. Dennehy. *Bipolar Disorder: The Latest Assessment and Treatment Strategies.* Kansas City: Compact Clinicals, 2005.

Suppes, Trisha, and Paul E. Keck Jr. *Bipolar Disorder: Treatment and Management.* Kansas City: Compact Clinicals, 2005.

VandenBos, Gary R., ed. *APA Dictionary of Psychology.* Washington, DC: American Psychological Association, 2007.

PERIODICALS

American Psychiatric Association. *Diagnostic and Statistical Manual of Mental Disorders.* 4th ed, text rev. Washington, DC: American Psychiatric Association, 2000.

Simon, Naomi, et al. "Anxiety Disorder Comorbidity in Bipolar Disorder Patients: Data From the First 500 Participants in the Systematic Treatment Enhancement Program for Bipolar Disorder (STEP-BD)." *American Journal of Psychiatry* December 2004: 2222–29.

Ghaemi, S. Nassir, et al. "Pharmacological Treatment Patterns at Study Entry for the First 500 STEP-BD Participants." *Psychiatric Services* May 2006: 660–65.

Miklowitz, David J., et al. "Psychotherapy, Symptom Outcomes, and Role Functioning Over One Year Among Patients With Bipolar Disorder." *Psychiatric Services* July 2006: 959–65.

Nierenberg, Andrew, et al. "Treatment-Resistant Bipolar Depression: A STEP-BD Equipoise Randomized Effectiveness Trial of Antidepressant Augmentation With Lamotrigine, Inositol, or Risperidone." *The American Journal of Psychiatry* February 2006: 210–16.

Perlis, Roy, et al. "Predictors of Recurrence in Bipolar Disorder: Primary Outcomes From the Systematic Treatment Enhancement Program for Bipolar Disorder (STEP-BD)." *The American Journal of Psychiatry* February 2006: 217–24.

Tamminga, Carol A., et al., eds. *Deconstructing Psychosis: Refining the Research Agenda for DSM-V.* Arlington, VA: American Psychiatric Association, 2010.

WEBSITES

"Questions and Answers About the STEP-BD Acute Depression Medication Trial." National Institute of Mental Health. (March 18, 2010). http://www.nimh.nih.gov/trials/practical/step-bd/questions-and-answers-about-the-step-bd-acute-depression-medication-trial.shtml (accessed August 30, 2011).

"Systematic Treatment Enhancement Program for Bipolar Disorder (STEP-BD)." National Institute of Mental Health. (March 31, 2011). http://www.nimh.nih.gov/trials/practical/step-bd/index.shtml (accessed August 30, 2011).

ORGANIZATIONS

American Psychiatric Association, 1000 Wilson Boulevard, Suite 1825, Arlington, VA, 22209-3901, (703) 907-7300, apa@psych.org, http://www.psych.org.

American Psychological Association, 750 First St. NE, Washington, DC, 20002-4242, (202) 336-5500, (800) 374-2721, http://www.apa.org.

American Sociological Association, 1430 K St. NW, Ste. 600, Washington, DC, 20005, (202) 383-9005, Fax: 1(202) 638-0882, http://www.asanet.org.

Depression and Bipolar Support Alliance, 730 N Franklin St., Ste. 501, Chicago, IL, 60654-7225, Fax: (312) 642-7243, (800) 826-3632, http://www.dbsalliance.org.

National Alliance on Mental Illness, 3803 N Fairfax Dr., Ste. 100, Arlington, VA, 22203, (703) 524-7600, Fax: (703) 524-9094, (800) 950-6264, http://www.nami.org.

National Institute of Mental Health, 6001 Executive Blvd., Rm. 8184, MSC 9663, Bethesda, MD, 20892-9663, (301) 443-4513, Fax: (301) 443-4279, (866) 615-6464, nimhinfo@nih.gov, http://www.nimh.nih.gov.

Substance Abuse and Mental Health Services Administration, PO Box 2345, Bethesda, MD, 20847-2345, Fax: (240) 221-4292, (877) 726-4727, SAMHSAInfo@samhsa.hhs.gov, http://www.samhsa.gov.

Stephanie N. Watson
William A. Atkins

Stereotypic movement disorder

Definition

Stereotypic movement disorder is characterized by repeated, rhythmic, purposeless movements or activities such as head banging, nail biting, or body rocking. These movements either cause self-injury or severely interfere with normal activities. Until 1994, the **American Psychiatric Association** referred to stereotypic movement disorder as stereotypy/habit disorder.

Demographics

Stereotypic movement disorder is most strongly associated with severe or profound intellectual disabilities, especially among people who are institutionalized and perhaps deprived of adequate sensory stimulation. It is estimated that 1%–3% of people with moderate **intellectual disability** living in the community have stereotypic movement disorder. About 25% of all people with intellectual disabilities who are institutionalized have the disorder. Among those with severe or profound intellectual disability, the rate is between 40% and 60%, with 15% showing behavior that causes self-injury.

Stereotypic movements are common among children with **pervasive developmental disorders,** such as **autism**, childhood degenerative disorder, and **Asperger syndrome**. These movements also can be seen in people with **Tourette syndrome** or with tics. Head banging is estimated to affect about 5% of children, with boys outnumbering girls three to one, although other stereotypic behaviors appear to be distributed equally between males and females. Despite its association with psychiatric disorders, there are some people with normal intelligence and who develop stereotypic movement disorder.

Description

Stereotypic movements were first described as a psychiatric symptom in the early 1900s. Since then, they have been recognized as a symptom of both psychotic and neurological disorders. They may also arise from unexplained causes. These movements may include:

- head banging
- nail biting
- playing with hair (but not hair pulling, which is considered the separate disorder of trichotillomania)
- thumb sucking
- hand flapping
- nose picking
- whirling
- body rocking
- picking at the body
- self-biting
- object biting
- self-hitting
- compulsive scratching
- eye gouging
- teeth grinding (bruxism)
- breath holding
- stereotyped sound production

The precise definition of stereotypic movement disorder changed between 1990 and 2010. The new definition limits the disorder to repetitive movements that cause physical harm or severely interfere with normal activities. These movements cannot be better described by another psychiatric condition such as anxiety disorder, a general medical condition such as Huntington's disease, or as the side effect of a medication or illicit drug (for example, **cocaine** use).

Stereotypic movements occur in people of any age, including the very young, but they are most prevalent among adolescents. People may exhibit only one particular stereotyped movement or several. The movements may be slow and gentle, fast and frenetic, or varied in intensity. They typically increase with boredom, tension, or frustration, and it appears that the movements are self-stimulatory and sometimes pleasurable. The root causes are unknown.

Stereotypic movements are common in infants and toddlers. Some estimates suggest that 15–20% of children under age three exhibit some kind of rhythmic, repetitive movements. Thumb sucking and body rocking are common self-comforting mechanisms in the very young. This type of repeated movement is temporary and usually ends by age three or four. It is not the same as stereotypic movement disorder.

Causes and symptoms

Although the root causes are unknown, inadequate caregiving and institutionalization are implicated as contributing factors in many cases. The symptoms are noted for their excessive and obsessive nature and for the tendency of individuals to hurt themselves.

KEY TERMS

Autism—A syndrome characterized by a lack of responsiveness to other people or outside stimulus, often in conjunction with a severe impairment of verbal and nonverbal communication skills.

Huntington's disease—A hereditary disease that typically appears in midlife, marked by gradual loss of brain function and voluntary movement. Some of its symptoms resemble those of schizophrenia.

Obsessive-compulsive disorder (OCD)—An anxiety disorder in which a person cannot prevent himself from dwelling on unwanted thoughts, acting on urges, or performing repetitious rituals, such as washing his hands or checking to make sure he turned off the lights.

Trichotillomania—A disorder characterized by compulsive hair pulling.

Causes

Causes of stereotypic movements include the following:

- sensory deprivation (blindness or deafness)
- drug use (cocaine, amphetamines)
- brain disease (seizures, infection)
- major psychiatric disorders (anxiety disorder, obsessive-compulsive disorder, autism)
- intellectual disability

It has also been suggested that inadequate caregiving may cause the disorder. Although many situations can give rise to stereotypic movements, the root causes of stereotypic movement disorder are unknown. Different theories propose that the causes are behavioral, neurological, and/or genetic. Although there are many theories to account for this disorder, as of 2011 no evidence clearly supported one line of reasoning or specific cause.

Symptoms

Symptoms of stereotypic movement disorder include all the activities listed above. It should be noted that many of these activities are normal in infants. They usually begin between 5 and 11 months and disappear on their own by age 3. About 55% of very young children grind their teeth. These passing phases of repetitive movement are not the same as stereotypic movement disorder. They do not cause harm and often serve the purpose of self-comforting or helping the child learn a new motor skill.

People with stereotypic movement disorder often hurt themselves. They may pick their nail cuticles or skin until they bleed. They may repeatedly gouge their eyes or bite or hit themselves causing bleeding, bruising, and sometimes, as in the case of eye gouging or head banging, even more severe damage. Some people develop behaviors such as keeping their hands in their pockets, to prevent these movements. In other cases, those who hurt themselves appear to welcome, rather than fight, physical restraints that keep them safe. However, when these restraints are removed, they return to their harmful behaviors.

Diagnosis

Stereotypic movements are diagnosed by the presence of the activities mentioned above. Young children rarely try to hide these movements, although older children may, and the first sign of them may be the physical harm they cause (bleeding skin, chewed nails). Often parents mention these repetitive movements when the physician takes a history of the child.

The difficulty in diagnosing stereotypic movement disorder comes from distinguishing it from other disorders where rhythmic, repetitive movements occur. The disorder may be classified as either with self-injurious behavior or without self-harm. To be diagnosed

QUESTIONS TO ASK YOUR DOCTOR

- Are the repetitive movements normal for a child this age?
- Can you recommend a specialist who has experience dealing with repetitive movement disorders?
- Is there an underlying medical disorder that may explain the repetitive movements?
- Will my insurance pay for the assistance of a behavioral or other therapist?
- Could the repetitive movements be the side effect of a medication?

with stereotypic movement disorder, the following conditions must be met.

- The patient must show repeated, purposeless motor behavior.
- The patient must experience physical harm from this behavior, or it must seriously interfere with activities.
- If the patient is intellectually disabled, the behavior must be serious enough to require treatment.
- The behavior must not be a symptom of another psychiatric disorder.
- The behavior must not be a side effect of medicinal or illicit substance use.
- The behavior must not be caused by a diagnosed medical condition.
- The behavior must last at least four weeks.

This definition of stereotypic movement disorder rules out many people who show repetitive movement because of autism or other pervasive developmental disorders. It also rules out those with **obsessive-compulsive disorder**, among whom movements are apt to be ritualistic and follow rigid rules or patterns. In addition, specific disorders such as **trichotillomania** (hair pulling) do not receive the **diagnosis** of stereotypic movement disorder nor do developmentally appropriate self-stimulatory behaviors among young children, such as thumb-sucking, rocking, or transient head banging.

Treatment

There are few successful treatments for stereotypic movement disorder. When the behaviors are harmful to the patient, physical restraints may be required. In less severe situations, behavioral modification techniques may help decrease the intensity of the behavior. Drugs that have been used with some success to treat stereotypic movement disorder are **clomipramine** (Anafranil), **desipramine** (Norpramin), **haloperidol** (Haldol), and **chlorpromazine** (Thorazine).

Prognosis

Stereotypic movements peak in adolescence, then decline, and sometimes disappear. Although **behavior modification** may reduce the intensity of the stereotypic movements, rarely does it eliminate them. **Stress** and physical pain may bring on these movements, which may come and go for years, especially among those patients with severe intellectual disability.

Prevention

Stereotypic movement disorder cannot be prevented. Interventions should be made to prevent self-injury.

Resources

BOOKS

Larsen, Barbara J., ed. *Movement Disorders: Causes, Diagnoses, and Treatments.* Hauppauge, NY: Nova Science Publishers, 2010.

Schapira, Anthony H. V., Anthony E. T. Lang, and Stanley Fahn. *Movement Disorders.* 4th ed. Philadelphia: Saunders/Elsevier, 2010.

Watts, Ray L., David G. Standarett, and Jose A. Obeso, eds. *Movement Disorders.* 3rd ed. New York: McGraw-Hill, 2011.

PERIODICALS

Freeman, Roger D., Atefeh Soltanifar, and Susan Baer. "Stereotypic Movement Disorder: Easily Missed." *Developmental Medicine and Child Neurology* 52, no. 8 (August 2010):733–38.

Singer, Harvey S. "Movement Stereotypies." *Seminars in Pediatric Neurology* 16, no. 2 (June 2009): 77–81.

Zinner, Samuel H., and Jonathan W. Mink. "Movement Disorders I: Tics and Stereotypies." *Pediatrics in Review* 31, no. 6 (June 2010): 223–33.

ORGANIZATIONS

American Association on Intellectual and Developmental Disabilities, 501 3rd St. NW, Ste. 200, Washington, DC, 20001, (202) 387-1968, (800) 424-3688, Fax: (202) 387-2193, http://www.aaidd.org.

The Arc, 1660 L St. NW, Ste. 301, Washington, DC, 20036, (202) 534-3700, (800) 433-5255, Fax: (202) 534-3731, info@thearc.org, http://www.thearc.org.

Movement Disorder Society, 555 E Wells St., Ste. 1100, Milwaukee, WI, 53202, (414) 276-2145, Fax: (414) 276-3349, info@movementdisorders.org, http://www.movementdisorders.org.

Tish Davidson, AM

Steroids

Definition

Steroids constitute a large class of naturally occurring and synthetic chemicals, including sterols, such as cholesterol, and various corticosteroid and sex hormones that have wide-ranging effects. There are five classes of steroid hormones: mineralocorticoids, glucocorticoids, estrogens, progestins, and androgens. However, the term "steroid" commonly refers to anabolic-androgenic steroids (AASs), which are synthetic derivatives of the male sex hormone testosterone.

Purpose

Anabolic-androgenic steroids are growth inducers. They were first developed in Europe in the 1930s to treat malnourishment and to promote healing following surgery. They are most commonly prescribed for hormone-replacement therapy, but may also prescribed for several other conditions, including muscle wasting (cachexia), anemia, and malnutrition, among others.

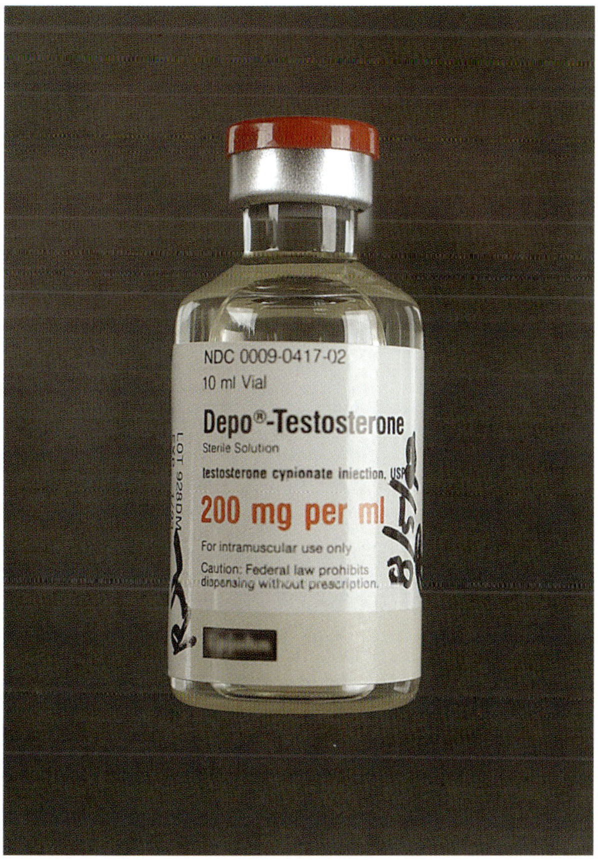

Depo-Testosterone, 10 mL. *(U.S. Drug Enforcement Administration)*

In addition to their legitimate medical uses, AASs are widely abused for building muscle, increasing strength, losing fat, enhancing athletic performance, and otherwise engaging in high-risk behavior. Their anabolic effects build muscle and their androgenic effects develop male sexual characteristics in both males and females. At medically prescribed dosages, the growth effects of anabolic steroids are slow or unnoticeable. However, at high abusive doses, muscles increase rapidly in size and strength, and AAS may increase energy and libido.

Competitive weightlifters began using AASs in the 1950s, and their use gradually spread to other sports. Most major athletic competitions, including the Olympic Games, the Wimbledon tennis tournament, the Tour de France bicycle race, and major-league professional sports teams, now routinely screen athletes for steroid use. Some steroids are easily detectable with a urine screen; the products of steroid metabolism can be identified in the urine for six months or longer after the drugs are discontinued. However, the technology for detecting steroids in blood or urine—and distinguishing the use of AASs from the products of normal metabolism or legitimate medications—is often one step behind the design of new steroid drugs.

Description

Steroids are chemicals containing a steroid nucleus that consists of four rings of 17 carbon atoms. They are fat-soluble compounds found in both plants and animals that function as hormones, or chemical messengers. In humans, steroids are produced from cholesterol in the endocrine glands, such as the adrenal cortex and the gonads (ovary and testis). Glands secrete the hormones directly into the bloodstream, where they are transported to distant parts of the body and control various vital physiologic functions ranging from suppressing inflammation to regulating physiological changes during pregnancy.

Anabolic-androgenic steroids have three mechanisms of action:

- protein metabolism
- increased synthesis of skeletal muscle tissue
- athletic endurance (allowing athletes to train harder and longer)

Common AASs preparations include:

- testosterone esters—testosterone propionate, cypionate, and enanthate
- testosterone derivatives—methyltestosterone (which is rarely used), methandrostenolone, and fluoxymesterone (which is rarely used clinically but is abused)
- nandrolone derivatives—nandrolone decanoate, ethylestrenol, and trenbolone

- dihydrotestosterone (DHT) derivatives—oxandrolone, stanozolol, and oxymetholone

AASs are taken orally as tablets or capsules, injected into muscles, or applied through the skin via ointments or transdermal patches. They are sometimes combined with creatine, protein powders, and/or various antioxidant formulations. These are considered to be ergogenic aids—substances that enhance the body's production, use, or recovery of energy and provide athletes with a competitive advantage.

U.S. brand names

AASs that are prescribed for medical purposes in the United States include:

- Depo-Testosterone (testosterone cypionate) for low testosterone levels
- Android (methyltestosterone) for treating hot flashes in postmenopausal women
- nandrolone decanoate, an injectable preparation available only as a generic and relatively safe at clinical doses for treating osteoporosis, but one of the most widely abused AASs
- Oxandrin (oxandrolone), oral tablets prescribed for HIV/AIDS-related conditions, bone pain from osteoporosis, to prevent certain side effects of corticosteroids, and sometimes abused by female athletes
- Anadrol-50 (oxymetholone), oral tablets that are abused worldwide and are considered to be carcinogenic

In the past, steroidal supplements such as androstenedione ("Andro") were commercially available in the United States. They were declared illegal in 2004 in an amendment to the Controlled Substances Act. The only remaining legal steroidal supplement in the United States is dehydroepiandrosterone (**DHEA**), which may or may not be converted to testosterone in the body.

Many athletes and other people obtain and use AASs illegally. Estimates of steroid abuse in the general adult population of the United States range from 0.5–5%. Although most anabolic steroid users are adult males, misuse is increasing among women and adolescents.

Street names for veterinary steroids that are abused include:

- Abolic
- Dianabol
- Equipoise
- Finajet/Finaject
- Parabolin
- Trenbolone
- Winstrol V

Street names for oral steroids that are abused include:

- Anadrol
- Anavar
- Maxibolin
- Methyltestosterone
- Parabolin
- Primbolin
- Primobolin
- Proviron
- Winstrol

Street names for abused injectable steroids include:

- Anatrofin
- Bolasterone
- Deca-Duabolin
- Delatestryl
- Depo-testosterone
- Dihydrolone
- Durabolin
- Dymethzine
- Enoltestovis
- Methatriol
- Primbolin
- Primobolin
- Quinolone
- Sustanon 250
- Therobolin
- Trophobolene

So-called designer steroids include:

- THG (tetrahydrogestrinone)
- Madol (desoxymethyltestosterone)
- Genabol (norbolethone)
- Equipoise and others (boldenone undecylenate)

Canadian brand names

Canadian AASs include Deca-Durabolin (nandrolone decanoate) and Anapolon 50 (oxymetholone).

International brand names

There are thousands of international brand names for AASs, and in some countries they are available over the counter. Methandrostenolone (Dianabol, Danabol, DBOL, Reforvit-b) and ethylestrenol (Maxibolin) have been discontinued in the United States but are still manufactured internationally. Trenbolone, a veterinary drug in the United States, is a widely abused

KEY TERMS

Anabolic—Causing muscle and bone growth and a shift from fat to muscle in the body.

Androgenic—Causing testosterone-like, masculinizing effects.

Angioedema—Patches of swelling of the skin, subcutaneous layers, mucus membranes, and sometimes internal organs.

Cachexia—Physical wasting and malnutrition, usually from chronic disease.

Cholesterol—A steroid alcohol in cells and body fluids that serves as a precursor for hormones and other steroids.

Corticosteroid—A steroid, such as cortisone, produced by the adrenal cortex.

Creatine—A nitrogen-containing substance found in muscle.

Estrogen—The primary female sex hormone.

Hormones—Chemical messengers that are carried by the bloodstream to various organs where they affect functioning, often by stimulatory action.

Sex hormones—Hormones that are responsible for sexual characteristics and reproductive functioning.

Steroids—A class of hormones and drugs that includes sex and stress hormones and anti-inflammatory medications, contraceptives, and growth-promoting substances.

Sterols—Steroid alcohols, such as cholesterol, that are widely distributed in the body.

Testosterone—The primary male sex hormone.

European prescription drug. Winstrol (stanozolol) is marketed internationally as well as in the United States, comes in both oral and injectable forms, and is widely abused.

Recommended dosage

Dosages used by AAS abusers are often 50–100 times higher than those for treating medical conditions. In one survey of 500 AAS users, more than half reported taking 1,000 mg or more every week. In addition 13% acknowledged using unsafe injection practices such as sharing needles, reusing needles, or sharing multi-dose vials of steroids.

In addition to higher doses, AAS abusers may practice:

- stacking—taking two or more AASs together, using more than one route of administration, or mixing AASs with other drugs such as stimulants or painkillers
- cycling—alternating periods of steroid use with periods of abstinence
- pyramiding—cycling of increasing doses over several weeks followed by decreasing doses

Some users believe that cycling and pyramiding maximize the desirable effects of steroids while reducing the undesirable effects, although there is no scientific evidence to support this claim, and cycling may build tolerance, requiring higher dosages.

Precautions

Although AASs are considered to be relatively safe at the usual prescribed dosages, at abusive dosages they can result in a wide range of serious health problems:

- abnormal lipid profiles
- early heart attacks
- strokes
- kidney failure
- severe liver problems including jaundice, tumors, and cancer
- depression
- severe psychiatric disturbances

Unsafe injection of AASs can result in HIV and hepatitis B and C infections. It has also been suggested that steroids may be gateway drugs for narcotics abuse, and it is possible to become psychologically addicted to them.

Withdrawal from high doses of AASs may require:

- medication to relieve withdrawal symptoms
- antidepressants
- hormones to restore normal hormonal function

Pediatric

AASs should be used with extreme caution in children. They can cause early puberty and lead to premature cessation of bone growth, resulting in permanent short stature.

QUESTIONS TO ASK YOUR DOCTOR

- When should I take this medication?
- Should I take it with food?
- What if I miss a dose?
- What side effects might I experience?
- Can I become addicted to this drug?

A 2008 survey by the National Institute on Drug Abuse found that 1.4% of eighth graders, 1.4% of tenth graders, and 2.2% of twelfth graders had used AASs. Some were athletes attempting to increase their strength and size; others were simply attempting to speed up their growth to keep pace with their peers. Many teenagers are also attracted by the psychological rush that comes with steroid abuse. Prevention programs often target school- or community-sponsored athletic teams, team leaders, and coaches. It has been recommended that educational prevention programs start with middle-school athletes.

Side effects

AASs usually have few side effects at medical dosages. However, at the much higher doses used to improve **body image** or athletic performance, side effects can be serious and sometimes irreversible. Excessive use can cause harmful imbalances in hormones and body chemistry. Side effects of AAS abuse can include:

- shrinking testicles, falling sperm counts, gynecomastia (swelling and enlargement of the breasts), increased urination, and enlarged prostate glands in males
- virilization in females, including hirsutism (growth of body and facial hair), male-pattern baldness, cessation of menstruation, decreased breast size, deepening of the voice, and abnormal enlargement of the clitoris
- an increase in "bad" cholesterol (LDL) and a decrease in "good" cholesterol (HDL)
- water retention leading to high blood pressure and stroke
- heart attacks
- liver and kidney tumors
- insomnia
- drastic mood swings ranging from mania to depression
- aggression, paranoia, irritability, delusions, hostility, psychosis

Treatment

Treatment of steroid abuse may include counseling to address the reasons for steroid use and medications to alleviate any symptoms associated with withdrawal. Hormones may be used to restore normal hormonal functioning in the body, and **antidepressants** may be used to alleviate **depression** that can occur when steroid use is terminated.

Resources

BOOKS

Fourcroy, Jean L., ed. *Pharmacology, Doping, and Sports: A Scientific Guide for Athletes, Coaches, Physicians, Scientists, and Administrators.* New York: Routledge, 2009.

Freedman, Jeri. *Steroids: High-Risk Performance Drugs.* New York: Rosen, 2009.

Kiesbye, Stefan. *Steroids.* Detroit: Greenhaven Press, 2007.

Thompson, Teri, et al. *American Icon: The Fall of Roger Clemens and the Rise of Steroids in America's Pastime.* New York: Alfred A. Knopf, 2009.

Walker, Ida. *Steroids: Pumped Up and Dangerous.* Philadelphia: Mason Crest, 2008.

PERIODICALS

Dines, Josh, and Rock Positano. "Steroid Talk Rages On." *New York Daily News* (June 21, 2009): 55.

Kokkevi, A., et al. "Daily Exercise and Anabolic Steroids Use in Adolescents: A Cross-National European Study." *Substance Use and Misuse* 43, no. 14 (2008): 2053–65.

Talih, F., et al. "Anabolic Steroid Abuse: Psychiatric and Physical Costs." *Cleveland Clinic Journal of Medicine* 74, no. 5 (2007): 341–52.

WEBSITES

Kishner, Stephen. "Anabolic Steroid Use and Abuse." Medscape Reference. Last updated July 6, 2011. http://emedicine.medscape.com/article/128655-overview (accessed August 15, 2011).

Mayo Clinic staff. "Performance-Enhancing Drugs: Are They a Risk to Your Health?" MayoClinic.com. December 23, 2010. http://www.mayoclinic.com/print/performance-enhancing-drugs/HQ01105/METHOD=print (accessed August 15, 2011).

National Institute on Drug Abuse. "Anabolic Steroid Abuse." http://www.steroidabuse.org (accessed August 15, 2011).

———. "Steroids (Anabolic-Androgenic)." *NIDA InfoFacts,* July 2009. http://www.drugabuse.gov/infofacts/steroids.html (accessed August 15, 2011).

ORGANIZATIONS

American College of Sports Medicine, PO Box 1440, Indianapolis, IN, 46202-1440, (317) 637-9200, Fax: (317) 634-7817, http://www.acsm.org.

National Institute on Drug Abuse, 6001 Executive Blvd., Rm. 5213, Bethesda, MD, 20892-9561, (301) 443-1124, information@nida.nih.gov, http://www.drugabuse.gov/NIDAHome.html.

Jill U. Adams
Margaret Alic, PhD

Stigma

Definitions

Stigma (plural, stigmas) is a Greek word that in its origins referred to a kind of tattoo mark that was cut or burned into the skin of criminals, slaves, or traitors in order to visibly identify them as blemished or morally polluted persons. These individuals were to be avoided or shunned, particularly in public places. The word was later applied to other personal attributes that are considered shameful or discrediting.

Social psychologists have distinguished three large classes, or categories, of stigma:

- Physical deformities. These include extremes of height and weight and such conditions as albinism and facial disfigurements or missing limbs. In the developed countries, this category also includes such signs of aging as gray hair, wrinkles, and stooped posture.
- Weaknesses or defects of individual character. This category includes biographical data that are held to indicate personal moral defect, such as a criminal record, addiction, divorce, unemployment, suicide attempts, or psychiatric disorders.
- Tribal stigma. This type of stigma refers to a person's membership in a race, ethnic group, religion, or (for women) gender that is thought to devalue all members of the group.

The second category, weaknesses or defects of an individual's character, is particularly relevant to treatment for mental illness. The 1999 report on mental health by the Surgeon General of the United States was regarded as a landmark document in the United Kingdom as well as the United States because of its straightforward identification of the stigma associated with mental illness as the chief obstacle to effective treatment of persons with mental disorders. Chapter 1 of the report noted that "Stigma leads others to avoid living, socializing or working with, renting to, or employing people with mental disorders... It reduces patients' access to resources and opportunities (e.g., housing, jobs) and leads to low self-esteem, isolation, and hopelessness. It deters the public from seeking, and wanting to pay for, care. In its most overt and egregious form, stigma results in outright discrimination and **abuse**. More tragically, it deprives people of their dignity and interferes with their full participation in society."

The report attributed the stigma attached to mental illness in the United States to three major factors:

- A misguided philosophical separation of mind and body going back to René Descartes (1596–1650) in the seventeenth century that led to a tendency to regard mental health issues as completely separate from physical disorders.
- Separation of treatment systems in which the mentally ill were isolated from the rest of society in "asylums" or mental hospitals.
- Fear of violent behavior on the part of the mentally ill. The report stated that public perception of those diagnosed with psychotic disorders in particular as dangerous was much stronger in the late 1990s than in the 1950s, even though the general public appeared to have a better understanding of the various causes of mental disorders than had been the case in the 1950s.

Psychiatrists who have studied the social stigma associated with mental illness maintain that it is important to distinguish two types of stigma: public stigma, which they define as prejudice and discrimination on the part of the general population against those diagnosed with mental disorders, and self-stigma, which is a person's internalization of public discrimination and disapproval.

The nature of stigma

Origins

One explanation for the origin of stigmas is that it is rooted in humans' concern for group survival at earlier times in their evolutionary journey. According to this theory, stigmatizing people who were perceived as unable to contribute to the group's survival, or who were seen as threats to its well-being, were stigmatized in order to justify isolating or forcing them out of the group.

The group survival theory is also thought to explain why certain human attributes seem to be universally regarded as stigmas, while others are specific to certain cultures or periods of history. Mental illness appears to be a characteristic that has nearly always led to the stigmatization and exclusion of its victims. The primary influences on Western culture, the classical philosophical tradition of Greece and Rome, and the religious traditions of Judaism and Christianity, indicate that mental illness was a feared affliction that carried a heavy stigma.

Contemporary contexts

The core feature of stigma in the modern world is defined by social psychologists as the possession of an attribute "that conveys a devalued social identity within a particular context." Context is important in assessing the nature and severity of **stress** that a person suffers with regard to stigma. Certain attributes, such as race, sex, level of education, or occupation, affect an individual's interactions with other people in so many different situations that they have been termed "master status attributes." These have become the classic identifying characteristics of the person who possesses them.

Other forms of devalued social identity are relative to specific cultures or subcultures. In one social context, a person who is stigmatized for an attribute devalued by a particular group may find acceptance in another group that values that particular attribute. One common example is that of an artistically or athletically talented child who grows up in a family that values only intellectual accomplishment. When the youngster is old enough to leave the family of origin, he or she can find a school or program for other students who share the same interest. A less marked contrast, but one that is relevant to the treatment of mental illness, is the cultural differences with regard to the degree of response to certain symptoms of mental illness. A study of **dementia** patients from minority ethnic groups reported in 2011 that members of these groups were much slower to seek **diagnosis** and treatment than members of the general public, in large measure because of the greater stigma attached to dementia in the ethnic minority communities.

One additional complicating feature of stigma is the issue of overlapping stigmas. Many people belong to several stigmatized groups or categories, and it is not always easy to determine which category triggers the unkind or discriminatory treatment encountered. For example, one study of the inadequate medical treatment that is offered to most HIV-positive Native Americans noted that the stigma of Acquired Immune Deficiency Syndrome (AIDS) provides a strong motivation for not seeking treatment. The study protocol, however, did not seek to investigate whether young Native American men are afraid of being stigmatized for their sexual orientation, their race, their low socioeconomic status, or all three. A later Canadian study, however, did attempt to account for the overlapping layers of stigma in this population.

Stigma and mental illness

Stigma and specific disorders

The stigma that is still attached to mental illness in the developed countries does not represent a simple or straightforward problem. Public health experts who have studied the stigmatization of mental illness in recent years have noted that the general public's perception of mental illness varies according to the nature of the disorder. While in general the stigma of mental illness in contemporary society is primarily associated with the second of the three categories of stigma, supposed character failings, it also spills over into the first category, physical deformities. Mental disorders that affect a person's physical appearance, particularly weight gain, are more heavily stigmatized than those that do not. Obese persons are also a stigmatized group even without the context of a mental disorder.

The stigma related to certain types of mental disorders has declined since the 1950s, most notably in regard to **depression** and **anxiety disorders**. It is thought that the reason for this change is that people are now more likely to attribute these disorders to stress, with which most people can identify. Moreover, there has been greater awareness and education about mental disorders and their treatments in the past decade. On the other hand, the stigma associated with psychotic disorders appears to be worse than it was in the 1950s. Changes in public attitude are also reflected in age-group patterns in seeking or dropping out of treatment for mental disorders. One study demonstrated that older adults being treated for depression were more likely than younger adults to drop out of treatment because they felt stigmatized. The difference in behavior is related to public attitudes toward mental illness that were widespread when the older adults were adolescents.

The types of mental disorders that carry the heaviest stigma fall into the following categories:

- Disorders associated in the popular mind with violence and/or illegal activity. These include schizophrenia, mental problems associated with HIV infection or other sexually transmitted diseases, and substance abuse disorders. Veterans of military service are particularly likely to be stigmatized by treatment for PTSD as well as substance abuse.
- Disorders in which the patient's behavior in public may embarrass family members. These include dementia in the elderly, borderline personality disorder or schizophrenia in adults, and the autistic spectrum disorders in children.
- Disorders treated with medications that cause weight gain, facial puffiness, tardive dyskinesia, or other visible side effects. Pharmacy students in particular are reported to hold strongly negative opinions of persons diagnosed with these disorders.
- Disorders treated with medications that can be abused for mood alteration. One survey of U.S. college students reported in 2011 that 13% of the students surveyed admitted to misusing psychiatric medications to improve studying (usually stimulants) or to get "high" (usually benzodiazepine tranquilizers).

Role of the media

The role of the media in perpetuating the stigmatization of mental illness has received increasing attention from public health researchers, particularly in Great

Britain. In 1998, the Royal College of Psychiatrists launched a five-year campaign intended to educate the general public about the nature and treatment of mental illness. Surveys conducted among present and former mental patients found that they considered media coverage of their disorders to be strongly biased toward the sensational and the negative. One-third of patients said that they felt more depressed or anxious as a result of news stories about the mentally ill, and 22% felt more withdrawn. The main complaint from mental health professionals, as well as patients, is that the media presented mentally ill people as "dangerous time bombs waiting to explode" when in fact 95% of murders in the United Kingdom are committed by people with no mental illness. The proportion of homicides committed by the mentally ill has decreased by 3% per year since 1957, but this statistic goes unreported. Much of the same unfair stigmatization in the media occurs in the United States according to a 1999 report of the Surgeon General.

Physicians' attitudes toward mental illness

Physicians' attitudes toward the mentally ill are also increasingly recognized as part of the problem of stigmatization. The patronizing attitude of moral superiority toward the mentally ill in the early 1960s, specifically in mental hospitals, has not disappeared. This was reported by Erving Goffman in his classic study. An American physician who specializes in the treatment of substance addicts cites three reasons for the persistence of stigmatizing attitudes among his colleagues: their tendency to see **substance abuse** as a social issue, rather than a health issue; their lack of training in detecting substance abuse; and their mistaken belief that no effective treatments exist. A similar lack of information about effective treatments characterizes many psychiatrists' attitudes toward **borderline personality disorder**.

Negative attitudes on the part of physicians toward the mentally ill can be found in Europe and Asia as well as North America. For example, a survey of Turkish medical students reported in 2011 that 90% would not want a person with a history of **suicide** attempts to care for their children, and 73% would not rent a room to such a person.

Stigma as cause of mental illness

It is significant that researchers in the field of social psychology have moved in recent years to analyzing stigma in terms of stress. Newer studies in this field now refer to membership in a stigmatized group as a stressor that increases a person's risk of developing a mental illness. The physiological and psychological effects of stress caused by racist behavior, for example, have been documented in African Americans. Similar studies of obese people have found that the stigmatization of obesity is the single most important factor in the psychological problems of these patients. To give still another example, the high rates of depression among postmenopausal women have been attributed to the fact that aging is a much heavier stigma for women than for men in contemporary society.

Stigma has a secondary effect on rates of mental illness in that members of stigmatized groups have less access to educational opportunities, well-paying jobs, and adequate health care. They are therefore exposed to more environmental stressors in addition to the stigma itself.

Stigma as effect

Stigma resulting from mental illness has been shown to increase the likelihood of a patient's **relapse**. Since a mental disorder is not as immediately apparent as race, sex, or physical disabilities, many people with mental disorders undergo considerable strain trying to conceal their condition from strangers or casual acquaintances. More seriously, the stigma causes problems in the job market, leading to stress caused by lying to a potential employer and fears of being found out. Erving Goffman, a sociologist who wrote a landmark study of mental institutions, reported in the 1960s that one common way around the dilemma involved taking a job for about six months after discharge from a mental institution, then quitting that job and applying for another with a recommendation from the first employer that did not mention the history of mental illness.

The stigmatization of the patient with mental illness extends to family members, partly because they are often seen, or see themselves, as the source of the patient's disorder. A study done in Israel reported in 2011 that the parents of individuals with severe mental illness carry a heavy burden of self-stigma. An editorial published in the *Journal of the American Medical Association* in 2001 tells the story of two sets of parents coping with the stress caused by other people's reactions to their children's mental illness, and the different responses they received when the children's disorders were thought to be a physical problem. The writer also recounts the problems encountered by the parents of an autistic child. The writer stated that family excursions were difficult, and continued, "My friend's wife was reprimanded by strangers for not being able to control her son. The boy was stared at and ridiculed. The inventive parent, fed up with the situation, bought a wheelchair to take the child out. The family was now asked about their child's disability. They were praised for their tolerance of his physical hardship and for their courage; the son was commended for his bravery. Same parents, same child, different view."

Results of stigma

The stigmatization of mental disorders has a number of consequences for the larger society. Patients' refusal to seek treatment, noncompliance with treatment, and inability to find work carry a high price tag. Disability related to mental illness accounts for fully 15% of the economic burden caused by *all* diseases in developed countries.

Seeking treatment

Stigmatization of mental illness is an important factor in preventing persons with mental disorders from asking for help. This factor affects even mental health services on university campuses; interviews with Harvard students following a 1995 murder in which a depressed student killed a classmate found that students hesitated to consult mental health professionals because many of their concerns were treated as disciplinary infractions rather than illnesses. The tendency to stigmatize mental disorders as character faults is as prevalent among educators as among medical professionals. Another institution in which persons are reluctant to seek help is the military, including veterans as well as service personnel on active duty; many soldiers, sailors, and airmen mention the possible effect of mental health treatment records on promotion or career advancement as a major reason for not seeking help.

In addition, studies of large corporations indicate that employees frequently hesitate to seek treatment for depression and other stress-related disorders for fear of receiving negative evaluations of job performance and possible termination. These fears are especially acute during economic downturns and periods of corporate downsizing.

Compliance with treatment

Another link between mental disorders and stigma is the low rates of treatment **compliance** among patients. To a large extent, patient compliance is a direct reflection of the quality of the doctor-patient relationship. Other reasons for low compliance with treatment regimens are related to stigmatized side effects. Many patients, particularly women, discontinue medications that cause weight gain because of the social stigma attached to obesity in females.

Social and economic consequences

Persons with a history of treatment for mental disorders frequently encounter prejudice in the job market and the likelihood of long periods of unemployment; this can result in lower socioeconomic status as well as loss of self-esteem. These problems are not limited to North America. In 1990, the U.S. Congress included mental disorders (with a few exceptions for disorders related to substance abuse and compulsive sexual behaviors) in the anti-discriminatory provisions of the Americans with Disabilities Act (ADA). As of 2011, mental disorders constituted the third-largest category of discrimination claims against employers.

Stigmatization of mental disorders also affects funding for research into the causes and treatment of mental disorders. Records of recent debates at the federal and state levels indicate that money for mental health research was still apportioned as of 2011. Increasing such funding is one of the goals of the National Consortium on Stigma and Empowerment (NCSE), an organization of mental health researchers founded in the late 1990s.

Future prospects

The stigma of mental illness will not disappear overnight. Slow changes in attitudes toward other social issues have occurred in the past three decades, giving

KEY TERMS

Asylum—An older term for psychiatric hospitals; it is rarely used except in historical studies of psychiatric treatment.

Master status attribute—A term used in sociology for a characteristic that is the most important definer of an individual's social status or identity; one that overshadows other traits and affects the person's behavior in most situations. Common master status attributes are race, sex, sexual orientation, level of education, age, and mental illness or disability.

Medical model of mental illness—An approach to psychiatric diagnosis and treatment patterned on the process of diagnosis and treatment of physical disease.

Self-stigma—Loss of self-esteem and personal effectiveness that develops when a person being treated for a mental health issue internalizes public prejudice against people diagnosed with mental disorders.

Tardive dyskinesia—A disorder characterized by involuntary and repetitive body movements that sometimes develops after long-term use of antipsychotic medications.

QUESTIONS TO ASK YOUR DOCTOR

- Do you think people still fear being stigmatized if they seek help for mental health problems?
- Have you ever had difficulty referring a patient to a psychiatrist because they were afraid of stigma?
- Do you think that the situation is gradually improving and that the general public is more understanding of mental health issues?
- What is your opinion of media treatment of people with mental disorders?

hope to the lessening of stigma borne by people with mental illness. In addition, the stigmatizing of mental conditions has become a major topic of sociological as well as psychiatric research and publication since the early 2000s. However, economic limitations are an ongoing reason for concern. As the economic "pie" has to be divided among a larger number of advocacy groups, causing stiffer competition for public funding, persons with mental disorders will need skilled and committed advocates if their many serious needs are to receive adequate attention and help. Such groups as the National Alliance on Mental Illness (NAMI), which has launched a "StigmaBusters" campaign, have stepped up their efforts to educate the public as well as press for increases in funding to reduce the stigma of mental illness.

Another approach to reducing the stigma of mental illness is setting up education groups for caregivers of patients diagnosed with such severe disorders as **schizophrenia** and **Alzheimer's disease**; the groups include helping caregivers cope with the stigma of their loved one's illness as well as providing direct care for him or her. Online courses for caregivers as well as some for patients themselves are also available; these resources appear to be particularly useful to high school and college students with mental health problems. Readers interested in educating themselves about stigma or in advocacy at the local community level can find resources on the NAMI website as well as on the website of the National Consortium on Stigma and Empowerment (NCSE), listed under Organizations below.

The proposed change in the definition of a mental disorder for DSM-5 may also help to reduce the stigma associated with mental health problems. The new definition represents a move away from the traditional medical model of mental disorders by referring to them as "behavioral or psychological syndrome[s] or pattern[s] that occur in an individual" and that reflect "an underlying psychological dysfunction." One of the rationales given for the new definition is the growing recognition that human behavior and psychology cannot be separated from the biological dimension of human beings. This recognition is a clear rejection of the Cartesian separation of mind and body noted earlier.

Resources

BOOKS

Arboleda-Flórez, Julio, and Norman Sartorius, eds. *Understanding the Stigma of Mental Illness: Theory and Interventions*. Hoboken, NJ: John Wiley and Sons, 2008.

Corrigan, Patrick William, David Roe, and Hector W.H. Stang. *Challenging the Stigma of Mental Illness: Lessons for Therapists and Advocates*. Hoboken, NJ: John Wiley and Sons, 2011.

Goffman, Erving. *Asylums: Essays on the Social Situation of Mental Patients and Other Inmates*. New York: Anchor Books, 1961.

Goffman, Erving. *Stigma: Notes on the Management of Spoiled Identity*. New York: Simon and Schuster, Inc., 1963.

PERIODICALS

Barnes, E., et al. "Developing an Online Education Package for Bipolar Disorder." *Journal of Mental Health* 20 (February 2011): 21–31.

Emul, M., et al. "The Attitudes of Preclinical and Clinical Turkish Medical Students toward Suicide Attempters." *Crisis* 32 (January 1, 2011): 128–133.

Galletly, C., and C. Burton. "Improving Medical Student Attitudes towards People with Schizophrenia." *Australian and New Zealand Journal of Psychiatry* 45 (June 2011): 473–476.

Gorman, L.A., et al. "National Guard Families after Combat: Mental Health, Use of Mental Health Services, and Perceived Treatment Barriers." *Psychiatric Services* 62 (January 2011): 28–34.

Hasson-Ohayon, I., et al. "Insight into Mental Illness, Self-stigma, and the Family Burden of Parents of Persons with a Severe Mental Illness." *Comprehensive Psychiatry* 52 (January-February 2011): 75–80.

Horgan, A., and J. Sweeney. "Young Students' Use of the Internet for Mental Health Information and Support." *Journal of Psychiatric and Mental Health Nursing* 17 (March 2010): 117–123.

Mill, J., et al. "Accessing Health Services While Living with HIV: Intersections of Stigma." *Canadian Journal of Nursing Research* 41 (September 2009): 168–185.

Mukadam, N., et al. "A Systematic Review of Ethnicity and Pathways to Care in Dementia." *International Journal of Geriatric Psychiatry* 26 (January 2011): 12–20.

O'Reilly, C.L., et al. "Consumer-led Mental Health Education for Pharmacy Students." *American Journal of Pharmaceutical Education* 74 (November 10, 2010): 167.

Riley, G., et al. "Carer's Education Groups for Relatives with a First Episode of Psychosis: An Evaluation of an Eight-week Education Group." *Early Intervention in Psychiatry* 5 (February 2011): 57–63.

Schomerus, G., et al. "The Stigma of Alcohol Dependence Compared with Other Mental Disorders: A Review of Population Studies." *Alcohol and Alcoholism* 46 (March-April 2011): 105–112.

Skidmore, W.C., and M. Roy. "Practical Considerations for Addressing Substance Use Disorders in Veterans and Service Members." *Social Work in Health Care* 50 (January 2011): 85–107.

Stone, A.M., and L.J. Merlo. "Attitudes of College Students toward Mental Illness Stigma and the Misuse of Psychiatric Medications." *Journal of Clinical Psychiatry* 72 (February 2011): 134–139.

Vogt, D. "Mental Health-related Beliefs as a Barrier to Service Use for Military Personnel and Veterans: A Review." *Psychiatric Services* 62 (February 2011): 135–142.

Weissman, Myrna M. "Stigma." *Journal of the American Medical Association* 285 (January 17, 2001): 261.

WEBSITES

American Psychiatric Association. DSM-5 Development. "Definition of a Mental Disorder." http://www.dsm5.org/ProposedRevisions/Pages/proposedrevision.aspx?rid=465 (accessed May 23, 2011).

Mental Health: A Report of the Surgeon General, Chapter 1, "Introduction and Themes," section 5, "The Roots of Stigma." http://www.surgeongeneral.gov/library/mentalhealth/chapter1/sec1.html#roots_stigma (accessed May 29, 2011).

National Alliance on Mental Illness (NAMI). "The ADAAmericans with Disabilities Act." http://www.nami.org/Template.cfm?Section=Helpline1&template=/ContentManagement/ContentDisplay.cfm&ContentID=47065 (accessed May 29, 2011).

ORGANIZATIONS

American Psychiatric Association (APA), 1000 Wilson Blvd., Ste. 1825, Arlington, VA, 22209-3901, (703) 907-7300, apa@psych.org, http://www.psych.org

National Alliance on Mental Illness (NAMI), 3803 N Fairfax Dr., Ste. 100, Arlington, VA, 22203, (703) 524-7600, Fax: (703) 524-9094, (800) 950-NAMI, http://www.nami.org

National Consortium on Stigma and Empowerment (NCSE), Illinois Institute of Technology, Institute of Psychology, 3424 S State St., First Fl., Chicago, IL, 60616, (312) 567-6751, Fax: (312) 567-6753, corrigan@iit.edu, http://www.stigmaandempowerment.org

National Institute of Mental Health (NIMH), 6001 Executive Blvd., Rm. 8184, MSC 9663, Bethesda, MD, 20892-9663, (301) 443-4513, Fax: (301) 443-4279, (866) 615-6464, nimhinfo@nih.gov, http://www.nimh.nih.gov/index.shtml

Rebecca J. Frey, Ph.D.

Stockholm syndrome

Definition

Stockholm syndrome refers to a group of psychological symptoms that occur in some persons in a captive or hostage situation. It has been used to explain the behavior of such well-known kidnapping victims as Patty Hearst (1974) and Elizabeth Smart (2002). The term takes its name from a bank robbery in Stockholm, Sweden, in August 1973. The robber took four employees of the bank (three women and one man) into the vault with him and kept them hostage for 131 hours. After the employees were finally released, they appeared to have formed a paradoxical emotional bond with their captor; they told reporters that they saw the police as their enemy rather than the bank robber and that they had positive feelings toward the criminal. The syndrome was first named by Nils Bejerot (1921–1988), a medical professor who specialized in **addiction** research and served as a psychiatric consultant to the Swedish police during the standoff at the bank. Stockholm syndrome is also known as Survival Identification Syndrome.

Description

Stockholm syndrome is considered a complex reaction to a frightening situation and experts do not agree completely on all of its characteristic features or on the factors that make some people more susceptible than others to developing it. One reason for the disagreement is that it would be unethical to test theories about the syndrome by experimenting on human beings. The data for understanding the syndrome derive from actual hostage situations since 1973 that differ considerably from one another in terms of location, number of people involved, and time frame. Another source of disagreement concerns the extent to which the syndrome can be used to explain other historical phenomena or more commonplace types of abusive relationships. Many researchers believe that Stockholm syndrome helps to explain certain behaviors of survivors of World War II concentration camps, members of religious cults, battered wives, incest survivors, and physically or emotionally abused children, as well as persons taken hostage by criminals or terrorists.

Most experts, however, agree that Stockholm syndrome has three central characteristics:

- The hostages have negative feelings about the police or other authorities.
- The hostages have positive feelings toward their captor(s).
- The captors develop positive feelings toward the hostages.

Causes & symptoms

Stockholm syndrome does not affect all hostages (or persons in comparable situations); in fact, a Federal Bureau of Investigation (FBI) study of more than 1,200 hostage-taking incidents found that 92% of the hostages did *not* develop Stockholm syndrome. FBI researchers then interviewed flight attendants who had been taken hostage during airplane hijackings, and concluded that three factors are necessary for the syndrome to develop:

- The crisis situation lasts for several days or longer.
- The hostage takers remain in contact with the hostages; that is, the hostages are not placed in a separate room.
- The hostage takers show some kindness toward the hostages or at least refrain from harming them. Hostages abused by captors typically feel anger toward them and do not usually develop the syndrome.

In addition, people who often feel helpless in other stressful life situations or are willing to do anything in order to survive seem to be more susceptible to developing Stockholm syndrome if they are taken hostage.

People with Stockholm syndrome report the same symptoms as those diagnosed with **post-traumatic stress disorder** (PTSD): **insomnia**, nightmares, general irritability, difficulty concentrating, being easily startled, feelings of unreality or confusion, inability to enjoy previously pleasurable experiences, increased distrust of others, and flashbacks.

Diagnosis

Stockholm syndrome is a descriptive term for a pattern of coping with a traumatic situation rather than a diagnostic category. Most psychiatrists would use the diagnostic criteria for **acute stress disorder** or post-traumatic **stress** disorder when evaluating a person with Stockholm syndrome.

Treatment

Treatment of Stockholm syndrome is the same as for PTSD, most commonly a combination of medications for short-term sleep disturbances and **psychotherapy** for the longer-term symptoms.

Prognosis

The prognosis for recovery from Stockholm syndrome is generally good, but the length of treatment needed depends on several variables. These include the nature of the hostage situation; the length of time the crisis lasted; and the individual patient's general coping style and previous experience(s) of **trauma**.

KEY TERMS

Coping—In psychology, a term that refers to a person's patterns of response to stress. Some patterns of coping may lower a person's risk of developing Stockholm syndrome in a hostage situation.

Flashback—The re-emergence of a traumatic memory as a vivid recollection of sounds, images, and sensations associated with the trauma. The person having the flashback typically feels as if they are reliving the event. Flashbacks were first described by doctors treating combat veterans of World War I (1914–1918).

Identification with an aggressor—In psychology, an unconscious process in which a person adopts the perspective or behavior patterns of a captor or abuser. Some researchers consider it a partial explanation of Stockholm syndrome.

Regression—In psychology, a return to earlier, usually childish or infantile, patterns of thought or behavior.

Syndrome—A set of symptoms that occur together.

Prevention

Prevention of Stockholm syndrome at the level of the larger society includes further development of **crisis intervention** skills on the part of law enforcement, as well as strategies to prevent kidnapping or hostage-taking incidents in the first place. Prevention at the individual level is difficult, because researchers have not been able to identify all of the factors that may place some persons at greater risk than others; in addition, they disagree on the specific psychological mechanisms involved in Stockholm syndrome. Some regard the syndrome as a form of regression, while others explain it in terms of emotional paralysis ("frozen fright") or identification with the aggressor.

Resources

BOOKS

Ledwig, Marion. *Emotions: Their Rationality & Consistency.* New York: Peter Lang, 2006.

McMains, Michael J. *Crisis Negotiations: Managing Critical Incidents and Hostage Situations in Law Enforcement and Corrections.* Newark, NJ: LexisNexis, 2006.

PERIODICALS

Bejerot, Nils. "The Six-Day War in Stockholm." *New Scientist* 61, no. 886 (1974): 486–487. http://www.nilsbejerot.se/sexdagar_eng.htm (accessed October 27, 2011).

Grady, Denise. "Experts Look to Stockholm Syndrome on Why Girl Stayed." *The New York Times* March 17, 2003. http://www.dannyhaszard.com/smartbackup.htm (accessed October 27, 2011).

ORGANIZATIONS

American Psychiatric Association, 1000 Wilson Blvd., Ste. 1825, Arlington, VA, 22209-3901, (703) 907-7300, apa@psych.org, http://www.psych.org.

Federal Bureau of Investigation, 935 Pennsylvania Ave. NW, Washington, DC, 20535-0001, http://www.fbi.gov.

Rebecca Frey, PhD

Strattera *see* **Atomoxetine**

Stress

Definition

Stress is defined as an organism's total response to physical, mental, emotional, or environmental demands or pressures. A stressor is defined as the stimulus or event that provokes a stress response. Stressors can be categorized as acute or chronic and as external or internal to the organism.

Demographics

Nearly everyone experiences stress in their lives at some time. One study found that about 75% of those surveyed reported experiencing at least some stress in the previous two weeks. Occasional stress is an expected part of life for most people, and while often unpleasant, it does not lead to long-term negative outcomes. In some cases, however, severe or prolonged stress can lead to illness.

Work plays a highly visible role in the stress burden among Americans; in a 2010 survey conducted by the **American Psychological Association**, 70% of those surveyed included work as a top source of stress, with the other top two being money (76%) and the economy (65%). Forty-nine percent of workers cited job insecurity as a major source of stress, and only 32% felt their employers helped them attain a satisfactory work-life balance. Only one-third of respondents felt they were successful in managing their stress levels.

Primary sources of stress, by generation

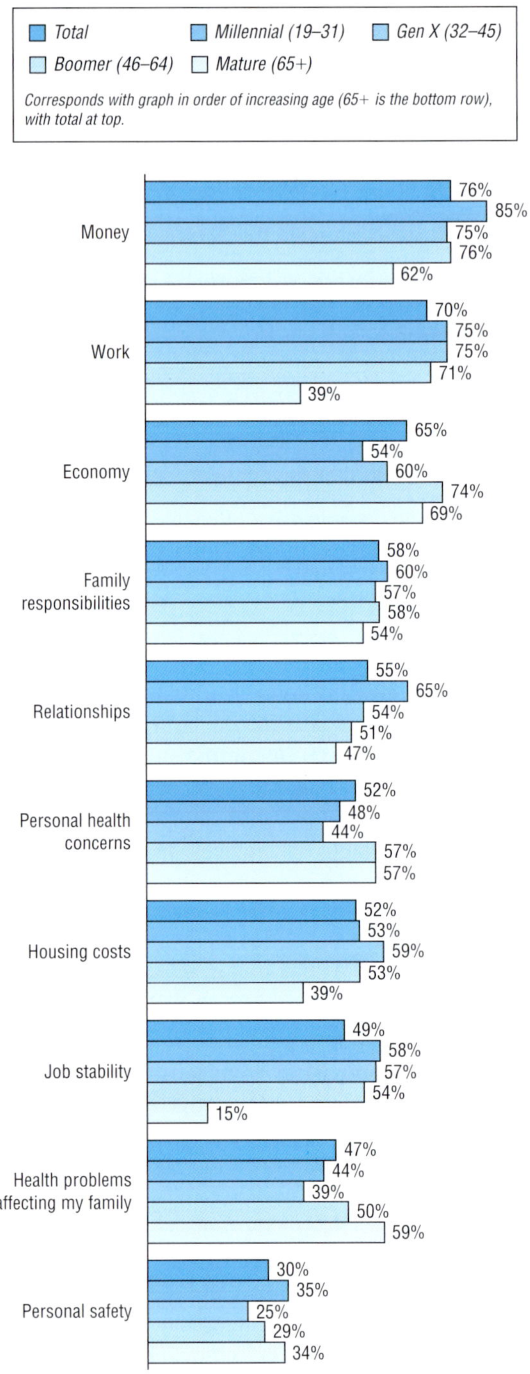

SOURCE: American Psychological Association, *Stress in America Findings* (November 2010).

Report available online at http://www.apa.org/news/press/releases/stress/index.aspx. *(Graph by PreMediaGlobal. © 2012 Cengage Learning.)*

Possible consequences of stress

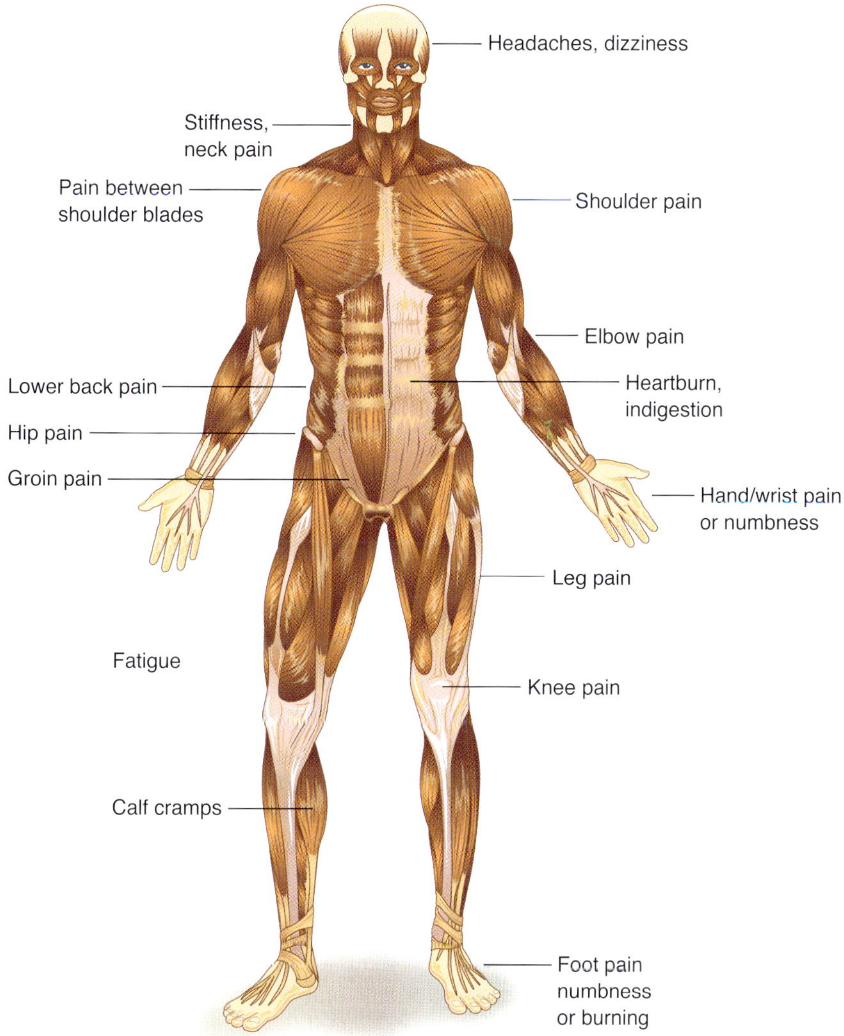

Stress reduction techniques:

- Identify your stressors
- Don't fret over small details
- Try and find positive solutions to stressful situations
- Turn to friends and family for help and support
- View stress as a challenge to be overcome, rather than as a roadblock

Activities that help manage stress:

- T'ai chi
- Massage therapy
- Yoga
- Meditation
- Guided imagery
- Breathing exercises
- Cognitive behavioral therapy

(Illustration by Electronic Illustrators Group. Reproduced by permission of Gale, a part of Cengage Learning.)

Description

Stress results from interactions between persons and their environment that are perceived as straining or exceeding the individuals' adaptive capacities or threatening their well-being. A certain degree of stress is a normal part of life; it comprises individuals' responses to inevitable changes in their physical or social environment. Moreover, positive as well as negative events can generate stress. Graduating from college, for example, is accompanied by stress related to the challenge of finding employment or saying good-bye to friends and family, as well as feelings of positive accomplishment. Some researchers refer to stress associated with positive events as eustress.

Stress may be acute or chronic. Acute stress is defined as a reaction to something believed to be an immediate threat. Acute stress reactions can occur to a falsely perceived danger as well as to a genuine threat; they can also occur in response to memories. For example, a war veteran who hears a car backfire may drop to the ground because the noise triggers vivid memories, called flashbacks, of combat experience. Common acute stressors are loud, sudden noises; being in a crowded space, such as an elevator; being cut off in heavy traffic; and being exposed to dangerous weather. Chronic stress is a reaction to a stressful situation that is ongoing, such as financial insecurity or caring for a dependent elderly parent.

Stress-related disease results from chronic stress resulting from excessive and prolonged demands on an individual's ability to cope with the stressor(s). Canadian researcher Hans Selye (1907–1982), a pioneer in studying stress, observed that an increasing number of people, particularly in developed countries, died of so-called diseases of civilization, or degenerative diseases, which are primarily caused by stress.

The role of perception in identifying stressors indicates that human stress responses reflect differences in personality, as well as differences in physical strength or general health. Selye affirmed that stress in humans depends partly on people's evaluation of a situation and their emotional reaction to it; thus, an experience that one person finds stimulating and exciting, for example, bungee jumping, may produce harmful stress in another.

One recurrent disagreement among researchers concerns the definition of stress in humans. The debate centers on whether stress is primarily an external response that can be measured by changes in glandular secretions, skin reactions, and other physical functions or a solely an internal interpretation of, or reaction to, a stressor. Perhaps, in some cases, it is both.

Risk factors

Risk factors for stress-related illnesses are a mix of personal, interpersonal, and social variables. These factors include lack or loss of control over one's physical environment and lack or loss of social support networks. People who are dependent on others, such as children, the elderly, or those who are socially disadvantaged, are at greater risk of developing stress-related illnesses. Other risk factors are feelings of helplessness, hopelessness, extreme fear or anger, and cynicism or distrust of others.

Research indicates that some vulnerability to stress is genetic. Scientists at the University of Wisconsin and King's College London discovered that people who inherited a short, or stress-sensitive, version of the **serotonin** transporter gene were almost three times as likely to experience **depression** following a stressful event as people with the long version of the gene. Further research is likely to identify other genes that affect susceptibility to stress.

Stress and mental disorders

The ***Diagnostic and Statistical Manual of Mental Disorders***, fourth edition, text revised (*DSM-IV-TR*) specifies two major categories of mental disorders directly related to stress: the post-traumatic syndromes and **adjustment disorders**. Proposed changes for the *Diagnostic and Statistical Manual of Mental Disorders*, fifth edition (*DSM-5*), scheduled for publication in 2013, combine these categories into one: trauma- and stressor-related disorders. Stress is closely associated with depression and can worsen the symptoms of most other disorders.

POST-TRAUMATIC DISORDERS. **Post-traumatic stress disorder** (PTSD) and **acute stress disorder** (ASD) are defined by their connection to a traumatic event in an individual's life, whether experienced or witnessed. The post-traumatic disorders are characterized by a cluster of anxiety and dissociative symptoms and by their interference with the patient's normal level of functioning. **Magnetic resonance imaging** (MRI) studies have shown that the high levels of sustained stress in some PTSD patients cause demonstrable damage to the hippocampus. Excessive amounts of stress hormones in **brain** tissue cause the nerve cells, or neurons, in parts of the hippocampus to wither and eventually die. One group of Vietnam veterans with PTSD lost as much as 8% of the tissue in the hippocampus.

SUBSTANCE ABUSE DISORDERS. Stress is related to **substance abuse** disorders in that chronic stress frequently leads people to self-medicate with drugs of abuse or alcohol. Substance abuse disorders are associated with a specific type of strategy for dealing with stress called emotion-focused coping. Emotion-focused coping strategies concentrate on regulating painful emotions related to stress, as distinct from problem-focused coping strategies, which involve efforts to change or eliminate the impact of a stressful event. Persons who handle stress from a problem-oriented perspective are less likely to turn to mood-altering substances when they are under stress.

ADJUSTMENT DISORDERS. The *DSM-IV-TR* defines adjustment disorders as psychological responses to stressors that are excessive given the nature of the stressor or that result in impairment of a person's academic, occupational, or social functioning. The most important difference between the post-traumatic disorders and adjustment disorders is that most people would not regard stressors involved in the latter disorder as traumatic. Adjustment disorders appear to be more common following divorce, the birth of a child, or retirement from work.

Causes and symptoms

The human stress response began as a biologically conditioned set of reactions that was necessary during earlier points in human evolution but is now less adaptive under the circumstances of modern life. In humans, the biochemical response to acute stress is known as the fight-or-flight reaction. It begins with the activation of a section of the brain called the hypothalamic-pituitary-adrenal system, or HPA. This system first activates the release of steroid hormones, which are also known as glucocorticoids. These hormones include cortisol, the primary stress hormone in humans.

Following the stress hormones, the HPA system releases a set of **neurotransmitters** known as catecholamines, which include **dopamine**, norepinephrine, and epinephrine (also known as **adrenaline**). Catecholamines have three important effects:

- They activate the amygdala, an almond-shaped structure in the limbic system that triggers an emotional response of fear.
- They signal the hippocampus, another part of the limbic system, to store the emotional experience in long-term memory.
- They suppress activity in parts of the brain associated with short-term memory, concentration, and rational thinking. This suppression allows a human to react quickly to a stressful situation, but it also lowers ability to deal with complex social or intellectual tasks that may be part of the situation.

In reaction to stress, heart rate, blood pressure, and breathing intake rise, allowing the lungs to take in more oxygen. Blood flow to the muscles, lungs, and brain may triple or quadruple. The spleen releases more blood cells into circulation, which increases the blood's ability to transport oxygen. The immune system redirects white blood cells to the skin, bone marrow, and lymph nodes, where injury or infection are most likely to occur.

At the same time, nonessential body systems shut down. The skin becomes cool and sweaty as blood is drawn away toward the heart and muscles. The mouth becomes dry, and the digestive system slows.

After the crisis passes, the levels of stress hormones drop, and the body's various organ systems return to normal, a process known as the relaxation response. Some people are more vulnerable to stress than others because their hormone levels do not return to normal after a stressful event. An absent or incomplete relaxation response is most likely to occur in professional athletes and in people with a history of depression.

Causes

Any event or occurrence that puts pressure on a person's coping mechanisms or resources can produce stress. Events such as a job interview, work-related presentation, or final exam can cause significant stress. Persons who dread a future event may experience an increased level of agitation and fretfulness. They may visualize the event negatively, worrying about what may go wrong. It is often hard to stop thinking about the event. This type of stress can take a significant toll if it persists for a long time.

Stress also may be caused by negative world news. Events such as the terrorist attacks on the United States, on September 11, 2001, are believed to increase stress both among Americans and people living elsewhere in the world. Events like terrorist attacks can prompt people to worry about the safety of family members and to fret about potential future attacks. These kinds of worries, when they occur over a long period of time, can produce chronic stress and related negative symptoms.

One study conducted telephone interviews following the September 11 terrorist attacks to assess stress reactions among the general U.S. population. The team found that the single most important factor was not geographical location relative to the attacks but the amount of time spent watching televised reports of the attacks. The interviewers discovered that 49% of the adults had watched at least eight hours of television on September 11, and the researchers considered extensive television viewing a reaction to stress.

Experiencing directly or witnessing a traumatic event such as a car accident, earthquake, or an attack of physical violence can cause severe stress. In these cases, an individual may mentally relive the event repeatedly. This is a normal response to a traumatic event, but if it persists for more than a short time or does not seem to get better, the individual may have PTSD or ASD.

Stress can also be caused by the presence of issues and problems that are upsetting or frustrating in day-to-day life. These can include worries about money, pressure at work, and problems in a relationship. Events such as divorce or the death of a loved one can also cause stress for many months or years but are not generally suggestive of PTSD or ASD.

Other causes of stress can include:

- social changes, such as living far away from family members or growing apart from childhood friends
- economic issues, such as a recession or lowered socioeconomic status
- technology, including constant access to news and events or feeling tied to work via e-mail or mobile devices
- environmental changes, such as pollution or nuclear disasters apparently due to chronic emotional stress rather than physiological exposure to harmful chemicals or radioactivity
- changes in mainstream beliefs and attitudes

Symptoms

The symptoms of stress can be physical, psychological, or both. Physical symptoms may include problems sleeping, indigestion, stomach pain or chest pain, **fatigue**, headache, back or neck pain, and many others. Psychological signs of stress include anxiety, frustration, irritability, and even depression. These symptoms may not be problematic if they occur for a brief time, but in cases of chronic stress, the body's organ systems do not have the opportunity to return fully to normal functioning. Different organs become under- or overactivated on a long-term basis. In time, these abnormal levels of activity can damage an organ or organ system.

In the workplace, stress-related illness often takes the form of burnout, a loss of interest in or ability to perform one's job due to long-term high stress levels. For example, palliative care nurses are at high risk of burnout due to their inability to prevent their patients from dying or even to relieve their physical suffering in some circumstances.

Effects of chronic stress on body systems

CARDIOVASCULAR SYSTEM. Stress has a number of negative effects on the heart and circulatory system. Acute, sudden stress increases the heart rate but also causes the arteries to narrow, which may block the flow of blood to the heart. The emotional effects of stress can alter the rhythm of the heart. In addition, stress triggers an inflammatory response in the blood vessels that can ultimately result in injury to the lining of the arteries. Markers of inflammation, linked to the development of cardiovascular disease, are also markers of the acute-phase response to stress. Stress also can cause a change in cholesterol levels, increasing fats in the blood that can eventually lead to clogged arteries and heart attack or **stroke**.

GASTROINTESTINAL SYSTEM. The effects of chronic stress on the gastrointestinal system include diarrhea, constipation, bloating, and irritable bowel syndrome. Although stress does not cause ulcers, which arise from an infection with *Helicobacter pylori* bacteria, it can exacerbate them. Stress can also influence inflammatory bowel disease, stimulating colon spasms and possibly interacting with the immune system in producing flare ups.

Stress is the cause of abnormal weight loss in some people and of weight gain in others, largely related to stress-related inability to eat or to control eating. It is thought that stress related to the physical and emotional changes of puberty is a major factor in the development of eating disorders.

REPRODUCTIVE SYSTEM. Stress affects sexual desire in both men and women and can cause impotence in men. It appears to worsen the symptoms of **premenstrual syndrome** (PMS) in women. Stress affects fertility because the high levels of cortisol in the blood can affect the hypothalamus, which produces hormones related to reproduction. Very high levels of cortisol can cause amenorrhea or cessation of menstrual periods.

In pregnancy, stress has been strongly associated with miscarriage during the earliest weeks of gestation; in one study, 90% of women with high cortisol levels experienced a miscarriage in the first three weeks of pregnancy, compared to 33% of women with normal cortisol levels. High stress levels of the mother during pregnancy are also related to higher rates of premature births and babies of lower-than-average birth weight; both are risk factors for infant mortality. In addition, stress during pregnancy is also associated with negative effects that persist after the baby is born.

MUSCULOSKELETAL SYSTEM. Stress intensifies the chronic pain of arthritis and other joint disorders. It also produces tension headaches, caused by the tightening of the muscles in the neck and scalp. Research indicates that people who have frequent tension headaches have a biological predisposition for converting emotional stress into muscle contraction.

BRAIN. The physical effects of stress hormones on the brain include interference with memory and learning. Acute stress interferes with short-term memory, although this effect goes away after the stress is resolved. People who are under severe stress are unable to concentrate and may become physically inefficient and accident prone. In children, the brain's biochemical responses to stress hampers the ability to learn.

KEY TERMS

Adjustment disorder—A psychiatric disorder marked by inappropriate or inadequate responses to a change in life circumstances. Depression following retirement from work is an example of adjustment disorder.

Biofeedback—A technique in which patients learn to modify certain body functions, such as temperature or pulse rate, with the help of a monitoring machine.

Burnout—An emotional condition, marked by fatigue, loss of interest, or frustration, that interferes with job performance. Burnout is usually regarded as the result of prolonged work-related stress.

Stress hardiness—A personality characteristic that enables persons to stay healthy in stressful circumstances. It includes belief in one's ability to influence the situation; commitment to or full engagement with one's activities; and a positive view of change.

Stress management—A category of popularized programs and techniques intended to help people deal more effectively with stress.

Stressor—A stimulus, or event, that provokes a stress response in an organism. Stressors can be categorized as acute or chronic and as external or internal to the organism.

Chronic stress appears to be a more important factor than aging in the loss of memory in older adults. Older people with low levels of stress hormones perform as well as younger people in tests of cognitive (knowledge-related) skills, but those with high levels of stress hormones test between 20% and 50% lower than the younger test subjects.

IMMUNE SYSTEM. Chronic stress affects the human immune system and increases a person's risk of getting an infectious disease. Several research studies have shown that people under chronic stress have lower-than-normal white blood cell counts and are more vulnerable to colds and influenza. Men with HIV infection and high stress levels progress more rapidly to AIDS than infected men with lower stress levels.

Diagnosis

To identify a stress-related illness, doctors take a careful medical history that includes stressors in the patient's life (e.g., family or employment problems, other illnesses, recent major life changes). Many physicians evaluate patients' personality as well, in order to assess their coping resources and emotional response patterns. Many clinicians think that differences in attitudes toward stressful events are the single most important factor in assessing individuals' vulnerability to stress-related illnesses. The ability to cope with stress depends in part on a person's perception of the stressor. The person's resources, previous physical and psychological health, and previous life experiences all affect this interpretation. Someone who has had good experiences of overcoming hardships is more likely to develop a positive interpretation of stressful events than someone who has repeatedly faced traumas and discouragement in solving problems.

There are several personality inventories and psychological tests that doctors can use to help diagnose the amount of stress that the patient experiences and the coping strategies that the patient uses to deal with them. Doctors also try to identify what the patient perceives as threatening and stressful.

The ways in which people cope with stress can be categorized according to two different sets of distinctions. One is the distinction between emotion-focused and problem-focused styles of coping. Problem-focused coping is believed to lower the impact of stress on health; people who use problem-focused coping have fewer illnesses, are less likely to become emotionally exhausted, and report higher levels of satisfaction in their work and feelings of personal accomplishment. Emotion-focused coping, in contrast, is associated with higher levels of interpersonal problems, depression, and social isolation. Although some studies reported that men are more likely to use problem-focused coping and women to use emotion-focused coping, other research done in the early 2000s found no significant gender differences in coping styles.

The second set of categories distinguishes between control-related and escape-related coping styles. Control-related coping styles include direct-action behaviors that can be done alone, help-seeking behaviors that involve social support, and positive thinking. Escape-related coping styles include avoidance of or resignation from the stressful event and substance abuse.

Stress-related illness can be diagnosed by primary care doctors, as well as by those who specialize in psychiatry. The doctor will need to distinguish between adjustment disorders and anxiety or mood disorders, and between psychiatric disorders and physical illnesses that have psychological side effects (e.g., abnormal thyroid activity).

Treatment

Advances in the understanding of the many complex connections between the human mind and body have

QUESTIONS TO ASK YOUR DOCTOR

- Are there any lifestyle changes that I can make to reduce stress?
- How can I tell the difference between a symptom of stress and being sick with an illness?
- What type of support is there to help me handle the stressors in my life?
- Can you recommend any support groups for me and my family?

produced a variety of mainstream approaches to treating stress and stress-related illness. Present treatment regimens may include one or more of the following:

- Medications may include drugs to control blood pressure or other physical symptoms of stress, as well as drugs that affect the patient's mood (antianxiety drugs or tranquilizers, antidepressants).
- Stress management programs may be either individual or group treatments and usually involve analysis of the stressors in the patient's life. They often focus on job or workplace-related stress.
- Behavioral approaches include relaxation techniques, breathing exercises, and physical exercise programs, including walking.
- Cognitive therapies teach patients to reframe or mentally reinterpret the stressors in their lives in order to modify the body's physical reactions. Anger management techniques are recommended for people who have stress-related symptoms due to chronic anger.

Alternative treatment

Treatment of stress is one area in which the boundaries between traditional and alternative therapies have changed in recent years, in part because some forms of physical **exercise** (**yoga**, tai chi, aikido) that were once associated with the counterculture have become widely accepted as useful parts of mainstream **stress reduction** programs. **Meditation**, **music therapy**, and relaxation techniques have been clinically proven to alleviate symptoms of stress. Other alternative therapies for stress that are occasionally recommended are **aromatherapy**, **dance therapy**, **biofeedback**, nutrition-based treatments (including dietary guidelines and nutritional supplements), **acupuncture**, homeopathy, pranayama (controlled breathing), massage and other **bodywork therapies**, and herbal medicine. Eating a well-balanced diet, exercising regularly, and receiving adequate sleep each night promote good health in general but may also provide stress relief.

Prognosis

The prognosis for recovery from a stress-related illness is dependent on a wide variety of factors in a person's life, many of which are genetically determined (e.g., race, sex, illnesses that run in families) or beyond the individual's control (e.g., economic trends, cultural stereotypes and prejudices, death of a loved one). It is possible, however, for individuals to learn new responses to stress and, thus, change their perceptions and experiences. A person's ability to remain healthy in stressful situations is sometimes referred to as stress hardiness. Stress-hardy people have a cluster of personality traits that strengthen their ability to cope. These traits include believing in the importance of what they are doing, believing that they have some power to influence their situation, and viewing life's changes as positive opportunities rather than as threats.

Prevention

Complete prevention of stress is neither possible nor desirable because stress is an important stimulus of human growth and creativity, as well as an inevitable part of life. Specific strategies for stress prevention vary widely from person to person, depending on the nature and number of the stressors in an individual's life and the amount of control he or she has over these factors. In general, a combination of attitudinal and behavioral changes works well for most patients. An important form of prevention may be parental **modeling** of healthy attitudes and behaviors within the family.

Resources

BOOKS

Al' Absi, Mustafa. *Stress and Addiction: Biological and Psychological Mechanisms.* Boston: Academic Press, 2007.

Greenberg, Jerrold S. *Comprehensive Stress Management.* Boston: McGraw-Hill, 2010.

Miller, Allen R. *Living with Stress.* New York: Facts on File, 2010.

Romas, John A., and Sharma, Manoj. *Practical Stress Management: A Comprehensive Workbook for Managing Change and Promoting Health.* 5th ed. San Francisco: Pearson Benjamin Cummings, 2010.

Seaward, Brian Luke. *Essentials of Managing Stress.* 2nd ed. Sudbury, MA: Jones and Bartlett, 2010.

ORGANIZATIONS

American Institute of Stress, 124 Park Ave., Yonkers, NY, 10703, (914) 963-1200, Fax: (914) 965-6267, Stress125@optonline.net, http://www.stress.org.

Centers for Disease Control and Prevention, 1600 Clifton Rd., Atlanta, GA, 30333, (404) 639-3534, 800-232-4636, inquiry@cdc.gov, http://www.cdc.gov.

National Institute of Mental Health, 6001 Executive Blvd., Rm. 8184, MSC 9663, Bethesda, MD, 20892-9663, (301) 443-4513, (866) 615-6464 TTY (866) 415-8051, Fax: (301) 443-4279, nimhinfo@nih.gov, http://www.nimh.nih.gov/index.shtml.

Rebecca J. Frey, PhD
Tish Davidson, AM
Laura Jean Cataldo, RN, EdD

Stress management/reduction

Definition

Stress management and stress reduction comprise a set of techniques and programs intended to help people deal more effectively with stress by identifying and analyzing the specific stressors that affect them and taking positive actions to minimize the effects of these stressors. Most organized stress management programs deal with job stress and workplace issues.

Purpose

The purpose of stress management and reduction is to protect the physical and mental health of people; within businesses and large organizations, it has the additional purpose of reducing employee burnout and turnover.

Demographics

Stress affects the lives of most adults in developed countries in many ways. It is a major factor in rising healthcare costs; one public health expert maintains that 90% of all diseases and disorders in the United States are stress-related. Stress plays a part in many social problems, such as child and **elder abuse**, workplace violence, juvenile crime, **suicide**, substance **addiction**, "road rage," and the like.

Stress also affects the productivity of businesses and industries. One nationwide survey conducted in the early 2000s reported that 80% of workers experience stress on the job; 53% of American workers name their job as the greatest single source of stress in their lives; nearly half report that they need help in learning how to manage

Preferred forms of stress management, by generation

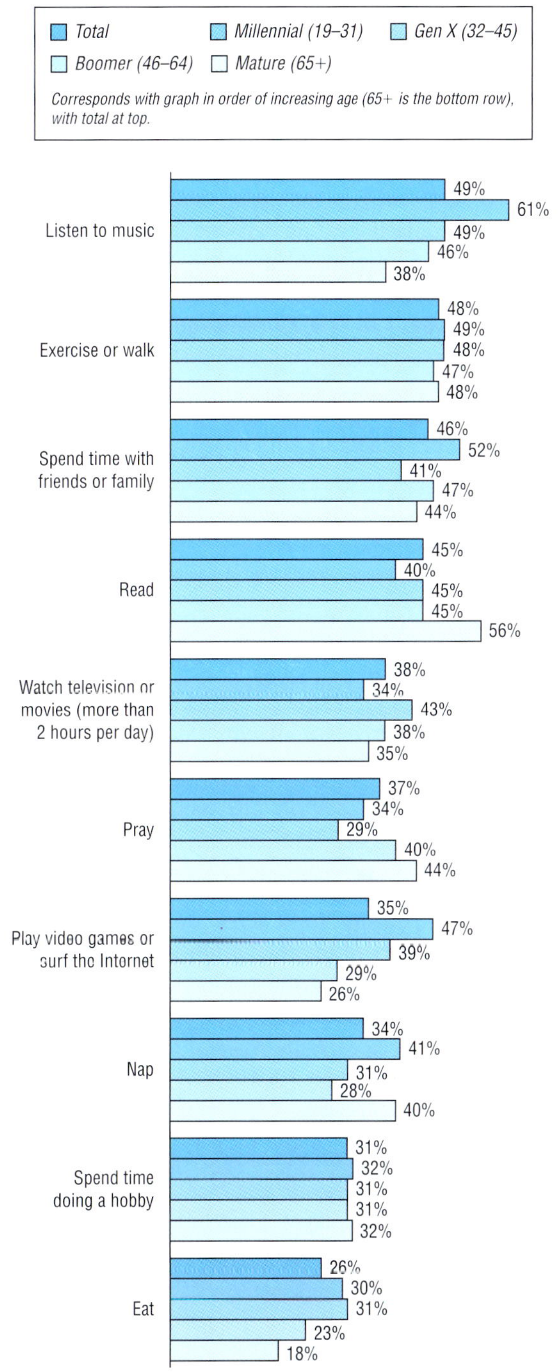

SOURCE: American Psychological Association, *Stress in America Findings* (November 2010).

Report available online at http://www.apa.org/news/press/releases/stress/index.aspx. *(Graph by PreMediaGlobal. © 2012 Cengage Learning.)*

stress; 42% say their coworkers need such help; 25% have felt like screaming or shouting because of job stress; 10% are concerned about an individual at work they fear could become violent; and 9% know of an assault or violent act in their workplace within the past year.

Precautions

People considering a stress management program or technique on their own should inform themselves about its basic approach and underlying assumptions, and consult their physician if it is a movement-oriented therapy. Those participating in a workplace stress management program may wish to question the organizers or trainers conducting the program about the types of stress reduction techniques the program will involve and whether there is a choice of activities.

Description

In order to understand stress management and stress reduction programs and techniques, it is important to understand the nature of stress, its effects on the human organism, and the ways people try to cope with it prior to learning about stress reduction.

What stress is

Most researchers consider the human stress response a biologically conditioned set of reactions that was a necessary adaptation at earlier points in human evolution but is less adaptive under the circumstances of modern life. In humans, the biochemical response to acute stress is known as the "fight-or-flight" reaction. It begins with the activation of a section of the **brain** called the hypothalamic-pituitary-adrenal system, or HPA. This system first activates the release of steroid hormones, which include cortisol, the primary stress hormone in humans.

The HPA system then releases a set of **neurotransmitters** known as catecholamines. The catecholamines include **dopamine**, norepinephrine, and epinephrine (also known as **adrenaline**). Catecholamines have three important effects:

- They activate the amygdala, an almond-shaped structure in the limbic system that triggers an emotional response of fear.
- They signal the hippocampus, another part of the limbic system, to store the emotional experience in long-term memory.
- They suppress activity in parts of the brain associated with short-term memory, concentration, and rational thinking. This suppression allows a human to react quickly to a stressful situation, but it also lowers the person's ability to deal with complex social or intellectual tasks that may be part of the situation.

Heart rate and blood pressure rise; the person breathes more rapidly, which allows the lungs to take in more oxygen. Blood flow to the muscles, lungs, and brain may increase 3–4 times the at rest pace. The spleen releases more blood cells into the circulation, which increases the blood's ability to transport oxygen. The immune system redirects white blood cells to the skin, bone marrow, and lymph nodes. At the same time, nonessential body systems shut down. The skin becomes cool and sweaty as blood is drawn away from it toward the heart and muscles. The mouth becomes dry, and the digestive system slows down.

After the crisis passes, the levels of stress hormones drop and the body's various organ systems return to normal. This return is called the relaxation response. In chronic stress, the organ systems of the body do not have the opportunity to return fully to normal levels. Different organs become under- or overactivated on a long-term basis. In time, these abnormal levels of activity can damage an organ or organ system.

Ways of coping

Psychologists define coping is as a person's habitual patterns of response to stress. Many clinicians think that differences in attitudes toward and approaches to stressful events are the single most important factor in assessing a person's vulnerability to stress-related illnesses. A person's ability to cope with stress depends in part on that person's interpretation of the event. One person may regard a stressful event as a challenge that can be surmounted, whereas another views it as a problem with no solution. Interpretation of the event in turn is affected by the person's resources, previous physical and psychological health, and previous experience. Someone who has benefited from overcoming setbacks and hardships is more likely to develop a positive interpretation of stressful events than someone who has been repeatedly beaten down by **abuse** and traumas.

People cope with stress in basically two ways. One is a distinction between emotion-focused and problem-focused styles of coping. Emotion-focused coping strategies focus on changing painful emotions related to stress, whereas problem-focused coping strategies involve efforts to change or eliminate the impact of a stressful event. Persons who handle stress from a problem-oriented perspective are less likely to turn to mood-altering substances when they are under stress.

The second way distinguishes between control-related and escape-related coping styles. Control-related coping styles include such behaviors as direct action (behavior that the person can carry out alone), help-seeking (behavior that involves social support), and positive thinking. Escape-related coping styles include avoidance or resignation (distancing oneself from the stressful event) and alcohol or drug use.

Some specific approaches to stress management

Most contemporary approaches to stress management involve various mind/body interventions associated with complementary and alternative medicine as well as mainstream cognitive behavioral techniques. Some people look into stress management techniques on their own, as there are a number of books and workbooks designed for the general public; others participate in **clinical trials** of various stress reduction techniques; and still others may enroll in workplace stress management programs. These programs have become increasingly widespread in large corporations since the 1980s; most combine education about the nature of stress and its effects on the body with training in some specific stress reduction techniques, including tai chi, massage, and relaxation techniques.

No single approach to stress management, prevention, or reduction works for everyone. Just as people vary in their reactions to stressful events and situations, they vary in what they find calming or relaxing.

COGNITIVE-BEHAVIORAL THERAPY. **Cognitive-behavioral therapy** (CBT) is the most common form of **psychotherapy** used in stress management. Sometimes called cognitive restructuring, CBT begins with the premise that a person's perceptions of a stressor are a major factor in that person's ability to cope and that perceptions are often distorted by dysfunctional thoughts and emotions. Typical thought distortions include overgeneralization (one mistake on the job means that the person cannot do anything right); catastrophizing (assuming that minor errors will always lead to major disasters); and selective abstraction (a minor detail becomes the focus of attention while the larger context is ignored).

By learning to identify and correct their distorted thinking, individuals can then move on to challenge their dysfunctional thinking and substitute positive thoughts and beliefs. Behavioral changes then follow as individuals feel less overwhelmed by the stressors in their life and adopts a problem-solving style of coping rather than an emotion-driven one. A CBT therapist typically gives homework assignments so that participants can practice their new behaviors and coping strategies. CBT therapy is one of the most commonly recommended approaches to stress management and appears to be particularly helpful in treating children and adolescents.

STRESS INOCULATION TRAINING. Stress inoculation training (SIT) is a technique of stress management developed by Donald Meichenbaum, a Canadian researcher and teacher. Like CBT, SIT is based on the assumption that individuals' thoughts about and perceptions of a stressor are a critical element in the way they cope. The SIT approach is intended to help people expand their present repertoire of coping skills, acquire greater flexibility in their application of these skills, gain confidence in their overall ability to cope with stressors, and practice applying their new skills. SIT has been used with families and groups as well as individuals. A recent development in SIT methods is the use of virtual reality for practice exercises in coping with stress.

RELAXATION TECHNIQUES. Many relaxation techniques are based on the work of Herbert Benson (1935–), a professor of medicine at Harvard who published *The Relaxation Response* in 1975, a book now considered a classic in mind/body medicine. *The Relaxation Response* outlines six simple steps that people can take to relax when under stress:

- sit quietly in a comfortable position
- close the eyes
- deeply relax all muscles and keep them relaxed
- breathe through the nose and focus on the breathing. While breathing out, silently say the word "one" (or any other one-syllable word). Breathe easily and naturally.
- continue for 10–20 minutes. One may open the eyes to check the time but an alarm should not be used. When the time is up, sit quietly for a few minutes, at first with eyes closed and later with eyes open. Do not stand up right away.
- avoid worrying about the depth of the relaxation. Relaxation comes at its own pace. When distracting thoughts occur, one should not dwell on them but simply return to repeating "one" on each exhalation.

Other relaxation techniques include autogenic training; deep breathing exercises; self-hypnosis; **biofeedback**; progressive muscle relaxation; and visualization.

MOVEMENT-RELATED MIND/BODY INTERVENTIONS. Many stress management programs incorporate movement-related CAM therapies into their activities even when the primary focus of the program may be cognitive-behavioral or mindfulness practice. Research indicates that active mind/body techniques such as **yoga**, tai chi, qigong, or gentle stretching are more effective in reducing stress than passive bodywork techniques such as massage therapy, shiatsu, or chiropractic.

KEY TERMS

Amygdala—An almond-shaped brain structure in the limbic system that is activated in acute stress situations to trigger the emotion of fear.

Autogenic training—A relaxation technique with parallels to hypnosis and meditation. It consists of six exercises in which the person uses visualization and verbal cues to relax the body.

Biofeedback—A technique for helping a user gain control over such body processes as heart rate, blood pressure, skin temperature, and muscle tension by obtaining real-time information about these processes and using thoughts and will to influence them.

Burnout—An emotional condition that interferes with job performance, marked by tiredness, loss of interest, or frustration. Burnout is usually regarded as the result of prolonged stress.

Catecholamines—A set of neurotransmitters released by the hypothalamic-pituitary-adrenal system in the brain in response to acute stress. The catecholamines include dopamine, norepinephrine, and epinephrine.

Coping—In psychology, a term that refers to a person's patterns of response to stress.

Hippocampus—A curved ridge in the mammalian brain that is part of the limbic system. The hippocampus stores long-term memories of stressful experiences.

Homeostasis—The tendency of the physiological system in humans and other mammals to maintain its internal stability by means of a coordinated response to any stimulus that disturbs its normal condition. The term was invented by Walter Cannon.

Johrei—A form of energy therapy that originated in Japan in the 1920s. It emphasizes the channeling of spiritual energy to heal people of the toxins that accumulate in their physical bodies through raising their spiritual vibrations.

Limbic system—A group of structures in the brain that includes the amygdala, hippocampus, olfactory bulbs, and hypothalamus. The limbic system is associated with homeostasis and the regulation of emotions.

Progressive muscle relaxation—A technique for lowering stress-related anxiety by alternately tensing and relaxing the muscles.

Relaxation response—The body's inactivation of stress responses and return of stress hormone levels to normal after a threat has passed.

Stressor—A stimulus or event that provokes a stress response in an organism. Stressors can be categorized as acute or chronic and as external or internal to the organism.

Visualization—A technique that employs the imagination to visualize specific events or behaviors occurring in one's life. An example of visualization in stress management is picturing oneself handling a stressful situation in the present with confidence and competence.

SPIRITUAL APPROACHES. Spiritual approaches to stress management include traditional Western prayer and worship rituals, both corporate and private, and Eastern forms of mindfulness **meditation**. Some Christian churches have special healing services that appeal to members suffering from stress-related illnesses as well as other injuries and disorders.

Mindfulness meditation originated in Buddhism centuries ago. The application of mindfulness practice to stress management is usually credited to Jon Kabat-Zinn (1944–), the founding director of the Stress Reduction Clinic and the Center for Mindfulness in Medicine, Health Care, and Society at the University of Massachusetts Medical School. The center conducts programs in mindfulness-based stress reduction, or MBSR. Since 1976, over 18,000 people have completed the program. The central notion of the program is that people can reduce the impact of stress on their lives by paying attention to what is going on inside and outside them in the moment, rather than reacting mindlessly to the outside world and living on automatic pilot, so to speak.

Origins

Modern interest in stress and its effects on the body began with Walter Cannon (1871–1945), a Harvard physiologist who used animal studies to measure the effects of stress related to thirst, heat and cold, and prolonged restraint. Hans Selye (1907–1982), a Canadian researcher, continued Cannon's work by extending it to humans. Selye defined stress as essentially the rate of wear and tear on the body. He observed that an increasing number of people, particularly in developed countries, die of so-called diseases of civilization, or degenerative diseases, which are primarily caused by stress. Selye also observed that stress in humans depends partly on a person's evaluation of a situation and that person's emotional reaction to it; thus an experience that one person finds stimulating and exciting—for example, bungee jumping—may produce harmful stress in another.

In 1967 psychiatrists Thomas Holmes and Richard Rahe devised a scale to measure the impact of life events as stressors on humans. The Holmes and Rahe Stress Scale is still used to evaluate the likelihood of a person's becoming physically ill as the result of accumulating too many stressors in the course of a calendar year. Holmes and Rahe graded the death of a spouse as 100 life change units or LCUs, imprisonment as 73, job loss as 47, down to Christmas, which rated 12 LCUs. A person who scores 300 or higher on this scale has "a high or very high risk of becoming ill in the near future"; a score between 150 and 299 carries a moderate risk; and a score below 150 carries a low risk. Holmes and Rahe's work has since been modified by researchers who argue that the specific stressors are less important than the individual's perceptions of and responses to them. For example, some people may be more relieved than upset by the loss of a spouse if the marriage itself had been stressful or if the spouse was suffering slowly in a terminal affliction.

Preparation

Preparation for a mainstream stress management or reduction program usually includes an evaluation of individuals using the Holmes and Rahe scale or a similar instrument, the nature of the stressors in their life or workplace, and their typical ways of coping with stress.

Risks

There are few risks to participation in a well-designed stress management program led or conducted by a competent professional. Movement-oriented mind/body interventions that are used in stress management programs are usually gentle, slow-paced, and unlikely to lead to physical injury.

Results

Most stress management techniques are helpful to at least some of those who try them. The degree of success, however, depends in part on whether individuals are using an approach that appeal to them and is well suited to their circumstances.

QUESTIONS TO ASK YOUR DOCTOR

- How are the stresses in my life affecting my physical and mental health?
- Would you recommend a formal stress management program for me? If so, what type?
- What is your opinion of CAM approaches to stress management and stress reduction?
- Are there any forms of stress management that you consider unproven or risky?

Healthcare team roles

Healthcare team roles in stress management and reduction may include a baseline physical examination by the participant's primary care physician to evaluate his or her general health status and possibly identify specific stress-related symptoms or disorders. The participant may also be evaluated by a clinical **psychologist** or **psychiatrist** to analyze his or her habitual responses to stress, preferred coping styles, and the types of situations or experiences that the person finds particularly stressful.

Research & general acceptance

There is a high level of interest among researchers in stress management and stress reduction programs and techniques, reflected in the fact that there were at least 429 clinical trials under way in early 2010. A number of different modalities of stress reduction are represented in these studies, ranging from cognitive-behavioral and relaxation training approaches to biofeedback, yoga, mindfulness meditation, Johrei, anger management, mantra repetition, self-hypnosis, and Healing Rhythms meditation.

Caregiver concerns

Caregivers of seniors or others in their care who are interested in stress management should consult with the person's doctor to make sure that the technique(s) chosen are taught or guided by certified or licensed instructors and are appropriate to the person's overall health status.

Resources

BOOKS

Greenberg, Jerrold S. *Comprehensive Stress Management*. 12th ed. New York: McGraw-Hill, 2010.

Meichenbaum, Donald. "Stress Inoculation Training: A Preventative and Treatment Approach." In *Principals and*

Practices of Stress Management. 3rd ed. New York: Guilford Press, 2007.

Olpin, Michael, and Margie Hesson. *Stress Management for Life: a Research-based Experiential Approach*. 2nd ed. Belmont, CA: Wadsworth/Cengage Learning, 2009.

Oxington, Kimberly V., ed. *Psychology of Stress*. New York: Nova Science Publishers, 2008.

Romas, John A., and Manoj Sharma. *Practical Stress Management: A Comprehensive Workbook for Managing Change and Promoting Health*. 5th ed. San Francisco, CA: Pearson Benjamin Cummings, 2009.

Selye, Hans. *The Stress of Life*. 2nd ed. New York: McGraw-Hill, 1978.

PERIODICALS

Agee, D., et al. "Comparing Brief Stress Management Courses in a Community Sample: Mindfulness Skills and Progressive Muscle Relaxation." *Explore* (NY) 5, no. 2 (March–April 2009): 104–09.

Esch, T., et al. "Mind/body Techniques for Physiological and Psychological Stress Reduction: Stress Management via Tai Chi Training—A Pilot Study." *Medical Science Monitor* 13, no. 11 (November 2007): CR488–CR497.

Lucini, D., et al. "Complementary Medicine for the Management of Chronic Stress: Superiority of Active versus Passive Techniques."*Journal of Hypertension* 27, no. 12 (December 2009): 2421–2428.

McKee, M.G. "Biofeedback: An Overview in the Context of Heart-brain Medicine." *Cleveland Clinic Journal of Medicine* 75 Suppl. 2 (March 2008): Suppl. 2, S31–S34.

Oman, D., et al. "Meditation Lowers Stress and Supports Forgiveness among College Students: A Randomized Controlled Trial." *Journal of American College Health* 56, no. 5 (March–April 2008): 569–78.

Ruzek, J., et al. "Cognitive-Behavioral Psychology: Implications for Disaster and Terrorism Response." *Prehospital and Disaster Medicine* 23, no. 5 (September–October 2008): 397–410.

Sierpina, Victor, John Astin, and James Giordano. "Mind-Body Therapies for Headache." *American Family Physician* 76, no. 10 (November 15, 2007): 1518–22. http://www.aafp.org/afp/2007/1115/p1518.html (accessed October 27, 2011).

Stetz, M.C., et al. "Stress, Mental Health, and Cognition: A Brief Review of Relationships and Countermeasures." *Aviation, Space, and Environmental Medicine* 78, Suppl. 1 (May 2007): B252–B260.

Wethington, H.R., et al. "The Effectiveness of Interventions to Reduce Psychological Harm from Traumatic Events among Children and Adolescents: A Systematic Review." *American Journal of Preventive Medicine* 35, no. 3 (September 2008): 287–313.

WEBSITES

American Institute of Stress. *Stress Reduction, Stress Relievers*. http://www.stress.org/topic-reduction.htm (accessed October 27, 2011).

Center for Mindfulness in Medicine, Health Care, and Society. *Stress Reduction Program*. http://www.umassmed.edu/uploadedFiles/cfm2/SRP_for_desktop_printing.pdf (accessed October 27, 2011).

Consortium for Research on Emotional Intelligence in Organizations. "Stress Management Training." http://www.eiconsortium.org/model_programs/stress_management_training.html (accessed October 27, 2011).

Health.com. "Autogenic Training." June 30, 2009. http://www.health.com/health/library/topic/0,ta7045spec_tp21225,00.html (accessed October 27, 2011).

Holmes, Thomas, and Richard Rahe. "The Holmes and Rahe Stress Scale: Understanding the Impact of Long-Term Stress." Mind Tools, Ltd. 1967. http://www.mindtools.com/pages/article/newTCS_82.htm (accessed October 27, 2011).

Mayo Clinic. "In-Depth: Stress Management." http://www.mayoclinic.com/health/stress-management/MY00435/TAB=indepth (accessed October 27, 2011).

ORGANIZATIONS

American Institute of Stress, 124 Park Ave., Yonkers, NY, 10703, (914) 963-1200, Fax: (914) 965-6267, stress125@optonline.net, http://www.stress.org.

Benson-Henry Institute for Mind/Body Medicine, 151 Merrimac St., 4th Fl., Boston, MA, 02114, (617) 643-6090, Fax: (617) 643-6077, mindbody@partners.org, http://www.massgeneral.org.

Center for Mindfulness in Medicine, Health Care, and Society, University of Massachusetts Medical School, 55 Lake Ave. N., Worcester, MA, 01655, (508) 856-2656, Fax: (508) 856-1977, mindfulness@umassmed.edu, http://www.umassmed.edu.

Rebecca J. Frey, PhD

Stroke

Definition

A stroke, also called a cerebral vascular accident (CVA), is the sudden death of cells in a specific area of the **brain** due to inadequate blood flow.

Demographics

According to the U.S. Centers for Disease Control and Prevention (CDC), stroke is one of the leading causes of death in the United States and is responsible for about 130,000 deaths each year. About 795,000 Americans have strokes each year, with 610,000 having a stroke for the first time and 185,000 having a second or third stroke. Of these cases, approximately 87% are ischemic strokes. The total cost of stroke to the American economy in 2010 was approximately $53.9 billion. By the year 2025, the annual number of strokes is expected to reach 1 million. According

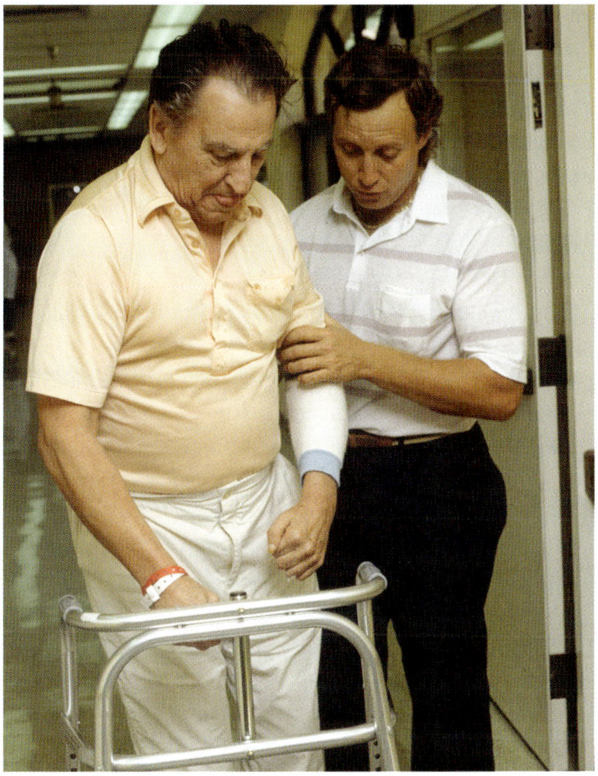

A male therapist works with a stroke victim. *(© Custom Medical Stock Photo, Inc. Reproduced by permission.)*

to the National Stroke Association, more than 7 million people in the United States are stroke survivors. Worldwide, the World Health Organization estimates that 15 million people suffer a stroke each year, resulting in 5 million deaths and 5 million permanently disabled survivors.

About 50,000 Americans have a transient ischemic attack (TIA) in an average year; of this group, 35% will have a severe stroke at some point in the future.

Strokes can affect people in any age group; however, the risk increases sharply in people over 55 years of age. Seventy-five percent of all strokes in Canada and the United States occur in people over 64. Men are 1.25 times more likely to have strokes than women; however, women are more likely to die of stroke because they are usually older when they have their first stroke.

Strokes in children are rare—about 6 cases per 100,000 children per year in North America. About a third of these cases are in newborns.

African Americans have an increased risk of stroke compared to other racial and ethnic groups in the United States, and they are also more likely to suffer a stroke at younger ages. Hispanics are at lesser risk of stroke than African Americans, but they also tend to have strokes at relatively young ages. African Americans between the ages of 45 and 55 die from stroke 4–5 times more often that Caucasians in the same age group.

Description

A stroke occurs when blood flow is interrupted to a part of the brain, either when an artery bursts or becomes closed when a blood clot lodges in it. Blood circulation to the area of the brain served by that artery stops at the point of disturbance, and the brain tissue beyond that is damaged or dies. (Brain cells need blood to supply oxygen and nutrients and to remove waste products.) Depending on the region of the brain affected, a stroke can cause paralysis, loss of vision, speech impairment, memory loss and reasoning ability, coma, or death. The effects of a stroke are determined by how much damage occurs, and which portion of the brain is affected.

About a third of all strokes are preceded by transient ischemic attacks (TIAs), or mini-strokes, that temporarily interrupt blood flow to the brain. While TIAs cause similar symptoms (such as sudden vision loss or temporary weakness in a limb), they abate much more quickly than full-fledged strokes, usually within a few hours and sometimes as quickly as a few minutes.

Stroke is a medical emergency requiring immediate treatment. Prompt treatment improves the chances of survival and increases the degree of recovery that may be expected. A person who may have suffered a stroke should be seen in a hospital emergency room without delay. Treatment to break up a blood clot, the major cause of stroke, must begin within three hours of the stroke to be most effective. Improved medical treatment of all types of stroke has resulted in a dramatic decline in death rates in recent decades. In 1950, 9 in 10 stroke victims died, compared to slightly less than 1 in 3 today. However, about two-thirds of stroke survivors will have disabilities ranging from moderate to severe.

Risk factors

Risk factors for stroke involve:

- Age and sex—the risk of stroke increases with age, doubling for each decade after age 55. Men are more likely to have a stroke than women.
- Heredity—people with a family history of stroke have an increased risk of stroke themselves. In addition, African Americans, Asians, and Hispanics all have higher rates of stroke than whites, related partly to higher blood pressure.
- Diseases—people with diabetes, heart disease (especially atrial fibrillation), high blood pressure, or prior

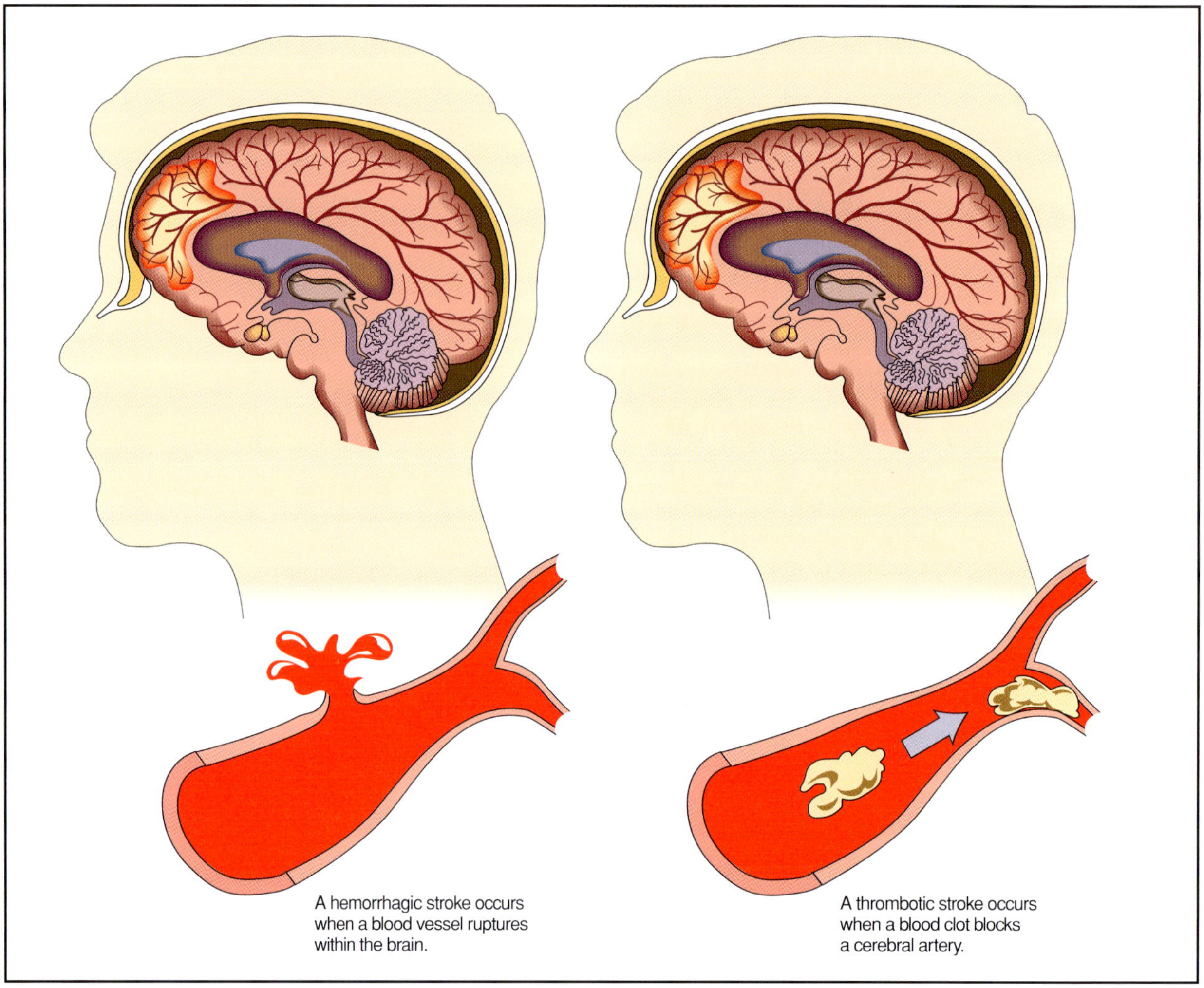

Illustration of a hemorrhagic and a thrombotic stroke. *(Illustration by Hans & Cassady.)*

stroke are at greater risk for stroke. Patients with one or more TIAs have ten times the risk.

- Other medical conditions—stroke risk increases with obesity, high blood cholesterol, or high red blood cell count.
- Lifestyle choices—stroke risk increases with cigarette smoking (especially if combined with the use of oral contraceptives), a sedentary lifestyle, alcohol consumption above two drinks per day, and/or the use of cocaine or intravenous drugs.

Causes and symptoms

Causes

There are four main types of stroke: cerebral thrombosis, cerebral embolism, subarachnoid hemorrhage, and intracerebral hemorrhage. Cerebral thrombosis and cerebral embolism, known as ischemic strokes, are caused by blood clots that block an artery supplying the brain, either in the brain itself or in the neck. They account for 70%–80% of all strokes. Subarachnoid hemorrhage and intracerebral hemorrhage are hemorrhagic strokes, which occur when a blood vessel bursts around or in the brain, either from **trauma** or excess internal pressure. Hypertension (high blood pressure) and atherosclerosis are usually contributing factors in these types of strokes.

CEREBRAL THROMBOSIS. Cerebral thrombosis, the most common type of stroke, occurs when a blood clot, or thrombus, forms within the brain itself, blocking blood flow through the affected vessel. This is usually due to atherosclerosis (hardening) of brain arteries, caused by a buildup of fatty deposits inside the blood vessels. Cerebral thrombosis occurs most often at night or early in the morning, and is often preceded by a TIA. Recognizing the occurrence of a TIA and seeking immediate treatment is an important step in stroke prevention.

CEREBRAL EMBOLISM. Cerebral embolism occurs when a blood clot from elsewhere in the circulatory system breaks free. If it becomes lodged in an artery supplying the brain, either in the brain or in the neck, it can cause a stroke. The most common cause of cerebral embolism is atrial fibrillation, which occurs when the upper chambers (atria) of the heart beat weakly and rapidly, instead of slowly and steadily. Blood within the atria does not empty completely, and may form clots that can then break off and enter the circulation. Atrial fibrillation is a factor in about 15% of all strokes, but this risk can be dramatically reduced with daily use of anticoagulant medication (such as Heparin or Coumadin).

SUBARACHNOID HEMORRHAGE. In this type of stroke, blood spills into the subarachnoid space between the brain and cranium. As fluid builds up, pressure on the brain increases, impairing its function. Hypertension is a frequent cause of these types of stroke, but vessels with preexisting defects, such as an aneurysm, are also at risk for rupture. Aneurysms are most likely to burst when blood pressure is highest, and controlling blood pressure is an important preventive strategy. Subarachnoid hemorrhages account for about 7% of all strokes.

INTRACEREBRAL HEMORRHAGE. Representing about 10% of all strokes, intracerebral hemorrhage affects vessels and tissue within the brain itself. As with subarachnoid hemorrhage, bleeding deprives affected tissues of blood supply, and the accumulation of fluid within the inflexible skull creates pressure on the brain that can quickly become fatal. Despite this, recovery may be more complete for a person who survives hemorrhage than for one who survives a clot, because the effects of blood deprivation are usually not as severe.

Symptoms

Knowing the symptoms of stroke is as important as knowing those of a heart attack. Patients with stroke symptoms should seek emergency treatment without delay, which may mean dialing 911 rather than their family physician. Specific symptoms of a stroke depend on the type, but all types share some characteristics in common.

An embolic stroke usually comes on quite suddenly and is intense right from the start, while symptoms of a thrombotic stroke come on more gradually. Symptoms for these ischemic strokes may include:

- blurring or decreased vision in one or both eyes
- severe headache, often described as "the worst headache of my life"
- weakness, numbness, or paralysis of the face, arm, or leg, usually confined to one side of the body
- dizziness, loss of balance or coordination, especially when combined with other symptoms

Hemorrhagic strokes are somewhat different. An intracranial hemorrhage exhibits any or all of the following symptoms:

- loss of consciousness
- altered mental state
- seizure
- vomiting or severe nausea
- extreme hypertension
- weakness, numbness, or paralysis, especially on one side of the body
- sudden, severe headache

Symptoms of a subarachnoid hemorrhage include:

- severe headache that begins suddenly
- nausea or vomiting
- stiff neck
- light intolerance
- loss of consciousness

In addition, the American Stroke Association has a quick symptom checklist called "Give Me 5" that can be used by a friend, relative, coworker, or caregiver, as well as by a person who thinks they may be having a stroke:

- Walk: Is the person having trouble with balance or coordination?
- Talk: Is speech difficult or slurred? Is the person's face drooping?
- Reach: Is one side of the body weak or numb?
- See: Is vision partly or entirely lost?
- Feel: Does the person have a sudden severe headache with no obvious cause?

If any of these symptoms are observed and stroke is suspected, call 911 immediately.

Diagnosis

Diagnosing a stroke begins with a careful medical history, especially concerning the onset and distribution of symptoms and presence of risk factors; in this way, other possible causes are excluded. The next step is a complete physical and neurological examination to rule out the possibility that the patient's symptoms are being caused by a brain tumor. The examination has several purposes: checking the patient's airway, breathing, and circulation; identifying any neurological deficits; identifying the potential cause(s) of the stroke; and identifying any comorbid conditions the patient may have. The neurologist may use the National Institutes of Health Stroke Scale (NIHSS), which is a checklist that allows the doctor to record the patient's level of consciousness; visual function; ability to move; ability to feel sensations; ability to move the facial muscles; and ability to talk.

Once stroke is suspected, imaging technology is used to determine what type the patient has suffered—a critical distinction that guides therapy. A noncontrast **computed tomography** scan (CT scan) can reliably identify hemorrhagic strokes, caused by uncontrolled bleeding in the brain. **Magnetic resonance imaging** (MRI), on the other hand, particularly diffusion-weighted imaging, can detect ischemic strokes, caused by blood clots, earlier and more reliably than CT scanning.

Blood and urine tests are also run to look for possible abnormalities. Other investigations that may be performed to guide treatment include electrocardiogram, angiography, ultrasound, and electroencephalogram.

Treatment

When brain cells die during a stroke, they release toxic chemicals that can trigger a chain reaction that can injure or kill other nearby cells. Damage from stroke may be significantly reduced by emergency treatment, a significant factor in how fully a patient will recover.

Emergency treatment

Emergency treatment of an ischemic stroke attempts to dissolve the clot. This "thrombolytic therapy" is performed most often with tissue plasminogen activator (t-PA), which must be administered within three hours of the stroke event. (Patients who awaken with stroke symptoms are ineligible for this type of therapy, since the time of onset cannot be reliably determined.) t-PA therapy has been shown to improve recovery and decrease long-term disability in patients. It carries a 6.4% risk of inducing a cerebral hemorrhage, however, and is not appropriate for patients with bleeding disorders, very high blood pressure, known aneurysms, any evidence of intracranial hemorrhage, or incidence of stroke, head trauma, or intracranial surgery within the past three months. Patients with clot-related stroke who are ineligible for t-PA treatment may be treated with heparin or other blood thinners, or with aspirin or other anticlotting agents in some cases.

Emergency treatment of hemorrhagic stroke is aimed at controlling intracranial pressure that accompanies these types of strokes. New surgical techniques can effectively relieve the pressure, especially when begun soon after the stroke event occurs. Surgery for hemorrhage due to aneurysm may be performed if the aneurysm is close enough to the cranial surface to allow access. Ruptured vessels are closed off to prevent rebleeding. For aneurysms that are difficult to reach surgically, endovascular treatment, in which a catheter is guided from a larger artery up into the brain to reach the aneurysm, may be effective. Small coils of wire are discharged into the aneurysm, which plug it up and block off blood flow from the main artery.

Rehabilitation

Rehabilitation refers to a comprehensive program designed to regain as much function as possible and compensate for permanent losses. Approximately 10% of stroke survivors recover without any significant disability and are able to function independently. Another 10% are so severely affected that they must remain institutionalized for severe disability. The remaining 80% can return home with appropriate therapy, training, support, and care.

Rehabilitation is coordinated by a team of medical professionals and may include the services of a neurologist, a physician who specializes in rehabilitation medicine, a physical therapist, an occupational therapist, a speech-language pathologist, a nutritionist, a mental health professional, and a social worker. Rehabilitation services may be provided in an acute care hospital, rehabilitation hospital, long-term care facility, outpatient clinic, or at home.

The rehabilitation program is based on the patient's individual deficits and strengths. Strokes on the left side of the brain primarily affect the right half of the body, and vice versa. In addition, in left brain–dominant people, who constitute a significant majority of the population, left-brain strokes usually lead to speech and language deficits, while right-brain strokes may affect spatial perception. Patients with right-brain strokes may also deny their illness, neglect the affected side of their body, and behave impulsively.

Rehabilitation may be complicated by cognitive losses, including diminished ability to understand and follow directions. Poor results are more likely in patients whose strokes left them with significant or prolonged cognitive changes, sensory losses, language deficits, or incontinence.

PREVENTING COMPLICATIONS. Rehabilitation begins with prevention of medical complications, including stroke recurrence, using many of the same measures used to prevent stroke, such as **smoking cessation** and getting hypertension under control.

One of the most common medical complications following stroke is deep venous thrombosis, in which a clot forms within a limb immobilized by paralysis. Clots can also become lodged in an artery feeding the lungs, a condition called pulmonary embolism, that is a common cause of death in the weeks following a stroke. Resuming activity within a day or two after the stroke is an important preventive measure, along with use of elastic

KEY TERMS

Aneurysm—A symptomless bulging of a weak arterial wall that can rupture, leading to stroke.

Angiography—A procedure in which a contrast medium is injected into the bloodstream (through an artery in the neck) and its progress through the brain is tracked. This illustrates where a blockage or hemorrhage has occurred.

Anticoagulant—A medication (such as warfarin [Coumadin], or Heparin) that decreases the blood's clotting ability preventing the formation of new clots. Although anticoagulants will not dissolve existing clots, they can stop them from getting larger. These drugs are commonly called blood thinners.

Atrial fibrillation—A disorder in which the upper chambers (atria) of the heart do not completely empty with each contraction (heartbeat). This can allow blood clots to form and is associated with a higher risk of stroke.

Electrocardiogram—(EKG) A test that measures the electrical activity of the heart as it beats. An abnormal EKG can indicate possible cardiac disease.

Electroencephalogram—(EEG) A test that measures the electrical activity of the brain by means of electrodes placed on the scalp or on or in the brain itself. It may be used to determine whether or not a stroke victim has had a seizure.

Hypertension—High blood pressure, often brought on by smoking, obesity, or other causes; one of the major causes of strokes.

Pressure ulcers—Also known as pressure sores or bed sores, these can develop in stroke patients who are unable to move. If not treated properly, they can become infected.

Tissue plasminogen activator (tPA)—A drug that is sometimes given to patients within three hours of a stroke to dissolve blood clots within the brain; also used to treat heart attack victims.

Ultrasound—A noninvasive test in which high-frequency sound waves are reflected off a patient's internal organs allowing them to be viewed. In stroke victims, a cardiac ultrasound, or echocardiogram, allows the beating heart to be examined.

stockings on the lower limbs. Drugs that prevent clotting may also be given, including intravenous heparin and oral warfarin.

Weakness and loss of coordination of the swallowing muscles may impair swallowing (dysphagia), and allow food to enter the lower airway. This may lead to aspiration pneumonia, another common cause of death shortly after a stroke. Dysphagia may be treated with retraining exercises and temporary use of pureed foods.

Other medical complications include urinary tract infections, pressure ulcers, falls, and **seizures**. **Depression** occurs in 30–60% of stroke patients; its severity is usually related to the level of permanent functional impairment. Depression may be treated with **antidepressants** and **psychotherapy**.

TYPES OF REHABILITATIVE THERAPY. Brain tissue that dies in a stroke cannot regenerate. In some cases, however, rehabilitation training can help other brain regions perform the same functions of that tissue. In other cases, compensatory actions may be developed to replace lost abilities.

Physical therapy is used to maintain and restore range of motion and strength in affected limbs, and to maximize mobility in walking, wheelchair use, and transferring (from wheelchair to toilet or from standing to sitting, for instance). The physical therapist advises patients on mobility aids such as wheelchairs, braces, and canes. In the recovery period, a stroke patient may develop muscle spasticity and contractures (abnormal muscle contractions) that can be treated with a combination of stretching and splinting.

Occupational therapy improves self-care skills, such as feeding, bathing, and dressing, and helps develop effective compensatory strategies and devices for activities of daily living. A speech-language pathologist focuses on communication and swallowing skills. When dysphagia is a problem, a nutritionist can advise alternative meals that provide adequate **nutrition**.

Psychological therapy can help treat depression or loss of thinking (cognitive) skills. A social worker may help coordinate services and ease the transition out of the hospital back into the home. Both **social workers** and mental health professionals help counsel the patient and family during the difficult rehabilitation period. Caring for a person affected with stroke requires a new set of skills and adaptation to new demands and limitations. Home caregivers may develop **stress**, anxiety, and depression—caring for the caregiver is an important part of the overall stroke treatment program. **Support groups** can provide an important source of information, advice, and comfort for stroke patients and caregivers; joining one can be an important step in the rehabilitation process.

Prognosis

The prognosis of stroke depends on the person's age, the type and location of the stroke, and the amount of time elapsed between **diagnosis** and treatment. In general, patients with ischemic stroke have a better prognosis than those with hemorrhagic stroke. In one study in the Boston area, 19% of patients with ischemic stroke died within the first 30 days of the attack compared to 35% with hemorrhagic stroke.

Stroke is fatal for about 26% of white males, 51% of African American males, 39% of white females, and 39% of African American females. However, recent research suggests that African Americans may have a better chance of survival following acute ischemic stroke. Those who do survive a stroke may be left with significant deficits. Emergency treatment and comprehensive rehabilitation can significantly improve both survival and recovery. One recent study found that treating stroke survivors with certain antidepressant medications, even if they were not depressed, could increase their chances of living longer. People who received the treatment were less likely to die from cardiovascular events than those who did not receive antidepressant drugs.

About 10% of stroke patients recover enough function to live independently without help; another 50% can remain at home with outside assistance. The remaining 40% require long-term care in a nursing home.

Stroke in children can be devastating. Between 20% and 35% of newborns who survive a stroke will go on to have a second stroke. More than 66% of older children who suffer strokes will have cognitive deficits, seizures, behavioral problems, changes in personality, or physical disabilities. Unlike adult survivors, children who survive strokes may develop intellectual disabilities, epilepsy, or cerebral palsy.

Prevention

The risk of stroke can be reduced by quitting smoking, controlling blood pressure, exercising regularly, maintaining a healthy weight, avoiding excessive alcohol consumption, getting regular checkups, and following physician advice regarding diet and medications.

Use of high-estrogen dose oral contraceptives increase the chances for developing stroke, particularly in women who smoke and/or who are over 35. Currently, there are low-estrogen dose oral contraceptives, for which a clear relationship with stroke development is unclear.

Treatment of atrial fibrillation may also significantly reduce the risk of stroke. Preventive anticoagulant therapy may benefit those with untreated atrial fibrillation. Warfarin (Coumadin) has proven to be more effective than aspirin for those with higher risk. Warfarin is, however, complicated to use because it interacts with a large number of other drugs and requires frequent monitoring by the patient's physician.

Screening for aneurysms may be an effective preventive measure in those with a family history of aneurysms or autosomal polycystic kidney disease, which tends to be associated with aneurysms.

People with no previous history of stroke may be given certain drugs as preventive measures. These drugs include statins (drugs that lower blood cholesterol levels) and platelet antiaggregants (medications intended to prevent platelets in the blood from forming clumps that may lead to clots).

A recent innovation is the use of computer technology to allow stroke experts in one hospital to evaluate and diagnose a patient in another hospital that might not have a specialist available. Called TeleStroke, the network allows a patient to be evaluated for ischemic stroke within the three-hour time limit for the effective use of tPA. More recently, stroke specialists have proposed an updated version of TeleStroke called TeleStroke 2.0, which would be a Web-based system that could be accessed from any desktop or laptop computer, not just those connected to videoconferencing equipment.

Resources

BOOKS

American Heart Association. *American Heart Association Family Guide to Stroke Treatment, Recovery, and Prevention*. New York: Clarkson Potter, 1996.

Duthie, Edmund H., Jr., and Paul Katz. *Practice of Geriatrics*. 3rd ed. Philadelphia: W. B. Saunders, 2007.

Goetz, Christopher G. *Textbook of Clinical Neurology*. Philadelphia: W. B. Saunders Company, 2003.

McEwen, Mark. *Change in the Weather: Life after Stroke*. New York: Gotham Books, 2008.

Warlow, C. P., et al. *Stroke: A Practical Guide to Management*. Boston: Wiley-Blackwell, 2008.

Williams, Olajide. *Stroke Diaries: A Guide for Survivors and Their Families*. New York: Oxford University Press, 2010.

PERIODICALS

Alvarez-Sabin, J., et al. "Therapeutic Interventions and Success in Risk Factor Control for Secondary Prevention of Stroke." *Journal of Stroke and Cerebrovascular Diseases* 18, no. 6 (November–December 2009): 460–65.

Krishnan, K. Ranga Rama. "Depression as a Contributing Factor in Cerebrovascular Disease." *American Heart Journal* 140, no. 4 Suppl. (October 2000): 70–76.

Mathews, M.S., et al. "Safety, Effectiveness, and Practicality of Endovascular Therapy within the First 3 Hours of Acute Ischemic Stroke Onset." *Neurosurgery* 65, no. 5 (November 2009): 860–65.

Xian, Ying, et al. "Racial Differences in Mortality Among Patients with Acute Ischemic Stroke: An Observational Study." *Annals of Internal Medicine* 154, no. 3 (January 2011): 152–159.

WEBSITES

Jausch, Edward C. "Acute Management of Stroke." Medscape Reference. http://emedicine.medscape.com/article/1159752-overview (accessed October 27, 2011).

Mayo Clinic. "Stroke." July 2010. http://www.mayoclinic.com/health/stroke/DS00150 (accessed October 27, 2011).

U.S. Centers for Disease Control and Prevention."Stroke." http://www.cdc.gov/stroke/index.htm (accessed October 27, 2011).

U.S. National Institute of Neurological Disorders and Stroke. "Stroke: Hope through Research." http://www.ninds.nih.gov/disorders/stroke/detail_stroke.htm (accessed October 27, 2011).

ORGANIZATIONS

American Academy of Neurology, 1080 Montreal Ave., St. Paul, MN, 55116, (651) 695-2717, (800) 879-1960, Fax: (651) 879-2791, memberservices@aan.com, http://www.aan.com.

American Stroke Association, 7272 Greenville Ave., Dallas, TX, 75231, (800) 242-8721, http://www.heart.org.

Brain Aneurysm Foundation, 269 Hanover St., Bldg. 3, Hanover, MA, 02339, (781) 826-5556, Fax: (781) 826-5566, office@bafound.org, http://www.bafound.org.

National Heart, Lung, and Blood Institute, Health Information Center, PO Box 30105, Bethesda, MD, 20824-0105, (301) 592-8573; TTY: (240) 629-3255, Fax: (240) 629-3246, nhlbiinfo@nhlbi.nih.gov, http://www.nhlbi.nih.gov.

National Institute of Neurological Disorders and Stroke, PO Box 5801, Bethesda, MD, 20824, (301) 496-5751; TTY: (301) 468-5981, (800) 352-9424, http://www.ninds.nih.gov.

National Stroke Association, 9707 E Easter Ln., Ste. B, Centennial, CO, 80112, (800) 787-6537, Fax: (303) 649-1328, Info@stroke.org, http://www.stroke.org.

Laith Farid Gulli, M.D.
Bilal Nasser, M.D.

Structured Clinical Interview for DSM-IV

Definition

The Structured Clinical Interview for *DSM-IV* (SCID) is the generic term for a series of **psychological assessment** instruments used by clinicians and researchers to make diagnoses of mental disorders listed in the ***Diagnostic and Statistical Manual of Mental Disorders***, fourth edition (*DSM-IV*), produced by the **American Psychiatric Association**. Its primary authors are Michael First and Robert L. Spitzer. Dr. Spitzer was the primary author of an earlier version of the SCID created in 1990 for the third edition of the *DSM* (*DSM-III*).

Purpose

The primary purpose of the SCID is the differential **diagnosis** of mental disorders according to *DSM-IV* categories. There are two parts to the SCID. The choice of which part is administered depends on what general type of disorder is suspected in the patient. The SCID-I is designed for use by clinicians to accurately and consistently diagnose 37 of the most frequently seen *DSM-IV* Axis I clinical disorders. The disorders fall into the following categories:

- disorders usually first diagnosed in infancy, childhood, or adolescence (excluding intellectual disability)
- delirium, dementia, and amnestic and other cognitive disorders
- mental disorders due to a general medical condition
- substance-related disorders
- schizophrenia and other psychotic disorders
- mood disorders
- anxiety disorders
- somatoform disorders
- factitious disorders
- dissociative disorders
- sexual and gender identity disorders
- eating disorders
- sleep disorders
- impulse-control disorders not elsewhere classified
- adjustment disorders
- other conditions that may be a focus of clinical attention

The SCID-II is designed to measure disorders that are part of Axis II (**personality disorders**) of the *DSM-IV*. These are:

- paranoid personality disorder
- schizoid personality disorder
- schizotypal personality disorder
- antisocial personality disorder
- borderline personality disorder
- histrionic personality disorder
- narcissistic personality disorder

KEY TERMS

Reliability—The ability of a psychological test or diagnostic instrument to consistently measure the concept or entity that it has been designed to measure.

Structured interview—A type of interview often used by researchers to gather data, in which subjects are asked a series of standardized questions in the same order with the same wording. The questions are usually closed-ended (the choice of answers is fixed in advance), although some structured interviews include a few open-ended questions.

Validity—The ability of a test or instrument to measure accurately what it is supposed to measure.

- avoidant personality disorder dependent personality disorder
- obsessive-compulsive personality disorder
- personality disorder not otherwise specified

In addition, the SCID-II is designed to diagnose depressive personality disorder, passive-aggressive personality disorder, and **dependent personality disorder**. Neither the SCID-I nor the SCID-II diagnoses disorders included on Axis III (general medical conditions) or Axis IV (psychosocial and environmental problems) as defined in *DSM-IV*.

Description

The SCID is designed to help clinicians and researchers consistently and accurately diagnose mental disorders and to avoid making a premature diagnosis based on insufficient data or preconceived notions. The SCID uses a standard set of questions that are asked in patient interviews. The diagnosis is made on the basis of the answers to these questions.

The SCID has been translated into numerous other languages, including Chinese (Mandarin), Danish, Dutch, French, German, Greek, Hebrew, Italian, Persian, Portuguese, Romanian, Russian, Spanish, Swedish, and Turkish. Depending on the complexity of the patient's psychiatric history and his or her ability to clearly describe episodes and symptoms, it takes approximately one to two hours to complete the SCID-I and 30 minutes to an hour to complete the SCID-II. These times tend to be shorter than for other comprehensive assessment instruments of this type.

A version of the SCID for use with children-the KID-SCID-was developed by Dr. Fred Matzner in 1993 and is available to researchers on request from Dr. Matzner at 718-920-9362. This version includes most of the disorders included on the SCID-I and SCID-II (with questions rewritten for applicability to children) as well as many childhood disorders, including disruptive behavior disorders and separation **anxiety disorders**. The author expects to add eating disorders and **Tourette syndrome** to the KID-SCID at some point in the future. The KID-SCID has not been formally published as of mid-2011.

Reliability and validity

When determining whether a psychological assessment instrument such as the SCID is useful for the purpose for which it is designed, two factors should be considered: the instrument's reliability and its validity. Reliability is the ability of the assessment instrument to consistently measure the idea or concept it has been designed to measure. Validity is the ability of the instrument to accurately measure what it is intended to measure. Unless a test is reliable, it cannot be valid.

Research studies investigating the reliability of the SCID-I and the SCID-II have shown wide variation in the reliability of the SCID, ranging from poor to good. These findings may be due to such factors as the varying designs of research studies, level of training of the individuals administering the SCID, and the types of disorders represented in those interviewed.

To determine the validity of such assessment instruments as the SCID, researchers typically look at the agreement between diagnoses made using the instrument and diagnoses using an objective standard. Unfortunately, such an objective standard for mental disorders has yet to be developed. However, given the fact that the reliability of the SCID is not consistent, the validity of the instrument must also be called into question.

Versions of the SCID

There are several different versions of the SCID:

- Clinician version (SCID-CV). The clinician version of the SCID is a streamlined form of the research version of the SCID that omits some disorders and covers the remainder in less detail than the research version.
- Research version (SCID-I-RV). This is the standard version of the SCID and comes in three forms: a patient edition (SCID-I-RV/P), for use with subjects who are psychiatric patients; an abridged patient version that includes screening for psychotic disorders; and a nonpatient edition (SCID-I-RV/NP) for use

with subjects who are not psychiatric patients (community samples, family studies, etc.)

- Clinical trials version (SCID-CT). The SCID-CT is a streamlined form of the research version designed for use in clinical trials, particularly trials of medications for mental disorders. There are forms of the SCID-CT available to test drugs for major depressive disorder, bipolar disorder, schizophrenia, and generalized anxiety disorder.
- Electronic versions. There are computer-assisted versions of the SCID-CV that require a clinician to be present while the subject answers the questions on a computer. A computer-assisted version of the SCID-I-RV was in development as of 2011.

A series of revisions and fixes of the various versions of the SCID has been posted on the instrument's website. The latest entry, made in January 2010, covers all changes made since October 2008. The details are available at http://cpmcnet.columbia.edu/dept/scid/revisions/jan10.html.

There was no information available as of 2011 about whether the SCID will be updated or altered for the forthcoming fifth edition of *DSM* (*DSM-5*), scheduled for publication in 2013.

Preparation

There is no specific preparation required on the patient or research subject's part for receiving the SCID.

Aftercare

There is no aftercare necessary for the SCID.

Risks

The only significant risk regarding the SCID is receiving the interview from an untrained or unqualified interviewer. While most interviewers who administer the SCID are physicians, psychologists, or other mental health professionals with advanced degrees who have been trained to use the instrument, in some cases, research assistants without clinical experience have been trained to administer the SCID. The less clinical experience the potential interviewer has had, the longer the training period required. According to the authors of the SCID, at least 20 hours of training are required to learn how to administer the instrument.

Results

While the SCID is used in many diagnostic situations, it is not the only assessment instrument available. Other instruments include the Personality Disorder Examination, Structured Clinical Interview for DSM-IV Personality, Diagnostic Interview for Personality Disorders, Brief Psychiatric Rating Scale, Composite International Diagnostic Interview, and Present State Examination. Researchers and clinicians should choose which assessment instrument to use, based on what they are trying to measure and the comparative strengths and weaknesses of the instruments. Note, however, that the lack of objective standards against which to measure validity affects the veracity of the results from all of these instruments, and the problems attendant with using human interviewers affect all interview techniques.

Some clinicians have found that the **depression** module of the SCID has drawbacks for use with depressed patients in that they are likely to leave some questions unanswered, leading to a missed diagnosis.

QUESTIONS TO ASK YOUR DOCTOR

- What is your opinion of the SCID? Is it a reliable diagnostic test?
- Have you ever administered the SCID?

Resources

BOOKS

American Psychiatric Association. *Diagnostic and Statistical Manual of Mental Disorders*. 4th ed., Text rev. Washington, DC: American Psychiatric Association, 2000.

Benjamin, Lorna Smith, and Michael B. First. *Structured Clinical Interview for DSM-IV Axis II Personality Disorders (SCID-II), User's Guide*. Arlington, VA: American Psychiatric Publishing, 1997.

First, Michael B., ed. *Standardized Evaluation in Clinical Practice*. Washington, DC: American Psychiatric Publishing, 2003.

First, Michael B., et al. *Structured Clinical Interview for DSM-IV Axis I Disorders (SCID-I), Clinician Version, User's Guide*. Arlington, VA: American Psychiatric Publishing, 1997.

First, Michael B., and Alan Tasman. *Clinical Guide to the Diagnosis and Treatment of Mental Disorders*. Hoboken, NJ: Wiley, 2006.

Kupfer, David J., Michael B. First, and Darrel A. Regier, eds. *A Research Agenda for DSM-V*. Washington, DC: American Psychiatric Association, 2002.

Phillips, Katharine A., Michael B. First, and Harold Alan Pincus, eds. *Advancing DSM: Dilemmas in Psychiatric Diagnosis*. Washington, DC: American Psychiatric Association, 2003.

VandenBos, Gary R., ed. *APA Dictionary of Psychology.* Washington, DC: American Psychological Association, 2006.

PERIODICALS

Galione, J., and M. Zimmerman. "A Comparison of Depressed Patients with and without Borderline Personality Disorder: Implications for Interpreting Studies of the Validity of the Bipolar Spectrum." *Journal of Personality Disorders* 24 (December 2010): 763–772.

Gjerdingen, D., et al. "Problems with a Diagnostic Depression Interview in a Postpartum Depression Trial." *Journal of the American Board of Family Medicine* 24 (March-April 2011): 187–193.

Lobbestael, J., et al. "Inter-rater Reliability of the Structured Clinical Interview for DSM-IV Axis I Disorders (SCID I) and Axis II Disorders (SCID II)." *Clinical Psychology and Psychotherapy* 18 (January 2011): 75–79.

Sharifi, V., et al. "A Persian Translation of the Structured Clinical Interview for Diagnostic and Statistical Manual of Mental Disorders, Fourth Edition: Psychometric Properties." *Comprehensive Psychiatry* 50 (January 2009): 86–91.

Torres, L.R., et al. "Diagnosing Co-occurring Substance-related Disorders: Agreement between SCID, Hispanic Clinicians, and Non-Hispanic Clinicians." *Journal of Clinical Psychiatry* 68 (November 2007): 1655–1662.

WEBSITES

American Psychiatric Association. DSM-5 Development Home Page. http://www.dsm5.org/Pages/Default.aspx (accessed May 12, 2011).

SCID. "SCID-Frequently Asked Questions." http://www.scid4.org/faq/scidfaq.html (accessed May 17, 2011).

ORGANIZATIONS

American Psychiatric Association (APA), 1000 Wilson Blvd., Ste. 1825, Arlington, VA, 22209-3901, (703) 907-7300, apa@psych.org, http://www.psych.org.

SCID, c/o Biometrics Research Department, Columbia University at NYSPI, 1051 Riverside Dr., Unit 60, New York, NY, 10032, (212) 543-5524, Fax: (212) 543-5525, scid4@columbia.edu, http://www.scid4.org.

Ruth A. Wienclaw, Ph.D.
Rebecca J. Frey, Ph.D.

Stuttering

Definition

There is no standard definition of stuttering (sometimes called "stammering"), but most attempt to define stuttering as blockages, discoordination, or fragmentations of the forward flow of speech (fluency). These stoppages, referred to as "disfluencies," are often excessive and characterized by specific types, such as repetitions of sounds and syllables, prolongation of sounds, and blockages of airflow. Individuals who stutter are often aware of their stuttering and feel a loss of control when they are disfluent. Both children and adults who stutter expend an excessive amount of physical and mental energy when speaking. Older children and adults who stutter show myriad negative reactive behaviors, feelings, and attitudes. These behaviors, referred to as "secondary behaviors," make the disorder more severe and difficult.

Demographics

Stuttering is a relatively low-prevalence disorder. According to the National Institute on Deafness and Other Communication Disorders (NIDCD), about three million people in the United States stuttered as of 2011, or about 1% of the population. Worldwide estimates total approximately 60 million. This figure differs from incidence, or the number of individuals who have been diagnosed with stuttering at some point in their lives. Research suggests that roughly 5% of the U.S. population has been diagnosed with a stuttering disorder at some point during their lifespan. This difference suggests that a significant number of individuals who stutter develop through or outgrow the problem.

Stuttering is most common in children between the ages of two and five, the period when they are learning to speak. The majority of these children will eventually stop stuttering. In adults, approximately three times as many men stutter as women. The sex ratio seems to be lower in early childhood, with a similar number of girls and boys stuttering. The ratio of boys to girls appears to increase as children become older. This phenomenon suggests that males are more likely to continue to stutter than females.

Description

Stuttering is a confusing and often misunderstood developmental speech and language disorder. Before discussing stuttering, it is important to understand the concepts of speech fluency and disfluency. Fluency is generally described as the forward flow of speech. For most speakers, fluent speech is easy and effortless. It is free of any interruptions, blockages, or fragmentations. Disfluency is defined as a breakdown or blockage in fluency. For all speakers, some occurrence of disfluency is normal. For example, people may insert short sounds or words, referred to as "interjections" or "fillers" when speaking; examples include "um," "like," or "uh." Also, speakers might repeat phrases, revise words or phrases, or sometimes repeat whole words for the purpose of clarification. For young children, disfluency is a part of the normal development of speech and language, especially during the preschool years (between the ages of two and five years).

The occurrence of disfluency is not the same as stuttering, though stuttered speech is characterized by an excessive amount of disfluency. The disfluencies produced by people who stutter will often be similar to those in the speech of individuals who do not stutter; however, certain types of disfluent behavior are likely to appear only in the speech of people who stutter. These disfluencies are sound and syllable repetitions (e.g., ca- ca-ca-cat), sound prolongations (e.g., "sssss–salad," "ffffff-fish"), and complete blockages of airflow. These behaviors, often referred to as "stuttering-type disfluencies," distinguish stuttered speech from nonstuttered speech.

Stuttering behaviors can develop and vary throughout the lifespan. Sometimes, children will experience periods when stuttering appears to go away for a time, only to return in a more severe pattern. Many children (estimates range between 50% and 80%) will develop normal fluency after periods of stuttering. For those who continue to stutter during late childhood, adolescence, and into adulthood, stuttering can become a chronic problem. Lifelong efforts are needed to cope successfully with the behavior.

Unlike speakers who do not stutter, most people who stutter react negatively to their disfluencies. A person may develop a number of physical reactions, including tension of the muscles involved in speech (in the tongue, jaw, lips, or chest, for example) and tension in muscles not related to speech (such as shoulders, limbs, and forehead). In addition to these physiological reactions, people who stutter often have negative emotional reactions to the disorder. Among the emotions reported by people who stutter are embarrassment, guilt, and frustration. Many who stutter develop a number of negative attitudes and beliefs regarding themselves and speaking, because of their stuttering. These may be negative attitudes and beliefs in certain speaking situations, with people with whom they interact, and in their own abilities. These physiological, emotional, and attitudinal (cognitive) reactions to stuttering, described as secondary stuttering behaviors, are often very disruptive to the communication process and the person's life.

Due to the effect that stuttering has on communication, the person who stutters may experience difficulty in other parts of his or her life. These problems might result from internal or external factors, such as self-doubt or society's attitudes toward stuttering and other barriers. The 2010 Oscar-winning film *The King's Speech* drew widespread attention to the social stigma that accompanies stuttering, which places undue pressure on the speaker. The film profiles King George VI and his stammer. Persons who stutter may feel increased **stress** or anxiety when faced with speaking situations. Many report difficulties in social settings and as a result may withdraw from social environments to avoid having to speak. Children who stutter often experience teasing and other social penalties that carry through to adolescence and adulthood. Academic settings may be difficult for children who stutter because of the emphasis most schools place on verbal performance in the classroom.

There is some evidence that people who stutter confront barriers in employment, at least for jobs that require interacting with the public. These barriers may take the form of inability to do certain tasks easily (talking on the phone, for example), limitations in job choices, and discrimination in the hiring and promotion processes.

Risk factors

According to the Stuttering Foundation of America (SFA), the following are known risk factors for stuttering:

- Family history of stuttering.
- Gender. Boys are at greater risk of stuttering than girls.
- Age when stuttering begins. Children who begin to stutter before age three are more likely to outgrow it than those who begin to stutter later.
- Time elapsed since onset of stuttering. Children who have been stuttering longer than six months are less likely to outgrow the condition.

As far as was known as of 2011, race, ethnicity, and native language are not risk factors for stuttering. The rate of stuttering and sex ratio are thought to be similar throughout the world, although some researchers believe that rates of stuttering are higher in Africa than elsewhere. What does seem to vary most widely from country to country is cultural attitude toward stuttering.

DSM-5

Stuttering is classified as a mental disorder in the ***Diagnostic and Statistical Manual of Mental Disorders*** (*DSM*), the clinical reference manual used by mental health professionals. Previously listed as a disorder usually diagnosed in infancy, childhood, and adolescence, proposed changes for the fifth edition (*DSM-5*, 2013) refer to stuttering as childhood onset fluency disorder, a neurodevelopmental communication disorder. Other communication disorders include language impairment, late language emergence, **social communication disorder**, speech sound disorder (**phonological disorder**), and voice disorder.

Causes and symptoms

Although research has not identified a single cause of stuttering, there appear to be several factors that are viewed as being important to the onset and development of stuttering. Therefore, stuttering is often described as multifactorial and having possibly multiple causes. First, there is a genetic predisposition to stutter, as evidenced by studies of families and twins. Approximately 60% of children who stutter have family members with the same condition. In 2010, researchers at NIDCD identified three specific genes—one on chromosome 12 and two on chromosome 16—that are linked to stuttering. The genes are known as GNPTAB, GNPTG, and NAGPA.

A second important factor in stuttering the onset of stuttering is the physiological makeup of people who stutter. Research suggests that the brains of people who stutter may function abnormally during speech production. These differences in functioning may lead to breakdowns in speech production and to the development of disfluent speech.

Third, there is some evidence that speech and language development is an important issue in understanding the development of stuttering. Studies have found some evidence that children who show stuttering-type behaviors may also have other difficulties with speech-language. Additionally, children with speech-language delays often show stuttering-type behaviors. Finally, environmental issues have a significant impact on the development of stuttering behaviors. An environment that is overly stressful or demanding may cause children to have difficulties developing fluent speech. Although the environment, in particular parental behaviors, does not cause stuttering, it is an important factor that might adversely affect a child who is operating at a reduced capacity for developing fluent speech.

There is no evidence that stuttering is secondary to a psychological disturbance. It is reasonable to assume that stuttering might have some effect on psychological adjustment and a person's ability to cope with speaking situations. People who stutter might experience a lower self-esteem, and some might report feeling depressed. These feelings and difficulties with coping are most likely the result and not the cause of stuttering. In addition, several research studies have reported that many people who stutter report high levels of anxiety and stress when they are talking and stuttering. These feelings, psychological states, and difficulties with coping are most likely the result and not the cause of stuttering.

Generally, children begin to stutter between the ages of two and five years. This type of stuttering is categorized as developmental stuttering. Another major category of stuttering is called "neurogenic stuttering." Neurogenic stuttering results from **brain** damage, such as a **stroke**, a traumatic injury to the brain, or a degenerative neurological disease. In other cases, stuttering may be secondary to a psychological **conversion disorder** due to a psychologically traumatic event. When stuttering has abrupt onset secondary to a psychological **trauma**, it is described as "psychogenic stuttering." This is considered the least common type.

KEY TERMS

Developmental—Referring to a speech problem or other disorder that arises during a specific stage in human development.

Disfluency—Any difficulty in fluent speech, including stuttering.

Neurogenic—Referring to a disorder associated with damage to the central nervous system.

Psychogenic—Referring to a disorder associated with mental or emotional conflict. At one time, most stuttering was considered psychogenic, but recent research indicates that psychogenic stuttering is the least common form.

The primary symptoms of stuttering include excessive disfluency, both stuttering and normal types (core behaviors), as well as physical, emotional, and cognitive reactions to the problem. These behaviors vary in severity across people who stutter, from very mild to very severe. Additionally, behaviors will vary considerably across different speaking situations. There are specific situations when people tend to experience more stuttering (such as talking on the phone or with an authority figure) or less stuttering (speaking with a pet or to themselves, for example). It is likely that this variability might even extend to people having periods (days and even weeks) when they can maintain normally fluent or nonstuttered speech.

Other symptoms that may be associated with stuttering in children include eye blinking, tremor in the lips or jaw, and tension or movement of the face or upper body.

Diagnosis

The *DSM* diagnostic criteria for stuttering requires that disfluencies persist over time; be incongruous with the patient's age and language ability; impede communication and/or social, academic, or occupational performance; and not be brought on by trauma, injury, or

malingering. One or more of the following characteristics must also be present:

- repetitions of sounds and syllables
- prolongation of letter pronunciation
- pauses within spoken words
- general pauses in speech, with or without sound
- avoidance of problematic words
- physical tension when speaking
- repetitions of monosyllabic words (e.g., "I," "a")
- anxiety over, and avoidance of, speaking

Examination

Speech-language pathologists (SLPs) are responsible for making the **diagnosis** and managing the treatment of adults and children who stutter. Preferably, a board-certified speech-language pathologist should be sought for direct **intervention** or consulting. Diagnosis of stuttering, or identifying children at risk for stuttering, is difficult because most children show excessive disfluencies in their speech. With children, diagnostic procedures include the collection and analysis of speech and disfluent behaviors in a variety of situations. In addition, the child's general speech-language abilities will be evaluated.

Finally, the speech-language pathologist will interview parents and teachers regarding the child's general development and speech-language development, and their perceptions of the child's stuttering behaviors. For adults and older children, diagnostic procedures will also include gathering and analyzing speech samples from a variety of settings. In addition, the speech-language pathologist will conduct a lengthy interview with the person about their stuttering and history of their stuttering problem. Finally, the person who stutters might be asked to report his or her attitudes and feelings related to stuttering, either while being interviewed or by completing a series of questionnaires.

Tests

In some cases, the child may be referred to an otolaryngologist (specialist in ear, nose, and throat disorders) or a neurologist to rule out the possibility that abnormalities in the structure of the child's tongue or mouth, or a brain disorder, are related to the stuttering.

Treatment

Traditional

GENERAL CONSIDERATIONS. Experts generally accept the view that conducting interventions with children and families early in childhood (preschool) is the most effective means of total recovery from stuttering. Up to 80% of children recover from stuttering if treated between the ages of two and five. The chances for a person to recover fully from stuttering by obtaining near-normal fluency are reduced as the person ages. This is why early intervention is critical. For older children and adults for whom stuttering has become a chronic disorder, the focus of therapy is on developing positive coping mechanisms for dealing with the problem. This therapy varies in success based on the individual.

YOUNG CHILDREN. Treatment of young children generally follows one of two basic approaches. These approaches may also be combined into a single treatment program. The first type of approach, often referred to as "indirect therapy," focuses on altering the environment to allow the child opportunities to develop fluent speech. With this approach, counseling parents regarding the alteration of behaviors that affect fluency is the focus. For example, parents may be taught to reduce the amount of household stress or the level of speech-language demands being placed on the child. In addition, parents may be advised to change characteristics of their speech, such as their speech rate and turn-taking style; this is done to help their children develop more fluent speech.

The other basic approach in treatment with young children targets the development of fluent speech. This type of approach, often referred to as "direct therapy," teaches children to use skills that will help them improve fluency, and they are sometimes given verbal rewards for producing fluent speech.

OLDER CHILDREN AND ADULTS. Treatment approaches for older children and adults usually take one of two forms. These approaches target either helping the person to modify his or her stuttering or fluency. Approaches that focus on modifying stuttering usually teach individuals to reduce the severity of their stuttering behaviors by identifying and eliminating all of the secondary or reactive behaviors. Individuals also work to reduce the amount of emotional reaction toward stuttering.

Finally, the speech-language pathologist will help the individual to learn techniques that allow them to stutter in an easier manner. Therapy does not focus on helping the individual to speak fluently, although most individuals will attain higher levels of fluency if this approach is successful. The other groups of approaches focus on helping adults and children who stutter to speak more fluently. This type of therapy, which focuses less on changing secondary and emotional reactions, helps the person to modify their speech movements in a specific manner that allows for fluent-sounding speech. These procedures require the individual to focus on developing new speech patterns. This often requires a significant amount of practice and skill. The successful outcome of these approaches is nonstuttered, fluent-sounding speech. Many therapists integrate stuttering modification and fluency shaping approaches into more complete treatment programs. In addition, psychological counseling may be used to supplement traditional speech therapy.

Drugs

There is no drug that has been approved by the U.S. Food and Drug Administration (FDA) for the treatment of stuttering as 2011. Although various medications used to treat epilepsy, **depression**, and **anxiety disorders** have been tried as therapy for stuttering, all of these agents have problematic side effects, and none has been particularly successful in treating stuttering. There are, however, isolated case studies of successful treatment of neurogenic stuttering using antipsychotic drugs, such as **asenapine**. In 2011, the FDA was conducting a clinical trial on the anxiolytic (antianxiety) drug pagoclone, after a pilot trial produced positive results, though its sample size was too small to consider as substantial evidence. The trial was expected to finish at the end of 2011. With no FDA-approved medications, the NIDCD advises utilizing therapy or similar methods.

Another method of therapy for stuttering is the use of electronic devices to improve fluency. One type of device fits into the ear like a hearing aid and digitally replays the child's voice so that it sounds as if the child is speaking in unison with someone else. Another type of device, called "delayed auditory feedback," forces the child to speak more slowly so that his or her voice will not sound distorted through the machine. NIDCD researchers maintain that the evidence about the success of these devices is mixed, as it is not clear how long the effects will last or whether the devices are practical.

Prognosis

The prognosis for developmental stuttering is generally good. About 65% of preschool children who stutter outgrow the condition, and 74% recover by their early teens. In general, girls have a better prognosis than boys.

According to the American Speech-Language-Hearing Association (ASHA), no single factor can be used to estimate a given child's prognosis for full recovery from stuttering. Complete recovery from severe stuttering is most likely when children and their families receive treatment close to the time of onset. Thus, early identification and treatment of stuttering is critical. For older children and adults, stuttering becomes a chronic problem that requires a lifetime of formal and self–directed therapy. For individuals who show this more chronic form of the disorder, internal motivation for change and support from significant others will be an important part of recovery.

Friends, an association for young people who stutter, was founded in 1997 by John Ahlbach, an adult who stutters, and Lee Caggiano, a speech-language therapist who specializes in stuttering and is the mother of a son who stutters. Friends offers online support to young people who stutter, their parents, and speech-language professionals who work with them. The group also publishes books and a bi-monthly newsletter as well as holding an annual convention.

Prevention

With the exception of the small number of cases in which stuttering is caused by a **traumatic brain injury**, the condition is not preventable.

Resources

BOOKS

Guitar, Barry, and Rebecca McCauley, eds. *Treatment of Stuttering: Established and Emerging Approaches*. Baltimore, MD: Lippincott Williams and Wilkins, 2010.

Harrison, Alan E., ed. *Speech Disorders: Causes, Treatment and Social Effects*. Hauppauge, NY: Nova Science Publishers, 2009.

Ramig, Peter R., and Darrell Dodge. *The Child and Adolescent Stuttering Treatment and Activity Resource Guide*, 2nd ed. Clifton Park, NY: Delmar Cengage Learning, 2010.

PERIODICALS

Catalano, G., et al. "Olanzapine for the Treatment of Acquired Neurogenic Stuttering." *Journal of Psychiatric Practice* 15 (November 2009): 484–88.

Changsoo, Kang, et al. "Mutations in the Lysosomal Enzyme-Targeting Pathway and Persistent Stuttering." *New England Journal of Medicine* 362, no. 8 (February 25, 2010): 677–685.

Iverach, L., et al. "The Relationship between Mental Health Disorders and Treatment Outcomes among Adults Who Stutter." *Journal of Fluency Disorders* 34 (March 2009): 29–43.

Jenkins, H. "Attitudes of Teachers towards Dysfluency Training and Resources." *International Journal of Speech–Language Pathology* 12 (June 2010): 253–58.

Kang, C., et al. "Mutations in the Lysosomal Enzyme–targeting Pathway and Persistent Stuttering." *New England Journal of Medicine* 362 (February 25, 2010): 677–85.

Maguire, G., et al. "Exploratory Randomized Clinical Study of Pagoclone in Persistent Developmental Stuttering: the Examining Pagoclone for peRsistent dEvelopmental

Stuttering Study [EXPRESS].” *Journal of Clinical Psychopharmacology* 30, no. 1 (February 2010): 48–56.
Menzies, R.G., et al. “Cognitive Behavior Therapy for Adults Who Stutter: A Tutorial for Speech-Language Pathologists.” *Journal of Fluency Disorders* 34 (September 2009): 187–200.
Prasse, J.E., and G.E. Kikano. “Stuttering: An Overview.” *American Family Physician* 77 (May 1, 2008): 1271–76.
Prins, D., and R.J. Ingham. “Evidence-based Treatment and Stuttering—Historical Perspective.” *Journal of Speech, Language, and Hearing Research* 52 (February 2009): 254–63.

WEBSITES

American Speech–Language–Hearing Association (ASHA). “Stuttering.” http://www.asha.org/public/speech/disorders/stuttering (accessed September 23, 2010).
Friends: The National Association of Young People Who Stutter. “Friends Stuttering Presentation Guide.” http://www.friendswhostutter.org/pdfs/FRIENDS_Stuttering_Presentation_Guide.pdf (accessed September 23, 2010).
Guitar, Barry, and Edward G. Conture. “If You Think Your Child Is Stuttering . . . ” http://www.stutteringhelp.org/Default.aspx?tabid=6 (accessed September 23, 2010).
Mayo Clinic. “Stuttering.” http://www.mayoclinic.com/health/stuttering/DS01027 (accessed September 23, 2010).
National Institute on Deafness and Other Communication Disorders (NIDCD). “Stuttering.” http://www.nidcd.nih.gov/health/voice/stutter.html (accessed September 23, 2010).

ORGANIZATIONS

American Academy of Otolaryngology—Head and Neck Surgery, 1650 Diagonal Rd., Alexandria, VA, 22314-2857, (703) 836-4444, http://www.entnet.org.
American Speech–Language–Hearing Association (ASHA), 2200 Research Blvd., Rockville, MD, 20850-3289, (301) 296-5700, http://www.asha.org/default.htm.
Friends: The National Association of Young People Who Stutter, [c/o Lee Caggiano] 38 South Oyster Bay Rd., Syosset, NY, 11791, (866) 866-8335, LCAGGIANO@aol.com, http://www.friendswhostutter.org.
International Stuttering Association (ISA), [c/o Joseph Lukong Tardzenyuy, Secretary] PO Box 9598, Douala, Cameroonadmin@stutterisa.org, http://www.stutterisa.org/index.html.
National Institute on Deafness and Other Communication Disorders (NIDCD), 31 Center Dr., MSC 2320, Bethesda, MD, 20892-2320, (800) 241-1044, Fax: (301) 770–8977, nidcdinfo@nidcd.nih.gov, http://www.nidcd.nih.gov/index.asp.
Stuttering Foundation of America (SFA), 3100 Walnut Grove Rd., Suite 603, Memphis, TN, 38111-0749, (901) 452-7343, (800) 992-9392, Fax: (901) 452-3931, info@stutteringhelp.org, http://www.stutteringhelp.org/Default.aspx?tabid=4.

Rodney Gabel, PhD
Rebecca J. Frey, PhD

Substance Abuse and Mental Health Services Administration

Definition

The **Substance Abuse** and Mental Health Services Administration (SAMHSA) is an agency of the U.S. Department of Health and Human Services. It was established by an act of Congress in 1992 to focus attention, programs and funding on improving the lives of people with or at risk for mental and substance abuse disorders.

Description

SAMHSA began as part of a realignment of federal antidrug services centered on the Alcohol, Drug, and Mental Health Administration (ADAMHA). ADAMHA, was originally founded in the early 1970s as a direct response to the awareness of the growing problem of illegal drug abuse. The ADAMHA Reorganization Act in 1992 created SAMHSA to take over the prevention and treatment functions related to mental health and substance abuse. ADAMHA’s three research institutes—the National Institute on Alcohol Abuse and Alcoholism, the National Institute on Drug Abuse, and the National Institute of Mental Health— were placed under the National Institutes of Health (NIH) to carry out research. The newly formed SAMHSA had a clear focus for providing resources and leadership in coordination with the states’ efforts to prevent and treat mental disorders and substance abuse.

Program centers

The three original centers of SAMHSA are the Center for Mental Health Services, the Center for Substance Abuse Prevention, and the Center for Substance Abuse Treatment. In the early 2000s, a fourth center was added, the Center for Behavioral Health Statistics and Quality to replace the managerial division the Office of Applied Studies.

CENTER FOR MENTAL HEALTH SERVICES. The Center for Mental Health Services (CMHS) has the stated mission of preventing and treating mental illness. The goal of the Center is to work with local service providers through the state to identify the causes of mental illness and to undermine the effect of negative influences. When prevention is not possible, the appropriate treatment is recommended to ease the effect of the mental illness. The CMHS provides funding for services and program development mainly by offering block grants.

Even in states not receiving funding, CMHS influences mental health services by setting goals for mental health prevention and advising on improving treatment. The CMHS has advisors available to the states for training staff and improving services. The CMHS also serves as an advocate for the mentally ill and their families. In fulfilling its mandate to provide timely information on mental health promotion, the center maintains a clearinghouse of publications and documents related to its mission. While the CMHS sponsors its own research conferences, the center also sends experts to other relevant conferences.

CENTER FOR SUBSTANCE ABUSE PREVENTION. The Center for Substance Abuse Prevention (CSAP) was instituted to be the federal leader in providing services and information regarding substance problems. The goal of the Center is to be the primary driver of actions promoting the reduction in the problem use of alcohol, tobacco, and drugs. To this end, CSAP advises legislators and federal agencies on the issues of substance use, while providing services and programs to states in the form of models and block grants.

A main program of CSAP is the Strategic Prevention Framework, which is a community-based model encouraging the implementation of research on effective prevention. The framework takes into consideration the challenges of youth among all lifespan development stages. The problems specific to youth include challenges to self esteem and self autonomy when facing peer pressure. Other problems include the adolescent tendency for risk taking.

CENTER FOR SUBSTANCE ABUSE TREATMENT. The Center for Substance Abuse Treatment (CSAT) is charged with identifying and providing effective treatment for those with substance-based disorders by providing grants for the development of treatments to the states and communities. The center also manages a referral service to help those seeking treatment to find appropriate help. The referral service provides detailed information to address individual situations such as lack of insurance or court-ordered treatment.

In funding and promoting community-based treatment, CSAT emphasizes flexibility of delivery. As the needs of the community and individuals vary, the processes of the funded programs must be matched to the identified needs. The treatment models recommended by CSAT are those that have been found by research to be effective for most people. However, to encourage innovation, CSAT also promotes and funds evaluation of new programs.

CENTER FOR BEHAVIORAL HEALTH STATISTICS AND QUALITY. The Center for Behavioral Health Statistics and Quality (CBHSQ) disseminates information and statistics regarding substance abuse, including the number and types of medical situations involving drug abuse. The CBHSQ collects data from various sources. While the center analyzes its own data, it also has access to substance abuse data analysis from outside sources. Abuse data include not only legal substances, such as alcohol, tobacco, and prescription drugs, but also illegal drugs. The center's information includes the availability, growth, and use of substance abuse treatment.

Typical reports updated regularly include topics such as the level of substance abuse among various ethnic groups. The data systems producing reports include Drug and Alcohol Service Information System, Drug Abuse Warning network, National Survey on Drug Use and Health. The CBHSQ also provides independent analysts appropriate data related to substance abuse and mental health.

Strategic initiatives

In an effort to improve behavioral health services in a community setting, SAMHSA has identified eight strategic initiatives. These strategic initiatives provide a means to focus agency resources in areas that have the greatest need or the greatest chance for impact. Each

KEY TERMS

Behavioral health—A broad term for any condition related in any way to mental health.

Community-based—Used to describe any organization or initiative stemming from non-government, local, and independent sources.

Mental disorder—Any illness interfering with perceptions, consciousness, and adjustment.

Mental health—Appropriate adaptation to everyday psychosocial challenges.

Prevention—Successful encouragement of individuals and communities to avoid the use of substances that lead to abuse or dependence.

Recovery—State of being in which someone has changed lifestyle and dependency to the point of not using the previous addictive substance.

Substance abuse—The illicit use of drugs or other psychotropic chemicals to change cognitive or emotional perceptions.

Treatment—The process of helping those with a mental disorder to adapt to life challenges by changing lifestyle and dependency.

strategic initiative provides funding and expertise in the assigned area.

PREVENTION OF SUBSTANCE ABUSE AND MENTAL ILLNESS. The Prevention of Substance Abuse and Mental Illness initiative is predominantly covered through the efforts of CSAP. The goal of this initiative is to encourage community based organizations to promote the education and **intervention** necessary to avoid and reduce substance abuse. These organizations include schools, workplaces and faith-based organizations. All qualified groups are invited to apply for grants to support their efforts and to accept SAMHSA's programs in this effort. The main thrust of this effort is toward prevention among children and adolescents.

TRAUMA AND JUSTICE. The **trauma** and justice initiative, which is covered by all the centers, is focused on efforts to reduce the effects of violence and the resulting trauma. The main effort is directed toward sharing important research on dealing with trauma with all health and mental services. Related to sharing information to offset unexpected crisis is the effort to negotiate in the justice system to protect the rights of the mentally ill, promoting treatment rather than harsh punishments for these persons, particularly when crimes stem from a person's disorder.

MILITARY FAMILIES. The military families initiative, which is predominantly covered by CMHS, aims to promote mental health and adjustment in military families facing crises. The CMHS primarily ensure that military families have community services available when needed and that these families are aware of what is available. When mental illness results from the constant challenges of the military families, CMHS informs through community services that treatment is available and follows up to be sure that the treatment is effective.

HEALTH REFORM IMPLEMENTATION. The health reform implementation initiative is a cross-center effort to assure that any healthcare reform legislation includes coverage for mental conditions and substance abuse treatment. Beyond influencing legislation, the effort is on informing mental health consumers of their rights and opportunities when facing funding problems for mental health treatment. In negotiating with insurance and healthcare providers, SAMHSA centers address the disparity between coverage for mental health care and other conditions.

RECOVERY SUPPORT. The recovery support initiative, which is predominantly covered by CMHS, aims to encourage follow-up treatment for those with a mental or substance use disorder. The follow-up treatment is especially important to help those who are in recovery avoid conditions leading to a **relapse**. The importance of avoiding relapse is stressed through this initiative to all levels of the behavioral health system. Other support covers access to housing education and employment coordinated with a decrease of social barriers.

HEALTH INFORMATION TECHNOLOGY. The health information technology initiative is predominantly handled by CSAT. The goal of this initiative is to promote the use of electronic systems for maintaining and updating health records. The concept behind this initiative is that with an accessible electronic file system of behavioral health records, service to individuals will be less complex and less redundant. The two systems promoted by this initiative are Health Information Technology and Electronic Health Records.

DATA, OUTCOMES, AND QUALITY. The data, outcomes, and quality initiative is predominantly covered by CBHSQ. The goal of this initiative is to disseminate timely, accurate information to the public and to policy makers. The data are collected from many sources; they are analyzed within SAMHSA but made available for analysis by independent researchers. Information regarding program evaluation and effectiveness is also collected and circulated. With greater availability of information, it is hoped that better policy will lead to greater improvement in the behavioral healthcare system.

PUBLIC AWARENESS AND SUPPORT. The public awareness and support initiative is a cross-center effort to communicate and market the information and approaches to better improve behavioral health services. One of the tools used in this effort is the strategic communications framework that is designed to coordinate the many information services within SAMHSA. The Office of Communication within SAMHSA operates a blog on SAMHSA's website. The blog is updated as necessary, usually once a week. This initiative is in support of the others, particularly in advertising innovations and successes.

Resources

BOOKS

Hanson, Glen R., et al. *Drugs and Society.* Burlington, MA: Jones & Bartlett Learning, 2011

Levin, Bruce Lebotsky, et al. *Mental Health Services: A Public Health Perspective.* New York: Oxford University Press, 2010.

PERIODICALS

Knopf, Alison. "Senate Appropriations Committee Rejects SAMHSA's 'New Vision'." *Alcoholism & Drug Abuse Weekly* (October 3, 2011). http://www.alcoholismdrugabuseweekly.com/sample-articles/senate-committee-rejects-samhsa-vision.aspx (accessed October 27, 2011).

Torrey, E. Fuller. "Bureaucratic Insanity." *National Review Online* (June 29, 2011). http://www.freerepublic.com/focus/f-news/2742321/posts (accessed October 27, 2011).

ORGANIZATIONS

Substance Abuse and Mental Health Services Administration Referral Resource, 1 Choke Cherry Rd., Rockville, MD, 20857, (877) SAMHSA-7 (726-4727), (800) TTY: 487-4889, Fax: (240) 221-4292, SAMHSAInfo@samhsa.hhs.gov, http://www.samhsa.gov.

U.S. Department of Health & Human Services, 200 Independence Ave. SW, Washington, DC, 20201, (202) 619-7800, (877) 696-6775, http://www.hhs.gov.

Ray F. Brogan, PhD

Substance abuse and related disorders

Definition

Substance abuse, also referred to as alcoholism, **addiction**, drug abuse, or drug misuse, is the continued, compulsive use of mind-altering substances despite personal, social, and/or physical problems caused by the use. Such use, which may involve illegal or legal substances, is for nontherapeutic or nonmedical purposes. Chronic abuse may lead to substance dependence, meaning that the user is physically dependent on the substance and often requires increased amounts of the abused substance to achieve the desired effect or level of intoxication. If use of the substance is suddenly ceased, the user will undergo a period of withdrawal.

Substance abuse and dependence

Approximately 22.1 million people* were classified as having a substance dependence or abuse disorder in 2010.

Dependence on specific drugs included:

Alcohol	17.0 million**
Marijuana	4.5 million
Pain relievers	1.9 million
Cocaine	1.0 million
Tranquilizers	521,000
Hallucinogens	397,000
Heroin	359,000
Stimulants	357,000
Sedatives	162,000
Inhalants	161,000

*Aged 12 and older
**Users may have abused more than one substance, so the number of users of each substance may be higher than the total estimated number of people with a substance abuse disorder.

SOURCE: Substance Abuse and Mental Health Services Administration, Office of Applied Studies, *Results from the 2010 National Survey on Drug Use and Health: Summary of National Findings* (September 2011).

Report available online at http://oas.samhsa.gov/NSDUH/2k10NSDUH/2k10Results.htm. *(Table by PreMediaGlobal.*

Demographics

In 2010, in the United States, approximately 22.6 million people (8.9% of the U.S. population) were using illegal drugs, according to the *National Survey on Drug Use and Health* performed by the **Substance Abuse and Mental Health Services Administration** (SAMHSA), an agency of the U.S. Department of Health and Human Services (HHS). The number of persons receiving treatment for abuse is much lower, estimated at 2.6 million.

Marijuana is the most commonly used drug, with 17.4 million Americans using it in 2010, compared to 14.4 million in 2007. Use of other substances has dropped, however, with an estimated 353,000 people using **methamphetamine** (down from 731,000 in 2006) and 1.5 million using **cocaine** (down from 2.4 million in 2006). Still, there is a substantial problem in the United States, with drug use among 18- to 25-year-olds rising from 19.6% in 2008 to 21.5% in 2010.

Substance abuse and dependence cut across all lines of race, culture, education, and socioeconomic status. In addition to the toll that substance abuse can take on a person's physical health, substance abuse is considered an important factor in a wide variety of social problems, affecting rates of crime, domestic violence, sexually transmitted diseases (including human immunodeficiency virus/acquired immune deficiency syndrome [HIV/AIDS]), unemployment, **homelessness**, teen pregnancy, and failure in school. One study estimated that 20% of the total yearly cost of health care in the United States is spent on the effects of drug and alcohol abuse.

Description

According to the mental health clinician's handbook, the ***Diagnostic and Statistical Manual of Mental Disorders*** (*DSM*), substance-related disorders include disorders of use and abuse, intoxication, and withdrawal, as well as the various mental states (e.g., **dementia**, **psychosis**, anxiety, mood disorder) that the substance may induce when it is used. Intoxication is the direct effect of the substance; different substances produce different reactions, but some common effects include impaired judgment, emotional instability, increase or decrease in appetite, and altered sleep habits.

Substance abuse is commonly defined as the use of illegal drugs or misuse of prescribed drugs. If a person consistently abuses a drug for a period of time, they will become physically dependent on it. A substance-dependent person must have a particular dose or concentration of the substance in his or her bloodstream at any given moment in order to avoid the unpleasant symptoms associated with withdrawal from that substance. This amount of the dosage increases as the person becomes tolerant of the substance; as his or her body adapts to the presence of the substance, higher amounts are needed to produce the same effects. If the substance-dependent person abruptly stops using the substance, his or her body will respond by overcompensating for the substance's absence. Functions slowed by the abused substance will be suddenly sped up, while previously stimulated functions will be suddenly slowed. This results in a number of unpleasant effects, known as "withdrawal symptoms." Withdrawal symptoms vary with the substance, but common symptoms include increased heart rate, tremor, **insomnia**, **fatigue**, and irritability.

"Substance addiction" refers to the mind-state of a person who reaches a point where he or she must have a specific substance, despite any negative social, physical, and legal consequences (e.g., deteriorating health or loss of relationships, employment, or housing). "Craving" refers to an intense hunger for a specific substance, to the point where this need essentially directs the individual's behavior. Craving is usually seen in both dependence and addiction and can be so strong that it overwhelms a person's ability to make decisions that will deprive him or her of the substance. Drug possession and use become the most important goals, and other forces (including the law) have little effect on the individual's substance-seeking behavior.

Common classes of substances of abuse include:

- alcohol, such as beer, liquor, and wine
- amphetamines, such as 3,4-Methylenedioxymethamphetamine (MDMA, commonly called "Ecstasy"), ephedrine, and methamphetamine
- barbiturates, such as amobarbital (Amytal), pentobarbital (Nembutal), and secobarbital (Seconal)
- benzodiazepines, including prescription drugs used for treating anxiety, such as diazepam (Valium), and baclofen (Kemstro, Lioesal, and Gablofen)
- caffeine, contained in coffee, tea, and energy drinks
- cannabinoid drugs obtained from the hemp plant, including marijuana and hashish
- cocaine-based drugs (also called "crack" or "coke")
- hallucinogenic or "psychedelic" drugs, including lysergic acid diethylamide (LSD), phencyclidine (PCP, or angel dust), and other PCP-type drugs
- inhalants, including gaseous drugs used in the medical practice of anesthesia, as well as such common substances as paint thinner, gasoline, and glue
- methamphetamines, also called "meth," "ice," "speed," or "crystal"
- methaqualone, such as Quaaludes
- nicotine, such as contained in cigarettes
- opioids, including such prescription pain killers as morphine and Demerol, as well as illegal substances such as heroin
- prescription medications, including other types of sedatives ("downers," such as tranquilizers) and stimulant drugs ("uppers," such as methylphenidate [Ritalin])

The *DSM* does not recognize caffeine abuse or dependence, but it does recognize the effects of caffeine intoxication (e.g., restlessness, nervousness, or excitement after caffeine consumption), caffeine-induced anxiety disorder (feelings of anxiety or panic attacks after caffeine consumption), and caffeine-induced sleep disorder (usually insomnia, but some may experience excessive sleepiness when caffeine is not consumed), and caffeine withdrawal.

In May 2013, the next edition of *DSM* will be available (*DSM-5*). Proposed changes include combining the former categories of substance abuse and substance dependence into one category, *substance use;* adding caffeine and **cannabis** withdrawal disorders; adding non-substance addictions, such as **gambling disorder** (formerly considered an impulse-control disorder); and adding to the list of substance-induced disorders, including substance-induced **obsessive-compulsive disorder** and mild or major neurocognitive disorder associated with substance use.

Causes and symptoms

Causes

It is generally believed that there is not one single cause of substance abuse, though scientists are increasingly convinced that certain people possess a genetic predisposition that can affect the development of addictive behaviors, along with a number of other biological, psychological, and social factors. One theory holds that a particular nerve pathway in the **brain** (dubbed the "mesolimbic reward pathway") holds certain chemical characteristics, which can increase the likelihood that substance use will ultimately lead to substance addiction. Certainly, however, other social factors are involved, including family problems and peer pressure. Primary mood disorders (**bipolar disorder**), **personality disorders**, and the role of learned behavior can be influential on the likelihood that a person will become substance dependent.

Research from the late 2000s and early 2010s continues to investigate the causes of substance abuse. Although concrete facts have yet to determine an exact cause, or causes, of substance abuse, researchers contend that certain risk factors predispose some children early in their developmental years to be more likely to abuse substances later in life, compared to the general population. Medical research has found that the presence of substance abuse disorder is higher for children who come from families where it is already present, making genetics a potential contributing factor for causing such disorders. Common risk factors, within the home and outside, found to increase the presence of substance abuse include:

- disorganized or chaotic home environment
- ineffective parenting skills
- insufficient nurturing and parental attachment
- aggressive or shy behavior
- poor coping skills in society
- general perception that drug and alcohol use is acceptable
- poor school achievement and performance
- association with children showing deviant or socially inappropriate behaviors

Symptoms

The symptoms of substance abuse may be related to its social effects as well as its physical effects. The social effects of substance abuse may include dropping out of school or losing a series of jobs, engaging in fighting or violence in relationships, and legal problems (ranging from driving under the influence to the commission of crimes designed to obtain the money needed to support a drug habit).

Physical effects of substance abuse are related to the specific drug being abused:

- Opioid drug users may appear slowed in their physical movements and speech, lose weight, exhibit mood swings, and have constricted (small) pupils.
- Benzodiazepine and barbiturate users may appear sleepy and slowed, with slurred speech, small pupils, and occasional confusion.
- Amphetamine users may have excessively high energy, inability to sleep, weight loss, rapid pulse, elevated blood pressure, occasional psychotic behavior, and dilated (enlarged) pupils.
- Marijuana users may be sluggish and slow to react, exhibiting mood swings, changes in weight, and red eyes with dilated pupils.
- Cocaine users may have wide variations in their energy level, severe mood disturbances, psychosis, paranoia, and a constantly runny nose. "Crack" cocaine use may cause aggressive or violent behavior.
- Hallucinogenic drug users may display bizarre behavior due to hallucinations (imagined sights, voices, sounds, or smells that seem completely real to the individual experiencing them) and dilated pupils. LSD use can cause flashbacks.

Other symptoms of substance abuse may be related to the form in which the substance is used. For example, heroin, certain other opioid drugs, and certain forms of cocaine may be injected using a needle and a hypodermic syringe. A person abusing an injectable substance may have "track marks," outwardly visible signs of the site of an injection, with possible redness and swelling of the vein in which the substance was injected. Furthermore, poor judgment brought on by substance use can result in the injections being made under dirty conditions. These unsanitary conditions and the use of shared needles can cause infections of the injection sites, major infections of the heart, infection with HIV (the virus that causes AIDS), certain forms of hepatitis (a liver infection), and tuberculosis.

Cocaine is often taken as a powdery substance that is "snorted" through the nose. This can result in frequent nosebleeds, sores in the nose, and even erosion (an eating away) of the nasal septum (the structure that separates the two nostrils). Other forms of cocaine include smokable or injectable forms, such as freebase and crack cocaine.

Overdosing on a substance is a frequent complication of substance abuse. Drug overdose can be purposeful (with **suicide** as a goal) or the result of carelessness, such as when purchasing from street dealers, where the strength or composition of the drugs are unpredictable; when mixing more than one type of substance or mixing a substance with alcohol; or because of the ever-increasing doses the person must take once he or she has become tolerant. A substance overdose can be a life-threatening emergency, with the specific symptoms dependent on the type of substance used. Substances with depressive effects may dangerously slow the breathing and heart rate, drop the body temperature, and result in general unresponsiveness. Substances with stimulatory effects may dangerously increase the heart rate and blood pressure, increase body temperature, and cause bizarre behavior. With cocaine, there are risks of **stroke** and heart attack.

Diagnosis

The most difficult aspect of **diagnosis** involves overcoming the patient's **denial**. Denial is a psychological trait whereby a person is unable to allow himself or herself to acknowledge the reality of a situation. This may lead a person to completely deny his or her substance use, or it may cause the person to greatly underestimate the degree of the problem and its effects on his or her life.

The *DSM-5* diagnostic criteria for a substance use disorder requires a person to display two or more of the following symptoms within a 12-month period:

- an inability to fulfill obligations, including work, school, and home or family responsibilities
- repeated use of the substance in dangerous situations (e.g., driving under the influence)
- recurrent use despite a negative effect on personal and social life or physical health
- tolerance—either a need for increased amounts of the substance to achieve the intended effect, or loss of effect when continuing to take the same amount
- withdrawal syndrome or continuing use to avoid withdrawal
- substance is taken in higher doses or continued for longer than originally intended
- unsuccessful attempts or intention to cut down on use
- significant time is spent around the substance or activity (obtaining, participating/using, recovering)
- substance use is favored over other activities, including work, hobbies, or social outings
- persistent craving to use substance

Fulfillment of criteria may be revealed during a physical examination or psychiatric test, or suspected abuse may be brought up by the patient's family member or friend. Meeting two or three criteria is considered moderate abuse, while four or more signifies severe substance abuse.

Examination

A physical examination may reveal signs of substance abuse in the form of needle marks, **trauma** to the inside of the nostrils from snorting drugs, or unusually large or small pupils. With the person's permission, substance use can also be detected by examining blood, urine, or hair in a laboratory. Drug testing is affected by drug sensitivity, specificity, and the time elapsed since the person last used the drug.

Tests

One of the simplest and most common screening tools that practitioners use to begin the process of diagnosing substance abuse is the CAGE questionnaire. CAGE (Cut, Annoyed, Guilty, Eye) refers to the first letters of each word that forms the basis of the four questions in the screening examination:

- Have you ever tried to cut down on your substance use?
- Have you ever been annoyed by people trying to talk to you about your substance use?
- Do you ever feel guilty about your substance use?
- Do you ever need an eye opener (use of the substance first thing in the morning) in order to start your day?

Longer questionnaires exist to assess the severity and effects of a person's substance abuse. It is also relevant to determine whether anyone else in the user's family has ever suffered from substance or alcohol addiction.

Treatment

Treatment is difficult if the abuser does not believe they have a problem. Most substance abusers think they can stop using drugs without outside help. However, only a small minority are successful on their own. Medical research shows that the brains of long-time substance abusers are altered due to their habit, resulting in cravings, withdrawal symptoms, and difficulty quitting without help. Therefore, treatment has several goals, which include helping a person deal with the uncomfortable and possibly life-threatening symptoms associated with withdrawal from an addictive substance (called "detoxification"), helping an abuser deal with the social effects that substance abuse has had on his or her life, and working to prevent **relapse** (resumed use of the substance).

Traditional

Detoxification is the halting of substance use, a process that may take from several days to many weeks. It can be accomplished "cold turkey," by complete and immediate cessation of all substance use, or by slowly decreasing (tapering) the dose that a person is taking, to minimize the side effects of withdrawal. Individual or group **psychotherapy** is often recommended and is likely to be important after detoxification.

The most important part of treatment is preventing the abuser from relapsing back to his or her former habits. Behavioral therapies help people cope with their drug cravings and develop strategies so as to not return to using substances. Sometimes the person with the substance abuse disorder also has mental disorders that are exaggerating the problem. Treatment then involves treating the mental disorder(s) with psychiatric medications and/or psychotherapy, along with the substance abuse problem.

Because substance abuse has severe effects on the functioning of the user's family, and because research has shown that family members can accidentally develop behaviors that inadvertently support a person's substance habit, most successful treatment programs will involve family members or close friends to help ensure the patient's recovery.

Drugs

Some abused substances absolutely must be tapered back, because "cold turkey" methods of detoxification are potentially life threatening. Alternatively, a variety of medications may be utilized to combat the unpleasant and threatening physical symptoms of withdrawal. A substance (such as **methadone** in the case of heroin addiction, or **nicotine** patches with cigarette smokers) may be substituted for the original substance of abuse, with gradual tapering of this substituted drug. In practice, many patients may be maintained on methadone and lead a reasonably normal lifestyle. Because of the rebound effects of wildly fluctuating blood pressure, body temperature, and heart and breathing rates, as well as the potential for bizarre behavior and hallucinations, a person undergoing withdrawal must be carefully monitored.

Pharmacological remediation is being investigated for the treatment of stimulant abuse disorders. In the same way that medications are prescribed to treat the cognitive deficits present in psychiatric disorders, research is ongoing as to whether this same theory can be applied to substance abuse disorders. As of 2011, a vaccine was in development (TA-CD, or Therapy for Addiction—Cocaine Addiction) with the goal of helping cocaine addicts reduce consumption by at least half. A similar vaccine is also being developed for nicotine use (TA-NIC).

Prognosis

After a person has successfully withdrawn from substance use, the even-more-difficult task of recovery begins. "Recovery" refers to the lifelong efforts of a person to avoid returning to substance use. Cravings can continue for years after the initial withdrawal and might never completely cease. Triggers for relapse include any number of life stresses (problems on the job or in the marriage, loss of a relationship, death of a loved one, financial stresses) in addition to exposure to a place or an acquaintance associated with previous substance use. While some people remain in counseling indefinitely as a way of maintaining contact with a professional to help monitor behavior, others find that various **support groups** or 12-step programs, such as Alcoholics Anonymous (AA) and Narcotics Anonymous (NA), are the most helpful in monitoring the recovery process and avoiding relapse.

KEY TERMS

Addiction—The state of being both physically and psychologically dependent on a substance.

AIDS—Acquired immunodeficiency syndrome.

Dependence—A state in which a person requires a steady concentration of a particular substance in order to avoid experiencing withdrawal symptoms.

Detoxification—A process whereby an addict is withdrawn from a substance.

HIV—Human immunodeficiency virus.

Street drug—A substance purchased from a drug dealer. It may be a legal substance, sold illicitly (without a prescription and not for medical use), or it may be a substance that is illegal to possess.

Tolerance—A phenomenon whereby a drug user becomes physically accustomed to a particular dose of a substance and requires ever-increasing dosages in order to obtain the same effects.

Withdrawal—Those side effects experienced by a person who has become physically dependent on a substance, upon decreasing the substance's dosage or discontinuing its use.

Prevention

Prevention is best aimed at childhood or adolescence. Teenagers are at very high risk for substance experimentation. Education regarding the risks and consequences of substance use, as well as teaching methods of resisting peer pressure, are both important components of a prevention program. Such education includes teaching the penalties associated with substance abuse, along with the social, physical, and psychological harm that it can cause an individual. Substance abuse efforts should occur in schools and communities, and parents should be actively involved in such programs to better communicate the risks to their children. Misperceptions about readily available

QUESTIONS TO ASK YOUR DOCTOR

- What treatment options are available?
- Where can I find support groups in my area?
- Will my insurance handle the expenses of treatment?
- Would you recommend seeing a therapist?

substances such as cigarettes and alcohol can be quickly corrected with proper communication. Furthermore, it is important to identify children at higher risk for substance abuse (including victims of physical or **sexual abuse**; children of parents who have a history of substance abuse, especially alcohol; and children with school failure and/or attention deficit disorder). These children may require a more intensive prevention program.

See also Alcohol use and related disorders; Amnestic disorders; Amphetamines and related disorders; Anti-anxiety drugs and abuse-related disorders; Caffeine and related disorders; Cannabis and related disorders; Cocaine and related disorders; Disease concept of chemical dependency; Hallucinogens and related disorders; Inhalants and related disorders; Nicotine and related disorders; Opioids and related disorders; Phencyclidine and related disorders; Polysubstance dependence; Sedatives and related disorders; Substance Abuse Subtle Screening Inventory; Substance-induced anxiety disorder; Substance-induced psychotic disorder; Wernicke-Korsakoff syndrome

Resources

BOOKS

Ferri, Fred, ed. *Ferri's Clinical Advisor 2010,* 1st ed. Philadelphia: Mosby Elsevier, 2009.

Goldman L, and D. Ausiello, eds. *Cecil Textbook of Internal Medicine,* 23rd ed. Philadelphia: Saunders, 2008.

Kaminer, Yifrah, and Ken C. Winters, eds. *Clinical Manual of Adolescent Substance Abuse Treatment.* Washington, DC: American Psychiatric, 2011.

Rakel, R. *Textbook of Family Medicine,* 7th ed. Philadelphia: Saunders Elsevier, 2007.

Rakel, R.E., and E.T. Bope. *Conn's Current Therapy,* 60th ed. Philadelphia: Saunders Elsevier, 2009.

Stern, T.A., et al. *Massachusetts General Hospital Comprehensive Clinical Psychiatry,* 1st ed. Philadelphia: Mosby Elsevier, 2008.

Wilson, Richard, and Cheryl A. Kolander. *Drug Abuse Prevention: A School and Community Partnership.* Sudbury, MA: Jones and Bartlett, 2011.

PERIODICALS

Hylton, Hilary. "A Drug to End Drug Addiction." *New York Times,* January 9, 2008. http://www.time.com/time/health/article/0,8599,1701864,00.html (accessed September 16, 2011).

Vocci, Frank J. "Cognitive Remediation in the Treatment of Stimulant Abuse Disorders: A Research Agenda." *Experimental and Clinical Psychopharmacology* 16, no. 6 (2008): 484–97.

OTHER

Substance Abuse and Mental Health Services Administration. *Results from the 2010 National Survey on Drug Use and Health: Summary of National Findings.* NSDUH Series H-41, HHS Publication no. (SMA) 11-4658. Rockville, MD: Substance Abuse and Mental Health Services Administration, 2011. http://oas.samhsa.gov/NSDUH/2k10NSDUH/2k10Results.htm (accessed September 16, 2011).

WEBSITES

Mayo Clinic staff. "Drug Addiction." MayoClinic.com (October 2, 2009). http://www.mayoclinic.com/health/drug-addiction/DS00183 (accessed July 19, 2011).

MedlinePlus. "Drug Abuse." U.S. National Library of Medicine, National Institutes of Health. http://www.nlm.nih.gov/medlineplus/drugabuse.html (accessed September 16, 2011).

National Institute on Drug Abuse. "Drugs, Brains, and Behavior: The Science of Addiction." August 2010. http://www.nida.nih.gov/scienceofaddiction (accessed September 16, 2011).

Office of Applied Studies. "Substance Abuse and Mental Health Statistics." Substance Abuse and Mental Health Services Administration (SAMHSA). http://oas.samhsa.gov (accessed September 16, 2011).

"Substance Abuse Treatment Facility Locator." SAMHSA. http://dasis3.samhsa.gov (accessed September 16, 2011).

American Psychiatric Association. "Substance Use and Addictive Disorders." DSM-5 Development. http://www.dsm5.org/ProposedRevision/Pages/SubstanceUseandAddictiveDisorders.aspx (accessed September 16, 2011).

Times Health Guide. "Drug Abuse." *New York Times.* http://health.nytimes.com/health/guides/specialtopic/drug-abuse/overview.html (accessed September 16, 2011).

ORGANIZATIONS

National Council on Alcoholism and Drug Dependence, Inc. (NCADD), 244 E 58th St., 4th Fl., New York, NY, 10022, (800) 622-2255, (212) 269-7797, Fax: (212) 269-7510, national@ncadd.org, http://www.ncadd.org.

National Institute on Drug Abuse, 6001 Executive Blvd., Rm. 5213, Bethesda, MD, 20892, (301) 443-1124; Spanish: (240) 221-4007, information@nida.nih.gov, http://drugabuse.gov.

Substance Abuse and Mental Health Services Administration (SAMHSA), 1 Choke Cherry Rd., Rockville, MD, 20857, (877) SAMHSA-7 (786-4727), TTY: (800) 487-4889, Fax: (240) 221-4292, SAMHSAInfo@samhsa.hhs.gov, http://www.samhsa.gov.

Substance Abuse Subtle Screening Inventory

Definition

The **Substance Abuse** Subtle Screening Inventory is also referred to as the SASSI. Dr. Glenn A. Miller developed the SASSI as a screening questionnaire for identifying people with a high probability of having a substance dependence disorder.

Purpose

The SASSI is intended for gathering information, organizing it, and using it to help make decisions about the likelihood of an individual having a substance dependence disorder, even if the individual does not acknowledge symptoms of the disorder or misuse of substances. Guidelines are available for professionals to flag individuals with a potential substance abuse disorder for further evaluation. Interpreting the results of the SASSI helps professionals understand their clients better and plan their treatment.

Precautions

When used by trained professionals, the SASSI can be an important tool in the assessment of substance use disorders. The SASSI is not intended to prove or diagnose an individual as an alcoholic or addict; it is intended to screen for a person who has a "high probability of having a substance dependence disorder." It should be kept in mind that a thorough assessment integrates other available information, such as self-report and family history, and is done by a skilled professional. This comprehensive assessment is required to determine if an individual meets the accepted standards in the mental health professional's handbook, **diagnosis** of a substance-related disorder.

The accuracy rate of the SASSI is 94%. Although that is very high, this means that there is a 6% probability that an individual will be misclassified based on SASSI scores. While the SASSI is a popular and widely used screening questionnaire, independent research on it has been limited. Some researchers have questions about the SASSI regarding the extent to which subscales measure what they are intended to measure and the accuracy of classification based on direct versus indirect scales. In addition, the SASSI is not to be used to discriminate against individuals, including disqualifying job applicants. It would be a violation of the Americans With Disabilities Act to eliminate a job applicant based on SASSI scores.

Description

The SASSI is a simple, brief one-page paper-and-pencil questionnaire that can be answered in 10 to 15 minutes. The SASSI is easy to administer, to individuals or groups, and can be objectively scored by hand and interpreted, based on objective decision rules, in a minute or two. Optical scanning equipment is available for mass scoring and interpretation. The SASSI does not require a high level of reading ability. The SASSI may be used by a variety of programs and professionals, including school counselors, student assistance programs, employee assistance programs, vocational counselors, psychotherapists, medical personnel, criminal justice programs, and other human service providers.

The SASSI went through rigorous scientific development over a 16-year period before it was first published in 1988. Two new scales were added, and the SASSI-2 was published in 1994. In 1997 the SASSI-3 was published with a new scale and increased accuracy. Items on the SASSI were selected based on established research methods and statistical analysis. Items were included that identified individuals with substance dependence disorders. The selected items were consistently answered differently by individuals with a substance dependence disorder compared to individuals without a substance dependence disorder.

In 1996, a Spanish version was made available. In addition to the paper and pencil format, computer versions of the SASSI, in several formats, are available.

Some questions on the SASSI ask how frequently clients have had certain experiences directly related to alcohol and other drugs. These are answered on a four-point scale, ranging from never to repeatedly. Some items that may appear to be unrelated to substance use (indirect or subtle items) are in a true/false format. Overall, the items make up 10 subscales. The results are reported on a profile form that is discussed with the client. There are separate profile forms for males and females. The objective scoring system results in a yes or no answer about whether the client has a high probability of having a substance dependence disorder. The SASSI-3 has been empirically tested and can identify substance dependence disorder with an overall accuracy of 94%. More specifically, the SASSI identifies individuals with a substance dependence disorder with 94% accuracy, and it identifies those without a substance dependence disorder with 94% accuracy. The accuracy of the SASSI is not significantly affected by gender, age, socioeconomic status, ethnicity, occupational status, marital status, educational level, drug of choice, and general level of functioning. Research is ongoing to improve the accuracy and usefulness of the SASSI.

Since 1990 an adolescent version of the SASSI has been available. The second version of the Adolescent SASSI (SASSI-A2) has a 94% overall accuracy of identifying an adolescent with a substance dependence disorder, including both substance abuse and substance dependence. The SASSI-A2 is designed to screen individuals who are 12 to 18 years old. The accuracy of the SASSI-A2 is not affected by the respondent's gender, age, ethnicity, education, employment status, living situation, prior legal history, or general level of functioning.

Results

A profile of the SASSI results will be reviewed with the client. The actual scores are plotted on a profile graph in comparison to a sample of people who were not being evaluated or treated for addictions or other clinical problems (also called a normative sample). Feedback is then given in terms of whether the individual has a high or low probability of having a substance dependence disorder. Individual scale scores may be used to come up with ideas or hypotheses for further evaluation and treatment. This information is based on clinical experience with the SASSI. The results may indicate issues that are important for treatment (such as difficulty acknowledging personal shortcomings, or primarily focusing on others' needs while unaware of one's own needs). The results may suggest an approach to take with the client (such as increasing awareness, or acknowledging and validating their feelings). The results may suggest a treatment plan that the client may respond to (such as addiction self-help groups or an education-focused program). Finally, the results may indicate appropriate treatment goals for the client (anger management and/ or social skills, for example). The goal of providing feedback about SASSI results is to have a two-way sharing and understanding of information that is descriptive and not judgmental.

Resources

BOOKS

Laux, John M., and Kathleen M. Salyers. "The SASSI-3 Face Valid Other Drugs Scale: A Psychometric investigation." *Psychology* 26 (October 2005) 15–22.

PERIODICALS

Gray, B. Thomas. "A Factor Analytic Study of the Substance Abuse Subtle Screening Inventory (SASSI)." *Educational and Psychological Measurement* 61 (2001): 102–118.

OTHER

U.S. National Institute of Alcohol Abuse and Alcoholism. "Substance Abuse Subtle Screening Inventory (SASSI)." http://pubs.niaaa.nih.gov/publications/Assesing%20 Alcohol/InstrumentPDFs/66_SASSI.pdf (accessed October 30, 2011).

WEBSITES

One Click Pharmacy.com "Substance Abuse Subtle Screening Inventory—Mental Health." http://www.oneclick pharmacy.co.uk/product_article_detail.php?id=6098 (accessed October 27, 2011).

Joneis Thomas, Ph.D.

Substance-induced anxiety disorder

Definition

A substance-induced anxiety disorder occurs when prominent anxiety symptoms (e.g., generalized anxiety, panic attacks, obsessive-compulsive symptoms, or phobia symptoms) are caused by the effects of a psychoactive substance. A substance may induce anxiety symptoms during intoxication (while the individual is under the influence of the drug) or during withdrawal (after an individual stops using the drug).

Demographics

Little is known regarding the demographics of substance-induced **anxiety disorders**. About 40 million American adults have an anxiety disorder, but there are not any reliable statistics indicating what percentage of these individuals have an anxiety disorder induced by substance use. However, it is clear that anxiety disorders occur more commonly in individuals who abuse alcohol or illicit drugs.

Description

A substance-induced anxiety disorder is subtyped or categorized based on whether the prominent feature is generalized anxiety, panic attacks, obsessive-compulsive symptoms, or phobia symptoms. In addition, the disorder is subtyped based on whether it began during intoxication on a substance or during withdrawal from a substance. A substance-induced anxiety disorder that begins during substance use can last as long as the drug is used. A substance-induced anxiety disorder that begins during withdrawal may first manifest up to four weeks after an individual stops using the substance.

Causes and symptoms

Substance-induced anxiety disorder is caused by the effects of certain drugs and alcohol, and the symptoms may look like other anxiety disorders except that in these cases, the conditions are linked to drug use or withdrawal.

Causes

A substance-induced anxiety disorder, by definition, is directly caused by the effects of drugs, including alcohol, prescription medications, illicit drugs, and toxins. Anxiety symptoms can result from intoxication on alcohol, **amphetamines** (and related substances), caffeine, **cannabis** (marijuana), **cocaine**, **hallucinogens**, **inhalants**, phencyclidine (PCP) and related substances, and other or unknown substances. Anxiety symptoms also can result from withdrawal from alcohol, **sedatives**, hypnotics, and anxiolytics (**antianxiety drugs**), cocaine, and other known or unknown substances.

Prescription drugs that may induce anxiety symptoms include anesthetics, analgesics, sympathomimetics (e.g., epinephrine or norepinephrine), bronchodilators, anticholinergic agents, anticonvulsants, antihistamines, insulin, thyroid preparations, oral contraceptives, antihypertensive and cardiovascular medications, antiparkinsonian medications, corticosteroids, **antidepressants**, **lithium carbonate**, and antipsychotic medications. Heavy metals and toxins, such as fuel, paint, organophosphate insecticides, nerve gases, carbon monoxide, and carbon dioxide may also induce anxiety.

Symptoms

The **diagnosis** is made only when the anxiety symptoms are above and beyond what would be expected during intoxication or withdrawal and when the symptoms are severe. The following list comprises the criteria necessary for the diagnosis of a substance-induced anxiety disorder as listed in the ***Diagnostic and Statistical Manual of Mental Disorders***, fourth edition, text revision (*DSM-IV-TR*):

- prominent anxiety, panic attacks, or obsessions or compulsions
- symptoms developing during or within one month of intoxication or withdrawal from a substance or medication known to cause anxiety symptoms
- symptoms not part of another anxiety disorder (such as generalized anxiety disorder, phobias, panic disorder, or obsessive-compulsive personality disorder) and not substance induced (For instance, if the anxiety symptoms began prior to substance or medication use, then another anxiety disorder is likely.)
- symptoms not occurring only during delirium
- symptoms causing significant distress or impairment in functioning.

KEY TERMS

Analgesic—Medicine used to relieve pain.

Anticonvulsants—A class of drugs given to control seizures.

Corticosteroid—A steroid hormone produced by the adrenal gland and involved in metabolism and immune response.

Corticosteroid drug—A medication that acts like a type of hormone (cortisol) produced by the adrenal gland of the body. Corticosteroids produced by the body stimulate specific types of functional activity. As a drug, a corticosteroid (sometimes just called steroid) helps treat inflammation, infection, or trauma to the body.

Insulin—A hormone made by the pancreas that controls blood glucose (sugar) levels by moving excess glucose into muscle, liver, and other cells for storage.

Diagnosis

Diagnosis of a substance-induced anxiety disorder requires the case being differentiated from an anxiety disorder due to a general medical condition. Some medical conditions (e.g., hyperthyroidism, hypothyroidism, and hypoglycemia) also can produce anxiety symptoms. Since individuals are likely to be taking medications for these conditions, it can be difficult to determine the cause of the anxiety symptoms. If the symptoms are determined to be due to the medical condition, then a diagnosis of an anxiety disorder due to a general medical condition is warranted. Substance-induced anxiety disorders also need to be distinguished from **delirium**, **dementia**, primary psychotic disorders, and substance intoxication and withdrawal.

Clinical history and physical examination are the best methods to help diagnose anxiety disorders in general; however, appropriate laboratory testing will most likely be necessary to specifically identify substance-induced anxiety disorder. Lab tests may include:

- complete blood count (CBC)
- chemistry panels
- serum and/or urine screens for drugs

Treatment

The underlying cause of the anxiety symptoms, as well as the specific type of symptoms, determine course of treatment. Treatment often is similar to that

QUESTIONS TO ASK YOUR DOCTOR

- Could any of my medications be causing my anxiety symptoms?
- What programs can you recommend to help me stop using the substance causing my anxiety?
- Can you refer me to a mental health professional?
- Will my insurance cover an alternative medication if this one is causing anxiety symptoms?
- What other steps can I take to help reduce my anxiety?
- Are there any support groups in this area that might be right for me?

used to treat a primary anxiety disorder such as **generalized anxiety disorder**, phobias, **panic disorder**, or **obsessive-compulsive disorder**. Appropriate treatment usually includes medication (e.g., antianxiety or antidepressant medication). Additional treatment may be needed to address symptoms of withdrawal when substance use is stopped, a process that should be conducted under the care of a physician.

Prognosis

Anxiety symptoms induced by substance intoxication usually subside once the substance responsible is eliminated. The length of time symptoms persist depends on how long it takes before the substance is no longer present in an individual's body (intoxication-induced anxiety) or how long it takes the body to adjust to no longer having the substance (withdrawal-induced anxiety). Symptoms, therefore, can persist for hours, days, or weeks after a substance is last used. Obsessive-compulsive symptoms induced by substances sometimes do not disappear, even though the substance inducing them has been eliminated. More intensive treatment for the obsessive-compulsive symptoms is then necessary and typically includes a combination of medication and behavioral therapy.

Prevention

Little is documented regarding the prevention of substance-induced anxiety disorder. However, abstaining from illicit drugs and alcohol sharply reduces the risk of developing this disorder. In addition, taking medication under the supervision of an appropriately trained physician should reduce the likelihood of a medication-induced anxiety disorder. Finally, reducing one's exposure to toxins and heavy metals reduces the risk of toxin-induced anxiety disorder.

Resources

BOOKS

Daitch, Carolyn. *Anxiety Disorders: The Go-To Guide for Clients and Therapists.* New York: Norton, 2011.

Doctor, Ronald M., Ada P. Kahn, and Christine Adamec. *The Encyclopedia of Phobias, Fears, and Anxieties,* 3rd ed. New York: Facts on File, 2008.

Fisher, Gary L., and Nancy A. Roget, eds. *Encyclopedia of Substance Abuse Prevention, Treatment, and Recovery.* Los Angeles: SAGE, 2009.

PERIODICALS

Leeies, Murdoch, et al. "The Use of Alcohol and Drugs to Self-Medicate Symptoms of Post-traumatic Stress Disorder." *Depression and Anxiety* 27, no. 8 (August 2010):731–36.

Torrens, Marti, et al. "Psychiatric Comorbidity in Illicit Drug Users: Substance-Induced versus Independent Disorders." *Drug and Alcohol Dependence* (2011).

ORGANIZATIONS

American Psychiatric Association, 1000 Wilson Blvd., Ste. 1825, Arlington, VA, 22209-3901, (703) 907-7300, apa@psych.org, http://www.psych.org.

American Psychological Association, 750 1st St. NE, Washington, DC, 20002-4242, (202) 336-5500; TDD/TTY: (202) 336-6123, (800) 374-2721, http://www.apa.org.

National Council on Alcoholism and Drug Dependence, Inc., 244 E 58th St., 4th Fl., New York, NY, 10022, (212) 269-7797, (800) NCA-CALL, Fax: (212) 269-7510, national@mcadd.org, http://www.ncadd.org.

Substance Abuse and Mental Health Services Administration Referral Resource, 1 Choke Cherry Rd., Rockville, MD, 20857, (877) SAMHSA-7 (726-4727), (800) TTY: 487-4889, Fax: (240) 221-4292, SAMHSAInfo@samhsa.hhs.gov, http://www.samhsa.gov.

Jennifer Hahn, PhD
Tish Davidson, AM

Substance-induced persisting amnestic disorder *see* **Amnesia and amnestic disorders; Wernicke-Korsakoff syndrome**

Substance-induced psychotic disorder

Definition

The primary feature of a substance-induced psychotic disorder is prominent psychotic symptoms (i.e., hallucinations and/or **delusions**) determined to be caused by the effects of a psychoactive substance. A substance may induce psychotic symptoms during intoxication (while the individual is under the influence of the drug) or during withdrawal (after an individual stops using the drug.

Demographics

Little is known regarding how common substance-induced **psychosis** is across all substances. Approximately 3% of individuals who are dependent on alcohol experience psychosis at some time, either while severely intoxicated or during withdrawal. Substance-induced first episodes of psychosis are more common in men than women. Approximately 51% of individuals experiencing a first episode of psychosis caused by non-medication substance use report having used marijuana. The next most common substance to induce psychosis is alcohol, at 43%, with other substances accounting for the remaining 6% of instances.

Description

A substance-induced psychotic disorder is subtyped or categorized based on whether the prominent feature is delusions or hallucinations. Delusions are fixed, false beliefs. Hallucinations are seeing, hearing, feeling, tasting, or smelling things that are not there. In addition, the disorder is subtyped based on whether it began during intoxication on a substance or during withdrawal from a substance. A substance-induced psychotic disorder that begins during substance use can last as long as the drug is used. A substance-induced psychotic disorder that begins during withdrawal may first manifest up to four weeks after an individual stops using the substance.

Causes and symptoms

Substance-induced psychotic disorder is caused by using certain substances or withdrawing from that use. Symptoms are of two basic sorts: delusions or hallucinations.

Causes

A substance-induced psychotic disorder, by definition, is directly caused by the effects of drugs, including alcohol, illicit drugs, prescription medications, or toxins. Psychotic symptoms can result from intoxication on alcohol, **amphetamines** (and related substances), **cannabis** (marijuana), **cocaine**, **hallucinogens**, **inhalants**, **opioids**, phencyclidine (PCP) and related substances, **sedatives**, hypnotics, anxiolytics, and other or unknown substances. Psychotic symptoms can also result from withdrawal from alcohol, sedatives, hypnotics, anxiolytics, and other or unknown substances.

Medications that may induce psychotic symptoms include anesthetics and analgesics, anticholinergic agents, anticonvulsants, antihistamines, antihypertensive and cardiovascular medications, antimicrobial medications, antiparkinsonian medications, chemotherapeutic agents, corticosteroids, gastrointestinal medications, muscle relaxants, nonsteroidal anti-inflammatory medications, other over-the-counter medications, antidepressant medications, and **disulfiram**. Toxins that may induce psychotic symptoms include anticholinesterase, organophosphate insecticides, nerve gases, carbon monoxide, carbon dioxide, and volatile substances (such as fuel or paint).

The speed of onset of psychotic symptoms varies depending on the type of substance. For example, a large quantity of cocaine can produce psychotic symptoms within minutes. In contrast, psychotic symptoms may result from **alcohol use** only after days or weeks of intensive use.

The type of psychotic symptoms also tends to vary according to the type of substance. For instance, auditory hallucinations (specifically, hearing voices), visual hallucinations, and tactile hallucinations are most common in an alcohol-induced psychotic disorder, whereas persecutory delusions and tactile hallucinations (especially formication, which is the sensation that bugs are crawling on the skin) are commonly seen in a cocaine- or amphetamine-induced psychotic disorder.

Symptoms

The **diagnosis** is made only when the psychotic symptoms are above and beyond what would be expected during intoxication or withdrawal and when the psychotic symptoms are severe. The following are criteria necessary for diagnosis of a substance-induced psychotic disorder as listed in the ***Diagnostic and Statistical Manual of Mental Disorders***, fourth edition, text revision (*DSM-IV-TR*):

- Presence of prominent hallucinations or delusions.
- Hallucinations and/or delusions developing during, or within one month of, intoxication or withdrawal from a substance or medication known to cause psychotic symptoms.
- Psychotic symptoms not part of another psychotic disorder (such as schizophrenia, schizophreniform disorder, schizoaffective disorder) that is not substance induced. For instance, if the psychotic symptoms began before substance or medication use, then another psychotic disorder is likely.

KEY TERMS

Dementia—A chronic condition in which thinking and memory are progressively impaired. Other symptoms may also occur, including personality changes and depression.

Hallucination—A false or distorted perception of objects, sounds, or events that seems real. Hallucinations usually result from drugs or mental disorders.

Huntington's chorea—An hereditary disease that typically appears in midlife, marked by gradual loss of brain function and voluntary movement. Some of its symptoms resemble those of schizophrenia.

Schizophrenia—A severe mental disorder in which a person loses touch with reality and may have illogical thoughts, delusions, hallucinations, behavioral problems, and other disturbances.

- Psychotic symptoms not only occurring during delirium.

Diagnosis

Diagnosis of a substance-induced psychotic disorder must be differentiated from a psychotic disorder due to a general medical condition. Some medical conditions (such as temporal lobe epilepsy or Huntington's chorea) can produce psychotic symptoms, and, since individuals are likely to be taking medications for these conditions, it can be difficult to determine the cause of the psychotic symptoms. If the symptoms are determined to be due to the medical condition, then a diagnosis of a psychotic disorder due to a general medical condition is warranted.

Substance-induced psychotic disorder also needs to be distinguished from **delirium**, **dementia**, primary psychotic disorders, and substance intoxication and withdrawal. While there are no absolute means of determining substance use as a cause, a thorough patient history, including a careful assessment of onset and course of symptoms, along with that of substance use, is imperative. Often, the patient's testimony is unreliable, necessitating the gathering of information from family, friends, coworkers, employment records, medical records, and the like. Differentiating between substance-induced disorder and a psychiatric disorder may be aided by the following:

- Time of onset: If symptoms began before substance use, it is most likely a psychiatric disorder.
- Substance use patterns: If symptoms persist for three months or longer after substance is discontinued, a psychiatric disorder is probable.
- Consistency of symptoms: If symptoms are more exaggerated than one would expect with a particular substance type and dose, then the condition most likely is a psychiatric disorder.
- Family history: A family history of mental illness may indicate a psychiatric disorder.
- Response to substance abuse treatment: Clients with both psychiatric and substance use disorders often have serious difficulty with traditional substance abuse treatment programs and relapse during or shortly after treatment cessation.
- Client's stated reason for substance use: Those with a primary psychiatric diagnosis and secondary substance use disorder will often indicate they "medicate symptoms," for example, drink to dispel auditory hallucinations, use stimulants to combat depression, or use depressants to reduce anxiety or soothe a manic phase. While such substance use most often exacerbates the psychotic condition, it does not necessarily mean the client has a substance-induced psychotic disorder.

Unfortunately, psychological tests are not always helpful in determining if a psychotic disorder is caused by substance use or is being exacerbated by it. However, evaluations, such as the MMPI-2 MAC-R scale or the Wechsler Memory Scale—Revised, can be useful in making a differential diagnosis.

Treatment

Treatment is determined by the underlying cause and severity of psychotic symptoms. However, treatment of a substance-induced psychotic disorder often is similar to treatment for a primary psychotic disorder such as **schizophrenia**. Appropriate treatments may include psychiatric **hospitalization** and antipsychotic medication. Concurrent treatment will also be conducted for the **substance abuse** problem.

Prognosis

Psychotic symptoms induced by substance intoxication usually subside once the substance is eliminated. Symptoms persist depending on how long it takes before the substance is no longer present in an individual's system. Symptoms, therefore, can persist for hours, days, or weeks after a substance is last used.

QUESTIONS TO ASK YOUR DOCTOR

- Is the psychosis likely to be the result of substance use?
- Could changing a medication reduce the psychosis symptoms?
- Will my insurance pay for a rehabilitation center?
- Can you recommend a psychiatrist or other specialist experienced in treating this disorder?
- Are there any support groups that might be appropriate for me in this area?
- If I stop using the substance, how long can I expect the symptoms to last?
- Where can I find help for my substance use?

Prevention

There is very little documented regarding prevention of substance-induced psychotic disorder. However, abstaining from drugs and alcohol or using these substances only in moderation clearly reduces the risk of developing this disorder. In addition, taking medication under the supervision of an appropriately trained physician should reduce the likelihood of a medication-induced psychotic disorder. Finally, reducing one's exposure to toxins reduces the risk of toxin-induced psychotic disorder.

Resources

BOOKS

Fisher, Gary L., and Nancy A. Roget, eds. *Encyclopedia of Substance Abuse Prevention, Treatment, and Recovery.* Los Angeles: SAGE, 2009.

Meaden, Alan, and David Hacker. *Problematic and Risk Behaviours in Psychosis: A Shared Formulation Approach.* Hove, East Sussex: Routledge, 2010.

Stern, Theodore A., et al., eds. *Massachusetts General Hospital Handbook of General Hospital Psychiatry,* 6th ed. Philadelphia: Saunders/Elsevier, 2010.

PERIODICALS

Jordaan, Gerhard P., et al. "Alcohol-Induced Psychotic Disorder: A Comparative Study on the Clinical Characteristics of Patients with Alcohol Dependence and Schizophrenia." *Journal of Studies on Alcohol and Drugs* 70, no. 6 (November 2009):870–76.

Pierre, Joseph M. "Psychosis Associated with Medical Marijuana: Risk vs. Benefits of Medical Cannabis Use." *American Journal of Psychiatry* 167, no. 5 (May 2010): 598–99.

Torrens, Marti, et al. "Psychiatric Comorbidity in Illicit Drug Users: Substance-Induced versus Independent Disorders." *Drug and Alcohol Dependence* (2011).

ORGANIZATIONS

American Psychiatric Association, 1000 Wilson Blvd., Ste. 1825, Arlington, VA, 22209-3901, (703) 907-7300, apa@psych.org, http://www.psych.org.

American Psychological Association, 750 1st St. NE, Washington, DC, 20002-4242, (202) 336-5500; TDD/TTY: (202) 336-6123, (800) 374-2721, http://www.apa.org.

National Council on Alcoholism and Drug Dependence Inc., 244 E 58th St., 4th Fl., New York, NY, 10022, (212) 269-7797, (800) NCA-CALL, Fax: (212) 269-7510, national@mcadd.org, http://www.ncadd.org.

Substance Abuse and Mental Health Services Administration Referral Resource, 1 Choke Cherry Rd., Rockville, MD, 20857, (877) SAMHSA-7 (726-4727), (800) TTY: 487-4889, Fax: (240) 221-4292, SAMHSAInfo@samhsa.hhs.gov, http://www.samhsa.gov.

Jennifer Hahn, PhD
Tish Davidson, AM

Suicide

Definition

Suicide is defined as the intentional taking of one's own life. In some European languages, including German, the word for suicide translates into English as "self-murder." In Latin, suicide is derived from *suicidium*, or "to kill oneself." Until approximately the end of the twentieth century, suicide was considered a criminal act; legal terminology used the Latin phrase *felo-de-se*, which means "a crime against the self." Much of the social **stigma** that is still associated with suicide derives from its former connection with legal judgment as well as with religious condemnation.

Demographics

In the United States, the rate of suicide has continued to rise since the 1950s. More people in the general population die from suicide than homicide in North America. There are 11.3 suicide deaths each year for every 100,000 people living in the United States, according to the **National Institute of Mental Health** (NIMH), and for every suicide, there are approximately 11.5 attempts. In any given year, there are approximately 40,000 suicide-based deaths, along with up to 500,000 suicide attempts. The U.S. Centers for Disease Control

Suicidal thoughts and behaviors in the past year among adults, by age group: 2008 and 2009

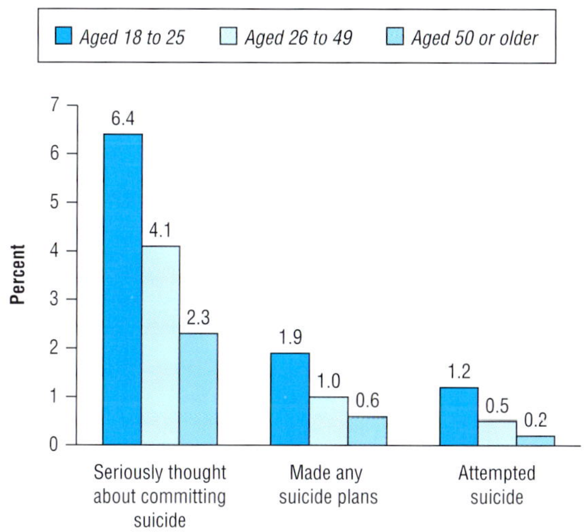

SOURCE: Substance Abuse and Mental Health Services Administration, Center for Behavioral Health Statistics and Quality, "Suicidal Thoughts and Behaviors among Adults: 2008 and 2009," *The NSDUH Report* (December 21, 2010).

Report available online at http://www.oas.samhsa.gov/2k10/212/SuicidalThoughts.htm. *(Graph by PreMediaGlobal. © 2012 Cengage Learning.)*

and Prevention (CDC) states that in 2009, suicide was the tenth-leading cause of death in the United States. According to the U.S. Department of Defense/Veterans Affairs website, more years of life are lost due to suicide than to any other single cause except for heart disease and cancer. Substance abuse is a major factor associated with suicide. Statistics show that substance abuse is thought to be involved in as many as one-half of all suicide cases. In fact, the abuse of alcohol is involved with about 20% of all suicide attempts. Completed suicides are most likely to involve a man over the age of 45 years who is suffering from depression or alcoholism.

By state, region

The demographics of suicide in the United States vary considerably from state to state, with rates higher than the national average in the West and lower in the Midwest and Northeast. Some states, like Alaska, have suicide rates that are almost twice the national average; others, such as Massachusetts, have notably lower rates.

Age and gender

These variations from state to state, and region to region, result in part from differences in age and ethnic distributions and gender ratios among the states. In 2008, suicide was the eighth-leading cause of death among males and sixteenth-leading cause of death among females. Males are four times more likely than females to succeed in their suicide attempts, but females report attempting suicide at some point in their lives three times as often as men do. An increase in the overall suicide rate in the United States between 1999 and 2009 was due primarily to an increase in suicides among Caucasians aged 40–64 years, with white middle-aged women experiencing the largest annual increases.

In terms of age, the highest number of suicides are committed by people under age 40 years, but suicide rates (percentages in a given group) increase with age. People over age 65 years have high suicide rates, with men outnumbering women who commit suicide nearly four to one.

SENIORS. The incidence of suicide and attempted suicide among seniors is widely perceived as a growing public health problem in the United States; in 2009, older adults represented about 13% of the U.S. population but accounted for 20% of suicides. According to the NIMH, the highest suicide rate in the nation is for Caucasian men aged 85 years and older, at 65.3 deaths per 100,000 persons—about six times the national U.S. rate of 10.8 per 100,000.

The ratio of attempted suicides to completed suicides among people over 65 is thought to be around 4:1. According to the National Strategy for Suicide Prevention (NSSP), seniors are more likely than are younger persons to use highly lethal means of suicide. According to a Canadian study published in 2008, seniors are most likely to use firearms to commit suicide, followed by hanging, self-poisoning, and leaping from heights.

YOUNG PEOPLE. The overall rate of suicide among young people has declined slowly since 1992, but it still remains the third-leading cause of death in age groups spanning children 10 years old to young adults up to age 24. Suicidal behavior is rare in prepubertal children, probably because of their relative inability to plan and execute a suicide attempt. Children as young as 5 years, however, have succeeded in killing themselves by leaping out of windows or shooting themselves—as happened with one five-year-old who witnessed his mother kill herself with a gun and imitated her behavior several months later. According to the NIMH, the rates of suicide for American youth in 2007 (the most recent data available) were as follows:

- children between the ages of 10 and 14: 0.9 suicides per 100,000

- teenagers between the ages of 15 and 19: 6.9 per 100,000
- young adults between the ages of 20 and 24: 12.7 per 100,000

Race or ethnicity

In 2007, the NIMH reported the highest suicide rates among American Indians and Alaska Natives, at 14.3 per 100,000, and Non-Hispanic whites, at 13.5 per 100,000. The lowest suicide rates were found among Hispanics, at 6.0 per 100,000; Non-Hispanic blacks, at 5.1 per 100,000; and Asian and Pacific Islanders, at 6.2 per 100,000. Suicide rates among American Indian and Alaskan natives between 15 and 34 years are almost twice the national average for this age range. Young Hispanic females make significantly more suicide attempts than their male or non-Hispanic counterparts.

In the military

In 2008, the rate of suicides in the U.S. Army surpassed the civilian (non-military) rate (19.2 per 100,000), hitting an all-time high of 20.2 suicides per 100,000 people. In that year, at least 128 soldiers committed suicide (with other deaths being investigated as possible suicide cases); suicide deaths numbered 115 and 102 in the two years prior, respectively.

According to 2009 data, five members of the military were unsuccessful in their suicide attempt for every one that was successful. The U.S. Veterans Affairs Department (VA) reported in 2010 that the suicide rate for 17–29 year old male veterans increased by 26% from 2005 to 2007. Statistics show that one of the major causes of suicide within these military personnel was substance abuse (drug or alcohol). Between 2005 and 2009, the use of drugs or alcohol contributed to over 45% of unsuccessful suicide attempts and 30% of suicide deaths. The Defense Survey of Health-Related Behaviors found that 12% of military personnel had the presence of "dangerous levels" of alcohol or illicit drugs within their bodies. Relationship problems were also a major cause of suicide, with 58% of suicide deaths in 2009 believed caused by such stressful situations.

International

Suicide has become a major social and medical problem around the world, not just in North America. Worldwide suicide rates have increased by 60% since 1960. The World Health Organization (WHO) reports that nearly one million people worldwide die annually from suicide, more than the number of people murdered or killed in war. That number of suicides breaks down to 16 deaths per 100,000 people, or one death every 40 seconds. According to WHO, more suicides occur in Asia than in any other region of the world, with China, Japan, and India accounting for 40% of the world's suicides. China is also the only country in the world where more women than men take their own lives, with female suicides representing 58% of the total.

Rates among young people have risen even faster, to the point where they are now the age group at highest risk in 35% of the world's countries. Among people 10 to 24 years of age, suicide is the third-leading cause of death in the world, and it is the second-leading cause in persons aged 15 to 44 years. For every 20 attempted tries at suicide, there is one death. In Europe and North America, mental disorders are particularly high in the cause of suicides. All over the world, suicide involves a complex play of biological (genetic), cultural, environmental, psychological, and social factors.

Description

Suicidal behavior is most commonly regarded—and responded to—as a psychiatric or medical emergency, one often committed due to a mental disorder such as **bipolar disorder**, **depression**, **schizophrenia**, or **substance abuse**. At other times, suicide may be contemplated due to pressures in life, such as financial or legal difficulties or a troubling interpersonal relationship such as a crumbling marriage. Law enforcement personnel may be involved in preventing an attempted suicide or taking suicidal individuals to a hospital emergency department but not in arresting these persons for breaking the law.

Historical background

Attitudes toward suicide have varied throughout history. The ancient Greeks considered it an offense against the state, which was deprived of contributions by potentially useful citizens. The Romans, by comparison, thought that suicide could be a noble form of death, although they legislated against persons taking their own lives before an impending criminal conviction in order to insure their families' financial inheritance. Early Christianity, which downplayed the importance of life on Earth, was not critical of suicide until the fourth century, when Algerian philosopher St. Augustine (354–430) condemned it as a sin because it violated the sixth commandment ("Thou shalt not kill."). Eventually, the Roman Catholic Church excommunicated and even denied funeral rites to people who killed themselves. The view of suicide as a sin prevailed in Western societies for hundreds of years, and many people are still influenced by it, either consciously or unconsciously. For instance, suicide was a felony and attempted suicide a misdemeanor in England until 1961.

Austrian neurologist Sigmund Freud (1856–1939) provided the first theory that addressed suicide in terms of a person's inner mental and emotional state. In *Mourning and Melancholia* (1917), he proposed that suicide was the result of turning hostility toward a loved one back on oneself. In *Man against Himself* (1936), American **psychiatrist** Karl Menninger (1893–1990) extended Freud's contribution to the psychodynamic study of suicide, relating it to such other forms of self-destructive behavior as alcoholism or drug abuse. Some people still refer to such behavior as "slow-motion suicide."

Types of suicidal behavior

Some mental health professionals distinguish five levels of suicidal behavior: completed suicide; suicide attempts, which are potentially fatal; suicide gestures, which involve acting-out behavior that is not necessarily lethal; suicide gambles; and suicidal ideation, or thinking about suicide. An example of a suicide gesture would be cutting one's wrist just deeply enough to draw blood from the skin but not deeply enough to sever veins and arteries. The suicide gamble is a type of suicidal behavior in which the person takes the risk that he or she will be discovered in time and that the discoverer will save them. The suicide of American poet Sylvia Plath (1932–1963) is considered an example of a suicide gamble. Plath gassed herself in the kitchen by turning on her oven without lighting it, but left a note on the door for her children's new nanny, had opened the windows in the children's bedroom to protect them, and had sealed the door to the kitchen with dish towels.

Suicidal ideation, or thinking about suicide, is even more common than suicide gestures or attempted suicide. Suicidal ideation spans a continuum from nonspecific thoughts such as "life is not worth living" to specific ideation. Community surveys indicate that 12%–25% of primary and high school children have some form of suicidal ideation, whereas 5%–10% combine suicidal ideation with a plan or intent to make a suicide attempt. Specific ideation is more closely associated with risk for attempted suicide and frequently occurs in combination with other risk factors.

Risk factors

Some factors increase a person's risk of suicide:

- male gender
- age over 75 years
- family history of suicide or mental illness
- history of suicide attempts
- Caucasian race
- history of abuse
- traumatic experiences after childhood
- recent stressful events, such as separation or divorce, job loss, or death of spouse
- dealing with homosexuality in an unsupportive environment
- lack of a support network, poor relationships with parents or peers, and feelings of social isolation
- chronic medical illness—patients with acquired immune deficiency syndrome (AIDS) have a rate of suicide 20 times that of the general population
- chronic, severe, or intractable pain
- loss of mobility or independence
- access to a firearm—death by firearms accounts for the majority of suicides in the United States
- alcohol or substance abuse—while mood-altering substances do not cause a person to kill himself or herself, they do weaken impulse control
- high blood cholesterol levels
- presence of a psychiatric illness

More than 90% of Americans who commit suicide have a mental illness. Major depression accounts for 60% of suicides, followed by schizophrenia, alcoholism, substance abuse, **borderline personality disorder**, Huntington's disease, and epilepsy. The lifetime mortality due to suicide in psychiatric patients is 15% for major depression, 20% for bipolar disorder, 18% for alcoholism, 10% for schizophrenia, and 5–10% for borderline and certain other **personality disorders**. In children and adolescents, the most common triggers of suicidal behavior involve interpersonal conflict or loss, most frequently with parents or romantic attachment figures. Family discord, physical or **sexual abuse**, and an upcoming legal or disciplinary crisis are also commonly associated with completed and attempted suicides. The most serious suicide attempts involve suicide notes, evidence of planning, and an irreversible method. Most adolescent suicide attempts are of relatively low intent and lethality, and only a minority actually want to die. Usually, children and adolescents who attempt suicide want to escape psychological pain or unbearable circumstances, gain attention, influence others, or communicate such strong feelings as rage or love.

Factors that lower the risk of suicide include:

- significant friendship network outside the workplace
- religious faith and practice, especially those that discourage suicide and value life
- stable marriage
- close-knit extended family
- strong interest in or commitment to a project or cause that brings people together—community service,

environmental concerns, neighborhood associations, animal rescue groups, etc.

Ethical issues related to suicide

Several ethical issues related to suicide have emerged as public policy matters in the early twenty-first century. The most controversial of these are the notion of a "right to suicide" and the question of assisted suicide.

RIGHT TO SUICIDE. The idea that suicide is a right among the elderly or those with terminal illnesses surfaced with the 1991 publication of English-born American journalist Derek Humphry's (1930–) *Final Exit*, a controversial book described by its author as a how-to manual for suicide and assisted suicide. Humphry is the founder of the Euthanasia Research and Guidance Organization (ERGO), known until 2003 as the Hemlock Society. Humphry maintains that people have a right to choose the time, place, and method of their death and that rational suicide is a legitimate and even reasonable choice.

People who are often overlooked in discussions of the right to commit suicide, however, are the relatives and friends who are bereaved by the suicide. It is estimated that each person who commits suicide leaves six survivors to deal with the aftermath. On the basis of this figure, there are at least 4.5 million survivors of suicide in the United States. In addition to the **grief** that ordinarily accompanies death, survivors of suicide often struggle with feelings of guilt and shame as well. Some people have blamed Humphry and his book for their loved one's decision to commit suicide.

ASSISTED SUICIDE. Questions pertaining to the legalization of assisted suicide for persons suffering from a terminal illness are connected in part to increases in the average lifespan. Physician-assisted suicide (also known as physician-assisted death or PAD) was legalized in the Netherlands in April 2001, and in the states of Oregon, Washington, and Montana. As of 2011, it was also legal in Belgium and Luxembourg and was practiced openly in Switzerland. It is important to distinguish between physician-assisted suicide and euthanasia, or "mercy killing." Assisted suicide, which is called "self-deliverance" in Britain, refers to individuals bringing about their own death with the help of another person. Because the other person is often a physician, the act is often called doctor-assisted suicide.

Euthanasia strictly speaking means that the physician or other person is the one who performs the last act that causes death. For example, if a physician injects a patient with a lethal dose of a pain-killing medication, the physician is performing euthanasia. If the physician leaves the patient with a loaded syringe and the patient injects himself or herself with it, the act is an assisted suicide. Euthanasia is illegal in all 50 states.

Causes and symptoms

Causes

One model that has been used by clinicians to explain why people suffering under the same life stresses respond differently is known as the stress/diathesis model. Diathesis is a medical term for a predisposition that makes some people more vulnerable to thoughts of suicide. In addition to factors at the individual level, factors in the wider society have been identified as contributing to the rising rate of suicide in the United States, including:

- Stresses on the nuclear family, including more frequent divorce and economic hardship.
- Loss of a set of moral values held in common by the entire society.
- Weakening of churches, synagogues, neighborhood associations, and other mid-range social groups outside the family. In the past, these institutions often provided a sense of belonging for people from troubled or emotionally distant families.
- Frequent geographical moves, which makes it difficult for people to make and keep long-term friendships outside their immediate family.
- Sensationalized treatment of suicide in the mass media. A number of research studies have shown that there is a definite risk of "contagion" or copycat suicides from irresponsible reporting, particularly among impressionable adolescents. One group of researchers has estimated that as many as 6% of all suicides in the developed countries are copycat suicides.
- Development of medications that allow relatively painless suicide. For most of human history, the available means of suicide were uncertain, painful, or both.
- Easy availability of lethal methods of suicide, most notably firearms, and so-called suicide magnets such as bridges or tall buildings that do not have suicide barriers and are easy to reach. The Golden Gate Bridge in San Francisco, California, is the most notorious public suicide location in the United States; others include the Aurora Bridge in Seattle, Washington, the Sunshine Skyway Bridge in Florida, and the Duke Ellington Bridge in Washington, DC. Other popular suicide locations elsewhere

in the world include the Aokigahara Forest at the base of Mount Fuji in Japan, and Beachy Head in the United Kingdom.

The role of the Internet in the rate of adolescent suicide has been debated. On the one hand, there are websites and chat rooms that foster preoccupation with suicide and offer detailed descriptions of suicide methods. There are even instances of adolescents recruiting other adolescents over the Internet to join them in a suicide pact. For instance, seven young people who had met via the Internet committed group suicide by inhaling carbon monoxide from a charcoal burner inside a locked van. Other websites attack psychiatry and mental health professionals, which may steer some vulnerable young people away from seeking help. On the other hand, there are many supportive websites for teens that offer resources (including peer counseling) and contact information for getting help if they are considering suicide.

Media treatment of suicide

In 1989, the CDC sponsored a national workshop to address the connection between sensationalized media treatments of suicide and the rising rate of suicide among American youth. The CDC and the American Association of Suicidology subsequently adopted a set of guidelines for media coverage of suicide intended to reduce the risk of copycat suicides.

The CDC guidelines point out that the following types of reporting may increase the risk of copycat suicides:

- Presenting oversimplified explanations of suicide, when in fact many factors usually contribute to it. One example concerns the suicide of the widow of a man who was killed in the collapse of the World Trade Center on September 11, 2001. Most newspapers that covered the story described her death as due solely to the act of terrorism, even though she had a history of depressive illness.
- Giving excessive, ongoing, or repetitive coverage of the suicide.
- Sensationalizing the suicide by including morbid details or dramatic photographs.
- Giving "how-to" descriptions of the method of suicide.
- Referring to suicide as an effective coping strategy or as a way to achieve temporary fame or other goals.
- Glorifying the act of suicide or the person who commits suicide.
- Focusing on the person's positive traits without mentioning his or her problems.

Symptoms

Potential warning signs of suicidal thinking may include:

- reading a lot of books or articles on death and suicide
- talking a lot about death or suicide or expressing feelings of hopelessness
- stockpiling medications
- refusing to take care of oneself
- sudden interest in guns
- giving away cherished possessions, writing long letters, or making other elaborate farewells
- disrupted sleep patterns
- hurriedly revising a will
- increased intake of alcohol or prescription drugs

Diagnosis

The **diagnosis** of a suicide attempt is often made when the patient either goes to the emergency room of a hospital to seek help or is taken there by family members or first responders. In many cases, the patient will have written a suicide note, talked about his or her intention, or begun to carry out a plan to kill him- or herself. If the patient is not conscious, the doctor will obtain as much information as possible from family members or first responders.

Treatment

Suicide attempts are treated as a psychiatric emergency by police or other rescue personnel. Treatment in a hospital emergency room includes a complete psychiatric evaluation, a **mental status examination**, and a detailed assessment of the circumstances surrounding the attempt. The physician will interview the person's relatives or anyone else who accompanied the patient in order to obtain as much information as possible. Some questions that the physician will ask include whether the patient had a detailed plan for suicide; whether he or she had the means of suicide at hand; what the patient hoped to gain by killing themselves (freedom from pain, reunion with a dead loved one, solution to financial problems, etc.); and whether the patient had any tendencies toward homicide. As a rule, suicide attempts requiring advance planning and the use of violent or highly lethal methods are regarded as the most serious. The patient will be kept under observation while decisions are made about the need for **hospitalization**.

People who have attempted suicide and who are considered a serious danger to themselves or to others can be legally hospitalized against their will. The doctor bases the decision on the severity of the patient's depression or agitation; the presence of other suicide risk factors, including a history of previous suicide attempts, substance abuse, recent stressful events, and symptoms of **psychosis**; and the availability of friends, relatives, or other social support. If the attempt is judged to be a nonlethal suicide gesture, and the patient has adequate support outside the hospital, he or she may be released after the psychiatric assessment is completed.

Traditional

People who survive a suicide attempt are usually treated with a combination of antidepressant medications and **psychotherapy**.

Drugs

In 2003, the Food and Drug Administration (FDA) approved the use of **clozapine** (Clozaril), an antipsychotic medication, for the treatment of patients with schizophrenia who have attempted suicide.

Treatment of suicide survivors

In addition to the grief that ordinarily accompanies death, survivors of a friend or relative's suicide often struggle with feelings of guilt and shame as well. In spite of a general liberalization of social attitudes since World War II (1939–1945), suicide is still stigmatized in many parts of Europe and the United States. Survivors often benefit from group or individual psychotherapy in order to work through such issues as wondering whether they could have prevented the suicide or whether they are at increased risk of committing suicide themselves. Increasing numbers of clergy as well as mental health professionals are trained in counseling survivors of suicide.

Prognosis

The prognosis for a person who has attempted suicide is generally favorable, although further research needs to be done. Many different studies have followed individuals who attempted suicide to determine how likely they are to die by suicide. These studies have generally found that the likelihood is less than 10%. A doctor who studied 515 people who attempted suicide between 1937 and 1971 found that 94% were still alive at the time of his study or had died of natural causes. In general, individuals who attempt suicide and rate highly on intent to commit suicide and hopelessness may be more likely to commit suicide later. These findings may indicate that suicidal behavior is more likely to be a passing response to an acute crisis than a reflection of a permanent state of mind.

KEY TERMS

Assisted suicide—A form of self-inflicted death in which individuals voluntarily bring about their own death with the help of another, usually a physician, relative, or friend. Assisted suicide is sometimes called physician-assisted death (PAD).

Cortisol—A hormone released by the cortex (outer portion) of the adrenal gland when a person is under stress. Such levels are now considered a biological marker of suicide risk.

Diathesis—The medical term for predisposition. The stress/diathesis model is a diagram that is used to explain why some people are at greater risk of suicidal behavior than others.

Euthanasia—The act of putting individuals or animals to death painlessly or allowing them to die by withholding medical services, usually because of an incurable disease.

Frontal cortex—The part of the human brain associated with aggressiveness and impulse control. Abnormalities in this part of the brain are associated with an increased risk of suicide.

Self-deliverance—Another term for assisted suicide, more commonly used in Great Britain than in the United States.

Serotonin—A chemical that occurs in the blood and nervous tissue and functions to transmit signals across the gaps between neurons in the central nervous system. Abnormally low levels of this chemical are associated with depression and an increased risk of suicide.

Suicide gesture—Attempted suicide characterized by a low-lethality method, low level of intent or planning, and little physical damage; sometimes called pseudocide.

Suicide magnet—A bridge, tall building, or geographic location that acquires a reputation for attracting people who want to commit suicide and attempt it.

Prevention

One reason that suicide is such a tragedy is that most self-inflicted deaths are potentially preventable. Many suicidal people change their minds if they can be

QUESTIONS TO ASK YOUR DOCTOR

- There have been a number of suicides in my family. Does that mean that I am at increased risk of suicide?
- How can I help a depressed friend who says that he or she has nothing to live for?
- How can I tell the difference between an occasional blue spell and the kind of depression that can lead to suicide?
- What would you recommend as good ways to deal with occasional thoughts of suicide?

helped through their immediate crisis; Dr. Richard Seiden, from the University of California at Berkeley, a specialist in treating survivors of suicide attempts, puts the high-risk period at 90 days after the crisis. Some potential suicides change their minds during the actual attempt; for example, a number of people who survived jumping off the Golden Gate Bridge told interviewers afterward that they regretted their action even as they were falling and that they were grateful they survived.

Brain research is an important means of suicide prevention. Known biological markers for an increased risk of suicide may be correlated with personality profiles linked to suicidal behavior under **stress** to help identify individuals at risk. Brain **imaging studies** using **positron emission tomography (PET)** are being used to detect abnormal patterns of **serotonin** uptake in specific regions of the brain. Genetic studies are also yielding new information about inherited predispositions to suicide.

Research is ongoing to discover better methods of treating depression and other disorders that may influence a person's decision to commit suicide. Primary care physicians are continually learning how to better identify and intervene when treating suicidal patients. An estimated 67% of all adults and 80% of seniors who complete suicide have seen a physician within a month of their death, placing primary care physicians in a good position to evaluate patients for signs of depression. The good news is that depression in adults in any age group is highly treatable, particularly when antidepressant medications are combined with psychotherapy.

People who are concerned about a friend or relative at risk of self-harm should take the following steps:

- Become educated about warning signs and risk factors.
- Identify physicians and other healthcare professionals who know the person and can provide help.
- Talk openly with the person about his or her feelings—although many people are afraid to ask whether someone is thinking about suicide for fear of angering them or giving them an idea, in many cases honest concern is welcomed by the individual.
- Call the local hospital emergency department or 911 if the person seems to be at immediate risk of suicide.

Resources

BOOKS

American Psychiatric Association. *Diagnostic and Statistical Manual of Mental Disorders*. 4th ed., text rev. Washington, DC: American Psychiatric Association, 2000.

Beers, Mark H., and Robert Berkow, eds. *Merck Manual of Geriatrics*. 3rd ed. Whitehouse Station, NJ: Merck, 2005.

Giddens, Sandra. *Suicide*. New York: Rosen Publishing, 2007.

Goldney, Robert D. *Suicide Prevention*. New York: Oxford University Press, 2008.

Kutcher, Stanley P., and Sonia Chehil. *Suicide Risk Management: A Manual for Health Professionals*. Malden, MA: Blackwell Publishing, 2007.

Paris, Joel. *Half in Love with Death: Managing the Chronically Suicidal Patient*. Mahwah, NJ: Lawrence Erlbaum Associates, 2007.

PERIODICALS

Ajdacic-Gross, V., et al. "Methods of Suicide: International Suicide Patterns Derived from the WHO Mortality Databse." *Bulletin of the World Health Organization* 86 (September 2008): 726–32.

Alao, A. O., M. Soderberg, E. L. Pohl, and A. L. Alao. "Cybersuicide: Review of the Role of the Internet on Suicide." *Cyberpsychology and Behavior* 9 (August 2006): 489–93.

American Academy of Hospice and Palliative Medicine. "Position Statement on Physician-Assisted Death." *Journal of Pain and Palliative Care Pharmacotherapy* 21 (April 2007): 55–57.

Apter, A., and R. A. King. "Management of the Depressed, Suicidal Child or Adolescent." *Child and Adolescent Psychiatric Clinics of North America* 15 (October 2006): 999–1013.

Beyer, J. L. "Managing Depression in Geriatric Populations." *Annals of Clinical Psychiatry* 19 (October/December 2007): 221–38.

Centers for Disease Control and Prevention (CDC). "Alcohol and Suicide among Racial/Ethnic Populations—17 States, 2005–2006." *Morbidity and Mortality Weekly Report* 58 (June 19, 2009): 637–41.

———. "Increases in Age-Group-Specific Injury Mortality—United States, 1999–2004." *Morbidity and Mortality Weekly Report* 56 (December 14, 2007): 1281–84.

Coryell, William H. "Clinical Assessment of Suicide Risk in Depressive Disorder." *CNS Spectrums* 11, no. 6 (2006): 255–461. http://www.cnsspectrums.com/aspx/articledetail.aspx?articleid=474 (accessed November 13, 2011).

Friend, Tad. "Jumpers: The Fatal Grandeur of the Golden Gate Bridge." *New Yorker* (October 13, 2003). http://www.newyorker.com/archive/2003/10/13/031013fa_fact?currentPage=all (accessed July 20, 2011).

Fu, K. W., et al. "Estimating the Risk for Suicide Following the Suicide Deaths of 3 Asian Entertainment Celebrities: A Meta-Analytic Approach." *Journal of Clinical Psychiatry* 70 (June 2009): 869–78.

Guthmann, Edward, et al. "Lethal Beauty." *San Francisco Chronicle* (October 30, 2005). http://www.sfgate.com/cgi-bin/article.cgi?f=/c/a/2005/10/30/MNG2NFF7KI1.DTL (accessed July 20, 2011).

Jelinek, Pauline, and Kimberly Hefling. "Army Suicide Rates Hit Record High." *Huffington Post* (January 29, 2009). http://www.huffingtonpost.com/2009/01/30/army-suicide-rates-hit-re_n_162484.html (accessed July 20, 2011).

Jokinen, A., et al. "HPA Axis Hyperactivity and Attempted Suicide in Young Adult Mood Disorder Inpatients." *Journal of Affective Disorders* 116 (July 2009): 117–20.

Liu, X., A. L. Gentzler, P. Tepper, et al. "Clinical Features of Depressed Children and Adolescents with Various Forms of Suicidality." *Journal of Clinical Psychiatry* 67 (September 2006): 1442–50.

Voaklander, D. C., et al. "Medical Illness, Medication Use, and Suicide in Seniors: A Population-Based Case Control Study." *Journal of Epidemiology and Community Health* 62 (February 2008): 138–46.

Yip, P.S., et al. "Years of Life Lost from Suicide in China, 1990–2000." *Crisis* 29 (March 2008): 131–36.

OTHER

Centers for Disease Control and Prevention. "Deaths: Preliminary Data for 2009." *National Vital Statistics Report* 59, no. 4 (March 16, 2011). http://www.cdc.gov/nchs/data/nvsr/nvsr59/nvsr59_04.pdf (accessed July 20, 2011).

WEBSITES

American Academy of Child and Adolescent Psychiatry. "Teen Suicide." *Facts for Families* 10 (May 2008). http://www.aacap.org/cs/root/facts_for_families/teen_suicide (accessed July 20, 2011).

American Association of Suicidology. "Fact Sheets." http://www.suicidology.org/web/guest/stats-and-tools/fact-sheets (accessed July 20, 2011).

———. "If You Are Considering Suicide." http://www.suicidology.org/web/guest/thinking-about-suicide (accessed July 20, 2011).

American Foundation for Suicide Prevention. "About Suicide: Frequently Asked Questions." http://www.afsp.org/index.cfm?fuseaction=home.viewPage&page_id=052618D2-02D2-04B4-00EDA31CFC336B63 (accessed July 20, 2011).

Andrew, Louise B. "Depression and Suicide." Medscape Reference. May 9, 2011. http://emedicine.medscape.com/article/805459-overview (accessed July 20, 2011).

Centers for Disease Control and Prevention. "National Suicide Statistics: At a Glance." September 30, 2009. http://www.cdc.gov/violenceprevention/suicide/statistics/index.html (accessed July 20, 2011).

National Institute of Mental Health. "Suicide Prevention." July 20, 2011. http://www.nimh.nih.gov/health/topics/suicide-prevention/index.shtml (accessed July 20, 2011).

———. "Suicide in the U.S.: Statistics and Prevention." September 30, 2009. http://www.nimh.nih.gov/health/publications/suicide-in-the-us-statistics-and-prevention/index.shtml (accessed July 20, 2011).

Soreff, Stephen. "Suicide." Medscape Reference. January 11, 2011. http://emedicine.medscape.com/article/288598-overview (accessed July 20, 2011).

U.S. Department of Defense and Veterans Administration. "About Suicide." DoD/VA Suicide Outreach. http://www.suicideoutreach.org/about_suicide (accessed July 20, 2011).

ORGANIZATIONS

American Academy of Child and Adolescent Psychiatry, 3615 Wisconsin Ave. NW, Washington, DC, 20016-3007, (202) 966-7300, Fax: (202) 966-2891, http://www.aacap.org.

American Association of Suicidology, 5221 Wisconsin Ave. NW, Washington, DC, 20015, (202) 237-2280, Fax: (202) 237-2282, http://www.suicidology.org/web/guest/home.

American Foundation for Suicide Prevention, 120 Wall St., 29th Fl., New York, NY, 20016-3007, (212) 363-3500, (888) 333-2377, Fax: (212) 363-6237, inquiry@afsp.org, http://www.afsp.org.

American Psychiatric Association, 1000 Wilson Blvd., Ste. 1825, Arlington, VA, 22209, (703) 907-7300, apa@psych.org, http://www.psych.org.

Mental Health America, 2000 N Beauregard St., 6th Fl., Alexandria, VA, 22311, (703) 684-7722, Fax: (703) 684-5968, (800) 969-6642, http://www1.nmha.org.

National Alliance on Mental Illness, 3803 N Fairfax Dr., Ste. 100, Arlington, VA, 22203, (703) 524-7600, Fax: (703) 524-9094, http://www.nami.org.

National Institute of Mental Health, 6001 Executive Blvd., Rm. 8184, MSC 9663, Bethesda, MD, 20892-9663, (301) 443-4513, (866) 615-6464, Fax: (301) 443-4279, nimhinfo@-nih.gov, http://www.nimh.nih.gov.

National Suicide Prevention Lifeline, (800) 274-TALK (8255), http://www.suicidepreventionlifeline.org.

U.S. Department of Veterans Affairs (VA), 810 Vermont Ave. NW, Washington, DC, United States 20420, (800) 827-1000; Mental health crisis line: (800) 273-8255 (press 1), http://www.va.gov.

Rebecca J. Frey, PhD
David A. Brent, MD
William A. Atkins, BB, BS, MBA

Support groups

Definition

Support groups are an informal resource that attempts to provide healing components to a variety of problems and challenges. An informal support outside of family, friends, or professionals often provides greater understanding, more similarity (from individuals experiencing similar life events), an opportunity for empathy and altruism, and a sense of identity for participants. Learning new ways to handle challenges, cope with changes, and maintain new behaviors are all important aspects of the support group experience.

A characteristic unique to support groups is the mutual support members are able to provide one another. This support and validation from other group members help facilitate personal growth and change in a way that individual therapy cannot. Although experts and professionals can provide support and positive direction, the mutual exchange of information between group members is a powerful experience that often induces lasting change.

Description

Most support groups are facilitated or led by lay persons, often in conjunction with existing organizations (such as the National Alliance on Mental Illness [NAMI] or Alcoholics Anonymous [AA]). Support groups usually have a set meeting time (generally weekly or monthly), and an open format. Open format means that the groups are ongoing, and members have the option of attending when it is convenient for them. This is in contrast to other types of structured treatment or psycho-educational groups that may meet for a certain number of sessions, with the expectation that participants attend every meeting. The open format allows members to feel some degree of anonymity, and to participate as they are comfortable. For some people, simply attending meetings and listening to the experiences of others can be helpful.

The healing power of groups is well documented, and support groups offer many of the same therapeutic characteristics as more structured groups. These factors include: altruism (chance to help others), belongingness, universality (there are others who struggle with similar challenges), interpersonal learning, guidance, catharsis,

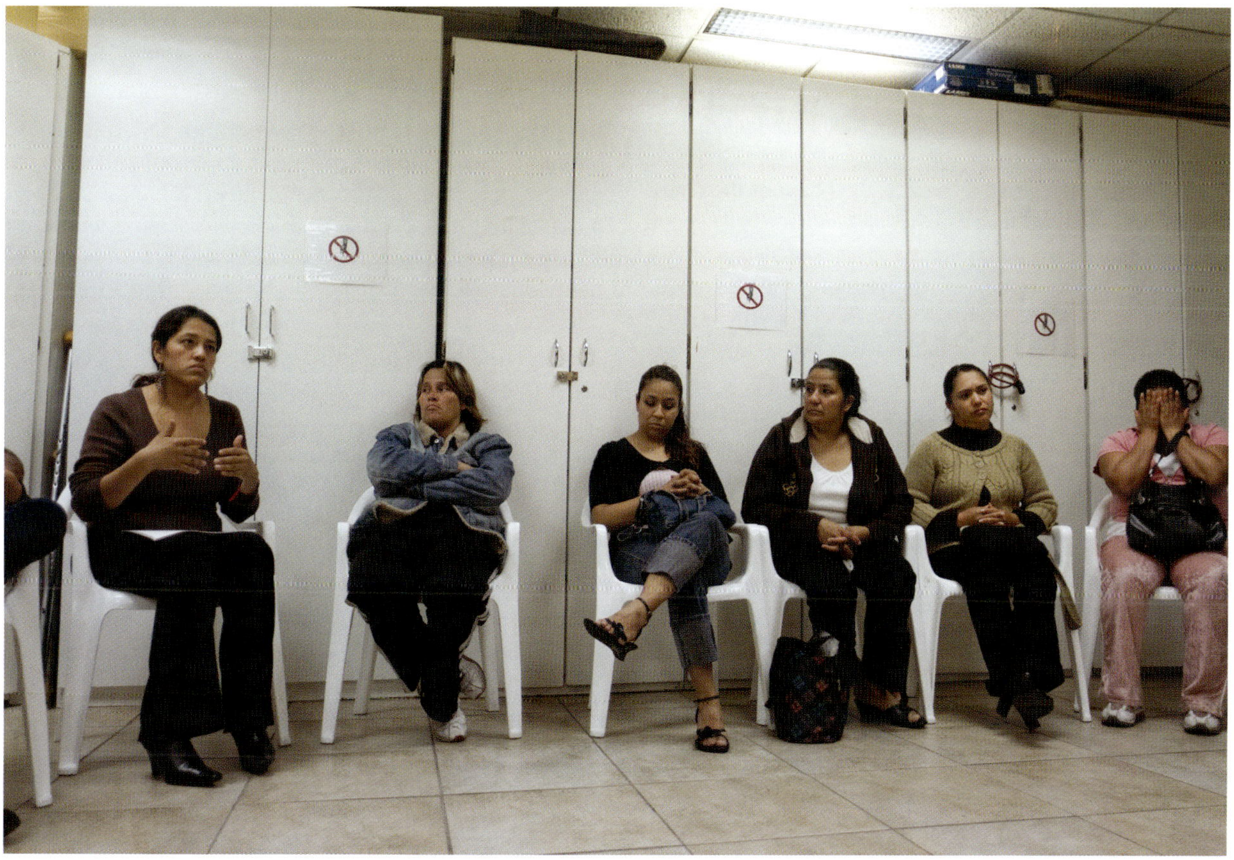

A group of women listen to another woman speak at a support group for victims of domestic violence. *(© Lynn Johnson/ National Geographic Image Collection/Alamy)*

identification, self-understanding, instillation of hope, and existential factors (such as the search for larger meaning in life). Each of these factors is directly related to the mutual support that members provide one another.

Support groups are generally less structured than psycho-educational groups or therapy groups, however, as each group usually sets its own norms, rules, and schedules. Some groups, such as AA, traditionally reserve time for individual members to discuss their own challenges and progress in front of the group. Others bring in speakers periodically to provide information about disorders or specific coping skills. However, the strength of support groups lies in its members, and their willingness to share their own experiences, challenges, and solutions in the context of the group.

In addition to these traditional, face-to-face support groups, technology has had an impact on the functioning and availability of support groups. There are many listserves, e-mail groups, and chat groups that provide information about specific life problems (adoption of children outside the United States, for example), certain types of mental illness, and specific health problems. While there is always the risk of communicating with others who are not honest, many people benefit from these Internet interactions. Some individuals are actually more comfortable participating in Internet support groups due to the greater anonymity they offer.

There are a variety of problems and challenges that are addressed in support groups. Generally speaking, the severity of the symptom, as well as the phase of the illness or disorder, will determine whether participation in a support group is appropriate. For more severe types of mental illness, such as **schizophrenia**, or **depression** with psychotic episodes, a support group is probably not the optimal **intervention**, particularly at initial onset. After stabilization through therapy and medication (as appropriate), a support group may offer an important addition to more formal treatment. In these cases, the socialization, interpersonal relationships, and social support that can be gained through the group may not be available elsewhere, and as such, it can be a very positive experience for the participant. In a group situation, a participant can learn how to express feelings in a healthy and positive way, practice assertive communication, receive feedback about appropriate and inappropriate content for conversation, receive feedback about nonverbal communication, learn new ways to ask for help from others, be able to help others, learn how to form friendships, and learn new coping skills and behaviors.

Types of support groups

Various types of support groups exist. Some groups provide support for very specific types of loss, illness, or life adjustment. A representative sample is listed below.

BEREAVEMENT/GRIEF COUNSELING GROUPS. Bereavement and **grief counseling** groups provide support to people who have experienced a loss. There are groups for people who have lost a spouse or partner, parents, children, or pets. There are specific groups for people who have lost a loved one due to homicide, **suicide**, SIDS, cancer, or miscarriage. These groups help individuals adjust to the death of a family member or friend, learn how to accept the loss, honor the memory of their loved one, and adjust to life after the loss.

MEDICAL SUPPORT GROUPS. Medical support groups may be more short-term than other types of support groups, depending on the specific disorder. Some groups are formed to help patients adjust to specific treatments, such as chemotherapy or radiation, while others focus on longer-term adjustment and recovery issues, such as a breast cancer support group. These groups may have a stronger educational component to help members understand physical changes they may be experiencing as a result of their medical procedures.

WEIGHT LOSS GROUPS. Although these groups are very specific in their focus, their individual structures can vary greatly. Some weight loss support groups are actively involved in the process of losing weight, and may include monitoring of diet and **exercise**, while others focus on maintaining weight loss, and, therefore, may focus more on social support.

MENTAL HEALTH/ILLNESS SUPPORT GROUPS. These groups usually focus on specific disorders, such as bipolar or eating disorders. Members of these support groups are often at different phases in dealing with their illnesses, and, therefore, the needs and contributions of individual members may vary greatly from meeting to meeting.

FAMILY SUPPORT GROUPS. Family support groups, such as CHADD for parents of children with ADD or NAMI for families with members who struggle with any type of mental illness, provide support from other parents and children who may be feeling the same level of frustration and exasperation. Meeting others who truly understand one's experience has a very powerful effect. For many parents, participation in a support group is the first opportunity to learn that there are other parents who are experiencing the same challenges and frustrations.

LIFE TRANSITIONS GROUPS. Life transitions groups include divorce and aging support groups. Support groups for children of divorce also exist in many communities and schools.

ADDICTIONS SUPPORT GROUPS. Traditional **addiction** support groups include Alcoholics Anonymous (AA), Narcotics Anonymous (NA), and Gambler's Anonymous (GA). Many of these groups follow the traditional "12-step" program of working through various aspects of the addiction, and, as such, are more structured than many other types of support groups.

Support group locations

Support groups meet in many different locations within a community. Hospitals and medical centers may provide meeting locations for medical support groups. **Community mental health** centers, inpatient psychiatric programs, and residential treatment centers are common locations for mental health and mental illness-related support groups. Life transition groups are often provided through schools, senior centers, and daycare centers. **Bereavement** groups and addiction support groups often meet in churches, community meeting rooms of local businesses, and mental health agencies.

Structure of support groups

Support groups are most successful when composed of persons close in age who are experiencing similar life challenges. Support groups are usually led by members of the group, such as the chapter president or another member of the organizing group. Some support groups may be led by paraprofessionals if they are offered as part of an aftercare program associated with a treatment facility.

Support groups usually have explicit norms and expectations for member participation, such as respecting members' feelings and opinions, and coming to meetings free from drugs or alcohol. Due to the open nature of most support groups, members typically feel free to miss a session here or there, which is usually not acceptable in a treatment or therapy group.

Conclusion

Group experiences can be very powerful in changing behavior and maintaining that change. The support group becomes part of the individual's daily life, and promotes healthy functioning by providing reminders about change and support when he or she is feeling down or is drawn toward old patterns. It also provides opportunities to own one's change by helping others. These factors contribute to the positive prognosis for most who participate in a group experience. However, a person could be harmed by a group experience as well. Much of this risk is dependent on the characteristics of individual members, particularly in support groups that operate without professional guidance. For example, if certain individuals dominate the group with their own agenda, perhaps at the expense of other group members, then the experience may have a negative impact on more vulnerable individuals.

See also Grief counseling

Resources

BOOKS

Giuseppe, R., and G. Riva, eds. *Towards Cyberpsychology: Mind, Cognition and Society in the Internet Age* Amsterdam, Netherlands: IOS Press, 2001.

Kaduson, H.G., and Schaefer, C.E., eds. *Short-term Play Therapy for Children*. 2nd ed. New York: The Guilford Press, 2009.

Yalom, I.D. *The Theory and Practice of Group Psychotherapy*. 5th ed. New York: Basic Books, Inc., 2005.

PERIODICALS

Evans, J., J. Jones, and I. Mansell. "Supporting Siblings: Evaluation of Support Groups for Brothers and Sisters of Children with Learning Disabilities and Challenging Behavior." *Journal of Learning Disabilities* 5, no. 1 (March 2001): 69–78.

Gottlieb, B.H. "Self-help, Mutual Aid, and Support Groups Among Older Adults." *Canadian Journal on Aging* 19, Suppl 1 (Summer 2000): 58–74

Martin, D.J., et al. "Support Group Participation, HIV Viral Lead and Sexual Risk Behavior." *American Journal of Health Behavior* 25, no. 6 (November–December 2001): 513–527.

Montazeri, A., et al. "Anxiety and Depression in Breast Cancer Patients Before and After Participation in a Cancer Support Group." *Patient Education & Counseling* 45, no. 3 (December 2001): 195–198.

Sansone, R. A. "Patient-to-Patient E-mail: Support for Clinical Practices." *Eating Disorders* 9, no. 4 (Winter 2001): 373–375.

ORGANIZATIONS

Children and Adults with Attention Deficit/Hyperactivity Disorder, 8181 Professional Pl., Ste. 150, Landover, MD, 20785, (301) 306-7070, Fax: (301) 306-7090, http://www.chadd.org.

National Alliance on Mental Illness, 3803 N Fairfax Dr., Ste. 100, Arlington, VA, 22203, (703) 524-7600, http://www.nami.org.

Deanna Pledge, Ph.D.

Surmontil *see* **Trimipramine**

SVR-20 *see* **Sexual Violence Risk-20**

Sycrest *see* **Asenapine**

Symmetrel *see* **Amantadine**

Systematic desensitization

Definition

Systematic desensitization is a technique used to treat phobias and other extreme or erroneous fears based on principles of **behavior modification**.

Purpose

Systematic desensitization is used to help the client cope with phobias and other fears, and to induce relaxation. In progressive relaxation, one first tightens and then relaxes various muscle groups in the body. During the alternating clenching and relaxing, the client should be focusing on the contrast between the initial tension and the subsequent feelings of relaxation and softening that develop once the tightened muscles are released. After discovering how muscles feel when they are deeply relaxed, repeated practice enables a person to recreate the relaxed sensation intentionally in a variety of situations.

After learning relaxation skills, the client and therapist create an "anxiety hierarchy." The hierarchy is a catalogue of anxiety-provoking situations or stimuli arranged in order from least to most distressing. For a person who is frightened by snakes, the anxiety hierarchy might start with seeing a picture of a snake, eventually move to viewing a caged snake from a distance, and culminate in actually handling a snake. With the therapist's support and assistance, the client proceeds through the anxiety hierarchy, responding to the presentation of each fearful image or act by producing the state of relaxation. The person undergoing treatment stays with each step until a relaxed state is reliably produced when faced with each item. As tolerance develops for each identified item in the series, the client moves on to the next. In facing more menacing situations progressively, and developing a consistent pairing of relaxation with the feared object, relaxation rather than anxiety becomes associated with the source of their anxiety. Thus, a gradual desensitization occurs, with relaxation replacing alarm. Several means of confronting the feared situations can be used. In the pre-computer era, the exposure occurred either through imagination and visualization (imagining a plane flight) or through actual real-life—or so-called *in vivo*—encounters with the feared situation (going on an actual plane flight). More recently, during the 1990s, virtual reality or computer simulated exposure has come to be utilized in lieu of *in vivo* exposure. Research findings indicate that mental imagery is the least effective means of exposure; *in vivo* and virtual reality exposure appear to be indistinguishable in terms of effectiveness.

Description

Systematic desensitization is a therapeutic **intervention** which reduces the learned link between anxiety and objects or situations that are typically fear-producing. The aim of systematic desensitization is to reduce or eliminate fears or phobias that sufferers find are distressing or that impair their ability to manage daily life. By substituting a new response to a feared situation—a trained contradictory response of relaxation which is irreconcilable with an anxious response—phobic reactions are diminished or eradicated.

This behavior modification technique, which is founded on the principles of classical conditioning, was developed by Joseph Wolpe in the 1950s. Some of the most common fears treated with desensitization include fear of public speaking, fear of flying, stage fright, elevator phobias, driving phobias and animal phobias. Relaxation responses are trained to occur through *progressive relaxation training*, a technique initially perfected by Edmund Jacobson during the 1930s.

KEY TERMS

Behavior modification—An approach to therapy based on the principles of operant conditioning. Behavior modification seeks to replace undesirable behaviors with preferable behaviors through the use of positive or negative reinforcement.

Classical conditioning—In psychology, a process in which a previously neutral stimulus eventually produces a specific response by being paired repeatedly with another stimulus that produces that response. The best-known example of classical conditioning is Pavlov's dogs, who were conditioned to salivate when they heard a bell ring (the previously neutral stimulus) because the sound had been paired repeatedly with their feeding time.

Precautions

Because of the potential for extreme panic reactions to occur, which can increase the phobia, this technique should only be conducted by a well-qualified, trained professional. Also, the relaxation response should be thoroughly learned before confronting the anxiety-provoking hierarchy.

Results

Desensitization is an effective form of therapy. Individuals who have a positive response are enabled to resume daily activities that were previously avoided. The majority of persons undergoing this treatment show symptom reduction.

Resources

BOOKS

Craighead, W. Edward, and Michael J. Mahoney. *Behavior Modification: Principles, Issues, and Applications*. New York: Houghton Mifflin, 1981.

Wolpe, Joseph. *The Practice of Behavior Therapy*. Tarrytown, NY: Pergamon Press, 1990.

PERIODICALS

North, M.M., S.M. North, and J.R. Coble. "Virtual Reality Therapy: An Effective Treatment for Psychological Disorders." *Student Health Technology and Information* 44 (1997), 59–70.

Rothbaum, B., et al. "A Controlled Study of Virtual Reality Exposure Therapy for the Fear of Flying." *Journal of Consulting and Clinical Psychology* 68, no. 6 (December 2000), 1020–1026.

Deborah Rosch Eifert, Ph.D.

T

Tacrine

Definition

Tacrine is a drug used to treat **dementia** associated with **Alzheimer's disease**. It was sold in the United States under the brand name Cognex but is no longer widely prescribed due to the risk of liver toxicity; however, it remains on the market.

Purpose

Tacrine is used to treat symptoms of Alzheimer's disease in people with mild to moderate illness. The drug may result in mild improvements in thinking for a short period. Tacrine does not cure or stop the progression of Alzheimer's disease.

Description

The U.S. Food and Drug Administration (FDA) approved tacrine in 1993 for treating Alzheimer's disease. In Alzheimer's disease, some cells in specific regions of the **brain** die. Because of this cell death, some brain cells lose their ability to transmit nerve impulses. Brain cells normally transmit nerve impulses by secreting various chemicals known as **neurotransmitters**.

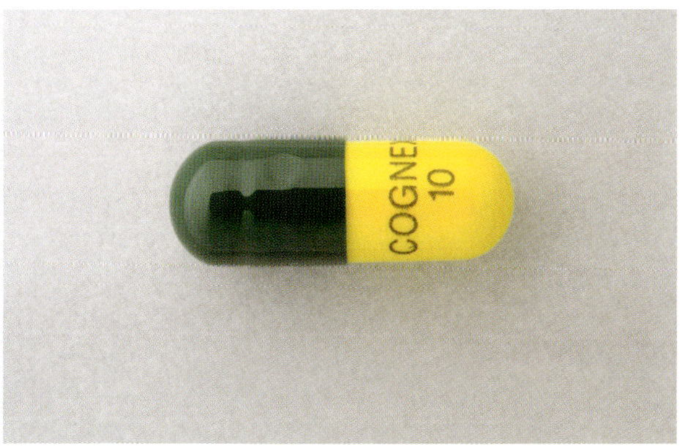

Cognex (tacrine), 10 mg. *(© Custom Medical Stock Photo, Inc. Reproduced by permission.)*

Brain cells that make and secrete a neurotransmitter called acetylcholine are affected early in the course of Alzheimer's disease. Tacrine helps prevent the breakdown of acetylcholine in the brain, thus temporarily increasing its concentration. In doing so, tacrine may improve the thinking process by facilitating nerve impulse transmission within the brain.

Recommended dosage

Tacrine is available as capsules in several different strengths. Tacrine is broken down (metabolized) in the liver.

The proper dose of tacrine will be different for different people. An initial dosage of tacrine is usually 10 mg taken four times per day. This dose should be continued for four weeks while liver function is monitored. If no adverse liver effects are detected, the dosage should be increased to 20 mg taken four times per day. Higher dosages such as 30–40 mg given four times per day may also be used. Liver function must be monitored every other week during the first 16 weeks of treatment. After 16 weeks of tacrine therapy, liver function can be assessed every three months. Dosage increases should not occur more often than every four weeks. Tacrine should be taken on an empty stomach between meals, but if stomach upset occurs, it may be taken with food.

If problems in liver function arise, tacrine may be stopped, or the dosage reduced, until liver function returns to normal. Very specific guidelines should be followed by physicians with regard to dosage adjustments based upon the severity of liver effects. Newer drugs that work in the same manner as tacrine are not as toxic to the liver and may be preferred for patients just beginning therapy for Alzheimer's-type dementia.

Precautions

Tacrine may cause liver damage. It may not be the best drug to treat symptoms of Alzheimer's disease in people with known liver damage. If these individuals take tacrine, their liver function should be closely monitored. Tacrine may also slow heart rates, increase acid secretion in the stomach, make urination difficult, cause breathing difficulties, or contribute to **seizures**. As a result, it should be used carefully in people with certain heart conditions, those who are prone to stomach ulcers, people with bladder obstruction, individuals with asthma, and those with a history of seizure disorders.

People should not stop taking tacrine suddenly, as this could cause behavioral disturbances. The drug may be stopped slowly if improvements are not noted by caregivers or physicians.

Side effects

The most common side effect of tacrine is impaired liver function. This causes 8% of people to stop taking the drug. Other common side effects occurring in at least 5% of people and at twice the rate of placebo are stomach upset (nausea, vomiting, diarrhea, indigestion, or anorexia), muscle aches, and difficulty walking. Side effects affecting the stomach appear to be more severe at higher dosages.

Side effects that occur less often are behavioral disturbances, abnormal thinking, hostility, tremor, inability to sleep, slow heart rates, changes in blood pressure, urinary difficulties, rash, flushing, aggravation of asthma, or cold-like symptoms.

Healthcare providers should be informed immediately if nausea, vomiting, loose stools, or diarrhea occur soon after the dose of tacrine is increased or if rash, jaundice (yellow tinge to eyes or skin), or changes in stool color occur at any time.

Interactions

Many drugs can alter the effects of tacrine. Some drugs such as dicyclomine may lessen the effects of tacrine. Other drugs such as **propranolol**, cimetidine, ciprofloxacin, **fluoxetine**, **fluvoxamine**, neostigmine, or bethanechol may increase some of tacrine's side effects. **Rivastigmine** may interact with some of the drugs used to relax muscles during surgery. The interaction increases the effects of both drugs.

Tacrine may also diminish the effects of levodopa and increase the side effects of theophylline. Smoking cigarettes may reduce the effectiveness of tacrine.

KEY TERMS

Acetylcholine—A naturally occurring chemical in the body that transmits nerve impulses from cell to cell. Generally, it has opposite effects from dopamine and norepinephrine; it causes blood vessels to dilate, lowers blood pressure, and slows the heartbeat. Central nervous system well-being is dependent on a balance among acetylcholine, dopamine, serotonin, and norepinephrine.

Dementia—A group of symptoms (syndrome) associated with a progressive loss of memory and other intellectual functions that is serious enough to interfere with a person's ability to perform the tasks of daily life. Dementia impairs memory, alters personality, leads to deterioration in personal grooming, impairs reasoning ability, and causes disorientation.

Neurotransmitter—A chemical in the brain that transmits messages between neurons, or nerve cells.

Placebo—An inactive substance or preparation used as a control in experiments with human subjects to test the effectiveness of a drug or herbal preparation. Some patients may experience a medicinal response or experience side effects to a placebo simply because they have faith in its powers even though it contains no medicine.

Resources

BOOKS

Ellsworth, Allan J., et al. *Mosby's Medical Drug Reference*. St. Louis, MO: Mosby, 2007.

Physicians' Desk Reference 2011. 66th ed. Montvale, NJ: PDR Network, 2011.

Wolters Kluwer Health. *Drug Facts and Comparisons 2012*. 66th ed. St. Louis: Lippincott, Williams & Wilkins, 2011.

OTHER

Alzheimer's Association. "FDA-Approved Treatments for Alzheimer's." July 2007. http://www.alz.org/national/documents/topicsheet_treatments.pdf (accessed November 13, 2011).

ORGANIZATIONS

U.S. Food and Drug Administration, 10903 New Hampshire Ave., Silver Spring, MD, 20993-0002, (888) INFO-FDA (463-6332), http://www.fda.gov.

Kelly Karpa, RPh, Ph.D.

Tai chi *see* **Bodywork therapies**

Talk therapy

Definition

Talk therapy is an alternate name for the various forms of **psychotherapy** that emphasize the importance of the client or patient speaking to the therapist as the main means of expressing and resolving issues.

Purpose

The purpose of talk therapy is to foster verbal exchange and expression between a client and a therapist. Talk therapy may be conducive in helping individuals work through a variety of feelings, thoughts, and memories.

Description

Psychoanalysis, the first modern form of psychotherapy, was called the "talking cure," and the many varieties of therapy practiced today are still characterized by their common dependence on a verbal exchange between the counselor or therapist and the person seeking help. Some of these therapies that are characterized by the verbal exchange include: **cognitive-behavioral therapy**, behavior therapy, **couples therapy**, **family therapy**, **grief counseling** and therapy, **group therapy**, **interpersonal therapy**, **person-centered therapy**, **psychodynamic psychotherapy**, and **rational emotive therapy**. Both **self-help groups** and **support groups** also rely on the discussion of an issue as a main part of the cure.

Benefits

Talk therapy may allow an individual to candidly describe thoughts, feelings, and concerns relating to fears, memories, upcoming events, or anxiety-provoking situations. In addition, the exchange of verbal communication allows the individual to listen to feedback from the therapist, who may offer insightful advice and further direction to the individual.

Precautions

Most commonly practiced talk therapy is safe and free of side effects.

Preparation

Talk therapy should take place in a quiet, relaxing atmosphere in which the person has a comfortable place to sit or recline. Some people find that quiet background music improves their talk therapy sessions. If an instructional audiotape or videotape is to be used, the appropriate equipment should be available.

The talk therapy session, which can last anywhere from a few minutes to an hour, should be uninterrupted. Taking the phone off the hook, turning off cell phones, and asking family members for privacy and silence can ensure a more successful talk therapy session.

Aftercare

Aftercare may be provided through informal support systems, which may include family and friends, as well as support groups.

Risks

On occasion, individuals may find some discussion during talk therapy to be emotionally forthright and intense; however, there are no risks associated with talk therapy.

Resources

BOOKS

Burns, Donna M. *When Kids Are Grieving: Addressing Grief and Loss in School.* Thousand Oaks, CA: Corwin Press, 2010.

James, John W., and Russell Friedman. *The Grief Recovery Handbook,* 20th Anniversary ed. New York: Harper Paperbacks, 2009.

Jeffreys, J. Shep. *Helping Grieving People—When Tears Are Not Enough: A Handbook for Care Providers,* 2nd ed. New York, NY: Routledge, 2011.

Meier, Scott T., and Susan R. Davis. *The Elements of Counseling,* 7th ed. Belmont, CA: Brooks Cole, 2010.

Noel, Brook., and Pamela D. Blair. *I Wasn't Ready to Say Goodbye: Surviving, Coping and Healing After the Sudden Death of a Loved One.* Naperville, IL: Sourcebooks, 2008.

ORGANIZATIONS

American Psychiatric Association, 1000 Wilson Blvd., Ste. 1825, Arlington, VA, 22209-3901, (703) 907-7300, apa@psych.org, http://www.psych.org.

American Psychoanalytic Association, 309 East 49th Street, New York City, NY, 10017, (212) 752-0450, Fax: (212) 593-0571, info@aspa.org, http://www.apsa.org.

American Psychological Association, 750 1st St. NE, Washington, DC, 20002-4242, (202) 336-5500; TDD/TTY: (202) 336-6123, (800) 374-2721, http://www.apa.org.

Paula Ford-Martin
Laura Jean Cataldo, RN, Ed.D.

Tardive dyskinesia

Definition

Tardive dyskinesia is a neurological disorder consisting of abnormal, involuntary body movements. It usually is associated with taking antipsychotic medications, although it can occur in the absence of drug administration.

Demographics

Tardive dyskinesia is much more common in clinical populations than in the general population. It has been identified as a rare disorder by the National Organization for Rare Disorders. Diseases and disorders are classified as "rare" if they affect fewer than 200,000 individuals in the United States. Prevalence rates are believed to be approximately the same for populations outside the United States.

The majority of individuals with tardive dyskinesia are receiving antipsychotic medications. Estimates of the percentage of individuals in clinical populations with tardive dyskinesia vary widely, from as low as 5.9% to as high as 65%. Risk is greater in older patients, who exhibit a prevalence rate that is five or six times higher than that of people under 50 years of age. Post-menopausal women taking antipsychotics are believed to be at the greatest risk for developing the disorder. The risk of tardive dyskinesia is greater for individuals taking antipsychotic medications for more than three months than for individuals taking the medications for shorter durations.

Description

Tardive means "late" and *dyskinesia* means "abnormal movements." The term refers to abnormal body movements that occur usually after a person has been taking an antipsychotic medication for a long time. The symptoms can sometimes arise even after the medication has been discontinued. In the early stages, the movements may be so subtle that neither the person nor others notice them. For instance, the person may blink rapidly or lick his or her lips often. In later stages, the movements become noticeable and may affect the person's physical abilities.

Other subtypes of tardive dyskinesia can occur. In tardive dystonia, there are abnormal contractions of the neck and shoulder muscles. In tardive akathisia, the person feels restless all the time.

Causes and symptoms

The cause of tardive dyskinesia is uncertain. Because antipsychotics block the proteins that recognize and transmit the signals from **dopamine**, a neurotransmitter, hypotheses about the causes of tardive dyskinesia center on these dopamine pathways in the **brain**. The leading hypothesis is that after an extended period of blocked dopamine signaling, nerves become hypersensitive to dopamine, and stimulation by even a small amount of dopamine results in abnormal movements. The parts of the brain that send signals to the muscles and use dopamine signaling may be affected.

Causes

The types of drugs most commonly associated with the development of tardive dyskinesia are:

- Antipsychotic drugs used to treat schizophrenia and other psychoses. These are also known as neuroleptic medicines. "First-generation" or older versions of these drugs were strongly linked to tardive dyskinesia and other movement disorders. With "second-generation" or so-called atypical antipsychotics, which generally block dopamine receptors more weakly and briefly, clinicians expected to see a reduction in the incidence of tardive dyskinesia. Although a reduction in other motor symptoms related to antipsychotics was observed, it has not yet been clearly established whether tardive dyskinesia rates have fallen. It does appear, however, that the atypical neuroleptics carry a lower risk.
- L-dopa, which is used to treat Parkinson's disease (although paradoxically, high doses of L-dopa may actually help control tardive dyskinesia).
- Antiemetic drugs used to control nausea and vomiting.
- Tricyclic antidepressants used to treat depression and other mood disorders.
- Other drugs that block dopamine signaling.

Symptoms

Symptoms of tardive dyskinesia include:

- involuntary movements of the face (orofacial dyskinesia), including frowning, blinking, smiling, lip licking, mouth puckering, biting or chewing, clenching the jaw, and tongue thrusting or rolling the tongue around in the mouth
- involuntary movements of the hands, arms, feet, or legs, such as twitching the hands or tapping the feet
- trunk movements, such as rocking, twisting, or squirming
- grunting or trouble speaking because of involuntary movements of the diaphragm

Movements may be rapid or slow and complicated. They usually are irregular and do not follow a pattern.

KEY TERMS

Antiemetic—A preparation or medication given to stop vomiting.

Antipsychotic—A drug used to treat symptoms of schizophrenia or other psychotic disorders.

Dopamine—A neurochemical made in the brain that is involved in many brain activities, including movement and emotion.

Neurotransmitter—One of a group of chemicals secreted by a nerve cell (neuron) to carry a chemical message to another nerve cell, often as a way of transmitting a nerve impulse. Examples of neurotransmitters are acetylcholine, dopamine, serotonin, and norepinephrine.

Orofacial dyskinesia—Involuntary movements of the face.

Tardive akathisia—A disorder in which the individual continuously feels restless.

Tardive dystonia—Involuntary, abnormal movements of the neck and shoulder muscles.

Diagnosis

The **diagnosis** of TD is suspected upon observation of involuntary movements of the head, neck, face, and tongue in individuals who have a history of antipsychotic drug prescription.

Treatment

Each case is treated differently. In some cases, the drug causing the problem can be stopped, reduced, or changed. However, most people taking antipsychotic drugs cannot stop taking them because of the high risk that their **psychosis** will return. The atypical antipsychotic drug associated with the lowest incidence of tardive dyskinesia is **clozapine** (Clozaril, Fazaclo). The atypical antipsychotics that have been more frequently associated with tardive dyskinesia are **risperidone** (Risperdal) and **olanzapine** (Zyprexa); in the case of risperidone, its longer history of clinical use may be an explanation. It may be possible to lower the dose to a level that does not cause the movements. One study has found that low-potency first-generation antipsychotics taken at moderate doses may carry no increased risk of eliciting tardive dyskinesia compared to second-generation drugs. There is controversy about whether so-called "drug holidays" reduce the likelihood of developing tardive dyskinesia. Drug holidays are planned periods in which the person goes off the medicine, then later resumes it.

QUESTIONS TO ASK YOUR DOCTOR

- Is it likely that my symptoms are being caused by a medication I am taking?
- Is there an alternative medication I could try that has a lower risk of tardive dyskinesia?
- Could my involuntary movements be caused by another underlying medical condition?
- Could we try reducing the dosage of my medication?
- Are there any vitamins or supplements that might help reduce my symptoms?

Vitamin E has been shown to be helpful in patients, especially those who have had the problem for less than five years. L-dopa and some other medicines are sometimes helpful.

Prognosis

The earlier the problem is noticed and treatment is begun, the better chance of eliminating abnormal movements. Reports indicate that in most cases, tardive dyskinesia is not progressive and can be reversed. Most patients have a noticeable improvement in their symptoms within 18 months; however, some abnormal movements may remain. People who are over age 60 have a greater chance of having the problem go away on its own.

Resources

BOOKS

Mignon, Laurence, ed. *Antipsychotics.* New York: Cambridge University Press, 2009.

Rothschild, Anthony J. *The Evidence-Based Guide to Antipsychotic Mediations.* Washington, DC: American Psychiatric Publishing, 2010.

Watts, Ray L., David G. Standarett, and Jose A. Obeso, eds. *Movement Disorders,* 3rd ed. New York: McGraw-Hill, 2011.

PERIODICALS

Chan, Hung-Yu, et al. "A Randomized Controlled Trial of Risperidone and Olanzapine for Schizophrenic Patients with Neuroleptic-Induced Tardive Dyskinesia." *Journal of Clinical Psychiatry* 71, no. 9 (September 2010): 1226–33.

Peritogiannis, V., and S. Tsouli. "Can Atypical Antipsychotics Improve Tardive Dyskinesia Associated with Other

Atypical Antipsychotics?" *Journal of Psychopharmacology* 24, no. 7 (July 2010): 1121–25.

Tenback, D.E., et al. "Incidence and Persistence of Tardive Dyskinesia and Extrapyramidal Symptoms in Schizophrenia." *Journal of Psychopharmacology* 24, no. 7 (July 2010):1031–35.

ORGANIZATIONS

American Psychiatric Association, 1000 Wilson Blvd., Ste. 1825, Arlington, VA, 22209-3901, (703) 907-7300, (888) 35-PSYCH (357-7924), apa@psych.org, http://www.psych.org.

American Psychological Association, 750 1st St. NE, Washington, DC, 20002-4242, (202) 336-5500; TDD/TTY: (202) 336-6123, (800) 374-2721, apa@psych.org, http://www.apa.org.

Movement Disorder Society, 555 East Wells St., Ste. 1100, Milwaukee, WI, 53202, (414) 276-2145, Fax: (414) 276-3349, info@movementdisorders.org, http://www.movementdisorders.org.

National Organization for Rare Diseases, PO Box 1968, Danbury, CT, 06813-1968, (203) 744-0100, (800) 999-NORD (6673), orphan@rarediseases.org, http://www.rarediseases.org.

Jody Bower, MSW
Tish Davidson, AM

TAT *see* **Thematic Apperception Test**

Tegretol *see* **Carbamazepine**

Temazepam

Definition

Temazepam is a drug that belongs to a family of drugs known as **benzodiazepines**. Temazepam is sold under the brand name Restoril in the United States and is also available under its generic name.

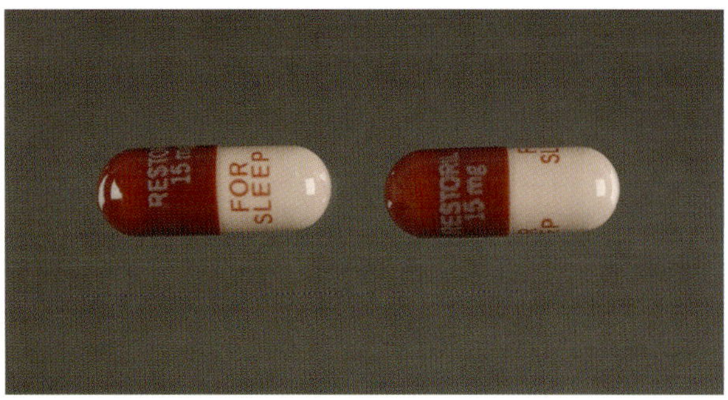

Temazepam (Restoril), 15 mg. *(U.S. Drug Enforcement Administration)*

Purpose

Temazepam is given to patients with sleeping problems. It is often prescribed for **insomnia** characterized by frequent awakening during the night or by awakening early in the morning.

Description

Temazepam is one of several drugs in the class known as benzodiazepines. These drugs produce a variety of effects, but most cause some degree of drowsiness (sedation). Temazepam is used almost exclusively as a hypnotic, or drug given to help people fall asleep. It is nearly always taken just before bedtime. The drug works by slowing down certain impulses in the **brain**, allowing the patient to fall asleep.

Recommended dosage

The typical starting dose for adults is 7.5–15 mg taken just before bedtime. The maximum recommended dose is 30 mg. Elderly patients and those in a weakened condition may need only 7.5 mg. The doctor should determine the dose in children 18 years of age and younger on an individual basis.

Precautions

Patients taking this drug should be monitored by their physicians to ensure that significant side effects do not develop. Insomnia that lasts longer than 7–10 days may point to a significant medical problem that should be thoroughly evaluated. Temazepam should not be combined with alcohol or other drugs that lower the level of activity in the central nervous system. Examples of such drugs include prescription pain medications, antihistamines, **barbiturates**, and muscle relaxants. Some persons may develop dizziness, lightheadedness, and clumsiness after taking temazepam. These side effects are especially common in the elderly.

Persons with a history of anemia, liver disease, kidney disease, drug abuse, serious psychological disorders, and **suicide** attempts should be given temazepam only after being thoroughly evaluated by their physician. This caution also applies to persons with a history of lung disease, seizure disorders, and narrow-angle glaucoma.

People who are taking temazepam should not stop taking it abruptly. Instead, the dose should be reduced gradually. Withdrawal symptoms, including depressed mood, sweating, abdominal cramps, muscle cramps, vomiting, **seizures**, and shakiness can develop if the medication is stopped suddenly.

Although patients are instructed to take temazepam in the evening before bedtime, they often experience side effects the next day, particularly drowsiness and loss of coordination or clumsiness. Pregnant women should not use this drug because it increases the risk of birth defects in the baby. Nursing mothers should not be given temazepam because it can make their babies drowsy and unable to nurse properly. Patients should not operate heavy machinery or drive a car while they are taking temazepam or any other benzodiazepine.

Side effects

Temazepam is a relatively safe drug, safer than most of the benzodiazepines. Its less serious but more common side effects include clumsiness or unsteady behavior, dizziness, drowsiness, and slurred speech. Some patients taking temazepam experience abdominal cramps, dry mouth, constipation, diarrhea, headache, nausea, vomiting, a giddy sense of well-being, and changes in sexual drive.

A small number of patients taking temazepam have experienced anger outbursts, confusion, mental **depression**, unusually low blood pressure, memory difficulties, nervousness, irritability, and muscle weakness. Symptoms of a temazepam overdose include extreme drowsiness, significant confusion, breathing difficulties, a very slow heartbeat, and staggering.

Rebound insomnia is one of the more common side effects of tapering a patient's dose of temazepam. Rebound insomnia is a reaction characterized by the recurrence of the symptom that the drug was originally given to suppress, namely problems with falling or staying asleep. When a person takes a medication for sleep on a regular basis, the body adjusts to the presence of the drug. As a result, when the person stops taking the sleeping medication, the body will take a few nights to return to its normal condition. During this period of readjustment, the person may experience a few sleepless hours each night. People often mistake the rebound insomnia for regular insomnia and consider it a good reason to continue taking temazepam, even though the drug is no longer needed.

People can also develop withdrawal symptoms even when they are gradually decreasing their dose of temazepam, particularly if the original dose was high. The more common withdrawal symptoms include sleeping difficulties, irritability, and nervousness. Less common withdrawal side effects include abdominal cramps, confusion, sweating, nausea, trembling, increased heart rate, and mental depression.

Interactions

Patients should always inform any healthcare provider that they see—doctors, dentists, nurses, and others—about all the medications they are taking, including temazepam. Temazepam interacts with certain other drugs, including cimetidine (an antihistamine), **disulfiram** (a drug given to help patients control cravings for alcohol), and **clozapine** (an antipsychotic medication). Rifampin, which is an antibiotic, may decrease the effectiveness of the temazepam if the two are taken together. Persons taking temazepam should not eat grapefruit or drink grapefruit juice, as the fruit may inhibit the metabolism of the drug, resulting in potentially toxic levels. Also, patients should avoid drinking alcohol or taking other medications that cause drowsiness (such as antihistamines) while taking temazepam, because these substances will intensify the drug's sedative effects. Heavy smoking interferes with the effectiveness of temazepam.

KEY TERMS

Antihistamine—A medication used to alleviate allergy or cold symptoms such as runny nose, itching, hives, watering eyes, or sneezing.

Barbiturates—A class of medications that causes sedation and drowsiness. They may be prescribed legally but are also used as drugs of abuse.

Generic—A term that refers to a medication that is not protected by a registered trademark.

Hypnotic—A type of medication that induces sleep.

Insomnia—A chronic inability to sleep or to remain asleep throughout the night.

Narrow-angle glaucoma—An eye disorder caused by a buildup of fluid pressure inside the eyeball due to an abnormally small angle between the iris (the colored portion of the eye) and the cornea (the transparent front part of the eye).

Rebound—A physical reaction to stopping a medication characterized by the reappearance of the symptom(s) that the medication was given to suppress. For example, people who stop taking temazepam may experience rebound excitability and sleeping problems.

Sedation—A state of emotional or physical relaxation. The term is usually used to refer to this condition when it is produced by a medication.

Withdrawal—Symptoms experienced by a person who has become physically dependent on a drug, experienced when the drug use is discontinued.

Resources

BOOKS

Brunton, Laurence, Bruce Chabner, and Bjorn Knollman. *Goodman & Gilman's The Pharmacological Basis of Therapeutics* 12th ed. New York: McGraw-Hill, 2010.

Consumer Reports and American Society of Health-System Pharmacists. *Consumer Reports Complete Drug Reference.* Yonkers, NY: Consumers Reports, 2009.

Ellsworth, Allan J., et al. *Mosby's Medical Drug Reference.* St. Louis, MO: Mosby, 2007.

Venes, Donald. *Taber's Cyclopedic Medical Dictionary.* 21st ed. Philadelphia: F.A. Davis Company, 2009.

WEBSITES

PubMed Health. "Temazepam." U.S. National Library of Medicine. http://www.ncbi.nlm.nih.gov/pubmedhealth/PMH0000808 (accessed November 13, 2011).

ORGANIZATIONS

U.S. Food and Drug Administration, 10903 New Hampshire Ave., Silver Spring, MD, 20993-0002, (888) INFO-FDA (463-6332), http://www.fda.gov.

Mark Mitchell, M.D.

Tenex *see* **Guanfacine**

Thematic Apperception Test

Definition

The Thematic Apperception Test, or TAT, is a projective measure intended to evaluate a person's patterns of thought, attitudes, observational capacity, and emotional responses to ambiguous test materials. In the case of the TAT, the ambiguous materials consist of a set of cards that portray human figures in a variety of settings and situations. The subject is asked to tell the examiner a story about each card that includes the following elements: the event shown in the picture; what has led up to it; what the characters in the picture are feeling and thinking; and the outcome of the event.

Because the TAT is an example of a *projective* instrument—that is, it asks the subject to project his or her habitual patterns of thought and emotional responses onto the pictures on the cards—many psychologists prefer not to call it a "test," because it implies that there are "right" and "wrong" answers to the questions. They consider the term "technique" to be a more accurate description of the TAT and other projective assessments.

Purpose

Individual assessments

The TAT is often administered to individuals as part of a battery, or group, of tests intended to evaluate personality. It is considered to be effective in eliciting information about a person's view of the world and his or her attitudes toward the self and other persons. As persons taking the TAT proceed through the various cards and tell stories about the pictures, they reveal their expectations of relationships with peers, parents or other authority figures, subordinates, and possible romantic partners. In addition to assessing the content of the stories that the subject is telling, the examiner evaluates the subject's manner, vocal tone, posture, hesitations, and other signs of an emotional response to a particular story picture. For example, a person who is made anxious by a certain picture may make comments about the artistic style of the picture, or remark that he or she does not like the picture; this is a way of avoiding telling a story about it.

The TAT is often used in individual assessments of candidates for employment in fields requiring a high degree of skill in dealing with other people and/or ability to cope with high levels of psychological stress—such as law enforcement, military leadership positions, religious ministry, education, diplomatic service, etc. Although the TAT should not be used in the differential **diagnosis** of mental disorders, it is often administered to individuals who have already received a diagnosis in order to match them with the type of **psychotherapy** best suited to their personality. Lastly, the TAT is sometimes used for forensic purposes in evaluating the motivations and general attitudes of persons accused of violent crimes. For example, the TAT was recently administered to a 24-year-old man in prison for a series of sexual murders. The results indicated that his attitudes toward other people are not only outside normal limits but are similar to those of other persons found guilty of the same type of crime.

The TAT can be given repeatedly to an individual as a way of measuring progress in psychotherapy or, in some cases, to help the therapist understand why the treatment seems to be stalled or blocked.

Research

In addition to its application in individual assessments, the TAT is frequently used for research into specific aspects of human personality, usually including needs for achievement, fears of failure, hostility and aggression, and interpersonal object relations. "Object relations" is a phrase used in psychiatry and psychology to refer to the ways people internalize their relationships with others and the emotional tone of their relationships. Research into object relations using the TAT investigates a variety of different topics, including the extent to which people are emotionally involved in relationships with others; their ability to understand the complexities of human relationships; their ability to distinguish between their viewpoint on a situation and the perspectives of others involved; their ability to control aggressive impulses; self-esteem issues; and issues of personal identity. For example, one recent study compared responses to the TAT from a group of psychiatric inpatients diagnosed with **dissociative disorders** with responses from a group of non-dissociative inpatients, in order to investigate some of the controversies about **dissociative identity disorder** (formerly called multiple personality disorder).

Precautions

Students in medicine, psychology, or other fields who are learning to administer and interpret the TAT receive detailed instructions about the number of factors that can influence a person's responses to the story cards. In general, they are advised to be conservative in their interpretations, and to err "on the side of health" rather than of psychopathology when evaluating a subject's responses. In addition, the 1992 Code of Ethics of the **American Psychological Association** requires examiners to be knowledgeable about cultural and social differences, and to be responsible in interpreting test results with regard to these differences.

Experts in the use of the TAT recommend obtaining a personal and medical history from the subject before giving the TAT, in order to have some context for evaluating what might otherwise appear to be abnormal or unusual responses. For example, frequent references to death or **grief** in the stories would not be particularly surprising from a subject who had recently been bereaved. In addition, the TAT should not be used as the sole examination in evaluating an individual; it should be combined with other interviews and tests.

Cultural, gender, and class issues

The large number of research studies that have used the TAT have indicated that cultural, gender, and class issues must be taken into account when determining whether a specific response to a story card is "abnormal" strictly speaking, or whether it may be a normal response from a person in a particular group. For example, the card labeled 6GF shows a younger woman who is seated turning toward a somewhat older man who is standing behind her and smoking a pipe. Most male subjects do not react to this picture as implying aggressiveness, but most female subjects regard it as a very aggressive picture, with unpleasant overtones of intrusiveness and danger. Many researchers consider the gender difference in responses to this card as a reflection of the general imbalance in power between men and women in the larger society.

Race is another issue related to the TAT story cards. The original story cards, which were created in 1935, all involved Caucasian figures. As early as 1949, researchers who were administering the TAT to African Americans asked whether the race of the figures in the cards would influence the subjects' responses. Newer sets of TAT story cards have introduced figures representing a wider variety of races and ethnic groups. It is not known, however, whether a subject's ability to identify with the race of the figures in the story cards improves the results of a TAT assessment.

Multiplicity of scoring systems

One problem in assessing the TAT is the absence of a normative scoring system for responses. The original scoring system devised in 1943 by Henry Murray, one of the authors of the TAT, attempted to account for every variable that it measures. Murray's scoring system is time-consuming and unwieldy, and as a result has been little used by later interpreters. Other scoring systems have since been introduced that focus on one or two specific variables, for example hostility or **depression**. While these systems are more practical for clinical use, they lack comprehensiveness. No single system presently used for scoring the TAT has achieved widespread acceptance. The basic drawback of any scoring system in evaluating responses to the TAT story cards is that information that is not relevant to that particular system is simply lost.

Computer scoring

A recent subject of controversy in TAT interpretation concerns the use of computers to evaluate responses. While computers were used initially only to score tests with simple yes/no answers, they were soon applied to interpretation of projective measures. A computerized system for interpreting the **Rorschach**, for example, was devised as early as 1964. There are no computerized systems for evaluating responses to the TAT; however, users of the TAT should be aware of the controversies in this field. Computers have two basic limitations for use with the TAT: the first is that they cannot observe and record the subject's vocal tone, eye contact, and other aspects of behavior that a human examiner can note. Second, computers are not adequate for the interpretation of unusual subject profiles.

Description

The TAT is one of the oldest projective measures in continuous use. It has become the most popular projective technique among English-speaking psychiatrists and psychologists, and is better accepted among clinicians than the Rorschach.

History of the TAT

The TAT was first developed in 1935 by Henry Murray, Christiana Morgan, and their colleagues at the Harvard Psychological Clinic. The early versions of the TAT listed Morgan as the first author, but later versions dropped her name. One of the controversies surrounding the history of the TAT concerns the long and conflict-ridden extramarital relationship between Morgan and Murray, and its reinforcement of the prejudices that existed in the 1930s against women in academic psychology and psychiatry.

It is generally agreed, however, that the basic idea behind the TAT came from one of Murray's undergraduate students. The student mentioned that her son had spent his time recuperating from an illness by cutting pictures out of magazines and making up stories about them. The student wondered whether similar pictures could be used in therapy to tap into the nature of a patient's fantasies.

Administration

The TAT is usually administered to individuals in a quiet room free from interruptions or distractions. The subject sits at the edge of a table or desk next to the examiner. The examiner shows the subject a series of story cards taken from the full set of 31 TAT cards. The usual number of cards shown to the subject is between 10 and 14, although Murray recommended the use of 20 cards, administered in two separate one-hour sessions with the subject. The original 31 cards were divided into three categories, for use with men only, with women only, or for use with subjects of either sex. Recent practice has moved away from the use of separate sets of cards for men and women.

The subject is then instructed to tell a story about the picture on each card, with specific instructions to include a description of the event in the picture, the developments that led up to the event, the thoughts and feelings of the people in the picture, and the outcome of the story. The examiner keeps the cards in a pile face down in front of him or her, gives them to the subject one at a time, and asks the subject to place each card face down as its story is completed. Administration of the TAT usually takes about an hour.

Recording

Murray's original practice was to take notes by hand on the subject's responses, including his or her nonverbal behaviors. Research has indicated, however, that a great deal of significant material is lost when notes are recorded in this way. As a result, some examiners now use a tape recorder to record subjects' answers. Another option involves asking the subject to write down his or her answers.

Interpretation

There are two basic approaches to interpreting responses to the TAT, called *nomothetic* and *idiographic* respectively. Nomothetic interpretation refers to the practice of establishing norms for answers from subjects in specific

KEY TERMS

Apperception—The process of understanding through linkage with previous experience. The term was coined by one of the authors of the TAT to underscore the fact that people don't "perceive" the story cards in a vacuum; rather, they construct their stories on the basis of past experiences as well as present personality traits.

Battery—A number of separate items (such as tests) used together. In psychology, a group or series of tests given with a common purpose, such as personality assessment or measurement of intelligence.

Forensic—Pertaining to courtroom procedure or evidence used in courts of law.

Idiographic—An approach to interpreting the results of a projective test within the context of the individual subject's record.

Nomothetic—An approach to interpreting the results of a projective test in which the subject's answers are measured against a normative comparison sample.

Object relations—In psychology, a phrase that refers to the way in which a subject describes relationships with other people in their environment, and the ways in which he or she has internalized interpersonal relationships.

Projective test or projective measure—A type of psychological evaluation that assesses a person's thinking patterns, observational ability, feelings, and attitudes on the basis of responses to ambiguous test materials. Projective measures are not intended to diagnose psychiatric disorders, although they are often used in outcome studies to compare the effectiveness of different forms of psychotherapy.

Rorschach test—A commonly administered projective measure in which subjects are asked to describe a series of black or colored inkblots.

age, gender, racial, or educational level groups and then measuring a given subject's responses against those norms. Idiographic interpretation refers to evaluating the unique features of the subject's view of the world and relationships. Most psychologists would classify the TAT as better suited to idiographic than nomothetic interpretation.

In interpreting responses to the TAT, examiners typically focus their attention on one of three areas: the content of the stories that the subject tells; the feeling tone of the stories; or the subject's behaviors apart from responses. These behaviors may include verbal remarks (for example, comments about feeling stressed by the situation or not being a good storyteller) as well as nonverbal actions or signs (blushing, stammering, fidgeting in the chair, difficulties making eye contact with the examiner, etc.) The story content usually reveals the subject's attitudes, fantasies, wishes, inner conflicts, and view of the outside world. The story structure typically reflects the subject's feelings, assumptions about the world, and an underlying attitude of optimism or pessimism.

Results

The results of the TAT must be interpreted in the context of the subject's personal history, age, sex, level of education, occupation, racial or ethnic identification, first language, and other characteristics that may be important. "Normal" results are difficult to define in a complex multicultural society like the contemporary United States.

Resources

BOOKS

Aronow, Edward, Kim Altman Weiss, and Marvin Reznikoff. *A Practical Guide to the Thematic Apperception Test: The TAT in Clinical Practice*. Philadelphia, PA: Taylor and Francis, 2001.

Dana, Richard H. "Thematic Apperception Test." In *International Encyclopedia of Psychiatry, Psychology, Psychoanalysis, & Neurology*, edited by Benjamin B. Wolman. New York: Aesculapius Publishers, Inc., 1983.

Douglas, Claire. *Translate This Darkness: The Life of Christiana Morgan*. Princeton,NJ: Princeton University Press, 1997.

Geiser, Lon, and Morris I. Stein. *Evocative Images: The Thematic Apperception Test and the Art of Projection*. Washington, DC: American Psychological Association, 1999.

Maddox, Taddy. *Tests: A Comprehensive Reference for Assessments in Psychology, Education, and Business*. 4th ed. Austin, TX: Pro Ed, 1997.

PERIODICALS

Hatayama, Toshiteru, et al. "Guilt and Shame in Japan: Data Provided by the Thematic Apperception Test in Experimental Settings." *North American Journal of Psychology* 8, no. 1 (2006): 85.

Pica, M., et al. "The Responses of Dissociative Patients on the Thematic Apperception Test." *Journal of Clinical Psychology* 57, no. 7 (July 2001): 847–864.

Porcerelli, J.H., et al. "Object Relations and Defense Mechanisms of a Psychopathic Serial Sexual Homicide Perpetrator: A TAT Analysis." *Journal of Personality Assessment* 77, no. 1 (August 2001): 87–104.

Schultheiss, O.C., and J.C. Brunstein. "Assessment of Implicit Motives with a Research Version of the TAT: Picture Profiles, Gender Differences, and Relations to Other Personality Measures." *Journal of Personality Assessment* 77, no. 1 (August 2001): 71–86.

ORGANIZATIONS

American Psychological Association, 750 1st Street NE, Washington, DC, 20002-4242, (202) 336-5500; TDD/TTY: (202) 336-6123, (800) 374-2721, http://www.apa.org.

Rebecca J. Frey, Ph.D.

Thioridazine

Definition

Thioridazine is a potent antianxiety and antipsychotic agent. It is a member of the phenothiazine family of compounds. In the United States, thioridazine is sold under the brand name of Mellaril and is also available under its generic name.

Purpose

Thioridazine is used to manage psychotic disorders, such as **schizophrenia**. It reduces excitement, abnormal levels of energy, excessive movements (hypermotility),

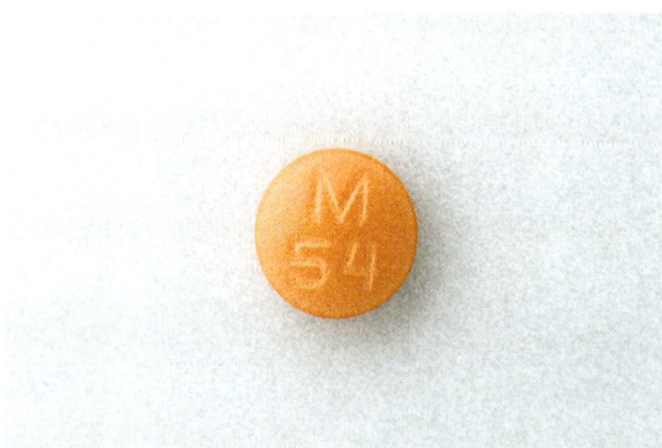

Mellaril (thioridazine), 10 mg. *(© Custom Medical Stock Photo, Inc. Reproduced by permission.)*

and agitation. It is also used in the short-term treatment of **depression** when accompanied by anxiety, sleep disturbances, agitation, and tension, and in children who display seriously inappropriate responses to exciting stimuli. Because of a number of serious side effects associated with thioridazine use, it is only prescribed when other medications have been unsuccessful or when the benefits significantly outweigh the risks.

Description

Thioridazine is used in treating anxiety and **psychosis**. When used for the treatment of schizophrenia, thioridazine reduces the symptoms of emotional withdrawal, anxiety, tension, hallucinations, and suspiciousness. Compared to other phenothiazine drugs, it is less likely to cause vomiting and Parkinson-like symptoms.

Recommended dosage

The dosage of thioridazine is determined based on the individual. The usual initial dosage for adults is 50 to 100 mg three times a day. This may be gradually increased to a maximum of 800 mg per day. Once the desired therapeutic effect has been achieved, the dosage should be stabilized. A typical maintenance dosage is 200 to 800 mg per day, given in three to four doses.

The usual initial dosage for adults being treated for symptoms of anxiety is 25 mg three times per day. After reaching equilibrium and controlling undesired symptoms, the typical maintenance dosage is 20 to 200 mg per day divided into three or four doses.

For children between the ages of 2 and 12, the usual daily dosage of thioridazine is 0.5 to 3.0 mg per 2 lb (1 kg) of body weight. Severely psychotic children who are hospitalized may receive 25 mg twice each day.

Precautions

Thioridazine may cause dangerous heart arrhythmias (irregular heartbeat) that can be fatal. Patients with a history of heart disease or a heart condition, low or high blood pressure, or low levels of potassium in the blood are particularly at risk. If a person taking thioridazine experiences irregular heartbeat, dizziness, light-headedness, or fainting, the patient should call his or her doctor immediately.

It is dangerous to give thioridazine to persons in a comatose state. **Seizures** due to thioridazine therapy have been reported but are unusual. A sudden decrease in blood pressure due to a change in body position (orthostatic hypotension) with accompanying lightheadedness, may occur in people who have taken the drug. This is more common among women than among men.

Thioridazine is not approved for use in treating the behavioral symptoms of dementia in elderly adults. Patients taking thioridazine for this purpose are at an increased risk of death during treatment.

Thioridazine increases the level of prolactin in the blood; prolactin is a hormone that stimulates the mammary glands in the breast. This is a potential problem for persons with a personal or family history of breast cancer and may increase the risk of breast cancer. Thioridazine is also associated with malignant hyperthermia, vision and urinary problems, and blood dyscrasias (abnormal levels of blood cells).

Some babies born to mothers who took thioridazine during pregnancy exhibited withdrawal symptoms, including increased agitation and trouble breathing; women who are pregnant or planning to become pregnant should not take thioridazine.

Long-term use of thioridazine increases the probability of developing **tardive dyskinesia** (TD). Because of the many serious side effects associated with thioridazine, the risks and benefits of thioridazine must be carefully explained and understood before the drug is started.

Side effects

A common side effect of thioridazine is drowsiness and lack of physical and mental alertness. This side effect is especially noticeable early in therapy. Patients taking thioridazine should refrain from performing hazardous activities requiring mental alertness or coordination. Other common side effects include greater sensitivity to the sun and increased risk of serious sunburn, dry mouth, constipation, and urinary retention. Urinary retention (difficulty starting a urine flow or passing urine,) is a particular problem in men with enlarged prostates.

Thioridazine use may lead to the development of symptoms that resemble Parkinson's disease, but which are not caused by Parkinson's. These symptoms may include a taut or mask-like expression on the face, drooling, tremors, pill-rolling motions in the hands, cogwheel rigidity (abnormal rigidity in muscles, characterized by jerky movements when the muscle is passively stretched), and a shuffling gait. Taking the anti-Parkinson drugs **benztropine** mesylate or **trihexyphenidyl** hydrochloride along with thioridazine usually readily controls these symptoms.

Thioridazine has the potential to produce a serious side effect called tardive dyskinesia. This syndrome consists of involuntary, uncoordinated movements that may not disappear or may only partially improve after the drug is stopped. Tardive dyskinesia involves involuntary

KEY TERMS

Orthostatic hypotension—A sudden decrease in blood pressure due to a change in body position, as when moving from a sitting to standing position.

Prolactin—A hormone that stimulates milk production and breast development.

Schizophrenia—A severe mental illness in which a person has difficulty distinguishing what is real from what is not real. It is often characterized by hallucinations, delusions, language and communication disturbances, and withdrawal from people and social activities.

Tardive dyskinesia—A condition that involves involuntary movements of the tongue, jaw, mouth or face or other groups of skeletal muscles that usually occurs either late in antipsychotic therapy or even after the therapy is discontinued. It may be irreversible.

movements of the tongue, jaw, mouth or face or other groups of skeletal muscles. The incidence of TD increases with patient age and higher doses. It may also appear after thioridazine use has been discontinues. Women are at greater risk than men for developing TD. There is no known effective treatment for tardive dyskinesia, although gradual (but rarely complete) improvement may occur over a long period.

An occasionally reported side effect of thioridazine is **neuroleptic malignant syndrome**. This is a complicated and potentially fatal condition characterized by muscle rigidity, high fever, alterations in mental status, and cardiac symptoms such as irregular pulse or blood pressure, sweating, tachycardia (fast heartbeat), and arrhythmias (irregular heartbeat). People who think they may be experiencing any side effects from this or any other medication should talk to their physician promptly.

Interactions

Thioridazine increases the effect of drugs and substances that depress the central nervous system. This class of drugs includes anesthetics, opiates, **barbiturates**, atropine, and alcohol. These substances should be avoided or used sparingly by people taking thioridazine.

Propranolol increases the concentration of thioridazine. Concurrent administration of pindolol also increases the concentration of thioridazine, and thioridazine increases the concentration of pindolol in the body. Thioridazine may interact with other drugs used to treat mental disorders. People planning to take this drug should let their physicians know of all other drugs they are taking, including amiodarone (Cordarone), cisapride (Propulsid), disopyramide (Norpace), dofetilide (Tikosyn), erythromycin (E.E.S., E-Mycin, Erythrocin), fluoxetine (Prozac, Sarafem), **fluvoxamine** (Luvox), moxifloxacin (Avelox), **paroxetine** (Paxil, Pexeva), **pimozide** (Orap), pindolol (Visken), procainamide, propranolol (Inderal), quinidine, and sotalol (Betapace, Betapace AF), any of which may be dangerous if used in combination with thioridazine.

Resources

BOOKS

Jacobson, J. L., and A. M. Jacobson. *Psychiatric Secrets*. 2nd ed. Philadelphia: Hanley & Belfus, 2001.

Stern, T. A., et al.*Massachusetts General Hospital Comprehensive Clinical Psychiatry*. 1st ed. Philadelphia: Mosby Elsevier, 2008.

PERIODICALS

Dallaire, S. "Thioridazine (Mellaril) and Mesoridazine (Serentil): Prolongation of the QTc Interval." *Canadian Medical Association Journal* 164, no 1 (2001): 91–95.

Pisani, F., et al. "Effects of Psychotropic Drugs on Seizure Threshold." *Drug Safety* 25, no. 2 (2002): 91–110.

Ray, W. A., et al. "Antipsychotics and the Risk of Sudden Cardiac Death." *Archives of General Psychiatry* 58, no. 12 (2001): 1161–67.

WEBSITES

PubMed Health. "Thioridazine." U.S. National Library of Medicine. http://www.ncbi.nlm.nih.gov/pubmedhealth/PMH0000584 (accessed November 13, 2011).

ORGANIZATIONS

U.S. Food and Drug Administration, 10903 New Hampshire Ave., Silver Spring, MD, 20993-0002, (888) INFO-FDA (463-6332), http://www.fda.gov.

L. Fleming Fallon, Jr., M.D., Dr.P.H.

Thiothixene

Definition

Thiothixene is in a class of drugs called antipsychotics. It is available with a prescription under the generic name of thiothixene or the brand name Navane.

Purpose

Thiothixene is a drug used to treat symptoms of **schizophrenia**. It is also sometimes used to calm severely agitated people.

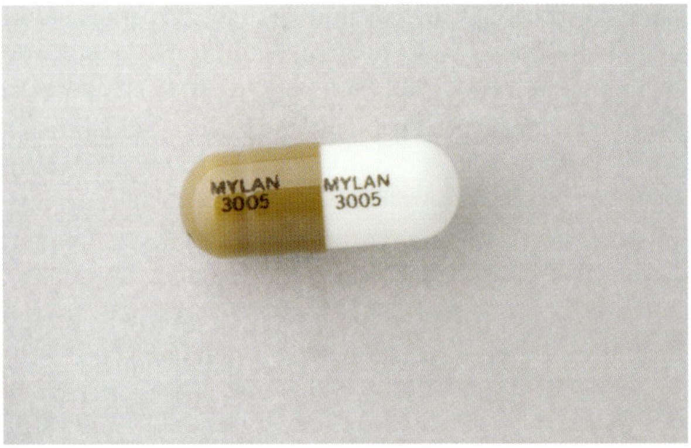

Thiothixene, 5 mg. *(© Custom Medical Stock Photo, Inc. Reproduced by permission.)*

Description

Thiothixene has been used in the United States for many years as a treatment for schizophrenia. It is believed to modify the balance of naturally occurring chemicals in the **brain** called **neurotransmitters** that regulate the transmission of nerve impulses from cell to cell. The proper balance between neurotransmitters is responsible, in part, for maintaining mental well-being. Thiothixene is thought to alter the balance among neurotransmitters in a way that improves symptoms of schizophrenia.

Thiothixene is available in several different strengths as capsules, as an injection, and as a concentrated liquid form taken by mouth. It is broken down by the liver and eliminated from the body by the kidneys.

Recommended dosage

The dosage of thiothixene varies widely from one individual to another. Initially, 2 mg of thiothixene taken by mouth three times daily is used in milder cases. This dosage may be increased slowly. Fifteen to 30 mg per day is often an effective range.

For more severe cases, 5 mg taken by mouth twice per day is a common starting dosage, with slow increases to 20–30 mg per day. Up to 60 mg of thiothixene may be taken daily. Doses greater than 60 mg per day usually do not provide any additional benefit and may increase side effects.

Precautions

Thiothixene may alter the rhythm of the heart. As a result, it should not be used by people with a history of irregular or prolonged heart rhythms (long QT syndrome), those with heart failure, or people who have recently had a heart attack. People with other heart conditions should discuss with their physician whether thiothixene is the right antipsychotic drug for them.

Thiothixene may increase the tendency to have **seizures**. People who have had seizures in the past, including alcohol or drug-induced seizures, should take thiothixene only after discussing the risks and benefits with their physician. People taking thiothixene should call their doctor immediately if they experience any abnormal, involuntary muscle movements, because this adverse effect may be permanent. The risk of abnormal, involuntary muscle movements is believed to increase with long-term use of thiothixene and high dosages.

Thiothixene may increase body temperatures to dangerously high levels. People who **exercise** strenuously, those exposed to extreme heat, individuals taking drugs with anticholinergic effects (this includes many common **antidepressants**), and persons prone to dehydration should be alert to increased body temperatures and dehydration-related side effects. Fevers, difficulty moving muscles, irregular heartbeats, rapid heartbeats, or excessive sweating are warning signs of possible overheating that should be addressed by a physician immediately.

Thiothixene is not approved by the U.S. Food and Drug Administration (FDA) for use in treating the behavioral symptoms of elderly patients with dementia; patients taking thiothixene for this purpose are at an increased risk of death during treatment.

People taking thiothixene should have regular eye examinations, since use of thiothixene has been associated with abnormalities of the retina, the light-sensitive layer of the eye. Thiothixene may also alter reproductive hormone levels causing irregular menstrual periods, difficulty getting pregnant, enlarged breasts, and breast milk production. Thiothixene can cause enlarged breasts and breast milk secretion in men as well as women. People who have had breast cancer should not take thiothixene unless the benefits of this drug substantially outweigh the risks.

Thiothixene may cause drowsiness. People should not perform hazardous tasks that require mental alertness and until they see how the drug affects them. This side effect usually diminishes with continued use of the drug. Thiothixene may make it more difficult to make a patient vomit after a drug overdose or accidental poisoning. Because there is a high incidence of **suicide** in all patients with psychotic illnesses, people using thiothixene should be observed carefully for signs of suicidal behavior. Women who are pregnant or breast-feeding should not take thiothixene; some babies born to mothers who took thiothixene during pregnancy exhibited withdrawal symptoms, including increased agitation and respiratory problems.

KEY TERMS

Anticholinergic—Related to the ability of a drug to block the nervous system chemical acetylcholine. When acetylcholine is blocked, patients often experience dry mouth and skin, increased heart rate, blurred vision, and difficulty in urinating. In severe cases, blocking acetylcholine may cloud thinking and cause delirium.

Antihistamine—A medication used to alleviate allergy or cold symptoms such as runny nose, itching, hives, watering eyes, or sneezing.

Antipsychotic—A medication used to treat psychotic symptoms of schizophrenia such as hallucinations, delusions and delirium. May be used to treat symptoms in other disorders, as well.

Neurotransmitter—A chemical in the brain that transmits messages between neurons, or nerve cells.

Schizophrenia—A severe mental illness in which a person has difficulty distinguishing what is real from what is not real. It is often characterized by hallucinations, delusions, language and communication disturbances, and withdrawal from people and social activities.

Side effects

Common side effects associated with the use of thiothixene include abnormal muscle movements and muscle stiffness, muscle tremors, weight gain, sleepiness, dry mouth, dry eyes, difficulty urinating, constipation, and sudden decreases in blood pressure that cause dizziness when standing up suddenly. Other side effects that may occur when using thiothixene are headaches, seizures, high blood pressure, rapid heartbeats, blurred vision, liver changes, irregular menstrual periods, abnormal blood cell counts, difficulty breathing, and rash.

Uncommon and serious side effects include **neuroleptic malignant syndrome** and **tardive dyskinesia**. Neuroleptic malignant syndrome is an unusual but potentially life-threatening condition. The person with this syndrome becomes extremely rigid, has a high fever, rapid heart rate, and abnormalities on blood tests. The affected person also may have a difficult time breathing and may sweat, and will need to be admitted to the hospital. Tardive dyskinesia (TD) is a condition that may occur after a long period of using antipsychotic medications. TD is characterized by involuntary movements of the facial muscles and tongue, and may also involve muscles in the trunk or hands or feet. TD may disappear as soon as the medication is stopped, but if it does not, it is difficult to treat. All potential side effects should be discussed with the patient's doctor before starting treatment with thiothixene.

Interactions

When thiothixene is used with drugs such as bethanechol, **propranolol**, levodopa, and some antidepressants, some of the side effects associated with thiothixene may increase. Use of narcotic drugs with thiothixene may cause blood pressure to fall to dangerously low levels. If thiothixene is used with levodopa, the actions of levodopa with be diminished.

When thiothixene is used with **barbiturates** or lithium, thiothixene may be less effective. Because thiothixene may cause sleepiness, it should rarely be used with other drugs that also cause drowsiness, such as antidepressants, antihistamines, some pain relievers, and alcohol.

Resources

BOOKS

Stern, T. A., et al. *Massachusetts General Hospital Comprehensive Clinical Psychiatry*. Philadelphia: Mosby Elsevier, 2008.

WEBSITES

PubMed Health. "Thiothixene." http://www.ncbi.nlm.nih.gov/pubmedhealth/PMH0000797 (accessed November 13, 2011).

ORGANIZATIONS

U.S. Food and Drug Administration, 10903 New Hampshire Ave., Silver Spring, MD, 20993-0002, (888) INFO-FDA (463-6332), http://www.fda.gov.

Kelly Karpa, RPh, Ph.D.

Thorazine *see* **Chlorpromazine**

Tic disorders

Definition

Tic disorders are characterized by the persistent presence of abrupt, repetitive involuntary movements and sounds (tics) that have been described as caricatures of normal physical acts. The revised fourth edition of the ***Diagnostic and Statistical Manual of Mental Disorders*** (*DSM-IV-TR*) lists three main types of tic disorders: **Tourette syndrome**, chronic motor or vocal tic disorder, and transient tic disorder. The best known of these disorders is Tourette syndrome, named after Georges Gilles de la Tourette (1857–1904), who first described its symptoms in 1885.

Demographics

An estimated 200,000 Americans have the most severe form of Tourette syndrome, but as many as one in 100 people exhibit minor tics. Tourette syndrome is three-to-five times more common in males than females. Tic disorders have been reported in people of all races, ethnic groups, and socioeconomic classes, but they appear to occur more frequently in Caucasians than African Americans.

Description

Tics are sudden, painless, nonrhythmic behaviors that are either motor (related to movement) or vocal and that appear out of context—for example, knee bends in science class. They are fairly common in childhood; in the vast majority of cases, they are temporary conditions that resolve on their own. In some children, however, the tics persist over time, becoming more complex and severe.

Tics may be simple (using only a few muscles or simple sounds) or complex (using many muscle groups or full words and sentences). Simple motor tics are brief, meaningless movements like eye blinking, facial grimacing, head jerks, or shoulder shrugs. They usually last less than one second. Complex motor tics involve slower, longer, and more purposeful movements like sustained looks, facial gestures, biting, banging, whirling or twisting around, or copropraxia (obscene gestures).

Simple phonic tics are meaningless sounds or noises like throat clearing, coughing, sniffling, barking, or hissing. Complex phonic tics include syllables, words, phrases, and such statements as "Shut up!" or "Now you've done it!" The child's speech may be abnormal, with unusual rhythms, tones, accents, or intensities. The echo phenomenon is a tic characterized by the immediate repetition of one's own or another's words. Coprolalia is a tic made up of obscene, inappropriate, or aggressive words and statements. It occurs in fewer than 10% of people with tic disorders.

Children under the age of 10 with simple tics find them to be difficult to suppress, or control. Many older patients and children with complex tics describe feeling strong sensory urges in their joints, muscles, and bones that are relieved by the performance of a motor tic in that particular body part. These patients also report inner conflict over whether and when to yield to these urges. A sensation of relief and reduction of anxiety frequently follows the performance of a tic. Unless the tic disorder is very severe, most people with tics can suppress them for varying periods of time.

Motor and vocal tics may be worsened by anxiety, **stress**, boredom, **fatigue**, or excitement. Some people have reported that tics are intensified by **premenstrual syndrome**, additives in food, and stimulants. The symptoms of tic disorders may be lessened while the patient is asleep. **Cannabis** (marijuana), alcohol, relaxation, playing a sport, or concentrating on an enjoyable task are also reported to reduce the severity and frequency of symptoms.

Tics are the core symptom shared by transient tic disorder, chronic motor or vocal tic disorder, and Tourette syndrome. The age of onset for these disorders is between two and 15 years. It is the severity and course that distinguishes these disorders from one another. Tourette symptoms typically appear before the age of 18. In most patients, Tourette symptoms subside after adolescence.

Causes and symptoms

Causes

Emotional factors were once viewed as the cause of tics, but this explanation has been largely discounted. The search for causes now focuses on biological, chemical, and environmental factors. No definitive cause of tics has yet been identified.

There appear to be both functional and structural abnormalities in the brains of people with tic disorders. While the exact neurochemical cause is unknown, it is believed that abnormal **neurotransmitters** (chemical messengers within the **brain**) contribute to the disorders. The affected neurotransmitters are **dopamine**, **serotonin**, and cyclic AMP. Researchers have also found changes within the brain itself, for example in the basal ganglia (an area of the brain concerned with movement) and the anterior cingulate cortex. Functional imaging using **positron emission tomography (PET)** and single photon emission computerized tomography (SPECT) has highlighted abnormal patterns of blood flow and metabolism in the basal ganglia, thalamus, and frontal and temporal cortical areas of the brain. **Magnetic resonance imaging** (MRI) has identified a reduction in frontal lobe tissue in patients with Tourette. Researchers have also shown a correlation between reduced corpus callosum size and the severity of tics in children with Tourette.

Evidence from twin and family studies suggests that vulnerability to tic disorders is genetic, or transmitted within families. Several genes have been suspected as contributing to the development of Tourette, including variations to the SLITRK1 gene. Gender-related inheritance patterns play a role in determining symptoms. Males are more likely to develop tics, while females are more likely to develop the related **obsessive-compulsive disorder**. Researchers have not found a pattern suggesting that certain types of parenting or childhood experiences lead to the development of tic disorders, although some think that there is an interaction between genetic and environmental factors. Researchers are paying close attention to prenatal factors, which are thought to influence the development of the disorders. Some research has indicated that maternal smoking increases the severity of symptoms in Tourette syndrome.

In some cases, tic disorders appear to be caused or worsened by recreational drugs or prescription medications. The drugs most commonly involved are such psychomotor stimulants as **methylphenidate** (Ritalin), **pemoline** (Cylert), **amphetamines**, and **cocaine**. It is not clear whether tics would have developed in these cases if stimulants had not been used. In a smaller percentage of cases, antihistamines, tricyclic **antidepressants**, antiseizure medications, and **opioids** have been shown to worsen tics.

Some forms of tics may be triggered by the environment. A cough that began during an upper respiratory infection may continue as an involuntary vocal tic. New tics may also begin as imitations of normally occurring events, such as mimicking a dog barking. How these particular triggers come to form enduring symptoms is a matter for further study.

Tourette syndrome often occurs together with obsessive-compulsive disorder (OCD) and **attention deficit hyperactivity disorder** (ADHD). People with Tourette syndrome are about 20 times more likely than those in the general population to develop OCD. Tic disorders are also associated with behaviors such as **depression**, rage, sexual aggressiveness, and anxiety.

In some cases, neuropsychiatric disorders, such as tic disorders and obsessive-compulsive disorder, have been shown to develop after streptococcal infection. No precise mechanism for this connection has been determined, although it appears to be related to the autoimmune system. There are other illness-related causes of tics, though they appear to be rare. These include the development of tics after head **trauma**, viral encephalitis, or **stroke**.

Symptoms

The diagnostic criteria of all tic disorders specify that the symptoms must appear before the age of 18 and that they cannot result from ingestion of such substances as stimulants or from such general medical conditions as Huntington's disease. Tic disorders can be seen as occurring along a continuum of severity in terms of disruption and impairment, with transient tic disorder being the least severe and Tourette disorder being the most severe.

Tics increase in frequency when a person is under any form of mental or physical stress, even if it is of a positive nature (e.g., excitement about a party). Some people's tics are most obvious when the person is in a relaxed situation, such as quietly watching television. Tics tend to diminish when the person is placed in a new or highly structured situation, such as a doctor's office—a factor that can complicate **diagnosis**. When the symptoms of a tic are present over long time periods, they do not remain constant but will wax and wane in their severity.

Transient tic disorder occurs in approximately 4–24% of schoolchildren. It is the mildest form of tic disorder, and may be underreported because of its temporary nature. In transient tic disorder, there may be single or multiple motor and/or vocal tics that occur many times a day nearly every day for at least four weeks, but not for longer than one year. If the criteria have been met at one time for Tourette disorder or for chronic motor or vocal tic disorder, transient tic disorder may not be diagnosed.

Chronic motor or vocal tic disorder is characterized by either motor tics or vocal tics, but not both. The tics occur many times a day nearly every day, or intermittently for a period of more than one year. During that time, the patient is never without symptoms for more than three consecutive months. The severity of the symptoms and functional impairment is usually much less than for patients with Tourette disorder.

Tourette is defined by the *DSM-IV-TR* as the presence of both vocal and motor tics for a period of more than one year. The tics occur many times a day, usually in bouts, nearly every day or intermittently. The patient is never symptom-free for more than three months at a time.

Children and adolescents with Tourette disorder frequently experience additional problems including aggressiveness, self-harming behaviors, emotional immaturity, social withdrawal, physical complaints, conduct disorders, affective disorders, anxiety, panic attacks, **stuttering**, **sleep disorders**, migraine headaches, and inappropriate sexual behaviors.

Tics seem to worsen during the patient's adolescence, although some clinicians think that the symptoms become more problematic rather than more severe, because the patient experiences more embarrassment than he or she did before. The symptoms do become more unpredictable from day to day during adolescence. Many teenagers may refuse to go to school when their tics are severe. Coprolalia (uttering obscene, hostile, or inappropriate words) often appears first in adolescence; this symptom causes considerable distress for individuals and their families.

Behavioral problems also become more prominent in adolescence. There is some evidence that temper tantrums, aggressiveness, and explosive behavior appear in preadolescence, intensify in adolescence, and gradually diminish by early adulthood. Aggression appears to increase at approximately the same time that the tics decrease in severity.

Diagnosis

There are no diagnostic laboratory tests to screen for tic disorders. Except for the tics, the results of the patient's physical and neurological examinations are normal. The doctor takes a complete medical history including a detailed account of prenatal events, birth history, head injuries, episodes of encephalitis or meningitis, poisonings, and medication or drug use. The patient's developmental, behavioral, and academic histories are also important. Measurement of thyroid-stimulating hormone levels can be helpful, because tics are often associated with hyperthyroidism (overactive thyroid gland). Also, a strep-A test is useful if the patient suddenly developed tic symptoms after a throat or ear infection.

There is an average delay of 5 to 12 years between the initial symptoms of a tic disorder and the correct diagnosis. This delay is largely related to the misperception that tics are caused by anxiety and should be treated by **psychotherapy**. This misperception in turn is fueled by the fact that tics tend to increase in severity when the affected person is angry, anxious, excited, or fatigued. It is also common for the patient to manifest fewer tics in a doctor's office than at home, leaving parents feeling frustrated and undermined and physicians confused. In addition, children quickly learn to mask their symptoms by converting them to more socially acceptable movements and sounds. The diagnosis of a tic disorder can be aided in some cases by directly observing, videotaping, or audiotaping the patient in a more natural setting.

Clinicians can also become confused by such additional symptoms of tic disorders as touching, hitting, jumping, smelling hands or objects, stomping, twirling, and doing deep-knee bends. They disagree, however, as to whether such symptoms should be classified as tics or compulsions. There appears to be a significant overlap between the symptoms of tic disorders and those of obsessive-compulsive disorder (OCD).

Abnormal obsessive-compulsive behavior has been found in 40% of patients with Tourette disorder between the ages of 6 and 10 years. Obsessions are persistent ideas, thoughts, impulses, or images that are experienced as intrusive, inappropriate, senseless, and repetitive. Compulsions are defined as repetitive behaviors performed to reduce the anxiety or distress caused by the obsessions. For those diagnosed with OCD, common obsessions have to do with dirt, germs, and contamination. Patients with Tourette disorder often have obsessions that involve violent scenes, sexual thoughts, and counting; their compulsions are often related to symmetry (e.g., lining things up and getting them "just right"). OCD symptoms occur considerably later than tics and appear to worsen with age. Some theorists have suggested that obsessive thoughts are cognitive tics.

Tic disorders can be differentiated from **movement disorders** by the following characteristics: they are suppressible; they tend to persist during sleep; they are preceded by sensory symptoms; they have both phonic and motor components; and they wax and wane.

Dual diagnoses

Children and adults with tic disorders are at increased risk for depression and other mood disorders, as well as **anxiety disorders**. This comorbidity may be due to the burden of dealing with a chronic, disruptive, and often stigmatizing disorder. The energy and watchfulness required to suppress tic symptoms may contribute to social anxiety, social withdrawal, self-preoccupation, and fatigue. Low self-esteem and feelings of hopelessness are common in patients diagnosed with tic disorders.

While OCD behaviors have been noted in as many as 80% of individuals with tic disorders, only 30% meet the full criteria for OCD. Distinguishing complex tics from simple compulsions can be difficult. Touching compulsions appear to be characteristic of the tic-related type of OCD. Compared to obsessive-compulsive disorder in persons without a history of tics, there will likely be an earlier age of onset, a greater proportion of male sufferers, a more frequent family history of chronic tics, and a poorer therapeutic response to **selective serotonin reuptake inhibitors** (SSRIs)—although the addition of a neuroleptic to the treatment regimen sometimes brings about improvement.

More than 25% of children with Tourette syndrome also have ADHD, including a short attention span, restlessness, poor concentration, and diminished impulse control. On average, ADHD will manifest two-and-a-half years before the tics appear. A dual diagnosis of ADHD and tic disorder is associated with more severe tics and greater social impairment than for tic disorder by itself. Over time, the problems caused by the inattention, impulsivity, motor overactivity, and the resultant underachievement in school associated with ADHD are often more disabling than the tics themselves.

Children with tic disorders are five times as likely as other children to require special education programs. The tics may be disruptive and mistakenly interpreted by teachers as intended to disturb the class. Often, children with tic disorders have underlying learning disabilities as well. While there does not appear to be any impairment in general intellectual functioning, researchers have identified patterns of specific learning problems in children with tic disorders. These problems include abnormal visual-perceptual performance, reduced visual-motor skills, and discrepancies between verbal and performance IQ. Many of these learning difficulties are also commonly found in children with ADHD.

Increasing numbers of children with tic disorders are also diagnosed with a **conduct disorder**. Children with conduct disorder show inappropriate and sometimes severe aggression toward people and animals. They may also act out other destructive impulses. Unfortunately, some of these children grow up to develop a personality disorder.

Treatment

A holistic approach is recommended for the treatment of tic disorders. A multidisciplinary team should work together with the affected child's parents and teachers to put together a comprehensive treatment plan. Treatment should include:

- Educating the patient and family about the course of the disorder in a reassuring manner.
- Completion of necessary diagnostic tests, including self-reports (by child and parents); clinician-administered ratings; and direct observational methods.
- Comprehensive assessment, including the child's cognitive abilities, perception, motor skills, behavior and adaptive functioning.
- Collaboration with school personnel to create a learning environment conducive to academic success.
- Therapy, most often behavioral or cognitive-behavioral, though other modalities may be appropriate.
- If necessary, evaluation for medication.

Behavioral and cognitive-behavioral therapy

Habit reversal is the most commonly used technique, combining relaxation exercises, awareness training, and contingency management for positive **reinforcement**. This method shows a 64–100% success rate. Adding a cognitive component to habit reversal involves the introduction of flexibility into rigid thinking, and confronting the child's irrational expectations and unrealistic anticipations. The specific cognitive technique of distraction has been shown to help patients resist sensory urges and to restore the patient's sense of control over the tic.

Massed negative practice is a behavioral therapy technique used in the treatment of children with tic disorder. The patient is asked to deliberately perform the tic movement for specified periods of time interspersed with brief periods of rest. Patients have shown some decrease in tic frequency, but the long-term benefits of massed negative practice are unclear.

Contingency management is another behavioral treatment. It is based on positive reinforcement, usually administered by parents. Children are praised and rewarded for not performing tics and for replacing them with alternative behaviors. Contingency management, however, appears to be of limited use outside of such controlled settings as schools or institutions.

Self-monitoring consists of having the patient record tics by using a wrist counter or small notebook. It is fairly effective in reducing some tics by increasing the child's awareness.

Medications

Medication is the main treatment for motor and vocal tics. Because medications can cause side effects, patients and their families should be evaluated fully and use other treatment methods in conjunction with medication. Because the symptoms of tic disorders overlap those of OCD and ADHD, it is essential to determine which symptoms are causing the greatest concern and impairment, and treat the patient according to the single diagnostic category that best fits him or her, whether it is a tic disorder, OCD, or ADHD.

These medications may be prescribed for patients with tic disorders.

- Typical neuroleptics (antipsychotic medications), including haloperidol (Haldol), risperidone (Risperdal), and pimozide (Orap). Neuroleptics can have significant side effects, which include concentration problems, cognitive blunting, sedation, and, more rarely, tardive dyskinesia (a movement disorder that consists of lip, mouth, and tongue movements).
- Alpha-adrenergic receptor agonists, including clonidine (Catapres) and guanfacine (Tenex). Clonidine has fewer and milder side effects than the neuroleptics in

general, with the most common being sedation. Sedation occurs in 10–20% of cases and can often be controlled by adjusting the dosage.

- The phenothiazines may be used when haloperidol or pimozide has proven ineffective.
- Atypical antipsychotics such as aripiprazole (Abilify) and other agents that block dopamine receptors including risperidone (Risperdal) and clozapine (Clozaril).
- Tetrabenazine is a promising new medication with fewer side effects than other typical neuroleptics. It can be used in combination with the older antipsychotic medications, allowing for lower doses of both medications with substantial relief. However, it may cause depression and Parkinson's-like symptoms.
- Selective serotonin reuptake inhibitors (SSRIs), which include medications such as fluoxetine (Prozac) and sertraline (Zoloft), can be used to treat the obsessive-compulsive behaviors associated with Tourette disorder. They can also be helpful with depression and difficulties with impulse control, though they must be given at higher dosages for OCD than for depression. The SSRIs, however, can cause gastric upset and nausea.
- Benzodiazepines are used in some cases to decrease tic severity and lower the patient's anxiety level, but are often avoided because they can cause dependence and tolerance.
- Nicotine chewing gum appears to reduce tics when added to ongoing treatment with haloperidol, but is in need of further study.
- Calcium channel blockers, such as verapamil (Calan) and nifedipine (Adalat) may ease symptoms by reducing the release of neurotransmitters in the brain.

Surgical treatments

Surgery to the frontal lobe (prefrontal lobotomy) and limbic system (limbic lencotomy) have not been shown effective in treating tic disorders. However, deep brain stimulation—the high-frequency stimulation of the brain with electrodes—has been shown in studies to reduce tic severity by 70%.

Alternative therapies

There is growing interest in dietary changes and nutritional supplements to prevent and manage the symptoms of tic disorders, although formal studies have not yet been conducted in this area. Some theorists have suggested that hidden food and chemical allergies or nutritional deficiencies may influence the development and maintenance of tic disorders. Recommendations include eating organic food and avoiding pesticides, taking antioxidants, increasing intake of folic acid and the B vitamins, eating foods high in **zinc** and magnesium, eliminating caffeine from the diet, and avoiding artificial sweeteners, colors and dyes.

Prognosis

There is presently no cure for tic disorders, and there is no evidence that early treatment alters prognosis. When a child is first evaluated, it is not possible to determine whether the tics will be chronic or transient, mild or severe.

As recently as twenty years ago, tic disorders were considered to be lifelong conditions, with remissions believed to be rare. There is now a general consensus that if a tic disorder is the only diagnosis, the prognosis is favorable. Up to 73% of patients report that their tics decreased markedly or disappeared as they entered the later years of adolescence or early adulthood.

In a small number of patients, the most severe and debilitating forms of a tic disorder occur in adult life. In addition, stress in later life can cause tics to re-emerge. The tics may be new developments in adulthood, a phenomenon that may be more common than previously thought. Remission rates for tic disorders are difficult to pinpoint among this seldom-studied population, but appear to be extremely low.

Although the tics themselves may decline, the associated problems often continue into adult life. Obsessive-compulsive symptoms and other behavioral problems, as well as learning disabilities, may grow worse. Obsessive-compulsive behaviors become most pronounced at age 15 and remain at that level. Panic attacks, depression, **agoraphobia**, and alcoholism are most significant in the early adult years, while a tendency toward obesity increases steadily with age, particularly in women.

In adulthood, a patient's repertoire of tics is reduced and becomes predictable during periods of fatigue and heightened emotionality. Some studies suggest remission rates, with the complete cessation of symptoms, to be as high as 50%. Cases of total remission appear to be related to the family's treatment of the patient when he or she was a child. Persons who were punished, misunderstood and stigmatized because of their tics experience greater functional impairment as adults than those who were supported and understood as children.

Prevention

There are few preventive strategies for tic disorders. There is some evidence that maternal emotional stress

KEY TERMS

Atypical antipsychotics—A group of medications for the treatment of psychotic symptoms that were introduced in the 1990s. The atypical antipsychotics include clozapine, risperidone, quetiapine, ziprasidone, and olanzapine. They are sometimes called serotonin dopamine antagonists, or SDAs.

Basal ganglia—A group of masses of gray matter located in the cerebral hemispheres of the brain that control movement as well as some aspects of emotion and cognition.

Behavioral therapy—An approach to treatment that focuses on extinguishing undesirable behavior and replacing it with desired behavior.

Benzodiazepines—A group of central nervous system depressants used to relieve anxiety or to induce sleep.

Cognitive-behavioral therapy—An approach to psychotherapy that emphasizes the correction of distorted thinking patterns and changing one's behaviors accordingly.

Comorbidity—Association or presence of two or more mental disorders in the same patient. A disorder that is said to have a high degree of comorbidity is likely to occur in patients diagnosed with other disorders that may share or reinforce some of its symptoms.

Compulsion—A strong impulse to perform an act, particularly one that is irrational or contrary to one's will.

Coprolalia—A vocal tic characterized by uttering obscene, hostile, or inappropriate words. A motor tic characterized by obscene gestures is called copropraxia.

Cyclic AMP—A small molecule of adenosine monophosphate (AMP) that activates enzymes and increases the effects of hormones and other neurotransmitters.

Dopamine—A chemical in brain tissue that serves to transmit nerve impulses (is a neurotransmitter) and helps to regulate movement and emotions.

Holistic—A treatment approach that is comprehensive and respectful of a person's emotional, social, cognitive, and interpersonal needs.

Neuroleptic—Another name for the older antipsychotic medications, such as haloperidol (Haldol) and chlorpromazine (Thorazine).

Neurotransmitter—A chemical in the brain that transmits messages between neurons, or nerve cells.

Obsession—A persistent image, idea, or desire that dominates a person's thoughts or feelings.

Onset—The point in time at which the symptoms of a disorder first became apparent.

Phenothiazines—A class of drugs widely used in the treatment of psychosis.

Remission—In the course of an illness or disorder, a period of time when symptoms are absent.

Serotonin—A widely distributed neurotransmitter that is found in blood platelets, the lining of the digestive tract, and the brain, and that works in combination with norepinephrine. It causes very powerful contractions of smooth muscle, and is associated with mood, attention, emotions, and sleep. Low levels of serotonin are associated with depression.

Stigma—A mark or characteristic trait of a disease or defect; by extension, a cause for reproach or a stain on one's reputation. Tic disorders are sometimes regarded as a stigma by the patient's family.

Tardive dyskinesia—A condition that involves involuntary movements of the tongue, jaw, mouth, or face or other groups of skeletal muscles that usually occurs either late in antipsychotic therapy or even after the therapy is discontinued. It may be irreversible.

Thalamus—The middle part of the diencephalon (a part of the human forebrain), responsible for transmitting and integrating information from the senses.

Tic—A sudden involuntary behavior that is difficult or impossible for the person to suppress. Tics may be either motor (related to movement) or vocal, and may become more pronounced under stress.

during pregnancy and severe nausea and vomiting during the first trimester may affect tic severity. Attempting to minimize prenatal stress may possibly serve a limited preventive function.

Similarly, because people with tic disorders are sensitive to stress, efforts to maintain a low-stress environment can help minimize the number or severity of tics (e.g., reducing the number of social gatherings, which can provoke anxiety). This approach cannot prevent tics altogether, and must be undertaken with an awareness that it is neither healthful nor advisable to attempt to eliminate all stressful events in life.

Resources

BOOKS

American Psychiatric Association. *Diagnostic and Statistical Manual of Mental Disorders*. 4th ed., text rev. Washington, DC: American Psychiatric Publishing, 2000.

Chowdhury, Uttom, and Isobel Heyman. *Tics and Tourette Syndrome: A Handbook for Parents and Professionals*. London: Jessica Kingsley Publishers, 2004.

Kurlan, Roger, ed. *Handbook of Tourette's Syndrome and Related Tic and Behavioral Disorder*. New York: Marcel Dekker, 2005.

Woods, Douglas W., and Raymond G. Miltenberger, eds. *Tic Disorders, Trichotillomania, and Other Repetitive Behavior Disorders: Behavioral Approaches to Analysis and Treatment*. New York: Springer, 2006.

PERIODICALS

Balen, George M., et al. "An overview of the treatment of Tourette's disorder and tics." *Journal of Child and Adolescent Psychopharmacology* 20, no. 4 (2010): 249.

Fan, Wenqing, et al. "Association between antipsychotics and body mass index when treating patients with tics." *Journal of Child and Adolescent Psychopharmacology* 20, no. 4 (2010): 277.

Gilbert, Donald L., Elana Harris, and Steve W. Wu. "Tic suppression: the medical model." *Journal of Child and Adolescent Psychopharmacology* 20, no. 4 (2010): 263.

Otto, M. Alexander. "Habit reversal training can bring end to tics: treatment sometimes works as a 'useful adjunct' to drug therapy and can be 'good place to start.'" *Clinical Psychiatry News*. (March 2011): 20.

Piacentini, John C., John T. Walkup, and Douglas W. Woods. "Comprehensive behavioral intervention for tics in children with Tourette syndrome." *Communique* (Oct. 2010): 1.

ORGANIZATIONS

Association for Comprehensive Neurotherapy, PO Box 2198, Broken Arrow, OK, 34688-1967, (561) 798-0472, Fax: (561) 798-9820, acn@latitudes.org, http://www.latitudes.org.

National Institute of Neurological Disorders and Stroke, PO Box 5801, Bethesda, MD, 20824, (301) 496-5751; TTY: (301) 468-5981, (800) 352-9424, http://www.ninds.nih.gov.

Tourette Syndrome Association, Inc, 42-40 Bell Blvd., Bayside, NY, 11361-2861, (718) 224-2999, http://www.tsa-usa.org.

Holly Scherstuhl, M.Ed.
Stephanie N. Watson

Tofranil *see* **Imipramine**

Toilet phobia

Definition

Toilet phobia is an often debilitating psychological condition that affects an individual's ability to urinate or defecate in public facilities. It is an inclusive term that encompasses two different phobias—paruresis, the fear of urinating in public places (also referred to as "bashful bladder syndrome," "shy bladder syndrome," or "pee-phobia") and parcopresis, the fear of having a bowel movement in a public place or when other people are nearby. Many psychologists consider toilet phobias to be a form of social anxiety disorder.

Demographics

An estimated 7%, or 17 million Americans, experience paruresis. Although paruresis can occur in both men and women, approximately 90% of those who seek treatment for the condition are male. This may be because public men's restrooms are much more open (urinals, rather than closed stalls) than women's restrooms. The severity of paruresis can vary widely. It is estimated that between 1 and 2 million Americans have such severe paruresis that it has a significant negative effect on their daily personal and professional lives.

Description

Many people occasionally experience difficulty urinating or having a bowel movement. Often, these difficulties stem from an underlying medical condition, such as a blockage in the urinary system, constipation, illness, or a side effect of medication. However, when an individual is able to urinate or defecate normally at home but not in a public facility, the cause is likely psychological (paruresis or parcopresis). Individuals with these conditions feel embarrassed at the thought that they might be heard or criticized while using the toilet, and their anxiety can gradually worsen as the inability to use public bathrooms persists.

Different degrees of toilet phobias exist. People who have the most severe form are totally unable to use a public restroom and may even be unable to use the bathroom at the home of a friend or family member. Other people with toilet phobias can only use a public restroom if no one else is using it at the same time. Still others can go in a public facility if they are enclosed in a private stall rather than standing at a urinal.

To prevent the urge to urinate when away from home, individuals with toilet phobia may restrict fluids or take medications that prevent them from going to the bathroom. They may refuse to attend social functions and avoid traveling, for fear that they will be unable to find an empty restroom.

Young children may experience phobias during toilet training. The primary causes of toilet phobias in children are the fears of passing a painful bowel movement or being punished for making a mess. In

KEY TERMS

Biofeedback—A technique in which patients learn to modify certain body functions, such as temperature or pulse rate, with the help of a monitoring machine.

Obsessive-compulsive disorder (OCD)—An anxiety disorder in which a person cannot prevent himself from dwelling on unwanted thoughts, acting on urges, or performing repetitious rituals, such as washing his hands or checking to make sure he turned off the lights.

Parcopresis—Fear of having a bowel movement in a public place.

Paruresis—Fear of urinating in a public place.

Prostate—A gland found in men that surrounds the neck of the bladder and secretes fluid that when mixed with sperm becomes semen.

Sympathetic nervous system—The part of the autonomic nervous system that is concerned especially with preparing the body to react to situations of stress or emergency; it contains chiefly adrenergic fibers and tends to depress secretion, decrease the tone and contractility of smooth muscle, and increase heart rate.

most people with paruresis, the condition develops during the adolescent or teenage years, although it can arise at any time.

Causes and symptoms

Toilet phobias are believed to have genetic, physical, and psychological components. The symptoms include various levels of inability in using public toilets.

Causes

Paruresis and parcopresis tend to occur in families, as do social anxiety disorder and **depression**, which also commonly coexist in those individuals with toilet phobias.

The physical component of the disorder occurs when an individual experiences anxiety using a public restroom. That anxiety awakens the sympathetic nervous system, which causes smooth muscles in the urinary tract to contract, shutting off the flow of urine. The level of anxiety the person feels may grow with each subsequent attempt to use a public restroom.

Theories regarding the psychological triggers for toilet phobias include:

- memories of harassment, bullying, or teasing during a childhood or adolescent bathroom experience
- sexual abuse
- a subconscious association between using the bathroom and sexuality
- obsessive-compulsive disorder connected to a fear of contamination
- critical parents or an upbringing that associated shame with the toileting process

Because of the embarrassment involved with toilet phobias, most people who experience them do not seek professional help for their condition.

Symptoms

The following are symptoms of toilet phobias:

- limiting or avoiding fluids
- taking medication to prevent urination or a bowel movement
- avoiding travel, social situations, and jobs that require the use of a public restroom
- having a distended bladder from holding in urine for long periods of time or having other bladder or kidney problems
- feeling sweaty, dizzy, faint, or shaky when attempting to use a public restroom
- being embarrassed or ashamed of using the toilet and of the phobia itself

Diagnosis

Individuals with toilet phobias are often referred to a urologist for an initial evaluation. The urologist will do a series of tests to identify whether the problem stems from a condition such as diabetes or an enlarged prostate gland or is the side effect of a medication. The doctor may do a urodynamic evaluation, which measures urine flow rate, bladder pressure, and residual urine volume to see how well the bladder is filling and emptying. If the urological assessment is negative, the patient may be referred to a **psychiatrist**. For a **diagnosis** of toilet phobia to be made, the phobia must be significant enough to affect the individual's daily life. For example, the person must be going out of his or her way to avoid public restrooms.

Treatment

Several treatments have been proposed for toilet phobias, including **cognitive-behavioral therapy**, **hypnotherapy**, **biofeedback**, medication, and self-

QUESTIONS TO ASK YOUR DOCTOR

- Can you refer me to a therapist or other mental health professional?
- What tests are necessary to rule out an underlying physical condition?
- Is medication to treat anxiety appropriate for me?
- Is there a support group available for this problem?
- Do you have anyone on staff experienced in treating this condition?
- Is cognitive-behavior therapy right for me?

catheterization. The most commonly used treatment for paruresis is graduated behavior therapy, in which patients learn to overcome their phobia by progressing through increasingly public bathroom scenarios. For example, someone may first urinate in a private bathroom while someone is standing in another room in the house and gradually work their way up to voiding while in a public bathroom with someone right outside the stall.

Toilet phobias also may be treated with medication, although no clinical evidence exists to prove its effectiveness. Sometimes the drug **diazepam** (Valium) can relax the pelvic floor muscles to relieve urinary retention. **Selective serotonin reuptake inhibitors (SSRIs)** may be used to treat the underlying anxiety that is causing the toilet phobia.

For children who experience toilet phobias, several possible interventions can be used. If the child fears having a painful bowel movement, stool softeners can help ensure that the bowel movement is not uncomfortable. Parents can reassure their child about using the toilet or use small rewards and incentives. If the phobia stems from anxiety or depression, the child may require counseling from a psychiatrist or **psychologist**.

Prognosis

Although cognitive-behavioral therapy, **psychotherapy**, and other treatments are not effective in every case, these techniques help some people overcome toilet phobias. No randomized, controlled studies have been done to evaluate toilet phobia treatments; however, surveys and case studies suggest that behavioral therapies can at least improve symptoms in more than half of patients and can have complete success in many cases.

Prevention

There is no sure way to prevent toilet phobias. However, treatments such as graduated behavior therapy may be effective in reducing the anxiety associated with using public restrooms.

Resources

BOOKS

Axelby, Clayton P., ed. *Social Phobia: Etiology, Diagnosis, and Treatment.* New York: Nova Biomedical Books, 2009.

Olmert, Carol. *Bathrooms Make Me Nervous: A Guidebook for Women with Urination Anxiety (Shy Bladder).* Walnut Creek, CA: CJOB, 2008.

Robinson, Theresa M., ed. *Social Anxiety: Symptoms, Causes, and Techniques.* Hauppauge, NY: Nova Science, 2010.

PERIODICALS

Soifer, S., J. Himle, and K. Walsh. "Paruresis (Shy Bladder Syndrome): A Cognitive-Behavioral Treatment Approach." *Social Work in Health Care* 49, no. 5 (May 2010): 494–507.

Soifer, Steven, et al. "Paruresis or Shy Bladder Syndrome: An Unknown Urologic Malady?" *Urologic Nursing* 29, no. 2 (March/April 2009): 87–94.

ORGANIZATIONS

Anxiety Disorders Association of America, 8730 Georgia Ave., Ste. 600, Silver Spring, MD, 20910, (240) 485-1001, http://www.adaa.org.

International Paruresis Association, PO Box 65111, Baltimore, MD, 21209, (800) 247-3864, http://www.paruresis.org.

National Institute of Mental Health, 6001 Executive Blvd., Rm. 8184, MSC 9663 , Bethesda, MD, 20892-9663, (301) 443-4513, Fax: (301) 443-4279, (866) 615-6464; TTY: (301) 443-8431; TTY tollfree: (866) 415-8051, http://www.nimh.nih.gov.

Stephanie N. Watson
Tish Davidson, AM

Token economy system

Definition

A token economy is a form of **behavior modification** designed to increase desirable behavior and decrease undesirable behavior with the use of tokens. Individuals receive tokens immediately after displaying desirable behavior. The tokens are collected and later exchanged for a meaningful object or privilege.

Purpose

The primary goal of a token economy is to increase desirable behavior and decrease undesirable behavior. Often token economies are used in institutional settings (such as psychiatric hospitals or correctional facilities) to manage the behavior of individuals who may be aggressive or unpredictable. However, the larger goal of token economies is to teach appropriate behavior and social skills that can be used in one's natural environment. Token economies are often used in special education (for children with developmental or learning disabilities, hyperactivity, attention deficit, or behavioral disorders), regular education, colleges, various types of **group homes**, military divisions, nursing homes, **addiction** treatment programs, occupational settings, family homes (for marital or parenting difficulties), and hospitals. Token economies can be used individually or in groups.

Description

Several elements are necessary in every token economy:

- Tokens: Anything that is visible and countable can be used as a token. Tokens should preferably be attractive, easy to carry and dispense, and difficult to counterfeit. Commonly used items include poker chips, stickers, point tallies, or play money. When an individual displays desirable behavior, he or she is immediately given a designated number of tokens. Tokens have no value of their own. They are collected and later exchanged for meaningful objects, privileges or activities. Individuals can also lose tokens (response cost) for displaying undesirable behavior.
- A clearly defined target behavior: Individuals participating in a token economy need to know exactly what they must do in order to receive tokens. Desirable and undesirable behavior is explained ahead of time in simple, specific terms. The number of tokens awarded or lost for each particular behavior is also specified.
- Back-up reinforcers: Back-up reinforcers are the meaningful objects, privileges, or activities that individuals receive in exchange for their tokens. Examples include food items, toys, extra free time, or outings. The success of a token economy depends on the appeal of the back-up reinforcers. Individuals will only be motivated to earn tokens if they anticipate the future reward represented by the tokens. A well-designed token economy will use back-up reinforcers chosen by individuals in treatment rather than by staff.
- A system for exchanging tokens: A time and place for purchasing back-up reinforcers is necessary. The token value of each back-up reinforcer is pre-determined based on monetary value, demand, or therapeutic value. For example, if the reinforcer is expensive or highly attractive, the token value should be higher. If possession of or participation in the reinforcer would aid in the individual's acquisition of skills, the token value should be lower. If the token value is set too low, individuals will be less motivated to earn tokens. Conversely, if the value is set too high, individuals may become easily discouraged. It is important that each individual can earn at least some tokens.
- A system for recording data: Before treatment begins, information (baseline data) is gathered about each individual's current behavior. Changes in behavior are then recorded on daily data sheets. This information is used to measure individual progress, as well as the effectiveness of the token economy. Information regarding the exchange of tokens also needs to be recorded.
- Consistent implementation of the token economy by staff: In order for a token economy to succeed, all involved staff members must reward the same behaviors, use the appropriate amount of tokens, avoid dispensing back-up reinforcers for free, and prevent tokens from being counterfeited, stolen, or otherwise unjustly obtained. Staff responsibilities and the rules of the token economy should be described in a written manual. Staff members should also be evaluated periodically and given the opportunity to raise questions or concerns.

Initially tokens are awarded frequently and in higher amounts, but as individuals learn the desirable behavior, opportunities to earn tokens decrease. (The amount and frequency of token dispensing is called a **reinforcement** schedule.) For example, in a classroom, each student may earn 25 to 75 tokens the first day, so that they quickly learn the value of the tokens. Later, students may earn 15 to 30 tokens per day. By gradually decreasing the availability of tokens (fading), students should learn to display the desirable behavior independently, without the unnatural use of tokens. Reinforcers that individuals would normally encounter in society, such as verbal praise, should accompany the awarding of tokens to aid in the fading process.

Advantages of token economies are that behaviors can be rewarded immediately, rewards are the same for all members of a group, use of punishment (response cost) is less restrictive than other forms of punishment, and individuals can learn skills related to planning for the future. Disadvantages include considerable cost, effort, and extensive staff training and management. Some professionals find token economies to be time-consuming and impractical.

Risks

Risks involved in token economies are similar to those in other forms of behavior modification. Staff members implementing the therapy may intentionally or

KEY TERMS

Back-up reinforcer—A desirable item, privilege, or activity that is purchased with tokens and serves as a delayed reward and subsequent motivation for target (desired) behavior.

Baseline data—Information regarding the frequency and severity of behavior, gathered before treatment begins.

Behavior modification—An approach to therapy based on the principles of operant conditioning. Behavior modification seeks to replace undesirable behaviors with preferable behaviors through the use of positive or negative reinforcement.

Fading—Gradually decreasing the amount or frequency of a reinforcer so that the target behavior will begin to occur independent of any rewards.

Reinforcement schedule—The frequency and amount of reinforcers administered.

Reinforcer—Anything that causes an increase of a particular behavior.

Response cost—A behavioral technique that involves removing a stimulus from an individual's environment so that the response that directly precedes the removal is weakened. In a token economy system, response cost is a form of punishment involving loss of tokens due to inappropriate behavior, which consequently results in decreased ability to purchase back-up reinforcers.

Target behavior—The specific behavior to be increased or decreased during treatment.

Therapeutic value—The potential benefit of an object or situation, in terms of its ability to enhance functioning (social, emotional, intellectual, occupational, etc.) in an individual.

Token—Any item that can be seen and collected (such as stickers or points in a point tally) that has no value of its own, but is used as an immediate reward for desirable behavior that is later exchanged for back-up reinforcers.

unintentionally neglect the rights of individuals receiving treatment. Token economies should never deprive individuals of their basic needs, such as sufficient food, comfortable bedding, or reasonable opportunities for leisure. If staff members are inadequately trained or there is a shortage of staff, desirable behaviors may not be rewarded or undesirable behaviors may be inadvertently rewarded, resulting in an increase of negative behavior. Controversy exists regarding placing individuals in treatment against their will (such as in a psychiatric hospital), and deciding which behaviors should be considered desirable and which should be considered undesirable.

Results

Ideally, individuals will use the skills learned in a token economy in their everyday surroundings. They will display the undesirable behavior less frequently or not at all. They will also engage in positive, adaptive behaviors more often.

If the token economy was ineffective, or time spent in the token economy was limited, individuals may show either no changes or even increases in the undesirable behavior.

Resources

BOOKS

Martin, Garry. *Behavior Modification: What It Is and How to Do It*. 9th ed. Upper Saddle River, New Jersey: Prentice-Hall, 2010.

Miltenberger, Raymond G. *Behavior Modification: Principles and Procedures*. 5thed. Belmont, California: Wadsworth/Thomson Learning, 2011.

Reinke, Wendy M., Keith C. Herman, and Randy Sprick. *Motivational Interviewing for Effective Classroom Management: The Classroom Check-Up*. New York: The Guilford Press: 2011.

Young, Ellie L., Paul Caldarella, Michael J. Richardson, and K. Richard Young. *Positive Behavior Support in Secondary Schools: A Practical Guide*. New York: The Guilford Press: 2011.

PERIODICALS

Fortson, Beverly L., et al. "Managing Classroom Behavior of Head Start Children Using Response Cost and Token Economy Procedures." *The Journal of Early and Intensive Behavioral Intervention* 2, no. 1 (2005): 28.

Moore, James W., et al. "Restructuring an Existing Token Economy in a Psychiatric Facility for Children." *Child & Family Behavior Therapy* 23, no. 3 (2001): 53–59.

Nelson, Karl G. "Exploration of Classroom Participation in the Presence of a Token Economy." *Journal of Instructional Psychology* 37, no. 1 (2010): 49.

ORGANIZATIONS

Association for Behavioral Analysis International, 550 West Centre Ave., Ste. 1, Portage, MI, 49024, (269) 492-9310, Fax: (269) 492-9316, http://www.abainternational.org.

Cambridge Center for Behavioral Studies, PO Box 7067, Cummings Center, Ste. 340F, Beverly, MA, 01915, (978) 369-2227, Fax: (978) 369-8584, http://www.behavior.org.

Sandra L. Friedrich, M.A.

Tourette syndrome

Definition

Tourette syndrome (TS) is an inherited disorder of the nervous system that typically appears in childhood. The main features of TS are repeated movements and vocalizations called tics. TS can also be associated with behavioral and developmental problems.

Demographics

Tourette syndrome is a relatively common disorder found in all populations and all ethnic groups. TS is three to four times more common in males than females. The exact incidence of Tourette syndrome is unknown, but it is estimated to affect 1–10 per 1,000 children. According to the National Institute for Neurological Disorders and Stroke (NINDS), an estimated 200,000 Americans have the most severe form of TS, and as many as one in 100 have milder symptoms such as chronic motor or vocal tics. Early TS symptoms are almost always noticed first in childhood, with the average onset between 7–10 years.

Description

Tourette syndrome is a variable disorder with onset in childhood. Though symptoms can appear anywhere between 2–18 years of age, typical onset is around age 6 or 7. Tics, which may be motor or vocal, tend to wax and wane (increase and decrease) in severity over time. The first references in the literature to what might today be classified as TS largely describe individuals who were wrongly believed to be possessed by the devil. In 1885 Gilles de la Tourette, a French neurologist, provided the first formal description of this syndrome, which he described as an inherited neurological condition characterized by motor and vocal tics.

Although vocal and motor tics are the hallmark of Tourette syndrome, other symptoms such as the expression of socially inappropriate comments or behaviors, obsessive compulsive disorder, attention deficit disorder, self injuring behavior, **depression**, and anxiety also appear to be associated with Tourette syndrome. Symptoms usually intensify during teenage years and diminish in late adolescence or early adulthood. Patients may also develop co-occurring behavioral disorders, namely **obsessive-compulsive disorder** (OCD), **attention deficit hyperactivity disorder (ADHD)** or attention deficit disorder (ADD), poor impulse control, or **sleep disorders**. Though some children have learning disabilities, intelligence is not impaired. TS is not degenerative and life span is normal.

Risk factors

TS risk factors are unknown, and researchers are studying risk factors before and after birth that may contribute to this complex disorder. Some of the suggested factors are severe psychological **trauma**, recurrent daily stresses, extreme emotional excitement, PANDAS (pediatric autoimmune neuropsychiatric disorder with streptococcal infection), and drug abuse.

Causes and symptoms

A variety of genetic and environmental factors likely play a role in causing TS. Studies suggest that the tics in Tourette syndrome are caused by an increased amount of a neurotransmitter called **dopamine**. A neurotransmitter is a chemical found in the **brain** that helps to transmit information from one brain cell to another. Other studies suggest that the defect in Tourette syndrome involves the neurotransmitter **serotonin** or involves other chemicals required for normal functioning of the brain.

Genetic factors are believed to play a major role in the development of TS. Several chromosomal regions have been identified as possible locations of genes that confer susceptibility to TS. Some family studies have indicated that TS may be inherited in an autosomal dominant manner, but other studies have shown that this is not the case. Mutations involving the SLITRK1 gene have been identified in a small number of TS patients. This gene provides instructions for making a brain protein called SLITRK1. This protein probably plays a role in the development of nerve cells, including the growth of axons and dendrites that allow each nerve cell to communicate with nearby cells. It is unclear how mutations in the SLITRK1 gene can lead to this disorder. The inheritance pattern of Tourette syndrome remains unknown. Although the features of TS can cluster in families, many genetic and environmental factors are likely to be involved. Some researchers believe that Tourette syndrome has different causes in different individuals or is caused by changes in more than one gene. Further research is needed to establish the cause of Tourette syndrome.

Motor and vocal tics

The principal symptoms of Tourette syndrome are simple and complex motor and vocal tics. Simple motor tics are characterized by brief muscle contractions of one or more limited muscle groups. An eye twitch is an example of a simple motor tic. Complex motor tics tend to appear more complicated and purposeful than simple tics and involve coordinated contractions of several muscle groups. Some examples of complex motor tics are the act of hitting oneself and jumping. Copropraxia, the involuntary display of unacceptable or obscene gestures, and echopraxia, the imitation of the movement of another individual, are other examples of complex motor tics.

Vocal tics are actually manifestations of motor tics that involve the muscles required for vocalization. Simple vocal tics include **stuttering**, stammering, abnormal emphasis of part of a word or phrase, and inarticulate noises such as throat clearing, grunts, and high-pitched sounds. Complex vocal tics typically involve the involuntary expression of words. Perhaps the most striking example of this is coprolalia, the involuntary expression of obscene words or phrases, which occurs in fewer than one-third of people with Tourette syndrome. The involuntary echoing of the last word, phrase, sentence or sound vocalized by oneself (palilalia) or of another person or sound in the environment (echolalia) are also classified as complex tics.

The type, frequency, and severity of tics exhibited varies tremendously among individuals with Tourette syndrome. Tourette syndrome has a variable age of onset, and tics can start anytime between infancy and age 18. Initial symptoms usually occur before the early teens, and the mean age of onset for both males and females is approximately seven years of age. Most individuals with symptoms initially experience simple muscle tics involving the eyes and the head. These symptoms can progress to tics involving the upper torso, neck, arms, hands, and occasionally the legs and feet. Complex motor tics are usually the latest onset muscle tics. Vocal tics usually have a later onset then motor tics. In some rare cases, people with Tourette syndrome suddenly present with multiple, severe, or bizarre symptoms.

Not only is there extreme variability in clinical symptoms among individuals with Tourette syndrome, but individuals commonly experience a variability in type, frequency, and severity of symptoms within the course of their lifetime. Adolescents with Tourette syndrome often experience unpredictable and variable symptoms, which may be related to fluctuating hormone levels and decreased **compliance** in taking medications. Adults often experience a decrease in symptoms or a complete end to symptoms.

A number of factors appear to affect the severity and frequency of tics. **Stress** appears to increase the frequency and severity of tics while concentration on another part of the body that is not taking part in a tic can result in the temporary alleviation of symptoms. Relaxation, following attempts to suppress the occurrence of tics, may result in an increased frequency of tics. An increased frequency and severity of tics can also result from exposure to drugs such as **steroids**, **cocaine**, **amphetamines**, and caffeine. Hormonal changes such as those that occur prior to the menstrual cycle can also increase the severity of symptoms.

KEY TERMS

Attention deficit disorder (ADD)—Disorder characterized by a short attention span, impulsivity, and in some cases hyperactivity.

Autosomal dominant—A pattern of genetic inheritance where only one abnormal gene is needed to display the trait or disease.

Axon—The long extension of a nerve fiber that generally conducts impulses away from the body of the nerve cell.

Coprolalia—The involuntary expression of obscene words or phrases.

Copropraxia—The involuntary display of unacceptable/obscene gestures.

Decreased penetrance—Individuals who inherit a changed disease gene but do not develop symptoms.

Dendrites—Fibers of a brain cell that receive signals from other brain cells.

Dysphoria—Feelings of anxiety, restlessness, and dissatisfaction.

Echolalia—Involuntary echoing of the last word, phrase, or sentence spoken by someone else or sound in the environment.

Echopraxia—The imitation of the movement of another individual.

Neurotransmitter—Chemical in the brain that transmits information from one nerve cell to another.

Obsessive compulsive disorder (OCD)—Disorder characterized by persistent, intrusive, and senseless thoughts (obsessions) or compulsions to perform repetitive behaviors that interfere with normal functioning.

Palilalia—Involuntary echoing of the last word, phrase, sentence, or sound vocalized by oneself.

Tic—Brief and intermittent involuntary movement or sound.

Other associated symptoms

People with Tourette syndrome are more likely to exhibit socially inappropriate behaviors such as expressing insulting or socially unacceptable comments or socially unacceptable actions. It is not known whether these symptoms stem from a more general dysfunction of impulse control that might be part of Tourette syndrome.

Tourette syndrome appears to also be associated with attention deficit disorder (ADD). ADD is characterized by a short attention span and impulsivity and in some cases hyperactivity. Researchers have found that 21%–90% of individuals with Tourette syndrome also exhibit symptoms of ADD, whereas 2%–15% of the general population exhibit symptoms of ADD.

People with Tourette syndrome are also at higher risk for having symptoms of obsessive-compulsive disorder (OCD). OCD is characterized by persistent, intrusive, and senseless thoughts (obsessions) or compulsions to perform repetitive behaviors that interfere with normal functioning. A person with OCD, for example, may be obsessed with germs and may counteract this **obsession** with continual hand washing. Symptoms of OCD are present in 1.9%–3% of the general population, whereas 28%–50% of people with Tourette syndrome have symptoms of OCD.

Self-injurious behavior (SIB) is also seen more frequently in those with Tourette syndrome. Approximately 34%–53% of individuals with Tourette syndrome exhibit some form of self-injuring behavior. The SIB is often related to OCD but can also occur in those with Tourette syndrome who do not have OCD.

Symptoms of anxiety and depression are also found more commonly in people with Tourette syndrome. It is not clear, however, whether these symptoms are symptoms of Tourette syndrome or occur as a result of having to deal with the symptoms of moderate to severe Tourette syndrome.

People with Tourette syndrome may also be at increased risk for having learning disabilities and **personality disorders** and may be more predisposed to behaviors such as aggression, antisocial behaviors, severe temper outbursts, and inappropriate sexual behavior. Further controlled studies need to be performed, however, to ascertain whether these behaviors are symptoms of Tourette syndrome.

Diagnosis

The TS **diagnosis** is made through observation and interview of the patient and discussions with other family members. The diagnosis of Tourette syndrome is complicated by a variety of factors. The extreme range of symptoms of this disorder makes it difficult to differentiate Tourette syndrome from other disorders with similar symptoms. Diagnosis is further complicated by the fact that some tics appear to be within the range of normal behavior. For example, an individual who only exhibits tics such as throat clearing and sniffing may be misdiagnosed with a medical problem such as allergies. In addition, bizarre and complex tics such as coprolalia may be mistaken for psychotic or "bad" behavior. Diagnosis is also confounded by individuals who attempt to control tics in public and in front of healthcare professionals and deny the existence of symptoms. Although there is disagreement over what criteria should be used to diagnose Tourette syndrome, one aide is the ***Diagnostic and Statistical Manual of Mental Disorders*** (*DSM-IV*). The *DSM-IV* outlines suggest diagnostic criteria for a variety of conditions including Tourette syndrome:

- presence of both motor and vocal tics at some time during the course of the illness
- occurrence of multiple tics nearly every day through a period of more than one year, without a remission of tics for a period of greater than three consecutive months
- symptoms cause distress or impairment in functioning
- age of onset is prior to 18 years of age
- symptoms not due to medications or drugs and are not related to another medical condition

Some physicians criticize the *DSM-IV* criteria, citing that they do not include the full range of behaviors and symptoms seen in Tourette syndrome. Others criticize the criteria because it limits the diagnosis to those who experience a significant impairment, which may not be true for individuals with milder symptoms. For this reason many physicians use their clinical judgment as well as the *DSM-IV* criteria as a guide to diagnosing Tourette syndrome.

Tests

Patients may undergo blood tests, **imaging studies** such as **magnetic resonance imaging** (MRI), or an electroencephalogram (EEG) scan in order to rule out other possible explanations for the symptoms.

Treatment

There is no cure for Tourette syndrome, and treatment involves the control of symptoms through educational and psychological interventions and/or medications. The treatment and management of Tourette syndrome varies from patient to patient and is typically focused on the alleviation of the symptoms that are most bothersome to the patient or that cause the most interference with daily functioning.

Traditional

Psychological treatments such as counseling are not generally useful for the treatment of tics but can be beneficial in the treatment of associated symptoms such as obsessive-compulsive behavior and attention deficit disorder. Counseling may also help individuals to cope better with the symptoms of this disorder and to have more positive social interactions. Psychological interventions may also help people cope better with stressors that can normally be triggers for tics and negative behaviors. Relaxation therapies may, however, increase the occurrence of tics. Treatment is crucial in helping the affected person avoid depression, social isolation, and strained family relationships. The education of family members, teachers, and peers about Tourette syndrome can be helpful and may help to foster acceptance and prevent social isolation.

Drugs

Many people with mild symptoms of Tourette syndrome never require medications. Those with severe symptoms may require medications for all or part of their lifetime. No single or combination drug therapy offers complete cessation of symptoms without adverse effects. The most effective treatment of tics associated with Tourette syndrome involves the use of drugs such as **Haloperidol**, **Pimozide**, Sulpiride, and Tiapride, which decrease the amount of dopamine in the body. Unfortunately, the incidence of side effects, even at low dosages, is quite high. The short-term side effects can include sedation, dysphoria, weight gain, movement abnormalities, depression, and poor school performance. Long-term side effects can include phobias, memory difficulties, and personality changes. These drugs are therefore better candidates for short-term rather than long-term therapy.

Tourette syndrome can also be treated with other drugs such as **clonidine**, **clonazepam**, and **risperidone**, but the efficacy of these treatments is unknown. In many cases, treatment of associated conditions such as ADD and OCD is often more of a concern than the tics themselves. Clonidine used in conjunction with stimulants such as Ritalin may be useful for treating people with Tourette syndrome who also have symptoms of ADD. Stimulants should be used with caution in individuals with Tourette syndrome since they can sometimes increase the frequency and severity of tics. OCD symptoms in those with Tourette syndrome are often treated with drugs such as Prozac, Luvox, Paxil, and Zoloft.

In many cases the treatment of Tourette syndrome with medications can be discontinued after adolescence. Trials should be performed through the gradual tapering off of medications and should always be done under a doctor's supervision.

Alternative

Clinical trials for the treatment of Tourette syndrome are often sponsored by the National Institutes of Health (NIH) and other agencies. Clinical trial information is constantly updated by NIH, and the most recent information on Tourette syndrome trials can be found at http://clinicaltrials.gov.

Prognosis

The prognosis for Tourette syndrome in individuals without associated psychological conditions is often quite good, and only approximately 10% of Tourette syndrome individuals experience severe tic symptoms. Approximately 30% of people with Tourette syndrome experience a decrease in the frequency and severity of tics, and another 30–40% experience a complete end of symptoms by late adolescence. The other 30–40% continue to exhibit moderate to severe symptoms in adulthood. There does not appear to be a definite correlation between the type, frequency, and severity of symptoms and the eventual prognosis. Patients with severe tics may experience social difficulties and may isolate themselves from others for fear of shocking and embarrassing them. People with Tourette syndrome who have other symptoms such as obsessive compulsive disorder, attention deficit disorder, and self-injurious behavior usually have a poorer prognosis.

Prevention

There is no known way to prevent Tourette syndrome.

Resources

BOOKS

Buffolano, Sandra. *Coping with Tourette Syndrome: A Workbook to Help Kids With Tic Disorders.*Oakland, CA: Instant Help Books (New Harbinger), 2008.

Buzbuzian, Denise. *Victory Over Tourette's Syndrome and Tic Disorders.* Truro, NS: Woodland Publishing, 2007.

Chowdhury, Uttom, and Isobel Heyman. *Tics and Tourette Syndrome: A Handbook for Parents and Professionals.* London: Jessica Kingsley Publishers, 2004.

Marsh, Tracy L., ed. *Children with Tourette Syndrome: A Parent's Guide,* 2nd ed. Bethesda, MD: Woodbine House, 2006.

Peters, Dylan. *Tic Talk: Living with Tourette Syndrome: A 9–Year–Old Boy's Story in His Own Words.* Chandler, AZ: Little Five Star, 2009.

Woods, Douglas W., et al. *Managing Tourette Syndrome: A Behavioral Intervention Adult Workbook.* New York: Oxford University Press, 2008.

PERIODICALS

Altman, G., J.D. Staley, and P. Wener. "Children with Tourette Disorder: A Follow-up Study in Adulthood." *Journal of Nervous and Mental Disease* 197, no. 5 (May 2009): 305–310.

Bernard, B. A., et al. "Determinants of Quality of Life in Children with Gilles de la Tourette Syndrome." *Movement Disorders* 24, no. 7 (May 2009): 1070–1073.

Cavanna, A. E., et al. "The Behavioral Spectrum of Gilles de la Tourette Syndrome." *Journal of Neuropsychiatry and Clinical Neurosciences* 21, no. 1 (Winter 2009): 13–23.

Hedderick, E. F., C. M. Morris, and H. S. Singer. "Double-blind, Crossover Study of Clonidine and Levetiracetam in Tourette Syndrome." *Pediatric Neurology* 40, no. 6 (June 2009): 420–425.

Jimenez-Shahed, J. "Tourette Syndrome." *Neurologic Clinics* 27, no. 3 (August 2009): 737–755.

Verdellen, C. W., et al. "Habituation of Premonitory Sensations during Exposure and Response Prevention Treatment in Tourette's Syndrome." *Behavior Modification* 32, no. 2 (March 2008): 215–227.

OTHER

National Tourette Syndrome Association. "Facts About Tourette Syndrome." http://www.tsa-usa.org/aPeople/LivingWithTS/Images/Fact_Sheet.pdf (accessed October 27, 2011).

WEBSITES

Genetics Home Reference, Lister Hill National Center for Biomedical Communications. "Tourette Syndrome." U.S. National Library of Medicine, National Institutes of Health. http://ghr.nlm.nih.gov/condition=tourettesyndrome (accessed October 27, 2011.)

MedlinePlus. "Tourette Syndrome." U.S. National Library of Medicine, National Institutes of Health. http://www.nlm.nih.gov/medlineplus/tourettesyndrome.html (accessed October 27, 2011)

U.S. Centers for Disease Control. "Tourette Syndrome (TS)." http://www.cdc.gov/ncbddd/tourette/default.htm (accessed October 27, 2011).

ORGANIZATIONS

National Institute of Neurological Disorders and Stroke, PO Box 5801, Bethesda, MD, 20824, (301) 496-5751; TTY: (301) 468-5981, (800) 352-9424, http://www.ninds.nih.gov.

Tourette Syndrome Association, 42-40 Bell Blvd., Bayside, NY, 11361, (718) 224-2999, http://www.tsa-usa.org.

Tourette Syndrome Foundation of Canada, 5945 Airport Rd., Suite 195, Mississauga, ON, L4V 1R9, (905) 673-2255, (1-800) 361-3120, Fax: (905) 673-2638, http://www.tourette.ca.

Lisa Maria Andres, MS, CGC
Dawn J. Cardeiro, MS, CGC
Monique Laberge, PhD

Tranquilizers *see* **Antianxiety drugs and abuse; Sedatives and related disorders**

Transcranial magnetic stimulation

Definition

Transcranial magnetic stimulation (TMS) is a noninvasive experimental procedure that gently stimulates the **brain** using short bursts of electromagnetic energy.

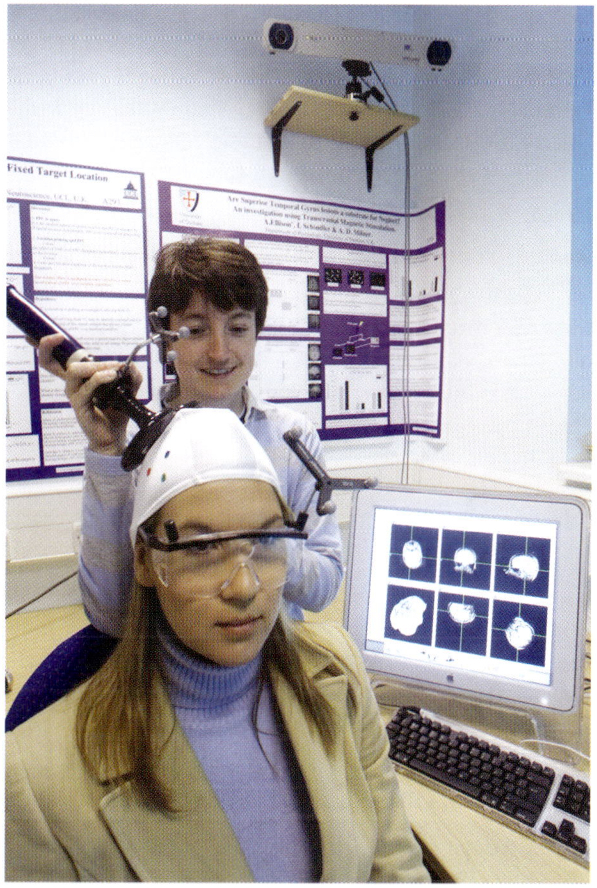

A woman undergoes transcranial magnetic stimulation (TMS). *(© Simon Fraser/University of Durham/Photo Researchers, Inc.)*

Purpose

Originally, TMS was a research tool used to map the brain and to study the differences between a normal brain and a brain with pathology. TMS has been used to study how various functions, such as perception, memory, or attention, are organized in the brain.

More recently, TMS research has also begun to focus on practical applications for the technology in the treatment of various disorders. In October 2008, the Food and Drug Administration (FDA) cleared the first transcranial magnetic stimulation device for treating **depression** in adults who failed to respond favorably to **antidepressants**. Called the NeuroStar device (from a company called Neuronetics), patients receiving TMS would not require sedation (the method is noninvasive) and would have treatment administered on an outpatient basis.

Description

TMS uses specialized electromagnets that are placed on the patient's scalp. The magnets generate short bursts of magnetic energy of approximately the same strength as a **magnetic resonance imaging** (MRI) scanner, but over a more focused area. These pulses produce electrical currents in the brain that change the brain's activity in the area of focus. Repetitive transcranial magnetic stimulation (rTMS) is treatment using a series of TMS pulses.

Use of TMS in the treatment of depression

Much of the application research in TMS has focused on its effectiveness in the treatment of severe and treatment-resistant depression. Although antidepressants, **psychotherapy**, and **electroconvulsive therapy** (ECT) are usually effective in the treatment of depression, not all cases can be successfully treated using these methods. In **clinical trials**, TMS has been found to be effective in many, but not all, of the more difficult cases.

Since the use of antidepressants in children and adolescents is not recommended due to safety issues, TMS offers a promising alternative treatment. However, most research studies to date have focused only on depression in adults. The effectiveness of TMS for children and adolescents cannot be assumed to be the same.

Use of TMS in the treatment of other illnesses

Although most research in the clinical application of TMS and rTMS is focused on the treatment of depression, experimental research and clinical case studies also point to the possibility of TMS being an effective treatment in a number of other disorders. Among these are:

- chronic pain
- epilepsy
- migraine
- obsessive-compulsive disorder
- panic disorder
- Parkinson's disease
- post-traumatic stress disorder
- rehabilitation following a stroke
- tinnitus
- Tourette syndrome
- various psychiatric symptoms, particularly auditory hallucinations associated with schizophrenia

Further research is needed in neuroimaging technology, as well as advances in our understanding of neurocircuitry in mental disorders and how TMS shifts or alters circuitry in the brain.

KEY TERMS

Depression—A mental state characterized by feelings of sadness, despair, and discouragement.

Electroconvulsive therapy (ECT)—Therapy for mood disorders that involves passing electrical current through the brain in order to create a brief convulsion.

Hallucination—To hear, see, or otherwise sense things that are not real. Hallucinations can result from nervous system abnormalities, mental disorders, or the use of certain drugs.

Magnetic resonance imaging (MRI)—An imaging technique that uses a large circular magnet and radio waves to generate signals from atoms in the body. These signals are used to construct images of internal structures.

Psychotherapy—The treatment of mental and behavioral disorders by support and insight to encourage healthy behavior patterns and personality growth.

Seizure—A convulsion, or uncontrolled discharge of nerve cells that may spread to other cells throughout the brain.

Tinnitus—Perceived ringing, buzzing, whistling, or other noise heard in one or both ears that has no external source. A number of conditions may cause this.

Tourette syndrome—An abnormal condition that causes uncontrollable facial grimaces and tics and arm and shoulder movements. Tourette syndrome is perhaps best known for uncontrollable vocal tics that include grunts, shouts, and use of obscene language (coprolalia).

Risks

At this time, it is generally thought that there are no harmful side effects to TMS or rTMS. The main risk of treatment with TMS is of inducing a seizure. Even in cases where **seizures** resulted from TMS, the seizures occurred either during the treatment or immediately thereafter and did not lead to the development of epilepsy. In general, the research shows this risk to be low, and safety guidelines have been put in place to minimize seizure risk.

Although there is the potential risk of TMS to affect the normal functioning of the brain, the literature to date reports few side effects. Unlike the potential memory loss, inability to concentrate, and similar side effects

QUESTIONS TO ASK YOUR DOCTOR

- What are the indications that I should have transcranial magnetic stimulation performed?
- What kind of results can occur with the use of transcranial magnetic stimulation?
- Should I have other procedures in addition to transcranial magnetic stimulation? If so, what other procedures should I have done?

often associated with ECT, the side effects of TMS tend to be very rare, mild, and transient.

Potential side effects of TMS include neckaches or headaches. These tend to be mild reactions that respond well to common over-the-counter analgesics. rTMS has been shown to cause tinnitus or temporary hearing loss. However, the use of earplugs during the treatment prevents this risk. The long-term risks of rTMS treatment are unknown.

Precautions

Individuals with increased risk of seizure—including those with epilepsy or a seizure disorder, a history of seizures, or a family history of epilepsy or a seizure disorder—should not receive TMS. Other people at increased risk for seizures, such as those with increased intracranial pressure due to **trauma** or other causes, those taking medications that increase the risk or seizures, or anyone with serious heart disease, should not receive TMS.

The magnetic force generated by TMS will attract metallic objects and repel magnetic objects. Therefore, individuals with intracranial metallic or magnetic objects such as shrapnel or plates, screws, or clips from surgical procedures should not receive TMS unless the effects of the magnetic force on the object are known. Similarly, individuals with cardiac pacemakers, electrodes inside the heart, or implanted medication pumps should not receive TMS. Pregnant women or those who might be pregnant should not receive TMS.

Resources

BOOKS

Albers, Lawrence J., MD, Rhoda K. Hahn, MD, and Christopher Reist, MD. *Handbook of Psychiatric Drugs.* Laguna Hills, CA: Current Clinical Strategies Publishing, 2010.

American Psychological Association. *Publication Manual of the American Psychological Association,* 6th ed. Washington, DC: American Psychological Association, 2009.

Eisenberg, Ronald, JD MD FACR., and Alexander Margulis, MD.*A Patient's Guide to Medical Imaging.* New York, NY: Oxford University Press, 2011.

Graham, George. *The Disordered Mind: An Introduction to Philosophy of Mind and Mental Illness.*New York, NY: Routledge, 2010.

Marcolin, M. A., and F. Padberg, eds. *Transcranial Brain Stimulation for Treatment of Psychiatric Disorders.* Basel, Switzerland: Karger Publishers, 2007.

Virani, Adil S., et al., eds. *Clinical Handbook of Psychotropic Drugs,* 19th ed. Cambridge, MA: Hogrefe Publishing, 2011.

PERIODICALS

Barrett, Anna M., Elizabeth E. Galletta, and Paul R. Rao. "Transcranial magnetic stimulation (TMS): potential progress for language improvement in aphasia." *Topics in Stroke Rehabilitation* 18, no. 2 (2011): 87.

Bishnoi, Ram, et al. "Utility of repetitive transcranial magnetic stimulation as an augmenting treatment method in treatment-resistant depression." *Indian Journal of Psychiatry* 53, no. 2 (2011): 145.

Dannon, Pinhas, et al. "Deep transcranial magnetic stimulation for the treatment of auditory hallucinations: a preliminary open-label study." *Annals of General Psychiatry* 10 (2011): 3.

ORGANIZATIONS

American College of Physicians, 190 N. Independence Mall West, Philadelphia, PA, 19106-1572, (215) 351-2600, (800) 523-1546, http://www.acponline.org.

American Medical Association, 515 N. State Street, Chicago, IL, 60610, (312) 464-5000, http://www.ama-assn.org.

American Psychiatric Association, 1000 Wilson Boulevard, Suite 1825, Arlington, VA, 22209, (703) 907-7300, apa@psych.org, http://www.psych.org.

Mental Health America (NMHA), 2000 N. Beauregard Street, 6th Floor, Alexandria, VA, 22311, (703) 684-7722, (800) 969-6642, Fax: (703) 684-5968, http://www1.nmha.org.

National Alliance on Mental Illness (NAMI), Colonial Place Three, 2107 Wilson Blvd., Suite 300, Arlington, VA, 22201, (703) 524-7600, (800) 950-NAMI (6264) Fax: (703) 524-9094, http://www.nami.org/Hometemplate.cfm.

National Institutes of Health (NIH), 9000 Rockville Pike, Bethesda, MD, 20892, (301) 496-4000, http://www.nih.gov/index.html.

National Institute of Mental Health (NIMH), 6001 Executive Boulevard, Room 8184, MSC 9663, Bethesda, MD, 20892, (301) 443-4513, (866) 615-6464, Fax: (301) 443-4279, nimhinfo@nih.gov, http://www.nimh.nih.gov/index.shtml.

U.S. Food and Drug Administration (FDA), 10903 New Hampshire Ave., Silver Spring, MD, 20993, (888) 463-6332, http://www.fda.gov.

U.S. National Library of Medicine, 8600 Rockville Pike, Bethesda, MD, 20894, http://www.nlm.nih.gov/medlineplus/medlineplus.html.

Ruth A. Wienclaw, PhD
Laura Jean Cataldo, RN, EdD

Transient tic disorder *see* **Tic disorders**
Transsexualism *see* **Gender identity disorder**

Transvestic fetishism

Definition

Transvestic **fetishism**, or transvestic disorder, is characterized by the desire to dress in clothing traditionally attributed to the opposite sex. It is classified by the mental health professional's handbook, the ***Diagnostic and Statistical Manual of Mental Disorders*** (*DSM*), as a paraphilia. The **paraphilias** are a group of mental disorders characterized by **obsession** with unusual sexual practices or with sexual activity involving nonconsenting or inappropriate partners (such as children or animals). Paraphilias are not inherently causes for psychiatric diagnoses, but when the paraphilia causes distress, harm, or otherwise impairs everyday functioning for the person or others, it is considered a disorder. The essential feature of transvestic fetishism is recurrent intense sexual urges and sexually arousing fantasies involving dressing in clothing associated with members of the opposite sex. A **diagnosis** of transvestic fetishism is made only if an individual has acted on these urges and is markedly distressed by them. In other systems of psychiatric classification, transvestic fetishism is considered a sexual deviation.

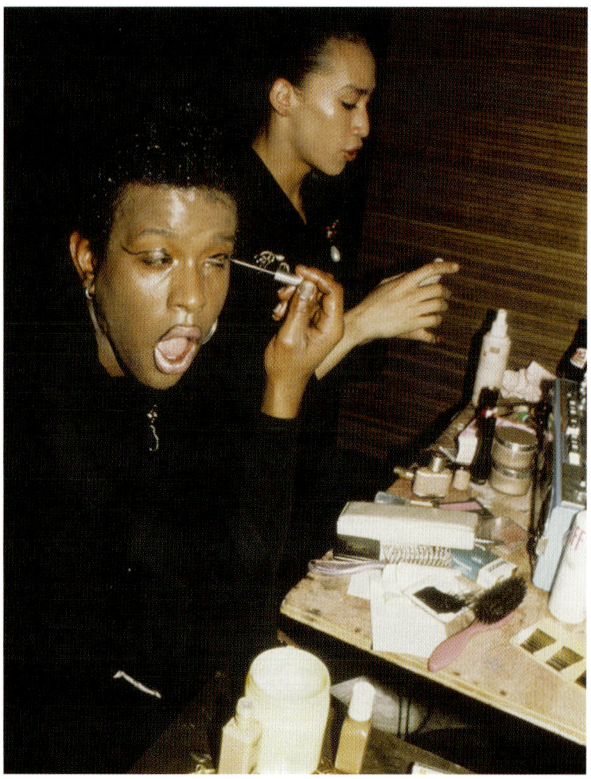

A transvestite male applies makeup. *(© Custom Medical Stock Photo, Inc. Reproduced by permission.)*

Demographics

Except for **sexual masochism**, in which the gender ratio is estimated to be 20 males for each female, paraphilias such as transvestic fetishism are practically never diagnosed in females, although a few cases have been reported. This lopsided gender ratio may be partly due to the fact that contemporary Western societies allow women to dress in a wide range of clothing styles influenced by menswear, whereas the reverse is not the case. While it is not at all unusual to see women wearing jeans, tailored trousers, Western-style boots, or even tuxedos in some circumstances, men wearing dresses or high-heeled shoes look distinctly out of place. Virtually no information is available on family patterns of the disorder.

Description

A person with a transvestic fetish derives sexual gratification from dressing in clothing appropriate for a member of the opposite sex. The participation in transvestism usually is gradual. Over time, a person with a transvestic fetish assumes the role and appearance of a member of the opposite gender and may be difficult to distinguish from members of the opposite sex. A so-called mature transvestic fetish involves adopting all of the mannerisms, clothing, materials and other items associated with persons of the opposite sex. It is important to note that this activity is closely associated with achieving sexual gratification rather than a desire to actually be of the opposite gender (gender dysphoria).

Though transvestic fetishism primarily occurs in males, proposed changes for the fifth edition of the *DSM* (*DSM-5*) account for different types of transvestic disorder, including if the person is sexually aroused only by the clothing (fetishism), by the thought of being a female if a male (autogynephilia), or by the thought of being a male if a female (autoandrophilia).

Causes and symptoms

Causes

The basis for a transvestic fetish is obtaining sexual gratification by dressing in clothing appropriate for the opposite sex. The cause may begin as adolescent curiosity. A person with a transvestic fetish may not be aware of its roots. Transvestic fetishism sometimes begins when a young boy dresses up in the clothes of an older sister or his

KEY TERMS

Cognitive-behavioral therapy—A type of psychotherapy in which people learn to recognize and change negative and self-defeating patterns of thinking and behavior.

Gender dysphoria—A disorder in which an individual experiences prolonged, significant distress or dissatisfaction with his or her biologic gender.

Orgasmic reorientation—A form of behavioral therapy that attempts to help people learn to respond sexually to culturally appropriate stimuli.

Paraphilias—A group of mental disorders characterized by obsession with unusual sexual practices or with sexual activity involving nonconsenting or inappropriate partners.

mother. The activity is continued because it is enjoyable, but the reasons for the enjoyment remain unconscious. In some cases, a boy's mother may initiate the cross-dressing by dressing him as if he were a girl.

A transvestic fetish is not an indication of a person's sexual orientation. According to the revised fourth edition of the *DSM* (*DSM-IV-TR*), most men who practice cross-dressing are basically heterosexual in their orientation, though some do have occasional sexual encounters with other men.

Symptoms

Early symptoms of transvestic fetishism involve touching or wearing items of clothing that are considered typically feminine. This initial interest may progress to wearing undergarments or other items that can be hidden from the view of others while providing arousal to the wearer. Over time, the extent of dressing in women's clothing expands, sometimes to the point of dressing as a woman on a regular basis. A developed transvestic fetish often involves feminine hair styling and the use of women's cosmetics and accessories.

In some individuals diagnosed with transvestic fetishism, the motivation for cross-dressing may change over time from a search for sexual excitement to simple relief from **stress**, **depression**, or anxiety.

In some cases, individuals with a transvestic fetish discover that they are unhappy with their biological sex, a condition known as gender dysphoria. They may elect to have hormonal and surgical procedures to change their bodies. Some may choose to have gender reassignment surgery. The incidence of gender dysphoria and subsequent gender reassignment among persons diagnosed with transvestic fetishism is not known.

Diagnosis

Individuals with transvestic fetishism may or may not seek **psychotherapy** on their own account. In some instances, the person has agreed to consult a **psychiatrist** because his wife or girlfriend is distressed by the cross-dressing. The actual diagnosis of transvestic fetishism is most commonly made by taking a history or by direct observation. The diagnosis is made only if the individual has been markedly distressed by an inability to dress in such a manner or if the disorder is interfering with his education, occupation, or social life. The DSM diagnostic criteria also requires the behavior to occur for at least six months; dressing in women's clothing for such occasions as Halloween or a costume party is not sufficient for a diagnosis of transvestic fetishism.

Treatment

In the earliest period of behavior therapy, transvestic fetishes were narrowly viewed as inappropriate behavior that was confined to a limited range of situations. Sometimes they were treated with **aversion therapy**, usually with electric shocks. This approach was largely unsuccessful. Individuals with fetishes also have been treated by using a form of behavioral therapy known as orgasmic reorientation, which attempts to help people learn to respond sexually to culturally appropriate stimuli. This treatment also has had limited success.

Most people who have a transvestic fetish never seek treatment from professionals. Most are capable of achieving sexual gratification in culturally appropriate situations. Their preoccupation with cross-dressing is viewed as essentially harmless to others, since transvestism is not associated with criminal activities. American society has developed more tolerance for persons with a transvestic fetish, thus further reducing the demand for professional treatment.

Prognosis

The prognosis for treatment of transvestic fetishism is poor, as most persons with this disorder do not desire to change. Most cases in which treatment was demanded by a spouse as a condition of continuing in a marriage have not been successful. The prognosis for personal adjustment is good, however, as a person with a transvestic fetish and his related activities do not usually disturb others.

Prevention

The classification of transvestic fetishism as a mental disorder is highly controversial, as is the need for treatment and prevention. To address these concerns, revisions for the *DSM-5* acknowledge that transvestic behavior should only be considered a disorder if it causes a person significant distress; the behavior in itself is not considered a disorder.

In cases where transvestic fetishism may arise out of parental pressures, such as may be the case when parents wish they had a child of the opposite gender and treat their child as such, experts agree that providing gender-appropriate guidance in culturally appropriate situations will prevent the formation of a transvestic fetish. The origin of some cases of transvestism may be a random association between clothing inappropriate for a person's gender and sexual gratification. There is no reliable way to predict the formation of such associations. Supervision during childhood and adolescence, combined with acceptance of a child's biological sex, may be the best deterrent that parents can provide.

Resources

BOOKS

Clinton, Tim, and Laaser, Mark. *The Quick-Reference Guide to Sexuality and Relationship Counseling*. Grand Rapids, MI: Baker Books, 2010.

Laws, D. Richard, and O'Donohue, William T., eds. *Sexual Deviance: Theory, Assessment, and Treatment*. 2nd ed. New York, Guilford Press, 2008.

Rowland, David, and Luca Incrocci. *Handbook of Sexual and Gender Identity Disorders*. Hoboken, NJ: John Wiley & Sons, 2008.

PERIODICALS

Blanchard, Ray. "The DSM Diagnostic Criteria for Transvestic Fetishism." *Archives of Sexual Behavior,* 39, no. 2 (April 2010): 363–372.

Wright, Susan. "Depathologizing Consensual Sexual Sadism, Sexual Masochism, Transvestic Fetishism, and Fetishism." *Archives of Sexual Behavior,* 36, no. 6 (December 2010): 1229–1230.

ORGANIZATIONS

American Psychiatric Association, 1000 Wilson Blvd., Suite 1825, Arlington, VA, 22209-3901, (703) 907-7300, apa@psych.org, http://www.psych.org.

American Psychological Association, 750 1st Street NE, Washington, DC, 20002-4242, (202) 336-5500; TDD/TTY: (202) 336-6123, (800) 374-2721, http://www.apa.org.

Gay, Lesbian, Bisexual, and Transgender National Help Center, 2261 Market Street, PMB #296, San Francisco, CA, 94114, (415) 355-0003, Fax: (415) 552-5498, info@GLBTNationalHelpCenter.org, http://www.glbtnationalhelpcenter.org.

L. Fleming Fallon, Jr., MD
Tish Davidson, AM

Tranxene *see* **Clorazepate**

Tranylcypromine

Definition

Tranylcypromine is classified as a monoamine oxidase inhibitor (MAOI). It is used to treat serious **depression**. In the United States, tranylcypromine is sold under the brand name Parnate and under its generic name.

Purpose

Tranylcypromine is used primarily to treat depression that does not respond to other types of drug therapy. It is also used occasionally to treat **panic disorder**, **agoraphobia**, and **bulimia nervosa**, though these uses are not approved by the U.S. Food and Drug Administration (FDA).

Description

Tranylcypromine is a member of a class of drugs called **monoamine oxidase inhibitors**. Monoamine oxidase, or MAO, is an enzyme found throughout the body. In the **brain**, MAO breaks down norepinephrine and **serotonin**, two naturally occurring chemicals that are important for maintaining mental well-being and preventing depression. Monoamine oxidase inhibitors such as tranylcypromine reduce the activity of MAO, resulting in more norepinephrine and serotonin left in the brain, which helps alleviate depression.

Tranylcypromine is especially effective for treating complicated types of depression that have not responded to more traditional **antidepressants**. However, tranylcypromine affects the MAO enzyme in many other areas of the body, not just the brain, which results in a large number of serious side effects and drug interactions.

Recommended dosage

The typical starting dosage of tranylcypromine in adults is 10 mg taken twice per day. This dosage is sometimes increased to 30 mg per day after a two-week period. The maximum recommended amount is 60 mg per day. Those over age 60 are usually started on a dose of 2.5 mg per day. After this, their doctors will make an individualized decision about increasing the dosage. Older adults typically take smaller doses and do not take more than 45 mg per day. A doctor must make an individual determination of whether to give tranylcypromine to youths under the age of 18 years, because guidelines for this age group have not been developed.

The benefits of this drug may not become apparent for several weeks. Patients should be aware of this and

KEY TERMS

Depression—A mental state characterized by feelings of sadness, despair, and discouragement.

Norepinephrine—A chemical messenger in the brain thought to play a role in mood regulation.

Schizophrenia—A major mental illness marked by psychotic symptoms, including hallucinations, delusions, and severe disruptions in thinking.

Seizure—A convulsion, or uncontrolled discharge of nerve cells that may spread to other cells throughout the brain.

Serotonin—A chemical messenger in the brain thought to play a role in mood regulation.

continue taking the drug as directed, even if they do not see an immediate improvement.

Precautions

People taking tranylcypromine should not eat foods rich in tyramine. These foods include yeast or meat extracts, fermented sausage, overripe fruit, sauerkraut, cheese, and fava beans. Alcohol should not be consumed, and the same holds true for alcohol-free beer and wine. Large amounts of caffeine-containing food and beverages, such as chocolate, tea, coffee, and cola should be avoided. The treating doctor needs to approve the use of any drug, including prescription, over-the-counter drugs, and herbal treatments, that patients take while taking tranylcypromine.

Tranylcypromine should be used with great caution in pregnant and nursing women only after the risks and benefits of treatment have been assessed. The drug may not be appropriate for people with a history of **seizures**, children under age 18 years, people at risk for **suicide**, those with severe depression, or persons with a history of **schizophrenia**. The drug should also be used with caution in patients with glaucoma or diabetes mellitus. People with these conditions should discuss the risks and benefits of this drug with their physicians, and a decision to treat should be made on an individual basis. People with a history of high blood pressure, congestive heart failure, severe liver disease, severe kidney disease, severe heart disease, and blood vessel problems in the brain should not take tranylcypromine.

Children and adults up to age 24 are at an increased risk for developing suicidal thoughts and actions when taking antidepressant drugs, including tranylcypromine. Patients of any age taking an antidepressant medication should be monitored for signs of worsening depression or changes in behavior.

Tranylcypromine should not be stopped suddenly. Instead, the dose should be gradually reduced, then discontinued.

Side effects

Tranylcypromine should be stopped if symptoms of unusually high blood pressure develop. These symptoms include severe chest pain, severe headache, nausea, vomiting, stiff or sore neck, enlarged pupils, and significant changes in heart rate. If these symptoms develop, it should be considered an emergency. Patients should get medical help immediately. Generally, these serious side effects are rare.

More common but less serious side effects include light-headedness or dizziness when arising from a sitting position. These symptoms need to be reported to a doctor but are not considered an emergency. Less common symptoms that should be reported include pounding heartbeat, swelling of the lower extremities, nervousness, and diarrhea. Rare but reportable symptoms include fever, skin rash, dark urine, slurred speech, yellowing of the eyes or skin, and staggering when walking. Common but not serious side effects include decreased sexual performance, increased appetite, muscle twitching, trembling, blurred vision, and reduced urine output.

Overdose symptoms include confusion, seizures, severe dizziness, hallucinations, severe headache, severe drowsiness, significant changes in blood pressure, difficulty in sleeping, breathing difficulties, and increased irritability.

Interactions

Tranylcypromine interacts with a long list of drugs. Some of these interactions can cause death. Patients must make sure every healthcare professional who takes care of them (for example, doctors, dentists, podiatrists, optometrists, pharmacists, nurses) knows that they take tranylcypromine, as well as all of the other prescription or nonprescription drugs and herbal remedies that they take.

The combination of tranylcypromine with any type of stimulant can increase the risk of developing serious increases in blood pressure. Tranylcypromine when taken with antidiabetic drugs can reduce blood sugar levels to far below normal. The combination of tranylcypromine with **barbiturates** can prolong the effects of the barbiturate drug.

Tranylcypromine should never be combined with other antidepressant drugs, especially the **selective serotonin reuptake inhibitors (SSRIs)**, because of potentially severe or fatal reactions, including increased risk of dangerously high blood pressure. Patients taking tranylcypromine should stop the drug, then wait at least 14 days before starting any other antidepressant. The

QUESTIONS TO ASK YOUR DOCTOR

- What kind of changes can I expect to see or feel with this medication?
- Does it matter what time of day I take this medication?
- Should I take this medication with or without food?
- What are the side effects associated with this medication?
- Will this medication interact or interfere with other medications I am currently taking?
- What symptoms or adverse effects are important enough that I should seek immediate treatment?

same holds true when discontinuing another antidepressant and starting tranylcypromine.

Dangerously high blood pressure has resulted from the combination of **MAOIs** and antianxiety (anxiolytic) drugs such as **buspirone** (BuSpar). Patients taking tranylcypromine should stop the medication and wait at least ten days before starting buspirone.

Alcohol combined with tranylcypromine can lead to significantly increased blood pressure. Tranylcypromine combined with the blood pressure drug guanethidine (Ismelin) can reduce the beneficial effects of the guanethidine. When tranylcypromine is combined with levodopa (Dopar, Larodopa), a drug used to treat Parkinson's disease, severely increased blood pressure can develop. Tranylcypromine combined with lithium can cause fever. Meperidine (Demerol), when combined with tranylcypromine, can cause fever, seizures, increased blood pressure, and agitation. Tranylcypromine combined with norepinephrine can cause increased response to norepinephrine. Tranylcypromine combined with reserpine (Serpalan, Serpasil) can produce greatly increased blood pressure. When tranylcypromine is combined with the migraine drug sumatriptan (Imitrex), significantly increased concentrations of the latter drug develop that can produce potentially toxic effects.

Resources

BOOKS

Albers, Lawrence J., Rhoda K. Hahn, and Christopher Reist. *Handbook of Psychiatric Drugs*. Laguna Hills, CA: Current Clinical Strategies Publishing, 2010.

American Society of Health-System Pharmacists. *AHFS Drug Information 2011*. Bethesda, MD: American Society of Health-System Pharmacists, 2011.

Graham, George. *The Disordered Mind: An Introduction to Philosophy of Mind and Mental Illness*. New York: Routledge, 2010.

Holland, Leland Norman, and Michael Patrick Adams. *Core Concepts in Pharmacology*. 3rd ed. New York: Prentice Hall, 2011.

North, Carol, and Sean Yutzy. *Goodwin and Guze's Psychiatric Diagnosis*. New York: Oxford University Press, 2010.

Preston, John D., John H. O'Neal, and Mary C. Talaga. *Handbook of Clinical Psychopharmacology for Therapists*. 6th ed. Oakland, CA: New Harbinger Publications, 2011.

PERIODICALS

Frieling, Helge, and Stefan Bleich. "Tranylcypromine: New Perspectives on an 'Old' Drug." *European Archives of Psychiatry and Clinical Neuroscience* 256, no. 5 (Aug. 2006): 268–73.

McGrath, Patrick J., et al. "Tranylcypromine Versus Venlafaxine Plus Mirtazapine Following Three Failed Antidepressant Medication Trials for Depression: A STAR*D Report." *American Journal of Psychiatry* 163, no. 9 (Sept. 2006): 1531–41.

Thase, Michael E. "Bipolar Depression: Issues in Diagnosis and Treatment." *Harvard Review of Psychiatry* 13, no. 5 (Sept.–Oct. 2005): 257–71.

Tulen, Joke H. M., et al. "Sustained Effects of Phenelzine and Tranylcypromine on Orthostatic Challenge in Antidepressant-Refractory Depression." *Journal of Clinical Psychopharmacology* 26, no. 5 (Oct. 2006): 542–44.

Valenstein, Marcia. "Keeping Our Eyes on STAR*D." *American Journal of Psychiatry* 163, no. 9 (Sept. 2006): 1484–86.

ORGANIZATIONS

American Psychiatric Association, 1000 Wilson Boulevard, Suite 1825, Arlington, VA, 22209, (703) 907-7300, apa@psych.org, http://www.psych.org.

Mental Health America, 2000 N. Beauregard Street, 6th Floor, Alexandria, VA, 22311, (703) 684-7722, (800) 969-6642, Fax: (703) 684-5968, http://www1.nmha.org.

National Alliance on Mental Illness (NAMI), Colonial Place Three, 2107 Wilson Blvd., Suite 300, Arlington, VA, 22201, (703) 524-7600, (800) 950-NAMI (6264), Fax: (703) 524-9094, http://www.nami.org/Hometemplate.cfm.

National Institute of Mental Health (NIMH), 6001 Executive Boulevard, Room 8184, MSC 9663, Bethesda, MD, 20892, (301) 443-4513, (866) 615-6464, Fax: (301) 443-4279, nimhinfo@nih.gov, http://www.nimh.nih.gov/index.shtml.

U.S. Food and Drug Administration, 10903 New Hampshire Ave., Silver Spring, MD, 20993-0002, (888) INFO-FDA (463-6332), http://www.fda.gov.

Mark Mitchell, MD
Ruth A. Wienclaw, Ph.D.
Laura Jean Cataldo, RN, Ed.D.

Trauma

Definition

The English word *trauma* (plural, traumata) is simply the Greek word for "wound" written in the letters of the Roman rather than the Greek alphabet. It is used to refer to both physical and psychological injuries. In medicine, trauma is a physical wound or injury, often sudden, resulting from a violent blow or accident. In psychiatry, the term refers to damage to the mind and emotions resulting from a single event or series of experiences that overwhelm a person's ability to cope or to integrate the memories and feelings associated with the traumatic event(s).

Demographics

Physical trauma is the sixth-leading cause of death worldwide and accounts for 10% of all human deaths. In the United States, traumatic injury is the leading cause of death for persons between the ages of 1 and 44, with about 180,000 trauma deaths each year. About two-thirds of these deaths are accidental.

Psychological traumata vary widely in frequency and severity in the general population. It is estimated that between 50% and 90% of people in North America will undergo a traumatic experience at some point in life, but only 7%–8% will develop **post-traumatic stress disorder** (PTSD) or a complex post-traumatic syndrome. The lifetime prevalence of rape and sexual assault is estimated at 15%–20% for women and 3%–5% for men, although many researchers maintain that rapes for both sexes are under-reported. With regard to child **sexual abuse**, between 15% and 25% of women in North America and 5% to 15% of men report being sexually abused in childhood. In terms of combat-related trauma, about a quarter of the men and women deployed to Iraq and Afghanistan and during the Gulf War met or still meet the criteria for **acute stress disorder** (ASD) or PTSD.

Mass traumata, such as major industrial explosions, severe natural disasters, the loss of a large airplane or ship, or large-scale terrorist attacks, are rare but may have a disproportionate impact on survivors and first responders. Mass traumata are also more likely to lead to survivor guilt, a condition in which a person feels that they did something wrong or should feel guilty about surviving a disaster when others did not.

Description

Psychological or psychiatric trauma has two dimensions, objective and subjective. It may or may not be associated with physical trauma; in general, physical traumata that cause permanent damage to the senses or other body functions, or that result in disfigurement (particularly to the face), are more likely to have psychological sequelae than those that heal completely. The objective aspect of psychological trauma is its external description or definition, such as "rape," "airplane crash," or "earthquake." The subjective

Common symptoms following exposure to trauma

Behavioral	Cognitive/mental	Emotional	Physical
Antisocial acts	Change in alertness	Agitation	Chills
Change in activity	Confusion	Anxiety	Difficulty breathing
Change in appetite	Hypervigilance	Apprehension	Dizziness
Change in communication	Increased or decreased awareness of surroundings	Denial	Elevated blood pressure
Change in sexual functioning	Intrusive images	Depression	Fainting
Change in speech pattern	Memory problems	Emotional shock	Fatigue
Emotional outbursts	Nightmares	Fear	Grinding teeth
Inability to rest	Placing blame on others	Feeling overwhelmed	Headaches
Increased alcohol consumption	Poor abstract thinking	Grief	Muscle tremors
Intensified startle reflex	Poor attention	Guilt	Nausea
Pacing	Poor concentration	Inappropriate emotional response	Pain
Suspiciousness	Poor decision making	Irritability	Profuse sweating
Social withdrawal	Poor problem solving	Loss of emotional control	Rapid heart rate
			Twitches
			Weakness

SOURCE: Department of Veterans Affairs and Department of Defense, Management of Post-Traumatic Stress Working Group, *VA/DoD Clinical Practice Guideline for Management of Post-Traumatic Stress*, 2010.

Guidelines provided by the Department of Veterans Affairs and available online at http://www.healthquality.va.gov/PTSD-FULL-2010c.pdf. *(Table by PreMediaGlobal. © 2012 Cengage Learning.)*

dimension is the survivor's experience of being overwhelmed and rendered helpless by the event or incident. It is the individual's subjective experience that defines the event as traumatic for that person.

Causes and symptoms

Different people tend to respond differently to the same traumatic event; for example, some survivors may develop PTSD, some may have a time-limited **stress** reaction, and others may appear to be unaffected. The type of traumatic event or incident, however, may have some effect on the victims' response:

- Intentional human-caused traumata (e.g., war, criminal assault, rape, or torture) can be more distressing than technological accidents (e.g., transportation disasters, oil spills, plant explosions) or natural disasters (e.g., floods, hurricanes, tornadoes, blizzards, earthquakes, or volcanic eruptions).
- Repeated stressors, such as physical or sexual abuse, domestic violence, and military combat, are more likely to lead to PTSD than single episodes of trauma, as are stressors of long duration (e.g., kidnapping, some natural disasters, or warfare). The National Cancer Institute (NCI) maintains that the duration of the illness and its treatment helps to explain the emergence of PTSD in cancer patients.
- Multifaceted traumata may be a greater risk factor for experiencing a trauma-related disorder than simple traumata. For example, a person caught in a tornado may witness the death of, or injury to, loved ones in addition to suffering the loss of their home and personal possessions, and possibly their job, as well as physical injury to their own body.
- Traumata experienced in childhood are more likely to have long-term effects than those experienced in adult life.
- Unpredictable traumata (e.g., most industrial accidents, airplane and railroad crashes, or terrorist attacks) are more shocking than those that could be at least partly predicted or foreseen (e.g., hurricanes, tornadoes, or some epidemics) and thus may produce a more severe traumatic response.
- Traumata inflicted by a parent, caregiver, or other trusted adult may have a more serious effect on the victim than would similar actions inflicted by a stranger.

Post-traumatic stress disorder and acute stress disorder

PTSD and ASD are two of the more common disorders associated with trauma. Although the conditions are distinct, they do share some similar symptoms, including:

- flashbacks or recurring nightmares of the traumatic event
- avoidance of persons, places, or things that might spark a memory of the event
- a constant state of hyperarousal, a condition characterized by irritability, anxiety, insomnia, lack of concentration, and extreme startle response
- detachment from people or surroundings

Complex trauma

Complex trauma is a term with two different meanings, depending on whether it is applied to children or adults. According to the National Child Traumatic Stress Network, the term refers to a child's "exposure to multiple or prolonged traumatic events and the impact of this exposure on their development." Complex trauma in children may be either sequential or simultaneous and may include psychological maltreatment, **neglect**, physical and sexual abuse, and domestic violence. This type of trauma is chronic, begins in early childhood, and occurs within the primary caregiving system. It is estimated that about 30% of children nationwide in North America are exposed to complex trauma, and as many as 50% of children in some distressed communities; however, only about 12% of these children receive treatment. Rates of **self-mutilation** and nonsuicidal self-injury are as high as 62% among these children. Developmental trauma disorder (DTD) appears to be increasingly used as a synonym for complex trauma in children.

Complex trauma is also sometimes used to describe a condition in adults more accurately referred to as complex PTSD or C-PTSD. C-PTSD is a concept that Judith Herman developed in the 1997 edition of her book *Trauma and Recovery*. Herman maintained that the *DSM-IV* criteria for PTSD did not adequately account for the symptoms of survivors of chronic repetitive trauma, such as domestic violence, hostage situations, other forms of captivity, torture, or other abusive situations from which escape is difficult. Herman identified psychological fragmentation; the loss of a sense of safety, trust, and self-worth; a tendency to be revictimized; and insecure or disorganized forms of attachment to others as the symptoms that most clearly differentiate C-PTSD from PTSD. She also described three phases in the recovery of adults with C-PTSD: re-establishing a sense of safety, remembering and mourning what was lost in the traumatic experience, and reconnecting with the survivor's community and the larger society. Although some medical journals have published papers on C-PTSD, the disorder was not recognized by *DSM-IV*, although it is possible that *DSM-5* could include it under the category of "Other specified trauma- or stressor-related disorder."

Rape trauma syndrome

Rape trauma syndrome (RTS) is a term first coined by Ann Burgess and Lynda Holmstrom in 1974 to describe a complex form of psychological trauma to a rape victim (male or female) reflected in disruptions of the survivor's emotional, cognitive, physical, and interpersonal behaviors. RTS is a syndrome with two phases, an acute phase that lasts from several days to several weeks after the assault, and a longer "reorganization phase." Survivors react in different ways during the acute phase. Some survivors are expressive, meaning that they show their emotions by crying, yelling, or being openly angry. Others are controlled; they may be completely silent about the rape and go about their daily routines as if nothing has happened. Neither type of response is considered superior to the other.

The second phase of RTS is the reorganization phase, in which the survivor tries to recover the sense of safety and ability to trust others that he or she had before the rape. The survivor must cope with intense feelings of guilt and shame as well as fear and anxiety. In some cases, the survivor may feel disconnected or dissociated from her or his body. Male survivors are more likely than females to have questions about their sexual identity and orientation; they are also more likely to postpone or avoid treatment. One study of 100 male rape survivors found that the average time interval between the assault and seeking therapy was 16 years.

In addition to the emotional symptoms of RTS, many survivors also experience a variety of physical symptoms ranging from tension headaches and generalized muscle pain to specific symptoms in the parts of the body that were penetrated during the assault. Survivors of oral rape may have a variety of mouth and throat complaints, nausea and vomiting, and bulimia or anorexia, while survivors of vaginal or anal rape may suffer from abdominal cramping, dysmenorrhea, constipation, or diarrhea.

Indirect trauma

Indirect trauma, also called vicarious trauma or empathic strain, is a condition that may develop in therapists and others who work with trauma survivors over long periods of time. The symptoms of indirect trauma are similar to those of survivors; the care provider may experience nightmares, intrusive thoughts, intense anxiety, avoidance behaviors, **sleep disorders**, difficulty regulating emotions, and disruptions in personal or professional relationships. Indirect trauma may also involve a form of survivor guilt, such as when first responders feel that they are to blame for not having rescued everyone from a disaster, or when a therapist feels guilty about not being able to relieve a patient's suffering quickly.

Diagnosis

The subjective aspect of psychological trauma complicates assessment and evaluation of trauma survivors. A person who thinks that he or she may have PTSD or another trauma-related disorder should consult a **psychiatrist** or other health care provider with special training in the assessment of trauma survivors. In addition, the person should ask whether the doctor specializes in the type of trauma that the survivor underwent, and whether the doctor is also experienced in assessing members of the survivor's age group. There are different tests or question sets that can be used to evaluate adult and child survivors for symptoms of a disorder, and it requires specialized training to decide which test to administer in a given case and then interpret the results.

DSM-IV and DSM-5

The fourth edition of the ***Diagnostic and Statistical Manual of Mental Disorders***, first published in 1994 and revised in 2000, defined two trauma-related disorders—PTSD and ASD—under the larger category of anxiety disorders. A third disorder associated with trauma, adjustment disorder, was placed in a separate category of its own. The *DSM-5*, slated for publication in 2013, has revised this classification, introducing a new category, titled Trauma- and Stressor-Related Disorders, which includes the three trauma-related disorders defined by *DSM-IV* plus five new diagnostic categories, three of which are restricted to children.

The eight disorders listed under the proposed *DSM-5* category are as follows:

- Reactive attachment disorder of infancy or early childhood. This disorder was moved from the *DSM-IV* category of "Disorders Usually First Diagnosed in Infancy, Childhood, or Adolescence" to the new diagnostic category.
- Disinhibited social engagement disorder. Previously defined as a subtype of reactive attachment disorder in *DSM-IV*, the diagnosis describes children who lack the normal ability to select appropriate attachment figures

and demonstrate excessive familiarity with, or closeness to, relative strangers.

- Post-traumatic stress disorder in preschool children. This disorder is essentially a form of PTSD as found in children below the age of six years. Some of the criteria are similar to those for developmental trauma disorder, another proposed new diagnostic category.
- Acute stress disorder (ASD). The major revisions proposed for *DSM-5* are the division of symptoms into four categories (intrusive, dissociative, avoidance, and arousal); the addition of "learning that the [traumatic] event(s) occurred to a close relative or close friend" as well as witnessing or experiencing the event oneself; and the specifier that "[the criterion of exposure] does not apply to exposure through electronic media, television, movies or pictures, unless this exposure is work-related."
- Post-traumatic stress disorder (PTSD). As with ASD, proposed changes include the addition of "learning that the [traumatic] event(s) occurred to a close relative or close friend" as well as witnessing or experiencing the event oneself; and the specifier that "[the criterion of exposure] does not apply to exposure through electronic media, television, movies or pictures, unless this exposure is work-related."
- Adjustment disorders. The major difference between the *DSM-IV* definition of adjustment disorder and the proposed changes for *DSM-5* is the addition of a distinct subtype called *bereavement-related disorder*.
- Other specified trauma- or stressor-related disorder.
- Unspecified trauma- or stressor-related disorder.

Developmental trauma disorder

The *DSM-5* working group lists developmental trauma disorder (DTD) among the "Conditions Proposed by Outside Sources." The new diagnostic category has been discussed among experts in **child abuse** since the 1980s, on the grounds that the criteria for PTSD in adults fail to detect the symptoms of recurrent traumata in childhood, and that as a result, affected children do not receive proper treatment. Only 5%–10% of children exposed to interpersonal abuse, domestic violence, and other recurrent dangers meet criteria for PTSD; however, over 50% of such children have problems with affect regulation, attention and concentration, negative self-image, impulse control, aggression, and risk-taking. As a result, the children are usually diagnosed as having one or more of a set of unrelated conditions, including **bipolar disorder**, **attention deficit hyperactivity disorder (ADHD)**, **conduct disorder**, phobic anxiety, reactive attachment disorder, and separation anxiety, and they are usually treated with medications only, rather than **psychotherapy**. The diagnostic category of "developmental trauma disorder" would allow clinicians to effectively recognize and treat the core symptoms in these children—impaired capacity for emotional and behavioral regulation, and attachment-related difficulties.

A tentative set of criteria for the disorder was drawn up by Bessel van der Kolk in 2005 and revised by the National Child Traumatic Stress Network (NCTSN) in 2009. There are seven criteria in the present proposal:

- A. Exposure. The child or adolescent has experienced or witnessed multiple or prolonged adverse events over a period of at least one year beginning in childhood or early adolescence, including direct experience or witnessing of repeated and severe episodes of interpersonal violence and disruption of protective caregiving as the result of repeated changes in primary caregiver, repeated separation from the primary caregiver, or exposure to severe and persistent emotional abuse.
- B. Affective and emotional dysregulation. The child or adolescent exhibits at least two of the following: inability to recover from states of fear, shame, or anger, including prolonged tantrums or immobility; problems with such bodily functions as eating, sleeping, and elimination; diminished awareness of emotions, sensations, or bodily states; and inability to vocalize emotions or sensations.
- C. Attentional and behavioral dysregulation. The child experiences at least three of the following: inability to focus attention appropriately; preoccupation with threats or, conversely, a failure to perceive them; active thrill-seeking or risk-taking; lack of goal-directed behavior; and repeated or habitual acts of self-harm.
- D. Self- and relational dysregulation. The child demonstrates at least three of the following: impaired sense of identity; preoccupation with caregiver's safety; extreme distrust of, or aggressive action toward, others; inappropriate attempts to seek intimacy with adults or peers, including, but not limited to, sexual or physical contact; excessive reliance on others for safety or reassurance; inability to show empathy for others in pain or, conversely, showing excessive distress.
- E. Post-traumatic symptoms. The child shows at least one symptom in two of the three symptom clusters of adult PTSD (criteria B, C, and D).
- F. Duration. The symptoms in criteria B, C, D, and E must be present for at least six months.
- G. Functional impairment. The child suffers clinically significant distress or impaired function in at least two of six areas: academic, family, peer group, legal

system, physical health, and vocational preparation or planning.

Treatment

Treatment for trauma-related disorders usually involves a combination of approaches rather than a single form of treatment. In addition, a person in an ongoing traumatic situation, such as a violent family situation or abusive relationship, needs to be removed from the traumatic environment prior to therapy in order for treatment to be effective.

Traditional

There are several different forms of psychotherapy that are used in the treatment of trauma survivors. According to the **National Institute of Mental Health** (NIMH), psychotherapy for adults with PTSD and acute stress disorder usually lasts about 6–12 weeks but may take longer. Therapies include:

- Cognitive-behavioral therapy (CBT). CBT may include exposure therapy, in which the survivor is exposed in a safe place to situations or images that they are avoiding, as reminders of the trauma; cognitive restructuring (sometimes called "cognitive processing" therapy when used to treat survivors of PTSD), in which the survivor learns to reframe memories of the traumatic event, particularly those that lead to feelings of guilt or shame; and stress inoculation training, in which the survivor learns to identify the cues that trigger traumatic memories and to cope with them by using relaxation and deep-breathing techniques.
- Psychodynamic psychotherapy. This approach is helpful to survivors with unresolved issues from childhood or adolescence that resurfaced as a result of the traumatic experience. It may be combined with CBT.
- Group therapy and family therapy. These approaches are often recommended for survivors of specific traumata (e.g., rape, combat, workplace violence, or accidents) or mass disasters.
- Supportive therapy. *Supportive therapy* refers to any form of treatment intended to relieve the patient's symptoms rather than to bring about changes in the patient's behaviors or basic character structure.

There were 120 **clinical trials** underway as of mid-2011 for various medications and psychotherapy in the treatment of psychological trauma, and an additional eight studies of medications (topiramate and **risperidone**) or cognitive processing therapy for women with rape trauma syndrome.

Therapists and other healthcare providers affected by indirect trauma are advised to consult a supervising therapist or another specialist in trauma treatment if self-care—activities such as getting adequate rest; eating a healthful diet; balancing their trauma work with other work; getting support from friends, family, and colleagues; and acknowledging the difficulties of the work—do not help.

Drugs

Medications for trauma- and stressor-related disorders include the **selective serotonin reuptake inhibitors (SSRIs)**; mood stabilizers like valproate (Depakote), **carbamazepine** (Tegretol), and topiramate (Topamax) to treat flashbacks, nightmares, and other symptoms of hyperarousal; and benzodiazepine tranquilizers to treat sleep disorders. The only two **SSRIs** specifically approved by the U.S. Food and Drug Administration (FDA) for the treatment of PTSD are **sertraline** (Zoloft) and **paroxetine** (Paxil). Other SSRIs that may be prescribed include **fluoxetine** (Prozac) and **citalopram** (Celexa). However, it is important for trauma survivors with a coexisting **substance abuse** disorder to be treated for that before being given any psychoactive drugs.

Alternative

One form of complementary therapy that is often recommended to trauma survivors is relaxation training. Sometimes called "anxiety management training," relaxation training includes breathing exercises and similar techniques intended to help the patient prevent hyperventilation and relieve the muscle tension associated with the fight-or-flight reaction of anxiety. **Yoga**, aikido, tai chi, and other forms of movement therapy are also reported to help patients work with the physical as well as the emotional tensions that are associated with trauma-related anxiety.

Other complementary therapies that are reported to relieve the symptoms of PTSD and other trauma-related disorders include massage therapy, **art therapy**, journaling, and **music therapy**. However, there is little research support for these therapies.

Some trauma survivors benefit from spiritual or religious counseling. Because traumatic experiences often affect people's spiritual views and beliefs, counseling with a trusted religious or spiritual advisor may be part of a treatment plan. A growing number of pastoral counselors in the major Christian and Jewish bodies in North America have advanced credentials in trauma therapy. Native Americans are often helped to recover from PTSD by participating in traditional tribal rituals for

KEY TERMS

Affect—In psychology, an observed emotional expression or response.

Cognitive processing therapy—A term that is sometimes used for the cognitive restructuring aspect of cognitive-behavioral therapy as it is applied to treatment for PTSD.

Cue—In psychology, a sensory stimulus or signal that can be extracted or distinguished from surrounding stimuli by a perceiver.

Dissociation—Partial or complete disruption of a person's normal memory and psychological functioning. Dissociative symptoms are commonly experienced by persons with PTSD.

Exposure therapy—An approach to treating trauma survivors that helps them to cope with trauma-related thoughts, feelings, and situations by exposing them to these reminders of the trauma in a safe situation.

Indirect trauma—A term used to refer to symptoms of trauma in therapists, first responders, and others who treat trauma survivors. It is sometimes called *vicarious trauma.*

Polytrauma—The medical term for injury to more than one part of the body or more than one type of injury (such as burn injuries in addition to broken bones).

Post-traumatic stress disorder (PTSD)—A psychological reaction that continues long after a highly stressful event and is characterized by depression, anxiety, flashbacks, and nightmares.

Psychoactive—Referring to any substance that crosses the blood-brain barrier and acts primarily upon the central nervous system, leading to changes in mood, perception, thinking, feeling, or behavior.

Sequela (plural, sequelae)—In medicine, a pathological condition resulting from a disease, injury, or other trauma. For example, PTSD may be a sequela of rape or abuse.

Supportive therapy—An approach to psychotherapy that seeks to encourage the patient or offer emotional support to him or her rather than attempt behavioral changes.

Survivor guilt—A mental condition in which a person feels that he or she did something wrong by surviving a disaster in which others died. It can also affect therapists and first responders who feel that they did not do enough to rescue or help people caught in a disaster.

Syndrome—A group of signs or symptoms that occur together and characterize or define a particular disease or disorder.

cleansing memories of war and other traumatic events. These rituals may include sweat lodges, prayers and chants, or consultation with a shaman or tribal healer.

Treatment of mass trauma

Treatment of survivors of a mass accident or disaster is different from treating survivors of an individual or small-scale attack or event. While most people in mass critical events can be helped by getting to safety, obtaining food and water, getting medical help if injured, contacting loved ones, and getting accurate information about what is being done to help, some survivors do not get better on their own after a mass disaster and may even find their **depression** or PTSD becoming worse with time. One reason for this phenomenon is widespread destruction of the community's infrastructure (e.g., buildings, roads, bridges, railroads, water supply, or airports), often involving loss of jobs, schools, and basic housing as well as difficulty finding health care, purchasing food, or paying bills. In many cases, families may have to move to a different location hundreds of miles away. Hospitals and trauma centers in the affected area may be overwhelmed by the scale of the disaster, meaning that some survivors do not receive the psychological or physical care they need in a timely fashion, especially when doctors and other healthcare providers may be struggling with their own injuries, lack of supplies and transportation, and emotional reactions to the situation.

One approach to psychotherapy following mass trauma that is still considered experimental is the use of Internet- and phone-based therapy to treat survivors who could not be assessed immediately following the disaster.

Prognosis

There is considerable discussion among psychiatrists and other therapists regarding the classification of different types of psychological traumata, particularly in regard to complex forms of traumatization and the specification of the age group affected. There is a growing recognition that trauma affects the development

QUESTIONS TO ASK YOUR DOCTOR

- Will therapy help me cope with my experience?
- Can you recommend a support group for trauma survivors?
- Do you think that medication will help my symptoms?
- Are there any side effects to medications?
- Will I experience any long-term effects as a result of my trauma?
- How can I help my child cope with the aftereffects of trauma?
- How can I tell the difference between a healthy reaction to trauma and an abnormal reaction to trauma?

and maturation of children and adolescents in a variety of ways; that symptoms in children and adolescents differ from those in adults; and that proper **diagnosis** of young survivors is essential to effective treatment. At present, however, researchers have not reached agreement on the most appropriate names for trauma-related disorders, their diagnostic criteria, or their relationship to other mental disorders.

Resources

BOOKS

American Psychiatric Association. *Diagnostic and Statistical Manual of Mental Disorders*. 4th ed., text rev. Washington, DC: American Psychiatric Association, 2000.

Arnold, Cheryl, and Ralph Fisch. *The Impact of Complex Trauma on Development*. Lanham, MD: Jason Aronson, 2011.

Courtois, Christine A., and Julian D. Ford, eds. *Treating Complex Traumatic Stress Disorders: An Evidence-Based Guide*. New York: Guilford Press, 2009.

Ledray, Linda, Ann Wolbert Burgess, and Angelo P. Giardino, eds. *Medical Response to Adult Sexual Assault: A Resource for Clinicians and Related Professionals*. St. Louis, MO: STM Learning, 2011.

Mendelsohn, Michaela, et al. *The Trauma Recovery Group: A Guide for Practitioners*. New York: Guilford Press, 2011.

PERIODICALS

Argentero, P., and I. Setti. "Engagement and Vicarious Traumatization in Rescue Workers." *International Archives of Occupational and Environmental Health* 84 (January 2011): 67–75.

Beaudoin, C.E. "Hurricane Katrina: Addictive Behavior Trends and Predictors." *Public Health Reports* 126 (May-June 2011): 400–409.

Beck, C.T. "Secondary Traumatic Stress in Nurses: A Systematic Review." *Archives of Psychiatric Nursing* 25 (February 2011): 1–10.

Carlson, E.B., et al. "Development and Validation of a Brief Self-Report Measure of Trauma Exposure: the Trauma History Screen." *Psychological Assessment* 23 (June 2011): 463–77.

Chard, K.M., et al. "A Comparison of OEF and OIF Veterans and Vietnam Veterans Receiving Cognitive Processing Therapy." *Journal of Traumatic Stress* 23 (February 2010): 25–32.

Cukor, J., et al. "Prevalence and Predictors of Posttraumatic Stress Symptoms in Utility Workers Deployed to the World Trade Center Following the Attacks of September 11, 2001." *Depression and Anxiety* 28 (March 2011): 210–17.

Hall, B., and M. Place. "Cutting to Cope—A Modern Adolescent Phenomenon." *Child Care, Health and Development* 36 (September 2010): 623–29.

Keogh, A. "Rape Trauma Syndrome: Time to Open the Floodgates?" *Journal of Forensic and Legal Medicine* 14 (May 2007): 221–24.

Lewis, S.P., et al. "The Scope of Nonsuicidal Self-Injury on YouTube." *Pediatrics* 127 (March 2011): e552–e557.

Liberman, Moishe, et al. "The History of Trauma Care Systems from Homer to Telemedicine." *McGill Journal of Medicine*, Spring 2004. http://www.med.mcgill.ca/mjm/issues/v07n02/feature_rev/feature_rev.htm (accessed August 2, 2011).

Raphael, B., and H. Ma. "Mass Catastrophe and Disaster Psychiatry." *Molecular Psychiatry* 16 (March 2011): 247–51.

Shalev, A.Y., et al. "Barriers to Receiving Early Care for PTSD: Results From the Jerusalem Trauma Outreach and Prevention Study." *Psychiatric Services* 62 (July 2011): 765–73.

Wolmer, L., et al. "Preventing Children's Posttraumatic Stress after Disaster with Teacher-Based Intervention: A Controlled Study." *Journal of the American Academy of Child and Adolescent Psychiatry* 50 (April 2011): 340–48.

OTHER

van der Kolk, Bessel, et al. "Proposal to Include a Developmental Trauma Disorder Diagnosis for Children and Adolescents in DSM-V." http://www.cathymalchiodi.com/dtd_nctsn.pdf (accessed August 11, 2011).

WEBSITES

American Academy of Experts in Traumatic Stress (AAETS). "Rape Trauma Syndrome." http://www.aaets.org/article210.htm (accessed August 12, 2011).

American Psychiatric Association. "Conditions Proposed by Outside Sources." DSM-5 Development. http://www.dsm5.org/ProposedRevisions/Pages/ConditionsProposedbyOutsideSources.aspx (accessed August 7, 2011).

———. "Trauma- and Stressor-Related Disorders." DSM-5 Development. http://www.dsm5.org/proposedrevision/pages/traumaandstressorrelateddisorders.aspx (accessed August 7, 2011).

Center for the Study of Traumatic Stress (CSTS). "Dealing with the Effects of Trauma—A Self-Help Guide." http://www.centerforthestudyoftraumaticstress.org/csts_items/SHG_Effects_of_trauma.pdf (accessed August 8, 2011).

International Society for Traumatic Stress Studies (ISTSS). "Self-Care for Providers: Indirect Trauma." http://www.istss.org/SelfCareForProviders/3050.htm (accessed August 7, 2011).

National Center for PTSD. "Cognitive Processing Therapy: Effective Treatment for Veterans with PTSD." This is a 15-minute video about CPT. http://www.ptsd.va.gov/public/videos/CPT/cpt_dvd.asx (accessed August 11, 2011).

———. "Coping with Traumatic Stress Reactions." U.S. Department of Veterans Affairs. http://www.ptsd.va.gov/public/pages/coping-traumatic-stress.asp (accessed August 29, 2011).

———. "FAQs about PTSD Assessment." http://www.ptsd.va.gov/public/pages/faqs-ptsd-assessment.asp (accessed August 11, 2011).

———. "Prolonged Exposure Therapy for PTSD." http://www.ptsd.va.gov/public/pages/prolonged-exposure-therapy.asp (accessed August 11, 2011).

———. "PTSD Overview." http://www.ptsd.va.gov/public/pages/fslist-ptsd-overview.asp (accessed August 3, 2011).

National Institute of Mental Health (NIMH). "Coping with Traumatic Events." This is a gateway page that includes two video presentations and links to NIMH publications about trauma-related disorders. http://www.nimh.nih.gov/health/topics/coping-with-traumatic-events/index.shtml (accessed August 8, 2011).

Sidran Institute. "What Is Psychological Trauma?" http://www.sidran.org/sub.cfm?contentID=88&sectionid=4 (accessed August 9, 2011).

ORGANIZATIONS

American Academy of Experts in Traumatic Stress (AAETS), 203 Deer Road, Ronkonkoma, New York, United States 11779, (631) 543-2217, Fax: (631) 543-6977, info@aaets.org, http://www.aaets.org/index.htm

Center for the Study of Traumatic Stress (CSTS), Uniformed Services University of the Health Sciences (USU), 4301 Jones Bridge Road, Bethesda, MD, United States 20814, (301) 295-2470, Fax: (301) 319-6965, cstsinfo@usuhs.mil, http://www.centerforthestudyoftraumaticstress.org/index.php

International Society for Traumatic Stress Studies (ISTSS), 111 Deer Lake Road, Suite 100, Deerfield, IL, United States 60015, (847) 480-9028, Fax: (847) 480-9282, http://www.istss.org/Home.htm

National Center for PTSD, 810 Vermont Avenue, NW, Washington, DC, United States 20420, (802) 296-6300, ncptsd@va.gov, http://www.ptsd.va.gov/index.asp

National Child Traumatic Stress Network (NCTSN), National Center for Child Traumatic Stress (NCCTS), University of California, Los Angeles, 11150 W. Olympic Blvd., Suite 650, Los Angeles, CA, United State 90064, (310) 235-2633, Fax: (310) 235-2612, http://www.nctsn.org/about-us/contact-us, http://www.nctsn.org/

National Institute of Mental Health (NIMH), 6001 Executive Boulevard, Room 8184, MSC 9663, Bethesda, MD, United States 20892-9663, (301) 443-4513, Fax: (301) 443-4279, (866) 615-6464, nimhinfo@nih.gov, http://www.nimh.nih.gov/index.shtml

Sidran Institute, PO Box 436, Brooklandville, MD, United States 21022-0436, (410) 825-8888, Fax: (410) 560-0134, info@sidran.org, http://www.sidran.org/index.cfm

Rebecca J. Frey, Ph.D.

Traumatic brain injury

Definition

Traumatic **brain** injury (TBI) is a physical injury to brain tissue that temporarily or permanently impairs brain function. TBI is sometimes known as acquired brain injury. TBIs can be evaluated as mild, moderate, or severe, depending on whether the person was knocked out and how long they were unconscious. In a mild TBI, also known as a concussion, the person either does not lose consciousness at all or is unconscious for 30 minutes or less. In a moderate TBI, the person is unconscious longer than 30 minutes but less than 6 hours. Unconsciousness lasting longer than 6 hours indicates a severe TBI.

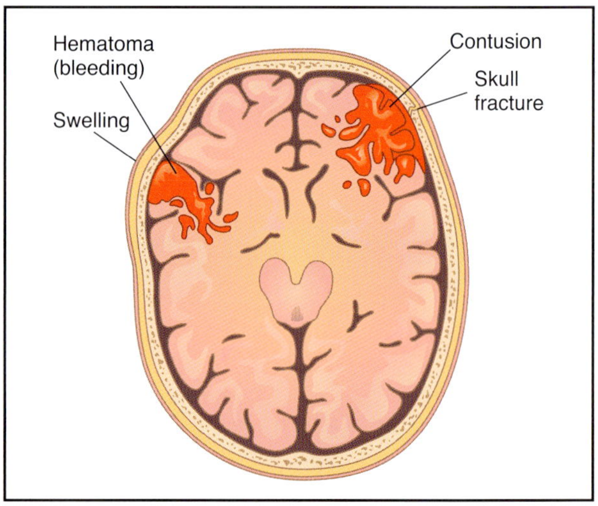

Possible signs of a traumatic brain injury include brain swelling, hematoma (bleeding), a contusion (bruise), or a skull fracture. *(Illustration by Electronic Illustrators Group. © 2012 Cengage Learning.)*

Demographics

Estimates for the number of Americans affected by TBI vary. One source estimates that the number of persons in the United States who have had a TBI ranges between 2.5 and 6.5 million, making it a major public health problem that costs the country more than $48 billion annually. Yearly estimates range from 180 to 220 cases per 100,000 population, or 600,000 TBIs annually. As many as 10% of these injuries are fatal, resulting in almost 550,000 persons hospitalized annually in the United States with head injuries. According to the U.S. Centers for Disease Control and Prevention (CDC), 52,000 individuals die from traumatic brain injuries each year in the United States, with almost twice that number suffering permanent disability. TBI is a contributing factor in 30% of all injury-related deaths in North America. Since 75% of head injuries are classified as mild, it is likely that many mild injuries go unreported.

With regard to sex and race, in North America, males are twice as likely to be hospitalized for a TBI as females. This sex ratio in found worldwide. African Americans and Native Americans have higher rates of TBIs than other ethnic groups in the United States. With regard to age, half of all hospital admissions for TBIs involve people 24 years of age or younger.

Infants, children under five years of age, and adults 75 years and older are also at higher risk for TBI than the general population because they are most susceptible to falls around the home. Other factors predisposing the very young and the very old to TBI include physical **abuse**, such as violent shaking of an infant or toddler known as shaken baby syndrome.

Description

No two brain injuries are exactly the same; TBIs vary greatly in regard to changes in brain structure as well as severity. Mild TBIs may produce only microscopic changes in the structure of the brain, while severe TBIs may produce gross (major) damage. The nature and extent of injury depend on the mechanism of the injury and the amount of force involved. There are three main types of brain injuries: contusions (bruising of the brain tissue), axonal injuries (injuries to the axons, the long slender projects of nerve cells that carry nerve impulses away from the body of the cell), and hematomas (bleeding in the brain).

Immediate complications of TBI may include **seizures**, enlargement of the fluid-filled chambers within the brain (hydrocephalus or post-traumatic ventricular enlargement), leaks of cerebrospinal fluid, infection, injury to blood vessels or to the nerves supplying the head and neck, pain, bed sores, failure of multiple organ systems, and trauma to other areas of the body.

Long-term survivors of a TBI may suffer from persistent problems with behavior, thinking, and communication disabilities, as well as epilepsy; loss of sensation, hearing, vision, taste, or smell; ringing in the ears (tinnitus); coordination problems; and/or paralysis. Recovery from cognitive deficits is most dramatic within the first six months after TBI, and less apparent subsequently.

Risk factors

Risk factors for TBIs include:

- age—children younger than 4 years, adolescents between 16 and 19, and adults over 65 are at increased risk.
- male sex
- African American, Native American, or Hispanic ethnicity
- participation in contact sports, diving, or mountain climbing
- employment in construction, mining, and other occupations requiring blasting or wearing a hard hat
- frontline military combat
- drug or alcohol abuse
- driving under the influence of drugs or alcohol

Causes and symptoms

Causes

The causes of TBIs are commonly classified as either closed- or open-head injuries. Either type of injury may cause direct damage to brain tissue (crushing or tearing of brain tissue itself), or the damage may result from the cascade of events resulting from the original injury. In some cases, there is increased intracranial pressure (ICP), resulting from the fact that the skull is a closed space filled with cerebrospinal fluid that cannot be compressed and brain tissue that allows only minimal compression. Any swelling from edema or a hematoma inside the skull leads to a rise in the ICP. This process reduces the amount of blood flow to the brain, which in turn can lead to ischemia (inadequate blood supply) of the brain tissue.

CLOSED-HEAD INJURIES. A closed head injury is a type of TBI in which the head is hit by or strikes an object without breaking the skull. In a penetrating head injury, an object such as a bullet fractures the skull and enters brain tissue.

Diffuse brain damage associated with closed head injury may result from back-and-forth movement of the brain against the inside of the bony skull. This is sometimes called coup-contrecoup injury. "Coup," French for "blow," refers to the brain injury directly under the point of maximum impact to the skull. "Contrecoup," French for "opposite the blow," refers to the brain injury opposite the point of maximum impact. Coup-contrecoup injury may occur in a rear-end collision, with high-speed stops, or with violent shaking of a baby, because the brain and skull are of different densities and therefore travel at different speeds. The impact of the collision causes the soft, gelatinous brain tissue to jar against bony ridges on the inside of the skull.

Because of the movement of these injuries and the position of the brain within the skull, the frontal lobes (behind the forehead) and temporal lobes (underlying the temples) are most susceptible to this type of diffuse damage. These lobes house major brain centers involved in speech and language, so problems with communication skills often follow closed head injuries of this type.

Depending on which areas of the brain are injured, other symptoms of closed head injury may include difficulty with concentration, memory, thinking, swallowing, walking, balance, and coordination; weakness or paralysis; changes in sensation; and alteration of the sense of smell.

The consequences of a TBI can be relatively subtle or completely devastating, depending on the severity and mechanism of injury. Diffuse axonal injury (DAI), or shear injury, may follow contrecoup injury even when there is no damage to the skull or obvious bleeding into the brain tissue. A DAI involves damage to the axon, which is the part of the nerve that communicates with other nerves. The injured axon degenerates and releases harmful substances that can damage neighboring nerves. DAI is typically the underlying injury in shaken baby syndrome.

SKULL FRACTURES. Skull fractures caused by severe blunt trauma are considered a type of open-head injury. When the skull cracks or breaks, the resulting skull fracture can cause a contusion—an area of bruising of brain tissue associated with swelling and blood leaking from broken blood vessels. A depressed skull fracture occurs when fragments of the broken skull sink or are pushed downward from the skull surface and press against the surface of the brain. In a penetrating skull fracture, bone fragments enter brain tissue. Either type of skull fracture can cause bruising of the brain tissue, called a contusion. Contrecoup injury can also lead to brain contusion.

Some skull fractures are likelier than others to lead to a severe TBI. They include:

- Skull fractures in persons who already have a neurological disorder or impairment.
- Depressed skull fractures.
- Fractures of the occipital bone and the basilar bones of the skull. The basilar bones are strong, thick bones that require a very strong impact to break them, which implies a force strong enough to cause significant damage to the brain tissue itself.
- Fractures in infants. There is a risk of the fracture widening as the baby's skull is still growing.
- Fractures involving the carotid canal. The carotid canal is a passageway through the temporal bone of the skull that allows the internal carotid artery to enter the skull. A fracture in the area of the carotid canal can result in dissection of the carotid artery.

HEMATOMAS. If the physical trauma to the head ruptures a major blood vessel, the resulting bleeding into or around the brain is called a hematoma. Bleeding between the skull and the dura, the thick, outermost layer covering the brain, is termed an epidural hematoma. When blood collects in the space between the dura and the arachnoid membrane, a more fragile covering underlying the dura, it is known as a subdural hematoma. An intracerebral hematoma involves bleeding directly into the brain tissue.

All three types of hematomas can damage the brain by putting pressure on vital brain structures. Intracerebral hematomas can cause additional damage as toxic breakdown products of the blood harm brain cells, cause swelling, or interrupt the flow of cerebrospinal fluid around the brain.

EXTERNAL CAUSES. Transportation accidents involving automobiles, motorcycles, bicycles, and pedestrians account for half of all TBIs and for the majority of TBIs in individuals under the age of 75. At least half of all TBIs are associated with **alcohol use**. Sports injuries cause about 3% of TBIs; other accidents leading to TBI may occur at home, at work, or outdoors.

In those aged 75 and older, falls are responsible for most TBIs. Other situations leading to TBI at all ages include violence, implicated in about 20% of TBIs. Firearm assaults are involved in most violent causes of TBI in young adults, whereas **child abuse** is the most common violent cause in infants and toddlers. In shaken baby syndrome, a baby is shaken with enough force to cause severe countrecoup injury.

Symptoms

Symptoms, complaints, and neurological or behavioral changes following TBI depend on the location(s) of the brain injury and on the total volume of injured brain. Usually, TBI causes focal brain injury involving a single area of the brain where the head is struck or where an object such as a bullet enters the brain. Although damage is typically worst at the point of direct impact or entry, TBI may also cause diffuse brain injury involving several other brain regions.

The symptoms of TBI may occur immediately or they may develop slowly over several hours, especially if there is slow bleeding into the brain or gradual swelling. Depending on the cause, mechanism, and extent of the injury, the severity of immediate symptoms of TBI can be mild, moderate, or severe, ranging from mild concussion to deep coma or even death.

With concussion, the injured person may experience a brief or transient loss of consciousness, much like fainting or passing out, or merely an alteration in consciousness described as "seeing stars" or feeling dazed or "out of it." At the other extreme, coma refers to a profound or deep state of unconsciousness in which the individual does not respond to the environment in any meaningful way.

Approximately 40% of patients with TBI develop postconcussion syndrome within days to weeks, with symptoms including headache, dizziness or a sensation of spinning (vertigo), memory problems, trouble concentrating, sleep disturbances, restlessness, irritability, **depression**, and anxiety. This syndrome may persist for a few weeks, especially in patients with depression, anxiety, or other psychiatric symptoms before the TBI.

With more severe injuries, there may also be immediate numbness or weakness of one or more limbs, blindness, deafness, inability to speak or understand speech, slurred speech, lethargy with difficulty staying awake, persistent vomiting, loss of coordination, disorientation, or agitation. In addition to some of these symptoms, young children with moderate to severe TBI may also experience prolonged crying and refusal to nurse or eat.

When a person with a TBI regains consciousness, some symptoms are immediately apparent, while others are not noticed until several days or weeks later. Symptoms that may be obvious right away after mild TBI include headache, changes in vision such as blurred vision or tired eyes, nausea, dizziness, lightheadedness, ringing in the ears, bad taste in the mouth, or altered sense of smell, which is usually experienced as loss of the sense of taste.

While the injured person is preoccupied with headache or pain related to other physical trauma, symptoms such as difficulty in thinking or concentrating may not be evident. Often these more subtle symptoms may appear only when the individual attempts to return to work or to other mentally challenging situations. Similarly, personality changes, depression, irritability, and other emotional and behavioral problems may initially be attributed to coping with the **stress** of the injury, and their severity may not be fully recognized until the individual is recuperating at home. Other symptoms that may appear immediately or that may be noticed only while the individual is returning to usual activities are confusion, **fatigue** or lethargy, altered sleep patterns, and trouble with memory, concentration, attention, and finding the right words or understanding speech. Seizures may occur soon after a TBI or may first appear up to a year later, especially when the damage involves the temporal lobes.

Diagnosis

Diagnosis of a TBI is suspected on the basis of the clinical signs and symptoms and confirmed by diagnostic imaging.

Examination

Recognizing a serious head injury, starting basic first aid, and seeking emergency medical care can help the injured person avoid disability or even death. When encountering a potential TBI, helpers on the scene should try to find out what happened from the injured person, from clues at the scene, and from any eyewitnesses. Because spinal cord injury often accompanies serious head trauma, it is prudent to assume that there is also injury to the spinal cord and to avoid moving the person until the paramedics arrive. Spinal cord injury is a challenging diagnosis; nearly one-tenth of spinal cord injuries accompanying TBI are initially missed.

Signs apparent to the observer that suggest serious head injury and mandate emergency treatment include shallow or erratic breathing or pulse; a drop in blood pressure; broken bones or other obvious trauma to the skull or face such as bruising, swelling, or bleeding; one pupil being larger than the other; or clear or bloody fluid drainage from the nose, mouth, or ears.

Symptoms reported by the injured person that should also raise red flags include severe headache, stiff neck, vomiting, paralysis or inability to move one or more limbs, blindness, deafness, or inability to taste or smell. Other ominous developments may include initial improvement followed by worsening symptoms, deepening lethargy or unresponsiveness, personality changes including irritability or unusual behavior, or loss of coordination.

When emergency personnel arrive, they will stabilize the patient, evaluate the patient's signs and symptoms, and assess the nature and extent of other injuries, such as broken bones, spinal cord injury, or

KEY TERMS

Closed-head injury—A head injury in which the skull is not cracked or fractured.

Coma—A decreased level of consciousness with deep unresponsiveness.

Computed tomography (CT) scan—A neuroimaging test that generates a series of cross-sectional x rays of the head and brain.

Concussion—Injury to the brain causing a sudden but temporary impairment of brain function.

Contrecoup—An injury to the brain opposite the point of direct impact.

Contusion—A focal area of swollen and bleeding brain tissue.

Dementia pugilistica—A term for "punch-drunk" syndrome of brain damage caused by repeated head trauma.

Depressed skull fracture—A fracture in which pieces of broken skull press into brain tissue.

Diffuse axonal injury (DAI; also called shear injury)—Traumatic damage to individual nerve cells resulting in breakdown of overall communication between nerve cells in the brain.

Epidural hematoma—Bleeding into the area between the skull and the dura, the tough, outermost brain covering.

Executive functions—An umbrella term for the group of mental processes responsible for planning, abstract thinking, logical deduction, choosing appropriate behaviors and inhibiting inappropriate behaviors, and distinguishing between relevant and irrelevant sensory information.

Glasgow coma scale—A measure of the level of consciousness and neurological functioning after TBI.

Hematoma—Bleeding into or around the brain caused by trauma to a blood vessel in the head.

Intracerebral hematoma—Bleeding within the brain caused by trauma to a blood vessel.

Ischemia—An inadequate flow of blood to a part of the body, caused by narrowing or blockage of the blood vessels supplying it.

Penetrating head injury—TBI in which an object pierces the skull and enters brain tissue.

Post-concussion syndrome—A complex of symptoms including headache following mild TBI.

Post-traumatic amnesia (PTA)—Difficulty forming new memories after TBI.

Post-traumatic dementia—Persistent mental deterioration following TBI.

Sequela (plural, sequelae)—In medicine, a pathological condition resulting from a disease, injury, or other trauma. For example, PTSD may be a sequela of a traumatic brain injury.

Shaken baby syndrome (SBS)—A severe form of TBI resulting from shaking an infant or small child forcefully enough to cause the brain to jar against the skull.

Stabilization—A set of procedures for preventing shock in an injured person by protecting the airway, controlling bleeding (if any), keeping the person warm, and preventing injury to the spinal cord.

Subdural hematoma—Bleeding between the dura and the underlying brain covering.

Syndrome—A group of signs or symptoms that occur together and characterize or define a particular disease or disorder.

Ventriculostomy—Surgery that drains cerebrospinal fluid from the brain to treat hydrocephalus or increased intracranial pressure.

damage to other organ systems. Medical advances in early detection and treatment of associated injuries have improved the overall outcome in TBI. Severely injured victims transported rapidly by helicopter or ambulance have better outcomes compared to those who cannot be transported quickly.

When possible, persons with severe head injuries are taken to a hospital with a dedicated trauma center. Such centers have specialized staff and equipment, and their patients have better outcomes compared to those taken to general hospitals. The initial evaluation measures vital signs such as temperature, blood pressure, pulse, and breathing rate, while the neurological examination assesses reflexes, level of consciousness, ability to move the limbs, and pupil size, symmetry, and response to light.

Neurological features are standardized using the Glasgow Coma Scale (GCS), a test scored from 1 to 15 points. Each of three measures (eye opening, best verbal response, and best motor response) is scored separately, and the combined score helps determine the severity of TBI. A total score of 3 to 8 reflects a severe TBI, 9 to 12 a moderate TBI, and 13 to 15 a mild TBI. The lowest possible score, 3, usually indicates a fatal injury. There is a modified version of the GCS for use with infants and children.

Tests

Definitive diagnosis of a TBI is provided by **imaging studies**. Sophisticated imaging tests can help differentiate the variety of unconscious states associated with TBI and can help determine their anatomical basis. Until neck fractures or spinal instability have been ruled out with skull and neck x rays, or with head and neck **computed tomography** (CT) scans for more severe injuries, the patient should remain immobilized in a neck and back restraint.

By constructing a series of cross-sectional slices, or x-ray images through the head and brain, CT scans can diagnose bone fractures, bleeding, hematomas, contusions, swelling of brain tissue, and blockage of the ventricular system that circulates cerebrospinal fluid around the brain. In later stages after the initial injury, scans may also show shrinkage of brain volume in areas where neurons have died.

Using magnetic fields to detect subtle changes in brain tissue related to differences in water content, **magnetic resonance imaging** (MRI) scans show more detail than x rays or CT. However, MRI takes more time than CT and is not as readily available, making it less suited for routine emergency imaging.

For patients with seizures or for those with more subtle episodic symptoms thought to be seizures, an electroencephalogram (EEG) may reveal abnormalities in the electrical activity of the brain, or brain waves. Other diagnostic techniques that may be helpful include cerebral angiography, transcranial Doppler ultrasound, and **single photon emission computed tomography** (SPECT).

Treatment

Although no specific treatment may be needed for a mild head injury, it is crucial to watch the person closely for any developing symptoms over the next 24 hours. Over-the-counter pain relievers like acetaminophen or ibuprofen may be used for mild headache. Aspirin should not be given, however, because it can increase the risk of bleeding.

If the person is sleeping, he or she should be awakened every two to three hours to determine alertness and orientation to name, time, and place. Immediate medical help is needed if the person becomes unusually drowsy or disoriented, develops a severe headache or stiff neck, vomits, loses consciousness, or behaves abnormally.

Emergency care and surgery

Treatment for moderate or severe TBI should begin as soon as possible by calling 911 and beginning emergency care until the EMT team arrives. This care includes stabilizing the head and neck by placing the hands on both sides of the person's head to keep the head in line with the spine and prevent movement, which could worsen spinal cord injury. Bleeding should be controlled by firmly pressing a clean cloth over the wound. If a skull fracture is suspected, it should be covered with sterile gauze dressing without applying pressure. If the person is vomiting, the head, neck, and body should be rolled to the side as one unit to prevent choking without further injuring the spine.

Although the initial brain damage caused by trauma is often irreversible, the goal is to stabilize the patient and prevent further injury. To achieve these goals, the treatment team must insure adequate oxygen supply to the brain and the rest of the body, maintain blood flow to the brain, control blood pressure, stabilize the airway, assist in breathing or perform CPR if necessary, and treat associated injuries. Recent research has found that increasing the patient's caloric intake by 50% during the first two weeks after the TBI helps reduce inflammation and gives the brain the energy it needs to heal.

About half of severe head injuries require neurosurgery for hematomas or contusions. Swelling of the injured brain may cause increased intracranial pressure (ICP) within the closed skull cavity. ICP can be measured with an intraventricular probe or catheter inserted through the skull into the fluid-filled chambers (ventricles) within the brain. Placement of the ICP catheter is usually guided by CT scan. If ICP is elevated, ventriculostomy may be needed. This procedure drains cerebrospinal fluid from the brain and reduces ICP. Drugs that may decrease ICP include mannitol and **barbiturates**.

Drugs

Although some patients need medication for psychiatric and physical problems resulting from the TBI, prescribing drugs may be problematic, because TBI patients are more sensitive to side effects.

Rehabilitation

Both in the immediate and later stages of TBI, rehabilitation is vital to optimal recovery of the patient's ability to function at home and in society. Rehabilitation is a highly individualized process and is based on each patient's specific strengths and abilities.

Problems with orientation and thinking and communication problems should be addressed early, often during the hospital stay. The focus is typically on improving alertness, attention, orientation, speech understanding, and swallowing problems.

As the patient improves, rehabilitation should be modified accordingly. Physical therapy, occupational therapy, speech or language therapy, physiatry (physical medicine), psychology or psychiatry, and social support should all play a role in TBI rehabilitation. Appropriate settings for rehabilitation may include the patient's home, the hospital outpatient department, inpatient rehabilitation centers, comprehensive day programs, supportive-living programs, independent-living centers, and school-based programs. Families should become involved in rehabilitation, in modifying the home environment if needed, and in **psychotherapy** or counseling as indicated.

Prognosis

The prognosis of TBIs is highly individualized and varies with their severity and cause: 91% of TBIs caused by firearms (two-thirds of which may represent suicide attempts) are fatal, compared with only 11% of TBIs from falls.

Following TBI, patients may be at increased risk of such other long-term problems as Parkinson's disease, **Alzheimer's disease**, "punch-drunk" syndrome (**dementia** pugilistica), and post-traumatic dementia. Some patients may have difficulty returning to work following TBI, as well as problems with school, driving, sports, housework, and social relationships.

Mental health issues

Mental disorders and behavioral problems are common sequelae of TBIs. The most common are depression and behavioral problems. A report published in the August 2011 edition of the journal *Schizophrenia Bulletin* found that persons with TBIs may also be at risk for developing schizophrenia, being 1.6 times more likely to develop the disorder than persons in the general population. A major reason for the development of mental disorders after TBI is that the parts of the brain most susceptible to traumatic injury—the frontal and temporal lobes—are the portions of the brain that are responsible for executive functions (judgment, reasoning, decision making, evaluating a situation, processing information, etc.). These portions of the brain contain such structures as the hippocampus, which helps to form long-term memory; Broca's and Wernicke's areas, which govern speech; and the amygdala, which processes emotions and is also responsible for memory consolidation. Thus, damage to the frontal and temporal lobes can have long-term behavioral and psychiatric consequences.

DEPRESSION. Depression is a common mood disorder that affects TBI patients; about half of all persons with a TBI will be diagnosed with major depression within a year after injury. Many TBI patients with depression also have concurrent **anxiety disorders**. Depression following a TBI usually results from a combination of factors that include physical changes in the brain after injury; emotional reactions to such changes as job or role loss, short- or long-term disability, loss of self-sufficiency and other losses; a personal or family history of depression; and genetic susceptibility to mood disorders.

Depression following a TBI is treated in the same way as depression in the general population, most often with a combination of antidepressant medications and cognitive behavioral or **group therapy**. Some patients with depression following a TBI report being helped by **yoga**, other gentle forms of **exercise**, **acupuncture**, and **biofeedback**.

Behavioral problems

Behavioral problems are another common sequela of a TBI. The problematic behaviors most frequently encountered in TBI patients are agitation, impulsive behaviors, loss of inhibition, and loss of motivation. Aggressive outbursts toward others, cursing, yelling, inappropriate sexual behaviors, self-injury, property destruction, and noncompliance with treatment can all hinder relationships with family members, return to work, and reintegration within the larger community. Assessment of the frequency and severity of behavioral problems is an important part of evaluation. For example, occasional temper tantrums in the home are one matter, but aggression may evolve to violence, placing friends and family in dangerous situations. Although some problem behaviors may not be physically dangerous to others, having them repeated literally hundreds of times a day can damage family relationships as well as the possibility of employment.

One way to understand behavioral problems in patients with TBIs is that they result from a combination of changes in the functioning of the patient's brain and negative feedback from the surrounding environment. The affected person may not be able to detect and respond to the social cues and feedback that remind most people of the limits of acceptable behavior. In return, healthcare workers as well as family members may respond to the problem behaviors by reprimanding or punishing the individual, which often makes the behavioral problems worse.

An additional complication in addressing problem behaviors in patients with TBIs is that there is no consensus regarding the best therapeutic approach. There are many different schools of psychiatry and psychotherapy, and treatment recommendations based on one theory of human behavior may vary considerably from recommendations based on a different theory. No two TBIs are identical, nor are the patients affected by them. Some general recommendations for treating behavioral problems are as follows:

- The individual should have a complete neurological examination and imaging studies to determine as precisely as possible which parts of the brain have been injured, along with the severity of the damage.
- Mild behavioral problems can often be managed in community settings or outpatient clinics with a combination of behavioral therapy and medications. The patient should be involved in the design of the treatment plan as much as possible.
- Some behavioral problems can also be managed by changing the patient's environment to minimize confusion and frustration.
- Severe behavioral problems often require inpatient treatment. The patient's family or friends, however, should make sure that the facility is staffed by physicians, psychologists, speech pathologists, and other therapists with extensive training and specific expertise in treating behavior problems resulting from TBIs. Other concerns include the safety of the facility (to prevent self-injury) and its security (to prevent the patient's wandering away).

Cognitive dysfunction

Cognition refers to a set of mental functions that include attention, memory, language, problem solving, logic, and decision making. Memory itself is a complex set of active storage processing that encodes information rather than just passively storing it. Cognitive skills assist memory by identifying what is important to remember in a given situation and by rearranging what is stored in memory when a person learns new information. In many cases, what appears to be memory loss in patients with TBIs is really a consequence of other cognitive deficits, such as difficulty concentrating or damage to vision and other forms of sensory perception.

In general, cognitive deficits are most noticeable immediately after the person emerges from coma (if they have lost consciousness). Although there are exceptions, a common rule of thumb is that recovery of cognition is most rapid in the first 6 to 12 months after injury, and proceeds at a slower pace for the next one to three years. With regard to assessment of the person's cognitive abilities, most doctors recommend waiting until the person's condition has stabilized sufficiently to allow them to participate in a meaningful assessment.

Cognitive assessments serve several purposes, including identification of specific cognitive abilities and deficits, evaluating treatment outcomes, monitoring the patient's recovery, designing a treatment program, assessing the person's educational and occupational future, and documenting symptoms for legal purposes, particularly for decisions about the person's competency or applying for Medicaid or Social Security benefits. The cognitive assessment is usually repeated, as it is not unusual for new symptoms to appear as previous symptoms resolve. An example would be the appearance of difficulties with impulse control after the patient's initial loss of interest in activity has disappeared.

There are different treatment strategies for different cognitive deficits, although most involve long-term therapy; recovery of cognitive skills is a slow process that usually takes years, not months. Assistive technologies, such as wristwatches that beep to remind the person of a task or computer software that helps with organizing and managing complex information, are useful to many patients. Those with low mental stamina or difficulties with concentration may be helped by fatigue management strategies or by medications that have been shown to improve alertness and the ability to focus attention. With regard to impairment-specific treatments, speech-language therapy and treatment for loss of visual/spatial coordination have yielded better results than memory training strategies. Deficits in executive skills have been effectively treated by a combination of individualized psychotherapy and coaching in real-life situations, including the workplace.

Veterans' issues

TBI has been described as the "signature" injury of the conflicts in Iraq and Afghanistan; the rate of such injuries is higher in veterans of Iraq and Afghanistan compared to Vietnam veterans (12%). Veterans' advocates believe that between 10% and 20% of Iraq veterans (150,000 to 300,000 men and women) have some level of TBI. Among wounded troops, the rate of TBI is as high as 33%. The major causes of TBIs in recent veterans are blasts, motor vehicle accidents, and gunshot wounds. Unfortunately, TBI is underdiagnosed and therefore undertreated in military personnel. In 2008, the U.S. Department of Defense awarded a four-year grant to the Brain Trauma Foundation (BTF) to develop an eye-tracking device that can be used in the field to instantly

QUESTIONS TO ASK YOUR DOCTOR

- Do you know of any nearby rehabilitation facilities that specialize in treating TBIs?
- What are my best treatment options?
- Will my TBI have long-term effects?

determine if a soldier or airman has suffered any brain damage as a result of blast injury or another type of head injury.

Because many veterans with TBIs have coexisting PTSD or **substance abuse** disorders, they typically take longer than civilians to recover from these head injuries. Women veterans with TBIs are more likely than male veterans to be diagnosed with concurrent depression. Veterans with TBIs are also almost twice as likely to attempt **suicide** as veterans who did not suffer such injuries. Treatment for TBIs in veterans is similar to that for civilians, with rehabilitation programs that address **cognitive retraining**, psychosocial adjustment, communication and leisure skills, and vocational issues. The U.S. Veterans Administration (VA) maintains 4 polytrauma rehabilitation centers and 21 polytrauma network sites for veterans with the most severe TBIs.

Prevention

Not all accidents or other causes of TBIs can be prevented. People can, however, lower their risk by taking the following safety measures:

- Athletes should wear protective headgear for such sports as mountain climbing, martial arts, football, baseball, bicycling, motorcycling, rollerblading, and skateboarding. They should make sure their helmets and other protective gear are properly fitted. Coaches should insist that players are taught the rules of safe play and that they follow them. Players should report all head injuries to the team doctor even if they seem minor at the time.
- Adults and children should be careful when diving in shallow water, particularly in bodies of water with rocky shores and bottoms.
- Drivers and passengers should always wear seat belts when traveling in a motor vehicle, and people should never drive when under the influence of alcohol or other drugs.
- People in occupations requiring hardhats should wear them at all times, particularly in mining and construction work. Even a small object dropped from the upper floors of a building can cause a serious head injury.
- Elderly persons or parents of small children should check their house or apartment for loose rugs, poor lighting, slippery floors, and other problems that increase the risk of falls, which are a common cause of TBIs in the very old and very young.

Resources

BOOKS

Erdman, John, Maria Oria, and Laura Pillsbury. *Nutrition and Traumatic Brain Injury: Improving Acute and Subacute Health Outcomes in Military Personnel.* Washington, DC: National Academies Press, 2011.

Kerpelman, Larry C. *Pieces Missing: A Family's Journey of Recovery from Traumatic Brain Injury.* Minneapolis, MN: Two Harbors Press, 2011.

Phillips, Joseph R. *Hidden Wounds: Traumatic Brain Injury and Post Traumatic Stress Disorder in Service Members.* New York: Nova Science Publishers, 2011.

Roberts, Richard J., and Mary Ann Roberts. *Mild Traumatic Brain Injury: Episodic Symptoms and Treatment.* San Diego, CA: Plural Publishing, 2011.

Silver, Jonathan M., Thomas W. McAllister, and Stuart C. Yudofsky, eds. *Textbook of Traumatic Brain Injury.* 2nd ed. Arlington, VA: American Psychiatric Publishing, 2011.

Stone, C. Keith, and Roger L. Humphries, eds. *Current Diagnosis and Treatment: Emergency Medicine.* 6th ed. New York: McGraw-Hill, 2008.

PERIODICALS

Farrer, T. J., and D. W. Hedges. "Prevalence of Traumatic Brain Injury in Incarcerated Groups Compared to the General Population: A Meta-Analysis." *Progress in Neuro-Psychopharmacology and Biological Psychiatry* 35 (March 30, 2011): 390–94.

Gould, K. R., et al. "The Nature, Frequency and Course of Psychiatric Disorders in the First Year after Traumatic Brain Injury: A Prospective Study." *Psychological Medicine* 41 (October 2011): 2099–109.

Hart, T., et al. "Major and Minor Depression after Traumatic Brain Injury." *Archives of Physical Medicine and Rehabilitation* 92 (August 2011): 1211–19.

Hettich, T., et al. "Case Report: Use of the Immediate Post Concussion Assessment and Cognitive Testing (ImPACT) to Assist with Return to Duty Determination of Special Operations Soldiers Who Sustained Mild Traumatic Brain Injury." *Journal of Special Operations Medicine* 10 (Fall 2010): 48–55.

Iverson, K. M., et al. "Psychiatric Diagnoses and Neurobehavioral Symptom Severity among OEF/OIF VA Patients with Deployment-related Traumatic Brain Injury: A Gender Comparison." *Women's Health Issues* 21 (July–August 2011), Suppl. 4: S210–S217.

Max, J. E., et al. "Anxiety Disorders in Children and Adolescents in the First Six Months after Traumatic Brain

Injury." *Journal of Neuropsychiatry and Clinical Neurosciences* 23 (Fall 2011): 29–39.

Meares, S., et al. "The Prospective Course of Postconcussion Syndrome: The Role of Mild Traumatic Brain Injury." *Neuropsychology* 25 (July 2011): 454–65.

Reeves, R. R., and R. L. Panguluri. "Neuropsychiatric Complications of Traumatic Brain Injury." *Journal of Psychosocial Nursing and Mental Health Services* 49 (March 2011): 42–50.

Simpson, G. K., et al. "Suicide Prevention after Traumatic Brain Injury: A Randomized Controlled Trial of a Program for the Psychological Treatment of Hopelessness." *Journal of Head Trauma Rehabilitation* 26 (July–August 2011): 290–300.

Weeks, D. L., et al. "Association of Antidepressant Medication Therapy with Inpatient Rehabilitation Outcomes for Stroke, Traumatic Brain Injury, or Traumatic Spinal Cord Injury." *Archives of Physical Medicine and Rehabilitation* 92 (May 2011): 683–695.

Williams, W. H., et al. "Self-reported Traumatic Brain Injury in Male Young Offenders: A Risk Factor for Re-offending, Poor Mental Health and Violence?" *Neuropsychological Rehabilitation* 20 (December 2010): 801–12.

Zafonte, R. "Diagnosis and Management of Sports-Related Concussion: A 15-year-old Athlete with a Concussion." *Journal of the American Medical Association* 306 (July 6, 2011): 79–86.

Zatzick, D.F., and D.C. Grossman. "Association between Traumatic Injury and Psychiatric Disorders and Medication Prescription to Youths Aged 10–19." *Psychiatric Services* 62 (March 2011): 264–271.

OTHER

Centers for Disease Control and Prevention (CDC). "Traumatic Brain Injury in Prisons and Jails: An Unrecognized Problem." http://www.cdc.gov/traumaticbraininjury/pdf/Prisoner_TBI_Prot-a.pdf (accessed August 29, 2011).

Veterans Administration (VA). "Traumatic Brain Injury: A Guide for Patients." http://www.mentalhealth.va.gov/docs/tbi.pdf (accessed August 29, 2011).

WEBSITES

Brain Injury Association of America (BIAA). "Brain Injury in the Community." http://biausa.fyrian.com/brain-injury-community.htm (accessed August 29, 2011).

Brain Trauma Foundation (BTF). "More about Concussion." https://www.braintrauma.org/more-about-concussion (accessed August 26, 2011).

Centers for Disease Control and Prevention (CDC). "Traumatic Brain Injury." http://www.cdc.gov/TraumaticBrainInjury/index.html (accessed August 27, 2011).

Crippen, David W. "Head Trauma." http://emedicine.medscape.com/article/433855-overview (accessed August 27, 2011).

Mayo Clinic staff. "Traumatic Brain Injury." MayoClinic.com. http://www.mayoclinic.com/health/traumatic-brain-injury/DS00552 (accessed August 26, 2011).

Merck Manual Online. "Traumatic Brain Injury." http://www.merckmanuals.com/professional/sec22/ch330/ch330a.html (accessed August 27, 2011).

Olson, David A. "Head Injury." Medscape Reference. http://emedicine.medscape.com/article/1163653-overview (accessed July 5, 2011).

National Center for PTSD. "Traumatic Brain Injury and PTSD." http://www.ptsd.va.gov/public/pages/traumatic_brain_injury_and_ptsd.asp(accessed August 4, 2011).

National Institute of Neurological Disorders and Stroke (NINDS). "Traumatic Brain Injury Information Page." http://www.ninds.nih.gov/disorders/tbi/tbi.htm *accessed August 26m 2011).

Rettner, Rachael. "Head Trauma may Boost Schizophrenia Risk." MSNBC.com. (August 19, 2011). http://www.msnbc.msn.com/id/44202899/ns/health-mental_health (accessed November 13, 2011).

Research Channel. "Living with Traumatic Brain Injury" [half-hour video from the University of Washington Medical Center]. http://www.youtube.com/watch?v=FgtHvBF4t-E&feature=related (accessed August 28, 2011).

ORGANIZATIONS

American Academy of Neurology (AAN), 1080 Montreal Ave., Saint Paul, MN, United States 55116, (651) 695-2717, (800) 879-1960, Fax: (651) 695-2791, http://www.aan.com.

American College of Emergency Physicians (ACEP), PO Box 619911, Dallas, TX, United States 75261-9911, (972) 550-0911, (800) 798-1822, Fax: (972) 580-2816, http://www.acep.org.

Brain Injury Association of America (BIAA), 1608 Spring Hill Rd., Ste. 110, Vienna, VA, United States 22182, (703) 761-0750, (800) 444-6443, Fax: (703) 761-0755, http://www.biausa.org.

Brain Trauma Foundation (BTF), 7 World Trade Center, 34th Fl., 250 Greenwich St., New York, NY, United States 10007, (212) 772-0608, http://www.braintrauma.org/contact/, http://www.braintrauma.org.

National Center for PTSD, 810 Vermont Ave. NW, Washington, DC, United States 20420, (802) 296-6300, ncptsd@va.gov, http://www.ptsd.va.gov/index.asp.

National Institute of Mental Health, 6001 Executive Boulevard, Room 8184, MSC 9663, Bethesda, MD, United States 20892-9663, (301) 443-4513, (866) 615-6464, Fax: (301) 443-4279, nimhinfo@nih.gov, http://www.nimh.nih.gov/index.shtml.

National Institute of Neurological Disorders and Stroke (NINDS), PO Box 5801, Bethesda, MD, United States 20824, (301) 496-5751, (800) 352-9424, http://www.ninds.nih.gov.

Rebecca J. Frey, Ph.D.

Trazodone

Definition

Trazodone is an oral antidepressant. It is sold in the United States under the brand name Desyrel and is also available under its generic name.

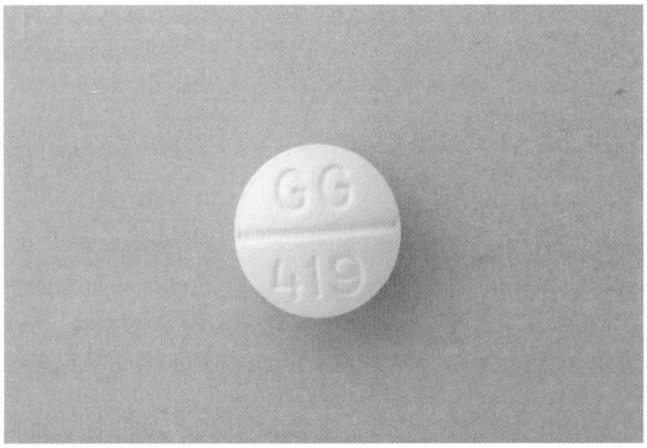

Trazodone, 50 mg. *(© Custom Medical Stock Photo, Inc. Reproduced by permission.)*

Purpose

Trazodone is used to treat **depression** and to treat the combination of symptoms of anxiety and depression. Like most **antidepressants**, trazodone has also been used in limited numbers of patients to treat **panic disorder**, **obsessive-compulsive disorder**, **attention deficit hyperactivity disorder**, **enuresis** (bed-wetting), eating disorders such as **bulimia nervosa**, **cocaine** dependency, and the depressive phase of **bipolar disorder**, but it should be noted that trazodone is not approved by the U.S. Food and Drug Administration (FDA) for these uses.

Description

Trazodone acts to change the balance of naturally occurring chemicals in the **brain** that regulate the transmission of nerve impulses between cells. Its action primarily increases the concentration of norepinephrine and **serotonin** (both chemicals that stimulate nerve cells) and, to a lesser extent, blocks the action of another brain chemical, acetylcholine. Trazodone is classified as an atypical antidepressant, but it shares many of the properties of tricyclic antidepressants (**amitriptyline**, **clomipramine**, **desipramine**, **doxepin**, **imipramine**, **nortriptyline**, **protriptyline**, and **trimipramine**). It also shares some of the properties of **selective serotonin reuptake inhibitor** (SSRI) antidepressants (such as **fluoxetine**, **paroxetine**, and **sertraline**).

The therapeutic effects of trazodone, like other antidepressants, appear slowly. Maximum benefit is often not evident for at least two weeks after starting the drug. People taking trazodone should be aware of this and continue taking the drug as directed even if they do not see immediate improvement.

Recommended dosage

As with any antidepressant, the dosage of trazodone must be carefully adjusted to produce the desired therapeutic effect. Trazodone is available as 50 mg, 100 mg, and 150 mg film-coated tablets that cannot be divided, as well as in 150 mg and 300 mg oral tablets that can be split. Therapy is usually started at a total of 150 mg per day divided into two or three doses. This dose is increased by 50 mg every three or four days until the desired effects are seen. Daily doses may be increased to a maximum of 400 mg per day in outpatients and up to 600 mg per day in hospitalized patients. In cases of extreme depression, daily doses of up to 800 mg have been used in hospitalized patients. To minimize daytime drowsiness, a major portion of the daily dose can be given at bedtime.

Precautions

Children and adults up to age 24 are at increased risk of developing suicidal thoughts and actions when taking antidepressant drugs, including trazodone. Patients of any age taking an antidepressant medication should be monitored for signs of worsening depression or changes in behavior. Trazodone is not approved for use in children younger than 18.

Although lower in anticholinergic side effects than the tricyclic antidepressants, trazodone should be used cautiously and with close physician supervision in people, especially the elderly, who have benign prostatic hypertrophy, urinary retention, and glaucoma, especially angle-closure glaucoma (the most severe form). Before starting treatment, people with these conditions should discuss the relative risks and benefits of treatment with their doctors to help determine if trazodone is the right medication for them.

Trazodone may increase heart rate and **stress** on the heart. Trazodone is associated with an increased risk of death in patients with heart disease. In rare cases where patients with cardiovascular disease must take trazodone, they should be monitored closely for cardiac rhythm disturbances and signs of cardiac stress or damage. Trazodone is also associated with an increased risk of bleeding, especially internal bleeding within the gastrointestinal tract.

The most common problem with trazodone is sedation (drowsiness and lack of mental and physical alertness). This side effect is especially noticeable early in therapy. In most patients, sedation decreases or disappears entirely with time, but until then patients taking trazodone should not perform hazardous activities requiring mental alertness or coordination, including driving or operating machinery. The sedative effect is increased when trazodone is taken with other central nervous system depressants, such as alcoholic beverages, sleeping medications, other **sedatives**, or antihistamines. It may be dangerous to take trazodone in combination with these substances.

Side effects

Trazodone shares side effects common to many antidepressants. The most frequent of these are dry mouth, constipation, and urinary retention, though these are less common than with tricyclic antidepressants. Increased heart rate, sedation, irritability, dizziness, and decreased coordination can also occur. As with most side effects associated with antidepressants, the intensity is highest at the beginning of therapy and tends to decrease with continued use.

Dry mouth, if severe to the point of causing difficulty in speaking or swallowing, may be managed by dosage reduction or temporary discontinuation of the drug. Patients may also chew sugarless gum or suck on sugarless candy in order to increase the flow of saliva. Some artificial saliva products may give temporary relief.

Men with prostate enlargement who take trazodone may be especially likely to have problems with urinary retention. Symptoms include having difficulty starting a urine flow and more difficulty than usual passing urine. In most cases, urinary retention is managed with dose reduction or by switching to another type of antidepressant. In extreme cases, patients may require treatment with bethanechol, a drug that reverses this particular side effect. In rare cases, trazodone has also been known to cause priapism, a prolonged and painful penile erection. People who think they may be experiencing any side effects from this or any other medication should tell their physicians.

Interactions

Because both trazodone and members of the class of antidepressants known as **monoamine oxidase inhibitors (MAOIs)** may increase serotonin levels in the brain, the combination of these drugs can lead to a serious condition known as **serotonin syndrome**. Symptoms of serotonin syndrome include a prolonged rapid heart rate, hypertension (high blood pressure), flushing of the skin, hallucinations, tremors, and hyperthermia (increased body temperature). It is dangerous to take trazodone in combination with MAOIs, such as **phenelzine** (Nardil) or **tranylcypromine** (Parnate). The same holds true when combining trazodone with an SSRI antidepressant, such as fluoxetine (Prozac), paroxetine, or sertraline.

Trazodone may increase the blood pressure–lowering effects in patients who are taking antihypertensive medications. Patients who take these drugs together should have their blood pressure monitored regularly so that their antihypertensive medications can be adjusted if their blood pressure becomes too low.

The sedative effects of trazodone are increased by medications used for other mental disorders such as **schizophrenia**. The anticholinergic effects of trazodone may be additive with other anticholinergic drugs such as **benztropine**, **biperiden**, **trihexyphenidyl**, and antihistamines.

KEY TERMS

Acetylcholine—A naturally occurring chemical in the body that generally produces effects that are the opposite of those produced by dopamine and norepinephrine. Central nervous system well-being is dependent on a balance between acetylcholine, serotonin, dopamine and norepinephrine.

Anticholinergic—Related to the ability of a drug to block the nervous system chemical, acetylcholine. When acetylcholine is blocked, patients often experience dry mouth and skin, increased heart rate, blurred vision, and difficulty urinating. In severe cases, blocking acetylcholine may cloud thinking and cause delirium.

Benign prostatic hypertrophy—Enlargement of the prostate gland.

Norepinephrine—A neurotransmitter in the brain that acts to constrict blood vessels and raise blood pressure. It works in combination with serotonin.

Serotonin—A widely distributed neurotransmitter that is found in blood platelets, the lining of the digestive tract, and the brain, and that works in combination with norepinephrine. It causes very powerful contractions of smooth muscle, and is associated with mood, attention, emotions, and sleep. Low levels of serotonin are associated with depression.

Resources

BOOKS

American Society of Health-System Pharmacists. *AHFS Drug Information 2008*. Bethesda, MD: American Society of Health-System Pharmacists, 2008.

PERIODICALS

Jayaram, Geetha, and Pravin Rao. "Safety of Trazodone as a Sleep Agent for Inpatients." *Psychosomatics* 46, no. 4 (July–August 2005): 367–69.

Luparini, Maria Rita, et al. "A Cortical GABA-5HT Interaction in the Mechanism of Action of the Antidepressant Trazodone." *Progress in Neuro-Psychopharmacology & Biological Psychiatry* 28, no. 7 (November 2004): 1117–27.

Mayers, Andrew G., and David S. Baldwin. "Antidepressants and Their Effect on Sleep." *Human Psychopharmacology: Clinical and Experimental* 20, no. 8 (December 2005): 533–59.

McNeill, Alisdair. "Chorea Induced by Low-Dose Trazodone." *European Neurology* 55, no. 2 (2006): 101–102.

Mendelson, Wallace B. "A Review of the Evidence for the Efficacy and Safety of Trazodone in Insomnia." *Journal of Clinical Psychiatry* 66, no. 4 (April 2005): 469–76.

Mizoguchi, Yoshito, and Akira Monji. "Low-Dose-Trazodone-Induced Disorganized Type Psychosis." *Journal of Neuropsychiatry & Clinical Neurosciences* 17, no. 2 (May 2005): 253–4.

WEBSITES

Drugs.com "Trazodone (Trazodone hydrochloride)." http://www.drugs.com/pro/trazodone.html (accessed October 27, 2011).

PubMed Health. "Trazodone." http://www.ncbi.nlm.nih.gov/pubmedhealth/PMH0000530 (accessed November 13, 2011).

ORGANIZATIONS

National Institute of Mental Health, 6001 Executive Blvd., Rm. 8184, MSC 9663, Bethesda, MD, 20892-9663, (301) 433-4513; TTY: (301) 443-8431, Fax: (301) 443-4279, (866) 615-6464; TTY: (866) 415-8051, nimhinfo@nih.gov, http://www.nimh.nih.gov.

U.S. Food and Drug Administration, 10903 New Hampshire Ave., Silver Spring, MD, 20993-0002, (888) INFO-FDA (463-6332), http://www.fda.gov.

Jack Raber, Pharm.D.
Ruth A. Wienclaw, PhD

The Treatment for Adolescents with Depression Study (TADS)

Definition

The Treatment for Adolescents with Depression Study (TADS) was a clinical trial sponsored by the National Institutes of Health that examined the effectiveness of short- and long-term medication and **psychotherapy** treatments for teenagers (aged 12–17) with **major depressive disorder** (MDD).

MDD is a mood disorder also known as major depression, clinical depression, or unipolar depression. A person with MDD has experienced at least five of the nine symptoms below for two weeks or more, for most of the time almost every day, and this is a change from their prior level of functioning. One of the symptoms must be either (a) depressed mood, or (b) loss of interest. Recurrent MDD is diagnosed when two or more of these depressive periods occur with at least two months between episodes.

- Depressed mood (may be manifested as irritable mood).
- A significantly reduced level of interest or pleasure in most or all activities.
- A considerable loss or gain of weight (may also be an increase or decrease in appetite).
- Difficulty falling or staying asleep (insomnia), or sleeping more than usual (hypersomnia).
- Behavior that is agitated or slowed down (observable by others).
- Feeling fatigued, or having diminished energy.
- Thoughts of worthlessness or extreme guilt (not about being ill).
- Ability to think, concentrate, or make decisions is reduced.
- Frequent thoughts of death or suicide (with or without a specific plan), or suicide attempt.

It is estimated that 3 to 5% of adolescents in the United States have MDD. Depression occurs both in boys and in girls, although it is more prevalent in girls, and it is one of the most common disorders of adolescence. MDD frequently interferes with home, school, and family life, and often causes a high degree of family **stress**. **Suicide** is the third leading cause of death among teenagers, with approximately 50% of the deaths associated with depression.

Description

TADS was conducted at 13 academic and community clinics across the United States and enrolled 439 participants. The first participant entered TADS in the spring of 2000 and the last one in the summer of 2003. The initial findings were gathered from data from the first 12-week treatment period. The study showed that the antidepressant **fluoxetine** and **cognitive-behavioral therapy** combined produced the best success rate in treating depression in adolescents; 71% of participants receiving both medication and cognitive-behavioral therapy improved at the end of 12 weeks of treatment. Medication alone was also an effective treatment; 61% of participants improved; cognitive-behavioral therapy alone improved 44% of the cases; and 35% percent of the subjects improved with clinical management and placebo combined. Cognitive behavioral therapy taught the adolescent participant and their family skills to help relieve the depression.

TADS participants were randomly assigned to four treatment arms: 1) fluoxetine medication alone, 2) clinical management with placebo, 3) cognitive behavior therapy (CBT, talking with a therapist), and 4) combination of medication and CBT. The treatment phase was conducted in stages. Stage I lasted 12 weeks and included 6–14 visits to the clinic.

At the end of the first 12-week stage participants were advised of the treatment group to which they were assigned. Participants in the placebo group who did not improve during the first 12 weeks, or whose depression returned within 3 months, were offered any one of the other three treatments in the study—active medication, CBT, or both. The placebo condition was used only in stage I. During stage II (6 weeks, 2–6 clinic visits) and stage III (18 weeks, 3 clinic visits) participants received one of three treatments: 1) fluoxetine alone, 2) CBT alone, or 3) fluoxetine with CBT. Only participants who responded to one of the active treatments in stage I continued with treatment in stages II and III. Participants who responded well in stage I continued with their original treatment in stage II and later in stage III.

Fluoxetine is the generic name for Prozac, a selective **serotonin** reuptake inhibitor (SSRI). **SSRIs** primarily affect serotonin, a neurotransmitter in the **brain** that plays a pivotal role in depression. **Neurotransmitters** modulate mood, emotion, sleep, and appetite. Fluoxetine is the only medication approved by the FDA to treat depression in adolescents. However, since the TADS study, more recent studies suggest that antidepressant use in adolescents may be associated with a higher incidence of suicidal behavior and suggest close observation and caution.

CBT is a form of psychotherapy that emphasizes modifying everyday thoughts and behaviors, with the aim of positively influencing emotions. The precise therapeutic techniques vary according to particular client and issue, but commonly include keeping a diary of significant events and associated feelings, thoughts, and behaviors; questioning and testing assumptions or habits of thoughts that might be unhelpful and unrealistic; gradually facing activities that may have been avoided; and trying out new ways of behaving and reacting. Relaxation and distraction techniques are also commonly used.

Results

The study determined that the combination of fluoxetine with CBT was significantly better than fluoxetine alone or CBT alone in treating the symptoms of depression in adolescents. Fluoxetine alone was found to be a superior treatment to CBT alone. Clinically significant suicidal thinking, which was present in 29% of the sample at the beginning of the study, while improved significantly in all four treatment arms, was most improved in the fluoxetine with CBT group. The data suggest that the combination of fluoxetine with CBT offered the most favorable tradeoff between benefit and risk for adolescents with MDD.

Resources

BOOK

American Psychiatric Association. *Diagnostic and Statistical Manual of Mental Disorders.* 4th ed., text rev. Washington, DC: American Psychiatric Association, 2000.

PERIODICALS

Bhatia, S. K., and S. C. Bhatia. "Childhood and Adolescent Depression." *American Family Physician* 75, no. 1 (2007): 73–80.

Emslie, G., et al Columbia Suicidality Classification Group; TADS Team. "Treatment for Adolescents with Depression Study (TADS): Safety Results." *Journal of the American Academy of Child and Adolescent Psychiatry* 45, no. 12 (2006):1440–55.

March, J., S. Silva, and B. Vitiello. TADS Team. "The Treatment for Adolescents with Depression Study (TADS): Methods and Message at 12 Weeks." *Journal of the American Academy of Child and Adolescent Psychiatry* 45, no. 12 (2006): 1393–1403.

Simon, G. E. "The Antidepressant Quandary: Considering Suicide Risk when Treating Adolescent Depression." *New England Journal of Medicine* 355, no. 26 (2006): 2722–23.

Vitiello, B., et al. TADS Team. "Functioning and Quality of Life in the Treatment for Adolescents with Depression Study (TADS)." *Journal of the American Academy of Child and Adolescent Psychiatry* 45, no. 2 (2006): 1419–26.

ORGANIZATIONS

National Institute of Mental Health, 6001 Executive Blvd., Rm. 8184, MSC 9663, Bethesda, MD, 20892-9663, (301) 433-4513; TTY: (301) 443-8431, Fax: (301) 443-4279, (866) 615-6464; TTY: (866) 415-8051, nimhinfo@nih.gov http://www.nimh.nih.gov.

National Institutes of Health, 9000 Rockville Pike, Bethesda, MD, 20892, (301) 496-4000; TTY: (301) 402-9612, http://www.nih.gov.

Andrew J. Bean, PhD

Triazolam

Definition

Triazolam is a hypnotic drug. It is a member of the benzodiazepine family of drugs. In the United States, it is

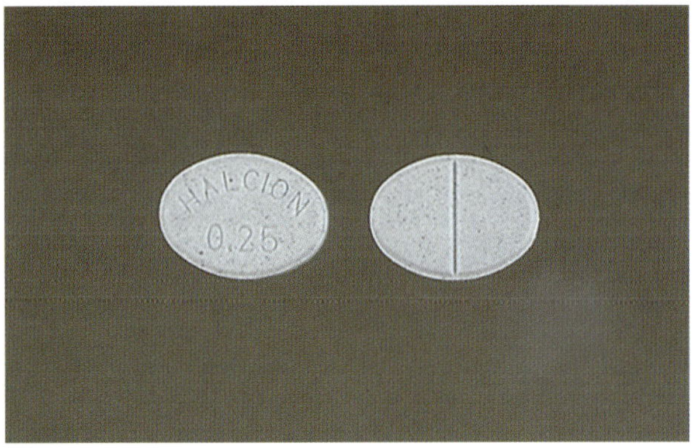

Halcion (triazolam), 25 mg. *(U.S. Drug Enforcement Administration)*

sold under the brand name Halcion as well as under its generic name.

Purpose

Triazolam is used for the short-term (generally seven to ten days) treatment of **insomnia**. Continued usage for more than two to three weeks requires a complete re-evaluation of the person receiving the drug.

Description

Triazolam increases the speed with which people achieve sleep, increases the duration of sleep, and decreases the likelihood of being awakened during sleep. The effect of triazolam decreases after 14 days of continuous use. In such cases, sleep patterns frequently return to those experienced prior to beginning use of triazolam; sometimes they are worse. This is called rebound insomnia.

Recommended dosage

The recommended dose of triazolam is 0.25 mg before going to bed. People with smaller body masses and older individuals can receive a comparable effect with 0.125 mg of triazolam. The lowest effective dosage of the drug should be used to minimize adverse reactions.

Precautions

Because of problems with rebound insomnia, patients should not receive triazolam for more than seven consecutive days. Daytime anxiety may occur after as few as 10 days of continuous usage. If this occurs, triazolam use should be discontinued.

Triazolam can cause serious birth defects. Women should not take this medicine if they are pregnant, think they may be pregnant, or are trying to get pregnant.

People using triazolam should exercise caution when driving or using power tools or machinery, due to the drug's sedative effects. People who use triazolam to reduce jet lag on long flights should be aware of a condition sometimes called "traveler's amnesia." This is a condition in which the traveler completes the flight and carries on with normal activities, including driving, but never fully awakens and has no memory of these activities. The period of **amnesia** may last for a few minutes or a few hours. Traveler's amnesia is most common when the traveler has had too little sleep or has been drinking alcohol.

KEY TERMS

Amnesia—A general medical term for loss of memory that is not due to ordinary forgetfulness. Amnesia can be caused by head injuries, brain disease, or epilepsy as well as by dissociation.

Euphoria—A feeling or state of well-being or elation.

Hypnotic—A type of medication that induces sleep.

Insomnia—A chronic inability to sleep or to remain asleep throughout the night.

Tachycardia—A pulse rate above 100 beats per minute.

Side effects

Triazolam has relatively few side effects. Those that have been reported include drowsiness, headache, dizziness, nervousness, a feeling of being light-headed, problems with coordination, nausea, and vomiting.

Less frequent side effects include euphoria, tachycardia, **fatigue**, confusion, impaired memory, muscle cramping, pain, and **depression**.

Interactions

Triazolam increases the effect of drugs and substances that depress the central nervous system. This class of drugs includes anesthetics, narcotics, **sedatives** and other sleeping pills, atropine, and alcohol.

Some drugs and foods increase the effects of triazolam and may also increase the chances of having side effects. These include cimetidine, isoniazid, oral contraceptives, and grapefruit juice.

Resources

BOOKS

Adams, Michael, and Norman Holland. *Core Concepts in Pharmacology*. 3rd ed. Upper Saddle River, NJ: 2010.

Foreman, John C., and Torben Johansen. *Textbook of Receptor Pharmacology*. 2nd ed. Boca Raton, FL: CRC Press, 2002.

Page, Clive P., et al. *Integrated Pharmacology*. 3rd ed. St. Louis, MO: Elsevier, 2006.

PERIODICALS

Mintzer, Miriam Z., et al. "Dose Effects of Triazolam on Brain Activity During Episodic Memory Encoding: A PET Study." *Psychopharmacology* 188, no. 4 (November 2006): 445–61.

Vansickel, Andrea R., Lon R. Hays, and Craig R. Rush. "Discriminative-Stimulus Effects of Triazolam in Women and Men." *American Journal of Drug and Alcohol Abuse* 32, no. 3 (2006): 329–49.

OTHER

Pfizer, Inc. *Halcion (Triazolam Tablets U.S.P.)*. http://www.pfizer.com/pfizer/download/uspi_halcion.pdf (accessed October 28, 2011).

WEBSITES

PubMed Health. "Triazolam." http://www.ncbi.nlm.nih.gov/pubmedhealth/PMH0000809 (accessed November 13, 2011).

ORGANIZATIONS

American Academy of Clinical Toxicology, 6728 Old McLean Village Drive, McLean, VA, 22101, (703) 556-9222, Fax: (703) 556-8729, admin@clintox.org, http://www.clintox.org.

American Academy of Family Physicians, 11400 Tomahawk Creek Parkway, Leawood, KS, 66211-2672, (913) 906-6000, (800) 274-2237, Fax: (913) 906-6075, contactcenter@aafp.org, http://www.aafp.org.

American Medical Association, 515 N State Street, Chicago, IL, 60610, (312) 464-5000, (800) 621-8335, http://www.ama-assn.org.

American Psychiatric Association, 1000 Wilson Blvd., Ste. 1825, Arlington, VA, 22209-3901, (703) 907-7300, apa@psych.org, http://www.psych.org.

American Society for Clinical Pharmacology and Therapeutics, 528 North Washington Street, Alexandria, VA, 22314, (703) 836-6981, http://www.ascpt.org.

American Society for Pharmacology and Experimental Therapeutics, 9650 Rockville Pike, Bethesda, MD, 20814-3995, (301) 634-7060, Fax: (301) 634-7061, http://www.aspet.org.

L. Fleming Fallon, Jr., MD, Dr.P.H.
Ruth A. Wienclaw, PhD

Trichotillomania

Definition

Individuals with trichotillomania repetitively pull out their own hair. Trichotillomania is an impulse-control disorder, although some researchers view it as a type of affective or **obsessive-compulsive disorder**. Nail-biting, skin-picking, and thumb-sucking are considered to be related conditions.

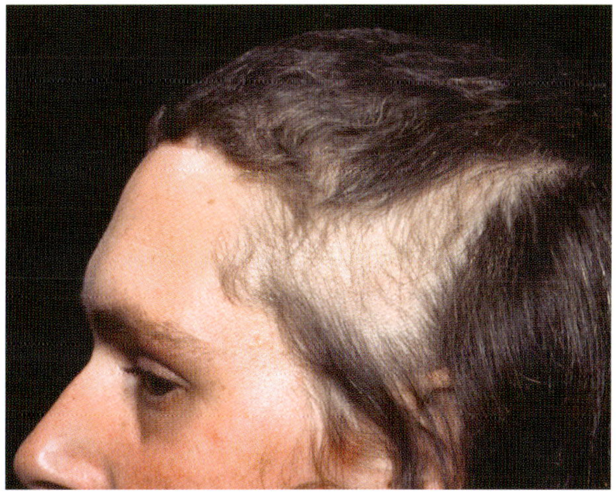

The bald patch on this man's scalp shows the effects of trichotillomania. *(© Custom Medical Stock Photo, Inc. Reproduced by permission.)*

Demographics

Once regarded as rare, trichotillomania is now considered more common, affecting 1–4% of people in the general population. When the tension-release requirement is excluded, trichotillomania occurs in adult females (3.4%) more often than adult males (1.5%). Among children, both genders are affected equally. Nonclinical levels of hair-pulling behavior may be as high as 15.3% among university students.

Description

Trichotillomania involves hair pulling episodes that result in noticeable hair loss. Although any area of the body can be a target, the most common areas are the scalp, followed by the eyelashes, eyebrows, and pubic region. Hair-pulling can occur without the individual's awareness but is frequently preceded by a sense of increasing tension and followed by a sense of relief or gratification, common features of behavioral **addiction** disorders. The resulting hair loss can be a source of embarrassment or shame. Because of a tendency to hide symptoms and because professionals are relatively unfamiliar with the disorder, individuals either may not seek or are not offered treatment. Untreated trichotillomania can result in impaired social functioning, reduced quality of life, and medical complications.

Causes and symptoms

Causes

Psychoanalytic theories explain compulsive hair-pulling behavior as a way of dealing with unconscious conflicts or childhood **trauma** (such as **sexual abuse**). Behavioral theories assume that symptoms are learned, that a child may imitate a parent who engages in hair-pulling. The behavior may also be learned independently if it serves a purpose. For example, hair-pulling may begin as a response to **stress** and then develop into a habit. Biological theories address a genetic basis. For instance, people with trichotillomania often have a first-degree relative with an obsessive-compulsive spectrum disorder.

Researchers have also evaluated similarities between trichotillomania and **Tourette syndrome**. One group at Duke noted that the parent of a patient with Tourette syndrome in one of their studies displayed symptoms of trichotillomania. The researchers identified a link between mutations in a specific gene and the incidence of Tourette syndrome among the families in this study. Intrigued because the parent carried the mutation but did not exhibit symptoms of Tourette, the researchers completed a study analyzing the potential link between carrying the gene and having trichotillomania. They confirmed a link between the hair-pulling behavior and the mutant form of the gene, called SLITRK1, which is involved in the formation of connections among **brain** cells (called neurons). Two mutations in this gene appear to be linked to trichotilloma-nia, and the researchers suggested that the mutant protein that results may cause missed connections among neurons, leading to the hair-pulling urges.

Symptoms

According to the **diagnosis** of trichotillomania:

- noticeable hair loss (alopecia) due to recurrent hair-pulling
- tension immediately before hair-pulling, or when attempting to resist hair-pulling
- reduction of tension, or a feeling of pleasure or gratification, immediately following hair-pulling
- significant distress or impairment in social, occupa-tional, or other important areas of functioning

In addition, the *DSM-IV-TR* requires that the patient's hair-pulling not be due to another medical or mental disorder. The tension-release requirement is controversial because 17% of people who otherwise qualify for this diagnosis do not experience this.

Symptoms usually emerge in early adolescence. Episodes may last a few minutes or a few hours during periods of stress or relaxation. Those with trichotilloma-nia may prefer hairs with unique textures or qualities. The pulling may include rituals, such as twirling hair off or examining the root. Half of those individuals with trichotillomania engage in oral behaviors—running hair across the lips or through the teeth, biting off the root (trichophagy), or eating hair (trichophagia). They usually try to control their behavior in the presence of others and may hide the affected areas. Symptoms may come and go for weeks, months, or years at a time.

Diagnosis

Other possible causes of symptoms must first be ruled out. Hair loss may have a medical cause, such as a dermatological condition. Hair-pulling may have another psychological cause, such as a delusion or **hallucination** in **schizophrenia**.

If individuals deny symptoms, hair-pulling behav-ior can be assessed by objective measures such as the presence of short, broken hairs or damaged follicles. Some **psychological assessment** instruments are also available. These include the Massachusetts General Hospital Hair Pulling Scale (MGH-HPS), a seven-item, self-report measure of the symptoms of hair-pulling. Also the Alopecia Rating assesses the level of hair loss, and the Trichotillomania Interference Checklist interviews patients to assess the effects of pathological hair-pulling on various quality-of-life and health parameters.

Severity of symptoms is also important. Twisting or playing with hair when nervous does not qualify as trichotillomania. If symptoms are minor or undetectable, a diagnosis should be given only if the individual expresses significant distress. Children should be given the diagno-sis only if symptoms persist because hair-pulling may be a temporary phase, much like thumb-sucking.

Treatment

Treatment usually starts by determining the current frequency and severity of symptoms. This information, which serves as a measure of progress, is gathered by (a) self-report, (b) reports from significant others, (c) objec-tive measures, such as saving pulled hairs, videotapes, or measuring areas of hair loss, or (d) a combination of these methods.

Primarily, three categories of therapy have been used in the treatment of trichotillomania:

- Psychoanalysis focuses on childhood experiences and unresolved conflicts during early development.
- Medications. Those typically used are antidepressants with serotonergic properties (also used with obsessive-compulsive disorders). Clomipramine (Anafranil) has proven most effective. The **selective serotonin reuptake inhibitors** (SSRIs) have had mixed results. Some researchers recommend low doses of antipsychotic drugs (neuroleptics) in conjunction with SSRIs. Medications are usually combined with behavior therapy.

KEY TERMS

Alopecia—Hair loss.

Selective serotonin reuptake inhibitors (SSRIs)—Commonly prescribed drugs for treating depression. SSRIs affect the chemicals that nerve cells in the brain use to send messages to one another. These chemical messengers (neurotransmitters) are released by one nerve cell and taken up by others. Neurotransmitters not taken up by other nerve cells are taken up by the same cells that released them. This process is termed "reuptake." SSRIs work by inhibiting the reuptake of serotonin, an action that allows more serotonin to be taken up by other nerve cells.

Serotonergic—Containing, activating, or otherwise involving serotonin, which is a chemical that aids in the transmission of nerve impulses.

Trichobezoar—A hairball that results from a buildup of swallowed hairs becoming lodged in the digestive system.

Trichophagia—Eating hair.

Trichophagy—Biting hair.

- Behavior therapy. Habit-reversal training is the most accepted approach. It teaches individuals to monitor their hair-pulling and substitute it for healthier behaviors. Alternative forms of behavior therapy include biofeedback and hypnosis.

Prognosis

The effects of trichotillomania can be very serious. Associated feelings of shame may result in avoidance of social situations; chewing hair can result in dental erosion; and eating hair may result in hairballs (trichobezoars) becoming lodged in the stomach or large intestine, which can lead to anemia, abdominal pain, nausea and vomiting, hematemesis (vomiting blood), or bowel obstruction or perforation.

Studies show low success rates with medications and traditional **psychoanalysis**. Behavioral therapy has reported long-term success rates of 90% or more. Follow-up sessions are encouraged to prevent **relapse**. A major issue in prognosis is whether an individual receives treatment. Professionals may not recognize or know how to treat trichotillomania effectively. Conversely, individuals with the disorder may be too embarrassed to address their symptoms.

Prevention

No specific information is available regarding prevention.

Resources

BOOKS

American Psychiatric Association. *Diagnostic and Statistical Manual of Mental Disorders*. 4th ed., text rev. Washington, DC: American Psychiatric Publishing, 2000.

Franklin, Martin E., and David F. Tolin. *Treating Trichotillomania: Cognitive-Behavioral Therapy for Hairpulling and Related Problems*. New York: Springer: 2010.

Grant, Jon E., and Dan J. Stein, Douglas Woods, and Nancy J. Keuthen. *Trichotillomania, Skin Picking, and Other Body-Focused Repetitive Behaviors*. Washington, DC: American Psychiatric Publishing: 2011.

PERIODICALS

Dia, David A. "'I Can't Stop Pulling my Hair!' Using Numbing Cream as an Adjunct Treatment for Trichotillomania." *Health and Social Work* 33, no. 2 (2008): 155.

Edson, Aubrey L., Martin E. Franklin, and Jennifer B. Freeman. "Behavior Therapy for Pediatric Trichotillomania: Exploring the Effects of Age on Treatment Outcome." *Child and Adolescent Psychiatry and Mental Health* 4 (2010): 18.

Parakh, Preeti, and Mona Srivastava. "The Many Faces of Trichotillomania." *International Journal of Trichology* 2, no. 1 (2010): 50.

WEBSITES

Duke Center for Human Genetics. "Trichotillomania." 2005. http://www.chg.duke.edu/diseases/ttm.html (accessed October 28, 2011).

Duke Medicine News and Communications. "Hair-pulling Disorder Caused by Faulty Gene in Some Families." September 27, 2006. Available online at DukeHealth.org: http://www.dukehealth.org/news/9887 (accessed November 10, 2011).

ORGANIZATIONS

Trichotillomania Learning Center, Inc, 207 McPherson Street, Ste. H, Santa Cruz, CA, 95060, (831) 457-1004, Fax: (831) 426-4383, info@trich.org, http://www.trich.org.

Sandra L. Friedrich, MA
Emily Jane Willingham, PhD

Trifluoperazine

Definition

Trifluoperazine is a phenothiazine antipsychotic agent. In the United States, this drug is sold under the brand name Stelazine.

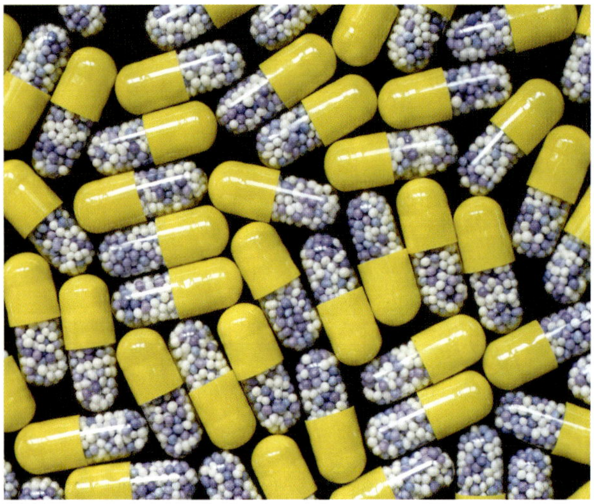

Stelazine (trifluoperazine), 2 mg. *(© Adam Hart-Davis/Photo Researchers, Inc.)*

KEY TERMS

Anxiety—An abnormal and overwhelming sense of apprehension and fear often marked by physiological signs (as sweating, tension, and increased pulse), by doubt concerning the reality and nature of a threat, and by self-doubt about the capacity to cope with an issue.

Hallucination—An occurrence when a person sees or hears things that are not really there. Hallucinations can result from nervous system abnormalities, mental disorders, or the use of certain drugs.

Schizophrenia—A major mental illness marked by psychotic symptoms, including hallucinations, delusions, and severe disruptions in thinking.

Purpose

Trifluoperazine is a drug used to treat **schizophrenia**. It may also be used to treat anxiety in persons who have not had success with other medications.

Description

Trifluoperazine is an effective agent in treating symptoms of psychotic behavior. When used for the treatment of **schizophrenia**, trifluoperazine reduces the symptoms of emotional withdrawal, anxiety, tension, hallucinations, and paranoia.

Recommended dosage

The dosage of trifluoperazine should be adjusted to the lowest level needed to control symptoms. The drug may be given orally or by intramuscular injection (a shot).

A useful initial dosage of trifluoperazine for psychotic adults is 2–5 mg two times each day. A common total dosage is 15–20 mg per day. Some people may require up to 40 mg or more per day. When using deep intramuscular injection, 1–2 mg every four to six hours is usually sufficient to control symptoms within 24 hours. Total intramuscular trifluoperazine should not exceed 10 mg per day.

Control of psychotic symptoms in children between the ages of 6 and 12 can usually be achieved with 1–2 mg per day, given in 1 mg increments. Trifluoperazine is not recommended for use in children younger than 6.

Precautions

Trifluoperazine may cause bone marrow and blood disorders. It has also been associated with sudden cardiac death (heart attack). Some newborns born to mothers who took trifluoperazine during pregnancy displayed symptoms of withdrawal, including increased agitation and trouble breathing; women who are pregnant or planning to become pregnant should not take trifluoperazine.

Trifluoperazine is not approved by the U.S. Food and Drug Administration (FDA) for use in treating the behavioral symptoms of dementia in elderly patients. Patients taking trifluoperazine for this purpose are at increased risk of death during treatment.

Trifluoperazine increases the level of prolactin in the blood, a hormone that stimulates the mammary glands in the breast. This is a potential problem for people with a personal or family history of breast cancer and may increase the risk of breast cancer. For this reason and the other serious side effects associated with trifluoperazine, health professionals must carefully evaluate the benefits and risks of the drug before administering it.

Side effects

Relatively common side effects that accompany trifluoperazine include drowsiness, dizziness, rash, dry mouth, **insomnia**, **fatigue**, muscular weakness, anorexia, blurred vision, some loss of muscular control, and amenorrhea (lack of menstruation) in women.

Dystonia (difficulty walking or moving) may occur with trifluoperazine use. This condition may subside in 24 to 48 hours even when the person continues taking the drug, and it usually disappears when trifluoperazine is discontinued.

Trifluoperazine use may lead to the development of symptoms that resemble Parkinson's disease. These symptoms may include a tight or mask-like expression

QUESTIONS TO ASK YOUR DOCTOR

- What kind of changes can I expect to see or feel with this medication?
- Does it matter what time of day I take this medication?
- Should I take this medication with or without food?
- What are the side effects associated with this medication?
- Will this medication interact or interfere with other medications I am currently taking?
- What symptoms or adverse effects are important enough that I should seek immediate treatment?

on the face, drooling, tremors, pill-rolling motions in the hands, cogwheel rigidity (abnormal rigidity in muscles characterized by jerky movements when the muscle is passively stretched), and a shuffling gait. Taking the anti-Parkinson drugs **benztropine** mesylate or **trihexyphenidyl** hydrochloride along with the trifluoperazine usually controls these symptoms.

Trifluoperazine has the potential to produce a serious side effect called **tardive dyskinesia**. This syndrome consists of involuntary, uncoordinated movements that may appear late in therapy and may not disappear even after the drug is discontinued. Tardive dyskinesia involves involuntary movements of the tongue, jaw, mouth, face, or other groups of skeletal muscles. The incidence of tardive dyskinesia increases with age and with increasing dosage of trifluoperazine. Women are at greater risk than men for developing tardive dyskinesia. There is no known effective treatment for tardive dyskinesia, although gradual (but rarely complete) improvement may occur over a long period.

An occasionally reported side effect of trifluoperazine is **neuroleptic malignant syndrome**. This is a complicated and potentially fatal condition characterized by muscle rigidity, high fever, alterations in mental status, and cardiac symptoms such as irregular pulse or blood pressure, sweating, tachycardia (fast heartbeat), and arrhythmias (irregular heartbeat). People who think they may be experiencing any such side effects from this or any other medication should tell their physicians immediately.

Interactions

Trifluoperazine may reduce the effectiveness of oral anticoagulant (blood-thinning) drugs. It should not be taken with the drug metoclopramide (Reglan). The blood concentration of the drug phenytoin is increased by trifluoperazine, which may lead to phenytoin toxicity. **Propranolol** increases theconcentration of trifluoperazine. The blood pressure–lowering effects of guanethidine may be diminished by trifluoperazine. The use of diuretics with trifluoperazine may cause a sudden decrease in blood pressure often accompanied by dizziness due to a change in body position (known as orthostatic hypotension).

Trifluoperazine increases the effect of drugs and substances that depress the central nervous system. These drugs include anesthetics, opiates, **barbiturates**, atropine, and alcohol. These substances should be avoided or used sparingly by people taking trifluoperazine.

Several herbal supplements may interact with trifluoperazine; patients should inform their doctors of all drugs and supplements they are currently taking.

Resources

BOOKS

Albers, Lawrence J., MD, Rhoda K. Hahn, MD, and Christopher Reist, MD. *Handbook of Psychiatric Drugs.* Laguna Hills, CA: Current Clinical Strategies Publishing, 2010.

American Society of Health-System Pharmacists. *AHFS Drug Information 2011.* Bethesda: American Society of Health-System Pharmacists, 2011.

Graham, George. *The Disordered Mind: An Introduction to Philosophy of Mind and Mental Illness.*New York, NY: Routledge, 2010.

Holland, Leland Norman, and Michael Patrick Adams. *Core Concepts in Pharmacology,*3rd ed. New York, NY: Prentice Hall, 2011.

North, Carol, and Sean Yutzy. *Goodwin and Guze's Psychiatric Diagnosis.* New York, NY: Oxford University Press, 2010.

Preston, John D., John H. O'Neal, and Mary C. Talaga. *Handbook of Clinical Psychopharmacology for Therapists,* 6th ed. Oakland, CA: New Harbinger Publications, 2011.

WEBSITES

PubMed Health. "Trifluoperazine." http://www.ncbi.nlm.nih.gov/pubmedhealth/PMH0000585 (accessed November 13, 2011).

ORGANIZATIONS

American Psychiatric Association, 1000 Wilson Boulevard, Suite 1825, Arlington, VA, 22209, (703) 907-7300, apa@psych.org, http://www.psych.org.

Mental Health America, 2000 N. Beauregard Street, 6th Floor, Alexandria, VA, 22311, (703) 684-7722, (800) 969-6642, Fax: (703) 684-5968, http://www1.nmha.org.

National Alliance on Mental Illness (NAMI), Colonial Place Three, 2107 Wilson Blvd., Suite 300, Arlington, VA, 22201, (703) 524-7600, (800) 950-NAMI (6264), Fax: (703) 524-9094, http://www.nami.org/Hometemplate.cfm.

National Institute of Mental Health (NIMH), 6001 Executive Boulevard, Room 8184, MSC 9663, Bethesda, MD, 20892, (301) 443-4513, (866) 615-6464, Fax: (301) 443-4279, nimhinfo@nih.gov, http://www.nimh.nih.gov/index.shtml.

U.S. Food and Drug Administration, 10903 New Hampshire Ave., Silver Spring, MD, 20993-0002, (888) INFO-FDA (463-6332), http://www.fda.gov.

L. Fleming Fallon, Jr., MD, Dr.P.H.
Ruth A. Wienclaw, Ph.D.
Laura Jean Cataldo, RN, Ed.D.

Trihexyphenidyl

Definition

Trihexyphenidyl is classified as an anti-parkinsonian agent. It is sold in the United States under the brand name Artane and is also available under its generic name.

Purpose

Trihexyphenidyl is used to treat a group of side effects (called parkinsonian side effects) that includes tremors, difficulty walking, and slack muscle tone. These side effects may occur in patients who are taking antipsychotic medications used to treat mental disorders such as **schizophrenia**.

Description

Some medicines, called antipsychotic drugs, that are used to treat schizophrenia and other mental disorders can cause side effects that are similar to the symptoms of Parkinson's disease. Such patients do not have Parkinson's disease, but they may experience shaking in muscles while at rest, difficulty with voluntary movements, and poor muscle tone. These symptoms are similar to the symptoms of Parkinson's disease.

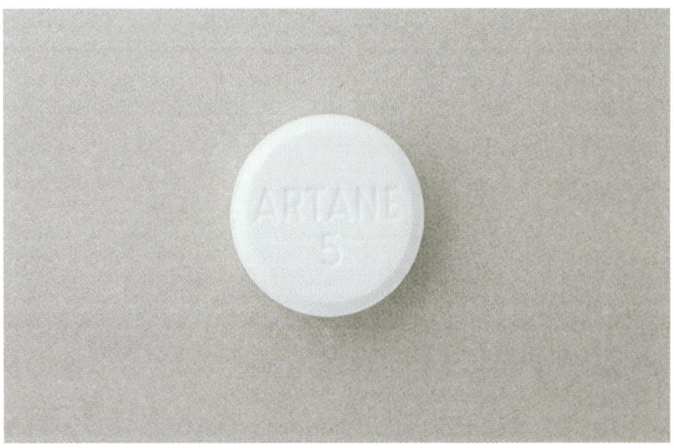

Artane (trihexyphenidyl), 5 mg. *(© Custom Medical Stock Photo, Inc. Reproduced by permission.)*

One way to eliminate these undesirable side effects is to stop taking the antipsychotic medicine. Unfortunately, the symptoms of the original mental disorder usually come back, so in most cases simply stopping the antipsychotic medication is not a reasonable option. Some drugs such as trihexyphenidyl that control the symptoms of Parkinson's disease also control the parkinsonian side effects of antipsychotic medicines.

Trihexyphenidyl works by restoring the chemical balance between **dopamine** and acetylcholine, two neurotransmitter chemicals in the **brain**. Taking trihexyphenidyl along with the antipsychotic medicine helps to control symptoms of the mental disorder, while reducing parkinsonian side effects. Trihexyphenidyl is in the same family of drugs (commonly known as anticholinergic drugs) as **biperiden** and **benztropine**.

Recommended dosage

Trihexyphenidyl is available in 2 mg and 5 mg tablets and an elixir containing 2 mg per teaspoonful. For the treatment of tremors, poor muscle tone, and similar side effects, trihexyphenidyl should be started at a dose of 1 to 2 mg orally two to three times daily or as needed, to a maximum daily dose of 15 mg per day. Parkinson's-like side effects caused by antipsychotic drugs may come and go, so trihexyphenidyl may not be needed on a regular basis. Trihexyphenidyl may also be prescribed to prevent these side effects before they actually occur. This is called prophylactic (preventative) therapy.

Precautions

Trihexyphenidyl should never be used in children under age three. It should be used cautiously and with close physician supervision in older children and in people over age 60. Trihexyphenidyl, like all anticholinergic drugs, decreases sweating and the body's ability to cool itself. People who are unaccustomed to being outside in hot weather should take care to stay as cool as possible and drink extra fluids. People who are chronically ill, have a central nervous system disease, or who work outside during hot weather may need to avoid taking trihexyphenidyl.

People who have the following medical problems may experience increased negative side effects when taking trihexyphenidyl. People with these problems should discuss their conditions with their physicians before starting the drug:

- glaucoma, especially closed-angle glaucoma
- intestinal obstruction
- prostate enlargement
- urinary bladder obstruction

Although rare, some patients experience euphoria while taking trihexyphenidyl and may abuse it for this reason. Euphoria can occur at doses only two to four times the normal daily dose. Patients with a history of drug abuse should be observed carefully for trihexyphenidyl abuse.

Side effects

Although trihexyphenidyl helps to control the side effects of antipsychotic drugs, it can produce side effects of its own. A person taking trihexyphenidyl may have some of the following reactions, which may vary in intensity:

- dry mouth
- dry skin
- blurred vision
- nausea or vomiting
- constipation
- disorientation
- drowsiness
- irritability
- increased heart rate
- urinary retention

Dry mouth, if severe to the point of causing difficulty speaking or swallowing, may be managed by reducing or temporarily discontinuing trihexyphenidyl. Chewing sugarless gum or sucking on sugarless candy may also help to increase the flow of saliva. Some artificial saliva products may give temporary relief.

Men with prostate enlargement may be especially prone to urinary retention. Symptoms of this problem include having difficulty starting a urine flow and more difficulty passing urine than usual. This side effect may be severe and require discontinuation of the drug. Urinary retention may require catheterization. People who think they may be experiencing any side effects from this or any other medication should tell their physicians.

Patients who take an overdose of trihexyphenidyl are treated with forced vomiting, removal of stomach contents and stomach washing, activated charcoal, and respiratory support if needed. They are also given physostigmine, an antidote for anticholinergic drug poisoning.

Interactions

When drugs such as trihexyphenidyl are taken with **antidepressants** such as **amitriptyline**, **imipramine**, **trimipramine**, **desipramine**, **nortriptyline**, **protriptyline**, **amoxapine**, and **doxepin** or with many antihistamines that also have anticholinergic properties, the effects and side effects of trihexyphenidyl are usually intensified.

Drugs such as trihexyphenidyl decrease the speed with which food moves through the stomach and intestines. Because of this, the absorption of other drugs taken may be enhanced by trihexyphenidyl. Patients receiving trihexyphenidyl should be alert to unusual responses to other drugs they might be taking and report any changes to their physician.

Resources

BOOKS

American Society of Health-System Pharmacists. *AHFS Drug Information 2008*. Bethesda, MD: American Society of Health-System Pharmacists, 2008.

PERIODICALS

Nappo, Solange Aparecida, et al. "Trihexyphenidyl (Artane): A Brazilian Study of Its Abuse." *Substance Use and Misuse* 40, no. 4 (2005): 473–82.

Jack Raber, Pharm.D.
Ruth A. Wienclaw, PhD

Trilafon *see* **Perphenazine**

Trileptal *see* **Oxcarbazepine**

Trimipramine

Definition

Trimipramine is an oral tricyclic antidepressant. It is sold in the United States under the brand name Surmontil.

Purpose

Trimipramine is used primarily to treat **depression** and to treat the combination of symptoms of anxiety and depression. Like other **antidepressants** of this chemical and pharmacological class, trimipramine has also been used in limited numbers of patients to treat **panic disorder**, **obsessive-compulsive disorder**, **attention deficit**

hyperactivity disorder, **enuresis** (bed-wetting), eating disorders such as **bulimia nervosa**, **cocaine** dependency, and the depressive phase of bipolar (manic-depressive) disorder, although not all of these uses are approved by the U.S. Food and Drug Administration (FDA).

Description

Tricyclic antidepressants act to change the balance of naturally occurring chemicals in the **brain** that regulate the transmission of nerve impulses between cells. Trimipramine acts primarily to increase the concentration of norepinephrine and **serotonin** (both chemical messengers in nerve cells) and, to a lesser extent, to block the action of another brain chemical, acetylcholine. Trimipramine shares most of the properties of other tricyclic antidepressants, such as **amitriptyline**, **amoxapine**, **clomipramine**, **desipramine**, **imipramine**, **nortriptyline**, and **protriptyline**. Studies comparing trimipramine with these other drugs have shown that trimipramine is no more or less effective than other antidepressants of its type. Its choice for treatment is as much a function of physician preference as any other factor.

The therapeutic effects of trimipramine, like other antidepressants, appear slowly. Maximum benefit is often not evident for at least two weeks after starting the drug. People taking trimipramine should be aware of this and continue taking the drug as directed even if they do not see immediate improvement.

Recommended dosage

The recommended dosage can vary based on the patient's age and situation. The initial dose of trimipramine for depression in an adult begins at 75 mg per day. This dosage can be increased as necessary, usually plateauing at a maximum of 200 mg a day. For patients who are hospitalized, the dose may exceed the 200 mg per day cutoff. This drug is not recommended for children and teenagers, but if it is prescribed, the recommended dosage for teenagers is an initial 50 mg per day that may be gradually increased by the doctor to a typical maximum of 100 mg per day. For children age 12 years and younger, the dose will be determined by the doctor. For the elderly, the initial dose is 50 mg per day, which can be increased as the doctor deems necessary, but typically no higher than 100 mg per day.

Precautions

Like all tricyclic antidepressants, trimipramine should be used cautiously and with close physician supervision in people, especially the elderly, who have benign prostatic hypertrophy, urinary retention, and glaucoma, especially angle-closure glaucoma (the most severe form). Before starting treatment, people with these conditions should discuss the relative risks and benefits of treatment with their doctors to help determine if trimipramine is the right antidepressant for them.

Some studies have shown that children and teenagers up to age 24 who take antidepressants such as trimipramine may have an increased risk of committing self-harm or **suicide**. Children under the age of 18 should not normally take this drug; if a child is prescribed the drug, parents or caregivers should closely monitor the child, as serious symptoms can develop suddenly. Any signs that a patient is considering self-harm or suicide warrants an immediate call to the doctor. These signs might include worsening depression, panic attacks, difficulty falling asleep, irritability, planning to engage in self-harm or to attempt suicide, or abnormal excitement.

Trimipramine may increase the possibility of having **seizures**. Patients should tell their physician if they have a history of seizures, including seizures brought on by the abuse of drugs or alcohol. These people should use trimipramine only with caution and be closely monitored by their physician. Trimipramine may also increase heart rate and **stress** on the heart. It may be dangerous for people with cardiovascular disease, especially those who have recently had a heart attack, to take this drug or other antidepressants in the same pharmacological class. In rare cases where patients with cardiovascular disease must receive trimipramine, they should be monitored closely for cardiac rhythm disturbances and signs of cardiac stress or damage.

A common problem with tricyclic antidepressants is sedation (drowsiness, lack of physical and mental alertness). This side effect is especially noticeable early in therapy. In most patients, sedation decreases or disappears entirely with time, but until then patients taking trimipramine should not perform hazardous activities requiring mental alertness or coordination. The sedative effect is increased when trimipramine is taken with other central nervous system depressants, such as alcoholic beverages, sleeping medications, other **sedatives**, or antihistamines. It may be dangerous to take trimipramine in combination with these substances.

Side effects

Trimipramine shares side effects common to all tricyclic antidepressants, including dry mouth, constipation, urinary retention, increased heart rate, sedation, irritability, dizziness, and decreased coordination. As with most side effects associated with tricyclic antidepressants, the intensity is highest at the beginning of therapy and tends to decrease with continued use.

Dry mouth, if severe to the point of causing difficulty speaking or swallowing, may be managed by dosage reduction or temporary discontinuation of the drug. Patients may also chew sugarless gum or suck sugarless candy to increase the flow of saliva. Some artificial saliva products may give temporary relief.

Men with prostate enlargement who take trimipramine may be especially likely to have problems with urinary retention. Symptoms include having difficulty starting a urine flow and more difficulty than usual passing urine. In most cases, urinary retention is managed with dose reduction or by switching to another type of antidepressant. In extreme cases, patients may require treatment with bethanechol, a drug that reverses this particular side effect. People who think they may be experiencing any side effects from this or any other medication should tell their physicians.

Interactions

Dangerously high blood pressure has resulted from the combination of tricyclic antidepressants, such as trimipramine, and members of another class of antidepressants known as **monoamine oxidase inhibitors (MAOIs)**. Because of this, trimipramine should never be taken in combination with **MAOIs**. Patients taking any MAOIs, for example **phenelzine** (Nardil) or **tranylcypromine** (Parnate), should stop taking the MAOI and wait at least 14 days before starting trimipramine or any other tricyclic antidepressant. The same holds true when discontinuing trimipramine and starting an MAOI.

Trimipramine may decrease the blood pressure–lowering effects of **clonidine**. Patients who take both drugs should be monitored for loss of blood pressure control and the dose of clonidine increased as needed.

The sedative effects of trimipramine are increased by other central nervous system depressants such as alcohol, sedatives, sleeping medications, or medications used for other mental disorders such as **schizophrenia**. The anticholinergic effects of trimipramine are additive with other anticholinergic drugs such as **benztropine**, **biperiden**, **trihexyphenidyl**, and antihistamines.

Resources

BOOKS

Stahl, Stephen. *The Prescriber's Guide: Antidepressants; Stahl's Essential Psychopharmacology*. 4th edition. New York: Cambridge University Press: 2011.

WEBSITES

PubMed Health. "Trimipramine." U.S. National Library of Medicine. http://www.ncbi.nlm.nih.gov/pubmedhealth/PMH0000191 (accessed November 12, 2011).

ORGANIZATIONS

American Society of Health-System Pharmacists, 7272 Wisconsin Ave., Bethesda, MD, 20814, (866) 279-0681, custserv@ashp.org, http://www.ashp.org.

U.S. National Library of Medicine, 8600 Rockville Pike, Bethesda, MD, 20894, http://www.nlm.nih.gov.

United States Food and Drug Administration, 10903 New Hampshire Ave., Silver Spring, MD, 20993, (888) 463-6332, http://www.fda.gov.

Jack Raber, Pharm.D.
Emily Jane Willingham, PhD

Trisomy 21 *see* **Down syndrome**

Tryptophan *see* **Serotonin**

U

Undifferentiated somatoform disorder

Definition

Undifferentiated somatoform disorder occurs when a person has physical complaints for more than six months that cannot be attributed to a medical condition. If there is a medical condition present, the complaints must be far more severe than can be accounted for by the presence of the medical problem.

Demographics

Undifferentiated somatoform disorder is relatively common. It is estimated that between 4% and 11% of the population experience the disorder at some time in their lives. Women are more likely than men to have undifferentiated somatoform disorder, as are the elderly and people of lower socioeconomic backgrounds. Young women who have low socioeconomic status are the most likely group to have undifferentiated somatoform disorder. Fifty percent of the people with this disorder have other psychological or psychiatric disorders as well, such as anxiety or depression.

Description

The physical complaints that are expressed by people with undifferentiated somatoform disorder are many and varied. The similarity between all physical complaints associated with undifferentiated somatoform disorder is an absence of medical evidence for the symptoms or for their severity.

The physical complaints usually begin or worsen when the patient is under **stress**. People with undifferentiated somatoform disorder experience problems functioning in their daily lives due to the physical symptoms that they experience. Seeing multiple doctors in an effort to find a physical cause for the reported symptoms is typical of people with this disorder. Undifferentiated somatoform disorder is also sometimes referred to as somatization syndrome.

Causes and symptoms

The symptoms of undifferentiated somatoform disorder vary widely from person to person. Some of the most common physical complaints are pain, **fatigue**, appetite loss, and various gastrointestinal problems. The physical complaints generally last for long periods. Patients with undifferentiated somatoform disorder tend to complain of many different physical problems over time.

No matter what symptoms a person complains about, the overarching characteristic of the complaints is that no physical reason can be found for them. Laboratory tests and thorough examinations by doctors will reveal no medical reason for the pains or problems the person is having. The physical problems, however, persist after the person has been told no explanation can be found.

The causes of undifferentiated somatoform disorder are not clear. Some experts believe that problems in the family when the affected person was a child may be related to the development of this disorder. **Depression** and stress are thought to be other possible causes. In people who worry about even minor medical conditions, paying obsessive attention to any minor changes or sensations that their bodies experience may be a factor in developing the disorder. They give the feelings undue weight and worry unnecessarily about them.

Diagnosis

A person with undifferentiated somatoform disorder usually begins by visiting physicians looking for treatments for physical complaints. Later, he or she may be referred to a mental health professional. Referring physicians may continue to see the patient, however, so that a trusting relationship can be established and so the patient does not continue to bounce from doctor to doctor.

Mental health professionals use the handbook called the ***Diagnostic and Statistical Manual of Mental Disorders*** to diagnose mental disorders. The book lists diagnostic criteria for undifferentiated somatoform disorder and requires that the following conditions be met in order for the clinician to diagnose this disorder:

- There must be no underlying medical cause evident that could explain the patient's physical complaints. If there is a medical condition that could be related to the complaints, the symptoms reported must be far worse than any that could be explained by the existing medical problems.
- The unexplained physical symptoms must persist for at least six months.
- The symptoms must cause problems in the patient's daily life or relationships or interfere with the patient achieving his or her goals.
- There cannot be another mental disorder that accounts for the complaints.
- The patient cannot knowingly make false complaints of physical distress.

Somatization disorder

Somatization disorder is very similar to undifferentiated somatoform disorder, and the two can be easily confused. The symptoms are the same, but the diagnostic criteria are much more specific for somatization disorder. To be diagnosed with somatization disorder, the patient must have four different pain symptoms, two gastrointestinal symptoms, one sexual symptom, and one pseudoneurological symptom. These symptoms can occur at different times. The symptoms must be present for several years and must have begun before the patient was 30 years old. Just as with undifferentiated somatoform disorder, the complaints must not be traceable to any medical cause.

Hypochondriasis

Patients with hypochondriasis usually have a specific **diagnosis** in mind when they visit a doctor, unlike most patients with undifferentiated somatoform disorder who have complaints but do not have a cause in mind.

Treatment

Most treatments of undifferentiated somatoform disorder focus on treating any underlying psychological problems or stresses that may be causing the disorder. When the disorder occurs in conjunction with another mental health problem such as depression, treating that problem often helps to resolve or lessen the symptoms of undifferentiated somatoform disorder. Some studies indicate that **antidepressants** are effective in treating this disorder. Patients also may benefit from programs intended to teach them how to manage stress and to understand the correlation between psychological stressors and physiological symptoms. These programs also teach people how to cope with criticism and how to stop negative behavior patterns.

Prognosis

For many people, undifferentiated somatoform disorder is a lifelong disorder. Often, the physical complaints increase or decrease in relation to stressors in the affected person's life. Many people with this disorder are eventually diagnosed with another mental disorder or with a legitimate medical problem. For some people, treatment can be successful at lessening or completely resolving symptoms.

Prevention

There are no known ways to prevent undifferentiated somatoform disorder; it is possible, however, for people who appear to be developing the disorder to enroll in programs designed to teach them coping strategies and about the relationship between psychological factors and physical symptoms.

Resources

BOOKS

American Psychiatric Association. *Diagnostic and Statistical Manual of Mental Disorders*. 4th ed., text rev. Washington, DC: American Psychiatric Publishing, 2000.

PERIODICALS

Koh, K. B., E. H. Choi, Y. J. Lee, and M. Han. "Serotonin-Related Gene Pathways Associated with Undifferentiated Somatoform Disorder." *Psychiatry Research* 189, no. 2 (2011): 246–50.

Koh, K. B., J. I. Kang, J. D. Lee, and Y. J. Lee. "Shared Neural Activity in Panic Disorder and Undifferentiated Somatoform Disorder Compared with Healthy Controls." *Journal of Clinical Psychiatry* 71, no. 12 (2010): 1576–81.

Tish Davidson, A.M.

V

Vaginismus

Definition

Vaginismus occurs when the muscles around the outer third of the vagina contract involuntarily when vaginal penetration is attempted during sexual intercourse.

Demographics

Although many women experience sexual disorders, it is hard to gather accurate data regarding the frequency of specific problems. Many cases go unreported. Vaginismus is thought to occur most often in women who are highly educated and of high socioeconomic status.

Description

Vaginismus is a reflex response to pressing on the vagina. Women with vaginismus do not intentionally contract their vaginal muscles; rather, the muscles of the outer vagina tighten automatically, often causing pain. Vaginismus can occur with any type of attempted vaginal penetration such as by a penis, speculum, tampon, or other object. Sometimes it occurs with mere touching. Pushing harder increases the pain and most women with vaginismus cannot tolerate sexual intercourse. Vaginismus does not affect a woman's desire for sexual intercourse. Most women with vaginismus enjoy sexual activity that does not involve penetration and many have orgasms through clitoral stimulation.

There are different types of vaginismus:

- Lifelong vaginismus is the most common type and begins the first time vaginal penetration is attempted.
- Acquired vaginismus begins after a period of normal sexual functioning, often after a physical condition causes an episode of painful intercourse or after a woman has intercourse while emotionally distressed.
- General vaginismus occurs whenever vaginal penetration is attempted.
- Situational vaginismus occurs only in specific situations, such as with a certain sexual partner or during a gynecological examination.

Causes and symptoms

According to the health professional's handbook, the ***Diagnostic and Statistical Manual of Mental Disorders*** (fourth edition, or *DSM-IV-TR*), in order for a condition to be diagnosed as vaginismus, the response must be due to psychological factors or a combination of psychological and medical factors, but not to medical factors alone. This entry focuses on the psychological causes and treatments of vaginismus.

Causes

There are many possible causes of vaginismus. One example is an upbringing in which sex was considered wrong or sinful—as in the case of some strict religious backgrounds. This is common among women with this disorder. Concern that penetration is going to be painful, such as during a first sexual experience, is another possible cause. It is also thought that women who feel threatened or powerless in their relationship may subconsciously use this tightening of the vaginal muscles as a defense or silent objection to the relationship. A traumatic childhood experience, such as sexual molestation, may cause lifelong vaginismus. Acquired-type vaginismus is often the result of sexual assault or rape.

Symptoms

The major symptom of vaginismus is the severe contraction of the outer vaginal muscles as the vagina is about to be penetrated. This may completely prevent penetration or make it difficult and painful. Women with vaginismus may be unable to consciously relax their vaginal muscles even when they truly desire to have sexual intercourse or allow penetration. Pelvic examinations may also be painful, and some women cannot tolerate inserting a tampon.

Diagnosis

Diagnosing sexual disorders such as vaginismus can often be very difficult. This is mainly due to the discomfort many people feel when discussing sexual relations, even with their physicians. Cultural norms and taboos often deter women from seeking help when they are experiencing problems. When a physician or gynecologist is consulted, involuntary spasm during pelvic examination can confirm the **diagnosis** of vaginismus, and a complete physical exam and medical and sexual history will rule out any physiological causes for the condition. When psychological causes are suspected, the patient should be referred to a **psychiatrist**, **psychologist**, or sex therapist.

DSM-IV-TR

The *DSM-IV-TR* criteria require that for a diagnosis of vaginismus, the spasm of the muscles in the outer third of the vagina must be involuntary and recurring or persistent and must interfere with sexual intercourse; the symptoms must cause physical or emotional distress or problems with relationships; and the symptoms must exist independently of another disorder, mental or physical, that could account for them.

DSM-5

Proposed changes for the *DSM-5* (fifth edition, 2013) subsume the diagnoses of vaginismus and **dyspareunia** (pain associated with sexual intercourse) into one condition, known as genito-pelvic pain/penetration disorder. A diagnosis will require that the patient experience one or more of the following symptoms over a six-month period:

- inability to have sexual intercourse
- vulvovaginal or pelvic pain during intercourse attempts
- anxiety or fear resulting from the pain or the act of intercourse
- significant tension of the pelvic floor muscles during attempted penetration

The subtypes of lifelong vs. acquired and generalized vs. situational will still apply.

Treatment

There are many different treatments of vaginismus. Therapists may use behavioral, hypnotic, psychological, educational, or **group therapy** techniques. Multiple techniques are often used simultaneously for the same patient. Unless physical causes are present, treatment is aimed at reducing the anxiety and fear associated with penetration.

Traditional

PSYCHOTHERAPY. There are three settings in which psychological treatment can occur. These are in individual, couple, or group settings. Individual therapy often focuses on identifying and resolving underlying causes for vaginismus, such as childhood **trauma** or rape. When a woman has a trusting relationship with her therapist, insecurities or fears around sex resulting from factors such as parental attitudes or religious upbringing can often be revealed and successfully resolved.

Couples therapy, or dual-sex therapy, is based on the concept that any sexual problems should be addressed by the couple, rather than by the affected individual alone. The therapist interacts with the partners individually and as a couple, addressing the couple's sexual history and any other relationship problems. Confronting these issues may help to reveal and resolve the causes of vaginismus, especially when the disorder represents a nonverbal form of protest against some aspect of the relationship. The couple is educated about the condition and taught various activities that may be helpful in overcoming the disorder.

Group therapy also can be effective for treating vaginismus. Couples or individuals who have the same or similar sexual disorders are brought together in a group. This setting can provide comfort and support for women or couples who feel embarrassed or ashamed of the disorder. Witnessing others discussing sex and sexual problems in an open and honest forum can encourage patients to become more open and honest themselves. Group therapy also exerts a certain amount of positive pressure and encouragement to open up and express oneself and to follow through with "homework," which may include masturbation or certain kinds of foreplay.

HYPNOTHERAPY. Hypnotherapy is effective for some patients with vaginismus. Hypnotherapy tends to focus on overcoming the condition itself, rather than resolving any underlying causes or conflicts. It often entails a number of sessions during which the patient and therapist define the goals of hypnotherapy. When the actual hypnosis occurs, suggestions are aimed at resolving underlying fears or concerns and at alleviating symptoms. For example, the patient may be told that she can have intercourse without pain and that she will be able to overcome her muscle spasms. During hypnosis, the problems causing the vaginismus may be explored, or an attempt may even be made to reverse the feelings or fears causing the disorder. Exploring causal relationships, as well as suggesting to the woman she can overcome her vaginal muscle spasms, can be very effective for certain patients.

OTHER TREATMENTS. Behavioral therapy, including **cognitive-behavioral therapy** (CBT), is also used to treat vaginismus. When behavioral therapy is chosen, it is assumed that the vaginismus is a learned behavior that can be unlearned. Behavioral therapy generally involves desensitization. Patients are exposed to situations that they find create a mild sense of psychological discomfort or anxiety. Once these situations are conquered, the patient is exposed to sexual situations that they find more threatening, until eventually coitus is achieved without difficulty.

Another type of treatment for vaginismus involves desensitization over a period of time using systematic vaginal dilation. In the beginning of the treatment, the woman touches near or inserts a small object into her vagina. Over time, she inserts larger and larger vaginal dilators. Eventually, a dilator the size of a penis can be inserted comfortably and sexual intercourse can be achieved. There is some debate about this procedure, as it treats the symptoms and not the underlying causes of the vaginismus disorder.

Desensitization procedures are somewhat controversial because they address the symptoms but not the cause of vaginismus. The exercises should be pursued under the direction of an experienced therapist or other healthcare provider. They should involve the sexual partner and gradually include intimate contact before culminating in sexual intercourse.

Prognosis

Vaginismus is one of the most treatable sexual disorders, with a success rate of at least 63%. Because the causes of vaginismus vary, different treatments are successful with different women. In general, a treatment plan that combines two or more therapeutic techniques supervised by a specialist in sex therapy has the greatest likelihood of success. Untreated vaginismus can lead to unsatisfying sexual relationships, tension, and emotional distress between partners.

Prevention

There are no known preventions for vaginismus; however, maintaining open and honest communication within a sexual relationship may help prevent the disorder. Seeking prompt treatment if vaginismus does occur can minimize problems.

KEY TERM

Coitus—Sexual intercourse.

Resources

BOOKS

American Psychiatric Association. *Diagnostic and Statistical Manual of Mental Disorders*. 4th ed., text rev. Washington, DC: American Psychiatric Publishing, 2000.

Goldstein, Andrew, Caroline F. Pukall, and Irwin Goldstein, eds. *Female Sexual Pain Disorders*. Hoboken, NJ: Wiley-Blackwell, 2009.

Meana, Mart. "Painful Intercourse: Dyspareunia and Vaginismus." In *Systemic Sex Therapy*, edited by Katherine M. Hertlein, Gerald R. Weeks, and Nancy Gambescia. New York: Routledge, 2009.

Sadock, Benjamin J., and Virginia A. Sadock, eds. *Comprehensive Textbook of Psychiatry*. Vol. 2. 7th ed. Philadelphia: Lippincott Williams and Wilkins, 2000.

PERIODICALS

Binik, Yitzchak M. "The DSM Diagnostic Criteria for Vaginismus." *Archives of Sexual Behavior* 39, no. 2 (April 2010): 278–91.

Kleinplatz, Peggy J. "Sex Therapy for Vaginismus: a Review, Critique, and Humanistic Alternative." *The Journal of Humanistic Psychology* 38, no. 2 (Spring 1998): 51–82.

Sadovsky, Richard. "Management of Dyspareunia and Vaginismus." *American Family Physician* 61, no. 8 (April 15, 2000): 2511.

Ter Kuile, Moniek M., et al. "Therapist-Aided Exposure for Women With Lifelong Vaginismus: A Replicated Single-Case Design." *Journal of Consulting and Clinical Psychology* 77, no. 1 (February 2009): 149–59.

ORGANIZATIONS

American College of Obstetricians and Gynecologists, PO Box 96920, Washington, DC, 20090-6920, (202) 638-5577, http://www.acog.org.

American Psychological Association, 750 1st Street NE, Washington, DC, 20002-4242, (202) 336-5500; TDD/TTY: (202) 336-6123, (800) 374-2721, http://www.apa.org.

Tish Davidson, A.M.

Vagus nerve stimulation

Definition

Vagus nerve stimulation (VNS) is a type of adjunctive therapy that involves electrical stimulation of the vagus nerve, which is the tenth of the twelve

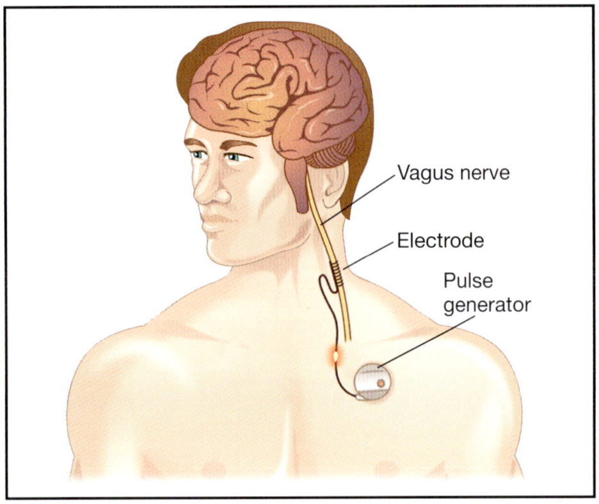

In vagus nerve stimulation, a device called a pulse generator is implanted in the chest. The device sends electrical pulses via a lead wire to the vagus nerve. *(Illustration by Electronic Illustrators Group. © 2012 Cengage Learning.)*

cranial nerves. It arises from the medulla (the lower part of the **brain** stem) and controls such varied functions as heart rate, sweating, the rhythmic contractions of the intestines (peristalsis), speech, and keeping the airway open for breathing. The name *vagus* comes from the Latin word for "wandering" because the nerve takes a roundabout course through the body from the brain stem to the digestive tract. The vagus nerve is also known as "cranial nerve X" and the "pneumogastric nerve" because it has branches that innervate both the lungs and the stomach.

The most common form of VNS in current use involves the surgical implantation of a battery-powered stimulator. The procedure was approved by the Food and Drug Administration (FDA) to treat partial-onset epilepsy in 1997 and treatment-resistant **depression** in 2005. The VNS device is sometimes referred to as a "pacemaker for the brain." It is placed under the skin on the chest wall, and a wire runs from it to the vagus nerve in the neck.

A newer, noninvasive form of VNS known as transcutaneous vagus nerve stimulation (t-VNS) was developed by a German company, Cerbomed, founded in 2005. In 2009, the company conducted a pilot test of a new device called NEMOS, which consists of a stimulator and an electrode that the patient attaches to the ear and wears like an earphone for four to five hours per day. Intended for patients with treatment-resistant epilepsy, t-VNS is based on the fact that a branch of the vagus nerve runs directly under the skin of portions of the outer ear. This branch of the nerve can be stimulated transcutaneously (through the skin) with electrical impulses. No surgery is necessary to use the device. NEMOS was presented at the Fourth International Epilepsy Colloquium in Marburg, Germany, at the end of June 2011. The device had not been approved by the FDA for use in the United States as of late 2011; however, the company has applied for several U.S. patents. Investigational applications of t-VNS include treatment of chronic tinnitus (ringing in the ears), migraine headaches, and **schizophrenia**.

Purpose

The goal of VNS is to change the functioning of various brain and somatic systems by reducing the frequency of **seizures** in the case of epilepsy or by inducing a more positive mood in the case of treatment refractory depression (TRD). In epilepsy, treatment has been concurrent with pharmaceuticals used to reduce seizures. Although approved by the FDA in 2005 for use in treating major depression that has not responded to at least four depression treatments, solid evidence for the efficacy of VNS in depression had not been established as of 2011.

Clinical applications of VNS that were still considered investigational as of 2011 are the treatment of such inflammatory conditions as arthritis, colitis, myocardial infarction, and congestive heart failure. In 2000, a researcher in New York discovered that stimulation of the vagus nerve reduces the release of cytokines, small cell-signaling protein molecules that help to regulate the immune system. Slowing the release of cytokines produced in the spleen helps to protect against organ damage resulting from excessive cytokine production. Thus, it may be possible to use VNS instead of drugs like infliximab (Remicade) or etanercept (Enbrel) to treat rheumatoid arthritis and other autoimmune diseases associated with inflammation.

Description

Research has not been able to establish exactly how VNS works, except to note a multiplicity of effects on the brain and body by stimulating the vagus nerve. That nerve, the tenth cranial nerve, originates in the brain and travels through the mid-brain. Branching into left and right vagus nerves, it runs down the neck and to the thorax and abdomen. The functions of the vagus nerve are many and various, ranging from the stimulation and release of **neurotransmitters** in the brain to issues related to breathing, swallowing, and the vocal chords, to the functioning of the digestive tract. The vagus nerve has been shown to create changes in the functioning of the hypothalamus, the amygdala, and the cingulate gyrusstructures that affect neurotransmitter release and reuptake; mood; and seizure activity, among other things. Because the vagus nerve runs through the middle of the brain, it influences many areas of the brain indirectly, so that while some brain cells increase their activity with VNS, others decrease in synaptic activity. The manufacturers of the only FDA-approved VNS treatment in the United States for epilepsy and depression have used the omnipresent effects of vagus nerve stimulation to bolster their claims as to its efficacy as a treatment for those two disorders.

Implantation and maintenance

VNS involves the surgical implantation of an electrical stimulation device alongside the vagus nerve in the area of the carotid artery, located in the neck. The pulse generator device, which is about the size of a pocket watch, is implanted on the left side of the body, just below the collarbone. Electrodes from the pulse generator are then implanted on the left side of the neck and wrapped around the left vagus nerve. The electrodes are connected to the pulse generator by a wire. The surgical procedure takes about an hour and is usually done as an outpatient procedure.

After implantation, the surgeon tests the device and closes the incisions. Further changes are made with the use of a special wand, a software package, and a portable computer, so patients need not undergo any more invasive procedures related to adjusting the intensity of the electrical impulse. The device is usually set to stimulate the vagus nerve for 20 seconds every five minutes. As an additional control, patients are provided with a strong handheld magnet. When the magnet is held over the skin covering the pulse generator, it prevents it from operating. If patients experience problems with the pulse, they can use the magnet to control it until they get to the physician. The patented collection of pulse generator, leads, software, and programming devices was at one time called the NeuroCybernetic Prosthesis System, or NCP, but the name appears to have been dropped after the FDA sent the manufacturer, Cyberonics, a warning letter in 2001. The FDA had received reports of 83 deaths and several dozen infections linked to the NeuroCybernetic Prosthesis System. The FDA accused the company of improperly reporting and recording the adverse events and of failing to investigate the causes of the deaths.

The pulse generator, which contains a battery with a lifespan of one to 16 years, sends out an electrical impulse whose strength, frequency, and duration are determined by the physician. The impulse travels through the wire to the electrodes, which transmit the pulse to the vagus nerve. VNS was originally used for patients with refractory episodic epilepsy who were deemed unsuitable for epilepsy surgery, but it has been increasingly prescribed for patients whose illnesses are less severe.

Origins and history

VNS was first described in the medical literature as a treatment for epilepsy in 1990. The first VNS implant for treatment-resistant depression was performed in the United States in 1998. Physicians using VNS for patients with epilepsy had reported that patients seemed more alert, and combining anecdotal observations with the fact that some anticonvulsant drugs have also been used in depression treatment, the manufacturer of the VNS system decided to test its efficacy as a treatment for treatment-resistant depression.

As of 2011, about 60,000 patients worldwide had received implanted VNS devices for the treatment of epilepsy. The reported VNS depression research to date has had low numbers of participants, and much research has been directly or indirectly funded by Cyberonics, leaving reported findings open to debate. In fact, in May 2006, the Public Citizen's Health Research Group sent a letter to the FDA requesting that the organization require Cyberonics to withdraw its advertisement from WebMd.com and issue a corrective statement. The group said that the Cyberonics ad "greatly exaggerated" the findings from the clinical studies, and called the advertisement "false and misleading." The nonprofit then pointed out 10 items in a two-paragraph advertisement, explaining why they were false, exaggerated, or both. In September 2006, the group followed up with a second letter to the FDA, requesting denial of Medicare reimbursement for the VNS device when implanted to treat depression.

In another case, one journal editor resigned over having failed to disclose that he and eight other researchers had been funded by Cyberonics in regards to a published study on VNS. Other researchers have included statements in their published papers on VNS, acknowledging that they received funding from the company. In view of the company's legal problems, it is significant that the Mayo Clinic's description of VNS as a treatment for depression urges caution: "For most people, vagus nerve stimulation doesn't significantly ease depression symptoms [although] it does seem to make a significant difference for some people. Some mental health experts don't recommend its use for depression at all, and most health insurance companies don't cover the procedure for depression treatment."

Transcutaneous VNS

Transcutaneous VNS, or t-VNS, is a noninvasive form of VNS. NEMOS, the device currently undergoing **clinical trials** in Europe, will be marketed in Germany for the treatment of epilepsy in September 2012. It consists of an electrode worn over the ear that is attached to a stimulator unit. The ear electrode stimulates a branch of the vagus nerve that runs below the skin of the concha of the ear. The patient uses the device for three one- or two-hour sessions each day, in the morning, at noon, and in the evening. The small size of the device allows it to be used unobtrusively in the workplace as well as at home.

The stimulator unit records data as well as sending electrical impulses to the ear electrode; this data collection allows the patient's physician to fine-tune the strength of the impulses and otherwise supervise the therapy. In addition to its portability and ease of use, NEMOS eliminates the risk of infection from a surgically implanted VNS.

Benefits

The benefits of VNS are partial or (in some cases) complete relief of the symptoms of the condition for which it was implanted. It is not a cure for either epilepsy or depression.

Precautions

The physician's manual published by the VNS manufacturer contains in the introduction a document subtitled *Indications, Contraindications, Warnings and Precautions*. This 20-page document must be considered the primary resource for precautionary information, as there is not yet much research available beyond that which the manufacturer, Cyberonics, has funded. Precautionary information for this section has been taken from this document, which can be found online at http://www.vnstherapy.com/depression/hcp/Manuals/default.aspx.

The difference among contraindications, warnings, and precautions as published by the manufacturer seem unclear, as they combine VNS requirements, pre-existing health conditions, procedures that cannot be performed on people using VNS, age limitations, and therapeutic devices that cannot be used in conjunction with VNS. The VNS system is only to be used on the left vagus nerve and is approved for children over the age of 12 in cases of epilepsy and for patients over the age of 18 for depression.

Procedures and devices that can damage the implant, the patient's tissue, or both, and consequently that should not be used with VNS:

- diathermy, or cauterization; causes a concentration of heat in the implant, which can damage the implant, destroy tissue, and even lead to death
- radiation therapy
- external and internal defibrillation devices
- electrosurgery
- therapeutic ultrasound
- full-body MRI

Pre-existing conditions under which VNS should not be prescribed:

- having only one vagus nerve
- having metal plates or other implants such as pacemakers
- pregnancy
- dysphagea (problems with swallowing)
- obstructive sleep apnea (OSA) (a condition that causes patients to stop breathing while asleep)
- previous heart attacks and other cardiac abnormalities
- respiratory illness such as asthma or dyspnea
- brain injury
- injury to the central nervous system (CNS)
- dysautonomis (disease of the autonomic nervous system)
- vasovagal syncope (a condition in which the blood vessels dilate and the heart rate slows, causing fainting)
- ulcers
- hoarseness
- having other concurrent forms of brain stimulation treatments
- suicidal thoughts or ideas
- bipolar disorder
- schizophrenia or schizoaffective disorders
- delusional disorders

With regard to t-VNS, the German manufacturer lists only four contraindications:

- age below 18
- pregnancy
- skin infection or open wound on the part of the ear where the electrode is worn
- use of a pacemaker or other active implanted device

Preparation

Patients must be informed of the risks of the procedure, and those with contraindicated health conditions must be ruled out before surgery. Patients who elect to have VNS should have the procedure and equipment

KEY TERMS

Adjunctive therapy—Any treatment that is secondary or subordinate to a primary therapy.

Concha—The hollow shell-shaped portion of the external ear nearest the ear canal.

Cytokine—Any of a group of small protein molecules (including interferon, interleukin, and tumor necrosis factor) secreted by certain cells in the immune system that modulate certain functions associated with the immune response.

Obstructive sleep apnea—A disorder caused by obstruction of the upper airway during sleep and characterized by repeated pauses in breathing during sleep despite efforts to breathe. It is sometimes a side effect of VNS.

Tinnitus—A ringing or buzzing sensation in the ear in the absence of an external cause or stimulus. It is not a disease by itself but a symptom that may have a number of different causes.

Transcutaneous—Through the skin.

thoroughly explained, and will be taught the use of the handheld magnet in case it is needed.

Aftercare

The surgical procedure takes about an hour, but there are two incisions and, as with any implant, risk of infection. Wound care must be addressed, and patients require follow up appointments with their physicians to monitor the effects of the treatment and adjust the strength or frequency of the electrical impulse. Changes in patients' health also need to be monitored, as so many conditions are contraindicated in the use of VNS. For example, in the case of treatment-resistant depression, if a depressed patient becomes suicidal or experiences a **manic episode**, use of VNS is contraindicated.

Obese patients and others with a history of **sleep disorders** should be monitored for signs of obstructive sleep apnea during postsurgical follow-up.

Risks

With regard to surgically implanted VNS devices, along with the risk of infection there is the potential for breakage, migration, or corrosion. The first 1990 report on the device noted that the electrodes had to be redesigned after the first group of devices showed an unacceptably high rate of breakage. Other issues may have to do with irritation to the vagus nerve, which can result in hoarseness or permanent nerve damage. Because VNS affects the rate of respiration during sleep, patients with an implanted device are at increased risk of developing obstructive sleep apnea. Some psychiatrists have also reported manic episodes in depressed patients treated with VNS. According to the Mayo Clinic, other side effects of VNS implantation include difficulty swallowing, nausea, tingling, neck pain, chest pain or spasms, breathing problems during **exercise**, and paralysis of the vocal cords. Because of these risks, it is imperative that the surgeon receive specialized training for implanting the VNS.

People who have cardiac arrhythmia are at risk, and occurrences of bradycardia (slowed heartbeat) or asystole (heart stoppage) during or after implantation have been reported. The manufacturer states that safety has not been established for patients who suffer bradycardia or asystole during implantation. Although there is implant information for cardiac patients, it is listed under the heading of contraindications.

Patients should be warned to avoid anything that may generate a strong electrical or magnetic field, as the field could affect the functioning of the VNS system. This includes strong magnets, hair clippers, and anti-shoplifting tag deactivators. The magnet used with the VNS can affect televisions, credit card strips, and computer disks. The pulse generator in the VNS is said to affect pocket transistor radios and hearing aids.

Another consideration is the high cost of an implanted VNS device. According to an article published in the *New York Times* in 2006, the device itself costs about $15,000, with implantation surgery costing an additional $10,000.

With regard to t-VNS, the German manufacturer reports a 10% risk of itchy skin and an 8% risk of numbness or localized discomfort at the point where the electrode is placed on the ear. No serious adverse affects had been reported as of late 2011.

Research and general acceptance

According to published studies, VNS has a fairly low rate of success in epilepsy patients as well as in patients with major depression. According to the manufacturer, 40% to 50% of patients report a reduction of seizures of 50% or more, 18 months after implantation. The rate of complete freedom from seizures in patients with partial-onset epilepsy that cannot be managed by medications is less than 10%.

Even though the benefits of VNS as a treatment for depression have not been established, as of 2011 there were

QUESTIONS TO ASK YOUR DOCTOR

- What is your opinion of VNS as a treatment for epilepsy?
- What is your opinion of VNS as a treatment for depression?
- Have you ever treated a patient with an implanted VNS device? Did they find it helpful?
- Do you think that transcutaneous VNS is a promising new development?

nine clinical trials under way of VNS as a treatment for the disorder, along with 10 studies of VNS as a treatment for epilepsy. VNS was also being studied as a treatment for vegetative states following **traumatic brain injury**, heart failure, ischemic heart disease, rheumatoid arthritis, fibromyalgia, and obesity. Four additional clinical trials were under way of transcutaneous vagus nerve stimulation (t-VNS) as a treatment for schizophrenia, chronic pain, tinnitus, and treatment-refractory epilepsy.

Resources

BOOKS

Donovan, Charles E., III. *Out of the Black Hole: A Patient's Guide to Vagus Nerve Stimulation and Depression.* St Louis, NC: Wellness Publishers, 2006.

Higgins, Edmund S., and Mark S. George. *Brain Stimulation Therapies for Clinicians.* Washington, DC: American Psychiatric Pub., 2009.

Rey, Joseph M., and Boris Birmaher, eds. *Treating Child and Adolescent Depression.* Philadelphia: Wolters Kluwer Health/Lippincott Williams and Wilkins, 2009.

PERIODICALS

Burakgazi, A.Z., et al. "The Correlation between Vagus Nerve Stimulation Efficacy and Partial Onset Epilepsies." *Journal of Clinical Neurophysiology* 28 (August 2011): 380–382.

Elliott, R.E., et al. "Vagus Nerve Stimulation for Children with Treatment-resistant Epilepsy: A Consecutive Series of 141 Cases." *Journal of Neurosurgery. Pediatrics* 7 (May 2011): 491–500.

Gerson, R., et al. "Mania Following Vagus Nerve Stimulation: A Case Report and Review of the Literature." *Epilepsy and Behavior* 20 (January 2011): 138–140.

Gigante, P.R., and R.R. Goodman. "Alternative Surgical Approaches in Epilepsy." *Current Neurology and Neuroscience Reports* 11 (August 2011): 404–408.

Grimm, S., and M. Bajbouj. "Efficacy of Vagus Nerve Stimulation in the Treatment of Depression." *Expert Review of Neurotherapeutics* 10 (January 2010): 87–92.

Howland, R.H., et al. "The Emerging Use of Technology for the Treatment of Depression and Other Neuropsychiatric Disorders." *Annals of Clinical Psychiatry* 23 (February 2011): 48–62.

Noe, K.H., et al. "Treatment of Depression in Patients with Epilepsy." *Current Treatment Options in Neurology* 13 (August 2011): 371–379.

Parhizgar, F., et al. "Obstructive Sleep Apnea and Respiratory Complications Associated with Vagus Nerve Stimulators." *Journal of Clinical Sleep Medicine* 7 (August 15, 2011): 401–407.

Terry, R., et al. "An Implantable Neurocybernetic Prosthesis System." *Epilepsia* 31 (1990), Suppl. 2: S33–S37.

Wozniak, S.E., et al. "Vagal Nerve Stimulator Infection: A Lead-Salvage Protocol." *Journal of Neurosurgery. Pediatrics* 7 (June 2011): 671–675.

OTHER

Feder, Barnaby. "Battle Lines in Treating Depression." *New York Times*, September 10, 2006. http://www.nytimes.com/2006/09/10/business/yourmoney/10cyber.html?adxnnl=1&pagewanted=all&adxnnlx=1316484059-Xd/Wuk7s5DZ8YrhgFUqE7w (accessed September 18, 2011).

Food and Drug Administration (FDA). *Summary of Safety and Effectiveness Data.* http://www.fda.gov/ohrms/dockets/ac/04/briefing/4047b1_02_Summary%20of%20Safety%20and%20Effectiveness.pdf (accessed September 17, 2011).

WEBSITES

Cerbomed Gmbh. "NEMOS: Frequently Asked Questions." http://www.cerbomed.com/index.php?lang=en#faq (accessed September 17, 2011).

Cyberonics, Inc. "VNS Therapy." http://us.cyberonics.com/en/vns-therapy (accessed September 17, 2011).

Mayo Clinic. "Vagus Nerve Stimulation for Depression." http://www.mayoclinic.com/health/vagus-nerve-stimulation/MY00183 (accessed September 17, 2011).

Medscape. "Epilepsy and Seizures." http://emedicine.medscape.com/article/1184846-overview (accessed September 17, 2011).

Public Citizen's Health Research Group. "Letter Requesting the Halt of Ads for Vagus Nerve Stimulator Device," May 18, 2006. http://www.citizen.org/Page.aspx?pid=636 (accessed September 18, 2011).

Public Citizen's Health Research Group. "Letter Requesting that Medicare Deny Reimbursement for Vagus Nerve Stimulation Device for Treatment-Resistant Depression," September 6, 2006. http://www.citizen.org/Page.aspx?pid=632 (accessed September 18, 2011).

WebMD. "Epilepsy: Vagus Nerve Stimulation (VNS)." http://www.webmd.com/epilepsy/guide/vagus-nerve-stimulation-vns (accessed September 17, 2011).

ORGANIZATIONS

Cerbomed Gmbh, Henkestrasse 91, Erlangen, Germany 91052, +49 9131 9202 76 0, Fax: +49 9131 9202 76 92, info@cerbomed.com, http://www.cerbomed.com/index.php?lang=en.

Cyberonics, Inc, 100 Cyberonics Boulevard, Houston, TX, 77058, Fax: (281) 218-9332, (800) 332-1375, http://us.cyberonics.com/en.

National Institute of Neurological Disorders and Stroke (NINDS), PO Box 5801, Bethesda, MD, 20824 (301) 496-5751, (800) 352-9424, http://www.ninds.nih.gov.

Public Citizen, Inc, 1600 20th Street NW, Washington, DC, 20009, (202) 588-1000, hrg1@citizen.org, http://www.citizen.org/Page.aspx?pid=183.

U.S. Food and Drug Administration (FDA), 10903 New Hampshire Ave., Silver Spring, MD, 20993, (888) 463-6332, http://www.fda.gov/default.htm.

Lorena S. Covington, M.A.
Rebecca J. Frey, Ph.D.

Valerian

Description

Valerian (*Valeriana officinalis*) is one of at least 300 species of the Valerianaceae family. This plant is native to Europe and west Asia; it is naturalized throughout North America. A common name for this hardy perennial is garden heliotrope. Valerian has been valued for its soothing qualities for at least a millennium. The name valerian may have come from the Latin *valere* meaning "to be strong" or "to be in good health." Chaucer (c. 1343–1400) called the herb setewale. Other common names are all-heal, vandal root, and Capon's tail.

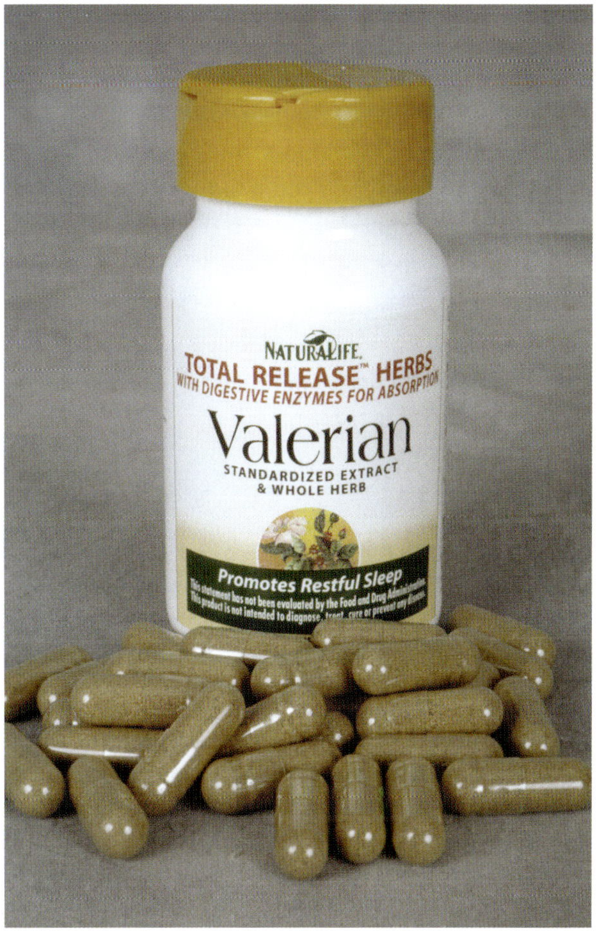

Bottle of valerian supplements. *(© Custom Medical Stock Photo, Inc. Reproduced by permission.)*

Purpose

Valerian has been used as a medicinal herb for more than a thousand years, especially for mild cases of **insomnia**. Research shows that proper use of valerian promotes sleep, reduces night awakenings, and increases dream recall in most people. A team of pharmacologists in Argentina reported that they had isolated two flavonoids, 6-methylapigenin and hesperidin, as the compounds in valerian with sedative and sleep-enhancing properties. A German study of more than 900 children suffering from pathological restlessness and/or difficulty falling asleep reported in 2006 that a twice-daily dose of 160 mg of valerian and 80 mg of lemon balm significantly decreased restlessness and difficulty falling asleep. The researchers suggested this combination may be a safer and more practical alternative to prescription medications.

Historically, valerian has been highly regarded as a tranquilizer that acts without narcotic effects. It has been thought to act as a pain reliever, antispasmodic, sedative, and carminative, but only its use in treating insomnia has been shown the most effective in **clinical trials**, and even those results have been conflicting.

Description

Valerian grows in lime-rich soil near streams or in damp, low meadows where it may reach a height of 5 ft. (1.5 m). It is also found in drier environments at higher elevations, where it grows to just 2 ft. (0.6 m). Roots harvested from the drier environment may be more medicinally potent. This variety is sometimes known as sylvestus.

Valerian's short vertical rhizome is dark yellow-brown in color and has round rootlets. These rootlets produce hollow, fluted stems with opposite leaves and a single leaflet at the tip, with as many as ten pairs of toothed leaflets. The upper leaves are attached at their base and emerge from a white sheath along the stem. The stems remain erect and unbranched until the very top, where the small, white flowers, tinged with pink, bloom in clusters in the middle of summer.

Preparations

Valerian's rhizome and root make up the medicinal part of this herb. Fresh root will produce the highest quality of medicinal extract and should be harvested in the autumn of its second year. Valerian works well in combination with other tranquilizing herbs such as **passionflower** (*Passiflora incarnata*) to safely induce sleep or skullcap (*Scutellaria laterifolia*) to relieve nervous tension. The somewhat bitter, unpleasant taste of the tea may be masked by adding peppermint oil, or the user can take the herb in capsule form. Combinations contain equal parts of each herb. The herb may be drunk as an herbal tea, used as a tincture, or swallowed in capsule form one hour before bedtime.

It is important to note that there is no standard dosage for valerian and that the potency of valerian products can vary drastically from brand to brand. In 2006, ConsumerLab.com tested 16 brands of valerian products and found that most had a lower potency than what was printed on the label and/or contained contaminants. One of the products was contaminated with lead, which can damage almost every system in the human body, and two others were contaminated with cadmium, a heavy metal that can cause kidney damage.

Precautions

Valerian should not be used in large doses or for an extended period. People should not take it continuously for more than two to three weeks. Users of valerian may become tolerant to its effects with prolonged use. Increasing the dose of the herb to achieve desired effects may result in negative side effects. Prolonged use, according to some research, could result in liver damage and central nervous system impairment. Women who are pregnant or breast-feeding should not use valerian, as the herb's effects on the fetus or infant have not yet been tested. Patients undergoing surgery should stop taking valerian at least two weeks before their procedure.

Side effects

Large doses of valerian may occasionally cause headache, muscle spasm, heart palpitations, dizziness, gastric distress, sleeplessness, and confusion. Uninterrupted use may cause **depression**.

KEY TERMS

Carminative—A medication or preparation that prevents the formation of intestinal gas or allows it to be expelled.

Flavonoid—Any of a group of plant compounds with an aromatic nucleus, often found as a pigment.

Rhizome—A fleshy plant stem that grows horizontally under or along the ground; roots are sent out below this stem and leaves or shoots are sent out above it.

Interactions

Although valerian has been regarded as a relatively safe herb, it should not be used with other **sedatives**, including alcoholic beverages, **benzodiazepines**, **barbiturates**, or antihistamines. Long-term safety studies (longer than one month) of valerian had not been conducted as of early 2011.

Resources

BOOKS

Barnes, Joanne, Linda A. Anderson, and J. David Phillipson. *Herbal Medicines (Includes CD-ROM)*. 3rd. ed. London: Pharmaceutical Press, 2007.

PDR for Nonprescription Drugs, Dietary Supplements, and Herbs 2009. Montvale, NJ: PDR Network, 2009.

Woolven, Linda, and Ted Snider. *Healthy Herbs: Everyday Guide to Medicinal Herbs and Their Use*. Markham, ON, Canada: Fitzhenry & Whiteside, 2006.

PERIODICALS

Bone, Kerry. "Valerian: A Safe and Effective Herb for Sleep Problems." *Townsend Letter for Doctors and Patients* (April 2005): 44.

Brown, Donald. "Valerian and Lemon Balm Safely and Effectively Treat Restlessness and Dyssomnia in Children" *Original Internist* (December 2006).

Castleman, Michael. "Rest Assured: Valerian, a Safe and Effective Herbal Sleep Aid, Will Help You Close the Door on Insomnia." *Natural Health* (March 2007): 98.

WEBSITES

National Center for Complementary and Alternative Medicine. "Valerian." National Institutes of Health. http://nccam.nih.gov/about/ataglance (accessed December 18, 2011).

ORGANIZATIONS

American Institute of Homeopathy, 101 South Whiting Street, Suite 16, Alexandria, VA, 22304, (888) 445-9988, admin@homeopathyusa.org, http://homeopathyusa.org.

Homeopathic Medical Council of Canada, 31 Adelaide Street East, Box 605, Toronto, ON, M5C 2J8, (416) 788-4622, Ontario@HMCC.ca, http://www.hmcc.ca.

National Center for Complementary and Alternative Medicine, 9000 Rockville Pike, Bethesda, MD, 20892, info@nccam.nih.gov, http://nccam.nih.gov.

U.S. Food and Drug Administration, 10903 New Hampshire Ave., Silver Spring, MD, 20993, (888) 463-6332, http://www.fda.gov.

Clare Hanrahan
Ken R. Wells

Valium *see* **Diazepam**

Valproic acid

Definition

Valproic acid is an anticonvulsant (antiseizure) drug. In the United States, valproic acid is also known as valproate and is sold under brand name Depakene.

Purpose

The U.S. Food and Drug Administration (FDA) recognizes valproic acid for the treatment of epilepsy and for mania that occurs with **bipolar disorder**. Valproic acid is also approved for the prevention of migraine headaches.

Description

Valproic acid's properties in preventing **seizures** were first discovered in Europe in 1963. The medication was first used clinically in the United Stated in 1978.

Valproic acid is effective in treating a variety of seizure types, which include simple and complex absence seizures, partial seizures, and tonic-clonic seizures (grand mal seizures). Valproic acid is also effective in treating the manic episodes of patients with bipolar disorder. Patients who have bipolar disorder resulting from a head injury and patients who do not respond to or who cannot tolerate conventional lithium therapy (normally the therapy of choice for bipolar disorder) can be treated with valproic acid. In addition, valproic acid provides a 50% or greater reduction in the frequency of migraine headaches. Valproic acid is also safe and effective in preventing headaches that arise as a side effect of taking a class of drugs known as **selective serotonin reuptake inhibitors** (SSRIs). These drugs include **sertraline** (Zoloft), **paroxetine** (Paxil), **fluoxetine** (Prozac), **fluvoxamine** (Luvox), and **citalopram** (Celexa).

Valproic acid comes in 250 mg gelatin capsules and in a 250 mg/5mL syrup.

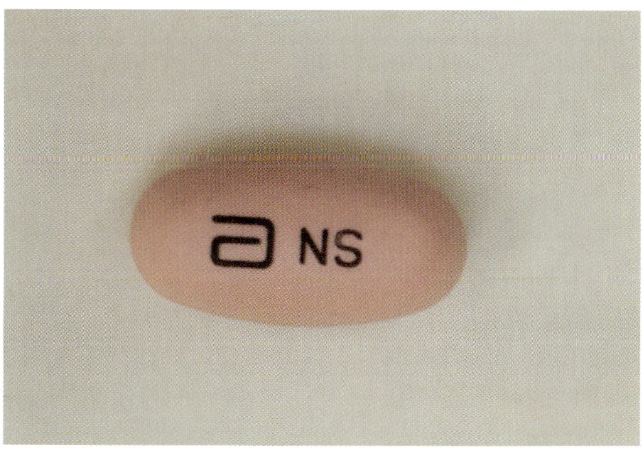

Depakote (valproic acid), 500 mg. *(© Custom Medical Stock Photo, Inc. Reproduced by permission.)*

Recommended dosage

The dosage of valproic acid used to treat epilepsy depends on the type of seizures the patient has. The doses are determined based on the patient's weight.

The initial dose of valproic acid used to treat mania is 750 mg daily. This dose is then reduced to the lowest dose that will achieve the desired effects. Another dosage strategy is based on patient weight. The starting dose is 30 mg per 2 lb (1 kg) of body weight on days one and two followed by 20 mg per kg of body weight taken daily on days three through ten.

For prevention of migraine headaches, a dose of 250 mg twice daily is beneficial. It may take up to 1,000 mg of valproic acid to control migraine attacks.

Precautions

Valproic acid may cause life-threatening damage to the liver and pancreas. Before starting valproic acid therapy, every patient should have a blood test to assess his or her liver function. The risk of valproic acid causing liver damage is greatest during the first six months of treatment. Liver function tests should be done once a month during the first three months, then every three to six months for as long as the patient continues to take the drug. Vomiting, lethargy, anorexia, and jaundice (yellowing of the skin) may precede signs of liver damage. If a patient develops severe or unusual abdominal pain, this may be a sign of pancreatitis (inflammation of the pancreas). Pancreatitis can occur in both children and adults. It can develop shortly after valproic acid is started or after several years of use.

Patients who are younger than two years old should not take valproic acid. When it is necessary for children

KEY TERMS

Absence seizure—Absence (petit mal) seizures usually begin with a brief loss of consciousness and last between one and 10 seconds. People having a petit mal seizure become very quiet and may blink, stare blankly, roll their eyes, or move their lips. A petit mal seizure lasts 15–20 seconds. When it ends, the individual resumes whatever he or she was doing before the seizure began, and may not realize that anything unusual happened.

Anorexia—Loss of appetite.

Tonic-clonic seizure—This is the most common type of seizure among all age groups and is categorized into several phases beginning with vague symptoms hours or days before an attack. These seizures are sometimes called grand mal seizures.

under age two to take valproic acid, the drug should be used cautiously and with close physician monitoring.

Pregnant women or women who are planning to become pregnant should not take valproic acid, as the drug is harmful to the fetus and may cause birth defects, including **intellectual disability**.

Side effects

Side effects of valproic acid may include nausea, vomiting, indigestion, and either diarrhea or constipation. Headaches, dizziness, lack of coordination, confusion, **fatigue**, tremor, drowsiness, and seizures have also been associated with the use of valproic acid. Behavioral changes associated with the drug including irritability, longer and deeper sleep, hyperactivity, increased sociability, increased sadness, happiness or aggression, are seen more often in children than in adults taking valproic acid.

Less than 1% of patients experience appetite changes. These changes may include either diminished or increased appetite. Skin rash, photosensitivity, (acute sensitivity to the sun) hair loss, and other hair changes have also been reported in people using valproic acid.

Interactions

Using valproic acid with other anticonvulsant drugs, such as phenobarbital, **clonazepam**, and **lamotrigine** may cause excessive sedation (drowsiness and lack of physical and mental alertness). Valproic acid may diminish the benefits of phenytoin, another commonly used anticonvulsant. Severe central nervous **depression** has been reported with the use of valproic acid and another anticonvulsant called primidone.

Taking aspirin during valproic acid therapy may cause valproic acid levels to increase to toxic (poisonous) levels. Other medications that may cause valproic acid toxicity are the antibiotic erythromycin and the antidepressant **amitriptyline**. Drugs that can decrease the effectiveness of valproic acid include **carbamazepine** and cholestyramine. **Ginkgo biloba**, an herbal supplement commonly available in the United States, may be prepared with a chemical called 4′-O-methylpyridoxine. If this chemical remains in the herbal preparation, it can cause seizures and reduce the effectiveness of valproic acid.

Resources

BOOKS

Lacy, Charles F. *Drug Information Handbook with International Trade Names Index*. Hudson, OH: Lexi-Comp, Inc. 2011.

Sadock, Benjamin J., and Virginia A. Sadock, eds. *Comprehensive Textbook of Psychiatry*. Vol. 2. 7th ed. Philadelphia: Lippincott Williams and Wilkins, 2000.

WEBSITES

PubMed Health. "Valproic Acid." http://www.ncbi.nlm.nih.gov/pubmedhealth/PMH0000677 (accessed November 13, 2011).

ORGANIZATIONS

U.S. Food and Drug Administration, 10903 New Hampshire Ave., Silver Spring, MD, 20993-0002, (888) INFO-FDA (463-6332), http://www.fda.gov.

Ajna Hamidovic, Pharm.D.

Vascular dementia

Definition

Vascular **dementia** is a group of disorders characterized by the severe loss of mental functioning resulting from cerebrovascular disease. Vascular dementia is often caused by repeated strokes.

Demographics

In most countries, vascular dementia is a much less common form of dementia than **Alzheimer's disease**

(AD), though the reverse is true in Japan, where it is more common than AD. Overall, vascular dementia is the second most common form of dementia, after AD. About 10%–20% of patients who experience dementia have the vascular form of the disorder. The difference in prevalence in different countries may result from different lifestyle factors rooted in the culture.

About 1.5% of individuals are affected by vascular dementia in the United States. Vascular dementia is more common in men than in women, which may be because men are more likely than women to suffer from strokes. Vascular dementia becomes increasingly prevalent as people grow older. The number of people affected by vascular dementia rises dramatically during and after age 70. Vascular dementia usually occurs at a younger age than AD.

Description

Vascular dementia is caused by cerebrovascular disease and occurs almost always in the elderly. People with vascular dementia generally experience a decline in thought processes (cognitive function) that follows specific steps. This decline is often punctuated by small strokes—ruptures of tiny blood vessels in the **brain**. People experiencing vascular dementia often have problems with memory, abstract thinking, object identification or recognition, speech creation, speech comprehension, and motor activities.

Causes and symptoms

Vascular dementia is thought to be caused by small strokes that interfere with blood flow to the brain. Usually, vascular dementia is caused by many small strokes over time, rather than one large **stroke**. Sometimes this is referred to as multi-infarct dementia (MID). If the vascular dementia is caused by one large stroke, or develops in less than three months, then it is called acute onset vascular dementia. Acute onset vascular dementia is rare.

The signs of dementia often begin with impaired memory function. Sometimes a person has difficulty learning new things or remembering new events, and sometimes the person has difficulty recalling events or things that he or she used to know. Other signs of dementia include impairment in other areas of thought processing. Sometimes a person with vascular dementia may have difficulty producing coherent speech or may have other language impairments, such as problems understanding spoken or written language. The signs of vascular dementia are similar to those of Alzheimer's disease.

KEY TERMS

Acute onset vascular dementia—Vascular dementia caused by a single stroke or with an onset of fewer than three months.

Alzheimer's disease—An incurable disease of older individuals that results in the destruction of nerve cells in the brain and causes gradual loss of mental and physical functions.

Delirium—A disturbance of consciousness marked by confusion, difficulty paying attention, delusions, hallucinations, or restlessness. It can be distinguished from dementia by its relatively sudden onset and variation in the severity of the symptoms.

Dementia—A chronic condition in which thinking and memory are progressively impaired. Other symptoms may also occur, including personality changes and depression.

Hypertension—Persistently high blood pressure.

Multi-infarct dementia (MID)—Dementia caused by a series of many small strokes over a period longer than three months.

Difficulty with motor activities is a problem for some people with vascular dementia. Things that require hand-eye coordination, such as tying shoes or undoing buttons, are examples of motor activities that may be impaired. People with vascular dementia may also have difficulty recognizing familiar objects or may be unable to name them. Problems organizing things, putting events in sequence, or performing other types of abstract thinking may be present.

Some people with vascular dementia exhibit neurological signs that indicate the presence of cerebrovascular disease. They may have weakness of the arms or legs, abnormal reflexes, or abnormalities in the way they walk (gait abnormalities). Some people also exhibit behavioral disturbances related to the dementia, such as violence or aggression, often toward his or her caretaker. The patient may act impulsively and irritably or sometimes scream.

Diagnosis

The first step in the **diagnosis** of vascular dementia is to verify that dementia is present. The ***Diagnostic and Statistical Manual of Mental Disorders***, fourth edition, text revision (*DSM-IV-TR*), the handbook used by medical professionals in diagnosing mental disorders, indicates that impairments to memory must be present for a diagnosis of vascular dementia. Memory problems can include difficulties in learning and retaining new information or problems remembering past events or things that were learned before dementia took root.

In addition to memory impairment, the *DSM-IV-TR* specifies that one or more other impairments must be present. These impairments can include language problems, such as not being able to form speech and/or not being able to understand language, either spoken or written; problems performing activities that require hand-eye coordination, such as tying shoes, even though motor function is normal; problems recognizing or identifying objects, although the person is able to use his or her sense organs fully; problems doing tasks such as organizing, planning events, or putting things into sequence; or problems thinking abstractly. To meet the criteria for diagnosis, the memory problems and other impairments must cause the patient either significant distress or must impair his or her functioning in activities of daily life, such as by affecting the person's job or relationships with family or friends. The *DSM-IV-TR* specifies that the symptoms must show a decline in cognitive functioning and that the problems cannot occur during the course of an event that is categorized as **delirium**. There must be evidence that the problem is a result of cerebrovascular disease.

If dementia occurs without any other significant signs or symptoms, then it is classified as uncomplicated. There are three other possible *DSM-IV-TR* classifications based on the predominant feature of the dementia: vascular dementia with delirium, vascular dementia with **delusions**, and vascular dementia with depressed mood. If there are significant behavioral disturbances occurring as a result of the dementia, then the disturbances are specified.

Vascular dementia and AD are similar in many ways and can be confused. The most significant difference between the two is that vascular dementia can be diagnosed using physiological evidence of cerebrovascular disease. Also, AD generally occurs first as a slow loss of memory function, and then as a gradual decline into eventual dementia. Vascular dementia, however, generally occurs suddenly. The patient often declines in a stepwise fashion, with each step occurring after a small stroke.

Treatment

The treatments for vascular dementia focus on attempts to slow or halt the progression of the disorder and alleviate some of the symptoms. The disorder cannot be cured or reversed. The most common way to treat vascular dementia is to try to prevent further strokes. Treatments include diet and drug treatment for hypertension (high blood pressure), aspirin therapy, **smoking cessation**, avoidance of heavy **alcohol use**, and **stress reduction**. Some drugs that are used to treat mild AD are being studied for their effectiveness in treating vascular dementia.

QUESTIONS TO ASK YOUR DOCTOR

- Are my symptoms such as memory loss signs of dementia?
- Is the dementia vascular dementia or Alzheimer's disease?
- What steps can I take to help slow or halt the progression of the disease?
- Are there dietary changes that could help reduce the risk of additional strokes?
- Is there any light-to-moderate exercise you could recommend to help reduce the risk of additional strokes?

Prognosis

Vascular dementia is a disorder that cannot be reversed. The progression of the disorder can, however, be slowed. Using drugs along with lifestyle changes to prevent more strokes from occurring may help slow the progression of vascular dementia.

Prevention

Vascular dementia is generally associated with a series of strokes causing increasing mental impairment. Measures generally recommended by physicians to prevent strokes may be effective in helping to prevent vascular dementia. These include such things as quitting smoking, decreasing cholesterol levels, treating hypertension by reducing sodium (salt) intake, decreasing alcohol consumption, and making other lifestyle changes. Some studies have shown that drinking moderate daily amounts of alcohol, particularly red wine, may help to prevent dementia, but further research is needed.

Resources

BOOKS

Banejee, Sube, and Lawrence, Vanessa. *Managing Dementia in a Multicultural Society*. Hoboken, NJ: John Wiley and Sons, 2010.

Jacobsen, Sarah R., ed. *Vascular Dementia: Risk Factors, Diagnosis, and Treatment*. Hauppauge, NY: Nova Science, 2011.

Wahlund, Lars-Olof, Timo Erkinjuntti, and Serge Gauthier. *Vascular Cognitive Impairment in Clinical Practice*. New York: Cambridge University Press, 2009.

PERIODICALS

Aarsland, Dag, et al. "Is Physical Activity a Potential Preventive Factor for Vascular Dementia? A Systematic Review." *Aging and Mental Health* 14, no. 4 (May 2010): 386–395.

Heyanka, Daniel J., et al. "Distinguishing Alzheimer's Disease from Vascular Dementia: An Exploration of Five Cognitive Domains." *International Journal of Neuroscience* 120, no. 6 (June 2010): 409–414.

Yeager, Catherine A., et al. "Alzheimer's Disease and Vascular Dementia: The Complex Relationship Between Diagnosis and Caregiver Burden." *Issues in Mental Health Nursing* 31, no. 6 (June 2010): 376–384.

ORGANIZATIONS

American Aging Association, 2103 Cornell Rd., Room 5125, Cleveland, OH, 44106, (216) 368-3671, Fax: (216) 368-8964, americanaging@case.edu, http://www.americanaging.org.

American Association of Cardiovascular and Pulmonary Rehabilitation, 401 North Michigan Ave., Suite 2200, Chicago, IL, 60611, (312) 321-5146, Fax: (312) 673-6924, aacvpr@aacvpr.org, http://www.aacvpr.org.

National Institute on Aging, Bldg. 31, Rm. 5C27, 31 Center Drive, MSC 2292, Bethesda, MD, 20892, (301) 496-1752, (888) TTY: (800) 222-4225, Fax: (301) 496-1072, http://www.nia.nih.gov.

Tish Davidson, AM

Venlafaxine

Definition

Venlafaxine is an antidepressant available in the United States under the trade name of Effexor or Effexor XR.

Purpose

Venlafaxine is used to treat **depression** and **generalized anxiety disorder**. It has also been used to treat **obsessive-compulsive disorder** and irritable bowel syndrome.

Description

Venlafaxine is an antidepressant. It has actions common to both the cyclic **antidepressants**, such as **imipramine** (Tofranil) and **amitriptyline** (Elavil), and the **selective serotonin reuptake inhibitors (SSRIs)**, such as **fluoxetine** (Prozac), **sertraline** (Zoloft), and **paroxetine** (Paxil). It is believed that venlafaxine works by increasing levels of the neurotransmitters norepinephrine and **serotonin** in the **brain**.

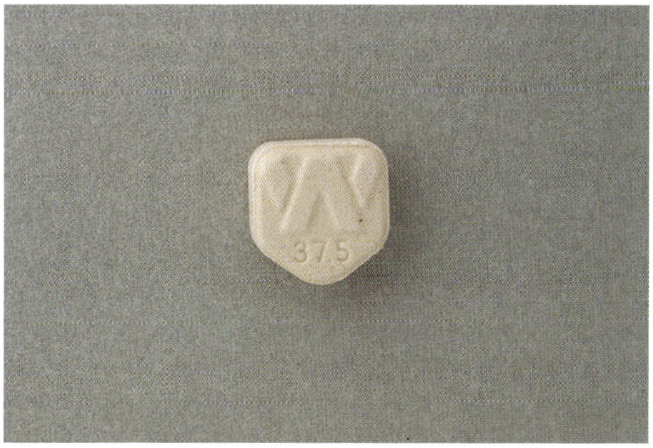

Effexor (venlafaxine), 37.5 mg. *(© Custom Medical Stock Photo, Inc. Reproduced by permission.)*

The therapeutic effects of venlafaxine, like other antidepressants, appear slowly. Maximum benefit is often not evident for at least two weeks after starting the drug. People taking venlafaxine should be aware of this and continue taking the drug as directed even if they do not see immediate improvement.

Venlafaxine is available in 25 mg, 37.5 mg, 50 mg, 75 mg, and 100 mg rapid-release tablets and 75 mg and 150 mg extended-action capsules.

Recommended dosage

The recommended initial dose of venlafaxine is 75 mg daily taken as two or three equal doses. The dose may be increased in 75 mg increments every four days as needed until symptoms of depression or anxiety resolve. Most commonly, dosages range between 150 mg to 225 mg daily, although in severe situations 375 mg per day may be needed. Once patients are stabilized using the rapid-acting tablets, they may be converted over to the appropriate dose of extended-release capsules.

Venlafaxine is broken down by the liver and eliminated from the body by the kidneys. As a result, the dose of venlafaxine must be lowered in people with liver or kidney disease. In people with liver disease, the daily dosage of venlafaxine should be cut in half. In patients with kidney disease, the daily dosage of venlafaxine should be reduced 25%–50%, depending upon the extent of kidney damage. When stopping venlafaxine, the dosage should be reduced gradually over a period of at least two weeks before the drug is totally stopped.

Precautions

Patients taking venlafaxine should be monitored closely for **insomnia**, anxiety, mania, significant weight loss, **seizures**, and thoughts of **suicide**. Children and adults up to age 24 are at increased risk for developing suicidal thoughts and behaviors when taking an antidepressant drug, including venlafaxine. Patients of any age who are taking antidepressants should be monitored for signs of worsening depression or changes in behavior.

Caution should also be exercised when prescribing venlafaxine to patients with impaired liver or kidney function, the elderly (over age 60), children, individuals with **bipolar disorder** or a history of seizures, people with diabetes, persons with narrow-angle glaucoma, and individuals expressing ideas of committing suicide. People with diabetes should monitor their blood or urine sugar more carefully, since venlafaxine may affect blood sugar.

Care should be taken to weigh the risks and benefits of this drug in women who are or wish to become pregnant, as well as in breast-feeding mothers.

Until individuals understand the effects that venlafaxine may have, they should avoid driving, operating dangerous machinery, or participating in hazardous activities. Alcohol should not be used while taking venlafaxine.

Side effects

More common side effects include decreased sexual drive, restlessness, difficulty sitting still, skin rash, hives, and itching. Less common side effects include fever and/or chills and pain in joints or muscles.

Rare side effects include pain or enlargement of breasts and/or abnormal milk production in women, seizures, fast heart rate, irregular heartbeats, red or purple spots on the skin, low blood sugar and its symptoms (anxiety, chills, cold sweats, confusion, difficulty concentrating, drowsiness, excess hunger, rapid heart rate, headache, shakiness or unsteadiness, severe **fatigue**), low blood sodium and its symptoms (including confusion, seizures, drowsiness, dry mouth, severe thirst, decreased energy), **serotonin syndrome** (characterized by at least three of the following symptoms: diarrhea, fever, sweatiness, mood or behavior changes, overactive reflexes, fast heart rate, restlessness, shivering or shaking), excitability, agitation, irritability, pressured talking, difficulty breathing, and odd body or facial movements.

QUESTIONS TO ASK YOUR DOCTOR

- What kind of changes can I expect to see or feel with this medication?
- Does it matter what time of day I take this medication?
- Should I take this medication with or without food?
- What are the side effects associated with this medication?
- Will this medication interact or interfere with other medications I am currently taking?
- What symptoms or adverse effects are important enough that I should seek immediate treatment?

Interactions

Venlafaxine interacts with a long list of other medications. Anyone starting this drug should review the other medications they are taking with their physician and pharmacist for possible interactions. Patients should always inform all of their healthcare providers, including dentists, that they are taking venlafaxine.

Dangerously high blood pressure has resulted from the combination of antidepressants, such as venlafaxine, and members of another class of antidepressants known as **monoamine oxidase inhibitors** (MAOIs). Because of this, venlafaxine should never be taken in combination with MAOIs. Patients taking any MAOIs, for example **phenelzine** (Nardil) or **tranylcypromine** (Parnate), should stop taking the MAOI and wait at least 14 days before starting venlafaxine or any other antidepressant. When stopping treatment with venlafaxine, patients should wait five weeks before taking an MAOI.

Some other drugs such as **trazodone** (Desyrel), sibutramine (Meridia), and sumatriptan (Imitrex) also interact with venlafaxine and cause a syndrome known as **neuroleptic malignant syndrome**, characterized by irritability, muscle stiffness, shivering, muscle spasms, and altered consciousness.

KEY TERMS

Depression—A mental state characterized by excessive sadness. Other symptoms include altered sleep patterns, thoughts of suicide, difficulty concentrating, agitation, lack of energy, and loss of enjoyment in activities that are usually pleasurable.

Generalized anxiety disorder—A general form of fear that can dominate a person's life.

Insomnia—A sleep disorder characterized by waking in the middle of the night and having difficulty returning to sleep, or waking too early in the morning.

Mania—An elevated or euphoric mood or irritable state that is characteristic of bipolar disorder.

Narrow-angle glaucoma—An eye disorder caused by a buildup of fluid pressure inside the eyeball due to an abnormally small angle between the iris (the colored portion of the eye) and the cornea (the transparent front part of the eye).

Norepinephrine—A chemical messenger in the brain thought to play a role in mood regulation.

Obsessive-compulsive disorder—A disorder in which affected individuals have an obsession (such as a fear of contamination, or thoughts they do not like to have and cannot control) and feel compelled to perform certain acts to neutralize the obsession (such as repeated hand washing).

Seizure—A convulsion, or uncontrolled discharge of nerve cells that may spread to other cells throughout the brain.

Serotonin—A chemical messenger in the brain thought to play a role in mood regulation.

Serotonin syndrome—A condition characterized by at least three of the following symptoms: diarrhea, fever, extreme perspiration, mood or behavior changes, overactive reflexes, fast heart rate, restlessness, shivering, or shaking. The condition occurs when there is too much serotonin in the body.

The sedative effects (drowsiness or lack of mental clarity) of venlafaxine are increased by other central nervous system depressants such as alcohol, **sedatives**, sleeping medications, or other medications used for mental disorders such as **schizophrenia**. Patients taking blood thinners, including aspirin, are at risk for increased bleeding when taking venlafaxine.

Resources

BOOKS

Albers, Lawrence J., Rhoda K. Hahn, and Christopher Reist. *Handbook of Psychiatric Drugs*. Laguna Hills, CA: Current Clinical Strategies Publishing, 2010.

American Society of Health-System Pharmacists. *AHFS Drug Information 2011*. Bethesda: American Society of Health-System Pharmacists, 2011.

Graham, George. *The Disordered Mind: An Introduction to Philosophy of Mind and Mental Illness*. New York: Routledge, 2010.

Holland, Leland Norman, and Michael Patrick Adams. *Core Concepts in Pharmacology*. 3rd ed. New York: Prentice Hall, 2011.

North, Carol, and Sean Yutzy. *Goodwin and Guze's Psychiatric Diagnosis*. New York: Oxford University Press, 2010.

Preston, John D., John H. O'Neal, and Mary C. Talaga. *Handbook of Clinical Psychopharmacology for Therapists*. 6th ed. Oakland, CA: New Harbinger Publications, 2011.

PERIODICALS

Baca, Enrique, et al. "Venlafaxine Extended-Release in Patients Older than 80 Years with Depressive Syndrome." *International Journal of Geriatric Psychiatry* 21, no. 4 (April 2006): 337–43.

Davidson, Jonathan, et al. "Treatment of Posttraumatic Stress Disorder with Venlafaxine Extended Release." *Archives of General Psychiatry* 63, no. 10 (Oct. 2006): 1158–65.

Johnson, Ellyn M., et al. "Cardiovascular Changes Associated With Venlafaxine in the Treatment of Late-Life Depression." *American Journal of Geriatric Psychiatry* 14, no. 9 (Sept. 2006): 796–802.

Kim, Tae-Suk, et al. "Comparison of Venlafaxine Extended Release Versus Paroxetine for Treatment of Patients with Generalized Anxiety Disorder." *Psychiatry and Clinical Neurosciences* 60, no. 3 (June 2006): 347–51.

McGrath, Patrick J, et al. "Tranylcypromine Versus Venlafaxine Plus Mirtazapine Following Three Failed Antidepressant Medication Trials for Depression: A STAR*D Report." *American Journal of Psychiatry* 163, no. 9 (Sept. 2006): 1531–41.

Montgomery, Stuart A. "Escitalopram Versus Venlafaxine XR in the Treatment of Depression." *International Clinical Psychopharmacology* 21, no. 5 (Sept. 2006): 297–309.

Nemeroff, Charles B., and Michael E. Thase. "A Double-Blind, Placebo-Controlled Comparison of Venlafaxine and Fluoxetine Treatment in Depressed Outpatients." *Journal of Psychiatric Research* 41, nos. 3–4 (April–June 2007): 351–59.

Post, R. M., et al. "Mood Switch in Bipolar Depression: Comparison of Adjunctive Venlafaxine, Bupropion and Sertraline." *British Journal of Psychiatry* 189, no. 2 (Aug. 2006): 124–31.

Tiihonen, Jari, et al. "Antidepressants and the Risk of Suicide, Attempted Suicide, and Overall Mortality in a Nationwide Cohort." *Archives of General Psychiatry* 63, no. 12 (Dec. 2006): 1358–67.

Yazicioglu, Bengi, et al. "A Comparison of the Efficacy and Tolerability of Reboxetine and Sertraline Versus Venlafaxine in Major Depressive Disorder: A Randomized, Open-Labeled

Clinical Trial." *Progress in Neuro-Psychopharmacology & Biological Psychiatry* 30, no. 7 (Sept. 2006): 1271–76.

WEBSITES

PubMed Health. "Venlafaxine." U.S. National Library of Medicine. http://www.ncbi.nlm.nih.gov/pubmedhealth/PMH0000947 (accessed November 13, 2011).

ORGANIZATIONS

American Psychiatric Association, 1000 Wilson Boulevard, Suite 1825, Arlington, VA, 22209, (703) 907-7300, apa@psych.org, http://www.psych.org.

National Alliance on Mental Illness (NAMI), Colonial Place Three, 2107 Wilson Blvd., Suite 300, Arlington, VA, 22201, (703) 524-7600, (800) 950-NAMI (6264), Fax: (703) 524-9094, http://www.nami.org/Hometemplate.cfm.

National Institute of Mental Health (NIMH), 6001 Executive Boulevard, Room 8184, MSC 9663, Bethesda, MD, 20892, (301) 443-4513, (866) 615-6464, Fax: (301) 443-4279, nimhinfo@nih.gov, http://www.nimh.nih.gov/index.shtml.

U.S. Food and Drug Administration, 10903 New Hampshire Ave., Silver Spring, MD, 20993-0002, (888) INFO-FDA (463-6332), http://www.fda.gov.

Kelly Karpa, R.Ph.,Ph.D.
Ruth A. Wienclaw, Ph.D.
Laura Jean Cataldo, RN, Ed.D.

Veterans' mental health *see* **Military mental health**

Violence *see* **Mental health and violence**

Vivactil *see* **Protriptyline**

Vivitrol

Purpose

Vivitrol (**naltrexone** for extended-release injectable suspension) is a once-monthly injection used in the treatment of alcohol dependence in patients who are able to abstain from alcohol at least seven to ten days prior to treatment.

Description

Naltrexone, the active ingredient in Vivitrol, is an opioid antagonist that blocks the effects of alcohol; it is not an aversive therapy that pairs a strong feeling of dislike or disgust with alcohol. Naltrexone has few, if any, intrinsic actions other than as an opioid antagonist. It produces withdrawal symptoms in patients physically dependent on **opioids**. Vivitrol should be used as only one component of a comprehensive alcoholism management program that includes counseling, self-help **support groups**, or other psychosocial support.

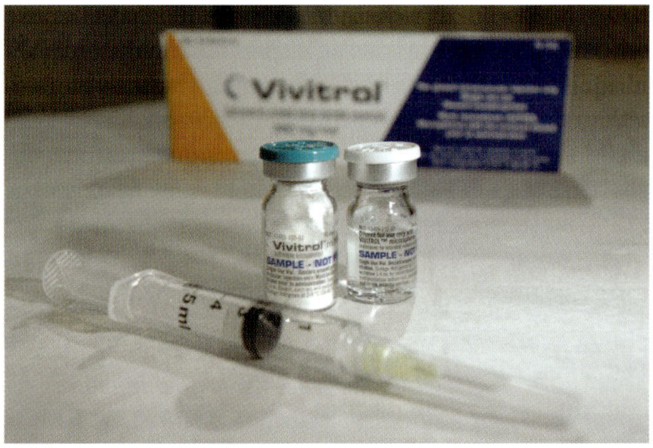

Vivitrol injection. *(© Mark Dye/Star Ledger/Corbis)*

Recommended dosage

The recommended dosage of Vivitrol is 380 mg once a month. Vivitrol is delivered by intramuscular gluteal injection and should not be administered intravenously. Patients missing a dose should be given the next dose as soon as possible. Vivitrol must be administered by a healthcare professional.

Before starting treatment with Vivitrol, the patient should abstain from alcohol in an outpatient setting, not be actively drinking, not be in acute opiate withdrawal, and be opioid free for at least seven to ten days.

Precautions

In excessive doses, naltrexone has been found to cause liver damage. Therefore, Vivitrol is not recommended for use in cases of acute hepatitis or liver failure. Careful consideration should be given before administering Vivitrol to patients with liver disease. Vivitrol should be discontinued in the event of signs of acute hepatitis.

Vivitrol should not be given to patients with a physiological dependence on opioids or who are in opioid withdrawal. To prevent withdrawal, Vivitrol should not be administered to patients receiving opioid analgesics. In cases where Vivitrol blockade needs to be reversed for pain management, patients should be monitored in a setting enabled for cardiopulmonary resuscitation.

Side effects

Vivitrol counteracts the effects of opioid-containing medications, including analgesics, cough and cold medications, and antidiarrheal preparations.

Vivitrol is generally well tolerated. In **clinical trials**, serious adverse reactions occurred in patients receiving Vivitrol at a similar rate to patients receiving a placebo. Mild to moderate adverse events were seen in most patients. The most common of these were nausea, vomiting, headache, dizziness, **insomnia**, **fatigue**, and injection site reaction.

In clinical trials, suicidal tendencies (including thoughts of **suicide**, suicide attempts, and completed suicides), although infrequent, occurred more often in patients treated with Vivitrol (1%) than in patients receiving a placebo (0). Similarly, depression-related events were higher for patients taking Vivitrol (1%) than for those taking a placebo (0). Patients taking Vivitrol should be monitored for **depression** or suicidal thinking.

Side effects and other reactions reported include:

- blood and lymphatic system disorders (e.g., swollen, firm, or possibly tender lymph nodes; increased white blood cell count)
- cardiac disorders (e.g., palpitations, atrial fibrillation, myocardial infarction, angina pectoris, angina unstable, congestive heart failure, atherosclerosis)
- eye disorders (e.g., conjunctivitis)
- gastrointestinal disorders (e.g., constipation, toothache, flatulence, gastroesophageal reflux disease, hemorrhoids, colitis, gastrointestinal hemorrhage, paralysis/obstruction of the intestine, perirectal abscess)
- general disorders (e.g., fever, lethargy, rigors, chest pain or tightness, weight loss)
- liver disorders (e.g., gallstones)
- infections and infestations (e.g., influenza, bronchitis, urinary tract infection, gastroenteritis, tooth abscess, pneumonia)
- immune system disorders (e.g., seasonal allergy, hypersensitivity reaction)
- injection site reactions (e.g., pain, tenderness, skin reactions)
- metabolism and nutrition disorders (e.g., anorexia, appetite disorders, increased appetite, heat exhaustion, dehydration, elevated blood cholesterol)
- musculoskeletal and connective tissue disorders (e.g., pain in limbs, muscle spasms, joint stiffness)
- nausea, particularly after initial injection
- nervous system disorders (e.g., headache and migraine, dizziness, fainting, sleepiness, abnormality of the sense of taste, disturbance in attention, mental impairment, convulsions, ischemic stroke, cerebral arterial aneurysm)

KEY TERMS

Alcohol dependence—A chronic disease with both neurological and genetic factors. Diagnostic criteria include increased tolerance for alcohol, withdrawal symptoms, loss of control over the use of alcohol, and/or impaired function. Alcohol dependence is distinguished from alcohol abuse, alcohol withdrawal syndrome, and other alcohol-induced syndromes.

Analgesic—A medication to reduce or eliminate pain.

Opioid—A synthetic narcotic that resembles natural opiates.

Placebo—A preparation without pharmacological effect that is given in place of a drug in clinical trials to determine the effectiveness of the drug under study; a "sugar pill."

- psychiatric disorders (e.g., irritability, decreased libido, abnormal dreams, alcohol withdrawal syndrome, agitation, euphoric mood, delirium)
- respiratory, thoracic, and mediastinal disorders (e.g., shortness of breath, sinus congestion, chronic obstructive airways disease)
- skin and subcutaneous tissue disorders (e.g., increased sweating, night sweats)
- vascular disorders (e.g., elevated blood pressure, hot flushes, deep venous thrombosis, pulmonary embolism)

Interactions

Although Vivitrol is a powerful drug with prolonged effects for blocking the action of opioids, the blockade can be overcome. However, such action is extremely dangerous. Any attempt by the patient to overcome the blockage by taking higher amounts of opioids or large dose of heroin while on Vivitrol could lead to serious injury, coma, or death.

A number of drugs may interact with Vivitrol. Patients should inform their doctor of all drugs they are currently taking before starting treatment. It has been shown, however, that patients treated simultaneously with Vivitrol and antidepressant medications (e.g., **sertraline**, **citalopram**, **paroxetine**, **fluoxetine**, trazodone, **bupropion** hydrochloride) had similar safety profiles to patients taking Vivitrol without **antidepressants**.

Resources

BOOKS

American Psychiatric Association. *Diagnostic and Statistical Manual of Mental Disorders*. 4th ed., text rev. Washington, DC: American Psychiatric Publishing, 2000.

WEBSITES

Cephalon, Inc. "U.S. Government Organizations Release Positive Information About VIVITROL for the Treatment of Alcoholism." http://investors.cephalon.com/phoenix.zhtml?c=81709&p=irol-newsArticle&ID=1000756&highlight= (accessed October 29, 2011).

Cephalon, Inc. "Vivitrol (naltrexone for extended-release injectable suspension): Prescribing Information." 2010. http://www.vivitrol.com/pdf_docs/prescribing_info.pdf (accessed October 29, 2011).

Hilt, Emma. "Naltrexone Extended-Release Prescribing Information Strengthened." Medscape Medical News. May 5, 2010. http://www.medscape.com/viewarticle/721288 (accessed October 29, 2011).

Ruth A. Wienclaw, Ph.D.

Vocational rehabilitation

Definition

Vocational rehabilitation (VR) is a set of services offered to individuals with mental or physical disabilities. These services are designed to enable participants to attain skills, resources, attitudes, and expectations needed to compete in the interview process, get a job, and keep a job. Services offered may also help an individual retrain for employment after an injury or mental disorder has disrupted previous employment.

Purpose

Vocational rehabilitation services prepare qualified applicants to achieve a lifestyle of independence and integration within their workplace, family, and local community. This transition is achieved through work evaluation and job readiness services, job counseling services, and medical and therapeutic services. For individuals with psychiatric disabilities, situational assessments are generally used to evaluate vocational skills and potential.

Precautions

Vocational rehabilitation as operated by state agencies is not an entitlement program. Only individuals considered eligible can receive VR services. Eligibility criteria require that an individual be at least 16 years old, unemployed or under-employed, and have a physical or mental disability that results in a substantial barrier to employment, such as psychotic disorders, alcohol and other drug abuse dependence, mental and emotional disorders, attention deficit disorders, specific learning disabilities, or physical or sensory disabilities. In addition, the individual must be able to benefit from VR services. An individual must also need help to prepare for, find, and succeed in paid employment. When resources are limited, individuals with the most significant disabilities must be served first.

Description

Vocational rehabilitation services are based on individual needs and defined as any goods or services an individual might need to be employable, such as assistive technology devices and services. For instance, a person who is blind would need screen reading software to access a computer and people with a cognitive or mental disability might need a talking electronic reminder device programmed to prompt them when it is time to perform certain tasks.

Vocational rehabilitation can be provided by private organizations, but is not typically funded under **managed care** arrangements. Thus, most people apply to state vocational rehabilitation agencies that are funded through federal and state monies. Typically, state agencies have offices in their state's major cities and towns. State VR agencies do not necessarily offer the same services or deliver services in the same way in every state, so individuals seeking services must learn how to access the VR program in their own state. The federal VR component is administered by the U.S. Department of Education Rehabilitation Services Administration and authorized by the Rehabilitation Act of 1973 as amended in the 1988 reauthorization.

Most vocational rehabilitation services are free for eligible applicants; however, applicants may be asked to use other benefits, such as insurance, Pell grants or other financial aid for training or higher education, to pay part of program costs.

Best practices in vocational rehabilitation include individual choice, person-centered planning, integrated setting, natural supports, rapid placement, and career development. The term *integrated setting* refers to placing individuals in usual employment situations rather than making placements into sheltered workshops or other segregated settings. Natural supports are the person's already existing support network, including family members, service providers, and friends, who can help the person reach a goal, such as the employment of their choice. Person-centered planning is a technique in which a plan for a person's future is developed by a team consisting of the person and his or her natural supports, and the team develops a practical plan based on the person's wishes and dreams. Each teammember agrees to perform certain tasks identified in the plan to help the person reach goals. Unfortunately, not all VR programs incorporate all of these best practices.

Preparation

Vocational rehabilitation transition planning services are required for all public and private education students aged 16 and over, who have Individualized Education Plans (IEPs) or Rehabilitation Act Section 504 Plans. Transition services help students make the transition from school to employment, training or higher education. Older individuals who have acquired disabilities and are applying for VR services must undergo medical and psychological assessments at their local VR office to determine the extent of their disabilities, except for individuals receiving SSDI or SSI who are presumed eligible without assessments. Applicants may receive treatment and counseling, if needed, before training and employment. All VR services are described in an applicant's Individualized Plan for Employment (IPE). Applicants may design the IPE either on their own or with the assistance of their assigned VR counselor, usually a person with a master's degree in rehabilitation counseling.

Aftercare

A vocational rehabilitation counselor will help applicants access an employment agency to help locate a job. Counselors may provide support (supported employment programs) if applicants need support to keep a job. This support may include job coaching, which includes working with the person in the workplace until the person is comfortable with the work. The counselors also act as resources if a job does not work out by assessing what happened and counseling the person on how to improve performance or change habits that were not looked on with favor in the workplace.

KEY TERMS

IEP (Individualized Education Plan)—Under federal law governing special education, every child in public schools who is determined through assessment to have special mental disability needs has an IEP. An IEP is typically developed by a team of professionals that may include special education teachers; physical, occupational and speech therapists; psychologists; parents or guardians; and others who may be called on to provide expertise. The team meets at least once a year to set goals for the next school year and to assess progress on already established goals. Parents who are not satisfied with school-based assessments have the right to ask for independent assessments that must be paid for by the school system.

Integrated setting—Placing individuals in usual employment situations rather than making placements into sheltered workshops or other segregated settings.

Natural supports—Using a person's already existing support network to help the person reach a goal, such as the employment of their choice.

Person-centered planning—A technique in which a plan for a person's future is developed by a team consisting of the person, family members, service providers and friends (natural supports). The team develops a practical plan based on the person's wishes and dreams. Each team member agrees to perform certain tasks identified in the plan to help the person reach goals.

Section 504—This section of the Rehabilitation Act of 1973 provides that no person may be discriminated against because of a physical disability—for instance, a child who uses a wheelchair. If a science class is on the second floor and the building has no elevator, the school must find a way to ensure that children in wheelchairs have access to that science class. An educational plan for a child who has both cognitive and physical disabilities is developed under an IEP.

Risks

Applicants may not be satisfied with the pace of progress toward their employment goal through VR, or they may not believe their wishes or talents and skills are being taken seriously. Applicants wanting to start their own businesses or engage in telecommuting may not be successful in receiving vocational rehabilitation assistance. Applicants may find that VR counselors tend to recommend low-level and low-paying jobs traditionally recommended for VR applicants, such as food service and janitorial work. Applicants may also be turned away by VR counselors because the counselors decide the applicant's disability is too severe for the person to benefit from VR services. An additional risk for individuals with mental disorders is a usual lack of coordination between VR and mental health systems.

To address these problems in the VR system, the U.S. Congress passed the Ticket To Work Act in 1999. Under this Act, persons with mental or physical disabilities receive a ticket worth a certain amount of money. They may take this ticket to any private or public entity that provides job training and placement, including state VR programs. The entities providing the employment-related services are able to redeem the tickets for payment only after the person has been gainfully employed for a certain period of time.

Results

Individuals with mental or physical disabilities will receive the assessments, counseling, training, placement, accommodations and long-term supports needed to allow them to engage in the gainful employment of their choice.

Resources

PERIODICALS

Cook, Judith A. "Research-Based Principles of Vocational Rehabilitation for Psychiatric Disability." University of Chicago National Reserach and Training Center on Psychiatric Disability. Issue 4 (September 1999).

Harding, Courtney. "Some Things We've Learned about Vocational Rehabilitation of the Seriously and Persistently Mentally Ill." Presented at the Boston University Colloquium, Brookline, MA: April 17, 1996.

Lehman, Anthony F. "Vocational Rehabilitation in Schizophrenia." *Schizophrenia Bulletin* 21, no. 4 (1995): 645–56.

MacDonald-Wilson, K., et al. "Unique Issues in Assessing Work Function Among Individuals with Psychiatric Disabilities." *Journal of Occupational Rehabilitation* 11, no. 3 (2001): 217–32.

Maronne, J., et al. "If You Think Work Is Bad for People with Mental Illness, Then Try Poverty, Unemployment, and Social Isolation." *Psychiatric Rehabilitation Journal* 23, no. 2 (2000): 187–193.

WEBSITES

Office of Special Education and Rehabilitation Services. "Rehabilitation Services Administration (RSA) Programs and Projects." http://www2.ed.gov/about/offices/list/osers/rsa/programs.html (accessed December 18, 2011).

U.S. Social Security Administration. "About Ticket to Work." http://ssa.gov/work/aboutticket.html (accessed December 18, 2011).

ORGANIZATIONS

Association for Persons in Supported Employment, PO Box 1280, Rockville, MD, 20849, (301) 279-0060, Fax: (301) 251-3762, http://www.apse.org.

Office of Special Education and Rehabilitative Services, Rehabilitation Services Administration, 400 Maryland Ave., SW, Washington, DC, 20202-2800, (202) 245-7488, http://rsa.ed.gov.

State Rehabilitation Councils, 1902 Market Street, Camp Hill, PA, 17011, (888) 250-5175, http://www.parac.org.

Geoffrey Grimm, Ph.D., LPC

Voyeurism

Definition

Voyeurism is a psychosexual disorder in which a person derives sexual pleasure and gratification from looking at naked bodies and genital organs or observing the sexual acts of others. The voyeur is usually hidden from view of others. Voyeurism is a form of paraphilia. Other **paraphilias** include **exhibitionism**, **fetishism**, and **pedophilia**.

A variant form of voyeurism involves listening to erotic conversations. This is commonly referred to as telephone sex, although it is usually considered voyeurism primarily in the instance of listening to unsuspecting people.

Demographics

Voyeurism is more common in men but does occasionally occur in women. However, the prevalence of voyeurism is not known. Contemporary society in the United States is increasingly voyeuristic (as illustrated by the popularity of reality television); however, **diagnosis** is made only when voyeurism is a preferred or exclusive means of sexual gratification. Paraphilias in total are generally believed to occur much more frequently in men than women, with about 20 men diagnosed for each woman diagnosed.

Description

The object of voyeurism is to observe unsuspecting individuals who are naked, in the process of undressing, or engaging in sexual acts. The person being observed usually is a stranger to the observer. The act of looking or peeping is undertaken for the purpose of achieving sexual excitement. The observer generally does not seek to have sexual contact or activity with the person being observed.

If orgasm is sought, it is usually achieved through masturbation. This may occur during the act of observation or later, relying on the memory of the act that was observed.

Frequently, a voyeur may have a fantasy of engaging in sexual activity with the person being observed. In reality, this fantasy is rarely acted out.

A number of states have statutes that render voyeurism a crime. Such statutes vary widely regarding definitions of voyeurism. Most states specifically prohibit anyone from photographing or videotaping another person without consent while observing that person in the privacy of his home or some other private place.

Causes and symptoms

Professionals do not agree about the causes of voyeurism, but its symptoms are generally accepted as having to do with violating the privacy of others for personal sexual gratification.

Causes

There is no scientific consensus concerning the basis for voyeurism. Some experts attribute the behavior to an initially random or accidental observation of an unsuspecting person who is naked, in the process of disrobing, or engaging in sexual activity. Successive repetitions of the act tend to reinforce and perpetuate the voyeuristic behavior.

Other experts view this and other paraphilias as having an obsessive-compulsive element, and some findings describe these behaviors in a category of compulsive-impulsive sexual behaviors or behaviors that fit in the inclusive term of **process addiction**. For example, those with symptoms of compulsive-impulsive sex behavior related to process addiction may have frequent, intrusive thoughts about sex and engage repeatedly in sex behaviors that can spiral out of control.

Single case studies have suggested some effectiveness in treating paraphilic behaviors with drugs used to treat **bipolar disorder**, implying a potential link to bipolar disorders. People with pedophilia, which is also characterized as a paraphilia, have abnormalities in **brain imaging studies** that are similar to those observed in imaging studies of people with **obsessive-compulsive disorder**. Disruption of the pathways of **dopamine** and **serotonin** (both nerve-signaling molecules) is implicated in these disorders. People who engage in paraphilic behavior may also have a higher rate of substance use, novelty seeking, and sexual risk-taking behaviors.

Symptoms

The act of voyeurism is the repeated observation of an unsuspecting person who is naked or who is in the process of disrobing or engaging in sexual activity that provides sexual arousal to the viewer, who usually remains hidden from the individual being observed. The onset of voyeuristic activity is usually before the age of 15.

Diagnosis

According to the handbook used by mental health professionals to diagnose mental disorders, the *Diagnostic and Statistical Manual of Mental Disorders* (*DSM*), two criteria are required to make a diagnosis of voyeurism:

- An individual must experience recurrent, intense, and sexually arousing fantasies, urges, or behaviors that involve the act of observing a person who is naked, disrobing, or engaging in sexual activity, and who is unaware of being observed.
- The actions must cause significant distress or impairment in areas of everyday functioning, or the person must have sought sexual stimulation from observing three or more persons on at least three separate occasions.

Revisions for the fifth edition of the *DSM* (*DSM-5*) proposed changing voyeurism to voyeuristic disorder, in order to help differentiate between paraphilias and paraphilic disorders. Paraphilias are not inherently causes for psychiatric diagnoses, but when the paraphilia causes distress, harm, or otherwise impairs everyday functioning for the person or others, it is considered a disorder.

Treatment

For treatment to be successful, a person with voyeuristic disorder must want to modify existing patterns of behavior. This initial step is difficult for most patients to admit and then take, and usually individuals must be compelled to accept treatment, often as the result of a court order.

KEY TERMS

Bipolar disorder—A psychiatric disorder characterized by periods of mania alternating with periods of depression.

Dopamine—A neurochemical made in the brain that is involved in many brain activities, including movement and emotion.

Paraphilia—A group of sexual disorders involving fantasies, desires, or behaviors with uncommon objects or in uncommon situations generally not found sexually arousing by others and that are not generally accepted by society.

Serotonin—5-Hydroxytryptamine; a substance that occurs throughout the body with numerous effects, including neurotransmission. Low serotonin levels are associated with mood disorders, particularly depression and obsessive-compulsive disorder.

QUESTIONS TO ASK YOUR DOCTOR

- Could my behavior or sexual preferences indicate voyeurism?
- Can you recommend a mental health professional who is experienced in treating this disorder?
- Will my insurance cover treatment for this disorder?
- Are there any support groups in this area?
- What are the laws concerning voyeuristic behavior in this state?

Behavioral therapy is commonly used to try to treat voyeurism. The voyeur must learn to control the impulse to watch nonconsenting victims and acquire more acceptable means of sexual gratification. Outcomes of behavioral therapy are not known. There are no direct drug treatments for voyeurism.

Voyeurism is a criminal act in many jurisdictions. It is usually classified as a misdemeanor. As a result, legal penalties are often minor. The possibility of exposure and embarrassment may deter some persons from engaging in voyeurism. It is not easy to prosecute cases of voyeurism, as intent to watch is difficult to prove. In defense statements, perpetrators of voyeurism usually claim that the observation was accidental.

Prognosis

Once voyeuristic activity is undertaken, it commonly does not stop. Over time, it may become the main form of sexual gratification for the voyeur. Its course tends to be chronic.

The prognosis for completely eliminating voyeuristic actions is poor, largely because most persons with voyeuristic disorder have no desire to change their pattern of behavior. Because voyeurism involves nonconsenting partners and is against the law in many jurisdictions, the possibility of embarrassment may deter some individuals.

Prevention

Most experts agree that providing guidance regarding culturally acceptable behavior will help to prevent the development of a paraphilia such as voyeurism. The origin of some instances of voyeurism may be accidental observation with subsequent sexual gratification. There is no way to predict when such an event and association may occur.

Members of society can reduce the incidence of voyeurism by drawing curtains, dropping blinds, or closing window curtains. Reducing opportunities for voyeurism may reduce the practice.

Resources

BOOKS

Clinton, Tim, and Mark Laaser. *The Quick-Reference Guide to Sexuality and Relationship Counseling.* Grand Rapids, MI: Baker Books, 2010.

Hock, Roger R. *Human Sexuality,* 2nd ed. Upper Saddle River, NJ: Prentice Hall, 2010.

Laws, D. Richard, and William T. O'Donohue, eds. *Sexual Deviance: Theory, Assessment, and Treatment,* 2nd ed. New York, Guilford Press, 2008.

Rowland, David L., and Luca Incrocci, eds. *Handbook of Sexual and Gender Identity Disorders.* Hoboken, NJ: John Wiley and Sons, 2008.

PERIODICALS

Hinderliter, Andrew C. "Disregarding Science, Clinical Utility and the DSM's Definition of Mental Disorder: The Case of Exhibitionism, Voyeurism, and Frotteurism." *Archives of Sexual Behavior* 39, no. 6 (December 2010): 1235–37.

Langstrom, Niklas. "The DSM Diagnostic Criteria for Exhibitionism, Voyeurism, and Frotteurism." *Archives of Sexual Behavior* 39, no. 2 (April 2010): 317–24.

ORGANIZATIONS

American Academy of Child and Adolescent Psychiatry, 3615 Wisconsin Ave. NW, Washington, DC, 20016-3007, (202) 966-7300, Fax: (202) 966-2891, http://www.aacap.org.

American Psychological Association, 750 1st St. NE, Washington, DC, 20002-4242, (202) 336-5500; TDD/TTY: (202) 336-6123, (800) 374-2721, apa@psych.org, http://www.apa.org.

L. Fleming Fallon, Jr, MD
Tish Davidson, AM

Vyvanse *see* **Lisdexamfetamine**

W

Wechsler Intelligence Scales

Definition

The Wechsler Intelligence Scales are a series of **intelligence tests** used to assess general cognition in children and/or adults. The series of tests consists of the Wechsler Preschool and Primary Scale of Intelligence (WPPSI) for children from three to seven years of age, the Wechsler Intelligence Scale for Children (WISC) for children from six to 16 years of age, and the Wechsler Adult Intelligence Scale (WAIS) for adults 16 years and older.

Purpose

The purpose of the Wechsler Scales is to test cognitive abilities (intelligence) in children and adults by providing various index scores that indicate different verbal and non-verbal (performance) abilities.

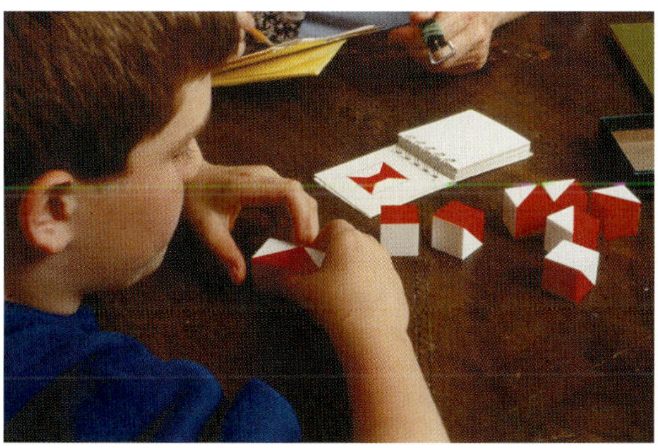

A five-year-old child is assessed using the Wechsler Intelligence Scale for Children. *(© Custom Medical Stock Photo, Inc. Reproduced by permission.)*

Description

Origins

The Wechsler Intelligence Scales were developed by Romanian-born American **psychologist** David Wechsler (1896–1981). In 1939, Dr. Wechsler developed the first of his tests, the Wechsler Adult Intelligence Scale, while working at the Bellevue Hospital Center in Manhattan, New York City. In 1949, he developed the Wechsler Intelligence Scale for Children, and in 1967, the Wechsler Preschool and Primary Scale of Intelligence. These tests were originally developed by Wechsler as a way to learn more about his patients at Bellevue after he realized that existing intelligence tests were not adequate for his purposes and, especially, that those tests did not provide very much validity for older children and adults.

Wechsler believed that intelligence was based on performance and not on capacity. As such, he viewed intelligence as an individual's ability to solve problems. He stated in 1944, "Intelligence is the aggregate or global capacity of the individual to act purposefully, to think rationally and to deal effectively with his environment." Wechsler developed his Scales by introducing two parts for the testing in intelligence: Verbal and Performance (non-verbal). Each part was then subdivided into subtests. He assigned an arbitrary value of 100 to the mean intelligence, to stand for the average or expected value of intelligence. Wechsler then added or subtracted 15 points from 100 for each standard deviation above or below the mean, respectively.

Components

As a widely used series of intelligence tests developed by clinical psychologist David Wechsler, their most distinctive feature is a division into a verbal section and a nonverbal (or "performance") section, with separate scores available for each one. Verbal intelligence—the component most often associated with academic accomplishment—implies the ability to reason abstractly in terms using either words or mathematical symbols.

Performance intelligence suggests the ability to perceive relationships and piece individual parts together logically into a whole. The inclusion of the performance section in the Wechsler scales is especially helpful in assessing the cognitive ability of non-native speakers and children with speech or language disorders. The test can be of particular value to school psychologists screening for specific learning disabilities because of the number of specific subtests that make up each section.

For all of the Wechsler scales, separate verbal and performance scores, as well as a total score, are computed. These are then converted using a scale divided into categories (such as average and superior), and the final score is generally given as one of these categories rather than as a number or percentile ranking.

WPPSI

The Wechsler Preschool and Primary Scales of Intelligence (WPPSI) has traditionally been geared toward children ages four to six years of age, although the newest version of the test (WPPSI-III, publication year: 2002) broadens the age range downward to two years, six months, and upward to seven years, three months. The younger age limit allows earlier testing for such children. Originally developed in 1967, it has been revised in 1989 (WPPSI-II) and 2002 (WPPSI-III).

WPPSI-III provides subtests and related scoring in verbal and performance (non-verbal), along with a composite scoring that assesses general intellectual ability. Two age divisions are included in the test. The test takes 30 to 45 minutes to administer for children from two years, six months, to three years, eleven months, and 45 to 60 minutes for children from four years to seven years, three months. Compared to older children, younger children take fewer subtests that measure verbal comprehension and perceptual organization skills, and processing speed skills. In both groups, less acquired knowledge is required of the child test takers when compared to earlier versions of the test. In addition, the third edition of the WPPSI contains more simplified instructions and scoring procedures that enhance the ability of the administrator to examine children.

In all, 14 subtests are provided. These are:

- Block Design (recreate one- or two-color blocks)
- Information (Performance: respond to question by selecting one picture from four options; Verbal: respond to question from general-knowledge topics)
- Matrix Reasoning (fill in incomplete matrix from four or five response options)
- Vocabulary (Performance: name pictures displayed; Verbal: give definitions for words verbally stated by administrator)
- Picture Concepts (choose one picture from rows of pictures with common characteristic)
- Symbol Search (decide whether target symbol matches any symbol in group)
- Word Reasoning (identify common concept in series of clues)
- Coding (copy symbols paired with geometric shapes)
- Comprehension (answer questions based on general principles and social situations)
- Picture Completion (look at pictures, and indicate what important parts are missing)
- Similarities (find missing part of an incomplete sentence containing two concepts)
- Receptive Vocabulary (select one of four pictures based on what the administrator says)
- Object Assembly (arrange pieces of puzzle within a time limit)
- Picture Naming (name pictures as displayed in book)

The Verbal section includes the five subtests of Information, Vocabulary, Comprehension, Object Assembly, and Picture Naming. The Performance section includes all 14 subtests as with the Verbal section.

The scoring of the WPPSI-III includes a Verbal IQ score and a Performance IQ score, along with a Full Scale IQ score. In addition, a score for Processing Speed Quotient is produced for children from four years to seven years, three months. A General Language Composite score is available for children from both age divisions.

WISC

The Wechsler Intelligence Scale for Children (WISC), now in its third revision (WISC-IV, publication year 2003), is designed for children and adolescents from the ages of six years to 16 years, 11 months. Each version is re-standardized to compensate for the Flynn Effect, to ensure that the biases against women and minorities are eliminated, and to ensure that the administration of the test is as easy as possible. Originally developed in 1949, it has been revised in 1974 (WISC-R) and 1991 (WISC-III). The current version is WISC-IV, which was first produced in 2003. It takes approximately 60 to 90 minutes to administer the core subtests, and about 10 to 15 minutes for each supplemental test.

In all, 15 subtests are provided. They are divided into: Verbal Comprehension (VCI), Perceptual Reasoning

(PRI), Processing Speed (PSI), and Working Memory (WMI). For VCI, the five subtests are:

- Vocabulary (define words)
- Similarities (state why two words are alike or different)
- Comprehension (answer questions pertaining to social situations or well-known concepts)
- Information (supplemental subtest; answer questions pertaining to general knowledge)
- Word Reasoning (supplemental subtest; solve clues that help to identify word)

For PRI, the four subtests are:

- Block Design (arrange red-and-white blocks based on pre-provided pattern)
- Picture Concepts (select which pictures (one from each row) go together from two or three rows of pictures)
- Matrix Reasoning (select one picture (from a choice of five) that fits an array of pictures with one missing spot)
- Picture Completion (supplemental subtest; identify missing part from common art objects)

For WMI, the three subtests are:

- Digit Span (repeat sequence of numbers stated by administrator, either as stated or in reverse order)
- Letter-Number Sequencing (repeat sequence of numbers and letters stated by administrator, in predetermined order)
- Arithmetic (supplemental subtest; complete problems orally stated by administrator)

For PSI, the three subtests are:

- Coding (children under eight years: mark rows of shapes with different lines according to particular code; children over eight: transcribe digit-symbol code)
- Symbol Search (mark whether target symbols appear in rows of symbols or not)
- Cancellation (supplemental, answer based on visual-perceptual speed)

A Full Scale score (FSIQ) is generated from the subtests. Scores are also generated from the four indices (VCI, PRI, WMI, and PSI).

WAIS

The Wechsler Adult Intelligence Scale (WAIS), now in its third revision (WAIS-IV, publication year 2008), is designed for adolescent and adult intelligence. Each version is re-standardized to compensate for the Flynn Effect, to ensure that the biases against women and minorities are eliminated, and to ensure that the administration of the test is as easy as possible. Originally developed in 1955, it has been revised in 1974 (WISC-R) and 1991 (WISC-III). The current version is WISC-IV, which was first released in 2008. It takes approximately 60 to 90 minutes to administer the core subtests, and about 10 to 15 minutes for each supplemental test.

The WAIS-IV consists of 10 core subtests and five supplemental subtests. Four index scores are included: Verbal Comprehension Index (VCI), Perceptual Reasoning Index (PRI), Working Memory Index (WMI), and Processing Speed Index (PSI).

For VCI, the five subtests (which are similar in meaning but not exactly the same as in the WISC) are:

- Similarities (asks such questions as "In what ways are a cat and dog similar?")
- Vocabulary (asks questions such as "What is an airplane?")
- Information ("What is the capital of the United States?")
- Comprehension (supplemental subtest; "What does *The sky is as thick as pea soup* mean?")

For PRI, the five subtests are:

- Block Design (abstract problem solving and spatial perception)
- Matrix Reasoning (inductive reasoning and nonverbal problem solving)
- Visual Puzzles (nonverbal reasoning)
- Picture Completion (supplemental subtest; ability to see details quickly)
- Figure Weights (supplemental subtest; analogical and quantitative reasoning)

For WMI, the three subtests are:

- Digit Span (repeat sequence of numbers in different ways, such as *Repeat 7-9-3-5 in reverse order*)
- Arithmetic (mathematics problems using memory, such as administrator may ask "How much money do you have if you are given two quarters, three dimes, and four five-dollar bills?")
- Letter-Number Sequencing (supplemental subset; repeat sequence of numbers and letters stated by administrator, but in a different order, such as "State 7-A-Z-9-3-5-T but, first, the numbers in numerical order and, second, the letters in alphabetical order.")

For PSI, the three subtests are:

- Symbol Search (ability to perceive a situation visually and to do it quickly)

KEY TERMS

IQ—The acronym for intelligence quotient.

Percentile—A statistical measure that shows, on a scale of 100, whether a distribution is below or above it.

Standard deviation—A statistical measure of the difference to an arithmetical mean.

- Coding (mental speed and visual-motor coordination)
- Cancellation (supplemental, visual-perceptual speed).

A Full Scale score (FSIQ) is generated from the subtests. Scores are also generated from the four indices (VCI, PRI, WMI, and PSI).

Preparation

Preparation for the Wechsler Intelligence Scales is neither needed nor recommended.

Risks

The Wechsler Intelligence Scales are some of the most frequently used tests by psychologists and other professionals to assess general intellectual ability. Analysis and research into the way they are administered, however, indicates that errors are sometimes made in scoring and administering the tests. Such errors lessen the accuracy of the Wechsler tests. For instance, sometimes professionals place more emphasis on differences between the Verbal IQ and Performance IQ scores than they should. In other cases, they make conclusions regarding **brain** damage based only on the test, when other screening instruments should be included. Research has also shown that the ethnicity of the administrator may have an effect on the scoring of individual of minority groups.

Despite criticisms, the Wechsler Intelligence Scales remain a good way to access general intelligence when performed by a trained, unbiased professional.

Results

Administering and scoring of the three Wechsler Scales are very similar. Each of the three tests has a series of subtests grouped into two general areas: Verbal Scales and Performance Scales. The Verbal Scales measure general knowledge, reasoning, language, and memory skills, and the Performance Scales assess problem solving, spatial, and sequencing abilities.

The tests are administered by trained professionals. Raw scores are first generated and then converted to standard scores with a mean and standard deviations from that average. In addition, scores in the Verbal battery are summed and converted to a Verbal IQ score; the same is done for the Performance scores, providing the Performance IQ score. The Verbal and Performance IQ scores are added together and are then converted to an overall Full Scale IQ score. The Verbal, Performance, and Full Scale IQ scores are considered "normative" IQ scores, which means, in this specific case, that they have a mean of 100 and a standard deviation of 15.

A Full Scale IQ score higher than 130 indicates that the test taker is in the highest intelligence category. Scores in the 120s are considered very high in intelligence, and in the 110s they are above normal, while scores from 90 to 109 are considered normal-average, and in the high 80s low-average. Scores below 85 are considered low in mental functioning, with the lower the score the less ability to function mentally.

Resources

BOOKS

Drummond, Robert J. *Assessment Procedures for Counselors and Helping Professionals.* Boston: Pearson, 2010.

Green, Susan K. and Robert L. Johnson. *Assessment is Essential.* Boston: McGraw-Hill Higher Education, 2010.

Hart, Diane. *Authentic Assessment: A Handbook for Educators.* Menlo Park, CA: Addison-Wesley, 1994.

McAfee, Oralie, and Deborah J. Leong. *Assessing and Guiding Young Children's Development and Learning.* Upper Saddle River, NJ: Pearson, 2011.

McCullough, Virginia E. *Testing and Your Child: What You Should Know about 150 of the Most Common Medical, Educational, and Psychological Tests.* New York City: Plume, 1992.

Mindes, Gayle. *Assessing Young Children.* Boston: Pearson, 2011.

Walsh, W. Bruce, and Nancy E. Betz. *Tests and Assessment*, 4th ed. Upper Saddle River, NJ: Prentice Hall, 2001.

Wechsler, David. *Manual for the Wechsler Adult Intelligence Scale.* New York: The Psychological Corporation, 1955.

Wechsler, David. *Manual for the Wechsler Intelligence Scale for Children.* New York: The Psychological Corporation, 1949.

Wechsler, David. *Manual for the Wechsler Preschool and Primary Scale of Intelligence.* New York: The Psychological Corporation, 1967.

WEBSITES

David Wechsler (1896–1981) Psychologist. Human Intelligence, Indiana University. (July 25, 2007), http://www.indiana.edu/~intell/wechsler.shtml (accessed October 28, 2010).

Wechsler Adult Intelligence Scale—Fourth Edition (WAIS—IV). Pearson. http://www.pearsonassessments.com/HAIWEB/Cultures/en-us/Productdetail.htm?Pid=015-8980-808(accessed October 28, 2010).

Wechsler Intelligence Scale for Children™—Fourth Edition (WISC™—IV). Pearson. http://www.pearsonassessments.com/HAIWEB/Cultures/en-us/Productdetail.htm?Pid=015-8979-044 (accessed October 27, 2010).

Wechsler Preschool and Primary Scale of Intelligence™—Third Edition (WPPSI™—III. Pearson. http://www.pearson assessments.com/haiweb/cultures/en-us/productdetail.htm?pid=015-8989-317 (accessed October 27, 2010).

William Arthur Atkins

Wellbutrin *see* **Bupropion**

Wernicke-Korsakoff syndrome

Definition

Wernicke-Korsakoff syndrome is a severe memory disorder usually associated with chronic excessive alcohol consumption, although the direct cause is a deficiency in the B vitamin thiamin.

The *Diagnostic and Statistical Manual of Mental Disorders,* fourth edition, text revision (DSM-IV-TR), the professional handbook that aids clinicians in diagnosing patients' mental disorders, refers to Korsakoff syndrome as alcohol-induced persisting amnestic disorder and includes it under the category of substance-induced persisting amnestic disorders.

Demographics

When **diagnosis** is based on postmortem findings, the estimated prevalence of Wernicke-Korsakoff syndrome is between 1% and 2% of the population. The classic presentation with acute onset of Wernicke's encephalopathy is fairly rare, about 0.05% of all hospital admissions, although this does not account for patients who do not seek medical attention. Wernicke-Korsakoff syndrome usually follows many years of chronic alcoholism or malnutrition and is seldom seen among people under 20. Most patients are 40 years of age or older. The disorder is apparently more common in alcoholic individuals who are particularly vulnerable to malnutrition such as indigent or homeless people.

Description

The disorder was first identified in the late nineteenth century. The first phase of the condition, called Wernicke's encephalopathy, was described by German neurologist and **psychiatrist** Karl Wernicke in 1881. He noted three key symptoms in three patients—two with alcoholism and one who had swallowed sulfuric acid. These patients suffered from mental confusion, eye **movement disorders**, and ataxia (poor motor coordination). A few years later, S. S. Korsakoff, a Russian psychiatrist, began publishing reports describing a syndrome of anterograde amnesia—an inability to form new memories—and confabulation in individuals with severe alcoholism or certain medical illnesses. (Confabulation refers to the practice of filling in gaps in memory by fabrication.) By 1900, researchers and clinicians studying alcoholism recognized a connection between the two conditions. The typical syndrome begins with acute Wernicke's encephalopathy, with Korsakoff syndrome emerging when the acute phase resolves. The symptoms of Wernicke's encephalopathy appear suddenly. The most prominent symptom initially is mental confusion including memory problems. On examination, patients have difficulty moving their eyes to follow a visual stimulus due to paralysis of the muscles controlling eye movements. For instance, patients may have trouble looking upward or to the side with one or both eyes. Problems maintaining balance while standing or walking, a condition known as ataxia, are frequently observed as well. If left untreated, most of these symptoms may resolve spontaneously, but the severe memory disorder characteristic of Korsakoff syndrome remains.

The typical person with Korsakoff syndrome appears fairly normal on first impression. Intelligence is intact and individuals with the syndrome can carry on a conversation quite naturally. They are usually able to recall and talk about incidents that took place before the onset of the disorder and recognize family members and old friends without much difficulty. The ability to form new memories is nearly absent, however. In the course of conversation, people with Korsakoff syndrome may repeat comments or questions several times. They will fail to recognize people they met minutes before or greet a friend with excitement and surprise after a brief trip to another room. These are the characteristics of anterograde **amnesia**. Research shows that anterograde amnesia results from a failure of memory formation and storage. New information is processed normally but almost immediately forgotten, never making it into the regions of the **brain** where memories of the past are stored. People with Korsakoff syndrome thus have no memories of events that happened after the onset of the illness. Many previously stored memories are still available, however, explaining why individuals with Korsakoff syndrome can usually remember the distant past quite well.

Causes and symptoms

Causes

Wernicke-Korsakoff syndrome is caused by thiamin deficiency. It is most commonly observed in people with alcoholism because heavy drinkers often eat poorly, and alcoholism interferes with absorption of nutrients from the digestive system. It can also occur in people who are malnourished for other reasons, including hyperemesis gravidarum (excessive vomiting during pregnancy) or an eating disorder. Thiamin helps produce the energy-containing molecules needed to make neurons function properly. Insufficient thiamin can lead to damage to or death of neurons.

Thiamin deficiency damages regions of the brain, particularly the thalamus and the mammillary bodies. The thalamus is a structure deep within the brain that serves many important functions. It is often called the major relay station of the brain, and many neurons make connections in the thalamus. The mammillary bodies are part of the hypothalamus, located just below the thalamus. The mammillary bodies receive many neural connections from another part of the brain called the hippocampus, which appears to be the primary part of the brain involved in the formation of memories. Neurons in the mammillary bodies make connections with the thalamus, which in turn makes connections with the cortex of the brain, where long-term memories are stored. This may explain why damage to the mammillary bodies and thalamus can lead to anterograde amnesia. Memories formed in the hippocampus are never stored since connections between hippocampus and cortex are disrupted.

Eye movement disorders observed in the acute phase of the condition are probably due to damage to other nearby brain regions that make connections to the nerves controlling eye muscles. These nerves emerge from the brainstem located right below the thalamus and mammillary bodies. Nerves involved in balance also make connections with other nerves in the brain stem, but a separate part of the brain called the cerebellum may also contribute to ataxia.

Symptoms

Mental confusion, eye movement disturbances, and ataxia are the primary symptoms of Wernicke's encephalopathy—the first, acute stage of Wernicke-Korsakoff syndrome. At first glance, confusion and ataxia may resemble the effects of severe alcohol intoxication, but they persist after intoxication wears off. Some patients with Wernicke's encephalopathy will recover completely without residual memory deficits, particularly if they are treated quickly with thiamin. Patients with this acute phase may not be recognized because they may not necessarily exhibit all three "classic" symptoms; therefore, their cases may be overlooked.

About 80%–90% of alcoholics with Wernecke's go on to develop Korsakoff's **psychosis**, the chronic stage of Wernicke-Korsakoff syndrome. This stage is distinguished by anterograde amnesia, and most untreated patients with Wernicke's encephalopathy will develop this severe memory disorder, which prevents them from forming lasting memories of events or information encountered after the onset of the initial symptoms. Symptoms of Korsakoff syndrome may also develop spontaneously in many patients who never show signs of Wernicke's encephalopathy. Once patients develop Korsakoff's amnesia, recovery is unlikely.

Loss of memory for past events is called retrograde amnesia. Many people with Korsakoff syndrome have some retrograde amnesia in addition to anterograde amnesia, particularly for events that occurred shortly before the onset of illness, but most can recall the distant past without difficulty.

Immediate memory is not affected. For instance, an individual with Korsakoff syndrome could repeat a sentence or string of numbers immediately after hearing them, although this information would likely be forgotten within half a minute. Preservation of immediate memory allows individuals with Korsakoff syndrome to interact with others and respond to questions. Implicit memory is also preserved, so people with Korsakoff syndrome can learn new motor skills or develop conditioned reactions to stimuli. For example, individuals who play computer games can show improved performance each time they play, even if they cannot explicitly remember having played the game before.

Confabulation is another striking feature of Korsakoff syndrome, although it is not always observed. Confabulation refers to falsification of memory. The individual appears to be making up stories to cover up for inability to remember. Confabulation often seems to involve a confusion of the past and present. For example, if patients with Korsakoff syndrome are asked why they are in the hospital, they may say they just had a baby, are recovering from pneumonia, undergoing medical tests, or even applying for a job.

Patients with Wernicke-Korsakoff syndrome may also show signs of **apathy** and a lack of spontaneous behavior. Emotional expression may be lacking as well.

Autopsies often reveal brain lesions characteristic of Wernicke-Korsakoff syndrome in alcoholic patients who showed general cognitive problems like those seen in **dementia**, but who never developed anterograde amnesia. These findings suggest that onset may be gradual in some patients, or, as some experts suspect, that there is a genetic component to susceptibility and manifestation of the disorder.

Diagnosis

Wernicke's encephalopathy is diagnosed when patients seek medical attention and have the classic trio of signs: mental confusion, eye movement disorders, and ataxia, although not every patient will exhibit all three signs. The diagnosis of Korsakoff syndrome is given when anterograde amnesia is present in an individual with a history of chronic, heavy drinking or malnutrition. When Korsakoff syndrome follows Wernicke's encephalopathy, the entire Wernicke-Korsakoff syndrome diagnosis is appropriate. The diagnosis is supported by neuroimaging or autopsy findings showing degeneration of the thalamus and mammillary bodies and loss of brain volume in the area surrounding the fourth ventricle—a fluid-filled cavity near the brain stem.

Although the *DSM-IV-TR* criteria for alcohol-induced persisting amnestic disorder apply to most people with Wernicke-Korsakoff syndrome, there are some differences between the two diagnoses. Despite research findings suggesting that severe amnesia is not a necessary symptom of Wernicke-Korsakoff syndrome, the *DSM-IV-TR* requires the presence of either anterograde or retrograde amnesia for a diagnosis of alcohol-induced persisting amnestic disorder. One additional cognitive symptom is also required. Symptoms listed in the *DSM-IV-TR* include language disturbance (aphasia), inability to carry out motor activities (apraxia), inability to recognize objects (agnosia), or deficits in planning, initiation, organization, and abstraction (executive functions). Individuals with Wernicke-Korsakoff syndrome frequently demonstrate problems with executive functions that contribute to the symptoms of confabulation and apathy. Aphasia, apraxia, and agnosia are not common signs of Wernicke-Korsakoff syndrome.

The *DSM-IV-TR* also requires that memory impairment must significantly impair a person's ability to perform normal activities and functions, and it must represent a decline from a previous level of functioning. Amnesia cannot occur exclusively during states of **delirium**, alcohol intoxication, or withdrawal, or be exclusively associated with dementia. Both of these requirements are consistent with the usual presentation of Wernicke-Korsakoff syndrome.

Finally, the *DSM-IV-TR* requires evidence that amnesia is caused by use of alcohol. Such evidence can include an extensive history of heavy drinking; or physical examination or laboratory findings revealing other signs of heavy **alcohol use**, such as abnormal liver function tests. Despite this *DSM-IV-TR* requirement, Wernicke-Korsakoff syndrome can occur in the absence of heavy alcohol use. Emergence of the disorder in people without alcoholism is much less common today than it was in the past, however, since vitamins are now added to many foods. In practice, most people who show the hallmark symptoms of Wernicke-Korsakoff syndrome also qualify for the *DSM-IV-TR* diagnosis.

Treatment

Nutritional

Individuals with signs of Wernicke's encephalopathy should be treated with thiamin immediately. In many cases, prompt administration of thiamin reverses the symptoms and prevents amnesia from developing. Thiamin can be administered intravenously or directly into the digestive system. Unfortunately, thiamin is less effective in the chronic phase of the condition. Based on autopsy findings suggesting the presence of Wernicke-Korsakoff syndrome in people with milder cognitive problems who do not show the classic signs of the disorder, researchers have examined the usefulness of thiamin treatment in people with alcohol dependence who are at risk of developing the syndrome. Results suggest that thiamin treatment improves performance on memory tests in this group, and that higher thiamin doses are associated with better performance. These findings suggest that thiamin treatment can help prevent Wernicke-Korsakoff syndrome in heavy drinkers. Other nutritional treatments may include use of magnesium sulfate to address magnesium deficits common in people with alcoholism, and potassium acid phosphate to address potassium deficiencies.

Medication

Recent reports suggest that **donepezil** and **rivastigmine**, drugs used to treat **Alzheimer's disease**, may improve memory in patients with Wernicke-Korsakoff syndrome. Both drugs affect the action of the neurotransmitter acetylcholine, which is important for the formation of memories. Patients treated with these drugs showed improvements on memory tests and were more able to recognize hospital staff and family members. Although improvements appear to be rather modest, these drugs may be useful for patients who do not respond to thiamin. **Antidepressants** that increase levels of **serotonin** may also be helpful, although the reasons why are not clear since these drugs are not effective with other memory disorders.

Conditioning

The fact that implicit memory is not affected by Wernicke-Korsakoff syndrome has led some researchers

KEY TERMS

Anterograde amnesia—Amnesia for events that occurred after a physical injury or emotional trauma but before the present moment.

Apathy—Lack of feelings or emotions.

Cognitive—Pertaining to the mental processes of memory, perception, judgment, and reasoning.

Encephalopathy—Brain disease that causes damage or degeneration.

Explicit memory—Consciously recalled memory for facts or events.

Implicit memory—Unconsciously recalled memory for skills, procedures, or associations.

Neurons—Nerve cells in the brain that produce nerve impulses.

Neurotransmitter—A chemical in the brain that transmits messages between neurons, or nerve cells.

Retrograde amnesia—Amnesia for events that occurred before a traumatic injury.

Serotonin—A widely distributed neurotransmitter that is found in blood platelets, the lining of the digestive tract, and the brain, and that works in combination with norepinephrine. It causes very powerful contractions of smooth muscle, and is associated with mood, attention, emotions, and sleep. Low levels of serotonin are associated with depression.

Syndrome—A group of symptoms that together characterize a disease or disorder.

to explore the use of classical conditioning procedures in helping patients to remember specific people. In classical conditioning, animals and people learn to associate a stimulus with an outcome. The most famous example is the pairing of a ringing bell with food. Dogs naturally salivate when given food. In a famous experiment, Ivan Pavlov rang a bell immediately before serving food to dogs. After doing this repeatedly, Pavlov found that the dogs salivated upon hearing the bell ring even when the food was not presented. This form of learning does not rely on the hippocampus and cortex but appears to involve neurons in other parts of the brain. Patients with Wernicke-Korsakoff syndrome who are given specific rewards for correctly choosing a picture of a face that matches a face they have seen previously are more able to choose the correct face than those who do not receive the rewards. Although these individuals do not explicitly remember the face they saw previously, they are still able to make the correct choice. Working with patients in this way could enable them to recognize familiar people and differentiate them from strangers.

Prognosis

The prognosis for full recovery from Wernicke-Korsakoff syndrome is poor. Once chronic Korsakoff's amnesia ensues, approximately 80% of patients will never fully recover the ability to learn and remember new information. Because they cannot learn from experience, individuals with Wernicke-Korsakoff syndrome almost always require some form of custodial care. They are usually unable to work, although some can perform simple tasks they learned prior to onset of the condition if closely supervised. The mortality rate is between 10% and 20%, usually from liver failure or infection, but sometimes as a result of the irreversible effects of prolonged thiamin deficiency.

Prevention

Wernicke-Korsakoff syndrome can be prevented with a nutritious diet containing sufficient thiamin. Because severe chronic alcoholism is the most common cause of thiamin deficiency, treatment of alcohol dependence is extremely important. To prevent Wernicke-Korsakoff syndrome among people who are unable to stop drinking or among particularly vulnerable individuals like homeless drinkers, some researchers and clinicians have advocated supplementing alcoholic beverages with thiamin.

Resources

BOOKS

American Psychiatric Association. *Diagnostic and Statistical Manual of Mental Disorders.* 4th ed., text rev. Washington, DC: American Psychiatric Publishing, 2000.

Hochhalter, Angela K., et al. "Using Animal Models to Address the Memory Deficits of Wernicke-Korsakoff Syndrome." In *Animal Research and Human Health: Advancing Human Welfare Through Behavioral Science,* edited by Marilyn E. Carroll and J. Bruce Overmier. Washington, DC: American Psychological Association, 2001.

Mesulam, M.-Marsel. *Principles of Behavioral and Cognitive Neurology.* 2nd ed. Oxford: Oxford University Press, 2000.

Nolte, John. *The Human Brain: An Introduction to Its Functional Anatomy.* 6th ed. St. Louis: Mosby, 2008.

Walsh, Kevin, and David Darby. *Neuropsychology: A Clinical Approach.* 5th ed. Edinburgh: Churchill Livingstone, 2005.

PERIODICALS

Ambrose, Margaret L., Stephen C. Bowden, and Greg Whelen. "Thiamin Treatment and Working Memory Function of Alcohol-dependent People: Preliminary Findings." *Alcoholism: Clinical and Experimental Research* 25, no. 1 (January 2001): 112–16.

Angunawela, Indira I., and Andrew Barker. "Anticholinesterase Drugs for Alcoholic Korsakoff Syndrome." *International Journal of Geriatric Psychiatry* 16, no. 3 (2001): 338–39.

Cochrane, M., et al. "Acetylcholinesterase Inhibitors for the Treatment of Wernicke-Korsakoff Syndrome: Three Further Cases Show Response to Donepezil." *Alcohol and Alcoholism* 40, no. 2 (March/April 2005): 151–54.

Harding, Antony, et al. "Degeneration of Anterior Thalamic Nuclei Differentiates Alcoholics with Amnesia." *Brain* 123, no. 1 (2000): 141–54.

Iga, Jun-Ichi, et al. "A Case of Korsakoff's Syndrome Improved by High Doses of Donepezil." *Alcohol and Alcoholism* 36, no. 6 (2001): 553–55.

WEBSITES

Martin, Peter R., Charles K. Singleton, and Susanne Hiller-Sturmhoefel. "The Role of Thiamine Deficiency in Alcoholic Brain Disease." U.S. National Institute of Alcohol Abuse and Alcoholism, 2004. http://pubs.niaaa.nih.gov/publications/arh27-2/134-142.htm (accessed October 29, 2011).

Memory Disorders Project. "Memory Loss and the Brain" Rutgers University. http://www.memorylossonline.com (accessed October 29, 2011).

U.S. National Institute of Neurological Disorders and Stroke. "Wernicke-Korsakoff Syndrome Information Page." http://www.ninds.nih.gov/disorders/wernicke_korsakoff/wernicke-korsakoff.htm (accessed October 29, 2011).

U.S. National Institute on Alcohol Abuse and Alcoholism. "Alcohol's Damaging Effects on the Brain." http://pubs.niaaa.nih.gov/publications/aa63/aa63.htm (accessed October 29, 2011).

Xiong, Glen L. "Wernicke-Korsakoff Syndrome." Medscape Reference. http://emedicine.medscape.com/article/288379-overview (accessed October 29, 2011).

ORGANIZATIONS

Family Caregiver Alliance, 180 Montgomery Street, Ste. 900, San Francisco, CA, 94104, info@caregiver.org, http://www.caregiver.org.

Medical Council on Alcohol, 5 St. Andrew's Place, London, UKNW1 4LB, (020) 7487-4445, Fax: (020) 7935-4479, mca@medicalcouncilalcol.demon.co.uk, http://www.m-c-a.org.uk.

National Institute on Alcohol Abuse and Alcoholism, 5635 Fishers Lane, MSC 9304, Bethesda, MD, 20892-9304, http://www.niaaa.nih.gov.

Danielle Barry, MS
Emily Jane Willingham, PhD

Wide range achievement test

Definition

The Wide Range Achievement Test (WRAT) is an achievement test that measures basic abilities to read, spell, and comprehend writing and to solve mathematics calculations and problems. Achievement tests refer to skills that individuals learn through direct instruction or intervention. In addition, the WRAT is a screening test that can be administered to determine if a more comprehensive achievement test is needed. The WRAT is currently in its fourth edition: WRAT-4.

Purpose

The WRAT-4, the latest edition of the test, measures basic skills in reading, arithmetic, spelling, and comprehension. The test covers ages from five to 94 years and takes approximately 15 to 45 minutes to administer, dependent primarily on the age of the test taker (15 to 25 minutes for those from five to seven years of age, and 35 to 45 minutes for those eight years or older).

The fourth edition has four subtests: Sentence Comprehension, Word Reading, Spelling, and Math Computation. The Sentence Comprehension subtest is new to this latest edition of the WRAT, providing for a way to assess reading comprehension in test takers. Overall, the WRAT-4 provides reliable measurement for fundamental academic skills, along with **diagnosis** of learning disabilities, progression of academic ability over time, evaluation of achievement discrepancies, progression of remedial learning, and evaluation of instructional needs.

Description

American psychologists Sidney William Bijou (1908–2009) and Joseph Jastak first developed the WRAT in 1941. Its various editions have been used

KEY TERMS

Achievement test—Any of a number of tests that assess developed knowledge or skill.

Arithmetic—The branch of mathematics involving problems of addition, subtraction, multiplication, and division.

Psychometric—The branch of psychology that deals with the measurement of mental capacities, traits, and processes.

widely as a measure of basic academic skills used for learning, thinking, reading, spelling, and calculating of arithmetic.

The WRAT-4 has two alternative, but equivalent, testing forms (Green and Blue). One form is administered with the second form available if needed. Both Green and Blue testing forms can be administered together, if necessary, as a pre-test and a post-test arrangement, using either one at the start. When both tests forms are used, a combined scored is obtained and a more comprehensive evaluation is provided. Each testing form consists of one Word Reading subtest, one Math Computation (arithmetic) subtest, one Spelling subtest, and one Sentence Comprehension subtest. The Word Reading and Sentence Comprehension subtests can be administered individually, but the other two tests, the Spelling and Math Computation subtests, may be given in groups.

The Word Reading subtest consists of various letters and individual words that the examinee is asked to name or pronounce. The Spelling subtest consists of writing one's name, various letters, and numerous words dictated to the examinee and used in a sentence. The spelling items increase with difficulty. The Math Computation subtest consists of counting, reading number symbols, and solving simple arithmetic problems that are verbally presented to the examinee. It also consists of using paper and a pencil to calculate up various arithmetic problems. The Sentence Comprehension subtest assesses reading comprehension through the use of various sentences.

Preparation

Preparation by the test taker is not necessary nor advised.

Risks

Although screening instruments may save time, these instruments can sometimes have misleading results. For instance, the scores may overestimate or underestimate a person's skills or the test does not measure other important achievement abilities.

Precautions

To obtain a more in-depth result of an examinee's abilities, a more comprehensive achievement test must be administered. For example, the WRAT-4 does not provide assessment of fundamental skills such as reading comprehension, writing abilities, and applying mathematical concepts to real-life situations. Finally, psychometric testing requires a clinically trained examiner. Therefore, the test should only be administered and interpreted by a trained examiner.

QUESTIONS TO ASK YOUR DOCTOR

- Do you know of a properly trained administrator for the WRAT?
- If I should need additional assessment, what are other appropriate tests to use after the WRAT is completed?
- Will health insurance cover the test in whole or part?

Results

The WRAT-4 is an easy and sound measure of fundamental academic skills. It was standardized on a representative sample of the U.S. population using approximately 3,000 people from the ages of five to 94 years. It was improved over the previous edition, WRAT-3, by adding grade-based norms, which helps to assess students in grades kindergarten through twelfth grade. In addition, the new edition has been improved with respect to age-based norms, allowing test takers up to the age of 94 years, as opposed to a maximum of 75 years in edition three.

Scoring consists of a "1" for a correct answer and a "0" for an incorrect answer. The raw scores are converted to standard scores. These are scores that allow the examiner to compare the individual's score to other people who have taken the test. Additionally, by converting raw scores to standard scores the examiner has uniform scores and can more easily compare an individual's performance on one test with the individual's performance on another test. The average score for each test of the WRAT-4 is 100. An examiner can also obtain grade-equivalent scores, percentile ranks, and normal curve equivalents. A poor performance in any of the three areas assessed by this instrument can indicate the need for further testing.

Specifically, the WRAT-4 uses the following: a score summary table, which provides raw scores and standard scores, along with confidence intervals, percentile ranks, grade equivalents, and other such measures; a standard score profile, which provides a graphic representation of standard scores and confidence intervals; and a standard score comparison table, which provides relative performance data on subtests.

Resources

BOOKS

Boyer, Bret A., and M. Indira Paharia, editors. *Comprehensive Handbook of Clinical Health Psychology.* Hoboken, NJ: John Wiley and Sons, 2008.

Groth-Marnat, Gary. *Handbook of Psychological Assessment.* 4th edition. Hoboken, NJ: John Wiley and Sons, 2003.

Hersen, Michel, editor. *Comprehensive Handbook of Psychological Assessment.* Hoboken, NJ: John Wiley and Sons, 2004.

Kellerman, Henry, and Anthony Burry. *Handbook of Psychodiagnostic Testing: Analysis of Personality in the Psychological Report.* New York: Springer, 2007.

Leeming, David A., Kathryn Madden and Stanton Marlan, eds. *Encyclopedia of Psychology and Religion.* New York: Springer, 2010.

Sattler, Jerome M. *Assessment of Children: Cognitive Foundations.* San Diego, CA: J.M. Sattler, 2008.

PERIODICALS

"Sidney W. Bijou, Child Psychologist, Is Dead at 100." *New York Times*, (July 21, 2009). http://www.nytimes.com/2009/07/22/science/22bijou.html?_r=1 (accessed January 7, 2011).

WEBSITES

"Reynolds Intellectual Assessment Scales/Wide Range Achievement Test 4 Discrepancy Interpretive Report (RIAS/WRAT4-DIR)." Par. (2010), http://www4.parinc.com/Products/Product.aspx?ProductID=RIAS/WRAT4/DIR (accessed January 7, 2011).

"Wide Range Achievement Test 4 (WRAT4)." Western Psychological Services. http://portal.wpspublish.com/portal/page?_pageid=53,118660&_dad=portal&_schema=PORTAL (accessed January 7, 2011).

ORGANIZATIONS

American Psychiatric Association, 1000 Wilson Blvd., Ste. 1825, Arlington, VA, 22209-3901, (703) 907-7300, apa@psych.org, http://www.psych.org.

American Psychological Association, 750 1st St. NE, Washington, DC, 20002-4242, (202) 336-5500; TDD/TTY: (202) 336-6123, (800) 374-2721, http://www.apa.org.

National Association of School Psychologists, 4340 East West Highway, Ste. 402, Bethesda, MD, 20002, (301) 657-0270, (866) 331-5277, Fax: (301) 657-0275, http://www.nasponline.org.

Keith Beard, Psy.D.

Wilson disease

Definition

Wilson disease, or WD, is a rare inherited disorder that causes excess copper to accumulate in the body. It is also known as hepatolenticular degeneration. Steadily increasing amounts of copper circulating in the blood are deposited primarily in the **brain**, liver, kidneys, and the cornea of the eyes. WD is fatal if it is not recognized and treated. It is named for a U.S. neurologist, Samuel A. K. Wilson, who first described it in 1912.

Demographics

Wilson disease affects approximately 1 in 30,000 to 1 in 100,000 individuals and can affect people from many different populations. Approximately one in 90 individuals are carriers of the gene for Wilson disease.

Description

Under normal conditions, copper that finds its way into the body through the diet is processed within the liver. This processed form of copper is then passed into the gallbladder, along with the other components of bile (a fluid produced by the liver, which enters the small intestine in order to help in digestive processes). When the gallbladder empties its contents into the first part of the small intestine (duodenum), the copper in the bile enters and passes through the intestine with the waste products of digestion. In healthy individuals, copper is then passed out of the body in stool.

In Wilson disease, copper does not pass from the liver into the bile, but rather begins to accumulate within the liver. As copper levels rise in the liver, the damaged organ begins to allow copper to flow into the bloodstream, where it circulates. Copper is then deposited throughout the body, building up primarily in the kidneys, the brain and nervous system, and the eyes. Wilson disease, then, is a disorder of copper poisoning occurring from birth.

Causes and symptoms

Causes

Wilson disease is inherited in an autosomal recessive manner. Autosomal recessive refers to the pattern of inheritance where each parent carries a gene for the disease on one of his or her chromosome pairs. When each parent passes on the chromosome with the gene for Wilson disease, the child will be affected with the disease. Both males and females can be affected with Wilson disease. If an individual is a carrier of the Wilson disease gene, they do not have any symptoms of this disease. In order to be affected, an individual must inherit two copies of the gene, one from each parent. Many cases of Wilson disease may not be inherited but occur as a spontaneous mutation in the gene.

The gene for Wilson disease is located on chromosome number 13. The name of the gene is called ATP7B and is thought to be involved in transporting copper. More than 200 different mutations of this gene have been identified, making **diagnosis** by genetic testing difficult.

Symptoms

Symptoms typically present between the ages of 3 and 60, with age 17 considered to be the average age at diagnosis. About half of all patients experience their first symptoms in the liver. The illness causes swelling and tenderness of the liver, sometimes with fever, mimicking more common disorders, such as viral hepatitis and infectious mononucleosis. Abnormal levels of circulating liver enzymes reveal that the liver is being seriously damaged. This form of damage is referred to as fatty degeneration. Without medical **intervention**, the liver damage will progress to actual cirrhosis. An often-fatal manifestation of liver disease is called fulminant hepatitis. This extremely severe inflammation of the liver (hepatitis) results in jaundice, fluid leaking into the abdomen, low protein circulating in the blood, abnormalities of the blood clotting system, swelling of the brain, and anemia due to the abnormal destruction of red blood cells.

Neurological symptoms are the first to occur in half of all patients due to copper accumulation in the brain and nervous system. The average age of onset for neurological symptoms is 21. These symptoms include tremors of the hands, uncontrollable movements of the limbs, stiffness, drooling, difficulty swallowing, difficulty talking, and headache. There is no change in patient's intelligence.

About one-third of all patients with Wilson disease have a variety of psychiatric symptoms as the first signs of the disease. These symptoms include inability to cope, **depression**, irritability, increased anger, and inappropriate behavior. Often times patients have trouble completing tasks at work or in school.

Other symptoms that can affect patients with Wilson disease, and that may occur before or after a diagnosis has been made, include joint disorders, symptoms of arthritis, and skeletal problems such as osteoporosis. Patients have occasionally been affected with kidney stones and abnormal handling of glucose in their body, and women may have menstrual cycle irregularities including stopping their regular cycle temporarily.

Diagnosis

The diagnosis of Wilson disease can be performed relatively easily through several different tests; however, because Wilson disease is so rare, diagnosis is often unfortunately delayed. The tests used to diagnose Wilson disease can be performed on patients who have and who have not already shown symptoms of the disease. It is extremely important to make a diagnosis as soon as possible, since liver damage can occur before there are any signs of the disease.

An easy way to diagnose Wilson disease is to measure the amount of a glycoprotein found in the blood called ceruloplasmin. Low levels of ceruloplasmin can diagnose the disease in about 80% of affected patients. This procedure is not as effective for women taking birth control pills, pregnant women, or infants younger than six months of age.

A second test involving an eye examination to detect a characteristic ring of copper deposited in a membrane of the cornea (referred to as Kayser-Fleischer rings) is very easy to perform and is very useful in diagnosing patients who have already exhibited symptoms. This test is not as effective in persons without symptoms. This diagnostic test cannot be used by itself to make a diagnosis because some patients with liver disease but not Wilson disease will test positive.

A third test for diagnosing Wilson disease involves measuring the amount of copper in the liver. This can be accomplished by sampling a portion of the liver, called a biopsy. This is one of the most effective ways to diagnose Wilson disease, but the procedure itself is more difficult to perform than the others.

Other tests are also useful, such as measuring the amount of copper passed into the urine daily (high in Wilson disease). Another lab test measures the ability of a patient's ceruloplasmin to bind with a form of copper (decreased in Wilson disease). Some patients can be diagnosed through a DNA test to determine whether or not they carry two genes for Wilson disease. This test does not always prove to be useful in certain patients and is of most use when used to test the brothers and sisters of affected patients.

Molecular genetic testing is not particularly valuable in diagnosing Wilson disease because of the large number of possible gene mutations.

Treatment

Treatment involves life-long administration of either D-penicillamine (Cuprimine, Depen) or trientine hydrochloride (Syprine). Both of these drugs remove copper deposits throughout the body by binding to the copper which then leaves the body in the urine. This type of treatment is called chelation therapy. **Zinc** acetate (Galzin) and a low-copper diet are other ways in which to treat Wilson disease.

Penicillamine has a number of serious side effects:

- joint pain
- neurological problems
- systemic lupus erythematosus
- decreased production of all blood elements
- interference with clotting
- allergic reactions

Careful monitoring is necessary. When patients have side effects from penicillamine, the dose can sometimes be lowered to an effective level that causes fewer difficulties. Alternatively, steroid medications may be required to reduce certain sensitivity reactions. Trientine has fewer potential side effects, but must still be carefully monitored.

KEY TERMS

Anemia—A blood condition in which the level of hemoglobin or the number of red blood cells falls below normal values. Common symptoms include paleness, fatigue, and shortness of breath.

Bile—A substance produced by the liver, and concentrated and stored in the gallbladder. Bile contains a number of different substances, including bile salts, cholesterol, and bilirubin.

Biopsy—The surgical removal and microscopic examination of living tissue for diagnostic purposes.

Cell—The smallest living units of the body which group together to form tissues and help the body perform specific functions.

Ceruloplasmin—A protein circulating in the bloodstream that binds with copper and transports it.

Chelation therapy—A method of removing copper or other heavy metals from the body by giving medications that bind to the metal and allow it to be excreted.

Chromosome—A microscopic thread-like structure found within each cell of the body and consists of a complex of proteins and DNA. Humans have 46 chromosomes arranged into 23 pairs. Changes in either the total number of chromosomes or their shape and size (structure) may lead to physical or mental abnormalities.

Cirrhosis—A chronic degenerative disease of the liver, in which normal cells are replaced by fibrous tissue. Cirrhosis is a major risk factor for the later development of liver cancer.

Deoxyribonucleic acid (DNA)—The genetic material in cells that holds the inherited instructions for growth, development, and cellular functioning.

Gallbladder—A small, pear-shaped organ in the upper right hand corner of the abdomen. It is connected by a series of ducts (tube-like channels) to the liver, pancreas, and duodenum (first part of the small intestine). The gallbladder receives bile from the liver and concentrates and stores it. After a meal, bile is squeezed out of the gallbladder into the intestine, where it aids in digestion of food.

Gene—A building block of inheritance, which contains the instructions for the production of a particular protein, and is made up of a molecular sequence found on a section of DNA. Each gene is found on a precise location on a chromosome.

Glucose—One of the two simple sugars, together with galactose, that makes up the protein, lactose, found in milk. Glucose is the form of sugar that is usable by the body to generate energy.

Hepatitis—A viral disease characterized by inflammation of the liver cells (hepatocytes). People infected with hepatitis B or hepatitis C virus are at an increased risk for developing liver cancer.

Jaundice—Yellowing of the skin or eyes due to excess of bilirubin in the blood.

Toxic—Poisonous.

Treatment with zinc acetate is also an effective way to remove excess copper from the body. Zinc is a metal that works to block copper absorption and bind copper in the intestinal cells until it is all released into the stool approximately one week later. The benefit of treatment with zinc is there are no toxic side effects; however, the zinc is a slower acting agent than the other drugs. It takes four to eight months for the zinc to be effective in reducing the overall amount of copper in the body.

Patients with Wilson disease are encouraged to follow a diet low in copper, with an average copper intake of 1 mg per day. Foods to be avoided for the high levels of copper include liver and shellfish. Patients are also instructed to monitor their drinking water for excess levels of copper and drink distilled water instead.

Patients may be given a liver transplant in the event of liver failure as a complication of Wilson disease. Liver transplantation has been reported to have a relatively favorable outcome, in some cases decreasing the patient's neurologic symptoms.

Prognosis

Without treatment, Wilson disease is always fatal. With treatment, symptoms may continue to worsen for the first six to eight weeks. After this time, definite improvement should begin to be seen. However, it may take several years (two to five) of treatment to reach maximal benefit to the brain and liver. Even then, many patients are not returned to their original level of functioning. Patients with Wilson disease need to maintain some sort of anticopper treatment for the rest of their lives in order to prevent copper levels from rising in the body. Interruptions in treatment can result in a **relapse** of the disease which is not reversible and can ultimately lead to death.

Resources

BOOKS

Porter, Robert S., and Justin L. Kaplan, eds. *The Merck Manual of Diagnosis and Therapy*. 19th ed. Whitehouse Station, NJ: Merck Research Laboratories, 2011.

PERIODICALS

Daniel, K.G., et al. "Copper Storage Diseases: Menkes, Wilsons, and Cancer." *Frontiers in Bioscience* 9 (September 1, 2004): 2652–2662.

Georghe, L., et al. "Wilson's Disease: A Challenge of Diagnosis. The 5-Year Experience of a Tertiary Centre." *Romanian Journal of Gastroenterology* 13, no. 3 (September 2004): 179–185.

Velez-Pardo, C., et al. "New Mutation (T1232P) of the ATP-7B Gene Associated with Neurologic and Neuropsychiatric Dominance Onset of Wilson's Disease in Three Unrelated Colombian Kindred." *Neuroscience Letters* 367, no. 3 (September 9, 2004): 360–364.

ORGANIZATIONS

American Liver Foundation, 39 BRd.way, Suite 2700, New York, NY, 10006, (212) 669-1000, Fax: (212) 483-8179, http://www.liverfoundation.org.

National Organization for Rare Disorders, PO Box 1968, Danbury, CT, 06813-1968, (203) 744-0100, (800) 999-6673, Fax: (203) 798-2291, http://www.rarediseases.org.

Wilson Disease Association, 5572 North Diversey Blvd., Milwaukee, WI, 53217, (414) 961-0533, (866) 961-0533, info@wilsonsdisease.org, http://www.wilsonsdisease.org.

Katherine S. Hunt, MS

Rebecca J. Frey, PhD

WISC *see* **Wechsler intelligence scales**

Women's mental health *see* **Gender issues in mental health**

XY

Xanax *see* **Alprazolam**

Yoga

Definition

Yoga is an ancient system of breathing practices, physical exercises and postures, and **meditation** intended to integrate the practitioner's body, mind, and spirit. It originated in India several thousand years ago, and its principles were first written down by the scholar Patanjali in the second century B.C. The word *yoga* comes from a Sanskrit word *yukti* and means "union" or "yoke." In modern times, yoga is practiced both as directed by its ancient foundations and as a way to maintain fitness and health. In fact, some people use yoga to help relieve certain mental and physical conditions, such as **stress**, anxiety, and injuries. Yoga has not been medically verified to be beneficial for some of these problems. It is recommended to consult with a medical professional before trying yoga for such medical problems.

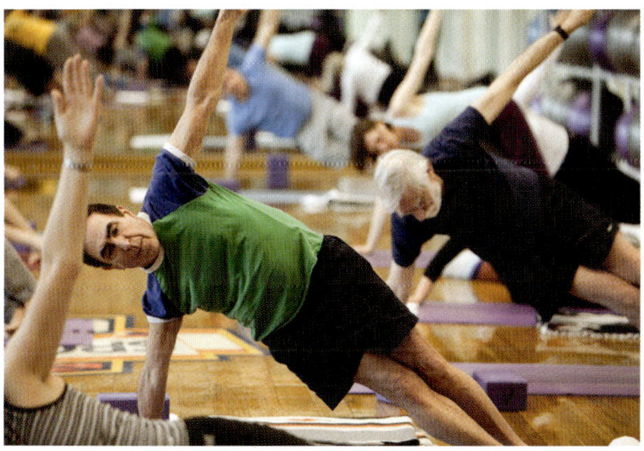

Adults in a yoga class. *(© Ira Block/National Geographic Image Collection/Alamy)*

Purpose

Traditionally, yoga is a method joining the individual self with the Divine, Universal Spirit, or Cosmic Consciousness. Physical and mental exercises are designed to help achieve this goal, also called self-transcendence or enlightenment. On the physical level, yoga postures, called *asanas*, are designed to tone, strengthen, and align the body. Flexibility to the back, shoulders, hips, and hamstring muscles are improved with yoga, providing greater range of motion to these muscles and joints and others. These postures are performed to make the spine supple and healthy and to promote blood flow to all the organs, glands, and tissues. Many yoga postures require that individuals support their own weight, which also helps to improve balance and strength in the legs (such as with the tree pose) or the arms (such as with the downward facing dog pose).

Yoga uses breathing techniques (*pranayama*) and meditation (*dyana*) to quiet, clarify, and discipline the mind. Mental calm can be achieved with yoga and its practice of controlling the breathing process. Overall, such physical activity and mental focus in yoga help to relieve stress. In essence, yoga can be a **stress management** technique as participants become more aware of their body and mind.

Yoga can also be used as an aerobic type of **exercise** for staying fit and healthy. Rather than as a series of slow movements, a form of yoga taught in Western countries is called power yoga. Also called by the Sanskrit term *Vinyasa Yoga*, power yoga consists of a series of slower moves at the beginning to warm up the body. Later, more active poses are performed, which are not as long as the other types of yoga but are quicker in movement for the participants and more challenging to their muscles.

Demographics

In 2008, the Harris Interactive Service Bureau conducted a poll for the magazine *Yoga Journal*. The survey, called "Yoga in America," found that 6.9% of adults, or 16.5 million people, practice yoga in the United

States. Of these, 77.1% are female and 22.9% are male. According to age, 29.1% are 18–34 years, 41.6% are 35–54 years, and 18.4% are 55 years or older.

Description

There are six major branches of yoga: hatha, raja, karma, bhakti, jnana, tantra and raja. Hatha yoga is the type most familiar to Westerners. Karma yoga emphasizes selfless work as a service to others. Bhakti yoga, also called devotional yoga, is the path of cultivating an open heart and single-minded love of God. It is one of the most popular types of yoga in India. Jnana yoga is the sage or philosopher's approach; it cultivates wisdom, intellect, and discernment, and is considered the most difficult type of yoga. Tantra yoga emphasizes transcending the self through religious rituals, including sacred sexuality. Raja yoga, or royal yoga, is a spiritual path of self-renunciation and simplicity. It is a combination of bhakti, karma, and jnana yogas.

Hatha yoga

Hatha yoga, sometimes called physical yoga, is the best-known form of yoga in the West because it is often taught as a form of physical therapy. A typical hatha yoga practice consists of a sequence of asanas, or physical poses, designed to exercise all parts of the body in the course of the practice. The asanas incorporate three basic types of movement: forward bends, backward bends, and twists. Practitioners of hatha yoga have over 200 asanas to choose from in creating a sequence for practice. The postures have traditional Indian names, such as eagle pose, half moon pose, or mountain pose. There are steps for entering and leaving the pose, and the student is taught to concentrate on proper form and alignment. The pose is held for a period of time (usually 10–20 seconds), during which the practitioner concentrates on breathing correctly. Mental focus and discipline are necessary in order to maintain one's poise and balance in the asana. At the close of the practice, most students of yoga rest in a position that allows for a period of meditation. Most yoga practices take about an hour, although some are as short as 20 minutes.

Different styles of hatha yoga are taught in the United States, the best known being iyengar, bikram, kripalu, and ashtanga yoga. Iyengar yoga, which was developed by Indian yoga teacher B.K.S. Iyengar (1918–), also called bellur krishnamachar sundararaja iyengar, emphasizes attention to the details of a pose and the use of such props as blocks and belts to help students gain flexibility. It puts strict emphasis on form and alignment, and the props make it easier for beginners to get into the yoga postures. Bikram yoga, taught on the West Coast by Indian yoga guru Bikram Choudhury (1946–), is practiced in heated rooms intended to make participants sweat freely as they warm and stretch their joints and muscles. Kripalu yoga, sometimes called the yoga of consciousness, emphasizes breathing exercises and the proper coordination of breath and movement. It also teaches awareness of one's psychological and emotional reactions to the various poses and movements of the body. Ashtanga yoga, developed by Indian yoga teacher Sri Krishna Pattabhi Jois (1915–2009), is the basis of so-called power yoga. Ashtanga yoga is a physically demanding workout that is not suitable for beginners.

A typical hatha yoga routine consists of a sequence of asanas designed to work all parts of the body, with particular emphasis on making the spine supple and healthy and increasing circulation. Hatha yoga asanas utilize three basic movements: forward bends, backward bends, and twisting motions. Each asana is named for a common object or creature it resembles, like the cobra, locust, bow, eagle, and tree poses. A pose is held for some time, depending on its level of difficulty and one's strength and stamina, and the practitioner is also usually aware of when to inhale and exhale at certain points in each posture, as breathing properly is another fundamental aspect of yoga. Breathing should be deep and through the nose. Mental concentration in each position is also important, which improves awareness, poise, and posture. During a yoga routine there is often a position in which to perform meditation, if deep relaxation is one of the goals of the sequence.

Yoga routines can take anywhere from 20 minutes to two or more hours, with one hour being a good time investment to perform a sequence of postures and a meditation. Some yoga routines, depending on the teacher and school, can be as strenuous as the most difficult workout, while others merely stretch and align the body, keeping the breath and heart rate slow and steady. Yoga achieves its best results when it is practiced as a daily discipline and can be a lifelong exercise routine, offering deeper and more challenging positions as a practitioner becomes more adept. The basic positions can increase a person's strength, flexibility, and sense of well-being almost immediately, but it can take years to perfect and deepen them, which is an appealing and stimulating aspect of yoga.

Yoga as complementary therapy

One of the advantages of yoga as a complementary therapy is its adaptability to patients with a wide variety of physical and psychiatric conditions. There are a number of different schools of yoga—over 40, according to one expert in the field—and even within a particular school or tradition, the asanas and breathing exercises can be tailored to the patient's needs. One can find special yoga courses for children; for people over 50 years of age; for people with fibromyalgia, arthritis, or back problems; for cancer patients; and for people who are overweight or obese (extremely overweight). Although most people who participate in yoga attend classes, it is possible to learn the basic postures and breathing techniques at home from beginners' manuals or videos. Patients who feel self-conscious about exercising in the presence of others may find yoga appealing for this reason. In addition, yoga does not require expensive equipment or special courts, tracks, or playing fields. An area of floor space about 6 feet by 8 feet (1.8 m by 2.4 m), a so-called sticky mat to keep the feet from slipping, and loose clothing that allows the wearer to move freely are all that is needed.

Origins

Yoga originated in ancient India and is one of the longest surviving philosophical systems in the world. Some scholars have estimated that yoga is as old as 5,000 years; artifacts detailing yoga postures have been found in India dating from 3000 B.C. Yoga masters (*yogis*) claim that it is a highly developed science of healthy living that has been tested and perfected through the centuries. Yoga was first brought to the United States in the late 1800s when Swami Vivekananda (1862–1902), an Indian teacher and yogi, presented a lecture on meditation in Chicago, Illinois.

Yoga slowly began gaining followers and flourished during the 1960s when there was a surge of interest in Eastern philosophy. After that, yoga knowledge in the United States became more extensive, with many students going to India to study and many Indian experts coming to the United States to teach, resulting in the establishment of a wide variety schools. Yoga practice remains popular in the United States, and teachers and practitioners are easily located across the country.

Millions of Americans do yoga regularly or occasionally. Physical therapists and professional sports teams use yoga stretches, and movie stars and *Fortune* 500 executives tout the benefits of yoga. Many prestigious schools of medicine have studied and introduced yoga techniques as proven therapies for illness and stress. Some medical schools, such as the one at the University of California at Los Angeles (UCLA), even offer yoga classes as part of their physician training program.

Benefits

Yoga is often recommended as an adjunct to **psychotherapy** or standard medical treatments. Its integration of the mental, physical, and spiritual dimensions of being is helpful to patients struggling with distorted cognitions or pain syndromes. The stretching, bending, and balancing involved in the asanas help to align the head and spinal column; stimulate the circulatory system, endocrine glands, and other organs; and keep muscles and joints strong and flexible. Yoga programs have been shown to reduce the risk of heart disease by lowering blood pressure and anxiety levels. The breath control exercises emphasize slow and deep abdominal breathing. They benefit the respiratory system, help to induce a sense of relaxation, and are useful in pain management. The meditation that is an integral part of classical yoga practice has been shown to strengthen the human immune system. In addition, pain relief can be achieved with the use of yoga. When the body is more flexible and strong, many types of pain are relieved, such as pain in the back.

Yoga also guides the individual toward self-control (*yama*), involving abstinence, truthfulness, honesty, and not doing harm to other living things. In addition, the individual is instructed in contentment and austerity and in devotion to the Supreme Being, what is called *niyama*. Yoga also helps individuals to look inward into the soul (what is called restraint of the senses, or *pratyahara*); to concentrate on one object, such as a body part, in order to avoid being sensitive to external disturbances (*dharana*); and to achieve complete contemplation (*samadhi*). It should be remembered that yoga is not a religion, but a way of living, with health and peace of mind as its aims.

Yoga provides the same benefits as any well-designed exercise program, increasing general health and stamina, reducing stress, and improving those conditions brought about by sedentary lifestyles. Yoga has the added advantage of being a low-impact activity that uses only gravity as resistance, which makes it an excellent physical therapy routine.

Meditation has been much studied and approved for its benefits in reducing stress-related conditions. The landmark book, *The Relaxation Response* (1975), by Harvard University cardiologist Herbert Benson (1935–), showed that meditation and breathing techniques for relaxation could have the opposite effect of stress, reducing blood pressure and other indicators. Since that publication, much research has reiterated the benefits of meditation for **stress reduction** and general health. The American Medical Association recommends meditation techniques as a first step before medication for treating borderline hypertension.

Modern psychological studies have shown that even slight facial expressions can cause changes in the involuntary nervous system; yoga utilizes the mind/body connection. That is, yoga practice contains the central ideas that physical posture and alignment can influence a person's mood and self-esteem and also that the mind can be used to shape and heal the body. Yoga practitioners claim that the strengthening of mind/body awareness can bring eventual improvements in all facets of a person's life.

Yoga exercises are also recommended as a way to tone muscles and nerves, as a way to reduce weight, and as an overall way to improve health and prolong life.

Preparation

Yoga can be performed by those of any age and condition, although not all poses should be attempted by everyone. Yoga is also an accessible form of exercise; all that is needed is a flat floor surface large enough to stretch out on, a mat or towel, and enough overhead space to extend the arms. It is a good activity for those who cannot go to gyms, who do not like other forms of exercise, or have busy schedules. Yoga should be done on an empty stomach, and teachers recommend waiting at least two to three hours after meals to engage in yoga. Loose and comfortable clothing should be worn, and the feet are usually left bare.

Risks

Most reported injuries in yoga result from lack of concentration or attempts to perform difficult poses without working up to them. People who have consulted a physician before starting yoga and practice under the supervision of an experienced teacher are unlikely to suffer injury. Beginners sometimes report muscle soreness and **fatigue** after performing yoga, but these side effects diminish with practice.

Patients with a history of heart disease, severe back injuries, inner ear problems or other difficulties with balance, glaucoma, or recent surgery should consult a physician before beginning yoga. Certain yoga positions should not be performed with a fever or during menstruation. Pregnant women are usually advised to modify their yoga practice during the first trimester.

People diagnosed with a dissociative disorder should not attempt advanced forms of pranayama (yogic breathing) without the supervision of an experienced teacher. Some yogic breathing exercises may trigger symptoms of derealization or **depersonalization** in these patients.

Beginners should exercise care and concentration when performing yoga postures and not try to stretch too much too quickly, as injury could result. A stretch or posture should be stopped if there is pain, dizziness, or fatigue. Some advanced yoga postures, such as headstand and full lotus position, can be difficult and require strength, flexibility, and gradual preparation, so beginners should get the help of a teacher before attempting them.

One additional precaution is often necessary for Westerners. Yoga is not a competitive sport, and a "good" practice is defined as whatever one's body and mind are capable of giving on a specific day. Westerners are, however, accustomed to pushing themselves hard, comparing their performances to those of others, and assuming that exercise is not beneficial unless it hurts—an attitude summed up in the phrase "no pain, no gain." Yoga teaches a gentle and accepting attitude toward one's body rather than a punishing or perfectionistic approach. A person should go into the stretches and poses gradually, not forcibly or violently. Stretching should not be done past the point of mild discomfort, which is normal for beginners; frank pain is a warning that the body is not properly aligned in the pose or that the joints are being overstressed. Most people beginning yoga will experience measurable progress in their strength and flexibility after a week or two of daily practice.

The mental component of yoga is just as important as the physical postures. Concentration and awareness of breath should not be neglected. While performing the yoga of breathing (pranayama) and meditation (dyana), it is best to have an experienced teacher, as these powerful techniques can cause dizziness and discomfort when done improperly.

QUESTIONS TO ASK YOUR DOCTOR

- How do you think yoga will benefit me?
- Do I have any physical limitations that would prohibit my undertaking yoga?
- What tests or evaluation techniques will you perform to see if yoga has been beneficial for me?
- What other treatment options do you recommend for me?
- Will yoga interfere with my current medications?
- What symptoms or behaviors are important enough that I should seek immediate treatment?

KEY TERMS

Asana—A position or stance in yoga.

Dyana—The yoga term for meditation.

Hatha yoga—A form of yoga using postures, breathing methods, and meditation.

Meditation—Technique of concentration for relaxing the mind and body.

Pranayama—Yogic breathing techniques.

Yogi (feminine, yogini)—A trained yoga expert.

Research and general acceptance

Although Western medical researchers have been studying yoga only since the 1970s, **clinical trials** in the United States have demonstrated its effectiveness in treating stress-related illnesses, anxiety, **premenstrual syndrome**, and mood disorders. Other reports indicate that yoga merits further research in the treatment of **obsessive-compulsive disorder** (OCD) and **substance abuse**. Studies done in Germany have focused on the psychological benefits of yoga. Many have been randomized, controlled studies, which are the most strenuous ones available to prove or disprove the validity of a hypothesis.

In 2008, researchers from the University of Utah studied yoga and its association with reducing pain. Forty-two participants were studied: 12 were experienced in yoga, 14 had fibromyalgia (hypersensitivity to pain), and 16 were overall healthy individuals. All of the participants were subjected to the pain caused by pressing down with a thumbnail. Functional magnetic resonance image (fMRI) scans were performed on each person to measure activity within the **brain** caused by the pain. The people with fibromyalgia showed the most pain response with the least amount of pressure. By contrast, the yoga practitioners reported the least amount of pain when compared to the other two groups. The researchers concluded that yoga can help individuals control their stress levels when pain is present.

The Harvard University Medical School also reports that yoga is being studied for people with **post-traumatic stress disorder** (PTSD), such as sometimes found among military combatants. One such study looked at military veterans from Australia who had fought in Vietnam. All of the participants were taking at least one type of antidepressant on a daily basis and were also considered daily heavy drinkers of alcohol. Some of the veterans were enrolled in a five-day course that included yoga, along with education on stress reduction. A control group did not receive this training.

Using the Clinician Administered PTSD Scale (CAPS), the researchers found that scores dropped from 57 (moderate to severe symptoms) to 42 (mild to moderate symptoms), on average, after six weeks. The veterans were re-evaluated six months later and it was found that their scores remained at these lower levels. The control group did not show improvement during this period. Based on this study and others, the Walter Reed Army Medical Center in Washington, DC, started offering yoga classes to U.S. service men and women returning from combat in Iraq and Afghanistan in the hope that it would help to counter PTSD. Studies are ongoing to determine the results of this treatment.

Other studies performed in the 2000s and early 2010s showed that yoga is helpful with **depression**, stress, fatigue, headaches, back pain, sleep problems, and symptoms of **schizophrenia** and **bipolar disorder**. Further studies showed improvements in mood and quality of life for breast cancer survivors, patients with epilepsy, the elderly, and people caring for patients with **dementia**.

Training and certification

Yoga is usually best learned from a yoga teacher or physical therapist, but yoga is simple enough that one can learn the basics from good books on the subject, which are plentiful. Yoga classes are generally inexpensive, averaging around ten dollars per class, and students can learn basic postures in just a few classes. Many Young Men Christian Associations (YMCAs), colleges, and community health organizations offer beginning yoga classes as well, often for nominal fees. If yoga is part of a physical therapy program, its cost can be reimbursed by insurance.

Resources

BOOKS

Butera, Robert J. *The Pure Heart of Yoga: Ten Essential Steps for Personal Transformation.* Woodbury, MN: Llewellyn, 2009.

Christensen, Alice. *The American Yoga Association's Easy Does It Yoga.* New York: Fireside/Simon & Schuster, 1999.

Coulter, David H. *Anatomy of Hatha Yoga: A Manual for Students, Teachers, and Practitioners.* Honesdale, PA: Body and Breath, 2010.

Iyenger, B. K.S. *Yoga Wisdom & Practice.* New York: DK, 2009.

Rountree, Sage. *The Athlete's Pocket Guide to Yoga: 50 Routines for Flexibility, Balance, and Focus.* Boulder, CO: VeloPress, 2009.

Williams, Nancy. *Yoga Therapy for Every Special Child: Meeting Needs in a Natural Setting.* Philadelphia: Jessica Kingsley, 2010.

WEBSITES

"Yoga for Anxiety and Depression." Harvard Health Publications Harvard Medical School. http://www.health.harvard.edu/newsletters/Harvard_Mental_Health_Letter/2009/April/Yoga-for-anxiety-and-depression (accessed August 16, 2011).

Yoga Journal Releases 2008 "Yoga in America" Market Study. Yoga Journal. (February 26, 2008). http://www.yogajournal.com/advertise/press_releases/10 (accessed July 21, 2011).

Mayo Clinic staff. "Yoga: Tap into the Many Health Benefits." MayoClinic.com, January 16, 2010. http://www.mayoclinic.com/health/yoga/CM00004 (accessed August 16, 2011).

ORGANIZATIONS

American Yoga Association, PO Box 19986, Sarasota, FL, 34276, info@americanyogaassociation.org, http://www.americanyogaassociation.org.

International Association of Yoga Therapists, PO Box 12890, Prescott, AZ, 86304, (928) 541-0004, mail@iayt.org, http://www.iayt.org.

Yoga Science Foundation, 759 South State St., No. 24, Ukiah, CA, 95482, http://www.yrec.org.

Rebecca J. Frey, PhD
William A. Atkins, BB, BS, MBA

Z

Zaleplon

Definition

Zaleplon is classified as a hypnotic drug. Such drugs help people sleep. Zaleplon is available in the United States under the brand name Sonata.

Purpose

Zaleplon is a drug that is used to treat short-term **insomnia**.

Description

The U.S. Food and Drug Administration approved Zaleplon in 1999 to treat short-term sleep problems. Zaleplon is thought to act by mimicking a chemical in the **brain** that helps to facilitate sleep. It is different from other sleeping pills in that it begins to work almost immediately and its effects are rather short-lived (a few hours). These properties make it beneficial both for people who have troubling falling asleep at bedtime and for people who awaken in the middle of the night and have trouble falling back to sleep. Zaleplon may be taken in the middle of the night so long as the person can sleep at least four more hours before having to awaken.

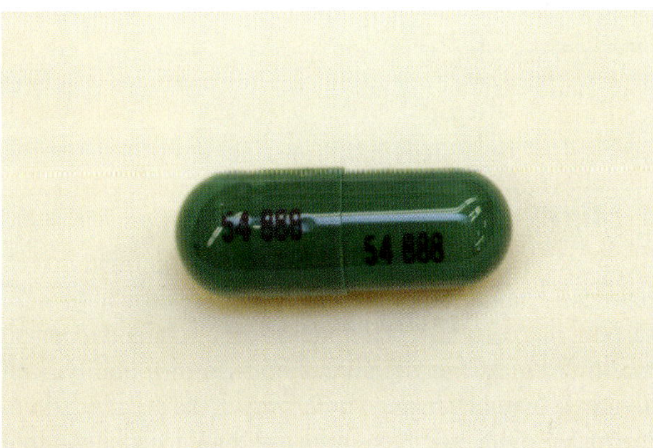

Zaleplon, 10 mg. *(© Custom Medical Stock Photo, Inc. Reproduced by permission.)*

Zaleplon is available as capsules. The drug is broken down by the liver. It is a controlled substance and can be habit-forming.

Recommended dosage

The usual dose of zaleplon for adults is 5–20 mg. For healthy adults, 10 mg is a common dosage. However, people over age 65, small adults with low body weight, and people with serious health problems (especially liver disease) should take a dose at the low end of this range (usually 5 mg). Zaleplon is taken immediately before bedtime. It usually takes only about 30 minutes for the sleep-inducing actions of zaleplon to be felt, and sleep-facilitating effects appear to last only a few hours. If zaleplon is taken with a meal, it will take longer to work. For the fastest sleep onset, it should be taken on an empty stomach. The maximum dose for one day is 20 mg. Under no circumstances should a person take more than 20 mg in one day.

Precautions

Zaleplon should be taken exactly as directed by a physician. A person who forgets a dose of zaleplon should skip the dose and take the next dose at the regularly scheduled time.

Because zaleplon is used to help people fall asleep, it should only be taken when the patient is preparing for a full night's sleep (seven to eight hours). Some patients taking sleep medications have engaged in sleep-related behaviors, including eating, talking, and even driving while asleep, with no recollection of the events. Zaleplon should not be used with other drugs (over-the-counter or prescription) that also cause drowsiness. It should be used only with close physician supervision in people with liver disease and in the elderly because these individuals are especially sensitive to the sedative properties of zaleplon. Zaleplon should not be used before driving, operating machinery, or performing other activities that require mental alertness. People with a history of drug abuse, psychiatric disorders, or **depression** should be carefully monitored when using zaleplon, since the drug may worsen symptoms of some psychiatric disorders and can become a drug of abuse.

If zaleplon is needed for more than seven to ten days, patients should be re-evaluated by a physician to determine whether another disorder is causing their difficulty sleeping. When zaleplon or other sleeping pills are used every night for more than a few weeks, they begin to lose their effectiveness, and/or people may become dependent upon them to fall asleep. Zaleplon can be addictive. People using zaleplon should not suddenly stop taking the drug because withdrawal symptoms, including sleep disturbances, may occur even if zaleplon has been used for only a short time.

Side effects

There is a risk of severe allergic reaction upon taking a sleep medication for the first time. Some sleeping pills such as zaleplon can cause aggressiveness, agitation, hallucinations, and **amnesia** (memory problems). A patient experiencing these side effects should call a physician immediately. A physician should also be called immediately if a person taking zaleplon develops a fast or irregular heartbeat, chest pains, skin rash, or itching.

The most common side effects of zaleplon are less serious and include dizziness, drowsiness, impaired coordination, upset stomach, nausea, headache, dry mouth, and muscle aches. Other side effects that may occur include fever, tremor, or eye pain. Many side effects appear worse at higher doses so it is important to use the lowest dose that will induce sleep.

Interactions

Any drug that causes drowsiness may lead to substantially decreased mental alertness and impaired motor skills when taken with zaleplon. Examples include alcohol, **antidepressants** such as **imipramine** or **paroxetine**, antipsychotics like **thioridazine**, and some antihistamines.

Because zaleplon is broken down by the liver, it may interact with other drugs also broken down by the liver. For example, the drug rifampin, which is used to treat tuberculosis, may cause zaleplon to be less effective. Alternatively, cimetidine (Tagamet), a drug commonly used to treat heartburn, may cause people to be more sensitive to zaleplon.

Resources

BOOKS

Preston, John D., John H. O'Neal, and Mary C. Talaga. *Handbook of Clinical Psychopharmacology for Therapists*. 5th ed. Oakland, CA: New Harbinger Publications, 2008.

Wolters Kluwer Health. *Drug Facts and Comparisons 2012*. 66th ed. St. Louis: Lippincott, Williams & Wilkins, 2011.

PERIODICALS

Bain, Kevin T. "Management of Chronic Insomnia in Elderly Persons." *American Journal of Geriatric Pharma cotherapy* 4, no. 2 (June 2006): 168–92.

Conn, David K., and Robert Madan. "Use of Sleep-Promoting Medications in Nursing Home Residents: Risks versus Benefits." *Drugs and Aging* 23, no. 4 (2006): 271–87.

Glass, Jennifer, et al. "Sedative Hypnotics in Older People with Insomnia: Meta-Analysis of Risks and Benefits." *British Medical Journal* 331, no. 7526 (November 2005): 1–7.

McCall, W. "Diagnosis and Management of Insomnia in Older People." *Journal of the American Geriatrics Society* 53, no. 7 Suppl. (July 2005): S272–S277.

Rosenberg, Russell P. "Sleep Maintenance Insomnia: Strengths and Weaknesses of Current Pharmacologic Therapies." *Annals of Clinical Psychiatry* 18, no. 1 (January–March 2006): 49–56.

Kelly Karpa, R.Ph., PhD
Ruth A. Wienclaw, PhD

Zinc

Definition

Zinc (chemical symbol Zn) is a mineral and a metal that is essential for a healthy immune system, production of certain hormones, wound healing, bone formation, and clear skin. It is required in very small amounts and is thus known as an essential trace element. Despite this low requirement, zinc is found in nearly every cell of the body and is key to the proper function of more than 300 enzymes.

Purpose

Zinc is vital for the body to function normally, both physically and mentally, and has been shown to help sustain intellectual (cognitive) function, mood control, healthy skin, strong vision, blood-clotting ability, cell division, wound repair, and proper taste and smell. Normal growth and development cannot occur without zinc. Zinc is also important in promoting mental health and has increasingly been found to reduce symptoms of certain mental disorders. Research has found that

Recommended Dietary Allowance (RDA) of zinc

Age group	RDA
Children, 0–6 months	2 mg
Children, 7–12 months	3 mg
Children, 1–3 years	3 mg
Children, 4–8 years	5 mg
Children, 9–13 years	8 mg
Teenage females, 14–18 years	9 mg
Teenage males, 14–18 years	11 mg
Adult females (19+)	8 mg
Adult males (19+)	11 mg
Pregnant teenage females	12 mg
Pregnant adult females	11 mg
Breast-feeding teenage females	13 mg
Breast-feeding adult females	12 mg

SOURCE: Office of Dietary Supplements, National Institutes of Health.

(Table by PreMediaGlobal. Reproduced by permission of Gale, a part of Cengage Learning.)

symptoms of **schizophrenia**, **autism**, **attention deficit hyperactivity disorder (ADHD)**, **Down syndrome**, Wilson's disease, and other mental health problems may be reduced with zinc supplementation. However, too much zinc can be harmful to persons with other mental illnesses, such as **Alzheimer's disease**.

Description

Zinc deficiency is a serious health problem in the world, although it is relatively uncommon in the United States. The World Health Organization (WHO) estimates that zinc deficiency affects about one-third of the world's population. Although this deficiency is considered to be mild to moderate in most cases, it can result in mental health problems, such as **depression**.

General symptoms of zinc deficiency include:

- depression
- impotence in men, low fertility in men and women
- poor growth in infants and children, along with delayed sexual maturation in adolescents
- night blindness
- pale skin, along with skin problems, such as acne
- eye sores
- lowered alertness levels
- poor hair growth, along with hair loss
- diarrhea
- lack of menstrual period
- frequent infections, such as pneumonia
- loss of appetite, weight loss
- reduced ability to taste or smell
- poor wound healing

Symptoms of too much zinc in the body include:

- nausea
- vomiting
- loss of appetite
- stomach cramping
- diarrhea
- headaches
- lower immunity levels
- low levels of high-density lipoprotein (HDL) cholesterol—the so-called "good cholesterol"

Many of these symptoms could be signs of other medical problems. It is wise to see a medical professional if such symptoms are present.

Zinc and mental health

Over the past 40 years, research has found a correlation between mental health and zinc. American physician and biochemist Carl Curt Pfeiffer (1908–1988) discovered in the 1970s that low amounts of zinc and manganese (Mn) in children can adversely affect their learning ability, as well as lead to an increased risk of **intellectual disability**. Pfeiffer also reported that zinc and vitamin B_6 supplements helped to control pyroluria-type schizophrenia (a type of schizophrenia characterized by an abnormal number of pyrroles in the body) in the vast number of cases he studied. Since the Pfeiffer-led study, many people with pyroluria-type schizophrenia are successfully treated with a combination of zinc and vitamin B_6.

Zinc has also been found to help symptoms of **ADHD**. Studies performed in the last quarter of the twentieth century showed that children with low levels of zinc, manganese, and vitamin B_6 (along with excessive amounts of copper [Cu] and lead [Pb]) were hyperactive. Canadian **psychiatrist** and biochemist Abram Hoffer (1917–2009) showed that zinc, along with other vitamins and minerals, helped children minimize symptoms associated with autism and ADHD. A separate study performed at Capella University, in Minneapolis, Minnesota, concluded that zinc supplements given along with **methylphenidate** (Ritalin), an ADHD medication, showed positive results in treating the symptoms of attention deficit and hyperactivity in ADHD children. In 2005, a study published in the *Journal of Child and Adolescent Psychopharmacology* further correlated that a relationship exists between zinc and inattentiveness in children. Other studies have supported the evidence that zinc can improve symptoms of ADHD, such as impulsiveness and hyperactivity, in children who regularly take zinc along with their traditional ADHD treatment.

Additionally, zinc may play a role in helping people with Down syndrome (DS). Studies showed that a deficiency of zinc adversely affects the nervous, neuroendocrine, and immune systems of people with DS. A 2004 study reported in the journal *Down Syndrome Research and Practice* that zinc levels in the hair of children with DS were significantly less than in other children. The researchers concluded that some of the problems found in DS children could be due to low levels of zinc. Since this study, others have suggested that oral zinc supplements be used to correct immune and endocrinological disorders associated with DS.

In 2008, American clinical **psychologist** Ann M. DiGirolamo, an assistant professor at Rollins School of Public Health (Emory University), and Guatemalan physiologist Manuel Ramirez-Zea, a principle investigator at the Institute of **Nutrition** of Central America and Panama (Guatemala City), reported that low levels of zinc increase the risk of depression and ADHD, especially in people already at high risk for these two mental illnesses. Their study, based on 30 years of research, was published in the *American Journal of Clinical Nutrition*.

Wilson's disease, or hepatolenticular degeneration, is a neurodegenerative disease that is caused by the inability of the body to metabolize copper. In this disease, copper builds up to abnormally large levels in the **brain**, liver, and other organs. Symptoms often include depression, clumsiness, difficulty speaking, problems walking, and involuntary shaking. For its treatment, medications are prescribed that reduce the amount of copper in the body. Chelating agents are used for this reduction method. This process allows copper to be taken into the bloodstream so that it can be released through urine. Two chelating agents are penicillamine (Cuprimine, Depen) and trientine (Syprine). To prevent a buildup of copper into the body from the foods that are eaten, zinc is used.

In the 2010s, zinc has often been promoted as an aid for memory. This may be true to the extent that vitamin B_6 and **neurotransmitters** are not properly utilized without it. However, in the case of people with Alzheimer's disease (AD), zinc can cause more harm than good. Some experiments indicate that zinc actually decreases intellectual function of patients with AD. Under these circumstances, it is best to adhere to the recommended dietary allowance (RDA) for zinc of 11 mg for adult males and 8 mg for adult females.

Overall, zinc has been found to generally help in reducing symptoms associated with some mental health problems when used in conjunction with conventional treatments. When used alone, zinc has not been found to be as beneficial. Further studies are warranted to better learn about zinc's role in helping with mental health conditions.

Recommended dosage

For treating symptoms of ADHD, the U.S. National Institutes of Health (NIH) recommends using from 55 mg of zinc sulfate (15 mg elemental zinc) to 150 mg (40 mg elemental) each day. It has also been suggested that zinc may promote weight gain and improve symptoms of depression in patients with **anorexia nervosa**; the NIH recommended dosage for this purpose is 100 mg of zinc gluconate per day. Exact dosage amounts should be confirmed with a physician. Without medical supervision, the daily tolerable upper intake levels (UL) of zinc are:

- children under the age of 6 months, 4 mg
- children aged 7 to 12 months, 5 mg
- children aged 1 to 3 years, 7 mg
- children aged 4 to 8 years, 12 mg
- children aged 9 to 13 years, 23 mg
- adolescents aged 14 to 18 years (including pregnancy and lactation), 34 mg
- adults aged 19 years and older (including pregnancy and lactation), 40 mg

Natural sources

Oysters are tremendously high in zinc. Some sources, such as whole grains, beans, and nuts, have good zinc content, but the fiber in these foods prevents it from being absorbed well. Foods with high amounts of zinc include red meat; poultry, such as chicken and turkey; crabs and lobsters; fortified breakfast cereals; and dairy products such as milk, cheese, and yogurt. Pure maple syrup also is a good source of zinc.

Supplemental sources

Zinc supplements are available as oral tablets in various forms as well as lozenges. Zinc gluconate is the type most commonly used in lozenge form to kill upper respiratory viruses. Consumers should look for brands that do not use citric acid or tartaric acid for flavoring, as these appear to impair the effectiveness. The best-absorbed oral types of zinc may include zinc citrate, zinc acetate, or zinc picolinate. Zinc sulfate is the most likely to cause stomach irritation. Topical formulations are used for acne and skin injuries. Oral zinc should not be taken with foods or substances that will reduce its absorption, such as coffee, bran, protein, phytates, calcium, or phosphorus. Supplements should be stored in a cool, dry location, away from direct light, and out of the reach of children.

Precautions

It is not uncommon to have mild to moderately low levels of zinc, although serious deficiency is rare. Symptoms can include an increased susceptibility to infection, rashes, hair loss, poor growth in children, delayed healing of wounds, rashes, acne, male infertility, poor appetite, decreased sense of taste and smell, and possible swelling of the mouth, tongue, and eyelids.

A more serious, chronic deficiency can cause severe growth problems, including dwarfism and poor bone maturation. The spleen and liver may become enlarged. Testicular size and function both tend to decrease. Cataracts may form in the eyes, the optic nerve can become swollen, and color vision is sometimes affected by a profound lack of zinc. Hearing is sometimes affected as well.

Since meats are the best sources of zinc, people on a restricted diet, such as strict vegetarians and vegans, are among the groups more likely to be deficient. The absorption of zinc is inhibited by high-fiber foods, so people who have **diets** that are very high in whole grain and fiber need to take supplements separately from the fiber. Zinc is needed in larger amounts for women who are pregnant, lactating, or breastfeeding. Deficiency during pregnancy may lower fetal birth-weight, as well as increase maternal risk of toxemia. A good prenatal vitamin is likely to contain an adequate amount of zinc. People over the age of 50 years do not absorb zinc as well as younger people, nor do they generally have adequate intake, and they may require a supplement. Alcoholics generally have poor nutritional status to begin with, and alcohol also depletes stored zinc.

There is an increased need for most vitamins and minerals for people who are chronically under high **stress**. Those who have had surgery, severe burns, wasting illnesses, or poor nutrition may require larger amounts of zinc than average.

Interactions

The absorption of vitamin A is improved by zinc supplements, but they may interfere with the absorption of other minerals taken at the same time, including calcium (Ca), magnesium (Mg), iron (Fe), and copper (Cu). Supplements of calcium, magnesium, and copper should not be taken at the same time as the zinc. Iron should only be taken if a known deficiency exists.

KEY TERMS

Acrodermatitis enteropathica—Hereditary metabolic problem characterized by dermatitis, diarrhea, and poor immune status. Oral treatment with zinc is curative.

Enzyme—A biological catalyst that increases the rate of a chemical reaction without being used up in the reaction.

Hemochromatosis—A hereditary condition that results in excessive storage of iron in various tissues of the body.

Pyrrole—A heterocyclic aromatic organic compound with chemical formula C_4H_4NH.

RDA—The abbreviation for "recommended dietary allowance," which is the amount of vitamins and minerals needed to provide adequate nutrition in most healthy people; the amount varies depending on age, gender, and physical conditions, such as pregnancy; sometimes RDA is called "daily value" (DV) in the United States.

Schizophrenia—A severe mental illness in which a person has difficulty distinguishing what is real from what is not real. It is often characterized by hallucinations, delusions, and withdrawal from people and social activities.

Sickle cell anemia—An inherited disorder in which red blood cells contain an abnormal form of hemoglobin, a protein that carries oxygen. The abnormal form of hemoglobin causes the red cells to become sickle-shaped. The misshapen cells may clog blood vessels, preventing oxygen from reaching tissues and leading to pain, blood clots, and other problems.

Thiazide and loop diuretic medications, sometimes used for people with high blood pressure, congestive heart failure, or liver disease, increase the loss of zinc. Levels are also lowered by oral contraceptives. Zinc can decrease the absorption of tetracycline and quinolone class antibiotics, antacids, soy, or manganese, and should not be taken at the same time of day.

Drinking coffee at the same time as taking zinc can reduce the absorption by as much as half. Even moderate amounts of alcohol impair zinc metabolism and increase its excretion. Chelation with ethylenediaminetetraacetic acid (EDTA) can deplete zinc, so patients undergoing chelation need to supplement with zinc, according to the instructions of the health care provider.

QUESTIONS TO ASK YOUR DOCTOR

- In what way do you think zinc will benefit me?
- Will zinc interfere with my current medications?
- What symptoms or adverse effects are important enough that I should seek immediate treatment?

Make sure to inform the medical professional who regularly makes regular physical examinations as to any dietary supplements and medicines that are being taken. Zinc can interact with many over-the-counter or prescription medications.

Complications

Some diseases increase the risk of zinc deficiency. Sickle cell anemia, diabetes, and kidney disease can all affect zinc metabolism. People with Crohn's disease, sprue (celiac disease), chronic diarrhea, or babies with acrodermatitis enteropathica (a metabolic disorder affecting the absorption of zinc) also have an increased need for zinc. People who are anorexic also are at increased risk of having insufficient amounts of zinc within the body, as are people with hookworm, cirrhosis, chronic renal disease, and severe **trauma**. Consult a health care provider for appropriate supplementation instructions.

Toxicity can occur with excessively large doses of zinc supplements and can produce symptoms including fever, cough, abdominal pain, nausea, vomiting, diarrhea, drowsiness, restlessness, and gait abnormalities. If doses greater than 100 mg per day are taken chronically, anemia, immune insufficiency, heart problems, and copper deficiency can result. High doses of zinc can also cause a decrease in high-density lipoprotein (HDL), or "good" cholesterol.

People who have hemochromatosis, are allergic to zinc, or are infected with human immunodeficiency virus (HIV) should not take supplemental zinc. Ulcers in the stomach or duodenum may be aggravated by supplements as well. Those with glaucoma should use caution if using eye drops containing zinc. Overuse of supplemental zinc during pregnancy can increase the risk of premature birth and stillbirth, particularly if the supplement is taken in the third trimester. This increase in adverse outcomes has been documented with zinc dosages of 100 mg taken three times daily.

Zinc may cause irritation of the stomach and is best taken with food in order to avoid nausea. The lozenge form used to treat colds has a strong taste and can alter the sense of taste and smell for up to a few days.

Resources

BOOKS

Marian, Mary J., Pamela Williams-Mullen, and Jennifer Muir Bowers. *Integrating Therapeutic and Complementary Nutrition.* Boca Raton, FL: CRC, 2006.

Micozzi, Marc S. *Fundamentals of Complementary and Alternative Medicine.* New York: Saunders, 2010.

Pelletier, Kenneth R. "Western Herbal Medicine: Nature's Green Pharmacy." Chapter 6 in *The Best Alternative Medicine.* New York: Simon and Schuster, 2007.

Physician's Desk Reference. *PDR for Nonprescription Drugs, Dietary Supplements, and Herbs 2009,* 30th ed. New York: Physician's Desk Reference, 2008.

Purchon, Nerys. *The Essential Natural Health Bible: The Complete Home Guide to Herbs and Oils, Natural Remedies and Nutrition.* NSW, Australia: Millennium House, 2011.

Therapeutic Research Faculty. *Natural Medicines Comprehensive Database 2007.* Stockton, CA: Natural Medicines Database, 2006.

Ulbricht, Catherine E. *Davis's Pocket Guide to Herbs and Supplements.* Philadelphia: F.A. Davis, 2011.

PERIODICALS

Yenigun, Ayse, et al. "Hair Zinc Level in Down Syndrome." *Down Syndrome Research and Practice* 9, no. 2 (2004): 53–57. http://dx.doi.org/10.3104/reports.292 (accessed September 2, 2011).

WEBSITES

Mayo Clinic staff. "Wilson's Disease." MayoClinic.com (September 24, 2009). http://www.mayoclinic.com/health/wilsons-disease/DS00411 (accessed August 30, 2011).

Mayo Clinic staff. "Zinc Supplement." MayoClinic.com (November 1, 2010). http://www.mayoclinic.com/health/drug-information/DR602313 (accessed August 30, 2011).

"Zinc." Office of Dietary Supplements, National Institutes of Health. http://ods.od.nih.gov/factsheets/Zinc-Health Professional (accessed August 30, 2011).

ORGANIZATIONS

American Botanical Council, 6200 Manor Road, Austin, TX, 78723, (512) 926-4900, Fax: (512) 926-2345, abc@herbalram.org, http://abc.herbalgram.org.

American Psychiatric Association, 1000 Wilson Boulevard, Suite 1825, Arlington, VA, 22209, (703) 907-7300, apa@psych.org, http://www.psych.org.

National Center for Complementary and Alternative Medicine Clearinghouse, 9000 Rockville Pike, Bethesda, MD, 20892, info@nccam.nih.gov, http://nccam.nih.gov.

Natural Standard, One Davis Square, Somerville, MA, 02144, (617) 591-3300, Fax: (617) 591-3399, http://naturalstandard.com.

Office of Dietary Supplements, National Institutes of Health, 6100 Executive Boulevard, Room 3B01, MSC 7517, Rockville, MD, 20892-7517, (301) 435-2920, Fax: (301) 480-1845, ods@nih.gov, http://ods.od.nih.gov.

United States Pharmacopoeia, 12601 Twinbrook Parkway, Rockville, MD, 20852-1790, (800) 227-8772, http://www.usp.org.

Judith Turner
Teresa G. Odle
William A. Atkins

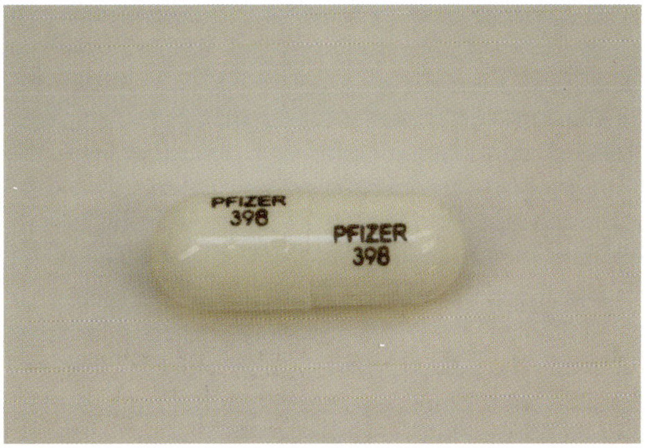

Geodon (ziprasidone), 60 mg. *(© Custom Medical Stock Photo, Inc. Reproduced by permission.)*

Ziprasidone

Definition

Ziprasidone is an atypical antipsychotic drug used to treat **schizophrenia**. It is also used to treat acute manic or mixed episodes associated with **bipolar disorder**. It is available with a prescription under the brand name Geodon.

Purpose

Ziprasidone is in a class of drugs called antipsychotics. It is used to control symptoms of schizophrenia, or for acute symptoms associated with bipolar disorder. It may also be used in conjunction with lithium or valproate (Depakote) as maintenance treatment for bipolar disorder. Ziprasidone is one of the newer antipsychotic drugs—often called atypical antipsychotics—that is less likely to cause significant adverse side effects than conventional antipsychotic medications.

Description

The U.S. Food and Drug Administration (FDA) approved ziprasidone for treatment of schizophrenia in 2001, for treatment of acute manic or mixed episodes associated with bipolar disorder in 2004, and as maintenance treatment of bipolar disorder in 2009. In people with schizophrenia or bipolar disorder, chemical systems in the **brain** are out of balance. Mental well-being is partially related to maintaining a balance between naturally occurring chemicals called **neurotransmitters**. Ziprasidone is thought to modify the actions of several neurotransmitters and restore appropriate function to the chemical systems.

Recommended dosage

The dosage of ziprasidone varies widely from one individual to another. A common initially dosage is 20 mg of ziprasidone taken twice daily. The dosage is gradually increased until symptoms of schizophrenia subside. Dosages of up to 100 mg may be taken twice daily. Dosing for treatment of bipolar disorder generally ranges from 40–80 mg twice daily. Ziprasidone should be taken with food.

For acute treatment of agitation in schizophrenia, ziprasidone may be administered intramuscularly (as an injection) at a dose of 10–40 mg (maximum) per day.

Precautions

Ziprasidone may interact with other medications to caused altered heart rhythms (arrhythmia). It should not

QUESTIONS TO ASK YOUR DOCTOR

- What kind of changes can I expect to see or feel with this medication?
- Does it matter what time of day I take this medication? If so, what is the recommendation?
- What are the side effects associated with this medication?
- Will this medication interact or interfere with other medications I am currently taking?
- What symptoms or adverse effects are important enough that I should seek immediate treatment?

KEY TERMS

Delusions—Irrational beliefs that defy normal reasoning and remain firm even when overwhelming proof is presented to dispute them. Delusions are distinct from culturally or religiously based beliefs that may be seen as untrue by outsiders.

Neurotransmitter—One of a group of chemicals secreted by a nerve cell (neuron) to carry a chemical message to another nerve cell, often as a way of transmitting a nerve impulse. Examples of neurotransmitters include acetylcholine, dopamine, serotonin, and norepinephrine.

Schizophrenia—A major mental illness marked by psychotic symptoms, including hallucinations, delusions, and severe disruptions in thinking.

Seizure—A convulsion, or uncontrolled discharge of nerve cells that may spread to other cells throughout the brain.

Serotonin—A chemical messenger in the brain thought to play a role in mood regulation.

be taken by people with a history of irregular or prolonged heart rhythms (long QT syndrome), those with heart failure, or individuals who have recently had a heart attack. People with a history of heart disease should discuss the risks and benefits of treatment with their doctor before starting ziprasidone. Ziprasidone may also lower blood pressure to dangerously low levels, possibly causing a person to faint. It should not be taken by people who have slow heartbeats or low levels of potassium or magnesium in their blood; people taking medication to regulate their blood pressure should have their blood pressure monitored and their treatment modified as needed.

Individuals with a history of **seizures**, even seizures brought on by drug or alcohol abuse, should use ziprasidone cautiously and with close physician supervision, as it may increase the risk of seizures. Ziprasidone may also increase body temperatures to dangerously high levels. People who **exercise** strenuously, those exposed to extreme heat, individuals taking drugs with anticholinergic effects (this includes many common **antidepressants**), and persons prone to dehydration should use the drug cautiously and be alert to dehydration-related side effects.

Elderly persons with increased risk of developing pneumonia should be carefully monitored while taking ziprasidone. Because there is a high incidence of **suicide** in all patients with psychotic illnesses, people using ziprasidone should be observed carefully for signs of suicidal behavior. Women who are pregnant or breast-feeding should not take ziprasidone, as it may harm the fetus. Some newborns born to mothers who had taken ziprasidone during pregnancy exhibited withdrawal symptoms, including respiratory problems and tremor.

In June 2008, the FDA announced a requirement for manufacturers of ziprasidone (and other antipsychotic drugs) to issue a warning label regarding the adverse effects of using ziprasidone to treat behavioral problems in older individuals with dementia-related **psychosis**, including death. Studies showed that older adults with **dementia** taking antipsychotics such as ziprasidone were at increased risk of having a **stroke** or mini-stroke during treatment and, in some cases, an increased chance of death during treatment, though the reason for the finding was unclear. The use of ziprasidone in treating older adults with dementia-related psychosis is not approved by the FDA.

Side effects

The most common reason that ziprasidone is stopped is the development of a rash. Another common side effect is drowsiness. This side effect is usually worse when starting the drug and becomes less severe with continued use. People performing tasks that require mental alertness such as driving or operating machinery should refrain from doing so until they see how the drug affects them. Other side effects that may occur are abnormal, involuntary twitching (5%) and respiratory disorders (8%). Nausea, constipation, indigestion, and dizziness due to low blood pressure occur in more than 5% of people taking ziprasidone.

Other less common side effects include rapid heartbeat, low blood pressure, agitation, tremor, confusion, **amnesia**, dry mouth, increased salivation, joint pains, and abnormal vision.

The incidence of some adverse effects such as low blood pressure, loss of appetite, abnormal involuntary movements, sleepiness, tremor, cold symptoms, rash, abnormal vision, dry mouth, or increased salivation appears to increase at higher dosages.

People taking ziprasidone should alert their healthcare provider immediately if they develop a rash or hives, since this could indicate a potentially serious adverse reaction. Patients should also notify their health care provider right away if they experience any abnormal involuntary muscle movements. People who think they may be experiencing side effects from this or any other medication should tell their physicians.

Interactions

Ziprasidone interacts with many other drugs, and patients should let their physician know of all the other medications they are taking before starting treatment with ziprasidone. Ziprasidone may produce irregular heart rhythms and other cardiac problems when used with other drugs, including quinidine, dofetilide, **pimozide**, sotalol, erythromycin, **thioridazine**, moxifloxacin, and sparfloxacin; these drugs should not be taken in combination with ziprasidone.

Drugs that cause drowsiness, such as antidepressants, antihistamines, some pain relievers, and alcohol, may increase the sedative effects of ziprasidone. Individuals taking **zolpidem** (Ambien, Ambien CR) concomitantly with ziprasidone should be monitored for central nervous system effects such as respiratory **depression** and should avoid activities requiring mental alertness and motor coordination.

Other drugs taken in combination with ziprasidone may alter the effects of ziprasidone. Drugs such as **carbamazepine**, used to treat seizures, increases liver metabolism and may cause ziprasidone to be less effective. Alternatively, drugs such as ketoconazole, used to treat fungal infections, slow liver metabolism and may increase negative side effects associated with ziprasidone. Ziprasidone may also decrease the effects of drugs used to treat Parkinson's disease such as levodopa.

Resources

BOOKS

Albers, Lawrence J., Rhoda K. Hahn, and Christopher Reist. *Handbook of Psychiatric Drugs*. Laguna Hills, CA: Current Clinical Strategies Publishing, 2010.

American Society of Health-System Pharmacists. *AHFS Drug Information 2011*. Bethesda: American Society of Health-System Pharmacists, 2011.

Graham, George. *The Disordered Mind: An Introduction to Philosophy of Mind and Mental Illness*. New York: Routledge, 2010.

Holland, Leland Norman, and Michael Patrick Adams. *Core Concepts in Pharmacology*. 3rd ed. New York: Prentice Hall, 2011.

North, Carol, and Sean Yutzy. *Goodwin and Guze's Psychiatric Diagnosis*. New York: Oxford University Press, 2010.

Preston, John D., John H. O'Neal, and Mary C. Talaga. *Handbook of Clinical Psychopharmacology for Therapists*. 6th ed. Oakland, CA: New Harbinger Publications, 2011.

PERIODICALS

Barak, Yoram, Doron Mazeh, Igor Plopski, and Yehuda Baruch. "Intramuscular Ziprasidone Treatment of Acute Psychotic Agitation in Elderly Patients with Schizophrenia." *American Journal of Geriatric Psychiatry* 14, no. 7 (July 2006): 629–33.

Frederickson, Anne M., John M. Kane, and Peter Manu. "Does Antipsychotic Polypharmacy Increase the Risk For Metabolic Syndrome?" *Schizophrenia Research* 89, no. 1–3 (2007): 91–100.

Gentile, Salvatore. "Extrapyramidal Adverse Events Associated With Atypical Antipsychotic Treatment of Bipolar Disorder." *Journal of Clinical Psychopharmacology* 27, no. 1 (2007): 35–45.

Ginsberg, David L. "Ziprasidone-Induced Torsade de Pointes." *Primary Psychiatry* 13, no. 8 (2006): 27–29.

Glick, Ira D. "Understanding the Results of CATIE in the Context of the Field." *CNS Spectrums* 11, no. 7 (July 2006): 40–47.

Harvey, Philip D., Christopher R. Bowie, and Antony Loebel. "Neuropsychological Normalization with Long-Term Atypical Antipsychotic Treatment: Results of a Six-Month Randomized, Double-Blind Comparison of Ziprasidone vs. Olanzapine." *Journal of Neuropsychiatry and Clinical Neurosciences* 18, no. 1 (2006): 54–63.

Joyce, Amie T., et al. "Effect of Initial Ziprasidone Dose on Length of Therapy in Schizophrenia." *Schizophrenia Research* 83, no. 2–3 (2006): 285–92.

Kane, John M., Sumant Khanna, Sunita Rajadhyaksha, and Earl Giller. "Efficacy and Tolerability of Ziprasidone in Patients with Treatment-Resistant Schizophrenia." *International Clinical Psychopharmacology* 21, no. 1 (Jan. 2006): 21–28.

Kinon, Bruce J., et al. "A 24-Week Randomized Study of Olanzapine Versus Ziprasidone in the Treatment of Schizophrenia or Schizoaffective Disorder in Patients with Prominent Depressive Symptoms." *Journal of Clinical Psychopharmacology* 26, no. 2 (2006): 157–62.

Malhotra, Anil K., et al. "Ziprasidone-Induced Cognitive Enhancement in Schizophrenia: Specificity or Pseudospecificity?" *Schizophrenia Research* 87, no. 1–3 (2006): 181–84.

Stroup, T. Scott, et al. "Effectiveness of Olanzapine, Quetiapine, Risperidone, and Ziprasidone in Patients with Chronic Schizophrenia Following Discontinuation of a Previous Atypical Antipsychotic." *American Journal of Psychiatry* 163, no. 4 (2006): 611–22.

Ziegenbein, Marc, and Iris T. Calliess. "Clozapine and Ziprasidone: A Useful Combination in Patients With Treatment-Resistant Schizophrenia." *Journal of Neuropsychiatry and Clinical Neurosciences* 18, no. 2 (Spring 2006): 246–47.

ORGANIZATIONS

American Psychiatric Association, 1000 Wilson Boulevard, Suite 1825, Arlington, VA, 22209, (703) 907-7300, apa@psych.org, http://www.psych.org.

National Alliance on Mental Illness (NAMI), Colonial Place Three, 2107 Wilson Blvd., Suite 300, Arlington, VA, 22201, (703) 524-7600, (800) 950-NAMI (6264), Fax: (703) 524-9094, http://www.nami.org/Hometemplate.cfm.

National Institute of Mental Health (NIMH), 6001 Executive Boulevard, Room 8184, MSC 9663, Bethesda, MD, 20892, (301) 443-4513, (866) 615-6464, Fax: (301)

443-4279, nimhinfo@nih.gov, http://www.nimh.nih.gov/index.shtml.

U.S. Food and Drug Administration, 10903 New Hampshire Ave., Silver Spring, MD, 20993-0002, (888) INFO-FDA (463-6332), http://www.fda.gov.

Kelly Karpa, RPh, PhD
Ruth A. Wienclaw, PhD
Laura Jean Cataldo, RN, EdD

Zoloft *see* **Sertraline**

Zolpidem

Definition

Zolpidem is classified as a hypnotic drug. These drugs help people sleep. In the United States, zolpidem is sold as tablets under the brand name Ambien.

Purpose

Zolpidem is a drug that is used to treat **insomnia**. Zolpidem is especially helpful for people who have trouble falling asleep. However, once individuals have fallen asleep, zolpidem also helps them continue to sleep restfully. Zolpidem should be used only for short periods, approximately seven to ten days. If sleeping pills are needed for a long period, an evaluation by a physician is recommended to determine if another medical condition is responsible for the insomnia.

Description

Although the way zolpidem helps people sleep is not entirely understood, it is believed to mimic a chemical in

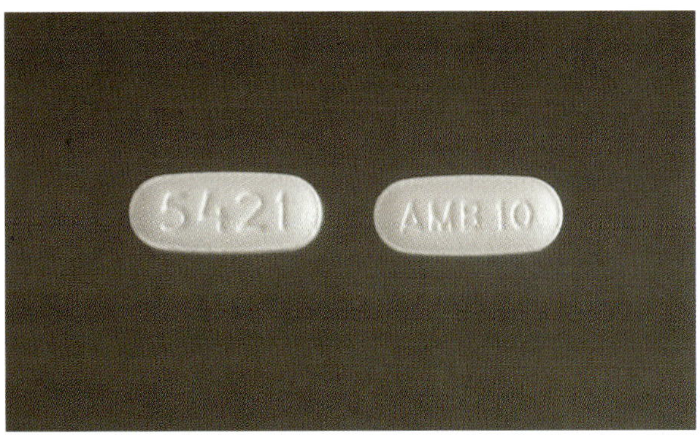

Zolpidem (Ambien), 10 mg. *(U.S. Drug Enforcement Administration)*

the **brain** called gamma-aminobutyric acid (GABA) that naturally helps to facilitate sleep. Zolpidem is a central nervous system depressant, which means that it slows down the nervous system. Unlike some sleeping pills, zolpidem does not interfere with the quality of sleep or usually leave the user feeling sedated in the morning. As a result, most people using zolpidem usually awake feeling refreshed.

Recommended dosage

The usual dose of zolpidem in adults is 5–10 mg. For healthy adults, 10 mg is commonly recommended. However, people taking other drugs that cause drowsiness; people who have severe health problems, especially liver disease; and older people (over age 65) should take a lower dose usually 5 mg. Zolpidem should be taken immediately before bedtime and only if the person can count on getting seven or eight hours of uninterrupted sleep. It usually takes only about 30 minutes for the sleep-inducing actions of zolpidem to be felt. Unlike some sleeping pills, the sleep-facilitating effects appear to last six to eight hours.

If zolpidem is taken with a meal, it will take longer to work. For the fastest sleep onset, it should be taken on an empty stomach. The maximum dose for one day is 10 mg. People who miss a dose of zolpidem should skip the missed dose and take the next dose at the regularly scheduled time. Under no circumstances should a person take more than 10 mg in one day. Zolpidem should be taken exactly as directed by the prescribing physician.

Precautions

Because zolpidem is used to help people fall asleep, it should not be used with other drugs (either over-the-counter, herbal, or prescription) that also cause drowsiness (for example, antihistamines or alcohol). Zolpidem should be used only with close physician supervision in people with liver disease and in the elderly, because these individuals are especially sensitive to the sedative properties of zolpidem. Zolpidem should not be used before driving, operating machinery, or performing activities that require mental alertness. People with a history of drug abuse, psychiatric disorders, or **depression** should be carefully monitored when using zolpidem since zolpidem may worsen symptoms of some psychiatric disorders.

If zolpidem is needed for more than seven to ten days, patients should be reevaluated by a physician to determine if another disorder is causing their difficulty in sleeping. When zolpidem or other sleeping pills are used every night for more than a few weeks, they begin to lose their effectiveness, and people may become dependent upon them to fall asleep. Zolpidem can be habit-forming when taken over a long period. People using zolpidem should

KEY TERMS

Antidepressant—A medication used to treat the symptoms of depression.

Antihistamine—A medication used to alleviate allergy or cold symptoms such as runny nose, itching, hives, watering eyes, or sneezing.

Antipsychotic—A medication used to treat psychotic symptoms of schizophrenia such as hallucinations, delusions, and delirium. May be used to treat symptoms in other disorders as well.

not stop taking the drug suddenly but should gradually reduce the dose over a few days before quitting, even if zolpidem has been used only for a short time.

Side effects

Some sleeping pills such as zolpidem can cause aggressiveness, agitation, hallucinations, **amnesia** (partial or complete loss of memory), rapid heartbeat, and chest pains. These side effects are rare but patients should call their physician immediately if such side effects occur. Other serious side effects include anaphylaxis (severe allergic reaction) and angioedema (facial swelling).

Some patients taking sleep medications have engaged in sleep-related behaviors, including eating, talking, and even driving while asleep, with no recollection of the events. More common side effects include headache, nausea, muscle aches, and drowsiness. Although drowsiness is desired when trying to fall asleep, a few people continue to feel drowsy the next day. Daytime drowsiness may cause people, especially the elderly, to be less coordinated and more susceptible to falls. Other less common side effects include anxiety, confusion, dizziness, and stomach upset.

Interactions

Any drug that causes drowsiness may lead to substantially decreased mental alertness and impaired motor skills when taken with zolpidem. Some examples include alcohol, **antidepressants** such as **imipramine** or **paroxetine**, antipsychotics such as **thioridazine**, and antihistamines (commonly found in allergy and cold medications).

The effectiveness of zolpidem may be reduced if taken with rifampin, an antibiotic that is commonly used to treat tuberculosis infections.

Resources

BOOKS

Physicians' Desk Reference 2011. 66th ed. Montvale, NJ: PDR Network, 2011.

Preston, John D., John H. O'Neal, and Mary C. Talaga. *Handbook of Clinical Psychopharmacology for Therapists*. 5th ed. Oakland, CA: New Harbinger Publications, 2008.

Wolters Kluwer Health. *Drug Facts and Comparisons 2012*. 66th ed. St. Louis: Lippincott, Williams & Wilkins, 2011.

PERIODICALS

Conn, David K., and Robert Madan. "Use of Sleep-Promoting Medications in Nursing Home Residents: Risks versus Benefits." *Drugs and Aging* 23, no. 4 (2006): 271–87.

Glass, Jennifer, et al. "Sedative Hypnotics in Older People with Insomnia: Meta-Analysis of Risks and Benefits." *British Medical Journal* 331, no. 7526 (November 2005): 1–7.

Hajak, G., et al. "Continuous versus Non-Nightly Use of Zolpidem in Chronic Insomnnia: Results of a Large-scale, Double-blind, Randomized, Outpatient Study." *International Clinical Psychopharmacology* 17, no. 1 (January 2002) 9–17.

Hart, Carl L., et al. "Combined Effects of Methamphetamine and Zolpidem on Performance and Mood During Simulated Night Shift Work." *Pharmacology, Biochemistry and Behavior* 81, no. 3 (July 2005): 559–68.

Lucchesi, Lígia M., et al. "Acute Neurophysiological Effects of the Hypnotic Zolpidem in Healthy Volunteers." *Progress in Neuro-Psychopharmacology and Biological Psychiatry* 29, no. 4 (May 2005): 557–64.

Meléndez, Jaime, et al. "Zolpidem and Triazolam Do Not Affect the Nocturnal Sleep-Induced Memory Improvement." *Psychopharmacology* 181, no. 1 (August 2005): 21–26.

Moen, Marit D., and Greg L. Plosker. "Zolpidem Extended Release in Insomnia: Profile Report." *Drugs and Aging* 23, no. 10 (2006): 843–46.

Rosenberg, Russell P. "Sleep Maintenance Insomnia: Strengths and Weaknesses of Current Pharmacologic Therapies." *Annals of Clinical Psychiatry* 18, no. 1 (January–March 2006): 49–56.

Staner, Luc, et al. "Next-Day Residual Effects of hypnotics in DSM-IV Primary Insomnia: A Driving Simulator Study with Simultaneous Electroencephalogram Monitoring." *Psychopharmacology* 181, no. 4 (October 2005): 790–98.

Wesensten, Nancy Jo, et al. "Daytime Sleep and Performance Following a Zolpidem and Melatonin Cocktail." *Sleep: Journal of Sleep and Sleep Disorders Research* 28, no. 1 (January 2005): 93–103.

Kelly Karpa, R.Ph., PhD
Ruth A. Wienclaw, PhD

Zyban *see* **Bupropion**

Zyprexa *see* **Olanzapine**

ORGANIZATIONS

The following is an alphabetical compilation of relevant organizations listed in the *Resources* sections of the main body entries. Although the list is comprehensive, it is by no means exhaustive. It is a starting point for gathering further information. U.S. government organizations and agencies are alphabetized under the first letter of the primary name (e.g., U.S. Food and Drug Administration is listed under "F"). Many of the organizations listed provide information for multiple disorders and have links to additional related websites. E-mail addresses and web addresses listed were provided by the associations; Gale, Cengage Learning is not responsible for the accuracy of the addresses or the content of the websites.

A

Academy for Eating Disorders
111 Deer Lake Rd., Ste. 100
Deerfield, IL 60015
Phone: (847) 498-4274
Fax: (847) 480-9282
E-mail: info@aedweb.org
Web site: http://www.aedweb.org

U.S. Administration on Aging
1 Massachusetts Ave. NW
Washington, DC 20001
Phone: (202) 401-4634
Web site: http://www.aoa.gov

AGS Foundation for Health in Aging
40 Fulton St., 18th Fl.
New York, NY 10038
Phone: (212) 755-6810
Fax: (212) 832-8646
Toll free: (800) 563-4916
Web site: http://www.healthinaging.org

Albert Ellis Institute
45 E 65th St.
New York, NY 10021
Phone: (212) 535-0822
Fax: (212) 249-3582
Toll free: (800) 323-4738
E-mail: info@albertellis.org
Web site: http://www.rebt.org

Alzheimer Europe
145, route de Thionville
Luxembourg, L-2611
Phone: +352 29 79 70
Fax: +352 29 79 72
E-mail: info@alzheimer-europe.org
Web site: http://www.alzheimer-europe.org

Alzheimer's Foundation of America
322 8th Ave., 7th Fl.
New York, NY 10001
Fax: (646) 638-1546
Toll free: (866) 232-8484
E-mail: info@alzfdn.org
Web site: http://www.alzfdn.org

American Academy of Addiction Psychiatry (AAAP)
400 Massasoit Ave., Ste. 307, 2nd Fl.
East Providence, RI 02914
Phone: (401) 524-3076
Fax: (401) 272-0922
Web site: http://www.aaap.org

American Academy of Child and Adolescent Psychiatry
3615 Wisconsin Ave. NW
Washington, DC 20016-3007
Phone: (202) 966-7300
Fax: (202) 966-2891
Web site: http://aacap.org

American Academy of Clinical Toxicology
6728 Old McLean Village Dr.
McLean, VA 22101
Phone: (703) 556-9222
Fax: (703) 556-8729
E-mail: admin@clintox.org
Web site: http://www.clintox.org

American Academy of Experts in Traumatic Stress (AAETS)
203 Deer Rd.
Ronkonkoma, NY 11779
Phone: (631) 543-2217
Fax: (631) 543-6977
E-mail: info@aaets.org
Web site: http://www.aaets.org

American Academy of Family Physicians
11400 Tomahawk Creek Pkwy.
Leawood, KS 66211-2672

Phone: (913) 906-6000
Fax: (913) 906-6075
Toll free: (800) 274-2237
E-mail: contactcenter@aafp.org
Web site: http://www.aafp.org

American Academy of Medical Acupuncture
1970 E Grand Ave.
El Segundo, CA 90245
Phone: (310) 364-0193
E-mail: administrator@medicalacupuncture.org
Web site: http://www.medicalacupuncture.org

American Academy of Neurology (AAN)
1080 Montreal Ave.
Saint Paul, MN 55116
Phone: (651) 695-2717
Fax: (651) 695-2791
Toll free: (800) 879-1960
E-mail: memberservices@aan.com
Web site: http://www.aan.com

American Academy of Pain Medicine
4700 W. Lake
Glenview, IL 60025
Phone: (847) 375-4731
Fax: (847) 375-6477
E-mail: info@painmed.org
Web site: http://www.painmed.org

American Academy of Pediatrics (AAP)
141 Northwest Point Blvd.
Elk Grove Village, IL 60007-1098
Phone: (847) 434-4000
Fax: (847) 434-8000
Web site: http://www.aap.org

American Academy of Private Practice in Speech-Language Pathology and Audiology
7349 Topanga Canyon Blvd.
Canoga Park, CA 91303
Web site: http://www.aappspa.org

American Academy of Psychiatry and the Law (AAPL)
PO Box 30, One Regency Dr.
Bloomfield, CT 06002
Phone: (860) 242-5450
Fax: (860) 286-0787
Toll free: (800) 331-1389
E-mail: http://www.aapl.org/contact.htm
Web site: http://www.aapl.org

American Academy of Sleep Medicine
2510 N Frontage Rd.
Darien, IL 60561
Phone: (630) 737-9700
Fax: (630) 737-9790
E-mail: inquiries@aasmnet.org
Web site: http://www.aasmnet.org

American Aging Association
2103 Cornell Rd., Rm. 5125
Cleveland, OH 44106
Phone: (216) 368-3671
Fax: (216) 368-8964
E-mail: americanaging@case.edu
Web site: http://www.americanaging.org

American Art Therapy Association
225 N Fairfax St.
Alexandria, VA 22314
E-mail: info@arttherapy.org
Web site: http://www.americanarttherapyassociation.org

American Association of Acupuncture and Oriental Medicine
PO Box 162340
Sacramento, CA 95816
Fax: (916) 443-4766
Toll free: (866) 455-7999
Web site: http://www.aaaomonline.org

American Association of Cardiovascular and Pulmonary Rehabilitation
401 N Michigan Ave., Ste. 2200
Chicago, IL 60611
Phone: (312) 321-5146
Fax: (312) 673-6924
E-mail: aacvpr@aacvpr.org
Web site: http://www.aacvpr.org

American Association for Clinical Chemistry
1850 K St. NW, Ste. 625
Washington, DC 20006
Fax: (202) 887-5093
Toll free: (800) 892-1400
Web site: http://www.aacc.org

American Association for Geriatric Psychiatry (AAGP)
7910 Woodmont Ave., Ste. 1050
Bethesda, MD 20814-3004
Phone: (301) 654-7850
Fax: (301) 654-4137
E-mail: main@aagponline.org
Web site: http://www.aagponline.org

American Association on Intellectual and Developmental Disabilities (AAIDD)
501 3rd St. NW, Ste. 200
Washington, DC 20001
Phone: (202) 387-1968
Fax: (202) 387-2193
Toll free: (800) 424-3688
Web site: http://www.aaidd.org

American Association for Marriage and Family Therapy (AAMFT)
112 S Alfred St.
Alexandria, VA 22314-3061
Phone: (703) 838-9808
Fax: (703) 838-9805
Web site: http://www.aamft.org

American Association of Naturopathic Physicians
4435 Wisconsin Ave. NW, Ste. 403
Washington, DC 20016
Phone: (202) 237-8150
Fax: (202) 237-8152
Toll free: (866) 538-2267
Web site: http://www.naturopathic.org

American Association of Neuromuscular and Electrodiagnostic Medicine
2621 Superior Dr. NW
Rochester, MN 55901
Phone: (507) 288-0100

E-mail: aanem@aanem.org
Web site: http://www.aanem.org

American Association of Sexuality Educators, Counselors, and Therapists (AASECT)
1444 I St. NW, Ste. 700
Washington, DC 20005
Phone: (202) 449-1099
Fax: (202) 216-9646
E-mail: info@aasect.org
Web site: http://www.aasect.org

American Association of Sleep Technologists
2510 N Frontage Rd.
Darien, IL 60561
Phone: (630) 737-9704
Fax: (630) 737-9788
E-mail: AAST@aastweb.org
Web site: http://www.aastweb.org

American Association of Suicidology
5221 Wisconsin Ave. NW
Washington, DC 20015
Phone: (202) 237-2280
Fax: (202) 237-2282
Web site: http://www.suicidology.org

American Board of Psychiatry and Neurology
2150 E Lake Cook Rd., Ste. 900
Buffalo Grove, IL 60089
Phone: (847) 229-6500
Fax: (847) 229-6600
E-mail: questions@abpn.com
Web site: http://www.abpn.com

American Board of Registration for Electroencephalographic Technologists
2509 W Iles Ave., Ste. 102
Springfield, IL 62704
Phone: (217) 726-7980
Fax: (217) 726-7989
E-mail: abreteo@att.net
Web site: http://www.abret.org

American Botanical Council
6200 Manor Rd.
Austin, TX 78723
Phone: (512) 926-4900
Fax: (512) 926-2345
Toll free: (800) 373-7105
E-mail: abc@herbalram.org
Web site: http://abc.herbalgram.org

American Chronic Pain Association
PO Box 850
Rocklin, CA 95677
Fax: (916) 632-3208
Toll free: (800) 533-3231
E-mail: ACPA@pacbell.net
Web site: http://www.theacpa.org

American College of Neuropsychopharmacology
5034-A Thoroughbred Ln.
Brentwood, TN 37027
Phone: (615) 324-2360
Fax: (615) 523-1715
E-mail: acnp@acnp.org
Web site: http://www.acnp.org/default.aspx

American College of Physicians
190 N Independence Mall W
Philadelphia, PA 19106-1572
Phone: (215) 351-2400
Toll free: (800) 523-1546
Web site: http://www.acponline.org

American Council for Drug Education
50 Jay St.
Brooklyn, NY 11201
Phone: (646) 505-2061
E-mail: acde@phoenixhouse.org
Web site: http://www.acdc.org

American Dance Therapy Association
10632 Little Patuxent Pkwy., Ste. 108
Columbia, MD 21044
Phone: (410) 997-4040
Fax: (410) 997-4048
Web site: http://www.adta.org

American Epilepsy Society
342 N Main St.
West Hartford, CT 06117-2507
Phone: (860) 586-7505
Fax: (860) 586-7550
Web site: http://www.aesnet.org

American Foundation for Suicide Prevention
120 Wall St., 29th Fl.
New York, NY 20016-3007
Phone: (212) 363-3500
Fax: (212) 363-6237
Toll free: (888) 333-2377
E-mail: inquiry@afsp.org
Web site: http://www.afsp.org

American Geriatrics Society (AGS)
40 Fulton St., 18th Fl.
New York, NY 10038
Phone: (212) 308-1414
Fax: (212) 832-8646
E-mail: info.amger@americangeriatrics.org
Web site: http://www.americangeriatrics.org

American Health Assistance Foundation
22512 Gateway Center Dr.
Clarksburg, MD 20871
Fax: (301) 948-4403
Toll free: (800) 437-2423
E-mail: info@ahaf.org
Web site: http://www.ahaf.org

American Hospice Foundation
2120 L St. NW, Ste. 200
Washington, DC 20037
Phone: (202) 223-0204
Fax: (202) 223-0208
Toll free: (800) 347-1413
Web site: http://www.americanhospice.org

American Hospital Association
325 7th St. NW
Washington, DC 20004-2802
Phone: (202) 638-1100
Web site: http://www.aha.org

American Institute of Homeopathy
101 S Whiting St., Ste. 16
Alexandria, VA 22304
Toll free: (888) 445-9988
E-mail: admin@homeopathyusa.org
Web site: http://homeopathyusa.org

American Institute of Stress
124 Park Ave.
Yonkers, NY 10703
Phone: (914) 963-1200
Fax: (914) 965-6267
E-mail: Stress125@optonline.net
Web site: http://www.stress.org

American Lung Association
1301 Pennsylvannia Ave. NW, Ste. 800
Washington, DC 20004
Phone: (202) 785-3355
Fax: (202) 452-1805
E-mail: info@lungusa.org
Web site: http://www.lung.org

American Massage Therapy Association
500 Davis St., Ste. 900
Evanston, IL 60201-4695
Phone: (847) 864-0123
Fax: (847) 864-5196
Toll free: (877) 905-0577
E-mail: info@amtamassage.org
Web site: http://www.amtamassage.org

American Medical Association (AMA)
515 N State St.
Chicago, IL 60610
Phone: (312) 464-5000
Toll free: (800) 621-8335
Web site: http://www.ama-assn.org

American Music Therapy Association
8455 Colesville Rd., Ste. 1000
Silver Spring, MD 20910
Phone: (301) 589-3300
Fax: (301) 589-5175
Web site: http://www.musictherapy.org

American Neurological Association
5841 Cedar Lake Rd., Ste. 204
Minneapolis, MN 55416
Phone: (952) 545-6284
E-mail: ana@llmsi.com
Web site: http://www.aneuroa.org

American Neuropsychiatric Association
700 Ackerman Rd., Ste. 625
Columbus, OH 43202
Phone: (614) 447-2077
E-mail: anpa@osu.edu
Web site: http://www.anpaonline.org/home.php

American Organization for Bodywork Therapies of Asia
1010 Haddonfield-Berlin Rd., Ste. 408
Voorhees, NJ 08043-3514
Phone: (856) 782-1616
Fax: (856) 782-1653
E-mail: office@aobta.org
Web site: http://www.aobta.org

American Physical Therapy Association
1111 N Fairfax St.
Alexandria, VA 22314-1488
Phone: (703) 684-APTA (2782); TDD: (703) 683-6748
Toll free: (800) 999-APTA (2782)
Web site: http://www.apta.org

American Polarity Therapy Association
122 N. Elm St., Ste. 512
Greensboro, NC 27401
Phone: (336) 574-1121
Fax: (336) 574-1151
E-mail: aptaoffices@polaritytherapy.org
Web site: http://www.polaritytherapy.org

American Psychiatric Association (APA)
1000 Wilson Blvd., Ste. 1825
Arlington, VA 22209-3901
Phone: (703) 907-7300
Toll free: (888) 357-7924
E-mail: apa@psych.org
Web site: http://www.psych.org

American Psychoanalytic Association
309 E 49th St.
New York, NY 10017
Phone: (212) 752-0450
Fax: (212) 593-0571
E-mail: info@aspa.org
Web site: http://www.apsa.org

American Psychological Association (APA)
750 1st St. NE
Washington, DC 20002-4242
Phone: (202) 336-5500; TDD/TTY: (202) 336-6123
Toll free: (800) 374-2721
E-mail: apa@psych.org
Web site: http://www.apa.org

American Psychotherapy Association
2750 E Sunshine St.
Springfield, MO 65804
Phone: (417) 823-0173
Toll free: (800) 205-9165
Web site: http://www.americanpsychotherapy.com

American Sleep Apnea Association
6856 Eastern Ave. NW, Ste. 203
Washington, DC 20012
Phone: (202) 293-3650
Fax: (202) 293-3656
Web site: http://www.sleepapnea.org

American Sleep Association
614 S 8th St., Ste. 282
Philadelphia, PA 19147
Phone: (443) 593-2285
E-mail: sleep@1sleep.com
Web site: http://www.sleepassociation.org

American Society of Addiction Medicine
4601 N Park Ave., Upper Arcade #101
Chevy Chase, MD 20815
Phone: (301) 656-3920
Fax: (301) 656-3815
E-mail: email@asam.org
Web site: http://www.asam.org

American Society of Clinical Hypnosis
140 N Bloomingdale Rd.
Bloomingdale, IL 60108
Phone: (630) 980-4740
Fax: (630) 351-8490
E-mail: info@asch.net
Web site: http://www.asch.net

American Society for Clinical Pharmacology and Therapeutics
528 N Washington St.
Alexandria, VA 22314
Phone: (703) 836-6981
E-mail: info@ascpt.org
Web site: http://www.ascpt.org

American Society of Electroneurodiagnostic Technologists
402 E Bannister Rd., Ste. A
Kansas City, MO 64131-3019
Phone: (816) 931-1120
Fax: (816) 931-1145
E-mail: info@aset.org
Web site: http://www.aset.org

American Society of Health-System Pharmacists
7272 Wisconsin Ave.
Bethesda, MD 20814
Toll free: (866) 279-0681
E-mail: custserv@ashp.org
Web site: http://www.ashp.org

American Society for Pharmacology and Experimental Therapeutics
9650 Rockville Pike
Bethesda, MD 20814-3995
Phone: (301) 634-7060
Fax: (301) 634-7061
Web site: http://www.aspet.org

American Sociological Association
1430 K St. NW, Ste. 600
Washington, DC 20005
Phone: (202) 383-9005
Fax: (202) 638-0882
Web site: http://www.asanet.org

American Speech-Language-Hearing Association (ASHA)
2200 Research Blvd.
Rockville, MD 20850-3289
Phone: (301) 296-5700; TTY: (301) 296-5650
Fax: (301) 296-8580
Toll free: (800) 638-8255
Web site: http://www.asha.org

American Stroke Association
7272 Greenville Ave.
Dallas, TX 75231
Toll free: (800) 242-8721
Web site: http://www.heart.org

American Thyroid Association
6066 Leesburg Pike, Ste. 550
Falls Church, VA 22041
Phone: (703) 998-8890
Fax: (703) 998-8893
E-mail: thyroid@thyroid.org
Web site: http://www.thyroid.org

American Yoga Association
PO Box 19986
Sarasota, FL 34276
E-mail: info@americanyogaassociation.org
Web site: http://www.americanyogaassociation.org

Angelman, Rett & Prader-Willi Syndromes Consortium (ARPWSC), Rare Diseases Clinical Research Network
University of Alabama at Birmingham
Birmingham, AL 35294-1150
Phone: (205) 934-1130
Fax: (205) 975-6330
E-mail: jlane@uab.edu
Web site: http://rarediseasesnetwork.epi.usf.edu/arpwsc

Anxiety Disorders Association of America
8730 Georgia Ave.
Silver Spring, MD 20910
Phone: (240) 485-1001
Fax: (240) 485-1035
E-mail: information@adaa.org
Web site: http://www.adaa.org

The Arc
1660 L St. NW, Ste. 301
Washington, DC 20036
Phone: (202) 534-3700
Fax: (202) 534-3731
Toll free: (800) 433-5255
E-mail: info@thearc.org
Web site: http://www.thearc.org

ARCH National Respite Network and Resource Center, Chapel Hill Training-Outreach Project
800 Eastowne Dr., Ste. 105
Chapel Hill, NC 27514
Phone: (919) 490-5577
Fax: (919) 490-4905
Web site: http://www.chtop.com

Art Therapy Credentials Board
3 Terrace Way
Greensboro, NC 27403-3660
Phone: (336) 482-2856
Fax: (336) 482-2852
Toll free: (877) 213-2822
E-mail: atcb@nbcc.org
Web site: http://www.atcb.org

Assertive Community Treatment Association
PO Box 2428
Brighton, MI 48116
Phone: (810) 227-1859
Fax: (810) 227-5785
E-mail: acta@actassociation.org
Web site: http://www.actassociation.org

Associated Bodywork & Massage Professionals
25188 Genesee Trail Rd.
Golden, CO 80401
Fax: (800) 667-8260
Toll free: (800) 458-2267
Web site: http://www.abmp.com

Association for the Advancement of Behavior Therapy
305 7th Ave., 16th Fl.
New York, NY 10001
Phone: (212) 647-1890

Fax: (212) 647-1865
Web site: http://www.abct.org

The Association for the Advancement of Gestalt Therapy
Web site: http://www.aagt.org

Association for Applied Psychotherapy and Biofeedback
10200 W 44th Ave., Ste. 304
Wheat Ridge, CO 80033
Phone: (303) 422-8436
Toll free: (800) 477-8892
E-mail: aapb@resourcecenter.com
Web site: http://www.aapb.org

Association for Behavioral Analysis International
550 W Centre Ave., Ste. 1
Portage, MI 49024
Phone: (269) 492-9310
Fax: (269) 492-9316
Web site: http://www.abainternational.org

Association for Behavioral and Cognitive Therapies
305 7th Ave., 16th Fl.
New York, NY 10001
Phone: (212) 647-1890
Fax: (212) 647-1865
Toll free: (866) 615-6464
Web site: http://www.abct.org

Association for Comprehensive Neurotherapy
PO Box 2198
Broken Arrow, OK 34688-1967
Phone: (561) 798-0472
Fax: (561) 798-9820
E-mail: acn@latitudes.org
Web site: http://www.latitudes.org

Association for the Development of the Person-Centered Approach
Web site: http://www.adpca.org

Association for Frontotemporal Degeneration
290 King of Prussia Rd., Radnor Station Bldg. 2, Ste. 320
Radnor, PA 19103
Phone: (267) 514-7221
Toll free: (866) 507-7222
Web site: http://www.theaftd.org

Association for Persons in Supported Employment
PO Box 1280
Rockville, MD 20849
Phone: (301) 279-0060
Fax: (301) 251-3762
Web site: http://www.apse.org

Association for Play Therapy, Inc
3198 Willow Ave., Ste. 110
Clovis, CA 93703
Phone: (599) 294-2128
Fax: (559) 294-2129
E-mail: info@a4pt.org
Web site: http://www.a4pt.org

Association for the Treatment of Sexual Abusers
4900 SW Griffith Dr., Ste. 274
Beaverton, Oregon 97005
Phone: (503) 643-1023
Fax: (503) 643-5084
E-mail: atsa@atsa.com
Web site: http://www.atsa.com

Association for Treatment and Training in the Attachment of Children
PO Box 533
Lake Villao, IL 60046
Phone: (847) 453-8224
Fax: (847) 356-7856
E-mail: questions@attach.org
Web site: http://www.attach.org

Attention Deficit Disorder Association (ADDA)
PO Box 7557
Wilmington, DE 19803-9997
Toll free: (800) 939-1019
E-mail: info@add.org
Web site: http://www.add.org

Augustine Fellowship, Sex and Love Addicts Anonymous
PO Box 119, New Town Branch
Boston, MA 02258
Phone: (617) 332-1845

Autism Network International (ANI)
PO Box 35448
Syracuse, NY 13235-5448
Web site: http://autreat.com

Autism Society
4340 East-West Hwy., Ste. 350
Bethesda, MD 20814
Phone: (301) 657-0881
Toll free: (800) 3-AUTISM (328-8476)
Web site: http://www.autism-society.org

Autism Speaks
1 E 33rd St., 4th Fl.
New York, NY 10016
Phone: (212) 252-8584
Fax: (212) 252-8676
Toll free: (888) AUTISM2 (288-4762)
E-mail: contactus@autismspeaks.org
Web site: http://www.autismspeaks.org

B

The Balanced Mind Foundation (formerly the Child & Adolescent Bipolar Foundation)
820 Davis St., Ste. 520
Evanston, IL 60201
Phone: (847) 492-8510
E-mail: info@thebalancedmind.org
Web site: http://www.thebalancedmind.org

The Bazelon Center for Mental Health Law
1101 15th St. NW, Ste. 1212
Washington, DC 20005
Phone: (202) 467-5730
E-mail: info@bazelon.org
Web site: http://www.bazelon.org

Beck Institute for Cognitive Therapy and Research
One Belmont Ave., Ste. 700
Bala Cynwyd, PA 19004-1610

Phone: (610) 664-3020
Fax: (610) 664-4437
E-mail: beckinst@gim.net
Web site: http://www.beckinstitute.org

Benson-Henry Institute for Mind Body Medicine
151 Merrimac St., 4th Fl.
Boston, MA 02114
Phone: (617) 643-6090
Fax: (617) 643-6077
E-mail: mindbody@partners.org
Web site: http://www.massgeneral.org/bhi

Better Sleep Council
501 Wythe St.
Alexandria, VA 22314-1917
Web site: http://www.bettersleep.org

Biofeedback Certification International Alliance
10200 W 44th Ave., Ste. 310
Wheat Ridge, CO 80033
Phone: (303) 420-2902
Fax: (303) 422-8894
Toll free: (866) 908-8713
E-mail: info@bcia.org
Web site: http://www.bcia.org

Borden Institute
1546 Porter St., Ste. 207
Fort Detrick, MD 21702
Phone: (301) 619-3470
Fax: (301) 619-3471
E-mail: bordeninfo@amedd.army.mil
Web site: http://www.bordeninstitute.army.mil/index.html

Brain Aneurysm Foundation
269 Hanover St., Bldg. 3
Hanover, MA 02339
Phone: (781) 826-5556
Fax: (781) 826-5566
E-mail: office@bafound.org
Web site: http://www.bafound.org

Brain and Behavior Research Foundation
60 Cutter Mill Rd., Ste. 404
Great Neck, NY 11021
Phone: (516) 829-0091
Fax: (516) 487-6930
E-mail: info@bbrfoundation.org
Web site: http://www.bbrfoundation.org

Brain Injury Association of America (BIAA)
1608 Spring Hill Rd., Ste. 110
Vienna, VA 22182
Phone: (703) 761-0750
Fax: (703) 761-0755
Toll free: (800) 444-6443
Web site: http://www.biausa.org

Brain Trauma Foundation (BTF)
7 World Trade Center, 34th Fl., 250 Greenwich St.
New York, NY 10007
Phone: (212) 772-0608
Web site: http://www.braintrauma.org

British Columbia Institute Against Family Violence
74640 Kitsilano RPO
Vancouver, British Columbia V6K 4P4
Canada
Phone: (604) 669-7055
Toll free (within Canada): (877) 755-7055
E-mail: ngrunberg@bcifv.org

Bureau of Justice Assistance
810 7th St. NW, 4th Fl.
Washington, DC 20531
Phone: (202) 616-6500
Fax: (202) 305-1367
Toll free: (866) 859-2687
Web site: http://www.ojp.usdoj.gov/BJA/index.html

C

Callier Center for Communication Disorders
University of Texas at Dallas
1966 Inwood Rd.
Dallas, TX 75235
Phone: (214) 905-3000
Fax: (214) 905-3022
Web site: http://www.utdallas.edu/calliercenter

Cambridge Center for Behavioral Studies
PO Box 7067
Cummings Center, Ste. 340F
Beverly, MA 01915
Phone: (978) 369-2227
Fax: (978) 369-8584
Web site: http://www.behavior.org

Canadian Movement Disorder Group
Web site: http://www.cmdg.org

Canadian Symposium for Parental Alienation Syndrome (CS-PAS)
150 Hollidge Blvd., Ste. 252
Aurora, Ontario L4G 8A3
Canada
Phone: (647) 476-3170
E-mail: info@cspas.ca
Web site: http://cspas.ca

Center for Brain and Cognition, University of California, San Diego
0109 Mandler Hall, 9500 Gilman Dr.
La Jolla, CA 92093-0109
Phone: (858) 534-6240
Fax: (858) 534-7190
E-mail: ramalab@ucsd.edu
Web site: http://cbc.ucsd.edu/index.html

Center for Internet Addiction Recovery
PO Box 72
Bradford, PA 16701
Phone: (814) 451-2405
Fax: (814) 368-9560
Web site: http://www.netaddiction.com

Center for Mind-Body Medicine
5225 Connecticut Ave. NW, Ste. 415
Washington, DC 20015
Phone: (202) 966-7338
Fax: (202) 966-2589
Web site: http://www.cmbm.org

Center for Mindfulness in Medicine, Health Care, and Society
University of Massachusetts Medical School
55 Lake Ave. N
Worcester, MA 01655
Phone: (508) 856-2656
Fax: (508) 856-1977
E-mail: mindfulness@umassmed.edu
Web site: http://www.umassmed.edu/cfm/home/index.aspx

Center for Psychological Studies, Nova Southeastern University
3301 College Ave.
Fort Lauderdale-Davie, FL 33314-7796
Toll free: (800) 541-6682, ext. 25700
Web site: http://www.cps.nova.edu

Center for Science in the Public Interest
1220 L St. NW, Ste. 300
Washington, DC 20005
Phone: (202) 332-9110
Fax: (202) 265-4954
Web site: http://www.cspinet.org

Center for Studies of the Person
1150 Silverado, Ste. 112
La Jolla, CA 92037
Phone: (858) 459-3861
Web site: http://www.centerfortheperson.org

Center for the Study of Anorexia and Bulimia
1841 Broadway, 4th Fl.
New York, NY 10023
Phone: (212) 333-3444
Fax: (212) 333-5444
E-mail: casb@icpnyc.org
Web site: http://www.csabnyc.org

Center for the Study of Traumatic Encephalopathy
Boston University
Phone: (617) 638-6143
E-mail: cbaugh@bu.edu
Web site: http://www.bu.edu/cste

Center for the Study of Traumatic Stress (CSTS)
Uniformed Services University of the Health Sciences (USU)
Department of Psychiatry
4301 Jones Bridge Rd.
Bethesda, MD 20814
Phone: (301) 295-2470
Fax: (301) 319-6965
E-mail: cstsinfo@usuhs.mil
Web site: http://www.centerforthestudyoftraumaticstress.org/index.php

U.S. Centers for Disease Control and Prevention
1600 Clifton Rd.
Atlanta, GA 30333
Phone: (404) 639-3534
Toll free: 800-232-4636
E-mail: inquiry@cdc.gov
Web site: http://www.cdc.gov

U.S. Centers for Medicare & Medicaid Services
7500 Security Blvd.
Baltimore, MD 21244-1850
Toll free: (800) 633-4223
Web site: http://www.medicare.gov

Centre for Addiction and Mental Health
33 Russell St.
Toronto, Ontario M5S 2S1
Canada
Phone: (416) 535-8501
Toll free: (800) 463-6273
Web site: http://www.camh.net

Children and Adults with Attention Deficit/Hyperactivity Disorder (CHADD)
8181 Professional Pl., Ste. 150
Landover, MD 20785
Phone: (301) 306-7070
Fax: (301) 306-7090
Toll free: (800) 233-4050
Web site: http://www.chadd.org

Cocaine Anonymous World Services
21720 S Wilmington Ave., Ste. 304
Long Beach, CA 90810-1641
Phone: (310) 559-5833
Fax: (310) 559-2554
E-mail: cawso@ca.org
Web site: http://www.ca.org

Colorado Learning Disabilities Research Center (CLDRC)
Institute for Behavioral Genetics, University of Colorado Boulder
1480 30th St.
Boulder, CO 80303
Phone: (303) 492-7362
Fax: (303) 492-8063
E-mail: info@ibg.colorado.edu
Web site: http://ibgwww.colorado.edu/cldrc

Compassionate Friends
PO Box 3696
Oak Brook, IL 60522
Phone: (630) 990-0010
Fax: (630) 990-0246
Toll free: (877) 969-0010
Web site: http://www.compassionatefriends.org

U.S. Consumer Product Safety Commission
4330 East-West Hwy.
Bethesda, MD 20814
Phone: (301) 504-7923
Web site: http://www.cpsc.gov

Council of State Governments Justice Center
100 Wall St., 20th Fl.
New York, NY 10005
Phone: (212) 482-2320
Web site: http://www.justicecenter.csg.org

D

U.S. Department of Health & Human Services
200 Independence Ave. SW
Washington, DC 20201
Phone: (202) 619-7800
Toll free: (877) 696-6775
Web site: http://www.hhs.gov

U.S. Department of Housing and Urban Development
451 7th St. SW
Washington, DC 20410
Phone: (202) 708-1112
Web site: http://www.hud.gov

U.S. Department of Veterans Affairs (VA)
810 Vermont Ave. NW
Washington, DC 20420
Toll free: (800) 827-1000; Mental health crisis line: (800) 273-8255 (press 1)
Web site: http://www.va.gov

Depression and Bipolar Support Alliance (DBSA)
730 N Franklin St., Ste. 501
Chicago, IL 60654-7225
Fax: (312) 642-7243
Toll free: (800) 826-3632
E-mail: info@dbsalliance.org
Web site: http://www.dbsalliance.org

Disaster Psychiatry Outreach
One Gustave L. Levy Pl., PO Box 1228
New York, NY 10029-6574
Phone: (646) 233-1215
E-mail: info@disasterpsych.org
Web site: http://www.disasterpsych.org.

Dougy Center
PO Box 86852
Portland, OR 97286
Phone: (503) 775-5683
Toll free: (866) 775-5683
E-mail: help@dougy.org
Web site: http://www.grievingchild.org

U.S. Drug Enforcement Administration
Mailstop AES
8701 Morrissette Drive
Springfield, VA 22152
Toll free: (800) 882-9539
Web site: http://www.justice.gov/dea

Dual Recovery Anonymous
PO Box 8107
Prairie Village, KS 66208
Phone: (913) 991-2703
Web site: http://www.draonline.org/index.html

E

Emotions Anonymous
PO Box 4245
St. Paul, MN 55104-0245
Phone: (651) 647-9712
Fax: (651) 647-1593
Web site: http://www.emotionsanonymous.org

Epilepsy Foundation
8301 Professional Pl.
Landover, MD 20785-7223
Fax: (301) 577-2684
Toll free: (800) 332-1000
E-mail: contactus@efa.org
Web site: http://www.epilepsyfoundation.org

Eunice Kennedy Shriver National Institute of Child Health and Human Development (NICHD)
Bldg 31, Rm. 2A32, MSC 2425, 31 Center Dr.
Bethesda, MD 20892
Fax: (866) 760-5947
Toll free: (800) 370-2943; TTY: (888) 320-6942
E-mail: NICHDInformationResourceCenter@mail.nih.gov
Web site: http://www.nichd.nih.gov

European College of Neuropsychopharmacology (ECNP)
PO Box 85410
Utrecht 3508 AK
The Netherlands
Phone: +31 30 2538567
Fax: +31 30 2538568
E-mail: secretariat@ecnp.eu
Web site: http://www.ecnp.eu

F

Families for Depression Awareness
395 Totten Pond Rd., Ste. 404
Waltham, MA 02451
Phone: (781) 890-0220
Fax: (781) 890-2411
Web site: http://www.familyaware.org

Family Caregiver Alliance
180 Montgomery St., Ste. 900
San Francisco, CA 94104
Phone: (415) 434-3388
Toll free: (800) 445-8106
E-mail: info@caregiver.org
Web site: http://www.caregiver.org

Federation of Families for Children's Mental Health
9605 Medical Center Dr.
Rockville, MD 20850
Phone: (240) 403-1901
Fax: (240) 403-1909
E-mail: ffcmh@ffcmh.org
Web site: http://ffcmh.org.

Fetal Alcohol Spectrum Disorders Center for Excellence
2101 Gaither Rd., Ste. 600
Rockville, MD 20850
Toll free: (866) 786-7327
E-mail: fasdcenter@samhsa.hhs.gov
Web site: http://www.fascenter.samhsa.gov

Fetal Alcohol Syndrome (FAS) World Canada
2448 Hamilton Rd.
Bright's Grove, Ontario N0N 1C0
Canada
Phone: (519) 869-8026
Web site: http://www.faslink.org

Fisher Center for Alzheimer's Research Foundation
One Intrepid Square, W 46th St. & 12th Ave.
New York, NY 10036
Toll free: (800) 259-4636
Web site: http://www.alzinfo.org

U.S. Food and Drug Administration (FDA)
10903 New Hampshire Ave.
Silver Spring, MD 20993

Toll free: (888) 463-6332
Web site: http://www.fda.gov

Freedom from Fear
308 Seaview Ave.
Staten Island, NY 10305
Phone: (718) 351-1717
E-mail: help@freedomfromfear.org
Web site: http://www.freedomfromfear.org

Friends: The National Association of Young People Who Stutter
c/o Lee Caggiano, 38 S Oyster Bay Rd.
Syosset, NY 11791
Toll free: (866) 866-8335
E-mail: LCAGGIANO@aol.com
Web site: http://www.friendswhostutter.org

Fuqua Center for Late-Life Depression
Wesley Woods Health Center, 4th Fl., 1841 Clifton Rd. NE
Atlanta, GA 30329
Phone: (404) 728-6948
Web site: http://www.fuquacenter.org

G

Gamblers Anonymous, International Service Office
PO Box 17173
Los Angeles, CA 90017
Phone: (626) 960-3500
Fax: (626) 960-3501
Toll free: (888) GA-HELPS (424-3577)
E-mail: isomain@gamblersanonymous.org
Web site: http://www.gamblersanonymous.org

Gay, Lesbian, Bisexual, and Transgender National Help Center
2261 Market St., PMB #296
San Francisco, CA 94114
Phone: (415) 355-0003
Fax: (415) 552-5498
E-mail: info@GLBTNationalHelpCenter.org
Web site: http://www.glbtnationalhelpcenter.org

Genetic Alliance
4301 Connecticut Ave. NW, Ste. 404
Washington, DC 20008-2369
Phone: (202) 966-5557
Fax: (202) 966-8553
E-mail: info@geneticalliance.org
Web site: http://www.geneticalliance.org

Geriatric Mental Health Foundation
7910 Woodmont Ave., Ste. 1050
Bethesda, MD 20814
Phone: (301) 654-7850
Fax: (301) 654-4137
E-mail: web@GMHFonline.org
Web site: http://www.gmhfonline.org

Global and Regional Asperger's Syndrome Partnership
135 E 15th St.
New York, NY 10003
Phone: (646) 242-4003
E-mail: info@grasp.org
Web site: http://www.grasp.org.

GROWW (Grief Recovery Online)
11877 Douglas Rd., #102-PMB101
Alpharetta, GA 30005
Web site: http://www.groww.org

H

Hazelden Foundation
PO Box 11
Center City, MN 55012-0011
Phone: (651) 213-4200
Toll free: (800) 257-7810
E-mail: info@hazelden.org
Web site: http://www.hazelden.org

Hoarding of Animals Research Consortium (HARC)
c/o Gary Patronek, Animal Rescue League of Boston, 10 Chandler St.
Boston, MA 02116
Phone: (617) 426-9170
Fax: (617) 426-3028
E-mail: cfapp@tufts.edu
Web site: http://www.tufts.edu/vet/hoarding

Homeopathic Medical Council of Canada
31 Adelaide St. E, Box 605
Toronto, Ontario M5C 2J8
Canada
Phone: (416) 788-4622
E-mail: Ontario@HMCC.ca
Web site: http://www.hmcc.ca

The Hormone Foundation
8401 Connecticut Ave., Ste. 900
Chevy Chase, MD 20815-5817
Fax: (301) 941-0259
Toll free: (800) 467-6663
E-mail: hormone@endo-society.org
Web site: http://www.hormone.org

I

I CAN [children's communication charity]
8 Wakley St.
London, United Kingdom, EC1V 7QE
Phone: 0845 225 4071 or 020 7843 2510
Fax: 0845 225 4072 or 020 7843 2569
E-mail: info@ican.org.uk
Web site: http://www.ican.org.uk

Imagery International
1574 Coburg Rd. #555
Eugene, OR 97401
Toll free: (800) 494-9985
E-mail: information@imageryinternational.com
Web site: http://imageryinternational.org

Insight Meditation Society
1230 Pleasant St.
Barre, MA 01005
Phone: (978) 355-4378
Web site: http://www.dharma.org

Institute for Traditional Medicine
2017 SE Hawthorne Blvd.
Portland, OR 97214
Phone: (503) 233-4907
Web site: http://www.itmonline.org

International Association of Yoga Therapists
PO Box 12890
Prescott, AZ 86304
Phone: (928) 541-0004
E-mail: mail@iayt.org
Web site: http://www.iayt.org

International Center for Alcohol Policies
1519 New Hampshire Ave. NW
Washington, DC 20036
Phone: (202) 986-1159
Fax: (202) 986-2080
E-mail: info@icap.org
Web site: http://www.icap.org

International Dyslexia Association (IDA)
40 York Rd., 4th Fl.
Baltimore, MD 21204
Phone: (410) 296-0232
Fax: (410) 321-5069
E-mail: http://www.interdys.org/ContactUs.htm
Web site: http://www.interdys.org

International League Against Epilepsy
342 N Main St.
West Hartford, CT 06117-2507
Phone: (860) 586-7547
Fax: (860) 586-7550
Web site: http://www.ilae-epilepsy.org

International Neuropsychiatric Association
INA Secretariat Office Neuropsychiatric Institute Euroa Centre
The Prince of Wales Hospital, NSW Australia 2031
Phone: 612 93823816
Fax: 612 93823774
E-mail: angie.russell@unsw.edu.au
Web site: http://www.inawebsite.org

International Neuropsychological Society
700 Ackerman Rd., Ste. 625
Columbus, OH 43202
Phone: (614) 263-4200
Fax: (614) 263-4366
Web site: http://www.the-ins.org

International OCD Foundation Hoarding Center
PO Box 961029
Boston, MA 02196
Phone: (617) 973-5801
Fax: (617) 973-5803
E-mail: info@ocfoundation.org
Web site: http://www.ocfoundation.org/hoarding

International Paruresis Association
PO Box 65111
Baltimore, MD 21209
Toll free: (800) 247-3864
Web site: http://www.paruresis.org

International Psychoanalytical Association
Broomhills, Woodside Ln.
London, United Kingdom N12 8UD
Phone: +44 20 8446 8324
Phone: +44 20 8445 4729
E-mail: ipa@ipa.org.uk
Web site: http://www.ipa.org.uk

International Psychogeriatric Association (IPA)
550 Frontage Rd., Ste. 3759
Northfield, IL 60093
Phone: (847) 501-3310
Fax: (847) 501-3317
Web site: http://www.ipa-online.org

International Rett Syndrome Association
4600 Devitt Dr.
Cincinnati, OH 45246
Fax: (513) 874-2520
Toll free: (800) 818-7388
Web site: http://www.rettsyndrome.org

International Society for ECT and Neurostimulation (ISEN)
5454 Wisconsin Ave., Ste. 1220
Chevy Chase, MD 20815
Phone: (301) 951-7220
Fax: (301) 299-4918
E-mail: contact@isen-ect.org
Web site: http://www.isen-ect.org

International Society for Interpersonal Psychotherapy
University of Iowa, Department of Psychiatry, 1-293 Medical Education Bldg.
Iowa City, IA 52242
Phone: (391) 353-4230
Fax: (391) 353-3003
E-mail: scott-stuart@uiowa.edu
Web site: http://interpersonalpsychotherapy.org

International Society for Mental Health Online (ISMHO)
E-mail: https://www.ismho.org/contact.asp
Web site: https://www.ismho.org/home.asp

International Society of Psychiatric Genetics (ISPG)
5034-A Thoroughbred Ln.
Brentwood, TN 37027
Phone: (202) 336-5500
Web site: http://www.ispg.net

International Society for the Study of Personality Disorders
University of Michigan Health System, Psychiatry MCHC-6, Box 5295, 1500 E Medical Center Dr.
Ann Arbor, MI 48109-5295
Phone: (734) 936-8316
Fax: (734) 936-9761
Web site: http://www.isspd.com

International Society for the Study of Subtle Energies and Energy Medicine
2770 Arapahoe Rd., Ste. 132
Lafayette, CO 80026
Phone: (303) 425-4625
Fax: (866) 269-0972
Web site: http://www.issseem.org

International Society for the Study of Trauma and Dissociation
8400 Westpark Dr., 2nd Fl.
McLean, VA 22102
Phone: (703) 610-9037

Fax: (703) 610-0234
Web site: http://www.isst-d.org

International Society for Traumatic Stress Studies (ISTSS)
111 Deer Lake Rd., Ste. 100
Deerfield, IL 60015
Phone: (847) 480-9028
Fax: (847) 480-9282
Web site: http://www.istss.org

International Stuttering Association (ISA)
c/o Joseph Lukong Tardzenyuy, Secretary, 1018 S Payne St.
New Ulm, MN 56073
E-mail: admin@stutterisa.org
Web site: http://www.stutterisa.org

J

Jin Shin Do Foundation for Bodymind Acupressure
PO Box 416
Idyllwild, CA 92549
Phone: (951) 659-5707
Web site: http://www.jinshindo.org

The Johns Hopkins Hospital, Sexual Behaviors Consultation Unit
600 N Wolfe St., Meyer 144
Baltimore, MD 21287
Phone: (410) 583-1661
Fax: (410) 583-2693
Web site: http://www.hopkinsmedicine.org/psychiatry/specialty_areas/sexual_behaviors

Johns Hopkins University Center for Epigenetics in Common Human Disease
855 N Wolfe St.
Baltimore, MD 21205
Phone: (410) 614-3489
Web site: http://www.hopkinsmedicine.org/epigenetics

K

The Kempe Foundation for the Prevention and Treatment of Child Abuse and Neglect
The Gary Pavilion at Children's Hospital Colorado
Anschutz Medical Campus
13123 E 16th Ave., B390
Denver, CO 80045
Phone: (303) 864-5300
Web site: http://www.kempe.org

Kleine-Levin Syndrome Foundation
PO Box 5382
San Jose, CA 95150-5382
Phone: (408) 265-1099
Fax: (408) 269-2131
E-mail: facts@klsfoundation.org
Web site: http://www.klsfoundation.org

Kristin Brooks Hope Center
615 7th St., NE
Washington, DC 20002
Phone: (202) 536-3200
Toll free: (800) 442-4673
Web site: http://www.hopeline.com

L

Leadership Council on Child Abuse and Interpersonal Violence
c/o Joyanna Silberg, PhD, 6501 N Charles St., PO Box 6815
Baltimore, MD 21285-6815
E-mail: desk1@leadershipcouncil.org
Web site: http://www.leadershipcouncil.org/index.html

Learning Disabilities Association of America (LDA)
4156 Library Rd.
Pittsburgh, PA 15234-1349
Phone: (412) 341-1515
Fax: (412) 344-0224
E-mail: http://www.ldanatl.org/contact/contact.cfm
Web site: http://www.ldanatl.org

M

MAAP Services for Autism, Asperger Syndrome, and PDD
PO Box 524
Crown Point, IN 46308
Phone: (219) 662-1311
Fax: (219) 662-0638
E-mail: info@maapservices.org
Web site: http://www.maapservices.org

March of Dimes Foundation
1275 Mamaroneck Ave.
White Plains, NY 10605
Phone: (914) 997-4488
Web site: http://www.marchofdimes.com

Matrix Institute on Addictions
Web site: http://www.matrixinstitute.org

Medical Council on Alcohol
5 St. Andrew's Place
London, United Kingdom NW1 4LB
Phone: 011 4420 7 7487 4445
Fax: 011 4420 7 7935 4479
E-mail: mca@medicalcouncilalcol.demon.co.uk
Web site: http://www.m-c-a.org.uk

Mental Health America
2000 N Beauregard St., 6th Fl.
Alexandria, VA 22311
Phone: (703) 684-7722
Fax: (703) 684-5968
Toll free: (800) 969-6642
E-mail: infoctr@mentalhealthamerica.net
Web site: http://www.mentalhealthamerica.net

Mental Health Foundation
PO Box 322
Albany, NY 12201
E-mail: info@mentalhealthfoundation.net
Web site: http://www.mentalhealthfoundation.net

Movement Disorder Society
555 E Wells St., Ste. 1100

Milwaukee, WI 53202
Phone: (414) 276-2145
Fax: (414) 276-3349
E-mail: info@movementdisorders.org
Web site: http://www.movementdisorders.org

Munchausen by Proxy Survivors Network
PO Box 806177
St. Clair Shores, MI 48080

N

Narcolepsy Network
110 Ripple Ln.
North Kingstown, RI 02852
Phone: (401) 667-2523
Fax: (401) 633-6567
Toll free: (888) 292-6522
E-mail: narnet@narcolepsynetwork.org
Web site: http://www.narcolepsynetwork.org

Narcotics Anonymous
PO Box 9999
Van Nuys, CA 91409
Phone: (818) 773-9999
Fax: (818) 700-0700
E-mail: fsmail@na.org
Web site: http://www.na.org

National Academy of Neuropsychology
7555 E Hampden Ave., Ste. 525
Denver, CO 80231
Phone: (303) 691-3694
Fax: (303) 691-5983
E-mail: office@nanonline.org
Web site: http://nanonline.org

National Alliance on Mental Illness (NAMI)
3803 N Fairfax Dr., Ste. 100
Arlington, VA 22203
Phone: (703) 524-7600
Fax: (703) 524-9094
Toll free: (800) 950-NAMI (6264)
Web site: http://www.nami.org

National Aphasia Association
350 7th Ave., Ste. 902
New York, NY 10001
Toll free: (800) 922-4622
E-mail: naa@aphasia.org
Web site: http://aphasia.org

National Association of Anorexia Nervosa and Related Eating Disorders, Inc.
PO Box 640
Naperville, IL 60566
Phone: (630) 577-1330
E-mail: anadhelp@anad.org
Web site: http://www.anad.org

National Association of Cognitive-Behavioral Therapists
PO Box 2195
Weirton, WV 26062
Phone: (304) 723-3982
Toll free: (800) 853-1135
E-mail: nacbt@nacbt.org
Web site: http://www.nacbt.org

National Association for Continence
PO Box 1019
Charleston, SC 29402-1019
Toll free: (800) 252-3337
Web site: http://www.nafc.org

National Association for Holistic Aromatherapy
PO Box 1868
Banner Elk, NC 28604
Phone: (828) 898-6161
Fax: (828) 898-1965
E-mail: info@naha.org
Web site: http://www.naha.org

National Association of School Psychologists
4340 East-West Hwy., Ste. 402
Bethesda, MD 20002
Phone: (301) 657-0270
Fax: (301) 657-0275
Toll free: (800) 331-5277
Web site: http://www.nasponline.org

National Association on Sexual Addiction Problems
22937 Arlington Ave., Ste. 201
Torrance, CA 90501
Phone: (213) 546-3103

National Association of Social Workers
750 First St. NE, Ste. 700
Washington, DC 20002-4241
Phone: (202) 408-8600
Web site: http://www.naswdc.org

National Black Association for Speech-Language and Hearing
700 McKnight Park Dr., Ste. 708
Pittsburgh, PA 15237
Phone: (412) 366-1177
Fax: (412) 366-8804
E-mail: NBASLH@nbaslh.org
Web site: http://www.nbaslh.org

National Cannabis Prevention and Information Centre (NCPIC)
PO Box 684
Randwick, NSW Australia 2031
Phone: +612 9385 0208
E-mail: info@ncpic.org.au
Web site: http://ncpic.org.au

National Center for Complementary and Alternative Medicine (NCCAM)
9000 Rockville Pike
Bethesda, MD 20892
E-mail: info@nccam.nih.gov
Web site: http://nccam.nih.gov

National Center on Elder Abuse (NCEA)
University of California—Irvine, Program in Geriatric Medicine
101 The City Dr. S
200 Building
Orange, CA 92868
Fax: (714) 456-7933
Toll free: (855) 500-ELDR (3537)
E-mail: ncea-info@aoa.hhs.gov
Web site: http://www.ncea.aoa.gov

National Center for Learning Disabilities (NCLD)
381 Park Ave. S, Ste. 1401
New York, NY 10016
Phone: (212) 545-7510
Fax: (212) 545-9665
Toll free: (888) 575-7373
E-mail: ncld@ncld.org
Web site: http://www.ncld.org

National Center for Posttraumatic Stress Disorder, U.S. Department of Veterans Affairs
810 Vermont Ave. NW
Washington, DC 20420
Phone: (802) 296-6300
E-mail: ncptsd@va.gov
Web site: http://www.ncptsd.va.gov

National Center for Responsible Gambling
1299 Pennsylvania Ave. NW, Ste. 1175
Washington, DC 20004
Phone: (202) 552-2689
Fax: (202) 552-2676
E-mail: info@ncrg.org
Web site: http://www.ncrg.org

National Center on Sleep Disorders Research
6701 Rockledge Dr.
Bethesda, MD
Phone: (301) 435-0199
Fax: (301) 480-3451
Web site: http://www.nhlbi.nih.gov/sleep

National Certification Commission for Acupuncture and Oriental Medicine
76 S Laura St., Ste. 1290
Jacksonville, FL 32202
Phone: (904) 598-1005
Fax: (904) 598-5001
Web site: http://www.nccaom.org

National Child Traumatic Stress Network (NCTSN)
University of California, Los Angeles
11150 W. Olympic Blvd., Ste. 650
Los Angeles, CA 90064
Phone: (310) 235-2633
Fax: (310) 235-2612
E-mail: http://www.nctsn.org/about-us/contact-us
Web site: http://www.nctsn.org

National Chronic Fatigue Syndrome and Fibromyalgia Association
PO Box 18426
Kansas City, MO 64133
Phone: (816) 737-1343
Web site: http://www.ncfsfa.org

National Clearinghouse on Alcohol and Drug Information
PO Box 2345
Rockville, MD 20847
Fax: (240) 221-4292
Toll free: (877) SAMHSA-7; Spanish: (877) 767-8432; TDD: (800) 487-4889
Web site: http://ncadi.samhsa.gov

National Coalition Against Domestic Violence
1120 Lincoln St., Ste. 1603
Denver, CO 80203
Phone: (303) 839-1852; TTY: (303) 839-1681
Fax: (303) 831-9251
Web site: http://www.ncadv.org

National Coalition for the Homeless
2201 P St. NW
Washington, DC 20037
Phone: (202) 462-4822
Fax: (202) 462-4823
E-mail: info@nationalhomeless.org
Web site: http://www.nationalhomeless.org

National Coalition for Homeless Veterans
333 1/2 Pennsylvania Ave. SE
Washington, DC 20003-1148
Phone: (202) 546-1969
Fax: (202) 546-2063
Toll free: (800) 838-4357
E-mail: info@nchv.org
Web site: http://www.nchv.org

National Committee for the Prevention of Elder Abuse
151 1st Ave., No. 93
New York, NY 10003
Fax: (212) 420-6026
Toll free: (800) 677-1116
Web site: http://www.preventelderabuse.org

National Consortium on Stigma and Empowerment (NCSE)
Illinois Institute of Technology, Institute of Psychology
3424 S. State St.
Chicago, IL 60616
Web site: http://www.stigmaandempowerment.org

National Council on Alcoholism and Drug Dependence, Inc. (NCADD)
244 E 58th St., 4th Fl.
New York, NY 10022
Phone: (212) 269-7797
Fax: (212) 269-7510
Toll free: (800) 622-2255
E-mail: national@ncadd.org
Web site: http://www.ncadd.org

National Council for Community Behavioral Healthcare
1701 K St. NW, Ste. 400
Washington, DC 20006
Phone: (202) 684-7457
Fax: (202) 386-9391
E-mail: communications@thenationalcouncil.org
Web site: http://www.thenationalcouncil.org

National Council of Juvenile and Family Court Judges (NCJFCJ)
PO Box 8970
Reno, NV 89507
Phone: (775) 784-6012
Fax: (775) 784-6628
E-mail: staff@ncjfcj.org
Web site: http://www.ncjfcj.org

National Dissemination Center for Children with Disabilities
1825 Connecticut Ave. NW, Ste. 700
Washington, DC 20009
Phone: (202) 884-8200
Fax: (202) 884-8441

Toll free: (800) 695-0285
E-mail: nichcy@aed.org
Web site: http://www.nichcy.org

National Down Syndrome Society (NDSS)
666 Broadway, 8th Fl.
New York, NY 10012
Fax: (212) 979-2873
Toll free: (800) 221-4602
E-mail: info@ndss.org
Web site: http://www.ndss.org/index.php

National Eating Disorders Association
165 W 46th St.
New York, NY 10036
Phone: (212) 575-6200
Fax: (212) 575-1650
Toll free: (800) 931-2237
E-mail: info@NationalEatingDisorders.org
Web site: http://www.nationaleatingdisorders.org

National Education Alliance for Borderline Personality Disorder
PO Box 974
Rye, NY 10580
E-mail: info@neabpd.com
Web site: http://www.borderlinepersonalitydisorder.com

National Family Caregivers Association
10400 Connecticut Ave., Ste. 500
Kensington, MD 20895-3944
Phone: (301) 942-6430
Fax: (301) 942-2302
Toll free: (800) 896-3650
E-mail: info@thefamilycaregiver.org
Web site: http://www.nfcacares.org

National Health Care for the Homeless Council
PO Box 60427
Nashville, TN 37206-0427
Phone: (615) 226-2292
Fax: (615) 226-1656
Web site: http://www.nhchc.org

National Human Genome Research Institute (NHGRI)
Bldg. 31, Rm. 4B09, 31 Center Dr., MSC 2152, 9000 Rockville Pike
Bethesda, MD 20892-2152
Phone: (301) 402-0911
Fax: (301) 402-2218
Web site: http://www.genome.gov

National Institute on Aging (NIA)
Bldg. 31, Rm. 5C27, 31 Center Dr., MSC 2292
Bethesda, MD 20892
Phone: (301) 496-1752
Fax: (301) 496-1072
Toll free: (800) 222-2225; TTY: (800) 222-4225
Web site: http://www.nia.nih.gov

National Institute on Alcohol Abuse and Alcoholism (NIAAA)
5635 Fishers Ln., MSC 9304
Bethesda, MD 20892-9304
Phone: (301) 443-3860
Web site: http://www.niaaa.nih.gov

National Institute of Biomedical Imaging and Bio-engineering
31 Center Dr., 1C14
Bethesda, MD 20892-8859
Phone: (301) 469-8859
Web site: http://www.nibib.nih.gov

National Institute on Deafness and Other Communication Disorders (NIDCD)
31 Center Dr., MSC 2320
Bethesda, MD 20892-2320
Phone: (301) 496-7243
Fax: (301) 770-8977
Toll free: (800) 241-1044
E-mail: nidcdinfo@nidcd.nih.gov
Web site: http://www.nidcd.nih.gov

National Institute on Drug Abuse (NIDA)
6001 Executive Blvd., Rm. 5213
Bethesda, MD 20892
Phone: (301) 442-1124; Spanish: (240) 221-4007
E-mail: information@nida.nih.gov
Web site: http://www.nida.nih.gov

National Institute of Justice (NIJ)
810 7th St. NW
Washington, DC 20531
Web site: http://www.nij.gov

National Institute of Mental Health (NIMH)
6001 Executive Blvd., Rm. 8184, MSC 9663
Bethesda, MD 20892
Phone: (301) 443-4513
Fax: (301) 443-4279
Toll free: (866) 615-6464
E-mail: nimhinfo@nih.gov
Web site: http://www.nimh.nih.gov

National Institute of Neurological Disorders and Stroke (NINDS)
NIH Neurological Institute, PO Box 5801
Bethesda, MD 20824
Phone: (301) 496-5751; TTY: (301) 468-5981
Toll free: (800) 352-9424
Web site: http://www.ninds.nih.gov

National Lead Information Center
422 S Clinton Ave.
Rochester, NY 14620
Fax: (585) 232-3111
Toll free: (800) 424-5323
Web site: http://www.epa.gov/lead/nlic.htm

U.S. National Library of Medicine
8600 Rockville Pike
Bethesda, MD 20894
Web site: http://www.nlm.nih.gov

National Mental Health Consumers' Self-Help Clearinghouse
1211 Chestnut St., Ste. 1207
Philadelphia, PA 19107
Phone: (215) 751-1810
Fax: (215) 636-6312
Toll free: (800) 553-4539
E-mail: info@mhselfhelp.org
Web site: http://mhselfhelp.org

National Organization on Fetal Alcohol Syndrome
1200 Eton Ct. NW, 3rd Fl.
Washington, DC 20007
Phone: (202) 785-4585
Fax: (202) 466-6456
E-mail: information@nofas.org
Web site: http://www.nofas.org

National Organization for Rare Disorders
55 Kenosia Ave., PO Box 1968
Danbury, CT 06813-1968
Phone: (203) 744-0100
Fax: (203) 798-2291
Toll free: (800) 999-6673
Web site: http://www.rarediseases.org

National Organization for the Reform of Marijuana Laws (NORML)
1600 K St. NW
Washington, DC 20006
Phone: (202) 483-5500
Fax: (202) 483-0057
E-mail: norml@norml.org
Web site: http://norml.org

National Psychological Association for Psychoanalysis
40 W 13th St.
New York, NY 10011
Phone: (212) 924-7440
Fax: (212) 989-7543
E-mail: info@npap.org
Web site: http://www.npap.org

National Resource Center on ADHD
8181 Professional Pl., Ste. 150
Landover, MD 20785
Toll free: (800) 233-4050
Web site: http://www.help4adhd.org

National Safety Council
1121 Spring Lake Dr.
Itasca, IL 60143-3201
Phone: (630) 285-1121
Fax: (630) 285-1315
Toll free: (800) 621-7615
E-mail: customerservice@nsc.org
Web site: http://www.nsc.org

National Schizophrenia Foundation
403 Seymour Ave., Ste. 202
Lansing, MI 48933
Phone: (517) 485-7168
Fax: (517) 485-7180
Toll free: (800) 482-9534
E-mail: inquiries@nsfoundation.org

National Sexual Violence Resource Center (NSVRC)
123 N Enola Dr.
Enola, PA 17025
Phone: (717) 909-0710
Fax: (717) 909-0714
Toll free: (877) 739-3895
E-mail: resources@nsvrc.org
Web site: http://www.nsvrc.org

National Sleep Foundation
1010 N Glebe Rd., Ste. 310
Arlington, VA 22201
Phone: (703) 243-1697
E-mail: nsf@sleepfoundation.org
Web site: http://www.sleepfoundation.org

National Stroke Association
9707 E Easter Ln., Ste. B
Centennial, CO 80112
Fax: (303) 649-1328
Toll free: (800) 787-6537
E-mail: info@stroke.org
Web site: http://www.stroke.org

National Suicide Prevention Lifeline
Toll free: (800) 274-TALK (8255)
Web site: http://www.suicidepreventionlifeline.org

Natural Standard
One Davis Sq.
Somerville, MA 02144
Phone: (617) 591-3300
Fax: (617) 591-3399
E-mail: questions@naturalstandard.com
Web site: http://naturalstandard.com

Neuroleptic Malignant Syndrome Information Service
Box 1069
Sherburne, NY 13460-1069
Phone: (607) 674-7920
Fax: (607) 674-7910
E-mail: info@nmsis.org
Web site: http://www.nmsis.org

New York Online Access to Health
Web site: http://www.noah-health.org/en/mental

New York State Psychiatric Institute, Columbia University Medical Center
1051 Riverside Dr.
New York, NY 10032
Phone: (212) 543-6000
Web site: http://www.nyspi.org

North American Family Institute
26 Howley St.
Peabody, MA 01960
Phone: (978) 538-0286
Fax: (978) 531-9313
Web site: http://www.nafi.com

O

Obsessive Compulsive Foundation
PO Box 961029
Boston, MA 02196
Phone: (617) 973-5801
Web site: http://www.ocfoundation.org

OCD Center of Los Angeles
11620 Wilshire Blvd., Ste. 890
Los Angeles, CA 90025
Phone: (310) 824-5200
E-mail: http://www.ocdla.com/contactus.html
Web site: http://www.ocdla.com/index.html

U.S. Office of Dietary Supplements, National Institutes of Health
6100 Executive Blvd., Rm. 3B01, MSC 7517
Rockville, MD 20892-7517
Phone: (301) 435-2920
Fax: (301) 480-1845
E-mail: ods@nih.gov
Web site: http://ods.od.nih.gov

Office of Fair Housing and Equal Opportunity, U.S. Department of Housing and Urban Development
451 7th St. SW
Washington, DC 20410
Web site: http://portal.hud.gov/hudportal/HUD?src=/program_offices/fair_housing_equal_opp

Office of Juvenile Justice and Delinquency Prevention, U.S. Department of Justice
810 7th St. NW
Washington, DC 20531
Phone: (202) 307-5911
Web site: http://www.ojjdp.gov

Office of Special Education and Rehabilitative Services, U.S. Department of Education
400 Maryland Ave., SW
Washington, DC 20202-2800
Phone: (202) 245-7488
Web site: http://rsa.ed.gov

Office on Women's Health, U.S. Department of Health and Human Services
200 Independence Ave., SW
Washington, DC 20201
Toll free: (800) 994-9662; TDD: (888) 220-5446
Web site: http://www.womenshealth.gov

Olweus Bullying Prevention Program
Toll free: (800) 328-9000
E-mail: olweusinfo@hazelden.org
Web site: http://www.olweus.org/public/index.page

Overeaters Anonymous
PO Box 44020
Rio Rancho, NM 87174-4020
Phone: (505) 891-2664
Fax: (505) 891-4320
Web site: http://www.oa.org

P

PAIRS Foundation
1675 Market St., Ste. 207
Weston, FL 33326
Toll free: (877) PAIRS-4U (724-7748)
E-mail: info@pairs.com
Web site: http://www.pairs.com

Parents Anonymous, Inc
675 W Foothill Blvd., Ste. 220
Claremont, CA 91711-3475
Phone: (909) 621-6184
Fax: (909) 625-6304
E-mail: Parentsanonymous@parentsanonymous.org
Web site: http://www.parentsanonymous.org

The Partnership at Drugfree.org
352 Park Ave. S, 9th Fl.
New York, NY 10010
Phone: (212) 922-1560
Fax: (212) 922-1570
Web site: http://www.drugfree.org

Personality Disorders Awareness Network
490 Sun Valley Dr., Ste. 205
Roswell, GA 30076
Phone: (770) 642-4236 x61
Fax: (770) 642-4239
E-mail: info@bpdan.org
Web site: http://www.bpdan.org

Pick's Disease Support Group
E-mail: info@pdsg.org.uk
Web site: http://www.pdsg.org.uk

Postpartum Support International
PO Box 60931
Santa Barbara, CA 93160
Phone: (805) 967-7636
Toll free: (800) 944-4773
Web site: http://www.postpartum.net

President's Committee for People with Intellectual Disabilities, Administration for Children and Families, U.S. Department of Health and Human Services
Aerospace Center, Ste. 210, 370 L'Enfant Promenade SW
Washington, DC 20447
Phone: (202) 619-0634
Fax: (202) 205-9519
Toll free: (800) 424-3688
Web site: http://www.acf.hhs.gov/programs/pcpid

Prevent Child Abuse America
228 S Wabash Ave., 10th Fl.
Chicago, IL 60604
Phone: (312) 663-3520
Fax: (312) 939-8962
E-mail: mailbox@preventchildabuse.org
Web site: http://www.preventchildabuse.org

Public Citizen, Inc
1600 20th St. NW
Washington, DC 20009
Phone: (202) 588-1000
E-mail: hrg1@citizen.org
Web site: http://www.citizen.org/Page.aspx?pid=183

Q

Qigong Human Life Research Foundation
PO Box 5327
Cleveland, OH 44101

R

Rape, Abuse & Incest National Network (RAINN)
2000 L St. NW, Ste. 406
Washington, DC 20036

Phone: (202) 544-1034
Toll free: (800) 656-HOPE
E-mail: info@rainn.org
Web site: http://www.rainn.org

Rational Recovery
Box 800
Lotus, CA 95651
Phone: (530) 621-2667
Fax: (530) 621-4374
Web site: https://rational.org/index.php?id=1

ReSTART
1001 290th Ave. SE
Fall City, WA 98024-7403
Phone: (425) 417-1715
Toll free: (800) 682-6934
E-mail: restart@netaddictionrecovery.com
Web site: http://www.netaddictionrecovery.com

Restless Legs Syndrome Foundation
1904 Banbury Rd.
Raleigh, NC 27608-4428
Phone: (919) 781-4428
Web site: http://www.rls.org

S

Schizophrenia.com
Web site: http://www.schizophrenia.com

Selective Mutism Group—A Division of Childhood Anxiety Network, Inc.
Web site: http://www.selectivemutism.org

Sensory Processing Disorder Foundation
5420 S. Quebec St., Ste. 135
Greenwood Village, CO 80111
Phone: (303) 794-1182
Fax: (303) 322-5550
Web site: http://www.sinetwork.org

Sex Addicts Anonymous
PO Box 70949
Houston, TX 77270
Toll free: (800) 477-8191
E-mail: info@saa-recovery.org
Web site: http://www.sexaa.org

Sexuality Information and Education Council of the United States
1706 R St., NW
Washington, DC 20009
Phone: (202) 265-2405
Fax: (202) 462-2340
Web site: http://www.aasect.org

SHARE Pregnancy and Infant Loss Support
402 Jackson St.
St. Charles, MO 63301
Fax: (636) 947-7486
Toll free: (800) 821-6819
Web site: http://www.nationalshare.org

Shyness Research Institute
4201 Grant Line Rd.
New Albany, IN 47150
Phone: (812) 941-2295
Fax: (812) 941-2591
E-mail: bcarducc@ius.edu
Web site: http://www.ius.edu/shyness

Sidran Institute
PO Box 436
Brooklandville, MD 21022-0436
Phone: (410) 825-8888
Fax: (410) 560-0134
E-mail: info@sidran.org
Web site: http://www.sidran.org/index.cfm

SIDS Alliance
1314 Bedford Ave., Ste. 230
Baltimore, MD 21208
Toll free: (800) 221-SIDS
Web site: http://www.sidsalliance.org

Society for Clinical and Experimental Hypnosis
PO Box 252
Southborough, MA 01772
Phone: (508) 598-5553
Fax: (866) 397-1839
E-mail: info@sceh.us
Web site: http://www.sceh.us

Society for the Exploration of Psychotherapy Integration
E-mail: geostricker@gmail.com
Web site: http://sepiweb.org

Society for Light Treatment and Biological Rhythms
824 Howard Ave.
New Haven, CT 60610
E-mail: sltbrinfo@gmail.com
Web site: http://www.sltbr.org

Society for the Psychological Study of Men and Masculinity (Division 51), American Psychological Association
750 1st St. NE
Washington, DC 20002-4242
Phone: (202) 216-7602
Fax: (202) 218-3599
E-mail: kcooke@apa.org
Web site: http://www.apa.org/about/division/div51.aspx

Stanford University School of Medicine Center for Narcolepsy
450 Broadway St., Pavilion B, 2nd Fl.
Redwood City, CA 94063
Phone: (650) 725-6517
Fax: (650) 725-4913
Web site: http://med.stanford.edu/school/Psychiatry/narcolepsy

The Stanley Medical Research Institute, Research on Schizophrenia and Bipolar Disorder
E-mail: info@stanleyresearch.org
Web site: http://www.stanleyresearch.org/dnn

State Rehabilitation Councils
1902 Market St.
Camp Hill, PA 17011
Toll free: (888) 250-5175
Web site: http://www.parac.org

STOP Cyberbullying
Phone: (201) 463-8663

E-mail: parry@aftab.com
Web site: http://www.stopcyberbullying.org/index2.html

Structured Clinical Interview for DSM Disorders (SCID)
c/o Biometrics Research Department, Columbia University at NYSPI
1051 Riverside Dr., Unit 60
New York, NY 10032
Phone: (212) 543-5524
Fax: (212) 543-5525
E-mail: scid4@columbia.edu
Web site: http://www.scid4.org

Stuttering Foundation of America (SFA)
3100 Walnut Grove Rd., Ste. 603
Memphis, TN 38111-0749
Phone: (901) 452-7343
Fax: (901) 452-3931
Toll free: (800) 992-9392
E-mail: info@stutteringhelp.org
Web site: http://www.stutteringhelp.org/Default.aspx?tabid=4

Substance Abuse and Mental Health Services Administration (SAMHSA)
1 Choke Cherry Rd.
Rockville, MD 20857
Fax: (240) 221-4292
Toll free: (877) SAMHSA-7 (726-4727); TTY: (800) 487-4889
E-mail: SAMHSAInfo@samhsa.hhs.gov
Web site: http://www.samhsa.gov

T

Therapeutic Touch International Association
PO Box 419
Craryville, NY 12521
Phone: (518) 325-1185
Fax: (509) 693-3537
E-mail: nhpai@therapeutic-touch.org
Web site: http://www.therapeutictouch.org

Tourette Syndrome Association, Inc.
42-40 Bell Blvd.
Bayside, NY 11361-2861
Phone: (718) 224-2999
Web site: http://www.tsa-usa.org

Tourette Syndrome Foundation of Canada
5945 Airport Rd., Ste. 195
Mississauga, Ontario L4V 1R9
Canada
Phone: (905) 673-2255
Fax: (905) 673-2638
Toll free: (800) 361-3120
Web site: http://www.tourette.ca

Tragedy Assistance Program for Survivors
1777 F St. NW, Ste. 600
Washington, DC 20006
Phone: (202) 588-TAPS (8277)
Fax: (202) 509-8282
Toll free: (800) 959-TAPS (8277)
E-mail: info@taps.org
Web site: http://www.taps.org

Treatment Advocacy Center
200 N Glebe Rd., Ste. 730
Arlington, VA 22203
Phone: (703) 294-6001
Fax: (703) 294-6010
E-mail: info@treatmentadvocacycenter.org
Web site: http://www.treatmentadvocacycenter.org

Treatment and Research Advancements Association for Personality Disorder
23 Greene St.
New York, NY 10013
Phone: (212) 966-6514
Toll free: (888) 4-TARA-APD
E-mail: tara4bpd@gmail.com
Web site: http://www.tara4bpd.org

Trichotillomania Learning Center, Inc.
207 McPherson St., Ste. H
Santa Cruz, CA 95060-5863
Phone: (831) 457-1004
Fax: (831) 426-4383
E-mail: info@trich.org
Web site: http://www.trich.org

U

Uniformed Services University of the Health Sciences (USU)
4301 Jones Bridge Rd.
Bethesda, MD 20814
Phone: (301) 295-1219
Fax: (301) 295-3757
Toll free: (800) 515-5257
Web site: http://www.usuhs.mil

United States . . . For U.S. agencies, see specific agency name (e.g., Food and Drug Administration).

United States Pharmacopoeia
12601 Twinbrook Pkwy.
Rockville, MD 20852-1790
Toll free: (800) 227-8772
Web site: http://www.usp.org

University of Minnesota Clinic, Center for Sexual Health
1300 S 2nd St.
Minneapolis, MN 55454
Phone: (612) 624-7821
Web site: http://www.fm.umn.edu/phs/clinic/home.html

University of North Carolina School of Medicine, Department of Psychiatry
110 Conner Dr., Ste. 4
Chapel Hill, NC 27514
Phone: (919) 929-7449
Web site: http://www.psychiatry.unc.edu

V

Vipassana Meditation Center
PO Box 24
Shelbourne Falls, MA 01370

Phone: (413) 625-2160
Web site: http://www.dhamma.org/en/schedules/schdhara.shtml

W

Weight-control Information Network
1 WIN Way
Bethesda, MD 20892-3665
Phone: (202) 828-1025
Fax: (202) 828-1028
Toll free: (877) 946-4627
E-mail: win@info.niddk.nih.gov
Web site: http://win.niddk.nih.gov/index.htm

Wellesley Centers for Women (WCW)
Wellesley College, 106 Central St.
Wellesley, MA 02481-8203
Phone: (781) 283-2500
E-mail: wcw@wellesley.edu
Web site: http://www.wcwonline.org

Wilson Disease Association
5572 N Diversey Blvd.
Milwaukee, WI 53217
Phone: (414) 961-0533
Toll free: (866) 961-0533
E-mail: info@wilsonsdisease.org
Web site: http://www.wilsonsdisease.org

Workplace Bullying Institute (WBI)
PO Box 29915
Bellingham, WA 98228
E-mail: http://www.workplacebullying.org/aboutwbi/contact/
Web site: http://www.workplacebullying.org

World Association for Person-Centered and Experiential Psychotherapy and Counseling
PO Box 142
Ross-on-Wye, United Kingdom HR9 9AG
Phone: 011 44 1989 763 901
Web site: http://www.pce-world.org

World Professional Association for Transgender Health (WPATH)
1300 S 2nd St., Ste. 180
Minneapolis, MN 55454
E-mail: wpath@wpath.org
Web site: http://www.wpath.org

Worldwide Education and Awareness for Movement Disorders (WE MOVE)
5731 Mosholu Avenue
Bronx, NY 10471
E-mail: wemove@wemove.org
Web site: http://www.wemove.org

Y

Yoga Science Foundation
759 S State St., No. 24
Ukiah, CA 95482
Web site: http://www.yrec.org

GLOSSARY

The glossary is an alphabetical compilation of terms and definitions listed in the *Key Terms* sections of the main body entries. Although the list is comprehensive, it is by no means exhaustive.

A

A1 ALLELE. An allele related to reward deficiency syndrome (RDS).

A1 D2. A chromosome sequence related to reward deficiency syndrome (RDS).

ABSENCE SEIZURE. A seizure characterized by a short-term (15–20 seconds) but abrupt lack of conscious activity. Individuals become very quiet and may blink, stare blankly, roll their eyes, or move their lips, but once the seizure ends, they may not even realize that anything unusual happened. Also called a petit mal seizure.

ABSTINENCE. Refraining from sexual intercourse for a period of time.

ABSTRACT REASONING. The ability to analyze information and solve problems.

ABUSE. Physical, emotional, or sexual harm.

ACAMPROSATE. Also called Campral, a medication used since 1989 in Europe and since 2004 in the United States to reduce the craving for alcohol.

ACETYLCHOLINE. A naturally occurring chemical in the body that transmits nerve impulses from cell to cell. Acetylcholine causes blood vessels to dilate, lowers blood pressure, and slows the heartbeat. Central nervous system well-being is dependent on a balance among the neurotransmitters acetylcholine, dopamine, serotonin, and norepinephrine.

ACETYLCHOLINESTERASE. The chemical responsible for the breakdown of acetylcholine.

ACHIEVEMENT TEST. Any of a number of tests that assess developed knowledge or skill.

ACRODERMATITIS ENTEROPATHICA. Hereditary metabolic problem characterized by dermatitis, diarrhea, and poor immunity. Oral treatment with zinc is curative.

ACTIVITIES OF DAILY LIVING (ADLs). A general term for routine activities of self-care (e.g., brushing teeth, dressing, bathing) and independent functioning (e.g., managing money, preparing meals, cleaning house).

ACUPOINT. A pressure point stimulated in acupressure.

ACUPRESSURE. A form of massage in which certain points of the body are pressed with the fingers and hands to produce a desired effect.

ACUTE. Having a sudden onset and lasting a short time.

ACUTE ONSET VASCULAR DEMENTIA. Vascular dementia caused by a single stroke or with an onset of fewer than three months.

ADAPTIVE BEHAVIOR. A person's ability to accomplish tasks and adapt to and function in an environment.

ADAPTIVE FUNCTIONING. A term used to describe a person's having the intellectual, social, and practical skills needed to live independently.

ADDICTION. A strong physical or psychological dependence on a physical substance.

ADDICTIVE DISORDER. A disorder involving repeated participation in a certain activity, despite negative consequences and/or attempts to stop the behavior. Alcohol abuse is an example.

ADDICTIVE PERSONALITY. The concept that addiction is the result of a pre-existing character disposition.

ADENOSINE. A nucleoside that plays multiple physiological roles in energy transfer and molecular signaling, as a component of ribonucleic acid (RNA), and as an inhibitory neurotransmitter that promotes sleep.

ADHD. Attention deficit hyperactivity disorder.

ADJUNCT THERAPY. A form of treatment that is not strictly necessary but is helpful to a therapy regimen (e.g., music or art therapy).

ADJUSTMENT DISORDER. A disorder defined by the development of significant emotional or behavioral symptoms in response to a stressful event or series of events. Symptoms may include depressed mood, anxiety, and impairment of social and occupational functioning.

ADRENAL GLAND. A small gland located above each kidney that produces many different hormones, including estrogen, progesterone, and stress hormones.

ADRENALINE ADDICTION. A drug-like dependency on the physiological effects of participating in activities that trigger adrenaline release (such as skydiving or gambling).

AEROBIC EXERCISE. Activity that increases the body's requirement for oxygen, thereby increasing respiration and heart rate.

AFFECT. In psychology, an observed emotional expression or response, such as through facial expressions, hand gestures, or tone of voice. Types of affect include flat (inanimate, no expression), blunted (minimally responsive), inappropriate relative to the context, and labile (abrupt changes in type and intensity of emotion).

AFFECTIVE DISORDER. A disorder involving an inappropriate or unexpected emotional experience or reaction relative to the circumstance (for example, feeling sad when there is no easily identifiable reason, as in depression).

AGE OF CONSENT. The minimum age at which a person is considered legally competent to consent to sexual acts. It should not be confused with the voting age, driving age, legal drinking age, or marriageable age. In most jurisdictions in the United States, the age of consent is 16 or 18, but it may be set as low as 12 or as high as 21.

AGE-ASSOCIATED MEMORY IMPAIRMENT (AAMI). A condition in which an older person suffers some memory loss and takes longer to learn new information. AAMI is different than dementia because it is not progressive and does not represent a serious decline from the person's previous level of functioning. Benign senescent forgetfulness is another term for AAMI.

AGITATION. Excessive restlessness or emotional disturbance that is often associated with anxiety, psychosis, or other mental disorder (such as Alzheimer's disease).

AGNOSIA. Inability to recognize familiar people, places, and objects.

AGONIST. Any chemical that binds to a receptor on a cell surface and stimulates that cell to respond.

AGORAPHOBIA. An anxiety disorder characterized by fear of crowds, open or public spaces, or situations that might trigger panic attacks, and from where exits (or help) may be inaccessible or impeded.

AIDS. Acquired immunodeficiency syndrome.

AKATHISIA. Agitated or restless movement, usually affecting the legs. Movement is accompanied by a sense of discomfort and an inability to sit, stand still, or remain inactive for periods of time. Akathisia is a common side effect of some neuroleptic (antipsychotic) medications.

ALCOHOL. An organic chemical and the active agent in beer, wine, and liquor; chemically known as ethanol.

ALCOHOL POISONING. A potentially life-threatening condition caused by consuming large amounts of alcohol within a short time period, negatively affecting heart rate, breathing, and the gag reflex.

ALCOHOL USE DISORDERS INVENTORY TEST (AUDIT). A test for alcohol use developed by the World Health Organization (WHO). Its ten questions address three specific areas of drinking over a 12-month period: the amount and frequency of drinking, dependence upon alcohol, and problems that have been encountered due to drinking alcohol.

ALCOHOLIC ENERGY DRINK. Caffeinated alcoholic beverages; malt liquors that, in addition to high alcohol content, have added caffeine and sometimes other stimulants.

ALCOHOLISM. Chronic and compulsive use of alcohol that interferes with everyday life.

ALIENATOR. In parental alienation disorder, the alienator is the parent attempting to negatively affect the child's opinion of the other (targeted or alienated) parent.

ALLELE. One member of a pair or a series of genes that occupies a specific position on a specific chromosome.

ALLERGIC REACTION. A physiological reaction to certain substances, such as ragweed or grass, that occurs when susceptible persons come into close proximity with the substance.

ALOPECIA. Hair loss (also, loss of feathers or wool in animals).

ALS. Amyotrophic lateral sclerosis.

ALTER. An alternate or secondary personality in a person with dissociative identity disorder. Each alter has a unique way of looking at and interacting with the world.

ALTRUISM. An unselfish willingness to help others.

ALVEOLAR. Pertaining to alveoli, which are tiny air sacs at the ends of the small air passages in the lungs.

ALZHEIMER'S DISEASE. A progressive, neurodegenerative disease characterized by loss of function and death of nerve cells in several areas of the brain, leading to loss of mental functions, including memory and learning. Alzheimer's disease is the most common cause of dementia.

AMBIVALENCE. A state of having conflicting feelings about a person or situation.

AMBULATION. Ability to walk.

AMENORRHEA. Abnormal absence of menstrual periods in a woman.

AMNESIA. Partial or complete loss of memory, or gaps in memory, that is not due to ordinary forgetfulness. Amnesia can be caused by diseases, seizures, medications, tumors, physical injuries, and emotional traumas (dissociation).

AMNESTIC. Having to do with, or related to, amnesia.

AMPHETAMINES. A group of powerful and highly addictive substances that stimulate the central nervous system. Amphetamines may be prescribed for various medical conditions but are often purchased illicitly and abused.

AMYGDALA. An almond-shaped brain structure in the limbic system that is activated in acute stress situations to trigger the emotion of fear.

AMYLOID. A waxy translucent substance, composed mostly of protein, that forms plaques (abnormal deposits) in the brain.

AMYOTROPHIC LATERAL SCLEROSIS (ALS). A degenerative disease that affects nerves of the brain and spinal cord, resulting in eventual paralysis; also known as Lou Gehrig's disease.

ANABOLIC. Causing muscle and bone growth and a shift from fat to muscle in the body.

ANALGESIC. A medication used to reduce or eliminate pain.

ANANKASTIC PERSONALITY DISORDER. The European term for obsessive-compulsive personality disorder.

ANCILLARY. Subordinate or secondary.

ANDROGENIC. Causing testosterone-like, masculinizing effects.

ANDROGYNY. The condition of having the characteristics of both a man and a woman, or not being clearly identified as male or female. Androgyny may refer to a person's physical characteristics, to psychological characteristics, or to behavior.

ANECDOTAL. Based on personal experience or reported individual observations, as opposed to controlled experiments or proven facts.

ANEMIA. A blood condition in which the level of hemoglobin or the number of red blood cells falls below normal values. Common symptoms include paleness, fatigue, and shortness of breath.

ANESTHESIA. A drug-induced loss of sensation or feeling. General anesthesia produces total unconsciousness, whereas local anesthesia produces numbness only around the site where the drug was introduced.

ANEURYSM. A symptomless bulging of a blood vessel, due to a weak arterial wall. Ruptured aneurysms can result in stroke or even death.

ANGINA. Severe pain and a feeling of constriction around the heart.

ANGIOEDEMA. Patches of swelling of the skin, subcutaneous layers, mucus membranes, and sometimes internal organs.

ANGIOGRAPHY. A procedure used to investigate the condition of blood vessels, usually via a combination of radiological imaging (x ray) and injection of a contrast medium, which highlights its path through the body. Angiography is used to check for blockage, bleeding, or any other abnormality.

ANOREXIA. Loss of appetite or unwillingness to eat. Can be caused by medications, depression, or many other factors.

ANOREXIA NERVOSA. A serious eating disorder characterized by a pathological fear of gaining weight. Anorexia nervosa causes disturbed eating behaviors and can lead to severe weight loss and malnutrition.

ANOXIA. Lack of oxygen.

ANTABUSE. Trade name for disulfiram (DSF), a chemical used to treat alcoholism by causing a severe physiological reaction to any amount of alcohol.

ANTAGONIST. A substance whose actions counteract the effects of, or work in the opposite way from, another chemical or drug.

ANTERIOR. Situated toward the head or front.

ANTEROGRADE AMNESIA. A type of amnesia characterized by the inability to form new memories, with existing memories left unaffected.

ANTICHOLINERGIC. Related to the ability of a drug to block the neurotransmitter acetylcholine. When acetylcholine is blocked, patients often experience dry mouth and skin, increased heart rate, blurred vision, and difficulty urinating. In severe cases, blocking acetylcholine may cloud thinking and cause delirium.

ANTICHOLINERGIC TOXICITY. A poisonous effect brought about by ingestion of medications or other toxins that block acetylcholine receptors. When these receptors are blocked, the person taking the medication may find that he or she gets overheated, has dry mouth, has blurry vision, and retains urine.

ANTICHOLINERGICS. Drugs that block the action of acetylcholine, a naturally occurring chemical that is involved in communication between nerve cells.

ANTICOAGULANT. A medication (such as warfarin [Coumadin] or Heparin) that decreases the blood's clotting ability, preventing the formation of new clots. Although anticoagulants do not dissolve existing clots, they can stop them from getting larger. These drugs are commonly called blood thinners.

ANTICONVULSANT. A drug used to relieve or prevent seizures.

ANTIDEPRESSANT. Any of a group of medications given to relieve mood disorders, including anxiety disorders as well as major depression. Antidepressants include monoamine oxidase inhibitors (MAOIs), tricyclic (TCAs) and tetracyclic (TeCAs) antidepressants, selective serotonin reuptake inhibitors (SSRIs), and serotonin-norepinephrine reuptake inhibitors (SNRIs).

ANTIEMETIC. A preparation or medication given to stop vomiting.

ANTIHISTAMINE. A medication used to alleviate allergy or cold symptoms such as runny nose, itching, hives, watering eyes, or sneezing.

ANTIHYPERTENSIVE. A drug used to treat hypertension (high blood pressure).

ANTIOXIDANT. A substance that protects the body from damaging reactive oxygen molecules (free radicals). These reactive oxygen molecules can come from inside the body or from environmental pollution and are thought to play a role in the aging process and the development of degenerative disease.

ANTIOXIDANT ENZYME. An enzyme that can counteract the damaging effects of oxygen in tissues.

ANTIPSYCHOTIC. A drug used to treat serious mental disorders that cause hallucinations or delusions, such as schizophrenia or psychosis.

ANTISEPTIC. A substance that inhibits the growth of microorganisms.

ANTISOCIAL BEHAVIOR. Behavior that differs significantly from the norms of society and is considered harmful to society.

ANTISOCIAL PERSONALITY. A personality characterized by attitudes and behaviors at odds with society's customs and moral standards, including illegal acts.

ANTISOCIAL PERSONALITY DISORDER. A psychological condition in which a person appears to be unaware of, or indifferent to, the feelings of others and to normal social rules and standards.

ANTISPASMODIC. A medication or preparation given to relieve muscle or digestive cramps.

ANXIETY. A psychological state characterized by strong feelings of worry, nervousness, apprehension, or agitation; may also be accompanied by physical symptoms, including sweating, tension, and increased pulse.

ANXIETY DISORDERS. A group of disorders characterized by anxiety, including generalized anxiety disorder, panic disorder, and post-traumatic stress disorder (PTSD).

ANXIOLYTIC. Any of a group of medications prescribed to relieve anxiety. Also called tranquilizers, anxiolytics include benzodiazepines, some of the selective serotonin reuptake inhibitors (SSRIs), barbiturates, and buspirone.

APATHY. Lack of feelings or emotions.

APHASIA. Loss of previously acquired ability to speak or understand written or spoken language.

APHONIA. Inability to speak caused by a functional disturbance of the voice box or vocal cords.

APNEA. A brief suspension or interruption of breathing.

APOLIPOPROTEIN E (APOE). A protein that transports cholesterol throughout the body. One form of this protein, APOE e4, is associated with a 60% risk of late-onset Alzheimer's disease.

APOTEMNOPHILIA. A word coined by John Money in 1977 to describe the condition now known as body integrity identity disorder (BIID).

APPERCEPTION. The process of understanding something in terms of previous experience.

APRAXIA. An inability to perform purposeful movements that is not caused by paralysis or loss of feeling.

ARITHMETIC. The branch of mathematics involving problems of addition, subtraction, multiplication, and division.

ARRHYTHMIA. Any disturbance in the normal rhythm of the heartbeat.

ARSON. The deliberate setting of fires for criminal purposes, usually to collect insurance money or to cover up evidence of another crime. It is distinguished from pyromania by its connection with planning and forethought rather than failure of impulse control.

ART THERAPY. The use of art to assess or treat an individual's development, abilities, personality, interests, concerns, or conflicts.

ARTERIOSCLEROSIS. A chronic condition characterized by a thickening and hardening of the arteries and the build-up of plaque on the arterial walls. Arteriosclerosis can slow or impair blood circulation.

ASANA. A position or stance in yoga.

ASPERGER SYNDROME. A developmental disorder that is similar to mild autism. It is characterized by impaired social interaction, repetitive patterns of behavior, and restricted interests, but with normal language and cognitive development and often above-average abilities in a narrow field.

ASSERTIVE. Confidently self-assured; able to express oneself constructively and directly.

ASSERTIVE COMMUNITY TREATMENT (ACT). A service-delivery model for providing comprehensive, highly individualized, and locally based treatment directly to patients with serious and persistent mental illness.

ASSISTED SUICIDE. A form of suicide in which individuals voluntarily bring about their own death with the help of another person, usually a physician, relative, or friend. Assisted suicide is sometimes called physician-assisted death (PAD).

ASTRINGENT. A substance or compound that causes contraction or constriction of soft tissue.

ASYLUM. An older term for psychiatric hospitals; it is rarely used except in historical studies of psychiatric treatment.

ATAQUE DE NERVIOS. A culture-specific anxiety syndrome found among some Latin American groups in the United States and in Latin America. It resembles panic disorder in some respects but also includes dissociative symptoms and frequently occurs in response to stressful events.

ATRIAL FIBRILLATION. A condition in which the upper chambers (atria) of the heart contract rapidly instead of pumping in an organized way. The irregular contractions do not allow the chambers to empty of blood, which can allow blood clots to form and is associated with a higher risk of stroke.

ATROPHY. Shrinkage or deterioration.

ATTACHMENT. The bond developed between an infant and his or her primary caregiver within the first 12 to 18 months of life.

ATTACHMENT DISORDER. A general term used to describe emotional and behavioral problems in children or adults that result from a failure to form healthy attachments in early childhood to parents or other primary caregivers.

ATTENTION DEFICIT HYPERACTIVITY DISORDER (ADHD). A condition characterized by lack of concentration, impulsive or inappropriate behavior (relative to age level), and hyperactivity.

ATYPICAL ANTIPSYCHOTICS. A group of medications for the treatment of psychotic symptoms that were introduced in the 1990s. The atypical antipsychotics include clozapine, risperidone, quetiapine, ziprasidone, and olanzapine. They are sometimes called serotonin dopamine antagonists, or SDAs.

AUDIOLOGIST. A healthcare professional with special training in testing people for hearing loss or other hearing disorders.

AUDITORY. Pertaining to the sense of hearing.

AURA. An energy field that is thought to emanate from the human body and to be visible to people with special psychic or spiritual powers.

AURICULAR ACUPUNCTURE. Acupuncture using only points found on the ears.

AUTISM. A severe developmental disorder that usually begins before three years of age and affects a child's social as well as intellectual development; often includes impairment of verbal and nonverbal communication skills.

AUTISM SPECTRUM DISORDER (ASD). One of a group of disorders with similar symptoms, including an impaired ability to communicate and form normal social relationships, with symptoms ranging in severity depending on the condition. ASDs include (in order of severity) Asperger syndrome, autism, pervasive developmental disorder not otherwise specified, and childhood disintegrative disorder.

AUTISTIC PSYCHOPATHY. The original name for Asperger syndrome; it is still used occasionally as a synonym for the disorder.

AUTOGENIC TRAINING. A relaxation technique with parallels to hypnosis and meditation. It consists of six exercises that use visualization and verbal cues to relax the body.

AUTOIMMUNE DISEASE. A condition in which the immune system's antibodies or T cells attack the body's own molecules, cells, or tissues as if they were foreign invaders.

AUTOMATIC BEHAVIOR. Activities that are carried out while a person is partially awake but is not conscious of his or her behavior and cannot recall the event afterward; occurs with some sleep disorders.

AUTOMATIC THOUGHTS. Thoughts that automatically come to mind when a particular situation occurs. Cognitive-behavioral therapy seeks to challenge automatic thoughts.

AUTONOMIC NERVOUS SYSTEM. The part of the nervous system that governs the heart, involuntary muscles, and glands.

AUTOSOMAL DOMINANT. A pattern of genetic inheritance where only one abnormal gene is needed to display the trait or disease.

AVERSANT. A chemical or medication with unpleasant effects that is used to deter a person from engaging in a specific activity; used in aversion therapy.

AVERSION. A strong feeling of unpleasantness, dislike, or disgust toward a certain object or activity.

AVERSION THERAPY. An approach to treatment in which an unpleasant or painful stimulus is linked to a behavior in order to condition the patient to dislike or avoid the behavior.

AXON. The long extension of a nerve fiber that generally conducts impulses away from the body of the nerve cell.

AYURVEDIC MEDICINE. The traditional medical system of India. Ayurvedic treatments include specialized diets, exercises, herbal treatments, meditation, massage, and breathing techniques.

B

BACK-UP REINFORCER. In a token economy system, a desirable item, privilege, or activity that is purchased with tokens and that serves as a delayed reward and as motivation to display a target (desired) behavior (which is how tokens are earned).

BACTERICIDAL. An agent that destroys bacteria (e.g., *Staphylococci aureus, Streptococci pneumoniae, Escherichia coli, Salmonella enteritidis*).

BARBITURATES. A class of medications that cause sedation and drowsiness. They may be prescribed legally but are also used as drugs of abuse.

BASAL GANGLIA. Masses of gray matter located in the cerebral hemispheres of the brain that control movement as well as some aspects of emotion and cognition.

BASELINE DATA. Information regarding the frequency and severity of behavior, gathered before treatment begins.

BATTERY. A number of separate items (such as tests) used together. In psychology, refers to a group or series of tests given with a common purpose, such as personality assessment or measurement of intelligence.

BEHAVIOR DISORDERS. Disorders characterized by disruptive behaviors, such as conduct disorder, oppositional defiant disorder, and attention deficit hyperactivity disorder.

BEHAVIOR MODIFICATION. An approach to therapy based on the principles of operant conditioning. Behavior modification seeks to replace undesirable behaviors with preferable behaviors through the use of positive or negative reinforcement.

BEHAVIORAL. Related to the way a person acts.

BEHAVIORAL CONTRACT. A behavioral contract is a written agreement that defines the behaviors to be performed and the consequences of the specified behaviors.

BEHAVIORAL COUPLES THERAPY (BCT). Traditional behavioral couples therapy (TBCT); relationship therapy based on behavioral psychology models.

BEHAVIORAL HEALTH. A broad term for any condition related in any way to mental health.

BEHAVIORAL INHIBITION. A set of behaviors that appear in early infancy and that are displayed when the child is confronted with a new situation or unfamiliar people. These behaviors include agitated movement, crying, and general irritability, followed by withdrawing from the situation and seeking comfort from a familiar person. Such behaviors are associated with an increased risk of social phobia and panic disorder in later life. Behavioral inhibition in children appears to be linked to anxiety and mood disorders in their parents.

BEHAVIORAL MEDICINE. The branch of medicine that studies mind-body relationships.

BEHAVIORAL THERAPY. An approach to treatment that focuses on learning how to replace an undesirable behavior with a desired behavior.

(LA) BELLE INDIFFÉRENCE. A psychiatric symptom sometimes found in patients with conversion disorder, in which the patient shows a surprising lack of concern about the nature or implications of his or her physical symptom(s).

BEM SEX ROLE INVENTORY (BSRI). A 60-item self-administered test that researchers often use to measure psychological androgyny in test subjects. It was devised in 1971 by Sandra Bem.

BENIGN PROSTATE HYPERTROPHY. Enlargement of the prostate gland.

BENZENE. A colorless toxic liquid with a chemical formula of C_6H_6, where C stands for carbon and H for hydrogen.

BENZODIAZEPINES. A group of central nervous system depressants used to relieve anxiety or to induce sleep.

BEREAVEMENT. The emotional experience of loss after the death of a friend or relative.

BETA BLOCKERS. Drugs that block beta-adrenergic receptors in the central nervous system, reducing the action of adrenaline, the body's natural fight-or-flight chemical. When these sites are blocked, heart rate, blood pressure, and anxiety levels decrease.

BETA-AMYLOID PLAQUES. Senile plaques; structures in the brain, composed of dead or dying nerve cells and cell debris surrounding deposits of beta-amyloid protein, that are diagnostic of Alzheimer's disease. Beta-amyloid forms when amyloid precursor protein (APP) is not broken down properly.

BEZOAR. A hard ball of hair or vegetable fiber that may develop in the stomach of humans as the result of ingesting nonfood items.

BIAS. A point of view, preference, or judgment.

BIBLIOTHERAPY. The use of books (usually self-help or problem-solving) to improve understanding of personal problems and/or to heal painful feelings.

BILE. A substance produced by the liver and concentrated and stored in the gallbladder. Bile contains a number of different substances, including bile salts, cholesterol, and bilirubin.

BINGE DRINKING. Consumption of multiple alcoholic beverages in a short time frame, with the goal of intoxication.

BINGEING. An excessive amount of food consumed in a short period of time. Usually, while a person binge eats, he or she feels disconnected from reality and feels unable to stop. The bingeing may temporarily relieve depression or anxiety, but after the binge, the person usually feels guilty and depressed.

BIOFEEDBACK. A technique in which patients learn to control certain body functions, such as temperature or pulse rate, in response to external stimuli, such as stress.

BIOFIELD THERAPIES. A subgroup of energy therapies that make use of energy fields (biofields) thought to exist within or emanate from the human body. Biofield therapies include such approaches as Reiki, therapeutic touch, qigong, and polarity balancing.

BIOLOGICAL MARKER. An indicator or characteristic trait of a disease that facilitates differential diagnosis (the process of distinguishing one disorder from other similar disorders).

BIOLOGICAL PSYCHIATRY. An approach to psychiatry that attributes mental disorders to biochemical or other biological malfunctions of the central nervous system, rather than factors such as environment or experience; it tends to favor drug treatments for mental disorders rather than psychotherapies.

BIOPSY. The surgical removal and microscopic examination of living tissue for diagnostic purposes.

BIOPSYCHOSOCIAL HISTORY. A history of experiences and other factors that influence behavior, including medical, educational, occupational, and interpersonal histories, as well as any alcohol or drug use or criminal activity.

BIOPSYCHOSOCIAL MODEL. An approach to human health that holds that a combination of biological, psychological, and social factors should be taken into account when evaluating a patient, rather than physical factors alone.

BIOSOCIAL. A psychological model that asserts that both social and biological factors contribute toward the development of personality.

BIPOLAR DEPRESSION. Depression with the presence of at least one manic episode.

BIPOLAR DISORDER. A mood disorder marked by alternating episodes of extremely low mood (depression) and exuberant highs (mania); formerly known as manic-depressive disorder.

BLADDER. A muscular sac in the lower abdomen that holds urine until it is discharged from the body.

BLENDED FAMILY. A family formed by the remarriage of a divorced or widowed parent. It includes a new husband and wife, plus some or all of their children from previous marriages.

BLOGGING. Creating and maintaining an online personal blog, in most cases allowing readers to add comments. The term comes from the word weblog, or online diary.

BLOOD ALCOHOL CONCENTRATION OR CONTENT (BAC). A measure of the amount of alcohol in the body; in most states, legal alcohol intoxication is defined as a BAC of at least 0.08 grams per deciliter of blood.

BLOOD-BRAIN BARRIER. A specialized, semi-permeable layer of cells around the blood vessels in the brain that controls which substances can leave the circulatory system and enter the brain.

BLUNTED AFFECT. A lack of display of emotion or feelings, including monotone voice and expressionless face.

BODY DYSMORPHIC DISORDER. A psychiatric disorder marked by preoccupation with an imagined physical defect.

BODY IMAGE. A person's perceptions of, beliefs about, and emotional attitudes toward his or her body.

BODY MASS INDEX, OR BMI. A measure of body fat, calculated as weight in kilograms over the square of height in meters.

BODYWORK. Any technique involving hands-on massage or manipulation of the body.

BORDERLINE PERSONALITY DISORDER. A severe and usually lifelong mental disorder characterized by violent mood swings and severe difficulties in sustaining interpersonal relationships.

BOTULINUM TOXIN. Any of a group of potent bacterial toxins or poisons produced by different strains of the bacterium *Clostridium botulinum*. The toxins cause muscle paralysis and force the relaxation of a muscle in spasm.

BRADYCARDIA. Slow heartbeat, defined as a rate of less than 60 beats per minute.

BRAIN STEM. The part of the brain consisting of the midbrain, pons, and medulla oblongata. The brain stem connects the forebrain and cerebrum to the spinal cord and regulates heart and respiratory function, the sleep cycle, and the nerves that convey sensory information to the face and neck.

BRAIN-DERIVED NEUROTROPHIC FACTOR (BDNF). A brain protein that helps maintain nerves and promotes the growth of new nerve cells (neurons).

BRIEF PSYCHOTIC DISORDER. An acute, short-term episode of psychosis lasting no longer than one month. This disorder may occur in response to a stressful event.

BRONCHIOLES. Tiny tubes in the lungs.

BRUXISM. Habitual, often unconscious, grinding of the teeth.

BULIMIA NERVOSA. A serious eating disorder characterized by compulsive overeating followed by purging, usually by way of self-induced vomiting or the use of laxatives or diuretics.

BULLYCIDE. Suicide attributed to the victim's having been bullied.

BUPRENORPHINE. A medication that blocks some of the withdrawal effects during heroin detoxification.

BURNOUT. An emotional condition marked by fatigue, loss of interest in a job or activity, or frustration. Burnout is usually regarded as the result of prolonged stress.

C

CACHEXIA. Physical wasting and malnutrition, usually from chronic disease.

CAGE. A four-question assessment used to detect alcoholism.

CAPD. Central auditory processing disorder; the inability to differentiate, recognize, or understand sounds, though hearing and intelligence are normal.

CARCINOID SYNDROME. The pattern of symptoms (often including asthma and diarrhea) associated with carcinoid tumors of the digestive tract or lungs.

CARMINATIVE. A medication or preparation that prevents the formation of intestinal gas or allows it to be expelled.

CARRIER OIL. An oil used to dilute essential oils for use in massage and other skin care applications.

CASE MANAGER. A professional who designs and monitors implementation of comprehensive care plans for individuals seeking mental health or social services.

CASTRATION. Desexing a person or animal by surgical removal of the testes (in males) or ovaries (in females).

CATAPLEXY. Sudden episode of muscle weakness (often causing a person to fall), usually triggered by intense emotion. It is regarded as a diagnostic sign of narcolepsy.

CATATONIA. Psychomotor disturbances that can include stupor, rigidity, muteness, or purposeless and bizarre movements.

CATATONIC SCHIZOPHRENIA. Schizophrenia accompanied by catatonic symptoms.

CATECHOLAMINES. A set of neurotransmitters released by the hypothalamic-pituitary-adrenal system in the brain in response to acute stress. The catecholamines include dopamine, norepinephrine, and epinephrine.

CATHA EDULIS. Leaves of an East African bush that can be chewed for their stimulant effect.

CATHARSIS. A powerful emotional release, usually preceded by emotional tension and followed by a feeling of great relief.

CATHETERIZATION. Placing a tube in the bladder so that it can be emptied of urine.

CELL. The smallest living unit of the body, which groups together with other cells to form tissues and help the body perform specific functions.

CENTRAL NERVOUS SYSTEM. The part of the nervous system that includes the brain and spinal cord.

CENTRAL NERVOUS SYSTEM DEPRESSANT. Any drug that lowers the level of stimulation or excitement in the central nervous system.

CENTRAL NERVOUS SYSTEM STIMULANT. Any drug that raises the level of activity in the central nervous system.

CEREBELLUM. The part of the brain between the brain stem and back of the cerebrum, consisting of two lateral lobes and a median lobe and involved especially in muscle coordination and maintenance of bodily equilibrium.

CEREBRAL CORTEX. The convoluted gray matter on the surface of the cerebrum that coordinates motor and sensory information and cognitive function.

CEREBRAL PALSY. A movement disorder caused by a permanent brain defect or injury present at birth or shortly after. It is frequently associated with premature birth. Cerebral palsy is not progressive, meaning that it does not worsen with age.

CEREBROSPINAL FLUID (CSF). The fluid that circulates through the central nervous system to maintain uniform pressure on the brain and spinal cord.

CEREBRUM. The largest area of the brain, consisting of the two cerebral hemispheres and connecting structures. The cerebrum is responsible for conscious mental processes, including movement and language.

CERULOPLASMIN. A protein circulating in the bloodstream that binds with and transports copper.

CERVIX. The neck or narrow lower end of a woman's uterus.

CHAKRA. One of the seven major energy centers in the body, according to traditional Indian yoga.

CHARACTER. An individual's set of emotional, cognitive, and behavioral patterns learned and accumulated over time.

CHARLES BONNET SYNDROME (CBS). A disorder characterized by visual hallucinations following a sudden age-related deterioration in a person's vision, most commonly glaucoma or macular degeneration. CBS is named for a Swiss doctor who first described it in his visually impaired grandfather in 1780.

CHELATION THERAPY. A method of treating heavy metal poisoning by giving medications that remove heavy metals from the bloodstream. The medications that are used are called chelating agents.

CHI. The traditional Chinese term for vital energy or the life force. The word is also spelled "ki" or "qi" in English translations of Japanese and Chinese medical books.

CHOLESTEROL. A steroid alcohol in cells and body fluids that serves as a precursor for hormones and other steroids.

CHOLINESTERASE INHIBITORS. Drugs that may slow the progression of Alzheimer's disease by inhibiting the enzymes that break down the neurotransmitter acetylcholine.

CHOREATHETOID MOVEMENTS. Repetitive dance-like movements that do not have any type of rhythm.

CHORIONIC VILLUS SAMPLING (CVS). A prenatal test that involves taking a small sample of the placenta, the organ that forms inside the uterus during pregnancy and supplies the baby with oxygen and nutrients carried by the blood. The placental tissue is then tested for chromosome abnormalities or other genetic diseases.

CHROMOSOME. A microscopic thread-like structure found within each cell of the body that consists of proteins and DNA. Humans have 46 chromosomes arranged into 23 pairs. Changes in either the total number of chromosomes or their shape and size (structure) may lead to physical or mental abnormalities.

CHRONIC. A disease or condition that progresses slowly but persists or reoccurs over time.

CHRONOTHERAPY. A sleep disorder treatment that involves adjusting sleep and wake times to help reset the patient's biological clock.

CIMETIDINE. A drug that decreases the amount of acid in the stomach, used to treat conditions such as ulcers, gastroesophageal reflux disease, and heartburn.

CIRCADIAN RHYTHM. Any physiological, mental, or behavioral activity that recurs in 24-hour cycles. The sleep-wake cycle is an example of a circadian rhythm.

CIRRHOSIS. A chronic degenerative disease of the liver, in which normal cells are replaced by fibrous tissue. Cirrhosis is a major risk factor for the later development of liver cancer.

CIVIL COMMITMENT. The involuntary confinement of persons who cannot care for themselves, as determined by a court of law.

CLASSICAL CONDITIONING. In psychology, a process in which a previously neutral stimulus eventually produces a specific response by being paired repeatedly with another stimulus that produces that response. The best-known example of classical conditioning is Pavlov's dogs, who were conditioned to salivate when they heard a bell ring (the previously neutral stimulus) because the sound had been paired repeatedly with their feeding time.

CLEFT PALATE. A failure of the two sides of the palate within the mouth to meet during fetal development.

CLINICAL. Pertaining to or founded on observation and treatment of participants, as distinguished from theoretical or basic science.

CLINICAL TRIAL. A controlled scientific experiment designed to investigate the effectiveness of a drug or treatment in curing or lessening the symptoms of a disease or disorder.

CLITORIS. The most sensitive area of the external genitals. Stimulation of the clitoris causes most women to reach orgasm.

CLONUS. Muscular spasm involving repeated, rhythmic contractions. Clonus may be spontaneous or inducible and may involve major body muscles or eye muscles.

CLOSED-HEAD INJURY. A head injury in which the skull is not cracked or fractured.

CLOZAPINE. An atypical antipsychotic medication used to treat schizophrenia. Clozapine is often given to patients who are not seeing improvement with other medications or who are developing adverse side effects (such as tardive dyskinesia).

CLUSTER SUICIDE. Refers to the phenomenon of additional suicides being attempted or completed after one suicide has occurred within a small community, such as a high school.

COGNITION. Conscious intellectual activity, including thinking, imagining, reasoning, remembering, and learning.

COGNITIVE. Associated with conscious intellectual activity.

COGNITIVE DISSONANCE. A conflict of anxiety resulting from the difference in personal beliefs and actions.

COGNITIVE PROCESSING THERAPY. A term that is sometimes used for the cognitive restructuring aspect of cognitive-behavioral therapy, especially in treatment for post-traumatic stress disorder (PTSD).

COGNITIVE RESTRUCTURING. An approach to psychotherapy that focuses on helping clients examine distorted patterns of perceiving and thinking in order to change their emotional responses to people and situations.

COGNITIVE STYLE. The way in which individuals process and use information to perform cognitive tasks, such as reasoning, learning, thinking, understanding, making decisions, and using memory.

COGNITIVE THERAPY. A form of psychotherapy that focuses on changing clients' emotional reactions by correcting distorted patterns of thinking and perception.

COGNITIVE-BEHAVIORAL THERAPY (CBT). A type of psychotherapy in which people learn to recognize and change negative and self-defeating patterns of thinking and behavior.

COITUS. Sexual intercourse.

COLD TURKEY. A slang term for suddenly and completely stopping the use of a substance or engagement in an activity.

COLIC. Excessive crying and irritability in babies, which may be caused by numerous problems such as stomach discomfort.

COMA. A state of prolonged unconsciousness.

COMBAT STRESS REACTION. A general term for mental health symptoms experienced after combat, such as depression, fatigue, dissociative symptoms, lack of concentration, or irritability. It is not identical to post-traumatic stress disorder (PTSD) but may be a precursor of it.

COMMAND HALLUCINATION. A type of auditory hallucination in which a person hears voices ordering him or her to perform a specific act.

COMMUNITY MENTAL HEALTH CENTERS. Organizations that manage and deliver a comprehensive range of mental health services, education, and outreach to residents of a given community.

COMMUNITY MENTAL HEALTH CENTERS ACT OF 1963. Federal legislation that provides grants for the operation of community mental health centers and related services.

COMMUNITY MENTAL HEALTH CLINIC (CMHC). A community-based provider of mental health services.

COMMUNITY-BASED. Used to describe any organization or initiative stemming from non-government, local, and independent sources.

COMORBID PSYCHOPATHOLOGY. The presence of other mental disorders in a patient together with a primary disorder that is the immediate focus of therapy.

COMORBIDITY. The presence of one or more diseases or disorders in a patient in addition to a primary disease or disorder.

COMPLIANCE. Adherence to a treatment plan or medication regimen.

COMPLICATED GRIEF. An abnormal response to bereavement that includes unrelieved yearning for the deceased, the total loss of positive beliefs or worldview, and general dysfunction.

COMPULSION. A strong impulse to perform an act, particularly one that is irrational or contrary to a person's disposition.

COMPULSIVE GAMBLING DISORDER. An impulse control disorder in which an individual cannot resist gambling despite repeated losses.

COMPUTED TOMOGRAPHY. An imaging technique in which cross-sectional x rays of the body are compiled to create a three-dimensional image of the body's internal structures; also referred to as a CT or CAT scan.

CONCHA. The hollow shell-shaped portion of the external ear nearest the ear canal.

CONCUSSION. Injury to the brain causing a sudden but temporary impairment of brain function.

CONDUCT DISORDER. A behavioral and emotional disorder of childhood and adolescence in which children display physical aggression and infringe on or violate the rights of others. Youths diagnosed with conduct disorder may set fires, exhibit cruelty toward animals or other children, sexually assault others, or lie and steal for personal gain.

CONFABULATION. Using false or imagined details to explain physical phenomena or to fill in memory gaps.

CONFLICT RESOLUTION. Various methods used by psychologists and other such professionals to eliminate sources of conflict in clients.

CONGENITAL. Present at birth.

CONSERVATOR. Legal guardian.

CONTACT DERMATITIS. Skin irritation as a result of contact with a foreign substance.

CONTRACEPTIVE. Birth control; an object or medication intended to prevent conception and pregnancy.

CONTRECOUP. An injury to the brain opposite the point of direct impact.

CONTROL GROUP. A group in a research study that does not receive the treatment being tested. For example, in an experiment testing the effectiveness of a new drug, the control group might receive the current drug of choice while the experimental group receives the new drug under investigation.

CONTUSION. A focal area of swollen and bleeding brain tissue.

CONVERSION. In psychiatry, a process in which a repressed feeling, impulse, thought, or memory emerges in the form of a bodily symptom.

CONVERSION DISORDER. A type of somatoform disorder in which unconscious psychological conflicts or other factors manifest as physical symptoms.

CONVULSION. An uncontrollable motion of a limb of the body or the body itself.

CO-OCCURRING DISORDERS. Sets of mental illnesses—usually substance abuse and at least one other disorder—that appear together in a single individual.

Also referred to as dual diagnosis or co-morbidity disorders.

COPING. In psychology, a term that refers to how a person responds to stress.

COPROLALIA. A vocal tic characterized by the uttering of obscene, hostile, or inappropriate words.

COPROPRAXIA. A motor tic characterized by the display of unacceptable or obscene gestures.

COROLLARY DISCHARGE. A mechanism in the brain that allows persons to distinguish between self-generated and external stimuli or perceptions.

CORONARY OCCLUSION. Blockage of the arteries supplying the blood to the heart.

CORPORA CAVERNOSA. The pair of columns of erectile tissue on either side of the penis that, together with the corpus spongiosum, produce an erection when filled with blood.

CORPUS CALLOSUM (PLURAL, CORPORA CALLOSA). A thick bundle of nerve fibers lying deep in the brain that connects the two cerebral hemispheres and coordinates their functions.

CORPUS SPONGIOSUM. The column of erectile tissue in the penis that contains the urethra.

CORTEX. The outer layer of the cerebrum in the brain, where sensation and perception are processed and integrated into thoughts, memories, and abilities and where actions are planned and initiated.

CORTICAL. Regarding the cortex, or the outer layer of the brain.

CORTICOSTEROID. A steroid hormone produced by the adrenal gland and involved in metabolism and immune response.

CORTICOSTEROID DRUG. A medication that acts like a type of hormone (cortisol) produced by the adrenal gland of the body. Corticosteroid drugs (also just called steroids) help treat inflammation, infection, or trauma to the body.

CORTISOL. A steroid hormone produced by the adrenal gland that is released in response to stress. Cortisol suppresses the immune system and slows down bone formation.

COVERT. Concealed, hidden, or disguised.

COVERT SENSITIZATION OR CONDITIONING. A form of aversion therapy in which a patient imagines or views images of an undesirable behavior, followed by imagining or viewing images of an aversive (negative) consequence.

C-REACTIVE PROTEIN (CRP). A protein whose levels in blood rise rapidly in response to inflammation. It can be measured to test for the presence of inflammation and response to treatment; it is also used as a rough indication of a patient's risk of heart disease.

CREATINE. A nitrogen-containing substance found in muscle.

CREUTZFELDT-JAKOB DISEASE. A degenerative disease of the central nervous system caused by a prion, or "slow virus."

CRIMINAL JUSTICE SYSTEM. The system instituted by federal, state, and local governments to control and deter crime and to punish persons who violate laws.

CRIMINALIZATION. The de facto societal trend over several decades of sending people with mental disabilities to jails and prisons instead of to treatment institutions.

CRITICAL INCIDENT. An event that is stressful enough to overwhelm the coping skills of a person or group; also known as a "crisis event."

CROSS-DRESSING. Wearing clothes and other accessories associated with the opposite sex.

CUE. Any behavior or event in a person's environment that stimulates a particular response. For example, the smell of liquor may be a cue for some people to pour themselves a drink.

CYBERBULLYING. The use of electronic devices, including computers, cell phones, and other mobile devices, to bully by means of hurtful messages, spreading rumors, or misusing social media.

CYCLIC AMP. A small molecule of adenosine monophosphate (AMP) that activates enzymes and increases the effects of hormones and other neurotransmitters.

CYCLOTHYMIA. A milder form of bipolar disorder characterized by alternating hypomania and less severe depressive episodes.

CYCLOTHYMIC DISORDER. A mood disorder in which hypomanic episodes and depressive episodes both occur over the course of at least two years, with symptom-free periods lasting no more than two months.

CYTOCHROME P450 (CYP450). Enzymes present in the liver that metabolize drugs.

CYTOGENETICS. The branch of genetics concerned with the structure and function of the individual cell, particularly its chromosome content.

CYTOKINE. Any of a group of small protein molecules (including interferon, interleukin, and tumor necrosis factor) secreted by certain cells in the immune system that modulate specific functions associated with the immune response.

D

D1, D2, ETC. Dopamine receptor proteins.

DAWN SIMULATION. A form of light therapy in which the patient is exposed while asleep to gradually brightening white light over a period of an hour and a half.

DE FACTO. Acting as; fulfilling a role, even though the occupation of the role is not legally recognized.

DECISION TREE. A decision support model used in medical and psychiatric diagnosis that consists of a tree-like chart or diagram listing various symptoms, tentative diagnoses, and diagnostic decisions and their possible consequences.

DECOCTION. An herbal extract produced by mixing an herb with cold water, bringing the mixture to a boil, and letting it simmer to evaporate the excess water. Decoction is usually chosen over infusion when the botanical or herb in question is a root, seed, or berry.

DECONDITIONING. Loss of physical strength or stamina resulting from bed rest or lack of exercise.

DECREASED PENETRANCE. Individuals who inherit a changed disease gene but do not develop symptoms.

DEFENSE. An unconscious mental process that protects the conscious mind from unacceptable or painful thoughts, impulses, or desires. Examples of defenses include denial, rationalization, projection, and repression.

DEFENSE MECHANISMS. Indirect strategies used to reduce anxiety rather than directly facing the issues causing the anxiety.

DEINSTITUTIONALIZATION. A movement to close public mental institutions and transfer patients to community treatment programs, with the goal of better serving people with mental disabilities. The movement shifted the responsibility for care from large (often governmental) agencies to families and community organizations.

DELIRIUM. A disturbance of consciousness marked by confusion, difficulty paying attention, delusions, hallucinations, or restlessness. It can be distinguished from other conditions by its relatively sudden onset and variation in the severity of the symptoms.

DELUSION. A false belief that persists despite evidence to the contrary.

DELUSIONAL DISORDER. A mental illness characterized by the presence of nonbizarre delusions (situations that could occur in real life) in the absence of other mood or psychotic symptoms.

DELUSIONAL DISORDER OF THE PERSECUTORY TYPE. A psychotic disorder characterized by a patient's belief that others are conspiring against him or her.

DEMENTIA. A disease characterized by the progressive deterioration of intellectual functions, such as memory, reasoning, and language. Other symptoms include changes in personality, deterioration in personal grooming, and disorientation. Alzheimer's disease is a type of dementia.

DEMENTIA PUGILISTICA. A delayed-onset form of dementia caused by repeated head injury; often occurs in boxers.

DENDRITES. Fibers of a brain cell that receive signals from other brain cells.

DENIAL. A psychological defense mechanism that reduces anxiety by excluding recognition of a problem or stressor from the conscious mind.

DEOXYRIBONUCLEIC ACID (DNA). The genetic material in cells that holds the inherited instructions for growth, development, and cellular functioning.

DEPENDENCE. A state in which a person requires a steady concentration of a particular substance in order to avoid withdrawal symptoms.

DEPENDENT PERSONALITY DISORDER. Personality disorder characterized by a constant, unhealthy need to be liked and appreciated by others at all costs.

DEPERSONALIZATION. A dissociative symptom in which a patient feels that his or her body is unreal, is changing, or is dissolving.

DEPERSONALIZATION NEUROSIS. Another name for depersonalization disorder.

DEPRESSANT. Any psychoactive substance that lowers the function or activity level of a specific part of the body or brain. Depressants are sometimes referred to as "downers." These include anxiolytics, sedatives, antipsychotics, opioids, and anesthetics as well as such nonprescription substances as alcohol.

DEPRESSED SKULL FRACTURE. A fracture in which fragment pieces of broken skull press into brain tissue.

DEPRESSION. A mental state characterized by excessive sadness and loss of interest in life; other symptoms may include altered sleep or eating patterns, loss of concentration, agitation, lack of energy, and, in severe cases, attempts at self-harm or suicide.

DEREALIZATION. A dissociative symptom in which a person's external environment is perceived as unreal or dreamlike.

DERMATITIS ARTEFACTA. A disorder characterized by the deliberate and conscious self-infliction of skin lesions.

DERMATOLOGIST. A physician who specializes in the diagnosis and treatment of disorders of the skin, scalp, hair, and nails.

DESENSITIZATION. The reduction or elimination of an overly intense reaction to a cue, achieved by controlled repeated exposures to the cue.

DESIGNER AMPHETAMINES. Substances close in chemical structure to classic amphetamines that provide both stimulant and hallucinogenic effects.

DETOXIFICATION. A process in which toxins (including drugs and alcohol) are eliminated from the body. In cases of substance abuse, the symptoms of withdrawal may be treated concurrently.

DEVELOPMENTAL. Referring to human development.

DEVELOPMENTAL DAMAGE. A term that some therapists prefer to personality disorder, on the grounds that it is more respectful of the patient's capacity for growth and change.

DEVELOPMENTAL DISABILITIES. Disabilities that are present from birth and that delay or prevent normal development, such as intellectual disability or autism.

DEVOTEE. With regard to body integrity identity disorder, someone who is sexually attracted to amputees or disabled persons.

DIABETES. Also called diabetes mellitus, a disease characterized by an inability to process sugars in the diet, due to a decrease in or total absence of insulin production. Type 1 diabetes (juvenile diabetes) involves failure of the body to produce insulin, while type 2 diabetes (adult-onset diabetes) involves failure of the body's cells to use insulin properly.

DIABETIC NEUROPATHY. Condition existing in people with diabetes in which their nerve endings, particularly in the legs and feet, become less sensitive. Minor injuries, such as blisters or callouses, are not felt and can thus become infected and develop into more serious problems.

***DIAGNOSTIC AND STATISTICAL MANUAL OF MENTAL DISORDERS* (DSM).** The handbook published by the American Psychiatric Association that mental health professionals use to diagnose mental disorders.

DIALECTICAL BEHAVIOR THERAPY (DBT). A type of cognitive-behavioral therapy designed specifically to treat borderline personality disorder.

DIATHESIS. The medical term for predisposition.

DIENCEPHALON. The "between brain" or "interbrain," located beneath the cerebral hemispheres and consisting of the thalamus and hypothalamus.

DIFFERENTIAL DIAGNOSIS. Comparing and contrasting the signs, symptoms, and laboratory findings of two or more diseases to determine which is causing a patient's condition.

DIFFERENTIATION. The ability to retain one's identity within a family system while maintaining emotional connections with the other members.

DIFFUSE AXONAL INJURY (DAI). Traumatic damage to individual nerve cells resulting in breakdown of overall communication between nerve cells in the brain; also called a shear injury.

DIFFUSION TENSOR IMAGING (DTI). A refinement of magnetic resonance imaging (MRI) that allows doctors to measure the flow of water and track the pathways of white matter in the brain. DTI can detect abnormalities in the brain that do not show up on standard MRI scans.

DIGRAPH. A pair of letters that represents a single speech sound. In English, the *th* in "thumb" and the *ei* in "vein" are examples of digraphs.

DIMINISHED CAPACITY. The inability of a person to understand the nature of his or her behavior when committing a criminal act.

DIPLOPIA. A disorder of vision in which a single object appears double (double vision).

DISENFRANCHISED GRIEF. Grief that is not openly expressed because the bereavement cannot be publicly acknowledged.

DISFLUENCY. Any difficulty in fluent speech, including stuttering.

DISINGENUOUS. Insincere, deceitful, dishonest.

DISORDER OF SEX DEVELOPMENT (DSD). The term that is increasingly preferred for an atypical pattern of chromosomal, genital, or gonadal development; also known as disorder of sex differentiation.

DISRUPTIVE BEHAVIOR DISORDER. A broader term that includes two similar disorders: oppositional defiant disorder and conduct disorder.

DISSOCIATION. A psychological mechanism in which the mind splits off certain aspects of an event (usually traumatic) from conscious awareness. Dissociation can affect the person's memory, sense of reality, and sense of identity.

DISSOCIATIVE AMNESIA. A dissociative disorder characterized by loss of memory for a period or periods of time in a person's life; may occur as a result of a traumatic event.

DISSOCIATIVE DISORDERS. Medical disorders characterized by disruptions or breakdowns of awareness, identity, memory, and/or perception.

DISSOCIATIVE IDENTITY DISORDER (DID). Also called multiple personality disorder, a mental condition in which a person displays multiple distinct personalities (alter egos).

DISULFIRAM. A medication that helps reinforce abstinence in people who are recovering from alcohol abuse. If a person taking disulfiram (Antabuse) drinks even a small amount of alcohol, he or she experiences facial flushing, headache, nausea, and vomiting.

DIURETIC. A substance that removes water from the body by increasing urine production.

DNA (DEOXYRIBONUCLEIC ACID). The hereditary material that makes up genes and influences the development and functioning of the body.

DNA METHYLATION. The imprinting process of introducing methyl into a gene, suppressing its usual function.

DO NOT RESUSCITATE ORDER (DNR). A directive specifying that if a patient's heart stops, he or she should not receive cardiopulmonary resuscitation (CPR).

DONEPEZIL HYDROCHLORIDE. A drug that increases the levels of acetylcholine in the brain; sold under the trade name Aricept.

DOPAMINE. A chemical in brain tissue that serves to transmit nerve impulses (a neurotransmitter) and helps to regulate movement, emotions, concentration, impulse control, judgment, attention span, and psychostimulation; may be involved in disease states such as addiction, ADHD, and depression.

DOPAMINE AGONIST. A drug that binds to dopamine receptors and produces effects that are similar to dopamine.

DOPAMINE ANTAGONIST. A substance that binds to dopamine receptors, preventing dopamine from binding and triggering its response.

DOUBLE ANXIETY. Acute anxiety from a recent stressful event combined with underlying persistent anxiety associated with generalized anxiety disorder.

DOUBLE-BLIND PLACEBO-CONTROLLED STUDY. A study in which patients are divided into two groups—those who will receive a medication, and those who will receive a placebo (a pill that looks like the medication but has no active ingredients). Neither the patients nor their physicians know which pill any specific patient is receiving.

DOUBLE-BLIND STUDY. A research study in which neither the participants nor the researchers know whether the subjects are receiving the experimental treatment or a placebo or control treatment.

DOWN SYNDROME. A genetic disorder characterized by an extra chromosome 21 (trisomy 21), intellectual disability, and susceptibility to early-onset Alzheimer's disease.

DREAM ANXIETY DISORDER. Another name for nightmare disorder.

DRUG ABUSE. Repeated use of controlled substances, prescription or over-the-counter drugs, or alcohol despite damage to personal health, thought processes, relationships, or functioning at work or school; also, using a substance for purposes other than which it is intended.

DSM. *Diagnostic and Statistical Manual of Mental Disorders.*

DYANA. The yoga term for meditation.

DYSARTHRIA. Difficulty talking and speaking caused by impairment of the muscles used in speech, often as a result of damage to the brain or nerves.

DYSCALCULIA. Difficulty in performing mathematical computations; also called mathematical learning disorder.

DYSFUNCTIONAL. Degraded ability or inability to function emotionally.

DYSGRAPHIA. A writing disorder characterized by illegible handwriting.

DYSKINESIA. Difficulty in performing voluntary muscular movements.

DYSLEXIA. A variable learning disability that is usually characterized by difficulty reading, writing, and spelling; also called developmental reading disorder (DRD) or specific reading disability.

DYSMENORRHEA. Painful menstruation.

DYSPAREUNIA. Painful sexual intercourse.

DYSPHORIA. A persistent mood of sadness, discomfort, or general unease. The English word comes from two Greek words meaning "difficult" or "hard" and "to bear."

DYSPRAXIA. Developmental dyspraxia is an impairment or immaturity of the organization of movement. It is a defect in the way the brain processes information, resulting in messages not being correctly or fully transmitted. The term dyspraxia comes from the word "praxis," meaning "doing" or "acting." Dyspraxia is associated with problems of perception, language, and thought.

DYSSOMNIA. A type of sleep disorder characterized by problems with the amount, quality, or timing of sleep.

DYSTHYMIA. A less severe but chronic (ongoing) form of depression.

DYSTHYMIC DISORDER. A mood disorder that is less severe than depression but usually more chronic.

DYSTONIA. A neurological disorder characterized by involuntary muscle spasms. The spasms can cause a painful twisting of the body and difficulty walking or moving.

E

EATING DISORDERS. Psychological disorders characterized by disturbances in eating patterns, abnormal attitudes toward food, and unhealthy efforts to control weight. Types of eating disorders include anorexia nervosa, binge eating disorder, and bulimia nervosa.

ECHOLALIA. Involuntary repeating the last word, phrase, or sentence spoken by someone else (or heard in the surrounding environment).

ECHOPRAXIA. The imitation of the movement of another individual.

ECSTASY. A drug that produces both stimulant and hallucinogenic effects; also known as MDMA.

EGO. In Freudian psychology, the conscious, rational part of the mind that experiences and reacts to the outside world.

EGO-SYNTONIC. Consistent with one's sense of self, as opposed to ego-alien or dystonic (foreign to one's sense of self).

EJACULATION. The discharge of semen by the male reproductive organs.

ELECTROCARDIOGRAM (EKG). A test that measures the electrical activity of the heart as it beats. An abnormal EKG can indicate possible cardiac disease.

ELECTROCONVULSIVE THERAPY (ECT). A psychological treatment in which a series of controlled electrical impulses are delivered to the brain in order to induce a seizure. ECT is used to treat major depression and severe mental illnesses that do not respond to other forms of treatment.

ELECTROENCEPHALOGRAPHY (EEG). A diagnostic test that measures electrical activity in the brain.

ELECTROLYTES. Ions—such as sodium, potassium, calcium, magnesium, chloride, phosphate, bicarbonate, and sulfate—that are dissolved in bodily fluids such as blood and that regulate or affect most metabolic processes.

ELECTROMAGNETIC RADIATION. Radiation including gamma rays, x rays, ultraviolet light, visible light, infrared radiation, microwaves, and radio waves.

ELIMINATION. The medical term for expelling waste from the body.

EMETIC. A medication that causes vomiting.

EMMENAGOGUE. A medication or substance given to bring on a menstrual period.

EMOTIONALLY FOCUSED THERAPY FOR COUPLES (EFT-C). A widely used, evidence-based system of therapy that emphasizes the individual emotions of each partner.

EMPIRICAL. Based on information gathered by scientific observation or experiments, as distinct from pure theory.

ENCEPHALITIS. Inflammation of the brain.

ENCEPHALOPATHY. An abnormality in the structure or function of tissues of the brain.

ENDOCRINE DYSFUNCTION. A problem relating to inadequate or excessive production of hormones.

ENDOGENOUS DEPRESSION. Depression arising from causes within a person, such as chemical or hormonal imbalances.

ENDOMETRIOSIS. A condition in which the tissue that is normally present in the lining of the uterus grows elsewhere in the body.

ENDORPHINS. A group of peptide compounds released by the body in response to stress or traumatic injury; may also be produced during exercise. Endorphins react with opiate receptors in the brain to reduce or relieve pain and improve mood.

ENDOTRACHEAL INTUBATION. The insertion of a flexible tube into the trachea for purposes of anesthesia, airway protection, and mechanical lung ventilation.

ENFLEURAGE. A technique for extracting essential oils from flower petals by placing them on a layer of purified fat.

ENTEROCHROMAFFIN CELLS. Specialized cells in the thin layer of tissue lining the cavity (lumen) of the digestive tract. Also known as Kulchitsky cells, enterochromaffin cells provide about 90% of the human body's supply of serotonin.

ENTRAINMENT. The patterning of body processes and movements to the rhythm of music.

ENURESIS. Involuntary urination.

ENVIRONMENTAL INFLUENCE. Any component of the cause of a behavior or condition that is perceived to be developed from experience.

ENZYMES. Proteins that trigger chemical reactions in the body.

EOSINOPHILIA MYALGIA SYNDROME (EMS). A chronic, painful disease of the immune system that causes joint pain, fatigue, shortness of breath, and swelling of the arms and legs. EMS can be fatal.

EPHEBOPHILIA. Sexual desire on the part of an adult for youths in the early stages of puberty, as distinct from prepubertal children.

EPHEDRINE. An amphetamine-like substance used as a nasal decongestant.

EPICANTHIC FOLD. A fold in the inner corner of the skin of the upper eyelid, found in about half of children with Down syndrome.

EPIDEMIOLOGY. A field of medical science dealing with the incidence, distribution, and control of disease in a population.

EPIDURAL HEMATOMA. Bleeding into the area between the skull and the dura, the tough, outermost brain covering.

EPIGENETICS. The study of heritable changes in an organism's appearance or gene expression, caused by chemical reactions and factors other than changes in the organism's DNA sequences.

EPIGENOME. A collection of chemical compounds (from food, medications, and other sources) that marks the human genome (a person's complete set of DNA) in certain ways, determining whether certain genes will be turned "on" (active) or "off" (inactive).

EPILEPSY. A neurological disorder characterized by recurrent seizures. Seizures are caused by a disturbance in the electrical activity in the brain and can cause loss of consciousness, muscle spasms, rhythmic movements, abnormal sensory experiences, or altered mental states.

EPINEPHRINE. Also known as adrenaline, the hormone secreted by the adrenal glands in response to stress.

EROTOMANIA. The false belief that a person is the object of another person's love or sexual desire.

EROTOMANIC DELUSIONS. Erotomanic delusions involve the mistaken belief that someone is in love with the delusional person. Often, the other person is a public figure of some prominence, such as an actress, rock star, or political figure.

ESSENTIAL OIL. A volatile oil extracted from the leaves, fruit, flowers, roots, or other components of a plant and used in aromatherapy, perfumes, and foods and beverages.

ESSENTIAL TREMOR. An uncontrollable (involuntary) shaking of the hands, head, and face; also called familial tremor if it is inherited.

ESTROGEN. The primary female sex hormone.

ETHANOL. The chemical name for beverage alcohol. It is also sometimes called ethyl alcohol or grain alcohol to distinguish it from isopropyl or rubbing alcohol.

ETHICS. The branch of philosophy that deals with questions of morality (good and evil, right and wrong).

ETIOLOGY. The cause or origin of a disease or disorder. The word is also used to refer to the study of the causes of disease.

EUGEROIC. A type of medication that promotes wakefulness.

EUNUCH. A castrated male, often one castrated at an early age with noticeable hormonal consequences.

EUPHORIA. A feeling or state of well-being or elation.

EUTHANASIA. The act of putting humans or animals to death painlessly or allowing them to die by withholding medical services, usually because of an incurable disease.

EUTHYMIA. A feeling of well-being often associated with individuals with bipolar disorder when they are not having a manic or a depressive episode.

EXCESSIVE DAYTIME SLEEPINESS (EDS). A condition characterized by a persistent sense of mental cloudiness, lack of energy, depressed mood, or extreme state of exhaustion.

EXCORIATION. The medical term for abrasion of the upper layer of skin caused by mechanical means, most often scratching or picking.

EXECUTIVE FUNCTIONS. An umbrella term for the group of mental processes responsible for planning, abstract thinking, logical deduction, self-control, and prioritization.

EXISTENTIAL FACTORS. Realities of life including death, isolation, freedom, and meaninglessness that must be faced by all individuals.

EXPLICIT MEMORY. Consciously recalled memory for facts or events.

EXPOSURE THERAPY. A form of cognitive-behavioral therapy in which individuals with phobias are exposed to their fears while accompanied by the therapist. The length of exposure is gradually increased until the association between the feared situation and the individual's experienced panic symptoms is no longer present.

EXTENDED FAMILY FIELD. A person's family of origin plus grandparents, in-laws, and other relatives.

EXTERNALIZING DISORDERS. Disorders in which a person acts out inner turmoil or conflict on the external environment. The three major characteristics of externalizing disorders are disruptive, hyperactive, and aggressive behaviors.

EXTINCTION. The elimination or removal of a person's reaction to a cue as a result of exposure treatment.

EXTRAPYRAMIDAL. Related to the motor system in the brain.

EXTRAPYRAMIDAL SYMPTOMS (EPS). A group of side effects associated with antipsychotic medications and characterized by involuntary muscle movements, including contraction and tremor.

F

"FACEBOOK DEPRESSION." A term used to describe a mood disorder associated with low self-esteem and depressed mood triggered by excessive concern with online social media.

FACTITIOUS DISEASES. Conditions in which symptoms are deliberately manufactured by patients in order to gain attention and sympathy. Patients with factitious diseases do not fake symptoms for obvious financial gain or to evade the legal system.

FACTITIOUS DISORDER. A false or exaggerated disorder in which the physical or psychological symptoms are controlled or produced by the patient.

FADING. In a token economy system, refers to gradually decreasing the amount or frequency of a reinforcer so that the target behavior will begin to occur independent of any rewards.

FAIR HOUSING ACT OF 1968. Federal legislation regarding access to housing that prohibits discrimination based on race, color, national origin, sex, religion, disability, or familial status.

FAMILY SYSTEMS THEORY. An approach to treatment that emphasizes the interdependency of family members rather than focusing on individuals in isolation from the family. This theory underlies the most influential forms of contemporary family therapy.

FARADIC. A type of discontinuous alternating electric current sometimes used in aversion therapy; named for the nineteenth-century British physicist Michael Faraday.

FASCIA (PLURAL, FASCIAE). A band or sheath of connective tissue that covers, supports, or connects the muscles and the internal organs.

FAST FOURIER TRANSFORM (FFT). A mathematical process used in the analysis of electroencephalograms (EEGs) to investigate the composition of an EEG signal.

FATHERS' RIGHTS MOVEMENT. A social movement that emerged in the 1980s in response to what members consider gender bias in favor of women in family law.

FAT-SOLUBLE VITAMIN. A vitamin that dissolves and can be stored in body fat or the liver.

FECES. Waste products eliminated from the large intestine; excrement.

FELONY. A major crime, such as sexual assault, aggravated assault and battery, grand theft, rape, burglary, arson, and similar acts.

FEMALE ATHLETE TRIAD. A group of three disorders often found together in female athletes, consisting of disordered eating, amenorrhea (absence of menstrual periods), and osteoporosis.

FETAL ALCOHOL SPECTRUM DISORDERS. A range of birth defects, including intellectual disability, poor growth, nervous system dysfunctions, and malformations, that result from heavy maternal alcohol consumption during pregnancy.

FETAL TISSUE TRANSPLANTATION. A method of treating Parkinson's and other neurological diseases by grafting brain cells from human fetuses onto the basal ganglia. Human adults cannot grow new brain cells but developing fetuses can; grafting fetal tissue stimulates the growth of new brain cells in affected adult brains.

FETUS. The stage of development between embryo and newborn.

FIBROMYALGIA. A chronic condition in which patients experience widespread musculoskeletal pain and fatigue.

"FIGHT-OR-FLIGHT" RESPONSE. A function of the autonomic nervous system that prepares the brain to make an immediate decision to deal with a sudden threat.

FINE MOTOR SKILLS. Control of the smaller muscles of the body, especially in the hands, feet, and head, for activities such as writing and crafts.

FLASHBACK. The reemergence of a memory as a vivid recollection of sounds, images, and sensations associated with the (often traumatic) event. The person having such a memory typically feels as if he or she is reliving the event.

FLAVONOIDS. Plant pigments that have a variety of effects on human physiology (such as anti-inflammatory, anticarcinogenic, or antioxidant effects).

FLOODING. A type of exposure treatment in which patients are exposed to anxiety-provoking or feared situations all at once and until the anxiety and fear subside.

FLUNITRAZEPAM (ROHYPNOL). A central nervous system depressant that is not legal in the United States but that is used illegally as a date-rape drug.

FOOD ALLERGY. An abnormal reaction to a food.

FOOD FREQUENCY QUESTIONNAIRE. A listing of how often a person consumes foods from certain food groups in a given period of time.

FORENSIC. Pertaining to courtroom procedures or evidence used in courts of law.

FORMICATION. The medical term for the sensation of insects crawling on or under the skin.

FRAGILE X SYNDROME. A genetic condition related to the X chromosome that affects mental, physical, and sensory development.

FREE RADICALS. Reactive molecules created during cell metabolism that can cause tissue and cell damage like that which occurs in aging and diseases such as cancer.

FREE-FLOATING. A term used in psychiatry to describe anxiety that is unfocused or lacking an apparent cause or object.

FREUDIAN ANALYSIS. A psychological treatment based on the theories developed by Sigmund Freud, in which the therapist seeks to help the patient resolve conflicts and traumas buried in the subconscious.

FRONTAL CORTEX. The part of the human brain associated with aggressiveness and impulse control.

FRONTAL LOBE. A part of the brain that is involved in processes such as muscle movement, speech production, working memory, planning, reasoning, and judgment.

FROTTAGE. The act of touching or rubbing against the body or genitals of a nonconsenting individual.

FROTTEURISM. The practice of rubbing one's pelvis or (for males) erect penis against a nonconsenting person for sexual gratification. Frotteurism is a type of paraphilia and is considered a form of sexual assault.

FUGUE. A dissociative experience during which those affected develop amnesia regarding their past and identity, and as a result travel far from home.

FUNCTIONAL MAGNETIC RESONANCE IMAGING (FMRI). A special type of magnetic resonance imaging (MRI) scan that measures changes in blood flow and blood oxygenation within the body.

G

GADOLINIUM. A very rare metallic element useful for its sensitivity to electromagnetic resonance, among other things. Traces of it can be injected into the body to enhance magnetic resonance imaging (MRI) scans.

GALACTORRHEA. Lactation occurring in the absence of pregnancy.

GALANIN. A neurotransmitter with roles in various physiological processes, including regulation of the stress response.

GALLBLADDER. A small, pear-shaped organ in the upper right-hand corner of the abdomen. It is connected by a series of ducts (tube-like channels) to the liver, pancreas, and duodenum (first part of the small intestine). The gallbladder receives bile from the liver and concentrates and stores it. After a meal, bile is squeezed out of the gallbladder into the intestine, where it aids in digestion of food.

GAMMA CAMERA. A device inside the machine used in single-photon emission computed tomography

(SPECT) that forms images of the gamma rays emitted by the radionuclides used in tracers in nuclear medicine.

GAMMA HYDROXYBUTYRATE (GHB). A central nervous system depressant that has been abused in the United States for euphoric, sedative, bodybuilding, and date-rape purposes.

GAMMA RAYS. Extremely short-wavelength electromagnetic radiation released during the process of radioactive decay.

GAMMA-AMINOBUTYRIC ACID (GABA). A neurotransmitter that helps to lower or reduce the level of excitement in the nerves, leading to muscle relaxation, calmness, sleep, and the prevention of seizures.

GANSER SYNDROME. A rare subtype of factitious disorder accompanied by dissociative symptoms. It is most often seen in male patients under severe stress in prison or courtroom settings.

GASTRITIS. Inflammation of the lining of the stomach.

GASTROSTOMY. A surgical opening into the stomach.

GENDER DYSPHORIA. A disorder in which an individual experiences prolonged, significant distress or dissatisfaction with his or her biological gender.

GENE. The basic unit of genetic material carried in a particular place on a chromosome. Genes are passed on from parents to child during conception and determine how traits such as blood type are inherited and expressed.

GENERALIZATION. A person's ongoing use of new behaviors that were previously modeled for him or her. Generalization is also called transfer of training or maintenance.

GENERALIZED ANXIETY DISORDER. An anxiety disorder characterized by daily irrational worry that is often excessive and uncontrolled.

GENERIC. A term that refers to a medication that is not protected by a registered trademark.

GENETIC DISEASE. A disease caused by genes inherited from one or both parents.

GENETIC INFLUENCE. Any component of the cause of a behavior or condition that is inherited biologically from a person's parents.

GENITALS. The reproductive organs in either sex, especially the external reproductive organs.

GENOGRAM. A family tree diagram that represents the names, birth order, sex, and relationships of the members of a family. Therapists use genograms to detect recurrent patterns in the family history and to help the members understand their problems.

GENOME. The complete set of DNA in a cell.

GERM CELL. A cell involved in reproduction. In humans, the germ cells are the sperm (male) and egg (female). Unlike other cells in the body, germ cells contain only half the standard number of chromosomes.

GESTALT THERAPY. A therapeutic approach that focuses on increasing awareness of feelings and impulses in the present.

GILLBERG'S CRITERIA. A six-item checklist for Asperger syndrome developed by Christopher Gillberg, a Swedish researcher. It is widely used as a diagnostic tool.

GINKGO. An herb from *Ginkgo biloba*, a shade tree native to China with fan-shaped leaves and fleshy seeds with edible kernels.

GLANS. The tip of the penis.

GLASGOW COMA SCALE. A measure of level of consciousness and neurological functioning after a traumatic brain injury (TBI).

GLAUCOMA. A group of eye diseases characterized by increased pressure within the eye, significant enough to damage eye tissue and structures. If untreated, glaucoma results in blindness.

GLIAL CELLS. The support cells of nervous tissue, especially in the brain, spinal cord, and ganglia, interspersed between signal-transmitting neurons. There are three main types of neuroglia: astrocytes, oligodendrocytes, and microglia.

GLUCOSE. One of the two simple sugars (the other being galactose) that makes up the protein lactose, found in milk. Glucose is the form of sugar that is used by the body to generate energy.

GLUTAMATE. An excitatory amino acid neurotransmitter that carries messages to and from nerve cells in the brain.

GLUTAMATERGIC SYSTEM. The neurotransmitter system in the central nervous system that plays a role in memory formation and information processing; it is also believed to play a role in depression and other mood disorders.

GLYCOGEN. The form of glucose (sugar) that is stored in the liver and muscles.

GONAD. The organ that makes gametes (germ cells). The gonads in males are called testicles and produce sperm; those in females are called ovaries and produce eggs.

GONADOTROPIN-RELEASING HORMONE. A hormone produced by the brain that stimulates the pituitary gland to release hormones that trigger ovulation.

GRANDIOSE DELUSIONS. Grandiose delusions are delusions that magnify a person's importance; the person experiencing the delusion may believe him- or herself to be a famous person, to have magical superpowers, or to be someone in a position of enormous power (such as a king or president).

GRANDIOSITY. Exaggerated and unrealistic self-importance; inflated self-assessment.

GRIEF REACTION. The normal depression felt after a traumatic major life occurrence, such as the loss of a loved one.

GROOMING. Deliberately establishing an emotional connection with someone in order to manipulate them psychologically.

GROSS MOTOR SKILLS. Control of the large muscles of the body, including the arms, legs, back, abdomen, and torso, for activities such as sitting, crawling, walking, and running.

GROUP PSYCHOTHERAPY. A form of therapy in which a small, carefully selected group of individuals meets regularly with a therapist to assist each individual in emotional growth and personal problem solving.

GROUP THERAPY. Therapy based on group interaction and designed to provide support, constructive criticism, and a forum for consultation and reference.

GUANETHIDINE. An antihypertensive drug used to treat high blood pressure.

GUIDED IMAGERY. A relaxation technique where individuals actively imagine themselves in a scene (usually a different location, such as a relaxing beach, or a trigger situation, such as handling a problem situation successfully), typically guided by another person describing the scene.

GUSTATORY. Pertaining to the sense of taste.

GYRI. Convoluted ridges between the sulci, or grooves on the surface of the brain.

H

HABITUATION. The reduction of a person's emotional or behavioral reaction to a cue by repeated or prolonged exposure.

HALLUCINATIONS. False sensory perceptions, such as hearing sounds or seeing people or objects that are not there. Hallucinations can also affect the senses of smell, touch, and taste.

HALLUCINOGEN. A drug or other substance that induces hallucinations.

HAPTIC. Pertaining to the sense of touch; sometimes called tactile hallucinations.

HATHA YOGA. A form of yoga that focuses on postures, breathing methods, and meditation.

HEALTH MAINTENANCE ORGANIZATION (HMO). A healthcare organization that provides managed care group health insurance, in which members pay a stated amount on a regular basis and in turn receive medical care from participating physicians, hospitals, and other providers.

HEBEPHILIA. Sexual attraction on the part of an adult to children in the early stages of puberty.

HEMATOMA. An accumulation of blood, often clotted, in a body tissue or organ, usually caused by a break or tear in a blood vessel.

HEMIPLEGIA. Paralysis of one side of the body.

HEMOCHROMATOSIS. A hereditary condition that results in excessive storage of iron in various tissues of the body.

HEPATITIS. A viral disease characterized by inflammation of the liver cells (hepatocytes).

HEREDITARY ATAXIA. One of a group of hereditary degenerative diseases of the spinal cord or cerebellum. These diseases cause tremor, spasm, and wasting of muscle.

HERITABILITY. The effects of differences in genetics (among the population) in producing differences in behavior.

HERTZ. A unit of frequency equal to one cycle per second.

HIERARCHY. In exposure therapy, a list of feared items or situations, ranked from least fearsome to most fearsome.

HIGH-DENSITY SEX OFFENSES. Several offenses within a short period of time.

HIGH-FUNCTIONING AUTISM (HFA). A subcategory of autistic disorder consisting of children diagnosed with IQs of 70 or higher.

HIPPOCAMPUS. A part of the brain's limbic system that is involved in forming, storing, and processing memories and in regulating mood.

HISTAMINE. Substance released during allergic reactions.

HISTONE. A type of protein that serves as a "spool" for wrapping DNA within a chromosome.

HISTRIONIC. Very dramatic or excessive in behavior; theatrical.

HIV. Human immunodeficiency virus.

HOLISTIC. In medicine, a practice that focuses on treating the patient as a whole (rather than just treating the disease); addresses the physical, social, emotional, and spiritual needs of a patient.

HOMEOSTASIS. The tendency of a system to maintain its internal stability and resist change.

HOMOCYSTEINE. An amino acid with the chemical formula $HSCH_2CH_2CH(NH_2)CO_2H$.

HORMONE. A chemical messenger produced by the body that is involved in regulating specific bodily functions such as growth, development, reproduction, metabolism, and mood.

HOST. The dominant or main alternate personality in a person with dissociative identity disorder (DID).

HUMAN TRAFFICKING. Illegal trade in human beings, whether adults or children, for the purposes of reproductive slavery, prostitution, other forms of sexual exploitation, or forced labor.

HUMANISTIC THERAPY. Sometimes also called "humanistic psychology," a perspective that stresses that people are basically good but deviate from that tendency through mental and social problems. It uses a holistic approach that focuses on individual potential and growth, along with self-actualization.

HUMORAL. A term describing a hormonal substance secreted by an endocrine gland (such as the thyroid).

HUNTINGTON'S DISEASE. A midlife-onset inherited disorder characterized by progressive loss of brain function and control over voluntary movements. It is sometimes called Huntington's chorea.

HYDROCEPHALUS. The excess accumulation of cerebrospinal fluid around the brain, often causing enlargement of the head.

HYDROGEN. The simplest, most common element known in the universe. It is composed of a single electron (negatively charged particle) circling a nucleus consisting of a single proton (positively charged particle).

HYDROTHERAPY. This term literally means "water treatment" and involves the use of water in physical therapy as well as treatment of physical and emotional illness.

HYMEN. A membrane that partially or completely covers the vaginal opening in females prior to first intercourse.

HYPERACTIVITY. Describes activity that is unusually active and restless, accompanied by an inability to concentrate for any extended period.

HYPERALIMENTATION. A method of refeeding persons with anorexia by infusing liquid nutrients and electrolytes directly into central veins through a catheter.

HYPERAROUSAL. A state of increased emotional tension and anxiety, often including jitteriness and a heightened startle response.

HYPEREMESIS. Severe vomiting during pregnancy. Hyperemesis appears to increase a woman's risk of postpartum depression.

HYPERSEXUALITY. A clinically significant level of desire to engage in sexual behaviors; usually associated with lowered sexual inhibitions.

HYPERSOMNIA. An abnormal increase of 25% or more in time spent sleeping. Patients usually have excessive daytime sleepiness.

HYPERSOMNOLENCE. Excessive daytime sleepiness in spite of sufficient nighttime sleep.

HYPERTENSION. High blood pressure.

HYPERTENSIVE CRISIS. A steep rise in blood pressure that can lead to brain hemorrhage or heart failure.

HYPERTHERMIA. Elevated body temperature.

HYPERTHYROIDISM. Condition resulting from the production of excess thyroid hormone, causing an increased basal metabolic rate and an increased need for food to meet the demand of the metabolic activity; generally, however, weight loss results.

HYPERVIGILANCE. A state of abnormally intense wariness or watchfulness that is often found in survivors of trauma or long-term abuse.

HYPERVIGILANT. Extreme attention and focus to both internal and external stimuli.

HYPNAGOGIC. Pertaining to drowsiness.

HYPNAGOGIC HALLUCINATIONS. Auditory or visual hallucinations that occur while falling asleep.

HYPNOPOMPIC. Persisting after sleep.

HYPNOSIS. The means by which a state of extreme relaxation and suggestibility is achieved.

HYPNOTIC. A medication that causes sleep.

HYPOCHONDRIASIS. An anxiety disorder in which the individual believes that real or imagined symptoms are indicative of a serious or life-threatening illness or condition.

HYPOCRETINS. A pair of closely related neuropeptide hormones that promote wakefulness, secreted by a small group of cells in the hypothalamus. The hypocretins are also called orexins and are identified as hypocretin-1 (orexin-A) and hypocretin-2 (orexin-B).

HYPOGONADISM. Functional incompetence of the male gonads, with impaired production of hormones and sperm cells.

HYPOKALEMIA. Abnormally low levels of potassium in the blood. Hypokalemia is a potential medical emergency, as it can lead to disturbances in heart rhythm.

HYPOKINESIA. A condition of abnormally diminished motor activity.

HYPOMANIA. A milder form of mania that is characteristic of bipolar II disorder.

HYPOPNEA. Shallow or excessively slow breathing, usually caused by partial closure of the upper airway during sleep, leading to disruption of sleep.

HYPOTENSION. Low blood pressure.

HYPOTHALAMIC-PITUITARY-ADRENAL (HPA) SYSTEM. A part of the brain involved in the human stress response. The HPA system releases cortisol, the primary human stress hormone, and neurotransmitters that activate other brain structures associated with the body's fight-or-flight reaction.

HYPOTHALAMUS. A part of the forebrain that controls heartbeat, thirst, hunger, body temperature and pressure, blood sugar levels, and other functions.

HYPOTHESIS. An assumption, proposition, or educated guess that can be tested empirically (verified by scientific fact or observation).

HYPOTHYROIDISM. A disorder in which the thyroid gland produces too little thyroid hormone, causing a decreased rate of metabolism.

HYPOTONIA. The medical term for poor muscle tone.

HYPOVENTILATION. An abnormally low level of blood oxygenation in the lungs.

HYPOXIA. Oxygen deficiency.

HYSTERIA. In nineteenth-century psychiatric use, a neurotic disorder characterized by violent emotional outbursts and disturbances of the sensory and motor (movement-related) functions. The term "hysterical neurosis" is still used by some psychiatrists as a synonym for conversion disorder.

I

ICTAL EEG. A type of electroencephalogram (EEG) done to determine the type of seizure characteristic of a person's disorder. During this EEG, seizure medicine may be discontinued in an attempt to induce a seizure during the testing period.

ID. A construct in Freudian psychodynamic theory that represents the irrational, self-centered aspects of human thought.

IDENTIFICATION WITH AN AGGRESSOR. In psychology, an unconscious process in which a person adopts the perspective or behavior patterns of a captor or abuser.

IDENTIFIED PATIENT (IP). In a family unit, the member whose symptom has emerged or is most obvious.

IDENTITY DIFFUSION. A character formation that is scattered or spread around rather than an identity that becomes solidified or consolidated.

IDIOGRAPHIC. An approach to interpreting the results of a projective test within the context of the individual subject's record.

IDIOPATHIC. Arising spontaneously or from an unknown or obscure cause.

IEP (INDIVIDUALIZED EDUCATION PLAN). Under federal law governing special education, every child in public schools who is determined through assessment to have special mental disability needs has an IEP. An IEP is typically developed by a team of professionals that may include special education teachers; physical, occupational, and speech therapists; psychologists; parents or guardians; and others who may be called on to provide expertise.

ILLUSION. A false interpretation of a real sensory image or impression.

IMITATIVE BEHAVIOR. Behaviors of a therapist or group member that are imitated, consciously or unconsciously, by other group members.

IMMUNOSUPPRESSANT. Medications that suppress or lower the body's immune system, primarily used to help the body accept a transplanted organ.

IMPAIRMENT. A physical or mental defect at the level of a major body system or organ.

IMPLICIT MEMORY. Unconsciously recalled memory for skills, procedures, or associations.

IMPULSE CONTROL DISORDERS. A group of emotional disorders characterized by the repeated inability to refrain from performing a particular action that is harmful either to oneself or others.

IN VIVO. A Latin phrase that means "in life."

INCEST. Unlawful sexual contact between people who are biologically related. Many therapists also use the term to refer to inappropriate sexual contact between members of a family unit, including stepparents and stepsiblings.

INCIDENCE. A measurement of the risk of developing a specific disease or disorder within a given time period in a specific population.

INCONTINENCE. The inability to control the release of urine or feces.

INDIRECT TRAUMA. A term used to refer to symptoms of trauma in therapists, first responders, and other persons who treat trauma survivors. It is sometimes called vicarious trauma.

INDIVIDUAL PSYCHOTHERAPY. A relationship between therapist and patient designed to foster the patient's emotional growth and personal problem-solving skills.

INFORMATION GIVING. Imparting of information about a disease or condition as part of the therapeutic process.

INFUSION. The most potent form of extraction of a herb into water. Infusions are steeped for a longer period of time than teas.

INHALANT. A substance a person can sniff, or inhale, to get high.

INSANITY DEFENSE. The common term for the defense that an accused person makes to argue against his or her actions having criminal intent because of an underlying mental illness.

INSIDIOUS. Progressing gradually and inconspicuously but with serious effects.

INSOMNIA. A chronic inability to sleep or to remain asleep throughout the night.

INSULIN. A hormone made by the pancreas that controls blood glucose (sugar) levels by moving excess glucose into muscle, liver, and other cells for storage.

INSULIN RESISTANCE. A condition in which a person's natural insulin becomes less effective in lowering the blood sugar level.

INTEGRATED SETTING. Placing individuals with disabilities in usual employment situations rather than making placements into sheltered workshops or other segregated settings.

INTEGRATIVE BEHAVIORAL COUPLES THERAPY (IBCT). A widely used and highly individualized form of behavioral couples therapy, developed by Andrew Christensen and Neil Jacobson in the 1990s.

INTELLECTUAL DISABILITY. Significant impairment in intellectual function, usually associated with an intelligence quotient (IQ) below 70.

INTERICTAL. Occurring between seizures.

INTERMEDIATE CARE FACILITY. An inpatient facility that provides periodic nursing care.

INTERMITTENT EXPLOSIVE DISORDER. A personality disorder in which an individual is prone to intermittent episodes of aggression and rage, particularly when the response is deemed inappropriate or extreme for the situation.

INTERNALIZING DISORDERS. Disorders related to issues within the self; depression and the anxiety disorders are two common types of internalizing disorders.

INTEROCEPTIVE. Referring to stimuli or sensations that arise inside the body.

INTERPERSONAL LEARNING. Learning that takes place via feedback from others.

INTERPERSONAL THERAPY. Also called "talking therapy," this type of psychological counseling is focused on determining how dysfunctional interpersonal relationships of the affected individual may be causing or influencing symptoms of depression.

INTER-RATER RELIABILITY. The degree to which judgments about a person are consistent among raters or diagnosticians.

INTERSEX. A term that is sometimes used to refer to having a sexual anatomy that is not standard for either a male or a female. It covers a number of different conditions but is considered a convenient umbrella term for discussing disorders of sex development.

INTERVENTION. A confrontation of a substance abuser by a group of interested people who propose immediate medical treatment. An intervention is also a method of treatment used in therapy.

INTOXICATION. The presence of significant behavioral or psychological changes following ingestion of a substance.

INTRACEREBRAL HEMATOMA. Bleeding within the brain caused by trauma to a blood vessel.

INTROJECTION. The unconscious incorporation of another person's ideas or attitudes into one's personality.

ION. Charged molecule, such as sodium or chloride, used in neuronal signaling in the brain.

ION CHANNEL. Physical opening on the surface of neurons that allows the passage of charged ions.

IONIZING RADIATION. Electromagnetic radiation that can damage living tissue by disrupting and destroying individual cells. All types of nuclear decay radiation (including x rays) are potentially ionizing. Radio waves do not damage the organic tissues they pass through.

IQ. Intelligence quotient, or a measure of the intelligence of an individual based on the results of a standardized test.

IRRITABLE BOWEL SYNDROME. Disorder involving dysfunction of the gastrointestinal tract that may include symptoms of constipation, diarrhea, or both.

IRRITATIVE HALLUCINATIONS. Hallucinations caused by abnormal electrical activity in the brain.

ISCHEMIA. An inadequate flow of blood to a part of the body, caused by a narrowing or blockage of the blood vessels supplying it.

J

JAUNDICE. Yellowing of the skin or eyes due to excess bilirubin in the blood.

JET LAG. A temporary disruption of the body's sleep-wake rhythm following high-speed air travel across several time zones. Jet lag is most severe in people who have crossed eight or more time zones in 24 hours.

JOHREI. A form of energy therapy that originated in Japan in the 1920s. It emphasizes the channeling of spiritual energy to heal people of toxins by raising their spiritual vibrations.

JOINT CONTRACTURES. Stiffness of the joints that prevents full extension.

JUNGIAN ANALYSIS. A psychological treatment based on the theories of Carl Jung, in which the patient strives to understand the internal, often mythical images in thoughts and dreams.

K

KARYOTYPE. The number and appearance of a complete set of chromosomes in a species or an individual organism. The arrangement of microphotographs of the chromosomes in a standard photographic format is called a karyogram.

KAVALACTONES. Medically active compounds in kava root that act as local anesthetics in the mouth and as minor tranquilizers.

KAVAPYRONES. Compounds in kava root that act as muscle relaxants and anticonvulsants.

KEGEL EXERCISES. Repetitive contractions to tone the pubococcygeus muscle of the pelvic floor for enhancing sexual response during intercourse or controlling incontinence.

KETAMINE. An anesthetic, used predominately by veterinarians to treat animals, that can be abused or used as a date-rape drug.

KI. The Japanese spelling of *qi*, the traditional Chinese term for vital energy or the life force.

KILOGRAM. A metric unit of weight equaling 2.2 lb.

KLEINE-LEVIN SYNDROME. A disorder that occurs primarily in young males and is marked by episodes of hypersomnia, hypersexual behavior, and excessive eating, occurring three or four times a year.

KLEPTOMANIA. A disorder of impulse control characterized by repeated stealing or shoplifting of items that the person does not need or that are of little or no value.

KORO. A culture-specific syndrome involving the belief that a person's external genitalia are shrinking or retracting and may disappear; it occurs primarily in Southeast Asia.

KUNDALINI. In Indian yoga, a vital force or energy at the base of the spine that is activated or released by certain yoga postures or breathing techniques. This release is called the "awakening" of the kundalini. Some Westerners have had kundalini experiences that were diagnosed as psychotic episodes or symptoms of schizophrenia.

L

LABIA. The outside folds of tissue that surround the clitoris and the opening of the urethra in women.

LABILE AFFECT. A display of frequently changing emotion or mood.

LANUGO. A soft, downy body hair that develops on the chest and arms of women with anorexia.

LAPSE. A single, isolated occurrence of a symptom or negative behavior.

LARYNGOSPASM. Spasms that close the vocal apparatus of the larynx (the organ of voice production).

LAXATIVE. Substance or medication that encourages a bowel movement.

LEARNED HELPLESSNESS. The tendency to give up on solving a problem when efforts appear to bring no results.

LEARNING DISORDER. A condition characterized by difficulty in learning that has an unknown cause.

LEAST RESTRICTIVE ENVIRONMENT. Refers to care options that involve the least amount of restraint and the greatest degree of independence possible, while still meeting the individual's needs and maintaining safety.

LESION. Any abnormality in or injury to body tissue.

LEVODOPA (L-DOPA). A substance used in the treatment of Parkinson's disease. Levodopa can cross the blood-brain barrier that protects the brain. Once in the brain, it is converted to dopamine and thus can replace the dopamine lost in Parkinson's disease.

LEWY BODIES. Areas of injury found on damaged nerve cells in certain parts of the brain associated with dementia.

LEWY BODY DEMENTIA. A type of dementia characterized by the presence of abnormal, sphere-shaped clumps of protein in nerve cells in the brain. Lewy body resembles Alzheimer's disease but progresses more rapidly. Common symptoms include confusion and recurring visual hallucinations.

LEXICAL. Relating to the individual words that make up a language.

LIBIDO. Sex drive; level of sexual desire.

LIDOCAINE. A local anesthetic.

LIMBIC SYSTEM. A group of structures in the brain that includes the amygdala, hippocampus, olfactory bulbs, and hypothalamus. The limbic system is associated with homeostasis and the regulation of emotions.

LOFEXIDINE. A medication approved for use in Great Britain to aid in the opioid detoxification process.

LOW AFFECT. Severe lack of interest and emotions; emotional numbness.

LUTEAL PHASE. The period of time between ovulation and menstruation.

LUX. The International System (IS) unit for measuring illumination, equal to one lumen per square meter.

LYSERGIC ACID DIETHYLAMIDE (LSD). The first synthetic hallucinogen, discovered in 1938.

M

MACERATION. A technique for extracting essential oils from plant leaves and stems by crushing the plant parts and soaking them in warm vegetable oil.

MACROSOCIAL. Pertaining to the wider society, as distinct from such smaller social groupings as families, neighborhoods, etc.

MAGNETIC FIELD. A region around a magnetized body or a current-carrying circuit, in which a magnetic force can be detected.

MAGNETIC RESONANCE IMAGING (MRI). An imaging technique that uses electromagnetic radiation and a strong magnetic field to obtain detailed images of soft tissues such as the brain.

MAGNETOENCEPHALOGRAPHY (MEG). A newer form of brain imaging that captures and records the brain's magnetic fields, produced by electrical currents occurring naturally in brain tissue. MEG can identify split-second changes in brain activity.

MAJOR DEPRESSION. A psychological condition in which a person experiences one or more disabling attacks of depression lasting two or more weeks.

MAJOR DEPRESSIVE DISORDER. A clinical psychiatric diagnosis of chronic depressed mood that interferes with normal life activities.

MALADAPTIVE. Unsuitable or counterproductive; for example, maladaptive behavior is inappropriate to a given situation.

MALADROITNESS. Another word for awkwardness or clumsiness.

MALINGERING. Pretending to be physically or mentally ill in order to be relieved of an unwanted duty or obtain some other obvious benefit.

MANIA. An elevated or euphoric mood or irritable state that is characteristic of bipolar disorder. Mania is characterized by mental and physical hyperactivity, disorganization of behavior, and inappropriate elevation of mood.

MANIC. Referring to mania, a state characterized by excessive activity, excitement, or emotion.

MANTRA. A sacred word or formula repeated over and over to concentrate the mind.

MAO-B INHIBITORS. Inhibitors of dopamine or noradrenaline reuptake by monoamine oxidase.

MAOIs. Monoamine oxidase inhibitors.

MASOCHISM. A condition in which people obtain sexual satisfaction through pain or humiliation inflicted by themselves or by another person. The term is sometimes used more generally to refer to a tendency to find pleasure in submissiveness or self-denial.

MASTER STATUS ATTRIBUTE. A term used in sociology for a characteristic that is the most important definer of an individual's social status or identity, one that overshadows other traits and affects the person's behavior in most situations. Common master status attributes are race, sex, sexual orientation, level of education, age, and mental illness or disability.

MATRIX. In statistics, variables that may influence a particular outcome are placed into a grid (matrix), either in columns or in rows. Statistical calculations can be performed that assign different weights to each variable, and the differential weighting of variables can be seen to affect the outcome (positive or negative).

MEDICAID. A program jointly funded by state and federal governments that reimburses hospitals and physicians for the care of individuals who cannot pay for their own medical expenses. These individuals may be in low-income households or may have chronic disabilities.

MEDICAID HOME AND COMMUNITY BASED-WAIVER. Legislation regarding the use of Medicaid funds for care services; allows certain federal requirements to be bypassed so that states can use the funds more flexibly for accessing home- and community-based services, rather than using hospitals or intermediate-care facilities.

MEDICAL MODEL OF MENTAL ILLNESS. An approach to psychiatric diagnosis and treatment patterned on the process of diagnosis and treatment of physical disease.

MEDICARE. A federal health insurance program in the United States that provides medical care and hospital treatment for people over a certain age (usually 65 years).

MEDITATION. Technique of concentration for relaxing the mind and body.

MEDROXYPROGESTERONE ACETATE (MPA). A female hormone that may be prescribed for male patients with sexual sadism or other paraphilias. MPA helps to control sexual urges in men by speeding up the clearance of testosterone from the bloodstream.

MELATONIN. A hormone involved in regulation of the sleep-wake cycle and other circadian rhythms.

MENARCHE. The first menstrual period.

MENINGES. The three membranes that enclose the brain and spinal cord, consisting of the dura mater, arachnoid mater, and pia mater.

MENOPAUSE. A period of decreasing hormonal activity in women, when ovulation stops and conception is no longer possible.

MENTAL DISORDER. A psychiatric disorder of mental faculties.

MENTAL HEALTH. Appropriate adaptation to everyday psychosocial challenges.

MENTAL ILLNESS. Any psychiatric disorder that causes unusual (atypical) behavior.

MENTAL STATUS EXAMINATION (MSE). A clinical evaluation in which the doctor assesses a patient's external appearance, attitude, behavior, mood and affect, speech, thought processes, thought content, perception, cognition, insight (or lack thereof), and judgment.

MERIDIANS. In traditional Chinese medicine, a network of pathways or channels that convey *qi* (also sometimes spelled *chi*), or vital energy, through the body.

MERYCISM. Another name for rumination disorder.

MESOLIMBIC PATHWAY. The "reward pathways" of the brain.

METABOLISM. All of the physical and chemical changes that occur in cells to allow growth and maintain body functions. These include processes that break down substances (such as food) to yield energy and processes that build up other substances necessary for life.

METABOLITE. Chemical compound that occurs as a result of a parent drug being broken down and metabolized in the body. A metabolite may be a medically active or inactive compound, depending on the drug in question.

METFORMIN. A drug developed to treat type 2 diabetes that has been used experimentally to treat weight gain in patients with schizophrenia.

METHADONE. A drug often prescribed legally as a replacement for heroin. It induces a slight high but blocks heroin from producing a more powerful euphoric effect. It may be used in heroin detoxification to ease the process, or it may be used daily after detoxification as maintenance therapy. Methadone maintenance therapy is controversial.

METHAMPHETAMINE. A drug that is approved by the U.S. Food and Drug Administration to treat attention deficit hyperactivity disorder but that is also the most common illegally produced amphetamine.

METHYLATION. A process in which chemical tags called "methyl groups" (made of one carbon and three hydrogen atoms) attach themselves to a DNA molecule in specific locations, affecting the level of a gene's activity.

METHYLPHENIDATE. A mild central nervous system stimulant that is used to treat hyperactivity.

MICROSLEEP. A brief episode of sleep lasting from a fraction of a second to 30 seconds. It may result from sleep deprivation, sleep apnea, or oxygen deprivation as well as from narcolepsy.

MILD COGNITIVE IMPAIRMENT (MCI). A transitional phase of memory loss in older people that precedes dementia or Alzheimer's disease.

MILLIGRAM (MG). One-thousandth of a gram. A gram is the metric measure that equals about 0.035 ounces.

MILLON CLINICAL MULTIAXIAL INVENTORY (MCMI-II). A self-report instrument designed to help clinicians assess *DSM-IV*-related personality disorders and clinical syndromes. It provides insight into 14 personality disorders and 10 clinical syndromes.

MINERAL. An inorganic substance found in the earth that is necessary in small quantities for the body to maintain health. Examples: zinc, copper, iron.

MINNESOTA MULTIPHASIC PERSONALITY INVENTORY (MMPI-2). A comprehensive assessment tool widely used to diagnose personality disorders.

MISDEMEANOR. A minor crime, such as petit larceny (petty theft), that is punishable by not more than one year in prison.

MIXED MANIA. A mental state in which symptoms of both depression and mania occur simultaneously.

MODALITY. The medical term for a method of treatment.

MODELING. A behavioral therapy technique in which a patient first observes and then imitates a desired behavior.

MONOAMINE OXIDASE INHIBITORS (MAOIs). A group of antidepressant drugs that decrease the activity of monoamine oxidase, a neurotransmitter found in the brain that affects mood.

MOOD DISORDER. Any of a group of mental disorders involving a disturbance of mood, along with either a full or partial excessively happy (manic) or extremely sad (depressive) syndrome not caused by any other physical or mental disorder. Mood refers to a prolonged emotion.

MORPHEME. The smallest meaningful speech sound.

MORTALITY RATE. A measure of the number of deaths in a specific population, usually expressed per 1,000 per year.

MOSAIC. A term referring to a genetic situation in which a person's cells do not have the exact same composition of chromosomes.

MOTIVATIONAL ENHANCEMENT THERAPY. Therapy that focuses on increasing motivation for change by empathically comparing and contrasting the consequences and benefits of changing or not changing.

MOTIVATIONAL THERAPY. An approach to treatment for learning disorders that emphasizes problem-solving skills, the ability to set and attain goals, and ways to counteract negative thinking and poor self-image.

MOTOR SKILLS. Skills pertaining to or involving muscular movement.

MOURNING. The public expression of bereavement, including funerals and other rituals, special clothing, and symbolic gestures.

MOVEMENT EDUCATION. The active phase of bodywork, in which clients learn to move with greater freedom and to maintain the proper alignment of their bodies.

MOXIBUSTION. An acupuncture technique that involves burning of the herb moxa or mugwort.

MULTIAXIAL. Refers to a type of classification system that involves numeric measurement along more than one dimension and that is not based on assignment to mutually exclusive categories.

MULTI-INFARCT DEMENTIA (MID). Dementia caused by a series of many small strokes over time; also called vascular dementia.

MULTIMODAL. Involving several types of therapeutic interventions, such as heat or ice packs, electrical stimulation, or ultrasound; sometimes refers to a mix of physical and psychological therapies.

MULTIPLE PERSONALITY DISORDER (MPD). An older term for dissociative identity disorder (DID).

MULTIPLE SCLEROSIS. A disease characterized by patches of hardened tissue in the brain or spinal cord, paralysis, and/or muscle tremors.

MUTATION. A change in a gene. A gene mutation may alter a trait or characteristic of an individual or may manifest as a disease; the mutation can also be transmitted to offspring.

MUTISM. The inability or refusal to speak.

MYASTHENIA GRAVIS. A chronic disease with symptoms that include muscle weakness and sometimes paralysis.

MYELIN. A white, fatty substance that covers and protects nerves.

MYOCARDIAL DISEASE. Disease of the muscular layer of the heart wall.

MYOCARDIUM. The specialized involuntary muscle tissue found in the walls of the heart.

MYOCLONUS. An abrupt spasm or twitching in a muscle or group of muscles.

N

NALTREXONE. A medication originally developed to treat addiction to heroin or morphine that is also used to treat alcoholism. It works by reducing the craving for alcohol rather than by producing vomiting or other unpleasant reactions.

NARCISSISTIC PERSONALITY DISORDER. Personality characterized by continually exaggerating one's own positive qualities and refusing to recognize personal defects or flaws.

NARCISSISTIC PERSONALITY INVENTORY (NPI). The most widely used English-language diagnostic instrument for narcissistic personality disorder. Based on the *DSM-III* criteria for NPD, the NPI is frequently used in research studies as well as patient assessment.

NARCOLEPSY. A disorder characterized by frequent and uncontrollable attacks of deep sleep.

NARCOTHERAPY. A form of psychotherapy that involves the administration of a drug that makes the patient drowsy.

NARCOTIC. A drug derived from opium or compounds similar to opium. Such drugs are potent pain relievers and can affect mood and behavior. Long-term use of narcotics can lead to dependence and tolerance.

NARROW-ANGLE GLAUCOMA. An eye disorder caused by a buildup of fluid pressure inside the eyeball due to an abnormally small angle between the iris (the colored portion of the eye) and the cornea (the transparent front part of the eye).

NASOGASTRIC INTUBATION. A process in which a tube is inserted down the throat and into the stomach.

NATURAL SUPPORTS. Existing relationships that can serve as part of a person's support network to help that person reach a goal.

NEGATIVE SYMPTOMS. Symptoms of schizophrenia characterized by the absence or elimination of certain behaviors, such as initiative, speech, or affect.

NEGATIVISM. Behavior characterized by resistance, opposition, and refusal to cooperate with requests, even reasonable ones.

NEPHRITIS. Inflammation of the kidney.

NERVOUS TIC. A repetitive, involuntary action, such as the twitching of a muscle or repeated blinking.

NEURALGIA. Pain that extends along the course of a nerve.

NEUROENDOCRINE SYSTEM. The part of the autonomic nervous system responsible for growth and hormonal regulation.

NEUROFIBRILLARY TANGLES. Accumulations of twisted protein fragments inside nerve cells in the brain that are diagnostic of Alzheimer's disease.

NEUROGENESIS. The development of new nerve cells in the brain, whether before birth or during adulthood.

NEUROGENIC. Referring to a disorder associated with damage to the central nervous system.

NEUROLEPTIC DRUGS. Antipsychotic drugs, including major tranquilizers, used in the treatment of psychoses such as schizophrenia.

NEUROLEPTIC MALIGNANT SYNDROME. An unusual but potentially serious complication that develops in some patients who have been treated with antipsychotic medications. NMS is characterized by changes in blood pressure, altered states of consciousness, rigid muscles, and fever. Untreated NMS can result in coma and death.

NEUROLEPTIC-INDUCED ACUTE DYSTONIA. A severe form of neurological movement disorder, caused by the use of neuroleptic drugs.

NEUROLEPTIC-INDUCED AKATHISIA. A disorder characterized by physical restlessness (the inability to sit still, for example) and excessive movement, caused by the use of neuroleptic drugs; research indicates it is likely the most common of neuroleptic-induced movement disorders.

NEUROLEPTIC-INDUCED PARKINSONISM. Symptoms similar to Parkinson's disease that may appear in people taking neuroleptic (antipsychotic) medications. These symptoms include tremors in muscles and a shuffling gait.

NEUROLEPTIC-INDUCED TARDIVE DYSKINESIA. A potentially irreversible neurological disorder caused by the use of antipsychotic/neuroleptic medications, with symptoms involving uncontrollable movement of various body parts.

NEUROLEPTICS. Drugs that treat psychosis, such as hallucinations.

NEUROLOGICAL. Relating to neurology, or the branch of medicine dealing with the function and structure of the nervous system, along with its associated diseases and disorders.

NEUROLOGICAL CONDITIONS. A condition that has its origin in some part of the patient's nervous system.

NEURONAL SIGNALING. The pathway by which neurons communicate, which can be electrical or chemical.

NEURONS. Nerve cells in the brain that produce nerve impulses.

NEUROPATHIC. Relating to neural damage.

NEUROPATHIC PAIN. State of pain related to the nervous system; also known as neurogenic pain.

NEUROPROTECTIVE. Conveying some form of protection to the nervous system from injury.

NEUROPSYCHOLOGICAL. Relating to neuropsychology, or the branch of neurology that studies behavior disorders such as memory loss, speech impairment, epilepsy, and others.

NEUROTRANSMITTER. A naturally occurring chemical in the body that carries chemical messages to nerve cells, often by transmitting nerve impulses. Central nervous system well-being is dependent on a balance among the neurotransmitters acetylcholine, dopamine, serotonin, and norepinephrine.

NEUROTRANSMITTER RECEPTOR. A physical recipient for chemicals called neurotransmitters. Receptors sit on the surface of cells that make up body tissues, and once bound to the neurotransmitter, they initiate the chemical signaling pathway associated with neurotransmitters.

NICOTINE. A colorless, oily chemical found in tobacco that makes people physically dependent on smoking. It is poisonous in large doses.

NIGHT TERROR. Commonly called sleep terror disorder; a disorder in which a person wakes up fearful and anxious but with no recollection of the source of the fear.

NIGHTMARE. A frightening dream that occurs during REM (rapid eye movement) sleep.

NIMBY PHENOMENON. Acronym for "Not In My Backyard," describing the common opposition displayed by citizens toward the placement of group homes or other social service facilities in their neighborhoods.

NOCTURNAL MYOCLONUS. A disorder in which a person is awakened repeatedly during the night by cramps or twitches in the calf muscles; sometimes called periodic limb movement disorder (PLMD).

NOMOTHETIC. An approach to interpreting the results of a projective test in which the subject's answers are measured against a normative comparison sample.

NON-AMBULATORY. Unable to walk.

NONDISJUNCTION. Nonseparation of a chromosome pair during either meiosis or mitosis.

NON-RAPID EYE MOVEMENT (NREM) SLEEP. The first phase of a sleep cycle, in which there is little or no eye movement.

NONSTEROIDAL ANTI-INFLAMMATORY DRUGS (NSAIDs). A class of pain relief medications that also decreases inflammation, such as ibuprofen (Advil), naproxen (Aleve) and acetylsalicylic acid (Aspirin).

NONVERBAL LEARNING DISABILITY (NLD). A learning disability syndrome identified in 1989 that may overlap with some of the symptoms of Asperger syndrome.

NORADRENERGIC. Acts similarly to norepinephrine.

NOREPINEPHRINE. Also called noradrenaline, a chemical messenger in the brain that regulates attention and that powers the "fight-or-flight" stress response; precursor of epinephrine.

NUCLEAR FAMILY. The basic family unit, consisting of father, mother, and their biological children.

NUCLEAR MEDICINE. A branch of medicine that makes use of radioisotopes (also called radionuclides) to evaluate the rate of radioactive decay in diagnosing and treating various diseases.

NUCLEOTIDES. Building blocks of genes, which are arranged in specific order and quantity.

NUCLEUS ACCUMBENS. A structure deep inside and near the center of the brain that makes up a major part of the pathway of pleasure and reward and that is implicated in addictive behavior.

O

OBJECT RELATIONS. In psychology, a phrase that refers to the way in which a subject describes relationships with other people in their environment, and the ways in which he or she has internalized interpersonal relationships.

OBSESSION. A persistent image, idea, or desire that dominates a person's thoughts or feelings.

OBSESSIVE THINKING. Thoughts that overcome a person's thought processes; a compulsive way of thinking in which the same thought repeats, preventing other thoughts.

OBSESSIVE-COMPULSIVE DISORDER. A disorder in which affected individuals have an obsession (such as a fear of contamination, or thoughts they do not like to have and cannot control) and feel compelled to perform certain acts to neutralize the obsession (such as repeated hand washing).

OBSTRUCTIVE SLEEP APNEA. A disorder caused by obstruction of the upper airway during sleep and characterized by repeated pauses in breathing during sleep despite efforts to breathe.

OCCIPITAL BONE. The bone that forms the back part of the skull.

OFF-LABEL. The use of a prescription medication to treat conditions outside the indications approved by the U.S. Food and Drug Administration (FDA). It is legal for physicians to prescribe these drugs, but it is not legal for pharmaceutical companies to advertise drugs for off-label uses.

OLFACTORY. Pertaining to the sense of smell.

OLFACTORY NERVE. The cranial nerve that regulates the sense of smell.

ONSET. The point in time at which the symptoms of a disorder first became apparent.

OPERANT. Conditioning in which the desired response is reinforced by an introduced stimulus.

OPERANT CONDITIONING. A psychological process in which a desired behavior is followed with positive or rewarding stimuli.

OPIATE BLOCKER. A type of drug that blocks the effects of natural opiates in the system. This type of drug makes some people appear more responsive to their environment.

OPIATES. A class of drugs that is either derived from opium (e.g., morphine, hydromorphone, oxymorphone, heroin, codeine, hydrocodone, oxycodone) or resembles these opium derivatives (such as meperidine); commonly referred to as narcotics.

OPIOID. Any of a group of potent pain-relieving drugs derived from the opium poppy or synthesized in the laboratory.

OPIOID ANTAGONIST. A type of receptor antagonist (drug) that acts on opioid receptors.

OPPOSITIONAL DEFIANT DISORDER. A psychiatric disorder characterized by an ongoing pattern of excessively hostile, angry, and disobedient behavior that is directed toward authority figures.

ORAL PHASE. The first of Freud's psychosexual stages of development in which satisfaction is focused on the mouth and lips. During this stage, sucking and eating are the primary means of gratification.

OREXINS. Another name for the hypocretins.

ORGANIC BRAIN DISORDER. An organic brain disorder refers to impaired brain function due to damage or deterioration of brain tissue.

ORGANIC BRAIN SYNDROME. A class of disorders characterized by progressive deterioration of mental processes caused by temporary brain dysfunction or permanent brain damage. Symptoms include delusions, dementia, amnesia, and delirium that are not caused by drugs, alcohol, or as a side effect of medication.

ORGANIC ILLNESS. A physical, biologically based illness.

ORGASM. Another word for sexual climax.

ORGASMIC REORIENTATION. A form of behavioral therapy that attempts to help people learn to respond sexually to culturally appropriate stimuli.

OROFACIAL DYSKINESIA. Involuntary movements of the face.

ORTHOSTATIC HYPOTENSION. A sudden decrease in blood pressure due to a change in body position, as when moving from a sitting to standing position.

OSTEOPATHY. A system of medical practice that believes that the human body can make its own remedies to heal infection. It originally used manipulative techniques but also includes surgical, hygienic, and medicinal methods when needed. Doctors of osteopathy are referred to as osteopaths or DOs.

OSTEOPOROSIS. The thinning of bone and loss of bone density.

OVERCOMPENSATION. An attempt to overcome or correct a behavior by going too far in the opposite direction.

OXIMETRY. The measurement of blood oxygen levels.

P

PAIN STATES. Refers to the four-way classification of pain disorder as being (1) acute with psychological factors, (2) acute with psychological factors and a general medical condition, (3) chronic with psychological factors, or (4) chronic with psychological factors and a general medical condition.

PALILALIA. Involuntary echoing of the last word, phrase, sentence, or sound vocalized by oneself.

PANIC ATTACK. A period of intense fear or discomfort combined with a feeling of doom and a desire to escape. Panic attacks may be unexpected or triggered by specific internal or external cues.

PANIC DISORDER. An anxiety disorder in which an individual experiences sudden, debilitating attacks of intense fear.

PARADIGM. The commonly accepted foundations among a group of similar theories, usually derived from a philosophy, including assumptions, terminology, measurements, and expectations.

PARAMETER. A characteristic or factor that is measured during a test of a complex process or activity like sleep.

PARANOIA. An unwarranted sense of suspicion or of being persecuted, sometimes reaching delusional proportions.

PARANOID PERSONALITY DISORDER. A personality disorder characterized by unwarranted suspicion, jealousy, hypersensitivity, social isolation, and a tendency to detect malicious intent in the words and actions of others.

PARAPHILIA. The medical term for a condition in which a person is sexually aroused by nonhuman objects, animals, corpses, children and other nonconsenting partners, or other individuals or situations that are not part of normative stimulation.

PARASOMNIA. A type of sleep disorder characterized by abnormal changes in behavior or body functions during sleep, specific stages of sleep, or the transition between sleeping and waking.

PARCOPRESIS. Fear of having a bowel movement in a public place.

PARENS PATRIAE. The legal concept by which the state has the responsibility to protect those with mental disabilities from self-harm.

PARESTHESIA. An abnormal sensation of tingling or "pins and needles."

PARIETAL LOBE. The middle portion of each cerebral hemisphere of the brain; associated with bodily sensations.

PARIETAL-OCCIPITAL. Relating to the parietal and occipital bones or lobes.

PARKINSONIAN. Related to symptoms associated with Parkinson's disease.

PARKINSON'S DISEASE. A disease of the nervous system most common in people over age 60, characterized by a shuffling gait, muscle stiffness, and tremors.

PARTIAL AGONIST. A substance that partially activates a receptor in the brain, while blocking the neurotransmitter for that receptor from binding to it.

PARURESIS. Fear of urinating in a public place.

PATHOLOGICAL. Uncontrollable in nature; relating to disease.

PAVOR NOCTURNUS. Another term for sleep terror disorder.

PEDOPHILIA. A sexual perversion in which children are the preferred sexual object.

PELVIS. The basin-like cavity in the human body below the abdomen, enclosed by a framework of four bones.

PENETRATING HEAD INJURY. A type of traumatic brain injury in which an object pierces the skull and enters brain tissue.

PENIS. The external male sex organ.

PERCENTILE. A statistical measure that shows, on a scale of 100, whether a distribution is below or above it.

PERINEAL. An anatomical area located between the external genitals and the anus.

PERIODIC LIMB MOVEMENTS IN SLEEP (PLMS). Random movements of the arms or legs that occur at regular intervals of time during sleep.

PERIPHERAL NERVE. A nerve in a distant location from the brain that receives information in the form of an impulse from the brain and spinal cord.

PERIPHERAL NERVOUS SYSTEM. The part of the nervous system that lies outside the brain and spinal cord. It connects the central nervous system with sensory organs, muscles, blood vessels, and glands.

PERISTALSIS. Waves of muscular contraction in the intestines that push food along during the process of digestion.

PERSEVERATION. Continuous involuntary repetition of speech or behavior.

PERSISTENT PULMONARY HYPERTENSION (PPHN). A life-threatening disorder seen in newborn babies in which blood does not properly enter the lungs.

PERSONALITY. The organized pattern of behaviors and attitudes that makes a human being distinctive. Personality is formed by the ongoing interaction of temperament, character, and environment.

PERSONALITY DISORDER. A maladaptive pattern of behavior, affect, and/or cognitive style displayed in a broad range of settings. The pattern deviates from the accepted norms of the individual's culture and can occur over a lifetime.

PERSONALITY INVENTORY. A type of psychological test that is designed to assess a client's major personality traits, behavioral patterns, coping styles, and similar characteristics. The MMPI-2 is an example of a personality inventory.

PERSONALITY TEST. Various standardized tasks that are used to determine aspects of personality or emotional status.

PERSONALIZATION. The tendency to relate large-scale events or general patterns of events to the self in inappropriate ways. For example, a person who regards the loss of a loved one in an accident as punishment for having quarreled with that person before the accident is said to be personalizing the event. This tendency increases a person's risk of developing acute stress disorder or post-traumatic stress disorder after a traumatic event.

PERSON-CENTERED PLANNING. A technique in which a plan for a person's future is developed by a team consisting of the person, family members, service providers, and friends (natural supports). The team develops a practical plan based on the person's wishes and dreams. Each team member agrees to perform certain tasks identified in the plan to help the person reach his or her goals.

PERSON-CENTERED THERAPY. A therapeutic approach that believes the client's own drive toward growth and development is the most important factor in healing.

PERVASIVE DEVELOPMENTAL DISORDERS (PDDs). A group of five disorders—including Asperger syndrome, autism, Rett disorder, childhood disintegrative disorder (CDD), and pervasive developmental disorder not otherwise specified (PDD-NOS)—that are characterized by developmental delays or impairments.

PHARMACODYNAMICS. The study of the effects of drugs on the human body.

PHARMACOKINETICS. The study of the absorption, distribution, and elimination of drugs from the body.

PHENOMENOLOGICAL THERAPY. A therapeutic approach that focuses on the interpretations individuals place on their experiences.

PHENOTHIAZINES. A class of drugs widely used in the treatment of psychosis.

PHENOTYPES. Observable traits or characteristics.

PHENYLKETONURIA (PKU). An enzyme deficiency present at birth that disrupts metabolism and causes brain damage. If left untreated, the disease progresses into intellectual disability.

PHOBIA. An intense, abnormal, or illogical fear of something specific, such as heights or open spaces.

PHONEME. The smallest detectable sound within a spoken word.

PHONICS. A method of teaching reading and spelling based on the phonetic interpretation of single letters, letter combinations, and syllables.

PHONOLOGICAL DISORDER. A developmental disorder of childhood in which the child fails to use speech sounds that are appropriate for his or her age level and native language or dialect.

PHOSPHODIESTERASE-5 (PDE5). An enzyme that is involved in the loss of penile erection.

PHOTOMULTIPLIER. A device that is designed to be extremely sensitive to electromagnetic radiation, especially within the ultraviolet, visible, and near-infrared ranges of the electromagnetic spectrum.

PHOTON. The smallest amount of electromagnetic radiation that possesses both particle and wave properties.

PHOTOTHERAPY. Also called light therapy, a therapy in which the patient is exposed to a bright light to compensate for reduced exposure to sunlight.

PHOTOTOXIC. Causes a harmful skin reaction when exposed to sunlight.

PHYSIOLOGIC. Describes physiology, particularly normal, healthy, physical functioning.

PHYSOSTIGMINE. A short-acting drug that enhances levels of acetylcholine (a neurotransmitter) between neurons in the brain.

PICA. An abnormal appetite or craving for non-food items, often such substances as chalk, clay, dirt, laundry starch, or charcoal.

PICK'S DISEASE. A rare type of primary dementia that affects the frontal lobes of the brain. It is characterized by a progressive loss of social skills, language, and memory, leading to personality changes and sometimes loss of moral judgment.

PILATES. An exercise regimen specifically designed to improve overall physiological and mental functioning.

PINEAL GLAND. A small endocrine gland in the brain that produces melatonin.

PITUITARY GLAND. A small endocrine organ in the brain that is associated with various hormones that control and regulate other endocrine organs. The pituitary affects most basic bodily functions, including growth and development.

PLACEBO. An inactive substance or preparation given to a control group in a clinical trial to test the effectiveness of the real medication or treatment; usually study participants do not know if they are receiving the drug or the placebo.

PLAQUE. A sticky cholesterol-containing substance that builds up on the walls of blood vessels, reducing or blocking blood flow.

PLATELET. A small, irregularly shaped cell fragment that plays an important role in blood clotting. Platelets are also called thrombocytes.

POINT-OF-SERVICE. A healthcare organization that provides managed-care group health insurance and has characteristics of both health maintenance organizations (HMOs) and preferred provider organizations (PPOs).

POLYGENIC. A trait or disorder that is determined by several different genes. Most human characteristics, including height, weight, and general body build, are polygenic, as is the development of certain diseases.

POLYPHARMACY. The use of a number of different medications by the same patient. Polypharmacy is most common among the elderly and those taking psychiatric medications.

POLYSOMNOGRAPHY. Laboratory measurement of a patient's basic physiological processes during sleep, used to diagnose sleep disorders. Polysomnography usually measures heart rate, eye movements, brain waves, muscle activity, breathing, changes in blood oxygen concentration, and body position.

POLYTRAUMA. The medical term for injury to more than one part of the body or more than one type of injury (such as burn injuries in addition to broken bones).

PORNOGRAPHY. Sexually explicit pictures, writings, or other material produced for the purpose of sexual arousal.

PORPHYRIA. A disease of the metabolism characterized by skin lesions, urine problems, neurologic disorders, and/or abdominal pain.

POSITIVE AFFIRMATION STATEMENTS. Statements repeated to oneself, either aloud or mentally, that reflect positive attitudes of self-worth.

POSITIVE REINFORCEMENT. A procedure or response that rewards a desired behavior.

POSITIVE SYMPTOMS. Symptoms that are characterized by the production or presence of abnormal or excessive behaviors, including hallucinations and thought-process disorder.

POSITRON. A positively charged particle; also called an "antielectron," the antimatter counterpart of the electron.

POSITRON EMISSION TOMOGRAPHY (PET). A medical imaging technique that allows for the scanning of the metabolic activity of the body's organs, which is useful to diagnosis cancer, locate brain tumors, and investigate other disorders.

POST-CONCUSSION SYNDROME. A complex of symptoms, including headache, following a mild traumatic brain injury.

POST-DEPLOYMENT SYNDROME (PDS). A term developed to describe a constellation of mental disorders found in veterans of the conflicts in Iraq and Afghanistan. PDS includes post-traumatic stress disorder, generalized anxiety disorder, major depression, chronic pain, and traumatic brain injury.

POSTPARTUM. Following childbirth.

POST-TRAUMATIC AMNESIA (PTA). Difficulty forming new memories after a traumatic brain injury.

POST-TRAUMATIC DEMENTIA. Persistent mental deterioration following a traumatic brain injury.

POST-TRAUMATIC STRESS DISORDER (PTSD). A condition that develops in response to a highly stressful or traumatic event, typically characterized by depression, anxiety, flashbacks, nightmares, and avoidance of reminders of the traumatic experience.

POSTURAL TREMOR. A continuous quiver that affects body posture and movement.

PRADER-WILLI SYNDROME. A rare genetic disorder that causes a constant feeling of hunger.

PRAGMATIC LANGUAGE IMPAIRMENT (PLI). A term that is used by some researchers as an equivalent to social communication disorder. PLI was previously known as semantic pragmatic disorder (SPD).

PRAGMATICS. A subfield of linguistics that explores the ways in which context contributes to the meaning of language. In ordinary usage, pragmatics refers to a person's ability to know what is appropriate to say, where and when to say it, and the give-and-take nature of conversation.

PRANAYAMA. Yogic breathing techniques.

PREFERRED PROVIDER ORGANIZATION (PPO). A healthcare organization that provides managed-care group health insurance and that has contracted with a group of doctors, hospitals, and other providers to provide health care at reduced rates for its clients.

PREFRONTAL CORTEX. Area of the brain involved in attention span, judgment, response to external stimuli, memory, motor function, and impulse control.

PREMENSTRUAL MOLIMINA. The normal signs that indicate that menses will soon occur.

PRENATAL EXPOSURE. Coming in contact with a fetus during pregnancy.

PRESENILE DEMENTIA. The original name for Alzheimer's disease.

PRESENILIN (PSEN). Proteins that are involved in processing amyloid precursor protein (APP). Mutations in the genes encoding these proteins can cause early-onset Alzheimer's disease.

PRESSURE ULCERS. Also known as pressure sores or bed sores, these can develop in patients who are unable to move. If not treated properly, they can become infected.

PRETENDER. With regard to body integrity identity disorder (BIID), a person who uses assistive devices or other props in public in order to appear disabled.

PREVALENCE. The number of cases of a disease or disorder existing in a specific population at a given point in time.

PRIAPISM. Painful involuntary penile erection that persists over long periods of time.

PRIMARY ENURESIS. Bed-wetting in a child who has not yet developed bladder control.

PRIMARY GAIN. In psychiatry, the principal psychological reason for the development of a patient's symptoms.

PRIMARY NARCISSISM. Sigmund Freud's term for a normal phase in early childhood development in which the infant has not yet learned to distinguish between itself and its world, seeing other people and things in its environment as extensions of itself.

PRIMARY PERSONALITY. The core personality of a patient with dissociative identity disorder.

PRIMARY PROGRESSIVE APHASIA. A disorder in which there is progressive loss of language skills.

PRIMARY SLEEP DISORDER. A sleep disorder that cannot be attributed to a medical condition, another mental disorder, prescription medications, or other substances.

PRION. An infectious agent consisting of protein in a misfolded form. Its name is a combination of "protein" and "infection."

PROCESS ADDICTION. A term used to describe addiction to an activity or behavior rather than a substance; also known as behavioral addiction or non-substance-related addiction.

PRODROMAL. The early stage or the start of a disease, before specific or characteristic symptoms occur.

PRODRUG. The inactive form of a drug that is metabolized into an active compound inside the body.

PROGRESSIVE MUSCLE RELAXATION. Relaxation exercises that involve slowly tensing and then relaxing each muscle group in the body separately in a systematic order.

PROGRESSIVE SUPRANUCLEAR PALSY. A rare disease that gradually destroys nerve cells in the parts of the brain that control eye movements, breathing, and muscle coordination. The loss of nerve cells causes palsy, or paralysis, that slowly gets worse as the disease progresses. The palsy affects ability to move the eyes, relax the muscles, and control balance.

PROJECTION. A psychological process in which a person unconsciously attributes unacceptable feelings to someone else.

PROJECTIVE TEST. A psychological test for assessing thinking patterns, observational abilities, attitudes, and feelings based on open-ended responses to ambiguous (having more than one meaning) stimuli; often used to evaluate personality disorders.

PROLACTIN. A hormone that stimulates milk production and breast development.

PROPRIOCEPTION. A person's normal sense of posture, balance, direction of movement, and location in space.

PROPRIOCEPTIVE. Pertaining to proprioception.

PROSTAGLANDINS. A group of unsaturated fatty acids involved in the contraction of smooth muscle, control of inflammation, and many other body processes.

PROSTATE. A walnut-shaped gland surrounding the urethra in males at the base of the urinary bladder. The prostate gland secretes the fluid that combines with the male sperm cells to form semen.

PROXY. An individual who makes decisions on behalf of another.

PSEUDODEMENTIA. A term for a type of depression with symptoms resembling those of dementia. The term "dementia of depression" is now preferred.

PSEUDOSEIZURE. A fit that resembles an epileptic seizure but is not associated with abnormal electrical discharges in the patient's brain.

PSYCHIATRIC. Relating to psychiatry.

PSYCHIATRIC BOARDING. The practice of holding patients with mental illness in emergency department corridors and waiting areas because of the lack of hospital beds or other facilities.

PSYCHIATRIC DISORDERS. Any behavioral or psychological condition that impairs basic bodily functions and increases the risk of death and disability.

PSYCHIATRIST. A medical doctor who has completed specialized training in the diagnosis and treatment of mental illness. Psychiatrists can diagnose mental illnesses, provide mental health counseling, and prescribe medications.

PSYCHIC. Relating to the mind rather than the body.

PSYCHIC NUMBING. An inability to respond emotionally to people or situations; this numbing affects positive as well as negative emotions.

PSYCHOACTIVE. Referring to any substance that crosses the blood-brain barrier and acts primarily upon the central nervous system, leading to changes in mood, perception, thinking, feeling, or behavior.

PSYCHOANALYSIS. The study of human psychological functioning and behavior.

PSYCHOANALYTIC. Understanding human motivations, emotions, and mental processes according to theories and concepts originally developed by Sigmund Freud.

PSYCHOANALYTIC THERAPY. Therapy based on the psychodynamic theory of Sigmund Freud.

PSYCHODIAGNOSTIC. Various methods used to examine and analyze the factors that form human behavior, especially abnormal behavior.

PSYCHODRAMA. A form of group therapy that has group members act out parts of important people in the lives of individual group members.

PSYCHODYNAMIC. Referring to the mental, emotional, or motivational forces or processes that form human attitudes and behaviors, especially unconscious processes that develop in early childhood.

PSYCHODYNAMIC GROUPS. Psychotherapy groups that utilize the principles of unconscious needs and motivations developed by Sigmund Freud.

PSYCHODYNAMIC PSYCHOTHERAPY. A therapeutic approach to helping persons find relief from emotional pain.

PSYCHODYNAMIC THEORISTS. Therapists who believe that the origins of mental problems lie in a person's internal conflicts and complexes.

PSYCHODYNAMIC THERAPY. A therapeutic approach that assumes that dysfunctional or unwanted behavior is caused by unconscious, internal conflicts and focuses on gaining insight into and resolving these conflicts.

PSYCHOGENIC. Originating in the mind, or in a mental process or condition. The term "psychogenic" is sometimes used as a synonym for "conversion."

PSYCHOLOGICAL. Refers to mental processes, including thoughts, feelings, and emotions.

PSYCHOLOGICAL ASSESSMENT. A process of gathering and synthesizing information about a person's psychological makeup and history for a specific purpose, which may be educational, diagnostic, or forensic.

PSYCHOLOGIST. A mental health professional who treats mental and behavioral disorders by providing support and insight to encourage healthy behavior patterns and personality growth. Psychologists also study the brain, behavior, emotions, and learning.

PSYCHOMETRIC PSYCHOLOGY. A branch of psychology that deals with measurement of mental capacities, processes, and traits.

PSYCHONEUROIMMUNOLOGY. The study of the relationships among the mind, nervous system, and immune response.

PSYCHOPATHOLOGY. The study of the causes and development of psychiatric disorders in humans.

PSYCHOPATHY. A serious personality disorder characterized by antisocial, aggressive, and violent behavior and thoughts, along with a lack of empathy for personal actions.

PSYCHOSEXUAL CONFLICTS. In Freudian categories, internal conflicts related to problems at a particular stage of childhood development. Freud associated each developmental stage with a particular part of the human body, such as the mouth or the phallus.

PSYCHOSIS. A general psychiatric term for a condition in which the patient loses touch with reality. It is marked by such symptoms as hallucinations, delusions, personality changes, and disordered thinking. Psychosis is usually one feature of an overarching disorder, not a disorder in itself.

PSYCHOSOCIAL. A term that refers to the emotional and social aspects of psychological disorders.

PSYCHOSOMATIC. A type of physical illness caused by mental factors.

PSYCHOSTIMULANT. A type of drug that increases the activity of the parts of the brain that produce dopamine.

PSYCHOTHERAPEUTIC DRUGS. Drugs used to treat psychiatric disorders, such as tranquilizers, sedatives, analgesics, and stimulants.

PSYCHOTHERAPY. The treatment of mental and behavioral disorders by providing support and insight to encourage healthy behavior patterns and personality growth.

PSYCHOTIC. Relating to psychosis, or a psychiatric disorder characterized by hallucinations, a distorted view of reality, and other such mental problems.

PSYCHOTIC DISORDER. Any psychiatric disorder involving a loss of touch with reality, made evident by such symptoms as hallucinations, delusions, and incoherence; examples of psychotic disorders include schizophrenia and mania.

PSYCHOTROPIC DRUG. A drug that acts on or influences the activity of the mind.

PSYCHOTROPIC MEDICATION. Medication that has an effect on the mind, brain, behavior, perceptions, or emotions. Psychotropic medications are used to treat mental illnesses because they affect a patient's moods and perceptions.

PTOSIS. Drooping of the upper eyelid.

PUNITIVE. Concerned with, or directed toward, punishment.

PURGING. Inappropriate actions taken to prevent weight gain, often after bingeing, including self-induced vomiting or the misuse of laxatives, diuretics, enemas, or other medications.

PYROMANIA. An impulse control disorder characterized by repeatedly setting fires.

PYRROLE. A heterocyclic aromatic organic compound with chemical formula C_4H_4NH.

Q

QI. The traditional Chinese term for vital energy or the life force. The word is also spelled *ki* or *chi* in English translations of Japanese and Chinese medical books.

QIGONG. An exercise practice derived from traditional Chinese medicine and designed to facilitate energy flow throughout the body.

QUALITATIVE. Relating to quality.

QUANTITATIVE. Relating to quantity.

QUANTITATIVE REASONING. The ability to complete mathematical problems and to apply mathematics on a practical level.

QUICKENING. A term that refers to the movements or other signs of life of a fetus in the womb.

R

RADIO WAVES. Electromagnetic energy of the frequency range corresponding to that used in radio communications, usually 10,000 cycles per second to 300 billion cycles per second. Radio waves are the same as visible light, x rays, and all other types of electromagnetic radiation but are of a higher frequency.

RADIOACTIVE. Relating to radiation emitted by certain substances.

RADIONUCLIDE. An atom with an unstable nucleus that emits gamma rays during the process of its radioactive decay. Radionuclides, also known as radioisotopes, are used to make the tracers used in some imaging studies.

RADIOPHARMACEUTICAL. A radioactive drug.

RANDOMIZATION. The process of randomly assigning participants in an experiment to the various treatment groups, so that each individual has an equal chance of being assigned to any of the groups.

RAPHE NUCLEI. A group of nine pairs of compact clusters of nerve cells found in the brainstem that secrete serotonin for use in the brain.

RAPID CYCLING. Four or more manic, hypomanic, mixed, or depressive episodes within a 12-month period.

RAPID EYE MOVEMENT (REM) SLEEP. A stage of sleep during which the sleeper's eyes move back and forth rapidly. Most dreams occur during REM sleep.

RAPPORT. A relation of empathy and trust between a therapist and patient.

RATIONAL EMOTIVE THERAPY. A form of psychotherapy developed by Albert Ellis and other psychotherapists based on the theory that emotional response is based on the subjective interpretation of events, not on the events themselves.

RAYNAUD'S SYNDROME. A disorder of the circulatory or vascular system characterized by abnormally cold hands and feet because of constricted blood vessels in these areas.

RDA. The abbreviation for recommended dietary allowance, which is the amount of vitamins and minerals needed to provide adequate nutrition in most healthy people. The amount varies depending on age, gender, and physical conditions, such as pregnancy; sometimes RDA is called "daily value" (DV) in the United States.

REALITY TESTING. A phrase that refers to a person's ability to distinguish between subjective feelings and objective reality.

REBOUND EFFECT. A physical reaction to stopping a medication characterized by the reappearance of the symptom(s) that the medication was given to suppress.

REBUS. A puzzle in which syllables of words and names are represented by pictures of objects that sound similar or by letters.

RECEPTOR. In biochemistry, a substance (usually a protein) found on the surface of a cell that interacts with specific other molecules, drugs, hormones, or antibodies.

RECIDIVISM. A tendency to return to a previous activity or behavior, especially criminal or deviant behavior.

RECREATIONAL DRUGS. The use of a drug with the intention of creating a psychoactive (heightened) mental experience; for the most part, such use is illegal.

REFOCUSING TECHNIQUES. Techniques that direct a person's attention away from overwhelming, negative thoughts and emotions by focusing on inner peace and managing one issue at a time.

REGIMEN. A regulated course of treatment for a medical or mental disorder.

REGISTERED DIETITIAN. A person who has met certain education and experience standards and is well-qualified to provide nutrition counseling.

REGRESSION. In psychology, a return to earlier, usually childish or infantile, patterns of thought or behavior.

REGURGITATION. The return of partly digested food from the stomach to the mouth. Regurgitation may be either an intentional act or an involuntary physical reaction.

REHABILITATE. To restore; to put back into good condition.

REINFORCEMENT. In behavioral therapy, the ability of a behavior to produce effects that will make the user want to perform the behavior again. In modeling, reinforcement refers to rewarding the model's demonstration of a skill or the client's performance of the newly acquired skill in practice or in real-life situations.

REINFORCEMENT SCHEDULE. The frequency and amount of reinforcers administered.

REINFORCER. Anything that causes an increase of a particular behavior.

RELAPSE. A recurrence of symptoms after a period of improvement or recovery.

RELATIVE DEPRIVATION. A feeling of deprivation based on comparison with neighbors and relatives.

RELAXATION RESPONSE. The body's inactivation of stress responses and return of stress hormone levels to normal after a threat has passed.

RELAXATION TECHNIQUES. Techniques used to relieve stress. Exercise, biofeedback, hypnosis, and meditation are all effective relaxation tools. Relaxation techniques are used in cognitive-behavioral therapy to teach patients new ways of coping with stressful situations.

RELEASE HALLUCINATIONS. Hallucinations that develop after partial loss of sight or hearing and that represent images or sounds formed from memory traces rather than present sensory input. They are called "release" hallucinations because they would ordinarily be blocked by incoming sensory data.

RELIABILITY. The ability of a test to yield consistent, repeatable results.

REM. Rapid eye movement; a stage of the normal sleep cycle characterized by rapid eye movements, increased forebrain and midbrain activity, and dreaming.

REM LATENCY. After a person falls asleep, the amount of time it takes for the first onset of REM sleep.

REMEDY ANTIDOTE. Certain foods, beverages, prescription medications, aromatic compounds, and other environmental elements that counteract the efficacy of homeopathic remedies.

REMISSION. In the course of an illness or disorder, a period of time when symptoms are absent.

REMOTE THERAPY. A general term for therapy delivered by electronic communication technologies; includes Internet-based therapy along with telephone therapy and videoconferencing.

REPETITIVE STRESS INJURY (RSI). A type of injury to the musculoskeletal and nervous systems associated with occupational strain or overuse of a specific part of the body. Bodywork therapies are often recommended to people suffering from RSIs.

RESILIENCE. In psychiatry, the ability of a person to respond positively to, or bounce back from, trauma or hardship. Resilience is considered a process of interaction between the person and his or her environment rather than a one-time action.

RESPITE CARE. Temporary care of a patient to provide the usual caregivers with a period of physical, mental, and emotional rest.

RESPONSE COST. A behavioral technique that involves removing a stimulus from an individual's environment so that the response directly preceding the removal is weakened. In a token economy system, response cost is a form of punishment involving loss of tokens due to inappropriate behavior, which consequently results in decreased ability to purchase back-up reinforcers.

RESPONSE TO INTERVENTION (RTI). An approach to diagnosis of learning disorders based on a child's response (or lack of response) to early interventions with learning problems.

RESPONSE-CONTINGENT. An approach to treatment in which rewards or punishments are given in response to a particular behavior, in order to encourage or correct the behavior.

RESTLESS LEGS SYNDROME (RLS). A neurological disorder characterized by aching, burning, or creeping sensations in the legs that can only be relieved by moving the legs, often resulting in insomnia.

RETROGRADE AMNESIA. Amnesia for events that occurred before the onset of an amnestic disorder.

RETROPERITONEAL. The anatomical area between the peritoneum (lining of the abdominal cavity) and the muscular and connective tissues of the abdominal wall.

RETT SYNDROME. An inherited progressive neurodevelopmental disorder that affects females, usually beginning in infancy. Rett syndrome is characterized by cognitive and motor deterioration, slow brain growth, and intellectual disability.

REVIEW OF SYSTEMS (ROS). A systematic checklist of the various organ systems in the human body—ear, nose, and throat; respiratory; cardiovascular; gastrointestinal; genitourinary; musculoskeletal; skin and hair; and neurological—used to ensure that all relevant physical signs and symptoms have been taken into account during a medical or psychiatric evaluation.

RHIZOME. A fleshy plant stem that grows horizontally under or along the ground; roots are sent out below this stem and leaves or shoots are sent out above it.

RISK ASSESSMENT. The process of gathering and interpreting data useful in estimating the probability that an individual will display a certain behavior.

RISK MANAGEMENT. Using the results of a risk assessment to tailor intervention strategies intended to reduce the likelihood that an individual will demonstrate a certain behavior.

ROLE. The set of customary or expected behavior patterns associated with a particular position or function in society.

ROLE PLAYING. A technique used in therapy in which participants act out roles relevant to real-life situations in order to change their attitudes and behaviors.

ROLE TRANSITION. Life changes that require an adjustment in social or occupational status or self-image.

RORSCHACH TEST. A popular projective psychological test, in which a subject's interpretations of a series of ten standard inkblots are used to assess personality and emotional traits and diagnose disorders; also known as the Rorschach psychodiagnostic test.

RUMINATE. To chew or rechew regurgitated food.

RUNNER'S HIGH. A feeling of exhilaration that occurs when a period of strenuous exercise activates the release of endorphins. While typically associated with long-distance runners, the experience of such a high has been reported by dancers and athletes in other sports.

RUSSELL'S SIGN. Scraped or raw areas on a patient's knuckles caused by self-induced vomiting.

S

SADISM. A mental disorder in which sexual arousal and gratification are obtained by inflicting pain or humiliation on another person.

"SATISFACTION WITH LIFE." Term coined by psychologist Ed Diener as a level of satisfaction determined by acceptance of the past, contentment with the present, and optimism for the future.

SCABIES. A contagious skin infection in humans and other animals caused by a tiny parasite that burrows under the skin and causes intense itching.

SCALE. A subset of test items from a multi-item test.

SCAPEGOATING. The emergence of behavioral problems in one family member, usually the identified patient, who is often punished for problems within the entire family.

SCHEMAS. Fundamental core beliefs or assumptions that are part of the perceptual filter people use to view the world. Cognitive-behavioral therapy seeks to change maladaptive schemas.

SCHIZOAFFECTIVE DISORDER. Having symptoms of both schizophrenia and bipolar disorder.

SCHIZOPHRENIA. A severe mental illness in which a person has difficulty distinguishing what is real from what is not real. It is often characterized by hallucinations, delusions, language and communication disturbances, and withdrawal from people and social activities.

SCHIZOPHRENIFORM DISORDER. A short-term variation of schizophrenia that has a total duration of one to six months.

SCINTILLATOR. A material that exhibits the property of luminescence (also called "scintillation") when it is excited by ionizing radiation.

SCREENING TEST. A test given as a preliminary tool that helps to later target a more thorough analysis.

SEASONAL AFFECTIVE DISORDER (SAD). A mood disorder characterized by depression, weight gain, and sleepiness during the winter months.

SECONDARY ENURESIS. Bed-wetting in a child who had previously established bladder control but has begun to wet the bed again, usually as the result of emotional stress.

SECONDARY GAIN. In conversion disorder, a term that refers to other benefits that a patient obtains from a conversion symptom. For example, a patient's loss of function in an arm might require other family members to do the patient's share of household chores, or they might give the patient more attention and sympathy than he or she usually receives.

SECTION 504. The section of the Rehabilitation Act of 1973 that provides that no person may be discriminated against because of a physical disability For example, if a child uses a wheelchair, his or her school must find a way to ensure that children in wheelchairs have access to all classes.

SEDATION. A state of emotional or physical relaxation. The term is usually used to refer to this condition when it is produced by a medication.

SEDATIVE. A medication that induces relaxation and sleep.

SEIZURE. A sudden attack, spasm, or convulsion.

SELECTIVE SEROTONIN NOREPINEPHRINE REUPTAKE INHIBITORS (SSNRIs). Drug class that acts to specifically inhibit the reuptake of serotonin and norepinephrine with little effect on other types of neurotransmitters, thereby decreasing side effects associated with broader-acting drugs.

SELECTIVE SEROTONIN REUPTAKE INHIBITORS (SSRIs). A class of antidepressants that works by blocking the reabsorption of serotonin in brain cells, raising the level of the chemical in the brain.

SELF-DELIVERANCE. A term for assisted suicide, more commonly used in Great Britain than in the United States.

SELF-HELP GROUPS. Groups that fall outside the realm of psychotherapy groups but that offer help to individuals with a particular problem or concern. These groups are typically not led by professionals.

SELF-STIGMA. Loss of self-esteem and personal effectiveness that develops when a person being treated for a mental health issue internalizes public prejudice against people diagnosed with mental disorders.

SEMANTIC DEMENTIA. A disorder in which there is progressive loss of knowledge about words and word meanings.

SEMANTICS. A subfield of linguistics that focuses on the meaning of words; in ordinary usage, the ability to use words correctly and understand their meanings.

SEMEN. A thick whitish fluid containing sperm, produced by the male reproductive organs.

SEMINAL FLUID. Fluid composed of semen from the testes and prostatic secretions.

SEMINAL VESICLES. Sac-like structures that border the male urethra and serve as storage depots for the seminal fluid.

SEMI-STRUCTURED INTERVIEW. A type of psychiatric interview in which the interviewer can ask new questions in the course of the interview, depending on the interviewee's answers to previous questions (does not follow a set format).

SENSITIZATION. To make sensitive or susceptible.

SENSORIMOTOR. Relating to sensory and motor coordination of the nervous system.

SEQUELA (PLURAL, SEQUELAE). In medicine, a pathological condition resulting from a disease, injury, or other trauma.

SEROTONERGIC. Containing, activating, or otherwise involving serotonin.

SEROTONIN. 5-Hydroxytryptamine; a substance that occurs throughout the body with numerous effects, including neurotransmission. Low serotonin levels are associated with mood disorders, particularly depression and obsessive-compulsive disorder.

SEROTONIN SYNDROME. A potentially life-threatening drug reaction involving an excess of the neurotransmitter serotonin, usually occurring when too many medications that increase serotonin are taken together.

SEROTONIN TRANSPORTER (SERT). A protein that removes serotonin from the spaces between neurons (synaptic clefts) and thus terminates its action. In effect, SERT recycles serotonin by returning it to the neuron that originally released it (the presynaptic neuron).

SEX HORMONES. Hormones that are responsible for sexual characteristics and reproductive functioning.

SEXUAL ASSAULT NURSE EXAMINER (SANE). A nurse with specialized training in the care and forensic examination of victims of sexual assault.

SEXUAL VIOLENCE. Actual, attempted, or threatened sexual contact with a person who is nonconsenting or unable to give consent.

SHAKEN BABY SYNDROME (SBS). A severe form of traumatic brain injury resulting from shaking an infant or small child forcefully enough to cause the brain to jar against the skull.

SHAMAN. In certain indigenous tribes or groups, a person who acts as an intermediary between the natural and supernatural worlds. Shamans are regarded as having the power or ability to cure illnesses.

SHARED PSYCHOTIC DISORDER. Also known as *folie à deux,* shared psychotic disorder is an uncommon disorder in which the same delusion is shared by two or more individuals, one of whom has no established mental illness.

SHIATSU. Japanese form of acupressure massage.

SHIFT. The transition of control from one personality to another in a person with dissociative identity disorder. Usually shifts occur rapidly, within seconds, but in some cases a more gradual changeover is observed. Also referred to as a switch.

SIBLING RIVALRY. Competition among brothers and sisters in a nuclear family.

SICKLE CELL ANEMIA. An inherited disorder in which red blood cells contain an abnormal form of hemoglobin, a protein that carries oxygen. The abnormal form of hemoglobin causes the red cells to become sickle shaped. The misshapen cells may clog blood vessels, preventing oxygen from reaching tissues and leading to pain, blood clots, and other problems.

SKILLED NURSING FACILITY. An inpatient facility that provides 24-hour nursing services to individuals in need of extended care.

SLEEP APNEA. A condition in which a person temporarily stops breathing during sleep.

SLEEP CYCLE. A period of NREM (non-rapid eye movement) sleep followed by a shorter phase of REM (rapid eye movement) sleep. Most adults have four to six sleep cycles per night.

SLEEP DISORDER. Any condition that interferes with sleep.

SLEEP DRUNKENNESS. A condition associated with primary hypersomnia in which the person has an abnormally prolonged period of transition from sleep to wakefulness; is disoriented, drowsy, and uncoordinated; and may behave in an excited or violent fashion.

SLEEP HYGIENE. Beneficial behavior and environmental choices that precede sleep and tend to help produce a good night's sleep.

SLEEP LATENCY. The amount of time that it takes to fall asleep. Sleep latency is measured in minutes and is important in diagnosing depression.

SLEEP PARALYSIS. An abnormal episode of sleep in which the patient cannot move for a few minutes, usually occurring on falling asleep or waking up. It is often found in patients with narcolepsy.

SLEEP TERROR DISORDER. A sleep disorder in which a person wakes up fearful and anxious but with no recollection of the source of the fear.

SOCIAL COMMUNICATION DISORDER. A communication disorder in which persons have trouble understanding the pragmatics of conversation, or the appropriate use of language depending on the context or social situation.

SOCIAL LEARNING THEORY. A subset of learning theories based on the concept that human behavior originates in and is affected by the interplay among the person's learned experiences, previous behaviors, and environmental influences.

SOCIAL MEDIA. A general term for both Web-based and mobile technologies that facilitate social (as distinct from commercial or academic) interaction online.

SOCIAL MODELING. A process of learning behavioral and emotional-response patterns from observing one's parents or other adults.

SOCIAL PHOBIA. An anxiety disorder characterized by a strong and persistent fear of social or performance situations.

SOCIALIZATION. The process through which a person learns his or her roles in society. It includes the society's customs, traditions, and professional roles as well as gender roles.

SOCIOECONOMIC STATUS. Perceived status of an individual, family, or community based on average income, education level, and social status.

SODOMY. Anal sex; the term is sometimes used to describe anal rape.

SOLUTION-FOCUSED THERAPY. A type of therapy that involves concrete goals and an emphasis on future direction rather than past experiences.

SOMATIC. Relating to the body, rather than the mind.

SOMATIC CONCERN. Excessive concern about the body, particularly in relation to illness.

SOMATIC EDUCATION. The integration of bodywork with self-awareness, intelligence, and imagination.

SOMATIZATION. When mental or emotional distress manifests as physical symptoms.

SOMATIZATION DISORDER. A disorder in which patients seek medical treatment for physical ailments with no discernible organic cause.

SOMATOFORM DISORDERS. A category of psychiatric disorders characterized by physical complaints that appear to be medical in origin but that cannot be explained in terms of a physical disease, the results of substance abuse, or by another mental disorder.

SOMNAMBULISM. Another term for sleepwalking.

SPECIFIC PHOBIA. A type of phobia in which the object or situation that arouses fear is clearly identifiable and limited. An older term for specific phobia is simple phobia.

SPEECH-LANGUAGE PATHOLOGIST. A professional with special training in the evaluation and treatment of persons with voice, speech, and language disorders.

"SPEED RUN." The episodic bingeing on amphetamines.

SPHENOIDAL ELECTRODES. Fine wire electrodes that are implanted under the cheek bones, used to measure temporal seizures.

SPLITTING. In regards to narcissistic personality disorder, a psychological process that occurs during childhood, in which the child separates aspects of him- or herself that the parents value from those that they disregard.

SPONTANEOUS REMISSION. Recovery from a disease or disorder that cannot be attributed to medical or psychiatric treatments.

SPORADIC. Occurring at random in persons with no known risk factors or genetic mutations.

SNRI. Selective serotonin norepinephrine reuptake inhibitor.

SSRI. Selective serotonin reuptake inhibitor.

STABILIZATION. Preventing shock in an injured person by protecting the airway, controlling bleeding (if any), keeping the person warm, and preventing injury to the spinal cord.

STALKING. The willful and repeated following, watching, and/or harassing of another person, usually with the intent of forcing the victim into a dating or sexual relationship.

STANDARD DEVIATION. A statistical measure of dispersion; that is, how much a set of values differs from an arithmetic mean.

STANDARDIZATION. The administration of a test to a sample group of people for the purpose of establishing scoring norms.

STANDARDIZED TEST. A test that follows a regimented structure, with each individual's scores compared to others within a group.

STATE CHILDREN'S HEALTH INSURANCE PROGRAM (SCHIP; CHIP). A state-administered health insurance program for lower- and middle-income children who are without private health insurance and whose family incomes are above the Medicaid eligibility limits.

STATUTORY RAPE. Sexual activity, often coercive, in which one party is below the age of consent.

STEAM DISTILLATION. A process of extracting essential oils from plant products through a heating and evaporation process.

STEROIDS. A class of hormones and drugs that includes sex and stress hormones and anti-inflammatory medications, contraceptives, and growth-promoting substances.

STEROLS. Steroid alcohols, such as cholesterol, that are widely distributed in the body.

STIGMA. Any attribute that is generally perceived as negative by society (regardless of fact).

STIMULANT. A type of psychoactive substance that increases alertness or wakefulness. Stimulants may be prescribed to treat disorders such as autism or attention deficit hyperactivity disorder but are also illegally abused.

STIMULANT ABUSE DISORDERS. Also called stimulant use disorders, any disorder that involves the abuse of stimulant drugs.

STIMULUS. An agent that directly elicits a response, such as a thought, emotion, or action, including images, smells, sounds, words, or ideas.

STIMULUS FADING. A form of behavior modification in which goals of gradually increasing difficulty are set for the client.

STOOLS. Feces; bowel movements.

STREET DRUG. A substance purchased from a drug dealer. It may be a legal substance sold illicitly (without a prescription and not for medical use), or it may be a substance that is illegal to possess.

STRESS. A physical and psychological response that results from being exposed to a demand or pressure.

STRESS HARDINESS. A personality characteristic that enables persons to stay healthy in stressful circumstances. It includes belief in one's ability to influence the situation, commitment to or full engagement with one's activities, and a positive view of change.

STRESS MANAGEMENT. A category of popularized programs and techniques intended to help reduce or eliminate stress.

STRESSOR. A stimulus or event that provokes a stress response in an organism. Stressors can be categorized as acute or chronic and as external or internal to the organism.

STRIATUM. Area of the brain involved in psychostimulation and addiction.

STROKE. A temporary loss of normal blood flow to an area of the brain, caused by blockage or rupture of a blood vessel.

STRUCTURAL INTEGRATION. Term used to describe the method and philosophy of life associated with Rolfing, a type of bodywork therapy.

STRUCTURED INTERVIEW. A type of interview often used by researchers to gather data, in which subjects are asked a series of standardized questions in the same order with the same wording. The questions are usually closed-ended (the choice of answers is fixed in advance), although some structured interviews may include a few open-ended questions.

STUPOR. A state of sluggishness or impaired consciousness.

SUBDURAL ELECTRODES. Strip electrodes that are placed under the dura mater (the outermost, toughest, and most fibrous of the three membranes [meninges] covering the brain and spinal cord) to locate the foci of epileptic seizures prior to epilepsy surgery.

SUBDURAL HEMATOMA. Active bleeding or a blood clot inside the dura (leathery covering of the brain). This causes swelling of the brain and if left untreated can cause death.

SUBJECTIVE. Referring to a person's unique internal thoughts and feelings, as distinct from the objects of those thoughts and feelings in the external world.

SUBJECTIVE UNITS OF DISTRESS (SUDS) SCALE. A scale used by patients during exposure treatment to rate their levels of fear and anxiety with numbers from 0–100.

SUBSTANCE ABUSE. Illicit or excessive use of a drug or other substance that has a pronounced effect on the mind or body without any therapeutic application.

SUBTHRESHOLD. A term used in psychiatry to describe a condition that has significant clinical features but does not meet the full criteria of any major disorder.

SUICIDE GESTURE. Attempted suicide by way of a low-lethality method, low level of intent or planning, and little physical damage; sometimes called pseudocide.

SUICIDE MAGNET. A bridge, tall building, or geographic location that acquires a reputation as a location for suicide attempts.

SULCI. The furrows or grooves on the surface of the brain between convolutions.

SUNSETTING. Confusion or agitation in the evening; also called sundowning.

SUPEREGO. According to Freud, the part of the mind that represents traditional parental and societal values. The superego is the source of guilt feelings.

SUPERIOR MESENTERIC ARTERY SYNDROME. A condition in which a person vomits after meals due to blockage of the blood supply to the intestine.

SUPPORT GROUP. A group whose primary purpose is to provide empathy and emotional support to its members. Support groups are less formal and less goal-directed than group therapy sessions.

SUPPORTIVE THERAPY. An approach to psychotherapy that seeks to encourage the patient or offer emotional support rather than attempt behavioral changes.

SUPRACHIASMATIC NUCLEUS (SCN). A pair of nerve clusters in the hypothalamus in the brain that receives light input from the retina via the optic nerve and regulates circadian rhythms.

SURVIVOR'S GUILT. A psychological reaction in trauma survivors that takes the form of guilt feelings for having survived or escaped a trauma without serious injury when others did not.

SYDENHAM'S CHOREA. A serious manifestation of acute rheumatic fever that commonly occurs in children ages 7 through 14, peaking at age 8. This disease of the central nervous system is characterized by emotional instability, purposeless movements, and muscular weakness.

SYMPATHETIC NERVOUS SYSTEM. The part of the nervous system that prepares the body to react to situations of stress or emergency; physical effects include increased heart rate and blood pressure, sweating, and pupil dilation.

SYNAPSE. A connection between a neuron (nerve cell) and another cell (which may be a neuron or another type of cell) that allows the neuron to transmit a chemical or electrical signal to the receiving cell.

SYNCOPE. A brief lapse of consciousness caused by a temporarily insufficient flow of blood to the brain.

SYNDROME. A group of signs or symptoms that occur together and characterize or define a particular disease or disorder.

SYSTEMIC LUPUS ERYTHEMATOSUS (SLE). A chronic inflammatory autoimmune disorder.

SYSTOLIC. Referring to the rhythmic contraction of the heart (systole) as the blood in the chambers is forced out. Systolic blood pressure is blood pressure measured during the systolic phase.

T

TACHYCARDIA. A pulse rate above 100 beats per minute.

TACTILE. The perception of touch.

TAI CHI. A martial art involving controlled movements specifically designed to improve physical and mental well-being.

TARDIVE AKATHISIA. A disorder in which an individual continuously feels restless.

TARDIVE DYSKINESIA (TD). A disorder characterized by involuntary and repetitive body movements that sometimes develops after long-term use of antipsychotic medications.

TARDIVE DYSTONIA. Involuntary, abnormal movements of the neck and shoulder muscles.

TARGET BEHAVIOR. The specific behavior to be increased or decreased during the course of a treatment.

TAU PROTEIN. A protein involved in maintaining the internal structure of nerve cells. Tau protein is damaged in Alzheimer's disease and forms neurofibrillary tangles.

TEMPERAMENT. A person's natural or genetically determined disposition.

TEMPORAL. Relating to the temples.

TEMPORAL LOBE. A part of the brain that is involved in processing auditory and visual information, emotion and motivation, and understanding language.

TEMPOROMANDIBULAR JOINT DYSFUNCTION. A condition resulting in pain in the head, face, and jaw. Muscle tension or abnormalities of the bones in the area of the hinged joint (the temporomandibular joint) between the lower jaw and the temporal bone are usually the cause.

TERATOGEN. An agent or chemical that causes a birth defect.

TERMINATION. The process of ending a therapy group; an important part of a group therapy.

TERRITORIAL AGGRESSION. The response of aggressively defending a defined space perceived as being threatened by a member of the same species.

TEST ANXIETY. A name for the stress and intensity of emotional upset that students experience before they take exams.

TESTOSTERONE. The primary male sex hormone.

THALAMUS. The middle part of the diencephalon (a part of the human forebrain), responsible for transmitting and integrating information from the senses.

THANATOLOGIST. A specialist in the study of death and the psychological mechanisms for coping with death.

THEMATIC APPERCEPTION TEST (TAT). A clinical psychology projective test where patients make up stories or descriptions for a set of pictures; used for diagnostic, psychodynamic, and personality assessments.

THERAPEUTIC ALLIANCE. The technical term for the cooperative relationship between a therapist and a client, considered essential for successful psychotherapy.

THERAPEUTIC VALUE. The potential benefit of an object or situation in terms of its ability to enhance functioning (social, emotional, intellectual, occupational, etc.) in an individual.

THERAPEUTIC WRITING. A treatment technique in which patients are asked to write an account of a traumatic event and their emotional responses to it.

THERMISTOR. An electrical device whose resistance decreases with rises in temperature.

THOUGHT DISORDER. A condition characterized by incomprehensible language, either written or spoken.

THROMBOCYTOPENIA. A condition involving abnormally low numbers of platelets (blood-clotting agents) in the blood; usually associated with hemorrhaging (bleeding).

THUJONE. A natural chemical compound found in sage as well as in wormwood and certain other spices. In large quantities, it can cause hallucinations and convulsions.

THYROID. A gland in the neck that produces the hormone thyroxine, which is responsible for regulating metabolic activity in the body.

TIC. A sudden involuntary behavior that is difficult or impossible for the person to suppress. Tics may be either motor (related to movement) or vocal and may become more pronounced under stress.

TINCTURE. An alcohol-based herbal extract prepared by soaking parts of the plant in a mixture of alcohol and water.

TINNITUS. Perceived ringing, buzzing, whistling, or other noise heard in one or both ears that has no external source. It is not a disease by itself but a symptom that may have a number of different causes.

TISSUE PLASMINOGEN ACTIVATOR (tPA). A drug that is sometimes given to patients within three hours of a stroke to dissolve blood clots within the brain; also used to treat heart attack victims.

TOKEN. In a token economy system, any item that can be seen and collected (such as stickers or points in a point tally) that has no value on its own but that is used as an immediate reward for desirable behavior to later be redeemed for a larger reward.

TOLERANCE. A progressive decrease in the effectiveness of a drug with long-term use, requiring higher doses to achieve the desired effect.

TOMOGRAPHY. A scanning technique that uses electromagnetic radiation (such as gamma rays or x rays) or ultrasound to produce a three-dimensional image of a structure.

TONIC. A preparation or medicine that invigorates, strengthens, or restores tone to body tissues.

TONIC-CLONIC SEIZURE. A seizure involving the entire body, characterized by unconsciousness, muscle contraction, and rigidity; also called grand mal or generalized seizures.

TONIFICATION. Acupuncture technique for strengthening the body.

TORPOR. Sluggishness or inactivity.

TOURETTE SYNDROME. A neurological disorder characterized by involuntary motor or vocal tics.

TOXIC. Poisonous.

TOXOCARIASIS. Infection with roundworm larvae, commonly transmitted by the feces of dogs and cats.

TOXOPLASMOSIS. A parasitic infection caused by the intracellular protozoan *Toxoplasmosis gondii.* Humans are most commonly infected by swallowing the oocyte form of the parasite in soil (or kitty litter) contaminated by feces from an infected cat or by swallowing the cyst form of the parasite in raw or undercooked meat.

TRACER. A substance containing a radioisotope, injected into the body and followed in order to obtain information about various metabolic processes in the body.

TRACHEOSTOMY. A surgical procedure in which an artificial opening is made in the patient's windpipe to relieve airway obstruction.

TRAIT ANXIETY. A type of persistent anxiety found in some patients with generalized anxiety disorder. Trait anxiety is regarded as a feature (trait) of a person's temperament.

TRANQUILIZER. A medication that induces a feeling of calm and relaxation; also known as an anxiolytic.

TRANSABLED. A word coined by people with body integrity identity disorder (BIID) to express their need to be disabled.

TRANSCENDENTAL MEDITATION. A meditation technique based on Hindu practices that involves the repetition of a mantra (positive affirmation).

TRANSCUTANEOUS. Through the skin.

TRANSIENT ISCHEMIC ATTACK (TIA). Temporary blockage of blood flow to the brain often resulting in slurred speech, vision disturbances, and loss of balance. The episode is brief and the damage is often short-term (not permanent); also called mini-stroke or warning stroke.

TRANSLOCATION. The transfer of one part of a chromosome to another chromosome during cell division. A balanced translocation occurs when pieces from two different chromosomes exchange places without loss or gain of any chromosome material. An unbalanced translocation involves the unequal loss or gain of genetic information between two chromosomes.

TRANSVESTIC FETISHISM. A paraphilia in which a person is sexually aroused by wearing the clothing of the other sex (as distinct from cross-dressing for a theater role or costume party).

TRAUMA. A severe injury or shock to a person's body or mind.

TRAUMATIC GRIEF. Grief resulting from bereavement under traumatic circumstances, such as natural or transportation disasters, acts of terrorism, and murder.

TREATMENT. In reference to mental disorders, the process of helping persons adapt to and overcome the challenges of their disorder.

TREMOR. Involuntary shaking.

TREPANATION. An operation in which a hole is cut through the skull in order to access the brain.

TRIAGE. A process for determining the order and priority of emergency treatment for injured people (civilians or military personnel), the order and priority of emergency transport, and the injured person's transport destination.

TRIANGLING. A process in which two family members diminish the tension between them by drawing in a third member.

TRICHOBEZOAR. A hairball that results from a buildup of swallowed hairs becoming lodged in the digestive system.

TRICHOPHAGIA. Eating hair.

TRICHOTILLOMANIA. A disorder marked by repeated pulling and tugging of one's hair, usually resulting in noticeable hair loss on the scalp or elsewhere on the body.

TRICHURIASIS. Infection with the larvae of roundworms. These parasites may live for 10–20 years in humans.

TRICYCLIC ANTIDEPRESSANTS (TCAs). An older group of antidepressant drugs.

TRIGEMINAL NEURALGIA. A disorder of the trigeminal nerve that causes severe facial pain.

TRIGGER. Any situation (people, places, times, events, etc.) that causes a person to experience a negative emotional reaction, which is often accompanied by a display of symptoms or problematic behavior.

TRIGLYCERIDES. A type of fat in the blood. High levels of triglycerides can increase the risk of coronary artery disease.

TRISOMY. The condition of having three identical chromosomes, instead of the normal two, in a cell.

TRYPTOPHAN. An essential amino acid produced in the body by the action of trypsin (a digestive enzyme) on protein molecules.

TSUBO. In shiatsu, a center of high energy located along one of the body's meridians. Stimulation of the *tsubos* during a shiatsu treatment is thought to rebalance the flow of vital energy in the body.

TUBAL LIGATION. A surgical procedure in which a woman's fallopian tubes are cut or blocked to prevent an egg from reaching the uterus for fertilization.

TUBEROUS SCLEROSIS. A genetic disease that causes skin problems, seizures, and intellectual disability.

TUMOR. An abnormal growth of body cells, which may be malignant (harmful) or benign (harmless).

24-HOUR RECALL. A listing of the type and amount of all foods and beverages consumed by a person in a 24-hour period.

TWIN STUDY. Research studies that use pairs of twins to study the effects of heredity and environment on behavior or another characteristic.

TYRAMINE. Intermediate product between the chemicals tyrosine and epinephrine in the body and a substance normally found in many foods, especially in protein-rich foods that have been aged or fermented, pickled, or bacterially contaminated, such as cheese, beer, yeast, wine, and chicken liver.

TYROSINE. The amino acid from which epinephrine is synthesized.

U

ULTRASOUND. A noninvasive test in which high-frequency sound waves are reflected off a patient's internal organs, allowing them to be viewed.

UNIVERSALITY. The feeling of being isolated, unique, and separate from others, often experienced by therapy group members.

UNNA SLEEVE. A dressing made of gauze impregnated with glycerin, zinc oxide, and calamine that can be used to protect skin injured by compulsive picking from further injury. It is named for the German dermatologist who invented it.

URETHRA. The tube that discharges urine (and in males, semen) from the bladder to the outside of the body.

URETHRITIS. Inflammation of the urethra.

URINARY INCONTINENCE. Inability to control urination.

URINARY RETENTION. Excessive storage of urine in the body.

URINARY SYSTEM. The kidney, urethra, bladder, and associated organs that process urine and eliminate it from the body.

U.S. FOOD AND DRUG ADMINISTRATION (FDA). The U.S. Department of Health and Human Services agency responsible for ensuring the safety and effectiveness of all drugs, biologics, vaccines, and medical devices. The FDA also works with the blood banking industry to safeguard the nation's blood supply.

UTERUS. The hollow muscular sac in which a fetus develops; sometimes called the womb.

V

VAGINA. The part of the female reproductive system that opens to the exterior of the body and into which the penis is inserted during sexual intercourse.

VAGINISMUS. An involuntary tightening of the vaginal muscles that makes sexual intercourse painful, difficult, or impossible.

VAGUS NERVE STIMULATION (VNS). An experimental treatment for depression that involves implanting a stimulator device that sends electrical impulses at timed intervals to the left vagus nerve.

VALIDITY. The ability of a test to measure accurately what it claims to measure.

VASCULAR. Pertaining to the bloodstream (arteries, veins, and blood vessels).

VASOCONGESTION. A pooling of blood in dilated blood vessels.

VASOCONSTRICTOR. Any substance that causes blood vessels to narrow or tighten.

VENTRAL TEGMENTAL AREA. Produces dopamine and signals to the nucleus accumbens and the rest of the striatum.

VENTRICULAR SYSTEM. The system of small cavities in the brain that forms, circulates, and drains the cerebrospinal fluid.

VENTRICULOSTOMY. Surgery that drains cerebrospinal fluid from the brain to treat hydrocephalus or increased intracranial pressure.

VERBAL REASONING. The ability to understand and reason using concepts involving words (within a particular language).

VESTIBULAR. Pertaining to the vestibule; regarding the vestibular nerve of the ear, which is linked to the ability to hear sounds.

VESTIBULAR SYSTEM. The system that helps to maintain balance and orient the body.

VETERAN'S ADMINISTRATION (VA) HOSPITALS. Medical facilities operated by the federal government explicitly for veterans of the U.S. military.

VICARIOUS. Acquired through imagined participation in the experience of others. Modeling is a form of vicarious learning.

VIPASSANA. A Buddhist meditative practice that emphasizes deep attentiveness to the present moment.

VIRTUAL REALITY. A realistic simulation of an environment, produced by a computer system using interactive hardware and software.

VISUALIZATION. A technique that employs the imagination to visualize specific events or behaviors.

VISUAL-MOTOR. The ability to coordinate vision and bodily movements.

VISUAL-SPATIAL. The ability to see how objects relate within the "big picture."

VISUOMOTOR. Pertaining to visual and motor processes.

VOLATILE. Something that vaporizes or evaporates quickly when exposed to air.

VOYEURISM. A paraphilia that involves watching unsuspecting people, usually strangers, undress or engage in sexual activity.

VULVAR VESTIBULITIS SYNDROME (VVS). Vulvar vestibulitis syndrome is thought to be the most frequent cause of dyspareunia in premenopausal women. A chronic, persistent clinical syndrome, VVS is characterized by severe pain on vestibular touch or attempted vaginal entry.

W

WANNABE. In reference to body integrity identity disorder, a person who feels a need for an amputation or impairment.

WEIGHT CYCLING. Repeatedly gaining and losing weight.

WELFARE-TO-WORK. Several American public reforms of the late 1990s and early 2000s designed to move individuals from public assistance programs to paying jobs.

WERNICKE-KORSAKOFF SYNDROME. A condition of the brain caused by alcohol abuse coupled with malnutrition; also called alcohol encephalopathy.

WILSON'S DISEASE. An inborn defect of copper metabolism in which free copper may be deposited in a variety of areas of the body. Deposits in the brain can cause tremor and other symptoms of Parkinson's disease.

WITHDRAWAL SYMPTOMS. A group of physical or mental symptoms that may occur when a drug is discontinued after prolonged regular use.

WRAPAROUND PROGRAMS. A form of mental health service delivery that strives to accommodate all family members based on self-defined needs, flexibly incorporating both formal and informal community services.

X

X RAY. A type of electromagnetic radiation, between gamma rays and ultraviolet, with a wavelength of between 0.01 and 10 nanometers.

Y

YIN/YANG. Universal characteristics used to describe aspects of the natural world.

YOGA. A physical, mental, and meditative discipline and practice that began in India.

YOGI (FEMININE, YOGINI). A trained yoga expert.

Z

ZEN MEDITATION. A discipline that teaches the mind to relax. Zen meditation involves sitting in prescribed positions in order to calm the body and mind, with the goal of slowing heart rate and breathing to reach a reflective meditative state.

ZOONOSIS (PLURAL, ZOONOSES). Any contagious disease that can be transmitted from nonhuman animals to humans or from humans to nonhuman animals. Zoonoses include viral, bacterial, parasitic, fungal, and prion diseases.

ZYGOMATIC ARCH. Cheekbone. A quadrilateral bone forming the prominence of the cheek. It articulates (touches or moves) with the frontal, sphenoid, maxillary, and temporal bones.

INDEX

In the index, references to individual volumes are listed before colons; numbers following a colon refer to specific page numbers within that particular volume. **Boldface** references indicate main topical essays. Photographs and illustration references are highlighted with an *italicized* page number. Tables are also indicated with the page number followed by a lowercase, italicized *t*.

A

B

C

D

E

F

G

H

I

J

K

L

M

N

O

P

Q

R

S

T

U

V

W

X

Y

Z